Brunner and Suddarth's Textbook of

MEDICAL·SURGICAL NURSING

Suzanne C. Smeltzer, RN, C, MS, EdD, FAAN

Associate Professor and Nurse Researcher
Department of Nursing
Thomas Jefferson University
Philadelphia, Pennsylvania

Brenda G. Bare, RN, MSN

Assistant Vice President, Medical–Surgical Nursing
The Alexandria Hospital
Alexandria, Virginia

With 39 Contributors

Brunner and Suddarth's Textbook of
MEDICAL·SURGICAL NURSING

SEVENTH EDITION

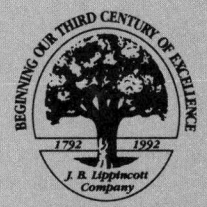

J. B. Lippincott Company

Philadelphia

New York   London   Hagerstown

Acquisitions Editor: **David P. Carroll**
Developmental Editor: **Marian A. Bellus**
Coordinating Editorial Assistant: **Amy R. Stonehouse**
Project Editors: **Lorraine Smith and Grace R. Caputo**
Indexer: **Ann Cassar**
Designer: **Doug Smock**
Production Manager: **Helen Ewan**
Production Coordinator: **Maura C. Murphy**
Compositor: **Tapsco, Inc.**
Printer/Binder: **Courier Book Company/Westford**
Cover Photograph: **Walter Plotnick**

7th Edition

6   5   4   3

Library of Congress Cataloging-in-Publication Data

Brunner and Suddarth's textbook of medical–surgical nursing.—7th
    ed./[edited by] Suzanne C. Smeltzer, Brenda G. Bare, with 39
    contributors.
        p.   cm.
    Rev. ed. of: Textbook of medical–surgical nursing/[edited by]
Lillian Sholtis Brunner, Doris Smith Suddarth. 6th ed. c1988.
        Includes bibliographical references and index.
        ISBN 0-397-54797-8
        1. Nursing.   2. Surgical nursing.   I. Smeltzer, Suzanne C.
O'Connell.   II. Bare, Brenda G.   III. Brunner, Lillian Sholtis.
IV. Suddarth, Doris Smith.   V. Textbook of medical–surgical nursing.
VI. Title: Textbook of medical–surgical nursing.   VII. Title:
Medical–surgical nursing.
        [DNLM: 1. Nursing Care.   2. Surgical Nursing.   WY 150 B8972]
RT41.T46   1992
610.73—dc20
DNLM/DLC
for Library of Congress   91-40902
                                                                        CIP

Unit photography by Tom Ferentz, in cooperation with the Bothin Burn Center, Saint Francis Memorial Hospital, San Francisco; the Herbert C. Moffitt Hospital, University of California, San Francisco; Joseph M. Long Hospital, University of California, San Francisco; the Children's Hospital, San Francisco; and the San Francisco General Hospital.

To Lillian Sholtis Brunner and Doris Smith Suddarth:

With appreciation for the many years you have helped countless nursing students and practitioners in the art and science of nursing.

Contributors

Margaret Ahearn-Spera, RN, C, MSN
Director, Clinical Nursing, Danbury Hospital, Danbury, Connecticut; and Assistant Clinical Professor, Yale University School of Nursing, New Haven, Connecticut
> *Chapter 57: Management of Patients With Neurologic Disorders*

Debra A. Bancroft, RN, BSN
Specialty Coordinator—Rheumatology, Midwest Arthritis Treatment Center, Columbia Hospital, Milwaukee, Wisconsin
> *Chapter 50: Management of Patients With Rheumatic Disorders*

Cynthia A. Blank, RN, MSN, CEN
Trauma Program Coordinator, Department of Nursing, Hospital of the Medical College of Pennsylvania, Philadelphia, Pennsylvania
> *Chapter 55: Assessment of Neurologic Function*

Linda J. Burns, PhD, RN
NIRA Project Coordinator, Somerset Medical Center, Somerville, New Jersey; formerly Assistant Professor, School of Nursing, Trenton State College, Trenton, New Jersey
> *Chapter 20: Preoperative Nursing Management*
> *Chapter 21: Intraoperative Nursing and Anesthesia*
> *Chapter 22: Postoperative Nursing Management*

Patricia Ann Cady, PhD, RN, CCRN
Clinical Nurse III, Beth Israel Hospital, Boston, Massachusetts
> *Chapter 4: Ethical Issues in Medical–Surgical Nursing*

Gladys E. Deters, RN, MSN
Assistant Professor, The University of Virginia School of Nursing, Charlottesville, Virginia
> *Chapter 51: Management of Patients With Dermatologic Problems*

Kathleen Kelleher Furniss, RN, C, MSN
Women's Health Care Nurse Practitioner, Wayne Obstetrical Group, Wayne, New Jersey; and Project Coordinator, Domestic Violence Prevention Project, University of Medicine and Dentistry of New Jersey, Newark, New Jersey
> *Chapter 44: Management of Problems Related to Female Physiologic Processes*
> *Chapter 45: Management of Patients With Disorders of the Female Reproductive System*
> *Chapter 46: Assessment and Management of Patients With Breast Disorders*

David B. P. Goodman, MD, PhD
Professor and Department Chief, Department of Pathology and Laboratory Medicine, Hospital of the University of Pennsylvania, Philadelphia, Pennsylvania
> *Appendix: Diagnostic Studies and Their Meanings*

Patricia M. Griffith, RN, MSN
Clinical Nurse Specialist, National Institutes of Health, Bethesda, Maryland
> *Chapter 32: Assessment and Management of Patients With Hematologic Disorders*

Doreen Chaffinch Grzelak, MSN, RN
Nursing Education, HCA Reston Hospital Center, Reston, Virginia
> *Chapter 34: Assessment and Management of Patients With Ingestive Problems and Upper Gastrointestinal Disorders*
> *Chapter 36: Management of Patients With Gastric and Duodenal Disorders*

Gail P. Hamilton, RNC, MSN, DSW
Associate Professor, Department of Nursing, College of Allied Health Professions, Temple University, Philadelphia, Pennsylvania
> *Chapter 12: Health Care of the Older Adult*

Lois M. Hoskins, PhD, RN
Dean, School of Nursing, The Catholic University of America, Washington, DC
> *Chapter 8: Homeostasis and Pathophysiologic Processes*
> *Chapter 9: Stress and Adaptation*

Ann N. Hotter, RN, MSN, CCRN, CS
Clinical Nurse Specialist, Critical Care, St Mary's Hospital, Rochester, Minnesota
> *Chapter 25: Respiratory Care Modalities*

Ryan R. Iwamoto, RN, CS, MN
Clinical Nurse Specialist, Section of Radiation Oncology, Virginia Mason Clinic, Seattle, Washington
> *Chapter 47: Management of Patients With Disorders of the Male Reproductive System*

Connie Rae Jarlsberg, BSN, MSN
Former Patient Care Coordinator, Burn Center, Detroit Receiving Hospital, Detroit, Michigan
> *Chapter 52: Management of Patients With Burn Injury*

Katherine J. Kaut, RN, MSN, CCRN
Critical Care Clinical Nurse Specialist, The Fairfax Hospital, Falls Church, Virginia

Chapter 31: Assessment and Management of Patients With Vascular Disorders and Problems of Peripheral Circulation

Dorothy B. Liddel, MSN, RN, ONC
Assistant Professor, Edyth T. James Department of Nursing, Columbia Union College, Takoma Park, Maryland

Chapter 14: Principles and Practices of Rehabilitation
Chapter 58: Assessment of Musculoskeletal Function
Chapter 59: Management Modalities for Patients With Musculoskeletal Dysfunction
Chapter 60: Management of Patients With Musculoskeletal Trauma
Chapter 61: Management of Patients With Musculoskeletal Disorders

Martha V. Manning, RN, MSN
Clinical Nurse Specialist, Cardiopulmonary Rehabilitation, The Alexandria Hospital, Alexandria, Virginia

Chapter 33: Assessment of Digestive and Gastrointestinal Function
Chapter 37: Management of Patients With Intestinal and Rectal Disorders

Diana J. Mason, PhD, RN, C, FAAN
Associate Director of Nursing for Education and Research, Beth Israel Medical Center, New York, New York

Chapter 16: Human Rhythms in Health and Illness

Shawn M. McCabe, RN, MSN, CCRN
Clinical Nurse Specialist—Trauma, University of Medicine and Dentistry of New Jersey/University Hospital, Newark, New Jersey

Chapter 56: Management of Patients With Neurologic Dysfunction

Norma M. Metheny, PhD, RN, FAAN
Professor of Nursing, St Louis University, St Louis, Missouri

Chapter 18: Fluids and Electrolytes: Balance and Disturbances

Kathleen Miller, RN, MBA, MSN, CCRN, CNA
Assistant Vice President, Critical Care Nursing, The Alexandria Hospital, Alexandria, Virginia

Chapter 63: Emergency Nursing

Kathleen Collins Monahan, RN, MSN
Nursing Education Department, Yale–New Haven Hospital, New Haven, Connecticut

Chapter 27: Assessment of Cardiovascular Function

Nancy A. Morrissey, MSN, RNC
Director of Nursing Care, Surgical Unit, The Alexandria Hospital, Alexandria, Virginia

Chapter 35: Gastrointestinal Intubation and Special Nutritional Management

Martha A. Mulvey, RN, MS, CS
Clinical Nurse Specialist—Surgery, University of Medicine and Dentistry of New Jersey, Newark, New Jersey

Chapter 49: Assessment and Management of Patients With Allergic Disorders

Anne Gallagher Peach, RN, MSN
Director of Health Care Education/Continuing Medical Education, Orlando Regional Medical Center, Orlando, Florida

Chapter 23: Management of Patients With Conditions of the Upper Respiratory Airway
Chapter 24: Assessment of Respiratory Function
Chapter 26: Management of Patients With Conditions of the Chest and Lower Respiratory Tract

Janice Smith Pigg, BSN, RN, MSN
Nurse Consultant—Rheumatology, Director of Musculoskeletal Service, Columbia Hospital, Milwaukee, Wisconsin

Chapter 50: Management of Patients With Rheumatic Disorders

Kathryn A. Pollon, RNC, MSN
Mental Health Therapist, Northwest Center for Community Mental Health, Reston, Virginia

Chapter 10: Human Response to Illness
Chapter 53: Assessment and Management of Patients With Vision Problems and Eye Disorders

Margaret Rafferty, RN, MA, MPH, CS
Assistant Professor, Long Island College Hospital—School of Nursing, Brooklyn, New York

Chapter 13: Homelessness in America: A Major Health Problem

Priscilla V. Rivera, RN, MS, CNA
Clinical Supervisory Nurse, Nursing Department, Heart, Lung and Blood Nursing Service, The National Institutes of Health Clinical Center, Bethesda, Maryland

Chapter 32: Assessment and Management of Patients With Hematologic Disorders

Susan A. Rokita, RN, MS
Clinical Nurse Specialist—Oncology, University Hospital, The M.S. Hershey Medical Center, Hershey, Pennsylvania

Chapter 19: Oncology: Nursing the Patient With Cancer

Carol S. Rosenberg, MSN, RN, CDE
Diabetes Clinical Nurse Specialist, Bay Shores Medical Group, Torrance, California; formerly Diabetes Clinical Specialist, Cedars-Sinai Medical Center, Los Angeles, California

Chapter 39: Assessment and Management of Patients With Diabetes Mellitus

Linda H. Schakenbach, RN, MSN, CCRN, CS
Clinical Nurse Specialist, Cardiovascular Critical Care, The Fairfax Hospital, Falls Church, Virginia

Chapter 30: Management of the Cardiac Surgery Patient

Mona B. Shevlin, MA, PhD
Professor, Department of Education, The Catholic University of America, Washington, DC; and Director, Counseling Center for Greater Washington, McLean, Virginia

> Chapter 11: Developmental Concepts of the Adult Life Phase

Loretta Spittle, RN, MS, CCRN
Doctoral Student, The University of Virginia, Charlottesville, Virginia

> Chapter 28: Management of Patients With Cardiac Disorders
> Chapter 29: Management of Patients With Complications of Cardiac Disorders

Cindy Stern, RN, MSN, OCN
Oncology Clinical Specialist, Thomas Jefferson University Hospital, Philadelphia, Pennsylvania

> Chapter 19: Oncology: Nursing the Patient With Cancer
> Chapter 48: The Immune System, Immunopathology, and Immunodeficiency

Laurel J. Sutherland, RN, MSN
Education Coordinator, Critical Care, The Alexandria Hospital, Alexandria, Virginia

> Chapter 62: Management of Patients With Infectious Diseases

Betty Temples-Mill, PhD, RN
Assistant Professor of Nursing, George Mason University, Fairfax, Virginia

> Chapter 54: Assessment and Management of Patients With Hearing Problems and Ear Disorders

Beverly Whipple, PhD, RN, FAAN
Associate Professor, College of Nursing, Rutgers, The State University of New Jersey, Newark, New Jersey

> Chapter 17: Human Sexuality

The authors would like to acknowledge the contributions of the following individuals who contributed to the previous edition of this text:

Elizabeth W. Bayley, RN, MS

> Chapter 52: Management of Patients With Burn Injury

Ellen K. Boyda, RN, MS, CCRN

> Unit 6 (Chapters 23–26): Oxygen–Carbon Dioxide Exchange and Respiratory Function

Mary Jo Boyer, RN, MSN

> Unit 8 (Chapters 33–37): Digestive and Gastrointestinal Function
> Chapter 50: Management of Patients With Rheumatic Disorders

Josephine Messer, RN, MS

> Chapter 13: Human Sexuality

Rita Nemchik, RN, MS

> Chapter 39: Assessment and Management of Patients With Diabetes Mellitus

Foreword

The first six editions of the *Textbook of Medical–Surgical Nursing* have been a collaborative effort reflecting an *effective* partnership. The continuing support of nursing educators, practitioners, and students has allowed us the greatest satisfaction and joy that come from studying, learning, and writing about the human response to health problems, which are the very heart of nursing.

We are pleased that Suzanne Smeltzer and Brenda Bare are the authors and editors of the seventh edition of this book. We have worked with Suzanne and Brenda for several editions and can attest to their integrity, intellectual ability, and commitment of time, energy, and focused purpose that publishing such a book requires. They understand the im-

portance and complexities of searching the literature, applying nursing research to practice, selecting *qualified* contributors, and scrutinizing each chapter for state-of-the-art information and accuracy.

We are grateful for the loyal support and encouragement of the nurses who have used our book. We now pass the torch to Suzanne and Brenda with the assurance that they are dedicated to the pursuit of excellence that is the hallmark of the *Textbook of Medical–Surgical Nursing*.

Lillian Sholtis Brunner, RN, MSN, ScD, LittD, FAAN
Doris Smith Suddarth, RN, BSNE, MSN

Preface

As we move toward the 21st century, professional health care literature abounds with predictions about what our world and, more specifically, our health care system will be like in the decades ahead. It is not unusual to read titles of articles and books that contain phrases such as "the demographics of the 21st century," "futuristic health care," and "the changing face of the health care delivery system." Likewise, many authors have sought to describe "nursing in the 21st century."

When one decade ends and another begins, predictions about the future are commonplace. The opportunity to proceed into a new century, however, presents a novel experience for futuristic thinking and the forecasting of events to come. As nurses and nursing approach the 21st century, preparations must be made for facing and meeting the challenges, changes, and forces that will confront the health care industry and the nursing profession. Knowledge of present trends and anticipation of future events and directions will allow nurses to shape their own professional destiny as they prepare to practice in the health care arena of the forthcoming century.

Anticipating and planning for the future present many challenges for nurses in both the academic and the clinical practice settings. The foundation for all of these challenges is commitment to excellence—academic excellence, professional practice excellence, and excellence of service to the American people.

In response to this commitment to excellence, the seventh edition of *Brunner and Suddarth's Textbook of Medical–Surgical Nursing* is designed to foster excellence of professional nursing practice for today's nursing students and nursing practitioners. The emphasis on pathophysiologic concepts, scientific rationale, available research findings, and state-of-the-art clinical nursing principles and practices that has served as the hallmark of previous editions continues here. The principles of the physical, biologic, and social sciences as well as nursing theory and biomedical technology are combined with the art of caring to delineate the broad scope of medical–surgical nursing and its many components.

The nursing process is the central, unifying framework of the book. Within this framework emphasis is placed on gerontologic considerations, pharmacotherapeutics, patient education, home health care, and preventive modalities. Health maintenance, health promotion, and self-care are integrated throughout. Focus is directed toward the care of adults with acute or chronic health conditions and the distinct roles of the nurse in providing and facilitating this care: practitioner, teacher, counselor, patient advocate, and coordinator of care, services, and resources.

Topics that reflect current concerns and developments in the field of health care have been expanded. Ethical issues that are now commonplace in nursing are described. Health care needs of the growing numbers of elderly people, homeless people, persons with AIDS and other immune disorders, and individuals who are living longer with chronic illnesses are presented in detail.

Special emphasis is given to nursing research. Annotated reviews of pertinent nursing research articles are presented in Nursing Research Profiles; nursing implications are identified. In the bibliographies, nursing research citations are designated by asterisks. Bibliographic citations were carefully selected to reflect state-of-the-art knowledge and practice.

The approach to care of patients continues to be eclectic, because this realistic approach allows students and practitioners to adapt what they are learning to their own philosophy, theory, or concept of nursing. The material presented in this textbook can be used within any framework of nursing practice.

A flexible approach to gender identification has been maintained in the interest of clarity and readability and in no way reflects sexism. The use of masculine and feminine gender pronouns is kept to a minimum, but in some instances the use of such pronouns serves to ensure a clearer presentation of the material and to preserve the flow of the text. Thus, the pronoun *he* is used to designate both male and female recipients of care, and *she* is used in referring to both male and female nurses. Those receiving care are identified as patients and are always portrayed as individuals whose desire for autonomy and independence should be respected and fostered by the nurse.

As society and health care continue to change with the approach of the new century, the caring values of nursing remain the hallmark of nursing's unique contribution to health care. This seventh edition of *Brunner and Suddarth's Textbook of Medical–Surgical Nursing*, with its focus on a holistic approach to the care of patients, reflects those caring values in delineating the art and the science of nursing.

Suzanne C. O'Connell Smeltzer, RN, MS, EdD, FAAN
Brenda G. Bare, RN, MSN

Acknowledgments

C. Renae Baker, RN, MSN
Vice-President, Nursing and Support Services, The Alexandria Hospital, Alexandria, Virginia

Carolyn F. Beck, RN
Clinician IV, Surgical Ophthalmic Specialist, The Fairfax Hospital, Falls Church, Virginia

Christen Berman, RD
Registered Dietician, Cedars-Sinai Medical Center, Los Angeles, California

Kathleen M. Bury, RN
Coordinator, IV Services, The Alexandria Hospital, Alexandria, Virginia

Mayer B. Davidson, MD
Director, Diabetes Program, Cedars-Sinai Medical Center; and Professor of Medicine, University of California, Los Angeles, Los Angeles, California

Christine L. Holland, MD
Clinical Professor, Allergy and Immunology, University of Medicine and Dentistry of New Jersey

Nina S. McCleskey, MLS
Director, Medical Library, The Alexandria Hospital, Alexandria, Virginia

Raymond Scarpa, RNC, BSN
Research Nurse Clinician, New Jersey Cancer Center at University Hospital, University of Medicine and Dentistry of New Jersey, Newark, New Jersey

Maryann W. Simpson, RN, BSN, CETN
Formerly Enterostomal Therapy Nurse, University Hospital, University of Medicine and Dentistry of New Jersey, Newark, New Jersey

Ronald K. Smeltzer, PhD

Robert P. Steinfeld, MD, FACS
Wayne, New Jersey

The authors wish to thank the following individuals who helped to make the 7th edition of Brunner and Suddarth's **Textbook of Medical–Surgical Nursing** *possible:*

Diana Intenzo
Publisher

David Carroll
Senior Editor

Marian Bellus
Developmental Editor

Grace Caputo and Lorraine Smith
Senior Project Editors

Amy Stonehouse
Editorial Assistant

Contents

unit 3
Biophysical and Psychosocial Concepts Related to Health and Illness

unit 4
Concepts and Challenges in Patient Management

unit 5
Perioperative Management of the Surgical Patient

unit 6

Oxygen–Carbon Dioxide Exchange and Respiratory Function

unit 7

Cardiovascular, Circulatory, and Hematologic Function

unit 8
Digestive and Gastrointestinal Function

unit 9
Metabolic and Endocrine Function

unit 10
Urinary and Renal Function

unit 11
Sexual and Reproductive Function

unit 12
Immunologic Function

unit 13
Integumentary Function

unit 14
Sensorineural Function

unit 15
Musculoskeletal Function

unit 16
Other Acute Problems

Brunner and Suddarth's Textbook of

MEDICAL·SURGICAL
NURSING

unit 1
Health Maintenance and Health Needs

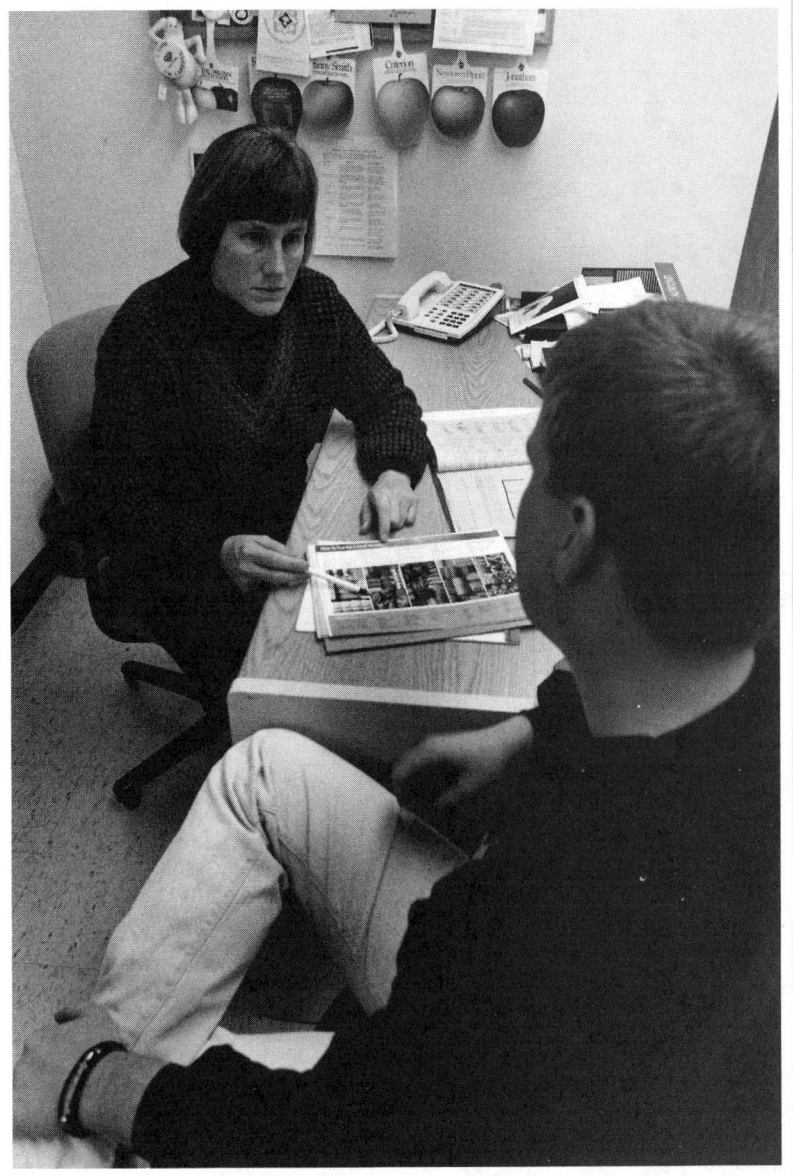

1

Nursing in Today's World: Concepts and Implementation

Learning Objectives

On completion of this chapter, the learner will be able to:

1. Develop a definition of nursing, with consideration given to the holistic nature of the patient
2. Discuss the significance of concept formation in nursing
3. Describe the concept of health maintenance within the context of the current health care delivery system
4. Identify the effects of diagnosis-related groups on health care and nursing practice
5. Describe the significance of quality assurance in the health care delivery system
6. Specify the expanded roles of the nurse
7. Describe the practitioner, leadership, and research roles of the nurse
8. Use Maslow's hierarchy of needs as a framework for assessing the needs of a patient
9. Describe primary nursing, case management, and collaborative practice

The health care delivery system of the 1990s reflects a century in which there were unprecedented demographic, sociological, and technological changes. As one century ends and another begins, health care professionals are faced with an aging population whose needs are increasingly more acute and more complex. New diseases continue to be identified and cures remain problematic. Solutions to drug abuse, homelessness, and chronic diseases and mental illness elude even the most sophisticated of health care systems and health care technologies. The resulting demands are compounded by skyrocketing costs of health care and shortages of personnel, not the least of which is the shortage of nurses—a shortage that is expected to continue past the turn of the century.

The changes occurring in the health care system make change in nursing inevitable. Nursing is a major contributor to health care delivery and is an important force in shaping its future.

Nursing Defined

Nursing leaders for decades have been attempting to articulate a universally accepted definition of nursing that identifies the uniqueness of the profession and has meaning for all practitioners of nursing as well as for the members of other professions involved in the delivery of health care. Such a definition has been slow in coming because nursing has lacked a clearly defined body of scientific knowledge. Historically, nursing practice has been based on tradition. Only in recent years have nurses accepted the challenge to demonstrate that nursing is indeed a profession with its own unique body of knowledge. Nurse theorists are using scientific methods to describe, explain, and predict nursing practice and its outcomes. As theory development proceeds, it will continue to be refined. An objective of this research is to validate nursing practice and provide society with a definition of nursing that will foster the autonomy of the profession.

Since the time of Florence Nightingale, who wrote in 1858 that the real goal of nursing was "to put the patient in the best condition for nature to act upon him," nursing leaders have defined nursing as both an art and a science. In the earlier years, they tended to emphasize the nursing services that are directed toward the care of the sick. More recently, the maintenance and promotion of health as well as the prevention of illness have also been stressed.

One of the classic definitions of nursing, as formulated by Virginia Henderson (1966), delineates the unique function of the nurse as follows:

> . . . to assist the individual, sick or well, in the performance of those activities contributing to health or its recovery (or to peaceful death) that he would perform unaided if he had the necessary strength, will or knowledge. And to do this in such a way as to help him gain independence as rapidly as possible.*

Review of the literature since the time of Henderson's definition of nursing reveals numerous attempts at further defining the unique function of the nurse—unique with regard to the functions of other health care disciplines. Most of these formulations have attempted to define nursing as a profession directed toward meeting both the health and illness needs of "man," who is viewed holistically as having physical, emotional, psychologic, intellectual, social, and spiritual needs.

More recently, the American Nurses Association published *Nursing: A Social Policy Statement* (1980), which provided a description of the social context of nursing and a definition of the nature and scope of nursing practice. Nursing was defined as "the diagnosis and treatment of human responses to actual or potential health problems."

An illustrative list of human responses that are the focus for nursing intervention was presented as follows:

Self-care limitations
Impaired functioning in areas such as rest, sleep, ventilation, circulation, activity, nutrition, elimination, skin, and sexuality
Pain and discomfort

Emotional problems related to illness and treatment, life-threatening events, or daily experiences, such as anxiety, loss, loneliness, and grief
Distortion of symbolic functions, reflected in interpersonal and intellectual processes, such as hallucinations
Deficiencies in decision making and ability to make personal choices
Self-image changes required by health status
Dysfunctional perceptual orientations to health
Strains related to life processes, such as birth, growth and development, and death
Problematic affiliative relationships

This definition of the nature and scope of nursing practice reflects a view of man as an integrated whole—a biopsychosocial being. In this holistic concept of health, the various aspects of human functioning are seen as interrelated, interdependent, and of equal importance. Nurses have a responsibility to demonstrate and be accountable for their role as defined in the social policy statement. They must also comply with the nurse practice act of the state within which they practice and with the guidelines established by the International Council of Nurses (ICN) and the American Nurses Association (ANA) in their respective codes for nurses.

As nursing investigations continue to be directed toward the advancement of nursing's body of knowledge and improvements in nursing practice, Schlotfeldt (1987) stated that the appropriate focus for any definition of nursing is a human health-seeking perspective:

> Nursing can be accurately and succinctly defined to reflect its long-established social mission and goal, to guide the preparation of professionals, and to identify the phenomena about which theories are now and likely henceforth will be needed as: "Nursing is the appraisal and the enhancement of the health status, health assets, and health potentials of human beings."*

Conceptual Models in Nursing

If nurses are to accomplish the goals of nursing as defined by nursing leaders, there must be a body of theoretic knowledge on which to base practice. Great strides toward "theory building" in nursing have been made in recent years.

In the past, nursing has used theories from various biopsychosocial sciences. Only within the past several decades have nurses made concerted efforts toward identifying a circumscribed body of knowledge that is unique to nursing and that can serve as the theoretic basis for the practice of nursing. Such a theoretic basis, when more fully developed, will consist of scientifically derived general principles that are applied consistently in nursing practice. Nursing theories will provide a guide for viewing nursing holistically and for determining the probable results of nursing actions in advance of their implementation. However, only as these theories of nursing evolve and mature and as they are tested and retested will a general theory of nursing be possible.

* Henderson V. *The Nature of Nursing.* New York, Macmillan, 1966.

* Schlotfeldt RM. *Defining nursing: A historic controversy.* Nurs Res 1987 Jan/Feb; 36(1):64–67.

Much of the progress that has been accomplished in the pursuit of a scientific theory of nursing has been in the areas of concept formation and model construction. Because nursing is a practice-oriented discipline, concepts of nursing have been evolving over the years. However, only in recent years have nurses attempted to articulate these concepts, to propose that they be used as the framework for nursing practice, and to test and validate them. Many concepts that have their foundations in the biopsychosocial sciences have been found to be particularly applicable to nursing and now serve as useful components of frameworks for nursing practice.

Several of the broad concepts that have been used extensively as frameworks for nursing curricula and for nursing practice throughout the country include (1) the wellness–illness continuum, (2) developmental processes throughout the life cycle, and (3) stress-adaptation.

The *wellness–illness continuum* provides a means by which the nurse focuses on the patient's positive health attributes and characteristics within the dimensions of his illness or potential illness situation. The individual is recognized as a holistic being who interacts with his internal and external environments. With such a focus and view of the individual, the nurse uses the nursing process to assist the patient to use his attributes in attaining and maintaining the highest level of wellness possible within his physical and psychosocial limitations. Dunn's (1961) concept of high-level wellness serves as the basis for this framework for nursing.

The *developmental processes* approach to nursing provides a frame of reference that emphasizes the complexity of variables that are involved in each of the developmental stages of the life cycle. Such a framework provides direction for the nurse in assisting the patient to accomplish his developmental tasks as they are affected by his state of health and wellness. The theories of Havighurst, Erickson, and Piaget serve as the bases for the developmental processes approach to nursing. Havighurst's developmental tasks emphasize the effects of physical and social developmental changes and events on the individual; Erikson's eight stages of human development emphasize the successful completion of psychosocial tasks necessary for attaining and maintaining one's identity; Piaget's stages of cognitive development emphasize development of cognitive abilities and related sensorimotor skills.

The *stress-adaptation framework* emphasizes the role of the nurse in assessing the patient's behavioral responses to the demands of his internal and external environments. Nursing interventions are then directed toward assisting the patient to strive toward adaptive behavior that promotes health and prevents illness. The general adaptation syndrome as described by Selye and the fight-or-flight syndrome as described by Cannon serve as the bases for the stress-adaptation framework.

These broad concepts and other related concepts, while serving as useful frameworks for nursing practice, are not in and of themselves unique to nursing. Therefore, nursing leaders have attempted to develop, more fully, concepts that are inherent within nursing itself and to construct models that describe the relationships between these concepts and their subconcepts. Four such conceptual models of nursing are the *life processes model* developed by Rogers (1970), the *self-care model* as advocated by Orem (1971, 1980, 1985, 1991), the *adaptation model* as formulated by Roy (1980), and the *behavioral systems model* developed by Johnson (1980).

These are certainly not the only conceptual models of nursing that have been developed, nor is it our intent to suggest that nurses should subscribe to any one of these models, forsaking other models that may also serve as valuable frameworks for the practice of nursing. However, it is our intent to present these models as examples of contemporary models of nursing, with the hope that they will generate interest, enthusiasm, and inquiry into the present status and future potential of conceptual frameworks of nursing and the state of theory building in nursing.

Life Processes Model

The life processes model of nursing focuses on the wholeness of the human organism in the person who is the recipient of nursing care. It is Rogers's belief that the purpose of the scientific body of knowledge of nursing is to describe, explain, and make predictions about mankind. Such knowledge leads to the evolution of theories that serve to guide nursing practice. Rogers identified fundamental human attributes that constitute the following basic assumptions on which nursing science is built:

1. Man is a unified whole possessing his own integrity and manifesting characteristics that are more than and different from the sum of his parts.
2. Man and the environment are continuously exchanging matter and energy with one another.
3. The life process evolves irreversibly and unidirectionally along the space–time continuum.
4. Pattern and organization identify man and reflect his innovative wholeness.
5. Man is characterized by the capacity for abstraction and imagery, language and thought, and sensation and emotion.

The qualities of the life processes as described in these assumptions include wholeness, openness, unidirectionality, pattern and organization, and sentience and thought. The underlying principles describe man as a dynamic entity who interacts mutually and simultaneously with his environment. The changes that occur during this interaction are irreversible, non-repeatable, and rhythmical, increasing in complexity and proceeding by the continual repatterning of man and his environment.

- With such a view of man, the goal of nursing becomes that of promoting the person's interaction with his environment in such a way that the maximum state of health that is possible is realized by the utilization of the individual's own energies and potential.

This holistic concept of human functioning serves as the basis for making predictions about nursing intervention. Data gathered for making nursing diagnoses are derived from the total pattern of events that have influenced the extent to which man is achieving his maximum health potential. These data then serve as the basis for the establishment of short-term and long-term health goals for the individual, his family, and society and for the implementation of nursing actions directed toward the achievement of these goals. These nursing actions are aimed at helping the individual to repattern his relationship with himself and his environment so that his maximum health potential can be attained. A conceptual model of nursing such as that proposed by Rogers contributes to the pursuit of a scientific theory of nursing. Testing, retesting, and validation of the model will no doubt serve to further the science of nursing.

Self-Care Model

Orem has developed a concept of nursing that places emphasis on the person's need for self-care—those activities that an individual practices for the purpose of maintaining life, health, and well-being. It is the concern of nursing to provide for and promote the person's self-care actions in an attempt to promote life and health and to assist him to recover from disease and injury or to cope with their effects. The need for nursing exists when an adult is unable to satisfactorily meet his self-care requisites or when a parent is unable to meet these demands for a child.

- Nursing is responsible for assisting the person to overcome those circumstances that interfere with self-care and that cause self-care limitations and deficits.

There are three broad categories of self-care requisites: universal, developmental, and those related to health deviation. *Universal self-care requisites* are those that are required of all individuals to maintain integrated human functioning. *Developmental self-care requisites* are those that occur as a result of developmental processes (*e.g.*, pregnancy) or of conditions that can affect human development (*e.g.*, loss of loved ones). *Health-deviation self-care requisites* are those that occur as a result of disease, injury, disfigurement, disability, or medical diagnoses and treatment and that require that changes be made in the person's routine of self-care depending on the nature and extent of the requisites. Self-care activity is purposeful, deliberate action that is goal-directed, self-initiated, and self-directed and is affected by the person's values and goals. When it is effective, it promotes the structural integrity, functioning, and development of the person.

Orem identifies three systems of nursing activities that are designed to meet the individual's self-care requirements, according to the extent to which self-care action is disrupted: the wholly compensatory system, the partly compensatory system, and the supportive–educative (developmental) system. The *wholly compensatory system* is used when the person is unable to assume an active role in his care and the nurse assists him by acting for and doing for him. The *partly compensatory system* is used when the nurse and the patient participate in accomplishing therapeutic self-care actions. The major responsibility for the performance of these actions may be assumed by the nurse or by the patient, depending on the patient's actual or medically prescribed limitations, his knowledge and skills, and his psychologic readiness to accomplish such activities. The *supportive–educative system* is used when the patient is capable of performing, or learning to perform, those measures that are necessary to accomplish his self-care requisites but for which he needs assistance in the form of support, guidance, provision of a developmental environment, and teaching.

Thus, as the health status of the patient changes, his needs for nursing activity may demand a change in the nursing system that is appropriate to meet his needs. Such a conceptual model of nursing can serve as a framework for guiding and directing nursing care. Currently, the framework is used within various nursing education and nursing service settings. However, further validation of the concept is necessary for the continuation of nursing's pursuit of a sound theoretic base.

Adaptation Model

The adaptation model of nursing developed by Roy is a systems model that incorporates interactionist concepts. *Adaptation* is defined as the process of change, a universal phenomenon of man. Within the model, man is viewed as a biopsychosocial being who is in constant interaction with his environment—an interaction that requires him to make continual adaptations. The capacity for adaptation depends on the stimuli to which he is exposed and the level of his adaptation. The adaptive level is determined by the effect of three classes of stimuli: (1) focal stimuli, or those with which the person is immediately confronted; (2) contextual stimuli, which include all other stimuli that are present; and (3) residual stimuli, or stimuli that the person has experienced in the past, such as beliefs, attitudes, and traits. Humans have four modes of adaptation: physiologic, self-concept, role function, and interdependence relations. Thus, adaptive or positive responses to stimuli serve to maintain the total integrity of the individual.

- The role of nursing is that of promoting adaptation in all four modes during health and illness by using the five components of the nursing process: assessing, nursing diagnosis, planning, implementing, and evaluating.

During the assessment phase of the nursing process, the person's position on the health–illness continuum is identified and the effectiveness of his ability to cope with the stimuli with which he is confronted is evaluated. The planning phase of the nursing process involves the establishment of goals for changing maladaptive behavior to adaptive behavior. Then, the nursing process is completed by the implementation and evaluation of a plan of nursing action directed toward promoting adaptation. The adaptation model of nursing is in operation in several schools of nursing and nursing service departments in hospital settings. However, it continues to require further validation as a framework for the practice of nursing.

Behavioral Systems Model

The behavioral systems model for nursing developed by Johnson describes man as a behavioral system that continually strives to maintain balance through adjustments and adaptations to his ever-changing internal and external environments. His behavior is orderly, purposeful, and predictable, and most of the time it is functionally efficient and effective. The behavioral system has seven subsystems (related to affiliation, dependency, ingestion, elimination, sexuality, aggression, and achievement), each of which has a specialized task or function that promotes integrated performance of the system as a whole.

The need for nursing arises when the balance of the system is disturbed or is likely to be disturbed sufficiently to warrant external assistance. Nursing is viewed as an external regulatory force directed toward preventing disturbance in the system and preserving or restoring optimal organization and integration of the patient's behavior.

- The goal of nursing is to assist the patient to modify his behavioral patterns in such a way that he is able to meet the demands of the elements in his life that cannot be modified.

During the assessment phase of the nursing process, the patient's ability to adapt to his actual or perceived threat without resultant instability is identified. In cases in which instability exists or is expected, an in-depth assessment of the involved subsystems is performed. Identification and validation of dysfunctional behaviors lead to the development of nursing diagnoses. Nursing intervention is then directed toward the promotion of regularity in the patient's behavior so that balance is maintained or attained in each subsystem. The nursing process is completed when expected behavioral outcomes have been measured and the plan of care has been revised as necessary to further promote stability of the behavioral system, adjustment to the situation, and adaptation to stress.

The behavioral systems model has been used in various settings to provide direction for nursing practice, education, and research. However, the empiric and theoretic knowledge base for the model needs further development, and the model requires further testing and validation.

In summary, these are only four of the available models of nursing that can serve as frameworks for nursing practice. Nurses throughout the country are using these models, adapting them to meet their own individual needs, following other models of nursing, or developing new models. A curriculum based on a conceptual model provides the student and the graduate with a framework for nursing practice within which she can function while providing nursing care and can be guided in furthering her nursing education experiences. It is our belief that students and graduates who use any of the various nursing models can appropriately incorporate into their own frameworks of nursing practice the information about health, illness, and specific disease entities included in this book. Only with knowledge of the physiologic as well as the psychosocial needs of the individual who has a right to health but who experiences the threat of illness can practitioners of nursing fulfill the expectations that are centered in them by society and by the nursing profession.

Nursing and the Health Care Delivery System

Health Defined

The nursing profession exists to meet the health needs of the people. Hence, as health needs change, so must health care. Unprecedented changes have occurred in the structure of our society, in life-styles, and in scientific and technological advances. These changes have altered the pattern of disease and the traditional therapeutic approaches as well as the concept of health care and the expectations that society has of the

health professions. Today, health is considered more than a basic human right; it has become a matter of public concern, national priority, and political action.

Our health system has traditionally been a disease-oriented system. However, the current trend is to emphasize health and its promotion. Health has been defined by the World Health Organization (WHO) as a "state of complete physical, mental, and social well being and not merely the absence of disease and infirmity."* However, such a definition of health does not allow for any variation in the degrees of wellness or illness. The concept of a health–illness continuum (as first described by Dunn [1961]) has markedly affected the purposes of the health professions. By viewing health and illness on a graduated continuum, a person is seen as having neither complete health nor complete illness. Instead, a person's state of health is ever changing and has the potential for ranging from high-level wellness to extremely poor health and imminent death. Thus, a person is viewed as simultaneously possessing degrees of both health and illness. A person who has a chronic illness cannot meet the expectations of health as defined by the WHO definition of health. However, according to the health–illness continuum, the person with a chronic illness can attain a high level of wellness if he is successful in meeting his health potential within the limits of his chronic illness.

During the past 50 years, the health problems of the American people have changed significantly. The majority of such problems are no longer infectious and acute but instead are chronic. Almost 50% of the U.S. population have one or more chronic conditions.

The elderly population has increased significantly, and this increase will continue. In 1989, the nation's 33 million elderly constituted 12% of the population; it is predicted that the number will reach 60 million by the year 2010. Many of the elderly suffer from multiple chronic conditions that are exacerbated by acute episodes. Their health care needs are complex and demand significant investments, both professional and financial, by the health care industry.

With these changes in the health status of the American people has come an increasing emphasis on health, health promotion, wellness, and self-care. Emphasis has shifted from a focus on cure to a focus on prevention and health maintenance. Health is seen as resulting from a life-style that is oriented toward wellness. The result has been the evolution of a wide range of health promotion techniques and programs, including multiphasic screening, lifetime health monitoring programs, environmental and mental health programs, accident prevention, and nutrition and health education. A growing interest in self-care skills is evidenced by the myriad health and medical care publications, conferences, and workshops designed for the lay public. Organized self-care education programs emphasize health promotion, disease prevention, management of illness, self-medication, and use of the professional health care system. In addition, well over 500,000 self-help groups exist for the purpose of developing and sharing self-care with peers who have common chronic disease or disability problems.

Special efforts are being made by health care professionals to reach and motivate members of various cultural and socioeconomic groups concerning life-style and health practices.

---

* *Preamble of the Constitution of the World Health Organization.*

The main thrust is to design a health care delivery system that makes comprehensive health care available to all the people at a tolerable cost. Of course, this type of health care has broad political and sociological implications as organizers, consumers, politicians, and health care providers become involved in the planning.

Concept of Promotion of Wellness and Health Maintenance

Members of health care delivery systems need to gain a vision of the concept of wellness, of what society could accomplish if it were freed from the burdens of illness. Each person should be approached in terms of what his potential state of health should and could be. Inherent in this concept is the understanding that health has to be developed, maintained, and cherished by a continuum of effort. After all, it is not a static state of being; instead, it requires that energy be expended toward reaching an ever higher potential.

It was suggested in the early 1970s (Hoffman, 1972) that "the next major advance in the health of this nation will come through health education, not through more doctors or more hospitals or new discoveries. . . . We must persuade the American people that next to genetics the single most important factor in health is life-style. That even more important than environmental pollution is personal pollution." This suggestion still holds true. Stress, improper diet, lack of exercise, risky sexual practices, smoking, drugs, accidents, and poor hygiene are all related to this concept of how life-style affects health. Health workers, then, should be concerned with encouraging behavior that promotes health. The goal is to motivate people so that they will make improvements in the way they live, in other words, to prompt them toward health behavior changes.

The Health Care Delivery System

The Changing Scene

The health care delivery system is rapidly changing as society's health needs and expectations change. Societal and legislative factors are significant motivators of the changing patterns of health care. Changes in the population in general are affecting the need for and the delivery of health care. It is estimated that by the year 2000 there will be over 300 million people in the United States. This population expansion has in part been attributed to improved public health services and improved nutrition. Not only is the population increasing, but the composition of the population also is changing. With the decline in birth rate since the mid 1950s and the increase in life span that has resulted from improved health care, there are fewer school-age children and more senior citizens. Likewise, the mobility of the population is changing. The advent of sophisticated transportation systems has allowed for increased mobility. The majority of the population reside in highly congested urban areas. Along with this trend toward urbanization, there has been a steady migration of minority groups to the inner cities and a migration of middle-class persons to suburban areas. The number of homeless people has reached significant proportions. Because of such population changes, the need for health care for specific age-groups and for persons within specific geographic localities is altering the effectiveness of the traditional means of providing health care and is necessitating far-reaching changes in the overall health care delivery system.

Technological advances have occurred in greater numbers during the past several decades than in all other epochs of human civilization. This is an era of sophisticated electronic machines, which have revolutionized the labor force by performing many tasks that previously were accomplished by humans. This is also an era of sophisticated communication systems connecting most parts of the world. A variety of systems have been devised for storing, retrieving, and disseminating information. Such scientific and technological advances are themselves precipitating rapid change as well as rapid obsolescence.

Public Concern for Cost-Effective, Quality Care

The general public has become increasingly interested in and knowledgeable about health care and health maintenance. This interest and knowledge have been stimulated by television, newspapers, magazines, and other communications media. The public has become more health conscious and has in general begun to subscribe strongly to the belief that health and health care constitute a basic right, not a privilege for a chosen few. Members of the health care professions have become increasingly aware of the public's beliefs about health and health care. One indication of such awareness is the time-honored Patient's Bill of Rights prepared by the American Hospital Association in 1973, which is directed toward the promotion of more effective patient care and patient satisfaction (Chart 1-1).

The National League for Nursing (NLN) has also issued a statement on patients' rights, which "specifies ways in which a respect for patients' rights and a commitment to safeguarding them can be incorporated into nursing education programs and upheld and reinforced by those in nursing service. In many cases, nurses can directly involve themselves in assuring specific rights; in others, they can make their influence felt indirectly" (Chart 1-2).

Awareness of the public's beliefs and concerns about health and health care has also been acknowledged by Congress. Comprehensive health planning legislation was enacted during the 1960s. The National Health Planning and Resources Act of 1974 emphasized the need for planning and providing quality health care for all Americans by means of coordinated health services, manpower, and facilities at the national, state, and local levels. Medically underserved populations were the target for primary care services provided for by this act. However, growing adherence to the philosophy that comprehensive, quality health care should be provided for all citizens has prompted governmental concern about spiraling health care costs and wide variations in costs among providers. These concerns led to the Medicare prospective payment system.

Diagnosis-Related Groups.   In 1983, Congress enacted the most significant health legislation since the Medicare program in 1965. The government was no longer able to afford retrospective reimbursement of hospitals. Thus, it approved a prospective payment system for hospital inpatient services. The Diagnosis-Related Groups (DRGs) system of reimbursement was adopted as the rate-setting method used for Medicare payments

Chart 1-1
AHA's Patient's Bill of Rights

1. The patient has the right to considerate and respectful care.
2. The patient has the right to obtain from his physician complete current information concerning his diagnosis, treatment, and prognosis in terms the patient can be reasonably expected to understand. When it is not medically advisable to give such information to the patient, the information should be made available to an appropriate person in his behalf. He has the right to know, by name, the physician responsible for coordinating his care.
3. The patient has the right to receive from his physician information necessary to give informed consent prior to the start of any procedure and/or treatment. Except in emergencies, such information for informed consent should include but not necessarily be limited to the specific procedure and/or treatment, the medically significant risks involved, and the probable duration of incapacitation. Where medically significant alternatives for care or treatment exist, or when the patient requests information concerning medical alternatives, the patient has the right to such information. The patient also has the right to know the name of the person responsible for the procedures and/or treatment
4. The patient has the right to refuse treatment to the extent permitted by law and to be informed of the medical consequences of his action.
5. The patient has the right to every consideration of his privacy concerning his own medical care program. Case discussion, consultation, examination, and treatment are confidential and should be conducted discreetly. Those not directly involved in his care must have the permission of the patient to be present.
6. The patient has the right to expect that all communications and records pertaining to his care should be treated as confidential.
7. The patient has the right to expect that within its capacity a hospital must make reasonable response to the request of a patient for services. The hospital must provide evaluation, service, and/or referral as indicated by the urgency of the case. When medically permissible, a patient may be transferred to another facility only after he has received complete information and explanation concerning the needs for and alternatives to such a transfer. The institution to which the patient is to be transferred must first have accepted the patient for transfer.
8. The patient has the right to obtain information as to any relationship of his hospital to other health care and educational institutions insofar as his care is concerned. The patient has the right to obtain information as to the existence of any professional relationships among individuals, by name, who are treating him.
9. The patient has the right to be advised if the hospital proposes to engage in or perform human experimentation affecting his care or treatment. The patient has the right to refuse to participate in such research projects.
10. The patient has the right to expect reasonable continuity of care. He has the right to know in advance what appointment times and physicians are available and where. The patient has the right to expect that the hospital will provide a mechanism whereby he is informed by his physician or a delegate of the physician of the patient's continuing health care requirements following discharge.
11. The patient has the right to examine and receive an explanation of his bill regardless of source of payment.
12. The patient has the right to know what hospital rules and regulations apply to his conduct as a patient.

(Reprinted with the permission of the American Hospital Association.)

for hospital services. Hospitals receive payment at a fixed rate for patients in specific DRGs. A fixed payment has been predetermined for over 460 possible diagnostic categories, which cover the majority of medical diagnoses of all patients admitted to the hospital. Thus, hospitals receive the same payment for every patient with a given DRG. If the cost of the patient's care is lower than the payment, the hospital gains a profit; if the cost is higher, the hospital incurs a loss. In order to qualify for Medicare reimbursement, hospitals must contract with peer review organizations (PROs) to perform quality and utilization review. The PROs monitor admission patterns, lengths of stay, transfers, and the quality of services, and validate DRG coding. The burden is now on hospitals to reduce costs, utilization, and lengths of patient stay.

The DRG system provides hospitals with an incentive to cut unnecessary costs and to discharge patients as quickly as possible. The importance of an effective discharge planning program along with utilization review and quality assurance programs is unquestionable. The impact of these initiatives on nurses is that they must assume responsibility with other health care team members for maintaining quality care while facing pressures to discharge patients and decrease staffing costs. Consequently, nurses in hospitals are caring for patients who are older and sicker and require more nursing services, and nurses in the community are caring for patients who have been discharged earlier and need acute care services, high technology and long-term care.

Quality Assurance.   Quality assurance programs in health care agencies are required for reimbursement of services and for accreditation by the Joint Commission on Accreditation of Healthcare Organizations (JCAHO).

- The concept of quality assurance refers to the accountability of the health professions to society for the quality, quantity, appropriateness, and costs of health services provided.

The impetus for the establishment of quality assurance programs by the health professions was provided by the enactment of the Social Security Amendments of 1972, which

---

Chart 1–2
NLN's *Statement on Patient's Rights*

According to the NLN statement, nurses have a responsibility to uphold the following rights of patients:

- To health care that is accessible and that meets professional standards, regardless of the setting.
- To courteous and individualized health care that is equitable, humane and given without discrimination as to race, color, creed, sex, national origin, source of payment, or ethical or political beliefs.
- To information about their diagnosis, prognosis, and treatment—including alternatives to care and risks involved—in terms they and their families can readily understand, so that they can give their informed consent.
- To informed participation in all decisions concerning their health care.
- To information about the qualifications, names, and titles of personnel responsible for providing their health care.
- To refuse observation by those not directly involved in their care.
- To privacy during interview, examination, and treatment.
- To privacy in communicating and visiting with persons of their choice.

- To refuse treatment, medications, or participation in research and experimentation, without punitive action being taken against them.
- To coordination and continuity of health care.
- To appropriate instruction or education from health care personnel so that they can achieve an optimal level of wellness and an understanding of their basic health needs.
- To confidentiality of all records (except as otherwise provided for by law or third party payer contracts) and all communications, written or oral, between patients and health care providers.
- To access to all health records pertaining to them, and the right to challenge and correct their records for accuracy, and the right to transfer alll such records in the case of continuing care.
- To information on the charges for services, including the right to challenge these.
- To be fully informed as to all their rights in all health care settings.

(National League for Nursing. Nursing's Role in Patient's Rights. New York, The League, 1977. Used with permission.)

---

provided for the creation of professional standards review organizations (PSROs) as a system for evaluating the quality of health care delivered. Since the advent of DRGs, hospitals must contract with PROs for review of quality and appropriateness of care. Subsequently, the Joint Commission has become a significant force in promoting and requiring ongoing quality assurance programs nationwide.

The Joint Commission's "Agenda for Change" for the 1990s requires that health care organizations show evidence that the care they provide results in desired patient health status changes. To ensure this, a generic model was developed that requires monitoring and evaluation of quality and appropriateness of care (Table 1-1).

The model is operational within health care institutions and agencies through an organization-wide quality assurance (QA) program and reporting system. Many aspects of the program may be centralized in a quality assurance department. In addition, each patient care and patient services department is responsible for developing its own plan for monitoring and evaluation. The plans are communicated through the organization's QA structure and committees.

Once responsibility for monitoring and evaluation has been assigned according to the organizational plan, the scope of care or service is defined for each department that provides patient care or services. This includes the range of conditions and patient populations served, treatments provided, procedures performed, locations where and times when services are provided, and the disciplines and specialties of professionals who provide the services. This scope of care then forms the basis for identifying the important aspects of care—those activities or services that are identified as high-volume, high-risk, and/or problem-prone.

Objective and measurable indicators that are appropriate for monitoring the quality of the important aspects of care are then identified. Indicators may measure structure (resources), process (events or activities), or outcome of care or services; a combination of these elements may be used to measure one aspect of care.

The threshold for evaluation is established for each indicator. This is a pre-established level of performance that, when reached, indicates that in-depth evaluation is necessary. Once data are collected, organized, and interpreted, it becomes evident whether or not the threshold for evaluation has been reached; if so, the quality and/or appropriateness of care is reviewed and assessed to determine if there is a problem or an opportunity to improve care. Appropriate action plans are then developed. Once these action plans have been imple-

TABLE 1-1. *JCAHO Ten-Step Model for Monitoring and Evaluation of Quality and Appropriateness of Care*

1. Assign responsibility
2. Delineate the scope of care or service
3. Identify important aspects of care or service
4. Identify indicators
5. Establish thresholds for evaluation
6. Collect and organize data
7. Evaluate
8. Take actions to resolve identified problems
9. Assess the actions and document improvement
10. Communicate relevant information to the organizationwide quality assurance program

mented, the results are assessed to determine if further action is needed. Because monitoring and evaluation activities are ongoing (*e.g.*, weekly, monthly), indications of whether or not action plans are effective quickly become evident.

Results of the monitoring and evaluation activities are documented and communicated as defined by the organization's QA program. The organization then, through objective measurable criteria, can communicate to the public the quality and appropriateness of the care that it provides.

Alternatives to Traditional Health Care: Managed Health Care

In the early 1970s, steadily rising health care costs led to the emergence of new alternative health care delivery systems. The first of these, the health maintenance organization (HMO), provided the first radical change in the provider–insurer relationship and in the traditional fee-for-service system. HMOs provide a means for the delivery of primary health care with emphasis on the adequacy of distribution and the quality of the care provided. They are prepaid group health practice systems designed to deliver comprehensive health care services to a defined group of voluntarily enrolled individuals. HMOs are based on the holistic concept of care—providing ambulatory and inpatient facilities that meet the health care needs of the whole person. The goal of HMOs is to give comprehensive health care that is of the best quality and quantity for the money available while eliminating fragmentation and duplication of services. As HMOs have grown, they have expanded to include specialist services and programs for Medicare and Medicaid populations.

Studies have shown that HMOs are cost-effective and that the quality of care provided by these health care delivery systems is comparable to the care provided elsewhere in the same communities.

HMOs paved the way and served as the model for the preferred provider organizations (PPOs) of the 1980s. In contrast to the HMO, the PPO is not a distinct entity. Rather, it is a business arrangement between a group of providers, usually hospitals and physicians, who contract to provide health care to subscribers, usually businesses, for a negotiated fee that usually is discounted. PPOs allow businesses to decrease their expenses for employee health care benefits, and they allow hospitals and physicians to market their services to employers.

The HMOs and PPOs of the 1970s and 1980s have given rise to a much broader pattern of reimbursement and cost control—*managed health care*. Managed care is considered by many to be the greatest trend in health care and the dominant theme of the 1990s. The failure of the regulatory efforts of the 1970s to cut costs and the resulting escalation of health care costs to 11% of the gross national product (GNP) in 1989 and a predicted 15% to 22% of the GNP by the year 2000 are stimuli that prompted business, labor, and government to assume greater control over financing and delivery of health care. The result is significant expansion of managed health care to the point that distinctions between HMOs, PPOs, exclusive provider arrangements (EPAs), managed indemnity plans, and self-insured managed care are blurring. Their commonalities of prenegotiated payment rates, mandatory precertification, utilization review, limited choice of provider, and fixed-price reimbursement characterize them all as managed care. The scope of managed care has broadened from in-hospital services to include ambulatory, long-term, and home care as well as related diagnostic and therapeutic services.

The results of managed care are already evident: dramatic reduction in in-patient days, continuing expansion of ambulatory care, fierce competition, and marketing strategies that appeal to consumers as well as to insurers and regulators. Hospitals are faced with declining census, increased acuity, and shorter lengths of stay. As patients return to the community, they have more health care needs than ever before, and many of these needs are complex. The demand for home health care services is escalating by leaps and bounds. Whether or not managed care is successful in managing the costs and use of health services will determine its future. If it is not successful, the age-old concept of a national health system may again be considered.

The Nurse as a Health Care Provider

Professional nursing is adapting to meet changing health needs and expectations. One such adaptation can be noted in the *expanded role of the nurse*. This has been a response to the need to improve the distribution of health care services and to decrease the cost of health care. The nurse who functions in an expanded role provides direct care to patients through independent practice, team or interdependent practice, or practice within a health care agency or with a physician. Specialization has evolved within the expanded roles of nursing, a result of the recent explosion of technology.

Nurses now receive advanced education in such specialties as intensive care, coronary care, respiratory care, oncological care, neonatal intensive care, renal dialysis care, trauma care, transplant care, and gerontological care, to name just a few. With the expanded role of the nurse, various titles have emerged that attempt to specify the functions as well as the educational preparation of nurses. Two of these titles are nurse practitioner and clinical nurse specialist.

Although initially the educational preparation for nurse practitioners was in certificate programs, at present both nurse practitioners and clinical nurse specialists are prepared at the master's degree level. These two graduate programs differ in scope and in the definition of the role component. However, despite these differences, comparison of the two roles reveals that there are many areas of overlap.

Nurse practitioners are, for the most part, prepared as generalists (*e.g.*, pediatric nurse practitioner, geriatric nurse practitioner). They define their role in terms of the direct provision of a broad range of services to patients and families. The focus is on providing direct patient care in an environment that promotes a significant degree of autonomy and collaboration with other health professionals. They practice in both acute and nonacute care settings.

Clinical nurse specialists, on the other hand, are prepared as specialists who practice within a circumscribed area of care (*e.g.*, cardiovascular clinical nurse specialist, oncology clinical nurse specialist). They define their role as having four major components: clinical practice, education, consultation, and research. Studies have shown that in reality the focus is often on the education and consultation roles: Education and counseling of patients and families, and education, counseling, and consultation with nursing staff. Although they may practice in a variety of settings, most often their practice is within the acute care hospital setting.

Through the commitment to clinical practice, both the nurse practitioner role and the clinical nurse specialist role have made significant contributions to the advancement of nursing practice. The body of clinical nursing knowledge and skills has been advanced, and clinical practice has been supported as the central focus for advanced practice and the expanded role of the nurse.

With the expanded role of the nurse has come a continuing effort by state nursing associations to more clearly define the practice of nursing. Nurse practice acts have been amended to give nurses the authority to perform functions that were previously restricted to the practice of medicine. These functions include nursing diagnosis, treatment, performance of invasive procedures, and prescription of medications and treatments. Regulations regarding these functions are stipulated by the board of nursing in each state, which defines the education and experience required and the clinical situations in which a nurse may perform these functions.

In general, initial care, ambulatory health care, and anticipatory guidance are all becoming increasingly important in nursing practice. The expanding roles will enable the nurse to function interdependently with other health care professionals and will help to establish a more collegial relationship between physician and nurse.

With the advent of DRGs, the role of the nurse in home care agencies has greatly expanded. Because of early discharge of patients from hospitals, complex care and specialized treatments and procedures are often required. The nurse caring for patients in the home must be skilled in the physical assessment of individuals of all ages. In addition, she must have acute care technological skills and the ability to coordinate the services of a variety of health care providers.

Because nursing services are being provided outside as well as within the hospital, nurses have a choice of practicing in a variety of health delivery settings: acute medical centers, ambulatory care settings, clinics, urgent care centers, outpatient departments, neighborhood health centers, home health care agencies, independent or group nursing practices, and managed care agencies. The expanding scope of nursing practice requires expert skills in interviewing, in observing, in physical assessment and examination, in practicing new clinical techniques, in understanding behavioral patterns, in gathering data, and in promoting the problem-solving skills of individuals, families, and groups. In addition, the nurse must be skillful in decision making, evaluation of the outcomes of care, and measures to promote cost containment and cost reduction. In order to acquire and maintain the necessary clinical expertise, the nurse is responsible for self-development and continuing education during her professional lifetime.

Roles of the Nurse

The professional nurse in both institutional and community health care settings assumes three roles. These may be defined as the *practitioner role*, the *leadership role*, and the *research role*. Although each role carries specific responsibilities, various aspects of each role interrelate with one another and are found in all nursing positions. Accomplishment of each of these roles is designed to meet the immediate and future health care and nursing needs of the patients who are the recipients of nursing care.

Practitioner Role

The *practitioner role* of the nurse involves those actions that the nurse takes when assuming responsibility that is primarily directed toward meeting the health care and nursing needs of individual patients, their families, and significant others. This role is the dominant role of nurses in primary, secondary, and tertiary health care settings. It is a role that can be achieved only through utilization of the nursing process, the basis for all nursing practice.

Within the practitioner role in acute care and long-term care settings, the nurse functions in the interdisciplinary role of *discharge planner*. She collaborates with other health care professionals to ensure timely discharge while promoting positive health outcomes. The discharge planning process is directed toward promotion of continuity of care and maximization of patients' self-care potentials after discharge.

Because the nursing process serves as the basis of nursing practice, and because the teaching–learning process is a significant, integral part of the nursing process, Chapters 2 and 3 have been devoted to the study of these two interrelated processes. Careful study of these chapters will promote increased skill in the practitioner role of nursing.

Clinical Ladders.   Clinical ladders provide practitioners of nursing an opportunity to advance in clinical practice while at the same time maintaining contact with patients. Clinical expertise is evaluated, recognized, and rewarded. By demonstrating increasing clinical competence, knowledge, and expertise, nurses have the opportunity to advance clinically while continuing to provide direct patient care.

Certification for Practice.   Recognition and prestige in nursing practice can also be attained through certification. Certification is voluntary except when required for expanded roles such as nurse anesthetist and nurse midwife. For the most part, it is administered by professional nursing organizations and requires varying amounts of experience and education. Certification provides a mechanism for validating nurses' expertise and demonstrating accountability to the public. The American Nurses Association offers certification in many generalist and specialist nursing areas.

Leadership Role

The leadership role of the nurse has traditionally been perceived as a specialized role assumed only by those nurses who have titles that suggest leadership and who are the leaders of large groups of nurses, related health care professionals, or patients. However, the definition of nursing leadership developed by Yura, Ozimek, and Walsh (1981) gives a broader scope to the concept and identifies leadership as a role that is inherent within all nursing positions. The leadership role of the nurse involves those actions that the nurse accomplishes when assuming responsibility for affecting the actions of others that are directed toward goal determination and achievement. Nursing leadership is a process that involves four behavioral components: deciding, relating, influencing, and facilitating. Each of these components is directed toward change and the ultimate outcome of goal achievement. Basic to the entire process is communication, the effectiveness of which determines the accomplishment of the process. Thus, the leadership process in nursing can be said to be an interpersonal process in which the nurse as a leader uses interpersonal skills to effect change in the behavior of those to whom she relates.

The leadership role that a nurse assumes may or may not involve a large number of people. The nurse uses the leadership process in a variety of circumstances: when assisting a single patient or his family to make changes in their health-related behaviors, when assisting groups or communities to alter their health practices, and when assisting groups of nurses or other health care professionals to affect the actions of patients, groups of patients, or communities with regard to the achievement of desirable health behaviors. The nurse may even be in a position to use the leadership process for assisting specific sectors of the public or the public in general to alter health-related behaviors through such means as legislation, campaigns, and health-oriented public service programs. Thus, the potential scope of the leadership role of the nurse is vast.

Each nurse assumes a leadership role whether she is focusing her practice on one single patient, groups of nurses or other health care professionals, communities, or society in general. The role is a significant one that goes hand in hand with and complements the practitioner role of the nurse.

Patient Advocate. Within an acute care hospital facility, where the nurse is involved in actuating her practitioner role for a single patient or a group of patients, the role of the nurse as a leader may be rather subtle. She may serve primarily as the patient's advocate, anticipating and meeting the needs that he is unable to meet for himself. She must not only be acutely aware of the patient's needs but be able to communicate his needs to other health care professionals involved in his care and to coordinate the efforts of all of these persons in an effort to promote goal achievement.

In the role of patient advocate, the nurse recognizes and respects each patient as a unique individual; within this framework she assists the patient to be autonomous and an informed decision maker. It is the nurse's responsibility to ensure that the patient has all the information he needs to make informed decisions about his health care.

Outside the hospital setting, the persons served by nurses are more independent and usually more capable of making decisions about their health and the health behaviors they strive to achieve. For this reason, the leadership role of the nurse in such a setting may be different from that in the hospital setting. The leadership skills are the same as those used within the hospital setting, but they must be adapted to the environmental variables that affect the patient population, specifically those variables that affect health needs and how they can be met. Environmental variables such as cultural values, attitudes, resources, and the influence of community leaders are just a few of the factors that must be considered by the nurse when attempting to effect changes in the health behaviors of persons within a community.

Research Role

The research role of the nurse has traditionally been assumed only by academicians, nurse scientists, graduate nursing stu-

dents, and researchers from other disciplines. Only recently have nurses in general recognized the acute need for nursing research. Likewise, nurses have just begun to appreciate the significant contributions that can be made to nursing research by nurses in clinical practice.

The primary task of nursing research is to contribute to the scientific base of nursing practice. Studies are needed to determine the actual effects of nursing intervention and nursing care. Without such research efforts, the science of nursing will not grow and a scientifically based rationale for making changes in nursing practice will not be generated.

It is the responsibility of all nurses to become involved in nursing research—to accept their research role. Nurses who have preparation in research methodology can use their research knowledge and skills to initiate and implement timely studies of nursing. This is not to say that nurses who do not initiate and implement nursing research studies do not play a significant role in nursing research. Every nurse has valuable contributions to make to nursing research and a responsibility to make these contributions. All nurses must constantly be alert for nursing problems and important questions about the practice of nursing, which can serve as the basis for the identification of researchable problem areas. Those nurses directly involved in patient care are often in the best position to identify such problems and questions. Their clinical insights are invaluable. Nurses also have a responsibility to become actively involved in ongoing research studies. This participation may involve facilitating the data collection process, or it may involve the actual collection of data. Explaining the study to other health care professionals or to patients and their families is often of invaluable assistance to the nurse who is conducting the study.

Above all, nurses must use research findings in their nursing practice. Research for the sake of research is meaningless. Only with the use of research findings in nursing practice will the science of nursing be furthered. Research findings can be substantiated only through utilization, validation, and dissemination. Nurses must be continually aware of studies that are directly related to their own area of clinical practice. The attitude of every health care agency and every nursing unit within such an agency should be one of interest in the progress of nursing research and of enthusiasm in the utilization of research findings. It must also be remembered that communication and dissemination of research findings are imperative. When findings of studies are not made available to other nurses, the impact of the findings on nursing practice is diminished.

Thus, research is an inherent part of nursing. The future of nursing science depends on the active involvement of nurses in the implementation and utilization of nursing research. Nurses must cultivate their curiosity about nursing practice and their belief in the worth of the practice of nursing by accepting their research role and responsibility. Only with questioning minds can nurses generate nursing research. The scientific basis of nursing depends on the research efforts of all nurses, practitioners and researchers alike.

The National Center for Nursing Research, legislated in 1985 and established at the National Institutes of Health, represents a triumph for the profession. Its purpose is to promote research pertinent to nursing with a focus on the health needs and well-being of the total person. It is the responsibility of practitioners of nursing to become cognizant of the research supported by the center and to incorporate the findings into clinical practice.

The Patient/Client: Consumer and Recipient of Health Care

The term *patient*, which is derived from the Latin verb meaning "to suffer," has traditionally been used to describe those persons who are recipients of nursing care. The connotation commonly attached to the word is one of dependence. For this reason, many nurses prefer to use the term *client*, which is derived from the Latin verb meaning "to lean" and which connotes alliance and interdependence. For the purposes of this book, the term *patient* will be used throughout, but with appreciation for each nurse's prerogative to choose the term that seems more suitable.

The central figure in health care services is, of course, the patient. The patient who presents at the hospital or health care facility with a health problem or problems (increasing numbers of patients have multiple health problems) also comes as an individual, a member of a family, and a citizen of the community. Depending upon the problem, associated circumstances, and past experiences, patients' needs will vary. One of the nurse's important functions is to identify the patient's immediate needs and take measures to alleviate them. Utilization of a basic needs approach to nursing care is appropriate.

The Patient's Basic Needs

Certain basic needs are common to *all* humans and demand satisfaction accordingly. Such needs are dealt with on the basis of priority, meaning that certain needs are more pressing than others. However, once an essential need is met, a person moves to a need on a higher level. Approaching needs according to priority reflects Maslow's hierarchy of needs, in which human needs may be ranked as follows: physiologic needs; safety and security; belongingness and affection; esteem and self-respect; and self-actualization, which includes self-fulfillment, desire to know and understand, and aesthetic needs.* Lower-level needs always remain, but because there is a reduction in need tension, the person is able to move to higher-level needs. A person's pursuit of higher-level needs indicates that he is moving toward psychologic health and well-being. Such a hierarchy of needs is a useful organizational framework that can be used with the various nursing models for assessment of patients' strengths, limitations, and need for nursing interventions (Fig. 1-1).

Physiologic Needs

Physiologic needs predominate in the motivation of human behavior and drive the mechanisms that maintain *homeostasis*—the constancy of the internal environment of an organism (see Chap. 8). They involve the regulation of respiratory, nutritive, and excretory functions, as well as maintenance of the water content of tissues, adjustments of body temperature, and the operation of numerous protective mechanisms. Also included as physiologic needs are the need for rest and sleep, and the avoidance of pain. Sex is considered a basic drive but is not essential for survival.

Maslow AH. Motivation and Personality. New York, Harper & Row, 1970.

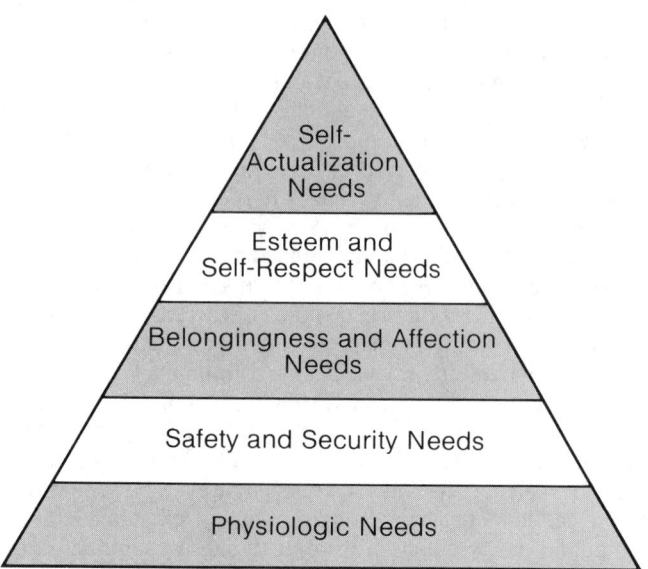

Figure 1-1. This scheme of Maslow's hierarchy of human needs shows how a person moves from basic need fulfillment to higher levels of needs, with the ultimate goal of integrated human functioning and health.

These physiologic needs are powerful; unless satisfied, they dominate the conscious mind. For example, if a patient is obliged to restrict his fluid intake for therapeutic reasons, thirst may absorb his thoughts. He may discuss nothing but drinking, complain incessantly of thirst, and repeatedly question his nurse and physician about when fluids will be forthcoming. During this period he is not likely to be too concerned about his environment. As soon as his thirst is quenched, he becomes aware of other needs; for example, now he may be disturbed by the absence of privacy.

Safety Needs and Security Needs

If the physiologic needs are satisfied, the concern for safety and security emerges—psychologic as well as physical safety. The normal adult is able to protect himself and usually does not feel endangered. He is relatively "safe" from death. His job is "safe." His insurance program and his savings furnish a sense of economic security.

Illness naturally poses a threat. The sick person may be apprehensive in response to the many different persons with unfamiliar functions who enter his room. Diagnostic tests and therapeutic procedures may contribute to his fears. He wants to feel safe and secure. Although he may not express his feelings in these terms, he wants the health team members to be aware of his insecurity. To help protect the patient from harm, the nurse must know the nature of his illness and be cognizant of any possible complications. If complications should occur, she must be able to provide intelligent, appropriate care. The nurse's role in promoting the psychologic safety of the patient is discussed in Chapter 10.

Need for Belongingness and Affection

Once the patient's physiologic and safety needs have been satisfied, his needs for belongingness and affection will become apparent. Every person, sick or well, desires the companionship and recognition of others. A sick person wants and needs his family or, in their absence, friends. Thus, any signs of genuine interest and kindness are usually appreciated. The wise nurse is constantly aware of this need and of its importance in relation to the patient's morale. One way to achieve this end is to help the family members feel that they have a definite contribution to make to the patient's recovery. Assessment and interpretation of the patient's behavior are essential for identification of indicators of his unmet need for belongingness and affection. He may be quiet, uncomplaining, and eager to please. Or, he may demand attention by constantly making requests, asking questions, or being generally disruptive. By accurately interpreting such behaviors, the nurse can intervene in ways that will promote the patient's feeling of acceptance and belonging. Mutual goal setting is important in assuring the patient and his family that they are important members of the health care team.

Need for Esteem and Self-Respect

Man is by nature a social being, abhorring isolation. Illness removes him from his relatively convivial world and transplants him into a strange environment, an environment that is entirely unsought and unfamiliar, one in which he feels incompetent and alone. Previously an actively contributing member of society, he now must accept a position of dependency. The patient needs to preserve his self-esteem. He needs to be recognized as an individual, a distinct personality. The professional nurse, imbued with the concept of the individual worth and dignity of man, sees to it that this need is fulfilled. She takes time to listen to the patient. To the extent that he desires it and opportunity permits, she joins him in conversation. She exhibits interest in all matters that seem important to him; her attentiveness, thoughtfulness, and kindness convey that he is respected and that his needs and problems are recognized.

Unmet esteem and self-respect needs are exhibited by feelings of dependency and lack of confidence, competence, and ability. Patient education that focuses on the patient's acquisition of skills and knowledge is helpful in increasing the patient's self-esteem and self-respect.

Need for Self-Actualization

Maslow estimated that only about 1% of the adult population ever reaches the level of self-actualization. Self-actualization may not be possible for persons in poverty-stricken or emotionally deprived environments. Additionally, many people are satisfied with meeting lower-level needs and do not strive for self-actualization.

Need for Self-Fulfillment.   Once the patient's physiologic needs have been met and he is feeling secure, esteemed, and wanted, his creative impulses may now emerge. During the course of a short hospital stay, this need is not likely to be frustrated. However, the patient with a long-term illness must be assured an opportunity to express himself creatively and to feel useful.

Need to Know and Understand.   The need to know and understand is a strong drive. The intelligent person seeks information, organizes it, analyzes it, and searches for its meaning. In general, patients want to know what is in store for them, and they are thwarted by explanations that are too brief or vague. Many patients know a surprising amount about the bodily functions. However, while some of their information may be factual, some of it is likely to be inaccurate, and correction or clarification may be necessary. Instruction is the responsibility of the nurse, and the teaching of patients is one of the most important nursing functions. To teach correctly and effectively,

the nurse must have a thorough knowledge of the subject, be skilled in communication, and be cognizant of the basic principles of teaching and learning. The explanations, while simple for the sake of comprehension, must be meaningful if they are to be accepted by the patient. His physical and emotional status, intelligence, experience as a patient, and awareness of the situation, as well as the urgency of his need to know and understand, must be given consideration. The nurse must also consider the possible implications of her intended remarks and guard with equal care against inaccuracies on her part and misunderstandings on the part of the patient.

Aesthetic Needs.   Aesthetic needs vary in importance from person to person, but for all patients the most salutary environment is one that is orderly and one in which there is beauty. The patient with highly developed aesthetic sensibilities will be distressed by unpleasant sights, sounds, odors, and disarray. He may crave flowers, books, or music—amenities that, when supplied, add immeasurably to his well-being.

In summary, it may be pointed out that most of the needs of the average individual, ill or well, can be satisfied only in part. Moreover, the nurse, whose responsibility and privilege it is to help the patient meet his needs and resolve his problems, must recognize the fact that some problems can be neither eliminated nor solved. In relation to the patient with such a problem, the nurse's role is to help him make a mature, objective, and compensatory adjustment to its continued existence or to its imperfect solution, if this solution is the best that can be achieved.

Approach to the Patient

In the process of searching for ways to fulfill patient needs, nursing has devised various methods of approaching the patient. During the 1950s and 1960s, the concept of team nursing came to the fore. Subsequently, questions were raised concerning the effectiveness of team nursing. In recent years, primary nursing has been advocated and implemented in many hospital settings. Some studies have shown that primary nursing, when compared with team nursing, significantly increases the quality of patient care and is more cost-effective. However, more research is needed to substantiate these findings.

Primary Nursing

Primary nursing, not to be confused with primary health care that deals with first-contact general health care, refers to comprehensive, individualized care that is provided with continuity. Individualized total care is provided to the patient by the same nurse from the time of the patient's admission until his discharge. This type of nursing care eliminates the fragmented care that typified team nursing. It allows the nurse to give direct patient care rather than manage and supervise the functions of others who care for the patient. In essence, it allows the nurse the opportunity to implement her practitioner role and her leadership role within the framework of rendering direct patient care.

The focus of primary nursing is the patient. The primary

nurse accepts total 24-hour responsibility for quality nursing care for the patient. This nursing care is directed toward meeting his total, individualized nursing needs—his biopsychosocial needs. The primary nurse is responsible and accountable for involving the patient and his family directly in all facets of his care. The primary nurse has autonomy that allows her to make decisions with the patient and his family concerning his care. Thus, she is a facilitator of family-centered as well as patient-centered nursing care. Communications with other members of the health team regarding the patient and his health care are made by the primary nurse. This allows the nurse to provide for continuity of care and to promote collaborative efforts directed toward the assurance of quality care. It provides the other health care professionals with the opportunity to communicate directly with the nurse who is responsible for the patient's care.

Ideally, the number of patients for whom the nurse acts as the primary nurse is limited to three or four. However, this number may range from one to ten depending on the extent of the nursing needs of the patients. The nurse meets the patient as soon as possible after his admission to the health care facility. This allows her to begin to establish a relationship with the patient, which will continue until discharge and, in some cases, after discharge. It allows the patient to identify with the nurse who will be responsible for his care. Each day that the primary nurse works she cares for the patient. She is aware of problems and needs as they arise, and she assumes responsibility for securing the means to solve the problems and meet the needs. Prior to the patient's discharge to another health care facility or to his home, the primary nurse assumes the responsibility for making the appropriate referrals and for ensuring that all relevant information is provided to those persons who will be involved in his care. Throughout the entire admission, the nurse continually strives to involve the patient's family in his care and in the preparations that are made for his discharge.

During the times when the primary nurse is not scheduled to work, she is assisted by an associate nurse, or co-nurse. This associate nurse implements the nursing care plan and provides feedback to the primary nurse that is invaluable in evaluation of the care plan. However, it remains the responsibility of the primary nurse to make sure that the patient's needs are met and that continuity of care is not lost when she is not present to render the care herself.

Within the concept of primary nursing, the nurse manager (head nurse) functions as a consultant for the primary nurses, and she strives toward providing opportunities for these nurses to continually improve their clinical expertise. The nurse manager initiates the nurse–patient relationship by assigning the primary nurse to her designated patients. This is done with knowledge of the primary nurse's capabilities and her particular areas of nursing expertise. The nurse manager then serves as a resource person for the primary nurse when she is confronted with patient problems or needs that she is unable to resolve. Periodic evaluation of the primary nurse's performance is her responsibility. Frequent interaction with the primary nurse and her patients gives her much information that can be used positively in assisting the primary nurse to use her capabilities to their utmost and to make strides toward overcoming limitations. The nurse manager may also function as a primary nurse for a small group of patients. By assuming such responsibility, she uses her clinical expertise in giving direct patient care and serves as a role model for the primary nurses.

Nursing students, practical nurses, and nursing assistants function within the primary nursing framework. The responsibility for maintaining continuity of total individualized nursing care remains with the primary nurse. However, when direct patient care is not given by the primary nurse, other members of the health care team assume this responsibility. They implement the plan of care developed by the primary nurse and consult with the primary nurse when changes in the plan of care seem warranted. In such instances, the primary nurse serves as a valuable consultant and teacher for associate nurses and other personnel. Nursing care conferences provide a means for the exchange of information. In these conferences, the quality of care rendered to the patient is the focus, and continuity of individualized total patient care is the goal.

Primary nursing has been designed to increase the accountability and responsibility of the nurse to the patient. Studies conducted at selected hospitals that have implemented primary nursing reveal that primary nurses recognize greater enrichment from their jobs because of the high degree of autonomy, identity, significance, and variety afforded them by the primary nursing system of delivering care.

The long-term survival of primary nursing as it is currently implemented is not known. As cost-containment measures accelerate and patient acuity increases, staffing ratios of patients to nurses are increasing. Many nursing service departments and agencies are meeting the increased workload demands by making modifications in their approach to primary nursing or by reverting to team or functional systems for delivering care. Others are changing their staffing mixes and redesigning their models of practice to accommodate nurse extender roles. Still others are changing to more innovative systems such as case management.

Case Management

Within recent years, with the myriad changes that have occurred in the health care environment, case management has gained interest among nurses as a means for providing coordination of services. The case management process dates back to the public health programs of the early 1900s, and it has always been the dominant role of public health nursing. Over the years, the process has varied in form and function, but the basic theme has remained: responsibility for meeting patient needs rests with one individual or team whose purpose is to provide the patient with access to required services and to evaluate the effectiveness of these services.

Although nurses within health care institutions have not traditionally functioned as case managers, a significant cadre of nursing leaders are expanding their models of practice from primary nursing to case management. The stimuli for this change in many cases include the decrease in in-patient length of stay coupled with the rapid and frequent inter-unit transfers from specialty care units to standard care units and the shortage of nurses to serve as primary nurses. In many cases, primary nurses are no longer able to meet the complex needs of patients during the shortened stay on a given unit.

The case manager role, instead of focusing on direct patient care, focuses on managing the care of an entire caseload of patients and managing the personnel who care for the patients. In most instances, the caseload is limited in scope to patients with similar diagnoses, needs, and therapies, and the case managers function across units. They are experts in their specialty areas and function to coordinate the in-patient and outpatient services needed by patients. The goals of this co-ordination include quality, appropriateness, and timeliness of services as well as cost reduction. The case manager follows the patient after discharge in an effort to access health care services that will avert or delay rehospitalization.

Chapter Summary

Throughout this chapter, the evolution of the profession of nursing has been explored. Many references have been made to the significance of nurses as members of the health care team. Over the years, nurses have strived to change their role from one of subservience to other members of the health care team, particularly the physician, to one that is collegial. As nursing practitioners and researchers make advances in the area of concept formalization and theory building, the unique competencies of the profession of nursing become more clearly articulated. It becomes increasingly more evident that nursing provides certain health care services that are unique to this profession. However, nursing continues to recognize the importance of collaboration with other health care disciplines in meeting all of the health care needs of patients.

In some institutions the *nurse–physician collaborative practice model* is used. Within a decentralized organizational structure and with a primary nursing care delivery system, nurses and physicians function collaboratively in making clinical decisions. A joint practice committee with equal representation from both professions functions at the unit level to monitor, support, and foster collaborative relations. Collaborative prac-

tice is further enhanced with integration of the clinical record and with joint patient care record reviews. Figure 1-2 compares the traditional model with the collaborative practice model. The Secretary of Health and Human Services Commission on Nursing, in its report in 1988, recognized the essential nature of collaborative practice to health care delivery by recommending that employers of nurses and the medical profession foster collaboration between members of the health care team.

The collaborative model or a variation of it should be a primary goal for nursing—a venture that would promote shared participation, responsibility, and accountability in a health care environment that is striving to meet the complex health care needs of the public.

Bibliography

Books

American Nurses Association. Issues in Professional Nursing Practice. Kansas City, MO, American Nurses Association, 1984.

Barnum BS. Nursing Theory: Analysis, Application, Evaluation. Glenview, IL, Scott Foresman/Little, Brown Higher Education, 1990.

Birmingham JJ. Home Care Planning Based on DRGs: Functional Health Pattern Model. Philadelphia, JB Lippincott, 1986.

Cabinet on Nursing Research. Education for Participation in Nursing Research. Kansas City, MO, American Nurses Association, 1989.

Cabinet on Nursing Research. Human Rights Guidelines for Nurses in Clinical and Other Research. Kansas City, MO, American Nurses Association, 1985.

Chinn P and Jacobs MK. Theory and Nursing: A Systematic Approach. St Louis, CV Mosby, 1991.

Curtin LL and Zurlage MA. DRGs: The Reorganization of Health. Chicago, S-N Publications, 1984.

Duldt BW and Giffin K. Theoretical Perspectives for Nursing. Boston, Little, Brown & Co, 1985.

Dunn HL. High-Level Wellness. Arlington, VA, RW Beatty, 1961.

Ellis JR and Hartley CL. Nursing in Today's World: Challenges, Issues, and Trends. Philadelphia, JB Lippincott, 1988.

England DA. Collaboration in Nursing. Rockville, MD, Aspen Systems Corporation, 1986.

Fawcett J. Analysis and Evaluation of Conceptual Models of Nursing. Philadelphia, FA Davis, 1989.

Fitzpatrick JJ and Whall AL. Conceptual Models of Nursing: Analysis and Application. Norwalk, CT, Appleton and Lange, 1989.

George JB. Nursing Theories. The Base for Professional Nursing Practice. Norwalk, CT, Appleton and Lange, 1990.

Grippando GM. Nursing Perspectives & Issues. Albany, NY, Delmar Publishers, 1989.

Hamric AB and Spross JA (eds): The Clinical Nurse Specialist in Theory and Practice. Philadelphia, WB Saunders, 1989.

Healthy People 2000. U.S. Dept of Health and Human Services. Public Health Services, Washington, DC, 1990.

Henderson V. The Nature of Nursing. New York, Macmillan, 1966.

Johnson DE. The behavioral system model in nursing. In Riehl JP and Roy C (eds). Conceptual Models for Nursing Practice. New York, Appleton-Century-Crofts, 1980.

King IM. A Theory for Nursing: Systems, Concepts, Process. New York, John Wiley & Sons, 1981.

Leddy S and Pepper JM. Conceptual Bases of Professional Nursing. Philadelphia, JB Lippincott, 1989.

Maslow AH. Motivation and Personality. New York, Harper & Brothers, 1970.

Mayer GG and Madden MJ. Patient Care Delivery Models. Rockville, MD, Aspen Systems Corporation, 1990.

Meleis AI. Theoretical Nursing: Development and Progress. Philadelphia, JB Lippincott, 1991.

Moloney MM. Professionalization of Nursing: Current Issues and Trends. Philadelphia, JB Lippincott, 1986.

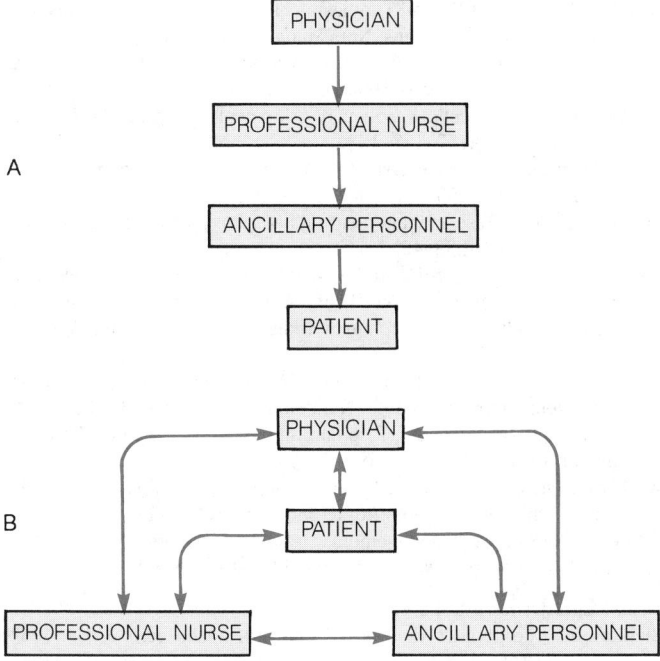

Figure 1–2. Comparison of traditional practice model (**A**) and collaborative practice model (**B**).

Neuman B. The Neuman Systems Model: Application to Nursing Education and Practice. Norwalk, CT, Appleton and Lange, 1989.

Nightingale F. Notes on Nursing: What It Is, and What It Is Not. New York, D Appleton, 1860.

Norris CM. Concept Clarification in Nursing. Rockville, MD, Aspen Systems Corporation, 1982.

Nursing. A Social Policy Statement. Kansas City, MO, American Nurses Association, 1980.

Nursing Case Management. Kansas City, MO, American Nurses Association, 1988.

Nursing's Vital Signs. Shaping the Profession for the 1990s. Battle Creek, Michigan, 1990.

Orem DE. Nursing: Concepts of Practice. St Louis, CV Mosby–Year Book, 1991.

Riehl JP and Roy C. Conceptual Models for Nursing Practice. New York, Appleton and Lange, 1989.

Rogers ME. An Introduction to the Theoretical Basis of Nursing. Philadelphia, FA Davis, 1970.

Styles MM. On Nursing: Toward a New Endowment. St Louis, CV Mosby, 1982.

Torres G. Theoretical Foundations of Nursing. Norwalk, CT, Appleton-Century-Crofts, 1986.

Yura H, Ozimek D, and Walsh MB. Nursing Leadership: Theory and Process. New York, Appleton-Century-Crofts, 1981.

Journals

Asterisks indicate nursing research articles.

Theories and Concepts of Nursing

Buchanan BF. Conceptual models: An assessment framework. J Nurs Adm 1987 Oct; 17(10):22–26.

Christmyer CS et al. Bridging the gap: Theory to practice—Part I, Clinical applications. Nurs Manage 1988 Aug; 19(8):42–50.

Cull–Welby BL and Pepin JI. Towards a coexistence of paradigms in nursing knowledge development. J Adv Nurs 1987 Apr; 12(4):515–521.

* Derdiarian AK. The relationships among the subsystems of Johnson's behavioral system model. Image: Journal of Nursing Scholarship 1990 winter; 22(4):219–225.

Fawcett J and Carino C. Hallmarks of success in nursing practice. Adv Nurs Sci 1989 Jul; 11(4):1–8.

Fruehwirth SES. An application of Johnson's behavioral model: A case study. J Community Health Nurs 1989; 6(2):61–71.

Geger JA et al. Roy adaptation model: ICU application. Dimens Crit Care Nurs 1987 Jul/Aug; 6(4):215–224.

* Hoch CC. Assessing delivery of nursing care. J Gerontol Nurs 1987 Jan; 13(1):10–17.

Schlotfeldt RM. Defining nursing: A historic controversy. Nurs Res 1987 Jan/Feb; 36(1):64–67.

Roles of Nurses

Becker KL et al. A nurse practitioner job description. Nurs Manage 1989 Jun; 20(6):42–44.

Bock LR. From research to utilization: Bridging the gap. Nurs Manage 1990 Mar; 21(3):50–51.

Bone LR et al. Improving patient care through a collaborative discharge planning instrument. Nursing Connections 1988 Winter; 1(4):57–66.

Brodie B. A commitment to care: The development of clinical specialization in nursing. ANNA J 1989 May; 16(3):181–186.

Corcoran S. Toward operationalizing an advocacy role. J Prof Nurs 1988 Jul/Aug; 4(4):242–248.

Cronin CJ and Maklebust J. Case-managed care: Capitalizing on the CNS. Nurs Manage 1989 Mar; 20(3):38–47.

* Dittmann EE and Gould MT. Refinement of nursing diagnosis skills: The effect of clinical nurse specialist teaching and consultation. J Contin Educ Nurs 1987 Sep/Oct; 18(5):157–159.

Doyen L. The ally too many nurses ignore. RN 1988 Nov; 51(11):40–41.

Harkness GA. Using research principles in nursing practice. Nursing Scan in Research 1989 Sep/Oct; 2(5):1–2.

Jassak PF and Ryan MP. Ethical issues in clinical research. Semin Oncol Nurs 1989 May; 5(2):102–108.

Jernigan M. Nursing and research: Some ethical concerns. Nursing Scan in Research 1989 Jan/Feb; 2(1):1–3.

Keen-Payne R. Consumerism in nursing. J Nurs Staff Dev 1988 Fall; 4(4): 169–173.

Kibbee P. An emerging professional: The quality assurance nurse. J Nurs Adm 1988 Apr; 18(4):30–33.

Meisenhelda JB. Essential ingredients for research in the clinical setting. Nursing Scan in Research 1990 May/Jun; 3(3):1–3.

Moore C. Need for a patient advocate. JAMA 1989 Jul 14; 262(2):259–260.

Murray JT. Credentialing: A pathway to quality. J Nurs Adm 1987 May; 17(5):33.

Stanford D. Nurse practitioner research: Issues in practice and theory. Nurse Pract 1987 Jan; 12(1):64–75.

Teasley D. Situational leadership for nurses. Nurs Manage 1987 Nov; 18(11): 112–113.

* Thibodeau J and Hawkins J. Nurse practitioners: Factors affecting role performance. Nurse Pract 1989 Dec; 14(12):47, 50–52.

Nursing Delivery Models

Beyers M. Future of nursing care delivery. Nurs Adm Q 1987 Winter; 11(2): 71–80.

Bowers L. The significance of primary nursing. J Adv Nurs 1989 Jan; 14(1): 13–19.

Bradford R. Obstacles to collaborative practice. Nurs Manage 1989 Apr; 20(4):72I–72P.

Clifford JC. Will the professional practice model survive? J Prof Nurs 1988 Mar/Apr; 4(2):77–78.

Crowley S and Wallner I. Collaborative practice: A tool for change. Oncol Nurs Forum 1987; 14(4):59–63.

Del Togno-Armanasco V, Olivas GS, and Harter S. Developing an integrated nursing case management model. Nurs Manage 1989 Oct; 20(10): 26–30.

Ethridge P and Lamb GS. Professional nursing case management improves quality, access and costs. Nurs Manage 1989 Mar; 20(3):30–35.

Executive Summary of Secretary's Commission on Nursing Report. Nurs Econ 1989 Jan/Feb; 7(1):57–59.

Franklin JL et al. An evaluation of case management. Am J Public Health 1987 Jun; 77(6):674–678.

Glandon GL, Colbert KW, and Thomasma M. Nursing delivery models and RN mix: Cost implications. Nurs Manage 1989 May; 20(5):30–33.

Jacoby J and Terpstra M. Collaborative governance: Model for professional autonomy. Nurs Manage 1990 Feb; 21(2):42–44.

Jovie EM et al. The practical aspects of primary nursing. ANNA J 1988 Jun; 15(3):157–158, 192.

Jovie EM et al. Theoretical basis for primary nursing practice. ANNA J 1988 Jun; 15(3):155–156.

Knollmueller RN. Case management: What's in a name? Nurs Manage 1989 Oct; 20(10):38–42.

Loveridge CE, Cummings SH, and O'Malley J. Developing case management in a primary nursing system. J Nurs Adm 1988 Oct; 18(10):36–39.

Magargal P. Modular nursing: Nurses rediscover nursing. Nurs Manage 1987 Nov; 18(11):96–104.

McKenzie CB, Torkelson NG, and Holt MA. Care and cost: Nursing case management improves both. Nurs Manage 1989 Oct; 20(10):30–34.

Mowry MM and Korpman RA. Hospitals, nursing, and medicine: The years ahead. J Nurs Adm 1987 Nov; 17(11):16–22.

Wolf GA, Lesic LK, and Leak AG. Primary nursing. The impact on nursing costs within DRGs. J Nurs Adm 1986 Mar; 16(3):9–11.

Zander K. Nursing case management: Strategic management of cost and quality outcomes. J Nurs Adm 1988 May; 18(5):23–30.

Health Care Delivery System

Blendon RJ. The public's view of the future of health care. JAMA 1988 Jun; 259(24):3587–3593.

Buchanan JR. Educational impacts of new care systems. J Med Educ 1987 Feb; 62(2):100–108.

* Bull MJ. Influence of diagnosis-related groups on discharge planning, professional practice, and patient care. J Prof Nurs 1988 Nov/Dec; 4(6):415–421.

Califano JA. Guiding the forces of the health care revolution. Nurs Health Care 1987 Sep; 8(7):401–404.

Carter S and Moward L. Is nursing ready for consumerism? Nurs Adm Q 1988 Spring; 12(3):74–78.

Coile RC. Health care 1990: Top 10 trends for the year ahead. Hospital Strategy Report 1989 Dec; 2(2):1–8.

Halloran EJ, Kiley M, and England M. Nursing diagnosis, DRGs, and length of stay. Appl Nurs Res 1988 May; 1(1):22–26.

Kramer M and Schmalenberg C. Magnet hospitals talk about the impact of DRGs on nursing care—Part II. Nurs Manage 1987 Oct; 18(10): 33–40.

Merrill J. The buck stops here. RN 1989 Oct; 52(10):28–36.

Moccia P. 1989: Shaping a human agenda for the nineties. Nurs Health Care 1989 Jan; 10(1):15–17.

Porter-O'Grady T. Restructuring the nursing organization for a consumer-driven marketplace. Nurs Adm Q 1988 Spring; 12(3):60–65.

Povar G and Moreno J. Hippocrates and the health maintenance organization. A discussion of ethical issues. Ann Intern Med 1988 Sep; 109: 419–424.

Sederer LI and St. Clair RL. Managed health care and the Massachusetts Experience. Am J Psychiatry 1989 Sep; 146(9):1142–1146.

Shaffer FA. DRGs: A new era for health care. Nurs Clin North Am 1988 Sep; 23(3):453–463.

Smith GR. The new health care economy: Opportunities for nurse entrepreneurs. Nurs Outlook 1987 Jul/Aug; 35(4):182–184.

Thompson JD and Diers D. Management of nursing intensity. Nurs Clin North Am 1988 Sep; 23(3):473–492.

Quality Assurance

Beyers M. Quality: The banner of the 1980s. Nurs Clin North Am 1988 Sep; 23(3):617–623.

Cassidy DA and Friesen MA. QA: Applying JCAHO's generic model. Nurs Manage 1990 Jun; 21(6):22–27.

Coons M et al. Unit or service standards. Nurs Clin North Am 1988 Sep; 23(3):639–648.

Coyne C and Killien M. A system for unit-based monitors of quality of nursing care. J Nurs Adm 1987 Jan; 17(1):26–32.

Donabedian A. The quality of care. How can it be assessed? JAMA 1988 Sep; 260(12):1743–1748.

* Erikson LR. Patient satisfaction: An indicator of nursing care quality? Nurs Manage 1987 Jul; 18(7):31–35.

Esper PS. Discharge planning—A quality assurance approach. Nurs Manage 1988 Oct; 19(10):66–68.

Harris SH, Krefer SM, and Davis MZ. A problem-focused quality assurance program. Nurs Manage 1989 Feb; 20(2):54–60.

Kanar RJ. Standards of nursing practice assessed through the application of the nursing process. J Nurs Qual Assur 1987 Feb; 1(2):72–78.

Lanza ML. Research and quality assurance: Similarities and differences. Nursing Scan in Research 1990 Mar/Apr; 3(2):1–3.

Matthais SM, Greenlee KK, and Proctor D. Developing unit-specific standards. Dimens Crit Care Nurs 1988 Nov/Dec; 7(6):364–368.

McAllister M. A nursing integration framework based on standards of practice. Nurs Manage 1990 Apr; 21(4):28–31.

New NA and New JR. Quality assurance that works. Nurs Manage 1989 Jun; 20(6):21–24.

O'Brien B. QA: A commitment to excellence. Nurs Manage 1988 Nov; 19(11):33–40.

Patterson CH. Standards of patient care: The Joint Commission focus on nursing quality assurance. Nurs Clin North Am 1988 Sep; 23(3):625–638.

Porter AL. Assuring quality through staff nurse performance. Nurs Clin North Am 1988 Sep; 23(3):649–655.

Robbins CL and Robbins WA. What nurse managers should know about sampling techniques. Nurs Manage 1989 Jun; 20(6):46–48.

Schroeder P. Directions and dilemmas in nursing quality assurance. Nurs Clin North Am 1988 Sep; 23(3):657–664.

Short NM and Baer L. Standards of care: Practicing what we preach. Nurs Manage 1990 Jun; 21(6):32–39.

Smith TC and Powers BA. An integrative approach to quality assurance. Nurs Manage 1990 Jun; 21(6):28–30.

Westfalt UE. Standards of practice: Nursing values made visible. J Nurs Qual Assur 1989 Feb; 1(2):21–30.

2

The Nursing Process

Learning Objectives

On completion of this chapter, the learner will be able to:

1. Define the components of the nursing process
2. Identify the variables involved in effectively conducting a nursing history and a health assessment
3. Describe the significance of nursing diagnosis to the profession of nursing
4. Describe the process of developing a nursing diagnosis
5. Describe the collaborative role of the nursing team, the patient and his family, and resource persons from health care and community agencies in meeting the patient's health care needs
6. Identify the purposes and essential components of the nursing care plan
7. Develop a nursing care plan for a patient
8. Identify the purposes of the problem-oriented health record system
9. Identify the appropriate information to be included in each section of the progress notes (SOAPIE)
10. Use the problem-oriented health record for documentation

The nursing process has been accepted as the essence of nursing. It is a deliberate, problem-identification, and problem-solving approach to meeting the health care and nursing needs of patients. Although the steps of the nursing process have been delineated in various ways by many nursing leaders, the commonalities found in all definitions are assessment, nursing diagnosis, planning, implementation, and evaluation. These fundamental components can be used to define the nursing process as follows:

1. *Assessment*—systematic collection of data to determine the patient's health status and to identify any actual or potential health problems. (Analysis of data is included as part of the assessment. For those who wish to emphasize its importance, analysis may be identified as a separate step of the nursing process.)

2. *Nursing Diagnosis*—identification of actual or potential health problems that are amenable to resolution by means of nursing actions.

3. *Planning*—development of goals and a plan of care designed to assist the patient in resolving the nursing diagnoses.

4. *Implementation*—actualization of the plan of care through nursing interventions or supervision of others to do the same.

5. *Evaluation*—determination of the patient's responses to the nursing interventions and the extent to which the goals have been achieved.

• Thus, the nursing process is a data-collecting, decision-making process that incorporates evaluation and subsequent modification as feedback mechanisms that promote the ultimate resolution of the patient's nursing diagnoses.

Division of the nursing process into five distinct components or steps serves to emphasize the critical nursing actions that must be accomplished when the nurse assumes responsibility for resolving the patient's nursing diagnoses. However, the nurse must remember that the divisions are artificial and that the process as a whole is cyclic, the steps being interrelated, interdependent, and recurrent (Fig. 2-1).

Assessment

The assessment component of the nursing process begins with the nurse's first encounter with the patient. It involves the systematic collection of data about the patient's health status, analysis of the data to determine his actual and potential health needs, and use of the data to formulate nursing diagnoses.

• The nursing diagnoses then become the basis for the nursing care plan.

Sensitive and continuous nursing assessment by means of the health history and the health assessment is essential to

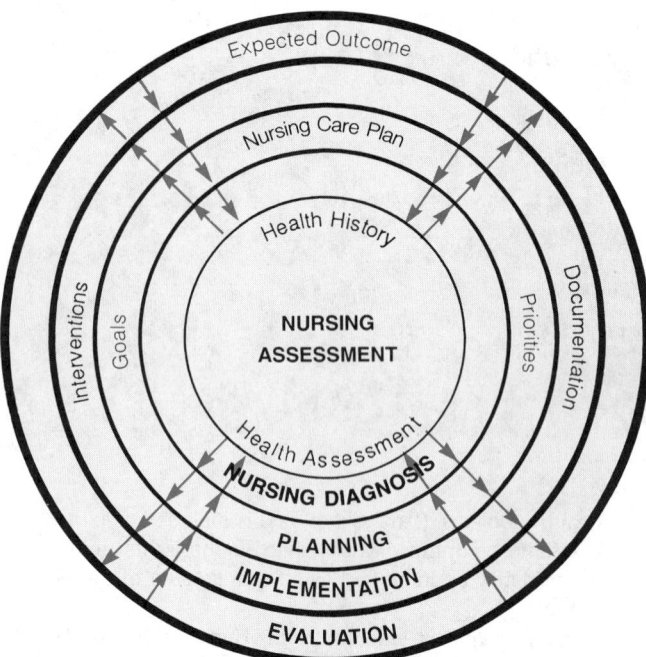

Figure 2–1. The nursing process is depicted schematically in this circle. Starting from the innermost circle, nursing assessment, the process moves outward through the formulation of nursing diagnoses, planning, the setting of goals and priorities, establishing the nursing care plan, and actual implementations health and documentation, and arrives at the ongoing process of evaluation and expected outcomes.

maintain an awareness of the patient's needs and the effectiveness of the nursing care that he receives.

Health History

The health history is carried out for the purpose of determining the patient's state of wellness or illness and is best accomplished as part of a planned interview. The interview is a dialogue between the patient and the nurse and is a very personal experience. Interviewing is a process that requires wisdom, judgment, tact, and experience. It involves the sensitive direction of a conversation with a patient in order to obtain information about him. The nurse's approach to the patient will largely determine the amount and quality of information that is received. Achieving a relationship of mutual trust and respect requires the ability to communicate a sincere interest in the patient. The patient is made as comfortable as possible and afforded privacy for the interview.

The skills involved in interviewing a patient include the following:

1. Listening and questioning
2. Observing and interpreting
3. Synthesizing
4. Incorporating what is learned into a plan of care

To learn about a patient, one must talk little and listen a lot. The nurse listens to the patient with "hearing ears" and asks herself, "What is he saying?" Because an ill person is so suggestible (easily influenced), it is best not to put words into his mouth. As he tells his story in his own words, he may discuss many topics. Usually if he is allowed time to talk without interruptions, his major concerns will become evident. The nurse, as she listens, is attentive not only to his verbal expressions but also to his nonverbal behavior, which may be exhibited in such subtle forms as gestures, posture, and facial expressions.

Anxiety is present in almost every patient; it may be well concealed, but it is there. The nurse anticipates the patient's anxieties and tries to relieve them during the interview. She attempts to convey to the patient that his words and feelings are being understood.

The use of a health history guide may help the nurse to obtain pertinent information and to facilitate the course of the interview. A variety of health history guides have been developed by individual nurses and committees of nurses. Many nursing divisions/departments have developed guides that are specifically directed toward obtaining the information that is most essential for their particular patients. Guides that are standard for a particular nursing division are based on the nursing model used by the division and its specific philosophy and concept of man, nursing, and health. These health history guides are just that—guides. They are designed to guide the interview but must be adapted to the individual responses, problems, and needs of the patient.

As the nurse gains expertise in conducting a health history, she strives toward developing her own format, one that allows for adaptability and flexibility while still obtaining the essential information. This essential information must reflect an assessment of the total patient with regard to his basic human needs and his state of wellness or illness. A variety of models can serve as frameworks for the assessment of basic needs. Functional health patterns (Gordon, 1987), Maslow's hierarchy of needs, and Erikson's eight stages of man are examples of frameworks that provide bases for the assessment of the total needs of the client—his physical, psychologic, emotional, intellectual, developmental, social, cultural, and spiritual needs.

The questions in Chart 2-1 are offered as guidelines for interviewing, but the questions actually asked are determined by the reaction of the individual patient.

In some instances it may be appropriate for the patient to fill out the health history form. If this technique of history taking is used, it remains the responsibility of the nurse to verify and clarify the information provided by the patient and to seek any additional information that is necessary to identify the patient's nursing needs.

Throughout the interview, the nurse has the opportunity to interact with the patient not only for the purpose of data collection but also for the purpose of establishing an effective nurse–patient relationship. Such a relationship is facilitated by the use of therapeutic communication techniques. Table 2-1 summarizes these techniques.

Chart 2-1
Suggestions for Interviewing Patients

Current Health Status

Nursing Focus: At the beginning of the interview, focus on what is most troublesome to the patient.

Suggested Initial Statement: "Please tell me what brought you to the hospital."*
- What is causing you the most discomfort?
- When did the symptoms appear?
- What did you do when you noticed these symptoms?
- Does anything seem to relieve these symptoms?
- Do you believe you are getting better or worse? (the directional trend: improvement or deterioration)
- How do you feel now?
- What do you know about your illness or condition?
- What do you do for yourself at home when you are sick?
- How has the illness affected your way of life? For how long?
- What factors aggravate or help your condition?
- Are you taking any medications?
- Do you have any allergies? (food, drugs)
- What is your greatest concern?
- What have you been told about the treatment or tests that have been planned for you?
- Who or what has been your chief source of information?

Past Health History

Nursing Focus: Learn about the patient's background and experience in order to determine his needs.†

Suggested Initial Statement: "It will be helpful if you will tell me about your past health history."*
- Would you tell me a little about yourself, your family, your way of life?
- What types of things do you do to try to stay healthy?
- How do you usually react to being ill?
- Whom do you usually turn to for help?
- What type of work do you do?
- Has your illness interfered with your work?
- How do you like to be treated when you are ill?
- What activities, hobbies, and forms of recreation do you enjoy?

Nursing Needs

Nursing Focus: Ascertain what can be done to support the patient and help him to make the best use of his resources.

Suggested Initial Statement: "Please tell me what you think your needs are, your strengths, and your limitations."*
- What would you like to be able to do to help yourself get better?
- What kinds of help do you need?
- Who do you think could provide this help?
- What aspects of your life are being disrupted by your illness?
- How do you think your illness will affect your family?
- What do you think will be the hardest part of the situation?
- What are your food preferences? Dislikes?
- What are your sleeping habits?
  Regular retiring time?
  Do you like a night light?
  How many pillows do you use?
- What are your elimination habits (bowel and urinary)?
- Do you have any limitations of seeing? hearing? walking?
- Would it be helpful to have a family member or friend stay with you?
- What annoys you most about being in the hospital?
- What do you miss the most in the hospital?
- How long do you think you will stay?
- What do you not understand as well as you would like to?
- What could the nursing staff do that would be most helpful for you?

---

* General requests for information often prompt the patient to discuss his health status, his problems, and his needs openly and fully; if such requests result in complete and appropriate sharing of information, more specific questions are often unnecessary.
† Social, cultural, developmental, and educational levels and the patient's readiness to learn can be assessed throughout the interview.

TABLE 2-1.   Summary of Therapeutic Communication Techniques

Technique	Definition	Therapeutic Value
Listening	An active process of receiving information and examining one's reaction to the messages received	Nonverbally communicates to patient nurse's interest in patient.
Silence	Periods of no verbal communication among participants	Nonverbally communicates nurse's acceptance of patient
Establishing guidelines	Statements regarding roles, purpose, and limitations for a particular interaction	Helps patient to know what is expected of him
Open-ended comments	General comments asking the patient to determine the direction the interaction should take	Allows patient to decide what material is most relevant and encourages him to continue
Reducing distance	Diminishing physical space between the nurse and patient	Nonverbally communicates that nurse wants to be involved with patient
Acknowledgment	Recognition given to a patient for contribution to an interaction	Demonstrates the importance of the patient's role within the relationship
Restating	Repeating to the patient what the nurse believes is the main thought or idea expressed	Asks for validation of nurse's interpretation of the message
Reflecting	Directing back to the patient his ideas, feelings, questions, or content	Attempts to show patient the importance of his own ideas, feelings, and interpretations
Seeking clarification	Asking for additional inputs to understand the message received	Demonstrates nurse's desire to understand patient's communication
Seeking consensual validation	Attempts to reach a mutual denotative and connotative meaning of specific words	Demonstrates nurse's desire to understand patient's communication
Focusing	Questions or statements to help the patient develop or expand an idea	Directs conversation toward topics of importance
Summarizing	Statement of main areas discussed during interaction	Helps patient to separate relevant from irrelevant material: serves as a review and closing for the interaction
Planning	Mutual decision making regarding the goals, direction, and so on, of future interactions	Reiterates patient's role within relationship

(Reprinted with permission from Sundeen SJ et al. Nurse–Client Interaction: Interpreting the Nursing Process. St Louis, CV Mosby, 1989.)

The Health Assessment

The health assessment of the patient may be carried out prior to, during, or following the health history, depending on the patient's physical and emotional state, his response to his illness and hospitalization, and the immediate priorities of his illness situation.

The purpose of the health assessment is to identify those parameters of physical, psychologic, and emotional functioning that indicate that a nursing need exists. It requires the use of the senses of sight, hearing, touch, and smell as well as the appropriate interview skills and techniques. Physical exami-

nation techniques as well as techniques and strategies for assessing behaviors and role changes are used.

The physical examination is designed to determine the patient's physical alterations and limitations and also to determine his strengths and assets, which may serve to compensate for his limitations.

- To accomplish the purposes of the physical examination, the nurse must be skilled in the techniques of inspection, palpation, percussion, and auscultation; she must also have a sound basic knowledge of anatomy and physiology and of the symptomatology of the disease process with which the patient presents.

Because the physical examination is such an important part of the health assessment component of the nursing process, and because it involves specific technical skills that must be learned and continuously refined, Chapter 7 is devoted to the study of the basic techniques of the physical examination. Significant observations that should be made for specific clinical conditions appear in the chapters in which the conditions are discussed. Careful study is required because the nurse must learn to observe with "seeing" eyes, hear with "hearing" ears, feel with "feeling" hands, and interpret the findings of the examination.

At the completion of the health history and the health assessment, the patient is told how the data will be used, the conclusions that will be drawn, and that he and his family or significant others will be involved in developing the plan for his care. He also knows who his nurse is and how he can communicate with her.

Other Components of the Data Base

Following the health history and the health assessment, the nurse seeks additional relevant information from the patient's family or significant others, from other members of the health team, and from the patient's health record or chart. Depending on the patient's immediate illness needs, this information may have been obtained prior to the nursing history and the health assessment. Whatever the sequence of events, the nurse uses all available sources of pertinent data to complete the nursing assessment. It is imperative that she study the patient's health record to determine the problem that caused the patient to seek help.

A tentative medical diagnosis has usually been formulated by the physician on the patient's admission to the hospital. It is absolutely essential to understand the pathophysiologic processes underlying this diagnosis. "Therapeutic conversation" is no substitute for knowing the effects of altered physiology, rationale of treatment, and potential complications. This knowledge helps the nurse to anticipate problems that may evolve, to formulate a nursing approach to their solution, and to participate with other members of the health care team in providing coordinated and collaborative health care.

Recording the Data Base

After completion of the health history and health assessment, the information obtained must be recorded in the patient's permanent record. The problem-oriented health record provides a systematic method of organizing all the information needed to diagnose the patient's needs and to meet these needs. The scientific method of problem solving is used. The components of the record are the data base, the patient problem list, the patient progress notes, and the discharge summary. The record provides a means of communication between the members of the health care team and facilitates coordinated planning and continuity of care. The record fulfills other functions as well:

- It serves as the business and legal record for the hospital and for the professional staff responsible for the patient's care.
- It serves as a basis for evaluating the quality and appropriate-

ness of care as well as for reviewing the effective use of patient care health practices.
- It provides data useful in research, education, and short- and long-range planning.

The information that is recorded first on the patient's record is the *data base,* which is a compilation of all of the data obtained at the time of his entry into the health care system. It consists of the health history and health assessment as well as the history and physical examination obtained by the physician and patient profiles from other sources, such as the social worker, pharmacist, nutritionist, dentist, physical therapist, and respiratory therapist. It also includes laboratory and radiologic data and any other data or profiles from other members of the health care team involved in the patient's care. The form and content of the data base are determined by the agency. Although many disciplines may participate in collecting different parts of the information, all of the data should be placed together in the same section of the health record. When all disciplines are not using the problem-oriented system, it is not always possible to achieve an integrated data base. In this case, the nursing department should determine what information is needed about all patients and seek to avoid duplication as much as possible.

Experience with the problem-oriented record system has shown that definite time limits need to be established by the agency so that the patient's problems are identified as soon after admission as possible. An example of a nursing data base form is found on pp. 26–29.

Nursing Diagnosis

The assessment component of the nursing process is followed by the formulation of the nursing diagnoses. As soon as possible after the completion of the nursing history and the health assessment, the nurse organizes, analyzes, synthesizes, and summarizes the data collected and determines the patient's need for nursing care.

- Those actual or potential health problems that are amenable to resolution by nursing actions are identified as nursing diagnoses.

Nursing, unlike medicine, does not yet have a complete taxonomy of diagnostic labels that convey the same meaning to all nurses. Until recent years, the nursing literature has contained little substantive work on the classification of nursing diagnoses. The 1970s brought a surge of professional activity aimed at making nursing diagnosis a function for which the nurse is held legally responsible and accountable. A large number of nurse practice acts were revised to include nursing diagnosis as a nursing function. Nursing diagnosis was included in the American Nurses Association Standards of Nursing Practice (1973) and in the standards developed by many nursing specialty organizations.

The National Conferences on the Classification of Nursing Diagnoses held regularly since 1973 have provided an impetus for the identification and classification of nursing diagnoses according to symptomatology. At the fifth conference, held in 1982, a major step was taken toward coordinating the work

(text continues on page 30)

ALEXANDRIA HOSPITAL

UNIT	DATE & TIME ARRIVED

MR 24-00

NURSING DATA BASE
☐ SHORT STAY   SIDE ONE

ADMITTED FROM	DIAGNOSIS	ALLERGIES/RESPONSE

ARMBAND ON	ALLERGY BAND	B/P	PULSE	RESPIRATIONS	TEMPERATURE	P.O.	Ax.	r
☐ YES	☐ YES ☐ NKDA	R L				☐	☐	☐

PHYSICAL ASSESSMENT

CARDIOVASCULAR SYSTEM

Skin: ☐ pale   ☐ cyanotic   ☐ flushed   ☐ warm & dry   ☐ cold
☐ clammy   ☐ mottled   other: _____

Edema: ☐ None   Location/Degree (1+ to 3+) _____

Heart Sounds: ☐ S₁S₂ (NL) ☐ Other: _____

Heart Rhythm: ☐ Regular   ☐ Irregular   ☐ Other: _____

Distal Pulses: Dorsalis Pedis: R ___ L ___

Radial: R _____ L _____ Other: _____

Other: _____

{ B = Bounding
N = Normal
W = Weak
D = Doppler only
A = Absent }

Capillary Refill: ☐ Brisk (NL)   ☐ Delayed: (›1 sec)

Neck Veins: ☐ Flat   ☐ Distended (HOB ☛ 30°)

Vascular Access: ☐ None   Type _____ Location _____
☐ Bruit/Thrill Present _____

IV: ☐ None - Describe _____
Other: _____

RESPIRATORY SYSTEM

Rhythm: ☐ Regular   ☐ Irregular/Description _____

Breath Sounds: _____

Cough: ☐ None   ☐ Productive   ☐ Non-productive

Sputum: ☐ None   Color/Consistency: _____

Oxygen: ☐ None   Type _____ FiO₂ _____

Dyspnea: ☐ None   Degree: MILD/MODERATE/SEVERE

Chest Tube: ☐ None   Location _____

Air Leak: ☐ None   Cm Suction _____
☐ Yes   Drainage _____

Other: _____

NERVOUS SYSTEM

LOC: ☐ Awake/alert   Other: _____

Motor Strength/All extremities: ☐ Normal Deficit _____

Deficit: _____

Pupils (indicate number):

Size: Right ____ Left ____   pin 2 3 4 6 mm

Reaction: **Right:**   Brisk/Sluggish/Fixed
(circle one) **Left:**   Brisk/Sluggish/Fixed

Orientation: (yes or no) Person _____ Place _____ Time _____

Describe: _____

Behavior/Emotional State: _____

Other: _____

MUSCULO-SKELETAL SYSTEM

Orthopedic Devices: ☐ None   Type/Location: _____

Limitations in ROJM: ☐ None   Location/Severity: _____

Other: _____

RENAL SYSTEM

Catheter: ☐ None   Type/Size _____

Urine Color _____

Other: _____

REPRODUCTIVE SYSTEM
Female:

Vaginal Discharge/Bleeding: ☐ None

Color/Amount: _____
Male:

Penile discharge ☐ None Color/Amount: _____

Other: _____

GASTROINTESTINAL SYSTEM

Nasogastric Tube: ☐ Yes   ☐ No   ☐ Position Check

Gastric Contents: ☐ None Color _____ Amount _____

Emesis: ☐ None Color _____ Amount _____

Bowel Sounds: (Circle one) Normal/ hyperactive/ hypoactive/ absent

Abdomen: ☐ Soft ☐ Firm ☐ Flat ☐ Distended

Tubes/Drains: ☐ None

Type	Location	Describe	Suction
			☐ Yes ☐ No

Other: _____

INTERGUMENTARY SYSTEM   ☐ BLACK   ☐ WHITE   ☐ OTHER

MARK DRAWING WITH APPROPRIATE LETTER AT EXACT LOCATION:

B-BURN   A-AMPUTATION
BR-BRUISE   L-LACERATION
P-PRESSURE   R-RASH
D-DRY PATCHES   S-SCAR
DS-DRESSING

OTHER COMMENTS/DESCRIPTION: _____

STAGES
0-POTENTIAL
1-REDDENED AREAS
2-DISRUPTION/ULCERATION
3-COMPLETE DESTRUCTION OF SKIN LAYERS (EXPOSED FAT, MUSCLE, BONE)
4-INVASION BY ULCERATION OF BONE STRUCTURE

Skin: pressure sore ☐ None   Location: _____

Size: _____ ☐ Stage (I-IV) _____

Areas @ risk for breakdown: ☐ None _____

Wound/incision: ☐ None Description/location: _____

Other: _____

Addressograph

_____ _____
R.N. Signature   Date/Time Completed

ADMISSION NURSING HISTORY

NUTRITION:
–MEALS ☐ Breakfast ☐ Lunch ☐ Dinner ☐ Snacks ☐ Special Diet type _____ ☐ Recent Change in Diet Other: _____

Dentures: ☐ None ☐ Upper ☐ Lower ☐ Chewing/Swallowing Problems Comments:

SLEEP/REST PATTERNS:
☐ No Difficulty ☐ Hx of Insomnia
Hours/Night _____ Naps: ☐ None _____ Sleep Aids: ☐ None _____
Comments: _____ ☐ Hx Orthopenea # of Pillows _____

CIGARETTE SMOKING: ☐ Denies Pack/Day: _____ Number of Years: _____ Quit: _____

ETOH: ☐ Denies Daily Intake (daily, weekly) _____ Quit: _____

STREET DRUGS: ☐ Denies Amount/Frequency _____ Type: _____

ELIMINATION GI/GU

GI INCONTINENCE: ☐ None ☐ Urinary ☐ Fecal

CONSTIPATION: ☐ None Duration: _____

DIARRHEA: ☐ None Frequency: _____ Duration: _____

USE OF LAXATIVES/ANTIDIARRHEALS/ANTACIDS: ☐ None Type/Frequency/Reason: _____

ABDOMINAL PAIN: ☐ None Location/Severity (1-10 Scale) _____

Last Bowel Movement Date _____

NAUSEA/VOMITING: ☐ None Frequency/Duration: _____

OSTOMY APPLIANCE: ☐ None Location/Type/Size: _____

COMMENTS: _____

GU

PAIN SEVERITY SCALE
1=least severe
10=most severe

RENAL PAIN: ☐ None Location/Severity (1-10 Scale) _____

FREQUENCY/BURNING: ☐ None Duration: _____ ☐ Nocturia

COMMENTS: _____

CARDIOVASCULAR

CHEST PAIN Hx ☐ None Location/Duration/Severity (1-10 Scale): _____

TREATMENT: _____ COMMENTS: _____

VASCULAR PAIN Hx ☐ None Location/Duration/Severity (1-10 Scale): _____

RESPIRATORY

DYSPNEA Hx ☐ None Degree/Precipitating Factors: _____

OTHER: ☐ Trach ☐ Mouth Breathing

PAIN: ☐ None Location/Severity: (1-10 Scale) _____

COMMENTS: _____

REPRODUCTIVE
FEMALE:
Last PAP Smear
Date: _____ LMP: _____ Pregnancy G _____ P _____

☐ Change in Menstrual Cycle-type: _____ length of time: _____

☐ Vaginal Discharge Hx _____ ☐ Performs Self Breast Exam ☐ Breast Changes Hx

☐ Contraceptive Related Hx: type _____ length of time _____

MALE: ☐ Prostate Problems Hx Comments: _____

PHYSICAL MOBILITY NEEDS:

☐ None ☐ Cane ☐ Prosthesis ☐ Walker ☐ WC ☐ Exercise Program

☐ Siderails ● × 2 ☐ × 4 ☐ Side Rail release form signed ☐ Arthritis _____
LOCATION

FALL RISK FACTORS

☐ AT RISK FOR FALLS IS HIGH

Level of Consciousness	CIRCLE	Age	CIRCLE	TOTAL SCORE RISK FACTOR (CIRCLE ONE)
a. Oriented/Cooperative	0	i. Under 50	0	0 — 6 Nil
b. Oriented/Uncooperative	2	j. 50—60 Years of age	2	7 — 24 High
c. Oriented with an Independent Personality	4	k. 60—70 Years of age	4	**ACTION:** (Circle One)
d. Confused/Disoriented	6	l. Over 70	6	Standard Safety Measures

Mobility		Medication		
e. Ambulatory without assistance	0	m. PRN Sedation	2	
f. Ambulatory with assistive device	2	n. Routine Sedation	4	Implement Fall Prevention Program
g. Ambulatory with assistant	4	o. Sleepers, Narcotics	6	
h. Patient has fallen before	6	p. Laxatives/Diuretics	4	
		TOTAL		

GERIATRIC FUNCTIONAL ASSESSMENT

☐ N/A < 60 Years Old   One week prior to Admission their ability for the following (S=Self, A=Assist, T=Total- CIRCLE ANSWER)

BATHING FREQUENCY _____

BATHING – S A T   TOILETING – S A T   GROOMING – S A T   FEEDING – S A T
DRESSING – S A T   TRANSFERS – S A T   STAIRS/AMBULATION – S A T

GENERAL PHYSICAL OBSERVATION

Height: _____ Weight: _____

☐ Unable to weigh - reason: _____

Estimate Weight: _____

History of Unintentional Weight Loss/Gain ☐ None ☐ Obese

_____ lbs. over _____ weeks/months

(Continued)

VALUES/BELIEFS/REQUIRED REQUEST:

Are there spiritual/cultural/family traditions impacting hospitalization? ☐ NONE

*Are you an organ donor? ☐ Yes ☐ No   Would you like information on organ donation? ☐ Yes ☐ No   Information provided ☐   Living Will ☐ Yes ☐ No   ☐ If yes, copy on chart

COMMUNICATION

PRIMARY LANGUAGE _____   REQUIRES AN INTERPRETER: ☐ YES ☐ NO

Vision: ☐ No difficulty ☐ Blurred ☐ Diplopia ☐ Blind ☐ Glasses ☐ Contact Lenses ☐ Artificial Eye ☐ L ☐ R

Hearing: ☐ No difficulty ☐ Limited ☐ Deaf ☐ Tinnitus ☐ Hearing Aide

Speech: ☐ No difficulty ☐ Slurred ☐ Aphasic ☐ Cataracts

☐ UNABLE TO READ   ☐ UNABLE TO WRITE   ☐ OTHER _____

PERTINENT MEDICAL HISTORY

Patient's Understanding of Reason for Hospitalization: _____

Previous illness/surgery/ current treatment: ☐ None ☐ Diabetes Hx ☐ Seizure Hx ☐ Depression
☐ Cancer ☐ Heart Disease ☐ Hepatitis ☐ Liver Disease

_____
_____
_____
_____
_____
_____

SIGNIFICANT OTHER(S)

Name(s): _____   Relationship: _____

Phone #: _____   Information Obtained from _____

SUPPORT SYSTEM: _____

Usual Coping Mechanisms: _____

EDUCATIONAL NEEDS

1. ☐ Patient   ☐ Family/Significant Other

2. Type:
☐ Diet   ☐ Skin Care
☐ Medications   ☐ Home Care
☐ Pre-op Procedure/Teaching
☐ Patient Education Flowsheet Initiated
☐ Post Operative Routine

DISCHARGE INFORMATION

☐ KARDEX COMPLETED

_____
_____
_____
_____
_____
_____

PRESENT MEDICATIONS

LIST PRESCRIPTION & OVER-THE-COUNTER: ☐ None

DISPOSITION OF MEDICATIONS: ☐ Sent to Pharmacy ☐ Sent Home/At Home

← MEDICATIONS AT BEDSIDE PER ORDER

*	DRUG DOSE/NAME/FREQUENCY	ROUTE	LAST DOSE TAKEN	

HOSPITAL ORIENTATION: ☐ Side Rails ☐ Lights ☐ Telephone ☐ TV

☐ Hospital Booklet   ☐ Bathroom Call Light   ☐ Chaplain Services
☐ Electrical Equipment   ☐ Call System   ☐ Bed Controls
☐ Bedside Medications   ☐ Visiting Hours ☐ Bathroom ☐ Meal Times

VALUABLES: ☐ VALUABLES FORM COMPLETED

_____
R.N. Signature   Date/Time Completed

(Continued)

ALEXANDRIA HOSPITAL

DATE	TIME	ADMITTING NURSING DIAGNOSES IN ORDER OF PRIORITY:
		1. CLINICAL:
		2.
		3.
		4. EDUCATIONAL:
		5. PSYCHOSOCIAL:
		SOAP ADMISSION NOTE:

NURSES NOTES

61499 R 9/90

(Continued)

of developing nursing diagnoses—a new organization, the North American Nursing Diagnosis Association (NANDA), was created.

In 1986, NANDA approved its first taxonomy for classification of nursing diagnoses; this taxonomy continues to be further developed. In 1989, efforts began toward preparing the taxonomy for possible inclusion into the World Health Organization's tenth revision of the International Classification of Diseases (ICD-10). In 1990, at the NANDA Biennial Conference, the association officially adopted a definition for nursing diagnosis:

> A nursing diagnosis is a clinical judgment about individual, family, or community responses to actual or potential health problems/life processes. Nursing diagnoses provide the basis for selection of nursing interventions to achieve outcomes for which the nurse is accountable.

The diagnostic categories identified by the conference groups are gaining general acceptance by nurses but require further validation and expansion. They are not yet complete or mutually exclusive. More research is needed to determine the predictive and prognostic attributes of the diagnostic labels. As this research continues, as the efforts of the NANDA group continue, and as nurses continue to use and validate nursing diagnoses, the profession as a whole continues to grow. The development of autonomy and accountability is fostered. The scope of nursing practice is delineated. Standards of practice are more definitive, and collaboration of nursing with other disciplines is facilitated. A list of accepted nursing diagnoses from the ninth Conference on the Classification of Nursing Diagnoses is shown in Chart 2-2.*

In spite of the need for research on the diagnostic process itself and on the diagnostic nomenclature, the term *nursing diagnosis* will be used in sections of this book where we have applied the nursing process to specific illness conditions. Both nurses and nursing students have a unique opportunity to use currently accepted nursing diagnoses and to develop additional diagnoses that describe actual or potential health problems that are amenable to nursing care. Only through clinical use and research of nursing diagnostic labels can these labels be validated and expanded.

When developing the nursing diagnoses for a particular patient, the nurse must first identify the commonalities among the assessment data collected. These common features lead to the categorization of related data that reveal the existence of a problem and the need for nursing intervention. *The patient's nursing problem is then defined as the nursing diagnosis.*

It must be remembered that nursing diagnoses are *not* medical diagnoses; they are *not* medical treatments prescribed by the physician; they are *not* diagnostic studies; they are *not* the equipment used to implement medical therapy; and they are *not* the problems that the nurse experiences while caring for the patient. They *are* the patient's actual or potential health problems that are amenable to resolution by nursing actions.

---

* *Every effort has been made to adhere to the official list of NANDA nursing diagnoses throughout this text. However, because nursing diagnoses continue to evolve, certain areas have not yet been addressed. Thus some of the diagnoses discussed in this text will not be found on the official NANDA list. In addition, the notation "potential for" has been added to some accepted diagnoses to alert nurses to the need to monitor the patient's condition for possible complications.*

Nursing diagnoses that are succinctly stated in terms of the specific problems of the patient will guide the nurse in the development of the nursing care plan.

In order to give additional meaning to the diagnosis, the characteristics and the etiology of the problem must be identified and included as part of the diagnosis. For example, the nursing diagnoses and their defining characteristics and etiology for a patient who has rheumatoid arthritis may include:

- Impaired physical mobility related to restricted joint movement
- Self-care deficits (feeding, bathing, dressing, toileting) related to fatigue and joint stiffness
- Self-esteem disturbance related to loss of independence
- Altered nutrition (less than body requirements) related to fatigue and inadequate food intake

With such specific diagnoses identified, the nurse is ready to record them and to plan nursing care directed toward their resolution.

Recording the Nursing Diagnoses

The patient's nursing diagnoses are recorded on the nursing care plan as well as in the patient problem list. The patient problem list serves as the "index" or "table of contents" to the record. A *problem* is defined as anything that concerns the patient, endangers his health, requires management, and concerns any member of the health care team.

If all professionals are using the problem-oriented system, then they all contribute to the same problem list. The problems are numbered and used by all concerned for writing progress notes.

Planning

Once the nursing diagnoses have been identified, the planning component of the nursing process is developed. This phase involves the following:

1. The assignment of priorities to the nursing diagnoses
2. The specification of immediate, intermediate, and long-term goals of nursing action
3. The identification of specific nursing interventions appropriate for attaining the goals
4. The identification of interdependent interventions
5. The specification of expected outcomes
6. The documentation of the nursing diagnoses, goals, nursing interventions, and expected outcomes on the nursing care plan

Also, during this phase of the nursing process it is the responsibility of the nurse to communicate to appropriate persons any assessment data indicative of health needs that can best be met by other members of the health care team.

Setting Priorities

The assignment of priorities to the nursing diagnoses is a joint effort by the nurse and the patient or his family members. Any disagreement about the priorities is resolved in a way that is

Chart 2–2
NANDA* Approved Nursing Diagnoses—1990

(Alphabetical)

Activity Intolerance
Activity Intolerance, High Risk for
Adjustment, Impaired
Airway Clearance, Ineffective
Anxiety
Aspiration, High Risk for
Body Image Disturbance
Body Temperature, High Risk for Altered
Breastfeeding, Effective
Breastfeeding, Ineffective
Breathing Pattern, Ineffective
Communication, Impaired Verbal
Constipation
Constipation, Colonic
Constipation, Perceived
Decisional Conflict (Specify)
Decreased Cardiac Output
Defensive Coping
Denial, Ineffective
Diarrhea
Disuse Syndrome, High Risk for
Diversional Activity Deficit
Dysreflexia
Family Coping, Compromised, Ineffective
Family Coping, Disabling, Ineffective
Family Coping: Potential for Growth
Family Processes, Altered
Fatigue
Fear
Fluid Volume Deficit
Fluid Volume Deficit, High Risk for
Fluid Volume Excess
Gas Exchange, Impaired
Grieving, Anticipatory
Grieving, Dysfunctional
Growth and Development, Altered
Health Maintenance, Altered
Health-Seeking Behaviors (Specify)
Home Maintenance Management, Impaired
Hopelessness
Hyperthermia
Hypothermia
Incontinence, Bowel
Incontinence, Functional
Incontinence, Reflex
Incontinence, Stress
Incontinence, Total
Incontinence, Urge
Individual Coping, Ineffective
Infection, High Risk for
Injury, High Risk for

Knowledge Deficit (Specify)
Noncompliance (Specify)
Nutrition: Less than Body Requirements, Altered
Nutrition: More than Body Requirements, Altered
Nutrition: Potential for More than Body Requirements, Altered
Oral Mucous Membrane, Altered
Pain
Pain, Chronic
Parental Role Conflict
Parenting, Altered
Parenting, High Risk for Altered
Personal Identity Disturbance
Physical Mobility, Impaired
Poisoning, High Risk for
Post-Trauma Response
Powerlessness
Protection, Altered
Rape-Trauma Syndrome
Rape-Trauma Syndrome: Compound Reaction
Rape-Trauma Syndrome: Silent Reaction
Role Performance, Altered
Self-Care Deficit, Bathing/Hygiene
Self-Care Deficit, Feeding
Self-Care Deficit, Dressing/Grooming
Self-Care Deficit, Toileting
Self-Esteem, Chronic Low
Self-Esteem, Situational Low
Self-Esteem Disturbance
Sensory/Perceptual Alterations (Specify) (Visual, auditory, kinesthetic, gustatory, tactile, olfactory)
Sexual Dysfunction
Sexuality Patterns, Altered
Skin Integrity, Impaired
Skin Integrity, High Risk for Impaired
Sleep Pattern Disturbance
Social Interaction, Impaired
Social Isolation
Spiritual Distress (Distress of the Human Spirit)
Suffocation, High Risk for
Swallowing, Impaired
Thermoregulation, Ineffective
Thought Processes, Altered
Tissue Integrity, Impaired
Tissue Perfusion, Altered (Specify Type) (Renal, cerebral, cardiopulmonary, gastrointestinal, peripheral)
Trauma, High Risk for
Unilateral Neglect
Urinary Elimination, Altered
Urinary Retention
Violence, High Risk for: Self-directed or directed at others

* NANDA—North American Nursing Diagnosis Association

mutually acceptable. Consideration must be given to the urgency of the problems, the most critical problems receiving the highest priorities. Maslow's hierarchy of needs provides a useful framework for the determination of priority problems. The use of this hierarchy requires that high priority be given to physical needs. Subsequent to the resolution of physical needs, priorities are reassigned according to the urgency of needs at other levels of the hierarchy (see pp. 14–15).

Establishing Goals for Nursing Action

After the priorities of the nursing diagnoses have been established, the immediate, intermediate, and long-term goals and the nursing actions appropriate for attainment of the goals are identified. The patient and his family are included in the establishment of the goals of the nursing actions. The immediate goals are those that can be reached in a short period of time. The intermediate and long-term goals require a longer period of time for their accomplishment and usually involve prevention of complications and further health problems, health education, and rehabilitation. For example, goals for a diabetic patient with a nursing diagnosis of "knowledge deficit relative to the prescribed diet" may be stated as follows:

Immediate goal: Oral intake and tolerance of 1500-calorie diabetic diet spaced in three meals and one snack
Intermediate goal: Planning of meals for 1 week based on diabetic exchange system
Long-term goal: Adherence to prescribed diabetic diet

The patient and his family are included whenever possible in the decisions about the nursing interventions to meet the goals. Involvement of the patient and his family in the planning of nursing interventions promotes their cooperation in the implementation of nursing care. The identification of appropriate nursing interventions and their related goals depends on the nurse's recognition of the strengths and potential of the patient and his family; her understanding of the pathophysiologic alterations that he experiences; and her sensitivity to his emotional, psychologic, and intellectual response to his illness state. Likewise, the nurse's knowledge of nursing, her clinical experience, and her awareness of available supporting resources influence the validity of the nursing interventions that she identifies as appropriate for resolving the patient's nursing diagnoses.

Establishing Expected Outcomes

Expected outcomes of the nursing interventions are stated in terms of the patient's behaviors. They must be realistic and measurable. Standard outcome criteria established by the health care agency for the target population applicable to the patient should be used whenever possible. However, it may be necessary to adapt these outcome criteria so that they are realistic in terms of the specific patient's potential for resolution of his problems. The critical time period within which the outcomes should be demonstrated by the patient are also identified.

- The outcomes that define the expected behavior of the patient will indicate problem resolution or progress toward resolution

and will serve as the basis for evaluation of the effectiveness of the nursing interventions.
- The critical time periods provide a time frame for determining the effectiveness of the nursing interventions and the existence of a need for additional or altered nursing care.

Team Planning

Ideally, the accomplishment of all aspects of the planning phase of the nursing process is a group effort. The nurse collaborates with other members of the nursing team, with the patient and his family, and with appropriate resource persons from the health care agency and community agencies. The physician initiates the medical regimen and is a valuable counselor, teacher, and resource person. A clinical nurse specialist, when available, can make significant contributions.

Because the plan revolves around the patient, he should have a part in it. The ultimate goal is to help the patient to help himself. This means that the patient is accepted as an individual and his right to self-determination is respected. Because the plan is oriented in terms of the patient's goals and capabilities, he has every right to express his feelings and voice his opinions about his care. He should be kept informed about his current health status (when feasible), any change in plans, the roles of health care personnel, and the resources available to him.

It is also important to remember that the patient is part of a family. The family members have needs that arise from the patient's illness. They may be included in the planning by questioning them about the patient's reactions and informing them about the nursing care plan and the expected results of treatment. The family may also make pertinent observations and offer effective suggestions.

Another aspect of care planning takes into account the fact that the patient comes from the community. Community agencies have an interest in the patient and are involved in planning. This means that the nurse must be aware of the community services that may be offered a patient following discharge from the hospital. These agencies can be informed of the goals to be reached, and decisions can then be made regarding the type of services that will be needed. Many communities have a directory listing all community resources available. These include community health and visiting nurse services, homemaking services, meals on wheels, and social and recreational services. A knowledge of these resources and the methods of referral is invaluable in helping patients to cope with long-term health needs.

Because discharge from the hospital has been accelerated with the advent of DRGs, many patients are leaving the hospital with complex needs, many of which require advanced technologies. For this reason, discharge planning must begin when the patient is first admitted to the hospital so that appropriate home health care services are available to him and his family when he is ready for discharge. It is imperative that this discharge planning be accomplished with interdisciplinary efforts.

Formulating the Nursing Care Plan

The entire planning phase of the nursing process culminates in the formulation of the patient's nursing care plan by the professional nurse. The nursing care plan serves to communicate the following information to all members of the nursing team:

1. The nursing diagnoses and their priorities
2. The goals of the nursing interventions
3. The nursing interventions, which are expressed in the form of nursing orders
4. The expected outcomes, which identify the expected behavioral responses of the patient
5. The critical time period within which each outcome is expected to be met

The information incorporated into the nursing care plan is written in a concise, systematic manner that facilitates its use by all nursing personnel. Space must be provided in the care plan for documentation of the patient's response to the nursing interventions—the outcomes. It must be remembered that the care plan is subject to change as the patient's problems change, as the priorities of the problems shift, as resolution of problems occurs, and as additional information about the patient's state of health is collected. As the nursing interventions are implemented, the patient's responses are evaluated and documented, and the care plan is changed accordingly. A well-developed, continuously updated nursing care plan is the patient's greatest assurance that his nursing diagnoses will be addressed and his basic needs will be met (see pp. 34–35).

Implementation

The implementation phase of the nursing process follows the formulation of the nursing care plan. Implementation refers to carrying out the proposed plan of care. The nurse assumes responsibility for the implementation but includes the patient and his family and other members of the nursing team and the health care team as appropriate. The activities of all persons involved in implementation are coordinated by the nurse.

- The nursing care plan serves as the basis for implementation.
- The immediate, intermediate, and long-term goals are used as a focus for the implementation of the designed nursing interventions.
- While implementing nursing care, the nurse continually assesses the patient and his response to the nursing care.
- Alterations are made in the care plan as the patient's condition, problems, and responses change and as a reassignment of priorities is required.

Implementation includes all of the nursing interventions that are directed toward resolution of the patient's nursing diagnoses and meeting his health needs. Some of these needs have already been discussed (see pp. 14–15). Needs specific to certain conditions are presented in the chapter in which the particular condition is discussed.

General Categories of Nursing Interventions

Included among nursing interventions are hygienic care; promotion of physical and psychologic comfort; support of respiratory and elimination functions; facilitation of the ingestion of food, fluids, and nutrients; environmental management;

health teaching; promotion of a therapeutic relationship; and a host of therapeutic nursing activities. The nurse uses judgment and decision-making skills in the selection of appropriate nursing interventions that are based on physiologic principles.

- All nursing interventions are patient-focused and goal-directed. They are based on scientific principles and are implemented with compassion, confidence, and a willingness to accept and understand the patient's responses.

Many nursing actions are independent. Others are interdependent, such as carrying out physicians' prescriptions for medications and therapies and collaborating with other health care team members to accomplish specific expected outcomes. Such interdependent functioning is just that—interdependent. Requests from other health care team members should not be followed blindly but should be assessed critically and questioned as necessary.

Delegating Nursing Actions

The nurse may delegate certain specific actions to other members of the nursing team. When delegating, the nurse must know the capabilities and limitations of the members of the nursing team, select the most appropriate person to implement the actions, and supervise the performance of the actions. The nursing team member is provided with all of the information that he or she needs to perform the actions in such a way that the patient remains the focus of the actions at all times.

Many members of the health care team may become involved in the patient's care. In order to provide for coordination and continuity of care, information about the patient's responses to his care and any changes that must be made in the plan of care must be communicated verbally and in writing to the appropriate persons. Continual updating of the care plan is of paramount importance in ensuring coordination and continuity.

Recording Outcomes

The implementation phase of the nursing process is concluded when the nursing interventions have been completed and the patient's responses to them have been recorded. Recordings are made concisely, precisely, and objectively. The recordings:

- Relate to the nursing diagnoses
- Describe the nursing interventions and the patient's responses to the interventions
- Include any additional pertinent data

Only with accurate recording can evaluation be accomplished. Documentation of information provides the basis for the measurement of the patient's behavioral response to the nursing interventions—his accomplishment of the defined outcome criteria.

Patient Progress Notes. The progress notes are written in a format that not only clearly and unmistakably relates them to the numbered problem—in the case of nursing, to the nursing diagnosis—but also uses the scientific method of problem solving on a day-by-day basis (see p. 36). Progress notes are written in a narrative form, using the acronym SOAPIE:

Example of an Individualized Nursing Care Plan

Mr. John Lee, a 50-year-old management consultant, was admitted to the nursing unit from his physician's office. A routine physical examination 3 months previously had revealed essential hypertension with BP 170/110 and decreased urine creatinine clearance. During the subsequent 3 months the blood pressure elevation did not respond to diet therapy. Mr. Lee admitted that he had not been successful in adhering to the low-sodium, low-cholesterol, weight-reduction diet that had been prescribed for him. He stated "my life is just too busy—I work all hours of the day and night." He indicated that in addition to his work he and his wife share the responsibility for raising their two teenage daughters. He drinks five to seven cups of coffee daily and drinks alcohol only at social occasions. Admission physical examination revealed BP 162/112, P 96, R 20, T 37°C, height 5'10", weight 210 lbs, and slight edema of the ankles and feet. Mr. Lee stated that his feet are "always puffy at night." A brief hospitalization was planned for thorough evaluation and initiation of therapy. The physician's orders on admission included: activity as desired; Lasix, 40 mg bid; monitor vital signs every 4 hours while awake; 1500 calorie, 1 g sodium, low cholesterol diet.

Nursing Diagnoses

1. Altered health maintenance related to hypertension, stress, obesity, and caffeine
2. Ineffective individual coping relative to role responsibilities at work and home
3. Noncompliance with dietary regimen

Goals

Immediate: Gradual decrease in blood pressure
Intermediate: Initiation of life-style alterations to decrease stress
Long-term: Alteration of life-style to reduce emotional and environmental stressors
        Compliance with dietary regimen

Nursing Interventions	Expected Outcomes	Outcomes
Monitor BP lying, sitting, and standing every 4 hr	Experiences no further increase in BP	BP range of 162/112–138/98 since admission No variation greater than 5 mm Hg in systolic or diastolic pressures with position changes No variation between right and left arms Maximum BP from 24 hr after admission to time of discharge: 138/98
Monitor fluid status: I&O	Urinary output adequate in relation to oral intake	Intake: 1850 ml Output: 1685 ml
Peripheral edema	No evidence of peripheral edema	Minimal edema of feet late in evening
Promote atmosphere conducive to physical and mental rest: Encourage alternation of rest and activity	Alternates periods of rest and activity	Rests in bed 1 hr in morning and 2 hr in afternoon; disconnects phone during rest periods Awake at intervals during night: 8 hr of uninterrupted sleep at night after initiation of 30 mg Dalmane at bedtime
Encourage limitation of visitors and interactions that are stress-producing	Limits visitors to family in the evenings	Wife and daughters visit 2 hr in evening; patient calm and relaxed after visits
	Avoids stress-producing interactions	Wife and daughters aware of need to decrease stress: they consult with patient about regular family activities
Assist patient to alter life-style to decrease stress: Discuss relationship between emotional stress and physiologic functioning	Describes stress as a precursor to alteration in physiologic functioning	Accurately described relationship between stress and hypertension

(continued)

Example of an Individualized Nursing Care Plan *(continued)*

Nursing Interventions	Expected Outcomes	Outcomes
Encourage patient to identify stress-producing stimuli	Identifies life-style factors that produce stress	Identified the following stressors: Self-imposed demands of job; unwillingness to refer clients Excessive involvement in daughters' school and recreational activities
Encourage patient to identify adjustments necessary to reduce stress	Identifies life-style adjustments necessary to reduce stress	Verbalized plans to make more referrals Identified need to decrease work hours to maximum of 8 hr per day
	Discusses life-style adjustments with family	Consulted with wife and daughters; will alternate with wife in attending daughters' activities; all family members supportive
Encourage patient to identify obesity and caffeine as stressors and aggravators of hypertension	Identifies harmful effects of obesity and caffeine	Accurately described effects of obesity and caffeine on blood pressure
	Makes plans for losing weight	Plans to go to Weight Watchers; has had success with this program in the past
	Makes plans for decreasing caffeine intake	Drinks 1 cup of coffee for breakfast; uses decaffeinated coffee at mid morning, lunch, and dinner; expressed satisfaction with this plan
Promote compliance with therapeutic regimen	(See teaching plan, p. 46)	

S Subjective data (symptoms that the patient describes)
O Objective data (signs that the professional observes)
A Assessment (the professional's conclusion about the subjective and objective data)
P Plan (immediate or future, including patient education)
I Intervention (nursing action done to, for, or with the patient)
E Evaluation (patient outcomes)

Flow sheets are used to follow or monitor a problem or response that does not lend itself to a single note or that requires measurement of multiple parameters at frequent intervals. They also may be used for the documentation of nursing and patient activities, such as treatments and daily care.

• The progress notes are the most critical part of the problem-oriented system. They are the mechanism that provides for ongoing assessment of the patient's problem. They provide feedback about problem identification and the effectiveness of the plan of care. If all professionals are recording on integrated progress notes, the patient has a greater chance of receiving continuity of care.

The progress notes always begin with the date, time, and problem number and title, and they continue, using the following format.

Subjective Data.   The subjective or symptomatic data are obtained from the patient's or family's point of view. When subjective data are recorded, the following are considered: onset (date, time, type), intensity, quality, location, radiation, number of episodes, time of day of episodes, sources of relief (rest, position, medication), precipitating factors, factors that make the problem worse, other associated symptoms existing at the same time, overall course, and the degree to which the symptoms have affected the patient's life-style.

Objective Data.   These include actual clinical observations or laboratory findings appropriate to the problem. When objective data are recorded, the following are included: location, size, shape, color, temperature, moisture, and consistency. Also, the presence or absence of swelling, movement, weakness, and associated pain with movement or touch is noted. Many nurses record their nursing actions in this section; others add their immediate interventions to the plan component of the progress notes.

Assessment.   This is the portion of the progress notes that deals with the subjective and objective data just collected and that presents the health care provider's conclusion, based on that information. If the data are consistent with the problem statement, little needs to be said here. One way of considering assessment in relation to patient progress is a comparison with the previous documentation, using such terms as *improved, worse, deteriorating, same,* and *stable.* If the problem is a new one, the subjective and objective data should support a new assessment of what is going on with the patient. If the problem statement and the subjective and objective data are

PATIENT CHART
Progress Notes

Date 4/16	Problem	Progress Notes

Time **3 pm**
Problem **2**

Problem: *Ineffective coping related to role responsibilities @ work & home*

Progress Notes:

S: "I hope I'm able to go home in 3 days; my family needs me & I need to get back to work."

O: Anxious after phone call from wife. Pacing in room; requested coffee BP 160/110; P 100; R 28

A: Emotional stress increased when faced c̄ responsibilites of work & home.

P: 1) Encourage periods of rest.
2) Discuss c̄ wife the necessity for decreasing stress-producing interaction c̄ husband.
3) Be available to let patient verbalize feelings.
4) Suggest relaxation techniques.

I: 1) Encouraged patient to rest in room and read.
2) Discussed c̄ wife the need to decrease stress-producing interactions.

E: Patient resting in room 1 hour later; visibly less anxious; BP 142/102

B. Brown, R.N.

Each Progress Note consists of the number and title of the problem stated on the Problem Lists and any or all of the following components:

S – Subjective data (Symptoms)
O – Objective data (Observable)
A – Assessment (Conclusion)
P – Plan (Immediate or future, including education)
I – Intervention (Nursing Action)
E – Evaluation (Patient outcomes)

not consistent, one can quickly assess the logic or accuracy of the information recorded.

Plan. The original or initial plan, if well thought out and developed, will continue to be followed or will be modified as new information is obtained. The plan will always consider the three areas described earlier: the need for more information, management and treatment, and patient and family education.

Intervention and Evaluation. Nurses use the same problem-oriented procedure as other health professionals to document their practice. However, there are two components that many nurses have added in order to comply with the requirements of the nursing process and of some regulatory agencies for documenting nursing practice. These components are labeled *I,* for the nursing intervention that was carried out immediately (*e.g.,* raise the head of the bed, perform postural drainage), and *E,* for evaluation of the nursing intervention (was it effective or ineffective?) as documented by patient outcomes. Some-

times the evaluation will appear in the next progress note because more time is needed to observe the patient's response to the nursing intervention.

One can see that when the plan is incorporated in the patient progress notes, it readily becomes a permanent part of the legal record.

Points to keep in mind when writing problem-oriented progress notes are summarized in Chart 2-3.

Evaluation

Evaluation is the final component of the nursing process and is directed toward determining the patient's response to the nursing interventions and the extent to which the goals have

Chart 2–3
Writing Problem-Oriented Progress Notes

Reminders to Consider Before Writing Problem-Oriented Progress Notes

1. Have the patient's problem list in front of you.
2. Think about your patient in light of each problem listed in the active column. Are there any new problems to be added or considered as a result of your observations or interactions with the patient today?
3. Read the immediately preceding notes so that you will not unnecessarily repeat information already recorded and so that you will be aware of plans that are in progress.
4. Decide which are the most important problems for you to discuss; always consider life-threatening or major problems first (*e.g.*, although a myocardial infarction may be a very threatening problem, if it is realtively stable or has recently been discussed, the patient's acute anxiety may be a more pertinent topic; it may have a significant impact on his well-being).
5. A follow-up note on data-base information or on your plans identified in previous notes may be appropriate if the data are now available; describe the effectiveness or ineffectiveness of your plan (*e.g.*, vital signs, weight, response to nursing measures).
6. Always begin your note with the date, time, problem number, and title. List the subjective or objective data, using the factors suggested in this chapter. Record both follow-up data and any new information you have gathered.

7. Write an assessment for each problem considered, stating your thoughts at the level at which you actually understand the information. If you want to write about specific observations or responses to medications or treatments with which you have had little experience, look them up first; you may find valuable information that will help all members of the health care team, or you might learn that your idea does not logically follow from the data you have available.
8. Review the plan for each problem listed, or initiate a new plan if you have identified a new problem. Always consider the following three factors:
   a. The *need for more information*, such as specific observations that might help clarify the problem
   b. *Nursing intervention*, such as specific nursing measures you can order or initiate to resolve the problem (*e.g.*, have patient turn, cough, and take deep breaths every hour for 24 hours)
   c. *Patient or family teaching* that is planned or that has already occurred.
9. Write a progress note when there is something pertinent to say, such as when there has been a change. Some days several notes for the day or for the shift may be indicated, whereas on other days *no* notes will be appropriate for some problems.

Some Don'ts When Recording on the Progress Notes

DON'T include comments on nonproblem item (*e.g.*, bed baths, h.s. care given, doing well).
DON'T include comments on normal physiologic functions unless they are pertinent to a particular problem (*e.g.*, the daily bowel movements should be recorded on a routine care flow sheet unless a problem exists).
DON'T use the progress notes to record *routine* tests performed or care given (these can be checked off on the Kardex care plan or considered recorded when the laboratory or x-ray reports are charted).

---

been achieved. The nursing care plan provides the basis for evaluation; the nursing diagnoses, goals, nursing interventions, and expected outcomes provide the specific guidelines that dictate the focus of the evaluation.

Evaluation will answer the following questions:

- Were the nursing diagnoses accurate?
- Did the patient reach the expected outcomes?
- Did the patient attain the expected outcomes within the critical time periods?
- Have the patient's nursing diagnoses been resolved?
- Have the patient's nursing needs been met?
- Should the nursing interventions be retained, altered, or discontinued?
- Have new problems evolved for which nursing interventions have not been planned or implemented?
- What factors influenced the achievement or lack of achievement of the goals?
- Do priorities need to be reassigned?
- Should changes be made in the goals and expected outcomes?

Objective data that answer these questions must be collected from all available sources (*i.e.*, patient, family or significant others, nursing and other health care team members). These data should be available in the patient's record and must be substantiated by direct observation of the patient.

Outcome Criteria

All methods used to accomplish the evaluation component of the nursing process are directly related to the nursing care plan. Evaluation of the patient's response to nursing interventions is accomplished by comparing the patient's behavioral outcomes with the established outcome criteria. This information then serves as a basis for modification of the nursing care plan.

The question is asked, "What should be done to improve the nursing care?" Other nursing interventions may have to be tried. Goals may have to be redesigned. Priorities may have to be reassigned. Outcome criteria may have to be made more realistic. There must be a continuous and thorough scrutiny of

Chart 2-4
Steps of the Nursing Process

Assessment

1. Conduct the health history.
2. Perform the health assessment.
3. Interview the patient's family or significant others.
4. Study the health record.
5. Organize, analyze, synthesize, and summarize the collected data.

Nursing Diagnosis

1. Identify the patient's nursing problems.
2. Identify the defining characteristics of the nursing problems.
3. Identify the etiology of the nursing problems.
4. State nursing diagnoses concisely and precisely.

Planning

1. Assign priority to the nursing diagnoses.
2. Specify the goals.
   a. Develop immediate, intermediate, and long-term goals.
   b. State the goals in realistic and measurable terms.
3. Identify nursing interventions appropriate for goal attainment.
4. Establish expected outcomes.
   a. Make sure that the outcomes are realistic and measurable.
   b. Identify critical times for the attainment of outcomes.
5. Develop the written nursing care plan.
   a. Include nursing diagnoses, goals, nursing interventions, expected outcomes, and critical times.
   b. Write all entries precisely, concisely, and systematically.
   c. Keep the plan current and flexible to meet the patient's changing problems and needs.
6. Involve the patient, his family or significant others, nursing team members, and other health team members in all aspects of planning.

Implementation

1. Put the nursing care plan into action.
2. Coordinate the activities of the patient, his family or significant others, nursing team members, and other health team members.
3. Record the patient's responses to the nursing actions.

Evaluation

1. Collect objective data.
2. Compare the patient's behavioral outcomes with the expected outcomes. Determine the extent to which the goals were achieved.
3. Include the patient, his family or significant others, nursing team members, and other health care team members in the evaluation.
4. Identify alterations that need to be made in the nursing diagnoses, goals, nursing interventions, and expected outcomes.
5. Continue all steps of the nursing process: assessment, nursing diagnosis, planning, implementation, and evaluation.

the care provided. Then changes are made, plans are altered, and a course of action is initiated that will be most supportive to the patient.

Chapter Summary

The nursing process is a deliberate, problem-identification, and problem-solving approach to meeting the health care and nursing needs of patients. The cyclic and recurrent steps of the nursing process are assessment, nursing diagnosis, planning, implementation, and evaluation. Each step is ongoing and is related to all other steps. Continuous evaluation provides the means for maintaining the viability of the entire nursing process and for demonstrating accountability for the quality of nursing care rendered.

For an overall view of the steps of the nursing process, see Chart 2-4.

Bibliography
Books

Alfaro R. Applying Nursing Diagnoses and Nursing Process: A Step-by-Step Guide. Philadelphia, JB Lippincott, 1989.
Bates B. A Guide to Physical Examination and History Taking. Philadelphia, JB Lippincott, 1991.
Bowers AC and Thompson JM. Clinical Manual of Health Assessment. St Louis, CV Mosby, 1988.
Carpenito LJ. Handbook of Nursing Diagnosis 1989–90. Philadelphia, JB Lippincott, 1989.
Carpenito LJ. Nursing Care Plans: Nursing Diagnoses and Collaborative Problems. Philadelphia, JB Lippincott, 1991.
Carpenito LJ. Nursing Diagnosis: Application to Clinical Practice. Philadelphia, JB Lippincott, 1989.
Carroll–Johnson RM (ed). Classification of Nursing Diagnoses. Proceedings of the Eighth Conference, North American Nursing Diagnosis Association. Philadelphia, JB Lippincott, 1989.
Gordon M. Manual of Nursing Diagnosis 1988–1989. St Louis, CV Mosby, 1989.
Gordon M. Nursing Diagnosis: Process and Application. New York, McGraw–Hill, 1987.

3

Patient Education/Health Teaching

Learning Objectives

On completion of this chapter, the learner will be able to:

1. Describe the purposes and significance of health education
2. Describe the concept of adherence to a therapeutic regimen
3. Identify factors that influence adherence behavior
4. Identify variables that influence the elderly person's adherence to a therapeutic regimen
5. Describe the variables that affect learning readiness
6. Describe strategies that facilitate elderly patients' learning abilities
7. Specify the relationship of the teaching–learning process to the nursing process
8. Develop a teaching plan for a patient

Health Education Today

Health promotion and self-care are concepts that have become a part of the American way of life. Inherent within them is the concept of health education. One of the greatest challenges facing members of the nursing profession today is that of meeting the health education needs of the American public. In this respect, nurses are becoming increasingly sensitive to and conscious of their role as teachers. Health education is considered to be an independent function of nursing practice and a primary responsibility of the nursing profession. Teaching, as a function of nursing, is included in many state nurse practice acts as well as in the American Nurses Association Standards of Nursing Practice.

- Health education is an essential component of nursing care and is directed toward promotion, maintenance, and restoration of health and toward adaptation to residual effects of illness.

The emphasis placed on the need for health education during recent years perhaps stems in part from the belief of many health care leaders that the American public has the right to expect and receive comprehensive health care, including health education. It also reflects the emergence of a better-informed American public, who are asking more significant questions about health, health care, and the services offered by the health care delivery system. Because of the emphasis that the American culture places on health and the responsibility of each individual for the maintenance and promotion of his own health, it is the obligation of the members of the health care delivery system and, specifically, of nurses to make health education available to the American public.

One of the largest groups of people in need of health education today are persons with chronic illnesses. As the life span of our population continues to increase, the number of people with such illnesses will also increase. It is the belief of many health care leaders that persons with chronic illness are entitled to as much health care information as they can handle in order that they may actively participate in and assume responsibility for much of their own care. Health education can aid the individual in adapting to his illness, in cooperating with his prescribed therapy, and in learning to solve problems when confronted with new situations. Health education can prevent rehospitalization for the same condition, which is a frequent result when a person does not understand how to care for his chronic condition.

- The goal of health education is teaching people to live life to its healthiest—that is, to strive toward achieving one's maximum health potential.

Every contact that a nurse has with a patient, whether he is ill or not, should be considered an opportunity for patient teaching. It is the patient's right to decide whether or not he will learn, but it is the nurse's responsibility to present him with the information that he needs to make the decision and to motivate him to appreciate the need for learning.

With the changes that have occurred in the health care delivery system in the past decade, resulting in competition for patients and increased emphasis on cost reduction and cost containment, patient education has taken on new significance. It is viewed as a strategy for cost reduction when it is directed toward decreasing length of stay and facilitating earlier discharge. It is viewed as a public relations tool when it increases patient satisfaction and stimulates patient self-referrals. It is viewed as a cost-avoidance strategy for those who believe that satisfactory staff–patient relations avert malpractice suits and that an emphasis on patient education promotes such relations.

Many health care agencies are directing their educational efforts not only toward their patient populations but also toward the community in general. A wide variety of health promotion programs are offered either free of charge or for a minimal fee. It is not unusual for health care agencies to offer programs that promote weight reduction, smoking cessation, and exercise, as well as prenatal classes, classes for grandparents, babysitter classes, classes for adults with aging parents, and classes and support groups for patients with chronic illnesses such as diabetes, cardiac conditions, and cancer. Many of these classes are presented by nurses who have expertise in health promotion.

Adherence to the Therapeutic Regimen

Inherent within the area of patient teaching is the concern for the promotion of the patient's adherence to his therapeutic regimen. The term *compliance* is often used to describe this behavior—he changes his behavior because he has been told to do so. However, this term suggests that the patient's role is passive. The term *adherence* implies that the patient assumes a more active role in self-determination and altering his health behaviors.

Adherence to a therapeutic regimen requires that the patient make one or more changes in his life-style. The patient may need to take medications, adhere to a diet, restrict his activities, observe himself for signs and symptoms of illness, practice specific hygienic measures, seek periodic evaluation of his health status, and attend to a host of other therapeutic and preventive measures. The fact that many patients do not adhere to their prescribed regimens cannot be ignored or min-

imized. The rates of patient adherence to therapeutic and preventive regimens are generally very low, especially when the regimens are complex or of long duration. The characteristics of nonadherent patients and their reasons for not adhering to their prescribed therapy have been the subjects of many studies. For the most part, the findings have been inconclusive. No one factor has been found to be the predominant cause of nonadherence. Instead, it seems that a wide range of variables interacting with one another influence the degree of adherence.

The factors influencing adherence include the following:

- Demographic variables, such as age, sex, race, socioeconomic status, and education
- Illness variables, such as the severity of the illness and the relief of symptoms afforded by the therapy
- Therapeutic regimen variables, such as the complexity of the regimen and uncomfortable side effects
- Psychosocial variables, such as intelligence, attitudes toward health professionals, acceptance or denial of illness, religious or cultural beliefs, and the costs involved in actuating the regimen

Knowledge alone concerning health and health promotion and illness and illness prevention has not been found to be a sufficient stimulus to motivate total adherence. However, it has been found that some degree of adherence in some patients is obviously enhanced by the use of teaching programs and by methods directed toward stimulating motivation to adhere to a regimen. The problem of nonadherence to therapeutic regimens is a substantial one that needs to be remedied to assist patients to participate in self-care and to achieve their maximum health potential.

Written contracts between patients and nurses have been found to promote motivation toward adherence for some patients. Contracting is based on the principles of positive reinforcement and behavior modification. Small, easily attainable goals are used to help the patient shape his behavior and then move to more complex goals.

The role of the nurse in teaching and directing patients toward adherence behavior is a significant one. It is the responsibility of the nurse to assess all variables that may have an effect on the patient's adherence and to use this information when developing and implementing the patient's teaching plan.

Gerontologic Considerations

The problem of nonadherence to therapeutic regimens is a particularly significant problem among the elderly. Elderly persons frequently have one or more chronic illnesses that are periodically complicated by acute episodes and managed with numerous medications. Besides these problems, they also often present with other variables that affect adherence to therapeutic regimens, such as increased sensitivity to drugs and their side effects, difficulty in adjusting to change and stress, financial constraints to costly therapies, forgetfulness, inadequate support systems, lifetime habits of self-medication with over-the-counter drugs, visual impairments, hearing impairments, and mobility limitations.

To promote adherence to therapeutic regimens by the elderly, time and effort must be taken to assess all variables that may affect this health behavior. In addition, the patient's strengths as well as limitations must be assessed so that his strengths can be capitalized on to minimize his limitations. Above all, continuous coordinated care must be provided for him. Otherwise, the efforts of one health care professional may be negated by the efforts of another.

The Nature of Teaching and Learning

When learning is defined as the acquiring of knowledge, attitudes, or skills, and teaching is defined as helping another person to learn, it becomes evident that the teaching–learning process is an active one. It requires the active involvement of both the teacher and the learner in the effort to reach the desired outcome—change in behavior. The teacher does not give knowledge to the learner but instead serves as a facilitator of learning. In general, there is a lack of knowledge about how learning occurs and is affected by teaching. No single theory of learning suffices to explain how learning occurs. However, some specific principles of learning and some guidelines for teaching have been identified.

Learning Readiness

There are many variables, both internal and external, that affect the learner and the learning situation. One of the most significant of these factors is the learner's readiness to learn—his physical, emotional, and experiential readiness to learn.

Physical readiness is of vital importance because until a patient is physically capable of learning, attempts at teaching and learning may be both futile and frustrating. A patient who is experiencing acute pain is unable to focus his attention away from the pain long enough to concentrate on learning. Likewise, a patient who is short of breath will concentrate his energies on breathing rather than on learning.

- Maslow's hierarchy of needs is helpful in considering the concept of physical readiness for learning.

Emotional readiness involves the patient's motivation to learn. Until the person has begun to accept his illness or to accept the fact that illness is a threat to him, he may not be motivated to learn. If his therapeutic regimen is not acceptable to him or is in conflict with his life-style, he may consciously avoid learning. Until he recognizes the need to learn and his own ability to learn, teaching efforts may be thwarted. However, it is not always wise to wait for the patient to become emotionally ready to learn—this time may never come unless efforts are made by the nurse to stimulate the patient's motivation to learn. Illness and the threat of illness are usually accompanied by anxiety and stress. The nurse who recognizes the patient's reactions to his illness or threatened illness can use simple explanations and instructions to alleviate his anxieties and to further motivate him to learn. It must be remembered that because learning involves changes in behavior, it normally produces mild anxiety. Such anxiety is often a useful motivating factor.

Emotional readiness can be promoted by creating a warm, accepting, positive atmosphere and by establishing realistic learning goals with the patient so that he can realize success and a feeling of accomplishment, which in themselves are motivators of learning.

Feedback about progress also serves to motivate learning. Such feedback should be presented in the form of positive reinforcement when the patient is successful and in the form of constructive suggestions for improvement when he is unsuccessful.

Experiential readiness to learn refers to the patient's past experiences that enable him to learn what is being taught. Previous educational experiences and life experiences in general are significant determinants of the patient's approach to learning. A person who has had little or no formal education may not be able to understand the instructional materials presented to him—although this is not always true. The person who has experienced difficulty in learning in the past may be hesitant to make new attempts to learn. Many behaviors required for meeting one's maximum health potential demand a rather extensive background of knowledge, physical skills, and attitudes. If the person does not have this background on which to build, learning may be very difficult and very slow for him. For example, until a patient understands the basics of normal nutrition, he may not be able to understand the restrictions of a special diet. Also, a person who is not future-oriented will be unable to appreciate many aspects of preventive health teaching. And a person who does not view the desired learning as meaningful to himself and his life-style will reject teaching efforts.

Thus, experiential readiness is closely related to emotional readiness, because motivation tends to be stimulated by one's appreciation for the need to learn and by those learning tasks that are familiar, interesting, and meaningful.

- Prior to initiating a teaching–learning program, the nurse must assess the patient's physical and emotional readiness to learn as well as his level of attainment of those behaviors that are prerequisites to learning what is being taught. This information then becomes the basis for the goals to be established, goals that in themselves can motivate the patient to learn.
- Involvement of the patient in the establishment of goals that are mutually acceptable to him and to the nurse serves the purpose of encouraging the patient to be actively involved in the learning process and to share the responsibility for his learning progress.

The Learning Atmosphere

Although a teacher is not always necessary, most patients who are attempting to learn new or altered health behaviors will need the services of a nurse-teacher at least part of the time. The interpersonal interaction between the patient and the nurse who is attempting to meet the patient's learning needs may be formal or informal, depending on the method and techniques of teaching that are found to be most appropriate for the individual patient.

The nurse facilitates learning by manipulating those external variables that affect the patient's learning. For example, the physical environment should be such that it is conducive to learning. That is, the room temperature, lighting, noise levels, and so on, should be appropriate to the learning situation. Also, the time selected for teaching should be suited to the patient's needs. Scheduling a teaching session at a time of day when the patient is fatigued, when he is anticipating diagnostic or therapeutic procedures about which he is anxious, or when he has visitors does not provide a conducive learning environment. Timing of teaching may also be determined by visits of the family members if they are to be included in the teaching plan.

Teaching Techniques

The nurse also facilitates learning by selecting teaching techniques and methods that are most appropriate to meet the individual patient's needs.

The *lecture or explanation* method of teaching is commonly used but should always be accompanied by discussion. The discussion is important because it affords the patient an opportunity to express his feelings and concerns, to ask questions, and to receive clarification of any misinformation or misunderstandings that he may have.

Group teaching is appropriate for some patients because it allows them not only to receive the information that is needed but also to experience security through being a member of a group. Patients with similar problems or learning needs have the opportunity to identify with each other and thus to gain moral support and encouragement. However, it must be remembered that all patients do not relate well in groups and therefore may not benefit from such experiences. It must also be remembered that if group teaching is used, assessment and follow-up of each individual patient is imperative to ensure that each patient gains the knowledge and skills that he needs.

Demonstration and practice are often essential ingredients of the patient's teaching program, especially when skills are to be learned. The nurse first demonstrates the skill to the patient and then allows him ample opportunity to practice the skill. When special equipment is necessary to perform the skill, such as insulin syringes, colostomy bags or dressings, it is important that the nurse provide the patient with the same equipment that he will be using after he leaves the hospital. Learning to perform a skill with one kind of equipment and then having to change to a different kind of equipment is more than should be expected of most patients.

Teaching aids are available to supplement the abilities of the nurse to help the patient to learn. These include books, pamphlets, pictures, films, slides, audio and video tapes, models, programmed instruction, and computer-assisted learning modules. Such teaching aids are invaluable when used appropriately, and they can save a significant amount of personnel time and related cost. However, it is the responsibility of the nurse to review all such aids before presenting them to patients to be sure that they are designed to meet the individual patient's learning needs.

Reinforcement and follow-up are also important factors to consider, because learning takes time. The patient must be allowed ample time to learn and to have his learning reinforced. A single teaching session is never adequate. Follow-up sessions are imperative to promote the patient's confidence in his ability to follow through with what he has learned. Such sessions also give the nurse the opportunity to evaluate the patient's progress and to plan for additional teaching sessions as required. It is also important to realize that the patient may not be able to transfer what he has learned in the hospital to his home setting. Thus, arrangements for follow-up after discharge are often essential for ensuring that the full benefits of the previous teaching program have been realized.

Gerontologic Considerations

The nurse caring for elderly patients must be aware of how normal aging changes affect learning abilities and how the patient can be assisted to adjust to these. Above all, she must recognize the fact that just because a person is elderly does not mean that he cannot learn. Many studies have shown that older adults can learn *and* remember if the information to be learned is paced appropriately, is relevant, and is followed by appropriate feedback, strategies that apply to all learners. The nurse must also be aware that aging changes vary significantly among elderly persons. Therefore, it is essential that thorough assessment of each patient's level of physiologic and psychologic functioning be conducted prior to the beginning of teaching.

Changes in cognition resulting from age include slowed cognitive functioning, decreased short-term memory, decreased abstract thinking and concentration abilities, and increased reaction time. These changes are often accentuated by the host of disease conditions that cause the elderly to seek health care in the first place. Teaching strategies that are often effective include a slowly paced presentation of small amounts of material at a time, frequent repetition of information, and the use of reinforcement techniques such as audiovisual and written materials and repeated practice sessions. The teaching environment must be one in which distracting stimuli are minimized as much as possible.

Sensory changes associated with aging also affect teaching and learning. Teaching strategies to accommodate decreased visual acuity include large-print, easy-to-read materials that are printed on nonglare paper. Because color discrimination is often impaired, the use of color-coded or highlighted teaching materials may not be effective. To maximize hearing, the teacher speaks distinctly in a normal or lowered pitch voice, facing the patient so he can lip read. Visual cues are often helpful to reinforce verbal teaching.

Family members are involved in teaching sessions when possible. They provide another source for reinforcement of material and can help the patient to recall instructions later. They can also provide valuable information about the patient's living situation and related learning needs.

When the nurse, other involved health care professionals, and the patient's family members work collaboratively to facilitate the patient's learning, the chances of success will be maximized. Successful learning for the elderly patient should result in improved self-care abilities, enhanced self-esteem, and future attempts to continue to learn.

▶ Nursing Process
The Nursing Process in Patient Teaching

The teaching–learning process is an integral part of the nursing process. With a focus on learning and with regard for the principles, variables, techniques, and strategies of teaching and learning, the steps of the nursing process—assessment, nursing diagnosis, planning, implementation, and evaluation—are used for the purpose of meeting the teaching and learning needs of the patient and his family.

▷ Assessment

Assessment in the teaching–learning process is comparable to that component of the nursing process. It is directed toward the systematic collection of data about the patient's learning needs and readiness to learn and about the family's learning needs. All internal and external variables that affect the patient's readiness to learn are assessed. A learning assessment guide may be helpful in obtaining pertinent information about the patient's need to learn and his readiness to learn. Some of the learning assessment guides available are very general and are directed toward the assessment of general health information. Others are specific to common medication regimens or disease processes. An example is the *Diabetes Mellitus Assessment Guides* published by the American Diabetes Association, North Carolina Affiliate, Inc. These assessment guides are designed for the assessment of the learning needs of the person with diabetes with regard to all aspects of the diabetic regimen. Such guides serve to facilitate the assessment but must be adapted to the individual responses, problems, and needs of the patient. As soon as possible after completing the assessment, the nurse organizes, analyzes, synthesizes, and summarizes the data collected and determines the patient's need for teaching.

Nursing Diagnosis

Nursing diagnoses that specifically relate to the patient's learning needs are then succinctly stated and serve to guide the nurse in the development of the teaching plan.

Planning

Once the nursing diagnoses related to the patient's need for learning have been identified, the planning component of the teaching–learning process follows. This plan follows the same sequence used in the nursing process:

1. Assigning priorities to the diagnoses
2. Specifying the immediate, intermediate, and long-term goals of learning
3. Identifying specific teaching strategies appropriate for attaining goals
4. Specifying the expected outcomes
5. Documenting the diagnoses, goals, teaching strategies, and expected outcomes on the teaching plan

As in the nursing process, the assignment of priorities to the diagnoses should be a joint effort by the nurse and the patient or his family members. Consideration must be given to the urgency of the patient's learning needs, the most critical needs receiving the highest priority.

After the priorities of the diagnoses have been established, the immediate, intermediate, and long-term goals and the teaching strategies appropriate for attaining the goals are identified. Studies have indicated that teaching is most effective when the patient's goals and the nurse's goals are in agreement. Goal-directed learning begins with the establishment of goals that are appropriate to the situation and that are realistic in terms of the patient's ability to achieve them. Goals are individualized according to the needs of the patient, specifically the needs perceived by the patient, and must be acceptable to the nurse, the patient, and the family. Involving the patient and his family in establishing goals and the subsequent planning of teaching strategies promotes their cooperation in the implementation of the teaching plan.

Expected outcomes of the teaching strategies are stated in terms of the patient's behaviors. Every effort is made to develop outcomes that are realistic and measurable. The critical time periods within which the outcomes should be demonstrated by the patient are also identified. The outcomes and the critical time periods will serve as a basis for evaluation of the effectiveness of the teaching strategies.

During the planning phase, the nurse gives consideration to the sequence in which the subject matter will be presented to the patient when each of the teaching strategies is implemented. An outline is often helpful for arranging subject matter and for ensuring that all necessary information is included. Also during this time, the nurse selects and secures the appropriate teaching aids to be used in implementing the teaching strategies.

The entire planning phase of the teaching–learning process is concluded with the formulation of the patient's teaching plan by the nurse. This teaching plan communicates the following information to all members of the nursing team.

1. The nursing diagnoses that specifically relate to the patient's learning needs and the priorities of these diagnoses
2. The goals of the teaching strategies
3. The teaching strategies, which are expressed in the form of teaching orders
4. The expected outcomes, which identify the expected behavioral responses of the patient
5. The critical time period within which each outcome is expected to be met
6. The patient's behavioral responses (must be documented on the teaching plan)

The same rules that apply to writing and revising the nursing care plan apply to the teaching plan. (For a sample teaching plan, see Chart 3-1. Note that it is not different from but is simply a continuation of the nursing care plan.)

Implementation

The implementation phase of the teaching–learning process follows the formulation of the teaching plan. The patient, his family, and other members of the nursing team and the health care team are included in the implementation. The activities of all of these persons are coordinated by the nurse, and the teaching plan serves as the basis for implementation.

- It is important to remain flexible during the implementation phase of the teaching–learning process and to continuously assess the patient's responses to the teaching strategies and to make alterations in the teaching plan as necessary.

It is highly desirable that the nurse use her creativity to the fullest to promote and sustain the patient's motivation to learn; she should anticipate teaching needs that may arise after the patient's discharge from the hospital that are not foreseen by the patient while he is still in the hospital. Then, and only then, can she assist the patient in transferring knowledge from the hospital to his home. The implementation phase is concluded when the teaching strategies have been completed and when the patient's responses to the actions have been recorded. This record serves as the basis for the evaluation of the patient's accomplishment of the defined goals and expected outcomes.

Evaluation

Evaluation is the final component of the teaching–learning process and is directed toward the determination of the patient's response to the teaching strategies and the extent

Chart 3-1
Example of a Teaching Plan*

Assessment of Mr. Lee's teaching and learning needs revealed the following:

Basic knowledge about the relationship between stress and physiologic functioning
Life-style conducive to excessive stress
Irregularity of meals
Previous noncompliance with dietary regimen
Inadequate knowledge about diet restrictions

Nursing Diagnosis

Potential noncompliance with dietary regimen related to knowledge deficit and life-style

Goals

Immediate: Demonstrates knowledge of dietary regimen
Intermediate: Adheres to the dietary regimen
Long-term: Alters life-style to reduce emotional and environmental stressors

Teaching Strategies	Expected Outcomes	Outcomes
Provide consultation with dietitian		
Reinforce instructions given by dietitian regarding: 1500-calorie diet 1-g sodium diet Low-cholesterol diet	Explains purposes of diet restrictions in relation to own condition Identifies ways in which his diet can be compatible with family's diet	Related explanation accurately. Wife planned meals for family for 1 week that included modifications compatible with dietary restrictions Patient identified need to plan schedule to accommodate regularity of meals Called Weight Watchers and made plans to begin in 1 week
Discuss necessity for life-style alterations with patient and wife	Decreases daily and weekend work hours Plans for daily periods of rest and relaxation Shares, with wife, responsibilities related to daughters' activities	Patient and wife working together to begin life-style alterations that will promote stress reduction; daughters included in plans Patient and wife developed schedule of daily and weekend activities, incorporating plans for designated periods of rest and relaxation; aware of desirability of a flexible schedule
Notify physician's office nurse of patient's need for reinforcement of teaching plan	Demonstrates compliance with dietary regimen	

* For background information, see Example of an Individualized Nursing Care Plan, pp. 34–35.

---

to which the goals have been achieved. Evaluation for the teaching–learning process will answer the same question as that used for the nursing process but with specific regard to teaching and learning. An important phase in evaluation remains: "What should be done to improve the teaching?" Answers to this question will dictate changes that must be made in the teaching plan.

It should never be assumed that an individual has learned because he has been taught. Learning does not automatically follow teaching. A variety of measurement techniques can be used to measure changes in behavior that give evidence of learning. These include direct observation of behavior, using rating scales, checklists, or anecdotal notes to document the behaviors, and indirect measures, such as oral questioning and written tests. Measurement of actual behavior (direct measurement) is the most accurate and appropriate technique in many patient teaching situations. However, it should be supplemented with indirect measurements whenever possible. When more than one measurement technique is employed, the reliability of the resultant data is enhanced because each individual measurement technique carries with it a potential source of error.

The use of measurement techniques is only the beginning of evaluation. It is followed by the interpretation of the data and the making of value judgments about learning and teaching. Such evaluation should be done periodically throughout the teaching–learning program, at its conclusion, and at varying periods subsequent to the program. Evaluation of learning after hospitalization is highly desirable but is not always feasible in terms of time, economics, and nursing personnel required for such evaluation. However, coordination of efforts and sharing of information between hospital-based and community-based nursing personnel serve to facilitate such posthospital evaluation.

- It should always be remembered that evaluation is not the end step in the teaching–learning process. The information gathered during evaluation should be used to redirect teaching actions with the goal of improving the patient's responses and outcomes that result from the teaching actions.

Chapter Summary

The goal of health education is to teach people to strive toward achievement of their maximum health potentials. The teaching–learning process is an integral part of the nursing process and consists of the same cyclic and recurrent steps: assessment, nursing diagnosis, planning, implementation, and evaluation. Each step is ongoing and is related to all other steps. Continuous evaluation provides the means for maintaining the viability of the entire teaching–learning process and for demonstrating accountability for the quality of the teaching provided. Chart 3-2 is intended to assist in the nurse's use of the teaching–learning process.

Chart 3-2
A Guide to Patient Teaching

Assessment

1. Assess the patient's readiness for health education.
   a. What are the patient's health beliefs and behaviors?
   b. What psychosocial adaptation is the patient making?
   c. Is the patient ready to learn?
      Is he able to learn these behaviors?
      What additional information about him is needed?
      What are his expectations?
      What does he want to learn?
2. Organize, analyze, synthesize, and summarize the collected data.

Nursing Diagnosis

Formulate the nursing diagnoses that relate to the patient's learning needs.
1. Identify the patient's learning needs, their characteristics, and etiology.
2. State nursing diagnoses concisely and precisely.

Planning

1. Assign priority to the nursing diagnoses that relate to the patient's learning needs.
2. Specify the immediate, intermediate, and long-term nurse-patient established learning goals.
3. Identify teaching strategies appropriate for goal attainment.
4. Establish expected outcomes.
5. Develop the written teaching plan.
   a. Include diagnoses, goals, teaching strategies, and expected outcomes.
   b. Put the information to be taught in logical sequence.
   c. Write down the key points.
   d. Select appropriate teaching aids.
   e. Keep the plan current and flexible to meet the patient's changing learning needs.
6. Involve the patient, his family or significant others, nursing team members, and other health care team members in all aspects of planning.

Implementation

1. Put the teaching plan into action.
2. Know the material to be presented.
3. Use language the patient can understand.
4. Use appropriate teaching aids.
5. Use the same equipment that the patient will use after discharge.
6. Encourage the patient to actively participate in learning.
7. Record the patient's responses to the teaching actions.
8. Give feedback.

Evaluation

1. Collect objective data.
   a. Observe the patient.
   b. Ask questions to determine if the patient understands.
   c. Use rating scales, checklists, anecdotal notes, and written tests when appropriate.
2. Compare the patient's behavioral responses with the expected outcomes. Determine the extent to which the goals were achieved.
3. Include the patient, his family or significant others, nursing team members, and other health care team members in the evaluation.
4. Identify alterations that need to be made in the teaching plan.
5. Make referrals to appropriate sources or agencies for reinforcement of learning after discharge.
6. Continue all steps of the teaching process: assessment, nursing diagnosis, planning, implementation, and evaluation.

Bibliography

Books

Haggard A. Handbook of Patient Education. Rockville, MD, Aspen Publishers, 1985.

Pender NJ. Health Promotion in Nursing Practice. Norwalk, CT, Appleton and Lange, 1987.

Rankin SH and Stallings KD. Patient Education: Issues, Principles, Practices. Philadelphia, JB Lippincott, 1990.

Redman B. The Process of Patient Education. St Louis, CV Mosby, 1988.

Journals

Asterisks indicate nursing research articles.

Alywahby NF. Principles of teaching for individual learning of older adults. Rehabil Nurs 1989 Nov/Dec; 14(6):330–333.

Armstrong ML. Orchestrating the process of patient education: Methods and approaches. Nurs Clin North Am 1989 Sep; 24(3):597–604.

Ashby L and Travis S. Teach yourself how to teach an older patient. RN 1988 Apr; 53(4):25–27.

Bailey-Allen AM. Who is responsible for patient teaching? Orthop Nurs 1989 Jan/Feb; 8(1):53–54.

Baker K, Kuhlmann T, and Magliaro BL. Homeward bound. Discharge teaching for parents of newborns with special needs. Nurs Clin North Am 1989 Sep; 24(3):655–664.

Barr WJ. Teaching patients with life-threatening illnesses. Nurs Clin North Am 1989 Sep; 24(3):639–644.

Barron S. Documentation of patient education. Patient Educ Couns 1987 Feb; 9(1):81–85.

Bartlett EE. Patient education can lower costs, improve quality. Hospitals 1989 Nov 5; 63(21):88.

Breeze W. Educational readiness in hospitalized adults. Today's OR Nurse 1987 July; 9(7):28–32.

Brillhart B and Steward A. Education as the key to rehabilitation. Nurs Clin North Am 1989 Sep; 24(3):675–680.

Close A. Patient education: A literature review. J Adv Nurs 1988 Mar; 13(2):202–213.

Criteria for the development of health promotion and education programs. Am J Public Health 1987 Jan; 77(1):89–92.

DeMuth JS. Patient teaching in the ambulatory setting. Nurs Clin North Am 1989 Sep; 24(3):645–654.

Derdiarian AK. Effects of information on recently diagnosed cancer patients' and spouses' satisfaction with care. Cancer Nurs 1989 Oct; 12(5):285–292.

Diehl LN. Client and family learning in the rehabilitation setting. Nurs Clin North Am 1989 Mar; 24(1):257–264.

Dobberstein K. Computer-assisted patient ed. Am J Nurs 1987 May; 87(5):697.

Duffy MM. Selecting educational materials for patients with limited reading abilities. ANNA J 1988 Apr; 15(2):114–117.

Ewing G. The nursing preparation of stoma patients for self-care. J Adv Nurs 1989 May; 14(5):411–420.

Foster SD. Evaluating patient learning. MCN 1987 Mar/Apr; 12(2):131.

Foster SD. The role of education in discharge planning. MCN 1988 Nov/Dec; 13(6):403.

Fulton ML and Coulter SJ. Alternative means of patient education. Nurs Manage 1989 Nov; 20(11):58–60.

Gessner BA. Adult education. The cornerstone of patient teaching. Nurs Clin North Am 1989 Sep; 24(3):589–595.

* Gilden JL. The effectiveness of diabetes education programs for older patients and their spouses. J Am Geriatr Soc 1989 Nov; 37(11):1023–1030.

Harrison LL. The patient education bridge. MCN 1989 Jan/Feb; 14(1):51.

Hicks S. The nurse and the patient: Partners in education. Can Crit Care Nurs J 1987 Sep/Oct; 4(3):18–22.

Higgins MG. Learning style assessment: A new patient teaching tool? J Nurs Staff Dev 1988 Winter; 4(1):14–18.

Hussey LC and Gilliland K. Compliance, low literacy, and locus of control. Nurs Clin North Am 1989 Sep; 24(3):605–611.

Johnson EA and Jackson JE. Teaching the home care client. Nurs Clin North Am 1989 Sep; 24(3):687–693.

Kick E. Patient teaching for elders. Nurs Clin North Am 1989 Sep; 24(3):681–686.

Lemphers C. Adult education strategies important for nurses. AARN News Lett 1989 Jan; 45(1):14–15.

Luker K and Caress A. Rethinking patient education. J Adv Nurs 1989 Sep; 14(9):711–718.

MacIssac AM, Rivers R, and Adamson CB. Multiple medications. Is your patient caught in the storm? Nursing 1989 Jul; 19(7):60–64.

Marchiondo K and Kipp C. Establishing a standardized patient education program. Crit Care Nurse 1987 May/Jun; 7(3):58, 60–64, 66.

McCabe BJ et al. A strategy for designing effective patient education materials. J Am Diet Assoc 1989 Sep; 89(9):1290–1292, 1295.

Molzahn AE and Northcott HC. The social bases of discrepancies in health/illness perceptions. J Adv Nurs 1989 Feb; 14(2):132–140.

* Mooney MA. Use of adult education principles in medication instruction. J Contin Educ Nurs 1987 May; 18(3):89–92.

Morrow D, Leirer V, and Sheikh J. Adherence and medication instructions. Review and recommendations. J Am Geriatr Soc 1988 Dec; 36(12):1147–1159.

* Murray PJ. Rehabilitation information and health beliefs in the post-coronary patient: Do we meet their information needs? J Adv Nurs 1989 Aug; 14(8):686–693.

Oberst MT. Perspectives on research in patient teaching. Nurs Clin North Am 1989 Sep; 24(3):621–628.

Ruzicki DA. Realistically meeting the educational needs of hospitalized acute and short-stay patients. Nurs Clin North Am 1989 Sep; 24(3):629–637.

Sansivero GE and Murray SA. Safe management of chemotherapy at home. Oncol Nurs Forum 1989 Sep/Oct; 16(5):711–713.

Siegel H. Nurses improve hospital efficiency through a risk assessment model at admission. Nurs Manage 1988 Oct; 19(10):38–40, 42, 44, 46.

Smith CE. Overview of patient education. Opportunities and challenges for the twenty-first century. Nurs Clin North Am 1989 Sep; 24(3):583–587.

Smith CE. Patient teaching. It's the law. Nursing 1987 Jul; 17(7):67–68.

Speers AT. Patient education: Theory and practice. J Nurs Staff Dev 1989 May/Jun; 5(3):121–126.

Stewart RB and Caranasos GJ. Medication compliance in the elderly. Med Clin North Am 1989 Nov; 73(6):1551–1563.

Stone S et al. Comparison between videotape and personalized education for anticoagulant therapy. J Fam Pract 1989 Jul; 29(1):55–57.

Taylor RA. Making the most of your time for patient teaching. RN 1987 Dec; 52(12):20–21.

* Tilley JD, Gregor FM, and Thiessen V. The nurse's role in patient education: Incongruent perceptions among nurses and patients. J Adv Nurs 1987 May; 12(3):291–301.

Tripp-Reimer T and Afifi LA. Cross-cultural perspectives on patient teaching. Nurs Clin North Am 1989 Sep; 24(3):613–619.

Weinrich SP, Boyd M, and Nussbaum J. Adapting strategies to teach the elderly. J Gerontol Nurs 1989 Nov; 15(11):17–21.

Wilson-Barnett J. Patient teaching or patient counseling? J Adv Nurs 1988 Mar; 13(2):215–222.

4

Ethical Issues in Medical–Surgical Nursing

Learning Objectives

On completion of this chapter, the learner will be able to:

1. Define ethics and nursing ethics
2. Identify several ethical dilemmas common to the medical–surgical area of nursing practice
3. Specify strategies that can be helpful to nurses in ethical decision making

In recent years, there has been a growing interest in ethical issues in all facets of daily life. Specifically in the health care milieu, the factors that led to the growth in ethical problems are diverse. Some of the common factors include increased technologic sophistication, increased life span, decreased resources, and the changing role of the professional nurse. In the past, medicine had few ways to combat disease; thus, the nurse's role was primarily one of support and comfort. Today, sophisticated technology can frequently prolong life indefinitely. Questions recently have been raised about whether it is always appropriate to use this technology, and if it is not appropriate to do so, why not? Who should make these decisions? The enhancement of technologic support has sparked controversy at both ends of the continuum of life. Benefits include a new chance at life for premature infants and an increase in the average life expectancy. However, the increased technologic sophistication has been a "mixed blessing." While many individuals are afforded a better quality of life, there is also the predicament of prolonging the dying process with additional

suffering, as well as additional cost. Presently, approximately 11% of the gross national product (GNP) is spent on health care expenditures. With diminished resources, the elderly population has been cited as one group where advanced technology has been inappropriately used. This raises the question of whether rationing health care based on the criterion of age alone is a sound concept.

Finally, the accepted definition of professional nursing has inspired a new advocacy role for nurses. A definition of nursing provided by the American Nurses Association in the publication *Nursing: A Social Policy Statement* (1980) defines nursing as "the diagnosis and treatment of human responses to actual or potential health problems." This definition supports the claim that nurses must be actively involved in the ethical decision-making process because the ethical concerns surrounding health care are human responses. However, this belief may come in conflict with administrators in health care settings where the traditional roles of the nurse are delineated within a bureaucratic environment. Health care settings in which nurses are valued members of the health care team promote multidisciplinary communication and may enhance patient care. To practice effectively in these settings, nurses must be aware of the ethical issues and assist patients in voicing their moral concerns.

Over the past decade, schools of nursing have included the topic of ethics within their curricula; however, the teaching modalities are varied in time and content. Understandably, nurses focus their initial training on learning the necessary technologic skills to provide safe and competent patient care upon graduation. However, as the practitioner becomes more experienced, it is frequently the ethical rather than the technical issues that become problematic. The focus of this chapter will be to provide an overview of ethical inquiry. A review of common terminology and ethical theories will be included to provide a background for more advanced investigation. Understanding the role of the professional nurse in ethical decision making will assist nurses in utilizing the identified steps in the analytic decision-making model and articulating ethical positions. Initially, ethical decision making appears overwhelming because it involves a different "language" than customary; however, one must remember that making these ethical decisions is a skill that can be learned.

Definition of Ethical Terms

Ethics Versus Morality

When one hears the terminology *ethics* and *morality,* it is usually within the context of some belief about right and wrong human conduct and various guidelines for action. The word "ethics" comes from the Greek language, whereas the origin of "morality" is Latin. It is unclear whether the meaning of these two words differs.

Ethics refers to the philosophical study of morality, and one relies on formal theory, rules, principles, or codes of conduct to determine the "right" course of action. In contrast, morality describes one's personal commitment to values, and these values are frequently influenced by societal norms and expectations. For example, children learn from their parents that it is wrong to steal. Society has fostered the belief that stealing is wrong; thus, an individual may incorporate these social mores into his own value hierarchy. With an ethical inquiry, individuals would analyze why it is wrong to steal and may base their arguments on the fact that stealing violates fundamental moral principles such as respect for persons, justice, and fidelity (promise keeping). Thus, one distinction is that ethics is the more formal, systematic study of moral beliefs, while morality is the adherence to informal personal values. Because the distinction between the two is slight, and many authors use them interchangeably, ethics and morality will be used synonymously in this chapter.

Approaches to Ethics

There are generally four ways to systematically study ethics, which can be classified under two headings: nonnormative and normative.

In a *nonnormative* approach, one subgroup is entitled *metaethics.* In metaethics, philosophers are concerned with understanding concepts and linguistic terminology. For example, what does it mean to be "good," "virtuous," or "right"? The description given above on the linguistic differences between morality and ethics is typical of a metaethical approach. An example of metaethics in the health care environment would be the analysis of the concept of "informed consent." Nurses are aware that patients must give consent prior to surgery, but sometimes nurses question whether the patient is truly informed; thus, delving deeper into the whole concept of informed consent would be a metaethical inquiry.

Another subgroup of nonnormative ethics is called *descriptive ethics.* In this category, philosophers or researchers seek to identify various behaviors and beliefs. There is no attempt to place a judgment on the practices; thus, it may be described as ethically neutral. This type of approach is frequently used by historians, anthropologists, or sociologists as they study the behavior of different groups of individuals. For example, in studies of the American Eskimos, it was found that a common practice was placing the elderly on ice rafts and allowing them to die when they were no longer productive members of society. With this type of descriptive research, there is no attempt to debate if this form of euthanasia is morally acceptable; rather, it is merely stating "the way it is." As the field of nursing ethics develops, nurse researchers may employ descriptive ethics to gain a better perspective of the ethical beliefs held by practicing nurses.

Normative ethics is the branch of moral philosophy one usually associates with ethics. When one hears the words "ought" or "should," it is in reference to identifying the morally correct course of behavior, using a systematic approach of moral theory and moral principles to answer the normative question, "What should I (we) do in this situation?" When this approach is used to identify global problems that transcend all fields, it is referred to as *general normative ethics.* For example, how should governments interact to obtain world peace? These questions are usually asked within a specific discipline and are referred to as *applied ethics.* Various disciplines utilize the frameworks of general ethical theories and moral principles and apply them to specific problems within their domain. Bioethics is the study of ethical problems in biology and medicine, although it may also be referred to as medical, clinical, or health care ethics. Nursing ethics may be considered a distinct form of applied ethics because there are many moral situations specific to the nursing profession. The ethical problems that may develop within the nursing profession may also be so broad as to fall under the realm of health care ethics; a clear line of demarcation between the two is difficult to identify. However, because the nursing profession is a "caring" rather than a predominantly "curing" profession, with its own professional code of ethics, it is imperative that one not equate nursing ethics solely with medical ethics.

Moral Situations

There are many different words to describe a moral situation. The most common word is *dilemma.* It is important to clarify the precise meaning of this word: what may appear to be a dilemma may actually be a moral problem. With a moral dilemma, there is a clear conflict of two or more moral principles, or competing moral claims. The choice of one action over another may lead to an unpleasant outcome, and the person must choose "the lesser evil of the two." For example, in a severely ill patient, adhering to the principle of sanctity of life may require the use of prolonged life-sustaining treatment. On the other hand, one may feel that the life-sustaining equipment only prolongs the patient's suffering. In this case, both alternatives are unpleasant: to continue treatment with the possibility of prolonged suffering versus discontinuing treatment and the patient's probable death. This example poses a true moral dilemma if the patient is incompetent (not able to make his own decisions). However, if the patient voices his own views and makes the statement "I want to live . . . do everything you can," then even if the nurse feels it is morally wrong to continue treatment, it should be continued. A competent adult has the right to make these decisions, and his wishes take precedence. This latter scenario depicts a moral problem rather than a moral dilemma because there is no conflict of moral principles. By adhering to the principle of respect for autonomy, there is only one morally correct choice of action—continuing treatment.

Jameton (1984) identified two other possible moral situations the nurse may encounter in practice. One is moral *uncertainty*. In this situation, one cannot accurately define what the moral situation is or what moral principles may apply, but there is a strong feeling that something is not right. Consider the example of an elderly person who undergoes surgery and does not do well. One may hear the comment, "The surgery was a success, but because he has so many other problems he is not getting better." Frequently, this type of patient requires significant nursing care. Prolonged bed rest may have resulted in the patient becoming dependent on others for ambulation, skin care, or other activities of daily living. There may be minimal medical intervention needed at this time, but the patient is not ready to be discharged. Gradually, this patient receives less attention than the other sicker and "more interesting" patients. Nurses may be aware that this particular patient is not receiving the necessary attention, but the precise moral situation is difficult to identify.

The second moral situation identified by Jameton is moral *distress*. In this situation, the nurse is aware of the correct action, but institutional constraints prevent the nurse from pursuing this action. For example, a patient asks a nurse if he has cancer. The surgeon and family have made the decision not to tell the patient the diagnosis. From a moral perspective, patients should be told their diagnoses if they specifically ask. Ideally, this information should come from the physician, with the nurse present to assist the patient in understanding the terminology and to assess the patient's responses to the information. The nurse could experience moral distress if the hospital threatens her with job termination if she discloses the information without agreement of the physician and/or the family.

In all situations, it is important to make the distinction between the medical and moral sphere. All relevant medical facts should be clearly separated from the moral perspectives. With medical education, the focus is on disease prevention and cure; this education alone does not make a physician a moral expert. Likewise, with a nursing assessment, the nurse may uncover different perspectives of the patient's values and beliefs, and she must separate them from her own values. It is essential that nurses freely engage in dialogue concerning moral situations. It is important to emphasize that such dialogue is difficult for everyone involved. Improved interdisciplinary communication is supported when all members of the health care team can voice their concerns and come to an understanding of the moral situation.

In summary, ethical terms help clarify the realm of moral philosophy. From a broad perspective, there are different approaches to the study of ethical issues. When one is attempting to answer questions regarding a specific course of action, one is engaging in normative ethics. Applied ethics utilizes ethical discussion to arrive at a morally correct decision in a specific discipline.

Classical Ethical Theories

When philosophers refer to ethical theory, the goal is to justify the question "What should be done?" by adherence to specific ethical frameworks. Ethical theories are broad frameworks consisting of moral rules and principles. Thus, ethical theories serve as the foundation for normative judgments or courses of action.

There are two major types of ethical theory: teleological and deontological. A brief overview of both types will be presented to assist the nurse in distinguishing between the two frameworks used in ethical decision making. For a more in-depth review of ethical theory, the reader should refer to the references at the end of the chapter.

Teleological Theory

Teleological comes from the Greek word *telos*, meaning "ends." This theory is also commonly referred to as consequentialism. With this framework, one is predominantly concerned with the consequences or end points of actions. The most famous formulation of consequentialism is called utilitarian theory. One commonly hears the slogan "the greatest good for the greatest number" in reference to utilitarian theory. Therefore, one's moral choice is the decision that maximizes the good consequences over the bad or at least attempts to balance the bad consequences overall.

A strong supporter of utilitarianism was the philosopher John Stuart Mill. In his work, Mill proposed that the foundation of moral judgments is the principle of utility, which is also referred to as the "Greatest Happiness Principle." For Mill, "actions are right in proportion as they tend to promote happiness, wrong as they tend to produce the reverse of happiness."* The desirable end points are freedom and absence of pain. This utilitarian perspective may apply to specific moral acts or rules. When using moral rules, one should apply the principle of utility to the specific moral rules that lead to the greatest possible happiness for all people. Although Mill's theory may be classified as hedonistic, the principle of pleasure or utility probably means more than pleasure in the common usage

---

* *Mill JS. Utilitarianism. In Reiser S, Dyck A, and Curran W (eds). Ethics in Medicine: Historical Perspectives and Contemporary Concerns. Cambridge, MA, MIT Press, 1871/1977.*

of the term. Nonetheless, other utilitarian philosophers favor other intrinsic values in addition to pleasure, such as knowledge, health, or friendship, as the goal for the attainment of the aggregate good.

There are many criticisms of a teleological moral framework based on consequences. The most obvious flaw in this type of approach is the uncertainty and difficulty in measuring various intrinsic values. How can one accurately measure and compare happiness, pleasure, or values such as health and friendship? In addition, basing one's moral actions on "the greatest good for the greatest number" may be problematic in certain situations. How can one morally justify decisions that may adversely affect individuals within minority groups? And, finally, teleological theory has been criticized because of its reliance on consequences. If the overall consequences are morally good, does this justify attainment of these goals by nonmoral actions or behavioral means? These questions certainly raise some issues within a teleological framework. An alternative approach delineated below attempts to address these issues.

Deontological Theory

The word deontology comes from the Greek word *deon*, which means duty or obligation. One may gain a better appreciation of deontological or formalist theory when it is viewed in contrast to utilitarian theory. Rather than focusing on the consequences of the act, a deontology framework argues that there are moral standards that exist independently of the ends. These moral standards refer to the various universal moral principles (see Chart 4-1 for some common ethical principles). The distinguishing feature among formalist thinkers is that one's justification of moral actions is more important than the specific consequences or results of the actions.

Similar to teleological theory, there is great diversity among

---

Chart 4-1
Common Ethical Principles

Common ethical principles one may use to validate moral claims.

Autonomy
Derived from the Greek words *autos* ("self") and *nomos* ("rule" or "law"), thus refers to self-rule. In contemporary discourse it has broad meanings, including individual rights, privacy, and choice. Autonomy entails the ability to make a choice free from external constraints.

Beneficence
The duty to do good and the active promotion of benevolent acts (for example, goodness, kindness, and charity). May also include the injunction not to inflict harm (see *Nonmaleficence*).

Confidentiality
This principle relates to the concept of privacy. Information obtained from an individual will not be disclosed to another unless it will benefit the person or there is a direct threat to the social good.

Double Effect
A principle that may morally justify some actions that may produce both good and evil effects. All four of the following criteria must be fulfilled:
1. The action itself is good or morally neutral.
2. The agent sincerely intends the good and not the evil effect (the evil effect may be foreseen but not intended).
3. The good effect is not achieved by means of the evil effect.
4. There is a proportionate or favorable balance of good over evil.

Fidelity
Promise keeping. The duty to be faithful to one's commitments. It includes both explicit and implicit promises to another.

Justice
From a broad perspective, justice states that like cases should be treated alike. A more restricted version of justice is distributive justice, which refers to the distribution of social benefits and burdens. Various theories of distributive justice may include the following notions: That each person receive
    A. Equally
    B. According to need
    C. According to effort
    D. According to societal contribution
    E. According to merit or
    F. According to legal entitlement.
Retributive justice is concerned with the distribution of punishment.

Nonmaleficence
The duty not to inflict as well as to prevent and remove harm. May be included within the principle of beneficence, in which case nonmaleficence would be more binding.

Paternalism
The intentional limitation of another's autonomy justified by an appeal to beneficence or the welfare or needs of another. Thus, the prevention of any evils or harm is greater than any potential evils caused by the interference of the individual's autonomy or liberty.

Respect for Persons
Frequently used synonymously with autonomy. However, it goes beyond accepting the notion or attitude that people have autonomous choice to treat others in such a way that enables them to make the choice.

Sanctity of Life
The perspective that life is the highest good. Thus, all forms of life, including mere biological existence, should take precedence over external criteria for judging quality of life.

Veracity
The obligation to tell the truth and not to lie or deceive others.

philosophers within the formalist tradition. One distinguishing feature among philosophers is whether there is only one moral principle that takes precedence (a monistic perspective) or several moral principles (a pluralistic perspective). Examples of each will be highlighted to illustrate this diversity.

Immanual Kant, an 18th century German philosopher, was an influential philosopher within the formalist perspective. Kant held that morality must ultimately be founded on principles of reason that all rational people possess. It is essential that individuals possess a "good will" that chooses actions *for the sake of duty*, not merely *in accordance with duty*. Therefore, the motives that compel one to act must be identified. For example, if a nurse reveals a medication error solely because of fear of punitive action if the error is later discovered, rather than because of concern for the potential harmful effects to the patient, she is not acting within a moral perspective. Although the action of revealing the medication error is correct, the motives behind the action are different.

Kant's perspective is considered monistic (an adherence to one moral principle or imperative) because he advances one essential test of rationality called the *categorical imperative*, which is absolute and universal without exception. Although the categorical imperative does not espouse a single moral principle *per se*, it provides the logical test for any acceptable moral principle. Within the categorical imperative, Kant* espoused various formulations. For example: "Act only according to that maxim whereby you can at the same time will that it should become a universal law." This formulation is similar to "the Golden Rule" espoused in theological beliefs and is also similar to the moral principle of respect for persons. Another formulation of his categorical imperative is "Act in such a way that you treat humanity, whether in your own person or in that of another, always at the same time as an end and never simply as a means." This perspective may be sharply contrasted to the utilitarian approach, where the consequences of the action are of primary importance. Kant was predominantly concerned with this latter formulation. This distinction is important to clarify in the area of health care research. For example, even though the goal of patient participation in a research study is to advance scientific knowledge, patients are not being used merely as a means to obtain this goal provided that they are truly informed and participate freely in the research.

A major criticism of Kant's theory is that it does not specify which moral principles take precedence or what to do when two or more actions (duties) are in conflict. Other formalist philosophers have attempted to resolve this issue.

W. D. Ross, a 20th century British philosopher, espoused a deontological framework based on a pluralism of moral rules. Ross identified two types of duties: *prima facie* and actual. The term *prima facie* may be roughly translated as *conditional*, or *all other things being equal*. A *prima facie* duty must be acted upon unless it comes in conflict with another equal or stronger duty. For example, it is a moral wrong to tell a lie; however, one may on occasion justify this action if there is a more compelling duty (for example, avoiding harm to another).

* Kant I. Grounding for the metaphysics of morals. In Ellington JW (trans). Kant's Ethical Philosophy. Indianapolis, Hackett Publishing, 1983. (Original work published 1785.)

The major criticism of Ross's theory, along with other formalist approaches, is that it does not specify which moral principles are the most important and/or take precedence.

Virtue Ethics

In contrast to the teleological and deontological theories discussed above, which focus on specific principles, actions, and the consequences of one's actions, ethics based on virtues focuses on the character traits of the individual. This approach is consistent with the writings of Aristotle and Plato, which espoused that moral conduct was directly related to the cultivation of virtuous character behaviors. Virtues are seen as specific habits or dispositions that a person possesses or aspires to possess. Thus, for Aristotle the moral question was "What shall I be?" rather than "What shall I do?" However, virtues may take many forms. For example, faith, hope, love, and charity are frequently expressed as virtues within religious writings. The question must then be asked, "Which virtues are moral?" One response may be that moral virtues are those specific traits that enable one to act morally and responsibly. Because this response is vague, some philosophers are reluctant to classify virtue ethics as a primary specific moral theory. Rather, they view virtue ethics as fundamental corollaries to the other normative ethical theories. Their reasoning is that many of the virtues inherently correspond to the various moral principles. For example, the virtues of benevolence and fairness correspond to the principles of beneficence and justice, respectively. However, it is necessary to have a basic understanding of the ethics of virtue because recent descriptive research based on moral reasoning has reemphasized this alternative moral perspective.

Ethical Pluralism

By delineating moral theory into contrasting frameworks, the aim is to illustrate how moral philosophy has evolved within the philosophical domain. While some philosophers would advocate that one's ethical reasoning should be consistent with one particular framework, in actual practice this is difficult to uphold. In the applied discipline of health care ethics, one frequently hears comments that reflect this notion of diversity. The ethical problem of allocation of scarce resources may serve as an illustration. Consider the situation in which a hospital is questioning whether to allocate funds to initiate a heart–lung transplant program. The hospital anticipates that in the first year there will be five candidates for this surgical procedure. However, the costs for implementing this program are substantial; therefore, to subsidize the program the hospital will close four community health clinics. The board of directors decides to vote against the transplant program. Their reasoning is that more people will benefit from the community health centers. In this example, a utilitarian framework based on the consequences of "the greatest good for the greatest number" was the moral basis for the claim to maintain the health clinics. Thus, on the "macro" level, utilitarian theory has substantial merit.

But consider another example. One of the patients in the intensive care unit is an 87-year-old woman with congestive heart failure. The physician in charge of the unit would like to transfer this patient to the general unit so that a younger, "more viable" patient may be admitted. Because the elderly woman continues to require the intensive care resources, her immediate caretakers argue that she should remain in the intensive care unit. The moral basis for their claims are the principles of respect for persons and nonmaleficence (do no harm). In this case, a formalist approach based on universal moral principles was the foundation of the moral decision. It is clear, then, in different moral situations one's moral reasoning may depend on the context of the moral problem. It should not be presupposed that one moral framework is inherently "better" than another. One general rule of thumb is that on the "macro" level (broad policy decisions), utilitarian theory is very useful, and on the "micro" level, where one particular patient is the focus of decision making, a formalist approach has particular merit.

It is essential to highlight the perspective of moral pluralism to clarify some misconceptions frequently held by students studying ethics. Initially, students may become frustrated if they attempt to strictly adhere to a particular moral framework. Rather, it may be more effective to take into consideration various frameworks. This may entail understanding the moral principles and applying them to specific moral situations as well as questioning what virtues or behaviors the student as a member of society wants to espouse. For nurses, one approach in assessing the ethical issues in the discipline of nursing may be taking into consideration a variety of perspectives.

In summary, historically there are two common types of ethical theory: teleological or utilitarianism, which is predominantly concerned with the consequences of the action, and deontological or formalism, which is concerned with the adherence to moral principles. Within these two frameworks there are a variety of perspectives espoused by different philosophers. In practice, many people use a combination of these two approaches. Combining these methods is called ethical pluralism. With a pluralistic framework, individuals incorporate the universal moral principles in the moral reasoning process, but they will also take into consideration various virtues or behaviors as well as the ethos of the profession as they attempt to answer the normative question, "What should I do in this situation?"

Domain of Nursing Ethics

There is a reciprocal relationship between the nursing profession and society: nurses provide continuing care to all human beings regardless of disease or social status, and society recognizes the profession's expectation that members act responsibly and according to a code of ethics. In this context, some ethical dilemmas confronting professional nurses may be considered applied ethics.

As a profession, nursing is accountable to society. Nursing with other health professions has accepted the American Hospital Association's Patient's Bill of Rights (Chart 1-1, p. 9). This document reflects societal beliefs about health and health care. Another means for a profession to achieve accountability is its professional Code of Ethics, and the profession's explicit values and goals. The American Nurses Association adopted the Code for Nurses in 1950 (Chart 4-2). The Code consists of 11 statements with interpretive statements; the latter are periodically revised. In the most recent revision, the interpretive statements incorporate the universal moral principles. The Code with interpretive statements is an excellent framework for nurses to use to assist them in ethical decision making. The Code could

---

Chart 4–2
American Nurses Association Code for Nurses

1. The nurse provides services with respect for human dignity and the uniqueness of the client, unrestricted by considerations of social or economic status, personal attributes, or the nature of the health problems.
2. The nurse safeguards the client's right to privacy by judiciously protecting information of a confidential nature.
3. The nurse acts to safeguard the client and the public when health care and safety are affected by the incompetent, unethical, or illegal practice of any person.
4. The nurse assumes responsibility and accountability for individual nursing judgments and actions.
5. The nurse maintains competence in nursing.
6. The nurse exercises informed judgment and uses individual competence and qualifications as criteria in seeking consultation, accepting responsibilities, and delegating nursing activities to others.
7. The nurse participates in activities that contribute to the ongoing development of the profession's body of knowledge.
8. The nurse participates in the profession's efforts to implement and improve standards of nursing.
9. The nurse participates in the profession's efforts to establish and maintain conditions of employment conducive to high-quality nursing care.
10. The nurse participates in the profession's effort to protect the public from misinformation and misrepresentation and to maintain the integrity of nursing.
11. The nurse collaborates with members of the health professions and other citizens in promoting community and national efforts to meet the health needs of the public.

(Reprinted with permission from American Nurses Association. Code for Nurses with Interpretive Statements. Kansas City, MO, American Nurses' Association, 1985.)

be considered a pluralistic framework because it espouses a variety of universal principles and the virtues of professional behavior.

The ethical dilemmas a nurse may encounter in the medical–surgical arena are numerous and diverse. However, in order to reason through these dilemmas, nurses must be aware of the underlying philosophic domain in order to apply these concepts in their professional practice. Because ethical reasoning can be enhanced through a basic understanding of moral philosophy, a significant portion of this chapter has been devoted to these philosophic concepts.

The factors mentioned earlier in the introduction have been instrumental in the explosion of ethical discourse. Certainly, it is often the "life and death" issues that serve as an impetus for the nurse to question the ethical dimension. However, paying attention to only the sensationalism of life and death dilemmas represents a narrow view of ethical inquiry. Levine states:

> There are overlooked ethical challenges in the mundane, everyday routine activities of professional practice, and these have largely gone unexamined. Ethical behavior is *not* the display of one's moral rectitude in times of crises. It is the day-by-day expression of one's commitment to other persons and the ways in which human beings relate to one another in their daily interactions.*

This perspective fosters the ethos of the nursing profession, an ethic of care. Nursing theories that incorporate the bio-psycho-social-spiritual dimensions portray a holistic framework with humanism or caring as the core. For nurses to embrace this professional ethos, it is necessary to be aware of not only major ethical dilemmas but also those daily interactions with patients that frequently are overlooked. Some of these daily interactions that occur in the medical–surgical area will be addressed. These examples may heighten nurses' awareness for other situations where a moral dilemma is not as easily identified.

Frequently, the principle of confidentiality is overlooked in practice. When a nursing assessment is performed, the patient should be informed of the purpose of the assessment and should be told that it will be recorded in the patient record. Occasionally, patients will provide information that is extraneous to either the medical or nursing diagnosis. If the information is not pertinent to the case, the nurse should question if it is prudent to record it in the patient's chart. In the practice setting, discussion of the patient with other members of the health care team is often necessary. However, these discussions should occur in a private area, not in the cafeteria or an elevator, when there is a strong possibility that the information could be overheard. In addition, the widespread use of computers has also raised questions about confidentiality. Patient information is easily obtainable, but only those individuals associated with direct patient care should be able to review the patient data.

Moral situations may also occur when nurses think they know "what is best" for the patient. A brief example from practice can highlight this situation: The patient was a diabetic on a strict diet. On her birthday, the nurses decided to surprise her with a birthday cake. In order for the patient to have some

cake, the nurses asked the dietary department to send half her sandwich at lunchtime. When the patient received her lunch, she became furious. The nurses then brought in the cake, and the patient immediately became embarrassed with her outburst. Although this example illustrates an everyday occurrence that may not be initially perceived as an ethical situation, an important lesson was learned. A different strategy that would have incorporated the principles of autonomy and respect for persons would have been to wish the patient a "Happy Birthday" in the morning and mention to her that a cake had been ordered for lunch. In this context, the patient would have the choice of either the sandwich or cake. Her choice, which may not have been apparent to the nurses, may have been to have the full sandwich and to offer the birthday cake to friends and staff.

The use of restraints is another area where nurses may not perceive a moral dilemma. Nurses should carefully weigh the risks of limiting a person's autonomy by the use of restraints (both physical and pharmacologic measures) against safety concerns. Often the use of restraints can have an unexpected effect and the patient becomes more agitated or confused. Nurses should evaluate the risk factors, which include the physiologic and behavioral data that may necessitate the need for restraints. Strategies to consider prior to restraints include soliciting family members or volunteers to sit with confused patients, manipulating the environment, or using diversionary activities. Concerns for safety, which include the potential injury to self or others, should be incorporated in the decision making.

Two moral situations that may occur in medical–surgical practice that come in direct conflict with the principle of veracity (truth telling) are the use of placebos and revealing a diagnosis to the patient. Inherent in the nurse–patient relationship is trust. To foster trust, there must be the understanding that both the patient and the nurse will be truthful to one another. In practice, the use of placebos has been declining, but when they are used, the attempt is to justify their use with the principle of paternalism. The subsequent deception that may occur with the use of placebos severely undermines the nurse–patient relationship. Consequently, the use of placebos should be considered only when the patient is involved in the decision-making process and is aware that this may be one approach used in the treatment regimen.

Informing patients of their diagnoses historically has been identified as a moral situation in nursing practice. Frequently, physicians and families withhold such information from patients for fear of additional distress for the patient, thus justifying their decisions on the principle of paternalism. Patients often are aware of their diagnosis, and their specific questions are indications that they are ready to hear the information. However, evasive comments by the nursing staff often are used as a means to maintain professional relationships with other health practitioners. This area is indeed complex because it challenges the nurse's integrity. Some strategies the nurse could consider in this situation include:

1. Not lying to the patient
2. Providing all information related to nursing procedures and diagnosis
3. Communicating to the family and physician the patient's requests for information

Families often are unaware of the patient's repeated questions to the nurse. With a better understanding of the situation,

---

* Levine M. Nursing ethics and the ethical nurse. Am J Nurs 1977 May; 77(5):845–847.

families may change their perspective. Finally, although providing the information may be the morally appropriate behavior, the context of the delivery is important. Nurses should remember to be compassionate and caring while informing patients; disclosure of information merely for the sake of patient autonomy does not convey respect for others.

Dilemmas that revolve around death and dying issues are prevalent in medical–surgical practice and frequently initiate moral reflection. The dilemmas may be enhanced by the fact that nursing is still influenced by the curing role in health care. With advanced technology, it may be difficult to accept the fact that "nothing more can be done" or that technology may prolong life, but at the expense of patient suffering. Focusing on the caring, as well as the curing, role may assist nurses in dealing with these difficult moral situations.

The do not resuscitate (DNR) order is frequently an area of concern. When a patient is competent to make decisions, his choice for a DNR order should be honored, justified by the principles of autonomy or respect for persons. However, it should be clear to nurses that a DNR order does *not* mean do not treat. Frequently these patients have significant medical and nursing needs, all of which demand attention. Physicians are often reluctant to write DNR orders in fear that the patient will receive less nursing attention. An unfortunate occurrence in practice is that patient assignments sometimes are made with the unstated belief that a DNR patient requires less nursing time. All patients deserve the care and comfort of nursing interventions regardless of their resuscitation status.

The use of narcotics to alleviate pain in patients with DNR orders is another dilemma for nurses. Patients with excruciating pain may require large dosages of pain medication. As a result, patients may have a decrease in respiratory function. Fear of respiratory depression should not prevent nurses from attempting to alleviate pain. In this situation, the actions may be justified by the principle of double effect. The intent or goal of nursing interventions is to alleviate pain and suffering while promoting comfort. The risk of respiratory depression is not the intent of the actions and should not be used as an excuse for withholding pain medication for DNR patients. However, the patient's respiratory status should be carefully monitored; any signs of respiratory depression are reported to the physician.

The moral situation relating to food and hydration has been receiving significant attention. Many individuals feel that food and hydration are basic human needs and are not considered "invasive measures"; thus, they should always be maintained. However, some consider food and hydration as a means of prolonging suffering. In evaluating this issue, nurses must take into consideration the potential harm as well as the benefit to the patient. Evaluation of harm necessitates a careful review of the reasons patients request the withdrawal of food and hydration. Although the principle of autonomy has considerable merit and is supported by the Code for Nurses, there may be situations where the request for withdrawal of food and hydration cannot be upheld. For patients who are not competent, the issues are more complex. This complexity is apparent in the many court cases that have been focused on this issue. Presently, individual states have different case-law precedents. At present, there are no firm guidelines to assist nurses in this area. In general, the provision of food and hydration is usually in the patient's best interest. However, there may be situations where food and hydration are futile attempts

to maintain life. This situation is one of the most perplexing issues confronting health care professionals and needs careful scrutiny. As professionals, we must protect the vulnerable members of society while balancing the inherent rights of individuals.

In summary, moral situations are common and diverse in the medical–surgical setting. Often, it is the larger, more sensational issues that initially cause nurses to reflect on the moral domain. Because the ethos of the nursing profession is one of care, the everyday human interactions should not be overlooked. Although the moral situations can vary, the fundamental philosophic principles remain. Nurses should become familiar with these concepts and use them as a basis for all moral reflection. As nurses become used to this process, they will gain the understanding that there are no clear solutions to these dilemmas. The process of moral reflection will help nurses to justify their moral actions. This discussion has merely highlighted a few of the many situations a nurse may encounter in practice. Chart 4-3 outlines the steps of an ethical analysis. The references at the end of this chapter can be consulted for in-depth coverage.

Preventive Ethics

As previously mentioned, a dilemma refers to a conflict between two unpleasant alternatives, and one's moral decision is to choose the "lesser evil" of the two. However, there are various strategies available to assist nurses in ethical decision making. These strategies may be referred to as "preventive" because they may be helpful in a current situation, or the knowledge derived may be beneficial in future ethical situations.

Frequently, dilemmas occur when the health care practitioners are unsure of the patient's wishes. A patient may enter the hospital as a competent decision-maker, but changes in his physiologic condition or cognitive status may affect his decision-making capabilities. An initial nursing assessment that includes a discussion of the patient's values and beliefs could elicit this relevant information.

Advance directives may also provide valuable information and may assist health care providers in decision making. Advance directives are legal documents that specify the patient's wishes prior to hospitalization. A *living will* is one type of advance directive. In most situations, living wills are limited to situations where the patient's medical condition is deemed terminal. Because it is difficult to accurately define "terminal," the living will is not always honored. Another potential drawback to the living will is that these documents are frequently written when the patient is in good health. It is not unusual for patients to change their perspective as their illness progresses. Therefore, the patient maintains the option to nullify the document. Another type of advance directive is the *durable power of attorney* (PA). With the PA, the patient has identified another individual to make the decisions on his behalf. In this type of decision making, the patient may have clarified his wishes concerning a variety of medical situations. As such, the power of attorney is a less restrictive advanced directive. These advance directives vary among state jurisdictions. However, even in states where these documents are not legally binding, they

Chart 4–3
Steps of an Ethical Analysis

The following are guidelines to assist nurses in ethical decision making. These guidelines reflect an active process in decision making, similar to the nursing process detailed in Chapter 2.

Assessment

1. Assess the ethical/moral situations of the problem.
   This step entails the recognition of the ethical, legal, and professional dimensions of the situation.
   A. Does the situation entail *substantive* moral problems? (Conflicts among ethical principles or professional obligations?)
   B. Are there *procedural* conflicts? (For example, who should make the decisions? Any conflicts among the health care providers, family, guardians, and patient?)
   C. Identify the significant people involved and those affected by the decision.

Planning

2. Collect information.
   A. Include the following information: the medical facts, treatment options, nursing diagnoses, legal data, and the values, beliefs, and religious components.
   B. Make a distinction between the factual and the values/beliefs.
   C. Validate the patient's capacity, or lack of capacity, to make decisions.
   D. Identify any other relevant information that should be elicited.
   E. Identify the ethical/moral issues and the competing claims.

Implementation

3. List the alternatives.
   Compare alternatives with applicable ethical principles and professional code of ethics. May choose either framework below, or follow both and compare outcomes.

Utilitarian Approach

   A. Predict the consequences to the alternatives.
   B. Assign a positive or negative value to each consequence.
   C. Choose the consequence that predicts the highest positive value or "the greatest good for the greatest number."

Deontological Approach

   A. Identify the relevant moral principles.
   B. Compare alternatives with moral principles.
   C. Appeal to the "higher level" moral principle if there is a conflict.

Evaluation

4. Decide and evaluate decision.
   A. What is the best or morally correct action?
   B. Give the ethical reasons for your decision.
   C. What are the ethical reasons against your decision?
   D. How do you respond to the reasons against your decision?

provide helpful information. They assist health care practitioners in determining the patient's prior expressed wishes in situations where this information can no longer be obtained directly from the patient.

Another strategy for nurses to consider is the availability of *institutional ethics committees*. In recent years, many hospitals have formed these multidisciplinary committees to assist practitioners with ethical dilemmas. The purpose of the com-

mittee may vary among institutions. In some hospitals, the committee exists solely for the purpose of developing policies. In other hospitals, the committee may have a strong educative or consultative focus. Because these committees usually are comprised of individuals with some advanced background in ethical decision making, nurses can consult with the committee members if available.

The heightened interest in ethical decision making has

Chart 4–4
Case Analysis

Guidelines that can be used in ethical decision making are outlined in Chart 4–3 and illustrated in the example that follows.

Mr. G. is a 68-year-old male admitted to the medical–surgical unit with a one-month history of abdominal pain and a recent history of nausea, vomiting, and blood in his stools for the last 48 hours. Mr. G. is a retired manager who lives with his wife; his three children are all grown and living on their own. He states he has kept busy in his retirement years by playing golf, volunteering at the church, and "tinkering around the house."

A complete GI workup revealed a colon mass and possible perforation. He is scheduled for immediate exploratory surgery. Prior to the surgery he appears quite anxious and states to the nurse that he is scared. In addition he states that "I hope they don't find anything bad, even though there is a good probabiity that they

may. I don't know what I would do. My brother died in the hospital two years ago and that was horrible. I never want to die the way he did, with all those machines and tubes hooked up to him. And my wife, I do not want her to be alone, but I'm reluctant to talk to her about this and get her all nervous and upset. I'll just pray that everything will go okay. Luckily, I've always had faith in the church."

The surgery revealed advanced carcinoma with metastasis. The surgery was palliative to remove the obstruction with a transverse colostomy, but there is a high probability of sepsis from the perforation. Mr. G. returns to the unit from the recovery room with intravenous fluids, antibiotics, and narcotic orders, along with a do not resuscitate (DNR) order. The nurse questioned the DNR order but was told "there is nothing more we can do for him."

Assessment

1. Are there substantive moral problems?

Yes. In this case there appears to be a conflict among the moral principles of autonomy, respect for persons, beneficence, and paternalism.

2. Are there procedural conflicts?

Yes. Between the physician and the nurse. The concern is that the patient was not included in the decision-making process.

Planning

Facts: Advanced cancer with metastases. Physician feels that chemotherapy is not an option because of the advanced stage of the disease. States he is ordering the other treatments because "this would be the best for this patient."

Legally, the patient is competent to make the decisions.

Although the nurse agrees with the intent of the DNR order, her concern is that the patient was not consulted. She feels that the comment by the physician that "this would be the best for this patient" is a value judgment that needs to be clarified. The nurse feels that it is essential to assess Mr. G.'s perspectives of his health situation and his personal values and beliefs. Al-

though she feels Mr. G. would agree to the DNR order, she also thinks that including Mr. G. will allow him to determine how much pain medication he needs, which in turn will allow him to be alert enough to discuss the situation with his family and clergy.

Moral Claims

Physician: Maintain the DNR order, it would be in the patient's best interests not to cause him additional distress. (*Alternative 1*)

Nurse: Include the patient and family in the decision-making process. (*Alternative 2*)

Implementation

The two alternatives to the moral problem are delineated above under the moral claims. In assessing the interventions, it is essential to evaluate the alternatives in light of the universal moral principles.

Alternative 1: This is based on the principles of paternalism and beneficence. In essence, limiting Mr. G.'s autonomy is justified by the benevolent acts of doing good and not inflicting additional harm. In this case, the ratio of benefit/harm is such that greater harm could result with the additional distress of allowing Mr. G. to make this difficult decision when there is no more medical treatment available to benefit him.

Alternative 2: This claim is based on the principles of autonomy, respect for persons, and beneficence. The nurse feels that because Mr. G. is a competent adult, he has the individual right to make this personal decision. The principle of respect for persons goes beyond admitting that the person has the choice, but also

enables the person to make the choice free from external constraints. In addition, the nurse feels that the benefit/burden ratio is weighted in the opposite direction. It would be more beneficial to allow Mr. G. to participate in the decision-making process because he could solicit the support from his clergy and family. Finally, the nurse substantiates her claim with Statement 1 of the Code of Ethics, which states, "The nurse provides services with respect for human dignity and the uniqueness of the client, unrestricted by considerations of social or economic status, personal attributes, or the nature of the health problems." Because each patient is unique, health providers cannot assume that all patients will respond in the same manner of distress with the additional information. Thus, patients should be given the information and the choice to make their own decisions. The nursing interventions would be to evaluate the patient's *responses* to the information and provide supportive services.

(continued)

Chart 4–4 *(Continued)*

Evaluation

This case poses a difficult moral dilemma. Some may argue that there is only one valid claim (including the patient in the decision making) because the patient is a competent adult. However, the physician's claim not to inflict additional harm is valid and based on universal principles. If the physician had not included these principles but had relied on his previous comments that "it would be the best for this patient," then the claim would not be valid because it would be based on his personal values and beliefs.

However, when the two alternatives or moral claims are valid, one must appeal to the "higher order" principle. In this case, the principles of autonomy and respect for persons are more influential than paternalism. Although the principle of beneficence is con-

sidered a strong moral principle, in this case it would hold less weight than autonomy or respect for persons because Mr. G. continues to have the mental capacity to make decisions. Consequently, Alternative 2 would be the morally correct decision.

Because the morally correct course of action is not always apparent, this case underscores how moral decision making must occur among all the health care providers actively involved in the case. Moral decisions are typically difficult decisions for everyone involved, and it is essential that all members of the health care team listen and respect the views of others. Through an open, nonjudgmental dialogue, the course of action that reflects the "best interests" of the patient will usually emerge.

---

resulted in many continuing education programs. These programs range from small seminars or workshops to full-semester courses. Nurses can consult with local colleges or professional organizations to determine the availability of these offerings.

Finally, within the last ten years there has been a significant increase in literature focusing on clinical ethics. The nursing journals frequently have articles on ethical issues. There are also numerous textbooks devoted to clinical ethics in general, or more specifically to nursing ethics. These books are valuable resources for nurses because they cover the ethical theory and dilemmas of practice in greater depth. The American Nurses Association also has publications available to assist nurses in this emergent field of inquiry.

Chapter Summary

Studying the domain of ethics is both challenging and complex. Once the philosophic terminology and frameworks are understood, the process of ethical decision making becomes easier. As the field of clinical ethics progresses, there is more information available to assist practitioners. The use of this information will help nurses understand and clarify ethical situations that may occur in the future. It is imperative that nurses actively participate in ethical decision making to foster patient advocacy, an essential role for professional nursing. Chart 4-4 illustrates the guidelines used in ethical decision making.

Bibliography

Books
Philosophical and Clinical Ethics
American Hospital Association: Report of the Special Committee on Biomedical Ethics. Values in Conflict: Resolving Ethical Issues in Hospital Care. American Hospital Association, 1985.

Beauchamp T and Childress J. Principles of Biomedical Ethics, 3rd ed. New York, Oxford University Press, 1989.

Beauchamp T and Walters LR (eds). Contemporary Issues in Bioethics, 3rd ed. Belmont, CA, Wadsworth Publishing, 1989.

Callahan D. Setting Limits: Medical Goals in an Aging Society. New York, Simon and Schuster, 1987.

Cranford R and Doudera AE (eds). Institutional Ethics Committees and Health Care Decision Making. Ann Arbor, MI, Health Administration Press, 1984.

Doudera AE and Peters JD (eds). Legal and Ethical Aspects of Treating Critically Ill Patients. Ann Arbor, MI, Aupha Press, 1982.

Engelhardt HT. The Foundations of Bioethics. New York, Oxford University Press, 1986.

Fletcher J, Quist N, and Jonsen A. Ethics Consultation in Health Care. Ann Arbor, MI, Health Administration Press, 1989.

Frankena W. Ethics, 2nd ed. Englewood Cliffs, NJ, Prentice–Hall, 1973.

Friedman E (ed). Making Choices: Ethical Issues for Health Care Professionals. American Hospital Publishing, 1986.

Gert B. Morality: A New Justification of the Moral Rules. New York, Oxford University Press, 1988.

Kant I. Grounding for the metaphysics of morals. In Ellington JW (trans). Kant's Ethical Philosophy. Indianapolis, IN, Hackett Publishing, 1983. (Original work published 1785)

Lynn J (ed). By No Extraordinary Means: The Choice to Forego Life-Sustaining Food and Water. Bloomington, IN, Indiana University Press, 1986.

MacIntyre A. After Virtue. Notre Dame, IN, Notre Dame Press, 1984.

Macklin R. Mortal Choices: Ethical Dilemmas in Modern Medicine. Boston, Houghton Mifflin, 1987.

Mill JS. Utilitarianism. In Reiser S, Dyck A, and Curran W (eds). Ethics in Medicine: Historical Perspectives and Contemporary Concerns. Cambridge, MA, MIT Press, 1871/1977.

Office of Technology Assessment: U.S. Congress. Life-Sustaining Technologies and the Elderly. Washington, DC, U.S. Government Printing Office, 1987.

Pellegrino E and Thomasma D. For the Patient's Good: The Restoration of Beneficence in Health Care. New York, Oxford University Press, 1988.

President's Commission for the Study of Ethical Problems in Medicine and Biomedical and Behavioral Research. Deciding to Forego Life-Sustaining Treatment. Washington, DC, U.S. Government Printing Office, 1983.

President's Commission for the Study of Ethical Problems in Medicine and Biomedical and Behavioral Research. Making Health Care Decisions, Vol 1: Report. Washington, DC, U.S. Government Printing Office, 1983.

President's Commission for the Study of Ethical Problems in Medicine and

Biomedical and Behavioral Research. Securing Access to Health Care, Vol 1: Report. Washington, DC, U.S. Government Printing Office, 1983.

Reich W. Encyclopedia of Bioethics. New York, Free Press, 1978.

Ross WD. The Right and the Good. Oxford, Clarendon Press, 1930.

Stout J. Ethics After Babel: The Languages of Morals and Their Discontents. Boston, Beacon Press, 1988.

The Hastings Center. Guidelines on the Termination of Life-Sustaining Treatment and the Care of the Dying. New York, The Hastings Center, 1987.

Veatch R. A Theory of Medical Ethics. New York, Basic Books, 1981.

Weir R. Abating Treatment with Critically Ill Patients. New York, Oxford University Press, 1989.

Wong C and Swazey J (eds). Dilemmas of Dying: Policies and Procedures Not to Treat. Boston, GK Hall Medical Publishers, 1981.

Moral Reasoning

Belenky M, Clinchy B, Goldberger N, and Tarule J. Women's Ways of Knowing. New York, Basic Books, 1986.

Brabeck M (ed). Who Cares? Theory, Research, and Educational Implications of the Ethic of Care. New York, Praeger, 1989.

Gilligan C. In a Different Voice: Psychological Theory and Women's Development. Cambridge, MA, Harvard University Press, 1982.

Gilligan C, Ward J, and Taylor J (eds). Mapping the Moral Domain. Cambridge, MA, Harvard University Press, 1988.

Ketefian S. Moral Reasoning and Ethical Practice in Nursing: An Integrative Review. New York, National League for Nursing, 1988.

Kittay E and Meyers D (eds). Women and Moral Theory. Rowman & Littlefield Publishers, 1987.

Kohlberg L. Essays on Moral Development, Vol 1: The Philosophy of Moral Development. San Francisco, Harper & Row, 1981.

Kohlberg L. Essays on Moral Development, Vol 2: The Psychology of Moral Development. San Francisco, Harper & Row, 1984.

Noddings N. Caring: A Feminine Approach to Ethics & Moral Education. Berkeley, CA, University of California Press, 1984.

Rest J. Moral Development: Advances in Research and Theory. New York, Praeger, 1986.

Nursing Ethics

American Nurses Association. Nursing: A Social Policy Statement. Kansas City, MO, American Nurses Association, 1980.

American Nurses Association. Ethics in Nursing Practice and Education. Kansas City, MO, American Nurses Association, 1980

American Nurses Association. Ethics References for Nurses. Kansas City, MO, American Nurses Association, 1982.

American Nurses Association. Code for Nurses with Interpretive Statements. Kansas City, MO, American Nurses Association, 1985.

American Nurses Association. Ethical Dilemmas Confronting Nurses. Kansas City, MO, American Nurses Association, 1985.

American Nurses Association. Ethics in Nursing: Position Statements and Guidelines. Kansas City, MO, American Nurses Association, 1988.

Bandman E and Bandman B. Nursing Ethics in the Life Span. Norwalk, CT, Appleton–Century–Crofts, 1985.

Benjamin M and Curtis J. Ethics in Nursing. New York, Oxford University Press, 1981.

Benner P and Wrubel J. The Primacy of Caring: Stress and Coping in Health and Illness. Menlo Park, CA, Addison-Wesley Publishing, 1989.

Curtin L and Flaherty J. Nursing Ethics: Theories and Pragmatics. Bowie, MD, Robert J Brady, 1982.

Davis A and Aroskar M. Ethical Dilemmas and Nursing Practice. New York, Appleton–Century–Crofts, 1978.

Fowler M and Levine-Ariff J. Ethics at the Bedside. Philadelphia, JB Lippincott, 1987.

Jameton A. Nursing Practice: The Ethical Issues. Englewood Cliffs, NJ, Prentice-Hall, 1984.

Ketefian S. Moral Reasoning and Ethical Practice in Nursing: An Integrative Review. New York, National League for Nursing, 1988.

* Leininger M. The phenomenon of caring: Importance, research questions and theoretical considerations. In Leininger M (ed). Caring: An Essential Human Need. Detroit, Wayne State University Press, 1988.

Murphy C. The moral situation in nursing. In Bandman E and Bandman B (eds). Bioethics and Human Rights. Boston, Little, Brown, and Co, 1978.

Murphy C and Hunter H. Ethical Problems in the Nurse–Patient Relationship. Boston, Allyn and Bacon, 1983.

Paterson J and Zderad L. Humanistic Nursing. New York, National League for Nursing, 1988.

Pence T. Ethics in Nursing: An Annotated Bibliography. New York, National League for Nursing, 1983.

Thompson J and Thompson H. Bioethical Decision Making for Nurses. Norwalk, CT, Appleton–Century–Crofts, 1985.

Veatch R and Fry S. Case Studies in Nursing Ethics. Philadelphia, JB Lippincott, 1987.

Watson J. Nursing: Human Science and Human Care. New York, National League for Nursing, 1988.

Journals

Asterisks indicate nursing research articles.

Annas G. Do feeding tubes have more rights than patients? The Hastings Center Report 1986 Feb; 16(1):26–28.

Aroskar M. Anatomy of an ethical dilemma: The theory. Am J Nurs 1980 Apr; 80(4):658–660.

Bedell S and Delbanco J. Survival after cardiopulmonary resuscitation in the hospital. N Engl J Med 1983 Sep; 309(10):569–575.

Bedell S and Delbanco J. Choices about cardiopulmonary resuscitation in the hospital. N Engl J Med 1984 Apr; 310(17):1089–1093.

Brennan T. Do-not-resuscitate orders for the incompetent patient in the absence of family consent. Law, Medicine & Health Care 1986; 14(1):13–19.

Cassel C. Care of the dying: The limits of law, the limits of ethics. Law, Medicine & Health Care 1989 Fall; 17(3):232–233.

* Cassells J and Redman B. Preparing students to be moral agents in clinical nursing practice: Report of a National Study. Nurs Clin North Am 1989 Jun; 24(2):463–473.

* Crisham P. Measuring moral judgment in nursing dilemmas. Nurs Res 1981 Mar/Apr; 30(2):104–110.

Crowley M. Feminist pedagogy: Nurturing the ethical ideal. Adv Nurs Sci 1989 Apr; 11(3):53–61.

Cunningham N and Hutchinson S. Myths in health care ethics. Image: Journal of Nursing Scholarship 1990 winter; 22(4):235–238.

Davis A. Ethics rounds with intensive care nurses. Nurs Clin North Am 1979 Mar; 14(1):45–55.

Davis A. Helping your staff address ethical dilemmas. J Nurs Adm 1982 Feb; 12(2):9–13.

* Davis A. Clinical nurses' ethical decision making in situations of informed consent. Adv Nurs Sci 1989 Apr; 11(3):63–69.

Davis A. New developments in international nursing ethics. Nurs Clin North Am 1989 Jun; 24(2):571–577.

Donovan C. Toward a nursing ethics program in an acute care setting. Top Clin Nurs 1983 Oct; 5(3):55–62.

Ellison P and Walwork E. Withdrawing mechanical support from the brain-damaged neonate. Dimens Crit Care Nurs 1986 Sep/Oct; 5(5):284–293.

Engelhardt HT and Rie MA. Intensive care units, scarce resources, and conflicting principles of justice. JAMA 1986 Mar 7; 255(9):1159–1164.

Evans R. Health care technology and the inevitability of resource allocation and rationing decisions: Part 1. JAMA 1983 Apr 15; 249(15):2047–2052.

Evans R. Health care technology and the inevitability of resource allocation and rationing decisions: Part 2. JAMA 1983 Apr 22; 249(16):2208–2219.

Gadow S. Clinical subjectivity: Advocacy with silent patients. Nurs Clin North Am 1989 Jun; 24(2):535–541.

* Gaul A. Ethics content in baccalaureate degree curricula: Clarifying the issues. Nurs Clin North Am 1989 Jun; 24(2):475–483.

Grady C. Ethical issues in providing nursing care to human immunodeficiency virus–infected populations. Nurs Clin North Am 1989 Jun; 24(2):523–534.

* Jameton A and Fowler M. Ethical inquiry and the concept of research. Adv Nurs Sci 1989 Apr; 11(3):11–24.

* Ketefian S. Critical thinking, educational preparation, and development of moral judgment among selected groups of practicing nurses. Nurs Res 1981 Mar/Apr; 30(2):98–103.

* Ketefian S. Moral reasoning and moral behavior among selected groups of practicing nurses. Nurs Res 1981 May/Jun; 30(3):171–176.

Ketefian S. Moral reasoning and ethical practice in nursing: Measurement issues. Nurs Clin North Am 1989 Jun; 24(2):509–521.

Knox L. Ethical issues in nutritional support nursing: Withholding and withdrawing nutritional support. Nurs Clin North Am 1989 Jun; 24(2):427–436.

Levine M. Nursing ethics and the ethical nurse. Am J Nurs 1977 May; 77(5):845–847.

Lumpp Sister F. The role of the nurse in the bioethical decision-making process. Nurs Clin North Am 1979 Mar; 14(1):13–21.

Micetich K, Steinecker P, Thomasma D. Are intravenous fluids morally required for a dying patient? Arch Intern Med 1983 May; 143:975–978.

Miller T. Do-not-resuscitate orders: Public policy and patient autonomy. Law, Medicine & Health Care 1989 Fall; 17(3):245–255.

Mitchell C. Code gray: Ethical dilemmas in nursing. Nurs Life 1986 Jan/Feb; 6(1):18–23.

Mitchell C. Ethical dilemmas in nursing: Part 2. Nurs Life 1986 Mar/Apr; 6(2):26–30.

Murphy P. The role of the nurse on hospital ethics committees. Nurs Clin North Am 1989 Jun; 24(2):551–556.

Omery A. Values, moral reasoning and ethics. Nurs Clin North Am 1989 Jun; 24(2):499–508.

Paris J and Reardon F. Court responses to withholding or withdrawing artificial nutrition and fluids. JAMA 1985 Apr 19; 253(15):2243–2245.

Parker RS. Measuring nurses' moral judgments. Image: Journal of Nursing Scholarships 1990 winter; 22(4):213–218.

Rabkin M, Gillerman G, and Rice N. Orders not to resuscitate. N Engl J Med 1976 Aug; 295(7):364–366.

Reed P. Nursing theorizing as an ethical endeavor. Adv Nurs Sci 1989 Apr; 11(3):1–9.

Salladay S and McDonnell Sr. M. Spiritual care, ethical choices, and patient advocacy. Nurs Clin North Am 1989 Jun; 24(2):543–549.

Smith S and Davis A. Ethical dilemmas: Conflicts among rights, duties and obligations. Am J Nurs 1980 Aug; 80(8):1463–1466.

Suber D and Tabor W. Withholding of life-sustaining treatment from the terminally ill, incompetent patient: Who decides? Part 2. JAMA 1982 Nov 19; 248(19):2431–2432.

Swartz M. The patient who refuses medical treatment: A dilemma for hospitals and physicians. Am J Law Med 1985; 11(2):147–194.

Symposium of Bioethical Issues in Nursing. Nurs Clin North Am 1979 Mar; 14:1–91.

Theis EC. Ethical issues: A nursing perspective. N Engl J Med 1986 Nov 6; 315(19):1222–1224.

Twomey J. Analysis of the claim to distinct nursing ethics: Normative and nonnormative approaches. Adv Nurs Sci 1989 Apr; 11(3):25–32.

Wise CT. Understanding advance directives. Virginia Nurse 1991 Spring; 59(1):8–11.

Wurzbach ME. The dilemma of withholding or withdrawing nutrition. Image: Journal of Nursing Scholarship 1990 winter; 22(4):226–230.

Yarling R. Ethical analysis of a nursing problem: Part 1. Supervisor Nurse 1978 May; 9:40–50.

Yarling R. Ethical analysis of a nursing problem: Part 2. Supervisor Nurse 1978 Jun; 9:28–34.

Yarling R and McElmurry B. Rethinking the nurse's role in "do not resuscitate" orders: A clinical policy proposal in nursing ethics. Adv Nurs Sci 1983 Jul; 5(4):1–12.

Yeo M. Integration of nursing theory and nursing ethics. Adv Nurs Sci 1989 Apr; 11(3):33–42.

5

Health Promotion

Learning Objectives

On completion of this chapter, the learner will be able to:

1. Define the concepts of health, wellness, and health promotion
2. Describe the health promotion principles of self-responsibility, nutrition, stress management, and exercise
3. Specify the variables that affect health promotion activities for children, young and middle-aged adults, and elderly adults
4. Describe the role of the nurse in health promotion

In recent years, there has been a virtual explosion of health promotion activities. Health care professionals who have traditionally focused on the curing of disease are turning their attention to prevention. Their focus is on improvement of health by altering life-style and by modifying factors that predispose to undesirable alterations in health.

The concept of health promotion has evolved from a changing definition of health and from an awareness that wellness exists on a continuum that extends from premature death at one extreme to optimal health at the other extreme. The definition of health as the mere absence of disease or as the quality of a person's physiologic functioning is no longer accepted. Today, *health* is regarded as a composite of physical, psychologic, emotional, social, and spiritual functioning that allows the person to carry out his roles and responsibilities and to move toward self-fulfillment in a variety of situations. Health is viewed as a dynamic, ever-changing condition, the status of which is measured in terms of how well the person uses his skills and abilities to strive toward functioning at his optimum potential at any given point in time. The ideal health status is one in which the person is successful in achieving his full potential regardless of any disabilities he may have.

The concept of wellness expands on the idea of health. *Wellness* is a process with many possible levels or degrees. It involves a conscious and deliberate approach toward maximizing one's health. Wellness does not just happen—it requires planning and conscious commitment. It is the result of life-style behaviors that are designed for the purpose of attaining one's highest potential for well-being. Wellness is not the same for every person. The person with a chronic illness or disability can have the same or a greater level of wellness as a person without such an illness or disability. The key to wellness is whether or not the person is functioning at his highest potential within the limitations over which he has no control.

A significant amount of research has shown that people, by virtue of what they do or what they fail to do, influence their own health. Today, many of the major causes of illnesses are chronic diseases that have been closely related to life-style behaviors (*e.g.*, heart disease, lung and colon cancer, chronic obstructive pulmonary diseases, hypertension, cirrhosis, peptic ulcers, and human immunodeficiency virus [HIV] infection). Thus, a person's health status to a large extent reflects his style of living.

In 1979, the nation's first public health agenda was described. Goals for improving the health of all Americans were delineated. This agenda was quickly followed in 1980 by a list of objectives referred to as "the 1990 health objectives." These identified improvements that need to be made in health status, reduction of risks, public awareness, health services, and protective measures. Progress has been made in accomplishing these objectives, but improvement is still needed. Thus, the "Year 2000 Objectives for the Nation" were formulated. The priorities identified include health promotion, health protection, and preventive services. Increased emphasis was placed on prevention of disability and morbidity, greater attention to improvements in the health status of specific groups that are at highest risk for premature death, and increased provision for early detection of asymptomatic disease conditions in an attempt to prevent disability and early death. These objectives are directed toward meeting the World Health Organization's goal of "health for all by the year 2000."

Definition of Health Promotion

Health promotion can be defined as activities that, by accentuating the positive, assist the person to develop those resources that will maintain or enhance his well-being and improve the quality of his life. It refers to the activities that a person does for himself in the absence of symptoms in an attempt to remain healthy; these activities do not need the assistance of a member of the health care team. The purpose of health promotion is to focus on the person's potential for wellness and to encourage him to alter his personal habits, life-style, and environment in ways that will enable him to enhance his health and well-being. Health promotion is an active process, that is, it is not something that can be prescribed or dictated. It is up to the individual to decide for himself whether he will make the changes that will help him to enhance his own health status and attain a higher level of wellness. Choices must be made, and only the person himself can make these choices.

A variety of health appraisal tools have been developed to facilitate the health promotion process. These tools generally are used to collect information about the person's health habits and life-style and related information such as age, sex, race, past health history, and family health history. The information is then used to determine the strengths and limitations of the individual's life-style and health habits, providing a basis for counseling him in making choices about his health behaviors.

The concepts of health, wellness, and health promotion have been extensively addressed in the lay literature and news media as well as in professional journals. The result has been a public outcry for health information and a tremendous response by health care professionals and agencies to provide this information. Health promotion programs that were once limited to hospital settings have now moved into the community in settings such as schools, churches, businesses, and industry. The workplace is quickly becoming an important site for health promotion programs. The goal of the employers who offer such activities is to reduce costs associated with absenteeism, hospitalization, disability, excessive turnover of personnel, and early death.

Health Promotion Principles

Health promotion as a concept and as an active process is built on the principles of self-responsibility, nutritional awareness, stress reduction and management, and physical fitness.

Self-Responsibility

Self-responsibility is the key to successful health promotion. It involves the recognition that the individual, and only the individual, has control over his life. He and only he can make those choices that determine whether his life-style is one that promotes health. As more people are recognizing the significant effect that life-style behaviors have on health, they are assuming responsibility for avoiding high-risk behaviors such as smoking, abusing alcohol and drugs, overeating, driving while intoxicated, risky sexual practices, and other unhealthy practices. They are also assuming responsibility for developing practices that have been found to be positive influences in promoting health, such as engaging in regular exercise, wearing a seat belt, and following a balanced diet.

A variety of different techniques have been used to try to encourage people to accept responsibility for promoting their health. These have ranged from extensive educational programs to reward systems and contracts. Studies have not shown any one technique to be superior to any other. Instead, it seems that self-responsibility for health promotion is very individualized and depends on the person's desires and inner motivations. Health promotion programs are important tools for offering encouragement to the individual to assume responsibility for his health and to develop behaviors that positively affect health.

Nutrition

Nutrition as a component of health promotion has received more attention and publicity than any other component. There is a vast array of books and magazine articles that address the topics of special diets, natural foods, and the hazards of certain substances such as sugar, salt, cholesterol, and food additives. Good nutrition has been suggested as the single most significant factor in determining health status and longevity.

Nutritional awareness involves an understanding of the importance of a properly balanced diet that supplies all of the essential nutrients and an understanding of the relationship between diet and disease. A diet that promotes health is thought to be one that substitutes natural foods for processed and refined ones and that reduces the intake of sugar, salt, fat, caffeine, alcohol, and food additives and preservatives.

Chapter 7 of this text, Physical Assessment and Nutritional Assessment, contains detailed information on the assessment of the individual's nutritional status. Physical signs indicating nutritional status, anthropometric measurements, assessment of food intake (food record, 24-hour recall), the basic four food groups, recommended daily dietary allowances, and ideal-weight tables are covered in the text and in tables.

Stress Management

Stress management and stress reduction have become important aspects of health promotion as studies have shown the deleterious effects of stress on health and a cause-and-effect relationship between stress and infectious diseases, traffic accidents, and some chronic illnesses. Stress is a part of the American way of life. It has become inevitable in our "high-tech," urban society in which self-imposed demands for productivity have become excessive. Thus, more and more emphasis is placed on encouraging people to manage their stress appropriately and to reduce stress that is counterproductive. Techniques such as relaxation training, exercise, and modification of stress-producing situations are often included in health promotion programs that deal with stress. The reader is referred to Chapter 9, Stress and Adaptation, for further information on stress management, including health risk appraisal and stress reduction methods such as biofeedback and the relaxation response.

Exercise

Physical fitness is another important component of health promotion. The relationship between health and physical fitness has been studied closely. It has been found that a regular exercise program can promote health by improving functioning of the circulatory system and the lungs, decreasing cholesterol and low-density lipoproteins, lowering body weight by increasing calorie expenditure, delaying degenerative changes such as osteoporosis, and improving flexibility and overall muscle strength and endurance. Despite these benefits, exercise can be harmful if it is not started gradually and increased slowly in accordance with the individual's response. An exercise program should be designed specifically for the individual, with consideration given to age, physical condition, and any known cardiovascular risk factors. An appropriate exercise program can have a significant positive effect on the individual's performance capacity, appearance, and general state of health.

Health Promotion Throughout the Life Span

Health promotion as a concept and a process is not limited to any particular age-group. Instead, it extends throughout the life span. Studies have shown that the health of a child can be affected, either positively or negatively, by the health practices of the mother during the prenatal period. Thus, health promotion starts before birth and extends through childhood, adulthood, and old age.

Children

For many years, health screening has been an important aspect of childhood health care. The goal has been to detect health problems at an early age so that they can be remedied and the child's health status can be improved. Today, health promotion goes beyond the mere screening of children for disabilities. Extensive efforts are made to promote positive health practices at a very young age. Because health habits and practices are in the formative stages during the years of childhood, children are more susceptible to influences that promote positive health attitudes at this time than they are in the adult years. For this reason, more and more programs are being offered to school-age children to help them develop good health habits. The emphasis is not so much on the negative results of such practices as smoking, risky sexual activities, alcohol and drug abuse, and poor nutrition as on values training, building of self-esteem, and healthy life-style practices. The programs are designed to appeal to the particular age-group, with emphasis on learning experiences that are fun and interesting.

Young and Middle-Aged Adults

The emphasis placed on health promotion for young and middle-aged adults is greater than that for any other age-group. These groups, as a whole, are interested in health and health promotion. They have responded positively and enthusiastically to studies that show how life-style practices affect health. Those who are highly motivated are self-sufficient in changing their life-styles in ways that are believed to enhance health and wellness. More often than not, however, adults who wish to improve their health turn to health promotion programs to assist them in making the desired changes in their life-styles. They respond in overwhelming numbers to programs that focus on such topics as general wellness, smoking cessation, exercise, physical conditioning, weight control, and stress management. Because of the nationwide emphasis on health during the reproductive years, young adults actively seek out programs that address prenatal health, parenting, family planning, and women's health issues. Programs that provide health screening, such as those that screen for cancer, hypertension, diabetes, and hearing impairments, are quite popular with adults. Programs that deal with health promotion for people with specific chronic illnesses such as cancer, diabetes, heart disease, and pulmonary disease are also popular. It is becoming more and more evident that chronic disease does not preclude health and wellness; rather, positive health attitudes and practices can promote optimal health for persons who must live with the limitations imposed by the chronic nature of their illnesses.

Because a person's motivation does not always suffice to encourage him to strive toward optimal health, health promotion programs are being offered in a variety of settings. For many adults, it is too much to expect that they will spend excessive time after a day at work traveling to an inconvenient place to exercise, learn about health risks, or perhaps join a smoking cessation group. Thus, health promotion programs have subscribed to the outreach approach. Although many programs are still available in centrally located health care agencies, more and more are becoming available in neighborhood settings. Common sites are elementary schools, high schools, community colleges, recreation centers, and churches. Health fairs are common in civic centers and shopping malls. The outreach idea for health promotion programs has served to meet the needs of many adults who otherwise would not avail themselves of opportunities to strive toward a healthier life-style.

Health promotion has also entered the realm of business and industry. Employers are becoming increasingly concerned about the rising costs of health care to treat illnesses that are related to life-style behaviors. They are also concerned about increased absenteeism and lost productivity. For these reasons, many businesses are instituting health promotion programs in the workplace. Some employ health promotion specialists to develop and implement the program for them, while others purchase packaged programs that have already been developed by health care agencies or private health promotion corporations. The programs that are offered at the workplace usually include employee health screening and counseling, physical fitness, nutritional awareness, work safety, and stress management and reduction. Efforts are made to promote a safe and healthy work environment. Many large businesses provide exercise facilities for their employees and offer their health promotion programs to retirees. If employers can show cost-containment benefits from such programs, their dollars will be considered well spent, and more businesses will provide health promotion programs as a benefit of employment.

Elderly Adults

Health promotion is as important for the elderly as it is for other age-groups. Despite the fact that 80% of people over the age of 65 have one or more chronic illnesses and about 50% of the aged population have activity limitations, the elderly as a group have been found to experience significant gains from health promotion. Studies have shown that the elderly are very health-conscious and that most view their health positively and are willing to adopt practices that will improve their health and well-being. Although their chronic illnesses and disabilities cannot be eliminated, these adults can benefit from activities that help them to achieve an optimal level of health.

Activities directed toward health promotion for the elderly are the same as those for other age-groups: physical fitness and exercise, nutrition, safety, and stress management and reduction. Physical fitness and exercise have not enjoyed as much popularity among the elderly as they have among younger people, but they are slowly catching on. Studies have shown that more than half of all people over the age of 65 do not exercise on a regular basis. However, this figure is slowly decreasing because the elderly are becoming more aware of the benefits of exercise for them, such as improved cardiovascular function, increased ventilatory capacity, reduced body fat, and enhanced muscle strength, endurance, and flexibility. Exercise programs

for the elderly, as for other people, are based on each person's physical abilities. They are begun slowly and, when appropriate, with medical advice. Programs that meet the needs of older people confined to wheelchairs or beds are not uncommon.

The importance of adequate nutrition for the elderly is paramount. Nutritional deficiencies are common among the elderly and have been found to be a factor in causing depression, confusion, headache, fatigue, and irritability. There is a significant need for nutritional counseling that does not simply stress those foods that are to be avoided but that presents information about what constitutes a healthy diet. Consideration must be given to physiologic factors such as impaired senses of taste or smell and dental health. Nutritional deficiencies can sometimes be easily remedied with properly fitting dentures. Psychosocial variables such as income, cultural influences, and food habits must also be considered.

The safety aspect of health promotion is as important, if not more important, for the elderly as for younger people. The elderly are particularly prone to injuries resulting from falls and automobile accidents. In many cases, falls could be prevented if the person's home environment were altered to include appropriate safety features. Many older people can benefit from knowing that their visual acuity is impaired at night because of the decreased ability of the eye to adapt to the darkness. In such cases, the use of nightlights and the restriction of automobile driving to the daytime hours can help to prevent accidents. Encouragement of the elderly to use seat belts in automobiles is also important, because only 10% of elderly people report that they use seat belts on a regular basis. Proper use of medications is another aspect of safety that is important for the elderly, who are heavy consumers of medications. They often do not take drugs as prescribed and mix prescription with nonprescription drugs. Community programs directed toward health promotion for the elderly are beginning to focus on the various aspects of safety that are particularly important to this age-group.

Finally, stress management and reduction are not reserved for younger age-groups but must be considered equally important for the elderly. The stresses confronted by the elderly are varied and can include difficulty coping with retirement, financial insecurity, health problems, unwanted change of residence, loss of a spouse, and feelings of helplessness and despair. Some strides have been made in helping people plan for their later years in an attempt to decrease these stresses. It seems that health promotion that starts during the young and middle years and that focuses on making plans for the later years is more successful than are efforts directed toward stress reduction after the elderly person is already faced with stress-provoking situations that seem insurmountable. Many businesses offer preretirement programs designed to help their employees prepare for the life-style changes that accompany retirement. As the population of older Americans continues to increase, more and more of these programs are needed. Health care and community groups are also recognizing this need and are beginning to offer such programs. The focus of these programs is the idea that aging is not synonymous with illness and uselessness and that focusing on wellness while growing old can promote control over one's health and state of well-being.

Many health promotion programs have been developed to meet the needs of older Americans. Many of these began within the Department of Health and Human Services. Both public and private organizations have been responsive to this initiative, and more programs that serve the elderly are emerging. Many of these are offered by health care agencies, churches, recreational centers, senior citizen residences, and a variety of other organizations.

Health Promotion Programs

Considering the fact that health promotion encompasses the entire life span and is applicable to both sexes, to people of all socioeconomic and cultural backgrounds, and to people who have no health problems as well as those with chronic illnesses and disabilities, the numbers and types of health promotion programs that have been developed are extensive. These can be categorized as health screening, wellness, safety, disease management, and various others. Examples of each of

these categories of programs are presented in Chart 5-1. The formats for these programs vary from lectures to workshops, support groups, health fairs, and computer-assisted programs. The settings vary depending on the needs of the target group. Some are presented in schools, churches, businesses, day-care centers, recreational centers, and shopping malls. As the health promotion movement continues to grow, more and more programs and activities will move out of the health care agencies into the community where larger numbers of people can be reached and served.

Implications for Nursing

By virtue of their expertise in health and health care and with their long-established credibility with consumers, nurses are playing a vital role in health promotion. In many instances they have stimulated the development of health promotion pro-

Chart 5-1
Health Promotion Programs

Health Screening

Cancer
Diabetes
Growth and development
Heart disease
Hypertension
Self-examination (of breasts, testes)
Speech and hearing

Wellness

Aerobic exercise
Aging
Alcohol abuse prevention
Cancer prevention
Childbirth preparation
Drug abuse prevention
Exercise
General wellness
Heart disease prevention
Mental health
Nutrition
Physical fitness and conditioning
Planning for retirement
Prenatal classes
Smoking cessation
Stress reduction and management
Stroke prevention
Weight control and management
Women's health issues

Safety

Accident prevention
Child safety
First aid
Infant safety
Medication use
Poison prevention
Safe sexual practices
Sports injury prevention

Disease Management

Alcohol abuse
Arthritis
Cancer
Diabetes
Drug abuse
Heart disease
Hypertension
Pain
Pulmonary disease

Miscellaneous

Babysitter classes
Cardiopulmonary resuscitation
Caregiver classes
Family planning
Grandparenting
Parenting
Sex education
Sibling classes

grams. In other cases they have been sought out by consumers to lead interdisciplinary teams in developing and providing wellness services in a variety of settings.

As health care professionals, nurses have a responsibility to promote activities that foster well-being, self-actualization, and personal fulfillment. Accomplishment of this is possible through a focus on those activities that promote health. Every interaction with consumers of health care must be viewed as an opportunity to promote positive health attitudes and behaviors.

Future Trends

With the current progress that is being made in health promotion, future trends can be anticipated. It is expected that the government and employers will become more aggressive in their efforts to decrease health care costs. More emphasis will be placed on health promotion in the workplace. Insurance policies will offer incentives for wellness. The government will further increase the regulations on the health care industry, requiring health promotion and wellness programs as a way of controlling costs.

Two specific groups who will have a significant impact on health promotion are children and the elderly. It is expected that a large proportion of heath promotion programs will be aimed at school-age children, particularly those between the ages of 8 and 12. The purpose of this is to promote good health practices at an early age. In the long run, it is believed that this will pay off by increasing the health of future generations and thus controlling the monies that are spent on medical care.

It is anticipated that the growing population of older people will provide a major market for health promotion programs. The number of Americans over the age of 65 is expected to increase to about 20% of the population by the middle of the 21st century. This generation of senior citizens is expected to be more self-sufficient, more responsible for their own health, and more demanding of means to promote their health and wellness. They are a prime target group for health promotion programs and activities.

Health promotion is certainly not the only answer to the health problems that exist in this country, but it is one answer. Without it, the health problems of this nation will not be solved. It is one opportunity to be used to strive toward meeting the health needs of individuals and of our society in general.

Chapter Summary

Health promotion is an active process, the purpose of which is to focus on the person's potential for wellness and to encourage him to alter his personal habits, life-style, and environment in ways that will enable him to enhance his health and well-being. It involves the principles of self-responsibility,

nutritional awareness, stress reduction and management, and physical fitness. It is not limited to any particular age-group but extends throughout the life span for people of both sexes and all socioeconomic and cultural backgrounds, and for those who have no health problems as well as those with chronic illnesses and disabilities. Two specific groups that are quickly becoming major markets for health promotion programs and activities are children and the elderly.

Nurses are assuming vital roles in health promotion. They are involved in developing programs and in leading interdisciplinary teams in providing wellness services. In addition, the promotion of positive health attitudes and behaviors has become an integral component of nursing care in all practice settings.

Bibliography
Books
Creek SF and Mettler M. A Healthy Old Age: A Source Book for Health Promotion with Older Adults. New York, Haworth Press, 1984.

Edelman C and Mandle CL. Health Promotion Throughout the Lifespan. St Louis, CV Mosby, 1990.

Ewies L and Simnett I. Promoting Health: A Practical Guide to Health Education. New York, John Wiley & Sons, 1985.

Greene WH and Simons-Morton BG. Introduction to Health Education. New York, Macmillan, 1984.

Kar SB. Health Promotion Indicators and Actions. New York, Springer Publishing Co, 1989.

Murray RB and Zentner JP. Nursing Assessment and Health Promotion Through the Life Span. Englewood Cliffs, NJ, Prentice–Hall, 1989.

O'Donnell MP and Ainsworth TH. Health Promotion in the Workplace. New York, John Wiley & sons, 1984.

Journals
Asterisks indicate nursing research articles.

Anderson RC and Fox R. Ethical issues in health promotion and health education. AAOHN J 1987 May; 35(5):220–223.

Armstrong DM. Nursing leads wellness promotion: Overview. Nurs Admin Q 1987 Spring; 11(3):13–14.

* Brown MA and Waybrant KM. Health promotion, education, counseling, and coordination in primary health care nursing. Public Health Nurs 1988 Mar; 5(1):16–23.

Califano JA. America's health care revolution: Health promotion and disease prevention. J Am Diet Assoc 1987 Apr; 87(4):437–440.

Criteria for the development of health promotion and education programs. Am J Public Health 1987 Jan; 77(1):89–92.

Duffy ME. Health promotion in the family: Current findings and directives for nursing research. J Adv Nurs 1988 Jan; 13(1):109–117.

Duffy ME and Pender NJ (eds). Conceptual Issues in Health Promotion. Proceedings of a Wingspread Conference. Racine, WI, Sigma Theta Tau International, Honor Society of Nursing.

Fielding JE and Piserchia PV. Frequency of worksite health promotion activities. Am J Public Health 1989 Jan; 79(1):16–20.

Fries JF, Green LW, and Levine S. Health promotion and the compression of morbidity. Lancet 1989 Mar 4; 1(8636):481–483.

Hoffman S. Wellness promotion in women's health care. Nurs Admin Q 1987 Spring; 11(3):38–40.

Larson EB. Health promotion and disease prevention in the older adult. Geriatrics 1988 Dec; 43:31–39.

Lindberg SC. Adult preventive health screening: 1987 update. Nurse Pract 1987 May; 12(5):19–32.

Maglacas AM. Health for all: Nursing's role. Nurs Outlook 1988 Mar/Apr; 36(2):66–71.

Matheis-Kraft C and York L. The hospital as wellness educator. Nurs Manage 1989 Jan; 20(1):72.

Pender NJ et al. Development and testing of the health promotion model. Cardiovasc Nurs 1988 Nov/Dec; 24(6):41–43.

Platakis J. Promoting health and wellness in the elderly. Nurs Admin Q 1987 Spring; 11(3):42–43.

Progress toward achieving the 1990 national objectives for physical fitness and exercise. JAMA 1989 Aug 11; 262(6):746, 748, 753.

Pruitt RH. Economics of health promotion. Nurs Econ 1987 May/Jun; 5(3): 118, 119–123.

Rielly PA, Gunn JL, and Sadowski AJ. Health and life styles: Employee wellness. Nurs Admin Q 1987 Spring; 11(3):29–35.

Surgeon General's workshop on health promotion and aging: Summary recommendations of the medication working group. JAMA 1989 Oct 6; 262(13):1755.

Tzirides E. Health outreach program: Marketing the "Health Way." Nurs Manage 1988 Apr; 19(4):55–57.

* Walker SN et al. Health-promoting life styles of older adults: Comparisons with young and middle-aged adults, correlates and patterns. Adv Nurs Sci 1988 Oct; 11(1):76–90.

Wilson RW, Patterson MA, and Alford DM. Services for maintaining independence. J Gerontol Nurs 1989 Jun; 15(6):31–37.

Year 2000 national health objectives. JAMA 1989 Oct 13; 262(14):1919, 1923.

Nursing Research Profile for Unit 1

Health Maintenance and Health Needs

In recent years, nursing leaders have stressed the need for research that demonstrates and helps to articulate the body of scientific knowledge that is unique to the profession. Consequently, nurse researchers are becoming more and more involved in studies that seek to determine the effects of nursing interventions on patient outcomes. The goal of such research is to describe, explain, and predict nursing practice and to validate the science of nursing.

The following studies are presented as examples of recent research that focuses on nursing models, nursing diagnosis, and the effectiveness of nursing interventions. Although subject populations are in some cases small and restricted in scope, and generalization of the findings is not always possible, the nursing implications warrant consideration and further study.

▷ Hoch CC. *Assessing delivery of nursing care.* J Gerontol Nurs 1987 Jan; 13(1):10–17.

The purpose of this study was to compare the utilization of the Roy Adaptation Model and the Neuman Health-Care Systems Model with regard to effectiveness in decreasing depression and increasing life satisfaction for retired individuals. Forty-eight residents of a large suburban senior citizen center volunteered to participate in the study. Random assignment to one of three groups—Roy group, Neuman group, and control group—resulted in each group having 16 members with similar mean age and length of retirement.

Protocols for group work directed toward decreasing depression and increasing life satisfaction were developed for each of the treatment groups; one was based on the Roy Adaptation Model, one was based on the Neuman Health-Care Systems Model, and one was not supported by a theoretic framework. Each protocol focused on assessment, stressor identification, goal establishment, and goal attainment consistent with the model. Six weekly group meetings were conducted by the same clinical nurse specialist for each group. The Depression Adjective Check List Form and the Life Satisfaction Index were used for pretesting and post-testing.

The post-test findings revealed a decrease in depression scores for both the Roy and Neuman groups and an increase for the control group; there was no significant difference in the scores of the Roy group and the Neuman group. Likewise, both the Roy and Neuman groups had significantly higher post-intervention life satisfaction scores than the control group, with no significant difference between the Roy and Neuman groups. Limitations of the study included the restricted sample population from one suburban senior citizen center and the fact that only one clinical specialist was used to apply the treatment interventions.

Nursing Implications. (1) Both the Roy and the Neuman models are useful as frameworks for planning and implementing nursing care. (2) Planned, purposeful nursing intervention based on a theoretic framework may be more effective than interventions without an organizing framework.

▷ Dittmann EE and Gould MT. *Refinement of nursing diagnosis skills: The effect of clinical nurse specialist teaching and consultation.* J Contin Educ Nurs 1987 Sep/Oct; 18(5): 157–159.

The researchers focused on the effectiveness of the role of the clinical nurse specialist and two strategies for assisting staff nurses to improve and refine their skills in using nursing diagnoses. Twelve registered nurses who were using nursing diagnosis in their practice on two medical units participated in the study; they were assigned to two groups based on the medical unit on which they worked. Thirty SOAP notes written by the nurse participants were used for the purposes of the study. The Nursing Diagnosis Audit Tool was developed to assess 12 criteria for the documentation of nursing diagnoses in the SOAP notes; this tool was used as a pretest and as a post-test.

Two clinical nurse specialists presented to both groups of study participants five 30-minute classes about the use of nursing diagnoses; these were followed by practice sessions. Results revealed that one group of nurses scored lower on the pretest than the other group and improved significantly on the post-test following the classes; the other group did not demonstrate a significant pretest/post-test change. Members of this second group then received individual consultation from the clinical nurse specialists; their second post-test scores revealed significant improvement.

Nursing Implications. (1) Thorough assessment of nurses' skills should be conducted prior to planning classes for skill improvement. (2) Because the skills of individual nurses may vary from one hospital unit to another, educational programs should be developed to meet the specific unit's needs. (3) Clinical nurse specialists can be used as effective change agents.

▷ Johnson CF and Hales LW. *Nursing diagnosis anyone? Do staff nurses use nursing diagnosis effectively?* J Contin Educ Nurs 1989 Jan/Feb; 20(1):30–35.

Although nursing diagnosis has gained wide acceptance as an essential component of the nursing process, the researchers sought to determine if there is a difference between this acceptance and the actual use of nursing diagnoses. Patterns of usage of nursing diagnoses were studied for 82 newly hired nurses in three clinical areas (medical–surgical, maternal child, and critical care) of a metropolitan hospital.

Each of the participants attended a 4-hour education program that focused on the nursing process and the importance of nursing diagnosis. An instrument that measured both theoretic and operational nursing application was used as a pretest and post-test. Post-test results indicated a significant increase in knowledge and a willingness to utilize and promote the nursing process in clinical practice.

Four to six weeks following the education program, an audit of three charts per nurse was conducted; the charts were audited for completeness of documentation of the nursing process on the nursing assessment form, the patient problem list, the patient progress notes, and the flow sheet. Although there was overall improvement in utilization and documentation of the nursing process, there was underutilization of each of the documentation forms. In comparing nurses from the three clinical areas, nursing diagnosis was used to a greater extent by maternal child nurses, followed by critical care nurses; medical-surgical nurses scored lowest.

Nursing Implications. (1) Staff education programs are effective strategies for promoting knowledge, attitudes, and the use of nursing diagnosis. (2) Differences in the extent of utilization of nursing diagnoses by nurses in the various clinical areas should be assessed in an attempt to identify learning needs and strategies for improvement.

▷ Eriksen LR. *Patient satisfaction: An indicator of nursing care quality?* Nurs Manage 1987 Jul; 18(7):31–35.

A descriptive correlational study was conducted to examine the relationship between the quality of the nursing care and patient satisfaction with nursing care; the former was measured by The Methodology for Monitoring Quality of Nursing Care (MMQNC), and the latter was measured by The Patient Satisfaction with Nursing Care Check List (PSWNC).

The sample population consisted of 136 randomly selected inpatients of a large medical center. Criteria for selection included orientation to person, place, and time, at least 21 years of age, ability to respond to a questionnaire in the English language, and minimum inpatient stay of 24 hours.

The results did not support the presence of strong positive and significant relationships between the study variables. However, some interesting findings were revealed. The areas in which the relationships between quality of nursing care and patient satisfaction with that care were most positive included social courtesy, orientation to surroundings, and attention to the need for oxygen. Negative relationships emerged relative to physical care and teaching patients to deal with illness and health status.

Nursing Implications. (1) Patient satisfaction should not be used as the sole criterion for evaluation of quality of nursing care. (2) The necessity for nursing interventions that have the potential for causing physical discomfort or emotional distress and conflict must be explained to patients; individualization of

nursing care is essential. (3) Social courtesy and attention to the patient's environment are important in promoting patient satisfaction.

▷ Bull MJ. *Influence of diagnosis-related groups on discharge planning, professional practice, and patient care.* J Prof Nurs 1988 Nov/Dec; 4(6):415–421.

The researcher reported the findings of a study on how eight hospitals in a Midwest health system adapted to diagnosis-related groups (DRGs). Discharge planning was used as the indicator of the hospitals' responses to DRGs. Open-ended interviews were conducted with health care personnel (administrators, nurses, social workers) and physicians affiliated with small, midsized, and large hospitals and with health care professionals from home health agencies and extended care facilities that were part of the hospitals' discharge planning network. The interviews focused on the process of implementation of DRGs and related changes in routines and practices; specific questions were asked about changes in discharge planning practices and the resulting implications for the home health agencies and extended care facilities. A total of 118 persons were interviewed. Findings of the study revealed that DRGs have a significant influence on discharge planning, professional practice, and patient care. Discharge planning was marked by initiation of regular rounds for all patients and increased communication and collaboration between health care professionals and patients and family members. Professional practice was affected by increased acuity of inpatients and outpatients and by the need for health care professionals to become involved in teaching the public about DRGs. Patient care was affected positively by greater family involvement in discharge planning and increased focus on self-care and independence. Negative effects included early discharge of patients with complex needs that resulted in increased family stress and the need for more extensive home and extended health care services than ever before. Health care professionals reported experiencing conflict between meeting patients' needs and complying with hospital regulations relative to decreasing length of patient stay.

Nursing Implications. (1) Assessment of discharge planning needs must include the needs of the patient's family as well as the needs of the patient. (2) Nurses must be knowledgeable about DRGs and serve as patient advocates in the clinical setting. (3) Conflict resolution should become an integral part of nursing education and staff development curricula.

▷ Tilley JD, Gregor FM, and Thiessen V. *The nurses's role in patient education: Incongruent perceptions among nurses and patients.* J Adv Nurs 1987 May; 12(3):291–301.

This study was directed toward describing the perceptions of patients and nurses concerning the nurse's role in patient education and evaluating the amount of congruence between these perceptions. The convenience sample of nurses and patients was selected from two university teaching hospitals in Canada. Thirty-eight matched nurse–patient dyads were recruited. Twenty-three were from a cardiology unit in one hospital; fifteen were from a general medical unit of the other hospital. All but three patients from the general medical unit had been hospitalized with the diagnosis of acute myocardial infarction; the three exceptions had the diagnosis of a respiratory disease.

A Nurse Questionnaire and a Patient Interview Schedule

were developed with complementary sets of questions: one set to measure nurses' perceptions of how much and what kind of patient education they perform and should perform, the other set to measure patients' perceptions of the same.

The results of the study suggested that incongruities existed between the nurses' and the patients' perceptions of the role of the nurse in patient education. Patients identified nurses as sources of information; however, when asked whom they preferred to have teach them specific information related to their conditions, they most frequently chose the physician. Nurses most frequently chose a nurse. Another incongruity was related to the appropriate time period for patient teaching. Nurses identified the time just prior to discharge; patients identified the early part of their hospitalization, indicating a need for information about what had happened to them rather than a need for discharge information. A third incongruity identified was a tendency of nurses to incorrectly assume that their desires relative to patient education were shared by their patients.

Nursing Implications. (1) Nurses must not assume that their perceptions about the need for patient education are the same as patients' perceptions; assessment of patients' perceptions of their learning needs is essential. (2) Type and timing of information desired by hospitalized patients must be assessed and information provided must be individualized accordingly. (3) Nurses need to clearly define their roles as patient educators.

unit 2

Health Assessment
of the Client/Patient

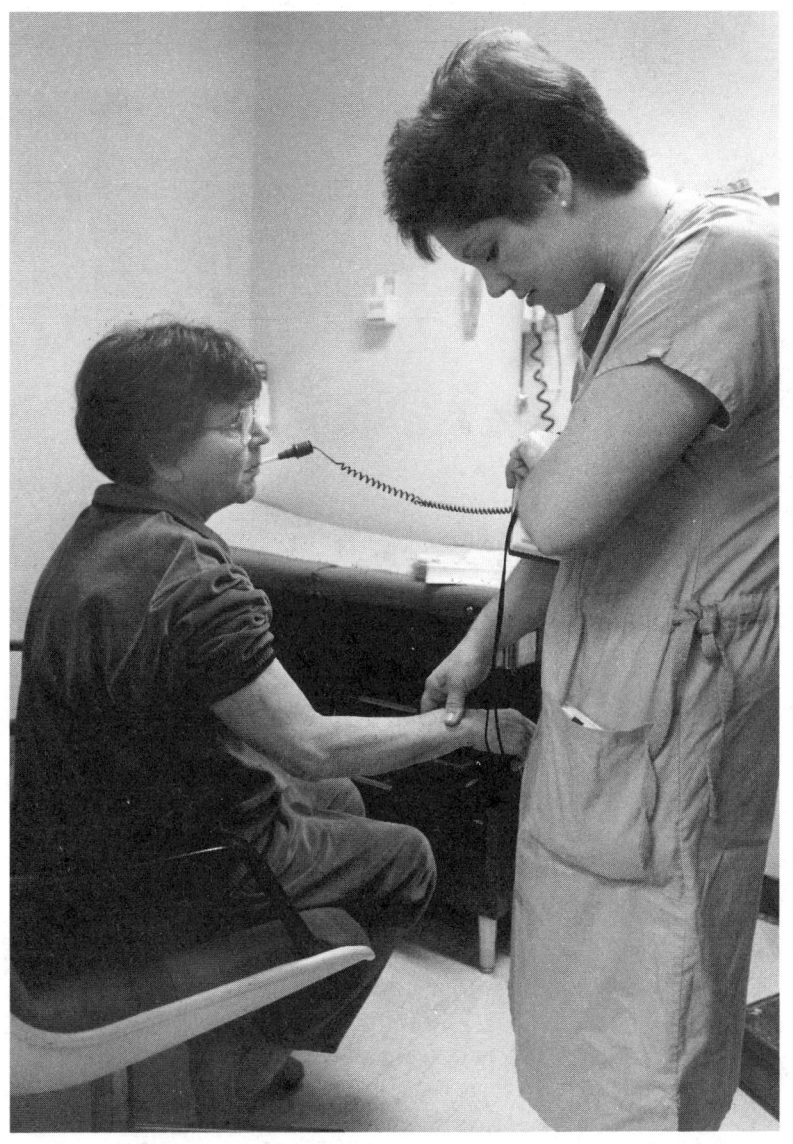

6

Clinical Interviewing: The Health History

Learning Objectives

On completion of this chapter, the learner will be able to:

1. Describe the role of the nurse in obtaining the patient's health history
2. Identify ethical considerations necessary for protection of the patient's rights related to data collected for health assessment
3. Identify environmental factors that are conducive to effective data collection
4. Describe effective use of the health history form
5. Specify the essential components of the data base
6. Discuss the patient's cultural, ethnic, religious, socioeconomic, and educational backgrounds as significant variables in the interview process
7. Describe specific modifications that may be necessary in obtaining a health history from an elderly patient
8. Conduct a patient interview for the purpose of obtaining a data base

The clinical interview is one of the most important facets of the nurse–patient relationship. It is through this process that the quality of the relationship is established, information sufficient to provide a thorough assessment of the patient's health status is obtained, and the foundation for nursing diagnoses is made. Behaviors appropriate to the interview and the techniques required to elicit appropriate information are not part of our everyday social lives. These behaviors and techniques must be learned. Interviewing skills require careful development and are refined through experience.

The Role of the Nurse

The role of the nurse in the provision of health care is an ever-changing one. The scope of nursing practice includes not only those functions for which the nurse has traditionally been prepared but also many activities once reserved for physicians and other members of the health care team. In order to facilitate the nursing process, nurses employ skills that include gathering the patient data base and performing a physical examination.

The concept that only the physician diagnoses patient problems and plans appropriate interventions has also changed.

Intrinsic to the concept of the health care team is the interdependence of health professionals, including physicians, nurses, nutritionists, social workers, and others, each maximizing his or her skills in contributing to the resolution of patient problems. Traditionally, nursing assessments and nursing histories have been present in a variety of styles, lengths, and focuses. Institutions and agencies have developed tools that address particular philosophies and concerns. The data base obtained by the nurse is ideally complementary to the data bases obtained by other members of the health care team yet focuses on nursing's concerns for the patient.

The Health History

Throughout the nursing assessment, and particularly in the history, interest is centered on the patient's psychosocial and cultural patterns. The interpersonal and physical environments, as well as the patient's life-style and activities of daily living, are explored in depth. Many nurses are also responsible for gathering a data base that includes a detailed history of the patient's current health problems, his past medical history, his family history, and a review of body systems. These areas, which constitute the focus of a medical history, were previously explored only by the physician. The inclusion of these categories within the context of the nursing history, the history obtained by the nurse, has resulted in a total health profile that focuses on health as well as illness and is more appropriately called a health history rather than a medical or a nursing history. The format of the health history is a combination of the traditional medical history and the nursing assessment. Both the review of systems and patient profile are expanded to include individual and family relationships, life-style patterns, health practices, and coping strategies. These components of the health history are the backbone of the nursing assessment and can easily be adapted to address the philosophy of nursing at a particular institution or agency and the needs of a particular patient population.

The consolidation of the medical history format and the nursing history format within one health history avoids a duplication of information, minimizes efforts on the part of the patient to provide this information, and encourages collaborative effort between the nurse and physician who share in the collection and interpretation of the data base.

In order to contribute significantly to the health history, the nurse must be cognizant of (1) ethical considerations in data collection, (2) communication skills and techniques of the interviewing process, and (3) the content of the health history.

Ethical Considerations in Data Collection

Whenever information is elicited from a person, that person has the right to know why the information is sought and how it will be used. For this reason, the nurse not only identifies herself and her role but also explains in detail what a health history is, how the information is elicited, and how it will be used.

It is important that the patient be fully informed of all aspects of the data collection process and that his decision to participate be freely made. A private setting for the interview promotes an atmosphere of trust between the patient and the nurse and encourages open, honest communication.

Following the interview, the nurse selectively records information that is pertinent to the patient's health status on the health history form. Isolated personal facts and highly sensitive information (arrest record, illegal drug use) are not initially entered in the health record but are discussed with the head nurse, supervisor, or physician. Occasionally, a patient will share very confidential matters with the nurse, and the responsibility for the disposition of such information is best shared.

When the interview is completed and the data recorded, the written record is maintained in a secure place and made available only to those health professionals directly involved in the care of the patient. This is another method of ensuring confidentiality and maintaining a high standard of nursing care and professional conduct.

Basic Guidelines for the Interviewer

- The interviewer approaches the patient as a unique individual. The interviewer puts the patient at ease and provides for his comfort.

The person who seeks health care for a specific problem is almost invariably anxious. He may not fully understand the significance of his symptoms. Anxiety is compounded by fears related to potential disruption of the person's life-style and perhaps by apprehension about the costs of health care. Given this set of circumstances, the person feels helpless, for he perceives that the outcome with respect to both his health and his economic well-being lies in the hands of others.

To minimize the patient's anxieties, the nurse introduces herself to the patient, defines her role on the health care team, and explains what the health history is. The nurse further explains that the health history will be used to identify areas of concern to the patient and the nurse regarding his health status. The patient is reassured that all the information shared is confidential and that only health professionals directly involved in his care will have access to that information.

The nurse ensures a private setting for the interview. If visitors are present, they are asked to leave, because the patient may find it difficult to communicate when visitors (even close relatives) are present. However, if the patient expresses a desire to have a family member present during the interview, this is acceptable and may generate additional information that the patient might otherwise forget or be unable to share. Distractions, such as those caused by radios or television sets, are reduced or eliminated.

The interview is conducted with consideration for the patient's comfort and self-respect. Before beginning, the nurse sees that the person is comfortable. If the interview is taking place in a hospital room, the nurse asks the patient if he would like another pillow or would prefer to be seated in a chair rather than in bed. The patient who is short of breath may be more comfortable in a sitting position than he would be if supine. If the patient is in pain or in urgent need of going to the bathroom, his discomfort is attended to before the interview begins.

- The interviewer permits the individual to express himself fully.

The goal of the clinical interview is to obtain all of the facts that will ultimately influence both the nursing diagnoses and the plan of care. This is best achieved in an atmosphere that encourages spontaneity on the part of the patient. Such spontaneity is influenced by the physical setting and by the behavior of the nurse. Even the simple act of the nurse's sitting during the interview conveys an important message to the patient.

It is important to put the patient at ease as much as possible and to encourage an open and honest description of the problem by the patient. Nonverbal communication on the part of the nurse is a critical element in promoting full expression by the patient. The nurse may actively encourage the patient to elaborate or continue by a nod of the head or by repeating the last few words if the patient appears hesitant. A puzzled look will encourage the patient to clarify apparent inconsistencies in the story.

Questions posed are frequently open-ended. "How can we help you?" "Tell me about it." "How did it feel?" are all appropriate questions. Examples of inappropriate questions are: "Was it a sharp pain?" "Did it happen only on weekdays?" Such questions presume the answer and "lead" the patient's response. Although one certainly wishes to obtain this information, it is sought in a more open-ended way. Otherwise, the patient attempts to "help" the nurse by providing the answer he thinks the nurse wants to hear.

However, the use of open-ended questions is not a technique to be employed throughout the entire interview. In order to refine the details that are important to the analysis of symptoms, some degree of direct questioning is necessary. Such questions provide the patient with options for his response. For example, the question "Does the pain have any relationship to meals?" gives the person the option of answering yes or no. Similarly, the question "Does the pain come before the meal, during the meal, or after the meal?" gives the person the opportunity to select from among several options. This more direct line of questioning is deferred until later in the interview when the patient has had an opportunity to express himself as fully as possible and has developed trust and confidence in the nurse.

It is not assumed that the approach to every patient will be the same. Clearly, the nurse will have to be more directive with certain patients. The sophistication that allows modification of the interview technique comes only with experience.

- The interviewer uses a health history form to guide the interview and adjusts the sequence of questions to coincide with the flow of conversation.

The health history form is a tool designed to assist the nurse in the collection of data relevant to the patient's health status. For this reason, the form is not memorized or rigidly adhered to at the expense of the individual. For example, if the person is sharing information about a particular problem and the nurse interrupts to ask direct questions about occupation, education, or family relationships, the flow of information may be broken and important facts overlooked.

It is also essential to *listen* to the patient as he answers the questions. Brief note-taking during the interview is acceptable, but when overdone it is highly distracting to the person being interviewed. It also limits eye contact and conveys an impersonal message.

- The interviewer demonstrates an understanding of the nature and intensity of the patient's problem.

The interviewing process does not consist entirely of questions and answers. The manner in which the nurse responds nonverbally to the patient and her ability to listen convey a genuine interest in the patient's concerns. Such behavior is often very reassuring, and thus the interview becomes therapeutic.

When the patient becomes silent during the interview, he may be emotionally overcome or may be attempting to formulate an accurate description of events. Such silences need not be interrupted by the nurse. Tearful episodes are also not interrupted, and the urge to tell the patient that matters are going to be all right or to provide similar verbal reassurances is resisted. Things may not be all right, and the reassurance may appear false. Moreover, the nurse has much to learn by exploring the patient's fears and anxieties. Sometimes, open-ended statements such as "You look sad" or "You seem frightened" will encourage the person to elaborate on his feelings and at the same time convey the nurse's empathy.

The nurse also makes every attempt to convey an understanding of and a respect for the patient's beliefs and attitudes. This is done in spite of the fact that such beliefs and attitudes may differ sharply from those held by the nurse. There is no place in the interview for a comment such as "You don't really believe that, do you?" If the person does not believe it, it is unlikely that he would state it candidly to the health professional conducting the interview. A nonjudgmental attitude is especially necessary when dealing with matters related to sexuality, drug and alcohol use, and cultural patterns.

- The interviewer takes into account the person's cultural background.

Cultural attitudes about family relationships, the role of women, and the meaning of health are accepted at face value, just as attitudes toward pain, illness, and hospitalization are accepted. These beliefs and attitudes are derived from personal experiences, which vary according to the person's cultural background.

- The interviewer is aware of his or her own feelings and attitudes.

Patient behavior that the nurse might find offensive in herself, her family, or her friends may arouse hostility, anger, anxiety, or even, at times, revulsion. The professional cannot allow this to be conveyed to the patient. Quite unconsciously, the nurse might convey irritation, boredom, or disbelief. Similarly, the nurse, because of her own fears, may be acutely uncomfortable when dealing with people who have certain kinds of illnesses. The nurse's own ethical and moral sense may make it difficult to develop relationships with alcoholic or drug-dependent patients, or those whose illness is a result of certain sexual practices or life-styles. It is a frequent failing of health professionals to view self-inflicted illness with disdain, hostility, and anger. Feelings are intensified when the patient is under the influence of alcohol or drugs, and the nurse may return hostility for hostility. The first step in dealing effectively with such patients is to understand the inner compulsions that cause the interviewer to reject the patient.

- The interviewer is attuned to nonverbal communication and learns to recognize gestures that convey defensiveness, hostility, confidence, impatience, and so on.

The nurse learns to respond to body language the same way she responds to the spoken word. Frequently, the body language and the patient's verbal expression are at variance. Often, this is obvious—as when the patient describes a seemingly happy event yet appears to be on the verge of tears. The interviewer might respond to such inconsistencies by drawing them to the patient's attention.

- The interviewer communicates in a manner that is consistent with the individual's level of understanding.

It is important for the nurse to take into consideration the patient's educational background and language. Patients whose first language is other than English and those who have had little or no contact with the health care system may be unfamiliar with terms commonly used by health care professionals. Therefore, the nurse phrases questions in such a way that they are easily understood by the patient; in counseling, she uses as few technical terms as possible. If the patient does not understand the language being used, it is unlikely that he will interrupt for clarification, largely out of fear that he will appear ignorant. Careful questioning may reveal the level of the patient's understanding of an issue that has just been discussed.

A second factor influencing the patient's level of understanding is cultural background. For example, a woman of another culture may have a perception of personal health different from that of a mother born and raised in an American suburb. Pregnancy is not something for which she would seek care and attention until labor begins. Thus, she may not understand the need for prenatal care as advocated by health professionals. In addition, a woman from a culture in which obesity is a way of life and admired by men would not understand the need for diet and weight control. Similarly, some women of Asian background not accustomed to complaining of pain, even when it is severe, might not consider taking analgesics. All such differences in outlook must be taken into account when dealing with members of other cultures.

Even differences in the life experiences of those who are well educated and from the same cultural background must be considered. An only child of an urban or suburban family may be less able to deal with the problems of being a mother than a woman from a rural society who was reared in a family of eight children and participated in rearing younger siblings.

- The interviewer terminates the interview in an appropriate manner that summarizes the information obtained and ensures that the patient has understood major points discussed.

Before ending the interview, the nurse inquires whether the patient has any questions. The nurse specifically searches for areas of misunderstanding by briefly summarizing the patient's responses. This gives the patient the opportunity to correct misinformation and also to add facts that he may have forgotten to mention earlier.

Content of the Interview

When the patient is seen for the first time by the health team (except in the emergency care situation), the first requisite is to obtain a *data base*. The nurse may be responsible for all or a part of that data base, but in either case she must be familiar with all of its facets. The data base contains the following components:

1. Biographical data
2. Informant
3. Chief complaint
4. History of present illness (or present health concern)
5. Past medical history
6. Review of systems
7. Family history
8. Patient profile
9. Physical examination
10. Radiologic and laboratory information
11. Problem formulation (medical and nursing diagnoses)

Biographical Data

Biographical or introductory identifying information helps to put much of the history in context. This information includes the name, address, age, sex, marital status, occupation, and ethnic origins of the patient. Some people prefer a full patient profile at this juncture, but most believe a full profile to be inappropriate until the interviewer has obtained the trust and confidence of the patient. Moreover, a patient in pain, or with an equally urgent problem for which he seeks attention, is unlikely to put a great deal of confidence in an interviewer who is more concerned with his marital or occupational status than with quickly addressing the problem for which the patient seeks help.

The Informant

The informant may not always be the patient, as is the case if the patient is a child or a disoriented or confused person or is unconscious, in a coma, or suffering a severe psychiatric disturbance. The interviewer assesses the reliability of the informant and the usefulness of the information provided. For example, hysterical or depressed patients are unlikely to provide a reliable data base, while patients who abuse drugs and alcohol are likely to use denial as part of their operating mechanism. It is reasonable for the interviewer to make such judgments (based on the context of the entire interview) and to incorporate them in the record.

Chief Complaint

The chief complaint is the issue that brings the patient to seek help. Questions such as "What brings you to the health center today?" or "Why have you been admitted to the hospital?" usually elicit the chief complaint. Frequently, the patient appears without a specific complaint, seeking an ongoing relationship with a health care team or requesting a "checkup." If this is the case, it is noted in lieu of a chief complaint. Once the patient has expressed his concern, his exact words are recorded in quotation marks. However, a statement such as "Doctor Smith sent me" is not a chief complaint. Although such information can be included as part of the introductory patient profile, the patient should be asked why he sought Dr. Smith's attention, and this reason should be entered as the chief complaint. If the patient has been admitted for a specific purpose, it is so stated (*e.g.,* "for cholecystectomy").

Frequently, the patient will have more than one problem and, therefore, more than one chief complaint. These are listed in terms of the patient's priorities and then explored as separate entities, if they represent separate problems, or as a single present illness if they are multiple manifestations of one cohesive problem.

History of Present Illness

Exploration of the facts related to a present illness frequently requires substantial knowledge of the pathophysiology and natural history of disease. If one does not know, for example, the manifestations of an acute myocardial infarction, it is difficult to subtly extract information that will ultimately lead to the diagnosis. The history of any illness is the single most important factor in assisting the health professional to arrive at a diagnosis. The physical examination is helpful but usually reveals manifestations that are expected consequences of the story that has unfolded. Occasionally, laboratory and radiologic information can be helpful; only rarely do they establish the diagnosis. On the other hand, a careful history assists in correct selection of appropriate diagnostic tests.

The present illness may well be but one episode in a sequence that is contained within a single disease process. An episode of insulin shock, for example, is only one event in a series of occurrences that define the natural history of diabetes. In such an instance, the entire course of the diabetic illness is unfolded in order to put the current complaint in context. Although the episode of insulin shock gains prominence in the delineation of the story, the description of it is obtained in the context of the natural history of the disease and communicated to the record in a similar manner. After all the facts have been obtained from the patient, the details of the present illness, or health concern, from onset until the time of contact with the health care team, are constructed. These facts are recorded in *chronologic order,* beginning with, for example, "The patient was in good health until . . ." or "The patient first experienced nausea 2 months prior to admission 11/4/91."

The history of the present illness is a compact, complete story rather than a statement of numerous disconnected facts. It includes such information as the date and manner (sudden, gradual) of the onset of the problem, the setting in which the problem developed (at home, at work, after an argument, after exercise), manifestations of the problem, and the course of the illness or problem. The course of the illness or problem includes self-treatment, medical interventions, progress and effects of treatment, and the patient's perceptions of the cause or meaning of the problem.

Specific symptoms (pain, headache, fever, change in bowel habits) are delineated in detail. Critical to the analysis of a symptom is its location and radiation (if pain), quality, severity, and duration. The interviewer also pursues the persistence or intermittence of the symptom, factors that aggravate or alleviate it, and any associated manifestations of which the patient may be aware.

Associated manifestations are symptoms that occur simultaneously with the chief complaint. The presence or absence of associated symptoms may shed light on the origin or extent of the patient's problem, as well as on the diagnosis. These symptoms are referred to as significant positive or negative findings and are derived from a review of systems directly related to the chief complaint. For instance, if the patient is complaining of a vague symptom, such as fatigue or weight loss, all body systems are reviewed and included in the history of the present illness. If, on the other hand, the patient's chief complaint is chest pain, only the cardiopulmonary and gastrointestinal systems would be included in the history of the present illness. In either situation, both positive and negative findings are recorded in order to further define the problem.

Health History

A detailed summary of the patient's health history is a valuable component of the data base. After obtaining a statement about the patient's general health in the past, the nurse proceeds in an orderly fashion to inquire about the patient's immunization status and any known allergies to drugs or other substances. The dates of immunization, along with the type of allergy and adverse reactions, are recorded. The patient is asked to provide information, if known, about his last physical examination, chest x-ray film, electrocardiogram (ECG), eye examination, hearing examination, dental checkup, and Papanicolaou smear (if female). The patient is then interviewed about previous illnesses. Negative as well as positive responses are recorded. Dates, or the age of the patient at the time of illness, as well as the names of the physician and hospital, the diagnosis, and the treatment are also recorded. A history of the following areas is elicited.

- Childhood illness—rubeola, rubella, polio, whooping cough, mumps, chickenpox, scarlet fever, rheumatic fever, strep throat
- Adult illnesses
- Psychiatric illnesses
- Injuries—burns, fractures, head injuries
- Hospitalizations
- Operations
- Current medications—prescription, over-the-counter, home remedies
- Use of alcohol and other drugs

If a particular hospitalization or major medical intervention is related to the present illness, it need not be repeated; rather, the nurse makes a reference such as "see history of present illness" or "see HPI" on the data sheet.

Family History

The age and health status, or the age and cause of death, of first-order relatives (parents, siblings, spouse, children) and second-order relatives (grandparents, cousins) are elicited to identify diseases that may be hereditary, communicable, or possibly environmental. The nurse specifically inquires about such conditions as cancer, hypertension, heart disease, diabetes, epilepsy, mental illness, tuberculosis, kidney disease, arthritis, allergies, asthma, alcoholism, and obesity. One of the easiest methods of recording such data is by using the family tree or genogram (Fig. 6-1).

Review of Systems

The review of systems includes a complete inventory of major body organ systems in terms of the presence or absence of symptoms past or present. It serves as a check and balance to prevent the interviewer from overlooking any relevant data. Negative as well as positive responses are recorded. If the patient responds positively, that symptom is analyzed according to the process outlined under History of Present Illness. Illnesses that have been previously described in the history of the present illness or the past medical history need not be repeated. Reference is made to the appropriate location of relevant information. The system review includes an overview of general health as well as symptoms related to each body system. A review of systems can be organized in a formal checklist, which becomes a part of the health history. One asset of the checklist process is that it is easily audited and less subject to error than is relying on the memory of the interviewer, who must obtain detailed information relevant to each organ system. One such format is outlined in Chart 6-1.

Patient Profile

The patient profile is an amplification of the biographical data elicited at the beginning of the interview. A complete composite, or profile, of the patient is critical to an analysis of his

problem, his capacity to deal with the problem, and the health care team's capacity to provide assistance.

The information elicited at this point in the interview is highly personal and subjective. During this stage, the nurse encourages the patient's open and uninhibited expression of feelings, values, and personal experiences. Usually, the nurse begins with general open-ended questions and then moves to direct questioning when specific facts are needed. The patient is often less anxious when the interview progresses from information that is less personal (birthplace, occupation, education) to information that is more personal (sexuality, body image, coping abilities).

A general patient profile consists of six content areas:

1. Past development
2. Education and occupation
3. Environment (physical, spiritual, interpersonal)
4. Life-style (patterns and habits)
5. Self-concept
6. Stress response

The patient profile is outlined in Chart 6-2.

Past Development.   The patient profile begins with a brief life history. Questions about the patient's place of birth and places where he has lived in the past help him to focus on the earlier years of his life. Personal experiences during childhood or adolescence that have special significance to the patient may be elicited by asking, "Was there anything that you experienced as a child or adolescent that would be helpful for me to know about?" The interviewer's intent is to encourage the patient to make a quick review of his earlier life, highlighting an event or circumstance of particular significance. Sometimes the person will not be able to recall anything that he believes is meaningful to share with the nurse. On the other hand, he may take the opportunity to share information such as a per-

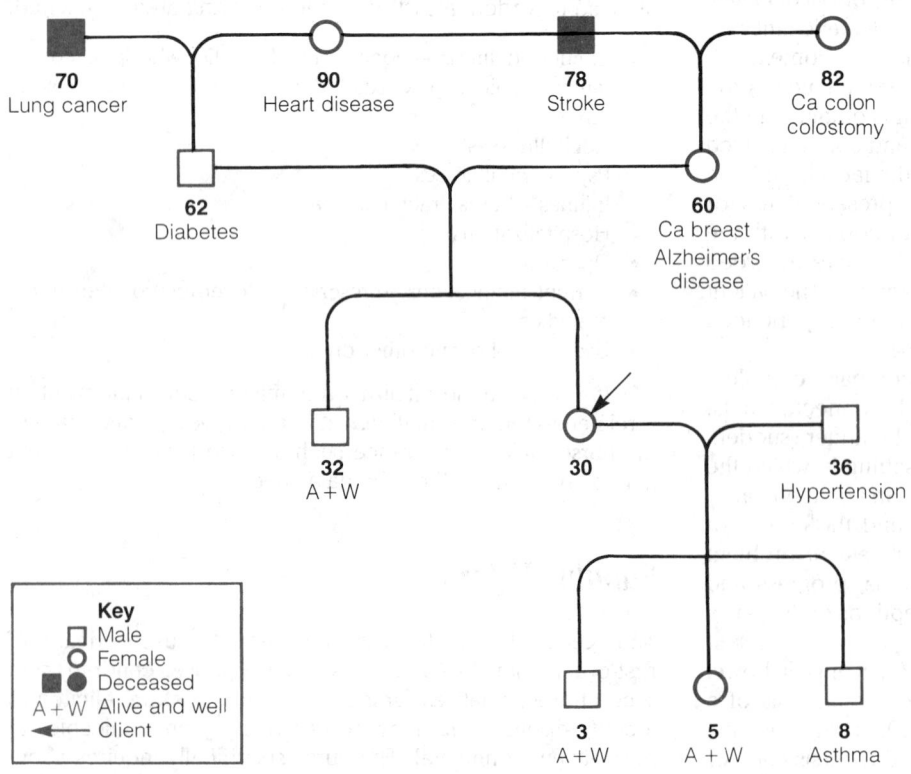

Key
□ Male
○ Female
■ ● Deceased
A + W Alive and well
◄— Client

Figure 6-1. Sample recording of family history as a "family tree." Grandparents, parents, siblings, spouse, and children are identified.

Chart 6-1
Review of Systems

Positive responses are circled and described in detail. Negative responses are underlined to indicate the absence of the symptom.

General

Usual weight	Weakness
Weight change	Fatigue
Appetite change	Fever
Night sweats	

Skin

Rash	Pruritus
Color change	Growths or masses
Dryness	Hair changes
Nail changes	

Head

Headache	Dizziness
Trauma	

Eyes

Vision (near and far)	Blurring
Glasses or contacts	Pain
Photophobia	Infection
Diplopia	Itching

Ears

Hearing	Hygiene practices
Pain	Tinnitus
Infection	Vertigo
Excessive cerumen	

Nose and Sinuses

Discharge	Epistaxis
Allergies	Pain
Obstruction	Frequent colds

Mouth and Throat

Sore throats	Dentures or partial plate
Difficulty swallowing	Hoarseness
Taste	Lesions (lips, tongue, mucosa)
Gums	Hygiene practices
Dentition	

Neck

Stiffness	Limited motion
Swelling	"Swollen glands"
Pain	Thyroid disease

Breasts

Pain	Nipple discharge
Swelling	Dimpling
Self-examination practices	

Musculoskeletal

Muscular pain or cramps	Back pain or history of injury
Pain, swelling, or redness of joints	Limitation of movement
Trauma	Ability to perform ADL

Endocrine

Heat or cold intolerance	Excessive thirst, hunger, or urination
Excessive sweating	
Changes in hair pattern	

Respiratory

Cough	Sputum (color, quantity)
Shortness of breath	Asthma
Hemoptysis	Recurrent upper respiratory tract infection
Wheezing	

Cardiovascular

Shortness of breath	Phlebitis
Dyspnea on exertion	Coldness or numbness of extremities
Orthopnea	
Chest pain	Edema
Palpitations	Varicosities
Paroxysmal nocturnal dyspnea	Claudication

Gastrointestinal

Anorexia	Hematemesis
Nausea	Melena
Vomiting	Jaundice
Indigestion	Food intolerance
Diarrhea	Change in bowel pattern
Pain	Hemorrhoids
Constipation	

Genitourinary

Nocturia	Dysuria
Incontinence	Dribbling
Infection	Frequency
Urgency	Hematuria

(continued)

Chart 6-1 *(Continued)*

Genitoreproductive

Female

Menses (menarche, cycle, duration, amount, cramps, intermittent bleeding, last menstrual period [LMP])

Number of pregnancies, live births, abortions (G__P__Ab__)

If menopausal: age of menses cessation, symptoms of menopause, postmenopausal bleeding

Vaginal discharge

Dyspareunia

Contraception practices

Pruritus

Sexually transmitted disease

Male

Pain	Sores
Discharge	Sexually transmitted disease
Swelling	Contraception practices

Neurologic

Syncope	Numbness or tingling
Seizures	Problems with speech or gait
Paralysis	
Weakness	Tremors
Dizziness	Memory loss
Vertigo	Loss of sensation

Hematologic

Blood transfusions	Easy bruising or bleeding
Anemia	

---

sonal achievement, a failure, a developmental crisis, or an instance of physical or emotional abuse.

Education and Occupation. Questions related to economic status and educational preparation can be threatening to the patient and are approached indirectly through a focus on his current occupation. If the patient is employed, a statement such as "Tell me about your job" often elicits information about his role, job tasks, and satisfaction with the position. It may be necessary to interject direct questions about past employment and career goals if the person does not initially provide this information.

Asking the person what kind of educational requirements were necessary to attain his present job is a more sensitive approach to educational background than asking whether he graduated from high school. It is rarely necessary to know the actual numerical value of the person's salary; the information needed is whether his income is sufficient to meet his expenses and support the life-style to which he is accustomed. Questions such as "Do you have any financial concerns at this time?" or "Sometimes there just doesn't seem to be enough money to make ends meet. Are you finding this true?" may be helpful. Inquiry about the person's insurance coverage and plans for health care payment are also appropriate.

Environment. The person's physical environment and its potential hazards, his spiritual awareness, and his cultural background, interpersonal relationships, and support system are included in the concept of environment.

Physical Environment. The type of housing (apartment, duplex, single family) in which the person lives, its location, and information related to safety and comfort within the person's home and neighborhood are elicited. The nurse attempts to identify environmental hazards, such as isolation, inadequate protection, potential fire risks, pollution (noise, air, water), and inadequate sanitation facilities.

Spiritual Environment. To be thoughtful or contemplative about one's existence, to accept challenges in one's life, and to seek and find answers to personal questions is to be "spiritual." For many persons, this spirituality is expressed through identification with a particular religion. Like cultural influences, spiritual values and beliefs direct a person's behavior and his approach to health problems and the health care system in general. A person's spirituality is often challenged during the experience of an illness or a developmental crisis. The patient may experience considerable turmoil about the meaning of this problem or crisis in his life. He is challenged to new perceptions and spiritual growth, and he may find this difficult. A brief spiritual assessment by the nurse is important; it focuses on three areas:

1. The extent to which religion is a part of the person's life
2. Religious beliefs related to the person's perception of health and illness
3. Religious practices

The following questions can be used in a spiritual assessment:

- Is religion or God important to you?
  If yes, in what way?
  If no, what is the most important thing in your life?
- Are there any religious practices that are important to you?
- Do you have any spiritual concerns because of your present health problem?

Interpersonal Environment. Cultural influences, relationships with family and friends, and the presence or absence of a support system are all a part of the interpersonal environment.

Ethnic Background. The beliefs and practices that have been shared from generation to generation are known as cultural or ethnic patterns. They are expressed through language,

Chart 6-2
Patient Profile

Past Development

Place of birth
Places lived
Significant childhood/adolescent experiences

Education and Occupation

Jobs held in past
Current position/job
Length of time at position
Educational preparation
Work satisfaction and career goals
Financial resources
Insurance coverage

Environment

Physical

Living arrangements (type of housing, neighborhood, presence of hazards)

Spiritual

Extent to which religion is a part of individual's life
Religious beliefs related to perception of health and illness
Religious practices

Interpersonal

Ethnic background (language spoken, customs and values held, folk practices used to maintain health or to cure illness)
Family relationships (family structure, roles, communication patterns, support system)
Friendships (quality of relationship)

Life-Style

Patterns

Sleep (time individual retires, hours per night, comfort measures, awakens rested?)
Exercise (type, frequency, time spent)
Nutrition (24-hour diet recall, idiosyncrasies, restrictions)
Recreation (type of activity, time spent)

Caffeine (coffee, tea, cola, chocolate)—kind, amount
Smoking (cigarette, pipe, cigar, marijuana)—kind, amount per day, number of years, desire to quit
Alcohol—kind, amount, pattern over past year
Drugs—kind, amount, route of administration

Self-Concept

View of self in present
View of self in future
Body image (level of satisfaction, concerns)
Sexuality—Perception of self as a man or woman
Quality of sexual relationships
Concerns related to sexuality or sexual functioning

Stress Response

Major concerns or problems at present
Daily "hassles"
Past experiences with similar problems
Past coping patterns and outcomes
Present coping strategies and anticipated outcomes
Individual's expectations of family/friends and health care team in problem resolution

---

dress, dietary choices, and role behaviors, in perceptions of health and illness, and in health-related behaviors. The influence of these beliefs and customs on the patient's experience with a health problem and his relationship with the health care team cannot be underestimated. For this reason, a patient's ethnic identity (cultural and social) and his racial identity (biologic) are determined. The following questions may assist the nurse in obtaining relevant information:

* Where did your parents or ancestors come from? When?
* What language do you speak at home?
* Are there certain customs or values that are important to you?
* Is there anything special you do to keep in good health?
* Do you have any specific practices for treating illness?

Family Relationships and Support System.   An assessment of family structure (members, ages, roles), patterns of communication, and the presence or absence of a support system is an integral part of the patient profile. Although the traditional "family" is recognized as a mother, father, and children, it is important to keep in mind that there are many different types of living arrangements within our society. "Family" may be interpreted to mean two or more people bound by emotional ties or commitments. Such an open definition of "family" encompasses the couple who live together but are not married, the college student whose dormitory companions provide a "family" structure, and the single person who lives alone but has significant relationships and a support system.

Life-Style.   The life-style section of the patient profile provides the nurse the opportunity to gain information about health-related behaviors. These behaviors include patterns of sleep, exercise, nutrition, and recreation, as well as personal habits of smoking and the use of drugs, alcohol, and caffeine. Most people have little difficulty sharing particulars about their sleeping patterns or recreational choices. On the other hand, many people are quite sensitive to questions about their smoking, alcohol use, and drug use. The person may fear the nurse's scrutiny and thus may minimize the extent of his habit. For this reason, the nurse may be able to elicit more information by asking, "What kind of alcohol do you enjoy drinking at a party" rather than "Do you drink?" Describing the person as a "social drinker" is vague and not recommended. Instead, the nurse identifies specifically the type of alcohol and the amount ingested per day or per week (*e.g.*, 1 pint of whiskey daily for 2 years).

When the nurse suspects that alcohol abuse may be a problem, additional information may be obtained by asking, "Has anyone ever said that drinking might be causing a problem for you?" or "Have you ever considered cutting down your alcohol intake?" In a similar fashion, the nurse elicits information related to smoking and caffeine consumption.

Questions about drug use follow naturally after questions about smoking, caffeine consumption, and alcohol use. A non-judgmental approach will make it easier for the patient to truthfully and factually discuss his use of illicit drugs. It is often helpful to ask questions that require responses other than a simple "yes" or "no." Because the names or terms used for different illicit drugs and their method of administration change over time, it may be necessary to ask the patient for clarification of these terms.

Self-Concept.   The self-concept is a product of relevant experiences with others and is the result of others' reactions to the "self." It is the impression one has of oneself, the product of years of input and interpretation by the individual. Sometimes the interviewer can assess a person's self-concept by asking him about his view of the present ("How do you feel about your life in general?") and his outlook for the future ("What will your life be like in the future?" or "How do you see yourself in a few years?").

Health concerns may threaten the way a person perceives himself. His body image, the mental picture he has of himself, is vulnerable during normal developmental crises (adolescence, pregnancy, aging) and also as a result of certain medical and surgical interventions. Simply being hospitalized can alter a person's perception of himself. Suddenly he sees himself as weak, helpless, and impotent. Surgical alterations such as a colostomy or a mastectomy pose an even greater threat to body image. It is therefore important for the nurse to be aware of the person's perceptions of himself and his body. The following questions may elicit useful information:

- What do you like most about yourself?
- What would you change about yourself if you could?
- Do you have any particular concerns about your body?

Sexuality.   No area of assessment is more personal than a sexual history. Because of anxiety on the part of the interviewer, this area of the patient profile is often overlooked or inadequately assessed. A lack of knowledge related to sexuality combined with anxiety about her own sexuality may hinder the nurse's effectiveness. The nurse may be perplexed about how or when to elicit this information in a sensitive way.

Sexual assessment can be approached at the end of the interview along with the interpersonal or life-style assessment, or it can be a part of the genitourinary history within the review of systems. The nurse may find it easier to approach a discussion of sexuality following a discussion of menstruation, for instance. A similar discussion with the male patient would follow questions related to the urinary system.

It is advisable to begin the assessment with a general question that takes into consideration the developmental stage of the person and the presence or absence of intimate relationships. For instance, when discussing sexuality with an adolescent, one or two of the following questions may be helpful:

- Do you have a special friend, a close relationship right now? Tell me about this closeness.
- Some teenagers are interested in having a sexual relationship at this age . . . how do you feel about that?

Such questions may lead to a discussion of concerns related to sexual expression, to the quality of a relationship, or to questions about contraception.

Whether the person is young or old, the nurse determines whether he is sexually active before exploring issues related to sexual identity, contraception, or the quality of the sexual relationship. The nurse is careful to avoid making assumptions related to fidelity, heterosexuality, or sexual practices. Questions are worded in such a way that the person feels free to discuss his sexuality regardless of his marital status or sexual preference. Direct questions are usually less threatening when prefaced with such statements as "Most people feel that. . ." or "Many people worry about. . ." This suggests the normalcy of such feelings or behavior and encourages the person to share information that he might otherwise leave out because he believes that his behavior or feelings are objectionable or different.

The needs of the patient direct the flow of the interview at all times. If the patient is abrupt with his responses and indicates that he does not wish to carry the discussion any further, the nurse proceeds to another part of the data collection. By introducing the subject of sexuality, however, the nurse has indicated to the person that a discussion of sexual concerns is acceptable and that she will be approachable in the future. (See also Chap. 17, Human Sexuality.)

Stress Response.   Every person handles a stressful event in a manner that is intended to eliminate or minimize the stress. Each individual's adaptive ability hinges on his capacity to cope effectively with the stressful situation. Exploring past coping patterns, as well as perceptions of current stresses and anticipated outcomes, assists the nurse in identifying the person's overall ability to handle stress. It is especially important to identify expectations that the person may have of his family, friends, and the health care team in helping him resolve his problems.

Other Health History Formats

The health history format presented and discussed above is only one possible format that is useful in obtaining and organizing information about a patient's current and past health status. Some nurses believe that this traditional format is appropriate for physicians but inappropriate for nurses because it does not focus exclusively on the assessment of human responses to actual or potential health problems. Several attempts have been made to create an assessment format and data base with this focus in mind. One example is the nursing data base prototype based on the North American Nursing Diagnosis Association's (NANDA) Unitary Person Framework and its nine human response patterns: exchanging, communicating, relating, valuing, choosing, moving, perceiving, knowing, and feeling. Although there is some support in nursing for this new approach to obtaining the data base, there is no consensus that this approach is superior to others.

The National Center for Health Services Research of the U.S. Department of Health and Human Services and other groups from the public and private sectors have focused on assessing not only biological health but other dimensions of health as well. These dimensions include physical, functional, emotional, mental, and social aspects of health. Modern efforts to assess health status have focused on the impact of the patient's disease or disability on *functional status*, the ability of the person to function normally and perform his usual physical, mental, and social roles or functions. An emphasis on functional assessment is viewed as a more holistic view of health than the traditional health or medical history. Instruments to assess health status in these ways may be of considerable assistance to nurses who use them along with their own clinical assessment skills to address the impact of illness, disease, disability, and health problems on functional status.

As was previously mentioned, the patient profile section of the traditional data base constitutes the major component of the nursing assessment and represents the nursing profession's strongest contribution to the data base. The education of the nurse and the focus of nursing practice clearly demonstrate this. The extent of the patient profile is usually determined by the patient's needs and the philosophy of nursing at a particular institution or agency. For all patients, however, a general assessment of the categories outlined provides a significant composite profile of the patient. Such a profile is appropriate whether the health problem is acute or chronic and whether the setting is inpatient, outpatient, a long-term care facility, or the patient's home.

Health concerns that usually are not complex (earache, tonsillectomy) and can be resolved in a short period of time usually do not require the depth or detail that is required when one is confronted with a person who is experiencing a major illness or health concern. Additional assessments that go beyond the general patient profile may be employed when the patient's health problems are acute and complex or when the illness is chronic. Regardless of the format used, the nurse's focus during collection of data about the patient's health is different from that of the physician and other health team members; however, it is complementary and encourages collaboration among the health care providers as each member brings his or her own expertise and focus to the situation.

Gerontologic Considerations

When obtaining a health history from the elderly patient, it is carried out in a calm, unrushed manner. Because of the increased incidence of impaired hearing and sight in the elderly, attention is paid to providing adequate lighting without glare and reducing distracting sounds from the environment. The interviewer positions herself so as to enable the patient to read lips and facial expressions; the patient with impaired hearing is asked to use his hearing aid during the interview.

The elderly patient often assumes that new physical prob-

lems are a result of age rather than a treatable illness; additionally, signs and symptoms of illness in the elderly are often very different from those in younger patients. Therefore, the interviewer inquires about subtle physical symptoms and recent changes in function and well-being. Particular care is taken in obtaining a complete history and account of the elderly patient's medications because of the frequent use of multiple medications in this population. Although it should not be assumed that the elderly patient is unable to provide an adequate history, it is often useful to interview the patient's family members (*i.e.*, spouse, adult child, sibling, or caretaker) to validate information and provide missing details. Further details about assessment of the elderly are provided in Chapter 12.

The Remainder of the Data Base

Following the health history, a physical examination is performed. The basic techniques and skills required for performing the physical examination are presented in Chapter 7. Special observations and assessments that must be made in specific clinical situations are described in the chapters in which these conditions are discussed. Based on the information elicited from the history and the physical examination, radiologic and laboratory tests may be indicated and prescribed. Problem identification, the formulation of nursing diagnoses, and the development of nursing care plans are discussed in Chapter 2, The Nursing Process.

Chapter Summary

The process of eliciting a health history is a complex one that requires new knowledge and understanding, clinical laboratory learning, and reinforcement in the practice setting. There is no one way to approach a patient or to elicit a health history. The nurse is encouraged to develop a style of interviewing that complements her personality and a health history format that is flexible, to accommodate the practice setting and the patient's needs. The health history format and interviewing techniques outlined in this chapter are presented as guidelines for the nurse in her acquisition of the initial components of the data base.

Bibliography

Books

Clinical Interviewing

Bates B. A Guide to Physical Examination and History Taking, 5th ed. Philadelphia, JB Lippincott, 1991.

Bernstein L and Bernstein RS. Interviewing: A Guide for Health Professionals, 4th ed. New York, Appleton and Lange, 1985.

DeGowin E and DeGowin R. Bedside Diagnostic Examination, 5th ed. New York, Macmillan, 1987.

Enlow A. Interviewing and Patient Care. New York, Oxford University Press, 1986.

Gordon M. Manual of Nursing Diagnosis 1988–1989. St Louis, CV Mosby, 1989.

Gordon M. Nursing Diagnosis. Process and Application. New York, McGraw-Hill, 1987.

Guzzetta CE et al. Clinical Assessment Tools for Use with Nursing Diagnosis. St Louis, CV Mosby, 1989.

Hagopian GA, Hymovich DP, and Lynaugh JE. Clinical Assessment: A Guide for Study and Practice. Philadelphia, JB Lippincott, 1987.

Malasanos L, Barkauskas V, and Stoltengerg–Allen K. Health Assessment, 4th ed. St Louis, CV Mosby, 1990.

Seidel H et al. Mosby's Guide to Physical Examination. St Louis, CV Mosby, 1990.

Journals

Applegate WB, Blass JP, and Williams TF. Instruments for the functional assessment of older patients. N Engl J Med 1990 Apr 26; 322(17): 1207–1214.

Barry PP and Ibarra M. Multidimensional assessment of the elderly. Hosp Pract [Off] 1990 Apr 15; 25(4):117–121, 124, 127–128.

Brown MD. Functional assessment of the elderly. J Gerontol Nurs 1988 May; 14(5):13–17.

Herth KA. The root of it all. Genograms as a nursing assessment tool. J Gerontol Nurs 1989 Dec; 15(12):32–37.

Hoeman SP. Cultural assessment in rehabilitation nursing practice. Nurs Clin North Am 1989 Mar; 24(1):277–287.

Holloran EJ. Computerized nurse assessments. Nurs Health Care 1988 Nov/Dec; 9(9):497–499.

Pinholt EM et al. Functional assessment of the elderly. Arch Intern Med 1987 Mar; 147(3):484–488.

Scher BB. Are checklists replacing good care? Nursing 1988 Jan; 18(1): 47.

Tompkins ES. In support of the discipline of nursing: A nursing assessment. Nurs Connect 1989 Fall; 2(3):21–29.

7

Physical Assessment and Nutritional Assessment

Learning Objectives

On completion of this chapter, the learner will be able to:

1. Describe the physical examination processes of inspection, palpation, percussion, and auscultation
2. Use inspection, palpation, percussion, and auscultation to perform physical assessment of the major body systems
3. Describe the importance of proper physical, emotional, and educational preparation of the patient for physical assessment
4. Use clinical examination, anthropometric measurements, biochemical assessment, and assessment of food intake to assess a person's nutritional status
5. Describe factors that may contribute to altered nutritional status in the elderly

---

Physical assessment, or the physical examination, is an integral part of the nursing assessment. The basic techniques and tools typically used in performing a physical examination are described in this chapter. The detailed discussion required for the thorough examination of specific systems, including special maneuvers, is found in appropriate chapters throughout the book. Because the patient's nutritional status is an important element of his total health profile, a section on nutritional assessment is included in this chapter.

The Physical Assessment

The physical examination is usually performed after the health history is taken. To facilitate this portion of the data collection process, the examiner performs the assessment in a well-lighted, warm area. The patient is undressed and draped appropriately so that only the area to be examined is exposed. The physical and psychologic comfort of the patient is considered at all times; procedures and their rationale are fully explained. If a particular maneuver may cause discomfort, an explanation of what to expect precedes that part of the examination. The examiner's hands are washed prior to and immediately following the examination. Fingernails are kept short to avoid injuring the patient.

The key to obtaining appropriate data in the least possible amount of time is an organized and systematic examination. Such an approach refines physical assessment skills and encourages cooperation and trust on the part of the patient.

The patient's health history provides the examiner with a complete health profile that guides all aspects of the physical examination. It helps to focus on body organs and systems that are of particular concern to the patient.

The complete physical examination usually proceeds in a logical head-to-toe sequence, as follows:

- Skin
- Head and neck
- Thorax and lungs
- Breasts
- Cardiovascular system
- Abdomen
- Rectum
- Genitalia
- Neurologic system
- Musculoskeletal system

In actual practice, all relevant organ systems are tested in the course of the physical examination, but not necessarily in the sequence described. For example, when the face is examined, it is appropriate at the same time to check for facial asymmetry and, thus, for the integrity of the seventh cranial nerve; one does not return to this point later, as part of a neurologic examination. When systems are combined in this manner, the patient is spared the sequence of sitting up, lying down, sitting up, and so forth, which can be exhausting and time-consuming.

A "complete" physical examination is not a "routine." Many of the elements fall in the category of "subroutines," which are selectively addressed as a function of the patient's particular problem. If, for example, a healthy 20-year-old college student reports for an examination in order to satisfy a requirement to play basketball and reports no history of neurologic abnormality, the requirements for an adequate survey of the neurologic system are minimal. Conversely, a complaint of transient numbness and diplopia usually necessitates a complete neurologic investigation. Similarly, a person with pleuritic chest pain receives a much more intensive examination of the chest than the person with, for instance, leg cramps.

The process of physical examination is a thoughtful one. Attempts to elicit physical findings are based on all the information available at the time the examination is conducted. In general, it is the patient's health history that directs the examiner in efforts to obtain additional data for a complete patient profile.

The process of learning physical examination requires memorization, skill repetition, and reinforcement in a clinical setting. Only after basic physical assessment techniques are mastered and integrated into a complete examination can the examiner tailor the routine screening examination to include thorough assessments of a particular system, including special maneuvers.

The basic tools of the physical examination are the human senses of vision, hearing, touch, and smell. These human tools may be augmented by special instruments or tools (*e.g.*, stethoscope, ophthalmoscope) to permit a better definition of visual and acoustic details, but these tools should be recognized only as extensions of the human senses; they are simple instruments that anyone can learn to use well. Expertise comes with practice, and sophistication comes with the interpretation of what is seen and heard.

The Process of Physical Examination

Four fundamental processes are employed in the examination of the patient: *inspection, palpation, percussion,* and *auscultation.*

Inspection

The first fundamental process is inspection. The power to observe is one that must be cultivated. General inspection is carried out at the first moment of contact with the patient. The examiner introduces herself to the patient and may shake hands with him, and they exchange the first words of communication. Many impressions register in this exchange, and numerous valuable observations can be made. The patient is old or young (how old? how young? does his appearance correspond to his/her stated age?); the patient is thin or obese; the patient is anxious or depressed; the patient's body structure is normal or perhaps deformed in some way (what way? how different from normal?).

It is essential to pay attention to the details of observation. Vague general statements, which are often used, are a poor substitute for specific descriptions based on careful observation:

1. *The patient looks sick.* In what way does the patient look sick? Is he pale; is his skin clammy; is he grimacing in pain; is he dyspneic; is the skin jaundiced or cyanotic; does he have edema? What specific physical features or behavioral manifestations convey that he is "sick"?
2. *The patient appears chronically ill.* In what way does the patient appear chronically ill? Does he appear to have lost weight? Patients who lose weight secondary to malignancy or other muscle-wasting disease appear different from those who are merely thin. The distribution of their weight loss takes a different form. Does the skin have the appearance of chronic illness? That is, is it pale, or does it give the appearance of dehydration or loss of subcutaneous tissue? These are important observations that health professionals frequently fail to note on the record.

Among general observations that should be noted in the initial examination of the patient are posture and stature, body movements, nutrition, speech pattern, and body temperature.

Posture and Stature.   The posture that a patient assumes often provides valuable information about his illness. Patients with the dyspnea of cardiac disease prefer to sit and may complain of "smothering" if forced to lie down for even brief periods of time. Persons with emphysema not only sit upright but also assume a posture that is quite characteristic. They thrust their arms forward and laterally onto the edge of the bed (tripod position) in order to place accessory muscles of respiration at an optimum mechanical advantage for respiratory assistance. Patients with abdominal pain due to peritonitis prefer to lie perfectly still. Even slight jarring of the bed by the examiner will incite agonizing pain. On the other hand, patients with abdominal pain due to renal or biliary colic are very restless. They may writhe in bed or even get up and pace the room. Patients with meningeal irritation associated with headache cannot bend the head or flex the knees without aggravating their pain.

Body Movements.   Abnormalities of body movement may be of two general kinds: generalized discontinuity of voluntary or involuntary movement and asymmetry of movement. The former category includes tremors of a wide variety; some may occur at rest (Parkinson's disease), while others occur only on voluntary movement (cerebellar ataxia). Other tremors may exist during both rest and activity (alcohol withdrawal delerium, thyrotoxicosis). Some voluntary or involuntary movements are fine, others quite coarse. At the extreme are the convulsive movements of epilepsy or tetanus and the gross choreiform movements of patients with rheumatic fever or Huntington's disease.

Asymmetry of movement is seen in patients with disease of the central nervous system (CNS), principally in those who have had cerebral vascular accidents. The patient may manifest drooping of one side of the face or be incapable of normal movement of the right or left upper and lower extremities. Strength is impaired on the involved side, and the patient walks with a foot-dragging gait.

Nutrition.   Nutritional status is important to note. Obesity may be generalized as a function of excessive intake of calories or may be specifically localized to the trunk in patients with endocrine disorders (Cushing's disease) or those who have been taking steroid drugs for long periods of time. Loss of weight may be generalized as a function of caloric deprivation or may be reflected more strikingly in loss of muscle mass in patients whose diseases interfere with protein synthesis. A more detailed discussion of nutritional assessment is presented later in this chapter.

Speech Pattern.   Speech may be slurred because of CNS disease or because of incapacity to articulate as a result of damage to cranial nerves. Damage to the recurrent laryngeal nerve will produce hoarseness, as will those diseases that produce edema or swelling of the vocal cords. Speech may be halting or interrupted in flow in some CNS disorders (multiple sclerosis).

Body Temperature.   The recording of body temperature is a part of every physical examination. Fever is an increase in body temperature above normal. A normal oral temperature for most persons is an average of 37.0°C (98.6°F). It should be recognized that there is some variation that is still within the range of normal. Some persons' temperatures are quite normal at 36.6°C (98°F) and others at 37.3°C (99°F). Children playing hard during summer months quite regularly run temperatures as high as 37.7°C (100°F), and occasionally higher, but this should decrease quickly with rest. Moreover, it should be recognized that there is a normal diurnal variation of a degree or two in body temperature throughout the day. Most persons achieve their low early in the morning. Body temperature rises during the day to 37.3° to 37.5°C (99° to 99.5°F) and then subsides through the night.

Palpation

Palpation is a vital part of the physical examination. Many structures of the body, although not visible, are accessible by the hand and may be assessed through touch. Examples include superficial blood vessels, lymph nodes, the thyroid, the organs of the abdomen and pelvis, and the rectum. It should be noted that in examining the abdomen, auscultation is performed *before* palpation and percussion to avoid altering bowel sounds.

Sounds generated within the body, if within specified frequency ranges, also may be detected through touch. Thus, certain murmurs generated in the heart or within blood vessels (thrills) may be detected. Thrills cause a sensation to the hand much like the purring of a cat. Voice sounds are transmitted along the bronchi to the periphery of the lung. These may be perceived by touch and will be altered by certain disease states within the lung. The phenomenon is called *tactile fremitus* and is useful in assessing diseases of the chest.

Percussion

The technique of percussion translates the application of physical force into sound. It is a difficult skill to perfect but one capable of yielding much information about disease processes in the chest and abdomen. The principle is to set the chest wall or abdominal wall into vibration by striking it with a firm object. The sound produced is reflective of the density of the underlying structure. Certain densities produce sounds that can be identified as percussion notes. These sounds, listed in a sequence that proceeds from the least to the most dense, are called *tympany*, *hyperresonance*, *resonance*, *dullness*, and *flatness*. The pitch of the sound progresses from lowest for tympany to highest for flatness; the duration of the sound ranges from long to short.

Tympany is the drumlike sound produced by percussing the air-filled stomach. *Resonance* is the sound elicited over air-filled lungs. *Hyperresonance* is audible when one percusses over inflated lung tissue of the patient with emphysema. Percussion of the liver produces a dull sound, while percussion of the thigh results in flatness.

The procedure (for right-handed persons; hands should be reversed if the examiner is left-handed) is conducted as follows (Fig. 7-1): The distal phalanx (distal portion of finger) of the left middle finger is placed firmly against the chest wall. The other fingers should be held away from the chest wall, because any pressure they might exert against the thorax would

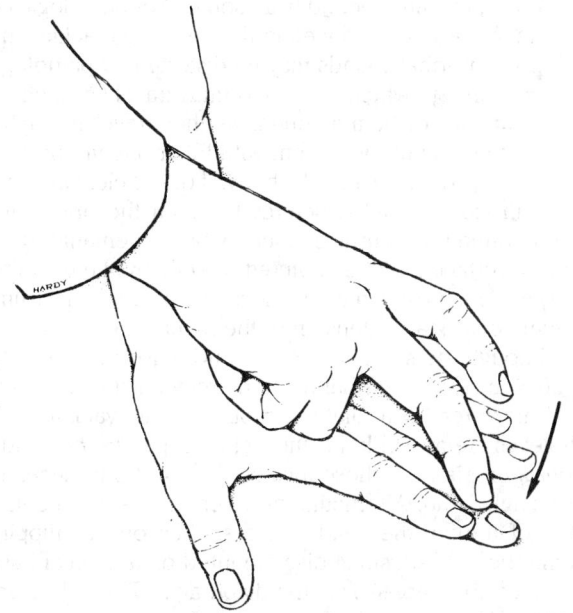

Figure 7–1. Percussion technique. The middle finger of the right hand strikes the terminal phalanx of the middle finger of the left hand. Care should be taken that only the terminal part of the middle finger of the left hand is in contact with the area to be percussed. The middle finger of the right hand should be held rigidly. It is properly a wrist action, and the intensity and clarity of the note will be a function of the quickness with which it is performed.

tend to mute or dampen the sound produced. The right hand now becomes the striking object. The middle finger of the right hand is used to strike the terminal phalanx of the middle finger of the left hand just behind the nail bed. If performed sharply, a brief resonant tone will be produced. The motion of the right hand should be dominantly a wrist action. The forearm itself should be held steady. The clarity of the sound produced is dependent on the brevity of the action. The intensity is a function of the force used.

Percussion gives one the capacity to assess such normal anatomic details as the degree to which the diaphragm descends during inspiration. The sound over lung tissue is normally resonant; the sound over the diaphragm is dull. One may percuss the border of the heart. One may determine the level of pleural effusion or the location of pneumonic consolidation or atelectasis of a lobe of the lung. Further application of the technique is discussed under examination of the thorax and abdomen.

Auscultation

Sound is produced within the body either by the movement of air through hollow structures or by the forces set up by the movement of columns of fluid that set solid structures in motion. Examples of clinically important acoustic phenomena include the movement of air through the trachea and bronchi (breath sounds), the movement of air past functioning vocal cords (spoken voice), the movement of air through the intestines (bowel sounds), the movement of blood through vascular structures that provide critical resistance to flow (murmurs), and the impedance to flowing blood provided by closed valves and the heart wall (heart sounds). Physiologic sounds may be normal (*e.g.*, first and second heart sounds) or pathologic (*e.g.*, murmurs in diastole produced in the heart, or crackles in the lung). Some normal sounds may be distorted by pathology of structures through which the sound must travel (*e.g.*, changes in the character of breath sounds as they travel through the consolidated lung of the patient with lobar pneumonia).

Sound produced within the body, if of sufficient amplitude, will set in vibration all structures between the origin of the sound and the body surface. Sound vibration emanating from the body surface may be captured directly by the examiner's ear or, more appropriately, by the stethoscope, an instrument that functions as an extension of the human ear.

Although the stethoscope does not have the capacity to amplify sound, it does channel it, thereby making physiologic sound more readily available for our critical evaluation. Two end-pieces are available for the stethoscope: the *bell* and the *diaphragm.* Many stethoscopes come with both pieces built into a single head. Alternating between the pieces becomes a matter of turning the head of the stethoscope or flipping a switch. The bell is a small disc mounted on a conical base; it is attached to a larger disc, the diaphragm. The bell is better suited for the transmission of very low frequency sounds. It is important to place the bell so that the entire surface of the disc rests lightly on the skin surface, to avoid flattening the skin and reducing audible vibratory sensations. The diaphragm, the larger disc, is constructed for the reception of high-frequency sounds. It is placed firmly against the skin for optimal transmission of sound.

The head of the stethoscope is held between the index and middle fingers to provide a firm contact with the skin surface. Care is taken to avoid touching the tubing or rubbing other surfaces (hair, clothing) during auscultation to minimize extraneous noises. The earpieces of the stethoscope should fit snugly into the ear canals, and the tubing should not be more than 20 cm in length. Dual tubing transmits sound more faithfully than single tubing.

Sound produced by the body, like any other sound, is characterized by intensity, frequency, and quality. The *intensity*, or loudness, associated with physiologic sound is low. Rarely may sounds of the body, except for speech, be heard without direct application of the ear or the stethoscope to the body surface. With respect to *frequency*, or pitch, it may be said that physiologic sound is in reality "noise," in that most sounds consist of a frequency spectrum as opposed to single-frequency sounds that we associate with music or the tuning fork. The frequency spectrum may be quite low, yielding a rumbling noise, or comparatively high, producing a harsh or blowing sound. The third feature of sound is *quality*. This relates to overtones and is the characteristic of sound that allows one to differentiate sound produced by the piano from that produced by the violin. Sound quality enables the examiner to distinguish between the musical quality of high-pitched wheezing and the low-pitched rumbling of a diastolic murmur.

Special applications of the fundamental processes of inspection, palpation, percussion, and auscultation with respect to specific organ systems and parts of the body are discussed in appropriate chapters throughout this book.

The Nutritional Assessment

Nutrition plays an important role in maintaining health and preventing disease. Although diseases of nutritional deficiency are less frequent than they once were, they have been replaced in frequency by diseases of dietary excess and imbalance, which contribute to the leading causes of illness and death in the U.S. today. Examples of health problems associated with dietary excess, imbalance, or inadequate consumption of specific nutrients include obesity, coronary artery disease, osteoporosis, cirrhosis, and diverticulitis. When illness or injury occurs, nutrition is an essential factor in promoting healing and reinforcing resistance to infection. Assessment of the person's nutritional status provides information on obesity, undernutrition, weight loss, malnutrition, deficiencies in specific nutrients, metabolic abnormalities, the effects of medications on nutrition, and special problems of the hospitalized patient.

Certain signs and symptoms that suggest possible nutritional deficiency are easy to note because they are specific. However, there are physical signs that have no relation to poor diet and that must be carefully distinguished from nutritional deficiencies. Some of the physical signs may be the result of other factors, such as poor hygiene or exposure to the sun or, possibly, systemic disorders. A physical sign that suggests a nutritional abnormality should be considered a clue rather than a diagnosis and as such should be pursued further. For example, certain signs that may appear to indicate nutritional deficiency may actually reflect other conditions, such as endocrine disorders, infectious disease, or disorders affecting digestion and absorption capacity or the excretion or storage of nutrients in the body.

Nutritional status can be determined by one or more of the following methods:

- Health history and clinical examination
- Anthropometric measurements
- Biochemical tests
- Dietary intake

Clinical Examination

The state of nutrition is reflected in a person's appearance. Although the most obvious physical sign of good nutrition is a normal body weight with respect to height, body frame, and age, other tissues can serve as indicators of general nutritional status and adequate intake of specific nutrients; these include the hair, skin, teeth, gums, mucous membranes, mouth and tongue, skeletal muscles, abdomen, lower extremities, and thyroid gland (Table 7-1).

Anthropometric Measurements

The most common anthropometric measurements include height, weight, and the circumferences of the upper arm and arm muscle. When anthropometric measurements are gathered as part of data collection, standardized equipment and procedures are used, as well as standard measurement guides. Although such measurements focus on undernutrition, they also detect obesity. See Table 7-2 for ideal adult weight. Table 7-3 provides a guide to use to determine frame size. Measurement of skinfold thickness and arm and muscle circumference is described under Nutritional Assessment of the Hospitalized Patient, later in this chapter (see Table 7-8).

Biochemical Assessment

Biochemical assessment reflects both the tissue level of a given nutrient and any abnormality of metabolism in the utilization of nutrients. These determinations are made from blood studies (serum protein, serum albumin and globulin, transferrin hemoglobin, serum vitamin A, carotene, and vitamin C) and from urine studies (creatinine, thiamine, riboflavin, niacin, and iodine). Some of these tests, while reflecting recent intake of the elements detected, can also identify suboptimal levels when there are no clinical symptoms of deficiency. (See Table 7-4 for a suggested guide for the interpretation of blood data.)

Assessment of Food Intake

The appraisal of food intake considers quantity and quality of diet and also frequency of consumption of certain food items in order to determine current or customary intake of nutrients. Commonly used methods of determining individual consumption include the food record and estimation of adequacy of the intake by 24-hour recall. These methods are discussed with the patient and explained during the taking of the diet history.

Food Record. The food record is used most often in nutritional status studies. The person is asked to keep a record of food actually consumed over a period of time, varying from 3 to 7 days. Some instructions are given for accuracy in estimating and describing the specific foods consumed. This method appears to be fairly accurate, depending on the subject's willingness to provide factual information and ability to estimate quantity of food.

24-Hour Recall. The 24-hour recall method is, as the name implies, recall of food intake over a 24-hour period. The subject is asked by the interviewer to recall all food eaten during the previous day and to estimate the quantities of the

TABLE 7–1.   *Physical Signs Indicative of Nutritional Status*

Body Area	Signs of Good Nutrition	Signs of Poor Nutrition
Hair	Shiny, lustrous; firm, healthy scalp	Dull and dry, brittle, depigmented, easily plucked
Face	Skin color uniform; healthy appearance	Skin dark over cheeks and under eyes, skin flaky, face swollen
Eyes	Bright, clear, moist	Eye membranes pale, dry (xerophthalmia); increased vascularity, cornea soft (keratomalacia)
Lips	Good color (pink), smooth	Swollen and puffy; angular lesion at corners of mouth (cheilosis)
Tongue	Deep red in appearance; surface papillae present	Smooth appearance, swollen, beefy red, sores, atrophic papillae
Teeth	Straight, no crowding, no cavities, bright	Cavities, mottled appearance (fluorosis), malpositioned
Gums	Firm, good color (pink)	Spongy, bleed easily, marginal redness, recession
Glands	No enlargement of the thyroid	Thyroid enlargement (simple goiter)
Skin	Smooth, good color, moist	Rough, dry, flaky, swollen, pale, pigmented; lack of fat under skin
Nails	Firm, pink	Spoon-shaped, ridged
Skeleton	Good posture, no malformation	Poor posture, beading of ribs, bowed legs or knock knees
Muscles	Well developed, firm	Flaccid, poor tone, wasted, underdeveloped
Extremities	No tenderness	Weak and tender; presence of edema
Abdomen	Flat	Swollen
Nervous system	Normal reflexees	Decrease in or loss of ankle and knee reflexes

TABLE 7–2.   Ideal Weights Derived From Life Insurance Statistics: 1983 Metropolitan Height and Weight Tables*

Men				Women			
Height Feet + Inches	Small Frame	Medium Frame	Large Frame	Height Feet + Inches	Small Frame	Medium Frame	Large Frame
5'2"	128–134	131–141	138–150	4'10"	102–111	109–121	118–131
5'3"	130–136	133–143	140–153	4'11"	103–113	111–123	120–134
5'4"	132–138	135–145	142–156	5'0"	104–115	113–126	122–137
5'5"	134–140	137–148	144–160	5'1"	106–118	115–129	125–140
5'6"	136–142	139–151	146–164	5'2"	108–121	118–132	128–143
5'7"	138–145	142–154	149–168	5'3"	111–124	121–135	131–147
5'8"	140–148	145–157	152–172	5'4"	114–127	124–138	134–151
5'9"	142–151	148–160	155–176	5'5"	117–130	127–141	137–155
5'10"	144–154	151–163	158–180	5'6"	120–133	130–144	140–159
5'11"	146–157	154–166	161–184	5'7"	123–136	133–147	143–163
6'0"	149–160	157–170	164–188	5'8"	126–139	136–150	146–167
6'1"	152–164	160–174	168–192	5'9"	129–142	139–153	149–170
6'2"	155–168	164–178	172–197	5'10"	132–145	142–156	152–173
6'3"	158–172	167–182	176–202	5'11"	135–148	145–159	155–176
6'4"	162–176	171–187	181–207	6'0"	138–151	148–162	158–179

* Weights at ages 25–59 based on lowest mortality. Weight in pounds according to frame (in indoor clothing weighing 5 lbs for men and 3 lbs for women; shoes with 1" heels).
(Revised Height–Weight Tables derived from life insurance statistics prepared by the Metropolitan Life Insurance Company: men and women. Copyright 1983, Metropolitan Life Insurance Company.)

food consumed. Information obtained by this method is not always representative of usual intake. For this reason, at the end of the interview the subject is asked if the previous day's food intake was a typical one. To obtain supplementary information about the typical diet, the interviewer should also ask how frequently foods from certain food groups are eaten.

The dietary and biochemical data for most nutrients provide more information than the clinical examination. The clinical examination is not sensitive enough to detect subclinical deficiencies unless such deficiencies become so advanced that overt signs develop. A low dietary intake of nutrients over a

period of time may lead to low biochemical levels and, without nutritional intervention, may result in characteristic and observable signs and symptoms.

Conducting the Interview

As was indicated in the chapter on interviewing techniques, it is important that the interviewer establish rapport with the patient in order to promote respect and trust. The success of the interviewer in eliciting pertinent information for dietary assessment depends on the quality of communication established at the outset.

In the initial stages of the interview, the interviewer introduces and explains the purpose of the interview. The rest of the session is conducted in a nondirective and exploratory way, allowing the respondent to express his feelings and thoughts. At the same time, the respondent is encouraged to respond specifically to the questions asked.

The manner in which a question is asked will influence the extent to which the respondent will cooperate. To this end, the interviewer should be nonjudgmental and avoid expressing disapproval, either directly by comment or indirectly by facial expression. For example, if the respondent says, "We eat rattlesnake meat as an appetizer," the reviewer should not express amazement or disgust by making faces or saying anything negative.

Sometimes several questions are necessary to elicit the information needed. Consider the following exchange:

Interviewer: "What time did you get out of bed yesterday?"
Respondent: "I got up at six o'clock in the morning to prepare breakfast for my husband, and I had a cup of coffee with him."

TABLE 7–3.   Determination of Frame Size by Elbow Breadth

Men		Women	
Height in 1" Heels	Elbow Breadth	Height in 1" Heels	Elbow Breadth
5'2"–5'3"	2½"–2⅞"	4'10"–4'11"	2¼"–2½"
5'4"–5'7"	2⅝"–2⅞"	5'0"–5'3"	2¼"–2½"
5'8"–5'11"	2¾"–3"	5'4"–5'7"	2⅜"–2⅝"
6'0"–6'3"	2¾"–3⅛"	5'8"–5'11"	2⅜"–2⅝"
6'4"	2⅞"–3¼"	6'0"	2½"–2¾"

To Make an Approximation of Frame Size . . . Extend arm and bend the forearm upward at a 90° angle. Keep fingers straight and turn the inside of the wrist toward the body. If you have a caliper, use it to measure the space between the two prominent bones on either side of your elbow. Without a caliper, place thumb and index finger of your other hand on these two bones. Measure the space between your fingers against a ruler or tape measure. Compare it with these tables that list elbow measurements for medium-framed men and women. Measurements lower than those listed indicate you have a small frame. Higher measurements indicate a large frame.
(Data from Metropolitan Life Insurance Company, copyright 1983.)

TABLE 7–4. *Biochemical Assessment of Nutritional Status*

	Acceptable	*Low*	*Deficient*
Plasma retinol (mg/100 ml)	>20.0	10–20.0	<10.0
Serum folate (ng/ml)	>6.0	3–6.0	<3.0
Red cell folate (ng/ml)	>150	100–150	<100
Serum vitamin B_{12} (pg/ml)	>200	100–200	<100
Serum vitamin B_6 (ng/ml)	>4.0	3–4.0	<3.0
Red cell vitamin B_6 (ng/ml)	>14.0	12–14.0	<12.0
Serum ascorbic acid (mg/100 ml)	>0.30	0.20–0.29	<0.20
Leukocyte ascorbic acid (mg/100 ml)	>15	8–15	<8

(Adapted from Roe DA. Nutritional assessment of the elderly. World Rev Nutr Diet 48:107, 1986 by Nelson R. Nutrition and Aging. Med Clin North Am 73[6]:1541, 1989.)

Interviewer: "Did you put anything in your coffee?"
Respondent: "Only a teaspoon of sugar, nothing else."
Interviewer: "Did you have anything else with your coffee?"
Respondent: "No, not at that time. I had breakfast later, around eight o'clock in the morning."

When attempting to elicit information about the kind and quantity of food eaten at a particular time, the interviewer should not ask a leading question, such as "Did you put sugar or cream in your coffee?" Also, assumptions should not be made about the size of servings. Instead, questions should be phrased so that quantities are more clearly determined. For example, to help determine the size of one hamburger eaten, the following question may be asked: "How many hamburgers were prepared out of the pound of ground meat you bought?" Another approach to determining quantities is to use food models of known sizes in estimating portions of meat, cake, or pie or to record quantities in common measurements, such as cups or spoonfuls (or according to the size of containers, when discussing intake of bottled beverages).

In recording a particular combination dish, such as Spanish rice or stew, it is useful to ask for the ingredients in the recipe, recording the largest quantities first. When recording quantities of ingredients, one notes if the quantity of the food item was raw or cooked and the number of servings provided by the recipe. When the client has finished listing the foods for the recall questionnaire, it may be helpful to read the list of foods back and ask if anything was forgotten, such as fruit, cake, candy, between-meal snacks, or cocktails.

Additional information obtained during the interview should include methods of preparing food, sources available for food (donated foods, food stamps), food-buying practices, vitamin and mineral supplements, and income range.

Evaluating the Dietary Information

Once the dietary information has been obtained, the diet must be evaluated for its nutritive value. The first method is to use acceptable food composition tables, like those issued by the Department of Agriculture. The diet is then calculated in terms of grams and milligrams of specific nutrients. The total nutritive value is then compared with the Recommended Dietary Allow-

ances, or RDAs (Table 7-5), and the nutritional evaluation is expressed in terms of percentage of adequacy for each nutrient.

A second method of evaluation is to compare the diet data with recommendations based on foods selected from various food groups for various age levels, such as the "Basic Four Food Groups: The Guide to Good Eating" (Table 7-6).

The choice of a method for dietary evaluation depends on the purpose of the assessment. If the health counselor is interested in knowing about the intake of specific nutrients, such as vitamin A, iron, or calcium, then the food record method would be the one to use. The food intake would be analyzed by consulting an official publication listing foods according to composition and nutrient content. This analysis would then be compared with the RDAs (Table 7-5) and the nutrient intake evaluated in terms of percentage of adequacy in reference to that standard.

Interpreting the 24-Hour Recall Form. An example of a 24-hour recall form is detailed in Table 7-7. This sample con-

TABLE 7-5. *Food and Nutrition Board, National Academy of Sciences: National Research Council Recommended Daily Dietary Allowances for Adults, Revised 1989*

Nutrient	*Male*	*Female*
Vitamin B_6	2.0 mg	1.6 mg
Vitamin B_{12}	2.0 μg	2.0 μg
Calcium (over age 25)	800 mg	800 mg
Calcium (under age 23)	1200 mg	1200 mg
Vitamin C	60 mg	60 mg
Folate	200 μg	180 μg
Vitamin K	80 μg	65 μg
Iron	10 mg	15 mg
Magnesium	350 mg	280 mg
Selenium	70 μg	55 μg
Zinc	15 mg	12 mg

(Data from National Research Council. Recommended Dietary Allowances, 10th ed. Washington, DC, National Academy Press, 1989. Copyright 1989 by the National Academy of Sciences.)

TABLE 7–6.   Basic Four Food Groups: The Daily Guide to Good Eating

Food Groups	Recommended Amounts		
MILK GROUP		*8-ounce cups:*	
Milk, cottage cheese, ice cream, yogurt		Children under 9	2 to 3 cups
		Children 9–12	3 to 4 cups
		Adolescents	4 or more cups
		Adults	2 or more cups
		Pregnant women	3 or more cups
		Nursing mothers	4 or more cups
MEAT GROUP	2- to 3-ounce serving; cooked, without bone; 2 servings total		
Lean beef, veal, pork, lamb, poultry, fish			
Alternatives:			
Dried beans, peas, lentils	1-cup serving, cooked		
Peanut butter	4-tablespoons serving		
Eggs	2		
VEGETABLES, FRUITS	½-cup serving, 1 piece fruit; 4 servings total		
Dark green or yellow	1 serving, vitamin A rich		
Citrus fruit or vegetable	1 serving, vitamin C rich—or 2 servings of a fair source		
Other vegetables and fruits	2 or more servings		
BREADS AND CEREALS	4 servings total		
Bread, rolls, biscuits, muffins	1 slice or small piece		
Ready-to-eat cereals	1-ounce serving		
Cooked cereal, cornmeal, grits, macaroni, noodles, rice, spaghetti	½- to ¾-cup serving, cooked		
MISCELLANEOUS GROUP			
Cream, bacon, butter, margarine, shortening, oil, salad dressing, olives, jam, jelly, sugar, candy, cake, pie, carbonated beverages, relishes, alcoholic beverages, snack foods, pretzels, potato chips, etc.	Provide mostly calories for the day's total intake		

tains dietary information about Mrs. Brown, a 24-year-old housewife, indicating the different kinds of food she consumed, the times during the day when she consumed them, and the quantities she consumed, as measured in household units. The questionnaire indicates that Mrs. Brown's diet is adequate with respect to the bread and cereal group and foods rich in vitamin A, low in food sources of calcium and vitamin C, and only slightly lacking in servings of protein foods. On the other hand, Mrs. Brown's 24-hour recall record shows an excessive intake of high-calorie foods from the miscellaneous food group. This food consumption practice is reflected in her weight, which is 19% over acceptable normal standards—enough to characterize her as obese.

A plan of action for nutritional intervention is based on the results of the dietary assessment and the client's profile. Two main objectives derived from the nutritional assessment and evaluation are:

- Appropriate food selection for a balanced diet
- Appropriate food intake for weight control

Nutritional Assessment of the Hospitalized Patient

Many disease conditions produce metabolic alterations that result in *negative nitrogen balance* (when nitrogen output exceeds nitrogen intake). When these conditions are coupled with anorexia, they can lead to malnutrition. It is known that malnutrition interferes with wound healing, increases susceptibility to infection, and contributes to prolonged bed confinement in the hospital population.

A poor nutritional status has been identified as a problem that may occur during hospitalization. Additionally, it has been identified as a significant factor in determining the outcome of illness and hospitalization in many patients. The factors that contribute to poor nutritional status of hospitalized patients include:

- Prolonged use of glucose and saline IV therapy
- Withholding of meals because of diagnostic tests

TABLE 7–7. *24-Hour Recall Questionnaire for Adults*

Name: *Mrs. Brown*	Date of recall: *3/4*	Day of recall: *Tuesday*	
Age: *24 Years*	Male _____	Female ✓	Occupation: *Housewife*
Height (in): *64*	Weight (lb): *148*	Ideal weight (lb): *124*	% of ideal: *119%*

Ingestion Period	Kinds of Foods and Description	Amount in Household Units	Frequency of Consumption of Various Foods	Times per Day-Week-Month		
				×D	×W	×M
6:00 AM	Coffee	1 cup	Milk, whole		4	
	Sugar	1 tsp	Milk, skin			
	Cream	2 tbsp	Yogurt		3	
			Cheese		3	
8:00 AM	Cornflakes	1 cup	Ice cream		5	
	Milk, whole	½ cup	Beef		4	
			Pork			1
12:00 NOON	Sandwich		Lamb			1
	Bread, white	2 slices	Fish		1	
	Peanut butter	2 tbsp	Poultry		3	
	Apple	1 small	Eggs		5	
	Coffee	1 cup	Cream	3		
	Sugar	1 tsp	Butter		3	
	Cream	2 tbsp	Margarine	3		
			Oil	1		
3:00 PM	Coca-Cola, regular	1 (12-ounce can)	Salad dressings	1		
	Almond Joy bar	1½ ounces	Vegetables			
			Green-yellow	1		
6:30 PM	Fried filet of sole	3 ounces	Citrus fruits		3	
	Green beans	½ cup	Legumes			
	Boiled potato	1 medium	Beans		1	
	Lettuce salad	1 cup	Chick peas			1
	French dressing	2 tbsp	Lentils			
	Muffin	1 small	Potatoes	1		
	Coffee	1 cup	Breads	3		
	Sugar	1 tsp	Pastas		4	
	Cream	2 tbsp	Rice			
			Cakes	1		
10:30 PM	Chocolate cake (8″ diam.)	1/16 cake	Pies		4	
	Coca-Cola, regular	1 (12-ounce can)	Candy bars	1		
			Jams-jellies		5	
			Sugar	3		
			Alcoholic beverage			
			Carbonated beverage	3		
			Coffee, tea	3		
			Snack foods	1		
			Vitamin supplement			
			Mineral supplement			

- Use of tube feedings in inadequate amounts and of uncertain composition
- Failure to recognize increased nutritional needs resulting from injury or illness

Many medications also influence the nutritional status of patients. Some of these medications may have a specific appetite depressant effect, may irritate the mucosa, or may cause nausea and vomiting. Others may influence bacterial flora in the intestine or directly affect nutrient absorption so that secondary malnutrition results.

The body in starvation may convert protein to glucose for energy; the result is persistent loss of muscle tissue. One sensitive indicator of the body's gain or loss of protein is its *nitrogen balance*. An adult is said to be in *nitrogen equilibrium* when the nitrogen intake (from food) equals the nitrogen output (in urine, feces, and perspiration); it is a sign of health. A *positive nitrogen balance* exists when nitrogen intake exceeds nitrogen output and indicates tissue growth, such as occurs during pregnancy, childhood, recovery from surgery, and rebuilding of wasted tissue. Negative nitrogen balance indicates that tissue is breaking down faster than it is being replaced. It can be

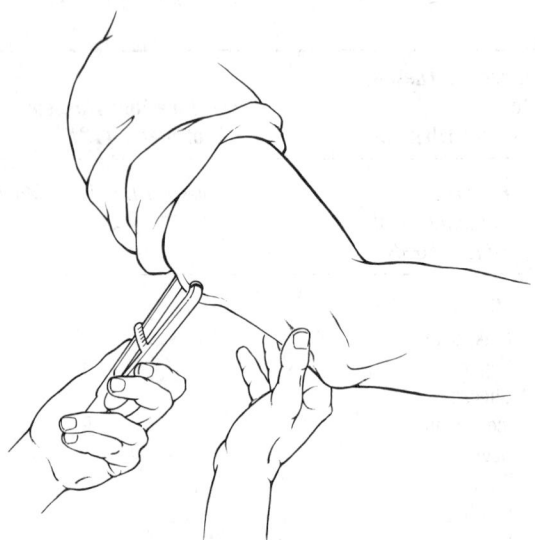

Figure 7-2. Skinfold calipers for measurement of skinfold thickness.

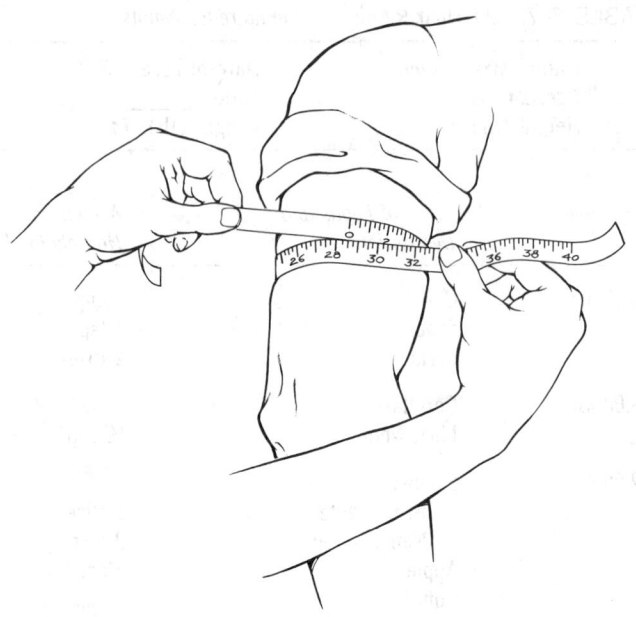

Figure 7-3. Measurement of arm muscle circumference.

brought about by fever, surgery, burns, and other debilitating diseases, as well as by starvation. For instance, each gram of nitrogen loss in excess of intake represents the depletion of 6.25 g of protein or 25 g of muscle tissue. Therefore, a negative nitrogen balance of 10 g/day for 10 days could mean the wasting of 2.5 kg (5.5 pounds) of muscle tissue.

The hospital may have a metabolic nutrition support unit, with a specially trained team consisting of a physician, a pharmacist, a nurse, and a dietitian. The following parameters are used for nutritional assessment of the hospitalized patient:

1. Anthropometric measurement
   Weight/height
   Triceps skinfold thickness
   Mid-arm and arm muscle circumferences
2. Biochemical measurements
   Albumin
   Transferrin
   Total lymphocyte count
   Creatinine/height index
   Urinary tests (sodium, potassium, urea, creatinine)

Weight loss is an extremely important measurement because it reflects inadequate calorie intake. In the semistarved patient, weight loss indicates an increased loss of protein from the body cell mass. With respect to *anthropometric measurements* for protein–calorie malnutrition, the best available indicators are triceps skinfold thickness (Fig. 7-2), which indicates fat stores, and muscle circumference (Fig. 7-3), which indicates the state of muscle protein (Table 7-8).

Low serum albumin and *transferrin* levels are useful measures of visceral protein deficits in adults and are expressed as percentages of normal values (Table 7-9). Both are indicators of the degree of malnutrition. Serial measurements of these, as well as prealbumin levels, are used to assess the results of nutritional therapy.

Reduced numbers of lymphocytes in hospitalized patients who become acutely malnourished as a result of stress and low-calorie feeding are associated with impairment of cellular immunity.

TABLE 7-8.   *Standard Values and Deficiency Levels for Anthropometric Measurements for Adults*

	Standard	90% of Standard	80% of Standard	70% of Standard	60% of Standard
MID-ARM CIRCUMFERENCE (cm)					
Male	29.3	26.3	23.4	20.5	17.6
Female	28.5	25.7	22.8	20.0	17.1
TRICEPS SKINFOLD (mm)					
Male	12.5	11.3	10.0	8.8	7.5
Female	16.5	14.9	13.2	11.6	9.0
MID-ARM MUSCLE CIRCUMFERENCE (cm)					
Male	25.3	22.8	20.2	17.7	15.2
Female	23.2	20.9	18.6	16.2	13.9

(Dudek SG, Nutrition Handbook for Nursing Practice. Philadelphia, JB Lippincott, 1987.)

TABLE 7-9. *Standards for Laboratory Indices*

Serum Values	Percent Deficiency		
	Mild	Moderate	Severe
Albumin (g/dl)	3.2–3.5	2.8–3.2	<2.8
Transferrin (mg/dl)	180–200	160–180	<160
Total lymphocyte count (n/mm^3)	1800–5000	900–1500	<900

(Adapted from Steffee WP. Nutritional support of elderly patients. Clin Consult Nutr Support 2:5, 1982 by Nelson R. Nutrition and Aging. Med Clin North Am 73[6]:1541, 1989.)

Information about *electrolyte balance* provides an assessment of kidney function as a metabolic response to infused electrolytes. The creatinine/height index calculated over a 24-hour period assesses the metabolically active tissue and indicates the degree of protein depletion, comparing expected body mass for height and actual body cell mass.

The nurse is in a position to take part in nutrition screening of her patients by devising her own nutrition record as a tool, if the hospital does not have a separate screening form. Such a brief assessment guide can help to identify patients who need more intensive nutritional evaluation. The findings can then be communicated to the dietitian and the rest of the team for further assessment and for clinical nutrition intervention.

Diagnostic Categories of Malnutrition

After the data for nutritional assessment have been collected, determination of the category of malnutrition that applies to the individual patient becomes the first consideration in order to plan an effective regimen for nutritional support of the hospitalized patient. Table 7-9 indicates the three categories of nutritional deficiency or malnutrition.

Gerontologic Considerations

The goal of diet therapy in the elderly is to maintain nutrition and replace nutrient losses within the framework of the patient's condition and environment. This may take patience and creativity.

Elderly persons may take excessive and inappropriate medications. The number of adverse reactions increases proportionately with the number of prescribed and over-the-counter drugs taken. Age-related physiologic and pathophysiologic changes may alter the metabolism and elimination of many drugs. Consequently, drugs can influence food intake by producing side effects such as nausea, vomiting, and decreased appetite. They may alter nutrient metabolism by interfering with distribution, utilization, and storage of nutrients. Disorders affecting any part of the gastrointestinal tract can be expected to alter nutritional requirements and health status in patients of any age; however, they are likely to occur quickly and more frequently in the elderly.

Furthermore, in the elderly, nutritional problems often occur or are precipitated by such infectious illnesses as pneumonia, urinary tract infections, and herpes zoster. Like malnutrition, acute and chronic diseases may affect the metabolism and utilization of nutrients, which already are altered because of the aging process. The goal obviously is to prevent infections or to shorten such illnesses by prescribing antibiotics and using available vaccines.

Even the well elderly may be nutritionally at risk because of limited ability to shop and cook, financial hardship, and the fact that they often eat alone. Additionally, reduction in physical exercise with age without concomitant changes in carbohydrate intake places the elderly at risk of obesity.

Chapter Summary

Physical assessment involves the use of many of the nurse's senses—touch, sight, hearing, smell—and effective communication skills to obtain data for further action. Repeated practice or use of these skills will improve the nurse's ability to pick up subtle deviations from normal and changes from the patient's usual baseline.

Assessment of the patient's nutritional status may provide information about the patient's previous dietary intake, his understanding of the principles of good nutrition, and the availability of resources for purchase and consumption of an adequate diet. Nutritional assessment may identify those patients who are poorly nourished and at risk for complications of illness and hospitalization because of poor nutrition. Early detection of these risks enables the nurse to intervene to prevent their occurrence or minimize their severity.

Bibliography
Books
Bates B. A Guide to Physical Examination and History Taking, 5th ed. Philadelphia, JB Lippincott, 1991.

Bernstein L and Bernstein RS. Interviewing: A Guide for Health Professionals, 4th ed. New York, Appleton and Lange, 1985.

Bowers AC and Thompson JM. Clinical Manual of Health Assessment. St Louis, CV Mosby, 1988.

DeGowin E and DeGowin R. Bedside Diagnostic Examination, 5th ed. New York, Macmillan, 1987.

Dudek SG. Nutrition Handbook for Nursing Practice. Philadelphia, JB Lippincott, 1987.

Gordon M. Manual of Nursing Diagnosis 1988–1989. St Louis, CV Mosby, 1989.

Gordon M. Nursing Diagnosis: Process and Application. New York, McGraw-Hill, 1987.

Guzzetta CE et al. Clinical Assessment Tools for Use with Nursing Diagnosis. St Louis, CV Mosby, 1989.

Hagopian GA, Hymovich DP, and Lynaugh JE. Clinical Assessment: A Guide for Study and Practice. Philadelphia, JB Lippincott, 1987.

Lohr KN and Mock GA (eds). Advances in Assessment of Health Status. Washington, DC, National Academy Press, 1989.

Malasanos L, Barkauskas V, and Stoltengerg–Allen K. Health Assessment, 4th ed. St Louis, CV Mosby, 1989.

Murray RB and Zentner JP. Nursing Assessment and Health Promotion Strategies Through the Life Span. East Norwalk, CT, Appleton and Lange, 1989.

National Research Council. Recommended Dietary Allowances, 10th ed. Washington, DC, National Academy Press, 1989.

Seidel H et al. Mosby's Guide to Physical Examination. St Louis, CV Mosby, 1990.

U.S. Department of Health and Human Services. Public Health Service. Surgeon General's Report on Nutrition and Health. Washington, DC, U.S. Government Printing Office, 1988.

Journals

General Assessment

Applegate WB, Blass JP, and Williams TF. Instruments for the functional assessment of older patients. N Engl J Med 1990 Apr 26; 322(17): 1207–1214.

Barry PP and Ibarra M. Multidimensional assessment of the elderly. Hosp Pract [Off] 1990 Apr 15; 25(4):117–121, 124, 127–128.

Barry PP. Primary care evaluation of the elderly for elective surgery. Geriatrics 1987 Apr; 42(4):77–85.

Becker KL and Stevens SA. Performing in-depth abdominal assessment. Nursing 1988 Jun; 18(6):59–64.

Becker KL and Stevens SA. Get in touch and in tune with cardiac assessment, Part 1. Nursing 1988 Mar; 18(3):51–55.

Brady PF. Labeling of confusion in the elderly. J Gerontol Nurs 1987 Jun; 13(6):29–32.

Brown MD. Functional assessment of the elderly. J Gerontol Nurs 1988 May; 14(5):13–17.

Buchanan BF. Functional assessment: Measurement with the Barthel Index and PULSES Profile. Home Healthcare Nurse 1986 Nov/Dec; 4(6): 11, 14–17.

Daly MP. The medical evaluation of the elderly preoperative patient. Med Clin North Am 1989 Jun; 16(2):361–376.

Engstrom JL. Assessment of the reliability of physical measures. Res Nurs Health 1988 Dec; 11(6):383–389.

Heath JM. Comprehensive functional assessment of the elderly. Med Clin North Am 1989 Jun; 16(2):305–327.

Henderson ML. Altered presentations. Assessing the elderly, system by system, Part 2. Am J Nurs 1985 Oct; 85(10):1104–1106.

Hoeman SP. Cultural assessment in rehabilitation nursing practice. Nurs Clin North Am 1989 Mar; 24(1):277–287.

Holloran EJ. Computerized nurse assessments. Nurs Health Care 1988 Nov/Dec; 9(9):497–499.

Jess LW. Investigating impaired mental status—An assessment guide you can use. Nursing 1988 Jun; 18(6):42–49.

Kallman H and May HJ. Mental status assessment in the elderly. Med Clin North Am 1989 Jun; 16(2):329–347.

Linderborn KM. The need to assess dementia. J Gerontol Nurs 1988 Jan; 14(1):35–39.

McConnell EA. Getting the feel of lymph node assessment. Nursing 1988 Aug; 18(8):55–57.

McEwan RT. Issues in evaluation: Evaluating assessments of elderly people using a combination of methods. J Adv Nurs 1989 Feb; 14(2):103–110.

Miracle VA. Get in touch and in tune with cardiac assessment, Part 2. Nursing 1988 Apr; 18(4):41–47.

Moreland BJ. A nursing form for gynecology patient assessment. Oncol Nurs Forum 1987 Mar/Apr; 14(2):19–23.

Morrison EG. Nursing assessment: What do nurses want to know? West J Nurs Res 1989 Aug; 11(4):469–476.

Murray JL. Health maintenance. Med Clin North Am 1989 Jun; 16(2):289–303.

National Institutes of Health. National Institutes of Health Consensus Development Conference Statement: Geriatric assessment methods for clinical decision-making. J Am Geriatr Soc 1988 Apr; 36(4):342–347.

Nesbitt B. Nursing diagnosis in age-related changes. J Gerontol Nurs 1988 Jul; 14(7):7–12.

Ramsdell JW et al. The yield of a home visit in the assessment of geriatric patients. J Am Geriatr Soc 1989 Jan; 37(1):17–24.

Runciman P. Health assessment of the elderly at home: The case for shared learning. J Adv Nurs 1989 Feb; 14(2):111–119.

Santo–Novak DA. Seven keys to assessing the elderly. Nursing 1988 Aug; 18(8):60–63.

Smith CE. Assessing bowel sounds—More than just listening. Nursing 1988 Feb; 18(2):42–43.

Stark JL. A quick guide to urinary tract assessment. Nursing 1988 Jul; 18(7): 56–58.

Stevens SA and Becker KL. How to perform picture-perfect respiratory assessment. Nursing 1988 Jan; 18(1):57–63.

Stevens SA and Becker KL. A simple, step-by-step approach to neurological assessment, Part 1. Nursing 1988 Sep; 18(9):53–61.

Stevens SA and Becker KL. A simple, step-by-step approach to neurological assessment, Part 2. Nursing 1988 Oct; 18(10):51–58.

Tompkins ES. In support of the discipline of nursing: A nursing assessment. Nursing Connections 1989 Fall; 2(3):21–29.

Utley R. Mid-arm circumference. Estimating patients' weight. Dimens Crit Care Nurs 1990 Mar/Apr; 9(2):75–81.

Nutritional Assessment

Berger S. The implementation of dietary guidelines—Ways and difficulties. Am J Clin Nutr 1987 May; 45(Suppl 5):1383–1389.

Cashman MD and Wightkin WT. Geriatric malnutrition: Recognition and prevention. Compr Ther 1987 Mar; 13(3):45–51.

Collinsworth R and Boyle K. Nutritional assessment of the elderly. J Gerontol Nurs 1989 Dec; 15(12):17–21.

Curtas S, Chapman G, and Maguid MM. Evaluation of nutritional status. Nurs Clin North Am 1989 Jun; 24(2):301–313.

Fahey PJ, Boltri JM, and Monk JS. Key issues in nutrition. Supplementation through adulthood and old age. Postgrad Med 1987 May 1; 81(6): 12–125, 128.

Nelson RC and Franzi LR. Nutrition and aging. Med Clin North Am 1989 Nov; 73(6):1531–1550.

Nixon DW. Nutrition and cancer: American Cancer Society guidelines, programs, and initiatives. CA 1990 Mar/Apr; 40(2):71–75.

Schlundt DG. Accuracy and reliability of nutrient intake estimates. J Nutr 1988 Dec; 118(2):1432–1435.

Simopoulos AP. Nutrition and fitness. J Am Med Assoc 1989 May 19; 261(19):2862–2863.

Suter PM and Russel RM. Vitamin requirements of the elderly. Am J Clin Nutr 1987 Mar; 45(3):501–512.

U.S. Department of Health and Human Services. Diet, nutrition, and cancer prevention: The good news. (NIH Publication No. 87–2878.) National Institutes of Health, 1986.

Zheng JJ and Rosenberg IH. What is the nutritional status of the elderly? Geriatrics 1989 Jun; 44(6):57–58, 60, 63–64.

Documentation

Amino PA. Perioperative nursing documentation. Developing the record and using care plans. AORN J 1987 Jul; 46(1):73–86.

Bergerson SR. More about charting with a jury in mind. Nursing 1988 Apr; 18(2):51–55.

Cline A. Streamlined documentation through exceptional charting. Nurs Manage 1989 Feb; 20(2):62–64.

Eggland ET. Charting: Document your care daily and fully. Nursing 1988 Nov; 18(11):76–84.

Haller KB. Systematic documentation of practice. MCN 1987 Mar/Apr; 12(2):152.

Herth KA. The root of it all. Genograms as a nursing assessment tool. J Gerontol Nurs 1989 Dec; 15(12):32–37.

Morrisey-Ross M. Documentation. If you haven't written it, you haven't done it. Nurs Clin North Am 1988 Jun; 23(2):363–371.

unit 3

Biophysical and Psychosocial Concepts Related to Health and Illness

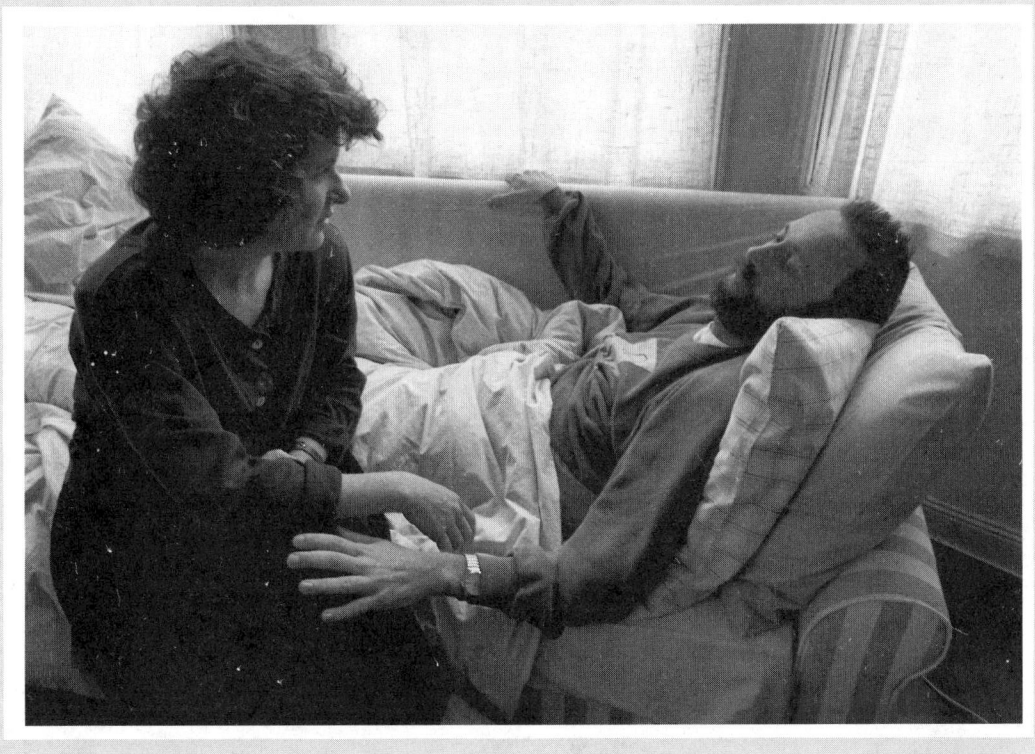

8

Homeostasis and Pathophysiologic Processes

Learning Objectives

On completion of this chapter, the learner will be able to:

1. Relate the principles of internal constancy, homeostasis, and adaptation to the concept of steady state
2. Identify the significance of the body's compensatory mechanisms in the promotion of adaptation and the maintenance of the steady state
3. Describe the relationship of the process of negative feedback to the maintenance of the steady state
4. Relate the concept of biofeedback to the maintenance of the steady state
5. Compare the adaptive processes of hypertrophy, atrophy, hyperplasia, and metaplasia
6. Identify external and internal environmental factors that can cause cellular injury and cellular death
7. Describe the inflammatory and reparative processes
8. Compare healing by regeneration to healing by replacement
9. Assess the health patterns of an individual and their effects on maintenance of the steady state
10. Assess a patient with regard to the stressors to which he is exposed and his physiologic responses to these stressors

When the body is threatened or suffers an injury, its response may involve functional and structural changes; these changes may be adaptive or maladaptive. The defense mechanisms that the body can mount will determine the difference between adaptation and maladaptation, health and disease. Physiology is the study of the functional activities of the living organism and its parts. *Pathophysiology* is the study of *disordered* function of the body. *Mechanisms* are patterns of action performed by different parts of the body to serve a common goal. These mechanisms may be compensatory to restore a lost balance, such as hyperpnea to correct an oxygen deficit and lactic acid excess following running. Or, they may be pathophysiologic, such as failure of the heart, leading to sodium and water retention and high venous pressure, which contribute to further disorder. These mechanisms give rise to signs that may be observed by the nurse or symptoms that may be reported by the patient. Based on these observations and a knowledge of the physiologic processes involved, the nurse can determine the existence of a problem and plan her course of action to treat it.

Dynamic Balance: The Steady State

Physiologic mechanisms must be understood in the context of the body as a whole. Man, as a living system, has both an internal and an external environment. Information and matter are continuously exchanged between one environment and the other. Within the body itself, each organ, tissue, and cell is also a system or subsystem of the whole, each with its own internal and external environment, each exchanging information and matter (Fig. 8-1). The goal of the interaction of the body's subsystems is to produce a dynamic balance or steady state, so that all are in harmony with each other, just as man, as an individual, seeks harmony with those with whom he interacts. For a better understanding of the concept of steady state, the development of the principles of internal constancy, homeostasis, and adaptation will be described.

Internal Constancy, Homeostasis, and Adaptation

Claude Bernard, a French physiologist in the 19th century, developed the biologic principle that for a "free life" there must be a *constancy* or "fixity of the internal milieu," despite changes in the external environment. The internal milieu he addressed was the fluid that bathes the cells, and the constancy was maintained by physiologic and biochemical processes; his principle implied a static process.

Later, Walter B. Cannon coined the term *homeostasis* to refer to this stability of the internal environment, which he said was coordinated by homeostatic or compensatory processes that responded to changes in the internal environment. Any change within the internal environment initiated a righting response or a response to minimize the change. These processes sought physiochemical balance and were under involuntary control.

Dubos (1965) took the change or dynamic nature of responses one step further. He stated that there are two complementary concepts: homeostasis and adaptation. Homeostasis refers to the necessary adjustments that the body can make *rapidly* to maintain its internal composition within an acceptable range, while adaptation refers to the adjustments that develop *over time*. Dubos also emphasized that there are acceptable ranges of response to stimuli and that these will vary for different individuals; "absolute constancy is only a concept of the ideal." Homeostasis and adaptation are both necessary for survival in a changing world.

Maintenance of the Steady State

The terms *steady state* and *dynamic equilibrium*, terms derived from general systems theory, describe this condition of internal constancy and harmony with the external environment. This harmony and constancy are necessary for a state of good health. When a change or stress occurs that produces a deviation in any body parameter from its stable range (disrupts the constancy), adjustment processes are initiated to restore and maintain the dynamic balance. When these adjustment processes, or compensatory mechanisms, are not adequate, the steady state is threatened, function will become disordered, and pathophysiologic mechanisms will become operative. The pathophysiologic mechanisms can lead to disease, and they are also active during disease. *Disease* is a threat to the steady state and is defined as any process or event that promotes a change in the internal environment that results in loss or disruption of cell function and thus limits man's freedom to act in the external world.

An analogy can be made to the pendulum of a clock. As it swings to and fro, maintaining correct time, it is in dynamic balance, or a steady state. Someone tips the clock, and the pendulum swings a bit to one side but is still able to maintain reasonably accurate time. The clock is tipped more; now the pendulum swings more to one side than the other, and with each swing the pendulum's own weight increases the erratic movement. The clock's functional ability to provide accurate time is damaged and, if nothing intervenes, may be destroyed altogether.

Nursing Implications

It is important for the nurse to realize that the optimal point of intervention to promote health is during the stage when the individual's own compensatory processes are still functioning. It is therefore imperative to be able to relate the presenting signs and symptoms to the physiology they represent. This makes it possible to identify the individual's position on the continuum of function, from health and compensation to pathophysiology and disease. Thus, if a middle-aged woman presented for a checkup and was found to be overweight, with a blood pressure of 130/85 mm Hg, the nurse would most likely counsel her with respect to diet and activity. She would encourage weight loss; question her intake of salt, which affects her fluid balance, and her intake of caffeine, for its stimulant effect; and discuss ways to decrease the stress in her life. The ultimate goal of her activities would be to control her blood pressure and prevent hypertension.

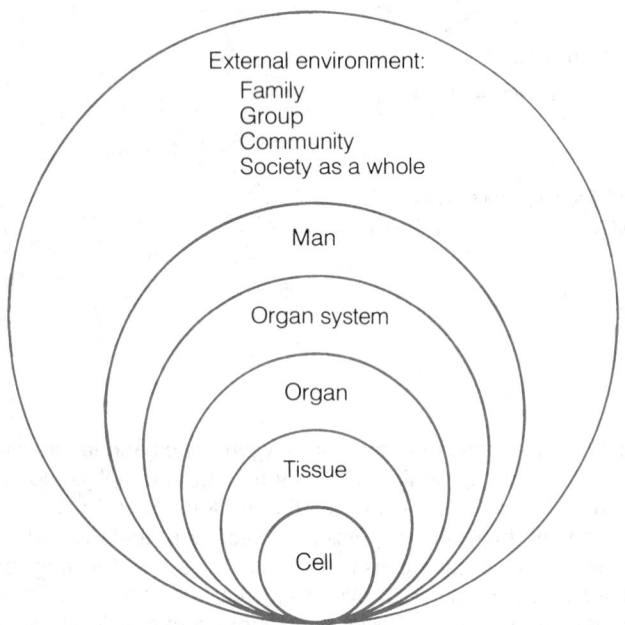

Figure 8–1.   Constellation of systems. Each system is a subsystem of the larger system (suprasystem) of which it is a part. In this figure the cell is the smallest system, being a subsystem of all other systems.

Another reason for becoming well versed in symptomatology and physiology is that there are many diseases, too numerous to memorize. However, the number of physiologic processes is limited. Having a knowledge of these processes makes it possible to detect the abnormalities or the degree of risk involved and to intervene effectively.

Pathophysiologic Processes at the Cellular Level

The processes described may occur at all levels of the biologic organism. (They also occur in society and populations, but in this chapter we will focus on the physiology of the individual.) If the cell is considered the smallest unit or subsystem (tissues being aggregates of cells, organs aggregates of tissues, etc.), the processes of health and disease, adaptation and maladaptation may all occur at the cellular level. Indeed, pathologic processes are described at the subcellular or molecular level. The cell may then be described as existing on a continuum of function and structure, from the normal cell, to the adapted cell, to the injured or diseased cell, to the dead cell (Fig. 8-2).

Nature of Changes

Changes from one state to another may occur rapidly and may not be readily detectable, because each state does not have distinct or discrete boundaries, and disease represents an extension and distortion of normal processes. For example, tanning of the skin is an adaptive, morphologic response to exposure to the rays of the sun. If the exposure is continued, however, sunburn and injury may occur, and some cells may die, as is evidenced by "peeling."

The earliest changes occur at the molecular or subcellular level and are not easily detectable. Not until steady-state functions or structures are altered do changes become apparent. With cell injury some changes may be reversible, whereas others are lethal and lead to death. Also, the adapted state is generally at a lower functional level in that it is maintained by the use of additional energy or reserves or by a morphologic change of tissue cells into a less specific, or less differentiated, cell type.

Responses to Stimuli/Stressors

Different cells and tissues respond to stimuli with different patterns and rates of response, some being more vulnerable to one type of stimulus or stressor than another. Thus, cardiac muscle cells respond to hypoxia (inadequate oxygenation) more quickly than smooth muscle cells. The cell involved, its ability to adapt, and its physiologic state are determinants of the response.

Other determinants of the response are the type or nature of the stressor, its duration, and its severity. For example, a drug tolerance to regular small amounts of a barbiturate may develop, but one large dose may result in unconsciousness and death.

Nursing Implications

Organs are capable of a wide range of activity, for example, the normal heart rate and the normal respiratory rate and volume can vary markedly; thus, the ability of the body to compensate and adapt to different situations and environmental conditions is remarkable. When injury does occur, it may be reversible up to a point; the earliest morphologic changes may be regarded as "fingerprints of disease; when the damage is slight the prints can be erased" (Boyd and Sheldon, 1988). For the health of the patient, it is imperative to detect these early changes.

Control of the Steady State: Control Systems

The concept of the cell on a continuum of function and structure (Fig. 8-2) includes the relationship of the "normal cell" and the "adapted cell" to compensatory mechanisms. These mechanisms include the adjustment processes that are continuously occurring in the body to maintain the dynamic balance, or steady state. These processes are primarily regulated by the autonomic nervous system and the endocrine system, and control is achieved through negative feedback.

Negative Feedback Process

Through the process of negative feedback, deviations from a predetermined set point or range of adaptability are detected,

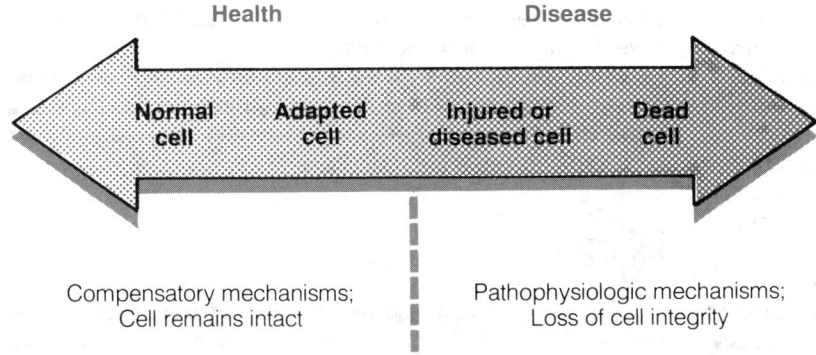

Figure 8–2. The cell on a continuum of function and structure. Changes in the cell are not as easily discerned as the diagram depicts. The point at which compensation is lost and pathophysiology begins is not clearly defined.

and these trigger a response in which the action offsets the deviation. Blood pressure, acid–base balance, blood glucose level, body temperature, and fluid and electrolyte balance are examples of parameters regulated through such compensatory mechanisms. Each of these parameters has a range for optimal function. If there is either an excess or a deficiency, negative feedback will trigger activity to cause a return to the optimal level.

A familiar illustration of the negative feedback process in a simple control system is the control of room temperature. The door is opened and a cold draft reduces room temperature, which is detected by a thermometer and relayed to a thermostat. The thermostat compares this temperature with a preset reference point. Detecting that the room is cooler, it sends a message to the furnace to fire up, with the effect of heating the room air. The new temperature is fed into the thermostat, and if it is equal to the reference point, the furnace is signaled to shut off. This is *negative feedback*, which is a series of actions in which the goal is to counter the influence of an initiating stimulus or disturbance. It does not change the disturbance, only its effect. In this case, the door was not closed, but its cooling effect was offset by the heating action of the furnace.

Organs of Homeostasis or Adjustment.   Most of the human body's control systems are integrated at the level of the brain in the nervous and endocrine systems. Control activities involve detecting deviations from the predetermined reference point and stimulating compensatory responses in the muscles and glands of the body. The major organs affected are the heart, lungs, kidneys, liver, gastrointestinal tract, and skin. When stimulated, these organs alter the rate of their activity or the amount of secretions they produce. They have been called the organs of homeostasis or adjustment.

Local Responses: Feedback Loops.   In addition to the responses controlled by the above system, there are local responses that consist of small feedback loops in a group of cells or tissues. The cells detect a change in their immediate environment and initiate an action to counteract its effect. For example, the accumulation of lactic acid in an exercised muscle will stimulate dilation of blood vessels in the area to increase blood flow and improve the delivery of oxygen and removal of waste products.

The net result of the activities of the control system through feedback loops is a dynamic equilibrium, a steady state achieved by the continuous, variable action of the organs of adjustment along with continuous small exchanges of chemical substances between cells, interstitial fluid, and blood throughout the body. For example, an increase in the carbon dioxide concentration of the extracellular fluid leads to increased pulmonary ventilation, which in turn decreases the carbon dioxide level. The increased carbon dioxide raises the hydrogen ion concentration of the blood. This is detected by chemosensitive receptors in the respiratory control center of the medulla. This stimulates an increase in the rate of discharge of the inspiratory neurons, which innervate the diaphragm and intercostal muscles, and increase the rate of respiration. Excess carbon dioxide is exhaled, the hydrogen ion concentration returns to normal, and the chemically sensitive neurons are no longer stimulated.

Positive Feedback.   Before concluding this discussion, another type of feedback, positive feedback, should be mentioned. Positive feedback perpetuates the chain of events set in motion by the original disturbance. Compensation does not occur, and the system becomes more out of balance; disorder and disintegration occur. (There are some exceptions to this: blood clotting in humans, for example, is an important positive feedback mechanism.)

Cellular Adaptation and Injury

Cells are complex units dynamically responding to the changing demands and stresses of daily life. They possess a maintenance function and a specialized function: the maintenance function refers to the activities the cell must perform with respect to itself; specialized functions are those that the cell performs in relation to the tissues and organs of which it is a part. Individual cells may cease to function without posing a threat to the organism; however, as the dead cells multiply, the specialized functions are altered and the individual's health is threatened.

Common Adaptations

Cells can adapt to environmental stress by structural and functional changes. A number of these adaptations are common and include hypertrophy, atrophy, hyperplasia, and metaplasia (Table 8-1).

Hypertrophy and Atrophy.   Hypertrophy and atrophy lead to changes in the size of cells and hence the size of the organs they form. Compensatory hypertrophy resulting in an enlarged muscle mass commonly occurs in skeletal and cardiac muscle under prolonged, increased workloads. Atrophy can be the consequence of a disease or of disuse but is more readily associated with aging. There is a decrease in cell and organ size that affects, principally, skeletal muscle, secondary sex organs, the heart, and the brain.

Hyperplasia.   Hyperplasia is an increase in the number of new cells in an organ or tissue; as cells multiply, volume increases. It is a mitotic response, but it is reversible when the stimulus is removed. This distinguishes it from neoplasia or malignant growth, which continues after the stimulus is removed. Hyperplasia may be hormonally induced.

Metaplasia.   Metaplasia is a cell transformation in which a highly specialized cell changes to a less specialized cell. This serves a protective function, because the less specialized cell is more resistant to the stress that stimulated the change. In smokers, the ciliated columnar epithelium lining the bronchi is replaced by squamous epithelium. The squamous cells can survive; however, loss of the cilia and protective mucus can have damaging consequences.

Thus, the adaptations allow the survival of the organism. They reflect changes in the normal cell in response to stress. If the stress continues, the function of the adapted cell may succumb and cell injury will occur.

Injury

Injury is defined as a disorder in steady-state regulation; any stressor that alters the ability of the cell or system to maintain

TABLE 8-1. *Cellular Adaptation*

Change	Stimulus	Example
HYPERTROPHY Increase in cell size, leading to increase in organ size	Increased workload	Leg muscles of runner Arm muscles of tennis player Cardiac muscle in person with hypertension
ATROPHY Shrinkage in size of cell, leading to decrease in organ size	Decrease in: 1. Use 2. Blood supply 3. Nutrition 4. Hormonal stimulation 5. Innervation	Secondary sex organs in aging person Extremity immobilized in plaster cast
HYPERPLASIA Increase in number of new cells (increase in mitosis)	Hormonal influence Tissue removal or destruction	Breast changes of a girl in puberty or of a pregnant woman Regeneration of liver cells New red blood cells in blood loss
METAPLASIA Transformation of one adult cell type to another (reversible)	Stress applied to highly specialized cell	Changes in epithelial cells lining bronchi in response to smoke irritation (cells become less specialized)

the optimal balance of its adjustment processes will lead to injury. Structural and functional damage then occurs, which may be reversible, permitting recovery, or irreversible, leading to death. Homeostatic adjustments are concerned with the small, minute-by-minute changes within the body's systems. With adaptive changes, compensation occurs and a steady state is achieved, although it may be at new levels; with injury, steady-state regulation is lost and changes in functioning ensue.

Causes of disorder and injury in the system (cell, tissue, organ, body) may arise from the external or internal environment of the system (Fig. 8-3). Causes may include the following: physical agents, chemical agents, infectious agents, immune mechanisms, genetic defects, hypoxia, and nutritional imbalance.

The most common causes are hypoxia, chemical injury, and infectious agents. An additional factor is that the presence of one injury makes the system more susceptible to another; for example, inadequate oxygenation and nutritional deficiencies make the system vulnerable to infection. These agents act at the cellular level by damaging or destroying the following:

- The integrity of the cell membrane, necessary for ionic balance
- The cell's ability to transform energy (aerobic respiration, production of adenosine triphosphate [ATP])
- The cell's ability to synthesize enzymes and other necessary proteins
- The cell's ability to grow and reproduce (genetic integrity)

Hypoxia

Inadequate cellular oxygenation, hypoxia, interferes with the cell's ability to transform energy. Hypoxia may be caused by a decrease in blood supply to an area; by a decrease in the oxygen-carrying capacity of the blood (decreased hemoglobin); by a ventilation–perfusion or respiratory problem, reducing the amount of oxygen available in the blood; or by a problem in the cell's enzyme system, making it unable to use the oxygen delivered to it. The usual cause is *ischemia*, or deficient blood supply. This is commonly seen in myocardial cell injury, in which arterial blood flow is decreased because of atherosclerosis. Intravascular clots (thrombi, emboli) interfering with blood supply are a common cause of cerebrovascular accidents. The length of time different tissues can survive without oxygen varies: brain cells may succumb in 3 to 6 minutes (sources vary). If the condition leading to hypoxia is slowly progressive, collateral circulation to the area may develop; however, this mechanism is not highly reliable.

Nutritional Imbalance

Nutritional imbalance refers to a relative or absolute deficiency or excess of one or more essential nutrients. This may be manifested as undernutrition, in which there is an inadequate consumption of food or calories, or as overnutrition, in which there is a caloric excess. Caloric excess to the point of obesity, in which the person is 20% or more above his ideal weight, over-

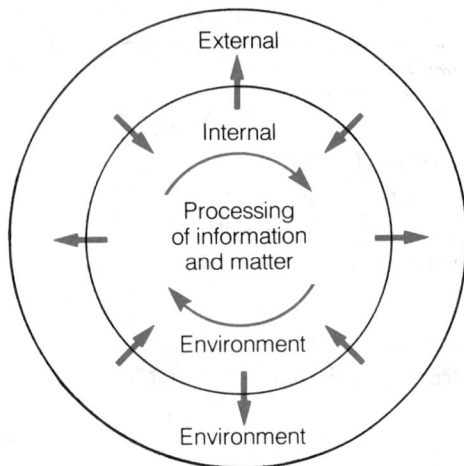

Figure 8–3. Influences leading to disorder may arise from the internal environment and the external environment of the system. Excesses or deficits of information and matter may occur or there may be faulty regulation of processing.

loads cells in the body with lipids. By requiring more energy to maintain the extra tissue, obesity places a strain on the body and has been associated with the production of disease, especially pulmonary and cardiovascular disease.

Specific deficiencies arise when an essential nutrient is deficient or when there is a disproportion of nutrients. Protein deficiencies and avitaminosis are examples.

An energy deficit leading to cell injury can occur when there is insufficient glucose or insufficient oxygen to transform the glucose into energy. A lack of insulin, or the inability to utilize insulin, may also prevent glucose from entering the cell from the blood. This is the problem in diabetes mellitus, which represents a metabolic disorder, leading to nutritional deficiency.

Physical Agents

Physical agents, including extremes of temperature, radiation, electrical shock, and mechanical trauma, may cause injury to the cells or the entire body. The duration of exposure and the intensity of the stressor determine the severity of damage.

Extremes of High Temperature. When temperatures are elevated, irrespective of cause, hypermetabolism occurs: the respiratory rate, heart rate, and basal metabolic rate increase. Eventually, the high temperature causes coagulation of cell proteins, and the cells die. With fever induced by infections, the hypothalamic thermostat may be reset at a higher temperature. Thus, the person responds to external heat and cold with a new setpoint of perhaps 40°C (104°F), just as he did with the normal setpoint of 37°C (98.6°F). When the fever breaks, the thermostat returns to normal. With fever from heat stroke, the function of the thermoregulatory center breaks down, and temperature soars. It is imperative that the body be cooled rapidly to prevent brain damage.

The local response to thermal injury is similar. There is an increase in metabolic activity, and as heat increases, protein is coagulated, enzyme systems are destroyed, and, in the extreme, charring or carbonization occurs. Burns of the epithelium are classified as partial-thickness burns if epithelializing elements remain to support healing; full-thickness burns lack such elements and must be grafted for healing. The amount of body surface involved determines the prognosis for the patient. If severe, the entire body system becomes involved, and hypermetabolism will develop as a pathophysiologic response.

Extremes of Low Temperature. Extremes of low temperature or cold cause vasoconstriction; blood flow becomes sluggish, and clots may form, leading to ischemic damage in the involved tissues. With still lower temperatures, ice crystals may form, and the cells may burst.

Radiation. Radiant energy may be used for diagnosis and treatment of diseases. In excessive amounts, it causes injury by its ionizing action. Electrical shock may produce burns as a result of the heat generated when electric current travels through the body. It may also stimulate nerves abnormally; for example, fibrillation of the heart may occur.

Mechanical Trauma. Mechanical trauma can result in wounds that disrupt the cells and tissues of the body. The severity of the wound, the blood loss, and the nerve damage are significant factors in the outcome.

Chemical Agents

Chemical injuries may be caused by known poisons, such as lye, which has a corrosive action on epithelial tissue, or by heavy metals, such as mercury, arsenic, and lead, each with its own specific destructive action. Many other chemicals may be toxic in certain amounts, in certain people, and in certain tissues; these include compounds of extrinsic and intrinsic origin. Too much hydrochloric acid can damage the stomach lining; large amounts of glucose can cause osmotic shifts, affecting the fluid and electrolyte balance; and too much insulin can cause hypoglycemia and lead to coma. Drugs, including medications prescribed by the physician, may cause chemical poisoning. Some individuals are less tolerant of drugs than others and manifest toxic reactions at customary dosages. Aging tends to decrease tolerance to drugs. Polypharmacy, the taking of many medications at one time, also often occurs in the aging population. It is a problem because of the unpredictable effects of the resulting drug interactions.

Alcohol (ethanol) is a chemical irritant. In the body, alcohol is broken down into acetaldehyde, which has a direct toxic effect on liver cells that leads to a variety of liver abnormalities, including cirrhosis in susceptible individuals. Disordered liver cell function leads to complications in other organs of the body.

Infectious Agents

Biologic agents known to cause disease in humans are viruses, bacteria, rickettsiae, mycoplasmas, fungi, protozoa, and nematodes. The severity of the infectious disease depends on the number of microorganisms entering the body, their virulence, and the host's defenses, such as health, age, and immune defenses. Some bacteria, such as those in tetanus and diphtheria, produce exotoxins that circulate and create cell damage; some, such as the gram negative bacteria, produce endotoxins when they are killed; and others, such as the tubercle bacillus, induce an immune reaction. Viruses, as the smallest living organisms, survive as parasites of the living cells they invade. Viruses infect specific cells; through a complex mechanism, they replicate within the cells they invade and then burst out to invade other cells and continue to replicate. An immune response is mounted by the body to eliminate the viruses, and the cells harboring the viruses can be injured in the process.

Typically, an inflammatory response and immune reaction are the pathophysiologic responses of the body to the presence of infection.

Immune Mechanisms

The immune system is an exceedingly complex system; its purpose is to defend the body from invasion by any foreign object or foreign cell type, such as cancerous cells. This is a steady-state mechanism, but like other adjustment processes it can become disordered, and cell injury occurs. Basically, the immune response detects foreign bodies or distinguishes nonself from self and destroys nonself entities. The entrance of an antigen (foreign body) into the body evokes the production of antibodies that attack and destroy the antigen (antigen–antibody reaction). The immune system can be hypoactive or hyperactive. When it is hypoactive, immunodeficiency diseases occur; when it is hyperactive, hypersensitivity disorders arise.

In hypersensitivity disorders, the antigen reacts with the cells of immunity (lymphocytes, macrophages, neutrophils, antibodies, or complement) in such a way that "self" or normal cells are injured.

For example, a person with seasonal allergic rhinitis due to pollen hyperreacts to the foreign protein by producing a sensitivity (Fig. 8-4). IgE, the immunoglobulin normally produced as an antibody against such an allergen, is produced in excessive amounts. This antibody attaches to the skin surfaces of the nasal mucosa. When the foreign protein, pollen, is inhaled again, an antigen–antibody reaction occurs at the site. Histamine and other irritating chemical substances are released and cell injury occurs, as is indicated by copious secretions, edema of the mucosa, sneezing because of secretions, and local itching. Basically, the immune response is the process of inflammation described below amplified by the participation of antibodies and sensitized lymphocytes.

Genetic Disorders

Genetic defects as causes of disease are of intense interest as more environmental pollutants are formed and their effects on genetic structure are studied. Many of these produce mutations

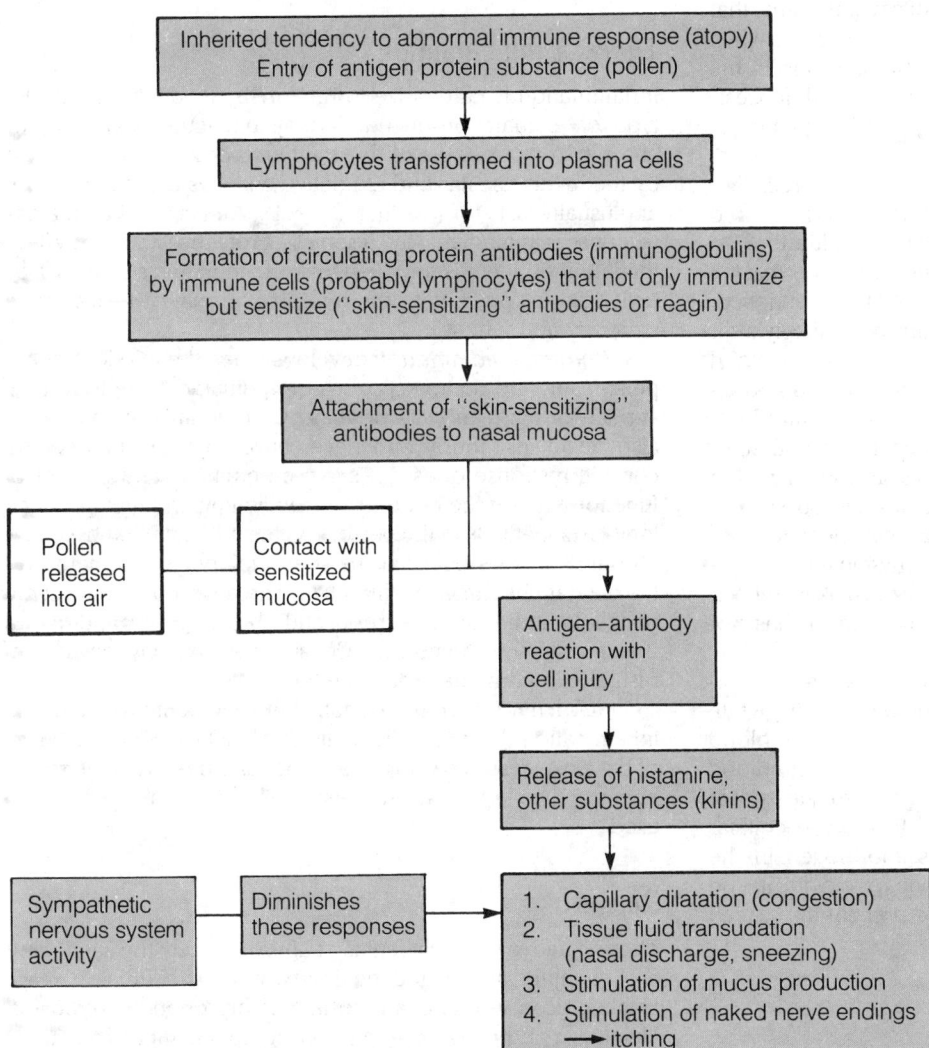

Figure 8–4. Pathophysiology of seasonal allergic rhinitis due to pollen.

that have no recognizable effect, such as lack of a single enzyme; others contribute to more obvious congenital abnormalities, such as Down's syndrome. Sickle cell disease, the hemophilias, and phenylketonuria are examples of diseases arising from genetic defects.

Response to Injury: Inflammation

Cells or tissues of the body may be injured or killed by any of the agents (physical, chemical, infectious) just described. When this happens there is a naturally occurring response in the healthy tissues adjacent to the site of injury. This is called the *inflammatory response*, or *inflammation*. It is a defensive reaction the intent of which is to neutralize, control, and/or eliminate the offending agent and to prepare the site for repair. It is a nonspecific response (not dependent on a particular cause) meant to serve a protective function. For example, inflammation may be observed at the site of a bee sting, in a sore throat, in a surgical incision, and in a burn. Inflammation also occurs in more serious cell injury events such as strokes and myocardial infarctions.

It is important to distinguish between inflammation and infection. An infectious agent is only one of several agents that may trigger an inflammatory response. An infection exists when the infectious agent is living, growing, and multiplying in the tissues and is able to overcome the body's normal defenses.

Regardless of the cause, there is a general sequence of events that can be described as the local inflammatory response. This sequence involves changes in the microcirculation in the area of the injury that include vasodilation, increased vascular permeability, and leukocytic cellular infiltration. As these changes take place, *five cardinal signs of inflammation* are produced: redness, heat, swelling, pain, and loss of function.

A transient vasoconstriction that occurs immediately after injury is followed by vasodilation and an increased rate of blood flow through the microcirculation. Local heat and redness result. Next, vascular permeability increases, and plasma fluids (including proteins and solutes) leak into the inflamed tissues, producing swelling. The pain produced is attributed to the pressure of fluids (swelling) on nerve endings and possibly to direct irritation of nerve endings by chemical mediators released at the site. Bradykinin is one of the chemical mediators suspected of causing pain. Loss of function is most likely related to the pain and swelling, but the exact mechanism has not been explained.

As the blood flow increases and fluid leaks into the surrounding tissues, the formed elements (red blood cells, white blood cells, and platelets) remain in the blood and the blood becomes more viscous and sluggish. Leukocytes (white blood cells) collect in the vessels, exit, and migrate to the site of injury to engulf offending organisms and to remove cellular debris in a process called phagocytosis. Fibrinogen in the leaked plasma fluid coagulates, forming fibrin for clot formation that serves to wall off the injured area and prevent the spread of infection.

Chemical Mediators

Injury initiates the inflammatory response, but chemical substances released at the site induce the vascular changes. Foremost among these are histamine and the kinins. Histamine is present in many tissues of the body but is concentrated in mast cells. It is released when injury occurs and is responsible for the early changes in vasodilation and vascular permeability. Kinins increase vasodilation and vascular permeability; they also attract neutrophils to the area. Prostaglandins, another group of chemical substances, are also suspected of causing increased permeability.

The process described is complex. Although it has phases, once started they may all occur at the same time. The process may be modified by different variables, the most important of which are (1) the nature and intensity of the injury, (2) the site and tissue affected, and (3) the resistance of the host.

The inflammatory response may be confined to the site, and only local signs may appear. On the other hand, systemic responses may also occur. Fever is the most common sign of a systemic response to injury. It is most likely caused by endogenous pyrogens released from neutrophils and macrophages (specialized forms of leukocytes). These substances reset the hypothalamic thermostat controlling body temperature and produce fever. Leukocytosis, an increase in the synthesis and release of neutrophils from bone marrow, may occur. Constitutional symptoms may develop, including malaise, loss of appetite, aching, and weakness.

Types of Inflammation

Inflammation is categorized primarily by its duration and the type of exudate produced. It may be acute, subacute, or chronic. A typical case of *acute inflammation* is characterized by the local vascular and exudative changes described above and usually lasts for less than 2 weeks. An acute inflammatory response is immediate, and it serves a protective function. When the injurious agent is removed, the inflammation subsides, and healing takes place with the return of normal or near-normal structure and function.

Chronic inflammation develops when the injurious agent persists and the acute response is perpetuated. Symptoms may appear for many months or years. Chronic inflammation may also begin insidiously and never have an acute phase. The chronic response does not serve a beneficial and protective function but, on the contrary, is debilitating and may produce long-lasting effects in the person. As the inflammation becomes chronic, changes occur at the site of injury and the nature of the exudate becomes proliferative. There is a continuing cycle of cellular infiltration, necrosis, and fibrosis (repair and breakdown occur simultaneously). Considerable scarring may occur, resulting in permanent damage to tissues.

Subacute inflammation falls between acute and chronic inflammation. There are elements of the active exudative phase of the acute response, and simultaneously there is some repair occurring, as in the chronic response. The term is not widely used.

Repair

The reparative process begins at approximately the same time as the injury and is indeed interwoven with inflammation. Healing proceeds after the inflammatory debris is removed. Healing may be by *regeneration*, in which there is gradual repair of the defect by proliferation of cells of the same type as those destroyed. Or, it may be by *replacement* with cells of another type, usually connective tissue, resulting in scar formation.

Healing by Regeneration.   The ability of cells to regenerate depends on whether they are labile, stable, or permanent. *Labile* cells include those that multiply constantly to replace cells worn out by normal physiologic processes; these include epithelial cells of the skin and those lining the gastrointestinal tract. *Permanent* cells include neurons—the nerve cell bodies, not their axons. Destruction of a neuron is a permanent loss, but axons may regenerate. If normal activity is to return, tissue regeneration must occur in a functional pattern, especially in the growth of several axons. *Stable* cells have a latent ability to regenerate. Under normal physiologic processes, they are not shed and do not need replacement, but if they are damaged or destroyed, they are able to regenerate. These include functional cells of the kidney, liver, pancreas, and other organs of the body.

Healing by Replacement.   Healing may be by primary intention or secondary intention. In *primary intention healing*, the wound is clean and dry and the edges are approximated, such as may occur in a surgical wound. Little scar formation occurs, and the wound is usually healed in a week. In *secondary intention healing*, the wound or defect is larger and gaping and has more necrotic material. The wound fills from the bottom upward with granulation tissue. The process of repair takes longer and results in more scar formation with loss of specialized function. Persons who have recovered from myocardial infarctions will have abnormal electrocardiographic (ECG) tracings because the electrical signal cannot be conducted through the connective tissue that replaces the defect.

As has been stated many times in this chapter, the condition of the host, the environment, and the nature and severity of the injury affect the processes and outcomes—in this case, the processes of inflammation and repair.

Cell Death

Any of the injuries discussed can lead to death of the cell. Essentially, the cell membrane becomes impaired, resulting in a nonrestricted flow of ions. Sodium and calcium enter the cell, followed by water, which leads to edema, and energy transformation ceases. Nerve impulses are no longer transmitted; muscles no longer contract. As the cells rupture, lysosomal enzymes that destroy tissues escape; cell death and necrosis occur.

A Representative Pathophysiologic Process: Hypertensive Heart Disease

Hypertensive heart disease is presented here as a representative pathophysiologic process. Unfortunately, words and figures can only partly portray the patient's condition, moment by moment or day by day in acute illness, or week by week in chronic illness. The influence of physiologic changes, of social adjustments between patient and health care personnel or family, of unknown or expressed concern and anxiety, and of the patient's total life experience in the development and course of disease is well recognized by the health care team. These variables cannot be inserted into a flow diagram, yet they may be major factors governing the course of the disease.

Mechanisms of Blood Pressure Regulation

A brief summary of selected mechanisms for regulating blood pressure will facilitate the understanding of hypertensive heart disease. The regulation of arterial pressure involves complex nervous system and hormonal controls that interrelate to affect the cardiac output and peripheral resistance. This relationship is expressed in the following equation:

$$\text{mean arterial pressure} = \text{cardiac output} \times \text{total peripheral resistance}$$

Cardiac output is determined by the stroke volume and the heart rate. Peripheral resistance is determined by the diameter of the arterioles. If the diameter is decreased (vasoconstriction), peripheral resistance increases; if the diameter is increased (vasodilation), peripheral resistance decreases.

Primary regulation of arterial pressure is effected by the baroreceptors in the carotid sinus and aortic arch, which relay impulses to the sympathetic nervous centers in the medulla. These impulses act to inhibit the stimulation of the sympathetic nervous system. When the arterial pressure is increased, the baroreceptor endings are stretched. They fire, inhibiting the sympathetic center. This reduces the discharge of the sympathetic center, with the result that the heart rate is decreased, the arterioles dilate, and the arterial pressure returns to its former level. The reverse happens with a fall in arterial pressure. The baroreceptors control only temporary changes in blood pressure.

One other mechanism, which has a longer-term effect, will be described. Renin, produced by the kidneys when their blood flow is decreased, leads to the formation of angiotensin I, which converts to angiotensin II. Angiotensin II elevates the blood pressure by direct constriction of arterioles. It also indirectly stimulates the release of aldosterone, which leads to renal retention of sodium and water. The latter increases the extracellular fluid volume, which in turn increases the flow of blood returned to the heart, thereby raising the stroke volume and cardiac output. The kidneys also have an intrinsic mechanism to increase sodium and water retention.

When a *persistent* disturbance that causes arteriolar constriction occurs, total peripheral resistance is increased and the mean arterial pressure rises. In the face of the persistent disturbance, cardiac output must increase to maintain balance in the system (see equation). This is necessary to overcome the peripheral resistance, so that delivery of oxygen and nutrients to the cells and removal of cellular waste products will be maintained. To increase the cardiac output, the sympathetic nervous system stimulates the heart to beat faster; it also increases the stroke volume by causing a selective vasoconstriction in peripheral organs, thus returning more blood to the heart. With chronic hypertension, the baroreceptors are reset at a higher level, and they respond as though the new level were normal.

Initially, this mechanism is compensatory. This adaptive mechanism, however, exacts a toll by creating an increased workload for the heart. At the same time, degenerative changes take place in the arterioles that are subjected to continuous high pressure. These changes occur in organs throughout the body, including the heart, which may contribute to a depleted blood supply in the myocardium. To eject blood, the heart must exert enough force to overcome the pressure reflected back to the aortic inlet. In response to this workload, the muscle of the left ventricle hypertrophies. Eventually, it dilates, and the heart becomes enlarged. These two structural changes are adaptive; they improve the stroke volume delivered by the heart. At rest, these compensatory mechanisms may be effective, but on exertion, the heart cannot meet the demands of the body; the patient is easily fatigued and becomes short of breath.

The point at which compensation ends and injury and failure begin is not continuous or discrete. With the increased demands, there are changes in the distribution of blood flow that result in a reduced flow to the kidneys. This stimulates the renin–angiotensin–aldosterone mechanism. This mechanism, once compensatory, now aggravates the failing heart by increasing the extracellular fluid volume and the peripheral resistance. The heart becomes engorged with blood that it cannot pump out, and left ventricular heart failure occurs. Failure of the left ventricle has both forward and backward effects. The forward effects are due to low output, which decreases the perfusion of tissues of the body. The decreased perfusion activates sodium and water retention mechanisms in the kidneys and glands, giving positive feedback to the failing heart. The backward effects are due to the decreased emptying of the left ventricle, which raises the end-diastolic pressure. This rise in pressure is reflected back into the left atrium and the pulmonary veins, and congestion occurs in the pulmonary capillaries. Gas exchange is disrupted, and fluid exudes from the capillaries into the alveolar spaces, leading to pulmonary edema. Crackles will be heard when the lungs are auscultated; severe dyspnea and orthopnea will be present; coughing will occur; and, with pulmonary edema, pink, frothy sputum may be present. Eventually, this backward progression will affect the right side of the heart and lead to right-sided heart failure accompanied by congestion in the veins and organs drained by the venae cavae. The system is in total failure, and death is imminent.

The initial disturbance that caused the increased peripheral resistance may be unknown, as is the case in primary or essential hypertension, although a number of agents have been postulated as being contributory. The pathologic mechanism was hypoxia due to failure of the blood transportation system. In the latter stages, oxygen saturation of the blood was also decreased by the pulmonary edema.

Nursing Implications

In the assessment of the patient who seeks health care, objective signs will be the primary indicators of the physiologic processes that are occurring. The following questions are answered during the assessment: Are the heart rate, respiratory rate, and temperature normal? If not, is any change only a temporary one? Are there other indicators of steady-state deviation? What is the patient's blood pressure, height, and weight? Are there any problems in movement or sensation? Does the patient demonstrate any problems in orientation or memory? Are there

obvious lesions or deformities? Further signs of internal processes are indicated in laboratory data, including electrolytes, blood urea nitrogen (BUN), blood glucose, and urinalysis. In making a nursing diagnosis, the nurse must compare the symptoms or complaints expressed by the patient with the physical signs present.

Specific problems and their nursing treatment are addressed in greater depth in other chapters. It has been reiterated many times in this chapter that the state of the host and the environment are two of the three predictors of the health outcome in all situations. These two are directly related to the health patterns of the individual. The nurse has a significant role and responsibility in identifying the health patterns of the patient treated. If those patterns are not achieving balance for the patient physiologically, psychologically, and socially, the nurse is obligated—with the assistance and agreement of the patient—to seek ways to promote balance. This chapter is physiologically oriented; in that context, the nutrition–metabolism pattern, elimination pattern, activity–exercise pattern, and sleep–rest pattern would be specifically analyzed. However, the way one copes with stress, the way one relates to others, and the values and goals held are interwoven in those physiologic patterns. Similarly, who you eat with, when you eat, and how much money you have for food are directly related to what you eat and how much you eat. To evaluate the patient's health patterns and to intervene if a problem exists requires a total assessment of the patient.

Chapter Summary

This chapter discusses man as an integral part of dynamic external and internal environments. Man has an elaborate system for maintaining a steady state or internal constancy amid changing environments. Two components of this system are homeostasis and adaptation. Homeostasis refers to the adjustments that the body must make *rapidly* to maintain constancy within a changing environment; adaptation, in contrast, refers to changes that must take place over time to maintain constancy. The presence or absence of homeostasis or adaptation often is the difference between health and disease.

When homeostasis cannot be maintained, disordered functioning of the body occurs. If not checked, disordered functioning can lead to various states of disease. The body has a system of predictable responses to disordered functioning that assists in maintaining a steady state and alerts the organism that something is wrong. These responses can be categorized into signs and symptoms of disease states. Signs are those responses that may be objectively evaluated; symptoms are those responses that are subjectively evaluated.

Principles of maintaining a steady state can be applied to the functioning of each individual cell. Cells possess both maintenance and specialized functions. Maintenance functions are those required by the individual cell for viability; specialized functions are those functions important to the tissue or organ of which the cell is a part. Cells are capable of adapting to environmental stress by changing structure and function. Some of the most common adaptations are hypertrophy, atrophy, hyperplasia, and metaplasia.

Injury to the cell may arise from the internal and external

environments. Some examples of substances or events that can cause injury include: physical agents, chemical agents, infectious agents, immune mechanisms, genetic defects, hypoxia, and nutritional imbalance. These substances and events interfere with the cell's metabolic processes.

A naturally occurring response to agents that may damage or destroy cells is the inflammatory response. The inflammatory response is a defensive reaction that occurs in the healthy tissue adjacent to the injured tissue. The purpose of the reaction is to neutralize, control, and/or eliminate the noxious agent and prepare the site for repair. The sequence of events that occurs results from changes in microcirculation at the site of injury. Redness, heat, swelling, pain, and loss of function are the five cardinal signs that are predictably produced by inflammation. Inflammation may be described by its duration and/or type of exudate produced.

Cell death can also occur as a response to injury and is generally undesirable. When cell death does not occur, the reparative process ensues. Repair occurs by either regeneration or replacement of tissue.

The concepts of homeostasis and adaptation are important to nurses' understanding of man's response to illness; nursing implications are described throughout the chapter.

Bibliography

Books

Boyd W and Sheldon H. Boyd's Introduction to the Study of Disease, 10th ed. Philadelphia, Lea & Febiger, 1988.

Bullock BL and Rosendahl PP. Pathophysiology: Adaptations and Alterations in Function, 2nd ed. Glenview, IL, Scott Foresman & Co, 1988.

Dubos R. Man Adapting. New Haven, CT, Yale University Press, 1965.

Frohlich ED (ed). Pathophysiology, Altered Regulatory Mechanisms in Disease. Philadelphia, JB Lippincott, 1984.

Groer MW and Shekleton ME. Basic Pathophysiology, A Conceptual Approach, 3rd ed. St Louis, CV Mosby, 1989.

Guyton AC. Textbook of Medical Physiology. Philadelphia, WB Saunders, 1986.

Harrison TR, Braunwald E et al (eds). Harrison's Principles of Internal Medicine, 11th ed. New York, McGraw-Hill, 1988.

Kent TH and Hart MN. Introduction to Human Disease, 2nd ed. Norwalk, CT, Appleton-Century-Crofts, 1987.

Kissane JM. Anderson's Pathology, 9th ed. St Louis, CV Mosby, 1989.

Porth C. Pathophysiology: Concepts of Altered States, 3rd ed. Philadelphia, JB Lippincott, 1990.

Price SA and Wilson LM. Pathophysiology, Clinical Concepts of Disease Processes. New York, McGraw-Hill, 1986.

Robbins SL and Kumar V. Basic Pathology, 4th ed. Philadelphia, WB Saunders, 1987.

Robbins SL, Cotran RS, and Kumar V. Pathologic Basis of Disease, 4th ed. Philadelphia, WB Saunders, 1989.

Vander AJ, Sherman JH, and Luciano DS. Human Physiology: The Mechanisms of Body Function. New York, McGraw-Hill, 1985.

Weiner H and Fawzy FI. An integrative model of health, disease, and illness. In Cheren S (ed). Psychosomatic Medicine: Theory, Physiology, and Practice (2 vols). Madison, CT, International Universities Press, Inc, 1989.

Journals

Crosby LJ. Stress factors, emotional stress and rheumatoid arthritis disease activity. J Adv Nurs 1988 Jul; 13(4):452–461.

Ninemann JL. Trauma, sepsis, and the immune response. J Burn Care Rehab 1987 Nov/Dec; 8(6):462–468.

9

Stress and Adaptation

Learning Objectives

On completion of this chapter, the learner will be able to:

1. Define stress and adaptation
2. Identify physiologic and psychosocial stressors
3. Compare the sympathetic–adrenal–medullary response to stress to the hypothalamic–pituitary response to stress
4. Describe the influence of social support on coping with stress
5. Describe the General Adaptation Syndrome as a theory of adaptation to biologic stress
6. Identify ways in which maladaptive responses to stress can increase the risk of illness and cause disease
7. Describe the nursing implications of health risk appraisal
8. Identify measures that are useful for reduction of stress
9. Specify the functions of social networks and support groups in the reduction of stress

---

Stress is a term that is difficult to define: it is used loosely and means different things to different people. Some use it to describe an *upset feeling* or *response*; others use it to describe the *source* or *stimulus* for their feeling upset. It has even been suggested that the term is so confusing it should not be used. Cannon, in 1936, described the "fight or flight" response that prepared the individual to cope with immediate danger. Selye (1976), who is sometimes called the "father of stress," described it as essentially the wear and tear on the body, and he stated that there is eustress, or good stress, and distress, or bad stress. Later (1976), he spoke of stress as being a "nonspecific response," meaning that regardless of the stimulus producing the stress, the physiologic response of the body was

always the same. Other research has demonstrated that the body actually has different patterns of response to different threats, most likely related to how emotionally aroused the person becomes (Mason, 1975). These researchers have concentrated on the physiologic reactions of the body in response to stress.

Psychologists have been more concerned with predisposing factors and with the mental processes involved in stress. Engel (1960), studying psychosomatic illness, defined psychologic stress as referring to

all processes, whether originating in the external environment or within the person, which impose a demand or requirement upon

115

the organism, the resolution or handling of which necessitates work or activity of the mental apparatus before any other system is involved or activated.*

Lazarus and Folkman (1984, p 19) have developed a transactional theory of stress in which they define psychologic stress as a "particular *relationship* between the person and the environment that is appraised by the person as taxing or exceeding his or her resources and endangering his or her well-being." This theory has been used by many nurse researchers.

Other psychosocial researchers have concentrated on the stimuli or sources of stress, particularly looking at stressful life events or life changes that can be associated with stress. Thus, study in the field of stress has been pursued by scientists in different disciplines, with each evolving his own particular theories.

In nursing, such scientists as Shaver (1985) and Sutterley and Donnelly (1981) have developed models that link the environment, the mind, and the body. They provide a holistic approach, which reflects the view that the body, mind, and spirit of a person are an integral unit. An individual's characteristic behavior patterns reflect this unity. Although the particular behavior pattern (physiologic, psychologic, social) can be assessed, it must be realized that it reflects the whole person. Neumann's theory of nursing focuses on the client and on stress and adaptation; Roy's theory emphasizes the adaptive system of the person (Marriner, 1986).

The process of stress, the adaptive responses to stress, some of the maladaptive outcomes, and the nursing implications associated with the process are described in this chapter.

Stress and Adaptation Defined

Stress

Stress is a state produced by a change in the environment that is perceived as challenging, threatening, or damaging to the person's dynamic equilibrium. There is an actual or perceived imbalance in the person's capability to meet the demands of the new situation. The change or stimulus that evokes this state is the *stressor*. The nature of the stressor is variable: an event or change that will produce stress in one person will be neutral for another, and an event that may produce stress at one time and place for one person may not do so for the same person at another time and place. A person appraises and copes with changing situations. The desired goal is adaptation, or adjustment to the change, so that the person is again in equilibrium and has the energy and ability to meet new external demands. This is the stress-coping process, a compensatory process with both physiologic and psychologic components.

Adaptation

Adaptation is a constant, ongoing process that occurs along the time continuum, beginning with birth and ending with death. Also existing along this lifetime continuum are the dimensions

of health and illness. Health and illness are relative concepts. As a person traverses the life continuum, he encounters stressors that challenge his ability to meet his needs and maintain equilibrium. Successful positive adaptation to these stressors represents health; illness is an unsuccessful or maladaptive outcome. According to Dubos (1965), "Health in the case of human beings means more than a state in which the organism has become physically suited to the surrounding physiochemical conditions through passive mechanisms; it demands that the personality be able to express itself creatively." Dubos described human life as the interplay of three classes of determinants: the universal characteristics of man's nature, "which are inscribed in his flesh and bone"; the conditions of any given situation; and man's ability to make choices and control his own actions.

Because both stress and adaptation may exist at different levels of a system, it is possible to study them at cell, tissue, and organ levels. The biologist's study is mainly concerned with subcellular components or with subsystems of the total body. Stress and adaptation may also be studied in individuals, families, groups, and societies; thus, the sociologist speaks of the adaptation of groups, in the sense that their organization is modified to meet the requirements of the social and physical environment in which they exist. Adaptation is a continuous process of seeking harmony in an environment. The desired end goals of adaptation for any system are growth and reproduction. A major nursing objective is to support and promote the efforts of each patient to achieve a healthy adaptation.

Stress-Coping Model. Perception of the stressor is coordinated by structures of the brain and may be a conscious or unconscious process. Initially, following perception, there is a *global response*, a generalized state of anxiety involving psychoneuroendocrine activation. A *more specific response* develops as the person has more time to appraise the stressor and the resources available to cope with it. Anxiety will change from a diffuse reaction to a specific emotion: joy–sadness, fear–anger, acceptance–distrust, surprise–anticipation; the endocrine responses will become more specific. In all, there will be a more defined pattern of emotional and physiologic responses. Perception and response are intertwined and occur simultaneously; they cannot be singled out, except for the purposes of discussion as presented here. The stress response has both physiologic and psychologic, or emotional, components, and manifestations of these are demonstrated in a person's behaviors: signs, symptoms, and self-reports. As the person copes with the situation, reappraisal will occur. Coping and reappraisal will become a circular activity providing feedback to the perception of the situation. If the person is successful in his activity, adaptive outcomes will occur; if unsuccessful, a pattern of maladaptive responses to specific situations may develop, or one of the so-called diseases of adaptation may occur. This is also a period when the person is particularly vulnerable to other stressors. The sequence of processes described is diagrammed in Figure 9-1.

Stressors: The Sources of Stress

Each person operates at a certain level, or within a range, that may be considered his adaptation level. A certain amount of

* Engel G. Health and disease. Perspect Biol 1960 Summer; 3(4):459–485.

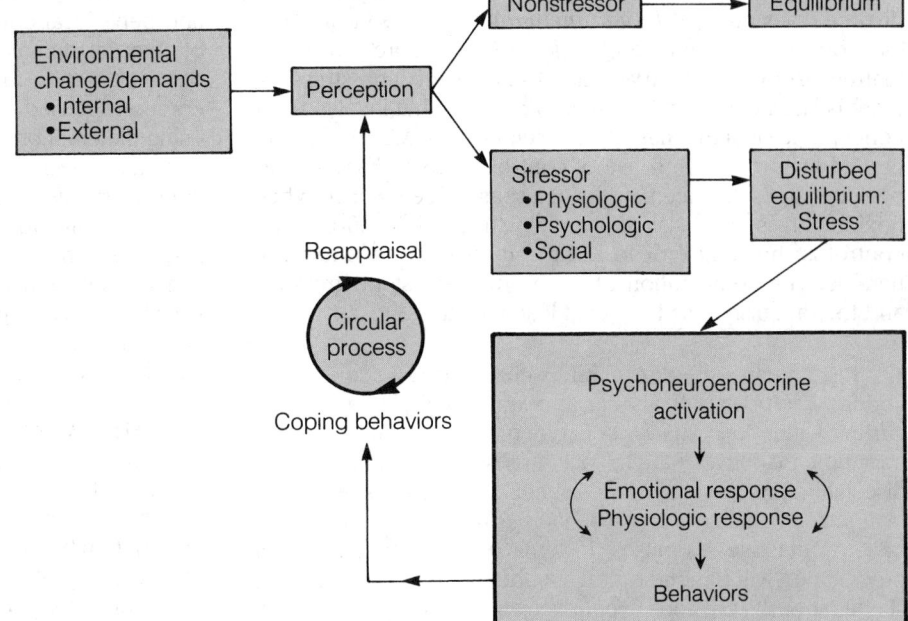

Figure 9–1. The stress-coping model. When an environmental change is perceived by the brain as stressful, psychoneuroendocrine activation occurs, which elicits emotional and physiologic responses in the individual. These are manifested in objective and subjective behaviors. As the individual copes, using his own resources and social supports, reappraisal will recur again and again, providing feedback to the perception of the situation.

change is encountered regularly: it is expected, it contributes to growth, and it enhances life. This healthy state can be upset by a number of stressors. This leads to imbalance in the person's physiologic or psychologic state, or both, resulting in responses that, if prolonged or severe, may lead to illness. Sources of stress may be broadly categorized into physiologic stressors and psychosocial stressors.

Physiologic Stressors. The following agents may be considered as primarily physiologic stressors: chemical agents (drugs, poisons, alcohol), physical agents (heat, cold, radiation, electrical shock, trauma), infectious agents (viruses, bacteria, fungi), faulty immune mechanisms, genetic disorders, nutritional imbalance, and hypoxia. All stressors have both a general effect and a specific effect. The specific effect of these agents and the pathophysiology they incur are the subjects of another chapter and thus are not described further here. The general effect is the subject of the stress response in this chapter.

Psychosocial Stressors. The list of sources of psychosocial stress is extensive and for convenience can be broken down into three groups: (1) day-to-day stressors, or commonly occurring frustrations; (2) major complex occurrences that may involve large groups, even entire nations; and (3) stressors that fall in between, that occur less frequently and involve fewer people. The first group, the day-to-day stressors, includes such common occurrences as getting caught in a traffic jam, running out of ribbon on the typewriter, having an argument with a spouse or roommate, and feeling lonely. These experiences vary in effect; for example, a rainstorm while one is vacationing at the beach will most likely evoke a more negative response than it might at another time. These less dramatic, frustrating, and irritating events, called "daily hassles," have been shown to affect health more strongly than major life events.

Some stressors influence not only the individual but also larger groups, possibly even entire nations of people. These include events of history such as terrorism and war, which are threatening situations brought into the living room through live news coverage and dramatization by the mass media. The changes occurring in society, such as demographic, economic, and technologic changes, are stressors. The stress produced is sometimes an effect not only of the change itself but also of the rapidity of the change.

The third group of stressors has been studied most frequently and deals with relatively infrequently occurring situations that directly affect the individual. This category includes the influence of life events, such as death, birth, marriage, divorce, and retirement. It includes the psychosocial crises described by Erikson as occurring in the life-cycle stages of the human experience. More enduring chronic stressors have also been placed in this category. The latter may include having a permanent functional disability or the burden associated with providing long-term care to a frail elderly parent.

Relating life events to illness has been a major focus of psychosocial studies and can be traced to Adolph Meyer, who in the 1930s used "life charts" of his patients from which he observed a linkage between illnesses and critical life events. Harold Wolff, following this line of research, concluded that people under constant stress had a high incidence of psychosomatic disease. More recently, Holmes and Rahe (1967) have developed life events scales that assign numerical values to typical life events. They call these *life-change units.* By checking off the number of recent events and deriving a total score, one can predict the likelihood of illness. The items reflect events that require a change in the person's life pattern; the variable of change is important because it requires adjustment. The Recent Life Changes Questionnaire (RLCQ) contains 118 items related to events such as death, birth, marriage, divorce, promotions, serious arguments, and vacations. The events listed include both desirable and undesirable happenings.

Stressors can also be categorized according to their *duration.* They may be *acute,* time-limited stressors, such as awaiting surgery or a final examination. They may be *stressor sequences* consisting of a series of events over a period of time that result from some initiating event such as job loss or divorce. They may be *chronic intermittent* (hassles fall into this category) or they may be *chronic enduring* sources of stress that persist over time. In addition to life events and stressors, there is another step in the etiology of stress that involves self-concept, particularly mastery and self-esteem. Mastery is concerned with the same sense of control a person has over his own life, and self-esteem refers to a sense of self-worth. When noxious stressors persist, unaltered by the person's efforts, and control is threatened or lost, the self-concept becomes vulnerable. The combination of life events, persistent stressors, and the diminished self-concept leads to stress.

In summary, stressors create a change in a person's equilibrium. Each person has a range of adaptability. Changes occurring within this range produce demands that fall within his existing capability. Changes falling outside this range lead to disequilibrium and require readjustment; such readjustment may lead to a new adaptation level, increasing the person's repertoire of adaptive responses. In terms of stressors, the stress precipitated will depend on the number of stressors occurring simultaneously, previous experience with the stressor, the type of stressor, and its magnitude and duration.

Mediating Resources: Internal and External

The resources used to mediate or intervene in the stress process are internal, or characteristics of the individual, and external, most commonly social support. Both resources are used to reduce, avoid, or eliminate stress and the conditions that produce stress. The theory developed by Lazarus emphasizes cognitive appraisal of the stressful situation and coping strategies to manage the situation.

Appraisal and Coping.   Cognitive appraisal (Lazarus and Folkman, 1984) is a process through which an event is evaluated with respect to what is at stake (primary appraisal) and what coping resources and options are available (secondary appraisal). During primary appraisal, the situation may be identified as either nonstressful or stressful. If nonstressful, the situation is irrelevant or benign-positive. A stressful situation may be one of three kinds: (1) those in which harm or loss has occurred; (2) those that are threatening, in that harm or loss is anticipated; and (3) those that are challenging, in that some opportunity or gain is anticipated. The degree of stress is determined by a comparison of what is at stake and what resources the person has for coping with it (a sort of risk–benefit analysis). Reappraisal also occurs and refers to a changed appraisal based on new information.

There is an emotional response as an outcome of the appraisal process. Negative emotions such as fear, anger, and resentment accompany harm/loss appraisals, while positive emotions such as excitement and eagerness accompany challenge. To illustrate this concept, an unexpected quiz in the classroom might be judged as threatening by the unprepared student, and fear, anger, and resentment might be felt. These emotions might be expressed by outwardly hostile behavior or comments.

Coping, according to Lazarus, consists of the cognitive and behavioral efforts made to manage the specific external or internal demands that tax a person's resources. Coping can be emotion-focused or problem-focused. Coping that is emotion-focused seeks to make the person feel better by lessening the emotional distress felt. Problem-focused coping aims to manage the problem causing the distress. Both types of coping usually occur in a stressful situation.

The ability to cope effectively is influenced by a person's resources. These include such internal capabilities as the person's health and energy, his problem-solving skills, and his social skills. Having a sense of control or power in a situation is also important. Important external resources include money and the services and materials that money can buy. A valuable external resource is social support.

External Resource: Social Support   The nature of social support and its influence on coping has been studied extensively, and it has been demonstrated to be an effective moderator of life stress. Cobb (1976) defined social support as information belonging to one or more of three categories. The first category of information leads the subject to believe that he is cared for and loved. This appears most often in a relationship between two people in which mutual trust and attachment are expressed by helping one another meet their needs. Such expressions, sometimes called *emotional support*, are most commonly thought of in the marital relationship but also occur between a nurse and patient.

The second category of information leads the subject to believe that he is esteemed and valued. This is most effective when it is announced in public and thus demonstrates the favorable position the individual has in the group. It elevates his sense of self-worth; this is called *esteem support*.

The third category of information leads the subject to believe that he belongs to a network of communication and mutual obligation. Information is shared by the members of the network, they all know what it is, and they are all aware that it is shared. This information is of two types. One is communications, which are "the essence of history"—what is going on, who is affected, and so forth. Another communication in this category is the knowledge that goods and services are available to the members on demand; for example, a person can call on a close friend in an emergency. Cobb emphasized that social support encourages independent behavior; it does not lead to dependency.

Social support begins *in utero;* it is fostered through maternal and paternal attachment behavior and develops through family, peer, and community relationships as the person grows. A number of sociologic and family theories attest to the production of stress and illness when the family structure is disrupted so that there is no stable hierarchy or authority, territorial limits are not well defined, and strong attachment behavior is lacking.

Social support facilitates the coping behaviors of a person; however, this is conditional on the nature of the social support. People can have extensive relationships and interact frequently, but the necessary support comes only when there is a deep level of involvement and concern, not when people merely touch the surface of each other's lives. The critical qualities within the network are the exchange of intimate communications and the presence of solidarity and trust. Recognizing the value of social support theory to nursing, Brandt and Weinert

(1981) and Norbeck and associates (1983) have developed questionnaires to identify the social support used by patients.

Physiologic Response

Interpretation of Stimuli by the Brain.   The perception of stress involves taking in a sensation and giving meaning to it; this occurs in the brain. The brain has been compared to an international casino visited by people from all over the world. Each person comes to the casino with his own currency; to gamble, he must change it into the currency of the casino. In a similar fashion, all sensations, internal and external, coming into the brain must be converted into electrochemical impulses that are the "currency of the brain." Different stimuli are reg-

istered in different areas of the brain in different patterns, and the brain interprets these patterns and responds to them. In this way, it controls and regulates the activities of the body.

A model to explain the functional organization of the brain for the interpretation of stimuli is presented in Figure 9-2. This may be considered a communication and control hierarchy for the pituitary–adrenal system. There are three functional levels: interpretation of basic drive or need states occurs at the lowest level; emotions are interpreted at the intermediate level; and cognitions are interpreted at the highest level.

The hypothalamus sits in the center of the brain, surrounded by the limbic system and the cerebral hemispheres. It integrates autonomic mechanisms that maintain the chemical constancy of the internal environment of the body. With the limbic system, the hypothalamus also regulates emotional and instinctive behavior. The hypothalamus is made up of a number of nuclei, and the limbic system contains the amygdala, hip-

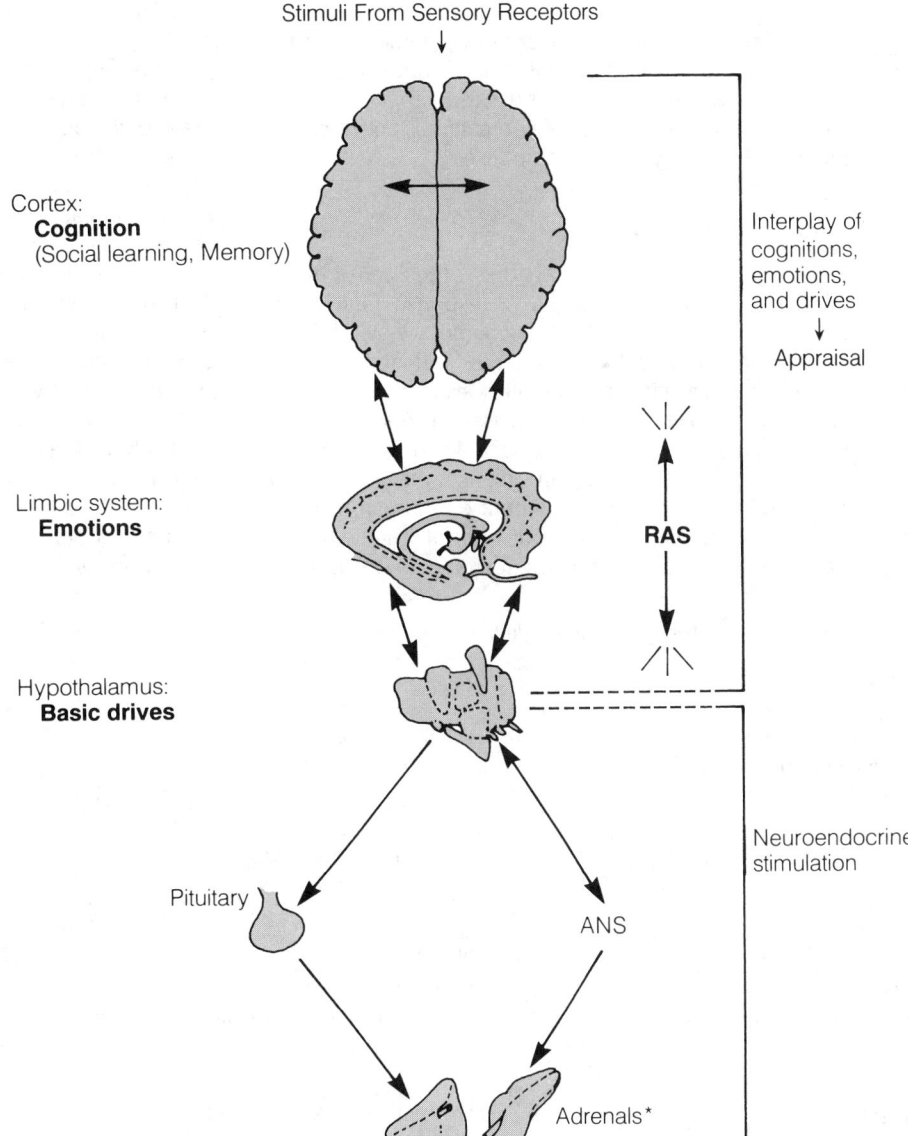

Figure 9–2.   Functional organization of the brain. In the process of appraisal of environmental change, different levels of the brain are involved. The highest level, the cortex, has evolved more than the other two levels and can exert control over emotional states and basic drives. The reticular-activating system (RAS) is a network of cells that forms a two-way communication system extending from the brain stem into the midbrain and limbic system. The lower half of the diagram depicts the response, neuroendocrine stimulation (hypothalamus controls pituitary, autonomic nervous system [ANS]) in the presence of perceived threat.

*Other glands are also affected by pituitary hormones; however, the adrenal glands play a greater role in stress.

pocampus, and septal nuclei, along with other structures. Research supports the concept that these structures each respond differently to stimuli, and each has its characteristic response. The cerebral hemispheres are concerned with cognitive functions: thought processes, learning, and memory. The limbic system has connections with both the cerebral hemispheres and the brain stem. In addition, the reticular activating system (RAS), which is a network of cells that forms a two-way communication system, extends from the brain into the midbrain and limbic system. This network controls the alert or "waking" state of the body; it sends signals that are relayed up to the cortex and relays signals from the cortex downward. Its signals are capable of modifying ongoing input and processing.

In the process of appraising environmental change to determine whether a stressor is present, cognition, emotion, and drive states interact. Emotions are complex and are described as having both mental and physical components: there is the feeling itself, or affect; there is an awareness of the feeling and possibly its cause, or cognition; there is an urge to take action; and there are physical changes. The cognitive appraisal of the potential stressor contributes to the type of emotional response and its intensity.

Whatever the outcome of the primary appraisal, the response is integrated in the hypothalamus. Either there is no stressor and the hypothalamus continues to maintain a steady state, or there is a stressor and the hypothalamus activates the sympathetic and pituitary adrenal responses.

Neuroendocrine Response

Neural and neuroendocrine pathways under the control of the hypothalamus are activated in the stress response. First, there is a sympathetic nervous system discharge followed by a sympathetic–adrenal–medullary discharge, and finally, if the stress persists, the hypothalamic–pituitary system is activated.

Sympathetic Nervous System Response. The sympathetic nervous system response is rapid and short-lived. Norepinephrine is released at nerve endings in direct contact with their respective end organs to cause an increase in function of the vital organs and a state of general body arousal. The heart rate is increased. Peripheral vasoconstriction occurs, raising the blood pressure. Blood is also shunted away from abdominal organs. The purpose of these activities is to provide better perfusion of vital organs (brain, heart, skeletal muscles). Blood glucose is increased and supplies more readily available energy. The pupils are dilated, and mental activity is increased; a greater sense of awareness exists. Constriction of the blood vessels of the skin limits bleeding in the event of trauma. Subjectively, the person is likely to experience cold feet, clammy skin and hands, chills, palpitations, and a knot in the stomach. Typically, the person appears tense, with the muscles of the neck, upper back, and shoulders tightened; respirations may be rapid and shallow, with the diaphragm tense.

Sympathetic–Adrenal–Medullary Response. In addition to its direct effect on major end organs, the sympathetic nervous system (SNS) stimulates the medulla of the adrenal gland to release the hormones epinephrine and norepinephrine into the bloodstream. The action of these hormones is similar to that of the SNS and has the effect of sustaining and prolonging its actions. Epinephrine and norepinephrine together also stimulate the nervous system and produce metabolic effects that increase the blood glucose level and stimulate the metabolic rate. The effect of the sympathetic and adrenal–medullary responses is summarized in Table 9-1. This effect is called the "fight or flight" reaction.

Hypothalamic–Pituitary Response. The longest-acting phase of the physiologic response, which is more likely to occur in persistent stress, involves the hypothalamic–pituitary pathway. The hypothalamus secretes corticotropin-releasing factor, which stimulates the anterior pituitary to produce adrenocorticotropic hormone (ACTH). ACTH in turn stimulates the adrenal cortex to produce glucocorticoids, primarily cortisol. Cortisol stimulates protein catabolism, releasing amino acids; stimulates liver uptake of amino acids and their conversion to glucose (gluconeogenesis); and inhibits glucose uptake (anti-insulin action) by many body cells but not those of the brain and heart. These cortisol-induced metabolic effects provide the body with a ready source of energy during a stressful situation. There are some important implications to this effect: a person with diabetes who is under stress, such as an infection, will need more insulin than usual; any patient who is under stress (illness, surgery, prolonged psychologic stress) will ca-

TABLE 9-1.   *Sympathetic–Adrenal–Medullary Response*

Effect	Goal	Mechanism
↑ Heart rate ↑ Blood pressure	Better perfusion of vital organs	Increased cardiac output due to increased myocardial contractility and heart rate; also, increased venous return (peripheral vasoconstriction)
↑ Blood glucose	Increased available energy	Increased liver and muscle glycogen breakdown; also, increased breakdown of adipose tissue triglycerides
↑ Mental activity	Alert state	
Dilated pupils	Increased awareness	
↑ Tension of skeletal muscles	Preparedness for activity, decreased fatigue	Excitation of muscles; also, increase in amount of blood shunted to the muscles from the abdominal viscera
↑ Ventilation (may be rapid and shallow)	Provision of oxygen for energy	
↑ Coagulability of blood	Prevention of hemorrhage in event of trauma	Vasoconstriction of surface vessels

tabolize body protein and need supplements; and children subjected to severe stress will have retarded growth.

The glucocorticoids also depress the immune system. When they are present in high concentrations, there is a reduction in the inflammatory response to injury or infection. The steps of the inflammatory process are inhibited, lymphocytes are destroyed in lymphoid tissues, and antibody production is decreased. As a result, the ability of the person to resist infections is reduced. The inhibition of the inflammatory response can also be used to advantage pharmacologically in the prescription of cortisol to treat the inflammatory and allergic responses in arthritis, asthma, and transplant rejection.

The relationship of stress to the immune response is a subject of new fields of study called behavioral immunology, psychoneuroimmunology, and neuroimmunomodulation. Studies of animals have shown that extreme psychologic stress can have a profound effect on immune competence. Studies in humans have not been as conclusive (partially because of problems in experimental design and control), but investigators believe that the mind influences immune responses with consequences that can be harmful to the host (Cohen, 1985).

The actions of the catecholamines (epinephrine and norepinephrine) and cortisol are most important in the general response to stress. Other hormones that are also released are antidiuretic hormone (ADH) from the posterior pituitary and aldosterone from the adrenal cortex. ADH and aldosterone promote sodium and water retention, which is an adaptive mechanism in the event of hemorrhage or loss of fluids through excessive perspiration. ADH has also been shown to influence learning and so may facilitate coping in new and threatening situations. Growth hormone and glucagon are secreted and stimulate the uptake of amino acids by cells helping to mobilize energy resources. The secretion of other hormones is also affected, but their adaptive function is less clear.

The production of endorphin, an endogenous opiate, is also increased during stress and enhances the threshold for tolerance of painful stimuli. It may also affect mood. It has been implicated in the so-called "high" that long-distance runners experience.

In summary, the initial components of the physiologic response to stress, the sympathetic response, and the sympathetic–adrenal–medullary response occur in practically all stressful situations. The observable behaviors (*e.g.*, blood pressure, pulse) may vary, but the essential neuroendocrine response is the same. With the onset of the more chronic phase, there is a great deal of variability. The hypothalamic–pituitary–adrenal–cortical response will be activated in most cases, but the total pattern of the endocrine response will vary with the nature, duration, and severity of the chronic stressor. With continued exposure to the same stressor, the response will be attenuated.

Selye and the General Adaptation Syndrome

Because of his profound influence on the scientific development of the study of stress and the manner in which he has popularized the concept, it is important to understand Hans Selye's theory. In 1936, Selye first described a syndrome consisting of enlargement of the adrenal cortex; shrinkage of the thymus, spleen, lymph nodes, and other lymphatic structures; and the appearance of deep, bleeding ulcers in the stomach and duodenum. He identified this as a nonspecific response to diverse, noxious stimuli. From this beginning, he developed a theory of adaptation to biologic stress, which he named the general adaptation syndrome (GAS).

Phases of the GAS. The GAS has three phases: alarm, resistance, and exhaustion. During the acute phase, or alarm reaction, the sympathetic fight or flight response is activated with release of adrenal medullary hormones, and the ACTH–adrenal cortical response begins. The alarm reaction is defensive and anti-inflammatory but self-limited. Because it is impossible to live in a continuous state of alarm (death would ensue), the person moves into the second stage, resistance. During this stage, adaptation to the noxious stressor occurs. Cortisol activity is still increased. If exposure to the stressor is prolonged, exhaustion sets in, and endocrine activity increases, producing deleterious effects on the body systems (especially circulatory, digestive, and immune) that can lead to death. Stages one and two of this syndrome are repeated, in different degrees, throughout life as the person encounters stressors.

Selye also compared the GAS with the life process. During childhood, there have been few encounters with stress to promote the development of adaptive functioning, and the child is vulnerable. During adulthood, the person has encountered a number of life's stressful events and has developed a resistance or adaptation. During the later years, the accumulation of life's stressors and the wear and tear on the organism again deplete the person's ability to adapt, resistance falls, and eventually death ensues.

Local Adaptation Syndrome. According to Selye's theory, there is also a local adaptation syndrome (LAS). The syndrome includes the inflammatory response and repair processes that occur at the local site of tissue injury. The LAS occurs in small, topical injuries, such as bee stings; in the case of emotional arousal, the cerebral cortex is involved. "Even if the target area is not a small area but instead the cerebral cortex, the general metabolism, or the reticuloendothelial system, there is a primary topical response" (Selye, 1976b). Depending on the severity of the injury, stimuli are sent to the nervous system to elicit the hypothalamic–pituitary–adrenocortical response; this results in the GAS or systemic stress response. Cortical hormones are released and then superimpose their effect on the LAS.

Selye emphasized that stress is the nonspecific response common to all stressors, regardless of whether they are physiologic, psychologic, or social. The fact that different demands are interpreted by different people as stressors is explained by the many conditioning factors in each person's environment. Conditioning factors also account for differences in the tolerance of different persons for stress. Some may develop diseases of adaptation, such as hypertension and migraine headaches, while others appear to be unaffected.

Recent Views. In his early research, Selye used extremes of physical stressors. With newer hormone detection techniques, a variety of stressors of differing intensities have been used, and multihormonal patterns of response are being detected. These studies indicate that there are different patterns of response to different stimuli, *stimulus specificity*, and that each person develops a characteristic pattern of autonomic response that carries over from one type of stress to another, *individual response specificity*. It has been suggested that the nonspecific response is not elicited by a diverse number of stimuli but rather by one factor, emotional arousal, and that it is the degree of the arousal that affects the intensity of the hormonal response and thus the manifestations displayed by the individual.

Maladaptive Responses

The mechanisms identified by Cannon and Selye serve as adaptations to meet threatening situations. These can be both beneficial and harmful. Dubos (1965) stated that these are traits retained from the human evolutionary past that "no longer fit the needs of life in civilized societies." The fight or flight response, for example, is an anticipatory response that mobilized the bodily resources of our ancestors to deal with predators and other harsh exigencies of the environment. This same mobilization comes into play in response to emotional stimuli unrelated to danger.

> Whatever the life situation, whether it corresponds to an actual physical danger or merely to an emotional crisis, the nature and intensity of the anticipatory changes the symbol elicits in the body have remained much the same in modern man as they were in his Paleolithic ancestor.*

When the body has been prepared physiologically to act and does not do so, the result is likely to be frustrating and injurious to the person's health. For example, consider the father waiting outside the delivery room for his wife to deliver their first baby. He may be as exhausted at the end of labor as the mother. Anxiety prepared him for fight or flight; when he could not do either, conflict developed, frustration appeared, tension became obvious, and pacing, perspiration, and other behaviors occurred that used up as much energy as the physical labor. In this case, the father was rewarded; in instances in which that might not be true, the conflict and frustration would be intensified.

The fight or flight and rage responses stimulate sympathetic adrenal–medullary activity. In instances in which this is prolonged or excessive, a state of chronic arousal develops, leading to high blood pressure, arteriosclerotic changes, and cardiovascular disease. When the production of the adrenal cortical hormone is prolonged or excessive, behavior patterns of withdrawal and depression are seen. In addition, the immune response is decreased, and infections and tumors may develop. Two behavior patterns have been observed and correlated with the two extremes in endocrine activity just described: excessive dominance and excessive subordination.

Risk-Inducing Coping Processes

Coping itself can add to social, psychologic, and physiologic malfunction that increases the risk of illness. One way in which it does this is by direct damage to tissues. For example, the use of alcohol or drugs to alleviate stress may create liver damage; social relationships and psychologic welfare may also be affected. Coping by smoking may create lung damage. Over-

eating or undereating may have serious nutritional effects; psychosocial welfare may also be harmed. All of these increase the vulnerability of the body to further disease.

A second way in which coping increases the risk of illness is more indirect and can best be understood through an example. Type A people are driving, competitive, and achievement-oriented. The pattern they have developed reflects a socialization process that emphasizes the work ethic. Mobilization of type A behavior requires the increased output of catecholamines, the adrenal-medullary hormones. One might say the life of a type A person is a series of fight or flight responses.

A third way in which coping can increase health risk is called palliative. This is typified by the woman who feels a lump in her breast but denies its seriousness and delays seeking medical attention. The intention of palliative coping methods is to control the threat to life, but in the end they increase the risk of developing more severe illnesses because of their delaying action.

Ego defenses are "basically a coping strategy to deal with conflicts over a particular emotion." For example, if you are angry with someone, rather than create a scene that may lead to threats and retaliation, which would endanger your self-concept, you are likely to pick a less dangerous scapegoat or possibly work the anger out in physical exercise. Ego defenses imply an unconscious aspect in that usually the behavior is not the result of a deliberate thinking process, although some of it may be. Continual internal conflict and repression of emotions can lead to psychopathology.

Indices of Stress

Laboratory measurements of indicators of stress have significantly improved since the early experiments in the field and are daily adding to the understanding of this complex process. Among the measures, blood and urine analyses can be used to demonstrate changes in hormonal levels and hormonal breakdown products. Reliable measures of stress include blood levels of catecholamines, corticoids, ACTH, and a drop in eosinophils. The blood creatine/creatinine ratio and elevations of cholesterol and free fatty acids can also be measured. Immunoglobulin assays may be done. (With the growth of neuroimmunology, improved laboratory measures are likely to follow.)

The electroencephalogram may be used to measure brain activity. Galvanic skin resistance, which measures the electrical conductivity of the skin, may be performed. This is primarily a measure of sweat excretion, which rises in stress, and is typically used in lie detector tests. Rises in blood pressure and heart rate can also be measured.

In addition to these measurable signs, there are a number of other indices of stress that may be observed by others or by the person himself; they are listed in Chart 9-1. Over time, each person tends to develop a characteristic pattern of behavior in stress that is a warning that the system is out of balance. Researchers have developed many questionnaires to identify the *state* of stress in people and also the tendency toward stress, a *trait* of the personality.

Diseases of Adaptation: Maladaptation

The autonomic and endocrine responses to stress serve an adaptive function; their purpose is to restore equilibrium in the

---

* Dubos R. *Man Adapting*, p 30. New Haven, *Yale University Press, 1965.*

Chart 9–1
Indices of Stress

General irritability, hyperexcitation, or depression	Pounding of the heart
Dryness of the throat and mouth	Impulsive behavior, emotional instability
Overpowering urge to cry or run and hide	Inability to concentrate
Easily fatigued, loss of interest	Feelings of unreality, weakness, or dizziness
"Floating anxiety"—do not know exactly why or what	Tension, alertness
Easily startled	Trembling, nervous tics
Stuttering or other speech difficulties	Nervous laughter
Hypermotility: pacing, moving about, cannot sit still	Grinding of teeth
Gastrointestinal signs and symptoms: "butterflies" in the stomach, diarrhea, vomiting	Insomnia
Change in menstrual cycle	Perspiring
Loss of or excessive appetite	Increased frequency of urination
Increased use of legally prescribed drugs, such as tranquilizers or psychic energizers	Muscle tension and migraine headaches
	Pain in the neck or lower back
Accident proneness	Increased smoking
Disturbed behavior	Alcohol and drug addiction
	Nightmares

(Based on Selye H. Stress in Health and Disease. Stoneham, MA, Butterworths, 1976. Reprinted by permission of the publisher.)

individual. They may last minutes, hours, or days; the disturbance they cause is reversible. However, when we speak of "diseases of adaptation," we mean diseases in which the stress response plays the predominant etiologic role and irreversible pathology may be present. The preceding discussion has identified the mechanisms contributing to the formation of these diseases. Other chapters of the book discuss individual diseases in greater detail.

Selye (1976a) gives the following comprehensive list of disorders:

> High blood pressure, diseases of the heart and blood vessels, diseases of the kidney, eclampsia, rheumatic and rheumatoid arthritis, inflammatory diseases of the skin and eyes, infections, allergic and hypersensitivity diseases, nervous and mental diseases, sexual derangements, digestive diseases, metabolic diseases, cancer, and diseases of resistance in general.*

Some are due to an "excess of defensive, others to an over-abundance of submissive bodily reactions." It is important to retain the holistic concept in considering the multiple factors involved in these diseases. Emotional arousal may lead to the neuroendocrine responses. A pattern of positive feedback may develop that continues to stimulate the production of hormones, the bodily responses feed the emotional arousal, and a vicious cycle ensues. Other regulatory mechanisms, which have been on the periphery, become involved and contribute to further disturbances.

A Framework for the Concept of Stress

As we have seen, there is a long history in the study of stress and its relationship to illness, with many disciplines having presented theories to describe such a relationship. It has also become popular to associate stress with negative consequences and to spend a great deal of time and energy on methods to reduce stress, ignoring the potential positive effects (consider the positive effects of exercise). The National Academy of Science's Institute of Medicine convened a multidisciplinary group to study the research on stress and human health. The report (Elliot and Eisdorfer, 1982) reflected upon the diverse definitions of stress and developed a framework that incorporates multiple elements and can be used for the examination of stress by different fields. Three major elements are identified in the model: the potential activator, the reaction to that activator, and the resulting consequences (Fig. 9-3). (The reader will recognize these as incorporating concepts presented earlier in this chapter, more or less, forming a composite.)

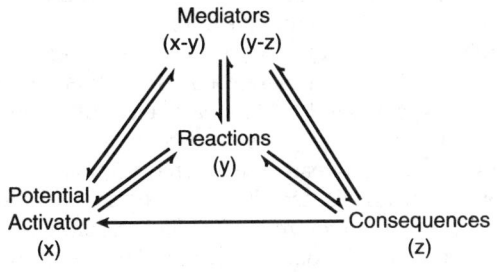

Figure 9–3. A framework for interactions between the individual and the environment. (Reproduced with permission from Elliott G and Eisdorfer C [eds]. Stress and Human Health. New York, Springer Publishing, 1982.)

* Selye H. The Stress of Life, pp 169–170. New York, McGraw-Hill, 1976.

An *activator* is "an internal and external environmental event or condition that alters one's physical and psychological state" (Elliott, 1989, p 51). The activator can be described by intensity, quantity, temporal pattern, and organizational level. Organizational level refers to the part of the body affected; it could be an enzyme, an organ, a system, or the whole psychologic state. A *potential activator* is one, such as a divorce or death of a loved one, for which a prediction can be made about the consequence. In this model, stressors are defined as a "subset of activators which are sufficiently intense or frequent to produce significant physical or psychological reactions" (Elliott, 1989, p 51).

Reactions are the physiologic and psychologic responses produced. They can be characterized by the same set of descriptors used for activators: intensity, quantity, temporal pattern, and organizational level. For example, being startled will lead to an immediate increase in heart rate, blood pressure, and respiratory rate, with increased vigilance, curiosity, and possibly fear.

Consequences may be confused with reactions but should be considered as cumulative and longer lasting, while reactions are transient. Not all consequences are relevant to one's health. They can be physiologic, psychologic, or sociologic, and they can be evaluated on the basis of their quality as good or bad, desirable or undesirable. In addition to the evaluation of quality, they are characterized by the same descriptors (*e.g.*, intensity, quantity) used for activators and reactions.

The model also incorporates *mediators* as those characteristics of the individual that influence the response to the activator. This includes not only coping abilities but also external supports. There is *dynamic interaction* among the elements of the model, with each part of the sequence continually changing and being affected by the other parts. This sequence occurs over and over, and different sequences occur simultaneously, such that the individual may be encountering the consequences of one event while another is being activated. Mediators, which help to determine the x-y-z sequence, are particularly affected by past experiences, or reactions and consequences.

A continuing problem in stress research has been to attribute the "cause" of an illness to stress; for example, stress on the job has led to a peptic ulcer, demands of the classroom have led to a migraine headache. In the x-y-z model, this is an x-z association and leaves out the intervening steps of reaction and mediation (x-y, y-z) or real causes. The x-z association can be very important in identifying risk factors, or stressors, that can be expected to lead to a particular consequence. For example, cigarette smoking has been demonstrated statistically to be associated with heart disease (more smokers than nonsmokers have heart disease). Determining that a factor is actually the cause requires reducing the incidence of the risk factor and analyzing the outcome (this is the case with cigarette smoking), or blocking the physiologic and psychologic reactions it produces.

Lowery (1987) has used the above x-y-z model to examine the state of stress research in the nursing field. Lyon and Werner (1987) have reviewed stress research in nursing from the conceptions of stress as a stimulus, as a response, and as a transaction. Both reviews concluded that there is great potential for nursing research in assessing stress and developing strategies for intervention. They also concluded that there have been serious methodologic issues in current nursing research in stress, not unlike those in other disciplines studying stress.

In summary, stress, like beauty, is in the eye of the beholder. Each person perceives and reacts to situations and change differently depending on his personal characteristics, abilities, and experiences, his external support systems, and characteristics of the stressor itself. The stress response produced may be elicited by real, potential, or imagined threats, leading to varied and multiple patterns of hormonal discharge. The goal is to mobilize the person's energy resources to cope with the stressor and to promote adaptive outcomes.

Stress Management

Stress or the potential for stress is ubiquitous: it can be everywhere and anywhere at once. Throughout this book, health problems will be identified that carry with them the potential for stress. Anxiety is the usual emotion accompanying stress. In the presence of anxiety, the customary activities of daily living may be disrupted; for example, sleep disturbance may be present and eating patterns altered. Coping patterns may be ineffective, thought processes may be impaired, and role relationships may suffer. It is obvious that many nursing diagnoses are possible.

Major factors that influence the development and impact of stress have been identified as the person's inner capabilities, his external resources, and the nature of the stressor itself. These are considered in discussing methods that nurses might use for reducing and controlling stress, not only in their patients but also in themselves. The need to prevent illness, improve the quality of life, and decrease the cost of health care makes efforts to promote health even more significant. The decrease of stress is an important goal.

Health Risk Appraisal

Health risk appraisal is an activity designed to promote health by examining the personal habits of the patient and recommending changes where health risk is indicated. Health risk questionnaires estimate the likelihood that a person with a given set of characteristics will become ill within a given time span. It is reasoned that if the patient is provided with this information, he will alter his activities (*e.g.*, stop smoking, have periodic screening examinations) to improve his health status. Questionnaires typically collect the following types of information:

1. Demographic data: age, sex, race, ethnic background
2. Personal and family history of certain diseases
3. Life-style factors
   - Eating, sleeping, exercise, smoking, drinking, and driving habits
   - Stressors on the job
   - Role relationships and associated stressors

4. Physical measurements
   - Blood pressure
   - Height, weight
   - Laboratory analyses of blood and urine
5. Membership or nonmembership in a high-risk group, such as a family with a history of cancer

The personal data are compared with average population risk data, and the risk factors are identified and weighted. From this analysis the person's chronologic age and risk age are determined, and a list of the person's major health hazards are identified. If the person makes suggested changes, further comparisons with population data can estimate how many years will be added to his life span (compliance age). Research so far has not demonstrated that providing people with such information ensures that they will change their habits.

Nursing Implications

Although the collection of data bases like the one just described is a common part of taking a nursing history, the controlled analysis of risk is not customary. The development of a *nursing* data base that supplies the essential information for making decisions about patient care is a necessity.

Health risk appraisal and patient education to improve health behavior are activities that nurses can perform to prevent health problems and reduce stress. In patients who *already* have health problems, there will be some degree of stress, and the nurse can *anticipate* changes based on the stress response. For example, the postsurgical patient will have fluid and electrolyte changes corresponding to the general neuroendocrine response. It should be mentioned that this response has a snowballing effect. Although it does not primarily affect the kidney, the vasoconstriction induced as part of the stress response may decrease the flow of blood to the kidney, which stimulates the renin–angiotensin mechanism, leading to an increase in aldosterone with sodium and water retention. Psychosocially, if the person typically withdraws and becomes nonexpressive in stress situations, that same behavior may be expected during this postsurgical period.

Coping Behaviors

It should be remembered that a person is in constant interaction with his environment, both internal and external. This implies that change is constant and necessary for optimal psychosocial and physiologic growth. Responding to change requires adaptive energy; the important issue is to regulate the use of energy so that there is an adequate store. This then becomes an issue of regulating one's own actions to reduce stress.

The functions of coping were listed earlier, as follows:

- *Emotion-focused:* directed at lessening emotional distress; include such strategies as avoidance, minimizing, distancing, selective attention
- *Problem-focused:* directed to management of the problem; include such strategies as defining the problem, finding alternative solutions, weighing them, and acting

Two commonly prescribed nursing interventions, the provision of sensory information and preoperative teaching, have the goal of improving the patient's coping ability. Major nursing research using these interventions has been conducted by Leventhal and Johnson (1983). They have tested the theory that people acquire a sense of control over events when they are given information that makes it possible for them to form a mental image of them. If people were provided with a description of the sensations they could expect to feel (*e.g.*, pulling, burning, pressure), if the routine of the procedure were described to them, and if they were given instructions in coping behaviors (deep breathing, coughing, turning, exercises), they would experience less distress and have better outcomes (less pain, better mood, fewer analgesics needed, more rapid recovery). In their work, the researchers have tested these techniques alone and in combination in different short-term and long-term threatening situations (diagnostic examinations and surgery). The outcomes have been complex and illustrate that individual differences in the perception of stress and its management must be taken into consideration.

Among their findings, Leventhal and Johnson discovered that the combination of sensory information and postoperative exercise instruction was not consistently effective. If the instruction provided the patient with a way of coping when he previously had none, it was more likely to be effective. If he already had an effective coping strategy, any new ones could be considered conflicting. In some instances, attempting to use the new strategy rather than relying on existing strategies was thought to delay recovery, particularly after the patient went home. Specific coping strategies were usually more effective in short-term than in long-term events. Individual differences were found to be significant.

The importance of this research lies in helping the nurse to decide who will benefit from the information provided, the goal to be achieved, and the specific outcome criteria to be used in evaluating the information.

Through health appraisals, nurses may identify patient stressors. However, stress control requires self-care and motivation, and therefore the patient must actively and willingly participate in appraising, identifying, and managing his sources of stress. At the same time, one should identify and capitalize on the patient's sources of strength. This helps to improve the patient's self-esteem and reinforces positive behavior patterns.

Stress-Reduction Methods

Numerous methods for reducing stress are available and being publicized. The important point to be remembered is that just as each person develops a particular pattern of stress response, so will each person have his preferred method of stress reduction. Bulechek and McCloskey (1985) described three nursing interventions for stress management: relaxation training, cognitive reappraisal, and music therapy. Sutterley and Donnelly (1981) identified categories of activities for the self-regulation of stress, including nutrition; exercise, physical activity, and recreation; muscle control and kinesiology; meditation and creative imagery; communication and time management; and group process and support systems.

Proper nutrition, adequate rest, and regular exercise improve one's well-being and help develop resistance to stressors. Regular exercise assists in weight control, decreases a sense of fatigue and monotony, and increases the exercise tolerance for some patients with angina pectoris and peripheral arterial disease. Some studies indicate that it may prevent heart attacks, and it may help to prevent premature atherosclerosis. The need for outside and diversionary activities for everyone has become a fact of life.

Biofeedback.   The purpose of biofeedback is to gain some degree of mental control over the autonomic nervous system and possibly decrease blood pressure, control heart rate, and prevent disorders such as migraine headache. Some form of electronic instrumentation is used to monitor a biologic function, such as measuring skin conductance with the galvanic skin responder. This information is amplified and sent back to the person, who then tries consciously to alter the output of the machine in some way. For example, by relaxing and decreasing the sweating of his palms, the person attempts to alter the tone generated by the machine. The activity that produces an altered tone in the machine alters the biologic functioning.

Through practice and reinforcement, the person learns how to control the activity without the machine. Some people suffering from migraine headaches have developed a technique of "thinking their hands hot" and theoretically have directed the blood flow from the head to the hands. The long-term efficacy of such techniques is still being tested.

Relaxation Response. The "relaxation response" is a calming state opposite to the arousal state of stress. Four elements are necessary to produce the relaxation response: a quiet environment, a comfortable position, a passive attitude, and a mental device or object, such as a word, sound, or phrase to occupy the mind and keep out thoughts. For example, the word *one* could be repeated silently or audibly. By sitting quietly and practicing relaxation 15 to 20 minutes once or twice a day, a person should be able to achieve positive results in lowering stress levels. Other techniques, such as meditation and yoga, also produce the relaxation response. Still others use the sound of pleasant music or a mountain stream in conjunction with relaxation techniques to help achieve the desired state. Progressive relaxation is a technique in which muscle groups are alternately tensed and relaxed in a systematic fashion so that the person can compare the two effects, and it culminates with a period of complete relaxation.

Other techniques, such as massage, may be used; the effectiveness of slow-stroke back massage in patients with high emotional and physiologic arousal has been demonstrated. Relaxation training might be used in the following nursing diagnoses: anxiety, sleep disturbance, ineffective breathing pattern, ineffective coping, and pain.

It is important for the nurse to determine what type of stress-reduction activities work best and to encourage their regular use.

Social Support. The importance of social support as a mediating resource in stress has already been identified. To reinforce that information, the function of social networks includes the following:

- The maintenance of positive social identity
- The provision of emotional support
- The provision of material aid and tangible services
- Access to information
- Access to new social contacts and new social roles

The emotions—anxiety, fear, guilt—that accompany stress are unpleasant, and often increase in a spiraling fashion without intervention. Emotional support from family and significant others provides a person with love and a sense of sharing the burden. Being able to talk with someone and express one's feelings openly may help one to gain mastery of the situation. Nurses can provide this source of support; however, it is important to identify the patient's social support system and encourage its use. People who are "loners" or isolated, or who withdraw in times of stress have a high risk of coping failure.

Anxiety may also distort a person's ability to process information. Perception is narrowed, thoughts may be unclear, and reality may be distorted. For a time, this cognitive blurring is adaptive and allows the person to tolerate a threat, perhaps some bad news. However, reality must be faced for the longer run. It helps to seek information and advice from others who can assist with analyzing the threat and developing a strategy to manage it. Again, this use of others helps the person to maintain mastery of a situation and to keep his self-esteem.

There is a growing awareness in the public of the need for support groups. Groups have been formed by parents of children with leukemia, ostomates, mastectomy patients (Reach to Recovery) and other cancer victims, and persons with other serious diseases. There are groups for single parents, and Alcoholics Anonymous and spouses of alcoholics, drug addiction groups, and child abuse groups meet for mutual support. Professional, civic, and religious support groups are active in the community. Being a member of a group with similar problems has a releasing effect on the person that promotes freedom of expression and exchange of ideas. There are also encounter groups, assertiveness training programs, and consciousness-raising groups to help people modify their usual behavior.

Human evolution has led to a brain that possesses neural networks characterized by a plasticity that permits behavior to be modified. This flexibility allows people to make choices and thereby exert some control over the strategies they select for survival. The nurse can play a significant role in influencing those choices.

Chapter Summary

Stress has been identified as being capable of producing psychologic and physiologic effects that are disruptive to health. When an individual is ill, some degree of stress is a usual accompaniment. In the patient care situation, it will be the nurse's role to appraise and diagnose the patient's health state (including life-style, self-care activities, health promotion, coping behaviors, and resources) and to support and instruct the patient in stress management or reduction techniques. Stress reduction techniques utilize relaxation and psychoeducational techniques to gain mental control. The use of support groups and health-promoting life-style practices also decrease the effects of stress.

Bibliography

Books

Asterita MF. The Physiology of Stress. New York, Human Sciences Press, 1985.

Bulechek GM and McCloskey JC. Nursing Interventions: Treatments for Nursing Diagnoses. Philadelphia, WB Saunders, 1985.

Cheren S (ed). Psychosomatic Medicine: Theory, Physiology, and Practice (2 vols). Madison, CT, International Universities Press, 1989.

Dubos R. Man Adapting. New Haven, CT, John Wiley & Sons, 1965.

Elliott G. Stress and illness. In Cheren S (ed). Psychosomatic Medicine: Theory, Physiology, and Practice (2 vols). Madison, CT, International Universities Press, 1989.

Elliott G and Eisdorfer C (eds). Stress and Human Health. New York, Springer Publishing Co, 1982.

Groer MW and Shekleton ME. Basic Pathophysiology: A Conceptual Approach, 3rd ed. St Louis, CV Mosby, 1989.

Guyton AC. Textbook of Medical Physiology. Philadelphia, WB Saunders, 1986.

Lazarus RS and Folkman S. Stress, Appraisal, and Coping. New York, Springer Publishing Co, 1984.

Leventhal H and Johnson JE. Laboratory and field experimentation: Development of a theory of self-regulation. In Wooldridge PJ et al (eds). Behavioral Science and Nursing Theory. St Louis, CV Mosby, 1983.

Marriner A (ed). Nursing Theorists and Their Work. St Louis, CV Mosby, 1986.

Milsum JH. Health, Stress, and Illness: A Systems Approach. New York, Praeger, 1984.

Monat A and Lazarus RS (eds). Stress and Coping. New York, Columbia University Press, 1985.

Pelletier KR. Mind as Healer, Mind as Slayer. New York, Dell, 1977.

Restak RM. The Brain. New York, Bantam Books, 1984.

Selye H. The Stress of Life. New York, McGraw–Hill, 1976a.

Selye H. Stress in Health and Disease. Boston, Butterworths, 1976b.

Selye H (ed). Selye's Guide to Stress Research. New York, Van Nostrand Reinhold, 1980.

Sutterley DC and Donnelly GF (eds). Coping with Stress. Rockville, MD, Aspen Systems, 1981.

Vander AJ, Sherman JH, and Luciano DS. Human Physiology: The Mechanisms of Body Function. New York, McGraw–Hill, 1985.

Weiner H and Fawzy FI. An integrative model of health, disease, and illness. In Cheren S (ed). Psychosomatic Medicine: Theory, Physiology and Practice (2 vols). Madison, CT, International Universities Press, 1989.

Wolf SW and Goodell H. Harold Wolff's Stress and Disease. Springfield, IL, Charles C Thomas, 1968.

Wooldridge PJ et al (eds). Behavioral Science & Nursing Theory. St Louis, CV Mosby, 1983.

Journals

Asterisks indicate nursing research articles.

* Brandt P and Weinert C. The PRQ—A social support measure. Nurs Res 1981 Sep/Oct; 30/(5):277–280.

Burckhardt CS. Coping strategies of the chronically ill. Nurs Clin North Am 1987 Sep; 22(3):543–551.

Cobb S. Social support as a moderator of life stress. Psychosom Med 1976 Sep/Oct; 38(5):300–314.

Cohen JJ. Stress and the human immune response: A critical review. J Burn Care Rehabil 1985 Mar/Apr; 6(2):167–173.

Crosby LJ. Stress factors, emotional stress and rheumatoid arthritis disease activity. J Adv Nurs 1988 Jul; 13(4):452–461.

Doswell WM. Physiological responses to stress. Annu Rev Nurs Res 1989; 7:51–70.

Fagin CM. Stress: Implications for nursing research. Image: Journal of Nursing Scholarship 1987 Spring; 19(1):38–42.

Folkman S and Lazarus RS. The relationship between coping and emotion: Implications for theory and research. Soc Sci Med 1988; 26(3):309–317.

Folkman S et al. Age differences in stress and coping processes. Psychol Aging 1987 Jun; 2(2):171–184.

Holmes TH and Rahe RH. The social readjustment rating scale. J Psychosom Res 1967 Aug; 11:213–218.

Illness and stress. ANS 1989; 11(2) (Entire issue).

Johnson JE and Lauver DR. Alternative explanations of coping with stressful experiences associated with physical illness. Adv Nurs Sci 1989; 11(2): 39–52.

Lambert CE and Lambert VA. Hardiness: Its development and relevance to nursing. Image: Journal of Nursing Scholarship 1987 Summer; 19(2): 92–95.

Lindeman CA. Patient education. Annu Rev Nurs Res 1989; 7:199–212.

Lowery BJ. Stress research: Some theoretical and methodological issues. Image: Journal of Nursing Scholarship 1987 Spring; 19(1):42–46.

Lyon BL and Werner JS. Stress. Annu Rev Nurs Res 1987; 6:3–22.

* Manfredi C et al. Perceived stressful situations and coping strategies utilized by the elderly. J Community Health Nurs 1987; 4(2):99–110.

Mason JW. A historical view of the stress field, Part I. J Hum Stress 1975a Mar; 1(1):6–12.

Mason JW. A historical view of the stress field, Part II. J Hum Stress 1975b Jun; 1(2):22–36.

*McNett S. Social support, threat, and coping responses and coping effectiveness in the functionally disabled. Nurs Res 1987 Mar/Apr; 36(2): 98–103.

Norbeck JS. Social support. Annu Rev Nurs Res 1988; 6:85–110.

Norbeck JS, Lindsey AM, and Carrieri VL. Further development of the Norbeck Social Support Questionnaire: Normative data and validity testing. Nurs Res 1983 Jan/Feb; 32(1):4–9.

Orshan SA. Pain and stress management in nursing: Controversy and theory. Holistic Nurs Pract 1988 May; 2(3):9–16.

Pearlin LI et al. The stress response. J Health Soc Behav 1981 Mar; 22: 337–356.

Pollock SE. Adaptation to chronic illness. Nurs Clin North Am 1987 Sep; 22(3):631–644.

Ryan MC and Austin AG. Social supports and social networks in the aged. Image: Journal of Nursing Scholarship 1989 Fall; 21(3):176–180.

Shaver, JF. A biopsychosocial view of human health. Nurs Outlook 1985 Jul/Aug; 33(4):186–191.

Social support. ANS 1988 Jan; 10(2).

Sutterley DC. Stress management: Grazing the clinical turf. Holistic Nurs Pract 1986 Nov; 1(1):36–53.

* Toth JC. Stressors affecting older versus younger AMI patients. Dimens Crit Care Nurs 1987 May/Jun; 6(3):147–157.

* Walker SN, Sechrist KR, and Pender NJ. The health-promoting lifestyle profile: Development and psychometric characteristics. Nurs Res 1987 Mar/Apr; 36(2):76–81.

Woods NF. Women's health. Annu Rev Nurs Res 1989; 7:209–236.

10

Human Response to Illness

Learning Objectives

On completion of this chapter, the learner will be able to:

1. Identify the stages of illness and the role of the nurse during each of these stages
2. Describe the significance of the patient's need for inclusion, control, and affection during his adaptation to illness
3. Specify nursing strategies that are appropriate for assisting patients to develop and maintain a positive self-image and body image
4. Explain the emotions of anxiety, anger, hostility, grief, mourning, and hope as related to illness adaptation
5. Use the nursing process as a framework for care of patients with emotional reactions to illness and treatment: anxiety, anger and hostility, grief, mourning, and hope
6. Assess the significance of role changes that result from illness
7. Identify nursing actions that promote effective coping strategies
8. Specify the significance of communication and the nurse–patient relationship in the promotion of effective coping with illness
9. Identify ways that nurses can resolve their own emotional reactions that result from dealing with patients and families during the crisis of illness
10. Specify nursing strategies appropriate for dealing with patients with problems of cognition, affect, and behavior and psychophysiologic interactions

Most people do not expect to get sick or have life-altering accidents. One of the most prominent hopes among Americans is that they and their families will have long and healthy lives. Yet, at any point along the life continuum they may be faced with difficult and painful changes in their health status.

The experience of illness precipitates many stressful feelings and reactions. These include frustration, anxiety, anger, denial, shame, grief, and uncertainty. Patients and their families have to adapt to the demands of the different stages of illness. Painful and disturbing symptoms lead to diagnostic tests and medical treatment. There are often dreaded questions about prognosis, body changes, and the reactions of others. Hospitalization is a major stress. Although necessary and often life-saving, it places people in an unfamiliar and often frightening environment, where they feel vulnerable and out of control. Acute illness calls for immediate action; chronic illness involves intricate changes in life-style with an uncertain future.

Sick people are often sensitive and vulnerable. Their whole lives are changed, at least temporarily. They struggle with the resurgence of past experiences as they cope with the present reality and the anticipated future. Issues of mortality, dependency, trust, and identity are raised.

The nurse is a central figure in the patient's immediate life. Through sensitive understanding and intelligent action, she provides many opportunities for patients to maintain basic security, self-esteem, and integrity. She helps patients and families to cope with the crisis of illness.

Serious illness or injury is always more than just physical pain and inconvenience. The life goals, family, work and income, mobility, body image, and life-style of a patient may be drastically altered. Whether the changes are temporary or permanent, the situation may develop into a crisis for the person— a crisis that affects family, friends, and professional helpers. Emotional demands on the nurse are often continuous and draining. Without proper understanding and coping skills, the cumulative effect may be overwhelming and may lead to professional and personal problems.

To be of optimal help to patients, families, staff, and themselves, the nurse needs to know the following:

- The usual stages of illness and various emotional responses
- The major tasks of adapting to significant illness or injury
- The typical coping strategies used by patients and families
- The psychologic and social factors that help or hinder coping
- Her own reactions to the various stresses and how to deal with them

Stages of Illness

The transition from health to illness is a complex and highly individualized experience. In addition to restoring physiologic balance, the two main tasks are (1) to modify the body image, concept of self, and relations to other people and work and (2) to readjust realistically to the limitations imposed by the condition. The two tasks begin in the setting in which the person is being treated for the health problem.

In the cycle of health and illness, most people go through three stages: (1) the transition from health to illness, (2) the period of "accepted" illness, and (3) convalescence. The duration and quality of the experience vary with differences in personality, the specific disorder, and the changes made in the person's life.

First Stage

The development of symptoms usually is accompanied by unpleasant sensations, loss of vigor and stamina, and a decrease in the ability to function. Certain symptoms, such as chest pain, indigestion, and headache, may increase in frequency and intensity. Anxiety often is present and is handled with the person's usual coping mechanisms. To ward off the prospect of illness, one person may plunge into activity, keeping late hours with extra work and social activities. Another may become passive

and withdrawn, hoping that the vague symptoms will go away. A person may put off seeking medical care for fear of the diagnosis, especially if something serious is suspected, such as cancer. Anxiety, guilt, shame, and denial are prominent during this initial period.

If the symptoms persist, the person seeks medical attention. He may have ambivalent feelings toward examination and diagnostic tests, which are reflected in canceled or missed appointments. He may not follow initial recommendations or take prescribed medication. Some patients go from physician to physician, hoping to learn "what's really the matter" or that a previous diagnosis was inaccurate.

When a person experiences a sudden catastrophe, such as heart attack or stroke, he is instantly shifted from health to illness. His immediate concern is that help will not arrive in time or that the medical strangers on whom he is suddenly so dependent will not be competent. Families experience similar fears but have no time to consider alternatives. Apprehension is expressed through excessive demands, denial that the problem exists, refusal to cooperate or accept the proposed treatment, withdrawal, and suspicion of the motives and methods of those trying to help. To offset this reaction, it is helpful for the nurse to contact close relatives, significant others, and the person's own physician, if possible. Calm explanation of the necessary procedures and demonstration of technical skill will convey to patients that they are being cared for adequately.

When patients and families are experiencing shock, disbelief, and denial of the condition, the nurse helps by listening. In a noncritical way, she does not support the denial but accepts the need to cope with the situation in this way at the present time. She establishes herself as a professional person who wants to understand and help. She orients patients to the immediate environment and answers questions to the best of her ability.

Second Stage

The second stage is a shift to the period of accepting illness. The patient recognizes and admits that he is sick and in need of help from others, especially from the medical and nursing staffs. Temporarily, he adopts the patient role. This includes abdication from usual responsibilities and cooperation in the task of getting well. In this stage, patients become preoccupied with themselves, their symptoms, and their treatment; interest in current events and even concern about family and friends may be quite limited. Increased dependency accompanies preoccupation with somatic concerns. This behavior is often described as regressive, because it is a return to earlier forms of acting, feeling, and relating to others.

A certain amount of regression is necessary so that patients can allow themselves to rest in bed, eat specified diets, sleep, and let their bodies heal. People who normally resist being dependent may find this very difficult. They are so threatened that they continue to deny their condition in part or refuse prescribed treatment. They push themselves beyond their physical limits and discontinue treatment prematurely. The other extreme of dependency problems is seen in patients who receive so much gratification from dependency that they attempt to continue it indefinitely; the terms *hospitalitis* and *secondary gain* refer to this.

When acutely ill, patients need a great deal of help from others. There must be a realistic evaluation of the stage of illness, the patient's need for dependency, and the need for a trusting, caring person. The nurse who cares for the same patients over long periods of time should evaluate her own needs for having others dependent on her. The nurse can help patients move through the stages of illness so that they become autonomous and able to care for themselves again.

During the stage of accepting illness, the patient may express anger, guilt, and resentment. He may be very critical of care and medical management, attacking the very people he depends on. The most helpful nursing approach is to view this reaction as the person's attempt to deal with the situation. The nurse tries to understand how patients and families feel. She encourages the expression of feelings without passing judgment, moralizing, or arguing. Labeling the feeling (*i.e.,* "This must be difficult to believe," or "You must be feeling a loss of control") will encourage patients to verbalize fears.

When sick, patients often feel helpless and hopeless. The nursing staff assumes responsibility for the care of patients, recognizing their individual differences and needs. They provide opportunities for the patient to make decisions and assume responsibility whenever indicated. As the patient's condition improves and he becomes more assured of the staff's availability, interest, and competence, he is less anxious and more able to relinquish dependency. During this period, the patient may be experiencing an acute sense of loss. The clinical picture is depression with sadness, hopelessness, and anger. He may be mourning the loss of health and vigor, the loss of a body part or function, or changes anticipated in job and family. He may be moving into the emotional reactions to dying (see the discussion of dying and death at the end of this chapter).

Third Stage

The third stage is the convalescent or restitution period. The return of health and physical strength often precedes the patient's feeling and acting "well." Just as a lag usually occurs in the initial stage between the appearance of physical symptoms and the emotional acceptance of illness, a reverse lag occurs in recovery. Getting well implies giving up a dependent, regressive position and resuming adult responsibilities and normal relations with others. Although some people are reluctant to give up the patient role, most are motivated toward health but are afraid or hesitant to try out new skills. This is particularly true if the illness and treatment require major changes in work and family relations.

The nurse helps patients in this stage by gradually relaxing protection and offering guidance, advice, and encouragement to progress. She quietly retires to the sidelines, ready to reassure but encouraging experimentation with new skills. She steps in only when gross errors in judgment occur. The patient senses the confidence of the nurse and is reassured by it, especially if ideal or perfect results are not expected.

During the convalescent stage, the nurse can stimulate the patient to renew his interest in the world, communicate better with family, and make plans for the future. For example, there are support groups for people who have had strokes, mastectomies, and other conditions. A member of one of these groups may be called in to talk to the patient both before and after an operation, to convey hope and to give realistic, firsthand information on coping with their common disability. At first, the patient may be overwhelmed by anxiety or grief and unable to use these services. During convalescence, he is reminded and encouraged to avail himself of this help. It is important to keep individual differences in mind because some patients do not want to affiliate with such groups. The connotation of being different, especially with a stigmatized condition, may be too painful to admit publicly.

Adapting to Illness

Just what is it that patients and families have to cope with when they become sick? The major tasks have been identified by Moos (1984) as follows:

- Dealing with the discomfort, incapacitation, and symptoms of the illness or injury
- Managing the stress of treatment procedures and hospitalization
- Developing and maintaining adequate relationships with the medical, nursing, and other caretaking staff
- Preserving a satisfactory self-image and maintaining a sense of competence and mastery
- Balancing the disturbing feelings aroused by illness and treatment
- Maintaining relationships with family and friends despite a changed role identity
- Preparing for an uncertain future in which further loss, death, or recovery are possibilities

These adaptive tasks often occur simultaneously or recur at different stages of the illness.

The stages of transition from health to illness and back to health are most clearly defined when a person has an acute condition that responds favorably to treatment. A similar series of steps takes place in adapting to a chronic condition. The stages are disbelief, developing awareness, reorganization, and resolution. In a successful adaptation to a chronic illness, the person can comfortably or resignedly regard himself as having a specific condition. He acknowledges and copes with the necessary changes in his life imposed by the condition. Although he may have gone through periods of despair, anger, and self-depreciation, he is able to regard himself as a worthwhile person who happens to need help in some form and degree.

Adaptation to chronic illness is a lengthy and continuous process. The extent of adaptation required depends on the type of illness, the degree of disability, and the patient's unique personality. Some chronic illnesses are relatively stable, with few changes; others have acute remissions and slow degeneration; some are terminal. Unpredictability is a hallmark of chronic illness, in terms of symptoms, effectiveness of treatment, hopes for future remissions and medical breakthroughs, and the reactions of others. Patients are often torn between living within their limitations and pushing for more.

Basic Emotional Needs

Everyone has the same basic emotional needs. These have been variously categorized as the need for love, trust, autonomy, identity, self-esteem, recognition, and security and are summarized by Schutz (1966) as the interpersonal need for inclusion, control, and affection. The nonrealization of a need leads to undesired feelings and behaviors. Feelings such as anxiety, anger, loneliness, and self-doubt are raised.

The interpersonal needs for inclusion, control, and affection are expressed in group as well as one-to-one situations. This is seen in relationships among patients on a unit and within their families. The needs are present in staff relationships and often make the difference in the morale of a unit as well as in how well it is managed.

These needs are overlapping and continuous. Inclusion is primarily related to the formation of a relationship, while control and affection are demonstrated within the relationship. Inclusion is feeling "in" or "out"; control is "top" or "bottom"; and affection is "remote" or "close." Generally, people establish equilibrium between themselves and others in these three areas. Illness with hospitalization disturbs this equilibrium, giving rise to a wide variety of new stresses.

Need for Inclusion

The need for inclusion is defined behaviorally as the need to establish and maintain satisfactory relationships with people with respect to association and interaction. It refers to the establishment and maintenance of a feeling of mutual interest in others. The need for inclusion is the need to feel that the self is significant and worthwhile. Inclusion behavior refers to association between individuals and is indicated by such words as *associate, interact, belong, join,* and *communicate*. Lack of inclusion is connoted by words such as *excluded, ignored, withdrawn, aloof,* or *isolated*. The need to be included is shown by the desire to attract attention and interest. The "demanding" patient who frequently signals and monopolizes the staff with extensive conversation may simply be indicating strong needs for inclusion. The nurse who feels personally slighted when a patient ignores her attempts at polite conversation or treats her like a servant rather than a professional person may be demonstrating her own inclusion needs.

The desire for prestige and status is a part of inclusion needs; the individual needs people to pay attention to him, know who he is, and distinguish him from others. Identity is closely related to inclusion. One is known as a distinct individual, who therefore deserves attention. The height of inclusion is to be understood, which implies that someone is interested enough to seek and discover a person's particular characteristics, likes, and dislikes.

When a person enters a hospital situation, his first crisis involves inclusion needs. Will the staff know who he is? Will he be treated like a person and not just another case—"room 111" or "the new cardiac"? Many routines of hospital admission strip the patient of outward signs of prestige and status. His clothes and belongings, even his dentures, may be taken away. He may be bombarded by a series of questions relating to the most intimate details of his life. He is expected to join the patient "group" but may be given little explanation or few guidelines about what to do. When it is necessary to place a patient in isolation, attention should be given to his inclusion needs—the nurse becomes a vital link in satisfying them.

Other ways to help a patient with his inclusion needs include giving him a thorough and considerate orientation to his physical surroundings. The nurse can inquire about the patient's questions and expectations related to treatment. She can give some guidelines about the scope of her professional responsibility, explaining that she will be available to help in a variety of ways.

The patient who is withdrawn and avoids association with other may have unmet inclusion needs. He may not talk to his roommates or the nurse and may spend long periods sleeping or with the curtains pulled. A certain amount of regression and isolation is often a necessary part of adaptation to illness and recovery, but extremes over a period of time may indicate the need for evaluation. Underneath an apparent indifference to others may lie a basic anxiety about relationships with others. The patient's worst fear may be that others will ignore him and show no interest in him, although the fear is disguised with a lack of interest in others and a seeming independence. Patients who feel abandoned and isolated from their families and friends, who believe that they are so changed now as to be unacceptable, or who feel rejected and ignored by the medical and nursing staff may give up the struggle. On the other hand, such patients may get lifesaving reassurance and support from the nurse who communicates her recognition of their individuality and worth.

Part of the decision of where to place a patient on the nursing unit is based on the need for inclusion. Will he do better in a room with other people? How close to the nursing station should he be? Patients who are together for long periods of time, such as in a rehabilitation facility, demonstrate a particularly wide variety of inclusion needs.

Need for Control

The second major need is control. This is the need to establish and maintain a satisfactory relation to others with regard to power, decision making, and authority. It has to do with the feeling of mutual respect for the competence and responsibility of oneself and others. Control needs are suggested by such words as *dominance, influence, boss, rebellion, submission, leader, noncooperation,* and *follower*. Control represents assumption of power over others and therefore over one's own future, whereas *being* controlled means giving up responsibility for oneself.

When a person comes to a hospital, he struggles with his need for control. In addition to the problems of inclusion, he may find other people making decisions for him that he would ordinarily make for himself—when to get up, what to eat, and when to go to the toilet. The rules of the hospital may take away his usual decision-making capacity. An extreme example of control behavior is the person who completely gives up or abdicates his own responsibility. He is a clinging, helpless patient who seeks direction from everyone about what to do and how to do it. This reinforces his conviction that he is incompetent, irresponsible, and powerless. Behind these beliefs often lie anxiety, hostility, and a lack of trust in others as well as oneself. Nursing interventions that help the patient to assume responsibility early for making decisions about his own care contribute to restoring control.

The other extreme in control behavior is reflected in actions of constant rebellion and domination. Although the patient's overt behavior may be that of a strong, competent, responsible person, his underlying feelings may be those of uncertainty in his own power. He takes every opportunity to disprove these fears and therefore has a great deal of difficulty in accepting the need for dependency in such matters as bed rest or following "doctor's orders." Nurses also need to examine their own needs for power and control in relation to patients, co-workers, and physicians.

Need for Affection

The third major need is that of affection. This represents the need to establish with another person a give-and-take relationship based on mutual liking. Affection is suggested by such words as *love, like, emotionally close, personal, friendship,* and *intimacy.* Lack of affection is connoted by *hate, dislike,* and *emotionally distant.* The need for affection usually is met by family members, spouses, and close friends. When a person is separated from these sources by illness or hospitalization, the need for affection may not be satisfied. Being emotionally close to another generally results in confiding to that person one's innermost anxieties, wishes, and feelings. In the hospital setting, the patient may turn to the nurse to share these things, especially if the family member is unavailable or too anxious to listen. One difference between a social and a professional relationship is that the former implies mutual need satisfaction, the latter, exclusive attention to the patient's needs. However, the need for affection in both patient and nurse must be considered, particularly when the relationship continues over a period of time.

Self-Image and Body Image

The person has a mental and social picture of himself that is based on multiple experiences in the past, present, and anticipated future. Serious illness and injury abruptly interfere with that self-concept. Adaptation to the changes imposed by illness can affect the person's sense of identity. People often rate themselves as courageous or cowardly in terms of how they handle pain; crying may be a sign of weakness to them. A major disability can be viewed as a limitation to be challenged. Other people regard themselves as cripples, which emphasizes the disability and is stigmatizing. An important aspect of the total self-image that is often affected by physical illness is body image.

Concept of Body Image

The concept of body image is useful in understanding the many complex reactions of people to changes in health status. Body image may be considered as the total, constantly changing and evolving perception of one's physical self as separate and distinct from all others. This perception is based on inner sensations and functionings as well as on information derived from the external environment. Society prescribes norms of physical appearance and behavior. The perception of body image operates on both conscious and unconscious levels.

Integration of experiences with use of the body takes place over a long period of time. The formative years of childhood are particularly significant in laying down the basic body image and its relation to the personality. While a child is being held, fondled, fed, played with, and toilet-trained, he gradually accumulates related concepts pertaining to ability to use his physical body, pride, and sense of identity. Through sensory impressions, mobility, and touch, he experiences pleasure, pain, shame, failure, or pride of accomplishment as he tests his boundaries and abilities. As the small child becomes aware of his separation from others, he grows increasingly conscious of his own body, its relation to others, and his ability to control his muscles in the acts of locomotion, bowel and bladder retention and release, motor coordination, and speech. During this period, he begins to master these abilities, and thus acquires pride and self-esteem. If he is not able to gain this mastery, because of loss of self-control and parental overcontrol, he may develop basic attitudes that lead him to regard his body as inadequate, worthless, and shameful. Illness, with enforced dependency and lack of body control, reactivates in people of all ages many of these early conflicts and perceptions of body image. Feeling ashamed of a disfigurement or deformity stems from early feelings of smallness, weakness, and ugliness as compared to others. The prominent sociocultural values of youth, physical attractiveness, health, and wholeness are incorporated early and reinforced throughout life.

Threats to Body Image. Threats to the body image, and hence to self-esteem, are recognizable in many nursing situations. Feelings of shame, inadequacy, and guilt may be precipitated, depending on the patient's assessment of the situation. Violation of modesty and invasion of privacy cause anxiety and embarrassment. Exposure of the body during physical examinations and such treatments as enemas and catheterizations may be upsetting, even though expected as part of the therapeutic regimen. Disturbances in usual elimination processes and the need for using a bedpan or talking about bowel and bladder habits threatens self-esteem. This is a major problem for people requiring the type of surgery that produces such drastic changes as a colostomy or ileostomy.

Major changes in the body image are brought about by amputation of any part or by surgery on the face, hands, and reproductive organs—these areas particularly are related to identity and self-esteem. Other parts of the body may have unconscious symbolic meanings for a person and may cause unexpected reactions to relatively minor external changes.

Besides the sudden changes in body structure and functioning that occur through accident or surgical intervention, subtle changes occur in progressive conditions such as arthritis, obesity, and multiple sclerosis. Even normal changes in the body, such as occur in puberty and pregnancy, pose a problem of altering the body image. During adolescence there is a sensitive, often painful awareness of the body and its many changes. Complexion, weight, and development of primary and secondary sexual characteristics are closely linked to feelings of worth and sexual desirability.

Changes in the body image may result from such side effects of medication as development of a moon face, changes in the secondary sex characteristics, and growth of facial hair. The reaction of the body to radiation treatment may further threaten the body image, as may changes in skin color, such as those that occur in jaundice.

Changes in medical technology require that nurses meet the challenge of new and different approaches to helping people. A person with chronic kidney damage extends his body image to include the "artificial kidney." Organ transplantation is another area that raises questions about body image. What does it mean to a person to have another person's heart beating in one's chest?

Nursing Implications. The first step in understanding the concept of body image is to become more aware of one's own attitude toward health, illness, disfigurement, and changes in body functioning. Anxiety, revulsion, disgust, and pity are often automatic responses to abnormal body appearance and functioning. To help patients who have these conditions, nurses must come to terms with their own feelings. A patient has a right to expect that nurses will be knowledgeable about his condition, impartial toward it, willing to help him, and concerned about him. A patient often uses the nurse's reactions as a test of whether he is still a worthwhile person in spite of his altered appearance or functioning.

The nurse needs to learn what alteration in the body can mean to the individual patient and what adjustments it will require. Both the patient and his family should be considered because, ideally, the adjustment that takes place is mutual. In formulating the nursing care plan for a particular patient, it is useful to include the ability of the family to help the patient cope with changes, orientation to reality, specific problems in coping and methods of coping, and nursing care. The nurse needs to determine how she can support the family and the steps she will take in response to the patient's positive moves. She can anticipate grief, mourning, and anger as reactions to changes in body appearance and functioning. The need for hope and steps toward full rehabilitation must be supported.

Social Adjustments.   Even after the patient has begun to alter his body image and feels worthwhile and accepted in the hospital setting, he is faced with adjusting to society. Many conditions of altered appearance and functioning are stigmatizing. Because of their close proximity to illness, nurses may lose sight of the fact that being disfigured or incapacitated still evokes negative responses and rejection by most of the population. Any such stigma implies that the person is not quite normal—that he is a disabled person, rather than a person having a specific disability. The tendency to stereotype denies the person's individuality. A person with an obvious physical disability has a challenge in handling tensions in interpersonal situations. He may be subjected to curiosity and stares. He may be asked intrusive questions about his condition or treated as if he were completely helpless.

If the condition is not readily visible, learning to exercise information control may help one to avoid being stigmatized. For instance, wearing a prosthesis following a mastectomy can keep one's radical surgery from becoming common knowledge. Talking about one's health status, body functioning, and difficulties in adjustment is appropriate with health personnel and close family and friends. With other people, excessive dwelling on these topics may lead to rejection and ostracism.

A person making necessary adjustments to alterations in his body often is faced with physical and social insecurity. A physically normal person has a general idea of how high the bus steps are and is able to read from a menu. However, the person with a physical impairment may have to make constant and vigilant adaptations to his physical world. The person who uses a wheelchair must find a restroom large enough to maneuver in; one with diabetes must calculate his allowed food intake at a cocktail party; a person with crutches may find a revolving door almost impossible to manage. Adaptation requires energy, ingenuity, and persistence. Sometimes a person limits his living space and activities in order to provide more predictable situations. Although this arrangement may be safer, it also limits a person's full participation in life.

Reactions of others toward a person with a disability are ambiguous and conflicting. Acceptance and rejection, sympathy and pity, trust and fear, curiosity and revulsion, valuation and devaluation face him in countless interpersonal situations. He is often unsure of where he stands, particularly with strang-

ers. He is also often unsure of himself, because the process of adaptation and self-acceptance is a dynamic one.

Emotional Reactions to Illness and Treatment

Many disturbing feelings are aroused by acute and chronic illnesses and the treatment they require. Some emotional reactions commonly experienced by patients and their families are anxiety, anger, grief, hope, shame, guilt, courage, pride, despair, love, depression, helplessness, envy, loneliness, and faith. Nursing staff members also experience these feelings. How they are experienced and expressed depends on the basic personality, the perception of the situation, and the amount of support from others. There is no right or wrong way to feel about serious illness. Nurses can anticipate patterns and help patients and families express feelings in a constructive way.

Anxiety

Anxiety is a normal reaction to stress and threat. It is an emotional reaction to the perception of danger, real or imagined, that is experienced physiologically, psychologically, and behaviorally. Anxiety and fear are often used synonymously; however, fear generally refers to a specific threat, anxiety to a nonspecific one. A person experiencing anxiety may feel uneasy and apprehensive and may have a vague sense of dread. Feelings of helplessness and inadequacy may be present along with a sense of alienation and insecurity. The intensity of these feelings may range from mild to severe enough to cause panic, and the intensity may be increased or diminished by interpersonal means.

Anxiety can be viewed as a process that includes the following steps: (1) an expectation exists; (2) the expectation is not met; (3) internal tension occurs; (4) relief behaviors are manifested; and (5) relief is experienced (Fig. 10-1). A typical example is that of a student taking an examination.

The student's expectation is that he will pass the exami-

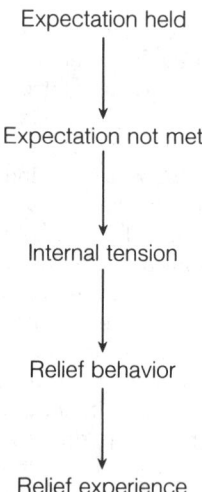

Figure 10–1. Operational definition of the anxiety process model. (Adapted from Anxiety: Concept and Manifestations [videocassette], 1977. Reproduced with permission from American Journal of Nursing.)

nation. This expectation is not met when he learns that he has failed. His internal tension rises and he experiences increased perspiration, palpitations, and abdominal discomfort. Relief behaviors are manifested, such as gum chewing, crying, or making an appointment to talk with the instructor. He experiences relief when he meets with the instructor and together they develop a structured study plan for him.

The anxiety process model can be used to facilitate nursing interventions. When a relief behavior is identified, the nurse can assist the patient to correlate the behavior with the increase in anxiety. Once this is accomplished, the nurse and the patient can explore what expectation was held and what occurred that prevented that expectation from being met. In doing this, the nurse helps the patient examine and handle future anxiety-producing situations in a healthier manner.

Anxiety is caused by a threat to the functioning of the organism—either to physical survival or to the integrity of the psychosocial self (self-image). Often, the threat affects both of these areas: a person who is anxious because of acute pain may also be anxious in response to his feelings about his levels of courage and dependency. Illness and hospitalization include the following anxiety-precipitating threats: general threat to life, health, and body integrity; exposure and embarrassment; discomfort from pain, cold, fatigue, and changes in diet; deprivation of sexual satisfaction; restriction of movement; isolation; interruption or loss of one's means of livelihood; precipitation of a financial crisis; dislike, rejection, or ridicule from others as the result of the condition; inconsistent and unpredictable behavior of the authority figures on whom one's welfare depends; frustration of goals and expectations; confusion and uncertainty about the present and the future; and separation from family and friends.

Physiologic reactions to anxiety are primarily reactions of the autonomic nervous system and are defensive. They include increases in pulse and respiratory rates; shifts in blood pressure and temperature; relaxation of the smooth muscles in the bladder and bowel; cold, clammy skin; increased perspiration; dilated pupils; and dry mouth. The bodily responses to mild anxiety initially promote learning and the ability to function, but

as the reaction increases in severity, learning decreases, perception is reduced or distorted, and the ability to concentrate is greatly diminished (Fig. 10-2). Nurses must be able to evaluate the level of anxiety in a patient so that it can be effectively reduced. An extremely anxious person is suffering and is very uncomfortable. He has difficulty giving or receiving information of any kind. He learns little about health matters and magnifies or distorts what he hears.

Characteristic manifestations of anxiety reflect a person's individuality. They include withdrawal, muteness, hyperactivity, swearing, talking and joking excessively, striking out verbally or physically, fantasizing, complaining, and crying. The specific means of coping with anxiety, whether successful or not, vary with individuals and with the situation. One disadvantage of enforced immobility and isolation is that a person who is accustomed to active approaches in handling anxiety is deprived of his usual means of coping and so must develop alternative strategies.

Nursing Interventions.   Nursing intervention directed toward reducing anxiety has four aspects:

1. The nurse recognizes that the patient is anxious. She is aware of situations that can potentially precipitate anxiety and is alert to physiologic, emotional, and behavioral clues.
2. The nurse verbally encourages the patient to recognize and express his feelings of anxiety.
3. If the source of the anxiety is external, such as poor orientation to the unit or disturbing noises and sights, the nurse takes steps to change these conditions or, if this is impossible, helps the patient to understand and cope with his reactions. She encourages the patient to share his immediate experience by open-ended statements such as "Tell me what happened," "What was going on?" or "What did you expect to happen?" Patients often need help in describing their reactions and thoughts. To ask initially, "Why are you anxious?" may or may not elicit the information. The person may be too afraid or unsure to tell you, he may not know why he is anxious, or he may resent the inquisition.
4. The nurse helps the patient to cope with what is now a specific

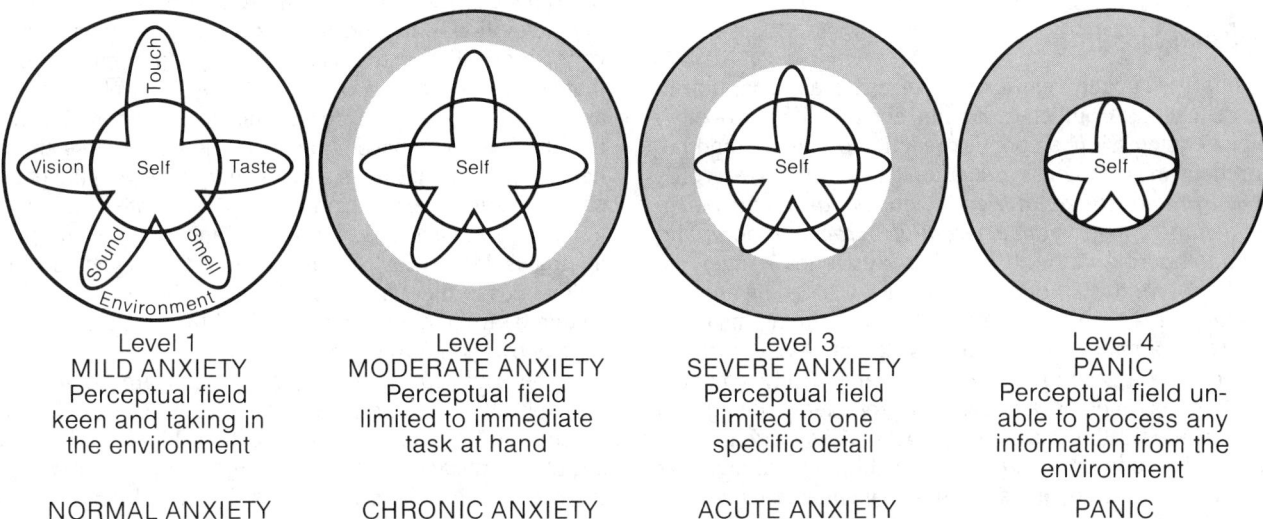

Figure 10-2. Levels of anxiety and the perceptual field. Shaded area indicates amount of environmental stimuli not attended to. (Reproduced with permission from Haber J et al. Comprehensive Psychiatric Nursing. New York, McGraw-Hill, 1987; copyright CV Mosby, St Louis.)

threat. The patient may be helped to reevaluate the situation and his reaction to it. Many times just the sharing of a feeling reduces its intensity. The nurse asks the patient what he usually does to handle anxious feelings and helps him to use similar or other means. The physical presence of the nurse may help, as well as the appropriate use of touch, physical care, and tone of voice.

The apprehension of patients recovering from surgery may be demonstrated by their anxiety about whether the operation was a success and whether they will survive the bewildering, painful, often uncertain postoperative period. The expert physical nursing care given in the recovery room or intensive care unit must take into consideration the patient's fears resulting from isolation; the unfamiliar noises and equipment attached to all parts of the body; the blinking, beeping monitor signaling the heart's functioning; and the periods of disorientation and loss of physical and emotional control. In this tense situation, the nurse must be constantly aware of her own behavioral manifestations of anxiety.

Illness and its treatment precipitate anxiety. For many people, early conflicts are revived. There is often a great deal of uncertainty about the future. Nurses sometimes are powerless to decrease the patient's anxiety at all, but they can avoid adding to it. For some patients, the thought of getting well and leaving the hospital produces anxiety. Nurses can be helpful to these people by encouraging them to mobilize their strengths and by encouraging decision making and the resumption of responsibility.

Nursing in almost all areas is a profession that deals continually with anxiety. The intimate association with life, death, and all the stages in between arouses within the nurse conscious and unconscious fears about her own vulnerability. Recognition, achievement, and attention are all important; she must be able to say that she did all that was possible. There are emotional high-risk situations in nursing, such as the intensive care unit and the emergency department, in which the nurse's understanding and management of her own anxiety as well as that of patients and their families are vital. See Nursing Care Plan 10-1 for an example of a nursing care plan for the patient with anxiety.

Anger and Hostility

In addition to anxiety, expressions of anger are common in nursing situations. Conflict, frustration, and loss of control often precipitate aggression, a complex reaction of feelings and behavior that varies in intensity, duration, and expression. Words such as *irritated, sullen, unfriendly, hostile, assertive, belligerent, defiant, uncooperative, resentful, enraged, furious,* and *indignant* describe various forms of aggressiveness. Anger, the general term for this emotion, is one way of handling anxiety, particularly in response to real or perceived threat, insult, or injury. To be a patient means to be sick, helpless, controlled by others, and assaulted—however therapeutically—by needles, catheters, enemas, and surgical procedures. Being told to wait for medication angers many patients who are in pain. Being awakened in the middle of the night to cough and take deep breaths taxes anyone's patience. Hospital rules and restrictions on visitors may arouse feelings of anger. When a patient is new to the hospital or clinic, he is often uncertain and anxious about his diagnosis, treatment, and prognosis; as a defense, he may lash out verbally at the nurse or withdraw

in sullen noncommunicativeness. Expressions of anger may decrease markedly as the element of the unknown is reduced and the patient becomes more familiar with his surroundings, the personnel, and the treatment program. On the other hand, anger may increase if the threat grows and the patient's needs are not met adequately. Allowing the patient choices provides for control by the patient and often helps reduce feelings of anger and frustration.

A person who has been angry, unhappy, and chronically dissatisfied with himself and others brings this behavior with him to the clinical setting. He may be argumentative, demanding, unappreciative, sarcastic, and unwilling to go along with nursing care. Extreme overfriendliness, ingratiation, and refusal to make any decision concerning one's care are also expressions of aggression. Occasionally, a patient is aggressive to the point of violence—throwing his dinner tray, shouting, cursing, doing or threatening to do physical harm. Nonverbal expressions of anger—glaring eyes, clenched fist, a sneer—can be equally as expressive. A patient's aggressive behavior may produce avoidance by the nurse, thus increasing feelings of distrust in the patient. The nurse then needs to make a conscious effort not to act on her feelings of avoidance but to be even more supportive to the patient.

Aggressive behavior that is ascribable to a toxic condition is acceptable; the patient can be excused because he was delirious or "not in his right mind." The continuously hostile patient who is fully conscious and in control is much harder to deal with and understand. The expression of anger in the clinical situation may reflect the person's best manner of coping with perceived threats. Anger may be an attempt to relieve feelings of helplessness and dependency. In other situations, anger is part of the grief process or emergence from apathy and depression. A patient's anger may vanish when someone helps him to identify what is frustrating or threatening him and to take steps toward successfully dealing with the threat.

It is not unusual for people to displace feelings of anger, that is, to express them toward someone or something other than the original source of frustration. When one believes oneself to be in a vulnerable position, it may not be safe to express dissatisfaction and anger directly. Therefore, one takes it out on somebody less likely to retaliate or less vitally important to one's emotional and physical well-being. A patient may be very angry with his physician but afraid to complain for fear that he will receive less attention. Instead, he yells at the nurse and later insists that she contact his doctor. Or, the nurse and the physician may have a covert misunderstanding; she finds herself snapping at others and being irritable with the patients. Generally, direct expressions of anger are not socially acceptable, and outbursts are followed by guilt, shame, and profuse apologies. Moreover, because of cultural and socioeconomic differences in the expression of anger, the nurse may be bewildered, insulted, and overwhelmed by behavior considered normal by another person.

The usual social responses to anger are counterattack, withdrawal, and avoidance of the situation. A nurse's initial reaction to an angry patient is to treat him as she would in social circumstances. Many times this is not appropriate from the therapeutic standpoint. The professional nursing responsibility is to try to help this person, even with and in spite of his anger. The nurse does this by first recognizing her own responses to angry behavior. It is not unusual for a nurse to experience feelings of irritation and annoyance. She may be

Nursing Care Plan 10–1

Care of the Patient With Anxiety

Mrs. Ann Stumpf, a 70-year-old widow, was taken to the emergency department following a fall in her apartment. She was alert and oriented but complained of pain in her right hip and inability to move her right leg. After examination in the emergency department, Mrs. Stumpf was admitted to the orthopedic unit with the diagnosis of fracture of the right hip.

Mrs. Stumpf was placed in Buck's traction with a trochanter roll. Her family was notified and she was scheduled for surgery the next day. Ms. Sabol, the primary nurse, entered Mrs. Stumpf's room to begin preoperative teaching. Mrs. Stumpf's vital signs were as follows: BP 138/98, P 100, R 28, and T 37.2°C (99°F). Her speech was rapid, she complained of pain in her hip, a dry mouth, excessive perspiration, increased restlessness, and her "heart pounding"; and she frequently requested the bedpan for urination. She had difficulty focusing on the information presented by Ms. Sabol as evidenced by her repeatedly asking, "What are you saying—I don't understand."

Nursing Diagnoses

1. Anxiety related to crisis situation and impending surgery
2. Pain related to fractured hip

Goals

1. Use of effective methods to cope with and lessen anxiety
2. Relief of pain

Nursing Interventions	Expected Outcomes	Outcomes

1. Establish relationship built on trust.
  a. Introduce self.
  b. Obtain patient's perception of problem.
	a. Acknowledges presence of nurse
	b. Verbalizes events leading to hospitalization and feelings about anticipated surgery and recovery
		• Called primary nurse by name
		• On admission, reconstructed events leading to hospitalization and events that followed; described feelings as "I don't know what will happen now"; unable to identify fears

c. Provide consistency in care and in approach to patient.
  d. Accept patient as an individual.
  e. Provide preoperative instructions in clear, simple manner.
	c–d. Exhibits behavior indicative of trust
	
	e. Focuses on preoperative instructions
		• One day after admission, expressed fears of unknown and anger at the situation; fearful about death, immobility, dependence
		• Verbalized that talking is helpful; asked when nurse will return; body posture relaxed. Provided accurate feedback of instructions

2. Assist patient to identify anxious feelings.
  a. Encourage patient to verbalize feelings of anxiety.
  b. Remain with patient.
	a. Verbalizes feelings of anxiety
	
	b. Anxiety decreases
		• Expressed anxiety about surgery, learning to walk, expenses of treatment, returning to apartment
		• Physiologic reactions to anxiety decreased (*i.e.*, mouth less dry, decreased perspiration, less urinary frequency, decreased restlessness)

c. Assist in identifying events that increase anxiety.	c. Identifies events that increase anxiety	• Identified the following as increasing anxiety: hurried atmosphere, pain when analgesic wears off, immobility
d. Discuss relationship between increased anxiety and physiologic functioning	d. Identifies increased anxiety as a precursor to altered physiologic function	• Accurately described relationship between anxiety and heart palpitations; reported fewer incidents of palpitations; reported increased salivation, decreased perspiration, decreased urinary frequency
e. Discuss relationship between increased anxiety and behavior patterns.	e. Identifies increased anxiety as a precursor to alterations in behavior	• Identified increased motor activity as a consequence of increased anxiety

(continued)

Nursing Care Plan 10–1 *(Continued)*

Care of the Patient With Anxiety

Nursing Interventions	Expected Outcomes	Outcomes
f. Note time and occasion of increased restlessness.	f. Decrease in restlessness	• Restlessness decreased; less adjustment of bed covers; able to process preoperative instructions; speech remained rapid at times
g. Promote use of effective coping measures to decrease anxiety.	g. Identifies effective coping mechanisms	• Identified the following as effective in decreasing anxiety: listening to music, visiting with family, reading magazines
h. Teach relaxation techniques.	h. Uses relaxation techniques to decrease anxiety	• Practiced relaxation techniques when feeling anxious; stated that relaxation techniques decreased feelings of anxiety
i. Encourage patient to use support systems.	i. Uses support of family	• Discussed impending surgery and fears about future with family
3. Relieve pain and discomfort.		
a. Administer analgesics as prescribed.	a. Experiences relief from pain	• Reported less discomfort 30 minutes after analgesic administered
b. Observe for side effects of analgesic.	b. Absence of side effects	• No evidence of side effects
c. Assess TPR, BP, q4h.	c. Vital signs normal	• Elevation of vital signs continues 24 hr after admission: T 37.4°C, P 90–100, R 22–26, BP 130/86–146/90
d. Observe right leg and foot for color, temperature, edema, position, sensation, ability to move foot/toes.	d. Absence of cyanosis, heat, edema, paralysis, abnormal sensation	• Swelling noted in right thigh; positioning maintained by traction and trochanter roll; color, temperature, sensation, and foot mobility normal

frightened, embarrassed, and hurt. When a patient lashes out verbally, she may feel inadequate and guilty, even if she has acted appropriately. She may feel helpless or immobilized to the extent that she dreads caring for the patient and begins to avoid him whenever possible. This kind of behavior may heighten the patient's frustration by leaving him isolated, helpless, and unable to depend on the nursing staff to meet his physical and emotional needs. Thus, a vicious circle is established.

Nursing Interventions. Therapeutic responses to angry patients are based on the attempt to understand the person and his situation. The nurse is aware of her own reaction to the patient and attempts to help him sort out the issues involved. She enables the patient to maintain his dignity, pride, and self-esteem so that his situation can be accepted as reality. She sets limits on his behavior so that he does not hurt himself or others and helps him to find more appropriate means of expressing his feelings. Although she may feel angry or frightened in reaction to the behavior, she uses her feelings for further problem solving, instead of giving way to retaliation or withdrawal. Helpful questions in arriving at a nursing care plan for patients who are angry and hostile include the following: When does the patient get angry and how does he show it? Does his anger interfere with his receiving the care he needs? Why does his behavior bother me? How do I react? Does he get angry with other people too? Is there someone who does get along with him? What does that person do that is different? Does the patient's hostility serve a useful purpose? How much of this

behavior reflects his usual way of reacting to people? How much is he willing to change? What realistic goals shall we work toward? Are there any other resources—physician, family, psychiatric nursing consultant, psychiatrist, occupational therapist, or other patients—that we could call in? If the patient stops expressing anger, will he develop more destructive patterns?

Learning to work therapeutically with angry, hostile patients is a challenging and rewarding part of nursing. Patients who disguise temporary fear and shame with anger appreciate the nurse who stands by them in the crisis without condemnation, rejection, or retaliation. Patients who have made a lifelong adjustment by means of hostile attack are also grateful, although they may never express it directly, to the nurse who refuses to be alienated and who applies herself to understanding and caring for them. Nursing Care Plan 10-2 is an example of a nursing care plan for the patient with anger and hostility.

Grief and Mourning

Grief is a complex of emotional responses to the anticipated or actual loss of someone or something valued. The loss may be that of a relative or friend, a part of the body, a job, health, or life. Feelings of anxiety, helplessness, hopelessness, guilt, anger, depression, remorse, sadness, and loneliness are part of grief. Mourning refers to the processes that follow the loss and ultimately result in overcoming the grief. Grief and mourning involve social responses that are best dealt with by the

Care of the Patient With Anger and Hostility

Following the reduction and internal fixation of Mrs. Stumpf's right hip, Ms. Sabol entered Mrs. Stumpf's room. Mrs. Stumpf became angry, sarcastic, and demanding. She complained that "no one has been in to check on me and I could have died—then all you nurses would be in trouble." She demanded that Ms. Sabol "take care of me just like the doctor said" and then told her to leave the room and "send someone else who knows what they're doing."

Nursing Diagnosis

1. Ineffective coping:
   a. Verbal abuse related to feelings of helplessness
   b. Uncooperative behavior related to feelings of loss of control

Goals

1. Restoration of appropriate communication
2. Verbalization of feelings
3. Participation in therapeutic regimen

Nursing Interventions	Expected Outcomes	Outcomes
1. Promote appropriate communications. a. Establish relationship built on trust (see Nursing Care Plan 10–1)		
b. Remain calm; do not take verbal abuse personally.	b. Communicates within normal limits of volume	• Voice raised only occasionally at 24 hr
c. Set and keep limits; withdraw attention as needed.	c. Communicates appropriately	• Requests, observations, questions expressed verbally in an appropriate manner
d. Encourage patient to express feelings.	d. Verbalizes feelings of anger, fear, frus-	• Verbalized frustration, fear, anger, and loss of control; expressed fear and concern over loss of independence
e. Do not argue with patient.	e. Verbalizes how anger affects her verbal communication	• Apologized for shouting and belittling behavior; verbalized ways in which she used anger to avoid dealing with loss of control and loss of independence
2. Promote verbalization of feelings. a. Encourage patient to express feelings about dependency.	a. Verbalizes feelings about dependency	• Described feeling dependent on nursing staff for satisfaction of basic needs
b. Allow patient to make as many choices as possible.	b. Maintains as much control as possible	• Established own schedule for ADL and dressing changes; consulted with physical therapist and chose time for therapy
c. Involve patient in goal establishment.	c. Verbalizes goals and expectations	• Identified realistic expectations for therapy, discharge, and rehabilitation; established goal for living situation. Identified changes that had occurred since hospital admission; expressed her perception of the effect of these changes on life-style; identified need to regain control and to learn to care for self
d. Discuss feelings of loss of control and helplessness.	d. Verbalizes feelings of loss of control and helplessness	
3. Promote participation in therapeutic regimen. a. Emphasize strengths and potential.	a. Identifies own strengths and potentials	• Identified social supports, age, physical condition, life-style, and stamina; expressed desire to talk with discharge planner to facilitate interim plan for extended care facility
b. Encourage involvement in self-care.	b. Accomplishes self-care activities	• After establishing schedule for ADL, began active participation in own care; self-sufficient in ADL by 72 hr

inclusion of others. There are many cultural factors involved in the specific way in which grief and mourning take place, from the extremes of stoic appearance to elaborate and ritualistic weeping and public display.

The intensity of grief and mourning depends on the significance and extent of the loss to the person. It is generally greater if the loss, especially through death, comes suddenly. If the survivor has been particularly dependent on the deceased person, or if in any way he feels responsible for the death, grief is intensified. A person who is very sensitive to separation as a result of early separations may be deeply affected. Ambivalence (mixed feelings) is present in all significant relationships. If the ambivalence is marked, grief may be particularly intense. Guilt and irrational ideas about the causation of the death may prevent a person from facing himself and mourning effectively.

The stages of mourning are similar to the stages of adaptation to illness—shock and disbelief, awareness, and restitution. On recognition of a loss, people often experience a sinking feeling, tightness in the throat, loss of appetite, fatigue, tension, and acute anxiety. The sensorium is altered, and there is a feeling of unreality and distance from people. There is a preoccupation with the deceased or lost object and a state of readiness for its return. Feelings of guilt may be present, and there may be soul-searching and remorse about things that could have been done differently. The grieving person's relationships with other people lack warmth and are characterized by irritation and the desire not to be bothered. He is likely to withdraw from activities, neglect personal care, or be restlessly and purposelessly busy. He may develop symptoms similar to those of the deceased person. Sometimes the shock of the loss is accepted intellectually and the person goes through the motions of making arrangements and caring for others. His emotional reaction is cut off in his attempt to protect himself from the pain of the loss.

In the stage of developing awareness, the person experiences pain, anguish, emptiness, and acute sadness. Crying or the desire to cry is common and often elicits support from others. Many people cannot allow themselves to cry in public and need privacy to handle their grief.

In the stage of restitution, the physical reality of the loss is emphasized. In the case of death, the funeral makes this fact unavoidable. In the case of amputation, the sight of the stump and the first attempt at using a prosthesis underline the reality. The mourner begins a long process of coping with the absence of the loved person or object. There may be repetitive talk about the person or object and there is a tendency to idealize, so that only pleasant memories are reinforced. Gradually, this assists in the task of achieving emotional detachment. As dependence on the lost object decreases, the person begins to develop new interests and invests energy in other people. He is able to remember the relationship more realistically, with its good and bad aspects, and can talk about it without emotional dependence on the memory of the relationship.

Nursing Interventions.   Nursing interventions to help patients and families with the experience of grief and mourning include anticipating reactions to loss, supporting the usual coping mechanisms, and allowing the expression of feelings. The nurse provides privacy and availability. When a body part or function is lost, the nurse designs specific nursing care and controls the environment to prevent additional loss of self-esteem. The nurse's presence and her willingness to participate in the painful experiences that accompany grief help to prevent

feelings of total abandonment. By being aware of the usual patterns of grief and mourning, the nurse can recognize maladaptive patterns and help evaluate the need for other types of therapeutic intervention, such as psychotherapy. Nursing Care Plan 10-3 is an example of a nursing care plan for the patient experiencing grief and mourning.

Hope

Hope is a complex human experience that has a relationship to health. It is a mixture of feelings and thoughts that center on the fundamental belief that there are solutions to significant human needs and problems. Most people have hoped for and expected a long and healthy life for themselves and significant others. Serious illness and injury raise questions of vulnerability and uncertainty about the future.

The purpose of hope is to ward off despair, which is characterized by mental anguish, disorganization, helplessness, and hopelessness. Loss of hope leads to giving-up behavior, which leads to physical and emotional disequilibrium. Death may result from the loss of the will to live or through suicide. Hope is a catalyst that activates the motivational system. It is reinforced by other people who give support and encouragement to continue the struggle. When patients see "the light at the end of the tunnel," they can persist in moving toward future goals of improved functioning. Even with patients who are dying, hope for relief of suffering and meaningful living in the present are important aspects that can be reinforced with nursing care.

Nursing Interventions.   To help patients and families maintain or restore hope, nurses contribute to a hopeful atmosphere that comes from themselves, other staff members, patients, and the physical environment. This is possible if individuals have faced and explored their views of the meaning of life, illness, and death. Feelings of hope, hopelessness, and helplessness are found in all nursing situations. Even while helping others with these feelings, nurses must deal with similar shifts in their own experience of hope. If they feel hopeless, they talk about feelings with others to get encouragement and a clearer picture of the reality of the situation. When hopes for the recovery of a patient are disappointed, staff members, along with families, feel bewildered, angry, and grief-stricken. Nursing Care Plan 10-4 is an example of a nursing care plan to assist the patient in restoring hope.

Role Changes

When people get sick, their role identities often change. This affects the ways in which others interact with them and relate to them; relationships with family and friends must be reestablished and maintained.

Some of the most important role changes are those that take place in the family when parents are no longer able to carry out their usual activities with their children. There may be role reversals, with children caring for their parents. In the usual life cycle, aging parents become increasingly dependent on their middle-aged children for help and direction; serious illness makes this even more evident.

Role changes in terms of occupational functioning may be drastically altered. When physicians and nurses become patients, they often find it very difficult to accept the patient

Nursing Care Plan 10–3

Care of the Patient Experiencing Grief and Mourning

As Mrs. Stumpf's hip began to heal and her rehabilitative therapy began, she verbalized feelings of loss and fear regarding change in independent functioning. She told Ms. Sabol, "You know—I've lived alone for quite a while now—I've never wanted to be a burden on my family and friends." When alone, Mrs. Stumpf was observed staring at a blank wall. She told her family and friends how much she missed her apartment and worried about who was caring for her plants.

Nursing Diagnosis

1. Anticipatory grieving related to change in independent functioning

Goals

1. Acceptance of loss
2. Alteration in life-style to accommodate loss

Nursing Interventions	Expected Outcomes	Outcomes
1. Encourage patient to identify meaning of loss.		
a. Establish relationship built on trust (see Nursing Care Plan 10–1).		
b. Encourage expression of feelings about loss.	b. Identifies feelings about loss	• Cried and talked about loss of independence
c. Encourage to identify effects of loss.	c. Identifies effects of loss on life-style	• Talked about decreased mobility and need to go to extended care facility for rehabilitation
d. Assist in decreasing depressive symptoms.	d. Experiences decrease in symptoms of depression	• Reported increase in appetite and extended periods of uninterrupted sleep; fewer periods of crying; increased ability to concentrate while reading a book; participating in ADL and physical therapy
e. Facilitate movement through the stages of grieving and loss	e. Resolves loss	• Talked positively about rehabilitation; expressed interest in actively participating in rehabilitative program; described family support system
f. Assist in altering life-style	f. Identifies necessary life-style changes	• Identified modifications that could be made to apartment and social supports available

role; staff members also have difficulty seeing them in a new light. This is true of persons who are considered VIPs. They may demand and get deferential treatment, which at times is detrimental to their best interests as well as disruptive to the unit. Many people base their sense of self-worth on the ability to work and be productive. If forced to convalesce or retire because of illness, some people tend to feel lost and bereft of important links with others. Vocational rehabilitation is an important part of health planning for patients who must make major alterations.

A difficult role for a patient to deal with and others to react to is that of a terminally ill patient, a dying person. For many people, this is an unfamiliar and frightening aspect of life. They do not know what is expected of them, what to talk about, and how to carry on in light of the poor prognosis. Health professionals may withdraw from patients once it is clear that they are not going to recover. Nurses play an im-

portant part in helping patients and families go through this period.

Persons with chronic illness struggle with the role of being impaired. They want to be as normal as possible, yet sometimes the conditions of illness interfere with this to a large degree. They must continually make decisions about how to act and what to tell others. This is especially true in social situations; some people simply withdraw and cut themselves off from others, which leads to loneliness and depression.

Coping Strategies

Patients, families, and staff strive to adapt to serious illness in many ways. These coping skills are generally the approaches

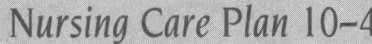

Nursing Care Plan 10–4

Assisting the Patient in Restoring Hope

Mrs. Stumpf made progress in learning to walk with a walker. She looked forward to her therapy sessions and worked hard during these sessions. She spoke to Ms. Sabol about her plans after discharge: "Of course I'll have to continue with therapy for a while and I think once I'm stronger I'll be able to leave the extended care facility and go back to my apartment. My family is supportive of the changes I'll have to make in my apartment. Things really do look hopeful."

Nursing Diagnoses

1. Disturbance in self-concepts: self-esteem, independence/dependence, role performance
2. Potential noncompliance with therapeutic regimen

Goals

1. Improvement in self-concept
2. Resumption of independent life-style
3. Compliance with therapeutic regimen

Nursing Interventions	Expected Outcomes	Outcomes
1. Increase self-esteem. a. Give positive feedback for progress made in self-care and ambulation	a. Accomplishes walking with walker	• Safely ambulated with walker
b. Help patient identify strengths and potentials.	b. Identifies strengths and potentials	• Made a list of physical activities she will be able to continue; identified supports within family and community; verbalized self-determination as an inner strength
c. Give positive feedback for progress made in accepting change in independent living.	c. Describes feelings about how independent living has changed	• Verbalized sadness related to loss of independence and put into perspective the effect of this loss on self and family; stated she was looking forward to returning to her apartment
2. Encourage efforts toward successfully altering life-style.	2. Makes necessary arrangements for promoting mobility	• Had safety equipment installed in her apartment • Arranged for Meals on Wheels to be delivered once she returned home
3. Encourage adherence to therapeutic regimen. a. Encourage participation in discharge planning.	a. Participates in making plans for discharge	• Attended discharge planning conference; consulted with physical therapist—therapy to be continued at nursing home
b. Provide patient with discharge instructions.	b. Exercises according to plan. Keeps appointments with physician, physical therapist	
c. Discuss nursing care plan with nursing home for transition to new care facility.	c. Transition to new level of care without incident; adjusts to new environment rapidly; participates in rehabilitative activities	• Adjusted to nursing home; actively participated in rehabilitative plan of care

that were used in other difficult periods. Moos (1984) described these as coping skills that can be learned and practiced. Although divided into seven categories, the skills are often used in different combinations and vary in appropriateness and helpfulness. At different stages of illness, one or more of the coping skills may predominate.

Denial

Denial involves denying or minimizing the seriousness of the crisis, as well as isolating or dissociating feelings connected with the condition. This approach downplays the symptoms as evidence of illness or disregards the seriousness of the diagnosis. The first reaction to loss is shock and disbelief. Denial or numbing of feelings gives one time to absorb the meaning and protects one from being overwhelmed by feelings. Denial and isolation are ego defense mechanisms that protect against anxiety by distorting reality. Generally, the increase or persistence of symptoms forces the person to abandon the denial in time.

As a coping skill, denying or minimizing the problem helps to maintain psychologic equilibrium. It can be harmful when it leads to such things as missing appointments, signing out of the hospital, and refusing appropriate treatment. Inappropriate cheerfulness and lack of concern about symptoms may indicate denial. If anxiety, depression, and anger are not expressed in situations where they are expected, the patient may be using denial for self-protection. However, sometimes patients act this way to protect others. This happens when patients are aware they are dying but perceive that the family would be more comfortable if the mutual deception were continued. They may be able to talk about fears and feelings with the staff, thereby lessening isolation.

Denial mechanisms operate in families as they try to protect themselves from recognizing the severity of the situation. Even when imminent death is discussed, the family may deny that this is possible.

Nursing Interventions. In dealing with denial of illness as a nursing problem, nurses assess the extent to which the denial is harmful and the ways in which it is beneficial. Generally, the defense of denial is not challenged directly, because such action tends to reinforce the position or leaves the person without necessary ego protection. The nurse does not support or encourage the denial and remains available. The nurse's use of gentle exploring questions may help the patient's acceptance of reality. When patients can relinquish denial, they need help in dealing with the difficult aspects of reality that they were attempting to ward off.

Denial is a coping skill that nurses use to handle their own feelings about illness, radical surgery, and death. Along with other health professionals, they may need this defense to keep working in high-risk areas. When nurses can talk about their feelings with others, they develop more realistic ways of dealing with the stresses and thus are better able to help patients and families face their difficult problems.

Seeking Information

The coping skill of seeking information involves (1) seeking relevant information that can relieve anxiety caused by misconceptions and uncertainty and (2) using one's intellectual resources effectively. Patients and families are often relieved by information about the illness, its treatment, and the course the illness is expected to take. This provides a framework in which plans can be made and effective action taken. Patients and their families are encouraged by hearing about successful treatment of others with the same condition. Worrying is decreased when correct facts and clarification of misconceptions and fears are provided. Giving a time dimension in which certain reactions are anticipated helps to decrease feelings of helplessness. Informed patients are better able to participate in their own treatment.

Requesting Emotional Support

Being able to request reassurance and emotional support from family, friends, and medical/nursing staff while maintaining a sense of personal competence is important. Patients are often frightened and anxious. They may feel very much alone. A valuable coping skill is being able to reach out for or receive the concern of others. This maintains hope through encouragement. Whether limitations are temporary or permanent, people need to have a sense of mastery over other functions.

Patients can be encouraged by other people with similar conditions. Support groups for patients and families are helpful in encouraging the expression of feelings, sharing practical problems, and passing along effective ways of coping. Patients are reassured by being told that their cooperation with the health team is helpful in fighting together against the difficult illness.

Sometimes, physicians and nurses use shaming and guilt-provoking tactics to get patients to adhere to treatment programs. These are generally ineffective and lead to the patient's being all the more demoralized or seeking health treatment elsewhere.

Learning Self-Care

Learning illness-related procedures confirms personal ability and effectiveness. People can learn to care for themselves even in the aftermath of catastrophic illness and injury. Helplessness is decreased because the sense of pride in accomplishments helps to restore or maintain self-esteem. Family members can often learn how to help a loved one during acute as well as chronic illness. Being able to participate often relieves anxiety and guilt. Patient teaching is an important aspect of nursing care.

Setting Concrete, Limited Goals

The overall tasks of adaptation to serious illness seem overwhelming, yet they can be accomplished. Breaking down the components into small, manageable goals will eventually lead to success. Motivation is maintained. The feelings of helplessness are decreased as patients experience the impact of action on outcome. Instead of just worrying about results and the future, the person takes action that is effective. Principles of learning are important in accomplishing the eventual long-term goals.

Rehearsing Alternative Outcomes

There are usually multiple alternatives in most situations. Recognizing this helps a person to feel less trapped and helpless. This is accomplished through mental preparation and discussion with others. Exploring options with the nurse and one's family helps to expand the reality base on which to make decisions. Anticipatory planning reduces helplessness by rehearsing "what will happen if. . . ."

This coping skill is often used in conjunction with information seeking. It helps to decrease anxiety by preparing for the future. Recalling how one has been able to manage other difficulties bolsters confidence.

When there is a choice of several treatment modalities, talking over the alternatives is a vital part of including the patient in self-determination. Health professionals do not always know what is best. They can give information based on knowledge and past experience; the patient and family are left with the final decision. Patients may have definite ideas about what they want done in the final stages of life.

Skill in rehearsing is very important for patients with altered body parts and functions. They may need to rehearse what to do in a variety of social situations. They use the staff as sounding boards. Groups of patients and other individuals may be helped by role-playing situations.

Finding Meaning in Illness

Illness is a human experience. Many people have found that serious illness was a turning point in their lives. This may reflect either a spiritual orientation or a philosophic approach to life. Patients find encouragement in the belief that their suffering may have some meaning or be helpful to others. They may participate in research projects or training programs to this end. Sensitive, poignant accounts of illness that convey hope and inspiration have been written by patients, families, and health professionals. Plays, movies, and television dramas have made it possible for millions of people to share in some of the finest moments of human caring, courage, and compassion.

Families may be brought together by illness in a painful but very meaningful way. People experience a sense of their basic worth as well as that of others. Many survivors of serious illness report that they experienced a change in values and priorities, greater concern for others, and a heightened appreciation for the beauty of nature. After serious illness, people may find meaning in helping others through support groups or political action or by entering one of the health professions.

Factors That Help or Hinder Coping

Serious physical illness is a potential life crisis for the patient and family. Crisis is that state in which the person feels that obstacles to important life goals are insurmountable and that the usual means of problem solving are not sufficient. New approaches are needed. Successful mastery leads to greater self-integration, understanding, and trust in others.

Stressors that disturb equilibrium are divided into biologic and psychosocial stressors. These are most often intertwined, because one system affects the other. The *biologic stressors* include illness and injury. Not only is the degree of impairment important, but so is the meaning of the condition to the individual. Lack of sleep, poor nutrition, dehydration, drug and alcohol use, and pain are biologic stressors that hinder coping with ongoing and new difficulties.

Psychosocial stressors include interpersonal problems with family and significant others, occupational situations, finances, living circumstances, and legal problems. The person's maturational age, especially childhood, adolescence, and aging,

specifically affects the impact of illness. Sometimes, psychosocial issues drop away in importance in the face of acute illness and possible death. In many instances, the coping abilities are stretched even more as new problems are created by the illness.

The *personal characteristics* of an individual include age, intelligence, basic personality style, religious and philosophic beliefs, and previous experiences in coping with difficulties, especially prior illness. These affect the person's perception of the illness and his resources for handling the problems.

Social, cultural, and situational supports affect the way in which a person copes with illness. These are primarily interpersonal supports—people to whom the distressed person turns. Close friends and understanding family members may be vital to maximal recovery. Isolated persons or patients whose family ties are chaotic and disturbed will be under even greater stress with illness. The professional health team is part of the support system. Because nurses are so close and necessary to the ongoing care of patients, they become vital supports during the uncertainty of illness and treatment. They are sensitive to the patient's need for additional help and are instrumental in arranging for this support from family, clergy, other patients, psychiatric and psychologic therapists, and social service agencies.

The *physical environment* may help or hinder coping. The problems of sensory overload, sensory deprivation, and isolation, along with the unfamiliar and frightening aspects of the hospital, all contribute to problems of adjustment. Sometimes, although little can be done about these problems, just recognizing that they cause stress can be reassuring to patients and families.

The patient's *basic coping mechanisms* may be altered because of the circumstances of the illness. Pain, fatigue, and immobility interfere with action methods of tension release. Important persons to whom the patient usually turns may not be available, and impaired mobility may restrict his ability to visit them. Generally, the families of seriously ill patients are also very anxious, which leaves them less able to respond to their loved one. An intensification of usual coping patterns may be seen in disturbed communication, behavior, and ways of interacting with others. Common patterns of disturbed behavior resulting from efforts to cope include excessive withdrawal, making demands, disorientation, depression, and manipulative behavior. Changes in a patient's perceptual field as the intensity of anxiety increases to a state of panic are illustrated in Figure 10-2.

Assessing Psychosocial Needs

Nurses encounter sick people at many stages of illness and treatment. They often see only a small part of the picture. When dealing with acute illness, they see patients and families in the crisis situation without knowing much about what preceded or followed the condition. Strauss (1984) regards sick persons as having at least three biographies that have meaning in their illness; they are (1) the person's chronological experience with the illness (2) treatment experiences with prior medical aid (legitimate or not), and (3) the social biography of the person's life history with family, friends, work colleagues, and strangers. Staff members often know little about these biographies; nurses need to learn more about them, because they may affect treatment and recovery in definite ways.

Psychosocial History

A psychosocial history is the organized assessment of the important events of a person's life; it is sometimes referred to as a *case history.* The psychosocial history is a specific biography of a person from before birth (heritage and heredity) through the important developmental stages to the present. The anticipated future is also part of this assessment. The psychosocial history touches on the turning points—the important milestones. Significant illnesses, physical and mental, experienced by the patient and family members have an important impact on the immediate situation.

The specific psychosocial history is obtained through initial interviewing and from additional contacts. Nurses should be familiar with the elements of a psychosocial assessment. It describes patients in the context of their lives and identifies major problems and assets. Nurses can obtain and use this information while they are providing other nursing care for patients. The nurse talks with patients in a goal-directed way to determine areas in which help is needed. For those patients too ill or young, the nurse may gather these data from family members and significant others.

In many instances, these are ongoing interviews. The contacts continue over the period of illness; the time spent corresponds to the needs of the patient. Critically ill patients will not be able to communicate much more than immediate needs. It is not necessary to get all this information at one time. As the nurse–patient relationship develops, patients feel more confident in talking about matters of serious concern to them. This is particularly true if the listener is interested, compassionate, and nonjudgmental. Nurses also talk with and assess the psychosocial needs of the family members. In the uncertainty and stress of illness, many persons want and need to talk with their professional helpers.

Mental Status Examination

In addition to the psychosocial history, nurses pay attention to the current mental status of the patient. The mental status examination assesses the ways in which a person is thinking, feeling, and acting. It is both a descriptive inventory of behavior and a method of organizing and recording observations of behavior. Problems are identified, and working diagnoses determine the treatment plan. Many of the aspects of the mental status examination are expressed in ongoing speech and behavior. Specific questions are necessary during a formal examination or when clarification, update, or additional information is needed. Patients with serious physical illness often show dramatic shifts in mental status when recovering from surgery, when delirious, or when experiencing changes in body temperature or reactions to medication. The patient with a history of mental illness may decompensate during the stress of illness. Confusion may escalate to extreme behavior unless it is recognized and treated along with the medical condition. Families may need reassurance about the changes in the psychologic state of their loved ones.

Aspects of Communication

Acute and chronic physical illness pose many problems to patients and their families. Nurses communicate with them to (1) identify health needs, (2) clarify misconceptions, and (3) help them verbalize fears and other reactions. Anxiety is lessened or channeled through sharing. Nurses are concerned with the impact of illness on the person's life. They are aware of the need to provide privacy while talking with the patient about his conditions in order to help him.

The basic nurse–patient relationship takes into account the physician, the family, other patients, the rest of the health team, and society at large. The relationship is established and maintained by the communication process—a complex, dynamic exchange of verbal and nonverbal messages.

Communication is based on mutually intelligible symbols. To be understood, a person must have a knowledge of himself and his needs, an ability to speak the language and express himself clearly, and a familiarity with the usual conventions of the situation. To understand others, he must be able to observe and evaluate behavior. To make oneself understandable and to understand others is vital to the establishment of relationships. The patient whose English is limited or who speaks a foreign language, or whose ability to express himself is markedly impaired through physical or psychologic causes, poses a challenge to the nurse.

The process of communication may be considered to consist of four segments: (1) *I* (2) *am communicating something* (3) *to you* (4) *in this situation.* Breakdowns in communication can be pinpointed by identifying the segment in which the interference is taking place.

The sender of the message, the *I,* is affected by such factors as age, sex, socioeconomic status, marital status, occupation, intelligence, physical condition (especially as related to the nervous system and the organs of communication), personality, and current emotional status.

The message *am communicating something* consists of both verbal and nonverbal elements that may be complementary or incongruous. The patient who says, "Oh, I'm fine. Nothing is the matter," while restlessly moving about, wringing his hands, and sighing, frequently illustrates the latter.

The receiver of the communication, *to you,* is influenced by the same factors as the sender with respect to behavior. The ability to hear or "read" a patient's behavior depends largely on the ability to listen openly and sensitively. The presence of stereotypes, misconceptions, and anxiety may prevent the nurse from correctly identifying the message from a particular patient.

The context of the communication, *in this situation,* refers to the sociocultural status of the patient, the context of illness, the social order of the hospital, and immediate environmental aspects. The importance of understanding the cultural background and the values of patients has gained recognition in all areas of nursing. When patients enter the hospital world, they may be overwhelmed and bewildered by the change in their status and role. The nurse plays a vital part in orienting patients to their new position. She also needs to acquaint them with the scope of her professional services. Many people do not know that the nurse is prepared and eager to assist with a wide variety of health needs. In addition to performing the traditional services related to physical needs, she offers help as a health teacher, a rehabilitation worker, a communications link with other professional services, and, in some instances, a psychotherapeutic counselor.

A person in the first stages of adapting to illness, who is taking the defensive measure of denying his illness, does not seek or welcome accurate information about his condition or treatment. A nurse who attempts to do effective health teaching will find her efforts of little avail at this time. The behavior of the patient, the questions he asks or avoids, and his reactions to the changes in his health status all give clues to his readiness and needs. In turn, the patient is also very sensitive to the reactions of the medical and nursing staff and seeks to interpret nonverbal messages with regard to his prognosis, especially when it is not favorable.

The expressive function of the nurse involves helping the patient to maintain equilibrium and motivation and supporting his attempts to cope with the experience of illness and treatment by providing direct gratifications that reduce his tension level. The provision of physical comfort and care is combined with such interpersonal activities as explaining, reassuring, understanding, protecting, and simply being with the patient. When a patient is acutely ill, communication generally takes place on a primitive, chiefly nonverbal level. A touch, a soft but reassuring tone of voice, and the presence of the nurse may convey to the patient that he is not alone and that he is being cared for. When it is anticipated that a patient will experience direct interference with communication patterns as a result of treatment, it is vital to set up a system of communication in advance. One patient reported, "The worst part about my laryngectomy was that I couldn't tell anyone what I needed—but the magic slate helped."

An important part of the development of interpersonal and communication tools is the nurse's understanding of herself, her interpersonal needs, and her usual patterns of communication. *As she becomes more aware of her own needs, she is better able to identify those of her patients and to know when her own perceptions and reactions are preventing her from accurately assessing the situation.* This is particularly true when the patient's behavior is frustrating, puzzling, hostile, or demanding. The nurse must be able to evaluate her own responses so that she does not retaliate with anger or rejection. The situations that lead to feelings of helplessness and hopelessness must be talked about and shared so that the nurse can maintain her own equilibrium and give optimal nursing care to patients with incurable, repulsive, or terminal conditions. The nurse's awareness of her own need for approval and recognition plays an important part in her reactions to patient behavior and to the behavior of co-workers, supervisors, and the medical staff.

Reactions of Nurses to Illness

Nurses have many personal emotional reactions to patients and families in the crisis of physical illness. Some common responses are frustration, anxiety, anger, hope, guilt, compassion, helplessness, love, hopelessness, disgust, envy, and pride. These are stimulated by the combination of the personal characteristics of the nurse, the professional tasks and obligations involved, and the intricacies of the patient's illness and personality. Nurses not only react emotionally to patients and families but also have important emotional interactions with other members of the health team. Illness in a patient may evoke emotional responses based on personal experiences or the experiences of close family members.

Nurses are faced with difficulties in adjusting to the many changes in the health status of their patients. This is particularly true with "difficult" patients, those who are not responding to treatment, and dying patients. A high-risk factor is involved in working in settings such as the emergency unit, intensive care unit, premature nursery, and medical units, where a high percentage of patients die. Nurses have to struggle with conflicts between the idealism instilled in nursing school and the reality of the usual work situation. Even when they recognize psychosocial needs, many nurses feel overwhelmed in helping patients—there is "no time." Yet, the ultimate recovery and maximal functioning of patients with serious illnesses depend on the nurse's ability to deal with multifaceted problems. Sensitive attention to the emotional needs of patients and families helps make hospitalization and treatment smoother, enhances health teaching, and contributes to the quality of life.

It is important for nurses to be aware of their emotional reactions to clinical situations so that they do not become overstressed and unable to cope. When this happens, they experience the phenomenon known as "burnout," which results in personal distress, in indifference to the suffering of others, and often in the decision to leave the job or profession. Nurses who are aware of their many reactions are better able to help others.

"Problem Patients"

Many patients cope with the difficult and often frightening tasks of adaptation to illness. Some inspire with their courage and dignity. Others simply do the best they can in the immediate situation and over the long period in which they convalesce and learn to live with a chronic illness.

Some patients stand out as not dealing with their illness and treatment in the usual expected ways. They may be called "difficult," "management problems," or, in exasperation, "impossible" or "crocks." These labels indicate the breakdown of usually effective coping patterns in both the staff and the patient. The staff need to talk together about the situation. Consultation is often indicated—with a psychiatrist, a consultation-liaison team, or a psychiatric nursing clinical specialist. These persons can help by clarifying the factors, suggesting alternative approaches, giving reassurance to the staff and patient, providing short-term psychotherapy, and evaluating the need for psychoactive drugs. *The principle underlying these approaches is that "problem patients" are patients with problems.*

Problems With Cognition, Affect, and Behavior

According to Groves (1982), problems of patients can be classified in three groups, although there is often overlap. These groups are as follows:

1. *Problems of cognition*—delirium, denial, psychosis, failure to process information
2. *Problems of affect*—anxiety, hostility, depression, apathy
3. *Problems of behavior*—noncompliance, withdrawal, dependency, aggressiveness, manipulation

Cognition refers to the ways in which people process information—their ways of thinking, and hence of responding. Perception, memory, understanding, and judgment are involved. Medical-surgical problems often affect these processes. This is seen particularly in *delirium* and *dementia*. The therapeutic approach consists largely in recognizing the nature of the impairment. When the source is identified, steps can be taken, such as clarifying the medical treatment, changing the environment, and readjusting the medication regimen.

Disturbances of affect (emotions) become problems in a medical–surgical situation when they are overwhelming or inappropriate. Disturbed behavior may result as an exacerbation of a previous mental illness or in response to the immediate situation, illness, or treatment. Excessive anxiety comes from many sources. The therapeutic approach consists of recognizing the causes of the disturbed feelings and helping to restore control. This is accomplished by talking with patients and families about the situation, making necessary changes, and prescribing medication if needed.

Disturbed behavior is directly related to disturbed cognition and overwhelming affects. Severe depression is very distressing to the patient and interferes with healing. It can also precede suicidal behavior. Misinterpretation of the environment leads to panic and aggressive behavior. Patients signal their unmet needs by such behavior as signing out of the hospital, refusing medical treatment, using drugs and alcohol on the unit, and inappropriate sexual behavior.

Extreme dependency leads to difficult patient–staff interactions. This is shown through clinging, demanding behavior in which the patient begs for reassurance yet is unrelieved by it. There may be ongoing demands for services and for pain medication beyond the expected need. Dependent patients are often manipulative and play staff members off against one another. They show anger and hostility both directly and covertly. Nurses feel frustrated, angry, and hopeless in working with these patients.

Nursing Interventions. The therapeutic approach to patients showing disturbed behavior begins with an assessment of the situation from the standpoint of both the staff and the patient. Clear communication is vital. Necessary limits are spelled out. Generally, long-standing personality styles and defenses are not challenged in the midst of a physical illness. The staff members are encouraged to meet needs as much as possible and to allow the patient to exert interpersonal control and distance without being punished or abandoned. During the crisis of illness, psychoactive medication, such as tranquilizers and antianxiety agents, can be used to help patients manage disturbed feelings and behavior.

A way of understanding and dealing with problem behavior is through learning theory. Behavior that is learned and continued is behavior that is reinforced (rewarded). There is a system of rewards and punishments (even if not acknowledged) in all social systems, including that of the hospital. Patients bring their learned behavior patterns and react to the new interpersonal environment accordingly.

If patients' behaviors tag them as "difficult," nurses should study the situation to identify (1) what constitutes the maladaptive behavior and how this interferes with care, progress, and rehabilitation; (2) how and by whom the behavior is reinforced; and (3) how the environment and reinforcers can be changed so that the behavior changes. This is the approach to behavior modification. Nurses should examine their own behavior to see if they are inadvertently playing a part in continuing the situation. Nursing behavior can influence patient behavior in either positive or negative directions. Positive reinforcers include spending time, smiling, showing interest in the conversation, providing food, giving medication as needed, giving back rubs, and granting extra privileges.

Psychophysiologic Interactions

Knowledge about the relationship between emotions and physical reactions is increasing. This is a highly complex and little understood matter that the mass media have simplified to the point at which the words *psychophysiologic, psychosomatic, neurotic, imaginary, faking, malingering, psychogenic,* and *somatopsychic* are used loosely and create confusion.

Anxiety is experienced as both emotional and physiologic reactions. Many people seek treatment for symptoms that are due to chronic, continued anxiety. The anxiety may represent a reaction to reality factors in the present, such as a job or a marriage, or to long-standing conflicts over sexuality, dependency, aggression, and other factors.

Psychophysiologic Illness. Anxiety reactions in which the symptoms center around one organ system are described in the nomenclature as psychophysiologic reactions having autonomic and visceral responses (*e.g.,* "psychophysiologic reaction, cardiovascular," if the symptoms are predominantly cardiac in nature). Any organ system can be affected. When actual structural changes do occur, the condition is described as a psychophysiologic illness that has resulted from a combination of emotional and physiologic factors. Common conditions that are generally considered to involve psychophysiologic factors are peptic ulcer, chronic ulcerative colitis, hyperthyroidism, bronchial asthma, essential hypertension, and neurodermatitis. The frequency and severity of these illnesses point to the need for greater understanding of the relationship between mind and body.

Hypochondriasis. Another manifestation of underlying emotional conflict that expresses itself in physical symptoms is hypochondriasis. A hypochondriacal patient may be totally absorbed in his body and its functioning and presents endless complaints and reports. Hypochondriasis may be used as a means of attempting to meet long-standing dependency needs. The nurse must evaluate her reactions to such a patient's complaints and demands. Frustration and anger are common responses to this type of patient. The nurse often resents someone who avoids adult responsibility so easily. Expressing this anger directly to the patient is not helpful, because he is struggling to maintain some kind of equilibrium. Not recognizing her own anger could result in the nurse's avoiding the patient and not caring for his realistic needs. If the nurse attempts to meet all of the patient's unsatisfied dependency needs, she soon finds that the patient is insatiable. Finding a reasonable middle ground is a challenge in working with these patients. Very little is known about successful nursing approaches to hypochondriacal patients. Excessive preoccupation with one's body accompanied by unusual ideation may be a sign of more severe emotional disorders, such as psychotic depression or schizophrenia. Through proper assessment of needs and evaluation of behavior, the nurse may help plan for more appropriate treatment.

Conversion Reactions.   Another group of physical reactions that have an emotional basis are conversion reactions. Conversion is an ego defense mechanism in which anxiety is eliminated or reduced by the production of a physical symptom. This symptom may be directly related to the emotional conflict; the hand that would strike out is paralyzed; the eyes that would look at the forbidden become blind. In most instances, the conflict and the symbolic meaning of the symptom are complex, disguised, and difficult to unravel. These patients come into a medical-surgical setting for differential diagnosis. A conversion reaction may develop after an organic illness has occurred, which tends to prolong the secondary gains of dependency and security.

Generally, the symptoms of conversion reactions simulate disturbances in the voluntary nervous system or in the organs of the special senses. Disturbances of sensation and motion are the most common. Sensation changes include anesthesia, paresthesia, and pain. Loss of hearing and sight are much more common than loss of the other special senses. Disturbances of motion include paralysis, usually of the extremities or speech mechanism, and uncontrolled movements, such as tics and nonorganic convulsions. If the symptom is diagnosed as a conversion reaction, the treatment is generally best directed by a psychiatrist. The nurse can help greatly by accurately observing the patient's behavior, including his reaction to other people. She must keep in mind that symptom formation in a person with a conversion reaction occurs on an unconscious level—the patient is not faking, and his symptoms are not imaginary. This is his way of coping with situations at the present time; with professional help he may be able to find more adequate ways of doing so.

Disturbances in Orientation.   Disturbances in orientation occur frequently in patients on medical–surgical services. Acute brain syndrome, which may be a reaction to anesthesia, infection, surgical or metabolic disturbances, overdose of drugs or alcohol, or assault of the brain, as in head injury, often produces delirium. *Delirium* is a state of altered consciousness or awareness manifested by disorientation and confusion. It is induced by interference with the metabolic processes of the brain and is generally acute in onset and reversible. The first signs are restlessness, anxiety, and suspicion, which quickly mount to agitation, excitement, and confusion. The patient often begins to hallucinate and experience delusions. These distortions of reality are extremely frightening, and the desperate behavior of the person experiencing them necessitates skilled nursing action. It is necessary to reduce the terror and extreme anxiety of these patients not only for emotional reasons but also to prevent overloading the body with more stress.

Nursing care for a delirious patient includes continual reorientation, a calm voice, and adequate lighting through the night. If possible, the same nurses should attend the patient much of the time, because they repeatedly demonstrate by familiar words and action that he is safe and cared for. It often helps to tell the patient that you know he is very frightened but that the things he is experiencing are a reaction to his illness that will go away. Hallucinations caused by organic processes are often vivid and threatening. Along with visual hallucinations, the patient may experience tactile hallucinations in which he feels he is being touched or bugs are crawling on him.

Acute brain syndrome is treated by alleviating the causative agents, and the nurse must be aware that proper hydration, nutrition, and medication are directed toward this end. Restraints may be necessary to keep the patient in bed, but they may also frighten and irritate him. The nurse must be aware of his distortion of reality and poor judgment in order to protect him from injuring himself or others. Patients have walked out of unprotected windows while delirious.

Following an episode of delirium, a person may experience anxiety and shame over his behavior when not in full control. He may fear that he has acted inappropriately, hurt someone, or said vulgar or obscene things. He may be afraid of having told confidences and secrets about himself. If the patient gives evidence of such concern, the nurse can encourage him to talk about his fears and then reassure him that his behavior was understandable in the situation and that his confidence will not be betrayed. This is a potentially shameful situation in which the rights, dignity, and privacy of the patient must be protected.

Chronic brain syndrome may result from damage to brain tissue sustained by the causes of acute brain syndrome; from long-term infections such as syphilis; from heavy-metal intoxication; from circulatory disturbances such as cerebral arteriosclerosis; from convulsive disorders; from disturbances of growth, metabolism, or nutrition; from intracranial neoplasm; from prenatal factors; and from diseases that affect the brain, such as Alzheimer's disease and AIDS. The behavior common to people with these conditions is described as *dementia*, and it represents chronic, irreversible brain damage with deterioration of intellectual capacities due to structural changes. Both delirium and dementia are characterized by loss of abilities—defects in memory, orientation (of time, place, and person), and judgment. In planning nursing care and long-term treatment, the nurse must evaluate the patient's strengths along with his limitations. Environmental manipulation and simplification may help him to live his life to the fullest.

Dying and Death

The manner in which a person dies is individual, just as his life was. One of the major problems in understanding death is that, in our culture, it is a taboo and unfamiliar experience. Dying often takes place in hospitals or nursing homes rather than as part of the life cycle at home. Death is a strange new experience that does not affect most people until their adult years. Many nursing students come into contact with death for the first time during the medical–surgical clinical experience.

For most people, just the thought of death is frightening and even impossible. Regardless of religious beliefs, it is difficult to imagine oneself not existing in the world. Nurses are deeply committed to life and health. The dying patient is a direct contradiction to that commitment. Sometimes the medical and nursing staff react to dying patients as if they represent a failure of their skill and care. Although nothing can be done to reverse the ultimate process, dying patients and their families can be helped during final days.

People face death in many ways. According to Kübler–Ross (1969), the emotional responses of a person facing death can be traced through five stages: denial and isolation, anger, bargaining, depression, and acceptance. These five stages do not always occur in sequence; they may be mixed or overlapping. Patients and their families move back and forth through the experience and may be at different stages at a given time.

Denial and Isolation

Recognition and acceptance of the fact that death is to be faced shortly is difficult; the common reaction is to insulate oneself until other defenses are marshaled. Denial permits hope to exist. Often, patients are ready to accept the fact that they are dying, but the family continues to express denial. This delays communication of concerns. Denial and isolation are interrupted when the patient begins to think about unfinished business—personal affairs, finances, arrangements for spouse, children, and others.

Anger

The next emotion expressed is anger. The question "Why me?" does not require an answer, but the patient is helped if the nurse is present to offer support and to listen. The behavior of patients in this stage is difficult because nothing can be done that seems to please. Nurses can expect this expression of anger and should not take it personally. Patients often want to express their sense of outrage and helplessness. When feelings have been vented, they are able to move on.

Bargaining

Bargaining is a phase of coping during which the dying person attempts to negotiate a trade. Usually, it involves a deal with God or fate: "If I can live long enough to attend my son's wedding, I'll be ready to die." If possible everything should be done to grant patients their requests.

Depression

The full impact of the inevitable is apparent to patients in this stage. Defense mechanisms are no longer effective; sadness and anguish are felt and expressed. By crying, they also elicit the support of loved ones and nurses. The resolution of this phase leads quietly into the final stage.

Acceptance

This is a time of relative peace. The patient seems to want to review the past and contemplate the unknown future. Often, patients do not talk a great deal but want others nearby. If pain is relieved, the person who has accepted death often wants to be comforted by having contact with those who are meaningful.

Nursing Interventions

To give maximal help to the dying, nurses should examine their own feelings about death. An underlying principle in nursing is that patients are individuals to be treated with respect and dignity regardless of their background or condition. However, studies have shown that social values determine reactions to the dying person. Such factors as age, attractiveness, socioeconomic status, and former accomplishments affect whether the patient is cared for or abandoned while dying. Many times, *nurses become the most important link with life for dying patients*. They promote physical comfort and emotional support. It is an emotional strain to attend people who are dying. Nurses assigned to areas in which death is a common occurrence need to share their feelings and reactions with others to obtain needed support.

Chapter Summary

Illness is an unpredictable event that has an impact on one's homeostasis and sense of well-being. Moving from health to illness is a process to which each individual adapts in stages based on his past coping behaviors.

To facilitate the patient's adaptation to illness or injury, the nurse must use effective communication. Communication is an essential mechanism by which the nurse can assess and intervene to meet mutually established goals.

The nurse needs to acknowledge and examine her own emotional response to patients and families. "Problem patients" engender a variety of responses in the nurse, and it is valuable to look at these responses to prevent "burnout" and provide optimal patient care. Caring for the dying patient allows the nurse to examine her own feelings about death and at the same time utilize the entire scope of her nursing knowledge and judgment to provide physical and emotional care and comfort.

Bibliography

Books

Aguilera DC and Messick JM. Crisis Intervention: Theory and Methodology, 6th ed. St Louis, CV Mosby, 1989.

Arnold E and Boggs K. Interpersonal Relationships: Professional Communication Skills for Nurses. Philadelphia, WB Saunders, 1988.

Bandman EL and Bandman B. Critical Thinking in Nursing. East Norwalk, CT, Appleton and Lange, 1988.

Barry P. Psychosocial Nursing Assessment and Intervention. Philadelphia, JB Lippincott, 1984.

Benner P and Wurbel J. The Primacy of Caring: Stress and Coping in Health and Illness. Menlo Park, CA, Addison-Wesley, 1989.

Bishop AH and Scudder JR (eds). Caring, Curing, Coping: Nurse, Physician,

Patient Relationships. Birmingham, AL, University of Alabama Press, 1985.

Bishop AH and Scudder JR (eds). The Practical, Moral, and Personal Sense of Nursing: A Phenomenological Philosophy of Practice. New York, State University of New York Press, 1990.

Brallier L. Successfully Managing Stress. Los Altos, CA, National Nursing Review, 1982.

Brown GW and Harris TO. Life Events and Illness. New York, Guilford Press, 1989.

Burgess AW. Psychiatric Nursing in the Hospital and the Community, 4th ed. Englewood Cliffs, NJ, Prentice-Hall, 1985.

Chesney MA and Rosenman RH (eds). Anger and Hostility in Cardiovascular and Behavioral Disorders. Washington, DC, Hemisphere Publishing Corp, 1985.

Clayton PJ and Barrett JE (eds). Treatment of Depression. New York, Raven Press, 1983.

Derogatis LR and Wise TN. Anxiety and Depressive Disorders in the Medical Patient. Washington, DC, American Psychiatric Press, 1989.

Dossey BM, Guzzetta CE, and Kenner CV. Essentials of Critical Care Nursing: Mind, Body, Spirit, 3rd ed. Philadelphia, JB Lippincott, 1990.

Friedman M. Family Nursing Theory and Assessment, 2nd ed. Norwalk, CT, Appleton-Century-Crofts, 1986.

Fritz P et al. Interpersonal Communication in Nursing. Norwalk, CT, Appleton-Century-Crofts, 1984.

Gallon RL. The Psychosomatic Approach to Illness. New York, Elsevier Biomedical, 1982.

Goldberg IK et al. Pain, Anxiety and Grief. New York, Columbia University Press, 1986.

Goodwin DW. Anxiety. New York, Oxford University Press, 1986.

Haber J et al. Comprehensive Psychiatric Nursing, 3rd ed. New York, McGraw-Hill, 1987.

Handly R. Anxiety and Panic Attacks. New York, Fawcett Crest, 1985.

Hawes C and Joseph D. Basic Concepts of Helping, 2nd ed. Norwalk, CT, Appleton and Lange, 1986.

Hill L and Smith N. Self-Care Nursing. East Norwalk, CT, Appleton and Lange, 1989.

Infante MS (ed). Crisis Theory: A Framework for Nursing Practice. Reston, VA, Reston Publishing Co, 1982.

Janoski EH and Daview JL. Psychiatric Mental Health Nursing, 2nd ed. Boston, Jones and Bartlett, 1989.

Janoski EH and Phipps LB. Life Cycle Group Work in Nursing. Monterey, CA, Wadsworth Health Services Division, 1986.

Keable D. The Management of Anxiety. New York, Churchill Livingstone, 1989.

Kendall PC and Watson D (eds). Anxiety and Depression: Distinctive and Overlapping Features. San Diego, Academic Press, 1989.

Kennerley H. Managing Anxiety. New York, Oxford University Press, 1990.

Kriegh H and Perka J. Psychiatric and Mental Health Nursing: A Commitment to Care and Concern. East Norwalk, CT, Appleton and Lange, 1988.

Kübler-Ross E. On Death and Dying. New York, Macmillan, 1969.

Lambert V and Lambert C. Psychosocial Care of the Physically Ill, 2nd ed. Englewood Cliffs, NJ, Prentice-Hall, 1985.

Lerner H. The Dance of Anger. New York, Harper & Row, 1985.

Lipp MR. Respectful Treatment: The Human Side of Medical Care, 2nd ed. New York, Harper & Row, 1986.

McCann-Flynn JB and Heffron PB. Nursing From Concept to Practice. Bowie, MD, Robert J. Brady, 1984.

Miller JF. Coping with Chronic Illness: Overcoming Powerlessness. Philadelphia, FA Davis, 1983.

Millon I et al (eds). Handbook of Clinical Health Psychology. New York, Plenum Press, 1982.

Millman H (ed). Therapies for Adults: Depressive, Anxiety and Personality Disorders. San Francisco, Jossey-Bass, 1982.

Moos R (ed). Coping with Physical Illness, vol. 2. New York, Plenum Medical Book Co, 1984.

Morce N and Robins P. The 36-Hour Day. Baltimore, Johns Hopkins University Press, 1981.

Murray RB and Zentner JP. Nursing Assessment and Health Promotion Strategies Through the Life Span. East Norwalk, CT, Appleton and Lange, 1989.

Norris CM (ed). Concept Clarification in Nursing. Rockville, MD, Aspen Systems, 1982.

Purtila R. Health Professional/Patient Interaction, 3rd ed. Philadelphia, WB Saunders, 1984.

Roberts S. Behavioral Concepts and the Critically Ill Patient, 2nd ed. Englewood Cliffs, NJ, Prentice-Hall, 1986.

Rowan D and Eayrs C. Fears and Anxieties. New York, Longman, 1987.

Rubin TA. The Angry Book. New York, Macmillan, 1969.

Salter M (ed). Altered Body Image. New York, John Wiley & Sons, 1988.

Schultz W. The Interpersonal Underworld. Palo Alto, CA, Science and Behavior Books, 1966.

Selzer R. Letters to a Young Doctor. New York, Simon and Schuster, 1982.

Simons RC. Understanding Human Behavior in Health and Illness, 3rd ed. Baltimore, Williams & Wilkins, 1985.

Strauss A. Chronic Illness and the Quality of Life, 2nd ed. St Louis, CV Mosby, 1984.

Sundeen SJ et al. Nurse-Client Interaction, Implementing the Nursing Process. St Louis, CV Mosby, 1989.

Wilkes E. The Dying Patient: The Medical Management of Incurable and Terminal Illness. Ridgewood, NJ, George A. Boyden and Son, 1982.

Williams JM and Mark G. The Psychological Treatment of Depression. New York, Free Press, 1984.

Wilson HS and Kneisl CR. Psychiatric Nursing, 3rd ed. Menlo Park, CA, Addison-Wesley, 1988.

Woods NF. Human Sexuality in Health and Illness, 3rd ed. St Louis, CV Mosby, 1984.

Journals

Asterisks indicate nursing research articles.

Anger

Antai-Otong D. When your patient is angry. Nursing 1988 Feb; 18(2):44–45.

Barnum B. Anger and creating one's world . . . nursing personality. Nurs Health Care 1989 May; 10(5):235.

Grainger RD. Anger within ourselves. Am J Nurs 1990 Jul; 90(7):12.

Medved R. Strategies for handling angry patients—and their families. Nursing 1990 Jan; 19(1):27–30.

Thomas SP. Is there a disease-prone personality? Iss Ment Health Nurs 1988; 9(4):339–352.

Thomas SP. Theoretical and empirical perspectives on anger. Issues Ment Health Nur 1990 Jul/Sep; 113):203–216.

Turnhull J et al. Turn it around: short term management for aggression and anger . . . training for nurses. J Psychosol Nurs Ment Health Serv 1990 Jun; 28(6):6–10, 13, 34–35.

Anxiety

Birrell J. Managing anxiety. Prof Nurse 1988 Apr; 3(7):243–246.

Boyd MD et al. Is your MI patient too scared to recover? RN 1988 May; 51(5):50–54.

* Brown SM. Quantitative measurement of anxiety in patients undergoing surgery for renal calculus disease. J Adv Nurs 1990 Aug; 15(8):962–970.

* Kaempf G et al. The effect of music on anxiety: A research study. AORN J 1989 Jul; 50(1):112, 114–118.

Kneisl CR. Combating anxiety. RN 1990 Aug; 53(8):50–54.

Martin P. A feeling that needs expressing: helping patients manage their anxiety. Prof Nurs 1990 Apr; 5(7):374–375.

* Nyamathi A et al. Preoperative anxiety: Its effect on cognitive thinking. AORN J 1988 Jan; 47(1):164–165, 167–170.

* Raleigh EH et al. Significant others benefit from preoperative information. J Adv Nurs 1990 Aug; 15(8):841–845.

* Taylor-Laughran AE et al. Defining characteristics of the nursing diagnosis fear and anxiety: A validation study. Appl Nurs Res 1989 Nov; 2(4):178–186.

Wheeler BR. Crisis intervention: Recognizing and helping patients overcome anxiety. AORN J 1988 May; 47(5):1241, 1244, 1246+.

Zimmerman LM et al. Effects of music on patient anxiety in coronary care units. Heart Lung 1988 Sep; 17(5):560–566.

Body Image

Janelli LM. The impact of health status on body image of older women. Rehabil Nurs 1988 Jul/Aug; 13(4):178–180.

Price BJ. A model for body-image care. J Adv Nurs 1990 May; 15(5):585–593.

Smith SA. Extended body image in the ventilated patient. Intensive Care Nurs 1989 Mar; 5(1):31–38.

* Utz SW et al. Perceptions of body image and health status in persons with mitral valve prolapse. Image: Journal of Nursing Scholarship 1990 Spring; 22(1):18–22.

* Wright JE. Self perception alterations with coronary artery by-pass surgery. Heart Lung 1987 Sep; 16(5):483–490.

Communication

Amenta MO et al. Communicating with dying patients. Nursing 1987 Mar; 17(3):100.

Haggerty LA. An analysis of senior nursing students' immediate responses to distressed patients. J Adm Nurs 1987 Jul; 12(4):451–461.

* Harrison TM et al. Assessing nurses' communication: A cross-sectional study. West J Nurs Res 1989 Feb; 11(1):75–91.

Kasch CR et al. Person-centered communication and social perspective taking. West J Nurs Res 1988 Jun; 10(3):317–326.

Maguire M. Storm signals. Nursing 1988 Oct; 18(10):64J.

Montgomery C. How to say "I care" when you have no time to talk. RN 1987 May; 59(5):21.

* Paxton R et al. Teaching nurses therapeutic conversation: A pilot study. J Adv Nurs 1988 May; 13(3):401–404.

Plowman FT. Straight talk. Am J Nurs 1990 Aug; 90(8):40–41.

Sarvimaki A. Nursing care as a moral, practical, communicative and creative activity. J Adm Nurs 1988 Jul; 13(4):462–467.

Thomas DO. How to make your point on paper. RN 1988 Aug; 51(8):14, 18.

Coping

Baker AF. How families cope. J Psychosoc Nurs Ment Health Serv 1989 Jan; 27(1):31–36.

Capp LA. The spectrum of suffering . . . An AJN Classic. Am J Nurs 1990 Aug; 90(8):35–39.

Christman NJ et al. Uncertainty, coping and distress following myocardial infarction: Transition from hospital to home. Res Nurs Health 1988 Apr; 11(2):71–82.

Conboy-Hill S. Coping with change. Int Nurs Rev 1989 Jan/Feb; 36(1):27–28.

de Chesnay M et al. How healthy families cope with stress. AAOHN J 1988 Sep; 36(9):361–365.

* Dewe PJ. Stressor frequency, tension, tiredness and coping: Some measurement issues and a comparison across nursing groups. J Adm Nurs 1989 Apr; 14(4):308–320.

Geach B. Pain and coping. Image: Journal of Nursing Scholarship 1987 Spring; 19(1):12–15.

Holmes BC. Psychological evaluation and preparation of the patient and family. Cancer 1987 Oct; 60(8):2021–2024.

Kallop S. Finding the ability to cope. Emergency 1990 Jul; 22(7):48–50.

* Long CG et al. Group coping skills training for anxiety and depression: Its application with chronic patients. J Adm Nurs 1988 May; 13(3):358–364.

* McNett SC. Social support, threat, and coping response and effectiveness in the functionally disabled. Nurs Res 1987 Mar/Apr; 36(2):98–103.

Mishel MH. Uncertainty in illness. Image: Journal of Nursing Scholarship 1988 Winter; 20(4):225–232.

* Roberts JG et al. Analysis of coping responses and adjustment: Stability of conclusion . . . burn injury. Nurs Res 1987 Mar/Apr; 36(2):94–97.

Walker JM et al. The nursing management of pain in the community: A theoretical framework. J Adv Nurs 1989 Mar; 14(3):240–247.

Culture

Hoeman SP. Cultural assessment in rehabilitation nursing practice. Nurs Clin North Am 1989 Mar; 24(1):277–289.

Major MB. Developing cultural sensitivity. Calif Nurs 1987 Mar; 83(2):5.

Martinelli AM. Pain and ethnicity: How people of different cultures experience pain. AORN J 1987 Aug; 46(2):273–274, 276, 278.

Nolde T et al. Planning and evaluation of cross-culture health education activities. J Adm Nurs 1987 Mar; 12(2):159–165.

Rothenburger RL. Transcultural nursing: Overcoming obstacles to effective communication. AORN J 1990 May; 5(5):1349–1354+.

Death

Burson N. Sharing death. Nursing 1987 Apr; 17(4):58–59.

Corcoran DK. Helping patients who've had near-death experiences. Nursing 1988 Nov; 8(11):34–39.

Darden J. Dying at home. AD Nurse 1988 Jan/Feb; 3(1):21–22.

Dugan DO. Death and dying: Emotional, spiritual, and ethical support for patients and families. J Psychosoc Nurs Ment Health Serv 1987 Jul; 25(7):21, 25–29.

Henderson KJ. Dying, God and anger. Comforting through spiritual care. J Psychosoc Nurs Ment Health Serv 1989 May; 27(5):17–21.

Lyons TAB. We gave Elizabeth her last trip home. RN 1988 Dec; 51(2):26–29.

Ufema J. Facing death: Look to the past. Nursing 1988 Nov; 18(11):93–94.

Ufema J. Insights on death and dying. Nursing 1988 Oct; 18(10):93–94.

Ufema J. Mrs. Murphy's strange behavior . . . "dying" talk. Nursing 1989 May; 19(5):84–85.

Welter KM. Night watch . . . a nurse reflects on how little—and how much—she can offer a dying patient. Nursing 1989 May; 19(5):105.

Zerwekh JV. Comforting the dying dyspneic patient. Nursing 1987 Nov; 17(11):66–69.

Depression

Beck A et al. An inventory for measuring depression. Arch Gen Psychiatry 1961; 4:561–571.

* Buckholter KC et al. Alleviating the discharge crisis: The effects of a cognitive–behavioral nursing intervention for depressed patients and their families. Arch Psychiatr Nurs 1987 Oct; 1(5):350–358.

* Davis T et al. Identifying depression in medical patients. Image: Journal of Nursing Scholarship 1988 Winter; 20(4):191–195.

Doan BD and Wadden NP. Relationships between depressive symptoms and descriptions of chronic pain. Pain 1989 Jan; 36(1):75–84.

Dreyfus JK. Depression: Assessment and interventions in the medically ill frail elderly. J Gerontol Nurs 1988 Sep; 14(9):27–36, 38–39.

Grainger RD. Dealing with feelings: depression. Am J Nurs 1990 May; 90(5):13–14.

* Gulesserian B et al. Coping resources of depressed patients. Arch Psychiatr Nurs 1987 Dec; 1(6):392–398.

Gull HJ. The chronically ill patient's adaptation to hospitalization. Nurs Clin North Am 1987 Sep; 22(3):593–560.

Kline PM et al. Heading off depression in the chronically ill. RN 1987 Oct; 50(10):44–49.

Koenig HG et al. Self-rated depression scales and screening for major depression in the older hospitalized patient with medical illness. J Am Geriatr Soc 1988 Aug; 36(8):699–706.

* Leja AM. Using guided imagery to combat postsurgical depression. J Gerontol Nurs 1989 Apr; 15(4):6–11, 40–41.

* Nickel JT et al. Depression and anxiety among chronically ill heart patients: Age differences in risk and predictors. Res Nurs Health 1990 Apr; 13(2):87–97.

Rosenbaum JN. Depression: Viewed from a transcultural nursing theoretical perspective. J Adm Nurs 1989 Jan; 14(1):7–12.

* Sneed NV et al. Anxiety, depression and hostility in cancer patients: differences based on age. Sci Nurse 1989 Spring; 4(1):26–27.

Tanner DC et al. Guidelines for treatment of chronic depression in the aphasic patient. Rehabil Nurs 1989 Mar/Apr; 14(2):70–80, 87.

Valente SM and Saunders JM. Dealing with serious depression in cancer patients. Nursing 1989 Feb; 19(2):44–47.

Grief

Allan JD and Hall BA. Between diagnosis and death: The case for studying grief before death. Arch Psychiatr Nurs 1988 Feb; 2(1):30–34.

Archer DN et al. Sorrow has many faces: Helping families cope with grief. Nursing 1988 May; 18(5):43–45.

* Carter SL. Themes of grief. Nurs Res 1990 Nov/Dec; 38(6):354–358.

Chard PS. Grief: Handling theirs and yours. Emerg Med Serv 1987 Jan/Feb; 16(1):36–38, 40–41.

Dubin WR et al. Sudden unexpected death: Managing the survivors. Emerg Med Serv 1987 Apr; 11(4):243–256.

Honer M. How you can ease a family's grief. RN 1987 Feb; 50(2):15–17.

Oerlemans–Bunn M. On being gay, single and bereaved. Am J Nurs 1988 Apr; 88(4):472–476.

Stephany T. Caregiver grief. Home Health Nurs 1989 Jan/Feb; 7(1):43–44.

Walker KL. "I don't know what to say" . . . Dealing with bereaved family members. Emerg Med Serv 1987 Jan/Feb; 16(1):3–4.

Hope

Buettner C. Where there is despair, hope . . . AD Nurse 1988 Sept/Oct; 3(5):24–25.

* Christman NJ. Uncertainty and adjustment during radiotherapy. Nurs Res 1990 Jan/Feb; 39(1):17–20, 47.

Mader JP. The importance of hope. RN 1988 Dec; 51(12):17–18.

* Miller JF et al. Development of an instrument to measure hope. Nurs Res 1988 Jan/Feb; 37(1):6–10.

* Parse RR. Parse's research methodology with an illustration of the lived experience of hope. Nurs Sci Q 1990 Spring 3(1):9–17.

Urbanowicz GR. Hardened by death, heartened by hope. J Emerg Med Serv 1987 July; 12(7):11.

"Problem Patients"

Cerchini JAL. Mr. Tanner knew what he wanted . . . Getting a patient to cooperate. Nursing 1987 Oct; 17(10):62–64.

Cellary C. When the patient is ready for independence. RN 1988 Sep; 51(9):23–24, 26.

Jones MK. Caring for the patient who makes caring difficult. Nursing 1986 May; 16(5):44–46.

Lewen–Pitz L. Violence . . . in patients. AD Nurse 1986 Nov/Dec; 1(6):9–13.

McLean RM. Mrs. Elliot wasn't just over-hearing . . . she was over-whelming. Nursing 1989 Jun; 19(6):60–62.

Montgomery CL. How to set limits when a patient demands too much. Am J Nurs 1987 Mar; 87(3):365–368.

Morrison JL. The special needs of the special patient . . . your med/surg patient is also mentally retarded. RN 1986 Jul; 49(7):49–50.

Navis ES. Controlling violent patients before they control you. Nursing 1987 Sep; 17(9):52–54.

Pelletier LR et al. Strategies for handling manipulative patients. Nursing 1989 May; 19(5):82–85.

* Podrasky DL et al. Nurses' reactions to difficult patients. Image: Journal of Nursing Scholarship 1988 Spring; 20(1):16–21.

Reale J. Life changes: Can they cause disease? Nursing 1987 Jul; 17(7):52–55.

Sarsany SL. Violent behavior. RN 1988 Sep; 51(9):66, 68.

Valinoti E. More than a garden . . . Anne focused all her fury on her nurses. Nursing 1987 Jun; 17(6):120.

Psychosocial Aspects of Illness

Allen JK. Physical and psychosocial outcomes after coronary artery bypass graft surgery. Heart Lung 1990 Jan; 19(1):49–55.

* Baillie V et al. Stress, social support, and psychological distress of family caregivers of the elderly. Nurs Res 1988 Jul/Aug; 37(4):217–222.

Beadieson–Baird M et al. Reminiscing: Nursing actions for the acutely ill geriatric patient. Issues Ment Health Nurs 1988; 9(1):83–94.

Bluhm J. Helping families in crisis hold on. Nursing 1987 Oct; 17(10):44–46.

Cohen LJ. A modern parable . . . a man's faith in life. Am J Nurs 1987 Aug; 87(8):1043.

Gadow S. The ethics of care and the ethics of cure: Synthesis in chronicity. Covenant without cure: Letting go and holding on in chronic illness. National League for Nursing, 1988; #15-2237:5–14.

Groves C et al. Nursing grand rounds: ICU psychosis; helping your patient return to reality. Nursing 1982 Jan; 12(1):58–63.

Johnson JE and Lauver DR. Alternative explanations of coping with stressful experiences associated with physical illness. ANS 1989 Jan; 11(2):39–52.

* Lowery BJ et al. On the prevalence of causal search in illness situations. Nurs Res 1987 Mar/Apr; 36(2):88–93.

* Miller JF. Hope-inspiring strategies of the critically ill. Appl Nurs Res 1989 Feb; 2(1):23–29.

* Mishel MH and Braden CJ. Finding meaning: Antecedents of uncertainty in illness. Nurs Res 1988 Mar/Apr; 37(2):98–103, 127.

* Pollock SE. Adaptation to chronic illness: Analysis of nursing research. Nurs Clin North Am 1987 Sep; 22(3):631–644.

* Thorne SE and Robinson CA. Health care relationships: The chronic illness perspective. Res Nurs Health 1988 Oct; 11(5):293–300.

Van Riper S. Helping your patient to emotional recovery. Nursing 1988 Apr; 18(4):32C, 32F.

Watson J and Ray MA. The ethics of care and the ethics of cure: Synthesis in chronicity. National League for Nursing, 1988; #15-2237:1–64.

Wicker P. The ethics of care and the ethics of cure: Synthesis in chronicity. Discussion group summary: When caring doesn't mean curing. National League for Nursing, 1988; #15-2237:53–55.

Psychosocial Support

* Gardner KG et al. Patients' perception of support. West J Nurs Res 1987 Feb; 9(1):115–131.

Gilpatrick DM. Moving clients toward wellness: Behavioral change. Clin Nurs Spec 1989 Spring; 3(1):25–28.

Hamilton J. Comfort and the hospitalized chronically ill. J Gerontol Nurs 1989 Apr; 15(4):28–33.

Jennings BM. Social support: A way to a climate of caring. Nurs Admin Q 1987 Summer; 11(4):63–71.

* Tilden VP et al. Social support and the chronically ill individual. Nurs Clin North Am 1987 Sep; 22(3):613–620.

Woods NF et al. Supporting families during chronic illness. Image: Journal of Nursing Scholarship 1989 Spring; 21(1):46–50.

Self-Care

Bertram M. A self-care project. The use of landmarks. J Gerontol Nurs 1989 Feb; 15(2):6–8.

* Braden CJ. A test of the self-help model: learned response to chronic illness experience. Nurs Res 1990 Jan/Feb; 39(1):42–47.

Connelly CE. Self-care and the chronically ill patient. Nurs Clin North Am 1987 Sep; 22(3):621–629.

Cypress M et al. Let patients be partners in their care. RN 1989 Feb; 52(2):17, 20.

* Denyes MJ. Orem's model used for health promotion: Directions from research. ANS 1988 Oct; 11(1):13–21.

Keegan L. Holistic nursing: An approach to patient and self-care. AORN J 1987 Sep; 46(3):499–500, 502, 504.

Keegan L. Self-care: Maintaining meaningful relationships. Part 2. AORN J 1987 Apr; 47(4):996–997, 1000.

Kirkpatrick MK. Self care guide for hypertensive risk reduction. AAOHN J 1987 Jun; 36(6):254–257.

* Lucas MD et al. Exercise of self-care agency and patient satisfaction with nursing care. Nurs Admin Q 1988 Spring; 12(3):23–30.

Walker LO et al. Designing and testing self-help interventions. Appl Nurs Res 1989 May; 2(2):96–99.

Self-Concept

Grainger RD. The standards of perfection. Am J Nurs 1990 Aug; 90(8):14, 17.

Husted GL et al. 5 ways to build your self esteem. Nursing 1990 May; 20(5):152, 154.

McGonigle D. Making self-talk positive. Am J Nurs 1988 Mar; 88(5):725–726.

* Muhlenkamp AF et al. Self-esteem, social support and positive health practices. Nurs Res 1986 Nov/Dec; 35(6):334–338.

Phippon ML. Patient shame; implication for perioperative nursing. AORN J 1987 Jul; 46(1):88–89, 92–94.

* Valden C et al. The relationship of age, gender, and exercise practices to measures of health, life-style, and self-esteem. Appl Nurs Res 1990 Feb; 3(1):20–26.

Stress

* Bargagliothi LA et al. Differences in stress and coping findings: A reflection of social realities or methodologies? Nurs Res 1987 May/Jun; 36(3): 170–173.

* Barnfather JS et al. Construct validity of an aspect of the coping process: Potential adaptation to stress. Issues Ment Health Nurs 1989; 10(1): 23–40.

* Biley FC. Nurses' perception of stress in preoperative surgical patients. J Adm Nurs 1989 Jul; 14(7):575–581.

Clements I et al. Implementation of a course of holistic health practices in stress management. J Holistic Nurs 1987 Spring; 5(1):19–22.

Crickmore R. A review of stress in the intensive care unit. Intensive Care Nurs 1987 Mar; 3(1):19–27.

* Davis LL. Illness uncertainty, social support, and stress in recovering individuals and family care givers. Appl Nurs Res 1990 May; 3(2):69–71.

Doran MO. Managing ICU-induced stress. Am J Nurs 1988 Nov; 88(11): 1559–1560, 1562.

Fagin CM. Stress: Implications for nursing research. Image: Journal of Nursing Scholarship 1987 Spring; 19(1):38–41.

Flannery RB Jr. The stress-resistant person. Harv Med Sch Health Lett 1989 Feb; 14(4):5–7.

* Gurklis JA and Menke EM. Identification of stressors and use of coping methods in chronic hemodialysis patients. Nurs Res 1988 Jul/Aug; 37(4):236–239, 248.

* Holden–Lund C. Effects of relaxation with guided imagery on surgical stress and wound healing. Res Nurs Health 1988 Aug; 11(4):235–244.

* Knapp TR. Stress versus strain: A methodological critique. Nurs Res 1988 May/Jun; 37(3):181–184.

Leidy NK et al. Psychophysiological processes of stress in chronic physical illness: A theoretical perspective. J Adv Nurs 1990 Apr; 15(4):478–486.

* Leidy NK. A structural model of stress, psychosocial resources, and symptomatic experience in chronic physical illness. Nurs Res 1990 Jul/Aug; 39(4):230–236.

Linn BS et al. Effects of psychophysical stress on surgical outcome. Psychosom Med 1988 May/Jun; 50(3):230–244.

Michener J. Practical ways to snuff out stress. RN 1988 Mar; 51(3):18–21.

Reale J. Life changes: Can they cause disease? Nursing 1987 Jul; 17(7): 52–55.

* Wilson VS. Identification of stressors related to patients' psychologic responses to the surgical intensive care unit. Heart Lung 1987 May; 16(3):267–273.

Touch

* Estabrooks CA. Touch: A nursing strategy in the intensive care unit. Heart Lung 1989 Jul; 18(4):392–401.

Fink K. Therapeutic touch: A hands-off affair. Emerg Med Serv 1987 Jan/ Feb; 16(1): EMS Today:81, 84–85.

Ingham A. A review of the literature relating to touch and its use in intensive care. Intensive Care Nurs 1989 Jun; 5(2):65–75.

* Lane PL. Nurse–client perceptions: The double standard of touch. Issues Ment Health Nurs 1989; 10(1):1–13.

Payne MB. The use of therapeutic touch with rehabilitation clients. Rehabil Nurs 1989 Mar/Apr; 14(2):69–72.

Quinn JF. Building a body of knowledge: Research on therapeutic touch. J Holistic Nurs 1988; 6(1):37–45.

* Schoenhover SO. Affectional touch on critical care nursing: A descriptive study. Heart Lung 1989 Mar; 18(2):146–154.

Stone G. "High touch" is the focal point of this practice. Tar Heel Nurs 1989 Jan/Feb; 51(1):14.

Tovar MK et al. Touch: The beneficial effects for the surgical patient. AORN J 1989 May; 49(5):1356–1361.

Wright SM. The use of therapeutic touch in the management of pain. Nurs Clin North Am 1987 Sep; 22(3):705–714.

11

Developmental Concepts of the Adult Life Phase

Learning Objectives

On completion of this chapter, the learner will be able to:

1. *Identify the developmental tasks and conflicts characteristic of each stage of adulthood*
2. *Describe the role expectations, role losses, rewards, and stresses encountered during each stage of adulthood*
3. *Specify the significance of the developmental stages of adulthood to members of the health professions*

For almost a century, major efforts in research, theory building, and life stage development have been focused on and devoted to childhood, adolescence, and old age. The time of early adulthood, encompassing the chronologic ages of 18 to 35, and the time of middle adulthood, ages 36 to 60, until recently have been relatively uncharted and unexplored aspects of the life span. The main development attributed to this period in life consists of simultaneous processes of change and continuity. This chapter focuses on an overview of early, middle, and late adulthood, stressing aspects of developmental changes, transitions, and tasks, as well as themes and variations of human life.

Stages of Adulthood

Books, monographs, and reports on the concerns of early and middle adulthood began to appear in 1976. These efforts in research, theory building, and life stage development focused on the divisions of adulthood and the major question of what it means to be an adult. The divisions of adulthood, as developed by the theoreticians, have been subdivided into approximately 11 stages, as shown in Chart 11-1.

Note that there are overlapping age dates in the various stages; this is due to both differences in theories about stage

Chart 11-1
Stages of Adulthood

1. Early adulthood transition	17 to 22 years
2. Entering the adult world	22 to 28 years
3. Age 30 transition	28 to 33 years
4. Settling down period	33 to 40 years
5. Mid-life transition	35 to 45 years
6. Entering middle adulthood	45 to 50 years
7. Age 50 transition	48 to 55 years
8. Culmination of middle adulthood	55 to 60 years
9. Late adulthood transition	60 to 65 years
10. Late adulthood	65 to 80 years
11. Late late adulthood	80+ years

development and the difficulty involved in applying specific age classifications to all people.

The major question of what it means to be an adult is divided into several subquestions:

- What are the things that I can expect in my development?
- Is what is happening to me normal?
- Will there be order in my life throughout the adult years as there was during childhood and adolescence?
- How will I adjust to the losses and changes in my personal identity?

The issues and essential problems of adult life, as well as the sources of its disappointments, joys, griefs, and fulfillment, are all topics of research and investigation.

Interest in adult development was originally prompted by the increasing number of people entering this period of life. However, although interest was intensifying, there was also reluctance to explore this phase of life because of anxiety and the fear that deliberate and organized scrutiny would uncover many negative factors. Dread of the process of change, unfulfilled expectations, decline, and decay were ever present.

Early Adulthood Transition (17–22 Years)

The myth that "now that you are 21 you have all the attributes for success" is scary to many young adults. Although young adults are biologically and legally adults at 21, they receive conflicting messages from society. "You're only young once" heard simultaneously with "You should be getting on with your life" can produce confusion, indecision, impulsiveness, and sometimes irrational and destructive behavior patterns. Most people in early adulthood are fearful of leaving the pre-adult world. People in this age-group have been socialized to believe that they must separate from their parents financially, socially, and psychologically and learn to become independent. Yet, during this period of life, most young adults believe that they will always belong to their parents and that their parents will support them financially, psychologically, and socially, no matter what happens. They believe in their parents' world.

Parents are the bulwark of young adults. Many people in their late teens and early 20s think that only their parents will

keep them safe and that their parents represent the only "true" family they will ever have. Often, marriage at this time is a means of breaking away from the parents and gaining greater independence; however, in many cases such marriages result in greater dependence and are likely to fail. Marrying to get away from one's parents is one of the most common unstated reasons for marriage and one of the poorest foundations for its success.

At this time also, the young adult must pull away from adolescent peers and give up hero worship of teachers and adulation of significant others. The relinquishing of these once important experiences and the changes that result may produce a sense of loss, feelings of anxiety, and fear about one's personal future.

Entering the Adult World (22–28 Years)

The chronologic age period of 22 to 28, although described as relatively tranquil in comparison to early adulthood transition, is marked by many confrontations with reality and the collapse of childhood myths. This is a period described as "postponement." Young people are postponing traditional social responsibility and allowing themselves personal space.

Confronting Childhood Myths. In childhood, it was sufficient to tell adults in authority that one had tried, even if the effort was unsuccessful. The child received positive reinforcement for just making the effort. In adulthood, one must learn that trying is not enough and that it will not suffice to make excuses for one's efforts. Positive reinforcement will not be forthcoming for merely trying. Rewards will be given solely for meeting the standard of what the "prudent person," in whatever state of life, would do.

The adult in this period of life must discard the fallacious thinking that if one does all the right things, one will automatically be rewarded. The person must realize that following the activity patterns of one's parents does not guarantee success, and that one should not expect or anticipate parental intervention when one's projects are faltering. The idea that parents will always be available to rescue the young adult fosters dependence, which precludes growth toward adult maturity.

One of the most difficult myths to dispel is the belief that there is only one right way to do things. Black-and-white thinking must be shaded with gray in order to begin successful interaction in the adult world. The realization that fair treatment of others does not guarantee fairness in return is not easily accepted by this age-group. The idea that a rational approach toward and commitment to important life events will ensure the results that one wants must be abandoned. These beliefs, adopted in childhood and reinforced in adolescence, must be challenged and rethought in adulthood.

Rejecting one of the major premises of our society, that working hard will always bring success, is extremely difficult for the young adult, who has grown up hearing this prescription for succeeding in life. On the personal level, the young adult needs to realize that reliance on self and self-direction must supplant the expectation that his or her spouse or children will provide personal fulfillment. Failure to relinquish this expectation often leads to highly disturbed situations.

Establishing Relationships. The transition into early adulthood has two unique dimensions that must be noted. The first is that during this period many people establish a relationship with a mentor, an older and more experienced person who assists the young person in entering his or her chosen field of work. Initially, the mentor is superior to the young person, but gradually the relationship becomes equalized. Eventually, young adults give up their mentors in much the same way they gave up their parents.

The second relationship is formed with a special man or woman who brings out the young person's affectionate, romantic, and sexual feelings and simultaneously serves as a critic, guide, and sponsor as the person works toward his or her goals. This special person fulfills a transitional role by helping the young adult to move from dependency on father and mother toward autonomous independence.

Finding Oneself. In addition to the task of confronting childhood myths about how life is managed, this period requires extensive exploration of life structures and the making of tentative commitments that can be modified if necessary. It is a time for broadening one's experience and approaching life with a sense of adventure. However, later in this period some hard life choices must be faced. The person must consider whether or not to marry, whether to seek a job or a career, and how to establish goals to be pursued. During this period, both men and women confront conflicts inherent in trying to meet the contradictory demands of marriage and work. Premature commitments in one or both of these areas are often questioned at this time.

Age 30 Transition (28–33 Years)

The hallmark of the age 30 transition for many people is the growing awareness that if a change is to be made, it must be made soon; otherwise, one will be riveted to commitments made in the 20s, and future possibilities for desired change will be ruled out. This stage of aging is often characterized by a period of depression, which is usually alleviated when the person develops a different perspective of the world and its inhabitants. It can also be identified as a period of discovery (or rediscovery) of suppressed feelings, interests, aptitudes, talents, and goals that have been ignored or deeply hidden. A realistic understanding of one's strengths, abilities, and liabilities is a formidable task to be undertaken at this time. If the task is successfully completed, the person becomes aware of both the contradictory feelings competing within himself and similar feelings that originate in the outside world.

In the age 30 transition, there is a greater sense of urgency. Life is more serious, more restrictive, and more real. For many people, the age of 30 provides a long-awaited second chance to construct a more satisfactory life structure.

Settling Down (33–40 Years)

The transitional period of the late 20s and the early 30s is usually followed by a calmer period characterized as "settling down." Settling down is interpreted as that period in life when one takes a hard look at what is really important, becomes serious about a few major goals, and begins to build a life structure around the determined choices. Selecting and purchasing a home at this time fulfills the need of many people to establish roots and become more home-oriented. The need to establish a niche is further extended by a focus on child-

bearing, which often results in a decline in marital satisfaction. By this time, the romance of marriage may have lapsed into daily routine.

Consolidating One's Position. In the world of work, advancement becomes a major task. Conflict often occurs because the young person must challenge senior people in the establishment, the very people who have the power to grant or deny the bid for advancement. In this vulnerable position, the young adult often feels both oppressed by others and restrained by internal conflicts and inhibitions. Despite these difficulties, this is a period of extending and attempting to solidify one's position in the work force and at home.

Mid-Life Transition (35–45 Years)

The adage that life begins at 40 was heralded as a great positive statement of life; however, many adults secretly believe that life ends at 40 and that this age marks the end of a fulfilling, exciting, and self-directed life. Stereotypes of being 40 only add to internal confusion, because in the 40s individual differences are becoming more significant. Many people go through difficult changes in the 40s that are often compared with the changes of adolescence (labeled "middlescence"). Some people experience mild self-questioning. The true feelings of dread about entering middle age have kept this stage of life a well-guarded secret. The mid-life transition is a bridge between early and middle adulthood. It is a point in time when one begins to count the years that are left, rather than all those that are yet to come.

Reappraising the Past. The initial task of this transitional phase is to reappraise the past. The awareness of one's mortality is uppermost in the consciousness. One is confronted with a limited amount of time remaining and a desire to use that time wisely. This is a time when the person's previous life structure comes seriously into question, and answers must be found to questions that assume a new importance:

- How satisfactory is my present life structure—how meaningful to myself, how meaningful to the world?
- How shall that life structure be changed to provide a better basis for the future?

Discarding Illusions. One of the profound discoveries made at this time is the extent to which one's life has been based on illusion. A formidable task that must be undertaken is the process of "de-illusionment"—dealing with the recognition that many long-held and cherished assumptions about oneself and the world are not true. Although one may have been indulged in childhood to encourage imaginative development, as an adult, one is expected to be more realistic and practical. Dispensing with illusions is considered desirable and is anticipated as a natural step in attaining maturity. At the same time, it is also the process through which a person is stripped of most of his cherished values, beliefs, and opinions about life and people. The result may be feelings either of irreparable loss or of being liberated so that one may develop more flexible values, beliefs, and opinions. One may be able to look at oneself and others in a more genuine, less idealized manner.

Adapting to Change. As time passes in this life phase, a major task is to modify the life structure of the 30s transition so that it will become appropriate to middle adulthood. External changes at this time, such as distance in the marital relationship (sometimes better, sometimes worse), children grown and leaving home, and parents dead or dependent, have a specific impact on the role expectations of the person as a spouse, family member, son, or daughter.

Changes in a person's position in the work force have a profound impact. As the character of work changes, the person must respond to innovations or be left behind. World events, social movements, and economic conditions affect each person according to age and period of development.

The internal changes in a person's life structure are significant at this juncture. It is quite common to revise one's social outlook, personal values and goals, and career objectives. Many people describe a feeling of "internal slippage" at this time.

Coming to Terms With Mortality and Creative/Destructive Forces.
The mid-life transition activates one's awareness of death and destruction. The person becomes aware of his mortality as well as of the actual and impending death of significant others; he also realizes that significant persons in his life may have acted destructively toward him with both good and bad intentions in mind. He, in turn, has inflicted irrevocable hurt on parents, spouse, lovers, children, friends, and colleagues with the same mixed motivation. In middle adulthood, one becomes painfully aware of the ability to be simultaneously creative and destructive while working toward control of these powerful forces.

Achieving Individualization.
At mid-life, people must come to terms with the synchronous existence of masculine and feminine parts of the self. A man must integrate his powerful need for attachment to others with his antithetical but equally important need for separateness. A woman must integrate her new-found need for separateness and achievement with her lesser need for attachment. As the individualization process occurs, the person becomes a more differentiated and complex human; most important, he develops effective boundaries that link him to the external world with a more satisfying interaction process.

Entering Middle Adulthood (45–50 Years)

Mature adulthood is not a period of stability and certainty, but rather one of change. The changes that occur during this stage of life have no absolute chronologic or sequential order, although certain events are biologically, psychologically, and socially determined or expected. The impact of these changes, which often include new sets of relationships, new expectations, and altered or modified evaluations of self, inevitably involves the adult in transitions or turning points. The events of adult life entail either role gains or role losses. Getting married, having a child, acquiring a new home, obtaining a job, and receiving a promotion are usually perceived as role gains. Becoming separated, getting a divorce, being chronically ill, retiring from work, going through menopause, and being widowed are perceived as role losses.

The main themes of adulthood include stress, stock-taking and *locus of control*, shifts in time perspective, changes in biologic and psychologic functioning, generational roles, sex role reversal, and the evolution of careers and activities.

Stress.
The primary source of stress for middle-aged men is their work. For middle-aged women, stress is often a result of their concern for their husband's work and health or for their own work; their own health and physical appearance and the events in the lives of their children are a secondary cause.

Stock-Taking, Locus of Control.
Although adults of any age may go through the process of reassessment, the stock-taking of middle age is characterized by a focus on the inner self, a concern with self-development, and a reexamination and reevaluation of competency. The period of "middlescence" often causes people to see their children as capable of getting more enjoyment from sex, love, and life in general than they can; moreover, at the same time they are aware that their children view them as being on the decline. For some middle-aged people, the position of being "caught between two generations" intensifies a sense of loss and a fear of aging; it also confirms the feeling that they are no longer masters of their fates and their environments.

People inclined toward this view may be described as having an *external locus of control* in that they feel like puppets on a string, controlled by other people, impersonal social forces, or fate. On the other hand, people with an *internal locus of control* perceive themselves as having power over their own destinies. These are the people who view middle adulthood as a period of maximum capacity that underscores their ability to handle a highly complex environment and more challenging self-goals. For these people, stock-taking produces a renewed sense of self as they triumph over difficulties and develop new coping skills. For others, however, it is a time of feeling trapped, anxious, or panic-stricken by life events. Many of these people become immobilized and are unable to act, thus sinking into deeper depression.

Shift in Time Perspective.
One of the most startling events in middle age is a shift in time perspective; one starts thinking in terms of the time left to live, rather than the time lived since birth. This awareness of mortality appears to be somewhat more important to men than to women. Men become more conscious of their loss of strength and vitality, more preoccupied with their health, and more fearful that time is running out. Women become more concerned with the health of the significant people in their lives, particularly their spouses. Women may "rehearse for widowhood" by fantasizing about being on their own. However, like men, they become overwhelmingly aware that they have little time left.

The shift in time perspective brings a confrontation with death that is now a personal reality rather than something that happens to other people. An awareness that life in middle age is not progressing as smoothly as was expected may lead middle-aged adults to believe they are abnormal. They often do not realize that other adults experience the same self-doubts, feelings of helplessness, lost hopes, and sense of inadequacy that they are experiencing.

Changes in Biologic Functioning.
Although biologic decline for most people ordinarily occurs gradually, several minute changes often bring about a major qualitative drop in bodily function by the early 40s. It is necessary to exercise caution when making generalizations about physical changes during the adult years—not only about when they will happen, but whether they will, in fact, occur at all. There is no physical change that can be predicted to happen to all adults. It should be noted that the ages discussed are averages and not absolutes. People deviate widely from these averages at both ends. Some people die of "old age" in their 40s, whereas others live to be well over 100.

Generally, one has reached maximum strength by age 30. After this point in life, there is a slight but steady loss of strength through the adult years. The points of experienced weakness occur more in the back and leg muscles and less in the arm muscles. These weaknesses can be halted by individualized exercise that is undertaken on a regular basis.

The loss of physical attributes takes its greatest toll on people who derive their feelings of worth from their bodies. People who value themselves for their strength or beautiful bodies exhibit psychologic patterns of aging as soon as their bodies begin to age significantly. An overemphasis on physical development and beauty in childhood and adolescence can boomerang in maturity and later adult years.

Changes in health during adulthood are not all negative. Middle age does not necessarily bring poor health. Many people live all their adult years without ever being sick or incapacitated in any way. In general, adults can expect fewer acute illnesses, fewer accidents, and more chronic illness.

Sensory Acuity. In the area of the senses, the process of aging starts in infancy. Visual acuity for most people is best at about 20, remains relatively constant to 40, and then, barring gross organic difficulties, begins a slow decline. Hearing, like sight, seems to be at its peak at about 20; from about 20 on, a gradual loss occurs that affects high tones more than low tones and, after age 55, more men than women. Furthermore, after 50 there is a higher incidence of loss of ability to distinguish the finer nuances of taste, although the four basic tastes of sweet, sour, salt, and bitter remain constant. There also appears to be a sharp decrease in the sense of touch after 45.

Some theorists believe that sensitivity to pain tends to remain steady to approximately age 50 and then declines for different parts of the body, resulting in an increase in pain tolerance. Other theorists believe that the consciousness of pain increases after 50, making older people victims of wide pain sensitivity. The one sense that seems to retain a high level of effectiveness is balance, which is at its best between 40 and 50.

Physical Appearance and Health. One's physical appearance and physical health are probably the most important factors in determining how one approaches everyday life. The influence of physical appearance on physical health can be seen in the attention a person pays to nutrition, exercise, and relaxation. Although there is a minimal amount of physical change throughout early adulthood, middle age is often characterized by dramatic changes in appearance. Probably the most obvious change perceived by others is weight gain. Redistribution of body fat makes the body structure look like a diamond—narrow at both ends and heavy in the middle. The thinning and color change of hair are also noticeable physical changes. Many men in their 40s begin to experience hairline recession, reduced hair growth, and ultimate baldness. By the 50s, both women and men are at least gray, if not whitehaired. Women begin to experience some hair growth on their upper lips and chins at this time also.

For both men and women, the skin loses elasticity and becomes coarser and darker on the face, arms, and hands. Wrinkles and looseness of the skin also appear. The lower part of the face changes because of alterations in teeth, bone, muscles, and connective tissues. The voice loses timbre and quality and becomes more high-pitched. The physical movements of the body become less graceful because of joint stiffening and loss of resiliency in the muscles. The cumulative effects of these changes may make it painful for the middle-aged adult to look at himself in a mirror.

Psychologic Functioning. In the area of psychologic functioning, the middle-aged adult recognizes that of all age-groups, his is the most powerful. Despite the fact that society is oriented toward youth, it is controlled by the middle-aged. They set the standards and are the policy makers. Furthermore, middle age is generally a period of heightened sensitivity to one's position in a highly complex and confusing social environment. Assessing and reassessing oneself is a major and continual theme throughout this period of life.

Psychologically, the rewards associated with middle age are not as easily discerned as those of early adulthood and old age. In early adulthood, chronologic aging (*i.e.*, getting older) means becoming increasingly eligible for adult rewards, such as more status, power, and attractiveness, whereas advanced old age means receiving rewards for simply surviving; each additional year lived brings a mark of distinction. The middle-aged rely more on the functioning of their bodies, career status, and family cycles to determine their identities than on chronologic age. Because changes in these aspects of their lives are not synchronized or predictable, the middle-aged often experience intense conflict and confusion.

Relating to Other Generations. One of the major psychologic stresses is the distance the middle-aged experience from both the younger and the older generations. In general, the distance from the young is much greater; younger people can neither understand nor relate to the middle-aged because they lack the necessary life experience. The particular historical events of living create a bond between people who have lived through them together and a distance between those who have not. Although there is also a certain degree of distance between the middle-aged and the elderly, the sense of proximity and identification with them is more intense, because those who are older have experienced what it is like to be middle-aged. There is often a tendency to blur the differences between the middle-aged and the older generation.

Although most middle-aged people have become or are in the process of becoming aware of the finiteness of time, very few express a desire to be young again. Rather, they wish to have again the vigor and appearance of youth while enjoying the authority and autonomy they have acquired.

A special task of the middle-aged adult is to become more conscious of both the child and the older person within himself and others. Attention to this task allows him to transcend, at least in some degree, the barriers that tend to separate the generations. It is important because one of the major enrichments in life is learning how to be successful in relating in a fully human way to people of all ages.

Relationships between generations are important in all societies. Although most people are aware of profound differences between generations, one can concentrate on increasing positive interaction between them. At each stage of development, people carry within themselves aspects of every generation. However, it is difficult for the child and the adolescent to visualize the "older self" and to develop empathy for persons who are more than 10 years older than they are.

The concept of generation is, for the most part, poorly understood. Members of a given generation are classified at the same age level by contrasting them to both younger and older generations. As years pass, a young adult develops a sense of moving from one generation to the next and of establishing new relationships with the other generations in his world. During adulthood, other persons are roughly the same age if they are not more than 6 or 7 years older or younger. Thus, one's own generation covers a span of some 12 to 15 years. A half generation includes an age spread of from 8 to 15 years in either direction. An older person in a generational relationship maintains an implicit claim to greater authority in the relationship and is often viewed as an older sibling. As the age difference increases to 20 years and beyond, a full generation is marked, and the older person in the relationship carries a parental role. When the age difference is 40 years or more, there is a distance of two generations, and the older person is often viewed as a symbolic grandparent.

A new and troubling change in generational status begins in the late 30s and is usually well established by the middle 40s. People in their 40s are usually regarded by people in their 20s as a full generation removed and as part of the "establishment." Furthermore, the people in their 40s are often perceived as parental figures and, at a deeper level, as becoming "old," losing their place in society, and having lost their capacity for youthful adventures. More frightening to these people is the growing realization that they are leaving the youthful generation and entering the vaguest and most poorly defined of all generations—"the middle-aged."

Generativity Versus Stagnation.   The theory of the life cycle developed by Erik Erikson encompasses stages from early childhood to late adulthood. The stage that has the most relevance to the middle-aged is that of "generativity versus stagnation." Generativity means the ability to develop authority in younger persons and to establish mutuality with them. It also means offering leadership to younger people while simultaneously treating them as adults and encouraging them to develop greater independence and personal authority. Stagnation refers to the sense of not growing, that is, being static and bogged down in a life that is full of heavy obligations and devoid of self-fulfillment.

The middle-aged person, if generative, is becoming a senior member of the adult world and must learn to relate to persons in their 30s as junior but fully adult members who will succeed him in a few years. He must also be able to relate to people in their 20s as neophytes going through their initial formative period within the adult world.

A formidable but necessary task to be accomplished by the person in middle adulthood is to experience, endure, and fight against stagnation. Stagnation is not purely negative and should not be totally avoided. It is necessary to do battle with stagnation in order to recognize that one's own vulnerability is a source of wisdom that increases one's capacity for sympathy and compassion for others.

Sex Role Reversal.   Sex role reversal is a phenomenon in which women become more assertive, more autonomous, more oriented toward achievement in the work place, and more personally active, while men become more nurturant, more emotional, more home- and family-oriented, and more passive. The process of becoming more androgynous tends to be actualized during middle age. Androgeny involves allowing the development of *all* the male and female qualities in a person that have been socially identified as male or female. As sexual role stereotypes dissipate and drop away, people can become more truly human.

Evaluating Past Achievements and Setting New Goals.   Each segment of a person's life is variously mirrored in the relationship of the person to work, family, individual self, social self, life plans, and goals. In general, life has been divided into two halves, with the dividing point at about age 40. By age 40, one has an opportunity to build a personal life and, ideally, to realize the rewards of youthful endeavors. For most people, the 40s are a period of reexamination. Questions about what has been accomplished, what is yet to be done, and the value of the person's life to society as well as to others and to himself are posed. The reexamination culminates in coming to terms with the disparity between what a person is and what he had hoped to become.

Irrespective of what answers surface to these profound questions of living, a person must move forward. If one has not been successful in achieving early life goals, this reality must be accepted, and goals to rebuild one's life must be formulated. If one has achieved according to or in excess of expectations of early goals, the meaning and value of one's success must be considered. A few people may be satisfied with their present lives and may wish to continue as they are for the remainder of the life span. However, despite their satisfactory situations, there will be changes that cannot be anticipated at this point. Many people experience feelings of entrapment and meaninglessness when they realize that the attainment of their early adulthood goals has not provided the satisfaction they had hoped for. The lives of many people are relatively satisfactory in some respects and disappointing or destructive in others. Whatever the life condition at 40, each person must go through the process of sorting things out, coming to terms with personal limitations, reformulating goals, and moving forward through the life span.

Culminating Events.   Events of marked significance may occur in the late 30s and early 40s: promotion, demotion, firing, establishing a family unit, divorce, personal health breakdown, illness or death of significant others, loss of financial base, acquisition of considerable wealth, and lack of recognition or accolades from society. Any of these may serve as a culminating event. A culminating event represents a form of success or failure, necessitating movement forward or backward on the path of life. How the person deals with a culminating event dictates chances for the future.

The culminating event frequently makes one aware of the period of mid-life transition. If the precipitating event occurred at another stage of life, it would have different meanings and implications. During middle adulthood, the culminating event must be integrated with life reappraisal. One must look at the event as a factor in the possibilities for a better or worse life in the future. The successful handling of culminating events demands continuous self-renewal and creative involvement in one's own life, as well as in the lives of others.

One of the most important services rendered by members of the helping professions is to assure people who are struggling with the "crises" of middle age and aging that they are not alone in what they are feeling and that the process of handling culminating events is not outside the range of normal experience.

Age 50 Transition (48–55 Years)

At every point in adult life, crossing the threshold into the next stage represents a loss of youth, diminishing vitality, and, finally, a threat to life itself. Many people use the term *the big O* in referring to the transitions of the 20s, 30s, 40s, 50s, 60s, 70s, 80s, 90s, and 100s (*e.g.*, "the big four-O"). The age 50 transition is considered to include the ages of 48 to 55. This is a time to continue working on the tasks of the mid-life transition while anticipating and planning for the building of a second middle adult structure that will be the medium for completing middle adulthood.

One of the difficult aspects of the age 50 transition is the realization that one is neither young nor old but rather suspended in the middle. At 50, one cannot ignore the graying hair, the wrinkling skin, and the frequent pains, aches, and strained muscles occasioned by activities that in previous years would have caused only minimal physical stress.

One of the worst feelings at this period of transition is the contemplation of long and continuing years of a meaningless existence—a time when youthful passions have ceased, there is little opportunity for creative tasks, and one's contributions to society are minimal. This period evokes strong feelings of self-doubt that intensify as the person realizes he is moving toward being old and begins to fear disintegration, despair, and eventual death. There is often an inner voice that says, "There is little time left to enjoy life—the end is nearly here."

Achieving Immortality.   Two of the major tasks in the 50s are defining the ultimate value of life and defining how one is going to achieve a form of immortality. Successfully resolving these basic needs of life can help to ease the strong feelings of self-doubt, meaninglessness, and despair that so many people experience when entering this period of life. For most people, dealing with a form of immortality translates into a personal decision about the legacy they can or will bequeath to future generations.

Many people place the highest value on having and raising children and maintaining familial relationships, viewing these accomplishments as their most precious gifts to generations to come. Children take the places of their parents in the adult world. Whatever rewards, accomplishments, and satisfactions children receive are also regarded as gifts of the parents. Parents often feel that parts of them will live on in their children.

Another way of confronting mortality is to bequeath one's material possessions to charities and worthy causes. People often make sizable contributions to religious groups, colleges, unions, professional organizations, and community projects. These groups reflect continuance and enduring value. The giver's munificence is often accompanied by a pervasive need to guarantee personal immortality by means of a name registered or engraved on a worship bench or plaque.

The legacy of professional and artistic people to future generations can take the form of an enduring product, such as a book, statue, painting, or poem; or perhaps their work will contribute to improved health and better and more comprehensive education for future generations. Whatever the means of attempting to guarantee immortality, be it material possessions, creative products or enterprises, or influences on others, the process must be recognized and implemented for success in the transition of the 50s.

Culmination of Middle Adulthood (55–60 Years)

The end of middle adulthood occurs at approximately 55 to 60 years of age. This period has often been compared to the settling down period of early adulthood. The task of this period is completing middle adulthood and becoming ready for late adulthood. For most people, the decade of the 50s can be a period of great fulfillment if they can resolve the young/old conflict. This conflict suggests that one is both young and old at every age; moreover, the human starts becoming old at birth, yet often remains young in certain respects during old age.

The serenity of ending middle adulthood is achieved when one accepts that there are clearly advantages as well as disadvantages in growing older, just as there were in being young. At this time, the mature adult realizes that when he was young he was lively, growing, heroic, and full of potential, but at the same time impulsive, lacking in experience and wisdom, and imperfectly developed. While growing old, he can still be lively and full of potential as well as wise, psychologically and socially powerful, and accomplished.

At the culmination of middle adulthood, one should have struck a balance with the young/old continuum. Once the balance is struck, one can have a solid structure on which to base the use of considerable energy, imagination, and motivation for change. Middle adulthood is the core of the life cycle and the period of intense preparation for what is to come.

Late Adulthood Transition (60–65 Years)

We describe the period of late adulthood transition as the period from ages 60 to 65. It is often marked by the recognition and experience of physical decline. The fact that one becomes more forgetful, takes longer to complete tasks, and has more difficulty getting the body to move heralds the passage from middle to old age. Even if one is in relatively good health and remains physically active, he is constantly reminded of the tentativeness of his condition. Reminders of serious illness and death occur with increasing frequency in the experiences of family and friends. As one approaches 60, it seems that all traces of youth, even the last vestiges remaining from middle age, are about to vanish, leaving only the undetermined vagaries of old age. Not all these aspects of physical and mental change happen to all people, but all are likely to experience some changes and be affected by them.

A major task of the 60s is to maintain youthfulness in a new form appropriate to late adulthood. The process of termination and the modification of the earlier life must take place. As they enter this period, many people have not yet internalized the fact that they will become old; they are aware that old age comes to all people but somehow believe that this applies to everyone except them. The 60 transition signals the culmination of the strivings of middle age. One must begin to relinquish the role occupied in the center stage of one's world, reduce the heavy responsibilities of middle adulthood, and learn to live in a different relationship with one's society. The gradual loss of recognition, power, and authority can become traumatic.

Probably one of the most difficult changes to accept is the movement of one's generation out of the limelight into a position of subservience. To allow one's children to assume the power and authority of the family is necessary but difficult to accept. In the world of business, similar transitions are also taking place. An older person who has a great deal of authority and the power to make decisions must make way for the middle adult generation, who need to acquire the ultimate power and responsibility. If he tries to hold on to formal authority after

70, he is "out of sync" with his own generation and in conflict with the generation of middle adulthood.

Retirement from formal work endeavors does not mean the end of one's worth; instead, it is an opportunity to continue in valued work that stems from one's own creative energies rather than from societal pressures and financial need. At this point, a person who is in the young/old category has a series of options regarding the form of retirement available: *early retirement,* an option that requires sound financial planning and a secure economic base; *gradual retirement,* an option that allows a slow phasing out of a major career or shifting to a new, less demanding career or job; *traditional retirement,* an option that provides for the cessation of work in the marketplace at age 65; *late retirement,* an option that provides for the cessation of work at the now-legal age of 70; and the final option of *nonretirement,* which is to continue work until death. These several options are now available to more and more people. The "work" a retired person chooses may encompass play or, in other words, involve him in his own determined interests for financial gain or personal satisfaction. At this time of life, one should be relatively free from pressures of society and should be able to choose the activities, be they work, play, or a combination of both, that meet one's needs. Thus, the older person should be able to fulfill one of the primary developmental tasks of late adulthood—achieving a balance of involvement with society and self.

Late Adulthood (65–80 Years)

Late adulthood ushers in a period of decline as well as an opportunity for development. This is the period of life when many people must begin the process of rehearsal for or the actual experience of widowhood. Needs that have been met in marriage are no longer met. For many, this period of life is filled with loneliness, because widowhood is both a personal and a social loss. The social role of husband or wife, head of household or homemaker, no longer applies.

In late adulthood, chronic disease processes become more common. Also, sociogenic aging, that is, aging caused by social expectations, comes to the fore. If we act old, we physically decline, fulfilling our own prophecy. A further complication of sociogenic aging is hypokinetic disease, disease that occurs as a result of too little physical movement. Thus, one's attitude and expectations can influence biologic aging.

The person entering late adulthood senses that he has most probably completed the major part, if not all, of his life work. Whatever he was to do for society has been done, and his choice of a way to guarantee immortality has been made. At this time, the ultimate appraisal of life must be achieved. Finding meaning and value in life as a whole is necessary to avoid bitterness and despair in the final years. In striving to attain personal integrity, the person can come to terms with his own view of death. It is necessary for most people to realize that whatever values and expectations they had held dear are not likely to be fully realized. Each person must reconcile the imperfections and elements of destruction in his life. Making peace with oneself and with those who are perceived as having injured one is a necessary task of late adulthood. Most people at this stage of life continue to hold strong convictions but are more realistic about how these convictions can be carried out in daily life.

Late Late Adulthood (80 Years and Older)

Late late adulthood, the last period of life, encompasses ages 80 and beyond. People who survive beyond 80 generally experience myriad infirmities and at least one chronic condition. At this point, signs of aging are more evident than any signs of growth. The scope of life tends to be narrowed, and the individual focuses intently on a few significant relationships—the place where he lives, immediate bodily concerns, and personal comforts. The person has to fight diligently to avoid the feeling that life has no meaning or, worse, that he is simply being tolerated.

All other phases of the life cycle have focused on the development of strategies for a new beginning—a new basis for living. This era focuses on strategies to learn how to die. One approach is disengagement, in which the older person progressively withdraws from society, ceases caring about things and people, and becomes increasingly self-concerned. The second approach follows the activity theory, in which the older person engages in a high level of physical activity and social integration and follows a controlled nutrition regimen, all of which result in a healthy and involved late, late adulthood. To continue to live effectively, one must make peace with dying. If one can maintain a personal vitality, engagement in social life will continue. Most important, people at this stage of life can serve as models of wisdom, hope, integrity, and personal nobility. At this time, one reaches an ultimate involvement with self—an awareness that the final task of life is accepting and loving oneself and being ready to move on to the next stage, which is death.

Chapter Summary

This chapter describes the physiologic, psychologic, and sociologic events that can be expected during the adult life cycle. Emphasis is placed on developmental concepts from early adulthood years through the middle years and late adulthood. Developmental concepts of early childhood are not discussed. Concepts relative to late adulthood are further described in detail in Chapter 12.

The key events that occur in life, such as establishing relationships, developing an employment status, bearing children, and dealing with loss, are viewed from each stage of adulthood. Each developmental stage is given a name and an age range. The name describes the key event that can be expected to occur during a given age range. For example, the years 33–40 are described as settling down. The experience of settling down tends to fall somewhere in this 7-year range; however, some individuals may experience the process of settling down much earlier, much later, or not at all.

This information is of value to the nurse for purposes of patient care planning. Acquiring an understanding of normal adult development assists the nurse in establishing communication with patients and in understanding her own behaviors.

Bibliography

Books
Belsky JK. Here Tomorrow: Making the Most of Life After Fifty. Baltimore, Johns Hopkins University Press, 1988.

Berman PL (ed). The Courage to Grow Old. New York, Ballantine Books, 1989.

Critchton J. The Age Care Sourcebook; A Resource Guide for the Aging and Their Families. New York, Simon & Schuster, 1987.

Dychtwald K and Flower J. Age Wave: The Challenges and Opportunities of an Aging America. Los Angeles, JP Tarcher Publishers, 1989.

Gould J. Spirals: A Woman's Journey Through Family Life. New York, Random House, 1988.

Henig R. How a Woman Ages. New York, Ballantine Books, 1985.

Hughes FP. Human Development Across the Life Span. St Paul, West Publishing, 1985.

Kimmel DC. Adulthood and Aging: An Interdisciplinary Developmental View, 2nd ed. New York, John Wiley & Sons, 1980.

Le Shan E. Oh to Be 50 Again! On Being Too Old for a Midlife Crisis. Alexandria, VA, Time-Life Books, 1986.

Maddox GL and Busse EW. The Universal Human Experience. New York, Springer, 1987.

Okun BF. Working with Adults: Individual Family and Career Development. Monterey, CA, Brooks-Cole, 1984.

Pesmen C. How a Man Ages. New York, Ballantine Books, 1984.

Smith WJ. The Senior Citizens' Handbook: A Nuts and Bolts Approach to More Comfortable Living. Los Angeles, Price/Stern/Sloan, 1989.

Whitbourne SK. Adult Development, 2nd ed. New York, Praeger, 1986.

Journals/Magazines

Bennett H. Two of us is one too many. The New York Times Magazine 1989 Oct 22; 22, 24.

Brock AM and O'Sullivan P. From wife to widow: Role transition in the elderly. J Psychosoc Nurs Ment Health Serv 1985 Dec; 23(12):6–12.

Davis I. Sixteen—The third time around. The New York Times Magazine 1989 Dec 17; 22, 24.

Enos SF. "Husband is having a mid-life crisis." Ladies Home Journal 1988 Sep; 105:14, 18, 20, and 185.

Holahan CK, Holahan CJ, and Belk SS. Adjustment in aging: The roles of life stress, hassles and self-efficacy. Health Psychol 1984; 3(4):315–328.

Holahan CJ and Moos RH. Life stress and health: Personality, coping and family support in stress resistance. J Pers Soc Psychol 1985 Sep; 49(3):730–747.

Hoopes R. Working late: On the outside looking in. Modern Maturity 1989 Jun/Jul; 32(3):32–35, 38, 39.

Horn JC. Peaking after 65: Here's how. Psychology Today 1989 Jul/Aug; 23:33–34.

Hoyt MF. Women in the middle. Good Housekeeping 1988 Jan; 206:54.

Lakey B and Heller K. Response biases and the relation between negative life events and psychological symptoms. J Pers Soc Psychol 1985 Dec; 49(6):1662–1668.

Luciano L. Eight myths of retirement. Money 1990 Feb; 19(2):110, 111.

Luciano L. The joyful new music of aging. Money 1990 Feb; 19(2):113, 114, 116.

Luciano L. Pre-retirees; long on hope, short on readiness. Money 1990 Mar; 19(3):25.

Over 40 and fabulous. Harper's Bazaar 1988 Aug; 121:106–131, 138–141.

Over 40 and sensational. Harper's Bazaar 1989 Aug; 122:152–157, 190, 192, 194.

Prodigal parents: Family vs. the 80 hour work week. New Perspect Q 1990 Winter;7:2–62.

Stevenson JS. Adulthood: A promising focus for future research. Annu Rev Nurs Res 1986; 1:55–74.

Streff MD. Examining family growth and development: A theoretical model. ANS 1981 Jul; 3(4):61–69.

Topolnici DM. How you can find help for your elderly relative from afar. Money 1988 Dec; 17:199–200.

12

Health Care of the Older Adult

Learning Objectives

On completion of this chapter, the learner will be able to:

1. Develop a definition of aging based on developmental and sociologic theories of aging
2. Describe the aging American population based on demographic data, economic status, housing needs, and health care needs
3. Identify physiologic changes that occur with aging
4. Describe the significance of preventive health care and health promotion for the elderly
5. Specify the major causes of physical and mental health problems in the aged
6. Describe the special nursing needs of the elderly patient
7. Use the nursing process as a framework for care of patients with Alzheimer's disease
8. Specify nursing implications relative to medication therapy in the elderly
9. Compare the needs of the elderly in the community, in an acute care setting, and in a protected environment

The Study of Aging

Aging, the normal process of time-related change, begins with birth and continues throughout life. Old age is the final phase of the life span.

The older segment of the total population is increasing in size and will continue to do so for the next 50 years. With longer life, as indicated by increasing life expectancy, the helping professions must focus upon improving the quality of life for elderly persons. Regular mental, social, and physical activities must be available. Community-based support services provide essential help to the elderly to enable them to remain in a familiar setting with meaning and dignity.

Geriatrics, the study of old age, includes the physiology, pathology, diagnosis, and management of the diseases of older adults. The broader field of *gerontology* is the study of the aging process and includes the biologic, psychologic, and sociologic sciences. Because old age is a normal occurrence within the life span that encompasses all experiences of life, care and concern for the elderly cannot be limited to one discipline. Optimal care of elderly persons can best be provided through a cooperative effort. The *interdisciplinary team*, made up of specialists from many fields, can combine expertise and resources in contributing knowledge and research to provide insight into all aspects of the aging process.

Gerontologic or gerontic nursing is the field of nursing that specializes in care of the elderly. Standards and Scope of Gerontological Nursing Practice were originally developed in 1969 and revised in 1976 and 1987 by the American Nurses Association. The nurse gerontologist can be either a specialist or a generalist offering comprehensive nursing care to the older person. The basic nursing process of assessment, nursing diagnosis, planning, implementation, and evaluation is used in combination with a specialized knowledge of aging. Gerontologic nursing can be provided in acute, chronic, or community settings. Emphasis of care is placed on promoting, maintaining, and restoring health and independence. Strengths of older adults are identified and used to help them achieve optimal independence. The nurse helps the older person to maintain dignity and maximum autonomy despite physical, social, and psychologic losses. As a patient advocate, the nurse collaborates with the interdisciplinary team to provide non-nursing services and a holistic approach to care. The nurse can be creative in instituting interventions that will help the older person achieve positive physical and mental health.

Old Age Defined

The definition of old age varies with the individual's frame of reference. A parent of 35 years may be considered old by the child of 10 years and young by his parents of 65 years. The active person of age 65 may consider 75 years as the beginning of old age.

With the adoption of the retirement age of 65 years through Social Security legislation in the 1930s, American society accepted 65 years as the beginning of old age. This represents the chronologic definition of old age and is used by society. Functional and physiologic age differ with the individual and therefore cannot be standardized. Functionally, a professional basketball player is old at the age of 35 although he may be in superb physical health and physiologically young. Gerontologists have attempted to allow for individual differences by using the classification of young–old for 65 to 74 years, and old–old for 75 years and beyond.

Life Span Versus Life Expectancy

Life span is the maximum number of years a person can live under the best of conditions in the absence of disease. The longest verified life span is about 113 years. There has been little change in the life span in recorded history. *Life expectancy* is the average number of years that a person can be expected to live. In the twentieth century, life expectancy from birth has risen dramatically from an average of 47.3 years (1900) to 74.9 years (1988), with women (78.2 years) living about 7 years longer than men (71.2 years). Early in this century, increased life expectancy was attributed to the decreased death rates of infants and young people. Since 1970, however, increases in life expectancy have been due to decreased mortality among the middle-aged and elderly populations. In 1990, life expectancy differences between the sexes was 6.9 years at birth and 4.5 years at 65 years (Table 12-1).

It is predicted that in future years more people will live longer. Therefore, health professions will be challenged to make these added years healthy and productive ones.

Profile of an Aging America

The older population in America has been increasing steadily in proportion and numbers. Since 1900, the total population of persons 65 years and older has tripled (4.1% in 1900 to 12.5% in 1989; 3.1 million in 1900 to 31 million in 1989). This increase in numbers is due to the rise in longevity as well as to the high birth rate prior to 1920. A dramatic decline in the

TABLE 12-1.   *Projected Life Expectancy at Birth and Age 65 by Sex: 1990–2050*

| | At Birth | | At Age 65 | |
Year	Male	Female	Male	Female
1990	72.1	79	15	19.5
2000	73.5	80.4	15.7	20.4
2010	74.4	81.3	16.2	21.1
2020	74.9	81.8	16.6	21.5
2030	75.4	82.3	17	21.9
2040	75.9	82.8	17.3	22.3
2050	76.4	83.3	17.7	22.7

(Spencer G, U.S. Bureau of the Census. Projections of the Population of the United States, by Age, Sex, and Race: 1988 to 2080. Current Population Reports Series P-25, No. 1018, January 1989.)

birth rate after the tremendous growth in fertility between 1946 and 1964, the baby boom generation, has resulted in an ever-increasing proportion of older persons. The median age of the population has increased from 27.9 in 1970 to 33 in 1990. It will rise to 37 years by 2000 and to 44 years by 2030. The baby boom generation will begin to reach age 65 by 2010. U.S. Census Bureau projections indicate that by 2030 there will be a higher proportion of older persons over 65 years (23%) than younger persons under 18 years (18%) in the population. In 1989 there were 31 million Americans over age 65; presently, one in eight persons is over 65 years (Fig. 12-1). Those 85 and older constitute one of the fastest growing segments of the population. By the turn of the century, half of the older population will be age 75 and older. This will place greater demands for care upon the health care system.

In retirement years, older persons become financially dependent upon Social Security benefits in combination with asset income and earnings, pensions, and savings. Social Security is the major source of income for older families and individuals. Although there is a growing perception that the elderly are well off financially, they are economically vulnerable because of inflation and an increased threat to loss of independence and health. Economic status varies considerably within the older age group, with some older people holding substantial resources other than cash. However, approximately one fifth (19%) of the older population was either below or barely above the poverty level in 1989. (The 1989 poverty level was defined as $7501 for an older couple or $5947 for a single person.) Older consumers spent proportionately more of their incomes on housing, food, and health care than their younger counterparts.

Health Status of an Aging America

Although most older persons consider themselves to be in good health, many of them suffer from at least one chronic illness (Fig. 12-2). Acute conditions occur with less frequency, while chronic illnesses become more common. Progression of the disease process threatens independence and quality of

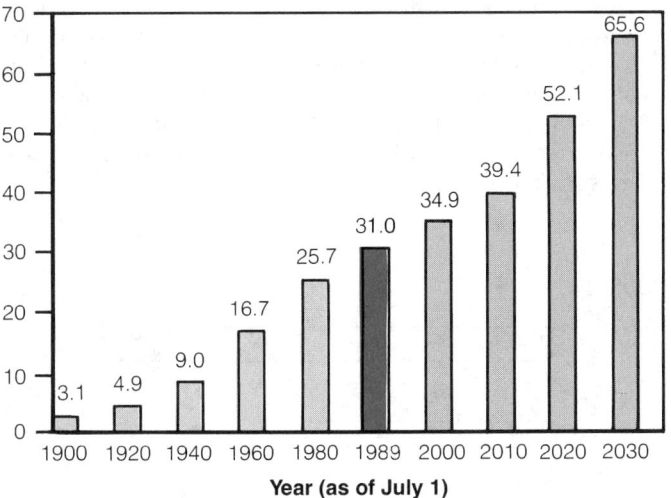

Figure 12-1. Increase in 65+ population (in millions: 1900–2030). Figures through 1989 are actual figures. Those after 1989 are projected. Note that increments in years on horizontal scale are uneven. (Based on data from U.S. Bureau of the Census.)

life by impeding ability to perform personal care and everyday tasks. Heart disease followed by cancer and stroke accounts for more than 75% of elderly deaths (Fig. 12-3; Table 12-2). Health care utilization is greatest among the oldest persons.

Psychosocial Aspects of Aging

Successful psychologic aging is reflected in the older person's ability to adapt to physical, social, and emotional losses and achieve contentment, serenity, and life satisfactions. Because changes in life patterns are inevitable over a lifetime, the person must show resiliency and coping skills when confronting stresses and change. The nurse can encourage participation in decision making, optimal independence, social activities, and involvement in productive, fulfilling activities. Flexibility, humor, and curiosity all contribute to the older person's social and psychologic adjustment. A positive self-image enhances risk taking and participation in new, untested roles.

The study of the psychosocial development of older adults has been an area of interest and research for gerontologists. Researchers are attempting to understand the complex process of successful aging. Psychologic adjustment is believed to be related to successful completion of developmental tasks as identified by Erikson, Havighurst, and others.

The societal position of the elderly is determined by culture. Certain roles are assigned to the older person. Although attitudes toward old people differ in ethnic subcultures of America, a subtle theme of ageism predominates. *Ageism* is a prejudice against a distinct group of people who are defined by age boundaries. *Stereotypes,* simplified and often untrue beliefs, reinforce society's negative image of the aged person. Elderly people make up an extremely heterogeneous group, yet negative stereotypes are attributed to all of them.

It is believed that this prejudice is based upon fear of aging and the inability for many to confront their own aging process. Retirement and perceived nonproductivity are also responsible for negative feelings. The younger working person may see the older person as one who is not contributing to society and is draining economic resources. This negative image is so common in American society that the elderly themselves often believe it. Stereotypes call for certain behaviors, and the elderly may adopt these expected roles. Thus, negative stereotypes are reinforced.

Health professionals may be instrumental in perpetuating a negative image. Nurses who care for sick old people see many problems that they may generalize to the entire elderly community. Only by understanding the aging process and respecting each person as an individual can the myths of aging be dispelled. If aged persons are treated with dignity and encouraged to make decisions and maintain autonomy, the quality of their lives should improve.

Developmental Theories

Erikson developed the concept of eight stages of man, each stage representing crucial turning points in the life span stretching from birth to death. He delineated the major developmental task of old age as ego integrity versus despair.

NUMBER PER 1,000 PERSONS

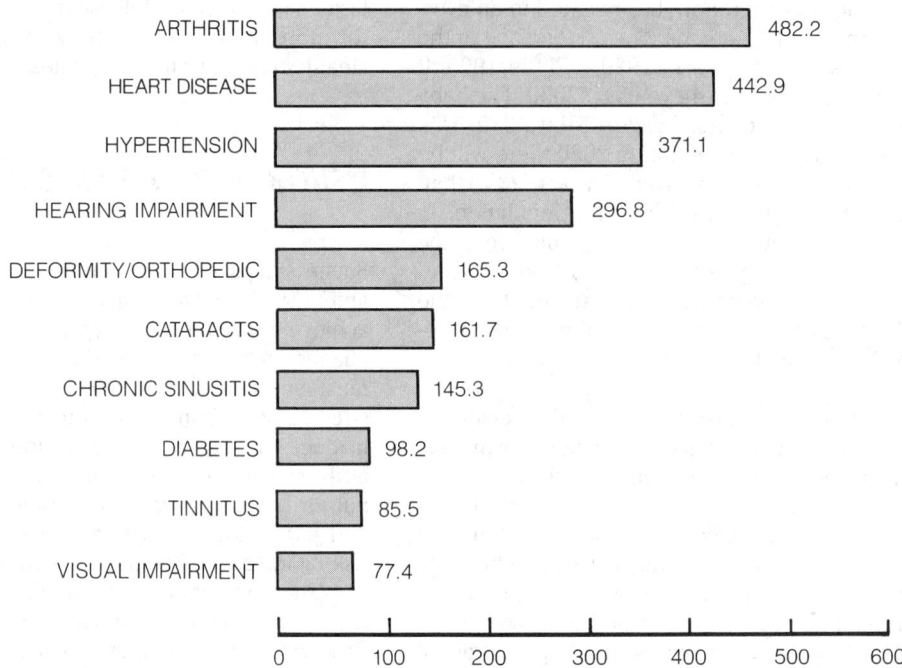

Figure 12–2. The top ten chronic conditions for persons 65+: 1987. (National Center for Health Statistics, Health Interview Survey, 1987.)

Ego integrity suggests an acceptance of one's life-style and a belief that choices made were the best that could be made at a particular time. One is still in control of one's life, a life of dignity. *Despair,* the opposite of ego integrity, implies that the older person feels dissatisfied and disappointed with his life. If given another chance, the person would live life differently.

Havighurst lists developmental tasks that occur during a lifetime. A person who completes the tasks successfully will feel contentment. These tasks of aging persons include adjusting to decreases of physical strength and health, retirement, reduced income, and death of a spouse; establishing affiliation with one's age group; adapting to social roles in a flexible way; and establishing satisfactory physical living arrangements.

Combining these concepts, the major developmental tasks are to: (1) maintain feelings of self-worth; (2) resolve old conflicts; (3) adjust to loss of power roles; (4) adjust to the deaths of significant others; (5) adapt to environmental changes; and (6) maintain an optimal level of wellness.

Sociologic Theories of Aging

Aged persons are influenced in their behavior and life-style by society. Gerontologists have proposed the following theories of aging to understand and predict the successful adjustments of elderly people.

The *disengagement theory* suggests that by withdrawing from society at the same time that society is withdrawing its support from his age-group, the elderly person achieves high morale and life satisfaction. This theory has been refuted by research findings showing that engaged, active persons achieve higher life satisfaction than disengaged, more passive people.

The *activity theory* proposes that life satisfaction in normal aging involves maintaining the active life-style of middle age. This theory reflects the majority thinking of middle-class America. It assumes that the older person will find satisfying replacements for activities.

RATE PER 100,000

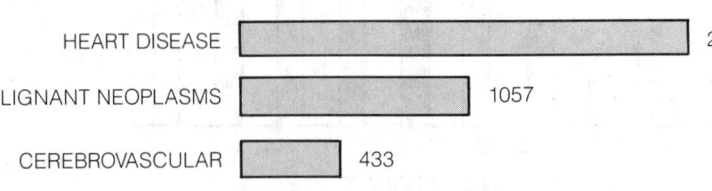

Figure 12–3. The top causes of death among older persons: 1986 and 1987. (National Center for Health Statistics, Annual Summary of Births, Marriages, Divorces, and Deaths: United States, 1987.)

TABLE 12-2. *Death Rates for Ten Leading Causes of Death Among Older People, by Age: 1986–1987*
(*Rates per 100,000 Population in Age-Group*)

Cause of Death	65 Plus	65 to 74	75 to 84	85 Plus
All causes	5070	2764	6266	15,406
Diseases of the heart	2085	1020	2556	7122
Malignant neoplasms	1058	846	1283	1632
Cerebrovascular diseases	433	153	563	1734
Chronic obstructive pulmonary disease	217	146	306	363
Pneumonia and influenza	206	57	235	1029
Diabetes	94	60	122	207
Accidents	87	50	103	259
Atherosclerosis	74	16	76	425
Nephritis, nephrotic syndrome, nephrosis	64	28	80	231
Septicemia	53	25	66	187
All other causes	701	362	876	2217

(*National Center for Health Statistics. Annual Summary of Births, Marriages, Divorces and Deaths: United States, 1987. Monthly Vital Statistics Report, Vol 36, No. 13, July 29, 1988, and unpublished data.*)

The *continuity theory* proposes that successful adjustment to old age rests with the ability of the person to continue life patterns across a lifetime. A person who adjusted well in earlier life will continue to do so in later life.

Cognitive Aspects of Aging

Intelligence

Stereotypes suggest that older people have slow thinking processes, forgetfulness, confusion, and senility. Many people erroneously believe that it is difficult, if not impossible, to introduce new learning to an older adult.

Intelligence tests measure the ability to accomplish intellectual tasks such as forming concepts, solving problems, acquiring information, and reasoning. When intelligence test scores from people of all ages are compared (cross-sectional testing), test scores for older adults show a progressive decline beginning in mid-life. Because older persons are slower in their responses and need more time to react, their scores may not reflect their actual ability. The presence of disease, predisease conditions, and stress may also negatively affect intellectual functioning.

Research studies, as well as demonstrations of creativity by older adults, show that creativity is found in all persons regardless of age. Creative performance in older adults is best manifested within a society that will provide stimulating opportunities and reward risk taking.

Learning and Memory

Many older persons continue to learn and participate in varied educational experiences. However, the ability to learn and re-

member efficiently may be negatively affected by the aging process. Mnemonics, a learned skill, has been shown to improve the effectiveness of memory. The process by which older adults learn is facilitated when the nurse

- uses visual, auditory, and other sensory cues
- encourages the learners to wear their glasses and hearing aids
- provides glare-free lighting
- provides a quiet, nondistracting environment
- sets short-term goals with input from the learning group
- keeps teaching periods short
- paces learning tasks according to the stamina of the group
- encourages verbal participation from the learners
- reinforces successful learning in a positive manner

Memory is a complex process that involves acquiring, storing, and retrieving or remembering information. Sensory losses, distractions, and disinterest interfere with acquiring information; age-related changes in the brain affect storing and remembering. Many older people are able to recall episodes from many years past with clarity and precision. These selected events were probably of great importance and recalled to memory many times.

Normal Physiologic Aging

Primary (Normal) Versus Secondary (Pathologic) Aging

Primary aging refers to those changes caused by the normal aging process and is characterized by being universal, progressive, decremental (gradually less), and intrinsic (from within the person). Universality is the major criterion that distinguishes primary (normal) aging from secondary (pathologic) aging. Using the above characteristics, the nurse can distinguish normal from pathologic aging. Secondary (pathologic) changes of aging result from influences outside the person. Illness and disease, air pollution, and sunlight are examples of pathologic factors that may hasten the aging process. The nurse can be instrumental in eliminating or retarding secondary aging processes.

Age-Related Cellular, Tissue, and Organ Changes

Cellular and extracellular changes of old age cause a deterioration of physical appearance and function. There are measurable changes in body shape and composition. The aged person is shorter, with diminished shoulder width and increased chest circumference, abdomen, and pelvic diameter. Skin appears thin and wrinkled. Lean body mass diminishes and fat mass increases. The fat (adipose tissue) is redistributed from subcutaneous tissues and the extremities to the trunk.

Maintenance of homeostasis within the body becomes increasingly difficult. Organ systems cannot function at full efficiency because of cellular and tissue deficits. Cells become less able to replace themselves. They accumulate a pigment known as lipofuscin. Within the connective tissue, a degradation of elastin and collagen causes tissues to become stiffer and less elastic.

Age-Related Body System Changes: Health Promotion

The well-being of an aged person depends on physical, mental, social, and environmental factors. A total assessment includes an evaluation of all major body systems, social and mental status, and the ability of the person to function independently despite the presence of a chronic illness. (See Table 12-3 for nursing assessment and interventions for age-related changes in body systems.)

Cardiovascular Changes

Heart disease is the leading cause of death for all age-groups including the aged (see Fig. 12-3). The mortality rate from cardiovascular disease also increases with age. The normal structural changes of aging that occur in the heart and vascular system reduce their ability to function efficiently. The heart valves become thicker and stiffer, and the heart and arteries lose their elasticity. Calcium and fat deposits accumulate within arterial walls. Veins become increasingly tortuous.

Although function is maintained under normal circumstances, the cardiovascular system has less reserve, and its ability to respond to stress is reduced. The resting cardiac output (heart rate [HR] × stroke volume) decreases about 1% annually after age 20. Under conditions of stress, both the maximum cardiac output and the maximum heart rate diminish

annually. The relationship between maximum heart rate and age is:

$$\text{maximum HR} = 220 - \text{age in years}$$

In the past it was believed that systolic hypertension was part of the normal aging process. Hypertension, although not universal, is a common problem in the older population. Therefore, it is a disease process. Hypertension has been shown to be a prominent risk factor at all ages for cardiovascular disease. Older people with a blood pressure reading of less than 140/90 mm Hg live longer than persons with higher readings. A diagnosis of hypertension should be made only after it has been confirmed by at least two subsequent readings. In older persons, the diagnosis of hypertension is classified as: (1) isolated systolic hypertension in which the systolic reading exceeds 160 mm Hg, with the diastolic measurement normal or near-normal; (2) essential hypertension in which the diastolic pressure is greater than or equal to 90 regardless of the systolic pressure; and (3) secondary hypertension or hypertension that can be attributed to an underlying cause. Reduction of systolic blood pressure to the range of 140 to 160 is the goal of treatment.

Cardiovascular dysfunction may become exaggerated and interfere with normal activities of daily living. The normal changes of aging, genetic factors, and life-style may contribute to major disorders that include cardiac dysrhythmias, congestive heart failure, coronary artery disease, arteriosclerosis, hypertension, intermittent claudication, myocardial infarction, peripheral vascular disease, and cerebrovascular accidents.

Promotion of Cardiovascular Health

Refer to Table 12-3 for details. The nurse must be alert for adverse responses to medication, including orthostatic hypotension, electrolyte imbalance, confusion, and depression. To avoid faintness and possible falls caused by orthostatic hypotension, the older person should be counseled to rise slowly from a lying, to a sitting, to a standing position.

Respiratory Changes

Age-related changes in the respiratory system that affect lung capacity and function include the following: an increase in the anteroposterior chest diameter, osteoporotic collapse of vertebrae resulting in kyphosis, calcification of the costal cartilages and reduced mobility of the ribs, diminished efficiency of the respiratory muscles, an increase in lung rigidity, and a decrease in alveolar surface area. The increased rigidity or loss of elastic recoil results in an increase in residual lung volume and a decrease in vital capacity. Gas exchange and diffusing capacity are diminished.

Decreased cough efficiency, reduced ciliary activity, and increased dead space make the older person more vulnerable to respiratory infections. Although older adults have sufficient respiratory function to carry out activities of daily living, there is a diminished ventilatory capacity. This results in a decreased tolerance for sustained exercise and a need for short rest periods during prolonged activity.

Promotion of Respiratory Health

Refer to Table 12-3 for details.

TABLE 12–3. *Body Systems: Normal Changes in Functional Status With Nursing Recommendations*

Normal Changes	Subjective and Objective Assessment	Health Promotion/ Nursing Recommendations
CARDIOVASCULAR SYSTEM Decreased cardiac output diminished ability to respond to stress; heart rate and stroke volume do not increase with maximum demand; slower heart recovery rate; increased blood pressure	Complaints of fatigue with increased activity Increased heart rate recovery time Normal BP = < 140/90 mm Hg	Exercise regularly; pace activities; avoid smoking; eat a low-fat, low-salt diet; participate in stress-reduction activities; check blood pressure regularly, medication compliance, weight control
RESPIRATORY SYSTEM Increase in residual lung volume; decrease in vital capacity; decreased gas exchange and diffusing capacity; decreased cough efficiency	Fatigue and breathlessness with sustained activity; impaired healing of tissues due to decreased oxygenation; difficulty coughing up secretions	Exercise regularly; avoid smoking; take adequate fluids to liquefy secretions; receive yearly influenza immunization; avoid exposure to upper respiratory tract infections
INTEGUMENTARY SYSTEM Decreased protection against trauma and solar exposure; decreased protection against temperature extremes; diminished secretion of natural oils and perspiration	Skin appears thin and wrinkled; complaints of injuries, bruises, and sunburn; complaints of intolerance to heat; bone structure is prominent; dry skin	Avoid solar exposure (clothing, sunscreen, stay indoors); dress appropriately for temperature; maintain a safe indoor temperature; bathe only 1–2 times weekly; lubricate skin
REPRODUCTIVE SYSTEM *Female:* Vaginal narrowing and decreased elasticity; decreased vaginal secretions *Male:* Decreased size of penis and testes *Male and female:* Slower sexual response	*Female:* Painful intercourse; vaginal bleeding following intercourse; vaginal itching and irritation; delayed orgasm *Male:* Delayed erection and achievement of orgasm	May require a prescription for estrogen/ antibiotic cream; use a lubricant with intercourse; seek health/sexual counseling if needed
GENITOURINARY SYSTEM *Male and female:* Bladder capacity decreased; delayed sensation to void *Male:* Benign prostatic hyperplasia *Female:* Relaxed perineal muscles	Urinary retention Difficulty voiding Urgency, frequency, and incontinence of urine	Seek regular medical supervision; have ready access to toilet; wear easily manipulated clothing; drink adequate fluids; maintain an acid urine; avoid bladder irritants (*e.g.*, caffeinated beverages, alcohol, sweeteners); practice pelvic floor muscle exercises; maintain perineal hygiene: skin clean and dry, absorbent pads, water-resistant skin cream, clean underclothes
GASTROINTESTINAL SYSTEM Decreased salivation; difficulty swallowing food; delayed esophageal and gastric emptying; reduced gastrointestinal motility	Complaints of dry mouth; complaints of fullness, heartburn, and indigestion; complaints of constipation, flatulence, and abdominal discomfort	Use ice chips, mouthwash; brush, floss, and massage gums daily; receive regular dental care; eat small, frequent meals; sit up and avoid heavy activity after eating; limit antacids; eat a high-fiber, low-fat diet; limit laxatives; toilet regularly; drink adequate fluids
MUSCULOSKELETAL SYSTEM Loss of bone density; loss of muscle strength and size; degenerated joint cartilage	Height loss; prone to fractures; kyphosis; complaints of back pain; loss of strength, flexibilty, and endurance; complaints of joint pain	Exercise regularly; eat a high-calcium diet; limit phoshorus intake; estrogens and calcium supplements may be prescribed

(continued)

TABLE 12-3.   *(Continued)*

Normal Changes	Subjective and Objective Assessment	Health Promotion/ Nursing Recommendations
NERVOUS SYSTEM		
Reduced speed in nerve conduction; increased confusion with physical illness and loss of environmental cues; reduced cerebral circulation (becomes faint, loses balance)	Slower to respond and react; learning takes longer; becomes confused with hospital admission; complaints of faintness; frequent falls	Pace teaching; with hospitalization, encourage visitors; enhance sensory stimulation; with sudden confusion, look for cause; encourage slow rising from a resting position; encourage use of a cane
SPECIAL SENSES		
Vision: Diminished ability to focus on close objects; inability to tolerate glare; difficulty adjusting to changes of light intensity; decreased ability to distinguish colors	Holds objects far away from face; complaints of glare; complaints of poor night vision; confuses colors	Wear eyeglasses; use sunglasses outdoors; avoid abrupt changes from dark to light; use adequate indoor lighting with area lights and night lights; use large-print books; use magnifier for reading; avoid night driving; use contrasting colors for color coding; avoid glare of shiny surfaces and direct sunlight
Hearing: Decreased ability to hear high-frequency sounds	Gives inappropriate responses; asks people to repeat words; strains forward to hear	Recommend a hearing examination; reduce background noise; face person; enunciate clearly; speak with a low-pitched voice; use nonverbal cues
Taste and smell: Decreased ability to taste and smell	Uses excessive sugar and salt	Encourage use of lemon, spices, herbs

Integumentary Changes

The functions of the skin include protection, temperature regulation, sensation, and excretion. With advanced age, intrinsic and extrinsic changes occur that affect function and appearance. The epidermis and dermis become thinner. There are fewer elastic fibers; collagen becomes stiffer. Subcutaneous fat diminishes, particularly in the extremities. A loss of capillaries in the skin results in a decreased blood supply. These changes result in a loss of resiliency and a wrinkling and sagging of the skin. Hair pigmentation decreases and hair becomes gray. The skin becomes drier and susceptible to irritations because of decreased activities of the sebaceous and sweat glands. Spotty and irregular distribution of pigment occurs, particularly in areas that have been exposed previously to sunlight. These changes in the integument reduce tolerance to extremes of temperature and solar exposure. Skin dryness makes the person susceptible to itching and skin irritation.

Promotion of Integumentary Health

See Table 12-3.

Reproductive Changes

Ovarian production of estrogen and progesterone ceases with menopause. Changes occurring in the female reproductive system include thinning of the vaginal wall with a narrowing in size and a loss of elasticity; decreased vaginal secretions resulting in vaginal dryness, itching, and decreased acidity; in-volution (atrophy) of the uterus and ovaries; and decreased pubococcygeal muscle tone resulting in a relaxed vagina and perineum. These changes contribute to vaginal bleeding and painful intercourse. In the male, the penis and testes decrease in size and levels of androgens diminish.

Promotion of Sexual Health

See Table 12-3. Sexual desire and activity declines, but does not disappear; nor should sexual activity be discouraged. Society often views older people erroneously as asexual. The nurse can explain that sexual activity varies individually but is related to sexual behavior at an earlier age.

Genitourinary Changes

The genitourinary system continues to function adequately although there is a loss in kidney mass due primarily to loss of nephrons. Changes in kidney function include decreased filtration rate, diminished tubular function with less efficiency in resorbing and concentrating the urine, and a slower restoration of acid–base balance in response to stress. The ureters, bladder, and urethra lose muscle tone. The bladder capacity decreases, and the older person may be unable to empty the bladder completely. Retention of urine increases the risk of infections. Frequency, urgency, and incontinence are also common problems. The female may have decreased perineal muscle tone resulting in stress incontinence and urgency. Benign prostatic hyperplasia is a common finding in older males. Enlargement of the prostate causes chronic urinary retention, frequency, and incontinence.

Health Promotion of the Genitourinary System

See Table 12-3. Adequate consumption of fluids is necessary to prevent bladder infections and to maintain fluid balance. Problems of urinary incontinence and frequency can be reduced if the older person

- has ready access to toilet facilities
- voids regularly
- practices pelvic floor exercises

These exercises, first described by Kegel, can be highly useful in reducing the symptoms of stress and urge incontinence. Because achievement of better muscle control takes at least several weeks to accomplish, the nurse must encourage the patient to persist regularly with the exercises. The patient is first taught to identify the pubococcygeus muscle. The patient can be taught that this muscle is the same one that is used to hold back flatus or to voluntarily stop the flow of urine. The abdomen, thighs, and buttocks are to remain relaxed. The pubococcygeus muscle is first tightened and then relaxed, each for ten seconds. These two exercises should be alternated and repeated ten times, four to six times a day. The patient can practice them when standing, sitting, or lying down. The nurse can suggest incorporating the exercises into other daily activities because they are undetectable by others. These exercises are also recommended for men with dribbling incontinence related to prostatic surgery. The nurse instructs the patient to tighten the rectal sphincter until the penis retracts. Frequent repetition produces the desired muscle tone.

Constipation can be a major factor contributing to urinary incontinence. The nurse encourages the patient to eat a high-fiber diet, drink adequate fluids, and increase mobility to promote regular bowel function.

Gastrointestinal Changes

The function of the gastrointestinal tract usually remains adequate throughout life. Nevertheless, many older people suffer from discomforts that are related to the sluggish passage of food or delayed motility. About half of the population have lost all their teeth by the age of 60. Although it is not an inevitable consequence of aging, periodontal disease leading to tooth decay and loss of teeth is common. Salivary flow diminishes, and the older person may experience a dry mouth.

Peristalsis in the esophagus is less efficient in the elderly. In addition, the gastroesophageal sphincter may fail to relax, leading to delayed esophageal emptying and dilation of the lower esophagus. Major complaints often center upon feelings of fullness, heartburn, and indigestion. Gastric motility may decrease, resulting in delayed emptying of stomach contents. Diminished secretion of acid and pepsin reduces the absorption of iron, calcium, and vitamin B_{12}.

Absorption of nutrients in the small intestine appears to be diminished but is adequate throughout life. The function of the liver, gallbladder, and pancreas is generally maintained, although there exist some inefficiencies in absorption and tolerance to fat. The incidence of gallstones and common bile duct stones increases progressively with advanced years. Abdominal surgery in persons 60 years and older is performed more frequently for gallbladder disease than for any other disorder.

Constipation is high on the list of complaints of aged persons. When mild, the symptoms involve abdominal discomfort and flatulence. However, more serious consequences include fecal impaction that contributes to diarrhea around the impaction, fecal incontinence, and obstruction. Predisposing factors for constipation include lack of dietary bulk, prolonged use of laxatives, ignoring the urge to defecate, side effects of medications, emotional problems, inactivity, insufficient fluid intake, and excessive dietary fat.

Health Promotion for the Gastrointestinal System

Refer to Table 12-3 for details.

Nutritional Health

The social, psychologic, and physiologic functions of eating influence the dietary habits of the aged person. Decreased physical activity and a slower metabolic rate reduce the number of calories needed by the older adult to maintain an ideal weight. Although fewer calories are desirable, the older person continues to require the same nutrients. Apathy, immobility, depression, loneliness, poverty, inadequate knowledge, lack of oral health, and lack of taste discrimination contribute to undesirable eating habits. Wasted, empty calories are found primarily in foods that are high in fats, cholesterol, and sugar.

The nurse encourages a diet low in sodium and saturated fats, with an emphasis on vegetables, fruits, and fish. The older adult requires a variety of foods to maintain balanced nutrition. Fats, particularly saturated fats, should be avoided because they are high in calories and contribute to atherosclerosis. No more than 20% to 25% of dietary calories should be consumed by fat intake. Sodium reduction has been shown to reduce levels of hypertension.

Protein intake should remain the same in later adulthood. Dried beans and peas are inexpensive and excellent sources of protein and fiber. Red meats, whole milk, eggs, and cheese should be replaced by chicken, fish, and low-fat dairy products to provide adequate protein and reduce fat intake.

Carbohydrates, a major source of energy, should supply the diet with 55% to 60% of the daily calories. Simple sugars should be avoided and complex carbohydrates encouraged. Potatoes, whole grains, brown rice, and fruit provide the person with minerals, vitamins, and fiber; eating these foods should be encouraged, even though they are more difficult to prepare and chew. Commercially processed foods often have a low nutritional and high-sodium content in proportion to the number of calories they contain.

Insufficient consumption of water leads to dehydration and constipation, common problems for aged persons. Adequate fluid balance is necessary to maintain peristalsis and urinary function. Eight glasses of water are recommended daily unless contraindicated by a medical condition.

Musculoskeletal Changes

A gradual, progressive decrease in bone mass begins before the age of 40 years. Excessive loss of bone density results in osteoporosis (see Chap. 61). This condition is most apparent in postmenopausal women and is associated with inactivity, inadequate calcium intake, and loss of estrogens. Its incidence is higher in northern Europeans and other whites and in the Chinese and Japanese. The danger of fracture due to bone resorption is especially high for the dorsal vertebra, humerus, radius, femur, and tibia. A loss of height occurs in later life. This shortening of the trunk is due to osteoporotic changes of the spine, kyphosis, and flexion of the hips and knees. These changes negatively affect mobility, balance, and internal organ function.

The muscles diminish in size and lose strength, flexibility, and endurance with decreased activity and advanced age. Back pain is common. Beginning in middle age, the cartilage of joints shows progressive deterioration. Degenerative joint disease is found in all older persons past the age of 70.

Health Promotion for Bones

See Table 12-3. Osteoporosis is a common problem in older women. The demineralization that occurs in osteoporosis is accelerated by the loss of estrogens, inactivity, and a low-calcium, high-phosphorus diet. The nurse can recommend:

- a high calcium intake (dairy products and dark green vegetables are excellent sources, as are soups and broths made with a soup bone and cooked with added vinegar to leach calcium from the bone)
- a low-phosphorus diet (a calcium:phosphorus ratio of 1:1 is ideal; red meats, cola drinks, and processed foods that are low in calcium and high in phosphorus are avoided)
- exercise (the pull of muscle insertions on the long bones strengthens them and retards calcium resorption)

Calcium supplements, vitamin D, fluoride, and estrogens are often prescribed for the person who is at high risk or who already has osteoporosis. Although osteoporosis cannot be reversed, the disease process can be prevented or arrested.

Health Promotion for Musculoskeletal Function

A program of regular exercise can be lifelong or begun in later life. The axiom "use it or lose it" is very relevant when considering the physical capacity of aged persons. A major barrier to exercise is societal attitude in general and a negative attitude of older people themselves. Old persons are considered to be frail and physically unfit. Many elderly believe that they need less exercise, that vigorous exercise has many risks, and that they have limited ability to perform exercise. They tend to stay indoors and often lack motivation to initiate or maintain physical activity. The nurse plays an important role by encouraging and challenging older adults to participate in a regular exercise program. Research shows that exercise enhances cardiovascular and respiratory efficiency. Regular exercise increases the strength and efficiency of heart contractions and improves oxygen uptake by cardiac and skeletal muscles. Exercise has been shown to reduce fatigue, increase energy, and reduce cardiovascular risk factors. Muscle endurance, strength, and flexibility, all outcomes of regular exercise, help to promote independence and psychologic well-being. Aerobic exercises are the foundation of programs of cardiovascular endurance conditioning. A physical examination by a physician is necessary prior to initiating an exercise program. The program is based on current health status and past activity with a warm-up and cool-down period before and after exercise. The older person should perform exercises in moderation and use short rests to avoid undue fatigue. Swimming and brisk walking are often recommended because they are managed easily and usually enjoyed by the older person.

Nervous System Changes

The structure and function of the nervous system change with advanced age. A progressive loss in brain mass is attributed to a loss of nerve cells that are not replaced. There is a reduction in the synthesis and metabolism of the major neurotransmitters. Nerve impulses are conducted more slowly, and therefore older persons take a longer time to respond and react. The autonomic nervous system performs less efficiently, and postural hypotension may occur. Cerebral ischemia with related lightheadedness may interfere with mobility and safety. Homeostasis is more difficult to maintain, but in the absence of pathologic changes the older person functions adequately and retains cognitive and intellectual abilities. Accompanying the nervous system changes is a reduction of cerebral blood flow. However, under ordinary circumstances, oxygen and glucose supply are adequate.

Health Promotion for the Nervous System

See Table 12-3. A slowed reaction time places the older person at risk for accidents and injury. Loss of consciousness or a feeling of faintness may occur when the person rises too rapidly from a lying or sitting position. The nurse advises the person to allow a longer time to respond to a stimulus and to move more deliberately. Mental function is threatened by physical or emotional stresses. A sudden onset of confusion may be the first symptom of an infection or change in physical condition (pneumonia, urinary tract infection, drug interactions, dehydration, and others).

Sensory Changes

The sensory organs of sight, hearing, taste, touch, and smell allow each person to communicate with the environment. Messages received from one's surroundings keep the person oriented, interested, and contented. Sensory losses with old age affect all sensory organs and threaten this interaction. This is a time of life when the older person is less able to perform physically and is sedentary. Sensory losses can be devastating to the person who cannot see to read or watch television, who cannot hear conversation well enough to communicate, or who cannot discriminate taste well enough to enjoy food.

Sensory Losses Versus Sensory Deprivation

The diminishing function of the sensory organs results in sensory losses that can often be helped by assistive devices such as glasses or hearing aids. Sensory deprivation is the absence of stimuli in the environment, or the inability to interpret existing stimuli (perhaps as a result of a sensory loss). This deprivation can lead to boredom, confusion, irritability, disorientation, and anxiety. Meaningful sensory stimulation offered to the older person is often helpful in correcting this problem. Although all old people have sensory losses and as a result are at high risk for sensory deprivation, all do not suffer from sensory deprivation. One sense can substitute for another in observing and interpreting stimuli. The nurse can enhance sensory stimulation in the environment with colors, pictures, textures, tastes, smells, sounds, and so forth. The stimuli are most meaningful when they are interpreted to the older person and if they are changed often. The confused person responds well to touching and to familiar songs.

Vision

As new cells form on the outside surface of the lens, the older central cells accumulate and become yellow, rigid, dense and cloudy. Thus, only the outer portion of the lens is elastic enough to change shape (accommodate) and focus at near and far distances. As the loss of lens flexibility progresses, the near point of focus gets farther away. This condition, presbyopia, usually begins in the 40s. Reading glasses for magnifying objects are required. In addition, the yellowing, cloudy lens causes light to scatter and therefore makes the older person susceptible to glare. The ability to discern blue from green declines. The pupil dilates slowly and less completely because of increased stiffness of the muscles of the iris. The older person takes longer to adjust when going to and from dark and light environments/settings and needs brighter light for close vision. Although pathologic visual conditions are not a part of normal aging, there is an increased incidence of eye disease in older persons. Those most commonly occurring include cataracts, glaucoma, senile macular degeneration, and diabetic retinopathy.

Hearing

Loss of the ability to hear high-frequency tones occurs in mid-life. This age-related hearing loss, called presbycusis, is attributed to irreversible inner ear changes. Older persons are often unable to follow conversation because tones of high-frequency consonants (letters *f, s, th; ch, sh; b, t, p*) all sound alike. Unable to communicate, they feel isolated and withdraw from social events. When hearing difficulties are suspected, the ears and hearing should be assessed. Wax buildup or other correctable problems may be responsible for major hearing difficulties. A properly prescribed and fitted hearing aid may be useful in reducing hearing deficits.

Hearing loss may cause the older person to respond inappropriately, to misunderstand conversation, and to avoid social interaction. This behavior may be interpreted as confused or "senile."

Touching

The sense of touch offers the most intimate of messages and is easiest to interpret. When other senses diminish, touching can reduce feelings of isolation and give a sense of well-being. Although sensory receptors dull with age, they do not disappear. Older persons are eager to touch and be touched. Reduced mobility and fewer social contacts often diminish such opportunities. The nurse can enhance touching contact by offering back rubs, foot massages, and hand pats. Companion animals are becoming popular in nursing homes with residents and staff. These pets offer many older persons love, warmth, and touching stimulation that vastly improve their quality of life.

Taste and Smell

The four basic tastes are sweet, sour, salty, and bitter. Of these, sweet tastes are particularly dulled in older persons. This ex-

plains why they tend to use sweets excessively. Blunted taste may contribute to the preference for salty, highly seasoned foods. Herbs, onions, garlic, and lemon are encouraged as substitutes for salt to flavor food.

Health Promotion for Sensory Disorders

Refer to Table 12-3 for details.

Mental Health Disorders

Mental health disorders are a major problem and threat to older adults and their families. It is estimated that as many as 15% to 20% of the elderly have a mental or psychiatric disorder that is significant enough to require evaluation and treatment. The major portion of these disorders can be helped with medications and psychologic counseling. (For mental status assessment see Chart 12-1.)

Mental health disorders are loosely classified as functional and organic. The functional disorders occur throughout life. Associated with them are no known pathologic changes in tissues or conditions of the brain. Symptoms often benefit from medication and psychotherapeutic counseling. Organic mental disorders are accompanied by abnormal mental and behavioral functioning and pathologic changes of the brain. Although the exact incidence of this disease is not known, it is estimated that 4% to 6% of persons over 65 and 20% of persons over 80 years have an organic mental disorder.

Age-Related Stress and Coping Mechanisms

Coping patterns and the ability to adapt to stress are developed over the course of a lifetime. In youth or mid-life, the recovery from grief or stress can be hastened by options that are made available by an active life-style. For example, a young widow may find happiness in a new marriage. A job loss can be replaced by a new opportunity. In later life, the coping mechanisms are consistent with earlier life. A flexible, well-functioning individual will probably continue as such. However, the same options may not be available to aged persons. Losses may accumulate within a short period of time and be overwhelming. The older person will have fewer choices and diminished resources to deal with stress. Common stressors of old age include normal aging changes that impair physical function, activities, and appearance; disabilities of chronic illness; social and environmental losses of income, roles, and activities; and the death of significant others.

Functional Disorders

Depression is the most common emotional disorder of old age. Signs of depression include sadness, low energy, diminished memory and concentration, sleeping disturbances, appetite disturbances, withdrawal, irritability, alcohol abuse, expressed feelings of helplessness and hopelessness, apathy, impaired attention span, and expression of suicidal wishes.

Chart 12–1
Mental Status Assessment

The mental status assessment is a narrative report that should incorporate observations from each of the following parameters with detailed descriptions where indicated.

Parameters That Require Simple Descriptions

Appearance
- neat
- untidy
- appropriate
- clean
- healthy
- apparent age

Attitude
- cooperative
- hostile
- suspicious
- fearful
- evasive

Activity Level
- restless
- slow
- appropriate
- threatening
- repetitive movement

Mood
- appropriate
- apathetic
- sad (crying)
- happy
- mood swing

Communication
- nonverbal (facial expression, body language)
- speech patterns
- word selection
- articulation of words
- flight of ideas
- rambling

Attention and Concentration
- distracted
- normal

Parameters That Require Active Interventional Testing

Orientation
- time (today's date)
- place (where are we?)
- person (what is your name?)

Remote Memory
- birthdate
- stories from childhood
- current U.S. president
- last U.S. president

Recent Memory
- what did you eat for lunch? (verify)

Retention Memory
- repeat the names of 3 items that you list (immediately and in 5 minutes)

General Intellect
- name 5 cities
- simple math ($3 \times 8 = ?$)

Attention and Concentration
- serial 7s ($100 - 7$ and continue)

Abstract Reasoning
- ask to explain "Don't cry over spilt milk" or "A stitch in time."

Judgment
- ask "What would you do with a stamped, addressed letter that you find on the sidewalk?"
- or "Why are criminals put into prison?"

Many depressed persons are often mistaken as confused or suffering from an organic mental disease. Depression is often treatable and reversible through use of antidepressant medications and counseling. Suicide attempts are a potential risk when depression exists. The suicide rate in older white males is higher than in any other age-group.

Other functional disorders include hypochondriasis and paranoia. *Hypochondriasis* is characterized by a preoccupation with body functioning and an overconcern with physical complaints. Loneliness, isolation, and sensory impairments may make the older person feel threatened and mistrustful of others, resulting in *paranoia*.

Organic Mental Disorders

Organic mental syndrome is a general term that refers to a group of mental symptoms found in specific organic mental disorders. The five major symptoms are loss of memory, loss of intellect, loss of judgment, impairment of orientation, and lability of affect (excessive or shallow emotional response). Two of the most commonly occurring syndromes characterized by some or all of these are delirium (usually acute) and dementia (usually chronic).

Delirium

Delirium, often called acute confusional state, begins with confusion and progresses to disorientation and change in the level of consciousness. The onset is rapid and often occurs in a hospital or other unfamiliar setting.

The brain dysfunction is secondary to any number of causes, including physical illness, drug or alcohol toxicity, dehydration, fecal impaction, malnutrition, infection, head trauma, lack of environmental cues, and sensory deprivation or overload. Older adults are particularly vulnerable to symptoms of delirium because of their marginal biologic reserve and the high number of medications that they take.

The major manifestation in delirium is disturbance in the level of consciousness, which may range from stupor to excessive activity. Thinking is disorganized, and the attention span is characteristically fleeting. Hallucinations, delusions, fear, anxiety, and paranoia may be evident. The course of this syndrome is short, usually lasting less than a week and no more than a month. If the symptoms go unrecognized and the underlying cause is not treated, permanent irreversible brain damage or death will follow.

Therapeutic interventions vary, depending on the reason for the symptoms. Because drug interactions and toxicity are often implicated, it is desirable that unessential medications be withdrawn. To increase orientation and provide familiar environmental cues, the nurse encourages family members or friends to touch and talk to the patient. With a newly admitted patient, the nurse questions the family carefully about his prior cognitive state. Ongoing mental status assessments using this baseline will be helpful in evaluating responses to treatment.

Dementia

Dementia (senile dementia, chronic brain syndrome) is a syndrome rather than a distinct disease entity. It is usually progressive and irreversible and is not a part of normal aging. It is characterized by a general decline in cognitive abilities that may include losses of memory, abstract reasoning ability, judgment, and impulse control as well as changes in personality. It is usually subtle in onset and often progresses slowly until the symptoms are very obvious and profoundly devastating. The three most common dementias are Alzheimer's disease, multi-infarct dementia, and a mixed Alzheimer's disease and multi-infarct dementia.

Alzheimer's Disease

Alzheimer's disease is sometimes called primary degenerative dementia or senile dementia of the Alzheimer's type (SDAT). It accounts for at least 50% of all the dementias suffered by the elderly. It is a progressive, irreversible, degenerative neurologic disease of unknown origin that begins insidiously. Alzheimer's disease is not found exclusively in old people, although old age is considered a risk factor. Its onset may be in the 40s and 50s, and it is then called *presenile dementia*. However, both presenile and senile dementias are considered to be clinically and pathologically identical. Epidemiologic studies suggest that as many as 50% of the cases are familial. Some researchers speculate that its cause is genetic.

A recent study of a defined community population showed that prevalence rates of Alzheimer's disease are strongly associated with age. In the 65 to 74 age-group, 3% were found to have Alzheimer's disease, compared with 18.7% of those 75 to 84 years old and 47.2% of those older than 85 years. This figure for the 85 and older group far exceeds previous estimates and suggests that Alzheimer's disease will have a considerable impact on our aging population. The life expectancy following the diagnosis varies from 6 to 20 years.

Pathophysiology

The etiology of the disease is unknown, but there are specific neuropathologic and biochemical changes. These include neurofibrillary tangles (a tangled mass of nonfunctioning neurons) and senile or neuritic plaques (deposits of amyloid protein and altered cell structures on the interneuronal junctions). This neuronal damage occurs primarily in the cerebral cortex and results in decreased brain size. These changes are found to a lesser extent in normal brain tissue of older adults. Cells principally affected by this disease are the ones that use the neurotransmitter acetylcholine. Biochemically, the enzyme active in producing acetylcholine is decreased. Acetylcholine is specifically involved in memory processing.

Diagnostic Evaluation

There has been a major research effort to develop a specific diagnostic test for Alzheimer's disease. Presently, many of the investigations focus on the amyloid protein. Although it was first believed that this protein was found only in the brain, researchers are trying to isolate the amyloid precursor protein elsewhere in the body. At present, the diagnosis is one of exclusion and is confirmed by autopsy. Clinical symptoms, electroencephalography (EEG), computed tomography (CT scan), magnetic resonance imaging (MRI), and examination of the blood and cerebrospinal fluid (CSF) may all refute or support a diagnosis. The EEG changes are not always specific. The CT and MRI scans are very useful for excluding hematoma, brain tumor, stroke, and atrophy but are not reliable in making a definitive diagnosis of Alzheimer's disease. Infections and chemical abnormalities can be excluded by examination of the blood and cerebrospinal fluid, but findings are not specific enough to make the diagnosis.

Clinical Manifestations

Symptoms of Alzheimer's disease are highly variable. Early in the disease, forgetfulness and subtle memory loss occur, but the patient has adequate cognitive function to hide the loss. Social skills and behavior patterns remain intact; problems are difficult to detect on casual observation. With further progression of the disease there is an inability to conceal the deficits. Forgetfulness is manifested in many daily actions. The patient may lose his way in a familiar environment. He may repeat the same stories because he forgets that he told them. Trying to reason with the patient and reality orientation by caretakers increase the patient's anxiety without increasing function, because this is also forgotten.

Conversation becomes difficult because the patient forgets what he was about to say or may not be able to remember words. The ability to formulate concepts and think abstractly disappears. The patient can interpret a proverb only in concrete terms. The patient is often unable to appreciate the consequences of his actions and will therefore exhibit impulsive behavior. For example, on a hot day he may decide to wade in the city fountain fully clothed. He will have difficulty with everyday activities such as operating simple appliances and handling money.

Personality changes are usually negative. The patient may become depressed, suspicious, paranoid, hostile, and even combative. Progression of the disease intensifies the symptoms. Speaking skills deteriorate to nonsense syllables; agitation and physical activity increase. A voracious appetite often develops because of the high activity level. The patient may wander at night for hours. Eventually he will need help in all areas of personal care, including toileting and eating; dysphagia occurs and incontinence develops. The terminal stage may last for months. The patient is usually immobile and requires total care. Occasionally the patient may recognize family or caretakers. Death occurs as a result of a complicating condition such as pneumonia, malnutrition, or dehydration.

Nursing Interventions

Interventions by the nurse are aimed at maintaining optimal cognitive function, promoting physical safety, reducing anxiety and agitation, improving communication, promoting independence in self-care activities, providing for the patient's needs for socialization and intimacy, maintaining adequate nutrition, managing sleep pattern disturbances, and supporting and educating family caregivers.

Support of Cognitive Function

As the patient's cognitive ability declines, the nurse provides a calm, predictable environment that helps him interpret his surroundings and activities. Environmental stimuli are limited and a regular routine is followed. The nurse's quiet, pleasant manner, clear and simple explanations, and the use of memory aids and cues help to minimize confusion and disorientation and give the patient a sense of security. A prominently displayed clock and calendar will enhance orientation to time. Color-coding his doorway will help the patient who has difficulty locating his room.

Promoting Physical Safety

A safe environment will allow the patient to move about as freely as possible and relieve the family of constant worry about his safety. To prevent falls and other accidents, all obvious hazards are removed. Night lights, a call light, and a low bed with half bed rails are used at bedtime. The nurse or family monitors the patient's intake of medications and food. Smoking is allowed only with supervision. A hazard-free environment allows the patient maximum independence and a sense of autonomy. Because of a short attention span and forgetfulness, wandering behavior can often be directed with gentle persuasion and distraction. Restraints are avoided because they may increase agitation. Doors leading from the house must be secured. Outside the home all activities must be supervised to protect the patient. The patient should wear an identification bracelet or neck chain in case he becomes separated from the caregiver.

Reducing Anxiety and Agitation

Despite profound cognitive losses, there will be times when the patient is aware of his rapidly diminishing abilities. He will need constant emotional support that will reinforce a positive self-image. When losses of skills occur, the nurse then adjusts goals to the patient's declining ability.

The nurse appreciates the importance of recreation and encourages the patient to enjoy simple activities. Realistic goals that provide satisfaction are appropriate. Hobbies and activities (walking, exercise, socializing) can improve the quality of life.

The nurse actively tries to keep the environment simple, familiar, and noise-free. Excitement and confusion can be upsetting and may precipitate a combative, agitated state known as a catastrophic reaction (overreaction to excessive stimulation). During such a reaction, the patient responds by screaming, crying, or becoming abusive (physical or verbal assault). This is his way of expressing his inability to deal with the environment. When this occurs, the nurse remains calm and unhurried. Measures such as listening to music, stroking, rocking, or distraction may quiet the patient. Frequently he forgets what triggered the reaction. Structuring activities is also helpful for this patient. Familiarity with his predicted responses to certain stressors helps the nurse avert similar situations.

Improving Communication

To promote the patient's interpretation of messages, the nurse remains unhurried and reduces noises and distractions. Clear, easy-to-understand sentences are used to convey messages because the meaning of words is frequently forgotten or there is difficulty with organizing and expressing a thought. Lists and simple written instructions can serve as reminders to the patient and are often helpful.

Sometimes the patient can point to an object or use nonverbal language to communicate. Tactile stimuli such as a hug or a hand pat are usually interpreted as signs of affection, concern, and security.

Promoting Independence in Self-Care Activities

Pathophysiologic changes in the cerebral cortex make it difficult for a patient with a self-care deficit to achieve physical independence. Efforts are directed toward helping him maintain independent functioning for as long as possible. One suggestion is to simplify daily activities by organizing them into short, achievable steps so that the patient can experience a sense of accomplishment. Frequently the occupational therapist is able to suggest ways to simplify tasks or recommend adaptive equipment. Direct patient supervision is sometimes necessary.

Maintaining personal dignity and autonomy is important for the patient with Alzheimer's disease. He is encouraged to make choices when appropriate and to participate in self-care activities as much as he can.

Providing for Socialization and Intimacy Needs

Socialization with old friends can be comforting. The nurse and family should encourage visits, letters, and phone calls. Visits should be brief and nonstressful; limiting visitors to one or two at a time is recommended.

The confused, lonely person may find stimulation, comfort, and contentment in the soft fur, melodious purr, or warm, wet tongue of a pet. The nonjudgmental friendliness of an animal can be helpful. Care of the pet by the patient can provide satisfying activity and an outlet for energy.

Alzheimer's disease does not eliminate the need for intimacy. The patient and his spouse may or may not continue to enjoy sexual activity. The nurse encourages the spouse to talk about any sexual concerns and suggests sexual counseling if necessary. Simple expressions of love, such as touching and holding, are often meaningful for this couple.

Inappropriate sexual behaviors seldom occur, but when they do they can cause extreme embarrassment to family members. For example, the patient may undress in a public place on a hot day or may masturbate publicly. The use of gentle distraction is recommended.

Promoting Adequate Nutrition

Mealtime can be a pleasant, social occasion, or it can become a time of upset and distress. Mealtime should be kept simple and calm without confrontations. The patient will prefer familiar foods that look appetizing and taste good. To avoid "playing," the nurse offers one dish at a time. Food is cut into small pieces to prevent choking. Liquids may be easier to swallow if they are converted to gelatin. Hot food and beverages are served warm; the nurse monitors the temperature to prevent burns.

When lack of coordination interferes with self-feeding, adaptive equipment is helpful. Some patients may do well eating with their fingers. If this is the case, an apron or a smock, rather than a bib, is used to protect clothing. As deficits progress, it may be necessary to feed the patient. Forgetfulness, disinterest, dental problems, incoordination, overstimulation, and choking can all provide barriers to good nutrition.

Promoting Balanced Activity and Rest

Many patients with Alzheimer's disease exhibit sleep disturbances and wandering behavior. These behaviors are most likely to occur when the patient is bored, restless, agitated, or disoriented, particularly in a new setting and frequently at night. The patient who wanders outside of the house is often unable to find his way home and is at risk for accident and injury. Family members and neighbors are frequently asked to search for the patient.

All Alzheimer's patients should wear some form of visible identification (bracelet or neck chain) at all times. Although the patient is allowed to walk around in a protected environment, his access to the outdoors should be blocked. If his sleep is disturbed or he is unable to go to sleep, music, warm milk, or a back rub may help him relax. During the day he should be given sufficient opportunity to participate in exercise activities, because a regular pattern of activity and rest will enhance nighttime sleep. Long periods of daytime sleeping are discouraged.

Support and Education of Family Caregivers

The emotional burden placed upon the family of a patient with Alzheimer's disease is enormous. The physical health of the patient is usually excellent, and the mental degeneration is gradual. Because the diagnosis is not specific, the family may cling to the hope that the diagnosis is incorrect and that the patient will improve if he tries harder. Aggression and hostility exhibited by the patient are often misunderstood by the caregiver or family, who feel unappreciated, frustrated, and angry. Feelings of guilt, nervousness, and worry contribute to caregiver fatigue, depression, and family dysfunction.

The multiple needs of family caregivers have been addressed by the Alzheimer's Association (formerly known as ADRDA). This national organization with more than 100 local chapters is a coalition of family members and professionals sharing the goals of family support and service, education, research, and advocacy. Family support groups, respite care, and adult day care are available through the Alzheimer's Association. Concerned volunteers are trained to provide structure to caregiver support groups. Through the use of respite care, a service commonly provided, the caregiver can get away from the home for short periods of time while someone else is tending to the patient's needs.

The nurse must be sensitive to the highly emotional issues that the family is confronting. Support and education of the caregivers are essential components of care. The family can contact the Alzheimer's Association or a comparable group to meet with others experiencing similar problems. (See Nursing Care Plan 12-1: Care of the Patient With Alzheimer's Disease.)

Multi-Infarct Dementia

Multi-infarct dementia (MID) is an organic mental disorder second only to Alzheimer's disease in incidence. About 15% of the cases of dementia are attributed to this disease. It is characterized by an uneven, downward decline in mental function. MID is sometimes confused with Alzheimer's disease, paranoia, or delirium because of its unpredictable clinical course. The diagnosis can sometimes be even more difficult because the patient may be suffering from both Alzheimer's disease and MID.

Cerebral damage occurs when blood supply to the brain is disrupted. Infarction, the death of brain tissue, occurs with striking rapidity. Multiple small cerebral infarctions, clinically manifested as small strokes, result in multi-infarct dementia. Instead of displaying the progressively downhill course of Alzheimer's disease, the progress of multi-infarct dementia is uneven. Every small infarct is followed by some recovery and a

(text continues on page 185)

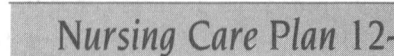

Nursing Care Plan 12-1

Care of the Patient With Alzheimer's Disease

Nursing Interventions	Rationale	Expected Outcomes

Nursing Diagnosis: Alterations in thought processes (altered cognition, perception, confusion, and disorientation) related to neuronal degeneration and progressive dementia

Goal: Maintenance of optimal cognitive functions

Nursing Interventions	Rationale	Expected Outcomes

1. Reduce environmental confusion.
  a. Approach patient in a pleasant, calm way.
  b. Be predictable in your manner and conversation.
  c. Keep the environment simple and pleasing.
  d. Maintain a regular daily schedule.
  e. Devise memory aids as needed (lists, reminding notes, labels on items, pictures, diagrams).
	1. Simple and limited stimuli will facilitate interpretation and reduce distortion of imput; predictable behavior is less threatening than nonpredictable behavior; memory aids will assist the patient to remember.	• Maintains optimal memory function.
		• Shows a reduction in confused behavior.
		• Demonstrates an appropriate response to tactile, visual, and auditory stimuli.
		• Verbalizes a sense of security and protection.

2. Increase environmental cues.
  a. Identify yourself when interacting with the patient.
  b. Address patient by name.
  c. Offer environmental cues for orientation to time, place, and person (pictures, photos, clock, calendar with crossed-off days, color-coded halls and doors).
  d. Provide hourglass timer if unable to tell time on clock.
  e. Interpret environmental stimulation as part of the conversation.
	2. Environmental cues will enhance orientation to time, place, and person by filling memory gaps and serving as reminders. As memory loss increases, it may be necessary to identify yourself at the beginning of every interaction with the patient.	• Demonstrates optimal orientation to time, place, and person.

Nursing Diagnosis: High risk for injury related to impulsive behavior, impaired judgment, lack of insight, and dysfunctional behaviors

Goal: Maintenance of physical safety

Nursing Interventions	Rationale	Expected Outcomes

1. Control the environment.
  a. Remove obvious hazards.
  b. Reduce injury potential from bedtime falls.
    (1) Use only half bedrails.
    (2) Keep bed in low position.
    (3) Use night lights.
    (4) Have accessible call light.
  c. Monitor medication regimen.
  d. Permit smoking only with supervision.
  e. Monitor food temperature.
  f. Supervise all activities outside of the home.
	1. A hazard-free environment will reduce the risk of injury and free the family from constant worry. Outside the home, everything is assumed to be a hazard.	• Complies with safety procedures
		• Moves freely and independently around the home.

2. Permit maximum independence and freedom.
  a. Allow freedom in the "safe" environment.
  b. Avoid use of restraints.
	a. This will give the patient a sense of autonomy.
	b. Restraints may increase agitation.
		• Verbalizes a sense of security and contentment.

(continued)

Nursing Care Plan 12-1 *(Continued)*

Care of the Patient With Alzheimer's Disease

Nursing Interventions	Rationale	Expected Outcomes
c. When wandering, distract rather than force.	c. Force will increase anxiety. Distraction is facilitated by immediate memory loss.	
d. Keep identification tag on patient.	d. A name and phone number will facilitate a safe return if the patient wanders away.	

Nursing Diagnosis: Anxiety related to cognitive losses and reduction in self-concept

Goal: Maintenance of an optimal level of psychologic functioning

Nursing Interventions	Rationale	Expected Outcomes

1. Reduce anxiety-provoking situations in daily routine.
  a. Keep reality orientation nonthreatening.
  b. Be patient with forgetfulness.
  c. Accept harmless eccentric behavior.
  d. Maintain a daily, regular routine.
  e. Keep stimuli simple.
  f. Distract rather than confront unacceptable behavior.
  g. When the patient demonstrates a negative attitude in interacting, leave patient and return in a short time.
  h. Avoid situations that have upset patient in the past.
  i. Reassure following a catastrophic reaction.
  j. Do not try to reason with the patient.
	a–c. Constant corrections will increase anxiety and may result in a highly agitated, angry, and combative state known as a catastrophic reaction.
	
	d–e. Simple, structured stimuli are easiest to interpret.
	f–g. Often forgets immediately and becomes involved in new activity.
	
	j. Unable to conduct abstract thinking.
		• Shows fewer episodes of catastrophic reactions, angry outbursts, and crying.
		• Demonstrates less restlessness, irritability, and agitation.
		• Verbalizes feelings of calmness and contentment.

2. Enhance the quality of life.
 	
  a. Offer multiple opportunities for fulfillment (music, pets, walks, exercise, old hobbies, simple chores).
  b. Provide comfort and security.
	2. Goals are minute-by-minute. The patient has the capacity to enjoy and experience happiness.	• Seeks out the companionship of others.
		• Participates in activities willingly.

3. Encourage positive feelings of self.
  a. Treat the patient as a person with feelings.
  b. Openly discuss his feelings of anxiety and offer encouragement.
  c. Praise appropriately.
  d. Do not infantilize (treat as a child) by using baby talk or child terms.
  e. When skills are lost, do not try to retrain.
	3. Acceptance will give support. This person is in the process of grieving over his profound losses; infantilization increases the anxiety; deterioration of the cognitive processes makes losses of skills inevitable.	• Shows a greater level of self-assurance in difficult situations.

(continued)

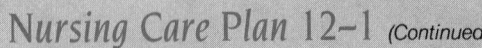

Nursing Care Plan 12-1 (Continued)

Care of the Patient With Alzheimer's Disease

Nursing Interventions	Rationale	Expected Outcomes

Nursing Diagnosis: Impaired verbal communication related to cognitive losses

Goal: Attainment of an optimal exchange of ideas between the patient and others

1. Implement strategies to promote the patient's interpretation of messages.
   a. Be calm, pleasant, and unhurried.
   b. Keep verbal messages short and simple.
   c. Avoid decision-making situations.
   d. Use nonverbal messages along with words.
   e. Be consistent in conversation.
   f. Avoid competing noises and distractions.
   g. Avoid complex issues.
   h. Write down simple instructions and lists.
   i. Observe patient's expression for signs that he understands.
   j. Talk to the patient even if he gives little response.

a-g. Simple, short messages are easiest to interpret.

h. Alternate methods for communication often are successful.
i. A good listener must be responsive to feedback.
j. The patient may not be indicating how much he understands of the conversation.

- Shows an improved ability to understand messages.
- Shows an improved ability to express himself verbally.
- Uses alternate methods of communication (writing, nonverbal).

2. Develop strategies to improve the patient's ability to express messages.

   a. Supply forgotten words when possible.
   b. Guess the message and confirm with the patient.
   c. Ignore mistakes.
   d. Allow adequate time for conversation.
   e. Encourage short, simple sentences.
   f. Ask yes/no questions.
   g. Provide alternative methods for communication (pointing, describing, pictures).
   h. Acknowledge the frustration that the patient is experiencing.

2. This will allow the patient to express his needs and feelings. Feelings of isolation are reduced.
   a-c. Active helpful listening can minimize frustrations when the patient needs help communicating his message.
   d-f. An unhurried attitude will enhance communication.

   g. Certain methods may be more successful than others.

   h. Acknowledging the patient's frustration communicates acceptance.

- Shows fewer frustrations when communicating.

Nursing Diagnosis: Self-care deficits related to confusion, cognitive losses, and dysfunctional behaviors

Goal: Maintenance of maximum independence in activities of daily living

1. Develop strategies to facilitate daily performance of activities.
   a. Provide adaptive devices.
   b. Maintain a regular daily schedule at a time convenient with the patient.
   c. Keep the environment simple and pleasant.

a-d. A regular schedule, adaptive equipment, and simple tasks will reduce confusion, enhance ability to care for self, and ensure safety.

- Performs activities of daily living at expected optimal level.

(continued)

Nursing Care Plan 12–1 *(Continued)*

Care of the Patient With Alzheimer's Disease

Nursing Interventions	Rationale	Expected Outcomes

d. Keep instructions simple and divide tasks into small parts.
e. Monitor function of body systems.
 	
2. Provide specific safeguards in bathing.
  a. Monitor bath water temperature.
 	
  b. Encourage use of safety devices (*e.g.,* handrails, rubber mats).
3. Allow patient autonomy and dignity while providing needed care.
  a. Encourage patient to make choices of selection (*e.g.,* clothing, foods, schedule).
  b. Provide adequate privacy.
4. Provide specific measures to encourage continency.
  a. Provide accessibility to the bathroom. If needed, color-code the door of bathroom.
  b. Use clothing that opens easily.
 	
  c. Maintain toileting schedule (every 2 hours and after meals).
  d. Encourage adequate fluids, fiber, and activity for regular bowel elimination.
  e. Recommend restricting fluids in evening hours.
	e. Supervision will promote optimal function and detect early problems.
	
	a. The patient is unreliable in adjusting bath temperature.
	b. Impulsive behavior increases a risk of accidents.
	3. Encouraging autonomy will enhance a sense of dignity and well-being.
	
	a. Visual stimuli can reinforce recognition.
	
	b. Facilitates continence when haste is necessary.
	c–d. Help to maintain normal elimination.
	
	e. Excessive fluids in the evening may interfere with the sleep–activity routine.
		• Demonstrates the ability to use adaptive equipment.
		• Uses safety measures to prevent injury.
		
		• Verbalizes an awareness of dignity and autonomy.

Nursing Diagnosis: Alterations in family processes related to care of a dysfunctional family member

Goal: Attainment of family adaptation and harmony

1. Initiate and enhance family knowledge of disease.
  a. Teach family about Alzheimer's disease.
  b. Encourage family members to read *The 36-Hour Day* and ask questions.
2. Acknowledge the emotional impact of the disease upon the family system.
  a. Elicit family reaction to patient's illness.
  b. Encourage family to talk about their worry, guilt, anger, and frustrations.
  c. Encourage use of stress-reduction techniques.
  d. Encourage family to share concerns and feelings with patient.
	1. If the family understands the disease, they will be better prepared to help the patient and adjust their style of living to his needs.
	
	2. This illness has profound effects upon the family. They will be frightened, frustrated, angry, and guilty and will feel helpless.
		The family will:
		• provide appropriate care and support to the patient
		
		• discuss feelings and frustrations with the nurse
		• seek appropriate help from community agencies
		• join a self-help group

(continued)

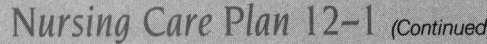

Nursing Care Plan 12–1 *(Continued)*

Care of the Patient With Alzheimer's Disease

Nursing Interventions	Rationale	Expected Outcomes
3. Initiate referrals to obtain community help.		
a. Assist family to contact community agencies to receive such support services as respite care, adult day care, visiting nurse services, and social work services.	a. Community services will provide respite care, suggestions for home management, financial advice, and nursing. These will help the family cope and manage this family crisis in the best possible way.	
b. Encourage the family to contact Alzheimer's Association and participate in a self-help group.	b. A support group will help the family better understand how others are dealing with similar problems.	

Nursing Diagnosis: Impaired social interaction related to cognitive impairment and dysfunctional behaviors

Goal: Enhancement of socialization and fulfillment of intimacy needs

Nursing Interventions	Rationale	Expected Outcomes
1. Encourage social encounters with family and friends. Encourage family and friends to:		• Participates in social events with family and friends.
a. Use touching to maintain contact with patient	a. Tactile stimulation is easiest to interpret.	• Increases touching behavior.
b. touch, hug, and demonstrate affection c. share feelings honestly and openly with patient	b–c. The patient continues to need love and affection.	• Verbalizes or demonstrates contentment when socializing and interacting with others.
d. react objectively to negative responses e. accept patient despite negative interactions	d–e. Positive interactions are best maintained if the family overlooks negative encounters.	
f. limit numbers of visitors to 2 or 3 at a time	f. Fewer visitors will help maintain simple stimuli and avoid a catastrophic reaction.	
g. provide a companion animal if possible and appropriate	g. Pets provide loving acceptance and opportunities for touching and are a catalyst to socialization.	
2. Provide opportunities for meeting intimacy needs and sexual expression: a. Encourage expressions of intimacy and tenderness with spouse. b. Encourage a sexual relationship with spouse if interests exist. c. Provide privacy if patient masturbates or exposes self.	2. Intimacy and sexual expression will provide a sense of contentment and fulfillment to the patient.	• Engages in sexual activity or intimate behavior with spouse. • Meets sexual needs privately in an acceptable manner.

Nursing Diagnosis: Alterations in nutrition related to confusion and imbalance of intake/activity

Goal: Maintenance of an optimal level of nutrition

Nursing Interventions	Rationale	Expected Outcomes
1. Monitor food intake and observe food habits. a. Note weight loss or gain. b. Encourage adequate fluid intake c. Provide regular mealtime schedule. 2. Maintain a favorable environment for eating.	1. Encouragement and reminders to eat will help this patient eat adequately and regularly.	• Eats a balanced diet and drinks needed fluids.

(continued)

Nursing Care Plan 12–1 (Continued)

Care of the Patient With Alzheimer's Disease

Nursing Interventions	Rationale	Expected Outcomes
a. Allow patient optimal independence.	a. Finger foods, adaptive equipment, and a large apron will facilitate independence if lack of coordination interferes with the patient's ability to use utensils.	• Demonstrates enjoyment and maximum independence at mealtime.
b. Maintain a calm, pleasant environment. c. Offer a menu choice. d. Offer familiar foods.	b–d. If mealtime is pleasant, with favorite and familiar foods, the patient will eat well with enjoyment.	
3. Promote regular mouth care. a. Encourage care of gums and teeth after meals. b. Encourage the patient's participation with care.	3. Healthy teeth and properly fitted dentures are important for maintaining nutritional health. A reminder may be necessary if patient forgets.	• Teeth and gums are brushed regularly.

Nursing Diagnosis: Sleep pattern disturbance related to anxiety, confusion, and activity/rest imbalance

Goal: Maintenance of a balance of sleep and activity

1. Reduce nighttime distractions. a. Indentify and reduce discomforts such as noise and anxiety. b. Avoid disturbing patient during the night for procedures or medications.	1. A nonstimulating environment will decrease confusion and minimize hyperactive behavior.	• Establishes rest and sleep patterns on a regular schedule. • Reduces wandering behaviors at night.
2. Take measures to increase safety a. Provide night lights. b. Block accessibilty to the outdoors. c. Distract, monitor, and confine patient to a safe area. d. Provide patient with identification bracelet.	2. These will enhance the patient's safety if he wanders at night.	• Verbalizes a feeling of safety and comfort at bedtime.
3. Enhance comfort if awake at night. a. Avoid the use of restraints. b. Provide comfort measures when awake at night (warm milk, bath, back rub, soft music, rocking, caressing pet).	3. A pleasant, nonrestrictive environment will enhance return to sleep, minimize anxiety, and increase the patient's sense of well-being.	
4. Design a balanced schedule of activity/sleep. a. Increase daytime wakefulness and encourage short rests rather than long naps. b. Encourage regular exercise and activity programs.	4. Daily activity and regular exercise reduce agitation and produce a calming effect.	• Establishes activity patterns on a regular schedule.

plateau until the next infarction occurs. Often the patient has a history of hypertension. The age of onset is between 50 and 70 years, and the condition occurs more frequently in men than in women.

Dizziness, headaches, and decreased mental and physical vigor are early signs of the disease. In more than half the cases, the disease appears acutely as sudden confusion. This is followed by gradual, spotty memory loss. The patient may hallucinate and display symptoms of delirium. Speech disturbances may be present. Early treatment of hypertension and vascular disease may prevent progression of the disease. In later stages, manifestations of the decline are similar to the signs discussed with Alzheimer's disease, and often they cannot be distinguished.

Medications and the Elderly

Elderly people use more medications than any other age-group, averaging more than 13 prescriptions and renewals a year. One of every four prescriptions is dispensed to a person over 65. Studies show that those persons who have symptoms of disease are the persons most likely to be taking medications. Medications have improved the health and well-being of older persons by alleviating symptoms of discomfort, treating chronic illnesses, and curing infectious processes. However, problems commonly occur because of drug interactions, multiple drug effects, multiple drug use (polypharmacy), and noncompliance. Those medications that are most frequently overprescribed and misprescribed are mind-affecting drugs (tranquilizers, sedatives, hypnotics, and antipsychotics), cardiovascular drugs, and gastrointestinal drugs.

In any medication regimen for the elderly, one must bear in mind that drugs are capable of altering the patient's nutritional status, which may already be compromised by a marginal diet and chronic disease and its treatment. Medications can depress the appetite, cause nausea and vomiting, irritate the stomach, cause constipation and diarrhea, and decrease absorption of nutrients. In addition, they can alter the electrolyte balance and carbohydrate and fat metabolism. A few examples of medications that are capable of altering the nutritional status are the antacids (produce thiamine deficiency), cathartics (diminish absorption), antibiotics and phenytoin (Dilantin) (reduce use of folic acid), and phenothiazines, estrogens, and steroid hormones (increase food intake and weight gain).

Physiologic Considerations

There is great variability in the absorption, distribution, metabolism, and excretion of medications in older patients (see Table 12-4 for altered drug responses in older people). In part, this is due to a reduced capacity of the liver and kidneys to metabolize and excrete the drugs and to lowered levels of circulatory and nervous system efficiency in coping with the effect of certain drugs. Many medications and their metabolites are excreted by the kidney.

However, in many older persons, both glomerular and tubular functions are reduced. In advanced old age there are decreases in body weight, total body water, lean body mass, and plasma albumin (protein) and an increase in body fat (see Table 12-5 for the effects of aging on pharmacologic response).

Nursing Implications

The nurse administering medications to older persons must be aware of the following:

- Those commonly used drugs that are removed from the body primarily by *renal excretion* remain in the body for a longer time. Drug dosages often must be reduced. Overdosage and drug toxicity at usual therapeutic dosages commonly occur.
- A decline in cardiac output may decrease the delivery rate to the target organ or storage tissue.

- The circulatory and central nervous systems of older persons are less able to cope with the effect of certain drugs even when blood levels are "normal."
- Medication dosages often must be reduced because overdosage and drug toxicity at usual therapeutic dosages may result.
- Paradoxical or unusual responses to drugs may be manifested in the form of toxic reactions and complications.
- As a result of a slowing *metabolism,* the drug levels may increase in the tissues and plasma, leading to prolonged drug action.
- Many elderly persons have multiple medical problems that require treatment with one or more medications. The possibility of interactions between drugs is further magnified if the older person is also taking one or more over-the-counter drugs.
- If for any reason the patient may be undependable about taking his medication, the nurse must be sure that the pill or capsule is actually swallowed and not retained between the cheeks and the gums or teeth.

Self-Administered Medications

In teaching self-administration of medication, the nurse throughout the teaching process can ask questions of the client and request return demonstrations to be sure learning has occurred. It is important to consider possible sensory and memory losses as well as decreased manual dexterity. To help the client manage his medications and improve patient compliance, the nurse can:

- explain the action, side effects, and dosage of each medication
- write out the drug schedule
- encourage the use of standard containers rather than safety lids
- destroy old, unused medications
- periodically review the medication schedule
- discourage the use of over-the-counter drugs without consulting a health professional
- encourage sips of water first, followed by several more swallows with the pill to help it go down more easily
- explain that capsules will dissolve better if the water is at room temperature rather than iced

HIV-Positive Infection and AIDS

Human immunodeficiency virus (HIV) culminating in the symptomatic acquired immune deficiency syndrome (AIDS) is transmitted from person to person by contact with body fluids, especially blood and semen. Considered to be asexual and removed from the IV drug abuse of their younger counterparts, the elderly are not expected to have the AIDS virus. Nonetheless, older persons have contracted AIDS. Homosexual behavior (particularly among males), IV drug use, and transfusion of blood products (particularly prior to the blood screening programs) have been shown to be modes of transmission for every age-group, including older adults. Diagnosis in older

TABLE 12-4. *Altered Drug Responses in Older People*

Age-Related Changes	Impact of Age-Related Change	Applicable Drugs
ABSORPTION		
Reduced gastric acid	Rate of drug absorption—possibly delayed	
Increased pH (less acid)	Extent of drug absorption—not affected	
Reduced GI motility		
Prolonged gastric emptying		
DISTRIBUTION		*Selected Highly Protein-Bound Drugs*
Decreased albumin sites	Serious alterations in drug binding to plasma proteins. (The unbound drug gives the pharmacologic response). Highly protein-bound drugs will have fewer binding sites, leading to increased effects and accelerated metabolism and excretion.	Oral anticoagulants (warfarin)
		Oral hypoglycemics (sulfonylureas)
		Barbiturates
		Calcium channel blockers
		Furosemide (Lasix)
		Nonsteroidal anti-inflammatory drugs
		Sulfonamides
		Quinidine
		Phenytoin (Dilantin)
Reduced cardiac output	Decreased perfusion of many bodily organs	
Impaired peripheral blood flow	Decreased perfusion	*Selected Fat-Soluble Drugs*
Increased percentage of body fat	Proportion of body fat increases with age and thus gives the body an increased ability to store fat-soluble drugs. This causes drug accumulation, prolonged storage, and delayed excretion.	Barbiturates
		Diazepam (Valium)
		Lidocaine
		Phenothiazines (antipsychotics)
Decreased lean body mass	Decreased body volume allows higher peak levels of drugs	Ethanol
		Morphine
METABOLISM		
Decreased cardiac output and decreased perfusion of the liver	Decreased metabolism and delay of breakdown of drugs resulting in prolonged duration of action, accumulation, and drug toxicity	All drugs metabolized by the liver
EXCRETION		*Selected Drugs With Prolonged Action*
Decreased renal blood flow	Decreased rates of elimination and increased duration of action	Aminoglycoside antibiotics
Loss of functioning nephrons		Cimetidine (Tagamet)
Decreased renal efficiency	Danger of accumulation and drug toxicity	Chlorpropamide (Diabinese)
		Digoxin
		Lithium
		Procainamide

adults may be delayed because the symptoms of AIDS are often similar to those of other, more common chronic illnesses. For instance, a dementia diagnosed as Alzheimer's disease may, in fact, be a manifestation of the AIDS virus.

Universal precautions established by the Centers for Disease Control (CDC) are usual practices within acute care settings, including those patients who are considered to be at risk for AIDS. Because the disease occurs in the older population in all environments, health care providers must practice uni-

versal precautions with all patients whether in a nursing home, the community, or the hospital. Proper hand washing before and after patient contact is effective and simple. Appropriate use of protective barriers includes gloves, protective clothing, and eyewear when there is danger of contact with blood and body fluids. Careful handling and disposal of needles are essential.

Problems dealing with this illness can be particularly difficult for older persons. They may find it painful to tell their

TABLE 12-5.   *The Effects of Aging on Pharmacologic Response*

Commonly Used Drugs	*Actions and Nursing Implications*
DIGITALIS GLYCOSIDES	Use with care. Reduced kidney and liver function and drug interactions increase danger of toxicity. Even small dosages can cause dysrhythmias and conduction disturbances. Toxicity and dysrhythmias are enhanced by the depletion of intracellular potassium. If taken with non-potassium-sparing diuretics, a high risk of digitalis toxicity exists. (Common signs of digitalis toxicity are fatigue, visual disturbances, muscle weakness, nausea, and anorexia.)
Digoxin	Excreted unchanged by kidney. Usual short half-life of 1½ days. With reduced kidney function, can accumulate. Increased action when taken with quinidine.
Digitoxin	Long-acting (half-life 7 days). Danger of accumulation and toxicity with small safety margin. Metabolized by liver so may be useful with kidney disease.
DIURETICS	Rapid effects may cause urge incontinence. May cause drug toxicities at usual therapeutic dosages (esp. digitalis and lithium). Dehydration, electrolyte disturbances (particularly hypokalemia), and impaired mental function may result.
Thiazides (Diuril, Hydrodiuril)	Thiazides may cause hyperglycemia, glucose intolerance, and symptoms of gout. May potentiate nondiuretic antihypertensive agents.
Furosemide (Lasix)	Potent non–potassium-sparing loop diuretic.
ANTIHYPERTENSIVES	Age-related impaired baroreceptor responses, decreased venous tone (varicose veins), and reduced cardiovascular and autonomic nervous system responses create a high potential for postural hypotension with usual dosages. May cause sexual impotence and depression.
RAUWOLFIA ALKALOIDS	Rauwolfia may induce mental depression.
ANTICOAGULANTS	
Heparin	An increased risk of bleeding occurs when heparin is used in combination with some nonsteroidal anti-inflammatory drugs
Warfarin (Coumadin)	Greater risk of bleeding with usual doses of warfarin in the elderly due to (1) greater inhibition of vitamin K synthesis at usual doses and (2) reduced protein binding and therefore increased amounts of circulating free drug. Highly interactive and may be potentiated by NSAIDs.
NARCOTIC ANALGESICS	Morphine, codeine, and meperidine hydrochloride (Demerol) are the drugs of choice. Enhanced effects are due to a higher pain threshold and greater sensitivity. Lower dosages are often sufficient. Withold prescribed opiates if the respiratory rate is lower than 14.
ANALGESICS	
Aspirin	See NSAIDs. Take with 6 oz. of water with upper body upright. Tinnitus occurs quickly with large doses. Inhibits platelet clumping: increases risk of bleeding after trauma or with surgery.
Acetaminophen (Tylenol)	Effective for mild pain. Overdosing can occur with liver and kidney insufficiency.
NONSTEROIDAL ANTI-INFLAMMATORY DRUGS	
Fenoprofen, ibuprofen, naproxen, Indocin, Clinoril, phenylbutazone, etc.	Highly protein-bound. Can potentiate oral hypoglycemics and warfarin (Coumadin); therefore, use cautiously in combination. Gastrointestinal irritation. Should not be given to anyone with active ulcer disease, liver disease, or kidney disease. Act as analgesics at lower dosages and as anti-inflammatory drugs at higher doses. Aspirin interferes with analgesia of other NSAIDs.
ANTIBIOTICS	Can cause superinfections and metabolic and neurologic toxicities. Dietary blue cheese replaces intestinal flora. May be newly allergic: monitor closely for anaphylactic shock, angioneurotic edema, and exfoliative dermatitis. Sodium- and potassium-containing penicillins may cause electrolyte imbalance.
SEDATIVES, HYPNOTICS, ANTIANXIETY DRUGS	Can lead to confusion, delusion, hallucinations, falls, habituation, agitation, and altered behavior. Give in smaller doses.

(continued)

TABLE 12-5.   *(Continued)*

Commonly Used Drugs	Actions and Nursing Implications
Barbiturates	Barbiturates should not be used in older persons. They cause paradoxical reactions, respiratory depression, agitation, and psychoses.
Benzodiazepine hypnotics (Dalmane, Halcion) Benzodiazepine antianxiety agents (Librium, Valium, Xanax, Ativan, Serax, etc.)	Sensitivity is heightened and adverse reactions are increased. These drugs remain in the body longer because of slower liver metabolism, reduced renal excretion, and increased tissue uptake. Smaller doses are usually sufficient. Tolerance can develop.
ANTIPSYCHOTIC DRUGS Phenothiazides (Mellaril, Thorazine, Prolixin, Compazine) Butyrophenones (Haldol)	Increased sensitivity to the effects of these drugs and slow excretion place elderly persons at a high risk for serious adverse effects such as parkinsonism and tardive dyskinesia. Because of the significant potential for toxicity, these drugs should be given cautiously and only to those persons exhibiting severe symptoms of agitation and psychosis.
TRICYCLIC ANTIDEPRESSANTS Elavil, Sinequan, Tofranil	May cause paradoxical effects and cause further depression. Take 1–2 weeks for therapeutic effect. Danger of drug overdose; use small doses. Contraindicated in patients with narrow-angle glaucoma.
MONAMINE OXIDASE INHIBITORS Marplan, Nardil, Parnate	Multiple adverse reactions in the central, autonomic, and cardiovascular systems preclude the use of these drugs in persons over 60 years of age or in debilitated patients.
LAXATIVES	May increase bowel motility and prevent absorption of other medications. Stool softeners and "bulk" laxatives must be accompanied by large quantities of water or they can cause impactions or large-bowel obstructions.

adult children or grandchildren about their diagnosis. Lack of a strong support network, reduced finances, and the presence of other chronic physical problems may all contribute to physical and emotional vulnerability. The nurse must be sensitive to the many issues that the older person and family are confronting. Along with providing physical and emotional caregiving, the nurse will teach the patient how to protect others from infection.

The Older Person in the Community

Ninety-five percent of the elderly live in the community; 75% own their homes. In 1989, 30% were living alone (80% women). In the 65 and older age-group, half as many women as men were married and living with their spouses (40% of women, 74% of men). Half of the women over age 65 (49%), but only 14% of the men, were widowed. This difference in marital status is due to several factors: women have a longer life expectancy than men, women tend to marry older men, and women remain widowed while men often remarry.

Family

Planning for care and understanding the psychosocial aspects of the older person must be accomplished within the context

of the family. When dependency needs occur, the spouse assumes the role of primary caregiver. In the absence of the surviving spouse, an adult child usually assumes caregiver responsibilities and eventually may need help in providing care and support. A widely held myth within American society is that adult children and their aged parents are socially alienated. Furthermore, many believe that adult children abandon their parents when health and other dependency problems arise. Extensive research refutes these beliefs. The family is an important source of support for older persons. Eighty-one percent of the elderly have living children. Of those living alone, three-fourths have at least one child living within 30 minutes of their home, and 64% see at least one adult child weekly.

Social attitudes and cultural values that prescribe an "etiquette of filial behavior" have been formulated. These rules and social expectations dictate that adult children should provide services and financial support, and assume the burden of care for their aged parents. Children of the aged are aware of these expectations and are profoundly influenced by their implications. Most people want to do the "right" thing and conform to the norms society has placed upon human behavior. Regardless of the amount of responsibility and love the adult child exhibits toward the dependent aged parents, strains will develop if care continues over a period of time. Research exploring the relationship between aged parents and their adult children shows that with poor health of the parent, the quality of the parent–child relationship declines. Under certain circumstances of high risk, strains in intergenerational relationships can result in elder abuse. *Elder abuse* is an active or passive act or behavior that is harmful to the elderly person. Such behavior includes physical violence, personal neglect, mental anguish, financial exploitation, violation of rights, denial of health care, and self-inflicted abuse. Before elder abuse occurs, when strains are evident, the nurse takes preventive action. Interdisciplinary team members can be enlisted to help the caregiver develop self-awareness, increased insight, and understanding of the aging process. At the same time, community resources may be useful for both the aged person and the caregiver. Independence of the elderly person should be encouraged and supported.

The Home Environment

Safety and Comfort

Accidents rank seventh as a cause of death for older people. *Falls*, the major cause of accidents in the elderly, are not often fatal but threaten health and the quality of life. Normal and pathologic consequences of aging that contribute to increased falls include visual changes, such as loss of depth perception, susceptibility to glare, loss of visual acuity, and difficulty in light accommodation; neurologic changes, including loss of balance, loss of position sense, and delayed reaction time; cardiovascular changes resulting in cerebral hypoxia and postural hypotension; cognitive changes, including confusion, loss of judgment, and impulsive behavior; and musculoskeletal changes, including altered posture and decreased muscle strength. Many medications, drug interactions, and alcohol use precipitate falls by causing drowsiness, incoordination, and postural hypotension.

There are life-style and environmental changes that the nurse can encourage the older adult and his family to adopt. Adequate lighting with minimal glare and shadow calls for small area lamps, indirect lighting, sheer curtains to diffuse direct sunlight, dull rather than shiny surfaces, and night lights. Sharply contrasting colors can be used to mark the edges of stairs. Grab bars by the tub and toilet are useful. Canes are excellent deterrents to falls, particularly outdoors where many hazards exist. Loose clothing, improperly fitting shoes, scatter rugs, small objects, and pets create hazards and increase the risk of accidents. A person will function best in familiar settings if furniture and objects remain unchanged. When the older person enters a new environment, he should be watched carefully, assisted often, and urged to use a cane because the potential for accidents is greater in unfamiliar spaces.

Personal Space

The older person needs a place of his own, a very special location that can offer him security, comfort, and privacy. This important "charted territory" can be a house, a room, or part of a room. It will contain treasures and mementos from a lifetime. The nurse can help the older person to maintain his own space. If he is moved, he will adjust more easily if he can establish a new area of privacy. Clutter is understandable if the space is small and the items are many. These articles can be touched, thought about, and enjoyed regularly to enhance the quality of life.

Chronic Illness and Common Disturbances of Well-Being

Urinary Incontinence

The older person often does not report this very common problem unless specifically asked about it. It can be acute and develop during an illness, or it can develop chronically over a period of years. Using the acronym DRIP, transient causes can be attributed to delirium, dehydration (D), restricted mobility (R), inflammation, infection, impaction (I), and pharmaceuticals or polyuria (P). Established incontinence may be due to neurologic or structural pathologies. Often these can be helped or corrected with nonsurgical interventions such as Kegel exercises or environmental manipulation (see Health Promotion of the Genitourinary System in Table 12-3). Certainly the patient with this problem should be urged to seek help from appropriate health personnel.

Fatigue

There is a well-circulated myth that older people should "take it easy" and avoid vigorous activity. Many of the elderly, therefore, may expect to feel tired and adopt an inactive role. Activity, however, is a desired state in older adults. Normal fatigue following strenuous or sustained exercise is expected with the aging process. A short rest usually restores vigor.

General chronic fatigue is not normal and may be a consequence of oversedation. Fatigue may be an indicator of depression or a symptom of physical illness such as anemia or heart disease.

Headaches

Most headaches are caused by incorrect posture and muscle strain around the head and neck. Heat, ice, massage, and exercise are used to relieve the symptoms. Serious organic disease such as brain tumor or hematoma may be the underlying cause and needs to be excluded. The patient should be encouraged to seek medical advice if headaches persist.

Back Pain

The common complaint of back pain can accompany a number of chronic problems requiring medical attention. Back pain may be a sign of osteoporosis; accompanying vertebral fractures may press on the spinal nerves, causing severe pain that radiates to the legs (sciatica). Other, less common causes of back pain include metastatic cancer and infection. Muscle spasms responsible for much of the discomfort can be relieved by heat, ice, and rest. When acute back pain subsides, recurrence can be prevented by initiating a low back muscle exercise program.

Sleep Disturbances

Drowsiness is often due to boredom, habit, depression, or organic disease. Sleep patterns change with advanced age. Stages 3 and 4 of the sleep cycle are the stages of deepest sleep when arousal is most difficult. These levels of deepest sleep occur with less frequency in later life. Many brief arousals are predominant in the sleep of older persons. This increased wakefulness, although brief, may create an impression of sleeplessness or insomnia. Daytime napping and inactivity contribute to reduced sleep at night. Arthritis, muscle aches, nocturia, and sleep apnea may cause interruption in sleep (see Chap. 16).

A positive and reassuring attitude is necessary when the nurse counsels older adults about sleep. Daytime physical activity is encouraged. Quiet activity and reading are fine alternatives if sleep does not come. Symptoms are dealt with individually and sedatives discouraged. Some people find a warm bath and a glass of milk at bedtime helpful.

Heartburn and Indigestion

Heartburn and indigestion occur as a result of a reflux of stomach acid into the esophagus. Common causes include overeating, an incompetent lower esophageal sphincter, hiatal hernia, side effects of medications, and organic disease.

The nurse can advise the older person to chew his food carefully, eat small meals, avoid heavy spices, and sit rather than recline after eating. Medical evaluation is necessary if symptoms persist.

Dyspnea

A normal decline in pulmonary function may be responsible for shortness of breath following physical exertion. Obesity, anemia, smoking, lung disease, respiratory infections, and heart disease are all causes of increased breathlessness. Because fever may not occur with respiratory infection in the older adult, increased respirations followed by increased pulse rate often are the first observable signs of acute illness.

Foot Problems

The feet of the older person should be given particular attention. Diminished subcutaneous fat reduces the protective padding and makes the skin more vulnerable to injury. Diminished blood supply as a result of circulatory impairment puts the older person at high risk for foot infections and subsequent complications. Ingrown toenails, corns, and calluses all cause discomfort and may lead to infection and tissue necrosis. Toenails often are thick and difficult to cut.

If the older person is unable to care for his toenails, the nurse can provide nail care. The feet are soaked in warm water and dried thoroughly. Debris around the cuticles and between the toes is removed with a soft towel. The nails are cut straight across beyond the nail grooves. Sharp edges are blunted with an emery board. Lotion is applied regularly. For the diabetic, only a podiatrist or other specially trained person should cut the nails.

Community Programs and Services

Hospital and health services are used more by the elderly than other age-groups in the population. In 1987, the elderly (12% of the population) accounted for 36% of total personal health care expenditures. Chronic rather than acute disease is the major cause of illness. Over 80% of people 65 and older have at least one chronic condition; multiple conditions are common. With advancing age, disabilities resulting from these chronic illnesses create the need for help with basic activities of daily living. Twenty-two percent of the elderly are limited to a point where they can no longer carry on regular daily activities. Community programs provide help beyond the capabilities of informal supports. Such valuable services as health care at home or in an adult day care center, opportunities for socialization, transportation, and home-delivered meals often keep the older person in the community and postpone or possibly eliminate the need for a nursing home.

Medicare and Medicaid

Medicare is a federal social insurance program designed to provide health care for elderly persons who are entitled to Social Security benefits. It has two parts: part A is hospital insurance and part B is medical insurance. All entitled persons receive part A, which provides limited coverage for hospital and posthospital nursing home care and unlimited visits for home health care. Part B is a voluntary program that costs a small additional monthly premium. Part B pays for limited outpatient medical services and doctor's visits. Major items not covered by either part include nonskilled home nursing care, ongoing nursing home care, prescription drugs, eyeglasses, and dental care. Medicare pays about 45% of the health costs of older people.

Medicaid is a health assistance program financed by state funds and matching federal grants. This program varies from state to state and is available only to the poor. It is the major source of public funding that provides nursing home care for the poor elderly. This program covers all the basic medical services and often covers such items as medications, eyeglasses, and dental care. Eligibility requirements prevent many low-income people from receiving financial support for health care.

Home Care

The older adult usually prefers to live independently, even if he has difficulty getting around the home. This may be against the wishes of his adult children. If the older person is capable of accepting responsibility for the personal risk involved and other persons are not endangered, the adult children should not interfere with this decision. There are many community supports that help the older person maintain independence. Informal sources of help such as family, friends, the mail carrier, church members, and neighbors can all keep an informal watch. Area agencies on aging (AAAs) perform many community services, including telephone reassurance, friendly visitors, home repair services, and home-delivered meals. Homemaker and chore services can be obtained on an hourly rate through AAAs or the local community nursing services. If the person is financially unable to pay, these services are subsidized through local and state funds. Nursing care and rehabilitation services requiring the expertise of a registered nurse and appropriate health professionals are paid by Medicare.

There are other community support services available to help the older person outside of his home. Senior centers have social and health promotion activities; some provide a nutritious noontime meal. Adult day care facilities offer daily nursing care and social opportunities. Family members can carry on daily activities while the older person is at the day care center.

Ethical and Legal Issues

Loss of rights, victimization, and other grave consequences face the person who has made no plans for personal and property management in the event of disability or death. The advice and services of a competent attorney regarding financial and personal issues can preserve future autonomy and self-determination. The nurse as an advocate can encourage the older person to give advance directives for future decision making in the event of incapacitation.

Power of attorney is a legal agreement that authorizes a person who is designated by the older person to act in specific, outlined purposes on behalf of the signer. This is a form of voluntary guardianship; permission is freely granted when the older person is competent. Unless stated otherwise, this power of attorney is invalidated upon the incapacity of the signer. A *durable power of attorney* is a similar agreement that continues even if the older person is disabled or incapacitated. This power can include financial and/or personal decisions depending upon the desires of the older person.

A *trust* is another option that the competent older person can consider. With a trust, the person designates someone to manage his property, stipulates how and under what circumstances the property will be managed, and designates a beneficiary. If incompetency or disability occurs, management of the property will be according to the person's wishes.

If no advance arrangement has been made, and the older person seems unable to make decisions, anyone can petition the court for an incompetency hearing. If the court rules that the person is incompetent, the judge will appoint a *guardian*, a third party who is given powers by the court to assume responsibility for making financial and/or personal decisions for that person. There are two kinds of guardians—guardian of the person and guardian of the estate. Because such a court action strips the civil liberties and constitutional rights from the older person, there is potential for great harm. Safeguards include (1) the older person must be given notice, (2) he must be given an opportunity to be legally represented, and (3) medical testimony can be cross-examined. A less restrictive

form of guardianship called the *limited guardianship* transfers to the appointed guardian only those powers or duties that the older person cannot exercise. Although this alternative is not widely used, it remains an option.

In the event of severe illness with no reasonable expectation of recovery, the older person may not want to have his life extended by heroic measures. Those who want to avoid technologic interventions can give an advance directive regarding medical treatment through the use of a *living will.* This written document must be signed by the individual and have two witnesses. It should be given to the physician and incorporated into the medical record. Many states have enacted legislation to accept such a document. The nurse can help the person keep this document current and encourage discussion with the physician. The doctor must write and sign a no-code or do not resuscitate (DNR) order. Otherwise, resuscitative measures are taken if a medical emergency occurs.

The Older Adult in an Acute Care Setting: Altered Responses to Illness

Pain and Fever

Altered physical, emotional, and systemic reactions to disease are attributed to age-related changes in the older person. Useful and reliable physical indicators of illness in the young and middle-aged person cannot be relied upon for the diagnosis of potential life-threatening problems in the older adult. The response to pain in the older person may be altered because of reduced acuity of touch, decreased speed of response, and diminished processing of sensory data. Research has demonstrated the absence of chest pain in 81% of older adults experiencing a myocardial infarction. Hiatal hernia or upper gastrointestinal distress is often responsible for chest pain in the elderly. Acute abdominal conditions such as mesenteric infarction and appendicitis often go unrecognized in elders because of atypical signs and absence of pain.

Fever may be absent or delayed in the older person with pneumonia or urinary tract infection. Elevations in temperature rarely exceed 39.5°C (103°F). The nurse must be alert to more subtle signs of infection: mental confusion, increased respirations, tachycardia, and changed facial appearance and color.

Emotional Impact

The emotional component of illness in older persons may differ from that of younger people. Many elderly equate good health with the absence of old age. "You are as old as you feel" is a belief of many. An illness that requires hospitalization or a change in life-style is an imminent threat to well-being. Admission to the hospital is often feared and actively avoided. Economic concerns and fear of becoming a burden to the family often lead to high anxiety in an older person. The nurse must recognize the implications of fear, anxiety, and dependency in the elderly patient. Autonomy and independent decision making are encouraged. A positive and confident demeanor from the nurse and the family help lift the mental outlook of the patient. In addition to anxiety and fear, older persons are at high risk for disorientation, confusion, change in levels of consciousness, and other symptoms of delirium when they are admitted to the hospital.

Systemic Impact

The systemic impact of illness upon the aged person has far-reaching effects. The decline in organ function that occurs in every system of the aging body eventually forces one or more body systems to function at full capacity. Illness places new demands upon body systems that have little or no reserve to meet this crisis. Homeostasis, the ability of the body to maintain an internal balance of function and chemical composition, is jeopardized. The older person may be unable to respond effectively to an acute illness, or, if he has a chronic health condition, he may be unable to sustain appropriate responses over a long period of time. Furthermore, the older person's ability to respond to definitive treatment is impaired.

The Older Adult in a Protected Environment

Many housing communities for older people will perform routine maintenance and provide opportunities for socialization and recreation. Easier access to shopping and health care may convince the person that a new location will solve many residential problems. When preparation time is sufficient and money, energy, and health are adequate, a move to a new home can be a positive life experience.

Retirement communities have living quarters of apartments, condominiums, and houses that are developed specifically for the older person. An independent life-style is enhanced with social and recreational events. Health services are not provided. *Life care (continuing care) communities* offer all the features of retirement communities plus health care and skilled nursing care units. When entering such a community, the resident must be capable of independent living.

Although only 5% of the elderly population live in nursing homes, the percentage ranges from 2% for persons 65 to 74 years to 23% for persons 85 and older. Nursing homes offer a variety of health and personal services that include skilled nursing care and rehabilitation. They do not provide acute care. Medicare will pay nursing home costs only for a limited number of days, and Medicare does not pay for personal care. The cost of nursing home care comes out of the family's funds. When money and all assets are totally depleted, the costs will be paid by Medicaid.

Often, a decision for a nursing home placement is made by the family without consulting the older person. Research indicates that successful adjustment to the nursing home is enhanced if the older person participates in the decision-making process. The nurse and social worker as advocates can emphasize this point and encourage a family decision that includes the patient. When this occurs, the patient selects the home of his choice and will enter with a positive mental attitude and a feeling of control. If the patient wants to remain in his home,

he might be able to manage with the help of community supports. Decisions made "for your own good" by the family may, in fact, not be. Placement in a nursing home against the wishes of the patient should be made only as a last resort when no other alternative is available.

Chapter Summary

The population over age 65 is growing in numbers and in average age. Health problems, particularly those associated with chronic illness, increase with age. To provide optimal care to elderly persons, nurses must provide holistic care and work cooperatively with other health disciplines. Emphasis of care must be on promotion of health and maximizing independence.

Ageism and negative false beliefs are found commonly in the United States. Older people know these beliefs, and many unconsciously adjust their behavior to correspond to these beliefs. *Adaptation* and styles of coping are learned in early life. The older adult is likely to use the same adaptation patterns to adjust to the losses of old age.

Mental health disorders of aging are divided into two categories. *Functional disorders* are emotional dysfunctions that show no brain damage. *Organic mental disorders* are cognitive and behavioral dysfunctions that reflect brain disease or systemic illness that is affecting the brain. *Depression* is the most common functional disorder. *Alzheimer's disease* is the most common organic mental disorder.

Normal age changes affect the absorption, distribution, metabolism, and elimination of drugs. The elderly are at high risk for *drug interactions* and *drug toxicities*. Caution must be used in providing medications to older persons. *Falls* are the major cause of accidents in older adults. Negative consequences of aging and environmental hazards can be modified to reduce the occurrence of falls.

Chronic illness is often accompanied by symptoms that cause discomfort. The nurse may be able to suggest *life-style changes* that will increase comfort.

Older adults manifest signs of acute illness in a manner different from that of younger persons. Physical, emotional, and systemic differences exist. Reserve capacity, the body's ability to continue efficiently in the presence of stress, is diminished. If at some point the older adult needs an alternative living arrangement, the family must allow him to share in the decisions if at all possible. Retirement communities, continuing care communities, and nursing homes are among the choices available. Finances, state of health, individual needs, and availability are all factors to be considered in the decision-making process. Prevention and planning ahead can ease the many transitions that are so evident in the life of the older adult.

Many older people lead satisfying and active lives. In the absence of illness, cognitive abilities and intelligence remain stable across a lifetime. There are normal losses in all the body systems, but in the absence of disease the body continues to function adequately. Many persons are able to stay in their own homes because community agencies offer supportive care and services. The family is the main source of social support for the older adult. Most elderly live close to at least one of their children. There is mutual support between the generations, and adult children care very much about the welfare of their parents.

Bibliography

Books

Aiken LR. Later Life, 3rd ed. Hillsdale, NJ, Lawrence Erlbaum Assoc, 1989.

Berg RL and Cassells JS (eds). The Second Fifty Years: Promoting Health and Preventing Disability. Washington, DC, National Academy Press, 1990.

Burggraf V and Stanley M (eds). Nursing the Elderly. Philadelphia, JB Lippincott, 1989.

Burnside IM. Nursing and the Aged, 3rd ed. New York, McGraw–Hill, 1988.

Butler RN and Lewis MI. Aging and Mental Health, 3rd ed. St Louis, CV Mosby, 1982.

Carcio HN. Manual of Health Assessment. Boston, Little, Brown and Co, 1985.

Carnevali DL and Patrick M. Nursing Management for the Elderly, 2nd ed. Philadelphia, JB Lippincott, 1986.

Cook–Deegan RM. Confronting Alzheimer's Disease and Other Dementias. Philadelphia, JB Lippincott, 1988.

Delafuente JC and Stewart RB (eds.). Therapeutics in the Elderly. Baltimore, Williams & Wilkins, 1988.

Dychtwald K. Wellness and Health Promotion for the Elderly. Rockville, MD, Aspen Systems Corp, 1986.

Eliopoulos C. Caring for the Elderly in Diverse Care Settings. Philadelphia, JB Lippincott, 1989.

Eliopoulos C. Gerontological Nursing, 2nd ed. Philadelphia, JB Lippincott, 1987.

Erikson EH. Childhood and Society, 2nd ed. New York, WW Norton, 1963.

Esberger KK and Hughes ST. Nursing Care of the Aged. Norwalk, CT, Appleton & Lange, 1989.

Fowles DG. A Profile of Older Americans: 1990. American Association of Retired Persons and the Administration on Aging, U.S. Department of Health and Human Services, 1990.

Havighurst R. Developmental Tasks and Education, 3rd ed. New York, David McKay, 1972.

Kenney RA. Physiology of Aging: A Synopsis, 2nd ed. Chicago, Year Book Medical Pub, 1989.

Lavizzo–Mourey R et al. Practicing Prevention for the Elderly. Philadelphia, Hanley & Belfus, 1989.

Mace NL and Rabins PV. The 36-Hour Day. Baltimore, The Johns Hopkins Press, 1981.

Matteson MA and McConnell ES. Gerontological Nursing: Concepts and Practice. Philadelphia, WB Saunders, 1988.

Malseed RT and Harrigan GS. Textbook of Pharmacology and Nursing Care. Philadelphia, JB Lippincott, 1989.

National Council on Patient Information and Education. Priorities and Approaches for Improving Prescription Medicine Use by Older Americans. Washington, DC, The National Council on Patient Information and Education, 1987.

Subcommittee on the 10th Edition of the RDAs Food and Nutrition Board, Commission on Life Sciences, National Research Council. Recommended Dietary Allowances. Washington, DC, National Academy Press, 1989.

Taira F. Independence: Building Upon the Strengths of Aging People. Lancaster, PA, Technomic Publishing Co, 1988.

U.S. Department of Health and Human Services. The Surgeon General's Report on Nutrition and Health. DHHS (PHS) Publication No. 88-50210, 1988.

U.S. Senate Special Committee on Aging. Aging America: Trends and Projections. Washington, DC, Department of Health and Human Services Serial No. 101-J, February 1990.

Wolfe SM et al. Worst Pills Best Pills. Washington, DC, Public Citizen Research Group, 1988.

Journals
Asterisks indicate nursing research articles.

Achenbaum WA and Levin JS. What does gerontology mean? Gerontologist 1989 Jun; 29(3):393–400.

Bayer AJ et al. Changing presentation of myocardial infarction with increasing old age. J Am Geriatr Soc 1986 Apr; 34(4):263–266.

Berryman E et al. Point by point: Predicting elders' falls. Geriatr Nurs 1989 Jul/Aug; 10(4):199–201.

Blazer D. Depression in the elderly. N Engl J Med 1989 Jan 19; 320(3):164–166.

* Brink C, Wells T, and Diokno A. Urinary incontinence in women. Public Health Nursing 1987 Jun; 4(2):114–119.

* Burgio LD, Jones LT, and Engel BT. Studying incontinence in an urban nursing home. J Gerontol Nurs 1988 Apr; 14(4):40–45.

Christian E, Dluhy N, and O'Neill R. Sounds of silence: Coping with hearing loss and loneliness. J Gerontol Nurs 1989 Nov; 15(11):4–9.

Clark NM et al. Development of self-management education for elderly patients. Gerontologist 1988 Aug; 28(4):491–494.

Coralli C, Raisz LG, and Wood CL. Osteoporosis: Significance, risk factors and treatment. Nurse Pract 1986 Sep; 11(9):16–35.

Cowart BJ. Age-related changes in taste and smell. Pride Institute J Long Term Home Health Care 1988 Winter; 7(1):23–32.

Denny MS, Koren ME, and Wisby M. Gynecological health needs of elderly women. J Gerontol Nurs 1989 Jan; 15(1):33–38.

Dieckmann L et al. The Alzheimer's disease knowledge test. Gerontologist 1988 Jun; 28(3):402–407.

Dreyfus JK. Depression assessment and interventions in the medically ill frail elderly. J Gerontol Nurs 1988 Sep; 14(9):27–36.

Duffy LM et al. A research agenda in care for patients with Alzheimer's disease. Image 1989 Winter; 21(4):254–257.

Ellickson EB. Bowel management plan for the homebound elderly. J Gerontol Nurs 1988 Jan; 14(1):16–19.

Evans DA et al. Prevalence of Alzheimer disease in a community population of older persons. JAMA 1989 Nov 10; 262(18):2551–2556.

Fawdry K and Berry ML. Fear of senility: The nurse's role in managing reversible confusion. J Gerontol Nurs 1989 Apr; 15(4):17–21.

Goldsmith SR and Marx S. Updated use of digitalis and nitrates in the elderly. Geriatrics 1988 Jan; 43(1):71–94.

* Gomez G and Gomez EA. Dementia? Or delirium. Geriatr Nurs 1989 May/Jun; 10(3):141–142.

Gueldner SH and Spradley J. Outdoor walking lowers fatigue. J Gerontol Nurs 1988 Oct; 14(10):1–12.

Hall GR. Alterations in thought process. J Gerontol Nurs 1988 Mar; 14(3):30–37.

Haight BK. Nursing research in long-term care facilities (1984–1988). Nurs Health Care 1989 Mar; 10(3):147–150.

Hommel PA and Wood EF. Guardianship. Aging 1990; 360:6–12.

Iverson-Carpenter MS et al. Fulfilling nutritional requirements. J Gerontol Nurs 1988 Apr; 14(4):16–24.

Jackson MF. High risk surgical patients. J Gerontol Nurs 1988 Jan; 14(1):8–15.

* Johnston L and Gueldner SH. Remember when . . . ? Using mnemonics to boost memory in the elderly. J Gerontol Nurs 1989 Aug; 15(8):22–26.

Job S and Anema MG. Elder care: Ethical dimensions. J Gerontol Nurs 1988 Dec; 14(12):16–19.

Kannel W et al. Prevention of cardiovascular disease in the elderly. J Am Coll Cardiol 1987 Aug; 10(2, Suppl A):25A–28A.

Kaplan H. Communication problems of the hearing-impaired elderly: What can be done? Pride Institute J Long Term Home Health Care 1988 Winter; 7(1):10–22.

Kolcaba K and Miller CA. Geropharmacology treatment: Behavioral problems extend nursing responsibility. J Gerontol Nurs 1989 May; 15(5):29–35.

Kurfees JF and Dotson RL. Drug interactions in the elderly. J Fam Pract 1987; 25(5):477–488.

Lamy PP. The elderly and drug interactions. J Am Geriatr Soc 1986 Aug; 34(8):586–592.

Levin WC. Age stereotyping. Res Aging 1988 Mar; 10(3):134–148.

Linderborn KM. The need to assess dementia. J Gerontol Nurs 1988 Jan; 14(1):35–39.

Lipowski ZJ. Delirium (acute confusional states). JAMA 1987 Oct 2; 258(13): 1789–1792.

Longino CF. Who are the oldest Americans? Gerontologist 1988 Aug; 28(4): 515–523.

Luxton L. Visual impairments in the elderly: A composite look. Pride Institute J Long Term Home Health Care 1988 Winter; 7(1):3–9.

Madson S. How to reduce the risk of postmenopausal osteoporosis. J Gerontol Nurs 1989 Sep; 15(9):20–24.

Marx JL. Brain protein yields clues to Alzheimer's disease. Science 1989 Mar 31; 243(31):1664–1666.

Mayeux R et al. Risk of dementia in first-degree relatives of patients with Alzheimer's disease and related disorders. Arch Neurol 1991 Mar; 48:1991.

McCormick KA, Schere AAS, and Leaky E. Nursing management of urinary incontinence in geriatric patients. Nurs Clin North Am 1988; 23(1): 231–264.

McShane RE and McLane AM. Constipation: Impact of etiological factors. J Gerontol Nurs 1988 Apr; 14(4):35–39.

Newbern VB. Is it really Alzheimer's? Am J Nurs 1991 Feb; 91(2):50–56.

Newman DK. The treatment of urinary incontinence in adults. Nurse Pract 1989 Jun; 14(6):21–32.

Newman DK and Smith DA. Incontinence: The problem patients won't talk about. RN 1989 Mar; 52(3):42–45.

Oesting HH and Manza RJ. Sleep apnea. Geriatr Nurs 1988 Jul/Aug; 9(4): 232–233.

O'Leary PA et al. Gerontological research: Is it useful for nursing practice? J Gerontol Nurs 1990 May; 16(5):28–32.

Palmer MH. Incontinence. Nurs Clin North Am 1988; 23(1):139–157.

* Patsdaughter CA and Pesznecker BL. Medication regimens and the elderly home care client. J Gerontol Nurs 1988 Oct; 14(10):30–34.

Penn C. Promoting independence. J Gerontol Nurs 1988 Mar; 14(3):14–19.

Resnick BM. Care for life. Geriatr Nurs 1989 May/Jun; 10(3):130–132.

Rossor M. Alzheimer's disease: The entity and its cause. Biochem Soc Trans 1989 Feb; 17(1):67–69.

Rozzini R et al. Depression, life events and somatic symptoms. Gerontologist 1988 Apr; 28(2):229–232.

Schafer SL. An aggressive approach to promoting health responsibility. J Gerontol Nurs 1989 Apr; 15(4):22–27.

* Schank MJ and Lough MA. Maintaining health and independence of elderly women. J Gerontol Nurs 1989 Jun; 15(6):8–11.

* Scura KW and Whipple B. Older adults as an HIV-positive risk group. J Gerontol Nurs 1990 Feb; 16(2):6–10.

Selkoe DJ. Aging, amyloid, and Alzheimer's disease. N Engl J Med 1989 Jun 1; 320(22):1484–1486.

Soderlind S. Weaving a safety net. Geriatr Nurs 1989 Jul/Aug; 10(4):187–189.

Spellbring AM et al. Improving safety for hospitalized elderly. J Gerontol Nurs 1988 Feb; 14(2):31–37.

Strumpf NE. A new age for elderly care. Nurs Health Care 1987 Oct; 8(10): 445–448.

Tideiksaar R and Kay AD. What causes falls? A logical diagnostic procedure. Geriatrics 1986 Dec; 41(12):32–50.

* Trice LB. Meaningful life experience to the elderly. Image: Journal of Nursing Scholarship 1990 Winter; 22(4):248–251.

* Wagnild G and Young HM. Resilience among older women. Image: Journal of Nursing Scholarship 1990 Winter; 22(4):252–255.

Webster JA. Key to health aging: Exercise. J Gerontol Nurs 1988 Dec; 14(12):8–15.

Whipple B and Scura KW. HIV and the older adult: Taking the necessary precautions. J Gerontol Nurs 1989 Sep: 15(9):15–19.

White J. Osteoporosis: Strategies for prevention. Nurs Pract 1986 Sep; 11(9):36–50.

Whiteman KF. Why bother about flu shots? Am J Nurs 1987 Nov; 87(11): 1408–1413.

Wright BA and Staats DO. The geriatric implications of fecal impaction. Nurse Pract 1986 Oct; 11(10):53–66.

Information/Resources

Agencies

Administration on Aging
 330 Independence Ave. SW, Room 4146, Washington, DC 20201, (202) 245-2158

Alzheimer's Association
 70 East Lake St., Suite 600, Chicago, IL 60601, (312) 853-3060

The American Association for International Aging
 1511 K Street NW, Suite 443, Washington, DC 20005, (202) 638-6815

American Association of Homes for the Aging
 1129 20 St. NW, Suite 400, Washington, DC 20036-3489, (202) 296-5960

American Association of Retired Persons
 1909 K St. NW, Washington, DC 20049, (202) 728-4200

American College of Health Care Administrators
 325 S. Patrick St., Alexandria, VA 22314, (703) 549-5822

American Council of the Blind
 1010 Vermont Ave. NW, Suite 1100, Washington, DC 20005, (202) 393-3666

American Federation for Aging Research (AFAR)
 725 Park Ave., New York, NY 10021, (212) 570-2090

American Foundation for the Blind
 1660 L St. NW, Suite 214, Washington, DC 20036, (202) 467-5996

American Geriatrics Society, Inc.
 770 Lexington Ave., Suite 400, New York, NY 10021, (212) 308-1414

American Health Care Association
 1201 L St. NW, Washington, DC 20005, (202) 842-8444

American Society on Aging
 833 Market St., Suite 516, San Francisco, CA 94130, (415) 543-2617

Association for Gerontology in Higher Education (AGHE), 600 Maryland Ave. SW, West Wing, Suite 204, Washington, DC 20024 (202) 484-7505.

Gerontological Society of America
 1275 K. St. NW, Suite 350, Washington, DC 20005-4006, (202) 842-1275

Gray Panthers
 311 S. Juniper St., Suite 601, Philadelphia, PA 19107, (215) 545-6555

Legal Research and Services for the Elderly
 925 15th St. NW, Washington, DC 20005, (202) 347-8800

National Clearinghouse on Technology and Aging
 University Center on Aging, University of Massachusetts Medical Center, 55 Lake Ave. North, Worcester, MA 01655, (617) 856-3662

National Council on the Aging, Inc.
 600 Maryland Ave. SW, West Wing 100, Washington, DC 20024, (202) 479-1200

13

Homelessness in America: A Major Health Problem

Learning Objectives

On completion of this chapter, the learner will be able to:

1. Describe homelessness as a major health and social problem
2. Identify the multiple health problems characteristic of adult and elderly homeless populations
3. Describe the nurse's role in meeting the health needs of the homeless

Homelessness in America is a major social problem that goes beyond mere lack of shelter. The homeless often have difficulty gaining access to health care and frequently experience multiple health problems. Their lack of shelter makes even standard health problems more serious, and once they become ill, the homeless often wait longer to seek medical care and deteriorate more quickly than do other patients. As a result, homeless persons have a high rate of morbidity and mortality.

Since the crisis of homelessness has erupted, nurses have pioneered health care services for the homeless poor. Today, nurses offer compassionate care in emergency shelters, model residences, and soup kitchens as well as on the streets through

outreach projects. Nurses in hospitals provide temporary care and relief from street life.

Delivering care to the homeless demands that nurses provide more than traditional clinical care. Nurses serving the homeless must have the flexibility to practice in innovative ways and perhaps atypical settings. Nurses must be prepared to deal with what can be an overwhelming set of complex problems presented by the homeless.

This chapter presents a synopsis of the health problems of the homeless and the nursing interventions and roles of the nurse working with the homeless. Although the homeless are a heterogeneous group that includes children and families, this chapter places particular emphasis on the health needs of homeless adults.

Describing the Problem and the Population

Size

Estimates of the number of homeless persons range from about a quarter million to more than 3 million. Counting the homeless is complicated by the absence of a clear operational definition of homelessness. The question of who is housed and who is not is difficult to define and assess. The boundary between who is "homeless" and who is "housed" is fluid. Some homeless advocates include in their definition of homeless those families on the edge of poverty who are doubled up in substandard housing. Others reject this definition and count only those living on streets or in shelters. Others include elderly hospitalized patients awaiting nursing home placement. Thus, the way homelessness is defined is arbitrary and colored by political or ideologic motives.

Causes

The causes of homelessness are complex and interrelated but include gentrification (the replacement of low-income housing with luxury housing), deinstitutionalization, unemployment, substance abuse, lack of affordable housing, the inadequacies of public welfare, a breakdown in the family, catastrophic illness, and economic factors.

Composition

The homeless are a heterogeneous group comprised of single adults, families, battered wives, runaway and homeless youth, and persons with HIV illness and other health care problems who have exhausted their resources. The composition of the group is shifting. The mentally ill "bag lady" may be the commonly perceived stereotype of a homeless person. However, families are the fastest growing segment among the homeless. Another segment that will increase exponentially in the near future is that of homeless persons with HIV illness.

Gender

Overall, about 75% of homeless single adults are men. Officially, 85% of homeless families are headed by single women, but common-law relationships are frequent. In one study, the number of runaways was equally divided between males and females (Shaffer and Caton, 1984).

Age

In the early 1970s, the median age of homeless men on skid row was 50 years. By the 1980s, the median age had declined dramatically to the mid-thirties. Homeless single mothers tend to be even younger and in their mid-twenties (Berne et al, 1990).

Ethnicity and Social Class

Blacks and Hispanics are disproportionately represented among the ranks of the homeless as compared with community samples. This finding is not surprising because in recent years lack of shelter has become an indicator of poverty, and blacks and Hispanics are over-represented among the poor.

The most frequently assessed indicator of social class is education. In general, the level of education of the homeless has been found to be slightly lower than that of the general public (Fischer et al, 1986). In another study, the homeless had less education than their parents. Most of the homeless were unemployed. When the homeless did work, most had low-paying service jobs offering little prestige. The same was true of their parents (Struening, 1986).

Geographic Area

Most studies of the homeless have been carried out in large urban areas. Homeless persons are nonetheless evident in rural areas also.

Marital Status

All studies indicate a high degree of disaffiliation among the homeless (Fischer et al, 1986; Rossi et al, 1987; Bassuk et al, 1984). Most are either separated, divorced, or widowed. The incidences of each of these categories are much higher in the homeless population than in the general public.

The Reality of Street Life

The homeless live on streets, under bridges, in bus terminals, and in abandoned buildings. They use soup kitchens, drop-in centers, shelters, hotels, emergency departments, hospitals, jails, inns, community mental health centers, inpatient psychiatric units, and state hospitals. The more fortunate are rehoused in model projects offering transitional or permanent housing. Other living arrangements may be only temporary. Some homeless persons move in with friends or relatives for a time and then return to the streets. Homeless women are often forced to have sexual intercourse in exchange for a place to stay.

The lives of the homeless are complex. Landmark studies describe the busy schedules and directed actions of the homeless (Baxter and Hopper, 1981; Strasser, 1978). Many homeless persons wake up early because the shelters where they may be staying often have other uses during the day. The homeless who live in public transportation terminals often are evicted by police prior to the "rush hour." Walking from soup kitchen to soup kitchen, securing a bed for the night, avoiding dangerous shelter residents, and arranging entitlements are all time-consuming. In addition, some homeless people have full-time jobs or participate in work programs.

Because the modern epidemic of homelessness has existed for some time now, society has mobilized a loose network of services to help those without shelter. These services include soup kitchens, hotels, shelters, street outreach, and model residences.

Soup Kitchens

Soup kitchens offer free food to the homeless. Most large urban cities have many soup kitchens available to the homeless. By word of mouth, the homeless become well versed about the time, location, and quality of the food. Soup kitchens are generally run by nonprofit groups that rely heavily on volunteers and have minimal budgets. They often use government surplus food and receive donations of bruised produce or damaged canned goods from grocery stores and day-old bread from bakeries. Some soup kitchens sponsor on-site health clinics and offer other services such as assistance in securing benefits or legal help.

Shelters

The original purpose of shelters was to provide temporary emergency housing; many shelters, however, have been operating for a decade or more. Shelters vary greatly in quality and size and in the support services available. Shelters can have a transient population, but often the "guests" include a core of long-term residents. Persons in shelters are usually segregated by gender. Some shelters have a variety of procedures to screen out persons who may be intoxicated or have other medical or psychiatric impairments. Nonetheless, taken as a whole, shelters house a number of dual-diagnosis clients (persons who have both a psychotic disorder and a substance abuse problem) who have been barred from residential programs and have essentially become permanent shelter residents. Shelters are often staffed by workers who have no formal training. Some shelters have on-site service teams consisting of nurses, social workers, doctors, and alcoholism counselors who provide health services.

Hotels

Some cities offer emergency housing in hotels. Run down and often located in marginal neighborhoods, these hotels may also be sites of rampant drug dealing and prostitution. In skid row areas, these hotels are called flophouses and are frequented by the older alcoholic homeless (Cohen et al, 1988). Less like dormitories than flophouses, but still dilapidated, are SRO (single-room occupancy) hotels.

Street Outreach

The primary objective of street outreach is to help the homeless person accept services and eventually make the transition to permanent housing. Most street outreach teams target the mentally ill segment of the population. Outreach workers travel through the community in vans and offer coffee, sandwiches, blankets, and, unfortunately, cigarettes as concrete symbols of their concern for the homeless.

Street outreach requires tremendous patience. The homeless mentally ill have difficulty accepting treatment and have priorities different from those of mental health professionals. The process of helping the homeless accept services is known as engagement (Rog, 1988). Once the homeless person comes to the team's office, work can begin to obtain benefits (i.e., social security, Medicaid, and public assistance), to provide money management assistance, and to initiate medical and psychiatric treatment. When a homeless person is harmful to either himself or others or in some jurisdictions meets the criteria for being "gravely impaired," the team initiates involuntary hospitalization (Cohen and Marcos, 1986).

Residential Care

Transitional and permanent residences are often the best housing options for providing humane care. Policymakers have developed a number of projects for specific subgroups of the homeless population. Although these projects differ in philosophy, they share many key elements. They generally offer affordable rent, on-site services, case management, money and medication management, socialization, and crisis intervention.

Other Forms of Social Support

Although the homeless are often socially isolated, they do have certain relationships or connections. They may have connections to other homeless people, shopkeepers, clergy, and even interested citizens. Sometimes several different mental health treatment centers provide treatment concurrently without knowledge of the others' treatment. For instance, one homeless man named Joe lived outside a hospital in New York City. Many members of the staff regularly gave him food and clothing as well as money. Staff frequently had conversations with him on their way to and from work. Joe was a frequent and popular visitor to the hospital's emergency department. The head nurse remarked that she had never received so many phone calls about one patient as when Joe was admitted to the ICU. When Joe was murdered and robbed of the $200 he had collected from hospital employees one payday, nurses took up a collection to pay for his funeral.

The Health Problems of Homeless People

The homeless often have multiple health problems and marginal health status. Health care is often inaccessible because most of the homeless do not have health care insurance. In one study, 81% reported having no health insurance, 7% had Medicaid, 4% had Medicare, 5% had private health insurance, and 2% had veterans' benefits (Robertson and Cousineu, 1986).

Co-morbidity, the existence of concurrent health problems, is especially prevalent among the homeless. In one study, almost half of the homeless subjects diagnosed with a major mental illness also had several physical problems (Breakey et al, 1989).

Physical Problems

Numerous studies have underscored the excess of morbidity and mortality that the homeless experience (Wright and Weber, 1987; Gelberg and Linn, 1989; Breakey et al, 1989). In one study, males had an average of 8.3 health problems and females had an average of 9.2 (Breakey et al, 1989). Other studies found that over one third of the subjects reported that they were in fair or poor health (Rossi et al, 1987; Robertson and Cousineu, 1986). The homeless can suffer from any of the health problems described elsewhere in this text. Common chronic health problems such as diabetes, hypertension, and heart disease are prevalent, and management of these problems is made more difficult by the patient's living on the street.

Many of the health problems the homeless experience are related in large part to their living conditions. Street life exposes the homeless to extremes of heat and cold. Lack of proper nutrition, clothing, and sleep compounds the risks to health that are posed by extremes of temperature. The homeless who patronize shelters frequently encounter overcrowded, unventilated, and dimly lit quarters that provide an ideal environment for the spread of tuberculosis and other respiratory diseases. Over 75% of homeless single adults smoke cigarettes, which adds further health risks. Some evidence exists that the homeless who live in shelters are somewhat healthier than those who live outdoors (Gelberg and Linn, 1989).

The homeless have high rates of trauma, tuberculosis, upper respiratory infection, poor nutrition and anemia, lice and scabies, peripheral vascular problems, sexually transmitted disease, dental problems, arthritis, hypothermia, and foot problems.

Trauma

Trauma is a major reason for visits of the homeless to medical emergency departments. Accidents are a major cause of death among the homeless (Wright and Weber, 1987). They are often victims of violent crime. In one study, almost three-quarters of the subjects reported that they had been victimized during the previous year (Gelberg and Linn, 1989). In another study, during a 1-year period, 26% had been robbed, 59% had had property stolen, 24% had been threatened with a gun, knife, or other weapon, and 18% had been beaten (Struening, 1986). Both homosexual and heterosexual rape is a common occurrence among the homeless (Institute of Medicine, 1988). In one study, one third of homeless single women reported that they had been raped (Breakey et al, 1989).

Tuberculosis

Rates of tuberculosis (TB) among the homeless are high. Living in close proximity to others in poorly ventilated spaces with the compounding factor of poor nutrition increases the risk of contracting TB. Thus, shelters provide an optimal environment

for the spread or reactivation of this disease. Rates of clinically active tuberculosis in homeless single adults are estimated to range between 1.6% and 6.8% (Schieffelbein and Snider, 1988). The prevalence of latent disease is even higher (Morris and Crystal, 1989). Because TB is contagious and can be fatal if untreated, case finding is important among this high-risk group. Patients with acquired immunodeficiency syndrome (AIDS) are particularly prone to tuberculosis. In one study, 87% of homeless men with active tuberculosis also had AIDS (Torres et al, 1990). It is important to realize that homeless patients with HIV infection can have false-negative TB skin tests (PPDs [purified protein derivative]) and chest radiographs because of a blunted immune response.

Treating tuberculosis is often difficult because the homeless person must take several medications over many months. One writer estimated that only one third of the homeless would independently comply with the full course of treatment (Ramsden et al, 1988). If homeless patients stop taking the medication prior to completing the course, they can develop resistant strains of the tubercle bacillus.

Many cities have set up supervised treatment programs in which workers visit the patients daily to administer medications. Other cities have used computers to track patients with the disease. The Centers for Disease Control (CDC) recommends an intensive 6-month, multidrug course of medication. The CDC also has several different protocols to treat tuberculosis on a 3- or 5-day-a-week schedule, if daily supervised dosing is impossible. Some authors recommend lifetime treatment for dormant TB in patients with HIV infection.

Efforts must be made to provide good ventilation and sunlight and to decrease crowding in shelters. Ultraviolet lights are recommended to prevent the spread of infection (Stead, 1989; Nardell, 1989). Shelter staff should be screened for tuberculosis through the administration of PPDs at least once a year.

Upper Respiratory Infection

As in the general population, upper respiratory infection is the most common health problem that health care providers encounter among the homeless (Wright and Weber, 1987).

Inadequate Nutrition

The homeless face overwhelming obstacles to good nutrition. The lack of shelter generally results in the absence of adequate means to store and prepare food. Many of the homeless panhandle and then buy "junk food" at fast-food restaurants or delicatessens. Others among the homeless who scavenge through garbage cans in search of food are at high risk for food poisoning. Even those who rely on soup kitchens may be at risk for tainted food if the soup kitchens they frequent do not maintain hygienic conditions. Not surprisingly, one study found that the diets of the homeless deviate substantially from RDA requirements (Luder et al, 1989). Another study found that 18% of homeless men and 35% of homeless women were anemic (Breakey et al, 1989).

Lice and Scabies

Lice and scabies are endemic in homeless populations. Inadequate access to bathing and washing facilities leads to poor hygiene. The homeless mentally ill may resist the nurse's attempts to encourage appropriate hygienic practices. Some homeless persons, lacking access to washers and dryers, wear their clothes for weeks at a time and then discard them when replacement clothing is obtained from a clothing bank. All of these problems lead to frequent infestation.

The degree of infestation can often be severe. The homeless patient can be literally covered with bugs. Treatment of infestation, which includes washing all clothing and bedding, is time-consuming and must be done correctly to ensure nonrecurrence. Furniture, including sofas and mattresses, must be sprayed with R&C Lice Control Spray, A-200, or a comparable pesticide spray to decontaminate them. These sprays are available without a prescription in drugstores. Shelters can prevent infestation by covering mattresses with plastic and avoiding cloth furniture.

Lindane (Kwell) is the treatment of choice for scabies and intractable cases of lice. The patient treated with lindane must wash it off after 12 to 24 hours because the medication can cause itching and is carcinogenic. Nurses who are pregnant should not apply lindane, because it penetrates the skin and can cause central nervous system toxicity. Staff hysteria may result from outbreaks of infestation and must be addressed.

Peripheral Vascular Problems

Peripheral vascular problems (varicosities, phlebitis, thrombosis, chronic edema, cellulitis, gangrene) were found to be 10 to 15 times more prevalent among the homeless than among housed persons in one nationwide sample (Wright and Weber, 1987). Another researcher found that one fourth of women and men had varicose veins, venous stasis, ulceration, or inflammation of the lower extremities (Breakey et al, 1989). Once the patient has developed peripheral vascular disease, the continued lack of shelter complicates recovery.

Sexually Transmitted Diseases

In one sample of homeless single adults, almost 8% of the men and 11% of the women had gonorrhea or syphilis, and one third reported previous infection (Breakey et al, 1989). The most serious sexually transmitted disease that is prevalent among the homeless is HIV infection.

Estimating the HIV seroprevalence among the homeless is difficult. Estimates of intravenous drug users (IVDU) that depend on self-reporting are unreliable. Estimates based on retrospective chart reviews of patients using a medical clinic introduce a sampling bias. The homeless persons who attend clinics because of medical complaints may not be representative of the entire homeless population.

There is no precise estimate of the number of homeless persons with HIV infection, but 26 states surveyed in one study reported that they had homeless persons with AIDS (National Coalition for the Homeless, 1990). Advocates in Washington, DC, estimate the seroprevalence to be between 12% and 30% (Gaines-Carter, 1990). A researcher in a South Bronx shelter estimates that between 35% and 40% of homeless men admit to current episodes of IV heroin use and another 5% are homosexual. Half of these users are estimated to be HIV-positive, and 20% show overt signs of AIDS (Joseph and Roman-Nay, 1988). In New York City, between 9% and 18% of hospitalized HIV patients are homeless (Torres et al, 1990). In another study, a retrospective chart review of 169 homeless men in a New

York City shelter who were at risk for HIV infection revealed a seroprevalence of 62% (Torres et al, 1990).

Street life is hazardous to someone who is immunosuppressed. Exposure to the elements and tainted foods are constant threats. Diarrhea is also a problem when there are inadequate toilet facilities. For homeless persons with HIV, living in a crowded shelter has its own liabilities. Other shelter guests may be suffering from infectious diseases to which those with HIV infection are especially vulnerable. For example, some patients in shelters have herpes zoster or tuberculosis, as previously discussed. In addition, persons with HIV infection and AIDS are often stigmatized because of their disease and thereby become the targets of violence. The probability of violence is even greater for patients who are HIV-positive and take zidovudine (AZT), because it is an expensive drug for which a thriving black market exists.

Apathy, lethargy, and social withdrawal can make survival in shelters difficult for those with AIDS dementia. The short-term memory loss associated with AIDS dementia presents particular problems for homeless persons living in the community. They are incapable of complying with public assistance paperwork requirements. Some are on as many as 16 different medications and lack the cognitive skills to comply with complicated medication schedules. The psychosis, delirium, memory loss, depression, and mania that they exhibit also present major management problems for shelter workers.

Some homeless people are knowledgeable about HIV infection and AIDS and despite enormous odds take care of themselves. One primary care clinic found that almost three fourths of the patients were compliant with HIV antibody tests, medication, and follow-up visits (Torres et al, 1990). For others, denial is a major problem. They fear the worst and postpone confronting their HIV status until hospitalized with their first bout of *Pneumocystis carinii* pneumonia (PCP).

Many IVDUs have difficulty with hospitalization. Homeless IVDUs often cannot cope with many of the invasive procedures associated with inpatient hospitalization. Despite years of injecting themselves with drugs, many IVDUs are terrified of needles and come close to panic attacks when venipuncture procedures are performed. Another complicating factor is that IVDUs generally have poor veins and a high tolerance for pain medication (Schmitz, 1990). Undermedication is a frequent, albeit unintended, result. When the stress of an initial diagnosis of HIV (which has long been denied) is added, "acting out" behaviors can easily occur. One survey characterized IVDU homeless patients as more likely to sign out against medical advice and less likely to comply with treatment (Torres et al, 1987).

Several model projects currently rehouse the homeless person with HIV. These projects offer patients their own rooms and supportive staff on site. Other models offer scatter-site apartments with supportive services. Taken together, these projects offer homeless persons with AIDS their best hope for humane care.

Dental Problems

In one survey, 98 out of 100 homeless persons needed dental attention. Eighteen percent had pain and infection, and almost 30% had not visited a dentist in 14 years (Bolden, 1990). Homeless people have difficulty getting dentures made and maintaining dentures once they are obtained. These dental problems can adversely affect food intake and result in nutritional deficiencies. In addition, missing teeth or poor dental hygiene contributes to poor personal appearance, which can compound preexisting feelings of low self-esteem.

Physical Disability

Shelters are often inaccessible to the physically disabled homeless person. Broken elevators, obstructed ramps, lack of bathing or toilet facilities, and inattentive shelter staff often make the streets a more inviting alternative for many of these persons (Nathan, 1987).

Foot Problems

The homeless have a high incidence of foot problems. Ill-fitting shoes, inadequate leg elevation, frostbite, and the constant movement endemic to life on the streets all take their toll and lead to a variety of foot disorders. Disorders common in the homeless include calluses, corns, long or dystrophic nails, infections, ingrown toenails, ulcers, grossly macerated skin, friction blisters, painful deformed feet, sprained ankles, peripheral neuropathy, fractures, and frostbite (Jones, 1990).

Mental Disorders

During the 1980s, the mental status of the homeless received enormous attention from researchers (Bassuk et al, 1984; Breakey et al, 1989; Fischer et al, 1986; Koegel et al, 1988; Rossi et al, 1987; Roth et al, 1985; Struening, 1986). The results of the research show that the homeless suffer disproportionately from psychiatric, drug, and alcohol disorders. Twenty-five to 33% of homeless single adults can be considered "chronically mentally ill" (Struening, 1986). Recent data point to the extent of dual and multiple diagnosis within the homeless population (Fischer and Breakey). In one study, most patients with major mental disorders also had a second disorder based on their alcohol or drug use (Breakey et al, 1989).

The nurse must recognize the limitations of the diagnosis-oriented medical model that uses psychiatric labels to describe behavior that may also be related to lack of social support, economic factors, and the stress of homelessness itself. The nurse must exercise particular sensitivity and caution in using these labels to describe the behavior of homeless persons as homelessness becomes more and more a part of what being poor means in the United States today.

Several studies based on structured or unstructured clinical interviews reported the incidence of psychiatric disorders by diagnosis (Breakey et al, 1989; Koegel et al, 1988; Bassuk et al, 1984). According to these studies, schizophrenia occurred in about 15% of the homeless. Rates for mood disorders averaged about 25% (Fischer and Breakey). Less than a third had an anxiety disorder, usually phobia, panic, or generalized anxiety (Breakey et al, 1989; Koegel et al, 1988).

Determining rates for personality disorders presents significant methodologic problems. In the studies that have attempted to assign a diagnosis, the incidence varies from 21% to 42%. The most frequently diagnosed persons are those who are paranoid, schizoid, and antisocial (Fischer and Breakey). Several studies found an incidence of cognitive impairment of 2% to 3% (Koegel et al, 1988; Breakey et al, 1989). Mental retardation, a topic not often studied, was found in up to 6% of the subjects of three samples (Fischer and Breakey).

Many studies have found substance abuse to be a major problem for the homeless (Lubran, 1989; Koegel et al, 1988; Rossi et al, 1987; Breakey et al, 1989; Susser et al, 1989). An estimated 50% of homeless men have a problem with alcohol abuse or dependence. Between 20% and 40% of homeless single adults abuse drugs (Susser et al, 1989; Koegel et al, 1988).

About 25% of the homeless had a history of psychiatric hospitalization (Rossi et al, 1987; Koegel et al, 1988; Fischer et al, 1986; Struening, 1986). Many homeless persons have contact with the criminal justice system, but 75% of their offenses are crimes related to homelessness, such as loitering, living in an abandoned building, stealing food, or sleeping on a park bench (Fischer, 1988).

The Nurse's Role in Meeting the Health Needs of the Homeless

The homeless are a heterogeneous group with greatly varying needs. Devising a single nursing care plan is therefore impossible. A 23-year-old IVDU who is HIV-positive requires an approach different from that of a 72-year-old schizophrenic patient with diabetes. The patient's lack of shelter nonetheless affects the nursing care plan in important ways.

One helpful way to conceptualize the role of the nurse working with the homeless is to begin with the framework of work roles developed by Peplau and adapted by Scharer (1979). Although Peplau developed her framework to explain the role of the psychiatric nurse, her model has relevance to nurses working with homeless patients, especially nurses who practice in nontraditional settings. Many homeless persons have primary psychiatric problems. Others have mental health needs because homelessness is a catastrophic event that causes enormous stress.

According to Peplau, the subroles of the psychiatric nurse are mother surrogate, technician, manager, socializing agent, counselor/nurse psychotherapist, and teacher (Scharer, 1979). The subrole of political advocate may be added when caring for homeless persons.

Mother Surrogate

Because many homeless persons are estranged from their families, the nurse becomes a mother substitute. In this subrole, the nurse performs "mothering acts" such as supporting, persuading, disciplining, reassuring, and comforting. When patients are unable to negotiate the clinic system by themselves, the nurse may escort them to the clinic for visits. In addition, the nurse functions as a supportive listener, helps resolve disputes, and sets limits on extreme behavior. Some patients appreciate knowing that a nurse is available, even if they never speak with the nurse.

The goal of the nurse is to create and maintain a positive and nurturing environment to the extent possible. This is easiest for nurses to achieve in model residences that rehouse the homeless. Nurses who practice in shelters should strive to make these often stark quarters "home" to their homeless guests. Similarly, nurses who practice in hospitals must endeavor to replace the frequently impersonal environment of the hospital with an atmosphere that is more "homelike." These nurses are aided by the fact that for many homeless patients a hospital stay represents a distinct improvement over their current living situation.

Nurses working in hospitals can fulfill the subrole of mother surrogate in a number of other ways. Helping patients who are unable to carry out the activities of daily living, such as bathing and feeding, is basic to this subrole. Setting limits on behavior is also important. Using strategies to ensure that patients do not injure themselves by refusing necessary medical treatment or by leaving the hospital is an important function of the nurse. One elderly schizophrenic man was hospitalized involuntarily after he neglected a cancerous lesion on his ear for over a year. He was ordered by the courts to have surgery, which he tolerated well. He was quite intent on leaving the hospital so that he could return to distributing his poetry on the streets of New York. Seeing that the patient does not leave the hospital with an open wound is obviously a nursing priority.

The hospital nurse also assists the patient and social worker during the discharge planning process. Some homeless patients are unaware of the services available to them. As a first step, the nurse must be familiar with the services that are available. Patients can then be aided in their decision making by providing the appropriate information with a sufficient level of concern and interest.

Many homeless people are aware of the services that their community has to offer. Some communities have an array of services, whereas others have little in the way of support for the homeless. Some homeless persons may already have an outreach worker in the community whom they can identify. These workers who work in shelters, soup kitchens, legal clinics, or religious organizations are often involved with the patient and want to know what has been accomplished in the hospital and the follow-up plans. The outreach worker may want to visit the patient in the hospital. The nurse can encourage such visits by being flexible with the visiting hours and meeting with the outreach worker during the visit to discuss the patient's care. A telephone call from the hospital nurse to the nurse at the shelter can be helpful to both caregivers and to patients. Written summaries that can be given to both the outreach worker and the patient may promote follow-up health care and compliance after hospitalization. The hospital nurse should consider giving the patient's discharge medication to the outreach worker if the patient is unreliable.

For a discharge plan to succeed, the patient needs to be fully invested in it. The nurse should therefore discuss the goal of the plan with the patient and attempt to obtain the patient's agreement with that goal. This is particularly important with the substance user. For example, if a criterion for admission to a residence is that the patient be motivated to become drug-free, the nurse cannot substitute her motivation for the patient's. Admission of an unmotivated substance user inevitably leads to a quick departure of this person from the residence. The residence is then unlikely to accept any more referrals because it will not trust the nurse's judgment.

A "homeless" discharge (discharge to streets and shelters) is inappropriate for any patient, but it is especially contraindicated for patients who are unable to function on the street because of organic mental disorders and for persons whose health problems require a lot of support (*e.g.*, patients on dialysis and those with complex drug regimens or orthopedic problems). The nurse works with homeless patients to help them accept the discharge arrangements if they are to be placed, for example, in a nursing home or adult home.

One option short of a permanent home is respite care for the homeless modeled on that offered by Christ House in Washington, DC. At Christ House, patients have a home in which they can recuperate when they are not sick enough to be in the hospital but are too sick to be on the street or in a shelter. This facility provides a cheerful, restful environment, nutritious meals, and the support of on-site health care services. Another option, although less ideal than respite care, is the treatment offered by the infirmaries located in some shelters.

Technician

Many technical functions are important in delivering nursing care to homeless patients. Administering medications, assessing vital signs, screening for TB, giving immunizations and flu shots, changing dressings, and administering first aid and treatments are just some techniques the nurse performs whether in an inpatient or community setting.

Because homeless patients can become acutely ill with multiple system failure, nurses in intensive care units often care for homeless patients. The technical functions of the nurse treating the homeless patient in the inpatient unit are the same as those she would exercise in treating any other patient on that unit.

In the community, noninvasive techniques such as foot soaks and blood pressure screening—procedures that the homeless may find nonthreatening—can provide an opportunity for developing rapport and giving important feedback to the patient. The nurse practicing in the community also provides emergency medical and psychiatric care. Working with ambulance and police personnel is an essential skill. Because scabies and lice are endemic in the homeless population, the nurse must learn to deal with these problems and the hysteria that can develop among the staff when these problems are discovered. Nurses may find themselves serving as consultants to kitchen personnel in shelters to ensure reasonably hygienic conditions. These consultations can be as basic as helping homeless assistants in the kitchen use correct hand-washing technique.

Manager

Coordination and management are important parts of the nurse's role whether the patient is in the community or in the hospital. Most homeless persons need help with making and keeping clinic appointments, interpreting the results of medical workups, and complying with treatment. They need someone who can mediate and advocate on their behalf and explain to them clearly what is occurring. The nurse is often the one who must take the lead in filling the roles of mediator, advocate, and interpreter of the therapeutic regimen prescribed by health care personnel from different specialty areas.

Management of on-site health clinics is also important. This responsibility involves a broad spectrum of tasks, including scheduling clinicians' time, managing records, overseeing the proper disposal of needle containers, and negotiating with laboratories for services.

The nurse also provides leadership to the paraprofessionals who perform the bulk of the work in community settings and provide support to nursing personnel in hospitals. These caregivers often have no formal training and require a great deal of supervision and support.

Socializing Agent

The homeless have many acquaintances but few actual friends. Thus, remembering birthdays and celebrating holidays (e.g., serving Thanksgiving dinner) become an integral part of the nurse's role in caring for homeless patients. These and other activities help the patient develop social skills, provide support to patients, and build patients' self-esteem. In the hospital, these patients often have no visitors, an experience that can be painful for them. Nurses can provide emotional support by encouraging patients to interact with other patients or by finding them compatible roommates while they are in the hospital.

Counselor/Nurse Psychotherapist

As the counselor/nurse psychotherapist, the nurse validates the difficulty of homelessness and supports the patients' positive coping mechanisms. Simply acknowledging their plight is important.

Providing 50-minute biweekly psychotherapy sessions for the patients is not realistic or appropriate for most of the homeless or formerly homeless. Nurses practicing in the community can perform this role through brief informal interactions with patients. Communicating with patients in the hall or at lunch provides a way of keeping in touch and saying hello while at the same time evaluating the clients' mental status.

When they are hospitalized, homeless or formerly homeless persons have many psychosocial needs. Like all hospitalized patients, they worry about a number of matters, including their prognosis and treatment. Unfortunately, an attitude persists among many in the health care professions that these patients do not have the same worth as middle-class or wealthy patients. Basic courtesy is often lacking. One emergency department physician told a homeless woman who was physically unable to talk that if "she didn't tell him what was wrong with her, he would become her worst nightmare." Soon afterward, fearful of the doctor's threat, she disconnected her IV and left the emergency department. Although this level of abuse may be unusual, more subtle discrimination abounds.

When homeless patients have a major mental illness such as schizophrenia, they may present a management problem on busy inpatient medical and surgical units. They may refuse medication, be delusional about hospital procedures, and have difficulty getting along with their roommates. For example, some psychotic patients may be attached to their "bags" and refuse to part with what everyone else considers garbage. If

these bags are not vermin-infested or too large, allowing the patient to store them in a patient storage area may be a reasonable compromise. One psychotic patient's delusion was that her skin would dissolve if she washed herself. As a result, she did not bathe for a year and become infested with lice. Allowing her to bathe with her boyfriend and distracting her during the bath helped her to get through the procedure without a panic attack. Consulting with a psychiatric clinical nurse specialist is often helpful in resolving these situations.

Many homeless patients have substance abuse problems. In caring for these patients, the basic tenets of substance abuse nursing still hold. By definition, these patients manipulate others and deny their problems. Their presence in a shelter indicates that they have reached a marked point of deterioration. The first night in a shelter for these patients can be critical for nursing intervention because these patients may be close to the point of realizing that they have "hit bottom."

The nurse must use the necessary "street smarts" in dealing with addicted patients. Some patients are dangerous, and the nurse should never be alone with them. Many shelters have a policy that when patients are under the influence of alcohol or drugs and are disruptive, they should be evicted from the shelter for the night or, if circumstances warrant, permanently evicted from the shelter.

Some facilities have started programs to deal with substance abuse problems. In one suburban New York county, persons applying for shelter undergo a mandatory 3-day evaluation prior to admission to the shelter system. Patients with addictions are offered drug rehabilitation. Other shelter residents must submit to a drug screen before admission. Some shelters have substance abuse counselors and sponsor chapters of Alcoholics Anonymous and Narcotics Anonymous on site.

Nurses who work in hospitals need to be aware of patients' illicit use of drugs during hospitalization. Barring visitors may be an appropriate action. Patients may discharge themselves against medical advice to obtain drugs. For substance-use patients who remain, nurses need to point out in a caring, nonjudgmental way the negative effects of substance abuse. For example, the nurse might say, "Your elevated liver enzymes show that your drinking has seriously damaged your liver. If you continue this behavior, I'm afraid that you are going to die." Comments like this can break through denial and help the patient become motivated for treatment.

The nurse working in the community with the homeless mentally ill needs a nontraditional unstructured approach, preferably using a "drop in" model for patients (Rog, 1988; Ferguson, 1989). Money and medication management, crisis intervention, activities, and concrete services are important components of "therapy" for the chronically mentally ill homeless.

Teacher

Health teaching is an important part of the nurse's role in caring for homeless patients. This is especially true as HIV infection and AIDS strike the homeless in epidemic proportions. Many homeless people have little reliable information about how AIDS is treated. One patient, on hearing that she was HIV-positive, thought that she would be dead in 2 weeks.

Training in simple social skills is also important, especially if the homeless person moves into a temporary or permanent residence. Teaching homeless patients how to do laundry, to shop, and to readjust to life indoors are just some of the simple social skills that merit the attention of the nurse as a teacher.

Sometimes deciding what to teach the patient is difficult because all the alternatives involve compromise. For example, a young type I diabetic with a major psychiatric disorder was taking insulin. She carried her insulin and syringes with her on the street, was able to inject herself, kept her clinic appointments faithfully, but was unable to follow her diabetic diet. The nurse in the clinic continued to work with the patient although she knew that the patient was unable to maintain the degree of control that is desirable for a diabetic patient. So, instead of concentrating on control, she focused on helping the patient to avoid dangerous levels of hypoglycemia and hyperglycemia. As a result, the patient was able to avoid diabetic ketoacidosis and severe hypoglycemia and eventually accepted placement in an adult home. Another homeless patient who was judged to be unreliable about eating or independent insulin administration was taken off insulin. Clearly, such complex clinical situations have no easy or right solutions; the ambiguity of these situations makes nurses feel uncomfortable regarding their decisions about the plan of care for their patients. Collaboration and consultation with other health care professionals are important parts of the problem-solving approach in such situations.

Teaching patients about particular regimens also involves careful judgments. For example, patients with tuberculosis must be carefully assessed for their ability to be compliant with a regimen of drug therapy. Tuberculosis patients in shelters can infect many others if they are not compliant with their medication. Some patients can be discharged with a supervised therapy program; others require long-term hospitalization.

The nurse must assess whether patients are ready for discharge and have the resources to comply with their treatment. Patients with peripheral vascular disease need shelters that stay open during the day so that they can elevate their legs. For some patients with vascular disease, the nurse has to make a judgment about the likelihood of their returning to have their Unna boots removed or their wearing the boots for several months. For some patients, simply stressing the importance of their returning to the clinic ensures their compliance.

Political Advocate

Nurses who work with the homeless quickly realize that solutions to the problem of homelessness require more than outreach health services or beds in a local shelter. Nurses must advocate for a change in the social conditions that have created homelessness in the first place. A multidimensional response that includes job training, low-income housing, welfare reform, daycare, early childhood and adult education, a more responsive mental health system, and more long-term residential treatment centers for substance abusers is needed to address the problem. Because their homeless patients lack the wherewithal and influence to make this agenda a political priority, some nurses have become advocates to give voice to their patients' concerns.

Not every nurse working full-time with the homeless can also be a full-time advocate, but opportunities abound for nurses to make a difference in the public arena. By virtue of their education, experience, and professional skills and judgment,

nurses have much to contribute to the lobbying effort. They have built coalitions with other advocates, testified at public hearings, educated the public about the problem of homelessness, and become members of government task forces to push for passage of legislation for the homeless.

Implications for Nurses Working With the Homeless in Hospitals and in the Community

Positive Aspects

Working with the homeless can be rewarding. Nurses in community settings enjoy tremendous autonomy, have chances to form collegial work relationships with co-workers from other professions and disciplines, and have numerous opportunities to conduct nursing research. Often they work with schools of nursing to provide clinical experiences; have opportunities to work with a variety of other "helpers," such as members of the clergy, lawyers, community organizers, and politicians; and have the satisfaction of knowing that they are helping to improve life for some of their most disadvantaged fellow citizens. Most nonprofit organizations that provide services to the homeless are small, personable organizations with fewer regulatory restraints than large health care institutions. In addition, nurses who work with the homeless have received recognition for their work both within the profession and in the media.

Hospital nurses who work with the homeless can justifiably take pride in their efforts to promote the well-being of these patients. Most homeless persons are hospitalized in city and county hospitals. In some city hospitals in New York City, most of the patients are homeless. Working at Bellevue Hospital has been likened to joining the Peace Corps in Manhattan.

Special Challenges

Poor Working Conditions

Poor working conditions are a fact of life in many community settings. Among the hardships that nurses and their co-workers endure are inadequate heat in the winter, poor or no air conditioning in the summer, broken plumbing, vermin infestation, scarcity of secure parking facilities, and high-crime neighborhoods. By definition, street outreach workers spend much of their day outdoors. Nurses who work in shelters may not even have a private room for examining patients. Every day they set up cloth screens in a corner of the shelter and must transport all their equipment.

Similarly, county or city hospitals sometimes operate under severe budgetary constraints and have inadequate staffing, supplies, and equipment. Working conditions are frequently overcrowded. Delivering nursing care to patients with complex needs under these circumstances is difficult. In addition, homeless people who often lack access to primary care come to the hospital emergency department with nonemergent complaints. Overworked nurses who see these patients as "not real emergencies" often feel frustrated.

Inability to See Steady Progress

Nurses often do not see measurable progress either in their homeless patients or in the response of the system to their plight. Although responsible for the care of patients, nurses may have little control over significant matters such as safety and nutrition and must often work without the support services that are available in most hospitals. When intervening, the nurse must devise a treatment plan that frequently requires compromise. To prevent her own burnout, the nurse must keep the goals of treatment at a realistic level and redefine success on the basis of lowered expectations.

Despite the nurse's effort as a caregiver or as an advocate, the problem of homelessness may worsen. Time and time again, the same patients may be admitted for care because of the lack of essential support services outside the hospital. Under these circumstances, many nurses understandably develop a sense of frustration.

Professional Isolation

Nurses who work with the homeless in the community may find themselves professionally isolated. Nurses practicing in teaching hospitals have more formal and informal opportunities for learning (*e.g.*, rounds and in-service education programs) than do nurses employed in small nonprofit corporations that serve the homeless. The projects and programs that these non-profit organizations sponsor may employ only one nurse, a small team that may include a single nurse and one or more non-nursing professionals, or a nurse and a number of paraprofessionals. To prevent professional isolation, nurses who work in these settings must deliberately seek out continuing education programs and professional relationships. Faculty practice has also proved to be an effective way of attracting seasoned nursing professionals to the clinical front lines, because this permits the nurse to maintain other professional interests.

Stigma

The high incidence of HIV infection, TB, and substance abuse among the homeless has left this population not only increasingly at risk but also increasingly stigmatized. The homeless are currently the object of a significant community backlash. Eviction from public transportation centers and community resistance to projects that rehouse the homeless are merely two manifestations of this backlash. To some degree, nurses share the stigma of those they serve. Under these circumstances, a heightened awareness of peace and social justice values inherent in working with the homeless can provide nurses with continuing validation of the importance of their work.

Gerontologic Considerations

The elderly homeless are so under-represented in the general homeless population that two studies defined elderly in the homeless population as those who are 55 years of age or older (Institute of Medicine, 1988). Why do so few elderly appear to be homeless? Shelter samples often under-represent this group because the elderly shun these potentially violent environments (Cohen et al, 1988; Institute of Medicine, 1988). Several authors have hypothesized that fewer elderly appear to be homeless because once they are homeless, the elderly succumb more quickly to disease (Institute of Medicine, 1988; Brickner et al, 1990). Others have hypothesized that the higher level of benefits available at age 65 provides a "safety net" for the elderly homeless (Institute of Medicine, 1988).

Few studies have focused attention on the geriatric homeless, but two studies conducted on older homeless men living on New York City's Bowery have found physical and mental health problems similar to those of their younger counterparts. Physically, the homeless elderly are in much worse shape than their housed counterparts. Almost one third had been hospitalized in the previous 12 months for a physical problem (Cohen et al, 1988). From a mental health perspective, 49% consumed alcohol daily, 23% had psychotic symptoms or a history of prior psychiatric hospitalization, one third were clinically depressed, and 5% had dementia (Cohen et al, 1988). Anecdotal evidence suggests a higher incidence of psychosis and a history of state psychiatric hospitalization among elderly homeless women.

Chapter Summary

This chapter focused on the medical–surgical and psychosocial problems of homeless single adults and the nurse's role in assisting the homeless in the hospital and in the community. It also presented an overview of the problem of homelessness in the United States and described the reality of street life. The nurse's role was described with use of the Peplau model of the work role of the psychiatric nurse. To the subroles of mother surrogate, technician, manager, socializing agent, counselor/ nurse psychotherapist, and teacher that Peplau identified was added the role of the nurse as political advocate. The rewards and special challenges for the nurse working with the homeless were also described.

Bibliography

Books

Brickner PW et al (eds). Health Care for the Homeless. New York, Springer Publishing, 1985.

Brickner PW et al (eds). Under the Safety Net. New York, WW Norton, 1990.

Caton CL. Homeless in America. New York, Oxford University Press, 1990.

Institute of Medicine. Homelessness, Health and Human Needs. Washington, DC, National Academy Press, 1988.

National Research Council. AIDS: The Second Decade. Washington, DC, National Academy Press, 1990.

U.S. Department of Health and Human Services. Healthy People 2000. Washington, DC, U.S. Government Printing Office, 1990.

Wright JD and Weber E. Homelessness and Health. Washington, DC, McGraw-Hill, 1987.

Journals

Bassuk EL, Rubin L, and Lauriat AS. Is homelessness a mental health problem? Am J Psychiatry 1984 Dec; 141(12):1546–1550.

Berne A et al. A nursing model for addressing the health needs of homeless families. Image: Journal of Nursing Scholarship 1990 Spring; 22(1): 8–13.

Breakey WR et al. Health and mental health problems of homeless men and women in Baltimore. JAMA 1989 Sep; 262(10):1352–1357.

Cohen C, Teresi J, and Holmes D. The mental health of old homeless men. J Am Geriatr Soc 1988 Jun; 36(6):492–501.

Cohen C et al. Survival strategies of older homeless men. Gerontologist 1988 Feb; 28(1):58–65.

Cohen N and Marcos L. Psychiatric care of the homeless mentally ill. Psychiatr Ann 1986 Dec; 16(12):729–732.

Ferguson MA. Psych nursing in a shelter for the homeless. Am J Nurs 1989 Aug; 89(8):1060–1062.

Fischer PJ. Criminal activity among the homeless: A study of arrests in Baltimore. Hosp Community Psychiatry 1988 Jan; 39(1):46–51.

Fischer PJ et al. Mental health and social characteristics of the homeless: A survey of mission users. Am J Public Health 1986 May; 76(5):519–524.

Fischer P and Breakey W. The epidemiology of alcohol, drug, and mental disorders among homeless persons. American Psychologist

Gelberg L and Linn LS. Assessing the physical health of homeless adults. JAMA 1989 Oct; 262(14):1973–1979.

Jones C. Foot care for the homeless. J Am Podiatr Assoc 1990 Jan; 80(1):41–44.

Koegel P, Burnam MA, and Farr RK. The prevalence of specific psychiatric disorders among homeless individuals in the inner-city of Los Angeles. Arch Gen Psychiatry 1988 Dec; 45(12):1085–1092.

Luder E et al. Assessment of the nutritional status of urban homeless adults. Public Health Rep 1989 Sep/Oct; 104(5):451–456.

Morris W and Crystal S. Diagnostic patterns in hospital use by an urban homeless population. West J Med 1989 Oct; 151(4):472–476.

Nardell E. Tuberculosis in homeless, residential care facilities, prisons, nursing homes, and other close communities. Semin Respir Infect 1989 Sep; 4(3):206–215.

Rafferty M. Standing up for America's homeless. Am J Nurs 1989 Dec; 89(12):1614–1619.

Ramsden SS, Baur S, and El Kabir DJ. Tuberculosis among the central London single homeless. J R Coll Physicians Lond 1988 Jan; 22(1):16–17.

Robertson M and Cousineu M. Health status and access to health services among the urban homeless. Am J Public Health 1986 May; 76(5):561–563.

Rossi P et al. The urban homeless: Estimating composition and size. Science 1987 Mar 13; 235:1336–1341.

Scharer K. Nursing therapy with abusive and neglectful families. J Psychosoc Nurs Ment Health Serv 1979 Sep; 17(9):12–21.

Schieffelbein C and Snider D. Tuberculosis control among the homeless population. Arch Intern Med 1988 Aug; 148(8):1843–1846.

Schmitz D. When IV drug abuse complicates AIDS. RN 1990 Jan; 53(1):60–67.

Stead W. Special problems in tuberculosis. Clin Chest Med 1989 Sep; 10(3):397–405.

Strasser J. Urban transient women. Am J Nurs 1978 Dec; 78(12):2076–2078.

Susser E, Struening EL, and Conover S. Psychiatric problems in homeless men. Arch Gen Psychiatry 1989 Sep; 46(9):845–850.

Torres R et al. Human immunodeficiency virus among homeless men in a New York City shelter. Arch Intern Med 1990 Oct; 150(10):2030–2036.

Torres R et al. Homelessness among hospitalized patients with the acquired immunodeficiency syndrome in New York City. JAMA 1987 Aug; 258(6):779–780.

Speeches

Bolden A. Delivering dental care in shelter-based programs. Presented at the 118th Annual Meeting of the American Public Health Association, New York, October 1990.

Reports

Barrow S et al. Effectiveness of programs for the mentally ill homeless: Final report. New York, New York State Psychiatric Institute, 1989.

Baxter E and Hopper K. Private lives, public spaces. New York, Community Service Society, 1981.

Joseph H and Roman-Nay H. The homeless intravenous drug abuser and the AIDS epidemic. Washington, DC, National Institute of Drug Abuse Monograph, 1988, pp 210–253.

National Coalition for the Homeless. Fighting to live: Homeless people with AIDS. New York, Coalition for the Homeless, 1990.

Rog D. Engaging homeless persons with mental illness into treatment. Alexandria, VA, National Mental Health Association, 1988.

Roth D et al. Homelessness in Ohio: A study of people in need. Columbus, Ohio Department of Mental Health, 1985.

Shaffer D and Caton CL. Runaway and homeless youth in New York City. New York, Report to the Ittelson Foundation, 1984.

Struening E. A study of residents of the New York City shelter system. New York, New York State Psychiatric Institute, 1986.

Newspaper Articles

Foderaro L. Queries first, aid later for a county's homeless. The New York Times, Sept 4, 1990, p B3.

Gaines-Carter P. AIDS adding to troubles of homeless. The Washington Post, Oct 22, 1990, p D5.

Nathan J. Disabled homeless are said to find shelters inaccessible. The New York Observer, Nov 30, 1987.

Newsletter

Lubran B. Alcohol and other drug problems among the homeless population. The Nation's Health 1989 Sep; 19(9):23–25.

Nursing Research Profile for Unit 3

Biophysical and Psychosocial Concepts Related to Health and Illness

Overview

Nursing research studies that focus on the psychosocial aspects of illness and aging are increasing in number and in scope. Those that have been directed toward studying illness behaviors have typically investigated the concepts of stress and anxiety in relation to medical or surgical events. Those that have focused on the area of gerontology have included investigations of health promotion and health maintenance issues for older persons as well as studies of the physical problems encountered by the elderly.

The following studies are presented as examples of the research that has been conducted in these areas. Although there are limitations to the generalizability of each of the studies, the nursing implications warrant consideration and further study.

Response to Illness

▷ **Nyamathi A and Kashiwabara A. Preoperative anxiety: Its effect on cognitive thinking. AORN J 1988 Jan; 47(1): 164–169.**

The researchers studied the relationships between preoperative anxiety levels and cognitive thinking in 60 patients scheduled for same-day surgery in an acute care community hospital. Patients excluded from the study were those who had diagnoses of cancer and those who had previous surgery within the past 6 months. The levels of preoperative anxiety were measured by use of the State Trait Anxiety Inventory; critical thinking abilities were measured by use of the Critical Thinking Appraisal Tool. Variables of age, gender, and education were correlated, and results revealed that there were no statistically significant correlations except for women undergoing gynecologic surgery. Results of the study showed that subjects who had high State Trait Anxiety Inventory scores also had low scores on the Critical Thinking Appraisal.

Nursing Implications. Patient teaching is a vital part of preoperative preparation. If the anxiety level of the patient is high, short-term memory may be impaired, perception of the environment may be narrowed, and cognitive thinking and the

ability to problem solve may be decreased. Therefore, nurses should not assume that because information has been shared with the patient learning has necessarily occurred. Having the patient repeat the information and reinforcing that behavior while helping the patient reduce his anxiety level can help him to make decisions, problem solve, and learn.

▷ **Davis T and Jensen L. Identifying depression in medical patients. Image: Journal of Nursing Scholarship 1988; 20(4): 191–194.**

The Beck Depression Inventory (BDI) and the Structured Clinical Interview for DSM-III: Major Depressive Episode Section (SCID) were compared in an effort to identify optimal methods of assessing depression in medical patients. The subjects selected for study were 52 patients with myocardial infarction who were assessed at hospital discharge and 8 weeks later. The results indicated that although the Beck Depression Inventory can be used to evaluate patients for depression, the Structured Clinical Interview for DSM-III is the better method for assessing depression in patients with medical illnesses.

Nursing Implications. Depression is seen in both physically ill patients and those of the general population who are not physically ill. Physically ill patients may demonstrate both normal and abnormal mood. It is vital for nurses to respond to patients with depressive symptoms. Nurses are encouraged to use the Major Depressive Episode Section of the Structured Clinical Interview for DSM-III to assess patients with medical illnesses for depression and depressive symptomatology.

▷ **Wilson V. Identification of stressors related to patients' psychologic responses to the surgical intensive care unit. Heart Lung 1987 May; 16(3):267–273.**

Transient delirium, or impaired psychologic response, is observed in surgical intensive care unit patients in varying degrees. Change in the mental status of the patient may occur as early as the first postoperative day or may not be seen until the fifth postoperative day. A change in mental status of postoperative patients occurs more frequently when the patients are in the surgical intensive care unit than when on a general surgical unit.

The purpose of Wilson's study was to determine the incidence of impaired psychologic response and the relationship between psychologic response to the surgical intensive care unit and self-identification of stressors. Thirty-eight patients in a surgical intensive care unit were studied. Results revealed that those patients who experienced changes in mental status while in the surgical intensive care unit were most affected by four identified stressors: too much noise, losing track of time, having doctors and nurses talk *about* them rather than *to* them, and being examined by several doctors and nurses.

Nursing Implications.   Nursing interventions should be directed toward primary, secondary, and tertiary prevention of stressors. Primary prevention includes decreasing noise made by machines, providing clocks and calendars, talking directly to patients, and assigning the same nurse to care for the patient while he is in the surgical intensive care unit. Secondary prevention involves assessment and early treatment of changes in mental status. Reorientation (to person, place, or time), explanation of activities, and reassurance are often helpful. Tertiary prevention focuses on continuous explanations, reeducation, and reinforcements for patients.

Health Care of the Elderly

▷ *Schank MJ and Lough MA. Maintaining health and independence of elderly women. J Gerontol Nurs 1989 Jun; 15(6):8–11.*

The purpose of this exploratory study was to identify the reported health status and social support of elderly women living in noninstitutionalized settings. One hundred community-residing older women were studied. Half of these (N = 50) lived in public housing for the elderly and half (N = 50) lived in private housing for the elderly. A structured interview questionnaire designed to measure health status and social support was used for data collection.

The study revealed that those women living in private housing showed significantly higher levels of education and finances than their counterparts in public housing. The older women living in private housing more frequently reported excellent or good health status and a more positive attitude toward life than those living in public housing. Those women reporting excellent or good health had a greater degree of social support than the respondents reporting fair or poor health.

Nursing Implications.   Nurses must include social support assessment as a component of health assessment. Then, with a knowledge of available social support systems, the nurse can promote use of these resources consistent with the clients' needs and interests.

▷ *Patsdaughter CA and Pesznecker BL. Medication regimens and the elderly home care client. J Gerontol Nurs 1988 Oct; 14(10):30–34.*

Adults take more prescription and nonprescription medications as they get older. Older persons often experience a variety of problems related to self-administration of medications. These problems include (1) incorrect dosage, (2) inability to read the label or open the container, (3) lack of knowledge about the purpose of the medication, (4) poor medication storage, (5) forgetfulness or confusion about the medication, (6) difficulty obtaining medications because of cost or transportation, (7) inability to distinguish medications, and (8) adverse reactions.

The purpose of this study was to describe nurses' assessment and intervention activities related to facilitating appropriate home self-administration of medications. Forty-eight nurses who worked in home health care agencies for the elderly participated in the study. Following assessment of the medication-taking behavior of a patient, each nurse tape recorded her responses to seven general questions about her assessment of the patient and subsequent interventions.

Analysis of the responses of the nurses revealed that the majority of their interventions focused on teaching patients and their families about the medications. No responses indicated that insurance or financial agencies had been contacted or that polypharmacy had been addressed; few responses indicated that sensory or functional aids for self-administration of medications had been initiated.

Nursing Implications.   As an adjunct to patient teaching, the nurse should use varied interventions where they are indicated. A full assessment of the individual within the home situation may reveal interfering problems that teaching alone will not resolve. Communication with other health professionals, counseling regarding barriers to compliance, and supportive activities related to sensory and functional deficits may be appropriate strategies.

▷ *Johnston L and Gueldner SH. Remember when . . . ? Using mnemonics to boost memory in the elderly. J Gerontol Nurs 1989 Aug; 15(8):22–26.*

Short-term memory loss, a common occurrence in older persons, can cause anxiety, loss of self-esteem, and social withdrawal. To improve memory efficiency, learned skills of mnemonics, including digital grouping, memory pegging, and paired association, have been shown to be useful.

The purpose of this study was to examine the effect of a structured mnemonic memory skills improvement course on memory and self-esteem of independent, community-based adults. All the study volunteers were aware of memory loss and had no more than moderate mental impairment as measured by the Pfeiffer Short Mental Status Questionnaire. Eleven males and 20 females, aged 50 to 70 years, constituted the study population. Fifteen of the subjects were assigned to an experimental group that received a four-session mnemonics instruction program. Pretesting was accomplished with the Wechsler Memory Scale and the Rosenberg Self-Esteem Scale; post-testing was conducted 2 weeks after the final session of the mnemonics instruction program. Post-test results revealed that the experimental group demonstrated significant improvement in both memory and self-esteem as compared with the control group. Following the study, the members of the control group were provided with the opportunity to receive the mnemonics instruction program.

Nursing Implications.   This simple, effective intervention can be used by nurses and other caregivers to help older persons cope with the effects of memory loss associated with aging. Increased self-esteem and allayed anxiety can promote independence and contribute to a higher quality of life for the older person.

Additional Studies

Berryman E et al. Point by point: Predicting elders' falls. Geriatr Nurs 1989 Jul/Aug; 10(4):199–201.

Brink C, Wells T, and Diokno A. Urinary incontinence in women. Public Health Nurs 1987 Jun; 4(2):114–119.

Burgio LD, Jones LT, and Engel BT. Studying incontinence in an urban nursing home. J Gerontol Nurs 1988 Apr; 14(4):40–45.

Gaspar PM. What determines how much patients drink? Geriatr Nurs 1988 Jul/Aug; 9(4):221–224.

Haight BK. Nursing research in long-term facilities (1984–1988). Nurs Health Care 1989 Mar; 10(3):147–150.

Hamilton GP. Prevent elder abuse: Using a family systems approach. J Gerontol Nurs 1989 Mar; 15(3):21–26.

Harrell JS et al. Do nursing diagnoses affect functional status? J Gerontol Nurs 1989 Oct; 15(10):13–19.

Horgan PA. Health status perceptions affect health-related behaviors. J Gerontol Nurs 1987 Dec; 13(12):30–33.

O'Leary PA et al. Gerontological research: Is it useful for nursing practice? J Gerontol Nurs 1990 May; 16(5):28–32.

Palmer MH, McCormick KA, and Langford A. Do nurses consistently document incontinence? J Gerontol Nurs 1989 Dec; 15(12):11–16.

Richter JM. Support: A resource during crisis of mate loss. J Gerontol Nurs 1987 Nov; 13(11):18–22.

Strumpf NE and Evans LK. Physical restraint of the hospitalized elderly: Perceptions of patients and nurses. Nurs Res 1988 May/Jun; 37(3): 132–137.

Weinberg AD et al. Death in the nursing home: Senescence, infection and other causes. J Gerontol Nurs 1989 Apr; 15(4):12–16.

Winger J and Schirm V. Managing aggressive elderly in long-term care. J Gerontol Nurs 1989 Feb; 15(2):28–33.

unit 4

Concepts and Challenges in Patient Management

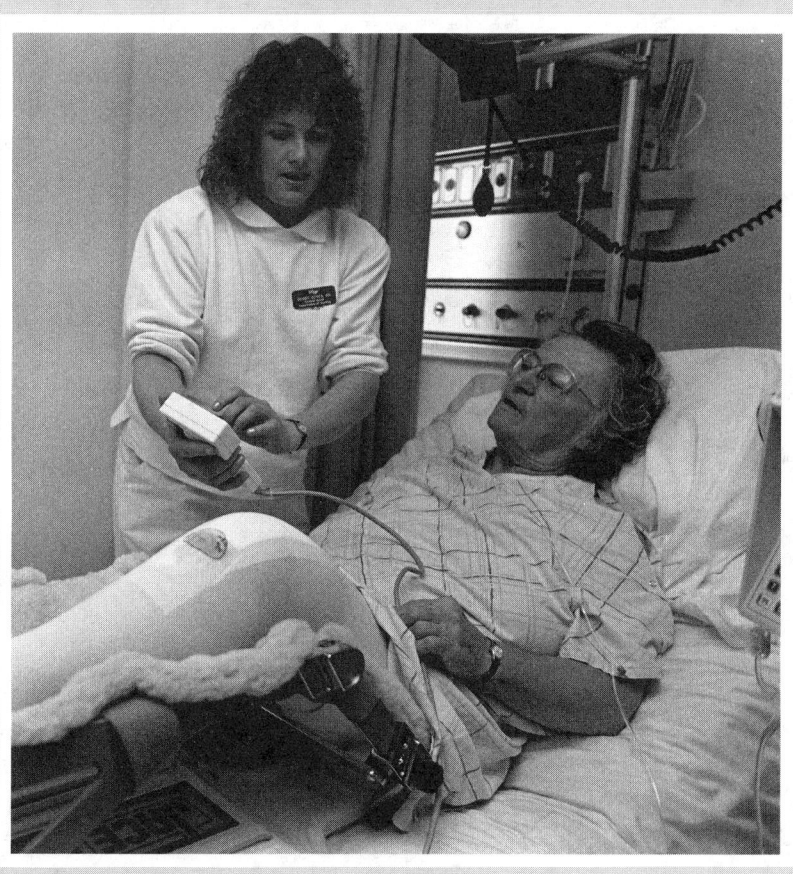

14

Principles and Practices of Rehabilitation

Learning Objectives

On completion of this chapter, the learner will be able to:

1. Describe the current philosophy of rehabilitation
2. Discuss the interdisciplinary approach to rehabilitation
3. Identify the usual series of emotional reactions exhibited by patients with newly acquired disabilities
4. Use the nursing process as a framework for care of patients with self-care deficits, impaired physical mobility, impaired skin integrity, and altered patterns of elimination
5. Describe nursing strategies appropriate for promoting self-care through activities of daily living
6. Describe nursing strategies appropriate for promoting mobility and ambulation and the use of assistive devices
7. Describe risk factors and related nursing measures to prevent development of pressure ulcers
8. Incorporate bladder training and bowel training into the plan of care for patients with problems of bladder and bowel incontinence
9. Describe the significance of continuity of care from the health care facility to the home or extended care facility for patients who need rehabilitative assistance and services

Philosophy of Rehabilitation

It is never how high one rises that determines one's merit, but rather how far one has come, considering his difficulties.
— Archibald Rutledge

Rehabilitation is a dynamic, health-oriented process that assists an individual who is ill or disabled to achieve his greatest pos-sible level of physical, mental, spiritual, social, and economic functioning. The rehabilitation process helps the person achieve an acceptable quality of life with dignity, self-respect, and independence. During rehabilitation, the individual is assisted to adjust to his disability by learning how to use his resources and to focus on existing abilities. *Abilities, not disabilities,* are emphasized. The individual learns how to live with residual, permanent disabilities. Genuine adjustment is an inner process and involves examination and possible reorientation of values.

Rehabilitation team members, recognizing the commonalities among all people and the uniqueness of individuals, work with the patient, helping him move from dependence to satisfying independence. The person is encouraged to be an active member of the rehabilitation team and to use the strength of his inner resources to develop a satisfying way of life. He is assisted in learning to cope with the problems and partake of the joys of life.

Rehabilitation is an integral part of nursing. Rehabilitation efforts should begin during the initial contact with the patient. Every major illness carries with it the threat of disability. *The principles of rehabilitation are basic to the care of all patients.* The emphasis of rehabilitation is on restoring the patient to independence or to regain his pre-illness/predisability level of function in as short a time as possible. If this is not possible, maximal independence within the limits of the disability and achievement of an acceptable quality of life are the overall aims. Realistic goals based on individual patient assessment are established to guide the rehabilitation program.

The patient must be an active participant in the rehabilitation goal setting and in the rehabilitation process. Only then can the individual achieve the desired level of self-sufficiency. Optimal functioning in his daily routine—the activities of daily living—is facilitated. The individual with a disability is encouraged to wear his own clothing during rehabilitation; this enhances self esteem and dignity and connotes health and wellness. The rehabilitation program motivates the patient and helps him to attain social independence and vocational reintegration when possible. It is through the support of the members of the rehabilitation team that the patient becomes all that he is capable of being.

Rehabilitation programs are designed for individuals with physical disabilities as well as mental and emotional handicaps. To focus on the needs of groups of people with specific conditions, special rehabilitation programs, such as cardiac and pulmonary rehabilitation, have been developed.

Rehabilitation services will be required by more people in the future, because advances in technology are saving the lives of the seriously ill and disabled. Every patient, regardless of age, socioeconomic status, or diagnosis, has a right to rehabilitation services. If individuals with disabilities are unable to receive needed rehabilitation services, recovery time is prolonged, existing abilities may not be developed, contractures and additional losses may occur that contribute to the disability, and the patient may experience additional pain and discomfort.

The economic advantage of rehabilitation is readily apparent; instead of being unemployed, the person is rehabilitated into employment. Instead of being dependent on society, he contributes to it.

Gerontologic Considerations

Dependency is the greatest concern of the aged. Doing even simple activities is very important to the frail elderly. Short-term rehabilitation goals must include maintaining independence. The health care personnel need to support independence and rehabilitative efforts. The older adult is encouraged to make decisions and to perform meaningful tasks. The older adult may require more time to learn self-care activities, exercises, transfer techniques, and independent mobility. Rehabilitation programs for the elderly must consider multiple pathologies, reduced physiologic reserve, impairments of mobility and balance, as well as mental status changes. The very old require an extensive support system.

Psychological Implications of a Disability

A physical disability has a direct impact on the patient's body image and often has a deep psychological significance to the patient. The patient may have the shattering realization that he can do less than formerly. The patient's shape and posture may have changed. His ability to socially interact with others may be altered. His position in the family, social system, and society may be different. The patient may perceive himself as a devalued person, a second-class citizen. In short, the patient may feel that he is different.

Depending on his premorbid personality, occupation, cultural background, and social status and on the support received from significant others, the disability may mean inconvenience, hardship, or tragedy to the individual. Self-concept, locus of control, hardiness, and social support are important factors in adaptation to a disability.

Emotional Reactions to Disability

A person usually goes through a series of emotional reactions to a newly acquired disability. The first reaction may be confusion, disorganization, and denial. The patient is in a state of conflict and faces problems of forced dependence, loss of self-esteem, and feelings that his personal and family integrity are threatened. The patient may refuse to accept these new limitations and at times has an unjustified overconfidence in speedy recovery. These false hopes lead the patient to hear only what he wants to hear. The patient may be self-centered and even childlike in his demands. The mechanism of denial is useful up to a certain point, but eventually the reality of the situation must be acknowledged.

The patient may progress to a stage of grief and depression in which he appears to mourn for the lost function or missing body part. (Depression may also be caused by sensory deprivation and restricted environmental stimulation.) There may be behavioral changes, particularly regression. This stage of grief appears to be a necessary phase in adapting to the disability. Grieving is part of the process of working through the meaning of the losses and is part of the emotional work of rehabilitation. Therefore, the patient should not merely be encouraged blithely to "cheer up." Such an approach can evoke extreme hostility and provoke behavior that will result in a "problem patient." Listening to the patient talk about his loss is important for healing.

The patient may go through a stage of anger in which he projects blame on others. This behavior frequently alienates the family and health care personnel, who may either capitulate to the patient's demands or withdraw from him.

Following the stages of depression, grief, and anger, there is generally a period of adaptation and adjustment. In time, the patient becomes more familiar with the condition and is able to tolerate it better. As the patient revises his body image and modifies his former picture of himself, the patient redirects his energies toward coping with his physical functioning.

The patient is able to accept a degree of dependency and not resent reliance on others for formerly easy or routine tasks. The patient begins to realize that hopelessness is futile and knows that he must adapt to the permanent aspects of the disability and modify his goals.

The acceptance of the limitations imposed by the disability and the total investment of the patient in his rehabilitation program is basic to adjustment. It is at this point in rehabilitation that the patient begins to look ahead and develop realistic goals for his future.

At the same time, it is important to realize that not all patients will progress in orderly fashion through the stages of grieving. Many frequently fluctuate between acceptance and grief, so that angry outbursts and depression may continue long after the usual period of mourning has supposedly passed. Each new situation (going home, starting vocational rehabilitation, entering a new relationship) reminds the patient anew of his limitations, changed body image, and the reality of the permanence of his situation. Satisfactory social experiences help renew a positive self-concept.

At the other end of the spectrum are those patients who do not accept their disability but instead waste emotional energy in rebelling futilely against unalterable damage. Or, there are those patients who ignore the disability and refuse to put forth any effort to adapt to everyday living. Still others may overreact and build a false reputation for being "cheerful and courageous." Although "ignoring" may seem healthy, often it involves a total rejection of the disability, which keeps the patient from doing those things that will be helpful to him. When a person fails to react at the appropriate time, it may indicate that he is not coping adequately. These patients may require assistance from a mental health professional. (The reader is referred to Chapter 10 for additional readings on responses to illness and coping strategies.)

Coping With Fatigue

Another problem faced by individuals with a disability is fatigue. Because it is uncomfortable and tiring to live with a physical disability, the disabled are vulnerable to fatigue. Physical disabilities have to be faced daily, and frustration brings weariness to mind and body. The fear of falling may always be present, and mobility often remains a minute-by-minute challenge fraught with difficulties. Walking with crutches or braces requires a high expenditure of energy.

The following may be useful in teaching patients how to reduce their energy output, thus conserving their strength to achieve a meaningful life-style.

Have well-defined goals and priorities.
- Keep priorities in order; eliminate nonessential activities.
- Plan and pace your activities.
    Plan each day.
    Distribute heavy work load throughout week.
    Organize work; have equipment within easy reach.
    Keep work in front of you.
- Rest before undertaking difficult tasks.
- Stop the activity before fatigue sets in.
- Continue with exercise conditioning program to strengthen muscles.

Control your environment.
- Try to be well organized.
- Place possessions in same place, so that they can be found with minimum of effort.
- Place equipment in box/basket (personal care, crafts, work).
- Use energy conservation and work simplification techniques.
- Use adaptive equipment, self-help aids, labor-saving devices.
- Take safety precautions.

Take control of your life.
- Face the reality of your disability.
- Emphasize areas of strength.
- Remain outward looking.
- Seek inventive ways to tackle problems.
- Maintain and improve general health.
- Plan for recreation.

Sexuality Issues

Sexuality involves not only biologic sexual activity but also the person's concept of his masculinity or her femininity and the way he reacts to others and is perceived by them. It takes many forms: caring, reaching out, sharing, and emotional intimacy. There is a growing recognition of the sexual needs and problems of the disabled.

Sexual matters are considered to be in the very private realm, and the patient is likely to be reticent about discussing his feelings. The professional person is focusing so intently on the rehabilitation of the patient (*i.e.*, helping him to gain independence) that there is a tendency to forget that sexuality is part of the patient's personality. Recognizing and dealing with sexual concerns are basic in establishing feelings of self-worth, which are essential to total rehabilitation. Professional personnel, family members, and the community must deal with the reality that disabled persons are sexual human beings with needs for social affiliation and sexual intimacy.

Problems faced by the disabled include limited access to information about sexuality, lack of opportunity to form friendships and loving relationships, impaired self-image and low self-esteem, and lack of social skills.

The sexuality concerns of the patient must be identified through an individual approach. The patient is encouraged to talk about his anxieties related to sex. The disabled person may need further sex education, communication, and social and assertiveness skills to develop relationships in general. The specialized services of a sex counselor are available to help those with specific sexual needs or conflicts. Classes, books, movies, and support groups are also useful. (The reader is referred to Chapter 17 for additional reading related to sexuality.)

The Rehabilitation Team

Rehabilitation is a creative, dynamic process that requires a team of professionals working together with the patient and his family. The team members represent a variety of disciplines, with each health professional making a unique contribution. Each health professional assesses the patient and identifies patient needs within the discipline's domain. Rehabilitative goals are set. Team members meet in group sessions at frequent intervals to collaborate, to evaluate progress, and to modify goals as needed to facilitate rehabilitation.

The *patient* is the key member of the rehabilitation team. He is the focus of the team effort and the one who determines the final outcomes of the process. The patient participates in goal setting, in learning to function using residual abilities, and in adjusting to living with disabilities. He is assisted in achieving independence, self-respect, and an acceptable quality of life.

The *patient's family* is incorporated into the team. The family is recognized as a dynamic system. Disability of one member affects other family members. Only by incorporating the family into the rehabilitation process can the family system adapt to the change in one of its members. The family provides ongoing support, participates in problem solving, and learns to provide necessary ongoing care.

The *rehabilitation nurse* develops a therapeutic and supportive relationship with the patient and his family. The nurse works with the patient, always emphasizing assets and strengths. During nurse–patient interactions, the nurse actively listens, encourages, and shares the patient's triumphs as he progresses in the program. The patient is praised for efforts to improve self-concept and self-care abilities.

Through application of the nursing process, the nurse develops a plan of care designed to facilitate rehabilitation, to restore and maintain optimum health, and to prevent complications. The nurse helps the patient to identify strengths and past successes and to develop new goals. Frequently, coping with the disability, self-care, mobility, skin care, and bowel and bladder management are areas for nursing intervention. The nurse assumes roles of caregiver, teacher, counselor, patient advocate, and consultant. Frequently the nurse is the case manager responsible for coordinating the total rehabilitative plan.

The *physician* is responsible for medical diagnosis and treatment. Included in this responsibility is the direction and coordination of the patient's therapeutic program.

The *physiatrist* is a physician-specialist in physical medicine and rehabilitation. The physiatrist's responsibilities include testing the patient's physical functioning, determining the potential functional goal, prescribing treatment for disorders of neuromusculoskeletal function, and supervising the physical medicine rehabilitation program.

The *physical therapist* uses multiple prescribed physical modalities and exercises to strengthen weak muscles, to relax spastic muscles, and to retrain muscles. Under the direction of the physical therapist, the patient learns how to transfer and maximize his mobility.

The *occupational therapist* assists the person with a disability to adapt to the challenges of daily living. Independent self-care and successful interaction with the environment are goals. The occupational therapist devises practical projects to improve the patient's strength and coordination, teaches energy conservation techniques, plans work simplification, fashions splints, and recommends adaptive equipment.

The *speech–language pathologist* helps the patient reestablish effective communication. In addition, the speech–language pathologist is involved in the diagnosis and treatment of swallowing disorders (dysphagia).

The *psychologist* assesses the patient's cognitive, perceptual, and behavioral status, as well as his motivation, values, and attitudes toward the disability. The psychologist helps the patient and his family cope with the problems that have occurred as a result of the patient's disability. Frequently the psychologist also works with the staff to help them manage the stress associated with patient care.

The *social worker* assesses the patient's socioeconomic status (*i.e.*, life-style, coping patterns, resources, support system). The social worker advises the patient and family about financial matters and disability benefits. The social worker assists in the transition from rehabilitation setting to home and community.

Career change may be necessary because of the nature of the disability. The *vocational counselor* tests the patient to determine his interests and aptitudes for vocational training. The vocational counselor advises the patient about appropriate vocational training, job modifications, and employment opportunities.

The *orthotist/prosthetist* designs and fabricates orthoses and prostheses (*e.g.*, extremity, joint, eye, breast). He is responsible for designing, fitting, and training the patient to use these.

The *rehabilitation engineer* uses science and technology to design and construct devices that help individuals with severe and multiple disabilities to function as independently and as productively as possible. There are a wide variety of electronic assistive devices designed to help the severely disabled person function with less dependence on others. Electronic devices include visual and mobility aids for the blind, aids for persons with hearing and tactile impairments, aids for those with communicative disorders, and manipulation and mobility aids.

The *sex counselor* assists the individual with a disability with problems related to sexuality. This role may be assumed by the psychologist, nurse, social worker, or certified sex therapist.

Assessment for Rehabilitation

Comprehensive assessment completed by the rehabilitation team members is the basis for formulation of a rehabilitation program. In addition to basic physiologic, psychological, and socioeconomic assessments, specific cognitive, behavioral, family, vocational, and functional ability assessments are completed.

Nursing assessment requires a holistic approach. Physical, mental, emotional, spiritual, social, and economic status must be assessed. The rehabilitation nurse focuses on coping patterns, functional ability, mobility, integrity of skin, and control of bowel and bladder function.

The nurse recognizes the patient as an individual and as a part of a family system. Because no two people react in the same way to a disability, the nurse must determine the patient's and family's perceptions of changes in body function or structure and coping patterns.

Functional ability assessment is another focus for rehabilitation nursing. Functional ability focuses on self-care: feeding, bathing/hygiene, dressing/grooming, toileting, and mobility. Functional ability depends on good joint motion, muscle strength, and an intact neurologic system. Disabilities most likely to produce loss of function are those involving the musculoskeletal, neurologic, and cardiovascular systems. Secondary problems related to the disability, such as muscle atrophy and deconditioning, that may affect functional ability are assessed. Residual strengths unaffected by disease or disability are evaluated.

The nurse assesses the ability of an individual to function by watching the person perform the activity (eating, dressing) and noting the degree of independence, the time taken, and the amount of assistance required. The nurse notes the patient's ability to move and his coordination and endurance.

There are numerous indexes and scales to evaluate the functional abilities of the patient. Generally these are used to assess the individual's ability to perform activities of daily living independently and ability to move as well as communicate. Rehabilitation centers use these indexes to initially assess the patient's abilities as well as to assess the patient's progress in independence.

The *PULSES* profile is used to assess *p*hysical condition (*e.g.*, health/illness status), *u*pper extremity functions (*e.g.*, eating, bathing), *l*ower extremity functions (*e.g.*, transfer, ambulation), *s*ensory functions (*e.g.*, vision, hearing, speech), *ex*cretory functions (*e.g.*, control of bowel/bladder), and *s*ituational factors (*e.g.*, social and financial support). Each of these areas is rated on a scale of 1 (independent) to 4 (greatest dependency).

The *Barthel Index* is used to measure the patient's level of independence in activities of daily living (feeding, bathing, dressing, grooming), continence, toileting, transfers, and ambulation (or wheelchair mobility). This scale does not consider communicative or cognitive abilities.

Functional Independence Measure (FIM) is used to assess the patient's level of independence in six areas, including communication and cognitive abilities. The six areas are self-care, sphincter management, mobility, locomotion, communication, and social cognition.

The *Patient Evaluation Conference System* (PECS) contains 15 categories. This comprehensive assessment scale includes the addition of such areas as medications, pain, nutrition, assistive devices, psychology, vocation, and recreation.

Other areas that require nursing assessment include potential for altered skin integrity and bowel and bladder control. For the individual to achieve maximal health, potential problems related to skin integrity must be identified. For the individual with a disability to achieve his highest level of functioning with dignity and self-respect, problems with bowel and bladder

control or management of incontinence must be identified and minimized.

▶ Nursing Process
Self-Care Deficit: Activities of Daily Living

Activities of daily living (ADLs) are those self-care activities that the patient must accomplish each day to meet his own needs and the demands of daily life. ADLs include personal hygiene/bathing, dressing/grooming, feeding, and toileting. Many patients are unable to perform these activities easily. An ADL program is started as soon as the rehabilitation process begins. The ability to perform ADLs is frequently the key to independence, return to the home, and reentry into the community.

◊ Assessment

The nurse must assess the patient's ability to perform ADLs to determine the level of independence in self-care and the need for nursing intervention. The nurse can do this by watching the patient perform an activity. The activity of bathing requires obtaining bath water and utensils, undressing, washing the body, and drying the body after bathing. Dressing requires selecting, putting on and taking off clothing, fastening the clothing, and combing the hair. Self-feeding requires selecting foods, using utensils to bring food to the mouth, and chewing and swallowing the food. The activity of toileting includes the ability to get to the toilet, removing clothing to use the toilet, getting on and off the toilet, cleansing self, redressing self, and performing hand hygiene. If the patient can sit up and raise his hands to his head, he probably can begin to bathe and feed himself. Balance and some muscle strength and coordination are required for dressing. Toileting requires transfer and dressing abilities.

One of the functional ability indexes may be useful in recording and tracking ADL abilities. In addition, the nurse needs to be aware of the patient's medical condition, functional capacity, and therapeutic goals. Assessment of the extent of assistance the family can provide is important in setting goals and in developing a plan of care.

◊ Nursing Diagnosis

Based on the assessment data, major nursing diagnoses for the patient may include the following:

- Self-care deficit: bathing/hygiene, dressing/grooming, feeding, toileting related to disability (*e.g.*, paralysis, amputation, neuromuscular impairment)

◊ Planning and Implementation

◊ *Goals:* The major goals of the patient include bathing/hygiene self independently or with assistance, using adaptive devices as appropriate; dressing/grooming self independently or with assistance, using adaptive devices as appropriate; feeding self independently or with assistance, using adaptive devices as appropriate; and toileting self independently or with assistance, using adaptive devices as appropriate.

Chart 14–1
Guidelines for Teaching the Activities of Daily Living

1. Define the goal of the activity with the patient. Be realistic. Set short-term goals that can be accomplished in the near future.
2. Identify several approaches to accomplish the task. (Example: There are several ways to put on a given garment.)
3. Select the approach most likely to succeed.
4. Specify the approach on the patient's care plan and the patient's level of accomplishment on the progress notes.
5. Identify the motions necessary to accomplish the activity. (Example: To pick up glass, extend arm; place open hand next to glass; flex fingers around glass; move arm/hand holding glass vertically; flex arm toward body.)
6. Focus on gross functional movements initially and gradually include activities that use finer motions (*e.g.*, buttoning clothes, eating with a fork).
7. Encourage the patient to perform the activity up to his maximal capacity within the framework of his disability.
8. Monitor the patient's tolerance.
9. Minimize frustration and fatigue.
10. Support the patient by giving appropriate praise for effort put forth and for acts accomplished.
11. Assist the patient to perform and practice the activity in real-life situation.

▷ Nursing Interventions

▷ *Self-Care: Bathing/Hygiene, Dressing/Grooming, Feeding, Toileting.* To effectively learn methods of self-care, the patient must be motivated. An "I'd rather do it myself" attitude is encouraged. The nurse must also help the patient identify the safe limits of independent activity. *Knowing when to ask for assistance is very important.*

The nurse teaches, guides, and supports the patient while he learns how to perform self-care activities. Consistency in instructions and assistance given by the caregiver facilitates the learning process. Recording the patient's performance provides data for evaluating progress and may be used as a source of motivation and for morale building. (See Chart 14–1: Guidelines for Teaching the Activities of Daily Living.)

Self-care techniques need to be adapted to accommodate the individual patient differences and life style. Often a simple maneuver requires concentration and the exertion of consid-

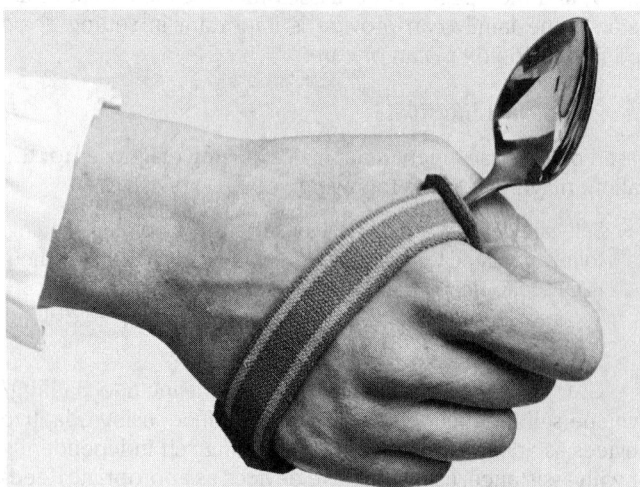

Figure 14–1. Universal ADL cuff. Eating utensils, toothbrush, comb, etc., can be inserted into cuff to promote independence for individuals with limited use of hands.

erable effort on the part of the individual with a disability. A great deal of common sense and a little ingenuity are frequently called for. It is important to remember that there is usually more than one way to accomplish a self-care activity. For example, if a person cannot quite reach his head, perhaps he will be able to do so by leaning forward.

If the patient has difficulty in performing an activity of daily living, an adaptive/assistive device (self-help device) may be useful. A large variety of assistive devices are available commercially or can be fabricated by the nurse, the occupational therapist, the patient, or the family. For example, the universal cuff (Fig. 14–1) is helpful for persons with limited use of the hands. Eating utensils, toothbrush, comb, and other essential items can be secured in the cuff, allowing independent use of the item. Long-handled combs and shoe horns are useful to many. "Building up" the handle on a spoon with a foam pad may be all that is necessary for independent eating. Automatic toothbrushes improve the oral hygiene of individuals with limited movements of the hands, wrists, and arms. Velcro fasteners on clothing and shoes are useful for those who have difficulty with buttons, zippers, and shoelaces. The nurse should be alert to "gadgets" coming on the market that may be useful to the individual with a disability. The nurse must exercise professional judgment and caution in recommending these to vulnerable patients.

A wide selection of computerized assistive devices is available or can be designed to help individuals with severe disabilities to function with less dependency. The Abledata System offers a computerized listing of commercially available aids and equipment for individuals with disabilities. Additional information is available from the National Rehabilitation Information Center.*

If a person is severely disabled, independent self-care may be an unrealistic goal. The individual with the disability may require a personal attendant to perform activities of daily living. Because of the roles one assumes in life, family members may

---

* *National Rehabilitation Information Center, 8455 Colesville Rd., Silver Spring, MD 20910-3319. Toll-free telephone number: 800-346-2742.*

not be appropriate for providing bathing/hygiene, dressing/grooming, feeding, and toileting assistance. A personal caregiver may need to be hired. The individual with the disability is assisted in accepting self-care dependency. Independence in other areas such as social interaction would be emphasized to promote self-concept: self-esteem, role performance, personal identity.

▷ Evaluation

Expected Outcomes

1. Demonstrates independent self-care in bathing/hygiene or with assistance, using adaptive devices as appropriate.
   a. Bathes self at maximal level of independence.
   b. Uses adaptive devices effectively.
   c. Reports satisfaction with level of independence in bathing.
2. Demonstrates independent self-care in dressing/grooming or with assistance, using adaptive devices as appropriate.
   a. Dresses/grooms self at maximal level of independence.
   b. Uses adaptive devices effectively.
   c. Reports satisfaction with level of independence in dressing/grooming.
   d. Demonstrates increased interest in appearance.
3. Demonstrates independent self-care in feeding or with assistance, using adaptive devices as appropriate.
   a. Feeds self at maximal level of independence.
   b. Uses adaptive devices effectively.
   c. Demonstrates increased interest in eating.
   d. Maintains adequate nutritional intake.
4. Demonstrates independent self-care in toileting or with assistance, using adaptive devices as appropriate.
   a. Toilets self at maximal level of independence.
   b. Uses adaptive devices effectively.
   c. Indicates positive feeling regarding level of toileting independence.
   d. Experiences adequate frequency of bowel and bladder elimination.
   e. Absence of incontinence, constipation, urinary tract infection, and other complications.

▶ Nursing Process
Impaired Physical Mobility

Individuals who are ill or injured are frequently placed on bed rest or have their activities limited. Problems frequently asso-

(text continues on page 224)

Chart 14–2
Range of Motion

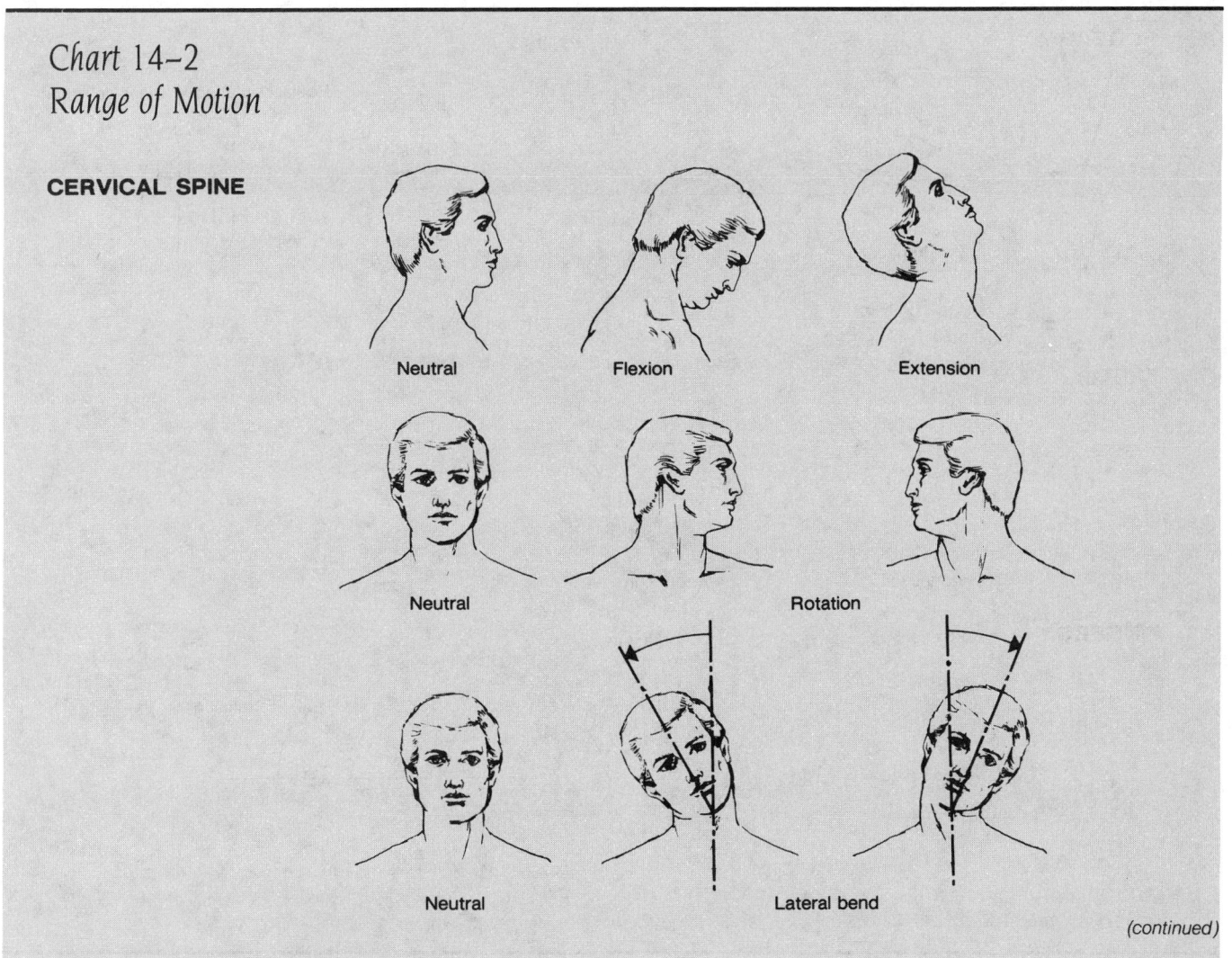

CERVICAL SPINE

Neutral   Flexion   Extension

Neutral   Rotation

Neutral   Lateral bend

(continued)

Chart 14-2 *(Continued)*

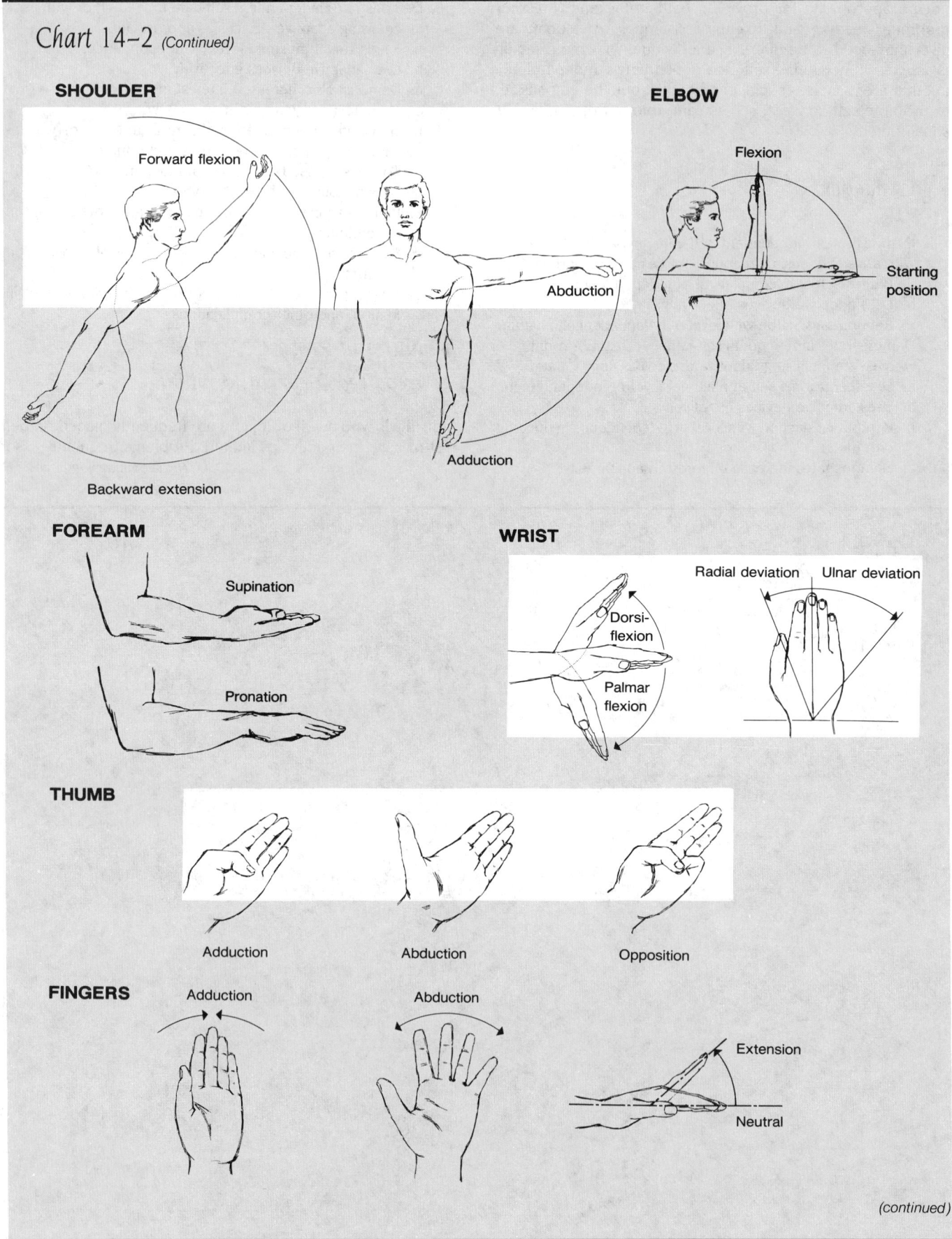

SHOULDER

Forward flexion

Abduction

Adduction

Backward extension

ELBOW

Flexion

Starting position

FOREARM

Supination

Pronation

WRIST

Radial deviation   Ulnar deviation

Dorsi-flexion

Palmar flexion

THUMB

Adduction

Abduction

Opposition

FINGERS

Adduction

Abduction

Extension

Neutral

(continued)

Chart 14-2 (Continued)

HIP

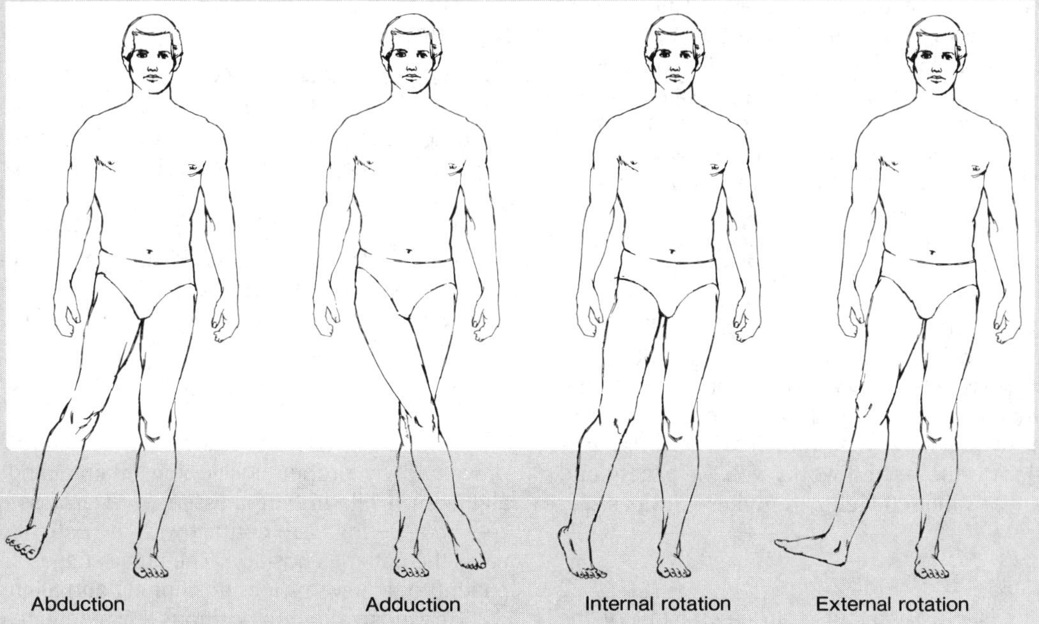

Abduction   Adduction   Internal rotation   External rotation

KNEE

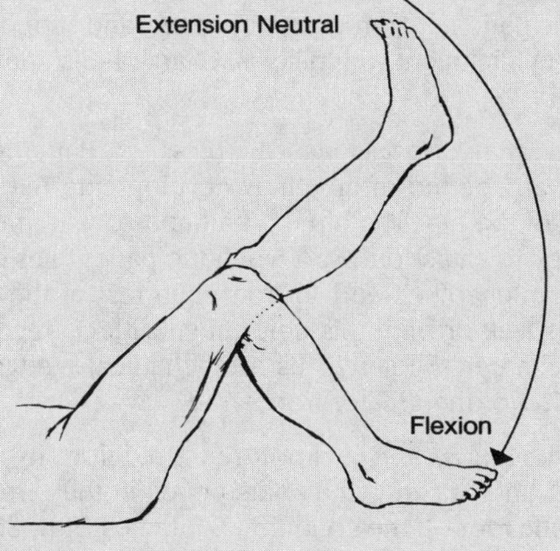

Extension Neutral

Flexion

ANKLE

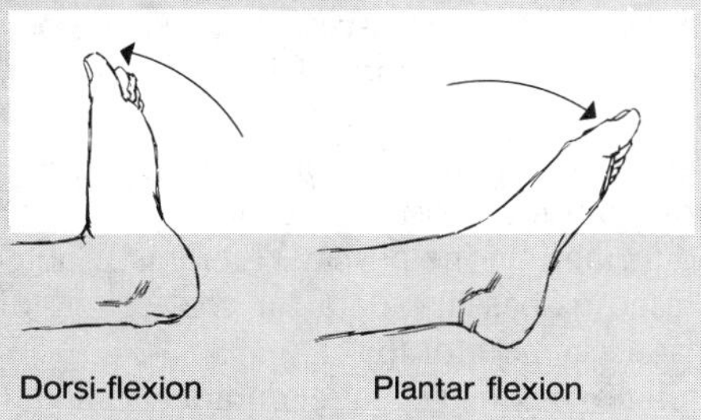

Dorsi-flexion   Plantar flexion

TOES

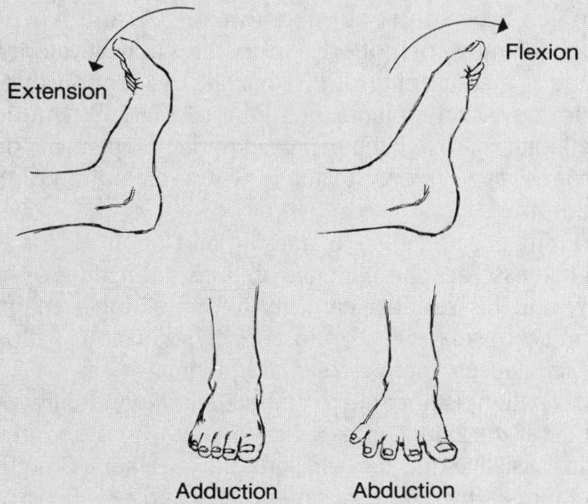

Extension   Flexion

Adduction   Abduction

FOOT

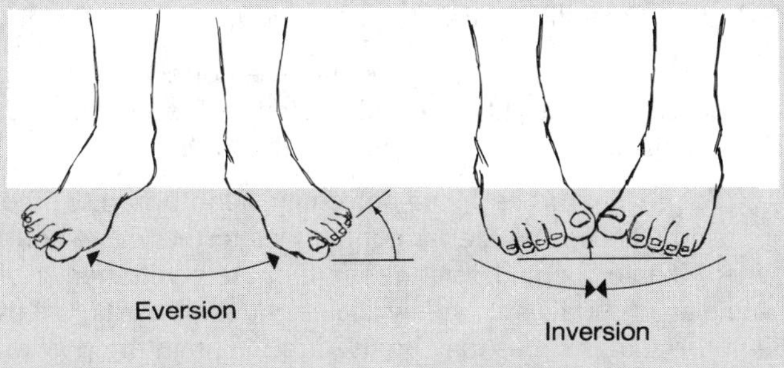

Eversion   Inversion

ciated with immobility include weakened muscles, joint contracture, and deformity. Each joint of the body has a normal range of motion (Chart 14–2). If the range is limited, the functions of the joint and of the muscles that move the joint are impaired and painful deformities may develop. Nurses must identify patients at risk for such complications.

Another problem frequently seen in rehabilitation nursing is an altered ambulatory/mobility pattern. The patient with a disability may be unable either temporarily or permanently to walk independently and unaided. The nurse assesses the mobility of the patient and designs care that promotes independent mobility within prescribed therapeutic limits.

At times an *orthosis*, an external appliance used to provide support and alignment, prevent or correct deformities, and improve the function of the body, must be used. Orthoses include braces, splints, collars, corsets, supports, or calipers designed and produced by an orthotist or prosthetist. Static orthoses (no moving parts) are used to stabilize joints and prevent contractures. Dynamic orthoses are flexible and are used to improve function by assisting weak muscles. The nurse recognizes the need for orthoses and works with the patient and orthotist to obtain maximum benefits from these devices.

Assessment

Included in the holistic assessment is an assessment of the patient's positioning, ability to move, muscular strength, joint function, and the prescribed mobility limits. At times an individual's mobility is restricted because of paralysis, loss of muscle strength, or the presence of an immobilizing device (*e.g.*, cast, brace).

Range of motion of joints can be measured using a goniometer (a protractor for measurement of joint motion). Generally this is performed by the physical therapist. Such determinations are used as baseline data for goal setting and for future comparisons to monitor for change.

Muscle strength, flexibility, and endurance testing may be performed by the physical therapist. Neurologic and muscle testing (*e.g.*, electromyogram, nerve conduction studies) may be conducted. The nurse reviews the results of these tests and gathers additional data by observing the patient move, noting his abilities and need for assistance.

When a person is not able to exercise and move joints through full range of motion, contractures may develop. A *contracture* is a shortening of the muscle and tendon that leads to deformity. Contractures limit joint mobility. When the contracted joint is moved, the patient experiences pain. In addition, it requires more energy to move when joints are contracted and deformed.

During position change, transfer, and ambulation activities, the nurse assesses the patient's abilities, the extent of his disability, and his residual capacity for physiologic adaptation. The nurse observes for orthostatic hypotension, pallor, diaphoresis, nausea, tachycardia, and fatigue.

If a patient is not able to ambulate independently, without assistance, the nurse assesses his ability to balance, transfer, and use assistive devices (*e.g.*, crutches, walker). Crutch walking requires a high energy expenditure and produces considerable cardiovascular stress. Older persons with reduced exercise capacity, decreased arm strength, and problems with balance due to age and multiple diseases may be unable to use crutches. A walker is more stable and may be a better choice for the older patient. The nurse assesses the patient's ability to use various devices that promote mobility.

If a patient uses an orthosis, the nurse monitors the patient for problems associated with its use.

Nursing Diagnosis

Based on the assessment data, major nursing diagnoses for the patient may include impaired physical mobility related to prescribed bed rest, neuromusculoskeletal disorder, immobilizing device, contracture, activity intolerance.

Planning and Implementation

Goals: The major goals of the patient may include absence of contracture and deformity, maintenance of muscle strength and joint mobility, independent mobility, and increased activity tolerance.

Nursing Interventions

Positioning. Deformities and contractures can often be prevented by proper positioning. Maintaining correct body alignment while in bed is essential regardless of the position selected. During each contact with the patient the nurse evaluates the patient's position. The nurse suggests and assists the patient to achieve proper positioning and alignment.

The most common positions that a patient assumes in bed are supine (dorsal), side-lying (lateral), and prone. The nurse helps the patient assume these positions and supports the body in correct alignment with pillows. Chart 14–3 summarizes these positions.

Preventing External Rotation of the Hip. Patients who are in bed for any period of time may develop external rotation deformity of the hip. The hip is a ball-and-socket joint and has a tendency to rotate outward when the patient lies on his back. A trochanter roll extending from the crest of the ilium to the midthigh will prevent this deformity. With correct placement, the trochanter roll serves as a mechanical wedge under the projection of the greater trochanter.

Preventing Footdrop. Footdrop is a deformity in which the foot is plantar flexed (the ankle bends in the direction of the sole of the foot). If the condition continues without correction, the patient will not be able to hold the foot in a normal position and will walk on his toes without touching the ground with the heel of his foot. The deformity is caused by contracture of both the gastrocnemius and the soleus muscles. Damage to the peroneal nerve may result in foot drop. It may also be produced by loss of flexibility of the Achilles tendon.

- Prolonged bed rest, lack of exercise, incorrect positioning in bed, and the weight of the bedding forcing the toes into plantar flexion are factors that contribute to footdrop.

To prevent this crippling deformity, a footboard or pillows are used to keep the feet at right angles to the legs when the patient is in a supine position. The feet are positioned so that both plantar surfaces are firmly against the footboard or pillows. High-top tennis shoes may be used to maintain the position.

The patient is encouraged to perform ankle exercises several times each hour. These exercises include dorsiflexion and plantar flexion of his feet, flexion and extension (curl and stretch) of the toes, and eversion and inversion of the feet at the ankles.

Chart 14-3
Positioning a Patient in Bed

Supine (Dorsal) Position

1. The head is in line with the spine, both laterally and anteroposteriorly.
2. The trunk is positioned so that flexion of the hips is minimized.
3. The arms are flexed at the elbow with the hands resting against the lateral abdomen.
4. The legs are extended with a small, firm support under the popliteal area.
5. The heels are supported off the mattress with a small pillow or towel roll at the ankle.
6. The toes are pointed straight up, supported by an adjusted foot board used to prevent footdrop.
7. Trochanter rolls are placed under the greater trochanter in the hip joint areas to prevent external rotation of the hip.

Side-Lying (Lateral) Position

1. The head is in line with the spine, supported by a pillow.
2. The body is in alignment and is not twisted.
3. Shoulders and elbows are flexed and the upper arm is supported by a pillow.
4. The uppermost hip joint is slightly forward and the leg is supported in a position of slight abduction by a pillow.
5. The feet are placed and supported in neutral dorsiflexion.
6. The back may be supported by a pillow.

Prone (on Abdomen) Position

1. The head is turned laterally and is in alignment with the rest of the body.
2. The arms are abducted and externally rotated at the shoulder joint; the elbows are flexed.
3. A small flat support is placed under the pelvis, extending from the level of the umbilicus to the upper third of the thigh.
4. The lower extemities remain in a neutral position.
5. The toes are suspended over the edge of the mattress.

▷ *Maintenance of Muscle Strength and Joint Mobility.* Exercise involves the function of muscles, nerves, bones, and joints as well as the cardiovascular and respiratory systems. *Return to function is dependent upon the strength of the musculature that controls the joints.* Both *range of motion exercises* and *therapeutic exercises* may be used to promote the rehabilitation of individuals with disabilities.

▷ *Range of Motion Exercises.* Range of motion is movement of a joint through its full range in all appropriate planes. (See Chart 14-2, Range of Motion. See also Chart 14-4, Definition of Terms.) To maintain or increase the motion of a joint, range of motion exercises (Chart 14-5) are initiated as soon as the patient's condition permits. The exercises are planned for the individual to accommodate the wide variation in the degrees of motion that persons of varying body build and age groups can attain.

Range of motion exercises may be *active* (performed by the patient under supervision of the nurse), *assisted* (the nurse helps the patient if unable to do exercise independently), or *passive* (performed by the nurse). Unless prescribed otherwise, a joint should be moved through its range of motion three times, at least twice a day. The joint should not be moved beyond its free range of motion. Therefore, the motion should be to the point of resistance and stopped at the point of pain. When muscle spasm is present, the joint should be moved slowly to the point of resistance, gentle steady pressure exerted until the muscle relaxes, and motion continued.

To perform assisted or passive range of motion exercises,

the patient must be in a comfortable supine position with arms at the sides and knees extended. Good body posture is maintained during the exercises. The nurse adjusts the bed to permit the use of good body mechanics during the exercise session.

When range of motion exercises are performed, the joint is supported, bones above the joint are stabilized, and the body part distal to the joint is moved through the range of motion of the joint. For example, when the elbow is taken through its range of motion, the humerus must be stabilized while the radius and ulna are moved through their ranges of motion at the elbow joint.

▷ *Therapeutic Exercises.* Therapeutic exercises are prescribed by the physician and performed with the assistance and guidance of a physical therapist or nurse.

The patient should have a clear understanding of what the prescribed exercise is to accomplish. Providing written instructions setting forth the frequency, duration, and number of repetitions, as well as simple line drawings of the exercise, help to assure adherence to the exercise program.

Exercise, when correctly performed, assists in (1) maintaining and building muscle strength, (2) maintaining joint function, (3) preventing deformity, (4) stimulating circulation, (5) building strength and endurance, and (6) promoting relaxation. Exercise is also valuable in helping restore the motivation and well-being of the patient. There are five types of exercise: passive, active assistive, active, resistive, and isometric. The description, purpose, and action of each of these exercises are summarized in Table 14-1.

Chart 14–4
Definition of Terms

Abduction—movement away from the midline of the body
Adduction—movement toward the midline of the body
Flexion—bending of a joint so that the angle of the joint diminishes
Extension—the return movement from flexion; the joint angle is increased
Rotation—turning or movement of a part around its axis
  Internal: turning inward, toward the center
  External: turning outward, away from the center
Dorsiflexion—movement that flexes or bends the hand back toward the body or foot toward the leg
Palmar flexion—movement that flexes or bends the hand in the direction of the palm
Plantar flexion—movement that flexes or bends the foot in the direction of the sole
Pronation—rotation of the forearm so that the palm of the hand is down
Supination—rotation of the forearm so that the palm of the hand is up
Opposition—touching thumb to each finger tip on same hand
Inversion—movement that turns the sole of the foot inward
Eversion—movement that turns the sole of the foot outward

▷ **Promoting Independent Mobility.** As soon as the patient's condition stabilizes and his physical condition permits, the patient is assisted to sit up on the side of the bed and then stand. The patient's tolerance of this activity is assessed.

Orthostatic (postural) hypotension may develop when the patient assumes a vertical position and, because of inadequate vasomotor reflexes, blood pools in the splanchnic (visceral) area and in the legs, resulting in inadequate cerebral circulation. If indicators of orthostatic hypotension (*i.e.*, pallor, diaphoresis, nausea, tachycardia, dizziness) are present, the activity is stopped and the patient is assisted to a supine position in bed.

Some disabilities, such as spinal cord injury, brain damage, and conditions that require extended periods in the recumbent position, prevent patients from assuming an upright position by the usual methods. A *tilt table*, a board that can be tilted in 5- to 10-degree increments from a horizontal to a vertical position, may be used to assist the patient to assume an upright position. In addition to promoting vasomotor adjustment to positional changes, the tilt table helps the patient with weight-bearing activities and standing balance and prevents disuse syndrome (*e.g.*, decalcification of the bones).

The patient is transferred from the bed to the tilt table, positioned so that he will not slide during standing, and secured to prevent falling. The feet are protected with a pair of proper fitting shoes.

The nurse stays with the patient during the tilting procedure and assesses his tolerance, monitoring for the development of orthostatic hypotension. The maximum angle of tilt is determined by the patient's tolerance and the desired amount of weight-bearing. The nurse monitors the patient's blood pressure and pulse and observes for pallor, diaphoresis, and complaints of dizziness or nausea. Drop in blood pressure, tachycardia, and signs and symptoms of cerebral insufficiency (*i.e.*, complaint of feeling faint and weakness) suggest intolerance of the upright position and the table is returned to the horizontal position. At times, in addition to gradual position change, a compression leotard or snug-fitting abdominal binder and elastic compression bandaging of the legs are needed to prevent orthostatic hypotension. Extended periods of standing are avoided because of venous pooling and pressure on the soles of the feet.

▷ **Assisting the Patient With Transfer.** A *transfer* is the movement of the patient from one place to another (*i.e.*, bed to chair, chair to commode, wheelchair to tub). As soon as the patient is permitted out of bed, transfer activities are started. The nurse assesses his ability to actively participate in the transfer.

While the patient is confined to bed, it is important that the patient maintain muscle strength and participate in "push-up" exercises to strengthen the arm and shoulder extensor muscles. The push-up exercise requires the patient to sit upright in bed; a book is placed under each of the patient's hands and he is instructed to push down on the book raising his body weight. It is desirable that the patient be able to raise and move his or her body in different directions by means of these push-up exercises.

If the muscles that the patient uses to lift himself off the bed are not strong enough to overcome the resistance of body weight, a polished lightweight board (transfer board; *sliding board*) may be used to bridge the gap between the bed and the chair. The patient slides across on the board. This board may also be used to transfer the patient from the chair to the toilet or bathtub bench. Safety is a primary concern during a transfer.

- Chairs and beds must be locked before the patient transfers.
- One end of the transfer board is placed under the patient's buttocks and the other end on the surface to which the transfer is being made (*i.e.*, the chair).
- The patient is instructed to push up with his hands to shift the buttocks and then to slide across the board to the other surface.

(text continues on page 230)

Chart 14–5
Range of Motion Exercises

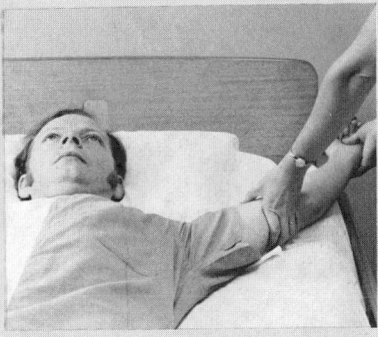

Abduction of shoulder. Move arm from side of body to above the head. Then return arm to side of body or neutral position (adduction).

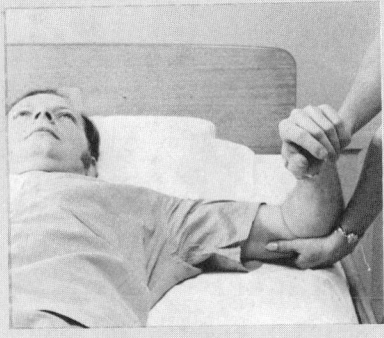

Internal rotation of shoulder. With arm at shoulder height, elbow bent at a 90-degree angle, and palm toward feet, turn upper arm until palm and forearm face backward.

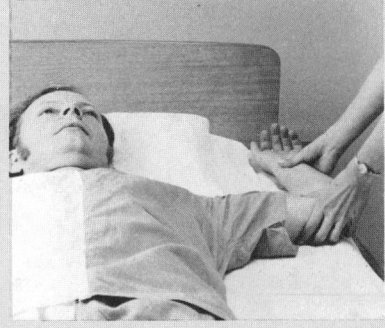

External rotation of shoulder. With arm at shoulder height, elbow bent at a 90-degree angle, and palm toward feet, turn upper arm until the palm and forearm face forward.

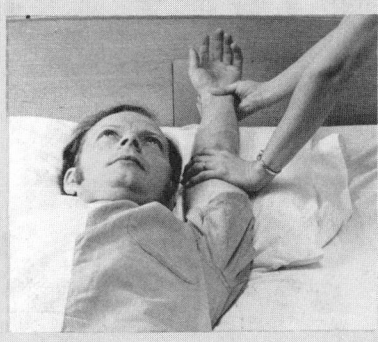

Forward flexion of shoulder. Move arm forward and upward until it is alongside of head.

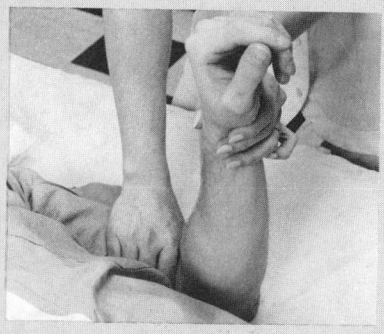

Pronation of forearm. With elbow at waist and bent at 90-degree angle, turn hand so that palm is facing down.

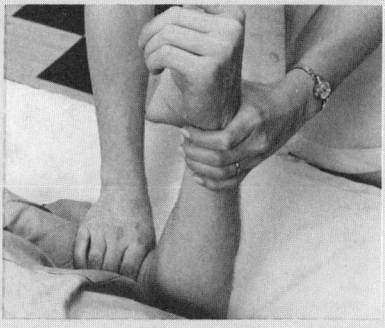

Supination of forearm. With elbow at waist and arm bent at 90-degree angle, turn hand so that palm is facing up.

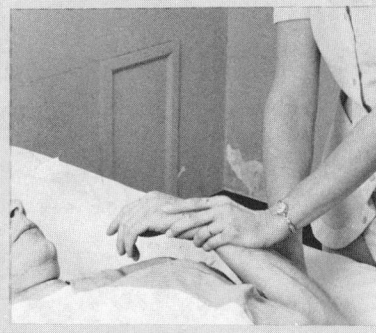

Flexion of elbow. Bend elbow, bringing forearm and hand toward shoulder. Then return forearm and hand to neutral position (arm straight).

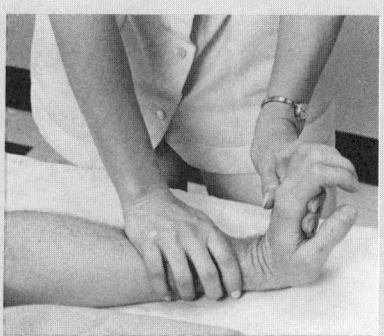

Wrist extension.

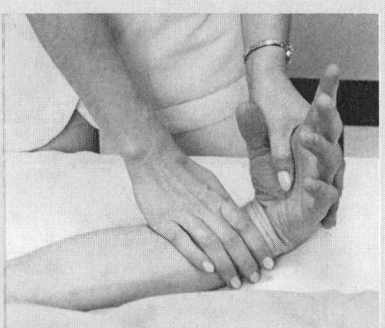

Flexion of wrist. Bend wrist so that palm is toward forearm. Straighten to a neutral position.

(continued)

Chart 14–5 (Continued)

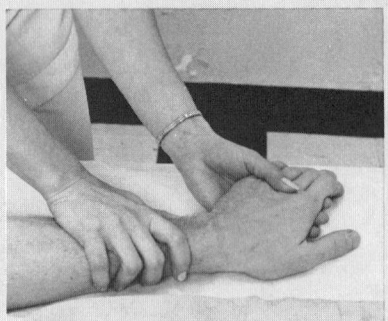

Ulnar deviation. Move hand sideways so that the side of hand on which little finger is located moves toward forearm.

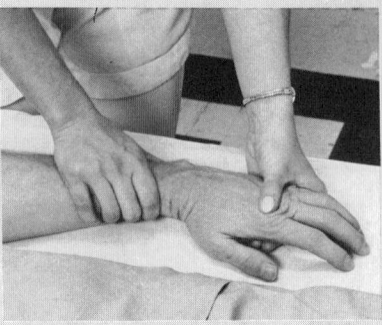

Radial deviation. Move hand sideways so that side of hand on which thumb is located moves toward forearm.

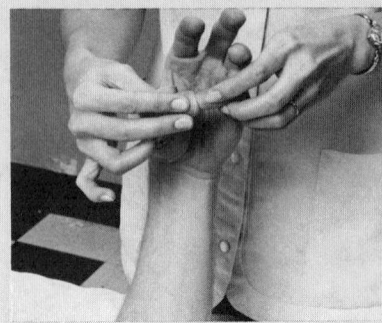

Thumb opposition. Move thumb out and around to touch little finger.

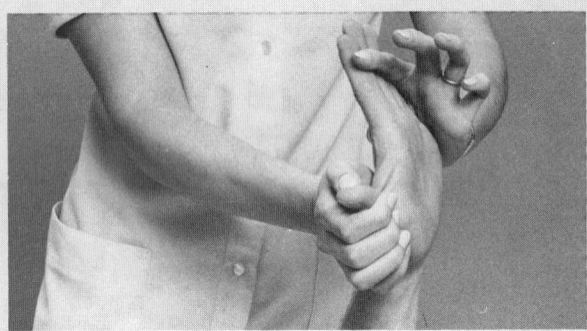

Extension of fingers.

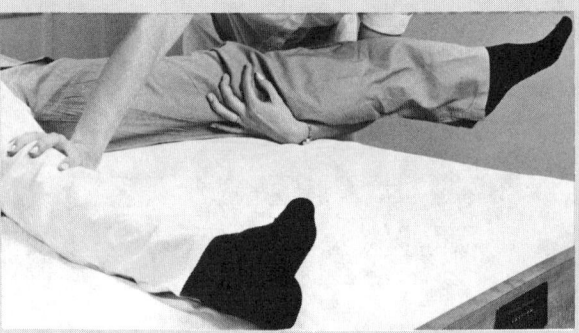

Abduction–adduction of hip. Move leg outward from the body as far as possible. Return leg from abducted position to neutral position and across the other leg as far as possible.

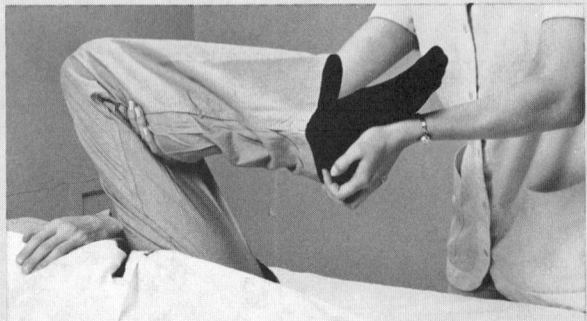

Flexion of hip and flexion of knee. Bend hip by moving the leg forward as far as possible. Return leg from the flexed position to the neutral position.

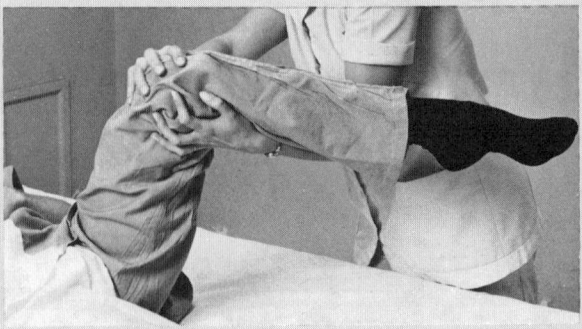

Internal–external rotation of hip. Turn leg in an inward motion so that toes point in. Turn leg in an outward motion so that toes point out.

(continued)

Chart 14–5 *(Continued)*

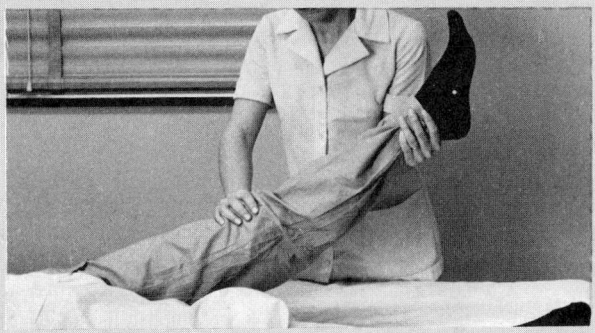

To stretch hamstring muscles, straighten leg and then raise the leg.

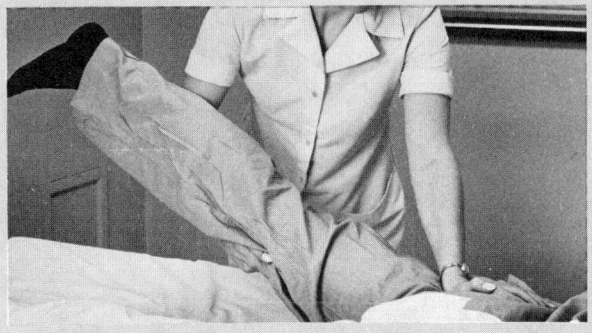

Hypertension of hip. Place the patient in a prone position, and move leg backward from the body as far as possible.

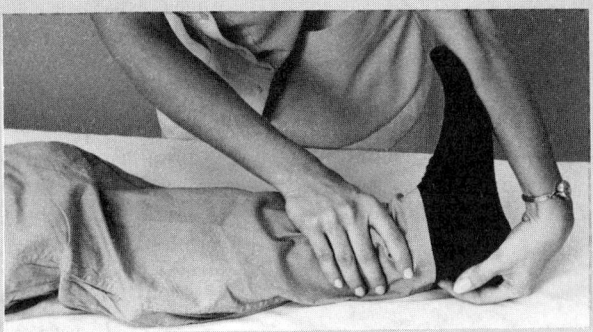

Dorsiflexion of foot. Move foot up and toward the leg. Then move foot down and away from the leg (plantar flexion).

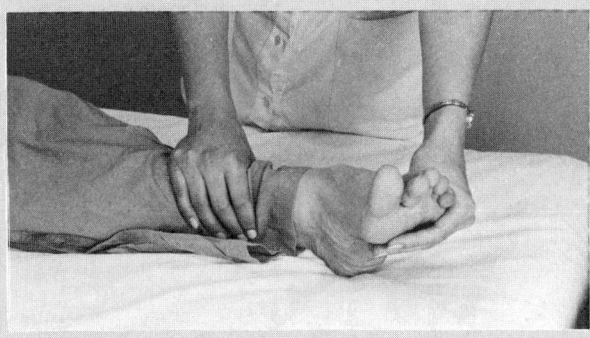

Inversion and eversion of foot. Move foot so that sole is facing outward (eversion). Then move foot so that sole if facing inward (inversion).

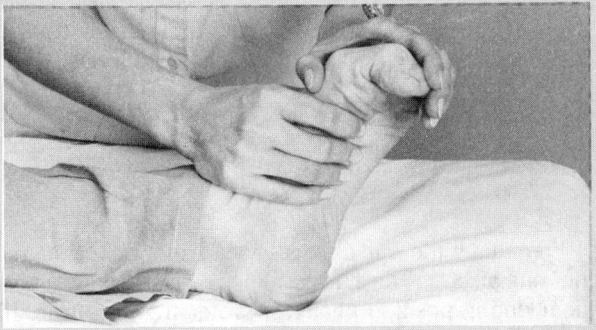

Flexion of toes. Bend the toes toward the ball of foot.

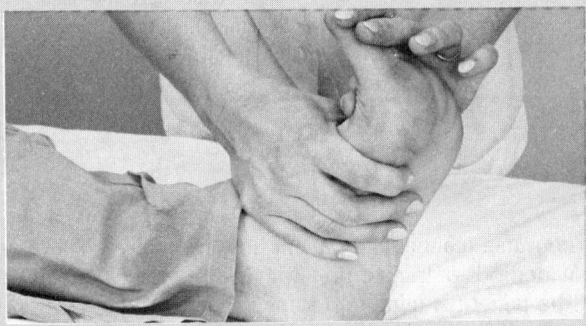

Extension of toes. Straighten toes and pull them toward the leg as far as possible.

TABLE 14-1.   *Therapeutic Exercises*

Exercise	Description	Purposes	Action
Passive	An exercise carried out by the therapist or the nurse without assistance from the patient	To retain as much joint range of motion as possible, to maintain circulation	Stabilize the proximal joint, and support the distal part. Move the joint smoothly, slowly, and gently through its full range of motion. Avoid producing pain.
Active assistance	An exercise carried out by the patient with the assistance of the therapist or the nurse	To encourage normal muscle function	Support the distal part, and encourage the patient to take the joint actively through its range of motion. Give no more assistance than is necessary to accomplish the action. Short periods of activity should be followed by adequate rest periods.
Active	An exercise accomplished by the patient without assistance, activities include turning from side to side and from back to abdomen and moving up and down in bed	To increase muscle strength	When possible, active exercise should be performed against gravity. The joint is moved through full range of motion without assistance. (Make sure that the patient does not substitute another joint movement for the one intended.)
Resistive	An active exercise carried out by the patient working against resistance produced by either manual or mechanical means	To provide resistance to increase muscle power	The patient moves the joint through its range of motion while the therapist resists slightly at first and then with progressively increasing resistance. Sandbags and weights can be used and are applied at the distal point of the involved joint. The movements should be performed smoothly.
Isometric or muscle setting	Alternately contracting and relaxing a muscle while keeping the part in a fixed position; this exercise is performed by the patient	To maintain strength when a joint is immobilized	Contract or tighten the muscle as much as possible without moving the joint, hold for several seconds, then let go and relax. Breathe deeply.

The nurse teaches the patient how to transfer. There are several methods of transferring from the bed to the wheelchair when the patient is unable to stand. The technique chosen is appropriate for the patient, considering his abilities and disabilities. It is helpful for the nurse to demonstrate the technique. If the physical therapist is involved in teaching the patient to transfer, the nurse and the physical therapist must collaborate so that consistent instructions are given to the patient. During transfer, the nurse assists and coaches the patient. Figure 14-2 shows weight-bearing and non–weight-bearing transfer.

Frequently the nurse assists weak and incapacitated patients out of bed. The nurse supports and gently assists the patient during position changes, protecting him from injury. The nurse avoids pulling on the weak or paralyzed upper extremity, which may result in dislocation of the shoulder. It is important for the nurse to be familiar with the techniques of moving the patient to the edge of the bed, sitting him on the edge of the bed, and assisting him to stand. The patient is always assisted to move toward his stronger side. Chart 14-6 outlines techniques for assisting the patient out of bed.

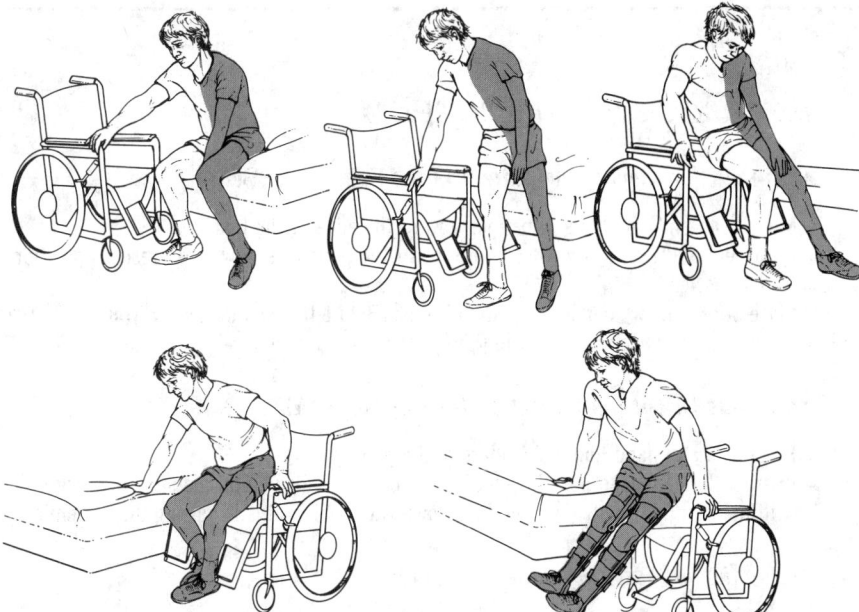

A. Weight-bearing transfer from bed to chair. The patient stands up, pivots until his back is opposite the new seat, and sits down.

B. (*Left*) Non–weight-bearing transfer from chair to bed. (*Right*) With legs braced.

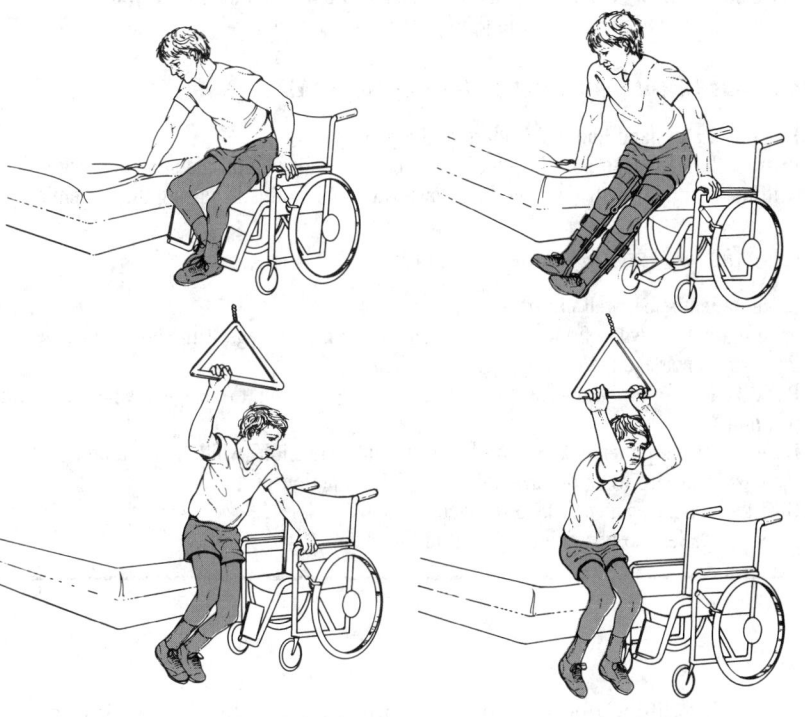

C. (*Left*) Non–weight-bearing transfer, combined method. (*Right*) Non–weight-bearing transfer, pull-up method.

Figure 14–2. Methods of transferring the patient from the bed to a wheelchair. The wheelchair is in a locked position. Shaded areas indicate non–weight-bearing body parts.

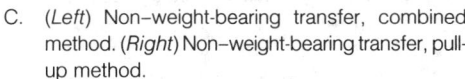

In the home setting, getting in and out of bed and performing chair, toilet, and tub transfers for persons with weak musculature and loss of hip, knee, and ankle motion are difficult. A rope attached to the headboard of the bed helps the patient to pull himself toward the center of the bed, and the use of a rope attached to the footboard facilitates getting in and out of bed. The height of a chair can be raised with hollowed-out blocks placed under the chair legs or with cushions on the seat. Bars can be attached to the wall near the toilet and tub to provide leverage and stability.

▷   *Preparing for Ambulation.*   Regaining the ability to walk is a prime morale builder. To be prepared for ambulation—whether with brace, walker, cane or crutches—the patient must strengthen the muscles required. *Exercise is the foundation of preparation.* The nurse instructs and supervises the patient in these exercises.

For ambulation, the quadriceps muscles and the gluteal muscles are strengthened. The quadriceps muscles stabilize the knee joint. To perform *quadricep setting exercises,* the patient contracts the quadriceps muscle by attempting to push the popliteal area against the mattress and at the same time raising the heel. The patient maintains the muscle contraction until a count of five and relaxes for a count of five. The exercise is repeated 10 to 15 times hourly. Exercising the quadriceps muscles prevents flexion contractures of the knee. In *gluteal setting*, the patient contracts or "pinches" the buttocks together until the count of five, relaxes for the count of five, and repeats 10 to 15 times hourly.

When ambulatory aids (*i.e.,* walker, cane, crutches) are used, the muscles of the upper extremities are exercised and strengthened. *Push-ups* are useful. While in a sitting position, the patient raises his body by pushing his hands against the chair seat or mattress. He should be encouraged to do push-ups while in a prone position also. *Pull-ups* on a trapeze, while lifting the body is another effective conditioner. The patient is taught to *raise his arms* above the head and lower them in a slow, rhythmic manner while holding weights. Gradually the poundage of the weights is increased. The hands are strengthened by *squeezing a rubber ball.*

The physical therapist designs exercises to help the patient develop sitting and standing balance, stability, and coordination needed for ambulation. After sitting and standing balance are achieved, the patient uses parallel bars. Under the supervision of the physical therapist, the patient practices shifting his weight

Chart 14-6
Assisting the Patient Out of Bed

Technique for Moving the Patient to the Edge of the Bed

- Move head and shoulders of patient toward the edge of the bed.
- Move feet and legs to the edge of the bed (The patient is now in a crescent position, which gives good range of motion to the lateral trunk muscles.)
- Place both arms well under the patient's hips (Before the next maneuver, you should tighten [set] the muscles of your back and abdomen.)
- Straighten your back while moving the patient toward you.

Technique for Sitting Patient on the Edge of the Bed

- Place arm and hand under shoulders of the patient.
- Instruct the patient to push his elbow into the bed while you lift his shoulders with one arm and swing his legs over the edge of the bed with the other. (Gravity pulls the legs downward, which aids in raising the patient's trunk.)

Technique for Assisting Patient to Stand

- Place patient's feet well under him.
- Face the patient while firmly grasping each side of his rib cage with your hands.
- Push your knee against one knee of the patient.
- Rock the patient forward as he comes to a standing position. (Your knee is pushed against the patient's knee as he comes to the standing position.)
- Ensure that the patient's knees are "locked" (full extension) while he is standing. (Locking the knees of the patient is a safety measure for those who are weak or have been in bed for a period of time.)
- Give the patient *enough time* to balance himself.
- Pivot the patient to position him to sit in the chair.

---

from side to side, lifting one leg while supporting his weight on the other, and then walking in the parallel bars.

▷ *Using Ambulatory Aids.* When the patient is ready to begin ambulation, he must be fitted with the appropriate ambulatory aid, instructed as to the prescribed weight-bearing limits (*e.g.*, non–weight-bearing, partial weight-bearing), and taught how to use the aid safely. The nurse continually assesses the patient for stability and protects him from falling. The patient should wear sturdy, well-fitting shoes. He should be advised of the dangers of wet and highly polished floors and shag rugs. The patient needs to learn how to ambulate on inclines, how to maneuver uneven surfaces, and how to manage stairs.

Crutches provide for support and balance and are a convenient method of getting from one place to another. Good balance and erect posture are essential for crutch walking. For safety, crutches should have large rubber suction tips and the patient should wear well-fitting shoes that have firm soles. Patients who are prescribed partial weight-bearing or non–weight-bearing ambulation may use crutches. The nurse or physical therapist determines if crutches are appropriate ambulatory aids for the patient.

Preparatory exercises are aimed at strengthening the shoulder girdle and upper extremity muscles, which bear the patient's weight when crutch walking.

The following muscle groups are important for crutch walking (Fig. 14–3*A*):

- Shoulder depressors—to stabilize the upper extremity and prevent shoulder hiking
- Shoulder adductors—to hold the crutch top against the chest wall
- Arm flexors, extensors, and abductors (at the shoulder)—to move crutches forward, backward, and sideward
- Forearm extensors—to prevent flexion or buckling; important in raising the body for swinging gait
- Wrist extensors—to enable weight-bearing on hand pieces
- Finger and thumb flexors—to grasp the hand piece

Crutches must be adjusted to the patient. Adjustable crutches allow for optimal individual fit.

Measuring for Crutches. To determine the approximate crutch length, the patient may be measured standing or lying, or the patient's height may be used.

To measure a standing patient for crutches, the patient is positioned against the wall with the feet slightly apart and away from the wall. Five centimeters (2 in) is marked out to the side from the tip of the toe. Fifteen centimeters (6 in) is measured straight ahead from the first mark and this point is marked. Five centimeters (2 in) is measured below the axilla to the second mark for the approximate crutch length.

If the patient has to be measured while lying down, measure from the anterior fold of the axilla to the sole of the foot,

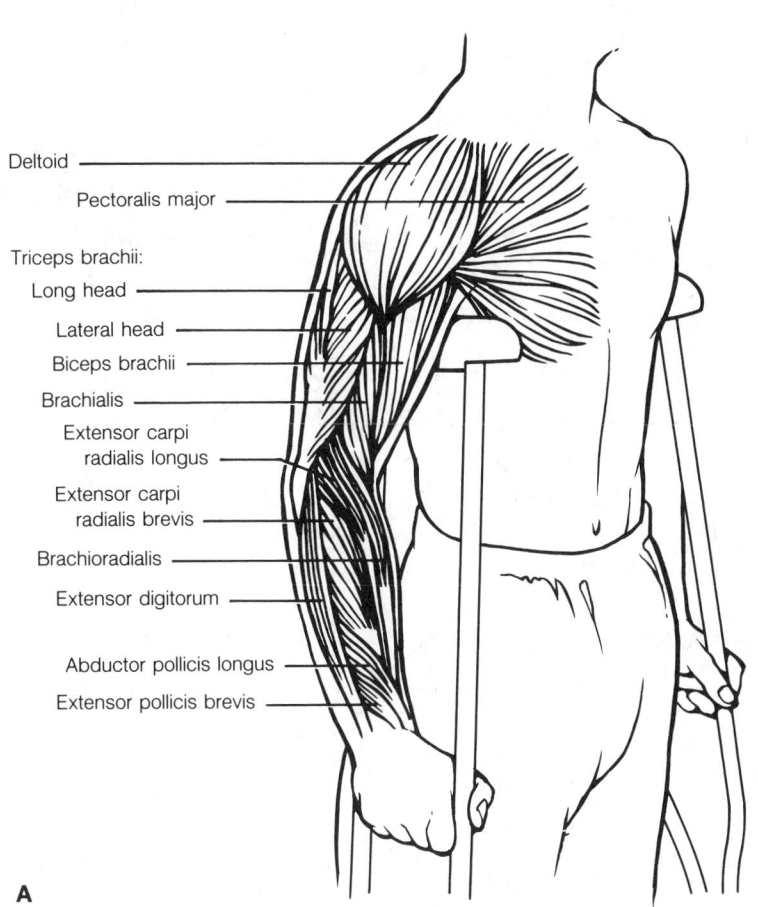

Deltoid
Pectoralis major
Triceps brachii:
Long head
Lateral head
Biceps brachii
Brachialis
Extensor carpi radialis longus
Extensor carpi radialis brevis
Brachioradialis
Extensor digitorum
Abductor pollicis longus
Extensor pollicis brevis

A

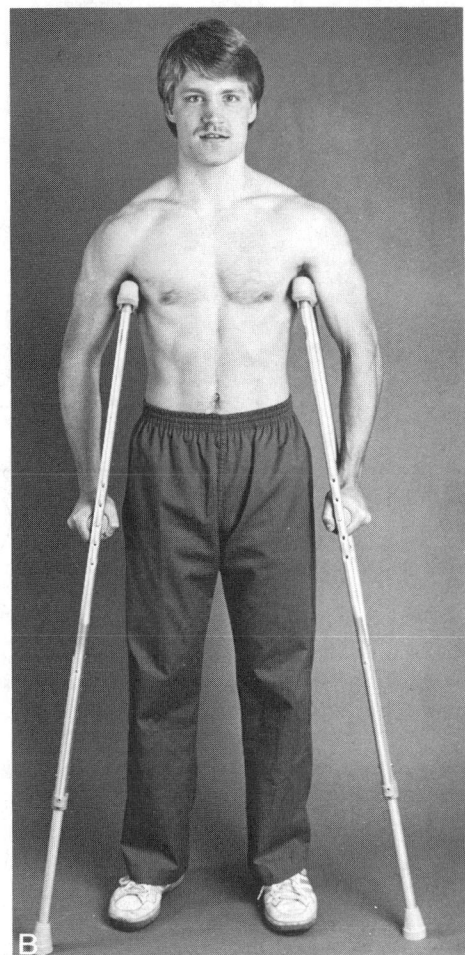

B

Figure 14–3. Crutch walking. (**A**) Muscle groups important for crutch walking. (**B**) The tripod position for the basic crutch stance.

and then add 5 cm (2 in). If the patient's height is used, subtract 40 cm (16 in) to obtain the approximate crutch length.

The hand piece should be adjusted to allow 20 to 30 degrees of flexion at the elbow. The wrist should be extended and the hand dorsiflexed. A foam rubber pad on the under arm piece may be used to relieve pressure of the crutch on the upper arm and thoracic cage.

▷ *Teaching the Patient to Ambulate With Crutches.* Because crutch walking is not an inherent skill, it must be taught. The nurse or physical therapist explains and demonstrates to the patient how he should manipulate his crutches before the patient attempts to do so. All patient education is individualized to meet the patient's learning needs. The patient should learn to stand by a chair on the unaffected leg to achieve balance. To help the patient maintain his balance, the nurse holds the patient near the waist or uses a transfer belt.

The patient is taught to support his weight on the hand pieces. (For individuals unable to support weight through the wrist and hand because of arthritis or fracture, platform crutches that support the forearm and allow the weight to be borne through the elbow are available.) If weight is borne on the

axilla, the pressure of the crutch can damage the brachial plexus nerves, producing "crutch paralysis."

Crutch Stance. For maximum stability, the patient learns to assume a *tripod position*. The crutches are placed approximately 20 cm to 25 cm (8 to 10 in) in front and to the side of the patient's toes (see Fig. 14–3*B*). This base of support is adjusted according to the height of the patient (*i.e.*, a tall patient requires a broader base of support than a short person).

Crutch Gaits. Before walking, the patient learns how to shift his weight and maintain his balance. The selection of the crutch gait depends on the type and severity of the disability and on the patient's physical condition, arm and trunk strength, and body balance. The patient should be taught two gaits so that he may change from one to another. Shifting crutch gaits relieves fatigue, as each gait requires the use of a different combination of muscles. (If a muscle is forced to contract steadily without relaxing, the circulation of the blood to the part is reduced.) A faster gait can be used for making speed, whereas a slower one is used in crowded places.

All gaits begin in the tripod position. The more common gaits are the four-point, the three-point, the two-point, and the

Chart 14–7
Crutch Gaits

Shaded areas are weight-bearing. ↑ indicates advance foot or crutch.

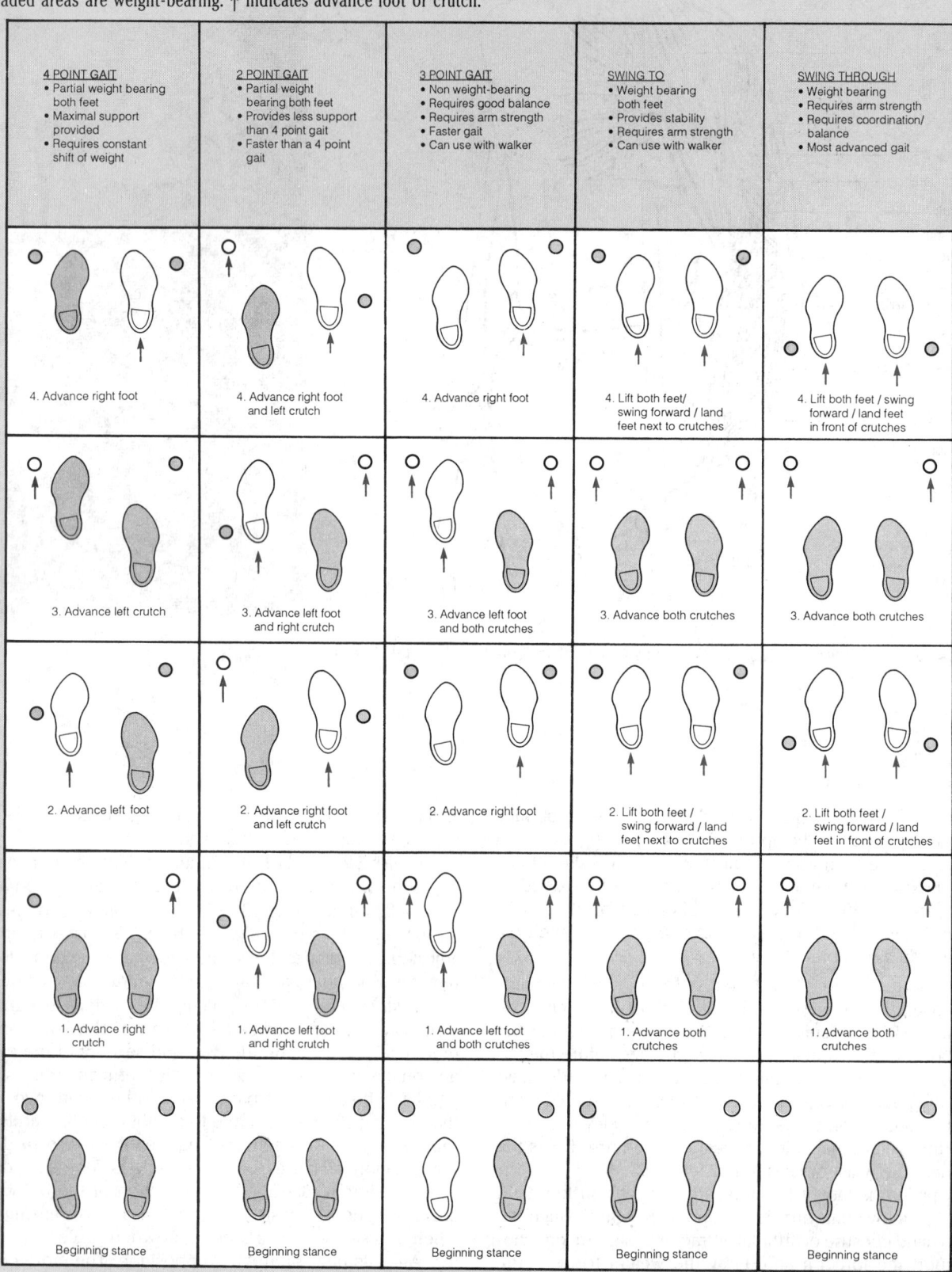

swinging-to and swinging-through gaits. The sequence of movements for each of these gaits is listed in Chart 14-7.

The nurse continually assesses the patient's stability and protects the patient from falls. The nurse walks with the patient, holding the patient at the waist as needed for balance.

The nurse monitors the patient's tolerance of crutch walking. Sweating and shortness of breath are indications that crutch walking practice should be stopped and the patient permitted to rest. Prolonged periods of bed rest and inactivity affect the patient's strength and endurance.

Other Crutch-Maneuvering Techniques. Before a patient is considered independent in crutch walking, he needs to learn to sit in a chair, stand from sitting, and go up and down stairs. The following instructions are given to the patient:

To Sit Down
1. Grasp the crutches at the hand pieces for control.
2. Bend forward slightly while assuming a sitting position.
3. Place the affected leg forward to prevent weight-bearing and flexion.

To Stand Up
1. Move forward to the edge of the chair with the strong leg slightly under the seat.
2. Place both crutches in the hand on the side of the affected extremity.
3. Push down on the hand piece while raising the body to a standing position.

To Go Down Stairs
1. Walk forward as far as possible on the step.
2. Advance crutches to the lower step. The weaker leg is advanced first and then the stronger one. In this way, the stronger extremity shares the work of raising and lowering the body weight with the patient's arms.

To Go Up Stairs
1. Advance the stronger leg first up to the next step.
2. Then advance the crutches and the weaker extremity. (Strong leg goes up first and comes down last.) A memory device for the patients is "up with the good; down with the bad."

▷ *Walker.* A walker provides more support than a cane or crutches. A walker does not permit a natural reciprocal walking pattern. It is useful for the patient who has poor balance and cannot use crutches. The patient should wear sturdy well-fitting shoes. The nurse continually assesses the patient's stability and protects the patient from falls. The nurse walks with the patient, holding the patient at the waist as needed for balance.

The height of the walker is adjusted to the patient. The patient's arms resting on the walker hand grips should exhibit 20 to 30 degrees of flexion at the elbows.

The patient is taught to ambulate with a walker as follows:

1. Patient must hold the walker on the hand grips for stability.
2. Lift the walker, placing it in front of you while leaning your body slightly forward.
3. Walk into the walker, supporting your body weight on your hands when advancing your weaker leg, permitting partial weight-bearing or non–weight-bearing as prescribed.
4. Balance yourself on your feet.
5. Lift the walker and place it in front of you again. Continue this pattern of walking.

▷ *Cane.* A cane is used to help the patient walk with greater balance and support and to relieve the pressure on weight-bearing joints by redistributing the weight. Quad canes (four-footed canes) provide more stability than straight canes.

The cane should be fitted with a gently flaring tip that has flexible and concentric rings, which gives optimal stability, functions as a shock absorber, and enables the patient to walk with greater speed and less fatigue.

To fit the patient for a cane, the patient is instructed to flex his elbow at a 30-degree angle, hold the handle of the cane approximately level with the greater trochanter, and place the tip of the cane 15 cm (6 in) lateral to the base of his fifth toe. Adjustable canes make individual adjustment easy.

The cane is held in the hand opposite to the affected extremity. In normal walking, the opposite leg and arm move together (reciprocal motion); such motion is to be carried through in walking with a cane.

The nurse continually assesses the patient's stability and protects the patient from falls. The nurse walks with the patient, holding him at the waist as needed for balance.

The patient is taught to ambulate with a cane as follows:

Cane-Foot Sequence
1. Hold the cane in the hand opposite the affected extremity to widen the base of support and to reduce the stress on the involved extremity. (If the patient for some reason is unable to use the cane in the opposite hand, the cane may be used on the same side.)
2. Advance the cane at the same time as the affected leg is moved forward.
3. Keep the cane fairly close to the body to prevent leaning.
4. Bear down on the cane when the unaffected extremity begins the swing phase.

To Go Up and Down Stairs Using the Cane
1. Step up on the unaffected extremity.
2. Then place the cane and affected extremity up on the step.
3. Reverse this procedure for descending steps. (Strong leg goes up first and comes down last.)

▷ *Assisting the Patient Using an Orthosis/Prosthesis.* Orthoses and prostheses are designed to facilitate mobilization and maximize the patient's quality of life. The nurse helps the patient develop an attitude of realistic hopefulness. After amputation, the nurse promotes tissue healing, uses compression dressings to promote residual limb shaping, and minimizes contracture formation. The nurse works with the patient and emphasizes the orthotist's/prosthetist's instructions related to skin care and care of the orthosis/prosthesis. Skin problems or pressure ulcers may develop if the device is applied too tightly or adjusted improperly. The patient is taught to examine the orthosis periodically to see that it fits as designed, its shape is not distorted, and the padding distributes pressure evenly.

Learning to successfully use a prosthesis requires the efforts of the patient, physical therapist, nurse, and prosthetist. Efforts are directed at acceptance of the prosthesis and using it to maximize one's mobility and quality of life.

▷ Evaluation

Expected Outcomes
1. Demonstrates improved physical mobility
   a. Maintains muscle strength and joint mobility

b. Does not develop contractures
c. Participates in exercise program
2. Transfers safely
a. Demonstrates assisted transfers
b. Performs independent transfers
3. Ambulates with maximum independence
a. Uses ambulatory aid safely
b. Adheres to weight-bearing prescription
c. Requests assistance as needed
4. Demonstrates increased activity tolerance
a. Does not experience orthostatic hypotension episodes
b. Reports absence of fatigue associated with ambulatory efforts
c. Gradually increases distance and speed of ambulation

▶ Nursing Process
Impaired Skin Integrity

Patients confined to bed for long periods, patients with motor or sensory dysfunction, and patients who experience muscular atrophy and reduction of padding between the overlying skin and the underlying bone are prone to *pressure ulcers*. Pressure ulcers are localized areas of infarcted soft tissue that occur when pressure applied to the skin over time is greater than normal capillary pressure (32 mm Hg). The initial sign of pressure is erythema (redness of the skin) due to reactive hyperemia. The tissue becomes ischemic or anoxic. The cutaneous tissues become broken or destroyed, leading to progressive destruction and necrosis of underlying soft tissue. The resulting pressure ulcer is painful and slow to heal.

Factors that have been identified as contributing to the development of pressure ulcers include immobility, decreased sensory perception, decreased tissue perfusion, decreased nutritional status, friction and shear forces, increased moisture, and age-related skin changes.

When a person is immobile and inactive, pressure is exerted on the skin and subcutaneous tissue by objects on which the person rests, such as a mattress, chair seat, or cast. Weight-bearing bony prominences are most susceptible to pressure ulcer development. These prominences are covered by skin and small amounts of subcutaneous tissue. Susceptible areas include the sacrum and coccygeal areas, ischial tuberosities (especially in persons who sit for prolonged periods), greater trochanter, heel, knee, malleolus, medial condyle of the tibia, the fibular head, scapula, and elbow (Fig. 14-4).

If the patient has suffered sensory loss, has an impaired level of consciousness, or has paralysis, he may not be aware of the discomfort associated with prolonged pressure on the skin. Therefore, the person will not reposition his body to relieve the pressure. This prolonged pressure impedes blood flow, reducing nourishment of the skin. A pressure ulcer may develop in a very short period.

Any condition that reduces the circulation and nourishment of the skin and subcutaneous tissue (altered peripheral tissue perfusion) increases the risk of pressure ulcer development. Persons with diabetes mellitus experience an alteration in microcirculation. Similarly, patients with edema have impaired circulation and poor nourishment of the skin tissue. Obese patients have large amounts of poorly vascularized adipose tissue, which is susceptible to breakdown.

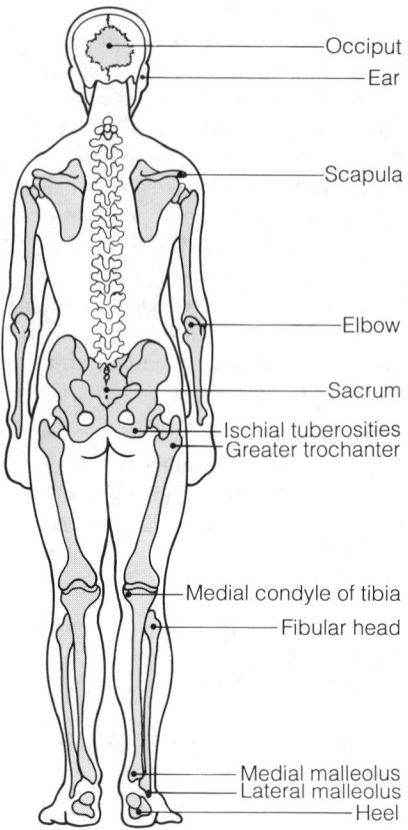

Occiput
Ear
Scapula
Elbow
Sacrum
Ischial tuberosities
Greater trochanter
Medial condyle of tibia
Fibular head
Medial malleolus
Lateral malleolus
Heel

Figure 14-4.   Areas susceptible to pressure ulcers.

Nutritional deficiencies, anemias, and metabolic disorders that diminish tissue health also contribute to pressure ulcer development. Anemia, regardless of its cause, decreases the blood's oxygen-carrying ability and predisposes to pressure ulcer formation. Patients who have low protein levels or who are in a negative nitrogen balance experience tissue wasting and inhibited tissue repair. Specific nutrients such as vitamin C and trace minerals are needed for tissue maintenance and repair.

Mechanical forces contribute to the development of pressure ulcers. *Friction* is the resistance to movement between two bodies (surfaces). Friction occurs when two surfaces are moved across each other. Rubbing damage to the skin surface results. *Shearing force* is created by the interplay of gravitational forces (forces that push the body down) and friction. When a patient slides down in bed, shearing forces are created (Fig. 14-5). With shearing, tissue layers slide over one another, blood vessels stretch and twist, and the microcirculation of the skin and subcutaneous tissue is disrupted. Pressure ulcers from friction and shearing forces occur when the patient slides down in bed or when patients are moved or positioned improperly (*e.g.*, incorrectly pulled up in bed). Spastic muscles and paralysis increase the patient's vulnerability to pressure ulcers related to friction and shearing forces.

Prolonged contact with moisture from perspiration, urine, feces, or drainage produces maceration (softening) of the skin. The skin reacts to the substances in the excreta or drainage and becomes irritated. The moist, irritated skin is more vulnerable to pressure breakdown.

Once the skin is broken, the area is invaded by microorganisms (*e.g.*, streptococci and staphyloccoci, *Pseudomonas*

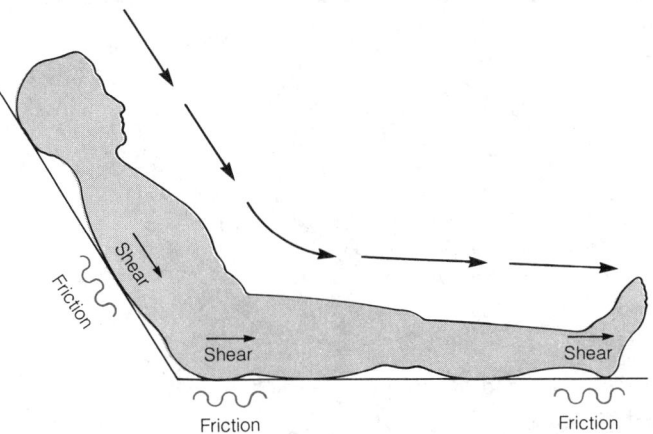

Figure 14–5. Mechanical forces contribute to pressure ulcer development. As the person slides down in bed, *friction* resists this movement. *Shearing* occurs when one layer of tissue slides over another, disrupting microcirculation of skin and subcutaneous tissue.

aeruginosa, Escherichia coli), and infection occurs. Foul-smelling infectious drainage is present. The lesion may enlarge and produce a continuous loss of serum, which may further deplete the body of essential protein needed for tissue repair and maintenance. The lesion may continue to enlarge and extend deep into the fascia, muscle, and bone, with multiple sinus tracts radiating from the pressure ulcer. With extensive pressure ulcers, systemic infections may develop, frequently from gram-negative organisms.

▷ *Gerontologic Considerations.* In the older adult, the skin has diminished epidermal thickness, dermal collagen, and tissue elasticity. The skin is drier as a result of diminished sebaceous and sweat gland activity. Cardiovascular changes result in decreased tissue perfusion. Muscles atrophy and bone structures become prominent. Diminished sensory perception and reduced ability to reposition oneself contribute to prolonged pressure on the skin. Therefore, the older adult is more susceptible to pressure ulcers, which cause pain and suffering and reduce quality of life.

An estimated 35% of the institutionalized older adults may be afflicted with pressure ulcers at any given time. The treatment of pressure ulcers is very time-consuming and costly.

▷ Assessment

In assessing the patient for potential risk for pressure ulcer development, the nurse assesses the patient's mobility, sensory perception and cognitive abilities, tissue perfusion, nutritional status, friction and shear forces, sources of moisture on the skin, and age (Chart 14-8, Risk Factors for Development of Pressure Ulcers). The nurse

> Assesses total skin condition at least twice a day
> Inspects each pressure site for erythema
> Assesses the areas for blanching response
> Palpates the skin for increased warmth
> Inspects for dry skin, moist skin, breaks in skin
> Notes drainage and odor
> Evaluates level of mobility
> Notes restrictive devices (*e.g.*, restraints, splints)
> Evaluates circulatory status (*e.g.*, peripheral pulses, edema)
> Assesses neurologic status

Chart 14–8
Risk Factors for Development of Pressure Ulcers

Prolonged pressures
Immobility, compromised mobility
Loss of protective reflexes, sensory deficit/loss
Poor skin perfusion: edema
Malnutrition, hypoproteinemia, anemia, vitamin deficiency
Friction, shearing forces, trauma
Incontinence of urine or feces
Altered skin moisture: excessively dry, excessively moist
Advanced age, debilitation
Equipment: casts, traction, restraints, bedding, chairs

> Determines presence of incontinence
> Evaluates nutritional and hydration status
> Reviews the patient's record for hematocrit, hemoglobin, and blood chemistry (serum albumin values)
> Notes present health problems
> Reviews current medications

If a pressure area is noted, the nurse notes its size and location and may use a grading system to describe its severity (Chart 14-9). Generally, a stage I pressure ulcer is an area of erythema, tissue swelling, and congestion, with the patient complaining of discomfort. The erythema blanches on pressure. The skin temperature is elevated because of the increased vasodilation. The redness progresses to a dusky, cyanotic blue–gray appearance, which is the result of the skin capillary occlusion and subcutaneous weakening. A stage II pressure ulcer exhibits a break in the skin through the epidermis and includes the dermis. Necrosis occurs. There is venous sludging and thrombosis and edema with cellular extravasation and infiltration. A stage III pressure ulcer extends into the subcutaneous tissues. A stage IV ulceration extends into the underlying structures, including the muscle and possibly the bone. The skin lesion may represent only the "tip of the iceberg," because a small surface ulcer may overlie a large undermining area.

The appearance of pus or foul odor suggests an infection. With an extensive pressure ulcer, deep pockets of infection are often present. Drying and crusting of exudate may be present. Infection of a pressure ulcer may advance to osteomyelitis, pyarthrosis (pus formation within a joint cavity), or generalized sepsis.

▷ Nursing Diagnosis

Based on the assessment data, major nursing diagnoses for the patient may include impaired skin integrity related to any of the following factors: immobility, decreased sensory perception, decreased tissue perfusion, decreased nutritional status, friction and shear forces, increased moisture, advanced age.

▷ Planning and Implementation

▷ *Goals:* The major goals of the patient may include relief of pressure, improved mobility, improved sensory perception, improved tissue perfusion, improved nutritional status, mini-

Chart 14-9
Assessment of Pressure Ulcer Stage

Stage I

- Area of erythema
- Erythema blanches with pressure
- Skin temperature elevated
- Tissue swollen and congested
- Patient complains of discomfort
- Erythema progresses to dusky, blue-gray

Stage II

- Skin breaks
- Edema persists
- Necrosis of tissue
- Ulcer drains
- Infection may develop

Stage III

- Ulcer extends into subcutaneous tissue
- Necrosis and drainage continue
- Infection develops

Stage IV

- Ulcer extends to underlying muscle and bone
- Deep pockets of infection develop
- Necrosis and drainage continue

mized friction and shear forces, dry surfaces in contact with skin, and healing of pressure ulcer, if present.

◊ Nursing Interventions

◊ *Relieving Pressure.*   The patient needs frequent changes of position to relieve and redistribute the pressure on the skin and to prevent prolonged reduced blood flow to the skin and subcutaneous tissues. This can be accomplished by turning and repositioning the patient, which allows the blood to flow back to the ischemic areas and helps the tissues recover from pressure.

- Thus, the patient should be turned at 1-hour or 2-hour intervals.

The patient should be positioned on all four sides (laterally, prone, dorsally) in sequence unless contraindicated. In addition to regular turning, there should be small shifts of body weight, such as repositioning an ankle, elbow, or shoulder. The skin is inspected at each position change and assessed for temperature elevation. If redness or heat is noted, pressure must be kept off that area.

In the aging patient, small shifts of body weight may be effective. Placing a small rolled towel or sheepskin under a shoulder or hip will allow a return of blood to the skin on which the patient is sitting or lying. The towel or sheepskin is moved around the patient's pressure points in a clockwise fashion. Other preventive measures to minimize risk factors are also included in the plan of care.

Another way to relieve pressure over bony prominences is the bridging technique accomplished through the correct positioning of pillows. Just as a bridge is supported on pillars to allow traffic to move underneath, so can the body be supported by pillows to allow for space between bony prominences and the mattress. For the feet and extremities, a footboard or pillows will support the bedding and thus reduce pressure. To protect the heels, 2.5 cm (1 in) of foam rubber may be placed between a well-laundered soft sheet and the mattress, or a commercial heel protector may be used.

At times, special equipment and beds may be needed to help relieve the pressure on the skin. These are designed to provide support for specific body areas or for distributing pressure evenly and uniformly.

Patients sitting in wheelchairs for prolonged periods should have wheelchair cushions fitted and adjusted on an individualized basis, using pressure measurement techniques as a guide to selection and fitting. The aim is to redistribute pressure away from areas at risk for developing sores. No cushion is able to eliminate excessive pressure, however. The patient should be reminded to shift his weight frequently and raise himself up for a few seconds every half hour while sitting in a chair (Fig. 14-6).

An alternating pressure pad mattress may be used in conditions in which the patient cannot turn. The alternating inflation and deflation of the pad produces constriction followed by dilatation of the superficial blood vessels of the skin. By such action, pressure on any one part is reduced and the blood supply is increased.

A polyurethane foam mattress (egg-crate mattress) distributes pressure evenly by bringing more of the patient's body surface in contact with the supporting surface. Properly inflated plastic convoluted air mattresses also distribute pressure evenly.

For patients susceptible to pressure on bony prominences, a variety of pads and supportive devices are available that can be placed on top of the traditional mattress. The gel-type flotation pad reduces pressure because the material is similar in consistency to human adipose tissue and "gives" with the patient's weight. Soft, moisture-absorbing padding is also useful because the softness and resilience of padding provides even distribution of pressure and the dissipation and absorption of moisture, along with freedom from wrinkles and friction. Bony prominences may be protected by inserting pieces of gel pads, sheepskin padding, or soft foam rubber beneath the sacrum, the trochanters, heels, elbows, scapulae, and the back of the head when there is pressure on the sites.

The use of the flotation mattress, or water bed, has been advocated for the prevention (and treatment) of pressure sores. As the patient's body sinks into the fluid, additional surface

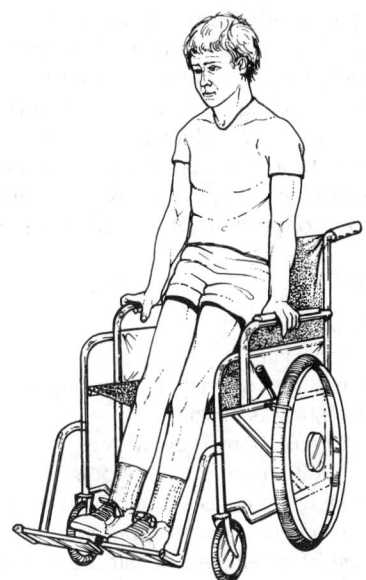

Figure 14–6. Wheelchair push-up to prevent ischial pressure ulcers. These push-ups should become an automatic routine (every 30 minutes) for the person with paraplegia. He should stay up, out of contact with the seat, for 60 seconds. The wheels are kept in the locked position during the exercise. (Adapted from Hirschberg GG, Lewis L, and Vaughan P. Rehabilitation: A Manual for the Care of the Disabled and Elderly, 2nd ed. Philadelphia, JB Lippincott, 1976.)

becomes available for weight-bearing, thereby further decreasing body weight per unit area. (Pascal's law states that the weight of the body floating on a fluid system is evenly distributed over the entire supporting surface.) Thus, there is less pressure on the body parts.

Specialized beds have been designed to prevent pressure on the skin. Air-fluidized beds float the patient, low-air-loss beds selectively support the patient, and kinetic (rocking) beds, which constantly move the patient to redistribute weight and stimulate circulation, are examples of special bed systems.

▷ *Improving Mobility.* The patient is encouraged to remain active. The patient is ambulated whenever possible. When sitting, the patient is reminded to change positions frequently to redistribute weight. Active and passive exercises increase muscular, skin, and vascular tone. Circulation is stimulated with activity, which relieves tissue ischemia, the forerunner of pressure ulcers.

For the patient at risk for pressure ulcers, turning schedules and exercise schedules are essential. *Repositioning must occur around the clock.*

▷ *Improving Sensory Perception.* The nurse helps the patient recognize and compensate for altered sensory perception. Depending on the origin of the alteration (*e.g.,* decreased level of consciousness, spinal cord lesion), specific interventions will be selected. Strategies to improve cognition and sensory perception may include stimulating the patient to increase awareness of self in the environment, encouraging the patient to participate in self-care, or supporting the patient's efforts toward active compensation for loss of sensation (*e.g.,* a paraplegic lifting himself from the sitting position every 30 minutes). The patient/caregiver is taught to visually inspect potential pressure areas, using a mirror if needed, for evidence of pressure ulcer development.

▷ *Improving Tissue Perfusion.* Exercise and repositioning improve tissue perfusion. When repositioning the patient, the nurse can improve tissue perfusion by gently massaging the healthy skin in potential pressure areas with a bland moisturizing lotion. Massage around bony prominences stimulates the blood flow in the skin, promotes venous return, reduces edema, and increases vascular tone.

- Reddened areas are *not* massaged, as this may increase the damage to already traumatized skin.

If the patient has evidence of compromised peripheral circulation such as edema, positioning and elevation of the edematous body part to promote venous return and diminish congestion will improve tissue perfusion. The nurse must be alert to environmental factors (*e.g.,* wrinkles in sheets, pressure of tubes) that may contribute to pressure on the skin and diminished circulation; the source of pressure *must* be removed.

▷ *Improving Nutritional Status.* The patient's nutritional status must be adequate and a positive nitrogen balance must be maintained. Pressure ulcers develop more quickly and are more resistant to treatment in patients suffering from nutritional disorders. A high-protein diet with protein supplements may be helpful. Iron preparations may be necessary to raise the hemoglobin level so that tissue oxygen levels will be maintained within acceptable limits. Ascorbic acid (vitamin C) is necessary for tissue vitality and healing.

Other nutrients associated with healthy skin include vitamin A, B vitamins, zinc, and sulfur. With balanced nutrition and hydration, the skin is able to maintain a healthy status and repair damaged tissues.

▷ *Reducing Friction and Shear Forces.* Shearing forces occur when the patient is pulled, allowed to slump, or moves by digging his or her heels or elbows into the mattress. Raising the head of the bed by even a few centimeters increases the shearing force over the sacral area. Therefore, the semireclining position is avoided for patients at risk. The patient can be protected from sliding down in bed by using a well-padded footboard and by placing extra protection on the heels. Proper positioning with adequate support is important when a patient is sitting in a chair. Polyester sheepskin pads are thought to reduce shearing and friction and may be used with at-risk patients.

- To avoid shearing forces when repositioning the patient, he must be lifted, not dragged.

▷ *Minimizing Moisture.* Continuous moisture on the skin must be prevented by meticulous hygienic measures. The soiled skin should be promptly washed with mild soap and water and blotted dry with a soft towel. The skin may be lubricated with a bland lotion to keep it soft and pliable. Drying agents and powders are avoided. A barrier cream may be helpful in protecting the skin of patients who are incontinent. Patients who are incontinent need to be checked and their wet linens changed promptly. Perspiration, urine, stool, and drainage must be removed from the skin promptly.

The linens must be kept clean and dry. Plastic sheets and waterproof incontinence pads must be avoided. All efforts should be made to keep the skin clean and dry.

▷ *Promoting Pressure Ulcer Healing.* Regardless of the stage of the pressure ulcer, the pressure on the area must be eliminated. The ulcer will not heal until all pressure is removed. The patient must not lie or sit on the pressure ulcer, even for a few minutes. Individualized positioning and turning schedules must be written in the nursing plan of care and followed meticulously.

In addition, inadequate nutritional status and fluid and electrolyte abnormalities must be corrected to promote healing. Wounds that drain body fluids and protein place the patient in a catabolic state and predispose him to hypoproteinemia and serious secondary infections. Protein deficiency must be corrected to heal the pressure ulcer. Carbohydrates are necessary to "spare" the protein and to provide an energy source. Vitamin C and trace elements, especially zinc, are necessary for collagen formation and wound healing.

To permit healing of stage I pressure ulcers, the pressure is removed to permit increased tissue perfusion, improved nutritional and fluid and electrolyte status, reduction of friction and shearing forces, and avoidance of moisture to the skin.

- The reddened skin must not be massaged as increased tissue damage may result.

Stage II pressure ulcers have broken skin. In addition to measures listed for stage I pressure ulcers, a moist environment is desired to aid wound healing. *A heat lamp is not used to dry the open wound.* Migration of epidermal cells over the ulcer surface occurs more rapidly in a moist environment. A semipermeable occlusive dressing or wet saline dressings are helpful in providing a moist environment for healing and in minimizing the loss of fluids and proteins from the body.

Stage III and IV pressure ulcers have extensive damaged tissue. In addition to measures listed for stage I, these advanced draining, necrotic pressure ulcers must be cleaned (debrided) to create an area that will heal. Necrotic, devitalized tissue favors bacterial growth, delays granulation, and inhibits healing. Wound cleaning and dressing are uncomfortable; therefore, the nurse must prepare the patient, explain the procedure, and administer prescribed analgesia when needed.

Debridement may be accomplished by wet-to-damp dressing changes, mechanical flushing of necrotic and infective exudate, application of prescribed enzyme preparations that dissolve necrotic tissue, or surgical dissection. If an eschar covers the ulcer, it is removed surgically to ensure a clean, vitalized wound. Exudate may be absorbed by dressings or special hydrophilic powders, beads, or gels. Cultures of infected pressure ulcers are obtained to guide selection of antibiotic therapy.

After the pressure ulcer is clean, a topical treatment is prescribed. The goal of therapy is to promote granulation. New granulation tissue must be protected from reinfection, drying, and damage to the granulating tissue. Care should be taken to prevent further trauma to the area. Dressings, solutions, and ointments applied to the ulcer should not disrupt the healing process. Multiple agents and protocols are used to treat pressure ulcers. Consistency is an important key to success. In addition, objective evaluation of the response of the pressure ulcer to the treatment protocol must be made every 4 to 6 days. It can take a long time to heal a pressure ulcer.

Surgical intervention is necessary when the ulcer is extensive, when potential complications (such as fistula) exist, and when the ulcer does not respond to treatment. Surgical procedures include incision and drainage, skin grafting, bone resection, skin flaps, and myocutaneous flaps.

Recurrence of pressure ulcers should be anticipated; therefore, continuing assessment is essential. The patient's tolerance for sitting/lying on the healed pressure area is built up

gradually; the time that pressure is allowed on the area is increased in 5- to 15-minute increments. The patient is taught to increase his mobility and to follow a regimen of turning, weight shifting, and repositioning. The patient teaching plan includes instruction on strategies to reduce the risk for developing pressure ulcers and methods to detect, inspect, and minimize pressure areas. Early recognition and intervention are keys to long-term management of potential impaired skin integrity.

◊ Evaluation

Expected Outcomes

1. Maintains intact skin
   a. Exhibits no areas of erythema at bony prominences
   b. Exhibits no breaks in skin
2. Avoids pressure on bony prominences
   a. Changes position every 1 to 2 hours
   b. Uses bridging techniques to remove pressure
   c. Uses special equipment as appropriate
   d. Raises self from seat/wheelchair every 30 minutes
3. Increases mobility
   a. Performs range of motion exercises
   b. Adheres to turning schedule
   c. Shifts weight frequently
4. Improves sensory and cognitive ability
   a. Demonstrates improved level of consciousness
   b. Inspects potential pressure ulcer areas
5. Demonstrates improved tissue perfusion
   a. Stimulates circulation with massage
   b. Elevates body parts susceptible to edema
6. Attains/maintains adequate nutritional status
   a. Verbalizes the importance of protein and vitamin C in diet
   b. Consumes balanced diet high in protein and vitamin C
   c. Hemoglobin level maintained at an acceptable level
   d. Is in positive nitrogen balance
7. Avoids friction and shearing forces
   a. Avoids semi-reclining position
   b. Uses sheepskin pad/heel protectors when appropriate
   c. Lifts body instead of sliding across surfaces
8. Maintains clean, dry skin
   a. Avoids prolonged contact with wet or soiled surfaces
   b. Keeps skin clean and dry
   c. Uses lotion to keep skin lubricated
9. Experiences healing of pressure ulcer
   a. Avoids pressure on area
   b. Improves nutritional status
   c. Participates in therapeutic regimen
   d. Demonstrates behaviors to prevent new pressure ulcers
   e. States early indicators of pressure ulcer development

▶ Nursing Process
Altered Elimination Patterns: Urinary/Bowel

Urinary and bowel incontinence are frequent problems in the disabled patient. Bladder and bowel control are important functions of the body and are influenced by prescribed social behavior. Incontinence curtails a person's independence, causing embarrassment, isolation, and often institutionalization of the elderly. It occurs in up to 15% of the community-based elderly population, whereas almost half of nursing home residents are either bowel or bladder incontinent or both.

In addition, constipation may be a problem for the person with a disability. Regularity is a goal. If a bowel routine is not established, the person may experience abdominal distention, small, frequent oozing of stool, or impaction.

▷ Assessment

Urinary incontinence may be classified as urge, reflex, stress, functional, or total incontinence. Urinary incontinence may result from multiple causes (*e.g.*, urinary tract infection, detrusor instability, bladder outlet obstruction/incompetence, neurologic impairment, bladder spasm/contracture, inability to reach the toilet in time). The cause of the incontinence must be determined. The nurse reviews the results of the diagnostic studies (*e.g.*, urinalysis, urodynamic tests, postvoiding residual volumes).

The nurse assesses previous and current voiding and fluid intake patterns. A time and amount voiding record is kept for at least 48 hours. Episodes of incontinence and associated activity (*e.g.*, coughing, sneezing, lifting), fluid intake time and amount, and medications are recorded. This record is analyzed for patterns and relationships.

The ability to get to the bathroom, manipulate clothing, and use the toilet are important functional factors that may be related to incontinence. Related cognitive functioning (perception of need to void, verbalization of need to void, and ability to learn to control urination) must be assessed.

Bowel incontinence and constipation may result from multiple causes (*e.g.*, diminished/absent sphincter control, cognitive/perceptual impairment, neurogenic factors, diet, immobility). The origin of the bowel problem must be determined.

The nurse assesses the patient's normal bowel patterns, nutritional patterns, use of laxatives, gastrointestinal problems (*e.g.*, colitis), bowel sounds, anal reflex and tone, and functional abilities. The character and frequency of bowel movements are recorded.

▷ Nursing Diagnosis

Based on the assessment data, major nursing diagnoses for the patient may include altered elimination pattern related to urinary incontinence, bowel incontinence, or constipation.*

▷ Planning and Implementation

▷ *Goals:* The major goals of the patient may include control of urinary incontinence, control of bowel incontinence, and regular bowel elimination pattern.

▷ Nursing Interventions

▷ *Promoting Urinary Continence.* Once the nature of the urinary incontinence has been identified, a nursing plan of care is developed based on analysis of the assessment data. Various approaches to promotion of urinary continence have been designed. Most approaches attempt to condition the body to successfully control urination or to minimize the occurrence of unscheduled urination. Selection of the approach depends on the cause of the patient's incontinence. For the program to be successful, the patient's participation and desire to avoid

---

* *Specific NANDA nursing diagnoses that may be appropriate for the individual with elimination problems are Constipation; Bowel incontinence; Functional incontinence; Reflex incontinence; Stress incontinence; Total incontinence; Urge incontinence; Self-care deficit, toileting; Altered urinary elimination; Urinary retention.*

incontinence episodes are crucial. An optimistic attitude with positive feedback for even slight gains is essential for success.

To maintain skin integrity, the skin is washed and dried thoroughly after each incontinent episode. Moisture barrier ointment may be needed for individuals with constant urinary leakage.

At no time should the fluid intake be restricted just to decrease frequency of urination. Sufficient fluid intake (2000 to 3000 ml/day according to patient needs) must be assured. To optimize the likelihood of voiding as scheduled, measured amounts of fluids may be given approximately 30 minutes before voiding attempts. Most of the fluids should be consumed before evening to minimize the need to void frequently during the night.

The goal of *bladder training* is to restore the bladder to normal function. It can be used with cognitively intact individuals experiencing urge incontinence. A voiding/toileting schedule is formulated based on analysis of the assessment data. The schedule specifies times for the patient to try to empty his bladder using a toilet or commode. Privacy should be provided during voiding efforts. The interval between voidings in the early phase of the bladder training period is short (1½ to 2 hours). The patient is encouraged to hold his urine until the specified voiding time. Voiding success and episodes of incontinence are recorded. As the patient's bladder capacity and control increase, the interval is lengthened. Usually there is a temporal relationship between drinking, eating, exercising, and voiding. The alert patient can participate in recording intake, activity, and voiding and can plan his schedule to achieve maximum continence.

Improved accessibility to the toilet and modification of clothing help the patient with functional incontinence to achieve self-care in toileting and continence.

Habit training attempts to keep the patient dry by strictly adhering to a toileting schedule. It may be successful with stress, urge, or functional incontinence. With a confused elderly person, the caregiver takes the person to the toilet according to the schedule before involuntary voiding occurs.

Biofeedback is a system through which the patient learns to contract excretory sphincters. Cognitively intact patients who have stress or urge incontinence may gain bladder control through biofeedback.

Pelvic floor exercises strengthen the pubococcygeus muscle. Daily practice is essential. These exercises are helpful for cognitively intact women who experience stress incontinence.

Clean intermittent catheterization is an appropriate approach for controlling incontinence associated with overflow incontinence.

Indwelling catheters are *avoided* if at all possible. The incidence of urinary tract infection with indwelling catheters is high. Short-term use may be needed during treatment of severe skin breakdown due to continued incontinence.

External catheters (condom catheters) to collect spontaneous voidings are useful for male patients with reflex or total incontinence. The appropriate design must be chosen for maximal success. The patient or caregiver must be taught how to apply the device, provide hygiene, including daily skin inspection, and care for the equipment.

Incontinence pads (diapers) are used only as a last resort. They conceal rather than solve the incontinence problem. Also they have the psychological effect of regression rather than progression. Every effort should be made to reduce the incidence of incontinence episodes through other methods that have been described. Incontinence pads may be useful at times for patients with stress or total incontinence to protect clothing, but should be avoided when possible.

▷ **Promoting Bowel Continence.**   The goals of a bowel training program are to develop regular bowel habits and to prevent uninhibited bowel elimination. *Regular complete emptying of the lower bowel results in bowel continence.* A bowel training program takes advantage of the patient's natural reflexes. Regularity, timing, nutrition and fluids, exercise, and correct positioning promote predictable defecation.

The nurse records defecation time, character of stool, nutritional intake, cognitive abilities, and functional self-care toileting abilities for 5 to 7 days. Analysis of this record helps design a bowel program for the individual with fecal incontinence.

Consistency in implementing the plan is essential. Attempts at evacuation should be made within 15 minutes of the same time daily. Natural gastrocolic and duodenocolic reflexes occur about 30 minutes after a meal. Therefore, after breakfast is one of the best times to plan for bowel evacuation. If the patient had a previously established habit pattern at a different time of day, it should be followed.

The anorectal reflex may be stimulated by rectal suppository (*e.g.,* glycerine) or mechanical stimulation (*e.g.,* digital stimulation with a lubricated gloved finger or anal dilator). The suppository should be inserted about 30 minutes before the scheduled bowel elimination time. The interval between insertion of suppository and defecation is noted for subsequent modification of the bowel program. Once the bowel routine is well established, stimulation with a suppository probably will not be necessary.

If at all possible the patient should assume the normal squatting position (knees higher than the hips) for defecation. Bedpans should be avoided if possible. The patient is instructed to bear down and to contract his abdominal muscles. If necessary, he can lean forward to increase intra-abdominal pressure and massage the abdomen right to left to facilitate movement of feces in the lower tract.

To promote regular bowel elimination, the diet should be high in fiber with adequate fluid (2000 to 2400 ml/day). Natural stimulants such as prunes, fruits, vegetables, and whole grains are preferred to laxatives.

▷ **Preventing Constipation.**   The record of bowel elimination, character of stool, food and fluid intake, level of activity, bowel sounds, medications, and other assessment data are reviewed to develop the plan of care. Multiple approaches may be used to prevent constipation.

The diet should be well balanced and include adequate intake of high fiber foods (vegetable, fruits, bran) to prevent hard stools and stimulate peristalsis. Fluid intake should be between 2 and 4 liters (2.1 to 4.2 quarts) per day unless contraindicated. Prune juice or fig juice (120 ml) taken 30 minutes before a meal once daily is helpful to some when constipation is a problem.

Physical activity and exercise are encouraged, as is self-care in toileting. A regular time for defecation is established. *The patient is encouraged to respond to the natural urge to defecate.* Privacy during toileting is provided.

Stool softeners, bulk-forming agents, mild stimulants, and suppositories may be prescribed to stimulate defecation and to prevent constipation.

▷ **Evaluation**

Expected Outcomes
1. Demonstrates control over excreta
   a. Experiences no episodes of incontinence
   b. Avoids constipation
   c. Achieves independence in toileting
2. Achieves urinary continence
   a. Uses therapeutic approach appropriate to type of incontinence
   b. Maintains adequate fluid intake
   c. Washes and dries skin after episodes of incontinence
3. Achieves bowel continence
   a. Participates in bowel program
   b. Verbalizes need for regular time for bowel evacuation
   c. Modifies diet to promote continence
   d. Uses bowel stimulators as prescribed and needed
4. Experiences relief of constipation
   a. Uses high-fiber diet, fluids, and exercise to promote defecation
   b. Responds to urge to defecate

Continuing Rehabilitation in the Community

An important goal of rehabilitation is to assist the person to return to his own environment after learning to manage his disability. A referral system maintains continuity of care when the patient is transferred to his home or to an extended care facility. The plan for discharge is formulated when the patient is first admitted to the hospital, and discharge plans are made with the patient's functional potential in mind.

The patient's support system (family, friends) is assessed. The attitudes of family and friends toward the patient, his disability, and his return home are important in successful transition to home.

Not all families are able to carry on the arduous programs of exercise and physical training that a patient may need. They may not have the resources or stability to care for a severely disabled family member. Even a stable family may be overwhelmed by the physical, emotional, economic, and energy strains of disabling disease. The family may require family therapy to allow them to discuss and explore their feelings and attitudes (rejection, aversion, avoidance) toward the disabled family member. Every effort is made for successful transition to home.

The family will need to know as much as possible about the patient's condition and care so that they will not fear his return home. The nurse plans with the patient and family methods for coping with problems that may arise. A skills checklist individualized for the patient and family can be developed to make certain that the family is proficient in assisting the patient with certain tasks.

The community health nurse visits the patient in the hospital, interviews the patient and family, reviews the ADL sheet, and gains first-hand knowledge of the activities the patient can perform. This helps ensure continuity of management and that the patient does not ''lose ground'' and instead maintains the independence gained while in the hospital. The family may need to purchase, borrow, or improvise needed equipment such as safety rails, raised toilet seat or commode, or tub bench. Ramps may have to be built or doorways widened to achieve full access.

Family members are taught how to use equipment and are given a copy of the manufacturer's instruction booklet, the names of resource persons, and lists of supplies and where these may be obtained. A written summary of the care plan is included in family teaching.

A network of support services and communication systems may be required to enhance opportunities for independent living. The nurse uses collaborative, administrative skills to coordinate these activities and pull the network of care together. The nurse also provides skilled care, initiates additional referrals when indicated, and serves as the patient's advocate and counselor when obstacles are encountered. She continues to reinforce the teaching that has been done and helps the patient to set and achieve attainable goals. The degree to which he adapts to his home and community environment depends on the confidence and self-esteem developed during the rehabilitation process and on the acceptance, support, and reactions of his family, employer, and community members.

There is a growing trend toward independent living by severely disabled people, either independently or in groups that share resources. Preparation for independent living should include training in managing a household and working with personal care attendants as well as training in mobility. The goal is integration into the community—living and working in the community with accessible housing, employment, public buildings, transportation, and recreation.

State rehabilitation administration agencies provide services to assist disabled persons in obtaining the help they need to engage in gainful employment. These services include diagnostic, medical, and mental health services. There are counseling, training, placement, and follow-up services available to help the individual with a disability select and attain a vocational objective.

If the patient is transferred to an extended care facility, the transition is planned to promote continued progress. Independence gained continues to be supported, and progress is fostered. Adjustment to the extended care facility is facilitated through communication. The family is encouraged to visit, to be involved, and to take the patient home on weekends and holidays if possible.

Chapter Summary

Rehabilitation is an integral part of nursing. It is a dynamic process that assists an individual, ill or disabled, in achieving his highest level of functioning and an acceptable quality of life with dignity, self-respect, and independence. Rehabilitation begins with the initial contact with the patient. Abilities, not disabilities, are emphasized. An interdisciplinary team approach is required. The individual with a disability is the key member of the rehabilitation team and an active participant in the rehabilitation process.

The rehabilitation nurse develops a therapeutic relationship with the patient. Within the nursing process, the nurse helps the individual with a disability identify his strengths and abilities, actively listens to the patient, encourages him, and shares in the rehabilitation process. The nursing assessment may include

a functional abilities index (*e.g.,* PULSES, Barthel Index, FIM, PECS). Based on the assessment and subsequent plan, the nurse will help the patient cope and adjust to the disability. The nurse focuses on facilitating self-care, improving mobility, promoting skin integrity, and managing bladder and bowel problems. The nurse in rehabilitation assumes many roles, including caregiver, teacher, counselor, client advocate, consultant, and case manager.

In facilitating self-care, the nurse teaches, guides, and supports the patient. The nurse encourages participation. Adaptive/assistive devices may be useful in attaining self-care goals. The patient is assisted in recognizing situations in which he needs assistance and in learning how to secure such assistance without overdependency.

A goal of rehabilitation is reentry into the community. Transitions between levels of health care and resumption of independent self-care (or with necessary and appropriate assistance) in the community are planned. The community health nurse works with the rehabilitation team, the patient, the patient's support system, and available community services to optimize the transition.

Bibliography
Books
American Nurses Association and Association of Rehabilitation Nurses. Standards of Rehabilitation Nursing Practice. Kansas City, MO. American Nurses Association, 1986.

Avillion A and Mirgon B. Quality Assurance in Rehabilitation Nursing: A Practical Guide. Rockville, MD, Aspen, 1989.

Basmajian JV and Wolf S (eds). Therapeutic Exercise. 5th ed. Baltimore, Williams & Wilkins, 1990.

Brandstater J and Basmajian J. Stroke Rehabilitation. Baltimore, Williams & Wilkins, 1987.

Carlson CE et al. Rehabilitation Nursing Procedure Manual. Rockville, MD, Aspen, 1990.

DeLisa J (ed). Rehabilitation Medicine: Principles and Practice, Philadelphia, JB Lippincott, 1988.

Dittmar S. Rehabilitation Nursing: Process and Application. St. Louis, CV Mosby, 1989.

England B et al. Quality Rehabilitation: Results Oriented Patient Care. Chicago, American Hospital Publishing Inc., 1989.

Ford J. Physical Management for the Quadriplegic Patient. 2nd ed. Philadelphia, FA Davis, 1987.

Fraser B et al. Physical Management of Multiple Handicaps: A Professional's Guide. Baltimore, Brookes, 1987.

Galias D. Rehabilitative Nursing Care of the Geriatric Resident. Des Moines, IA, Briggs Corp., 1988.

Goodgold J (ed). Rehabilitation Medicine. St. Louis, CV Mosby, 1988.

Heller B et al (eds). Psychosocial Interventions with Physically Disabled Persons. New Brunswick, NJ, Rutgers University Press, 1989.

Kottke F and Lehmann J (eds). Handbook of Physical Medicine and Rehabilitation. 4th ed. Philadelphia, WB Saunders, 1990.

Maloney FP, Burke JS and Ringel SP. Interdisciplinary Rehabilitation of Multiple Sclerosis and Neuromuscular Disorders. Philadelphia, JB Lippincott, 1985.

Matthews P and Carlson C. A Guide to Rehabilitation Nursing. Rockville, MD, Aspen, 1987.

Mumma C (ed). Rehabilitation Nursing: Concepts and Practice. 2nd ed. Evanston, IL, Rehabilitation Nursing Foundation, 1987.

O'Sullivan S and Schmitz T. Physical Rehabilitation: Assessment and Treatment. 2nd ed. Philadelphia: FA Davis, 1988.

Power P et al (ed). Family Interventions Throughout Chronic Illness and Disability. New York: Springer, 1988.

Rehabilitation Nursing Procedures Manual: the Nursing Division, the Rehabilitation Institute of Chicago. Rockville, MD, Aspen, 1989.

Schover L. Sexuality and Chronic Illness. New York: Guilford Press, 1988.

Sine R et al. Basic Rehabilitation Techniques: A Self-instructional Guide. 3rd ed. Rockville, MD, Aspen, 1988.

Singleton M and Branch E (ed). The Geriatric Patient: Common Problems and Approaches to Rehabilitation Management. New York, Haworth, 1989.

Journals

Asterisks indicate nursing research articles.

Rehabilitation

* Baillie V et al. Stress, social support, and psychological distress of family caregivers of the elderly. Nurs Res 1988 Jul/Aug; 37(4): 217–222.

Banja J. Independence and rehabilitation: A philosophic perspective. Arch Phys Med Rehabil 1988 May; 69(5): 381–382.

Burton W et al. Cost management of short term disability. AAOHN J 1987 Aug; 36(5): 224–227.

Caradoc-Davies T et al. Benefit from admission to a geriatric assessment and rehabilitation unit. J Am Geriatr Soc 1989 Jan; 37(1): 25–28.

Carlson R. Adult rehabilitation: Attitudes and implications. J Gerontol Nurs 1988 Feb; 14(2): 24–30.

Diehl L. Client and family learning in the rehabilitation setting. Nurs Clin North Am 1989 Mar; 24(1): 257–264.

Drayton-Hargove S et al. Rehabilitation and long term management of the spinal cord injured adult. Nurs Clin North Am 1986 Dec; 21(4): 599–610.

Evans RL et al. Prospective payment for rehabilitation: Effects on hospital readmission, home care, and placement. Arch Phys Med Rehabil 1990 Apr; 71(5): 291–294.

Fox B. Geriatric patient education: Issues and answers. J Contin Educ Nurs 1988 Jul/Aug; 19(4): 169–173.

* Gaynor SE. The long haul: The effects of home care on caregivers. Image J Nurs Sch 1990 winter; 22(4): 208–212.

Giberson T. Community liaison nursing. An expanded role for the rehabilitation nurse. Nurs Clin North Am 1989 Mar; 24(1): 165–170.

Gordon D (ed.) Rehabilitation. Nurs Clin North Am 1989 Mar; 24(1): 161–296.

Henderson S et al. Meet your colleague: The speech-language pathologist. Perspectives 1987 Spr; 11(1): 10–12.

Jaffe K. Home health care and rehabilitation nursing. Nurs Clin North Am 1989 Mar; 24(1): 171–178.

Kirchman M. Attitudes toward disability. Phys Occup Ther Geriatr 1987 Spr; 5(3): 51–63.

Malzer R. Patient performance level during inpatient rehabilitation: Therapist, nurse, and patient perspectives. Arch Phys Med Rehabil 1988 Mar; 69(5): 363–365.

* McNett SC. Social support, threat, and coping responses and effectiveness in functionally disabled. Nurs Res 1987 Mar/Apr; 36(2): 98–103.

Narain P et al. Predictions of immediate and 6-month outcomes in hospitalized elderly patients. J Am Geriatr Soc 1988 Sep; 36(9): 775–783.

Novak PP et al. Professional involvement in sexuality counseling for patients with spinal cord injuries. Am J Occup Ther 1988 Feb; 42(2): 105–112.

Powers J. Helping family and patients decide between home care and nursing home care. South Med J 1989 Jun; 82(6): 723–726.

Quigley R et al. Nurse's use of the terms compliance and non-compliance in rehabilitation nursing practice. Rehabil Nurs 1988 Mar/Apr; 13(2): 90–91.

Rubin M. The physiology of bed rest. Am J Nurs 1988 Jan; 88(1): 50–56.

Swanson B et al. The impact of psychosocial factors on adapting to physical disability: A review of research literature. Rehabil Nurs 1989 Mar/Apr; 14(2): 64–68.

* Waters K. Outcomes of discharge from hospital for elderly people. J Adv Nurs 1987 May: 12(3): 347–355.

* Watson P. Family participation in the rehabilitation process: The rehabilitator's perspective. Rehabil Nurs 1987 Mar/Apr; 12(2): 70–73.

* Willenbrink M. Rehabilitation nursing and the patient: Outside influences that affect the level of recovery. Rehabil Nurs 1990 Mar/Apr; 15(2): 90–92.

Assessment

Buchanan B. Functional assessment: Measurement with the Barthel Index and PULSES profile. Home Health Nurse 1986 Nov/Dec; 4(6): 11,14–17.

Brown M. Functional assessment of the elderly. J Gerontol Nurs 1988 May; 14(5): 13–17.

Gillies D. Family assessment and counseling by the rehabilitation nurse. Rehabil Nurs 1987 Mar/Apr; 12(2): 65–69.

* Harrell J et al. Do nursing diagnoses affect functional status? J Gerontol Nurs 1989 Oct; 15(10): 13–19.

Hoeman S. Cultural assessment in rehabilitation nursing practice. Nurs Clin North Am 1989 Mar; 24(1): 277–289.

Kane J et al. Diagnostic related groups: Their impact on an inpatient rehabilitation program. Arch Phys Med Rehabil 1987 Dec; 68(12): 833–836.

Ring C et al. Balance function in elderly people who have and have not fallen. Arch Phys Med Rehabil 1988 Apr; 69(4): 261–264.

Self-Care

Lenihan A. Identification of self-care behaviors in the elderly: A nursing assessment tool. J Prof Nurs 1988 Jul/Aug; 4(4): 285–288.

Lord J et al. Functional ability and equipment use among patients with neuromuscular disease. Arch Phys Med Rehab 1987 Jun; 68(6): 348–352.

Penn C. Promoting independence. J Gerontol Nurs 1988 Mar; 14(3): 14–19, 38–49.

Reich N et al. What to wear: A challenge for disabled elders. Am J Nurs 1987 Feb; 87(2): 98–103.

* Stride N. An investigation of the dependence of severely disabled people in a hospital. J Adv Nurs 1988 Sep; 13(5):557–564.

Mobility

Boies A. Management of contractures. Home Health Nurse 1987 Sep/Oct; 5(5): 40–41.

Gellman H et al. Late complications of the weight-bearing upper extremity in the paraplegic patient. Clin Orthop 1988 Aug; (233): 132–135.

Lane P and LeBlanc R. Crutch walking. Orthop Nurs 1990 Sep/Oct, 9(5): 31–38.

Maier P. Take the work out of range-of-motion exercises. RN 1986 Sep; 49(09): 46–49.

Mandzak-McCarron K and Drayton-Hargrove S. Ambulatory aids. Rehabil Nurs 1987 May/Jun; 12(3): 139–141.

Milde F. Impaired physical mobility. J Gerontol Nurs 1988 Mar; 14(3): 20–24, 38–40.

Selikson S et al. Risk factors associated with immobility. J Am Geriatr Soc 1988 Aug; 36(8): 707–712.

* Williams M et al. Efficacy of audiovisual tape versus verbal instructions on crutch walking: A comparison. J Emerg Nurs 1987 May/Jun; 13(3): 156–159.

Alteration in Skin Integrity

* Bergstrom N et al. The Braden Scale for predicting pressure sore risk. Nurs Res 1987 Jul/Aug; 36(4): 205–210.

Braden B and Bergstrom N. A conceptual schema for the study of the etiology of pressure sores. Rehabil Nurs 1987 Jan/Feb; 12(1):8–12, 16.

Brown EM et al. A strategy for the management of pressure ulcers in nursing homes. Ostomy Wound Management 1989 Spr; 22: 28–30, 32.

Ceccio CM. Understanding therapeutic beds. Orthop Nurs 1990 May/Jun; 9(3): 57–70.

Clark M. Measuring the pressure. Nurs Times 1988 Jun 22–28; 84(25): 72, 75.

* Copeland-Fields L and Hoshiko B. Clinical validation of Braden and Bergatrom's conceptual schema of pressure sore risk factors. Rehabil Nurs 1989 Sep/Oct; 14(5): 257–260.

* Dai V and Catanzaro M. Health beliefs and compliance with a skin care regimen, Rehabil Nurs 1987 Jan/Feb; 12(1): 13–16.

Gosnell D. Assessment and evaluation of pressure sores. Nurs Clin North Am 1987 Jun; 22(2): 399–416.

* Holmes R et al. Nutrition know how: Combating pressure sores nutritionally. Am J Nurs 1987 87 Oct; (10): 1301–1306.

Iverson-Carpenter M. Impaired skin integrity. J Gerontol Nurs 1988 Mar; 14(3): 38–40.

Kerbs L. Paralysis: Keeping bedsores at bay. RN 1987 Dec; 50(12): 30–31.

* LaMantia J et al. A program designed to reduce chronic readmissions for pressure sores. Rehabil Nurs 1987 Jan/Feb; 12(1): 22–25.

Melcher RE et al. Pressure sores in the elderly: a systematic approach to management. Postgrad Med 1988 Jan; 83(1): 299–308.

Mondoux L (ed). Pressure ulcers. Nurs Clin North Am 1987 Jun; 22(2): 357–492.

Moolten S. Prevention and treatment of decubitus ulcers. Hospital Medicine 1987 Aug; 23(8): 123–147.

Pressure ulcers prevalence, cost, and risk assessment: Consensus Development Conference. Decubitus 1989 May; 2(2): 24–28.

Rubin M. The physiology of bedrest. Am J Nurs 1988 Jan; 88(1): 50–58.

Tali C et al. User-friendliness of protective support surfaces in prevention of pressure sores. Rehabil Nurs 1989 Sep/Oct; 14(5): 261–263.

Waterlow J. Prevention is cheaper than cure. Nurs Times 1988 Jun 22–28; 84(25):69–70.

Altered Elimination

Abdellah FG. Incontinence: Implications for health care policy. Nurs Clin North Am 1988 Mar; 23(1): 291–298.

* Breakwell S et al. Differences in physical health, social interaction, and personal adjustment between continent and incontinent homebound aged women. J Community Health Nurs 1988; 5(1): 19–31.

Ellickson E. Bowel management plan for the homebound elderly. J Gerontol Nurs 1988 Jan/Feb; 14(1): 16–19.

Hahn K. Think twice about urinary incontinence. Nursing 1988 Jan; 18(1): 65–67.

Holmes P. Mind over bladder. Nurs Times 1990 Jan; 86(41): 16–17.

* Hu T et al. The cost effectiveness of disposable versus reuseable diapers; A controlled experiment in a nursing home. J Gerontol Nurs 1990 Feb; 16(2): 19–24, 36–37.

Jirovec MM, Brink CA, and Wells TJ. Nursing assessment in the inpatient geriatric population. Nurs Clin North Am 1988 Mar; 23(1): 219–230.

Johnson E et al. Dietary fiber intakes of nursing home residents and independent living older adults. Am J Clin Nutr 1988 Jul; 48(1): 159–164.

Kunin C et al. Morbidity and mortality associated with indwelling urinary catheters in elderly patients in a nursing home—Confounding due to the presence of associated diseases. J Am Geriatr Soc 1987 Nov; 35(11): 1001–1006.

McCormick K (ed). Urinary incontinence in the elderly. Nurs Clin North Am 1988 Mar; 23(1): 135–138.

McCormick KA, Scheve AAS, and Leahy E. Nursing management of urinary incontinence in geriatric inpatients. Nurs Clin North Am 1988 Mar; 23(1): 231–264.

Miller J. Assessing urinary incontinence. J Gerontol Nurs 1990 Mar; 16(3): 15–19, 34–35.

Morishita L. Nursing evaluation and treatment of geriatric outpatients with urinary incontinence. Nurs Clin North Am 1988 Mar; 23(1): 189–206.

Newman DK and Smith DA. Incontinence: The problem patients won't talk about. RN 1989 Mar; 52(3): 42–45.

Newman DK et al. Restoring urinary continence. Am J Nurs 1991 Jan; 91(1): 28–36.

Ouslander J et al. Clinical, functional, and psychosocial characteristics of an incontinent nursing home population. J Gerontol 1987 Nov; 42(6): 631–637.

Palmer MH. Incontinence: The magnitude of the problem. Nurs Clin North Am 1988 Mar; 23(1): 139–158.

Petrilli CO, Traughber B, and Schnelle JF. Behavioral management in the inpatient geriatric population. Nurs Clin North Am 1988 Mar; 23(1): 265–278.

Smith DAJ. Continence restoration in the homebound patient. Nurs Clin North Am 1988 Mar; 23(1): 207–218.

Wyman JF. Nursing assessment of the incontinent geriatric outpatient population. Nurs Clin North Am 1988 Mar; 23(1): 169–188.

15

The Person Experiencing Pain

Learning Objectives

On completion of this chapter, the learner will be able to:

1. Differentiate between acute and chronic pain
2. Describe existing theories of pain transmission and the role of endorphins in the perception of pain
3. Examine variables that affect the patient's response to pain
4. Describe how pain perception and response may differ in the elderly
5. Specify nursing interventions that are appropriate for managing anxiety related to pain
6. Incorporate noninvasive pain relief measures into the nursing care administered to patients with pain
7. Differentiate a preventive approach to pain management from an "as needed" approach to pain management
8. Explain the role of pain clinics, centers, and teams in the management of chronic pain
9. Write criteria appropriate for evaluation of the effectiveness of pain relief measures
10. Use the nursing process as a framework for care of patients with pain

---

Pain disables and distresses more people than any single disease entity. It is probably the most common reason for a person to seek health care. Most medical-surgical problems are associated with pain, resulting either from the disease process, diagnostic tests, or treatment modalities. (As a preliminary to this discussion, study Chart 15-1, Glossary of Terms.)

Until recently, little was known about pain. Most experts consider pain a phenomenon that defies precise definition. At

the very least, it appears to have three components: (1) a stimulus, physical or mental; (2) a bodily sensation of hurting; and (3) the reaction of the person experiencing it.

The nurse spends more time with the patient with pain than any other member of the health care team and therefore has the opportunity to make a significant contribution toward increasing the patient's comfort and relieving pain. The physician must seek to verify the patient's complaint of pain by

Chart 15-1
Glossary of Terms

Pain	A subjective, unpleasant sensory and emotional experience associated with actual or potential tissue damage.
Whatever the patient says it is, existing whenever the patient says it does.
Acute Pain	Pain that lasts 6 months or less and is most often associated with a specific injury.
Chronic Pain	Pain that lasts longer than 6 months and may or may not be associated with a specific cause; often unresponsive to treatment.
Nociceptor	A receptor sensitive to a noxious stimulus.
Noxious Stimulus	A stimulus that is damaging to normal tissues.
Pain Threshold	The least level of pain that a patient is able to detect.
Pain Tolerance	The greatest level of pain that a patient is able to tolerate.

establishing the cause and treating it. The nurse, in addition to collaborating with the physician toward this goal, also makes a major contribution to pain relief.

In clinical practice, when care is given to a patient with pain, it is essential that the nurse adopt the patient's point of view about his pain. A cardinal rule in the care of patients with pain is that *all pain is real*, regardless of its cause—even when the cause remains unknown. Therefore, the nurse's verification of pain is based simply on the patient's indication that it exists.

Within this context, *the nursing definition of pain is whatever bodily hurt the patient says he has, existing whenever he says it does.* This definition encompasses two important points that are ultimately relevant to assessment, intervention, and evaluation.

First, the nurse believes the patient when he indicates that he has pain. It is important to avoid concluding that the patient does not have pain because no physical origin can be identified. Although some painful sensations are initiated by or sustained by the patient's mental or psychological state, he actually feels a sensation of pain; he does not merely imagine that he has pain. Furthermore, painful states initiated by psychological states, such as anxiety, are usually accompanied by physical changes, such as decreased blood flow or muscle tension. Most painful sensations are the result of two sets of stimuli: physical and mental or emotional. Therefore, the assessment of a patient's pain involves obtaining information about the physical *and* mental or emotional causes of pain. Nursing intervention involves attempting to reduce or relieve both sources of pain.

The second point to keep in mind is that what the patient "says" about his pain is not limited to verbal statements. Some patients cannot or will not verbalize. Therefore, the nurse is also responsible for observing the many nonverbal behaviors that indicate the presence of pain.

Some patients deny pain, and they pose a different assessment problem. Although it is important to believe the patient who admits he has pain, it is equally important to be alert to patients who deny pain when they do in fact have pain. A very common reason for such denial is fear of becoming addicted to narcotics. If the nurse suspects pain in a patient who denies it, the nurse should explore with the patient his reason for suspecting pain, such as the fact that the disorder or pro-

cedure is usually painful, or that the patient grimaces when he moves, or avoids any movement. The nurse should also explore with the patient any reason that may cause him to deny pain, such as fear of addiction or further treatment.

Nursing Assessment

Assessment of the patient experiencing pain involves

- Determining whether the pain is acute or chronic
- Observing the patient's behavioral responses
- Identifying the factors that influence the pain and the patient's response to it

A thorough assessment is essential. To help the patient with his pain, the nurse must know that pain is occurring and how it affects the patient. This is not always obvious. The patient may try to hide his pain, or there may be a language barrier. Or, the patient may exhibit minimal responses to pain and, therefore, may appear not to experience pain.

Acute Versus Chronic Pain

The Commission on the Evaluation of Pain (1987) recognizes two basic categories of pain: acute pain and chronic pain. Acute pain is usually of recent onset and is most commonly associated with a specific injury. In the absence of residual damage or systemic disease, acute pain should subside as healing occurs; this takes place ordinarily in less than 6 months and usually occurs in less than 1 month. Chronic pain is constant or intermittent pain lasting for longer periods. It may or may not be associated with structural damage and may persist long after healing has occurred. Although acute pain is often thought to be useful in that it serves as a warning that something is wrong, chronic pain often becomes a problem in its own right and may not be an indication or warning of underlying impairment.

Acute Pain.   Acute pain is a very common occurrence. Generally, it indicates that some degree of damage has occurred within the body that requires some form of treatment or intervention. Usually organic disease or injury is present, although healing may also be accompanied by acute pain. As healing progresses, the pain subsides and gradually disappears.

Injuries or diseases that cause acute pain may require treatment or may heal spontaneously. For example, a prick of the finger may heal rapidly, the pain subsiding quickly, perhaps within a few minutes. In the case of a more drastic condition, such as appendicitis, surgery may be necessary. In these cases, the pain decreases with healing of the injury or surgical site.

Chronic Pain. Chronic pain is sometimes defined as pain that lasts for 6 months or longer, although 6 months is a rather arbitrary period for differentiating between acute and chronic pain. An episode of pain may assume the characteristics of chronic pain long before 6 months have elapsed, or some types of pain may remain primarily acute in nature for longer than 6 months. Nevertheless, after 6 months, the majority of pain experiences are accompanied by problems associated with chronic pain. Chronic pain serves no useful purpose, and if it persists, the pain itself may become the major disorder. Chronic pain persists beyond the expected healing time and often cannot be attributed to a specific cause of injury. It may not have a well-defined onset and usually does not respond to treatment methods directed at its cause.

The following are common types of chronic pain: (1) recurrent acute pain, (2) pain with obvious ongoing peripheral pathology, (3) chronic benign pain that may have peripheral or central pathology, and (4) chronic intractable benign pain syndrome.

Recurrent acute pain is intermittent pain. The patient has fairly well-defined episodes of pain interspersed with pain-free intervals. Because these episodes may recur over a period of years, recurrent acute pain is sometimes considered a type of chronic pain. Examples of recurrent acute pain are migraine headaches, sickle cell crises, and exacerbations of rheumatoid arthritis.

Pain with ongoing peripheral pathology may be of limited or unlimited duration. An example of time-limited pain with obvious ongoing peripheral pathology is the pain related to cancer. The pain may be of limited duration because the patient is eventually relieved after months of painful treatments, or the patient lives only a few months. In either case, the pain does not last for an extended period. An example of pain with ongoing peripheral pathology and unlimited duration is pain associated with degenerative arthritis.

Chronic benign pain (CBP) may be due to peripheral or central (brain and spinal cord) pathology. The pathology is often unclear, but it is not life threatening. (Benign means nonmalignant.) An example of CBP with central pathology is poststroke syndrome after a cerebral vascular accident (CVA). Tic douloureux is an example of central and peripheral pathology. Low back pain, a very common example of CBP, may be due to peripheral pathology, such as ischemic muscles, or central pathology, such as emotions causing muscle tension. As long as the patient functions well in daily life in spite of his pain, he usually remains classified in this category of CBP.

Chronic intractable benign pain syndrome (CIBPS) has the same characteristics as CBP, but the patient copes poorly. For example, the patient with low back pain may begin to use his pain to avoid dealing with marital or employment problems. Eventually, he may cope poorly with his job or marriage.

Although the last two categories describe pain that is benign, that is, not life-threatening, such pain can be destructive in terms of the patient's life-style or livelihood.

Assessment of Pain and the Patient's Behavioral Responses

The patient's responses to the pain may be any one or a combination of possible reactions. These may include physiologic manifestations, verbal statements, vocal behaviors, facial expressions, body movements, physical contact with others, or alterations in response to the environment. These behaviors vary greatly from one person to another and may differ within the same person from one time to the next.

The nurse observes the patient's behavioral response to identify the following:

- The *intensity* of the patient's pain. Whenever possible, the patient is asked to rate his pain on a verbal or numerical scale (*e.g.*, none, slight, moderate, severe, or very severe; or 0 to 10: 0 = no pain, 10 = worst possible pain) or a visual analogue scale. Use of such scales aids in identifying the pattern of pain and evaluating interventions.
- The patient's tolerance for this particular painful sensation. Pain *tolerance* may be defined as the maximum intensity or duration of pain the person is willing to endure.
- Characteristics of the painful sensation. These include *location* (see Fig. 15–1 for areas to which pain in various organs may be referred), *duration, rhythmicity* (periods of waxing and waning of the intensity or existence of pain), and *quality* (*e.g.*, pricking, burning, aching).
- Effects of pain on activities of daily living (*e.g.*, sleep, appetite, concentration, interactions with others, physical movement, work, and leisure activities). Acute pain is usually associated with anxiety, chronic pain with depression.
- What the patient believes will help him with his pain. Many patients have definite ideas about what will increase or decrease the intensity of their pain or what will make it more tolerable. These are often based on experience or trial and error.
- The patient's concern about his pain. This may include a wide variety of items, such as financial burdens, prognosis, interference with role performance, and body image changes.

Adaptation of Responses to Pain

Assessment of physiologic and behavioral indications of pain sometimes is difficult, if not impossible, during periods of adaptation. During this time, observable clues to the existence and nature of pain may be absent or minimal. An understanding of adaptation in contrast to the acute pain model will help one avoid the mistaken conclusion that a patient has no pain simply because "he doesn't act as though he has pain" (Fig. 15–2).

Most members of the health care team are more familiar with the acute pain model than the chronic pain model. It is not unusual for the nurse or physician to doubt the statement of a calm patient who says, "I have severe pain in my right leg," or of a patient who is able to sleep soundly immediately before or after reporting severe pain. One mistakenly tends to expect *all* patients with pain to exhibit some behavioral or physiologic responses associated with acute pain, including increased pulse and respiratory rates and the occurrence of

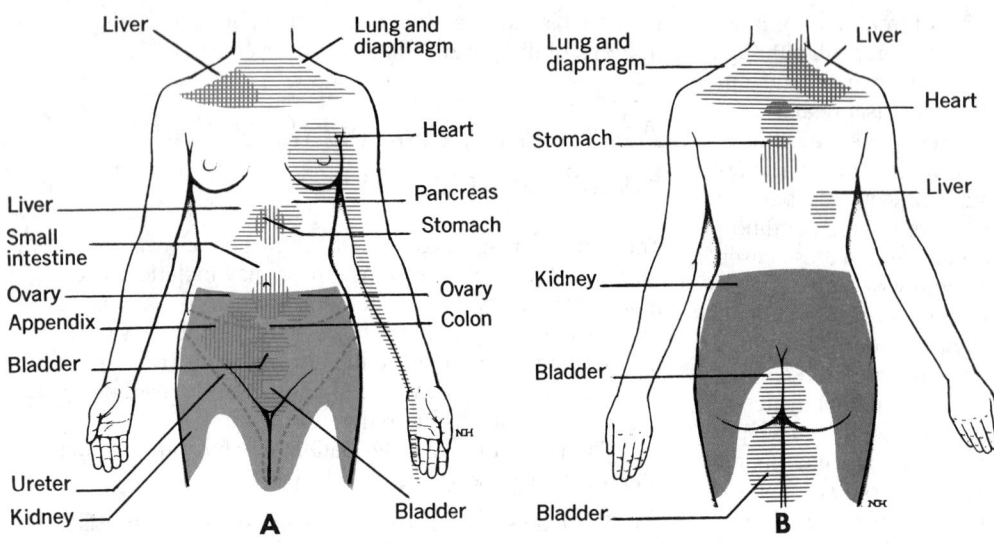

Figure 15–1. Referred pain. (**A**) Anterior view. (**B**) Posterior view. (Chaffee EE and Lytle IM. Basic Physiology and Anatomy, 4th ed. Philadelphia, JB Lippincott, 1980.)

pallor and perspiration. The patient in acute pain may also cry, moan, frown, immobilize a body part, clench his fist, or withdraw.

The responses a particular patient makes to the sudden onset of acute pain may not be the ones he makes when pain lasts more than a few minutes or when it becomes chronic. Because the body is unable to sustain an intense physiologic reaction to pain for weeks or years, or even several hours, a patient usually responds differently to acute and chronic pain.

Other behavioral manifestations of pain may also change drastically. The fatigue of being in pain may leave the patient too exhausted to moan or cry. He may sleep even when he has severe pain. The patient may appear relaxed and involved in activities because he has become a master at distracting

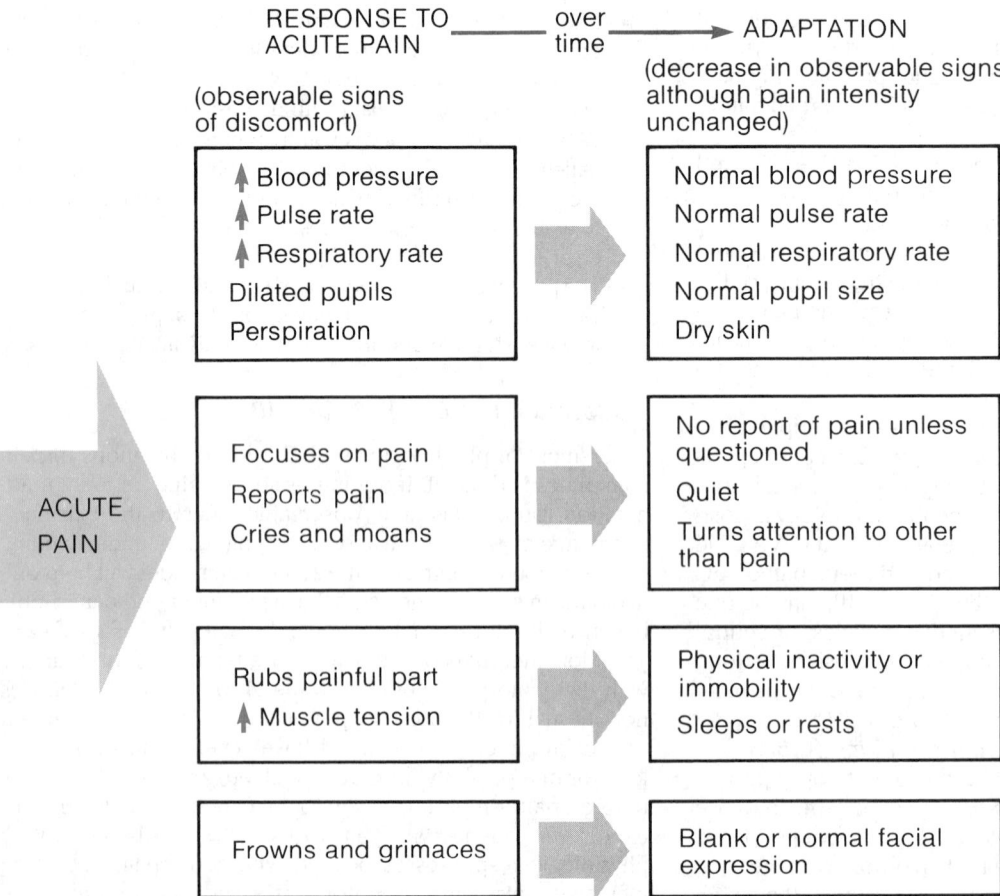

Figure 15–2. Adaptation to acute pain.

himself from pain. The patient who has succeeded in minimizing the effect of chronic pain on his life should be encouraged rather than discouraged from coping in this way.

Regardless of the type of adjustment made by the patient with chronic pain, pain over an extended period often produces behaviors typical of a disability. To some extent, the patient may be unable to continue the activities and interpersonal relationships he engaged in before pain began. This may range from merely having to curtail his participation in some vigorous physical activities to being unable to take care of his personal needs, such as dressing or eating.

Assessing the Harmful Effects of Pain

Special emphasis is placed on assessing the harmful effects of pain. Pain is often considered a helpful warning or signal that injury has occurred and that efforts must be taken to treat the injury or prevent further tissue damage. If, however, pain persists or ceases to be a warning of tissue damage, it becomes a distressing and often harmful experience. Prolonged or chronic pain may hamper rehabilitation from illness, or the pain itself may become a disability. Persistent, unrelieved pain may result eventually in depression, fatigue, sleep deprivation, weight gain or loss, decreased concentration, job loss, and divorce or other interpersonal problems.

Acute pain may result in problems that delay recovery from the acute illness associated with the pain, disturb the amount and quality of sleep, decrease appetite, reduce fluid intake, and cause nausea and vomiting. Adequate rest and nutrition are recognized as important factors in recovery from illness. When pain interferes with sleep and nutritional intake, the patient is deprived of important resources necessary for recovery and restoration of health. In addition, nausea, vomiting, and decreased fluid intake are potential threats to fluid and electrolyte balance.

Assessing the existence of pain, its nature, and its distressing and harmful effects requires that the nurse ask specific questions and make careful observations. Global, nonspecific questions are not sufficient because patients may give incomplete and inaccurate reports of their pain experience unless the nurse asks for details.

Assessment Tools

The initial assessment of pain may be accomplished using the assessment tool in Figure 15–3. If the location of pain is difficult to identify, the drawings in Figure 15–4 may also be used. Once completed, these forms may become a part of the health record or chart. As the nurse gains experience in the assessment of pain, it may be necessary to expand the assessment tool. Chart 15–2 provides guidelines for assessment of the patient with pain.

Information about pain is obtained from the patient and recorded on the pain assessment tool. The health record and the patient's family may supplement the information obtained from the patient. It is important to remember, however, that only the patient experiences the sensation of pain. Therefore, he is the only one who can rate it. Any verbal or numerical pain scale can be used, as long the same scale is used with that patient each time. The scale suggested on the assessment tool is 0 to 10 (0 = no pain, 10 = worst possible pain).

Factors Influencing the Pain Experience

The patient's pain experience is influenced by a large number of factors. These factors may increase or decrease the patient's perception of intensity of pain, increase or decrease his tolerance for pain, and produce a particular set of behavioral responses rather than other responses.

Some of these factors are situational, arising from the immediate circumstances. Others, discussed here, were already a part of the patient's physical and emotional makeup before the onset of pain. The following discussion focuses on only a

A.   NAME_____ DATE_____
LOCATION: Describe or point to area of pain. _____

QUALITY: What words best describe your pain?
_____

INTENSITY: Rate your pain on a scale of 0 (no pain) to 10 (worst pain possible)
    At present _____   1 hour after medication _____
    Worst it gets _____   Best it gets _____

ONSET: When did pain begin? _____   What time of day does it occur? _____
    How often does it occur? _____   How long does it last? _____

EFFECT OF PAIN: What relieves the pain? _____
What makes the pain worse? _____
What other problems/symptoms occur with the pain? _____
How does the pain affect your life and your activities? _____
_____

PLAN:
_____

B.   0   10
No pain   Visual Analogue Scale   Worst possible pain

Figure 15–3. (**A**) Pain assessment tool. (**B**) A 10-cm visual analogue scale. The patient is asked to indicate the intensity of his pain by marking the scale with an X.

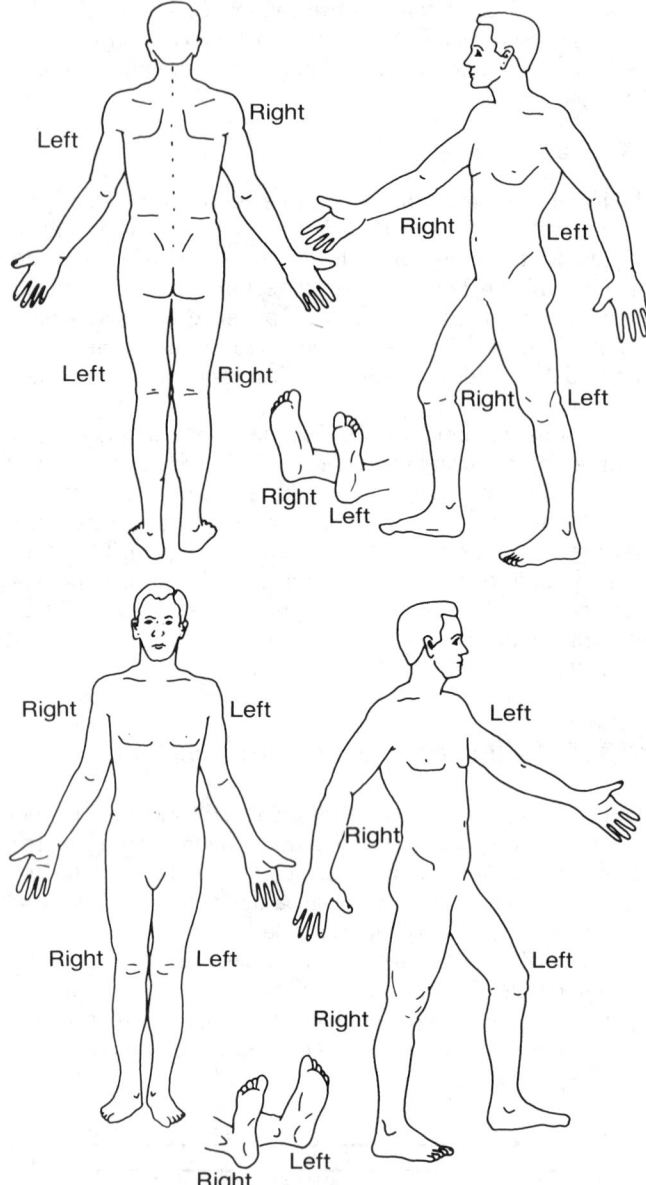

Figure 15–4. Pain assessment. The location of pain is noted and recorded on the figures as appropriate. (Melzack R [ed]. Pain Measurement and Assessment. New York, Raven Press.)

few of these preexisting factors that both influence the patient's pain experience *and* the nurse's understanding of it.

Neurophysiologic Mechanisms of Pain

Specific neuroanatomic structures are involved in the transformation of a stimulus into a sensation perceived as painful by the patient. This fact may lead to the erroneous conclusions that there is a direct and predictable relationship between a stimulus and the occurrence of pain and that all patients exposed to the same stimulus (*e.g.*, appendectomy) experience the same intensity of pain. This is *not* true; comparable lesions in different patients may result in very different sensations of pain. A nurse who does not realize this may expect the patient to have pain when he does not, or may believe that the patient

has little or no pain when he is actually experiencing severe pain.

There are many theories about the neurologic mechanisms that underlie a sensation of pain. Three commonly discussed theories are (1) the specificity theory, (2) the pattern theory, and (3) the gate control theory. These theories are not mutually exclusive, and none is considered entirely accurate or comprehensive. Each, however, makes a contribution to our understanding of what causes a person to perceive pain after a specific stimulus.

The *specificity theory* proposes that there are separate and specific receptors for pain and these transmit information to pain centers in the brain. Proponents of the *pattern theory* of pain state that pain receptors share nerve endings and pathways with other sensory modalities, but that different patterns of activity in the same neurons determine if sensations are perceived as painful or not painful. The *gate control theory* provides a particularly helpful basis for understanding the individuality of the pain experience. This theory proposes that there is interaction between pain and other sensory modalities and that stimulation of fibers that transmit nonpainful sensations are able to block the transmission of pain impulses through an inhibitory gating circuit.

Recent pain-related research has demonstrated that no single theory fully explains how pain is transmitted or perceived, nor does any theory adequately reflect the complexity of the neuroanatomic pathways that play a role in transmission of pain impulses, modulate the sensation of pain, explain individual differences in pain sensation, and enable us to distinguish between various types of pain.

Pain Transmission

Briefly, pain results when *nociceptors* (nerve endings) are stimulated by mechanical, thermal, or chemical factors. Nociceptive stimuli are those that have the potential to cause tissue damage. The impulse is transmitted from the nociceptors to the spinal cord along either A-delta fibers or C fibers (Fig. 15–5). Because they are covered with myelin, the A-delta fibers transmit painful impulses quickly. C fibers are small, unmyelinated fibers that conduct impulses more slowly. Impulses that are carried by the A-delta fibers are perceived as sharp, localized pain; those impulses carried by the smaller C fibers are perceived as diffuse, dull, aching pain. Nociceptive fibers enter the spinal cord through the dorsal horn, synapse in the spinal cord (in laminae I, II and V) and ascend as the spinothalamic tract. The spinothalamic tract has two divisions. One of these, the neospinothalamic tract, ascends to the thalamus and projects to the somatosensory cortex, where it transmits information about the quality, intensity, and location of the offending painful stimulus. Transmission along the second division, the paleospinothalamic tract, occurs at many synapses, transmits impulses through the reticular system, and terminates in the thalamus, with projections to the limbic and subcortical areas. The organization of this tract may explain why impulses conducted by the paleospinothalamic tract are perceived as more diffuse than those of the neospinothalamic tract.

Many substances currently under investigation have been found to have a significant influence on pain transmission. For example, substance P is a neuropeptide that facilitates the transmission of pain; whereas endorphins and enkephalins de-

---

Chart 15–2
Guidelines for Assessment of the Patient With Pain

1. Assess the characteristics of the patient's pain
   A. Severity of pain
   B. Quality, location, duration, and rhythmicity of pain
   C. Tolerance for pain
   D. Harmful effects of pain on patient's recovery
   E. Strategies that patient believes will help relieve pain
   F. Concerns the patient has about his pain
2. Assess the patient's behavioral responses to the pain experience
   A. Determine if the pain is acute or chronic
   B. Observe for the following behavioral responses
       (1) Physiologic manifestations (changes in pulse, blood pressure, respiratory rate, etc.)
       (2) Verbal statements
       (3) Vocal responses
       (4) Facial expressions
       (5) Body movements
       (6) Alteration in response to the environment
       (7) Physical contact with others
       (8) Adaptation of physiologic or behavioral responses
       (9) Effect of pain on ability to communicate and carry out usual activities of daily living
3. Assess factors that influence responses to pain
   A. Ethnic and cultural factors
   B. Previous pain experiences
   C. Meaning of the pain experience
   D. Patient's responses to pain relief strategies

---

crease the release of substance P and inhibit the transmission of painful impulses.

Endorphins and Enkephalins

The term *endorphin* is a combination of two words: *endogenous* and *morphine*. It means morphine within. Research has shown that the human body manufactures its own supply of endorphins and enkephalins, another morphine-like substance. When the body releases these substances, one effect is pain relief.

Endorphins and enkephalins are peptides that are found in heavy concentrations in the central nervous system. These substances relieve pain by the same mechanism as morphine and other narcotics. They are thought to inhibit impulses that would be experienced as painful by blocking their transmission in the brain and spinal cord.

The existence of these substances in the body has several possible implications in clinical practice. First, it helps explain why different people feel different amounts of pain from similar stimuli. There are individual differences in endorphin levels as well as situational factors, such as anxiety, that influence endorphin levels. People with more endorphin feel less pain, and those with less endorphin feel more pain.

Second, certain techniques may relieve pain at least in part because they cause the release of endorphins. Studies have suggested that placebos, acupuncture, and transcutaneous electric nerve stimulation may cause the release of endorphins.

Third, other methods of pain relief, such as mental imagery, may help the patient release his own endorphins.

Cultural Influences

Early in childhood a person learns what those around him expect and accept with respect to painful experiences. For example, the person may learn that an injury sustained during a sports activity is not expected to hurt as much as a comparable injury caused by an unexpected accident. Or, he may learn that the latter warrants a greater expression of pain than the former. He learns from others what stimuli are supposed to be painful and what kind of behavioral responses he should make. The people in his culture teach him this by their behavior toward him. They may ignore, punish, reward, or praise him, depending on his behavior and their beliefs. Because these beliefs vary from one culture to another, it is apparent that patients who experience the same intensity of pain may not necessarily report it or respond to it in the same ways.

Each person learns his own culture's expectations about pain throughout his life. Once these expectations are internalized, they are rarely altered by exposure to the opposing values of other cultures. Consequently, a person tends to grow up believing that his perceptions of and reactions to pain are the only correct and normal ones.

The values of the nurse's culture may conflict with the values of a patient from another culture. The nurse's cultural expectations and values may include avoiding overt expressions

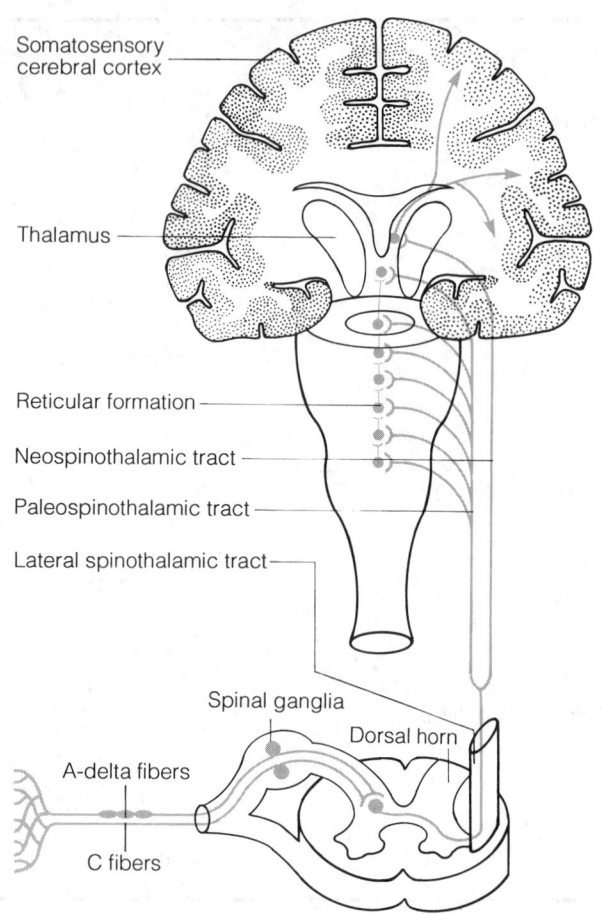

Figure 15-5. Pathways of transmission of nociceptive stimuli.

of pain, such as crying and moaning; seeking immediate relief from pain; giving complete descriptions of the pain; and having confidence in the health professions. A patient's cultural experiences may have taught him to moan and complain about pain, to refuse pain relief measures that do not cure the cause of the pain, to use adjectives like "unbearable" in describing his pain, and to be somewhat distrustful of the health care team. A patient from still another cultural background may behave differently, or he may behave similarly but for different reasons.

Many other attitudes and behaviors—a patient's preference for having visitors or being alone or his attitude toward his diagnosis—may vary from one culture to another. Recognizing the values of one's own culture and learning how these values differ from those of other cultures help the nurse avoid evaluating the patient's behavior on the basis of her own cultural expectations and values. It is equally important, however, to avoid stereotyping patients by culture. A nurse who recognizes cultural differences will have greater understanding of the patient's pain and will be more accurate in assessing pain and behavioral responses to it as well as more effective in relieving the patient's pain.

Past Experience With Pain

It is tempting to expect that a person who has had multiple or prolonged experiences with pain will be less anxious and more

tolerant of pain than a person who has not experienced much pain. For most patients, however, the reverse is true.

Often, the more experience the patient has had with pain, the more frightened he will be about subsequent painful events. He may also be less able to tolerate pain, that is, he wants relief from the pain sooner and at lower levels of intensity. This is understandable if we consider that many patients with pain receive unsatisfactory or inadequate pain relief from time to time. Thus, the patient with repeated pain experiences may learn to fear the escalation of pain and the possibility that he will not receive relief. Furthermore, once a patient experiences severe pain, he knows just how severe pain can become. Conversely, the patient who has never experienced severe pain may not have fear of such pain.

A patient's response to pain may be a consequence of many separate painful events during his life. For other patients, past pain may have been constant and unrelenting, as in prolonged or chronic and persistent pain. The patient who has pain for months or years may suffer additional effects from this experience and he may become irritable, withdrawn, and depressed.

The undesirable effects that may result from past experiences point to the need for the nurse to be aware of the patient's past experiences with pain. If the patient's pain is relieved promptly and adequately, he may be less fearful of future pain and more able to tolerate it. Table 15-1 presents and corrects many of the common misconceptions we have about pain and its assessment.

Gerontologic Considerations

Assessment of pain in the elderly may be difficult because of physiologic, psychological, and social characteristics found in the aged. Older persons may experience reduced sensory perception and an increased pain threshold because of degeneration of neurons in the dorsal column of the spinal cord. As a result, they may incur injury without being aware of it or may experience a painful condition in an atypical way. Acute pain may not be as sharply perceived in the elderly, although chronic pain may be more intense. The pain response and pattern may be different from those usually seen in younger patients, or the pain may be referred far from the site of injury or disease.

Although pain is one of the major reasons that many of the elderly seek health care, others are reluctant to seek help even if in severe pain because they think of pain as a problem expected in old age. It has been estimated that over 85% of older adults have at least one chronic health problem that could cause pain. The older adult tends to underreport pain and endure more pain for longer periods before reporting it or seeking health care. Others fail to seek care because they fear that the pain may indicate a serious illness or they fear loss of control. The patient may respond to pain by using over-the-counter medications or medications prescribed for other illnesses. The elderly person deals with pain according to his life-style, personality, and cultural background. Many elderly people are very fearful of addiction and as a result will not report that they are in pain or ask for pain medication.

Contrary to the views of the elderly as well as many health care providers, pain in the elderly is often *more* significant than in younger persons. For example, the onset of persistent headache in the elderly may be a symptom of serious intracranial bleeding. Appendicitis in the elderly may be overlooked be-

TABLE 15–1. Misconceptions About Assessment of Patients Who Indicate They Have Pain

Misconception	Correction
1. The health team is the authority about the existence and nature of the patient's pain sensation.	The person with pain is the only authority about the existence and nature of that pain, as the sensation of pain can be felt only by the person who has it.
2. Our personal values and intuition about the trustworthiness of others is a valuable tool in identifying whether a person is lying about pain.	Personal values and intuition do not constitute a professional approach to the patient with pain. The patient's credibilty is not on trial.
3. Pain is largely an emotional or psychological problem, especially in the patient who is highly anxious or depressed.	Having an emotional reaction to pain does not mean that pain is caused by an emotional problem. If anxiety or depression is alleviated, the intensity of pain will not necessarily be any less.
4. Lying about the existence of pain, malingering, is common.	Very few people who say they have pain are lying about it. Outright fabrication of pain is considered rare.
5. The patient who obtains benefits or preferential treatment because of pain is receiving secondary gain and does not hurt as much as he says or may not hurt at all.	The patient who uses his pain to his advantage is not the same as a malingerer and may still hurt as much as he says he does. Also, secondary gain may be an inaccurate diagnosis.
6. All real pain has an identifiable physical cause.	All pain is real, regardless of its cause. Almost all pain has both physical and mental components. Pure psychogenic pain is rare.
7. Visible signs, either physiologic or behavioral, accompany pain and can be used to verify its existence and severity.	Even with severe pain, periods of physiologic and behavioral adaptation occur, leading to periods of minimal or no signs of pain. Lack of pain expression does not necessarily mean lack of pain. How must the patient act for us to believe he has pain?
8. Comparable physical stimuli produce comparable pain in different people. The severity and duration of pain can be predicted accurately for everyone on the basis of the stimuli for pain.	Comparable stimuli in different people do *not* produce the same intensities of pain. Comparable stimuli in different people will produce different intensities of pain that last different periods. There is no direct and invariant relation between any stimulus and the perception of pain.
9. People with pain should be taught to have a high tolerance for pain. The more prolonged the pain or the more experience a person has with pain, the better is his tolerance for pain.	Pain tolerance is the individual's unique response, varying between patients and varying in the same patient from one situation to another. People with prolonged pain tend to have an increasingly low pain tolerance. Respect for the patient's pain tolerance is crucial for adequate pain control.
10. When the patient reports pain relief after a placebo, this means that the patient is a malingerer or that the pain is psychogenic.	There is not a shred of evidence anywhere in the literature to justify using a placebo to diagnose malingering or psychogenic pain.

(McCaffery M and Beebe A. Pain: Clinical Manual for Nursing Practice. St Louis, CV Mosby, 1989, p 17.)

cause of altered pain responses, delay in reporting symptoms, or blunted immune responses.

Nursing Interventions

Basic Care Plan

Once information about the patient is obtained, it provides a basis for designing individualized nursing care. *First, the nurse plans to alter factors that influence the nature of the pain sensation and factors that increase the intensity of the patient's behavioral responses to the pain experience.* Some influencing factors, however, cannot be altered. For example, if a painful sensation is being caused by pressure from an inoperable malignancy, it is not possible to alter this factor because the tumor cannot be removed. In some cases, positioning, chemotherapy, or irradiation may decrease the pressure.

Appropriate use of analgesic agents may relieve the pain. The influence of the patient's cultural expectations usually cannot be altered, and no attempt should be made to do so.

Because it may not be possible or desirable to alter some of the patient's responses to his pain experience, *the second part of the nurse's plan of care includes identifying appropriate ways to respond to the patient's behaviors and attitudes about pain.* For example, the patient's cultural and personal experiences may have taught him that the preferred and natural response to pain experiences is not to share his feelings and sensations with anyone. Another patient may feel quite the opposite, wanting to describe his feelings and pain in detail. Appropriate and helpful nursing approaches to these two patients will differ markedly.

After examining what can be done to assist the particular patient with his pain experience, *the third phase of the nurse's plan is to identify appropriate goals for nursing intervention and share or validate these goals with the patient.* For a few patients, the goal may be total elimination of the painful sensation. For many patients, this is not realistic. Other goals may include a decrease in intensity, duration, or frequency of pain and limitation of the detrimental effects of pain on the patient. For example, pain may decrease appetite or interfere with sleep and thereby hamper recovery from an acute illness. Thus, goals may be a good night's sleep and adequate nutritional intake. Prolonged pain may decrease the quality of life by interfering with work or interpersonal relationships. Thus, a goal may be to decrease time lost from work or increase the quality of interpersonal relationships.

These goals may be accomplished by pharmacologic or nonpharmacologic, noninvasive means. In the acute stages of illness, the patient may be less able to actively participate in relief measures, but when the patient has the mental and physical energy, he may learn self-management techniques for pain relief, such as relaxation imagery. Hence, as the patient progresses through the stages of recovery, a goal may be to decrease reliance on medication for pain relief and increase the patient's use of self-management and noninvasive pain relief measures.

Managing Anxiety Related to Pain

Anxiety may have a profound effect on the sensation and response to pain. Therefore, anxiety related to the anticipation of a painful experience, the painful experience itself, or the consequence or aftermath of the pain experience will be discussed.

Anticipation of Pain. It may be desirable for the patient anticipating a painful experience to have a moderate amount of anxiety about the impending pain so that he will be motivated to find methods of coping with it. It is not unusual for this patient to worry about his anticipated pain some of the time but not all of the time. Usually, this useful level of anxiety results from informing the patient about when his pain will occur, its locations, and the intensity and duration of pain that are expected. The nurse then channels this anxiety into helping the patient learn a variety of pain relief measures (see pp. 257–260).

During the phase of anticipation of pain, teaching the patient about the nature of the impending painful experience and what he can do to obtain relief usually minimizes the anxiety the patient will have when he actually feels the pain sensation. With this approach, the patient knows that he can do something about the pain when it occurs. Hence, anticipation of pain is less likely to increase anxiety as much as it would if the patient had no knowledge of what to do to reduce or cope with the pain. Learning about pain relief measures may give the patient a sense of control over sensations of pain, as he views pain as less threatening.

One of two extremes of reaction may occur when a patient is taught about a future painful event: intense anxiety or complete absence of anxiety. Anxiety-reducing techniques that may be effective with patients who appear to be highly anxious include focusing the patient's attention on a specific activity or eliminating a source of anxiety; for instance, by helping an anxious relative to become less anxious. Administering tranquilizing drugs, if prescribed, behavior modification, hypnosis, or consultation with a psychiatrist or psychiatric clinical nurse specialist may be indicated if anxiety is severe.

The person who shows little or no anxiety about impending pain may know from his past experiences that he has a high tolerance for pain. However, some patients who show low anxiety or no anxiety are denying the fact that they may have pain. When pain actually occurs, these patients tend to have considerable difficulty in coping with pain and are quite anxious. What can be done to assist these patients before the painful event is largely unknown. It is not known with certainty whether it is better to continue to give them information or to give them no information. When giving the patient specific information about pain does not result in moderate anxiety, further information probably should focus on pain relief measures; the information should be brief, essential, and general.

When the nurse suspects that the patient's lack of anxiety reflects an effort to deny information he receives about pain, the nurse explores with the patient whether he wants more information about either pain or its relief; the patient's wishes and decision should be respected. The patient should be closely observed for a marked increase in anxiety, however, as the time of the painful event approaches. The previous suggestions regarding interactions with patients with moderate and severe anxiety can then be employed, depending on the level of anxiety noted.

At times, the nurse may be tempted not to tell a patient that he may experience pain or that the pain may be much greater than he seems to think. The nurse may predict correctly that such knowledge will make the patient anxious. The prospect of pain usually arouses some anxiety in the patient. If the patient is to learn ways of coping with pain, however, he must first know that pain may occur. Failure to forewarn the patient of pain is probably a mistake *unless:* (1) previous experience shows that forewarning this patient produces such a high level of uncontrollable anxiety that the patient is unable to take positive steps to handle his pain; (2) the patient specifically requests that he not be forewarned, and this request has been thoroughly explored with the patient; or (3) previous experience shows that teaching this patient about pain and its relief impedes his coping mechanism of denial and that he has no other effective mechanism for coping with stress.

What the nurse tells the patient about the available pain relief measures and their effectiveness may also affect his anxiety. The nurse may prevent an increase in anxiety by explaining briefly to the patient the general type of pain relief he can expect from each pain relief measure. For example, if the patient expects distraction or medication to eliminate his pain totally, his anxiety may increase when this does not occur. These pain relief measures along with many others frequently do not eliminate the pain completely or reduce its intensity. Instead they tend to increase the patient's tolerance for pain or make the pain less bothersome to the patient.

The Sensation of Pain. When pain sensations are felt by the patient, it is desirable to reduce the patient's anxiety to as low a level as possible. When the patient is anxious about his pain, there is a tendency for him to perceive a greater intensity of pain or to be less tolerant of the pain. This in turn produces greater anxiety. Thus, a spiraling process is initiated in which the patient becomes more anxious and experiences greater pain or becomes progressively less tolerant of it.

It is important to interrupt this cyclical process as soon as possible to prevent escalation of the pain level. Low levels of anxiety or pain are easier to reduce or control than are higher levels. Consequently, *pain relief measures should be used before pain becomes severe.* Many patients believe that they should not request pain relief measures until pain approaches or exceeds the maximum level they are able to tolerate, making it difficult for mediations to provide adequate relief. Therefore, it is important to explain to all patients that pain relief or control is more successful if pain relief measures are used *before* pain becomes unbearable.

Anxiety during anticipation of pain or the pain experience itself may often be managed effectively by establishing a relationship with the patient and by patient teaching (see Nurse–Patient Relationship and Teaching). Almost all nursing interventions for pain relief contribute in some way toward decreasing anxiety.

Aftermath of a Painful Experience. When the pain sensation subsides, it is hoped that the patient's anxiety also will subside. When this does not happen, certain techniques may help the patient to integrate the pain experience (Table 15–2).

For many patients, the experience of pain continues after the sensation of pain ceases or subsides. Some patients continue to fear pain because they do not know that there is no longer any danger that pain will occur. Explaining that the noxious stimuli have been removed often reduces the patient's fear and anxiety.

Most patients do not forget about a painful experience as soon as pain decreases or disappears. The patient may be disturbed about his own behavior during the pain experience or be concerned about how others view his responses. He may have incorrect or somewhat frightening ideas about the cause of his pain or the treatment for it. His general sense of personal safety and control may be shaken by having felt more intense pain than he had imagined possible. The patient who is relieved of chronic pain may experience a crisis, fearing what he will be like without pain. The patient also may suddenly begin trembling, perspiring, or have nausea, vomiting, or chills. Some patients have nightmares about a painful experience for weeks and months after it is over. Obviously, the care of the patient with pain and management of anxiety extend beyond the actual episode of pain.

Noninvasive Pain Relief Measures

Because of the lack of knowledge or time, many patients and health team members tend to regard analgesics as the only method of pain relief. There are many nursing activities, however, that can be used to assist the patient with his pain experience. Various categories of such nursing activities are outlined in Table 15–2.

The purpose of the table is to introduce the nurse to the variety of nursing activities that may be used to help patients with their pain experiences. This brief synopsis is intended to introduce these measures. For help in acquiring additional knowledge, the nurse is referred to more complete sources of information (see Bibliography). Through reading and practice, the nurse may easily learn to use these activities with patients.

Some of the noninvasive nursing activities listed in Table 15–2 will be discussed here in more detail. *Noninvasive* simply means that no physical or bodily intrusion is involved. Noninvasive methods of pain relief entail very low risks. Although noninvasive pain relief measures are not a substitute for analgesics, a noninvasive technique may be all that is necessary or appropriate for brief episodes of pain lasting only seconds or minutes. In other instances, especially when there is severe

pain that lasts for hours or days, the use of some noninvasive techniques along with medications may be the most effective way to relieve pain.

Nurse–Patient Relationship and Teaching

The two nursing measures basic to all others in pain management are the nurse–patient relationship and patient teaching about pain and its relief. These activities may reduce pain in the absence of other pain relief measures. Each may enhance the effectiveness of other pain relief measures used. The nurse–patient relationship and teaching serve to reduce the patient's anxiety about pain and commonly result in pain relief, either by decreasing the intensity of pain or by making it more tolerable to the patient.

Trust is an important aspect of the nurse–patient relationship. Conveying to the patient the belief that he has pain often helps reduce his anxiety. Some patients spend considerable time and energy trying to convince others that they have pain. The presence of pain may be doubted by others because no cause can be found for it or because the person's behavior is not typical of what the health care team expects. This is particularly true for those patients whose coping strategies often result in minimal outward signs of pain or distress. To say to a patient, "I know you have pain [or discomfort], and I want to understand it better," often will set the patient's mind at rest. Occasionally, a patient who has feared that no one will believe that he has pain will feel gratitude and relief when he knows that he can trust the nurse and that the nurse believes him.

Whenever the nurse encounters a patient with pain, the nurse must convey to the patient that she wants to assist him to obtain pain relief. The patient may not know where to turn for help in relieving the pain; it is seldom that any one person on the health care team is explicitly responsible for providing pain relief. However, when the nurse says very simply, "Let me know when you begin to hurt so I can help you do something about it," the nurse conveys to the patient that she cares and assumes responsibility for helping with his pain.

The nurse also provides information, through patient teaching, about how pain can be controlled. The patient is informed, for example, that pain should be reported in the early stages. When the patient waits too long before reporting it, the pain may be intense and his anxiety may be very high. It is much easier to prevent severe pain and panic than to relieve them once they occur.

Cutaneous Stimulation

According to the gate control theory, stimulation of large-diameter nerve fibers in the skin may reduce the intensity of pain. Skin stimulation may also cause the release of endorphins. Such skin stimulation can be accomplished in a variety of ways. In devising methods of cutaneous stimulation for pain relief, the nurse considers which form of stimulation is to be used and the location, duration, and intensity of stimulation. The approach is one of trial and error, but common sense often is an effective guide.

Various forms of cutaneous stimulation are easily available at low cost. Although some form of cutaneous stimulation is usually acceptable, consultation with the patient's physician may be necessary, for some forms may be contraindicated because of the patient's medical diagnosis or physical condi-

TABLE 15-2. *Nursing Activities to Assist the Patient With His Pain Experience*

Category of Nursing Activity	Explanation	Example of Nursing Activity
1. Establishing a relationship with the patient with pain	Interacting with the patient as a total person, believing what the patient says he experiences, and respecting his reactions and attitudes regarding pain (see text)	Telling the patient you believe what he says about his pain experience
2. Teaching the patient about pain and its relief	Using a variety of the patient's sensory modalities for the purpose of conveying to him information about his pain experience (see text)	Explaining the quality and location of impending pain by applying pressure or lightly pinching the skin in the area where the patient will have an incision
3. Using the patient–group situation	Using the principles of small group functioning to teach the patient and family about the patient's pain experience	The nurse, two female patients with arthritis, and their husbands discussing modifications in homemaking activities after discharge from the hospital
4. Managing other people who come in contact with the patient	Assisting other people to reach their maximum potential for helping the patient with his pain experience	Talking alone with a patient's wife, who shows marked anxiety in the presence of her husband when he complains of his undiagnosed abdominal pain
5. Using cutaneous stimulation	Using various qualities, locations, durations, and intensities of stimuli in contact with the skin (see text)	Applying a hand-held vibrator to the scalp and back of the neck to relieve headache
6. Providing distraction from pain	Obtaining the patient's response to and participation in stimuli through the major sensory modalities (see text)	Helping the patient to use chant with breathing during a painful dressing change
7. Promoting relaxation	Using a variety of techniques to assist the patient to avoid fatigue and to achieve skeletal muscle relaxation	Helping the patient learn to use slow, rhythmic breathing
8. Using guided imagery	Assisting the patient to imagine a pleasant event as a substitute for the pain experience or to imagine a means of ridding his body of the pain (see text)	Helping the patient imagine that he is ridding himself of pain as he exhales slowly
9. Administering pharmacologic agents	Giving medications with pain-relieving potential to the patient and explaining the effects, assisting the physician in determining the patient's need for analgesics (see text)	Administering analgesics on a preventive basis
10. Decreasing noxious stimuli	Using a variety of techniques to reduce the transmission of pain signals to the cortex of the brain	Splinting an abdominal incision during coughing and deep breathing
11. Using the assistance of professionals	Assisting the patient, his family, and his physician to identify the need for additional help in dealing with pain; assisting the patient and his family to obtain this help and to use it to their best advantage	Suggesting to the patient that his clergyman may be able to counsel him about his concern (reduce anxiety) that his pain is punishment for a sin
12. Being with the patient	Identifying and responding to the patient who would benefit from the mere presence of the nurse or someone else	Getting a hospital volunteer to sit at the bedside of the patient who does not want to be alone with his pain experience
13. Conveying that the source of noxious stimuli has been removed or decreased	Conveying to the patient, when appropriate, that something has been done to diminish or eliminate a cause of his pain (see text)	Telling the patient undergoing lumbar puncture that the needle has just been removed and all that remains is to cleanse his back
14. Assisting with the assimilation of the painful experience	Identifying the patient's need for and assisting him with the intellectual and emotional incorporation of a painful experience (see text)	Discussing with the patient what sensations he felt and what he was thinking while experiencing the myocardial infarction on the previous day

(Adapted from McCaffery M. Nursing Management of the Patient With Pain, 2nd ed. Philadelphia, JB Lippincott)

tion. Different types of skin sensations may be elicited when the following measures are applied: pressure, vibration, heat, cold, bathing, lotion, menthol cream, and transcutaneous electric nerve stimulation (TENS). TENS has proved to be helpful in both acute and chronic pain relief, and its use is becoming more widespread. It consists of a battery-operated unit with electrodes that are applied to the skin to produce a tingling, vibrating, or buzzing sensation in the area of pain (Fig. 15–6.)

Local application of cold to a painful part is an underused but often highly effective method of relieving pain. Compared with local applications of heat, cold relieves pain faster, and pain relief may last longer. Contrary to popular belief, cold does not necessarily cause muscle contraction, but slows the conduction of impulses that maintain muscle tone and may cause muscle relaxation. Therefore, cold is not only indicated to reduce bleeding and swelling of a new injury but also may be continued for pain relief.

When cutaneous stimulation is used, it is applied to different areas of the body. Usually, stimulating the skin on or near the pain site is effective. In other instances, direct stimulation over the pain site must be avoided because it elicits more pain. If stimulation of the skin near the pain site is ineffective, painful, impossible, or contraindicated, the side of the body opposite the painful area may be stimulated for pain relief. This is called *contralateral stimulation*. For example, the pain of "tennis elbow" on the left side may be relieved as well or better by applying menthol cream to the right elbow rather than the left. This is especially helpful to remember when the site of pain is difficult to stimulate directly, such as when a cast has been applied over a painful area or when the entire extremity is injured or burned.

Stimulation of moderate intensity is usually applied. Mild stimulation tends to be ticklish or annoying, whereas intense stimulation may cause pain.

In general, the duration of cutaneous stimulation indicated and the intervals between its applications vary considerably.

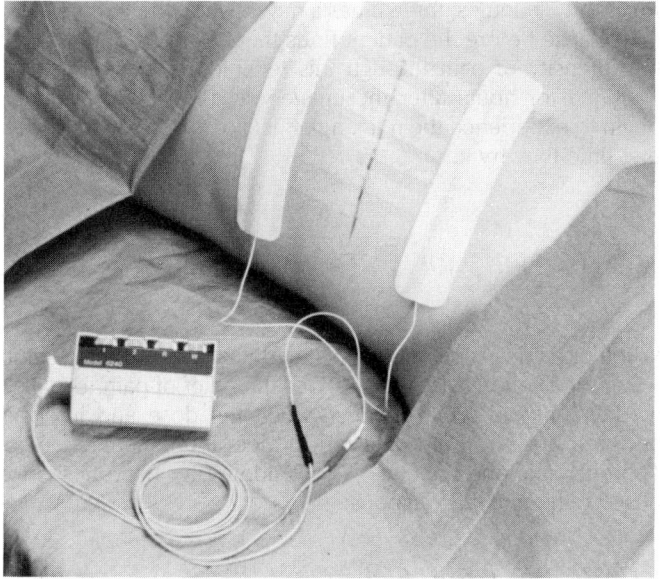

Figure 15–6. Transcutaneous electric nerve stimulation (TENS) being used for relief of incisional pain postoperatively. (Courtesy of Health Care Specialties Division/3M, St Paul, Minnesota.)

Some patients experience pain relief for hours or days after cutaneous stimulation. Others obtain relief only while stimulation is being applied. For these patients, use of a menthol cream or a TENS unit is an efficient means of providing continuous stimulation without interfering with the patient's activity. It takes only a few minutes to apply, but the cutaneous stimulation lasts for hours. The TENS unit may be worn 24 hours a day.

Distraction

Distraction, or focusing the patient's attention away from his painful sensations, may be an effective method of pain relief. It may decrease the perceived intensity of pain, or increase tolerance for pain, making it less bothersome. If the person is less aware of pain or pays less attention to it, he will be less bothered by pain and more tolerant of it.

There are many types of distraction, ranging from simply preventing monotony to the use of highly complex physical and mental activities. When environmental stimuli are deficient in amount, pattern, or variation, the person's centrally regulated thresholds for sensation tend to be lowered, resulting in increased sensitivity to input such as pain.

If the patient with pain is experiencing decreased environmental or sensory stimuli, pain may be reduced by the nurse's introducing environmental stimuli. This is a mild form of distraction that focuses the patient's attention away from his pain. The distraction may involve minimizing strange noises, making brief but frequent visits to the patient, bringing him a snack, or teaching him appropriate physical exercises.

More deliberate and intense forms of sensory stimulation may be necessary to distract the patient from brief episodes of severe pain, such as pain from bone marrow aspiration or wound debridement, or longer periods of moderate to severe pain. Some patients are able to use distraction effectively for hours for pain relief.

The value of distraction techniques for pain relief is frequently misunderstood by the health care team. A common misconception about distraction as a means of pain relief is that the patient who can be distracted from his pain does not have much pain. For example, the nurse may erroneously assume that the patient cannot have pain if he is laughing and talking with visitors. Distraction is a powerful method of pain relief, however, which should be encouraged. Doubting the patient's pain because he uses distraction effectively may result in the patient's discarding this effective way to cope with pain.

The effectiveness of distraction depends on the degree to which the patient is able to receive and create sensory input other than pain. As a rule, pain relief is increased in direct relation to the patient's active participation, the number of sensory modalities used, and the patient's interest in the stimuli. Therefore, stimulation of sight, sound, and touch is likely to be more effective in reducing pain than stimulation of a single sense.

Increasing the complexity of the distractor as pain increases will be effective in pain relief, however, only up to a certain level of pain intensity. With severe pain, the patient may be unable to concentrate well enough to engage in highly complicated mental or physical activities.

Many patients devise their own distraction strategies. The patient may hum, mentally calculate math problems, or choose an absorbing television program. The nurse may support these efforts and assist the patient to elaborate on them.

Under conditions of brief, severe pain, it may be effective to teach the patient a distraction strategy. A technique that may be taught quickly, even to patients who are debilitated, fatigued, sedated, or in severe pain, is to combine rhythmic rubbing with visual concentration. The patient is asked to open his eyes, stare at a specific spot on the wall or ceiling, and rub or massage a part of his body. The rubbing may be done initially by the nurse. Then the nurse may take the patient's hand and guide him in doing the rubbing. Rubbing with a firm, circular motion on bare skin may be effective. Use of these measures involves a steady source of sensory input through visual and tactile-kinesthetic modalities along with a focus of rhythm. If this is not distracting enough, another activity, such as breathing in and out slowly, may be added. The patient may repeat silently to himself, "Breathe in slowly, breathe out slowly." Sensory input through several modalities combined with rhythm and a focus on breathing are common characteristics of successful distraction techniques. (Massage of the legs is always contraindicated because of risk of formation and mobilization of emboli.)

Another distraction technique that is very useful with patients who are fatigued or sedated, or when pain lasts longer than several minutes, is "active listening." The patient may use a tape recorder with an earphone or headset, select a cassette of music, and listen to the music, while keeping time by tapping his finger or nodding his head. For visual input, he can focus on an object or close his eyes and imagine something about the music, such as dancing to the music. When the pain increases, the patient can increase the volume; when pain decreases, he decreases the volume. For example, a burned patient undergoing a painful dressing change might use this method of distraction to make the painful experience more tolerable.

Relaxation

Skeletal muscle relaxation may reduce the intensity of pain or increase pain tolerance. It can also be combined with other pain relief measures, such as analgesics or a heating pad, to enhance their effectiveness. Many people learn relaxation techniques for the purpose of dealing with life stresses. Community agencies offer adult education programs in transcendental meditation, yoga, hypnosis, music therapy, and a variety of other potentially relaxing activities. If a patient already knows a technique for relaxing, the nurse may need only suggest that he use it to reduce or to prevent increased pain.

Almost all patients with chronic pain need to learn some method of relaxing and to use it on a regular basis several times a day. Regular periods of relaxation are needed to combat the fatigue and muscle tension that occur with chronic pain tolerance or increase the intensity of the pain.

A simple relaxation technique for patients with acute or chronic pain consists of abdominal breathing at a slow, rhythmic rate. The patient may close his eyes and breathe slowly and comfortably (not too deeply) at about six to nine breaths per minute. The patient can maintain a constant rhythm by counting silently and slowly to himself as he inhales ("in, two, three") and as he exhales ("out, two, three"). The patient concludes this relaxation technique by taking another deep breath. When the nurse is teaching this technique to the patient, it is helpful to count out loud for him at first. Initially the patient may benefit from keeping his eyes open as the nurse breathes in coordination with him.

Slow, rhythmic breathing may also be used as a distraction technique. This, however, as well as other noninvasive pain relief measures, may require practice before the patient becomes skillful in using it.

A quick and easy method of helping the tense patient with severe pain to relax is to give the following instructions: "Clench your fists; breathe in deeply and hold it a moment. As you breathe out, feel yourself go limp. Now start yawning."

Guided Imagery

Therapeutic guided imagery may be defined as the use of one's imagination in an especially designed manner to achieve a specific positive effect. In this instance, the effects desired are relaxation and pain relief. Imagery of various types is capable of altering body functions over which we seem to have no direct or conscious control. Most people have experienced this in the form of increased cardiac rate (pounding heart) or perspiration when a distressing mental image comes to mind just before falling asleep. Although images of this sort seem to provoke a stress response, certain other images seem to evoke relaxation responses or pain relief. A considerable amount of time is usually required to teach and explain the technique of guided imagery. The patient must invest time and energy in practicing it. For these reasons, guided imagery most often is taught to patients with chronic pain, although it is effective with acute pain as well. To learn to use guided imagery, the patient must be able to concentrate, use his imagination, and follow directions. It is not advisable to try to teach it when the patient is fatigued, sedated, or in severe pain. One simple form of therapeutic guided imagery for relaxation and pain relief consists of combining the slow rhythmic breathing described as a relaxation technique with a mental image of relaxation and comfort. With eyes closed, the patient imagines that each time he exhales slowly he is breathing out muscle tension and discomfort, leaving behind a relaxed and comfortable body. Each time he inhales, he can imagine that the air sends healing energy to the area of discomfort. Each time he exhales, he can imagine that the exhaled air carries away the pain and tension.

Usually, the patient is asked to practice guided imagery for about 5 minutes, three times a day. Several days of practice may elapse before the patient finds that he or she can reduce the intensity of pain through this technique. Pain relief can continue for hours after the imagery is used. Many patients begin to experience the relaxing effects of guided imagery the first time they try it.

Medications for Pain Relief

Whether pain is acute or chronic, certain guidelines are useful when medications are indicated for the relief of pain. Usually, medications are most effective when the dose and interval between doses is individualized to meet the patient's needs. The only safe and effective way to administer narcotics is to observe the patient's response.

Preventive Approach

Using a preventive approach to pain relief means that medications (analgesics in particular) are given before the pain occurs, if it can be predicted, or at least before it reaches a severe intensity. If the patient's pain is expected to occur around the clock or for a great portion of the 24-hour period, a regular around-the-clock schedule of administration of analgesia may be indicated. Even if the analgesic is prescribed "as needed" or "prn," the nurse can administer the analgesic on a preventive basis before it is needed as long as the prescribed interval between doses is observed. This is preferable to the usual approach to a prn request, which may require that the patient have intense pain before requesting and receiving his medication.

A preventive approach has many advantages. It usually takes a smaller dose to relieve mild pain or prevent the occurrence of pain than it does to relieve pain that has escalated and become severe. Thus, a preventive approach may result in less medication over a 24-hour period. In addition to providing more effective pain relief, this helps prevent tolerance to analgesics and decreases the severity of side effects such as sedation and constipation. With a preventive approach, there need not be any peaks of severe pain and the patient spends less time in pain. With a prn approach to pain relief, the patient usually experiences pain, obtains his analgesic, and waits for it to take effect. Within a 24-hour period, this may result in his spending a total of several hours in pain.

Better pain control achieved with a preventive approach may reduce the likelihood of the patient's craving the drug. Some health care team members seem to feel that the frugal use of narcotics will help prevent addiction in the patient with acute pain. A patient who is in pain and has his analgesic withheld, however, is more likely to crave the medication than the patient whose pain is relieved before it becomes distressing to him.

Individualized Doses

Individualizing the dose and the interval between doses is necessary because patients metabolize and absorb medications at different rates and because adjustments are required for varying intensities of pain. It should not be surprising that a certain dosage of a narcotic given at specified intervals would be effective for one patient but totally inappropriate for another. Too often, however, analgesics, especially narcotics, are prescribed and given in a very standardized, inflexible manner. The nurse must remember that there are no magic numbers for milligrams or for hours between doses. For example, when a patient metabolizes 100 mg of meperidine (Demerol) intramuscularly (IM) in 2 hours, it should be understood that this is a well-documented physiologic phenomenon, not a drug abuse problem.

Because of the fear of promoting addiction or causing respiratory depression, there is a tendency to provide inadequate doses of narcotics in the treatment of acute pain or prolonged pain in the terminally ill. The result is needless suffering. Even prolonged administration of a narcotic is associated with less than 3% incidence of addiction. Furthermore, small doses are not necessarily safe doses. There have been reports of life-threatening respiratory depression in patients receiving 25 mg to 50 mg of meperidine IM, whereas other patients have not exhibited any sedation or respiratory depression after 200 mg of meperidine IM.

Therefore, it is mandatory for purposes of pain relief and

patient safety that the effects of narcotics be observed, especially when the first dose of a narcotic is given to a patient or when a change is made in dosage or frequency. A simple way to make these observations is to maintain a flow sheet, noting time and date, the patient's pain rating (scale of 0 to 10), the analgesic agent, other pain relief measures, side effects, and patient activity. At regular intervals, the patient is asked to rate his or her pain on a scale of 0 to 10. Respiratory rate and status are observed frequently, along with other physiologic changes of concern. For example, when a postoperative patient is given the first dose of meperidine, 75 mg IM, a pain rating and respiratory rate, along with other relevant physiologic parameters, should be noted. If 1 hour later the pain rating has not decreased, the patient is reasonably alert, and the respiratory status, blood pressure, and pulse rate are satisfactory, some change in analgesia is indicated. The meperidine dose is safe for this patient, but does not relieve the pain. Another dose of meperidine may be indicated; therefore, the nurse consults with the physician to determine what further action is warranted.

Gerontologic Considerations

Physiologic changes in the elderly make it imperative that analgesics are administered with caution. Drug interactions are more likely to occur in the elderly because of the higher incidence of chronic illness and increased use of prescription and over-the-counter drugs. Before administering narcotic and non-narcotic analgesics to the elderly, it is important to obtain a careful drug history to identify potential harmful drug interactions.

Absorption and metabolism of drugs are altered in the elderly patient because of decreased liver, renal, and gastrointestinal function. In addition, changes in body weight, protein stores, and distribution of body fluid alter the distribution of drugs in the body. As a result, drugs are not metabolized as quickly and blood levels of the drug remain higher for a longer period. The patient is more sensitive to drugs and is at increased risk of drug toxicity.

Narcotic and non-narcotic analgesics can be given effectively to the elderly, but must be used cautiously because of increased susceptibility to depression of the nervous system and respiratory system. Meperidine must be used with particular caution because decreased binding of the drug by plasma proteins results in blood concentrations of the drug twice those found in younger patients. Because the elderly are generally more sensitive to analgesics, it is advisable to begin with a smaller dose of a non-narcotic analgesic first, increasing the dose slowly, and adding additional drugs carefully. Frequent monitoring is necessary for safe, effective pain relief.

Routes of Administration for Moderate to Severe Pain

The route of administration of analgesics selected is based on the patient's condition and desired effect of the drug. For moderate to severe pain, the most common routes of administration of a narcotic are the intramuscular or subcutaneous routes. Parenteral administration of the medication produces more rapid analgesic effects than oral administration, but these effects are of shorter duration. Intravenous or rectal routes of administration may also be indicated if the patient is not permitted any oral intake or is vomiting. Postoperative pain, for example, has been effectively relieved with rectal suppositories of 10 mg of oxymorphone (Numorphan; two suppositories, totaling 10 mg, provide analgesia equivalent to that of 10 mg of morphine intramuscularly or 75 mg of meperidine intramuscularly). The rectal route may be indicated for patients with bleeding problems, such as hemophilia.

Intravenous narcotics may be administered by "push" (or "slow push," *e.g.*, over a 5- to 10-minute period) or by continuous drip using an infusion pump. The latter provides a more steady level of analgesia and is indicated when pain is to be controlled over a 24-hour period, such as postoperatively for the first day or so, or in a patient with prolonged cancer pain who cannot take medication by mouth. Studies show that the majority of patients do not absorb meperidine IM well during the first 8 hours postoperatively and that the intravenous (IV) route may be much safer and more effective in relieving pain. The amount of narcotic administered intravenously is calculated carefully to relieve pain without producing respiratory depression and other side effects.

If the patient can take medication by mouth, this route is preferred over all others because it is easy, noninvasive, and not painful, as are injections. Severe pain can be relieved with oral narcotics *if* the doses are high enough. Patients with prolonged pain should receive analgesics orally rather than by injection if at all possible. Many narcotics can be given effectively by mouth for severe pain. To be effective, however, dosage must be altered because of differences in absorption of drugs given by different routes. Oral doses of narcotics that are equal to 10 mg of morphine given intramuscularly are 30 to 60 mg of morphine and 4 to 8 mg of hydromorphone (Dilaudid). See Table 15–3 for a list of selected analgesics equivalent to 10 mg of morphine. In terminally ill patients with prolonged pain, doses may gradually become much higher because of increased pain with disease progression or tolerance to analgesia. In the majority of these patients, the higher doses provide additional pain relief (*i.e.*, there is no ceiling on the analgesia of the powerful narcotics; a "ceiling effect" means that once the pain-relieving effect has been achieved, increasing the dose further will not increase the pain relief effect further), and the higher doses are not lethal (the patient is tolerant to respiratory depression and sedation as well as analgesia). If

the patient's medication is changed from a parenteral dose to an oral narcotic at a dose that is not equivalent in strength (equianalgesic), the lesser dose of oral narcotic may result in a withdrawal reaction and the reappearance of pain and anxiety.

Sustained-release oral morphine (MS Contin, Roxanol) preparations with a duration of action of 8 to 12 hours have provided pain relief for patients with severe pain. Caution must be used in switching a patient from frequent IM injections to oral doses to provide adequate doses and adequate pain relief.

Alternate Routes and Approaches to Pain Management

Attention to the problem of acute and chronic pain has led to the development of alternate methods of pain relief. These methods of delivering analgesics include intraspinal infusion and patient-controlled analgesia.

Intraspinal Infusion of Analgesics. Intraspinal infusion of narcotics or local anesthetic agents has been effective in pain control in postoperative patients as well as those with chronic pain unrelieved by usual methods of pain relief. A catheter is inserted by the physician into the subarachnoid or epidural space in the thoracic or lumbar region for administration of narcotics or local anesthetics. Repeated infusion of these agents through the catheter results in pain relief without many of the side effects of systemic analgesia, including sedation.

If analgesics are required for a longer period or if the patient has persistent, severe pain secondary to a terminal disease (*i.e.*, cancer), the catheter may be tunneled through the subcutaneous tissue and the inlet or port placed under the skin in the abdominal region. The narcotic analgesic is injected through the skin into the outlet or port and catheter, which delivers the medication directly into the subarachnoid or epidural space. This method may require injection of the narcotic several times a day to maintain an adequate level of pain relief.

In those patients who are likely to require more frequent doses or continuous infusions of narcotics to keep them pain free, an implantable infusion device or pump may be used to administer the narcotic continuously. The dose of narcotic is administered at a small, constant dose at a preset rate into the epidural or subarachnoid space. The infusion device has a reservoir that stores the medication for slow release and needs to be refilled once every 1 or 2 months, depending on the patient's needs. This eliminates the need for repeated injections through the skin and reduces the number of trips to the hospital for frequent injections.

Very small doses of narcotic analgesics can be administered by these methods to block pain pathways with little effect on pulse, respiration, or blood pressure. The shortcomings of intramuscular administration of narcotic analgesia, such as delay in pain relief and need for frequent injections, are eliminated. Adverse side effects such as respiratory depression and sedation are reduced because of the small doses given by these methods. However, delayed onset of respiratory depression has been reported with use of intraspinal analgesia; therefore, the patient must be monitored and narcotic antagonists such as naloxone (Narcan) must be available for administration to reverse respiratory depression if it occurs. Although the highest incidence of respiratory depression is 6 to 12 hours after ad-

TABLE 15–3.   *Selected Analgesics and Their Equianalgesic Drug Doses**

Analgesics	Subcutaneous or Intramuscular Route (mg)	Oral Route (mg)
Morphine	10	60
Codeine	120	200
Dilaudid	1–2	8
Demerol	75–100	300
Buprenex	0.3	—

* Approximately equal to 10 mg of morphine sulfate.

ministration of epidural narcotics, it can occur earlier or up to 24 hours after the first injection. Therefore the patient is monitored very closely for at least the first 24 hours after the first injection and longer if changes in respiratory status or level of consciousness occur. The patient is also observed for urinary retention, pruritus, nausea, vomiting, and dizziness. Precautions must be taken to minimize the risk of infection at the catheter site and displacement of the catheter.

Subcutaneous Infusions of Analgesics. Continuous infusions of narcotic analgesia have been used effectively in patients who require frequent analgesia but are unable to tolerate oral administration or frequent intramuscular injections and do not have other access sites available. The analgesic agent is infused through a butterfly needle that has been inserted in the subcutaneous tissue. Use of an ambulatory infusion device permits maximal mobility while promoting a continuous level of pain relief. The patient is observed for systemic and local effects of the analgesic agent; the site of insertion is changed weekly. Use of the subcutaneous site has enabled patients to go home with adequate pain relief; however, close monitoring and careful instruction of the patient and his family are necessary for successful use of this route.

Patient-Controlled Analgesia. Patient-controlled analgesia (PCA) has been used effectively with postoperative patients, as well as in patients with chronic cancer pain. This method of pain management allows the patient who is able and willing to exercise control to administer his own medication within predetermined safety limits. PCA can be implemented with oral analgesics as well as continuous infusions of narcotic analgesics by intravenous, subcutaneous, or spinal routes. Ad-

ditionally, PCA can be used in the hospital or home setting. PCA pumps (Fig. 15-7) permit continuous infusion in addition to self-administered boluses of medication within limits of safety; therefore, the patient is able to administer extra medication with episodes of increased pain or initiation of painful activities. Use of PCA has resulted in a more consistent level of analgesia with few side effects; safety limits programmed into the pump to prevent inadvertent administration of overdoses and to insure adequate control of patients' pain have limited the number of side effects and pulmonary complications of narcotic analgesia. The amount of medication administered by the patient using PCA has not been greater than that administered in the traditional methods of pain relief. The patient who is receiving PCA needs to be instructed about administration of the medication and the preventive approach to pain management so that he administers additional doses before the pain becomes severe. If PCA is to be used in the patient's home, the patient and family are taught about the actions and side effects of the medication and need to be well versed in the operation of the PCA pump.

Drug Preferences

The American Pain Society has recommended a stepwise approach to management of cancer pain. The initial step is use of a non-narcotic analgesic such as nonsteroidal anti-inflammatory drugs (NSAIDs) and aspirin; these act on peripheral nerve endings and minimize pain by interfering with prostaglandins. If pain persists or increases, a weak narcotic agonist

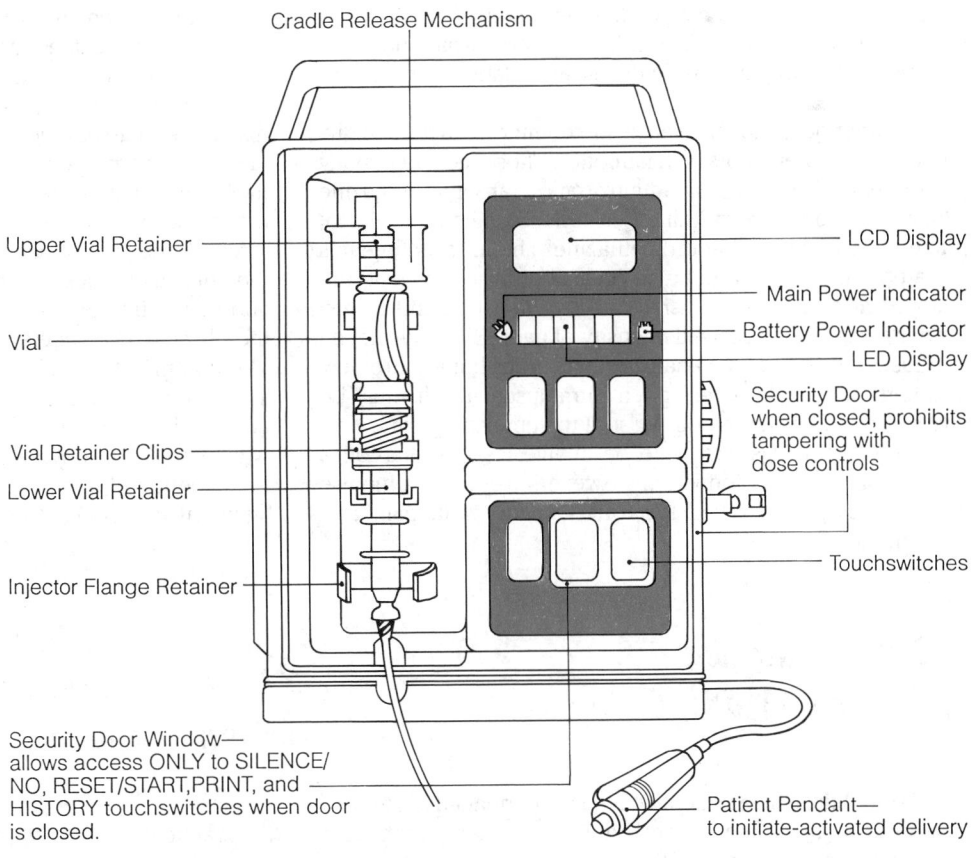

Figure 15-7. Patient-controlled analgesia pump.

Cradle Release Mechanism

Upper Vial Retainer

Vial

Vial Retainer Clips

Lower Vial Retainer

Injector Flange Retainer

LCD Display

Main Power indicator

Battery Power Indicator

LED Display

Security Door—when closed, prohibits tampering with dose controls

Touchswitches

Security Door Window—allows access ONLY to SILENCE/NO, RESET/START, PRINT, and HISTORY touchswitches when door is closed.

Patient Pendant—to initiate-activated delivery

such as codeine is added. Strong narcotics such as morphine are recommended for persistent or increasing severe pain.

With both acute and chronic pain, it is wise to use aspirin, acetaminophen (*e.g.,* Tylenol, Datril), or the more potent NSAIDs, such as ibuprofen (Motrin), to the extent possible. These drugs provide non-narcotic analgesia without the sedation and constipation that often accompany narcotics. Furthermore, when narcotics are necessary, it is logical to give the non-narcotic analgesic concurrently because their sites of actions differ: NSAIDs produce analgesia by action at the peripheral nervous system level, whereas narcotics act primarily at the central nervous system level. Side effects include GI disturbances and decreased renal function. Therefore, the lowest possible doses should be used that will result in adequate control of pain.

Chronic pain is often accompanied by depression. Therefore, the use of tricyclic antidepressants may be considered. These drugs have a sedative effect and may be given at bedtime; therefore, they assist in relieving sleep disturbances, a common problem in depression and chronic pain. Because these drugs have an analgesic effect after 10 days of regular administration, the patient may receive an added benefit of non-narcotic analgesia.

Probably the most commonly prescribed injectable narcotic is meperidine. There are several indications, however, that this practice should be reevaluated. Meperidine is short acting and very irritating to the tissues; therefore, adequate pain control may result in frequent (every 2 to 3 hours) injections of an irritating substance. Furthermore, meperidine is more toxic than was previously recognized. Neuropsychiatric effects, such as disorientation and hallucinations, are relatively intense with parenteral meperidine. Accumulation of the metabolite normeperidine, as a result of multiple doses of meperidine, especially in patients with compromised renal function, can result in excitatory effects, such as twitching, irritability, and seizures. These problems have not been observed with morphine, which is an acceptable alternative to meperidine.

Another potential problem is the common practice of giving so-called potentiators with narcotics. Those most frequently prescribed for parenteral administration are promethazine (Phenergan) and hydroxyzine (Vistaril). Studies and clinical practice have shown that promethazine is highly sedating; it is not a potentiator of narcotic analgesia but instead is a potentiator of respiratory depression and hypotension, and it may even increase the perceived intensity of pain. Hydroxyzine, by contrast, may have some analgesic properties but is extremely irritating and painful when given intramuscularly. It must be given by the Z-track method. Most of the time analgesia is best achieved with drugs known to be analgesics—the narcotics and nonnarcotics. Potentiators, however, may have some use in decreasing the nausea that often occurs with pain and meperidine.

Patient Education and Home Health Care

Acute Pain.   The patient who has experienced acute pain as a result of injury, illness, procedures, or surgery often fears its recurrence once he is discharged from the hospital. Fear

and anticipation of pain are further increased because nurses, physicians, and pain relief measures are less available to the patient for control of pain in the home. The patient may leave the hospital with the expectation that the pain will not recur and is very frightened if it returns unexpectedly or persists longer than expected. In preparation for hospital discharge, the patient and family members receive instruction and guidance about what type of pain or discomfort to expect, how long that discomfort is expected to last, and when the pain or discomfort signals a problem that should be reported. Additionally, they are prepared for home care by guidance about medication to be used in case of pain as well as its side effects. The patient is reminded that those pain relief strategies that were effective in the hospital can be used at home. The nurse gives support and reassurance to the patient and family that pain can be successfully managed at home.

Chronic Pain.   Inadequate control of pain in the outpatient is a common cause of readmission to the hospital. If chronic pain was the primary reason for the patient's initial hospitalization, the anxiety and fear of the patient and family are multiplied when the patient is about to return home. The patient and family are instructed in the techniques of pain assessment and administration of pain medications. These instructions are given verbally and in writing, and opportunities are provided for the patient and family member to practice administration of the medication until they are comfortable and confident with the procedure. They are instructed how to monitor respiratory status and to recognize central nervous system depression and other side effects of narcotic and non-narcotic analgesics. If the medications cause other predictable effects such as constipation, the patient and family are instructed about its treatment and prevention so that pain relief is not interrupted to resolve the problem.

If the patient is to receive analgesics at home by intramuscular or subcutaneous injection or intravenous or intraspinal infusions, a referral to a community health nurse is indicated. The community health nurse visits the patient in the home after discharge to assess the patient, to determine if the patient and family are carrying out the pain management program effectively, and if indicated, to evaluate the injection or infusion technique used by the patient and family for accuracy and safety. If the patient has an implanted infusion pump in place, the nurse examines the condition of the pump or injection site and may refill the reservoir with medication as prescribed by the physician or supervise family members in the procedure. The community health nurse assesses the patient for changes in his need for analgesic medications. She assists the patient and family in altering the medication dose in collaboration with the patient's physician. The nurse supports and encourages the patient and family members to use noninvasive pain management techniques to supplement analgesic therapy. These efforts enable the patient to obtain adequate pain relief while remaining in his own home and with his family.

Neurosurgical Methods of Pain Management

Several neurosurgical approaches are available and have been used successfully for patients whose pain cannot be relieved

Nursing Care Plan 15-1

Care of the Patient With Pain

Nursing Interventions	Rationale	Expected Outcomes
Nursing Diagnosis: Pain and discomfort		
Goal: Relief of pain and discomfort or decrease in intensity of pain and discomfort		
1. Assure patient that you know pain is real and will assist him in dealing with it	1. Fear that pain will not be accepted as real increases tension and anxiety and decreases pain tolerance	• Reports relief that pain is accepted as real and that he will receive assistance in pain relief
2. Use pain assessment scale to identify intensity of pain and discomfort	2. Provides baseline for assessing changes in pain level and evaluating interventions	• Reports lower intensity of pain and discomfort after interventions used
3. Assess and record pain and its characteristics: location, quality, frequency, duration	3. Assist in evaluation of pain and pain relief and identifying multiple sources and types of pain	• Reports less disruption from pain and discomfort after use of intervention
4. Administer analgesics to promote optimum pain relief within limits of physician's prescription	4. Analgesics are more effective when administered early in pain cycle.	• Accepts pain medication as prescribed
5. Assess patient's behavioral responses to pain and pain experience	5. Provides additional source of information about patient's pain	• Exhibits decreased physical and behavioral signs of pain and discomfort in *acute pain* (no grimacing, crying, is aware of surroundings, participates in events and activities)
6. Identify and encourage strategies of pain relief that patient has used successfully in previous pain experiences	6. Encourages success of pain relief strategies familiar to and accepted by patient	• Identifies effective pain relief strategies
7. Teach patient new strategies to relieve pain and discomfort: • Distraction • Imagery • Relaxation • Cutaneous stimulation	7. Increases number of options and strategies available to patient	• Demonstrates use of new strategies to relieve pain and reports their effectiveness
Nursing Diagnosis: Potential ineffective coping related to anticipation and stress of pain		
Goal: Increased effectiveness of coping		
1. Assess patient's coping strategies and factors that produce ineffective coping	1. Provides baseline for assessing interventions and allows patient and health care provider to identify factors that have hampered effective coping	• Identifies effective and ineffective coping strategies • Demonstrates use of effective strategies • Avoids destructive coping strategies (smoking, aggression, abuse of alcohol and drugs)
2. Teach patient appropriate and safe ways to use analgesics	2. Provide patient with alternate and safe coping strategies	• Explains safe and appropriate use of analgesics • Uses analgesics safely and appropriately • States side effects of analgesics and adequate pain relief • Exhibits absence of side effects of analgesics and adequate pain relief • Reports decreasing reliance on analgesics • Reports pain relief with less potent analgesics
3. Assist patient to identify and use effective coping strategies	3. Previous reliance on ineffective or less effective coping strategies indicates the need for assistance in identifying effective ones	• Verbally acknowledges need for new, more effective coping strategies

(continued)

Nursing Care Plan 15-1 *(Continued)*

Care of the Patient With Pain

Nursing Interventions	Rationale	Expected Outcomes
4. Assist patient to plan and participate in activities	4. Provides distraction for patient and assists patient, who may have decreased all participation in activities, to become involved	• Participates in family, social, and work activities • Exhibits awareness of events and environment • Reports ability to sleep and rest • Reports less preoccupation with pain • Converses about topics other than own pain experience. • Reports that life style is appropriate and acceptable to patient

or controlled satisfactorily with medications and other nonsurgical approaches without causing drug addiction or disabling sedation. These procedures, including those that interrupt neurological tracts that conduct pain sensation, are discussed in Chapter 56.

Pain Centers, Clinics, and Teams

Pain clinics have been established in the United States to help patients with chronic pain. They use a multidisciplinary approach and offer a variety of perspectives on the relief of pain. Therapy may include biofeedback, acupuncture, nerve blocks, hypnosis, autogenic training, group therapy, medication, physical therapy, nutritional counseling, and many others. Not all pain centers offer the same approaches to pain relief. Some clinics or centers treat the patient on an outpatient basis, whereas others admit the patient to a pain control unit.

When the patient is not able to obtain satisfactory pain relief, the physician may refer him to a pain center for evaluation and treatment. Some hospitals have identified teams of health care professionals on their staffs with expertise in assisting patients with their pain. Referral to these pain teams often can be initiated by a nurse, physician, or other health team member who requires assistance in helping a patient with unrelieved pain.

Hospice programs have been developed in many areas to give care and symptomatic relief to the dying patient. Pain control is one of their primary goals.

Evaluating the Effectiveness of Pain Relief Measures

To determine objectively the effectiveness of nursing activities designed to help the patient with his or her pain experience,

sponses. This assessment is repeated at appropriate intervals after the intervention.

The *comparison* of these assessments indicates the effectiveness of the pain relief measures. This provides a basis for continuing or modifying nursing intervention (Nursing Care Plan 15–1).

The expected outcome of nursing intervention for pain relief is usually one or more of the following possibilities, each having many possible manifestations:

 1. Achieves pain relief or decreased intensity of pain
   a. Rates pain at a lower intensity (on a scale of 0 to 10) after intervention
   b. Rates pain at a lower intensity for longer periods
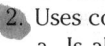 2. Uses coping strategies effectively
   a. Is alert and pain free enough to engage in activities important to recovery (*e.g.*, drinking fluids, coughing, ambulating)
   b. Sleeps all night
   c. Increases the amount of time spent out of bed
   d. Increases the amount of time spent engaged in activities of daily living: work, school, parenting, social interaction
   e. Says the pain does not bother him or her as much as it did before intervention
   f. Says he or she pays less attention to the pain
   g. Spends less time talking about pain

Chapter Summary

Pain—acute or chronic in nature—is the most frequent reason for individuals to seek health care. Pain may be disabling and may cause significant disability and time lost from work, school, and other routine activities. Although pain and discomfort are often associated with disease or injury, they may also occur with diagnostic testing and treatment. When significant pain occurs, it generally affects every aspect of a person's life.

Care of the patient with acute or chronic pain remains a challenge for the beginning nurse as well as the nurse with many years of nursing experience. Care of this patient provides an opportunity for the nurse to use her basic nursing skills to provide quality physical care for the patient; problem-solving skills to assist the patient to cope with the pain experience; and assessment, communication, interviewing, and evaluation skills to identify and modify those factors that affect the patient's response to pain. Caring for the patient with pain requires knowledge of the actions of a variety of analgesic agents as well as their side effects and strategies to reduce the side effects. Quality nursing care for the patient in pain requires the ability to suggest creative and innovative approaches and knowledge of a wide variety of pain management strategies.

Bibliography

Books

American Pain Society. Principles of Analgesic Use in the Treatment of Acute Pain and Chronic Cancer Pain. A Concise Guide to Medical Practice, 2nd ed. Skokie, IL, American Pain Society, 1989.

Malseed RT and Harrigan GS. Textbook of Pharmacology and Nursing Care. Philadelphia, JB Lippincott, 1989.

McCaffery M and Beebe A. Pain: Clinical Manual for Nursing Practice. St Louis, CV Mosby, 1989.

Porth CM. Pathophysiology: Concepts of Altered Health States, 3rd ed. Philadelphia, JB Lippincott, 1990.

Price D. Psychological and Neural Mechanisms of Pain. New York, Raven Press, 1988.

Sterbeck R. The Psychology of Pain. New York, Raven Press, 1986.

Taylor AG. Pain. In Fitzpatrick JJ and Taunton RL (eds). Annual Review of Nursing Research. New York, Springer, 1987.

US Department of Health and Human Services. Report of the Commission on the Evaluation of Pain. Washington, DC, Government Printing Office, 1987.

Wall PD and Melzack R (eds.) Textbook of Pain, 2nd ed. New York, Churchill Livingstone, 1989.

World Health Organization. Cancer Pain Relief. World Health Organization: Geneva, Switzerland, 1986 (reprinted 1988).

Journals

Asterisks indicate nursing research articles.

Amadio PC et al. A framework for management of chronic pain. Am Fam Physician 1988 Nov; 38(5): 155–160.

American Pain Society. Principles of analgesic use in the treatment of acute pain and chronic cancer pain. Am J Nurs 1988 Jun; 88(6): 815–826.

Arner S and Meyerson BA. Lack of analgesic effect of opioids on neuropathic and idiopathic forms of pain. Pain 1988 Apr; 33(1): 11–23.

Barkas G and Duafala ME. Advances in cancer pain management: A review of patient-controlled analgesia. J Pain Symptom Manage 1988 Summer; 3(3): 150–160.

Bragg CL. Interpleural analgesia. Heart Lung 1991 Jan; 20(1): 30–38.

Bruera E et al. Continuous sc infusion of narcotics for the treatment of cancer pain: An update. Cancer Treatment Reports. 1987 Oct; 71(10): 953–955.

Bruera E et al. Influence of the pain and symptom control team (PSCT) on the patterns of treatment of pain and other symptoms in a cancer center. J Pain Symptom Manage 1989 Sep; 4(3): 112–116.

* Burke SO and Jerrett M. Pain management across age groups. West J Nurs Res 1989 Apr; 11(2): 164–180.

* Cahill CA. Beta-endorphin levels during pregnancy and labor: A role in pain modulation? Nurs Res 1989 Jul/Aug; 38(4): 200–203.

* Camp LD. A comparison of nurses' recorded assessments of pain with perceptions of pain as described by cancer patients. Cancer Nurs 1988 Aug; 11(4): 237–243.

Christoph SB. Pain assessment: The problem of pain in the critically ill patient. Crit Care Nurs Clin North Am 1991 Mar; 3(1): 11–16.

Cicala RS et al. Side effects and complications of cervical epidural steroid injections. J Pain Symptom Manage 1989 Jun; 4(2): 64–66.

Cowan P and Lovasik DA. American Chronic Pain Association: Strategies for surviving chronic pain. Orthop Nurs 1990 Jul/Aug; 9(4): 47–49.

* Coyle N et al. Character of terminal illness in the advanced cancer patient: Pain and other symptoms during the last four weeks of life. J Pain Symptom Manage 1990 Apr; 5(2): 83–93.

Coyle N. Analgesics and pain: Current concepts. Nurs Clin North Am 1987 Sep; 22(3): 727–741.

* Dalton JA. Nurses' perceptions of their pain assessment skills, pain management practices, and attitudes toward pain. Oncol Nurs Forum 1989 Mar/Apr; 16(2): 225–231.

* Dalton JA et al. Pain relief for cancer patients. Cancer Nurs 1988 Dec; 11(6): 322–328.

* Dalton JA and Feuerstein M. Biobehavioral factors in cancer pain. Pain 1988 May; 33(2): 137–147.

* Davis GC. Measurement of the chronic pain experience: Development of an instrument. Res Nurs Health 1989 Aug; 12(4): 221–227.

* Davis GC. The clinical assessment of chronic pain in rheumatic disease: Evaluating the use of two instruments. J Adv Nurs 1989 May; 14(5): 397–402.

Dean RJ Jr. Regional anesthetic techniques for postoperative analgesia. Crit Care Nurs Clin North Am 1991 Mar; 3(1): 43–47.

Diekmann JM et al. Cancer pain control: One state's experience. Oncol Nurs Forum 1989 Mar/Apr; 16(2): 219–223.

* Donovan M et al. Incidence and characteristics of pain in a sample of medical-surgical inpatients. Pain 1987 Jul; 30(1): 69–78.

Doody SB, Smith C, and Webb J. Nonpharmacologic interventions for pain management. Crit Care Nurs Clin North Am 1991 Mar; 3(1): 69–75.

Edwards WT. Optimizing opioid treatment of postoperative pain. J Pain Symptom Manage 1990 Feb; 5(1 Suppl): S24–S36.

* Ferrell BR et al. Evolution and evaluation of a pain management team. Oncol Nurs Forum 1988 May/Jun; 15(3): 285–289.

* Ferrell B et al. Effects of controlled-release morphine on quality of life for cancer pain. Oncol Nurs Forum 1989 Jul/Aug; 16(4): 521–526.

Gaston-Johansson F et al. Similarities in pain descriptions of four different ethnic-culture groups. J Pain Symptom Manage 1990 Apr; 5(2): 94–100.

* Geden EA et al. Effects of music and imagery on physiologic and self-report of analogued labor pain. Nurs Res 1989 Jan/Feb; 38(1): 37–41.

Gilbert HC. Pain relief methods in the postanesthesia care unit. J Post Anesth Nurs 1990 Feb; 5(1): 6–15.

* Hargreaves A and Lander J. Use of transcutaneous electrical nerve stimulation for postoperative pain. Nurs Res 1989 May/Jun; 38(3): 159–161.

Hill CS. Relationship among cultural, educational, and regulatory agency influences on optimum cancer pain treatment. J Pain Symptom Manage 1990 Feb; 5(1 Suppl): S37–S45.

Hoffert MJ. The neurophysiology of pain. Neurol Clin 1989 May; 7(2): 183–203.

* Holm K et al. Effect of personal pain experience on pain assessment. Image J Nurs Sch 1989 Summer; 21(2): 72–75.

Jaros JA. The concept of pain. Crit Care Nurs Clin North Am 1991 Mar; 3(1): 1–10.

Jones NJ. Creative analgesic dosing in the elderly. Am J Nurs 1989 Oct; (10): 1285.

Kane NE et al. Use of patient-controlled analgesia in surgical oncology patients. Oncol Nurs Forum 1988 Jan/Feb; 15(1): 29–32.

Krause SJ et al. Pain distribution, intensity, and duration in patients with chronic pain. J Pain Symptom Manage 1989 Jun; 4(2): 67–71.

* Lange MP et al. Patient-controlled analgesia versus intermittent analgesia dosing. Heart Lung 1988 Sep; 17(5): 495–498.

* Lapin J et al. Cancer pain management with controlled-release oral morphine preparation. J Pain Symptom Manage 1989 Sep; 4(3): 146–151.

Lein DH Jr et al. Comparison of effects of transcutaneous electrical nerve stimulation of auricular, somatic, and the combination of auricular and somatic acupuncture points on experimental pain threshold. Phys Ther 1989 Aug; 69(8): 671–678.

Lisson EL. Ethical issues related to pain control. Nurs Clin North Am 1987 Sep; 22(3): 649–659.

Lisson EL. Ethical issues related to pain management. Semin Oncol Nurs 1989 May; 5(2): 114–119.

Lubenow TR and Ivankovich AD. Postoperative epidural analgesia. Crit Care Nurs Clin North Am 1991 Mar; 3(1): 25–32.

Lubenow TR and Ivankovich AD. Patient-controlled analgesia for postoperative pain. Crit Care Nurs Clin North Am 1991 Mar; 3(1): 35–41.

Madrid JL et al. Intermittent intrathecal morphine by means of an implantable reservoir: A survey of 100 cases. J Pain Symptom Manage 1988 Spring; 3(2): 67–71.

Massie MJ and Holland JC. The cancer patient with pain: Psychiatric complications and their management. Med Clin North Am 1987 Mar; 71(2): 243–258.

McCaffery M et al. Nurses' knowledge of opioid analgesic drugs and psychological dependence. Cancer Nurs 1990 Feb; 13(1): 21–27.

McCaffery M and Beebe A. Myths and facts . . . about chronic nonmalignant pain. Nursing 1990 Jan; 20(1): 18.

McCaffery M. When your patient is a drug abuser. Nursing 1988 Nov; 18(11): 49.

McCaffery M. Patient controlled analgesia: More than a machine. Nursing 1987 Nov; 17(11): 62–64.

McCaffery M. A postable chart of equianalgesic doses. Nursing 1987 Aug; 17(8): 56–57.

McCaffery M. Giving meperidine for pain: Should it be so mechanical? Nursing 1987 Apr; 17(4): 60–64.

McNair ND. Epidural narcotics for postoperative pain: Nursing implications. J Neurosci Nurs 1990 Oct; 22(5): 275–279.

Melzack R et al. Pain on a surgical ward: A survey of the duration and intensity of pain and the effectiveness of medication. Pain 1987 Apr; 29(1): 67–72.

Melzack R. The tragedy of needless pain. Sci Am 1990 Feb; 262(2): 27–33.

Nelson L et al. Improving pain management for hip fractured elderly. Orthop Nurs 1990 May/Jun; 9(3): 79–83.

Nitescu P et al. Epidural versus intrathecal morphine-bupivacaine: Assessment of consecutive treatments in advanced cancer pain. J Pain Symptom Manage 1990 Feb; 5(1): 18–26.

Nolan MF. Selected problems in the use of transcutaneous electrical nerve stimulation for pain control–An appraisal with proposed solution. Phys Ther 1988 Nov; 68(11): 1694–1698.

* Norvell KT et al. Pain description by nurses and physicians. J Pain Symptom Manage 1990 Feb; 5(1): 11–17.

Olsson GL et al. Nursing management of patients receiving epidural narcotics. Heart Lung 1989 Mar; 18(2): 130–138.

Paice JA. Intrathecal morphine infusion for intractable cancer pain: A new use for implanted pumps. Oncol Nurs Forum 1986 May/Jun; 13(3): 41–47.

Paice JA. New delivery systems in pain management. Nurs Clin North Am 1987 Sep; 22(3): 715–726.

Pasternak GW. Multiple morphine and enkephalin receptors and the relief of pain. JAMA 1988 Mar 4; 259(9): 1362–1367.

Patt RB and Jain S. Recent advances in the management of oncologic pain. Curr Probl Cancer 1989 May/Jun; 13(3): 135–195.

Payne R. Role of epidural and intrathecal narcotics and peptides in the management of cancer pain. Med Clin North Am 1987 Mar; 71(2): 313–327.

* Pearson BD. Pain control: An experiment with imagery. Geriatr Nurs (New York) 1987 Jan/Feb; 8(1): 28–30.

Portenoy RK. Continuous intravenous infusion of opioid drugs. Med Clin North Am 1987 Mar; 71(2): 133–241.

Portenoy RK. Optimal pain control in elderly cancer patients. Geriatrics 1987 May; 42(5): 33–40.

Portenoy RK. Practical aspects of pain control in the patient with cancer. CA 1988 Nov/Dec; 38(6): 327–352.

Portenoy RK. Mechanisms of clinical pain: Observations and speculations. Neurol Clin 1989 May; 7(2): 205–230.

Portenoy RK. Chronic opiod therapy in nonmalignant pain. J Pain Symptom Manage 1990 Feb; 5(1 Suppl): S46–S62.

Powell AH and Bova MB. How do you give continuous epidural fentanyl? Am J Nurs 1989 Sep; 89(9): 1197–1198, 1200

Puntillo KA. The phenomenon of pain and critical care nursing. Heart Lung 1988 May; 17(3): 262–273.

Rogers AG. Management of postoperative pain in patients on methadone maintenance. J Pain Symptom Manage 1989 Sep; 4(3): 161–162.

Rowland MA. Myths—and facts—about postoperative discomfort. Am J Nurs 1990 May; 90(5): 60–64.

Schug SA et al. Cancer pain management according to WHO analgesic guidelines. J Pain Symptom Manage 1990 Feb; 5(1): 27–32.

Smith IW, Airey S, and Salmond SW. Nontechnologic strategies for coping with chronic low back pain. Orthop Nurs 1990 Jul/Aug; 9(4): 26–32.

Storey P et al. Subcutaneous infusions for control of cancer symptoms. J Pain Symptom Manage 1990 Feb; 5(1): 33–41.

Swezey RL. Low back pain in the elderly: Practical management concerns. Geriatrics 1988 Feb; 43(2): 39–44.

* Taylor AG et al. Psychologic distress of chronic pain sufferers and their spouses. J Pain Symptom Manage 1990 Feb; 5(1): 6–10.

* Teter KA, Viellion G, and Keating EM. Patient controlled analgesia and GI dysfunction. Orthop Nurs 1990 Jul/Aug; 9(4): 51–56.

Thorsteinsson G. Chronic pain: Use of TENS in the elderly. Geriatrics 1987 Dec; 42(12): 75–82.

Vandenbosch TM. How to use a pain flow sheet effectively. Nursing 1988 Aug; 18(8): 50–51.

Ventafridda V et al. Clinical observations on controlled-release morphine in cancer pain. J Pain Symptom Manage 1989 Sep; 4(3): 124–129.

Vissering TR. Pharmacologic agents for pain management. Crit Care Nurs Clin North Am 1991 Mar; 3(1): 17–23.

Walker JM et al. The nursing management of pain in the community: A theoretical framework. J Adv Nurs 1989 Mar; 14(3): 240–247.

Walker VA et al. Evaluation of WHO analgesic guidelines for cancer pain in a hospital-based palliative care unit. J Pain Symptom Manage 1988 Summer; 3(3): 145–149.

* Watt-Watson JH and Graydon JE. Sickness impact profile: A measure of dysfunction with chronic pain patients. J Pain Symptom Manage 1989 Sep; 4(3): 152–156.

White PF. Use of patient-controlled analgesia for management of acute pain. JAMA 1988 Jan 8; 259(2): 243–247.

Whipple B. Methods of pain control: Review of research and literature. Image J Nurs Sch 1987 Fall; 19(3): 142–146.

* Wilkie DJ et al. Use of the McGill questionnaire to measure pain: A meta-analysis. Nurs Res 1990 Jan/Feb; 39(1): 36–41.

Wilkie DJ. Cancer pain management. State-of-the art nursing care. Nurs Clin North Am 1990 Jun; 25(2): 331–343.

Witte M. Pain control. J Gerontol Nurs 1989 Mar; 15(3): 32–37.

Zimmerman L et al. Effects of music in patients who had chronic cancer pain. West J Nurs Res 1989 Jun; 11(3): 298–309.

Pain Syndromes

Amadio PC. Pain dysfunction syndromes. J Bone Joint Surg 1988 Jul; 70A(6): 944–949.

Davidoff G et al. Pain measurement in reflex sympathetic dystrophy syndrome. Pain 1988 Jan; 32(1): 27–34.

Hodges DL and McGuire TJ. Burning and pain after injury. Is it causalgia or reflex sympathetic dystrophy? Postgrad Med 1988 Feb 1; 83(2): 185–188, 190, 192.

Schwartzman RJ and McLellan TL. Reflex sympathetic dystrophy: A review. Arch Neurol 1987 May; 44(5): 555–561.

Smith DL and Campbell SM. Reflex sympathetic dystrophy syndrome–Diagnosis and management. West J Med 1987 Sep; 147(3): 342–345.

Agencies

American Pain Society
    PO Box 186, Skokie, IL 60076
International Pain Foundation
    909 NE 43rd St, Room 306, Seattle, WA 98105
Commission on Accreditation of Rehabilitation Facilities (CARF)
    101 N Wilmot Rd, Suite 500, Tucson, AZ 85711, (602) 748-1212
    (Provides list of organizations accredited in chronic pain management)

16

Human Rhythms in Health and Illness

Learning Objectives

On completion of this chapter, the learner will be able to:

1. Describe the characteristics of human rhythms
2. Identify environmental factors that can influence human rhythms
3. Describe common rhythms that occur in humans
4. Discuss the implications of alterations in human rhythms for health and well-being
5. Identify parameters to be included in the assessment of a patient's rhythms
6. Discuss timing considerations for the nurse's assessment, planning, and interventions for patient care
7. Identify strategies to promote optimal sleep–wake/activity–rest in patients in health care institutions
8. Describe the changes in human rhythms that occur with aging
9. Identify strategies the nurse can use to minimize the detrimental effects of shift work

Glossary

acrophase—the phase of the rhythm as marked by the time of the peak value of the rhythm; it can be expressed in clock hours

amplitude—half the difference between the peak and the trough, or high and low points, of the rhythm

chronobiology—the study of the nature and mechanisms of the biologic time structure, including the rhythmic manifestations of life

chronopharmacology—pharmacology with a chronobiologic approach

circadian rhythms—rhythms that are about 24 hours in length

cycle—a complete pattern that is repeated at regular intervals

desynchronization—a loss of synchronization between two previously synchronized rhythms

entrainment—the synchronization and coupling of two oscillators or rhythms that have similar periods and fairly constant timing between their respective phases or peaks

frequency—the reciprocal of the period; the number of cycles occurring per unit of time

infradian—rhythms with periods longer than 24 hours

(continued)

Glossary (continued)

mesor—*the rhythm-adjusted mean*

period—*the time interval occupied by a wave, or one complete cycle*

phase—*the value of a rhythm at a fixed time*

phase advance—*change in the timing of a rhythm such that its peak occurs at an earlier time of day*

phase delay—*change in the timing of a rhythm such that its peak occurs later*

rhythms—*any set of changes that systematically recur with a predictable waveform*

synchronization—*the state that exists when two or more rhythms exhibit similar periods and have relatively constant phase relationships*

ultradian—*rhythms with periods shorter than 24 hours*

zeitgebers—*exogenous or environmental factors that are able to influence or synchronize the timing of endogenous or internal rhythms*

Life is characterized by a rhythmic patterning that is predictable and necessary for coordinated interaction between living systems and the environment. The temporal organization of humans is essential for optimum functioning, health, and well-being. The rhythmic patterning of life is universal. The day–night cycle repeats itself and shapes the daily routine of humans and other animals. Monthly menstrual periods are expected in women of childbearing age. And everyone knows that the cessation of the rhythm of one's heart is an indicator of death. Despite these and other obvious manifestations of the rhythmic nature of the universe, relatively little attention has been given to the role of these rhythms in nursing practice.

Records from the first century document the rhythmic movement of plants throughout the day. However, these rhythms were generally interpreted as passive responses to a rhythmic environment. In the eighteenth century, Jean Jacques d'Ortous de Mairan discovered that the daytime opening and nighttime closing of the leaves of a certain plant persisted when isolated from sunlight. He further noted that the sleep–wake cycle of bedridden patients persisted even when the patients did not know the time of day. The notion that living systems might possess inherent rhythmicities independent of the environment gradually came into acceptance. In the early 1900s, evidence accumulated demonstrating that living organisms have an internal timing mechanism that enables them to measure the passage of time. A major advance in this century was the recognition that human rhythms are manifestations of an internal timing system that provides temporal organization of biologic processes.

The research into rhythms has increased exponentially during the past 30 years by scientists from a variety of disciplines and reflects work on the subcellular through total organism levels. As a relationship between rhythmicity and health became apparent, nurses began to pay increasing attention to this aspect of human systems. Nurse scientists are increasingly studying changes in rhythmicity that occur with alterations in health and how nurses can promote rhythmic patterning. Nurses' attention to the rhythmic nature of humans and the human–environment interaction promises to improve the quality of nursing care and the health of individuals.

This chapter examines the rhythmic nature of human systems, alterations of human rhythms, how such alterations can affect health and well-being, and how nurses can promote rhythmic patterning to foster health.

Conceptual Bases for Human Rhythms

A vast body of research has documented the temporal nature of human beings. Although this research demonstrates a relationship between temporal organization and health, functioning, and well-being, more research is needed about the relationship between human rhythms and specific illnesses, as well as about therapies that promote health through manipulation of human rhythms.

Rhythms can be defined as any set of changes that systematically recur with a predictable waveform. The rhythm of a song provides the listener with the ability to anticipate the next beat and thus dance in concert with the music. Similarly, the predictability of the earth's rotation enables most individuals to maintain a day-active, night-sleep schedule. One can anticipate regular occurrences throughout the day in both the external and internal environments (*i.e.*, one can predict and prepare for a work schedule that begins every weekday at 9:00 AM, and one can anticipate and prepare for the body's need for nourishment at lunchtime).

Chronobiology is the study of the nature and mechanisms of the biologic time structure, including the rhythmic manifestations of life. The field of chronobiology has been developed by scientists from diverse disciplines, but until recently few nurses have been involved in the field. The conceptual underpinnings of chronobiology reflect predominantly the perspectives of biologists and physicians. Nurses can and are bringing new perspectives to this field. Differences between theoretic perspectives in nursing and traditional chronobiology becomes apparent in this chapter's section on human rhythms and aging.

The temporal nature of human beings has not been explicit in many of the conceptual frameworks and theories that nurses have used. Neither the medical model nor the systems model of human organization has been developed with the assumption that humans are temporal beings. However, Gordon's Functional Health Patterns and the nursing diagnosis classification system by NANDA (North American Nursing Diagnosis Association) are both organized around human patterns, which convey a sensitivity to the repeatable, predictable, and rhythmic aspects of human beings.

Conceptual systems based on adaptation can incorporate the concept of rhythm as an expected variation within the person's range of homeostasis. Disruption in normal biologic rhythms prompts the person to mobilize adaptive mechanisms. This framework is consistent with the chronobiologic perspective in which rhythms are seen as a reactive mechanism of homeostasis that allows the person (or animal or plant) to respond to challenge, and as a predictive mechanism of homeostasis that enables the anticipation of changes that occur over time.

The nurse theorist who most explicitly incorporates temporality into a nursing framework is Rogers (1970, 1986). She describes human and environmental energy fields that are in constant simultaneous interaction and are developing in the direction of greater complexity, diversity, and higher, shorter waveforms (higher frequencies). However, there are major differences in the underlying assumptions of chronobiology and Rogerian Nursing Science that make it difficult to appropriately and easily transfer findings from chronobiologic research to Rogerian Nursing Science, and vice versa. Despite this concern, critical analysis of chronobiologic research and its integration into nursing practice is necessary if nurses are to recognize and capitalize on the temporal nature of human beings.

This chapter presents findings from research conducted by both traditional chronobiologists and nurse researchers who may or may not identify themselves as chronobiologists. It also uses these findings and the principles of chronobiology to describe the implications of the temporal dimension of persons for nursing practice.

The Nature of Human Rhythms

Definitions of Rhythm Parameters

Rhythms can be described by certain parameters or standardized characteristics (Fig. 16-1).

The *period* of the rhythms is the time interval occupied by a wave, or one complete *cycle* (*i.e.*, a complete pattern that is repeated at regular intervals). The reciprocal of the period is the *frequency*, that is, the number of cycles occurring per unit of time. Franz Halberg, one of the pioneers in the field of chronobiology, coined the term *circadian* (*circa* meaning "about"; *dies* meaning "day") to refer to rhythms that are about 24 hours in length. The sleep–wake and rest–activity cycles are obvious examples of circadian rhythms. As is demonstrated throughout this chapter, the circadian period is the dominant rhythm of concern to human health and well-being. Indeed, almost all human physiologic variables that have been studied demonstrate a circadian rhythmicity.

Infradian rhythms are those with periods longer than 24 hours, such as the lunar month, menstrual cycles, and seasonal depression. *Ultradian* rhythms are those that are shorter than 24 hours. Ultradian rhythms include the heart and respiratory rhythms, the attention span, and the rhythmic variations that occur during sleep. This latter example demonstrates that rhythms can have multiple periods. For example, melatonin secretion, which has been related to seasonal affective depression, has a definite circadian rhythm that peaks during the night. It also has an ultradian rhythm with a period of about 5.5 hours in length, indicating that there are finer fluctuations in the secretion of this hormone that occur throughout the 24-hour period. In addition, the amount of light in the natural environment affects melatonin secretion such that during the winter months in northern climates, the reduction in sunlight can alter the circadian rhythm of melatonin and lead to depression. Such a seasonal fluctuation in the circadian pattern of melatonin secretion represents an infradian rhythm.

The *amplitude* of the rhythm is half the difference between the peak and the trough, or high and low points, respectively, of the rhythm. A zero amplitude indicates no rhythmicity (*i.e.*, little or no difference between the peak and trough). A "flattening" of a rhythm indicates a reduction in amplitude and occurs with shift rotation, jet lag, aging, and some illnesses.

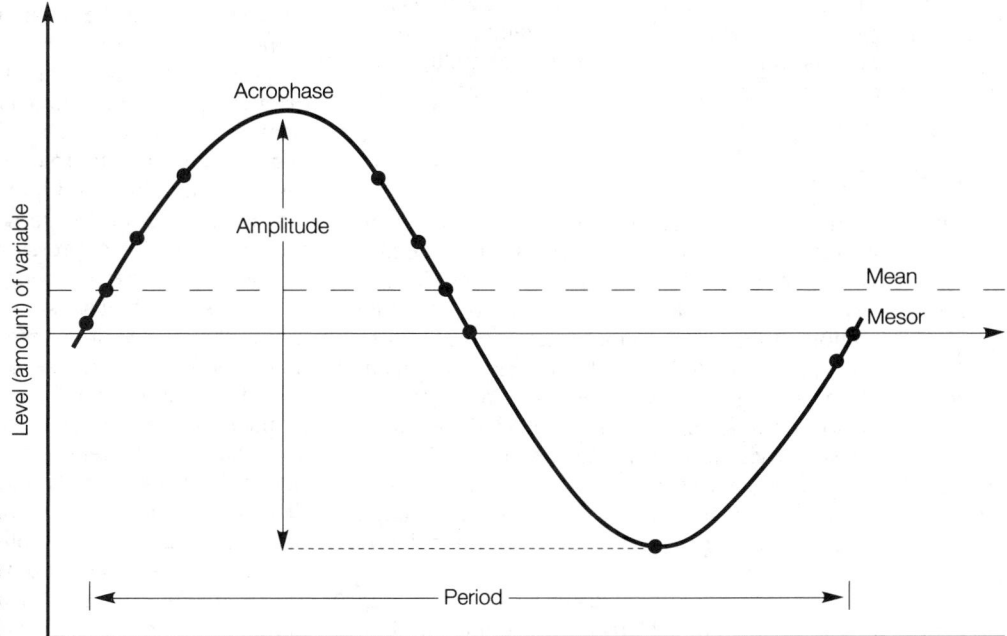

Figure 16–1. Rhythm parameters. The dots (●) represent actual measurements or data points. The solid line connecting the data points represents a symmetrical waveform that is fitted to the data points, or a cycle.

The *phase* is the value of a rhythm at a fixed time. Phase is usually discussed in terms of the *acrophase,* or the time of the peak value of the rhythm, and can be expressed in clock hours (usually using military time). For example, the peak in the rhythm of body temperature may occur in an individual at 1800 hours (6:00 PM). As will be seen, the acrophase holds great significance for the rhythmic health of individuals. It is important in terms of the relationship of the peak of a rhythm to the phases of other internal and external rhythms. For example, nurses who change shifts from days to nights experience an inversion of their activity–rest cycles in relation to the external environment's time of day. Their temperature and other physiologic circadian rhythms are also trying to shift to the new time structure. Changes in the timing of the acrophases of activity and body temperature can produce new *phase relationships* until the individual adapts to the new time schedule, which usually takes 7 to 10 days. Research has shown that such disruptions in phase relationships affect performance and well-being.

The *mesor* is defined as the rhythm-adjusted mean. For example, if Figure 16-1 is viewed as representing the circadian rhythms in body temperature, the data points represent actual temperature readings that were taken during the waking hours of the patient's day. These data points can be averaged to provide a mean. However, if a symmetric waveform is fitted to these data points to project the full 24-hour rhythm of the temperature (as has been done in the figure), the waveform provides a different, rhythm-adjusted mean (*i.e.,* the mesor).

Rhythm parameters provide a means for describing and discussing human rhythms and their alterations with specificity and accuracy.

Endogenous and Exogenous Bases for Human Rhythms

Two mechanisms have been identified as being responsible for the temporal organization of humans: (1) *endogenous* factors, or the individual's own genetically programmed internal clock or clocks that drive a system composed of multiple oscillators, and (2) *exogenous* factors, or environmental time cues that synchronize rhythms.

Endogenous Factors

Evidence that humans possess an internal genetic clock came from isolation studies in which all known environmental cues were removed so that the individual's rhythms were allowed to "free-run," or assume their natural internal period. To create isolation conditions, the individual must have no cues as to what time it is (*e.g.,* no knowledge of whether it is day or night [no windows, no one saying "good morning"], no access to radio or television or other media that would indicate what day or hour it is, no visible clocks, and no one telling the individual what meal to eat or when to go to bed or otherwise indicating time of day in conversation). As is discussed later, intensive care units sometimes unwittingly simulate isolation conditions.

Under isolation conditions, the individual's rhythms often assume a period that varies from the usual or entrained period. For example, under normal conditions, the body temperature and sleep–wake rhythms maintain strong circadian periods (*i.e.,* usually 24 hours in length). Under isolation conditions, the body temperature rhythm will free-run to a period that is about 25 hours long. The sleep–wake rhythm will also free-run to a period of about 25 hours and, if allowed to free-run for a long enough time, will separate or dissociate from the temperature rhythm and free-run to a period of 30 to 50 hours. Such studies demonstrate that human circadian rhythms have an endogenous or internal component. Moreover, these studies suggest that the two rhythms are driven by two different clocks or are coupled to two different oscillators or pacemakers, with one pacemaker driving the core body temperature rhythm and the other driving the sleep–wake rhythms. The two pacemakers influence each other under normal conditions. Most of the body's physiologic circadian rhythms are thought to be coupled to one of these two pacemakers.

Animal studies provide evidence that these endogenous rhythms are genetic and not merely learned responses. Successive generations of mice reared in constant isolation conditions continued to have circadian rhythms even though they had never experienced a light–dark cycle. Further evidence for an endogenous clock arose from animal studies in which different parts of the body and areas of the brain were systematically destroyed to determine which site resulted in loss of rhythmicity. These studies have isolated the superchiasmic nuclei in the hypothalamus as the site of one of the primary pacemakers. Observations of brain-damaged humans provided additional support for the proposition that there is an endogenous basis for human rhythms that is at least partially located in the superchiasmic nuclei.

Exogenous Factors

Human circadian rhythms (and the rhythms of most living organisms) are strongly influenced by exogenous or environmental factors. These factors are referred to as synchronizers or *zeitgebers,* meaning "time-giver." The strongest zeitgeber for most plants and animals is the light–dark cycle. *Diurnal* animals are those that maintain a day-active, night-rest pattern, whereas *nocturnal* animals maintain a night-active, day-rest pattern.

For a long time, light was known to be a strong synchronizer for plants and animals but was thought to play a less significant role in synchronizing human rhythms. Acknowledgement of a greater role for light as a synchronizer of human rhythms was stimulated largely by the observation that some individuals experience seasonal depression, also known as seasonal affective depression or disorder (SAD). These individuals are depressed during the winter months, when the period and strength of sunshine are at their lowest levels, but not during the bright summer months. One of the effective treatments for SAD is exposure to bright light. Increasingly, research is demonstrating that light can be a strong synchronizer in humans if it is of a great enough intensity. This intensity is 2500 lux, which is the intensity achieved shortly after sunrise and is out of the range of most indoor lighting. However, some individuals may be sensitive to less intense indoor lighting, particularly if it is incandescent or cool white fluorescent.

Among the strongest zeitgebers for humans are social cues. These include regularly scheduled activities such as mealtimes or administrations of medications, auditory cues such as alarm clocks, and other environmental influences that suggest a time of day or time of week. Those who work a Monday through

Friday schedule know that the environmental cues on the weekdays are different from those on the weekend. In fact, it has been suggested that the Monday morning "blues" or fatigue results from the individual's rhythms free-running on the weekend to a longer period (producing a later time of awakening than on weekdays), creating a phase-shifting of the body's circadian rhythms so that the individual's body seems to be awakening to an earlier time of day on Monday. Human interactions create a host of other social cues that act as zeitgebers. In isolation studies where individuals are isolated in groups, the group of individuals in one room will free-run to similar periods, but this period will differ from the period of another group in another room.

Synchronization of Endogenous and Exogenous Components of Rhythms

The synchronizing effect of zeitgebers is important in many respects. The zeitgebers enable the individual to be synchronized to the environment. Thus, they enable the individual to function in an environment that varies from day to night, although this can be problematic for shift workers. Second, the zeitgebers help to coordinate disparate endogenous rhythms. As will be seen, the relationship of the temperature rhythm to the sleep–wake rhythm determines the quality and amount of sleep an individual gets on any given night. Therefore, the zeitgebers help to maintain constant phase relations between the individual and the environment and among the individual's different physiologic, psychologic, and social rhythms.

Zeitgebers entrain the individual's rhythms. *Entrainment* is a synchronization and coupling of two oscillators or rhythms that have similar periods and fairly constant timing between their respective phases or peaks. This entrainment is determined by a variety of factors; these include the natural frequencies of the two oscillators (*e.g.*, the individual's endogenous rhythm and the zeitgeber), the strength of the zeitgeber, the sensitivity of the pacemaker to that zeitgeber, and the timing of the zeitgeber. The natural frequency is the frequency that the rhythm would assume if it were not entrained. For example, young and middle-aged adults are able to be entrained to a 21-hour day and a 27-hour day. Entrainment to shorter or longer periods is difficult. An example of the differentiating effect of the strength of the zeitgeber is the fact that light does not necessarily synchronize human rhythms unless it is at 2500 lux. However, this strength factor is relative; the elderly individual with failing hearing and vision may not perceive a zeitgeber as strongly as a young adult will. Sensitivity of the pacemaker to the zeitgeber varies according to the species, individual, and kind of zeitgeber. For example, cycles in the availability of food are strong zeitgebers in some animals but are less so in humans.

Studies of light stimuli have demonstrated that the timing of the zeitgeber can also influence its entraining effect. Exposure to bright light in the early morning can result in a *phase advance* in a rhythm, meaning that the rhythm shifts its peak to an earlier time of day. Conversely, the timing of a zeitgeber can cause a *phase delay* in the circadian timing system, and the acrophase of rhythms will occur later.

In summary, human rhythms are thus the result of an interaction between the individual's own internal rhythms and the rhythms of the external environment. The environmental cues or zeitgebers can influence both the period and timing of the individual's rhythms. An understanding of the role of zeitgebers in synchronizing an individual's rhythms can assist the nurse in designing interventions to prevent and restore synchronization in clients in and out of institutions, as is discussed later in this chapter.

The Nature of Selected Rhythms

There is a vast body of research that describes a variety of human physiologic, psychologic, and social rhythms. A description of all of these is beyond the scope of this chapter; however, Figure 16-2 provides an overview of a variety of human physiologic rhythms. The grid indicates the timing of the acrophase (with 95% confidence intervals) within the 24-hour span of the usual activity–rest cycle. Discussion of some of the rhythms gives the nurse a sense of the importance of investigating the rhythmic structure of various aspects of patients.

It should be noted that the descriptions that follow regarding the daily fluctuations of the various rhythms are applicable to about 80% of the young and middle-aged adult population. The other 20% fall into one of two extreme categories: "larks" or morning people who are extreme in their preference for early morning activity and "owls" or evening people who are extreme in their preference for late evening activity. For these individuals, the timing of the acrophases that are reported here is phase-advanced (*i.e.*, occur earlier for larks) or phase-delayed (*i.e.*, occur later for owls). However, even among the other 80% of the population, there are lark and owl tendencies that provide individual variations around the acrophase estimates.

Body Temperature

One of the most stable rhythms in humans is core body temperature. It has a strong endogenous component and is often used as a marker for assessing the whole circadian timing system in humans. Its daily rise and fall in individuals have been documented repeatedly and found to occur independent of such factors as fever, environmental temperature, and activity.

The stability of core body temperature is the result of an efficient thermoregulatory system responsible for balancing heat loss and heat production. Although skin temperature plays a role in regulating core body temperature, the circadian rhythm of skin temperature is weaker and differs from that of core body temperature and is even thought to be driven by a different pacemaker.

Although the body has its own endogenous temperature rhythm that free-runs to a period slightly longer than 24 hours, certain exogenous factors have been shown to influence this rhythm. Light is certainly one of these factors. The temperature rhythm is also influenced by the activity rhythm. For example, a drop in temperature is usually associated with naps, and a rise in temperature is associated with exercise. However, these two effects occur independent of the circadian periodicity of body temperature (*i.e.*, the temperature rhythm does not depend on activity for its rhythmicity). Individuals kept on bed rest or deprived of sleep maintain a circadian rhythm in core body temperature.

The usual diurnal rhythm of body temperature has a trough

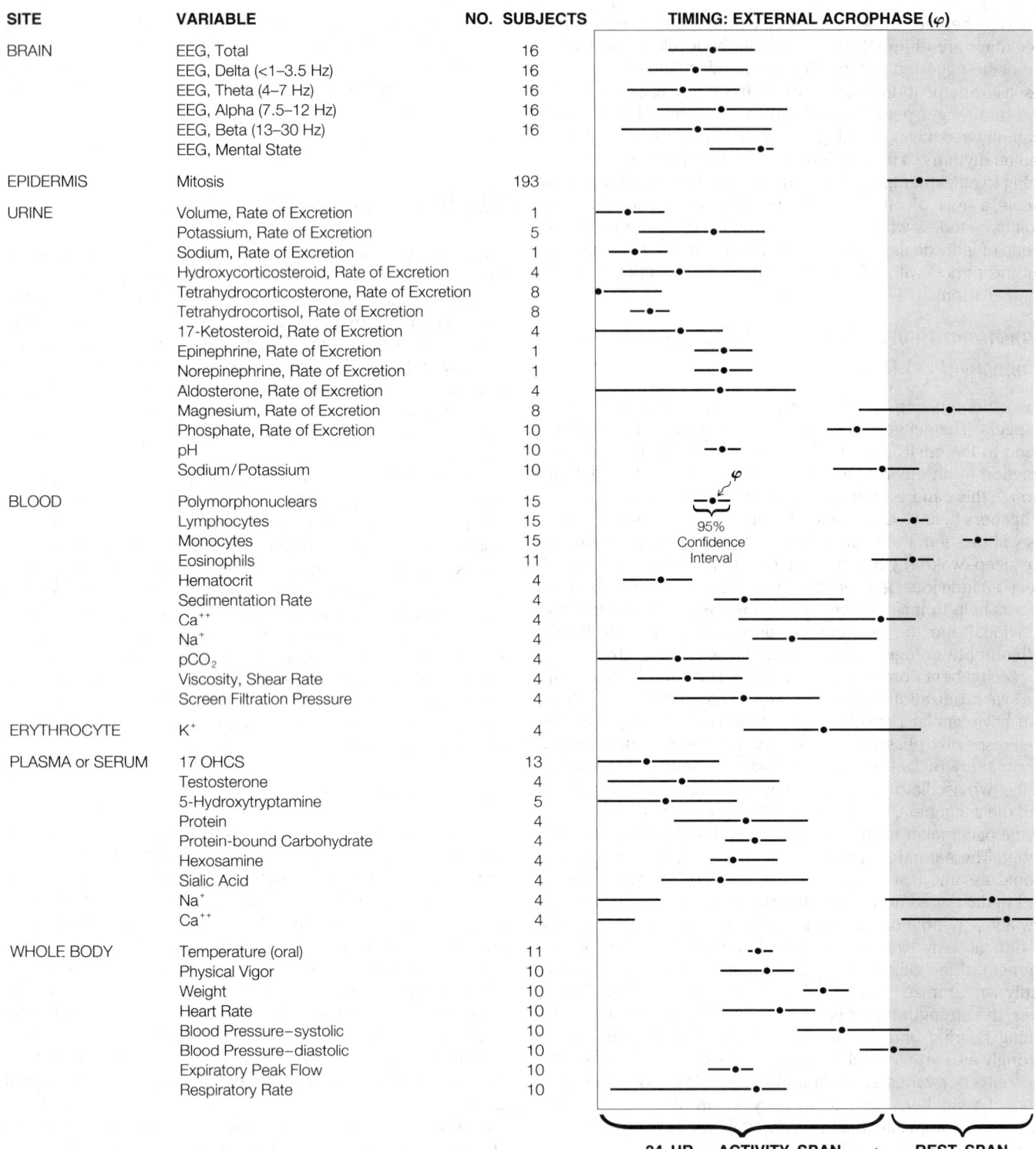

SITE	VARIABLE	NO. SUBJECTS
BRAIN	EEG, Total	16
	EEG, Delta (<1–3.5 Hz)	16
	EEG, Theta (4–7 Hz)	16
	EEG, Alpha (7.5–12 Hz)	16
	EEG, Beta (13–30 Hz)	16
	EEG, Mental State	
EPIDERMIS	Mitosis	193
URINE	Volume, Rate of Excretion	1
	Potassium, Rate of Excretion	5
	Sodium, Rate of Excretion	1
	Hydroxycorticosteroid, Rate of Excretion	4
	Tetrahydrocorticosterone, Rate of Excretion	8
	Tetrahydrocortisol, Rate of Excretion	8
	17-Ketosteroid, Rate of Excretion	4
	Epinephrine, Rate of Excretion	1
	Norepinephrine, Rate of Excretion	1
	Aldosterone, Rate of Excretion	4
	Magnesium, Rate of Excretion	8
	Phosphate, Rate of Excretion	10
	pH	10
	Sodium/Potassium	10
BLOOD	Polymorphonuclears	15
	Lymphocytes	15
	Monocytes	15
	Eosinophils	11
	Hematocrit	4
	Sedimentation Rate	4
	Ca^{++}	4
	Na^+	4
	pCO_2	4
	Viscosity, Shear Rate	4
	Screen Filtration Pressure	4
ERYTHROCYTE	K^+	4
PLASMA or SERUM	17 OHCS	13
	Testosterone	4
	5-Hydroxytryptamine	5
	Protein	4
	Protein-bound Carbohydrate	4
	Hexosamine	4
	Sialic Acid	4
	Na^+	4
	Ca^{++}	4
WHOLE BODY	Temperature (oral)	11
	Physical Vigor	10
	Weight	10
	Heart Rate	10
	Blood Pressure–systolic	10
	Blood Pressure–diastolic	10
	Expiratory Peak Flow	10
	Respiratory Rate	10

TIMING: EXTERNAL ACROPHASE (φ)

95% Confidence Interval

24 HR = ACTIVITY SPAN   +   REST SPAN

Figure 16–2. Acrophase diagram of human circadian system (Analyses from Chronobiology Laboratories, University of Minnesota, Minneapolis.) (Reproduced with permission from Harvey V. Samis and Salvatore Capobianco (Eds.), *Aging and Biological Rhythms.* New York: Plenum Press, 1978.)

or low point between 0400 and 0600 hours. It then begins a sharp rise until 1000 hours and gradually increases until it reaches its peak (acrophase) between 1700 and 2200 hours, coinciding with the end of the activity time. The temperature then drops rapidly over the late evening and night.

Sleep–Wake/Rest–Activity

Circadian Sleep–Wake Rhythm
The sleep–wake cycle is probably the circadian rhythm most obvious to individuals. Sleep is a complex physiologic and be-

havioral process. Webb (1988) describes the primary factors that affect sleep: sleep demand, circadian tendencies, and behavioral inhibitors and facilitators. Sleep demand is related to the time of wakefulness preceding sleep. The circadian factors relate to the timing of sleep within the 24-hour day. Behavioral facilitators are sleep-promoting, and inhibitors interfere with sleep. These behavioral factors can be voluntary (use of sleeping medication) or involuntary (environmental noise). These factors are interactive and mediated by the state of the individual, which can be altered by illness. The circadian factors are emphasized here; however, it will become clear how the other factors interact with circadian factors.

Most individuals have bedtimes between 2200 and 0100 hours and awaken between 0600 and 0900 hours, providing the individual with about 8 hours of uninterrupted sleep and 16 hours of wakefulness. However, this pattern is culturally determined and a reflection of the state of "modernization" of societies. Many "underdeveloped" countries incorporate a siesta, or midday nap, into their sleep–wake pattern. Controlled studies of human rhythms suggest that the siesta accommodates the body's natural tendency for a "postlunch dip" in energy that occurs independent of food intake and may reflect an ultradian, 12-hour rhythm of sleepiness. It has not yet been determined whether ignoring the body's natural inclination for this midday rest period is detrimental to health and well-being. However, it is an example of the strong role of social factors in modulating the endogenous circadian rhythms.

Under isolation conditions, the sleep–wake cycle will initially free-run a period of about 25 hours and then, if the free-running conditions persist long enough, will extend to a 30- to 50-hour period (*i.e.*, the individual will sleep once in a 30- to 50-hour period). Individuals who are owls tend to have longer sleep–wake periods than do larks. When the endogenous sleep–wake period is longer than the 24 hours, there is a tendency for the individual to want to stay up later each night. Maintaining a constant sleep–wake time will require continual adjustments by the human system. There is some speculation that this adjustment takes place on a regular basis, providing an infradian component of the sleep–wake cycle that may be about 3 or 4 days long.

An interaction between the sleep–wake and temperature rhythms influences the timing and nature of sleep. The duration of sleep is more dependent on the phase of the circadian rhythm of body temperature than on the length of prior wakefulness. Sleep duration and ease of sleep onset are maximized when sleep occurs around the time of the trough in body temperature. Wake episodes are more likely to occur when temperature is in its rising phase, whereas sleep is more likely when the temperature is in its declining phase.

Ultradian Sleep Rhythm

Sleep is composed of sleep stages that represent an ultradian rhythm (Fig. 16-3). These stages have been well defined and described predominantly through polysomnography, which consists of simultaneous recordings of an electroencephalogram (EEG) measuring brain wave activity, an electromyelogram (EMG) measuring muscle activity, and an electrooculogram (EOG) measuring eye movement. Sleep is characterized by a cyclical alternation between rapid eye movement, or REM, sleep and non-REM sleep with a period of 90 to 110 minutes. REM sleep is characterized by rapid eye movements, a loss of muscle tone, and dreaming. Non-REM sleep is comprised of

four stages (I to IV) that are characterized by increasing magnitude of the EEG waves and slower frequency until the deep, slow-wave sleep of stage IV sleep is reached. Stages III and IV differ primarily in the percentages of slow waves seen on EEG. Together, the two stages of slow-wave sleep are called delta sleep. Muscle tone is not lost in non-REM sleep, so periodic movements occur throughout the four stages. Although the young adult spends about 25% of sleep time in REM sleep, there is a gradual decline in REM sleep with aging.

Sleep usually begins with stage I sleep, a light level of sleep. REM sleep begins about 70 to 90 minutes later. REM sleep recurs at 90- to 110-minute intervals; however, the length of REM sleep periods increases throughout the night so that non-REM sleep predominates at the beginning of the sleep period and REM sleep predominates at the end. Both REM and non-REM sleep are essential for health and optimal functioning. Interruptions in sleep that interfere with the attainment of delta or REM sleep are particularly problematic if persistent, even if total sleep time is not reduced.

The ultradian rhythm of sleep persists under free-running conditions, suggesting a strong endogenous component. It is thought to operate independent of the circadian sleep–wake cycle but can be modulated by it. Increased daytime activity is associated with more slow-wave sleep. Posture also affects the ultradian rhythm. Although some non-REM sleep can occur with standing, REM sleep cannot because of the loss of muscle tone during this stage. Extremes in environmental temperature can influence both the circadian and ultradian sleep cycles. REM sleep is the stage that is most affected by circadian factors. The rising trend of REM sleep throughout the night is reversed to a declining one if sleep occurs between 0700 and 1500 hours (as might occur with night-shift workers). Naps earlier in the day have a larger amount of REM sleep than naps late in the day. When sleep is phase shifted, as occurs when shift workers rotate from days to nights, REM sleep readjusts only after several days. On the other hand, delta sleep is not greatly affected by circadian factors. The declining trend in delta sleep is maintained regardless of the time of sleep onset, and it adjusts immediately to phase shifting of the circadian sleep cycle.

Rest–Activity

The sleep–wake cycle is not synonymous with the rest–activity cycle, although the two are clearly related. One can rest without being asleep, and one can be asleep but active (as with leg movements or sleepwalking). Distinguishing between the two cycles is most objectively and reliably accomplished by polysomnography. Activity obviously is highest during the day for diurnal individuals. The acrophase for activity in young adults occurs around 1500 hours.

Hormones

The human timing system uses the endocrine system to communicate temporal information to the body and thus synchronize it internally as well as to the external environment. Most hormones have definitive circadian rhythms, although the parameters of these hormones differ. Most also have ultradian rhythms of varying length. In fact, the ultradian component of luteinizing hormone (LH) is stronger than its circadian component.

Cortisol secretion, along with body temperature, is con-

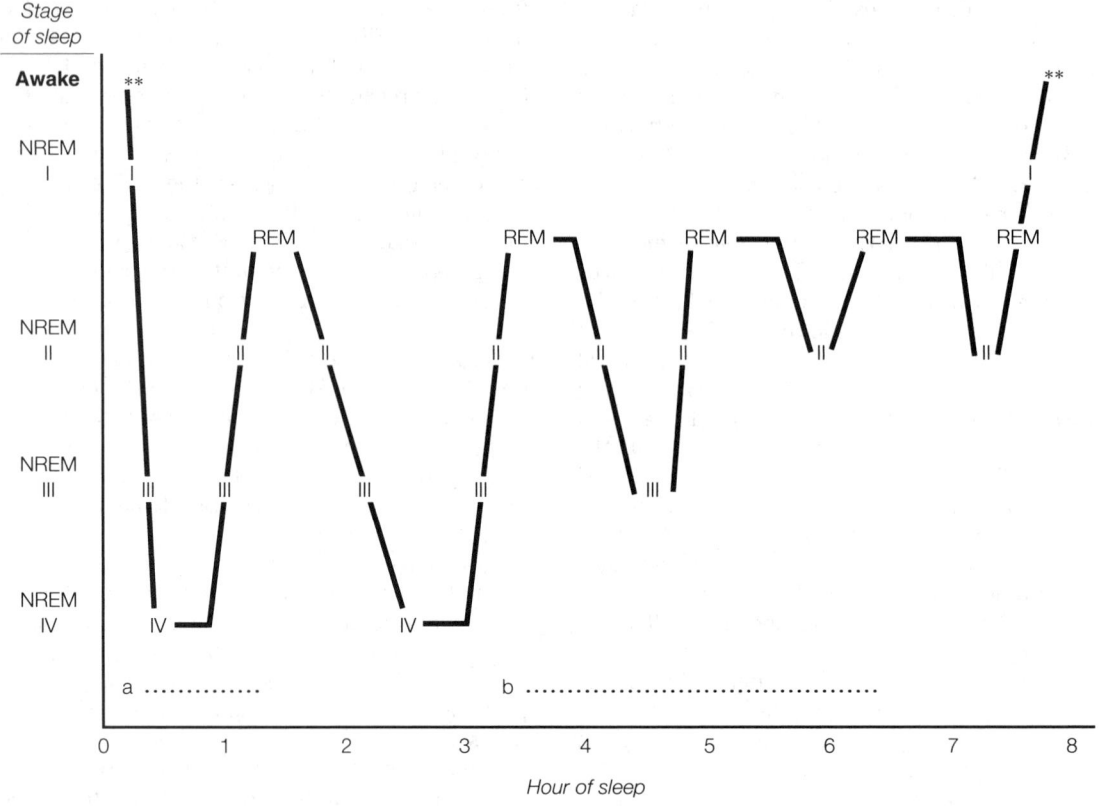

Notes:
a. *Progression of sleep through nonrapid eye movement (NREM) I-II-III-IV-III-II to precede first rapid eye movement (REM) phase.*
b. *REM phases lengthen somewhat as NREM III and IV are lost.*
c. *Figure depicts 5 REM phases.*

Figure 16–3. Normal adult sleeping pattern and the stages of sleep. (Reproduced with permission from Chuck Biddle and T.R.F. Oaster, "The Nature of Sleep," *ANNA J* 1990 Feb; 58(1);38.)

sidered a reliable indicator of the human circadian pacemaker. Plasma cortisol secretion is characterized by a surge and peak at around 0600 with a gradual decline throughout the day until its minimum is reached a couple of hours before sleep begins. There is also a circadian rhythm in the body's ability to secrete corticosteroids. For example, the body's susceptibility to a fever-producing substance is greatest during the evening when corticosteroid levels are low. Although mild stressors do not affect the circadian pattern of cortisol secretion, stronger stressors can. The circadian rhythm of corticosteroids is a persistent one with a strong endogenous component such that if the sleep–wake cycle is reversed, it takes about 3 weeks for the cortisol rhythm to invert.

The rhythms of other hormones, such as melatonin, growth hormone, aldosterone, testosterone, prolactin, thyrotropin, luteinizing hormone, and follicle-stimulating hormone, are well documented. Clear differences exist in their phases and amplitudes. For example, cortisol and growth hormone have high-amplitude rhythms (*i.e.*, they show a relatively large amount of variation). On the other hand, thyrotropin and testosterone have much less variation. Another example of the differences in hormone parameters is that growth hormone peaks during

the night, when plasma cortisol is at its minimum. The shape of the rhythms of hormones also varies.

Cardiovascular Functions

There is a definitive circadian variation in cardiovascular functioning that leaves humans in a vulnerable state in the early morning hours. A hypercoagulable tendency occurs between 0600 and 0900 hours, when there is a circadian peak in platelet aggregability. Fibrolytic activity is decreased in early morning and may be related to an increase in the circulating levels of tissue plasminogen inhibitor. The tendency for a hypercoagulable state may also be related to an early morning increase in hematocrit and blood viscosity.

Other variations in the cardiovascular system reflect the morning arousal state of awakening that is associated with sympathetic stimulation. With the predominance of vagal stimulation that occurs during sleep, the blood pressure and heart rate decline. On arising, both of these increase, as do the circulating levels of catecholamines. Furthermore, the rate of increase in blood pressure is maximal during the wake period. It begins to increase about an hour before waking and peaks

2 hours after arising. Changes in heart rate are also maximal during the first 2 hours after awakening; however, no increase prior to awakening is seen.

Performance and Cognitive Functioning

Performance is related to sleep and rest; however, circadian and ultradian rhythms of performance persist under conditions of sleep deprivation, suggesting a degree of independence from sleep. The neural processes controlling alertness and sleep produce an increased sleep tendency and diminished capacity to function between 0200 and 0700 hours. An ultradian factor results in another, albeit smaller, increase in sleep tendency and reduction in performance between 1400 and 1700 hours.

Rhythms in performance vary according to the nature of the task. The performance of tasks requiring little memory peaks at the maximum of body temperature (*i.e.,* in the early evening). Conversely, the performance of tasks requiring memorization peak near the minimum of body temperature (*i.e.,* in the early morning). General mental functioning shows an initial morning rise and then deteriorates throughout the day. Although this pattern holds for short-term memory efficiency, long-term memory (and information retention) is best when the material is presented in the afternoon.

Alterations in Rhythms

As the picture of humans as temporal beings unfolds, definitions of health that include temporal organization become necessary. Such definitions need to reflect the predictable rhythmic variations in physiologic, psychologic, and social functioning that have a variety of frequencies and fairly constant internal and external phase relationships. The factors of predictability and time relations reflect the fact that integrated human functioning is dependent on a rhythmic pattern among biologic functions.

Illness

Illness or deviations from health can also be expressed in temporal terms: an uncoupling of internal rhythms that results in a temporal disorganization of processes. Recovery then can be seen as a resynchronization of internal and external rhythms. The return of rhythmicities can become a criterion for evaluating the effectiveness of therapies or interventions.

Although certain illnesses have been associated with changes in circadian rhythms (*e.g.,* increased nighttime urination in congestive heart failure and the disturbed sleep–wake rhythm in depression and bipolar disease), whether the illness causes the rhythm change, results from it, or is merely associated with it has not been clearly established in most cases. Abnormal amplitudes or acrophases can be early indicators of developing disease.

Some illnesses are associated with abnormal rhythms of susceptibility to otherwise benign stimuli. For example, the circadian variation in airway resistance is usually of such a low amplitude that it has little or no effect on respiratory performance. However, in the individual with respiratory failure sec-

ondary to bronchial asthma, bronchial constriction increases in the early morning (0600 hours), causing an increased amplitude and exaggerated circadian rhythm. The frequency of respiratory arrest is greatest during this early morning period.

Variations in Morbidity and Mortality

The ultradian rhythms in performance, alertness, and sleepiness coincide with mortality rates from a variety of causes. Vehicular accidents due to "falling asleep behind the wheel" peak between 0100 and 0400 hours and show a smaller peak between 1300 and 1600 hours. Job performance errors, including major industrial accidents such as nuclear power plant accidents, are clustered between 0200 and 0400 hours, with a second peak between 1400 and 1600 hours. Mortality from all causes has shown an ultradian pattern that peaks between 0400 and 0600 hours and again to a lesser degree between 1400 and 1600 hours.

There is a well-documented circadian variation in cardiovascular morbidity and mortality that peaks in the early morning, including acute myocardial infarction, ischemia and anginal attacks, sudden death, dysrhythmias, and stroke. The incidence of these events peaks between 0600 and 1200 hours and reaches a minimum between midnight and 0600 hours. This pattern reflects the circadian variation in cardiovascular functioning that was described earlier and that accompanies the morning state of arousal (*e.g.,* hypercoagulability tendency and an increase in blood pressure, heart rate, and catecholamine secretion).

Spontaneous labor and births are also more likely to occur during the night, although it is not clear why. An infradian rhythm has also been documented that is connected to the phases of the moon, with more births and psychiatric admissions to the emergency room occurring on nights of a full moon. This finding is not so bizarre when one considers the effect of the moon on the tides and the role of the environment in influencing living systems.

Desynchronization

One principle of chronobiology is that an organism functions most effectively when it is synchronized to a period that is close to its own natural frequency. This was evident in one of the earliest human isolation studies. Aschoff (1965) reported that a subject studied under isolation conditions made diary notations on days when he felt especially well and fit, and these notations coincided with times when his dissociated free-running rhythms of temperature, activation, and other functions happened to be in phase with each other.

On the other hand, a lack of synchronization between the organism and the environment is associated with decrements in performance, functioning, health, and well-being. Plant and animal research has demonstrated that a persistent lack of synchronization between the organism and the environment can impair growth and longevity. This lack of synchronization is referred to as *desynchronization*. It occurs when two or more previously synchronized rhythms no longer exhibit the same period or acrophase.

This desynchronization can be external or internal. External desynchronization occurs when a biologic rhythm becomes desynchronized from an environmental rhythm. Internal desynchronization occurs when two or more biologic rhythms in the same entity become desynchronized from each other. These two types of desynchronization can occur simultaneously. For example, some blind individuals are unable to maintain a 24-hour sleep–wake cycle. This rhythm often free-runs so that the blind person moves in and out of phase with the environmental rhythm, and external desynchronization occurs. At the same time, the sleep–wake rhythm can uncouple from the temperature rhythm, creating a state of internal desynchrony.

The effect of light on the circadian pacemaker is thought to play a role in seasonal affective depression or disorder (SAD), in which symptoms (including sadness, anxiety, irritability, decreased energy and activity, excessive sleepiness and sleeping, increased appetite and weight gain, and difficulties with work and interpersonal relations) increase during the winter and abate or disappear during the summer. The prevalence of SAD increases with distance from the equator and under low-light conditions of climate. One survey, using a random sample of adults living in New York City with telephones, revealed that 25% of the adults suffered from some degree of SAD (Terman, 1989). Exposure to bright light has been shown to effectively treat SAD, particularly when high-intensity light is provided for mildly depressed clients in the early morning (Terman et al, 1989).

Desynchrony also occurs with transmeridian jet travel across multiple time zones and with shift work. The nurse who rotates from days to nights demonstrates a flattening of the temperature rhythm after about 3 days then a gradual reversal of the peak in temperature until it adapts to the new time structure and peaks during the nurse's subjective day (which is the night). This process takes about 7 to 14 days. If the nurse then rotates back to days, the same shifting of the temperature rhythm must take place to eventually bring the temperature back in phase with the nurse's subjective day. This process occurs to greater and lesser degrees with the individual's other physiologic and psychologic rhythms.

Well-being and optimal functioning are associated with fully developed, high-amplitude circadian patterns, the loss of which occurs with the desynchrony that is associated with shift work and jet lag. Shift workers have been reported to show impaired performance efficiency and accuracy, fatigue, mood changes, an increase in subjective estimates of distress, and decrements in subjective measures of physical, social, and mental well-being. Disturbances in body temperature that result from transmeridian flight (*i.e.*, across several time zones) result in impaired reaction time and information processing and an increase in subjective fatigue.

Sleep Disorders

Disturbances in some circadian rhythms can be of great subjective concern to individuals, with sleep disorders being particularly bothersome. Forty percent of the adult population are dissatisfied with the quality of their sleep; 15% to 20% of these adults consult a physician, and 50% of the physicians prescribe sedative hypnotics. The incidence of sleep problems is higher in people with chronic illnesses. The inappropriate use of seda-

tives has been a topic of growing concern, particularly in relation to the elderly.

Sleep disorders can be caused by exogenous and endogenous factors. Insomnia is any inability to sleep during the usual sleep period. There are different types of insomnia, but the most common type is sleep-onset insomnia, occurring in about 10% of the adult population. Sleep-onset insomnia is characterized by difficulty initiating sleep, with little or no difficulty maintaining sleep once it occurs. Sometimes referred to as delayed sleep phase insomnia, the only abnormality is the timing of sleep, often occurring around 0300 hours; the length and nature of the sleep are unchanged. However, if the individual must maintain a work or school schedule that requires him to arise at 0700 hours, for example, the individual gets too little sleep and usually experiences excessive daytime sleepiness to a degree that can impair performance. Studies of sleep-onset insomnia have demonstrated that individuals with this sleep disorder have a delayed phase in body temperature (*i.e.*, their temperature peak and trough occur about 2.5 hours later than those of normal sleepers) (Morris et al, 1990).

Early morning awakening insomnia (also called terminal insomnia) is characterized by a relatively rapid sleep onset, reasonably undisturbed sleep, and premature awakening with an inability to return to sleep. It has been suggested that this type of insomnia is related to an advance in the temperature rhythm (*i.e.*, the body temperature begins to rise at a time earlier than that of normal sleepers). Early morning insomnia is also one of the classic symptoms of depression.

Alcoholism is associated with altered sleep patterns, and even moderate evening drinking in the nonalcoholic can produce temporary nighttime arousals. Sleep–wake patterns can also become disrupted as a result of the fatigue that is associated with many illnesses. Inactivity and bed rest are associated with longer sleep, as are illnesses such as myocardial infarction and stroke. On the other hand, people who exercise regularly often report sleeping more poorly on days when they do *not* exercise, suggesting that some activity may be necessary for satisfactory sleep.

Alterations in the sleep–wake and other circadian rhythms have been noted in people with a variety of chronic and acute illnesses, including chronic renal failure. Relapses of multiple sclerosis have been associated with a loss of the circadian rhythm of somatostatin in the cerebrospinal fluid (Sorensen et al, 1987). Increased daytime sleep is associated with severe dementia, including Alzheimer's disease. An inversion of the sleep–wake cycle is characteristic of progression of Alzheimer's disease, suggesting that pathologic changes may be occurring in the circadian timing system with this disease. The inversion has a profound effect on both the individual with Alzheimer's disease and the family who is caring for him at home. The nighttime wanderings of the person with Alzheimer's become disruptive to the sleep cycle of the caregiver to the point that sleep deprivation, fatigue, and depression can occur in the caregiver. This often is the turning point for the family to decide to institutionalize the patient.

Restlessness

Norris (1986) has described restlessness as an early manifestation of the individual's adaptive response to a disturbance in rhythmicity. The restlessness itself may have a circadian pattern, as is evident in "sundown syndrome":

> As night falls, the patient who functioned well becomes disoriented. . . . The patient, with clothes or pillow in hand, is found searching the hall for his room. No matter how many times he is returned to the room that in the daytime he recognizes, the nurse finds him a little while later once again searching for "my room." When morning comes, this patient becomes reoriented, and restlessness disappears. (p 302)

Sundown syndrome is characterized by an increase in confusion and restlessness as night approaches.

Stress

Disruptions in circadian rhythms and the sleep–wake cycle can act as stressors and further compromise clients who are in poor health. On the other hand, stress has been shown to be able to delay rhythms and can have an indirect effect through interfering with the normal sleep–wake cycle (too much or too little). Surgery may act as a stressor; research has demonstrated that circadian rhythms are disrupted following surgery and that the extent of disruption may affect recovery (see Farr's study in Nursing Research Profile). Whether the disruption in rhythmicity is due to the surgery, the anesthesia, or an interaction between the two has not been clearly delineated.

Strong, synchronized rhythms are associated with health and well-being. Whether illness results from, leads to, or merely accompanies changes in rhythms, the various rhythmicities and temporal organization itself can vary in nonhealthy conditions. Nurses' considerations of this fact can assist with prevention of temporal disruptions and promotion of temporal organization.

Nursing Assessment of Human Rhythms

Nursing assessment of patients needs to routinely reflect the rhythmic nature of humans. This is accomplished in two ways: (1) by assessing the patient's rhythms and (2) by considering temporal factors when interpreting assessment data.

Assessing the Patient's Rhythms

Important information about the circadian system can be obtained by measuring body temperature every 2 to 4 hours for 3 days. However, the nurse should avoid awakening the patient at night to do this. Rather, the patient should be asked to ring for the nurse if he awakens at night, and the temperature should be taken then. In addition, temperature readings should be taken immediately on awakening and just before sleep. Measuring the temperature continuously with a rectal probe provides more measurements for objectively evaluating whether a rhythm disorder exists. Because the length and quality of sleep are enhanced when sleep occurs around the time of minimum body temperature, an examination of the patient's temperature rhythm can also provide important information about sleep problems.

Assessing sleep–wake patterns can provide additional information about the state of the circadian timing system and can also provide other information that the nurse can use to promote optimum sleep–wake patterns. The following questions can be used to assess these patterns:

- What is the client's usual sleep schedule? What are the patient's usual hours of sleeping and awakening? Is the patient a daytime or nighttime sleeper?
- How much sleep does the patient believe he needs each night? Does the patient consider himself to be a "good" or "poor" sleeper? What are the patient's perceptions of "normal" sleep?
- What are the patient's usual bedtime rituals (how does he usually prepare for bed)?
- Does the patient take naps? Frequency? Usual timing and length? Do they seem to interfere with nighttime sleep? Does the patient perceive naps to be restorative?
- Does the patient have any sleep problems, such as difficulty falling or staying asleep, or awakening too early? What does the patient do for these problems?
- Does the patient have a problem with excessive daytime sleepiness? Does the sleepiness vary throughout the day? At what times is sleepiness increased and decreased?

Having the patient keep a sleep–wake diary for a month is a simple way to evaluate circadian sleep–wake disorders in the clinic or homebound patient. The patient records times of going to sleep and waking and the timing of naps on a daily basis. Particular attention should be given to the individual who works evenings or nights and who now must undergo resynchronization to a day schedule.

Asking the patient whether he prefers the early morning hours or evening hours can indicate whether the patient is an owl or a lark. The nurse can ask, "What is your 'best' time of the day?" This information can be used to plan interventions, including patient teaching and rehabilitation.

Information about the timing of meals, exercise, urination, and bowel habits should also be assessed. For example, the patient who is accustomed to jogging in the morning may respond best to physical therapy that is planned for the morning, unless the patient has cardiovascular disease. Approximating the patient's routine daily schedule while he is in the hospital may promote synchronization.

As is discussed later, medications and dietary substances can also affect the circadian timing system. Thus, the nurse should assess what medications the patient is taking and when they are taken. The assessment should also include the use of alcohol and substances such as caffeine, which is found in coffee, tea, and soft drinks. These substances have both direct and indirect effects on circadian rhythms.

Chronobiologic Profile

Ideally, patients should have a temporal profile constructed while in good health. This profile can be performed in concert with an annual checkup and used as baseline information to evaluate deviations from health and progress with recovery. Such a profile may include rhythms of temperature, sleep–

wake, and corticosteroid secretion; rhythms of other blood constituents and urine, alertness, performance, and mood could also be included. Autorhythmometry, or the self-measurement of human rhythms, is commonly used in research on human rhythms and could be used for obtaining these individual profiles.

Timing Consideration for Assessments and Interpretation of Assessment Data

The timing of nursing assessment is an important consideration for several reasons: (1) to provide data to assess the circadian system itself, (2) to increase the efficiency and effectiveness of obtaining other information about the patient, and (3) to accurately interpret assessment data. As has already been discussed, repeated measures of variables such as body temperature can provide information about the status of the circadian system itself. These data can then be used to formulate nursing diagnoses related to alterations in rhythms.

Consideration of the timing of the nurse's assessment of any variable can also promote efficient, effective, and safe nursing care. For example, the early morning pattern of mortality, particularly from cardiovascular causes, suggests that the nurse be vigilant in monitoring patients between 0400 and 1000 hours. This is especially important on the night shift, when it may be assumed that clients require less attention if they are sleeping, and during the first hour after the patient awakes. Such attentiveness to timing of nursing assessments requires an understanding of the rhythmic nature of humans and their environment.

Interpretation of assessment data obtained from a physical examination (including observation) and from laboratory tests must include time-of-day considerations. If these considerations are ignored, normal circadian fluctuations may be misinterpreted as abnormal. For example, measurements of body temperature must be interpreted with an understanding of the normal circadian pattern. A temperature of 98.6°F in the early morning may actually represent a low-grade fever in some individuals, particularly the elderly.

Chronotherapeutic Nursing Interventions

Timing of Interventions

One of the major principles of chronobiology is that the organism's response to any stimulus depends on the time of day. The response to a stimulus applied during the morning may be different from the response to a stimulus applied at night. This means that nurses must consider the timing of their interventions. Because of the variation in the phases of different biologic rhythms, the timing depends on the nature of the intervention. For example, because long-term memory is best in the afternoon, patient teaching of young and middle-aged adults

should probably take place then (further research is needed to determine whether such timing is beneficial for older adults as well). On the other hand, scheduling physical therapy during the patient's "postlunch dip" can diminish the progress of the rehabilitation.

Knowing when to plan an intervention for optimal chronobiologic response may not always be clear-cut. However, an understanding of the temporal nature of humans and the environment can assist the nurse in evaluating the effectiveness of the intervention and determining whether timing alterations should be considered to improve the patient's response.

Light

The human circadian pacemaker can be reset to any desired phase by planned exposure to light for 2 or 3 days. Exposure to light for longer durations has been used effectively to treat seasonal affective depression. While researchers are continuing to study the effects of different dosages, timing, and type of light and individual sensitivities to variations in these factors, the nurse can begin to use light as a therapeutic and preventive intervention in some basic and practical ways.

First, institutional and home lighting should be assessed. Lighting designs that provide bright room light without glare should be encouraged. Architectural designs that eliminate windows should be avoided, because windows not only allow light into the room but provide synchronizing information about the time of day.

Second, room lighting should be regulated to simulate day–night when possible. For example, intensive care units should be designed so that room lights can be dimmed during the night and individual bedside lights can be used when a particular patient needs attention. Full lighting should then be restored at a fairly consistent time in the morning.

Finally, exposure to natural sunlight outside should be provided whenever possible. This could be accomplished by encouraging the family to take the patient outside in a wheelchair, if the patient is able and weather permits. Similarly, the visiting nurse can help the homebound patient arrange to be taken outdoors in the morning.

Other Institutional Factors

Studies have documented that hospitals are not conducive to rest and sleep (see Coss's study in Nursing Research Profile). Constant lighting and noise, lack of visible windows and clocks, shift-rotating workers, and nighttime staff and patient activity all interfere with the zeitgeber effect of the environment to the point that some clients may actually begin to free-run and become desynchronized while in the hospital.

The nurse's knowledge of exogenous factors that influence human rhythms can promote synchronization of rhythms. The regulation of lighting to simulate a day–night schedule has already been discussed. Noise levels can also be regulated. Daytime noise is expected; however, nighttime noise can be minimized. Discussions among staff should take place out of the range of the sleeping patient whenever possible. This may mean closing the doors of rooms near the nurses' station, often the center of staff noise and activity. Having calendars and clocks within the patient's view can promote orientation to date and time. Verbal reportings of time and date can reinforce this effect.

Whenever there is any routine modification of the institutional environment, it must be assumed that all or most of the patients are benefited by the schedule adopted by the institution. However, variations in circadian rhythms exist in the adult population, so that not everyone's schedule can be accommodated within an institution. The early morning routine that is standard in hospitals and nursing homes may be appropriate for most of the adult population. Some special accommodations may assist the patient who is an "owl": placement in a private room or in a room with other "owls," delayed wakening, the option of a cold breakfast that can be served after the delayed awakening, and providing a television or reading room for late-night patients.

Promoting Sleep–Wake/Activity–Rest Patterns

Manipulations of the institutional environment can promote synchronization of the individual's rhythms and foster fairly regular sleep patterns without the need for sleep-inducing medications. These can be augmented by minimizing sleep interruptions. For example, when the night nurse makes rounds, use of a flashlight can prevent awakening the patient; shining the flashlight directly in the client's face should be avoided. Furthermore, when a variety of procedures must be performed with a patient during the night, the procedures should be clustered together if at all possible, and efforts should be made to begin them when the patient stirs in his sleep. This is particularly possible in the intensive care unit, where the nurse can observe all patients from the nurse's station.

Sleep can also be promoted by allowing the patient to engage in his regular bedtime routines as much as possible. Such bedtime routines help to condition the body to prepare for sleep. For example, the patient who is accustomed to taking a shower right before bedtime may be conditioning the body to relax. When consistently done, it also signals the body to prepare for sleep. Allowing such a patient to take a shower at night may foster regular sleep without medication.

The typical treatment for sleep-onset insomnia has been the use of hypnotic drugs (see "Medications and Other Ingestible Substances," below). Although these provide initial symptomatic relief of the insomnia, they can have side effects such as withdrawal rebound insomnia, drug dependence, and daytime sedation, the latter being particularly dangerous for the elderly patient or for a person whose job requires a high degree of alertness. Recent research has demonstrated that individuals with particularly severe sleep-onset insomnia can be treated successfully by progressively delaying their bedtime by about 3 hours per night/day over the course of a week to 10 days until the desired bedtime is reached. This becomes difficult for the daytime worker who cannot sleep during the day for a few days; however, other routines can also be applied. Early morning exercise and exposure to bright light in the morning have been shown to advance the phase of the sleep–wake cycle. On the other hand, exposure to bright light in the evening has been shown to delay the circadian cycle. Furthermore, maintenance of a consistent bedtime routine can prevent some sleep disturbances. Maintaining a weekday sleep schedule on the weekends (including both sleep and arising times) can also help to synchronize sleep–wake rhythms.

Sleep deprivation is of particular importance to nurses who work in intensive care units, where constant lighting and activity can interfere with patient's sleep. Sleep deprivation is also known as ICU syndrome, ICU psychosis, postoperative delirium, cardiac psychosis, and cardiac delirium. It is associated with impaired performance and deterioration in mood. Severe sleep deprivation may also produce cognitive impairment and confusion and even hallucinations, particularly in the elderly patient who may be more prone to confusion. Decreases in lymphocyte and granulocyte functions can also occur. All of these manifestations can jeopardize the recovery and health of the patient in an intensive care unit.

Daytime sleepiness increases with partial or total nighttime sleep deprivation. It should be noted that subjective sleepiness may have a rhythm that is separate from the sleep rhythm. Sleepiness and alertness are seen as reciprocal and as a function of the circadian timing system and of prior sleep and wakefulness. Increases in subjective sleepiness (the individual's self-rating of felt sleepiness) have been related to self-reported increases in tension, confusion, fatigue, and sadness, as well as decrements in calmness and vigor. However, these effects do not necessarily occur with objective measurements of sleepiness (*e.g.*, how quickly one can fall asleep). Objective sleepiness does decline with adequate nocturnal sleep and is decreased by caffeine; however, subjective sleepiness does not correlate with nocturnal sleep and is less affected by caffeine. These differences suggest that one's subjective feelings of sleepiness should be expected to differ from objective indicators of sleepiness, but both are important to the well-being of the individual. Patient reports of sleepiness after a seemingly "good" night's sleep should not be doubted; the timing of the sleep and the patient's reports of midsleep awakenings should be explored.

General daytime activity and exercise are helpful in promoting uninterrupted sleep at night. They also augment the social cues that a person receives. Most individuals benefit from exercise and physical activity during the morning when the body's arousal is on the rise; however, it has been suggested that individuals who are prone to cardiac ischemia should exercise during the afternoon or evening hours, when cardiac vulnerability is not as great.

Rest that is appropriately integrated into the client's schedule can be helpful to both the sleep-deprived and recuperating patient. Because of the 12-hour ultradian rhythm in sleepiness that occurs in the early afternoon (postlunch dip), rest or a nap at this time of day may have a restorative effect. Although napping can provide some relief from poor nocturnal sleep, it can also interfere with subsequent nocturnal sleep, particularly for the patient who is not accustomed to napping. Because morning naps simulate early morning sleep in that they are mostly REM sleep, restless clients can be encouraged to take early morning naps if the restlessness is due to loss of REM sleep. On the other hand, afternoon naps, which promote delta sleep, can be encouraged for the elderly patient who complains of fatigue, because the nighttime sleep of the elderly is characterized by reduction of the deep slow-wave sleep.

Relaxation techniques can be used to facilitate both rest and sleep. These include abdominal breathing, progressive muscle relaxation, meditation, imaging, hypnosis, and biofeedback.

Medications and Other Ingestible Substances

Medications can affect human rhythms. Some have a direct effect; others have an indirect effect on rhythms. Furthermore, many drugs have been shown to have circadian rhythms of efficacy and of toxicity. *Chronopharmacology* is pharmacology with a chronobiologic approach.

Substances that can reset the circadian clock include methyl xanthines, theophylline, caffeine, phenobarbital, chloramphenicol, puromycin, and ethanol. Because caffeine and theophylline are present in some coffees, teas, and soft drinks, and ethanol is in alcoholic beverages, individuals may be constantly resetting their clocks with habitual use of these substances. Triazolam, a short-acting benzodiazepine, can phase-advance (*i.e.*, cause the peak to move to an earlier time) the circadian rhythms of luteinizing hormone and locomotor activity in animals and has been shown to facilitate the synchronization of endocrine rhythms after they have been disrupted by changes in the light–dark cycle. Triazolam is used predominantly for depression and anxiety, both of which are often accompanied by sleep disorders.

Some of the above substances can also have indirect effects on the circadian system. Caffeine increases alertness and enhances performance that has been impaired by fatigue or sleep loss. Psychoactive medications such as amphetamines may dampen the sleep–wake and alertness rhythms, particularly in older adults, by making the person feel groggy or "hungover" the next day. Whether direct or indirect in their effects, these and other substances can clearly have both positive and negative effects on the timing of the human circadian system.

Sleep problems are most often treated with medications. Although hypnotic medications can induce sleep better than placebos, long-term use of these sleep-inducing medications can reduce their efficacy and lead to rebound insomnia on withdrawal. This rebound insomnia can occur on the first night of sleep without the medication or several nights later. When the patient's concern about insomnia stems more from fear of poor performance the next day than from the loss of sleep itself, the hypnotics are not as effective because they have not been shown to improve daytime functioning. Whereas low doses of short half-life hypnotics do not impair next-day performance, long half-life hypnotics do. Hypnotics also can cause respiratory depression, which can exacerbate preexisting sleep apnea (frequent cessation of breathing during sleep), and they must be used with extreme caution in patients with this disorder. Benzodiazepines are currently the hypnotic drugs of choice for treating insomnia.

Because pain can interfere with sleep, the arthritic patient, postsurgical patient, or other patients with pain may need an analgesic prior to or during the sleep period. Some analgesics can interfere with the ultradian stages of sleep and even influence the circadian component (*e.g.*, daytime analgesia administration producing excessive daytime sleeping that interferes with the ability to fall asleep or stay asleep at night). Therefore, overmedicating should be avoided, and attention should be given to determining whether the disruptions from pain are greater than the disruptions from the medication. Overmedicating can be avoided by anticipating the circadian pattern of pain, which has been shown to peak at 2200 hours.

Although individual variations in this pattern must be assessed, an increase in the patient's pain in the early evening should alert the nurse to administer analgesics before the pain peaks and requires a higher dosage for relief.

The circadian variation in physiologic rhythms can have other implications for the timing of medications. Valle and Lemberg (1990b) have pointed out that clients on long-term nitrate (nitroglycerin) therapy for angina need a daily drug-free period of 10 to 12 hours to prevent tolerance. They suggest that this interval is tolerated better if it occurs during the afternoon and evening hours, rather than during the morning when individuals are particularly at risk for cardiovascular events. This provides nitrate coverage during the morning, when the greatest incidence of anginal attacks occurs. Furthermore, clients with hypertension and additional coronary risk factors would benefit from evening administration of alpha-2 agonists such as clonidine (Catapres), guanabenz (Wytensin), and guanfacine (Tenex), in long-acting or sustained-release form. This timing allows for maximum action during the early morning hours. Similar considerations should be given to the timing of other cardiovascular drugs to counteract the body's early morning vulnerability to cardiovascular problems.

The timing of administration of a variety of medications can be the crucial factor in how effective the drug is and whether the patient experiences side effects. A classic example of this is the administration of corticosteroids. For the individual who has adrenal insufficiency and needs hormone replacement, administration of a steroid medication in a manner that approximates the body's own circadian rhythm of corticosteroid secretion results in the greatest therapeutic effect and minimal side effects. This means administering the steroid in a single dose in the early morning hours (around 0600), or two thirds of the 24-hour dose at this time and one third in the afternoon. Such timing reduces the adverse effect of suppression of the adrenal cortex. However, if suppressed adrenal functioning is a therapeutic goal, administration of the steroid medication at a constant level throughout the day or in the evening and night results in the greatest suppression.

Variations in the body's response to medications are related to circadian rhythms in the rate of drug absorption, metabolism, and excretion and in tissue susceptibility. Cancer chemotherapy is increasingly administered with a sensitivity to circadian variations in therapeutic and side effects that reflect a circadian variation in the patient's sensitivity to the drugs. Cancer cells and normal cells often have different circadian rhythms of cell division such that they have different rhythms of susceptibility. Timing of the administration of chemotherapy is thus planned so that the drug peak coincides with the peak of the tumor cells' susceptibility. Studies of animals suggest that such considerations to timing can make the difference between life and death. Anesthetics, analeptics, antihistamines, some analgesics, and a variety of other medications also have marked rhythms of effectiveness and toxicity.

Gerontologic Considerations

A growing body of research is demonstrating that temporal organization changes as one ages. Studies of older adults have demonstrated decreased amplitudes (flattening of rhythms sometimes to the point of a loss of rhythmicity), decreased mesors, and changes in the timing of the acrophases of a variety of physiologic rhythms, compared with the rhythms of young and middle-aged adults. These are similar to the changes that occur with shift work and jet leg. There is also evidence that the period of circadian rhythms shortens with aging and that the circadian timing system itself becomes phase-advanced.

Theoretical Perspectives

Chronobiologists have proposed that the changes in rhythms that occur with aging are due to one or more causes. First, in accordance with theories of "programmed" aging, it has been proposed that aging is the result of a genetically predetermined program for temporal disorganization, which accounts for species-specific predictable life spans. A second proposition falls into the category of the "accumulated errors" theory of aging and holds that as the organism ages, disruptions in temporal organization result from the lifetime accumulation of assaults or mutations on cellular processes and structures. Because of the loss of adaptive capacity that occurs with aging, the cell or organism is unable to re-entrain such internal desynchronizations with the same efficiency and recovery seen in younger adults. Even slight desynchronizing that remains uncorrected will accumulate and lead to greater degrees of phase dissociation, resulting in a loss of coordination among various interdependent oscillating systems and a further loss of functional potential and adaptive capacity. Third, it has been suggested that the aging individual is less sensitive to zeitgebers. Because of the loss of sensory perception that occurs with aging, the individual is thought to be unable to sense the primary environmental time cues and consequently experiences desynchronization. Other life-style changes that may occur with aging, such as increased social isolation and lack of a regular work schedule, could compound this lack of entrainment.

The changes in rhythms that occur with aging have been assumed by chronobiologists to be detrimental; however, one nurse theorist offers an alternative explanation. Nurse theorist Martha Rogers (1970, 1986) holds that humans are energy fields that are continually interacting with environmental fields and changing in the direction of greater complexity, diversity, and higher-frequency waveforms. Rather than assuming that older adults have decrements in their temporal organization or their ability to perceive their environment, a Rogerian perspective would suggest that the older adults are evolving and thus perceiving their environment differently. Some support for this perspective comes from an isolation study of older and younger subjects (Weitzman et al, 1982). The finding that isolated, free-running adults demonstrate a shortened period in body temperature lends support to the idea that humans evolve to higher-frequency waveforms (*i.e.,* shortened periods). In addition, other studies of aging have suggested that there is greater intragroup variability in the rhythms of older adults compared with younger adults, lending support to the view of increasing diversity with human development. Thus, from a Rogerian viewpoint, changes in the temporal organization of older adults may be associated with high levels of well-being.

Changes in Rhythms With Aging

Although research has not yet determined whether Rogers or the chronobiologists are correct in their explanations of temporal aging, the debate is important for nurses to keep in mind as they care for older adults. For example, among the rhythms that often change with aging are the circadian and ultradian components of the sleep–wake cycle. Older adults, and some middle-aged adults, often arise earlier in the morning (a phase advance in the sleep–wake cycle) and experience changes in the internal construction of their sleep that may leave them feeling less rested. Delta sleep, the deep slow-wave sleep, is reduced, and stage IV sleep may be absent. Older adults often complain of more frequent nighttime awakenings and not sleeping as soundly. Because most people tend to evaluate the sleep of older person in terms of the norms for sleep in young adults, information about age-related changes in sleep may be helpful in reducing undue concern about such sleep changes and inappropriate use of sleeping medications.

Additional information about the changes in rhythms that are characteristic of the older adult can help the nurse to make adjustments in identifying both problems and interventions that reflect these changes. Contrary to the generally held perception that older adults are less active than young adults, a study of healthy young and older adults revealed that the elderly have higher overall levels of activity (measured as gross body movements) than younger individuals (Lieberman et al, 1989). The greatest difference in activity between the two groups was early in the morning, when the elderly were more active than the young adults. The acrophase for younger subjects occurred around 1500 hours, whereas the older adults' mean acrophase was close to 1330 hours. Although involvement in vigorous physical activity may decline with aging, this study suggests that maintenance of an active life-style that reflects the phase-advanced circadian system of many older adults may foster health in these individuals. Furthermore, the older adult without cardiovascular problems may respond best to exercise when it is performed in the morning hours. This study also demonstrated differences in the circadian pattern of sleepiness by age (and gender) (Fig. 16-4). Because alertness is the reciprocal of sleepiness, these findings indicate that patient teaching for the older patient may be most effective when provided between 0900 and 1100 hours.

Despite the maintenance of activity and alertness in healthy older adults, there is a need for increased rest and, to a lesser extent, increased sleep. Older adults tend to tire more easily than younger adults and to require longer rest periods to recuperate.

Because there is an increased variability in the rhythmic patterns among older adults, however, it is more difficult to define "normal" for the older adult based on group data. Thus, it is particularly important for nurses to obtain baseline data on individual older adults. For example, one study of circadian rhythms in healthy older women found that although some of the women were bothered by sleep disruptions, one older woman was not. She awoke during the night with great regu-

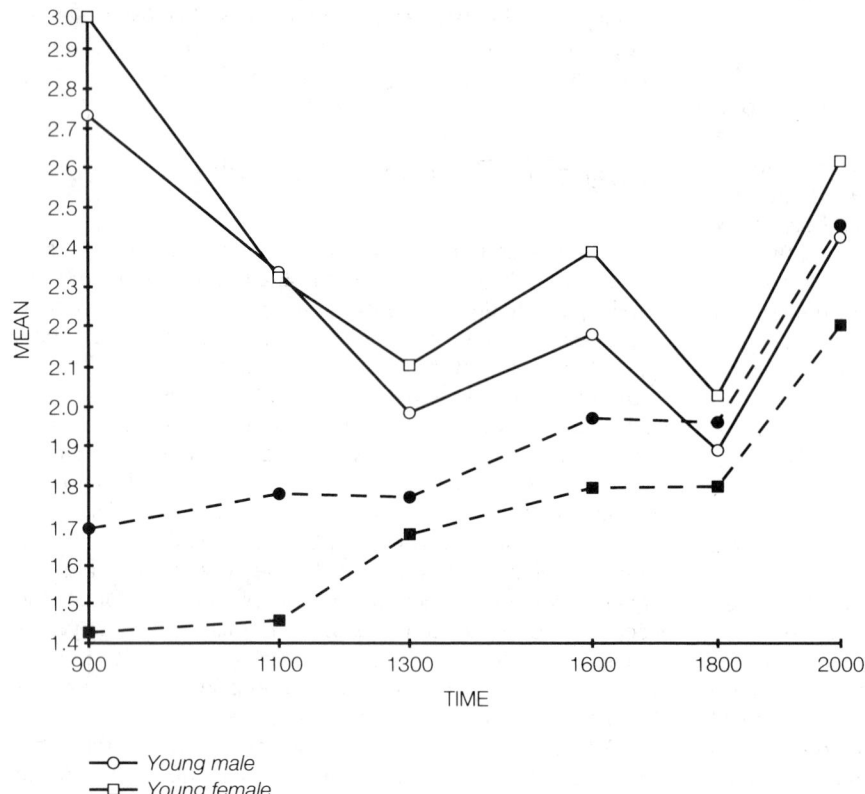

Figure 16–4. Mean self-reported sleepiness at various times of the day as assessed by the Stanford Sleepiness Scale. (Reproduced with permission from Harris R. Lieberman, Judith J. Wurtman, and Martin H. Teicher, "Circadian Rhythms of Activity in Healthy Young and Elderly Humans," *Neurobiology of Aging* 1989; 10:259–265.)

larity; however, because she was retired and did not have to arise at any particular time, she said she was not disturbed by these awakenings and would follow her body's endogenous tendency to sleep. If she awoke during the night and felt wide awake, she would often get out of bed and clean or engage in some other activity until she felt tired. Despite the sleep interruptions, she had a high level of subjective well-being and the strongest circadian rhythm of oral temperature of all subjects in the study (Mason, 1988; see Nursing Research Profile).

Nursing Implications

The above study and the differences in theoretic perspectives on the changes in rhythms that occur with aging raise some crucial issues regarding the extent to which the nurse should strengthen zeitgebers of patients in institutions (or recommend that the patient do so at home) or encourage the patient to follow his own body's rhythms. Until further research is available, several recommendations can be made for balancing these perspectives:

1. Determine what the older adult knows about the normal changes in rhythms that occur with aging, particularly in terms of the sleep–wake cycle, and provide education where necessary. If older adults continue to define "normal" sleep in terms of their sleep patterns in young adulthood, any change that is a normal occurrence of aging is likely to be interpreted as a problem. Education about normal changes can enable

the elderly patient to be satisfied with changes that are experienced and can perhaps prevent unnecessary use of medication. However, because the sleep changes that are seen with aging are also associated with anxiety, depression, and chronic illness, the older adult who complains of poor sleep should be assessed for these factors. Various medications (in addition to hypnotics), pain, and respiratory problems can compound the usual changes in sleep that are associated with aging and should also be considered.

2. Educate the older adult about the effects of the chronic use of hypnotics and mood/alertness-altering drugs on the quality of sleep. In addition, other medications that the patient is taking should be examined for their potential side effects on the circadian timing system or rhythms, particularly if the patient is manifesting a bothersome effect such as increased daytime sleepiness.

3. When alterations in the rhythms of the elderly patient occur, assess the patient's sensory capacity and the possibility of diminished social cues. Restoration of vision (*e.g.,* by cataract removal) or hearing (*e.g.,* through use of a hearing aid) may improve the patient's synchronization. The homebound patient is at particular risk for social isolation that can result in free-running rhythms. Regularly timed telephone calls from family or visits from neighbors can decrease the isolation and provide additional social cues for promoting synchronization.

4. When alternations in the rhythms of the elderly patient are subjectively or objectively detrimental, interventions that strengthen the patient's environmental cues should be tried. Examples of such interventions include pulling back dark cur-

tains so the patient can clearly detect night versus day, maintaining regular mealtimes, removing or inserting daytime naps if nighttime sleep or daytime sleepiness is a problem, or increasing the lighting during the day and dimming the lights at night. However, if the nurse or patient suspects that the rhythm disturbance arises from trying to force the older adult's rhythms into the 24-hour rhythm of the environment, the nurse might encourage the patient to follow the schedule dictated by the body's signals (*i.e.,* to free-run). This can be facilitated by providing the patient with the opportunity to be active during the night (without disturbing other patients, perhaps by having a night-active room in the nursing home or using the visitors' room in the hospital) and to sleep or nap during the day without undue disturbance. Meal adjustments may also be needed. Until comparative studies of the effects of such environmental flexibility on the health and well-being of older adults have been conducted, the nurse and the patient with disturbed rhythms can work together to try both zeitgeber-enhancing and zeitgeber-reducing strategies for the individual patient.

Rhythms and the Nurse

Because health care is provided on a 24-hour basis in hospitals, nursing homes, and in patients' homes, nurses are often required to work evening and night shifts. Even the traditional day shift of 0700 to 1500 hours can be a hardship for nurses who are owls or have evening tendencies, because the day shift requires an earlier than "normal" awakening for many young adults. Shift work has consequences not only for the nurse but also for the quality of care that patients receive.

Studies have shown that shift work is associated with sleep disorders and gastrointestinal disorders, including peptic ulcers, gastritis, and intestinal problems. Disruptions in mealtimes and the duration and quality of sleep are the major reasons for these disorders. Shift work also affects performance, because psychomotor and judgment errors peak during the night in unsynchronized workers. Sleep loss combined with a period of stress, such as responding to a patient in cardiac arrest, can foster personality changes and irrational behavior, as well as increases in job errors.

The negative effects of shift work can be minimized in several ways:

- Assess workers' shift preferences. Most individuals can identify which shift is preferable. Contrary to some expectations, not everyone will select day shift. Owls will prefer evenings and nights. Where some shift rotation is necessary, workers should be rotated to two of the three shifts that they identify as being preferable for them. Expecting everyone to be able to work nights or days is not conducive to the workers' health nor to safe, quality patient care.
- Avoid shift rotation whenever possible by using permanent shift assignments that are based on the workers' shift preferences.
- Shift rotation should always proceed in a forward manner (*i.e.,* from days to evenings, evenings to nights, nights to days). This rotation pattern takes into account the body's endoge-

nous tendency to a slightly longer circadian period, which is also why jet travel that lengthens the traveler's subjective day (from east to west) is easier to adjust to than travel that shortens the day (from west to east).

- If rotation is necessary, it should be done in either 3- or 4-week stretches or in 2-day stretches. One's circadian rhythms will begin to shift after a couple of nights and flatten out before they achieve a full reversal to the new time schedule 7 to 14 days after the beginning of the rotation. Thus, if the person is rotating to another shift at the end of 5 to 7 days, one's rhythms must adapt again, leaving the individual in a constant state of desynchronization. Many industries have gone to 2-day rotations to prevent this; however, one's circadian rhythm of performance will still dip between 0300 and 0500 hours, so caution must be taken during this time to prevent errors and accidents.
- Many of the problems related to night work are associated with disturbed sleep. Daytime sleep can be promoted by the following: use of dark blinds, taking the phone off the hook or getting an answering machine that can turn off the telephone ring but still record calls, maintaining an eating schedule that approximates what the individual's *subjective* day has become (*e.g.,* eating breakfast before going to work at night and making dinner the last major meal before sleeping; however, one should avoid eating any heavy meal within 2 hours of sleep), and maintaining one's routine awakening and bedtime rituals while working other shifts (*e.g.,* if one normally takes a shower before going to bed, this practice should be continued before the new "bedtime" when working nights).

While shift work may be necessary to provide the continuous care that patients need, it should be avoided if possible. When required, shift work can be planned to minimize the detrimental effects on the health of the nurse and on the quality of care. In addition, nurses can use their own patterns and modify environmental cues to promote adequate sleep.

Chapter Summary

Humans are temporal beings, characterized by a rhythmic variation in physiologic, psychologic, and social processes and functions. Human rhythms are influenced by a variety of factors, including environmental cues and medications. These factors can promote or alter rhythmicity. They should be assessed and manipulated by the nurse to foster rhythmicity. The nurse should be attentive to timing considerations for patient assessments, particularly in terms of interpreting laboratory and other physiologic data. Timing must also be considered when planning nursing interventions, because the individual's response to an intervention may depend on the time of day when the intervention occurs.

Attention to the individual's temporal organization can promote optimal functioning, well-being, and health in both nurses and their patients. Although much research still needs to be conducted in this area, sufficient information about human rhythms is available for the nurse to use in assessing, planning, and implementing care for patients. Such integration enhances the quality of nursing care that patients receive and can promote health and recovery.

Bibliography

Asterisks indicate nursing research articles.

Books

*Coss SJ. Factors affecting the sleep of patients on surgical wards in Scotland. In Funk SL et al (eds). Key Aspects of Recovery: Improving Nutrition, Rest, and Mobility. New York, Springer, 1990, pp 223–238.

Felton G. Human Biologic Rhythms. Annual Review of Nursing Research, Vol 6. New York, Springer, 1989, pp 71–93.

Fryger MH. Principles and Practice of Sleep Medicine. Philadelphia, WB Saunders, 1989.

Hobson AJ. Sleep. New York, Scientific American Library, 1989.

Mendelson WB. Human Sleep: Research and Clinical Care. New York, Plenum Medical Book Co, 1987.

Rogers M. An Introduction to the Theoretical Basis of Nursing. Philadelphia, FA Davis, 1970.

Rogers M. Science of unitary human beings. In Malinski VM (ed). Exploration of Martha Rogers' Science of Unitary Human Beings. Norwalk, CT, Appleton-Century-Crofts, 1986, pp 3–8.

Shaver JLF and Giblin EC. Sleep. Annual Review of Nursing Research, Vol 7. New York, Springer, 1989, pp 45–77.

Journals

Ancoli-Israel S et al. Sleep fragmentation in patients from a nursing home. J Gerontol 1989 Jan; 4(1):M18–M21.

Aschoff J. Circadian rhythms in man. Science 1965 Jun; 148(11):1427–1432.

Biddle C and Oaster TRF. The nature of sleep. AANA J 1990 Feb; 58(1):35–42.

Bliwise DL, Carroll JS, and Dement WC. Predictors of observed sleep/wakefulness in residents in long-term care. J Gerontol 1990 Jul; 45(4):M126–M130.

Borbely AA and Tobler I. Endogenous sleep-promoting substances and sleep regulation. Physiol Rev 1989 Apr; 69(2):605–670.

Broughton R et al. Chronobiologic aspects of SWS and REM sleep in extended night sleep of normals. Sleep Res 1988; 17:361.

Czeisler CA et al. Bright light induction of strong (type 0) resetting of the human circadian pacemaker. Science 1989 Jun; 244(4910):1328–1333.

Dinges DF et al. Temporal placement of a nap for alertness: Contributions of circadian phase and prior wakefulness. Sleep 1987 Aug; 10(4):313–329.

* Farr LA, Campbell-Grossman C, and Mack JM. Circadian disruption and surgical recovery. Nurs Res 1988 May/Jun; 37(3):1171–1174.

* Hansell H. The behavioral effects of noise on man: The patient with intensive care unit psychosis. Heart Lung 1984 Jan; 13(1):59–65.

Hauri PJ and Esther MS. Insomnia. Mayo Clin Proc 1990 Jun; 65(6):869–882.

* Hilton A. Noise in acute patient care areas. Res Nurs Health 1985 Sep; 8(3):283.

Hyyppa MT and Kronholm E. Quality of sleep and chronic illness. J Clin Epidemiol 1989; 42(7):633–638.

Johnson LC et al. Daytime sleepiness, performance, mood, nocturnal sleep: The effect of benzodiazepine and caffeine on their relationship. Sleep 1990 Apr; 13(2):121–135.

Levine B et al. Fragmenting sleep diminishes its recuperative value. Sleep 1987 Dec; 10(6):590–599.

Lieberman HR, Wurtman JJ, and Teicher MH. Circadian rhythms of activity in healthy young and elderly humans. Neurobiol Aging 1989 May/Jun; 10(3):259–265.

* Mason DJ. Circadian rhythms of body temperature and activation and the well-being of older women. Nurs Res 1988 Sep/Oct; 37(5):276–281.

Mitler MM et al. Catastrophes, sleep, and public policy: Consensus report. Sleep 1988 Feb; 11(1):100–109.

Monk TH. Subjective ratings of sleepiness: The underlying circadian mechanisms. Sleep 1987 Aug; 10(4):343–353.

Monk TH and Moline ML. Removal of temporal constraints in the middle-aged and elderly: Effects on sleep and sleepiness. Sleep 1988 Dec; 11(6):513–520.

* Moore MN. Development of a sleep-awake instrument for use in a chronic renal population. ANNA J 1989 Feb; 16(1):15–19.

Morris M, Lack L, and Dawson D. Sleep-onset insomniacs have delayed temperature rhythms. Sleep 1990 Feb; 13(1):1–14.

National Institutes of Health Consensus Statement: The treatment of sleep disorders of older people. 1990 Mar; 8(3):1–22.

Norris CM. Restlessness: A disturbance in rhythmicity. Geriatr Nurs 1986 Nov/Dec; 7(6):302–306.

* Richards KC and Bairnsfather L. A description of night sleep patterns in the critical care unit. Heart Lung 1988 Jan; 17(1):35–42.

Rivest RW et al. Difference between circadian and ultradian organization of cortisol and melatonin rhythms during activity and rest. J Clin Endocrinol Metab 1989 Apr; 68(4):721–729.

* Samples JF et al. Circadian rhythms: Basis for screening for fever. Nurs Res 1985 Nov/Dec; 34(5):377–379.

Sorensen KV et al. CSF somatostatin in multiple sclerosis: Reversible loss of diurnal oscillation in relapses. Neurology 1987 Jun; 37(6):1050–1053.

Terman M. On the question of mechanism in phototherapy for seasonal affective disorder: Considerations of clinical efficacy and epidemiology. J Biol Rhythms 1988 Summer; 3(2):155–172.

Terman M et al. Light therapy for seasonal affective disorder: A review of efficacy. Neuropsychopharmacology 1989; 2(1):1–22.

Turek F and Van Reeth O. Use of benzodiazepines to manipulate the circadian clock regulating behavioral and endocrine rhythms. Horm Res 1989; 31(1/2):59–65.

Valle GA and Lemberg L. Circadian influence in cardiovascular disease (part 1). Chest 1990a Jun; 97(6):1453–1457.

Valle GA and Lemberg L. Circadian influence in cardiovascular disease (part 2). Chest 1990b Jul; 98(1):218–221.

Webb WB. An objective behavioral model of sleep. Sleep 1988 Oct; 11(5):488–496.

Weitzman ED et al. Chronobiology of aging: Temperature, sleep-wake rhythms and entrainment. Neurobiol Aging 1982; 3:299–309.

Wever RA. Light effects on human circadian rhythms: A review of recent Andechs experiments. J Biol Rhythms 1989 Sep; 4(2):161–185.

17

Human Sexuality

Learning Objectives

On completion of this chapter, the learner will be able to:

1. Describe the significance of sexual self-assessment in assisting the nurse to identify her own strengths and limitations in the sexual aspects of clinical practice

2. Identify biologic, psychologic, and environmental variables that can alter sexual function

3. Describe the human sexual response pattern

4. Include sexual assessment as part of the health history of the hospitalized patient

5. Specify the relationship between body image and sexuality

6. Describe the significance of sexual counseling for preventing and treating sexual dysfunction resulting from health problems (i.e., myocardial infarction, mastectomy, spinal cord injury, diabetes mellitus, hypertension)

The topics of sexuality and sexual interactions are often avoided by nurses when caring for patients with medical problems or those who have undergone surgical interventions. We are all sexual beings, however, from the time of birth until the time of death. Every patient with whom the nurse comes in contact, therefore, no matter where he is on the health–illness continuum, is a sexual being.

The term *sexuality* refers to the totality of a being—to human qualities, not just to the genitals and their function. It includes all the components that make the person who he is—biologic, psychological, emotional, social, cultural, and spiritual. Individuals have the capacity to express their sexuality in any of these areas. An example of the psychological area would be a person's inner self-concept; that is, I am a man, or I am a women, or I am "half a man," or I am no longer attractive (Whipple & Gick, 1980).

To provide total patient care, it is important to have an adequate knowledge base about sexuality and sexual function and to feel comfortable with one's own sexuality and the sexuality of one's patients. A course in human sexuality that includes a sexual attitude reassessment (SAR) program helps the nurse to gain an adequate knowledge base and to become aware of and understand and accept his own attitudes, values, and feelings. A nurse cannot consider the patient's attitudes and feelings nonjudgmentally until she has come to terms with her own.

People in our society often have been taught to view any behavior that does not meet our standards of acceptable behavior as immoral, illegal, or culturally taboo. The role of culture, mores, religious beliefs, and familial values cannot be ignored; they help to determine who an individual is and how he accepts information about and expresses sexuality. The nurse may be called on to care for patients whose behavior or sexual orientation is different from or conflicts with her definition of "acceptable." To give total patient care, however, one has to be aware of how biases could have a negative impact on care; and one needs to be comfortable with one's own sexuality and the sexuality of patients.

The Role of the Nurse

The role of the nurse in the delivery of sexual health care is to provide a therapeutic environment conducive to sexual health. When acting as a sex educator and counselor, the nurse can assist the patient to acquire knowledge, validate normalcy, and prepare for changes in sexuality throughout the life cycle, in both health and illness. The nurse, using the nursing process, is able to carry out a meaningful assessment, identify problem areas, plan, implement, coordinate referral sources, and evaluate effectiveness of care.

Sexual Development

Sexual development begins at conception. The woman's ovum (egg) carries the X chromosome, and the male's sperm carries either an X or a Y chromosome. Thus, the sperm determines the sex of the offspring. An X chromosome paired with another X chromosome equals a female embryo; when X is paired with a Y chromosome in the presence of androgens, a male embryo develops. All embryos are female in sexual development until the sixth or seventh week of embryonic life, when androgens stimulate male sexual development in the XY fetus (Guyton, 1986). Deviations in early sexual development can occur due to chromosomal error or hormonal disturbances. After birth, sexual development is influenced by other people through the socialization process.

Basic to our development as sexual humans is our personal sense of maleness or femaleness and the way we perceive and express it. To provide clarity and consistency, several related terms are defined.

Biologic sex is defined as the basic anatomic and reproductive differences between males and females. The components are chromosomal differentiation, hormonal secretions, differentiation of internal sex organs, and external genitalia.

Gender is a behavioral term, a psychological phenomenon. The two components are biologic sex and gender identity.

Gender identity refers to the degree to which an individual perceives being a male or a female. To a great extent, this perception is culturally determined. The core of juvenile gender identity is established by 18 months. At the time of puberty, hormonal influences on pubertal morphology, eroticism, and body image lead to the development of adult gender identity. Gender identity becomes relatively immutable by the end of adolescence (Money & Ehrhardt, 1972).

Gender role refers to the way in which a person expresses gender identity. It is learned behavior through imitation of the same-sex parent and complementation of the opposite-sex parent. It is influenced by the complex interaction of parental

rewards and punishments. Gender role continues to be defined throughout the life cycle.

Traditionally, in our Western culture, masculinity and femininity referred to restrictive sex-role stereotyped behavior. "Masculine" was defined in terms of strong, aggressive, logical, and independent characteristics. "Feminine" was defined in terms of weak, submissive, dependent, and emotional characteristics. Gender roles have changed for both women and men over the past two decades. Gender role is now viewed on a continuum, so that having characteristics traditionally identified as male traits does not necessarily make a person less feminine, and vice versa. The term *androgenous* (unisex) refers to both masculine and feminine characteristics, providing more options for individuals and ultimately greater equality between sexes (Bem, 1974).

Sexual preference refers to choice of sexual partner: heterosexual (opposite sex), homosexual (same sex), bisexual (both sexes).

To provide anticipatory guidance throughout the life cycle, the nurse must be familiar with psychosexual development: developmental tasks, sexual growth, sexual behaviors, and common sexual concerns, problems, and areas of intervention.

Table 17–1 provides a summary of psychosexual development that may be used as a guideline for obtaining assessment data. The framework used has been provided by Erikson; however, in all cases, individual differences should be considered (Erikson, 1963).

Human Sexual Response Patterns

The findings of Masters and Johnson indicate that sexual response can be described as a cycle with four stages (Masters & Johnson, 1966). These stages follow a consistent pattern of progression, from excitement to plateau, then to orgasm and resolution. Two basic physiologic responses are responsible for the sexual response cycle: vasocongestion and myotonia.

Vasocongestion is the filling of blood vessels of the genitals and specific body regions, causing enlargement and color changes. *Myotonia* is increased muscle tension, voluntary and involuntary. Both are a result of sexual stimulation, begin during excitement, become more pronounced and reach a peak at orgasm, and subside during resolution.

Sexual desire preceding excitement is controlled by the limbic system in the brain and is greatly influenced by the hormone testosterone. Therefore, anything that inhibits testosterone production may inhibit sexual desire. Stress causes a decrease in testosterone levels; consequently, a person who perceives a threat, pain, or fear is not likely to experience sexual desire (Kaplan, 1974).

Only the sexual response patterns as described by Masters and Johnson (1966) will be discussed in detail in this chapter. Other researchers, however, report data that differ from Masters and Johnson's response cycle. Kaplan (1979) developed a model that divides the response patterns into two stages: excitement and orgasm. Zilbergeld and Ellison (1980) divide the sexual arousal and response cycle into five parts: desire, arousal, physiologic readiness, orgasm, and satisfaction. The

(text continues on page 294)

TABLE 17-1. *Summary of Stages of Psychosexual Development and Related Nursing Intervention*

Developmental Tasks	Sexual Growth	Sexual Behaviors	Sexual Concerns and Problems	Intervention
DEVELOPMENTAL STAGE: Infancy (0–18 Months) *DEVELOPMENTAL CRISIS: Trust Versus Mistrust*				
Develops a need for affection and to return affection	Sensitivity to a warm, loving environment	Cuddling, hugging, kissing	Touch deprivation	Reinforce the importance of close physical contact and related problems.
	Oral sensitivity, lips, tongue, mouth (oral stage)	Sucking	Oral deprivation (early weaning)	Explain the significance of early weaning and related problems.
Begins to interpret expectations of significant others	Genital sensitivity; erectile potential in males; orgasmic potential in males and females	Stimulation of genitals by self or others; erections in males; primitive orgasms	Parental concern Parental fear	Clarify parental attitudes and beliefs toward self. Explain the primitive nature of the response: higher brain centers not well developed. Reinforce that behavior is normal and cannot harm the infant.
Develops a communication system	Feels good/bad about body parts and functions	Labels body parts based on parental values, voice inflections	Body image	Stress the importance of relating to infant's body in a positive way.
Establishes separateness and becomes social; can differentiate between strange and familiar people	Distinguishes between self and others Reinforcement of gender identity	Begins to show maleness or femaleness Identifies with same sex parent	Blurred identity, restrictive sex role, stereotyping, coding (pink for girls, blue for boys), limiting play objects	Infant needs close contact with a person to develop gender identity. Sex-role stereotyping can be avoided by focusing on the infant as an individual.
DEVELOPMENTAL STAGE: Toddler (18 Months to 3 Years) *DEVELOPMENTAL CRISIS: Autonomy Versus Shame, Doubt*				
Begins to demonstrate toilet training	Learns control of bowel and bladder (anal stage)	Sensual pleasure derived from elimination	Strict toilet training	Relate problems identified with strict toilet training: compulsive behavior, castration anxiety. Provide alternative method of toilet training.
Begins to participate as a family member	Development of core of gender identity	Imitates behavior of parent of same sex	Anxiety about acceptable behavior for males and females	Avoid sex stereotyping by providing options: dress, playthings, focus on individual child.
Communicates with others outside family	Learns differences between male and female bodies	Shows an interest in bodies of other children	Parental concern	Clarify attitudes, values, and beliefs.
	Establishes concept of body image	Labels body parts and may ask questions	Poor self-image; may view sexual organs as "dirty"	Provide vocabulary that emphasizes acceptance of body: genitals, reproduction, elimination.
Develops autonomous behavior	Genital sensitivity Erection potential Orgasmic potential	Sensual, erotic behaviors; masturbation patterns of self-pleasure, toys, objects	Parental concern	Emphasize normal part of sexual development. Clarify values, attitudes, and beliefs.

(continued)

TABLE 17–1.   *(Continued)*

Developmental Tasks	Sexual Growth	Sexual Behaviors	Sexual Concerns and Problems	Intervention
DEVELOPMENTAL STAGE: Preschool (4–6 Years) *DEVELOPMENTAL CRISIS: Initiative Versus Guilt*				
Participates actively as a family member	Oedipal attachment to opposite sex parent: complementation— learns what to expect from opposite parent; identification with same sex parent; learns sex roles	Physically affectionate; interested in parents' bodies; fantasizes about parents; may dress in parents' clothing	Excessive attachment to parent; seductive behavior of parent toward child; hostility of same sex parent	Provide alternatives for seductive parent in a nonthreatening manner. Refer parents to parenting class (avoid confusing messages for child). Sexual variations may be related to seductive parent. Refer for counseling.
Responds to expectations of others; begins to understand and establish a sense of morality	Sexual curiosity; penis and clitoris become chief areas of erotic pleasure (phallic stage); capacity to perceive sexual odors	Self-play increases; "plays doctor," touches and sees other children's bodies; asks questions about genitals, reproduction	Parental concern; child may learn to suppress sexual feelings and behavior to be accepted by others.	Overreaction leads to guilt; anticipate sexual curiosity; stress importance of answering questions in a nonjudgmental manner. Use correct terms (*penis, vagina*) as appropriate terminology.
DEVELOPMENTAL STAGE: School Age (6–12 Years) *DEVELOPMENTAL CRISIS: Industry Versus Inferiority*				
Decreases dependency on family for total love and support; begins to understand peer relationships	Close contact with same sex peers; development of friendships	Homosexual experiences part of same sex relationships; also, sex play with opposite sex common	Parental overreaction; guilty child	Reassure parents that this is a normal part of psychosexual growth and development. Validate normalcy.
	Curiosity about sex (no latency)	Discussion of sex with peers	Confusing or frightening information	Clarify myths, giving accurate information about reproduction.
	Orgasm potential (males and females); some girls begin menarche	Mutual masturbation, self-stimulation	Fear from lack of information	
Acknowledges body changes	Increasing self-awareness; interest in body growth	Comparison of body growth with peers	Concerns over body growth	Elicit sexual history in a comfortable, confidential manner. What do you know about having babies? When you have questions about sex, who do you ask? Do you have questions about sex? Have you noticed changes in your body? How do you feel about changes in your body?

(continued)

TABLE 17–1.   *(Continued)*

Developmental Tasks	Sexual Growth	Sexual Behaviors	Sexual Concerns and Problems	Intervention
Relates to social, religious, or familial values, attitudes, and beliefs	Learns internal sexual value system; learns self-control	Learns to be secretive; may use slang for shock value	Testing behavior limits; obsessive, antisocial behavior; repression	Refer for counseling, family therapy. Attempts by parents to restrict may lead to low self-esteem. No limits delay internal value-system formation.
	Understands concepts of masculinity and femininity	Continues to define sex role in activities inside and outside family	Strict sex-role stereotyping by parents: male may be discouraged from developing "female" skills; females may be discouraged from sports activities	Provide alternatives to limitations of sex-role stereotyping. Focus on preferences of the individual child.

DEVELOPMENTAL STAGE: *Early Adolescence (12–15 Years) and Late Adolescence (15–18 Years)*
DEVELOPMENTAL CRISIS: *Identity Formation Versus Identity Diffusion*

Developmental Tasks	Sexual Growth	Sexual Behaviors	Sexual Concerns and Problems	Intervention
Acknowledges and accepts physical changes and body image	Female: menarche; development of breasts; distribution of fat to hips and thighs; increased size of uterus; pubic hair growth Male: ejaculation; testicular enlargement; growth of pubic hair and facial hair; voice change and nocturnal emissions	Comparison of body changes with same sex peers; sexual fantasies related to body	Anxiety over change in body image; embarrassment	Discuss relationship of body image and sexual growth and how these changes perceived by the individual are a reflection of self-image.
Develops close peer relationships with both sexes; develops deep personal relationship with opposite sex	Learns intimacy, heterosexual relationships; develops "crushes"	Heterosexual encounters: kissing, petting, mutual masturbation; heterosexual fantasies. One half of teenagers will have intercourse.	Performance; orgasm; virginity; anxiety.	Provide direct and confidential approach in eliciting sexual history: Are you sexually active? Frequency? How do you feel about it? Provide birth control counseling. STD risk-reduction counseling, Pap testing, BSE, TSE.
			Compulsive, mechanical masturbation	May represent escape from another problem; provide sex counseling.
Attains a male or female role	Increased awareness of sexual feelings integrated in self	Males group together in sports; females group together	Sexual variations may surface: homosexuality, transsexuality, bisexuality	Provide role clarification: What do you think it means to be a man or a woman? Validate normalcy. Refer to sex counseling if problems exist.

(continued)

TABLE 17–1.   *(Continued)*

Developmental Tasks	Sexual Growth	Sexual Behaviors	Sexual Concerns and Problems	Intervention
Seeks more of a peer relationship with parents	Expresses feelings about sexual self	Responds to parental limitations	Parental concern, communication breakdown; guilt	Communication is essential. Parents fail to take "crush" seriously. Problems related to double standard may surface. Restrictive limitations impede development.

DEVELOPMENTAL STAGE: Young Adult (20–45 Years)
DEVELOPMENTAL CRISIS: Intimacy Versus Self-Isolation

Developmental Tasks	Sexual Growth	Sexual Behaviors	Sexual Concerns and Problems	Intervention
Stabilizes self-image	Acceptance of one's body; pregnancy	Comfortable nude with intimate others	Male: anxiety over penis size. Female: anxiety over breast size. Both: self-consciousness; shame	Stress the fact that size of breasts or penis has little to do with sexual gratification. Negative body image may interfere with the establishment of sexual relationships.
Establishes sexual behavior patterns	Mature concept of sexual self; gender role continues to be defined; sexual orientation and sexual lifestyle established	Heterosexual adjustment—bisexuality, homosexuality, celibacy, masturbation, cohabitation, monogamy, marriage, extramarital sex	Ambivalence to gender role, identity, sexual orientation, "homosexual panic," feelings of being trapped by sex orientation	Elicit sexual history: How do you feel about gender identity, role, and orientation? Explore feelings about sex partner. Regardless of expression, intimacy versus isolation should be evaluated. Validate normalcy.
	Learns to give and receive pleasure	Experimentation with different forms of sexual expression	Boredom; fear of experimentation; inability to communicate sexual needs to partner; lack of information	Explain sexual response cycle. Discuss patterns of sexual behavior. Identify areas of concern. Possible referrals.
Determines desire for having family; protects reproductive integrity	Makes decisions about childbearing	Reproduction control; maintains integrity of sex organs; Pap screening, BSE, TSE-STD risk-reducing behaviors	Unwanted pregnancy; fear of physical exam—pelvic; lack of information about STDs or birth control	Elicit sexual history and birth control method, and provide alternatives. Explore feelings about childbearing, STD counseling, and risk reduction.
Formulates life philosophy and develops ethical standards	Develops sexual value system	Behavior reflects individual values, attitudes, and beliefs.	Sexual needs are not met because of strict, inflexible beliefs.	Values clarification is needed: absolutistic—sexuality for reproduction; hedonistic—pleasure; relativistic—acts judged on the basis of their effects.

(continued)

TABLE 17-1.   *(Continued)*

Developmental Tasks	Sexual Growth	Sexual Behaviors	Sexual Concerns and Problems	Intervention
DEVELOPMENTAL STAGE: Middle Age (45–65 Years) *DEVELOPMENTAL CRISIS: Generativity Versus Self-Absorption/Stagnation*				
Acknowledges and accepts physical and emotional changes	Declining hormonal production: menopause—vaginal atrophy and loss of vaginal mucosa; vasomotor symptoms—hot flashes; irritability, fatigue, external genitalia, and breast tissue changes; male climacteric—slower to attain erection, sustained shorter, and ejaculatory force lessens	Focus on quality of sexual encounter versus quantity; frequency may decline; intercourse expression of love and trust; reaffirmation of self-concept	Anxiety about losing youthfulness, vitality, sex appeal, and fear of loss of partner; may stop sexual activity because of dyspareunia caused by lack of vaginal secretions; self-image crisis; depression and denial; male concern: losing vigor and virility.	Give anticipatory guidance. Explain changes in sexual response with aging. Postmenopausal women: recommend vaginal lubricant. Regular sexual activity will increase capacity for sexual performance.
Adjusts to independence of grown children	Adjusts to "empty nest"; redefines sex roles	Spends time reestablishing primary relationship; develops and cultivates new joint activities; relinquishes control of children	Attempts to continue to control offspring	Focus on maintenance of relationship with spouse or intimate other.
DEVELOPMENTAL STAGE: Later Maturity (65+) *DEVELOPMENTAL CRISIS: Ego Integrity Versus Despair*				
Continues close, loving relationship with spouse	Accepts slowed sexual response cycle; development of alternative ways to achieve sexual satisfaction	Adjusts sexual activities; appropriate time may be AM, when less fatigued; oral or manual stimulation; fantasy; emphasis on sensual touching, holding, kissing	Conforms to prevailing societal myth of sex for procreation; lack of information; rigid stereotyped image of what older person should be	Sexual need for intimacy and sexual expression does not change with age. Explain physical changes in sexual response with aging.
Copes with illness or death of spouse or friend	Learns new social patterns; develops alternative ways to achieve sexual satisfaction	Cohabitation; homosexual or lesbian relationship; masturbation; heterosexual relationship; remarriage	Guilt; anxiety; depression; isolation; avoidance of sex altogether	Elicit sexual history: Are you sexually active? Assess sexual patterns and satisfaction. Values clarification needed. Give patient permission for sexual behavior.
Maintains an interdependent relationship with children	Maintaining control of developing relationships	Continues to meet sexual needs	Lack of privacy in environment; children's reactions; anxiety, jealousy, anger	Assist client in maintaining independence. Some grown children fear exploitation of parents. Some are "will watchers." Recommend premarital legal planning.

Singers (1978) proposed three types of female orgasm: vulval, uterine, and blended. The Singers' hypothesis was partially supported by the work of Perry and Whipple (1981, 1982). They reported a sensitive area felt through the anterior wall of the vagina which they named the Grafenberg spot. Stimulation of this area is reported by research subjects as being the "trigger point" for deeper or uterine orgasms (Perry & Whipple, 1981).

Excitement

Sexual excitement may be triggered by external stimuli (visual, auditory, tactile, and olfactory) or by internal stimuli (fantasy and memory).

Female Response

In women, the first sign of excitement begins with vaginal lubrication resulting from transudation of fluid from engorged vessels through the vaginal wall. The inner two thirds of the vagina lengthen and widen; the walls become dark purple and smooth. The uterus begins to be pulled upward in the lower abdomen. Labia majora become thin and flattened in a nulliparous woman. In a multiparous woman, the labia majora swell with blood and double in size, resulting from increased vascularization occurring with pregnancy. The labia minora swell and become engorged with blood, eventually serving to lengthen the vagina.

The nipples become erect due to involuntary contraction of muscle fibers in the areola. Venous blood trapped in the breasts causes an increase in size. The clitoris enlarges as it fills with blood. This process of tumescence is very similar to penile enlargement, although it occurs more slowly than it does in the penis.

In older women, the clitoris maintains its high degree of sensitivity. The vagina's ability to expand decreases. The walls become thin and smooth; consequently, there is less protection for the bladder and urethra during intercourse, predisposing the aging female to cystitis. Lubrication may be slower in developing or may be diminished, causing *dyspareunia* (painful intercourse). Water-soluble lubricant will help alleviate this symptom.

Male Response

During the excitement phase, the penis becomes tumescent (erect); this process takes from several seconds to several minutes. The scrotum tenses and thickens; at the same time, the testes elevate toward the perineum as the muscles associated with the spermatic cords contract.

In both men (25%) and women (74%), a skin flush causing a maculopapular sex flush due to superficial vasocongestive reaction in skin occurs late in excitement or early in plateau. The blood pressure and heart rate begin to accelerate.

Older men experience a slowing of the sexual response. If an older man is slow to reach erection, he can stimulate his partner and continue to maintain high levels of excitement. Erection takes longer in men over 50 years of age, and full erection may not be attained until orgasm. In both older men and women, vasocongestive and myotonic responses diminish, causing associated color changes to be less apparent.

Plateau

The length of plateau depends on the effectiveness of the stimulation, the age of the person, and the desire to attain orgasm. If there are any negative stimuli perceived by males or females, resolution can occur without orgasm. During plateau, muscular tension, heart rate, and blood pressure increase.

Female Response

The outer third of the vagina becomes distended and shortened. The clitoris retracts under the clitoral hood but maintains a high degree of sensitivity. The Bartholin's glands secrete a small amount of mucoid substance.

In older women, the engorgement of labia and ballooning of the vagina is decreased, but constriction responses assisting in the formation of the orgasmic platform continue.

Male Response

The penis increases in diameter, and the glans may darken. The testes elevate tightly against the perineum and increase in size as a result of vasocongestion. Preejaculatory fluid is secreted from the Cowper's glands.

In both men and women, myotonia increases, resulting in voluntary and involuntary contractions of arms, legs, neck, rectum, and buttocks. Carpopedal spasms of hands and feet may occur. Women may contract pubococcygeal muscles (Kegel exercises) to enhance sexual pleasure and to increase sexual response (Perry & Whipple, 1981). Hartman and Fithian (1984) report that men can do the Kegel exercises to learn to have multiple orgasms.

In older men, testicular elevation and scrotum changes diminish. Ejaculatory control increases; however, if erection is partially lost, there may be difficulty in attaining a full erection again, and resolution may occur without orgasm.

Orgasm

During orgasm, vasocongestion and myotonia reach a peak and are released during involuntary contractions throughout the body. Both male and female orgasms may be described as occurring in stages.

Female Response

Female orgasm begins with intense sexual awareness of the pelvic area with involuntary rhythmic contractions of the orgasmic platform and uterus. Whole body warmth as well as a throbbing sensation in the pelvis are felt.

The female orgasmic response is highly variable from individual to individual, as well as from orgasm to orgasm in the same woman. Recent research has indicated that some women ejaculate. Stimulation of the Grafenberg spot through the anterior wall of the vagina results in a secretion of prostatic-like fluid during orgasm in some women (Addiego et al, 1981; Belzer et al, 1984).

Multiple orgasms occur when sexual tensions do not fall below the plateau phase and stimulation is continued. Status orgasmus occurs when orgasmic levels can be maintained from 20 seconds to a minute.

Male Response

Male orgasmic response is described in two stages. In the first stage, the prostate seminal vesicles and ampullae contract rhythmically, expelling seminal fluid into the prostatic portion of the urethra and causing a feeling of ejaculatory inevitability. In the second stage, semen flows into the distended urethral meatus by a series of rhythmic contractions. The male is aware of urethral contractions, as well as fluid volume.

In both males and females, there are generalized muscular contractions of face, thighs, buttocks, and anal sphincter. Vital signs reach their peak: respiration—40/min; heart rate—110 to 180 beats/min. The systolic blood pressure increases 30 to 100 mm Hg; the diastolic blood pressure rises 20 to 50 mm Hg.

The orgasm decreases in duration in the older man and woman. In women, the number of contractions of both the orgasmic platform and the uterus decrease. In men, a single-stage expulsion of seminal fluid occurs, and ejaculatory emission and force decrease.

Resolution

Resolution is characterized by the release of muscular tension and the return of organs to the unstimulated state. There is a physiologic retreat through plateau and excitement that can take from 10 to 15 minutes. If orgasm has not been achieved, resolution may take about an hour or longer; however, this causes no harm to the individual. Superimposed on the resolution phase for males is a refractory period in which the man cannot attain another erection.

In both the aging man and woman, resolution occurs more rapidly. In the aging man, the mandatory refractory period is lengthened.

Alterations in Health and Effects on Sexuality

Alterations in sexual health occur as a result of the complex interaction between the individual and the environment. A holistic approach requires that biologic, psychological, and environmental variables be evaluated to achieve an accurate assessment of a person's level of sexual health.

Although sexual dysfunctions are usually a result of both organic and psychological problems, sexual dysfunctions may be due to purely organic factors. Biologic variables include anatomic or physiologic disruptions that inhibit any or all of the phases of the sexual response cycle. The desire phase (libido) of sexual response is affected by pain, fatigue, and depression, as well as damage to higher brain centers, specifically the limbic cortex. Any condition that alters the necessary hormonal environment (*i.e.,* blood-level androgens) will influence sexual desire.

Myotonia and vasocongestion may be impaired by disease or trauma that affects the autonomic nervous system and the cardiovascular system. Trauma, surgery, and acute and chronic illness all affect sexual response, either directly or indirectly.

Medications prescribed as part of the therapeutic regimen can affect sexual desire, vasocongestion, and myotonia by interfering with hormonal, neurologic, or circulatory mechanisms.

Some sexual dysfunctions are due to psychological causes. These include both intrapersonal and interpersonal factors. Intrapersonal factors include development, thought content and process, mood and affect, and body image. Interpersonal variables include communication, patterns of sexual expression, physical attraction to the sex partner, and conflicts with the sex partner (values, attitudes and beliefs, sex role, and preference). Problems arising from psychological variables can be precipitated by illness or can occur in healthy people. They affect sexual response by decreasing libido and inhibiting myotonia or vasocongestion, together or separately.

Environmental variables having a negative effect on sexual functioning can arise from life-style changes, life cycle changes, or life events. The hospitalized, institutionalized, or socially isolated person may have difficulty in meeting sexual needs. An older adult living with grown children in an environment shared with grandchildren may have limits placed on healthy sexual expression.

Death of a spouse or divorce may force an older adult to develop new patterns of sexual expression. Failure to adapt may cause a person to repress, avoid, or withdraw from sex altogether.

The combination of physical, psychological, and environmental variables is seen in patients in the health care setting. Therapeutic intervention is based on the identification of problems arising from the interaction of these variables.

Sexual Assessment and Counseling

A sexual assessment is initiated by collecting subjective and objective data. Essential information from health and sexual histories, physical examination, and laboratory findings all make significant contributions to the data base.

Sexual History

The sexual history is a tool that enables the nurse to discuss sexual matters openly and gives the patient permission to express sexual concerns to an informed professional. This information can be obtained in conjunction with the health history after the gynecologic/obstetric or genitourinary history is completed. By incorporating the sexual history into the general health history, the nurse is able to move from areas of lesser sensitivity to areas of greater sensitivity after establishing initial rapport.

The interviewing style should be nonjudgmental. If the patient perceives negative verbal or nonverbal communication, sensitive information is likely to be withheld. Language used during the interview should be appropriate to the person's age and background. Ambiguity should be avoided by not using euphemisms, which are inaccurate and imprecise and will inevitably lead to confusion (*i.e.,* a couple can make love without having intercourse, can have intercourse without sleeping together, and can sleep together without making love). Open-ended questions may be preferable as discussion starters. For example, when interviewing an adolescent, "How did you learn about masturbation?" is more appropriate than "Do you masturbate?"

Patients may experience considerable anxiety, guilt, and embarrassment during the sexual assessment. Therefore, the environment in which the interview takes place is extremely important. Comfort and privacy *without* interruption, as well as verbal and nonverbal assurances of confidentiality, are essential to establishing and maintaining rapport.

The sexual history of the adult can be initiated by the general open-ended question, "Are you sexually active?" If the answer is no, the nurse should explore

- Sexual experiences in the past and why they were discontinued
- Level of satisfaction with the present status

The person may be satisfied with the present status but still may have concerns about sexual attitudes or behaviors of family and friends. An invitation to ask questions about any aspect of sexuality is appropriate at this time. The nurse may provide anticipatory guidance or information related to the patient's developmental stage. Also, information about medications and illnesses and their effects on sexual functioning should be explored.

If the patient is sexually active, and if the setting and situation are appropriate, the nurse may explore the following:

1. Variety and frequency of sexual activity (includes choice of sex partner and degree of sex drive)
2. Current satisfaction with present sexual functioning (which includes sufficient stimulation and lubrication for women, the ability to obtain an erection and control ejaculation in men, and the ability of either party to have a satisfying orgasm without pain)
3. Partner function and satisfaction (which include all aspects of sexual and social compatibility)
4. Marital or relationship history
5. The effects of life events (*i.e.*, rape, death of spouse, aging, medication, illness, contraception) on sexual functioning
6. The need for information about sexual concerns

A more detailed history is required when the patient identifies a problem. This could include information about the following:

1. Early sexual development (*i.e.*, parental, peer, and religious influences on values, attitudes, and beliefs)
2. Adolescent sexual development and experiences (*i.e.*, puberty, masturbation, nocturnal emissions, menstruation, first intercourse, and sexual fantasies)
3. Premarital and postmarital sexual history (*i.e.*, dating, nonmarital sexual relationships, sexual techniques used, frequency of nonmarital sex, and frequency of marital sex and any changes)
4. History of the present problem (*i.e.*, onset, duration, severity, contributing factors, and alleviating factors)

This information should be recorded in the patient's own words.

Sexual history taking becomes a dynamic process in which there is an exchange of information between the person and the nurse. It provides the opportunity to clarify myths and explore areas of concern that the person may not have had permission to discuss in the past.

Physical Assessment

Similarly, the physical assessment affords the nurse an opportunity to provide role modeling and sex education, thus creating a therapeutic milieu.

The physical assessment provides an opportunity for the nurse to teach the woman about breast self-examination (BSE), Kegel exercises, the purpose of Papanicolaou (Pap) screening, effective contraception, and behaviors that reduce the risk of contracting sexually transmitted disease. Men are taught testicular self-examination (TSE), sexually transmitted disease risk reduction, contraception, and breast examination.

The attitude of the practitioner performing the physical assessment is of the utmost importance. Concerned practitioners can make the process of the physical assessment a wholesome, positive experience, taking care to afford comfort and privacy and explaining all procedures with sensitivity.

Persons at risk for sexual problems are those who are unaware of the effects of life cycle changes on sexuality, particularly during adolescence and middle age; those who have communication or behavioral problems; those who experience traumatic life events (*i.e.*, rape, death of a spouse); those who have changes in self-image (*i.e.*, surgery); those who have anatomic or physiologic disruptions (*i.e.*, trauma); those who are taking pharmacologic agents that affect sexuality; and those who have changes in life style (*i.e.*, hospitalized person).

Sexual Counseling

One frequently used sexual counseling method was developed by Annon (1974). He calls it the PLISSIT model. Level one is permission; level two is limited information; level three is specific suggestions; and level four is intensive therapy. Each succeeding level of the model requires increasing degrees of knowledge, training, and skill on the part of the nurse.

1. *Permission* basically involves letting the patient know that it is all right to continue doing what he has been doing. Receiving permission for thoughts, fantasies, sexual behavior, and so on may prevent a person from developing a significant problem and can also relieve guilt. This is primarily preventive intervention.
2. *Limited information* provides information specific to the person's needs. It can be preventive or therapeutic. An example is provision of anticipatory guidance to the adolescent to dispel misinformation and myths regarding sexually transmittable disease. The foregoing could then be reinforced by teaching sexually transmitted disease (STD) risk-reduction behaviors.
3. *Specific suggestions* refers to giving suggestions or a description of a therapeutic technique. For example, the specific suggestion of using a water-soluble lubricant for a postmenopausal woman with atrophic vaginitis is an appropriate nursing intervention.
4. *Intensive therapy* may be indicated as in the case of someone who has behavioral or communication problems resulting in a sexual dysfunction. The nurse can identify referral sources

by contacting the American Association of Sex Educators, Counselors, and Therapists (AASECT), Chicago, for the names of qualified professionals in the area.

Interventions for Specific Health Problems Affecting Sexuality

Changes in Body Image

In understanding the effects of illness on sexuality, one must understand the effects of illness on body image, common coping mechanisms, and the influence of the specific pathologic process on sexual response.

Body image, which is the self-perception of the body, begins in early childhood and continues to evolve throughout the life span. It is interwoven with sexual identity, sexual role, and patterns of sexual functioning.

In our society, we see idealized standards of the perfect body and face for men and women. A high value is placed on physical appearance. Conflict arises when self-image does not conform with idealized image. When there is a loss, perceived loss, or disfigurement of body structure or function, self-perception, environmental interaction, and interpersonal relationships may change.

Moving from levels of health to illness can threaten a person's sense of self, causing lowered self-esteem, a negative self-image, and insecurity. The result can be disturbances of mood and affect. Depression is commonly seen in people with alterations in body image and is recognized as part of the grieving process. Dependency occurring as an adjustment to the sick role can be accompanied by feelings of powerlessness and loss of control, influencing sexual interactions. Prolonged denial or guilt can prevent a person from revising his self-image to a more positive one.

Performance anxiety occurs when a person perceives the body change as having a negative impact on sexual role, identity, or functioning. Traditional male and female stereotyped roles may be incompatible with altered body structure or function. Traditional patterns of sexual functioning may no longer be possible. Myths, misinformation, and negative attitudes and values can inhibit a person from finding new ways of sexual expression, a change often required for those with altered body structure or function.

The severity of the reaction to altered body image is also influenced by the visibility of the affected part, the meaning of symbolism attached to it, and the person's perception of the way others view the change. Usually, the more visible the part, the more severe the emotional reactions. If the body part is strongly correlated with sexual identity, such as the breast and uterus, the impact on self-image may be profound. A person who perceives the sexual partner as reacting to the altered body image with disgust may fear rejection. The result may be avoidance of sex, withdrawal, and self-imposed isolation.

The relationship between sexual partners is a most important factor in sexual functioning after illness. In a sexual relationship, an unexplained decrease in sexual activity due to illness, lack of communication, or negative body image usually results in conflict, frustration, and irritability. The sexual partner may withdraw affection for fear that sexual intercourse may harm the patient. Anger and hostility can occur if this is not communicated.

Assessment of patients with body image changes includes evaluating the effects on self-concept and self-esteem; the impact on sex role, sexual identity, sexual functioning, and sexual relationships; and the person's coping mechanisms.

General goals of intervention include allowing the patient to ventilate negative feelings, clarifying misinformation and myths with the patient and spouse separately and together, encouraging recognition of sexual attributes and capabilities, and widening sexual repertoire through permission and education.

Several disorders that may alter sexuality are described below.

Myocardial Infarction

Although men and women can experience a myocardial infarction (MI), most of the research with MIs has been performed on men; thus, our discussion will refer to the male patient. The person who has had an MI is at risk for sexual dysfunction because of perceived body image changes. Fear of sudden death, fear of impotence, feelings of emasculation, increased dependency on the sick role, and decreased general activity may prevent a patient from returning to pre-infarction levels of sexual functioning.

The actual incidence of sudden death during intercourse post-MI is very low, although it is slightly higher with an unfamiliar partner in a stressful environment (*e.g.*, extramarital affair). The body's energy expenditure during intercourse is equated to that required to walk up two flights of stairs. Depending on the extent of cardiac damage, most post-MI patients can resume their normal level of sexual activity after exercise tolerance is assessed and results are evaluated—usually in 8 to 12 weeks.

Assessment factors include the usual or preferred type, time, and frequency of sexual activity; alcohol and food consumption associated with sexual activity; previous occurrences of angina; previous symptoms of fatigue; sleeplessness associated with sexual activity; and prescribed and over-the-counter medications.

Sexual counseling as a part of cardiac rehabilitation has a significant impact on the frequency and quality of subsequent sexual functioning. After the fear of death has passed, a patient may act out sexually toward the nurse. This situation can be used as an opportunity to begin sexual education and counseling. Permission begins by acknowledging the behavior as normal.

Counseling the patient and his sexual partner may be necessary to clarify myths and misinformation. Information about the normal sexual response cycle, extent of cardiac damage, and effects on sexual behaviors is included in the teaching plan.

The environment in which intercourse is initiated should be familiar, avoiding extremes of temperature. Alcoholic beverages should not be consumed for at least 3 hours before intercourse, because alcohol increases the heart rate and dilates blood vessels.

If angina is a concern, a nitroglycerin tablet may be taken

before sexual activity is begun. The patient and partner can be encouraged to begin with less strenuous forms of sexual activity.

The patient can be informed of self-assessment factors or warning signs to stop intercourse until a physician is consulted. These include angina during or after intercourse, prolonged palpitations 15 minutes after intercourse, sleeplessness or fatigue the following day, and elevated heart rate and respirations that continue 20 minutes after intercourse.

Medications that may be prescribed for the cardiac patient include antihypertensives, antidepressants, tranquilizers, and hypnotics. These may cause a decrease in sex drive or libido and impair vasocongestion and myotonia. The patient should be informed of these side effects (Table 17–2).

The patient who experiences sexual dysfunction after an MI (erectile dysfunction, premature ejaculation, orgasmic dysfunction) should be referred for further evaluation. Sexual dysfunction may be a result of impaired vasocongestion due to cardiovascular assault, prescribed medications, anxiety, depression, fear of failure, or fatigue.

Mastectomy

To many women, breasts are a symbol of femininity and are equated with sexual attractiveness and desirability. The reality of cancer, fear of death, change in body image, and fear of

TABLE 17–2. *Commonly Prescribed Medications That Have Adverse Effects on Sexual Response*

Drug	Probable Mechanism of Action	Possible Adverse Effects on Sexual Response
ANTIDEPRESSANTS		
Amitripyline (Elavil)	Central depression; peripheral blockade of nervous innervation of sex glands	
Desipramine (Norpramin, Pertofrane)		
Imipramine (Tofranil)		
Nortriptyline (Aventyl)		
Pargyline (Eutonyl)		
Phenelzine sulfate (Nardil)		
Protriptyline (Vivactil)		
Tranylcypromine sulfate (Parnate)		
ANTIHISTAMINES		
Chlorpheniramine maleate (Chlor-Trimeton)	Blockade of parasympathetic nervous innervation of sex glands	Depress libido and decrease vaginal lubrication
Diphenhydramine (Benadryl)		
Promethazine (Phenergan)		
ANTIHYPERTENSIVES		
Clonidine (Catapres)	Centrally acting anti-adrenergic; peripherally acting anti-adrenergic	May cause impotence, erectile dysfunction; orgasmic dysfunction in both men and women
Guanethidine (Ismelin)		
Methyldopa (Aldomet)		
Propranolol (Inderal)		
ANTISPASMODICS		
Glycopyrrolate (Robinul)	Ganglionic blockage of nervous innervation of sex glands	May cause erectile and vaginal lubrication problems
Hexocyclium methylsulfate (Tral)		
Methantheline bromide (Banthine)		
Poldine (Nacton)		
SEDATIVES AND TRANQUILIZERS		
Benperidol	Central sedation; blockage of autonomic innervation of sex glands; suppression of hypothalamic and pituitary function; tranquilization and relaxation	May cause loss of libido
Chlordiazepoxide (Librium)		
Chlorpromazine (Thorazine)		
Chlorprothixene (Taractan)		
Diazepam (Valium)		
Mesoridazine (Serentil)		
Methaqualone (Quaalude)		
Phenoxybenzamine (Dibenzyline)		

(continued)

TABLE 17-2. *(Continued)*

Drug	Probable Mechanism of Action	Possible Adverse Effects on Sexual Response
SEDATIVES AND TRANQUILIZERS Prochlorperazine (Compazine) Thioridazine (Mellaril)		
ETHYL ALCOHOL	Central depression; suppression of motor activity, diuresis; release of inhibitions; relaxation	
BARBITURATES	Central depression; suppression of motor activity; hypnosis	
NARCOTICS AND PSYCHOACTIVE DRUGS Amphetamines Cocaine	Central depression	Decreased libido; impaired potency
SEX-HORMONE PREPARATIONS Cyproterone acetate Methandrostenolone (Dianabol) Nandrolone phenproprionate (Durabolin) Norethandrolone (Nilevar)	Antiandrogenic effects on sexual function	Loss of libido; decreased potency Decreased erectile ability

(Adapted from Woods JS. Drug effects on human sexual behavior. In Woods NF. Human Sexuality in Health and Illness, 3rd ed. St Louis, CV Mosby, 1984; and Whipple B. Drugs that affect sexual functioning. In Francoeur RT. Becoming a Sexual Person. New York, John Wiley & Sons, 1982.)

rejection create multiple adjustment problems for a woman undergoing a mastectomy. Denial, depression, and anger are experienced as part of the grieving process. Guilt may also be experienced if the woman views the mastectomy as punishment for sexual activity that she believes is excessive or inappropriate, such as engaging in an extramarital affair. The partner may also experience guilt if he believes that he may have caused damage to the breast during sexual activity. The quality of the relationship before the mastectomy influences the subsequent postoperative relationship.

Supportive sexual counseling and enhancement of communication between partners during hospitalization can have a positive effect on postoperative sexual functioning.

Misinformation and myths can be clarified in preoperative counseling. The nurse validates that the woman's concerns are normal and reassures the patient that the mastectomy will not affect the capacity for sexual responsiveness. Assessment factors include the sexual relationship, the perceived effect of body image change on sex role and identity, the importance of the breast in sexual arousal during sexplay, the identification of support systems, the ability of the woman to express her sexual needs and concerns, and the sexual history. Using a person-centered approach, the nurse should identify whether the partner should be included in the initial assessment. If not, counseling the partner separately is recommended.

In the immediate postoperative period, the partner may be present, providing additional support and actively involved in postoperative care to prevent delaying confrontation or prolonged denial. Communication, touching, holding, and caressing should be encouraged early in the postoperative period.

The woman and her partner may fear wound disruption.

They should be informed that with proper positioning, intercourse usually can be resumed 1 week after discharge. Male superior and side-by-side positions are usually more comfortable. The use of a prosthesis during sexual activity is discouraged, to increase comfort and enhance self-acceptance.

Positive role modeling and additional support can be obtained by referral to Reach to Recovery. It may also dispel the myth that the surgery is unique.

A woman who does not have a partner may feel sexually unattractive and experience low self-esteem similar to that experienced by the married woman. She may lack the additional support system available to the married woman, however. It is especially important that this woman move through the stages of denial and establish a positive self-image early in rehabilitation to avoid feelings of abandonment when she goes home.

Specific suggestions to enhance positive body image include looking in the mirror nude and having the partner see the surgical site while the patient is still in the hospital. This helps to desensitize reactions and feelings about altered body image and can be explored by the couple alone or with the nurse.

Sensate focus or pleasuring exercises can enhance the establishment of a positive body image. Water play with a shower massage is a nonthreatening, self-pleasuring exercise that can increase sensory discrimination. Touching is also an important part of sensate focus.

Asking the client to draw a picture of herself may assist her in venting feelings of altered body image. The nurse can then provide feedback and stress positive aspects of body and sexual functioning.

Breast self-examination should be taught to the mastectomy patient. Because there is a three times greater chance of developing cancer in the other breast, early detection can decrease the risk of mortality.

Spinal Cord Injuries

Adolescents and young adults are frequently the victims of spinal cord injuries and represent a challenge to the delivery of comprehensive health care. The majority of these patients are male. The injury and consequential changes in self-esteem, self-image, sexual functioning, and interpersonal relationships pose a serious threat to a person's physical and psychological well-being. Sexual rehabilitation begins when the threat of death is no longer perceived by the person during hospitalization. It is essential that persons with spinal cord injuries receive information about sexual functioning before going home.

The two variables in planning sexual rehabilitation include the level of the injury and the number of fibers severed (complete or incomplete lesion). Patients with upper motor neuron lesions usually exhibit increased spasticity, hyperreflexia, and reflexogenic erections. Those with lower motor neuron lesions exhibit flaccidity and hyporeflexia. Psychogenic erections are possible, but are seen less frequently.

Reflexogenic erections can be stimulated by genital manipulation or a full bladder and occur during rapid eye movement sleep in healthy males. The stimulus is transmitted from the penis to the sacral area of the spinal cord by way of the autonomic nervous system to the pelvis. Women experience reflexogenic vaginal lubrication and pelvic engorgement from the stimulation of the perineal area.

Psychogenic erections are initiated in the higher brain centers and travel by way of thoracolumbar sympathetic nerves to the genitalia. Psychogenic erections are more common in lower motor neuron lesions because impulses pass down and leave the cord above the level of the injury. The reflex arc is interrupted, and reflexogenic erections are improbable with complete lower motor neuron lesions. The effects on sexual

response in complete spinal cord lesions are outlined in Table 17–3. It is essential that the patient have realistic expectations about the ability to meet his sexual needs.

The following assessment factors provided by Comarr and Gunderson (1975) can be used in distinguishing complete or incomplete upper motor neuron lesions from complete or incomplete lower motor neuron lesions after spinal shock subsides:

- *Complete upper motor neuron lesion:* No sensation or voluntary control of external rectal sphincter; evidence of external rectal sphincter tone and a positive bulbocavernosus reflex
- *Incomplete upper motor neuron lesion:* Positive light touch sensation of partially diminished responses to pinprick; the loss of voluntary control of external rectal sphincter; external rectal sphincter tone and a positive bulbocavernosus reflex
- *Complete lower motor neuron lesion:* No sensation or voluntary control or tone of the external rectal sphincter and no bulbocavernosus reflex
- *Incomplete lower motor neuron lesion:* Partial sensation; no voluntary control of external rectal sphincter; no sphincter tone or bulbocavernosus reflex

Persons who have incomplete lesions will experience less neurologic deficit and have a greater chance of successful coitus. Individual differences must be considered and should influence the approach to sexual rehabilitation.

A person with a spinal cord injury may be troubled by many myths regarding sexuality and sexual functioning after the injury. Counseling begins with validating concerns as normal and giving information to dispel myths and misinformation. Cultural, religious, and social taboos associated with anal intercourse or oral sex should be discussed. Counseling couples is recommended; if the patient objects, the partner can be counseled separately.

Several principles related to sexual response in spinal cord injuries should be incorporated into the teaching plan. Sexual

TABLE 17–3. *The Effects of Complete Spinal Cord Lesions on Sexual Response*

Phase of Sexual Response	C1–T12 Lesions	T12–S4 Lesions
Excitement (psychogenic)	No psychogenic erection	Psychogenic erection
	No vaginal lubrication	Vaginal lubrication
	Other manifestation activated by fibers above the lesion; change in BP, respirations pulse	Visual, auditory, olfactory, stimuli; dreams, memory, fantasy
	Breast changes, sex flush	
Plateau (reflexogenic)	Reflexogenic erection caused by stroking penis, catheter change, full bladder	No reflex response
	Reflexogenic vaginal lubication and pelvic engorgement with perineal stimulation.	Reflexes are interrupted
Orgasm	Ejaculation: rare	Ejaculation and orgasm occur more frequently
	Orgasms can occur as purely cerebral events	Ejaculatory force varies

(Adapted from Geiger RC. Neurophysiology of sexual response in spinal cord injury. In Bullard D and Knight V. Sexuality and Physical Disability. St Louis, CV Mosby, 1981.)

excitement occurring from thoughts, fantasies, or tactile stimulation in areas above the level of the lesion does not result in any genital response, and, conversely, reflexogenic genital responses occur without cognitive awareness.

Even though erections are more frequent in complete upper motor lesions, they may not produce sexual satisfaction. Orgasm, however, may occur as a purely cerebral event without either genital stimulation or manifestation of physical components of the human sexual response. Imagery, autosuggestion, and erotic visual or audio material can enhance the possibility of achieving an orgasm, which may be similar or different from a genital stimulation-produced orgasm.

Areas available for tactile stimulation are dependent on the level of the injury. Frequently, areas such as the neck, ears, and breasts, which may previously have been insensitive, become highly sensitive with increased stimulation. Areas of tactile hypersensitivity at the level of the lesion can induce profound sexual pleasure for the person with a spinal cord injury.

Infertility in the male is a common sequela to spinal cord injuries. Fertility in the female is usually not affected. The sensory level of the uterus is at T6, and if the injury is at that level, sensation of labor will be absent. More research concerning the sexual response of women with spinal cord injuries is needed.

Problems in meeting sexual needs can arise from the absence of a partner, from an inability to engage in traditional sexual patterns, from sexual inexperience before the injury, and from the perception of oneself as asexual.

Sexual assertiveness training can help alleviate some of these problems. Confidence and skillful communication are essential in establishing a new sexual relationship or altering a familiar one.

A person with a spinal cord injury can be encouraged to widen his sexual repertoire with new patterns of sexual functioning. Areas of hypersensitivity may be discovered through different approaches to stimulation. Enhanced communication will assist in expressing what feels good.

An indwelling catheter can be taped in place and left in during intercourse. Spasticity in clients can be reduced by administering antispasmodics before sexual activity, even though there may be a resultant decrease in sensation.

Excellent audiovisual materials are available that help people with spinal cord injuries realize that they are not alone and that there are many pleasurable activities available to them.

No matter what level of ability, patients are capable of expressing their sexuality and with education and training are able to achieve high levels of sexual satisfaction. Sexual rehabilitation depends on self-confidence, a willing sex partner, and a sensitive, knowledgeable health care team.

Diabetes Mellitus

Diabetes mellitus is a common health problem that has been related to disturbances in sexual function. One of the problems determining the cause of sexual dysfunctions is differentiating between an organic origin and a psychological cause. Many people who are diabetic have heard that they will have a problem with impotence or orgasm and thus these problems may be a self-fulfilling prophecy and not related to an organic cause. Other psychogenic factors may include adaptation to a chronic illness, dependency, depression, and low self-esteem, leading to performance anxiety.

The cause of sexual dysfunctions in people with diabetes mellitus is complex and uncertain; contributing factors include diabetic neuropathy, microangiopathies, a disruption of biochemical or hormonal balance, and psychogenic factors. Men may experience impotence and retrograde ejaculation (see Chapter 39 for further discussion). Women may experience orgasmic dysfunction, problems with vaginal lubrication, and dyspareunia. Dyspareunia in female diabetics is often a result of vaginitis, commonly caused by *Candida albicans*.

With advanced knowledge about diabetes, including improved glucose control and early detection and treatment of long-term complications, it is hoped that the incidence of sexual dysfunctions will be reduced.

Fertility problems seen in diabetic men are usually caused by retrograde ejaculation, ejaculatory dysfunction, and decreased sperm count and volume. Although usually not infertile, women with diabetes that is not well controlled have a higher number of stillborns, spontaneous abortions, and infants with high birth weight.

Assessment factors include sexual history, marital history, detailed physical assessment, present coping mechanisms, and laboratory tests to determine if there is a fertility or diabetes control problem.

Counseling begins with the sexual history. At this time, myths and misinformation should be dispelled and guilt alleviated if it is present, as is frequently the case. For those who are married, conjugal counseling is recommended. Information about genetic transmission of diabetes mellitus and its impact on fertility and sexual functioning may be discussed. Techniques to overcome intromission difficulties and to enhance stimulation may be explored if the couple is receptive.

For women with dyspareunia, a water-soluble lubricant can be suggested. In addition, any existing candidal infection should be treated. If poor control of diabetes is evident, the nurse can provide diabetic teaching. Referral to a physician may be indicated for changes in medical management of the disease.

The diabetic patient who experiences sexual dysfunction related to psychogenic or organic factors and who identifies the need for assistance with the problem may be referred for sexual therapy.

Hypertension

Hypertension alone has no documented negative effect on sexual response, and no restrictions on sexual activity are necessary.

Noncompliance with the therapeutic regimen seen in those who are hypersensitive is frequently attributed to drug-induced sexual dysfunction. Antihypertensive agents produce vasodilation and decreased cardiac output by acting on the sympathetic nervous system either peripherally or centrally. The effects on sexual response include decreased libido, erectile difficulty, retrograde ejaculation, and reduced orgasmic intensity. Several antihypertensives block ovulation and suppress menstruation, causing infertility in females.

A detailed sexual history and physical assessment are necessary to determine if the sexual dysfunction is due to the antihypertensive medication, other medication, other organic cause (*e.g.*, diabetes), or psychological factors. If the onset is related specifically to an increase in dosage or change of medication with no apparent psychogenic cause or organic pathology, the dysfunction is likely to be due to medication (Table 17–2).

A person experiencing sexual dysfunction as a result of antihypertensives should be counseled that the problem is reversible and that alternative medications are available. It is necessary to point out that adverse reactions concerning sexual response are highly individual.

Stress management techniques, such as deep relaxation, yoga, cardiovascular exercise, and compliance with the therapeutic diet, may decrease the necessity of high doses of antihypertensives and can enhance sexual response.

Sexually Transmitted Diseases

Although sexually transmitted diseases (STDs) are covered elsewhere (see Chaps. 45 and 62), it is important to emphasize that when caring for people with STDs, the nurse must be nonjudgmental in all phases of the nursing process. Not all nurses may feel comfortable caring for patients who have STDs or the symptoms of acquired immunodeficiency syndrome (AIDS) or whose behaviors are those that may challenge their biases or prejudices. Again, the nurse must deal with her own feelings and attitudes before dealing with the patient's feelings and behaviors. It is difficult to teach safer sex practices to a person with whom you are uncomfortable.

It is also important to emphasize that STDs including AIDS affect people of all ages, from newborn infants to people in their 80s and 90s. Older adults who are HIV-infected experience the same risks as people from other age groups (Scura & Whipple, 1990).

Sexual Dysfunction

Sexual response is controlled by the automatic nervous system with sympathetic and parasympathetic subsystems. Under stress and anxiety, the sympathetic system overpowers the parasympathetic system, making the relaxation required for sexual response impossible. Vasocongestion and myotonia may be inhibited together or separately. This type of dysfunction results in unsatisfactory sexual responses.

Masters and Johnson (1966) estimated that 50% of all couples may require some assistance with sexual dysfunctions. The cause is complex. Chart 17–1 summarizes some of the psychological causes of sexual dysfunction. It is important to keep in mind that there are both psychological and organic causes of sexual dysfunctions.

Sexual dysfunctions are categorized as primary or secondary. An individual who has never experienced a satisfactory response suffers from a *primary dysfunction. Secondary sexual dysfunction* occurs when a satisfactory sexual response was achieved at least once in the past. The onset of the dysfunction may be related to a specific time, event, or person.

There are a variety of individual responses within each dysfunction. They can be viewed on a continuum, depending on the frequency and severity of the inadequate response.

Male Sexual Dysfunctions

Erectile dysfunction occurs when the vasocongestion aspects of the sexual response are impaired. Varying responses include

---

Chart 17–1
Psychological Causes of Sexual Dysfunction

Predisposing Factors

Restrictive upbringing
Disturbed family relationships
Inadequate sexual information
Traumatic early sexual experiences
Early insecurity in psychosexual role

Precipitants

Childbirth
Discord in the general relationship
Infidelity
Unreasonable expectations
Dysfunction in the partner
Random failure
Reaction to organic factors
Aging
Depression and anxiety
Traumatic sexual experience

Maintaining Factors

Performance anxiety
Anticipation of failure
Guilt
Loss of attraction between partners
Poor communication between partners
Discord in the general relationship
Fear of intimacy
Impaired self-image
Inadequate sexual information; sexual myths
Restricted foreplay
Psychiatric disorder

(Hawton K. Sex Therapy: A Practical Guide. New York, Oxford University Press, 1985.)

the complete inability to attain an erection, a partial erection, or a firm extravaginal erection. The presence of a reflexogenic erection rules out organic cause.

Premature ejaculation occurs when a man is unable to voluntarily control the ejaculatory reflex and, once aroused, reaches orgasm before or shortly after intromission. It is the most common dysfunction in men.

Retarded ejaculation is the involuntary inhibition of the ejaculatory reflex. The varying responses include occasional ejaculation through intercourse or self-stimulation, or the complete inability to ejaculate under any circumstances.

Female Sexual Dysfunction

Orgasmic dysfunction occurs when involuntary control of the orgasmic reflex leads to the inability to achieve orgasm (similar to retarded ejaculation in men). Varying responses range from the complete inability to achieve orgasm under any circumstance to the ability to achieve orgasm only by either self-stimulation or stimulation by their partners.

Inhibited Sexual Desire

Inhibited sexual desire is persistent and pervasive inhibition of sexual desire. The inhibition may be selective; some people experience erection or lubrication and orgasm, but derive little pleasure from the physical feelings. Others have a desire that is at such a low ebb that they have no interest in self-stimulation or in participating in sexual interaction with another person. People with desire disorders tend to experience sexually related anxiety and, in some cases, considerable hostility toward their partners.

The nurse who identifies a person who is at risk for sexual dysfunction can use the PLISSIT model with the nursing process and identify the level of intervention that is needed. Education and counseling to dispel misinformation and to give permission, limited information, or specific suggestions may be all that is needed. If intensive therapy is needed, referral should be made to a certified sex therapist.

Sex therapists use a variety of techniques to help people have more satisfying sexual experiences. These include systematic desensitization, nondemand pleasuring, sensate focus, masturbation training, and other specific techniques, in addition to psychotherapy.

Follow-up on the success of the intervention will evaluate the person's satisfaction with the counselor or therapist, alleviation of the dysfunction, and enhancement of the sexual relationship.

Chapter Summary

In summary, sexuality has been acknowledged as a basic human need; however, it is a need that has not been fully addressed in nursing education or in the implementation of nursing care. Being informed about human sexuality and feeling comfortable talking about sexual concerns to patients are important for all nurses. Nurses who recognize that all individuals, no matter what their age or where they are on the health–illness continuum, are sexual beings with sexual needs will be better able to educate and counsel patients about sexual concerns.

Bibliography

Books

Allgeier AR and Allgeier ER. Sexual Interactions. Lexington, MA, DC Heath, 1988.

Annon JS. Behavioral Treatment of Sexual Problems. Vol I. Brief Therapy. Honolulu, Enabling Systems, Inc., 1974.

Bancroft J. Human Sexuality and Its Problems. New York, Churchill Livingstone, 1983.

Barbach L. For Each Other. New York, Doubleday, 1982.

Erikson EH. Childhood and Society, 2nd ed. New York, WW Norton, 1963.

Farber M. Human Sexuality: Psychosexual Effects of Disease. New York, Macmillan, 1985.

Francoeur RT. Becoming a Sexual Person. New York, Macmillan, 1991.

Guyton AC. Textbook of Medical Physiology. Philadelphia, WB Saunders, 1986.

Green R. Human Sexuality: A Health Practitioner's Text, 2nd ed. Baltimore, Williams & Wilkins, 1979.

Hartman W and Fithian M. Any Man Can. New York, St Martin Press, 1984.

Hawton K. Sex Therapy: A Practical Guide. New York, Oxford University Press, 1985.

Hogan R. Human Sexuality: A Nursing Perspective. New York, Appleton–Century-Crofts, 1985.

Johnson WR and Kempton W. Sex Education and Counseling of Special Groups. Springfield, IL, Charles C Thomas, 1981.

Kaplan HS. Disorders of Sexual Desire. New York, Simon & Schuster, 1979.

Kaplan HS. The New Sex Therapy. New York, Brunner–Mazel, 1974.

Kerfoot KM and Buckwalter KC. Sexual counseling. In Bulecheck GM and McCloskey JC (eds). Nursing interventions: Treatments for Nursing Diagnoses. Philadelphia, WB Saunders, 1985.

Kinsey AC et al. Sexual Behavior in the Human Male. Philadelphia, WB Saunders, 1948.

Kinsey AC et al. Sexual Behavior in the Human Female. Philadelphia, WB Saunders, 1953.

Ladas AK et al. The G Spot and Other Recent Discoveries About Human Sexuality. New York, Dell, 1983.

Masters W and Johnson V. Human Response. Boston, Little, Brown, 1966.

Money J and Ehrhardt A. Man, Woman, Boy and Girl. Baltimore, Johns Hopkins University Press 1972.

Perry JD and Whipple B. Multiple components of the female orgasm. In Graber B (ed). Circumvaginal Musculature and Sexual Function. New York, S Karger, 1982.

Simons RC. Understanding Human Behavior in Health and Illness, 3rd ed. Baltimore, Williams & Wilkins, 1985.

Singer J and Singer I. Types of female orgasm. In LoPiccolo J and LoPiccolo L (eds). Handbook of Sex Therapy. New York, Plenum, 1978.

Smith PB and Mumforf DM. Adolescent Reproductive Health: A Handbook for the Health Professionals. New York, Gardner Press, 1985.

Tallmer M (ed). Sexuality and Life-Threatening Illness. Springfield, IL, Charles C Thomas, 1984

Webb C. Sexuality, Nursing and Health. New York, John Wiley & Sons, 1985.

Weg RB (ed). Sexuality in Later Years. New York, Academic Press, 1983.

Weinstein E and Rosen E. Sexual Counseling. Pacific Grove, Brooks/Cole, 1988.

Whipple B. Female sexuality. In Leyson J (ed). Sexual Rehabilitation of the Spinal Cord Injured Patient. Clifton, NJ, Humana Press, 1990.

Whipple B and Ogden G. Safe Encounters: How Women Can Say Yes to Pleasure and No to Unsafe Sex. New York, McGraw–Hill, 1989.

Woods N. Human Sexuality in Health and Illness, 3rd ed. St Louis, CV Mosby, 1984.

Zilbergeld B and Ellison CR. Desire discrepancies and arousal problems in sex therapy. In Leiblum SR and Pervin LA (eds). Principles and Practice of Sex Therapy. New York, Guilford Press, 1980.

Journals

Asterisks indicates nursing research articles.

Adolescence and Sex

Alexander E. Counseling teenagers about sex. Medical Aspects of Human Sexuality 1989 Aug; 23(8): 26–36.

Brooks B. Sexually abused children and adolescent identity development. Am J Psychother 1985 Jul; 39(3):401–410.

Eisen M and Zellman GL. The role of health belief attitudes, sex education, and demographics in predicting adolescents' sexual knowledge. Health Educ Q 1986 Spring; 13(1):9–22.

Furstenberg FF Jr et al. Sex education and sexual experience among adolescents. Am J Public Health 1985 Nov; 75(11):1331–1332.

Howe CL. Developmental theory and adolescent sexual behavior. Nurse Pract 1986 Feb; 11(2):65, 68, 71.

Pestrak VA and Martin D. Cognitive development and aspects of adolescent sexuality. Adolescence 1985 Winter; 20(8):981–987.

Pietropinto A and Arora A. Medical problems in adolescence: Effects on sexual adjustment. Medical Aspects of Human Sexuality 1988 Jul; 22(7): 108–109.

Smith EA et al. Pubertal development and friends: A biosocial explanation of adolescent sexual behavior. J Health Soc Behav 1985 Sep; 26(3): 183–192.

Aging and Sexuality

Hobson KG. The effects of aging on sexuality. Health Soc Work 1984 Winter; 9(1):25–35.

McCracken AL. Sexual practice by elders: The forgotten aspect of functional health. Gerontol Nurs 1988 Oct; 14(10): 13–25.

Steinke EE and Bergen MB. Sexuality and aging. J Gerontol Nurs 1986 Jun; 12(6):6–10.

Walbroehl GS. Effect of medical problems on sexuality in the elderly. Medical Aspects of Human Sexuality 1988 Oct; 22(10):56–66.

Whipple B and Scura KW. HIV and the Older Adult: Taking the Necessary Precautions. Gerontol Nurs 1989 Sep; 15(9): 15–19.

Assessment

Conte HR. Multivariate assessment of sexual dysfunction. J Consult Clin Psychol 1986 Apr; 54(2): 149–157.

Hammond DC. Screening for sexual dysfunction. Clin Obstet Gynecol 1984 Sep; 27(3):732–737.

Hoon PW. Physiologic assessment of sexual response in women: The unfulfilled promise. Clin Obstet Gynecol 1984 Sep; 27(3):767–780.

Stoudemire A et al. Sexual assessment of the urologic oncology patient. Psychosomatics 1985 May; 26(5):405–408,410.

Waterhouse J and Metcalfe MC. Development of the sexual adjustment questionnaire. Oncol Nurs Forum 1986 May/Jun; 13(3):53–59.

Watters WW et al. An assessment approach to couples with sexual problems. Can J Psychiatry 1985 Feb; 30(1):2–11.

* White EJ. Appraising the need for altered sexuality information. Rehabil Nurs 1986 May/Jun; 11(3):6–9.

Cancer and Sexuality

Anderson BL et al. Sexual dysfunction and signs of gynecologic cancer. Cancer 1986 May 1; 57(9):1880–1886.

Kriss RT and Kramer HC. Efficacy of group therapy for problems with postmastectomy self-perception, body image, and sexuality. J Sex Res 1986 Nov; 22(4):438–451.

MacElveen-Hoehn P and McCorkle R. Understanding sexuality in progressive cancer. Semin Oncol Nurs 1985 Feb; 1(1):56–62.

Schain WS. Breast cancer surgeries and psychosexual sequelae: Implications for remediation. Semin Oncol Nurs 1985 Aug; 1(3):200–205.

Schwartz-Appelbaum J et al. Nursing care plans: Sexuality and treatment of breast cancer. Oncol Nurs Forum 1984 Nov/Dec; 11(6):16–24.

Walbroehl GS. Sexuality in cancer patients. Am Fam Physician 1985 Jan; 31(1): 153–158.

Wellisch DK. The psychologic impact of breast cancer on relationships. Semin Oncol Nurs 1985 Aug; 1(3):195–199.

Whipple B. Sexual counseling of couples after a mastectomy or myocardial infarction. Nurs Forum 1987/88; 23(3): 85–90.

Yarbro CH et al (eds). Sexuality and cancer. Semin Oncol Nurs 1985 Feb; 1(1):1–75.

Diabetes

Berstein G. Counseling the male diabetic patient with erectile dysfunction. Medical Aspects of Human Sexuality 1989 Apr; Special issue: 20–23.

Bhen-Auger N et al. Sexual response of the type I diabetic woman. Medical Aspects of Human Sexuality 1988 Oct; 22(10): 94–100.

Hollander P. The need to address sexual dysfunction in diabetes. Postgrad Med 1986 Apr; 79(5):15–16, 18.

House WC and Pendleton L. Sexual dysfunction in diabetes. Postgrad Med 1986 Apr; 79(5):227–235.

Jensen SB. Sexual dysfunction in insulin-treated diabetics: A six-year follow-up study of 101 patients. Arch Sex Behav 1986 Aug; 15(4):271–283.

Dysfunction

Avery-Clark C. Sexual dysfunction and disorder patterns of working and nonworking wives. J Sex Marital Ther 1986 Summer; 12(2):93–107.

Barlow DH. Causes of sexual dysfunction: The role of anxiety and cognitive interference. J Consult Psychol 1986 Apr; 54(2):140–148.

Berstein J et al. Assessment of psychological dysfunction associated with infertility. Journal of Obstetrical and Gynecological Nursing 1985 Nov/Dec; 14 (suppl 6): 63s–66s.

Hesford A. Sexual dysfunction in women. Nurs Times 1986 Apr 2–8; 82(14): 49–51.

LoPiccolo J and Stock WE. Treatment of sexual dysfunction. J Consul Clin Psychol 1986 Apr; 54(2): 158–167.

Newton W and Keith LG. Role of sexual behavior in the development of pelvic inflammatory disease. J Reprod Med 1985 Feb; 30(2): 82–88.

Pariser SF et al. Clinical sexuality. Reprod Med 1983; 3: 1–222.

Human Sexuality

*Addiego F et al. Female ejaculation: A case study. J Sex Res 1981 Feb; 17: 13–21.

*Belzer EG et al. On female ejaculation. J Sex Res 1984 Nov; 20(4): 403–406.

Bem S. The measurement of psychological androgyny. J Consult Clin Psychol 1974 Apr; 42(4): 155–162.

Chinn PL (ed). Sexuality and sex roles. ANS 1985 Apr; 7(3): 1–86.

Comarr A and Gunderson B. Sexual function in traumatic paraplegia and quadriplegia. Am J Nurs 1975 Feb; 75(2): 250–255.

Greener D and Reagan P. Sexuality: Knowledge and attitudes of student nurse-midwives. J Nurse Midwife 1986 Jan/Feb; 31(1): 30–37.

Hahn K. Sexuality and COPD. Rehabil Nurs 1989. Jul/Aug; 14(4): 191–195.

Leiblum S and Rosen R. Guidelines for taking a sexual history. Unpublished paper presented at course on human sexuality. Department of Psychiatry, CMDNJ, Rutgers Medical School, New Jersey, Jan 1980.

Perry JD and Whipple B. Pelvic muscle strength of female ejaculators: Evidence in support of a new theory of orgasm. J Sex Res 1981 Feb; 17(1): 22–39.

Rosenbaum J and Monaghan ML. A sexuality workshop: Increasing sexual self-awareness. Can J Psychiatr Nurs 1986 Apr; 27(2): 8–10.

Weisberg M. Physiology of female sexual function. Clin Obstet Gynecol 1984 Sep; 27(3): 697–705.

Whipple B. Sexuality education in a nursing curriculum: The whys and hows. Imprint 1989 Nov; 36(4): 55–56.

Whipple B and Gick R. A holistic view of sexuality: Education for the health professional. Topics Clin Nurs 1980 Jan; 1(4): 91–98.

Myocardial Infarction and Hypertension

* Baggs JG and Karch AM. Sexual counseling of women with coronary heart disease. Heart Lung 1987 Mar; 16(2): 154–159.

Dhubuwala C et al. Myocardial infarction and its influence on male sexual function. Arch Sex Behav 1986 Dec; 15(6):499–504.

MacKey FG. Sexuality in coronary artery disease: A problem-oriented approach. Postgrad Med 1986 Jul; 80(1): 58–69.

McCann ME. Sexual healing after heart attack. Am J Nurs 1989 Sep; 89(9): 1132–1140.

Moore K et al. The joy of sex after a heart attack: Counseling the cardiac patient. Nursing 1984 Apr; 14(4): 104–113.

Smith PJ and Talbert RL. Sexual dysfunction with antihypertensive and antipsychotic agents. Clin Pharm 1986 May; 5(5):378–384.

Whipple B. Sexual counseling of couples after a mastectomy or myocardial infarction. Nurs Forum 1987/88; 23(3): 85–90.

Spinal Cord Injury

Comarr AE. Sexuality and fertility among spinal cord and/or corda equina injuries. J Am Paraplegia Soc 1985 Oct; 8(4): 67–75.

Persaud DH. Assessing sexual function of the adult with traumatic quadriplegia. J Neurosci Nurs 1986 Feb; 18(1): 11–12.

Sexually Transmitted Diseases

*Scura KW and Whipple B. Older adults as an HIV positive risk group. J Gerontol Nurs 1990 Feb; 15(2): 6–10.

Shubin S. Caring for AIDS patients: The stress will be on you. Nursing 1989 Oct; 19(10): 43–47.

Agencies

American Association of Sex Educators, Counselors, and Therapists
435 North Michigan Ave, Suite 1717, Chicago, IL 60611-4067

Sex Information and Education Council of the US (SIECUS)
80 Fifth Avenue, Suite 801, New York, NY 10011

18

Fluids and Electrolytes: Balance and Disturbances

Learning Objectives

On completion of this chapter, the learner will be able to:

1. Differentiate between osmosis, diffusion, filtration, and active transport

2. Describe the role of the kidneys, lungs, and endocrine glands in regulation of the body's fluid composition
   and volume

3. Identify the effects of aging on fluid and electrolyte regulation

4. Use the nursing process as a framework for care of patients with the following imbalances:
   Fluid volume deficit and fluid volume excess
   Sodium deficit (hyponatremia) and sodium excess (hypernatremia)
   Potassium deficit (hypokalemia) and potassium excess (hyperkalemia)

5. Specify the etiology, clinical manifestations, management, and nursing interventions for the following
   imbalances:
   Calcium deficit (hypocalcemia) and calcium excess (hypercalcemia)

(continued)

Fundamental Concepts

Amount and Composition of Body Fluids

Factors that influence the amount of body fluid in humans are age, sex, and body fat content. As a general rule, younger people have a higher percentage of body fluid than do older people, and men have proportionately more body fluid than do women (Table 18–1). Obese people have less fluid than thin people, because fat cells contain little water.

The typical adult is approximately 60% fluid (water and electrolytes) by weight. Approximately two thirds of the body fluid in adults exists in the intracellular space (primarily in the skeletal muscle mass). The remaining one third is found in the extracellular space, between the cells and in the plasma.

As a preliminary to this discussion, consult Chart 18-1, Glossary of Terms.

Electrolytes

Electrolytes in body fluids are active chemicals (anions and cations) that unite in varying combinations. Therefore, electrolyte concentration in the body is expressed in terms of milliequivalents (mEq) per liter, a measure of chemical activity, rather than in terms of milligrams (mg), a unit of weight. More specifically, a milliequivalent is defined as being equivalent to the electrochemical activity of 1 mg of hydrogen.

Electrolyte concentrations in intracellular fluid (ICF) differ from those in extracellular fluid (ECF). Because special techniques are required to measure electrolyte concentrations in the ICF, it is customary to measure the electrolytes in the most accessible portion of body fluids, namely, the plasma.

Sodium ions in the ECF far outnumber other extracellular cations (Table 18–2). About 90% of the ECF osmolality is determined by the sodium concentration. As a result, sodium is important in the regulation of body fluid volume. Retention of sodium is associated with fluid retention; conversely, excessive sodium loss is usually associated with decreased body fluid volume.

TABLE 18–1.   Approximate Values of Total Body Fluid as a Percentage of Body Weight in Relation to Age and Sex

Age		Total Body Fluid (% body weight)
Full-term newborn		70%–80%
1 year		64%
Puberty to 39 years	Men:	60%
	Women:	52%
40 to 60 years	Men:	55%
	Women:	47%
More than 60 years	Men:	52%
	Women:	46%

(Metheny N. Quick Reference to Fluid Balance. Philadelphia, JB Lippincott, 1984.)

TABLE 18–2.   Plasma Electrolytes

Electrolytes	mEq/L
CATIONS	
Sodium (Na^+)	142
Potassium (K^+)	5
Calcium (Ca^{2+})	5
Magnesium (Mg^{2+})	2
Total cations	154
ANIONS	
Chloride (Cl^-)	103
Bicarbonate (HCO_3^-)	26
Phosphate (HPO_4^{2-})	2
Sulfate (SO_4^{2-})	1
Organic acids	5
Proteinate	17
Total anions	154

(Metheny N. Fluid and Electrolyte Balance: Nursing Considerations. Philadelphia, JB Lippincott, 1987.)

Chart 18-1
Glossary of Terms

Acidosis—an acid–base disturbance characterized by increased hydrogen ion concentration (decreased pH); may be due to increased production of acids or loss of base.

Alkalosis—an acid–base disturbance characterized by decreased hydrogen ion concentration (increased pH); may be due to loss of acids or increased production of base.

Diffusion—passive movement of particles from an area of high concentration to one of lower concentration.

Osmosis—movement of fluid through a semipermeable membrane from an area of low concentration to an area of high concentration of particles to equalize the concentration on both sides of the membrane.

Hydrostatic pressure—force exerted by a fluid against the walls of the container (in the body, the pressure of fluid against the walls of the blood vessels results from the weight of the fluid itself and the force resulting from cardiac contraction).

Osmolality—number of dissolved particles contained in a specific unit or volume of fluid (i.e., 1 kg of fluid).

Isotonic solution—solution in which the number of dissolved particles is equal to the number of particles dissolved in normal body fluids.

Hypotonic solution—one with fewer dissolved particles than another solution (i.e., fewer than the number of particles in normal body fluids).

Hypertonic solution—one with more dissolved particles than another solution (i.e., more than the number of particles in normal body fluids).

As shown in Table 18–3, the major electrolytes in the ICF are potassium and phosphate. Because the ECF can tolerate only small changes in potassium concentrations (approximately 5 mEq/L), release of large stores of intracellular potassium by trauma can be extremely dangerous. The body expends a great deal of energy maintaining the extracellular preponderance of sodium and the intracellular preponderance of potassium. It does so by means of cell membrane pumps, which exchange sodium and potassium ions. Normal movement of fluids through the capillary wall into the tissues depends on the force of the hydrostatic pressure (the pressure exerted by the fluid on the walls of the blood vessel) at both the arterial and the venous ends of the vessel and the osmotic pressure exerted by the protein of plasma. Direction of fluid movement depends on the differences in these two opposing forces. The ECF transports other substances, such as enzymes and hormones. It also carries blood components, such as red and white blood cells, throughout the body.

Regulation of Body Fluid Compartments

Osmosis

When two different solutions are separated by a membrane impermeable to the dissolved substances, a shift of water occurs through the membrane from the region of low solute concentration to the region of high solute concentration until the solutions are of equal concentration (Fig. 18–1). The magnitude of this force depends on the *number* of particles dissolved in the solutions and not on their weights. The number of dissolved particles contained in a unit of water determines the osmolality of a solution.

Diffusion

Diffusion is defined as the natural tendency of a substance to move from an area of higher concentration to one of lower concentration. It occurs through the random movement of ions and molecules. An example of diffusion is the exchange of oxygen and carbon dioxide between the pulmonary capillaries and alveoli.

Filtration

Hydrostatic pressure in the capillaries tends to filter fluid out of the vascular compartment into the interstitial fluid. An example of filtration is the passage of water and electrolytes from the arterial capillary bed to the interstitial fluid; in this instance, the hydrostatic pressure is furnished by the pumping action of the heart.

TABLE 18–3. *Approximation of Major Electrolyte Content in Cellular Fluid*

Electrolytes	mEq/L
CATIONS	
Potassium (K^+)	150
Magnesium (Mg^{2+})	40
Sodium (Na^+)	10
Total cations	200
ANIONS	
Phosphates / Sulfates	150
Bicarbonate (HCO_3^-)	10
Proteinate	40
Total anions	200

(Metheny N. Fluid and Electrolyte Balance: Nursing Considerations. Philadelphia, JB Lippincott, 1987.)

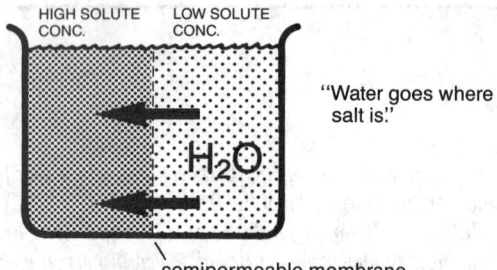

Figure 18–1. Osmosis. ("Water goes where salt is.") (Metheny N. Fluid and Electrolyte Balance: Nursing Considerations. Philadelphia, JB Lippincott, 1987.)

Sodium–Potassium Pump

As stated earlier, sodium concentration is greater in ECF than in ICF; because of this, there is a tendency for sodium to enter the cell by diffusion. This tendency is offset by the sodium-potassium pump, which is located in the cell membrane and actively moves sodium from the cell into the ECF. Conversely, the high intracellular potassium concentration is maintained by pumping of potassium into the cell. By definition, active transport implies that energy expenditure must take place for the movement to occur against a concentration gradient.

Routes of Gains and Losses

Water and electrolytes are gained in various ways. In health, one gains fluids by drinking and eating. In some types of illnesses, fluids may be provided by the parenteral route (intravenously or subcutaneously) or by means of an enteral feeding tube in the stomach or intestine. When fluid balance is critical, all routes of gain and all routes of loss must be recorded and the volumes compared. Organs of fluid loss include the kidneys, skin, lungs, and gastrointestinal tract.

Kidneys

The usual urine volume in the adult is between 1 and 2 liters each day. A general rule is that the output is approximately 1 ml of urine per kilogram of body weight per hour (1 ml/kg/hr) in all age groups.

Skin

Sensible perspiration refers to visible water and electrolyte loss through the skin by way of sweating. The chief solutes in sweat are sodium, chloride and potassium. Actual sweat losses can vary from 0 to 1000 ml or more every hour, depending on the environmental temperature. Continuous water loss by evaporation (approximately 600 ml/day) occurs through the skin as *insensible perspiration*, a nonvisible form of water loss. Fever greatly increases insensible water loss through the lungs and the skin, as does loss of the natural skin barrier through major burns.

Lungs

The lungs normally eliminate water vapor (insensible loss) at a rate of 300 to 400 ml every day. The loss is much greater with increased respiratory rate or depth, or both.

Gastrointestinal Tract

The usual loss through the gastrointestinal tract is only 100 to 200 ml every day, even though approximately 8 liters of fluid circulate through the gastrointestinal system every 24 hours (called the "gastrointestinal circulation"). Because the bulk of fluids is reabsorbed in the small intestine, it is obvious that large losses can be incurred from the gastrointestinal tract if diarrhea or fistulas occur.

In healthy persons, the 24-hour average intake and output of water are approximately equal (Table 18–4).

Homeostatic Mechanisms

The body is equipped with remarkable homeostatic mechanisms to keep the composition and volume of body fluid within narrow limits of normal. Organs involved in homeostasis include the kidneys, lungs, heart, adrenal glands, parathyroid glands, and pituitary gland.

Kidneys

Vital to the regulation of fluid and electrolyte balance, the kidneys normally filter 170 liters of plasma every day in the adult, while excreting only 1.5 liters of urine. They act both autonomously and in response to bloodborne messengers, such as aldosterone and antidiuretic hormone (ADH). Major functions of the kidneys in fluid balance homeostasis include the following:

- Regulation of ECF volume and osmolality by selective retention and excretion of body fluids
- Regulation of electrolyte levels in the ECF by selective retention of needed substances and excretion of unneeded substances
- Regulation of pH of ECF by retention of hydrogen ions
- Excretion of metabolic wastes and toxic substances

Given the above facts, it is readily apparent that renal failure will result in multiple fluid and electrolyte problems. Renal function declines with advanced age, as do muscle mass and daily exogenous creatinine production. Thus, high-normal and minimally elevated serum creatinine values may indicate substantially reduced renal function in the elderly.

TABLE 18–4. *Average Intake and Output in an Adult for a 24-Hour Period*

Intake		Output	
Oral liquids	1300 ml	Urine	1500 ml
Water in food	1000 ml	Stool	200 ml
Water produced by metabolism	300 ml	*INSENSIBLE*	
		Lungs	300 ml
Total	2600 ml	Skin	600 ml
		Total	2600 ml

(Metheny N. Fluid and Electrolyte Balance: Nursing Considerations. Philadelphia, JB Lippincott, 1987.)

Heart and Blood Vessels

The pumping action of the heart circulates blood through the kidneys under sufficient pressure for urine to form. Failure of this pumping action interferes with renal perfusion and thus with water and electrolyte regulation.

Lungs

The lungs are also vital in maintaining homeostasis. The lungs remove approximately 300 ml of water daily through exhalation in the normal adult. Abnormal conditions such as hyperpnea or continuous coughing increase this loss; mechanical ventilation with excessive moisture decreases it. The lungs also have a major role in maintenance of acid–base balance, which is discussed later in this chapter. Normal aging changes result in decreased respiratory function, causing increased difficulty in regulation of *p*H in elderly individuals experiencing major illness or trauma.

Pituitary Gland

The hypothalamus manufactures a substance known as antidiuretic hormone (ADH), which is stored in the posterior pituitary gland and released as needed. Sometimes referred to as the "water-conserving hormone," ADH makes the body retain water. Functions of ADH include maintenance of osmotic pressure of the cells by controlling renal water retention or excretion, and control of blood volume (Fig. 18–2).

Adrenal Glands

Aldosterone, a mineralocorticoid secreted by the zona glomerulosa (outer zone) of the adrenal cortex, has a profound effect on fluid balance. Increased secretion of aldosterone causes sodium retention (and thus water retention) and potassium loss. Conversely, a decreased secretion of aldosterone

causes sodium and water loss and potassium retention. Cortisol, another adrenocortical hormone, has only a fraction of the mineralocorticoid potency of aldosterone. When secreted in large quantities, however, it can also produce sodium and fluid retention and potassium deficit.

Parathyroid Glands

The parathyroid glands, embedded in the corners of the thyroid gland, regulate calcium and phosphate balance by means of parathyroid hormone (PTH). PTH influences bone resorption, calcium absorption from the intestines, and calcium reabsorption from the renal tubules.

Gerontologic Considerations

Normal physiologic changes of aging, including reduced renal and respiratory function/reserve and alterations in the ratio of body fluids to muscle mass, may alter the responses of the elderly patient to fluid and electrolyte changes and acid–base disturbances. In addition, the frequent use of medications in the elderly that affect renal and cardiac function and fluid balance increases the likelihood of fluid and electrolyte disturbances. Routine procedures, such as the vigorous administration of laxatives before colon x-rays, may induce serious fluid volume deficit in the elderly, necessitating intravenous fluids to prevent hypotension and other effects of hypovolemia.

Alterations in fluid and electrolyte balance that may initially produce minor changes in the young and middle-aged adult have the potential to produce profound changes in the elderly, accompanied by a rapid onset of signs and symptoms. In other elderly patients, the clinical manifestations of fluid and electrolyte disturbances may be subtle or atypical. For example, fluid deficit or hyponatremia may present as confusion in the elderly patient; in young and middle-aged patients increased thirst may be a common first sign of fluid deficit. Rapid infusion

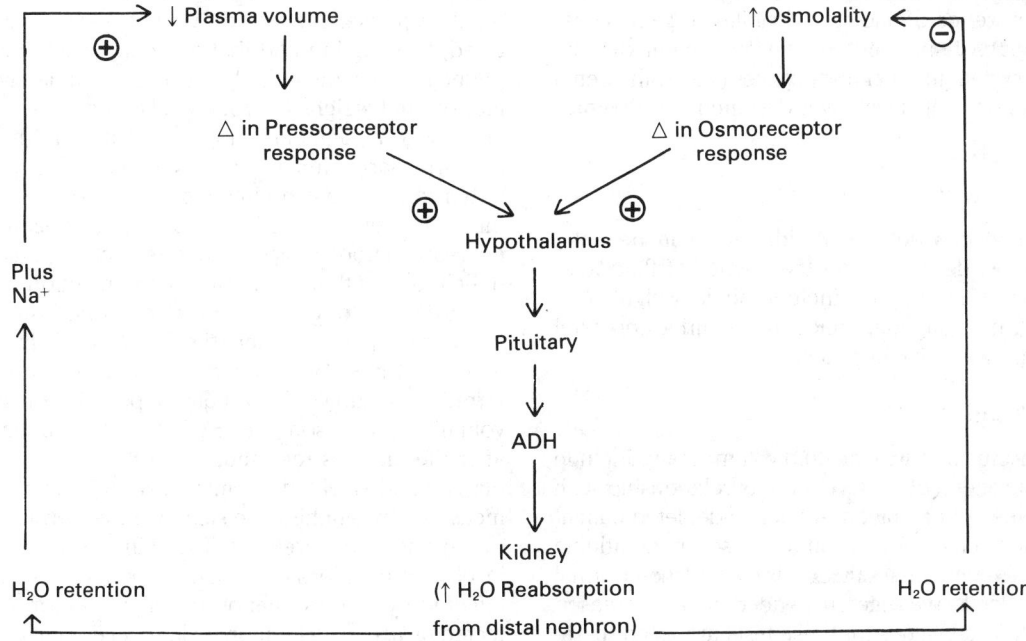

Figure 18–2. ADH-induced water retention. The major stimulus for ADH secretion is increased serum osmolality. A secondary stimulus is a severe decrease in extracellular volume.

of an excessive volume of intravenous fluids may produce fluid overload and cardiac failure in the elderly; these are likely to occur more quickly and with administration of a smaller volume of fluid than in healthy young and middle-aged adults because of decreased cardiac reserve and reduction of renal function with advancing age.

Increased sensitivity to fluid and electrolyte changes in the elderly necessitates careful assessment of elderly patients with attention to intake and output of fluids from all sources and changes in daily weight, careful monitoring of side effects and interactions of medications, and prompt reporting and management of disturbances. Additional gerontologic considerations are discussed in this chapter with specific fluid and electrolyte disturbances.

Fluid Volume Disturbances

Fluid Volume Deficit

Definition and Etiology

Fluid volume deficit (FVD) results when water and electrolytes are lost in the same proportion as they exist in normal body fluids, so that the ratio of serum electrolytes to water remains the same. It should not be confused with the term *dehydration*, which refers to loss of water alone with increased serum sodium levels. FVD may occur alone or in combination with other imbalances. Unless other imbalances are present concurrently, serum electrolyte concentrations remain essentially unchanged.

Fluid volume deficit results from loss of body fluids and occurs more rapidly when coupled with decreased fluid intake. It is possible to develop FVD on the basis of inadequate intake alone if the decreased intake is prolonged. Causes of FVD include abnormal fluid losses, such as resulting from vomiting, diarrhea, gastrointestinal suction, and sweating, and decreased intake, as in the presence of nausea or inability to gain access to fluids. Third-space fluid shifts, or the movement of fluid from the vascular system to other body spaces (*i.e.*, with edema formation in burns or ascites with liver dysfunction), also produce FVD.

Clinical Manifestations

Fluid volume deficit can develop rapidly and can be mild, moderate, or severe, depending on the degree of fluid loss. Important characteristics of FVD include acute weight loss, decreased skin turgor, oliguria, concentrated urine, postural hypotension, and a weak, rapid pulse.

Diagnostic Evaluation

Laboratory data useful in evaluating fluid volume status include the blood urea nitrogen (BUN) level and its relationship with the serum creatinine concentration. A volume-depleted patient has a BUN elevated out of proportion to the serum creatinine level ($>10:1$). Also, the hematocrit level is greater than normal as the red blood cells become suspended in a decreased plasma volume. Normal values for these tests are listed in Table 18–5.

Management

In planning correction of fluid loss for the patient with FVD, usual maintenance requirements and other factors (such as fever) that can influence fluid needs are considered. When the deficit is not severe, the oral route is preferred, provided the patient is able to drink. When fluid losses are acute or severe, however, the intravenous route is required. Isotonic electrolyte solutions (such as lactated Ringer's or 0.9% sodium chloride) are frequently used to treat the hypotensive patient with FVD, because such fluids expand plasma volume. As soon as the patient becomes normotensive, a hypotonic electrolyte solution (such as 0.45% sodium chloride) is often used to provide both electrolytes and free water for renal excretion of metabolic wastes. These, and additional fluids, are summarized in Table 18–6.

If the patient with severe FVD is oliguric, it must be determined whether the depressed renal function is the result of reduced renal blood flow secondary to FVD (prerenal azotemia) or, more seriously, to acute tubular necrosis due to prolonged FVD. The therapeutic test used in this situation is referred to as a fluid challenge test. Prompt treatment of FVD is imperative to prevent renal damage.

▶ Nursing Process
The Patient With Fluid Volume Deficit

▷ Assessment

To assess for the presence of FVD, fluid intake and output are measured and evaluated at least at 8-hour intervals; sometimes, hourly measurements are indicated. As FVD is developing, body fluid losses exceed fluid intake. This loss may be in the form of polyuria, diarrhea, vomiting, and so on. Later, after FVD has fully developed, the kidneys attempt to conserve needed body fluids, leading to a urinary output less than 30 ml/hr in an adult; urine in this instance is concentrated and represents a healthy renal response. Daily body weight measurements are monitored, keeping in mind that an acute weight loss of 0.5 kg (1 pound) represents a fluid loss of approximately 500 ml. (One liter of fluid weighs approximately 1 kg, or 2.2 pounds.)

The vital signs are closely monitored. The nurse should be particularly alert for a weak rapid pulse and postural hypotension (*i.e.*, a drop in the systolic pressure greater than 15 mm Hg when changed from a lying to a sitting position). A decrease in body temperature often accompanies fluid volume deficit, unless there is a concurrent infection.

Skin and tongue turgor are monitored on a regular basis. In a normal person, pinched skin will immediately fall back to its normal position when released. This elastic property, referred to as turgor, is partially dependent on interstitial fluid volume. In a person with FVD, the skin flattens more slowly after the pinch is released; when the FVD is severe, the skin may remain elevated for many seconds. Tissue turgor is best measured by pinching the skin over the sternum, inner aspects of the thighs, or forehead. The skin turgor test is not as valid in elderly people as in younger people, as skin elasticity is affected by age. Evaluation of tongue turgor, which is not affected by age, may be more valid than evaluation of skin turgor. In a normal person, the tongue has one longitudinal furrow.

TABLE 18–5.   *Laboratory Tests Used to Evaluate Fluid, Electrolyte, and Acid–Base Status*

Test	Usual Reference Range	SI Units
Serum sodium	135–145 mEq/L	135–145 mmol/L
Serum potassium	3.5–5.5 mEq/L	3.5–5.5 mmol/L
Total serum calcium	8.5–10.5 mg/dl (approximately 50% in ionized form)	2.1–2.6 mmol/L
Serum magnesium	1.5–2.5 mEq/L	0.80–1.2 mmol/L
Serum phosphorus	2.5–4.5 mEq/L	0.80–1.5 mmol/L
Serum chloride	100–106 mEq/L	100–106 mmol/L
Carbon dioxide content	24–30 mEq/L	24–30 mmol/L
Serum osmolality	280–295 mOsm/kg	280–295 mmol/L
Blood urea nitrogen (BUN)	10–20 mg/dl	3.5–7 mmol/L of urea
Serum creatinine	0.7–1.5 mg/dl	60–130 μmol/L
BUN: Creatinine ratio	10:1	
Hematocrit	Male: 44–52%	Volume fraction: 0.44–0.52
	Female: 39–47%	Volume fraction: 0.39–0.47
Serum glucose	70–110 mg/dl	3.9–6.1 mmol/L
Serum albumin	3.5–5.5 g/dl	3.5–5.5 g/L
Arterial blood gases		
pH	7.35–7.45	7.35–7.45
$PaCO_2$	38–42 mm Hg	38–42 mm Hg
HCO_3^-	22–26 mEq/L	22–26 mmol/L
Urinary sodium	80–180 mEq/day	80–180 mmol/day
Urinary potassium	40–80 mEq/day	40–80 mmol/day
Urinary chloride	110–250 mEq/day	110–250 mmol/day
Urinary specific gravity	1.003–1.035	1.003–1.035
Urine osmolality		
Extreme range:	50–1400 mOsm/L	40–1400 mmol/kg
Typical urine:	500–800 mOsm/L	500–800 mmol/kg
Urinary *p*H	4.5–8.0	4.5–8.0
Typical urine:	<6.6	<6.6

In the person with FVD, there are additional longitudinal furrows and the tongue is smaller, because of fluid loss. The degree of oral mucous membrane moisture is also assessed; a dry mouth may indicate either FVD or mouth breathing.

Urinary concentration is monitored; when available, a urinometer should be used to measure specific gravity (SG). In a volume-depleted patient, the urinary SG should be above 1.020 (indicating healthy renal conservation of fluid).

Severe volume depletion eventually affects the sensorium by decreasing cerebral perfusion. Decreased peripheral perfusion can result in cold extremities. In patients with relatively normal cardiopulmonary function, a low central venous pressure is indicative of hypovolemia. Patients with acute cardiopulmonary decompensation require more extensive hemodynamic monitoring with a device that measures pressures in both sides of the heart.

▷ Nursing Diagnosis

The nursing assessment and identification of patients at risk for this disturbance lead to a nursing diagnosis of fluid volume deficit. For example, in a patient with volume depletion secondary to uncontrolled diabetes mellitus, the diagnosis may be stated as fluid volume deficit related to osmotic diuresis.

▷ Planning and Implementation

▷ *Goals:*   A major goal is, of course, prevention of this common disturbance. Once the imbalance has developed, the goal is to correct the abnormal fluid volume status before renal damage results. More precise nursing goals vary with the cause of FVD and individual patient characteristics.

▷ Nursing Interventions

▷ *Prevention of* FVD.   To prevent FVD, one must be aware of patients at risk and take measures to minimize fluid losses. For example, if the patient has diarrhea, measures should be implemented to control the diarrhea while replacing fluids. These may include the administration of antidiarrheal medications and small volumes of oral fluids at frequent intervals.

TABLE 18–6.   *Selected Water and Electrolyte Solutions*

Solution	Comments
0.9% NaCl (Isotonic saline) Na⁺ 154 mEq/L Cl⁻ 154 mEq/L (308 mOsm/kg) Also available wtih varying concentrations of dextrose (the most frequently used is a 5% dextrose concentration)	• An isotonic solution that expands the extracellular fluid volume, used in hypovolemic states • Supplies an excess of Na⁺ and Cl⁻; can cause fluid volume excess and hyperchloremic acidosis if used in excessive volumes, particularly in patients with compromised renal function • Not desirable as a routine maintenance solution, as it provides only Na⁺ and Cl⁻ (and these are provided in excessive amounts) • Sometimes used to correct mild Na⁺ deficit • When mixed with 5% dextrose, the resulting solution becomes hypertonic in relation to plasma and, in addition to the above described electrolytes, provides 170 calories per liter
0.45% NaCl (half-strength saline) Na⁺ 77 mEq/L Cl⁻ 77 mEq/L (154 mOsm/L) Also available with varying concentrations of dextrose (the most common is a 5% concentration)	• A hypotonic solution that provides Na⁺, Cl⁻, and free water • Free water is desirable to aid the kidneys in elimination of solute • Lacking in electrolytes other than Na⁺ and Cl⁻ • When mixed with 5% dextrose, the solution becomes slightly hypertonic to plasma and in addition to the above-described electrolytes provides 170 calories
Lactated Ringer's solution (Hartmann's solution) Na⁺ 130 mEq/L K⁺ 4 mEq/L Ca²⁺ 3 mEq/L Cl⁻ 109 mEq/L Lactate (metabolized to bicarbonate) 28 mEq/L (274 mOsm/L) Also available with varying concentrations of dextrose (the most common is 5% dextrose)	• An isotonic solution that contains multiple electrolytes in roughly the same concentration as found in plasma (note that solution is lacking in Mg²⁺) • Used in the treatment of hypovolemia, burns, and fluid lost as bile or diarrhea • Lactate is rapidly metabolized into HCO₃⁻ in the body. Lactated Ringer's solution should not be used in lactic acidosis because the ability to convert lactate into HCO₃⁻ is impaired in this disorder.
5% dextrose in water (D₅W) No electrolytes 50 g of dextrose	• An isotonic solution that supplies 170 calories per liter and free water to aid in renal excretion of solutes • Should not be used in excessive volumes in the early postoperative period (when ADH secretion is increased due to stress reaction) • Should not be used solely in treatment of fluid volume deficit, because it dilutes plasma electrolyte concentrations.
3% NaCl (hypertonic saline) Na⁺ 513 mEq/L Cl⁻ 513 mEq/L (1026 mOsm/L)	• Grossly hypertonic solution used only in critical situations to treat hyponatremia

(Adapted from Metheny N. Fluid and Electrolyte Balance: Nursing Considerations. Philadelphia, JB Lippincott, 1987.)

Correction of FVD.   When possible, oral fluids are given to help correct FVD, keeping in mind the patient's likes and dislikes. Also, the type of fluid the patient has lost is considered and attempts are made to select fluids most likely to replace the lost electrolytes. If the patient is reluctant to drink because of oral discomfort, frequent mouth care is given and fluids that are nonirritating to the mucosa are provided. It is often helpful to offer small volumes of fluids at frequent intervals rather than a large volume all at once. If nausea is present, antiemetics may be needed before oral fluid replacement can be tolerated.

If the patient is unable to eat and drink, the physician may consider an alternative route (enteral or parental) for fluid in-

take. This intervention is important to prevent renal damage related to prolonged FVD.

Evaluation

Expected Outcomes
1. Exhibits normal turgor of skin and tongue
2. Excretes increased amount of urine with normal specific gravity
3. Exhibits return of pulse and blood pressure to normal
4. Exhibits clear sensorium; is oriented to time, person, and place

5. Drinks fluids as prescribed
6. Exhibits absence of precipitating risk factors (*e.g.*, excessive fluid loss, decreased fluid intake)

Fluid Volume Excess

Definition and Etiology

Fluid volume excess (FVE) refers to an isotonic expansion of the ECF caused by the abnormal retention of water and sodium in approximately the same proportions in which they normally exist in the ECF. It is always secondary to an increase in the total body sodium content, which, in turn, leads to an increase in total body water. Because there is isotonic retention of body substances, the serum sodium concentration remains essentially normal.

Fluid volume excess may be caused by simple fluid overloading or by diminished function of the homeostatic mechanisms responsible for regulating fluid balance. Causative factors can include congestive heart failure, renal failure, and cirrhosis of the liver. Overzealous administration of sodium-containing fluids to persons with impaired regulatory mechanisms particularly predisposes to serious fluid volume excess. Excessive ingestion of table salt (sodium chloride) or other sodium salts also predisposes to fluid overload.

Clinical Manifestations

The clinical manifestations of FVE stem from expansion of the ECF compartment and include edema, distended veins, increased venous pressure, bounding pulse, and crackles (abnormal lung sounds).

Diagnostic Evaluation

Laboratory data useful in the diagnosis of FVE include the BUN and hematocrit levels. In the presence of FVE, both of these values may be decreased because of plasma dilution. Other causes for abnormalities in these values include low protein intake and anemia.

Management

Management of FVE is directed at the causative factors. Symptomatic treatment consists of administration of diuretics, restriction of fluids, or both. When the fluid excess is related to excessive administration of sodium-containing fluids, discontinuing the infusion may be all that is needed. Because treatment almost always involves sodium restriction in the diet, concepts related to sodium-restricted diets are discussed below.

Sodium-Restricted Diets

An average daily diet not restricted in sodium contains 6 to 15 g of salt, whereas low-sodium diets can range from a mild restriction to as low as 250 mg of sodium per day, depending on the patient's needs. A mild sodium-restricted diet allows only light salting of food (about half the amount as usual) in cooking and at the table, and no addition of salt to commercially prepared foods that are already seasoned. Of course, foods high in sodium must be avoided. Because about half of ingested sodium is in the form of seasoning, use of substitute seasonings plays a major role in decreasing sodium intake.

Lemon juice, onion, and garlic are excellent substitute flavoring agents; however, some patients prefer salt substitutes. Most salt substitutes contain potassium and should be used cautiously by those patients taking potassium-sparing diuretics (*e.g.*, spironolactone, triamterene, and amiloride). They should not be used at all in patients with conditions associated with potassium retention, such as advanced renal disease. Salt substitutes containing ammonium chloride can be harmful to patients with liver damage.

In certain communities, the drinking water may contain too much sodium for a sodium-restricted diet. Depending on its source, water may contain as little as 1 mg or more than 1500 mg per quart. It may be necessary for patients to use distilled water when the local water supply is very high in sodium. Also, patients on sodium-restricted diets should be cautioned to avoid ''water softeners'' that add sodium to water in exchange for other ions, such as calcium.

▶ ## Nursing Process

The Patient With Fluid Volume Excess

▷ ### Assessment

To assess for FVE, the fluid intake and output are measured at regular intervals for indication of excessive fluid retention. The patient is weighed daily, and acute weight gain is noted. (Remember that an acute weight gain of 0.9 kg [2 pounds] represents a gain of approximately 1 liter of fluid.)

It is important to assess breath sounds at regular intervals in at-risk patients, particularly when parenteral fluids are being administered. The nurse monitors the degree of edema in the most dependent parts of the body, such as the feet and ankles in ambulatory patients and the sacral region in bedridden patients. The degree of pitting edema is assessed and the extent of peripheral edema is measured with a tape marked in millimeters.

▷ ### Nursing Diagnosis

Based on the nursing assessment and identification of the patient at risk for this disturbance, the nursing diagnosis is fluid volume excess. For example, in a patient with congestive heart failure, the nursing diagnosis might be stated as follows: fluid volume excess related to compromised regulatory mechanism (cardiac failure).

▷ ### Planning and Implementation

▷ *Goals:*   A major goal is the prevention of FVE in patients at risk. If prevention is not possible, the presence of FVE must be detected early so that therapeutic interventions can be implemented before the condition becomes severe. Specific goals vary with individual patients and their clinical conditions.

▷ ### Nursing Interventions

▷ *Prevention of FVE.*   Specific interventions vary somewhat with the underlying pathologic condition and the degree of FVE. Most patients, however, require sodium-restricted diets in some form. Therefore, adherence to the prescribed diet is encouraged. The patient is instructed to avoid ''over-the-counter" drugs without first checking with the health care provider, as these substances may contain sodium. When fluid retention persists despite adherence to a prescribed diet, one should consider hidden sources of sodium, such as the water supply or use of water softeners.

▷ *Detection and Control of FVE.* Detection of FVE is of primary importance before the condition becomes critical. Interventions include providing rest, sodium restriction, close monitoring of parenteral fluid therapy, and administration of appropriate medications. Some patients benefit from regular rest periods, as bed rest favors diuresis of edema fluid. The mechanism is probably related to diminished venous pooling and subsequent increase in effective circulating blood volume and renal perfusion. Sodium and fluid restriction should be instituted as indicated. Because most patients with FVE require diuretics, the patient's response to these drugs is monitored. The rate of parenteral fluids and the patient's response to the fluids are also closely monitored. If dyspnea or orthopnea is present, the patient is placed in semi-Fowler's position to favor lung expansion. The patient is turned and positioned at regular intervals, because edematous tissue is more prone to skin breakdown than normal tissue.

Because conditions predisposing to FVE are likely to be chronic, the patient is taught to monitor his own response to therapy by recording and evaluating fluid intake and output and body weight changes. The importance of adherence to the medical regimen is emphasized.

▷ Evaluation

Expected Outcomes
1. Exhibits normal skin turgor and absence of edema
2. Excretes increased amount of urine
3. Demonstrates return of body weight to normal
4. Demonstrates no distention of jugular veins
5. Adheres to diet with prescribed sodium intake
6. States rationale for dietary prescription
7. Exhibits normal breath sounds without adventitious sounds (crackles, wheezes)
8. Maintains bed rest when prescribed
9. Exhibits absence of precipitating risk factors (*e.g.*, fluid overload, high sodium intake)

Gerontologic Considerations

The percentage of elderly persons is increasing in our society. The aged have special nursing care needs because of their propensity for developing fluid and electrolyte problems. Fluid balance in the elderly is often marginal at best because of certain physiologic changes associated with the aging process. Some of these changes include reduction in total body water (associated with increased body fat content and decreased muscle mass), reduction in renal function resulting in decreased ability to concentrate urine, decreased cardiovascular and respiratory function, and disturbances in hormonal regulatory functions. Although these changes are viewed as normal in the aging process, they must be considered when the elderly person becomes ill, because they predispose to fluid and electrolyte imbalances.

Assessment of the elderly client should be modified somewhat from that of younger adults. For example, skin turgor is less valid as an assessment tool in the elderly because their skin has lost some of its elasticity; therefore, other assessment measures, such as slowness in filling of veins of the hands and feet, become more important in detecting fluid volume deficit. When skin turgor is tested in the elderly, it is best tested over the forehead or the sternum, because alterations in skin elasticity are less marked in these areas. As in any patient, skin turgor should be monitored serially to detect subtle changes.

The nurse should perform a functional assessment of the aged person's ability to determine his need for and to obtain adequate food and fluid intake. For example, is the patient mentally clear? Is he able to ambulate and use his arms and hands to reach fluids and foods? Is he able to swallow? All of these questions have direct bearing on how the patient will be able to manage his own need for fluids and foods. The nurse must, of course, provide for the patient when he is unable to provide for himself. Another concern is that some elderly patients deliberately restrict their fluid intake to avoid embarrassing episodes of incontinence. In this situation, the nurse needs to implement interventions to deal with the incontinence.

Sodium Imbalances

Disturbances in sodium balance occur frequently in clinical practice and can develop under simple and complex circumstances. Before discussion of disruptions in sodium balance, important facts about the role of sodium in physiologic activities are reviewed.

Functions of Sodium

Sodium is the most abundant electrolyte in the ECF; its concentration ranges from 135 to 145 mEq/L (SI: 135–145 mmol/L.) Because of this, it is the primary determinant of ECF concentration. The fact that sodium does not easily cross the cell-wall membrane, plus its dominance in quantity, accounts for its primary role in controlling water distribution throughout the body. In addition, sodium is the primary regulator of ECF volume. A loss or gain of sodium is usually accompanied by a loss or gain of water. Sodium also functions in the establishment of the electrochemical state necessary for muscle contraction and the transmission of nerve impulses.

Sodium Deficit (Hyponatremia)

Definition and Etiology

Hyponatremia refers to a serum sodium level that is below normal (less than 135 mEq/L; SI: 135 mmol/L). It may be due to an excessive loss of sodium or an excessive gain of water; in either event, it results in a relatively greater concentration of water than of sodium. This imbalance should not be confused with FVD, which refers to an isotonic or equivalent loss of sodium and water, resulting in an essentially normal serum sodium level. A hyponatremic state can, however, be superimposed on an existing FVD or FVE.

Sodium may be lost by way of vomiting, diarrhea, fistulas, or sweating, or it may be associated with diuretics, particularly in combination with a low-salt diet. A deficiency of aldosterone, as occurs in adrenal insufficiency, also predisposes the patient to sodium deficiency.

Water may be gained abnormally by the excessive parenteral administration of dextrose and water solutions, particularly during periods of stress. It may also be gained by compulsive water drinking (psychogenic polydipsia).

A special type of hyponatremia associated with excessive antidiuretic hormone (ADH) activity is referred to as the syndrome of inappropriate ADH secretion (SIADH). The basic physiologic disturbances in SIADH are excessive ADH activity, with water retention and dilutional hyponatremia, and inappropriate urinary excretion of sodium in the presence of hyponatremia. SIADH can be the result of either sustained secretion of ADH by the hypothalamus or production of an ADH-like substance from a tumor (aberrant ADH production). Conditions associated with SIADH include oat-cell lung tumors, head injuries, endocrine and pulmonary disorders, and use of drugs such as Pitocin, cyclophosphamide, vincristine, thioridazine, and amitriptyline.

Clinical Manifestations

Clinical manifestations of hyponatremia depend on the cause, magnitude, and rapidity of onset. Although nausea and abdominal cramping occur, most of the symptoms are neuropsychiatric and are probably related to the cellular swelling and cerebral edema associated with hyponatremia. As the extracellular sodium level decreases, the cellular fluid becomes relatively more concentrated and "pulls" water into the cells (Fig. 18–3). In general, those patients having acute decline in serum sodium levels have more severe symptoms and higher mortality rates than do those with more slowly developing hyponatremia.

Features of hyponatremia associated with sodium loss and water gain include anorexia, muscle cramps, and a feeling of exhaustion. When the serum sodium level drops below 115 mEq/L (SI: 115 mmol/L), signs of increasing intracranial pressure, such as lethargy, confusion, muscular twitching, focal weakness, hemiparesis, papilledema, and convulsions, may occur.

Diagnostic Evaluation

Regardless of the cause of hyponatremia, the serum sodium level is less than 135 mEq/L; it may be quite low, such as 100 mEq/L (SI: 100 mmol/L) or less, in SIADH. When hyponatremia is due primarily to sodium loss, the urinary sodium content is less than 10 mEq/L (SI: 10 mmol/L) and the specific gravity is low, such as 1.002 to 1.004. When hyponatremia is due to SIADH, however, the urinary sodium content is greater than 20 mEq/L and the urinary specific gravity is usually greater than 1.012. Although the patient with SIADH gains water abnormally and thus gains body weight, there is no peripheral edema; instead, the edema is inside the cells. This phenomenon is sometimes manifested as "fingerprinting" when the finger is pressed over a bony prominence, such as the sternum.

Management

The obvious treatment for hyponatremia is careful administration of sodium. This may be accomplished orally, by nasogastric tube, or parenterally. For patients who are able to eat and drink, sodium replacement is easily accomplished, because sodium is plentiful in a normal diet. For those unable to take sodium orally, lactated Ringer's solution or isotonic saline (0.9% sodium chloride) may be prescribed (see Table 18–6). The usual daily sodium requirement in adults is approximately 100 mEq, provided there are no abnormal losses.

When hyponatremia is present in a patient with normovolemia or hypervolemia, the treatment of choice is water restriction. This is far safer than sodium administration and is usually quite effective. When neurologic symptoms are present, however, it may be necessary to administer small volumes of a hypertonic sodium solution, such as 3% or 5% sodium chloride. Incorrect use of these fluids is extremely dangerous; this is understandable when one considers that a liter of 3% sodium chloride solution contains 513 mEq of sodium and a liter of 5% sodium chloride solution contains 855 mEq of sodium. Grossly hypertonic sodium solutions (3% and 5% sodium chloride) should be administered only in intensive care settings under close observation, because only small volumes are needed to elevate the serum sodium level from a dangerously low value. These fluids are administered slowly, in small volumes, while the patient is monitored closely for fluid overload.

▶ Nursing Process
The Patient With Sodium Deficit

▷ Assessment

It is important to identify patients at risk for hyponatremia so that they can be monitored. Early detection and treatment of this disorder are necessary to prevent serious consequences. For patients at risk, the nurse monitors fluid intake and output as well as daily body weight. Abnormal losses of sodium or gains of water are noted. Gastrointestinal manifestations, such as anorexia, nausea, vomiting, and abdominal cramping, are also noted. One is particularly alert for central nervous system changes, such as lethargy, confusion, muscular twitching, and convulsions. In general, more severe neurologic signs are as-

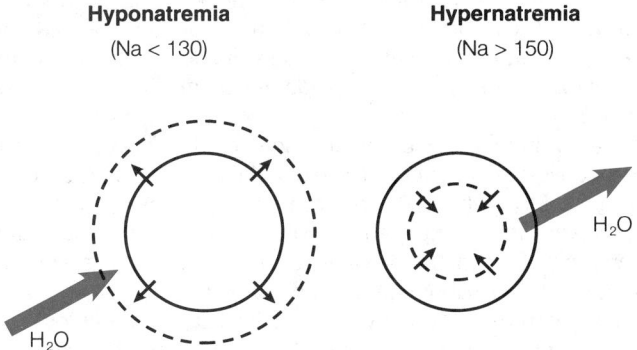

Hyponatremia
(Na < 130)

Hypernatremia
(Na > 150)

Cell size increases as water moves into the cell from the relatively hypotonic extracellular fluid.

Cell size decreases as water is pulled out by the relatively hypertonic extracellular fluid.

sociated with very low sodium levels that have fallen rapidly because of water overloading. It is most important to monitor serum sodium levels closely in patients at risk for hyponatremia. When indicated, urinary sodium levels and specific gravity are also monitored. Hyponatremia as a cause of confusion is an often overlooked problem in elderly patients. The elderly are at increased risk for hyponatremia because of changes in renal function and subsequent decreased ability to excrete excessive water loads. Administration of medications causing sodium loss or water retention is a predisposing factor.

◊ Nursing Diagnosis

The nursing assessment data and the presence of clinical manifestations associated with hyponatremia in a patient at risk lead to the appropriate nursing diagnosis. For example, in a patient with diarrhea who drinks large amounts of tap water to relieve thirst, the diagnosis might be stated as follows: alteration in sodium balance (hyponatremia) related to excessive sodium loss and water gain. Once the causative factors have been identified, therapeutic measures are taken to deal with the disturbance. Some of the nursing interventions for this imbalance are independent (such as increasing dietary sodium or limiting free water intake, as tolerated). Often, however, the nursing interventions are meshed with those of other disciplines, such as the safe parenteral administration of fluids containing sodium.

◊ Planning and Implementation

◊   *Goals:*   A major goal is the early detection of hyponatremia so that interventions can be implemented before the condition becomes severe. Once hyponatremia has developed, the goal is a safe return of the serum sodium level to normal. How quickly this can be accomplished depends on a number of variables, such as the cause and severity of the imbalance.

◊ Nursing Interventions

◊   *Early Detection and Control of Hyponatremia.*   One should be aware of patients at risk for hyponatremia and initiate measures to detect the disturbance before it becomes severe. For patients suffering abnormal losses of sodium, yet able to consume a general diet, foods and fluids with a high sodium content are encouraged and provided. For example, broth made with one beef cube contains approximately 900 mg of sodium, and 8 ounces of tomato juice contains approximately 700 mg of sodium.

It is important to be familiar with the sodium content of parenteral fluids (see Table 18–6). When administering fluids to patients with cardiovascular disease, one should monitor the patient for signs of circulatory overload, such as crackles, with auscultation of the lungs. As was stated earlier, extreme care is essential when administering grossly hypertonic sodium fluids (such as 3% or 5% sodium chloride), because these fluids can be lethal if they are infused carelessly.

For patients taking lithium, one should be alert for lithium toxicity when sodium is lost by an abnormal route. In such instances, supplemental salt and fluid are administered. Because diuretics promote sodium loss, patients taking lithium are instructed not to use diuretics unless under close medical supervision. For all patients on lithium therapy, an adequate salt intake should be ensured.

Excess water supplements are avoided in patients receiving isotonic or hypotonic tube feedings, particularly if abnormal sodium loss occurs or water is being abnormally retained (as in SIADH). Actual fluid needs are determined by evaluating the intake and output, urinary specific gravity, and serum sodium levels.

◊   *Safe Return of Serum Sodium Level to Normal.*   When the primary problem is water retention, it is safer to restrict fluid intake than to administer sodium. Administration of sodium to a patient with normovolemia or hypervolemia predisposes to fluid volume overload. As was stated previously, patients with cardiovascular disease receiving fluids containing sodium should be monitored very closely for signs of circulatory overload, such as crackles. In severe hyponatremia, the aim of therapy is to elevate the serum sodium level only enough to alleviate neurologic signs. For example, it has been recommended that the serum sodium concentration be raised to a level no higher than 125 mEq/L (SI: 125 mmol/L) with hypertonic saline.

◊ Evaluation

Expected Outcomes
1. Oriented to time, place, and person
2. Reports decreased muscle cramping and muscle twitching
3. Exhibits normal strength of upper and lower extremities
4. Reports decreased level of fatigue, exhaustion, and lethargy
5. Achieves normal body weight
6. Excretes normal urine volume with normal concentration and specific gravity
7. Demonstrates no seizure activity
8. Consumes food and fluids within prescribed fluid and sodium intake
9. Exhibits absence of precipitating risk factors (*e.g.,* gastrointestinal loss of sodium, diuretic therapy, excessive intake of electrolyte-free fluid)

Sodium Excess (Hypernatremia)

Definition and Etiology

Hypernatremia refers to a greater than normal serum sodium level, that is, a serum level greater than 145 mEq/L (SI: 145 mmol/L). It can be caused by a gain of sodium in excess of water or by a loss of water in excess of sodium. It can occur in patients with normal fluid volume or in those with FVD or FVE.

A common cause of hypernatremia is deprivation of water in unconscious patients who are unable to perceive or respond to thirst. Most often affected are very old, very young, and cognitively impaired patients who are unable to communicate their thirst. Administration of hypertonic tube feedings without adequate water supplements leads to hypernatremia, as does watery diarrhea and greatly increased insensible water loss (as in hyperventilation or denuding effects of burns). Diabetes insipidus leads to hypernatremia if the patient does not experience, or cannot respond, to thirst or if fluids are excessively restricted. Less common are heatstroke, drowning in sea water (which contains a sodium concentration of approximately 500 mEq/L), and malfunction of either hemodialysis or peritoneal dialysis proportioning systems.

Clinical Manifestations

The clinical manifestations of hypernatremia are primarily neurologic and are presumably the consequence of cellular dehydration. Hypernatremia results in a relatively concentrated ECF, causing water to be pulled from the cells (see Fig. 18–3). Clinically, these changes may be manifested by restlessness and weakness in moderate hypernatremia and by disorientation, delusions, and hallucinations in severe hypernatremia. Dehydration (hypernatremia) is often overlooked as the primary reason for behavioral changes in the elderly. If hypernatremia is severe, permanent brain damage can occur (especially in children). Brain damage is apparently due to subarachnoid hemorrhages that result from brain contraction.

A primary characteristic of hypernatremia is thirst. Thirst is so strong a defender of serum sodium levels in normal people that hypernatremia never occurs unless the person is unconscious or is denied access to water; unfortunately, ill people may have an impaired thirst mechanism. Other signs include dry, swollen tongue and sticky mucous membranes. A mild elevation in body temperature may occur, but on correction of the hypernatremia the body temperature should return to normal.

Diagnostic Evaluation

In hypernatremia the serum sodium level is greater than 145 mEq/L (SI: 145 mmol/L) and the serum osmolality is greater than 295 mOsm/kg (SI: 295 mmol/L). The urinary specific gravity is greater than 1.015 as the kidneys attempt to conserve water (provided the water loss is from a route other than the kidneys).

Management

Treatment of hypernatremia consists of a *gradual* lowering of the serum sodium level by the infusion of a hypotonic electrolyte solution (such as 0.3% sodium chloride). A hypotonic sodium solution is considered safer than 5% dextrose in water by many clinicians because it allows a gradual reduction in the serum sodium level and thus decreases the risk of cerebral edema. A rapid reduction in the serum sodium level temporarily decreases the plasma osmolality below that of the fluid in the brain tissue, causing dangerous cerebral edema.

There is not agreement about the exact rate at which serum sodium levels should be reduced. As a general rule, the serum sodium level is reduced at a rate no faster than 2 mEq/L/hr to allow sufficient time for readjustment through diffusion across fluid compartments.

▶ Nursing Process
The Patient With Sodium Excess

▷ Assessment

Fluid losses and gains are carefully monitored in patients at risk for hypernatremia. One should look for abnormal losses of water or low water intake and for large gains of sodium, as might occur with ingestion of proprietary drugs with a high sodium content (such as Alka-Seltzer). Also, it is important to obtain a drug history, as some prescription drugs may have a high sodium content.

The presence of thirst or an elevated body temperature is noted and evaluated in relation to other clinical signs. The patient is monitored for changes in behavior, such as restlessness, disorientation, and lethargy.

▷ Nursing Diagnosis

The nursing assessment and identification of the presence of clinical manifestations associated with hypernatremia in patients at risk for this disorder should lead to the appropriate nursing diagnosis. For example, in a confused elderly patient unable to respond to thirst, the nursing diagnosis might be alteration in sodium balance (hypernatremia) related to inadequate water intake.

▷ Planning and Implementation

▷ *Goals:* A major goal is to prevent hypernatremia in patients at risk. Once hypernatremia has developed, the primary goal is to return the serum sodium level to normal gradually, thus avoiding further cerebral changes.

▷ Nursing Interventions

▷ *Prevention of Hypernatremia.* The nurse attempts to prevent hypernatremia by offering fluids at regular intervals, particularly in debilitated patients unable to perceive or respond to thirst. If fluid intake remains inadequate, the nurse consults with the physician to plan an alternate route for intake, either by tube feedings or by the parenteral route. If tube feedings are used, sufficient water should be administered to keep the serum sodium and blood urea nitrogen levels within normal limits. As a general rule, the higher the osmolality of the tube feeding, the greater is the need for water supplementation.

For patients with diabetes insipidus, it is important to ensure adequate water intake. If the patient is alert and has an intact thirst mechanism, merely providing access to water may be sufficient. If the patient has a decreased level of consciousness, or other disability interfering with adequate fluid intake, however, parenteral fluid replacement may be prescribed. This therapy in patients with neurologic disorders, particularly in the early postoperative period, can be anticipated.

▷ *Safe Correction of Hypernatremia.* When hypernatremia is present and parenteral fluids are necessary for its management, the nurse monitors the patient's response to the fluids by reviewing serial serum sodium levels and by observing for changes in neurologic signs. With a gradual decrease in the serum sodium level, the neurologic signs should improve. As stated in the section on management, too rapid reduction in the serum sodium level renders the plasma temporarily hypoosmotic to the fluid in the brain tissue, causing dangerous cerebral edema.

▷ Evaluation

Expected Outcomes
1. Oriented to time, place, and person
2. Exhibits absence of delusions, hallucinations, and restlessness
3. Reports normal thirst
4. Exhibits moist skin and mucous membranes
5. Demonstrates normal body temperature
6. Excretes normal urinary volume with normal specific gravity
7. Consumes adequate fluid and adheres to low-sodium diet

8. States rationale for adequate fluid intake and sodium restriction
9. Reports decreased lethargy
10. Exhibits normal serum and urinary sodium levels
11. Exhibits absence of precipitating risk factors (*e.g.,* excessive fluid restriction, ingestion of hypertonic tube feedings, excess fluid loss from diabetes insipidus)

Potassium Imbalances

Disturbances in potassium balance are common, as they are associated with a number of disease and injury states. Unfortunately, they may also be induced by medications such as diuretics, laxatives, and certain antibiotics, as well as by therapies such as hyperalimentation and chemotherapy. It is helpful to review some pertinent facts about potassium before proceeding to a discussion of hypokalemia and hyperkalemia.

Functions of Potassium

Potassium is the major intracellular electrolyte; in fact, 98% of the body's potassium is inside the cells. The remaining 2% is in the ECF; it is this 2% that is all important in neuromuscular function. Potassium influences both skeletal and cardiac muscle activity. For example, alterations in its concentration change myocardial irritability and rhythm. Potassium is constantly moving in and out of cells according to the body's needs, under the influence of the sodium-potassium pump. The normal serum potassium concentration ranges from 3.5 to 5.5 mEq/L (SI: 3.5 to 5.5 mmol/L), and even minor variations are significant. Normal renal function is necessary for maintenance of potassium balance, because 80% of the potassium is excreted daily from the body by way of the kidneys. The other 20% is lost through the bowel and sweat glands.

Potassium Deficit (Hypokalemia)

Definition and Etiology

Hypokalemia refers to a below-normal serum potassium concentration. It usually indicates a real deficit in total potassium stores; however, it may occur in patients with normal potassium stores when alkalosis is present, as alkalosis causes a temporary shift of serum potassium into the cells. (See pp. 331–332 for a discussion of alkalosis.)

As stated earlier, hypokalemia is a common imbalance. Gastrointestinal loss of potassium is probably the most common cause of potassium depletion. Vomiting and gastric suction frequently lead to hypokalemia, partly because of actual potassium loss in gastric fluid, but largely because of increased renal potassium loss associated with metabolic alkalosis. Relatively large amounts of potassium are contained in intestinal fluids; for example, diarrheal fluid may contain as much as 30 mEq/L. Therefore, potassium deficit occurs frequently with diarrhea, prolonged intestinal suction, recent ileostomy, and villous adenoma (a tumor of the intestinal tract characterized by excretion of potassium-rich mucus).

Alterations in acid–base balance have a significant effect on potassium distribution. The mechanism involves shifts of hydrogen ions and potassium ions between the cells and ECF. Hypokalemia can cause alkalosis, and alkalosis can cause hypokalemia. For example, hydrogen ions move out of the cells in alkalotic states to help correct the high *p*H, and potassium ions move in to maintain electroneutrality. (See pp. 329–333 for a discussion of acid–base balance.)

Hyperaldosteronism increases renal potassium wasting and can lead to severe potassium depletion. Primary hyperaldosteronism is seen in patients with adrenal adenomas. Secondary hyperaldosteronism occurs in patients with cirrhosis, nephrotic syndrome, congestive heart failure, and malignant hypertension. Potassium-losing diuretics, such as furosemide, the thiazides, and ethacrynic acid, can certainly induce hypokalemia, particularly when given in large doses to patients with poor potassium intake. Other medications that can lead to hypokalemia include steroids, sodium penicillin, carbenicillin, and amphotericin B.

Entry of potassium into skeletal muscle and hepatic cells is promoted by insulin. Thus, patients with persistent insulin hypersecretion may experience hypokalemia; this is often seen in patients receiving high-carbohydrate parenteral fluids (as in hyperalimentation).

Patients unable or unwilling to eat a normal diet for a prolonged period are candidates for hypokalemia. This may occur in debilitated elderly people, alcoholics, and patients with anorexia nervosa. In addition to poor intake, people with bulimia frequently suffer increased potassium loss through self-induced vomiting and laxative and diuretic abuse.

Clinical Manifestations

Potassium deficiency can result in widespread derangements in physiologic function. Most important, severe hypokalemia can result in death through cardiac or respiratory arrest. Clinical signs rarely develop before the serum potassium level has fallen below 3 mEq/L (SI: 3 mmol/L) unless the rate of fall has been rapid. Manifestations of hypokalemia include fatigue, anorexia, nausea, vomiting, muscle weakness, decreased bowel motility, paresthesias, dysrhythmias, and increased sensitivity to digitalis. If prolonged, hypokalemia can lead to impaired renal concentrating ability, causing dilute urine, polyuria, nocturia, and polydipsia.

Diagnostic Evaluation

In hypokalemia, the serum potassium concentration is less than the lower limit of normal. Electrocardiographic changes can include flat T waves and ST segment depression (Fig. 18–4). Hypokalemia increases sensitivity to digitalis, predisposing to digitalis toxicity at lower digitalis levels. Metabolic alkalosis is

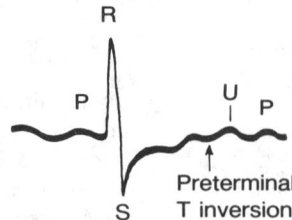

Figure 18–4. Electrocardiogram in hypokalemia. Note increased height of U wave.

frequently associated with hypokalemia. This is discussed further in the section on acid–base disturbances.

Management

The best treatment of hypokalemia is prevention. Potassium loss must be corrected daily; administration of 40 to 60 mEq/day of potassium is adequate in the adult if there are no abnormal losses of potassium. For patients at risk, a diet containing sufficient potassium should be provided; dietary intake of potassium in the average adult is 50 to 100 mEq/day. Foods high in potassium include raisins, bananas, apricots, oranges, avocados, beans, and potatoes. When dietary intake is inadequate for any reason, the physician may prescribe potassium supplements. Many salt substitutes contain 50 to 60 mEq of potassium per teaspoon and may be all the patient needs to supplement potassium intake.

When oral administration of potassium is not feasible, the intravenous route is indicated. In fact, the intravenous route is mandatory for patients with severe hypokalemia (such as a serum level of 2 mEq/L). Although potassium chloride is usually used to correct potassium deficits, the physician may prescribe potassium acetate or potassium phosphate.

▶ Nursing Process
The Patient With Potassium Deficit
▷ Assessment

Because hypokalemia can be life threatening, it is important to monitor for its early presence in patients at risk. The presence of fatigue, anorexia, muscle weakness, decreased bowel motility, paresthesias, or dysrhythmias should prompt one to examine the serum potassium concentration. When available, electrocardiograms may provide useful information. Patients receiving digitalis who are at risk for potassium deficiency should be monitored closely for signs of digitalis toxicity, because hypokalemia potentiates the action of digitalis. In fact, physicians usually prefer to keep the serum potassium level greater than 3.5 mEq/L (SI: 3.5 mmol/L) in digitalized patients.

▷ Nursing Diagnosis

The nursing assessment data and identification of patients at risk for this disturbance lead to the appropriate nursing diagnosis. For example, in a patient with diarrhea, the diagnosis might be stated as follows: alteration in potassium imbalance (hypokalemia) related to excessive potassium loss in diarrheal fluid. Once the etiologic factors have been identified, therapeutic measures are taken to deal with the imbalance.

▷ Planning and Implementation

▷ *Goals:* A major goal is the prevention of hypokalemia. Once it has developed, the goal of nursing management is to help correct the condition safely before serious derangements in cardiac or respiratory function occur.

▷ Nursing Interventions

▷ *Prevention of Hypokalemia.* Measures are taken to prevent hypokalemia when possible. Prevention may take the form of encouraging extra potassium intake for the patient at risk (when

the diet allows). See Table 18-7 for a list of high-potassium foods. When hypokalemia is due to abuse of laxatives or diuretics, patient education may help alleviate the problem. Part of the health history and assessment should be directed at identifying problems amenable to prevention through education.

▷ *Safe Correction of Hypokalemia.* Great care should be exercised when administering potassium intravenously. Concentrated potassium solutions are *never* administered without first diluting them as directed by the manufacturer. The usual concentration is 40 mEq/L of infusion solution, with 80 mEq/L as the maximum desired concentration. In general, concentrations greater than 60 mEq/L are not given in peripheral veins, because venous pain and sclerosis may occur. For routine maintenance needs, potassium is administered at a rate no faster than 10 mEq/hr, suitably diluted.

In critical situations, more concentrated solutions (such as 20 mEq/dl) may be administered through a central line. Even in extreme hypokalemia, it is recommended that potassium be administered no faster than 20 to 40 mEq/hr (suitably diluted); in such a situation, the patient must be monitored by electrocardiogram (ECG) and observed closely for other signs, such as changes in muscle strength.

Potassium should be administered only after adequate urine flow has been established. A decrease in urine volume to less than 20 ml/hr for 2 consecutive hours is an indication to stop potassium infusion until the situation is evaluated. Potassium is primarily excreted by the kidneys; therefore, when oliguria is present, administration of potassium can cause the serum potassium concentration to rise to dangerous levels.

Potassium replacement must be administered cautiously to the elderly because they have a lower lean body mass and total body potassium level and therefore lower potassium requirements. Additionally, with the physiologic loss of renal function with advancing years, administered potassium may be retained more readily than in younger persons.

▷ Evaluation

Expected Outcomes
1. Exhibits normal cardiac function with regular pulse rate, normal electrocardiogram, and absence of dysrhythmias
2. Demonstrates normal muscle strength of upper and lower extremities
3. Exhibits normal bowel sounds and gastrointestinal function
4. Reports decreased level of fatigue
5. Reports normal appetite without nausea or vomiting

TABLE 18-7. *Some High-Potassium Foods*

Food	Potassium (mg, approximate)
Apricots, raw, 3 medium	313
Bananas, raw, 1 medium	451
Orange, navel, raw, 1 medium	250
Potato, baked, without skin	610

(Adapted from Pennington J and Church H. Boxes and Church's Food Values of Portions Commonly Used, 15th ed. Philadelphia, JB Lippincott, 1989.)

6. Consumes prescribed foods high in potassium and potassium supplements.
7. Excretes adequate urine volume
8. Exhibits absence of precipitating risk factors (*e.g.,* diarrhea, vomiting, laxative and diuretic abuse)

Potassium Excess (Hyperkalemia)

Definition and Etiology

Hyperkalemia refers to a greater than normal serum potassium concentration. It seldom occurs in patients with normal renal function. Like hypokalemia, it is often due to iatrogenic (treatment-induced) causes. Although less common than hypokalemia, it is usually more dangerous because cardiac arrest is more frequently associated with high serum potassium levels.

Before considering real causes of hyperkalemia, one must be aware that there are a number of causes of factitious ("pseudo") hyperkalemia. The most common are the use of a tight tourniquet around an exercising extremity while drawing the blood sample and hemolysis of the sample before analysis. Other causes include marked leukocytosis or thrombocytosis and drawing blood above a site where potassium is infusing. Failure to be aware of factitious causes of hyperkalemia can result in aggressive treatment of nonexistent hyperkalemia, resulting in serious lowering of serum potassium levels. Thus, measurements of grossly elevated levels should be corroborated.

The major cause of hyperkalemia is decreased renal excretion of potassium. Thus, significant hyperkalemia is commonly seen in untreated patients with renal failure, particularly when potassium is being liberated from cells during infectious processes or exogenous sources of potassium are excessive, as in diet or medications. A deficiency of adrenal steroids causes sodium loss and potassium retention; thus, hypoaldosteronism and Addison's disease predispose to hyperkalemia.

Drug therapy has been implicated as a probable contributing factor in more than 60% of the hyperkalemic episodes identified through retrospective studies. Drugs commonly implicated are potassium chloride, captopril, nonsteroidal anti-inflammatory agents, and potassium-sparing diuretics. In most such cases, potassium regulation is compromised by renal insufficiency.

Although a high intake of potassium can cause severe hyperkalemia in patients with impaired renal function, the disorder rarely occurs in normal people. For all patients, however, improper use of potassium supplements predisposes to hyperkalemia, especially when salt substitutes are used. It should be remembered that not all patients receiving potassium-losing diuretics require potassium supplements. Certainly those patients receiving potassium-conserving diuretics should not receive supplements. Potassium supplements are extremely dangerous when patients have impaired renal function and thus decreased ability to excrete potassium. Even more dangerous is the intravenous administration of potassium to such patients, as serum levels can rise very quickly. Aged blood should not be given to patients with impaired renal function because the serum concentration of stored blood increases as storage time increases, a result of red blood cell deterioration. It is possible to exceed the renal tolerance of *any* patient with rapid intravenous potassium administration, as well as when large amounts of oral potassium supplements are ingested.

In the presence of acidosis, potassium leaks out of the cells into the ECF. This occurs as hydrogen ions enter the cells, a process that buffers the *p*H of the ECF. (See pp. 331 for further discussion of acidosis.) An elevated extracellular potassium level should be anticipated when extensive tissue trauma has occurred, as in burns, crushing injuries, or severe infections. Similarly, it can occur with lysis of malignant cells after chemotherapy.

Clinical Manifestations

By far the most clinically important effect of hyperkalemia is its effect on the myocardium. Cardiac effects of an elevated serum potassium level are usually not significant below a concentration of 7 mEq/L (SI: 7 mmol/L), but they are almost always present when the level is 8 mEq/L (SI: 8 mmol/L) or greater. As the plasma potassium concentration is increased, disturbances in cardiac conduction occur. The earliest changes, often occurring at a serum potassium level greater than 6 mEq/L (SI: 6 mmol/L), are peaked narrow T waves and a shortened QT interval. If the serum potassium level continues to rise, the PR interval becomes prolonged and is followed by disappearance of the P waves. Finally, there is decomposition and prolongation of the QRS complex (Fig. 18–5). Ventricular dysrhythmias and cardiac arrest may occur at any point in this progression.

Severe hyperkalemia causes muscle weakness and even paralysis, related to a depolarization block in muscle. Similarly, ventricular conduction is slowed. Although hyperkalemia has marked effects on the peripheral neuromuscular system, it has little effect on the central nervous system. Rapidly ascending muscular weakness leading to flaccid quadriplegia has been reported in patients with very high serum potassium levels. Paralysis of respiratory muscles and those required for phonation can also occur.

Gastrointestinal manifestations, such as nausea, intermittent intestinal colic, and diarrhea, may occur in hyperkalemic patients.

Diagnostic Evaluation

Serum potassium levels and electrocardiographic changes are crucial to the diagnosis of hyperkalemia. See the discussion of clinical manifestations.

Management

In nonacute situations, restriction of dietary potassium and potassium-containing medications may suffice. For example, eliminating the use of potassium-containing salt substitutes in the patient taking a potassium-conserving diuretic may be all that is needed to deal with mild hyperkalemia. Prevention of serious hyperkalemia by the administration of cation-exchange resins (such as Kayexalate) may be necessary in renal patients.

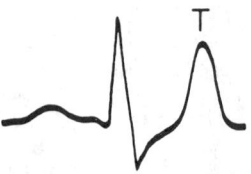

Figure 18–5. Electrocardiogram in hyperkalemia, showing widening QRS complex, decreased amplitude of P wave, and peaked T wave.

Emergency Measures

In emergency situations, it may be necessary to administer calcium gluconate intravenously. Within minutes after administration, calcium antagonizes the action of hyperkalemia on the heart. The ECG should be continuously monitored during administration; the appearance of bradycardia is an indication to stop the infusion. The myocardial protective effects of calcium are transient, lasting about 30 minutes. Extra caution is required if the patient has been digitalized, because parenteral administration of calcium sensitizes the heart to digitalis and may precipitate digitalis toxicity.

Intravenous administration of sodium bicarbonate may be necessary to alkalinize the plasma and cause a temporary shift of potassium into the cells. Also, sodium bicarbonate furnishes sodium to antagonize the cardiac effects of potassium. Effects of this therapy begin within 30 to 60 minutes and may persist for hours; however, they are only temporary.

Intravenous administration of regular insulin and hypertonic dextrose causes a temporary shift of potassium into the cells. Glucose and insulin therapy has an onset of action within 30 minutes and lasts for several hours.

The above stopgap measures only temporarily protect the patient from hyperkalemia. If the hyperkalemic condition is not transient, actual removal of potassium from the body is required; this may be accomplished by way of cation-exchange resins, peritoneal dialysis, or hemodialysis.

▶ Nursing Process
The Patient With Potassium Excess

◊ Assessment

Patients at risk for potassium excess should be identified so they can be monitored closely for signs of hyperkalemia. (See the section dealing with etiologic factors.) The nurse observes for signs of muscular weakness and dysrhythmias. The presence of paresthesias is noted, as are gastrointestinal symptoms such as nausea and intestinal colic. For patients at risk, serum potassium levels are measured periodically.

It is important to remember that elevated serum potassium levels may be erroneous; thus, grossly abnormal levels should be corroborated. To avoid false reports of hyperkalemia, prolonged use of a tourniquet while drawing the blood sample is avoided and the patient is cautioned not to exercise the extremity immediately before drawing of the sample. The blood sample is taken to the laboratory as soon as possible, because hemolysis of the sample results in a falsely elevated serum potassium level.

◊ Nursing Diagnosis

The nursing assessment data are used to identify the patient at risk for this disturbance and nursing diagnoses are identified. For example, in a patient with oliguric renal failure, the nursing diagnosis might be stated as alteration in potassium balance (hyperkalemia) related to decreased potassium excretion.

◊ Planning and Implementation

◊ *Goals:* A major goal in the care of patients at risk for hyperkalemia is prevention of the disorder. If the imbalance cannot be prevented, it must be detected early so that thera-

peutic interventions can be undertaken to safely restore potassium balance and prevent life-threatening effects including cardiac arrest.

◊ Nursing Interventions

◊ *Prevention of Hyperkalemia.* Measures are taken to prevent hyperkalemia in patients at risk, when possible, by encouraging the patient to adhere to the prescribed potassium restriction. Foods high in potassium to be avoided include coffee, cocoa, tea, dried fruits, dried beans, and whole grain breads. Milk and eggs also contain substantial amounts of potassium. Conversely, foods with minimal potassium content include butter, margarine, cranberry juice or sauce, ginger ale, gumdrops or jellybeans, lollipops, root beer, sugar, and honey.

◊ *Safe Restoration of Potassium Balance.* As stated earlier, it is possible to exceed the tolerance for potassium in any person if the substance is administered rapidly by the intravenous route. Therefore, great care should be taken to monitor potassium solutions closely, paying careful attention to the solution's concentration and rate of administration. When adding potassium to parenteral solutions, the added potassium is mixed with the fluid by inverting the bottle several times. Potassium chloride should *never* be added to a hanging bottle because it might result in the potassium being administered as a bolus (potassium chloride is heavy and settles to the bottom of the container).

It is important to caution patients to use salt substitutes sparingly if they are taking other supplementary forms of potassium or potassium-conserving diuretics. Also, potassium-conserving diuretics (such as spironolactone, triamterene, and amiloride), potassium supplements, and salt substitutes should not be administered to patients with renal dysfunction. Most salt substitutes contain approximately 60 mEq of potassium per teaspoon.

◊ Evaluation

Expected Outcomes

1. Exhibits normal cardiac function with normal pulse rate and no dysrhythmias on ECG
2. Excretes adequate urine volume
3. Exhibits normal thoracic excursion and normal respiratory function
4. Reports normal gastrointestinal function without diarrhea or abdominal cramping
5. Consumes foods low in potassium and avoids use of salt substitutes
6. States rationale for low-potassium diet
7. Exhibits normal serum potassium level
8. Exhibits absence of precipitating risk factors (*e.g.,* decreased renal function, excessive intake of potassium, extensive tissue trauma as in burns or crushing injuries)

Calcium Imbalances

Because many factors affect calcium regulation, both hypocalcemia and hypercalcemia are relatively common disturbances. To facilitate understanding of calcium disturbances, it is helpful to review factors affecting calcium balance.

Functions of Calcium

Over 99% of the body's calcium is concentrated in the skeletal system, where it is a major component of strong durable bones and teeth. About 1% of skeletal calcium is rapidly exchangeable with blood calcium; the rest is more stable and only slowly exchanged. The small amount of calcium located outside the bone circulates in the serum, partly bound to protein and partly ionized. Calcium helps hold body cells together. In addition, calcium exerts a sedative action on nerve cells and thus plays a major role in the transmission of nerve impulses. It helps regulate muscle contraction and relaxation, including normal heartbeat. Calcium is instrumental in activating enzymes that stimulate many essential chemical reactions in the body and also plays a role in blood coagulation.

The normal total serum calcium level is 8.5 to 10.5 mg/dl (SI: 2.1–2.6 mmol/L). About 50% of the serum calcium exists in an ionized form that is physiologically active and important for neuromuscular activity. The remainder of serum calcium exists bound to serum proteins, primarily albumin.

Calcium Deficit (Hypocalcemia)

Definition and Etiology

Hypocalcemia refers to a lower than normal serum concentration of calcium, which occurs in a variety of clinical situations. A patient, however, may have a total body calcium deficit (as in osteoporosis) and maintain a normal serum calcium level. Bed rest in the elderly person with osteoporosis is hazardous because impaired calcium metabolism with increased bone resorption is associated with immobilization.

A number of factors can cause hypocalcemia. Primary hypoparathyroidism results in this disturbance, as does surgical hypoparathyroidism. The latter is far more common. Not only is it associated with thyroid and parathyroid operations, but it can also occur after radical neck dissection and is most likely in the first 24 to 48 hours after surgery. Transient hypocalcemia can occur with massive administration of citrated blood (as in exchange transfusions in newborns), because citrate can combine with ionized calcium and temporarily remove it from the circulation.

Inflammation of the pancreas causes release of proteolytic and lipolytic enzymes; it is thought that calcium ions combine with the fatty acids released by lipolysis, forming soaps. As a result of this process, hypocalcemia is common in pancreatitis. It has also been suggested that hypocalcemia might be related to excessive secretion of glucagon from the inflamed pancreas, resulting in increased secretion of calcitonin (a hormone that lowers serum calcium).

Hypocalcemia is common in patients with renal failure because these patients frequently have elevated serum phosphate levels. Hyperphosphatemia usually causes a reciprocal drop in the serum calcium level. Other causes of hypocalcemia can include inadequate vitamin D consumption, magnesium deficiency, medullary thyroid carcinoma, low serum albumin levels, and alkalosis. Drugs predisposing to hypocalcemia can include aluminum-containing antacids, aminoglycosides, caffeine, cisplatin, corticosteroids, mithramycin, phosphates, isoniazid, and loop diuretics.

A condition referred to as osteoporosis is associated with prolonged low intake of calcium and represents a total body calcium deficit, even though serum calcium levels are usually normal. This disease strikes millions of Americans, mostly women. It is characterized by loss of bone mass, causing bones to become porous and brittle and, therefore susceptible to fracture (see Chap. 58).

Clinical Manifestations

Tetany is the most characteristic manifestation of hypocalcemia. Tetany refers to the entire symptom complex induced by increased neural excitability. These symptoms are due to spontaneous discharges of both sensory and motor fibers in peripheral nerves. Sensations of tingling may occur in the tips of the fingers, around the mouth, and, less commonly, in the feet. Spasms of the muscles of the extremities and face may occur. Pain may develop as a result of these spasms.

Trousseau's sign (Fig. 18–6) can be elicited by inflating a blood pressure cuff on the upper arm to about 20 mm Hg above systolic pressure; within 2 to 5 minutes carpal spasm will occur as ischemia of the ulnar nerve develops. Chvostek's sign consists of twitching of muscles supplied by the facial nerve when the nerve is tapped about 2 cm anterior to the earlobe, just below the zygomatic arch.

Seizures may occur because hypocalcemia increases irritability of the central nervous system as well as of the peripheral nerves. Other changes associated with hypocalcemia include an increased QT interval and mental changes such as emotional depression, impairment of memory, confusion, delirium, and even hallucinations. Chronic hypocalcemia in children can retard growth and reduce the IQ.

Diagnostic Evaluation

When evaluating serum calcium levels, one must consider several other variables, such as serum protein levels and arterial *p*H. Clinically, it is important to correlate the serum calcium concentration with the serum albumin level. Each fall (or rise) of the serum albumin level by 1 g/dl (beyond the normal range of 4 to 5 g/dl)(SI: 40 to 50 g/L) is associated with a fall (or rise) of serum calcium concentration of approximately 0.8 mg/

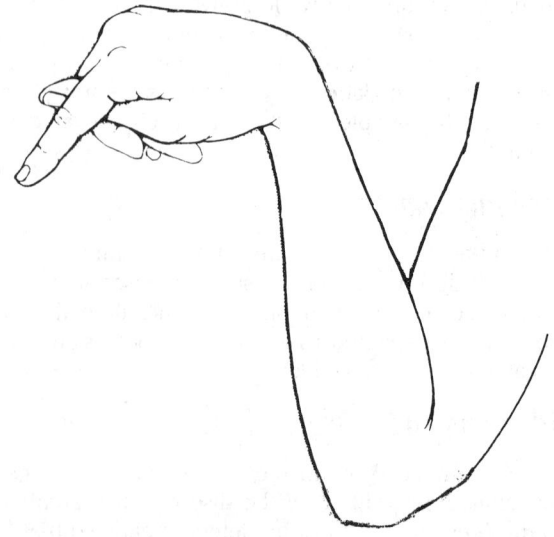

Figure 18–6. Trousseau's sign. Carpopedal spasm with hypocalcemia.

dl (SI: 0.2 mmol/L). For example, if a person with a total serum calcium level of 10 mg/dl, and a serum albumin value of 4 g/dl, develops a decrease in serum albumin level to 3 g/dl, the serum calcium value will drop to 9.2 mg/dl. Because of this, clinicians will often ignore a low serum calcium level in the presence of a similarly low serum albumin level. The ionized calcium level is usually normal in patients with reduced total serum calcium levels and concomitant hypoalbuminemia. When the arterial *p*H increases (alkalosis), more calcium becomes bound to protein. As a result, the ionized portion decreases. Symptoms of hypocalcemia often occur in the presence of alkalosis. Acidosis (low *p*H) has the opposite effect, that is, less calcium is bound to protein and thus more exists in the ionized form. Rarely will signs of hypocalcemia develop in the presence of acidosis, even when the total serum calcium level is lower than normal.

Ideally, the laboratory should measure the ionized level. In most laboratories, however, only the total calcium level is reported; thus, concentration of the ionized fraction must be estimated by simultaneous measurement of serum protein level and arterial *p*H.

Management

Acute symptomatic hypocalcemia is a medical emergency, requiring prompt intravenous administration of calcium. Parenteral calcium salts include calcium gluconate, calcium chloride, and calcium gluceptate. Although calcium chloride produces a significantly higher ionized calcium than an equimolar amount of calcium gluconate, it is not used as often because it is more irritating and can cause sloughing of tissue if allowed to infiltrate. Too rapid intravenous administration of calcium can induce cardiac arrest, preceded by bradycardia. Intravenous calcium administration is particularly dangerous in digitalized patients because calcium ions exert an effect similar to that of digitalis and can cause digitalis toxicity with adverse cardiac effects.

Nursing Interventions

It is important to observe for hypocalcemia in patients at risk. One should be prepared to take seizure precautions when hypocalcemia is severe. The condition of the airway is closely monitored because laryngeal stridor can occur. Safety precautions are taken, as indicated, if confusion is present. Persons at high risk for osteoporosis are instructed about the need for adequate dietary calcium intake; if not consumed in the diet, calcium supplements should be considered. Also, the value of regular exercise in decreasing bone loss should be emphasized, as should the effect of drugs on calcium balance. For example, alcohol and caffeine in high doses inhibit calcium absorption; and moderate cigarette smoking increases urinary calcium excretion.

Calcium Excess (Hypercalcemia)

Definition and Etiology

Hypercalcemia refers to an excess of calcium in the plasma. It is a dangerous imbalance when severe; in fact, hypercalcemic crisis has a mortality as high as 50% if not treated promptly.

The most common causes of hypercalcemia are malignant neoplastic diseases and hyperparathyroidism. Malignant tumors can produce hypercalcemia by a variety of mechanisms. The excessive parathyroid hormone secretion associated with hyperparathyroidism causes increased release of calcium from the bones and increased intestinal and renal absorption of calcium.

Bone mineral is lost during immobilization, sometimes causing elevation of total (and especially ionized) calcium in the bloodstream. Symptomatic hypercalcemia from immobilization, however, is rare; when it does occur it is virtually limited to persons with high calcium turnover rates (such as adolescents during a growth spurt). Most cases of hypercalcemia secondary to immobility occur after severe or multiple fractures or after extensive traumatic paralysis.

Thiazide diuretics may cause a slight elevation in serum calcium levels because they potentiate the action of parathyroid hormone on the kidneys, reducing urinary calcium excretion. The milk-alkali syndrome can occur in patients with peptic ulcer treated for a prolonged period with milk and alkaline antacids, particularly calcium carbonate.

Clinical Manifestations

As a rule, the symptoms of hypercalcemia are proportional to the degree of elevation of the serum calcium level. Hypercalcemia reduces neuromuscular excitability because it acts as a sedative at the myoneural junction. Symptoms such as muscular weakness, incoordination, anorexia, and constipation may be due to decreased tone in smooth and striated muscle.

Anorexia, nausea, vomiting, and constipation are common symptoms of hypercalcemia. Abdominal pain may also be present and at times may be so severe as to be mistaken for an acute abdominal emergency. Abdominal distention and ileus may complicate severe hypercalcemic crisis. Severe thirst may occur, secondary to the polyuria caused by the high solute (calcium) load. Patients with chronic hypercalcemia may develop symptoms similar to those of peptic ulcer because hypercalcemia increases the secretion of acid and pepsin by the stomach.

Mental confusion, impairment of memory, slurred speech, lethargy, acute psychotic behavior, or coma may occur. The more severe symptoms tend to appear when the serum calcium level is approximately 16 mg/dl or above. However, some patients may become profoundly disturbed with serum calcium levels of only 12 mg/dl. These symptoms resolve as serum calcium levels return to normal after treatment.

Polyuria due to disturbed renal tubular function produced by hypercalcemia may be present. Cardiac standstill can occur when the serum calcium is about 18 mg/dl. The inotropic effect of digitalis is enhanced by calcium; therefore, digitalis toxicity is aggravated by hypercalcemia.

Hypercalcemic crisis refers to an acute rise in the serum calcium level to 17 mg/dl or higher. Severe thirst and polyuria are characteristically present. Other findings may include muscular weakness, intractable nausea, abdominal cramps, obstipation (very severe constipation) or diarrhea, peptic ulcer symptoms, and bone pain. Lethargy, mental confusion, and coma may also occur. This condition is very dangerous and may result in cardiac arrest.

Diagnostic Evaluation

The serum calcium level is greater than 10.5 mg/dl (SI: 2.6 mmol/L). Cardiovascular changes may include a variety of dysrhythmias and shortening of the QT interval.

Management

Therapeutic aims in hypercalcemia include decreasing the serum calcium level and reversing the process causing hypercalcemia. General measures include administering fluids to dilute serum calcium and promote its renal excretion, mobilizing the patient, and dietary calcium restriction. Administration of 0.45% sodium chloride or 0.9% sodium chloride solutions intravenously dilutes the serum calcium level and increases urinary calcium excretion by inhibiting tubular reabsorption of calcium. Furosemide (Lasix) is often used in conjunction with saline administration; in addition to causing diuresis, furosemide increases calcium excretion. Calcitonin can be used to lower the serum calcium level and is particularly useful for patients with heart disease or renal failure who cannot tolerate large sodium loads.

For patients with malignant disease, treatment is directed at controlling the condition by surgery, chemotherapy, or radiation therapy. Corticosteroids may be used to decrease bone turnover and tubular reabsorption for patients with sarcoidosis, myelomas, lymphomas, and leukemias; patients with solid tumors are less responsive. Mithramycin, a cytotoxic antibiotic, inhibits bone resorption and thus lowers the serum calcium levels. This drug must be used cautiously because it has significant side effects, including thrombocytopenia, nephrotoxicity, and hepatotoxicity. Inorganic phosphate salts can be given orally or by nasogastric tube (in the form of Phospho-Soda or Neutra-Phos), rectally (as retention Fleet enemas), or intravenously. Intravenous phosphate therapy is used with extreme caution in the treatment of hypercalcemia because it can cause severe calcification in various tissues, including the vein through which it is administered.

Nursing Interventions

It is important to monitor for the occurrence of hypercalcemia in patients at risk for this disorder. Initiation of interventions, such as increasing patient mobility and encouraging fluids, can help prevent hypercalcemia, or at least minimize its severity. Hospitalized patients at risk for hypercalcemia are encouraged to ambulate as soon as possible; outpatients are informed of the importance of frequent ambulation. When encouraging oral fluids, the nurse considers the patient's likes and dislikes. Sodium-containing fluids should be given, unless contraindicated by other conditions, because sodium favors calcium excretion. Patients at home are encouraged to drink 3 to 4 quarts of fluid daily, if possible. Adequate bulk should be provided in the diet to offset the tendency for constipation. Safety precautions are taken, as necessary, when mental symptoms of hypercalcemia are present. The patient and family are informed that these mental changes are reversible with treatment.

Magnesium Imbalances

Functions of Magnesium

Next to potassium, magnesium is the most abundant intracellular cation. It acts as an activator for many intracellular enzyme systems and plays a role in both carbohydrate and protein metabolism. Magnesium balance is important in neuromuscular function. Because magnesium acts directly on the myoneural junction, variations in its serum concentration affect neuromuscular irritability and contractility. For example, an excess of magnesium diminishes excitability of the muscle cells, whereas a deficit increases neuromuscular irritability and contractility. Magnesium produces its sedative effect at the neuromuscular junction, probably by inhibiting the release of the neurotransmitter acetylcholine. It also increases the stimulus threshold in nerve fibers.

Magnesium exerts effects on the cardiovascular system, acting peripherally to produce vasodilation. Magnesium is thought to have a direct effect on peripheral arteries and arterioles, which results in a decreased total peripheral resistance.

Magnesium Deficit (Hypomagnesemia)

Definition and Etiology

Hypomagnesemia refers to a below normal serum magnesium concentration. The normal serum magnesium level is 1.5 to 2.5 mEq/L (or 1.8 to 3.0 mg/dl; SI: 0.75 to 1.25 mmol/L). Approximately one third of serum magnesium is bound to protein; the remaining two thirds exists as free cations (Mg^{2+}). Like calcium, it is the ionized fraction that is primarily involved in neuromuscular activity and other physiologic processes.

Hypomagnesemia is a common imbalance in critically ill patients, yet it is frequently overlooked. Magnesium deficit also occurs in other acutely ill patients, such as those experiencing withdrawal from alcohol and those receiving nourishment after a period of starvation, as in tube feedings or total parenteral nutrition.

An important route for magnesium loss is the gastrointestinal tract. Losses may take the form of drainage from nasogastric suction, diarrhea, or fistulas. Because fluid from the lower gastrointestinal tract is richer in magnesium (10 to 14 mEq/L) than is fluid from the upper tract (1 to 2 mEq/L), losses from diarrhea and intestinal fistulas are more likely to induce magnesium deficit than are those from gastric suction. Although magnesium losses are relatively small in nasogastric suction, hypomagnesemia will occur if losses are prolonged and parenteral fluids are magnesium free. Because the distal small bowel is the major site of magnesium absorption, any disruption in small bowel function, as in intestinal resection or inflammatory bowel disease, can lead to hypomagnesemia.

Alcoholism is currently the most common cause of symptomatic hypomagnesemia in the United States. It is particularly troublesome during treatment of alcohol withdrawal. Because of this, it is recommended that the serum magnesium level be measured every 2 or 3 days in hospitalized patients going through withdrawal from alcohol. Although the serum magnesium level may be normal on admission, it can fall as a result of metabolic changes associated with therapy, such as the intracellular shift of magnesium associated with intravenous glucose administration.

During nutritional repletion, the major cellular electrolytes are taken from the serum and deposited in newly synthesized cells. Thus, if the enteral or parenteral feeding formula is deficient in magnesium content, serious hypomagnesemia will occur. Because of this, serum levels of these primarily intracellular ions should be measured at regular intervals during the administration of total parenteral nutrition and even during enteral feedings, especially to patients who have undergone a period of starvation.

Other causes of hypomagnesemia include the administration of aminoglycosides, cyclosporine, cisplatin, diuretics, digitalis, and amphotericin and the rapid administration of citrated blood, especially to patients with renal or hepatic disease. Magnesium deficiency is often seen in patients with diabetic ketoacidosis; it is primarily the result of increased renal excretion of magnesium during osmotic diuresis and shifting of magnesium into the cells with insulin therapy.

Clinical Manifestations

Clinical manifestations of hypomagnesemia are largely confined to the neuromuscular system. Some of the effects are due directly to the low serum magnesium level; others are due to secondary changes in potassium and calcium metabolism. Symptoms do not usually occur until the serum magnesium level is less than 1 mEq/L (SI: 0.5 mmol/L).

Among the neuromuscular changes are hyperexcitability with muscular weakness, tremors, and athetoid movements (slow, involuntary twisting and writhing movements). Others include tetany, generalized tonic-clonic or focal seizures, laryngeal stridor, and positive Chvostek's and Trousseau's signs (see discussion on p. 324).

Magnesium deficiency predisposes to cardiac dysrhythmias, such as premature ventricular contractions, supraventricular tachycardia, and ventricular fibrillation. Increased susceptibility to digitalis toxicity is associated with low serum magnesium levels. This is an important consideration because patients receiving digoxin are also likely to be on diuretic therapy, predisposing to renal loss of magnesium.

Hypomagnesemia may be accompanied by marked alterations in mood. Apathy, depression, apprehension, or extreme agitation have been noted, as well as ataxia, vertigo, and a confusional state. At times, delirium and frank psychoses may occur, as may auditory or visual hallucinations.

Diagnostic Evaluation

On laboratory analysis, the serum magnesium level is less than 1.5 mEq/L or 1.8 mg/dl (SI: 0.75 mmol/L). Hypomagnesemia is frequently associated with hypokalemia and hypocalcemia.

Management

Mild magnesium deficiency can be corrected by diet alone. Principal dietary sources of magnesium are green vegetables, nuts, and legumes, and fruits such as bananas, grapefruits, and oranges. Magnesium is also plentiful in peanut butter and chocolate. When necessary, magnesium salts can be given orally to replace continuous excessive losses. Patients receiving total parenteral nutrition require magnesium in the intravenous solution to prevent the development of hypomagnesemia.

Overt symptoms of hypomagnesemia are treated with parenteral administration of magnesium. Magnesium sulfate is the most commonly used magnesium salt. Serial magnesium concentrations can be used to regulate the dosage.

Nursing Interventions

The nurse should be aware of patients at risk for hypomagnesemia and observe for its presence. Patients on digitalis are monitored closely because a deficit of magnesium predisposes to digitalis toxicity. When hypomagnesemia is severe, one should be prepared to take seizure precautions. Other safety precautions are instituted, as indicated, if confusion is present.

Because difficulty in swallowing may occur in magnesium-depleted patients, the ability to swallow should be tested with water before oral medications or foods are offered. Dysphagia is probably related to the athetoid or choreiform (rapid, involuntary, and irregular jerky movements) movements associated with magnesium deficit.

When magnesium deficit is due to misuse of diuretics or laxatives, patient education may help alleviate the problem. For patients on a general diet who are experiencing abnormal magnesium losses, the intake of magnesium-rich foods (*e.g.*, green vegetables, nuts and legumes, bananas and oranges) is encouraged.

Magnesium Excess (Hypermagnesemia)

Definition and Etiology

Hypermagnesemia refers to a greater than normal serum concentration of magnesium. A serum magnesium level can appear falsely elevated when blood specimens are allowed to hemolyze or are drawn from an extremity with an excessively tight tourniquet.

By far the most common cause of hypermagnesemia is renal failure. In fact, most patients with advanced renal failure have at least a modest elevation in serum magnesium levels. This condition is aggravated when such patients are given magnesium to control convulsions or inadvertently receive one of the many commercial antacids that contain magnesium salts. Patients with renal failure may also receive an exogenous magnesium load during hemodialysis, either because of inadvertent use of hard water or an error in manufacture of the concentrate used for preparing the dialysate.

Hypermagnesemia can occur in a patient with untreated diabetic ketoacidosis when catabolism causes release of cellular magnesium that cannot be excreted because of profound fluid volume depletion and resulting oliguria. An excess of magnesium can also result from excessive magnesium administration.

Clinical Manifestations

Acute elevation of the serum magnesium level depresses the central nervous system as well as the peripheral neuromuscular junction. At mildly elevated levels, there is a tendency for lowered blood pressure because of peripheral vasodilatation. Facial flushing and hypotension may occur, as well as sensations of warmth. At higher elevations, lethargy, dysarthria, and drowsiness can appear. Deep tendon reflexes are lost and muscular weakness and paralysis may supervene. The respiratory center is depressed when serum magnesium levels exceed 10 mEq/L. Coma and cardiac arrest can occur when the serum magnesium level is greatly elevated.

Diagnostic Evaluation

On laboratory analysis, the serum magnesium level is greater than 2.5 mEq/L or 3.0 mg/dl (SI: 1.25 mmol/L).

Management

The best treatment for hypermagnesemia is prevention. This can be accomplished by avoiding magnesium administration to patients with renal failure and by careful vigilance when magnesium salts are administered to seriously ill patients. In the presence of severe hypermagnesemia, all parenteral and oral magnesium salts are discontinued. When respiratory depression or defective cardiac conduction is present, emergency measures such as ventilatory support and intravenous administration of calcium are indicated. Hemodialysis with a magnesium-free dialysate is an effective treatment that should produce a safe serum magnesium level within hours.

Nursing Interventions

Patients at risk for hypermagnesemia are identified and assessed. When hypermagnesemia is suggested, the nurse should monitor the vital signs, noting the presence of hypotension and shallow respirations, and check for decreased patellar reflexes and changes in the level of consciousness. Care should be taken to avoid giving magnesium-containing medications to patients with renal failure or compromised renal function. Similarly, one should caution patients with renal failure to check with their health care providers before taking over-the-counter medications. Care should also be used when magnesium fluids are administered parenterally, particularly because parenteral magnesium solutions are packaged in greatly different sized containers (such as 2-ml ampules and 50-ml vials), all of which are sometimes loosely referred to as "amps."

Phosphorus Imbalances

Functions of Phosphorus

Phosphorus is a critical constituent of all the body's tissues. It is essential to the function of muscle, red blood cells, and the nervous system and to the intermediary metabolism of carbohydrate, protein, and fat. The normal serum phosphorus level ranges between 2.5 and 4.5 mg/dl (SI: 0.8 to 1.5 mmol/L) and may be as high as 6 mg/dl (SI:1.94 mmol/L) in infants and children. Serum phosphorus levels are presumably greater in children because of the high rate of skeletal growth.

Phosphorus Deficit (Hypophosphatemia)

Definition and Etiology

Hypophosphatemia is defined as a below normal serum concentration of inorganic phosphorus. Although it often indicates phosphorus deficiency, it may occur under a variety of circumstances in which total body phosphorus stores are normal. Conversely, phosphorus deficiency refers to an abnormally low content of phosphorus in lean tissues and may exist in the absence of hypophosphatemia.

Hypophosphatemia may occur during the administration of calories in normally required amounts to patients with severe protein-calorie malnutrition. It is most likely to occur with overzealous refeeding with simple carbohydrates. This syndrome can be induced in anyone with severe protein-calorie malnutrition (such as patients with anorexia nervosa, or alcoholism, or elderly debilitated patients unable to eat). Some sources indicate that as many as 50% of hospitalized chronic alcoholics suffer from hypophosphatemia.

Marked hypophosphatemia may develop in malnourished patients receiving total parenteral nutrition if correction of phosphorus loss is inadequate. Other causes of hypophosphatemia include prolonged intense hyperventilation, alcohol withdrawal, poor dietary intake, diabetic ketoacidosis, and major thermal burns.

Clinical Manifestations

Most of the signs and symptoms of phosphorus deficiency appear to result from deficiency of adenosine triphosphate (ATP), of 2,3-diphosphoglycerate (DPG), or of both. The former impairs cellular energy resources, and the latter impairs oxygen delivery to tissues.

A wide range of neurologic symptoms may occur, such as irritability, apprehension, weakness, numbness, paresthesias, confusion, seizures, and coma. Low levels of 2,3-DPG may reduce the delivery of oxygen to peripheral tissues, resulting in tissue anoxia.

It is thought that hypophosphatemia predisposes to infection. In laboratory animals, hypophosphatemia has been noted to produce depression of the chemotactic, phagocytic, and bacterial activity of granulocytes.

Muscle damage may develop as the ATP level in the muscle tissue declines. This is manifested clinically by muscle weakness, muscle pain, and, at times, acute rhabdomyolysis (disintegration of striated muscle). Weakness of respiratory muscles may greatly impair ventilation. Also, hypophosphatemia may predispose to an insulin-resistant state, and thus hyperglycemia.

Diagnostic Evaluation

On laboratory analysis, the serum phosphorus level will be less than 2.5 mg/dl (SI: 0.80 mmol/L) in adults. It is important to remember that glucose administration causes a slight decrease in the serum phosphorus level.

Management

As in any electrolyte imbalance, the best treatment is prevention. In patients at risk for hypophosphatemia, serum phosphate levels should be closely monitored and correction initiated before deficits become severe. Adequate amounts of phosphorus should be added to hyperalimentation solutions, and attention should also be paid to phosphorus levels in enteral feeding solutions.

Severe hypophosphatemia is dangerous and requires prompt attention. Aggressive intravenous phosphorus correction is usually limited to patients with serum phosphorus levels below 1 mg/dl (SI: 0.3 mmol/L). Possible dangers of intravenous administration of phosphorus include hypocalcemia and metastatic calcification from hyperphosphatemia. In less acute situations, oral phosphorus replacement is satisfactory.

Nursing Interventions

The nurse should identify patients at risk for hypophosphatemia and monitor for its presence. Because malnourished patients receiving hyperalimentation are at risk when calories are introduced too aggressively, prevention can take the form of gradual introduction of the feeding solution to avoid rapid shifts of phosphorus into the cells.

For patients with documented hypophosphatemia, careful attention should be paid to preventing infection because hypophosphatemia may produce changes in the granulocytes. For patients requiring correction of phosphorus losses, frequent monitoring of the serum phosphorus levels is indicated to augment clinical assessment.

Phosphorus Excess (Hyperphosphatemia)

Definition and Etiology

Hyperphosphatemia refers to a serum phosphorus level greater than normal. A variety of conditions can lead to this imbalance.

The most common cause of hyperphosphatemia is decreased renal phosphorus excretion in renal failure. Other causes include chemotherapy for neoplastic disease, high phosphate intake, profound muscle necrosis, and increased phosphorus absorption.

Clinical Manifestations

An elevated serum phosphorus level causes little in the way of symptoms. The most important long-term consequence is soft tissue calcification, which occurs mainly in patients with reduced glomerular filtration rates; the most important short-term consequence is tetany. High levels of serum inorganic phosphorus are harmful because they promote precipitation of calcium phosphate in nonosseous sites. Because of the reciprocal relationship between phosphorus and calcium, a high serum phosphorus level tends to cause a low calcium concentration in the serum. Tetany can result and can present as sensations of tingling in the tips of the fingers and around the mouth.

Diagnostic Evaluation

On laboratory analysis, the serum phosphorus level is greater than 4.5 mg/dl (SI: 1.5 mmol/L) in adults. Serum phosphorus levels are normally higher in children, presumably because of the high rate of skeletal growth.

Management

When possible, treatment is directed at the underlying disorder. For example, hyperphosphatemia related to tumor cell lysis might be lessened by prior administration of allopurinol to prevent urate nephropathy. For patients with renal failure, measures to decrease the serum phosphate level are indicated; these include the administration of phosphate-binding gels, dietary phosphate restriction, and dialysis.

Nursing Interventions

The nurse should be aware of patients at risk for hyperphosphatemia and monitor for its presence. When a low-phosphorus diet is prescribed, the patient is instructed to avoid foods high in phosphorus content. Such foods include hard cheese; cream; nuts; whole grain cereals, dried fruits; dried vegetables; special meats, such as kidneys, sardines, and sweetbreads; and foods made with milk. When appropriate, the nurse instructs the patient to avoid phosphate-containing substances, such as phosphate-containing laxatives and enemas.

In summary, disturbances of fluid and electrolyte balance are common in patients with any number of disorders. Additionally, they can occur in healthy individuals who fail to consume adequate fluids and dietary intake of electrolytes to meet the body's requirements. The hospitalized elderly patient may be at risk for fluid and electrolyte disturbance because of poor dietary intake, fluid losses that often occur with diagnostic procedures, and altered ability to respond quickly to changes in fluid and electrolyte status. Medications may also affect fluid and electrolyte balance. Although common in hospitalized patients, fluid and electrolyte disturbances can be severe and life threatening. Therefore, the nurse caring for *any* patient must be aware of the potential for these disturbances and must use astute assessment strategies to detect their occurrence and prevent their progression.

Major fluid and electrolyte imbalances are summarized in Table 18-8.

Acid–Base Disturbances

Regulation of Acid–Base Balance

There are four types of acid–base imbalances: metabolic acidosis and alkalosis and respiratory acidosis and alkalosis. The causes, characteristics, and management of each of these disorders are discussed here.

Remarkable homeostatic mechanisms exist to maintain plasma pH, an indicator of hydrogen ion (H^+) concentration, within the narrow normal range of 7.35 to 7.45. These consist of chemical buffering mechanisms, the kidneys, and the lungs. In review, pH is defined as H^+ concentration; the more hydrogen ions, the more acidic is the solution. The pH range compatible with life (6.8 to 7.8) represents a tenfold difference in hydrogen ion concentration in plasma.

Chemical Buffers

Chemical buffers are substances that prevent major changes in the pH of body fluids by removing or releasing hydrogen ions; they can act quickly to prevent excessive changes in hydrogen ion concentration. The body's major buffer system is the bicarbonate-carbonic acid (HCO_3^-–H_2CO_3) buffer system. Normally, there are 20 parts of bicarbonate to one part of carbonic acid. If this ratio is upset, the pH will change. It is the ratio that is important in maintaining pH, not absolute values. One must remember that carbon dioxide (CO_2) is a potential acid; when CO_2 is dissolved in water, it becomes carbonic acid ($CO_2 + H_2O = H_2CO_3$). Thus, when carbon dioxide is increased, the carbonic acid content is also increased and vice versa. If either bicarbonate or carbonic acid is increased or decreased so that the 20:1 ratio is no longer maintained, acid–base imbalance results.

Other less important buffer systems in the ECF include the inorganic phosphates and the plasma proteins. Intracellular buffers include proteins, organic and inorganic phosphates, and, in red blood cells, hemoglobin.

Kidneys

The kidneys regulate the bicarbonate level in ECF; they are able to regenerate bicarbonate ions as well as reabsorb them from the renal tubular cells. In the presence of respiratory acidosis, and most cases of metabolic acidosis, the kidneys excrete hydrogen ions and conserve bicarbonate ions to help restore balance. In the presence of respiratory and metabolic alkalosis,

TABLE 18–8.   *Summary of Major Fluid and Electrolyte Imbalances*

Imbalance	Causes	Clinical Signs and Symptoms
Fluid volume deficit	Loss of water and electrolytes, as in vomiting, diarrhea, fistulas, gastrointestinal suction, and third-space fluid shifts; and decreased intake, as in anorexia, nausea, and inability to gain access to fluid	Acute weight loss, decreased skin and tongue turgor, oliguria, concentrated urine, weak rapid pulse, and low central venous pressure
Fluid volume excess	Compromised regulatory mechanisms, such as renal failure, congestive heart failure, and cirrhosis; and overzealous administration of sodium-containing fluids	Acute weight gain, edema, distended veins, crackles, and elevated central venous pressure
Sodium deficit (hyponatremia)	Loss of sodium, as in use of diuretics, loss of gastrointestinal fluids, and adrenal insufficiency; Gain of water, as in excessive administration of D_5W and excessive water supplements for patients receiving hypotonic tube feedings; disease states associated with SIADH such as head trauma and oat cell lung tumor; and pharmacologic agents associated with water retention such as oxytocin and certain tranquilizers	Anorexia, nausea and vomiting, lethargy, confusion, muscle cramps, muscular twitching, seizures, papilledema, serum sodium < 135 mEq/L (SI: 145 mmol/L)
Sodium excess (hypernatremia)	Water deprivation in patients unable to drink at will, hypertonic tube feedings without adequate water supplements, diabetes insipidus, heatstroke, hyperventilation, and watery diarrhea	Thirst, elevated body temperature, swollen dry tongue and sticky mucous membranes, hallucinations, lethargy, irritability, focal or grand mal seizures, serum sodium > 145 mEq/L (SI: 145 mmol/L)
Potassium deficit (hypokalemia)	Diarrhea, vomiting, gastric suction, steroid administration, hyperaldosteronism, carbenicillin, amphotericin B, bulemia, and osmotic diuresis	Fatigue, anorexia, nausea and vomiting, muscle weakness, decreased bowel motility, dysrhythmias, paresthesias, and serum potassium < 3.5 mEq/L (SI: 3.5 mmol/L), and flat T waves on ECG
Potassium excess (hyperkalemia)	Pseudohyperkalemia (as in hemolysis of blood sample), oliguric renal failure, use of potassium-conserving diuretics in patients with renal insufficiency, acidosis	Vague muscular weakness, bradycardia, dysrhythmias, flaccid paralysis, paresthesias, intestinal colic, tall tented T waves on ECG, serum potassium > 5.8 mEq/L (SI: 5.8 mmol/L)
Calcium deficit (hypocalcemia)	Hypoparathyroidism, surgical hypoparathyroidism (may follow thyroid surgery or radical neck dissection), malabsorption, pancreatitis, and alkalosis	Numbness, tingling of fingers, toes, and circumoral region; Trousseau's sign; Chvostek's sign; convulsions; and serum calcium < 8.6 mg/dl (SI: 2.2 mmol/L) or ionized calcium < 50%
Calcium excess (hypercalcemia)	Hyperparathyroidism, malignant neoplastic disease, prolonged immobilization, and overuse of calcium supplements	Muscular weakness, constipation, anorexia, nausea and vomiting, polyuria and polydipsia, neurotic behavior, cardiac dysrhythmias, and serum calcium > 10.5 mg/dl (SI: 2.6 mmol/L)
Magnesium deficit (hypomagnesemia)	Chronic alcoholism, malabsorptive disorders, diabetic ketoacidosis, refeeding after starvation, and certain pharmacologic agents (such as gentamicin and cisplatin)	Neuromuscular irritability, dysrhythmias, disorientation, serum magnesium < 1.5 mEq/L (SI: <0.75 mmol/L)
Magnesium excess (hypermagnesemia)	Renal failure (particularly when magnesium-containing medications are administered), adrenal insufficiency, excessive magnesium administration	Flushing, hypotension, drowsiness, hypoactive reflexes, depressed respirations, cardiac arrest, and coma, and serum Mg > 2.5 mEq/L (SI: 1.25 mmol/L)

(continued)

TABLE 18-8. *(continued)*

Imbalance	Causes	Clinical Signs and Symptoms
Phosphorus deficit (hypophosphatemia)	Refeeding after starvation, alcohol withdrawal, diabetic ketoacidosis, respiratory alkalosis	Paresthesias, muscle weakness, muscle pain and tenderness, mental changes, cardiomyopathy, respiratory failure
Phosphorus excess (hyperphosphatemia)	Renal failure, excessive intake of phosphorus (as in phosphorus supplements and phosphate-containing laxatives)	Short-term consequences (symptoms of tetany, such as tingling of fingertips, and around mouth); long-term consequences (precipitation of calcium phosphate in nonosseous sites)

the kidneys retain hydrogen ions and excrete bicarbonate ions to help restore balance. The kidneys obviously cannot compensate for the metabolic acidosis created by renal failure. Renal compensation for imbalances is relatively slow (a matter of hours or days).

Lungs

The lungs, under the control of the medulla, control the carbon dioxide, and thus carbonic acid content of ECF. They do so by adjusting ventilation in response to the amount of carbon dioxide in the blood. A rise in the partial pressure of carbon dioxide in arterial blood ($PaCO_2$) is a powerful stimulant to respiration. Of course, the partial pressure of oxygen in arterial blood (PaO_2) also influences respiration. Its effect, however, is not as marked as that produced by the $PaCO_2$.

In the presence of metabolic acidosis, the respiratory rate is increased, causing greater elimination of carbon dioxide (to reduce the acid load). In the presence of metabolic alkalosis, the respiratory rate is decreased, causing carbon dioxide to be retained (to increase the acid load).

Metabolic Acidosis (Base Bicarbonate Deficit)

Definition and Etiology

Metabolic acidosis is a clinical disturbance characterized by a low *p*H (increased hydrogen concentration) and a low plasma bicarbonate concentration. It can be produced by a gain of hydrogen ion or a loss of bicarbonate. It can be divided clinically into two forms according to the values of the serum anion gap (AG): high anion gap acidosis and normal anion gap acidosis. Anion gap refers to the difference of anions (negatively charged electrolytes) and cations (electrolytes with a positive charge). The anion gap can be calculated by subtracting the sum of the serum chloride and bicarbonate concentrations (anions, or negatively charged electrolytes) from the serum sodium level (a cation, or positively charged electrolyte): AG = $Na^+ - (Cl^- + HCO_3^-)$. There are some unmeasured anions in the serum, such as sulfates, ketones, and lactic acid, that normally account for less than 16 mEq/L of the anion production. An anion gap greater than 16 mEq suggests excessive accumulation of unmeasured anions.

High anion gap acidosis results from excessive accumulation of fixed acid. It occurs in ketoacidosis, lactic acidosis, late phase of salicylate poisoning, uremia, methanol or ethylene glycol toxicity, and ketoacidosis with starvation. In all of these instances, abnormally high levels of anions flood the system, increasing the anion gap above normal limits.

Normal anion gap acidosis results from direct loss of bicarbonate, as in diarrhea and intestinal fistulas, or from excessive gain of chloride, as in the administration of large quantities of isotonic saline or ammonium chloride.

Clinical Manifestations

Signs and symptoms of metabolic acidosis vary with the severity of metabolic acidosis. They may include headache, confusion, drowsiness, increased respiratory rate and depth, nausea, and vomiting. Peripheral vasodilation and decreased cardiac output occur when the *p*H falls below 7.

Diagnostic Evaluation

Arterial blood gas measurements are valuable in the diagnosis of metabolic acidosis. Expected blood gas changes include a low bicarbonate level (less than 22 mEq/L) and a low *p*H (less than 7.35). Hyperkalemia may accompany metabolic acidosis, as a result of shift of potassium out of the cells. Hyperventilation decreases the carbon dioxide level as a compensatory action. As stated previously, calculation of the anion gap is helpful in determining the cause of metabolic acidosis.

Management

Treatment is directed at correcting the metabolic defect. If the cause of the problem is excessive intake of chloride, treatment is obviously elimination of the source of the chloride. When necessary, bicarbonate is administered.

Metabolic Alkalosis (Base Bicarbonate Excess)

Definition and Etiology

Metabolic alkalosis is a clinical disturbance characterized by a high *p*H (decreased hydrogen ion concentration) and a high plasma bicarbonate concentration. It can be produced by a gain of bicarbonate or a loss of hydrogen ions.

Probably the most common cause of metabolic alkalosis is vomiting or gastric suction with loss of hydrogen and chloride ions; it is particularly a problem in pyloric stenosis because only gastric fluid is lost in this disorder. Gastric fluid has an acid *p*H (usually 1 to 3); therefore, loss of this highly acidic fluid increases alkalinity of body fluids. Other situations predisposing to metabolic alkalosis include those associated with loss of potassium, such as potassium-losing diuretics (*e.g.,* thiazides, furosemide, and ethacrynic acid) and excessive adrenalcorticoid hormones (as in hyperaldosteronism and Cushing's syndrome). Hypokalemia produces alkalosis in two ways: (1) in the presence of hypokalemia, the kidneys conserve potassium and thus hydrogen ion excretion is increased, and (2) cellular potassium moves out of the cells into the ECF in an attempt to maintain near-normal serum levels (as potassium ions [K^+] leave the cells, hydrogen ions must enter to maintain electroneutrality). Excessive alkali ingestion, as of bicarbonate-containing antacids or sodium bicarbonate during cardiopulmonary resuscitation, can also cause metabolic alkalosis.

Clinical Manifestations

Alkalosis is primarily manifested by symptoms related to decreased calcium ionization, such as tingling of the fingers and toes, dizziness, and hypertonic muscles. The ionized fraction of serum calcium decreases in the presence of alkalosis as more calcium combines with serum proteins. Because it is the ionized fraction of calcium that influences neuromuscular activity, it is understandable why symptoms of hypocalcemia are often the predominant symptoms of alkalosis. Respirations are depressed as a compensatory action by the lungs.

Diagnostic Evaluation

Evaluation of arterial blood gases discloses a *p*H greater than 7.45 and a serum bicarbonate concentration greater than 26 mEq/L. The partial pressure of carbon dioxide will increase as the lungs attempt to compensate for the excess bicarbonate by retaining carbon dioxide. This hypoventilation is more pronounced in semiconscious, unconscious, or debilitated patients than in alert patients. The former may develop marked hypoxemia as a result of hypoventilation. Hypokalemia may accompany metabolic alkalosis.

Management

Treatment is aimed at reversal of the underlying disorder. Sufficient chloride must be supplied for the kidney to absorb sodium with chloride (allowing the excretion of excess bicarbonate). Treatment also includes restoration of normal fluid volume by administration of sodium chloride fluids (because continued volume depletion serves to maintain the alkalosis).

Respiratory Acidosis (Carbonic Acid Excess)

Definition and Etiology

Respiratory acidosis is a clinical disorder in which the *p*H is less than 7.35 and the $PaCO_2$ is greater than 42 mm Hg. It may be either acute or chronic.

Respiratory acidosis is always due to inadequate excretion of carbon dioxide with inadequate ventilation, resulting in elevated plasma carbon dioxide levels and thus elevated carbonic acid levels. In addition to an elevated $PaCO_2$, hypoventilation usually causes a decrease in PaO_2. Acute respiratory acidosis occurs in emergency situations, such as acute pulmonary edema, aspiration of a foreign object, atelectasis, pneumothorax, overdosage of sedatives, and severe pneumonia.

Chronic respiratory acidosis is associated with chronic disorders such as emphysema, bronchiectasis, and bronchial asthma.

Clinical Manifestations

Clinical signs are variable in acute and chronic respiratory acidosis. Sudden hypercapnia (elevated $PaCO_2$) can cause increased pulse and respiratory rate, increased blood pressure, mental cloudiness, and feeling of fullness in the head. An elevated $PaCO_2$ causes cerebrovascular vasodilation and increased cerebral blood flow, particularly when it is higher than 60 mm Hg. Ventricular fibrillation may be the first sign of respiratory acidosis in anesthetized patients.

The patient with chronic respiratory acidosis may complain of weakness, dull headache, and symptoms of the underlying disease process. Patients with chronic obstructive pulmonary disease who gradually accumulate carbon dioxide over a prolonged period (days to months) may not develop symptoms of hypercapnia because compensatory renal changes have had time to occur.

- *When the $PaCO_2$ is chronically above 50 mm Hg, the respiratory center becomes relatively insensitive to carbon dioxide as a respiratory stimulant, leaving hypoxemia as the major drive for respiration. Oxygen administration may remove the stimulus of hypoxemia, and the patient develops "carbon dioxide narcosis" unless the situation is quickly reversed. Therefore, oxygen must be administered with caution.*

Diagnostic Evaluation

Arterial blood gas evaluation discloses a *p*H less than 7.35 and a $PaCO_2$ greater than 42 mm Hg in acute respiratory acidosis. When compensation (renal retention of bicarbonate) has fully occurred, the arterial *p*H may be within the lower limits of normal.

Management

Treatment is directed at improving ventilation; exact measures vary with the cause of inadequate ventilation. Pharmacologic agents are used as indicated. For example, bronchodilators help reduce bronchial spasm; antibiotics are used for respiratory infections. Pulmonary hygiene measures are employed, when necessary, to rid the respiratory tract of mucus and purulent drainage. Adequate hydration (2 to 3 L/day) is indicated to keep the mucous membranes moist and thereby facilitate removal of secretions. Supplemental oxygen is used as necessary. A mechanical ventilator, used cautiously, may improve pulmonary ventilation. Overzealous use of a mechanical ventilator may cause such rapid excretion of carbon dioxide that the kidneys will be unable to eliminate excess bicarbonate with sufficient rapidity to prevent alkalosis and convulsions. For this reason, the elevated $PaCO_2$ must be decreased slowly.

Respiratory Alkalosis (Carbonic Acid Deficit)

Definition and Etiology

Respiratory alkalosis is a clinical condition in which the arterial *p*H is greater than 7.45 and the $PaCO_2$ is less than 38 mm Hg. As with respiratory acidosis, acute and chronic conditions can occur in respiratory alkalosis.

Respiratory alkalosis is always due to hyperventilation, which causes excessive "blowing off" of carbon dioxide and, hence, a decrease in plasma carbonic acid content. Causes can include extreme anxiety, hypoxemia, the early phase of salicylate intoxication, gram-negative bacteremia, and excessive ventilation by mechanical ventilators.

Diagnostic Evaluation

Analysis of arterial blood gases is needed to diagnose respiratory alkalosis. In the acute state, the pH is elevated above normal as a result of a low $PaCO_2$ and a normal bicarbonate level. (The kidneys cannot alter the bicarbonate level quickly.) In the compensated state, the kidneys have had sufficient time to lower the bicarbonate level to a suitable level.

Clinical Manifestations

Clinical signs consist of lightheadedness due to vasoconstriction and decreased cerebral blood flow, inability to concentrate, numbness and tingling due to decreased calcium ionization, tinnitus, and at times loss of consciousness.

Management

Treatment depends on the underlying cause of respiratory alkalosis. If due to anxiety, the patient should be made aware that the abnormal breathing pattern is responsible for the symptoms. Instructing the patient to breathe more slowly to cause accumulation of CO_2 or to breathe into a closed system (such as paper bag) is helpful. Usually a sedative is required to relieve hyperventilation in very anxious patients. Treatment for other causes of respiratory alkalosis is directed at correcting the underlying problem.

In summary, disturbances of acid–base balance range from those that are relatively mild problems (*i.e.*, respiratory alkalosis due to hyperventilation) that can be treated easily and quickly to severe, critical disturbances (*i.e.*, diabetic acidosis) that are life-threatening. An understanding of the mechanisms that regulate acid–base balance is essential in anticipating acid–base disturbances and in monitoring the patient for clinical manifestations of these disturbances. The nurse who thoroughly understands the regulatory mechanisms of the lungs, kidneys, and buffer systems can provide better care to patients with actual or potential acid–base disturbances.

A systematic approach to the analysis of acid–base disturbances helps to clarify acid–base concepts (Chart 18–2).

Parenteral Fluid Therapy

Purpose

The choice of an intravenous solution depends on the specific purpose for which it is intended. Generally, intravenous fluids are administered to achieve one or more of the following goals:

- To provide water, electrolytes, and nutrients to meet daily requirements
- To replace water and correct electrolyte deficits
- To provide a medium for intravenous drug administration

Chart 18–2
Systematic Assessment of Arterial Blood Gases

The following steps are recommended to evaluate arterial blood gas values. They are based on the assumption that the average values are

$pH = 7.4$ $PaCO_2 = 40$ mm Hg $HCO_3^- = 24$ mEq/L

1. First, look at the pH. It can be high, low, or normal:

   $pH > 7.4$ (alkalosis)

   $pH < 7.4$ (acidosis)

   $pH = 7.4$ (normal)

2. The next step is to determine the primary cause of the disturbance. This is done by evaluating the $PaCO_2$ and HCO_3^- in relation to the pH:

   $pH > 7.4$ (alkalosis):

   a. If the $PaCO_2$ is <40 mm Hg, the primary disturbance is respiratory alkalosis.

   b. If the HCO_3^- is >24 mEq/L, the primary disturbance is metabolic alkalosis.

   $pH < 7.4$ (acidosis):

   a. If the $PaCO_2$ is >40 mm Hg, the primary disturbance is respiratory acidosis.

   b. If the HCO_3^- is <24 mEq/L, the primary disturbance is metabolic acidosis.

3. The next step involves determining if compensation has begun. This is done by looking at the value other than the primary disorder. If it is moving in the same direction as the primary value, compensation is underway. Consider the following blood gases:

   a. pH 7.20 $PaCO_2 = 60$ mm Hg $HCO_3^- = 23$ mEq/L

   b. pH 7.40 $PaCO_2 = 60$ mm Hg $HCO_3^- = 37$ mEq/L

   In "a," respiratory acidosis is present. Note that the CO_2 level is high, whereas the bicarbonate is normal (uncompensated respiratory acidosis).

   In set "b," the CO_2 is still high, but the HCO_3^- has risen, allowing the pH to return to a normal level (compensated respiratory acidosis).

(Adapted from Metheny N. Fluid and Electrolyte Balance: Nursing Considerations. Philadelphia, JB Lippincott, 1987.)

Intravenous solutions contain dextrose or electrolytes mixed in various proportions with water. Pure or "free" water can never be administered intravenously because it rapidly enters red blood cells and causes them to burst.

Types of Intravenous Solutions

Solutions are often categorized as isotonic, hypotonic, or hypertonic, according to whether their total osmolality is the same as, less than, or greater than that of blood.

Some common water and electrolyte solutions are listed in Table 18–6, with comments about their use. Electrolyte solutions are considered isotonic if the total electrolyte content (anions plus cations) approximates 310 mEq/L. They are considered hypotonic if the total electrolyte content is less than 250 mEq/L and hypertonic if the total electrolyte content exceeds 375 mEq/L. The nurse must also consider a solution's osmolality, keeping in mind that the osmolality of plasma is approximately 300 mOsm/L (SI: 300 mmol/L). For example, a 10% dextrose solution has an approximate osmolality of 505 mOsm/L.

When administering parenteral fluids, it is important to monitor the patient's response to the fluids. One should consider the fluid volume, the content of the fluid, and the patient's clinical status.

Isotonic Fluids

Fluids that are classified as isotonic have a total osmolality close to that of ECF and do not cause red blood cells to shrink or swell. The composition of these fluids may or may not approximate that of ECF, however.

A solution of 5% dextrose in water has a serum osmolality of 252 mOsm/L. Once administered, the glucose is rapidly metabolized, and this initially isotonic solution then disperses as a hypotonic fluid, one third extracellular and two thirds intracellular. Therefore, 5% dextrose in water is mainly used to supply water and to correct an increased serum osmolality. One liter of 5% dextrose in water provides less than 200 kcal and is a minor source of calories for the body's daily requirements.

Normal saline (0.9% sodium chloride) has a total osmolality of 308 mOsm/L. Because the osmolality is entirely contributed by electrolytes, the solution remains within the extracellular compartment. For this reason, normal saline is often used to treat an extracellular volume deficit. Although referred to as normal, it contains only sodium and chloride and does not actually simulate ECF.

Several other solutions contain ions in addition to sodium and chloride and are somewhat more similar to ECF in composition. Ringer's solution contains potassium and calcium in addition to sodium chloride. Lactated Ringer's solution contains bicarbonate precursors as well. These solutions are marketed, with slight variations, under a variety of different trade names.

Hypotonic Fluids

One purpose of hypotonic solutions is to replace cellular fluid, because it is hypotonic as compared with plasma. Another is to provide free water for excretion of body wastes. At times, hypotonic sodium solutions are used to treat hypernatremia and other hyperosmolar conditions. Half-strength saline (0.45%

sodium chloride) is frequently used. Multiple-electrolyte solutions are also available.

Hypertonic Fluids

When 5% dextrose is added to normal saline or Ringer's solution, the total osmolality exceeds that of ECF. The dextrose is quickly metabolized, however, and only the isotonic solution remains. Therefore, any effect on the intracellular compartment is temporary: Similarly, 5% dextrose is usually added to hypotonic multiple-electrolyte solutions. Once the dextrose is metabolized, these solutions disperse as hypotonic fluids.

Higher concentrations of dextrose, such as 50% dextrose in water, are given to help meet calorie requirements. These solutions are strongly hypertonic and must be administered into central veins so that they can be diluted by rapid blood flow.

Saline solutions are also available in osmolar concentrations greater than that of ECF. These solutions draw water from the intracellular compartment to the extracellular compartment and cause cells to shrink. If given rapidly or in quantity, they may cause an extracellular volume excess and precipitate pulmonary edema. As a result, these solutions are given cautiously and usually only when the serum osmolality has decreased to dangerously low levels.

Other Substances Given Intravenously

When the patient's gastrointestinal tract cannot accept food, nutritional requirements are often met intravenously. Parenteral administration may include high concentrations of glucose, protein, or fat to meet nutritional requirements.

Many drugs are also delivered intravenously, either by infusion or directly into the vein. Because intravenous medications circulate rapidly, administration by this route is potentially very hazardous. Administration rates and recommended dilutions for individual medications are available in specialized texts pertaining to intravenous medications.

Nursing Management of the Patient Receiving Intravenous Therapy

Venipuncture

The ability to gain access to the venous system is an expected nursing skill in many settings. Components of this responsibility include knowledgeable selection of venipuncture site and type of cannula, and proficiency in the technique of vein entry.

Before proceeding with venipuncture, decisions must be made as to the most appropriate location and type of cannula for a particular patient. Factors influencing these choices include the type of solution to be administered, the expected length of intravenous therapy, the patient's general condition, and the availability of veins. The skill of the person initiating the infusion is also an important consideration.

Choice of Site

Many sites can be used for intravenous therapy, but ease of access and potential hazards vary among them. Veins of the extremities are designated as peripheral locations and are ordinarily the only sites used by nurses. Because they are relatively safe and easy to enter, upper extremity veins are most commonly used. Veins of the arm and hand are shown in Figure 18–7. Leg veins should rarely, if ever, be used, because of the high risk of thromboembolism. Central veins frequently cannulated by physicians include the subclavian and internal jugular veins. It is possible to enter these larger vessels even when peripheral sites have collapsed, and they allow administration of high-osmolar solutions. Hazards are much greater, however, including, for example, inadvertent entry into an artery or the pleural space.

Ideally, both arms and hands should be carefully inspected before a specific venipuncture site is chosen. A location should be selected that does not interfere with mobility. For this reason, the antecubital fossa is avoided, except as a last resort. The most distal site of the arm or hand is generally used first so that subsequent IVs can be moved progressively upward. The vein chosen should be palpated for elasticity and absence of hard knots that may indicate thromboses.

Venipuncture Devices

Three main types of cannulas are available: steel scalp vein needles, indwelling plastic catheters inserted over a steel needle, and indwelling plastic catheters inserted through a steel needle. Scalp vein or butterfly needles are short steel needles with plastic wing handles. These are easy to insert, but, because they are small and nonpliable, infiltrate easily (Fig. 18–8). Insertion of an over-the-needle catheter requires the additional step of advancing the catheter into the vein after venipuncture (Fig. 18–9). Because they are less likely to infiltrate, these devices are frequently preferred over scalp vein needles. Plastic

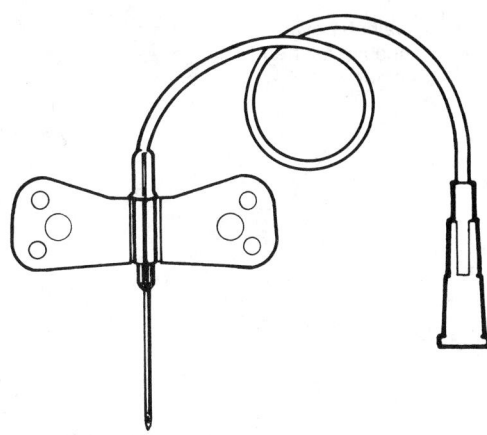

Figure 18–8. Scalp-vein needle: Winged infusion set. (Metheny N. Fluid and Electrolyte Balance: Nursing Considerations. Philadelphia, JB Lippincott, 1987, p 127.)

catheters inserted through a hollow needle are usually called intracatheters. They are available in long lengths and are well suited for placement in central locations. Because insertion requires threading the catheter through the vein for a relatively long distance, these are the most difficult catheters to place. (Fig. 18–10).

Informing the Patient

Except in emergency situations, a patient should be prepared in advance for having an intravenous infusion. A brief description of the venipuncture process, information about the expected length of infusion, and restrictions on activities are important topics. An opportunity should be given for the patient to verbalize concerns. For example, some patients believe they will die if small bubbles in the tubing enter their veins. After acknowledging this fear, the nurse can explain that usually only relatively large quantities of air administered rapidly are dangerous.

Preparation of Site

Because infection can be a major complication of intravenous therapy, the intravenous device must be sterile, as must the parenteral container and tubing. The insertion site should be scrubbed for 60 seconds, working from the center of the field to the periphery, using a 70% alcohol pledget. The nurse must wear nonsterile disposable gloves during the venipuncture procedure because the likelihood of coming into contact with the patient's blood is high.

Vein Entry

Guidelines and a suggested sequence for venipuncture are presented in Chart 18–3. For veins that are very small or particularly fragile, modifications in this technique may be necessary. Alternative methods can be found in journal articles or in specialized textbooks of intravenous therapy.

Monitoring Intravenous Therapy

Maintenance of an existing intravenous infusion is a nursing responsibility that demands knowledge of the solutions being administered and principles of flow. In addition, patients must be assessed carefully for both local and systemic complications.

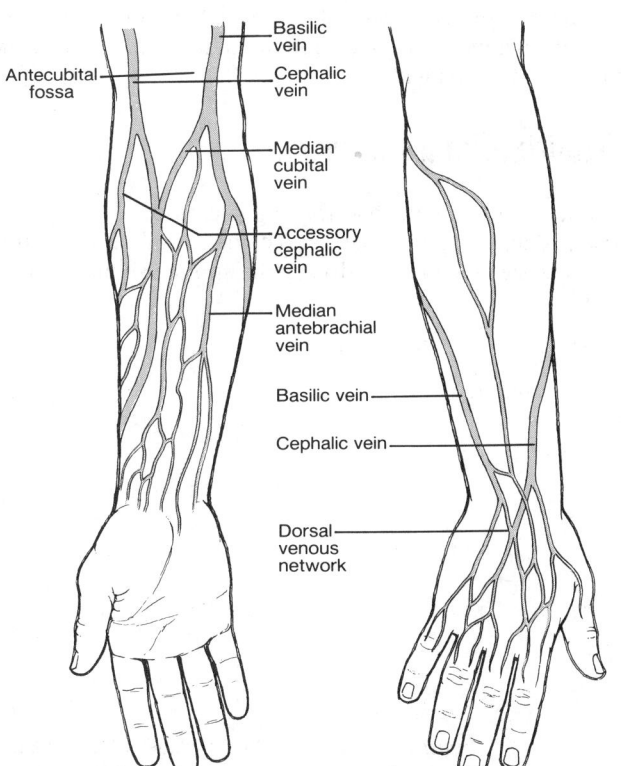

Figure 18–7. Sites of selection for the insertion of intravenous needles for the parenteral administration of fluids or for blood transfusion.

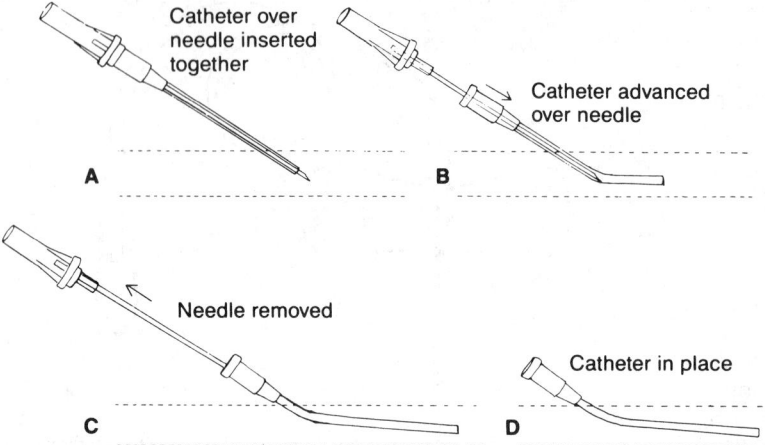

Figure 18–9. Insertion of catheter over a needle. (Textbook of Advanced Cardiac Life Support. Dallas, American Heart Association, 1987. Reproduced with permission of the American Heart Association, Inc.)

Factors Affecting the Gravity Flow of Intravenous Fluids

The flow of an intravenous infusion is subject to the same principles that govern fluid movement in general.

- *Flow is directly proportional to the height of the liquid column.* Raising the height of the infusion container will sometimes improve a sluggish flow.
- *Flow is directly proportional to the diameter of the tubing.* The clamp on IV tubing regulates the flow by changing the tubing diameter. In addition, the flow will be faster through cannulas of large gauge, as opposed to those of small gauge.
- *Flow is inversely proportional to the length of the tubing.* Adding extension tubing to an IV line will decrease the flow.
- *Flow is inversely proportional to the viscosity of a fluid.* Viscous intravenous solutions, like blood, require a larger cannula than do water or saline solutions.

Monitoring the Flow

Because so many factors influence the gravity flow, a solution does not necessarily continue to run at the speed originally set. Therefore, intravenous infusions must be monitored frequently to ascertain that the fluid is flowing at the intended rate. The IV flask or bag should be marked with tape to indicate at a glance whether the correct amount has infused. The flow rate should be calculated when the solution is originally hung, then rechecked at least hourly. To calculate the flow rate, the number of drops delivered per milliliter must be ascertained. This number varies with equipment and is usually printed on the solution set packaging. A formula that can be used to calculate the drop rate follows:

$$\frac{\text{gtt/ml of given set}}{60 \text{ (min in hour)}} \times \text{total hourly volume} = \text{gtt/min}$$

A variety of infusion pumps are available to assist in intravenous fluid delivery. These devices allow more accurate administration of fluids and medications than is possible with routine gravity-flow setups. Some pumps have flow rates calibrated in terms of milliliters/hour and are referred to as volumetric pumps (Fig. 18–11). Others are calibrated in drops/minute and are referred to as infusion controllers (Fig. 18–12). It is important to read the manufacturer's directions carefully before using any infusion pump or controller because there are many variations in available models. Use of these devices does not eliminate the need for frequent monitoring of the infusion and the patient.

Discontinuing an Infusion

The removal of an intravenous cannula is associated with two possible dangers: hemorrhage and catheter embolism. To prevent excessive bleeding, a dry, sterile sponge should be held

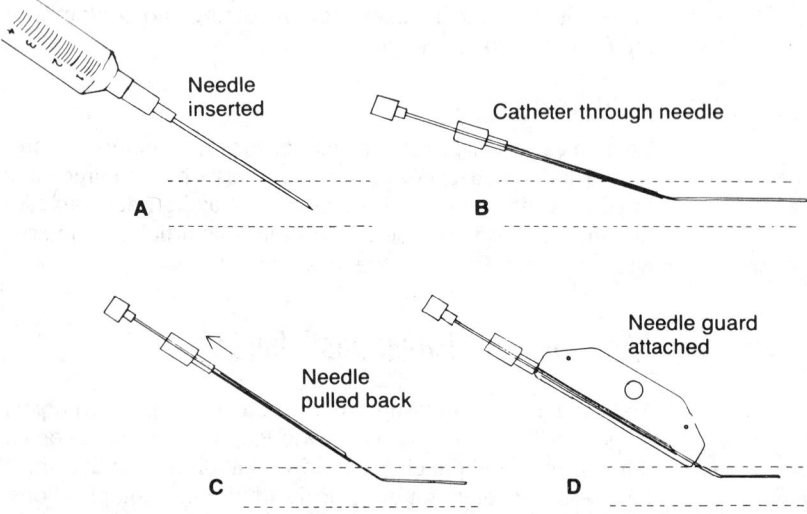

Figure 18–10. Insertion of catheter through a needle. (Textbook of Advanced Cardiac Life Support. Dallas, American Heart Association, 1987. Reproduced with permission of the American Heart Association, Inc.)

Chart 18–3
Guidelines for Starting an Intravenous Infusion

Nursing Action	Rationale
Preparation	
1. Verify order for IV therapy, check solution label, and identify patient.	1. Serious errors can be avoided by careful checking.
2. Explain procedure to patient.	2. Knowledge increases both patient comfort and cooperation.
3. Wash hands and put on nonsterile disposable gloves.	3. Asepsis is essential to prevent infection.
4. Choose site.	4. Careful site selection will increase likelihood of successful venipuncture and preservation of vein.
5. Choose IV cannula.	5. Length and gauge of cannula should be appropriate for both site and purpose of infusion.
6. Connect infusion flask or bag and tubing, and run solution through tubing to remove air; cover end of tubing.	6. Equipment must be attached immediately after successful venipuncture to prevent clotting.
7. Raise bed to comfortable working height and position for patient; adjust lighting.	7. Proper positioning will increase likelihood of success and provide comfort for patient.
Procedure	
1. Apply tourniquet 5 to 15 cm (2–6 inches) above injection site; check for radial pulse below tourniquet.	1. The tourniquet distends the vein and makes it easier to enter; it should never be tight enough to occlude arterial flow.
2. Prepare site by scrubbing with a 70% alcohol pledget for 60 seconds in circular motion, moving outward from injection site.	2. Strict asepsis and careful site preparation are essential to prevent infection.
3. With hand not holding needle, steady extremity and use finger or thumb to pull skin taut over vessel.	3. Applying traction to the vein helps to stabilize it.
4. Holding needle bevel up and at 45-degree angle, pierce skin to reach but not penetrate vein.	4. Bevel-up position usually produces less trauma to skin and vein.
5. Decrease angle of needle until nearly parallel with skin, then enter vein either directly above or from the side.	5. Two-stage procedure decreases chance of thrusting needle through posterior wall of vein as skin is entered.
6. If backflow of blood is visible, straighten angle and advance needle.	6. Backflow may not occur if vein is small; this position decreases chance of puncturing posterior wall of vein.
Additional steps for catheter inserted over needle:	
a. Advance needle 0.6 cm (¼ inch) after successful venipuncture.	a. Advancing the needle slightly makes certain the plastic catheter has entered the vein.
b. Hold needle hub, and slide catheter over the needle into the vein. *Never* reinsert needle into a plastic catheter or pull the catheter back into the needle.	b. Reinsertion of the needle or pulling the catheter back can sever the catheter, causing catheter embolism.
c. Remove needle, while pressing lightly on the skin over the catheter tip; hold catheter hub in place.	c. Slight pressure prevents bleeding before tubing is attached.
7. Release tourniquet, and attach infusion tubing; open clamp enough to allow drip.	7. Infusion must be attached promptly to prevent clotting in cannula.
8. Slip a sterile 2 × 2 inch gauze pad under the catheter hub.	8. The gauze acts as a sterile field.
9. Anchor needle firmly in place with a tape.	9. A stable needle is less likely to become dislodged or to irritate the vein.
10. Apply antimicrobial ointment over site and cover with Band-aid or sterile gauze; tape in place, but do not encircle limb.	10. Antimicrobial ointments somewhat decrease risk of infection; tape encircling extremity can act as tourniquet.
11. Tape a small loop of IV tubing onto dressing.	11. The loop decreases the chance of inadvertent cannula removal if the tubing is pulled.
12. Label dressing with type and length of cannula, date, and initials.	12. Labeling facilitates assessment and safe discontinuation.
13. Calculate drop rate, and regulate flow of infusion.	13. Infusion must be regulated carefully to prevent overinfusion or underinfusion
14. Document site, cannula type, and time in chart.	14. Documentation is essential to facilitate care and for legal purposes.

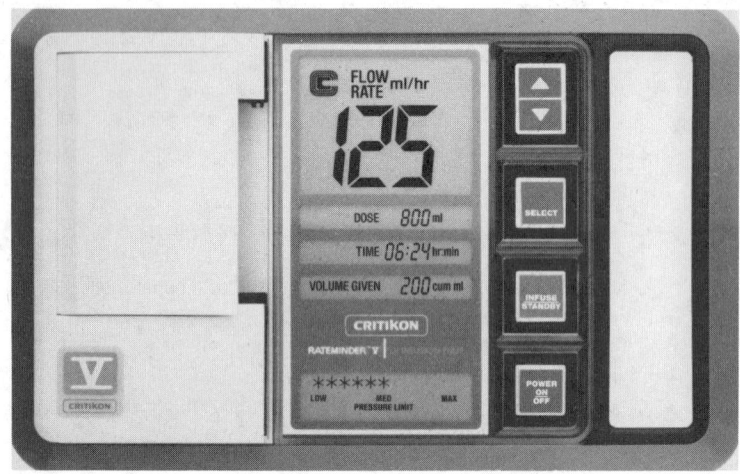

Figure 18–11. Volumetric pump. Flow rates calibrated in milliliters/hour. (Courtesy of Critikon, Inc.)

over the site as the cannula is removed. Firm pressure should then be applied until all bleeding has stopped. If a plastic IV catheter is severed, it can travel to the right ventricle and block the blood flow. To detect this complication during cannula removal, the expected length of the cannula is compared with its actual length. Plastic catheters should be withdrawn carefully and their length measured to make certain that no fragment has broken off. Great care must be exercised when using scissors around the dressing site. If severing of a catheter is detected immediately, an attempt can be made to occlude the vein above the site to prevent the catheter from entering the central circulation (until such time as surgical removal is possible). As always, however, it is better to *prevent* a potentially fatal problem than to deal with it after it has occurred. Fortunately, catheter embolism can easily be prevented by following simple rules, such as avoiding use of scissors near the catheter, and not withdrawing the catheter through the insertion needle.

Manufacturer's guidelines should be followed carefully, such as covering the needle point with the bevel shield to prevent severing of the catheter. Careful anchoring of the catheter will help prevent it from becoming liberated into the general circulation should it accidentally separate from the adapter.

Complications Associated With Parenteral Fluid Therapy

Unfortunately, intravenous therapy predisposes to numerous hazards; these include both local and systemic complications. Systemic complications occur less frequently but are often more serious than local complications and include circulatory overload, air embolism, febrile reaction, and infection.

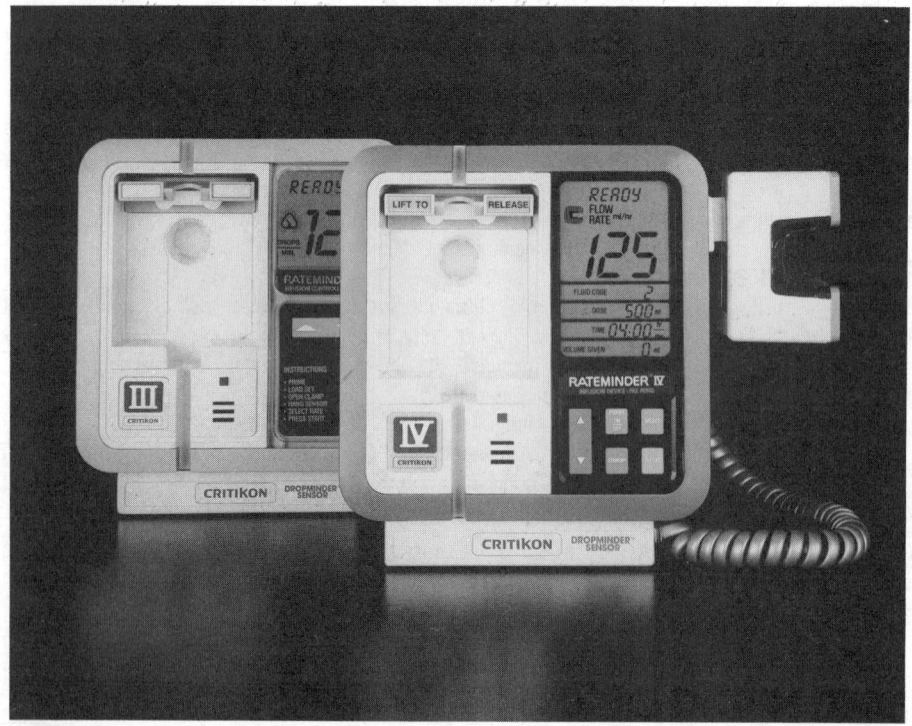

Figure 18–12. Infusion controller. Flow rates calibrated in drops/minute. (Courtesy of Critikon, Inc.)

Systemic Complications

Overloading the circulatory system with excessive intravenous fluids will cause increased blood pressure and central venous pressure and even severe dyspnea and cyanosis. This is particularly likely to occur in patients with cardiac disease and is referred to as *circulatory overload*.

The danger of *air embolism* is always present, even though it does not occur frequently. It is most often associated with cannulation of central veins. The presence of air embolism may be manifested by dyspnea and cyanosis, hypotension, weak rapid pulse, and loss of consciousness. The amount of air necessary to induce death in humans is not known. Apparently, the rate of entry is as important as the actual volume of air.

The presence of pyrogenic substances in either the infusion solution or the administration setup can induce a *febrile reaction*. With such a reaction, one might observe an abrupt temperature elevation shortly after the infusion is started, backache, headache, general malaise, and, if severe, vascular collapse.

Infection ranges in severity from local involvement of the insertion site to systemic dissemination of organisms through the bloodstream. Measures to prevent infection are essential at the time of insertion and throughout the entire period of infusion. Some of these include the following:

- Careful handwashing before every contact with any part of the infusion system or patient
- Examination of flasks or bags for cracks, leaks, or cloudiness, which may indicate a contaminated solution
- Strict asepsis
- Firm anchoring of the IV cannula to prevent to-and-fro motion
- Daily IV site inspection and replacement of sterile dressing (application of an antimicrobial ointment to the insertion site probably confers a slight additional benefit)
- Removal of the IV cannula at the first sign of local inflammation
- Replacement of the IV cannula every 48 hours, or as indicated
- Replacement of the IV cannula inserted during emergency conditions (with questionable asepsis) as soon as possible
- Replacement of the flask or bag every 24 hours and the entire administration set at least every 48 hours, and every 24 hours when blood or lipid products are being infused

Local Complications

Local complications of intravenous therapy include infiltration, phlebitis, and thrombophlebitis.

Dislodging of a needle and local infiltration of the solution into subcutaneous tissues is not uncommon. *Infiltration* is characterized by edema, discomfort, and coolness in the area of infiltration, and significant decrease in the flow rate. When the solution is particularly irritating, sloughing of tissue may result. Close monitoring of the insertion site is necessary to detect infiltration before it becomes severe. Infiltration is easily recognized if the insertion area is larger than an identical region in the opposite extremity. Infiltration, however, is not always so obvious. A common misconception is that a backflow of blood into the tubing proves that the cannula is properly placed within the vein. If the catheter tip has pierced the wall of the vessel, however, intravenous fluid will seep into tissues as well as flow into the vein. A more reliable means of confirming infiltration is to apply a tourniquet above or proximal to the infusion site and tighten it enough to restrict venous flow. If the infusion continues to drip despite the venous obstruction, infiltration is present.

Phlebitis is defined as inflammation of a vein and is evidenced by heat, redness, and swelling at the injection site. The incidence of phlebitis increases with the length of time the intravenous line is in place. *Thrombophlebitis* refers to the presence of a clot plus inflammation in the vein. It is evidenced by localized heat, redness, swelling, and hardness of the vein.

In summary, the administration of intravenous fluids is frequently managed by nurses. Although it is a common and extremely important form of treatment, intravenous therapy is associated with several serious hazards. These potential risks include infection, embolism, and fluid and electrolyte imbalances. By the use of aseptic technique during every contact with the apparatus, application of principles of flow, and frequent patient assessment, the nurse can reduce the likelihood of any of these complications.

Chapter Summary

Fluid and electrolyte disturbances and alterations in acid–base balance are common in ill and hospitalized patients and those undergoing surgical and diagnostic procedures. Serious disturbances in fluid and electrolyte and acid–base balance can occur even with mild illnesses characterized by fever, vomiting, or diarrhea. The risk of serious disturbances increases in those who are at the two extremes of the age spectrum and individuals who have pre-existing acute or chronic illnesses.

Because of their frequent occurrence and the speed with which fluid and electrolyte imbalances and acid–base disturbances can develop, it is important for the nurse to understand the functions of electrolytes and fluids in the body and the subtle as well as obvious signs that indicate changes in their status. The nurse must understand the physiologic mechanisms that are important in maintaining acid–base balance and must anticipate treatment strategies so that they can be implemented promptly.

Intravenous administration of fluids, electrolytes, medications, and other substances is commonplace today. Proper administration and maintenance of the infusion and the infusion site are the responsibility of the nurse caring for the patient receiving such infusions. Important observations of the nurse caring for such a patient include careful administration of the appropriate fluid or medication, observation and maintenance of the infusion site, monitoring of the patient for complications, and documentation of the patient's physiologic response and psychological reaction to treatments.

Bibliography

Books
Bray J et al. Lecture Notes on Human Physiology. 2nd ed. Oxford, Blackwell Scientific Publications, 1989.

Gahart B. Intravenous Medications. 6th ed. St. Louis, CV Mosby, 1990.

Goldberger E. A Primer of Water, Electrolyte & Acid–Base Syndromes. 7th ed. Philadelphia, Lea & Febiger, 1986.

Kim M et al. A Pocket Guide to Nursing Diagnoses. 3rd ed. St. Louis, CV Mosby, 1989.

Kokko J and Tannen R. Fluids and Electrolytes. 2nd ed. Philadelphia, WB Saunders, 1990.

MacFarland M and Grant M. Nursing Implications of Laboratory Tests. 2nd ed. New York, John Wiley & Sons, 1988.

Maxwell M et al. Clinical Disorders of Fluid and Electrolyte Metabolism. 4th ed. New York, McGraw–Hill, 1987.

Metheny N. Fluid and Electrolyte Balance: Nursing Considerations. Philadelphia, JB Lippincott, 1987.

Pennington J and Church H. Bowes and Church's Food Values of Portions Commonly Used. 15th ed. Philadelphia, JB Lippincott, 1989.

Pestano C. Fluids and Electrolytes in the Surgical Patient. 4th ed. Baltimore, Williams & Wilkins, 1989.

Plumer A. Principles and Practice of Intravenous Therapy. 4th ed. Boston, Little, Brown, 1986.

Rose B. Clinical Physiology of Acid–Base & Electrolyte Disorders. 3rd ed. New York, McGraw-Hill, 1989.

Scherer J. Lippincott's Nurses' Drug Manual. Philadelphia, JB Lippincott, 1985.

Schrier R. Renal and Electrolyte Disorders. 3rd ed. Boston, Little, Brown, 1986.

Shapiro B. Clinical Application of Respiratory Care. 3rd ed. Chicago, Year Book Medical Pub, 1985.

Ulrich B. Nephrology Nursing: Concepts and Strategies. Norwalk, CT, Appleton & Lange, 1989.

Journals

Asterisks indicate nursing research articles.

Abraham A et al. Magnesium in the prevention of lethal arrhythmias in acute myocardial infarction. Arch Intern Med 1987 147: 753–55.

* Adams F. Fluid intake: How much do elders drink? Geriatr Nurs (New York) 1988 Jul/Aug; 9(4): 218–221.

Ansari A. Hypokalemia and hyperkalemia: Diagnosis by electrocardiography. Primary Cardiol 1988; 14(4): 17–31.

Baicich R. Potassium supplementation. Nutritional Support Services 1987; 7(8): 29–31.

Barrus D and Danek G. Clinical controversy: Should you irrigate an occluded I.V. line? Nursing 1987 Mar; 17(3): 63–64.

* Bowman M et al. Effect of tube-feeding osmolality on serum sodium levels. Crit Care Nurse 1989; 9(1): 22–28.

Cagno J. Nursing care plan: Diabetes insipidus. Crit Care Nurse 1989; 9(6): 86–93.

Chazan J and McKay D. Acid–base abnormalities in cardiopulmonary arrest: Varying patterns in different locations in the hospital (letter). N Engl J Med 1989; 320(9): 597–598.

Cole M. Flushing heparin locks: Is saline flushing really cost- effective? J IV Nurs 1989; 12(1): 523–529.

* Coward D. Hypercalcemia knowledge assessment in patients at risk of developing cancer-induced hypercalcemia. Oncol Nurs Forum 1988; 15(4): 471–476.

Chernow B et al. Hypomagnesemia in patients in postoperative intensive care. Chest 1989; 95(2): 391–397.

Dudley D et al. Long-term tocolysis with intravenous magnesium sulfate. Obstet Gynecol 1989; 73(3): 373–377.

Garner B. Guide to changing lab values in elders. Geriatr Nurs 1989 May/Jun; 3: 144–145.

Hatjis C et al. Efficacy of combined administration of magnesium sulfate and ritodrine in the treatment of premature labor. Obstet Gynecol 1987; 69: 317.

Halevy J and Bulvik S. Severe hypophosphatemia in hospitalized patients. Arch Intern Med 1988; 148: 153–155.

Hazinski M. Fluid balance in the seriously ill child. Pediatr Nurs 1988; 14(3): 230–236.

Gershan JA et al. Fluid volume deficit: Validating the indicators. Heart Lung 1990 Mar; 19(2): 152–156.

Metheny NM. Why worry about IV fluids. Am J Nurs 1990 Jun; 90(6): 50–57.

Hoffman R. An "amp" by any other name: The hazards of intravenous magnesium dosing (letter). JAMA 1989 Jan 27; 261: 557.

Iqbal Z and Friedman E. Preferred therapy of hyperkalemia in renal insufficiency: Survey of nephrology training-program directors (letter). N Engl J Med 1989; 320(1): 60–61.

Johnson D. Fluid and electrolyte dysfunction in alcoholism. Crit Care Q 1986 Mar; 8(4): 53–64.

* Jordan L. Effects of fluid manipulation on the incidence of vomiting during outpatient cisplatin infusion. Oncol Nurs Forum 1989; 16(2): 213–218.

Kwan K and Barrett-Connor E. Dietary potassium and stroke-associated mortality. N Engl J Med 1987; 316: 235–240.

Ley J. Fluid therapy following intracardiac operation. Crit Care Nurse 1988; 8(1): 26–36.

Linas S. Potassium: Weighing the evidence for supplementation. Hosp Pract 1988 Dec 15; 23(12): 73–86.

Lunger D. Potassium supplementation: How and why? Focus Crit Care 1988; 15(5): 56–59.

* Mahon S. For the research record: Symptoms as clues to calcium levels. Am J Nurs 1987 Mar; 87(3): 354, 356.

Mathewson M. Intravenous therapy. Crit Care Nurse 1989; 9(2): 21–36.

Matz R. Hyperosmolar nonacidotic uncontrolled diabetes: Not a rare event. Clin Diabetes 1988; 6(2): 1, 30–37, 46.

* Metheny N et al. Electrolyte disturbances in tube-fed patients (Abstr). Thirteenth Annual Midwest Nursing Research Society Conference, Cincinnati, OH, April 2, 1989, p 220.

Moran T. AIDS: Current implications and impact on nursing. J IV Nurs 1989; 12(4): 220–226.

Murphy L and Lipman T. Central venous catheter care in parenteral nutrition: A review. J Parenteral Enteral Nutr 1987; 11(2): 190–201.

Pfister S and Bullas J. Interpreting arterial blood gas values. Crit Care Nurs 1986 Jul/Aug; 6(4): 9–14.

Poe C and Taylor L. Syndrome of inappropriate antidiuretic hormone: Assessment and nursing implications. Oncol Nurs Forum 1989; 16(3): 373–381.

Rimmer J et al. Hyperkalemia as a complication of drug therapy. Arch Intern Med 1987; 147(5): 867–869.

Ryan M. Diuretics and potassium/magnesium depletion: Directions for treatment. Am J Med 1987; 82(suppl 3A): 38–47.

Schrier R. Pathogenesis of sodium and water retention in high-output and low-output cardiac failure, nephrotic syndrome, cirrhosis, and pregnancy. N Engl J Med 1988; 319(16): 1065–1072.

Seligman M (ed). Potassium. Drug Therapy Review. Massachusetts General Hospital, 1986; 1–4.

Stein J. Hypokalemia: Common and uncommon causes. Hosp Pract 1988 Mar 30; 23(3A): 55–64, 66, 70.

* Thompson D et al. A trial of povidone-iodine antiseptic solution for the prevention of cannula-related thrombophlebitis. J IV Nurs 1989; 12(2): 99–102.

Todd B. Calcium: Should we supplement? Geriatr Nurs 1989 Mar/Apr; 2: 96–98.

Tucker S and Schimmel E. Postoperative hypophosphatemia: A multifactorial problem. Nutr Rev 1989; 47(4): 111–116.

Valle G and Lemberg L. Electrolyte imbalances in cardiovascular disease: The forgotten factor. Heart Lung 1988; 17(3): 324–329.

Wagman L et al. The effect of acute discontinuation of total parenteral nutrition. Ann Surg 1986; 204: 524–529.

Whang R. Magnesium deficiency: Pathogenesis, prevalence and clinical implications. Am J Med 1987; 82(suppl 3A): 24–29.

Whang R. Magnesium and potassium interrelationships in cardiac arrhythmias. Magnesium 1986; 5: 127–133.

Whang R. Routine serum magnesium determinations: A continuing unrecognized need. Magnesium 1987; 6: 1–4.

Young M and Flynn K. Third-spacing: When the body conceals fluid loss. RN 1988 Aug; 51: 46–48.

Zaloga G et al. A simple method for determining physiologically active calcium and magnesium concentrations in critically ill patients. Crit Care Med 1987; 15: 813–16.

Oncology: Nursing the Patient With Cancer

Learning Objectives

On completion of this chapter, the learner will be able to:

1. Compare the structure and function of the normal cell and cancer cell
2. Differentiate between benign and malignant tumors
3. Identify agents and factors that have been found to be carcinogenic
4. Describe the significance of health education and preventive care in decreasing the incidence of cancer
5. Differentiate between the purposes of surgical procedures used for cancer: treatment, diagnosis, prophylaxis, palliation, reconstruction
6. Describe the roles of surgery, radiation therapy, chemotherapy, hyperthermia, and biologic response modifiers in the treatment of cancer
7. Describe the special nursing needs of patients receiving chemotherapy
8. Describe common nursing diagnoses of patients with cancer
9. Use the nursing process as a framework for care of patients with cancer
10. Describe the concept of the hospice in providing care for patients with advanced cancer
11. Discuss the role of the nurse in assessment and management of common oncologic emergencies

Cancer nursing is an area of practice that covers all age groups and nursing specialties and is carried out in a variety of health care settings, including the home, community, acute care institutions, and rehabilitation centers. The field or specialty of cancer nursing, or oncology nursing, has paralleled the development of medical oncology and the major therapeutic advances that have occurred in the care of the person with cancer.

The scope, responsibilities, and goals of cancer nursing are as diverse and complex as those of any nursing specialty. There is a special challenge inherent in caring for people with cancer because the word *cancer* is often equated with pain and death in our society. To meet this challenge, the nurse must first identify her own reactions to cancer and realistically set goals that can be attained.

The nurse must be equipped to support the patient and his family through a wide range of physical, emotional, social, cultural, and spiritual crises. To accomplish the desired outcomes, the nurse provides realistic support to those in his care, using standards of practice and the nursing process as the basis of his care. The major areas of responsibility for the nurse caring for the patient with cancer are listed in Chart 19–1.

Incidence

Cancers affect every age group; however, most cancers occur in people over 65 years of age. Overall, men experience a higher incidence of cancer than do women.

At least 1,100,000 Americans are diagnosed each year with a cancer affecting one of various body sites (Fig. 19–1). Cancer incidence is higher in the industrialized nations of the world and in the industrial sectors of more developed countries.

Mortality Rates

Cancers are second only to cardiovascular disease as a leading cause of death in the United States. Each year, more than 476,000 Americans die of a malignant process. In the United States, in order of frequency, the leading causes of cancer deaths include cancers of the lung, colorectal area, and prostate in men and cancers of the lung, breast, and colorectal area in women. Relative 5-year survival rates in 1991 are 38% for black Americans and 52% for white Americans.

Pathophysiology of the Malignant Process

Cancer is a disease process that begins when abnormal cells arise from normal body cells as a result of some poorly understood mechanism of change. As the disease progresses locally, these abnormal cells proliferate, ignoring growth-regulating signals in the microenvironment surrounding the cell.

A stage is then reached, however, in which the cells acquire invasive characteristics, and changes occur in surrounding tissues. The cells infiltrate these tissues and gain access to lymph and blood vessels, by which they are transported to form *metastases* (cancer spread) in other parts of the body.

Although the disease can be described in the general terms just used, cancer is not a single disease with a single cause; rather it is a group of distinct diseases with different causes, manifestations, treatments, and prognoses.

Benign Versus Malignant Proliferative Patterns

During the life span, various body tissues normally experience periods of rapid or proliferative growth that must be distinguished from malignant growth activity. There are several patterns of cell growth, designated by the terms *hyperplasia*, *metaplasia*, *dysplasia*, and *neoplasia*, that may be described as follows.

Hyperplasia

Hyperplasia, an increase in the number of cells of a tissue, is a common proliferative process during periods of rapid body growth (*e.g.*, fetal and adolescent growth and development) and during epithelial and bone marrow regeneration. It is a normal cellular response when a physiologic demand exists and an abnormal response when growth exceeds the physiologic demand.

Metaplasia

Metaplasia occurs when one type of mature cell is converted to another type by means of an outside stimulus that affects the parent stem cell. Chronic irritation or inflammation, vitamin deficiency, and chemical exposure may be factors leading to

---

Chart 19–1
Responsibilities of the Nurse Caring for the Oncology Patient and Family

- Support the idea that cancer is a chronic illness that has acute exacerbations rather than one that is synonymous with death and suffering.
- Assess own level of knowledge relative to the pathophysiology of the disease process.
- Make use of current research findings and practices in the care of the patient with cancer and his family.
- Identify persons at high risk for the development of cancer.
- Participate in primary and secondary prevention efforts.
- Assess the nursing care needs of the person with cancer.
- Assess the learning needs, desires, and capabilities of the person with cancer.
- Identify nursing problems of the person and his family.

- Assess the social support networks available to the person.
- Plan appropriate interventions with the person and his family.
- Assist the person to identify his strengths and limitations.
- Assist the person to design short-term and long-term goals for care.
- Implement a nursing care plan that interfaces with the medical care regimen and that is consistent with the established goals.
- Collaborate with members of a multidisciplinary team to foster continuity of care.
- Evaluate the goals and resultant outcomes of care with the patient, his family, and the members of the multidisciplinary team.
- Reassess and redesign the direction of the care as determined by the evaluation.

1991 ESTIMATED CANCER INCIDENCE BY SITE AND SEX†

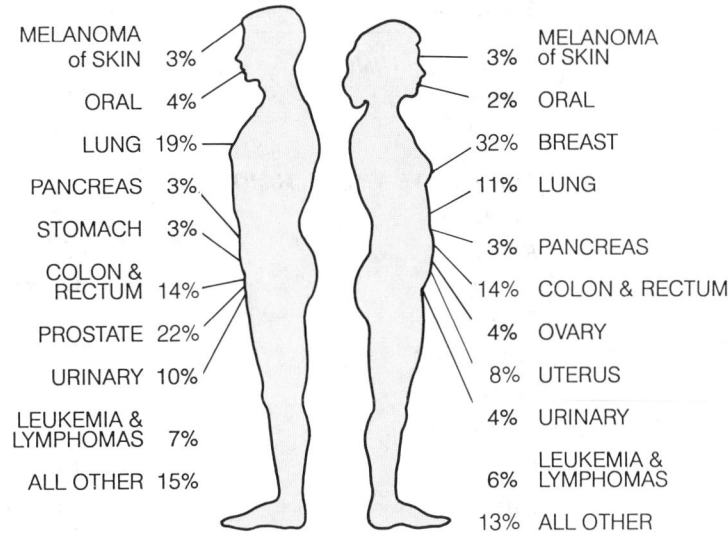

MELANOMA of SKIN	3%	3%	MELANOMA of SKIN
ORAL	4%	2%	ORAL
LUNG	19%	32%	BREAST
PANCREAS	3%	11%	LUNG
STOMACH	3%		
COLON & RECTUM	14%	3%	PANCREAS
		14%	COLON & RECTUM
PROSTATE	22%	4%	OVARY
URINARY	10%	8%	UTERUS
		4%	URINARY
LEUKEMIA & LYMPHOMAS	7%		
ALL OTHER	15%	6%	LEUKEMIA & LYMPHOMAS
		13%	ALL OTHER

†*Excluding nonmelanoma skin cancer and carcinoma in situ.*
A

1991 ESTIMATED CANCER DEATHS BY SITE AND SEX†

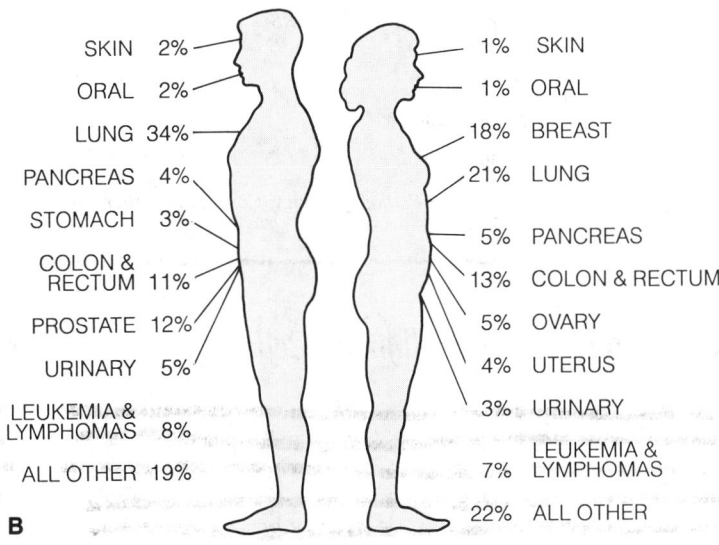

SKIN	2%	1%	SKIN
ORAL	2%	1%	ORAL
LUNG	34%	18%	BREAST
PANCREAS	4%	21%	LUNG
STOMACH	3%		
COLON & RECTUM	11%	5%	PANCREAS
		13%	COLON & RECTUM
PROSTATE	12%	5%	OVARY
URINARY	5%	4%	UTERUS
		3%	URINARY
LEUKEMIA & LYMPHOMAS	8%		
ALL OTHER	19%	7%	LEUKEMIA & LYMPHOMAS
		22%	ALL OTHER

B

Figure 19–1. (**A**) 1991 estimated cancer incidence by site and sex (excluding nonmelanoma skin cancer and carcinoma *in situ*). (**B**) 1991 estimated cancer deaths by site and sex. (Redrawn from Boring CC, Squires SS, and Tong T. Cancer statistics, 1991. CA 1991;41(1):19. Copyright 1991 CA—A Journal for Clinicians and the American Cancer Society, Inc.)

metaplasia. Metaplastic changes may be reversible or may progress to dysplasia.

Dysplasia

Dysplasia is bizarre cell growth resulting in cells that differ in size, shape, or arrangement from other cells of the same type of tissue. Dysplasia can occur from chemicals, radiation, or chronic inflammation or irritation. It can be reversible or can precede irreversible neoplastic change.

Anaplasia

Anaplasia is a lower degree of differentiation of dysplastic cells. (*Differentiation* refers to the extent to which the cells differ from their cells of origin and to their degree of maturity.) An

aplastic cells are poorly differentiated, irregularly shaped, or disorganized with respect to growth and arrangement. Anaplastic cells lack normal cellular characteristics and are nearly always malignant.

Neoplasia

Neoplasia, described as uncontrolled cell growth that follows no physiologic demand, can be either benign or malignant. Benign and malignant neoplastic growths are classified and named by tissue of origin (Table 19–1).

Benign and malignant cells differ in many cellular growth characteristics, as summarized in Table 19–2. The degree of anaplasia (lack of differentiation of cells) ultimately determines the malignant potential.

TABLE 19–1.   *Names of Selected Benign and Malignant Tumors According to Tissue Types*

Tissue type	Benign	Malignant
EPITHELIAL TUMORS		
Surface	Papilloma	Squamous cell carcinoma
Glandular	Adenoma	Adenocarcinoma
CONNECTIVE TISSUE TUMORS		
Fibrous	Fibroma	Fibrosarcoma
Adipose	Lipoma	Liposarcoma
Cartilage	Chondroma	Chondrosarcoma
Bone	Osteoma	Osteosarcoma
Blood vessels	Hemangioma	Hemangiosarcoma
Lymph vessels	Lymphangioma	Lymphangiosarcoma
MUSCLE TUMORS		
Smooth	Leiomyoma	Leiomyosarcoma
Striated	Rhabdomyoma	Rhabdomyosarcoma
NERVE CELL TUMORS		
Nerve cell	Neuroma	
Glial tissue		Glioma
Nerve sheaths	Neurilemoma	Neurilemic sarcoma
HEMATOLOGIC TUMORS		
Granulocytic		Myelocytic leukemia
Erythrocytic		Erythroleukemia
Plasma cells		Multiple myeloma
Lymphoid		Lymphocytic leukemia

(Porth CM. Pathophysiology: Concepts of Altered Health States. 3rd ed. Philadelphia, JB Lippincott, 1990.)

Characteristics of Malignant Cells

Despite their individual differences, all cancer cells share some common cellular characteristics. Cancer cells have altered cell membranes, which affects fluid movement in and out of the cell. The cell membrane of malignant cells also contains tumor-specific antigens, which develop as they become less differentiated (mature) over time. Malignant cellular membranes contain less fibronectin, a "cellular cement"; thus they have a decreased cohesiveness and adhesion to adjacent cells.

Nuclei of cancer cells are often large and irregularly shaped (pleomorphism). Nucleoli, structures within the nucleus that house ribonucleic acid (RNA), are larger and more numerous in malignant cells, perhaps because of increased RNA synthesis. Chromosomal abnormalities and fragility of chromosomes are commonly found on analysis of cancer cells. Mitosis (cell division) occurs more frequently in malignant cells than in normal cells. Additionally, cancer cells have altered amounts of cyclic adenosine monophosphate (AMP) and cyclic guanosine monophosphate (GMP). These substances, which are the building blocks of nucleic acids, facilitate the use of nutrients and the synthesis of RNA. As a result, cell growth and division are promoted, necessitating high glucose and oxygen availability. If these glucose and oxygen stores are unavailable, malignant cells will use anaerobic metabolic channels to produce energy.

Invasion and Metastasis

Malignancies have the ability to spread or transfer cancerous cells from one organ or body part to another by invasion and metastasis. *Invasion* involves the growth of the primary tumor into the surrounding host tissues. The process of invasion occurs in several ways. Mechanical pressure exerted by rapidly proliferating neoplasms may force fingerlike projections of tumor cells into surrounding tissue. Malignant cells may break off from the primary tumor and invade adjacent structures. Malignant cells are thought to possess specific destructive enzymes (lysosomal hydrolases or collagenases) that destroy surrounding tissue and facilitate invasion by malignant cells. The mechanical pressure of a rapidly growing tumor may enhance this process.

Metastasis is the dissemination of malignant cells from the primary tumor to distant sites by direct spread of tumor cells to body cavities or through lymphatic and hematogenous circulation. Tumors growing in or penetrating body cavities may shed cells or emboli that travel within the body cavity and "seed" the surfaces of other organs. This can occur in ovarian cancer when malignant cells enter the peritoneal cavity and seed peritoneal surfaces of abdominal organs such as the liver or pancreas.

The most common mechanism of metastasis is transport of tumor cells through the lymphatic circulation. Tumor emboli

TABLE 19–2. *Characteristics of Benign and Malignant Neoplasms*

Characteristics	Benign	Malignant
Cell characteristics	Well-differentiated cells that resemble normal cells of the tissue from which the tumor originated	Cells often bear little resemblance to the normal cells of the tissue from which they arose; there is both anaplasia and pleomorphism
Mode of growth	Tumor grows by expansion and does not infiltrate the surrounding tissues; usually encapsulated	Grows at the periphery and sends out processes that infiltrate and destroy the surrounding tissues
Rate of growth	Rate of growth is usually slow	Rate of growth is variable and is dependent on level of differentiation; the more anaplastic the tumor, the more rapid the rate of growth
Metastasis	Does not spread by metastasis	Gains access to the blood and lymph channels and metastasizes to other areas of the body
General effects	Is usually a localized phenomenon that does not cause generalized effects unless by its location it interferes with vital functions	Often causes generalized effects such as anemia, weakness, and weight loss
Destruction of tissue	Does not usually cause tissue damage unless its location interferes with blood flow	Often causes extensive tissue damage as the tumor outgrows its blood supply or encroaches on blood flow to the area; may also produce substances that cause cell damage
Ability to cause death	Does not usually cause death unless by its location it interferes with vital functions	Will usually cause death unless growth can be controlled

(Porth CM. Pathophysiology: Concepts of Altered Health States. 3rd ed. Philadelphia, JB Lippincott, 1990.)

enter the lymph channels by way of the interstitial fluid that communicates with lymphatic fluid. In addition, malignant cells may penetrate lymphatic vessels by invasion. After entering the lymphatic circulation, malignant cells either become lodged in the lymph nodes or pass between lymphatic and venous circulation. Tumors arising in areas of the body with rapid and extensive lymphatic circulation have a high risk of metastasis through lymphatic channels. Breast tumors frequently metastasize in this manner through axillary, clavicular, and thoracic lymph channels.

Hematogenous spread, or dissemination through the bloodstream, of malignant cells is less common than spread by other means. Few malignant cells are able to survive the turbulent nature of arterial circulation. In addition, the structure of most arteries and arterioles is far too secure to permit malignant invasion. Those malignant cells that do survive this hostile environment are able to attach to endothelium and attract fibrin, platelets, and clotting factors to seal themselves from immune surveillance. The endothelium will retract, allowing the malignant cells to enter the basement membrane and to secrete lysosomal enzymes to destroy surrounding body tissues, thus leading to implantation.

Malignant cells also have the ability to induce the growth of new capillaries from the host tissue to meet their needs for nutrients and oxygen. This process is referred to as *angiogenesis*. It is through this vascular network that tumor emboli may enter the systemic circulation and travel to distant sites. Large tumor emboli that become trapped in the microcirculation of distant sites may serve as the origin of growth for metastasis.

In summary, metastasis from the primary tumor to other sites is not a random process. The host provides a hostile environment that destroys most circulating tumor cells. Those successful cells that achieve metastasis are able to survive because of their virulence and adaptive abilities.

Since the late 1800s, investigators have recognized the tendency for malignancies of specific cell classifications to metastasize to specific organs.

Currently, investigators are focusing their attention on the following factors in metastasis: organ vascularity, immune defenses at the tissue level, surface recognition factors on tumor cells, and differing behavioral characteristics among cells within one tumor.

Carcinogenesis

Malignant transformation is thought to be at least a two-step cellular process. In the first or *initiation* step, initiators such as chemicals, physical factors, and biologic agents escape normal enzymatic mechanisms and cause alterations in the genetic structure of the cellular deoxyribonucleic acid (DNA). These alterations are irreversible, but usually are not of significance to cells until the second step of carcinogenesis occurs—*promotion*. During this step, repeated exposure to promoting agents causes the expression of abnormal or mutant genetic information. Cellular oncogenes, present in all mammalian systems, are responsible for the vital cellular functions of growth and differentiation. When these genes become mutated, rearranged, amplified, or lose regulatory capabilities, malignant transformation is allowed to occur.

Once this genetic expression occurs in cells, they begin to produce mutant cell populations that are different from their original cellular ancestors. Those agents that initiate or promote cellular transformation are referred to as *carcinogens*.

Etiology

Certain categories of agents or factors have been implicated in the carcinogenic process. These include viruses, physical agents, chemical agents, genetic or familial factors, dietary factors, and hormonal agents.

Viruses

Viral causation in human cancers is hard to ascertain because isolation of viruses is difficult. Infectious causes are considered when clusters of specific cancers are noted. Viruses are thought to incorporate themselves in the genetic structure of cells, thus altering future generations of that cell population—perhaps leading to a cancer. For example, the Epstein–Barr virus is highly suspect as a causative agent in Burkitt's lymphoma and nasopharyngeal cancers. Herpes simplex type II virus, cytomegalovirus, and papillomavirus have all been associated with dysplasia and malignancy of the uterine cervix; the hepatitis B virus has been implicated in hepatocellular carcinoma. Similarly, the human T-cell lymphotropic virus (HTLV-I) has been associated with some lymphocytic leukemias/lymphomas, especially among individuals in southern Japan.

Physical Agents

Physical factors associated with carcinogenesis include exposure to sunlight or to radiation, chronic irritation or inflammation, and tobacco use.

Excessive exposure to the ultraviolet radiation of the sun, especially in fair-skinned, blue- or green-eyed people, increases the risk of skin cancers. Exposure to ionizing radiation can occur with repeated diagnostic radiographic procedures of radiation therapy, from exposure to radioactive materials at nuclear weapon sites or nuclear power plants, and also from natural background radiation, which is essentially unavoidable. Those exposed to extensive radiation have a higher incidence of leukemia and cancers of the lung, bone, breast, thyroid, and other tissues.

Chronic irritation or inflammation is thought to damage cells, leading to abnormal cell differentiation. Cell mutations secondary to chronic irritation or inflammation are associated with lip cancers among pipe smokers. Oral cancers are associated with prolonged tobacco use or ill-fitting dentures. Melanomas are associated with chronically irritated moles, colorectal cancers with ulcerative colitis, and liver cancers with cirrhosis.

Chemical Agents

Eighty-five percent of all cancers are thought to be related to the environment around us. Tobacco smoke is a potent chemical carcinogen that accounts for at least 35% of cancer deaths. Smoking is also highly associated with cancers of the lung, head and neck, esophagus, pancreas, cervix, and bladder. Tobacco may also act synergistically with other substances such as alcohol, asbestos, uranium, and viruses to promote cancer development. Chewing tobacco is associated with cancers of the oral activity.

Many chemical substances found in the workplace have proved to be carcinogens or co-carcinogens in the cancer process. The extensive list of suspected chemical substances continues to grow. Chemical carcinogens include aromatic amines and analine dyes; arsenic, soots, and tars; asbestos; benzene; betel nut and lime; cadmium; chromium compounds; nickel ores; wood dust; and polyvinyl chloride.

Most hazardous chemicals produce their toxic effects by altering DNA structure in body sites distant from chemical exposure. The liver, lungs, and kidneys are the organ systems most often affected, presumably because of their roles in detoxification of chemicals.

Genetic and Familial Factors

Genetic factors also play a role in cancer cell development. If DNA damage occurs in cell populations where chromosomal patterns are abnormal, mutant cell populations may develop. Abnormal chromosomal patterns and cancer have been associated with extra chromosomes, too few chromosomes, or translocated chromosomes. Specific cancers with underlying genetic abnormalities include Burkitt's lymphoma, chronic myelogenous leukemia, meningiomas, acute leukemias, retinoblastomas, and skin cancers.

Some cancers of adulthood and childhood display familial predisposition. These cancers tend to occur at an early age and at multiple sites in one organ or pair of organs. Cancers associated with familial inheritance include retinoblastomas, nephroblastomas, pheochromocytomas, malignant neurofibromatosis, leukemias, and breast, endometrial, colorectal, stomach, prostate, and lung cancers.

Dietary Factors

Dietary factors are thought to be related to 40% to 60% of all environmental cancers. Dietary substances can be either proactive (protective) or carcinogenic or co-carcinogenic. The risk of cancer increases over long-term ingestion of carcinogens or co-carcinogens or chronic absence of proactive substances in the diet.

Dietary substances associated with an increased cancer risk include fats, alcohol, salt-cured or smoked meats, food containing nitrates and nitrites, and a high caloric dietary intake. Food substances that appear to reduce cancer risk include high-fiber foods, cruciferous vegetables (cabbage, broccoli, cauliflower, brussel sprouts, kohlrabi), and possibly vitamins A, E, and C, and selenium.

Hormonal Agents

Tumor growth may be promoted by disturbances in hormonal balance, by either the body's own (endogenous) hormone production or administration of exogenous hormones. Cancers of the breast, prostate, and uterus are considered to be dependent on endogenous hormonal levels for growth. Administration of oral contraceptives and diethylstilbestrol (DES) has been associated with hepatocellular carcinomas and vaginal carcinomas, respectively.

In summary, carcinogenesis can be caused by a variety of factors. Certain viruses, genetic characteristics, and hormonal status are thought to play a role in cancer etiology. Likewise, environmental factors such as chemical exposure, diet, and physical phenomena are also associated with cancer development. It is likely that a combination of several of these agents may be necessary to initiate and propagate malignant tumors.

The Role of the Immune System

In human beings, malignant cells are capable of developing on a regular basis. The surveillance function of the immune system is most often able to detect the development of malignant cells and destroy them before cell growth becomes uncontrolled. When the immune system fails to identify and stop the growth of malignant cells, clinical cancer develops. The increased incidence of malignancies in organ transplant recipients who receive immunosuppressive therapy to prevent rejection of the transplanted organ supports this theory. Patients receiving long-term chemotherapy to treat a malignancy are also at increased risk for the development of a second malignancy.

Patients with immunodeficiency diseases such as acquired immunodeficiency syndrome (AIDS) also have an increased incidence of malignancies. Most often these malignancies involve the lymphoreticular system.

Malignant cells undergo many changes in structure and function. As a result, new surface antigens, called tumor-associated antigens, are formed on cell membranes. These antigens are capable of stimulating the cellular and humoral immune responses. The T lymphocyte, the soldier of the cellular immune response, along with the macrophage, is responsible for the recognition of tumor cell antigens. When tumor antigens are recognized by T lymphocytes, other T lymphocytes toxic to the tumor cells are stimulated, proliferate, and are released into the circulation. In addition to possessing these cytotoxic properties, T lymphocytes are capable of stimulating other components of the immune system to rid the body of malignant cells. Certain *lymphokines*, which are substances produced by lymphocytes, are capable of killing or damaging various types of malignant cells. Other lymphokines are able to mobilize other cells such as macrophages that disrupt cancer cells. *Interferon*, a substance produced by the body in response to viral infection, also possesses some antitumor characteristics. Antibodies, produced by B lymphocytes of the humoral immune response, either alone or in combination with the complement system, also defend against malignant cells.

How is it, then, that malignant cells are able to survive and proliferate despite the immune system defense mechanisms? There are several theories about how tumor cells can overcome an apparently intact immune system. If the body fails to recognize the malignant cell as different from "self," the immune response may fail to be stimulated. The failure of the immune system to respond promptly to the malignant cells allows the tumor to grow to a size that is too large to be managed by normal immune mechanisms.

The tumor cells may actually suppress the patient's immune defenses. Tumor antigens may combine with the antibodies produced by the person and hide or mask themselves from normal immune defense mechanisms. These tumor antigen–antibody complexes can also depress further production of antibodies. Tumors are also capable of producing substances that impair usual immune defenses. These substances not only promote growth of the tumor, but also increase the patient's susceptibility to infection by a variety of pathogenic organisms.

As a result of prolonged contact with a tumor antigen, the patient's body may be depleted of the specific lymphocytes and no longer be able to mount an appropriate immune response.

Abnormal concentrations of host suppressor T lymphocytes may play a role in the development of malignancies. Suppressor T lymphocytes normally assist in the regulation of antibody production and diminish immune responses when they are no longer required. Studies have demonstrated that low levels of serum antibodies and high levels of suppressor cells have been found in patients with multiple myeloma, a malignancy associated with hypogammaglobulinemia (low amounts of serum antibodies). Carcinogens such as viruses or certain chemicals, including chemotherapeutic agents, may weaken the immune system and ultimately enhance tumor growth.

Finally, declining organ function, increased incidence of chronic diseases, and diminished immunocompetence associated with the aging process may contribute to an increased incidence of cancer in the later stages of the life cycle.

Detection and Prevention of Cancer

Nurses as well as physicians have traditionally been involved with *tertiary prevention*, the care and rehabilitation of the patient after cancer has been diagnosed and treated. In recent years, however, the American Cancer Society, the National Cancer Institute, clinicians, and researchers have placed greater emphasis on primary and secondary prevention of cancer. *Primary prevention* is concerned with reducing the risk or preventing the development of cancer in healthy people. *Secondary prevention* involves detection and screening efforts to achieve early diagnosis and prompt intervention to halt the cancerous process.

Nurses in all settings have an important role in cancer prevention. To participate in prevention of cancer, nurses must acquire the knowledge and skills necessary to provide the community with cancer prevention education about health-related behaviors, risk factors associated with the development of cancer, and screening and detection methods. Epidemiologic and laboratory studies have shown that dietary habits, sun exposure, tobacco use, and alcohol consumption can greatly influence the risk of developing cancer. Nurses also need teaching and counseling skills to foster client participation in cancer prevention programs and to promote healthy life styles.

To foster client participation in early detection and screening efforts, nurses have explored factors that influence behavior. Williams (1988) studied variables that influenced the practice of breast self-examination (BSE) in a population of older women. The findings suggest that women who engage in other health promotional activities are more likely to practice BSE.

Public awareness about health promotion can be increased in a variety of ways. Health education and health maintenance programs are sponsored by community organizations such as churches, senior citizen groups, and parent–teacher associations. Primary prevention programs may focus on the hazards of tobacco or the importance of nutrition. Secondary prevention programs may include breast and testicular self-examination and Papanicolaou tests. The American Cancer Society has developed a public education program, "Taking Control," that integrates diet, exercise, and general health habit tips that people can follow to reduce their risk of developing cancer (Table 19–3). Nurses in acute care settings can identify risks for patients and families and incorporate teaching and counseling in discharge planning.

Nurses also develop educational and counseling programs targeting patients and families with high incidences of cancer. Malignant melanoma and breast cancer are examples of malignancies often seen in more than one person in a family.

Screening of cancers for which there is a high incidence rate or in which early diagnosis plays a major role in improved survival rates is usually the focus of early detection efforts. Examples of these types of cancer include breast, colorectal, cervical, endometrial, testicular, skin, and oropharyngeal cancers.

Diagnosis of Cancer

The diagnosis of cancer is based on the assessment of physiologic and functional changes as well as on the results of the diagnostic evaluation. Patients with suspected cancer undergo extensive diagnostic testing to determine the presence of tumor and the extent of disease, to identify possible spread (metastasis) or invasion of other body tissues, to evaluate the function of involved as well as uninvolved body systems and organs, and to obtain tissue and cells for analysis of the cancer, including its stage and grade. Extensive testing most often includes a complete history and physical examination, radiologic, serologic, and other diagnostic and surgical procedures.

A patient undergoing extensive testing is usually fearful of the procedures themselves and anxious about the possible results of the testing. The patient and his family require information about the tests to be performed and the patient's role in the testing procedures. The nurse provides opportunities for the patient and family to verbalize their fears about the test results. She supports the patient and family throughout the period of diagnostic testing and reinforces and clarifies information conveyed to them by the physician. The nurse also encourages the patient and family members to communicate and share their concerns and to discuss their questions with each other.

Staging and Grading

A complete diagnostic evaluation includes identifying the stage and grade of malignancy. This must be accomplished before the initiation of treatment to provide for and maintain a systematic and consistent approach to diagnosis, treatment, and evaluation of interventions. Treatment options and prognosis are determined on the basis of staging and grading. This approach facilitates the exchange of information about similar types of cancer and their associated survival and response rates. Ultimately, these classifications can assist in ongoing cancer research.

Staging determines the size of the tumor and the existence of metastasis. Several systems exist for classifying the anatomic extent of disease. The *TNM system*, developed from the work of the International Union Against Cancer (IUCC) and the American Joint Committee for Cancer Staging and End Stage Reporting (AJCCS), is frequently used in describing malignancies such as breast, lung, or head and neck cancers. In this system, the *T* refers to the extent of the primary tumor, *N* refers to lymph node involvement, and *M* refers to the extent of me-

---

TABLE 19–3. *Ten Steps of Cancer Prevention*

Action	Rationale
PROTECTIVE FACTORS	
1. Increase consumption of fresh vegetables (especially those of the cabbage family).	Increase fiber intake; increase intake of vitamins.
2. Increase fiber intake.	High-fiber diets reduce risk of developing certain cancers (cancer of breast, prostate, and colon).
3. Increase intake of vitamin A.	Reduces risk of cancers (esophagus, larynx, and lung).
4. Increase intake of foods rich in vitamin C.	Citrus fruits and vegetables rich in vitamin C may protect against cancer of the stomach and esophagus.
5. Practice weight control.	Obesity is linked to cancers of the uterus, gallbladder, breast, and colon.
RISK FACTORS	
6. Reduce the amount of dietary fat.	A high-fat diet increases risk of developing breast, colon, and prostate cancers.
7. Reduce intake of salt-cured, smoked, and nitrate-cured foods.	Moderation in consumption of these foods is recommended, as they have been linked to cancers of the esophagus and stomach.
8. Stop cigarette smoking.	Smokers are at risk for lung cancer.
9. Reduce alcohol intake.	Drinking large amounts of alcohol increases the risk of liver cancer. Heavy drinkers who smoke are at greater risk for cancers of the mouth, throat, larynx, and esophagus.
10. Avoid overexposure to the sun.	Overexposure to the sun increases the risk of skin cancer. Protective clothing or use of a sunscreen reduces the risk.

(Modified from the Taking Control Program of the American Cancer Society.)

tastasis (Chart 19–2). A variety of other staging systems are available for cancers that do not lend themselves to the TNM system.

Grading refers to the classification of the tumor cells. Grading systems seek to define the origin of tissue of the tumor and the degree to which the tumor cells retain the functional and histologic characteristics of the tissue of origin.

This information assists in projecting the behavior and prognosis of various tumors. Grading is assigned a numeric value ranging from I to IV. Grade I tumors, also known as well-differentiated tumors, closely resemble the tissue of origin in structure and function. Tumors that do not clearly resemble the tissue of origin in structure or function are described as poorly or undifferentiated and are assigned a grade IV. These tumors tend to be more virulent and less responsive to treatment than well-differentiated tumors.

Management of Cancer

Treatment options offered to cancer patients should be based on realistic and achievable goals for each specific type of cancer. The range of possible treatment goals may include complete eradication of malignant disease (*cure*), prolonged survival with the presence of malignancy (*control*), or relief of symptoms associated with the cancerous disease process (*palliation*). It is imperative that the health care team, the patient, and the patient's family have a clear understanding of the treatment options and goals. Open communication and support are vital as the patient and his family periodically reassess treatment plans and goals when complications of therapy develop or disease progression occurs.

Multiple modalities are often employed in cancer treatment. A variety of therapies, including surgery, radiation therapy, chemotherapy, and biologic response modifier therapy may be used at various times during the course of treatment.

An understanding of the principles of each and how they interrelate is important in understanding the rationale and goals of treatment.

Surgery

Surgical removal of the entire cancer remains the best and most frequently used modality of treatment. The surgical approach, however, may be selected for a variety of reasons. Surgery may be selected as the primary method of treatment or it may diagnostic, prophylactic, palliative, or reconstructive.

Surgery as Primary Treatment

When surgery is used as the primary approach in the treatment of cancer, the goal is to remove the entire tumor (or as much as is feasible, a procedure often called *debulking*) and any involved surrounding tissue, including regional lymph nodes.

Two common surgical approaches used for the treatment of primary tumors are local and radical excisions. Local excision is warranted when the mass is small and tissue margins are safely accessible. Radical excisions include removal of the primary tumor, surrounding tissues, and lymph nodes. This surgical method can result in disfigurement and altered functioning. Radical excisions are considered, however, if the tumor can be completely removed and the chances of cure or control are optimal. A multidisciplinary approach is essential during and after the surgery. The effects on body image, self-esteem, and functional abilities are addressed. A plan for postoperative rehabilitation is made before the surgical intervention.

It is now recognized that the growth and dissemination of cancer cells have often produced distant micrometastases by the time the patient seeks treatment. Therefore, attempting to remove wide margins of tissue in the hopes of "getting all the cancer cells" is often not realistic. This reality substantiates the need for a coordinated multidisciplinary approach to cancer therapy. Once the surgery has been completed, one or more additional modalities may be chosen to increase the likelihood

---

Chart 19–2
TNM Classification System

T* subclasses

Tx—tumor cannot be adequately assessed
T0—no evidence of primary tumor
TIS—carcinoma *in situ*
T1, T2, T3, T4—progressive increase in tumor size and involvement

N† subclasses

Nx—regional lymph nodes cannot be assessed clinically
N0—regional lymph nodes demonstrably normal
N1, N2, N3, N4—increasing degrees of demonstrable abnormalities of regional lymph nodes

M‡ subclasses

Mx—not assessed
M0—no (known) distant metastasis
M1—distant metastasis present, specify site(s)

Histopathology

G1—well-differentiated grade
G2—moderately well-differentiated grade
G3, G4—poorly to very poorly differentiated grade

* T = Primary tumor.
† N = Regional lymph nodes.
‡ M = Distant metastasis.
(American Joint Committee on Cancer. Manual for Staging of Cancer. Chicago, American Joint Committee.)

of cancer cell destruction. There are, however, cancers that when treated surgically in the very early stages are considered to be curable (*e.g.*, skin cancers, testicular cancers).

Diagnostic Surgery

Diagnostic surgery is usually performed to obtain a biopsy (excision of a piece of tissue from a suspicious growth) to analyze the tissues and cells of the suggested malignancy. The three most common biopsy methods are the excisional, incisional, and needle methods. The *excisional method* is most frequently used for easily accessible tumors of the skin, breast, upper and lower gastrointestinal tract, and the upper respiratory tract. Often, removal of the entire tumor as well as surrounding normal tissue margins is possible. Removal of normal tissue beyond the area of the tumor decreases the possibility of residual microscopic disease that may lead to recurrence of the tumor. This approach not only provides the pathologist with the entire specimen but also decreases the chance of cellular seeding of the tumor. The *incisional method* is used if the tumor mass is too large to be removed. It is imperative that the biopsy be representative of the tumor mass so that the pathologist can provide an accurate diagnosis. Negative biopsy results do not guarantee absence of malignancy. Both of these approaches are often endoscopic procedures. Surgical incision is often required to determine the anatomic extent or stage of the tumor.

Needle biopsy is used to sample suspicious masses that are easily accessible, such as some growths in the breasts, lung, liver, and kidney. The procedure is fast, relatively inexpensive, easy to perform and generally requires only local anesthesia. In general, the patient experiences minimal and temporary physical discomfort. In addition, the degree to which the surrounding tissue is disturbed is kept to a minimum, thus decreasing the likelihood of disseminating cancer cells (seeding). There is, however, a chance that even the most skilled physician will obtain a biopsy specimen from such a small area that a full description of the cellular types is not possible.

The choice of biopsy to be performed takes into account many factors. Of greatest importance is the type of treatment anticipated if a diagnosis of cancer is confirmed. The surgical area includes the site of biopsy so that any cells that might have been dislodged during the procedure are excised at the time of surgery. In addition, the condition of the patient is considered. Assessment of nutritional, respiratory, renal, and hepatic systems is essential in determining the most appropriate method of treatment. If the biopsy requires general anesthesia, and subsequent surgery is likely, the effects of prolonged anesthesia on the patient are considered. The patient and his family are given an opportunity to discuss the available options before definitive plans are made. The nurse, as the patient's advocate, serves as a liaison between the patient and the physician to facilitate this process. Time should be set aside to minimize interruptions. Time for questions and for thinking through all that has been discussed should be provided.

Prophylactic Surgery

Prophylactic surgery involves the removal of lesions that are likely to develop into cancer, such as small tumors (polyps) that often grow in the colon. Recently, more aggressive surgical procedures have been performed as prophylactic measures. The two most common are colectomies and mastectomies in persons who are at a significantly high risk because of personal and family history. Because the long-term physiologic and psychologic effects are not known, these therapeutic approaches are offered selectively to patients. Preoperative information and counseling, as well as long-term follow-up, should be available.

Palliative Surgery

When cure of the cancer is not possible, the goal of treatment is to provide the patient with as much comfort as possible and a satisfying and productive life for as long as is possible. Whether the period is extremely short or lengthy, the major goal is a high quality of life—with quality defined by the patient and his family. Honest and informative communication with the patient and family about the goal of surgery is essential to avoid false hope and disappointment.

Palliative surgery is performed in an attempt to relieve complications of cancer, such as ulcerations, obstructions, hemorrhage, pain, or infection. This type of surgery includes nerve blocks and cordotomies designed to relieve intractable pain; tumor resection, to relieve obstruction that may occur if a segment of bowel is obstructed (this may result in ostomies, depending on the extent of invasion); and simple mastectomies for ulcerative breast disease.

Finally, surgical removal of hormone-producing glands that might enhance tumor growth is often performed. These glands include the pituitary, adrenals, ovaries, and testes.

Reconstructive Surgery

Reconstructive surgery may follow curative or radical surgery and is carried out in an attempt to produce a better return of function or a better cosmetic effect. It may be performed in one operation or in stages. Presurgery counseling and evaluation are recommended. The surgeon who is to perform the reconstructive surgery is often consulted preoperatively. For example, the woman who is to have breast reconstruction performed may see the surgeon before hospitalization for a mastectomy. This approach provides the woman with something positive to focus on, at a time when thoughts of disfigurement and death may be paramount. The physician performing the reconstructive surgery also benefits from seeing the way the woman's breasts appear normally and from establishing rapport with her. The nurse must be cognizant of the woman's sexual needs and the impact that an altered body image may have on her sexuality. Providing the woman and her family with opportunities to discuss these issues is imperative. The needs of the individual must be accurately assessed and validated in each situation for any type of reconstructive surgery.

Nursing Considerations

Nursing care for the patient undergoing surgery is discussed in Unit 5. The individual with cancer often has additional needs, however. These may include the existence of organ impairment, nutritional deficits, disorders of coagulation, and altered immunity that may lead to an increased incidence of postoperative complications. The use of combined modalities such as radiation and chemotherapy also contribute to postoperative complications such as infection, impaired wound healing, and the development of deep vein thrombosis. The nurse completes a thorough preoperative assessment for all factors that may affect patients undergoing surgical procedures.

The patient undergoing surgery for the diagnosis or treatment of cancer is often anxious about the surgical procedure, possible findings, postoperative limitations, changes in normal body functions, and prognosis. The patient and family require time and assistance to deal with the possible changes and outcomes.

The nurse provides education and emotional support by assessing patient and family needs. She explores fears and mechanisms of coping and allows patients and families to participate in decision making whenever possible.

The nurse who is asked about the results of diagnostic testing and surgical procedures is guided in her response by the information conveyed to the patient and family by the physician. She may be asked by the patient and family to explain and clarify information that was provided by the physician at a time when their level of anxiety kept them from understanding the information and its implications. It is important for the nurse to communicate frequently with the physician and other health care team members to be certain that a consistent approach is used.

After surgery, the nurse assesses the patient for responses to the surgical intervention and for possible complications such as infection, bleeding, thrombophlebitis, wound dehiscence, and organ dysfunction. The nurse also provides for patient comfort. Postoperative teaching includes wound care, activity, nutrition, and medications.

Plans for discharge and follow-up care and treatment are initiated as early as possible to ensure continuity of care from hospital to home or from a cancer referral center to the patient's local hospital and health care provider.

Radiation Therapy

Radiation therapy is the use of ionizing radiation to interrupt cellular growth. About half of patients with cancer receive a form of irradiation at some point in their course of treatment. This treatment modality may be chosen when the treatment goal is curative, such as in Hodgkin's disease, testicular seminomas, localized cancers of the head and neck, and cancers of the uterine cervix. Radiation therapy may also be used to control malignant disease when a tumor cannot be removed surgically or when local nodal metastasis is present, or prophylactically to prevent leukemic infiltration to the brain or spinal cord. Palliative irradiation is frequently used to relieve the symptoms of metastatic disease, especially when it has spread to brain, bone, or soft tissue.

Two types of ionizing radiation exist: electromagnetic rays (x-rays and gamma rays) and heavier particulate radiation (electrons [beta particles], protons, neutrons, and alpha particles). Either type can lead to tissue disruption by ionization. The most harmful tissue disruption is the alteration of the DNA molecule within the cells of the tissue. Ionizing radiation causes breakage among the strands of the DNA helix, leading to cell death. Ionizing radiation can also ionize body fluids, especially water, leading to the formation of free radicals, which also cause irreversible damage to DNA.

Cellular death may occur immediately if DNA repair does not occur, or at the time of cellular division when the damaged cell attempts mitosis and dies. Finally, a tumor cell may become sterile by the effects of radiation and die a natural death without the ability to produce progeny.

Cells are most vulnerable to the disruptive effects of radiation during DNA synthesis and mitosis (early S, G_2, and M phases of the cell cycle). Therefore, those body tissues that undergo frequent cell division are most sensitive to radiation therapy. These tissues include bone marrow, lymphatic tissue, epithelium of the gastrointestinal tract, and gonads.

Those tissues that are slower growing or at rest are relatively radioresistant; they include muscle, cartilage, and connective tissues. A *radiosensitive tumor* is one that can be destroyed by a dose of radiation that still allows for normal cell regeneration in the normal tissue. Tumors that are well oxygenated also seem to be more sensitive to radiation; therefore, radiation therapy might be enhanced if oxygen concentrations to tumors could be increased. In addition, if the radiation could be delivered at a time when most tumor cells were in either the S or M phases, the number of cancer cells destroyed ("cell kill") would be increased.

Radiation is delivered to tumor sites by either external or internal mechanisms. If external radiation therapy is used, one of several methods of delivery may be chosen, depending on

---

Chart 19–3
External Beam Radiation Therapy Equipment

Type of Radiation	Area of Maximum Dose	Indications
Kilovoltage		
Superficial radiation (10–125 Kv)	Skin surface	Superficial skin lesions
Orthovoltage radiation (125–400 Kv)	Skin surface (higher bone absorption)	Bony metastases
Gamma ray therapy		
Isotope source (cobalt or cesium)	0.5 cm below skin surface	Most malignant conditions
Megavoltage therapy		
Linear accelerators (x-rays or electrons)		
6-MV machines	1.5 cm below skin surface	Most malignant conditions; especially if
15-MV machines	3.0 cm below skin surface	deeply seated in the body
Particle beam therapy		
Cyclotrons (neutron beam therapy)	Increased uptake in fatty tissue	Late stage malignant disease; tumors that are large, anoxic, necrotic, and resistant to treatment

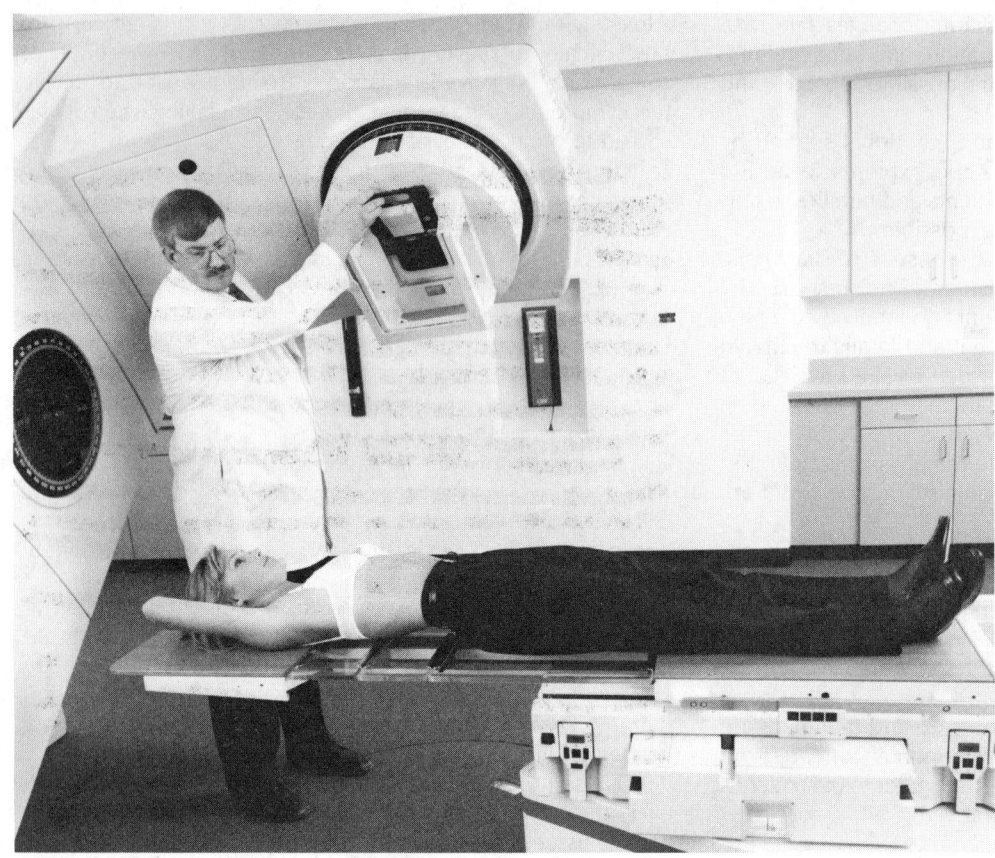

Figure 19-2. Mevatron, a linear electron accelerator used for radiotherapy. (Courtesy of Siemens Medical Laboratories, Inc.)

the depth of the tumor to be radiated (Chart 19-3). Kilovoltage therapy devices deliver the maximum radiation dose to superficial lesions such as lesions of the skin and breast, whereas gamma ray sources (cobalt-60 units) deliver the radiation dose to deeper body structures and spare the skin from possible adverse effects. Other radiation therapy machines, *linear accelerators* (Fig. 19-2) deliver their dosage to deeper structures without harming the skin and also create less scattering of radiation within the body tissues. A minimal number of centers nationwide treat more hypoxic, radioresistant tumors with cyclotrons that deliver neutron-beam therapy to the tumor.

Internal radiation implants are used to deliver a high dose of radiation to a localized area. The specific radioisotope for implantation is selected on the basis of its *half-life*, which is the time it takes for half of its radioactivity to decay. This internal radiation can be implanted by way of needles, seeds, beads, or catheters. With internal radiation therapy, as the distance from the radiation source increases, the dosage delivered to the patient decreases. This allows for sparing of tissue away from the local area. Patients receiving internal radiation emit radiation while the implant is in place. Principles of time, distance, and shielding must be used in planning care for these patients to minimize exposure of personnel to radiation.

Radiation Dosage

The radiation dosage is dependent on the sensitivity of the target tissues to radiation and the tumor size. The *lethal tumor dose* is defined as that dose that will eradicate 95% of the tumor yet preserve normal tissue.

The total radiation dose is delivered over several weeks to allow repair of healthy tissue and to achieve a greater cell kill by increasing the availability of a greater number of cells

in the early S, G$_2$, or M phases of the cell cycle. Repeated radiation treatments over time (fractioned doses) also allow time for the periphery of the tumor to be repeatedly reoxygenated, as tumors shrink from the outside inward. This increases the radiosensitivity of the tumor, thus increasing tumor cell death.

Toxicity

Toxicity of radiation therapy is usually localized to the region being irradiated. Local reactions occur when normal cells in the treatment area are also destroyed and cellular regeneration falls behind cellular death. Body tissues most frequently affected are those that normally proliferate rapidly; they include the skin, the epithelial lining of the gastrointestinal system, and the bone marrow. Alteration in skin integrity is a common effect and can include alopecia, erythema, and shedding of skin (desquamation). Once treatments have been completed, reepithelialization occurs. Alterations in oral mucosal membranes secondary to radiation therapy include stomatitis, dryness of the mouth (xerostomia), change and loss of taste, and decreased salivation. The entire gastrointestinal mucosa may be involved, and esophageal irritation with chest pain and dysphagia may result. Anorexia, nausea, vomiting, and diarrhea may occur if the stomach or colon is in the irradiated field. Symptoms subside and gastrointestinal reepithelialization occurs once treatments are complete. Bone marrow cells proliferate rapidly, and if bone marrow–producing sites are included in the field of irradiation, anemia, leukopenia, and thrombocytopenia may result. Patients are then at increased risk of infection and bleeding until blood cell counts return to normal. Chronic anemia may occur.

Certain systemic side effects are also commonly experienced by patients receiving radiation therapy. These manifestations, which are generalized, include fatigue, malaise, headache, nausea, and vomiting. This syndrome may be secondary to substances released when tumor cells break down. The effects are temporary and subside with the cessation of treatments.

Late effects of radiation therapy may also occur in various body tissues. These effects are chronic, usually produce fibrotic changes secondary to a decreased vascular supply, and are irreversible. These late effects can be most severe when they involve vital organs such as the lungs, heart, central nervous system, and bladder.

In summary, radiation therapy is a cancer treatment modality used to cure, control, or palliate malignant disease. Both internal and external means of radiation therapy are available for local delivery. Toxicity is very dependent on the area of the body radiated. Gastrointestinal, skin, and hematopoietic side effects continue to challenge nurses caring for patients receiving radiation therapy.

Nursing Considerations

The patient who is receiving radiation therapy and his family often have questions and concerns about its safety. The nurse is often in a position to answer questions and allay fears about its effects on others, on the tumor, and on the patient's normal tissues and organs. The actual procedure for delivering the radiation is explained, along with a description of the equipment to be used, the duration of the procedure (often minutes only), the possible need for immobilization of the patient during the procedure, and the absence of new sensations during the procedure. If the patient receives radiation therapy by means of a radioactive implant, he requires explanations about limitation of visitors and health care personnel and other radiation precautions. He also needs to understand his role before, during, and after the procedure.

Attention is given by the nurse to the patient's skin, nutritional status, and general feeling of well-being. The patient's skin and oral mucosa are assessed frequently for changes (particularly if radiation therapy is directed to these areas). The skin is protected from irritation, and the patient is advised to avoid using ointments, lotions, or powders on the area. Gentle oral hygiene is essential to remove debris and prevent irritation. If the patient experiences systemic changes such as weakness and fatigue, he may need assistance with activities of daily living and personal hygiene. Additionally, the nurse's explanation that these symptoms are a result of the treatment, and do not represent deterioration or disease progression, is often reassuring to the patient.

When a patient has a radioactive implant in place, the nurse also takes precautions to protect herself and other personnel as well as the patient from the effects of radiation. Pregnant staff, pregnant visitors, and children are discouraged from visiting and caring for patients with these implants.

Generally, the patient is either on bed rest or restricted to his room while the radioactive implant is in place. Specific instructions are frequently provided by the radiation safety officer from the radiology department and usually include the maximum amount of time to be spent in the patient's room, shielding equipment to be used, and special precautions and actions to be taken if the implant is dislodged. The patient is informed about the rationale for these precautions so that he does not feel unduly isolated.

Chemotherapy

Chemotherapy is the use of antineoplastic agents to promote tumor cell death by interfering with cellular functions and reproduction. It is used primarily to treat systemic disease rather than lesions that are localized and amenable to surgery or irradiation. Chemotherapy may be combined with surgery or radiation therapy, or both, to reduce tumor size preoperatively, to destroy remaining tumor cells postoperatively, or to treat some forms of leukemia. Goals of chemotherapy (cure, control, palliation) must be realistic, because they will define the medications to be used and the aggressiveness of the treatment plan.

Each time a tumor is exposed to a chemotherapeutic agent, a percentage of tumor cells (20% to 99%, depending on dosage) is destroyed. Repeated doses of drugs are necessary over a prolonged period to achieve regression of the tumor. Eradication of 100% of the tumor is nearly impossible, but a goal of chemotherapy is to eradicate enough of the tumor that the remaining tumor cells can be destroyed by the body's immune system.

Actively proliferating cells within a tumor (growth fraction) are the most sensitive to chemotherapeutic agents. Nondividing cells capable of future proliferation are the least sensitive to antineoplastic drugs and consequently are potentially dangerous. They must be destroyed, however, to eradicate a malignancy completely. Repeated cycles of chemotherapy are used to enhance tumor cell kill by destroying these nondividing cells as they are signaled into active proliferation. These effects are related to the phases of the reproductive cycle of the cell—the cell cycle. Reproduction of both healthy and malignant cells follows the cell cycle pattern (Fig. 19–3). The *cell cycle time* is the time required for one tissue cell to divide and re-

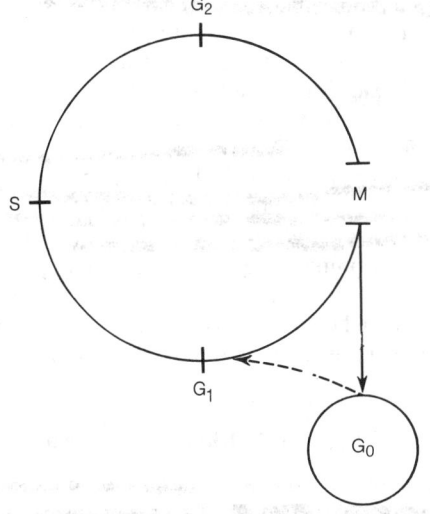

Figure 19–3. Phases of the cell cycle. The cycle represents the interval between the midpoint of mitosis to the subsequent end point in mitosis in a daughter cell. G_1 is the postmitotic phase during which RNA and protein synthesis is increased and cell growth occurs. G_0 is the resting or dormant phase of the cell cycle. The S phase represents synthesis of nucleic acids with chromosome replication in preparation for cell mitosis. During G_2, RNA and protein synthesis occurs as in G_1. (Porth CM. Pathophysiology: Concepts of Altered Health States, 3rd ed. Philadelphia, JB Lippincott, 1990.)

produce into two identical daughter cells. The cell cycle of any cell has four distinct phases, each with a vital underlying function: (1) G_1 phase—RNA and protein synthesis occurs; (2) S phase—DNA synthesis occurs; (3) G_2 phase—premitotic phase, DNA synthesis complete, mitotic spindle forms; and (4) mitosis—cell division occurs. The G_0 phase, the resting or dormant phase of cells, can occur after mitosis and during the G_1 phase. In the G_0 phase are those dangerous cells that are not actively dividing but have the future potential for replication. The administration of certain chemotherapeutic agents (as well as administration of some other forms of therapy) is coordinated with the cell cycle.

Classification of Chemotherapeutic Agents

Certain chemotherapeutic agents (cell cycle–specific drugs) destroy cells in specific phases of the cell cycle. Most cell cycle–specific drugs affect cells in the S phase by interfering with DNA and RNA synthesis. Others, such as the *vinca* or plant alkaloids, are specific to the M phase, where they halt mitotic spindle formation.

Those chemotherapeutic agents that act independently of the cell cycle phases are termed *cell cycle–nonspecific drugs*. These agents usually have a prolonged effect on cells, leading to cellular damage or death. Many treatment plans combine cell cycle–specific and cell cycle–nonspecific drugs to increase the number of vulnerable tumor cells killed during a treatment period.

Chemotherapeutic agents are also classified according to various chemical groups, each with a different mechanism of action. These include the alkylating agents, nitrosoureas, antimetabolites, antitumor antibiotics, plant alkaloids, hormonal agents, and miscellaneous agents. The classification, mechanism of action, common drugs, cell-cycle specificity, and common side effects of antineoplastic agents are listed in Table 19–4. Chemotherapeutic agents from each category may be used to enhance the tumor cell kill during therapy. Combinations of chemotherapy drugs used must also contain drugs of differing toxicities and with synergistic actions.

Investigational Drugs and Clinical Trials. Investigational antineoplastic drugs undergo thorough trials to test their toxicities and effectiveness. Before new chemotherapeutic agents are approved for clinical use in the treatment of cancer, they are subjected to rigorous and often lengthy evaluation to identify beneficial effects, side effects, and safety. Phase I clinical trials determine optimal drug dosing, scheduling, and toxicity. Phase II trials determine drug effectiveness with specific tumor types, and phase III clinical trials establish the effectiveness of new drug therapies as compared with conventional, established therapy.

Administration of Chemotherapeutic Agents

Routes of Administration. Chemotherapeutic drugs may be administered by topical, oral, intravenous, intramuscular, subcutaneous, arterial, intracavitary, and intrathecal routes. The route of administration is usually dependent on the type of drug, the required dose, and the type, location, and extent of tumor being treated.

Dosage. Dosage of antineoplastic agents is based primarily on the patient's total body surface area, previous response to chemotherapy or radiation therapy, and physical performance status.

Extravasation. Special care must be taken whenever intravenous vesicant agents are administered. *Vesicant drugs* are those agents that, if deposited into the subcutaneous tissue (extravasated), cause tissue necrosis and damage to underlying tendons, nerves, and blood vessels. Although the complete mechanism of tissue destruction is unclear, it is known that the *p*H of many antineoplastic drugs is responsible for the severe inflammatory reaction as well as the binding ability of drugs to tissue DNA. Sloughing and ulceration of tissue may be so severe that skin grafting may be necessary. The full extent of tissue damage may take several weeks to become apparent. Drugs classified as vesicant agents include dactinomycin, daunorubicin, doxorubicin (Adriamycin), nitrogen mustard, mithramycin, mitomycin, vinblastine, vincristine, and vindesine.

Only specially trained physicians and nurses are to be involved in the administration of vesicants. Careful selection of peripheral veins, skilled venipuncture, and careful drug administration are essential. Indications of extravasation during drug administration include loss of blood return from the intravenous device; resistance to intravenous fluid flow; and swelling, pain, or redness at the site. If extravasation is suspected, the drug administration is stopped immediately and ice applied to the site (except for *vinca* alkaloid extravasation). The physician may aspirate any infiltrated drug from the tissues and inject a neutralizing solution into the area to reduce tissue damage. Recommendations and guidelines for management of vesicant extravasation have been issued by individual drug manufacturers, pharmacies, and the Oncology Nursing Society, and differ from one drug to the next.

When frequent, prolonged administration of vesicant antineoplastic agents is anticipated, right atrial Silastic catheters or venous access devices may be inserted. These devices promote safety during drug administration and reduce problems with access to the circulatory system (Chart 19–4).

Toxicity

Toxicity associated with chemotherapy can be acute or chronic. Cells with rapid growth rates (*e.g.*, epithelium, bone marrow, hair follicles) are more susceptible to damage from these agents. Various body systems may be affected by these drugs and are discussed in the following paragraphs.

Gastrointestinal System. Nausea and vomiting are the most common side effects of chemotherapy and may persist for up to 24 hours after drug administration. Stimulation of the vomiting centers of the brain occurs by (1) stimulation of the chemoreceptor trigger zone of the medulla; (2) stimulation of peripheral autonomic pathways (gastrointestinal [GI] tract and pharynx); (3) stimulation of the vestibular pathways (inner-ear imbalances, labyrinth input); (4) cognitive stimulation (central nervous system [CNS] disease, anticipatory nausea and vomiting); and (5) a combination of factors. Use of phenothiazines, sedatives, steroids, and histamines, alone or in combination, is often effective in minimizing nausea and vomiting. Relaxation techniques and imagery can also help to decrease stimuli contributing to symptoms. Alterations in the patient's diet may reduce the frequency or severity of these symptoms.

Although the epithelium that lines the oral cavity quickly renews itself, its rapid rate of proliferation makes it susceptible to the effects of chemotherapy. As a result, stomatitis and anorexia are common. The entire gastrointestinal tract is suscep-

(text continues on page 358)

TABLE 19-4. *Classification, Actions, and Side Effects of Antineoplastic Agents*

Category	Mechanism of Action	Common Drugs	Cell Cycle Specificity	Common Side Effects
Alkylating agents	Alter DNA structure by • Misreading of DNA code • Breaks in DNA molecule • Cross-linking of DNA strands	Nitrogen mustard Cyclophosphamide Ifosfamide Melphalan Chlorambucil Thiotepa Carboplatin Cisplatin Busulfan	Cell cycle nonspecific	Bone marrow suppression, nausea, vomiting, cystitis (cyclophosphamide) stomatitis, alopecia, gonadal suppression renal toxicity (Cisplatin)
Nitrosoureas	Similar to alkylating agents; cross blood–brain barrier	Carmustine (BCNU) Lomustine (CCNU) Semustine (methyl CCNU) Streptozocin	Cell cycle nonspecific	Delayed and cumulative myelosuppression, especially thrombocytopenia; nausea, vomiting
Antimetabolites	Interfere with the biosynthesis of metabolites/nucleic acids necessary for RNA and DNA synthesis	Cytarabine 5-fluorouracil FUDR Methotrexate (MTX) Hydroxyurea 6-Mercaptopurine 6-Thioguanine 5-Azacytadine	Cell cycle specific (S phase)	Nausea, vomiting, diarrhea, myelosuppression, proctitis, stomatitis, renal toxicity (MTX), hepatotoxicity.
Antitumor antibiotics	Interfere with DNA synthesis by binding DNA; prevent RNA synthesis	Dactinomycin Bleomycin Daunorubicin Mithramycin Mitomycin Mitoxantrone Doxorubicin (Adriamycin)	Cell cycle nonspecific	Bone marrow suppression, nausea, vomiting, alopecia, anorexia, cardiac toxicity (Daunorubicin, Doxorubicin)
Plant alkaloids	Cause metaphase arrest by inhibiting mitotic tubular formation (spindle); inhibit DNA and protein synthesis	Vincristine (VCR) Vinblastine Vindesine VP-16 VM-26	Cell cycle specific (M phase)	Bone marrow suppression (mild with VCR), neuropathies (VCR), stomatitis
Hormonal agents	Bind to hormone receptor sites that alter cellular growth; block binding of estrogens to receptor sites (anti-estrogens); inhibit RNA synthesis	Androgens Estrogens Anti-estrogens Progesterone Steroids	Cell cycle nonspecific	Hypercalcemia, jaundice, increased appetite, masculinization, feminization, sodium and fluid retention, nausea, vomiting, hot flashes
Miscellaneous agents	Unknown; too complex to categorize	Asparaginase Procarbazine M-AMSA Hexamethylmelamine Dacarbazine (DTIC) Mitoxantrone Methyl-GAG	?	Anorexia, nausea, vomiting, myelosuppression, hepatotoxicity, anaphylaxis, hypotension, altered glucose metabolism

Chart 19-4
Vascular Access Devices

Frequent administration of intravenous chemotherapy, fluids, medications, blood products, parenteral nutrition, and frequent blood sampling often necessitate long-term central venous access for patients with cancer. Several varieties of venous access devices (VADs) available for use. The choice of device is dependent on patient preference, patient self-care abilities, type of treatment, mode of administration, longevity of the treatment, and the patient's financial resources. Two of the most commonly used VADs are summarized below.

Right Atrial Catheters

Right atrial catheters are made of a silicone silastic material that is flexible, nonirritating, and decreases the risk of thrombosis. These catheters are available with one or several lumens with comparable fluid-carrying capacities. The catheter is surgically placed under local anesthesia into a large vein (*i.e.*, cephalic, subclavian, or jugular)

and advanced until the distal tip is in the superior vena cava, just above the right atrium (Fig. 19-4). The proximal end of the catheter is tunneled through the subcutaneous tissue of the chest wall and brought out through an exit site on the chest midway between the clavicle and the nipple. Each catheter has a Dacron cuff that is embedded in the subcutaneous tissue just above the exit site on the chest wall. The cuff stabilizes the catheter and prevents micro-organisms from migrating up the catheter. The catheter is ready for use immediately after confirmation of placement by chest radiograph.

Cleansing and dressing of the exit site are performed in accordance with individual institutional policies. Examples of agents used for cleansing include alcohol, hydrogen peroxide, and povidine-iodine. Occlusive gauze or transparent dressings may be used to cover the exit site. Most commonly, cleansing and dressing changes are done every 24 to 72 hours. Routine catheter maintenance requires periodic heparin flushes to prevent catheter occlusion by a thrombosis. The frequency of flushing and the dosage of heparin vary according to

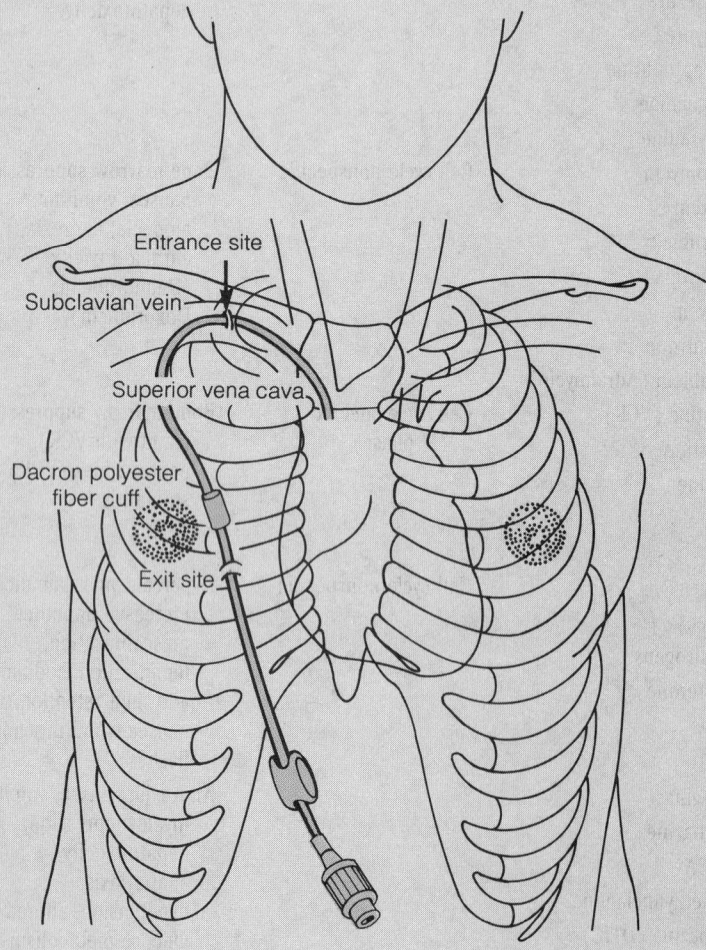

Entrance site

Subclavian vein

Superior vena cava

Dacron polyester fiber cuff

Exit site

Figure 19-4.   Right atrial catheter. The right atrial catheter is inserted into the subclavian vein and advanced until its tip is in the superior vena cava just above the right atrium. The proximal end is then tunneled from the entry site through the subcutaneous tissue of the chest wall and brought out through an exit site on the chest. The Dacron cuff helps to anchor the catheter in place and serves as a barrier to infection. (Redrawn from Viall CD. Your complete guide to central venous catheters. Nursing 1990 Feb; 20[2]:37.)

continued

Chart 19-4 *(Continued)*

individual institutional policies. Most catheters can be maintained by a daily or every other day flush with heparinized saline in a concentration of 100 units of heparin per 1 ml of normal saline in a volume of 2.5 to 3 ml. The catheter is also flushed after blood withdrawal or intermittent fluid administration. Patients and family members are taught to perform all aspects of catheter care at home. In addition, the nurse instructs patients and families to monitor for catheter-related infection. Signs and symptoms of infection include redness, drainage, swelling and pain at the exit site, and fever and chills. Other catheter-related complications include cuff extrusion, catheter occlusion, and catheter breakage.

Implanted Ports

An implanted port is a long-term VAD with no external parts. It consists of a polyurethane or silicone catheter that is attached to a self-sealing rubber septum encased in stainless steal, plastic, or titanium (Fig. 19-5*A*). Placement of an implanted VAD is similar to that of a right atrial catheter. A small incision is made over the selected vein and the catheter is advanced to the tip of the right atrium. A second incision is made on the anterior chest wall to create a pocket to house the port. The catheter is attached to the port once catheter position is confirmed with fluoroscopy. The port is sutured into place and the pocket is closed. All that can be seen externally is a slight bulge under the skin in the chest wall. Implanted ports are available for placement in the basilic or cephalic veins in the arm near the antecubital space and the femoral vein in the anterior thigh. Ports may also provide access to arterial circulation for arterial chemotherapy infusions such as those administered to the liver through the hepatic artery. Chemotherapy and analgesics are occasionally administered into the cerebral spinal fluid by ports that provide access to the subarachnoid space located along the spinal cord. For this type of drug administration, the port is located in the abdomen and connected to a catheter that extends into the subarachnoid space.

Depending on the manufacturer, access to the ports may be through top or side entry through the insertion of a special needle known as a *Huber needle* (see Fig. 19-5*B*). The design of the angled bevel of the Huber needle prevents coring of the rubber septum of the port and permits repeated needle insertion. Straight Huber needles are available for bolus injections and blood withdrawal from both top and side entry ports. A 90-degree angled Huber needle is used exclusively for top entry ports for prolonged continuous infusions of fluids or chemotherapy. A dressing is applied over the 90-degree needle to secure needle position and prevent infection. Heparin flushes, similar to those used for right atrial catheters, are required after completion of each infusion, blood withdrawal, or before removal of the Huber needle. Routine port maintenance requires heparin flushes every 3 to 4 weeks by the nurse or physician. Patients do not routinely need to learn how to flush this system or apply dressings because the needle is removed between port use. The patient and his family members are taught to monitor the site for signs of infection including pain, swelling, redness, or drainage. The patient is also instructed to monitor for fever and chills. Other complications include catheter occlusion and detachment of the catheter and the port.

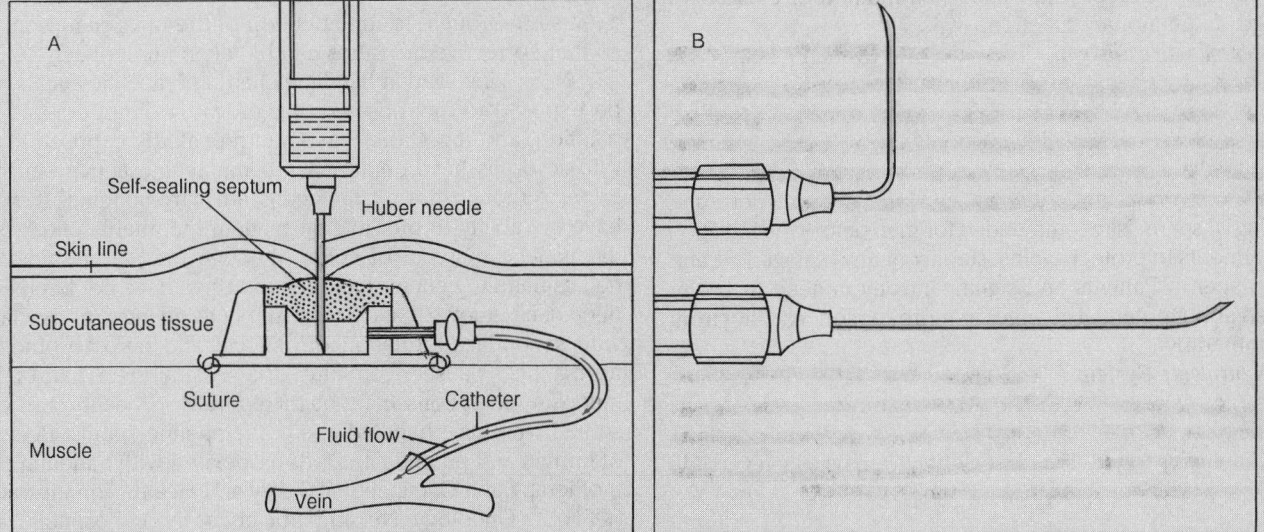

Figure 19-5. Implanted vascular access device. (**A**) A schematic diagram of an implanted vascular access device used for administration of medication, fluids, blood products and nutrition. The self-sealing septum permits repeated puncture by Huber needles without damage or leakage. (**B**) Two Huber needles used to enter the implanted vascular port. The 90-degree needle is used for top-entry ports for continuous infusions.

tible to mucositis (inflammation of the mucosal lining), with diarrhea a common result. Antimetabolites and antitumor antibiotics are the major culprits in mucositis and other gastrointestinal symptoms.

Hematopoietic System. Most chemotherapeutic agents depress bone marrow function (myelosuppression), resulting in decreased production of blood cells. Myelosuppression decreases the number of white blood cells or leukocytes (leukopenia), red blood cells (anemia), and platelets or thrombocytes (thrombocytopenia) and increases the risk of infection and bleeding. Depression of these cells is the usual reason for limiting the dose of the chemotherapeutic drugs. Frequent monitoring of blood cell counts is essential, and the patient must be protected from infection and injury, particularly while the blood cell counts are depressed.

Renal System. Chemotherapeutic agents can be harmful to the kidneys because of direct effects of the drugs during their excretion and the accumulation of end products after cell lysis. Cisplatin, methotrexate, and mitomycin are particularly toxic to the kidneys. Rapid cell lysis after chemotherapy results in increased urinary excretion of uric acid, which can lead to renal damage. Monitoring of blood urea nitrogen (BUN), serum creatinine, and creatinine clearance is essential. Adequate fluid hydration, alkalinization of the urine to prevent formation of uric acid crystals, and the use of allopurinol are frequently indicated to prevent these side effects.

Cardiopulmonary System. Antitumor antibiotics (daunorubicin and doxorubicin) are known to cause irreversible cumulative cardiac toxicities, especially when total dosage reaches 550 mg/m². Cardiac ejection fraction, electrocardiographic (ECG) tracings, and signs of congestive heart failure must be monitored closely. Bleomycin and busulfan are known for their cumulative toxic effects on lung function. Pulmonary fibrosis can be a long-term effect of prolonged dosage with these drugs. Therefore, the patient is monitored closely for changes in pulmonary function.

Reproductive System. Testicular and ovarian function can be affected by chemotherapeutic agents, resulting in possible sterility. Reproductive ability appears to be directly dependent on age and may return after chemotherapy; however, reproductive cells may have been damaged during treatment and result in chromosomal abnormalities in offspring. Therefore, banking of sperm is recommended for men before the initiation of treatments to protect against sterility or any mutagenic damage to sperm. Patients and significant others need to be informed about potential changes in reproduction resulting from chemotherapy.

Neurologic System. The plant alkaloids, especially vincristine, can cause neurologic damage with repeated doses. Peripheral neuropathies, loss of deep tendon reflexes, and paralytic ileus may occur. These side effects are usually reversible and disappear after completion of chemotherapy.

In summary, the use of chemotherapeutic agents in treating cancer is common, especially when cancer is viewed as a systemic disease with the potential of residual or microscopic disease in an individual. Using principles of cell renewal and the cell cycle, chemotherapy is capable of eradicating up to 99% of all malignant cells, allowing the immune system, it is hoped, to destroy remaining tumor. Toxicities both acute and chronic can be severe after chemotherapy, requiring health care professionals to possess astute assessment skills and to become creative in their management.

Nursing Considerations

The nurse has an important role in assessing and managing many of the problems experienced by the patient undergoing chemotherapy. Because of the systemic effects on normal as well as malignant cells, these problems are often widespread, affecting many body systems. Anorexia, nausea, vomiting, altered taste, and diarrhea put the patient at risk for nutritional and fluid and electrolyte disturbances. Changes in the mucosa of the gastrointestinal tract may lead to irritation of the oral cavity and intestinal tract, further threatening the patient's nutritional status. Therefore, it is important for the nurse to assess the patient's nutritional and fluid and electrolyte status frequently and to use creative ways to encourage an adequate fluid and dietary intake. Suppression of the bone marrow and immune system is an expected consequence of chemotherapy and frequently serves as a guide in determining appropriate chemotherapy dosage. However, this effect also increases the risk of anemia, infection, and bleeding disorders. Therefore, nursing assessment and care focus on identifying and modifying factors that further increase the patient's risk. Asepsis and gentle handling are indicated to prevent infection and trauma. Laboratory test results, particularly blood cell counts, are monitored closely. Untoward changes in blood test results and the occurrence of signs of infection and bleeding are reported promptly to the patient's physician. The patient and family members are instructed about measures to prevent these problems at home. (See Nursing Care Plan 19–1 for detailed nursing care.)

Local effects of the chemotherapeutic agent are also of concern. The patient is observed closely during its administration because of the risk and consequences of extravasation (particularly of vesicant agents or those that may produce tissue necrosis if deposited in the subcutaneous tissues). Local difficulties or problems with administration of chemotherapeutic agents are brought to the attention of the physician promptly so that corrective measures can be taken immediately.

Nurses involved in handling chemotherapeutic agents may be exposed to low doses of the drugs by direct contact, inhalation, and ingestion. Personnel repeatedly exposed to cytotoxic drugs have demonstrated mutagenic activity in their urine. Although not all mutagens are carcinogenic, they do have the ability to produce permanent inheritable changes in the genetic material of cells. Although long-term studies of nurses handling chemotherapeutic agents have not been conducted, it is known that chemotherapeutic agents are associated with secondary formation of cancers and chromosome abnormalities. Nausea, vomiting, dizziness, alopecia, and nasal mucosal ulcerations have been reported in health care personnel who have handled chemotherapeutic agents. Because of known and potential hazards associated with handling chemotherapy, the Occupational Safety and Health Administration (OSHA), Oncology Nursing Society (ONS), hospitals, and other health care agencies have developed specific precautions for those involved in preparation and administration of chemotherapy.

The guidelines from these organizations regarding the preparation and handling of antineoplastic agents recommend the following: (1) use of a biologic safety cabinet for the preparation of all chemotherapy drugs; (2) use of surgical latex gloves when handling drugs and the excretions of patients who received chemotherapy; (3) use of disposable, long-sleeved

(text continues on page 368)

Nursing Care Plan 19–1

Care of the Patient With Cancer

Nursing Interventions	Rationale	Expected Outcomes

Nursing Diagnosis: High risk for infection related to altered immunologic response

Goal: Prevention of infection

1. Assess patient for evidence of infection:
   a. Check vital signs every 4 hours.
   b. Monitor WBC count and differential WBC count each day.
   c. Inspect all sites that may serve as entry ports for pathogens (intravenous sites, wounds, skin folds, bony prominences, perineum, and oral cavity).
2. Report fever ≥ 101°F (38.3°C), chills, diaphoresis, swelling, heat, pain, erythema, exudate on any body surfaces.
3. Report change in respiratory or mental status, urinary frequency or burning, malaise, myalgias, arthralgias, rash, or diarrhea.
	1. Signs and symptoms of infection may be diminished in the immunocompromised host. Prompt recognition of infection and subsequent initiation of therapy will reduce morbidity and mortality associated with infection.	• Demonstrates normal temperature and vital signs.
		• Exhibits absence of signs of inflammation: local edema, erythema, pain, and warmth.
		• Exhibits normal breath sounds on auscultation.
		• Takes deep breaths and coughs every 2 hours to prevent respiratory dysfunction and infection.

4. Obtain cultures and sensitivities as indicated before initiation of antimicrobial treatment (wound exudate, sputum, urine, stool, blood).	4. These tests will identify organism and indicate most appropriate antimicrobial therapy. Use of inappropriate antibiotics will enhance proliferation of additional flora and encourage growth of antibiotic-resistant organisms.	• Exhibits absence of pathologic bacteria on cultures.

5. Initiate measures to minimize infection.
   a. Discuss with patient and family
 	
      (1) Placing patient in private room if absolute WBC count < 1000/mm³
      (2) Importance of patient avoiding contact with persons having known or recent infection or recent vaccination
   b. Instruct all personnel in careful handwashing before and after entering room.
   c. Avoid rectal or vaginal procedures (rectal temperatures, examinations, suppositories; vaginal tampons).
 	
   d. Use stool softeners to prevent constipation and straining.
   e. Assist patient in practice of meticulous personal hygiene.
   f. Instruct patient to use electric razor.
   g. Encourage patient to ambulate in room unless contraindicated.
	5. Exposure to infection is reduced.
	
	   b. Hands are significant source of contamination.
	
	   c. Incidence of rectal, perianal abscesses and subsequent systemic infection is high. Manipulation may cause disruption of membrane integrity and enhance progression of infection.
	
	   f. Minimizes skin breakdown.
	   g. Minimizes chance of skin breakdown and stasis of pulmonary secretions.
		• Patient avoids contact with others with infections.
		• Patient avoids crowds.
		• All personnel wash hands after each voiding and bowel movement.
		• Excoriation and trauma of skin is avoided.
		• Trauma to mucous membranes is avoided (avoidance of rectal temperatures, suppositions, vaginal tampons, perianal area trauma).
		• Patient uses recommended procedures and techniques if participating in management of invasive lines or catheters.
		
		• Patient uses electric razor.
		• Patient is without skin breakdown and stasis of secretions.

(continued)

Nursing Care Plan 19–1 (Continued)

Care of the Patient With Cancer

Nursing Interventions	Rationale	Expected Outcomes
h. Avoid fresh fruits, raw meat, fish, and vegetables if absolute WBC count < 1000/mm³, also remove fresh flowers and potted plants.	h. Fresh fruits and vegetables harbor bacteria not removed by ordinary washing. Flowers and potted plants are also sources of organisms.	• Adheres to dietary and environmental restrictions.
i. Each day: change drinking water, denture cleaning fluids, and respiratory equipment containing water.	i. Stagnant water is a source of infection.	
6. Assess intravenous sites every day for evidence of infection:	6. Nosocomial staphylococcal septicemia is closely associated with intravenous catheters.	• Exhibits no signs of septicemia or septic shock.
a. Change intravenous sites every other day.	a. Incidence of infection is increased when catheter is in place > 72 hr.	• Exhibits normal vital signs, cardiac output, and arterial pressures when monitored.
b. Cleanse skin with povidone-iodine before arterial puncture or venipuncture.	b. Povidone-iodine is effective against many gram-positive and gram-negtive pathogens.	
c. Change central venous catheter dressings every other day.		
d. Change all solutions and infusion sets every 48 hours.	d. Once introduced into the system, microorganisms are capable of growing in infusion sets despite replacement of container and high flow rates.	
7. Avoid intramuscular injections.	7. Risk of skin abcesses is reduced.	
8. Avoid insertion of urinary catheters; if catheters are necessary, use strict aseptic technique.	8. Rates of infection *greatly* increase after urinary catheterization.	

Nursing Diagnosis: High risk for injury related to bleeding problems

Goal: Prevention of injury and bleeding

1. Assess for potential for bleeding: monitor platelet count.	1. Mild risk: 50,000–100,000/mm³ (SI: 0.05–0.1 × 10¹²/L) Moderate risk: 20,000–50,000/mm³ (SI: 0.02–0.05 × 10¹²/L) Severe risk: less than 20,000/mm³ (SI: 0.02 × 10¹²/L)	• Signs and symptoms of bleeding are identified. • Exhibits no blood in feces, urine, or emesis. • Exhibits no bleeding of gums or of injection or venipuncture sites. • Exhibits no ecchymosis (bruising).
2. Assess for bleeding:		
a. Petechiae or ecchymosis	a. Indicates injury to microcirculation and larger vessels.	
b. Decrease in Hbg or Hct	b. Indicates blood loss.	
c. Prolonged bleeding from invasive procedures, venipunctures, minor cuts or scratches		
d. Frank or occult blood in any body excretion, emesis, sputum		
e. Bleeding from any body orifice		
f. Altered mental status	f. Indicates neurologic involvement.	
3. Instruct patient and family about ways to minimize bleeding:		• Patient and family identify ways to prevent bleeding.
a. Use soft toothbrush or toothette for mouth care.	a. Prevents trauma to oral tissues.	• Uses recommended measures to reduce risk of bleeding (uses soft toothbrush; shaves with electric razor only).

(continued)

Nursing Care Plan 19-1 *(Continued)*

Care of the Patient With Cancer

Nursing Interventions	Rationale	Expected Outcomes
b. Avoid commercial mouthwashes.	b. Contains high alcohol content that will dry oral tissues.	
c. Use electric razor for shaving.	c. Prevents trauma to skin.	
d. Use emery board for nail care.		
e. Avoid foods that are difficult to chew.	e. Prevents oral tissue trauma.	
4. Initiate measures to minimize injury related to bleeding.		• Exhibits normal vital signs. • Reports that environmental hazards have been reduced or removed.
a. Draw all blood for lab work with one daily venipuncture.	a. Minimizes trauma.	
b. Avoid taking temperature rectally or administering suppositories and enemas.	b. Prevents trauma to rectal mucosa.	
c. Avoid intramuscular injections; use smallest needle possible.	c. Prevents intramuscular bleeding.	
d. Apply direct pressure to injections and venipuncture sites for at least 5 minutes.		
e. Lubricate lips with petrolatum.	e. Prevents skin from drying.	
f. Avoid bladder catheterizations; use smallest catheter if necessary.	f. Prevents trauma to urethra.	
g. Maintain fluid intake of at least 3 L/24 hr unless contraindicated.	g. Hydration helps to prevent skin drying.	• Consumes adequate fluid.
h. Use stool softeners or increase bulk in diet.	h. Prevents constipation and straining that may injure rectal tissue.	• Reports absence of constipation.
i. Avoid medications that will interfere with clotting (*e.g.*, aspirin).	i. Minimizes risk of bleeding.	• Avoids substances interfering with clotting.
j. Recommend use of water-based lubricant before sexual intercourse.	j. Prevents friction and tissue trauma.	• Absence of tissue destruction.
5. When platelet count is less than 20,000/ mm^3, institute the following:	5. Platelet count of less than 20,000/mm^3 is associated with increased risk of spontaneous bleeding.	• Exhibits normal mental status and absence of signs of intracranial bleeding.
a. Bed rest with padded side rails.	a. Reduces risk of injury	• Avoids medications that interfere with clotting (aspirin).
b. Avoidance of strenuous activity.	b. Increases intracranial pressure and risk of cerebral hemorrhage.	
c. Platelet transfusions as prescribed; administer prescribed diphenhydramine hydrochloride (Benadryl) or hydrocortisone sodium succinate (Solu-Cortef) to prevent reaction to platelet transfusion.	c. Allergic reactions to blood products are associated with antigen–antibody reaction that causes platelet destruction.	
d. Supervise activity when out of bed.		
e. Caution against forceful noseblowing.	e. Prevents trauma to nasal mucosal and increased intracranial pressure.	• Absence of epistaxis and cerebral bleeding.

Nursing Diagnosis: Impaired skin integrity: erythematous/wet desquamation skin reactions

Goal: Maintenance of skin integrity

1. In erythematous areas, a. Avoid the use of soaps, cosmetics, perfumes, powders, lotions and ointments, deodorants.	1. Care to the affected areas must focus on preventing further skin irritation, drying, and damage	• Avoids use of soaps, powders, and other cosmetics on site of radiation therapy. • States rationale for special care of skin. • Exhibits minimal change in skin.

(continued)

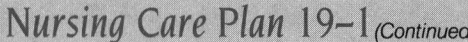

Nursing Care Plan 19–1 (Continued)

Care of the Patient With Cancer

Nursing Interventions	Rationale	Expected Outcomes
b. Use only lukewarm water to bathe the area. c. Avoid rubbing or scratching the area. d. Avoid shaving the area with a straight-edge razor. e. Avoid applying hot water bottles, heating pads, ice, and adhesive tape to the area. f. Avoid exposing the area to sunlight or cold weather. g. Avoid tight clothing in the area. Use cotton clothing. h. Apply vitamin A&D ointment to the area.		• Avoids trauma to affected skin region (avoids shaving, constricting and irritating clothing, extremes of temperature, and use of adhesive tape). • Reports change in skin promptly.
	g. Allows air circulation to affected area. h. Aids healing.	
2. If wet desquamation occurs. a. Do not disrupt any blisters that have formed. b. Avoid frequent washing of the area. c. Notify physician of blistering. d. Use *prescribed* creams or ointments. e. If area weeps, apply a thin layer of gauze dressing.	2. Open weeping areas are susceptible to bacteiral infection. Care must be taken to prevent introduction of pathogens. d. Decreases irritation and inflammation of the area. e. Enhances drying.	• Demonstrates proper care of blistered or open areas. • Exhibits absence of infection of blistered and opened areas.

Nursing Diagnosis: Alteration of oral mucous membranes: stomatitis

Goal: Maintenance of intact oral mucous membranes

1. Assess oral cavity daily.	1. Provides baseline for later evaluation	• States rationale for frequent oral assessment and hygiene.
2. Instruct patient to report oral burning, pain, areas of redness, open lesions on the lips, pain associated with swallowing or decreased tolerance to temperature extremes of food.	2. Identification of initial stages of stomatitis will facilitate prompt interventions, including modification of treatment as prescribed by physician.	• Identifies signs and symptoms of stomatitis to report to nurse or physician.
3. Encourage and assist in oral hygiene regimens. *Preventive* a. Avoid commercial mouthwashes. b. Brush with soft toothbrush; use nonabrasive toothpaste after meals and bedtime; floss every 24 hr.	 a. Alcohol content of mouthwashes will dry oral tissues and potentiate breakdown. b. Limits trauma and removes debris.	• Participates in recommended oral hygiene regimen: • Avoids mouthwashes with alcohol. • Brushes teeth and mouth with soft bristle toothbrush. • Uses lubricant to keep lips soft and nonirritated. • Avoids hard to chew, spicy, and hot foods.
Mild stomatitis (generalized erythema, limited ulcerations, small white patches: *Candida*) c. Use normal saline mouthrinses every 2 hr while awake; every 6 hr at night. d. Use soft toothbrush or toothette.	 c. Oxidizing action assists in removing debris, thick secretions, and bacteria. d. Minimizes trauma.	 • Exhibits clean, intact oral mucosa. • Exhibits no ulcerations or infections of oral cavity. • Reports absent or decreased oral pain.

(continued)

Nursing Care Plan 19–1 (Continued)

Care of the Patient With Cancer

Nursing Interventions	Rationale	Expected Outcomes

e. Remove dentures except for meals, be certain dentures fit well.
f. Apply lip lubricant.
 	
g. Avoid foods that are spicy or hard to chew and those with extremes of temperature.
Severe stomatitis (confluent ulcerations with bleeding and white patches covering more than 25% of oral mucosa)
h. Obtain cultures and sensitivities of areas of infection.
i. Assess ability to chew and swallow; assess gag reflex.
j. Oral rinses as prescribed or place patient on side and irrigate mouth; have suction available (may combine in solution saline, anti-*Candida* agent such as Mycostatin and topical anesthetic agent as described below).
k. Remove dentures.
l. Use toothette or gauze soaked with solution for cleansing.
m. Use lip lubricant.
n. Provide liquid or pureed diet.
o. Monitor for dehydration.
 	
4. Minimize discomfort.
   a. Consult physician for use of topical anesthetic such as dyclonine and diphenhydramine or viscous lidocaine.
   b. Administer systemic analgesics as prescribed.
   c. Perform mouth care as described.
	e. Minimizes friction and discomfort.
	f. Promotes comfort.
	
	g. Prevents local trauma.
	
	h. Assists in identifying need for antimicrobial therapy.
	i. Patient may be in danger of aspiration.
	j. Facilitates cleansing, provides for safety and comfort.
	
	l. Limits trauma, promotes comfort.
	m. Promotes comfort.
	n. Assures dietary intake.
	
	o. Decreased oral intake and ulcerations potentiate fluid deficits.
	
	a. Alleviates pain and increases sense of well-being; promotes participation in oral hygiene and nutritional intake.
	
	c. Promotes removal of debris, healing, and comfort.
		• Reports no difficulty swallowing.
		• Exhibits healing (re-epithelialization) of oral mucosa within 5 to 7 days if mild stomatitis has developed.
		• Exhibits healing of oral tissues within 10 to 14 days if severe stomatitis has developed.
		• Exhibits no bleeding or ulcerations of oral mucosa.
		• Consumes adequate fluid and food intake.
		• Exhibits absence of dehydration and weight loss.

Nursing Diagnosis: Impaired tissue integrity: alopecia

Goal: Maintenance of tissue integrity; coping with hair loss

1. Discuss potential hair loss and regrowth with patient and family. 2. Explore potential impact of hair loss on self-image, interpersonal relationships, and sexuality. 3. Prevent or minimize hair loss through the following: a. Scalp hypothermia/scalp tourniquets.	1. Provides information so patient and family can begin to prepare cognitively and emotionally for loss. 2. Facilitates coping. a. Decreases hair follicle uptake of chemotherapy (not used for patients with leukemia or lymphoma because tumor cells may be present in blood vessels or scalp tissue).	• Identifies alopecia as potential side effect of treatment. • Identifies positive and negative feelings and threats to self-image. • Verbalizes meaning that hair and possible hair loss have for him. • States rationale for modifications in hair care and treatment. • Uses mild shampoo and conditioner and shampoos hair only when necessary. • Avoids hair dryers, curlers, sprays, and other stresses on hair and scalp.

(continued)

Nursing Care Plan 19–1 *(Continued)*

Care of the Patient With Cancer

Nursing Interventions	Rationale	Expected Outcomes
b. Cutting long hair before treatment.	b–f. Minimizes hair loss due to the weight and pulling on hair.	
c. Avoiding excessive shampooing.		
d. Using mild shampoo and conditioner, gently pat dry.		
e. Avoiding use of electric curlers, curling irons, dryers, clips, barrettes, hair sprays, hair dyes, and permanent waves.		
f. Avoiding excessive combing or brushing; use of wide-toothed comb.		
4. Prevent trauma to scalp.		
a. Lubricate scalp with vitamin A&D ointment to decrease itching.	a. Assists in maintaining skin integrity.	• Wears hat or scarf over hair when exposed to sun.
b. Have patient use sunscreen or wear hat when in the sun.	b. Prevents ultraviolet light exposure.	
5. Suggest ways to assist in coping with hair loss:		
a. Purchase wig before hair loss.	a. Wig that closely resembles hair color and style is more easily selected if hair loss has not begun.	• Takes steps to deal with possible hair loss before it occurs; purchases wig or hair piece.
b. If hair loss is present, take photograph to wig shop to assist in selection.	b. Facilitates adjustment.	• Maintains hygiene and grooming. • Interacts and socializes with others.
c. Begin to wear wig before hair loss.		
d. Contact the American Cancer Society for donated wigs, or store that specializes in this product.		
e. Wear hat, scarf, or turban.	e. Conceals loss.	
f. Wear accessories that are attractive and stylish.	f. Redirects attention.	
6. Encourage patient to wear own clothes, retain social contacts, bring items of interest or special meaning to hospital room.	6. Assists in maintaining personal identity.	
7. Explain that hair growth usually begins again once therapy is completed.	7. Reassures patient that hair loss is usually temporary.	• States that hair loss and necessity of wig are temporary.

Nursing Diagnosis: Alteration in nutrition, less than body requirements, related to nausea/vomiting

Goal: Fewer episodes of nausea/vomiting before, during, and after chemotherapy administration

1. Adjust diet before and after drug administration according to patient preference and tolerance.	1. Each patient responds differently to food after chemotherapy. A diet containing foods that relieve the patient's nausea or vomiting is most helpful.	• Reports decrease in nausea. • Reports decrease in incidence of vomiting. • Consumes adequate fluid and food when nausea subsides.
2. Prevent unpleasant sights, odors, and sounds in the environment.	2. Unpleasant sensations can stimulate the nausea/vomiting center.	
3. Use distraction, relaxation techniques, and imagery before, during, and after chemotherapy.	3. Decreases anxiety, which can contribute to nausea/vomiting. Psychologic conditioning may also be decreased.	• Demonstrates use of distraction, relaxation, and imagery when indicated.

(continued)

Nursing Care Plan 19-1(Continued)

Care of the Patient With Cancer

Nursing Interventions	Rationale	Expected Outcomes
4. Administer prescribed antiemetics, sedatives, and corticosteroids as prescribed.	4. Combination drug therapy attempts to reduce nausea/vomiting through control of the various triggering pathways.	
5. Ensure adequate fluid hydration before, during, and after drug administration; assess intake and output.	5. Adequate fluid volume will dilute drug levels, decreasing stimulation of vomiting receptors.	• Exhibits normal skin turgor and moist mucous membranes.
6. Provide frequent oral hygiene.	6. Reduces unpleasant taste.	• Reports no additional weight loss.
7. Provide pain relief measures, if necessary.	7. Increased comfort will increase physical tolerance of symptoms.	

Nursing Diagnosis: Altered nutrition: less than body requirements, related to anorexia/cachexia/malabsorption

Goal: Maintenance of nutritional status and of weight within 10% of pretreatment weight

Nursing Interventions	Rationale	Expected Outcomes
1. Avoid unpleasant sights, odors, sounds in the environment during mealtime.	1. Anorexia can be stimulated or increased with noxious stimuli.	• Exhibits weight loss no greater than 10% of pretreatment weight. • Reports decreasing anorexia and increased interest in eating.
2. Provide foods preferred and well tolerated by the patient, preferably high-calorie/high-protein foods. Respect ethnic food preferences.	2. Foods preferred, well tolerated, and high in calories and protein will maintain nutritional status during periods of increased metabolic demand.	• Demonstrates normal skin turgor. • Identifies rationale for dietary modifications.
3. Provide adequate fluid intake, but limit fluids at mealtime.	3. Fluid levels are necessary to eliminate waste products and prevent dehydration. Increased fluid levels with meals can lead to early satiety.	• Participates in calorie counts and diet histories. • Uses appropriate relaxation and imagery before meals.
4. Provide smaller, more frequent meals.	4. Smaller feedings given more frequently are more easily tolerated because early satiety does not occur.	• Exhibits laboratory and clinical findings indicative of adequate nutritional intake: normal serum protein and transferrin levels, normal serum iron levels, normal hemoglobin, hematocrit, and lymphocyte levels, normal urinary creatinine levels.
5. Provide relaxed, quiet environment during mealtime with increased social interaction as desired.	5. A quiet environment promotes relaxation. Social interaction at mealtime increases appetite.	
6. If possible, serve wine at mealtime with foods.	6. Wine often stimulates appetite and adds calories.	
7. Offer cold foods, if desired.	7. Cold, high-protein foods are often more tolerable and less odorous than hot foods.	
8. Provide nutritional supplements, high-protein foods between meals.	8. Supplements/snacks add protein and calories to meet nutritional requirements.	• Consumes diet high in required nutrients.
9. Provide frequent oral hygiene.	9. Oral hygiene measures stimulate appetite and increase saliva production.	• Carries out oral hygiene before meals.
10. Provide pain relief measures.	10. Pain impairs appetite.	• Reports that pain does not interfere with meals.
11. Provide control of nausea/vomiting.	11. Nausea/vomiting increases anorexia.	• Reports decreasing episodes of nausea and vomiting.
12. Increase activity level as tolerated.	12. Increased activity promotes appetite.	• Participates in increasing levels of activity.
13. Decrease anxiety by encouraging verbalization of fears, concerns; use of relaxation techniques; imagery at mealtime.	13. Relief of anxiety may increase appetite.	

(continued)

Nursing Care Plan 19–1 *(Continued)*

Care of the Patient With Cancer

Nursing Interventions	Rationale	Expected Outcomes
14. Position patient properly at mealtime.	14. Proper body position and alignment are necessary to aid chewing and swallowing.	
15. Provide enteral tube feedings of commercial liquid diets, elemental diets or blenderized foods through Silastic feeding tubes as prescribed.	15. Tube feedings may be necessary in the severely debilitated patient who has a functioning gastrointestinal system.	• States rationale for use of tube feedings or hyperalimentation.
16. Provide parenteral hyperalimentation with lipid supplements as prescribed.	16. Parenteral hyperalimentation with supplemental fats supplies needed calories and proteins to meet nutritional demands, especially in the nonfunctional gastrointestinal system.	• Participates in management of tube feedings or hyperalimentation.

Nursing Diagnosis: Fatigue and activity intolerance

Goal: Increased activity tolerance and decreased fatigue level

1. Provide several rest periods during the day, especially before and after physical exertion.	1. During rest, energy is conserved and levels are replenished. Several shorter rest periods may be more beneficial than one longer rest period.	• Reports deceasing levels of fatigue. • Increases participation in activities gradually.
2. Increase total hours of nighttime sleep.	2. Sleep helps to restore body energy levels.	• Rests when fatigued. • Reports restful sleep.
3. Rearrange daily schedule and organize activities to conserve energy expenditure.	3. Reorganization of activities can reduce energy losses and reduce stressors.	
4. Allow/ask for others' assistance with necessary chores such as housework, child care, shopping, cooking.	4. Conserves energy.	• Requests assistance with activities appropriately.
5. Encourage reduced job workload, if possible, by reducing number of hours worked per week.	5. Reducing workload will decrease physical and psychologic stress and increase periods of rest/relaxation.	• Reports adequate energy to participate in activities important to him (visiting with family, hobbies, etc.)
6. Provide adequate protein and calorie intake.	6. Protein and calorie depletion decreases activity tolerance.	• Consumes diet with recommended protein and caloric intake.
7. Encourage use of relaxation techniques, mental imagery.	7. Promotion of relaxation and psychological rest will decrease physical fatigue.	• Uses relaxation exercises and imagery to decrease anxiety and promote rest.
8. Encourage participation in planned exercise programs.	8. Proper exercise programs will increase endurance and stamina.	• Participates in planned exercise program gradually. • Reports no breathlessness during activities.
9. Administer blood products as prescribed.	9. Lowered hemoglobin and hematocrit will predispose patient to fatigue due to decreased oxygen availability.	• Exhibits acceptable hemoglobin and hematocrit levels.
10. Assess for fluid and electrolyte disturbances.	10. May contribute to altered nerve transmission and muscle function.	• Exhibits normal fluid and electrolyte balance.
11. Assess for sources of discomfort.	11. Coping with discomfort requires energy expenditure.	• Reports decreased discomfort.
12. Provide strategies to facilitate mobility.	12. Impaired mobility requires increased energy expenditure.	• Exhibits improved mobility.

Nursing Diagnosis: Pain and discomfort

Goal: Relief of pain and discomfort

1. Assess pain and discomfort characteristics: location, quality, frequency, duration, etc.	1. Provides baseline for assessing changes in pain level and evaluation of interventions.	• Reports decreased level of pain and discomfort.

(continued)

▶ **Nursing Care Plan 19–1** *(Continued)*

Care of the Patient With Cancer

Nursing Interventions	Rationale	Expected Outcomes
2. Assure patient that you know that pain is real and will assist him in reducing it.	2. Fear that pain will not be considered real increases anxiety and reduces pain tolerance.	• Reports less disruption from pain and discomfort.
3. Assess other factors contributing to patient's pain: fear, fatigue, anger, etc.	3. Provides data about factors that decrease patient's ability to tolerate pain and increase pain level.	• Explains how fatigue, fear, etc., contribute to severity of his pain and discomfort.
4. Administer analgesics to promote optimum pain relief within limits of physician's prescription.	4. Analgesics tend to be more effective when administered early in pain cycle.	• Accepts pain medication as prescribed.
5. Assess patient's behavioral responses to pain and pain experience.	5. Provides additional information about patient's pain.	• Exhibits decreased physical and behavioral signs of pain and discomfort in *acute pain* (no grimacing, crying, moaning; displays interest in surroundings and activities around him).
6. Collaborate with patient, physician, and other health care team members when changes in pain management are necessary.	6. New methods of administration of analgesia must be acceptable to patient, physician, and health care team to be effective; patient's participation decreases his sense of powerlessness.	• Takes an active role in administration of analgesia.
7. Encourage strategies of pain relief that patient has used successfully in previous pain experience.	7. Encourages success of pain relief strategies accepted by patient and family.	
8. Teach patient new strategies to relieve pain and discomfort; distraction, imagery, relaxation, cutaneous stimulation, etc.	8. Increases number of options and strategies available to patient.	• Identifies additional effective pain relief strategies.
		• Uses alternative pain relief strategies appropriately.
		• Reports effective use of new pain relief strategies and decrease in pain intensity.
		• Reports that decreased level of pain permits participation in other activities and events.

Nursing Diagnosis: Grieving related to anticipatory loss; altered role functioning

Goal: Progression through grieving process appropriately

1. Encourage verbalization of fears, concerns and questions regarding disease, treatment, and future implications.	1. An increased and accurate knowledge base will decrease anxiety and dispel misconceptions.	• The patient and family will progress through the phases of grief as evidenced by increased verbalization and expression of grief.
2. Encourage active participation of patient or family in care and treatment decisions.	2. Active participation will maintain patient independence and control.	• The patient and family will identify resources available to aid coping strategies during grieving.
3. Visit family frequently to establish and maintain relationships and physical closeness.	3. Frequent contacts will promote trust and security and reduce feelings of fear and isolation.	• The patient and family use resources and supports appropriately.
		• The patient and family discuss the future openly with each other.
4. Allow for ventilation of negative feelings, including projected anger and hostility, within acceptable limits.	4. This allows for emotional expression without loss of self-esteem.	• The patient and family discuss concerns and feelings openly with each other.
5. Allow for periods of crying and expression of sadness.	5. These feelings are necessary for separation and detachment to occur.	• The patient and family use nonverbal expressions of concern for each other.
6. Involve clergy as desired by the patient and family.	6. This facilitates the grief process and spiritual care.	

(continued)

Nursing Care Plan 19–1(Continued)

Care of the Patient With Cancer

Nursing Interventions	Rationale	Expected Outcomes
7. Advise professional counseling as indicated for patient or family to alleviate pathologic grieving.	7. This facilitates the grief process.	
8. Allow for progression through the grieving process at the individual pace of the patient and family.	8. Grief work is variable. Not every person uses every phase of the grief process, and the time spent in dealing with each phase varies with every person. To complete grief work, this variability must be allowed.	

Nursing Diagnosis: Altered body image and self-esteem related to changes in appearance, function, and roles

Goal: Improved body image and self-esteem

Nursing Interventions	Rationale	Expected Outcomes
1. Assess patient's feelings about body image and level of self-esteem.	1. Provides baseline assessment for evaluating changes and assessing effectiveness of interventions.	• Identifies concerns of importance.
2. Identify potential threats to patient's self-esteem (*e.g.*, altered appearance, decreased sexual function, hair loss, decreased energy, role changes). Validate concerns with patient.	2. Anticipates changes and permits patient to identify importance of these areas to the patient.	
3. Encourage continued participation in activities and decision making.	3. Encourages/permits continued control of events and self.	• Takes active role in activities. • Maintains previous role in decision making.
4. Encourage patient to verbalize concerns.	4. Identifying concerns is an important step in coping with them.	• Verbalizes feelings and reactions to losses or threatened losses.
5. Individualize care for the patient	5. Prevents or reduces depersonalization and emphasizes patient's self-worth.	• Participates in self-care activities.
6. Assist patient in self-care when fatigue, lethargy, nausea, vomiting, and other symptoms prevent independence.	6. Physical well-being improves self-esteem.	• Permits others to assist in care when he is unable to be independent.
7. Assist patient in selecting and using consmetics, scarves, hair pieces, and clothing that increase his or her sense of attractiveness.	7. Promotes positive body image.	• Exhibits interest in appearance and uses aids (cosmetics, scarves, etc.) appropriately.
8. Encourage patient and partner to share concerns about altered sexuality/sexual function and to explore alternatives to their usual sexual expression.	8. Provides oppportunity for expressing concern, affection, and acceptance.	• Participates with others in conversations and social events and activities. • Verbalizes concern about sexual partner. • Explores alternative ways of expressing concern and affection.

gowns when preparing and administering chemotherapy drugs; (4) use of Luer-Lok fittings on all intravenous tubing used to deliver chemotherapy; (5) disposal of all equipment used in chemotherapy preparation and administration in appropriate, leak-proof, puncture-proof containers; and (6) disposal of all chemotherapy wastes as hazardous materials. When followed, these precautions greatly minimize the risk of exposure.

Hyperthermia

Hyperthermia (thermal therapy), the generation of temperatures greater than physiologic fever range (above 106.70°F [41.5°C]),

has been used for many years to elicit tumoricidal effects in human cancers. Research suggests that malignant cells are more sensitive than normal cells to the harmful effects of high temperatures for several reasons. Malignant cells lack enzymes for repair of DNA and cell membranes that are damaged by elevated temperatures. These cells are deficient in enzymes that generate adenosine triphosphate (ATP), which are necessary for a normal cellular response to the increased metabolic demands that occur with hyperthermia. Most tumor cells lack an adequate blood supply to provide needed oxygen during periods of increased cellular demand, such as during hyperthermia. Cancerous tumors lack blood vessels of adequate size for dissipation of heat. Research also suggests that the body's immune system may be indirectly stimulated when hyperthermia is used.

Hyperthermia is most effective when used in combination with radiation therapy or chemotherapy. Hyperthermia and radiation therapy are thought to work well together because hypoxic tumor cells and cells in the S phase of the cell cycle are more heat sensitive than radiosensitive; the addition of heat damages tumor cells so that they are unable to repair themselves after radiation therapy damage. Hyperthermia is thought to alter cellular membrane permeability when used with chemotherapy, allowing for an increased uptake of the chemotherapeutic drug. Also, hyperthermia is thought to inhibit cellular repair processes, enhancing tumor death.

Heat can be produced with the use of radiowaves, ultrasound, microwaves, magnetic waves, hot water baths, or even hot wax immersions. Hyperthermia may be local or regional, or it may include the whole body. Local or regional hyperthermia may be delivered to a cancerous extremity (for malignant melanoma) by regional perfusion, in which the affected extremity is isolated by a tourniquet and an extracorporeal circulator heats the blood flowing through the affected part. Hyperthermia probes may also be inserted around a tumor in a local area and attached to a heat source during the actual treatment period. Chemotherapeutic agents such as melphalan may also be heated and instilled into the regionally circulating blood. Local or regional hyperthermia may also include infusion of heated solutions into cancerous body organs. Whole body hyperthermia to treat disseminated disease may be achieved by extracorporeal circulation, immersion of patients in heated water or paraffin, or enclosure in heated suits.

Side effects of hyperthermia treatments include skin burns and tissue damage, fatigue, hypotension, peripheral neuropathies, thrombophlebitis, nausea, vomiting, diarrhea, and electrolyte imbalances. Resistance to hyperthermia may develop during the treatment because cells adapt to repeated thermal insult. Research into the efficacy of hyperthermia, its delivery, and its side effects is continuing.

Nursing Considerations

Although hyperthermia has been used for many years, many patients and their families are unfamiliar with this treatment for cancer. Consequently, they will need explanations about the procedure, its goals, and its effects. The patient is assessed for side effects, and efforts are made to reduce their occurrence and severity. Local skin care at the site of the implanted hyperthermia probes is also required.

Biologic Response Modifiers

Biologic response modifiers (BRMs) are agents or methods of treatment that have the ability to alter the immunologic relationship between the tumor and the cancer patient (host) to provide a therapeutic benefit. Although the mechanisms of action vary with each type of BRM, the goal is destruction or cessation of the malignant growth. Over the years we have come to understand the role of the body's natural immune defenses against cancer. The basis of BRM treatment lies in the restoration, stimulation, or augmentation of those natural immune defenses.

Some of the early investigations of the stimulation of the immune system involved nonspecific agents such as bacille Calmette–Guérin (BCG) and *Corynebacterium parvum*. These agents serve as antigens that stimulate an immune response when injected into the patient. It is hoped that the stimulated immune system will then be able to eradicate malignant growths. Extensive animal and human investigations with BCG have yielded some promising results, especially in the treatment of malignant melanoma and colorectal cancer. It is considered to be a standard form of treatment for localized bladder cancer. The exact role of these agents, however, requires further investigation.

Interferons are another example of BRMs with both antiviral and antitumor properties. When stimulated, all nucleated cells are capable of producing these glycoproteins, which are classified according to their biologic and chemical properties: α interferons are produced by leukocytes, β-interferons are produced by fibroblasts, and τ-interferons are produced by lymphocytes. The majority of clinical investigations have focused on the use of α-interferons. Interferons were first noted for their ability to inhibit viral infections.

Although the exact antitumor effects of interferons have not been thoroughly established, it is thought that they either stimulate the immune system or assist in prevention of tumor growth. Interferons enhance both lymphocyte and antibody production. They also facilitate the cytolytic role of macrophages and natural killer cells. Additionally, interferons are able to inhibit cell multiplication by increasing the duration of various phases of the cell cycle.

The effects of interferon have been demonstrated in a variety of malignancies. It is approved by the Food and Drug Administration (FDA) for the treatment of hairy cell leukemia and Kaposi's sarcoma. Other positive responses have been seen in the treatment of non-Hodgkin's lymphomas and malignant melanoma. Further efforts are underway to establish optimal dosing and methods of administration.

Monoclonal antibodies are another type of BRM; they became available through recent technologic advances that enabled investigators to grow and produce specific antibodies for specific malignant cells. The production of monoclonal antibodies involves injecting tumor cells into mice and harvesting the antibodies produced by the immune systems of the mice. The antibodies are then infused into the cancer patient.

Preliminary investigations of monoclonal antibodies in the treatment of hematologic malignancies and solid tumors have had limited success. More recent investigations are exploring the feasibility of conjugating or combining monoclonal antibodies with other substances such as radioactive materials, chemotherapy, hormones, lymphokines, and interferons. Immunoconjugate therapy combines multiple agents to enhance tumor destruction. Monoclonal antibodies are also being used as aids in diagnostic evaluations. By attaching a radioactive substance to the monoclonal antibody, physicians are able to detect both primary and metastatic tumors through radiologic techniques.

Lymphokines and *cytokines*, cell products of lymphocytes with known biologic roles in the normal immune response, are also the focus of current research efforts.

The most widely publicized agent is interleukin-2 (IL-2), which is known to stimulate the production and activation of several different types of T cell lymphocytes. When combined with IL-2, the null lymphocyte (lymphocyte lacking T or B markers on the surface membrane) becomes a lymphokine-activated killer cell (LAK cell) capable of destroying cancer cells. Clinical trials have combined infusions of both IL-2 and LAK cells in patients with cancers such as melanoma, sarcoma, and renal cell carcinoma. These trials are considered to be controversial by some clinicians because of the potential gravity of the toxic effects of IL-2. Future trials will examine optimal dosing regimens, antitumor effects, and management of toxicities. Other lymphokines under investigation include colony-stimulating factors, tumor necrosis factor, and transfer factor.

Colony-stimulating factors (CSFs) are hormone-like substances naturally produced by many cells within the immune system. CSFs of different types stimulate the production of all cells in the blood, including neutrophils, macrophages, monocytes, red blood cells, and platelets. Many CSFs are currently being examined for their role in helping to reverse the bone marrow–suppressing effects of chemotherapy. Additional studies are investigating the use of CSFs for patients with hematologic disorders to increase circulating levels of white blood cells, red blood cells, and lymphocytes.

Nursing Considerations

Patients receiving BRM therapy have many of the same needs as other cancer patients undergoing more conventional therapies. For many patients who have failed to respond to standard treatment modalities, however, BRM therapy may be viewed as a last chance effort. Consequently, it is essential that the nurse assess the need for education, support, and guidance for both the patient and family, and assist in planning and evaluating patient care. Nurses need to be familiar with each agent given and the potential adverse effects. Because of the investigational nature of these agents, the nurse will be administering them in a research setting. Accurate observations and careful documentation are essential components of the data collection process.

Unproven Methods

Forty-five percent of all cancer patients currently survive at least 5 years from the time of diagnosis and are potentially "cured" of their disease. Those patients who do not receive desired results from treatment, however, are susceptible targets for deceptive practices and quackery. Fear, ignorance, frustration, hopelessness, unmet needs, loss of control, desperation, and family and social pressures are major factors that motivate patients to seek unproven methods of cancer treatment. Unfortunately, such unconventional therapies may interfere with conventional approaches, cause increased financial burdens, and increase morbidity among cancer patients.

Most unproven cancer treatments can be categorized as machines and devices, drugs and biologicals, metabolic and dietary regimens, or mystical and spiritual approaches.

Machines and Devices.   Electrical gadgets and devices are commonly reputed to cure cancers. Most are operated by persons with questionable training who report incredulous success stories. Such machines are often decorated with elaborate lights and dials and produce vibrations or other sensations of currents or energy.

Drugs and Biologicals.   Medicinal agents, herbs, proteins, megavitamins, immune therapy, vaccines, enzymes, and sera have been frequent components of fraudulent cancer therapy.

These agents have included oral and external medications derived from weeds, flowers, and herbs and the blood and urine of patients and animals.

Metabolic and Dietary Regimens.   Metabolic and dietary regimens emphasize the ingestion of only natural substances to purify the body and retard cancerous growth. These regimens include the grape diet, the carrot juice diet, coffee colonic irrigations, and raw liver intake. Laetrile (vitamin B_{17}, amygdalin), one of the best-known forms of cancer quackery, was advocated as an agent to kill tumor cells by releasing cyanide, which is especially toxic to malignant cells. The National Cancer Institute, in response to public demand, investigated the effects of laetrile and reported no therapeutic benefits with its use. Many toxic effects (cyanide poisoning, fever, rash, headache, vomiting, diarrhea, and hypotension) were reported. Macrobiotic diets have also been advocated as cancer treatment to reestablish balance between the major forces in the universe, yin and yang. Persons adhering to macrobiotic diets tend to develop vitamin, mineral, and protein deficiencies; experience additional weight loss due to decreased calorie intake; and achieve no therapeutic benefits from the dietary manipulation.

Mystical and Spiritual Approaches.   Mystical or spiritual approaches to cancer therapy include such techniques as psychic surgery, faith healing, "laying on of hands," and invocation of mystical universal powers to kill cancerous growths. These techniques are difficult to disclaim because they are based on faith.

In summary, fraudulent cancer therapies may appear attractive to cancer patients who are not cured by conventional treatment modalities. Most unproven therapies contain machines/devices, drugs/biologicals, metabolic/dietary regimens, or mystical/spiritual approaches to treatment. Cancer patients turn to these therapies out of fear, hopelessness, and desperation for cure. Truthful and open communication by all health care professionals is essential to provide factual information regarding quackery and an understanding of patients' motivations toward quackery.

Nursing Considerations

A trusting relationship, supportive care, and promotion of hope in the patient and his family are the most effective means of protecting them from fraudulent therapy and questionable claims of cancer cures. Truthful responses given in a nonjudgmental manner to questions and inquiries about unproven methods of cancer treatments may alleviate the fear and guilt on the part of the patient and family that they are not "doing everything" to obtain a cure. Characteristics common to fraudulent therapy may be shared with patients and their families so that they are informed and cautious in evaluating other forms of "therapy" (Chart 19–5).

Nursing Care of the Patient With Cancer

The outlook for patients with cancer has greatly improved because of scientific and technological advances. As a result of the underlying malignancy or various treatment modalities, however, the patient with cancer may confront or experience

Chart 19–5
Common Characteristics Associated With Practitioners of Fraudulent Therapy

- They tend to be isolated from established scientific facilities or associates.
- They do not use regular channels of communication (current reputable scientific journals) for reporting scientific information. Physicians of this type tend to publish articles in journals that are not read by cancer specialists.
- They claim that prejudice or organized medicine hinders their efforts.
- They are prone to challenge established theories and attack prominent scientists with bitter criticism.
- They are quick to cite examples of physicians and scientists of the past who were forced to fight the rigid dogma of their day.
- They are often inclined to use complex jargon and unusual phraseology to embellish their writing.
- Their records are scanty or nonexistent.
- They often discourage, or even refuse, consultation with reputable physicians. If a scientific evaluation of their methods is made, they generally decline to accept the results, claiming that the "medical trust" is against them.

- Their method of treatment is often secret and is available only from them. Or, the mode of administration depends on special judgment that can be learned only from them.
- They discount biopsy verification in cancer diagnosis, sometimes by saying that it "spreads" the cancer. They may accept patients who have already been cured of cancer by orthodox means but fear they have not.
- They may use proven drugs or other methods of treatment as adjuvants to the unproven therapy, and if a favorable effect on cancer is shown, claim that it is the result of their unproven remedy.
- They may have multiple unusual degrees such as N.D. (Doctor of Naturopathy), Ph.N. (Philosopher of Naturopathy), or Ms.D. (Doctor of Metaphysics). These degrees may have been received from correspondence schools.
- The chief supporters tend to be prominent statesmen, actors, writers, lawyers, even members of state or national legislatures—persons not trained or experienced in the natural history of cancer, the care of patients with cancer, or in scientific methodology.

(Unproven Methods of Cancer Management. New York, American Cancer Society, 1982.)

---

a variety of secondary problems. Regardless of the type of cancer, treatment used, or prognosis, many patients with cancer are susceptible to these problems and complications. An important role of the nurse on the oncology team is to assess the patient for these problems and complications.

▶ Nursing Process
The Patient With Cancer

◊ Assessment

At all stages of cancer, the patient is assessed for those factors that predispose the patient to infection. Infection is the leading cause of mortality in the oncology population. Factors predisposing patients to infection are summarized in Table 19–5. The nurse monitors laboratory studies, particularly the complete blood cell count to detect early changes in white blood cells. Common sites of infection, such as the patient's pharynx, skin, perianal area, urinary tract, and respiratory tract, are assessed frequently. It is important to keep in mind, however, that the typical signs of infection (fever, swelling, redness, drainage, and pain) may be absent in the immunosuppressed patient. The patient is monitored for sepsis, particularly if invasive catheters or infusion lines are in place.

The functions of the white blood cells are often impaired in cancer patients. A decrease in circulating white blood cells (WBCs) is referred to as *leukopenia* or *granulocytopenia.* There are three types of WBCs: neutrophils, basophils, and eosinophils. The neutrophils, totaling 60% to 70% of all the body's WBCs, play a major role in combating infection through phagocytosis. Both the total WBC count and concentration of neutrophils are important in determining the patient's ability to fight infection. A differential count supplies the relative numbers of the various types of WBCs and permits tabulation of polymorphonuclear neutrophils (mature neutrophils, reported as "polys," PMNs, or "segs") and immature forms of neutrophils (reported as bands, metamyelocytes, and "stabs"). These numbers are compiled and reported as the absolute neutrophil count. The risk of infection rises as the absolute neutrophil count decreases.

The cancer patient is also monitored for factors that may contribute to bleeding. These include bone marrow suppression from chemotherapy, radiation, and other drugs that interfere with coagulation and platelet functioning such as aspirin, Persantine, heparin, or warfarin. Common sites assessed for bleeding include skin and mucous membranes, the intestinal, urinary, and respiratory tracts, and the brain.

Gross bleeding as well as oozing at injection sites, bruising (ecchymosis), and changes in mental status that may indicate intracranial bleeding are monitored and reported.

Skin and tissue integrity is at risk in cancer patients because of the effects of chemotherapy, radiation therapy, surgery, and invasive procedures for diagnosis and therapy. As part of the assessment, the nurse identifies which of these predisposing factors are present and assesses the patient for other risk factors, including nutritional deficits, bowel and bladder incontinence, immobility, immunosuppression, and changes related to aging. Skin lesions or ulceration secondary to the tumor are noted. Alterations in tissue integrity throughout the gastrointestinal tract are particularly bothersome to the patient. The oral mucous membranes and the appearance of lesions are noted, as is their effect on the patient's nutritional status and level of comfort. Hair loss (alopecia) is another form of tissue disruption common to cancer patients who receive radiation therapy or chemotherapy. In addition to noting its loss, the nurse also assesses the meaning of hair and hair loss to the patient and his family.

TABLE 19-5. *Factors Predisposing Cancer Patients to Infection*

Factors	*Underlying Mechanisms*
1. Impaired skin and mucous membrane integrity	• Loss of body's first line of defense against invading organisms.
2. Chemotherapy	• Many agents cause suppression of bone marrow, resulting in decreased production and function of white blood cells. Chemotherapy agents that cause mucositis impair skin and mucous membrane integrity. Organ damage associated with certain agents may also predispose patients to infection. Organ damage such as pulmonary fibrosis or cardiomyopathy that is associated with certain agents may also predispose patients to infection.
3. Radiation therapy	• Radiation involving sites of bone marrow production may result in bone marrow suppression. May also lead to impaired tissue integrity.
4. Biologic response modifiers	• Some BRMs may cause bone marrow suppression and organ dysfunction.
5. Malignancy	• Malignant cells may infiltrate the bone marrow and interfere with production of white blood cells and lymphocytes. Hematologic malignancies (leukemias and lymphomas) are associated with impaired function and production of blood cells
6. Malnutrition	• Results in impaired function and production of cells of the immune response. May contribute to impaired skin integrity.
7. Medications	• Antibiotics disturb the balance of normal flora, allowing them to become pathogenic. This process occurs most commonly in the gastrointestinal tract. Steroids and nonsteroidal anti-inflammatory drugs mask the inflammatory response.
8. Urinary catheter	• Creates port and mechanism of entry for organisms.
9. Intravenous catheter	• Results in impaired skin integrity and site of entry for organisms.
10. Other invasive procedures (surgery, paracentesis, thoracentesis, drainage tubes, endoscopies, mechanical ventilation)	• Creates port of entry and possible introduction of exogenous organisms into the system.
11. Contaminated equipment	• Environmental objects such as stagnant water in oxygen equipment are associated with growth of microorganisms.
12. Age	• Increasing age associated with declining organ function. Also associated with decreased production and functioning of the cells of the immune system.
13. Chronic illness	• Associated with impaired organ function and altered immune responses.
14. Prolonged hospitalization	• Allows increased exposure to nosocomial infection and colonization of new organisms.

Assessment of the patient's *nutritional status* is an important part of the nurse's role. Alterations in nutritional status and weight loss may be secondary to the effect of a local tumor, systemic disease, treatment-related side effects, or the emotional status of the patient. The patient's weight and caloric intake are monitored daily. Other information obtained through assessment includes diet history, frequency and duration of episodes of anorexia, changes in appetite, situations and foods that aggravate or relieve the anorexia, and medication history. Difficulty in chewing or swallowing is determined and the occurrence of nausea, vomiting, or diarrhea is noted. Clinical and laboratory data useful in assessing the patient's nutritional status include anthropometric measurements (triceps skin fold and mid upper arm circumference) serum protein levels (albumin and transferrin), lymphocyte count, hemoglobin levels, hematocrit, urinary creatinine levels, and serum iron levels.

Pain and discomfort in cancer may be related to the tumor or malignancy itself, to pressure exerted by the tumor, to diagnostic testing procedures, or to many of the cancer treatments that may be used. As in any other situation involving pain, the experience of cancer pain is affected by both physical and psychosocial influences. In addition to assessing the source and site of pain, the nurse also assesses those factors that increase the patient's perception of pain, such as fear and apprehension, fatigue, anger, and social isolation. Assessment scales for pain (see Chap. 15) are useful in assessing the patient's pain level before use of pain-relieving treatments and in evaluating the patient's response to them.

Although fatigue is a common experience for all individuals, it is often a chronic problem for individuals with cancer. The nurse assesses patients for feelings of weariness, weakness, lack of energy, and inability to carry out necessary and valued daily functions. Chronic fatigue may be characterized by patients exhibiting decreased interest, activity, motivation, and ability to concentrate. In addition, patients often provide slow and short responses to conversation and appear pale with relaxed facial musculature. The nurse assesses physiologic and psychological stressors that can contribute to fatigue. Pain, nausea, dyspnea, constipation, fear, and anxiety may be preceded, accompanied, or followed by fatigue.

Assessment of the cancer patient is not limited to the physiologic changes that may occur in the course of the disease but also focuses on the patient's *psychologic and mental status* as the patient and his family face this life-threatening experience, unpleasant diagnostic tests and treatment modalities, and progression of disease. The patient's mood and emotional reaction to the results of diagnostic testing and prognosis are assessed. His progression through stages of grief is assessed, as is his communication about his diagnosis and prognosis with his family.

Cancer patients are forced to cope with many *assaults to body image* throughout the course of disease and treatment. Entry into the health care system is often accompanied by depersonalization. Threats to self-concept are enormous as patients face the realization of illness, possible disability, and death. Many cancer patients are forced to alter their life styles to accommodate treatments or as a direct result of disease pathology. Priorities and value systems are often forced to change when body image is threatened and physical characteristics become less important. Disfiguring surgery, hair loss, cachexia, skin changes, altered communication patterns, and sexual dysfunction are some of the devastating results of cancer and its treatment that may threaten the patient's self-esteem and body image. During assessment, these potential threats are identified, as is the patient's ability to cope with these changes.

▷ Nursing Diagnoses

Based on the assessment data, nursing diagnoses of the patient with cancer may include the following:

- High risk for infection related to altered immunologic response
- High risk for injury related to bleeding disorder
- Impaired tissue integrity related to the effects of treatment and disease
- Alterations in nutrition: less than body requirements related to anorexia and gastrointestinal changes
- Pain and discomfort related to disease and treatment effects
- Fatigue related to physical and psychological stressors.
- Grieving related to anticipated loss and altered role function
- Body image disturbance related to changes in appearance and role functions

▷ Planning and Implementation

▷ *Goals:* The major goals of the patient may include prevention of infection, prevention of injury related to bleeding disorder, maintenance of tissue integrity, maintenance of nutrition, relief of pain, relief of fatigue, progression through grieving process appropriately, and improved body image.

▷ Nursing Interventions

▷ *Prevention of Infection.* Despite advances in the care of patients with cancer, infection remains the leading cause of death. Defense against infection is compromised in many different ways. Skin and mucous membrane integrity, the body's first line of defense, is challenged by multiple invasive diagnostic and therapeutic procedures, adverse effects of irradiation and chemotherapy, and the detrimental effects of immobility. Impaired nutrition resulting from anorexia, nausea, vomiting, diarrhea, and the underlying malignant process can alter the body's ability to combat invading organisms. Medications such as antibiotics disturb the balance of normal flora, allowing the overgrowth of pathogenic organisms. Other medications can also alter the immune response (see Chap. 48). Cancer itself may be immunosuppressive. Malignancies such as leukemia and lymphoma are often associated with defects in cellular and humoral immunity. Advanced cancer can lead to tumor obstruction of hollow viscera, blood, and lymphatic vessels, creating a favorable environment for proliferation of pathogenic organisms. In some patients, tumor cells infiltrate bone marrow and prevent normal production of white blood cells. Most often, however, a decrease in white blood cells is a result of bone marrow suppression after chemotherapy or irradiation.

Infections in the myelosuppressed or immunosuppressed patient are most often nosocomial, a result of organisms that have become part of the patient's resident flora after being acquired from the hospital environment. The most threatening pathogens are the gram-negative bacilli such as *Pseudomonas aeruginosa* and *Escherichia coli*. Gram-positive bacilli such as *Staphylococcus aureus* and fungal organisms such as *Candida albicans* can also contribute to serious infection.

Fever is probably the most important sign of infection in the immunocompromised patient. Although fever may be related to a variety of noninfectious conditions, including the underlying malignancy, any temperature elevation of 101°F (38.3°C) or above is reported and dealt with promptly. Antibiotic agents may be prescribed to treat infections after results of cultures and sensitivities of wound drainage, exudate, sputum, urine, stool, or blood specimens are obtained. Individuals who are granulocytopenic (decreased WBC count) are most often treated with broad-spectrum antibiotics before the cause of infection is identified. This is necessary because of the high incidence of mortality associated with untreated infection in this group of patients. Broad-spectrum antibiotic coverage or empiric therapy includes a combination of drugs that provide defense against the major pathogenic organisms.

An important component of the nurse's role is to administer these medications promptly according to the prescribed schedule to achieve adequate blood levels of the medications. Strict asepsis is essential when handling intravenous lines, catheters, and other invasive equipment. The patient is protected from exposure to others with active infections and is strongly advised to avoid crowds. Handwashing and appropriate hygiene are necessary to reduce exposure to potentially harmful bacteria and to eliminate environmental sources of contamination. Invasive procedures such as injections, vaginal or rectal examinations, rectal temperatures, and surgery are avoided. The patient is also encouraged to cough and take deep breaths frequently to prevent atelectasis and other potential respiratory problems.

Assessment of the patient for infection and inflammation is frequent and continues throughout the course of disease. Septicemia and septic shock are life-threatening complications that must be prevented or detected early in their course.

Signs and symptoms of septic shock include altered mental status, either subnormal or elevated temperature, cool and clammy skin, decreased urine output, hypotension, dysrhythmias, electrolyte imbalances, and impaired arterial blood gases. The patient and family members are instructed about signs of septicemia, preventive actions, and actions to take if infection or septicemia occurs.

▷ *Prevention of Injury Related to Bleeding Disorder.*   A decrease in the number of circulating platelets (thrombocytopenia) is the most common cause of bleeding in the patient with cancer. Thrombocytopenia is often a result of bone marrow depression after certain types of chemotherapy and radiation therapy. Tumor infiltration of bone marrow can also impair the normal production of platelets. In some cases, platelet destruction is associated with an enlarged spleen (hypersplenism) and abnormal antibody function that occur with leukemia and lymphoma.

Platelets are essential for normal blood clotting and coagulation (hemostasis). *Thrombocytopenia* is defined as a platelet count less than $100,000/mm^3$ (SI: $0.1 \times 10^{12}/L$). When the count falls to 20,000 to $50,000/mm^3$ (SI: 0.02 to $0.05 \times 10^{12}/L$), the risk for bleeding increases. Counts less than $20,000/mm^3$ (SI: $0.02 \times 10^{12}/L$) are associated with an increased risk for spontaneous bleeding and often require transfusion of platelets.

In addition to monitoring laboratory values, the nurse continues to assess the patient for evidence of bleeding. The nurse also takes steps to prevent trauma and minimize the risk of bleeding by replacing the patient's hard-bristled toothbrush with a soft-bristled one, by using an electric razor rather than a safety or straight-edge razor, and by avoiding unnecessary invasive procedures (*e.g.*, rectal temperatures, catheterization). The patient and family are assisted in identifying and removing environmental hazards that may lead to falls or other trauma. Soft foods, increased fluid intake, and stool softeners, if prescribed, may be indicated to reduce trauma to the gastrointestinal tract. The joints and extremities are handled and moved gently to minimize the risk of spontaneous bleeding.

▷ *Maintenance of Tissue Integrity.*   The person with cancer is at risk for the development of a variety of skin and mucous membrane impairments. The nurse in all health settings is in an ideal position to assess and assist the patient and family in the management of these problems. Some of the most frequently encountered disturbances include skin and tissue reactions to radiation therapy, stomatitis, alopecia, and metastatic skin lesions.

The patient who is experiencing skin and tissue reactions to radiation therapy requires careful skin care to prevent further skin irritation, drying, and damage. The skin over the affected area is handled gently; rubbing and use of hot or cold water, soaps, powders, lotions, and cosmetics are avoided. Trauma to the area is prevented by use of loosely fitting clothes that do not constrict, irritate, or rub the affected area. If blistering occurs, care is taken not to disrupt the blisters to reduce the risk of introducing bacteria. Aseptic wound care is indicated to minimize the risk of infection and sepsis.

Stomatitis.   Stomatitis is a common problem in cancer patients as a result of chemotherapy or radiation therapy. It is an inflammatory response of the oral tissues that may progress from mild erythema and edema to painful ulcerations, bleeding, and secondary infection. This condition most often develops within 5 to 14 days of the administration of certain chemotherapeutic agents such as doxorubicin and 5-fluorouracil. It may also occur with irradiation to the head and neck area. In very severe cases of stomatitis, chemotherapy may be temporarily halted until resolution of inflammation.

As a result of normal everyday wear and tear, the epithelial cells that line the oral cavity have a very rapid turnover or routinely slough off. Chemotherapy and irradiation interfere with the body's ability to replace those cells. An inflammatory response develops as denuded areas appear in the oral cavity. Myelosuppression as a result of the underlying malignancy or treatment predisposes the patient to oral bleeding and infection. Pain associated with ulcerated oral tissues can significantly interfere with nutritional intake and willingness to maintain oral hygiene. Soft-bristled toothbrushes and nonabrasive toothpaste prevent or reduce the trauma to the oral mucosa. Restriction of foods that are difficult to chew, too hot, or spicy may further reduce trauma and promote comfort. The patient's lips are lubricated to keep them soft. Topical antifungal agents and anesthetics may be prescribed to promote healing and minimize patient discomfort. The patient who experiences severe pain and discomfort with stomatitis requires encouragement and assistance to use these prescribed agents and to maintain an adequate fluid and food intake.

Alopecia.   The temporary or permanent thinning or complete loss of hair, referred to as *alopecia*, is a potential adverse effect of certain forms of radiation therapy and several chemotherapeutic agents. The extent of alopecia depends on the dose and duration of therapy. These treatment modalities cause alopecia by damaging stem cells and hair follicles. As a result, the hair is brittle and may fall out or break off at the surface of the scalp. Loss of other body hair is less frequent.

Many health professionals view hair loss as a minor problem when compared with the potential life-threatening consequences of the underlying malignancy. For many patients, however, hair loss poses a major threat to body image, arousing feelings of anxiety, sadness, anger, rejection, ridicule, and isolation. To patients and families, hair loss can serve as a constant reminder of cancer, interfering with coping abilities, interpersonal relationships, and sexuality. The nurse's role is to provide information about alopecia and to assist the patient and family in coping with hair loss and changes in body image. The patient is encouraged to acquire a wig or hairpiece before hair loss so that the replacement matches the patient's own hair. Use of attractive scarves and hats may make the patient feel more attractive. It is frequently of some comfort to patients that the hair usually begins to grow again after completion of the chemotherapy; however, the color and texture of the new hair may differ.

Malignant Skin Lesions.   Skin lesions may occur with local extension or tumor embolization into the epithelium and its surrounding lymph and blood vessels. Secondary growth of cancer cells into the skin may be characterized as erythematous areas progressing to wounds involving tissue necrosis and infection. The most extensive lesions are friable, purulent, and malodorous. In addition, these lesions are a source of considerable pain and discomfort. Although this type of wound is most often associated with breast cancer, it can also accompany lymphoma, leukemia, melanoma, and cancers of the head and neck, lung, uterus, kidney, colon, and bladder. The development of severe skin lesions is usually considered to be a poor prognostic sign for expected length of survival.

Ulcerating skin lesions usually indicate the presence of widely disseminated disease. Therefore, eradication of the problem is usually not feasible. The management of these lesions becomes a nursing priority. Nursing care includes careful assessment, cleansing, reduction of superficial bacterial flora, control of bleeding, reduction of odor, and protection against pain and further trauma to the skin. The patient and family require assistance and guidance to care for these skin lesions at home. Referral to a community health nurse is indicated to provide assistance and evaluation of wound care at home.

▷ *Maintenance of Nutritional Status.*   Most cancer patients experience some degree of weight loss during their illness. Anorexia, malabsorption, and cachexia are examples of nutritional problems commonly seen in cancer patients.

Anorexia.   There are many theories about the cause of anorexia in the cancer patient. Alterations in taste manifested by increased salty, sour, and metallic tastes and altered responses to sweet and bitter tastes lead to decreased appetite, decreased intake, and protein-calorie malnutrition in the cancer patient. Taste alterations may be due to deficiencies of minerals such as zinc, increases in circulating amino acids and cellular metabolites, and the administration of chemotherapeutic agents. Individuals undergoing radiation therapy to the head and neck may experience "mouth blindness," which is a severe impairment of taste. Alterations in the sense of smell also alter taste, which is a common experience of patients with head and neck cancers. Anorexia may be related to early satiety and a sense of fullness secondary to decreased digestive enzymes, abnormalities of glucose and triglyceride metabolism, and prolonged stimulation of gastric volume receptors. Psychologic distress such as fear, pain, depression, and isolation throughout illness may have a negative impact on appetite. Conditioned food aversions due to past experiences with nausea, vomiting, and treatment modalities may also contribute to anorexia.

Malabsorption.   Many cancer patients are unable to absorb nutrients from the gastrointestinal system secondary to tumor activity and cancer treatment. Tumors may impair enzyme production; create fistulas; secrete hormones and enzymes such as gastrin, which leads to increased gastrointestinal irritation, peptic ulcer disease, and decreased fat digestion; and interfere with protein digestion. Chemotherapy and irradiation can irritate and damage mucosal cells of the bowel, inhibiting absorption. Radiation therapy can cause sclerosis of the blood vessels in the bowel and fibrotic changes in the gastrointestinal tissue. Surgical intervention may change peristaltic patterns, alter gastrointestinal secretions, and reduce the absorptive surfaces of the gastrointestinal mucosa, all leading to malabsorption.

Cachexia.   Cachexia (wasting syndrome) is common in the cancer patient, especially in advanced disease states. Cancer cachexia is related to inadequate nutritional intake along with increasing metabolic demand, increased energy expenditure due to anaerobic metabolism of the tumor, impaired glucose metabolism, competition of the tumor cells for nutrients, altered lipid metabolism, and failure of appetite.

Creative dietary modification to overcome the factors contributing to anorexia must be carried out for each patient. Family members are included in the dietary plan of care to maintain consistency and aid compliance. Factors contributing to the patient's anorexia (unpleasant sights and odors) are eliminated. The patient's preferences as well as his physiologic and metabolic requirements are considered in selecting foods. Small, frequent meals are provided with additional supplements between meals. Oral hygiene and pain relief measures are offered before mealtime to make meals more pleasant.

Interventions to relieve malabsorptive states may include enzyme and vitamin replacement, changes in feeding schedule, use of elemental diets, and measures to relieve diarrhea. If malabsorption is severe, hyperalimentation may be necessary through a right atrial Silastic catheter, such as a Hickman or a Broviac catheter (Fig. 19–4 in Chart 19–4). These catheters are surgically placed and are maintained for long-term venous access. To prevent infection, these catheters are tunneled under the skin through the subcutaneous tissue before entering the superior vena cava and the right atrium. A Dacron cuff located just under the skin at the exit site anchors the catheter and prevents entry of bacteria. Maintenance of the catheter requires heparinization to prevent clotting and dressing changes at the exit site to prevent infection. Specific procedures for catheter care will vary among health care institutions. General nursing interventions include flushes with small doses of heparin in normal saline, infused every 24 to 48 hours or after each use of the catheter. The dressings are changed three times a week, and the exit site is assessed for redness, swelling, discharge, pain, or protrusion of the Dacron cuff. The site should be cleansed aseptically with alcohol followed by povidone-iodine (Betadine). An anti-infective topical agent is applied to the site, and an occlusive gauze or transparent dressing is applied. The infusion cap at the end of the catheter is changed weekly to prevent infection. Patient education is essential for prevention and management of potential complications, including catheter breakage, air emboli, and infection.

Interventions to reduce cachexia usually do not prolong survival but improve the quality of life. Creative dietary therapies, enteral (tube) feedings, or hyperalimentation may be chosen to deliver nourishment. Nursing care is also directed toward prevention of trauma, infection, and other complications that increase metabolic demands.

▷ *Relief of Pain.*   It is estimated that 60% to 96% of all individuals with progressive malignant disease experience pain. Although patients with cancer may have acute pain, their pain is more frequently characterized as chronic. (For a more detailed discussion of pain, see Chap. 15.) As in other situations involving pain, the experience of cancer pain is influenced by both physical and psychosocial factors.

Malignancies can cause pain in a variety of ways. Bone destruction as a result of tumor invasion is one of the most devastating sources of pain. Bone involvement is seen commonly in multiple myeloma and cancers of the breast and prostate. Infiltration or compression of nerves can cause pain that is described as sharp and burning. Vertebral metastasis involving spinal nerves may occur with breast and lung cancer. Tumors causing lymphatic or venous obstruction may lead to a dull, throbbing type of pain. This is often associated with lymphoma or Kaposi's sarcoma. Ischemic pain results from any tumor that occludes arterial circulation. Obstruction of hollow viscera is often associated with colon cancer. Patients with abdominal obstruction often complain of pain that is dull and poorly localized. Finally, tumors invading skin or mucous membranes may cause pain associated with inflammation, ulceration, infection, and tissue necrosis; this is common in patients with progressive head and neck malignancies and Kaposi's sarcoma.

Pain is also associated with various cancer treatment modalities. Acute pain is linked with trauma that results from surgical procedures. Tissue necrosis, peripheral neuropathies, and stomatitis are potential sources of pain that may occur with certain chemotherapeutic agents. Radiation therapy can cause inflammation of the skin or irradiated organs.

In today's society, most people expect pain to disappear or resolve quickly, and in fact it usually does. Although it is controllable, however, cancer pain is often irreversible and not quickly resolved. For many patients, pain is a signal of continued tumor progression and impending death. As anticipation and anxiety about the pain increase, the patient's perception of the pain is heightened, producing fear and additional pain. Chronic cancer pain, then, can be best described as a cycle progressing from pain to anxiety to fear and back to pain again.

Pain tolerance, the point past which pain can no longer be tolerated, varies among patients. Pain tolerance is decreased by fatigue, anxiety, fear of death, anger, powerlessness, social isolation, changes in role identity, loss of independence, and past experiences. Tolerance to pain is enhanced by adequate rest and sleep, diversion, mood elevation, empathy, antidepressants, antianxiety agents, and analgesics.

Successful management of cancer pain is based on a thorough and precise pain assessment that examines physical, psychosocial, environmental, and spiritual factors. A multidisciplinary team effort is essential to determine the most optimal approach for pain management. Prevention and reduction of pain serve to lessen anxiety and break the previously described pain cycle. These can be accomplished best by administering analgesics on a regularly scheduled basis (preventive approach to pain management) as prescribed and not as needed (prn). A variety of pharmacologic and nonpharmacologic approaches offer the best methods of providing for cancer pain management. No reasonable approaches, even those that may be somewhat invasive, should be overlooked because of a poor or terminal prognosis. Improving the quality of life is as valuable as preventing a painful death.

▷ *Decreasing Fatigue.* Nurses help patients and families to understand that fatigue is often an expected and temporary side effect of the cancer process and associated treatments. It does not always signify advancing disease or treatment failure. Many of the potential sources of fatigue are summarized in Table 19–6.

Nursing strategies are designed to minimize fatigue or help patients cope with existing fatigue. Energy conservation principles are used to help patients plan daily activities. Alternating periods of rest and activity is beneficial. Patients are encouraged to maintain as closely as possible their usual life style by including valued and enjoyable activities. Both patients and families are encouraged to plan for reallocation of responsibilities such as child care, cleaning, and meal preparation. Patients who are employed full time may need to reduce the number of hours worked each week.

Nurses also address factors that contribute to fatigue. Pharmacologic and nonpharmacologic strategies are used in

TABLE 19–6. *Potential Sources of Fatigue*

Pain, pruritus

Altered nutrition related to anorexia, nausea, vomiting, cachexia

Electrolyte imbalance related to vomiting, diarrhea

Altered protection related to neutropenia, thrombocytopenia, anemia

Impaired tissue integrity related to stomatitis, mucositis

Impaired physical mobility related to neurologic impairments, surgery, bone metastasis, pain and analgesic use

Knowledge deficit related to disease process, treatment

Anxiety related to fear, diagnosis, role changes, uncertainty of future

Ineffective breathing patterns related to cough, shortness of breath and dyspnea

Sleep pattern disturbance

managing pain. Nutritional counseling is used for patients with inadequate caloric and protein intake. Serum hemoglobin and hematocrit levels are monitored for deficiencies, and blood products are administered as per the physician's orders. Patients are monitored for alterations in oxygenation and electrolyte balances. Physical therapy and assistive devices are beneficial for patients with impaired mobility.

▷ *Progression Through the Grieving Process.* The diagnosis of cancer need not indicate a fatal outcome. Many forms of cancer are curable; many others achieve "cure" status if they are treated early. Despite these facts, many patients and their families view cancer as a fatal disease that is inevitably accompanied by pain, suffering, debility, and emaciation. Grieving is a normal response to these fears and to the losses anticipated or experienced by the patient with cancer. These may include loss of health, normal sensations, body image, social interaction, sexuality, and intimacy. The patient, his family, and friends may grieve the loss of quality time to spend with others, the loss of future and unfulfilled plans, and the loss of control over one's own body and emotional reactions.

The patient and his family who have just been informed by their physician about the diagnosis of cancer frequently respond with shock, numbness, and disbelief. It is often during this stage that the patient and family are called on to make important initial decisions about treatment and require the support of the physician, nurse, and other health care team members to make these decisions. An important role of the nurse is to answer the questions of the patient and family and clarify information provided by the physician. In addition to assessing the response of the patient and family to the diagnosis and planned treatment, the nurse assists them in framing their questions and concerns, identifying resources and support persons (*e.g.*, clergy, counselor), and communicating and sharing their concerns with each other.

As the patient and family progress through the grieving process, they may express feelings of anger, frustration, and depression. During this time, the nurse encourages the patient and family to verbalize their feelings in an atmosphere of trust and support. She continues to assess their reactions and provides assistance and support as they confront and learn to deal with new problems.

If the patient enters the terminal phase of disease, it may become obvious that the patient and family members are at different stages of the grieving process. Therefore, the nurse assists the patient and family at these different stages to come to grips with their reactions and feelings. Physical support, including holding the patient's hand or just being present at his bedside, frequently contributes to his feelings of trust and peace of mind. Maintaining contact with the surviving family members after death of the cancer patient may help them to progress through the process of grieving and to work through their feelings of loss.

▷ *Improved Body Image and Self-Esteem.*   A positive approach is essential when caring for the patient with an altered body image. Independence and continued participation in self-care and decision making are encouraged to help the patient retain control and a sense of self-worth. The patient is encouraged to express his feelings about threats to his body image. Assistance is provided to enable the patient to assume those tasks and participate in those activities of most importance and interest to him. The nurse serves as a good listener and counselor to the patient as well as to the family. Referral to a support group for cancer patients, their families, or both often provides additional assistance in coping with the changes resulting from cancer or its treatment.

The patient who is experiencing alterations in sexuality and sexual function is encouraged to share and discuss his concerns openly with his partner. Alternative forms of sexual expression are explored with the patient and partner to promote positive self-worth and acceptance. The nurse who identifies serious physiologic, psychological, or communication difficulties related to sexuality or sexual function is in a key position to assist the patient and partner to seek further counseling if necessary.

▷ *Collaborative Interventions.*   Hemorrhage may be related to a variety of underlying abnormalities such as thrombocytopenia and disorders of coagulation. These clinical situations are most often associated with the cancer process or the adverse effects of cancer treatments. Sites of hemorrhage may include the gastrointestinal, respiratory and genitourinary tracts, and the brain. Blood pressure, pulse, and respirations are monitored every 15 to 30 minutes when patients experience bleeding. The serum hemoglobin and hematocrit are followed carefully and compared with previous laboratory data for changes indicating blood loss. The nurse tests all urine, stool, and emesis for the presence of occult blood. Neurologic assessments are performed to detect changes in orientation and behavior. The nurse administers fluids and blood products as prescribed to replace patient losses. Vasopressor drugs are administered as prescribed to maintain blood pressure and ensure tissue oxygenation. Supplemental oxygen is used as necessary.

Septic shock is most often associated with overwhelming gram-negative bacterial infections. This type of shock is characterized by loss of hemodynamic stability and abnormalities of tissue oxygenation. Signs and symptoms of septic shock include altered mental status, either subnormal or elevated temperature, cool and clammy skin, decreased urine output, hypotension, dysrhythmias, electrolyte imbalances, and metabolic acidosis. The nurse monitors the patient's blood pressure, pulse, respirations, and temperature every 15 to 30 minutes. Neurologic assessments are completed to assess for changes in orientation and responsiveness. Fluid and electrolyte status is monitored by measuring fluid intake and output and serum electrolytes. Arterial blood gases are obtained to de-

termine tissue oxygenation. The nurse administers intravenous fluids, blood products, and vasopressor drugs as prescribed to maintain the patient's blood pressure and tissue perfusion. Supplemental oxygen is often necessary. Broad-spectrum antibiotics are administered as ordered to combat the underlying infection.

▷ ## Evaluation

Expected Outcomes.   (See Nursing Care Plan 19–1 for specific outcomes.)

1. Experiences no infection or inflammation
2. Exhibits no bleeding
3. Maintains adequate tissue (skin and mucous membrane) integrity
4. Maintains adequate nutritional status
5. Achieves relief of pain and discomfort
6. Demonstrates increased activity tolerance and decreased fatigue
7. Progresses through grieving process
8. Exhibits improved body image and self-esteem

Rehabilitation

Cancer is a chronic disease that affects the physical, psychological, social, and economic dimensions of individuals' lives. The diagnosis of cancer may be accompanied by emotional turmoil and changes in life style or daily habits. With advances in diagnosis and treatment, however, survival rates are improving. Many patients, including those who receive primary surgical treatment and adjuvant chemotherapy or irradiation, are returning to work and their usual activities of daily living. These patients may encounter a variety of problems, including coping with changes in functional abilities and attitudes of employers, co-workers, and families who still view cancer as a terminal, debilitating disease.

Nurses play an important role in the rehabilitation of the cancer patient. Cancer rehabilitation needs to begin early in the disease and treatment to maximize outcome. Assessment of body image changes as a result of disfiguring treatments is necessary to facilitate the patient's adjustment to changes in appearance or functional abilities. The nurse can refer the patient and family to a variety of support groups sponsored by the American Cancer Society, such as those for people who have had laryngectomies or mastectomies. Nurses also collaborate with physical and occupational therapists in improving the patient's abilities and use of prosthetic devices.

Some patients return to work and continue to receive either chemotherapy or radiation therapy for extended periods. These people may experience transient problems such as lethargy, easy fatigue, anorexia, nausea, or vomiting. Nurses assess for the existence of these problems and assist the patient in identifying strategies for coping with them. For patients with gastrointestinal disturbances after chemotherapy, altering work hours or receiving treatments in the evenings may prove to be helpful. Nurses collaborate with dietitians to help patients plan meals that will be acceptable and meet nutritional requirements. Nurses are also involved in the ongoing assessment of patients over time to detect any long-term sequelae of cancer treatment.

Discrimination against recovering cancer patients has been demonstrated in several forms. Often employers lack the understanding of the variability that exists in the diagnosis of cancer in terms of functional capacity and prognosis. As a result, employers may be hesitant to hire or continue employment of people with cancer, especially if continued treatment regimens might require adjustments in work schedules. Attitudes of co-workers can become a problem when related to communication impairments such as those experienced by some head and neck cancer patients. Finally, employers, co-workers, and families may continue to view the person as being "sick" despite ongoing recovery or completion of treatment.

Nurses can participate in efforts to educate employers and the public in general to ensure that the rights of patients with cancer are maintained. Whenever possible, nurses assist patients and families to resume preexisting roles. Nurses can encourage patients to regain the highest level of independence possible. In addition, the patient may be directed to vocational rehabilitation services of the American Cancer Society or other agencies. The diagnosis of cancer need not be a "death sentence." Many people can and do resume active roles in life.

In summary, as more cancer patients survive longer with their disease, nurses can promote quality of life for these individuals by incorporating rehabilitation principles into nursing care. Changes in functional abilities, attitudes of others, and societal discrimination challenge health care providers working toward rehabilitation of the cancer patient. Nurses working as educators, counselors, and advocates play a major role in the rehabilitation efforts, thus improving life satisfaction and quality for patients.

Gerontologic Considerations

Oncology nurses are working with increasing numbers of elderly patients. Approximately 55% of all cancers occur after 65 years of age. Common malignancies in the elderly include multiple myeloma, non-Hodgkin's lymphoma, oropharyngeal cancers, and cancers of the bladder, breast, colon, lung, and prostate.

It is important for oncology nurses working with this population to understand the normal physiologic changes that occur with aging. These changes include decreased skin elasticity; decreased skeletal mass, structure, and strength; decreased organ function and structure; impaired immune system mechanisms; alterations in neurologic function; and altered drug absorption, distribution, metabolism, and elimination. These changes ultimately influence the elderly patient's ability to tolerate treatment for cancer. In addition, many elderly patients have other chronic diseases that may also limit tolerance of treatment.

Potential toxicities associated with chemotherapeutic agents such as cisplatin may be increased by a decline in renal blood flow and creatinine clearance normally associated with the aging process. Cardiac toxicities associated with chemotherapy with doxorubicin may be more pronounced in the elderly patient who already has a decreased cardiac output as a result of normal physiologic aging.

The elderly person receiving radiation therapy may have a delayed recovery of normal tissues as a result of the changes in tissue repair associated with aging. The potential adverse effects involving the bone marrow, gastrointestinal tract, and skin may be enhanced, leading to an increased incidence and

severity of myelosuppression, skin impairments, anorexia, nausea, vomiting, and diarrhea.

The older patient is often slower to recover from surgical interventions. Decreased tissue healing capacity and pulmonary and cardiovascular functioning may increase the risk of the patient developing postoperative complications such as atelectasis, pneumonia, and wound infections.

The nurse must be aware of the increased risk of complications after cancer treatment in the elderly and carefully monitor for signs and symptoms of adverse effects. In addition, the elderly patient is instructed to report all symptoms to the physician. It is not uncommon for the elderly patient to delay reporting symptoms, attributing them to "old age." Many elderly persons do not want to report illness for fear of loss of independence, role functions, and financial security. The nurse acts as a patient advocate, encouraging independence and providing support when indicated.

Care of the Patient With Advanced Cancer

The patient with advanced cancer is likely to experience many of the problems previously described, but all to a greater degree. Symptoms of gastrointestinal disturbances, nutritional problems, weight loss, and cachexia make him more susceptible to skin breakdown, fluid and electrolyte problems, and infection. Although not all cancer patients experience pain, those who do often fear that it will not be adequately treated. Although treatment at this stage of illness is likely to be palliative rather than curative, prevention and appropriate management of problems can improve the quality of the patient's life considerably. For example, use of analgesia on a regular basis at set intervals rather than on an "as needed" basis frequently breaks the cycle of tension and anxiety associated with waiting until pain becomes severe and pain relief is inadequate once the analgesic is given. Working with the patient and family as well as other health care providers on a pain management program based on the patient's individual requirements frequently increases his comfort and sense of control. In addition, the dose of narcotic analgesic required is often reduced as pain becomes more manageable and other medications (*e.g.,* sedatives, tranquilizers, muscle relaxants) are added to assist in relieving pain.

The patient may be a candidate for radiation therapy or surgical intervention to relieve severe pain. The consequences of these procedures (*e.g.,* percutaneous nerve block, cordotomy) are explained to the patient and family, and measures are taken to prevent complications resulting from altered sensation, immobility, and changes in bowel and bladder function.

With the appearance of each new symptom, the patient often experiences dread and fear that the disease is progressing. However, one cannot assume that all symptoms are related to the cancer. The new symptoms and problems are evaluated and treated aggressively if possible to increase the patient's comfort and improve the quality of life.

Weakness, immobility, fatigue, and inactivity often occur in the advanced stages of cancer as a result of the tumor itself, treatment, inadequate nutritional intake, or dyspnea. The nurse works with the patient to set realistic goals and to provide rest balanced with planned activities and exercise. She assists the patient in identifying less energy-consuming methods of accomplishing tasks and activities that the patient values the most.

Efforts are made throughout the course of the disease to provide the patient with as much control and independence as he wants, but with assurance that support and assistance will be provided. Additionally, the health care team works with the patient and family to ascertain and adhere to the patient's wishes about treatment methods and care as he approaches the terminal phase of illness and death.

Hospice

For many years, society was unable to appropriately cope with patients in the most advanced stages of cancer, and patients were left in acute care settings to die rather than at home or in facilities specifically designed to manage the needs of patients with terminal disease. The needs of these persons do not require advanced technology or sophisticated equipment, but are best managed by a comprehensive multidisciplinary program that focuses on symptom relief and psychosocial and spiritual support for the patient and family when cure and remission are no longer possible. The concept of hospice, which originated in Great Britain, best addresses these needs. Most importantly, the unit of care is the family, not just the patient. Hospice may take several forms: free-standing hospices, hospital-based programs, and community or home-based programs.

Because of high costs associated with maintaining free-standing hospices, care is often provided by coordinating hospital-based and community services. Although physicians, social workers, clergy, dietitians, physical therapists, and volunteers are involved in patient care, nurses are most often the coordinators of all hospice activities. It is essential that community-based nurses possess advanced skill in the assessment and management of pain, nutrition, bowel dysfunction, and skin impairments.

In addition, hospice programs facilitate clear communication among family members and between health care providers. Most patients and families are informed of the prognoses and are encouraged to participate in decisions regarding pursuing or terminating treatment.

Community health nurses are also actively involved in bereavement counseling. Through collaboration with other support disciplines, nurses often assist patients and families to cope with changes in role identity, family structure, grief, and loss. In many instances, family support for survivors continues for a period of about 1 year.

Oncologic Emergencies

In addition to assessment and management of the previously described problems experienced by the patient with cancer, the nurse also has an important role in the prompt detection and management of complications of cancer that are considered oncologic emergencies. As a result of the underlying malignancy, its metastasis, or the effects of treatment, the oncology patient is at risk for the development of a unique group of acute conditions requiring immediate medical or surgical intervention. Common oncologic emergencies include superior vena cava syndrome, spinal cord compression, hypercalcemia, pericardial effusion, disseminated intravascular coagulation, and the syndrome of inappropriate secretion of antidiuretic hormone.

Superior Vena Cava Syndrome

The superior vena cava is the major site of venous drainage from the head, neck, arms, and upper thorax. Positioned within the rigid compartment of the mediastinum, it is closely surrounded by major structures, including the heart, lungs, vertebral bodies, and esophagus. Consequently, compression of the superior vena cava by tumor or enlarged lymph nodes can result in markedly impaired venous drainage of the head, neck, arms, and thorax. In most patients, the superior vena cava syndrome occurs with lung cancer, but it can also occur with lymphoma and metastasis from other sites.

The clinical manifestations of impaired venous drainage usually develop gradually over a period of 3 to 4 weeks, but they may also appear suddenly. Progressive shortness of breath, dyspnea, cough, and facial swelling are common. Edema of the neck, arms, hands, and thorax may develop with associated sensations of skin tightness and difficulty swallowing. The jugular, temporal, and arm veins may be engorged and distended. Dilated thoracic vessels often cause prominent venous patterns visible on the chest wall. Continued venous obstruction may lead to increased intracranial pressure, associated visual disturbances, headache, and altered mental status. If untreated, the superior vena cava syndrome may lead to cerebral anoxia, laryngeal edema, bronchial obstruction, and death.

Management

Prompt diagnosis and treatment are essential in managing this syndrome. Radiation therapy is the treatment of choice to decrease the tumor size and alleviate symptoms. Chemotherapy is used when the tumor is known to be responsive (lymphoma or small cell lung cancer). Other supportive measures such as oxygen therapy and diuretics may be used.

Nursing Interventions

Nursing care includes identifying patients at risk for developing superior vena cava syndrome. Clinical manifestations detected by the nursing assessment are reported to the physician and investigated promptly. Continued assessment of the patient's cardiopulmonary and neurologic status is essential. As a result of increasing difficulty in breathing and progressive edema, many patients become anxious and fearful of suffocating. Nursing care is directed toward facilitating breathing by positioning, promoting comfort, and reducing anxiety. Minimizing the patient's energy expenditure by energy conservation techniques may minimize shortness of breath. In addition, the patient's fluid volume status is monitored and fluids are administered cautiously to minimize edema.

Spinal Cord Compression

Malignancies such as breast, lung, kidney, and prostate cancers, myeloma, and lymphoma that metastasize to the spine may cause spinal cord compression. Most lesions develop in the space between the periosteum of the vertebrae and the dura of the spinal cord (extradural), leading to destruction of the vertebral bodies and epidural tissue. Less commonly, tumors develop in the spinal cord itself.

Spinal cord compression is characterized by pain that may be constant and exacerbated by movement, coughing, sneezing, or the Valsalva maneuver. The location and characteristics of the pain depend on the area of involvement of the spinal cord. Neurologic dysfunction develops when cord compression is prolonged or severe and may include motor and sensory deficit. Sensory deficits generally begin as loss of pinprick sensation, progressing to decreased vibratory sense and finally to loss of position sense. The sense of touch usually remains intact even when motor dysfunction is advanced. Motor loss (weakness and ataxia) is often present at the time of diagnosis. Progression of compression ultimately leads to flaccid paralysis. The occurrence of other dysfunctions such as urinary and fecal incontinence is dependent on the level of the lesion compressing the cord. Compression of upper motor neurons above S2 can lead to bladder-overflow incontinence. Cord compression at levels S3, S4, and S5 can result in flaccid sphincter tone and bowel incontinence.

Prompt neurologic assessment is essential if sensory and motor function is to be maintained or restored. Although a variety of diagnostic procedures may assist in identifying the compressing lesion, the myelogram is considered the most accurate means of localizing the site of compression. Once the diagnosis is established, medical intervention is quickly initiated because symptoms can progress within a relatively short period.

Management

Radiation therapy is most commonly used to reduce tumor size and halt disease progression. In most cases, surgical decompression is not used unless the symptoms progress despite irradiation or the patient has previously received a maximum amount of radiation to the area of the cord involved. Surgery may be indicated when the tumor involved is known to be insensitive or nonresponsive to radiation therapy. Steroids are often given in addition to radiation therapy to decrease the edema and inflammation at the site of compression. Recovery of neurologic function is influenced by promptness of diagnosis and treatment. Despite treatment, patients who develop complete paralysis usually do not regain neurologic function.

Nursing Interventions

Nursing interventions include ongoing assessment of neurologic function to identify existing and progressing dysfunction. Most patients will require both pharmacologic and nonpharmacologic measures to control pain. Because of pain and decreased functional abilities associated with spinal cord compression, patients are often at risk for the hazards of immobility such as skin breakdown, urinary stasis, thrombophlebitis, and decreased clearance of pulmonary secretions. Nursing measures are directed toward prevention of these problems and maintenance of muscle tone through range of motion exercises. For patients with bladder or bowel incontinence, intermittent urinary catheterization and bowel training programs are essential. Additionally, the patient and family require assistance in coping with pain and alterations in body functioning, life styles, roles, and level of independence.

Hypercalcemia

Hypercalcemia is a potentially life-threatening complication that is characterized by abnormal calcium metabolism, resulting in serum calcium levels in excess of 11 mg/dl (SI: 2.74 mmol/L) of blood. The skeletal system serves as the storage site for approximately 99% of all the calcium in the body. Hypercalcemia associated with cancer occurs when the release of calcium from the bones is more than the kidneys can excrete or the bones can reabsorb (see Chap. 18 for a discussion of normal calcium metabolism). Hypercalcemia is commonly seen in patients with multiple myeloma, and breast, squamous cell lung, and prostatic cancer. Less commonly, it develops in patients with leukemia, lymphoma, or renal cancer.

The underlying cause of hypercalcemia in the cancer patient varies. Approximately 70% of all cancer patients with hypercalcemia have metastatic bone disease. In this situation, direct invasion of the bone by tumor cells causes bone destruction and subsequent release of calcium. Hypercalcemia may also be caused by the production of *osteoclast-activating factor* and prostaglandins. These substances, produced by cancer cells, stimulate the breakdown of bone and the release of calcium. Hypercalcemia may also be caused by tumors that produce parathyroid-like substances and promote release of calcium from bones.

Factors unrelated to the underlying malignancy may contribute to hypercalcemia. These include immobility, dehydration, renal impairment and medications such as thiazide diuretics. In addition, hormonal medications used in the treatment of breast cancer may contribute to the development of hypercalcemia.

Management

The manifestations of hypercalcemia and its medical management are discussed in Chapter 18.

Nursing Interventions

Nursing care begins with identification of patients at risk for hypercalcemia. Careful nursing assessment will assist in identifying the signs and symptoms of hypercalcemia. These include fatigue, weakness, confusion, decreased level of responsiveness, hyporeflexia, nausea, vomiting, constipation, polyuria, polydipsia, dehydration, and dysrhythmias.

Assessment of the patient's and family's knowledge of hypercalcemia is essential because prevention and early detection can prevent potential fatality.

Patients at risk for developing hypercalcemia receive instructions concerning signs and symptoms to be aware of and to report. They are encouraged to maintain adequate fluid intake of 2 to 3 liters of fluid per day unless contraindicated by existing renal or cardiac disease. The importance of mobility must be emphasized to prevent demineralization and breakdown of bones. Patients with alterations in mental status and mobility as a result of hypercalcemia will require additional nursing measures to prevent the hazards of immobility and to promote safety.

Pericardial Effusion/Cardiac Tamponade

Cardiac tamponade is a cardiovascular disorder that occurs when fluid accumulates in the pericardial space and compresses the heart, impeding cardiac filling during diastole. Neoplastic disease or its treatment is the most common cause of cardiac tamponade. Pericardial disease secondary to neoplastic growth usually occurs by direct invasion from adjacent thoracic tumors (lung, esophagus, and breast cancers) or metastasis to the pericardium (lymphomas, leukemias, sarcomas, melanomas, and carcinomas of the GI tract). Fluid produced by the invasive tumor, metastatic lesion, or pericardial tissue in response to the malignant processes accumulates in the pericardial space, increases pressure on the myocardium, and impedes expansion of the ventricles. As ventricular volume and cardiac output fall, the cardiac pump fails and circulatory collapse develops. Radiation therapy of 4000 rad or more to the mediastinal area has also been implicated in pericardial fibrosis, pericarditis, and resultant cardiac tamponade, which may occur months or even years after the completion of radiation therapy.

Pericardial disease and cardiac tamponade may occur gradually or very rapidly. Gradual fluid accumulation allows the parietal (outer) layer of the pericardial space to stretch and compensate for the increased pressure. Therefore, large fluid volumes may accumulate before symptoms appear. When fluid accumulates rapidly, however, the pericardial pressures rise quickly and compensatory stretching cannot occur. Increased central venous pressures (CVP) and jugular distention develop. Distention of neck veins during inspiration (Kussmaul's sign) is suggestive of pericardial disease. Pulsus paradoxus (a decrease in systolic blood pressure of more than 10 mm Hg during inspiration with strengthening of the pulse on expiration) may be detected in moderate cardiac tamponade. Heart sounds become distant, and increased areas of cardiac dullness may be percussed. As cardiac output decreases, compensatory tachycardia and systemic vascular resistance occur. As tamponade progresses, the systolic blood pressure continues to fall and the diastolic pressure rises in compensatory effort, creating a narrow pulse pressure. Shortness of breath and tachypnea may also develop. Weakness, chest pain, orthopnea, anxiety, diaphoresis, lethargy, and altered consciousness due to decreased cerebral perfusion may result. Circulatory collapse with cardiac arrest is imminent if untreated.

Electrocardiographic tracings during pericardial effusion usually reveal nonspecific T-wave changes with reduced QRS voltage. Electrical alternans (QRS complexes that alternate in size) is common with tamponade. The chest x-ray film is not usually diagnostic with small-volume pericardial effusions. With larger effusions, however, a "water-bottle" heart appearance (obliteration of vessel contour and cardiac chambers) becomes apparent on x-ray. Echocardiography and computed tomography are valuable in the diagnosis of cardiac tamponade and evaluation of the effectiveness of treatment.

Management

The usual treatment of cardiac tamponade is *pericardiocentesis* (the aspiration of the pericardial fluid by a large-bore needle inserted into the pericardial space). Unfortunately, the benefits of pericardiocentesis in malignant effusions are only temporary, and fluid accumulation frequently recurs. Pericardial windows are often surgically created as a palliative measure to drain pericardial effusions into the pleural space. Catheters may also be placed in the pericardial space and sclerosing agents (such as tetracycline, bleomycin, 5-FU, or Thiotepa) may be injected to prevent effusive reaccumulation. Other therapeutic options such as radiation therapy or antineoplastic drugs are dependent on the sensitivity of the primary tumor. In mild effusions, prednisone and diuretics may be prescribed with careful monitoring of patient status.

Nursing Interventions

Nursing assessment includes frequent monitoring of vital signs; assessment for pulsus paradoxus; monitoring of ECG tracings; assessment of heart and lung sounds, neck vein filling, level of consciousness, respiratory status, and skin color and temperature; accurate monitoring of intake and output; and laboratory studies such as arterial blood gases and electrolytes.

Appropriate nursing actions may include elevation of the head of the patient's bed; minimization of physical activity to reduce oxygen requirements; supplemental oxygen as prescribed; frequent oral hygiene; turning, and encouraging the patient to cough and take deep breaths every 2 hours; reorientation, if needed; supportive measures; maintenance of patent intravenous access; and appropriate patient education.

In summary, pericardial effusion is an oncologic emergency resulting from constriction and impaired filling of the heart. It can result from direct invasion from tumor, fluid accumulation in the pericardium, or as a result of cancer treatment. Manifestations of pericardial effusion include distension of neck veins, increased CVP, decreased cardiac output, tachycardia, narrowing of pulse pressure, dyspnea, ECG changes, and finally, circulatory collapse with cardiac arrest. Treatment includes pericardiocentesis, formation of a pericardial window, or instillation of sclerosing agents through a pericardial catheter.

Disseminated Intravascular Coagulopathy

Disseminated intravascular coagulopathy (DIC, consumption coagulopathy) is the abnormal activation of both the coagulation and fibrinolytic mechanisms, resulting in the consumption of coagulation factors and platelets. DIC can occur with any malignant process; however, it is most commonly associated with cancers of the lung, gastrointestinal system, and prostate, and melanoma and the leukemias. Certain chemotherapeutic agents are also thought to precipitate DIC. These drugs include vincristine, methotrexate, 6-mercaptopurine, prednisone, and L-asparaginase. Certain disease processes commonly seen in the cancer patient may also initiate DIC, including sepsis, hepatic failure, and anaphylaxis.

Clot formation is initiated by triggering of the intrinsic or extrinsic mechanisms of normal coagulation. Malignant tumors stimulate the intrinsic coagulation pathway during metastasis when endothelial injury occurs. The extrinsic coagulation pathway is also activated by the release of thromboplastin (or thromboplastin-like substances) from tumor cells.

Chemotherapy-induced destruction of tumor cells triggers coagulation through the release of thromboplastin from the damaged cells. In the case of gram-negative sepsis, the release of endotoxins from bacterial cells stimulates the clotting cascade.

Once activated, the clotting cascade continues to consume clotting factors and platelets and forms fibrin clots in the microvasculature. These clots place the patient at high risk for thrombus formation, infarction, and bleeding. The last stage of the clotting cascade, fibrinolysis, also continues to occur at an abnormally high rate in DIC. Fibrinolysis, or clot dissolution, breaks down clots that have formed and places the patient at an even higher danger of hemorrhage.

Laboratory results indicative of DIC include prolonged prothrombin time (PT or protime) and partial thromboplastin time (PTT), decreased platelet counts and fibrinogen levels, and increased fibrin split products.

Chronic DIC may produce few or no observable symptoms. Patients may exhibit easy bruising, prolonged bleeding from venipuncture sites, gingival bleeding, and slow gastrointestinal bleeding. Acute DIC is associated with life-threatening hemorrhage and infarction. Clinical symptoms of this syndrome are varied and depend on the organ system involved in thrombus/infarct or bleeding episodes.

Management

Treatment of DIC centers on control of the underlying disease process. Chemotherapy is given for the treatment of the underlying malignancy. Antibiotics are used in the treatment of sepsis. Supportive measures with antithrombinolytic agents such as heparin or antithrombin III are often employed to decrease stimulation of the coagulation pathways. Transfusion with fresh frozen plasma or cryoprecipitates (which contain clotting factors and fibrinogen) may be used in conjunction with heparin therapy but is rarely effective when used alone. Antifibrinolytic agents such as aminocaproic acid (Amicar) are controversial forms of therapy and are associated with high incidence of thrombus formation.

Nursing Interventions

Indicated nursing assessments for the patient experiencing DIC include monitoring of vital signs; accurate intake and output measurements; assessment of skin color and temperature; assessment of lung, heart, and bowel sounds; assessment of level of consciousness; assessment of headache, visual disturbances, chest pain, decreased urinary output, and abdominal tenderness; assessments of all body orifices, tube insertion sites, incisions, and bodily excretions for bleeding; and monitoring of indicated laboratory test results.

Appropriate nursing interventions involve the minimization of physical activity to decrease risk of injury and oxygen requirements; increasing pressure to all venipuncture sites; minimization of invasive procedures; maintenance of adequate oral hygiene; assisting the patient to turn, cough, and take deep breaths every 2 hours; reorientation, if needed; maintenance of a safe environment; and appropriate patient education and supportive measures.

Syndrome of Inappropriate Secretion of Antidiuretic Hormone

The syndrome of inappropriate secretion of antidiuretic hormone (SIADH) is characterized by continuous, uncontrolled release of antidiuretic hormone (ADH). This leads to increased extracellular fluid volume with decreased osmolality, water intoxication, hyponatremia, increased urine osmolality, and increased excretion of urinary sodium. The most common cause of SIADH is malignancy, especially small cell cancers of the lung. It also occurs in patients with cancers of the pancreas, duodenum, brain, esophagus, colon, ovary, larynx, prostate, and nasopharynx and with Hodgkin's disease, thymomas, and lymphosarcomas. Antineoplastic drugs, vincristine, vinblastine, cisplatin, and cyclophosphamide, as well as the narcotic morphine, also stimulate ADH secretion leading to SIADH. Certain processes commonly seen in the cancer patient such as pain, stress, nausea, trauma, and hemorrhage are also associated with SIADH.

The ADH produced, stored, and released by tumor cells is identical to ADH normally produced by the posterior pituitary gland. When ADH is produced, the distal renal tubules and collecting ducts of the kidney conserve and reabsorb water. In SIADH, the posterior pituitary becomes unresponsive to the normal feedback mechanisms and water conservation continues despite decreasing serum osmolality and increasing urine osmolality. With continued absorption of fluid, circulatory volume increases, and sodium is actively excreted by the kidneys in compensation. If the serum sodium levels fall below 120 mEq/L (SI: 120 mmol/L), patients usually display symptoms of hyponatremia, which include personality changes, irritability, nausea, anorexia, vomiting, weight gain, fatigue, myalgia, headache, lethargy, and confusion. If serum sodium levels continue to fall below 110 mEq/L, seizure, abnormal reflexes, papilledema, coma, and death may result. Edema is rarely seen with SIADH.

Laboratory findings indicative of SIADH include (1) serum hyponatremia, (2) increased urine osmolality, and (3) increased urinary sodium. Decreased BUN, creatinine, and serum albumin levels secondary to dilution may also occur. Abnormal results of water load tests would also indicate the presence of SIADH.

Management

Treatment of SIADH depends on the severity of symptoms. With mild symptoms, fluids are limited to 500 to 1000 ml/day to increase the serum sodium level and decrease fluid overload. If water retention alone is not effective in correcting or controlling serum sodium levels, demeclocycline or lithium carbonate is often prescribed to interfere with the antidiuretic action of ADH. When neurologic symptoms are severe, parenteral sodium replacement and diuretic therapy are indicated. Electrolytes are monitored carefully during treatment because secondary magnesium, potassium, and calcium imbalances may occur.

After control of the symptoms of SIADH, the underlying malignancy is treated. If water excess continues despite oncologic treatment, pharmacologic intervention (urea and furosemide) may be indicated to control symptoms.

Nursing Interventions

Nursing assessment of the patient with SIADH includes accurate measurement of intake and output and assessment of level of consciousness, lung and heart sounds, vital signs, daily weight, and urine specific gravity. The patient is also assessed for nausea, vomiting, anorexia, edema, fatigue, and lethargy. The nurse monitors laboratory test results, including serum electrolytes, osmolality, BUN, creatinine, and urinary sodium and osmolality.

Indicated nursing interventions involve minimization of activity: appropriate oral hygiene measures; maintenance of environmental safety measures; reorientation, if necessary; fluid restriction, if necessary; and appropriate patient education and supportive measures.

In summary, SIADH is an oncologic emergency caused by the uncontrolled release of ADH, resulting in increased extracellular fluid volumes with decreased osmolality, water intoxication, hyponatremia, increased urine osmolality, and increased secretion of urinary sodium. Treatment of SIADH includes fluid restriction, parenteral sodium replacement, diuretic therapy, and use of pharmacological agents, which interfere with the action of ADH.

In summary, oncologic emergencies are serious complications of cancer that require prompt attention to maintain the patient's physical condition at as optimal a level as possible. These oncologic emergencies (superior vena cava syndrome, spinal cord compression, hypercalcemia, pericardial effusion, disseminated intravascular coagulation, and SIADH) require diligence in observation, skill in assessment, recognition of their consequences, and immediate attention to prevent deterioration of the patient's function or condition. The patient who experiences any of these complications also requires assistance to deal with the psychological reactions to them and to their treatment; their occurrence may produce anxiety, fear, depression, or even anger in a patient and his family. The nurse who understands that their occurrence may be seen as a serious setback to the patient is better able to assess and deal with these reactions.

Chapter Summary

Cancer is considered a systemic disease with multiple factors implicated in its etiology, including environmental, infectious, dietary, and hereditary influences. A major role of the nurse is in the area of prevention and screening. Teaching patients and consumers of nursing care about risk factors, early detection strategies (*i.e.*, breast self-examination and testicular examination), warning signs, and health promotion measures are important factors in cancer prevention and detection.

The patient diagnosed with cancer and his family confront a major crisis. Although they may equate cancer with inevitable pain and death, successful cure or long-term control of cancer is increasing with advances in therapeutic modalities. The patient may undergo surgery for diagnosis and staging, for excision of the tumor, or for relief of symptoms. Additional treatment with chemotherapy, radiation therapy, or other therapeutic modalities may be used. Although such treatment brings hope of eradication of the cancer, the therapy itself often causes significant side effects that are at least bothersome or inconvenient for the patient or severely disturbing and disabling. The patient who receives such treatments and his family require expert nursing care to deal effectively with the physiologic and psychologic consequences of cancer and its treatments.

Effective rehabilitation of the patient with cancer requires that the nurse consider the long- and short-term needs of the patient and his family. Support persons and groups can be consulted before surgery or initiation of treatment as well as after treatment begins. Representatives of Reach to Recovery, ostomy, or laryngectomy groups are often helpful by serving as successful role models for the patient and his family. Psychosocial and sexual needs of the patient and his family are as important as the physiologic needs and require attention and skill from the nurse and other members of the health care team.

For the patient with progressive disease, oncologic emergencies pose a significant threat to his well-being and survival. The nurse must be aware of the risks for these complications and knowledgeable and skilled in assessing their occurrence; early detection increases the likelihood of early and successful treatment.

Bibliography

Books

Baird S. Decision Making in Oncology Nursing. Toronto, BC Decker, 1988.

Billings JA. Outpatient Management of Advanced Cancer: Symptom-Control, Support, and Hospice-in-the-Home. Philadelphia, JB Lippincott, 1985.

Brager BL and Yasko JM. Care of the Client Receiving Chemotherapy. Reston, VA, Reston Publishing Co, 1984.

Carrieri VK et al (eds). Pathophysiological Phenomena in Nursing. Philadelphia, WB Saunders, 1986.

Chemecky CC and Ramsey PW. Critical Care Nursing of the Client With Cancer. Norwalk, CT, Appleton–Century–Crofts, 1984.

DeVita V et al (eds). Cancer: Principles and Practice of Oncology. Philadelphia, JB Lippincott, 1989.

Groenwald SL et al (eds). Cancer Nursing: Principles and Practice, 2nd ed. Boston, Jones and Bartlett, 1990.

Perez C and Brady L (eds). Principles and Practice of Radiation Oncology. Philadelphia, JB Lippincott, 1987.

Porth C. Pathophysiology: Concepts of Altered Health States, 2nd ed. Philadelphia, JB Lippincott, 1990.

Tenenbaum L. Cancer Chemotherapy: A Reference Guide. Philadelphia, WB Saunders, 1989.

Yasko JM. Guidelines for Cancer Care: Symptom Management. Reston, VA, Prentice–Hall, 1983.

Ziegfeld CR (ed). Core Curriculum for Oncology Nursing. Philadelphia, WB Saunders, 1987.

Journals

Asterisks indicate nursing research articles.

General

Aistars J. Fatigue in the cancer patient: A conceptual approach to a clinical problem. Oncol Nurs Forum 1987 Nov/Dec; 14(6): 25–30.

Anderson JL. The nurse's role in cancer rehabilitation. Cancer Nurs 1989 Apr; 12(2): 85–94.

Basch A. Changes in elimination. Semin Oncol Nurs 1987 Nov; 3(4): 287–292.

Boring CC, Squires TS, and Tong T. Cancer statistics: 1991. CA 1991 Jan/Feb; 41(1): 19–36.

* Curtis AE and Fernsler. Quality of life of oncology hospice patients: A comparison of patient and primary caregiver reports. Oncol Nurs Forum 1989 Jan/Feb; 16(1): 49–53.

Dudas S and Carlson CE. Cancer rehabilitation. Oncol Nurs Forum 1988 Mar/Apr; 15(2): 183–188.

Frank-Stromborg M and Welch-McCaffery D (eds). Cancer in the elderly. Semin Oncol Nurs 1988 Aug; 4(3): 155–306.

* Funkhouser SW and Grant MM. The 1988 ONS survey of research priorities. Oncol Nurs Forum 1989 May/Jun; 16(3): 413–416.

Herberth L and Gosnell DJ. Nursing diagnosis for oncology nursing practice. Cancer Nurs 1987 Feb; 10(1): 41–51.

McMillon SC. The relationship between age and intensity of cancer-related symptoms. Oncol Nurs Forum 1989 Mar/Apr; 16(2): 237–241.

Miaskowski C. The future of oncology nursing: A historical perspective. Nurs Clin North Am 1990 Jun; 25(2): 461–473.

Musgrave CF. The ethical and legal implications of hospice care. Cancer Nurs 1987 Aug; 10(4): 183–189.

Nail LM and King KB. Fatigue. Semin Oncol Nurs 1987 Nov; 3(4): 257–262.

Piper BF et al. Fatigue mechanisms in cancer patients: Developing nursing theory. Oncol Nurs Forum 1987 Nov/Dec; 14(6): 17–23.

Smith DB. Sexual rehabilitation of the cancer patient. Cancer Nurs 1989 Feb; 12(1): 10–15.

Yasko JM and Greesy P. Coping with problems related to cancer and cancer treatment. CA 1987 Mar/Apr; 37(2): 106–125.

Cancer Process/Epidemiology

Bakemeier AH. The potential role of vitamins A, C, and E and selenium in cancer prevention. Oncol Nurs Forum 1988 Nov/Dec; 15(6): 785–791.

Frank–Stromborg M. The epidemiology and primary prevention of gastric and esophageal cancer. Cancer Nurs 1989 Apr; 12(2): 53–64.

Lindsey AM et al. Endocrine mechanisms and obesity: Influences in breast cancer. Oncol Nurs Forum 1987 Mar/Apr; 14(2): 47–51.

Lovejoy NC. Precancerous lesions of the cervix. Cancer Nurs 1987 Feb; 10(1): 2–14.

Oleske DM. The epidemiology of lung cancer: An overview. Semin Oncol Nurs 1987 May; 3(3): 165–173.

Cancer Detection and Prevention

Beck S et al. The family high-risk program: Targeted cancer prevention. Oncol Nurs Forum 1988 May/Jun; 15(3): 301–306.

Cashavelly BJ. Cervical dysplasia. Cancer Nurs 1987 Aug; 10(4): 199–206.

d'Angelo and Gorrell CR. Breast reconstruction using tissue expanders. Oncol Nurs Forum 1989 Jan/Feb; 16(1): 23–27.

Fitzsimmons ML et al. Hereditary cancer syndromes: Nursing's role in identification and education. Oncol Nurs Forum 1989 Jan/Feb; 16(1): 87–94.

Foltz A. Nutritional factors in the prevention of gastrointestinal cancer. Semin Oncol Nurs 1988 Nov; 4(4): 239–245.

Frank–Stromborg M. The role of the nurse in cancer detection and screening. Semin Oncol Nurs 1986 Aug; 2(3): 191–199.

Lovejoy NC et al. Tumor markers, relevance to clinical practice. Oncol Nurs Forum 1987 Sep/Oct; 14(5): 75–83.

Rose MA. Health promotion and risk prevention: Applications for cancer survivors. Oncol Nurs Forum 1989 May/Jun; 16(3): 335–340.

* Rutledge DN and Davis GT. Breast self-examination compliance and the health belief model. Oncol Nurs Forum 1988 Mar/Apr; 15(2): 175-174.

Schleper JR. Prevention, detection and diagnosis of head and neck cancers. Semin Oncol Nurs 1989 Aug; 5(3): 139–149.

* Williams RD. Factors affecting the practice of breast self-examination in older women. Oncol Nurs Forum 1988 Sep/Oct; 15(5): 611–616.

Chemotherapy/Radiation Therapy

Brenner DE. Intraperitoneal chemotherapy: A review. J Clinical Oncol 1986 Jul; 4(7): 1135–1147.

Bujorian GA. Clinical trials: Patient issues in the decision-making process. Oncol Nurs Forum 1988 Nov/Dec; 15(6): 779–782.

* Caudell KA et al. Quantification of urinary nitrogens in nurses during potential antineoplastic agent exposure. Cancer Nurs 1988 Feb; 11(1): 41–50.

Cawley MN. Recent advances in chemotherapy: Administration and nursing implications. Nurs Clin North Am 1990 Jun; 25(2): 377–391.

Clark RA et al. Antiemetic therapy: Management of chemotherapy-induced nausea and vomiting. Semin Oncol Nurs 1989 May; 5(2 Suppl 1): 53–57.

Coons HL et al. Anticipatory nausea emotional distress in patients receiving cisplatin-based chemotherapy. Oncol Nurs Forum 1987 May/Jun; 14(3): 31–35.

Cotanch PH and Strum S. Progressive muscle relaxation as antiemetic therapy for cancer patients. Oncol Nurs Forum 1987 Jan/Feb; 14(1): 33–37.

Doig B. Adjuvant chemotherapy in breast cancer. Cancer Nurs 1988 Apr; 11(2): 91–98.

Dudjak LA. Mouth care for mucositis due to radiation therapy. Cancer Nurs 1987 Jun; 10(3): 131–140.

Eclers J et al. Development, testing, and application of the oral assessment guide. Oncol Nurs Forum 1988 May/Jun; 15(3): 325–330.

Fraser MC and Tucker MA. Late effects of cancer therapy: chemotherapy-related malignancies. Oncol Nurs Forum 1988 Jan/Feb; 15(1): 67–77.

Giaccone G et al. Scalp hypothermia in the prevention of doxorubicin-induced hair loss. Cancer Nurs 1988 Jun; 11(3): 170–173.

Glicksman AS. Radiobiologic basis of brachytherapy. Semin Oncol Nurs 1987 Feb; 3(1): 3–6.

Goodman M. Management of nausea and vomiting induced by outpatient cisplatin (Platinol) therapy. Semin Oncol Nurs 1987 Feb; 3(1 Suppl 1): 23–35.

Goodman M. Managing the side effects of chemotherapy. Semin Oncol Nurs 1989 May; 5(2 Suppl 1): 29–52.

Gullate MM and Graves T. Advances in antineoplastic therapy. Oncol Nurs Forum 1990 Nov/Dec; 17(6): 867–876.

Gullo SM. Safe handling of antineoplastic drugs: Translating the recommendations into practice. Oncol Nurs Forum 1988 Sep/Oct; 15(5): 595–601.

Hagle ME. Implantable devices for chemotherapy: Access and delivery. Semin Oncol Nurs 1987 May; 3(2): 96–105.

Haibeck SV. Intraoperative radiation therapy. Oncol Nurs Forum 1988 Mar/Apr; 15(2): 143–147.

Harris LL and Smith S. Chemotherapy in head and neck cancer. Semin Oncol Nurs 1989 Aug; 5(3): 174–181.

Hassey KM. Principles of radiation safety and protection. Semin Oncol Nurs 1987 Feb; 3(1): 23–29.

Hassey KM. Radiation therapy for rectal cancer and the implications for nursing. Cancer Nurs 1987 Dec; 10(6): 311–318.

* Headley JA. The influence of administration time on chemotherapy-induced nausea and vomiting. Oncol Nurs Forum 1987 Nov/Dec; 14(6): 43–47.

Hendrickson FR. The use of neutron beam therapy in the management of locally advanced nonresectable radioresistant tumors. CA 1988 Nov/Dec; 38(6): 353–361.

Hobbie WL and Schwartz CL. Endocrine late effects among survivors of cancer. Semin Oncol Nurs 1989 Feb; 5(1): 14–21.

Hogan, CM. Advances in the management of nausea and vomiting. Nurs Clin North Am 1990 Jun; 25(2): 475–497.

Hoff ST. Concepts in intraperitoneal chemotherapy. Semin Oncol Nurs 1987 May; 3(2): 112–117.

Holden S and Felde G. Nursing care of patients experiencing Cisplatin-related peripheral neuropathy. Oncol Nurs Forum 1987 Jan/Feb; 14(1): 13–19.

Hydzik CA. Late effects of chemotherapy: Implications for patient management and rehabilitation. Nurs Clin North Am 1990 Jun; 25(2): 423–446.

Jordan LN. Effects of fluid manipulation on the incidence of vomiting during outpatient cisplatin infusion. Oncol Nurs Forum 1989 Mar/Apr; 16(2): 213–217.

Keller JF and Blausey LA. Nursing issues and management in chemotherapy-induced alopecia. Oncol Nurs Forum 1988 Sep/Oct; 15(5): 603–607.

Kramer J and Moore IM. Late effects of cancer therapy on the central nervous system. Semin Oncol Nurs 1989 Feb; 5(1): 22–28.

Lewis F and Levita M. Understanding radiotherapy. Cancer Nurs 1988 Jun; 11(3): 174–185.

Lyndon J. Assessment of renal function in the patient receiving chemotherapy. Cancer Nurs 1989 Jun; 12(3): 133–143.

Lyndon J. Nephrotoxicity of cancer treatment. Oncol Nurs Forum 1986 Mar/Apr; 13(2): 68–77.

Maddock PG. Brachytherapy sources and applicators. Semin Oncol Nurs 1987 Feb; 3(1): 15–22.

Maran JN and Gray MA. Pulmonary laser therapy. Am J Nurs 1988 Jun; 88(6): 828–831.

Montrose PA. Extravasation management. Semin Oncol Nurs 1987 May; 3(2): 128–132.

Muller SA. Issues in cytotoxic drug handling safety. Semin Oncol Nurs 1987 May; 3(2): 133–141.

O'Rourke ME. Enhanced cutaneous effects in combined modality therapy. Oncol Nurs Forum 1987 Nov/Dec; 14(6): 31–35.

Ostehega Y et al. High-dose cisplatin-related peripheral neuropathy. Cancer Nurs 1988 Feb; 11(1): 23–32.

Pape LH. Therapy-related acute leukemia. Cancer Nurs 1988 Oct; 11(5): 295–302.

Parker R. The effectiveness of scalp hypothermia in preventing cyclophosphamide-induced alopecia. Oncol Nurs Forum 1987 Nov//Dec; 14(6): 49–53.

Rhodes VA et al. Patterns of nausea, vomiting, and distress in patients receiving antineoplastic drug protocols. Oncol Nurs Forum 1987 Jul/Aug; 14(4): 35–44.

Ruccione KR and Weinberg K. Late effects in multiple body systems. Semin Oncol Nurs 1989 Feb; 5(1): 4–13.

Schulmeister L. Developing guidelines for bleomycin test dosing. Oncol Nurs Forum 1989 Mar/Apr; 16(2): 205–207.

Shell JA and Carter J. The gynecological implant patient. Semin Oncol Nurs 1987 Feb; 3(1): 54–66.

Strohl RA. The nursing role in radiation oncology: Symptom management of acute and chronic reactions. Oncol Nurs Forum 1988 Jul/Aug; 15(4): 429–434.

Strohl RA. Radiation therapy for head and neck cancers. Semin Oncol Nurs 1989 Aug; 5(3): 166–173.

Strohl RA. Radiation therapy: Recent advances and nursing implications. Nurs Clin North Am 1990 Jun; 25(2): 309–329.

Valanis B and Shortridge L. Self protective practices of nurses handling antineoplastic drugs. Oncol Nurs Forum 1987 May/Jun; 14(3): 23–27.

Vizcarra C. Intraperitoneal Chemotherapy. J NITA 1988 May/Jun; 11(3): 184–187.

Wickham R. Managing chemotherapy-related nausea and vomiting: The state of the art. Oncol Nurs Forum 1989 Jul/Aug; 16(4): 563–574.

Witt ME et al. Adjuvant radiotherapy to the colorectum: Nursing implications. Oncol Nurs Forum 1987 May/Jun; 14(3): 17–21.

Yarbo CH (ed). Current concepts in emesis control. Semin Oncol Nurs 1990 Nov; 6(4): 1–22.

Yasko JM and Rust D. Trends in chemotherapy administration. Semin Oncol Nurs 1989 May; 5(2 Suppl 1): 3–7.

Biologic Response Modifiers

Baird SB and Irwin MM (eds). The biotherapy of cancer: IV. Oncol Nurs Forum 1990 May; 18(1): 1–30.

Creekmore SP and Longo DL. Biologic response modifiers, interferons, interleukins and other cytokines. Resident and Staff Physician 1988 Jul; 34(8): 23–28, 30–31.

Goldstein D and Laszlo J. The role of interferon in cancer therapy: A current perspective. CA 1988 Sep/Oct; 38(5): 1–20.

Haeuber D and DiJulio JE. Hemopoietic colony stimulating factors: An overview. Oncol Nurs Forum 1989 Mar/Apr; 16(2): 247–255.

Lynch M et al. Nursing care of AIDS patient participating a in phase I/II trial of recombinant human granulocyte-m colony stimulating factor. Oncol Nurs Forum 1988 Jul/Aug; 15(4): 403–469.

Mayer DK. Biotherapy: Recent advances and nursing implications. Nurs Clin North Am 1990 Jun; 25(2): 291–308.

Rieger PT. Monoclonal antibodies. Am J Nurs 1987 Apr; 87(4): 469–473.

Oncologic Emergencies

Baker WF. Clinical aspects of disseminated intravascular coagulation: A clinician's point of view. Semin Thromb Hemost 1989 Jan; 15(1): 1–57.

Barry SA. Septic shock: Special needs of patients with cancer. Oncol Nurs Forum 1989 Jan/Feb; 16(1): 31–35.

* Coward DD. Hypercalcemia knowledge assessment in patients at risk of developing cancer-induced hypercalcemia. Oncol Nurs Forum 1988 Jul/Aug; 15(4): 471–476.

Coward DD. Cancer induced hypercalcemia. Cancer Nurs 1986 Jun; 9(3): 125–132.

Germon K. Fluid and electrolyte problems associated with diabetes insipidus and syndrome of inappropriate antidiuretic hormone. Nurs Clin North Am 1987 Dec; 22(4): 785–796.

Glover DJ and Glick JH. Metabolic oncologic emergencies. CA 1987 Sep/Oct; 37(5): 302–320.

Green L and Bingenberg QS. Current concepts in the management of hypercalcemia of malignancy. Hospital Formulary 1988 Mar; 23(3): 268–287.

Helms SR and Carlson MD. Cardiovascular emergencies. Semin Oncol 1989 Dec; 16(6): 463–470.

Lazarus HM et al. Infectious emergencies in oncology patients. Semin Oncol 1989 Dec; 16(6): 543–560.

Mahon SM. Signs and symptoms associated with malignancy-induced hypercalcemia. Cancer Nurs 1989 Jun; 12(3): 153–160.

McCaffery DW. Metastatic bone cancer. Cancer Nurs 1988 Apr; 11(2): 103–111.

Poe CM and Taylor LM. Syndrome of inappropriate antidiuretic hormone: Assessment and nursing implications. Oncol Nurs Forum 1989 May/Jun; 16(3): 373–381.

Polomano RC and Miller SE (eds). Understanding and managing oncologic emergencies. Adria Laboratories 1987; 1–40.

Silverman P and Distelhorst CW. Metabolic emergencies in clinical oncology. Semin Oncol 1989 Dec; 16(6): 504–515.

Pain

American Pain Society. Relieving pain: An analgesic guide: Principles of analgesic use in the treatment of acute pain and chronic cancer pain. Am J Nurs 1988 Jun; 88(6): 815–826.

* Dalton JA. Nurses' perceptions of their pain assessment skills, pain management practices and attitudes toward pain. Oncol Nurs Forum 1989 Mar/Apr; 16(2): 225–231.

* Dalton JA et al. Pain relief for cancer patients. Cancer Nurs 1988 Dec; 11(6): 322–328.

* Dalton JA and Feuerstein M. Biobehavioral factors in cancer pain. Pain 1988 May; 33(2): 137–147.

* Donovan MI and Dillon P. Incidence and characteristics of pain in a sample of hospitalized cancer patients. Cancer Nurs 1987 Apr; 10(2): 85–92.

* Hill CS. Relationship among cultural, educational, and regulatory agency influences on optimum cancer pain treatment. Journal of Pain Symptom Management 1990 Feb; 5(1 Suppl): S37–S45.

Kane NE et al. Use of patient-controlled analgesia in surgical oncology patients. Oncol Nurs Forum 1988 Jan/Feb; 15(1): 29–32.

* Lapin J et al. Cancer pain management with a controlled-release oral morphine preparation. Journal of Pain Symptom Management 1989 Sep; 4(3): 146–151.

Levy MH. Pain management in advanced cancer. Semin Oncol 1985 Dec; 12(4): 394–410.

McCaffrey M. Patient-controlled analgesia: More than a machine. Nursing 1987 Nov; 17(11): 63–64.

Parce JA. The phenomenon of analgesic tolerance in cancer pain management. Oncol Nurs Forum 1988 Jul/Aug; 15(4): 455–460.

Patt RB and Jain S. Recent advances in the management of oncologic pain. Curr Probl Cancer 1989 May/Jun; 13(3): 135–195.

Wilkie DJ. Cancer pain management: State-of-the art nursing care. Nurs Clin North Am 1990 Jun; 25(2): 331–343.

Psychosocial Concerns

Benoliel JQ. Loss and terminal illness. Nurs Clin North Am 1985 Jun; 20(2): 439–448.

Blackmore C. The impact of orchiectomy upon the sexuality of the man with testicular cancer. Cancer Nurs 1988 Feb; 11(1): 33–40.

* Blank JJ et al. Perceived home care needs of cancer patients and their caregivers. Cancer Nurs 1989 Apr; 12(2): 78–84.

* Braum PJ and Katz LF. A study of burnout in nurses working in hospice and hospital oncology settings. Oncol Nurs Forum 1989 Jul/Aug; 16(4): 555–560.

* Foltz AT. The influence of cancer on self-concept and life quality. Semin Oncol Nurs 1987 Nov; 3(4): 303–312.

Gobel BH and Donovan MI. Depression and anxiety. Semin Oncol Nurs 1987 Nov; 3(4): 267–76.

Herman DC. Concerns for the dying patient and family. Semin Oncol Nurs 1989 May; 5(2): 120–123.

* Herth KA. The relationship between level of hope and level of coping response and other variables in patients with cancer. Oncol Nurs Forum 1989 Jan/Feb; 16(1): 67–72.

Holland JC. Managing depression in the patient with cancer. CA 1987 Nov/Dec; 37(6): 366–371.

Mount BM. Dealing with our losses. J Clin Oncol 1986 Jul; 4(7): 1127–1134.

Quigley KM. The adult cancer survivor: Psychosocial consequences of cure. Semin Oncol Nurs 1989 Feb; 5(1): 63–69.

Rice MA and Szopa TJ. Group intervention for reinforcing self-worth following mastectomy. Oncol Nurse Forum 1988 Jan/Feb; 15(1): 33–37.

Saunders JM and Valente SM. Cancer and suicide. Oncol Nurs Forum 1988 Sep/Oct; 15(5): 575–581.

Sodestrom KE and Martinson IM. Patients' spiritual coping strategies: A study of nurse and patient perspectives. Oncol Nurs Forum 1987 Mar/Apr; 14(2): 41–46.

Unproven Methods

Cassileth BR. The social implications of questionable cancer therapies. CA 1989 Sep/Oct; 39(5): 311–315.

Jarvis W. Helping your patients deal with questionable cancer treatments. CA 1986 Jul/Aug; 36(4): 293–301.

Uretsky S and Birdsall C. Quackery: A thoroughly modern problem. Am J Nurs 1986 Sep; 86(9): 1030–1033.

Nutrition

Chernoff R and Ropka M. The unique nutritional needs of the elderly patient with cancer. Semin Oncol Nurs 1988 Aug; 4(3): 189–197.

Grant M. Nausea, vomiting, and anorexia. Semin Oncol Nurs 1987 Nov; 3(4): 277–86.

Grant M et al. Nutritional management in the head and neck cancer patient. Semin Oncol Nurs 1989 Aug; 5(3): 195–204.

Simon RC. Small gauge central venous catheters and right atrial catheters. Semin Oncol Nurs 1987 May; 3(2): 87–95.

Tait N and Aisner J. Nutritional concerns in cancer patients. Semin Oncol Nurs 1989 May; 5(2 Suppl 1): 58–62.

Infection

Baird SB and Johnson J (eds). Prevention and management of neutropenia in the cancer patient. Oncol Nurs Forum 1990 Jan/Feb; 17(1): 1–24.

* Petrosino B et al. Infection rates in central venous dressings. Oncol Nurs Forum 1988 Nov/Dec; 15(6): 709–717.

Simonson GM. Caring for patients with acute myelocytic leukemia. Am J Nurs 1988 Mar; 88(3): 304–309.

Venous Access Devices

Moore CL et al. Nursing care and management of venous access ports. Oncol Nurs Forum 1986 May/Jun; 13(3): 35–39.

Simon RC. Small gauge central venous catheters and right atrial catheters. Semin Oncol Nurs 1987 May; 3(2): 87–95.

Viall CD. Your complete guide to central venous catheters. Nursing 90 1990 Feb; 20(2): 34–41.

Wickham RS. Advances in venous access devices and nursing management strategies. Nurs Clin North Am 1990 Jun; 25(2): 345–364.

Patient/Family Resources

Books

Bensen H. The Relaxation Response. New York, Times Books, 1984.

Boripenko J. Minding the Body With the Mind. New York, Bantam Books, 1988.

Burning N. Coping with Chemotherapy. New York, Doubleday, 1985.

Johnson J and Klein L. I Can Cope: Staying Healthy With Cancer. Minneapolis, The Wellness Series, 1988.

Petrek JA. A Woman's Guide to the Prevention, Detection and Treatment of Cancer. New York, Macmillan, 1985.

Seigel B. Love, Medicine and Miracles. New York, Harper and Row, 1986.

Organizations

American Cancer Society
777 Third Avenue, New York, NY 10017

American Academy of Otolarynggology
Head and Neck Surgery Inc, 1101 Vermont Avenue NW, Suite 302, Washington DC, 20005

Breast Cancer Advisory Center
11426 Rockville Pike, Suite 406, Rockville, MD 20857

Concern for Dying
250 West 57th Street, New York, NY 10107, (212) 246-6962

Leukemia Society of America
733 Third Avenue, New York, NY 10017, (212) 573-8484

Make Today Count
514 Tama Building, P.O. Box 303, Burlington, IN 52601

National Cancer Information Clearing House
Room 10A18 Building 31 NCI/NIH, Bethesda, MD 20205, (301) 496-4070

National Hospice Organization
1901 North Forth Meyer Drive, Suite 901, Arlington, VA 22209

United Ostomy Association Inc
2001 West Beverly Boulevard, Los Angeles, CA 90057

Support Groups: Check your local area.

Nursing Research Profile for Unit 4

Concepts and Challenges in Patient Management

Overview

The studies presented here demonstrate the contributions made by nurse researchers to many areas of nursing practice and patient care and illustrate the diversity of interests of nurse researchers. Nursing research has been conducted across the spectrum of nursing. Research highlighted here focuses on rehabilitation, pain assessment and management, human rhythms, issues in sexuality, detection and prevention of major fluid and electrolyte disorders, and complications of cancer and its treatment.

Rehabilitation

Because of their importance throughout nursing practice, concepts related to rehabilitation are addressed in a variety of clinical nursing and research journals. Specific patient problems (*e.g.*, mobility, skin integrity, and incontinence) and factors that influence rehabilitation have been the focus of many studies.

▷ Williams M and Manaske P. *Efficacy of audiovisual tape versus verbal instructions on crutch walking: A comparison.* J Emerg Nurs 1987 May/Jun; 13(3): 156–159.

The use of audiovisual tapes to provide consistent, cost-effective teaching of non–weight-bearing crutch walking was studied. Written and performance test scores were used to measure the efficacy of teaching methods (*i.e.*, individual nonstructured teaching by emergency department staff and a 13-minute audiovisual tape developed by the emergency department nurses).

A nonrandom, unmatched sample of 55 alert, visually and aurally competent adults who were first-time crutch users was selected from a midwestern acute care hospital emergency department during an 11-month period. The control group (N = 30) was selected first and was provided individual nonstructured teaching. The experimental group (N = 25) was provided audiovisual tape instruction. Subjects in both groups practiced crutch walking prior to individual testing.

The mean written, performance, and combined test scores were higher for the audiovisual tape instruction group. The combined total scores and performance scores of the experimental and control groups were statistically significant. Both patients and staff responded positively to the audiovisual instruction.

The researchers reported factors such as time of day (evening or night shift), presence of support person during teaching, and performance of testers as factors positively correlated with test scores. No interrater reliability was reported; however, the authors suggest that commitment to the project may have affected subjective scoring of the performance test. No relation was found between test score results and type of injury, location of injury, and age of the injury.

Nursing Implications. Generalization of the findings is limited by the convenience sample and nonrandom assignment to groups as well as interrater reliability and rival hypothesis issues. This study found that taped instructions for crutch walking are more effective than nonstructured staff instructions, reduce the need for reteaching, assure a specific level of instruction, and free the staff for other activities during the educational audiovisual viewing period. However, additional research is needed to determine the efficacy of audiovisual taped patient education and the effect of other variables on patient learning.

▷ Watson PG. *Family participation in the rehabilitation process: The rehabilitator's perspective.* Rehabil Nurs 1987 Mar/Apr; 12(2): 70–73.

This descriptive, retrospective study of 198 health professionals (30% nurses, 20% occupational therapists, 16% physical therapists, 34% other rehabilitators—speech therapists, social workers, physiatrists, and so forth) in free-standing rehabilitation hospitals describes family participation in the rehabilitation process. The Family in Rehabilitation Inventory measured the health professional's beliefs about family participation in rehabilitation and perceptions of family participation in the rehabilitation process. The findings of the study supported the notion that family participation is valuable and that opportunity for involvement had been provided. A high percentage of these health professionals indicated that family members should ask questions and express opinions, should participate in the rehabilitation program from the beginning to achieve better coping, and should follow the recommendations of health professionals.

The health professionals described a directive rehabilitation model with specific expectations for the family participation rather than a co-management participative model advocated by the rehabilitation literature. Respondents also indicated that families often have difficulty in understanding explanations about the family member's condition and may be fearful about participating in care. The nurse was identified as the rehabilitation team member who spent the most time with the patient and was most helpful to the family.

Nursing Implications.   Generalization of these descriptive study findings is limited by the nature of the sample and the study design. Additional research is needed to further understand family participation in rehabilitation in other settings (*i.e.*, acute rehabilitation settings). The rehabilitation literature describes the family and patient as co-managers in the rehabilitative process, whereas this study describes the actual use of a health professional–directed process for involvement of the patient and the family. The incongruency between the theoretic co-managers model for patient and family participation in rehabilitation and the practiced health professional–directed model needs further study. Finally, the value of nurse interactions with the family during the rehabilitative process needs to be recognized.

▷   *Holmes R et al. Combating pressure sores nutritionally. Am J Nurs 1987 Oct; 87(10): 1301–1303.*

Pressure ulcers are costly and diminish the well-being of the individual. Identification of patients at risk for developing pressure ulcers permits early preventive interventions. The authors report two studies.

The relation between nutritional status and pressure ulcer development was studied in a small convenience sample of six men and six women between 60 and 90 years of age who had pressure ulcers. The patients had low anthropometric measures, anemia, and low transferrin and serum albumin, indicators of protein depletion. Nine of them developed pressure ulcers while hospitalized and also experienced diminished nutritional status as demonstrated by low serum albumin, hemoglobin, and total lymphocyte count. These nutritional indices were statistically different from the patient's admission levels.

Nutritional support through enteral feedings or nutritional supplements improved the nutritional status of 11 of the patients. They experienced pressure ulcer healing. The nutritional status of one patient did not improve, and this subject did not experience ulcer healing.

In the second study, 36 consecutive medical-surgical patients between the ages of 30 and 95 years who were classified as at risk for pressure ulcer development were included. An individual's risk for developing a pressure ulcer was estimated with the Norton Scale, which scores general physical condition, mental status, activity, mobility, and incontinence. Within 2 weeks of admission, 20 of the subjects developed pressure ulcers. Admission nutritional assessment with the use of anthropometric measures and serum albumin levels was low in the subjects who subsequently developed pressure ulcers. The critical serum albumin level of 3.5 g/dl was identified as a predictor of pressure ulcer development. Early nutritional support was recommended to prevent further protein depletion.

Nursing Implications.   The findings of these studies suggest that assessment of nutritional status and assessment of the risk for pressure ulcer development must be included in the admission nursing assessment. Both the Norton Scale and serum albumin levels help to identify susceptible patients. If a patient is identified as at risk, interventions, including nutritional support, can be instituted early to reduce the incidence of pressure ulcers and promote healing of pressure ulcers.

▷   *Dai Y and Catanzaro M. Health beliefs and compliance with a skin care regimen. Rehabil Nurs 1987 Jan/Feb; 12(1): 13–16.*

Development of a pressure ulcer is a potential health problem for individuals who have experienced spinal cord injury. Compliance with skin care instructions was studied with use of the Health Belief Model as a framework. Individual beliefs concerning perceived susceptibility to pressure ulcers, perceived severity of pressure ulcers, perceived efficacy of skin care, and perceived barriers to skin care were studied.

The convenience sample of 20 spinal cord–injured, wheelchair-dependent men, who lived with their families and were able to independently perform routine skin care and manage their excretory function, was obtained through a Taiwan hospital clinic. The subjects completed health belief and multiple-choice knowledge questionnaires. Structured interviews were used to determine compliance with the skin care regimen.

Analysis of the data supported the hypotheses that subjects' perceived efficacy of skin care and perceived severity of pressure ulcers are correlated with compliance with the skin care regimen. Subjects' perceived susceptibility to pressure ulcers and perceived barriers to skin care did not correlate with their compliance.

Nursing Implications.   When working with individuals susceptible to pressure ulcers, the nurse can promote skin care through patient teaching emphasizing the effectiveness of the prescribed skin care regimen and the severity of pressure ulcers if they occur. If the person is unable to perform adequate skin care, alternative approaches to accomplish needed skin care must be instituted. Generalization of findings of this study is limited by the convenience sample. Replication in other settings is needed.

Pain

Pain assessment continues to be a major area of research for nurses and a focus of many nursing research studies. Although some intervention studies have appeared in the research literature, their number is limited in part by questions and concerns about the applicability of laboratory or simulated studies to actual clinical situations and the large number of variables in clinical situations that affect an individual's responses to pain.

▷   *Camp LD. A comparison of nurses' recorded assessments of pain with perceptions of pain as described by cancer patients. Cancer Nurs 1988 Aug; 11(4): 237–243.*

The purpose of this study was to assess agreement among nurses and patients about the pain experienced by the cancer patients. The sample included 30 nurse–patient dyads that consisted of cancer patients who experienced pain and the nurses providing care for them. The researcher used the factors contained in the McGill Pain Questionnaire to assess the following characteristics of the pain experienced by the cancer patients: location of pain, quality of pain, pattern of pain, relief of pain, factors that increase the pain, and the intensity of pain. Other areas assessed by the researcher included verbal statements about the pain by the patient and observations of nonverbal expression of pain. The nurses' notes were reviewed for pain assessment data recorded by the nurses in the patients' charts. The researcher's assessment of each patient's pain was compared to the documentation recorded in his chart by the nurse.

Nurses documented only 18.5% of patients' pain information and were in agreement with patients' descriptions less than 14% of the time. Although most cancer patients in the sample responded to seven of the eight categories of pain assessment used by the researcher, most nurses recorded only two of these eight categories: location of the pain and patients' verbal descriptions of pain.

Nursing Implications. Findings of this study indicate inadequate documentation of pain assessment data in nurses' notes. Although other aspects of patients' pain experience may have been assessed, if they were not documented, it could be assumed that they were not assessed. Attention must be given to adequate documentation of patients' pain for legal purposes and to provide other nurses and other members of the health care team with consistent data about patients' pain to provide adequate pain relief.

▷ Donovan M, Dillon P, and McGuire L. *Incidence and characteristics of pain in a sample of medical-surgical patients.* Pain 1987 Jul; 30(1): 69–78.

This study examined the incidence and characteristics of pain in patients hospitalized on a general medical-surgical unit and the type and perceived effectiveness of pain relief strategies. The sample included 353 patients who reported pain during their hospital stay; half of these patients reported that their pain was excruciating. Patients' pain was assessed with use of selected portions of the McGill Pain Questionnaire and an author-designed tool. Review of patients' reports and chart data regarding the administration of analgesia indicated that the analgesia administered was inadequate to achieve pain relief.

Although only 193 (43%) of the patients initially admitted to being in pain when asked if they were currently experiencing pain, an additional 46 patients reported that they too were in pain when they had the opportunity to rate their pain on a pain-rating scale. Despite a widespread problem of pain of moderate to severe intensity in this sample, only 45% of patients who experienced pain recalled that a nurse discussed their pain with them.

Methods perceived by patients to be most effective in reducing their pain were analgesics, sleep, immobilization, and distraction. Distraction was perceived as beneficial in reducing pain by a third of the patients who attempted to use it, regardless of the severity of the pain. Massage was reported to *increase* pain in 40 patients with noncancer pain.

Nursing Implications. Nurses along with other health care providers tend to underestimate the incidence and severity of pain in medical-surgical patients. The analgesia prescribed and administered is often insufficient for adequate pain relief, and subsequently patients suffer with unrelieved pain. The effectiveness of noninvasive methods of pain relief vary based on the severity and type of patients' pain. Further research of noninvasive methods of pain relief is warranted.

▷ Holm K et al. *Effect of personal pain experience on pain assessment.* Image: J Nurs Scholarship 1989 Summer; 21(2): 72–75.

The authors examined the effect of nurses' personal pain experiences on assessment of their patients' pain. A personal pain history questionnaire was completed by 134 nurses. They were asked to indicate their previous experience with 12 items commonly described as painful. They were also asked to indicate if a family member had experienced a painful condition in their presence. Additional questions regarded the nurses'

pain tolerance and actions taken when they experienced mild to moderate uncomfortable situations. A second instrument, the Standard Measure of Inferences of Suffering Questionnaire, was used; this questionnaire includes a series of vignettes describing patients' illness or injury as well as demographic characteristics of the patients. Nurses were asked to rate the degree of physical pain and psychologic distress likely in patients described in each vignette.

It was found that assessment of a patient's pain is significantly influenced by the intensity of the nurse's personal pain experience. Age, race, and sex of the patient in the vignette had little effect on nurses' assessment of patients' pain. Nurses who had previous experience with pain appeared to be more sympathetic to patients in pain than did those without such experiences.

Nursing Implications. Nurses need to be aware of their personal biases in their assessment of patients' pain. A major limitation of this study is the use of vignettes as a measure of nurses' assessments. Transfer or carryover of these biases into actual clinical practice cannot be assumed without further study.

▷ Ferrell B et al. *Effects of controlled-release morphine on quality of life for cancer pain.* Oncol Nurs Forum 1989 Jul/ Aug; 16(4): 521–526.

The purpose of this study was to compare the effects of controlled-release morphine and short-acting analgesia on the quality of life (QOL) of cancer patients. Eighty-three patients with cancer pain from oncology units of two hospitals were randomly assigned to two groups. One group received a short-acting analgesic; the second group received controlled-release analgesia (MS Contin). A third group, which served as a control, consisted of patients who had been receiving controlled-release morphine for at least 2 weeks and remained on that drug. QOL was assessed by five instruments: the Demographic Data Tool, the Pain Experienced Measure, the Present Pain Intensity Scale from the McGill–Melzack Pain Questionnaire, the Karnofsky Performance Status Scale, and the QOL Survey. Data were collected at the time of admission to the study and every 2 weeks for the next 6 weeks.

Data analysis indicated that patients assigned to the short-acting analgesia group consumed only 54% of the prescribed drug, whereas patients in the controlled-release morphine group consumed 92% of the prescribed group. Measures of pain intensity indicated that patients who received controlled-release morphine had a lower pain intensity and lower pain distress than those receiving short-acting analgesia. Results pertaining to the QOL indicated that patients in the controlled-release morphine group had greater QOL scores than those in the short-acting analgesia group, except for increased bowel disturbances and nausea. These were more frequent in the controlled-release morphine group than in the short-acting analgesia group. Trends in the data suggested that these problems decreased over time in the controlled-release morphine group.

Nursing Implications. The results of this study suggest that cancer patients in pain who receive controlled-release analgesia do better than those who receive short-acting analgesia on the traditional schedule of administration every 3 to 4 hours. Nursing care directed toward relieving gastrointestinal symptoms is indicated in the patient who begins controlled-release analgesia; attention to these symptoms has the potential to increase the cancer patient's quality of life further.

It is not clear whether it was necessary for patients in the short-acting analgesia group to ask for pain medication or whether it was self-administered. Furthermore, it is not clear whether the reason for the low consumption of analgesia in the short-acting analgesia group was because of patients' failure to ask for pain medication or because of unwillingness of nurses to administer the analgesia.

Human Rhythms

Nursing research studies have begun to address those factors that influence human rhythms, including circadian rhythms and sleep and activity rhythms, in healthy individuals and those ill or hospitalized.

▷ **Coss SJ. Factors affecting the sleep of patients on surgical wards in Scotland. In: Funk S et al (eds). Key Aspects of Recovery: Improving Nutrition, Rest, and Mobility. New York, Springer-Verlag, 1990, pp 223–238.**

This study examined the factors that affected the sleep of patients on surgical wards of two hospitals in Scotland. Using a convenience sample of 200 men and women patients, the researcher asked the subjects questions about their sleep at home and in the hospital. The reliability and validity of the interview instrument were not reported. Of the 200 patients, 122 thought that their sleep in the hospital was worse than their sleep at home; 54 believed that it was the same; and 24 claimed that it had improved with hospitalization. Differences between home and hospital sleep schedules were apparent, with the mean bedtime being almost a full hour earlier in the hospital. However, the time it took the patients to fall asleep (sleep onset latency) increased from about 24 minutes to 48 minutes; sleep duration decreased by almost 1 hour; and the number of nighttime awakenings increased from 1.4 to 2.3 per night.

In examining the factors that affected sleep, the researcher noted that: (1) patients who lived alone rated their hospital sleep more favorably than patients who lived with others, which may be due to the former group feeling more secure in the hospital than being sick at home and alone; (2) maintenance of the patients' home sleep rituals did not improve their hospital sleep, a situation that is suggested to be related to the many stressful stimuli in the hospital that negate the relaxing effect of bedtime rituals; (3) patients in small wards (2 to 4 beds) napped and slept longer with fewer nighttime awakenings than did patients in large wards (20 to 24 beds); (4) patients who took hypnotic sleep medications had a shorter sleep latency, a longer sleep duration, and reduced nighttime awakenings; (5) the quality of the mattress affected sleep duration; and (6) the reported causes of hospital sleep interruptions were pain (127 patients reported), noise (123), environmental temperature (113), bed problems such as plastic bed coverings or hard mattresses (87), needing to go to the bathroom (93), anxiety and worrying (73), discomfort (45), bad dreams (28), lighting (5), and treatments (5). Interestingly, most of the nurses' notes reported that the patients "slept well."

Nursing Implications.   Nurses should anticipate that hospitalized patients will often experience poorer sleep than they were accustomed to at home. Interventions that reduce pain and decrease noise should be instituted where appropriate. Nurses also should participate in hospital decisions regarding environmental control (temperature) and equipment (mattresses). Hypnotic medications may be useful as temporary interventions for those patients who are experiencing partic-

ularly problematic sleep. The researcher recommended that routine early morning assessments, medications, and meals should "only be adhered to when they are genuinely necessary for the care of the patients" (p 230). Routine nursing assessments on admission should include information about the patient's usual sleep. Nurses need to give patients the opportunity to say how they slept each night during hospitalization and should be sure to record sleep information in the patient's record. Sleep problems should be included in nurses' problem lists or nursing diagnoses so that plans can be developed for enhancing sleep.

▷ **Farr LA, Campbell-Grossman C, and Mack JM. Circadian disruption and surgical recovery. Nurs Res 1988 May/Jun; 37(3): 1171–1174.**

This study followed up an earlier study of Farr, Keene, Sampson, and Michael (Alterations in circadian excretion of urinary variables and physiological indicators of stress following surgery. Nurs Res 1984 May/Jun; 33[3]: 140–146) of changes in the circadian rhythms of urinary constituents and vital signs of postsurgical patients. Because of the difficulty in controlling data on rhythms and surgery in human subjects, the researchers used rats to examine circadian activity and temperature rhythms following abdominal surgery. Findings were similar to those of the human study, in which 23 adults experienced a 2- to 12-hour phase delay in circadian rhythms following abdominal surgery. Both studies found that the greater the circadian disruption, the longer the subject took to return to a normal circadian rhythm.

Nursing Implications.   Using the findings of both the earlier human study and the present rat study as a basis, the researchers made several recommendations for nursing practice. First, postoperative patients should be monitored for changes in circadian rhythmicity. Those who experience a high degree of circadian disruption should be closely monitored for signs and symptoms that can arise from desynchronization, including poor sleep, gastrointestinal problems, decreased vigilance and attention, and malaise. Second, a variation in the patient's needs should be anticipated; for example, the patient's need for pain medication may change as the circadian pattern of pain is altered. Third, on the basis of chronobiologic theory, the researchers suggest that strengthening environmental time cues may assist patients' resynchronization.

▷ **Mason DJ. Circadian rhythms of body temperature and activation and the well-being of older women. Nurs Res 1988 Sep/Oct; 37(5): 276–281.**

Eighteen healthy older women were studied in an attempt to discern whether the chronobiologic or Rogerian interpretations of the changes that occur in rhythmicity with aging are correct (*i.e.*, are the changes in rhythms that occur with aging unwanted detrimental correlates of aging that should be avoided, or are they a normal developmental phenomenon that should be supported?). Subjects who ranged in age from 65 to 80 years (mean, 71.6 years) took their temperature orally and completed a self-report instrument that measured activation (general bodily energy state) every 2 hours during the waking hours for 7 consecutive days. They also completed a daily well-being questionnaire. Although the results of the study were inconclusive, one finding did suggest that a Rogerian perspective may be valid. The subject with the strongest circadian rhythm in temperature and one of the highest levels of well-being was a woman who often awoke during the night, would often get up and clean her apartment or be active in some other way, and was not bothered by these nighttime disruptions. Some other interesting findings suggested the need for further study. Three subjects did not have circadian rhythms in body temperature. Two of these were among three subjects who stated that they had experienced disruptive events or life stressors within the past 2 months, supporting the possibility suggested in other chronobiologic research that stress can alter human rhythms. Further evidence for this was the finding that one of these subjects experienced a major emotional upset during the testing period and was the only one not to have circadian rhythms in both temperature and activation. The third subject without a circadian temperature rhythm stated that she awoke by her husband's alarm and followed his sleep–wake routine. This finding is consistent with work by Hoskins (1979) that demonstrated a dampening and lag in the circadian rhythms of married women.

Nursing Implications. Nurses should be aware of the variation in sleep–wake patterns in older adults, assess the patient's normal sleep–wake pattern and his perception of its "normalcy," and educate patients about the changes that can occur in the sleep–wake pattern with aging. Older adults who are experiencing a high degree of stress should be assessed for possible disruptions in circadian rhythms. Conversely, patients who are experiencing disruptions in circadian rhythms should be assessed for excessive stress.

▷ Moore MN. *Development of a sleep-awake instrument for use in a chronic renal population.* ANNA J 1989 Feb; 16(1): 15–19.

In this pilot study, a self-report instrument (the ESRD Sleep-Awake Questionnaire) to assess sleep–wake patterns of patients with end-stage renal disease was tested with nine ESRD patients. The subjects in this convenience sample had been on maintenance hemodialysis for 2 to 5 years but were without other significant preexisting disease or dialysis-related complications. They were all patients in an outpatient unit of a university medical center. More than half of the clients reported increases in the time required to go to sleep, the number of nighttime awakenings, the irregularity in sleep habits, and early morning awakenings, as well as self-reports of being "poor" sleepers. Mild to moderate depression was also reported by four subjects (using the Beck Depression Inventory). The investigator notes that further study is needed to describe the relations among ESRD, sleep–wake disturbances, and depression, and the effect of fatigue and dialysis on these variables.

Nursing Implications. While further study is needed before these findings can be generalized to the population of clients with end-stage renal disease, this study suggests that nurses working with chronic renal clients should be attentive to sleep–wake patterns in these clients. Other researchers have shown that sleep is important to the quality of life in ESRD, while disruption in the circadian sleep rhythm may act as a stressor.

▷ Richards KC and Bairnsfather L. *A description of night sleep patterns in the critical care unit.* Heart Lung 1988 Jan; 17(1): 35–42.

Sleep deprivation can be a severe problem for patients in an intensive care unit. The first three nights of sleep in an intensive care unit were examined in this study with use of the standard polysomnography (EEG, EMG, and EOG) and qualitative information about each subject. The 11 nonrandomly selected ICU patients who agreed to participate in the study ranged in age from 53 to 67 years, with a mean age of 59.6 years. A wide variation in the sleep patterns of the ICU patients

was found. A case study of each subject revealed factors that were associated with these differences: (1) closeness of bed to the nurses' station or supply closet; (2) acuity level of the patient, with the more acutely ill experiencing more awakenings for nursing care; (3) medications that affect sleep, such as theophylline compounds, morphine sulfate, hydrocortisone, diazepam, and triazolam; (4) daytime napping; and (5) whether the patient was usually a daytime or nighttime sleeper at home, with daytime sleeping arising from either shift work or chronic obstructive pulmonary disease (the latter patient reported being able to breathe more easily during the day and thus sleep more easily then).

Nursing Implications. Additional research is needed to adequately delineate the various factors that influence the sleep of the ICU patient and the relative strength of these factors. However, using the findings of this study as a basis, the researchers make several recommendations for nursing practice: (1) critical care units with individual patient rooms and observation windows should be designed to allow for door closing and reduced nighttime noise and light; (2) alarm systems on monitoring equipment, such as ventilators, that do not disturb the sleep of patients should be developed; (3) unnecessary waking of the ICU patient (*i.e.,* for a bath) should be avoided, and nursing care and other procedures should be clustered to avoid frequent sleep interruptions; (4) prehospital routines, including sleep schedules, should be assessed, and the patient's routine should be followed as much as possible; and (5) external stimuli should be provided to enhance the sleep–wake cycle (artificial lighting, sunlight, clocks).

▷ Samples JF et al. *Circadian rhythms: Basis for screening for fever.* Nurs Res 1985 Nov/Dec; 34(5): 377–379.

This study sought to determine whether circadian rhythms could be used as a basis for screening for fever. Subjects included 49 men aged 18 to 91 years and 58 women aged 19 to 87 years who were hospitalized for medical, diagnostic, or surgical treatments. The oral body temperature was measured with an electronic thermometer at 6 PM, 10 PM, 6 AM, 10 AM, 2 PM, and 6 PM. The researchers reported that 38 (36%) of the 107 subjects had fevers during the 24-hour period of measurement. No first fevers occurred at 6 AM or 10 AM. Of these 38, 23 (60%) were first febrile at the first 6 PM measurement; 9 (24%) at 10 PM; 3 (8%) at 2 PM; and 3 at the second 6 PM time. Of the 38 febrile subjects, 8 were not febrile at either of the 6 PM measurement times, and 6 of these had only one elevation during the testing time.

Nursing Implications. The researchers recommend that "one daily routine temperature recording at the peak of circadian thermal rhythm (5 to 7 PM) is adequate to screen for fever in adult hospitalized patients" (p 379). While this may promote efficiency in nursing practice, it overlooks the value that regular periodic temperature readings can have by providing an indication of the circadian timing system of the individual. It also should be noted that what is known from chronobiology suggests that what is "normal" must be defined according to the time of day. The researchers' interpretation that no one was febrile at 6 and 10 AM is based on the assumption that 98.6°F is the upper limits of normal regardless of time of day. The postsurgical patient who complains of not feeling well in the morning and whose "normal" body temperature at that time is 97.8°F could be considered febrile if his temperature were now 98.6°F, and he should be monitored more frequently.

Human Sexuality

There is a paucity of nursing research in the area of human sexuality and altered states of wellness. Because patients have concerns about their sexuality, this is an area that needs further investigations by nurse researchers.

▷ *Baggs JG and Karch AM. Sexual counseling of women with coronary heart disease.* Heart Lung 1987 Mar; 16(2): 154–159.

Baggs and Karch interviewed 58 women who had been admitted to the coronary care unit (CCU) with a diagnosis of myocardial infarction (MI), rule-out MI, or angina; they were alert, oriented, and English-speaking. The subjects were interviewed within 2 or 3 days of planned hospital discharge. The structured interview was designed by the researchers and administered by one of the investigators in the subject's hospital room. The interview included 25 questions; three fifths of the questions asked for fixed responses to obtain demographic data and specific information about sexual activity levels and sexual counseling. The remaining questions were open-ended to elicit individual responses relative to feelings and perceived needs relating to sexual counseling.

Information about returning to sexual activity was reported as being received during hospitalization by 33% of the women. Of these women, two had spoken with a health care provider and one woman and her partner had a counseling session with a CCU nurse who had initiated the counseling; the remainder (29%) had read one brief paragraph on sexual activity in the rehabilitation booklet given to most patients in this CCU. When asked if the health care worker should routinely initiate discussions about sexual activity, 76% of the subjects said yes. In this study, many married women were not sexually active, and many sexually active women were not married.

Nursing Implications.   The nurse cannot make assumptions about a patient's level of sexual activity or interest in sexual counseling based on marital status, age, or diagnosis. It is important to offer sexual counseling to all women who have coronary heart disease. Nurses should be educated to provide information about sexuality to all patients.

▷ *Scura KW and Whipple B. Older adults as an* HIV *positive risk group.* J Gerontol Nurs 1990 Feb; 15(2): 6–10.

Scura and Whipple conducted a retrospective review of hospital records at a 450-bed teaching hospital to identify patients 60 years of age and older who were HIV-positive to test the hypothesis that people 60 years of age and older may be at risk for infection with HIV. They identified nine men and three women with an average age of 69.3 years (range, 60 to 98 years) who were HIV-positive. Fifty-eight percent of these subjects were diagnosed as having AIDS. The older adults in this study who were HIV-infected fell into the same high-risk populations as did people from any other age group (*i.e.*, homosexual men, IV drug users, recipients of blood products, and unknown risk factors). However, the percentages for each risk group in this study did not support the figures for the national distribution of AIDS in people over 49 years of age as reported by the Centers for Disease Control.

Nursing Implications.   With the awareness that people of all ages are at risk for HIV infection, nurses must implement universal precautions with people of all ages and in all settings. The results of this study do not support the stereotypical judgment that older adults are asexual and thus not at risk for HIV infection.

▷ *White EJ. Appraising the need for altered sexuality information.* Rehabil Nurs 1986 May/Jun; 11(3): 6–9.

White demonstrated the need for an awareness of how patients communicate a readiness for information about altered sexuality. Although sexual counseling is an important part of rehabilitation, there had been no consensus on when it should begin. The ideal time to present information about sexuality is when the learner has the necessary skills, knowledge, and motivation to internalize the learning. Providing counseling to a client at the appropriate time is a function of recognizing readiness. In this study, White attempted to identify selected overt, measurable behaviors that 31 rehabilitation nurses believed to be a spinal cord–injured client's indicators of readiness for information on sexuality. The results of this exploratory survey indicated that this sample of rehabilitation nurses believes that people with spinal cord injuries communicate their needs for information in verbal and nonverbal ways. Common and socially accepted modes were those demonstrated most often, such as winking, rolling eyes, whistling, and making statements such as "I'm just not a man anymore."

Nursing Implications.   The appearance of verbal and nonverbal clues is identified as the time the client is ready to begin understanding his altered sexuality. Open, nonjudgmental actions on the part of the nurse can foster a positive curiosity about the emerging, changed sexual self and help to maximize the client's energy to develop a new and satisfying sexual identify.

Fluids and Electrolytes

Nursing research studies related to fluid and electrolyte balance are increasing. Factors that influence fluid and electrolyte status and indicators that signal disturbance of that balance have received attention by nurse researchers.

▷ *Adams F. Fluid intake*: How much do elders drink? Geriatr Nurs 1988 Jul/Aug; 9(4): 218–221.

This small descriptive study was designed to compare differences among institutionalized and noninstitutionalized elderly individuals in relation to fluid intake. Comparisons were made of the daily volume of fluid ingested by 30 subjects living in long-term care institutions and 30 elderly persons living at home; in addition, the types of fluids consumed and the patterns in which they were ingested were studied. It was found that elderly subjects living at home drank significantly more fluid each day than did the institutionalized group (2115 ml versus 1507 ml). It was suggested that the institutionalized group may have drunk less because of their dependence on nurses to offer fluid and perhaps because of their reluctance to ask for nursing assistance. An interesting finding was that the long-term care residents tended to drink the entire volume of fluid that was offered to them at the time of medications or meals. That is, if a 90-ml container was offered, the patient drank 90 ml; if 120 ml was offered, the patient drank 120 ml, and so on. Another interesting finding was that some subjects went without fluids for 15 hours and did not complain of thirst.

Although no difference was found in patterns of fluid intake, there were significant differences in the types of fluids consumed by the two groups. The institutionalized group drank only about half as much water as the noninstitutionalized group, even though water was available at all times. Milk intake was higher in subjects living in long-term care facilities; however, these individuals seemed to have less access to a variety of fluids, which may have affected their choice of beverage.

Nursing Implications. (1) Offer fluids at regular intervals to elderly persons; do not wait for complaints of thirst. (2) Offer fluids in larger containers at times of medication administration and at mealtimes to elderly persons requiring increased fluid intake. (3) Vary the types of fluids offered to elderly persons; consider individual likes and dislikes. (4) Offer to assist elderly subjects with regular trips to the bathroom (or other toileting needs) as additional fluids are consumed.

▷ *Coward D. Hypercalcemia knowledge assessment in patients at risk of developing cancer-induced hypercalcemia. Oncol Nurs Forum 1988 Jul/Aug; 15(4): 471–476.*

This study was designed to assess the knowledge level of patients at risk for cancer-induced hypercalcemia regarding the signs of hypercalcemia and measures to reduce the problem. A researcher-designed tool called the Hypercalcemia Knowledge Questionnaire (HKQ) was used to elicit data from a convenience sample of 22 hospitalized and 18 ambulatory patients. The tool contained 13 hypercalcemia knowledge items that were read to each subject by the investigator who recorded the responses. It was found that the patients' knowledge of hypercalcemia was poor. Socres on the HKQ ranged from 0 to 10 (out of a possible 13), with a mean of 1.8. Only 5 of the 40 subjects reported that they were told that hypercalcemia might occur. Most were unaware of the typical symptoms of hypercalcemia and the measures they could take to minimize the risk of hypercalcemia (such as drinking adequate amounts of liquids and staying as mobile as possible). The need to develop educational materials to enhance knowledge of hypercalcemia in patients at risk of developing this cancer-induced complication was emphasized, as was the need to research ways to enhance learning of this information.

Nursing Implications. (1) Teach patients at risk for cancer-induced hypercalcemia the signs and symptoms of this condition. Use printed materials and reinforce the information at regular intervals. (2) Instruct patients at risk for cancer-induced hypercalcemia to drink 2 to 3 qt of liquid daily to help the kidneys eliminate excess calcium through the urine. (3) Instruct patients at risk for cancer-induced hypercalcemia to remain as physically active as possible to help keep calcium in the bones.

▷ *Mahon S. Symptoms as clues to calcium levels. Am J Nurs 1987 Mar; 87(3): 254—256.*

A descriptive study was conducted to determine the incidence of symptoms of hypercalcemia in eight cancer patients. A total of 66 days in which serum calcium levels were greater than normal was noted among these eight subjects. Data were collected daily with use of a researcher-designed tool that assessed for symptoms of hypercalcemia. The most evident changes were those affecting mental status, such as reduced memory span, decreased ability to perform simple calculations, disorientation, and inappropriate behaviors. As serum calcium levels returned to normal with treatment, these symptoms decreased. In the presence of severe hypercalcemia, bowel movements were absent in some subjects for periods of 6 to 17 days, despite cathartics and enemas. Anorexia was noted to persist in other subjects until serum calcium levels returned to normal. One subject suffered cardiac arrest when her serum calcium level reached 17 mg/dl. Family members were interviewed to determine which symptoms of hypercalcemia were involved in causing admissions to the hospital. Among the most frequently cited causes were constipation, confusion, and anorexia.

Nursing Implications. (1) Teach patients at risk for hypercalcemia the expected symptoms of this condition; encourage them to seek help from health care providers as appropriate. (2) Teach patients and their significant others that the mental changes induced by hypercalcemia will diminish as serum calcium levels return to normal.

▷ *Bowman M et al. Effect of tube-feeding osmolality on serum sodium levels. Crit Care Nurse 1989 Jan; 9(1): 22–28.*

A retrospective chart review was conducted to investigate the effect of tube-feeding osmolality on serum sodium levels in elderly and nonelderly subjects. It was hypothesized that serum sodium levels would be higher in patients receiving hyperosmolal tube feedings and lower in those receiving hypo-osmolal formulas. Furthermore, it was hypothesized that elderly subjects would have a higher incidence of hypernatremia when receiving hyperosmolal feedings than would the nonelderly. The investigator reviewed 132 charts to obtain the following data: serum sodium levels, type of tube-feeding formula, and fluid intake and output volumes. However, only 55 charts contained sufficient serum sodium reports for comparison with concentrations of tube feedings. It was found that 60% of the subjects over 60 years of age receiving hyperosmolal tube feedings had hypernatremia (as compared to 10% and 13% for subjects receiving hypo-osmolal and iso-osmolal formulas). It was not possible to compare free water intake between the two groups because most charts contained inadequate records of intake and output.

Nursing Implications. (1) Consider the osmolality of tube feedings in relation to serum sodium levels when evaluating fluid needs for tube-fed patients. (2) Record all fluid intake and output in tube-fed patients; monitor for large discrepancies. (3) Assess for signs of hyponatremia or hypernatremia in tube-fed patients, particularly in elderly patients.

▷ *Thompson D et al. A trial of povidone-iodine antiseptic solution for the prevention of cannula-related thrombophlebitis. J IV Nurs 1989; 12(2): 99–102.*

Thrombophlebitis is a common complication of peripheral intravenous devices; it may be caused by either local infection or mechanical irritation induced by the cannula. A prospective study of 200 adult patients was conducted to determine the effectiveness of povidone-iodine antiseptic solution in preventing thrombophlebitis. In the test group of 97 subjects, the skin was cleansed with a solution of povidone-iodine that was allowed to dry prior to cannula insertion. Nothing other than 70% alcohol was applied to the insertion site of the 103 subjects in the control group. Daily inspections of the sites were performed until the cannulae were removed (either when signs of inflammation developed or when the patients were discharged from the unit). Inflammation at the site of cannulation was present in 40 of the 200 subjects; although the incidence was somewhat higher in the test group, there was no statistically significant difference between the test and control groups. It was found that inflammation was more likely to be present with increasing duration of cannulation, irrespective of whether the site had or had not been treated with povidone-iodine.

Nursing Implications. Results of this study indicate that scrubbing the venipuncture site with 70% alcohol prior to venipuncture is at least as effective as using povidone-iodine solution. Also, the authors suggested that limiting the duration of cannula placement to 48 hours (rather than the currently recommended 72 hours) per site may minimize the incidence of thrombophlebitis.

Oncology

Nursing research has examined physiologic and psychologic factors related to patient outcomes. Caregivers, who play an important role in care of the patient with cancer, have also been the focus of several nursing research studies.

▷   Herth KA. *The relationship between level of hope and level of coping response and other variables in patients with cancer.* Oncol Nurs Forum 1989 Jan/Feb; 16(1): 67–72.

Few empirically based studies exist that document hope and its relationship to coping in cancer patients. This study was conducted to examine the relationship between level of hope and level of coping in adult oncology patients. Other variables that play a role in hope and coping were also evaluated. These included treatment setting, family and job responsibilities, and religious convictions.

The sample for this study included 120 adult cancer patients who were receiving chemotherapy in either inpatient, outpatient or home settings. To control for stage of the disease, each group of 40 patients included 20 patients with local disease and 20 patients with metastatic disease. Each subject completed the Herth Hope Scale, the Jalowiec Coping Scale, and a demographic data form.

Results of this study illustrate a significant relationship between levels of hope and levels of coping. When the subjects' level of hope was high, their level of coping was high, and vice versa. A significant difference ($p = .05$) was also found in the mean levels of hope and coping for individuals receiving their chemotherapy in the inpatient or outpatient setting versus at home. More specifically, patients in this sample receiving their chemotherapy in either the inpatient or outpatient hospital setting had higher levels of hope and coping than did those receiving treatments at home. Mean levels of hope and coping were also significantly higher for individuals with little or no interference in performing family role responsibilities than they were for those indicating severe interference. Lastly, a significant difference was found between levels of hope and coping and strong religious convictions. Subjects who possessed a strong religious faith had higher levels of hope and coping than did those subjects with few religious convictions.

Nursing Implications.   This study supports the belief that enabling hope aids cancer patients in coping with their disease and its treatment. Also, findings support the dimension of spirituality as a need of some patients to assist them in developing coping strategies. This study also begins to assemble a body of knowledge to support environmental settings most conducive to cancer treatment.

▷   Blank JJ et al. *Perceived home care needs of cancer patients and their caregivers.* Cancer Nurs 1989 Apr; 12(2): 78–84.

The authors suggest that there is an increasing number of cancer patients being treated on an outpatient basis. Consequently, patients and families require greater home care skills and information concerning availability of community supports. The purpose of this exploratory descriptive study was to identify anticipated home care needs of caregivers and outpatients receiving treatment for cancer. Home care needs for each group

were identified as physical, psychologic, and health services requirements necessary to maintain optimal functioning at home. In addition to identifying the needs of patients and caregivers, the investigators sought to identify differences between the perceived home care needs of the two groups.

Neuman's General Systems Model served as the conceptual framework for this study. A convenience sample consisted of 16 subjects: 8 patients receiving treatment as outpatients and their 8 associated caregivers. Outpatient treatment consisted of radiation therapy or biologic response modifier therapy. The patients ranged in age from 59 to 73 years, with a mean age of 66.2 years. The diagnoses of the five female and three male patients included breast, mouth, abdominal, and pancreatic cancer. The functional abilities of the patients were assessed with the Eastern Cooperative Oncology Group (ECOG) performance scale, the Self-Maintenance Scale, and the Activities of Daily Living Scale. All revealed that the subjects were ambulatory and required little assistance with daily activity needs.

The caregivers consisted of four females and four males, seven of whom were married to and living with the patient. They ranged in age from 34 to 69 years, with a mean age of 56.7 years. The caregiver group had a mean of two health problems, indicating some compromise in health status.

Separate interviews of the patient and caregiver were conducted by trained research assistants. The tools used were developed by Neuman to assess the following categories of stressors for each group: intrapersonal (stressors occurring within the individual), interpersonal (stressors occurring between the individual and others), and extrapersonal (stressors occurring between the individual and the environment). Interviews were tape recorded for later analysis. Construct and content validity were established.

Intrapersonal stressors identified by patients included uncertainty about the course of treatment and potential outcomes; concerns regarding changes in physical abilities and role performance; and feelings of anger, depression, and isolation. Interpersonal stressors involved the need for support by friends and family. Extrapersonal stressors identified by patients revolved around finding a means of transportation for treatment and diagnostic procedures. Patients also identified concerns regarding financial support for treatment and daily living.

Caregivers identified the following intrapersonal stressors: treatment uncertainty, role conflict, new responsibilities, fear of being alone, and difficulties coping with the illness. Interpersonal stressors included lack of support, relationship with the patient, the physical needs of the patient, and lack of information concerning the disease. This group also identified finances and transportation as extrapersonal stressors.

The investigators found that patients and caregivers identified some of the same needs, including coping with role changes, need for information regarding treatment, need for social support, and concerns regarding finances and transportation. Needs unique to the patient group were related to coping with physical restrictions, anger, and depression. Needs unique to the caregiver group included coping with added responsibilities, fear of being alone, and guilt concerning recognition of own personal needs.

Nursing Implications.   Persons with cancer are living longer than they were previously. As a result of improved technology and changing financial reimbursement patterns, patients are leaving the hospital setting sooner than they were previously or are receiving active treatment as outpatients. Nurses in both inpatient and outpatient settings plan for the needs of patients and their caregivers. The stressors identified in this study can serve as a guide for nurses who are assessing and planning for patients receiving outpatient therapy. The authors also suggest that the results of this study can assist in providing baseline data for further refinement of needs-assessment tools.

▷ Bram PJ and Katz LF. *A study of burnout in nurses working in hospice and hospital oncology settings.* Oncol Nurs Forum 1989 Jul/Aug; 16(4): 555–560.

The aim of this study was to ascertain if nurses working with dying patients would experience different degrees of burnout based on the health care setting employed. This study also examined six work-related variables and their relationships among nurses experiencing burnout.

Fifty-seven nurses constituted the overall sample. Twenty-nine nurses worked in hospice settings and 28 nurses worked in hospital oncology units. All subjects completed the Staff Burnout Scale for Health Professionals, Corwin's Nursing Role Conception Scale, and a work-related questionnaire.

The results of this study showed a statistically significant difference ($p < .05$) between hospice nurses' level of burnout and hospital nurses' level of burnout, with the hospice nurse group displaying the lowest mean burnout scores. Results also indicated that different work-related variables correlated with burnout for each group. The one common variable among both groups that influenced burnout was perception of support in the workplace. Hospice nurses perceived a greater opportunity to express work-related feelings and discuss work-related problems than did hospital nurses, thus decreasing their mean burnout scores.

Nursing Implications. The implications of this study focus on the recruitment and retention, training, and communication patterns of nurses working with dying patients and their administrative supervisors. Study results suggest that nursing administrators should provide increased staff support to nursing personnel working with the dying. This finding supports the need to further investigate which environmental factors are most significant in preventing or contributing to burnout in oncology nursing.

▷ Petrosino B, Becker H, and Christian B. *Infection rates in central venous catheter dressings.* Oncol Nurs Forum 1988 Nov/Dec; 15(6): 709–717.

Infection control is of paramount importance in cancer patients with indwelling catheters being used for chemotherapy, parenteral nutrition, blood administration, and blood withdrawal. The purpose of this study was to examine the effects of local care and type of dressing on infection rates at central venous catheter sites.

Fifty-two subjects were randomly assigned to one of four dressing groups. These groups included use of a Tegaderm transparent dressing, an Op-Site transparent dressing, a gauze dressing, or no dressing. All subjects had indwelling single- or multiple-lumen tunneled catheters. Information regarding infection was gathered via site cultures taken 7 to 10 days, 26 to 30 days, and 60 days after catheter insertion; local site erythema (>3 cm); body temperature (>99°F); local site tenderness (>3 cm); and local site drainage. All patients, families, and nursing staff received verbal and written instructions regarding site care and dressing changes required for each group.

The results of this study did not show statistically significant results; however, the data trends did indicate that the Tegaderm and Op-Site transparent dressing groups may have a higher infection rate than the gauze dressing or no dressing groups. The lack of significance found with dressing technique suggests that other variables such as cleansing technique may be even more important.

Nursing Implications. This study has several implications for nursing practice. It stresses the need for meticulous cleansing techniques at the site of the indwelling catheter. It also suggests that costly dressings may not be necessary to prevent infection at catheter sites, and it may be acceptable to have no dressings once site healing has occurred.

Other Related Nursing Research Articles

Baillie V, Norbeck JS, and Barnes LEA. Stress, social support, and psychological distress of family caregivers of the elderly. Nurs Res 1988 Jul/Aug; 37(4): 217–222.

Caudell KA et al. Quantification of urinary mutagens in nurses during potential antineoplastic agent exposure. Cancer Nurs 1988 Feb; 11(1): 41–50.

Davis GC. Measurement of the chronic pain experience: Development of an instrument. Res Nurs Health 1989 Aug; 12(4): 221–227.

Davis GC. The clinical assessment of chronic pain in rheumatic disease: Evaluating the use of two instruments. J Adv Nurs 1989 May; 14(5): 397–402.

Geden EA et al. Effects of music and imagery on physiologic and self-report of analogued labor pain. Nurs Res 1989 Jan/Feb; 38(1): 37–41.

Hargreaves A and Lander J. Use of transcutaneous electrical nerve stimulation for postoperative pain. Nurs Res 1989 May/Jun; 38(3): 159–161.

Lange MP, Dahn MS, and Jacobs LA. Patient-controlled analgesia versus intermittent analgesia dosing. Heart Lung 1988 Sep; 17(5): 495–498.

Wilkie DJ et al. Use of the McGill questionnaire to measure pain: A meta-analysis. Nurs Res 1990 Jan/Feb; 38(1): 36–41.

Williams RD. Factors affecting the practice of breast self-exam in older women. Oncol Nurs Forum 1988 Sep/Oct; 15(5): 611–616.

unit *5*

Perioperative Management of the Surgical Patient

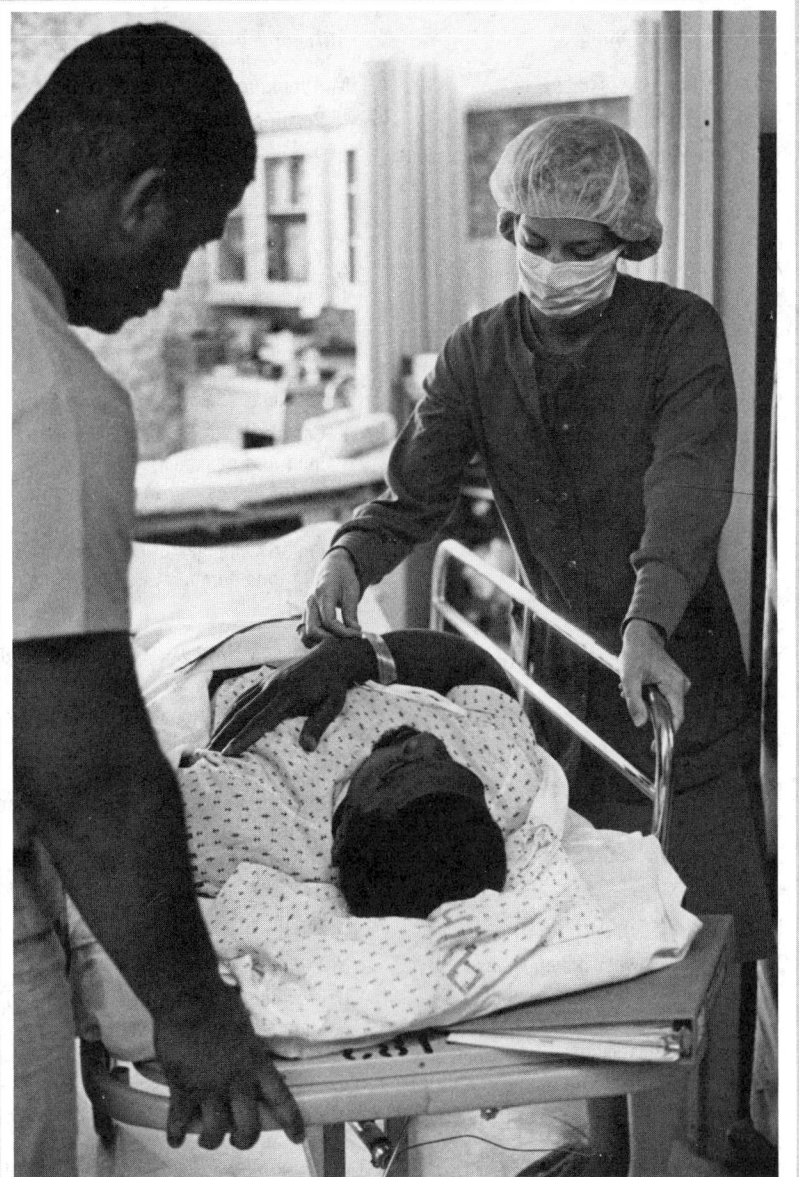

The person with a health care problem that requires surgical intervention usually undergoes a surgical procedure during which anesthesia is used. Anesthesia may also be used in certain nonsurgical procedures, such as closed reduction of a dislocation or fracture. Most surgical procedures are performed in a hospital operating room, although many simpler procedures that do not require hospitalization are carried out in surgicenters.

Recent technologic advances have led to more complex procedures, such as those requiring microsurgical techniques or the use of lasers, more sophisticated bypass equipment, and highly sensitive monitoring devices. Surgery has involved the transplantation of human organs and the implantation of mechanical devices. Concomitant advances have also been made in the development of anesthetic agents, pharmaceutical preparations, and nutritional supplements and in the establishment of more extensive and refined rehabilitation procedures. These technologic advances have focused attention on the essential "hi-tech, hi-touch" role of nursing personnel.

At the same time, the manner of delivering and paying for health care has changed, resulting in shorter hospital stays and cost-containment measures. As a result, many people scheduled for surgery undergo diagnostic and preoperative preparation before entering the hospital. They also leave the hospital sooner, increasing the need for home health care teaching and preparation for self-care. Since the advent of cost-containment measures, same-day surgery, and early discharge, it is not unusual for a patient to be admitted to the hospital on the day

Examples of Nursing Activities in the Perioperative Role

Preoperative Phase

Preoperative Assessment
Clinic/Telephone
1. Initiates initial preoperative assessment
2. Plans teaching methods appropriate to patient's needs
3. Involves family in interview
4. Verifies completion of preoperative testing
5. Assesses patient's need for postoperative transportation and care

Surgical Unit
1. Completes preoperative assessment
2. Coordinates patient teaching with other nursing staff
3. Explains phases in perioperative period and expectations
4. Develops a plan of care

Operating Room
1. Assesses patient's level of consciousness
2. Reviews chart
3. Identifies patient
4. Verifies surgical site

Planning
1. Determines a plan of care
2. Coordinates appropriate services and resources

Psychological Support
1. Tells patient what is happening
2. Determines psychological status
3. Gives warning of noxious stimuli
4. Communicates patient's emotional status to other appropriate members of the health care team

Intraoperative Phase

Maintenance of Safety
1. Positions the patient
   a. Functional alignment
   b. Exposure of surgical site
   c. Maintenance of position throughout procedure
2. Applies grounding device to patient
3. Provides physical support
4. Ensures that the sponge, needle, and instrument counts are correct

Physiologic Monitoring
1. Calculates effects on patient of excessive fluid loss or gain
2. Distinguishes normal from abnormal cardiopulmonary data
3. Reports changes in patient's pulse, respirations, temperature, and blood pressure

Psychologic Support (Before Induction and if Patient is Conscious)
1. Provides emotional support to patient
2. Stands near or touches patient during procedures and induction
3. Continues to assess patient's emotional status
4. Communicates patient's emotional status to other appropriate members of the health care team

Nursing Management
1. Provides physical safety for the patient
2. Maintains aseptic, controlled environment
3. Effectively manages human resources

Postoperative Phase

Communication of Intraoperative Information
1. States patient's name
2. States type of surgery performed
3. Describes intraoperative factors (*i.e.*, insertion of drains or catheters, occurrence of unexpected events)
4. Describes physical limitations
5. Reports patient's preoperative level of consciousness
6. Communicates necessary equipment needs

Postoperative Assessment
Recovery Area
   Determines patient's immediate response to surgical intervention

Surgical Unit
1. Evaluates effectiveness of nursing care in the OR
2. Determines patient's level of satisfaction with care given during perioperative period
3. Evaluates products used on patient in the OR
4. Determines patient's psychological status
5. Assists with discharge planning

Home/Clinic
1. Seeks patient's perception of surgery in terms of the effects of anesthetic agents, impact on body image, distortion, immobilization
2. Determines family's perception of surgery

he is scheduled for surgery, to receive general anesthesia and undergo a surgical procedure, and to be discharged home to the care of his family by noon of the same day.

Ambulatory, or same-day, surgery requires the nurse to have a solid knowledge of all aspects of surgical patient care. No longer is preoperative and postoperative nursing knowledge sufficient; complete care must include intraoperative nursing competency. This unit focuses on the application of the nursing process for the patient undergoing major surgery, same-day surgery, or surgery in a short-procedure unit. In each type of setting, the basic principles remain the same.

Perioperative Nursing

Perioperative nursing is the term used to describe the wide variety of nursing functions associated with the patient's surgical experience. The word ''perioperative'' is an encompassing term that incorporates the three phases of the surgical experience— preoperative, intraoperative, and postoperative. As shown in the chart Examples of Nursing Activites in the Perioperative Role, each of these phases begins and ends at a particular time in the sequence of events that constitute the surgical experience, and each includes a wide range of behaviors and nursing activities that the nurse performs using the nursing process and consistent with the standards of practice.

The *preoperative phase* of the perioperative nursing role begins when the decision for surgical intervention is made and ends with the transfer of the patient to the operating room table. The scope of nursing activities during this time can include establishing a baseline assessment of the patient in the clinical setting or at home, carrying out a preoperative interview, and preparing the patient for the anesthetic he is to receive and the surgery he is to undergo. Or the nursing activities may be limited to performing a preoperative patient assessment in the holding area or surgical suite.

The nursing functions included in the *intraoperative phase* begin when the patient is admitted or transferred to the surgery department and end when he is admitted to the recovery area. In this phase, the scope of nursing activity can include starting the IV infusion, administering IV medications, carrying out the full scope of physiologic monitoring throughout a surgical procedure, and providing for the patient's safety. Or the nursing activities can be limited to holding the patient's hand during general anesthesia induction, acting in the role of scrub nurse, or assisting in positioning the patient on the operating room table using basic principles of body alignment.

The *postoperative phase* begins with the admission of the patient to the recovery area and ends with a follow-up evaluation in the clinical setting or at home. The scope of nursing activities during this period may focus on assessing the postoperative status of the patient in terms of the effects of the anesthetic agents and the impact of surgery on body image or role function, as well as evaluating the family's perception of the surgery. Or these nursing activities may be limited to communicating pertinent information about the patient's surgery to personnel in the recovery area or surgical nursing unit.

Each phase is reviewed in more detail in this unit. Where pertinent and possible, the nursing process of assessment, nursing diagnosis, planning, intervention, and evaluation is described.

Gerontologic Overview

Surgery imposes physical and psychologic stress, but advances in assessment techniques, surgical procedures, anesthetic techniques, and monitoring capabilities allow older patients to tolerate elective surgery surprisingly well. The underlying principle that guides the preoperative assessment, surgery, and postoperative care is that the aged patient has *less physiologic reserve* (the ability of an organ to return to normal after a disturbance in its equilibrium) than the younger patient. The special requirements for optimum results following surgery on an elderly patient include (1) skillful preoperative assessment and treatment, (2) experienced and careful anesthesia and surgery, and (3) meticulous and competent postoperative management. The hazards of surgery for the aged are proportional to the number and severity of coexisting health problems and the nature and duration of the operative procedure.

20

Preoperative Nursing Management

Learning Objectives

On completion of this chapter, the learner will be able to:

1. Identify the causes of preoperative anxieties and nursing measures to allay anxiety
2. Use comprehensive preoperative assessment to identify surgical risk factors
3. Identify legal and ethical considerations related to the operative permit and informed consent
4. Describe preoperative nursing measures that decrease the risk for infection and other postoperative complications
5. Develop a preoperative teaching plan designed to promote the patient's recovery and to prevent postoperative complications
6. Describe the immediate preoperative preparation of the patient
7. Identify the nurse's responsibility in meeting the needs of the family of the preoperative/operative patient

Surgical Indications and Classifications

Surgery may be performed for a variety of reasons. It may be *diagnostic,* such as when a biopsy is obtained or an exploratory laparotomy is performed; it may be *curative,* such as when a tumor mass is excised or an inflamed appendix is removed; it may be *reparative,* such as when multiple wounds must be repaired; it may be *reconstructive* or *cosmetic,* such as when a mammaplasty or a face lift is performed; or it may be *palliative,* such as when pain must be relieved or a problem corrected—for example, when a gastrostomy tube is inserted to compensate for the inability to swallow food.

    Surgery may also be classified according to the degree of urgency involved, with use of the terms *emergency, urgent,*

required, elective, and *optional.* These terms are defined in Table 20-1, and examples of the types of surgery involved are provided.

▶ Nursing Process Overview

▷ Assessment

Assessment of the surgical patient involves evaluation of a wide range of physical and psychologic factors. Many parameters are considered in the overall assessment of the patient, and a variety of patient problems or nursing diagnoses can be anticipated or identified on the basis of the data. Detailed discussions of the psychosocial assessment and the physical examination of the surgical patient follow this section.

TABLE 20-1. *Categories of Contemplated Surgery Based on Urgency*

Classification	Indications for Surgery	Examples
I. Emergency—Patient requires immediate attention; disorder may be life-threatening	Without delay	Severe bleeding Bladder or intestinal obstruction Fractured skull Gunshot/stab wounds Extensive burns
II. Urgent—Patient requires prompt attention	Within 24–30 hr	Acute gallbladder infection Kidney or ureteral stones
III. Required—Patient needs to have operation	Plan within a few weeks or months	Prostatic hyperplasia without bladder obstruction Thyroid disorders Cataracts
IV. Elective—Patient should be operated upon	Failure to have surgery not catastrophic	Repair of scars Simple hernia Vaginal repair
V. Optional—Decision rests with patient	Personal preference	Cosmetic surgery

Nursing Diagnoses

Based on the assessment data, major preoperative nursing diagnoses of the surgical patient may include:

- Anxiety related to the surgical experience (anesthesia, pain) and the outcome of surgery
- Knowledge deficit regarding preoperative procedures and protocols and postoperative expectations

Planning and Implementation

Goals: The surgical patient's major goals may include relief of preoperative anxiety and increased knowledge of preoperative preparations and postoperative expectations.

Nursing Interventions

Reduction of Preoperative Anxiety.   Specific nursing interventions are discussed in detail under Psychosocial Nursing Assessment and Interventions.

Patient Education.   Specific nursing interventions are discussed in detail under Preoperative Patient Education. See also Preoperative Nursing Interventions and Immediate Preoperative Nursing Interventions.

Evaluation

Expected Outcomes

1. Anxiety is relieved
   a. Tells family/significant other he is looking forward to having problem corrected
   b. Queries anesthesiologist about concerns related to types of anesthesia and induction
   c. Verbalizes an understanding of the preanesthetic medication and general anesthesia
   d. Queries staff about last-minute concerns
   e. Verbalizes relief about hospital bills and other costs after talking with social worker, when appropriate
   f. Requests visit with member of clergy when appropriate
   g. Relaxes quietly after being visited by health team members
2. Prepares for surgical intervention
   a. Participates willingly in preoperative preparation
   b. Demonstrates and describes exercises he is expected to perform postoperatively
   c. Reviews information about postoperative care
   d. Accepts preanesthetic medication
   e. Remains in bed
   f. Relaxes during transportation to operating unit
   g. States rationale for use of side rails

Psychosocial Nursing Assessment and Interventions

Any surgical procedure is preceded by some type of emotional reaction in a patient, whether it is obvious or hidden, normal or abnormal. For example, preoperative anxiety is an anticipatory response to an experience that the patient may view as a threat to his customary role in life, body integrity, or even life itself. It is known that a mind that is not at peace directly influences the functioning of the body. Therefore, it is imperative to identify the anxieties that the patient is experiencing.

By taking a careful *health history,* the nurse elicits patient concerns that can have a direct bearing on the course of the surgical experience. Undoubtedly, a patient facing surgery is beset by fears; these may include fears of the unknown, of death, of anesthesia, of cancer. Concerns about loss of work time, the possible loss of job, the responsibility of family support, and the possibility of permanent incapacity further contribute to the enormous emotional strain created by the prospect of surgery. Less obvious concerns may occur because of previous experiences with the hospital and people the patient has known with the same condition. Consequently, the nurse must encourage verbalization, listen, be understanding, and provide information that helps to allay concerns.

The extent of the patient's reaction is based on many factors, including the discomforts and changes he anticipates—whether physical, financial, psychologic, spiritual, or social—and the surgical outcome he envisions. Will the operation improve his present condition? Will he be disabled? Is this just a temporary measure in a chronic condition?

An important part of the assessment is to determine the role of the patient's family or persons who are significant to him. The value and reliability of all available support systems are also determined. Other information, such as usual level of functioning and typical daily activities, may assist in the patient's care and rehabilitation plans.

Fear is expressed in different ways by different people. For example, fear may be expressed indirectly by the patient who asks a lot of questions, repeating them constantly even though answers were given previously. For another person, the reaction may be withdrawal—deliberately avoiding communication, perhaps by reading or watching television. Still others may talk incessantly about trivialities. Often such behavior ends abruptly as the patient turns to the nurse and says, ''I guess you can tell I'm a bit nervous about my operation.'' The need to keep the lines of communication open is never greater than at this time. To belittle the patient's fears by saying, ''Oh, there's nothing to be afraid of'' immediately closes the door and causes the patient to lapse into less effective means of coping with his worries.

Such breakdowns in communication may leave the patient upset, bewildered, and even unable to listen effectively. Something that was mentioned by a nurse or a physician may become exaggerated out of proportion to its importance. For example, if an operation is postponed because of a filled schedule, the patient who is merely told that ''something has come up'' may begin to worry that the reason for the delay is a deterioration in his condition.

A preoperative patient may experience a number of fears. *Fear of anesthesia* was justified years ago, when little was known about the control and the effect of anesthetic agents. But with refined methods, tested drugs, and skilled anesthesiologists, the hazards are minimized. The ease with which anesthesia is administered today is attributed to the adequacy of the physical and mental preparation that the patient receives. The price of poor preparation is a difficult period of induction, followed by an unpleasant emergence from the anesthetic agent. In her contact with each patient, the nurse can do much to dispel false conceptions and misinformation. When the anesthesiologist and the operating room nurse visit the patient the day before surgery, additional confidence is established, and the patient accepts the anesthetic more readily and is less fearful because the number of unknowns has been reduced.

Often the fear of the anesthetic is secondary to the *fear of pain or of death*. Will I feel the scalpel making the incision? What if the anesthesia wears off? The patient needs reassurance that the anesthesiologist will be in constant attendance to prevent these problems. Some surgeons will not operate on a patient who is convinced that he will die. This is a real fear, and it cannot be dismissed lightly. Good rapport between patient and nurse, together with tact on the nurse's part, may bring the patient to a realization that his fear is magnified. The patient's fears will be reduced if those responsible for his care enhance his confidence.

The *fear of the unknown* is often the most troubling. This fear stems partly from the patient's belief that he is not being told ''everything'' about his diagnosis or his illness. The more understanding one has of the probabilities for the future, the better is the adjustment. The nurse can do much to allay the patient's anxieties and induce a certain peace of mind. A patient frequently expresses fears and misgivings to the nurse but hides them from the surgeon. In such circumstances, the nurse privately communicates the patient's expression of anxiety to the surgeon.

The patient who has had a previous positive experience with surgery may not be apprehensive. However, an earlier negative experience can aggravate the person's fear. The nurse can help the patient to view the impending operation as a new and unique situation, not a repetition of the past.

The *fear of destruction of body image* occurs with radical surgery. However, with today's media emphasis on youth, the ''perfect'' body, and revealing fashions, it may also occur with minor surgery. Consequently, any surgical encroachment on the body, including the scar of a surgical incision, is viewed with distress by many patients.

Fear of separation from a loved one, from familiar support systems, and from former activities can also create anxieties.

In addition to the above fears, the average patient has many other worries. He may have financial problems, family responsibilities, and employment obligations, and he may fear a poor prognosis or the probability of disability in the future. These problems are investigated by the nurse. If the difficulty requires the assistance of a medical social worker, the aid of such a person is enlisted. If the worry stems from fear of what the prognosis is likely to be, the physician is informed.

When some of these fears have been addressed, it is beneficial to have the patient express his thoughts about the importance and the meaning of this surgery for the immediate future as well as the more distant future. Most fears are manifestations of concern over losing control over one's person, either physically or socially. The patient may be concerned about losing his independence, his integrity, and his control over his effectiveness in coping with his environment. As the nurse learns of patient concerns, it is important that she share them with the surgeon as they work together to prepare the patient for surgery.

Anxiety is not solely a negative activity. Psychologic preparation for subsequent stress includes permitting the patient some degree of worrying. This is more desirable than having little or no anticipatory fear. Moderately anxiety-producing information allows the patient to increase his tolerance for stress by developing effective ways of coping with his problems. Absence of worry deprives the patient of the motivation to prepare psychologically for a stressful experience, with the result that if a crisis develops he will have a low tolerance for stress.

The significance of *spiritual therapy* must not be forgotten. Regardless of the religious affiliation of the patient, the nurse recognizes that faith in a higher power can be as therapeutic as medication. Every attempt must be made to help the patient obtain the spiritual help that he requests. This may be accomplished by participating in prayer, by reading passages from the Scriptures, or by calling a member of the clergy. Faith has great sustaining power; thus, the beliefs of each individual patient should be respected and supported. Some nurses avoid the subject of a clergy visit on the premise that the suggestion may alarm the patient. Asking the patient if his minister, priest, or rabbi knows he is in the hospital is a caring, nonthreatening approach.

In some instances, the interval of time preparatory to surgery may become extended. *Cognitive control* in the form of recreation and diversion can be provided by such activities as reading, listening to the radio, watching television, engaging in handcrafts and games. The nurse can arrange for people with similar interests to meet. Many times, patients can help one another.

Perhaps the most valuable facility at the disposal of the nurse is the ability to *listen* to the patient, especially when obtaining the patient's history. By engaging in conversation and using the principles of interviewing, the nurse can acquire invaluable information and insight. An unhurried, understanding, and kind nurse invites confidence on the part of the patient.

Every patient must be treated as an individual who has fears and hopes quite distinct from the fears or hopes of the next person. Understanding and helping one patient may require an approach completely different from that used with another. Providing time to answer questions and offering psychologic support ensures a smoother postoperative course. The patient sleeps better, recalls fewer fearful images, needs less anesthetic and pain medication, recovers more rapidly, and is discharged from the hospital sooner.

Denial of Anxiety.   The preceding discussion of preoperative anxiety emphasizes the most common problems of the patient facing an operation. The opposite reaction, denying anxiety, can also provide obstacles to effective treatment, as in the case of a person who notices abnormal signs or symptoms but puts off seeking treatment. Denial is a reaction noted in many persons when they are suddenly confronted with potentially shocking information. Usually this reaction does not persist longer than a few days or a few weeks, but nevertheless such denial and delay may have serious consequences. The nurse's responsibility in this area extends to all members of the community. She should encourage anyone with a questionable abnormal physical finding or symptom to have it evaluated as soon as possible by a knowledgeable person in the health care field.

General Physical Assessment

Before treatment is initiated, a *health history* is obtained and a *physical examination* is performed during which vital signs are noted and a data base is established for future comparisons. Many diagnostic tests may be performed, such as blood analyses, x-ray studies, endoscopies, tissue biopsies, and stool and urine studies. In preparing the patient for these tests, the nurse is in a position to help the patient understand the need for the diagnostic studies. There is also an opportunity during the physical examination to note significant physical findings, such

as a rash or pressure ulcers, that may be contributing to the patient's condition.

These preliminary contacts with the staff during the health history, physical examination, and diagnostic testing provide the patient with opportunities to ask questions and to become acquainted with those who will be caring for him. In their efforts to establish rapport with the patient, the physician and nurse must respect the patient's feelings and needs.

Nutritional Status and Chemical Substance Use

Nutritional needs are determined by measuring the patient's height and weight, triceps skin fold, upper arm circumference, serum protein levels, and nitrogen balance. These measurements are discussed in detail in the nutritional assessment section of Chapter 7.

Nutritional Requirements.   Replacement of nutrients that are deficient is especially important with respect to protein and calorie malnutrition, because protein is essential for tissue repair. Protein deficiency may result from anorexia concomitant with the aging process, chronic debilitating illness, cancer, or frequent vomiting. Or it may be caused by poor food habits and a diet in which meats and eggs are almost absent. Protein may also be lost in severe burns, through draining abscesses or wounds, and through persistent losses from the gastrointestinal tract.

Protein replacement is a slow process and may take several days or weeks. The replacement may be accomplished by means of (1) a diet high in protein (meat, milk, eggs, and cheese), carbohydrates, and calories, but low in fat; (2) supplementary liquid feedings, such as milk enriched with skim milk powder; or (3) protein hydrolysates given orally or by infusion. Total parenteral nutrition may be administered through a polyethylene tubing inserted into a large vein, such as the subclavian vein. (See Total Parenteral Nutrition in Chap. 35.)

Vitamins are required for specific purposes. Thiamine (vitamin B_1) is necessary for oxidizing carbohydrates and maintaining normal gastrointestinal function. A deficiency in vitamin B_1 is noted in chronic gastrointestinal and liver diseases. Ascorbic acid (vitamin C) is required for wound healing and synthesis of collagen. Vitamin K is necessary for blood clotting and prothrombin production. These vitamins may be administered orally or parenterally.

Loss of body fluids results in electrolyte imbalances. The replacement of these fluids is discussed in Chapter 18. The nurse records all intake and output and keeps a daily record of the patient's weight.

Dental caries and poor mouth hygiene may contribute to general debilitation and should be corrected (see Chap. 34). Periodic evaluations are made to note the patient's progress and readiness for surgery. Readiness can be hindered by diagnostic testing. The patient, particularly if elderly, is a candidate for dehydration and decreased nutritional status when diagnostic tests require repeated food and fluid restrictions or enemas.

A nursing goal and challenge is to encourage the patient to eat by serving attractive and palatable meals of small, manageable servings. Patients on parenteral or enteral therapy or receiving gastrostomy feedings or infusions may need diversion and encouragement. The method of administering fluids depends on the type of replacement therapy. If a nasogastric tube is being used, liquids are given to the patient in a sitting position. If gastrostomy feedings are used, an upright or Fowler's position is used.

Dehydration, hypovolemia, and electrolyte imbalances are common and should be carefully documented. The degree of severity is often difficult to determine. When a patient is being prepared for surgery, additional time may be needed to correct deficits to promote the best possible preoperative condition.

Obesity. If the patient is overweight and if preoperative time permits, a prescribed and systematic program of weight reduction may be undertaken to reduce the surgical risk. Obesity greatly increases the risk and severity of complications. During surgery, fatty tissues are especially susceptible to infection. In addition, the surgeon faces increased technical and mechanical problems. Therefore, dehiscence (wound separation) and wound infections are more common. The obese patient is often more difficult to care for because of his weight; he breathes poorly when lying on his side and thus is subject to hypoventilation and postoperative pulmonary complications. In addition, abdominal distention, phlebitis, and cardiovascular, endocrine, hepatic, and biliary diseases are more common in obese patients. It has been estimated that for each 30 pounds of excess weight, about 25 additional miles of blood vessels are needed. The increased demands on the heart are obvious.

Narcotic, Drug, or Alcohol Use. People who have an addiction to drugs or alcohol frequently attempt to hide the habit. Often a variety of infections and trauma sites on the body can be noted. This situation calls for meticulous attention, patience, frank questions, and a nonjudgmental attitude on the part of the nurse who is assessing the patient.

The acutely intoxicated person is susceptible to injury. Therefore, surgery is postponed if possible. If emergency surgery is required, local or regional block anesthesia is used for minor surgery. Otherwise, the stomach must be intubated and aspirated before general anesthesia is administered to prevent vomiting and aspiration.

The person with a history of chronic alcoholism often suffers from malnutrition and other systemic problems that increase the surgical risk. Additionally, alcohol withdrawal delirium (delirium tremens) may be anticipated on the second or third day after alcohol withdrawal, and it is associated with a significant mortality rate when it occurs postoperatively.

Respiratory Status

The goal for potential surgical patients is to have optimum respiratory function. All patients are urged to stop smoking 4 to 6 weeks before an operation; those undergoing upper abdominal and chest surgery are taught breathing exercises and how to use an incentive spirometer.

Because it is necessary to maintain adequate ventilation during all phases of surgical treatment, surgery is usually contraindicated when the patient has a respiratory infection. Respiratory difficulties increase the possibility of atelectasis, bronchopneumonia, and respiratory failure when anesthetics are superimposed. Patients with pulmonary problems are evaluated by means of pulmonary function studies and blood gas analysis to note the extent of respiratory insufficiency. Antibiotics may be prescribed for infections.

Cardiovascular Status

The goal in preparing any patient for surgery is to have a well-functioning cardiovascular system to meet the oxygen, fluid, and nutritional needs throughout the perioperative period.

Because the margin of safety is lessened when a surgical patient exhibits signs of cardiovascular disease, this condition demands greater than usual diligence during all phases of management and care. Depending on the severity of symptoms, surgery may be deferred until maximal benefits have been obtained from medical treatment. At times, surgical treatment can be modified to meet the cardiac tolerance of the patient. For example, in an obese patient with acute obstructive cholecystitis and possible diabetes and coronary artery disease, simple gallbladder drainage with removal of calculi may be performed rather than a more extensive operation.

Of particular significance in the patient with cardiovascular disease is the necessity to avoid sudden changes of position, prolonged immobilization, hypotension or hypoxia, and overloading of the circulatory system with fluids or blood.

Hepatic and Renal Function

The goal is to have maximum functioning of the liver and urinary systems so that medications, anesthetic agents, and body wastes and toxins are adequately removed from the body.

The *liver* is important in the biotransformation of anesthetic compounds. Therefore, any disorder of the liver has an effect on anesthetic metabolism. Because acute liver disease is associated with a high surgical mortality, preoperative improvement in liver function is desired. Careful assessment is made with various liver function tests (see Chap. 38).

The *kidneys* are involved in the excretion of anesthetic drugs and their metabolites. Acid–base status and metabolism are also important considerations in anesthetic administration. Surgery is contraindicated when a patient has acute nephritis, acute renal insufficiency with oliguria or anuria, or other acute renal problems, unless the surgery is a lifesaving measure or is necessary to improve urinary function, as in an obstructive uropathy.

Endocrine Function

In uncontrolled diabetes, the chief life-threatening hazard is hypoglycemia, which may develop during anesthesia or from postoperative inadequate intake of carbohydrates or excessive administration of insulin. Other hazards that threaten the patient but occur less rapidly are acidosis and glucosuria. In general, the surgical risk of the patient with controlled diabetes is not greater than that of the nondiabetic patient; frequent monitoring of blood glucose levels is important before, during, and after surgery (see Chap. 39).

Patients receiving steroids are at risk for adrenal insufficiency; therefore, the use of steroid medications for any purpose must be reported to the anesthesiologist and surgeon.

Additionally, the patient is monitored for signs of adrenal insufficiency.

Immunologic Function

An important nursing goal is to determine the presence of a history of allergies, including previous allergic reactions. Particularly significant is the identification and documentation of sensitivities to certain medications and past adverse reactions to these agents. A list of substances that precipitated previous allergic reactions is obtained, including medications, blood transfusions, and contrast media. The signs and symptoms produced by these substances are explored and recorded. Current use of medications is recorded. A history of bronchial asthma is reported to the anesthesiologist.

Immunosuppression is common with corticosteroid therapy, renal transplantation, radiation therapy, and chemotherapy. The mildest symptoms or slightest temperature elevation must be investigated. Because these patients cannot tolerate breaks in technique, great care is taken to practice meticulous asepsis.

Previous Medication Therapy

Attention is given to the history of medication usage by the patient and should include the type and frequency of use of over-the-counter (OTC) preparations. Potent medications have an effect on physiologic functions; interactions of such medications with anesthetic agents have caused serious problems, such as arterial hypotension and circulatory collapse or depression.

The potential effects of prior medication therapy are evaluated by the anesthesiologist, who considers the length of time the patient has used the medications, his condition, and the nature of the proposed surgery. Medications that cause particular concern include the following:

Adrenal corticosteroids—Corticosteroids are not discontinued abruptly before surgery. Because the sudden termination of steroid therapy may cause cardiovascular collapse if therapy has been used for a chronic illness over a period of time, a bolus of steroid may be administered intravenously immediately before and after surgery.

Diuretics—Thiazide diuretics may cause excessive respiratory depression during anesthesia; this results from an associated electrolyte imbalance.

Phenothiazines—These medications may increase the hypotensive action of anesthetics.

Antidepressants—Monoamine oxidase (MAO) inhibitors increase the hypotensive effects of anesthetics.

Tranquilizers—Barbiturates, diazepam, and chlordiazepoxide may cause anxiety, tension, and even seizures if withdrawn suddenly.

Insulin—Interaction between anesthetics and insulin must be considered when a patient with diabetes is undergoing surgery.

Antibiotics—"Mycin" drugs such as neomycin, kanamycin, and, less frequently, streptomycin may present problems; when these medications are combined with a curariform muscle relaxant, nerve transmission is interrupted and apnea due to respiratory paralysis may result.

For the reasons cited, it is imperative that the patient's medication history be assessed by the nurse and anesthesiologist.

Gerontologic Considerations

An older person facing an operation may have a combination of chronic illnesses and health problems in addition to the specific one for which surgery is indicated. Elderly people frequently do not report symptoms, perhaps because they fear that a serious illness may be diagnosed or because they accept such symptoms as part of growing old. A high level of awareness of subtle clues alerts the nurse to underlying problems.

In general, the elderly are considered poorer surgical risks than younger patients. Cardiac reserves are lower, renal and hepatic function are depressed, and gastrointestinal activity is likely to be reduced. Dehydration, constipation, and malnutrition may be evident.

Sensory limitations such as dimming vision, impaired hearing, and reduced sensitivity of touch are often the reasons for accidents, injuries, and burns. Therefore, the nurse must be alert to maintaining a safe environment. Arthritis is common in older persons and may affect mobility, making it difficult for the patient to turn from one side to the other without discomfort. Protective measures include adequate padding for tender areas, moving the patient slowly, protecting bony prominences against prolonged pressure, and providing gentle massage to promote adequate circulation.

The condition of the mouth is important to assess because of the frequent presence of dental caries, dentures, and partial plates. Such findings are particularly significant to the anesthesiologist.

Decreased perspiration leads to dry, itchy skin. Such fragile skin is easily abraded, so added precautions are taken in moving an elderly person. Decreased subcutaneous fat makes older people less resistant to temperature changes. A lightweight cotton blanket is a desirable cover when an elderly patient is moved to and from the operating room.

The elderly person has had many experiences in his lifetime. He has been exposed to personal illness and life-threatening illnesses of friends and family. Consequently, he has fears about his own future that may not be obvious but nonetheless exist. Taking time to talk with him may encourage expression of his fears and make possible the relaxation and acceptance he needs.

In summary, the optimal goal is to have as many positive factors as possible. Every attempt is made to stabilize those conditions that otherwise hinder a smooth recovery. When negative factors dominate, the risks and postoperative complications increase (Chart 20-1).

Informed Consent

To attain the right to operate, it is necessary for the surgeon to obtain a voluntary and informed consent from the patient.

Chart 20-1
Risk Factors for Any Surgical Procedure

Systemic Factors

Hypovolemia
Dehydration or electrolyte imbalance
Nutritional deficits
Extremes of age
Extremes of weight
Infection and sepsis
Toxic conditions
Immunologic abnormalities

Pulmonary Disease

Renal Disease

Pregnancy

Diminished maternal physiologic reserve

Cardiovascular Disease

Coronary artery disease
Cardiac failure
Dysrhythmias
Hypertension
Prosthetic heart valve
Thromboembolism
Hemorrhagic diathesis
Cerebrovascular disease

Endocrine Dysfunction

Diabetes mellitus
Adrenal conditions
Thyroid malfunction

Hepatic Disease

Such written permission protects the patient against unsanctioned surgery and protects the surgeon against claims of an unauthorized operation. In the best interests of all parties concerned, sound medicolegal principles are followed.

The nurse's responsibility is to ensure that an *informed* consent has been obtained voluntarily from an informed and comprehending person (Table 20-2).

Before the patient signs the consent form, the surgeon should inform him in clear and simple terms what a reasonable person would want to be told and what the surgery will entail. The surgeon must also inform the patient of possible risks, complications, disfigurement, disability, and removal of body parts, as well as what to expect in the early and late postoperative periods.

Informed consent is necessary when

- The procedure is invasive, such as a surgical incision, a biopsy, a cystoscopy, or paracentesis
- Anesthesia is used
- A nonsurgical procedure is performed in which there is more than slight risk to the patient, such as an arteriogram
- A procedure is performed that involves radiation or cobalt therapy

TABLE 20-2. *Criteria for Valid Informed Consent*

Component	Comments
Consent voluntarily given	Valid consent must be freely given, without coercion.
Incompetent subject	Legal definition: individuals who are *not* autonomous and cannot give or withhold consent (*e.g.,* individuals who are mentally retarded, mentally ill, or comatose)
Informed subject	Consent form should be in writing (although law does not require written documentation). It should contain the following: Explanation of procedure and its risks Description of benefits An offer to answer questions about procedure Instructions that the patient may withdraw consent A statement informing the patient if the protocol differs from customary procedure
Subject able to comprehend	Information must be written and delivered in language understandable to the patient. Questions must be answered to facilitate comprehension if material is confusing.

(Adapted from Douglas S and Larson E. There's more to informed consent than information. Focus Crit Care 1986 Apr; 13[2]:44.)

The patient may sign his own consent form for operation if he is of legal age and mentally capable. If he is a minor or is unconscious or incompetent, permission must be obtained from a responsible family member or legal guardian. If he is an emancipated minor (married or independently earning his own living), he may sign his own permit. State regulations and agency policy must be followed. In an emergency, it may be necessary for the surgeon to operate as a lifesaving measure without the patient's informed consent. However, every effort must be made to contact the patient's family. In such a situation, contact can be made by telephone or telegram.

When the patient has doubts and has not had the opportunity to investigate alternative treatments, he is entitled to a second opinion. No patient should be forced to sign an operative permit. Refusing to have an operation is a person's legal right and privilege. However, such information must be documented and relayed to the surgeon so that other arrangements can be made; for instance, additional explanations may be offered to the patient and family, or the operation may be rescheduled at a more suitable time.

The consent process can be improved by providing audiovisual materials to supplement discussion, by ensuring that the wording of the consent form is understandable, and by using other strategies and resources as needed to help the patient understand.

- The informed consent is placed in a prominent place on the patient's chart and accompanies the patient to the operating room.

Preoperative Patient Education

The value of preoperative instruction to the patient has long been recognized. Each patient is taught as an individual, in terms of his anxieties, needs, and hopes. The background information of one patient is usually very different from that of other patients. Once these differences are recognized and par-

---

Chart 20–2
Preoperative Patient Instruction

A. Diaphragmatic Breathing

Diaphragmatic breathing refers to a flattening of the dome of the diaphragm during inspiration with resulting enlargement of the upper abdomen as air rushes in. During expiration, the abdominal muscles contract.

1. Practice in the same position you would assume in bed following surgery: a semi-Fowler's position, propped in bed with the back and shoulders well supported with pillows.
2. With the hands in a loose-fist position, allow the hands to rest lightly on the front of the lower ribs—fingernails against lower chest to feel the movement (Fig. 20–1).
3. Breathe out gently and fully as the ribs sink down and inward toward midline.
4. Then take a deep breath through your nose and mouth, letting the abdomen rise as the lungs fill with air.
5. Hold this breath for a count of five.
6. Exhale and let out *all* the air through the nose and mouth.
7. Repeat 15 times with a short rest after each group of five.
8. Practice this twice a day preoperatively.

B. Coughing

1. Lean forward slightly from a sitting position in bed, interlace the fingers together, and place the hands across the incisional site to act as a splint when coughing (Fig. 20–2).
2. Breathe with the diaphragm as described in *A.*
3. With the mouth slightly open, breathe in fully.
4. "Hack" out sharply for three short breaths.
5. Then, keeping the mouth open, take in a quick deep breath and immediately give a strong cough once or twice. This helps clear secretions from the chest. It may cause some discomfort but will not harm incision.

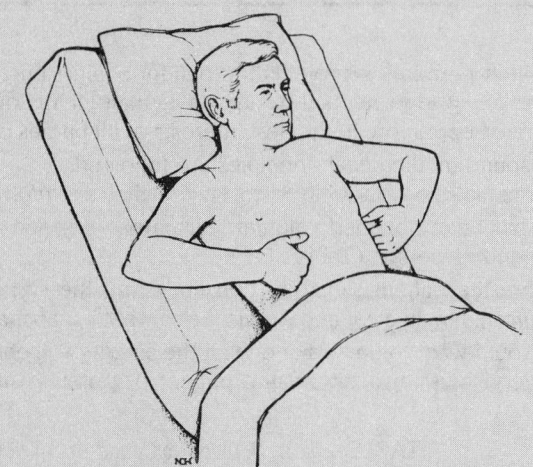

Figure 20–1. Diaphragmatic breathing.

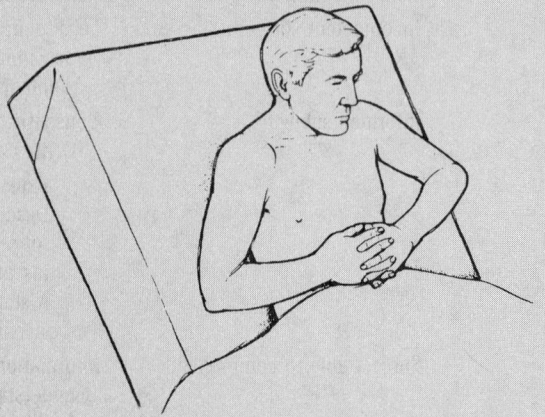

Figure 20–2. Splinting when coughing.

(continued)

ticular needs are assessed, a program of instruction can be planned and implemented at the proper time. If the patient is taught essential information several days before he needs it, he may not remember what he was told. If he is instructed too close to the time of surgery, he may not be in prime learning condition because of anxiety or the effect of the preanesthetic medication.

If instruction is offered at a time when the patient is most receptive and can participate in the learning process, the chances are that he will retain more of the information. Ideally, instruction is spaced over a period of time to allow the patient to assimilate information and to ask questions as they arise. Frequently, teaching sessions are combined with various preparation procedures to allow for an easy flow of information. In essence, the nurse must make a judgment about how much the patient wants and needs to know. In some instances, too much detail raises the patient's anxiety level.

Limiting teaching to a description of the various steps of a procedure is not as helpful as telling the patient what sensations he will experience. For example, telling the patient only that preoperative medication will relax him before the operation is not as effective as also informing him that the medication will make him feel lightheaded and sleepy. Once he knows what to expect, he can anticipate these reactions and thus attain a higher degree of relaxation than might otherwise be expected.

The ideal timing of preoperative teaching is not realistic in the surgicenter or same-day surgery setting. However, creative approaches used during the preadmission testing visit can provide a resource person for answering questions and the opportunity for learning and building rapport. During this visit, the patient can meet and ask questions of the liaison nurse, view audiovisuals, receive written materials, and be given the number to call as questions arise closer to the date of surgery.

Deep Breathing, Coughing, and Relaxation Skills

One goal of preoperative nursing care is to teach the patient how to promote lung ventilation and blood oxygenation following general anesthesia. This is accomplished by demon-

---

Chart 20-2 (Continued)

C. Leg Exercises

1. Lie in a semi-Fowler's position and perform the following simple exercises to improve circulation.
2. Bend the knee and raise the foot—hold it a few seconds, then extend the leg and lower it to the bed (Fig. 20–3).
3. Do this five times with one leg, then repeat with the other leg.
4. Then trace circles with the feet by bending them down, in toward each other, up, and then out (Fig. 20–4).
5. Repeat these movements five times.

D. Turning to the Side

1. Turn on your side with the uppermost leg flexed most and supported on a pillow.
2. Grasp the side rail as an aid to maneuver to the side.
3. Practice diaphragmatic breathing and coughing while on your side.

E. Getting Out of Bed

1. Turn on your side.
2. Push yourself up with one hand as you swing your legs out of bed.

F. Using the Urinal (for Male Patient)

When in bed for a time, have the nurse explain the method for using the urinal in bed.

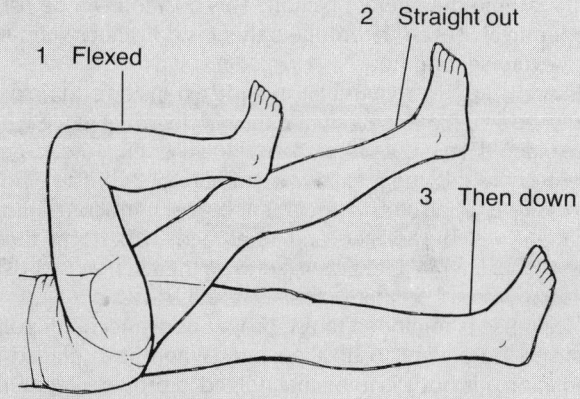

Figure 20–3. Leg exercises.

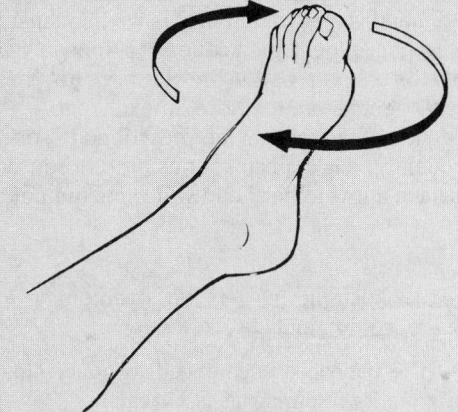

Figure 20–4. Foot exercise.

strating to the patient how to take a deep, slow breath (maximal sustained inspiration, MSI) and how to exhale slowly. The patient is placed in a sitting position to provide maximum lung expansion. After practicing deep breathing several times, he is instructed to breathe deeply, exhale through the mouth, take a short breath, and cough from deep in the lungs (Chart 20-2). In addition to enhancing respiration, these exercises make the patient more relaxed.

If there is to be a thoracic or abdominal incision, the nurse can demonstrate how the incision line can be splinted so that pressure is minimized and pain is controlled. The patient should put the palms of both hands together, interlacing the fingers snugly. Placing the hands across the incisional site acts as an effective splint when coughing. In addition, the patient needs to know that medications will be administered to control pain.

The goal in promoting coughing is to mobilize secretions so that they can be removed. When a deep breath is taken before coughing, the cough reflex is stimulated. If the patient does not cough effectively, hypostatic pneumonia and other lung complications may occur.

Turning and Active Body Movement

The goals of promoting deliberate body movement postoperatively are to improve circulation, to prevent venous stasis, and to contribute to optimal respiratory exchange.

The patient is shown how to turn from side to side and how to assume the lateral position. This position will be used postoperatively (even before the patient is conscious) and assumed every second hour.

Exercises of the extremities include extension and flexion of the knee and hip joints (similar to bicycle riding while lying on the side). The foot is rotated as though tracing the largest possible circle with the great toe (see Chart 20-2 C). The elbow and shoulder are also put through the range of motion. At first the patient will be assisted and reminded to perform these exercises, but later he is encouraged to do them himself. Muscle tone is maintained so that ambulation will be easier.

The nurse is reminded to use proper body mechanics and to instruct the patient to do the same. When he is placed in any position, his body is to be maintained in proper alignment.

Pain Control and Medications

The patient is informed that he will receive a preanesthetic medication to help him relax and perhaps feel sleepy. He is also informed that this medication may make him thirsty. Postoperatively, he can expect medications to reduce pain and keep him comfortable but not to prevent him from regaining activity and maintaining an adequate air exchange.

Prophylactic antibiotics may be prescribed in specific instances. Frequently, the cephalosporins are chosen because these agents have a low toxicity and wide spectrum of action.

Cognitive Control

Useful techniques for relieving tension, overcoming anxiety, and achieving relaxation include the following:

Imagery—The patient is encouraged to concentrate on a happy experience during his last vacation.
Distraction—The patient is encouraged to think of and recite several favorite sayings.

Optimistic self-recitation—Recitation of optimistic thoughts ("I know all will go well") is suggested.

Other Information

The patient feels more at ease when he knows at what point postoperatively he can expect a visit from family or friends. It helps him to know that the family will be kept informed about the acute phases of the surgical experience. He also appreciates knowing that a spiritual advisor of his preference will be available if he desires.

If the patient knows beforehand that he will be on assisted breathing via a ventilator and that drainage tubes will be in place along with any special equipment required, he is more likely to accept these postoperatively.

Preoperative Nursing Interventions

Nutrition and Fluids

When the operation is scheduled for the morning, the meal on the preceding evening may be an ordinary light diet. In dehydrated patients, and especially in older ones, fluids by mouth often are encouraged before an operation. In addition, fluids may be administered intravenously, as prescribed, especially in patients who are unable to take fluids by mouth. If the operation is scheduled to take place after noon and does not involve any part of the gastrointestinal tract, a soft breakfast may be prescribed. Most often, oral intake of food or water is withheld 8 to 10 hours before the operation.

The purpose of withholding food before surgery is to prevent aspiration. Aspiration occurs when food or fluid is regurgitated from the stomach and inhaled into the pulmonary system. Such inhaled material acts as a foreign substance, is irritating, and causes an inflammatory reaction, and at the same time, it interferes with adequate air exchange. Aspiration is a serious problem, with a high mortality rate (60% to 70%) when it occurs.

Intestinal Preparation

A warm cleansing enema or laxatives may be prescribed the evening before an operation and may be repeated if ineffectual. This is to prevent defecation during anesthesia or to prevent accidental trauma to the intestine during abdominal surgery. Unless the condition of the patient presents some contraindication, the toilet or bedside commode, rather than the bedpan, is used in evacuating the enema. In addition, antibiotics may be prescribed to reduce intestinal flora.

Preoperative Skin Preparation

The goal of preoperative skin preparation is to decrease bacterial sources without injuring the skin. When there is time, such as in surgery of a nonemergency nature, the patient may use a soap containing a detergent-germicide to cleanse the skin area for several days before surgery to reduce the number of skin organisms.

Before surgery, the patient should take a warm, relaxing bath or shower, using povidone-iodine (Betadine) soap. Although it is preferable that this be done on the day of surgery, the time scheduled for surgery may require that the shower be taken the night before. The purpose of the cleansing shower as close to the time of surgery as possible is to reduce the risk of skin contamination of the surgical wound. A shampoo the day before the operation is advisable unless the condition of the patient prevents it.

It is preferred that the skin at and around the operative site *not* be shaved. During shaving, the skin may be injured by the razor and become a portal of entry for bacteria; this injured tissue may act as a substrate for bacterial growth. In addition, the longer the interval between the shave and the operation, the higher the rate of postoperative wound infection. Skin that is well cleansed but unshaven is less often implicated in wound infections than is shaved skin.

Skin preparation is ordered by the surgeon, and protocols vary. Some surgeons prefer that hair be removed in and around the operative site. One approach involves the use of electrical clippers to remove hair to within 1 to 2 mm of the skin; in this way, skin is not abraded. The clippers must be thoroughly cleaned after use. Another approach is the use of a depilatory cream (see below).

If agency protocol or the surgeon requires that the skin be shaved, the patient is told about the shaving procedure, placed in a comfortable position, and not exposed unnecessarily. Any adhesive or grease may be readily removed with a sponge moistened in benzene or ether, if the odor and cold temperature are not objectionable to the patient.

Skin shaving may be performed by a special prep team, by the nurse assigned to the patient, or by a member of the operating room team. Scissors can be used to initially remove the longer hair.

An antimicrobial detergent can be used to raise a lather that makes hair easier to remove. The skin is held taut and shaved in the direction of hair growth. Long, continuous strokes are used. Scratches are avoided, and any potential sites of infection are reported. All actions and findings are documented.

Depilatory Cream. Chemical compounds (creams to remove hair) are safe for preparing the skin of the surgical patient. If there is question about the possibility of an allergic reaction, a test patch should be tried first. As an economic measure, long hairs may be cut before the cream is applied to reduce the amount of cream used.

The depilatory cream usually comes in a collapsible tube and is applied to the body surface. The cream is spread in a smooth layer of about 1.25 cm (½ inch) in depth over the entire operative site. A wooden tongue blade or a gloved hand can be used to apply the cream. After the cream has remained on the skin for 10 minutes (depending on directions), it is scraped off gently with the tongue blade or multiple moistened gauze sponges. When all cream and hair have been removed, the skin is washed with soap and water and patted dry.

There are several advantages to using a depilatory cream for preoperative skin preparation. The end result is a clean, smooth, and intact skin. Scrapes, abrasions, cuts, and inadequate hair removal are prevented. It is comfortable for the patient, and the patient may even apply the cream himself for

selected operative procedures. Depilatory creams are more effective and safer for use on uncooperative or agitated patients. This method is no more expensive than other methods. A disadvantage is that a few patients have had some transient skin reactions if depilatory cream is used near the rectal and scrotal areas.

Immediate Preoperative Nursing Interventions

The patient is dressed in a hospital gown that is left untied and open in the back. If the patient has long hair, it may be braided; hairpins are removed, and the hair is completely covered with a disposable paper cap.

The mouth is inspected, and dentures or plates, and chewing gum are removed. If left in the mouth, these items could easily fall to the back of the throat during induction of anesthesia and cause respiratory obstruction.

Jewelry is not worn to the operating room; even wedding rings should be removed. If a patient objects to the removal of a ring, a strip of narrow gauze can be looped through the ring and tied securely around the patient's wrist. All articles of value, including dentures and prosthetic devices, are labeled clearly with the patient's name and stored in a safe place according to agency policy.

When the gastrointestinal tract is the surgical site, a small prepackaged (Fleet's) enema may be prescribed and administered. Otherwise, cathartics are often prescribed. Routine tap water enemas are usually not suggested because of the possibility of creating an electrolyte imbalance.

All patients (except those with urologic problems) should void immediately before going to the operating room to maintain continence during low abdominal surgery and to make abdominal organs more accessible. Catheterization should not be resorted to, except in an emergency or when it is desirable to have an indwelling catheter in place to ensure an empty bladder. In this instance, such a catheter would be connected to a closed drainage system. The voided urine is measured, and the amount and the time of voiding are recorded on the preoperative record.

Preanesthetic Medication: Pharmacokinetics

A complete medication history on every patient scheduled for surgery is imperative because of possible problems of drug interaction. The history should include all the medications the patient has been taking or has taken within the past 2 months. (If steroids have been administered during the past year, this information is documented and brought to the attention of the anesthesiologist and the surgeon.) Note should be made of medication hypersensitivity, medication dosage, and the conditions for which medications were prescribed.

As with other management modalities, medication is prescribed on an individual basis to meet the needs of the particular patient.

Barbiturates/Tranquilizers. For sedation, barbiturates are commonly used—mainly pentobarbital (Nembutal) and secobarbital (Seconal Sodium)—as are hypnotics such as benzodiazepines (flurazepam, diazepam). However, it is worth noting that studies have shown that the reassuring visit of the anesthesiologist and operating room nurse prior to the operation has a more calming effect than the barbiturates. Nonetheless, the night before surgery a hypnotic is usually prescribed to allay insomnia.

Opiates.   Medications such as morphine and meperidine (Demerol) may be prescribed before an operation to reduce the amount of general anesthetic required. These medications can also be used to produce analgesia in patients who have pain before the operation. At the same time, it is important to realize that analgesic doses may depress respiration and the cough reflex and present an increased risk of respiratory acidosis and aspiration pneumonitis. Full doses may cause hypotension, nausea, vomiting, constipation, and abdominal distention.

Anticholinergics.   Anticholinergic medications may be prescribed to reduce respiratory tract secretions and to prevent or treat severe reflex slowing of the heart during anesthesia. They are administered also to counteract secretions that are anticipated with anesthetic induction and intubation. Atropine is frequently prescribed; however, it must be used with caution in patients with glaucoma, thyrotoxicosis, prostatic hyperplasia, or some forms of heart disease.

Because the belladonna alkaloids (atropine and scopolamine) have varying effects on pulse rate, as well as other shortcomings, a quaternary ammonium compound, glycopyrrolate (Robinul), is often used. It is an anticholinergic medication that is twice as potent an antisialagogue (reducing secretions) and acts three times as long.

Other Preanesthetic Medications.   Other medications used as preanesthetic medication are droperidol, fentanyl, or a combination of these. They should not be used with sedatives because they may cause respiratory or circulatory depression and may potentiate depressants.

Prophylactic antibiotics are administered when bacterial contamination is expected, or for the patient with a clean wound in which a prosthetic device is being inserted.

Timing of Administration of Medications.   Because preanesthetic medications should be given from 45 to 75 minutes before anesthesia is begun, it is most important that the nurse administer this medication precisely at the prescribed time; otherwise, its effect will have worn off, or it will not have begun to act when anesthesia is started.

After the preanesthetic medication is given, the patient is kept in bed because he will begin to feel lightheaded and drowsy. (If the patient is unattended, the side rails are placed in position.) If he receives atropine or glycopyrrolate (Robinul), he may be told it will make his mouth dry. During this time, the nurse observes the patient for any untoward reaction to the medications. His environment is kept quiet to assist in relaxing him.

Very frequently, operations are delayed or schedules are changed, and it becomes impossible to request that a medication be given at a specific time. In these situations, the preoperative medication is prescribed "on call from operating room." The nurse can have the medication ready to give and administer it as soon as a call is received from the operating room staff requesting that the medication be administered. It usually takes 15 to 20 minutes to prepare the patient for the operating room. If the nurse gives the medication before attending to the other details of preparing the patient, the patient will have at least partial benefit from the preoperative medication and will have a smoother and more pleasant anesthetic and operative course.

Preoperative Record

A preoperative checklist is shown in Figure 20-5. The completed chart accompanies the patient to the operating room. The informed consent form is also attached, as are all laboratory reports and nurses' records. Any unusual last-minute observations that may have a bearing on the anesthesia or surgery are to be placed at the front of the chart in a prominent place.

Transportation to the Presurgical Suite

The patient is transferred to the holding area or presurgical suite in a bed or on a previously prepared stretcher about 30 to 60 minutes before the anesthetic is to be given. The stretcher should be as comfortable as possible, with a sufficient number of blankets to ensure against chilling in air-conditioned rooms. A small pillow at the head is usually provided. The top covers of the stretcher should be long enough to tuck in around the patient at both feet and shoulders. Ideally, the nurse who has cared for the patient up to this time accompanies him to the operating room.

It is desirable to have the patient brought directly to a preoperative holding room or induction room, where he is greeted by name and made to feel that he is in safe hands. The area must be quiet if the preoperative medication is to have maximal effect. The patient should not hear undesirable sounds or conversations that might be misinterpreted or exaggerated.

- It is important that someone be with the preoperative patient at all times.

Even though he has had preoperative medication, appears to be dozing, and seems to be secure on the stretcher with a strap in place, he should not be left alone. Having someone with the patient provides reassurance as well as safety. Reassurance can be verbal as well as communicated by facial expression, manner, the warm grasp of a hand, and seeing a familiar face—the nurse who helped to prepare him before he was transferred to the operating unit, or the anesthesiologist who visited with him the day before and discussed anesthetic management.

Helping the Family Cope

Most hospitals have a special waiting room where the family can wait while the patient is undergoing surgery. This room may be equipped with comfortable chairs, television, telephones, and facilities for light refreshment. Volunteers may remain with the family, serve them coffee, and keep them informed of the patient's progress. After surgery, the surgeon may meet the family here and report his findings.

The family should never judge the seriousness of an operation by the length of time the patient is in the operating

1. Patient's name: _____ Date: _____ Height: _____ Weight: _____
   Identification band present: _____
2. Informed Consent signed: _____ Special permits signed: _____
   (Ex: Sterilization)
3. History & Physical Examination report present: _____ Date: _____
4. Laboratory records present: _____
   CBC: _____ Hb: _____ Urinalysis: _____ Hct: _____

5. Item	Present	Removed
a. Natural teeth	_____	_____
Dentures: upper, lower, partial	_____	_____
Bridge, fixed; crown	_____	_____
b. Contact lenses	_____	_____
c. Other prostheses—type: _____	_____	_____
d. Jewelry:		
Wedding band (taped/tied)	_____	_____
Rings	_____	_____
Earrings: pierced, clip-on	_____	_____
Neck chains	_____	_____
e. Make-up	_____	_____
Nail polish	_____	_____
6. Clothing		
a. Clean patient gown	_____	_____
b. Cap	_____	_____
c. Sanitary pad, *etc.*	_____	_____

7. Family instructed where to wait? _____
8. Valuables secured? _____
9. Blood available? _____ Ordered? _____ Where? _____
10. Preanesthetic medication given: _____
    Signature   Time
11. Voided: _____ Amount: _____ Time: _____ Catheter: _____
    Mouth care given: _____
12. Vital signs: Temperature: _____ Pulse: _____ Resp: _____ Blood Press: _____
13. Special problems/precautions: (Allergies, deafness, *etc.*): _____
14. Area of skin preparation: _____
15. _____ Date: _____ Time: _____
    Signature: Nurse releasing patient

Figure 20–5. Preoperative checklist.

room. He may be in surgery much longer than the actual operating time for several reasons:

- It is customary to send for the patient some time in advance of the actual operating time.
- Anesthesiologists often make additional preparations that may take from 30 to 60 minutes.
- Occasionally the surgeon takes longer than expected with the preceding case, which delays the start of the next operation.
- After surgery, the patient is taken to the recovery room to ensure satisfactory emergence from the anesthetic.

Those waiting to see the patient after the operation should be informed about the equipment that the patient may have in place when he returns to his room (*e.g.*, intravenous fluids, indwelling urinary catheter, nasogastric tube, suction bottles, air/oxygen lines, monitoring equipment, and blood transfusion lines). When the patient returns to his room, the nurse provides accurate assurances regarding the frequent postoperative observations. However, it is the responsibility of the surgeon, and not the prerogative or responsibility of the nurse, to relay the surgical findings and the prognosis, even when the findings are favorable.

Chapter Summary

Perioperative nursing involves the use of the nursing process during the patient's surgical experience and encompasses three phases: preoperative (before surgery), intraoperative (during surgery), and postoperative (after surgery).

The hallmarks of preoperative nursing are reduction of patient anxiety and patient education. Common fears that contribute to preoperative patient anxiety are fear of the unknown and of possible death, fear of anesthesia, and fear of change in body image. Listening and answering questions reduce anxiety. The content and teaching approach in patient education are individualized. Generally, preoperative patient education includes a description of the surgical procedure, the patient's role, a review of postoperative exercises, a discussion of preoperative and pain medication, and expectations of postoperative care.

The history and physical assessment performed in the preoperative phase provide the baseline for evaluating the intraoperative and postoperative courses. Data obtained from the review of systems, medication history, nutritional status, obesity, and age are collectively considered when assessing surgical risk factors and planning specific interventions.

Routine interventions include altering nutrition and fluid intake, skin preparation of surgical site, administration of preoperative medication, and completion of the preoperative checklist. Careful attention to psychologic and physical interventions prepares the patient optimally for the intraoperative phase.

Bibliography

See Bibliography for unit following Chapter 22.

21

Intraoperative Nursing and Anesthesia

Learning Objectives

On completion of this chapter, the learner will be able to:

1. Describe the interdisciplinary approach to the care of the patient during surgery
2. Describe the principles, protocols, and basic rules of surgical asepsis
3. Specify the role of the anesthesiologist in the preoperative and intraoperative care of the patient
4. Specify the risk factors related to surgery of elderly persons and nursing interventions to reduce risks to the elderly surgical patient
5. Compare the various types of anesthesia with regard to uses, advantages, disadvantages, and nursing responsibilities

Activity in the operating room centers on the patient who is undergoing a surgical procedure for the repair, correction, or relief of a physical problem. From the time the patient arrives in the operating room through the period when the anesthesia is administered, attention focuses on the psychologic as well as physiologic reactions of the patient.

Throughout the surgical experience, the nurse functions as the patient's chief advocate. The caring and concern of nursing management extend from the time when the patient is prepared for and instructed about the forthcoming operation, through the immediate preoperative period, into the operative phase and the recovery from anesthesia, and on through convalescence.

- Throughout this continuum, *priority is given to the patient, his safety, his understanding of the care he is receiving, and the biophysical and psychosocial needs he is experiencing.*

Because the operation is usually a stressful experience in the patient's life, he needs the security of knowing that someone is protecting his best interests at this time, especially when he is under anesthesia and unable to make decisions for himself.

A preoperative visit the day before (or the day of) surgery by the operating room nurse as well as the anesthesiologist/ nurse anesthetist has been documented as effective in promoting a smooth transition of the patient from the hospital unit to the operating room. Time is provided for the patient to become acquainted with what he will experience in the operating room; he is encouraged to ask questions. Later, seeing familiar faces when he is transported to surgery provides psychologic comfort.

When a patient arrives in the operating room, essentially three different groups of personnel are preparing for his care: (1) the anesthesiologist or nurse anesthetist, who administers the anesthetic agent and places the patient in the proper position on the operating table; (2) the surgeon and those assistants who scrub and perform the operation; and (3) the intraoperative nurses who manage the operating room are responsible for the safety and well-being of the patient, coordinate the many activities of the operating room personnel, and also provide care by performing scrub nurse and circulating activities during the surgery.

A recent addition has been made to the personnel of the operating room. *RN First Assistant (RNFA)* is a role that has been approved by the Association of Operating Room Nurses and endorsed by the American College of Surgeons. The practice of the RNFA depends on the scope of the state's Nurse Practice Act. Currently, the role of the RNFA is recognized as being within this scope in all but three states (New Jersey, Ohio, and Oklahoma). The RNFA practices under the direct supervision of the surgeon; responsibilities may include handling tissue, providing exposure at the operative field, using instruments, suturing, and providing hemostasis.

To ensure optimal patient care during the surgical procedure, information about the patient must be shared by the anesthesiologist or nurse anesthetist, the nurse, and the surgeon. In addition, any pertinent developments that are related to patient care in the recovery room (*e.g.*, hemorrhage, unexpected findings, fluid and electrolyte problems, shock, or respiratory difficulties) must be noted, documented, and relayed to the postanesthesia recovery room (PARR) staff.

Intraoperative Nursing Functions

Frequently, nursing functions in the operating room are described in terms of circulating and scrub activities.

The *circulating nurse* manages the operating room and protects the safety and health needs of the patient by monitoring the activities and state of the environment. She ensures cleanliness; proper temperature, humidity, and lighting; the safe functioning of equipment; and the availability of supplies and materials. The monitoring of aseptic practices to avoid breaks in technique continues as she coordinates the movement of related personnel (medical, x-ray, and laboratory). The circulating nurse also monitors the patient throughout the operative procedure to ensure that his needs are provided for and his rights upheld.

Scrub activities include scrubbing for the operation (Charts 21-1 through 21-4); setting up the sterile tables; preparing sutures, ligatures, and special equipment; assisting the surgeon and the surgical assistants during the surgical procedure by anticipating the required instruments, sponges, drains, and

(text continues on page 420)

Chart 21-1
Guidelines: Scrubbing for an Operation

Action

1. The nails are kept short and free of nail polish; special attention is given to the subungual space (beneath nail) with a sterile nail cleaner early in the scrub.
2. A soft but firm-bristled brush or one of the numerous polyurethane disposable sponges that are impregnated with soap is used for scrubbing.
3. There are many acceptable antiseptic detergents, such as the iodophors.
4. Hands and arms must be well lathered and rinsed frequently. No chemical agent can be relied upon as a substitute for conscientious mechanical cleansing of the skin.
5. The duration of the scrub may be determined by setting a time limit for the conscientious scrubbing of one part after another in a prescribed manner, or by counting a certain number of strokes per part. A practical, reliable, and effective procedure should be followed. Because the moisture and warmth present under surgical gloves provide an ideal growth medium for bacteria, it is essential that a prescribed scrub be performed between operations.
6. Following the scrub, hands and arms are rinsed thoroughly; soap and brush are left in sink or discarded in appropriate container. The elbow, knee, or foot is used to turn off the water. Hands are held higher than the elbows and away from the body.
7. When drying hands, care is taken to prevent the towel from touching the scrub dress or suit. One hand and then the arm are dried with a towel, proceeding from fingertips to elbow; the other hand and arm are dried in similar fashion using a dry segment of the towel.

Rationale

1. Scrubbing can cause nail polish to chip and peel; this would produce nicks in which microbes could breed.
2. The brush or special sponge facilitates removal of dead skin, soil, and resident organisms.
3. Broad-spectrum antimicrobial solution is preferred when gram-negative nosocomial infections predominate.
4. Microbes are removed by two actions:
   a. Physical mechanical separation
   b. Chemical antisepsis from action of antimicrobial solution
5. Individual conscientious attention to detail is important. Institutional policy is followed.
6. Holding hands higher than the elbows and away from the body allows water to run off at the elbow and prevents contaminated water (from above the elbow) from running down to the scrubbed hands.
7. Proceeding from the fingertips to the elbow prevents above-elbow sources of contamination from affecting scrubbed hands and lower arms.

Chart 21–2
Gowning

After the hands and arms are scrubbed with use of an antiseptic detergent, a sterile gown and gloves are put on. These are worn to allow the wearer to participate in or observe the surgical operation while maintaining a state of asepsis in as practical a way as possible.

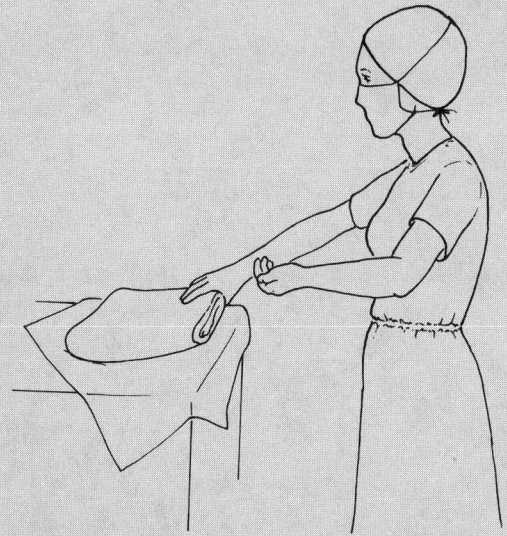

1. The sterile gown may be obtained from an open pack, or it may be handed by someone already scrubbed.

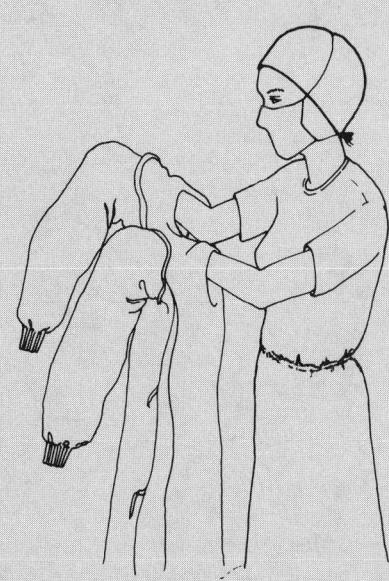

2. Because gowns are folded inside out (to eliminate the need to touch the outside of the garment), the gown can be held by the neckband and allowed to unfold from the extended hands. As the gown unfolds, the armholes should face the wearer. The hands are held upward and slipped into the armholes—but only as far as the sleeve cuff.

3. The circulating nurse can assist by reaching inside the gown and pulling the sleeves over scrubbed hands. (Sleeves are pulled to the hands, not over them, when the closed glove technique is to be used (see Chart 21–3).

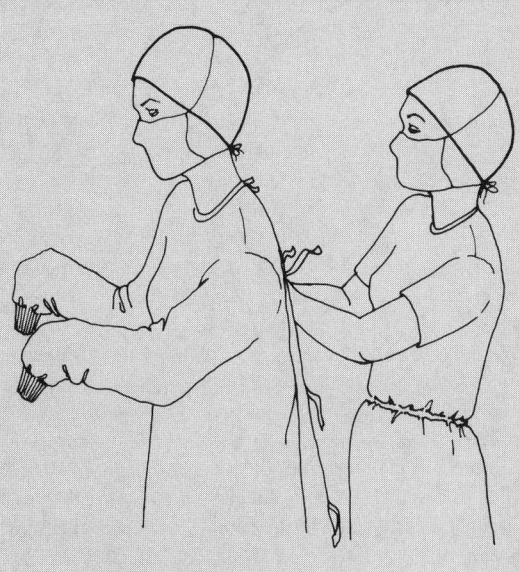

4. To secure the gown, the tapes at the back are tied. If the gown has tapes at the waist, the circulating nurse reaches for the ends of the tapes without touching the gown, draws the tapes back, and ties them. (Gowns may be fastened with Velcro, which eliminates the need for tapes.)

Note: A gown is sterile only as long as it is dry and not torn. If it is wet from perspiration or from any other cause, it is considered contaminated.

Chart 21–3
Putting on Sterile Gloves: Closed Method

When the gown is donned, the hands are slid into the sleeve only as far as the cuff seam, which is then grasped by the thumb and index finger through the fabric.

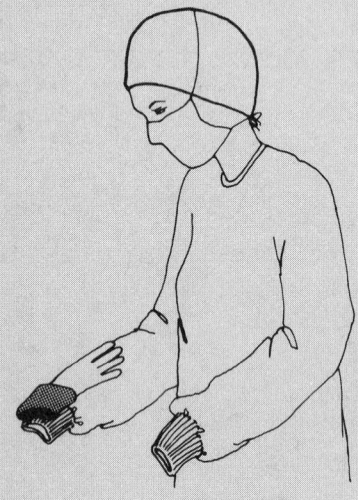

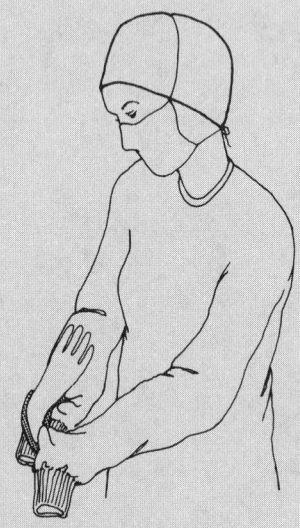

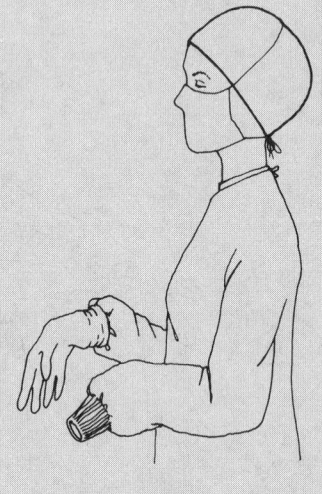

1. One glove is grasped (while the hand is still inside the sleeve) and placed thumbside down on the palmside of the other arm, with glove fingers pointing toward the shoulder. (Glove cuff lies over gown cuff.)*

2. The wrist edge of the glove that is against the sleeve is grasped with the finger that holds the seam, and the uppermost glove wrist edge is grasped with the sleeve-covered fingers of the other hand.

3. The glove wrist is pulled over the gown cuff. Care must be taken not to fold the gown cuff back or to expose the fingers inside it.

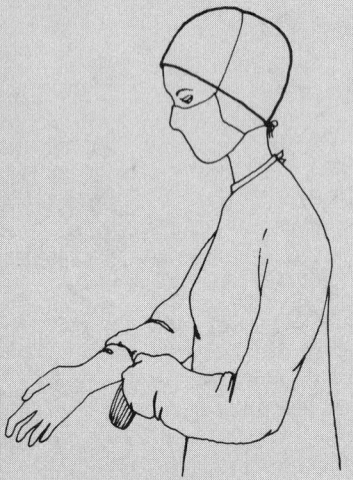

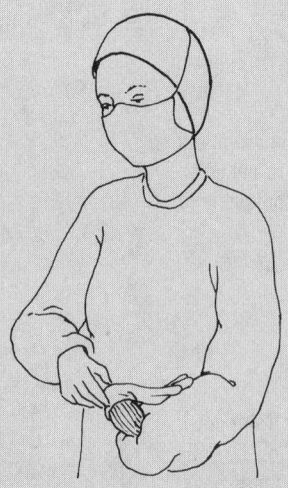

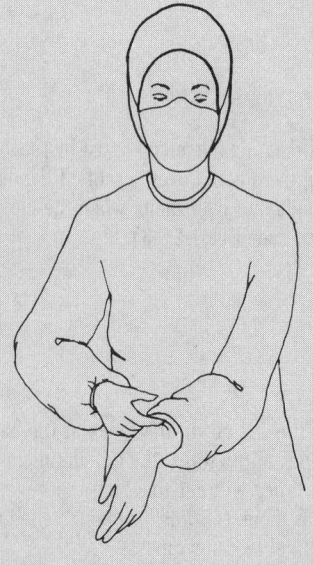

4. As the cuff is drawn onto the wrist, the fingers are directed into the glove, and the glove is adjusted to the hand.

5. The second glove is put on in the same manner, using the newly gloved hand to hold the glove.

* Shaded or crosshatched areas of the glove (representing the inside of glove) are considered unsterile.

Chart 21-4
Putting on Sterile Gloves: Open Method

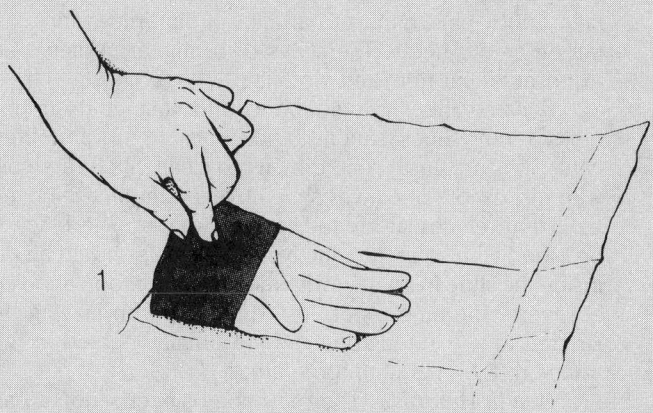

1. When the right glove is put on first, the cuff is grasped on the inside by the left hand.

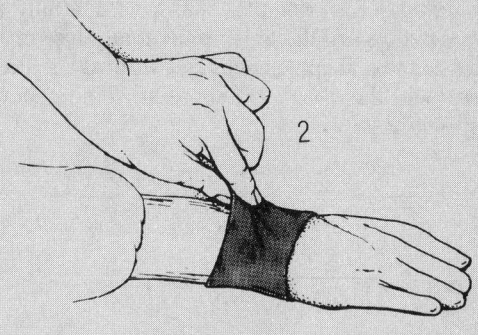

2. The right hand is inserted into the glove, which is then pulled into place with the left hand (the cuff is left in a turned-down position). The grasp is then released.

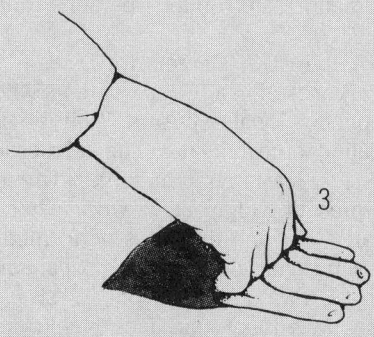

3. Now the right gloved hand can pick up the left glove by inserting the fingers under its cuff. (The outside is the sterile side.)

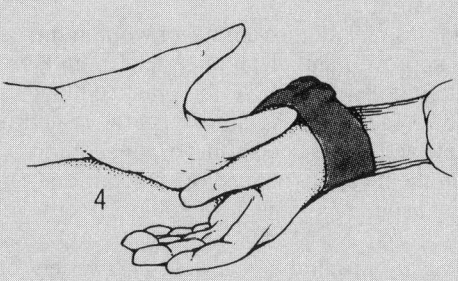

4. The left hand is inserted into the left glove and the glove is pulled into place. The cuff is left in a turned-down position.

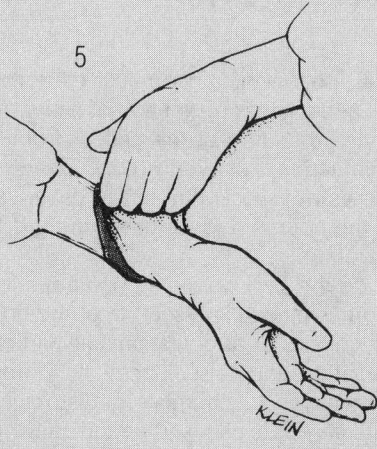

5. After folding the gown cuff snugly to the wrist, and while holding this fold in place with the sterile right gloved thumb, the fingers can safely pull the sterile glove cuff over the gown cuff.

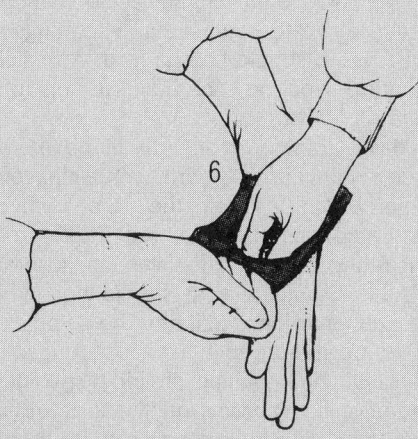

Another method: The scrub nurse holds the glove open for the person donning the gloves. The glove is held with the thumb facing the recipient. The top of the glove is spread wide so that the hand can be thrust into the glove without touching the person holding the glove. The glove cuff is pulled up over the gown cuff.

other equipment; and keeping the time the patient is under anesthesia and the time the wound is open to a minimum. Toward the end of the surgery, equipment and materials must be checked to ensure that all needles, sponges, and instruments are accounted for. In addition, specimens must be labeled and sent to the laboratory. The entire process requires a thorough understanding of the principles of asepsis, anatomy, and tissue care; an awareness of the objectives of the surgery; the knowledge and skill to anticipate needs and work as a skilled member of a team; and the ability to handle any emergency situation in the operating room.

Principles of Health and Operating Room Attire

Good health is essential for any person in the operating room. Colds, sore throats, and skin infections are sources of pathogenic organisms and must be reported. A series of wound infections in postoperative patients was traced in one instance to a mild throat infection in an operating room nurse. Therefore, the importance of reporting without delay any seemingly slight ailment is apparent.

Clothing.   Street clothes are never worn in the operating room. Only approved and clean operating room attire is permitted. Written policies describe the practice that all persons are required to follow. Dressing rooms are located near the operating suite and are reached from an outer corridor. Clothing is changed in the dressing room before entering and on leaving the operating room. Operating room attire is not worn out of the operating room.

Operating room attire is available in a variety of styles, including close-fitting cotton dresses, pants suits, and jumpsuits. When pants are worn, the ankles should have close-fitting cuffs (drawstring or knitted) to contain organisms shed from the perineum and legs. Shirts and waist drawstrings should be tucked inside the pants to prevent any accidental contact with sterile areas and again to contain skin sheddings. Garments that are wet or soiled should be changed. A fresh set of operating room attire is put on each time the person enters the operating room.

Mask.   Masks are worn at all times in the operating room for the purpose of minimizing airborne contamination. Droplets containing microorganisms from the oropharynx and nasopharynx must be contained and filtered. Therefore, the mask must be tight fitting and should cover the nose and mouth completely. At the same time, it should not interfere with breathing, speech, or vision, and it must be compact and comfortable. Forced expiration, such as that produced by talking, laughing, sneezing, and coughing, should be avoided because it deposits additional organisms on the mask. Effective disposable masks are available that have a high filtration efficiency of greater than 95%. Tests prove their superiority over gauze masks. Masks are changed at a minimum between patients and are not to be worn outside the surgery department.

Because the mask loses much of its effectiveness when it becomes moistened, it is changed between surgical procedures and more often if necessary. The mask is either on or off; it must not be allowed to hang around the neck. To prevent contamination of the hands, only the strings are handled when the mask is removed. Mask strings are tied snugly; top strings are tied at the back of the head, and bottom strings are tied at the back of the neck.

Headgear.   Headgear should completely cover the hair (head and neckline, including beard) so that single strands of hair, bobby pins, clips, or particles of dandruff or dust do not fall on sterile fields. The styles of headgear available are all disposable, lint-free, and clothlike.

Shoes.   Shoes should be comfortable and supportive; clogs, tennis shoes, sandals, and boots are not permitted because they are unsafe and difficult to clean. Shoes are covered with disposable or canvas shoe covers. Conductive covers establish an electrical ground for the wearer. The black strips provided with some conductive shoe covers should be placed inside the shoe in contact with the sole of the foot. Shoe covers are worn one time only and are removed on leaving the restricted area. Conductometers are usually located at the entrance to the operating room area.

Health Hazards.   The presence of occupational hazards in the operating room is not a new concept, but the characteristics of these hazards are changing. Internal monitoring of the operating room includes the analysis of swipe samples for infectious and toxic agents. In addition, policies and procedures for laser and radiation safety in the operating room have been established.

Since 1987, the CDC (Centers for Disease Control) has reported several cases of health care workers who contracted AIDS through occupational exposure. With the spread of the HIV virus, operating room attire has changed drastically. Double gloving is routine, at least in trauma surgery where sharp bone fragments are present. Goggles are worn when the surgical wound is irrigated or bone drilling is performed. In addition to the routine scrub suit and double gloves, some surgeons wear rubber boots, a waterproof apron, and sleeve protectors. In bloody cases, a wraparound face shield substitutes for goggles.

Principles of Perioperative Asepsis

Throughout all phases of the surgical experience, the main priority for all personnel is prevention of patient complications, which includes protection of the patient from infection. The possibility of infection is markedly reduced by strict adherence to the principles of asepsis during the patient's preoperative preparation, the course of the operation, and the healing of the surgical wound.

To provide the best possible conditions for surgery, the operating room is placed in a section of the hospital where it is free from such hazards as contaminating particles, dust, other pollutants, radiation, and noise. Electrical hazards, conductivity checks, emergency exit clearances, and storage of equipment and anesthetic gases are checked periodically by the state and the Joint Commission for the Accreditation of Healthcare Organizations (JCAHO).

In surgical practice, asepsis prevents the contamination of surgical wounds. Although postoperative wound infection may be caused by natural skin flora or a previously existing infection, it is the responsibility of the personnel in the operating room to use aseptic principles to minimize this risk. The following discussion on protocols illustrates how principles of asepsis are carried out in practice.

Protocols

Preoperative

Before the operation, all surgical material must be sterilized; this includes any instruments, needles, sutures, dressings, gloves, covers, and solutions that may come in contact with the wound and exposed tissues. In addition, the surgeon, surgical assistants, and nurses must prepare themselves by scrubbing their hands and arms with soap and water and donning long-sleeved, sterile gowns and gloves. Head and hair are covered with a cap, and a mask is worn over the nose and mouth to minimize the possibility of bacteria from the upper respiratory tract entering the wound. The patient's skin, over an area considerably larger than that requiring exposure during the course of the operation, also requires meticulous cleansing followed by the application of an antiseptic agent. The remainder of the patient's body is covered with sterile drapes.

Intraoperative

During the operation, the personnel who have scrubbed touch only those objects that were sterilized. Nonscrubbed personnel refrain from touching or contaminating anything that is sterile.

Postoperative

After the operation, the wound is protected from possible contamination by means of sterile dressings and by the use of sterile saline and antiseptics when the wound is cleansed and the dressings changed. Particular care is taken to protect the unhealed wound from coming in contact with anything that is not sterile.

When infection has already developed in tissues, antimicrobials specific for the offending organism are prescribed and heat is applied or drainage established to assist the body in eliminating the offending organisms. It may be necessary to remove and destroy microorganisms that are already in the tissues by removing, or débriding, devitalized tissues. To prevent subsequent infection from external sources, rigid aseptic technique must be followed during the course of treatment.

Environmental Controls

In addition to the above-mentioned protocols, the implementation of aseptic principles requires meticulous housekeeping in the operating room. Floors and horizontal surfaces are cleaned frequently with detergent soap and water or detergent germicide, and sterilizing equipment is inspected regularly to ensure optimal operation and performance. Prepackaged sterilized linens, drapes, and solutions are used; instruments are cleaned and sterilized in a unit near the operating room. Individually wrapped sterile items are used when additional individual items are needed.

Many operating rooms are equipped with laminar air flow systems that filter out a high percentage of dust and bacteria. Originally designed for spacecraft, these systems use high-efficiency particulate air (HEPA) filters to remove more than 99% of airborne particles measuring 0.3 μm or more. Laminar flow also exchanges air more effectively—about 200 times an hour—as compared with air conditioning, which exchanges air 12 times per hour.

Unfortunately, despite all these precautions, postoperative wound contamination may occasionally occur during an operation, appearing days or weeks later in the form of an incisional infection or abscess.

Constant surveillance and conscientious technique in carrying out aseptic practices must be stressed continually because errors and misjudgments can occur.

Basic Rules of Surgical Asepsis

General
- Sterile surfaces or articles may touch other sterile surfaces or articles and remain sterile; contact with unsterile objects at any point renders a sterile area contaminated.
- If there is any doubt about the sterility of an article or area, it is considered unsterile.
- Whatever is sterile for one patient (an opened sterile tray or tables with sterile supplies) can be used for this patient only. Unused sterile supplies must be discarded or resterilized if they are to be used again.

Personnel
- Scrubbed personnel remain in the area of the operation; if a scrubbed person leaves the room, that person's sterile status is lost. To return to the operation, this person is required to go through the procedure of scrubbing, gowning, and gloving.
- Only a small part of a scrubbed person's body is considered sterile: from front waist to the shoulder area; forearms and gloves. Therefore, the gloved hands must be kept in front between the shoulders and waistline.
- In some operating rooms, a special wraparound gown is worn, which extends the sterile area.
- The circulating nurse and any unscrubbed personnel remain at a safe distance to avoid contamination of any sterile area.

Draping
- During draping of a table or patient, the sterile drape is held well above the surface to be covered and is positioned from front to back.
- Only the top of the patient or table that is draped is considered sterile; drapes hanging over the edge are not regarded as sterile.
- Sterile drapes are kept in position by the use of clips or adherent material; drapes are not moved during the operation. A tear or puncture of the drape permitting access to an unsterile surface underneath renders the area unsterile. Such a drape must be replaced.

Delivery of Sterile Supplies
- Packages are wrapped or sealed in such a way that they can be opened easily without risk of contaminating contents.
- Sterile supplies, including solutions, are delivered to a sterile field or handed to a "scrubbed" person in such a way that sterility of the object or fluid remains intact.
- Edges of wrappers covering sterile supplies or outer lips of bottles or flasks containing sterile solutions are not considered sterile.
- The unsterile arm of the circulating nurse must not extend over a sterile area. Sterile articles are to be dropped onto the

sterile field, a reasonable distance from the edge of the sterile area.

Solutions

- Sterile solutions are poured from a point high enough to prevent accidental touching of the sterile receiving cup or basin, but not so high as to produce splashing. (When a sterile surface becomes wet, it is contaminated.)

The Patient Undergoing Anesthesia

The Patient and the Anesthesiologist

An *anesthesiologist* is a physician specifically trained in the art and the science of anesthesiology. After consulting with the surgeon, the anesthesiologist usually selects the anesthesia and deals with any technical problems relating to the administration of the anesthetic agent and supervision of the patient's condition during the operation.

An *anesthetist* is a qualified nurse, dentist, physician, or anesthesia assistant who administers anesthetics. Most anesthetists are nurses who have graduated from an accredited nurse anesthesia program and have passed certification by the American Association of Nurse Anesthetists to become certified registered nurse anesthetists (CRNA).

The surgical patient is usually interested in and concerned about the anesthesia that he is to receive. He has listened to the experiences and hearsay of friends and relatives, may have read about anesthesia, and has formed opinions about the merits or demerits of various methods in use. Therefore, it is helpful for the anesthesiologist/anesthetist to visit the patient in his room before the operation to inform, answer questions, and allay any fears that may exist in the patient's mind. Choice of anesthetic agent is discussed, and the patient has an opportunity to disclose previous reactions as well as to reiterate the medications he is currently taking that may affect the choice of an agent (see p. 406).

During this essential visit, the anesthesiologist assesses the condition of the patient's cardiovascular system and lungs and inquires about any preexisting pulmonary infections and the extent to which the patient smokes. The patient's general physical condition must also be assessed because it may affect the management of anesthesia (Table 21-1).

On the day of surgery, the patient is transported to the operating room and transferred to the operating table, where the anesthesiologist or nurse anesthetist again assesses his condition; blood pressure, pulse, and respiratory rate, in particular, are noted. Then induction of the anesthetic occurs.

During the course of surgery, the anesthesiologist monitors the patient's blood pressure, pulse, and respirations as well as the electrocardiogram, tidal volume, blood gas levels, blood pH, alveolar gas concentrations, and body temperature. Monitoring by electroencephalograph may be required in some instances. Anesthetic levels in the body can also be determined; a mass spectrometer is able to provide instant readouts of the critical concentration levels on strategically located display terminals.

After surgery when the patient is recovering from the anesthetic, the mass spectrometer can reveal the concentration of gaseous anesthetic still remaining in the patient. When he breathes on his own, the device assesses his ability to breathe unassisted and indicates the need for mechanical assistance.

Gerontologic Considerations

By the year 2000, it is estimated that there will be 35 million people over the age of 65 in the United States. As the percentage of the elderly population grows, increasing numbers of older patients are undergoing surgical procedures. Elderly patients face higher risks from anesthesia and surgery than do other adults. Statistically, perioperative risk increases with each decade over 60. However, with modifications tailored to the

TABLE 21-1. *Classification of Physical Status for Anesthesia Before Surgery*

Classification	Description	Example
1. Good	No organic disease, no systemic disturbance	Uncomplicated hernias, fractures
2. Fair	Mild to moderate systemic disturbance	Mild cardiac (I and II), mild diabetes
3. Poor	Severe systemic disturbance	Poorly controlled diabetes, pulmonary complications, moderate cardiac (III)
4. Serious	Systemic disease threatening life	Severe renal disease, severe cardiac disease (IV), decompensation
5. Moribund	Little chance of survival but submitting to operation in desperation	Massive pulmonary embolus, ruptured abdominal aneurysm with profound shock
E. Emergency	Any of the above when surgery is performed in an emergency situation	An uncomplicated hernia that is now strangulated and associated with nausea and vomiting; designation 1(E)
		If classification is 3 and an emergency, the designation is 3(E)

(American Society of Anesthesiology, Inc. Codes for the Collection and Tabulation of Data Relating to Anesthesia, Inhalation Therapy and Therapeutic Diagnostic Blocks.)

biologic changes that occur in the later decades of life (Fig. 21-1) and the application of research findings for this population, the risks are lowered. The following examples illustrate some of these changes and interventions.

With aging, the heart and blood vessels have a decreased ability to respond to stress. Cardiac changes include reduced cardiac output and limited cardiac reserve. With a reduced vascular bed, the elderly are prone to thermoregulatory problems and may require extra body covering to maintain body temperature. With diminished ciliary action and a less effective cough reflex, there is an increased risk of pneumonia. Reduced gas exchange adds to the risk of cerebral hypoxia.

In terms of surgery, an older person needs less anesthetic agent to produce anesthesia, and it takes longer to eliminate anesthetic drugs. One reason for reduction of anesthesia dosage is that, as people age, the percentage of fatty tissue steadily increases (from 20% to 30% at age 20, to 35% to 45% at age 60 to 70). Anesthetic agents that have an affinity for fatty tissue concentrate in body fat and the brain. In addition, there is a shrinkage of the body tissues that are made up predominantly of water and have a rich blood supply, such as skeletal muscle, liver, and kidney. Reduction in liver size decreases the rate at which the liver can inactivate many anesthetics. The decreased functioning of kidney cells reduces excretion of waste products and anesthetics.

Careful manipulation and positioning are required during surgery because of the normal bone loss in the elderly (25% in women; 12% in men). With intravenous infusions, an excessive amount or rapid rate may cause pulmonary edema. A sudden or prolonged drop in blood pressure may lead to cerebral ischemia, thrombosis, embolism, infarction, and anoxemia.

The reduced ability of the elderly to adjust rapidly to physical and emotional stress influences surgical outcomes. As expected, the mortality rate is higher with emergency surgery than it is with elective surgery. Consequently, continuous and careful monitoring with rapid intervention is essential for gerontologic surgical patients.

Anesthesia: An Overview

Anesthesia is a state of narcosis, analgesia, relaxation, and reflex loss. Inhalation anesthesia is the most popular because of its controllability. The intake and elimination of the agent is in large measure affected by pulmonary ventilation. Greater depth or plane of anesthesia requires greater concentration of the agent.

Anesthetics are divided into two classes according to whether they suspend sensation (1) in the whole body (general anesthesia) or (2) in parts of the body (local, regional, epidural, or spinal anesthesia).

General Anesthesia

General anesthesia is most commonly achieved by inhalation or by intravenous techniques.

Volatile liquid anesthetics produce anesthesia when their vapors are inhaled. Included in this group are halothane, enflurane, and isoflurane. All are administered with oxygen, and usually with nitrous oxide as well (Table 21-2).

Gas anesthetics are administered by inhalation and always combined with oxygen. This group of anesthetics includes nitrous oxide (Table 21-3).

The substances, when inhaled, enter the blood through the pulmonary capillaries and, when in sufficient concentration, act on the cerebral centers to produce loss of consciousness and sensation. When administration of the anesthetic is discontinued, the vapor or gas is eliminated by way of the lungs.

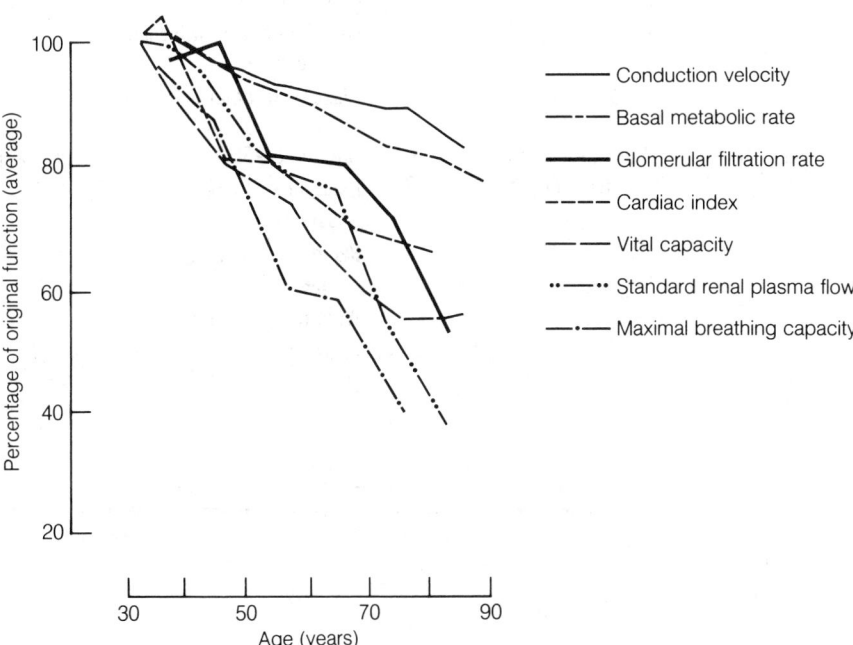

Figure 21-1. Decline in function as a result of age. (Adapted from Miller RD. Anesthesia for the elderly. New York, Churchill Livingstone.)

TABLE 21-2.   *Volatile Liquids as Agents of General Anesthesia*

Agent	Administration	Advantages	Disadvantages	Implications
Halothane (Fluothane)	Inhalation; special vaporizer	Not explosive or flammable Induction rapid and smooth Useful in almost every type of surgery Low incidence of postoperative nausea and vomiting	Requires skillful administration to prevent overdosage May cause liver damage May produce hypotension Requires special vaporizer for administration	In addition to observation of pulse and respiration postoperatively, it is important that blood pressure be monitored frequently.
Methoxyflurane (Penthrane)	Inhalation; special vaporizer	Nonflammable Seldom causes postoperative nausea and vomiting Analgesic action continues several hours after surgery Excellent muscle relaxation	Requires skillful administration Renal damage may occur Unpleasant odor	Prolonged postoperative depressant action calls for careful observation by recovery room personnel.
Enflurane (Ethrane)	Inhalation	Rapid induction and recovery Potent analgesic Not explosive or flammable	Respiratory depression may develop rapidly along with EEG abnormalities Not compatible with epinephrine	Observe for possible respiratory depression. Administration with epinephrine may cause ventricular fibrillation.
Isoflurane (Forane)	Inhalation	Rapid induction and recovery Muscle relaxants are markedly potentiated	This is a profound respiratory depressant.	Respirations must be monitored closely and supported when necessary.

TABLE 21-3.   *Gases as Agents of General Anesthesia*

Agent	Administration	Advantages	Disadvantages	Implications
Nitrous oxide (N_2O)	Inhalation (semiclosed method)	Induction and recovery rapid Nonflammable Useful with oxygen for short procedures Useful with other agents for all types of surgery	Poor relaxant Weak anesthetic May produce hypoxia	Most useful in conjunction with other agents with longer action Observe precautions with "other agents"
Cyclopropane (C_3H_6)	Inhalation (closed method)	Good relaxant Useful for all types of surgery Rapid induction and emergence Wide margin of safety Pleasant	Explosive Powerful depressant; therefore should be administered skillfully Frequently produces disturbances in heart rhythm May cause bronchospasm and acidosis	Use precautions against explosions. Because cyclopropane may be followed by hypotension, it is important to observe blood pressure postoperatively.

Physiologic and Physical Factors. General anesthetics produce anesthesia because they are delivered to the brain at high partial pressure. Relatively large amounts of anesthetic must be administered during induction and the early maintenance phases because the anesthetic is recirculated and deposited in body tissues. As these sites become saturated, smaller amounts of the anesthetic agent are required to maintain anesthesia because equilibrium or near equilibrium has been achieved between brain, blood, and other tissues. Anything that diminishes peripheral blood flow, such as vasoconstriction or a condition of shock, may cause only small amounts of anesthetic to be required. Conversely, when peripheral blood flow is unusually high, as in the muscularly active or the apprehensive patient, induction is slower and larger quantities of anesthetic are required because the brain receives a smaller quantity of anesthetic.

Methods of Administration. Liquid anesthetics may be administered by mixing the vapors with oxygen or nitrous oxide–oxygen and then having the patient inhale the mixture. The vapor is conducted to the patient via a tube and a mask.

The endotracheal technique for administering anesthetics consists of introducing a soft rubber or plastic endotracheal tube into the trachea by means of a flexible fiberoptic endoscope, either by exposing the larynx with a laryngoscope or by passing the tube "blindly." It may be inserted through either the nose or mouth (Fig. 21-2). When in place, the endotracheal tube seals the lungs off from the esophagus, so that if the patient vomits, none of the stomach contents enter the lungs.

Stages of General Anesthesia

Anesthesia consists of four stages, each of which presents a definite group of signs and symptoms. When narcotics and neuromuscular blockers (relaxants) are administered, several of the stages are absent.

Stage I: Beginning Anesthesia. As the patient breathes in the anesthetic mixture, he may have warmth, dizziness, and a feeling of detachment. He experiences a ringing, roaring, or buzzing in the ears and, though still conscious, is aware that he is unable to move his extremities easily. During this stage, noises are exaggerated; even low voices or minor sounds appear distressingly loud and unreal. For this reason, unnecessary noise or motion must be prevented when anesthesia is started.

Stage II: Excitement. The excitement stage—characterized variously by struggling, shouting, talking, singing, laughing, or even crying—frequently may be avoided by the smooth and rapid administration of the anesthetic. The pupils become dilated but contract if exposed to light; the pulse rate is rapid and respirations irregular.

Because of the uncontrolled movements of the patient during this stage, the anesthesiologist must always be attended by someone ready to help restrain the patient. A strap may be in place across the thighs of the patient, and the hands are secured to an armboard. The patient should not be touched except for purposes of restraint, but restraints should not be applied over the operative site. Manipulation increases circulation to the operative site, and therefore the potential for bleeding also increases.

Stage III: Surgical Anesthesia. Surgical anesthesia is reached by continued administration of the vapor or gas. The patient is unconscious, lying quietly on the table. The pupils are small but will contract on exposure to light. Respirations

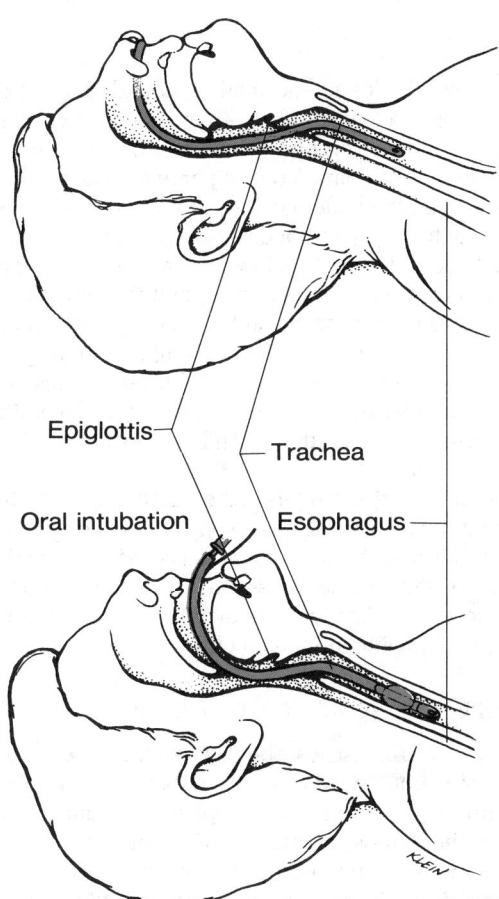

Intranasal intubation

Figure 21–2. Endotracheal anesthesia. (**Top**) Nasal endotracheal catheter in proper position. (**Bottom**) Oral endotracheal intubation; tube in position with cuff inflated. For both methods, the head is tilted back to permit the airway to be open.

are regular, pulse has a normal rate and volume; the skin is pink or slightly flushed. With proper administration of the anesthetic, this stage may be maintained for hours in one of several planes, ranging from light (1) to deep (4), depending on the depth of anesthesia needed.

Stage IV: Overdosage. This stage is reached when too much anesthesia has been administered. Respirations become shallow, the pulse weak and thready; the pupils become widely dilated and no longer contract when exposed to light. Cyanosis develops and, unless prompt action is taken, death follows rapidly. If this stage should develop, the anesthetic is discontinued immediately, and respiratory and circulatory support are necessary to prevent death. Stimulants, although rarely used, may be administered if an overdosage of anesthetic has been given. Narcotic antagonists can be used if overdosage is due to narcotics.

During smooth administration of an anesthetic there is, of course, no sharp division between the first three stages, and there is no Stage IV. The patient passes gradually from one stage to another, and it is only by close observation of the signs exhibited by the patient that an anesthesiologist can control the situation. The responses of the pupils, the blood pressure, and the respiratory and cardiac rates are probably the most reliable guides to the patient's condition.

Other Physiologic Changes

The administration of an anesthetic is attended by other physiologic activities. A few anesthetics may produce hypersecretion of mucus and saliva. This may be minimized by the preoperative administration of atropine. Vomiting or regurgitation may occur, especially when the patient comes to the operating room with a full stomach. If gagging occurs, the patient is turned to the side, the head of the table is lowered, and a basin is provided to collect the vomitus. A suction apparatus is always available and is used to remove saliva and vomited gastric contents.

During anesthesia, the patient's temperature may fall, and therefore every precaution must be taken against chilling. Warm, cotton blankets should be available (see Hypothermia). Glucose metabolism is reduced, and as a result, metabolic acidosis may develop.

In addition to the dangers of the anesthetic itself, the anesthesiologist must guard against asphyxia. This may be caused by foreign bodies in the mouth, spasm of the vocal cords, relaxation of the tongue, or aspiration of vomitus, saliva, or blood. These complications are avoided by the use of an endotracheal tube with an inflated cuff.

Intravenous Barbiturate Anesthesia

General anesthesia also can be produced by the intravenous injection of various substances, such as thiopental (Table 21-4). A short-acting barbiturate, thiopental sodium (Pentothal), is the anesthetic most commonly used for this purpose. This substance leads to unconsciousness within 30 seconds.

Advantages. The onset of anesthesia is pleasant; there is none of the buzzing, roaring, or dizziness known to follow administration of an inhalation anesthetic. For this reason, induction of anesthesia with an intravenous agent is preferred by patients who have experienced various methods. The duration of action is brief, and the patient awakens with little nausea or vomiting. Thiopental is often administered with other anesthetic agents in prolonged procedures.

Intravenous anesthetic agents have the advantages of being nonexplosive, requiring little equipment, and being easy to administer. The low incidence of postoperative nausea and vomiting makes the method useful in eye surgery, in which vomiting increases intraocular pressure and endangers vision in the operated eye. Intravenous anesthesia is useful for short procedures but is used less often for the longer procedure of abdominal surgery. It is not indicated for children, who have small veins and require intubation because of their susceptibility to respiratory obstruction.

Disadvantages. Thiopental is a powerful depressant of breathing, and its chief toxic effect results from this characteristic. It must be administered by skilled anesthesiologists and nurse anesthetists, and only when some method of giving oxygen is available immediately should difficulty arise. Sneezing, coughing, and laryngospasm are sometimes noted with its use.

Adjunctive Agents: Neuromuscular Blockers

Neuromuscular blockers (muscle relaxants) are agents that block transmission of nerve impulses at the neuromuscular junction of skeletal muscles. Goals in using muscle relaxants are to relax muscles in abdominal and thoracic surgery, relax eye muscles in certain kinds of eye surgery, facilitate endotracheal intubation, treat laryngospasm, and assist in mechanical ventilation.

Purified curare was the first widely used muscle relaxant; tubocurarine was isolated as the active principle. Succinylcholine was later introduced because it acts more rapidly than curare. Several other agents have since been introduced (Table 21-5). The ideal muscle relaxant has the following characteristics:

TABLE 21-4. *Intravenous Anesthetic Agents*

Agent	Administration	Advantages	Disadvantages	Implications
BARBITURATES				
Thiopental sodium (Pentothal)	Intravenous injection (or rectal)	Rapid induction Nonexplosive Requires little equipment Low incidence of postoperative nausea and vomiting	Powerful depressant of breathing Poor relaxant Sometimes produces coughing, sneezing, and laryngospasm Not useful for children because of small veins	Requires intelligent and close observation because of potency and rapidity of drug action.
NARCOTICS				
Meperidine hydrochloride (Demerol)	Intravenously Subcutaneously Intramuscularly	Prompt onset Because of spasmolytic effect, it is drug of choice for surgery of bile duct, distal colon, and rectum; easily detoxified and excreted	May slow rate of respirations Adverse reactions: dizziness, nausea, and vomiting	In some patients, histamine may be released; treatment is diphenhydramine (Benadryl).

(continued)

TABLE 21–4. *(Continued)*

Agent	Administration	Advantages	Disadvantages	Implications
NARCOTICS *(continued)*				
Morphine (high doses)	Intravenously	Not a myocardial depressant	Can depress arterial blood pressure by decreasing systemic vascular resistance Does not provide good amnesia Does not promote adequate muscular relaxation	Orthostatic hypotension may occur after morphine.

NEUROLEPTANALGESICS

The term *neuroleptanalgesic* refers to the combination of a short-acting synthetic narcotic agent (fentanyl) and a butyrophenone (droperidol). Patient becomes very drowsy; responds to voice command, although analgesia is profound. Of significance: The combination produces peripheral vasodilation followed by a decrease in arterial blood pressure. If administered rapidly, it may cause skeletal muscular rigidity and possibly respiratory impairment.

Agent	Administration	Advantages	Disadvantages	Implications
Fentanyl (Sublimaze; related chemically to meperidine)	Intravenously Transdermally	75–100 times more potent than morphine and about 25% of duration of morphine (IV) Little effect on cardiovascular system	In very high dosage, an alpha-adrenergic blocking effect Respiratory depression	Short duration of action is due to its more rapid redistribution and more active metabolism by liver than other narcotics.
Sufentanil	Injection	Onset, extremely rapid		Duration only about one third that of fentanyl.

DISSOCIATIVE AGENTS

When under dissociative analgesia, the patient appears not to be asleep or anesthetized, but rather dissociated from the surroundings.

Agent	Administration	Advantages	Disadvantages	Implications
Ketamine (Ketalar; Ketaject)	Intravenously Intramuscularly	Rapid induction and short action; often used to supplement nitrous oxide Useful when hypotension may be hazardous; can be administered as analgesic or anesthetic	May cause elevated blood pressure and depressed respirations Patient may experience hallucinations Vomiting and aspiration may occur	Avoid verbal, visual, or tactile stimulation because this may trigger psychic aberration. Droperidol or diazepam (see below) may eliminate such psychic phenomena. Observe for signs of respiratory depression. Keep resuscitation equipment nearby.

TRANQUILIZERS

Agent	Administration	Advantages	Disadvantages	Implications
Benzodiazepines Diazepam (Valium) Chlordiazepoxide (Librium)	Intravenously Orally Intramuscularly	Preoperative sedation Intraoperative tranquilization during regional anesthesia Production of hypnosis during anesthetic induction	Absorbed unpredictably when given intramuscularly	IV administration may produce thrombophlebitis (central vein therefore is preferred).
Droperidol (Inapsine)	Intravenously	Long duration of action	Weak antihistaminic action and alpha-adrenergic blocking action; inhibition of basic ganglionic dopaminergic pathways—may lead to extrapyramidal rigidity resembling parkinsonism	Major tranquilizer Keep IV fluids and vasopressors available for hypotension.

- Is nondepolarizing, with an onset time and duration of action similar to those of succinylcholine but without its problems of bradycardia and cardiac dysrhythmias
- Has a duration of action between those of succinylcholine and pancuronium
- Lacks cumulative and cardiovascular effects
- Is metabolizable and does not depend on the kidneys for its elimination

Regional Anesthesia

Regional anesthesia is a form of local anesthesia in which an anesthetic agent is injected around nerves so that the area supplied by these nerves is anesthetized. The effect depends on the type of nerve involved. Motor fibers are the largest and have the thickest myelin sheath. Sympathetic fibers are the smallest and have a minimal covering. Sensory fibers are intermediary. Thus, a local anesthetic blocks motor nerves least readily and sympathetic nerves most readily. An anesthetic cannot be regarded as having "worn off" until all three systems (motor, sensory, and autonomic) are no longer affected by the anesthetic.

The patient under spinal or local anesthesia is awake and aware of his surroundings. Careless conversation, unnecessary noise, and unpleasant odors must be avoided—these may be noticed by the patient in the operating room and may contribute to a negative view of the patient toward the surgical experience. A quiet environment is therapeutic. Even the diagnosis must not be stated aloud if the patient is not to know it at this time.

TABLE 21–5. *Muscle Relaxants*

Muscle Relaxant	Action	Advantages	Disadvantages	Uses and Comments
NONDEPOLARIZING NEUROMUSCULAR BLOCKING AGENTS				
Tubocurarine chloride (Tubarine)	Peaks at 30–60 min	50%–70% excreted unchanged in 3–6 hr	Histamine-like reaction; Hypotension; Increased airway resistance; Skin erythema	Contraindicated with history of allergy, asthma
Gallamine (Flaxedil)	1/5 as potent as curare; Lasts 25% shorter than curare; Blocks vagal ganglia in heart	All excreted unchanged	Tachycardia	Used well with cyclopropane or halothane
Pancuronium bromide (Pavulon)	Similar to curare but 5 times more potent; Duration, 60–85 min	Safe; stable; Good muscle relaxant; Reversible by neostigmine and atropine		Excellent for situations requiring complete relaxation; Avoid with myasthenia gravis or renal disease; Avoid with patients sensitive to bromide
Vecuronium bromide (Norcuron)	Blocks depolarization	Facilitates endotracheal intubation; good muscle relaxant	Prolonged dose-related apnea	Related to Pavulon; Well tolerated in patients with renal failure

DEPOLARIZING NEUROMUSCULAR BLOCKING AGENTS

These mimic the action of acetycholine at the neuromuscular junction.
Acetylcholine is discharged almost immediately on release → repolarization of muscle takes place. When depolarizing neuromuscular blocking agents are used, skeletal muscle depolarizes.

Succinylcholine (Anectine; Sucostrin)	Onset is rapid: 1 min; Duration: 4–8 min	Ideal for endotracheal intubation, fracture reduction; treatment of laryngospasm	Contraindicated for patients with low pseudocholinesterase; On second IV injection, bradycardia and various dysrhythmias; May cause fasciculations of the muscles and pain	Used to treat laryngospasm, status asthmaticus, and toxic reactions to local anesthetic drugs
Decamethonium bromide (Syncurine)	Onset: 30–40 sec; Duration: 15–20 min	Excreted unchanged by kidney	Some fasciculation of muscle: jaw masseter muscles; posterior calf muscles; Difficult to reverse its action	Produces depolarization of end plate region

Spinal Anesthesia

Spinal anesthesia is a type of extensive conduction nerve block that occurs by introducing a local anesthetic into the subarachnoid space at the lumbar level (usually L-2). It produces anesthesia of the lower extremities, perineum, and lower abdomen. For the lumbar puncture procedure, the patient lies on his side in a knee–chest position. With the use of sterile technique, a spinal puncture is made and the medication is injected through the needle. As soon as the injection has been made, the patient is placed on his back. If a relatively high level of block is sought, the head and shoulders are lowered. The spread of the anesthetic agent and the level of anesthesia depend on the amount of fluid injected, the rapidity with which it is injected, the positioning of the patient after the injection, and the specific gravity of the agent. If the specific gravity of the agent is greater than that of cerebrospinal fluid (CSF), the drug moves to the dependent position of the subarachnoid space; if the specific gravity is less than that of CSF, the drug moves away from the dependent portion. These boundaries are controlled by the anesthesiologist. Generally, the drugs used are procaine, tetracaine (Pontocaine), and lidocaine (Xylocaine) (Table 21-6).

In a few minutes, anesthesia and paralysis affect the toes and perineum and then gradually affect the legs and abdomen. If the anesthetic drug reaches the upper thoracic and cervical cord in high concentration, a temporary respiratory paralysis, partial or complete, may occur. Paralysis of the respiratory muscles is managed by maintaining artificial respiration until the effects of the drug on the respiratory nerves have worn off.

Nausea, vomiting, and pain may occur during surgery under spinal anesthesia. As a rule, these reactions result from traction on various structures, particularly those within the abdominal cavity. Such reactions may be avoided by the simultaneous intravenous administration of a weak solution of thiopental and inhalation of nitrous oxide.

Headache may occur as a postoperative complication. Several factors are involved in the incidence of headache: the size of the spinal needle used, the leakage of fluid from the subarachnoid space through the puncture site, and the degree of the patient's hydration. Measures that increase cerebrospinal pressure are helpful in relieving headache. These include keeping the patient flat, quiet, and well hydrated.

Nursing Assessment After Spinal Anesthesia. In addition to monitoring vital signs, the nurse observes these patients closely and records the time when motion and sensation of the legs and the toes return. When there is complete return of sensation in the toes (in response to pinprick), the patient may be considered to have recovered from the effects of the spinal drug.

Serial (Continuous) Spinal Anesthesia. The tip of a plastic catheter may be left in the subarachnoid space during operation so that more anesthetic may be injected as needed. Greater control of dosage is afforded by this technique. However, there is greater potential for postanesthetic headache because of the large-gauge needle used.

Conduction Blocks

There are many types of conduction blocks depending on the various nerve groups that are injected.

Epidural Block. Epidural anesthesia is obtained by the injection of a local anesthetic into the spinal canal in the space surrounding the dura mater. The neurologic sequelae, notably headache, that occasionally result from subarachnoid injection are avoided.

Advantages of epidural anesthesia are the absence of neurologic complications and slightly less disturbance of blood pressure. As a result, its use is increasing. One disadvantage lies in the greater technical challenge of introducing the anesthetic into the epidural rather than the subarachnoid space. Another is that the level of anesthesia is less controllable.

Brachial Plexus Block. A brachial plexus block produces anesthesia of the arm.

Paravertebral Anesthesia. Paravertebral anesthesia produces anesthesia of the nerves supplying the chest, abdominal wall, and extremities.

Transsacral (Caudal) Block. A transsacral block produces anesthesia of the perineum and, occasionally, the lower abdomen.

Local Infiltration Anesthesia

Infiltration anesthesia is the injection of a solution containing the local anesthetic into the tissues at the planned incision site. Often, it is combined with a local regional block by injection of nerves immediately supplying the area. The advantages of local anesthesia are as follows:

- It is simple, economical, and nonexplosive. The amount of equipment is minimal. Postoperative recovery is shortened.
- Undesirable effects of general anesthesia are avoided.
- It is ideal for short and superficial operations.

Local anesthesia is often administered in combination with epinephrine. Epinephrine causes constriction of blood vessels,

TABLE 21-6. *Spinal Anesthetic Agents*

Agent	Advantages of Spinal Anesthesia (Includes All Agents)	Disadvantages of Spinal Anesthesia (Includes All Agents)
Procaine (Novocaine) Tetracaine (Pontocaine) Lidocaine (Xylocaine)	Easily administered by a physician Inexpensive Minimum of equipment required Rapid onset Excellent muscular relaxation	Blood pressure may fall rapidly unless monitored carefully and treated with medications such as ephedrine. If the spinal anesthesia ascends to the chest, there may be respiratory difficulties. Occasionally postoperative complications occur, such as headache or, rarely, meningitis or paralysis.

which prevents rapid absorption of the anesthetic drug and thus prolongs its local action; rapid absorption into the bloodstream, which could cause convulsions, is also prevented. Different types of local anesthetic agents are listed in Table 21-7.

Contraindications.   Local anesthesia is the anesthesia of choice in any operation in which it can be used. However, it is contraindicated for operations on highly nervous, apprehensive patients, because surgery with local anesthesia may increase anxiety. A patient who begs to be put to sleep rarely does well under local anesthesia.

For some operations, local anesthesia is impractical because of the number of injections and the amount of anesthetic required—as in breast reconstruction, for example.

Technique.   The technique for the introduction of local infiltration requires the following:

- Solution of local anesthetic in various concentrations (0.5% to 2%)
- Sterile container
- Sterile syringes and needles
- Sterile sponges and drape

The skin is prepared as for any operation, and a small-gauge needle is used to inject a small amount of the anesthetic into the skin layers. This produces blanching or a wheal. The anesthetic then is carried ahead of the needle in the skin until an area the length of the proposed incision is anesthetized. A larger, longer needle then is used to infiltrate deeper tissues with the anesthetic. The action of the drug is almost immediate, so the operation may begin as soon as the injection is complete. Anesthesia lasts anywhere from 45 minutes to 3 hours, depending on the anesthetic and the use of epinephrine.

Patient Position on the Operating Table

The position in which the patient is placed on the operating table depends on the operation to be performed as well as on the physical condition of the patient (Fig. 21-3). Factors to consider include the following:

- The patient should be in as comfortable a position as possible, whether asleep or awake.
- The operative area must be adequately exposed.
- The vascular supply should not be obstructed by an awkward position or undue pressure on a part.
- There should be no interference with the patient's respiration

TABLE 21-7. *Local Anesthetic Agents*

Agent	Administration and Action	Advantages	Disadvantages	Implications and Use
AMIDES				
Lidocaine (Xylocaine) and mepivacaine (Carbocaine)	Topical or injection	Rapid Longer duration of action (compared with procaine) Free from local irritative effect	Occasional idiosyncrasy	Useful topically for cystoscopy Injected for use in dental work and surgery Observe for untoward reactions—drowsiness, depressed respiration
Bupivacaine (Marcaine)	Infiltration Peripheral nerve block Epidural	Duration is 2–3 times longer than lidocaine or mepivacaine	Use cautiously in persons with known drug allergies or sensitivities.	A period of analgesia persists after return of sensation; therefore, need for strong analgesics is reduced
Etidocaine (Duranest)	Infiltration Block			Greater potency and longer action than lidocaine
ESTERS				
Procaine (Novocain)	Subcutaneously, intramuscularly, intravenously, or spinal	Low toxicity Inexpensive	Some idiosyncrasies Skin rash Poor stability	Observe for reaction: hypotension, bradycardia, weak pulse Usually given with epinephrine, causing vasoconstriction, thereby slowing absorption and prolonging nerve-deadening effect
Tetracaine (Pontocaine)	Topical Infiltration Nerve block	Same as procaine	Same as procaine	More than 10 times as potent as procaine Usually administered with epinephrine

as a result of pressure of the arms on the chest or constriction of the neck or chest caused by a gown.

- Nerves must be protected from undue pressure. Improper positioning of the arms, hands, legs, or feet may cause serious injury or paralysis. Shoulder braces must be well padded to prevent irreparable nerve injury, especially when the Trendelenburg position is necessary.

- Precautions for patient safety must be observed, particularly with thin, elderly, or obese patients.
- The patient needs *gentle* restraint before induction, in case of excitement.

Dorsal Recumbent Position.   The usual position for surgery is flat on the back; one arm is at the side of the table, with the

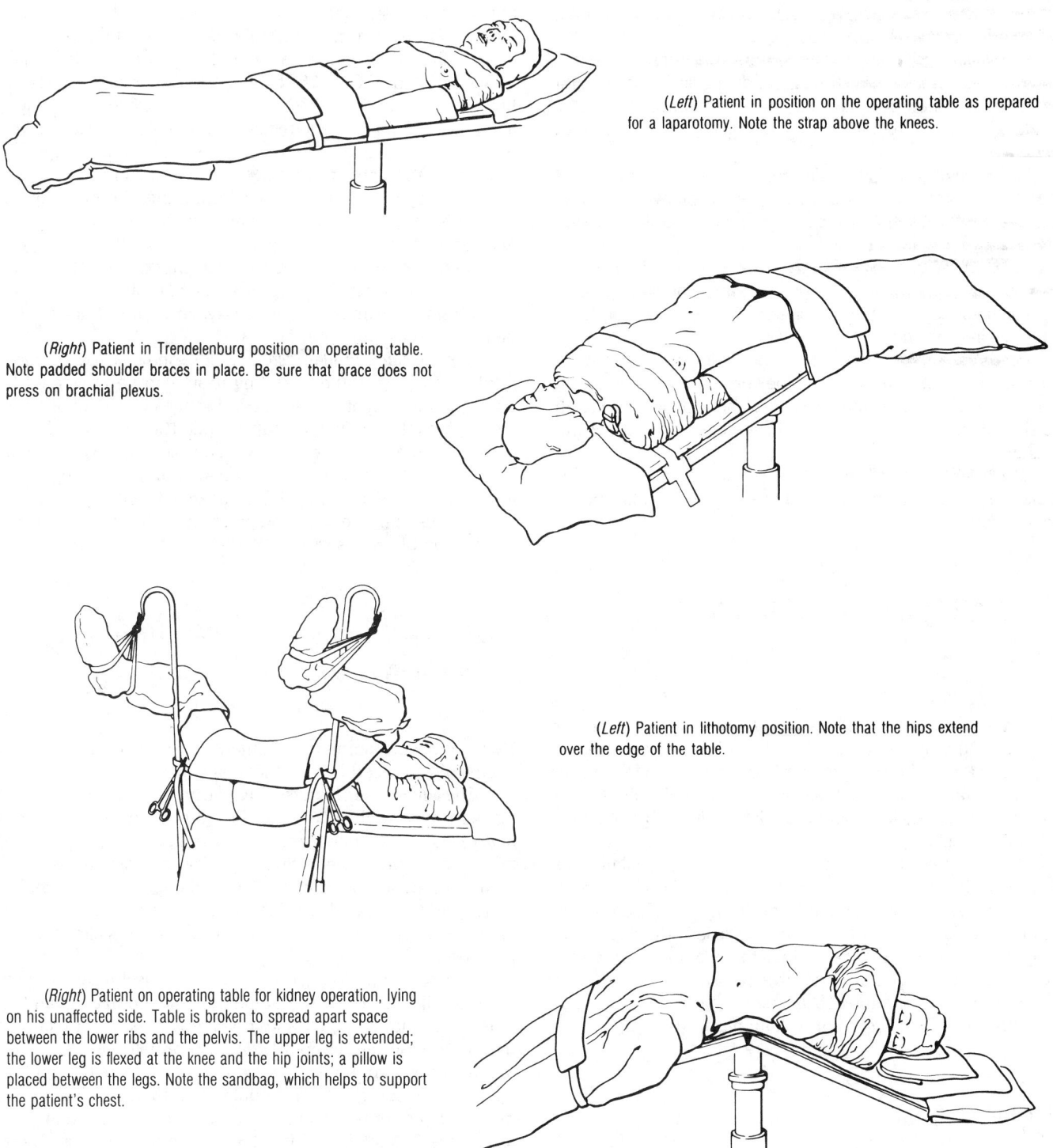

(*Left*) Patient in position on the operating table as prepared for a laparotomy. Note the strap above the knees.

(*Right*) Patient in Trendelenburg position on operating table. Note padded shoulder braces in place. Be sure that brace does not press on brachial plexus.

(*Left*) Patient in lithotomy position. Note that the hips extend over the edge of the table.

(*Right*) Patient on operating table for kidney operation, lying on his unaffected side. Table is broken to spread apart space between the lower ribs and the pelvis. The upper leg is extended; the lower leg is flexed at the knee and the hip joints; a pillow is placed between the legs. Note the sandbag, which helps to support the patient's chest.

Figure 21–3.   Positions on the operating table. Adjacent captions call attention to safety and comfort features. All surgical patients wear caps to completely cover the hair.

hand placed palm down; the other is carefully positioned on an armboard for intravenous infusion (see Fig. 21-3). This position is used for most abdominal operations, except for those on the gallbladder and the pelvis, and for the operations described below.

Trendelenburg Position.   The Trendelenburg position usually is used for operations on the lower abdomen and the pelvis to obtain good exposure by displacing the intestines into the upper abdomen. In this position, the head and body are lowered and the knees are flexed. The patient is held in position by padded shoulder braces (see Fig. 21-3).

Lithotomy Position.   In the lithotomy position, the patient is lying on his back with the legs and thighs flexed at right angles. The position is maintained by placing the feet in stirrups. Nearly all perineal, rectal, and vaginal operations require this posture (see Fig. 21-3).

For Kidney Operations.   The patient is placed on the non-operative side in Sims's position with an air pillow 12.5 to 15 cm (5 or 6 in) thick under the loin, or he is placed on a table with a kidney or back lift (see Fig. 21-3).

For Chest and Abdominothoracic Operations.   The position varies with the operation to be performed. The surgeon and the anesthesiologist place the patient on the operating table in the desired position.

Operations on the Neck.   Neck operations—for example, those involving the thyroid—are performed with the patient on his back, the neck extended somewhat by a pillow beneath the shoulders, and the head and chest elevated to reduce venous pressure.

Operations on the Skull and the Brain.   Such procedures demand special positions and apparatus, usually adjusted by the surgeon.

Induced Hypotension During the Operation

There are times during surgery when it is desirable to lower blood pressure in order to reduce bleeding at the operative site, because this allows for more rapid surgery with less blood loss. In operations such as brain surgery, radical neck dissection, and radical pelvic surgery, artificially induced hypotension has been used.

Deliberate hypotension is accomplished by inhalation or intravenous injection of medications that affect the sympathetic nervous system and peripheral smooth muscle. Halothane is the inhalation anesthetic agent commonly used. This anesthetic is supplemented with other measures to lower blood pressure, such as a head-up position, positive pressure applied to the airway, and administration of a ganglionic blocking agent such as pentolinium (Ansolysen) or sodium nitroprusside.

Hypothermia

Hypothermia is the state of core body temperature lowered below physiologic normal limits. *Normothermia* is 36.6° to 37.5°C (98.0° to 99.5°F). Inadvertent hypothermia may be experienced by the patient as a result of a low temperature in the operating room, infusion of cold fluids, inhalation of cold gases, open body wounds or cavities, decreased muscle activity, advanced age, or the pharmaceutical agents used (vasodilators, phenothiazines, general anesthetics). Hypothermia may also be intentionally induced in selected surgical procedures to reduce metabolic rate.

Treatment.   Prevention of hypothermia is a major objective; if it occurs, the goal of intervention is to minimize or reverse the physiologic process. With intentional hypothermia, the goal is safe return to normal body temperature.

Environmental temperature in the operating room should be set at 25° to 26.6°C (78° to 80°F). Intravenous and irrigating fluids are warmed to 37°C (98.6°F). Wet gowns and drapes are removed promptly and replaced with dry materials, because wet linens promote heat loss. Whatever methods are employed to rewarm the patient, warming must be accomplished gradually, not rapidly. Conscientious monitoring of core temperature, urinary output, ECG, blood pressure, arterial blood gases, and serum electrolytes is required.

Attention to hypothermia management extends into the postoperative period to prevent significant nitrogen loss and catabolism. Treatment includes oxygen administration, adequate hydration, and proper nutrition.

Gerontologic Considerations.   Studies indicate that heat loss in older patients in the operating room can be prevented by covering the head of the patient during anesthesia. An ordinary disposable plastic shower cap (applied after the patient is anesthetized and removed before consciousness is regained) can be effective and inexpensive. Also, the operating room temperature should be maintained at 26.6°C (80°F). Antiseptic solutions used in the initial preparation of the skin before the application of drapes should be comfortably warm, not cold.

Malignant Hyperthermia During General Anesthesia

Malignant hyperthermia is an inherited muscle disorder that is chemically induced by anesthetic agents.

Etiology and Pathophysiology.   During anesthesia, potent agents such as inhalation anesthetics (halothane, enflurane) and relaxants (succinylcholine) may trigger the symptoms of malignant hyperthermia. Such medications as sympathomimetics (epinephrine), theophylline, aminophylline, anticholinergics (atropine), and cardiac glycosides (digitalis) can also induce or intensify such a reaction. The process is also induced by stress.

The pathophysiology is related to muscle cell activity. Muscle cells are composed of inner fluid (sarcoplasm) and an outer surrounding membrane. Calcium, an essential factor in the process of muscle contraction, is normally stored in sacs in the sarcoplasm. When nerve impulses stimulate the muscle, calcium is released, allowing contraction to occur. A pumping mechanism returns calcium to the sacs so that relaxation can take place. In malignant hyperthermia, this mechanism is disrupted. Calcium ions are not returned and they accumulate, causing clinical symptoms of hypermetabolism, which in turn increases muscle contraction (rigidity), hyperthermia, and damage to the central nervous system.

With the mortality rate exceeding 50%, the identification of patients at risk is imperative. Persons susceptible to malignant hyperthermia include those with bulky, strong muscles, a history of muscle cramps or muscle weakness and unexplained temperature elevation, and an unexplained death of a family member during surgery that was accompanied by a febrile response.

Clinical Manifestations.   The initial symptoms of malignant hyperthermia are related to cardiovascular and musculoskeletal activity. Tachycardia (heart rate above 150/min) is often the earliest sign. Rigidity or tetany-like movements occur, often in the jaw, with the abnormal transport of calcium. In addition to the tachycardia, sympathetic nervous stimulation leads to ventricular dysrhythmia, hypotension, decreased cardiac output, oliguria, and, later, cardiac arrest. The rise in temperature is actually a late sign that develops rapidly, and it can increase 1° every 5 minutes.

Management.   Early recognition of symptoms by the circulating nurse and the prompt discontinuation of anesthesia are imperative. It is also necessary to monitor all vital signs, arterial blood gases, electrolytes, and the ECG. Goals of treat-

TABLE 21–8. *Pharmacologic Agents Used in Treating Malignant Hyperthermia*

Generic (Trade) Name	Action	Nursing Responsibilities
Dantrolene sodium (Dantrium)	Direct skeletal muscle relaxant Reduces release of calcium from sarcoplasmic reticulum, thus decreasing muscle contraction	Monitor ECG, temperature, BP, central venous pressure, serum potassium. Observe for infiltration to surrounding tissues. Maintain intravenous infusion until symptoms decrease. Mix with distilled water without bacteriostatic agents.
Sodium bicarbonate	Increases blood *p*H by buffering excess hydrogen ion concentration	Assess electrolytes. Monitor arterial blood gas values.
Regular insulin (Regular Iletin)	Increases glucose uptake into liver to meet hypermetabolic demands of body Forces potassium into cells	Observe for hypoglycemia.
Dextrose 50%	Increases movement of potassium from extracellular fluid back into cell	Monitor urine and blood glucose levels. Infuse via central venous catheter. Assess electrolytes.
Furosemide (Lasix)	Potent diuretic Enhances excretion of myoglobins, potassium, sodium, and magnesium	Monitor for hypotension. Observe urinary output. Assess BUN and creatinine. Assess electrolytes. Observe for dehydration. Weigh patient every day. Administer potassium supplements as prescribed.
Mannitol (Osmitrol)	Osmotic diuretic for excretion of excess fluid Increases urinary output to prevent renal failure	Monitor input and output. Weigh patient every day. Assess electrolytes. Maintain catheter patency.
Procainamide hydrochloride	Antidysrhythmic Decreases cardiac muscle excitability and slows conduction velocity	Monitor for hypotension. Monitor ECG, cardiac output. Check urine *p*H for drug toxicity.
Hydrocortisone sodium succinate (Solu-Cortef)	Given for its mineralocorticoid effect of potassium excretion and increased glomerular filtration rate Affects calcium absorption from gastrointestinal tract Used to reduce cerebral edema	Weigh patient every day. Do not use with salicylates. Monitor blood pressure. Observe for gastrointestinal bleeding. Assess electrolytes.
Heparin sodium	Anticoagulant to treat disseminated intravascular coagulopathy	Observe for bleeding. Monitor coagulation status. Check stool and urine for occult blood.

(Adapted from Caine R, Molla K, and Reynolds R. Malignant hyperthermia: A critical care challenge. Dimens Crit Care Nurs 1986 May/Jun; 5[3]:148.)

Chart 21-5
The Nursing Process in the Intraoperative Phase

Assessment

A. Use data from patient and the patient record to identify variables that can affect care and that serve as guidelines for developing an individualized plan of patient care.
  1. Identify patient.
  2. Validate necessary data with patient per department policy.
  3. Review patient record for:
    a. Correct informed surgical consent
    b. Completed records for health history and physical examination
    c. Results of diagnostic studies
    d. Completed nursing history and assessment
    e. Preoperative checklist
  4. Complete immediate preoperative nursing assessment.
    a. Physiologic status (*e.g.*, health–illness level, level of consciousness)
    b. Psychosocial status (*e.g.*, expressions of concern, anxiety level, verbal communication problems, coping mechanisms)
    c. Physical status (*e.g.*, operative site, skin condition and effectiveness of preparation, shave or depilatory; immobile joints)

Planning

A. Interpret common variables and incorporate them into the plan of care.
  1. Age, size, sex, surgical procedure, type of anesthesia planned, surgeon, anesthesiologist, and team members
  2. Availability of necessary equipment specific to procedure and surgeon
  3. Need for nonroutine medications, blood components, instruments, etc.
  4. Readiness of room for patient; completeness of physical setup; completeness of instrument, suture, and dressing setups.
B. Identify aspects of the operating room environment that may negatively affect the patient.
  1. Physical
    a. Room temperature and humidity
    b. Electrical hazards
    c. Potential contaminants (dust, blood, and discharge stains on floor or furniture; uncovered hair, faulty attire of personnel, jewelry worn by personnel, dirty footwear)
    d. Unnecessary traffic
  2. Psychosocial
    a. Noise
    b. Lack of recognition as a person
    c. Sense of abandonment—unchaperoned in waiting area
    d. Unnecessary conversation

Intervention

A. Provide nursing care based on priority of patient needs.
  1. Set up and maintain suction in working order.
  2. Set up invasive monitoring equipment.

Intervention

  3. Assist with line insertion (arterial, Swan–Ganz, CVP, IV)
  4. Initiate appropriate physical comfort measures for patient.
  5. Position patient correctly for anesthesia and surgical procedures; maintain functional body alignment.
  6. Follow steps in surgical procedure.
    a. Scrub/circulate competently.
    b. Respond to needs of patient by anticipating what supplies and equipment are required before they are requested.
    c. Assume role of RN First Assistant as required.
  7. Follow established procedures—for example:
    a. Care and use of blood and blood components
    b. Care and handling of specimens, tissue, and cultures
    c. Antiseptic skin preparation
    d. Donning gown—self; holding gown for surgeon
    e. Open and closed gloving
    f. Counts: sponge, instrument, needle, special
    g. Septic case technique
    h. Urinary catheter management
    i. Drainage/dressing management
  8. Communicate adverse situations to surgeon, anesthesiologist, or charge nurse, or act appropriately to control or reverse the situation.
  9. Use supplies judiciously for cost-effectiveness.
  10. Assist the surgeon and anesthesiologist in implementing their plans of care.
B. Act as the patient's advocate.
  1. Provide physical privacy.
  2. Maintain confidentiality.
  3. Act to provide physical safety and comfort.
C. Inform patient regarding his intraoperative experience.
  1. Describe any sensory stimulation he will experience.
  2. Use common, basic communication skills to reduce anxiety in the patient—for example:
    a. Touch
    b. Eye contact
    c. Assure the patient you will be with him in the operating room
    d. Realistic verbal reassurance
D. Coordinate activities of others involved in patient care:
  1. X-ray, laboratory, recovery or intensive care unit, surgical nursing unit
  2. Technicians—cast, laboratory, etc.
  3. Pharmacist
  4. Ancillary operating room personnel and nonprofessional staff
E. Operate and troubleshoot all equipment commonly used in the operating room and assigned specialty service (including autoclaves).
F. Participate in patient care conferences.
G. Document all observations and appropriate actions on the required forms, including patient's record.
H. Communicate, orally and in writing, with the recovery room and outpatient surgical nursing staff (as pertinent) regarding the health status of the patient on transfer from the operating room.

(continued)

> ## Chart 21-5 (Continued)
>
> ### Evaluation
>
> A. Evaluate the condition of the patient immediately prior to his discharge from the operating room—for example:
>   1. Respiratory condition: breathing easily (on his own or assisted)
>   2. Skin condition: color good; absence of abrasions, burns, bruises
>   3. Functioning of invasive tubing: IV, drains, catheters, nasogastric—no kinks or obstruction, functioning normally, etc.
>   4. Grounding pad site: good condition
>   5. Dressings: adequate for drainage, fastened securely, not too tight, etc.
> B. Participate in the identification of unsafe patient care practices and intervene appropriately.
> C. Participate in evaluating the safety of the environment—for example, equipment, cleanliness, etc.
> D. Report and document any adverse behavior or problem.
> E. Demonstrate understanding of principles of asepsis and technical nursing practices.
> F. Recognize the legal accountability of perioperative nursing.
>
> (Adapted from procedure and practices at Memorial Hospital Medical Center of Long Beach, California.)

ment are to decrease metabolism, reverse metabolic and respiratory acidosis, correct dysrhythmias, decrease body temperature, provide oxygen and nutrition to tissues, and correct electrolyte imbalance.

Although most instances occur about 10 to 20 minutes after induction, malignant hyperthermia can also occur in the first 24-hour postoperative period. As soon as the diagnosis of malignant hyperthermia is made, anesthesia and surgery are halted and the patient is hyperventilated with 100% oxygen. Dantrolene sodium, a skeletal muscle relaxant, and sodium bicarbonate are administered immediately. The pharmacologic agents used and the related nursing responsibilities are described in Table 21-8. Continued monitoring of all parameters is necessary to evaluate the patient's progress.

Although the condition happens infrequently, enough is now known about the problem that, if it does occur, it can be recognized. It is imperative that the nurse identify patients at risk, recognize the problem, have the appropriate medication and equipment available, and know the protocol to follow. This information may be lifesaving if malignant hyperthermia occurs.

Intraoperative Nursing: The Nursing Process

The nursing process as applied to intraoperative nursing is summarized in Chart 21-5.

Chapter Summary

The intraoperative phase, the second phase of perioperative nursing, focuses on the patient receiving anesthesia and undergoing surgery. The intraoperative nurse, anesthesiologist or nurse anesthetist, and surgeon work collaboratively to provide a safe outcome for the patient. Before surgery, the intraoperative nurse may visit the patient to establish rapport, discuss the experience, and answer questions. In the operating room, the nurse may assume a managing role as the circulating nurse or an assistant role as the scrub nurse. In either role, the intraoperative nurse maintains surgical asepsis by adhering to the operating room dress code and scrubbing procedure, identifying breaks in sterile technique, and using good health practices. The patient's safety needs are the primary concern and, for the elderly, involve considerations of higher risk including decreased response to stress, reduced gas exchange, and longer anesthetic effect.

The anesthesiologist or nurse anesthetist visits the patient before surgery to discuss the type of anesthetic agent, assess the patient's condition, and discuss any concerns expressed by the patient. During surgery, the anesthesiologist or nurse anesthetist administers anesthesia and monitors vital signs, cardiac status, anesthesia levels, and adequacy of respiratory exchange.

Anesthesia is classified as general or specific to a portion of the body. General anesthesia is usually administered by inhalation or intravenously; local anesthesia is injected directly into the tissues. General anesthesia is described in four stages of physiologic change: stages I, II, and III are normal, whereas stage IV is life-threatening. Intravenous anesthetic agents have a rapid onset of action and are used for short procedures or as adjuncts to inhalation anesthesia in surgery of longer duration. Local anesthetic agents are used in spinal, regional, and local anesthesia. Other agents include neuromuscular blockers that promote relaxation during surgery.

Following anesthesia, the nurse monitors the patient's vital signs and his return to mental and physical function. Assessment includes identifying signs of general anesthesia complications, including hypotension, hypothermia, and malignant hyperthermia. The nurse's observations, prompt reporting, and appropriate intervention in the intraoperative phase reduce the chance of complications and positively affect the postoperative course.

Bibliography

See Bibliography for unit following Chapter 22.

22

Postoperative Nursing Management

Learning Objectives

On completion of this chapter, the learner will be able to:

1. Describe the responsibilities of the recovery room nurse in the prevention of immediate postoperative complications
2. Use the nursing process as a framework for care of postoperative patients
3. Identify common postoperative discomforts and their management
4. Describe the gerontologic considerations related to postoperative management of patients
5. Describe variables that affect wound healing
6. Demonstrate sterile dressing technique
7. Identify assessment parameters appropriate for the early detection of postoperative complications
8. Describe the advantages and process of ambulatory surgery

During the postoperative period, the nursing process is directed toward the reestablishment of the patient's physiologic equilibrium, alleviation of pain, and prevention of complications. Careful assessment and immediate intervention assist the patient in returning to optimal function quickly, safely, and as comfortably as possible.

Considerable effort is directed toward anticipation and prevention of problems in the postoperative period. Prompt assessment prevents complications that prolong hospital stay or endanger the patient. In this respect, the nursing care of the patient after surgery is equal in importance to the operation itself.

Transferring the Patient to the Recovery Room

The transfer from the operating room to the recovery room involves special consideration of the patient's incision site,

vascular changes, and exposure. The site of the surgical incision is considered every time a new postoperative patient is moved. Many wounds are closed under considerable tension, and every effort is made to prevent further strain on the sutures. For example, in nephrectomy, the patient is not allowed to lie on the affected side because of the possibility of obstructing drains in the wound.

Serious arterial hypotension may occur when a patient is moved from one position to another, such as from a lithotomy position to a horizontal position, from a lateral to a supine position, or from a prone to a supine position. Even moving the anesthetized patient to the stretcher can precipitate this problem. Thus, the patient must be moved *slowly* and *carefully*.

As soon as the patient is placed on the stretcher or bed, the soiled gown is removed and replaced with dry gown. He is covered with lightweight blankets and secured with straps above the knees and elbows. The straps serve the double purpose of anchoring the blankets and restraining the patient should he pass through a stage of excitement as he recovers from the anesthetic. Side rails are raised to protect against falls.

Transfer of the postoperative patient from the operating room to the recovery room is the responsibility of the anesthesiologist, with a member of the surgical team in attendance. Additional assistance may be provided by a nurse assigned to this particular patient. The patient is transferred expediently with special attention paid in transit to his comfort, safety, and general condition. Tubes and drainage equipment are handled carefully for optimal function.

Postanesthesia Recovery Room

The postanesthesia recovery room (PARR) is a unit usually located adjacent to the operating rooms. Patients who are still under anesthesia or recovering from it are placed in this unit for easy access to (1) nurses who are especially prepared in caring for the immediate postoperative patient, (2) anesthesiologists and surgeons, and (3) monitors and special equipment, medications, and replacement fluids. In this setting, the patient is given the best care available by those best qualified to give it.

The room is kept quiet, clean, and free of unnecessary equipment. It should also have (1) walls and ceiling painted in soft, pleasing colors; (2) indirect lighting; (3) a soundproof ceiling; (4) equipment that controls or eliminates noise (*e.g.*, plastic emesis basins, rubber bumpers on beds and tables); and (5) isolated quarters (glass encased) for disruptive patients. These features are of psychological value to the patient to decrease anxiety.

Monitoring devices are available to provide accurate and instant appraisal of the patient's condition. Special equipment includes most types of breathing aids: oxygen, laryngoscopes, tracheotomy sets, bronchial instruments, catheters, mechanical ventilators, and suction equipment.

Other equipment is needed for meeting circulatory needs, such as blood pressure apparatus, parenteral equipment, universal donor blood, plasma expanders, intravenous trays and cutdown trays, cardiac arrest equipment, defibrillator, venous catheters, and tourniquets. Surgical dressing materials, narcotics, and emergency drugs are available, as well as catheterization sets and drainage equipment.

The recovery bed is one that provides easy access to the patient, is safe and easily movable, can readily be placed in shock position, and possesses features that facilitate care, such as intravenous poles, side guards, wheel brakes, and chart storage rack.

Room temperature should be 20° to 22.2°C (68° to 70°F), and the room should have good ventilation.

A patient remains in this unit until he has fully recovered from the anesthetic agent, that is, until he has a stable blood pressure, adequate respiratory function, and a reasonable degree of consciousness. Criteria to determine the degree of recovery are provided in detail in Figure 22-1.

The nursing management objectives of PARR are to care for the patient until he has recovered from the effects of anesthesia (*i.e.*, until return of motor and sensory functions), vital signs are stable, there is no evidence of hemorrhage, and he is oriented. If a problem arises, the proximity to the surgeon, anesthesiologist, and operating room provides assurance of immediate expert assistance. The patient who progresses un-

eventfully is transferred from the PARR to the surgical nursing unit.

Immediate Postoperative Assessment

The recovery room nurse who receives the patient reviews the following with the anesthesiologist:

1. Medical diagnosis and type of surgery performed
2. Patient's age and general condition: airway patency, vital signs, blood pressure
3. Anesthetic and other medications used (*e.g.*, narcotics, muscle relaxant, antibiotics)
4. Any problems that occurred in the operating room that might influence postoperative care (*e.g.*, extensive hemorrhage, shock, cardiac arrest)
5. Pathology encountered (if malignancy, whether the patient or family has been informed)
6. Fluid administered, blood loss and replacement
7. Any tubing, drains, catheters, or other supportive aids
8. Specific information about which the surgeon or anesthesiologist wishes to be notified

This preliminary assessment of the patient includes an evaluation of pulse volume and regularity, depth and nature of respirations, skin color, level of consciousness, and ability of the patient to respond to commands. The operative site is checked for drainage, hemorrhage, and clamped tubing that needs to be unclamped and connected to a drainage receptacle.

It is also essential for the nurse to know pertinent information from the preoperative history that may be significant at this time (*e.g.*, patient is hard of hearing, epileptic, diabetic, allergic to certain medications). This information may have been acquired in a preoperative visit with the patient.

Nursing Interventions

Vital signs are monitored and general physical assessment of the patient is performed at least every 15 minutes. In order of priority, patency of the airway and respiratory function are always evaluated first, followed by assessment of cardiovascular function (including vital signs), the condition of the surgical site, and function of the central nervous system.

- The primary objective is to maintain pulmonary ventilation and thus to prevent hypoxemia (reduced oxygen in blood) and hypercapnia (excess carbon dioxide in blood). These can occur if the airway is obstructed and ventilation is reduced (hypoventilation).

Shock can be avoided largely by the timely administration of intravenous fluids and blood, and medications that elevate blood pressure.

Respiratory Considerations. Respiratory difficulties are associated with specific types of anesthesia. Patients who received local anesthesia or nitrous oxide usually are awake within a few minutes of leaving the operating room. However, patients who have experienced prolonged anesthesia usually are unconscious, with all muscles relaxed. This relaxation extends to the muscles of the pharynx; therefore, when the patient lies on his back, the lower jaw and the tongue fall backward, and the air passages become obstructed (Fig. 22-2A). Signs of this difficulty include choking, noisy and irregular respirations, and, within minutes, a blue, dusky color (cyanosis) of the skin.

POSTANESTHESIA RECOVERY ROOM
Scoring

Patient:

Room:

Date:

Final Score:

Surgeon:

R.R. Nurse:

Area of Assessment	Point Score	Upon Admission	After		
			1 hr	2 hr	3 hr
Respiration:					
• Ability to breathe deeply and cough	2				
• Limited respiratory effort (dyspnea or splinting)	1				
• No spontaneous effort	0				
Circulation: Systolic arterial pressure					
• >80% of preanesthetic level	2				
• 50% to 80% of preanesthetic level	1				
• <50% of preanesthetic level	0				
Consciousness Level:					
• Verbally responds to questions/ oriented to location	2				
• Aroused when called by name	1				
• Failure to respond to command	0				
Color:					
• Normal skin color and appearance	2				
• Altered skin color: pale, dusky, blotchy, jaundiced	1				
• Frank cyanosis	0				
Muscle Activity: Moves spontaneously or on command:					
• Ability to move all extremities	2				
• Ability to move 2 extremities	1				
• Unable to control |any| extremity	0				
Totals:					

Required for Discharge from Recovery Room: 7-8 points

Time of Release

Signature of Nurse

Figure 22–1. Postanesthesia recovery room scoring chart. This may be used in the day surgery unit also.

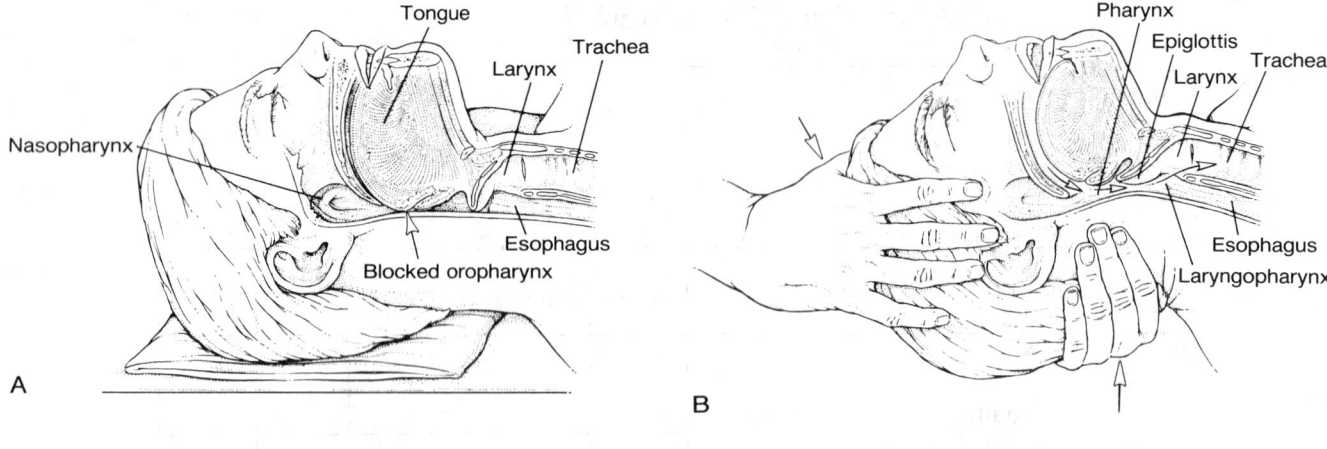

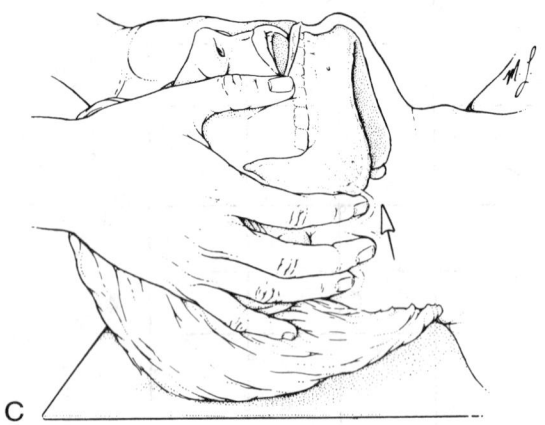

Figure 22–2. (**A**) A hypopharyngeal obstruction occurs when the flexing of the neck permits the chin to drop toward the chest; obstruction almost always occurs when the head is in the midposition. (**B**) Tilting the head back to stretch the anterior neck structure causes the base of the tongue to be lifted off the posterior pharyngeal wall. The directions of the arrows indicate the pressure of the hands. (**C**) Opening the mouth is necessary to correct valvelike obstruction of the nasal passage during expiration, which occurs in about 30% of unconscious patients. Open the patient's mouth (separate lips and teeth) and move the lower jaw forward so that the lower teeth are in front of the upper teeth. To regain backward tilt of the neck, lift with both hands at the ascending rami of the mandible.

- The only sure way of knowing whether a patient is breathing or not is to place the palm of the hand over the patient's nose and mouth to feel the exhaled breath. Movements of the thorax and the diaphragm do not necessarily mean that a patient is breathing.
- The treatment of hypopharyngeal obstruction involves tilting the head back and pushing forward on the angle of the lower jaw, as if to push the lower teeth in front of the upper teeth (see Fig. 22-2B,C). This maneuver pulls the tongue forward and opens the air passages.

Often the anesthesiologist leaves a hard rubber or plastic airway in the patient's mouth (Fig. 22-3) to maintain a patent airway. Such a device should not be removed until signs, such as gagging, indicate that reflex action is returning.

Occasionally, a patient may be brought to the recovery room with an endotracheal tube still in place and may require continued mechanical ventilation. The nurse then assists in the preparation of the ventilator and in the weaning and extubation procedures.

Clearing Secretions From the Airway.   Respiratory difficulty can result from excessive secretion of mucus. Turning the patient to one side allows the collected fluid to escape from the side of the mouth. If the patient's teeth are clenched, the mouth may be opened manually with a padded tongue blade. If vomiting occurs, the patient is turned to the side and the vomitus collected in the emesis basin. The face is wiped with gauze or paper wipes and the nature and amount of the vomitus are recorded.

Mucus or vomitus obstructing the pharynx or the trachea is suctioned with a pharyngeal suction tip or a nasal catheter introduced into the nasopharynx or the oropharynx. Wall suction or suction machines are available for this purpose. The catheter can be passed into the nasopharynx or the oropharynx safely to a distance of 15 to 20 cm (6 to 8 in) if secretions are obtained at this level. For aesthetic reasons, the same catheter can be passed from mouth to nose but not from nose to mouth.

If frequent aspiration of the nasopharynx and oropharynx is indicated, a clean aspirating catheter is used and a basin of water kept nearby to flush and clean the catheter. Caution is necessary in suctioning the throat of a patient who has had a tonsillectomy, because the operative area may become irritated, causing bleeding and added discomfort.

Positioning.   The bed is kept flat until the patient regains consciousness. Unless contraindicated, the unconscious patient is positioned on one side with a pillow at the back and with chin extended to minimize any danger of aspiration. Knees are flexed and a pillow positioned between the legs to reduce strain on abdominal sutures. If side-lying is contraindicated, just the head is turned to the side.

Psychologic Support.   The function of the recovery room nurse is not limited to bedside procedures, safety measures, and the relief of pain; an understanding of the significance of psychologic support is also important. The nurse who knows the patient and accompanies him through the immediate preoperative and operative experiences is in a unique position to offer valuable support. In the absence of such continuous care by one nurse, pertinent documentation on the chart helps the recovery room nurse to recognize the particular needs of each individual patient.

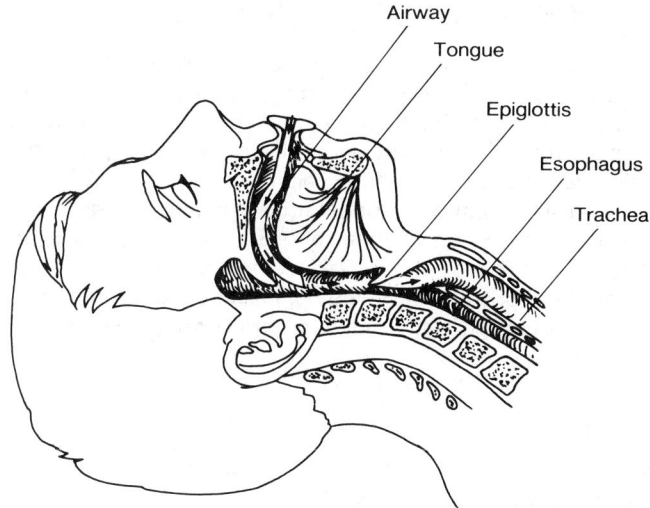

Figure 22–3. Diagrammatic view showing a method by which an airway prevents respiratory difficulty after anesthesia. The airway passes over the base of the tongue and permits passage of air into the pharynx in the region of the epiglottis. Patients are often brought from the operating room with an airway in place. This should remain in place until the patient recovers sufficiently to breathe normally. As the patient regains consciousness, the airway usually causes irritation; it should be removed.

Postanesthesia Recovery Room Criteria and Scoring Guide

Usually the following criteria are used to determine the patient's readiness for discharge from the PARR:

- Uncompromised pulmonary function
- Stable vital signs, including blood pressure
- Orientation to place, events, time
- Urine output not less than 30 ml/hr
- Nausea and vomiting under control; pain minimal

Many hospitals use a scoring system to determine the patient's general condition and readiness to be transferred from the recovery room. As the patient progresses through the recovery period, his physical signs are observed and evaluated by means of a scoring system based on a set of objective criteria. This evaluation guide, a modification of the Apgar scoring system used for evaluating newborns, makes possible a more objective assessment of the patient's physical condition in the PARR (see Fig. 22-1).

The patient's score is taken at stated intervals, such as every 15 or 30 minutes, and totaled on the assessment record. A patient with a total score of less than 7 must remain in the recovery room until his condition improves or he is transferred to an intensive care area.

Patient's Reception and Care on the Clinical Unit

The patient's unit is readied by assembling the equipment and supplies that are necessary to meet his specific needs: intra-venous pole, drainage receptacle holder, emesis basin, tissues, disposable pads (Chux), blankets, and postoperative charting sheets. When the call comes to the unit from the PARR, any additional items that might be needed are communicated.

The patient is transferred from the recovery room to the unit when the above criteria have been met and the PARR chart score (see Fig. 22-1) confirms the patient's responsiveness. The recovery room nurse reports the baseline data of the patient's condition to the receiving nurse. The report includes medications prescribed and administered for pain, the type and amount of fluids received, whether the patient has voided, and information that the patient and family have received about the patient's condition. Usually the surgeon speaks to the family after the operation and relates the general condition of the patient and what to expect when the patient arrives on the unit. Instructions and postoperative requests are also reviewed. The postoperative goals of the patient are established, and related nursing interventions are documented.

▶ Nursing Process
Caring for the Postoperative Patient

▷ Assessment

After the PARR report, the unit nurse performs an initial assessment and proceeds with any immediate nursing interventions. Usually the question "How are you feeling?" provides information about the patient's discomfort as well as the level of mental alertness. Often the physical transfer adds some temporary discomfort.

The nurse consults the patient's chart to determine when the pain medication can be given, and the patient is reminded of its availability. With current anesthetic agents and medications, it is less common for the postoperative patient to be nauseated; however, an emesis basin is kept nearby.

Immediate assessment of the surgical patient on returning to the clinical unit consists of the following:

Respiratory: Airway patency; depth, rate, and character; nature of breath sounds
Circulatory: Vital signs including blood pressure; skin condition
Neurologic: Level of responsiveness
Drainage: Presence; need to connect tubes to a specific drainage system; presence and condition of dressings
Comfort: Type of pain and location; nausea or vomiting; position change required
Psychological: Nature of patient's questions; need for rest and sleep; disturbance by noise, visitors; availability of call bell or call light
Safety: Need for side rails; drainage tubes unobstructed; IV sites properly splinted, if necessary
Equipment: Checked for proper functioning

▷ *Respiratory Assessment.* On admission to the clinical unit, the patient is observed for patency of the airway. The quality of respirations is noted, such as depth, rate, and sound. Often, because of medications given for pain, respirations are slow. Shallow and rapid respirations may be due to pain, constricting dressings, gastric dilatation, or obesity. Noisy breathing may be due to obstruction by secretions or the tongue (see p. 438).

Lung auscultation with accurate documentation is used as a baseline for later comparisons. Crackles may indicate secretions that should be mobilized. The patient is instructed and assisted to turn, cough, and deep breathe. Chest physical therapy may be prescribed if indicated.

▷ *Circulatory Assessment.* The basic consideration in assessment of cardiovascular function is monitoring the patient for signs of shock and hemorrhage. The chief guides are the patient's appearance and determinations of pulse, respiration, blood pressure, temperature, central venous pressure (CVP), and blood gases. CVP and blood gas values are monitored if the patient's condition requires such assessment.

Institutions have specific protocols for postoperative monitoring. Unless indicated more frequently, the pulse, blood pressure and respirations are recorded every 15 minutes for the first 2 hours, and every 30 minutes for the next 2 hours. Thereafter, they may be taken less frequently if they remain stable. The temperature is taken every 4 hours for the first 24 hours.

- A temperature above 37.7°C (100°F) or below 36.1°C (97°F), respirations over 30 or under 16 per minute, and a falling systolic blood pressure under 90 mm Hg are usually considered reportable at once. However, the patient's preoperative or baseline blood pressure is used to make informed postoperative comparisons.
- A previously stable blood pressure that shows a downward trend of 5 mm Hg at each 15-minute reading should also alert the nurse to a problem.

The general condition of the patient is assessed and recorded, including whether his color is good or cyanotic, his skin is cold and clammy or warm and moist, or there is excessive mucus in the throat and in the nostrils.

▷ Nursing Diagnoses

Based on the assessment data, major nursing diagnoses might include the following:

- Ineffective airway clearance related to depressant effects of medications and anesthetic agent
- Pain and other postoperative discomforts
- High risk for injury related to postanesthesia status
- Altered systemic tissue perfusion secondary to hypovolemia, peripheral blood pooling, and vasoconstriction
- High risk for fluid volume deficit
- Altered nutrition: Less than body requirement
- Altered urinary elimination related to decreased activity, effects of medications, and reduced intake of fluids
- Constipation related to decreased gastric and intestinal motility during intraoperative period
- Impaired skin integrity related to the surgical incision and drainage exits
- High risk for wound infection related to susceptibility to bacterial invasion
- Impaired physical mobility related to depressant effects of anesthesia, decreased activity tolerance, and prescribed activity restrictions
- Anxiety about postoperative diagnosis, possible changes in life-style, and alteration in self-concept

▷ Planning and Implementation

▷ *Goals:* The major goals of the patient may include optimal respiratory function, relief of pain and postoperative discomforts (nausea and vomiting, abdominal distention, hiccups), freedom from injury, maintenance of adequate tissue perfusion, maintenance of adequate fluid volume, maintenance of nutritional balance, return of normal urinary function, resumption of usual pattern of bowel elimination, maintenance of skin integrity and avoidance of infection, restoration of mobility within limitations of postoperative and rehabilitative plan, and reduction of anxiety and achievement of psychologic well-being.

▷ Nursing Interventions

▷ Ensuring Optimal Respiratory Function

Measures to maintain a patent airway are carried out as described earlier in this chapter.

▷ *Promoting Lung Expansion.* To encourage lung expansion and exchange of gas, a variety of measures may be followed. For example, having the patient yawn or take sustained maximal inspirations creates a negative intrathoracic pressure of minus 40 mm Hg and expands lung volume to total capacity.

At least every 2 hours, the patient is turned and encouraged to take deep breaths. Coughing is also encouraged to dislodge mucus plugs. Careful splinting of abdominal or thoracic incision sites helps the patient overcome the fear that the exertion of coughing might open the wound. Pain medications are administered to permit more effective coughing, and oxygen is administered to prevent or relieve hypoxemia or hypoxia. Coughing is contraindicated in patients who have head injuries or who have undergone head surgery (because of risk of increasing intracranial pressure), as well as in patients who have undergone eye surgery (because of increasing intraocular pressure) and in those who have had plastic surgery (because of increasing tension on delicate tissues).

Incentive Spirometry. Incentive spirometry is a method by which the patient performs sustained maximal inspirations and at the same time sees the results of his efforts as registered on the spirometer. Such motivation encourages the patient to continue to take deep breaths to maximize voluntary lung expansion. The patient is taught how to use the device for maximum effectiveness.

An example of this type of equipment is a device that shows the patient how well he is inhaling (Fig. 22-4). A goal is established toward which the patient strives. First he exhales; then he places his lips around the mouthpiece and slowly inhales, trying to drive the piston on the device to a marked goal. Such a device offers several advantages: (1) the patient is encouraged to participate actively in his own treatment; (2) because the device is present and prescribed, it ensures that the maneuver is physiologically appropriate and repeated; and (3) it is a cost-effective way of preventing complications.

▷ *Evaluation: Expected Outcomes.* The patient maintains optimal respiratory function.

1. Performs deep-breathing exercises
2. Displays clear breath sounds
3. Uses incentive spirometer as prescribed
4. Exhibits normal body temperature

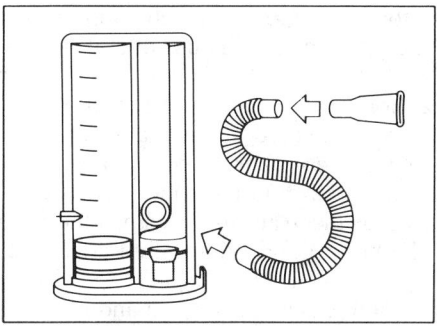

Remove components from package and attach mouthpiece to one end of tubing. Attach remaining free end of tubing to stem on front side of exerciser.

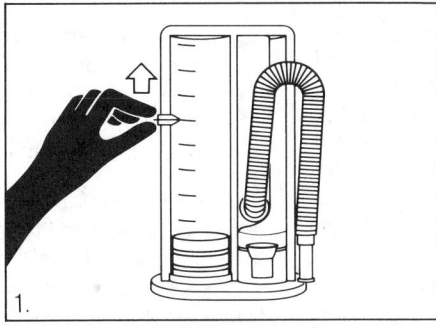

1. Slide the pointer of unit to prescribed volume level. Hold or stand exerciser in an upright position.

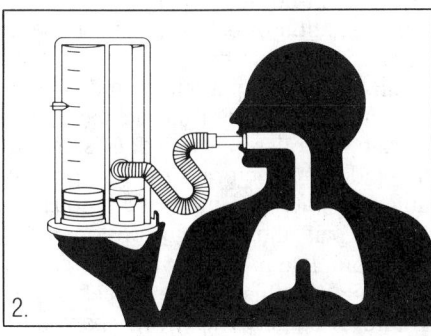

2. Exhale normally. Then place lips tightly around mouthpiece.

Figure 22–4. Volumetric Incentive Deep Breathing Exerciser (Voldyne). Follow instructions below each illustration. When inhalation is complete, remove mouthpiece, hold breath as prescribed, and exhale normally. Allow piston to return to bottom of chamber, rest, and repeat exercise. (Follow text for additional directives.)

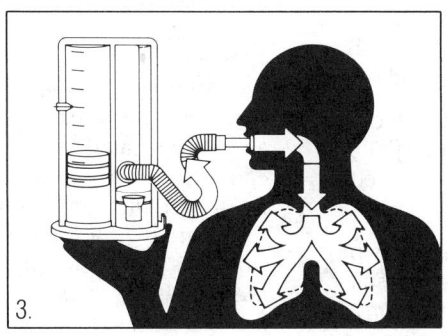

3. Inhale slowly, to raise the piston in the chamber.

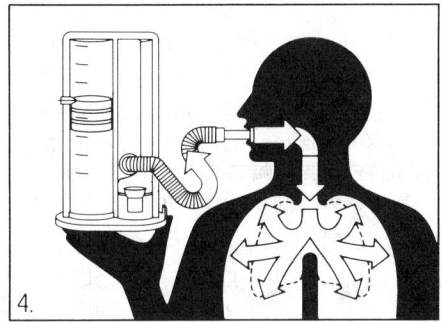

4. Continue inhaling and try to raise piston to prescribed level. Top of piston indicates level attained.

5. Maintains normal arterial blood gas values
6. Exhibits normal chest radiographs
7. Turns from one position to another as instructed
8. Coughs effectively to clear secretions
9. Exercises and ambulates as prescribed
10. Avoids persons with upper respiratory infections

◊ *Relief of Pain and Postoperative Discomforts*

◊ *Relief of Pain.* Many psychological factors (motivational, affective, cognitive, and emotional) influence the patient's total pain experience. Recent findings have led to a better understanding of how perception, learning, personality, ethnic and cultural factors, and environment can affect anxiety, depression, and pain. The degree and severity of postoperative pain depend on the physiologic and psychological makeup of the person, the subsequent tolerance level, the incision site, the nature of the operation, the extent of surgical trauma, and the type of anesthetic agent and how it was administered. The preoperative preparation received by the patient (including information about what to expect as well as reassurance and psychological support) is a significant factor in decreasing anxiety, apprehension, and even the pain experienced in the postoperative period.

With regard to the need for narcotics, about one third of patients complain of severe pain, one third of moderate pain, and one third of little or no pain. These statistics do not mean that the patients in the last group have no pain; rather, they appear to activate psychodynamic mechanisms that impair the registering of pain ("gate closing" theory and impaired nociceptive transmission).

Narcotic analgesics are often prescribed for pain and immediate postoperative restlessness. Although the minimum time between p.r.n. doses is prescribed, the time of administration is frequently the function of nursing judgment. However, pain in the first 24 hours after an operation requires relief by narcotics, and these medications should not be withheld when the patient is in pain.

Patient-controlled analgesia (PCA) permits the self-administration of pain medication via the intravenous or epidural route within time and dosage limits. Self-administration promotes patient participation in care and eliminates delayed pain medications. For thoracic and major abdominal surgery, certain narcotics may be administered by epidural infusion via an epidural catheter inserted in the operating room. PCA enables the patient to move, turn, cough, and take deep breaths without pain, thus reducing postoperative pulmonary problems.

Complete pain relief in the area of the surgical incision is seldom attainable for a few weeks, depending on the site and nature of surgery; however, changing the patient's position, using diversionary methods, applying cool washcloths to the face, and rubbing the back with a soothing lotion may be useful in relieving general discomfort temporarily and rendering the medication more effective when it is administered. In addition, the extremities may be stroked very lightly with alcohol or lotion.

- The legs should never be rubbed vigorously; vigorous rubbing may dislodge a thrombus and result in embolism and death.

Studies of the effectiveness of transcutaneous electrical nerve stimulation (TENS) in controlling pain show that patients using TENS have an easier time handling pain, which is reflected in less frequent requests for analgesics.

▷ *Relief of Restlessness.*   Postoperative restlessness may be a symptom that is significant. Restlessness may be a result of oxygen deficit or hemorrhage, which is also assessed through monitoring of vital signs. However, the most common cause is probably general discomfort resulting from the patient's lying in one position on the operating table, the surgeon's handling of tissues, and the body's reaction to recovery from the anesthetic. These discomforts may be relieved by administering the prescribed postoperative analgesics and changing the patient's position frequently. At the same time, the nurse assesses other possible causes of discomfort, such as tight, drainage-soaked bandages. Reinforcing or changing the dressing completely makes the patient more comfortable. Urinary output is noted, and the bladder is palpated for distention; urinary retention can cause restlessness. If possible, the patient should be helped to assume as normal a position as possible for voiding. Various techniques are used to encourage voiding before catheterization is performed.

▷ *Relief of Nausea and Vomiting.*   With the advent of newer anesthetic agents and antiemetic medications, vomiting has become a less common postoperative phenomenon, although inadequate ventilation during anesthesia can increase the incidence of vomiting. Also, the vomiting that occurs as the patient emerges from anesthesia is frequently an attempt to relieve the stomach of the mucus and saliva swallowed during the anesthetic period.

After surgery, simple symptomatic therapy is usually all that is required. Many authorities believe that most antiemetic medications (usually derivatives of phenothiazine) produce more undesirable effects, such as hypotension and respiratory depression. If a medication is required, short-acting barbiturates are often prescribed. Droperidol (Inapsine) may be prescribed for intravenous or intramuscular use to produce sedation and reduce the incidence of nausea and vomiting. The medication may be administered preoperatively and during surgery; its effects carry over into the postoperative period.

- At the slightest indication of nausea, the patient is turned completely on one side to promote mouth drainage.
- The most important nursing intervention required when vomiting occurs is to prevent aspiration of vomitus, which can cause asphyxiation and death (see Chap. 25).

When vomiting is likely because of the nature of surgery, a nasogastric tube is passed beforehand and remains in place throughout the operative procedure and the immediate postoperative period. The nasogastric tube is removed when peristalsis returns as indicated by the presence of bowel sounds and the passage of flatus.

Other causes of postoperative vomiting include an accumulation of fluid in the stomach, inflation of the stomach, and the ingestion of food and fluid before peristalsis returns. Psychologic factors also may play a role; the patient who expects to vomit postoperatively frequently does. Thus, helpful preoperative instruction can reduce the probability of vomiting after surgery.

After vomiting, the patient is assisted with oral hygiene; fluids may be withheld for a few hours. The main danger, as already indicated, is from aspiration of the vomitus. Thus, precautions are necessary even before the patient begins to vomit.

In an emergency situation, a patient may be brought to the operating room with food in his stomach. Some anesthesiologists administer preoperative oral antacids to counteract the acid-aspiration syndrome. Otherwise, if acid from the vomitus is aspirated into the lungs, it causes an asthma-like attack, with severe bronchial spasms and wheezing. Patients can subsequently develop pneumonitis and pulmonary edema and become extremely hypoxic.

Increasing medical attention is being paid to silent regurgitation of gastric contents because it occurs more frequently than was previously realized. The importance of pH in the etiology of acid aspiration is being studied, as is the value of preoperatively administering an H_2-receptor antagonist such as cimetidine.

▷ *Relief of Abdominal Distention.*   Postoperative distention of the abdomen results from the accumulation of gas in the intestinal tract. Manipulation of the abdominal organs during the operation may produce a loss of normal peristalsis for 24 to 48 hours, depending on the type and the extent of surgery.

Even though nothing is given by mouth, swallowed air and gastrointestinal secretions enter the stomach and the intestines; if not propelled by peristaltic activity, they collect in the intestines, producing distention and causing the patient to complain of fullness or pain in the abdomen. Most often the gas collects in the colon; hence, a rectal tube or catheter may provide relief (Fig. 22-5).

After major abdominal surgery, distention may be avoided by having the patient turn frequently, exercise, and, when permissible, ambulate. When postoperative distention is anticipated, a nasogastric tube may be inserted prior to surgery. Swallowing of air (often done by patients as part of an anxiety reaction) provides most of the gas that produces distention. The nasogastric tube may remain in place until full peristaltic activity (passage of flatus) has resumed. The nurse can determine when peristaltic bowel sounds return by listening to the abdomen with a stethoscope. The presence of bowel sounds is reported so that the proper diet modification can be prescribed.

◊ *Relief of Hiccups.* A hiccup is produced by intermittent spasms of the diaphragm and is manifested by a coarse sound (an audible "hic"), a result of the vibration of the closed vocal cords as the air rushes suddenly into the lungs. The cause of the diaphragmatic spasm may be any irritation of the phrenic nerve from its center in the spinal cord to its terminal ramifications on the undersurface of the diaphragm. This irritation may be (1) direct—such as stimulation of the nerve itself by a distended stomach, peritonitis or subdiaphragmatic abscess, abdominal distention, pleurisy, or tumors in the chest pressing on the nerves; (2) indirect—such as from toxemia or uremia that stimulates the center; or (3) reflexive—such as irritation from a drainage tube, exposure to cold, drinking very hot or very cold fluids, or obstruction of the intestines.

Hiccup occurs occasionally after abdominal operations. Often it occurs in mild transitory attacks that cease spontaneously or with very simple treatment. When hiccups persist, they may produce considerable distress and serious effects, such as vomiting, exhaustion, and possibly wound dehiscence.

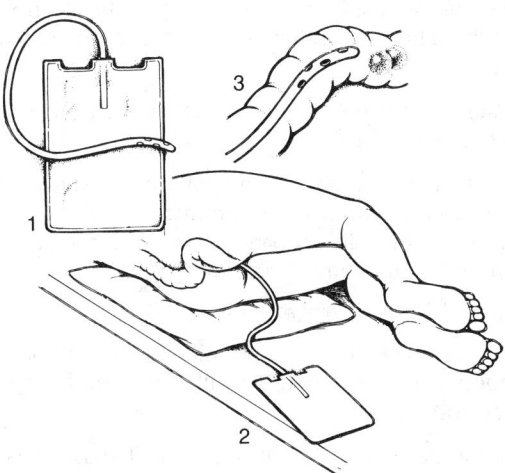

Figure 22-5. Relief of abdominal distention. (1) Rectal tube or catheter attached to plastic bag. (2) Tube or catheter in place, with patient lying on left side. (3) Enlargement of lower colon showing gas bubbles that will be tapped by rectal tube or catheter.

The multitude of remedies suggested for the relief of this condition is proof that no one treatment is effective in every situation. The best remedy is to eliminate causes, such as fluids that are too hot or too cold. Probably the most efficient of the older and simpler remedies is to hold the breath while taking swallows of water. Prescription of phenothiazine medications has been helpful on occasion. Another method is finger pressure on closed eyelids for several minutes. Induced vomiting has helped in some instances.

◊ *Evaluation: Expected Outcomes.* The patient experiences relief of pain and postoperative discomforts (restlessness, nausea and vomiting, abdominal distention, and hiccups).

1. Indicates that pain is decreased in intensity
2. Splints incision site when coughing to prevent pain
3. Participates in diversionary measures (*e.g.*, conversation, television)
4. Reports absence of nausea; no vomiting
5. Is free of abdominal distress and gas pains
6. Demonstrates the absence of hiccups

◊ **Freedom From Injury**

A patient emerging from anesthesia may display restless behavior. If at all possible, he should not be restrained, but he must be protected from injuring himself or interfering with IV therapy, tubes, and monitoring equipment. Analgesics and sedatives are administered as prescribed. Attention is given to possible causes of discomfort that can affect subconscious cognition, such as dressings that are too tight, pressure on a nerve due to improper positioning, irritating drainage, leakage of IV fluids, or a hot water bag that is too hot. Through careful monitoring as the patient emerges from the anesthetic, the nurse can detect problems before they cause injury.

1. Avoids injury
2. Accepts side rails in up position when required
3. Is free from injury related to faulty position, falling, other hazards
4. Attains normal sensorium

◊ **Maintenance of Adequate Tissue Perfusion**

The patient is monitored for any signs and symptoms suggesting diminished tissue perfusion: a decreasing blood pressure; rapid or labored respirations; resting pulse greater than 100 beats per minute; restlessness; slow responses; cold, clammy, pale, or cyanotic skin; diminished or absent peripheral pulses; or urine output less than 30 ml/hr. Any one of these signs and symptoms is reported.

Measures are initiated to maintain adequate tissue perfusion. Room temperature is kept comfortable and the patient is provided with sufficient clothing and blankets to prevent chilling, which causes vasoconstriction. The effects of fluid and blood component therapy are monitored. Activities are initiated to stimulate circulation, such as leg exercises learned preoperatively; the patient is encouraged to turn and change position slowly and to avoid positions that compromise venous return, such as a raised knee gatch or pillow under the knees, sitting for long periods, and dangling legs with pressure in back of the knees. The patient is assisted to get out of bed and walk if prescribed; antiembolic stockings are applied if prescribed but are removed during daily bathing.

▷ *Evaluation: Expected Outcomes.*   The patient maintains adequate tissue perfusion.

1. Exhibits normal vital signs
2. Displays absence of cyanosis of skin and mucous membranes
3. Is oriented to person, place, and time

▷ *Maintenance of Adequate Fluid Volume*

A considerable loss of body fluids occurs with surgery as a result of increased perspiration, increased mucus secretion in the lungs, and loss of blood. To combat the loss of fluids, solutions are prescribed intravenously for the first few hours after surgery. Even though an adequate amount of fluid is taken by this method, often it does not relieve thirst. Thirst is also a troublesome symptom after many general anesthetics, and even after local anesthesia. It stems largely from the dryness of the mouth and the pharynx caused by the inhibition of mucus secretion after the usual preoperative medication of atropine. Many patients who receive local anesthesia complain of thirst during the operation.

Because a sticky, dry mouth demands moisture, fluids may be given to most patients as soon as the postoperative nausea and vomiting have passed and bowel sounds are present. Sips of hot tea with lemon juice dissolve the mucus better than cold water does. As soon as the patient can take water by mouth in sufficient quantities, intravenous administration of fluids is discontinued.

The patient is observed for evidence of electrolyte imbalance: weakness, lassitude, nausea, vomiting, irritability, and possibly neuromuscular abnormalities. Monitoring of mental status, skin color, and temperature is continued, and the presence and quality of peripheral pulses are noted. Signs of decreasing tissue perfusion are reported. The elderly patient is especially at risk for fluid and electrolyte imbalances:

Signs of hypovolemia: Decreased blood pressure, tachycardia, reduced urinary output, CVP less than 4 cm H_2O
Signs of hypervolemia: Increased blood pressure, CVP greater than 15 cm H_2O, crackles in lung bases (wet), an S_3 gallop

▷ *Evaluation: Expected Outcomes.*   The patient maintains adequate fluid volume.

1. Increases fluid intake gradually
2. Maintains fluid balance; relieves thirst
3. Voids adequately without use of catheter
4. Displays no symptoms of hypovolemia

▷ *Maintenance of Normal Body Temperature*

Patients who have been anesthetized are susceptible to chills and drafts. If the patient underwent prolonged exposure to cold in the operating room and received large amounts of intravenous infusions, he is monitored for potential hypothermia, and signs of hypothermia are reported to the physician. The room is maintained at a comfortable temperature and blankets are provided to prevent chilling.

▷ *Evaluation: Expected Outcomes.*   The patient maintains normal body temperature.

1. Exhibits normal core body temperature
2. Reports absence of chills
3. Demonstrates no shivering

▷ *Maintenance of Nutritional Balance*

Following surgery, the more rapidly the patient can accept his usual diet, the more quickly will his normal gastrointestinal function resume. Taking food by mouth stimulates digestive juices and promotes gastric function and intestinal peristalsis. Exercise in bed or early ambulation also assists the digestive process and prevents such problems as distention, "gas pains," and constipation.

The return to a normal dietary pattern should proceed at the pace set by the individual patient. Of course, the nature of surgery and the type of anesthesia directly affect the rate of return. Once the patient has completely recovered from the effects of anesthesia and is no longer nauseated, steps are taken to restore a normal diet.

Liquids are usually the first substances desired and tolerated by the patient after surgery. Water, fruit juices, and tea may be given in increasing amounts if vomiting does not occur. The fluids administered should be cool, not ice cold or tepid. Because fluids supply relatively few calories, soft foods (gelatin, junket, custard, milk, and creamed soups) that supply additional calories and nutrients are added gradually after clear fluids have been tolerated. As soon as the patient tolerates soft foods well, solid food may be given.

A well-balanced diet is provided and includes foods that are selected and preferred by the patient. Usually it takes 2 to 3 days for appetite to return, so attractive trays are a therapeutic consideration.

* When surgery has been performed on the gastrointestinal tract, peristalsis takes longer to return.

Usually, a nasogastric or gastrointestinal tube is in place for the first 24 to 48 hours following gastrointestinal surgery. Such decompression tubes remove flatus and secretions. Attention is given to the maintenance of proper fluid and electrolyte balance, and parenteral fluids or total parenteral nutrition may be prescribed to provide nutrients, fluid, and electrolytes (see Chap. 35).

When nothing is given by mouth postoperatively, conscientious oral hygiene is required. A clean, refreshed mouth diminishes nausea and promotes the appetite when eating is resumed. Weighing the patient daily provides an indication of progress.

▷ *Evaluation: Expected Outcomes.*   The patient maintains nutritional balance.

1. Exhibits increased gastrointestinal motility and absence of paralytic ileus; bowel sounds normal
2. Resumes normal dietary patterns when appropriate
3. Gains weight to return to baseline

▷ *Return of Normal Urinary Function*

The time a patient may be permitted to go without voiding after surgery varies considerably with the type of surgical procedure performed.

* Generally, every effort is made to avoid the use of a catheter because of the risk of urinary tract infection.

All known methods to aid the patient in voiding should be tried (*e.g.*, letting water run, applying heat to the perineum). A bedpan should be warm; a cold bedpan causes discomfort and reflex muscle tightening (including urethral sphincter).

When a patient complains of not being able to use the bedpan, it may be permissible to use a commode rather than resort to catheterization. Male patients are often permitted to sit up or stand beside the bed to use the urinal, but safeguards should be taken to prevent him from falling or fainting.

- All urine, whether voided or obtained by catheterization, is measured and the amount noted on the nurse's record.
- An intake and output chart is kept on all patients following urologic or complex operative procedures and on all elderly patients.
- A urine output of less than 30 ml for each of 2 consecutive hours is reported.

▷ *Evaluation: Expected Outcomes.*   Normal urinary function returns.

1. Voids adequately without use of a catheter
2. Demonstrates absence of frequent small amounts in voiding (indicative of retention)
3. Assumes responsibility for adequate intake of fluids

▷ *Resumption of Usual Pattern of Bowel Elimination*

Preoperative bowel preparation, immobility, intestinal manipulation during surgery, and reduced oral intake can all affect bowel function. Increased fluid intake and early ambulation can facilitate the return of bowel sounds and peristalsis. Abdominal auscultation with a stethoscope assists the nurse in determining the presence of bowel sounds; if bowel sounds are heard, the patient's diet is gradually increased.

Paralytic ileus is a complication that may occur after intestinal or abdominal surgery. It is characterized by the absence of bowel sounds (no peristalsis) and discomfort and distention of the abdomen (denoted by complaints of abdominal tightness and increased abdominal girth). The condition may even result in reverse peristalsis, which causes nausea and vomiting, and possibly the vomiting of fecal material. Insertion of a nasogastric tube is ordered and, depending on the patient's condition, intravenous fluids or total parenteral nutrition may be indicated.

▷ *Constipation.*   The causes of constipation after operation may be minor or serious. Irritation and trauma to the bowel at the time of the operation may inhibit intestinal movement for several days, but usually peristalsis returns after the third day, following the combined effect of early ambulation, an increase in diet, and perhaps a simple enema. If constipation results from secondary conditions (*e.g.,* local inflammation, peritonitis, or abscess), treatment of the cause is indicated. Constipation has been described as difficult or infrequent passage of stools.

It is important to note that many people are constipated habitually and often give a history of daily laxative use for many years. Attempts should be made to correct their bowel habits as soon as is practical. However, in some instances, especially with elderly patients, these attempts may not be feasible. If fluids, roughage, and bulk laxatives are ineffective, enemas are used to evacuate the lower bowel. Cathartics are not given unless prescribed by the physician.

▷ *Evaluation: Expected Outcomes.*   The patient resumes normal bowel function.

1. Exhibits normal and effective bowel sounds on auscultation
2. Is free of abdominal distress, gas pains, and constipation
3. Demonstrates usual bowel elimination pattern

▷ *Maintenance of Skin Integrity and Avoidance of Infection*

Between 10% and 15% of surgical patients develop nosocomial (hospital-acquired) infections. Most of these are in one of four anatomic sites: surgical wound, urinary tract, bloodstream, or respiratory tract. The infections occur for several reasons:

- Intact skin and mucous membranes have been invaded by tubes and catheters, by the disease process, or by the surgical procedure.
- The effects of anesthesia and surgery reduce the resistance of the body to infection.
- The patient may be exposed to infectious agents during hospitalization.
- The organisms that are found in hospital-acquired infections are widespread and resistant (*e.g., Staphylococcus aureus, Escherichia coli, Serratia marcescens, Pseudomonas, Klebsiella pneumoniae,* and *Proteus*).
- There are breaks in aseptic technique and may be inadequate hand-washing practices.

When postoperative infections occur, healing is delayed, convalescence is prolonged, functional recovery may be impaired, and death may occur. These complications impose serious burdens on the patient, the family, other patients (cross-contamination and consequent cross-infections), hospital staff (the increased patient care and hospitalization required), and society as a whole (increased hospitalization, insurance costs, and loss of manpower).

Effective infection control is carried out postoperatively by encouraging the patient to cough and take deep breaths by frequent turning. These measures prevent secretions from being retained and possibly causing atelectasis, lung congestion, and pneumonia. The use of sterile equipment (needles, cannulae, dressings), including equipment for respiratory management, prevents transmission of pathogenic organisms. Antibiotics may be prescribed prophylactically by the physician when infections are encountered, and antimicrobials may be prescribed for specific identified organisms in established infections. The nurse plays a key role in infection control by practicing aseptic technique and by conscientiously monitoring and instructing others.

- Conscientious hand washing is essential for every person who comes in contact with patients and is performed before and after each patient contact.

Dressings are inspected periodically to detect signs of hemorrhage or abnormal drainage. When incisions are on the anterior part of the body, the posterior area is inspected for bleeding, because gravity enables seepage to accumulate in an area quite removed from the incision. Dressings should be reinforced if necessary, and the time of dressing changes noted on the patient's chart. (Dressings and care of the incision are discussed in detail on p. 452.)

Judicious control of upper respiratory infections and skin lesions must be practiced. A common cause of infections is contamination related to intravenous infusions (see p. 338 for methods of control).

▷ *Evaluation: Expected Outcomes.*   The patient maintains skin integrity and avoids infection following the normal healing process.

1. Shows evidence of minimal or no wound drainage
2. Has no skin breakdown or infection
3. Can identify initial symptoms of hematoma, injury, and infection
4. Applies medicated ointments as prescribed
5. Is afebrile with normal white blood cell (WBC) count

▷ *Restoration of Mobility*

Hampered by dressings, splints, or drainage apparatus, the patient frequently is unable to change position. Lying constantly in the same position may lead to pressure ulcers or hypostatic pneumonia, to mention only two of the more serious resulting complications.

- The patient with limited mobility must be turned from side to side at least every 2 hours, and his position must be changed as soon as he becomes uncomfortable.

▷ *Positioning.*   Following surgery, the patient may be placed in a variety of positions (depending on the nature of the surgical procedure) to promote comfort and ease pain.

Supine Position.   The patient lies on his back without elevation of the head. In most cases, this is the position in which the patient is placed immediately after surgery. Bed covers should not restrict the movement of the patient's toes and feet.

Lateral Position.   The patient lies on either side with the upper arm forward. The bottom leg is slightly flexed, while the upper leg is flexed at the thigh and the knee. The patient's head is supported on a pillow, and a second pillow is placed longitudinally between the legs. This position is used when it is desirable to have the patient change positions frequently; to aid in the drainage of cavities, such as the chest and abdomen; and to prevent postoperative respiratory and circulatory complications.

Fowler's Position.   Of all the positions prescribed for a patient, perhaps the most common, as well as the most difficult to maintain, is Fowler's position. The difficulty in most instances lies in trying to make the patient fit the bed rather than having the bed conform to the needs of the patient. The patient's trunk is raised to an angle of 60 to 70 degrees. This is a comfortable sitting position. Patients with abdominal drainage usually are put in Fowler's position as soon as they have recovered consciousness, but the head of the bed must be raised slowly to reduce the feeling of light-headedness.

- It is not unusual for a patient to feel faint after the head of the bed is raised; for this reason, pulse rate and color must be assessed frequently. If the patient complains of any dizziness, the bed must be slowly lowered. If the dizziness ends, the head of the bed may be raised again in 1 to 2 hours.

The nurse must determine whether the patient is in correct position and comfortable. Often, very short people are most uncomfortable in the ordinary hospital bed and must be supported by pillows. It is advisable to place a support against the feet to prevent the patient from slipping down in bed and to make the patient feel more secure. Even with these measures, it will be necessary to move the patient up in bed frequently and to readjust the pillows.

▷ *Ambulation.*   Most surgical patients are encouraged to be out of bed as soon as indicated. This is determined by the stability of a patient's cardiovascular and neuromuscular systems, his usual level of physical activity, and the nature of the surgery performed. Following spinal anesthesia, minor surgery, and same-day surgery, the patient ambulates the same day.

- The advantage of early ambulation is that it reduces the incidence of postoperative complications such as atelectasis, hypostatic pneumonia, gastrointestinal discomfort, and circulatory problems.

Atelectasis and hypostatic pneumonia are relatively infrequent when the patient is ambulatory, because ambulation increases respiratory exchange and aids in preventing stasis of bronchial secretions within the lung. Ambulation also reduces the possibility of postoperative abdominal distention because it helps to increase the tone of the gastrointestinal tract and the abdominal wall.

Thrombophlebitis or phlebothrombosis occurs less frequently because early ambulation prevents stasis of blood by increasing the rate of circulation in the extremities. Clinical research findings indicate that the rate of healing in abdominal wounds is more rapid when ambulation is started early; the occurrence of postoperative evisceration in a series of cases was actually less frequent when patients were allowed to be out of bed soon after operation. Studies also indicate that pain is decreased when early ambulation is allowed. Comparative records show that the pulse rate and the temperature return to normal sooner when the patient attempts to regain normal preoperative activity as quickly as possible. Finally, there is the further advantage to the patient of a shorter stay in the hospital, with the consequent lower expense.

Early ambulation should not exceed the patient's tolerance. The condition of the patient must be the deciding factor, and a progression of steps is followed in mobilizing the patient.

- First of all, with nursing support and encouragement, and with safety as the main concern, the patient moves gradually from the lying position to the sitting position until any evidence of dizziness has passed. This position can be achieved by raising the head of the bed.
- Then the patient may be placed completely upright and turned so that both legs hang over the edge of the bed.
- After this preparation, the patient may be helped to stand beside the bed.

When accustomed to the upright position, the patient may start to walk. The nurse should be at the patient's side to give physical support and encouragement. Care must be taken not to tire the patient, and the extent of the first few periods of ambulation varies with the type of surgical procedure and the patient's physical condition and age.

▷ *Bed Exercises.*   When early ambulation is not feasible because of circumstances already mentioned, bed exercises may achieve the same desirable results to some extent. General exercises should begin as soon after operation as possible—preferably within the first 24 hours—and are performed under supervision to ensure their adequacy and the patient's safety. The purpose of these exercises is to promote circulation and prevent the development of contractures as well as to permit the patient the fullest return of physiologic functions. Such exercises include the following:

- Deep-breathing exercises for complete lung expansion
- Arm exercises through full range of motion, with specific attention to abduction and external rotation of the shoulder

- Hand and finger exercises
- Foot exercises to prevent foot drop and toe deformities and to aid in maintaining good circulation
- Leg flexion and leg lifting exercises to prepare the patient for ambulation activities
- Abdominal and gluteal contraction exercises

▷ *Evaluation: Expected Outcomes.*   The patient resumes mobility within the limitations of the postoperative and rehabilitation plan.

1. Alternates periods of rest and activity
2. Progressively increases ambulation
3. Resumes normal activities within prescribed time frame
4. Performs activities related to self-care
5. Participates in a rehabilitation program (when appropriate)

▷ *Reduction of Anxiety and Achievement of Psychosocial Well-Being*

Almost all postoperative patients need psychological support during the immediate postoperative period. When the patient's condition permits, a close member of his family may see him for a few moments. Thus, the patient feels more secure and the family is reassured.

The questions posed by a patient in PARR often indicate his deep feelings and thoughts. Perhaps he shows concern about the outcome of the operation or about the future. Whatever the patient's concern, the nurse should be in a position to answer queries reassuringly without going into a discussion of details. The immediate postoperative period is not the time for discussion of operative findings or prognosis. On the other hand, these questions should not be dismissed lightly because they may offer clues to the patient's concerns.

As the patient moves through the early postoperative phases, measures are implemented to provide feelings of stability. This is accomplished by assuring the patient that a nurse is available at all times to talk with him, to reinforce the explanations of the physician, and to correct any misconceptions he may have. He is instructed in relaxation techniques and diversional activities. Significant others are included in instructional sessions to assist the patient when he leaves the hospital. Projections are made about his adjustment and needs when he leaves the hospital. The nurse encourages the patient to verbalize his concerns about the recovery phase and the resumption of his own care.

▷ *Evaluation: Expected Outcomes.*   The patient attains/maintains psychosocial well-being.

- Participates in self-care activities
- Takes time for grooming
- Talks positively about future plans
- Asks questions about resuming sexual relations
- Expresses anticipation about seeing friends and family

Documentation and Reporting of Data

Determining the significance of the signs and symptoms noted in assessing the patient is a matter of judgment. When viewed in isolation, one sign may be of little importance, but in the broader context it may be significant in assessment of the patient.

There are a few general guidelines that may assist in guiding the nurse to make accurate judgments. Of course, any severe symptom is always important.

- Any apparently minor symptom that tends to recur repeatedly or to increase in severity should be regarded as significant— for example, hiccups may or may not be of importance, depending on their duration.
- A symptom may seem insignificant in itself but when associated with other definite changes may signal danger. For example, a repeated sigh, when accompanied by increasing restlessness, pallor, and a rising pulse rate, may be one of the clinical signs of dangerous hemorrhage.
- Any steadily progressive decline in the general condition of the patient, even with no outstanding symptoms evident, is of grave importance.
- The patient's complaints and statements should never be dismissed without investigation.

Recording information accurately and concisely not only informs all medical and nursing personnel of the patient's condition but also satisfies medicolegal requirements.

If a physician is to be notified for any reason, all necessary information should be at hand before the physician is contacted by phone, including the latest vital signs. It is also advisable to take the patient's chart, including nursing records, to the telephone to refer to them should questions arise.

Gerontologic Considerations

The elderly patient is transferred from the operating room table to the bed *slowly* and *gently* while monitoring the effects of this action on blood pressure, observing facial expression (if the patient is awake), and observing for evidence of hypoxia. Special attention is given to keeping the patient warm, because body temperature in the elderly is labile. Position is changed frequently to stimulate respirations and circulation and to promote comfort, because lying in one position can be uncomfortable.

Immediate postoperative care for the elderly patient is the same as that for any surgical patient, but additional support is given if there is impaired function of the cardiovascular, pulmonary, or renal systems.

With invasive monitoring, it is possible to detect cardiopulmonary deficits before obvious signs and symptoms are apparent. Because of monitoring and improved individualized preoperative preparation, many older adults tolerate surgery and recover well.

Confusion is one of the most common experiences of an older postoperative patient. This is aggravated by social isolation, restraints, and sensory deprivation. Nighttime confusion can be reduced by frequent nursing attention and caution in the use of medications, especially narcotic analgesics and sedatives.

Early mobilization is instituted to prevent pneumonia, the most frequent respiratory complication in the elderly. Keeping the patient active also prevents atelectasis, irritation of pressure areas, deep venous thrombosis (DVT), and undue weakness. Sitting positions that promote venous stasis in the lower extremities are to be avoided. *Ambulation means that the patient walks, not sits in a chair.* Adequate assistance is required to prevent bumping into objects and falling.

Urinary incontinence can be prevented by providing easy access to the call bell and the commode and by prompted voiding. Early ambulation and familiarity with the room help the patient to become self-sufficient sooner. Postoperative distention, reduced peristalsis, and fecal impaction can be prevented by promoting adequate hydration and activity.

During the early postoperative days, the patient may complain of sore muscles. This is common and usually due to maintaining a constant position during the operation. Massaging aching muscles *gently* and providing support with pillows can ease the discomfort.

Fluid and electrolyte status is monitored to avoid the extremes of fluid overload and dehydration. The nurse compares previous documentation with current records to note changes in fluid balance, breath sounds, and weight. It may be necessary to recommend physical therapy and intensive rehabilitation for patients undergoing prolonged convalescence.

Encouragement and positive thinking are offered. The nurse gently challenges the older adult to recognize that participation in all activities can enhance recovery and prevent complications.

Care of the Wound

A *wound* may be described as a disruption in the continuity of cells; it follows, then, that *wound healing* is the restoration of that continuity.

When wounds occur, a variety of effects may result: (1) immediate loss of all or part of organ functioning, (2) sympathetic stress response, (3) hemorrhage and blood clotting, (4) bacterial contamination, and (5) death of cells. Careful asepsis is the most important factor in keeping these effects to a minimum and promoting the successful care of wounds.

Wound Classification

Wounds may be classified in two different ways: according to the mechanism of injury and the degree of wound contamination at the time of surgery.

Mechanism of Injury.   Wounds may be described as incised, contused, lacerated, or puncture.

- *Incised wounds* are made by a clean cut with a sharp instrument—for example, those made by the surgeon in every operation. Clean wounds (those made aseptically) are usually closed by sutures after all bleeding vessels have been ligated carefully.
- *Contused wounds* are made by blunt force and are characterized by considerable injury of the soft parts, hemorrhage, and swelling.
- *Lacerated wounds* are those with jagged, irregular edges, such as would be made by glass or barbed wire.
- *Puncture wounds* result in small openings in the skin—for example, those made by bullets or knife stabs.

Degree of Contamination.   Wounds may be described as clean, clean-contaminated, contaminated, or dirty or infected.*

---

* *Centers for Disease Control: Guidelines for Prevention of Surgical Wound Infection. Washington, DC, U.S. Department of Health and Human Services, 1985.*

- *Clean wounds* are uninfected surgical wounds in which there is no inflammation and the respiratory, alimentary, genital, or uninfected urinary tracts are not entered. Clean wounds are usually sutured closed; if necessary, a closed drainage system (*e.g.*, Jackson–Pratt) is inserted. The relative probability of wound infection is 1% to 5%.
- *Clean-contaminated wounds* are surgical wounds in which the respiratory, alimentary, genital, or urinary tract is entered under controlled conditions; there is no unusual contamination. The relative probability of wound infection is 3% to 11%.
- *Contaminated wounds* include open, fresh, accidental wounds, and operations with major breaks in aseptic technique or gross spillage from the gastrointestinal tract; in this category are also incisions in which there is acute, nonpurulent inflammation. The relative probability of wound infection is 10% to 17%.
- *Dirty or infected wounds* are those in which the organisms that caused postoperative infection were present in the operative field before surgery. These include old traumatic wounds with retained devitalized tissue and those that involve existing clinical infections or perforated viscera. The relative probability of wound infection is over 27%. (See Wound Sepsis, p. 456.)

Treatment.   Prophylactic antibiotics are administered when bacterial contamination is expected, or for the patient with a clean wound in which a prosthetic device is being inserted.

Infected wounds are not closed until every effort has been made to remove all devitalized and infected tissue. When infection is present, the procedure that removes infected and devitalized tissue is called débridement. Often a small drain is inserted before the wound is sutured to prevent lymph and blood from collecting and retarding the healing process.

Physiology of Wound Healing

Various continuous and overlapping cellular processes contribute to the restoration of a wound: cell regeneration, cell proliferation, and collagen production. The response of tissue to injury goes through several phases: inflammatory, proliferative, and maturation (Table 22-1). See also Chapter 8.

Inflammatory Phase.   Vascular and cellular responses occur immediately when tissue is cut or injured. Vasoconstriction of vessels occurs with a deposition of a fibrinoplatelet clot in an attempt to control bleeding. This lasts from 5 to 10 minutes and is followed by vasodilation of the venules. Microcirculation loses its vasoconstriction ability because norepinephrine is destroyed by the intracellular enzymes. Also, histamine is released, which increases capillary permeability.

When there is damage to microcirculation, blood elements such as antibodies, plasma proteins, electrolytes, complement, and water permeate the vascular space for 2 to 3 days, causing edema, warmth, redness, and pain.

Neutrophils are the first leukocytes to move into damaged tissue. Monocytes that transform to macrophages engulf the debris and transport it from the area. Antigen-antibodies also appear.

Basal cells at wound edges undergo mitosis, and the resulting daughter cells migrate. With this activity, proteolytic enzymes are secreted and dissolve the base of blood clots. The gap between both sides of the wound is progressively filled, and the sides eventually meet in 24 to 48 hours. At this

TABLE 22-1. *Phases of Wound Healing*

Phase	Also Called	Length of Time
Inflammatory	Lag Exudative	1-4 days
Proliferative	Fibroblastic Connective tissue	5-20 days
Maturation	Differentiation Resorptive Remodeling Plateau	21 days to months and even years

point, cell migration is enhanced by hyperplastic bone marrow activity.

Proliferative Phase.   Fibroblasts multiply and form a lattice framework for migrating cells. Epithelial cells form buds at the edges of the wound; these buds develop into capillaries, the nutritional source for the new granulation tissue.

Collagen is the primary component of replaced connective tissue. Fibroblasts initiate the synthesis of collagen and mucopolysaccharides. In a 2- to 4-week period, amino acid chains form into fibers of increasing length and diameter; these fibers become a well-structured pattern of packed bundles. The synthesis of collagen causes capillaries to decrease in number. Thereafter, collagen synthesis decreases in an attempt to balance the amount of collagen that is destroyed. Such synthesis and lysis result in increased tensile strength. However, after 2 weeks, the wound has only 3% to 5% of the original skin strength. By the end of a month, only 35% to 59% of wound

strength has been reached. Never more than 70% to 80% of strength is regained. Many vitamins, particularly vitamin C, aid in the metabolic process involved in wound healing.

Maturation Phase.   About 3 weeks after injury, fibroblasts begin to leave the wound. The scar appears large, until collagen fibrils reorganize into tighter positions. This, along with dehydration, reduces the scar but increases its strength. Such tissue maturation continues and reaches maximum strength in 10 or 12 weeks, but it never reaches the original strength of the prewound tissue.

Forms of Healing

In the surgical management of wound healing, wounds are described as healing by first, second, or third intention.

Healing by First Intention (Primary Union).   Wounds made aseptically, with a minimum of tissue destruction, and properly closed, as with sutures, heal with little tissue reaction "by first intention" (Fig. 22-6). When wounds heal by first intention, granulation tissue is not visible and scar formation is minimal.

Healing by Second Intention (Granulation).   In wounds in which pus formation (suppuration) has occurred or in which the edges have not been approximated, the process of repair is less simple and takes longer. When an abscess is incised it collapses partly, but the dead and the dying cells forming its walls are still being released into the cavity. For this reason, drainage tubes or gauze packing is often inserted into the abscess pocket to allow drainage to escape easily. Gradually the necrotic material disintegrates and escapes, and the abscess cavity fills with a red, soft, sensitive tissue that bleeds very easily. This tissue is composed of minute, thin-walled capillaries and buds that later form connective tissue. These buds, called granulations, enlarge until they fill the area left by the destroyed tissue (see Fig. 22-6). The cells surrounding the capillaries

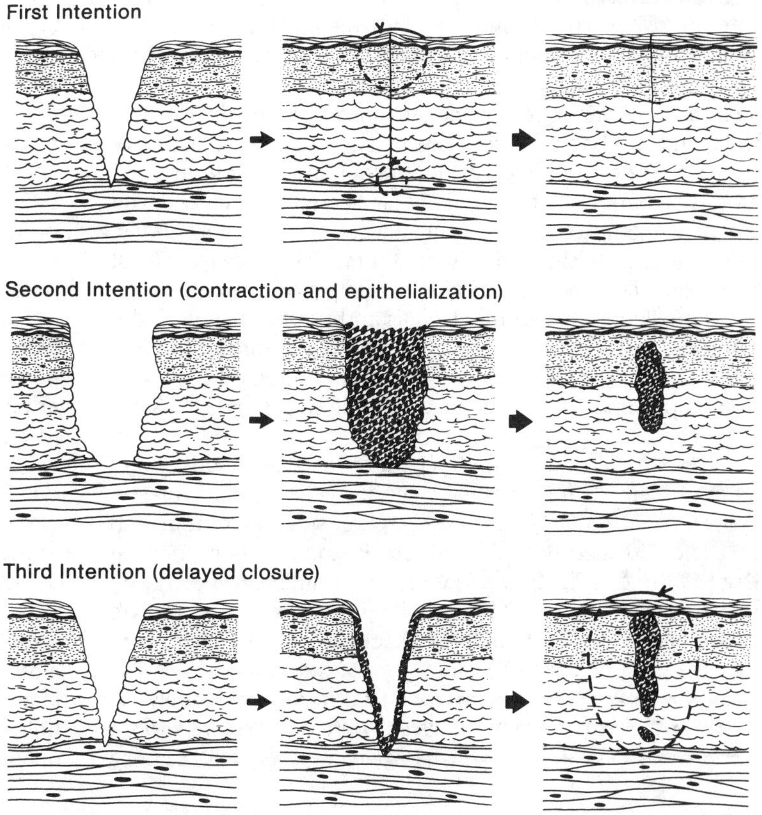

Figure 22-6.   Classification of wound healing. *First intention*—A clean incision is made with primary closure; there is minimal scarring. *Second intention* (contraction and epithelialization)—The wound is left open to granulate in with resultant large scab and abnormal dermal-epidermal junction. *Third intention* (delayed closure)—The wound is left open and closed secondarily when there is no evidence of infection. (Hardy JD. Hardy's Textbook of Surgery, 2nd ed. Philadelphia, JB Lippincott, 1988, p 107.)

change their round shape to become long, thin, and intertwined with each other to form a *scar* or *cicatrix*. Healing is complete when skin cells (epithelium) grow over these granulations. This method of repair is called *healing by granulation*, and it takes place whenever pus is formed or when loss of tissue has occurred for any reason.

Healing by Third Intention (Secondary Suture).   If a deep wound either has not been sutured early or breaks down and then is resutured later, two apposing granulation surfaces are brought together. This results in a deeper and wider scar (see Fig. 22-6).

Nursing Management and Its Effect on Wound Healing

As a wound undergoes the phases of healing, many elements, such as adequate nutrition, cleanliness, rest, and position, determine how quickly the process occurs. These factors are influenced by nursing interventions. Specific nursing assessments and interventions that address these factors and help to promote wound healing are presented in Chart 22-1. Methods for reducing the incidence of wound infection are described in Chart 22-2.

Dressings

The Purposes of an Effective Dressing

A dressing is applied to a wound for one or more of the following reasons: (1) to provide a proper environment for wound healing; (2) to absorb drainage; (3) to splint or immobilize the wound; (4) to protect the wound and new epithelial tissue from mechanical injury; (5) to protect the wound from bacterial contamination and soiling by feces, vomitus, and urine; (6) to promote hemostasis, as in a pressure dressing; and (7) to provide mental and physical comfort for the patient.

Many surgeons apply a dressing at the time of surgery and order dressing changes as needed. In addition to gauze dressings, gas- and vapor-permeable dressings that are impermeable to liquids and bacteria are available (Op-Site, Tegaderm, Bioclusive). These dressings, which resemble clear plastic film, are made of polyurethane film that is coated on one side with a hypoallergenic, water-resistant adhesive. Being highly elastic, they conform easily to body contours. They are used most commonly as coverings for arterial and venous catheter sites, pressure ulcers, skin around stomas and fistulas, skin graft donor sites, and surgical wounds. Their chief advantages are that the wound is visible, so infection can be detected early and treated promptly, and patients can bathe with these dressings in place.

The suture line is gently cleansed and swabbed at prescribed intervals until drainage ceases. When sutures are removed (before the seventh day), center sutures are removed first and replaced with steristrips to keep the tender incision line reinforced (Fig. 22-7). Thereafter, the incision line may be swabbed with tincture of benzoin for protection until complete healing has taken place. Sutures (black silk, nylon, or fine wire) or metal skin clips used to approximate the skin edges are of little value after the sixth or seventh day and are usually removed. After this, the dressings are purely protective from a functional point of view, but they give some patients a sense of security that is not present if wounds are treated without dressings.

Some surgeons prefer to eliminate dressings during the immediate postoperative period whenever feasible. Examples of circumstances in which dressings are not necessary are facial lacerations, pedicle flaps, or skin grafts on a smooth surface.

When the initial dressing on a clean, dry incision is removed, often it is not replaced. Generally, initial dressings on clean, dry incisions are left in place until the wound edges are sealed and the wound is healing (usually 24 hours for most wounds).

The advantages of not using any dressings include the following: (1) the conditions that promote growth of organisms (warmth, moisture, and darkness) are eliminated; (2) observation and early detection of the wound are enhanced; (3) bathing is easier; (4) reactions to tape are avoided; (5) patient comfort and activity are increased; (6) costs for dressings are reduced; and (7) psychological impact of the surgical incision is reduced.

Surgical Dressings—Nursing Interventions

Although all initial postoperative dressings are changed by the surgeon, subsequent dressings are usually changed by the nurse. A physician's order is not required to reinforce the dressing before the first dressing change. Reinforcement keeps the outer dressing layer dry and clean, thus reducing contamination. The condition of surgical dressings and wounds is documented as carefully as other pertinent observations.

Preparation of the Patient.   The patient is told that the dressing is to be changed and that changing the dressing is a simple procedure associated with little discomfort. The dressing change is scheduled for a suitable time. *Dressings should not be changed at mealtime.* If the patient is in an open unit, the curtains are drawn to ensure privacy; the patient should not be unduly exposed. The incision should not be referred to as a ''scar,'' because for some patients the term has negative connotations. Assurance is given that the incision will shrink as it heals and the redness will fade.

Removal of Adhesive Dressings.   The adhesive is removed by pulling it parallel with the skin surface and in the direction of hair growth, rather than at right angles (Fig. 22-8). Alcohol wipes or nonirritating solvents aid in removing adhesive tapes painlessly and quickly.

The old dressing and the pledgets used in cleaning the wound are removed by means of a forceps and are then deposited in a waterproof bag for easy disposal. Such dressings are never touched by ungloved hands because of the danger of transmitting pathogenic organisms. After instruments are used in the changing of dressings, they are placed in a bag or covered receptacle, not on surfaces where contamination of clean areas is possible. Disposable instruments are discarded in the proper receptacle.

A Simple Dressing.   The routine dressing requires cotton balls, dressings, and perhaps a solution container, along with such instruments as scissors, forceps, hemostat, and possibly a probe. When the tray has been properly opened, the person changing the dressing grasps a cotton ball with a forceps and holds it over the emesis basin as the assistant pours a small quantity of the desired antiseptic. After the wound and sur-

Chart 22–1
Factors Affecting Wound Healing

Factors	Rationale	Nursing Assessment/Interventions
Age of patient	The older the patient, the less resilient the tissues	Handle all tissues gently.
Handling of tissues	Rough handling causes injury and delayed healing	Handle tissues carefully and evenly.
Hemorrhage	Accumulation of blood creates dead spaces as well as dead cells that must be removed	Monitor vital signs. Observe incision site for evidence of bleeding and infection.
	The area becomes a growth medium for infection	
Hypovolemia	Insufficient blood volume leads to vasoconstriction and reduced oxygen and nutrients available for wound healing	Monitor for volume deficit (circulatory impairment). Correct by fluid replacement as prescribed.
Local factors Edema	Constricts blood supply by exerting increased interstitial pressure on vessels	Elevate part; apply cool compresses.
Inadequate dressing technique Too small	Permits bacterial invasion and contamination	Follow guidelines for proper dressing technique.
Too tight	Reduces blood supply carrying nutrients and oxygen	
Nutritional deficits	Insulin secretion may be inhibited, causing blood glucose to rise	Monitor blood glucose levels. Administer vitamin A & C supplements as prescribed.
	Protein-calorie depletion may occur	Correct deficits: this may require parenteral nutritional therapy.
Foreign bodies	Foreign bodies retard healing	Keep wounds free of dressing threads, talcum, and powder from gloves.
Oxygen deficit Tissue oxygenation insufficient Growth of microorganisms	Insufficient oxygen may be due to inadequate lung and cardiovascular function as well as localized vasoconstriction	Encourage deep breathing, turning, controlled coughing. Monitor portable and other closed drainage systems for proper functioning.
Drainage collection	Drainage secretion exceeds absorption	Institute measures to remove accumulated secretions.
Medications Steroids	May mask presence of infection by impairing normal inflammatory response to injury	Be aware of action/effect of medications patient is receiving.
Anticoagulants	May cause hemorrhage	
Broad-spectrum/specific antibiotics	Effective if administered immediately before surgery for specific pathology or bacterial contamination	
	If administered after wound is closed, ineffective because of intravascular coagulation	
Patient overactivity	Prevents approximation of wound edges Resting favors healing	Utilize measures to keep wound edges approximated: taping, bandaging, splints. Encourage rest.
Systemic disorders Hemorrhagic shock Acidosis Hypoxia Renal failure	These are depressants of cell function that directly affect wound healing	Be familiar with the nature of the specific disorder. Administer prescribed treatment. Cultures may be indicated to determine appropriate antibiotic.

(continued)

Chart 22–1 (Continued)

Factors	Rationale	Nursing Assessment/Interventions
Hepatic disease Sepsis Immunosuppressed state	Patient is more vulnerable to bacterial/viral invasion; defense mechanisms are reduced	Provide maximum protection to prevent infection. Restrict visitors with colds; institute mandatory hand washing of all attendants.
Wound stressors Vomiting Valsalva maneuver Heavy coughing Straining	Produce tension on wounds, particularly of the torso	Encourage frequent turning and ambulation, and administer antiemetic medications as prescribed.

Chart 22–2
Effective Methods of Lowering Incidence of Wound Infection

GOALS: Reduce risks that inhibit wound healing. Lower incidence of wound infections.

Interventions	Rationale
Preoperative	
Shorter preoperative hospitalization	Reduces exposure of patient to nosocomial infections.
Treatment of coexistent infections	Infections, such as respiratory, can initiate pulmonary complications.
Avoid shaving of hair; if necessary, remove hair with clippers or depilatories rather than a razor	The fewer nicks and cuts in the skin, the less opportunity for infection.
If shaving is requested, it is performed immediately before the surgical procedure	The longer the time between shaving and the operation, the greater the incidence of infection.
Thorough cleansing of operative site—povidone-iodine (Betadine) shower the evening before and repeated preoperative cleansing with antiseptic detergents	Resident bacteria and skin contaminants are reduced to a minimum.
Prophylactic antibiotics	
Intraoperative	
Thorough cleansing of operative site to remove superficial flora, soil, and debris	Reduces risk of contaminating the wound with patient's skin flora.
Flawless aseptic technique.	Any breaks in technique can initiate infection by introducing contaminants.
Powder or talcum washed off sterile gloves	Foreign particles in a wound, such as talcum or starch, will adversely affect the healing process.
Bleeding controlled with meticulous hemostasis	A clean wound heals without infection.
Drains eliminated in clean wounds	Drains are associated with higher wound infection rates.
Closure delayed in contaminated wounds	Permits healing from base of wound to exterior—otherwise, pocket of infection may develop.

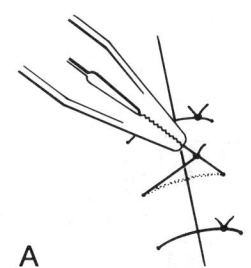 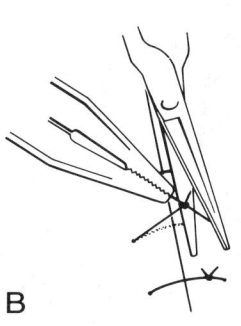 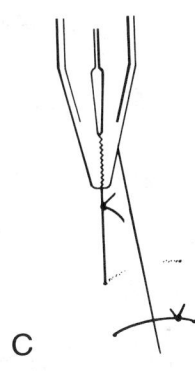

Figure 22-7. *Removing sutures.* (**A**) With the hemostat or forceps, lift the suture upward and away from the skin surface. This permits the blades of the scissors to slide under the suture (**B**) and cut it near the skin. (**C**) Using the hemostat, pull the freed suture up and out.

rounding skin are cleansed with an antiseptic, the new dressing is applied.

- All wound dressings are changed only with sterile gloves.
- If there is any doubt about the sterility of an instrument or a dressing, it is considered unsterile.
- The nurse must not touch soiled dressings with ungloved hands.

Tape is used to keep dressings in place. A variety of tapes are available for patients who are sensitive to the rubber base in adhesive tape. Many tapes are porous and thus permit ventilation and prevent maceration of the skin. Tension sutures are allowed to remain in place for a longer period of time in some instances.

The Dressing of Draining Wounds.   The risk of wound infection is reduced if there is adequate drainage. The wound needs to drain freely to release accumulated blood (clots), body fluids, pus, and necrotic material that otherwise collect in the wound and provide a rich growth medium for microorganisms. If a wound is draining, the skin is not completely closed, so a pathway exists for microorganisms to enter and cause infection. Therefore, closed drainage is preferred to open drainage.

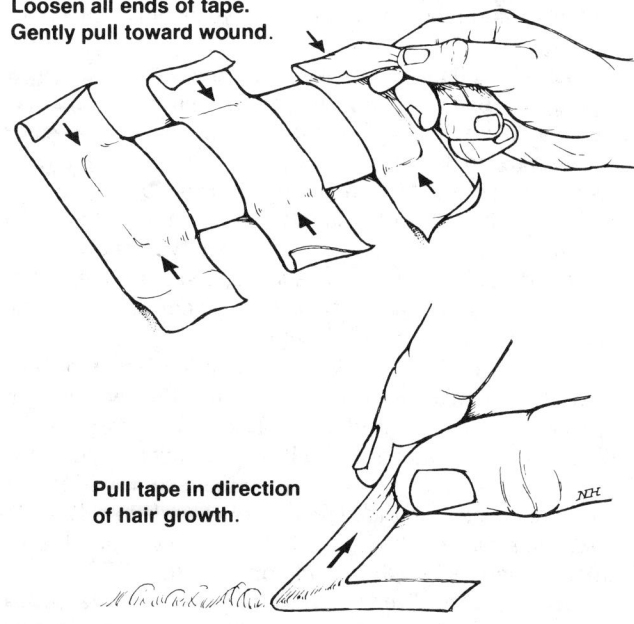

Loosen all ends of tape.
Gently pull toward wound.

Pull tape in direction
of hair growth.

Figure 22-8. Removing adhesive tape.

The drainage from an infected wound is frequently irritating to the surrounding skin. Often this situation can be avoided by the use of a protective ointment or dressing. Petrolatum gauze and zinc oxide ointment are effective preparations.

Portable Wound Suction.   The principle involved in portable wound suction is the use of gentle, constant suction to enhance drainage of serosanguineous fluid and to collapse the skin flaps against the underlying tissue. The *Hemovac* apparatus is a spring diaphragm evacuator for closed suction equipped with multiple small, perforated, inert polyethylene tubes. The tubes are inserted in the drainage areas in the operating room, and the wound is completely closed (Fig. 22-9). The *Surgivac* is a bellows-shaped evacuator for thicker drainage. These devices come in different sizes. *Redi-Vacette* is flat and canteen shaped.

Portable suction has several advantages: it is disposable, lightweight, inexpensive, silent, and space-saving and permits the patient to ambulate.

The Completion of a Dressing.   Dressings are held in place with tape that comes in many types and widths. If the patient is sensitive to adhesive material, hypoallergenic tape is used.

The correct way to apply tape is to place the tape at the center of the dressing and then press the tape down on both sides, applying tension evenly away from the midline (Fig. 22-10). The wrong method of applying tape—fixing one end of the tape to the skin and pulling it tight over the dressing—often wrinkles and pulls the skin in the process. The resulting continuous and forceful traction produces a shearing effect, causing the epidermal layer to slip sideways and become prematurely separated from the deeper dermal layers.

A commercial silicone aerosol is available that can be sprayed over the adhesive used to hold dressings in place; the silicone waterproofs the dressing so that the patient can bathe or swim, and it isolates the area from contamination. The spray is odorless, colorless, nonstaining, noninflammatory, heat-stable, and hypoallergenic.

Elastic adhesive bandage (Elastoplast, Microfoam-3M) is preferable for holding dressings in place over mobile areas, such as the neck or the extremities, or where pressure is required.

When the dressing is completed, the soiled dressings are placed in a waterproof bag and deposited in a covered utility can to await removal for final disposal.

Patient Education.   While changing the dressing, the nurse has an opportunity to teach the patient how to care for the wound at home. The nurse observes for readiness-to-learn clues, such as looking at the incision, expressing interest, or assisting in the dressing change. Information on self-care activities is summarized in Chart 22-3.

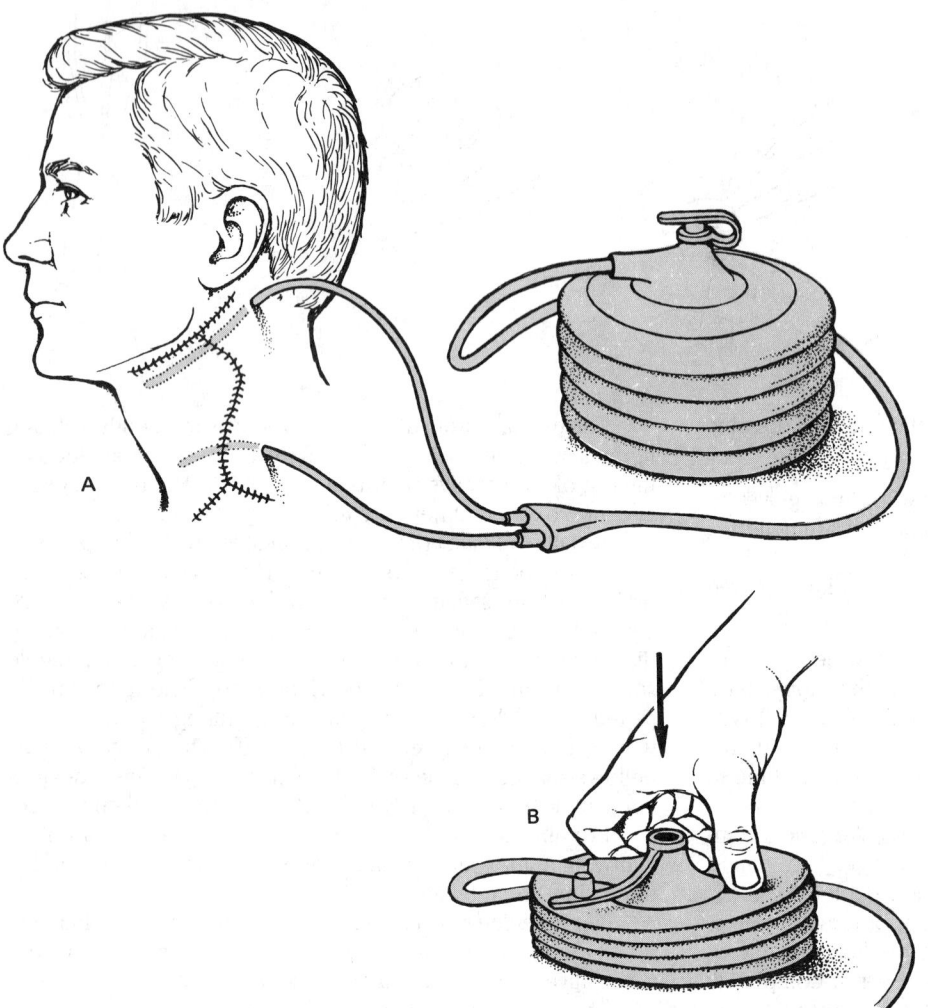

Figure 22–9. Portable wound suction. (**A**) Two perforated catheters are draining the incisional area following a radical neck resection. By means of a Y-tube, drainage is drawn into a portable wound suction receptacle. When full, open top plug of receptacle and empty. (**B**) To reestablish negative pressure, compress receptacle as indicated and replace plug; suction drainage will resume.

Wound Complications

Hematoma (Hemorrhage)

The nurse should know the location of the patient's incision so that the dressings may be inspected for hemorrhage at intervals during the first 24 hours after surgery. Any undue amount of bleeding is reported. At times, concealed bleeding occurs in the wound, beneath the skin. This hemorrhage usually stops spontaneously but results in clot formation within the wound. If the clot is small, it will be absorbed and need not be treated. When the clot is large, the wound usually bulges somewhat, and healing will be delayed unless it is removed. After several sutures are removed by the physician, the clot is evacuated and the wound is packed lightly with gauze. Healing occurs usually by granulation, or a secondary closure may be performed.

Infection (Wound Sepsis)

Surgical wound infections are the second most frequent nosocomial infections in hospitals. Risk factors for wound infections are listed in Chart 22-4. The most important area of prevention lies in meticulous wound management and surgical technique. In addition, cleanliness and environmental disinfection are important.

Staphylococcus aureus accounts for many postoperative wound infections. Other infections may result from *Escherichia coli*, *Proteus vulgaris*, *Aerobacter aerogenes*, *Pseudomonas aeruginosa*, and other organisms (see Nosocomial Infections, Chap. 62).

When the inflammatory process occurs, it usually causes symptoms in 36 to 48 hours. The patient's pulse rate and temperature increase, the WBC count rises, and the wound usually becomes swollen, warm, and tender with incisional pain. Local signs may be absent when the infection is deep.

When a diagnosis of wound infection in a postoperative wound is made, the surgeon usually removes one or more sutures and, under aseptic precautions, separates the wound edges with a pair of blunt scissors or a hemostat. Once the incision is opened, a drain is inserted.

Cellulitis is a bacterial infection that spreads into tissue planes. All the manifestations of inflammation are evident; streptococcus is frequently the responsible organism. Systemic antibiotics are usually effective. If an extremity is the site of the infection, elevation reduces dependent edema and the application of heat promotes local blood circulation. Rest decreases muscular contractions that could introduce the offending organisms into the circulatory system.

Abscess is a localized bacterial infection characterized by a collection of pus (bacteria, necrotic tissue, and WBCs). Usually a "point" develops that is tender. Because the area is under

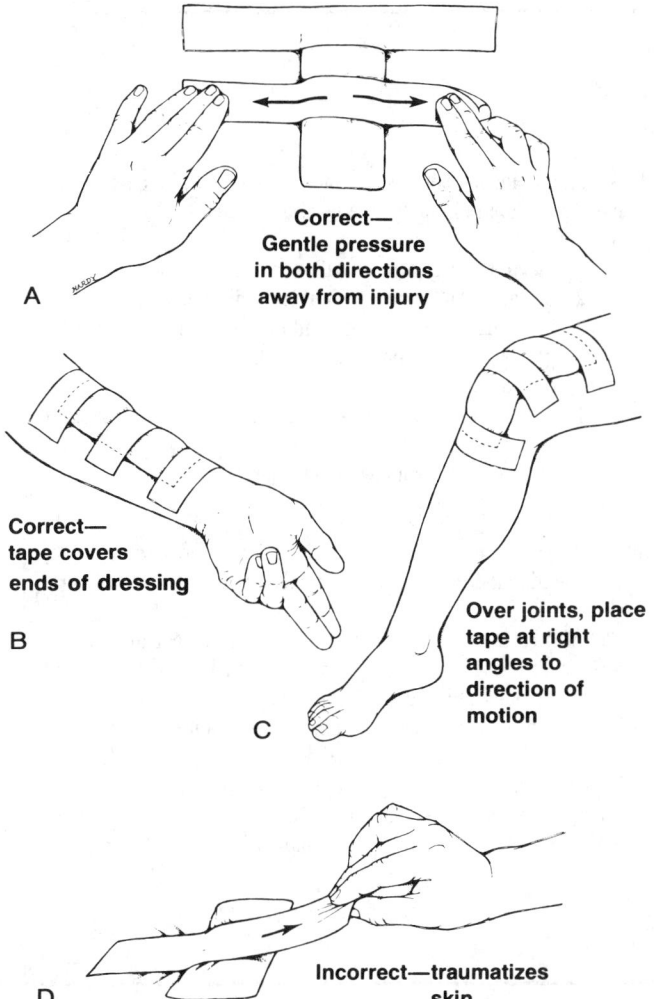

A

**Correct—
Gentle pressure
in both directions
away from injury**

**Correct—
tape covers
ends of dressing**

B

C

**Over joints, place
tape at right
angles to
direction of
motion**

D

**Incorrect—traumatizes
skin**

Figure 22–10. Application of tape. Views **A, B,** and **C** illustrate the correct method of application. The method shown in **D** is incorrect. (**A**) Pressure is applied evenly and directed away from the incision. (**D**) In the incorrect method, the tape is pulling against the skin and exerting pressure over the wound. (**B**) The proper way to cover the ends of a dressing for additional protection of the wound. (**C**) The correct way to position a dressing over a joint for maximum comfort and effectiveness.

pressure, there is a tendency for the infection to seed bacteria that may invade adjacent tissues (cellulitis) or vascular spaces (bacteremia, sepsis). Treatment is surgical drainage or excision and the administration of antibiotics. Recurrence is prevented by allowing the treated wound to drain. Rest, elevation of the part, and heat are helpful.

Lymphangitis is a spread of infection from a cellulitis or abscess to the lymphatic system. This is treated by rest and antibiotics.

Dehiscence and Evisceration

The complications of dehiscence (disruption of surgical wound) and evisceration (protrusion of wound contents) are especially serious when they involve abdominal wounds. These complications result from sutures giving way, from infection, and, more frequently, after marked distention or strenuous cough. They may also occur because of increasing age, poor nutritional

status, and the presence of pulmonary or cardiovascular disease in patients who undergo abdominal surgery.

When the wound edges separate slowly, the intestines may protrude gradually, or not at all, and the earliest sign may be a gush of serosanguineous peritoneal fluid from the wound. When the rupture of a wound occurs suddenly, coils of intestine may push out of the abdomen. Frequently, the patient may say that "something gave way." The evisceration causes pain and can be associated with vomiting.

- When disruption of a wound occurs, the surgeon is notified at once. The protruding coils of intestine are covered with sterile dressings moistened with sterile saline.

An abdominal binder, properly applied, is an excellent prophylactic measure against an evisceration of this kind, and often it is used along with the primary dressing, especially for operations on patients with weak or pendulous abdominal walls, or when rupture of a wound has occurred. Vitamin deficiency or lowered serum protein or chloride may require correction.

Keloid

Scar tissue that develops excessive growth is known as a keloid. Sometimes the entire scar is affected; at other times the condition is segmented. This keloid tendency is unexplainable, unpredictable, and unavoidable in some people.

Investigations of keloid prevention and cure have been conducted. Careful closure of the wound, complete hemostasis, and pressure support without undue tension on the suture lines are reported to combat this distressing wound complication.

Postoperative Complications

The danger inherent in surgery involves not only the risk of the operative procedure but also the hazard of postoperative complications that may prolong convalescence or adversely affect the surgical outcome. The nurse plays an important part in the prevention of these complications and in their early treatment, should they occur. The signs and symptoms of the more common postoperative complications are discussed below. In each instance, the most effective method of prevention and the usual treatment are emphasized.

Although specific complications are discussed, the nursing process involves the total patient and not just his particular surgical condition.

Shock

One of the most serious postoperative complications is shock, which may be described as inadequate cellular oxygenation accompanied by the inability to excrete waste products of metabolism. Shock can occur in association with many kinds of major illness, such as hemorrhage, trauma, burns, infection, and heart disease, and results from a failure of any one of the three aspects of circulation: the heart pump, peripheral resistance, and blood volume. Thus, while there are many kinds of shock, the basic definition centers on an inadequate blood flow to vital organs or the inability of the tissues of these organs to utilize oxygen and other nutrients.

Chart 22–3
Patient Education: Wound Care

Until Sutures Are Removed

1. Keep the wound dry and clean.
   a. If there is no dresssing, ask your nurse or physician if you can bathe or shower.
   b. If a dressing or splint is in place, do not remove it unless it is wet or soiled.
   c. If wet or soiled, change dressing yourself if you have been taught to do so; otherwise, call your nurse or physician for guidance.
   d. If you have been taught, instruction might be as follows:
      (1) Cleanse area *gently* with 70% isopropyl alcohol once or twice daily.
      (2) Cover with a sterile Telfa pad or gauze square—sufficiently large to cover wound.
      (3) Apply hypoallergenic Dermacel or paper tape (adhesive is not recommended because it is difficult to remove without possible injury to incision site).
2. Report immediately if any of these signs of infection occur:
   a. Redness, marked swelling (beyond 2.5 cm [½ in] from incision site), tenderness, increased warmth around wound
   b. Red streaks in skin near wound
   c. Pus or discharge, foul odor
   d. Chills or fever (over 37.7°C [100°F])
3. If soreness or pain is causing discomfort, apply a dry cool pack (containing ice or cold water) or take prescribed acetaminophen tablets (2) every 4–6 hours. Avoid aspirin without direction or instruction because bleeding may be enhanced with its use.

4. Swelling following surgery is common. To help reduce swelling, elevate the injured part to the level of the heart.
   a. Hand or arm
      (1) Sleep—elevate arm on pillow at side.
      (2) Sitting—place arm on pillow on adjacent table.
      (3) Standing—rest affected hand on opposite shoulder; support elbow with unaffected hand.
   b. Leg or foot
      (1) Sitting—place a pillow on a facing chair; provide support underneath the knee.
      (2) Lying—place a pillow under injured leg.

After Sutures Are Removed

Although the wound appears to be healed when sutures are removed, it is still tender and will continue to heal and strengthen for several weeks.

1. Follow directives of physician or nurse as to extent of activity.
2. Keep suture line clean; do not rub vigorously; pat dry. Wound edges may look red and be slightly raised. This is normal.
3. Massage around wound gently using a bland baby oil, petrolatum, or moisturizing cream (twice a day).
4. Report to the health care provider if after 8 weeks the site continues to be red, thick, painful to pressure. (This may be due to excessive collagen formation and should be checked.)

Chart 22–4
Risk Factors Contributing to Wound Sepsis

Local

Wound contamination
Foreign body
Faulty suturing technique
Devitalized tissue
Hematoma
"Dead" space

General

Debilitation
  Dehydration
  Malnutrition
  Anemia
Advanced age
Extreme obesity
Shock
Length of preoperative hospitalization
Length of operation
Associated diseases (*e.g.,* diabetes mellitus)

Pathophysiology

Catecholamines (epinephrine and norepinephrine) are elevated during shock and are the dominant hormones in response to severe shock. Their effect is to constrict arterioles in the skin, subcutaneous tissue, and kidneys; they dilate arterioles of skeletal muscles and the liver. Furthermore, the increase in heart rate, myocardial contractility, and venous return from the constriction of the great veins are responses that attempt to increase cardiac output. Shock stimulates corticotropin release from the pituitary gland and thereby increases plasma levels of glucocorticoids. Mineralocorticoids are elevated because of increased activity in the renin–angiotensin systems. Glucagon is released for energy, and antidiuretic hormone is released for maximum glomerular reabsorption of water.

Endorphins are released in conjunction with the release of corticotropin. Endorphins act like opiates, which may contribute to low blood pressure.

The effect of high levels of epinephrine, cortisol, and glucagon and insufficient levels of insulin stimulates catabolism. There is decreased oxygen utilization because of decreased cardiac output and insulin insufficiency. See Figure 22-11 in Chart 22-5 for microcirculatory changes in shock.

Classification

Shock may be classified as hypovolemic (oligemic), cardiogenic, neurogenic, or septic.

Chart 22–5
Pathophysiology of Shock

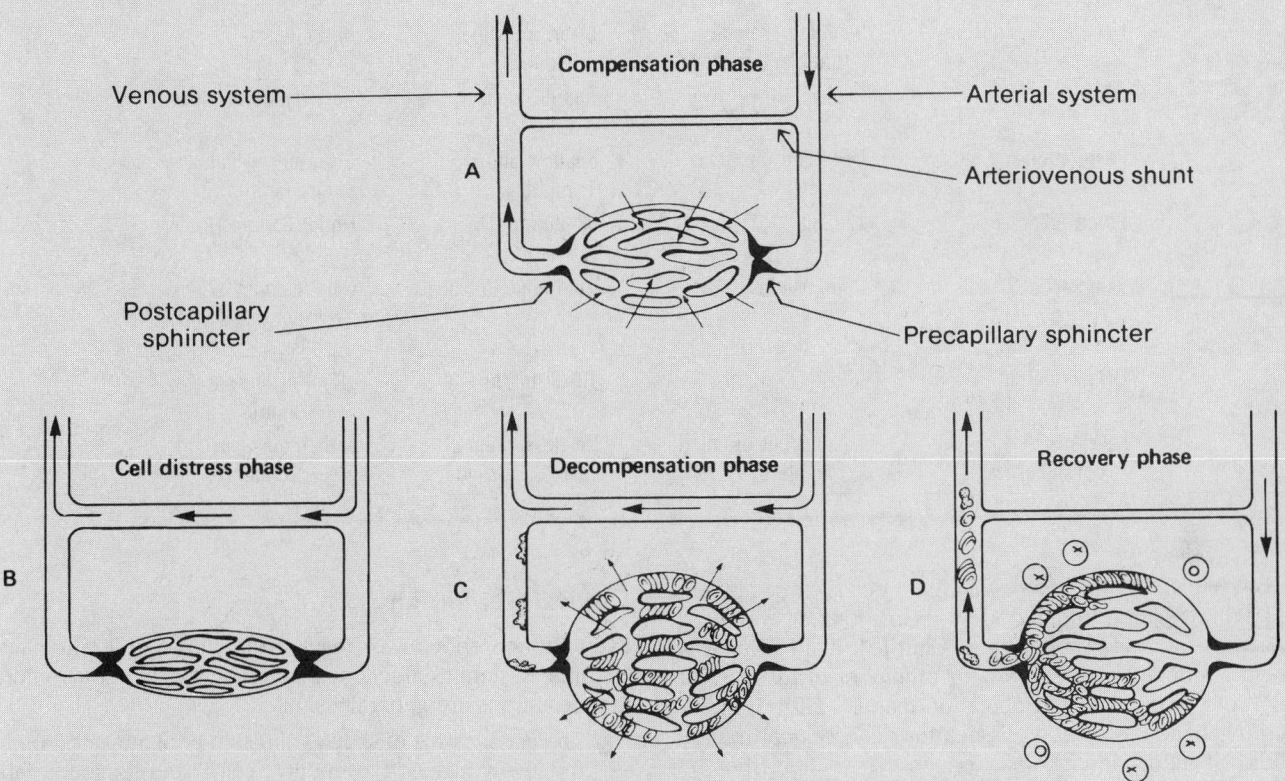

Figure 22–11. Microcirculatory changes in shock. (**A**) Compensation phase. (**B**) Cell distress phase. (**C**) Decompensation phase. (**D**) Recovery phase. (Dunphy JE and Way LW. Current Diagnosis and Treatment. Los Altos, California, Lange Medical Publishers.)

When the body sustains an insult, such as hemorrhage, extensive burns, or heart failure, a compensatory reaction occurs. The adrenal medulla releases catecholamines to constrict arterioles and venules in the major organs of the body (kidneys, liver, intestines) so that more blood is diverted to the brain and heart.

Pathophysiologic Consequences of Shock

The greatest impact of all types of shock is exerted on the microcirculation (arterioles, capillaries, venules—microvasculature), which reacts to shock in a series of steps. The first phase involves a response to the hypovolemia, as is seen in the contraction of the precapillary arteriole sphincters (Fig. 22–11*A*). This causes capillary pressure to fall, with the result that fluid moves into the vascular spaces and increases the blood volume. By such compensatory action, blood volume returns to normal and the precapillary sphincters relax. If shock is more prolonged, however, recovery is prevented and the next phase, cell distress, is entered (see Fig. 22–11*B*). In this phase, arteriovenous shunts open and divert arterial flow directly

back into the venous system. Meanwhile, the cells in the bypassed segment of microcirculation rely on anaerobic metabolism for energy. Glucose and oxygen are reduced markedly for the cells, and waste products such as lactate increase. Histamine is released and the postcapillary sphincter closes. Capillary flow is slowed considerably and the bed constricts with very few capillaries remaining open. In the decompensation phase (see Fig. 22–11*C*), just before the death of the cell, acidosis (decreasing serum *p*H) causes the precapillary sphincter to open. Fluid and protein are lost in the interstitial space, and the capillary expands with agglutinated red blood cells (sludge). White cells and platelets gather in the venules where acidosis is most profound. Arteriovenous circulation continues to supply essential oxygen to the vital areas of heart and brain. In the recovery phase (see Fig. 22–11*D*), if the blood volume is restored during the decompensation phase while the effects on microcirculation are still reversible, badly damaged cells can be repaired. Cell aggregates can be filtered out by the lungs and into the systemic circulation. If there is an overabundance of dead cells, however, this is not possible, and death results.

TABLE 22–2.   *Classification and Symptoms of Hypovolemic Shock*

	Mild	*Moderate*	*Severe*
Percentage of blood volume loss	Up to 20%	20%–40%	40% or more
Decreased perfusion	Skin, fat, skeletal muscle, bone	Liver, intestine, kidneys	Brain, heart
Pulse	Rapid	Rapid—weaker, thready	Very rapid, irregular
Respirations	Deep and rapid	Shallow and rapid	Even more shallow and rapid
Blood pressure	120/80	60–90 mm Hg systolic	Under 60 mm Hg systolic
Skin	Cool, pale	Cold, pale, moist	Cold, clammy, cyanotic lips and nails
Urinary output	Above 50 ml/hr	10–25 ml/hr	10 ml or less/hr → anuria
Level of consciousness	Anxious but oriented and alert	Restless, mentally fuzzy, vertigo	Lethargic → comatose

Hypovolemic Shock.   Hypovolemic shock is caused by decreased fluid volume from blood or plasma loss, or even fluid losses from prolonged vomiting or diarrhea. Fluid volume is frequently reduced after surgery for a number of reasons. At times, more blood is lost at operation than is realized. In addition, the handling of body tissues may cause local trauma and loss of blood and plasma from the circulation, thereby creating a decrease in the circulating blood volume. Hypovolemic shock is characterized by a fall in venous pressure, a rise in peripheral resistance, and tachycardia. For additional symptoms, see Table 22-2.

Cardiogenic Shock.   Cardiogenic shock results from cardiac failure or an interference with heart function (*i.e.,* diminished cardiac output from poor heart-pump function), as in myocardial infarction, dysrhythmias, tamponade, pulmonary embolism, advanced (late) hypovolemia, or epidural and general anesthesia. The signs are those of increased pressure in the venous bed and an increase in peripheral resistance.

Neurogenic Shock.   Neurogenic shock occurs as a result of a failure of arterial resistance (such as may be caused by spinal anesthesia or spinal cord injury). It is characterized by a fall in blood pressure due to pooling of blood in dilated capacitance vessels (those with the ability to change volume capacity). Heart activity increases and thus maintains a normal output (stroke volume); this helps to fill the dilated vascular system as it attempts to preserve perfusion pressure.

Septic Shock.   Although septic shock is caused by viruses, fungi, and gram-positive and gram-negative bacteria, it results most frequently from gram-negative septicemia (*e.g.,* infection, peritonitis). At first, the patient exhibits a fever, a rapid, strong pulse, rapid respirations, and normal or slightly decreased blood pressure. Skin is flushed, warm, and dry. However, if infection continues untreated, hypovolemic shock develops. These two phases may be referred to as *hyperdynamic septic shock* (the former) and *hypodynamic shock* (the latter, which is similar to hypovolemic shock). Hypovolemia develops along with depressed cardiac function (see Chap. 29).

Clinical Manifestations

Even though shock can result from many different causes (trauma, systemic infection, or cardiac dysfunction), clinical manifestations are generally similar.

- The classic signs of shock are pallor; cool, moist skin; rapid breathing; cyanosis of the lips, gums, and tongue; a rapid, weak, thready pulse; decreasing pulse pressure; and usually a low blood pressure and concentrated urine. See Table 22-2 for the progression of symptoms in relation to severity.

Diagnostic Assessment

Before treatment can be instituted promptly and intelligently, the *goal* in initial assessment is to determine the cause of volume loss and the status of vital functions. The initial assessment includes the following:

1. *Respirations.* Hyperventilation is an early sign of septic shock.
2. *Skin.* Cold, pale, moist skin indicates vasoconstriction with increased arteriolar resistance and is suggestive of hypovolemic shock. Warm, red skin indicates a decrease in arteriolar resistance and may be seen in septic and neurogenic shock.
3. *Pulse and blood pressure.* Alone, pulse and blood pressure may not be reliable guides to the severity of shock, but their progressive pattern is significant. That is, if each 10-minute interval shows a rise in pulse and a rise followed by a fall in blood pressure, then such signs are indicative of shock. A pulse of 80/min and a blood pressure of 120/80 are normal. When systolic pressure is between 90 mm Hg and 60 mm Hg (in the normotensive person), shock is well advanced. (For the hypertensive person, 30 mm Hg below the baseline systolic pressure is a sign of shock.) With a more rapid pulse rate, the amplitude is weaker and thready in hypovolemic and cardiogenic shock. Dysrhythmia may be noted in cardiogenic shock.
4. *Urinary output.* Because the output of urine is one of the most valuable indices of adequacy of vital organ perfusion,

an indwelling catheter is recommended for any patient at risk for shock. A drop in renal artery pressure and flow produces renal artery vasoconstriction and results in decreased glomerular filtration and decreased urine output. Normal urine flow is 50 ml/hr. An output of 30 ml/hr or less (oliguria or anuria) is suggestive of cardiac failure or inadequate volume replacement.

5. *Central venous pressure.* CVP is the pressure within the right atrium. It is a valuable guide to vascular volume replacement when other parameters (vital signs and cardiopulmonary status) are also considered. Average CVP is 5 to 12 cm water. Several readings are taken to determine the range; a reading near zero may indicate hypovolemia (if patient improves with rapid IV infusion, the patient was hypovolemic). Readings over 15 cm water may suggest hypervolemia, vasoconstriction, or congestive heart failure. Pulmonary artery pressure and pulmonary capillary wedge pressure are more accurate indications of the pumping ability of the left side of the heart (see Chap. 27).

6. *Arterial blood gases.* The partial pressures of oxygen pO_2 and carbon dioxide pCO_2 are useful indices in providing therapy. An arterial oxygen tension below 60 mm Hg indicates a marginal respiratory reserve. A pCO_2 over 45 mm Hg indicates serious hypoventilation. In shock, pCO_2 is usually within normal limits.

7. *Serum lactate.* In shock there is a close correlation between arterial blood lactate levels and survival. The higher the lactate level, the greater the oxygen need.

8. *Hematocrit.* Hematocrit is useful in determining the type of fluid to use in replacement. (Such a test must be repeated, because a few hours are required to reflect correctly the amount of blood loss.) If the hematocrit is over 55%, plasma and saline are administered. If the hematocrit is 20% or lower, blood is needed. The maximal oxygen-carrying capacity is best when the hematocrit is between 35% and 45%.

9. *Levels of consciousness.* Consciousness levels may range from alert in mild shock to mental cloudiness in moderate shock. As the condition worsens, the patient becomes lethargic and reacts only to noxious stimuli. Irreversible shock is suspected when the patient fails to react to stimuli.

Management and Nursing Interventions

Prevention. The best treatment for shock is prophylaxis. This consists of adequate preparation of the patient, mental as well as physical, and anticipation of any complication that may arise during or after surgery. Special equipment for the treatment of shock must be available. The proper type of anesthesia should be chosen by the anesthesiologist after careful consideration of the patient and the disorder. Blood and blood substitute should be available if indicated. Blood loss should be measured as accurately as possible.

- If the amount of blood loss exceeds 500 ml (especially if the loss is rapid), replacement is usually indicated.

Obviously, the individual patient and the particular circumstances must be considered in determining replacement therapy. An older, malnourished person is more likely to require this therapy than a patient whose health is generally good.

Surgical trauma should be kept at a minimum as the first step in avoiding shock. After the surgery, factors that may contribute to shock are avoided. Pain is controlled by making the

patient as comfortable as possible and by using narcotics judiciously. Exposure is avoided, and lightweight, unheated covers are used to prevent vasodilation. In the recovery room, the patient is monitored and cared for by nurses experienced in the recovery of patients from anesthesia. In addition, a quiet room helps to reduce stress. Any moving of the patient is done gently. He is placed in a supine position to facilitate circulation. Monitoring of vital signs is continued until the patient's recovery indicates that shock is unlikely.

Treatment. (See also Emergency Treatment of Shock, Chap. 63.) The patient is kept warm, but overheating is avoided to prevent cutaneous vessels from dilating and depriving vital organs of blood. An infusion of lactated Ringer's solution is started. The patient is placed flat in bed with legs elevated as shown in Figure 22-12. (The Trendelenburg position is avoided.) The patient's respiratory and circulatory status are monitored constantly: respiration, pulse, blood pressure, skin, urinary output, level of consciousness, CVP, pulmonary artery pressure, pulmonary capillary wedge pressure, and cardiac output.

The basic approach to the treatment of shock is to determine its cause and correct it if possible. Prevention strategies are described as follows:

1. *Ensure adequacy of airway and respiratory status.* Blood gas determinations are made to determine adequacy of pulmonary function, and the patient is given oxygen by intubation or nasal cannula if indicated.

2. *Restore blood/fluid volume.* The type of fluid and blood replacement depends on the type and amount lost as well as the condition of the patient. Fluids are administered intravenously immediately when the nature of loss is determined. Fluid replacement is modified accordingly. Under normal conditions, 20% of the total blood volume is in the capillaries, 10% is in the arterial system, and the balance is in the veins and heart. In shock there is dilatation of the capillary beds, so a considerable volume of blood can be accommodated.

   Two types of replacement fluids are used: crystalloids and colloids. *Crystalloids* are electrolyte solutions that diffuse into interstitial spaces. An example is lactated Ringer's injection, a buffering solution in which lactate is metabolized and excess hydrogen ions are neutralized.

   Three parts of crystalloids are lost to the extravascular space for every one part that remains in the vascular system. This means that for every 2000 ml given, 500 ml increase the vascular volume. For hemorrhagic shock, crystalloids are pre-

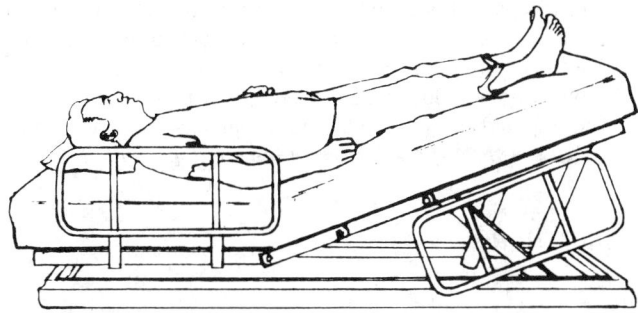

Figure 22-12. Proper positioning of the patient who shows signs of shock. The lower extremities are elevated to an angle of approximately 20 degrees; knees are straight, trunk is horizontal, and head is slightly elevated.

scribed initially to lower blood viscosity and aid in microcirculation.

Colloids include blood, artificial blood, blood substitutes, plasma, serum albumin, and plasma substitutes; these remain in the intravascular compartment. Blood of the same type as the patient's should be administered in preference to O-Rh-negative blood. Burn shock requires large amounts of colloid replacement.

3. *Drug therapy.* Cardiotonics are administered to correct dysrhythmias and improve cardiac efficiency. In addition to reducing fluid retention, diuretics are administered to reduce edema during and following neurosurgery. Vasodilators are prescribed to reduce peripheral resistance, which in turn decreases the work of the heart and increases cardiac output and tissue perfusion. The medication frequently used is sodium nitroprusside (Nipride), which stimulates myocardial contractility and lowers peripheral resistance. Some clinicians advocate the use of steroids, while others use combinations of pharmacotherapeutic agents. Some authorities believe that hypovolemic shock should not be treated with vasoactive medications. Their effect is to increase vascular resistance and decrease tissue perfusion, thus aggravating the effects of shock.

An infusion pump can be used to control the amount of sodium nitroprusside that is administered. Also available are monitors that measure the patient's blood pressure every 10 seconds and automatically adjust the drug dosage if there are any changes.

Nursing Interventions. The nurse assists the physician in carrying out the treatments just described. When vasodilators are prescribed, the patient's blood pressure requires constant monitoring. The patient is kept flat during the administration of these drugs. If the systolic blood pressure continues to fall, the medication is stopped and fluids are increased.

The following nursing measures are indicated:

1. *Psychologic support is provided, and the patient's energy expenditure is reduced.* The patient's reactions to treatment are assessed, and rest is promoted. Support and reassurance are provided to relieve apprehension. Sedatives are administered cautiously so that circulation is not further depressed. The patient is kept warm, because hypothermia decreases tissue oxygenation. Hypothermia also affects peripheral circulation. The patient is turned every 2 hours, and deep breathing is encouraged to promote optimal cardiopulmonary function.

2. *Complications are prevented.* All parameters are observed, and the patient is monitored closely in the 24-hour period following onset of shock because complications may develop. The most common complications are peripheral and pulmonary edema due to fluid overload, resulting from administering fluids faster than the body can accommodate them.

3. *All observations and interventions are documented.*

Hemorrhage

Classification

Hemorrhage is classified as (1) *primary,* (2) *intermediary,* and (3) *secondary.* Primary hemorrhage occurs at the time of the operation. Intermediary hemorrhage occurs during the first few hours after an operation when the rise of blood pressure to its normal level dislodges insecure clots from untied vessels. Sec-

ondary hemorrhage occurs some time after the operation when insecure tying, infection, or erosion of a vessel by a drainage tube results in the slipping of a ligature.

A further classification frequently is made according to the kind of vessel that is bleeding. *Capillary* hemorrhage is characterized by a slow, general ooze; *venous* hemorrhage bubbles out quickly and is dark in color; *arterial* hemorrhage is bright and appears in spurts with each heartbeat.

Hemorrhage is also characterized by its visibility: when the hemorrhage is on the surface and can be seen, it is *evident;* when it cannot be seen, as in the peritoneal cavity, it is *concealed.*

Clinical Manifestations

The clinical signs presented by hemorrhage depend on the amount of blood lost and the rapidity of its escape. The patient is apprehensive and restless, moves continually, and is thirsty; the skin is cold, moist, and pale. The pulse rate increases, the temperature falls, and respirations are rapid and deep, often of the gasping type spoken of as "air hunger." If the hemorrhage progresses untreated, cardiac output decreases, arterial and venous blood pressure and the hemoglobin of the blood fall rapidly, the lips and the conjunctivae become pallid, spots appear before the eyes, a ringing is heard in the ears, and the patient grows weaker but remains conscious until near death.

Management

Often the signs of hemorrhage after an operation are masked by the effects of the anesthetic or shock; therefore, the initial treatment of the patient is in a general way almost identical to that described for the patient with shock. (See previous section on shock.)

The patient is placed in the shock position (see Fig. 22-12), and sedatives or analgesics are administered as prescribed. The wound should always be inspected for bleeding. If bleeding is evident, a sterile gauze pad and a snug bandage are indicated, as is elevation, if possible.

- Giving a transfusion of blood or blood products and determining the cause of hemorrhage are the initial therapeutic measures.
- In giving fluids intravenously in cases of hemorrhage, it is important to remember that unless the hemorrhage has been well controlled, giving too large a quantity or too rapid administration of intravenous fluid may raise the blood pressure enough to start the bleeding again.

Deep Venous Thrombosis

DVT is a thrombosis of deep rather than superficial veins. Two serious complications of DVT are pulmonary embolism and postphlebitic syndrome (see p. 464).

Incidence

Postoperatively, those at greatest risk for DVT have been identified as follows*:

---

* *Consensus Development Conference Statement: Prevention of Venous Thrombosis and Pulmonary Embolism. Bethesda, MD, National Institutes of Health, March 1986.*

- Orthopedic patients having hip surgery, knee reconstruction, and elective lower extremity surgery
- Urologic patients having transurethral prostatectomy, and older patients having urologic surgery
- General surgical patients over age 40, obese, with malignancy, or having had prior DVT or pulmonary embolism, or those undergoing extensive complicated surgical procedures
- Gynecology (and obstetric) patients over age 40 with added risk factors (varicose veins, previous venous thrombosis, infection, malignancy, obesity)
- Neurosurgical patients, similar to other surgical high-risk groups (in stroke, for example, the risk of DVT in the paralyzed leg is as high as 75%)

Pathophysiology

A mild to severe inflammation of the vein occurs in association with a clotting of blood. The complication may result from a number of causes, including injury to the vein by tight straps or leg-holders at the time of surgery, pressure from a blanket roll under the knees, hemoconcentration from loss of fluid or dehydration, or, more commonly, the slowing of the blood flow in the extremity due to a lowered metabolism and depression of the circulation after operation. It is probable that several of these factors act together to produce thrombosis. The left leg is affected more frequently.

Clinical Manifestations

The first symptom of DVT may be a pain or a cramp in the calf (Fig. 22-13). Pressure there causes pain, and a day or so later a painful swelling of the entire leg occurs, often accompanied by a slight fever and sometimes chills and perspiration. The swelling is a soft edema that pits easily on pressure.

A milder form of the same disease is termed *phlebothrombosis*, to indicate intravascular clotting without marked inflammation of the vein. The clotting occurs usually in the veins of the calf, often with few symptoms except slight soreness of the calf. The danger from this type of thrombosis is that the clot may be dislodged, producing an embolus. It is believed that most pulmonary emboli arise from this source (see Fig. 22-13).

Medical and Nursing Management

The treatments of thrombophlebitis and DVT may be considered preventive and active.

Prevention. Efforts directed toward preventing the formation of a thrombus include such measures as leg exercises that can be taught before surgery (see Chap. 20, Chart 20-2). If the patient recognizes their significance in preventing circulatory complications, he often initiates his own exercises. To avoid thrombus formation, leg straps should not be fastened in the recovery room, particularly with stretchers that are equipped with side rails. Not only are the straps restrictive, but they can constrict and impair circulation.

The use of low-dose heparin until the patient is ambulatory is becoming increasingly common. This is prescribed subcutaneously. Low-dose warfarin is another possible anticoagulant. Dextran 40 and dextran 70 (low and high molecular weight, respectively) are plasma expanders that reduce the formation of microscopic clots triggered by hemoconcentration. Although comparable to anticoagulants in effectiveness, they are more expensive. External pneumatic compression and gradient elastic stockings can be used alone or in combination with low-dose heparin.

The adrenergic blocking agent dehydroergotamine has also been used with low-dose heparin; some claim that it is more efficacious, but the potential risks of vasoconstriction and its contraindications must be recognized. Aspirin alone has not been shown to be beneficial, and because aspirin increases the effect of anticoagulants, it should not be taken with them.

In addition to the nursing measures cited above, it is important to avoid the use of blanket rolls, pillow rolls, or any form of elevation that can constrict vessels under the knees. Even prolonged "dangling" (having the patient sit on the edge of the bed with legs hanging over the side) can be dangerous and is not recommended in susceptible individuals because pressure under the knees can impede circulation.

No one method is ideal, but prophylactic measures that are tailored to meet individual needs can be effective in markedly reducing what otherwise can be a serious and potentially lethal complication.

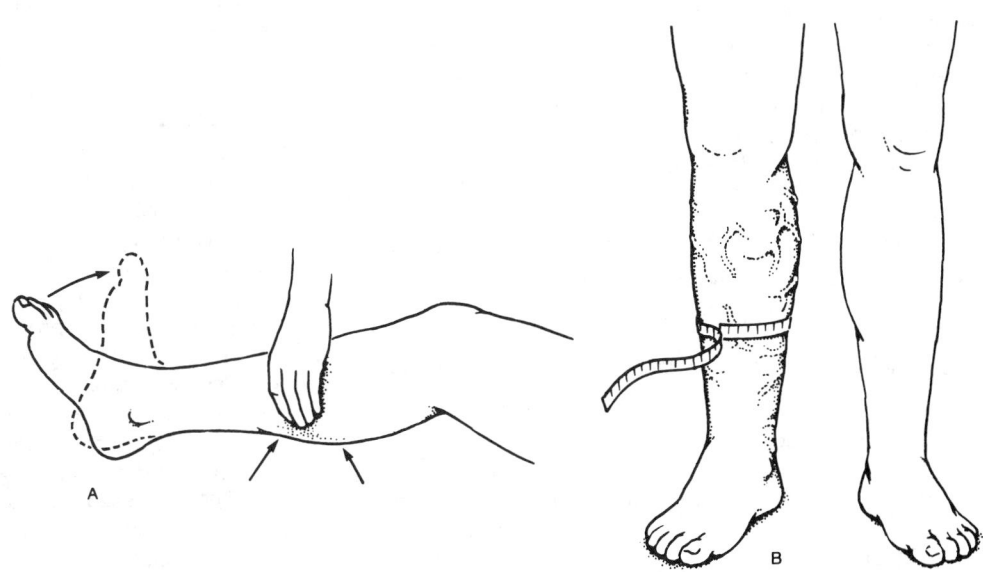

Figure 22-13. Assessment of signs and symptoms of phlebothrombosis. (**A**) With the knee flexed, the patient may complain of pain in the calf on dorsiflexion of foot (Homans' sign). This is a sign of early and subclinical thrombosis; it may or may not be present. Gentle compression reveals tenderness of the calf muscles (note arrow). (**B**) The affected leg may swell; veins are more prominent and may be palpated easily. (Suddarth DS. The Lippincott Manual of Nursing Practice, 5th ed. Philadelphia, JB Lippincott, 1991.)

Active Treatment.   Some surgeons believe that ligation of the femoral veins is an important therapeutic method. The rationale behind this method of therapy is to prevent pulmonary embolism by eliminating the cause (thrombi that could dislodge from the walls of the femoral veins and circulate in the blood).

Anticoagulant therapy has taken a prominent place in the treatment of phlebitis and phlebothrombosis. Heparin (a thrombin inactivator), prescribed intravenously by the drip method or subcutaneously, reduces the coagulability of the blood and is used most often when an immediate effect is desired. Repeated checks of the coagulation time or partial thromboplastin time of the blood are necessary to control its administration. Dicumarol or warfarin (Coumadin; a clotting factor inactivator) is used for the same purpose. It is given by mouth and does not become effective for about 24 hours. Daily dosage is controlled by daily estimations of the prothrombin time of the blood (see also p. 569).

High elastic stockings (toes to groin) have been used as an active treatment of phlebitis and thrombosis. These stockings prevent swelling and stagnation of venous blood in the legs and do much to relieve pain in the affected extremity. However, to be effective, elastic stockings must be used in combination with leg elevation and leg exercises. Early ambulation is helpful, but the nurse also needs to be aware of the problem that can result when a patient with a protruding abdomen walks a few steps and then sits with legs dependent; namely, the pressure of the abdomen can obstruct venous flow. Several research studies have questioned the value of elastic stockings, suggesting an actual danger when they are not applied correctly. Some clinics now do not advocate the use of elastic stockings for any surgical patient.

Pulmonary Embolism

An *embolus* is a foreign body (blood clot, air, fat) that becomes dislodged from its original site and is carried along in the bloodstream.

When the embolus travels to the right side of the heart and completely occludes the pulmonary artery, the symptoms are sudden and startling. A patient experiencing an apparently normal convalescence suddenly cries out with sharp, stabbing pains in the chest and become breathless, diaphoretic, anxious, and cyanotic. The pupils dilate, the pulse becomes rapid and irregular; sudden death may occur.

Fortunately, pulmonary embolism usually causes partial, rather than complete, occlusion of the pulmonary vasculature, and the patient has signs of mild dyspnea, dysrhythmia, or seemingly innocent chest pain. Alertness on the part of the nurse is necessary to detect these small embolic episodes so that early treatment may be initiated and further embolization avoided.

- Early postoperative ambulation reduces the risk of pulmonary embolism.

(See Chap. 26 for a full discussion of pulmonary embolus.)

Respiratory Complications

Respiratory complications are among the most frequent and serious problems encountered by the surgical patient (see Chart 22-6).

Chart 22-6
Risk Factors for Postoperative Pulmonary Complications

Type of surgery—Greater incidence following all forms of abdominal surgery when compared with peripheral surgery
Location of incision—The closer the incision to the diaphragm, the higher the incidence of pulmonary complications
Preoperative respiratory problems
Age—Greater risk after age 40 than before age 40
Sepsis
Obesity—Weight greater than 110% of ideal body weight
Prolonged bed rest
Duration of operation—More than 3 hours
Aspiration
Dehydration
Malnutrition
Hypotension and shock

Experience suggests that the incidence of these complications may be reduced by careful preoperative assessment and teaching and by taking precautions during and after the surgery. It is well known that patients who have respiratory dysfunction before operation are more likely to develop serious complications after surgery. Therefore, only emergency operations are performed when acute disease of the respiratory tract exists. The nurse reports a cough, sneezing, inflamed conjunctivae, nasal discharge, and abnormal breath sounds to the surgeon and anesthesiologist before the operation.

During and immediately after the operation, every effort is made to prevent chilling, which further lowers the patient's resistance. Suctioning of the nasopharynx in the recovery room removes secretions that would otherwise cause respiratory problems in the postoperative period. Occasionally, when secretions form that cannot be coughed up by the patient, aspiration of secretions may be carried out through an endotracheal tube or bronchoscope. In very debilitated patients in whom retained secretions are a complicating factor, a tracheostomy may be performed so that suctioning of the trachea is accomplished directly through the tube as necessary.

Respiratory complications are described briefly here and in more detail in Chapters 25 and 26.

Atelectasis.   When a mucus plug obstructs one of the bronchi entirely, there is a collapse of the pulmonary tissue beyond, and a massive atelectasis, an incomplete expansion of the lung results.

Bronchitis.   Bronchitis may appear at any time after surgery but usually occurs within the first 5 or 6 days. The symptoms vary according to the disease. Simple bronchitis is characterized by a productive cough but without marked temperature or pulse elevation.

Bronchopneumonia.   Bronchopneumonia is a frequent pulmonary complication. Along with a productive cough, there may be marked temperature elevation and an increase in the pulse and the respiratory rates.

Lobar Pneumonia.   Lobar pneumonia is a less frequent complication after surgery. Usually, it begins with a chill, followed by high temperature, pulse, and respiration. There may be little or no cough, but the respiratory distress, the flushed cheeks, and the obvious illness of the patient provide a combination of clinical signs that is distinctive. The disease runs its usual course but with the added demand of recovery from a surgical wound.

Hypostatic Pulmonary Congestion. Hypostatic pulmonary congestion is a condition that may develop in elderly or very weak patients. Its cause is a weakened heart and vascular system that permit a stagnation of secretions at the base of both lungs. It occurs most frequently in elderly patients who are not mobilized effectively. The symptoms are often vague—perhaps a slight elevation of temperature, pulse, and respiratory rate and a cough. However, physical examination reveals dullness and crackles at the base of the lungs. If the condition progresses, the outcome may be fatal.

Pleurisy. Pleurisy can occur after an operation. Its chief symptom is an acute, knifelike pain in the chest on the affected side that becomes excruciating when the patient takes a deep breath. Additionally, breath sounds are diminished or absent on the affected side. There is usually a slight fever and rise in pulse, and respirations are shallow and more rapid than normal.

Management

A most effective method of treating *bronchitis* is the inhalation of cool mist or steam, which may be administered by vaporizers as prescribed. The vaporizer must be kept filled with water, and precautions are taken to prevent the patient from being burned.

In *lobar pneumonia* and *bronchopneumonia*, the patient is encouraged to take fluids; expectorant and antibiotic medications are also prescribed. Breath sounds are assessed frequently to identify change before respiratory and cardiac embarrassment occur.

For *pleurisy*, analgesics may be prescribed, or the physician may perform a procaine intercostal block to provide symptomatic relief. A search is made to detect any possible underlying disease (pneumonia, infarction).

Pleurisy with effusion may result secondary to a primary pleurisy. In these patients, aspiration of the pleural space is frequently necessary.

Many times the pulmonary complication of *hypostatic pulmonary congestion* becomes more serious than the original surgical condition. In this case, the prime objective of therapeutic management is to treat the hypostatic pneumonia.

With the reduced aeration that occurs in many of the pulmonary complications, less oxygen reaches the blood, and treatment requires oxygen therapy. Principles and management are presented on pp. 523–526.

Superinfections. Superinfections can occur when antimicrobial agents alter the bacterial flora of the respiratory tract. Susceptible bacteria are killed, and resistant bacteria multiply. These infections must be treated aggressively.

Nursing Interventions

Awareness of the many possible respiratory complications enables the nurse to initiate the preventive measures cited in the previous discussion (pp. 442–443). Timely recognition of signs and symptoms allows the nurse to direct efforts toward combating specific respiratory difficulties. The patient requires close observation and careful management in the first postoperative week of recovery. The early signs of elevations in temperature, pulse, and respiratory rate are significant. Chest pain, dyspnea,

and cough may or may not accompany these elevations; however, the patient may seem to be restless and apprehensive. Such indications are important and should be reported and documented.

Measures to Promote the Full Aeration of the Lungs. Strategies to prevent respiratory complications include measures to promote full aeration of the lungs. The nurse instructs the patient to take at least five deep inhalations every hour. The use of an incentive spirometer is prescribed to expand the lungs fully (see p. 442 for fuller discussion). Turning the patient from side to side can trigger coughing and the expectoration of a mucous plug and thereby increase aeration of the lungs.

Early ambulation is one of the best prophylactic measures for pulmonary complications; having the patient ambulate increases metabolism and pulmonary aeration and, in general, improves all body functions. When his condition permits, the patient is usually allowed out of bed on the first or second day after surgery, and frequently on the day of surgery. This practice is especially valuable in preventing pulmonary complications in older patients.

Urinary Retention

Although urinary retention may follow any operation, it occurs most frequently after operations on the rectum, the anus, and the vagina, and after herniorrhaphies and surgery on the lower abdomen. The cause is thought to be a spasm of the bladder sphincter.

Nursing Interventions. Quite often patients are unable to void while lying in bed, but when allowed to sit or stand up they do so without difficulty. When standing or sitting is not contraindicated, male patients are allowed to stand by the side of the bed and female patients are allowed to sit on the edge of the bed with their feet on a chair or a stool. However, when sitting or standing is not possible, other means of encouraging urination must be tried. Some people cannot void with another person in the room. These patients should be left alone for a time after being provided with a warm bedpan or urinal.

Frequently the sound or sight of running water relaxes the spasm of the bladder sphincter. Using a bedpan containing warm water or irrigating the perineum with warm water frequently initiates urination for female patients. If the retention of urine continues for some hours and the patient complains of considerable pain in the lower abdomen, the bladder frequently can be palpated and seen in outline distending the lower anterior abdominal wall.

When all conservative measures have failed, catheterization becomes necessary. If the patient has voided just before surgery, this procedure may be delayed for 12 to 18 hours. Catheterization is avoided when possible because there is the possibility of infecting the bladder and producing cystitis and experience has shown that once a patient has been catheterized, often subsequent catheterizations are needed.

Many patients exhibit a palpable bladder, with lower abdominal discomfort, and still void small amounts of urine at frequent intervals. The nurse should not mistake this for normal functioning of the bladder. This voiding of 30 to 60 ml (1 to 2 oz) of urine at intervals of 15 to 30 minutes is, rather, a sign of an overdistended bladder, which allows the escape of small amounts of urine at intervals. The condition is called retention overflow. A catheter usually relieves the patient by draining 600 to 900 ml (20 to 30 oz) of urine from the bladder. Incontinence of retention overflow may be evidenced by a constant dribble of urine while the bladder remains overdistended. Because distention compromises the vascular supply of the bladder wall and increases risk of infection, catheterization is indicated.

At times the surgeon may anticipate voiding difficulties following extensive surgery, and an indwelling catheter is inserted before the patient emerges from anesthesia. The surgeon is notified if an amount less than 30 ml of urine per hour drains.

Gastrointestinal Complications

Nutritional Considerations

Surgery of the gastrointestinal tract frequently disrupts the normal physiologic processes of digestion and absorption. Complications arising from this disruption may take several forms, depending on the location and extent of surgery. For example, oral surgery may present problems of chewing and swallowing, requiring that diet be modified to accommodate the difficulty. Other surgical procedures, such as gastrectomy, small bowel resection, ileostomy, and colostomy, have a more drastic effect on the gastrointestinal system and require more extensive dietary considerations. These considerations are in Table 22-3.

Intestinal Obstruction

Intestinal obstruction is a complication that may follow abdominal operations. It occurs most often after operations on the lower abdomen and the pelvis, and especially after operations in which drainage has been necessary. The symptoms usually appear between the third and fifth days but may occur at any time, even years after the operation. The cause is some obstruction of the intestinal flow—frequently a loop of intestine that has become kinked from inflammatory adhesions or is involved with peritonitis or generalized irritation of the peritoneal surface.

Often there is no fever or pulse elevation, but there is discomfort. At first the pains are localized, which should be noted by the nurse because the localization of the early pains represents the loop of intestine that is just above the obstruction. The patient continues to have abdominal pains, with shorter and shorter intervals between waves of pain. When a stethoscope is placed on the abdomen, sounds may reveal extremely active intestinal movements, especially during an attack of pain. The intestinal contents, unable to move forward, distend the intestinal coils, are carried backward to the stomach, and are vomited. Thus, vomiting and increasing distention gradually become more prominent symptoms. Hiccup often precedes the vomiting in many patients. Defecation does not occur, and

TABLE 22–3.   *Dietary Support of Common Complications in Surgical Treatment*

Procedure	*Complications*	*Dietary Support*
Radical oropharyngeal surgery	Difficulty in mastication and swallowing	*Diet:* Liquid consistency—tube feedings Fluid by mouth—Fruit juices as tolerated Coffee, tea, gelatin, ice cream
Gastrectomy	*Small pouch:* "Dumping syndrome" Epigastric fullness, distention; pallor; sweating, tachycardia, hypotension, diarrhea	Low carbohydrate Moderate fat High protein Small, frequent feedings Periodic injections of vitamin B_{12}
Small bowel resection	Poor absorption Weight loss (absorptive capacity improves with time)	*Immediate support after surgery:* Total parenteral nutrition *Later:* oral intake of high-protein, high-calorie, low-fat diet Medium-chain triglycerides
Ileostomy or colostomy	Initial loss of water and electrolytes	Daily replacement of electrolytes, full liquid diet, high in protein
Bypass surgery	For intestinal obstruction Malabsorption syndrome Maldigestion, diarrhea	Feedings by oral route High protein, high vitamin C Adequate vitamins and minerals

(Valassi K. Nutritional management of cancer patients in a variety of therapeutic regimens. Arch Phys Med Rehab, Vol 58.)

enemas return nearly clear, showing that only a small amount of the intestinal contents has reached the large bowel. Unless the obstruction is relieved, the patient continues to vomit, distention becomes more pronounced, the pulse becomes rapid, and death can result.

Management. Sometimes the distention of the intestine above the obstruction can be relieved by the use of intermittent-suction drainage with a nasoenteral or simple nasogastric tube. Sometimes the inflammatory bowel reaction may subside with subsequent relief of the obstruction. However, at other times it is necessary to relieve the obstruction surgically. Intravenous infusions of prescribed solutions are usually prescribed as well. (See the section on intestinal obstruction for a more complete discussion of the treatment and postoperative care, pp. 944–947.)

Postoperative Psychosis

Postoperative psychosis (mental aberrations) may be physiologic or psychological in origin. Cerebral anoxia, thromboembolism, and fluid and electrolyte imbalances are recognized physical factors in postoperative central nervous system impairment and stress. Emotional factors such as fear, pain, and disorientation can contribute to postoperative depression and anxiety.

Older patients, particularly those with cerebrovascular atherosclerosis, are most susceptible to psychological disturbances. Usually these patients manage fairly well until they have been subjected to the anesthetic and surgery. Postoperatively they may become very disturbed and disoriented. Disfiguring surgery and operations for cancer also predispose the patient to intense emotional problems. Dressings that obscure vision or confinement in a body cast can result in behavioral changes because of the reduced sensory input.

Nursing Intervention: Preoperative and Postoperative. The patient should be thoroughly informed before the operation about what to expect after surgery. Opportunities need to be provided for the patient to express thoughts and fears; misinformation can be corrected and reassurance provided. High-risk patients as described above may require special attention and support. Judicious use of narcotics can also reduce confusion and disorientation.

Orienting the patient to time, day, and place can help him to accept unfamiliar surroundings. Studies have indicated that thorough preoperative briefing of both patient and family can usually diffuse many of the potential postoperative psychologic stresses. In addition, a positive attitude conveyed by all personnel who come in contact with the patient fosters positive feelings in the patient.

For overt psychosis, the patient may require a consultation, major tranquilizers, and therapy with mental health professionals. Because postoperative psychosis does occur, it is helpful when discussing this with family to indicate that it is transient. A patient with illusions or hallucinations is reassured that these aberrations are occasionally experienced and will resolve.

The patient's room should be lighted to reduce the incidence of visual hallucinations. It may be desirable to have a family member stay with the patient as much as possible, because the presence of another person has a reassuring and quieting effect.

Restraint. In the postoperative care of patients with psychologic disturbances, it is prudent for the nurse to explain the necessity for the patient's remaining in bed. Often, patients try to get out of bed to void or to get a drink of water rather than bother the nurse. This may lead to serious complications that a brief explanation can prevent. However, some patients, especially elderly patients and those who are disoriented, may find it impossible to grasp. For such patients, the simplest form of restraint is the use of beds with side rails or side protection. This permits patients to move about in bed but deters them from getting out of bed easily and injuring themselves.

To protect both patient and nurse, it often becomes necessary to apply some form of restraint in cases of delirium. These restraints require a physician's order. The psychological effect of being restrained can be severe; therefore, any form of restraint is applied *only as a last resort*. All other means of quieting the patient are tried first. If possible, he should be isolated from other patients. Any potentially harmful article in the patient's environment is removed.

When restraints are used, the patient should be in a comfortable and natural position, and care is taken that the part is not so constricted as to interfere with the circulation. Restraint to the chest is avoided. The appearance of cyanosis of the hand or foot indicates that the restraint is too tight. The restraint is padded carefully and placed so as to prevent chafing or pressure ulcers. The skin underneath the restraint is inspected frequently, bathed carefully, and massaged at least every 2 to 3 hours. Even though restraints are applied, the patient is never left unattended. Any patient requiring restraint should have constant and careful nursing attention. Consideration is given to respecting the patient as a person. He is experiencing changes in body image and self-esteem and needs understanding and support.

Delirium

Postoperative delirium occurs occasionally in several groups of patients. The most common types of delirium are toxic, traumatic, and alcohol withdrawal delirium (delirium tremens).

Toxic Delirium. Toxic delirium occurs in conjunction with the signs and symptoms of a general toxemia. The patient with toxic delirium is very ill, usually with a high temperature and rapid pulse rate. The face is flushed, and the eyes are bright and roving. The patient moves incessantly, often attempting to get out of bed. A marked degree of mental confusion is present. Toxic delerium is seen most often in patients with general peritonitis or other septic conditions.

In such patients, the intake of fluids is encouraged and the causative condition is treated by antimicrobial therapy. At times, however, the patient does not survive.

Traumatic Delirium. Traumatic delirium is a mental state resulting from sudden trauma of any sort. It often occurs in highly nervous people. The malady may take the form of wild, maniacal excitement, simple confusion with hallucinations and delusions, or depression. Sedative medications (chloral hydrate, paraldehyde, and morphine) are used in treatment. Usually traumatic delirium begins and ends suddenly.

Alcohol Withdrawal Delirium (Delirium Tremens). Individuals who have used alcohol habitually over a long period of time are poor surgical risks. Not only is their resistance lower than normal, but the effects of alcohol have most likely caused multiple organ damage. In addition, these patients react poorly to anesthesia.

After surgery, the alcoholic patient may do well for a few days, but the prolonged abstinence from alcohol causes him to become restless, nervous, and irritated easily by little things. Facial expression may change entirely. Sleep is poor and often disturbed by unreal dreams. When approached by the doctor or the nurse, the patient appears to wake suddenly, asks "Who are you?" and, when told where he is, appears to be fairly normal for a short time. These symptoms should be looked for in patients who use alcohol regularly; with intervention at this stage, the more violent delirium may be avoided.

Active alcohol withdrawal delirium may occur suddenly or gradually. After a period of restless, nervous semidelirium, the patient loses control of his mental functions. If attempts are made to restrain him, he may fight and injure himself and others.

Medical and Nursing Management. When possible, the treatment of patients with alcohol withdrawal delirium should begin 2 or 3 days before surgery with an increased fluid intake. These measures should be continued postoperatively, especially if any of the early signs of the condition develop. Sedatives or tranquilizers should be administered to keep the patient quiet. The chief cause of the symptoms in patients with chronic alcoholism has been shown to be a depletion of the carbohydrate stores of the body and an inadequate ingestion of vitamins. Therefore, glucose is prescribed intravenously and vitamins are administered in concentrated form by mouth and by injection and infusion.

Ambulatory Surgery

Although ambulatory surgery (same-day surgery, outpatient surgery) became popular in the 1970s, its recent growth is the product of advances in surgical practice and anesthesia techniques, prospective reimbursement, and government changes in Medicare–Medicaid provisions. Ambulatory surgery permits the patient to return home on the day of the operation, and it costs less than hospitalization.

The similarities of inpatient and outpatient perioperative nursing include perioperative standards that guide the practice, adherence to aseptic technique, and an emphasis on patient safety. The differences in outpatient perioperative nursing include telephone assessment and teaching environment and astute discharge planning skills.

Patient Assessment and Preoperative Preparation

The preoperative phase includes the preoperative testing, assessment interview, and teaching and usually occurs within 7 days of surgery. The interview may be conducted when the patient comes to the hospital or surgical center for testing or it may consist of a preoperative assessment telephone call. Preoperative teaching content may be presented in a group meeting, on a videotape, or during the preoperative interview. The instructions are presented in simple terms; for the elderly, the instructions should be in large print. The patient is told when and where to report, what to bring (insurance card, list of medications and allergies), what to leave at home (jewelry, watch, medications, contact lenses), and what to wear (loose-fitting, comfortable clothes; flat shoes). The last preoperative phone call is designed to remind the patient not to drink after midnight of the day before surgery; he may brush his teeth but is told not to swallow any fluids.

On the day of surgery, the nurse monitors the patient's vital signs and administers the preanesthetic medication. After voiding, the patient is accompanied to the anesthesia unit. Following surgery, the patient remains in the recovery unit until recovered sufficiently from the anesthetic to go home, accompanied safely by a responsible person. At this time, the patient demonstrates stable circulatory status, absence of bleeding, no nausea or vomiting, and no excessive pain. Postoperative orders, necessary prescriptions, and an information sheet are provided to the patient. Although recovery time varies, an example is 24 to 48 hours of "taking it easy." During this time, the patient is not to drive a vehicle, drink alcoholic beverages, or perform tasks that require energy or skill. Fluids may be consumed as desired, and smaller than normal amounts eaten at mealtime. The patient is cautioned not to make important decisions at this time because the medications, anesthesia, and surgery may affect his thinking.

Advantages of Ambulatory Surgery
- It is cost-effective for the patient, hospital, insurance carriers, and government agencies.
- There is less psychological stress for the patient.
- Hospital-acquired infections are prevented or reduced in incidence.
- Recovery time is more rapid.

Types of Procedures Handled as Ambulatory Surgery

Ambulatory procedures are usually of short duration, from 15 to 90 minutes, in which minimal bleeding and minor physiologic disturbances are anticipated, as in the following examples:

> General surgery—hernia repair, vasectomy, excision of small masses, lesions, or tumors
> Gynecology—dilation and curettage (D & C), tubal ligation, pregnancy termination, cervical diagnostic laparoscopy, biopsy, and conization
> Dermatology—excision of warts and condylomata
> Ophthalmology—cataract extraction, minor eye operations
> Ear, nose, and throat—myringotomy, adenoidectomy, nasal polypectomy, oral surgery
> Cardiac surgery—cardioversion, insertion and replacement of pacemakers
> Orthopedic surgery—carpal tunnel surgery, ganglionectomy

Patient Selection

The patient undergoing ambulatory surgery should be in stable medical condition and be free of infection. It may be more practical for the person with a mild systemic disease to have a surgical procedure in the short-term facility than to be exposed to the greater risk of hospitalization. Usually age is not a factor; however, it is desirable that the patient be psychologically willing to accept this mode of treatment.

The Elderly Surgical Outpatient. Third-party reimbursement policies often force the elderly into ambulatory surgery. If the elderly patient lives alone and expects self-care deficits related to his surgical experience, then strong family and friend support is necessary. In the careful assessment of the home environment, this support provides the basis for a realistic discharge plan.

Many elderly individuals have short-term memory loss and a chronic disease such as arthritis, hearing loss, hypertension, or a cardiac condition. These long-term conditions and the medications taken for them affect preoperative preparation, anesthesia, and surgical outcomes. Therefore, it is the collaborative effort of the patient and the operating room, recovery unit, and home health staffs that makes ambulatory surgery a successful experience.

Chapter Summary

The postoperative phase, the third and last phase of perioperative nursing, centers on the recovery of the patient following surgery. Critical nursing assessment and prompt intervention promote the patient's return to optimal function and decrease the occurrence of postoperative complications that delay recovery. Nursing management in the postoperative phase includes the following: (1) patient care in the PARR and in the surgical nursing unit, (2) wound care and wound complications, and (3) other postoperative complications.

Nursing management of the patient in the PARR focuses on adequate respiratory exchange, stabilization of vital signs, observation of the incision site, and comfort. In the PARR and after the patient's transfer from the PARR, nursing efforts focus on promotion of comfort, relief of pain, nausea and vomiting, and prevention or relief of abdominal and bladder distention.

Wound healing is promoted in the postoperative phase by meticulous wound care, aseptic dressing change, and attention to factors that influence wound healing and skin integrity. Nursing assessment and intervention focus on postoperative complications that can prolong recovery and adversely affect the surgical outcome: shock; hemorrhage; deep vein thrombosis; pulmonary embolism; respiratory, urinary, and intestinal dysfunction; and psychological disturbances.

The increasing emphasis on ambulatory surgery and short hospital stays has reduced the preoperative and postoperative time available for preparation of the patient for surgery and postoperative teaching and preparation for hospital discharge. Nurses are using new strategies to prepare patients for surgery and to assist them in planning for postoperative care at home.

Bibliography

Books

Altemeier WA et al. Manual on Control of Infection in Surgical Patients. Philadelphia, JB Lippincott, 1984.

American College of Surgeons. Care of the Surgical Patient. Vol 1. Critical Care. New York, Scientific American Inc, 1989.

American College of Surgeons. Care of the Surgical Patient. Vol 2. Elective Care. New York, Scientific American Inc, 1989.

AORN Standards and Recommended Practices for Perioperative Nursing. Denver, The Association of Operating Room Nurses, 1986.

Atkinson L. Berry and Kohn's Introduction to Operating Room Technique. New York, McGraw-Hill, 1986.

Barash PG, Cullen BF, and Stoelting RK. Clinical Anesthesia. Philadelphia, JB Lippincott, 1989.

Barret J and Nyhus LM. Treatment of Shock, 2nd ed. Philadelphia, Lea & Febiger, 1986.

Cameron J. Current Surgical Therapy, 2nd ed. St Louis, CV Mosby, 1986.

Cuschieri A, Giles GR, and Moossa AR. Essential Surgical Practice, 2nd ed. Boston, Wright, 1988.

Davis JE (ed). Major Ambulatory Surgery. Baltimore, Williams & Wilkins, 1986.

Deitel M (ed). Nutrition in Clinical Surgery, 2nd ed. Baltimore, Williams & Wilkins, 1985.

Dent TL et al (eds). Surgical Tips. New York, McGraw-Hill, 1989.

Dixon JA. Surgical Application of Lasers, 2nd ed. Chicago, Year Book Medical Publishers, 1987.

Drain CB and Christoph SS. The Recovery Room: A Critical Care Approach to Post Anesthesia Nursing. Philadelphia, WB Saunders, 1987.

Dripps RD, Eckenhoff JE, and Vandam LD. Introduction to Anesthesia, 7th ed. Philadelphia, WB Saunders, 1988.

Dudley HAF (ed). Scott: An Aid to Clinical Surgery. New York, Churchill Livingstone, 1989.

Eltringham R et al. Post-Anesthetic Recovery: A Practical Approach, 2nd ed. New York, Springer-Verlag, 1989.

Finkel ML. Surgical Care in the United States: A Policy Perspective. Baltimore, Johns Hopkins University Press, 1988.

Frost AME. Recovery Room Practice. St Louis, CV Mosby, 1985.

Greenfield LJ (ed). Complications in Surgery and Trauma, 2nd ed. Philadelphia, JB Lippincott, 1990.

Groah L. Operating Room Nursing: The Perioperative Role. Reston, VA, Reston Publishing Company, 1983.

Gruendemann BJ and Meeker MH. Alexander's Care of the Patient in Surgery, 8th ed. St Louis, CV Mosby, 1987.

Hathaway RC (ed). Nursing Care of the Critically Ill Surgical Patient. Rockville, MD, Aspen Systems, 1988.

Kirkwood EK. Guidelines for Preparing and Sterilizing Wrapped Packs. Erie, PA, American Sterilizer Company, 1983.

Kneedler JA and Dodge GH. Perioperative Patient Care. Boston, Blackwell Scientific, 1987.

Liechty RD and Soper RT. Fundamentals of Surgery. St Louis, CV Mosby, 1989.

McConnell EA. Clinical Consideration in Perioperative Nursing. Philadelphia, JB Lippincott, 1987.

McCredie JA. Basic Surgery, 2nd ed. New York, Macmillan, 1986.

Miller TA (ed). Physiological Basis of Modern Surgical Care. St Louis, CV Mosby, 1988.

Perry AG and Potter PA. Shock: Comprehensive Nursing Management. St Louis, CV Mosby, 1983.

Porter GA (ed). Acute Medical Problems in the Postoperative Patient. New York, Churchill Livingstone, 1987.

Ratz J. Lasers in Cutaneous Medicine and Surgery. New York, Year Book Medical Publishers, 1986.

Reed AP and Kaplan JA. Clinical Cases in Anesthesia. New York, Churchill Livingstone, 1989.

Rothrock J. RN First Assistant: An Expanded Perioperative Nursing Role. Philadelphia, JB Lippincott, 1987.

Sabiston D (ed). Textbook of Surgery, 13th ed. Philadelphia, WB Saunders, 1986.

Schrock TR (ed). Handbook of Surgery. Greenbrae, CA, Jones Medical Publishers, 1985.

Schwartz S et al. Principles of Surgery. New York, McGraw-Hill, 1989.

Seymour G. Medical Assessment of the Elderly Surgical Patient. Hagerstown, MD, Aspen Systems, 1986.

Zollinger RM and Zollinger RM Jr. Atlas of Surgical Operations, 6th ed. New York, Macmillan, 1988.

Articles

Asterisks indicate nursing research articles.

General

*Byra-Cook CJ, Dracup K, and Lazik AJ. Direct and indirect blood pressure in critical care patients. Nurs Res 1990 Sep/Oct; 39(5):285–288.

Davis AJ. Clinical nurses' ethical decision making in situations of informed consent. Adv Nurs Sci 1989 Apr; 11(3):63–69.

Edel EM et al. Perioperative documentation: Incorporating nursing diagnosis into the intraoperative record. AORN J 1989 Sep; 50(3):596–600.

*Llewellyn J et al. Analysis of falls in the acute surgical and cardiovascular surgical patient. Appl Nurs Res 1988 Nov; 1(3):116–121.

*OConnell M. Anxiety reduction in family members of patients in surgery and postanesthesia care: A pilot study. J Post Anesth Nurs 1989 Feb; 4(1):7–16.

Menyhert LR. Special considerations in geriatric care: An overview. J Post Anesth Nurs 1988 Jun; 3(3):162–164.

*Richards ML. Perioperative nursing research. Part 6. Postoperative phase. AORN J 1989 Jul; 50(1):120–122.

Stallard S and Prescott S. Postoperative urinary retention in general surgical patients. Br J Surg 1988 Nov; 75(11):1141–1143.

Stoughton A. Development of an interchange-of-gases assessment tool for the adult client. J Post Anesth Nurs 1988 Aug; 3(4):116–121.

Warner MA et al. Role of preoperative cessation of smoking and other factors in postoperative pulmonary complications: A blinded prospective study of coronary artery bypass patients. Mayo Clin Proc 1989 Jun; 64:609–616.

Weikel C. Informed consent: An ethical dilemma. Today's OR Nurse 1987 Jan; 9(1):10–15.

Perioperative Nursing

Alverson E. The preoperative interview: Its effect on perioperative nurses' empathy. AORN J 1987 May; 45(5):1158–1164.

Ammon-Gaberson KB. Adult learning principles: Applications for preceptor programs. AORN J 1987 Apr; 45(4):961–963.

Bailey SL. Electrical injuries: Considerations for the perioperative nurse. AORN J 1989 Mar; 49(3):773–787.

*Bargagliotti LA. Perioperative nursing research: Issues in perioperative nursing. Part 8. AORN J 1989 Sep; 50(3):613–617.

Berky PS. Combativeness: A treatable problem in the elderly patient. Today's OR Nurse 1987 Dec; 9(12):20–23.

Daly MP. The medical evaluation of the elderly preoperative patient. Med Clin North Am 1989 Jun; 16(2):361–376.

Dean AF. The aging surgical patient: Historical overview, implications, and nursing care. Periop Nurs Q 1987 Mar; 3(1):1–7.

Haddad AM. Ethics: Using principles of beneficence, autonomy to resolve ethical dilemmas in perioperative nursing. AORN J 1987 Jul; 46(1):120–124.

Hanowell LH and Boyle WA. Perioperative care of the hemodynamically unstable geriatric patient. Int Anesthesiol Clin 1988 Summer; 26(2):156–168.

Hart AL. Job satisfaction and personality: Are they related? AORN J 1988 Feb; 47(2):479–488.

Jackson MF. The elderly: High risk surgical patients. Prof Nurse 1987 May; 2(8):263–266.

Kleinbeck SV. Developing a nursing diagnosis for a perioperative care plan. AORN J 1989 Jun; 49(6):1613–1615.

Latz PA and Wyble SJ. Elderly patients: Perioperative nursing implications. AORN J 1987 Aug; 46(2):238–253.

Menyhert LR. Special considerations in geriatric care: An overview. J Post Anesth Nurs 1988 Jun; 3(3):162–164.

*Noriega L et al. Perioperative nursing research. Part 7. AORN J 1989 Aug; 50(2):379–381.

Sloane LA et al. Nursing care documentation: Creating a perioperative nursing record. AORN J 1989 Mar; 49(3):808–810, 812–813.

Wachstein J. Care of the elderly surgical patient. Geriatr Nurs Home Care 1987 Apr; 7(4):12–14.

*White et al. Body temperature in elderly surgical patients. Res Nurs Health 1987 Oct; 10(5):317–321.

Preoperative Nursing

Alverson E. The preoperative interview. AORN J 1987 May; 45(5):1158–1164.

*Biley C. Nurses' perception stress in preoperative surgical patients. J Adv Nurs 1989 Jul; 14(7):575–581.

Boghosian SG and Mooradian AD. Usefulness of routine preoperative chest roentgenograms in elderly patients. J Am Geriatr Soc 1987 Feb; 35(2):142–146.

Burke JF and Francos GC. Surgery in the patient with acute or chronic renal failure. Med Clin North Am 1987 May; 71(3):489–497.

Campbell IT and Gosling P. Preoperative biochemical screening. Br Med J 1988 Oct; 297(6652):803–804.

Charpak Y et al. Usefulness of selectively ordered preoperative tests. Med Care 1988 Feb; 26(2):95–104.

Charpak Y et al. Prospective assessment of a protocol for selective ordering of preoperative chest x-rays. Can J Anaesth 1988 May; 35(3):259–264.

*Devine EC et al. Clinical and financial effects of psychoeducational care provided by staff nurses to adult surgical patients in the post-DRG environment. Am J Public Health 1988 Oct; 78(10):1293–1297.

Dueholm S, Rubinstein E, and Reipurth G. Preparation for elective colorectal surgery: A randomized, blinded comparison between oral colonic lavage and whole-gut irrigation. Dis Colon Rectum 1987 May; 30(5):360–364.

Friedman LS and Maddrey WC. Surgery in the patient with liver disease. Med Clin North Am 1987 May; 71(3):453–476.

Galazka SS. Preoperative evaluation of the elderly surgical patient. J Fam Pract 1988; 27(6):622–632.

Gluck R, Munoz E, and Wise L. Preoperative and postoperative medical evaluation of surgical patients. Am J Surg 1988 Jun; 155:730–734.

Goldman DR. Surgery in patients with endocrine dysfunction. Med Clin North Am 1987 May; 71(3):499–509.

Goldmann L, Ogg TW, and Levey AB. Hypnosis and daycase anaesthesia: A study to reduce pre-operative anxiety and intra-operative anaesthetic requirements. Anaesthesia 1988 Jun; 43(6):466–469.

Gouma DJ et al. Preoperative total parenteral nutrition. (TPN) in severe Crohn's disease. Surgery 1988 Jun; 103(6):648–652.

Hathaway D and Powell S. An evaluation of a preoperative assessment program. Periop Nurs Q 1987 Jun; 3(2):56–64.

Jackson MF. High risk surgical patients. Today's OR Nurse 1988 Feb; 10(2):26–33.

Knight CG and Donnelly MK. Assessing the preoperative adult. Nurse Pract 1988 Jan; 13(1):6–8.

Leite JF et al. Value of nutritional parameters in the prediction of postoperative complications in elective gastrointestinal surgery. Br J Surg 1987 May; 74(5):426–429.

Leuze M and McKenzie J. Preoperative assessment: Using the Roy Adaptation Model. AORN J 1988 Feb; 47(2):537.

Manning FC. Preoperative evaluation of the elderly patient. Am Fam Physician 1989 Jan; 39(1):123–128.

McClay EF and Bellet RE. Preoperative evaluation of the oncology patient. Med Clin North Am 1987 May; 71(3):529–540.

McCleane GJ. Urea and electrolyte measurement in pre-operative surgical patients. Anaesthesiology 1988 May; 43(5):423–415.

*Gamotis PB et al. Inpatient vs outpatient satisfaction: A research study. AORN J 1988 Jun; 47(6):1424–1425.

Playforth MJ. Pre-operative assessment of fitness score. Br J Surg 1987 Oct; 74:890–892.

Rohrer MJ, Michelotti MC, and Nahrwold DL. A prospective evaluation of the efficacy of preoperative coagulation testing. Ann Surg 1988 Nov; 208(5):554–557.

*Rothrock JC. Perioperative nursing research: Preoperative psychoeducational interventions. Part 1. AORN J 1989 Feb; 49(2):597.

*Smith RC and Hartemink R. Improvement of nutritional measure during preoperative parenteral nutrition in patients selected by the Prognostic Nutritional Index: A randomized controlled trial. J Parenter Enteral Nutr 1988; 12(6):587–591.

Sue-Ling HM et al. Indicators of depressed fibrinolytic activity in preoperative prediction of deep venous thrombosis. Br J Surg 1987 Apr; 74(4):275–278.

*Takahashi JJ et al. Preoperative assessment: a research study. AORN J 1989 Nov; 50(5):1024–1032.

Tape TG and Mushlin AI. How useful are routine chest x-rays of preoperative patients at risk for postoperative chest disease? J Gen Intern Med 1988 Jan/Feb; 3(1):15–20.

Warner MA et al. Role of preoperative cessation of smoking and other factors in postoperative pulmonary complications: A blinded prospective study of coronary bypass patients. Mayo Clin Proc 1989 Jun; 64(6):609–616.

Wolff BG et al. A new bowel preparation for elective colon and rectal surgery: A prospective, randomized clinical trial. Arch Surg 1988 Jul; 123(7):895–900.

Yousif H et al. Preoperative myocardial ischaemia: Its relation to perioperative infarction. Br Heart J 1987 Jul; 58(1):9–14.

Intraoperative Nursing

*Bailes BK. Perioperative nursing research: intraoperative phase. Part 4.
AORN J 1989 May; 49(5):1397–1399.

Campbell K. Pressure point measures in the operating room. J Enterostomal
Ther 1989 May/Jun; 16(3):119–124.

Donnell SG. Coping during the wait: surgical nurse liason program aids
families. AORN J 1989 Nov; 50(5):1088–1092.

Miner D. Patient positioning. AORN J 1987 May; 45(5):1117–1127.

Moss VA. Burnout: Symptoms, causes prevention. AORN J Nov; 50(5):
1071–1076.

*Silo HM. Perioperative nursing research: intraoperative recommended
practices. Part 5. AORN J 1989 Jun; 49(6):1627–1636.

Williamson KM et al. Occupational health hazards for nurses. Part 2. Image
1988 Fall; 20(3):162–168.

Personnel and Communications

Bowen M and Davidhizar R. Anxiety in the operating room: The manager's
dilemma. Today's OR Nurs 1990 Jun; 12(6):32–33.

*Kneedler JA et al. Perioperative nursing research. Part 2. Intraoperative
chemical and physical hazards to personnel. AORN J 1989 Mar; 49(3):
829–836.

*Kneedler JA et al. Perioperative nursing research. Part 3. Potential intra-
operative biological hazard to personnel. AORN J Apr; 49(4):1066–
1067.

Langford RW and Harmon V. Self-image: Characteristics of operating room
nurses. AORN J 1987 Apr; 45(4):969–979.

Patterson P. OR managers face AIDS ethical dilemmas. Today's OR Nurs
1990 Jun; 12(6):31.

Scrubbing/Handwashing/Asepsis

Centers for Disease Control. Update: Universal precautions for prevention
of human immunodeficiency virus, hepatitis B virus, and other blood-
borne pathogens. Weekly Rep 1988; 37(24):377–390.

*Copp G et al. Covergowns and the control of operating room contami-
nation. Nurs Res 1986 Sep/Oct; 35(5):263–268.

*Korniewicz DM et al. Integrity of vinyl and latex procedure gloves. Nurs
Res 1989 May/Jun; 38(3):144–146.

Anesthesia and Surgery

Ivey DF. Local anesthesia: Implications for the perioperative nurse. AORN
J 1987 Mar; 3(1):682–689.

Osborn IP and Goldofsky S. Intrathecal and epidural narcotics. Progr Anesth
1989 Nov; 3(22):2–12.

Hypothermia and Malignant Hyperthermia

Burkle NL. Inadvertent hypothermia. Today's OR Nurse 1988 Jul; 10(7):
26–32.

*Erickson RS, Yount ST. Comparison of tympanic and oral temperatures
in surgical patients. Nurs Res 1991 Mar/Apr; 40(2):90–93.

Feroe DD and Augustine SD. Hypothermia in the PACU. Crit Care Nurs
Clin North Am 1991 Mar; 3(1):135–144.

Frederick C, Rosemann D, and Austin MJ. Malignant hyperthermia: Nursing
diagnosis and care. J Post Anesth Nurs 1990 Feb; 5(1):29–32.

*Heidenreich T and Guiffre M. Post-operative temperature measurement.
Nurs Res 1986 Jul/Aug; 39(3):153–155.

*Holtzclaw BJ. Effects of extremity wraps to control drug-induced shivering:
A pilot study. Nurs Res 1990 Sep/Oct; 39(5):280–284.

*Markin DA et al. Comparison between two types of body surface tem-
perature devices: Efficiency, accuracy and cost. J Post Anesth Nurs
1990 Feb; 5(1):33–37.

Newberry JE. Malignant hyperthermia in the postanesthesia care unit: A
review of current etiology, diagnosis and treatment. J Post Anesth
Nurs 1990 Feb; 5(1):25–28.

Norris MK. Action stat! Malignant hypothermia. Nurs 90 1990 Jun; 20(6):
33.

*White HE et al. Temperature in elderly surgical patients. Res Nurs Health
1987; 10:317–321.

Woody S. Malignant hyperthermia: Potential crisis in patient care. AORN
J 1989 Aug; 50(2):286–287.

Wlody GS. Malignant hyperthermia. Crit Care Nurs Clin North Am 1991
Mar; 3(1):129–134.

Postoperative Nursing

Biga CD and Bethel SA. Hemodynamic monitoring in postanesthesia care
units. Crit Care Nurs Clin North Am 1991 Mar; 3(1):83–93.

Creighton H. Recovery room nurses: Legal implications. Nurs Manage 1987
Jan; 18(1):22–23.

DeFazio-Matson DM. The formulation of standing orders in the PACU. J
Post Anesth Nurs 1988 Aug; 3(4):264–269.

Jones DH. Fluid therapy in the PACU. Crit Care Nurs Clin North Am 1991
Mar; 3(1):109–120.

Kochansky CY and Kochansky SW. Postanesthetic considerations for the
patient receiving ketamine. J Post Anesth Nurs 1988 Apr; 3(2):118–
120.

Lipov EG. Emergency delirium in the PACU. Crit Care Nurs Clin North Am
1991 Mar; 3(1):145–149.

Litwack K. Bleeding and coagulation in the PACU. Crit Care Nurs Clin
North Am 1991 Mar; 3(1):121–127.

Litwack K, Saleh D, and Schultz, P. Postoperative pulmonary complications.
Crit Care Nurs Clin North Am 1991 Mar; 3(1):77–82.

Tremblay DR et al. Arrhythmias in the PACU: A review. Crit Care Nurs
Clin North Am 1991 Mar; 3(1):95–108.

Van Sickel AD and Spadaccia K. Muscle relaxants and reversal agents. Crit
Care Nurs Clin North Am 1991 Mar; 3(1):151–158.

Pain

Dean RJ Jr. Regional anesthetic techniques for postoperative analgesia.
Crit Care Nurs Clin North Am 1991 Mar; 3(1):43–47.

Doddy SB, Smith C, and Webb J. Nonpharmacologic interventions for pain
management. Crit Care Nurs Clin North Am 1991 Mar; 3(1).

Eng JB and Sabanathan S. Postoperative wound pain. Br J Surg 1989 Jan;
76(10):101–102.

Gilbert HC. Pain relief methods in the postanesthesia care unit. J Post
Anesth Nurs 1990 Feb; 5(1):6–15.

*Hargraves A and Lander J. Use of transcutaneous electrical nerve stim-
ulation for postoperative pain. Nurs Res 1989 May/Jun; 38(3):159–
161.

Hussain SA and Hussain S. Incisions with knife or diathermy and postoperative pain. Br J Surg 1988 Dec; 75:1179–1180.

*Keen MF. Comparison of intramuscular injection techniques to reduce
site discomfort and lesions. Nurs Res 1986 Jul/Aug; 35(4):207–210.

Lubenow TR and Ivankovich, AD. Postoperative epidural analgesia. Crit
Care Nurs Clin North Am 1991 Mar; 3(1):25–32.

Lubenow TR and Ivankovich AD. Patient-controlled analgesia for postoperative pain. Crit Care Nurs Clin North Am 1991 Mar; 3(1):35–41.

Maurset A et al. Comparison of ketamine and pethidine in experimental
and postoperative pain. Pain 1989 Jan; 36(1):37–41.

Merrill DC. Clinical evaluation of FasTENS, an inexpensive, disposable
transcutaneous electrical nerve stimulator designed specifically for
postoperative electroanalgesia. Urology 1989 Jan; 33(1):27–30.

*Miller KM. Deep breathing relaxation: A pain management technique.
AORN J 1987 Feb; 45(2):484–488.

Nishino T et al. Breathing patterns during postoperative analgesia in patients
after lower abdominal operations. Anesth 1988 Dec; 69(6):967–972.

Stickley M, Jenkins PM, and Stebbins K. Postoperative blood pressure patterns in people 12 to 30 years old. J Post Anesth Nurs 1988 Oct;
3(5):332–335.

Vogelsang J. Opening the postanesthesia care unit to visitors. Dimens Crit
Care Nurs 1988 Jan/Feb; 7(1):40–47.

*Wilkie DJ. Use of the McGill Pain Questionnaire to measure pain: A meta-
analysis. Nurs Res 1990 Jan/Feb; 39(1):36–41.

Wounds and Infection

Hayek LJ, Emerson JM, and Gardner AM. A placebo-controlled trial of the
effect of two preoperative baths or showers with chlorhexidine detergent on postoperative wound infection rates. J Hosp Infect 1987
Sep; 10(2):165–172.

Lalyer J. Wound management in the home. Part II. Home Health Nurse 1988 May/Jun; 6(3):29–34.

Payman BC, Dampier SE, and Hawthorn PJ. Postoperative temperature and infection in patients undergoing general surgery. J Adv Nurs 1989 Mar; 14(3):198–202.

Troxler SH and Nichols RL. Surgical wound infections. Today's OR Nurse 1987 Mar; 9(3):16–22.

Ambulatory Surgery and Same-Day Surgery

Applegeet CJ. Nursing aspects of outpatient surgery. Urol Clin North Am 1987 Feb; 14(1):21–25.

Bean M. Preparation for surgery in an ambulatory surgery unit. J Post Anesth Nurs 1990 Feb; 5(1):42–47.

Burden N. The ambulatory surgical setting: Adding the caring touch. J Post Anesth Nurs 1988 Dec; 3(6):411–414.

Burden N. Handle with care: The geriatric patient in the ambulatory surgery environment. J Post Anesth Nurs 1989 Feb; 4(1):27–31.

Fehder WP. Help your patient get through outpatient surgery and anesthesia. Office Nurs 1989 May/Jun; 21–22.

Johnson H et al. Are routine preoperative laboratory screening tests necessary to evaluate ambulatory surgical patients? Surg 1988 Oct; 104(4): 639–645.

Keithley J et al. The cost effectiveness of same-day admission surgery. Nurs Econ 1989; 7(2):90–93.

Kempe AR. Ambulatory surgery: Patient education for the ambulatory surgery patient. AORN J 1987 Feb; 45(2):500–507.

Masterson C. Increasing volume and decreasing costs in the ambulatory surgery unit. J Post Anesth Nurs 1990 Feb; 5(1):38–41.

Mathias M. Same day surgery conference addresses risks, challenges, and advances. AORN J 1988 Jun; 47(6):1478–1480.

Omerod BJ. Perioperative nursing care of the elderly outpatient. Periop Nurs Q 1987; 3(2):22–26.

Parrinello KM. Accounting for patient acuity in an ambulatory surgery center. Nurs Econ 1987 Jul/Aug; 5(4):167–172.

Agencies

American Society of Anesthesiologists
    500 North Michigan Avenue, Chicago, IL 60611
American Society of Postanesthesia Nurses
    PO Box 11083, Richmond, VA 23230
Association of Operating Room Nurses, Inc
    10170 E. Mississippi Avenue, Denver, CO 80231
Malignant Hyperthermia Association of the United States (MHAUS)
    163 Waverly Street, Arlington, MA 02174

Nursing Research Profile for Unit 5

Perioperative Nursing

Overview

Nursing research in perioperative nursing has added to our knowledge of body temperature assessment, patient education and satisfaction, anxiety reduction, and the needs of the family.

Body Temperature Measurements

▷ *White HE, et al. Temperature in elderly surgical patients. Res Nurs Health 1987 Oct; 10(5):317–321.*

Because of their reduced cardiac reserves, elderly surgical patients are less tolerant of hypothermia than younger adults. Complications associated with hypothermia in older patients include prolonged postoperative recovery, ventricular fibrillation, and cardiac arrest. Mortality has been demonstrated to be associated with hypothermia in elderly surgical patients. White and colleagues investigated strategies that might prevent such complications in patients 60 years of age and older who were undergoing surgery. This quasi-experimental study specifically examined the effect of extra body coverings on thermal status of older surgical patients undergoing surgery for repair of a fractured hip. A convenience sample of subjects (N = 37) were randomly assigned either to a control group with the usual surgical covering (gown, flannelette blanket, and drape) or an experimental group that received the extra covering of head cap, stockinette on the unaffected leg, and heated flannelette blankets under and over the body. A tympanic membrane temperature probe was used to measure patient temperature 2 hours preoperatively and at 12-minute intervals during surgery and in the recovery room until the baseline temperature was reached.

The groups did not differ significantly in age, sex, length of surgery, medical status, preoperative medications, or preoperative temperature. Of the total of 37 subjects, 9 were hypothermic (defined in this study as having a temperature of 35°C or less). Of the 21 patients with usual coverings, 8 were hypothermic; of the 16 patients with extra coverings, 1 was hypothermic. Aural temperatures were significantly lower for the control group intraoperatively and in the recovery room.

Nursing Implications. Traditionally, assessment of blood pressure, pulse, and respirations has been used to evaluate the surgical patient. Because of risks of hypothermia in the elderly, temperature should also be monitored. The finding of signifi-

cant differences in the effect of coverings on intraoperative and postoperative body temperatures in this sample of elderly patients supports the need for more careful monitoring of body temperature during surgery and the use of strategies, such as extra coverings, to prevent hypothermia.

▷ *Heidenreich T and Giuffre M. Postoperative temperature measurement. Nurs Res 1990 May/Jun; 39(3):153–155.*

This study investigated the validity of axillary site temperature measurement in noncardiac, postoperative patients. The temperature measurements of 18 postoperative patients were taken with axillary electronic, axillary mercury, and rectal mercury thermometers and compared with the core temperatures obtained from the temperature-sensitive component of a pulmonary artery catheter.

Eleven men and seven women ranging in age from 53 to 86 years and who had pulmonary artery catheters in place for postoperative hemodynamic pressure monitoring constituted the sample. Values obtained from the different temperature measurements were compared with core readings. Correlations of all readings with core temperature readings were high; Pearson correlation coefficients ranged from .92 to .98. Rectal site measurements obtained by mercury thermometers were most closely correlated with core temperature readings; 10-minute mercury axillary temperature measurements were the second best indicator for core temperature. Findings also revealed that the older the patient, the cooler the patient on admission to the ICU, and that the longer the patient was in the operating room, the lower his or her body temperature.

Nursing Implications. The findings of this study further support the need for close monitoring of the temperature of elderly patients undergoing surgery. Further, rectal mercury thermometer readings are the best indicator of core body temperature and 10-minute axillary mercury temperature measurements provide the next best indicator. The findings further suggest the need to use and evaluate strategies to prevent hypothermia in elderly patients and those who have been in the operating room for extended periods.

Surgical Patient Satisfaction

▷ *Gamotis PB, et al. Inpatient vs. outpatient satisfaction. AORN J 1988 Jun; 47(6):1421–1425.*

In response to competition among health care facilities, providers are becoming more sensitive to the need to evaluate to what extent patients' health care needs are met. Studies on patient satisfaction exemplify this trend. The purpose of this study was to compare level of satisfaction with nursing care of surgical inpatients and surgical outpatients. The 183 subjects in the convenience sample had elective surgery as inpatients (N = 99) or outpatients (N = 84). Subjects' ages ranged from 18 to 65 years. They were asked to complete the Patient Satisfaction Instrument. This instrument contains three subscales: technical-professional relationship, education relationship, and trusting relationship. In the inpatient group, the questionnaire return rate was 56%, women outnumbered men by more than 2:1, and the mean age was 42.8 years. The outpatient group had a 99% return rate, consisted of 51 women and 33 men, and had a mean age of 56.7 years. Overall findings indicated that both groups were satisfied with their nurses and nursing care. When scores on the subscales were analyzed, outpatients were found to be more satisfied with technical professional skills than were inpatients. Analysis of the education relationship revealed a significant difference in the results: inpatients gave this the lowest rating of the three scales. Age and gender did not affect the responses for this subset. In the analysis of the trusting relationship, outpatients were more satisfied than were inpatients. Female inpatients and older inpatients rated the trusting relationship more positively than did outpatients and male and younger inpatients. There were no significant differences by age or gender in the outpatient results.

Nursing Implications. The fact that both inpatients and outpatients were satisfied with nurses and nursing care is encouraging. The low rating for inpatient education, wherein several nurses may provide aspects of the education for the same patient, suggests that different strategies for providing that education be considered. Further study is needed to contrast inpatient and outpatient satisfaction and to identify factors that are the most significant in determining patient satisfaction (*i.e.*, what aspects are the most important to the patient). Major limitations of this study included the different response rate and differences in demographic characteristics of the two groups, indicating that the two groups were not equivalent. Further, no comparisons were made for type of surgical procedure or patient risk factors.

Patient Education

▷ **Devine EC et al. Clinical and financial effects of psychoeducational care provided by staff nurses to adult surgical patients in the post-DRG environment. Am J Public Health 1988 Oct; 78(10):1293–1297.**

This study had two aims: (1) to determine whether the previously reported benefits of psychoeducational programs continue in the post-DRG environment and (2) to determine whether the results would be upheld when staff nurses, rather than researchers, were the educators. Staff nurses were provided with a 3-hour workshop on psychologic and educational interventions, and their effect on postsurgical outcomes for patients with elective surgery in a post-DRG environment were examined.

Surgical patients from two hospitals, an experimental and a control hospital, constituted the sample. Both hospitals were administered by the same corporation, had the same academic affiliation and many of the same surgeons, and had instituted prospective payment based on DRGs at the same time. Preworkshop and postworkshop groups of patients from both hospitals were studied. Patients hospitalized at each hospital during the 6-month period before the workshop were compared

with those hospitalized during the 7.5 months after the workshop.

The total sample consisted of 354 subjects who had undergone elective abdominal surgery, including cholecystectomies and other abdominal surgery, or transurethral resection of the prostate. The sample from the experimental hospital consisted of 148 patients; 74 subjects were studied in the preworkshop period and another 74 in the postworkshop period. The sample from the control hospital consisted of 206 patients; the preworkshop group in this hospital had 98 subjects, and the postworkshop group had 108 subjects.

The subjects in the experimental hospital group were interviewed by telephone the day after hospital discharge to determine the perceptions of their psychoeducational care. The remaining data were obtained from the health record. In the control hospital group, there was no patient contact; all data were obtained from health records.

The 3-hour workshop provided to nurses at the experimental hospital included information about psychoeducational care. Specific topics focused on providing patients with health-related information; information related to self-care, preoperative teaching, and psychosocial support to decrease patient anxiety and promote coping; and strategies to increase the levels of psychoeducational care. Data on the outcome variables were collected on patients in both hospitals before and after the workshop; these variables included postoperative length of stay and use of medications (analgesics, hypnotics, antiemetics, and sedatives).

When length of stay of preworkshop and postworkshop periods were compared, the length of stay decreased more in the experimental hospital. Postoperative use of sedatives and antiemetics was lower in the experimental group than in the control group. Use of analgesia by patients undergoing cholecystectomy was also decreased more in the experimental group than in the control group.

Nursing Implications. The findings of this study demonstrated that in a post-DRG environment, psychoeducational workshops and, presumably, implementation of psychoeducation with surgical patients resulted in shorter lengths of stays and decreased use of postoperative medication. The findings suggest that increasing nurses' knowledge and skill in psychoeducational strategies can affect patients' welfare and recovery positively. Because this study was surgery-specific, further research using other types of surgery in a variety of hospital settings is indicated.

Needs of the Family

▷ **O'Connell M. Special presentation. Anxiety reduction in family members of patients in surgery and postanesthesia care: A pilot study. Journal of Post Anesthesia Nursing 1989 Feb; 4(1):7–16.**

O'Connell investigated the relation between postanesthesia nurses' giving of information to family members and the family members' anxiety levels during the intraoperative and postanesthesia experience. It was hypothesized that the information given by postanesthesia nurses would reduce the anxiety level in family members. This was based on the theory that providing information would decrease fear of the unknown. "Information giving" was measured by the number of interactions between the postanesthesia nurse and family member while the patient was in the operating room, in the postanesthesia care unit, and just before transfer. Information included orienting the family to the waiting room and hospital surroundings (*e.g.,* location of coffee shop or cafeteria, restroom facilities); keeping the family informed about the status of the patient and progress of the surgery; explaining to family members equipment (*i.e.,* intravenous fluids, catheters, nasogastric tube, endotracheal tube, ventilator) in use; and repeating explanations and information as necessary. Family members' anxiety level was measured by Spielburger's State Anxiety Inventory. The inventory was administered to family members as they waited for patients undergoing surgery and again right before the patient was transferred to the patient unit.

The sample consisted of 43 family members of 36 patients undergoing surgery; 21 were females and 22 were males. Family members ranged in age from 19 to 80 years. The largest group of waiting family members was husbands. Several patients had more than one family member who completed the inventory. All but 7 of the patients were adults. Surgical procedures performed on adults varied from minor to major procedures.

State anxiety scores differed significantly from preinformation measurement to postinformation measurement, with anxiety levels significantly lower after information was received. No other significant relationships were found in analysis of the subjects' demographic data and level of anxiety.

Nursing Implications. This study indicated that family members waiting during the surgical experience benefited from the postanesthesia nurse's communication about the patient during surgery. Information given throughout the intraoperative and postanesthesia period reduced family anxiety. The limitations of this pilot study were the small sample size and the inability to control for other variables (*i.e.,* the physician's telling family members that the surgery went well).

Pain Management

▷ *Hargreaves A and Lander J. Use of transcutaneous electrical nerve stimulation for postoperative pain. Nurs Res 1989 May/Jun; 38(3):159–161.*

The purpose of this study was to examine the effects of transcutaneous electrical nerve stimulation (TENS) on incisional pain caused by cleaning and packing an abdominal surgical wound. The sample consisted of 75 patients who were randomly assigned to one of three groups: group 1 received TENS; group 2 received placebo TENS (the entire procedure except application of the electrical stimulation); group 3 received no treatment and served as a control group. The assigned treatment was applied during the dressing change 2 days after surgery. An 11-point visual analog pain scale was used by subjects to describe their pain during the dressing change.

Subjects who received the TENS reported significantly less pain than the other two groups; pain levels in groups 2 and 3 did not differ significantly. No other differences that could have accounted for the significant differences in pair ratings were found in the TENS group versus groups 2 and 3.

Nursing Implications. The use of TENS was found to be effective in reducing pain in postoperative patients undergoing procedures generally considered painful or at least uncomfortable. TENS is a safe, useful, and effective method of pain control. Easy to use, TENS is rarely contraindicated for patient use and produces analgesia without side effects. Studies using TENS with other types of procedural pain are indicated.

Bibliography

Other Related Nursing Research Articles

Erickson RS and Yount ST. Comparison of tympanic and oral temperatures in surgical patients. Nurs Res 1991 Mar/Apr; 40(2):90–93.

Holtzclaw BJ. Effects of extremity wraps to control drug-induced shivering: A pilot study. Nurs Res 1990 Sep/Oct; 39(5):280–284.

Keen MF. Comparison of intramuscular injection techniques to reduce site discomfort and lesions. Nurs Res 1986 Jul/Aug; 35(4):207–210.

Paymen BC, Dampier SE, and Hawthorn PJ. Postoperative temperature and infection in patients undergoing general surgery. J Adv Nurs 1989 Mar; 14(3):198–202.

Wilkie DJ. Use of the McGill Questionnaire to measure pain: A meta-analysis. Nurs Res 1990 Jan/Feb; 39(1):36–41.

unit 6

Oxygen–Carbon Dioxide Exchange and Respiratory Function

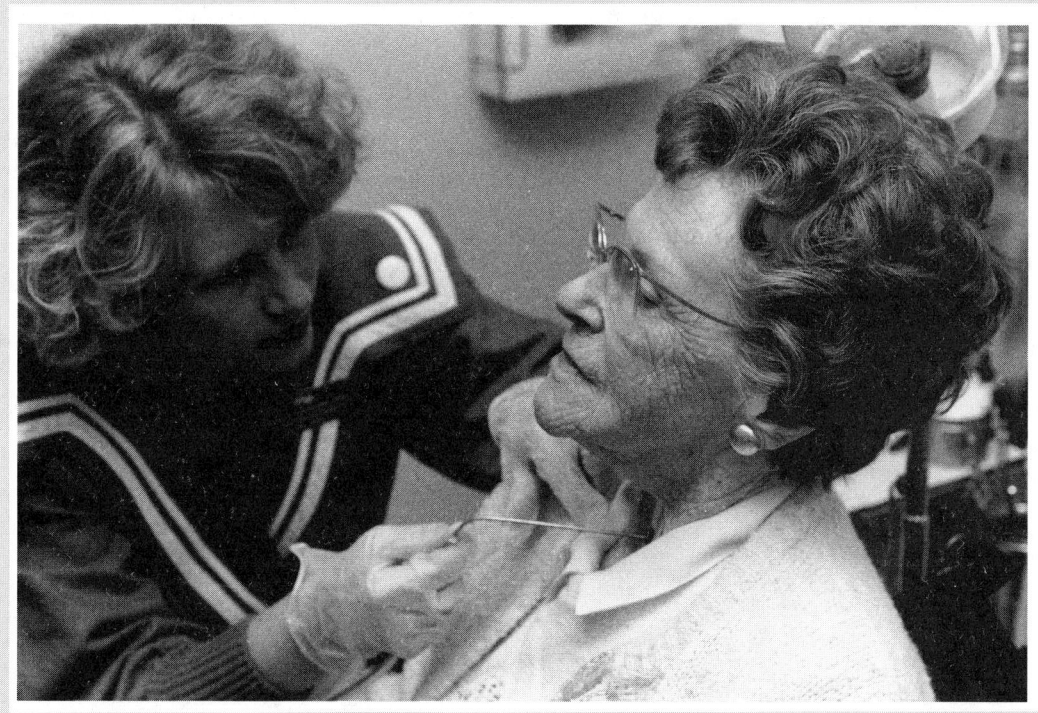

23

Management of Patients With Conditions of the Upper Respiratory Airway

Learning Objectives

On completion of this chapter, the learner will be able to:

1. Describe nursing assessment and management of patients with upper respiratory airway disorders
2. Compare the upper respiratory tract infections with regard to cause, incidence, clinical manifestations, management, and the significance of preventive health care
3. Use the nursing process as a framework for care of patients with upper airway infection
4. Describe nursing management of the patient with epistaxis
5. Use the nursing process as a framework for care of patients undergoing laryngectomy

Anatomy of the Upper Respiratory Airway

Nose

The nose is composed of an external and an internal portion. The external portion protrudes from the face and is supported by the nasal bones and cartilage. The anterior nares (nostrils) are the outside openings of the nasal cavities.

The internal portion of the nose is a hollow cavity separated into the right and left nasal cavities by a narrow vertical divider, the septum. Each nasal cavity is divided into three passageways by the projection of the turbinates (also called conchae) from the lateral walls. The nasal cavities are lined with highly vascular ciliated mucous membranes called the nasal mucosa. Mucus secreted continuously by goblet cells covers the surface of the nasal mucosa and is moved back to the nasopharynx by the action of the cilia.

The nose serves as a passageway for air to pass to and from the lungs. It filters impurities and humidifies and warms the air as it is inhaled into the lungs. It is responsible for olfaction (smell) because the olfactory receptors are located in the nasal mucosa. This function diminishes with age.

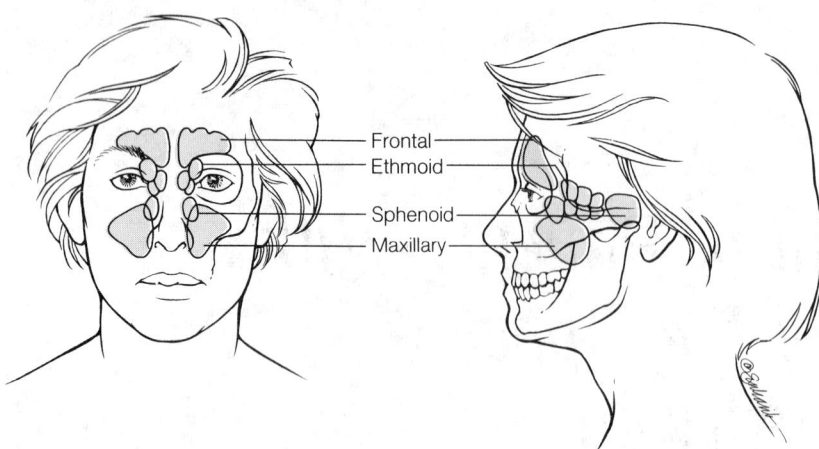

Figure 23–1. Paranasal sinuses.

The Paranasal Sinuses

The paranasal sinuses include four pairs of bony cavities that are lined with nasal mucosa and ciliated pseudostratified columnar epithelium. These air spaces are connected by a series of ducts that drain into the nasal cavity. The sinuses are named by their location, namely, frontal, ethmoidal, sphenoidal, and maxillary.

A prominent function of the sinuses is to serve as a resonating chamber in speech. The sinuses are a common site of infection (Fig. 23–1).

Turbinate Bones (Conchae)

The turbinate bones, or conchae (the name suggested by their shell-like appearance), are adapted by shape and position to increase the mucous membrane surface of the nasal passages and to slightly obstruct the current of air flowing through them.

The current of air entering the anterior nostrils is deflected upward to the roof of the nose and follows a circuitous route before it reaches the nasopharynx. On its way, it comes into contact with a large surface of moist, warm mucous membrane that catches practically all of the dust and germs in the inhaled air. This air is moistened and warmed to body temperature and brought into contact with sensitive nerves. Some of these nerves detect odors, and others provoke sneezing to expel irritating dust.

Pharynx, Tonsils, and Adenoids

The pharynx, or throat, is a tubelike structure that connects the nasal and oral cavities to the larynx. It is divided into three regions: nasal, oral, and laryngeal.

The nasopharynx is located posterior to the nose and is above the soft palate. The oropharynx houses the faucial, or palatine, tonsils. The laryngopharynx extends from the hyoid bone to the cricoid cartilage. The entrance of the larynx is formed by the epiglottis.

The adenoids, or pharyngeal tonsils, are located in the roof of the nasopharynx. The throat is encircled by the tonsils, the adenoids, and other lymphoid tissue. These structures are important links in the chain of lymph nodes guarding the body from invasion by organisms entering the nose and the throat. The function of the pharynx is to provide a passageway for the respiratory and digestive tracts.

Larynx

The larynx, or voice organ, is a cartilaginous epithelium-lined structure that connects the pharynx and the trachea (Fig. 23–2).

The major function of the larynx is to permit vocalization. It also protects the lower airway from foreign substances and facilitates coughing. It is frequently referred to as the voice box and consists of the following:

- *Epiglottis*—a valve flap of cartilage that covers the opening to the larynx during swallowing
- *Glottis*—the opening between the vocal cords in the larynx
- *Thyroid cartilage*—part of it forms the Adam's apple, the largest cartilage in the trachea
- *Cricoid cartilage*—the only complete cartilaginous ring in the larynx (located below the thyroid cartilage)

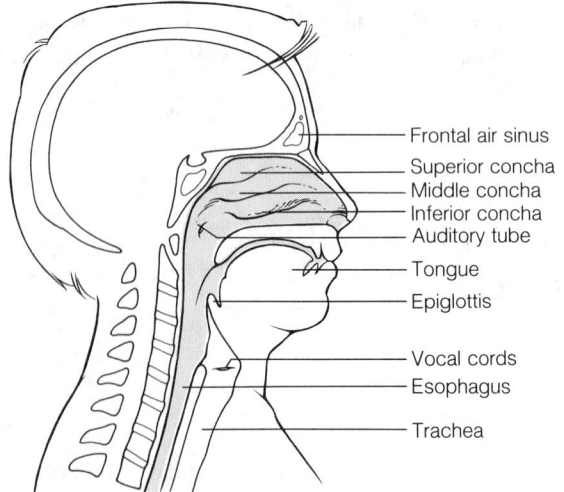

Figure 23–2. Sagittal section through face and neck. The nasal septum has been removed, exposing the lateral wall of the nasal cavity. Note the position of the conchae (turbinates).

- *Arytenoid cartilages*—used in vocal cord movement with the thyroid cartilage
- *Vocal cords*—ligaments controlled by muscular movements that produce vocal sounds; they are mounted in the lumen of the larynx

Assessment of the Upper Respiratory Airway

The Nose and Sinuses

The nose and sinuses are examined by inspection and palpation. For a routine examination, only a simple light source, such as a penlight, is necessary. A more thorough examination requires the use of a nasal speculum.

The external nose is inspected for lesions, asymmetry, or inflammation. The patient is then instructed to tilt his head backward while the examiner gently pushes the tip of the nose upward to examine the internal structures of the nose. The mucosa is inspected for color, swelling, exudate, or bleeding. The nasal mucosa is normally more red than the oral mucosa but may appear swollen and hyperemic in the presence of the common cold. Allergic rhinitis, however, is suggested when the mucosa appears pale and swollen.

The septum is inspected for deviation, perforation, or bleeding. A slight degree of septal deviation is present in most people. Actual displacement of the cartilage into either vestibule may produce nasal obstruction, but such deviation is usually asymptomatic.

With the patient's head tilted back, the examiner attempts to visualize the inferior and middle turbinates. In chronic rhinitis, nasal polyps may develop between the inferior and middle turbinates and are distinguished by their gray appearance. Unlike the turbinates, they are gelatinous and freely movable. The frontal and maxillary sinuses can be inspected by transillumination (passing a strong light through a body structure such as the sinuses to inspect the cavity).

The frontal and maxillary sinuses are palpated for tenderness. Using the thumbs, the examiner applies gentle pressure in an upward fashion at the supraorbital ridges (frontal sinuses) and in the cheek area adjacent to the nose (maxillary sinuses). Tenderness in either area suggests inflammation.

The Pharynx

A tongue blade, which often is used to depress the tongue for adequate visualization of the pharynx, is not always necessary. The patient is instructed to open his mouth wide and take a deep breath. Often this will flatten the posterior tongue and briefly expose a full view of the anterior and posterior pillars, tonsils, uvula, and posterior pharynx. These structures are inspected for color, symmetry, and evidence of exudate, ulceration, or enlargement. If a tongue blade is used to visualize the pharynx, it is pressed firmly beyond the midpoint of the tongue. Proper placement avoids a gagging response and minimizes the patient's aversion to future oral examinations.

The Trachea

The position and mobility of the trachea are usually noted by direct palpation. This is performed by placing the thumb and index finger of one hand on either side of the trachea just above the sternal notch. The trachea is highly sensitive, and palpating too firmly may incite a coughing or gagging response. The trachea is normally midline as it enters the thoracic inlet behind the sternum but may be deviated by masses in the neck or mediastinum. Pleural or pulmonary disorders, such as a significant pneumothorax, may result in displacement of the trachea.

Upper Airway Infections

Upper airway infections are common conditions that affect most people on occasion. Some of these conditions are acute, with symptoms that last several days; others are chronic, with symptoms that last a long time or occur repeatedly. Seldom do patients with these conditions require hospitalization; however, the nurse may encounter these infections in patients hospitalized for other reasons or in other nurse–client settings. Thus it is important to recognize the signs and symptoms and to provide appropriate nursing care.

Common Cold

The phrase *common cold* usually is used when referring to symptoms of an upper respiratory tract infection. Colds are highly contagious because patients shed virus for about 2 days before the symptoms appear and during the first part of the symptomatic phase. Colds prevail among 15% of the work population at any time during the winter and account for almost half of all work absences and one fourth of the total time lost from work.

Three waves of colds appear yearly in the United States— September, just after the opening of school; in late January; and toward the end of April. Immunity after recovery is variable and depends on many factors, including natural host resistance and the specific causative virus.

Clinical Manifestations.   The signs and symptoms of a cold are nasal discharge and obstruction, sore throat, sneezing, malaise, fever, chills, and often headache and muscle aching. As the cold progresses, cough usually appears. Most specifically, the term *cold* refers to an afebrile, infectious, acute inflammation of the mucous membranes of the nasal cavity. More broadly, the term refers to an acute upper respiratory tract infection, whereas terms such as *rhinitis, pharyngitis, laryngitis,* and *chest cold* distinguish the sites of the major symptoms.

The symptoms last 5 days to 2 weeks. If there is significant fever or more severe constitutional problems with the respiratory symptoms, it is no longer a common cold but one of the other acute upper respiratory tract infections. Many different viruses (over 100) are known to produce the signs and symptoms of the common cold, and about 10% of colds seem to be associated simultaneously with more than one virus. Also, allergic conditions affecting the nose can mimic the symptoms of a cold.

Management. There is no specific treatment for the common cold. Management of the common cold consists of adequate fluid intake, rest, prevention of chilling, aqueous nasal decongestants, vitamin C, and expectorants as needed. Warm salt water gargles soothe the sore throat, and aspirin or acetaminophen relieves the general constitutional symptoms. Antibiotics do not affect the virus or reduce the incidence of bacterial complications. They may be used prophylactically for high-risk respiratory patients.

Using disposable tissues and discarding them hygienically, covering the mouth when coughing, and avoiding crowds are important measures to prevent the spread of an upper respiratory airway infection.

Herpes Simplex Infection

The herpes simplex virus (HSV-1) most commonly produces the familiar *herpes labialis* (cold sore, fever blister, or canker). Small vesicles, single or clustered, may erupt on the lips, the tongue, the cheeks, and the pharynx. These soon rupture, forming sore, shallow ulcers that are covered with a gray membrane.

Herpes virus infections appear often in association with other febrile infections, such as streptococcal pneumonia, meningococcal meningitis, and malaria. The virus remains latent in cells of the lips or nose and is activated by febrile illnesses.

Management. The herpes virus may subside spontaneously in 10 to 14 days. If it does not, acyclovir, an antiviral agent, may be used to decrease the severity of symptoms and the duration or length of the flare-up. Analgesics, such as Tylenol with codeine or aspirin with codeine, are helpful in relieving pain and discomfort. Topical anesthetics, such as lidocaine (Xylocaine), Orabase, or dyclonine (Dyclone) give a measure of relief for oral pain. Applications of drying lotions or liquids may help to dry the lesions.

Sinusitis

The sinuses are involved in a high proportion of upper respiratory tract infections. If their openings into the nasal passages are clear, the infections resolve promptly. If their drainage is obstructed by a deviated septum or by hypertrophied turbinates, spurs, or polyps, however, sinusitis may persist as a smoldering secondary infection or flare up into an acute suppurative process.

Acute Sinusitis

The symptoms of acute sinusitis include pressure, pain over the sinus area, and purulent nasal secretions.

Acute sinusitis frequently develops as a result of a common cold, particularly a viral respiratory infection. Nasal congestion, caused by inflammation, edema, and transudation of fluid, leads to obstruction of the cavities. This provides an excellent medium for bacterial growth. Bacterial organisms account for over 60% of the cases of acute sinusitis, namely, *Streptococcus pneumoniae*, *Haemophilus influenzae*, and *Staphylococcus*

aureus. Dental infections also have been associated with acute sinusitis.

A careful history and diagnostic assessment are performed to rule out other local or systemic disorders, such as tumor, fistula, and allergy. Complications of sinusitis, although uncommon, include severe orbital cellulitis, subperiosteal abscess, cavernous sinus thrombosis, meningitis, and brain abscess.

Medical Management. The goals of treatment of acute sinusitis are control of the infection, shrinkage of the nasal mucosa, and relief of pain. The antibiotics of choice are amoxicillin (Augmentin) and ampicillin. Alternatives for patients allergic to penicillin include trimethoprim and sulfamathoxazole (Bactrim, Septra). Oral and topical decongestants may be administered. Heated mist and saline irrigation also may be effective for opening blocked passages, thereby allowing drainage of purulent discharge. The common oral decongestants are Drixoral and Dimetapp. Commonly used topical decongestants are Afrin and Otrivin. Topical decongestants should be administered with the patient's head back to promote maximum drainage.

Nursing Interventions. The nursing measures are directed toward facilitating drainage. Increased humidity, steam inhalation, increased fluid intake, and local heat application (hot wet packs) will assist in promoting drainage.

The nurse teaches the patient the early signs of a sinus infection and recommends preventive measures:

- Avoid allergens if allergies are suspected.
- Maintain general health so that the body's resistance is not lowered (eat properly, get plenty of rest and exercise).
- Avoid others with upper respiratory tract infections.
- Notify physician if pain in sinus areas persists or if nasal discharge is present and discolored.

Chronic Sinusitis

Clinical Manifestations. Chronic sinusitis usually is caused by chronic nasal obstruction due to discharge and edema of the nasal mucous membrane. The patient experiences cough, because of the constant dripping of the discharge backward into the nasopharynx, chronic headaches in the periorbital area, and facial pain, which are generally most pronounced on awakening in the morning. Fatigue is also common, as is nasal stuffiness.

Management. The medical management and nursing interventions of chronic sinusitis are the same as for acute sinusitis. Surgery may be indicated to correct structural deformities that obstruct the ostia (openings) of the sinus, including excision or cauterization of polyps, correction of a deviated septum, incision and drainage of the sinuses.

Some victims of severe chronic sinusitis obtain relief only by moving to a dry climate.

Rhinitis

Rhinitis is an inflammation of the mucous membranes of the nose. It may be caused by a variety of disorders, including viral rhinitis (common cold), bacterial rhinitis, and respiratory infections, namely, measles, tuberculosis, and nasal diphtheria. It also occurs as a result of intranasal foreign bodies and chronic use of vasoconstrictor drugs. Rhinitis may be a manifestation of an allergy (see Chap. 49), in which case it is referred to as "allergic rhinitis." It is estimated that between 10% and 20% of the population of the United States have allergic rhinitis. Rhinitis may be an acute or chronic condition (Fig. 23–3).

Clinical Manifestations. The signs and symptoms of rhinitis are nasal congestion, nasal discharge (purulent with bacterial rhinitis), nasal itchiness, and sneezing. Headache may occur, particularly if sinusitis is also present.

Medical Management. The management of rhinitis is dependent on the differential diagnosis. Particular attention is given to a complete history. Careful attention is given to home, environmental, and job-related exposure to allergens. The patient with suggested allergic rhinitis may be tested to identify allergens. Medication therapy may include antihistamines, decongestants, topical corticosteroids, and cromolyn sodium. The prescribed medications are usually used in some combination, depending on the patient's symptoms.

Nursing Interventions. The patient with allergic rhinitis is instructed to avoid allergens and irritants, such as dusts, fumes, odors, powders, sprays, and tobacco smoke. Saline nasal sprays may be helpful in soothing mucous membranes, softening crusted secretions, and removing irritants. The patient is instructed in the proper use and technique for administration of medications, particularly nasal sprays or aerosols. To achieve maximum relief, the patient is instructed to blow his nose before administration of any medication into the nasal cavity.

Acute Pharyngitis

Acute pharyngitis (strep throat) is a febrile inflammation of the throat that is caused by a viral organism 70% of the time. Group A streptococcus is the most common bacterial organism associated with acute pharyngitis.

Clinical Manifestations. The signs and symptoms of acute pharyngitis include a fiery red pharyngeal membrane, tonsils and lymphoid follicles that are swollen and flecked with exudate, and enlarged and tender cervical lymph nodes. Fever, malaise, and sore throat also may be present. Hoarseness, cough, and rhinitis are not uncommon.

Uncomplicated viral infections usually subside promptly, within 3 to 10 days after the onset. Pharyngitis caused by more virulent bacteria is a more severe illness during the acute stage, however, and far more important because of the incidence of dangerous complications. These complications include sinusitis, otitis media, mastoiditis, cervical adenitis, rheumatic fever,

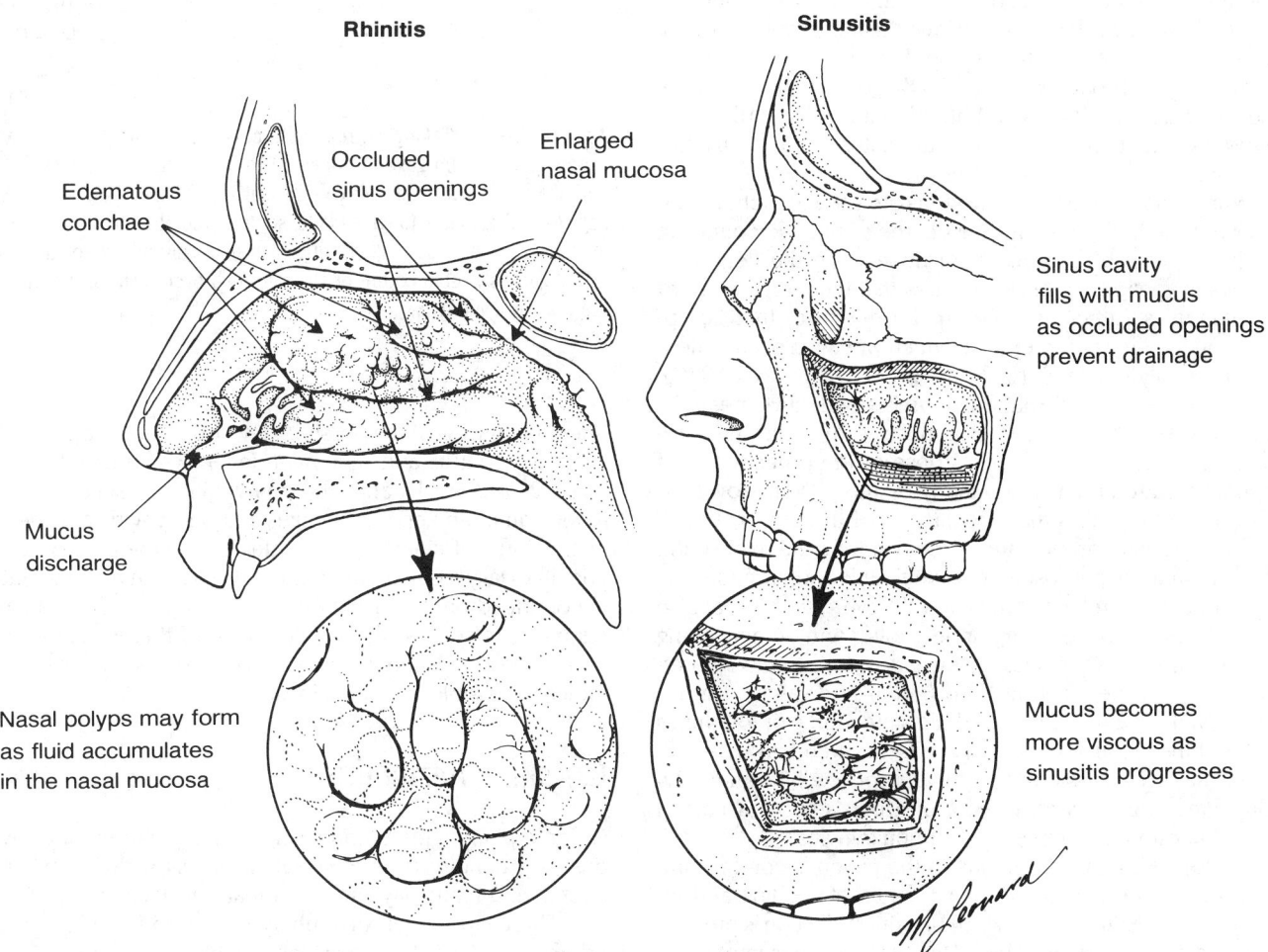

Figure 23–3. Rhinitis and sinusitis.

and nephritis. A throat culture is the chief means of determining the causative organism and, after it is obtained, proper therapy is prescribed.

Medical Management.   If a bacterial cause is suggested or demonstrated, treatment may include the administration of antimicrobial agents. For group A streptococci, penicillin is the drug of choice. For those patients who are allergic to penicillin and resistant to erythromycin (one fifth of group A streptococci and most *S. aureus* organisms are resistant to penicillin and erythromycin), tetracycline is the drug of choice. Antibiotics are administered for at least 10 days for optimal eradication of group A streptococci from the oropharynx.

A liquid or soft diet is provided during the acute stage of the disease, depending on the patient's appetite and the degree of discomfort caused by swallowing. Occasionally, the throat is so sore that liquids cannot be taken in adequate amounts by mouth; in this situation, fluids are administered intravenously. Otherwise, the patient is encouraged to drink to the limit of tolerance, with the minimum intake during the febrile stage exceeding, if possible, 2500 ml each day. Often, the patient can achieve this goal more easily if the rationale of therapy is explained to him. His personal tastes (in liquids) should be considered and indulged when possible.

Nursing Interventions.   The patient is kept in bed during the febrile stage of illness. When he is ambulatory, he needs periods of rest. Secretion precautions must be observed to prevent the spread of infection. The skin is examined once or twice daily for possible rash, because acute pharyngitis may precede some other communicable disease.

Aside from throat cultures (Fig. 23–4), it may be necessary to secure nasal swabbings and blood cultures for further laboratory investigation to determine the nature of the causative organism.

Warm saline gargles or irrigations are used, depending on the severity of the lesion and the degree of pain. Recognizing that the benefits of this treatment depend on the degree of heat that is applied, the nurse ensures that the temperature of the solution is sufficiently high to be effective, that is, approaching the limits of tolerance, which vary with each patient and are usually between 105° and 110°F (40.6° to 43.3°C). A properly performed throat irrigation is an effective means of reducing spasm in the pharyngeal muscles and relieving soreness of the throat. Unless the purpose of the procedure and its technique are understood clearly by the patient, however, the results may be less than satisfactory. If throat irrigation is a new experience for the patient, the nurse should explain the procedure and its purpose before beginning the procedure.

Symptomatic relief in patients with severe sore throat also may be afforded by applying an ice collar and administering analgesic drugs, as prescribed; for example, aspirin or acetaminophen can be given at 3- to 6-hour intervals and, if required, Tylenol with codeine is administered three or four times daily. Antitussive medication, in the form of codeine, dextromethorphan (Robitussin DM), or hydrocodone bitartrate (Hycodan), may be required to control a persistent and painful cough that often accompanies acute pharyngitis.

Mouth care may add greatly to the patient's comfort and may prevent the development of fissures of the lips and inflammation about the mouth when bacterial infection is present.

Patient Education and Home Health Care.   Resumption of activity is permitted gradually. Unusually conservative management is indicated in patients with hemolytic *Streptococcus*

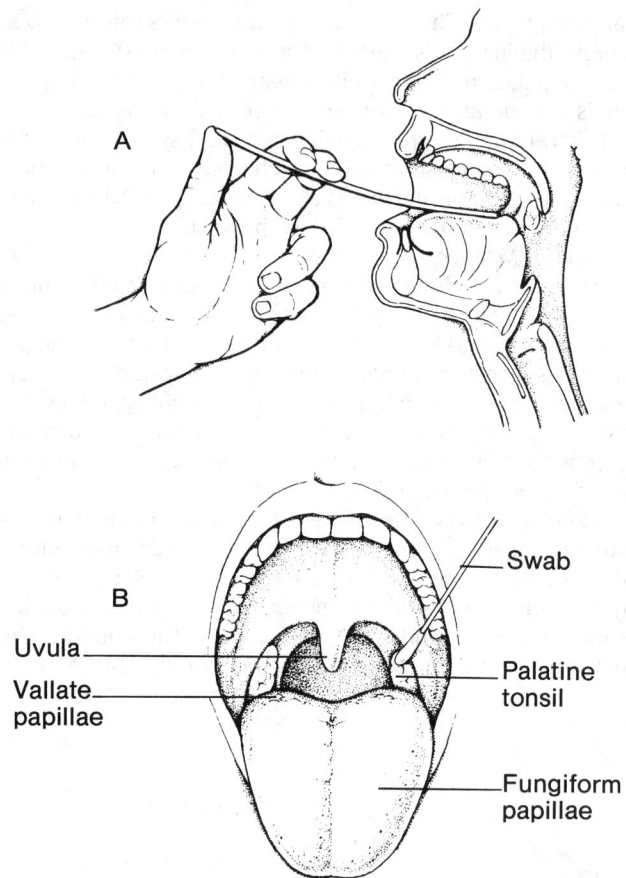

Figure 23–4.   Taking a throat culture. When obtaining a throat culture from a patient who gags, it is helpful to have him close his eyes. Since anticipation is lessened, the culture can be obtained with only a slight gag. (**A**) Grasp the tongue blade so that the thumb pushes the end upward (as a fulcrum) while the fingers push the middle section downward. (**B**) Vigorously rub a cotton or Dacron swab over each tonsilar area and the posterior pharynx.

infection in view of the possible development of complications such as nephritis and rheumatic fever, which may have their onset 2 or 3 weeks after the pharyngitis has subsided. Local extension of an apparently quiescent pharyngitis may develop in the form of sinusitis, otitis media, mastoiditis, or cervical adenitis. Daily assessment of morning and evening temperatures is continued until convalescence is complete. The patient or his family is advised that a full course of therapy is necessary and is informed about the symptoms to watch for that may indicate possible complications.

Chronic Pharyngitis

Chronic pharyngitis is common in adults who work or live in dusty surroundings, use the voice to excess, suffer from chronic cough, and habitually use alcohol and tobacco.

Three types of chronic pharyngitis are recognized: (1) hypertrophic, characterized by general thickening and congestion of the pharyngeal mucous membrane; (2) atrophic, probably a late stage of type 1 (the membrane is thin, whitish, glistening, and, at times, wrinkled); and (3) chronic granular ("clergyman's sore throat"), with numerous swollen lymph follicles on the pharyngeal wall.

Clinical Manifestations. Patients with chronic pharyngitis complain of a constant sense of irritation or fullness in the throat; of mucus, which collects in the throat and can be expelled by coughing; and of difficulty in swallowing.

Medical Management. The treatment of chronic pharyngitis is based on symptom relief, avoidance of exposure to irritants, and correction of any upper respiratory, pulmonary, or cardiac condition that might be responsible for a chronic cough.

Nasal congestion may be relieved by nasal instillations or sprays containing ephedrine sulfate (Afrin) or phenylephrine hydrochloride (Neo-Synephrine). If there is a history of allergy, one of the antihistamine decongestant drugs, such as Drixoral or Dimetapp, is administered orally every 4 to 6 hours. The attendant malaise is controlled effectively by aspirin or acetaminophen. Contact with others should be avoided, at least until the fever has subsided completely, to prevent the infection from spreading (see also Chap. 62).

Nursing Interventions. The nurse instructs the patient to avoid contact with others until the fever has subsided. The patient is instructed to avoid the use of alcohol, tobacco, secondhand smoke, and exposure to cold. Environmental/occupational pollutants should be avoided or minimized through the use of disposable masks, or scarfs. The patient is encouraged to drink plenty of fluids. Gargling with warm saline solutions may relieve throat discomfort. Lozenges will keep the throat moistened.

Tonsillitis and Adenoiditis

The tonsils are composed of lymphatic tissue and are situated on each side of the oropharynx. They frequently serve as the site of acute infection. Chronic tonsillitis is less common and may be mistaken for other disorders such as allergy, asthma, and sinusitis.

The adenoids consist of an abnormally large lymphoid tissue mass near the center of the posterior wall of the nasopharynx. Infection of the adenoids frequently accompanies acute tonsillitis.

Clinical Manifestations. The symptoms of tonsillitis include sore throat, fever, snoring, and difficulty in swallowing. Adenoid hypertrophy may cause mouth-breathing, earache, draining ears, frequent head colds, bronchitis, foul-smelling breath, voice impairment, and noisy respiration. Unusually enlarged adenoids may cause nasal obstruction. Extension of infection to the middle ears by way of the auditory (eustachian) tubes may result in acute otitis media, the potential complications of which include spontaneous rupture of the eardrums and further extension into the mastoid cells, causing acute mastoiditis. The infection also may reside in the middle ear as a chronic, low-grade, smoldering process that eventually may cause permanent deafness.

Diagnostic Evaluation. A thorough physical examination is performed, and a careful history is obtained to rule out related or systemic conditions. A culture of the organisms at the tonsillar site is performed to determine the presence of bacterial infection. In adenoiditis, if there are recurrent episodes of suppurative otitis media that are causing a hearing loss, it is im-

portant for the patient to have a comprehensive audiometric examination (see Chap. 54).

Tonsillectomy and Adenoidectomy

Appropriate antibiotic therapy is initiated for both tonsillectomy and adenoidectomy. Tonsillectomy is usually not performed unless medical treatment is unsuccessful and there is severe hypertrophy or peritonsillar abscess that occludes the pharynx, making swallowing difficult and endangering the airway. Enlargement of the tonsils is rarely an indication for their removal; most children normally have large tonsils, which decrease in size with age. Despite the continuing debate over the effectiveness of many tonsillectomies, the operation is still a common surgical procedure performed in the United States.

Tonsillectomy or adenoidectomy is performed only if the patient has had any of the following: repeated bouts of tonsillitis; hypertrophy of the tonsils and adenoids that could cause obstruction; repeated attacks of purulent otitis media; suspected hearing loss due to serous otitis media that has occurred in association with enlarged tonsils and adenoids; and some other conditions, such as an exacerbation of asthma or rheumatic fever. Laser surgery has been tried, but it prolongs anesthesia and causes other laser-related complications; therefore, in this situation laser surgery must be used judiciously.

Postoperative Nursing Interventions. Continuous nursing observation is required in the immediate postoperative and recovery period because of the significant risk of hemorrhage. After the operation, the most comfortable position is prone with the head turned to the side to allow for drainage from the mouth and pharynx. The oral airway is not removed until the patient demonstrates that his swallowing reflex has returned. An ice collar is applied to the neck, and a basin and tissues are provided for the expectoration of blood and mucus.

Bleeding may be bright red if the patient expectorates blood at once. Often, however, the blood is swallowed and immediately becomes brown because of the action of the acidic gastric juice.

- If the patient vomits large amounts of altered blood or spits bright blood at frequent intervals, or if the pulse rate and temperature rise and the patient is restless, the surgeon is notified immediately and the following items are made available to examine the surgical area for a bleeding site: a light, a head mirror, gauze, curved hemostats, and a waste basin.

Occasionally, it may be necessary to suture or ligate the bleeding vessel. In such cases the patient is taken to the operating room and placed under anesthesia. After ligation, continuous nursing observation and postoperative care are required, as in the initial postoperative period.

If there is no bleeding, water and cracked ice are given to the patient as soon as desired. He is instructed to refrain from too much talking and coughing, because this can produce throat pain. Alkaline mouthwashes and warm saline solutions are useful in coping with the thick mucus that may be present after a tonsillectomy. A liquid or semi-liquid diet is given for several days. Sherbet, gelatin desserts, and junkets are acceptable foods. Spicy, hot, cold, acidic, or rough foods are avoided. Milk and mild products (ice cream) may be restricted because they tend to increase the amount of mucus produced.

Patient Education and Home Health Care. On returning home, the patient needs to get plenty of rest, eat soft foods, drink fluids, and resume activity gradually. Any bleeding is reported to the physician; delayed hemorrhage may occur up to a week after surgery.

Peritonsillar Abscess

Peritonsillar abscess develops above the tonsil in the tissues of the anterior pillar and soft palate. As a rule, it occurs several days after an acute tonsillar infection and usually is caused by a group A streptococcus.

Clinical Manifestations.   The usual symptoms of an infection are present, together with such local symptoms as difficulty in swallowing anything other than liquids (dysphagia), thickening of the voice, drooling, and local pain. An examination shows marked swelling of the soft palate, often to the extent of half-occluding the orifice from the mouth into the pharynx.

Medical Management.   Antibiotics (usually penicillin) are extremely effective in the control of the infection in peritonsillar abscess. If antibiotics are prescribed early in the course of the disease, the abscess may be aborted and incision avoided. If antibiotics are not prescribed until later, the abscess must be drained, but improvement in the inflammatory reaction is rapid.

The abscess is evacuated as soon as possible. The mucous membrane over the swelling is first sprayed with a topical anesthetic and then injected with a local anesthetic. Single or repeated needle aspirations are performed to decompress the abscess. An incision and drainage is also a common treatment for peritonsillar abscess. These procedures are performed best with the patient in the sitting position, because this will make it easier for him to expectorate the pus and blood that accumulate in the pharynx. Almost immediate relief is experienced.

Some laryngologists advocate bilateral tonsillectomy for management of acute peritonsillar abscess to prevent recurrences and eliminate unsuspected asymptomatic pockets of infection.

Nursing Interventions.   Considerable relief may be obtained by throat irrigations or the frequent use of mouthwashes or gargles, using saline or alkaline solutions at a temperature of 105° to 110°F (40.6° to 43.3°C). The nurse instructs the patient to gargle at intervals of 1 or 2 hours for 24 to 36 hours.

Laryngitis

Inflammation of the larynx often occurs as a result of voice abuse, exposure to dust, chemicals, smoke, and other pollutants, or as part of an upper respiratory tract infection. It also may be caused by isolated infection involving only the vocal cords.

The cause of this inflammation is almost always a virus. Bacterial invasion may be secondary. Laryngitis usually is associated with acute rhinitis or nasopharyngitis. The onset of infection may be associated with exposure to sudden temperature changes, dietary deficiencies, malnutrition, and lack of immunity. Laryngitis is common in the winter and is readily transmitted.

Clinical Manifestations.   The signs and symptoms of acute laryngitis include hoarseness or complete loss of voice (aphonia) and severe cough. Chronic laryngitis is marked by persistent hoarseness. Laryngitis may be a complication of chronic sinusitis and chronic bronchitis.

Medical Management.   For acute laryngitis, the treatment is abstinence from talking (voice rest) and smoking, bed rest, and cool steam or aerosol therapy. If the laryngitis is part of a more extensive respiratory infection due to a bacterial organism or if it is severe, appropriate antibacterial therapy is instituted. The majority of patients recover with conservative treatment; however, laryngitis tends to be more severe in elderly patients and may be complicated by pneumonia.

For chronic laryngitis, the treatment includes voice rest, elimination of any primary respiratory tract infection that may be present, and restriction of smoking. Recently, the use of topical steroid preparations, such as beclomethasone dipropionate (Vanceril) inhalation, has been advocated. These preparations have no systemic or long-lasting effects and may reduce local inflammatory reactions. A well-humidified environment is important, and expectorants are helpful in thinning laryngeal secretions during acute episodes. A daily fluid intake of 3 liters is also necessary to thin secretions.

▶ Nursing Process
The Patient With Upper Airway Infection
▷ Assessment

The nurse obtains a complete history of the patient's problem. Signs and symptoms may include headache, sore throat, pain around the eyes and on either side of the nose, difficulty in swallowing, cough, hoarseness, fever, stuffiness, and generalized discomfort and fatigue. The nurse determines onset of the symptoms, what precipitated them, what relieves them, if anything, and what aggravates them. A history of allergy and the existence of a concomitant illness are identified.

On inspection, the nurse looks for swelling, lesions, or asymmetry of the nose as well as for any bleeding or discharge. The nasal mucosa is inspected for abnormal findings such as a reddened color, swelling, or exudate, and nasal polyps, which may develop in chronic rhinitis.

The frontal and maxillary sinuses are palpated for tenderness, which suggests inflammation. The throat is observed by having the patient open his mouth wide and take a deep breath. The tonsils and pharynx are inspected for the abnormal findings of reddened color, asymmetry, or evidence of drainage, ulceration, or enlargement.

The trachea is palpated for midline position in the neck, and any lumps or deformities are identified. The neck lymph nodes also are palpated for associated enlargement and tenderness.

▷ Nursing Diagnoses

Based on all the assessment data, the patient's major nursing diagnoses may include the following:

- Ineffective airway clearance related to excessive secretions secondary to an inflammatory process
- Pain related to upper airway irritation secondary to an infection
- Impaired verbal communication related to upper airway irritation secondary to an infection
- Fluid volume deficit related to increased fluid loss secondary to diaphoresis associated with a fever
- Knowledge deficit regarding prevention of upper respiratory infections

▷ Planning and Implementation

▷ *Goals:* The major goals for the patient may include maintenance of a patent airway, relief of pain, maintenance of effective means of communication, absence of fluid volume deficit, and knowledge of how to prevent upper airway infections.

▷ Nursing Interventions

▷ *Airway Clearance.* An accumulation of secretions can block the airway in many patients with an upper airway infection. Changes in the respiratory pattern result, and the work of breathing required to get beyond the blockage is increased. There are several measures that can be used to loosen thick secretions or to keep the secretions moist so that they can be easily expectorated. Increasing fluid intake provides systemic hydration, which is an effective expectorant. Humidifying the environment by room vaporizers or steam inhalations also loosens secretions and reduces inflammation of the mucous membranes. The patient is instructed about the best position to assume for facilitating drainage. This will depend on the location of the infection or inflammation. For example, drainage for sinusitis or rhinitis is achieved in the upright position. In some conditions, topical or systemic medications are administered as prescribed to relieve nasal or throat congestion.

▷ *Comfort Measures.* Upper respiratory tract infections usually produce localized discomfort. In sinusitis, pain may occur in the area of the sinuses or the patient may experience a headache. In pharyngitis, laryngitis, or tonsillitis, a sore throat occurs. The nurse can help to relieve this discomfort by administering analgesics, such as acetaminophen or Tylenol with codeine, as prescribed by a physician. Topical anesthetics provide symptomatic relief for herpes simplex blisters and sore throats. Hot packs help relieve the congestion of sinusitis and promote drainage. Warm water gargles or irrigations relieve the pain of a sore throat. An ice collar is applied in the immediate postoperative period after a tonsillectomy and adenoidectomy to reduce swelling and decrease bleeding. Encouraging the patient to rest will help relieve the generalized discomfort or fever that accompanies many upper airway conditions (especially rhinitis, pharyngitis, and laryngitis). The nurse instructs the patient in general oral and nasal hygiene techniques to help relieve localized discomfort and to prevent the spread of infection.

▷ *Communication.* Upper airway infections may result in hoarseness or loss of speech. The patient is instructed not to try to speak, but, instead, to communicate in writing if appropriate. Additional strain on the vocal cords may further delay return of full voice. Placing objects close to the patient minimizes unnecessary use of the voice to request items.

▷ *Fluid Intake.* In upper airway infections, the work of breathing and the respiratory rate increase as inflammation and secretions develop. This, in turn, may increase insensible fluid loss. An associated fever increases the metabolic rate, which results in diaphoresis and increased fluid loss.

Sore throat, malaise, and fever may interfere with a patient's willingness to eat. The patient is encouraged to drink 2 to 3 liters of fluid per day during his upper airway infection, unless contraindicated, to thin secretions and promote drainage. Liquids (hot or cold) may be soothing, depending on the illness.

▷ *Patient Education.* The prevention of most upper airway infections is difficult because there are many potential causes. The responsible pathogen usually cannot be identified, and vaccines are unavailable except in rare instances. Allergies, pathologic conditions of the septum and the turbinates, emotional problems, and various systemic illnesses may be predisposing factors in isolated cases.

The nurse instructs the patient about the following hygienic measures that support the body's defenses and reduce susceptibility to respiratory infections:

- Practice good health measures — nutritious diet, appropriate exercise, adequate rest and sleep, and hand washing.
- Avoid excesses in alcohol, smoke, and irritants.
- Correct air dryness by proper home humidification, especially during cold weather.
- Avoid irritants (dust chemicals, tobacco, and smoke) and allergens when possible.
- Avoid unnecessary chilling of the skin, especially the feet; chilling lowers resistance.
- Obtain influenza vaccination if advised by a physician. This is usually recommended for the elderly and those with chronic illness.
- Avoid crowds during flu season.
- Maintain adequate dental hygiene.

▷ Evaluation

Expected Outcomes

1. Maintains a patent airway by managing secretions
   a. Reports decreased congestion
   b. Uses room humidifier or vaporizer
   c. Assumes best position to facilitate drainage of secretions for the condition
   d. Verbalizes familiarity with use of medications (oral or nasal spray) to relieve nasal congestion
2. Is comfortable
   a. States that use of analgesics helps relieve localized pain or headache
   b. Demonstrates the application of hot packs for sinusitis, warm water gargles or irrigations for a sore throat, and an ice collar after a tonsillectomy and adenoidectomy
   c. Verbalizes an understanding of the need for rest at this time
   d. Demonstrates adequate oral hygiene
3. Is able to communicate
   a. Demonstrates ability to communicate needs, wants, level of comfort
   b. Uses paper and pencil as a method of communication
   c. Uses voice minimally
4. Maintains an adequate fluid balance
   a. States rationale for drinking plenty of fluids
   b. Demonstrates no significant weight loss
   c. Is not dehydrated
5. Identifies strategies to prevent upper airway infections and allergic reactions
   a. Eats a balanced diet daily
   b. Practices good hand washing
   c. Does not smoke
   d. Avoids enclosed areas polluted with smoke
   e. Stays away from crowded areas (shopping malls, crowded restaurants, movie theaters) during the flu season
   f. Contacts physician/clinic to receive a flu shot

g. Uses room humidifiers when necessary
h. Wears protective clothing (hat, scarf, gloves, boots) to keep warm and avoid chilling
i. Verbalizes understanding of irritants/allergens that precipitate upper airway reactions.

In summary, although rarely life-threatening, upper respiratory infections are significant because of the temporary disability they cause and the loss of time from work and school that accompanies these infections. Those individuals who are elderly or chronically ill may be at increased risk; therefore, upper respiratory infections in these individuals must be monitored closely. Preventive measures (*i.e.*, vaccination) are advised for the elderly and persons with chronic illnesses.

Obstruction and Trauma of the Upper Respiratory Airway

Epistaxis (Nosebleed)

A hemorrhage from the nose, referred to as *epistaxis*, is caused by the rupture of tiny, distended vessels in the mucous membrane of any area of the nose. Rarely does epistaxis originate in the densely vascular tissue over the turbinates. Most commonly, the site is the anterior septum, where three major blood vessels enter the nasal cavity: (1) the anterior ethmoidal artery on the forward part of the roof (Kesselbach's plexus), (2) the sphenopalatine artery in the posterosuperior region, and (3) the internal maxillary branches (the plexus of veins located at the back of the lateral wall under the inferior turbinate).

There are a variety of causes associated with epistaxis, including trauma, infection, drugs, cardiovascular diseases, blood dyscrasias, nasal tumors, low humidity, foreign body, and a deviated nasal septum. Additionally, vigorous nose-blowing and nose-picking have been associated with epistaxis.

Medical Management.   The management of epistaxis is dependent on locating the bleeding site. A nasal speculum or headlight may be used to determine the site of bleeding in the nasal cavity. The majority of nosebleeds originate from the anterior portion of the nose. Initial treatment may include applying direct pressure. The patient sits upright with the head tilted forward to prevent swallowing and aspiration of blood. The patient compresses the soft outer portion of the nose against the midline septum for 5 or 10 minutes continuously. If this is unsuccessful, additional treatment is indicated. In anterior nosebleeds, cauterization may be used, by chemical agents, such as a silver nitrate applicator and Gelfoam, or by electrocautery. Topical vasoconstrictors, such as adrenaline (1:1000), cocaine (0.5%), and phenylephrine may be prescribed.

If bleeding is occurring from the posterior regions, drug-moistened cotton pledgets may be inserted into the nostril to reduce the blood flow and improve the view. Suction can remove excess blood and clots from the field of inspection. The search should shift from the anteroinferior quadrant to the anterosuperior, then to the posterosuperior, and finally to the posteroinferior area. The field is kept clear by using suction and by shifting the cotton tampons. Only about 60% of the total nasal cavity can actually be seen, however.

When the origin of the bleed cannot be identified, the physician may pack the nose with gauze impregnated with petrolatum; a topical anesthetic spray and decongestant may be used to prepare the patient for insertion of the gauze packing. A postnasal packing may be inserted with a balloon-inflated catheter; other methods of applying pressure are shown in Figure 23–5. The packing may remain in place for 48 hours or up to 5 or 6 days if necessary to control bleeding.

Nursing Interventions.   The nurse monitors the vital signs and assists in the control of bleeding. Tissues and an emesis basin are provided to allow the patient to expectorate any excess blood.

It is not uncommon for patients to be anxious in response to a nosebleed. Blood loss on clothing and handkerchiefs can be frightening. The nasal examination and treatment are uncomfortable. The nurse reassures the patient and significant others that bleeding can be controlled. A calm, kind, efficient manner is maintained.

Discharge teaching includes reviewing ways to prevent epistaxis including: avoiding forceful nose blowing, straining, high altitudes, and nasal trauma (including nose-picking). Adequate humidification may prevent drying of the nasal passages. The patient is instructed how to apply direct pressure to the nose with the thumb and the index finger for 15 minutes in the case of a recurrent nosebleed. If recurrent bleeding cannot be stopped, the patient is instructed to seek additional medical attention.

Nasal Obstruction

The passage of air through the nostrils is frequently obstructed by a deflection of the nasal septum, hypertrophy of the turbinate bones, or the pressure of polyps, which are grapelike swellings that arise from the mucous membrane of the sinuses, especially the ethmoids. This obstruction also may lead to a condition of chronic infection of the nose and result in frequent attacks of nasopharyngitis. Very frequently, the infection extends to the sinuses of the nose (mucus-lined cavities filled with air that drain normally into the nose). When sinusitis develops and the drainage from these cavities is obstructed by deformity or swelling within the nose, pain is experienced in the region of the affected sinus.

Management.   The treatment of nasal obstruction requires the removal of the obstruction, followed by measures to overcome whatever chronic infection exists. In many patients the underlying allergy requires treatment. At times it is necessary to drain the nasal sinuses by a radical operation. The operations performed depend on the type of nasal obstruction found. Usually, they are performed using local anesthesia.

If a deflection of the septum is the cause of the obstruction, the surgeon makes an incision into the mucous membrane and, after raising it from the bone, removes the deflected bone and cartilage with bone forceps. The mucosa then is allowed to fall back in place and is held there by tight packing. Generally, the packing used is soaked in liquid petrolatum to facilitate its removal in 24 to 36 hours. This operation is called a *submucous resection* or septoplasty.

Nasal polyps are removed by clipping them at their base with a wire snare. Hypertrophied turbinates may be treated by astringent applications to shrink them close to the side of the nose.

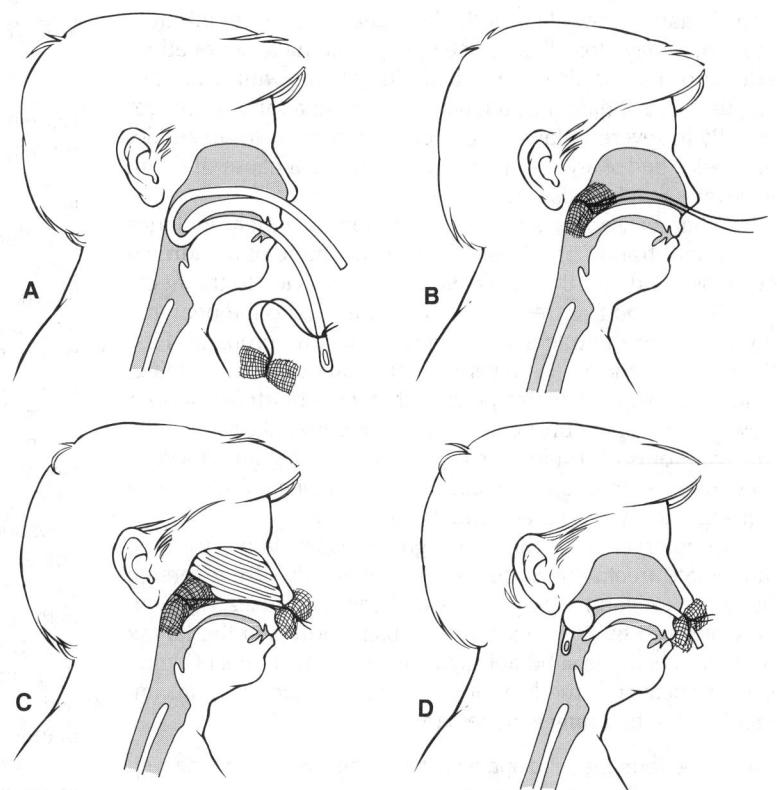

Figure 23–5. Packing to control bleeding from the posterior nose. (**A**) Catheter inserted and pack attached. (**B**) Pack drawn into position as catheter is removed. (**C**) Strip tied over a bolster to hold pack in place with anterior pack installed "accordion pleating" style. (**D**) Alternative method using balloon catheter instead of gauze pack. (Redrawn with permission from Way LW. Current Surgical Diagnosis and Treatment, 8th ed. Norwalk, Appleton & Lange, 1988.)

After these procedures, the head of the bed is elevated to promote drainage and to help in alleviating the patient's discomfort from edema. Frequent oral hygiene is given because the patient breathes through his mouth.

Fractures of the Nose

The location of the nose makes it susceptible to injury by a wide variety of causes. In fact, the nose sustains fractures more frequently than any other bone in the body. Fractures of the nose usually result from direct trauma. As a rule, no serious consequences result, but the deformity that may follow often gives rise to obstruction of the nasal air passages and to facial disfigurement.

Clinical Manifestations.   The signs and symptoms of a nasal fracture are bleeding from the nose externally and internally into the pharynx, swelling of the soft tissues adjacent to the nose, and deformity.

Assessment.   The nose is examined internally to rule out the possibility that the injury may be complicated by a fracture of the nasal septum and submucosal septal hematoma. If a hematoma develops and is not drained, it eventually may become an abscess with a dissolution of the septal cartilage. The familiar saddle deformity of the nose results.

Immediately after the injury there is usually considerable bleeding from the nose externally and internally into the pharynx. There is marked swelling of the soft tissues adjacent to the nose and, frequently, a definite deformity. Because of this swelling and bleeding, an accurate diagnosis can be made only after the swelling has subsided.

If there is clear fluid draining from either nostril, it suggests a fracture of the cribriform plate with leakage of cerebrospinal fluid. Because cerebrospinal fluid contains sugar, it can readily be differentiated from nasal mucus by using a dipstick (Dextrostix). Usually, careful inspection or palpation will disclose any deviations of the bone or disruptions of the nasal cartilages. An x-ray film may help to determine displacement of the fractured bones and help rule out extension of the fracture into the skull.

Medical Management.   As a rule, bleeding is controlled with the use of cold compresses. The nose is assessed for symmetry either before swelling has occurred or after it has subsided. The patient will be referred to a specialist for evaluation, usually 3 to 5 days after the injury to evaluate the need for realignment of the bones. Nasal fractures are reduced 7 to 10 days after the injury.

Nursing Interventions.   The nurse instructs the patient to apply ice packs to the nose for 20 minutes four times each day to decrease swelling.

In summary, the patient who experiences bleeding from the nose (epistaxis) because of injury or for unexplained reasons is usually frightened and anxious. The presence of packing to stop the bleeding may be uncomfortable and unpleasant; obstruction of the nasal passages by the packing forces the patient to breathe through his mouth; this in turn results in drying of the oral mucous membranes. Consequently the patient requires comfort measures to moisten the mucous membranes, to reduce the smell and taste of dried blood in the oropharynx and nasopharynx, and to relieve fear and anxiety about the bleeding.

Laryngeal Obstruction

Edema of the larynx is a serious, often fatal, condition. The larynx is a stiff box that will not stretch, and the space within it between the vocal cords (glottis), through which the air must pass, is narrow. Swelling of the laryngeal mucous membrane, therefore, may close this orifice tightly, leading to suffocation. Edema of the glottis occurs rarely in patients with acute laryngitis, occasionally in patients with urticaria, and more frequently in severe inflammations of the throat — for example, erysipelas and scarlet fever. It is an occasional cause of death in severe anaphylaxis (angioneurotic edema).

When caused by an allergic reaction, treatment includes the administration of subcutaneous epinephrine or an adrenal corticosteroid and the application of an ice pack to the neck.

Foreign bodies frequently are aspirated into the pharynx, the larynx, or the trachea and cause a twofold problem. First they obstruct the air passages and cause difficulty in breathing, which may lead to asphyxia; later they may be drawn farther down, entering the bronchi or one of their branches and causing symptoms of irritation, such as a croupy cough, blood or mucous expectoration, and paroxysms of dyspnea. The physical signs and x-ray results confirm the diagnosis.

In emergencies, when the signs of asphyxia are evident, immediate treatment is necessary. Frequently, if the foreign body has lodged in the pharynx and can be visualized, it can be dislodged by the finger. If the obstruction is in the larynx or the trachea, the subdiaphragmatic abdominal thrust (Heimlich) maneuver is tried. If all efforts are unsuccessful, an immediate tracheotomy is necessary.

- To perform the subdiaphragmatic abdominal thrust maneuver, one stands behind the person who is choking and places both arms around his waist, with one hand grasping the other fist. Then quickly and forcefully one exerts pressure against the victim's diaphragm, pressing slightly upward, just below the ribs 6 to 10 times or until the obstruction is cleared (Fig. 23–6).

The pressure will compress the lungs and expel the aspirated object. This is performed repeatedly until the object is expelled.

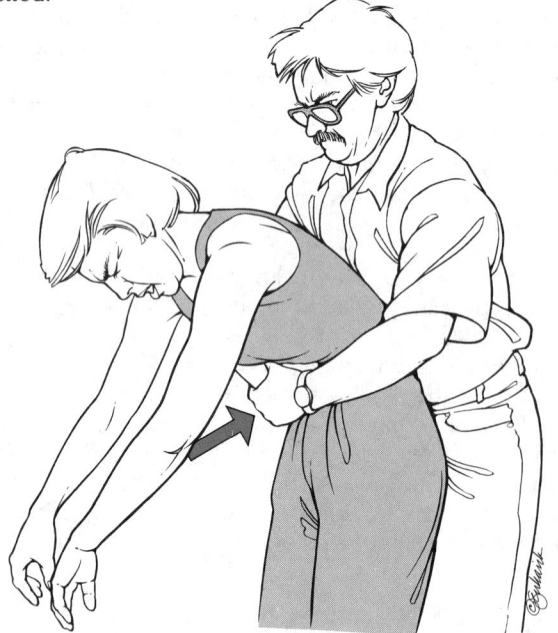

Figure 23–6. Subdiaphragmatic abdominal thrust (the Heimlich maneuver) administered to a conscious (standing) victim of foreign body airway obstruction. (American Heart Association. Instructor's Manual for Basic Life Support. Copyright 1987, American Heart Association.)

Cancer of the Larynx

Cancer of the larynx is potentially curable if detected early. It represents 1% of all cancers and occurs about eight times more frequently in men than in women and most commonly in men 50 to 65 years of age.

Each year in the United States, approximately 12,500 new cases are discovered and 3,650 persons with cancer of the larynx will die. Factors that contribute to laryngeal cancer are irritants, such as cigarette smoke and alcohol (and their combined effects), vocal straining, chronic laryngitis, industrial exposure, nutritional deficiencies, and family predisposition.

Clinical Manifestations.   A malignant growth may occur on the vocal cords (intrinsic) or on another part of the larynx (extrinsic). Hoarseness is noted early in the patient with intrinsic cancer because accurate approximation of the cords during phonation is interrupted by the presence of the tumor. Affected voice sounds are not early signs of extrinsic or supraglottic cancer; however, the patient may complain of pain and burning in the throat when drinking hot liquids and citrus juices. A lump may be felt in the neck. Later symptoms include dysphagia, dyspnea, hoarseness, and foul breath. Enlarged cervical nodes, weight loss, general debility, and the discomfort of pain radiating to the ear may be suggestive of metastasis.

Diagnostic Evaluation.   Direct laryngoscopic examination under general anesthesia is the primary method for evaluating the larynx. All areas of the larynx can be inspected and biopsies performed. The growth may involve any of the three areas (glottis, supraglottis, or subglottis) and varies in appearance. The precise involvement is determined, as this affects the treatment. Because many of these lesions are submucosal, biopsy may necessitate that an incision be performed with microlaryngeal techniques or laser to transect the mucosa and reach the tumor.

Mobility of the vocal cords is assessed; if normal movement is limited, the growth may affect muscle, other tissue, and even the airway. The lymph nodes of the neck and the thyroid gland are palpated to determine spread of the malignancy.

Computed tomography (CT scan) and laryngography are effective in determining the extent of tumor growth.

Management

Treatment varies with the extent of the malignancy. Precise determination of the exact location and involvement of the malignancy is performed by direct laryngoscopy, biopsy, and radiography before radiation therapy or surgery is prescribed.

If surgery is to be performed, thorough oral hygiene before the procedure is imperative. Antibiotics may be prescribed to reduce the possibility of infection. In men, preoperative shaving includes the beard and the hair on the neck and the chest down to the nipple line.

Radiation Therapy.   Excellent results have been achieved with radiation therapy in patients in whom only one cord is affected and is normally mobile (*i.e.*, moved with phonation). In addition, these patients retain a practically normal voice. A few may develop chondritis or stenosis; a small number may later require laryngectomy.

Partial Laryngectomy (Laryngofissure, Thyrotomy).   A hemilaryngectomy is recommended in the early stages, especially in intrinsic cancer of the larynx (limited to the vocal cords), and has a high cure rate. In this operation, the thyroid cartilage of the larynx is split in the midline of the neck, and the portion of the vocal cord that is involved with tumor growth is removed. A tracheostomy tube (see p. 532) sometimes is left in the trachea until the glottic airway is sufficient. It usually is removed after a few days and the stoma is allowed to close. There may be some changes in the voice quality and projection.

Supraglottic (Horizontal) Laryngectomy. A supraglottic laryngectomy is used in the management of certain extrinsic tumors. After adequate resection, sufficient normal larynx is left so that the cords remain intact and their function is maintained. During surgery, a radical neck dissection is also performed on the involved side. Postoperatively, the patient may experience some difficulty in swallowing for the first 2 weeks. The chief advantage of this operation is that it preserves the voice. The major problem is that there may be local recurrence; therefore, patients have to be selected carefully.

Total Laryngectomy. For extrinsic cancer of the larynx (extension beyond the vocal cords), the entire larynx is removed; this includes the thyroid cartilage, the vocal cords, and the epiglottis. Many surgeons recommend that a neck dissection be performed on the same side as the lesion even though no lymph nodes are palpable. The rationale for this approach is that many patients have had metastases to the cervical lymph nodes. The problem is more complex when a lesion involves midline structures or both vocal cords. With or without neck dissection, a total laryngectomy requires a permanent tracheal stoma (Fig. 23–7). This prevents aspiration of food and fluid into the lower respiratory tract, because the larynx that provides the protective sphincter is no longer present.

▶ Nursing Process
The Patient Undergoing Laryngectomy

◇ Assessment

The nurse assesses the patient for the following symptoms: hoarseness, sore throat, dyspnea, dysphagia, or pain and burning in the throat. The patient's neck is palpated for swelling.

If treatment includes surgery, it is important for the nurse to know the nature of the surgery to plan appropriate care. For example, some patients experience loss of speech. Once it has been determined that speech will be lost, a preoperative evaluation by the speech–language therapist is indicated.

In addition, the nurse determines the psychological preparedness of the patient. The idea of cancer is terrifying to most people; this is compounded by the potential for permanent loss of speech. The nurse evaluates the patient's coping methods to develop an effective approach to supporting him both preoperatively and postoperatively.

◇ Nursing Diagnoses

Based on all the assessment data, the patient's major nursing diagnoses may include the following:

• Knowledge deficit about the surgical procedure and postoperative course

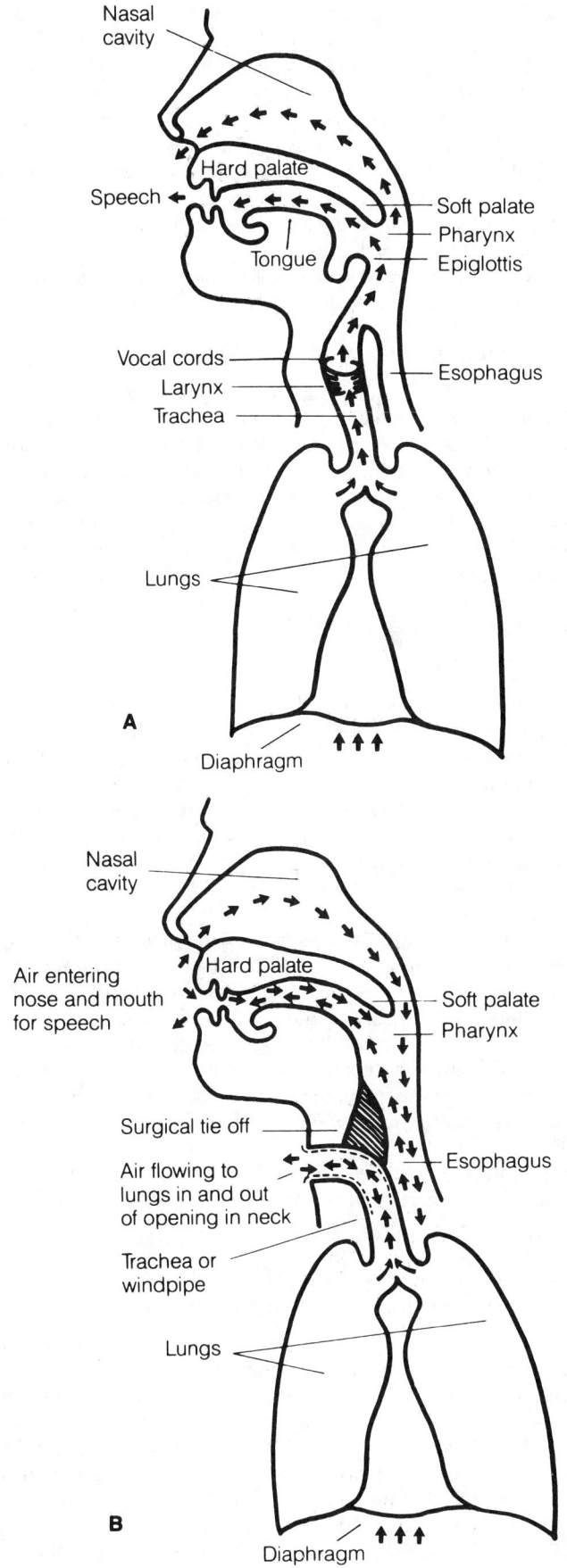

Figure 23–7. Direction of the air flow before (**A**) and after (**B**) total laryngectomy. (Courtesy of the American Cancer Society.)

- Anxiety related to the diagnosis of cancer and impending surgery
- Ineffective airway clearance related to surgical alterations in the airway
- Impaired verbal communication related to removal of larynx, and edema
- Altered nutrition: less than body requirements, related to swallowing difficulties
- Disturbance in body image, self-concept, and self-esteem related to major neck surgery
- Potential for noncompliance to rehabilitative program and home maintenance management

◊ Planning and Implementation

◊ *Goals:* The major goals for the patient may include attainment of an adequate level of knowledge, reduction in anxiety, maintenance of a patent airway (patient is able to handle own secretions), improvement in communication by use of alternative methods, attainment of optimal levels of nutrition and hydration, improvement in body image and self-esteem, adherence to rehabilitative program, and home maintenance management.

◊ Nursing Interventions

◊ Preoperative

◊ *Patient Education.*   The diagnosis of cancer of the larynx is associated with preconceived notions and fears. Many categorize it with other cancers and assume the worst. Others assume that loss of speech and disfigurement are inevitable with this condition. Once the physician explains the diagnosis to the patient, the nurse clarifies any misconceptions by identifying where the larynx is, what it does, what the particular procedure will be, and what effect surgery will have on the patient's speech.

If the patient is going to have a complete laryngectomy, he should know that he will lose his natural voice completely and that, with training, there are ways in which he can carry on a fairly normal conversation. (He will not be able to sing, laugh, or whistle.) Until the patient receives this training, he needs to know that the nurse can be reached by using the call light and that he can communicate in the immediate postoperative phase by writing. The nurse answers questions about the nature of the surgery and reinforces the physician's explanation that the patient will lose his ability to vocalize. He is assured that much can be done for him through a rehabilitation program.

Equipment and treatments that will be part of the postoperative care are reviewed. The patient's role in the postoperative and rehabilitative periods is explained.

◊ *Reduction of Anxiety and Depression.*   Because surgery of the larynx is performed most commonly for a tumor that is malignant, the patient has many questions: Will the surgeon be able to remove all of the tumor? Is it cancer? Will I die? Will I choke? Will I suffocate? Will I ever speak again? What will I look like? Therefore, the psychological preparation of the patient is as important as the physical preparation.

Any patient undergoing surgery may have many fears. (See Chap. 20 for further discussion.) The patient is given the opportunity to verbalize his feelings and share his perceptions. Any misconceptions the patient might have about his condition are addressed. He is given complete but concise answers to his questions. During the preoperative or postoperative period, a visit from an individual who has had a laryngectomy is often helpful in conveying to the patient that there are people available and willing to help him cope with his situation and that successful rehabilitation is possible.

◊ Postoperative

◊ *Airway Maintenance.* Respiratory effectiveness is promoted by positioning the patient in the semi-Fowler's or Fowler's position after recovery from anesthesia. The patient is observed for restlessness, labored breathing, apprehension, and increased pulse rate, because these suggest respiratory or circulatory problems. Medications that depress respirations are to be avoided. Like other surgical patients, the laryngectomy patient is encouraged to turn, cough, and take deep breaths; suctioning may be necessary. Early ambulation, also, aids in preventing atelectasis and pneumonia.

If a total laryngectomy was performed, a laryngectomy tube will most likely be in place. (In some instances a laryngectomy tube is not used, in others it is used temporarily, and in many it is used permanently.) The laryngectomy tube (which is shorter than a tracheostomy tube but has a larger diameter) is the only airway the patient has. The care of this tube is the same as for a tracheostomy tube (see p. 491).

The stoma is kept clean by daily cleansing with saline solution or prescribed solution; antibiotic ointment (of a non-oil base) may be prescribed and is applied around the stoma and suture line.

Wound drains may be in place to assist in removal of fluid and air from the dead space. Portable suction may also be used. Drainage is observed, measured, and recorded; when drainage is less than 50 to 60 ml/day, the physician usually removes the drains.

The laryngectomy tube may be removed when the stoma is well healed, usually within 3 to 6 weeks after the operation. Until that time, the patient will need to be taught how to clean and change the laryngectomy tube (see p. 493) and how to clear his airway of secretions. Through the postoperative period, the nurse must be alert for the possible serious complication of rupture of the carotid artery, particularly if wound infection is present. Should this occur, the nurse would apply direct pressure over the artery, summon assistance, and provide psychological support to the patient until the vessel can be ligated.

◊ *Communication and Speech Rehabilitation.*   The loss of speech or impaired speech is discussed preoperatively with the patient and family. Postoperatively, a system of communication with the nurse, physician, and family is established.

Because a "magic slate" often is used for communication, it is well to document which hand the patient uses for writing so that the opposite arm can be used for intravenous infusions. When notes are the means of communication, they should be destroyed to ensure the patient's privacy. If the patient is not able to write, a picture/word/phrase board or hand signals can be used.

An alternative to the call bell may be required, such as a hand bell. This system is reviewed preoperatively with the patient. The patient's ability to hear, see, read, and write is also assessed. Visual impairment and functional illiteracy may create additional problems and nursing considerations. The inability to speak can be very frustrating. It can be very time-consuming to have to write everything or communicate through gestures.

The patient may become impatient and angry when he is not understood. The nurse must be patient and understanding of such feelings. Other staff members should be alerted that the patient will be unable to use the intercom system.

The return of communication is generally the ultimate goal in the rehabilitation of the postlaryngectomy patient. Several methods of communication exist, such as writing, lip-speaking, and communication/word boards. The most commonly used and preferred methods at present, however, include esophageal speech, the electrolarynx, and tracheoesophageal puncture.

When the patient is informed that a laryngectomy procedure is required, it is likely to be quite traumatic. Although the patient is concerned about his health and survival, frequently, the most often asked question is, "Will I be able to talk again?" A speech–language pathologist is usually contacted before the laryngectomy procedure. This initial visit is to acquaint the patient with what can be done to facilitate communication after the laryngectomy and to provide support. Once the laryngectomy has been performed, the speech pathologist begins to work with the patient to establish the optimum communication method to be used.

As mentioned above, the most preferred methods of communication today are esophageal speech, the electrolarynx, and tracheoesophageal puncture (Fig. 23–8). All techniques may be used once medical clearance is obtained from the physician. Esophageal speech requires that the patient be able to compress air into the esophagus and expel it, setting off a vibration of the pharyngeal esophogeal segment.

This can be taught once the patient begins oral feedings or 1 week postoperatively. The patient first develops his ability to belch. An hour after he has eaten, the nurse reminds him to belch. This is practiced repeatedly. Later this conscious action is transformed into simple explosions of air from the esophagus for speech purposes. Thereafter, the speech–language pathologist works with him in an attempt to make his speech intelligible and as close to normal as possible.

If esophageal speech is not successful, or until the technique is mastered, an electric larynx may be used for communication. This apparatus projects sound into the oral cavity.

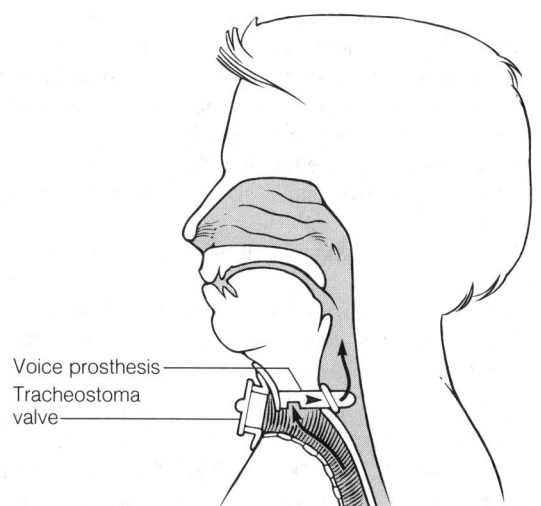

Figure 23–8. Schematic representation of tracheopharyngeal fistula speech. (Redrawn from Sofferman RA. Head and neck. In Davis JH et al. Clinical Surgery, Vol. 2. St Louis, CV Mosby, 1987.)

When words are formed by the mouth (articulated), the sound from the electric larynx becomes words that can be heard. The voice that is produced is obviously not the patient's normal voice, but he is able to communicate with relative ease.

Another form of communication that will help the patient be better understood is called tracheoesophageal puncture (TEP). In this method the voice is restored by diverting air, which travels from the lungs through a puncture in the posterior wall of the trachea, into the esophagus, and out of the mouth. Once the puncture is surgically created and has healed, a voice prosthesis (Blom–Singer) is fitted over the puncture site. The prosthesis is removed and cleaned when there is mucus buildup to prevent airway obstruction. The patient is given lessons in voice production by the speech–language pathologist, but the speech is produced just as before by moving the tongue and lips to form the sound into words.

▷ *Nutrition.* Postoperatively, the patient may be NPO (nothing by mouth) for 10 to 14 days. Alternative sources of nutrition and hydration must be provided, including intravenous fluids, enteral feedings through a nasogastric tube, and total parenteral nutrition.

Once the patient is ready to start oral feedings, the nurse explains to the patient that he will start with thick fluids, such as Ensure and Jello, which are easy to swallow. The patient is instructed to avoid sweet foods, which increase salivation and suppress the appetite. Solid foods are introduced as tolerated. In addition, the patient is instructed to rinse his mouth with warm water or mouthwash and to brush his teeth frequently.

▷ *Improved Body Image and Self-Esteem.* Disfiguring surgery and an altered communication pattern are a threat to a patient's self-concept, self-esteem, and body image. The reaction of family members is a major concern for the patient.

A positive approach is important when caring for the patient. The nurse allows the patient to participate in his care. The nurse reviews with the patient and family the tubes, dressings, and drains that are in place postoperatively. The patient is encouraged to express his feelings. The patient often experiences anger, depression, and isolation. The nurse is a good listener and support to the family. Referral to a support group, such as The American Laryngectomee Association and I Can Cope, may help the patient and family cope with the changes in their lives.

▷ *Patient Education.* The nurse has an important role in the rehabilitation of the laryngectomy patient. The patient will experience many emotions, physical changes, and changes in life style. The following patient education areas are addressed.

Tracheostomy and Stomal Care. The nurse conveys optimism to the patient, assuring him that he will be able to carry on most of his preoperative activities. The patient needs specific information about what to expect from his tracheostomy. He frequently will cough up rather large amounts of mucus through this opening. Because air passes directly into the trachea without being warmed and moistened by the upper respiratory mucosa, the tracheobronchial tree compensates by secreting excessive amounts of mucus. Therefore, the patient will have frequent coughing episodes and may be somewhat troubled by the brassy sounding, mucus-producing cough. He should be assured that these problems will diminish in time as the tracheobronchial mucosa adapts to the patient's altered physiology.

When the patient coughs, the orifice should be wiped clean and cleared of mucus. In addition, the skin around the stoma should be washed twice daily. If crusting occurs, the skin around the stoma is lubricated with a non–oil-based ointment (prescribed by the physician) and the crusts removed with sterile tweezers. It may be necessary that a bib be worn in front of the tracheostomy to keep the mucus from soiling the clothing. The bib may be a simple gauze dressing taped over the neck or one made of other porous fabric.

One of the most important factors in decreasing cough and mucus production as well as crusting around the stoma is to provide adequate humidification of the environment. Mechanical humidifiers and aerosol generators (nebulizers) are excellent sources of humidification and are absolutely essential for the patient's comfort. Some system of humidification should be set up in the home before the patient is discharged from the hospital. An air-conditioned atmosphere may be distressing to the newly laryngotomized patient, because the air may be too cool or too dry and thus too irritating.

Changes in Taste and Smell.   The patient can expect to have a diminished sense of taste and smell for a period after the operation. Because he is breathing directly into the trachea, air is not passing through the nose to the olfactory end organs. Because taste and smell are so closely connected, his taste sensations are altered. In time, however, the patient usually accommodates to this problem and his olfactory sensation adapts to meet his needs.

Hygienic and Recreational Measures.   Special precautions need to be taken in a shower to prevent water from entering the stoma. Wearing a loose-fitting plastic bib or simply holding one's hand over the opening is effective. Swimming is not recommended, however, because the patient with a laryngectomy can drown without getting his face wet. Barbers and beauticians need to be cautioned so that hair sprays, loose hair, and powder do not get near the stoma, because they could cause blockage, irritation, and possibly infection.

Recreation and exercise are important. Golf, bowling, bridge, spectator activities, and walking can be enjoyed safely. Moderation to prevent fatigue is important because, when tired, the laryngectomee has more difficulty speaking with his new voice. At such times he can easily become discouraged and depressed.

Follow-Up and Emergency Care.   The nurse encourages the person who has had a laryngectomy (laryngectomee) to visit his physician regularly for physical examinations and for advice concerning any problems relating to his convalescent program. He also should carry proper identification, such as a card, to alert a first-aider to the special requirements of resuscitation should this need arise. On the back of the card can be included the name of a responsible person to notify in the event of emergency.

◊ *Evaluation*

Expected Outcomes

1. Acquires an adequate level of knowledge
   a. Verbalizes an understanding of his specific surgical procedure
   b. States his role in his own care
   c. Performs self-care adequately
2. Experiences less anxiety and depression
   a. Describes the reason for his surgery and desires to work with staff

b. Verbalizes confidence that health care personnel will give him the care he needs
   c. Develops a sense of hope about his condition
   d. Expresses that he is comfortable with the support group
   e. Meets with someone from the Lost Chord or New Voice club
3. Maintains a clear airway and handles own secretions
   a. Demonstrates practical and correct technique involved in cleaning and changing the laryngectomy tube
   b. Demonstrates how to raise secretions from stoma or tube by coughing or by suctioning
   c. Is afebrile and eupneic (normal respiratory rate); has normal breath sounds
   d. Relates the significance of good hygienic measures in keeping mouth and stoma clean
   e. Covers stoma opening securely when shaving or showering
4. Acquires effective communication techniques
   a. Uses a "magic slate" until whispering is permitted
   b. Uses alternative communication techniques when voice is not audible; call bell, picture board, sign language, lip reading, computer aids
   c. Verbalizes how the vocal problem can be improved with adherence to the therapeutic plan, eventually mastering his very own program, whether it is esophageal speech or artificial larynx
   d. Communicates with family using newly learned speech techniques
   e. Practices the directives of the speech–language pathologist
5. Maintains balanced nutrition
   a. Verbalizes need to drink viscous fluids when experiencing swallowing difficulties
   b. Avoids sweet foods
   c. Tolerates solid foods
   d. Rinses mouth and brushes teeth frequently
6. Exhibits improved body image, self-esteem, and self-concept
   a. Expresses feelings and concerns about threats to body image and postoperative course
   b. Participates in self-care and decision making
   c. Accepts information about support group
7. Adheres to rehabilitation and home care program
   a. No longer smokes
   b. Practices recommended speech therapy in addition to keeping appointments with speech–language pathologist
   c. Demonstrates understanding of hygienic principles when caring for stoma and laryngectomy tube (if present)
   d. Involves spouse with his care activities
   e. Plans how to increase the humidity in his home
   f. Verbalizes understanding of symptoms that require medical attention
   g. Makes follow-up appointments with appropriate health care personnel
   h. Carries a card indicating procedures to follow in the event of an emergency, including the person to contact for assistance

In summary, if diagnosed and treated early, cancer of the larynx is potentially curable; many cases are also preventable. Treatment depends on the extent of the cancer. If extensive surgical resection with removal of the vocal cords is necessary, the patient's speech will be permanently lost. A permanent tracheotomy will be required with total laryngectomy. Because of the effects of these changes on the patient, the preoperative and postoperative care of the patient with cancer of the larynx requires collaboration among all members of the health care team. The patient and his family will assume major responsibility for care when the patient is discharged; therefore, it is imperative that they be well informed about the consequences of the surgical procedure and that they be considered vital members of the "team" when management decisions are made.

Chapter Summary

There are a variety of disorders that can affect the upper airway. These include upper airway infections, upper airway obstruction and trauma, and cancer of the larynx. Some of these disorders, such as upper airway infections, are more bothersome than threatening to life and well-being. Their high incidence and the time lost from usual activities because of upper airway infections make them clinically important. Although less common than infection, upper airway obstruction, trauma, and cancer of the larynx have serious implications for the health and well-being of the individual. The patient with cancer of the larynx faces potential major alterations in his ability to speak, alterations in life style, and often a prolonged rehabilitative phase. Nursing assessment and management are important in the preoperative, postoperative, and rehabilitative phases of care and focus on providing required treatment, comfort measures, support, and patient education.

Bibliography

Books

Braunwald E et al (eds). Harrison's Principles of Internal Medicine, 12th ed. New York, McGraw-Hill, 1991.

Davis JH et al. Clinical Surgery, Vol 2. St Louis, CV Mosby, 1987.

Fishman AP. Pulmonary Diseases and Disorders, 2nd ed, Vol 1. New York: McGraw-Hill, 1988.

Habal MB and Ariyan S. Facial Fractures. Philadelphia, BC Decker, 1989.

Jacobs C (ed). Cancers of the Head and Neck. Boston, Martinus Nijhoff, 1987.

Kitt S and Kaiser J. Emergency Nursing. Philadelphia, WB Saunders, 1990.

Murray JF and Nadel JA. The Textbook of Respiratory Medicine, 2nd ed. Vols 1 & 2. Philadelphia, WB Saunders, 1988.

Myers EN and Suen JY (eds). Cancer of the Head and Neck, 2nd ed. New York, Churchill Livingstone, 1989.

Pennington JE (ed). Respiratory Infections: Diagnosis and Management, 2nd ed. New York: Raven Press, 1989.

Schultz RC. Facial Injuries, 3rd ed. Chicago, Yearbook Medical Pub, 1988.

Tintinalli JE et al (eds). Emergency Medicine: A Comprehensive Study Guide, 2nd ed. New York, McGraw-Hill, 1988.

Journals

Altreuter RW. Nasal trauma. Emerg Med Clin North Am 1987 May; 5(2): 293–300.

Baker KH and Feldman JE. Cancers of the head and neck. Cancer Nurs 1987 Jun; 10(6): 293–299.

Berman BA. Allergic rhinitis: Mechanisms and management. J Allergy Clin Immunol 1988 May; 81(5): 980–983.

Biggs C. The cancer that can cost a patient his voice. RN 1987 Apr; 50(4): 44–51.

Cancer Facts and Figures—1991. American Cancer Society.

Feinstein D. What to teach the patient who's had a total laryngectomy. RN 1987 Apr; 50(4): 53–57.

Ganz NM et al. Questions and answers on sinusitis. Patient Care 1988 22(13): 53–60, 71–75.

Gray WC and Blanchard CL. Sinusitis and its complications. Am Fam Physician 1987 Mar; 35(3): 232–243.

Kulick MI. Craniofacial trauma (Part 2). Hosp Med 1990 Jan; 26(1): 41–56.

Loch WE et al. Sinusitis. Primary Care 1990 Jun; 17(2): 323–334.

Loos GD. Pharyngitis, croup and epiglottitis. Primary Care 1990 Jun; 17(2): 335–345.

Middleton E. Chronic rhinitis in adults. J Allergy Clin Immunol 1988 May; 81(5): 971–975.

Perretta LJ et al. Emergency evaluation and management of epistaxis. Emerg Med Clin North Am 1987 May; 5(2): 265–277.

Romm S. Cancer of the larynx: Current concepts of diagnosis and treatment. Surg Clin North Am 1986 Feb; 66(1): 109–118.

Simmons FER and Simmons KJH. Receptor antagonist treatment of chronic rhinitis. J Allergy Clin Immunol 1988 May; 81(5): 975–979.

Spofford B et al. An improved method for creating tracheoesophageal fistulas for Blom–Singer or Panje voice prostheses. Laryngoscope 1984, 94: 257–258.

Tanz RR and Shulman ST. Streptococcal pharyngitis: What's new. Postgrad Med 1988 Jan; 84(1): 203–206, 211–214.

Vogt HB. Rhinitis. Prim Care 1990 Jun; 17(2): 309–322.

Wilson EB and Malley N. Discharge planning for the patient with a new trachestomy. Crit Care Nurs 1990 Jul/Aug; 10(7): 73–79.

Information/Resources

Agencies

American Laryngectomee Association, Inc.
   American Cancer Society, Inc., 1599 Clifton Rd NE, Atlanta, GA 30329

"I Can Cope"
   American Cancer Society, Inc. (see above)

24

Assessment of Respiratory Function

Learning Objectives

On completion of this chapter, the learner will be able to:

1. *Describe ventilation, diffusion, perfusion, and shunting and the relationship of pulmonary circulation to these processes*
2. *Discriminate between normal and abnormal breath sounds*
3. *Use assessment parameters appropriate for determining the characteristics and severity of the major symptoms of respiratory dysfunction*
4. *Identify the nursing implications of the various procedures used for diagnostic assessment of respiratory function*

Physiologic Overview

The cells of the body derive the energy they need from the oxidation of carbohydrates, fats, and proteins. For this process, as for any type of combustion, oxygen is required. Certain vital tissues, such as those of the brain and the heart, cannot survive for long without a continuing supply of oxygen. As a result of oxidation in the body tissues, carbon dioxide is produced and must be removed from the cells to prevent buildup of acid waste products.

Oxygen is supplied to cells and carbon dioxide is removed from cells by way of the circulating blood. Cells are in close contact with capillaries, whose thin walls permit easy passage or exchange of oxygen and carbon dioxide. Oxygen diffuses from the capillary, through the capillary wall to the interstitial fluid, and then through the membrane of tissue cells, where it can be used by mitochondria for cellular respiration. The movement of carbon dioxide also occurs by diffusion and proceeds in the opposite direction, from cell to blood.

After these tissue capillary exchanges, blood enters the systemic veins (where it is called *venous blood*) and travels to the lung circulation. The oxygen concentration in blood within the lung capillaries is lower than it is in the lung gas spaces, which are called *alveoli*. As a result, oxygen diffuses from the alveoli to the blood. Carbon dioxide, which has a concentration in the blood higher than that in the alveoli, diffuses from the blood into the alveoli. Movement of air in and out of the airways (called *ventilation*) continually replenishes the oxygen and removes the carbon dioxide from the air spaces in the lung. This whole process of gas exchange between the atmospheric air and the blood and between the blood and cells of the body is called *respiration*.

Anatomy of the Lung

The lungs are elastic structures enclosed in the thorax, which is an airtight chamber with distensible walls. Ventilation involves movements of the walls of the thorax and of its floor, the diaphragm. The effect of these movements is alternately to increase and decrease the capacity of the chest. When the capacity of the chest is increased, air enters through the trachea, because of the lowered pressure within, and inflates the lungs. When the chest wall and diaphragm return to their previous positions, the elastic lungs recoil and force the air out through the bronchi and trachea.

The outer surfaces of the lungs are enclosed by a smooth, slippery membrane, the *pleura*, which also extends to cover the interior wall of the thorax and the superior surface of the diaphragm. *Parietal pleura* lines the thorax and *visceral pleura* covers the lungs. Between the two pleural surfaces is a small amount of fluid that lubricates the surfaces and allows them to slide freely during ventilation.

The *mediastinum* is the wall that divides the thoracic cavity into two halves. It is composed of two layers of pleura. All of the thoracic structures except the lungs are located between the two layers of pleura.

Each lung is divided into lobes. The left lung consists of upper and lower lobes, whereas the right lung has upper, middle, and lower lobes. Each lobe is further subdivided into two to five segments separated by fissures, which are extensions of the pleura. A schematic diagram of the airways and the lobes of the lungs is shown in Figure 24–1.

There are several divisions of the bronchi within each lobe of the lung. First are the lobar bronchi (three in the right lung and two in the left lung). Lobar bronchi divide into segmental bronchi (10 on the right and 8 on the left), which are the structures identified when choosing the most effective postural drainage position for a given patient. Segmental bronchi then divide into subsegmental bronchi. These bronchi are surrounded by connective tissue that contains arteries, lymphatics, and nerves. The subsegmental bronchi then branch into *bronchioles*, which have no cartilage in their walls. Their patency depends entirely on the elastic recoil of the smooth muscle that surrounds it and on the alveolar pressure. The bronchioles contain submucosal glands, which produce mucus that forms an uninterrupted covering for the inside lining of the airway. The bronchi and bronchioles are lined also with cells that have surfaces covered with short "hairs" called *cilia*. These cilia create a constant whipping motion that serves to propel mucus and foreign substances away from the lung toward the larynx.

The bronchioles then branch into *terminal bronchioles*, which do not have mucus glands or cilia. Terminal bronchioles then become *respiratory bronchioles*, which are considered to be the transition passageways between the conducting airways and the gas exchange airways. Up to this point, the conducting airways contain about 150 ml of air caught in the tracheobronchial tree that does not participate in gas exchange. The respiratory bronchioles then lead into alveolar ducts and alveolar sacs and then alveoli. Oxygen and carbon dioxide exchange takes place in the alveoli (Fig. 24–2).

The lung is made up of about 300 million alveoli, which are arranged in clusters of 15 to 20. So numerous are these alveoli that if their surfaces were united to form one sheet, it would cover an area 70 square meters (the size of a tennis court).

There are three types of alveolar cells. Type I alveolar cells are epithelial cells that form the alveolar walls. Type II alveolar

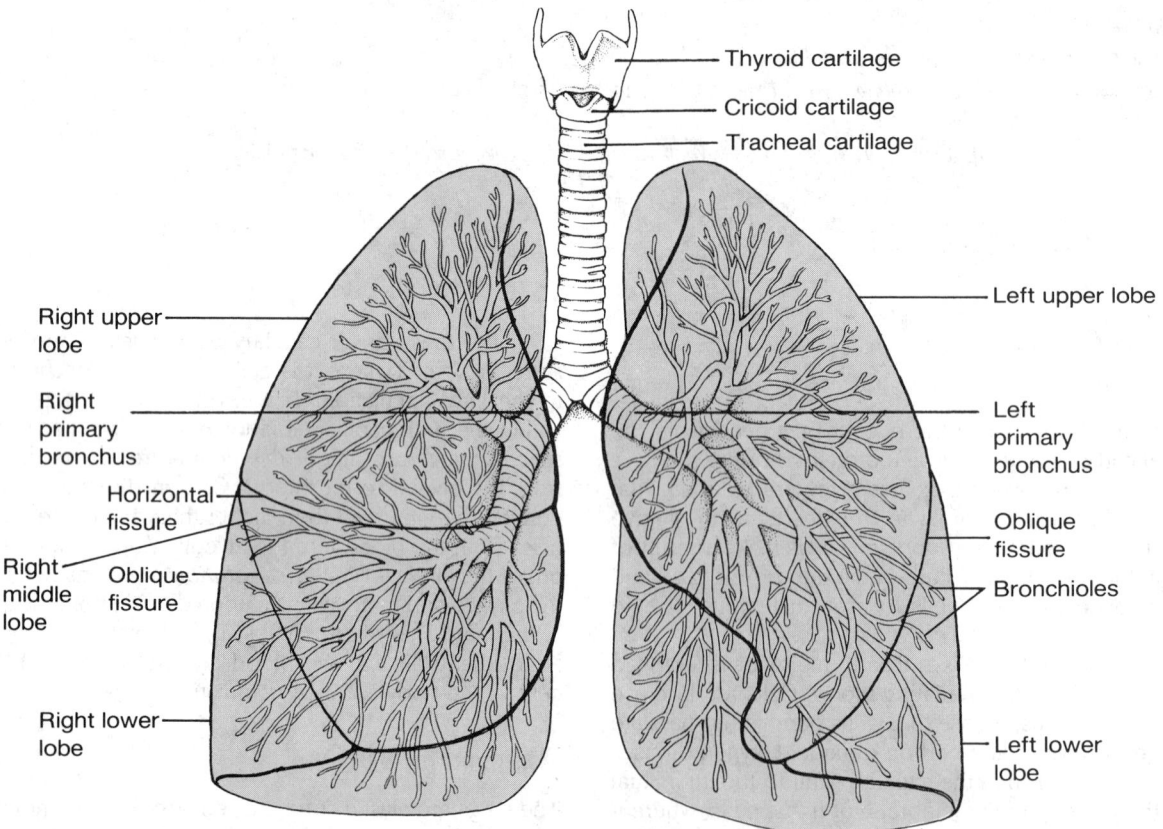

Figure 24–1. Larynx, trachea, and bronchial tree (anterior view). (Chaffee EE and Greisheimer EM. Basic Physiology and Anatomy. Philadelphia, JB Lippincott.)

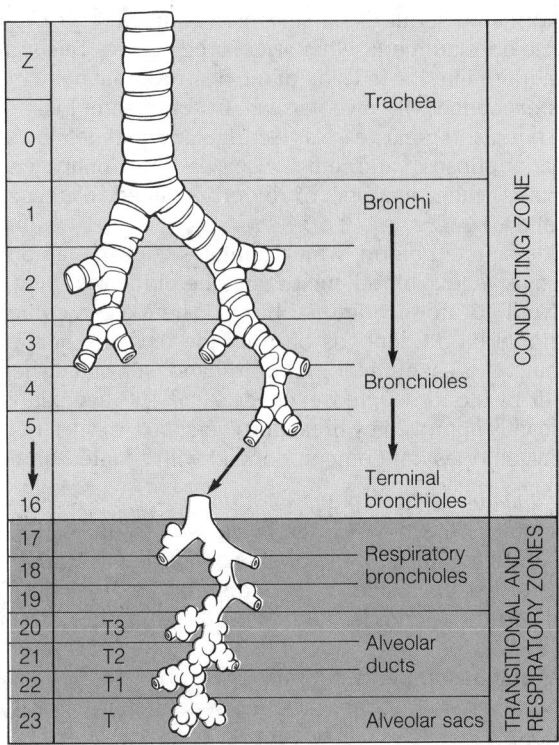

Figure 24-2. Airway branching in human lungs by regularized dichotomy from trachea (generation z = 0) to alveolar ducts and sacs (generations 20 to 23). The first 16 generations are purely conducting; transitional airways lead into the respiratory zone made of alveoli. (Redrawn from Fishman AP. Pulmonary Diseases and Disorders, 2nd ed, Vol 1. New York, McGraw-Hill, 1988.)

cells, metabolically active cells, secrete *surfactant*, which is a phospholipid that lines the inner surface of the alveoli. Type III, alveoli cell macrophages, are large phagocytic cells that ingest foreign matter (*e.g.*, mucus, bacteria) and act as an important defense mechanism.

Mechanics of Ventilation

During inspiration, air flows from the environment into the trachea, bronchi, bronchioles, and alveoli. During expiration, alveolar gas travels the same route in reverse.

The physical factors that govern air flow in and out of the lungs are collectively referred to as the mechanics of ventilation. Air flows from a region of higher pressure to a region of lower pressure. During inspiration, contraction of the diaphragm and other muscles of respiration enlarges the thoracic cavity and thereby lowers the pressure inside the thorax to a level below that of atmospheric pressure. Therefore, air is drawn through the trachea and bronchi into the alveoli.

During normal expiration, the diaphragm relaxes, and the lungs recoil, resulting in a decrease in the size of the thoracic cavity. The alveolar pressure then exceeds atmospheric pressure, and air flows from the lungs into the atmosphere.

Resistance is determined chiefly by the radius of the airway through which the air is flowing. Any process that changes bronchial diameter therefore will affect airway resistance and alter the rate of air flow for a given pressure gradient during respiration. Common factors that may alter bronchial diameter include contraction of bronchial smooth muscle, as in asthma;

thickening of bronchial mucosa, as in chronic bronchitis; or obstruction of the airway due to mucus, a tumor, or a foreign body. Loss of lung elasticity, such as is seen in emphysema, also may alter bronchial diameter, as the lung connective tissue encircles the airways and helps to keep them open during both inspiration and expiration. With increased resistance, greater than normal respiratory effort is required by the patient to achieve normal levels of ventilation.

The pressure gradient between the thoracic cavity and the atmosphere causes air flow in and out of the lungs and also stretches the lung tissue itself. The pressure required to stretch the lung is determined by the properties of its elastic tissue. A measure of how easily lungs can be expanded is called *lung compliance*. Compliance is usually measured under static conditions.

A compliant lung (high compliance) distends easily when pressure is applied, whereas a noncompliant lung (low compliance) requires greater than normal pressure to distend it. The major factors that determine lung compliance are connective tissue (collagen and elastin) and the surface tension in the alveoli. The surface tension at the surface of the alveoli is normally maintained at a low level by the presence of surfactant, which lines the alveoli. Increased connective tissue or increased alveolar surface tension results in low compliance. In adult respiratory distress syndrome, there is a surfactant deficiency and the lungs are stiff (low compliance). In pulmonary fibrosis, connective tissue proliferates and compliance is decreased. Lungs with low compliance require a greater than normal energy expenditure to achieve normal levels of ventilation.

The mechanics of ventilation can be measured to evaluate lung function (Fig. 24-3). Lung volumes and lung capacities are described in Table 24-1. Included in these measures are lung volumes and lung capacities.

In healthy upright lungs, ventilation is greatest in the lower regions of the lungs and decreases toward the apices. In addition to this regional inequality of ventilation, there is uneven ventilation among alveoli, permitting air to be distributed more evenly between them.

Diffusion and Perfusion

Diffusion is the process by which oxygen and carbon dioxide are exchanged at the air–blood interface. The alveolar–capillary membrane is ideal for diffusion because of its large surface area and thin membrane. In healthy lungs, oxygen and carbon dioxide travel across the alveolar–capillary membrane without difficulty.

Pulmonary perfusion is the actual blood flow through the pulmonary circulation. The blood is pumped into the lungs by the right ventricle through the pulmonary artery. The pulmonary artery divides into the right and left branches to supply both lungs. These two branches divide further to supply all parts of each lung. The pulmonary circulation is considered a low-pressure system because the systolic blood pressure in the pulmonary artery is 20 to 30 mm Hg and the diastolic pressure is 5 to 15 mm Hg. Because it is low, the pulmonary vasculature normally can vary its resistance to accommodate the blood flow it receives. When a person is in an erect position, however, the pulmonary artery pressure is not great enough to supply blood to the apex of the lung against the force of gravity. Thus, when a person is erect, the lung may be considered to be divided into three sections: an upper part with poor blood

STATIC LUNG VOLUMES

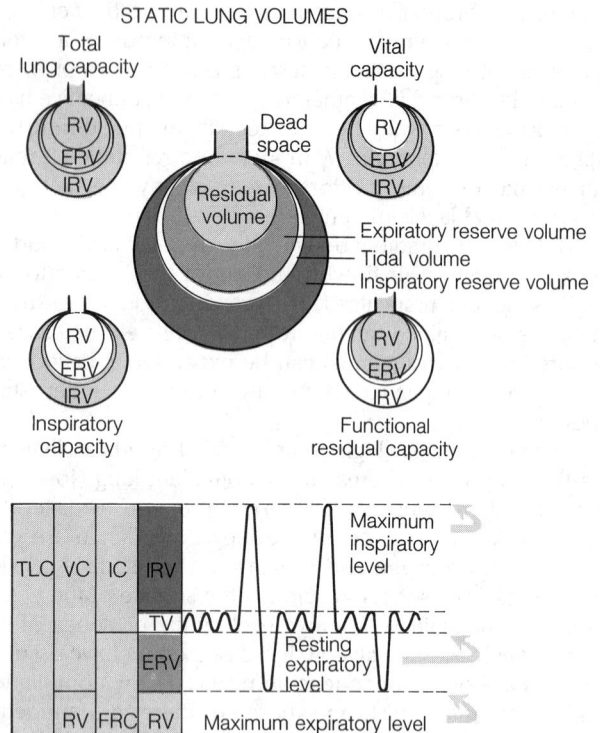

Figure 24–3. (**Above**) The large central diagram illustrates the four primary lung *volumes* and approximate magnitude. The outermost line indicates the greatest size to which the lung can expand; the innermost circle (residual volume), the volume that remains after all air has been voluntarily squeezed out of the lungs. Surrounding the central diagram are smaller ones; shaded areas in these represent the four lung *capacities.* The volume of dead space gas is included in residual volume, functional residual capacity and total lung capacity when these are measured by routine techniques. (**Below**) Lung volumes as they appear on a spiro-graphic tracing; shading in vertical bar next to tracing corresponds to that in central diagram above. (Comroe JH et al. The Lung: Clinical Physiology and Pulmonary Function Tests, 2nd ed. Chicago, Yearbook Medical Publishers, 1977.)

supply, a lower part with maximum blood supply, and the section in between the two with an intermediate supply of blood. When a person turns to one side, more blood passes to the dependent lung.

Perfusion is also influenced by alveolar pressure. The pulmonary capillaries are sandwiched between adjacent alveoli. If the alveolar pressure is sufficiently high, the capillaries will be squeezed. Depending on the pressure, some capillaries will be completely collapsed, whereas others will be narrowed.

Pulmonary artery pressure, gravity, and alveolar pressure determine the patterns of perfusion. In lung disease these factors vary and the perfusion of the lung may become very abnormal.

Ventilation–Perfusion Imbalances

A ventilation–perfusion (V/Q) imbalance occurs when there is an increase in *physiologic dead space* (adequate ventilation and no perfusion, as in pulmonary embolus) or with *shunting* (adequate perfusion and no ventilation, as in pulmonary edema, atelectasis, or chronic obstructive pulmonary disease [COPD]). Shunting is the most severe problem.

Normally, about 2% of the blood pumped by the right ventricle does not perfuse the alveolar capillaries. This *shunted blood* drains into the left side of the heart without participating in gas exchange with alveolar gas. In some pathologic states of the heart and great vessels (ventricular septal defect, patent ductus arteriosus) and lung diseases (pulmonary edema, atelectasis), the amount of blood shunted exceeds the normal 2%.

The shunted blood, which contains the same amount of oxygen as venous blood, mixes with the blood returning from the alveoli to produce arterial blood. The oxygen content of the arterial blood depends on both the oxygen content and the volume of each fraction. Severe hypoxia results when the amount of blood shunted exceeds 20%. The hypoxia is not significantly improved by breathing even 100% oxygen because the oxygen does not come in contact with shunted blood.

Distribution of Ventilation and Perfusion

Ventilation is the flow of gas in and out of the lungs, and perfusion is the filling of the pulmonary capillaries with blood. Adequate gas exchange is dependent on an adequate ventilation–perfusion ratio. In different areas of the lung, the ratio may vary.

Alterations in perfusion may occur with alteration in the pulmonary artery pressure, alveolar pressure, and gravity. Alteration in ventilation may occur with blockage of the airways, local changes in compliance of the lung, and gravity.

It is important for the nurse to understand the four possible ventilation–perfusion matches (Fig. 24–4).

- Normal—ventilation matches perfusion
    In the healthy lung, a given amount of blood bypasses an alveolus and is matched with an equal amount of gas. The ratio is 1:1 (ventilation matches perfusion).
- Low ventilation–perfusion ratio—shunt-producing disorders
    When perfusion exceeds ventilation, a shunt exists. Blood bypasses the alveoli without gas exchange occurring. This is seen with obstruction of the distal airways, such as with pneumonia, atelectasis, tumor, or a mucus plug.
- High ventilation–perfusion ratio—dead space-producing disorder
    When ventilation exceeds perfusion, dead space occurs. The alveoli have inadequate blood supply to allow gas exchange to occur. This is seen with a variety of disorders, including pulmonary emboli, pulmonary infarction, and cardiogenic shock.
- Silent unit—absence of ventilation and perfusion
    When there is limited ventilation and perfusion, a silent unit occurs. This is seen with pneumothorax and severe adult respiratory distress syndrome (ARDS).

Mismatching of ventilation and perfusion resulting in shunting of blood leads to hypoxia. It appears to be the main cause of hypoxia after thoracic or abdominal surgery and most types of respiratory failure. Its effects can be similar to those of shunts, or 100% oxygen can eliminate hypoxia, depending on the type of ventilation–perfusion mismatch.

Partial Pressure

Partial pressure is the pressure exerted by each type of gas in a mixture of gases. The partial pressure of a gas is proportional to the concentration of that gas in the mixture. The total pres-

TABLE 24-1. *Lung Volumes and Lung Capacities*

Term Used	Symbol	Description	Remarks
LUNG VOLUMES			
Tidal volume	V_T or TV	The volume of air inhaled and exhaled with each breath	The tidal volume may not vary, even with severe disease.
Inspiratory reserve volume	IRV	The maximum volume of air that can be inhaled after a normal inhalation	
Expiratory reserve volume	ERV	The maximum volume of air that can be exhaled forcibly after a normal exhalation	Expiratory reserve volume is decreased with restrictive disorders, such as obesity, ascites, pregnancy.
Residual volume	RV	The volume of air remaining in the lungs after a maximum exhalation	Residual volume may be increased with obstructive diseases.
LUNG CAPACITIES			
Vital capacity	VC	The maximum volume of air exhaled from the point of maximum inspiration	A decrease in vital capacity may be found in neuromuscular disease, body fatigue, atelectasis, pulmonary edema, and COPD patients.
Inspiratory capacity	IC	The maximum volume of air inhaled after normal expiration	A decrease in inspiratory capacity may indicate restrictive disease.
Functional residual capacity	FRC	The volume of air remaining in lungs after a normal expiration	Functional residual capacity may be increased with obstructive disease (COPD) and decreased in ARDS.
Total lung capacity	TLC	The volume of air in the lungs after a maximum inspiration and equal to the sum of all four volumes (V_T, IRV, ERV, RV)	Total lung capacity may be decreased with restrictive disease (atelectasis, pneumonia) and increased in obstructive disease (COPD)

sure exerted by the gaseous mixture is equal to the sum of the partial pressures.

The air we breathe is a gaseous mixture consisting mainly of nitrogen (78.62%) and oxygen (20.84%), with traces of carbon dioxide (0.04%), water vapor (0.05%), helium, argon, and so on. The atmospheric pressure at sea level is about 760 mm Hg. Based on these facts the partial pressure of nitrogen and oxygen can be calculated. Partial pressure of nitrogen is 79% of 760 (.79 × 760) = 600 mm Hg and that of oxygen is 21% of 760 (.21 × 760) = 160 mm Hg.

The following is a reference list of expressions related to partial pressure:

P = pressure
PO_2 — partial pressure of oxygen
PCO_2 — partial pressure of carbon dioxide
PAO_2 — partial pressure of alveolar oxygen
$PACO_2$ — partial pressure of alveolar carbon dioxide
PaO_2 — partial pressure of arterial oxygen
$PaCO_2$ — partial pressure of arterial carbon dioxide
PvO_2 — partial pressure of venous oxygen
$PvCO_2$ — partial pressure of venous carbon dioxide
P_{50} — partial pressure of oxygen when the hemoglobin is 50% saturated

Once the air enters the trachea, it becomes fully saturated with water vapor, which displaces some of the gases so that the air pressure within the lung may remain equal with the air pressure outside (760 mm Hg). Water vapor exerts a pressure of 47 mm Hg when it fully saturates a mixture of gases at the body temperature of 37°C (98.6°F). Nitrogen and oxygen are therefore now responsible for the remaining 713 mm Hg (760 − 47) pressure. Once this mixture enters the alveoli, it is further diluted by carbon dioxide. In the alveoli, the water vapor continues to exert a pressure of 47 mm Hg. The remaining 713 mm Hg pressure is now exerted as follows: nitrogen, 569 mm Hg (74.9%); oxygen, 104 mm Hg (13.6%), and carbon dioxide, 40 mm Hg (5.3%).

When a gas is exposed to a liquid, the gas will dissolve in the liquid until an equilibrium is reached. The dissolved gas also exerts a partial pressure. At equilibrium, the partial pressure of the gas in the liquid is the same as the partial pressure of the gas in the gaseous mixture. Oxygenation of venous blood in the lung illustrates this point. In the lung, venous blood and alveolar oxygen are separated by a very thin alveolar membrane. Oxygen diffuses across this membrane to dissolve in the blood until the partial pressure of oxygen in the blood is the same as that in the alveoli (104 mm Hg). Because carbon dioxide is manufactured in the cells, however, venous blood contains carbon dioxide at a higher partial pressure than that in the alveolar gas. In the lung, carbon dioxide diffuses out of venous blood into the alveolar gas. At equilibrium, the partial pressure of carbon dioxide in the blood and in alveolar gas is the same (40 mm Hg).

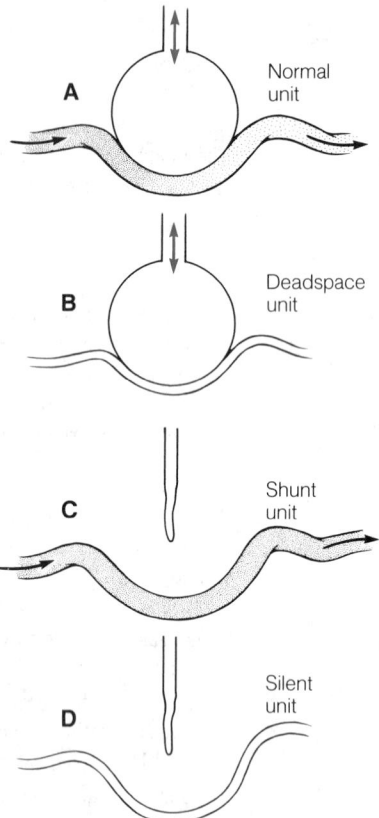

Figure 24–4. The theoretic respiratory unit. (**A**) Normal ventilation, normal perfusion. (**B**) Normal ventilation, no perfusion. (**C**) No ventilation, normal perfusion. (**D**) No ventilation, no perfusion. (After Shapiro BA, Harrison RA, and Walton JR. Clinical Application of Blood Gases, 3rd ed. Chicago, Mosby–Year Book, 1989.)

The entire sequence of changes in partial pressure readings (in milligrams) may be summarized as follows:

	Atmospheric Air	*Tracheal Air*	*Alveolar Air*
P_{H_2O}	3.7	47.0	47.0
P_{N_2}	597.0	563.4	569.0
P_{O_2}	159.0	149.3	104.0
P_{CO_2}	0.3	0.3	40.0
Total	760.0	760.0	760.0

Oxygen Transport

Oxygen and carbon dioxide are carried simultaneously by virtue of their abilities to dissolve in blood or to combine with some of the elements of blood. Oxygen is carried in the blood in two forms: (1) as physically dissolved oxygen in the plasma and (2) in combination with the hemoglobin of the red blood cells. Each 100 ml of normal arterial blood carries 0.3 ml of oxygen *physically dissolved* in the plasma and 20 ml of oxygen in combination with hemoglobin. Large amounts of oxygen can be transported in the blood because it forms an easily reversible combination with hemoglobin to oxyhemoglobin:

$$O_2 + Hb \rightleftarrows HbO_2$$

The volume of oxygen physically dissolved in the plasma varies directly with the PaO_2. The higher the PaO_2, the greater the oxygen dissolved. For example, it is found that at a PaO_2 of 10 mm Hg, 0.03 ml of oxygen is dissolved in 100 ml of plasma. At 20 mm Hg, twice this amount is dissolved in plasma, and at 100 mm Hg, ten times this amount is dissolved. Therefore, the amount of dissolved oxygen is directly proportional to the partial pressure, and this is true no matter how high the oxygen pressure rises. For example, in a hyperbaric chamber in which a subject is breathing oxygen at 3 atmospheres of pressure, the PaO_2 would be 2000 mm Hg. The dissolved oxygen would be 6 ml of oxygen per 100 ml of blood.

The volume of oxygen that combines with hemoglobin also depends on PaO_2, but only up to a PaO_2 of about 150 mm Hg. Above this PaO_2, hemoglobin is 100% saturated, by which it is meant that hemoglobin will not combine with any additional oxygen. When hemoglobin is 100% saturated, 1 g of hemoglobin will combine with 1.34 ml of oxygen. Therefore, in a person with 14 g/dl of hemoglobin, each 100 ml of blood will contain about 19 ml of oxygen associated with hemoglobin. If the PaO_2 is less than 150 mm Hg, the percentage of hemoglobin saturated with oxygen is lower. For example, at a PaO_2 of 100 mm Hg (normal value) saturation is 97%, and at a PaO_2 of 40 mm Hg, the saturation is 70%.

The oxygen dissociation curve of hemoglobin (Fig. 24–5) shows the relationship between the partial pressure of oxygen and the percentage saturation of the hemoglobin more clearly (SaO_2). The unusual shape of the oxygen dissociation curve is a distinct advantage to the patient for two reasons:

1. If the arterial PO_2 decreases from 100 to 80 mm Hg as a result of lung disease or heart disease, the hemoglobin of the arterial blood still will be almost maximally saturated (94%) and the tissues will not suffer from anoxia.
2. When the arterial blood passes into tissue capillaries and is exposed to the tissue tension of oxygen (about 40 mm Hg), hemoglobin gives up large quantities of oxygen for use by the tissues.

Oxygen Dissociation Curve

The oxygen dissociation curve demonstrates the relationship between the PaO_2 and the binding to hemoglobin. It indicates the methods used by the body to release oxygen to the tissues so that the oxygen obtained from the lungs is stored and then released to the tissues in amounts sufficient for their needs. The oxygen dissociation curve in Figure 24–5 is marked to show three levels of sufficiency: (1) normal levels — PaO_2 above 70 mm Hg; (2) relatively safe levels — PaO_2 45 to 70 mm Hg; and (3) dangerous levels — PaO_2 below 40 mm Hg.

Figure 24–5 shows that at a normal *p*H of 7.40, the steep part of the curve is between a PaO_2 of 40 mm Hg (75% hemoglobin saturation) and 20 mm Hg (33% hemoglobin saturation). P_{50} refers to the oxygen tension (27 mm Hg) at 50% hemoglobin saturation. When we talk about changes in PaO_2 and saturation, we talk about changes in P_{50}.

The oxygen–hemoglobin dissociation curve will shift to either the right or the left, depending on the presence of the following: CO_2, hydrogen ion concentration (acidity), temperature, and 2,3-diphosphoglycerate.

A rise in these factors will shift the curve to the right, so that more oxygen is then released to the tissues at the same PaO_2. A reduction in these factors will cause the curve to shift

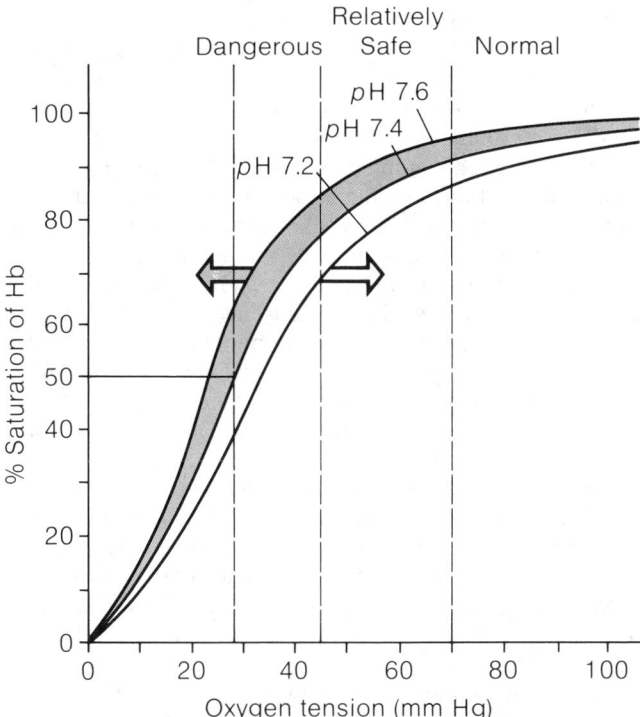

Figure 24–5. Oxygen–hemoglobin dissociation curve. The oxygen can attach to the hemoglobin more easily (higher SaO_2 per PO_2) but has more trouble coming off the hemoglobin at the tissues (less tissue oxygenation). Decreased oxygen affinity (shift to the right) means that it is more difficult for the oxygen to attach to the hemoglobin (lower SaO_2 per PO_2), but it can come off at the tissues more easily. P_{50} is normally 27 mm Hg. A shift to the right gives a higher P_{50}, and a shift to the left gives a lower P_{50}.

to the left, making the bond between oxygen and hemoglobin stronger, so that less oxygen is given up to the tissues at the same PaO_2. In Figure 24–3, the normal (middle) curve shows that 75% saturation occurs at a PaO_2 of 40 mm Hg. If the curve shifts to the right, the same saturation (75%) occurs at the higher PaO_2 of 57 mm Hg. If the curve shifts to the left, 75% saturation occurs at a PaO_2 of 25 mm Hg.

Clinical Significance

With a normal hemoglobin of 15 g/100 ml and a PaO_2 level of 40 mm Hg (oxygen saturation 75%), there is adequate oxygen available for the tissues, but there is no reserve. When a catastrophe occurs (*e.g.*, bronchospasm, aspiration, hypotension, or cardiac dysrhythmias) that reduces the intake of oxygen from the lungs, tissue hypoxia will result. The normal value of PaO_2 is 80 to 100 mm Hg (95% to 98% saturation). With this level of oxygenation, there is a 15% margin of excess oxygen available to the tissues.

An important consideration in the transport of oxygen is the cardiac output, which determines the amount of oxygen delivered to the body. If the cardiac output is normal (5 L/min), the amount of oxygen delivered to the body per minute will be normal. If cardiac output falls, the amount of oxygen delivered to the tissues also will fall. This is why cardiac output measurements are so important. Not all of the oxygen delivered to the body is used up. In fact, only 250 ml of oxygen is used up per minute. The rest of the oxygen returns to the right side

of the heart, and the PO_2 of venous blood drops to about 40 mm Hg.

Carbon Dioxide Transport

Simultaneously with the diffusion of oxygen from the blood into the tissues, carbon dioxide diffuses in the opposite direction (*e.g.*, from tissue cells to blood) and is transported to the lung for excretion. The amount of carbon dioxide in transit is one of the major determinants of the acid–base balance of the body. Normally, only 6% of the venous carbon dioxide is removed and enough remains in the arterial side to exert a pressure of 40 mm Hg. Most of the carbon dioxide (90%) enters the red blood cells, and the small portion (5%) that remains dissolved in the plasma (PCO_2) is the critical factor that will determine carbon dioxide movement in or out of the blood.

In summarizing respiratory gas transport, it is important to emphasize that the many processes described do not take place in intermittent stages but occur rapidly, simultaneously, and continuously.

Neurologic Control of Ventilation

The rhythmicity of breathing is controlled by respiratory centers located in the brain. The inspiratory and expiratory centers located in the medulla oblongata and pons control the rate and depth of ventilation to meet the body's metabolic demands.

The *apneustic center* in the lower pons possibly stimulates the inspiratory medullary center to promote deep, prolonged inspirations. In the upper pons is the *pneumotaxic center*, which possibly controls the pattern of respirations.

There are several groups of receptor sites that assist in the brain's control of respiratory function. The *central chemoreceptors* are located in the medulla and respond to chemical changes in the cerebrospinal fluid, which are in turn due to chemical changes in the blood. They respond to an increase or decrease in the *p*H and convey a message to the lungs to change the depth and then the rate of ventilation to correct the imbalance. The *peripheral chemoreceptors* are located in the aortic arch and the carotid arteries and respond first to changes in PaO_2, then to $PaCO_2$ and *p*H. The *Hering–Breuer reflex* is brought about by stretch receptors located in the alveoli. This reflex is stimulated when the lungs are distended and inhibits inspiration so that the lungs do not become overdistended. There are also *proprioceptors* in muscles and joints that respond to body movements such as exercise, causing an increase in ventilation. Thus, range of motion exercises in an immobile patient will stimulate breathing. *Baroreceptors*, also located in the aortic and carotid bodies, respond to an increase or decrease in arterial blood pressure and cause a reflex hypoventilation or hyperventilation.

Gerontologic Considerations

A gradual decline in respiratory function begins in early-middle adulthood and affects the structure as well as function of the respiratory system. During aging (40 years and over), changes in the alveoli reduce the surface area available for exchange of oxygen and carbon dioxide. At about age 50, alveoli begin to lose elasticity. The thickness of bronchial glands increases with age. The vital capacity of the lungs reaches a maximum at 20 to 25 years of age and decreases thereafter throughout life. A decrease in vital capacity occurs with loss of chest wall mobility, thus restricting tidal flow of air. The amount of respiratory dead space increases with age. These changes result in decreased diffusion capacity for oxygen with age, producing lower oxygen in the arterial circulation. Despite these changes, in the absence of chronic pulmonary disease, elderly persons are able to carry out activities of daily living, but they may have decreased tolerance for prolonged activity or excessive exertion and may require rest after prolonged or vigorous activity.

In summary, the lung is a series of branching airways. These airways begin at the trachea and branch to narrower and shorter tubes until they reach the alveoli. Blood is supplied to the lung by the right ventricle, which branches out in a series of capillaries, which surround the alveoli. Oxygen and carbon dioxide exchange occurs at the alveolar capillary level.

Many factors have an impact on adequate gas exchange, including intact respiratory and cardiovascular systems. Alteration in either system can lead to a ventilation–perfusion imbalance and, ultimately, inadequate gas exchange.

Assessment of Patients With Pulmonary Disease

History

The health history focuses on the physical and functional problems experienced by the patient and the effect of these problems on the patient's life and life-style. The reason for the patient's seeking health care often is related to one of the following: dyspnea, pain, the accumulation of mucus, wheezing, hemoptysis, edema of the ankles and feet, cough, and general fatigue/weakness. In addition to identifying the chief reason why the patient is seeking health care, it is important to determine when the health problem or symptom started, how long it lasted, if it was relieved at any time, and how relief was obtained. Information on precipitating factors, duration, severity, and associated factors or symptoms is collected. In a respiratory history, factors that may contribute to the patient's lung condition are assessed:

- Smoking (the single most important factor that contributes to lung disease)
- Previous personal or family history of lung disease
- Occupational history
- Allergens and environmental pollutants
- Hobbies

Psychosocial factors that may affect the patient's life are evaluated and include anxiety, role changes, family relationships, financial problems, and employment or unemployment. What are the patient's coping mechanisms? Is he exhibiting anxiety, anger, hostility, dependency, withdrawal, isolation, avoidance, noncompliance, acceptance, or denial? Finally, what are the support systems the patient uses to deal with the illness? Are supportive family members, friends, or community resources available?

Physical Assessment

If a patient has a known or suspected pulmonary condition, respiratory function must be assessed. Assessment of the thorax and lungs uses the skills of inspection, palpation, percussion, and auscultation. When these techniques are properly performed and the results logically interpreted, much can be learned that will help the nurse develop a care plan. When recording or communicating findings, it is customary to refer to known anatomic landmarks as points of reference.

With respect to the thorax, location is defined both horizontally and vertically. Horizontal reference is made in terms of the rib or the intercostal space overlying the examiner's fingers (Fig. 24–6). On the anterior surface, identifying the specific rib is facilitated by locating the angle at which the manubrium joins the body of the sternum in the midline. The second rib joins the sternum at this prominent landmark. Other ribs may be identified by counting down from the second rib. The intercostal spaces are referred to in terms of the rib immediately above the intercostal space.

Location of ribs on the posterior surface of the thorax is more difficult. The first step is to identify the spinous process. This is accomplished by finding the most prominent of the spinous processes, the seventh cervical vertebra (*vertebra prominens*). When the neck is slightly flexed, the seventh cervical spinous process stands out. Other vertebrae are then identified by counting down.

To identify thoracic findings in terms of vertical location, reference is made to several imaginary lines (Fig. 24–7). The *midsternal line* is drawn down through the center of the sternum. The *midclavicular line* is an imaginary line drawn from the middle of the clavicle. The point of maximum impulse of the heart most generally lies along this line on the left thorax. When the arm is abducted from the body at 90 degrees, imaginary vertical lines may be drawn from the anterior axillary fold, from the middle of the axilla, and from the posterior axillary fold. These lines are called, respectively, the *anterior axillary line,* the *midaxillary line*, and the *posterior axillary line*. A line drawn vertically through the superior and inferior poles of the scapula is called the *scapular line*, and a line drawn down the center of the vertebral column is called the *vertebral line*.

Using these landmarks, the examiner can easily be understood when referring to an area of dullness extending from the vertebral to the scapular line between the seventh and tenth ribs on the right.

Topographically, the lobes of the lung may be located on the surface of the chest wall in the following manner (Fig. 24–8): The line between the upper and lower lobes on the left begins at the fourth thoracic spinous process posteriorly, proceeds around to cross the fifth rib in the midaxillary line, and meets the sixth rib at the sternum. This line on the right divides the right middle lobe from the right lower lobe. The line dividing the right upper lobe from the middle lobe is an incomplete one that begins at the fifth rib in the midaxillary line, where it intersects the line between the upper and lower lobes and traverses horizontally to the sternum. Thus, the upper lobes are dominant on the anterior surface of the thorax and the lower lobes are dominant on the posterior surface. There is no presentation of the middle lobe on the posterior surface of the chest.

Inspection of the Thorax

Inspection of the thorax provides information about musculoskeletal structure, nutrition, and the status of the respiratory system. The skin over the thorax is observed for color and

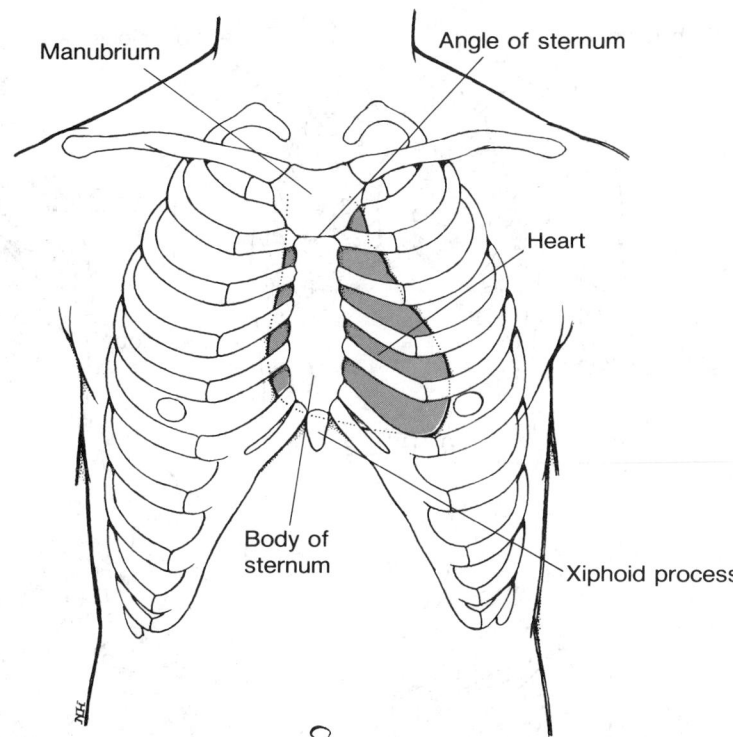

Figure 24-6. Topography of the anterior thorax.

turgor and for evidence of loss of subcutaneous tissue. Asymmetry, if present, is noted.

Chest Configuration

Normally, the anteroposterior diameter in proportion to the lateral diameter is 1:2. There are, however, four main deformities of the chest associated with respiratory disease: barrel chest, funnel chest (pectus excavatum), pigeon chest (pectus carinatum), and kyphoscoliosis.

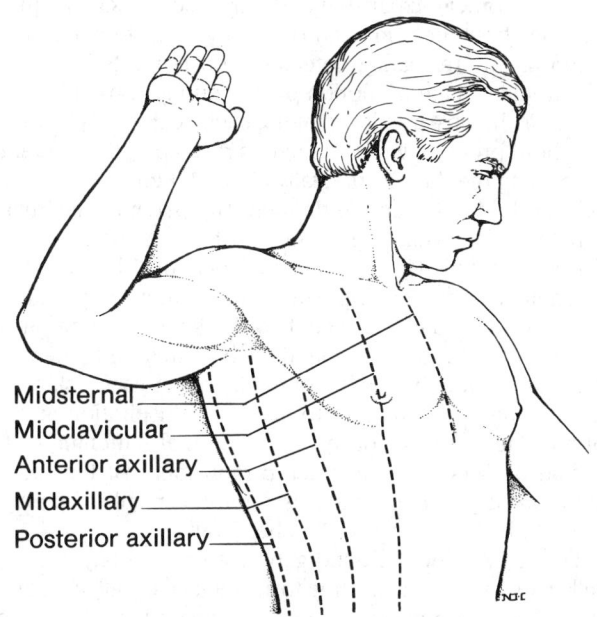

Figure 24-7. Topographic lines of the chest. Imaginary "longitudinal lines" permit verbal reference to the location of abnormalities over the chest wall.

Barrel Chest. Barrel chest occurs as a result of overinflation of the lungs. There is an increase in the anteroposterior diameter of the thorax. In a patient with emphysema, the ribs are more widely spaced and the intercostal spaces tend to bulge on expiration. The appearance of the patient with advanced emphysema is thus quite characteristic and allows the observer to detect its presence easily, even from a distance.

Funnel Chest. Funnel chest occurs when there is a depression in the lower portion of the sternum. This may compress the heart and great vessels, resulting in murmurs. This condition may occur with rickets, Marfan's syndrome, or as an occupational hazard (as in cobbler's chest.)

Pigeon Chest. A pigeon chest occurs as a result of displacement of the sternum. There is an increase in the anteroposterior diameter. This may occur with rickets, Marfan's syndrome, or severe kyphoscoliosis.

Kyphoscoliosis. A kyphoscoliosis appears with an elevation of the scapula, with a corresponding S-shaped curved spine. This deformity limits the lung within the thorax. This may occur with osteoporosis and other skeletal disorders that affect the thorax.

Breathing Patterns

Observation of the rate and depth of respiration is also important. In the adult, the normal respiratory rate is 12 to 18 breaths per minute; it is regular in depth and rhythm. An increase in the rate of respiration is called *tachypnea;* an increase in depth is called *hyperpnea.* An increase in both rate and depth that results in a lowered arterial P_{CO_2} is referred to as *hyperventilation.* At the extreme of hyperventilation is the marked increase in rate and depth, associated with severe acidosis of diabetic or renal origin, that is called *Kussmaul* respiration. Cheyne–Stokes respiration is characterized by alternating episodes of apnea (cessation of breathing) and periods of deep breathing. It most frequently is associated with heart

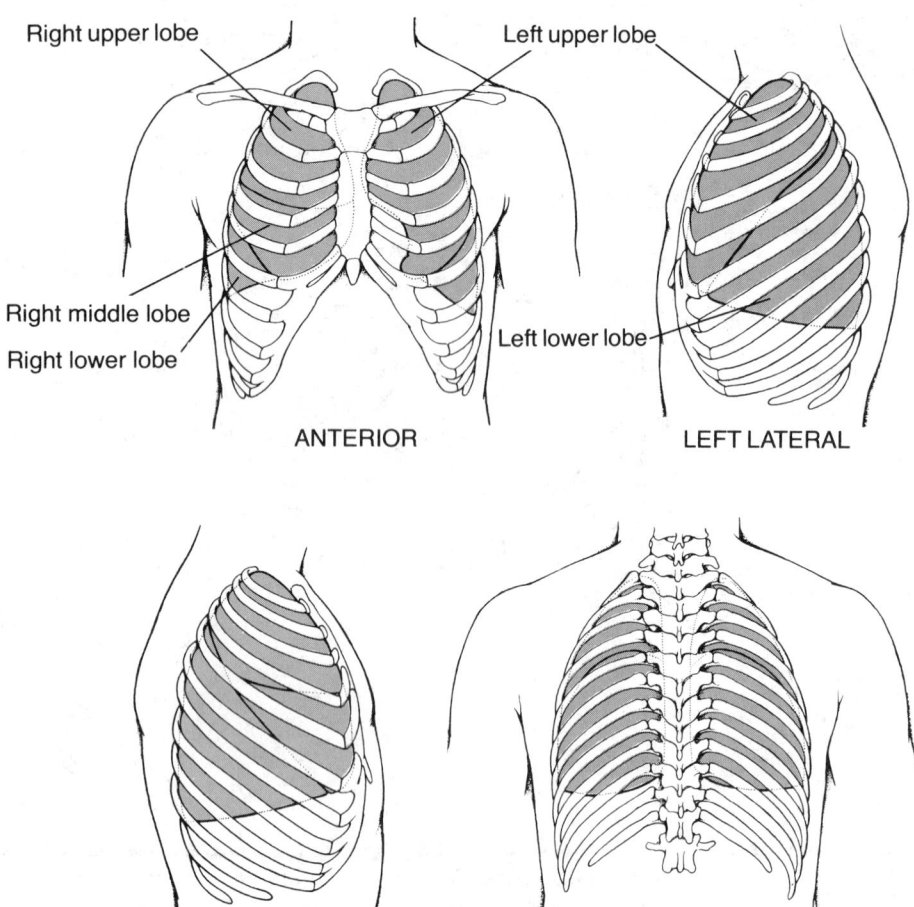

Right upper lobe   Left upper lobe

Right middle lobe

Right lower lobe   Left lower lobe

ANTERIOR   LEFT LATERAL

RIGHT LATERAL   POSTERIOR

Figure 24–8. Topographic relationship of the ribs to the lobes of the lung.

failure and damage to the respiratory center (drug-induced, tumor, trauma).

The inspiratory phase of respiration is the only one requiring energy in normal physiology. Expiration is passive. Inspiration occupies the first third of the respiratory cycle, expiration the latter two thirds. With rapid breathing, inspiration and expiration are nearly equal.

In thin persons, it is quite normal to note a slight retraction of the intercostal spaces during quiet breathing. Bulging during expiration implies obstruction of expiratory air flow, as in emphysema. Marked retraction on inspiration, particularly if asymmetric, implies blockage of a branch of the respiratory tree. Asymmetric bulging of the intercostal spaces, on one side or the other, is created by an increase in pressure within the hemithorax. This may be a result of air trapped under pressure within the pleural cavity where it does not belong (pneumothorax) or the pressure of fluid within the pleural space (pleural effusion).

The severe pain associated with pleurisy causes intercostal muscle spasm and a lag in respiration on the involved side.

Certain patterns of respiration are characteristic of specific disease states. Although the nurse may not recognize the specific pattern or its association with a disease state, she is expected to be able to describe abnormal patterns of rhythmicity and their deviation from normal.

Palpation of the Thorax

After inspection, the thorax is palpated for tenderness, masses, lesions, respiratory excursion, and vocal fremitus. If the patient has reported an area of pain, or if lesions are apparent, direct palpation with the fingertips (for skin lesions and subcutaneous masses) or with the ball of the hand (for deeper masses or generalized flank or rib discomfort) is performed.

Respiratory Excursion. Respiratory excursion is an estimation of thoracic expansion and may disclose significant information about the symmetry of breathing. Differences in expansion are more readily detectable on the anterior thorax, where a fuller range of motion occurs during respiration. The examiner's thumbs are placed along each costal margin, below the xiphoid process, while the hands rest along the lateral rib cage. Sliding the thumbs medially about 2.5 cm (1 in) raises a small skin fold between the thumbs. The patient is instructed to inhale deeply while the examiner observes the movement of the thumbs during inspiration and expiration. This movement is normally symmetric. A posterior assessment is performed by placing the thumbs adjacent to the spinal column at the level of the tenth ribs. The hands lightly grasp the lateral rib cage. Again, a medial motion of the thumbs raises a skin fold, and the patient is instructed to take a full inspiration and expiration. The examiner observes for normal flattening of the skin fold and feels the symmetric movement of the thorax. Respiratory lag or impairment is often the result of pleurisy, fractured ribs, or trauma to the chest wall.

Tactile Fremitus. Sound generated by the larynx travels distally along the bronchial tree to set the chest wall in resonant motion. This is especially true of consonant sounds. The capacity to *feel* sound on the chest well is called *vocal* or *tactile fremitus.*

There is a wide variation in normal fremitus. It is obviously influenced by the thickness of the chest wall, most especially if that thickness is muscular, although the increase in subcutaneous tissue associated with obesity has some influence. Lower-pitched sounds travel better through the normal lung and produce greater vibration of the chest wall. Thus, fremitus is more pronounced in men than in women because of the deeper male voice.

Normally, fremitus is most pronounced where the large bronchi are closest to the chest wall and least palpable as the examiner progresses from the major bronchi to the distant lung fields. Therefore, it is most palpable in the upper thorax anteriorly and posteriorly. To elicit tactile fremitus, the examiner instructs the patient to repeat the words *ninety-nine* or *one, two, three* with each movement of the examiner's hands. The vibrations are detected by placing the palmar surfaces of the fingers and hands, or the ulnar aspect of the extended hands, on the thorax. To facilitate comparison, only one hand is used as the examiner moves in sequence down the thorax. Corresponding areas of the thorax are compared (Fig. 24–9). Bony areas are not tested.

The physics of sound transmission through the lung require explanation. Air does not conduct sound well; solid substance (tissue) does, provided that it has elasticity and is not conglomerated into a nonresonant mass. Thus, an increase in solid tissue per unit volume of lung will enhance fremitus. An increase in air per unit volume of lung will impede sound. Patients with emphysema will exhibit almost no tactile fremitus. A patient with consolidation of a lobe of the lung due to pneumonia will have an increase in tactile fremitus over that lobe. Air in the pleural space will not conduct sound.

Percussion of the Thorax

Percussion sets the chest wall and underlying structures in motion, producing audible and tactile vibrations. The examiner uses percussion to determine whether underlying tissues are filled with air, fluid, or solid material. One also uses percussion to estimate the size and location of certain structures within the thorax (diaphragm, heart, liver).

Percussion usually begins with the posterior thorax. Ideally, the patient is in a sitting position with his head flexed forward and his arms crossed on his lap. This position separates the scapulae widely and exposes more lung area for assessment. The procedure is as follows: Percuss across each shoulder top, locating the 5-cm width of resonance overlying the lung apices (Fig. 24–10). Proceed down the posterior thorax, percussing symmetric areas at 5- to 6-cm (2- to 2½-in) intervals. The middle finger is positioned parallel to the ribs in the intercostal space; the finger is placed firmly against the chest wall before striking it with the middle finger of the opposite hand. Percussion over the scapulae or rib surfaces yields a dull sound and only confuses findings. Percussion over the anterior chest is performed with the patient in an upright position with shoulders arched backward and arms at the side. The examiner begins in the supraclavicular area and proceeds downward, from intercostal space to intercostal space. In the female patient, it is often necessary to displace the breasts for an adequate examination. Dullness noted to the left of the sternum between the third and fifth intercostal spaces is the heart and is a normal finding. Similarly, there is a normal span of liver dullness in the right thorax from the fifth intercostal space to the right costal margin at the midclavicular line.

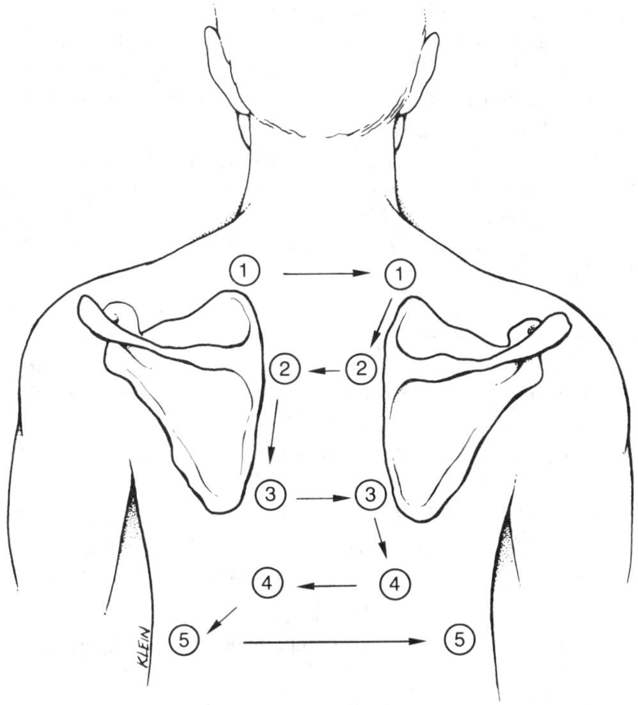

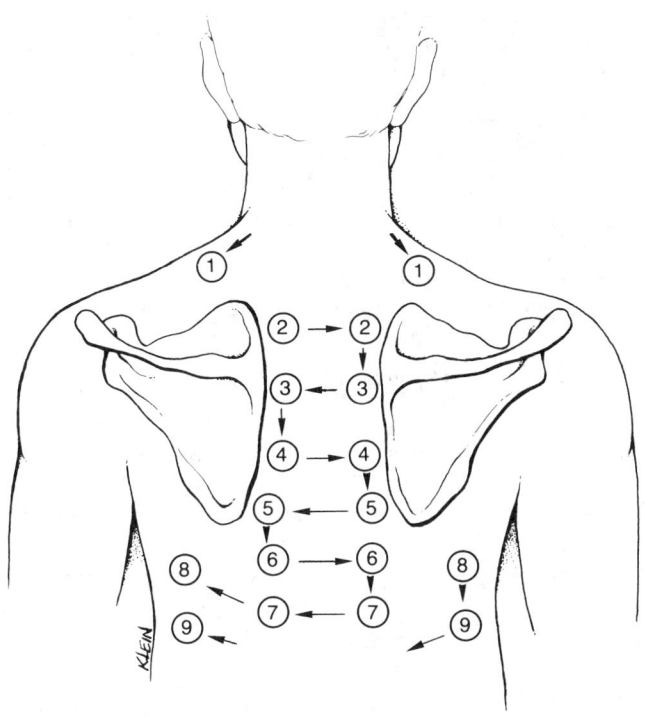

Figure 24–9. Palpation: Tactile fremitus. Numbers and arrows indicate sequence of examination. (Adapted from Bates B. A Guide to Physical Examination and History Taking, 5th ed. Philadelphia, JB Lippincott, 1991.)

Figure 24–10. Percussion of the posterior thorax. With the patient in a sitting position, symmetrical areas of the lungs are percussed at 5-cm intervals. This progression starts at the apex of each lung and concludes with percussion of each lateral chest wall. (Adapted from Bates B. A Guide to Physical Examination and History Taking, 5th ed. Philadelphia, JB Lippincott, 1991.)

The anterior and lateral thorax is examined with the patient in a supine position. If the patient is too ill or is unable to sit up, percussion of the posterior thorax is performed with the patient positioned on his side.

Indication of Disease. Dullness over the lung occurs when air-filled lung tissue is replaced by fluid or solid tissue. Examples include lobar pneumonia, in which alveoli are consolidated by cells, and accumulation of pleural fluid, blood, pus, fibrous tissue, or tumor in the pleural space. Pneumothorax produces a tympanic, or drumlike sound, whereas emphysema is perceived as hyperresonant (Table 24–2).

Diaphragmatic Excursion. The normal resonance of the lung stops at the diaphragm. The position of the diaphragm is different during inspiration than it is during expiration. For assessment of its position and motion, the patient is instructed to take a deep breath and hold it while the maximum descent of the diaphragm is percussed. This is performed along the midscapular lines bilaterally. The point at which the percussion note changes from resonance to dullness is noted. If desired, this point can be marked with a pen. The patient is then instructed to exhale fully and hold it while the examiner again percusses downward to the dullness of the diaphragm. This location is marked. The distance between the two markings indicates the range of motion of the diaphragm.

Maximum excursion of the diaphragm may amount to as much as 8 to 10 cm (3 to 4 in) in healthy, tall, young men. For most persons, it is usually 5 to 7 cm (2 to 2¾ in). The diaphragm is 2 cm (¾ in) or so higher on the right than on the left. This is because of the position of the heart and the liver above and below the left and right segments of the diaphragm, respectively. Decreased diaphragmatic excursion may be apparent in patients with pleurisy and emphysema. An increase in intra-abdominal pressure, such as occurs in pregnancy or ascites, may account for a diaphragm that is positioned high in the thorax.

Auscultation of the Thorax

Auscultation is useful in assessing the flow of air through the bronchial tree and in evaluating the presence of fluid or solid obstruction in the lung structures. To determine the condition of the lungs, the examiner auscultates for normal breath sounds, adventitious sounds, and voice sounds.

A thorough examination includes auscultation of the an-terior, posterior, and lateral thorax and is performed as follows: The diaphragm of the stethoscope is placed firmly against the chest wall as the patient breathes slowly and deeply through his mouth. Corresponding areas of the chest are auscultated in a systematic fashion from the apices to the bases and along midaxillary lines. The sequence of auscultation and the positioning of the patient are similar to those used for percussion. It often is necessary to listen to two full inspirations and expirations at each anatomic location to assure valid interpretation of the sound heard. Repeated deep breaths may result in symptoms of hyperventilation (*e.g.*, light-headedness) and can be avoided by having the patient rest and breathe normally once or twice during the examination.

Breath Sounds. Normal breath sounds are distinguished by their location over a specific area of the lung and are identified as vesicular, bronchial (tubular), and bronchovesicular breath sounds. Vesicular sounds are audible as quiet, low-pitched sounds that have a long inspiratory phase and a short expiratory phase. They are heard normally throughout the entire lung field, except over the upper sternum and between the scapulae. Bronchial breath sounds are usually louder and higher pitched than vesicular sounds. In comparison, the expiratory phase is longer than the inspiratory phase.

Bronchial sounds are heard over the trachea. Bronchovesicular sounds are heard over the main bronchus area; specifically, they can be heard between the scapulae and on either side of the sternum. Bronchovesicular breath sounds are medium in pitch; the inspiratory and expiratory phases are equal.

When bronchial and bronchovesicular sounds are audible elsewhere in the lungs, it is an indication of pathology, usually consolidation (for example, pneumonia, heart failure), and necessitates physician consultation (Table 24–3).

The quality and intensity of breath sounds are determined during auscultation. When air flow is decreased by bronchial obstruction (atelectasis) or when fluid (pleural effusion) or tissue (obesity) separates the air passages from the stethoscope, breath sounds are diminished or absent. For example, the breath sounds of the patient with emphysema are faint and often completely absent.

When heard, the expiratory phase is prolonged and may exhibit a high-pitched whistling tone called *wheezing*. This same sound is also heard in asthma and in any process associated with marked bronchoconstriction.

TABLE 24–2. *Percussion Sounds*

Note	Pitch	Intensity	Quality	Duration	Density	Examples of Location
Tympany	Very high	High	Musical	Long	More air than solid tissue	Gastric air bubble
Hyperresonance	Low	Moderately high	Slightly musical	Moderately long	More air than solid tissue	Emphysematous lung
Resonance	Moderately low	Moderate	Nonmusical	Moderate	Normal air to tissue ratio	Normal lung
Dull	Moderately high	Low	Nonmusical, muffled	Short	Fluid plus solid tissue	Liver, heart
Flat	High	Low	Soft thud	Short	Solid tissue	Bone, thigh

(Kinney MR et al [eds]. AACN's Clinical Reference for Critical Care Nursing. New York, McGraw-Hill, 1981; copyright CV Mosby, St Louis.)

TABLE 24-3. *Normal Breath Sounds*

Type	Normal Location	Pitch	Intensity	Inspiration: Expiration Ratio	Description	Graphic Illustration
Vesicular	Over most of chest except over central airways	Low	Moderate	3:1	"Breezy" (sound of wind in trees)	
Bronchial	Over major central airways	High	Great	2:3	Hollow, tubular	
Bronchovesicular	Over major central airways	Medium	Moderately great	1:1	"Breezy," tubular, tent-shaped	

(Adapted from Kersten LD. Comprehensive Respiratory Nursing: A Decision-Making Approach. Philadelphia, WB Saunders, 1989.)

Adventitious Sounds. The presence of an abnormal condition that affects the bronchial tree and alveoli may produce additional or adventitious sounds. Adventitious sounds are divided into two categories: discrete, noncontinuous sounds and continuous musical sounds. The duration of the sound is the important distinction to make in identifying the sound as noncontinuous or continuous. *Crackles* (formerly referred to as *rales*) are discrete, noncontinuous sounds that result from delayed reopening of deflated airways. *Fine crackles* are usually audible at the end of inspiration and originate from the alveoli. Their sound can be re-created by rubbing several pieces of hair next to one's ear. *Coarse crackles* have a gross, moist sound. They are produced in the large bronchi and are audible in early to mid-inspiration. Crackles may or may not be cleared by coughing. Crackles are a reflection of underlying inflammation or congestion and are often present in such conditions as pneumonia, bronchitis, congestive heart failure, and pulmonary fibrosis.

Wheezes (sibilant rhonchi) are continuous musical sounds that are longer in duration than crackles. They may be audible during inspiration, expiration, or both. These sounds result from the passage of air through narrowed or partially obstructed passages. Obstruction is often due to the presence of secretions or swelling, and hence wheezes may clear with coughing. Wheezes originate in the smaller bronchi and bronchioles; they are high pitched and whistling. Rhonchi originate in the larger bronchi or trachea and are lower pitched and sonorous. They are heard in patients with increased secretions. Wheezes are commonly heard in patients with asthma and emphysema.

Inflammation of pleural surfaces induces a crackling, grating sound that is usually heard in both inspiration and expiration. The sound is called a *friction rub*. It sounds quite close to the ear and is enhanced by applying pressure with the head of the stethoscope. The sound is imitated by rubbing the thumb and index finger together near the ear. The grating sound of a friction rub is not altered by coughing. If audible only during inspiration, it may be difficult to distinguish from crackles, which may be multiple and so frequent that a continuous sound is perceived. It is best heard over the lower lateral anterior surface (Table 24-4).

Voice Sounds. The sound heard through the stethoscope as the patient vocalizes is known as *vocal resonance*. The vibrations produced in the larynx are transmitted to the chest wall as they pass through the bronchi and alveolar tissue. During the process the sounds are diminished in intensity and altered so that syllables are not distinguishable. The spoken voice is usually assessed by having the patient repeat the phrase "ninety-nine" while the examiner listens with the stethoscope in corresponding areas of the chest from the apices to the bases.

If the vocal resonance is increased in intensity and clarity, *bronchophony* is said to be present. *Egophony* is best appreciated by having the patient repeat the letter *e*. The distortion produced by consolidation transforms the sound into a clearly heard "a" rather than "e."

Bronchophony and egophony have precisely the same connotation as bronchial breathing and an increase in tactile fremitus. Where one abnormality is detected, so should the others be. A change in tactile fremitus is more subtle and can be missed, but bronchial breathing and bronchophony present loudly and clearly to the examiner.

A very subtle finding, heard only in the presence of rather dense consolidation, is the phenomenon of *whispered pectoriloquy*. Transmission of high-frequency components of sound is so enhanced that even whispered words are heard, a circumstance not noted in normal physiology. The implication is the same as that of bronchophony.

A routine assessment of the thorax and lungs includes the following: inspection of the thorax and respirations, percussion of the posterior thorax, and auscultation of the thorax for breath sounds and the presence of adventitious sounds. Unless some facet of the history or a prior observation in the physical assessment leads the nurse to pursue additional information about respiratory status, palpation for fremitus and auscultation of voice sounds are omitted.

The physical findings for the most common respiratory diseases are summarized in Table 24-5.

Assessment of Respiratory Signs and Symptoms

The major signs and symptoms of respiratory disease are dyspnea, cough, sputum production, chest pain, wheezing, clubbing of the fingers, hemoptysis, and cyanosis. These clinical manifestations are related to the duration and severity of the disease.

TABLE 24–4. *Types of Adventitious Sounds*

Type	General Location	Associated Problem(s)	Characteristics	Graphic Illustration
Crackles (rales)	Peripheral airways and alveoli	Atelectasis Inflammation Excess fluid Excess mucus	Group of discrete crackles or popping sounds Discontinuous sound Usually inspiratory, may be inspiratory and expiratory	fine coarse
Rhonchi	Large airways	Inflammation Excess fluid Excess mucus	Coarse, low-pitched sonorous sounds Continuous sound Usually expiratory, may be inspiratory and expiratory Changes in quality and timing with coughing	
Wheeze	Large or small airways	Bronchoconstriction (airway narrowing) from bronchospasm, fluid, mucus, inflammatory by-products, obstructive lesion Airway instability	High- (sometimes low-) pitched musical sound Continuous sound Usually expiratory, may be inspiratory and expiratory	
Pleural friction rub	Pleural surfaces	Inflamed or roughened pleural surfaces (pleuritis)	Grating sound with continuous and discontinuous qualities May appear intermittently Variable duration; usually inspiratory, may be inspiratory and expiratory Sounds the same or louder with coughing	

(Kersten LD. Comprehensive Respiratory Nursing: A Decision-Making Approach. Philadelphia, WB Saunders, 1989.)

TABLE 24–5. *Physical Findings in Common Respiratory Problems*

Disease/Disorder	Tactile Fremitus	Percussion	Auscultation
Consolidation (*e.g.*, pneumonia)	Increased	Dull	Bronchial breath sounds, rales, bronchophony, egophony, whispered pectoriloquy
Bronchitis	Normal	Resonant	Normal to decreased breath sounds, wheezes, and rhonchi
Emphysema	Decreased	Hyperresonant	Decreased intensity of breath sounds, usually with prolonged expiration
Asthma (severe attack)	Normal to decreased	Resonant to hyperresonant	Wheezes and rhonchi
Pulmonary edema	Normal	Resonant	Rales at lung bases, possibly wheezes
Pleural effusion	Absent	Dull to flat	Decreased to absent breath sounds, bronchial breath sounds and bronchophony, egophony, and whispering pectoriloquy above the effusion over the area of compressed lung
Pneumothorax	Decreased	Hyperresonant	Absent breath sounds
Atelectasis	Absent	Flat	Decreased to absent breath sounds

(Kinney MR et al. AACN's Clinical Reference for Critical Care Nursing. New York, McGraw-Hill, 1981; copyright CV Mosby, St Louis.)

Dyspnea

Dyspnea (difficult or labored breathing) is a symptom common to many pulmonary and heart conditions, particularly when there is increased lung rigidity and airway resistance. The right ventricle of the heart will be affected ultimately by lung disease because it must pump blood through the lungs. Sudden dyspnea in a healthy person may indicate pneumothorax (air in the pleural cavity). Sudden shortness of breath in an ill patient or after surgery may denote pulmonary embolism. *Orthopnea* (ability to breathe only in an upright position) may be found in patients with heart disease and, occasionally, with patients with COPD. Shortness of breath with an expiratory wheeze is seen in COPD (asthma, bronchitis, emphysema). Noisy breathing may result from a narrowing of the airway or localized obstruction of a major bronchus by a tumor or foreign body. The presence of both inspiratory and expiratory wheezing usually signifies asthma, if the patient is not in congestive heart failure. Shortness of breath may be a significant clinical indicator. It may be the result of a cardiac or respiratory disease. In general, the acute diseases of the lungs produce a more severe grade of dyspnea than do the chronic diseases. The circumstance that produces the patient's dyspnea must be determined. It is important to ask the patient:

- How much exertion triggers shortness of breath?
- Is there an associated cough?
- Is dyspnea related to other symptoms?
- Was the onset of shortness of breath sudden or gradual?
- At what time of day or night does the dyspnea occur?
- Is the shortness of breath worse when the patient is flat in bed?
- Does the shortness of breath occur at rest? With exercise? Running? Climbing stairs?
- Is the shortness of breath worse while walking? If so, when walking how far?

The management of dyspnea depends on the success with which its cause can be alleviated. Relief of the symptom sometimes is achieved by placing the patient at rest with his head elevated and, in severe cases, by administering oxygen.

Cough

Cough results from irritation of the mucous membranes anywhere in the respiratory tract. The stimulus producing a cough may arise from an infectious process or from an airborne irritant, such as smoke, smog, dust, or a gas. The cough is the patient's chief protection against the accumulation of secretions in the bronchi and bronchioles.

Conversely, the presence of cough may indicate serious pulmonary disease. Of equal importance is the type of cough. A dry, irritative cough is characteristic of upper respiratory tract infection of viral origin. Laryngotracheitis causes an irritative, high-pitched cough. Tracheal lesions produce a brassy cough. A severe or *changing* cough may indicate bronchogenic carcinoma. Pleuritic chest pain accompanying coughing may indicate pleural or chest wall (musculoskeletal) involvement.

The character of the cough is evaluated. Is it dry? hacking? brassy? wheezing? loose? severe? The time of coughing is noted. Coughing at night may herald the onset of left-sided heart failure or bronchial asthma. A cough in the morning with sputum production is indicative of bronchitis. A cough that worsens when the patient is supine may indicate a postnasal drip (sinusitis). Coughing after food intake may indicate aspirated material in the tracheobronchial tree. A cough of recent onset is usually from an acute infectious process.

Sputum Production

A patient who coughs long enough almost invariably will produce sputum. Violent coughing causes bronchial spasm, obstruction, and further irritation of the bronchi and may result in syncope. A severe, repeated, or uncontrolled cough that is nonproductive is exhausting and potentially harmful. Sputum production is the reaction of the lungs to any constantly recurring irritant. It also may be associated with a nasal discharge. If there is a profuse amount of purulent sputum (thick and yellow or green) or a change in color of the sputum, the patient probably has a bacterial infection. Rusty sputum indicates the presence of bacterial pneumonia, if the patient has not received antibiotics. A thin, mucoid sputum frequently results from viral bronchitis. A gradual increase of sputum over time may indicate the presence of chronic bronchitis or bronchiectasis. Pink-tinged mucoid sputum is suggestive of a lung tumor, whereas profuse, frothy, pink material, often welling up into the throat, may indicate pulmonary edema. Malodorous sputum and bad breath point to the presence of lung abscess, bronchiectasis, or an infection caused by fusospirochetal or other anaerobic organisms.

If the sputum is too thick to raise, it is necessary to decrease its viscosity by increasing its water content through adequate hydration (drinking water) and inhalation of aerosolized solutions, which may be delivered by any type of nebulizer. Methods of assisting the patient to cough productively are discussed on p. 546.

Smoking is definitely contraindicated because it interferes with ciliary action, increases bronchial secretions, causes inflammation and hyperplasia of the mucous membranes, and reduces production of surfactant. Thus, bronchial drainage is impaired. If smoking is stopped, sputum volume will decrease and resistance to bronchial infections will improve.

The patient's appetite may be depressed because of the odor of the sputum and the taste it leaves in his mouth. Adequate oral hygiene, proper environment, and wise selection of food will stimulate appetite. After the patient's mouth is carefully cleansed and rinsed, sputum cups and emesis basins should be removed before the next meal arrives. Serving citrus juices at the beginning of the meal will make the mouth feel better and will help to make the patient more receptive to the rest of the meal.

Chest Pain

Chest pain or discomfort may be associated with pulmonary or heart disease.

Chest pain associated with pulmonary conditions may be sharp, stabbing, and intermittent or dull, aching, and persistent. The pain usually is felt on the side where the pathologic process is located, but it may be referred elsewhere, for example, to the neck, the back, or the abdomen. Chest pain is experienced by many patients with pneumonia, pulmonary embolism with lung infarction, and pleurisy, and is a late symptom of bronchogenic carcinoma. In carcinoma the pain may be dull and persistent because of invasion into the chest wall, mediastinum, or spine.

Lung disease does not always produce thoracic pain because the lungs and the visceral pleura lack sensory nerves and are insensitive to pain stimuli. But the parietal pleura has a rich supply of sensory nerves that are stimulated by inflammation and stretching of the membrane. Pleuritic pain due to irritation of the parietal pleura is sharp and seems to "catch" on inspiration; it is often described by patients as "like the stabbing of a knife." They are more comfortable when they lie on the affected side, a posture that tends to "splint" the chest wall, restrict the expansions and contractions of the lung, and reduce the friction between the injured or diseased pleurae on that side. Pain associated with cough may be lessened by manual splinting of the rib cage.

The quality, intensity, and radiation of pain are assessed and factors that precipitate it are identified and explored. Whether there is a relationship between pain and the patient's posture should be determined. Also, the inspiratory and expiratory phases of respiration and their effect on pain are evaluated.

Analgesic medications are effective in relieving chest pain, but care must be taken not to depress the respiratory center or a productive cough. The physician may perform a regional anesthetic block for relief of extreme pain. Procaine is injected along the intercostal nerves that supply the painful area.

Wheezing

Wheezing is often the major finding in a patient with bronchoconstriction or airway narrowing. It is heard with or without a stethoscope, depending on its location. Wheezing is a high-pitched, musical sound heard mainly on expiration (see p. 509 for assessment).

Clubbing of the Fingers

Clubbing of the fingers as a sign of lung disease is found in patients with chronic hypoxic conditions, chronic lung infections, and malignancies of the lung. This finding may be initially manifested as sponginess of the nailbed and loss of the nailbed angle (Fig. 24–11)

Hemoptysis

Hemoptysis (expectoration of blood from the respiratory tract) is a symptom of pulmonary or cardiac disorders. It varies from blood-stained sputum to a large, sudden hemorrhage and always merits investigation. The most common causes are (1) pulmonary infection, (2) carcinoma of the lung, (3) abnormalities of the heart or blood vessels, (4) pulmonary artery or vein abnormalities, and (5) pulmonary emboli and infarction. The onset of hemoptysis is usually sudden and may be intermittent or continuous. Several investigations are usually performed to determine the cause: blood examination, chest angiography, chest radiography, and bronchoscopy. A careful history and physical examination are necessary to establish a diagnosis of the underlying disease, irrespective of whether the bleeding produced involved a fleck of blood in the sputum or

CLUBBING OF THE NAILS

NORMAL

Normal angle 160°

The angle between the normal finger nail and the nail base is about 160°. When palpated, the nail base feels firm.

EARLY CLUBBING

Springy, floating   *Straightened angle (180°)*

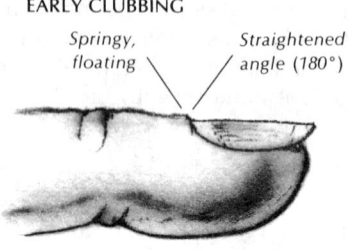

In early clubbing, the angle between nail and nail base straightens out. The nail base gives a springy or floating sensation when palpated. You can simulate this by squeezing your middle finger from each side between your thumb and ring finger of the same hand, just behind the nail. Then palpate the nail base with the index finger of the opposite hand.

LATE CLUBBING

Swollen, springy, floating   *Angle greater than 180°*

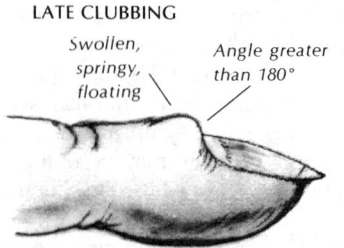

In late clubbing, the base of the nail becomes visibly swollen and the angle between nail and nail base exceeds 180°.

Clubbing has many causes, including hypoxia and lung cancer.

Figure 24–11. Nail clubbing. (Bates B. A Guide to Physical Examination and History Taking, 5th ed. Philadelphia, JB Lippincott, 1991.)

a massive hemorrhage. The amount of blood produced is not always indicative of the seriousness of the cause.

First it is important to determine the source of the bleeding: the gums, nasopharynx, lungs, or stomach. The nurse may be the only witness to the episode. The following points should be considered in making and recording observations. In patients whose bloody sputum originates from the nose or the nasopharynx, expectoration is usually preceded by considerable sniffing and blood may appear in the nares. Blood from the lung is usually bright red, frothy, and mixed with sputum. Initial symptoms include a tickling sensation in the throat, a salty taste, a burning or bubbling sensation in the chest, and perhaps chest pain, in which case the patient tends to splint the bleeding side. The term *hemoptysis* is reserved for the coughing up of blood arising from a pulmonary hemorrhage. This blood has an alkaline *p*H (greater than 7.0).

In contrast, if the hemorrhage is in the stomach, the blood is vomited (*hematemesis*) rather than coughed up. Blood that has been in contact with gastric juice is sometimes so dark that it is referred to as "coffeeground" material. This blood has an acid *p*H (less than 7.0).

Cyanosis

Cyanosis, a bluish coloring of the skin, is a very late indicator of *hypoxia*. For cyanosis to appear, there must be at least 5 g/dl of unoxygenated hemoglobin. A patient whose hemoglobin is 15 g/dl will not demonstrate cyanosis until 5 g/dl of that hemoglobin becomes unoxygenated, resulting in an effective circulating hemoglobin of two thirds of the normal level. This determines cyanosis even if the hemoglobin level is low or high (the anemic patient will rarely manifest cyanosis, and the polycythemic patient will look cyanotic even if adequately oxygenated). Therefore the presence of cyanosis is *not* a reliable sign.

Assessment of cyanosis is affected by room lighting, the patient's skin color, and depth of the vessels from the surface of the skin. In the presence of a pulmonary condition, central cyanosis is assessed by observing the color of the tongue and lips. This indicates a decrease in oxygen tension in the blood. Peripheral cyanosis results from decreased blood flow to a certain area of the body, as in vasoconstriction of the nail beds or ear lobes from exposure to cold, and does not necessarily indicate a central systemic problem.

Assessment of Breathing Ability

Tests of the patient's breathing ability are easily assessed at the bedside by measuring the respiratory rate, tidal volume, minute ventilation, vital capacity, inspiratory force, and compliance. These tests are particularly important for patients at risk of developing pulmonary complications, including those who have undergone chest or abdominal surgery, have experienced prolonged anesthesia, have preexisting pulmonary disease, or are elderly.

Patients whose chest expansion is limited by external restrictions such as obesity or abdominal distention and who are unable to breathe deeply because of postoperative pain or sedation produce low tidal volumes. Ventilation at low tidal volumes without sigh inflations can produce alveolar collapse or atelectasis. The functional residual capacity falls, lung com-

pliance is reduced, and the patient must breathe faster to maintain the same degree of tissue oxygenation. These events can be exaggerated in patients who have preexisting pulmonary diseases and in elderly patients whose airways are less compliant because of earlier closure of small airways during the expiratory cycle.

Respiratory Rate

The normal adult who is resting comfortably breathes at 12 to 18 breaths per minute. Except for occasional sighs, the breathing is regular.

- *Bradypnea*, or slow breathing, is associated with increased intracranial pressure, brain injury, and drug overdose.
- *Tachypnea*, or rapid breathing, is commonly seen in pneumonia, pulmonary edema, metabolic acidosis, septicemia, and rib fracture.

Tidal Volume

The volume of each breath is referred to as the tidal volume. The simplest instrument commonly used at the bedside to measure volumes is known as the Wright respirometer.

If the patient is breathing through an endotracheal tube or tracheostomy, the respirometer is directly attached to it and the exhaled volume is obtained from the dial. In others, the respirometer is attached to a face mask, which is placed to cover the nose and mouth so that it is airtight, and the exhaled volume is measured as before. Hand-held electronic respirometers that provide digital readouts of lung volumes are also available.

The tidal volume may vary from breath to breath. To make the measurement reliable, the volumes of several breaths are measured, and the range of tidal volumes together with the average tidal volume are noted. The normal tidal volume is 5 to 8 ml per kilogram of body weight.

Minute Ventilation

Tidal volume and respiratory rates alone are unreliable indicators of the adequacy of ventilation because both can vary widely from breath to breath. Together, however, the tidal volume and respiratory rate are important because they determine the minute ventilation, which is useful in the detection of respiratory failure. Minute ventilation ($\dot{V}_E$) is the volume of air expired per minute. It is equal to the product of the tidal volume (V_T) and respiratory rate or frequency (f) according to the following equation:

$$\dot{V}_E = V_T \times f$$

In practice, the minute ventilation is not calculated but is measured directly using a respirometer. Minute ventilation may be decreased by a variety of conditions, including those that

- Limit neurologic impulses transmitted from the brain to the respiratory muscles, such as spinal cord trauma, cerebrovascular accidents, tumors, myasthenia gravis, Guillain–Barré syndrome, polio, and drug overdose.
- Depress respiratory centers in the medulla, as with anesthesia and narcotic sedative overdose
- Affect the lungs by
  Limiting thoracic movement: kyphoscoliosis
  Limiting lung movement: pleural effusion, pneumothorax

Reducing functional lung tissue: chronic pulmonary diseases, severe pulmonary edema

When the minute ventilation falls, the amount of alveolar ventilation reaching the lungs also must decrease, and the $PaCO_2$ increases.

- One should not rely on visual inspection of the rate and depth of a patient's respiratory excursions to determine the adequacy of ventilation. Respiratory excursions may appear normal or exaggerated, but the patient may actually be moving only enough air to ventilate his dead space.

Vital Capacity

Vital capacity is measured by having the patient inspire maximally and exhale fully through a respirometer. The normal value depends on age, sex, body build, and weight.

- Most patients can generate a vital capacity twice their predicted tidal volume. If the vital capacity is less than 10 ml per kilogram of body weight, the patient will be too weak to sustain spontaneous ventilation and respiratory assistance will be required.

When the vital capacity is exhaled at a maximum flow rate, the forced vital capacity (FVC) is measured. Most patients can exhale at least 75% of their vital capacity in 1 second (forced expiratory volume in 1 second, or FEV_1) and almost all of it in 3 seconds (FEV_3). A reduction in the FEV_1 suggests abnormal pulmonary air flow. If a patient's FEV_1 and FVC are proportionately reduced, his maximum lung expansion is restricted in some way. If the reduction in FEV_1 greatly exceeds the reduction in FVC, the patient may have some degree of airway obstruction.

Inspiratory Force

Inspiratory force evaluates the effort a patient is making during inspiration. It does not require patient cooperation and hence is useful in the unconscious patient. The equipment needed for this measurement includes (1) a manometer that measures negative pressure and (2) adapters for connection to an anesthesia mask or a cuffed endotracheal tube. The manometer is attached and the airway is completely occluded.

This is continued for 10 to 20 seconds while the inspiratory efforts of the patient are registered on the manometer. The normal inspiratory pressure is -100 cm H_2O. If the negative pressure registered after 15 seconds of occluding the airway is less than -25 cm H_2O, mechanical ventilation is usually required, because the patient lacks sufficient muscle strength for deep breathing or effective coughing.

Compliance

Compliance is the distensibility or expandability of the lung. The healthy lung is usually said to be compliant. Compliance is calculated at the patient's bedside by measuring the tidal volume and airway pressure during inspiration. It also can be measured in the pulmonary laboratory using special instruments. When a patient is mechanically ventilated, his ease of breathing is quickly and easily estimated by measuring his compliance. This is accomplished by dividing the tidal volume delivered to the patient by the static pressure (pressure obtained during inspiratory hold, also referred to as static pressure)

measured minus the positive end-expiratory pressure (PEEP) value.

For example, if the tidal volume is 450 ml and the pressure is 15 cm H_2O, compliance is estimated to be $450 \div 15$ or 0.30 L/cm H_2O. If 20 cm H_2O is later required to deliver the same tidal volume, compliance has decreased ($450 \div 20 = 0.225$ L/cm H_2O).

If the pressure measurement is made while air is flowing into the lungs, it reflects changes in air flow resistance as well as lung and chest wall compliance (lung stiffness) and is termed *dynamic compliance.* Low compliance is a characteristic finding in pneumothorax, hemothorax, pleural effusion, pulmonary edema, atelectasis, and most acute illnesses of the lung. Compliance is useful in assessing the progress of the disease in adult respiratory distress syndrome.

- In general, a rapid reduction in static compliance suggests a pneumothorax. A gradual compliance reduction suggests progressive decreases in lung and chest wall compliance from conditions that restrict lung expansion, such as pleural effusion or atelectasis. A rapid reduction in dynamic compliance suggests air flow resistance, such as with accumulated secretions.

Atelectasis

Atelectasis refers to the collapse of an alveoli or a lobule or larger lung unit. It may be caused by obstruction of a bronchus; this impedes the passage of air to and from the alveoli communicating with it. The trapped alveolar air becomes absorbed into the bloodstream, and its replacement from the outside air is impossible because of the obstruction. The net result is that the isolated portion of the lung becomes airless and shrinks in size, causing the remainder of the lung to overexpand. Atelectasis may follow bronchial obstruction by a foreign body or a plug of thick exudate. Also, the supine position, splinting of the chest due to pain, respiratory depression from narcotics and relaxants, and abdominal distention increase the risk for atelectasis. Atelectasis resulting from bronchial obstruction by secretions is the usual cause of the "massive collapse" occasionally observed postoperatively and in debilitated, bedridden patients. In these patients, there is likely to be long, continued respiratory depression, together with inadequate respiratory excursion and retention of bronchial secretions.

Atelectasis may result from pressure on the lung tissue, which restricts normal lung expansion on inspiration. Such pressure may be produced by a variety of causes: fluid accumulation within the thorax (pleural effusion), air in the pleural space (pneumothorax), an extremely large heart, a pericardium distended with fluid (pericardial effusion), tumor growth within the thorax, or an elevated diaphragm that is displaced upward as the result of abdominal pressure. Atelectasis caused by pressure is often encountered in patients with pleural effusion due to cardiac failure or pleural infection. Atelectasis is often one of the first signs of a tumor of the bronchi.

Assessment.   If lung collapse occurs suddenly, and if sufficient lung tissue is involved, marked dyspnea, cyanosis, prostration, and pleural pain may be anticipated. Tachycardia and fever are common. The patient characteristically sits bolt upright in bed, is anxious, and has difficulty breathing. The chest wall on the affected side moves little, if at all, whereas the excursion appears excessive on the opposite side.

Management.   The goal is to improve ventilation and remove secretions. If atelectasis has resulted from a pleural effusion or pressure pneumothorax, the fluid or air may be removed by needle aspiration. If bronchial obstruction is the cause, it must be removed to permit air to enter the lung again. If respiratory care measures fail to remove the obstruction, a bronchoscopy is performed. Endotracheal intubation and mechanical ventilation may be necessary. Prompt treatment reduces the risk of pneumonia and lung abscess.

Nursing Interventions. Methods to relieve bronchial obstruction include aspirating secretions, encouraging the patient to cough, and using an aerosol nebulizer, followed by postural drainage and chest percussion. The patient should be turned frequently to stimulate coughing. If possible, the patient is ambulated to aid in mobilizing and in clearing secretions.

All stuporous, debilitated, and sedated patients are turned frequently in bed. Coughing and deep breathing (at least every 2 hours) assist in preventing and treating atelectasis. The use of incentive spirometry or voluntary deep breathing enhances inspiration and decreases the potential for airway closure. Nasopharyngeal and nasotracheal suction is also helpful in stimulating patients to cough, thereby removing tenacious secretions.

Diagnostic Assessment of Respiratory Function

A wide range of diagnostic studies, described on the following pages, may be conducted in patients with respiratory conditions.

Radiographic Examinations of the Chest

Normal pulmonary tissue is radiolucent; therefore, densities produced by tumors, foreign bodies, and other pathologic conditions can be detected by means of radiographic examination. A chest radiograph may reveal an extensive pathologic process in the lungs in the absence of symptoms. The routine chest radiograph consists of two views—the posteroanterior projection and the lateral projection. Chest radiographs are usually taken after full inspiration (deep breath) since the lungs are best visualized when they are well aerated. Also, the diaphragm is at its lowest level and the largest expanse of lung is visible. Radiographs taken on expiration may accentuate an otherwise unnoticed pneumothorax or obstruction of a major artery.

Tomography (Planigraphy). Tomography provides films of sections of the lungs at different planes within the thorax. It is valuable in studying patients with pulmonary TB, compressed lung, and lung abscess. Tomography can show cavities, nodular infiltrates, and bronchiectasis associated with pulmonary tuberculosis, solid lesions seen in bronchogenic carcinoma, calcification, and bronchial occlusion.

Computed Tomography. Computed tomography (CT) is an imaging method in which the lungs are scanned in successive layers by a narrow-beam x-ray. The images produced provide a cross-sectional view of the chest. A regular chest radiograph shows major contrast between body densities, such as bones, soft tissues, and air. CT scan, however, can distinguish fine tissue density.

It may be used to define pulmonary nodules and small tumors adjacent to pleural surfaces that are not visible on routine chest films, and to demonstrate mediastinal abnormalities and hilar adenopathy, which are difficult to visualize with other techniques.

Contrast material is most useful when evaluating the mediastinum and its contents. A computer printout may be obtained of the absorption values of the tissues in the plane that is being scanned.

Positron Emission Tomography. Positron emission tomography (PET) uses high-energy physics and sophisticated computer techniques to study the way cells function in a living person. The patient inhales or is injected with a short-lived radioactive version of an element that occurs naturally in the body (oxygen, nitrogen, carbon, fluorine). The radioisotope emits subatomic particles called *positrons* (a positively charged electron). When a positron encounters an electron, which it does just after emission, both are destroyed and two gamma rays are released. These bursts of energy are recorded by the PET scanner, and its computer determines where in the body the radioactive material is located. PET is particularly useful for quantitative measurements of regional pulmonary perfusion and for studying ventilation–perfusion relationships.

Fluoroscopy. Fluoroscopy is used to assist with invasive procedures, such as a chest needle biopsy or transbronchial biopsy, to identify lesions. It also may be used to study the movement of the diaphragm and regional variations in ventilation.

Barium Swallow. A barium swallow outlines the esophagus and shows displacement of the esophagus and encroachment on its lumen by the heart, lungs, or mediastinal structures.

Bronchography. Bronchography is rarely used today since the advent of fiberoptic bronchoscopy.

Angiographic Studies of the Pulmonary Vessels

Angiographic studies include pulmonary angiography, angiocardiography, aortography, bronchial arteriography, superior vena cava angiography, and azygography. Pulmonary angiography is most commonly used to investigate thromboembolic disease of the lungs and congenital abnormalities of the pulmonary vascular tree and to detect abnormal vasculature arising from tumors.

Pulmonary angiography is the rapid injection of a radiopaque medium into the vasculature of the lungs for radiographic study of pulmonary vessels. It can be performed by venous injection into one or both arms (simultaneously) or femoral vein, through a needle or catheter; by introducing a catheter into the main pulmonary artery or its branches; or by introducing a catheter into the great veins or heart proximal to the pulmonary artery.

Endoscopic Procedures

Bronchoscopy. Bronchoscopy is the direct inspection and examination of the larynx, trachea, and bronchi through either a flexible fiberoptic bronchoscope or a rigid bronchoscope. In current practice the fiberoptic scope is used more frequently.

The *diagnostic purposes* of bronchoscopy are (1) to examine tissues or collect secretions; (2) to determine the location and extent of the pathologic process and to obtain a tissue sample for diagnosis (by biting forceps, curettage, or brush biopsy); (3) to determine whether a tumor can be resected surgically; and (4) to diagnose bleeding sites (source of hemoptysis).

Therapeutically, bronchoscopy is used to (1) remove foreign bodies from the tracheobronchial tree, (2) remove secretions obstructing the tracheobronchial tree when the patient is unable to clear them, (3) provide postoperative treatment in atelectasis, and (4) destroy and excise lesions.

The *fiberoptic bronchoscope* is a thin, flexible bronchoscope that can be directed into the segmental bronchi (Fig. 24–12). Because of its smaller size, flexibility, and excellent optical system, it allows increased visualization of the peripheral airways and is ideal for diagnosing pulmonary lesions. Cytologic examinations can be performed without surgical intervention. Fiberoptic bronchoscopy is better tolerated by patients than rigid bronchoscopy, allows biopsy of previously inaccessible tumors, is safe to use in the very ill patient, and can be performed at the bedside or through endotracheal or tracheostomy tubes of patients on ventilators. Fiberoptic bronchoscopy allows direct intubation of the right upper lobe, which is impossible with the rigid bronchoscope.

The *rigid bronchoscope* is a hollow metallic tube with a light at its end; it is used mainly for the removal of foreign bodies, for suctioning thick secretions, or investigating the source of massive hemoptysis, or for endobronchial surgical procedures.

Possible complications of bronchoscopy include reaction to the local anesthetic, infection, aspiration, bronchospasm, hypoxemia, pneumothorax, bleeding, and perforation.

Nursing Interventions. An informed consent is obtained before the procedure. Food and fluids are withheld for 6 hours before the test to reduce the risk of aspiration when reflexes are blocked. The procedure is explained to the patient to reduce fear and correct misapprehensions. Preoperative medications (usually atropine and a sedative or narcotic) are administered as prescribed to inhibit vagal stimulation (thereby guarding against bradycardia, dysrhythmias, hypotension), suppress the cough reflex, sedate the patient, and relieve anxiety.

- *Caution:* Sedation given to patients with respiratory insufficiency may precipitate respiratory arrest.

Contact lenses, dentures, and other prostheses are removed. The examination is usually performed under local anesthesia, but general anesthesia may be given.

A topical anesthetic such as lidocaine (Xylocaine) may be sprayed on the pharynx or dropped on the epiglottis and vocal cords and into the trachea to reduce the cough reflex and pain. Diazepam (Valium) is administered as prescribed, intravenously, for additional sedation.

After the procedure, the patient is given nothing by mouth until the cough reflex returns, because the preoperative sedation and local anesthesia impair the protective laryngeal reflex and swallowing for several hours. Once the patient demonstrates that he can cough, ice chips and eventually fluids may be given. The nurse assesses for confusion and lethargy in the elderly, possibly due to large doses of lidocaine given during the procedure. Difficulty in breathing is observed for and reported promptly. The patient is observed for evidence of cyanosis, hypotension, tachycardia, dysrhythmias, hemoptysis, and dyspnea.

Esophagoscopy. Esophagoscopy is the viewing of the interior of the esophagus through a lighted tube. it is used in removing foreign bodies; in inspecting lesions of the esophagus, such as ulcers, diverticuli, and tumors; and for microscopic examination (biopsy). The care before and after the procedure is the same as for bronchoscopy.

Thoracoscopy. Thoracoscopy (pleuroscopy) is a diagnostic procedure in which the pleural cavity is examined with an endoscope. A small incision is made into the pleural cavity in an intercostal space; the location of the incision depends on clinical and radiologic findings. After aspiration of any fluid

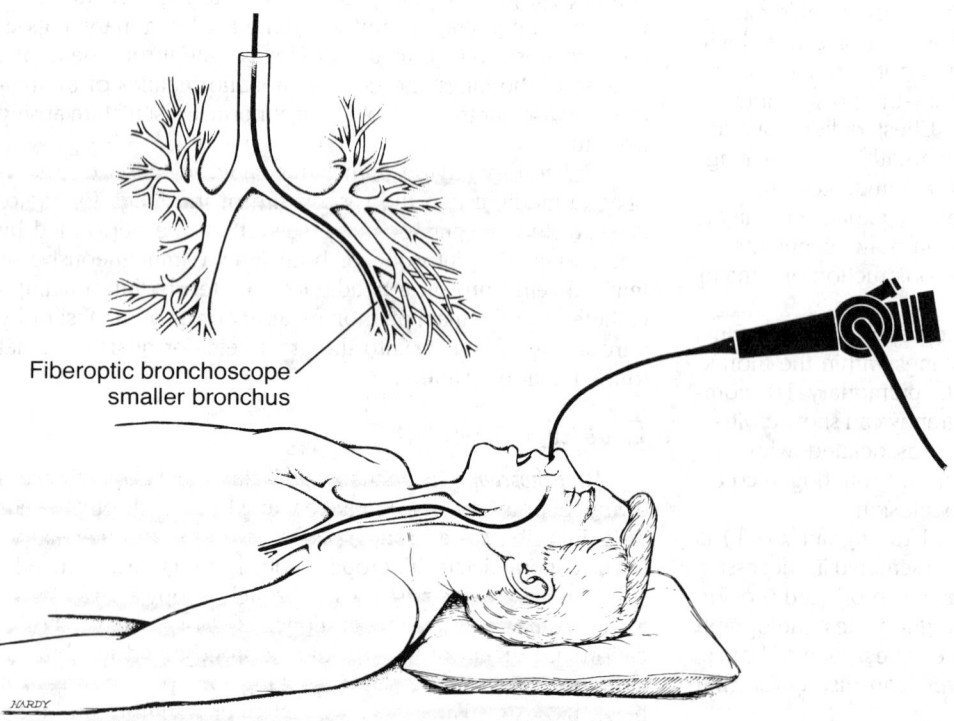

Fiberoptic bronchoscope smaller bronchus

Figure 24–12. Fiberoptic bronchoscopy.

present in the pleural cavity, the fiberoptic mediastinoscope is inserted into the pleural cavity and its surface is inspected through the instrument. Biopsies of the lesions can be performed under direct vision. After the procedure, a chest tube is inserted and the pleural cavity is drained by water-seal drainage.

Mediastinoscopy. See later discussion.

Sputum Studies

Sputum is obtained for study to identify pathogenic organisms and determine whether malignant cells are present. It also may be used to assess for hypersensitivity states (in which there is an increase of eosinophils). Periodic sputum examinations may be necessary for patients receiving antibiotics, steroids, and immunosuppressive drugs for prolonged periods, as these agents give rise to opportunistic infections. In general, sputum cultures are used in diagnosis, for drug sensitivity testing, and as a guide in treatment. Sputum can be obtained by expectoration. If the patient cannot raise the sputum spontaneously, he often can be induced to cough deeply by breathing an irritating aerosol of supersaturated saline, propylene glycol, or some other agent delivered with an ultrasonic nebulizer. Other methods of collecting sputum specimens include endotracheal aspiration, bronchoscopic removal, bronchial brushing, transtracheal aspiration, and gastric aspiration, usually for tuberculosis organisms (see Chap. 33). Generally, the deepest specimens are obtained in the early morning.

The patient is instructed to clear his nose and throat and rinse his mouth to decrease contamination of the sputum. He then takes a few deep breaths; coughs (rather than spits), using his diaphragm; and expectorates into a sterile container.

The specimen is sent to the laboratory immediately;

allowing it to stand for several hours in a warm room will result in the overgrowth of contaminant organisms and may make culture more difficult (especially for *Mycobacterium tuberculosis*).

Often a qualitative study is performed to determine whether the secretions are saliva, mucus, or pus. Usually, they separate into layers that are seen readily when a conical, glass container is used. A yellow-green color of the material expectorated usually implies infection (*i.e.*, pneumonia).

For quantitative studies, the patient is given a special container in which to expectorate. This is weighed at the end of 24 hours, and the amount and the character of the contents are described and recorded. Such a specimen is treated as biohazardous material and disposed of separately. To prevent odors, all sputum containers are covered. Malodorous mouth wipes are discarded and removed promptly, and good room ventilation is ensured. Frequent oral hygiene is a nursing priority for these patients.

Transtracheal aspiration of sputum is accomplished by transtracheal puncture through the cricothyroid membrane and by the introduction of a fine catheter through the needle into the trachea (Fig. 24–13). The needle is withdrawn, leaving the catheter in place. Sterile saline (2 to 5 ml) is injected into the catheter to loosen secretions and induce coughing. Then material is aspirated back through the catheter into a syringe. The contents of the syringe are expressed into a sterile culture tube. The catheter is withdrawn, and pressure is applied over the puncture site for 5 to 10 minutes to minimize bleeding and prevent subcutaneous emphysema.

This technique is used also to promote coughing and sputum production in thoracotomy patients and in those patients with an absent cough reflex. In this instance, the catheter is left in place for periodic instillation of saline to induce coughing.

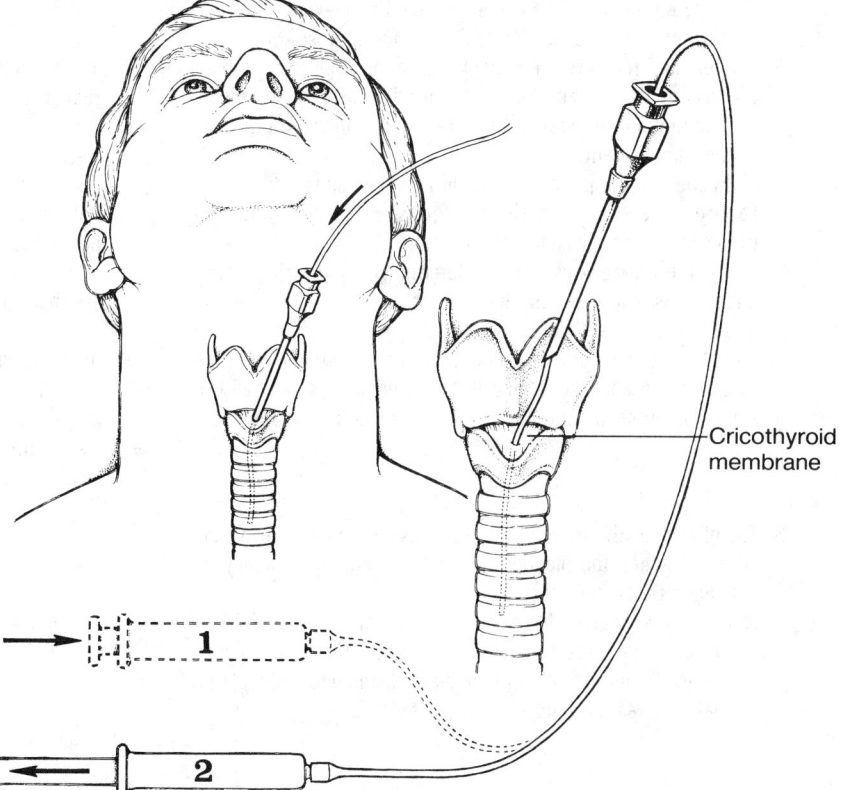

Figure 24–13. Transtracheal aspiration. After the catheter is positioned in the trachea, the needle is withdrawn, leaving the catheter in place. Sterile saline (2 to 5 ml) is injected into the catheter (1) to loosen secretions and induce coughing. Then the material is aspirated back through the catheter into a syringe (2).

Cricothyroid membrane

Chart 24–1
Guidelines for Assisting the Patient Having a Thoracentesis

A thoracentesis (aspiration of fluid or air from the pleural space) is performed on patients with various clinical problems. It may be a diagnostic or therapeutic procedure for

1. Removal of fluid and air from the pleural cavity
2. Diagnostic aspiration of pleural fluid
3. Pleural biopsy
4. Instillation of medication into pleural space

The responsibilities of the nurse in relation to the patient having a thoracentesis and the rationale for her participation are summarized below:

Nursing Activities

1. Ascertain in advance whether chest x-ray films have been prescribed and completed and the consent form has been signed.

2. Determine whether the patient is allergic to the local anesthetic agent to be used. Give sedation if prescribed.

3. Inform the patient about the procedure and indicate how he can be helpful. Explain the following:
   a. The nature of the procedure
   b. The importance of remaining immobile
   c. Pressure sensations to be experienced
   d. That no discomfort is anticipated after the procedure

4. Make the patient comfortable with adequate supports (see Fig. 24–14). If possible, place him upright and in one of the following positions:
   a. Sitting on the edge of the bed with the feet supported and his arms and head on a padded over-the-bed table
   b. Straddling a chair with his arms and head resting on the back of the chair
   c. Lying on his unaffected side with the bed elevated 30 to 45 degrees if he is unable to assume a sitting position

5. Support and reassure the patient during the procedure.
   a. Prepare the patient for cold sensation of skin germicide solution and of pressure sensation from infiltration of local anesthetic agent.
   b. Encourage the patient to refrain from coughing.

6. Expose the entire chest. The site for aspiration is determined from chest x-ray films and by percussion. If fluid is in the pleural cavity, the thoracentesis site is determined by the chest x-ray films, ultrasound scanning, and physical findings, with attention to site of maximal dullness on percussion.

7. The procedure is performed under aseptic conditions. After the skin is cleansed, a local anesthetic is injected slowly with a small-caliber needle into the intercostal space by the physician.

8. The physician advances the thoracentesis needle with the syringe attached. When the pleural space is reached, suction may be applied with the syringe.
   a. A 20-ml syringe with a three-way adapter (stopcock) is attached to the needle (one end of the adapter is attached to the needle and the other to the tubing leading to a receptacle that receives the fluid being aspirated).

Amplification/Rationale

1. Posteroanterior and lateral chest x-ray films are used to localize fluid and air in the pleural cavity and to aid in determining the puncture site. Ultrasound scanning is performed when fluid is loculated (isolated in a pocket of pleural fluid) to help select the best site for needle aspiration.

3. An explanation helps to orient the patient to the procedure, assists him to mobilize his resources, and gives him an opportunity to ask questions and verbalize anxiety.

4. The upright position facilitates the removal of fluid that usually localizes at the base of the chest. A position of comfort helps the patient to relax.

5. Sudden and unexpected movement by the patient can cause trauma to the visceral pleura with resultant trauma to the lung.

6. If air is in the pleural cavity, the thoracentesis site is usually in the second or third intercostal space in the midclavicular line. Air rises in the thorax because the density of the air is much less than the density of liquid.

7. An intradermal wheal is raised slowly; rapid injection causes pain. The parietal pleura is very sensitive and should be well infiltrated with anesthetic before the thoracentesis needle is passed through it. To minimize intercostal artery laceration, the needle is inserted into the intercostal space just above the lower rib.

   a. When a large quantity of fluid is withdrawn, a three-way adapter serves to keep air from entering the pleural cavity.

(continued)

Chart 24-1 *(Continued)*

Nursing Activities	*Amplification/Rationale*
b. If a considerable quantity of fluid is removed, the needle is held in place on the chest wall with a small hemostat.	b. The hemostat steadies the needle on the chest wall. Sudden pleuritic chest pain or shoulder pain may indicate that the visceral or diaphragmatic pleurae are being irritated by the needle point.
9. After the needle is withdrawn, pressure is applied over the puncture site and a small, sterile dressing is fixed in place.	
10. The patient is placed on bed rest. A chest x-ray film is obtained after thoracentesis.	10. A chest x-ray film verifies that there is no pneumothorax.
11. Record the total amount of fluid withdrawn and the nature of the fluid, its color, and its viscosity. If requested, prepare samples of fluid for laboratory evaluation. A specimen container with formalin may be needed if a pleural biopsy is to be obtained.	11. The fluid may be clear, serous, bloody, purulent, etc.
12. Evaluate the patient at intervals for increasing respiratory rate asymmetry in respiratory movement; faintness; vertigo; tightness in chest; uncontrollable cough; blood-tinged, frothy mucus; a rapid pulse, and signs of hypoxemia.	12. Pneumothorax, tension pneumothorax, subcutaneous emphysema, or pyrogenic infection may result from a thoracentesis. Pulmonary edema or cardiac distress can be produced by a sudden shift in mediastinal contents when large amounts of fluid are aspirated.

Transtracheal aspiration bypasses the oropharynx and thus avoids specimen contamination by mouth flora, particularly anaerobes. It is of special value to the immunocompromised patient with pneumonia who does not produce sputum.

The patient is observed for several hours after the procedure. Possible complications include intratracheal bleeding, hypoxemia, cardiac dysrhythmias, pneumomediastinum, subcutaneous emphysema, and infection.

Thoracentesis

A thin layer of pleural fluid normally remains in the pleural space. A sample of this fluid can be obtained by thoracentesis or by tube thoracotomy. Thoracentesis is the aspiration of pleural fluid for diagnostic or therapeutic purposes (Fig. 24-14).

A needle biopsy of the pleura may be performed at the same time. Guidelines for assisting the patient undergoing a thoracentesis are presented in Chart 24-1. Studies of pleural fluid include Gram stain culture and sensitivity, acid-fast staining and culture, differential cell count, cytology, pH, specific gravity, total protein, and lactic dehydrogenase.

Pleural Biopsy

Pleural biopsy is accomplished by needle biopsy of the pleura or by pleuroscopy, which is a visual exploration of the pleural space through a fiberoptic bronchoscope inserted into the pleural space. Pleural biopsy is performed when there is pleural exudate of undetermined origin and when there is need for pathologic tissue staining or tissue culture for tuberculosis and fungi.

Pulmonary Function Tests

Pulmonary function tests are performed to assess respiratory function and to detect and determine the extent of the abnormality. Such tests include measurements of lung volumes, ventilatory function, mechanics of breathing, diffusion, and gas exchange.

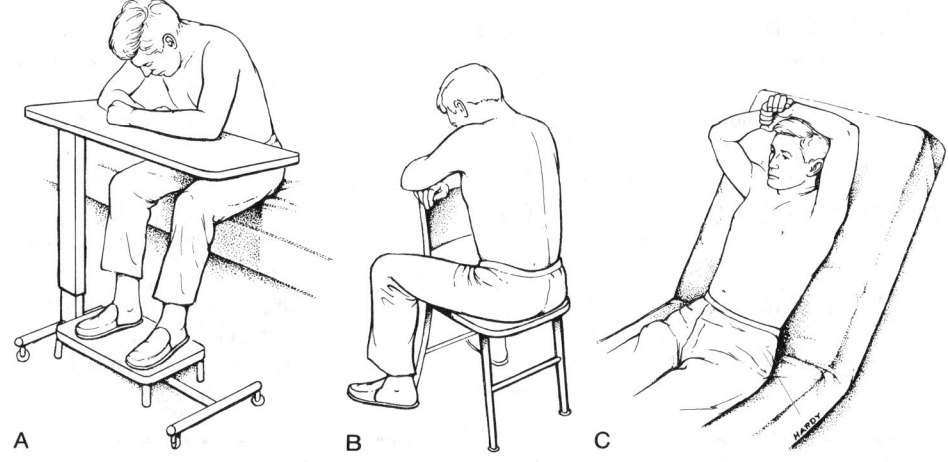

Figure 24-14. Positioning the patient for a thoracentesis. The nurse assists the patient to one of three positions, and offers comfort and support throughout the procedure. (**A**) Sitting on the edge of the bed with his head and arms on and over the bed table. (**B**) Straddling a chair with his arms and head resting on the back of the chair. (**C**) Lying on his unaffected side with the bed elevated 30 to 45 degrees. (Suddarth DS. The Lippincott Manual of Nursing Practice, 5th ed. Philadelphia, JB Lippincott, 1991.)

Pulmonary function tests are useful in following the course of a patient with established respiratory disease and assessing response to therapy. They are useful as screening tests in potentially hazardous industries, such as coal mining and those that involve exposure to asbestos and other noxious fumes, dusts, or gases. Preoperatively, they are useful for patients scheduled for thoracic and upper abdominal surgery, patients with a history of smoking and cough, obese patients, older patients, and patients with pulmonary disease.

Pulmonary function tests generally are performed by a technician. They require a spirometer that has a volume-collecting device attached to a recorder that demonstrates volume and time simultaneously. Pulmonary function testing is moving toward computerization; some systems measure multiple parameters. Smaller hospitals, by using a data transmitter, can send test information to a larger medical facility's computer for analysis.

A number of function tests are carried out because no single measurement provides a complete picture of pulmonary function. Usually, test results are interpreted on the basis of degree of deviation from normal, taking into consideration the patient's height, weight, age, and sex. Normal values have been established and are available in manufacturer's handbooks or with pulmonary function equipment.

Because there is a wide range of normal values, pulmonary function tests may not detect early localized changes. The patient with respiratory symptoms (dyspnea, wheezing, cough, sputum production) usually undergoes a complete diagnostic evaluation, even though the results of pulmonary function tests are ''normal.''

The most frequently used pulmonary function tests are described in Table 24–1 and Table 24–6.

Arterial Blood Gas Studies

Measurements of blood pH and of arterial oxygen and carbon dioxide tensions are obtained when managing patients with respiratory problems and in adjusting oxygen therapy as needed. The arterial oxygen tension (PaO_2) indicates the degree of oxygenation of the blood, and the arterial carbon dioxide tension ($PaCO_2$) indicates adequacy of alveolar ventilation. Arterial blood gas studies aid in assessing the degree to which the lungs are able to provide adequate oxygen and remove carbon dioxide and the degree to which the kidneys are able to reabsorb or excrete bicarbonate ions to maintain normal body pH. Serial blood gas analysis is also a sensitive indicator of whether the lung has been damaged after chest trauma. Arterial blood gases are obtained through an arterial puncture at the radial, brachial, or femoral artery or through an indwelling arterial catheter.

Radioisotope Diagnostic Procedures (Lung Scan)

There are three types of lung scans: perfusion scan, ventilation scan, and inhalation scan. They are used to detect normal lung functioning, pulmonary vascular supply, and gas exchange.

A *perfusion lung scan* is performed by injecting a radioactive agent (technetium) into a peripheral vein and then obtaining a scan of the chest and body to detect radiation. The isotope particles pass through the right side of the heart and are distributed into the lungs in amounts proportional to the

TABLE 24–6. *Pulmonary Function Tests*

Term Used	Symbol	Description	Remarks
Forced vital capacity	FVC	Vital capacity performed with a maximally forced expiratory effort	Forced vital capacity is often reduced in COPD because of air trapping.
Forced expiratory volume (qualified by subscript indicating the time intervals in seconds)	FEVt, usually FEV$_1$	Volume of air exhaled in the specified time during the performance of forced vital capacity	A valuable clue to the severity of the expiratory airway obstruction.
Ratio of timed forced expiratory volume to forced vital capacity	FEVt/FVC%, usually FEV$_1$/FVC%	FEVt expressed as a percentage of the forced vital capacity	Another way of expressing the presence or absence of airway obstruction.
Forced expiratory flow	FEF$_{200-1200}$	Mean forced expiratory flow between 200 and 1200 ml of the FVC	Formerly called maximum expiratory flow rate (MEFR). An indicator of large airway obstruction.
Forced midexpiratory flow	FEF$_{25\%-75\%}$	Mean forced expiratory flow during the middle half of the FVC	Formerly called maximum and midexpiratory flow rate. Slowed in small airway obstruction.
Forced end expiratory flow	FEF$_{75\%-85\%}$	Mean forced expiratory flow during the terminal portion of the FVC	Slowed in obstruction of smallest airways.
Maximal voluntary ventilation	MVV	Volume of air expired in a specified period (12 seconds) during repetitive maximal effort	Formerly called maximum breathing capacity. An important factor in exercise tolerance.

regional blood flow, making it possible to trace and measure the blood perfusion through the lung. This procedure is used clinically to measure the integrity of the pulmonary vessels relative to blood flow and to evaluate blood flow abnormalities as seen in pulmonary emboli. The nurse informs the patient that the imaging time is 20 to 40 minutes, that he will lie under the camera, and that a mask will be fitted over his nose and mouth during the test.

A *ventilation scan* is performed after the perfusion scan. The patient takes a deep breath of a mixture of oxygen and radioactive gas (xenon, krypton), which diffuses throughout the lungs. A scan is performed to detect ventilation abnormalities, especially in patients who have regional differences in ventilation. It may be helpful in the diagnosis of bronchitis, asthma, inflammatory fibrosis, pneumonia, emphysema, and lung cancer.

An *inhalation scan* is performed by administering droplets of radioactive material by a positive-pressure ventilator. This scan is helpful, particularly in visualizing the trachea and major airways.

The *gallium scan* is a radioisotope lung scan used to detect inflammatory conditions, abscesses, adhesions, and the presence, location, and size of tumors. It is used to stage bronchogenic cancer and record tumor regression after chemotherapy or radiation.

Lung Biopsy Procedures

When the chest x-ray film is inconclusive or shows pulmonary density (indicating an infiltrate or lesion), it is desirable to examine lung tissue to establish the nature of the lesion. There are several nonsurgical lung biopsy techniques that are used because they yield accurate information with low morbidity: (1) transcatheter bronchial brushing, (2) percutaneous (through the skin) needle biopsy, or (3) transbronchial lung biopsy.

In *transcatheter bronchial brushing,* a fiberoptic bronchoscope is introduced into the bronchus under fluoroscopy. A small brush is attached to the end of a flexible wire, which is inserted through the fiberscope. Under direct vision, the area under suspicion is brushed back and forth, causing cells to slough off and adhere to the brush. The bronchoscopic catheter may be irrigated with saline to secure material for additional studies. The brush is removed from the bronchoscope and a microscopic slide is made. Sometimes the brush is cut off and sent to the laboratory for pathologic tests.

This procedure is useful for cytologic evaluations of lung lesions and for the identification of pathogenic organisms (*Nocardia, Aspergillus, Pneumocystis carinii,* and other pathogens). It is especially useful in the immunologically compromised patient.

A consent form is signed before this procedure; the nurse provides explanations and clarifies questions that the patient may have. After the procedure, the patient may have a mild sore throat and transient hemoptysis. Fluids and food are withheld for several hours after the procedure. Possible complications include anesthetic reactions, laryngospasm, hemoptysis, and, rarely, pneumothorax.

Another method of bronchial brushing involves the introduction of the catheter through the transcricothyroid membrane by needle puncture. After this procedure, the patient is instructed to hold his thumb over the puncture site while coughing to prevent air from leaking into the surrounding tissues.

Percutaneous needle biopsy may be accomplished with a cutting needle or by aspiration with a spinal-type needle that provides a tissue specimen for histologic study. A *transbronchial lung biopsy* uses cutting forceps introduced by fiberoptic bronchoscope. This study is indicated when a lung lesion is suspected and routine sputum samples and bronchoscopic washings are negative.

A narcotic analgesic may be prescribed before the procedure. The skin over the biopsy site is cleansed and anesthetized, and a small incision is made. The biopsy needle is inserted through the incision into the pleura while the patient holds his breath in midexpiration. With flouroscopic monitoring, the surgeon guides the needle into the periphery of the lesion and obtains a tissue sample from the mass. Possible complications include pneumothorax, pulmonary hemorrhage, and empyema.

Lymph Node Biopsy

The scalene lymph nodes are enmeshed in the deep cervical pad of fat overlying the scalenus anterior muscle. They drain the lungs and mediastinum and may show histologic changes due to intrathoracic disease. When these nodes are palpable on physical examination, a biopsy may be in order. A biopsy of these nodes may be performed to detect lymph node spread of pulmonary disease and to establish a diagnosis or prognosis in such diseases as Hodgkin's disease, sarcoidosis, fungal disease, tuberculosis, and carcinoma.

Mediastinoscopy is the endoscopic examination of the mediastinum for exploration and biopsy of mediastinal lymph nodes that drain the lungs, without requiring a thoracotomy. Biopsy is usually performed through a suprasternal incision. Mediastinoscopy is carried out to detect mediastinal involvement of pulmonary malignancy and to obtain tissue for diagnostic studies of other conditions (*e.g.,* sarcoidosis).

An *anterior mediastinotomy* is thought to provide better exposure and diagnostic possibilities than a mediastinoscopy. An incision is made in the area of the second or third costal cartilage. The mediastinum is explored, and biopsies are performed on any lymph nodes found. Chest tube drainage is required after the procedure. This diagnostic modality is particularly valuable to determine whether a pulmonary lesion is resectable.

Laser Detection

Currently, the laser is used experimentally in the detection and photoradiation of early bronchogenic carcinoma. Two or three days after the intravenous injection of a hematoporphyrin derivative, the violet light of an argon or krypton laser can be used to detect early bronchogenic carcinoma.

Chapter Summary

In summary, diagnosis of respiratory diseases is determined after complete history, physical exam, and diagnostic studies. A variety of diagnostic tests may be performed to assist in the determination of respiratory conditions, including chest radiography, CT scan, PET scan, pulmonary angiography, bronchoscopy, thoracentesis, sputum studies, arterial blood gas studies, lung scan, and lymph node biopsy. After identifying critical portions of the history, alterations in the physical examination, and abnormal findings in diagnostic studies, the physician will make a determination of the underlying respiratory disease.

The patient undergoing extensive diagnostic evaluation for respiratory disorders is often short of breath, fatigued, and anxious about the results of the diagnostic tests. Support and psychological preparation for the tests often reduce the patient's fears and anxieties. Repeated tests may add to the patient's fatigue and discomfort; therefore, the patient may require assistance in performing activities of daily living.

Bibliography

Books

Bates B. A Guide to Physical Examination and History-Taking, 5th ed. Philadelphia, JB Lippincott, 1991.

Baum GL and Wolinsky E (eds). Textbook of Pulmonary Diseases, 4th ed. Boston, Little, Brown, 1983.

Burton GG and Hodgkin JE (eds). Respiratory Care: A Guide to Clinical Practice, 2nd ed. Philadelphia, JB Lippincott, 1984.

Comroe JH et al. The Lung, Clinical Physiology and Pulmonary Function Tests. 2nd ed. Chicago, Yearbook Medical Publishers, 1977.

Fishman AP. Pulmonary Diseases and Disorders, 2nd ed, Vol 1. New York, McGraw–Hill, 1988.

Guyton AC. Textbook of Medical Physiology, 7th ed. Philadelphia, WB Saunders, 1986.

Kersten LD. Comprehensive Respiratory Nursing. Philadelphia, WB Saunders, 1989.

Kinney MR et al. AACN's Clinical Reference for Critical Care Nursing, 2nd ed. New York, McGraw–Hill, 1988.

Murray JF and Nadel JA. The Textbook of Respiratory Medicine, 2nd ed. Vols 1 & 2. Philadelphia, WB Saunders, 1988.

Pennington JE (ed). Respiratory Infections: Diagnosis and Management, 2nd ed. New York, Raven Press, 1989.

Putman CE (ed). Lung Biology in Health & Disease: Diagnostic Imaging of the Lung, Vol 46. New York, Marcel Dekker, 1990.

Shapiro BA et al. Clinical Application of Respiratory Care, 3rd ed. Chicago, Year Book Medical Publishers, 1985.

Shapiro BA et al. Clinical Application of Blood Gases, 3rd ed. Chicago, Mosby–Year Book, 1989.

Thibodeau GA and Anthony CP. Structure and Function of the Body. St Louis, Times Mirror/Mosby College Publishing. 1988.

West JB. Respiratory Physiology, 4th ed. Baltimore, Williams & Wilkins, 1990.

Journals

Barbee RA. The medical history in pulmonary disease. Respir Care 1984 Jan; 29(1): 68–75.

Carrieri VK et al. The sensation of dyspnea: A review. Heart Lung 1984 Jul; 13(4): 436–447.

Clausen JL. Clinical interpretation of pulmonary function tests. Respir Care 1989 Jul; 34(7): 638–645.

Crapo RO. Reference values for lung function tests. Respir Care 1989 Jul; 34 (7) 626–633.

Gardner RM et al. Spirometry and flow volume curves. Clin Chest Med 1989 Jun; 10(2): 145–154.

Gift AG. Clinical measurement of dyspnea. Dimens Crit Care Nurs 1989 Apr; 8(4): 210–214.

Gift AG. Dyspnea. Nurs Clin North Am 1990 Dec; 25(4): 955–965.

Leitman BS and Naidich DP. Computerized tomography of the chest: Indications and basic interpretation (Part 1). Hosp Med 1990 Aug; 26(8) 114–128.

Leitman BS and Naidich DP. Computerized tomography of the chest: Indications and basic interpretation (Part 2). Hosp Med 1990 Sep; 26(9) 75–88.

Marini JJ. Lung mechanics determinations at the bedside: Instrumentation and clinical application. Respir Care 1990 Jul; 35(7): 669–696.

Mehta AC et al. Transbronchial needle aspiration for histology specimens. Chest 1989 Jun; 96(6): 1228–1332.

Munro NC et al. Chest pain in chronic sputum production: A neglected symptom. Respir Med 1989 Jul; 83(4): 339–341.

Pierson DJ. Measuring and monitoring lung volumes outside the pulmonary function laboratory. Respir Care 1990 Jul; 35(7): 660–668.

Raffin TA. Shortness of breath: Differential diagnosis. Hosp Med 1989 May; 25(5): 98–127.

Ries AL. Measurement of lung volumes. Clin Chest Med 1989 Jun; 10(2): 177–186.

Stevens RP. Flexible fiberoptic bronchoscopy. Hosp Med 1990 Jun; 26(6): 43–49.

Stoller JK. Pulmonary function-testing as a screening technique. Respir Care 1989 Jul; 34(7): 611–621.

Wilkins RL et al. Lung-sound terminology used by respiratory care practitioners. Respir Care 1989 Jan; 34(1): 36–41.

Wolkore N et al. The relationship between pulmonary function and dyspnea in obstructive lung disease. Chest 1989 Dec; 96(6): 1247–1251.

Information/Resources

Agencies
Governmental
National Heart, Lung and Blood Institute
National Institutes of Health, 900 Rockville Pike, Bldg 31, Bethesda, MD 20892, (301) 496-5166

Voluntary
American Association for Respiratory Care
1720 Regal Row, Dallas, TX 75235, (214) 630-3540
American Lung Association
1740 Broadway, New York, NY 10019, (212) 315-8700
American Thoracic Society
1740 Broadway, New York, NY 10019, (212) 315-8700

25

Respiratory Care Modalities

Learning Objectives

On completion of this chapter, the learner will be able to:

1. Describe the nursing management for patients receiving oxygen therapy, intermittent positive-pressure breathing, mini-nebulizer therapy, incentive spirometry, chest physiotherapy, and breathing retraining
2. Describe the nursing care for a patient with an endotracheal tube and for a patient with a tracheostomy
3. Demonstrate the procedure of tracheal suctioning
4. Use the nursing process as a framework for care of patients who are mechanically ventilated
5. Describe the significance of preoperative nursing assessment and patient teaching for the patient who is to have thoracic surgery
6. Explain the principles of chest drainage and the nursing responsibilities related to the care of the patient with water-seal drainage
7. Describe the patient education and home care considerations for patients who have had thoracic surgery

The Patient Requiring Specific Management of Respiratory Conditions

A wide variety of treatment modalities are used when caring for patients with different types of respiratory conditions. The choice of modality is based on the oxygenation disorder, that is, whether there is a problem with gas ventilation, diffusion, or both. Therapies range from simple, noninvasive ones (oxygen and nebulizer therapy, chest physiotherapy, breathing retraining) to complex, highly invasive ones (intubation, mechanical ventilation, surgery). Assessment and treatment of the respiratory patient is best accomplished when the approach is multidisciplinary and collaborative.

Oxygen Therapy

Oxygen therapy is the administration of oxygen at a concentration of pressure greater than that found in the environmental atmosphere. The concentration of oxygen in room air at sea level is 21%. The goal of oxygen therapy is to provide adequate transport of oxygen in the blood while decreasing the work of breathing and stress on the myocardium.

Oxygen transport to the tissues depends on factors such as cardiac output, arterial oxygen content, adequate concentration of hemoglobin, and metabolic requirements. All of these must be considered when oxygen therapy is considered. (Respiratory physiology and oxygen transport are discussed in Chap. 24.)

Assessment. A change in the patient's respiratory rate or pattern may be one of the earliest indicators of the need for oxygen therapy. The clinical signs of *hypoxemia* (a decrease in the arterial oxygen tension in the *blood*) include changes in mental status (progressing through impaired judgment, agitation, disorientation, confusion, lethargy, and coma) dyspnea, increase in blood pressure, changes in heart rate, dysrhythmias, central cyanosis (late sign), diaphoresis, and cool extremities. Hypoxemia usually leads to *hypoxia*, which is a decrease in oxygen supply to the *tissues*. Hypoxia, if severe enough, can be life-threatening.

The signs and symptoms of the need for oxygen may depend on how suddenly this need develops. With rapidly developing hypoxia there are changes in the central nervous system because the higher centers are more sensitive to oxygen deprivation. The clinical picture may resemble that of drunkenness, with the patient exhibiting incoordination and impaired judgment. Long-standing hypoxia (as seen in chronic obstructive pulmonary disease [COPD] and chronic congestive heart failure) may produce fatigue, drowsiness, apathy, inattentiveness, and delayed reaction time. The need for oxygen is assessed by arterial blood gas analysis (p. 519) as well as by clinical evaluation.

Types and Treatment of Hypoxia.   Hypoxia can occur from either severe pulmonary disease (inadequate supply) or from extrapulmonary disease (inadequate delivery) affecting gas exchange at the cellular level. The four general types of hypoxia are (1) hypoxemic hypoxia, (2) circulatory hypoxia, (3) anemic hypoxia, and (4) histotoxic hypoxia.

Hypoxemic hypoxia is a decreased oxygen level in the blood resulting in decreased oxygen diffusion into the tissues. It may be caused by hypoventilation, high altitudes, and pulmonary diffusion defects; it is corrected by increasing alveolar ventilation or providing supplemental oxygen.

Circulatory hypoxia is hypoxia from inadequate capillary circulation. It may be caused by decreased cardiac output, local vascular obstruction, low-flow states such as shock, or cardiac arrest. Although tissue partial pressure of oxygen (Po_2) is reduced, arterial Po_2 remains normal. Circulatory hypoxia is corrected by identifying and treating the underlying cause.

Anemic hypoxia is a result of decreased effective hemoglobin concentration, which causes a decreased oxygen-carrying capacity of the blood. It is rarely accompanied by hypoxemia. Because it reduces the oxygen-carrying capacity of hemoglobin, carbon monoxide poisoning, although similar, is not strictly anemic hypoxia because hemoglobin levels may be normal.

Histotoxic hypoxia occurs when a toxic substance, such as cyanide, interferes with the ability of tissues to use available oxygen.

Clinical Considerations.   As with other medications, oxygen is administered with care, and its effects on each patient are carefully assessed. Oxygen is a drug and except in emergency situations is prescribed by a physician.

In general, patients with respiratory conditions are given oxygen therapy only to raise the arterial oxygen pressure (PaO_2) back to the patient's normal baseline, which may vary from 60 to 95 mm Hg. Referring to the oxyhemoglobin dissociation curve (see p. 503), at these levels the blood is 80% to 98% (also written as 0.80 to 0.98) saturated; higher inspired oxygen flow (FiO_2) values will not add further significant amounts of oxygen to the red blood cells or plasma. Instead of helping, increased amounts of oxygen possibly may suppress ventilation in certain types of pulmonary patients.

Excessive oxygen may produce toxic effects on the lungs and central nervous system or may result in depression of ventilation. For example, in patients with COPD, the stimulus for respiration is a decrease in blood oxygen rather than an elevation in carbon dioxide levels. Thus, sudden administration of a high concentration of oxygen will remove the respiratory drive that has been created largely by the patient's chronic low oxygen tension. This decrease in alveolar ventilation can cause a progressive increase in arterial carbon dioxide pressure ($PaCO_2$), ultimately leading to death from carbon dioxide narcosis and acidosis (see p. 332).

When oxygen is administered by any method, the patient is assessed frequently for often subtle indications of inadequate oxygenation: confusion, restlessness progressing to lethargy, diaphoresis, pallor tachycardia, tachypnea, and hypertension.

Other precautions to be taken when administering oxygen involve the careful handling of the equipment. Because oxygen supports combustion, there is always a danger of fire when oxygen is used. "No smoking" signs must be posted when oxygen is in use. Oxygen therapy equipment is also a potential source of bacterial cross-infection and thus the tubing is changed frequently, depending on infection control policy and the type of oxygen delivery equipment.

Oxygen Toxicity.   Oxygen is a drug and can cause serious side effects, such as oxygen-induced hypoventilation (prevented by giving low-flow oxygen rates of 1 to 2 L/min) and atelectasis. Perhaps the most serious and insidious hazard is oxygen toxicity, which may occur when too high a concentration of oxygen (over 50%) is administered for an extended period (more than 48 hours).

The pathophysiology of oxygen toxicity is not fully understood, but is related to a destruction and decrease of surfactant, the formation of a hyaline membrane lining the lung, and the development of pulmonary edema that is not cardiac in origin. Signs and symptoms of oxygen toxicity include substernal distress, paresthesias, dyspnea, restlessness, fatigue, malaise, progressive respiratory difficulty, and an alveolar pattern on the chest x-ray.

Prevention of oxygen toxicity is achieved by using oxygen according to prescription. If high concentrations of oxygen are necessary, the duration of administration is kept to a minimum and reduced as soon as possible.

Methods of Oxygen Administration

Oxygen is dispensed from a cylinder or from a piped-in system. A reduction gauge is necessary to reduce the pressure to a working level, and a flowmeter regulates the control of oxygen in liters per minute. When oxygen is used at high flow rates, it may be moistened by passing it through a humidification system to prevent the mucous membranes of the respiratory tract from becoming dry.

There are many different oxygen devices; all will deliver oxygen if used as prescribed and if the devices are used and maintained correctly (Table 25–1). The amount of oxygen delivered is expressed as a percentage concentration (as in 70%). The appropriate form of oxygen therapy is best determined by arterial blood gas levels, which indicate the patient's oxygenation status.

TABLE 25–1. *Oxygen Administration Devices*

Device	Suggested Flow Rate (L/min)	O₂ Percentage Setting	Advantages	Disadvantages
Cannula	1–2 3–5 6	23–30 30–40 42	Lightweight, comfortable, inexpensive, continuous use with meals and activity	Nasal mucosal drying, variable FiO₂
Catheter	1–6	23–42	Inexpensive	Variable FiO₂, requires frequent change (q8h), gastric distention
Mask, simple	6–8	40–60	Simple to use, inexpensive	Poor fitting, variable FiO₂, must remove to eat
Mask, partial rebreather	8–11	50–75	Moderate O₂ concentration	Warm, poor fitting, must remove to eat
Mask, nonrebreather	12	80–100	High O₂ concentration	Poor fitting
Mask, Venturi	4–6 6–8	24, 26, 28 30, 35, 40	Provides low levels of supplemental O₂ Precise FiO₂, additional humidity available	Must remove to eat
Mask, aerosol	8–10	30–100	Good humidity, accurate FiO₂	Uncomfortable for some
Tracheostomy collar	8–10	30–100	Good humidity, comfortable, fairly accurate FiO₂	
T-piece, Briggs	8–10	30–100	Same as tracheostomy collar	Heavy with tubing
Face tent	8–10	30–100	Good humidity, fairly accurate FiO₂	Bulky and cumbersome

The *nasal cannula* is used when the patient requires a low-to-medium concentration of oxygen for which precise accuracy is not essential. This method is relatively simple and allows the patient to move about in bed, talk, cough, and eat without interruption of oxygen flow. Flow rates in excess of 6 to 8 L/min may lead to air swallowing and cause irritation and drying of the nasal and pharyngeal mucosa.

The *oropharyngeal catheter* is rarely used but may be prescribed for short-term therapy to administer low to moderate concentrations of oxygen. This method can lead to irritation of the nasal mucosa. When oxygen is administered nasally (cannula or catheter), the percentage of oxygen reaching the lungs varies with the depth and rate of respirations, particularly if the nasal mucosa is swollen or the patient is a mouth breather.

Simple masks are used for low to moderate concentrations of oxygen, whereas *partial or nonrebreathing masks* are used for moderate to high concentrations of oxygen. Although popular, these masks cannot be used for controlled oxygen concentrations and must be adjusted for proper fit. They should not press too tightly against the skin, as this may cause a sense of claustrophobia; adjustable elastic bands are provided to ensure comfort and security. Bags on partial and nonrebreather masks must remain inflated during both inspiration and expiration. This is accomplished by adjusting the flow so the bag does not collapse on inspiration.

The *Venturi mask* (Fig. 25–1) is the most reliable and accurate method for delivering precise oxygen concentration. The mask is constructed in such a way as to allow a constant flow of room air blended with a fixed flow of oxygen. It is used primarily for patients with COPD because it can provide low levels of supplemental oxygen, thus avoiding the risk of suppressing the hypoxic drive.

The Venturi mask employs the principle of air entrainment (trapping the air like a vacuum), which provides a high air flow with controlled oxygen enrichment. Excess gas leaves the mask through the perforated cuff, carrying with it the exhaled carbon dioxide. This method allows inhalation of a constant oxygen concentration regardless of the depth or rate of respiration.

The mask should fit snugly enough to prevent oxygen flow into the eyes, and the patient's skin is checked for irritation. The mask must be removed so that the patient may eat, drink, and take medications.

Aerosol masks, tracheostomy collars, and *face tents* are used with aerosol devices (nebulizers) that can be adjusted for oxygen concentrations in ranges from 27% to 100% (0.27 to 1.00). If the gas mixture flow falls below patient demand, room air will be pulled in, diluting the concentration. The aerosol mist must be available constantly for the patient during the entire inspiratory phase.

Oxygen concentrators are another means of providing varying amounts of oxygen, especially in the home setting. These devices are relatively portable, easy to operate, and cost effective. They also require more maintenance than tank or liquid systems, however, and probably cannot consistently deliver flows in excess of 4 liters (which provides an FiO₂ of approximately 36%).

Home Health Care. At times oxygen must be administered

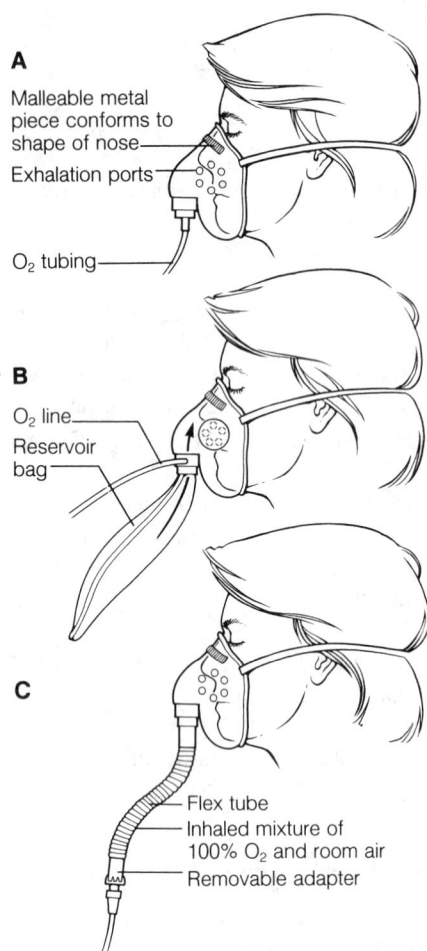

A
Malleable metal piece conforms to shape of nose
Exhalation ports
O₂ tubing

B
O₂ line
Reservoir bag

C
Flex tube
Inhaled mixture of 100% O₂ and room air
Removable adapter

Figure 25–1. Types of oxygen masks used to deliver varying concentrations of oxygen. (**A**) Simple face mask. (**B**) Partial rebreathing mask. The exhalation ports may be sealed to provide higher concentrations of oxygen. (**C**) Venturi mask.

to the patient at home. The patient or family should be instructed in the methods for administering oxygen and should be informed that oxygen is available in gas, liquid, and concentrated forms. The gas and liquid forms come in portable devices so that the patient can leave his home while receiving oxygen therapy. Humidity must be provided while oxygen is used (except with portable devices) to counteract the dry, irritating effects of compressed oxygen on the airway.

To maintain a consistent quality of care and to maximize the patient's financial reimbursement for home oxygen therapy, the nurse ensures that the physician's order includes the disorder, the prescribed oxygen flow, and conditions for use (*e.g.*, continuous use, nighttime use only).

Intermittent Positive-Pressure Breathing

Intermittent positive pressure breathing (IPPB) is the breathing of air or oxygen (or a combination of both) at a pressure higher than atmospheric pressure to produce air flow into the lungs during inhalation. IPPB is applied by a mechanical device that inflates the lungs through positive pressure, dispersing a pre-

scribed medication. When the patient inhales, the negative inspiratory force triggers the machine to deliver a positive-pressure breath; after a preset pressure is reached on the machine, the machine cycles off and there is passive exhalation. The IPPB machine may be powered by electricity or gas and may be connected with a mouthpiece, mask, or tracheostomy adapter.

Indications.   The use and indications for IPPB therapy have decreased in recent years, because of its inherent hazards. General indications include: difficulty in raising respiratory secretions, reduced vital capacity (VC) with ineffective deep breathing and coughing, or unsuccessful trials of simpler and cheaper methods of secretion mobilization, aerosol deposition, and lung expansion.

Complications of IPPB.   Intermittent positive-pressure breathing can cause pneumothorax, mucosal drying, increased intracranial pressure, hemoptysis, gastric distention, vomiting with possible aspiration, psychological dependency (especially with long-term use, as in COPD), hyperventilation, excessive oxygen administration and cardiovascular problems.

Mini-Nebulizer Therapy

The mini-nebulizer is a hand-held apparatus that disperses a liquid (medication) into microscopic particles and delivers it to the lungs as the patient inhales. The mini-nebulizer is usually air-driven by means of a compressor through connecting tubing. In some instances, the nebulizer is oxygen-driven rather than air-driven. To be effective, a visible mist must be available for the patient to inhale.

Indications.   The indications for use of a mini-nebulizer are similar to the indications for IPPB except that the patient must be able to generate a deep breath without the aid of the positive-pressure machine. Diaphragmatic breathing is helpful as a technique to prepare for the proper use of the mini-nebulizer. Mini-nebulizers frequently are used for patients with COPD to dispense inhaled medications and commonly are used at home on a long-term basis.

Nursing Considerations.   The patient breathes through his mouth, taking slow, deep breaths. The nurse instructs the patient to hold his breath for a few seconds at the end of inspiration to increase intrapleural pressure and reopen collapsed alveoli, thereby increasing functional residual capacity (see Chap. 24). The patient is encouraged to cough and to evaluate his progress with the therapy. He is instructed in proper cleaning and storing of the equipment if it is to be used at home.

Incentive Spirometry (Sustained Maximum Inspiration)

The incentive spirometer gives visual feedback to guide the patient to inhale slowly and deeply to maximize lung inflation (Fig. 25–2). The patient is placed in a sitting or semi-Fowler's position, as the diaphragmatic excursion is greater with this posture. This treatment may be performed with the patient in any position, however. Incentive spirometers may be one of two types: volume or flow. The tidal volume of the spirometer is set according to the manufacturer's instructions. The purpose

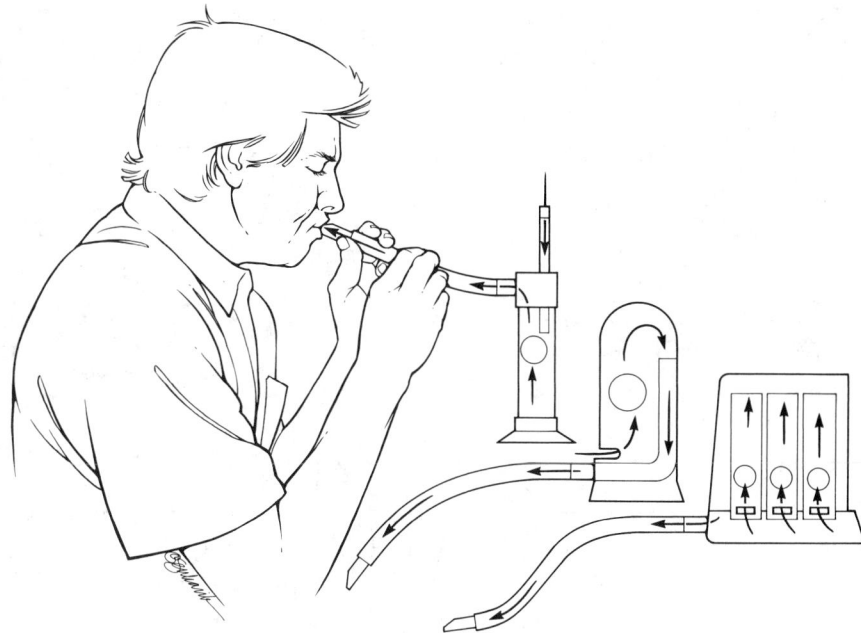

Figure 25–2. Flow incentive spirometer. Patients are instructed to inhale briskly to elevate the balls and to keep them floating for as long as possible. The volume inhaled is estimated and variable.

of the device is to measure a gradually increasing inhaled volume as the patient takes deeper and deeper breaths. The patient takes a deep breath through the mouthpiece, pauses at peak inflation, then relaxes and exhales. To avoid fatigue he should take several normal breaths before attempting another with the incentive spirometer. The volume is periodically increased as tolerated. A flow spirometer has the same purpose as a volume spirometer but the volume is not preset. Volume and flow are grossly estimated by the number of balls and length of time freely movable balls are held suspended in the air.

Indications. Incentive spirometry is used postoperatively, especially after thoracic and abdominal surgery to prevent or treat atelectasis. As prophylaxis, incentive spirometry may be more effective than IPPB because it maximizes inspiratory flow while maintaining relatively low airway pressures.

Nursing Considerations. Nursing management of the patient using incentive spirometry includes the following:

- Explaining the reason for therapy
- Assessing and medicating the patient for pain before beginning therapy.
- Positioning the patient in semi-Fowler's or an upright position (although any position is acceptable)
- Teaching the patient to use diaphragmatic breathing (p. 530)
- Instructing the patient to hold his breath at the end of inspiration (for 3 seconds), then to exhale slowly
- Encouraging coughing during and after each session
- Helping the patient splint the incision while coughing postoperatively
- Setting a reasonable volume and repetition goal (so as not to discourage the patient)
- Placing the spirometer within the patient's reach
- Beginning therapy immediately postoperatively (atelectasis can start within 1 hour after hypoventilation begins)
- Encouraging approximately 10 breaths with the spirometer per hour while awake

- Recording effectiveness and number of breaths achieved with the spirometer every 2 hours

Chest Physiotherapy

Chest physiotherapy includes postural drainage, chest percussion and vibration, breathing exercises/breathing retraining, and effective coughing. The goals of chest physiotherapy are removal of bronchial secretions, improved ventilation, and increased efficiency of the respiratory musculature.

Postural Drainage (Segmented Bronchial Drainage)

Postural drainage is the use of specific positions so the force of gravity can assist in the removal of bronchial secretions. The secretions drain from the affected bronchioles into the bronchi and trachea and are removed by means of coughing or suctioning. It is used to prevent or relieve bronchial obstruction due to secretions.

Because the patient is usually in an upright position, secretions are likely to accumulate in the lower parts of the lungs. When postural drainage is used, the patient is positioned sequentially in different postures (Fig. 25–3), so that the force of gravity helps to drain secretions from the smaller bronchial airways to the main bronchi and trachea. The secretions then are removed by coughing. Inhalation of prescribed bronchodilators and mucolytic agents before postural drainage assists in draining the bronchial tree.

Postural drainage exercises can be directed at any of the segments (bilateral) of the lung. The lower and middle lobe bronchi empty more effectively when the head is down; the upper lobe bronchi empty more effectively when the head is up. Frequently, the patient is placed in five positions, one for

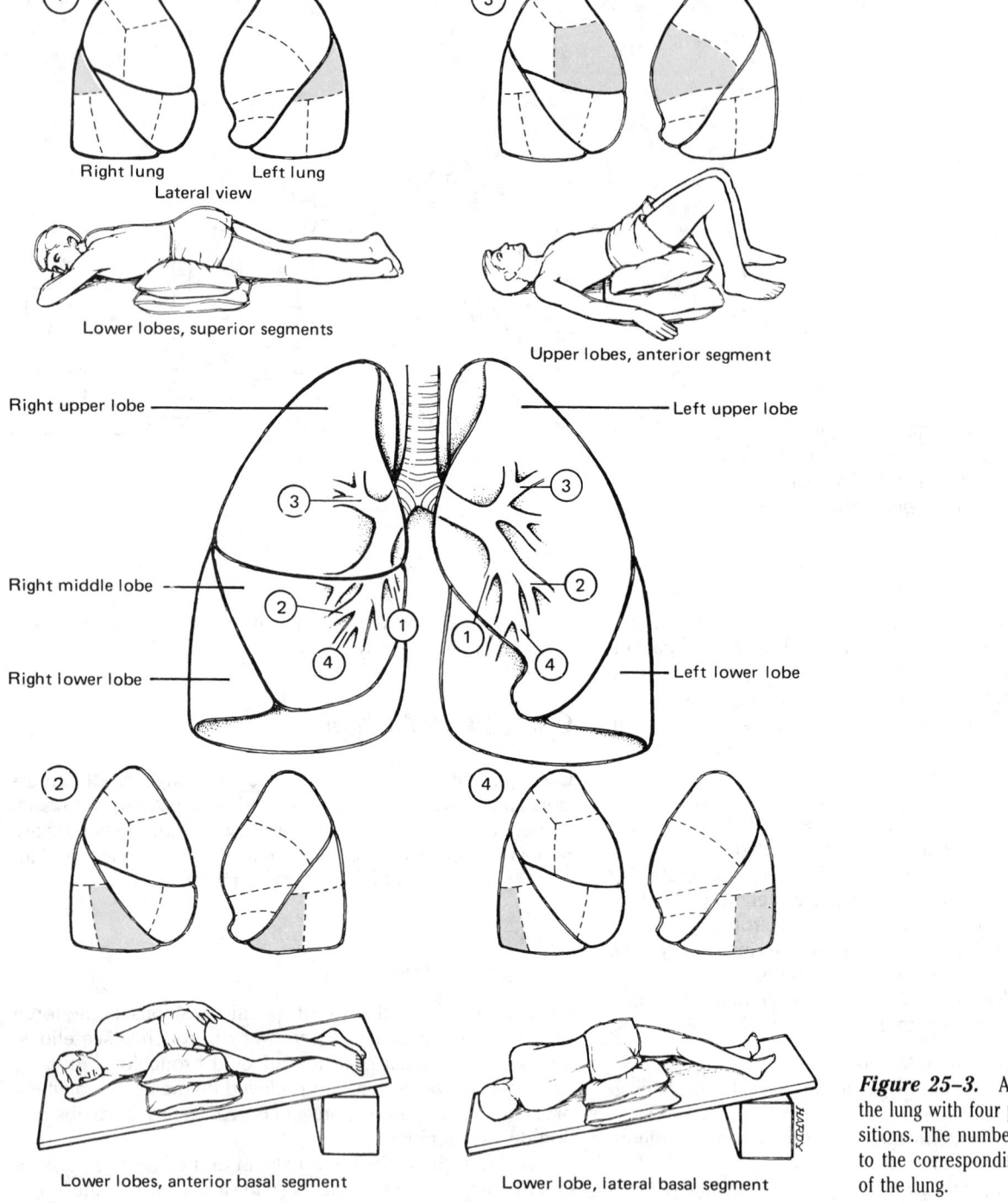

Figure 25–3. Anatomic segments of the lung with four postural drainage positions. The numbers relate the position to the corresponding anatomic segment of the lung.

drainage of each lobe: head down, prone, right and left lateral, and sitting upright.

Nursing Interventions.   The nurse should be aware of the patient's diagnosis as well as the lung lobes or segments involved, the cardiac status, and any structural deformities of the chest wall and spine. To identify the areas needing drainage and the effectiveness of treatment, the chest is auscultated before and after the procedure. This gives immediate feedback on the effectiveness of treatment.

Postural drainage is usually performed two to four times daily, before meals (to prevent nausea, vomiting, and aspiration) and at bedtime. If prescribed, bronchodilators, water, or saline may be nebulized and inhaled before postural drainage to dilate the bronchial tubes, reduce bronchospasm, decrease thickness of mucus and sputum, and combat edema of the bronchial walls. The patient is made as comfortable as possible in each position, and an emesis basin, sputum cup, and paper tissues are provided. The patient is instructed to remain in each position for 10 to 15 minutes and to breathe in slowly through his nose and then breathe out slowly through pursed lips to help keep airways open so that secretions can be drained while the various positions are assumed. If he cannot tolerate the position, he is helped to assume a modified posture. When the patient changes position, he is instructed to cough and remove secretions as follows:

1. Assume a sitting position and bend slightly forward because the upright position permits a stronger cough.
2. Keep the knees and hips flexed to promote relaxation and lessen the strain on the abdominal muscles while coughing.
3. Inhale slowly through the nose and exhale through pursed lips several times.
4. Cough twice during each exhalation while contracting (pulling in) the abdomen sharply with each cough.
5. Splint the incision, using pillow support, if necessary.

The secretions may need to be suctioned mechanically if the patient is unable to cough. It also may be necessary to use chest percussion and vibration to loosen bronchial secretions and mucus plugs that adhere to the bronchioles and bronchi and to propel sputum in the direction of gravity drainage.

After the procedure, the amount, color, viscosity, and character of the ejected sputum are noted; the patient's color and pulse are evaluated the first few times the procedure is performed. It may be necessary to administer oxygen during postural drainage.

If the sputum is foul smelling, postural drainage is carried out in a room away from other patients and deodorizers are used. After the procedure the patient may find it refreshing to brush his teeth and use a mouthwash before resting in bed.

Chest Percussion and Vibration

To aid in the loosening and removal of thicker secretions, the chest may be tapped (percussed) and vibrated by the therapist or nurse. Percussion and vibration help to dislodge mucus adhering to the bronchioles and bronchi.

Percussion is carried out by cupping the hands and lightly striking the chest wall in a rhythmic fashion over the lung segment to be drained. The wrists are alternately flexed and extended so that the chest is cupped or clapped in a painless manner (Fig. 25–4). A soft cloth or towel may be placed over the segment of the chest that is being cupped to prevent skin irritation and redness from direct contact. Percussion, alternating with vibration, is maintained for 3 to 5 minutes for each position. The patient uses diaphragmatic breathing during this procedure to promote relaxation (see Breathing Retraining) As a precaution, percussion over the sternum, spine, liver, kidneys, spleen, or breasts (in women) is avoided. Percussion is performed cautiously in the elderly because of their increased incidence of osteoporosis and risk of rib fracture.

Vibration is the technique of applying manual compression and tremor to the chest wall during the exhalation phase of respiration (see Fig. 25–4). This maneuver helps to increase the velocity of the expired tidal volume from the small airways, thus freeing the mucus. After three or four vibrations the patient is encouraged to cough, using his abdominal muscles. (Contracting the abdominal muscles increases the effectiveness of the cough.) A scheduled program of coughing and clearing sputum, together with hydration, will reduce sputum in the

majority of patients. The number of times the percussion and vibration cycle is repeated depends on the patient's tolerance and clinical response. Breath sounds are evaluated before and after the procedures.

Nursing Considerations

When performing chest physiotherapy, it is important to make sure the patient is comfortable, is not wearing restrictive clothing, and has not just eaten a meal. The uppermost areas of the lung are treated first. Medication is given for pain as prescribed before percussion and vibration, the incision is splinted, and pillows are used for support as needed. The positions are varied, but focus is placed on the affected areas. On completion of the treatment, the therapist returns the patient to a comfortable position. The treatment is stopped if any of the following untoward symptoms develop: increased pain, increased shortness of breath, weakness, light-headedness, or hemoptysis. Therapy is indicated until the patient has normal respirations, can mobilize secretions, and has normal breath sounds, and when the chest film is normal.

Patient Education and Home Health Care

Chest physiotherapy is frequently indicated at home for patients with COPD, bronchiectasis, and cystic fibrosis. The techniques are the same as described above, but gravity drainage is achieved by placing the hips over a stack of magazines, newspapers, or pillows (unless a hospital bed is available). The patient or family is instructed in the positions and the techniques of percussion and vibration, so that therapy can be continued throughout the day.

Breathing Retraining

Breathing retraining consists of exercises and breathing practices designed and carried out to achieve a more efficient and controlled ventilation, and to decrease the work of breathing. Breathing retraining is especially indicated in the patient with chronic obstructive pulmonary disease and dyspnea. These exercises enhance maximum alveolar inflation; promote muscle relaxation; relieve anxiety; eliminate useless, uncoordinated patterns of respiratory muscle activity; slow the respiratory rate; and decrease the work of breathing. Slow, relaxed, and rhythmic breathing also helps to control the anxiety that is present when the patient is dyspneic. Specific breathing exercises include diaphragmatic and pursed lip breathing (described below).

Breathing exercises may be practiced in several positions, because air distribution and pulmonary circulation vary according to the position of the chest. Many patients will require additional oxygen, using a low-flow method, while performing breathing exercises. Emphysema-like changes in the lung occur as part of the natural aging process of the lung; therefore, breathing exercises are appropriate for all elderly hospitalized patients regardless of whether they have primary lung disease.

Patient Education and Home Health Care

The patient is told to breathe slowly and rhythmically in a relaxed manner to permit more complete exhalation and emp-

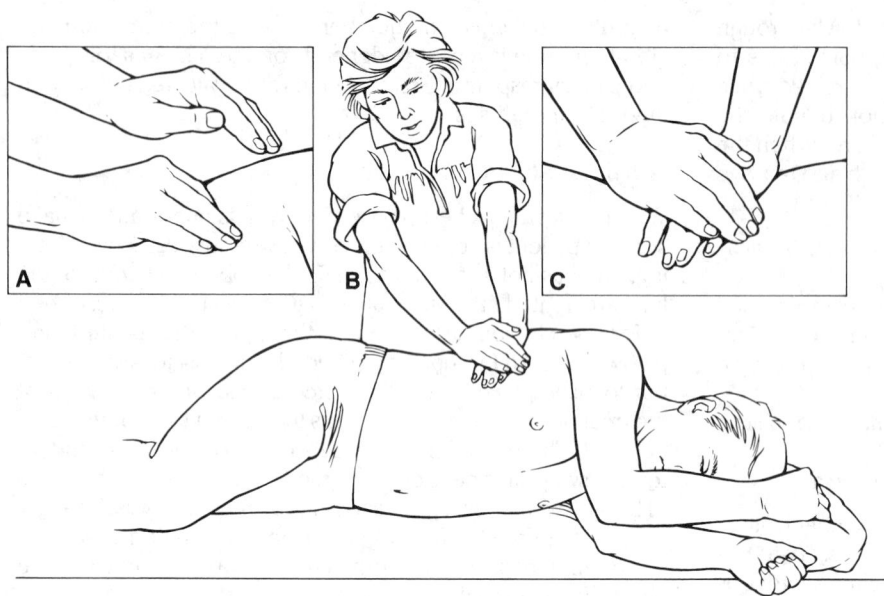

Figure 25–4. Percussion and vibration. (**A**) Proper hand positioning for percussion. (**B**) Proper technique for vibration. Note that the wrists and elbows are kept stiff and the vibrating motion is produced by the shoulder muscles. (**C**) Proper hand position for vibration.

tying of the lungs. He is instructed to always inhale through the nose because this filters, humidifies, and warms the air. If the patient becomes short of breath, he should concentrate on breathing slowly and rhythmically.

Diaphragmatic Breathing

The *goal* of diaphragmatic breathing is to use and strengthen the diaphragm during breathing. Diaphragmatic breathing can become automatic with sufficient practice and concentration. The patient is instructed to

1. Place one hand on the abdomen (just below the ribs) and the other hand on the middle of the chest. This increases awareness of the diaphragm and its function in breathing.
2. Breathe in slowly and deeply through the nose, letting the abdomen protrude as far as it will.
3. Breathe out through pursed lips while tightening (contracting) the abdominal muscles. Press firmly inward and upward on the abdomen while breathing out.
4. Repeat for 1 minute; follow by a rest period of 2 minutes. Work up to 5 minutes, several times a day (before meals and at bedtime).

Pursed Lip Breathing

Pursed lip breathing, which improves oxygen transport, helps to induce a slow, deep breathing pattern and assists the patient to control his breathing, even during periods of physical stress. This type of breathing helps prevent alveolar collapse secondary to loss of lung elasticity in emphysema.

The *goal* of pursed lip breathing is to train the muscles of expiration to prolong exhalation and increase airway pressure during expiration, thus lessening the amount of airway trapping and resistance.

The patient is instructed as follows:

1. Inhale through the nose while counting to 3, ("Smell a rose.") and exhale slowly and evenly against pursed lips while tightening the abdominal muscles. (Pursing the lips increases intratracheal pressure; exhaling through the mouth offers less resistance to expired air.)

2. Count to 7 while prolonging expiration through pursed lips. ("Blow out a candle.")
3. Sit in a chair and fold arms over the abdomen:
   • Inhale through the nose (count to 3). Exhale slowly through pursed lips while bending forward. Count to 7.
4. While walking:
   • Inhale while walking two steps.
   • Exhale through pursed lips while walking four or five steps.

The above steps may also be performed while practicing diaphragmatic breathing.

The Patient Requiring Airway Management

Adequate ventilation is dependent on free movement of air through the upper and lower airways. In many conditions the airway becomes narrowed or blocked as a result of disease process, bronchoconstriction (narrowing of airway by contraction of muscle fibers), a foreign body, or secretions. Maintaining a patent (open) airway is achieved through meticulous airway management, whether in an emergency situation, such as airway obstruction, or in long-term management, as in caring for a patient with an endotracheal or a tracheostomy tube.

Emergency Management of Upper Airway Obstruction

Upper airway obstruction has a variety of causes. Acute upper airway obstruction may be caused by food particles, vomitus, blood clots, or any other particle that enters and obstructs the larynx or trachea. It also may occur from enlargement of tissue in the wall of the airway, as in epiglottitis, laryngeal edema, laryngeal carcinoma, or peritonsillar abscess, or from thick secretions. Collapse of the walls of the airway, as occurs in retrosternal goiter, enlarged mediastinal lymph nodes, hematoma around the upper airway, and thoracic aneurysm also may result in upper airway obstruction.

The patient with an altered level of consciousness of any cause is at risk of obstructing the upper airway because he loses the protective reflexes (cough and swallowing) and the tone of the pharyngeal muscles, causing the tongue to fall back and block the airway.

The nurse makes the following observations to assess for signs and symptoms of upper airway obstruction:

Inspection. Is the patient conscious? Is there *any* inspiratory effort? Does the chest rise symmetrically? Is there use or retraction of accessory muscles? What is the skin color? Are there any obvious signs of deformity or obstruction (trauma, food, teeth, vomitus)? Is the trachea midline?

Palpation. Do both sides of the chest rise equally with inspiration? Are there any specific areas of tenderness, fracture or subcutaneous emphysema (crepitus)?

Auscultation. Is there any audible air movement, stridor (inspiratory sound), or wheezing (expiratory sound)? Are breath sounds present bilaterally in all lobes?

As soon as an upper airway obstruction is identified the following emergency measures are taken:

- Without hyperextension of the patient's neck, one hand is placed on his forehead, the chin is pulled up by grasping under the mandible to pull the tongue away from the back of the pharynx (Fig. 25–5).
- The patient is assessed by observing, listening, and feeling for movement of air.
- Using a cross-finger technique, the mouth is opened and observed for obvious obstructions such as secretions, blood clots, or food particles.
- If no passage of air is still possible, 6 to 10 quick, sharp abdominal thrusts are delivered, just below the xyphoid process to expel the obstruction (Heimlich maneuver). This procedure is repeated until the obstruction is expelled.
- If foreign objects causing obstruction are removed, and the patient is able to breathe spontaneously but unable to protect his airway with a cough, swallow, or gag reflex, an oral or nasopharyngeal airway is inserted.
- If assisted ventilation is required, a resuscitator bag and mask are used initially before intubation and mechanical ventilation. The mask is sealed onto the patient's face by placing the mask over the bridge of the nose with the left thumb while the mask is sealed firmly over the mouth. At the same time the rest of the fingers of the left hand pull on the chin and the angle of the mandible to maintain the head in extension (Fig. 25–6). The right hand inflates the lungs by periodically squeezing the bag to its full volume.
- If the patient is not breathing spontaneously, or if the upper airway obstruction is beyond the mouth or pharynx, assisted ventilation with a manual resuscitation bag or endotracheal intubation/crichothyroidotomy is necessary. Endotracheal intubation maintains a patent airway and prevents aspiration.

A self-inflating or resuscitation bag is also used after the patient is intubated. The mask on the resuscitation bag is removed, and the bag is squeezed in the same manner to its full volume. Head extension is not necessary because the upper airway is bypassed by the tube and thus is always open. Ventilation through a self-inflating bag can be accomplished by one person and is used not only for emergency ventilation but

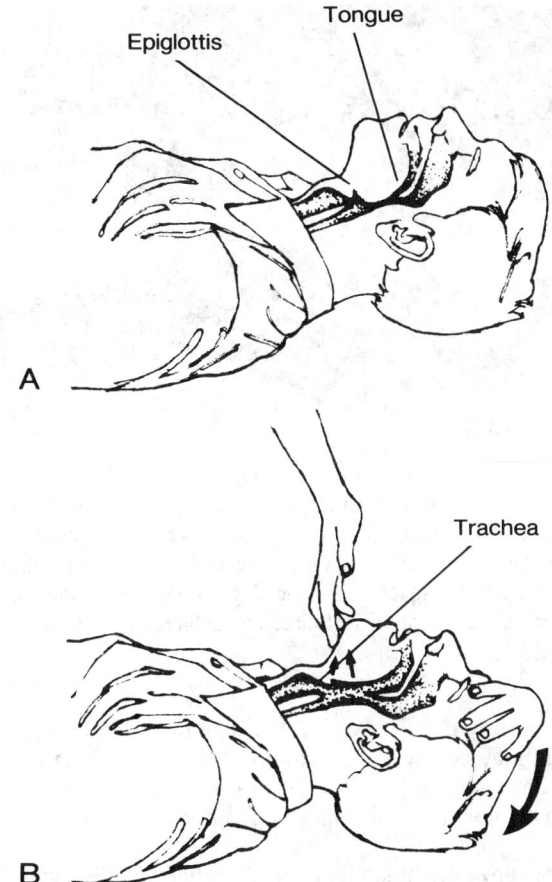

Figure 25–5. Opening the airway. (**A**) Airway obstruction produced by the tongue and epiglottis (**B**) Relief by head-tilt/chin-lift. (Reproduced with permission of the American Heart Association. Healthcare Provider's Manual for Basic Life Support. Copyright American Heart Association, 1988.)

also during suctioning procedures, ventilator maintenance, and transporting the patient on a ventilator.

Endotracheal Intubation

Endotracheal intubation refers to the passing of a tube through the mouth or nose into the trachea. Intubation provides a patent airway when the patient is having respiratory distress that cannot be treated by simpler methods. It is the method of choice in emergency care. Endotracheal intubation is used as a means of providing an airway for patients who cannot maintain an adequate airway on their own (comatose patients, those with upper airway obstruction), for mechanical ventilation, and provides an excellent means for suctioning secretions from the pulmonary tree.

An endotracheal tube usually is passed with the aid of a laryngoscope by medical, nursing, or respiratory therapy personnel who are specifically trained in this technique. Once the tube is inserted, a cuff around the tube is inflated to prevent leakage around the outer part of the tube and to minimize the possibility of subsequent aspiration and movement of the tube.

Suctioning of the tracheobronchial secretions is performed through the tube. Warm, humidified oxygen should always be introduced through the tube, whether the patient is breathing

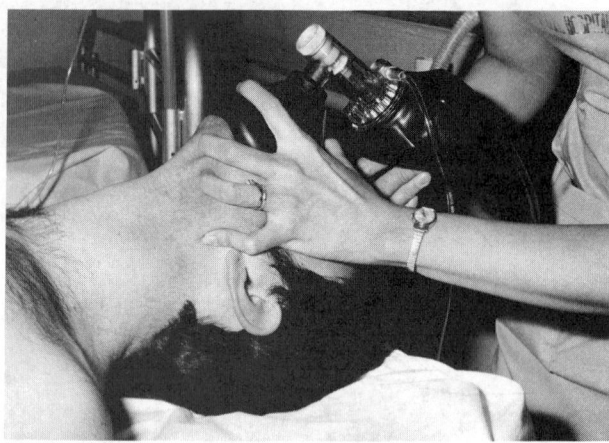

Figure 25–6. Bag and mask ventilation. The head is extended and the mask is sealed to the face by pressing the left thumb on the bridge of the nose and the index finger on the chin. The remaining three fingers pull the chin and mandible upward to maintain the head in extension. The right hand then squeezes the bag. Bag and mask ventilation should be performed only by specially trained and authorized personnel.

spontaneously or is on ventilatory support. Endotracheal intubation may be used for up to 2 weeks, at which time a tracheostomy must be considered to decrease irritation of and trauma to the tracheal lining and reduce mechanical dead space.

As in any other treatment modality, there are disadvantages associated with endotracheal or tracheostomy tubes. For one thing, the tube causes discomfort. In addition, the cough reflex is depressed because closure of the glottis is hindered. Secretions tend to become thicker because the warming and humidifying effect of the upper respiratory tract has been bypassed. The swallowing reflexes, composed of the glottic, pharyngeal, and laryngeal reflexes, are depressed because of prolonged disuse and the mechanical trauma of the endotracheal or tracheostomy tube. Ulceration and stricture of the larynx or trachea may develop.

Of great concern to the patient is his inability to talk and to communicate his needs. For nursing management of the patient with endotracheal intubation, see Chart 25–1.

Tracheostomy

A tracheotomy is a procedure in which an opening is made into the trachea. When an indwelling tube is inserted into the trachea, the term *tracheostomy* is used. A tracheostomy may be either temporary or permanent.

A tracheostomy is performed to bypass an upper airway obstruction, to remove tracheobronchial secretions, to permit the long-term use of mechanical ventilation, to prevent aspiration of oral or gastric secretions in the unconscious or paralyzed patient (by closing off the trachea from the esophagus), and to replace an endotracheal tube. There are many disease processes and emergency conditions that make a tracheostomy necessary.

The procedure is usually performed in the operating room or in an intensive care unit, where the patient's ventilation can be well controlled and optimal aseptic technique can be main-

tained. An opening is made in the second and third tracheal rings. After the trachea is exposed, a cuffed tracheostomy tube of an appropriate size is inserted (Fig. 25–7A) The cuff is an inflatable attachment to a tracheostomy or endotracheal tube that is designed to occlude the space between the trachea walls and the tube for mechanical ventilation.

The tracheostomy tube is held in place by tapes fastened around the patient's neck. Usually, a square of sterile gauze is placed between the tube and the skin to absorb drainage and prevent infection (see Fig. 25–7B).

Complications.   Complications may occur early or late in the course of tracheostomy tube management. They may even occur years after the tube has been removed. Immediately after the tracheostomy is performed there may be bleeding, pneumothorax, air embolism, aspiration, subcutaneous or mediastinal emphysema, recurrent laryngeal nerve damage, or posterior tracheal wall penetration. Long-term complications include airway obstruction due to accumulation of secretions or protrusion of the cuff over the opening of the tube, infection, rupture of the innominate artery, dysphagia, tracheoesophageal fistula, tracheal dilation, or tracheal ischemia and necrosis. Problems that may arise after the tube is removed include tracheal stenosis and vocal cord paralysis (secondary to laryngeal nerve damage).

Postoperative Nursing Interventions.   The patient requires continuous monitoring and assessment. The newly made opening must be kept patent by proper suctioning of secretions (see below). After the vital signs are stable, the patient is placed in a semi-Fowler's position to facilitate ventilation, promote drainage, minimize edema, and prevent strain on the suture lines. Analgesic and sedative drugs are administered with caution because it is undesirable to depress the cough reflex.

A major objective of nursing care is to alleviate the apprehension of the patient, and provide an effective means of communication. He needs this reassurance, as he may have a real fear that he will asphyxiate if unable to call for help.

Paper and pencil or a "magic slate" and the patient call light are kept within reach so that he has a means of communication.

Tracheal Suctioning (*Tracheostomy or Endotracheal Tube*)

When a tracheostomy or an endotracheal tube is present, it is necessary to suction the patient's secretions, because the effectiveness of his own cough mechanism is decreased. Tracheal suctioning is performed based on assessment of adventitious breath sounds or whenever secretions are obviously present. Unnecessary suctioning can initiate bronchospasm and cause mechanical trauma to the tracheal mucosa.

All equipment that comes into direct contact with the patient's lower airway must be sterile to prevent overwhelming pulmonary and systemic infections. The following equipment is used:

- Suction catheters
- Gloves
- 5- to 10-ml syringe
- Sterile normal saline poured in a cup for irrigation
- The patient's own self-inflating bag (hand resuscitator) with supplemental oxygen (the bag is changed daily to reduce infection)
- Suction machine

Chart 25–1
Nursing Management of the Patient With an Endotracheal Tube

Immediately After Intubation

1. Check symmetry of chest expansion
   a. Auscultate breath sounds of anterior and posterior chest bilaterally.
   b. Request order for chest radiograph to verify proper tube placement.
2. Ensure high humidity.
   A visible mist should be seen from the T-piece
3. Administer oxygen concentration as prescribed by physician.
4. Secure the tube to the patient's face with tape and mark the proximal end for position maintenance.
   a Cut proximal end of tube if it is longer than 7.5 cm (3 in) to prevent kinking.
   b. An oral airway or mouth bite may be inserted to prevent the patient from biting and obstructing the tube.
5. Use sterile suction technique and airway care to prevent iatrogenic contamination and infection.
6. Continue to reposition patient every 2 hours and as needed to prevent atelectasis and optimize lung expansion.
7. Provide oral hygiene and suction the oropharynx whenever necessary.

Extubation (Removal of Endotracheal Tube)

1. Explain procedure.
2. Have self-inflating bag and mask ready in case ventilatory assistance is required immediately after extubation.
3. Suction the tracheobronchial tree and oropharynx, remove tape, then deflate the cuff.
4. Give oxygen for a few breaths, then insert new, sterile suction catheter inside tube.
5. Have the patient inhale, and at peak inspiration remove the tube, suctioning the airway through the tube as it is pulled out.
Note: This procedure may also be performed by a respiratory therapist if permitted by hospital policy.

Care of Patient Following Removal of the Endotracheal Tube

1. Give heated humidity and oxygen by way of face mask.
2. Monitor respiratory rate and quality of chest excursions. Note stridor, color change, and change in mental alertness or personality.
3. Keep NPO or give only ice chips for next few hours.
4. Provide mouth care.
5. Instruct patient in coughing and deep-breathing exercises.

The steps in the tracheal suctioning procedure are as follows:

- Explain the procedure to the patient before beginning and reassure him during suctioning, as he may be apprehensive about choking and about his inability to communicate.

- Begin by washing hands thoroughly.
- Turn on suction source (pressure should not exceed 120 mm Hg).
- Open suction catheter kit.
- Fill basin with sterile normal saline.
- Put on sterile gloves.

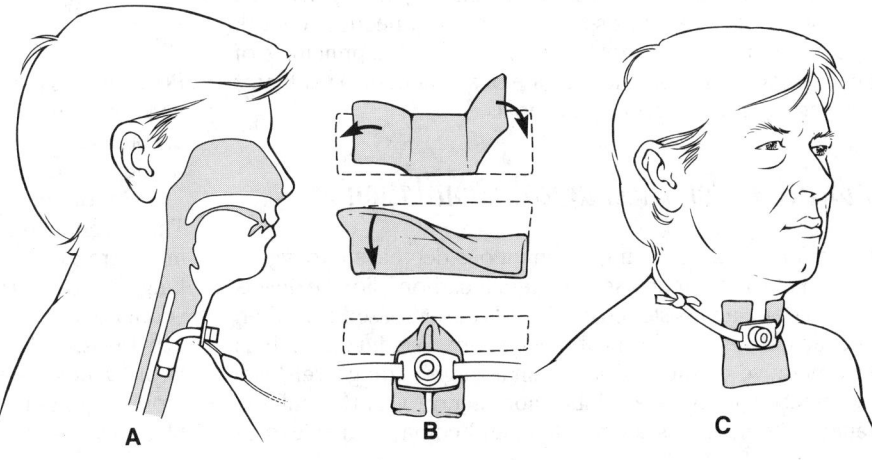

Figure 25–7. Tracheostomy tube dressing and tape changes. (**A**) The cuff of the tracheostomy tube fits smoothly within the tracheal wall. Pressure should be great enough to seal (above 20 cm H_2O) but not so great (below 25 cm H_2O) as to impair circulation. (**B**) How to fold a 4 × 4 gauze square so that it need not be cut (cut, frayed threads could be aspirated) and yet will provide a comfortable neck pad. (**C**) A precut gauze tracheostomy dressing. Dressings are changed as often as necessary. Note how the neck twill tapes are fastened to the openings in the neck plate of the trachestomy tube. Twill tapes should be tied to the side of the neck rather than in the back, eliminating the discomfort of lying on the knot.

- Pick up suction catheter in gloved hand and connect to suction.
- Instill 3 to 5 ml normal saline into the airway if secretions are thick.
- Hyperinflate/hyperoxygenate the patient's lungs for several deep breaths with a self-inflating bag.
- Insert catheter at least as far as the end of the tube without applying suction, just far enough to stimulate the cough reflex.
- Apply suction while withdrawing catheter, rotating catheter gently 360 degrees (no longer than 10 to 15 seconds, because patient can become hypoxic and develop dysrhythmias, which can lead to cardiac arrest).
- Reoxygenate and inflate the patient's lungs for several breaths.
- Repeat previous three steps until the airway is clear.
- Rinse catheter in basin with sterile normal saline between suction attempts if necessary.
- Suction oropharyngeal cavity after completing tracheal suctioning.
- Rinse suction tubing.
- Discard catheter, gloves, and basin.

Cuff Management.   As a general rule, the cuff on an endotracheal or tracheostomy tube should be inflated. The pressure within the cuff should be the lowest possible, however, to allow delivery of adequate tidal volumes and prevent pulmonary aspiration. Usually the pressure is maintained below 25 cm H_2O to prevent injury and above 20 cm H_2O to prevent aspiration. Cuff pressure is monitored at least every 8 hours by attaching a hand-held pressure gauge to the pilot balloon of the tube. With long-term intubation, higher pressures may be needed to maintain an adequate seal.

Tracheostomy Care.   The care of the patient with a tracheostomy tube is summarized in Chart 25–2.

The Patient Requiring Mechanical Ventilation

A mechanical ventilator is a positive- or negative-pressure breathing device that can maintain ventilation and oxygen delivery for a prolonged period.

Caring for a patient on mechanical ventilation has become an integral part of nursing care in critical care units, on general medical-surgical units, in extended care facilities, and even in the home. Nurses, physicians, and respiratory therapists must understand each patient's specific pulmonary needs and work together to set realistic goals. Understanding the principles of mechanical ventilation and the care of a patient on a ventilator is necessary for achieving these goals.

Indications for Mechanical Ventilation

If a patient is experiencing a continuous decrease in oxygenation (PaO_2), an increase in arterial carbon dioxide levels ($PaCO_2$), and a persistence of acidosis (a decreased pH), then mechanical ventilation may be necessary. Conditions such as postoperative thoracic or abdominal surgery, drug overdose, neuromuscular diseases, inhalation injury, COPD, multiple trauma, shock, multisystem failure, and coma all may lead to

respiratory failure and the need for mechanical ventilation. The criteria for mechanical ventilation (Chart 25–3) are guidelines for making the decision to place a patient on a ventilator. A patient with apnea that is not readily reversible is also a candidate for mechanical ventilation.

Classification of Ventilators

There are several types of mechanical ventilators. Ventilators are classified according to the manner in which they support ventilation. The two general categories are negative-pressure and positive-pressure ventilators.

By far the most common category in use today is the positive-pressure ventilator. Positive-pressure ventilators are also classified by the method of ending the inspiratory phase (volume-cycled, pressure-cycled, and time-cycled).

Negative-Pressure Ventilators

Negative-pressure ventilators exert a negative pressure on the external chest. By decreasing intrathoracic pressure during inspiration, air then flows into the lung, filling its volume. Physiologically, this type of assisted ventilation is similar to spontaneous ventilation. It is used mainly in chronic respiratory failure associated with neuromuscular conditions such as poliomyelitis, muscular dystrophy, amyotrophic lateral sclerosis, and myasthenia gravis. Its use is not appropriate for the unstable or complex patient, or one whose condition requires frequent ventilatory changes.

Negative-pressure ventilators are simple to use and do not require intubation of the airway. Indeed, their use is increasing in recent years, especially for the patient with borderline pulmonary function due to neuromuscular disease. Consequently, they are especially adaptable for home use. There are several types of negative-pressure ventilators: iron lung, body wrap, and chest cuirass.

Drinker Respirator Tank (Iron Lung).   The iron lung is a negative-pressure chamber used for ventilation. It was used extensively during polio epidemics in the past and currently is used by polio survivors and other neuromuscularly impaired patients.

Body Wrap (Pneumowrap) and Chest Cuirass (Tortoise Shell).   Both of these portable devices require a rigid cage or shell to create a negative-pressure chamber around the thorax and abdomen. Because of problems with proper fit and system leaks, these types of ventilators are infrequently used.

Positive-Pressure Ventilators

Positive-pressure ventilators inflate the lungs by exerting positive pressure on the airway, similar to a bellows mechanism, and thus force the alveoli to expand during inspiration. Expiration occurs passively.

Endotracheal intubation or tracheostomy is necessary. These ventilators are widely used in the hospital setting and are increasingly used in the home for patients with primary lung disease. There are three types of positive-pressure ventilators.

Pressure-Cycled Ventilators.   The pressure-cycled ventilator is a positive-pressure ventilator that ends inspiration when a preset pressure has been reached. In other words, the ventilator cycles on, delivers a flow of air until a certain predeter-

Chart 25–2
Care of the Patient With a Tracheostomy

Tracheostomy Care	Rationale

Tracheostomy Cuff

1. Cuffed tube (air injected into cuff) is required during prolonged mechanical ventilation.

The purpose of a cuffed tube is to prevent air from leaking during positive-pressure ventilation and to prevent tracheal aspiration of gastric contents. An adequate seal is indicated by the disappearance of any air leakage from the mouth or tracheostomy or disappearance of the harsh, gurgling sound of air coming from the throat.

2. Low-pressure cuff

Low-pressure cuffs exert minimal pressure on the tracheal mucosa and thus reduce the danger of tracheal ulceration and stricture.

Tracheostomy Tube and Skin Care

1. Wash hands.

The tracheostomy dressing is changed as needed to keep the skin clean and dry. Do not allow moist or soiled dressings to remain on the skin.

2. Explain procedure to patient.

A patient with a tracheostomy is apprehensive and requires ongoing assurance and support.

3. Wearing clean gloves, remove soiled dressing and discard.

Observing body substance isolation with contaminated dressings reduces cross-contamination.

4. Prepare sterile supplies, including hydrogen peroxide, normal saline or sterile water, cotton-tipped applicators, dressing.

Having necessary supplies and equipment readily available allows the procedure to be completed efficiently.

5. Put on sterile gloves.

Minimizes transmission of surface flora to sterile respiratory tract.

6. Cleanse wound and plate of tracheostomy tube with sterile applicators moistened with hydrogen peroxide. Rinse with sterile saline.

Hydrogen peroxide is effective in loosening crusted secretions. Rinsing prevents skin residue.

7. Use bacteriostatic ointment on the edge of the tracheostomy wound if prescribed.

Provides topical bacteriostatic protection.

8. If old tapes are soiled, place clean twill tapes in position to secure tracheostomy tube. Insert one end of tape through the side opening of the outer cannula. Wrap it around the patient's neck and thread it through the opposite opening of the outer cannula. Bring both ends around so that they meet on one side of the neck. Secure with a knot. Tighten until only two fingers can be comfortably inserted under tape.

This will provide a double thickness of tape around the neck. Tracheostomy tube can be dislodged by movement or forceful cough if left unsecured. It is difficult to reinsert the tracheostomy tube, and respiratory distress may occur if the tracheostomy tube is dislodged.

9. Remove old tapes and discard.

10. Use sterile tracheostomy dressing, and fit securely under the twill tapes and flange of tracheostomy tube so that the incision is covered (see Fig. 22-7).

Dressings that will shred are not used around a tracheostomy because of the danger that pieces of material, lint, or thread may get into the tube, and eventually into the trachea, causing obstruction or abscess formation. Special dressings that do not have a tendency to shred are used.

Chart 25–3
Indications for Mechanical Ventilation

$PaO_2 < 50$ mm Hg with $FIO_2 > 0.60$
$PaO_2 > 50$ mm Hg with $pH < 7.25$
Vital capacity < 2 times tidal volume
Negative inspiratory force < 25 cm H_2O
Respiratory rate > 35/min

mined pressure is reached, and then cycles off. The major limitation with this type of ventilator is that the volume of air or oxygen can vary as the patient's airway resistance or compliance changes. The result is an inconsistency in the amount of tidal volume delivered and a possible compromise of ventilation. Consequently, in adults, pressure-cycled ventilators are intended only for short-term use in the recovery room. The most common type is the IPPB machine.

Time-Cycled Ventilators. Time-cycled ventilators terminate or control inspiration after a preset time. The volume of air the patient receives is regulated by the length of inspiration and the flow rate of the air. Most ventilators have a rate control that determines the respiratory rate, but pure time-cycling is rarely used for adults. These ventilators are used in newborns and infants.

Volume-Cycled Ventilators.   By far, volume-cycled ventilators are the most commonly used positive-pressure ventilators in use today. With this type of ventilator, the volume of air to be delivered with each inspiration is preset. Once this preset volume is delivered to the patient, the ventilator cycles off and exhalation occurs passively. From breath to breath, the volume of air delivered by the ventilator is relatively constant, assuring consistent, adequate breaths despite varying airway pressures.

Features and Settings of Volume Ventilators

Numerous features are used in the management of the patient on a mechanical ventilator. The most crucial features and settings of a volume ventilator relative to nursing care are presented in Chart 25–4.

Adjustment on the Ventilator.   The ventilator is adjusted so that the patient is comfortable and "in sync" with the machine (Fig. 25–8). Minimal alteration of the normal cardiovascular and pulmonary dynamics is desired. If the volume ventilator is adjusted appropriately, the patient's arterial blood gas levels will be satisfactory and there will be little or no cardiovascular compromise. To determine how to achieve adequate mechanical ventilation for each patient, the following guidelines are recommended as initial ventilator settings for the patient:

1. Set the machine to deliver tidal volume required (10 to 15 ml/kg).

2. Adjust the machine to deliver the lowest concentration of oxygen to maintain normal PaO_2 (80 to 100 mm Hg). This setting may be set high and gradually reduced based on arterial blood gas results.

3. Record peak inspiratory pressure.

4. Set mode (assist-control or intermittent mandatory ventilation) and rate according to physician order. Modes of medical ventilation are described in Figure 25–9.

5. If patient is on assist-control mode, adjust sensitivity so that he can trigger the ventilator with a minimum effort (usually −2 mm Hg negative inspiratory force).

6. Record minute volume and measure carbon dioxide partial pressure (Pco_2), pH, and Po_2 after 20 minutes of continuous mechanical ventilation.

7. Adjust settings (FiO_2 and rate) according to results of arterial blood gases to provide normal values or those set by the physician.

8. In case of sudden onset of confusion, agitation, or unexplained "bucking the ventilator," the patient should be assessed for hypoxemia, and manually ventilated on 100% O_2 with a resuscitation bag.

▶ **Nursing Process**
Care of the Mechanically Ventilated Patient

◊ **Assessment**

The nurse has a vital role in assessing the patient's status and the functioning of the ventilator. In assessing the patient, the nurse evaluates the following:

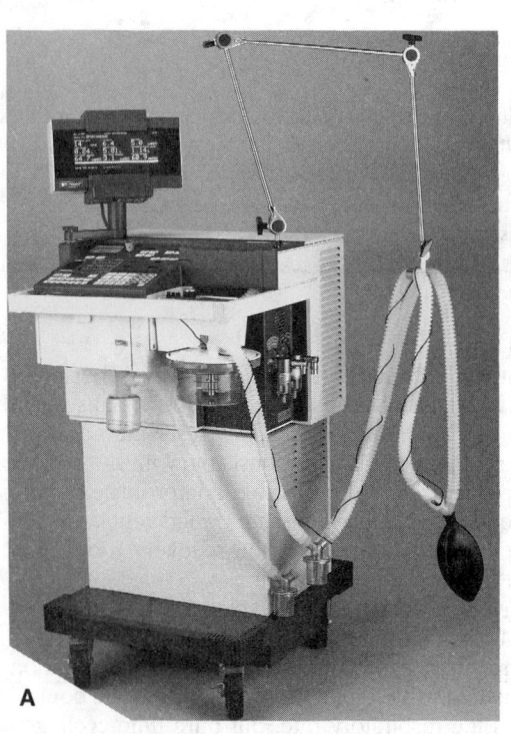

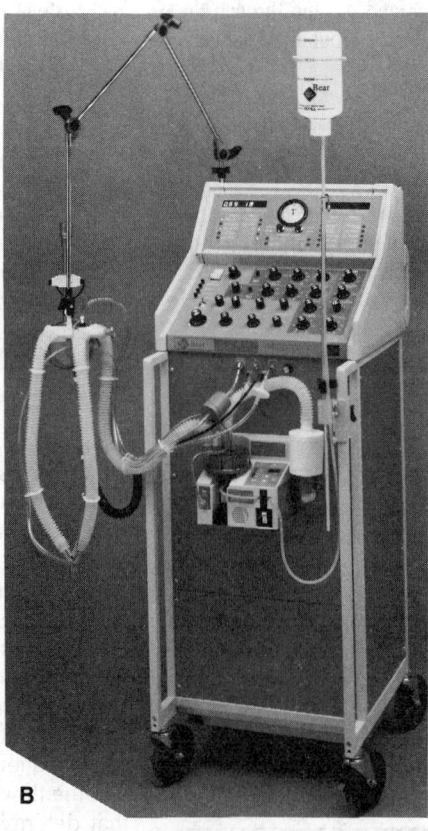

Figure 25–8. Two commonly used brands of volume-controlled ventilators: (**A**) Puritan-Bennett 7200A, (**B**) Bear 3 Adult. (**A** courtesy of Puritan Bennett Corp; **B** courtesy of Bear Medical Systems, Inc.)

A

B

Chart 25-4
Features and Settings of a Volume Ventilator

A volume-controlled ventilator (MAI, Bear, Servo) will deliver set tidal volume with varying pressures.

Fraction of Inspired Oxygen (FiO_2)

The concentration of oxygen delivered is dependent on patient need, as determined by the physician and evaluated by arterial blood gas levels.

Tidal Volume (V_T)

10–15 ml/kg body weight

Respiratory Rate

12–16/min

Sensitivity Setting

• The patient should not have to generate more than −2 cm H_2O to trigger the ventilator.

Type of Ventilation (see Fig. 25-9)

Controlled.   The machine completely controls the patient's ventilation according to set tidal volumes and respiratory rate. Because of problems with synchrony, it is rarely used.

Assist/Control.   The patient triggers the machine. If the patient fails to breathe, the machine will deliver a controlled breath at a minimum rate and volume already set.

Intermittent Mandatory Ventilation (IMV).   Machine allows patient to breathe spontaneously while providing preset FiO_2 and number of ventilator breaths to ensure adequate ventilation without fatigue.

Inspiration to Exhalation Ratio (I:E Ratio)

• Should be 1:3, 1:2, or more (1 second of inspiration to 3 seconds of exhalation, etc.), in keeping with normal respiratory pattern

Minute Volume ($\dot{V}_E$)

Tidal volume × respiratory rate/min
Normal = 6–8 L/min

Airway Pressure

Normal = 15–20 cm H_2O, but varies.
Low airway pressure is seen with air leak.
High airway pressure is seen in
• Increased secretions
• Airway obstruction
• Bronchospasms
• Pulmonary edema
• Pneumothorax
• Flail chest
• Patient exhaling when ventilator cycling

Sigh

• The lungs are hyperinflated periodically to open collapsed alveoli.
• Sigh volume is 1.5 times tidal volume 1–3 times/hr.
• Used only with assist-control mode.

Humidity and Temperature

• Heated humidity is provided for all intubated and tracheotomized patients to avoid thick secretions
• Daily clinical evaluation of the viscosity of the patient's secretions provides a guideline for the effectiveness of humidification and nebulization.

Positive End-Expiratory Pressure (PEEP)

• A positive pressure of 5 cm, 10 cm, or 15 cm H_2O is maintained at the end of exhalation instead of a normal 0 cm H_2O pressure.
• Increases functional residual capacity (opens collapsed alveoli) and improves oxygenation with lower FiO_2.

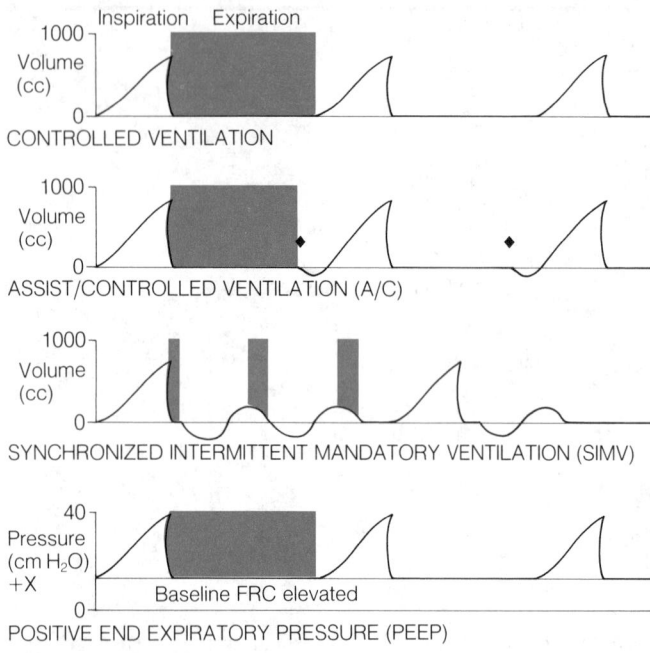

□ Inspiration
■ Exhalation
♦ Patient triggered breath

Figure 25–9. Modes of mechanical ventilation with air flow waveforms. (**A**) Flow in the controlled ventilation mode. A preset volume of gas is delivered to the patient under positive pressure while spontaneous patient respiratory effort is "locked out." (**B**) Gas flow in the assist/control ventilation mode. In this mode, a preset volume of gas is delivered to the patient at a preset rate, but the patient may trigger a ventilator breath with negative inspiratory effort. (**C**) Gas flow in the synchronized intermittent mandatory ventilation (IMV) mode. A preset minimum number of breaths are synchronously delivered to the patient, but the patient may also take spontaneous breaths of varying volumes. Note how inspiratory and expiratory pressures differ between spontaneous and ventilator breaths. (**D**) Airway pressure with varying levels of positive end expiratory pressure (PEEP). Note that at end expiration, the airway is not allowed to return to zero.

- Vital signs
- Evidence of hypoxia (restlessness, anxiety, tachycardia, increased respiratory rate, cyanosis)
- Respiratory rate and pattern
- Breath sounds
- Neurologic status
- Tidal volume, minute ventilation, forced vital capacity
- Nutritional status
- Suctioning needs
- Psychological status
- Patient's spontaneous ventilatory effort

▷ *Assessment of Cardiac Function.* Alterations in cardiac output may occur as a result of positive-pressure ventilation. The positive intrathoracic pressure during inspiration compresses the heart and great vessels, thereby reducing venous return and cardiac output. This is usually corrected during exhalation when the positive pressure is off.

To evaluate cardiac function, the nurse first looks for signs and symptoms of hypoxemia and hypoxia (restlessness, ap-

prehension, confusion, tachycardia, tachypnea, increased work of breathing, pallor progressing to cyanosis, diaphoresis, transient hypertension, and decreased urine output). If a pulmonary artery catheter is in place, cardiac output, cardiac index, and other hemodynamic values may be determined.

▷ *Assessment of Equipment.* The ventilator also needs to be assessed to make sure that it is functioning properly and that the settings are appropriate. Even though the nurse may not be primarily responsible for adjusting the settings on the ventilator or measuring ventilator parameters (usually the responsibility of the respiratory therapist), she is responsible for the patient and therefore needs to evaluate how the ventilator affects the patient. In monitoring the ventilator, the nurse should note the following:

- Type of ventilator (volume-cycled, pressure-cycled, negative-pressure)
- Controlling mode (control, assist/control, intermittent mandatory ventilation)
- Tidal volume and rate settings
- FiO_2 (fraction of inspired oxygen) setting
- Inspiratory pressure reached and pressure limit
- Sigh settings (usually 1½ times the tidal volume and range from 1 to 3/hr) if applicable
- Presence of water in the tubing, disconnection, or kinking of the tubing
- Humidification (humidifier filled with water)
- Alarms (functioning properly)
- PEEP (positive end-expiratory pressure) level, if applicable

Note: If a malfunction of the ventilator system occurs, and if the problem cannot be identified and corrected immediately, the nurse must be prepared to ventilate the patient with a manual resuscitation bag until the problem is resolved.

▷ ## Nursing Diagnoses

Based on the assessment data, the patient's major nursing diagnoses may include

- Impaired gas exchange related to underlying illness, or ventilator setting adjustment during stabilization or weaning.
  Note: The nursing diagnosis of impaired gas exchange is, by its complex nature, multidisciplinary and interdependent.
- Ineffective airway clearance related to increased mucus production associated with continuous positive-pressure mechanical ventilation
- High risk for injury or infection related to endotracheal intubation or tracheostomy
- Impaired physical mobility related to ventilator dependency
- Impaired verbal communication related to presence of endotracheal tube and attachment to ventilator
- Ineffective individual coping and powerlessness related to ventilator dependency

▷ ## Planning and Implementation

▷ *Goals:* The major goals of the patient may include the following:

- Optimal gas exchange
- Reduction of mucus accumulation
- Absence of injury or infection
- Attainment of optimal mobility

- Adjustment to nonverbal methods of communication
- Acquisition of successful coping measures

▷ *Nursing Interventions*

Nursing care of the mechanically ventilated patient requires unique technical and interpersonal skills. Nursing interventions are similar whether the patient is in an intensive care unit, a medical-surgical unit, or an extended care facility. The frequency of administering the care and the stability of the patient are the factors that vary from unit to unit.

▷ *Gas Exchange.* The entire purpose of mechanical ventilation is to optimize gas exchange by maintaining alveolar ventilation and oxygen delivery. The alteration in gas exchange may be due to the underlying illness or mechanical factors related to the adjustment of the machine to the patient. The nurse–physician–respiratory therapist team continually assesses the patient for adequacy of gas exchange, signs and symptoms of hypoxia, and response to treatment. It is imperative that there is free sharing of goals and information among team members. All subsequent goals listed below directly or indirectly relate to this primary goal.

Nursing interventions for the mechanically ventilated patient are not uniquely different from other pulmonary patients, yet the need for astute nursing observation and the establishment of a therapeutic nurse–patient relationship, is of paramount importance. The constellation of interventions used by the nurse is determined by the underlying disease process and the patient's response. For example, poor gas exchange can be related to a wide variety of factors: altered level of consciousness, atelectasis, fluid overload, incisional pain, or primary disease processes such as pneumonia or tuberculosis. As a result, nursing interventions to promote optimal gas exchange include judicious administration of pain medications to relieve pain but not significantly decrease the respiratory drive and frequent repositioning to diminish the pulmonary effects of immobility. The nurse also monitors for adequate fluid balance by assessing for the presence of peripheral edema, calculating daily intake and output, and monitoring daily weights. The nurse administers medications to control the primary disease and monitors for their potential side effects. Sterile suctioning of the lower airway combined with chest percussion, vibration, and lavage are other strategies to clear the airway of excessive secretions. Because of well-documented damage to the intima of the tracheobronchial tree, suctioning should be performed when clinically indicated rather than on a routine schedule.

Two general nursing interventions that are of particular importance to the mechanically ventilated patient are pulmonary auscultation and interpretation of arterial blood gases. The nurse is often the first to notice changes in physical assessment findings or significant trends in blood gases that signal the development of a significant problem (pneumothorax, tube displacement, pulmonary embolus).

▷ *Airway Management.* Continuous positive-pressure ventilation increases the production of secretions regardless of the patient's underlying condition. The nurse must identify the presence of secretions by lung auscultation at least every 2 to 4 hours. Measures to clear the airway of secretions include suctioning, chest physiotherapy, frequent position changes, and increased mobility as soon as possible. The sigh mechanism on the ventilator is adjusted to deliver at least 1 to 3 sighs per hour at 1.5 times the tidal volume if the patient is on assist-control. Because of the risk of hyperventilation and trauma to pulmonary tissue from excess ventilator pressure, these features are not being used as frequently in recent years. If the patient is on an intermittent mandatory ventilation (IMV) mode, the mandatory ventilations act as sighs because they are of greater volume than the patient's spontaneous breaths.

Periodic sighing prevents atelectasis and the further retention of secretions. Humidification by way of the ventilator is maintained to help liquefy secretions so they are more easily raised. Bronchodilators, either intravenous or inhaled, are administered as prescribed to dilate the bronchial tubes so that secretions are more easily mobilized.

▷ *Prevention of Injury and Infection.* Airway management must involve maintenance of the endotracheal or tracheostomy tube. The ventilator tubing is positioned so there is minimal pulling or distortion of the tube in the trachea. Cuff pressure is monitored every 8 hours to maintain the pressure under 25 cm H_2O. The presence of a cuff leak is evaluated at the same time. Tracheostomy care is performed at least every 8 hours and more frequently if indicated because of the increased risk of infection. Oral hygiene is administered frequently because the oral cavity is a primary source of contamination of the lungs in the intubated and compromised patient. The presence of a nasogastric tube and the use of antacids in the mechanically ventilated patient also have been shown to predispose the patient to nosocomial pneumonia from subclinical aspiration. The patient also should be positioned with the head elevated above the stomach as much as possible to decrease the potential for overt aspiration of gastric contents.

▷ *Promotion of Optimal Level of Mobility.* The patient's mobility is limited because of his attachment to the ventilator. If his condition is stable, he should get out of bed and to a chair as soon as possible. Mobility and muscle activity are beneficial because they stimulate respirations and improve morale. If the patient is not able to get out of bed, then active or passive range of motion exercises are performed every 8 hours to prevent muscle atrophy, contractures, and venous stasis.

▷ *Promotion of Optimal Communication.* Alternative methods of communication must be developed for the patient on a ventilator. The nurse assesses the patient's communication abilities:

- Is the patient conscious and able to communicate? (nod or shake head)
- Is his mouth unobstructed by tube for mouthing words?
- Is his hand strong and available for writing? (If he is right-handed, the intravenous line is placed in his left hand if possible.)

Once the patient's limitations are known, the nurse offers several appropriate communication approaches:

- Lip reading (use single key words)
- Pad and pencil or "magic slate"
- Communication board
- Gesturing
- Electric larynx
- Suggest use of "talking" or fenestrated trach to physician to allow the patient to talk while on the ventilator.

Additionally, eye glasses, a hearing aid, and translator are made available, if indicated, to enhance the patient's ability to communicate with others.

The patient must be assisted to find the communication method best suited for him. Some methods may be frustrating to the patient and they need to be identified and minimized. A speech–language pathologist can assist in determining the most appropriate method for the patient.

▷ *Promotion of Coping Ability.* Dependence on a ventilator is frightening to both the patient and his family and will disrupt even the most stable families. The patient and his family are assisted to verbalize their feelings about the ventilator, the patient's condition, and the environment in general. Explaining procedures every time they are performed will help to reduce anxiety and familiarize the patient with hospital routines. To restore a sense of control, the patient is encouraged to participate in decisions about his care, schedules, and treatment when possible. There is a tendency to become withdrawn or depressed during mechanical ventilation, especially if it is prolonged. Consequently, the patient is encouraged about his progress when appropriate. Diversion is provided by watching television, playing music, or taking a walk (if appropriate and possible). Stress-reduction techniques (a back rub, relaxation measures) help release tension and enable the patient to deal with his anxieties and fears about his condition and his dependence on the ventilator.

▷ Evaluation

Expected Outcomes

1. Exhibits adequate gas exchange
   a. Exhibits equal breath sounds bilaterally
   b. Has arterial blood gas values within acceptable level
   c. Heart rate, blood pressure, and pulmonary artery pressures within normal limits for patient
2. Manages ventilation with minimal mucus accumulation
   a. Exhibits clear lungs bilaterally
   b. Produces thin, white secretions
   c. Is afebrile
3. Is free of injury or infection.
   a. Assists with oral care if possible
   b. Tolerates tracheostomy care every 4 hours
   c. Is afebrile
   d. Exhibits normal white blood cell (WBC) count
4. Is mobile within limits of ability
   a. Gets out of bed to chair as soon as possible
   b. Exhibits no skin breakdown (especially oral mucosa) or contractures
   c. Performs range-of-motion exercises every 6 to 8 hours
5. Communicates effectively
   a. Writes messages as necessary
   b. Is able to use gestures to communicate
6. Copes effectively
   a. Verbalizes fears and concerns about his condition and the equipment
   b. Participates in decision making when possible
   c. Uses stress-reduction techniques when necessary
   d. Participates appropriately in care

Factors Causing the Patient to "Buck" the Ventilator

The patient is in synchrony with the ventilator when thoracic expansion coincides with the inspiratory phase of the machine and exhalation occurs passively. The patient "bucks" the ventilator when he is out of phase with the machine. This is manifested when the patient attempts to breathe out during the ventilator's mechanical inspiratory phase or when there is jerky and increased abdominal muscle effort. The following factors contribute to this problem: anxiety, hypoxia, increased secretions hypercarbia, inadequate minute volume, and pulmonary edema. These problems must be corrected before paralyzing agents are given to the patient, or else the underlying problem is masked and the patient's condition will continue to deteriorate.

Muscle relaxants, tranquilizers, analgesics, and paralyzing agents are not uncommon adjuncts to care of the mechanically ventilated patient. Their purpose is ultimately to increase the patient–machine synchrony by decreasing the patient's anxiety, hyperventilation, or excessive muscle activity. The selection and dose of the appropriate drug are determined carefully and are based on the individual patient's requirements and the cause of the patient's restlessness. Paralyzing agents (atracurium, vecuronium, and pancuronium) are always used as a last resort.

Problems With Mechanical Ventilation

Because of the seriousness of the patient's condition and the highly complex and technical nature of mechanical ventilation, a number of problems or complications can occur. Such situations basically fall into two categories: ventilator problems or actual patient problems. In either case, the patient must be supported while the problem is being identified and corrected. Frequently encountered problems or complications associated with mechanical ventilation are listed with probable causes and solutions in Table 25–2.

Weaning the Patient From the Ventilator

Weaning the patient from his dependence on the ventilator takes place in three stages. The patient is gradually weaned from the (1) ventilator, (2) tube, and (3) oxygen. Weaning from mechanical ventilation is performed at the earliest possible time consistent with patient safety. It is essential that the decision be made from a physiologic rather than from a mechanical viewpoint. A total understanding of the patient's clinical status is required in making this decision.

Weaning is started when the patient is recovering from the acute stage of his medical and surgical problems and when the cause of respiratory failure is sufficiently reversed.

The objective measurements of the patient's ventilatory capacities include the following:

1. An ability to generate a minimum vital capacity of 10 to 15 ml/kg of body weight or a vital capacity twice as large as the predicted normal resting tidal volume. The minimum required volume is usually in the range of 1000 ml in a normal adult.
2. A spontaneous inspiratory force of at least -20 cm H_2O pressure
3. A PaO_2 of greater than 60% with an FiO_2 of less than 40%
4. Vital signs that are stable

When the decision has been made that the patient has adequate ventilatory capacity, baseline measurements are noted: (1) vital capacity, (2) inspiratory force, (3) respiratory rate, (4) resting tidal volume, (5) minute ventilation (frequency times total volume, or $f \times V_T$), (6) arterial blood gases, and

TABLE 25–2. *Causes and Solutions of Ventilator Problems*

Problem	Cause	Solution
VENTILATOR		
Increase in peak airway pressure	Coughing or plugged airway tube	Lavage and suction airway for secretions, empty condensation fluid from circuit.
	Patient "bucking" ventilator	Adjust sensitivity.
		Manually ventilate patient.
		Assess for hypoxia or bronchospasm.
		Check blood gases.
		Sedate only if necessary
	Tubing kinked	Check tubing; reposition patient; insert oral airway if necessary.
	Pneumothorax	Manually ventilate patient; notify physician.
	Decrease in complications due to atelectasis or bronchospasm	Clear secretions.
Decrease in pressure or loss of volume	Increase in compliance	None.
	Leak in ventilator or tubing; cuff on tube/humidifier not tight	Check entire ventilator circuit for patency.
		Correct leak.
PATIENT		
Cardiovascular compromise	Decrease in venous return due to application of positive pressure to lungs	Assess for adequate volume status by measuring heart rate, blood pressure, central venous pressure, pulmonary capillary wedge pressure, and urine output. Notify physician if values are abnormal.
Barotrauma/pneumothorax	Application of positive pressure to lungs; high mean airway pressures lead to alveolar rupture.	Notify physician.
		Prepare patient for chest tube insertion.
		Avoid high pressure settings for patients with COPD, ARDS, or history of pneumothorax.
Pulmonary infection	Bypass of normal defense mechanisms; frequent breaks in ventilator circuit; decreased mobility; impaired cough reflex.	Meticulous aseptic technique.
		Frequent mouth care.
		Optimize nutritional status.

(7) FiO_2. It is important to follow the trend of these values as the weaning progresses, rather than to rely on isolated measurements.

Adequate psychological preparation is necessary before and during the weaning process. The patient needs to know what is expected of him during the procedure. He is frightened by having responsibility for his own breathing again and needs the reassurance that he is improving and is well enough to handle spontaneous breathing. The nurse explains what will happen during weaning and what his role in the procedure will be. The nurse emphasizes that someone will be with or near the patient at all times and allows time to answer any of his questions simply and concisely. A properly prepared patient can reduce the weaning time.

Methods of Weaning. Considerable effort has been devoted to finding the "best" method of weaning from mechanical ventilation. Actually, there is no "best" way. Success depends on the combination of adequate patient preparation, physician preference, unit protocols, available equipment, and knowledgeable health care personnel. The two most common weaning methods in use today are described below.

Traditional Method. The traditional method involves switching from the assist-control or IMV mode to one or more T-piece trials. This method of weaning is usually used when there is short-term ventilatory assistance (less than 2 days) *and* when the patient is awake, alert, breathing without difficulty, with good gag and cough reflexes, and hemodynamically stable. The patient breathes spontaneously with the aid of humidified oxygen. During the weaning process, the patient is maintained on the same or higher oxygen concentration than when he is on the ventilator.

While on the T-piece, the patient is observed for signs and symptoms of hypoxemia or increasing fatigue as manifested by the following: (1) tachycardia, premature ventricular contractions (PVCs), or any sign of increasing cardiac irritability; (2) restlessness; (3) a respiratory rate greater than 35/min; (4) use of accessory muscles, and (5) paradoxical chest movement. Fatigue or exhaustion is initially manifested by an increased respiratory rate associated with a gradual reduction in tidal volume. Later there is a slowing of the respiratory rate.

If the patient appears to be tolerating the T-tube trial, a second set of arterial blood gases is drawn 20 minutes after the patient has been on spontaneous ventilation at a constant FIO_2. (It takes 15 to 20 minutes for alveolar arterial equilibration to take place.)

Signs of exhaustion and hypoxemia correlated with a deterioration of the above measurements indicate the need for ventilatory support. The patient is placed back on the ventilator each time signs of fatigue or deterioration develop.

The patient usually can be extubated within 2 or 3 hours of weaning and allowed spontaneous ventilation by means of a mask with humidified oxygen. Patients who have had prolonged ventilatory assistance usually require more gradual weaning, which may take several days. They are weaned primarily during the day and placed back on the ventilator at night to rest.

Intermittent Mandatory Ventilation Method. Some patients are difficult to wean from mechanical ventilation. An IMV device incorporated into the ventilator will allow the patient to breathe spontaneously as desired but also delivers a mandatory ventilation at regular intervals. IMV is indicated if the patient satisfies all the criteria for weaning but cannot sustain adequate spontaneous ventilation for long periods.

Before the IMV method is initiated, the same weaning criteria are assessed and met as with the traditional method. The patient is assessed for symptoms of hypoxemia and cardiovascular compromise.

After initiation of IMV, serial determinations of the following are made and recorded: (1) respiratory rate, (2) minute volume ($\dot{V}_E$), (3) V_T of patient and machine, (4) FIO_2, and (5) arterial blood gas values.

If there is no deterioration in these parameters, and if the patient maintains adequate tidal volumes, the rate of the ventilator is progressively decreased and the patient is allowed to rely more on spontaneous respiration until weaning is complete.

Successful weaning from the ventilator is supplemented by intensive pulmonary care. The following are continued: (1) oxygen therapy, (2) arterial blood gas evaluation, (3) nebulizer therapy, (4) chest physiotherapy, (5) adequate hydration and humidification, and (6) incentive spirometry. These patients still have minimum pulmonary function and need vigorous supportive therapy before their respiratory status returns to normal.

Weaning From the Tube. The tracheostomy or endotracheal tube can be removed if the following criteria are present: (1) spontaneous ventilation is adequate; (2) the pharyngeal and laryngeal gag reflexes are active; (3) the patient is maintaining an adequate airway and can swallow, move his jaw, or clench his teeth; and (4) voluntary cough is effective in bringing up secretions. If these are ineffective, the tracheostomy tube is needed so that tracheobronchial secretions can be suctioned.

Before the patient is weaned from the tracheostomy tube, he is given a trial of mouth- or nose-breathing. This is accomplished by (1) changing to a smaller size tube to increase the resistance to air flow and plugging the tracheostomy (deflate the cuff) at the same time; (2) switching to a cuffless tracheostomy tube; (3) changing to a fenestrated tube (one with an opening or window in the bend of the tube), which permits air to flow around and through the tube to the upper airway and permits talking; (4) changing to a tracheostomy button; or (5) removing the tracheostomy tube completely.

Weaning From Oxygen. The patient has been weaned from the ventilator, cuff, and tube. His respiratory function has been checked, and oxygen has been given according to the result of the blood gas determinations. The FIO_2 then is gradually reduced until the PO_2 is in the 70 to 100 mm Hg range (9.31 to 13.30 kPa[a]) while the patient is breathing room air. If the PO_2 is less than 70 mm Hg (9.31 kPa[a]) on room air, supplementary oxygen is recommended.

Success in weaning the long-term ventilator-dependent patient also requires early, aggressive yet judicious nutritional support. Respiratory musculature (diaphragm and especially intercostals) quickly become weak or atrophied after just a few days of mechanical ventilation, especially if nutrition is not supported. High carbohydrate loads increase carbon dioxide production and thus may increase the work of breathing in patients with borderline pulmonary function. Consultation with a dietitian or nutrition team soon after admission to plan the best form of nutritional replacement may decrease the duration of mechanical ventilation and other complications, especially sepsis.

Research is underway in a number of areas related to the mechanically ventilated patient and strategies for weaning. Areas of particular interest are effectiveness of respiratory muscle training, nutritional support, modes and pressures of mechanical ventilation, suctioning frequency, and patient–nurse interactions.

Mechanical Ventilation in the Home

Under certain physiologic, psychological, or economic conditions, it is possible that the patient may not be completely weaned from the ventilator, from the tube, or from oxygen before leaving the hospital. Patients are being discharged to extended-care facilities or home on mechanical ventilators, with tracheostomy tubes, or on oxygen therapy. Patients on home ventilator care usually have neuromuscular conditions or COPD.

Mechanical ventilation in the home (or an extended-care facility) is increasing in frequency because of a number of influences:

1. Early diagnosis and treatment of pulmonary disorders has resulted in increased patient longevity.
2. Increasing numbers of health care professionals are becoming more proficient in providing rehabilitative and maintenance ventilator care in the home.
3. Prospective payment systems demand reductions in costs placed on the health care industry.
4. Concerned family members are willing to give necessary support care.
5. Recent technological advances have made ventilators simple, portable, versatile, compact, and safe for use by the homebound patient and his caregivers.

Caring for the patient with mechanical ventilator support at home can be accomplished quite successfully. Multiple factors are considered for this endeavor to work. The family must emotionally, educationally, and physically be able to assume the role of primary caregiver. A home care team consisting of nurse, physician, respiratory therapist, social service or home care agency, and equipment supplier needs to be available. The home itself is evaluated to determine if it is adequate for the safe operation of all electrical equipment. A summary of the basic assessment criteria needed for successful home care is presented in Chart 25–5.

Once the decision is made to initiate mechanical ventilation at home, the patient and his family are prepared for home care. Home health teaching includes information about the ventilator, suctioning, tracheostomy care, signs of pulmonary infection, cuff inflation and deflation, and assessment of vital signs. Family instruction begins in the hospital and continues in the home. Nursing responsibilities include evaluating the patient's and the family's understanding of the information presented.

Once the patient is at home, the community health nurse is involved in monitoring and evaluating the adaptation of the patient and family to the home environment. The adequacy of ventilation and oxygenation is assessed, as is airway patency. The nurse needs to solve any unique adaptation problems the patient may have. She listens to the patient's and the family's anxieties and frustrations and offers support and encouragement where appropriate. The nurse helps identify and contact appropriate community resources that may assist in home management of the patient with mechanical ventilation.

The technical aspects of the ventilator are managed by vendor follow-up. A respiratory therapist usually is assigned to the patient and makes frequent visits to evaluate the patient and perform a maintenance check of the ventilator.

Transportation services are identified to determine the procedure for providing patient transportation in an emergency. These arrangements need to be made before an emergency arises because of the uniqueness of the situation.

The family is taught cardiopulmonary resuscitation, including mouth-to-tracheostomy tube (instead of mouth-to-mouth) breathing. Handling a power failure is also explained. This involves the conversion of most ventilators from an electrical power source to a battery power source. Conversion is automatic in most types of home ventilators and lasts approximately 1 hour. The family also is instructed in the manual self-inflation technique should it be necessary.

Ultimately the patient/family responsibilities at home include the following:

Patient Care
- Monitor vital signs as directed.
- Observe physical signs such as color, secretions, breathing pattern, and state of consciousness.
- Perform physical care such as suctioning, postural drainage, and ambulation.
- Observe the tidal volume and pressure manometer regularly. Intervene when they are abnormal (ie, suction if airway pressure increases).
- Provide a communication method for the patient (*e.g.*, pad and pencil, electric larynx, talking trach)

Ventilator Care
- Check the ventilator settings twice each day and whenever the patient is removed from the ventilator.
- Adjust the volume and pressure alarms if needed.
- Fill humidifier as needed and check its level three times a day.
- Empty water in tubing as needed.

Ventilator Maintenance
- Use a clean humidifier when circuitry is changed.
- Keep exterior clean and free of any objects.
- Change external circuitry once a week or more.
- Report malfunction or strange noises right away.

Providing the opportunity for ventilator-dependent patients and their families to return home to live in familiar surroundings can be a rich, rewarding experience for all. The technical ability now exists to accomplish this. The ultimate goal for the patient on home ventilator therapy is to enhance life, not simply to support or prolong life.

In summary, a wide variety of devices, equipment, and systems may be used to assure adequate ventilation and delivery of oxygen to patients with compromised respiratory function. Although many of these devices are commonplace in the health care setting and are used routinely with postoperative patients as well as those with severe respiratory dysfunction, they are often frightening to patients and their families. Although methods to ventilate the patient and deliver oxygen can be life saving, they have potential side effects. Therefore, it is important for the nurse to work closely with other members of the health care team to assess the patient closely and monitor the functioning of the ventilator and oxygen delivery system. It is equally

---

Chart 25–5
Summary of Assessment Criteria for Successful Home Ventilator Care

1. The family members and professional staff are competent, dependable, and willing to spend the time required for proper training.
2. The patient is willing to go home.
3. The family understands the diagnosis and prognosis.
4. There is evidence of chronic underlying pulmonary abnormalities.
5. The patient's clinical pulmonary status is stable.
6. The family has sufficient financial/support resources.
7. A psychological consultation with the patient and family is made before the patient is discharged.
8. The home environment is conducive to accepting the patient.
9. The electrical facilities are adequate to operate all equipment safely.
10. The patient environment is controlled, preventing drafts in cold weather and ensuring proper ventilation in warm weather.
11. Equipment cleaning and storage space is available.

(Adapted from O'Ryan JA and Burns DG. Pulmonary Rehabilitation: From Hospital to Home. Chicago, Year Book Medical Publishers, 1984.)

important to focus on the patient's reactions and responses to treatment, his psychological status, and that of his family. Formal and informal education is an essential aspect of nursing care when these systems are part of the patient management.

The Patient Undergoing Thoracic Surgery

Assessment and management are particularly important in the patient undergoing thoracic surgery. Thoracic operations are performed for a wide variety of reasons; in addition, the patient may have obstructive pulmonary disease with compromised breathing. Preoperative management is important because there may be a narrow margin of safety in chest operations.

Fortunately, the lungs have a large functional reserve. Newer techniques of anesthesia, respiratory therapy, skillful surgery, and intensive postoperative care have made possible more extensive thoracic surgery.

The objectives of preoperative care are to ascertain the patient's functional reserve to determine if he can survive the operation and to ensure the optimal condition of the patient for surgery.

Diagnostic Evaluation

A number of preoperative tests are performed to determine the preoperative status of the patient and to assess his physical assets and limitations. The initial investigation starts with the history and physical examination—the foundation of preoperative evaluation. The general appearance of the patient, his behavior, and his mental alertness will indicate whether a significant surgical risk is involved.

The decision to perform any pulmonary resection is based on the patient's cardiovascular status and pulmonary reserve. Pulmonary function studies (especially lung volume and vital capacity) are performed to determine whether the contemplated resection will leave sufficient functioning lung tissue. Arterial blood gas values are assessed to provide a more complete picture of the functional capacity of the lung. Exercise tolerance tests have predictive value. Such tests are especially important to determine whether the patient who is a candidate for pneumonectomy can tolerate whole lung removal.

Preoperative studies are performed to provide a baseline for comparison during the postoperative period and to reveal any unsuspected abnormalities. These studies include chest radiography, electrocardiography (for arteriosclerotic heart disease, conduction defects), nutritional assessment including determination of blood urea nitrogen and serum creatinine (renal function), glucose tolerance or blood glucose (diabetes), assessment of blood electrolytes, serum protein studies, blood volume determinations, and complete blood cell count.

Operative Procedures

Lobectomy.   When the pathology is limited to one area of a lung, a lobectomy (removal of a lobe of a lung) is performed. This operation, which is more common than pneumonectomy, may be carried out for bronchogenic carcinoma, giant emphysematous blebs or bullae, benign tumors, metastatic malignant tumors, bronchiectasis, and fungus infections (Fig. 25–10).

A thoracotomy incision is used, its exact location depending on the lobe to be resected. When the pleura is entered, the involved lung collapses and the lobar vessels and the bronchus are ligated and divided. After the lobe is removed, the remaining lobes of the lung are re-expanded. Usually, two chest catheters are inserted for drainage (Fig. 25–11).

The upper tube is for the removal of air; the lower one is for drainage of fluid. Sometimes, only one catheter is needed. The chest tube is connected to a chest drainage apparatus for several days.

Pneumonectomy.   The removal of an entire lung (pneumonectomy) is performed chiefly for cancer when the lesion cannot be removed by a lesser procedure. It also may be performed for lung abscesses, bronchiectasis, or extensive unilateral tuberculosis. The removal of the right lung is more dangerous than the removal of the left, because the right lung has a larger vascular bed and its removal imposes a greater physiologic burden.

A posterolateral or anterolateral thoracotomy incision is made, sometimes with resection of a rib. The pulmonary artery and the pulmonary veins are ligated and severed.

The main bronchus is divided and the lung removed. The bronchial stump is stapled, and usually no drains are used because the accumulation of fluid in the empty hemithorax is the desired end result.

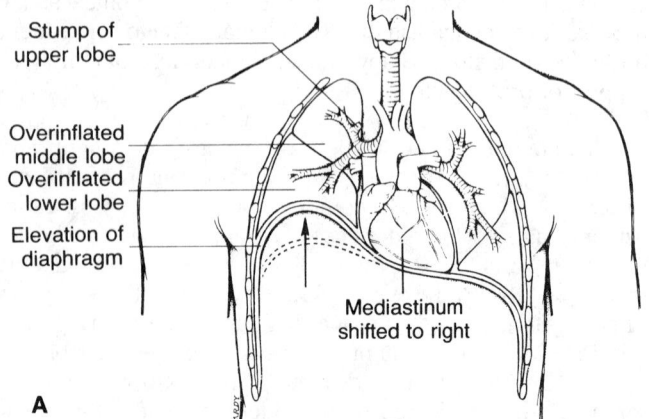

Stump of
upper lobe

Overinflated
middle lobe
Overinflated
lower lobe

Elevation of
diaphragm

Mediastinum
shifted to right

A

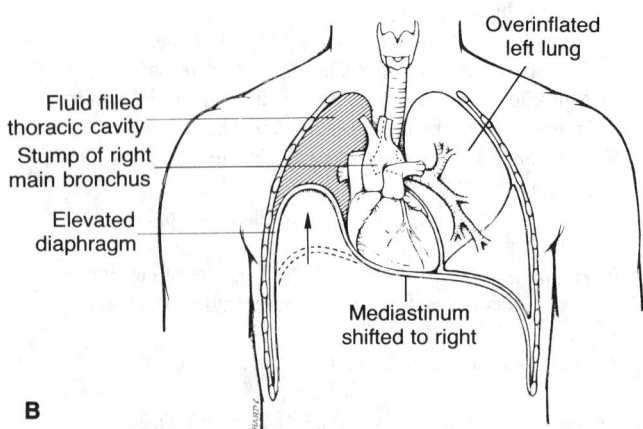

Overinflated
left lung

Fluid filled
thoracic cavity
Stump of right
main bronchus

Elevated
diaphragm

Mediastinum
shifted to right

B

Figure 25–10.   Operative procedures. (**A**) Lobectomy. (**B**) Pneumonectomy.

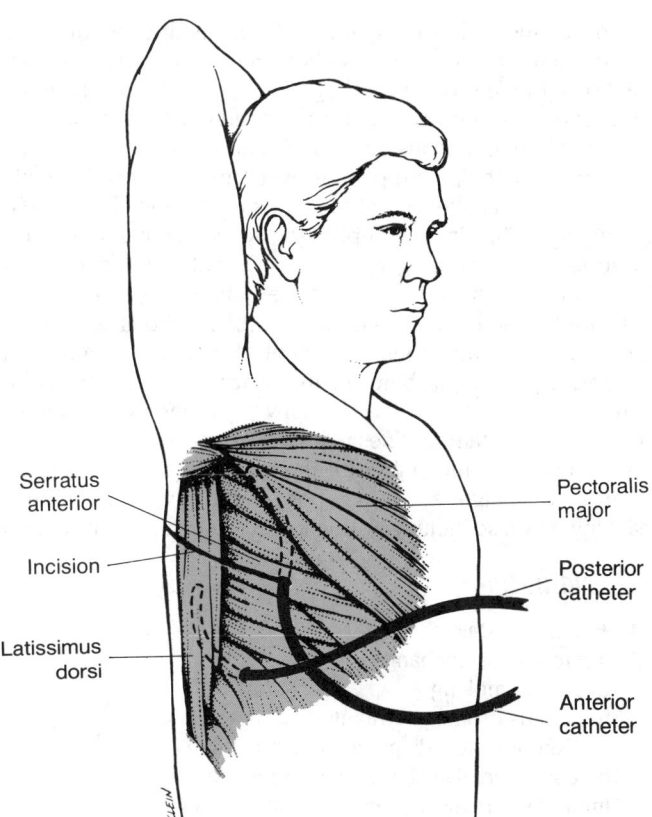

Serratus
anterior

Incision

Latissimus
dorsi

Pectoralis
major

Posterior
catheter

Anterior
catheter

KLEIN

Figure 25–11. Postoperative drainage of the chest. The upper drainage tube is used for the escape of air from leaks in the resected lung. The tip is anchored in the parietal pleura near the apex and brought out through the anterior end of the incision. The lower tube is usually for serosanguineous drainage.

Segmentectomy (Segmental Resection). Some lesions are located in only one segment of the lung. Bronchopulmonary segments are subdivisions of the lung that function as individual units (see Fig. 25–3). They are held together by delicate connective tissue; disease processes may be limited to a single segment. Care is used to preserve as much healthy and functional lung tissue as possible, especially in patients who already have a limited cardiopulmonary reserve. Single segments can be removed from any lobe, but the right middle lobe, because it has only two small segments, invariably is removed entirely. On the left side, corresponding to a middle lobe, is a "lingular" segment of the upper lobe. This can be removed as a single segment or by *lingulectomy*. This segment frequently is involved in bronchiectasis.

Wedge Resection. A wedge resection of a small, well-circumscribed lesion may be performed without regard for the location of the intersegmental planes. The pleural cavity usually is drained because of the possibility of an air or blood leak. This procedure is performed for random lung biopsy and for the excision of small peripheral nodules.

Bronchoplastic or Sleeve Resection. Bronchoplastic resection is a procedure in which only one lobar bronchus together with a part of the right or left bronchus is excised. The distal bronchus is reanastomosed to the proximal bronchus or trachea.

▶ Nursing Process
The Patient Undergoing Thoracic Surgery

◇ Preoperative Management

◇ Assessment

Chest auscultation provides an estimate of the intensity of breath sounds in the different regions of the lungs (see Chap. 24). When the chest is auscultated, it is important to note whether breath sounds are normal, indicating a free flow of air in and out of the lungs. (In the patient with emphysema, the breath sounds may be markedly decreased or even absent on auscultation.) Crackles, wheezes, and hyperresonance are noted, along with decreased diaphragmatic motion. Unilateral diminished breath sounds and rhonchi can be the result of occlusion of the bronchi by mucus plugs. Evidence of retained secretions is evaluated during auscultation by asking the patient to cough. Any signs of rhonchi or wheezing are noted. The nursing history and assessment include the following:

- What signs and symptoms are present—cough, sputum expectorated (amount), hemoptysis, chest pain, dyspnea?
- What is the smoking history? How long has the patient been smoking? How much is he currently smoking? Packs/day/years?
- What is the patient's cardiopulmonary tolerance while resting, eating, bathing, walking?
- What is his breathing pattern? How much exertion is required to produce dyspnea?
- Does he need to sleep in an upright position?
- What is the physiologic age of the patient—for example, general appearance, mental alertness, behavior, nutritional status?
- What other medical conditions exist—allergies, cardiac disorders, and so forth?
- What are his personal preferences and dislikes?

◇ Nursing Diagnoses

Based on the assessment data, the patient's major preoperative nursing diagnoses may include the following:

- Impaired gas exchange related to lung impairment
- Ineffective airway clearance related to lung impairment
- Knowledge deficit about the surgical procedure and self-care
- Anxiety related to diagnosis and surgical procedure

◇ Planning and Implementation

◇ *Goals:* The major goals for the patient may include improvement of gas exchange, improvement in airway clearance, acquisition of knowledge about the surgical procedure and self-care, and relief of anxiety.

◇ Nursing Interventions

◇ *Improvement of Gas Exchange.* An important preoperative goal is to improve alveolar ventilation, thereby enhancing gas exchange. The nurse assists in the delivery of care, which includes encouraging avoidance of bronchial irritants, especially cigarette smoking; drinking of more fluids and use of humidification to loosen secretions; administration of bronchodilators as prescribed to relieve bronchospasm; and instruction in diaphragmatic breathing for more effective ventilation. Incentive spirometry is initiated preoperatively to teach the patient the technique so that postoperatively he will be able to perform the maneuver without problems.

▷ *Improvement of Airway Clearance.* The underlying lung condition often is associated with increased respiratory secretions. Preoperatively, the airways are cleared of secretions to reduce the possibility of postoperative atelectasis or infection. This is accomplished through humidification, postural drainage, and chest percussion after the administration of bronchodilators, if prescribed. The volume of sputum is estimated in patients who expectorate large amounts of secretions. Such measurements are carried out to determine if the amount is decreasing. Antibiotics are administered as prescribed for infection, which may be causing the excessive secretions.

▷ *Understanding of the Surgical Procedure and Self-Care Techniques.* The patient is informed of what to expect in the postoperative period, that is, the possible presence of a chest tube or tubes and drainage bottles, the usual postoperative administration of oxygen to facilitate breathing, and the possible use of a ventilator. The importance of frequent turning to promote drainage of lung secretions is explained. Instruction in the use of incentive spirometry begins preoperatively to familiarize the patient with its correct use. Diaphragmatic and pursed lip breathing are taught and should be practiced at this time.

Because a coughing schedule will be necessary in the postoperative period to promote clearance or removal of secretions, the patient should be instructed in the technique of coughing and warned that the coughing routine may prove to be uncomfortable. He is taught to splint his incision with his hands, a pillow, or a folded towel.

The patient is taught coughing and huffing techniques as follows:

1. Sit upright with knees flexed and body bent slightly forward.
2. Splint the incisional area with firm hand pressure or support it with a pillow or rolled blanket while coughing. (The nurse can initially demonstrate this by using his hands).
3. Take three deep breaths followed by a deep inspiration (inhaling slowly and evenly through the nose).
4. Contract (pull in) the abdominal muscles and cough twice forcefully, with mouth open and tongue out.
5. If unable to sit, lie on one side with hips and knees flexed.

Forced Exhalation Technique (Huffing Technique). ''Huffing'' is the expulsion of air through an open glottis and may be helpful for the patient with diminished expiratory flow rates or for the patient in severe pain who refuses to cough. This type of forceful exhalation stimulates pulmonary expansion and assists in alveolar inflation.

1. Take a deep diaphragmatic breath and exhale forcefully against your hand. Exhale forcefully in a quick, distinct pant, or ''huff.''
2. Practice doing small huffs and progress to one strong huff during exhalation.

▷ *Relief of Anxiety.* Increasingly, patients are admitted only 1 or 2 days before or even on the day of surgery, which does not provide much time for the nurse to talk with the patient. To effectively use the time before surgery, the nurse listens to the patient to evaluate how he feels about his illness and pro-

posed treatment. The nurse also determines the patient's motivation to return to normal function. He may reveal significant reactions: the fear of hemorrhage because of bloody sputum, the fear of discomfort of a chronic cough and chest pain, or the fear of death because of dyspnea and tumor.

The nurse helps the patient overcome many of his fears and mobilize his intellectual functions to cope with the stress of surgery. This is accomplished by correcting any false impressions, by offering reassurance about the capability of the surgical team, by reassuring the patient that his incision will ''hold,'' and by dealing honestly with questions about pain and discomfort and their treatment. The management and control of pain begin before surgery when the patient is informed that he can overcome many postoperative problems by following certain routines related to deep breathing, coughing, turning, and moving. With the increasing use of patient-controlled analgesia (PCA) postoperatively, preoperative teaching may also include instruction in this treatment modality.

▷ Evaluation

Expected Outcomes

1. Improves gas exchange
   a. Stops smoking
   b. Avoids bronchial irritants
   c. Demonstrates diaphragmatic breathing
   d. Uses incentive spirometer correctly
2. Improves airway clearance
   a. Verbalizes importance of measures to improve airway clearance (humidification, postural drainage, chest percussion, bronchodilators)
   b. Collects sputum so that it can be measured
3. Attains knowledge of surgery and care
   a. Verbalizes what to expect in postoperative period, especially the presence of chest tubes
   b. Demonstrates effective breathing, coughing, and splinting techniques
4. Improves ability to cope
   a. Verbalizes that misconceptions have been clarified
   b. Demonstrates techniques to help control pain such as deep breathing, and splinting while coughing, turning, and moving

Postoperative Management

Potential Complications

Complications after thoracic surgery are always a possibility and must be identified and managed early. Pulmonary edema due to overinfusion of intravenous fluids is a significant danger. The early symptoms are dyspnea, crackles, bubbling sounds in the chest, tachycardia, and pink, frothy sputum. This constitutes an emergency and is reported immediately. In addition, the patient is monitored at regular intervals for signs of hemorrhage, mediastinal shift, bronchopulmonary fistula, infection, shock, atelectasis, pneumothorax, dysrhythmias, pleural effusion, and gastric distention.

Chest Drainage

A crucial intervention for improving gas exchange and breathing is the proper management of chest drainage. After thoracic surgery, chest tubes and a closed drainage system are used to re-expand the involved lung and to remove excess air and fluid (or blood).

The normal breathing mechanism operates on the principle of negative pressure (the pressure in the chest cavity is lower than the pressure of the atmosphere, causing air to move into the lungs during inspiration). Whenever the chest is opened, from any cause, there is a loss of negative pressure, which can result in the collapse of the lung. The collection of air, fluid, or other substances in the chest can compromise cardiopulmonary function and even cause collapse of the lung. Pathologic substances that collect in the pleural space include fibrin, or clotted blood; liquids (serous fluids, blood, pus, chyle); and gases (air from the lung, tracheobronchial tree, or esophagus).

Surgical incision of the chest wall almost always causes some degree of pneumothorax. Air and fluid collect in the intrapleural space, restricting lung expansion and reducing air exchange. It is necessary to keep the pleural space evacuated postoperatively and to maintain negative pressure within this potential space. Therefore, during or immediately after thoracic surgery, chest catheters are positioned strategically in the pleural space (see Fig. 25–11), sutured to the skin, and connected to a drainage apparatus to remove the residual air and drainage fluid from the pleural or mediastinal space. This results in the re-expansion of remaining lung tissue.

A chest drainage system must be capable of removing whatever collects in the pleural space so that a normal pleural space and normal cardiopulmonary function may be restored and maintained. Commercially available systems (*e.g.*, Pleur-Evac [Fig. 25–12]) are the most common method currently in use to provide water-seal drainage; these systems use the same principles as a three-bottle water-seal system. The chest tube or catheter is attached to the drainage system, using a one-way valve. Water in the second chamber acts as a seal and allows air and fluid to drain from the chest into the first chamber, but air cannot reenter the chest tube. Drainage accumulates in the first chamber and air exits from the second chamber. The water level fluctuates as the patient breathes; it moves up when the patient inhales and it moves down when the patient exhales. Suction may be added to the second chamber to create a negative pressure to promote drainage of fluid and removal of air. The addition of suction creates constant bubbling in the third chamber; if constant bubbling occurs in the absence of suction, there may be leakage of air from the lung or a leak in the system. Care of the patient with water-seal chest drainage is discussed in Chart 25–6.

To understand water-seal chest drainage, one-bottle, two-bottle, and three-bottle water-seal systems are described below. Their use has decreased, however, with the availability of self-contained, disposable commercial systems.

Single-Bottle Water-Seal System. The end of the drainage tube from the patient's chest is covered by a layer of water, which permits drainage of air and fluid from the pleural space

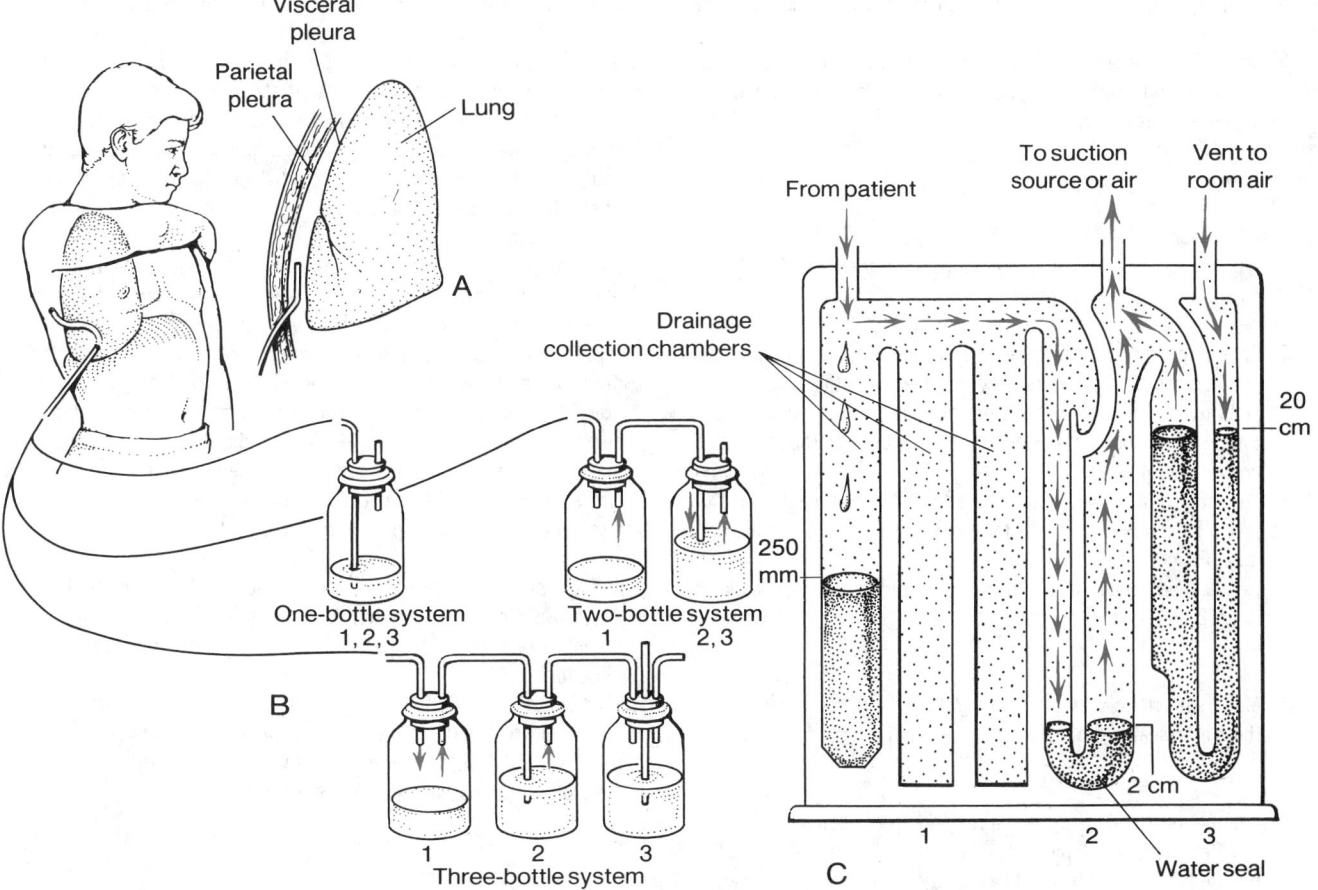

Figure 25–12. Chest drainage system. (**A**) Strategic placement of a chest catheter in the pleural space. (**B**) Three types of mechanical drainage systems. (**C**) A Pleur–Evac operating system: (1) the collection chamber, (2) the water seal chamber, and (3) the suction control chamber. The Pleur–Evac is a single unit with all three bottles identified as chambers.

Chart 25–6
Guidelines to the Nurse's Role in the Management of the Patient
With Water-Seal Chest Drainage*

An intrapleural drainage tube is used after most intrathoracic procedures. One or more chest catheters are held in the pleural space by suture to the chest wall and are attached to a drainage system. The purposes are
1. To remove solids, liquids, and gas from the pleural space or thoracic cavity and the mediastinal space
2. To bring about reexpansion of the lung and restore normal cardiorespiratory function after surgery, trauma, or medical conditions by establishing negative pressure in the pleural cavity

Procedure

Nursing Action	Rationale/Amplification
1. Fill the water-seal chamber with sterile water to the level equaling 2 cm H_2O.	Water-seal drainage provides for the escape of air and fluid into a drainage bottle. The water acts as a seal and keeps the air from being drawn back into the pleural space.
2. If suction is used, fill the suction control chamber with sterile water to the 20-cm level or as prescribed.	The water level will determine the degree of suction applied.
3. Attach the drainage catheter from the pleural space (the patient) to the tubing coming from the collection chamber of the water seal system. Tape securely.	In disposable units, the system is a closed system, with the only connection being the one to the patient's catheter.
4. If suction is used, connect the suction control chamber tubing to the suction unit. Turn on suction unit and increase pressure until slow but steady bubbling appears in the suction control chamber.	The degree of suction is determined by the amount of water in the suction control chamber and is *not* dependent on the rate of bubbling nor the pressure gauge setting on the suction unit.
5. Mark the original fluid level with tape on the outside of the drainage unit. Mark hourly/daily increments (date and time) at the drainage level.	This marking will show the amount of fluid loss and how fast fluid is collecting in the drainage bottle. It serves as a basis for blood replacement, if the fluid is blood. Grossly bloody drainage will appear in the bottle in the immediate postoperative period; it gradually becomes serous and if excessive may require reoperation or autotransfusion. Drainage usually declines progressively in the first 24 hours.
6. Ensure that the tubing is not looping or interfering with the movements of the patient.	Kinking, looping, or pressure on the drainage tubing can produce back-pressure, and may thus possibly force drainage back into the pleural space or impede drainage from the pleural space.
7. Encourage the patient to assume a position of comfort. Encourage good body alignment. When the patient is in the lateral position, make sure that the tubing is not compressed by the weight of the patient's body. Encourage the patient to change position frequently.	The patient's position should be changed frequently to promote drainage, and the body should be kept in good alignment to prevent postural deformities and contractures. Proper positioning helps breathing and promotes better air exchange. Pain medication may be needed to enhance comfort and deep breathing.
8. Put the arm and shoulder of the affected side through range of motion exercises several times daily. Some pain medication may be necessary.	Exercise helps to avoid ankylosis of the shoulder and assists in lessening postoperative pain and discomfort.
9. Gently "milk" the tubing in the direction of the drainage chamber every 2 hours or as needed.	"Milking" the tubing prevents it from becoming plugged with clots and fibrin. Constant attention to maintaining the patency of the tube facilitates prompt expansion of the lung and minimizes complications.
10. Make sure there is fluctuation ("tidaling") of the fluid level in the water-seal chamber.	Fluctuation of the water level in the tube shows that there is effective communication between the pleural cavity and the drainage bottle, provides a valuable indication of the patency of the drainage system, and is a gauge of intrapleural pressure.
11. Fluctuations of fluid in the tubing will stop when a. The lung has reexpanded. b. The tubing is obstructed by blood clots or fibrin, or kinking. c. A dependent loop develops. d. Suction motor or wall suction is not working properly.	

(continued)

Chart 25-6 (Continued)

Nursing Action	*Rationale/Amplification*
12. Observe for leaks of air in the drainage system as indicated by constant bubbling in the water-seal chamber.	Leaking and trapping of air in the pleural space can result in tension pneumothorax.
a. Assess chest tube system for correctable external leaks.	
b. Notify physician immediately of excessive bubbling in the water-seal chamber not due to external leaks.	
13. Observe and report immediately signs of rapid, shallow breathing; cyanosis; pressure in the chest; subcutaneous emphysema; symptoms of hemorrhage; significant changes in color or vital signs.	Many clinical conditions may cause these signs and symptoms, including tension pneumothorax, mediastinal shift, hemorrhage, severe incisional pain, pulmonary embolus, and cardiac tamponade. Surgical intervention may be necessary.
14. Encourage the patient to breathe deeply and cough at frequent intervals. If there are signs of incisional pain, adequate pain medication is indicated. Request order for PCA pump if appropriate. Instruct in use of incentive spirometry.	Deep breathing and coughing help to raise the intrapleural pressure, which allows emptying of any accumulation in the pleural space and removes secretions from the tracheobronchial tree, so that the lung expands and atelectasis is prevented.
15. If the patient has to be transported to another area, place the drainage system below the chest level, if he is lying on a stretcher. If the tube becomes disconnected, cut off the contaminated tips of the chest tube and tubing, insert a sterile connector in the chest tube and tubing, and reattach to the drainage system. Otherwise, do not clamp chest tube during transport.	The drainage apparatus must be kept at a level lower than the patient's chest to prevent backflow of fluid into the pleural space.
16. When assisting the surgeon in removing the tube:	
a. Instruct the patient to perform a gentle Valsalva maneuver or to breathe quietly.	The chest tube is removed as directed when the lung is reexpanded (usually 24 hours to several days) depending on the cause of the pneumothorax. During removal of the tube the chief priorities are prevention of entrance of air into the pleural cavity as the tube is withdrawn and prevention of infection.
b. The chest tube is clamped and quickly removed.	
c. Simultaneously, a small bandage is applied and made airtight with petrolatum gauze covered by a 4 × 4-inch gauze pad and thoroughly covered and sealed with adhesive tape.	

* There are commercial disposable chest drainage devices available that use the water-seal principle, and these guidelines refer to their use.

but does not allow air to move back into the chest. Functionally, drainage depends on gravity and on the mechanics of respiration. As the fluid level in the bottle increases, it becomes progressively more difficult for air and fluid to exit the chest. Therefore, suction may be added.

Two-Bottle System. The two-bottle system consists of the same water-seal chamber plus a fluid collection bottle. Drainage is similar to that of a single unit, except that when pleural fluid drains, the underwater seal system is not affected by the volume of drainage.

Effective drainage depends on gravity or on the amount of suction added to the system. When vacuum (suction) is added to the system from a vacuum source, such as wall suction, the connection is made at the vent stem of the underwater-seal bottle. The amount of suction applied to the system is regulated by the wall gauge.

Three-Bottle System. The three-bottle system is similar in all respects to the two-bottle system, except for the addition of a third bottle to control the amount of suction applied. The amount of suction is determined by the depth to which the tip of the venting glass tube is submerged. (For example, submersion to 10 cm below the surface of the water will equal 10 cm of water suction applied to the patient.)

In the three-bottle system (as in the other two), drainage depends on gravity or the amount of suction applied. The amount of suction in this system is controlled by the manometer bottle. The mechanical suction motor or wall suction creates

and maintains a negative pressure throughout the entire closed drainage system.

The third bottle regulates the amount of vacuum in the system. This depends on the depth to which the tube is submerged—the usual depth is 20 cm (7.6 in).

When the vacuum in the system becomes greater than the depth to which the tube is submerged, outside air is sucked into the system. This results in constant bubbling in the manometer (or pressure-regulator) bottle, which indicates that the system is functioning properly.

- **Note:** When the wall vacuum is turned off, the drainage system must be open to the atmosphere so that intrapleural air can escape from the system. This can be done by detaching the tubing from the suction port to provide a vent.

The commercially available systems are safer because they are self-contained, unbreakable, and disposable, and have no connections (except to the chest catheter) that may become loose. Nursing care is easier to provide, and the convenience of the systems encourages easier and earlier ambulation for the patient.

Assessment

The character and depth of the patient's respirations and his color serve as important criteria in evaluating whether the lungs are being adequately expanded. The heart rate and rhythm are monitored by auscultation and electrocardiography, because major dysrhythmic episodes are common after thoracic and cardiac surgery. Dysrhythmias can occur at any time, but frequently are seen between the second and sixth postoperative days. The rate of occurrence of dysrhythmias increases with patients over 50 years of age and with those undergoing pneumonectomy or esophageal surgery.

An arterial line is maintained to facilitate frequent monitoring of blood gases, serum electrolytes, hemoglobin and hematocrit values, and arterial pressure. Central venous pressure is monitored for the early recognition of fluid volume disturbances.

▷ Nursing Diagnoses

Based on the assessment data, the patient's major postoperative nursing diagnoses may include

- Impaired gas exchange related to lung impairment and surgery
- Ineffective airway clearance related to lung impairment, anesthesia, and pain
- Pain related to incision, drainage tubes, and the surgical procedure
- Impaired physical mobility of the upper extremities related to thoracic surgery
- Fluid volume imbalance related to the surgical procedure
- Anxiety related to outcomes of surgery, pain, technology
- Knowledge deficit about care procedures at home

▷ Planning and Implementation

▷ *Goals:*   The major goals for the patient may include improvement of gas exchange and breathing, improvement of airway clearance, relief of pain and discomfort, increased arm and shoulder mobility, maintenance of adequate fluid volume, decrease in anxiety to a manageable level, and understanding of self-care procedures.

▷ Nursing Interventions

▷ *Improvement of Gas Exchange and Breathing.*   Gas exchange is determined by evaluating oxygenation and ventilation. In the immediate postoperative period, this is achieved by measuring the blood pressure, pulse, and respirations every 15 minutes for the first 1 to 2 hours, then less frequently as the patient's condition stabilizes.

The diaphragmatic and pursed lip breathing taught preoperatively should be practiced every 2 hours to expand alveoli and prevent atelectasis. Another technique to improve ventilation is sustained maximal inspiratory (SMI) therapy or incentive spirometry (p. 527). This technique optimizes lung inflation, improves the cough mechanism, and provides for early assessment of acute pulmonary changes.

When the patient is oriented and his blood pressure stabilized, the head of the bed is elevated 30 to 40 degrees during the immediate postoperative period. This facilitates ventilation, promotes chest drainage from the lower chest tube, and helps residual air to rise in the upper portion of pleural space, where it can be removed through the upper chest tube.

The surgeon is consulted about individual patient positioning. The patient with limited respiratory reserve may not be able to turn on the unoperated side, as this limits ventilation of the operated side. The position is varied from horizontal to semi-upright, because remaining in one position tends to promote the retention of secretions in the dependent portion of the lungs. After a pneumonectomy, the operated side should be dependent so that fluid in the pleural space remains below the level of the bronchial stump, and the unoperative side can fully expand.

Turning Procedure
1. Instruct the patient to bend his knees and use his feet to push.
2. Have the patient shift his hips and shoulders to the opposite side of the bed while pushing with his feet.
3. Bring the patient's arm over his chest, pointing it in the direction toward which he is being turned and have him grasp the side rail with his hand.
4. Turn patient in "log roll" fashion to prevent twisting at the waist and possible pulling of the incision, which could be painful.

▷ *Improvement of Airway Clearance.*   Retained secretions are a threat to the thoracotomy patient postoperatively. Trauma to the tracheobronchial tree during operation, diminished lung ventilation, and diminished cough reflex all result in the accumulation of excessive secretions. If the secretions are not managed or removed, airway obstruction will occur, which causes air in the alveoli distal to the obstruction to become absorbed and the lung to collapse. Atelectasis, pneumonia, and respiratory failure may result.

There are a few techniques that are used to maintain a patent airway. First, secretions are suctioned from the tracheobronchial tree before the endotracheal tube is removed (this begins in the recovery room). Secretions continue to be removed by suctioning until the patient can cough up secretions effectively. Nasotracheal suctioning, although a difficult skill to master, may be useful to stimulate a deep cough and aspirate secretions that the patient is unable to cough up. It should be used only after other methods to raise secretions have been unsuccessful, however.

Technique for Nasotracheal Suctioning (Sterile technique is to be used.)

1. Explain procedure to the patient. Medicate patient for pain if necessary.
2. Place the patient in a sitting or semi-Fowler's position. Make sure the patient's head is not flexed forward. Remove excess pillows if necessary.
3. Oxygenate the patient several minutes before initiating the suctioning procedure. Have ready oxygen source nearby during procedure.
4. Put on sterile gloves.
5. Lubricate catheter with water-soluble gel.
6. Gently pass catheter through the patent nostril to the pharynx. Check the position of the tip of the catheter by asking the patient to open his mouth and inspecting; it should be in the lower pharynx.
7. Instruct the patient to take a deep breath or stick out his tongue. This opens the epiglottis and promotes downward movement of the catheter.
8. Advance the catheter into the trachea only during inspiration. Listen for cough or for passage of air through catheter.
9. Attach catheter to suction apparatus. Apply intermittent suction while slowly withdrawing the catheter. Do not let suction exceed 120 mm Hg.
10. Avoid suctioning for longer than 10 to 15 seconds, as dysrhythmias, bradycardia, or cardiac arrest may occur in patients with borderline oxygenation.

11. If another suctioning pass is needed, withdraw catheter. Reassure and oxygenate patient for several minutes before resuming.

Another measure that is used in maintaining a patent airway is the coughing technique. The patient is encouraged to cough effectively, as ineffective coughing will result in exhaustion and retention of secretions. To be effective, the cough must be low pitched, deep, and controlled. Because it is difficult to cough in a supine position, the patient is helped to a sitting position on the edge of the bed, with his feet resting on a chair. Coughing is carried out at least every hour (as described on p. 546) during the first 24 hours and when necessary thereafter. If audible crackles are present, it may be necessary to use chest percussion with the cough routine until the lungs are clear. Aerosol therapy is helpful in humidifying and mobilizing secretions so that they can be readily coughed up. To lessen incisional pain during coughing, the nurse supports the incision firmly over the operated side and against the opposite chest (Fig. 25–13).

After helping the patient to cough, the nurse should listen to both lungs, anteriorly and posteriorly, to determine whether there are any changes in breath sounds, as diminished sounds may indicate collapsed or hypoventilated alveoli.

The final technique for maintaining a patent airway is chest physiotherapy. If a patient is identified as being at high risk for developing postoperative pulmonary complications, then chest physiotherapy is started immediately (perhaps even preoperatively). The techniques of postural drainage, vibration, and percussion help to loosen and mobilize the secretions so that they can be coughed up or suctioned (see previous page).

▷ *Relief of Pain and Discomfort.*   Pain after a thoracotomy may be severe, depending on the type of incision and the patient's reaction to and ability to cope with pain. Deep inspiration is very painful after thoracotomy. Pain can lead to postoperative complications if it reduces the patient's ability to breathe deeply and cough and if it further limits chest excursions so that effective ventilation is decreased. Immediately after the surgical procedure and before the incision is closed, the surgeon may perform a nerve block with a long-acting local anesthetic, which can reduce postoperative pain. Small, intravenous doses of a narcotic are administered as prescribed and are titrated to relieve pain while still allowing the patient to cooperate in deep breathing, coughing, and mobilization efforts. It is important to avoid depressing the respiratory system with too much narcotic, however, as the patient should not be so somnolent that he does not cough.

Because of the need to maximize patient comfort without depressing the respiratory drive, newer methods of patient-controlled analgesia are increasing in popularity. Patient-controlled analgesia through an intravenous pump or epidural catheter allows the patient to control the frequency and total dose of narcotic. Preset limits are set on the pumps to avoid overdosage. With proper instruction, these methods are well tolerated and allow earlier mobilization and cooperation with the treatment regimen.

- **Note:** Do not confuse the restlessness of hypoxia with restlessness due to pain. Dyspnea, restlessness, increasing respiratory rate, increasing blood pressure, and tachycardia are warning signs of impending respiratory insufficiency.

▷ *Mobility and Shoulder Exercises.*   When the physician determines that the patient is ready for activity, the patient is encouraged and assisted to get out of bed. Often this occurs on the evening of the day of surgery. Although this may be painful initially, the earlier the patient moves, the sooner the pain will subside. In addition to getting out of bed, the patient begins arm and shoulder exercises (Fig. 25–14) to restore movement and prevent painful stiffening of the affected arm

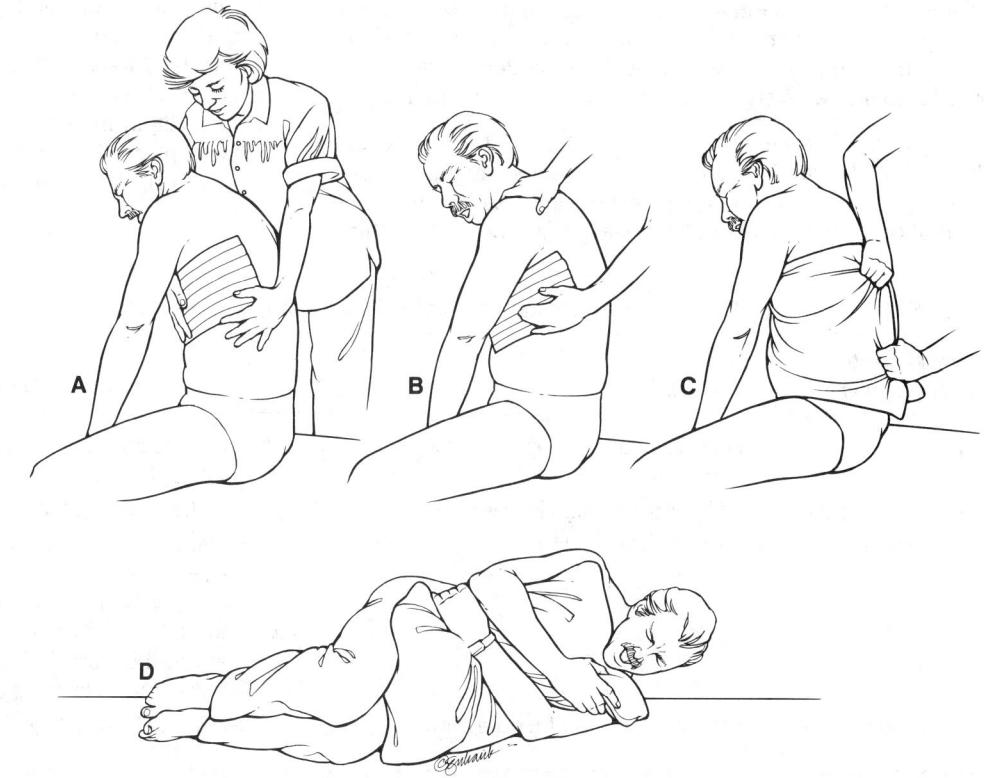

Figure 25–13. Techniques for support of incision while patient with thoracic surgery coughs. (**A**) The nurse's hands should support the chest incision anteriorly and posteriorly. The patient is instructed to take several deep breaths, inhale, and then cough forcibly. (**B**) With one hand, the nurse exerts downward pressure on the shoulder of the affected side while firmly supporting beneath the wound with the other hand. The patient is instructed to take several deep breaths, inhale, and then cough forcibly. (**C**) The nurse can wrap a towel or sheet around the patient's chest and hold the ends together, pulling slightly as the patient coughs, releasing as he takes deep breaths. (**D**) The patient can be taught to hold a pillow firmly against his incision while coughing. This can be done while lying down or sitting in an upright position.

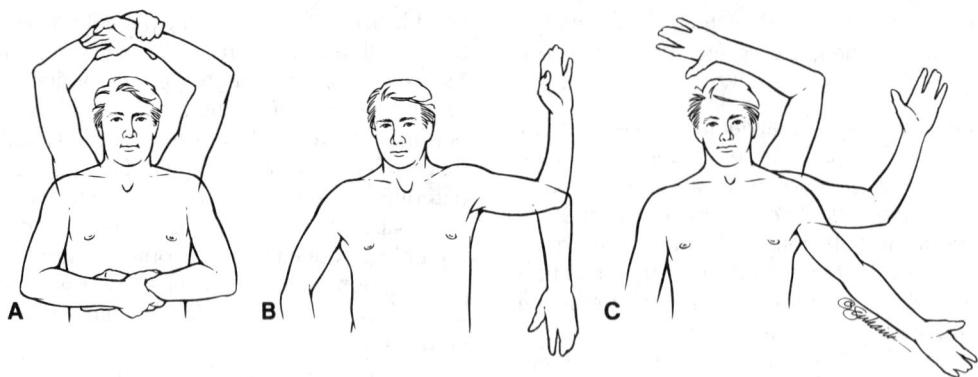

Figure 25–14. Arm and shoulder exercises are performed after thoracic surgery to restore movement, prevent painful stiffening of the shoulder, and improve muscle power. (**A**) Hold hand of the affected side with the other hand, palms facing in. Raise the arms forward, upward, and then overhead, while taking a deep breath. Exhale while lowering the arms. Repeat five times. (**B**) Raise arm sideward, upward, and downward in a waving motion. (**C**) Place arm at side. Raise arm sideward, upward, and over the head. Repeat five times. Both exercises can also be done while lying in bed.

and shoulder. Specific skeletal exercises designed to restore function after thoracic surgery are described in Table 25–3.

▷ *Fluid Volume and Nutritional Considerations.* During the operation or immediately after, the patient may receive a blood transfusion, followed by a continuous intravenous infusion. The rate of administration must be titrated (according to physician order) based on the nurse's assessment of patient tolerance, especially when there is evidence of limited cardiopulmonary reserve and when the pulmonary vascular bed has been greatly reduced, as in pneumonectomy. It is not unusual for patients undergoing thoracotomy to have poor nutritional status preoperatively, because of dyspnea, sputum production, and poor appetite.

It is especially important therefore that the patient's nutrition be supported as soon as feasible postoperatively. A liquid diet is provided as soon as there is evidence of bowel sounds. The patient is progressed to a full diet as soon as possible. Small, frequent, well-balanced meals are better tolerated and crucial to the recovery and maintenance of lung function.

▷ *Patient Education and Home Care Considerations.* Because large shoulder girdle muscles are transected during a thoracotomy, the arm and shoulder must be mobilized by full range of motion of the shoulder. This is accomplished by teaching

the patient exercises necessary to improve function and encouraging him to continue them on discharge. He is taught to extend his arm (stretch and reach) and then reach behind his head, and to do these exercises five times daily (see Fig. 25–14 and Table 25–3). This accelerates recovery of muscle function affected by incision, pain, and "splinting," and reduces long-term pain and discomfort and particularly the development of adhesions. All joints should be stretched and flexed. The patient is encouraged to assume a functional erect position to restore normal posture (preferably in front of a full-length mirror).

In addition to the arm and should exercises, the patient is instructed in the following on discharge:

1. Relieve intercostal pain that may occur by using local heat and oral analgesia.
2. Alternate walking and other activities with frequent rest periods. Be aware that weakness and fatigue are common for the first 3 weeks.
3. Practice breathing exercises for the first few weeks at home.
4. Avoid lifting more than 20 pounds until complete healing has taken place; the chest muscles and incision may be weaker than normal for 3 to 6 months after surgery.

(text continues on page 556)

TABLE 25–3.   *Skeletal Exercises Designed to Restore Function After Thoracic Surgery*

Muscle Affected by Thoracotomy	Function	Activities to Restore Function
Trapezius	Promotes arm extension, abduction, and reach extension	Extend the arm up and back, out to the side and back, down at the side and back.
Rhomboideus major	Adducts and slightly elevates scapula	Place hands in small of back. Push elbows as far back as possible.
Latissimus dorsi	Depresses the shoulder	Sit erect in an armchair: place the hands on the arms of the chair directly opposite either side of the body. Press down on hands, consciously pulling the abdomen in and stretching up from the waist. Inhale while raising the body until the elbows are extended completely. Hold this position a moment, and begin exhaling while lowering the body slowly to the original position.
Serratus anterior	Rotates scapula and fixes it against the rib cage	Reach over head and "push" in an upward and outward motion.

Nursing Care Plan 25–1

Care of the Patient Following Thoracotomy

Nursing Interventions	Rationale	Expected Outcomes

Nursing Diagnosis: Impaired gas exchange related to lung impairment and surgery

Goal: Improvement of gas exchange and breathing

Nursing Interventions	Rationale	Expected Outcomes
1. Monitor pulmonary status as directed and as needed: a. Auscultate breath sounds. b. Check rate, depth, and pattern of respirations. c. Evaluate patient's color for cyanosis. d. Assess blood gases for signs of hypoxemia or CO_2 retention.	1. Changes in pulmonary status indicate improvement or onset of complications.	• Lungs are clear on auscultation. • Respiratory rate is within normal range with no episodes of dyspnea. • Vital signs are stable. • Dysrhythmias are not present or are under control. • Demonstrates deep, controlled, effective breathing to allow maximal lung expansion. • Uses incentive spirometer every 2 hours while awake. • Demonstrates deep, effective coughing technique. • Lungs are expanded to capacity (evidenced by chest film).
2. Take and record blood pressure, apical pulse, and temperature every 2–4 hours, central venous pressure (if used) every 2 hours.	2. Aid in evaluating effect of surgery on cardiac status.	
3. Monitor continuous electrocardiogram for pattern and dysrhythmias.	3. Dysrhythmias are more frequently seen after thoracic surgery (especially atrial fibrillation and atrial flutter). A patient with total pneumonectomy is especially prone to cardiac irregularity.	
4. Elevate head of bed 30–40 degrees when patient is oriented and hemodynamic status is stable.	4. Maximum lung excursion is achieved when patient is as close to upright as possible.	
5. Encourage deep breathing exercises (see section Breathing Retraining, p. 529) and effective use of incentive spirometer (sustained maximal inspiration).	5. Helps to achieve maximal lung inflation and to open closed airways.	
6. Encourage and promote an effective cough routine to be performed every 1–2 hours during first 24 hours.	6. Coughing is necessary to remove retained secretions, which will be difficult to turn from operative side.	
7. Assess and monitor the water-seal system:* a. Assess for leaks and patency as needed. b. Monitor amount and character of drainage and document every 2 hours. Notify physician if drainage is 150 ml/hr or greater. c. See Chart 25-6 for summary of nurse's role in management of water-seal drainage.	7. System is used to eliminate any residual air or fluid after thoracotomy.	

(continued)

Nursing Care Plan 25–1 (Continued)

Care of the Patient Following Thoracotomy

Nursing Interventions	Rationale	Expected Outcomes

Nursing Diagnosis: Ineffective airway clearance related to lung impairment, anesthesia, and pain

Goal: Improvement of airway clearance and achievement of a patent airway

Nursing Interventions	Rationale	Expected Outcomes
1. Maintain an open airway.	1. Provides for adequate ventilation and gas exchange.	• Airway is patent. • Coughs effectively. • Splints incision while coughing. • Sputum is clear or colorless. • Lungs are clear on auscultation.
2. Perform endotracheal suctioning until patient is able to raise secretions effectively.	2. Endotracheal secretions are present in excessive amounts in post-thoracotomy patients due to trauma to the tracheobronchial tree during surgery, diminished lung ventilation, and cough reflex.	
3. Assess and medicate for pain. Encourage deep breathing and coughing exercises. Assist in splinting the incision during coughing.	3. Helps to achieve maximal lung inflation and to open closed airways. Coughing is painful; incision needs to be supported.	
4. Monitor amount, viscosity, color, and odor of sputum. Notify physician if sputum is excessive or contains bright red blood.	4. Changes in sputum suggest presence of infection or change in pulmonary status. Colorless sputum is not unusual; opacification or coloring of sputum may indicate dehydration or infection.	
5. Administer humidification and mini-nebulizer therapy as prescribed.	5. Secretions must be moistened and thinned if they are to be raised from the chest with the least amount of effort.	
6. Perform postural drainage, percussion, and vibration as prescribed. Do not percuss or vibrate directly over operative site.	6. Chest physiotherapy uses gravity to help remove secretions from the lung.	
7. Auscultate both sides of chest to determine changes in breath sounds.	7. Indications for tracheal aspirations are determined by chest auscultation.	

Nursing Diagnosis: Pain related to incision and surgical procedure

Goal: Relief of pain and discomfort

Nursing Interventions	Rationale	Expected Outcomes
1. Evaluate location, character, quality and degree of pain. Administer pain medication as prescribed and as needed. • Watch for respiratory effect of narcotic analgesic. Is patient too somnolent to cough? Are respirations depressed?	1. Pain limits chest excursions and thereby decreases ventilation.	• Asks for pain medication, but verbalizes that he expects some discomfort while deep breathing and coughing. • Verbalizes that he is comfortable and in no acute distress. • No signs of incisional infection evident.
2. Maintain care postoperatively in positioning the thoracotomy patient: a. Place patient in semi-Fowler's position. b. Patients with limited respiratory reserve may not be able to turn on unoperated side. c. Assist or turn patient every 2 hours.	2. If patient is comfortable and free of pain, he will be less likely to splint his chest while breathing. A semi-Fowler's position permits residual air to rise to upper portion of pleural space and be removed via the upper chest catheter.	
3. Assess incision area every 8 hours for signs of infection: redness, heat, induration, swelling, separation, and drainage.		
4. Request order for PCA pump if appropriate for patient.	4. Allowing patient control over frequency and dose improves comfort and compliance with treatment regimen.	

(continued)

Nursing Care Plan 25–1 *(Continued)*

Care of the Patient Following Thoracotomy

Nursing Interventions	Rationale	Expected Outcomes

Nursing Diagnosis: Anxiety related to outcomes of surgery, pain, technology

Goal: Reduction of anxiety to a manageable level.

1. Explain all procedures in simple terms before proceeding.	1. Explaining what can be expected in understandable terms decreases anxiety and increases cooperation.	• States that anxiety is at a manageable level.
2. Assess for pain (from both verbal and nonverbal cues) and medicate, especially before potentially painful procedures.	2. Premedication before painful procedures or activities improves comfort and minimizes undue anxiety.	• Participates with health care team in treatment regimen. • Uses appropriate coping skills (verbalization, pain relief, use of support systems such as family, clergy).
3. Silence all *unnecessary* alarms on technology (monitors, ventilators).	3. Unnecessary alarms increase the risk of sensory overload and may increase anxiety.	• Demonstrates basic understanding of technology used in care.
4. Encourage and support patient while increasing activity level.	4. Positive reinforcement and encouragement improve patient motivation and independence.	
5. Mobilize resources (family, clergy, social worker) to help patient cope with outcomes of surgery (diagnosis, change in functional abilities).	5. A multidisciplinary approach to anxiety relief serves to use the patient's strengths and coping mechanisms.	

Nursing Diagnosis: Impaired physical mobility of the upper extremities related to thoracic surgery

Goal: Absence of disability of the affected shoulder and arm

Assist patient with normal range of motion and function of shoulder and trunk.
  a. Teach breathing exercises to mobilize thorax.
  b. Encourage skeletal exercises to promote abduction and mobilization of shoulder (see Fig. 25–14).
  c. Assist out of bed to chair as soon as pulmonary and circulatory systems are compensated (usually by evening of surgery).
  d. Encourage progressive activities according to development of fatigue.
	Necessary to regain normal mobility of arm and shoulder and to speed recovery and minimize discomfort.	• Demonstrates arm and shoulder exercises and verbalizes intent to perform them on discharge.

Nursing Diagnosis: Fluid volume imbalance related to the surgical procedure

Goal: Maintenance of adequate fluid volume

1. Monitor and record hourly intake and output. Patient should excrete at least 30 ml of urine hourly after surgery.	1. Fluid management may be altered before, during, and after surgery, and patient's response to and need for fluid management must be assessed.	• Patient is adequately hydrated. as evidenced by: 1. Urine output greater than 30 ml/hr
2. Administer blood and parenteral fluids or diuretics as prescribed to restore and maintain fluid volume.	2. Pulmonary edema due to transfusion or fluid overload is an ever-present threat; after pneumonectomy, the pulmonary vascular system has been greatly reduced.	2. Vital signs stable, heart rate and CVP approaching normal. 3. No excessive peripheral edema

(continued)

Nursing Care Plan 25–1 (Continued)

Care of the Patient Following Thoracotomy

Nursing Interventions	Rationale	Expected Outcomes

Nursing Diagnosis: Knowledge deficit of care procedures at home

Goal: Ability to carry out care procedures at home

Nursing Interventions	Rationale	Expected Outcomes
1. Encourage patient to practice arm and shoulder exercises five times daily at home.	1. Exercise accelerates recovery of muscle function and reduces long-term pain and discomfort.	• Demonstrates arm and shoulder exercises.
2. Instruct patient to practice assuming a functionally erect position in front of a full-length mirror.	2. Practice will help restore normal posture.	• Verbalizes need to try to assume an erect posture.
		• Verbalizes the importance of relieving discomfort, alternating walking and rest, practicing breathing exercises, avoiding heavy lifting, avoiding undue fatigue, avoiding bronchial irritants, preventing colds or lung infections, getting flu vaccine, keeping follow-up visits, and stopping smoking.
3. Instruct patient in following aspects of home care:		
a. Relieve intercostal pain by local heat or oral analgesia.	a. Some soreness may persist for several weeks.	
b. Alternate activities with frequent rest periods.	b. Weakness and fatigability are common for the first 3 weeks.	
c. Practice the breathing exercises at home.	c. Effective breathing is necessary to prevent splinting of affected side, which may lead to atelectasis.	
d. Avoid heavy lifting until complete healing has occurred.	d. Chest muscles and incision may be weaker than normal for 3–6 months.	
e. Avoid undue fatigue, increased shortness of breath, or chest pain.	e. Undue stress may prolong the healing process.	
f. Avoid bronchial irritants.	f. The lung's resistance is lowered and more susceptible to irritant substances.	
g. Prevent colds or lung infection.	g. The lung is more susceptible during the recovery phase.	
h. Get annual influenza vaccine.	h. Vaccination helps prevent flu.	
i. Keep follow-up appointment with physician.		
j. Stop smoking.	j. Smoking will slow healing process by decreasing oxygen delivery to tissues and make lung susceptible to infection and other complications.	

*A patient with a pneumonectomy usually does not have water-seal chest drainage, because it is desirable that the pleural space fill with an effusion, which eventually obliterates this space. Some surgeons do use a modified water-seal system.

5. Walk at a moderate pace, and gradually extend walking time and distance. Be persistent.
6. Immediately stop any activity that causes undue fatigue, increased shortness of breath, or chest pain.
7. Avoid bronchial irritants (smoke, fumes, air pollution, aerosol sprays).
8. Prevent colds or lung infections.
9. Get an annual influenza vaccine. Also discuss vaccination against pneumonia with the physician.

10. Report for follow-up care by the surgeon or clinic as necessary.
11. Stop smoking.

◊ Evaluation

Expected Outcomes

1. Improves gas exchange
   a. Maintains adequate arterial blood gas values
   b. Demonstrates diaphragmatic and pursed lip breathing

c. Uses incentive spirometer hourly while awake

d. Verbalizes absence of dyspnea

2. Improves airway clearance
   a. Demonstrates deep, controlled coughing
   b. Verbalizes importance of humidity for keeping secretions moist
   c. Maintains clear breath sounds or decreases presence of adventitious sounds
   d. Produces thin, white, or clear sputum

3. Is relieved of pain and discomfort
   a. Verbalizes that pain is diminishing
   b. Splints incision during coughing
   c. Increases activity level, participates in activities of daily living

4. Improves mobility of shoulder and arm; demonstrates arm and shoulder exercises to relieve stiffening

5. Maintains adequate fluid intake and maintains nutrition for healing
   a. Drinks 6 to 8 glasses of water a day
   b. Eats well-balanced meals

6. States that anxiety is at a manageable level
   a. Participates with health care team in treatment regimen
   b. Uses appropriate coping skills (*e.g.*, verbalization, pain relief, use of support systems such as family, clergy)
   c. Demonstrates basic understanding of technology used in care

7. Adheres to therapeutic program and home care
   a. Demonstrates arm and shoulder exercises and the importance of practicing them five times a day
   b. Verbalizes the importance of alternating walking and rest, practicing breathing exercises, avoiding heavy lifting, relieving intercostal pain, avoiding bronchial irritants, preventing colds or lung infections, getting flu and pneumonia vaccines, keeping follow-up appointment, and stopping smoking

For a detailed plan of nursing care for the patient who has had a thoracotomy, see Nursing Care Plan 25-1 (pp. 553–556).

In summary, the patient who requires thoracic surgery experiences many threats to his comfort and sense of well-being. Breathing, a basic function necessary for life, may be assisted through insertion of an endotracheal tube and use of mechanical ventilation. Pain, anxiety, and threats to the patient's bodily integrity are common. The patient's usual mode of communication is temporarily impaired because of the endotracheal intubation; consequently he may be unable to express his concerns and even to convey to others his need for relief of pain and discomfort. Nursing care during the postoperative phase will focus on maintenance of the patient's airway and ventilatory function, monitoring of chest drainage and fluid and electrolyte status, and providing pain relief and comfort measures. Reducing the patient's fear and anxiety is essential during this time. The patient who has undergone thoracic surgery will require assistance and education to prepare for discharge and the possibility of subsequent treatment, depending on the reason for the surgery.

Bibliography

Books

Alspach JG and Williams SM. Core Curriculum for Critical Care Nursing, 3rd ed. Philadelphia, WB Saunders, 1985.

American Heart Association. Textbook of Advanced Cardiac Life Support. Dallas, American Heart Association, 1987.

Barton RO. Pulmonary Rehabilitation/Homecare: From Paper to Practice. Old Town, ME, Health Educator Publications, 1989.

Bone RC and Eubanks DH. Comprehensive Respiratory Care: A Learning System. St Louis, CV Mosby, 1985.

Burton GG and Hodgkin JE (eds). Respiratory Care: A Guide to Clinical Practice, 2nd ed. Philadelphia, JB Lippincott, 1984.

Carpenito LJ. Nursing Diagnosis: Application to Clinical Pratice. Philadelphia, JB Lippincott, 1991.

Downs JB and Douglas ME. Physiologic effects of respiratory therapy. In Shoemaker WB et al (eds). Textbook of Critical Care. Philadelphia, WB Saunders, 1989

Holloway NM. Nursing the Critically Ill Adult, 2nd ed. Menlo Park, CA, Addison–Wesley, 1988

Johanson BC et al. Standards for Critical Care, 2nd ed. St Louis, CV Mosby, 1985

Kersten LD. Comprehensive Respiratory Nursing: A Decision-Making Approach. Philadelphia, WB Saunders, 1989.

Kirby RR and Taylor RW. Respiratory Failure. Chicago, Year Book Medical Publishers, 1986.

Kirby RR et al. Mechanical Ventilation. New York, Churchill Livingstone, 1985.

Murray JF and Nadel JA. Textbook of Respiratory Medicine. Philadelphia, WB Saunders, 1988.

Roberts SL. Behavioral Concepts and the Critically Ill Patient, 2nd ed. Norwalk, CT, Appleton–Century–Crofts, 1986.

Waldhausen JA and Pierce WS. Johnson's Surgery of the Chest, 5th ed. Chicago, Year Book Medical Publishers, 1985.

Journals

Asterisks indicate nursing research articles.

Therapeutics

* Branstetter RD et al. Effect of nasogastric feedings on arterial oxygen tension in patients with symptomatic chronic obstructive pulmonary disease. Heart Lung 1988 Mar; 17(2): 170–173.

Carroll P. Safe suctioning. Nursing 1989 Sep; 19(9): 48–51.

* Chulay M and Graeber GM. Efficacy of a hyperinflation and hyperoxygenation suctioning intervention. Heart Lung 1988 Jan; 17(1): 15–22.

Chulay M. Arterial blood gas changes with a hyperinflation and hyperoxygenation suctioning intervention on critically ill patients. Heart Lung 1988 Nov; 17(6): 654–662.

Daschner F et al. Stress ulcer prophylaxis and ventilation pneumonia: Prevention by antibacterial cytoprotective agents. Infect Control Hosp Epidemiol 1988 Feb; 9(2): 59–65.

Fedorovich C and Littleton MT. Chest physiotherapy: Evaluating the effectiveness. Dimens Crit Care Nurs 1990 Mar/Apr; 9(2): 68–74.

Frye B and Hilton T. Preparing the caregiver to manage the ventilator-dependent patient at home. Rehabil Nurs 1988 Jan/Feb; 13(1): 38, 42.

Goodnough SKC. Reducing tracheal injury and aspiration. Dimens Crit Care Nurs 1988 Nov/Dec; 7(6): 324–331.

Harrison LL. Teaching parents to provide home-care for ventilator-dependent children. MCN 1989 Jul/Aug; 14(4): 281.

Hazlett DE. A study of pediatric home ventilator management: Medical, psychosocial, and financial aspects. J Pediatr Nurs 1989 Aug; 4(4): 284–294.

* Henneman EA. Effect of nursing contact on the stress response of patients being weaned from mechanical ventilation. Heart Lung 1989 Sep; 18(5): 483–489.

* Kleiber C et al. Acute histologic changes in the tracheobronchial tree associated with different suction catheter insertion techniques. Heart Lung 1988 Jan; 17(1): 10–14.

* Langlois PF et al. Accentuated complement activation in patient plasma during the adult respiratory distress syndrome: A potential mechanism for pulmonary inflammation. Heart Lung 1989 Jan; 18(1): 71–84.

* Lookinland S. Comparison of pulmonary vascular pressures based on blood volume and ventilator status. Nurs Res 1989 Mar/Apr; 38(2): 68–72.

Mularz L and Simandl-Gerr R. Caring for ventilator-dependent patients. Nurs Man 1989 Jun; 20(6): 26–28.

* Preusser BA et al. Effects of two methods of preoxygenation on mean arterial pressure, cardiac output, peak airway pressure, and postsuctioning hypoxemia. Heart Lung 1988 May; 17(3): 290–299.

* Renfroe KL. Effect of progressive relaxation on dyspnea and state anxiety in patients with chronic obstructive pulmonary disease. Heart Lung Jul; 17(4): 408–413.

Scharer K and Dixon DM. Managing chronic illness: Parents with a ventilator-dependent child. J Pediatr Nurs 1989 Aug; 4(4): 236–247.

Spector N. Nutritional support of the ventilator-dependent patient. Nurs Clin North Am 1989 Jun; 24(2): 407–414.

* Stone KS et al. Effects of lung hyperinflation on mean arterial pressure and postsuctioning hypoxemia. Heart Lung 1989 Jul; 18(4): 377–385.

Airway Management

Cuzzell JZ and Rodriquez LA. How to use a bag-valve-mask device for artificial ventilation. Am J Nurs 1989 Jul; 89(7): 932–933.

Montanari J and Spearing C. The fine art of measuring tracheal cuff pressure. Nursing 1986 Jul; 16(7): 46–49.

* Pierce JB and Piazza DE. Differences in postsuctioning arterial blood oxygen concentration values using two postoxygenation methods. Heart Lung 1987 Jan; 16(1): 34–38.

* Rogge JA et al. Effectiveness of oxygen concentrations of less than 100% before and after endotracheal suction in patients with chronic obstructive pulmonary disease. Heart Lung 1989 Jan; 18(1): 64–71.

Sinfield A et al. Airway obstruction from overinflation and herniation of tracheostomy tube balloon. Heart Lung 1989 May; 18(3): 260–262.

Siskind MM. A standard of care for the nursing diagnosis of ineffective airway clearance. Heart Lung 1989 Sep; 18(5): 477–482.

Mechanical Ventilation

Ashworth LJ. Pressure support ventilation/CE quiz. Crit Care Nurs 1990 Jul/Aug; 10(7): 20–25.

Acosta F. Biofeedback and progressive relaxation in weaning the anxious patient from the ventilator: A brief report. Heart Lung 1988 May; 17(3): 299–302.

* Bergbom-Engberg I et al. A retrospective study of patients' recall of respirator treatment: 1. Study design and basic findings. Intens Care Nurs 1988 Jun; 4(2): 56–61.

Brown LH. Pulmonary oxygen toxicity. Focus Crit Care 1990 Feb; 17(1): 68–75.

Celentano-Norton L. Mechanical ventilation strategies in adult respiratory distress syndrome. Crit Care Nurse 1986 Jul/Aug; 6(4): 71–74.

Colombo A et al. Hospital procedure and nursing for patients treated with synchronised independent lung ventilation (sILV). Intens Care Nurs 1987; 3(3): 117–124.

Drayton-Hargrove S and Mandzak-McCarron K. Portable ventilation. Rehab Nurs 1987 Sep/Oct; 12(5).

Fitch M. The patient's reaction to ventilation. Can Crit Care Nurs J 1989 Jun/Jul; 6(2): 13–16.

Goularte TA et al. Bacterial colonization in humidifying cascade reservoirs after 24 and 48 hours of continuous mechanical ventilation. Infect Control 1987 May; 8(5): 200–203.

Gries ML and Fernsler J. Patient perceptions of the mechanical ventilation experience. Focus Crit Care 1988 Apr; 15(2): 52–59.

Grossbach I. Troubleshooting ventilator and patient related problems/Part 1. Crit Care Nurse 1986 Jul/Aug; 6(4): 58–70.

Grossbach I. Troubleshooting ventilator and patient related problems/Part 2. Crit Care Nurse 1986 Sep/Oct; 6(5): 64–79.

* Gunderson LP, Stone KS, and Hamlin RL. Endotracheal suctioning-induced heart rate alterations. Nurs Res 1991 May/Jun; 40(3): 139–143.

Haynes N et al. Discharging ICU ventilator-dependent patients to home healthcare. Crit Care Nurse 1990 Jul/Aug; 10(7): 39–47.

* Henneman EA. Effect of nursing contact on the stress response of patients being weaned from mechanical ventilation. Heart Lung 1989 Sep; 18(5): 483–489.

Johnson MM and Sexton DL. Distress during mechanical ventilation: Patients' perceptions. Crit Care Nurse 1990 Jul/Aug 10(7): 48–52.

* Lookinland S and Appel PL. Hemodynamic and oxygen transport changes following endotracheal suctioning in trauma patients. Nurs Res 1991 May/Jun; 40(3): 133–138.

Loughran SC. High frequency ventilation: Application of nursing diagnosis. Dimens Crit Care Nurs 1987 Nov/Dec; 6(6): 328–334.

* Lush MT et al. Dyspnea in the ventilator-assisted patient. Heart Lung 1988 Sep; 17(5): 528–535.

Nett LM et al. Weaning from the ventilator: Weaning the unweanable. Am J Nurs 1987 Sep; 87(9): 1181–1184.

Nett LM et al. Weaning from the ventilator: In specific clinical situations. Am J Nurs 1987 Sep; 87(9): 1178–1180.

Nett LM et al. Weaning from the ventilator: Protocols that work. Am J Nurs 1987 Sep; 87(9): 1173–1177.

Richless CI. Current trends in mechanical ventilation. Crit Care Nurs 1991 Mar; 11(3): 41–50.

Robichaud-Ekstrand S. The ventilator and coping with relatives. Can Crit Care Nurs J 1989 Jun/Jul; 6(2): 9–12.

* Rogge JA et al. Effectiveness of oxygen concentrations of less than 100% before and after endotracheal suction in patients with chronic obstructive pulmonary disease. Heart Lung 1989 Jan; 18(1): 64–71.

* Shekleton M. Clinical indicators of the ability to sustain spontaneous ventilation: A pilot study. Chart 1989 Jan; 86(1): 6.

Smith SA. Extended body image in the ventilated patient. Intens Care Nurs 1989 Mar; 5(1): 31–37.

* Stone KS et al. The effect of lung hyperinflation and endotracheal suctioning on cardiopulmonary hemodynamics. Nurs Res 1991 Mar/Apr; 40(2): 76–85.

Storm DS and Baugartner RG. Achieving self-care in the ventilator-dependent patient: A critical analysis of a case study. Int J Nurs Stud 1987; 24(2): 95–106.

* Stovsky B et al. Comparison of two types of communication methods used after cardiac surgery with patients with endotracheal tubes. Heart Lung 1988 May; 17(3): 281–290.

Winters C. Monitoring ventilator patients for complication. Nursing 1988 Jun; 18(6): 38–41.

Thoracic Surgery

Armstrong D. Treatment of metastatic lung disease. Dimens Oncol Nurs 1985; 1(2): 7–9.

Brown SL. Practical points in the postanesthesia assessment and care of the patient undergoing thoracic surgery. J Post Anesth Nurs 1986 Nov; 1(4): 265–267.

Erickson RS. Mastering the ins and outs of chest drainage. Part 1. Nursing 1989 May; 19(5): 37–44.

Erickson RS. Mastering the ins and outs of chest drainage. Part 2. Nursing 1989 Jun; 19(6): 46–50.

Information/Resources

Agencies

Governmental

National Heat, Lung and Blood Institute
National Institutes of Health, 900 Rockville Pike, Bldg 31, Bethesda, MD 20892, (301) 496-5166

Voluntary

American Association for Respiratory Care
1720 Regal Row, Dallas, TX 75235, (214) 630-3540

American Lung Association
1740 Broadway, New York, NY 10019, (212) 315-8700

American Thoracic Society
1740 Broadway, New York, NY 10019, (212) 315-8700

Respiratory Nursing Society
5700 Old Orchard Rd, 1st Floor, Skokie, IL 60077

26

Management of Patients With Conditions of the Chest and Lower Respiratory Tract

Learning Objectives

On completion of this chapter, the learner will be able to:

1. Compare the various pulmonary infections with regard to causes, clinical manifestations, nursing management, complications, and prevention
2. Use the nursing process as a framework for care of the patient with pneumonia
3. Relate pleurisy, pleural effusion, and empyema to pulmonary infection
4. Discuss cigarette smoking and air pollution as causes of pulmonary disease
5. Compare and contrast chronic bronchitis, bronchiectasis, pulmonary emphysema, and asthma as chronic obstructive pulmonary diseases, and describe their relationship to pulmonary heart disease
6. Use the nursing process as a framework for care of the patient with chronic obstructive pulmonary disease (COPD)
7. Develop a teaching plan for patients with COPD
8. Describe risk factors and measures appropriate for prevention and treatment of pulmonary embolism
9. Specify preventive measures appropriate for controlling and eliminating the problem of occupational lung disease
10. Discuss the modes of therapy and related nursing management for patients with lung cancer
11. Describe the complications of chest trauma and their clinical manifestations and nursing management
12. Describe nursing measures to prevent aspiration
13. Relate the therapeutic management techniques of adult respiratory distress syndrome to the underlying pathophysiology of the syndrome

Respiratory Infections

Acute Tracheobronchitis

Acute tracheobronchitis is an acute inflammation of the mucous membranes of the trachea and the bronchial tree that often follows infections of the upper respiratory tract. A patient with a viral infection has a lessened resistance and can readily develop a secondary bacterial infection. Thus, the adequate treatment of upper respiratory tract infections is one of the major factors in the prevention of acute bronchitis. Aside from infection, inhalation of physical and chemical irritants, gases, and other air contaminants can also cause acute bronchial irritations.

Clinical Manifestations.   The signs and symptoms of acute tracheobronchitis result from the mucopurulent sputum that is secreted by the inflamed mucosa of the bronchi. Initially, the patient has a dry, irritating cough and expectorates a scanty amount of mucoid sputum. He complains of sternal soreness from coughing and has fever, headache, and general malaise. As the infection progresses, the patient may have inspiratory stridor and more profuse purulent sputum.

Examination including culture of the sputum is essential to identify the specific causative organism. Although *Streptococcus pneumoniae* and *Haemophilus influenzae* often cause this infection, tracheobronchitis is the most common clinical syndrome that results from infection from *Mycoplasma pneumoniae*.

Management.   The treatment is largely symptomatic. The patient is placed on bed rest. Moist heat to the chest will relieve the soreness and pain. Cool vapor therapy or steam inhalations are beneficial in relieving the laryngeal and tracheal irritation. Increasing the vapor pressure (moisture content) in the air will reduce irritation.

Cough depressants are not given or are prescribed only with caution when the cough is productive. Antihistamines may be excessively drying, making secretions more difficult to expectorate. Expectorants, such as Robitussin, may be prescribed, although their efficacy is subject to debate. Fluid intake is increased to "thin" the viscous and tenacious secretions. Antibiotic treatment is indicated when the sputum becomes purulent. If the patient is unable to handle or clear the copious, purulent secretions, the patient may be in danger of complete obstruction. Nasotracheal intubation may be required.

Nursing Interventions.   The nurse's observations are important in determining the therapeutic plan because care of the patient is largely symptomatic.

A primary nursing function is to encourage bronchial hygiene. The nurse cautions the patient against overexertion, which can induce a relapse or extension of the infection. The elderly patient can easily develop bronchopneumonia from acute tracheobronchitis if adequate care is not given. The patient is turned often and placed in a sitting position at frequent intervals to facilitate effective coughing and prevent retention of mucopurulent sputum. An adequate time is allowed for convalescence after the acute infection subsides to avoid recurrence.

Pneumonia

Pneumonia is an inflammatory process of the lung parenchyma that is commonly caused by infectious agents. Pneumonia is the most common infectious cause of death in the United States. It is classified according to its causative agent, if known: for example, it may be a *bacterial, viral, fungal, parasitic, or mycoplasma pneumonia*. It also may be caused by radiation therapy, ingestion of chemicals, and aspiration. Radiation pneumonia may follow radiation therapy for breast or lung cancer, usually 6 weeks or more after completion of treatment. Chemical pneumonia may occur after ingestion of kerosene or inhalation of irritating gases. Aspiration pneumonia is discussed on p. 598.

If a substantial portion of one or more lobes is involved, the disease is referred to as *lobar pneumonia. Bronchopneumonia* implies that the pneumonic process is distributed in a patchy fashion, having originated in one or more localized areas within the bronchi and extended to the adjacent surrounding lung parenchyma. Bronchopneumonia is more common than lobar pneumonia.

In general, patients with bacterial pneumonia usually have acute or chronic underlying disease that impairs host defenses. More often, pneumonia arises from endogenous flora of the patient whose resistance has been altered or from aspiration of mouth flora. Although most viral infections occur in previously healthy persons, when bacterial pneumonia occurs in a healthy person there is usually a history of preceding viral illness. In recent years there has been an increase in the number of patients who have deficient defenses against infections: those on corticosteroids or other immunosuppressive drugs, those on broad-spectrum antimicrobials, those with acquired immune deficiency syndrome (AIDS), and those requiring the use of life-support technology. These patients who have suppressed immune systems often acquire pneumonia from organisms of low virulence. In addition, there are increasing numbers of patients with impaired defenses who develop hospital-acquired pneumonia from gram-negative bacilli *(Klebsiella, Pseudomonas, Escherichia coli*, Enterobacteriaceae, *Proteus, Serratia)*. Gram-positive cocci, anaerobes, mycobacteria, nocardial species of bacteria, and viral, chlamydial, fungal, and parasitic agents can cause pneumonia. Commonly encountered pneumonias and their clinical features, treatment, and complications are presented in Table 26–1.

Prevention and Risk Factors

The nurse should be acquainted with the factors and circumstances that commonly predispose the person to pneumonia. Hence, the nurse is able to identify the patient at high risk and to engage in anticipatory and preventive nursing.

- Any condition that produces mucus or bronchial obstruction and interferes with normal drainage of the lung (cancer, chronic obstructive pulmonary disease [COPD]) renders the patient susceptible to pneumonia.
- Immunosuppressed patients are at risk.
- People who smoke are at risk because cigarette smoke disrupts both mucociliary and macrophage activity.
- Any patient who is permitted to lie passively in bed for prolonged periods, relatively immobile and breathing shallowly, is highly vulnerable to the risk of bronchopneumonia.
- Any person who has a depressed cough reflex (due to medications or weakness), has aspirated foreign material into the lungs during a period of unconsciousness (head injury, anesthesia), or has an abnormal swallowing mechanism is very likely to develop bronchopneumonia.
- Any hospitalized patient on a nothing-by-mouth regimen or

who is receiving antibiotics has increased pharyngeal colonization of organisms and is at risk. In very ill persons, the oropharynx is likely to be colonized by gram-negative bacteria.

- People who are intoxicated frequently are particularly susceptible to pneumonia, because alcohol suppresses the body's reflexes, white cell mobilization, and tracheobronchial ciliary motion.
- Any person scheduled to receive a sedative is observed for respiratory rate and depth before the drug is given; if respiratory depression is apparent, the medication should not be administered. Respiratory depression predisposes to the pooling of bronchial secretions and subsequent development of pneumonia.
- Frequent suctioning of secretions in patients who are unconscious or have poor cough and gag reflexes is an important preventive measure. This reduces the likelihood that secretions will be aspirated or accumulate in the lungs and induce bronchopneumonia.
- Elderly people are especially vulnerable to pneumonia because of depression of cough and glottic reflexes. Postoperative pneumonia should be anticipated in the elderly and forestalled by frequent mobilization, effective coughing, and breathing exercises.
- Anyone receiving treatment with respiratory therapy equipment can develop pneumonia if the equipment has not been properly cleaned.

Pneumonia has been known to be more prevalent with certain underlying disorders such as congestive heart failure, diabetes, alcoholism, and COPD. Certain diseases also have been associated with specific pathogens. For example, staphylococcal pneumonia has been noted after epidemics of influenza, and patients with COPD are at increased risk of developing pneumonia caused by pneumococci or *Haemophilus influenzae*.

Cystic fibrosis is associated with respiratory infection with *Pseudomonas* and *Staphylococcus*. *Pneumocystis carinii* pneumonia has been associated with AIDS. Pneumonias occurring in hospitalized patients often involve organisms not usually found in community-acquired pneumonias, including enteric gram-negative bacilli and *Staphylococcus aureus*.

Bacterial Pneumonia

Pneumonia caused by *Streptococcus pneumoniae* is the most common bacterial pneumonia and is most prevalent during the winter and spring, when upper respiratory tract infections are most frequent. It may occur as a lobar or bronchopneumonic form in patients of any age. A history of recent respiratory illness often can be elicited.

S. pneumoniae is a gram-positive, capsulated, nonmotile coccus that resides naturally in the upper respiratory tract. It commonly is referred to as the *pneumococcus*.

Pathophysiology. Bacterial pneumonia creates problems in both ventilation and diffusion. An inflammatory reaction initiated by pneumococci occurs in the alveoli and produces an exudate. This exudate, in turn, interferes with both movement and diffusion of oxygen and carbon dioxide. White blood cells, mostly neutrophils, also migrate into the alveoli, so that the lung segment assumes a more solid structure as the air-containing spaces become filled. Areas of the lung are not adequately ventilated because of secretions, mucosal edema, and bronchospasm. These conditions cause partial occlusion of the bronchi or alveoli, producing a drop in the alveolar oxygen

tension. Venous blood coming into the lungs passes through the underventilated area and goes out of the lung to the left side of the heart without being oxygenated. In essence, the blood is shunted from the right to the left side of the heart. This mixing of oxygenated and unoxygenated blood eventually results in arterial hypoxemia.

Clinical Manifestations. Classic bacterial (or pneumococcal) pneumonia usually starts with a sudden onset of shaking chills, rapidly rising fever (39.5° to 40.5°C [101° to 105°F]), and stabbing chest pain that is aggravated by respiration and coughing. The patient is severely ill with marked tachypnea (25 to 45/min) accompanied by respiratory grunting, nasal flaring, and the use of accessory muscles of respiration. He often lies on his affected side in an attempt to splint his chest. The pulse is rapid and bounding. It usually increases about 10 beats/min for every degree of Celsius temperature elevation. A relative bradycardia for the amount of fever should suggest viral infection, *Mycoplasma* infection, or infection with *Legionella* species. The cheeks are flushed, the eyes bright, and the lips and nail beds cyanotic. The patient prefers to be propped up in bed and leans forward, trying to achieve adequate gas exchange without trying to cough or breathe deeply. He perspires profusely. The sputum is purulent and not a reliable indicator of the etiologic agent. Rusty, blood-tinged sputum is produced in pneumococcal, staphylococcal, *Klebsiella*, and streptococcal pneumonia. *Klebsiella* pneumonia frequently also has viscous sputum. *H. influenzae* sputum is green.

Other signs occur in patients who suffer from a condition such as cancer or those who are undergoing treatment with immunosuppressants, which lower the resistance to infection and to organisms heretofore not considered serious pathogens. Such patients present with fever, crackles, and physical signs of lobar consolidation, including increased tactile fremitus, percussion dullness, bronchovesicular or bronchial breath sounds, egophony (change of patient's "ee" to "ay" sound on auscultation), and whispered pectoriloquy (whispered sounds heard louder and more clearly than normal on auscultation). These changes occur because sound is transmitted better through solid tissue (consolidation) than through normal tissue.

In older patients or those with COPD, the symptoms may develop insidiously. Purulent sputum may be the only sign of pneumonia in these patients. It is difficult to detect subtle changes in their conditions because they already have seriously compromised pulmonary function.

Diagnostic Evaluation. The diagnosis is made by history (particularly of recent respiratory tract infection), physical examination, chest x-rays, blood culture (bloodstream invasion, called *bacteremia*, occurs frequently), and sputum examination.

- To obtain an adequate sample of sputum, the patient rinses his mouth with water to minimize contamination by normal oral flora. He is told to breathe deeply several times and then to cough deeply and expectorate the raised sputum into a sterile container.

Sputum also may be obtained by transtracheal aspiration (p. 517) or fiberoptic bronchoscopy (p. 515) in patients who cannot raise sputum or those who are obtunded, have abnormal host defense mechanisms, or have developed pneumonia after antimicrobial therapy or while hospitalized.

Management. The treatment of pneumonia depends largely on administration of the appropriate antibiotic as determined by the results of the Gram stain. Penicillin G is clearly

(text continues on page 564)

TABLE 26–1.   *Commonly Encountered Pneumonias*

Type	Organism Responsible	Epidemiology
BACTERIAL PNEUMONIAS		
Streptococcal pneumonia	*Streptococcus pneumoniae*	Highest occurrence in winter months Incidence greatest in children less than 5 years of age and the elderly Accounts for 40% to 75% of community-acquired bacterial pneumonias Mortality rate: 10% to 15%
Staphylococcal pneumonia	*Staphylococcus aureus*	Incidence greatest in immunocompromised patients, IV drug users, and as a complication of epidemic influenza Accounts for 2% to 10% of community-acquired and 10% to 15% of hospital-acquired pneumonias Mortality rate: 25% to 60%
Klebsiella pneumonia	*Klebsiella pneumoniae* (Friedlander's bacillus—encapsulated gram-negative aerobic bacillus)	Incidence greatest in the elderly, alcoholics, patients with chronic disease, such as diabetes, congestive heart failure, chronic obstructive pulmonary disease, or prolonged institutionalization (*e.g.*, nursing home) Accounts for 2% to 5% of community-acquired and 10% to 30% of hospital-acquired pneumonias Mortality rate: 40% to 50%
Pseudomonas pneumonia	*Pseudomonas aeruginosa*	Incidence greatest in those with preexisting lung disease, cancer (particularly leukemia), those with homograft transplants, burns, debilitated persons; and patients receiving antimicrobial therapy and treatment such as tracheostomy, suctioning Accounts for 5% to 15% of hospital-acquired pneumonias Mortality rate: 40% to 60%
Haemophilus influenza	*Haemophilus influenzae*	Incidence greatest in alcoholics, diabetics, patients with chronic lung disease Accounts for 5% to 20% of community-acquired pneumonias Mortality rate: 33%
Legionnaires' disease	*Legionella pneumophila*	Highest occurrence in summer and fall May cause disease sporadically or as part of an epidemic Incidence greatest in middle-aged and older men, smokers, and patients with chronic diseases, receiving immunosuppressive therapy, or those in close proximity to excavation site Accounts for 0% to 20% of community-acquired pneumonia Mortality rate: 15% to 50%
Mycoplasma pneumonia	*Mycoplasma pneumoniae*	Highest occurrence in fall and early winter Responsible for epidemics of respiratory illness that occur every 4 years Incidence greatest in children and young adults Most common cause of nonbacterial pneumonia in young adults Mortality rate: less than 0.1%
NONBACTERIAL PNEUMONIAS		
Viral pneumonia	Influenza viruses types A, B, C	Incidence greatest in winter months Epidemics occur every 2 to 3 years

Clinical Features	Treatment	Complications
Herpes simplex often present on face. Usually involves one or more lobes.	Penicillin G IV Penicillin V PO Alternate drug therapy; erythromycin, clindamycin, cephalosporins, other penicillins, trimethoprim-sulfamethoxazole (Bactrim)	Shock Pleural effusion Superinfections Pericarditis Otitis media
Frequently requires hospitalization Staphalococcal pneumonia is a necrotizing infection. Treatment must be vigorous and prolonged because of disease's tendency to destroy the lungs. Organism may develop rapid drug resistance Prolonged convalescence expected.	Nafcillin, methicillin, oxacillin, vancomycin for methicillin-resistant organisms; cefazolin for penicillin-allergic patients.	Effusion/pneumothorax Lung abscess Empyema Meningitis Endocarditis
Tissue necrosis occurs rapidly in lungs, with cavity formation in some patients. May be rapidly fulminating, progressing to fatal outcome. Frequently requires hospitalization.	Gentamycin, tobramycin, Third-generation cephalosporins (cefotaxime, ceftizoxime, ceftriaxone) for long period.	Multiple lung abscesses with cyst formation Persistent cough with expectoration remains Empyema Pericarditis Pleural effusion
Usually requires hospitalization. Respiratory equipment may be contaminated with these organisms.	Gentamycin Piperacillin Ticarcillin combined with tobramycin or amikacin	Lung cavitation Has capacity to invade blood vessels, causing hemorrhage and lung infarction
Frequently insidious onset associated with upper respiratory tract infection 2 to 6 weeks before onset of illness. Usually involves one or more lobes.	Ampicillin, amoxicillin, cefaclor or cefuroxime for ampicillin-resistant organisms. Trimethoprim-sulfamethoxazole for penicillin-allergic patients. Clavulanic acid for ampicillin- or amoxicillin-resistant patients	Lung abscess Pleural effusion
Frequently requires hospitalization. Patients may also have gastrointestinal symptoms, including nausea, vomiting, diarrhea, and abdominal pain.	Erythromycin	Respiratory failure Hypotension Shock Acute renal failure
Onset is usually insidious. Patients not usually as ill as in other pneumonias. Sore throat, nasal congestion and coryza.	Erythromycin Tetracycline	Aseptic meningitis, meningoencephalitis, cerebral ataxia, Guillain-Barré syndrome, transverse myelitis
In majority of patients, influenza begins as an acute coryza; others have bronchitis, pleurisy, and so forth, and still others develop gastrointestinal symptoms.	Treated symptomatically Does not respond to treatment with presently available antimicrobials	May develop a superimposed bacterial infection Bronchopneumonia

(continued)

TABLE 26-1.   *(Continued)*

Type	Organism Responsible	Epidemiology
NONBACTERIAL PNEUMONIAS (continued)		
		Incidence greatest in pregnant women, the elderly, patients with heart disease, and those receiving immunosuppressive therapy Mortality rate: 0% to 30%
Pneumocystic carinii pneumonia	*Pneumocystis carinii*	Incidence greatest in patients with AIDS and patients receiving immunosuppressive therapy for cancer, organ transplants, and other disorders Mortality rate: 60%
Fungal pneumonia	*Aspergillus fumigatas*	Incidence greatest in neutropenic patients Mortality rate: 15% to 20%

the antibiotic of choice for infection with *S. pneumoniae*. Other effective drugs include erythromycin, clindamycin, the cephalosporins, other penicillins, and trimethoprim-sulfamethoxazole (Bactrim). Treatment for other types of pneumonia is outlined in Table 26-1.

The patient is placed on bed rest until infection shows signs of clearing. He is observed carefully and continually until his clinical condition improves.

The patient who is hypoxemic is given oxygen. Arterial blood gas analysis is performed to determine the need for oxygen and to evaluate oxygen effectiveness. A high concentration of oxygen is contraindicated in patients with COPD because it may worsen alveolar ventilation by removing the patient's only remaining ventilatory drive and lead to respiratory decompensation. Respiratory support measures such as endotracheal intubation, high inspiratory oxygen concentrations, mechanical ventilation, and positive end expiratory pressure (PEEP) may be required for some patients. These treatment modalities are discussed in Chapter 25.

▶ **Nursing Process**
The Patient With Pneumonia

▷ *Assessment*

The presence of a fever in any hospitalized patient should alert the nurse to the possibility of the development of bacterial pneumonia. Use of assessment skills will further identify the clinical manifestations of pain; tachypnea; use of accessory muscles; rapid, bounding pulse; coughing; and purulent sputum. The nurse determines the severity, location, and cause of the chest pain as well as what relieves it. Any changes in temperature, amount and color of secretions, frequency and severity of the cough, and degree of tachypnea or shortness of breath also are monitored. Consolidation is assessed by evaluating breath sounds (bronchial breathing, bronchovesicular or rhonchi rales), fremitus, egophony, whispered pectoriloquy, and the results of percussion (dullness in the chest area).

The elderly patient is assessed for unusual behavior, alterations in mental status, prostration, and congestive heart failure. A restless, excited delirium may be exhibited, especially in patients with alcoholism.

The potential complications of bacterial pneumonia are routinely evaluated so that intervention can begin early.

▷ *Complications.* Lethal complications may develop during the first few days of antibiotic treatment. The patient is observed for continuing or recurring fever. Inadequate lung drainage or insufficient blood supply to the involved lung may reduce the amount of antibiotic agent reaching the invading organism. Resistant or recurring fever may be due to drug allergy (assess for rash), drug resistance or slow response of the susceptible organism, superinfection, infected pleural effusion, or pneumonia caused by unusual organisms (such as *Pneumocystis carinii* or fungi). Failure of the pneumonia to resolve raises the suspicion of underlying carcinoma of the bronchus.

Patients usually respond to treatment within 24 to 48 hours after antibiotic therapy is initiated. Complications of pneumonia include sustained *hypotension and shock* and *respiratory failure* (especially in gram-negative bacterial disease in the elderly).

These complications are encountered chiefly in patients who have received no specific treatment, have received inadequate or delayed treatment, have received antimicrobial therapy to which the infecting organism is resistant, or are suffering from a preexisting disease that complicates the pneumonia.

To combat peripheral collapse and maintain arterial blood pressure, a vasopressor agent may be administered intravenously in the form of a constant infusion and at a rate that is readjusted constantly in accordance with the pressure response. Corticosteroid drugs may be administered parenterally to combat shock and toxicity in patients with pneumonia who are extremely ill and in apparent danger of succumbing to the infection. Patients may require endotracheal intubation and mechanical ventilation.

Atelectasis (from obstruction of a bronchus by accumulated secretions) may occur at any stage of acute pneumonia. Pleural effusion (p. 570) also is fairly common and may signal the beginning of empyema. A diagnostic thoracentesis is usually necessary to evaluate an effusion. A chest tube may be required to control pleural infection by establishing proper drainage of the empyema.

Clinical Features	Treatment	Complications
Risk of developing influenza related to crowding and close contact of groups of people.	Prophylactic vaccination recommended for high-risk persons (over 55, chronic cardiac or pulmonary disease, diabetes, and other metabolic disorders)	Pericarditis, endocarditis
Frequently associated concurrent infection by viruses (cytomegalovirus), bacteria, and fungi	Pentamidine methanesulfonate Trimethoprim-sulfamethoxazole	Patients are critically ill Prognosis guarded, as it usually is a complication of a severe underlying disorder
May develop *Aspergillus* as a superinfection.	Amphotericin B; ketoconazole Lobectomy in patients with severe hemoptysis	High fatality rate Invades blood vessels and destroys lung tissue by direct invasion and vascular infarction

Delirium is another possible complication and is considered a medical emergency when it occurs. It may be caused by hypoxia, meningitis, or the delirium tremens of alcoholism. The patient with delirium is given oxygen, adequate hydration, and mild sedation and is observed constantly. Congestive heart failure, cardiac dysrhythmias, pericarditis, and myocarditis are also complications of pneumonia.

Superinfection is an important complication that may occur with the administration of very large amounts of penicillin or with the use of combinations of antibiotics. If the patient improves and the fever diminishes after initial antibiotic therapy but subsequently there is a rise in temperature with increasing cough and evidence of spread of pneumonia, a superinfection has occurred. Antibiotics are changed appropriately or, in some cases, discontinued entirely.

The influenza vaccine is recommended yearly to all patients at risk (the elderly, cardiac and pulmonary disease patients), because pneumonia is a complication of influenza. The pneumococcal vaccine is recommended also for the same high-risk group, as well as for patients who have had a splenectomy and those with sickle cell disease or alcoholism. The vaccine provides specific prevention against pneumonia that is caused by major organisms.

Nursing Diagnoses

Based on the assessment data, the patient's major nursing diagnoses may include

- Ineffective airway clearance related to copious tracheobronchial secretions
- Activity intolerance related to altered respiratory function
- High risk for fluid volume deficit related to fever and dyspnea
- Knowledge deficit about the treatment regimen and preventive health measures

Planning and Implementation

Goals: The major goals for the patient may include improvement of airway patency, obtaining enough rest to conserve energy, maintenance of proper fluid volume, and an understanding of the treatment protocol and preventive measures.

Nursing Interventions

Improvement of Airway Patency. Retained secretions interfere with gas exchange and may cause slow resolution of the disease. A high level of fluid intake (2 to 3 L/day) is encouraged, as adequate hydration thins and loosens pulmonary secretions and also replaces fluid losses resulting from fever, diaphoresis, dehydration, and dyspnea. The air is humidified to loosen secretions and improve ventilation. A high-humidity face mask (using either compressed air or oxygen) delivers warm, humidified air to the tracheobronchial tree and liquefies secretions. The patient is encouraged to cough in the manner described for the postoperative patient (p. 546).

Chest physiotherapy is extremely important in loosening and mobilizing secretions. The patient is placed in the proper position to drain the involved lung, and then the chest is vibrated and percussed. After the lung has drained for 10 to 20 minutes (depending on tolerance), the patient is encouraged to breathe deeply and cough. If he is too weak to cough effectively, the mucus may have to be removed by nasotracheal suctioning or by bronchoscopic aspiration as determined by the physician.

If oxygen is prescribed, the nurse provides the necessary method of oxygen administration and monitors the effectiveness of the oxygen concentration by assessing for the clinical manifestations of hypoxia.

Rest and Energy Conservation. The patient is encouraged to rest and remain in bed to avoid overexertion and possible exacerbation of symptoms. He is placed in a comfortable position for resting and breathing (*e.g.*, semi-Fowler's) and encouraged to change position frequently.

If sedatives or tranquilizers are prescribed, the patient's sensorium is evaluated first. Restlessness, confusion, and aggression may be due to cerebral hypoxemia, in which case sedatives are contraindicated.

Proper Fluid Intake. The patient's respiratory rate increases because of dyspnea and fever. With an increased rate there is an increase in insensible fluid loss during exhalation. The patient can quickly become dehydrated. Therefore, fluids are encouraged (at least 2 L/day). Frequently, a patient who is dyspneic is also anorexic and will only take fluids. Fluids, then, are beneficial for volume replacement as well as nutrition.

▷ *Patient Education and Home Health Care.*   After the fever subsides, the patient may gradually increase his activities. Fatigue, weakness, and depression may be prolonged after pneumonia. Breathing exercises to clear the lungs and promote full lung expansion are encouraged. The patient is instructed to return to the clinic or physician's office for follow-up chest x-rays.

The nurse explains to the patient that it is wise to stop cigarette smoking because it destroys tracheobronchial ciliary action, which is the first line of defense of the lungs. Smoking also irritates the mucous cells of the bronchi and inhibits the function of alveolar macrophage (scavenger) cells. The patient is instructed to avoid fatigue, sudden changes in temperature, and excessive alcohol intake, which lower resistance to pneumonia. The nurse reviews with the patient the principles of adequate nutrition and rest, because one episode of pneumonia may make him susceptible to recurring respiratory tract infections. He is encouraged to obtain influenza vaccine at the prescribed times, because influenza increases susceptibility to secondary bacterial pneumonia, especially that caused by *Staphylococcus*, *H. influenzae*, and *S. pneumoniae*. The patient also is encouraged to seek medical advice about receiving vaccine (Pneumovax) against *S. pneumoniae*. The care plan for the patient with bacterial pneumonia is found in Nursing Care Plan 26–1.

▷ Evaluation

Expected Outcomes

1. Improves airway patency
   a. Maintains an arterial blood gas oxygen tension of 60 mm Hg or above
   b. Has a normal temperature
   c. Exhibits normal breath sounds
   d. Demonstrates effective coughing technique
   e. Adheres to humidification measures
2. Attains proper amount of rest
   a. Remains in bed while symptomatic
   b. Avoids the recumbent position
   c. Shows no signs of restlessness, confusion, or aggression
3. Achieves an adequate fluid intake
   a. Drinks at least 2 liters of fluid per day
   b. Verbalizes the importance of drinking at least 2 liters of fluid per day
   c. Has normal skin turgor
4. Complies with treatment protocol and prevention strategies
   a. Identifies factors that contribute to development of pneumonia
   b. Joins a support group to stop smoking
   c. Makes an appointment at clinic for follow-up chest film and influenza and pneumococcal vaccines
   d. Verbalizes that he will cope with fatigue by rest, alternating with increasing activity

Atypical Pneumonia Syndromes

Pneumonias associated with mycoplasmas, fungus, Q fever, Legionnaires' disease, and viruses are included in the atypical pneumonia syndromes. Pneumonias associated with myco-

plasmas, psittacosis, Q fever, Legionnaires' disease, and viruses are included in the atypical pneumonia syndromes (see Table 26–1).

Mycoplasma pneumoniae is the most common cause of primary atypical pneumonia. Mycoplasmas are small organisms surrounded by a triple-layered membrane without a cell wall. The organisms grow on a special culture medium but differ from viruses. Mycoplasma pneumonia occurs most frequently in older children and young adults.

It probably is spread by infected respiratory droplets, through person-to-person contact. Patients can be tested for mycoplasma antibodies.

The inflammatory infiltrate is primarily interstitial rather than alveolar. It spreads throughout the entire respiratory tract, including the bronchioles. Generally, it has the characteristics of a bronchopneumonia. Earache and bullous myringitis are common.

Clinical Manifestations.   Usually, the patient has had an upper respiratory tract infection, and the onset of his pneumonic symptoms is gradual. The predominant symptoms are a harassing and nonproductive cough, a feeling of tightness in the chest, and generalized aching and prostration, along with tracheal pain when coughing. After a few days, mucoid or mucopurulent sputum is expectorated. The patient complains of headache that is aggravated by the cough.

Nursing Interventions.   The goal of nursing care is to promote the patient's rest and comfort and to encourage the proper intake of prescribed drugs. *Mycoplasma* pneumonia responds to erythromycin and tetracycline. Other atypical pneumonias are viral in origin, and most do not respond to antimicrobials. *Pneumocystis carinii* responds best to pentamidine methanesulfanate and trimethoprim-sulfamethoxazole. Warm, moist inhalations are helpful in relieving bronchial irritation. The nursing care and treatment (with the exception of antimicrobial therapy) are the same as those given to the patient who has bacterial pneumonia.

Gerontologic Considerations

Pneumonia in the elderly patient may occur spontaneously or as a complication of a chronic disease process. Pulmonary infections in the elderly frequently are difficult to treat and are associated with a higher mortality than such infections in younger patients. The onset of pneumonia may be signaled by general deterioration, confusion, tachycardia, and increased respiratory rate. The classic symptoms of cough, chest pain, sputum production, and fever often are absent in the elderly patient.

The presence of some signs may be misleading. Abnormal breath sounds, for example, may be due to microatelectasis that occurs with aging. Because chronic congestive heart failure (CHF) is often seen in the elderly, chest radiography may be performed to assist in differentiating CHF from pneumonia as the cause of clinical signs and symptoms.

Supportive treatment includes increased fluid intake (with caution and frequent assessment in view of the risk of fluid overload in the elderly); oxygen therapy, and assistance with deep breathing, coughing, sputum production, and position changes are of particular importance in nursing care of the elderly patient with pneumonia.

To reduce or prevent serious consequences of pneumonia in the elderly, vaccination against pneumococcal and influenza

▶ Nursing Care Plan 26–1

Care of the Patient With Bacterial Pneumonia

Nursing Interventions	Rationale	Expected Outcomes

Nursing Diagnosis: Ineffective airway clearance related to tracheobronchial secretions

Goal: Improvement of airway patency

Nursing Interventions	Rationale	Expected Outcomes

1. Assist the patient to cough productively:
  a. Splint the patient's chest during coughing.
  b. Administer codeine as prescribed.
  c. Humidify air to loosen secretions and improve ventilation. Encourage increased fluid intake.
	1. Depression of the cough reflex may produce retention of pulmonary secretions and lead to atelectasis. Elderly patients have a diminished cough reflex and may require vigorous measures (suctioning, bronchoscopy) for removal of secretions. Adequate hydration thins mucus and serves as an effective expectorant.	• Demonstrates effective coughing techniques.
		• Verbalizes importance of drinking plenty of fluids.

2. Perform postural drainage, percussion, and vibration to mobilize secretions.	2. Postural drainage uses gravity to remove secretions from the lung.	• Airway is clear of secretions.

3. Use measures to reduce pleuritic pain:
  a. Apply heat and cold as directed.
  b. Assist with intercostal nerve block with procaine when indicated.
  c. Use prescribed analgesics with caution to prevent depression of cough reflex and central nervous system respiratory drive.
  d. Treat dry cough and laryngospasm with aerosol therapy.
	3. Pain and cough result from pleuritic invasion by pneumococci. The discomfort of pleuritic pain can interfere with the mechanics of ventilation and effective airway clearance.	• Uses appropriate methods to reduce pleuritic pain.
		• Verbalizes minimal pleuritic pain and uses methods to reduce it.

4. Administer prescribed antibiotic at correct time intervals.
  a. Penicillin is usually the drug of choice. Erythromycin or clindamycin can be prescribed if patient is allergic to penicillin.
  b. Observe patient for nausea, vomiting, diarrhea, anal pruritus, rash, and soft tissue reactions.
	4. Treatment is based on laboratory identification of the agent causing the infection and on the drainage of purulent secretions. Pneumococci are highly susceptible to the action of penicillin.	• Verbalizes importance of taking antibiotics at prescribed intervals and reports side effects.

5. Give oxygen as prescribed for dyspnea, circulatory disturbance, hypoxemia, or delirium. Monitor arterial blood gases to determine oxygen need and evaluate oxygen effectiveness.	5. Restlessness, confusion, and aggressiveness may be due to cerebral hypoxia.	• Arterial oxygen tension is 60 mm Hg or greater.

6. Monitor the patient's response to therapy.
  a. Monitor temperature, pulse, respiration, and blood pressure every 4 hours and more frequently if indicated. Observe for continuing and recurring fever from drug allergy, drug resistance, or slow response to therapy, inadequate/inappropriate antimicrobial therapy, superinfection, or failure of pneumonia to resolve.
  b. Auscultate chest for crackles, signs of consolidation, or pleural effusion.
	6. Lethal complications may develop during the early period of antimicrobial treatment. The temperature curve provides an index of the patient's response to therapy. Hypotension occurring early in the course of the illness may indicate hypoxia or bacteremia. Antipyretics are administered with caution, as they produce a decrease in temperature and thus interfere with evaluation of the temperature curve.	• Temperature is normal.
		• Pulse and respiration are within normal limits.
		• Is normotensive.
		• Breath sounds are normal.

(continued)

Nursing Care Plan 26–1 (Continued)

Care of the Patient With Bacterial Pneumonia

Nursing Interventions	Rationale	Expected Outcomes

Nursing Diagnosis: Activity intolerance related to altered respiratory function

Goal: Rest to conserve energy

1. Encourage patient to rest as much as possible	1. Rest decreases oxygen demand.	• Remains in bed as needed.
2. Assist patient to assume a comfortable position and to change position frequently.	2. A comfortable position promotes rest. Semi-Fowler's position is desirable if patient is dyspneic. Changing positions frequently prevents pooling of secretions in the lungs.	• Assumes best position for adequate breathing.
3. Evaluate sensorium before sedatives or tranquilizers are administered.	3. Restlessness, confusion, and aggression may indicate cerebral hypoxemia. If this is present, sedatives are inappropriate.	• Evidences a calm, appropriate affect.

Nursing Diagnosis: High risk for fluid volume deficit related to fever and dyspnea

Goal: Achieves adequate fluid balance

1. Give patient 2 to 3 liters of fluid per day.	Fever and tachypnea cause an increase in insensible volume loss. Patient may become dehydrated. A poor appetite during bacterial pneumonia increases the need for increased fluid intake.	• Verbalizes the importance of drinking 2 to 3 liters of fluid per day. • Is adequately hydrated.

Nursing Diagnosis: Knowledge deficit about the treatment protocol and methods of prevention

Goal: Acquisition of knowledge about the treatment protocol and preventive aspects

1. Teach the patient about preventive measures: a. Avoid smoking b. Maintain natural resistance (adequate rest and nutrition and proper exercise). c. Obtain influenza vaccine and pneumococcal vaccine at prescribed times. d. Avoid overfatigue, chilling, and excessive alcohol intake, which lower resistance to pneumonia. e. Report any signs and symptoms of a respiratory tract infection to physician. f. Have follow-up examinations after discharge from the hospital.	1. Cigarette smoking destroys tracheobronchial cilial action, stimulates mucosal cells, causes increased mucus production, and inhibits alveolar scavenger cells (macrophages). Susceptibility to recurring respiratory infections increases after initial exposure. Colds and upper respiratory tract infections may lead to bacterial invasion of the respiratory tract. Pneumonia frequently coexists with other pathologic pulmonary conditions, namely, cancer of the lung.	• Identifies factors that contribute to development of pneumonia. • Stops smoking. • Makes an appointment for a follow-up chest film and influenza and pneumococcal vaccinations. • Verbalizes that he will cope with fatigue by alternating rest periods with increasing activity.

viral infections has been recommended for persons over 50 years of age, nursing home residents, debilitated patients, and those with cardiovascular disease.

In summary, there are a variety of causative agents responsible for the development of pneumonia. The clinical presentation varies depending on the causative agent. The treatment will continue to change as organisms become resistant to different types of antimicrobial therapies. Although there have been tremendous strides in the diagnosis and treatment of pneumonia, little progress has been made in reducing morbidity and mortality. Prevention of pneumonia can be achieved by understanding the risk factors that contribute to transmission of the organisms and use of vaccines in certain patient populations.

Lung Abscess

Pathogenesis

A lung abscess is a localized necrotic lesion of the lung parenchyma containing purulent material; the lesion collapses and forms a cavity. Most lung abscesses occur because of aspiration of nasopharyngeal or oropharyngeal material.

Abscesses also may occur secondary to mechanical or functional obstruction of the bronchi, including tumor, foreign body, or bronchial stenosis; or they may be sequelae of necrotizing pneumonias, tuberculosis, pulmonary embolism, or chest trauma.

Patients with impaired cough reflexes and loss of glottal closure, or those who have swallowing difficulties, are at risk for aspiration of foreign material and abscess formation. Other at-risk patients include those with an altered state of consciousness from anesthesia, central nervous system disorders (seizure, stroke), drug addiction, alcoholism, or esophageal disease, as well as patients fed by nasogastric tube.

The site of the lung abscess is related to gravity and the position of the patient. The posterior segment of the upper right lobe is the most common site. The apical segments of both lower lobes are the next most frequent areas.

In the initial stages, the cavity in the lung may or may not communicate with a bronchus; eventually, however, it becomes surrounded, or *encapsulated*, by a wall of fibrous tissue, except at one or two points where the necrotic process extends until it reaches the lumen of some bronchus or the pleural space and thus establishes a communication with the respiratory tract, the pleural cavity, or both. In the first instance, its purulent contents are evacuated continuously in the form of sputum, whereas if a pleural exit is accessible, empyema (collection of pus in the pleural cavity) results; if both types of communication are present, the problem becomes one of *bronchopleural fistula*. The organisms most frequently associated with lung abscesses are *Klebsiella pneumoniae* and *S. aureus*.

Clinical Manifestations

The clinical presentations may vary from a mild productive cough to acute illness. Most patients are febrile, with a productive cough of moderate to copious amounts of foul-smelling sputum that is often bloody. Pleuritis, or dull chest pain, dyspnea, weakness, anorexia, and weight loss are common.

Diagnostic Evaluation

Physical examination of the chest may reveal dullness on percussion and decreased or absent breath sounds with an intermittent pleural friction rub. Crackles may be present. Confirmation of the diagnosis is made by chest radiograph, sputum culture, and bronchoscopy.

Management

The findings of the history, physical examination, chest radiograph, and sputum culture will indicate the type of organism and treatment required.

Antimicrobial therapy depends on the results of sputum culture and sensitivity and is administered for an extended period. Penicillin G is still the treatment of choice in most cases and often is supplemented by metronidazole (Flagyl) or clindamycin (Cleocin) if the patient is seriously ill. Large intravenous doses are generally required, because the antibiotic must penetrate necrotic tissue and abscess fluid.

Adequate drainage of the lung abscess often is achieved through postural drainage and chest physiotherapy. The use of bronchoscopy to drain an abscess is controversial. It can be useful to rule out a foreign body or a tumor or to locate the site of the draining bronchus.

A high-protein, high-calorie diet is necessary because chronic infection is associated with a catabolic state, necessitating increased intake of calories and protein to facilitate healing.

After the patient shows signs of improvement as demonstrated by normal temperature, lowering of white blood cell count, and improvement in the chest film (resolution of surrounding infiltrate, reduction in the size of the cavity, and absence of fluid), the antibiotic is administered orally rather than intravenously. If treatment is stopped too soon, a relapse may occur. The duration of antibiotic therapy may be from 6 to 16 weeks.

Surgical intervention is rare. Pulmonary resection (lobectomy) is performed when there is massive hemoptysis or a malignancy. A thoracotomy is performed for uncontrolled sepsis.

The following measures will reduce the risk of suppurative lung disease:

1. Patients who must have teeth extracted while their gums and teeth are infected may be given appropriate antibiotic therapy before any dental manipulations.
2. The patient is instructed to maintain adequate dental and oral hygiene, because anaerobic bacteria play a role in the pathogenesis of lung abscess.
3. Appropriate antimicrobial therapy is given to patients with pneumonia.

Nursing Interventions. The nurse administers the antibiotic and intravenous therapy as prescribed and monitors the patient for any adverse effects. Chest physiotherapy is initiated as prescribed to drain the abscess. The patient is taught deep breathing and coughing exercises to help expand the lungs. To ensure proper nutritional intake, a diet high in protein and calories is encouraged. Emotional support is provided because the abscess may take a long time to resolve.

Patient Education and Home Health Care. If surgery has been necessary, the patient most likely will return home before the wound closes entirely. It will be necessary to teach the patient or a caregiver how to change the dressings as needed to prevent skin excoriation and an offensive odor. Deep breathing and coughing exercises are to be performed every 2 hours during the day. Postural drainage and percussion techniques are taught to a caregiver so that lung secretions can be removed. Counseling is provided for attaining and maintaining an optimal state of nutrition.

Pleural Conditions

Pleurisy

Pleurisy (pleuritis) refers to inflammation of both the visceral and parietal pleurae. When these inflamed membranes rub together during respiration (particularly inspiration), the result is severe, sharp, "knifelike" pain. The pain may become minimal or absent when the breath is held, or it may be localized or radiate to the shoulder or abdomen. Later, as pleural fluid develops, the pain lessens. In the early period, when little fluid has accumulated, the pleural friction rub can be heard with the stethoscope, only to disappear later as fluid accumulates and separates the roughened pleural surfaces.

Pleurisy may develop with pneumonia or upper respiratory tract infection, tuberculosis, collagen disease, after trauma to the chest or pulmonary infarction or embolism, in primary and metastatic cancer, in the viral disease known as epidemic pleurodynia, and after thoracotomy.

Careful radiographic and sputum examinations and thoracentesis with pleural fluid examination and possibly pleural biopsy are indicated to discover the underlying condition.

Management. The objectives of treatment are to discover the underlying condition causing the pleurisy, and to relieve the pain. As the underlying disease (pneumonia, infection) is treated, the pleuritic inflammation usually resolves. At the same time it is necessary to watch for signs and symptoms of pleural effusion, such as shortness of breath, pain, and decreased local excursion of the chest wall.

Prescribed analgesics and applications of heat or cold will provide symptomatic relief. Indomethacin, a nonsteroidal anti-inflammatory drug, may provide pain relief while allowing the patient to cough effectively. If the pain is severe, a procaine intercostal block may be required.

Nursing Interventions. Because this patient has considerable pain on inspiration, the nurse can offer suggestions to enhance comfort, such as turning frequently on the affected side to splint the chest wall; this will lessen the stretch of the pleura. The nurse also can teach the patient to use his hands to splint the rib cage while coughing. Because pain on breathing produces anxiety, the patient will require support and understanding.

Pleural Effusion

Pleural effusion, a collection of fluid in the pleural space, is rarely a primary disease process but is usually secondary to other diseases. Normally, the pleural space may contain a small amount of fluid (5 to 15 ml) acting as a lubricant that allows the visceral and parietal surfaces to move without friction.

In certain intrathoracic and systemic diseases, fluid may accumulate in the pleural space to a point where it becomes clinically evident, and it is almost always of pathologic significance. The effusion can be a relatively clear fluid, which may be a transudate or an exudate, or it can be blood, pus, or chyle. A *transudate* (filtrates of plasma that move across intact capillary walls) occurs when factors influencing formation and reabsorption of pleural fluid are altered, usually by imbalances in hydrostatic or oncotic pressures. A transudate indicates that a condition such as ascites or a systemic disease such as congestive heart failure or renal failure underlies the fluid accumulation. An *exudate* (extravasation of fluid into tissues/cavity) usually results from inflammation by bacterial products or tumors involving the pleural surfaces.

In general, the differentiation is made on the basis of protein content and lactic dehydrogenase activity. Pleural effusion may be a complication of tuberculosis, pneumonia, congestive heart failure, pulmonary viral infections, and neoplastic tumors. Bronchogenic carcinoma is the most common malignancy associated with a pleural effusion.

Clinical Manifestations. Usually the clinical manifestations are those caused by the underlying disease; pneumonia will cause fever, chills, and pleuritic chest pain, whereas a malignant effusion may result in dyspnea and coughing. A large quantity of pleural effusion will cause shortness of breath with dullness or flatness to percussion over areas of fluid with minimal or absence of breath sounds. Egophony ("e" to "a" changes) will be present above the effusion (see p. 509). Tracheal deviation away from the affected side may occur with significant accumulation of pleural fluid.

The presence of fluid is confirmed by chest film, ultrasound, physical examination, and thoracentesis. Pleural fluid is analyzed by bacterial cultures, Gram stain, acid-fast bacillus stain (for tuberculosis), red and white blood cell counts, blood chemistry studies (glucose, amylase, lactic dehydrogenase, protein), and *p*H.

Management. The objectives of treatment are to discover the underlying cause to prevent fluid collection from recurring, and to relieve discomfort and dyspnea. Specific treatment is directed to the underlying cause (*e.g.*, congestive heart failure, cirrhosis).

Thoracentesis is performed to remove fluid, to collect a specimen for analysis, and to relieve dyspnea. If the underlying cause is a malignancy, however, the effusion may recur within a few days or weeks. Repeated thoracenteses result in pain, depletion of protein and electrolytes, and sometimes pneumothorax. In this event the patient may be treated with chest tube drainage connected to a water-seal drainage system or suction to evacuate the pleural space and re-expand the lung. Sometimes tetracycline, radioactive isotopes, or cytotoxic or other chemically irritating drugs are instilled in the pleural space to obliterate the pleural space and prevent further accumulation of fluid. After drug instillation, the chest tube is clamped and the patient is assisted to assume various positions to ensure uniform drug distribution and to maximize drug contact with the pleural surfaces. The tube is unclamped as prescribed, and chest drainage is usually continued several days longer to prevent reaccumulation of fluid and to facilitate obliteration of the pleural space by formation of adhesions between the visceral and parietal pleurae. Other modalities of treatment for malignant pleural effusions include radiation of the chest wall, surgical pleurectomy, and diuretic therapy. If the pleural fluid is an exudate, more extensive diagnostic procedures are performed to determine the cause. Treatment for the primary cause is then instituted.

Nursing Interventions. The nurse's role in the care of the patient with a pleural effusion involves implementing the medical regimen. The nurse prepares and positions the patient for thoracentesis and offers support throughout the procedure. Because the pleura is involved, there will be considerable pain; therefore, the patient is assisted to assume positions that are the least painful, and pain medication is administered as prescribed and as needed. If a chest tube drainage and water-seal system is used, the nurse is responsible for monitoring the system's function and recording the amount of drainage every 8 hours. Nursing care related to the underlying cause of the pleural effusion will be specific to that condition.

Empyema

Empyema is a collection of infected liquid or pus in the pleural cavity. At first, the pleural fluid is thin, with a low leukocyte count, but frequently it progresses to a fibropurulent stage and, finally, to a stage where it encloses the lung within a thick exudative membrane.

Clinical Manifestations. The patient has fever, night sweats, pleural pain, dyspnea, anorexia, and weight loss. Chest auscultation shows the absence of breath sounds and there is flatness to chest percussion, as well as decreased fremitus (vocal vibration detected on palpation). If the patient has received antimicrobial therapy, the clinical manifestations may be altered. The diagnosis is established on the basis of chest films and thoracentesis.

Management. The objectives of treatment are to drain the pleural cavity and to achieve full expansion of the lung. This is accomplished by adequate drainage and by appropriate antibiotics selected on the basis of the causative organism. Large doses of the drug are usually given.

Drainage of the pleural fluid or pus depends on the stage of the disease and is accomplished by:

- Needle aspiration (thoracentesis) if the fluid is not too thick
- Closed-chest drainage using a large-diameter intercostal tube attached to water-seal drainage (pp. 547–549)
- Open drainage by means of rib resection to remove the thickened pleura, pus, and debris and to resect the underlying diseased pulmonary tissue

If the inflammation has been long-standing, an exudate can form over the lung and interfere with its normal expansion. This will have to be removed surgically (decortication). The drainage tube is left in place until the pus-filled space is obliterated completely. The complete obliteration of the pleural space is monitored by chest radiograph, and the patient should be informed that this treatment may take a long time.

Nursing Interventions. Resolution of empyema is a prolonged process. The nurse helps the patient cope with the condition and instructs him in breathing exercises (pursed lip and diaphragmatic breathing), which help to restore normal respiratory function. The nurse also provides care specific to the method of drainage of the pleural fluid, such as needle aspiration, closed chest drainage, or rib resection and drainage. (See nursing management following a thoracotomy, pp. 553–556)

Chronic Obstructive Pulmonary Disease

COPD is a broad classification of disorders, including chronic bronchitis, bronchiectasis, emphysema, and asthma. It is an irreversible condition associated with dyspnea on exertion and reduced airflow not explained by specific infiltrative lung or heart disease. COPD is the fifth most common cause of death in the United States. It affects over 25% of the adult population.

Studies support the theory that COPD is a disease of genetics and environmental interaction. Cigarette smoking, air pollution, and occupational exposure (coal, cotton, grain) are important risk factors that contribute to its development, which may occur over a 20- to 30-year span. COPD has also been found in persons genetically lacking d-antitrypsin-deficient phenotypes (PiA, PiSZ). It appears to begin fairly early in life and is a slowly progressive disorder that is present many years before the onset of clinical symptoms and impairment of pulmonary function.

Gerontologic Considerations

COPD often presents during the middle adult years, but its incidence increases with age. Although there is a decrease in vital capacity and forced expiratory volume in 1 second (FEV_1) with age, COPD accentuates many of the physiologic changes associated with aging and results in airway obstruction (in bronchitis) and excessive loss of elastic lung recoil (in emphysema). Therefore, there are additional changes in ventilation–perfusion ratios in elderly patients with COPD.

▶ Nursing Process
The Patient With COPD

▷ Assessment

Data collection involves obtaining information about current symptoms as well as previous disease manifestations. The following is a list of questions that the nurse can use as a guide to obtain a clear history of the disease process:

- How long has the patient had respiratory difficulty?
- Does exertion increase the dyspnea? What type of exertion?
- What are the limits to his exercise tolerance?
- At what times during the day does he complain most of fatigue and shortness of breath?
- Have his habits of eating or sleeping been affected?
- What does he know about the disease and his condition?

Additional data are obtained through observation and examination; questions to consider in obtaining further data include:

- What are the pulse and the respiratory rates?
- Are the respirations even?
- Does the patient contract his abdominal muscles during inspiration?
- Does the patient have prolonged expiration?
- Is cyanosis evident?
- Are the patient's neck veins engorged?
- Does the patient have peripheral edema?
- Is he coughing?
- What are the color, amount, and consistency of the sputum?
- What is the status of the patient's sensorium?
- Is there increasing stupor? Apprehension?

▷ Nursing Diagnoses

Based on all the assessment data, the patient's major nursing diagnoses may include the following:

- Impaired gas exchange related to ventilation–perfusion inequality

- Ineffective airway clearance related to bronchoconstriction, increased mucus production, ineffective cough, and bronchopulmonary infection
- Ineffective breathing pattern related to shortness of breath, mucus, bronchoconstriction, and airway irritants
- Self-care deficit related to fatigue secondary to increased work of breathing and insufficient ventilation and oxygenation
- Activity intolerance due to fatigue, hypoxemia, and ineffective breathing patterns
- Ineffective individual coping related to less socialization, anxiety, depression, lower activity level, and the inability to work
- Knowledge deficit of self-care procedures to be performed at home

Planning and Implementation

▷ *Goals:*   The major goals for the patient may include improvement in gas exchange, achievement of airway clearance, improvement in breathing pattern, independence in self-care activities, improvement in activity tolerance, improvement in coping ability, and adherence to therapeutic program and home care.

Nursing Interventions

▷ *Improvement in Gas Exchange.*   Bronchospasm, which is present in many forms of pulmonary disease, causes reduction in the caliber of the small bronchi, resulting in stasis of secretions and infection. Bronchospasm is detected when wheezes are heard on auscultation with a stethoscope. Increased mucus production along with decreased mucociliary action contributes to further reduction in the caliber of the bronchi and results in decreased air flow and decreased gas exchange, which is aggravated by the loss of lung elasticity.

These changes in the airway demand that the nurse frequently assess the level of dyspnea and hypoxia in the patient. If bronchodilators are prescribed, the nurse must properly administer the medications and be alert for potential side effects. The relief of bronchospasm is confirmed by measuring improvement in expiratory flow rates and assessing whether the patient has a reduction in dyspnea.

Aerosol therapy helps loosen secretions so that they can be removed. Inhaled bronchodilators often are added to the nebulizer to provide direct bronchodilator action on the airways, thereby improving gas exchange. Nebulizer treatments should be given before meals to improve lung ventilation and thus reduce the fatigue that accompanies eating. After inhalation of nebulized bronchodilators, the patient is advised to inhale moisture to further liquefy secretions. Then expulsive coughing or postural drainage will aid him in expectorating secretions. The patient is helped to do this in a manner that is not exhausting to him.

Oxygen is prescribed by the physician when hypoxemia is present. The nurse must monitor the effectiveness of the oxygen therapy and ensure that the patient is compliant in his use of the oxygen delivery device. The nurse instructs him in the proper use of oxygen and cautions the patient and his family about the dangers of increasing the oxygen flow rate without explicit directions from the physician

- Because hypoxia is the stimulus for respirations in the patient with long-standing COPD and CO_2 retention, increasing the

oxygen flow rate may raise the oxygen level in the patient's blood and remove the stimulus for breathing.

Additionally, they are instructed that smoking with or near oxygen is extremely dangerous. In some cases, the patient may be discharged home with oxygen. Oxygen can be supplied to the home by compressed gas, liquid, or concentrator systems. Portable oxygen systems are available that allow the patient to work and travel. Patient education includes reassuring the patient that oxygen is not "addicting" and explaining the precautions involved in using oxygen (no smoking) and the necessity of having regular measurements of arterial blood gases.

Continuous oxygen therapy has been demonstrated to prolong life for those with arterial oxygen pressure (PaO_2) of 55 mm Hg (7.31 kPa[a]) or less on room air. Intermittent oxygen use has little value in the patient with COPD, except during an intensive exercise program or in the form of nocturnal therapy.

▷ *Removal of Bronchial Secretions.*   A major goal in the treatment of COPD is to diminish the quantity and viscosity of sputum to improve pulmonary ventilation and gas exchange. All pulmonary irritants must be eliminated, particularly cigarette smoking, which is the most persistent source of pulmonary irritation. A high fluid intake (6 to 8 glasses) daily is encouraged to liquefy secretions. An added reason for encouraging fluid intake is the tendency for the patient to breathe through his mouth, which accelerates water loss. Inhaling nebulized water also is helpful because it humidifies the bronchial tree, adding water to the sputum and decreasing its viscosity, so that evacuation of sputum is facilitated.

Postural drainage with percussion and vibration uses gravity to help raise secretions so that they can be coughed out or suctioned easily. When used in conjunction with aerosolized bronchodilators and aerosol by updraft or an intermittent positive-pressure breathing (IPPB) treatment, postural drainage should follow either of these therapies because drainage is facilitated after the tracheobronchial tree is dilated. The patient is instructed in effective breathing and coughing to help raise the secretions. Postural drainage usually is carried out when the patient wakes up, to remove secretions that have accumulated overnight, and before he retires, to promote sleep. The frequency of these measures throughout the day will be dictated by the patient's needs.

▷ *Prevention of Bronchopulmonary Infections.*   Bronchopulmonary infections must be controlled to diminish inflammatory edema and to permit recovery of normal ciliary action. Minor respiratory infections that are of no consequence to the person with normal lungs can produce fatal disturbances of pulmonary function in the person with COPD. The cough associated with bronchial infection introduces a vicious cycle with further trauma and damage to the lungs, further progression of symptoms, increased bronchospasm, and further increase in susceptibility to bronchial infection. Infection compromises lung function and is a common cause of respiratory failure.

In COPD, infection may be accompanied by subtle changes. The patient is instructed to report to the physician immediately if the sputum becomes discolored, because purulent expectoration or a change in the character, color, or amount of the sputum is evidence of infection. He is taught that any worsening of his symptoms (increased tightness of the chest, increase in dyspnea, and fatigue) is also suggestive of infection and must be reported. Viral infections are hazardous to these patients because they are so often followed by infections caused by *S. pneumoniae*, *H. influenzae*, and so on.

Patients with COPD are prone to respiratory infections and should be immunized against influenza and *S. pneumoniae*. During the spring when the pollen count is high or in areas with significant air pollution, these persons should avoid outdoor exposure because it may increase bronchospasm. Outdoor periods of high temperatures with high humidity should also be avoided.

▷ *Breathing Exercises and Retraining.*   Most people with COPD breathe shallowly from the upper chest in a rapid and inefficient manner. This type of upper chest breathing can be changed to diaphragmatic breathing with practice. Training in diaphragmatic breathing reduces the respiratory rate, increases alveolar ventilation, and sometimes causes a reduction of functional residual capacity (see p. 530 for technique).

Pursed-lip breathing slows expiration, prevents collapse of lung units, and helps the patient to control the rate and depth of respiration and to relax, which enables him to gain control of his dyspnea and feelings of panic.

A patient with COPD has definite periods of the day when his exercise tolerance is decreased. This is especially true on arising in the morning, because bronchial secretions and edema collect in the lungs during the night while he is lying on his back. The patient often will be unable to shave or bathe. Activities requiring the arms to be supported above the level of the thorax may produce distress. These activities may be tolerated better after the patient has been up and moving around for an hour or more. Because of these limitations, the patient must participate in planning his care with the nurse and in determining the best time for bathing and shaving. A hot beverage on arising, along with diaphragmatic breathing, will assist him to expectorate and will shorten the period of disability experienced on arising.

Another period of increased disability occurs immediately after meals, particularly the evening meal. Fatigue from the day's activities coupled with abdominal distention limits his exercise tolerance. The patient's chief complaint at this time is fatigue or dyspnea.

Once the patient has learned diaphragmatic breathing, a program of inspiratory muscle training may be initiated to help strengthen the muscles used in breathing. This device requires that the patient breathe against a resistance. The resistance is gradually increased and the muscles become better conditioned. Conditioning of the respiratory muscles takes a long time, and the patient is instructed to continue practicing at home.

▷ *Self-Care Activities.*   As gas exchange, airway clearance, and the breathing pattern improve, the patient is encouraged to assume some of his own care. He is taught to try to coordinate diaphragmatic breathing with activities such as walking, bathing, bending, or climbing stairs. The patient should begin to bathe, dress himself, and take short walks, resting as needed to avoid fatigue and excessive dyspnea. The inspiratory muscle trainer is used for 10 to 15 minutes every day. Fluids should be readily available, and the patient should begin to drink without encouragement. If the patient will be using postural drainage at home, he is instructed and supervised by the nurse before discharge.

▷ *Physical Conditioning.*   Physical conditioning techniques include breathing and general physical conditioning exercises intended to conserve and increase pulmonary ventilation. There is a close relationship between physical fitness and respiratory fitness. Graded exercises and physical conditioning programs employing treadmills, stationary bicycles, and measured level walks have been shown to improve symptoms and to increase work capacity and exercise tolerance. It is useful for the patient to have a physical activity that he can do on a regular sustained basis. A lightweight portable oxygen system is available for the ambulatory patient who requires oxygen therapy during physical activity to improve hypoxia. This type of rehabilitation improves the quality of life.

▷ *Coping Measures.*   Any factor that interferes with normal breathing quite naturally induces anxiety, depression, and changes in behavior. Many patients find the slightest exertion exhausting. Constant shortness of breath and fatigue may render the patient irritable and apprehensive to the point of panic. His enforced inactivity (and reversal of family roles due to loss of employment), the frustration of having to work to breathe, and the realization that he faces a prolonged, unrelenting disease may cause the patient to react with anger, depression, and demanding behavior. Sexual function may be compromised, which also diminishes self-esteem.

It is important for the nurse and other health care personnel to encourage the patient to remain active up to his level of symptom tolerance. Emphasis should be on controlling his symptoms and increasing self-esteem and sense of mastery and of well-being. Supportive medical and nursing care, ongoing patient teaching, exercise conditioning, and possibly group therapy sessions help to somewhat relieve an almost overwhelming burden.

The patient may also be directed to support groups conducted by the American Lung Association, to pulmonary rehabilitation programs where available, to smoking cessation programs (if still smoking), and to senior citizens' groups for social interaction. These groups will help to improve the patient's knowledge of his condition, his ability to cope with his disease, and his sense of self-worth.

▷ *Patient Education and Home Health Care.*   To help the patient with COPD live better, it is essential that he be educated about his disease process. One of the major teaching factors is helping the patient accept realistic short-term and long-range goals. If the patient is severely disabled, the objective of treatment is to preserve his present pulmonary function and relieve his symptoms as much as possible. If his disease is mild, the objective is to increase his exercise tolerance and prevent further loss of pulmonary function. The goals and expectations of treatment must be shared and planned with the patient. The patient and those caring for him need patience to achieve these goals.

The patient is instructed to avoid extremes of heat and cold. Heat increases the body temperature, thereby raising the oxygen requirements of the body; cold tends to promote bronchospasm. High altitudes aggravate the hypoxia. Bronchospasm may be initiated also by air pollutants such as fumes, smoke, dust, and even talcum, lint, and aerosol sprays.

Protection of the lung is basic for the preservation of lung function. Patients with COPD should be informed unequivocally that, for them, smoking is dangerous. Cigarette smoking depresses the activity of scavenger cells and affects the ciliary cleansing mechanism of the respiratory tract, the function of which is to keep the breathing passages free of inhaled irritants, bacteria, and other foreign matter. This is one of the major defense mechanisms of the body. When this cleansing mechanism is damaged by smoking, air flow is obstructed and air becomes trapped behind the obstructed airway. The air sacs greatly distend and the lung capacity is diminished. Cigarette smoking also irritates the goblet cells and mucous glands, causing an increased accumulation of mucus. The mucus accumulation produces more irritation, infection, and damage to the lung capacity. Frequently the patient is unaware of what is happening until he notices that extra physical effort produces respiratory distress. At this point the damage may be irreversible. Therefore, patients with COPD should definitely refrain from smoking. There is a wide variety of smoking control strategies, including prevention, cessation, and behavior modification.

Patients with COPD should restrict themselves to lives of moderate activity, ideally in a climate with minimal shifts in temperature and humidity. Stressful situations that might trigger a coughing episode or emotional disturbance should be avoided.

Patients may be directed to community resources such as pulmonary rehabilitation programs, smoking cessation programs, and other programs to help improve their ability to cope with their chronic condition and their therapeutic regimen and to give them a sense of worth, hope, and well-being.

⬦ Evaluation

Expected Outcomes

1. Improves gas exchange
   a. Verbalizes need for bronchodilators and for taking them on schedule
   b. Demonstrates ability to use and clean respiratory therapy equipment
   c. Uses oxygen equipment appropriately
   d. Evidences stable arterial blood gas values (but not necessarily normal due to chronic changes in gas exchange capability of the lung)
2. Achieves airway clearance
   a. States that 6 to 8 glasses of fluids per day are needed
   b. Identifies pollens, fumes, gases, dusts, and extremes of temperature and humidity as respiratory irritants to be avoided
   c. Stops smoking or agrees to attend a smoking cessation program
   d. Performs postural drainage correctly and reports that caregiver can do percussion/vibration
   e. Coughs less
   f. Knows signs of early infection and reason to notify physician at earliest sign of infection
   g. Is free of infection on discharge
   h. Verbalizes need to avoid crowds and people with colds during the flu season
   i. Plans to discuss flu and pneumonia vaccines with his physician to help prevent infection
3. Improves breathing pattern
   a. Practices pursed-lip and diaphragmatic breathing and uses them during activity and when short of breath

   b. Participates in inspiratory muscle training as instructed for prescribed time daily
   c. Shows signs of decreased respiratory effort
4. Performs self-care activities
   a. Paces activities of daily living with alternate rest periods to reduce fatigue and dyspnea
   b. Uses controlled breathing while bathing, bending to tie shoes, and so on
   c. Identifies ways to conserve energy
5. Achieves activity tolerance
   a. Performs activities with less shortness of breath
   b. Verbalizes need to exercise daily and demonstrates an exercise plan to be carried out at home
   c. Walks and gradually increases walking time and distance to improve physical conditioning
6. Acquires effective coping mechanisms
   a. Verbalizes activities or methods to ease shortness of breath
   b. Plans to join a support group
   c. Participates in a pulmonary rehabilitation program
7. Adheres to therapeutic program
   a. Is able to list those factors that improve his condition as well as those that make his condition worse
   b. Verbalizes the need to preserve existing lung function by adhering to treatment and rehabilitation program

Chronic Bronchitis

Clinical Manifestations and Pathophysiology

Chronic bronchitis is defined as the presence of a productive cough that lasts 3 months a year for 2 consecutive years. Chronic bronchitis is primarily associated with cigarette smoking or exposure to pollution. Smoke irritates the airways, resulting in hypersecretion of mucus and inflammation.

The patient's major problem is the protracted and abundant production of inflammatory exudate that fills and obstructs the bronchioles and is responsible for a persistent, productive cough and shortness of breath. This constant irritation causes hypertrophy of mucus-secreting glands, goblet cell hyperplasia, loss of cilia, and increased mucus production, leading to bronchial plugging and bronchial narrowing. Alveoli adjacent to the bronchioles may become damaged and fibrosed. Further bronchial narrowing follows as a result of these fibrotic changes in the airways. In time, irreversible lung changes may occur with resultant emphysema and bronchiectasis.

Patients with chronic bronchitis have increased susceptibility to recurring infections of the lower respiratory tract. A wide range of viral, bacterial, and mycoplasmal infections can produce acute episodes of bronchitis. Exacerbations of chronic bronchitis are most likely to occur during the winter. The inhalation of cold air produces bronchospasm in sensitive persons.

Preventive Measures.   Because of the disabling nature of chronic bronchitis, every effort is directed toward its prevention. An important feature is the avoidance of respiratory irritants (particularly tobacco smoke). People who are prone to respiratory tract infections should be immunized against common viral agents with vaccines for influenza and for *S. pneumoniae*. All patients with acute upper respiratory tract infections should receive proper treatment, including antimicrobial therapy based on cultures and sensitivity studies at the first sign of purulent sputum.

Management.   The main objectives of treatment are to maintain the patency of the peripheral bronchial tree, to facilitate removal of bronchial exudates, and to prevent disability. Changes in the sputum pattern (nature, color, amount, thickness) and in the cough pattern are important signs to note. Recurrent bacterial infections are treated with antibiotic therapy after the completion of culture and sensitivity studies.

To facilitate the removal of bronchial exudates, bronchodilators are prescribed to relieve bronchospasm and reduce airway obstruction; thus, gas distribution and alveolar ventilation are improved. Postural drainage and chest percussion after treatments are usually helpful. Water (given orally or parenterally if bronchospasm is severe) is an important part of therapy, because proper hydration helps the patient cough up secretions. Steroid therapy may be used when the patient fails to respond to more conservative measures, but its use is still controversial. When there is an underlying bronchiectasis, postural drainage is most important. The patient must stop smoking because smoke inhalation causes bronchoconstriction, paralysis of ciliary activity, and inactivation of surfactant. Smokers are also more susceptible to bronchial infection.

For nursing management and patient education, see Nursing Process: The Patient With COPD, pp. 571–574.

Bronchiectasis

Bronchiectasis is a chronic dilatation of the bronchi and bronchioles. Bronchial dilatation may be caused by a variety of conditions, including pulmonary infections and obstruction of the bronchus; aspiration of foreign bodies, vomitus, or material from the upper respiratory tract; and extrinsic pressure from tumors, dilated blood vessels, and enlarged lymph nodes. A person may be predisposed to bronchiectasis as a result of respiratory infection in early childhood, measles, influenza, tuberculosis, and immunodeficiency disorders. After surgery, bronchiectasis may develop when the patient's cough is ineffective, with the result that mucus obstructs the bronchi and leads to atelectasis.

Pathophysiology.   The infection damages the bronchial wall, causing loss of its supporting structure and producing thick sputum that ultimately may obstruct the bronchi. The walls become permanently distended by severe coughing. The infection extends to the peribronchial tissues, so that in the case of saccular bronchiectasis, each dilated tube virtually amounts to a lung abscess, the exudate of which drains freely through the bronchus. The lower lobes are most frequently involved.

The retention of secretions and obstruction ultimately lead to collapse of the distally situated lung (atelectasis). Inflammatory scarring or fibrosis replaces functioning lung tissue. In time the patient develops respiratory insufficiency with reduced vital capacity, decreased ventilation, and an increased ratio of residual volume to total lung capacity. There is impaired mixing of inspired gas (ventilation–perfusion imbalance) and hypoxemia.

Clinical Manifestations.   Characteristic symptoms of bronchiectasis include chronic cough and the production of

purulent sputum in copious amounts. The sputum has a characteristic quality of a "layering out" into three layers on standing: a frothy top layer, a middle clear layer, and a dense particulate bottom layer. A high percentage of patients with this disease experience hemoptysis. Clubbing of the fingers is also very common. The patient is likely to be subject to repeated episodes of pulmonary infection.

Many persons with bronchiectasis are not readily diagnosed because their symptoms are mistaken for those of simple chronic bronchitis. A definite clue is offered by the prolonged history of productive cough, with sputum consistently negative for tubercle bacilli. The diagnosis is established on the basis of bronchography and bronchoscopy (p. 515), and computed tomography. The results of these procedures demonstrate the presence or absence of bronchial dilatation.

Preventive Measures.   All respiratory infections should be treated promptly. Bronchial secretions can be removed (by expectorants, postural drainage, therapeutic bronchoscopy) to prevent bronchiectasis. If a child has a prolonged cough and fever, the family should be urged to seek medical treatment. Unconscious persons should be turned (prone position to lateral) to drain all bronchial segments. Patients should be vaccinated against influenza and pneumococcal pneumonia. (Immunization against pertussis and measles, which may lead to bronchiectasis, should be continued.)

Management.   The objectives of treatment are to prevent and control infection and to promote bronchial drainage to rid the affected portion of the lung or lungs of excessive secretions. Infection is controlled with antimicrobial therapy guided by results of sensitivity studies on organisms cultured from sputum. Patients may be put on a year-round regimen of antibiotics, alternating types of drugs at intervals. Some clinicians prescribe antibiotics throughout the winter or when acute upper respiratory tract infections occur.

Postural drainage of the bronchial tubes underlies all treatment considerations because draining the bronchiectatic areas by gravity reduces the amount of secretions and the degree of infection. (Sometimes mucopurulent sputum must be removed by bronchoscopy.) The affected chest area may be percussed or "cupped" to assist in raising secretions.

The patient is started out with short periods of postural drainage and its duration is increased steadily. Bronchodilators may be given to persons who also have obstructive airway disease. Patients with bronchiectasis almost always have associated bronchitis. β-Sympathomimetics may be used for bronchodilation and to increase the mucociliary transport of secretions.

To make sputum expectoration easier, the water content of the sputum is increased by aerosolized nebulizer treatments and by an increase in oral fluid intake. A face tent is ideal for providing extra humidification for aerosols. The patient should not smoke, as this impairs bronchial drainage by paralyzing ciliary action, increasing bronchial secretions, and causing inflammation of the mucous membranes, resulting in hyperplasia of the mucous glands.

Surgical intervention is used infrequently as treatment. It may be indicated for the patient who continues to expectorate fairly large amounts of sputum and experiences repeated bouts of pneumonia and hemoptysis in spite of a successful treatment regimen, provided the disease involves only one or two areas of the lung that can be removed without producing respiratory insufficiency. The goal of surgical treatment is to conserve normal pulmonary tissue and avoid infectious complications.

All diseased tissue is removed, provided that the postoperative lung function will be adequate. It may be necessary to remove a segment of a lobe (segmental resection), a lobe (lobectomy), or an entire lung (pneumonectomy). *Segmental resection* is the removal of an anatomic subdivision of a pulmonary lobe. The chief advantage is that only diseased tissue is removed, with greater conservation of healthy lung tissue. Bronchography aids in the delineation of the segment. The surgery is preceded by a period of preparation, which is exceedingly important. The objective is to obtain a dry (as dry as possible) tracheobronchial tree to prevent complications (atelectasis, pneumonia, bronchopleural fistula, and empyema). This is accomplished by means of postural drainage or, depending on the location of the abscess, by direct suction through a bronchoscope. A course of antibacterial therapy may be prescribed.

After the surgery, the care is the same as for any chest surgical patient, as is discussed on pp. 553–556.

Patient Education.   The patient is taught diaphragmatic breathing and postural drainage exercises. He is encouraged to have regular dental care and to avoid all pulmonary irritants (cigarette smoke, noxious fumes). He should monitor his sputum and report any change in its character or quantity. A decrease in sputum production is as significant as an increase. An important preventive aspect is immunization against influenza and pneumococcal pneumonia. Other aspects of health teaching are included under COPD on pp. 573–574.

Pulmonary Emphysema

Pulmonary emphysema is defined as a non-uniform pattern of abnormal permanent distention of the air spaces, distal to the terminal bronchioles with destruction of the alveolar septa. It appears to be the end stage of a process that has progressed slowly for many years. In fact, by the time the patient develops symptoms, pulmonary function often is irreversibly impaired. Along with chronic obstructive bronchitis, it is a major cause of disability.

Cigarette smoking is the major cause of emphysema. In a small percentage of patients, however, there is a familial predisposition to emphysema associated with a plasma protein abnormality, a deficiency of α_1-antitrypsin. The genetically susceptible person is sensitive to environmental influences (smoking, air pollution, infectious agents, allergens) and, in time, develops chronic obstructive symptoms. It is imperative that the carriers of this genetic defect be identified to permit genetic counseling and that the environmental factors be modified to delay or prevent overt symptoms of disease.

Pathophysiology.   In emphysema, there are several factors that cause airway obstruction, namely:

* Inflammation and swelling of bronchi
* Excessive mucus production
* Loss of elastic recoil of the airways
* Collapse of bronchioles and redistribution of functional alveoli

As the walls of the alveoli are destroyed (a process accelerated by recurrent infections), the alveolar–capillary surface continually decreases, causing an increase in dead space and impaired oxygen diffusion. Impaired oxygen diffusion results in hypoxemia. In the later stages of the disease, there is interference with carbon dioxide elimination and increased carbon dioxide tension in arterial blood (called hypercapnia), causing respiratory acidosis.

As the alveolar walls continue to rupture, the pulmonary capillary bed is reduced. The pulmonary blood flow is increased and the right ventricle is forced to maintain a higher blood pressure in the pulmonary artery. Thus, right-sided heart failure (cor pulmonale) is one of the complications of emphysema. The presence of leg edema (dependent edema), distended neck veins, or pain in the region of the liver suggests the development of cardiac failure.

Secretions are increased and retained, because the person is unable to generate a forceful cough to expel them. Chronic and acute infections thus persist in the emphysematous lungs, adding to the air transfer problem.

The person with emphysema has a chronic obstruction (marked increase in airway resistance) to the inflow and outflow of air from the lungs. The lungs are in a state of chronic hyperexpansion. To get air into and out of the lungs, negative pressure is required during inspiration and an adequate level of positive pressure must be attained and maintained during expiration. The resting position is one of inflation. Instead of being an involuntary passive act, expiration becomes a muscular active act. The patient becomes increasingly short of breath, the chest becomes rigid, and the ribs are fixed at their joints. The "barrel chest" of many of these patients is due to loss of lung elasticity in the presence of the continued tendency of the chest wall to expand (Fig. 26–1*A*).

In some instances, the barrel chest is due to kyphosis. Some patients bend forward to breathe, using the accessory muscles of respiration. There is also retraction of the supraclavicular fossae on inspiration (see Fig. 26–1*B*). In advanced disease, there is also contraction of the abdominal muscles on

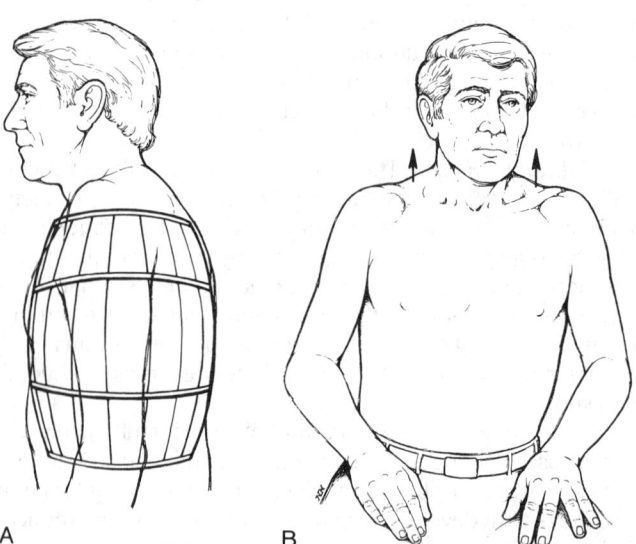

Figure 26–1.   Comparison of typical findings in the patient with pulmonary emphysema. (**A**) The common "barrel chest" condition of the patient with emphysema, showing characteristic increase of anteroposterior diameter. (**B**) Another posture of the patient with emphysema, showing elevation of shoulder girdle and retraction of the supraclavicular fossae on inspiration.

inspiration. There is a progressive reduction of the vital capacity. Normal exhalation becomes increasingly difficult and finally impossible. The total vital capacity (VC) may be normal, but the FEV_1/VC is low. The patient moves air more slowly and inefficiently and has to work hard to do it.

Classification. There are two main pathologic types of emphysema, which are classified on the basis of the type of changes taking place in the lung: (1) panlobular (panacinar) and (2) centrilobular (centriacinar).

In the *panilobular (panacinar) type,* there is destruction of the respiratory bronchiole, alveolar duct, and alveoli. All air spaces within the lobule are more or less enlarged, with little inflammatory disease. This patient typically has a hyperinflated chest and marked dyspnea on exertion, and weight loss. Sometimes he is referred to as a "pink puffer." This patient remains "pink," or well oxygenated, until the disease becomes terminal.

In the *centrilobular (centriacinar) form,* the pathologic changes take place mainly in the center of the secondary lobule, and the peripheral portions of the acinus are preserved. Frequently, there is a derangement of ventilation–perfusion ratios, producing chronic hypoxia, hypercapnia, and polycythemia and episodes of right-sided heart failure. This leads to cyanosis, peripheral edema, and respiratory failure. The patient is referred to as a "blue bloater." In addition to the management outlined below, the blue bloater usually receives diuretic therapy for edema. Both types of emphysema very often occur in the same patient.

Clinical Manifestations. Dyspnea is the presenting symptom in emphysema and has an insidious onset. The patient usually has a history of cigarette smoking and a long history of chronic cough, wheezing, and increasing shortness of breath and tachypnea, especially with respiratory infection. In time, even the slightest exertion, such as bending over to tie his shoelaces, produces dyspnea and fatigue (exertional dyspnea). The emphysematous lung is not contracted on expiration, and the bronchioles are not effectively emptied of their secretions.

The patient readily develops inflammatory reactions and infections due to the pooling of these secretions. After these infections, the patient experiences a prolonged wheezing expiration. Anorexia, weight loss, and weakness are common complaints. The neck veins may be distended during expiration. Physical examination discloses diminished breath sounds with rhonchi and prolonged expiration, hyperresonance with percussion, and a decrease in fremitus.

Diagnostic Evaluation. The patient's symptoms and the clinical findings on physical examination provide the initial clues to the patient's problem. Other aids in diagnosis include chest films, pulmonary function tests (particularly spirometry), blood gas studies (to assess ventilatory function and pulmonary gas exchange), and complete blood count (CBC).

Management. The major objectives of treatment are to improve the quality of life, to slow the progression of the disease process, and to treat the obstructed airways to relieve hypoxia. The therapeutic approach includes (1) treatment measures designed to improve ventilation and decrease the work of breathing, (2) prevention and prompt treatment of infection, (3) the use of physical therapy techniques to conserve and increase pulmonary ventilation, (4) maintenance of proper environmental conditions to facilitate breathing, (5) supportive and psychological care, and (6) an ongoing program of patient education and rehabilitation.

Bronchodilators. Bronchodilators are prescribed to dilate the airways, because they combat both bronchial mucosal edema and muscular spasm and help in reducing airway obstruction and improving gas exchange. These drugs include the β-adrenergic agonists (metaproterenol, isoproterenol) and the methylxanthines (theophylline, aminophylline), which produce bronchial dilatation by different mechanisms. Bronchodilator drugs may be administered orally, subcutaneously, intravenously, rectally, or by nebulization (conversion into a spray). Nebulized medications may be delivered by pressurized aerosols, hand-bulb nebulizers, pump-driven nebulizers, or IPPB. Bronchodilators may produce unwanted side effects, which include tachycardia, cardiac dysrhythmias, and central nervous system excitation. The methylxanthines may also produce gastrointestinal disturbances such as nausea and vomiting. Because side effects are common, the drug dosage is carefully adjusted for each patient in accordance with his tolerance and clinical response.

Aerosol Therapy. Aerosolization (the process of dispensing particles in a fine mist) of saline bronchodilators and mucolytics frequently is used to aid in bronchodilatation. The particle size in the aerosol mist must be small enough to allow the medication to be deposited deep within the tracheobronchial tree.

Nebulized aerosols relieve bronchospasm, decrease mucosal edema, and liquefy bronchial secretions. This facilitates the process of bronchial clearance, helps to control the inflammatory process, and improves ventilatory function. Hand-bulb nebulizers and metered-dose aerosol devices give the patient quick relief. Electrically powered nebulizers and air-powered nebulizers are useful if the patient has more marked ventilatory impairment. The improvement of the oxygen saturation of the arterial blood and the reduction of its carbon dioxide content assist in relieving the patient's hypoxia and give considerable relief from constant respiratory fatigue. Nebulizer treatments with oxygen must be given with extreme caution in patients who have chronically elevated carbon dioxide tensions and are breathing on hypoxic stimuli. There is a trend away from the use of IPPB, especially in the home-care setting.

Treatment of Infection. Patients with emphysema are susceptible to lung infections and must be treated at the earliest signs of infection. *Streptococcus pneumoniae, Haemophilus influenzae,* and *Branhamella catarrhalis* are the most common organisms involved. The physician usually prescribes antimicrobial therapy with tetracyclines, ampicillin, amoxicillin, or trimethoprim-sulfamethoxazole (Bactrim). An antimicrobial regimen is used at the first sign of respiratory infection, as evidenced by purulent sputum, increased cough, and fever.

Corticosteroids. Corticosteroids remain controversial in the treatment of emphysema. They are used after maximum bronchodilator and bronchial hygiene measures have been tried without success. Prednisone is usually prescribed.

The dosage is adjusted to keep the patient on the lowest possible dose. The side effects include gastrointestinal (GI) upset and increased appetite. Long term, the patient may develop peptic ulcer, osteoporosis, adrenal suppression, steroid myopathy, and cataract formation. See Chapter 40 for further description of the effects of corticosteroids.

Oxygenation. Oxygen therapy may increase survival in patients with severe emphysema. Severe hypoxemia is treated with low concentrations of oxygen to raise the PaO_2 to between 65 and 80 mm Hg. In severe emphysema, it is administered at least 16 hr/day, with 24 hours preferable. This modality may alleviate the patient's symptoms and improve the quality of life. Some patients require long-term home use of oxygen (Nursing Care Plan 26-2, pp. 579–582).

Asthma

Asthma is an intermittent, reversible, obstructive airway disease characterized by increased responsiveness of the trachea and bronchi to various stimuli. It is manifested by a narrowing of the airways, resulting in dyspnea, cough, and wheezing. The degree of airway narrowing may change either spontaneously or because of therapy. Asthma differs from other obstructive lung diseases in that it is a reversible process. Acute exacerbations may occur, which last from minutes to hours, interspersed with symptom-free periods. When asthma and bronchitis occur together, the obstruction is compounded and is called chronic asthmatic bronchitis.

Asthma can begin at any age; about half of the cases develop in childhood and another third before age 40. Approximately 17% of all Americans have had asthma at some time in their lives. Although asthma is rarely fatal, it affects school attendance, occupational choices, physical activity, and many other aspects of life.

Asthma is often characterized as allergic, idiopathic, nonallergic, or mixed. Allergic asthma is caused by a known allergen or allergens (*e.g.*, dust pollens, animals, molds, dander, food). Most of the allergens are airborne and seasonal. Patients with allergic asthma usually have a family history of allergies and a past medical history of eczema or allergic rhinitis. Exposure to the allergen triggers an asthmatic attack. Children with allergic asthma often outgrow the condition by adolescence.

Idiopathic or nonallergic asthma is not related to specific allergens. Factors, such as a common cold, respiratory tract infections, exercise, emotions, and environmental pollutants may trigger an attack. Some pharmacologic agents, such as aspirin and other nonsteroidal anti-inflammatory agents, coloring agents, beta-adrenergic antagonists, and sulfite agents (food preservatives), also may be factors. The attacks of idiopathic nonallergic asthma become more severe and frequent with time and can progress to chronic bronchitis and emphysema. Some patients will develop mixed asthma.

Mixed asthma is the most common form of asthma. It has characteristics of both the allergic and the idiopathic or nonallergic forms.

Pathophysiology. Asthma is a reversible diffuse airway obstruction. The obstruction is caused by one or more of the following: (1) contraction of muscles surrounding the bronchi, which narrows the airway; (2) swelling of membranes that line the bronchi; and (3) filling of the bronchi with thick mucus (Fig. 26–2). In addition, there is bronchial muscle enlargement, mucous gland enlargement, thick, tenacious sputum, and hyperinflation or air trapping in the alveoli. The exact mechanism for these changes is not known, but most of what is known involves the immunologic system and the autonomic nervous system.

Some persons with asthma develop exaggerated gamma E immunoglobulin (IgE) responses to their environments. This means that abnormally large amounts of IgE are produced in response to certain antigens and allergens. The IgE antibodies then attach to mast cells in the lung. Re-exposure to the antigen results in the antigen's binding to the antibody. This causes

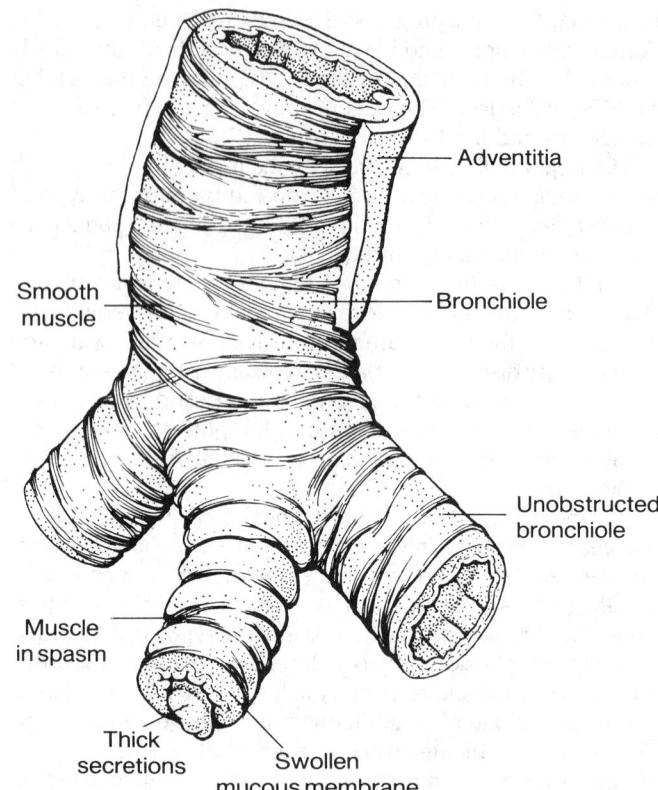

Figure 26–2. Obstruction of a bronchiole in asthma.

the release of mast cell products (called mediators) such as histamine, bradykinin, and prostaglandins and of the slow-reacting substance of anaphylaxis (SRS-A). The release of these mediators in the lung tissue affects the smooth muscle and glands of the airway, causing bronchospasm, mucous membrane swelling, and excessive mucus production.

The autonomic nervous system innervates the lung. Bronchial muscle tone is regulated by vagal nerve impulses through the parasympathetic system. In idiopathic or nonallergic asthma, when the nerve endings in the airway are stimulated by such factors as infection, exercise, cold, smoking, emotions, and pollutants, an increased amount of acetylcholine is released. This can directly cause bronchoconstriction as well as stimulate the production of the chemical mediators discussed above. A proposed theory is that persons with asthma have a low tolerance for parasympathetic responses.

In addition, α- and β-adrenergic receptors of the sympathetic nervous system are located in the bronchi. When the α-adrenergic receptors are stimulated, bronchoconstriction occurs; bronchodilation occurs when the β-adrenergic receptors are stimulated. The balance between α- and β-receptors is controlled primarily by cyclic adenosine monophosphate (cAMP). Alpha-receptor stimulation results in a decrease in cAMP, which leads to an increase in mast cell release of chemical mediators and bronchoconstriction. Beta-receptor stimulation results in increased levels of cAMP, which inhibits release of chemical mediators and causes bronchodilation. A proposed theory is that β-adrenergic blockade occurs in persons with asthma. Consequently, asthmatics are prone to an increased release of chemical mediators and constriction of smooth muscle.

(text continues on page 582)

Nursing Care Plan 26-2

Care of the Patient With Chronic Obstructive Pulmonary Disease

Nursing Interventions	*Rationale*	*Expected Outcomes*

Nursing Diagnosis: Impaired gas exchange related to ventilation–perfusion inequality

Goal: Improvement in gas exchange

1. Administer bronchodilators as prescribed:
  a. Can be given orally, intravenously, rectally, or by nebulization
  b. Administer oral or intravenous bronchodilators at alternate time to nebulizer or IPPB treatment to prolong the effectiveness of the medication.
  c. Observe for side effects: tachycardia, dysrhythmias, central nervous system excitation, nausea, and vomiting.
	1. Bronchodilators dilate the airways and help to combat bronchial mucosa edema and muscular spasm. Because side effects are common, the drug dosage is carefully adjusted for each patient, in accordance with his tolerance and clinical response.	• Verbalizes need for bronchodilators and for taking them on schedule.
		• Evidences minimal side effects; heart rate near normal, absence of dysrhythmias, normal mentation.

2. Evaluate effectiveness of mini-nebulizer or IPPB treatments.
  a. Assess for decreased shortness of breath, decreased wheezing or crackles, secretions loosened, decreased anxiety.
  b. Ensure that treatment is given before meals to avoid nausea and to reduce fatigue that accompanies eating.
	2. Combining medication with aerosolized bronchodilators is typically used to control bronchoconstriction. Improper administration of the treatment will render it ineffective. Aerosolization facilitates bronchial clearance, helps control the inflammatory process, and improves ventilatory function.	• Reports a decrease in dyspnea.
		• Shows an improved expiratory flow rate.
		• Demonstrates ability to use and clean respiratory therapy equipment as applicable.

3. Instruct and encourage patient in diaphragmatic breathing and effective coughing.	3. These techniques improve ventilation by opening airways and clearing the airways of sputum. Gas exchange is improved.	• Demonstrates diaphragmatic breathing and coughing.

4. Administer oxygen by the method prescribed.
  a. Explain importance to patient.
  b. Evaluate effectiveness; observe for signs of hypoxia. Notify physician if restlessness, anxiety, somnolence, cyanosis, or tachycardia is present.
  c. Analyze arterial blood gases and compare with baseline values. When arterial puncture is performed and a blood sample is obtained, hold puncture site for 5 minutes to prevent arterial bleeding.
  d. Explain that no smoking is permitted by patient or visitors while oxygen is in use.
	4. Oxygen will correct the hypoxemia. Careful observation of the liter flow or the percentage administered and its effect on the patient is needed. If the patient has chronic CO_2 retention, then hypoxia is his stimulus to breathe. Too much oxygen could suppress the hypoxic drive and death would occur. These patients generally need low-flow oxygen rates of 1 to 2 L/min. Periodic arterial blood gases help to evaluate adequacy of oxygenation.	• Uses oxygen equipment appropriately when indicated.
		• Evidences normal arterial blood gases.

Nursing Diagnosis: Ineffective airway clearance related to bronchoconstriction, increased mucus production, ineffective cough, and bronchopulmonary infection

Goal: Achievement of airway clearance

1. Give patient 6 to 8 glasses of fluids/day unless cor pulmonale is present.	1. Systemic hydration keeps secretions moist and easier to raise. Fluids must be given with caution if right-sided heart failure is present.	• Verbalizes need to drink 6 to 8 glasses of fluids/day.

(continued)

Nursing Care Plan 26–2 (Continued)

Care of the Patient With Chronic Obstructive Pulmonary Disease

Nursing Interventions	Rationale	Expected Outcomes
2. Teach and encourage the use of diaphragmatic breathing and coughing techniques.	2. These techniques will help to improve ventilation and to produce secretions without causing breathlessness and fatigue.	• Demonstrates diaphragmatic breathing and coughing.
3. Assist in administering nebulizer or IPPB treatments.	3. These treatments add water to the bronchial tree and to the sputum, decreasing its viscosity, so that evacuation of secretions is facilitated.	
4. Perform postural drainage with percussion and vibration in the morning and at night as prescribed.	4. Uses gravity to help raise secretions so they can be more easily coughed up or suctioned.	• Performs postural drainage correctly. • Coughs less.
5. Instruct patient to avoid bronchial irritants such as cigarette smoke, aerosols, extremes of temperature, and fumes.	5. Bronchial irritants cause bronchoconstriction and increased mucus production, which then interferes with airway clearance.	• Does not smoke. • Verbalizes that pollens, fumes, gases, dusts, and extremes of temperature and humidity are irritants to be avoided.
6. Teach early signs of infection that are to be reported to the physician immediately: a. Increased sputum b. Change in color of sputum c. Increased thickness of sputum d. Increased shortness of breath or tightness in chest or fatigue e. Increased coughing	6. Minor respiratory infections that are of no consequence to the person with normal lungs can produce fatal disturbances in the lungs of the person with emphysema. Early recognition becomes crucial.	• Identifies signs of early infection. • Is free of infection on discharge (no fever, no change in sputum, lessening of dyspnea). • Verbalizes need to notify physician at the earliest sign of infection.
7. Administer antibiotics as prescribed.		
8. Encourage patient to be immunized against influenza and *Streptococcus pneumoniae.*	8. People with respiratory conditions are prone to respiratory infections and are encouraged to be immunized.	• Verbalizes need to stay away from crowds in flu season or people with colds. • Plans to discuss flu and pneumonia vaccines with physician to help prevent infection.

Nursing Diagnosis: Ineffective breathing pattern related to shortness of breath, mucus, bronchoconstriction, and airway irritants

Goal: Improvement in breathing pattern

1. Teach patient diaphragmatic pursed lip breathing.—"Smell a rose"; "Blow out a candle."	1. Helps patient prolong expiration time. With these techniques, patient will breathe more efficiently and effectively.	• Practices pursed lip and diaphragmatic breathing and uses them when short of breath and with activity.
2. Encourage alternating activity with rest periods. Let patient make some decisions (bath, shaving) about his care based on his tolerance level.	2. Pacing activities will conserve patient's lung capacity and permit him to perform activities without excessive distress.	• Shows signs of decreased respiratory effort by pacing activities.
3. Teach the use of an inspiratory muscle trainer.	3. Strengthens and conditions the respiratory muscles.	• Uses inspiratory muscle trainer for 10 minutes every day.

Nursing Diagnosis: Self-care deficits related to fatigue secondary to increased work of breathing and insufficient ventilation and oxygenation

Goal: Independence in self-care activities

1. Teach patient to coordinate diaphragmatic breathing with activity (*e.g.,* walking, bending).	1. This will allow him to be more active and to avoid excessive fatigue or dyspnea during activity.	• Uses controlled breathing while bathing, bending, and walking. • Paces activities of daily living to alternate with rest periods to reduce fatigue and dyspnea.

(continued)

Nursing Care Plan 26-2 *(Continued)*

Care of the Patient With Chronic Obstructive Pulmonary Disease

Nursing Interventions	Rationale	Expected Outcomes
2. Encourage patient to begin to bathe self, dress self, walk, and drink fluids. Discuss energy conservation measures. 3. Teach postural drainage if appropriate.	2. As condition resolves, patient will be able to do more but needs to be encouraged or may become dependent. 3. Encourages patient to become involved in own care. Builds self-esteem and prepares patient to manage at home.	• Describes energy conservation strategies. • Can perform the same self-care activities as before admission. • Performs postural drainage correctly.

Nursing Diagnosis: Activity intolerance due to fatigue, hypoxemia, and ineffective breathing patterns

Goal: Improvement in activity tolerance

1. Support patient in establishing a regular regimen of exercise using treadmill and exercycle, walking or other appropriate exercises, such as mall walking. a. Assess the patient's current level of functioning and develop exercise plan from there. b. Suggest consultation with a physical therapist to determine an exercise program specific to the patient's capability. Have portable oxygen units available in case oxygen is needed during exercise.	1. Muscles that are deconditioned consume more oxygen and place an additional burden on the lungs. Through regular, graded exercise, these muscle groups become more conditioned, and the patient can do more without getting as short of breath. Graded exercise breaks this cycle of debilitation.	• Performs activities with less shortness of breath. • Verbalizes need to exercise daily and demonstrates an exercise plan to be carried out at home. • Walks and gradually increases walking time and distance to improve physical condition.

Nursing Diagnosis: Ineffective individual coping related to less socialization, anxiety, depression, lower activity level, and the inability to work

Goal: Attainment of an optimal level of coping

1. Adopt a hopeful and encouraging attitude toward patient.	1. Giving the patient a sense of hope will give him something to work toward, rather than a defeated, hopeless attitude.	• Expresses interest in the future. • Participates in the discharge plan.
2. Encourage activity to level of symptom tolerance.	2. Activity reduces tension and decreases degree of dyspnea as patient becomes conditioned.	• Discusses activities or methods that can be performed to ease shortness of breath.
3. Teach relaxation technique or provide a relaxation tape for patient.	3. Relaxation reduces stress and anxiety and helps patient to cope with disability.	• Uses relaxation techniques appropriately.
4. Enroll patient in pulmonary rehabilitation program where available.	4. Pulmonary rehabilitation programs have been shown to promote a subjective improvement in a patient's status and self-esteem as well as increased exercise tolerance and decreased hospitalizations.	• Expresses interest in a pulmonary rehabilitation program.
5. Suggest vocational counseling to explore alternative avenues of employment (if applicable).	5. Work modification may need to be made and appropriate resources used to achieve this goal.	• Explores resources available for work modification.

Nursing Diagnosis: Potential for noncompliance with recommended care procedures at home

Goal: Compliance with therapeutic program and home care

1. Help patient accept realistic short- and long-term goals.	1. Patient needs to see that there is a method and plan for his care in which	• Understands his disease and what affects his condition.

(continued)

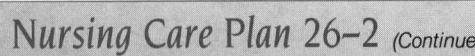

Nursing Care Plan 26–2 *(Continued)*

Care of the Patient With Chronic Obstructive Pulmonary Disease

Nursing Interventions	Rationale	Expected Outcomes
a. Teach the patient about his disease and care.	he plays a major role. He needs to know what to expect. Teaching him about his condition is one of the most important aspects of his care; it will prepare him to live and cope with his condition and improve his quality of life.	• Verbalizes that he must preserve existing lung function by adhering to his program.
2. Discuss the need to stop smoking. Provide information about resource groups. (*e.g.*, Smoke Enders, American Cancer Society).	2. Cigarette smoking causes definite damage to the lung and diminishes the lungs' protective mechanisms. Air flow is obstructed and lung capacity is reduced.	• Stops smoking or enrolls in a smoking cessation program.

Clinical Manifestations.   The three common symptoms of asthma are cough, dyspnea, and wheezing. It is interesting to note that cough may be the only symptom in some patients with asthma. Asthma attacks frequently occur at night. The causes are not completely understood, but may be related to circadian variations, which influence airway receptor thresholds.

The asthmatic attack starts suddenly with coughing and a sensation of tightness in the chest. Then slow, laborious, wheezy breathing begins. Expiration is always much more strenuous and prolonged than inspiration, which forces the patient to sit upright and use every accessory muscle of respiration. Obstructed air flow creates the sensation of dyspnea. The cough at first is tight and dry, but it soon becomes more forceful; a distinctive sputum of thin mucus containing small, round, gelatinous masses is coughed up with much difficulty. Later signs include cyanosis secondary to severe hypoxia, and symptoms of carbon dioxide retention, including sweating, tachycardia, and a widened pulse pressure. The attack may last from 30 minutes to several hours. Under certain circumstances, the attack may subside spontaneously, but this should not be assumed. Such attacks are rarely fatal. Occasionally, however, "status asthmaticus" occurs, in which therapeutic measures fail and the patient has repeated attacks or continuous asthma. This condition is life threatening (see p. 584).

Related Reactions.   Allergic reactions related to asthma include eczema (present at some time during life in 75% of patients with asthma), urticaria, and angioneurotic edema (present in 50% of patients). Asthmatic attacks may occur periodically after exposure to a specific allergen, occupational or environmental exposure, some pharmacologic agents, physical exertion, and emotional excitement.

Diagnostic Evaluation.   There is no single test that will confirm a diagnosis of asthma. A complete history, including a family, environmental, and occupational history may disclose factors or substances that precipitate asthma attacks. A positive wheal and flare reaction skin test identifies specific allergens.

A positive family history frequently is associated with allergic asthma. Environmental factors, including seasonal changes, high pollen counts, and mold also are associated with allergic asthma. Climate changes, particularly cold air and air pollution are primarily associated with nonallergic asthma. There are a variety of occupation-related chemicals and compounds that have been associated with the development of asthma, including metal salts, wood and vegetable dust, pharmacologic agents (aspirin, antibiotics, piperazine and cimetidine), industrial chemicals and plastics, biologic enzymes, including laundry detergents, animal and insect dusts, sera, and secretions.

During acute episodes, a chest radiograph may show hyperinflation and a flattened diaphragm. Sputum and blood studies may disclose eosinophilia. There is an elevation in serum levels of IgE in allergic asthma.

Sputum may be clear and foamy (allergic) or thick and white (nonallergic) and stringy (nonallergic).

Arterial blood gases reveal hypoxia during acute attacks. Initially, hypocapnia and respiratory alkalosis and low carbon dioxide partial pressure (PCO_2) are present. As the condition worsens and the patient becomes more fatigued, the PCO_2 may rise. A normal PCO_2 may be a signal of impending respiratory failure. Because PCO_2 is 20 times more diffusible than oxygen, it is rare for PCO_2 to be normal or elevated in the tachypneic patient.

Pulmonary function studies are usually normal between attacks. During an acute attack, there is an increase in the total lung capacity (TLC) and functional residual volume (FRV) secondary to air trapping. The forced expiratory volume (FEV), and forced vital capacity (FVC) are markedly decreased.

An alternate method of testing in a pulmonary function laboratory is the bedside portable spirometer, which can measure volumes, capacities, and flow rate.

Drug Therapy.   There are five categories of drugs used in the treatment of asthma:

• Beta agonists
• Methylxanthines
• Anticholinergics
• Corticosteroids
• Mast cell inhibitors

Beta Agonists.   The beta agonists (beta-adrenergic agents) are the initial drugs used in the treatment of asthma because they dilate bronchial smooth muscles. Adrenergic agents also increase ciliary movements, decrease the chemical mediators of anaphylaxis and can potentiate the bronchodilating effects of corticosteroids. The most commonly used adrenergic agents include epinephrine, albuterol, metaproterenol, isoproterenol and isoetharine, and terbutaline. They usually are administered parenterally or by inhalation. The inhalation route is the route of choice because of its bronchial selectivity and fewer side effects.

Methylxanthines.   Methylxanthines, such as aminophylline and theophylline, are used because of their bronchodilating effects. They relax bronchial smooth muscle, increase movement of mucus in the airways, and potentiate contraction of the diaphragm. Aminophylline is administered intravenously. Theophylline is given orally. Methylxanthines are not used in acute attacks because they are slower in onset than beta agonists. There are several factors that may alter the metabolism of methylxanthines, particularly theophylline, including cigarette smoking, heart failure, chronic liver disease, oral contraceptives, erythromycin, and cimetidine. Care should be taken when administering these medications intravenously. If given too rapidly, tachycardia or cardiac dysrhythmias may result.

Anticholinergics.   Anticholinergics, such as atropine, have not historically been used in the treatment of asthma routinely because of their systemic side effects, such as dryness of the mouth, blurred vision, urinary hesitancy, palpitations, and flushing. Their bronchodilator effects are similar to those of beta agonists. Newer quaternary ammonium derivatives, such as atropine methylnitrate and ipratropium bromide, have demonstrated excellent bronchodilator effects with minimal systemic side effects. These agents are given by inhalation. Anticholinergics may be particularly beneficial to asthmatics, who are not candidates for beta agonists and methylxanthines because of underlying cardiac disease.

Corticosteroids.   Corticosteroids are important in the treatment of asthma. These may be administered intravenously (hydrocortisone), orally (prednisone, prednisolone), or by inhalation (beclomethasone, dexamethasone). The mechanism of action is not certain; however, they are thought to reduce inflammation and reduce bronchoconstriction. Corticosteroids (*not* by inhalation) may be administered for an acute asthmatic attack that does not respond to bronchodilator therapy. Corticosteroids have proven effective in the treatment of asthma and COPD. Prolonged use of corticosteroids can result in the development of serious side effects, including peptic ulcers, osteoporosis, adrenal suppression, steroid myopathy, and cataracts.

Inhaled corticosteroids may be effective in the treatment of patients with steroid-dependent asthma. A major advantage of this mode of administration is reduction in systemic effects of corticosteroids. Throat irritation, coughing, dry mouth, hoarseness, and fungal infection of the mouth and pharynx may occur. Therefore, the patient is instructed to rinse his mouth and gargle immediately after using inhaled corticosteroids to decrease the incidence of fungal infection. He is instructed to report the incidence of redness or the presence of white patches in the mouth. Switching from systemic to inhaled corticosteroids puts the patient at risk for adrenal insufficiency. Therefore, the process must be accomplished gradually and under close supervision.

See Chapter 40 for detailed discussion of the effects of corticosteroids.

Mast Cell Inhibitors.   Cromolyn sodium, a mast cell inhibitor, is an integral part of the treatment of asthma. It is administered by inhalation. It prevents the release of chemical mediators of anaphylaxis, thereby resulting in bronchodilation and a decrease in airway inflammation. Cromolyn sodium is most beneficial between attacks or while the asthma is in remission. It may result in the reduction of use of other medications and overall improvement in symptoms.

Prevention.   In every patient with recurrent asthma, evaluation is conducted to identify foreign proteins that precipitate the attacks. If attacks occur chiefly at night, when the patient is in bed, skin tests are conducted with material from the mattress and pillows. If the test results are positive, then a mattress and pillow made from other materials are substituted. If attacks appear to be associated with the presence of a particular species of animal, such as a horse or a cat, similar skin tests are made with an antigen composed of hair or skin scrapings from the animal concerned. A seasonal incidence of attacks in a patient suggests an airborne allergen as the chief causative agent. In such cases, therapy may be attempted with pollen extracts. Air conditioning offers possibilities in the prevention of attacks, depending on the extent to which the patient can restrict his life to air-conditioned rooms during the pollen season. A complete change of climatic environment to a locality with different flora during that period is the most satisfactory solution, when feasible. The examiner should search for foci of bacterial infection (*e.g.*, of chronically infected sinuses or teeth) because their eradication may be strikingly beneficial in certain patients.

Exercise-induced asthma (EIA) can be prevented by inspiring air at 37°C (body temperature) and 100% relative humidity. Covering the nose and mouth with a mask necessitates rebreathing expired air that has been warmed and moistened by its passage through the respiratory tract. A simple face mask is an inexpensive, practical method for asthmatic ball players, runners, and skiers.

Associated Psychotherapeutic Modalities.   It is important to remember that asthmatic attacks, once started, may indicate that the patient will be susceptible to repeated attacks. In some patients, attacks may be induced by suggestion alone. Good general physical and mental health is most important.

Complications of Asthma.   The acute asthmatic attack per se is rarely life-threatening; however, death may occur as a result of respiratory failure, which is possible if sedatives are administered too freely.

Complications of asthma include a ruptured bleb, causing pneumothorax; mediastinal or subcutaneous emphysema; chronic and recurrent acute bronchitis; bronchiectasis; pulmonary hypertension; and hypertrophy of the right side of the heart with right-sided heart failure (pulmonary heart disease). Chronic hypoxia due to these complications may lead to symptoms and personality changes.

Airway obstruction, particularly during acute episodes, often results in hypoxemia, requiring the administration of oxygen and the monitoring of arterial blood gases. The administration of fluids is also important because persons with asthma are frequently dehydrated from diaphoresis and insensible fluid loss with hyperventilation.

Breathing exercises along with postural drainage and aerosol therapy are prescribed to aid in removing retained secretions. IPPB is not advocated for acute asthma attacks. If the patient's condition worsens to the point of acute respiratory failure, intubation and mechanical ventilation will be necessary.

Status Asthmaticus

Status asthmaticus is severe asthma that is unresponsive to conventional therapy and lasts longer than 24 hours. A vicious self-perpetuating cycle may occur as a result of infection, anxiety, overuse of tranquilizers, nebulizer abuse, dehydration, increased adrenergic block, and nonspecific irritants. An acute episode may be precipitated by hypersensitivity to aspirin.

Pathophysiology. A combination of factors, including constriction of the bronchiolar smooth muscle, swelling of bronchial mucosa, and thickened (inspissated) secretions, contribute to one pathologic problem—a decrease in the diameter of the bronchi. Another problem is the ventilation–perfusion abnormality that results from hypoxemia and respiratory acidosis or alkalosis.

There is a reduced PaO_2 and an initial respiratory alkalosis with a decreased $PaCO_2$ and an increased pH. As the severity of status asthmaticus increases, the $PaCO_2$ increases and the pH falls, reflecting respiratory acidosis.

Clinical Manifestations. The clinical manifestations are the same as those seen in severe asthma. There is no correlation between the severity of the attack and the amount of wheezes. With greater obstruction, wheezing may disappear, which is frequently a sign of impending respiratory failure.

Diagnostic Evaluation. Pulmonary function studies are the most accurate measurement of acute airway obstruction. The most frequent measurements are the FEV_1 or the peak expiratory flow rate (PEFR).

Arterial blood gases are useful if the patient is unable to perform pulmonary function maneuvers because of severe obstruction, fatigue, of if the patient does not respond to treatment. Respiratory alkalosis (low CO_2) is the most common finding in asthmatic patients. A rising PCO_2 (to normal levels or levels indicating respiratory acidosis) frequently is a danger signal of impending respiratory failure

Management. Asthmatic patients with an FEV of less than 1 liter or a PEFR of less than 100 to 125 L/min usually require hospitalization. Another indicator is worsening blood gases (respiratory acidosis), which may indicate that the patient is tiring and will require mechanical ventilation.

In the emergency room setting, the patient is treated initially with beta agonists, such as metaproterenol, terbutaline, and albuterol and glucocorticoids. The patient may also require *supplemental oxygen and intravenous fluids for hydration.*

To treat dyspnea, cyanosis, and hypoxemia, oxygen therapy is initiated on low-flow humidified oxygen, by either Venturi mask or nasal catheter. The amount is determined after blood gas determinations. The PaO_2 is maintained between 65 and 85 mm Hg (8.64 to 11.30 kPa^a). Sedatives are contraindicated. If there is no response to repeated treatments, the patient will require hospitalization. Most patients do not require mechanical ventilation. It is used most often when the patient is admitted to the emergency room in respiratory failure or in patients who tire and whose condition does not respond to initial treatment.

Nursing Interventions. Signs of dehydration are assessed by checking skin turgor. Fluid intake is essential to combat dehydration, to loosen secretions, and to facilitate expectoration. Intravenous fluids are administered as prescribed, up to 3000 to 4000 ml/day, unless contraindicated.

Constant monitoring of the patient by the nurse is important for the first 12 to 24 hours, or until status asthmaticus is halted. When it is necessary to question the patient, the nurse should try to phrase the questions so that he can answer in only one or two words. The room should be quiet and free of respiratory irritants, including flowers, cigarette smoke, perfumes, or odors of cleaning agents. The patient should have a nonallergenic pillow.

Patient Education and Home Health Care. Patient education is an important part of post-hospital care if recurrences are to be kept to a minimum. Patients are instructed as to which signs and symptoms require contact with their physician; for example, awakening during the night with an acute attack, incomplete relief from the inhaler, or respiratory infection. Bronchodilators may be required on an around-the-clock basis. Certain medications can be increased when asthmatic attacks occur. Adequate hydration must be maintained at home to keep secretions from thickening. The patient needs to recognize that infection is to be avoided, because it can trigger an attack.

Some patients can be instructed in self-care protocols designed with goals of (1) aborting severe attacks and (2) giving the patient with asthma a measure of independence. Included in this regimen is the administration of theophylline with a long-acting oral preparation. This is regulated within the narrow therapeutic ratio with careful instructions on the hazards of overuse. The patient gets a hand-held metered-dose inhaler that uses a β_2-selective adrenergic, such as metaproterenol or albuterol. This also is used within prescribed limitations. Should these bronchodilators fail, the patient is further instructed on beginning a corticosteroid drug (short, high dose), usually prednisone, at a prescribed dosage. He notifies the physician or nurse clinician of his progress.

Nursing Care Plan 26–2 provides a detailed review of the care of the patient with COPD (see pp. 579–582).

Gerontologic Considerations

Asthma may occur as a new problem in the elderly patient. Heart disease and other changes may complicate management of asthma in the elderly because of the cardiovascular effects of medications usually used to treat asthma.

In summary, COPD is a broad classification for a group of disorders, including chronic bronchitis, bronchiectasis, emphysema, and asthma. Reduced or obstructed airflow is common in each of these conditions.

COPD is a major cause of death and disability in this country. There are many preventable environmental factors associated with the development of COPD, including cigarette smoking, air pollution, and occupational exposure. COPD has been genetically linked to patients with little or no environmental exposure. The clinical course of the COPD depends on which disorder or combination of disorders is present. COPD is a slowly progressive disease that is associated with exacerbations and remissions. Education and early intervention during periods of exacerbations are critical in the control of the disease.

Pulmonary Hypertension

Pulmonary hypertension is a condition that is not clinically evident until late in its disease progression. Pulmonary hypertension exists when the systolic pulmonary arterial pressure exceeds 30 mm Hg and the mean pulmonary artery pressure is above 15 mm Hg. These pressures, however, cannot be measured indirectly as can systemic blood pressure, but must be measured during right-sided heart catheterization. In the absence of these measurements, clinical recognition becomes the only indicator for the presence of pulmonary hypertension.

There are two forms of pulmonary hypertension: primary (or idiopathic) and secondary. *Primary pulmonary hypertension* is an uncommon disease whose diagnosis is made by exclusion. The exact cause is unknown. The clinical presentation of pulmonary hypertension exists with no evidence of pulmonary and cardiac disease or pulmonary embolism. It occurs most often in women between 20 and 40 years of age and is usually fatal within 5 years of diagnosis.

Secondary pulmonary hypertension is more common and results from existing cardiac or pulmonary disease. Its prognosis depends on the severity of the underlying disorder and the changes in the pulmonary vascular bed. The most common cause of pulmonary hypertension is pulmonary artery constriction due to hypoxia from COPD (Chart 26–1).

Pathophysiology. Normally, the pulmonary vascular bed can handle the blood volume delivered by the right ventricle. It has a low resistance to blood flow and compensates for increased blood volume by dilation of unused vessels in the pulmonary circulation. If the pulmonary vascular bed is destroyed or obstructed, however, as in pulmonary hypertension, the ability to handle whatever flow or volume of blood it receives is lost and the increased blood flow then increases the pulmonary arterial pressures. As the pulmonary arterial pressure increases, the pulmonary vascular resistance also increases. Both pulmonary artery constriction (as in hypoxia or hypercapnia) and a reduction of the pulmonary vascular bed (which occurs with pulmonary emboli) result in an increase in pulmonary vascular resistance and pressure. This increased work load affects right ventricular function. The myocardium ultimately is unable to meet the increasing demands imposed on it, leading to right ventricular hypertrophy (dilatation) and failure (cor pulmonale).

Clinical Manifestations. Dyspnea is the main symptom of pulmonary hypertension associated at first with exertion and eventually at rest. Substernal chest pain is also common, affecting 25% to 50% of patients. Other signs and symptoms include weakness, fatigability, syncope, signs of right-sided heart failure (peripheral edema, ascites, distended neck veins, liver engorgement, crackles, heart murmur), electrocardiographic changes showing right ventricular hypertrophy, right axis deviation, tall peaked P waves in inferior leads, and decreased PaO_2 (hypoxemia).

Diagnostic Evaluation. A complete diagnostic evaluation includes a history, physical examination, chest x-ray, electrocardiogram (ECG), cardiac catheterization, perfusion lung scan and pulmonary function studies, and a lung biopsy. Cardiac catheterization of the right side of the heart will disclose elevated pulmonary arterial pressures. Pulmonary angiography will detect defects in pulmonary vasculature, such as pulmonary emboli. Pulmonary function studies will show an increased residual volume and total lung capacity and a decreased FEV_1 in obstructive pulmonary diseases and a decreased

---

Chart 26–1
Causes of Pulmonary Hypertension

Primary or Idiopathic

Altered immune mechanisms
Silent pulmonary emboli
Raynaud's phenomenon
Oral contraceptives
Sickle cell disease
Collagen diseases

Secondary

Pulmonary Vasoconstriction Due to Hypoxia
Chronic obstructive pulmonary disease
Kyphoscoliosis
Obesity
Smoke inhalation
High altitude
Neuromuscular disorders
Diffuse interstitial pneumonia

Reduction of the Pulmonary Vascular Bed (Must Impair 50% to 75% of the Vascular Bed)
Pulmonary emboli
Vasculitis
Widespread interstitial lung disease (sarcoidosis, systemic sclerosis)
Tumor emboli

Primary Cardiac Disease

Congenital (patent ductus arteriosus, atrial septal defect, ventricular septal defect)
Acquired (rheumatic valvular disease, mitral stenosis, myxoma, left ventricular failure)

vital capacity and total lung capacity in restrictive lung diseases. A lung biopsy will confirm the diagnosis of pulmonary hypertension.

Management.   The objective of treatment is to manage the underlying cardiac or pulmonary condition. Because hypoxia is the most common cause of pulmonary vasoconstriction leading to increased pulmonary vascular resistance and pulmonary hypertension, continuous oxygen therapy is the major component of management. In acute conditions, appropriate oxygen therapy (see Chap. 25, Table 25–1) will reverse the vasoconstriction and reduce the pulmonary hypertension in a relatively short time. In more chronic, progressive conditions, continuous oxygen therapy may be necessary to slow the progression of the disease. In the presence of cor pulmonale, treatment should include fluid restriction, cardiac glycosides such as digitalis to improve cardiac function, rest, and diuretics to decrease fluid accumulation. In primary pulmonary hypertension, vasodilators have been administered with variable success. Anticoagulants, such as coumadin, have been given to patients because of chronic pulmonary emboli. Heart–lung transplant has been successful in a number of patients with primary hypertension who have not been responsive to other therapies.

Nursing Interventions.   The major nursing goals are to identify those patients who are at high risk of developing pulmonary hypertension (*i.e.*, those with COPD, pulmonary emboli, congenital heart disease, and mitral valve disease); to be alert for signs and symptoms; and to administer oxygen therapy appropriately.

Pulmonary Heart Disease (Cor Pulmonale)

Cor pulmonale is a condition in which the right ventricle enlarges (with or without failure) as a result of diseases that affect the structure or function of the lung or its vasculature. Any disease that affects the lungs and has associated hypoxemia may result in cor pulmonale. The most frequent cause is COPD in which changes in the airway and retained secretions reduce alveolar ventilation. Other causes are conditions that restrict or compromise ventilatory function, leading to hypoxia or acidosis (deformities of the thoracic cage, massive obesity) or conditions that reduce the pulmonary vascular bed (primary idiopathic pulmonary arterial hypertension, pulmonary embolus). Certain disorders of the nervous system, respiratory muscles, chest wall, and pulmonary arterial tree may be responsible for cor pulmonale.

Pathophysiology.   Pulmonary disease can produce a chain of events that will in time produce hypertrophy and failure of the right ventricle. Any condition that deprives the lungs of oxygen can cause hypoxemia (decreased arterial oxygen tension) and hypercapnia (increased carbon dioxide in the blood), resulting in ventilatory insufficiency. Hypoxia and hypercapnia cause pulmonary arterial vasoconstriction. There may be associated reduction of the pulmonary vascular bed, as in emphysema or pulmonary emboli. The result is increased resistance in the pulmonary circuit, with a subsequent rise in pulmonary blood pressure (pulmonary hypertension). Pulmonary arterial mean pressures of 45 mm Hg or more may occur in cor pulmonale. Right ventricular hypertrophy may result and be followed by right ventricular failure. In short, cor pulmonale results from pulmonary hypertension that causes the right side of the heart to enlarge because of the increased work required to pump blood against high resistance through the pulmonary vascular system.

Clinical Manifestations.   Usually, the symptoms of cor pulmonale are those of underlying lung disease. COPD produces shortness of breath and cough. As the right ventricle fails, the patient develops edema of the feet and legs, distended neck veins, an enlarged, palpable liver, pleural effusion, ascites, and a heart murmur. Headache, confusion, and somnolence may be manifested as a result of carbon dioxide narcosis.

Management.   The objectives of treatment are to improve the patient's ventilation and to treat both the underlying lung disease and the manifestations of heart disease. In COPD the airways have to be dilated to improve gas exchange. With improved oxygen transport, the reactive pulmonary hypertension that leads to cor pulmonale is relieved. In short, the lung must be treated first. Oxygen is given to reduce pulmonary arterial pressure and pulmonary vascular resistance. Better survival and greater reduction in pulmonary vascular resistance have been reported with continuous (24 hr/day) oxygen therapy for patients with severe hypoxia. Substantial patient improvement may require 4 to 6 weeks of oxygen therapy. This is usually carried out at home. Assessment of arterial blood gases is necessary to determine adequacy of alveolar ventilation and to monitor the effectiveness of oxygen therapy.

Additional measures include bronchial hygiene and the administration of bronchodilators and chest physical therapy to improve ventilation. If the patient is in respiratory failure, endotracheal intubation and mechanical ventilation may be necessary. If the patient is in heart failure, the improvement of hypoxemia and hypercapnia will be necessary to improve cardiac action and output. In addition, he is placed on bed rest, and sodium restriction and diuretic therapy are employed judiciously to reduce peripheral edema (to lower pulmonary arterial pressure through a decrease in total blood volume) and the circulatory load on the right side of the heart. Digitalis may be given if the patient has coincident left ventricular failure, a supraventricular dysrhythmia, or right ventricular failure that does not respond to other therapy to relieve pulmonary hypertension. It is administered with extreme caution, because pulmonary heart disease appears to enhance susceptibility to digitalis toxicity.

Electrocardiographic monitoring is performed when necessary, as there is a high incidence of dysrhythmias in these patients. Respiratory infection must be treated, as it commonly precipitates pulmonary heart disease. The patient's prognosis depends on whether the hypertensive process is reversible. (The management of the patient with respiratory failure is discussed on p. 599.)

Patient Education and Home Health Care.   Because management of pulmonary heart disease is related to treating the underlying cause, it is often a long-term process. Consequently, most of the care and monitoring is performed in the home. The patient is advised to avoid those things that irritate the airway if he has COPD. If continuous oxygen is administered, the patient and his family are instructed in its use. Most important, the patient is urged to stop smoking. Nutrition counseling is necessary if the patient is on a sodium-restricted diet or is taking diuretics. The family is counseled that restlessness, depression, irritability, or atypical behavior may be encountered with hypoxemia or hypercapnia and should decrease as the arterial blood gas values improve.

Pulmonary Embolism

Pulmonary embolism refers to the obstruction of one or more pulmonary arteries by a thrombus (or thrombi) that originates somewhere in the venous system or in the right side of the heart, becomes dislodged, and is carried to the lung. It is estimated that over one half million patients develop pulmonary emboli, resulting in over 50,000 deaths each year. Pulmonary embolism is a common disorder and often is associated with advanced age, postoperative states, and prolonged immobility. It may occur in an apparently healthy person. Persons who are at risk of developing a pulmonary embolus are identified in Chart 26–2.

Most thrombi originate in the deep veins of the legs. Other sites include the pelvic veins and the right atrium of the heart. Stasis, or slowing of blood flow, secondary to damage to the blood vessel wall (particularly the endothelial lining) and changes in the blood coagulation mechanism, are factors favoring formation of venous thrombi.

Pathophysiology. After a complete or partial embolic obstruction of the pulmonary arteries by a thrombus, there is an increase in alveolar dead space because the area, although continuing to be ventilated, receives little or no blood flow. In addition, a number of vasoactive and bronchoconstrictive substances are released from the clot. These substances compound the ventilation–perfusion imbalance, causing venous admixture and shunting.

The hemodynamic consequences are increased pulmonary vascular resistance due to reduction in the size of the pulmonary vascular bed, resulting in an increase in pulmonary arterial pressure and, in turn, an increase in right ventricular work to maintain pulmonary blood flow. When the work requirements of the right ventricle exceed its capacity, right ventricular failure occurs. When this occurs, there is a decrease in cardiac output followed by a decrease in systemic blood pressure and the development of shock.

Clinical Manifestations. The symptoms of pulmonary embolism depend on the size of the thrombus and the area of the pulmonary artery occlusion. Chest pain is the most common symptom of a pulmonary embolism. It is usually sudden in onset and pleuritic in nature. It occasionally can be substernal and may mimic angina pectoris. Dyspnea is the second most common symptom, followed by tachypnea (respiratory rate greater than 16). Other symptoms include fever, tachycardia, apprehension, cough, diaphoresis, hemoptysis, and syncope.

A massive embolism occluding the bifurcation of the pulmonary artery can produce pronounced dyspnea, sudden substernal pain, rapid and weak pulse, shock, syncope, and sudden death.

Multiple small emboli can lodge in the terminal pulmonary arterioles, producing multiple small infarctions of the lungs. The clinical picture may simulate that of bronchopneumonia

---

Chart 26–2
Pulmonary Embolism: Risk Factors

The following events and conditions predispose to thrombophlebitis and pulmonary embolism.

Venous Stasis (slowing of blood flow in veins)

Prolonged immobilization (especially postoperative)
Prolonged periods of sitting/traveling
Varicose veins

Hypercoagulability (due to release of tissue thromboplastin after injury/surgery)

Injury
Tumor (pancreatic, GI, GU, breast, lung)
Increased platelet count (polycythemia, splenectomy)

Venous Endothelial Disease

Thrombophlebitis
Vascular disease
Foreign bodies (IV/central venous catheters)

Certain Disease States (combination of stasis, coagulation alterations, and venous injury)

Heart disease (especially congestive heart failure)
Trauma (especially fracture of hip, pelvis, spine, lower extremities)
Postoperative state/postpartum period
Diabetes mellitus
Chronic obstructive pulmonary disease
Previous pulmonary embolism

Other Predisposing Conditions

Advanced age
Obesity
Pregnancy
Oral contraceptive use
History of previous thrombophlebitis, pulmonary embolism
Constrictive clothing

or heart failure. In some instances, the disease presents in an atypical fashion with few signs and symptoms, whereas in other instances, it mimics various cardiopulmonary disorders.

Diagnostic Evaluation.   Because the clinical presentation of pulmonary embolism is not specific, a diagnostic workup is performed to rule out other diseases. Deep vein thrombosis is closely associated with the development of pulmonary embolism.

The diagnostic workup includes a chest radiograph, electrocardiogram, radiofibrinogen leg scanning, impedance plethysmography, arterial blood gases, ventilation–perfusion scan, and pulmonary angiography.

The chest radiograph is usually normal but may show pneumoconstriction, elevation of the diaphragm on the affected side, or great dilation of the pulmonary artery. The ECG usually shows tachycardia and may show right axis deviation or right ventricular strain. Radiofibrinogen leg scanning and impedance plethysmography are performed to determine the presence of deep vein thrombosis. Test results confirm or exclude the diagnosis of pulmonary embolism. Arterial blood gases will show hypoxemia and hypocapnia. A perfusion lung scan will indicate areas of diminished or absent blood flow. A ventilation scan will show whether there is also a perfusion abnormality present. If there is a ventilation–perfusion (V/Q) mismatch, there is a high probability of a pulmonary embolism. If lung scanning is not definitive, pulmonary angiography will confirm the diagnosis of pulmonary emboli.

Preventive Measures.   The most effective approach in preventing pulmonary embolism is to prevent deep vein thrombosis. Two strategies are recommended:

1. Anticoagulant therapy
2. Intermittent pneumatic leg compression devices

The American Heart Association recommends that patients who are over 40 and hemostatically competent, and who are undergoing major elective abdominothoracic surgery, be given low doses of heparin to diminish postoperative deep vein thrombus and pulmonary embolism. The heparin is administered subcutaneously 2 hours before surgery and continued every 8 to 12 hours until the patient is discharged. Low-dose heparin is thought to enhance the activity of antithrombin III, a major plasma inhibitor of clotting factor X. (This regimen is not recommended for patients who are experiencing an active thrombotic process or those undergoing major orthopedic surgery, open prostatectomy, or operations on the eye or brain.)

Coumadin also may be used prophylactically preoperatively to prevent the development of thromboembolism. Intermittent pneumatic leg compression devices are very useful in prevention of thromboembolism. The device inflates a bag that mechanically compresses the leg from the calf to the thigh, thereby improving venous return. It may be applied preoperatively and continued until the patient is ambulatory. The device is particularly useful for patients who are not candidates for anticoagulant therapy.

Emergency Interventions.   Massive pulmonary embolism is a true medical emergency; the patient's condition tends to deteriorate rapidly. The immediate objective of treatment is to stabilize the cardiorespiratory system. The majority of patients who die of massive pulmonary embolism do so in the *first 2 hours* after the embolic event. Emergency management consists of the following:

- Nasal oxygen is administered immediately to relieve hypoxemia, respiratory distress, and cyanosis.
- An infusion is started to establish an intravenous route for drugs or fluids that will be needed.
- Pulmonary angiography, hemodynamic measurements, arterial blood gas determinations, and perfusion lung scans are performed. A sudden rise in pulmonary resistance increases the work of the right ventricle, which can cause acute right-sided heart failure with cardiogenic shock.
- If the patient has suffered massive embolism and is hypotensive, an indwelling urethral catheter is inserted to monitor urinary output.
- Hypotension is treated by a slow infusion of isoproterenol (has a dilating effect on pulmonary vessels and bronchi) or dopamine.
- The ECG is monitored continuously for right ventricular failure, which may have a rapid onset.
- Sodium bicarbonate may be administered to correct metabolic acidosis. Digitalis glycosides, intravenous diuretics, and antidysrhythmic agents are administered when appropriate.
- Blood is drawn for serum electrolytes, blood urea nitrogen, complete blood count, and hematocrit.
- If clinical assessment and arterial blood gases indicate the need, the patient is placed on a volume-controlled ventilator.
- Small doses of intravenous morphine are given to relieve the patient's anxiety, to alleviate chest discomfort, to help him tolerate the endotracheal tube, and to ease his adaptation to the mechanical ventilator.

Management.   The treatment of pulmonary embolism may include a variety of modalities:

1. Anticoagulation therapy
2. Thrombolytic therapy
3. Surgical intervention

Anticoagulation Therapy.   Anticoagulant therapy (heparin, warfarin sodium) has traditionally been the primary method for management of acute deep vein thrombosis and pulmonary embolism.

Heparin is used to prevent recurrence of emboli but has no effect on emboli that are already present. It is administered as a loading dose followed by continuous infusion. The goal is to keep the partial thromboplastin time (PTT) 1.5 to 2 times normal. Heparin is administered for 7 to 10 days. Coumadin administration is started during heparin therapy and continued for 3 months. The prothrombin time (PT) is maintained at 1.5 times normal. Anticoagulation therapy is contraindicated in patients who are at risk for bleeding (GI, postoperative, or postpartum bleeding).

Thrombolytic Therapy.   Thrombolytic therapy (urokinase, streptokinase) also may be used in treatment of pulmonary embolism, particularly in patients who are severely compromised.

Thrombolytic therapy results in a more rapid resolution of the thrombi or emboli. It restores more normal hemodynamic functioning of the pulmonary circulation, resulting in a reduction of pulmonary hypertension. Bleeding, however, is a significant side effect. Consequently, thrombolytic agents are advocated only for patients with thrombi affecting the popliteal vein or deep veins of the thigh and pelvis, and for patients with massive pulmonary emboli affecting a significant area of blood flow to the lung.

Before the initiation of thrombolytic therapy, thrombin time (TT), activated partial thromboplastin time (APTT), PT, hematocrit values, and platelet counts are obtained. During therapy all but absolutely essential invasive procedures are avoided, with the exception of careful venipuncture with a 22- or 23-gauge needle for therapeutic monitoring. If necessary, fresh whole blood, packed red cells, cryoprecipitate, or frozen plasma is given to replace blood loss and reverse the bleeding tendency.

After completion of the thrombolytic infusion (which varies in duration according to the agent used and the condition being treated), the patient is placed on anticoagulants.

Other measures are initiated to support the patient's respiratory and vascular status. Oxygen therapy is administered to correct the hypoxia and to relieve the pulmonary vascular vasoconstriction and reduce the pulmonary hypertension. Venous stasis is reduced by use of elastic stockings, which compress the superficial venous system and increase the velocity of deep venous blood by redirecting the blood through the deep veins. Venous stasis is then reduced. Simple leg elevation (above the level of the heart) with flexion at the knees also increases venous flow, however. Some authorities believe elastic stockings are unnecessary if the patient's legs are elevated.

Surgical Intervention. If the patient has persistent hypotension, shock, and respiratory distress; if pulmonary artery pressure is greatly elevated; and if angiograms show obstruction of a large part of the pulmonary vasculature, embolectomy may be indicated. This requires a thoracotomy with cardiopulmonary bypass technique.

Another surgical technique used when pulmonary emboli recur, despite adequate medical therapy (or if the patient is intolerant of anticoagulant therapy), is an interruption of the inferior vena cava. This method prevents dislodged thrombi from being swept into the lungs while at the same time allowing adequate blood flow. This can be performed by total ligation or the use of Teflon clips applied to the vena cava to divide the caval lumen into small channels without occluding caval blood flow. The use of transvenous devices that occlude or filter the blood through the inferior vena cava is a fairly safe procedure for the prevention of recurrent pulmonary embolism. One such technique is the insertion of a filter (Greenfield filter) through a cervical incision in the internal jugular vein or common femoral vein (Fig. 26-3). This filter is advanced through the superior vena cava into the inferior vena cava, where it is brought into an open position. The perforated umbrella permits the passage of blood but prevents the passage of large thrombi.

Transvenous catheter embolectomy is a technique in which a vacuum-cupped catheter is introduced transvenously into the affected pulmonary artery. Suction is applied to the end of the embolus, and the embolus is aspirated into the cup. The surgeon maintains suction to hold the embolus within the cup, and the entire catheter is withdrawn through the right side of the heart and out the femoral venotomy. An inferior caval filter often is inserted at the same time to protect against a recurrence.

Nursing Assessment

The nurse examines each susceptible patient for a positive Homans' sign, which may or may not indicate impending thrombosis of the leg veins (see Chap. 31). Testing proceeds as follows:

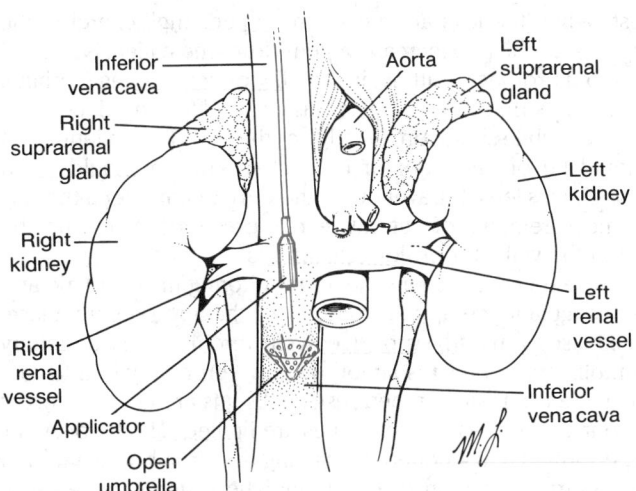

Figure 26-3. Insertion of umbrella filter in inferior vena cava to prevent pulmonary embolism. Filter (compressed within an applicator catheter) is inserted through an incision in the right internal jugular vein. The applicator is withdrawn when the filter fixes itself to the wall of the inferior vena cava after ejection from the applicator.

1. Position the patient on his back.
2. Lift the leg and dorsiflex the foot.
3. Note if there is pain in the calf during this maneuver (positive Homans' sign), which may indicate deep venous thrombosis.
4. Conduct another clinical assessment by tapping on the anterior tibial crest to see if this elicits pain.
5. Apply a blood pressure cuff around the patient's calf and inflate it. Pain on inflation of the cuff (80 to 100 mm Hg) is significant, as is tenderness along the course of a vein, pain in the calf or foot area, or edema in the ankle or calf area. It is best to compare both extremities.
6. Observe for swelling and palpable veins. Clinical evidence of phlebitis in one leg does not necessarily indicate that this is the site of the embolus; the other leg, even though normal on examination, may be the site.

The nurse's key role is to try to prevent the occurrence of pulmonary embolism in all patients and to identify those who are at high risk (see Chart 26-2). The nurse must have a high degree of suspicion for pulmonary embolism in any patient, but particularly those with conditions predisposing to slowing of venous return. Such conditions include trauma to the pelvis (especially surgical trauma) and lower extremities (especially hip fractures), obesity, history of thromboembolic disease, varicose veins, pregnancy, congestive heart failure, myocardial infarction, oral contraceptive use, and malignant disease; also, postoperative patients and the elderly often have a slower venous return.

Nursing Interventions

The nurse must be alert for the potential complication of shock or right ventricular failure subsequent to the effect of the pulmonary embolus on the cardiovascular system. Nursing activities for management of shock are found in Chapter 22.

Prevention of thrombus formation is a major nursing responsibility. Ambulation and active and passive leg exercises are encouraged to prevent venous stasis in patients on bed rest. When the legs are moved in a "pumping" exercise, the leg muscles help to increase venous flow. The patient is advised to avoid prolonged sitting, immobility, or constricting clothing. He is *not* permitted to "dangle" his legs and feet in a dependent position while sitting on the edge of the bed. The patient's feet should be on the floor or on a chair and he should avoid crossing his legs. Intravenous catheters (for parenteral therapy or measurements of central venous pressure) should not be left in the veins for prolonged periods.

The nurse is responsible for monitoring thrombolytic and anticoagulant therapy. Thrombolytic therapy (streptokinase, urokinase) causes lysis of deep vein thrombi and pulmonary emboli, promoting resolution. During thrombolytic infusion, the patient remains on bed rest, vital signs are assessed every 2 hours, and invasive procedures are limited. The PT or APTT is performed 3 to 4 hours after starting the thrombolytic infusion to confirm activation of the fibrinolytic systems. Because of the prolonged clotting time, only essential arterial blood gas studies are performed on the upper extremities, with digital compression of the puncture site for at least 30 minutes. The infusion is immediately discontinued if uncontrolled bleeding occurs. (See Chap. 31 for nursing management for the patient receiving anticoagulant therapy.)

When chest pain is present, it is usually pleuritic. The patient should be in semi-Fowler's position to allow for maximum ease in breathing and distribution of air. Narcotic analgesics are administered as prescribed for severe pain.

Careful attention is given to the proper use of oxygen. It is important to make sure that the patient understands the need for continuous oxygen therapy. The nurse assesses the patient frequently for signs of hypoxia as a means of evaluating the effectiveness of the oxygen therapy. Nebulizer therapy, incentive spirometry, or postural drainage is administered if there is an accumulation of secretions complicating the pulmonary embolism.

Coping With Anxiety. After the patient's condition stabilizes, he is encouraged to express his feelings and concerns about this condition. The patient's questions are answered concisely and accurately, the therapy is explained, and the patient is told how he can help by early recognition of untoward effects. The nurse reassures the patient of the competency of the health care personnel. On discharge, the patient is instructed how to prevent recurrence and what signs and symptoms should alert him to seek medical attention.

Postoperative Nursing Care. If surgery was performed, the patient's pulmonary arterial pressure and urinary output are measured. The insertion site of the arterial catheter is assessed for hematoma formation and infection. An adequate blood pressure must be maintained to ensure perfusion of the vital organs. To prevent peripheral venous stasis and lower extremity edema, the foot of the bed is elevated. Isometric exercises, elastic stockings, and walking are encouraged when the patient is permitted out of bed. Sitting is discouraged, because hip flexion causes compression of the large veins in the legs.

Patient Education and Home Health Care. The following patient instructions are intended to help prevent recurrences and side effects of treatment:

- When taking anticoagulants, look for bruising and bleeding; try to protect yourself from bumping into objects that can cause bruising.
- Use a toothbrush with soft bristles.

- Do not take aspirin or antihistamine drugs while receiving warfarin sodium (Coumadin). Always check with your physician before taking any medication, including over-the-counter medications.
- Continue to wear antiembolism stockings as long as directed.
- Avoid laxatives, because they affect vitamin K absorption.
- Avoid sitting with your legs crossed or sitting for prolonged periods.
- When traveling, change your position regularly, walk occasionally, and do active exercises of the legs and ankles while sitting. Drink plenty of liquids while traveling, to avoid hemoconcentration due to fluid loss.
- Report dark, tarry stools to your physician or clinic immediately.
- Wear an identification bracelet (or carry a card) stating that anticoagulants are being taken.

Breathing Disorders During Sleep

Respiratory abnormalities can occur during sleep. In patients with underlying respiratory disease, the effects can be profound. Some patients who have adequate blood oxygenation while awake develop hypoxemia while sleeping. There are a variety of respiratory disorders associated with sleep (Table 26–2). The most common disorder is sleep apnea syndrome. Sleep apnea syndrome is defined as cessation of air flow (apnea) to the nose or mouth during sleep. Sleep apnea is classified into three types: (1) obstructive—lack of air flow due to pharyngeal occlusion; (2) central—simultaneous cessation of both air flow and respiratory movements; and (3) mixed—a combination of central and obstructive apnea within one apneic episode.

The patient, usually male, snores loudly, stops breathing up to 10 seconds or more, and then awakens abruptly with a loud snort as his blood oxygen level drops. The patient may have more than ten apneic episodes per hour to several hundred per night. This can seriously tax the heart and lungs. Increasing age and obesity correlate positively with alterations in breathing and nocturnal oxygen desaturation. Other symptoms include excessive daytime sleepiness, morning headache, sore throat, intellectual deterioration, personality changes, behavioral disorders, and complaints by the bed partner that the patient snores loudly or is unusually restless during sleep (Chart 26–3).

TABLE 26–2. *Sleep-Related Respiratory Disorders*

Disorders related predominantly to sleep	Obstructive sleep apnea
	Periodic breathing and central sleep apnea
	Central alveolar hypoventilation syndromes
Underlying respiratory system disease	Respiratory neuromuscular disorders
	Chest wall abnormalities
	Bronchopulmonary disease

(Murray JF and Nadel JA. Textbook of Respiratory Disease. Philadelphia, WB Saunders, 1988.)

Management.   There are a variety of treatments used in the management of sleep apnea. In mild cases of obstructive sleep apnea, avoidance of alcohol and drugs that depress the upper airway and weight reduction may be effective measures. In more severe cases of obstructive sleep apnea, medications, such as tricyclic antidepressants (protriptyline), and supplemental oxygen may be required. Surgical procedures to correct the obstruction may be performed. As a last resort, a tracheostomy is performed to bypass the obstruction if the potential for life-threatening dysrhythmia exists. The tracheostomy is unplugged only at night.

The treatment of central sleep apnea includes use of respiratory stimulants. Nocturnal low-flow nasal oxygen can be beneficial for relieving hypoxemia in some patients. Pacemaker stimulation of the phrenic nerves may be helpful.

Sarcoidosis

Sarcoidosis is a multisystem granulomatous disease of unknown cause. It may involve almost any organ or tissue, but most commonly involves the lungs, lymph nodes, liver, spleen, skin, eyes, phalangeal bones, and parotid glands. The onset usually occurs between the second and fourth decades. Sarcoidosis is fairly common worldwide.

Patients with sarcoidosis may have a number of immunologic abnormalities. The first clinical manifestations are usually thoracic, with hilar gland enlargement. The clinical picture includes dyspnea, cough, hemoptysis, and congestion. Generalized symptoms include anorexia, fatigue, and weight loss. The chest film may show hilar adenopathy and disseminated miliary and nodular lesions in the lungs. The granulomas may disappear or gradually convert to fibrous tissue. Extrathoracic involvement includes uveitis, joint pain, fever, and granulo-

matous lesions of the skin, liver, spleen, kidney, and central nervous system. With multiple organ system involvement, the patient experiences fatigue, fever, anorexia, weight loss, and joint pain. The diagnosis is confirmed by biopsy of the skin and lymph nodes, which shows noncaseating granulomas. Pulmonary function tests are abnormal if there is restriction of lung function (reduction in total lung capacity). Arterial blood gases may be normal or may show hypocapnia and hypoxemia.

There is no specific treatment, because the natural course of the disease is toward resolution. Corticosteroid therapy may benefit some patients because of its anti-inflammatory effect, which relieves symptoms and improves organ function. It is useful for patients with ocular and myocardial involvement, extensive pulmonary disease with compromise of pulmonary function, and hypercalcemia. Isoniazid may be given to patients with positive tuberculin tests.

Occupational Lung Diseases

Diseases of the lungs can occur in a variety of occupations as a result of exposure to organic or inorganic (mineral) dusts and noxious gases (fumes and aerosols). The effect of inhaling these materials depends on the composition of the inhaled substance, its antigenic (precipitating an immune response) or irritating properties, the dose inhaled, the length of time inhaled, and the host's response (a person's susceptibility to the irritant). There are a growing number of occupational lung diseases due to new and untested industrial substances and chemicals (presumed to be harmless). The problem may be compounded by smoking, which appears to have a synergistic effect on occupational lung disease and may increase the risk of lung cancers in people exposed to asbestos.

Preventive Measures and Health Maintenance

First, every effort is made to reduce the exposure of the worker to industrial products. The work environment must be ventilated properly to remove the noxious agent from the worker's breathing zone. Dust control can prevent many of the pneumoconioses and includes ventilation, spraying an area with water to control release of dust, and effective and frequent floor cleaning. Air samples need to be monitored. Toxic substances should be enclosed to reduce their concentration in the air. Workers must wear protective devices (face masks, hoods, industrial respirators) to provide a safe air supply when in a toxic atmosphere. Every employee should be carefully screened and followed, especially the worker at high risk for developing occupational lung disease (hypersensitivity states, asthma). There is a risk of developing serious smoking-related illness (cancer) in industries in which there are unsafe levels of certain gases, dusts, fumes, fluids, and other toxic substances. Ongoing educational programs to teach the worker to bear responsibility for his own health, including smoking cessation and influenza vaccination, have a major role in the prevention of occupational lung disease.

The "Right to Know" law stipulates that employees must be informed about all hazardous and toxic substances in the workplace. Specifically, they must be educated about what substances they work with that are hazardous or toxic, what effect they could have on their health, and how they should protect themselves. The responsibility for implementation of these controls inevitably falls on the federal or state governments, as exemplified by the Coal Mine Health and Safety Act of 1969, the Occupational Safety and Health Act (OSHA) of 1970, and the Federal Mine Safety and Health Amendment Act of 1977. The workplace is currently monitored by the Mining Safety and Health Administration (MSHA) of the Department of Labor, the National Coal Workers' Health Surveillance Program of the National Institute for Occupational Safety and Health (NIOSH), as well as state and local agencies.

The Pneumoconioses

Pneumoconiosis refers to a nonneoplastic alteration of the lung resulting from exposure to inorganic dust (*e.g.*, "dusty lung"). The most common pneumoconioses are silicosis, asbestosis, and coalworker's pneumoconiosis.

Silicosis.   Silicosis is a chronic pulmonary disease caused by inhalation of silica dust (silicon dioxide particles). Because the earth's crust is composed of silica and silicates, exposure is encountered in almost any form of mining (*i.e.*, coal, tin, copper, silver, gold, uranium mining), quarrying (slate, sandstone), or tunneling operations. Stonecutting, the manufacture of abrasives and pottery, and foundry work are other occupations presenting exposure hazards. When the silica particles, which have fibrogenic properties, are inhaled, nodular lesions are produced throughout the lungs. With the passage of time and exposure, the nodules enlarge and coalesce. Dense masses form in the upper portion of the lungs, resulting in loss of pulmonary parenchymal volume. Restrictive lung disease (inability of the lungs to expand fully) and obstructive lung disease from secondary emphysema result. Cavity formation is likely to be the result of superimposed tuberculosis. Exposure of 10 to 20 years is usually required before the disease develops and shortness of breath is manifested. Fibrotic destruction of pulmonary tissue can lead to emphysema, pulmonary hypertension, and cor pulmonale.

There is no specific treatment, and therapy is directed at the complications of silicosis. Preventive measures must be directed at protecting workers from inhaling silica dust. With cavitary lesions or advanced fibrosis, many physicians treat the patient for tuberculosis, even when cultures are negative.

Asbestosis.   Asbestosis is a disease characterized by diffuse pulmonary fibrosis due to the inhalation of asbestos dust. The use of asbestos is almost indispensable in modern industry and there are thousands of applications for its use. Exposure occurs in numerous occupations, including asbestos mining and manufacturing, demolition work, and roofing. Materials such as shingles, cement, vinyl asbestos tile, fireproof paint and clothing, brake linings, and filters all contain asbestos. The risk appears to lie in the manufacture, cutting, and demolition of asbestos-containing materials.

The asbestos fibers are inhaled and enter the alveoli, which eventually are obliterated by fibrous tissue that surrounds the asbestos particles. There is fibrous pleural thickening and pleural plaque formation. The altered physiologic pattern is that of restrictive lung disease, with decrease in lung volume, diminished gas transfer, and hypoxemia. The patient has progressive dyspnea, mild to moderate chest pain, anorexia, and weight loss. Cor pulmonale and respiratory failure occur as the disease progresses. A significant proportion of workers exposed to asbestos dust die of lung cancer, especially those who smoke.

In addition to lung cancer and asbestosis, exposure to asbestos can produce nonmalignant pleural disease, diffuse malignant mesothelioma, and possibly neoplasms of other tissues. Avoidance, in general, is essential and *asbestos workers should stop smoking.*

There is no effective treatment for asbestosis. Management is directed at intercurrent infection and coexisting lung disease. In patients with severe gas transport abnormalities, continuous oxygen therapy may improve exercise tolerance.

Coal Worker's Pneumoconiosis.   Coal worker's pneumoconiosis ("black lung") includes a variety of respiratory diseases found in coal workers in which there is an accumulation of coal dust in the lungs causing a tissue reaction to its presence. Coal miners are exposed to dusts that are mixtures of coal, kaolin, mica, and silica. The first physiologic reaction to the deposition of coal dust in the alveoli and respiratory bronchioles is an increase of macrophages that engulf (by phagocytosis) the particles and transport them to the terminal bronchioles where they are removed by mucociliary clearance. In time, the clearance mechanisms are unable to handle the excessive dust load and the macrophages aggregate in the respiratory bronchioles and alveoli. Fibroblasts appear and a network of reticulin is laid down surrounding the dust-laden macrophages. The respiratory bronchioles and the alveoli become clogged with coal dust, dying macrophages, and fibroblasts, which leads to the formation of the coal macule, the primary lesion of the disorder. (Macules appear as blackish dots on the lungs.) As the macules enlarge, there is a dilation of the weakening bronchiole with subsequent development of a focal emphysema.

The patient with complicated coal worker's pneumoconiosis has massive lesions of dense fibrotic tissue containing black material. These masses eventually destroy blood vessels and the bronchi of the affected lobe. The patient develops dyspnea, cough, and sputum production with expectoration of varying amounts of black fluid (melanoptysis), particularly if he is a smoker. Eventually cor pulmonale and respiratory failure result. The treatment is symptomatic. (See also treatment of emphysema, p. 577.)

Tumors of the Chest

Tumors of the lung may be benign or malignant. A chest tumor that is malignant can be *primary*, arising within the lung or the mediastinum, or it may represent a *metastasis* from a primary tumor site elsewhere. Metastatic tumors of the lungs occur frequently because the bloodstream transports free cancer cells from primary cancers elsewhere in the body. Such tumors grow in and between the alveoli and the bronchi, pushing them apart as the tumor grows. This process may occur over a long period, causing few or no symptoms.

Many tumors of the chest arise from the bronchial epithelium. Bronchial adenomas are slow-growing, usually benign tumors, but they are very vascular and, therefore, produce symptoms of bleeding and bronchial obstruction. Bronchogenic carcinoma is a malignant tumor arising from the bronchus. Such a tumor is epidermoid, usually located in the larger bronchi, or is an adenocarcinoma, arising farther out in the lung. There are also several intermediate or undifferentiated types of lung cancer, identifiable by cell type.

Lung Cancer (Bronchogenic Carcinoma)

Lung cancer is the number one cancer killer among men in the United States. It is increasing at a greater rate in women than it is in men and now exceeds breast cancer as the most common cause of cancer death. Because in approximately 70% of patients the disease has spread to regional lymphatics and other sites at the time of diagnosis, the survival rate is low. It has been suggested that carcinoma tends to arise at sites of previous scarring (tuberculosis, fibrosis) in the lung.

Classification and Staging.   The four major cell types of lung cancer (which differ significantly) are epidermoid (squamous cell) carcinoma, small cell (oat cell) carcinoma, adenocarcinoma, and large cell (undifferentiated) carcinoma. The World Health Organization's classification of lung tumors by histologic type is shown in Chart 26-4. Many tumors contain more than one cell type. The different cell types display different biologic behavior and have prognostic significance. Therefore, different approaches to treatment may be indicated by the cell type.

The stage of the tumor refers to the anatomic extent of the tumor, spread to the regional lymph nodes, and metastatic spread. Staging is accomplished by tissue diagnosis, lymph node biopsy, and mediastinoscopy. It is important in determining whether tumor resection should be attempted. Prognosis appears most favorable for epidermoid and adenocarcinoma, whereas undifferentiated small cell (oat cell) tumors have a poor prognosis.

Risk Factors.   Bronchogenic cancer is ten times more common in cigarette smokers than in nonsmokers, with the prevalence being related to the length of time and the intensity of smoking. Epidermoid carcinoma, involving the larger bronchi, is thought to be almost entirely associated with heavy (one pack or more per day) cigarette smoking. Few cases of this type of cancer have been reported in nonsmokers. For reasons unknown, the incidence of adenocarcinoma is rising faster than that of other types.

Adenocarcinoma of the peripheral bronchi is not associated with any known cause and occurs equally in smokers and nonsmokers. Another risk factor is occupational exposure to asbestos, radioactive dusts, arsenic, and certain plastics alone or in combination with tobacco smoke. It is reported that the risk of lung cancer is 92 times greater for people exposed to tobacco smoke and asbestos dust. People at high risk who continue to smoke should have regular chest films and sputum examinations to increase their chances that lung cancer will be detected while it is still treatable.

Clinical Manifestations.   Tumors of the bronchopulmonary system may affect the lining of the respiratory tract, lung parenchyma, pleura, or chest wall. The disease begins insidiously (over several decades) and often is asymptomatic until late in its course. The signs and symptoms depend on the location and size of the tumor, the degree of obstruction, and the existence of metastases to regional or distant sites.

The most frequent symptom is cough, probably from irritation by the tumor mass. It is frequently ignored as a "cigarette cough." Starting as a hacking, nonproductive cough, it later progresses to a point where it produces a thick, purulent sputum as secondary infection occurs.

- A cough that changes in character should arouse suspicion of lung cancer.

A wheeze in the chest (occurs when a bronchus becomes partially obstructed by the tumor) is noted in about 20% of patients. The expectoration of blood-tinged sputum is common, particularly in the morning, and is due to the sputum's becoming

---

Chart 26-4
Histopathologic Types of Lung Tumors

I. Epidermoid carcinomas (squamous cell)
II. Small-cell anaplastic carcinomas
   A. Fusiform cell type
   B. Polygonal cell type
   C. Lymphocyte-like (oat cell) type
   D. Others
III. Adenocarcinomas
   A. Bronchogenic
      1. Acinar } with or without
      2. Papillary } mucin formation

   B. Bronchioloalveolar
IV. Large-cell carcinomas
   A. Solid tumors with mucinlike content
   B. Solid tumors without mucinlike content
   C. Giant cell carcinomas
   D. Clear cell carcinomas
V. Combined epidermoid and adenocarcinomas
VI. Carcinoid tumors

VII. Bronchial gland tumors
   A. Cylindromas
   B. Mucoepidermoid tumors
   C. Others
VIII. Papillary tumors of the surface epithelium
   A. Epidermoid
   B. Epidermoid with goblet cells
   C. Others
IX. Mixed tumors and carcinosarcomas
   A. Mixed tumors
   B. Carcinosarcomas of embryonal type (blastomas)
   C. Other carcinosarcomas
X. Sarcomas
XI. Unclassified
XII. Mesotheliomas
   A. Localized
   B. Diffuse
XIII. Melanomas

(Kreyberg L et al. Histological Typing of Lung Tumors. Geneva, World Health Organization.)

streaked with blood as it passes over the ulcerated tumor surface. In some patients, recurring fever due to a persisting infection in an area of pneumonitis distal to the tumor is the early symptom. In fact, cancer of the lung should be suspected in persons with repeated unresolved upper respiratory tract infections. Pain is a late manifestation and is often found to be related to bone metastasis. If the tumor spreads to adjacent structures and regional lymph nodes, the patient may present with chest pain and tightness, hoarseness (involvement of recurrent laryngeal nerve), dysphagia, head and neck edema, and symptoms of pleural or pericardial effusion. The most common sites of metastases are lymph nodes, bone, brain, contralateral lung, and adrenal glands. General symptoms of weakness, anorexia, weight loss, and anemia appear late.

Diagnostic Evaluation. If the patient with pulmonary symptoms is a heavy smoker, cancer of the lung is suspected. Chest radiography is performed to search for pulmonary density, a solitary peripheral nodule (coin lesion), atelectasis, and infection. Cytologic examination of fresh sputum obtained by cough or saline washings from a suggested bronchus is performed to search for malignant cells. Bronchoscopy with a flexible fiberoptic instrument allows a detailed study of the bronchial segments and identification of the source of malignant cells and of the probable extent of anticipated surgery. Fluorescent bronchofibroscopy is used to detect small, early bronchogenic cancers. Systematically injected hematoporphyrin is absorbed by malignant cells and presents a red fluorescent glow when examined under illumination by violet light.

Lung scans are part of the diagnostic workup. A bone scan or bone marrow study is performed for detection of bone metastasis, and liver scanning is used to verify metastatic spread to the liver. Detection of central nervous system metastases is accomplished by brain scanning, computed tomography, magnetic resonance imaging, and other neurologic diagnostic procedures. Mediastinoscopy may be used to evaluate tumor spread to hilar lymph nodes of the right lung, and the mediastinotomy gives access to the hilar lymphatics of the left lung.

Before surgery is performed, the patient is evaluated to determine whether the tumor is resectable and whether he can tolerate the physiologic impairment resulting from such surgery. Pulmonary function tests combined with split-function perfusion scans are performed to determine if the patient will have adequate pulmonary reserve after the procedure. The patient's ability to move air (vital capacity, FEV_1) is important because the ability to generate an effective cough is imperative in the postoperative period.

Gerontologic Considerations

Cancer of the lung is not unusual in the elderly; however, the presence of coronary artery disease or pulmonary insufficiency may be contraindications to surgical intervention. If the patient's cardiovascular status and pulmonary function are satisfactory, surgery is generally well tolerated.

Management

The objective of management is to provide the maximum likelihood of cure. The treatment depends on the cell type, the stage of the disease, and the physiologic status (particularly cardiac and pulmonary status) of the patient. In general, treatment may involve surgery, radiation therapy, chemotherapy, and immunotherapy, used separately or in combination.

Surgery. Surgical resection is the preferred method for patients with localized tumors with no evidence of metastatic spread and whose cardiopulmonary function is adequate. (Usually, surgery for small cell cancer of the lung is not advisable because this is a rapidly growing tumor that metastasizes early and widely.) Unfortunately, in a large number of patients with bronchogenic cancer the lesion is inoperable at the time of diagnosis. The usual operation for small, apparently curable tumor of the lung is lobectomy (removal of a lobe of the lung). An entire lung may be removed (pneumonectomy) in combination with other surgical procedures, such as resection of involved mediastinal lymph nodes. Before surgery, the cardiopulmonary reserve of the patient must be determined. (See pp. 544–557 for the preoperative and postoperative management of the patient undergoing chest surgery.)

Radiation Therapy. Radiation therapy may cure a small percentage of patients. It is useful in controlling radio-responsive neoplasms that cannot be resected. The small cell and epidermoid tumors are usually radiation sensitive. Radiation may be used as palliative treatment to decrease tumor size and relieve pressure on vital structures. It can control symptoms of spinal cord metastasis and superior vena cava compression. Also, prophylactic brain irradiation is used on certain patients to treat microscopic metastases to the brain. Respite may be obtained from cough, chest pain, dyspnea, hemoptysis, and bone and liver pain. Relief of symptoms may last from a few weeks to many months and is important in improving the quality of the remaining period of life.

With radiation therapy there is usually toxicity to normal tissue within the radiation field. Complications of radiation therapy include esophagitis, pneumonitis, and radiation lung fibrosis, which may impair ventilatory and diffusion capacity with a significant reduction in pulmonary reserve. Irradiation also can affect the heart.

Attention is paid to the patient's nutrition and psychological outlook. The patient should be monitored for signs of anemia and infection. (See pp. 351–353 for management of the patient receiving radiation therapy.)

Chemotherapy. At present chemotherapy is used to manipulate tumor growth patterns, to treat patients with distant metastases or with small-cell cancer of the lung, and in combination with surgery or radiation therapy. Combinations of two or more drugs may be more beneficial than single-dose regimens. A large number of drugs are reported to have some activity against lung cancer. Various combinations of doxorubicin hydrochloride (Adriamycin), cyclosphosphamide (Cytoxan) vincristine (Oncovin), and cisplatin (Platinol) are used. An effective drug in small-cell lung cancer is VP-16. It currently is used in combination with cisplatin. The choice depends on the growth of the tumor cell and the specificity of the drug for cell cycle phase. These agents are toxic and have a narrow margin of safety. Chemotherapy may provide palliation, especially of pain, but does not cure and rarely prolongs life. It is valuable in reducing pressure symptoms of lung cancer and in treating brain, spinal cord, and pericardial metastasis. (See p. 353 for chemotherapy for the patient with cancer.)

Nursing Interventions

Nursing care of the patient with lung cancer is similar to that of other cancer patients (see Chap. 19). Special attention is focused on the respiratory manifestations of the disease. Airway management is needed to maintain airway patency through the removal of secretions or exudate. As the tumor enlarges, there may be compression on a bronchus or involvement of a large area of lung tissue, resulting in impaired breathing pattern and poor gas exchange. Deep breathing and coughing, aerosol therapy, oxygen therapy, and mechanical ventilation may be necessary when there is respiratory impairment.

The psychological aspects of caring for the patient with lung cancer are extremely important. The patient will have to cope with many issues during the course of the disease (see Chap. 19).

In summary, cancer of the lung remains the most common cause of cancer deaths among men in the United States. Its incidence is increasing among women and it has surpassed breast cancer as the most frequent cause of cancer deaths in women. Early diagnosis and treatment improve the length of survival; treatment may include surgical resection, radiation therapy, and chemotherapy. Attention is given preoperatively and postoperatively to pain management, nutritional support, relief of shortness of breath, and maintenance of a patent airway. Psychological and emotional responses of the patient and his family to the diagnosis and prognosis of lung cancer require attention from all members of the health care team.

Tumors of the Mediastinum

Most mediastinal tumors are adjacent to vital structures and have an unpredictable manner of growth. They include neurogenic tumors, thymic tumors, and mesodermal and endocrine tumors. Thymic tumors have the highest percentage of malignancy.

Cysts of the mediastinum usually are small when benign. Dermoid cysts occasionally develop, and these may ulcerate into the air passages.

Clinical Manifestations.   Nearly all the symptoms of mediastinal tumors are due to the pressure of the mass against important intrathoracic organs. Among these pressure symptoms are chest pain; bulging of the chest wall; orthopnea (an early sign due to pressure against the trachea, a main bronchus, the recurrent laryngeal nerve, or the lung); cardiac palpitation, anginal attacks, and various other circulatory disturbances; cyanosis; superior vena caval syndromes (ie, swelling of the face, the neck, and the upper extremities) and the marked distention of the veins of the neck and the chest wall (evidence of the obstruction of large veins of the mediastinum by extravascular compression or intravascular invasion); and dysphagia from pressure against the esophagus.

Diagnostic Evaluation

Chest films are of great value in the diagnosis of mediastinal tumors and cysts. Lateral and oblique films and tomography are used to localize the tumor.

Computed tomography (CT) scans are used to detect occult thymomas as well as to define a mass lesion.

The biopsy of an enlarged lymph node removed from above the clavicle or one removed during mediastinoscopy may provide the diagnosis. Blood studies are of value in excluding leukemia, and sputum examinations aid in ruling out tuberculosis.

Management.   Many mediastinal tumors are benign and operable. The location of the tumor in the mediastinum will dictate the type of incision. Most incisions are median sternotomies. The care is the same as for any patient who is undergoing thoracic surgery (see pp. 544–557). The major complications, although infrequent, include hemorrhage, phrenic or recurrent laryngeal nerve injury, and infection. If the tumor is malignant and infiltrating, radiation therapy and chemotherapy are the therapeutic modalities used when complete surgical removal is not feasible.

Chest Trauma

Chest trauma accounts for approximately 25% of all trauma-related deaths in the United States and is closely associated with another 50% of trauma-related deaths involving multiple system injuries. The most common mechanisms of injury include automobile accidents, falls, crushing chest injuries, blast injuries, gunshot wounds, and stab wounds.

Injuries to the chest are often life threatening. There are five pathologic mechanisms that occur in chest trauma:

1. Loss of a patent airway
2. Alteration in intrathoracic pressure
3. Destruction of the chest wall and rib cage
4. Alteration in the central nervous system
5. Insufficient myocardial function

These mechanisms frequently result in impaired ventilation and perfusion leading to acute respiratory failure, hypovolemic shock, and death.

Immediate Assessment and Management

In treatment of chest trauma, time is critical. Patient history focuses on the time the injury occurred; identifying the mechanism of injury; if the patient is responsive, his specific complaints; the estimated blood loss; whether drugs or alcohol have been used; and the prehospital treatment. A physical examination includes inspection of the airway, thorax, neck veins, breathing, vital signs, and skin color for signs of shock. The thorax is palpated for tenderness, crepitus, and the position of the trachea. Breath sounds and heart sounds are auscultated. An initial diagnostic workup includes a chest x-ray, CBC, type and cross-match, urinalysis, arterial blood gases, and an ECG.

The goals of treatment are to restore and maintain a patent airway and cardiopulmonary function by aggressive airway management, fluid replacement, and chest tube placement.

Agitation, irrational behavior and hostility are signs of decreased oxygen delivery to the cerebral cortex. To restore and maintain cardiopulmonary function, an adequate airway is created and ventilation is initiated. This includes stabilizing and reestablishing chest wall integrity, correcting open pneumothorax, decompressing pneumothorax/hemothorax, and eliminating cardiac tamponade. Hypovolemia and low cardiac output are corrected. These treatment efforts, along with the control of hemorrhage, are usually carried out simultaneously by the emergency department team. The patient is completely undressed to avoid missing additional injuries. Many injuries involving the chest have associated head and abdominal injuries that require care. Ongoing assessment is essential to monitor the patient's response to treatment and to detect early signs of a deteriorating condition.

Principles of management are essentially those pertaining to care of the postoperative thoracic patient (see pp. 546–557).

Rib Fractures

Rib fractures are the most common type of chest trauma, occurring in over 60% of patients admitted with blunt chest injury. Fractures of the first three ribs are rare but can result in a high mortality because they are associated with laceration of the subclavian artery or vein. The fifth through ninth ribs are the most common sites of fractures. Fractures of the lower ribs are associated with injury to the spleen and liver.

If the patient is conscious, he will experience severe pain, tenderness, and muscle spasm over the area of fracture, which is aggravated by coughing, deep breathing, and motion. The area around the fracture will be ecchymotic. Subcutaneous crepitus may be palpated. To reduce the pain, the patient will breathe in a shallow manner and will avoid sighs, deep breaths, coughing, and moving. This results in diminished ventilation, collapse of unaerated alveoli (atelectasis), pneumonitis, and hypoxemia. Respiratory insufficiency and failure can be the outcomes of such a cycle. A diagnostic workup includes a chest x-ray, rib series, ECG, and arterial blood gases.

Management.   The goals of treatment are pain control, detection, and treatment of the injury. Sedation is used to relieve pain, and to allow deep breathing and coughing. Care must be taken to avoid oversedation and suppression of the respiratory drive. Other alternatives include intercostal nerve block and ice over the fracture site; a chest binder may decrease pain on movement. Usually the pain abates in 5 to 7 days and discomfort can be controlled with non-narcotic analgesia. Most rib fractures heal in 3 to 6 weeks. The patient is monitored closely for signs and symptoms of associated injuries.

Flail Chest

Flail chest occurs when two or more adjacent ribs are fractured at two or more sites, resulting in a free floating segment. There is a loss of stability of the chest wall with subsequent respiratory impairment, usually severe respiratory distress.

During inspiration, as the chest expands, the detached part of the chest (flail segment) will show a paradoxical movement in that it is pulled inward during inspiration. On expiration, because the intrathoracic pressure will exceed atmospheric pressure, the flail segment will bulge outward, impairing the patient's ability to exhale. This paradoxical action results in increased dead space ventilation, retained airway secretions, increased lung resistance, decreased compliance, and a reduction in alveolar ventilation. Lung contusion and atelectasis frequently accompany flail chest. As a result, blood oxygen content decreases and carbon dioxide content increases, producing respiratory acidosis. Often, hypotension, inadequate tissue perfusion, and metabolic acidosis follow as cardiac output decreases by the paradoxical motion of the mediastinum.

Management.   Several methods of management are available, depending on the degree of respiratory dysfunction. If only a small segment of the chest is involved, the objectives are to clear the airway (coughing, deep breaths, gentle suctioning) to aid in the expansion of the lung, and to relieve pain by intercostal nerve blocks, high thoracic epidural blocks, or careful use of intravenous narcotics.

For mild to moderate flail chest injuries, some clinicians advocate treating the underlying pulmonary contusion with fluid restriction, diuretics, corticosteroids, and albumin while relieving chest pain and by employing pulmonary physiotheraphy, combined with close and continuing patient monitoring.

When a severe flail is encountered, endotracheal intubation and mechanical ventilation with a volume-cycled ventilator and sometimes PEEP are used to splint the chest wall (internal pneumatic stabilization) and to correct abnormalities in gas exchange. This helps to treat the underlying pulmonary contusion, serves to stabilize the thoracic cage for healing of fractures, and improves alveolar ventilation and intrathoracic volume by decreasing the work of breathing. This treatment modality requires long-term endotracheal intubation and ventilator support.

Hemothorax and Pneumothorax

Severe chest injuries usually are accompanied by the collection of blood in the chest cavity (hemothorax) because of torn intercostal vessels, lacerations of the lungs, or the escape of air from the injured lung into the pleural cavity (pneumothorax). Often, both blood and air are found in the chest cavity (hemopneumothorax). Chest injury compresses lung tissue, resulting in interference with its normal function.

The seriousness of the problem depends on the amount and rate of thoracic bleeding. Needle aspiration (thoracentesis) or chest tube drainage of the blood or air allows decompression of the pleural cavity so that the lung is able to re-expand and again perform its function in respiration. A thoracotomy is performed when there is more than 1500 ml of blood aspirated initially by thoracentesis, 500 ml of drainage for more than an hour, or 200 ml for 5 to 6 hours. An emergency thoracotomy also may be performed in the emergency department if there is suggested cardiovascular injury secondary to chest or penetrating trauma.

Management.   A large-diameter chest tube (catheter) is inserted usually in the fourth through sixth intercostal space between the anterior and posterior line. This space is used because it is the thinnest part of the chest wall, minimizes the danger of contact with the thoracic nerve, and will leave a less visible scar. Prompt and effective decompression of the pleural cavity (drainage of blood or air) usually occurs. If there is an excessive amount of bleeding from the chest tube in a relatively short period, autotransfusion may be employed. This technique takes the patient's own blood that is drained from the chest, filters it, and then transfuses it back into the patient's vascular system.

Tension Pneumothorax

A tension pneumothorax is a life-threatening medical emergency that may result in death if not immediately treated. In some patients, air may be drawn into the pleural space from the lacerated lung or through a small hole in the chest wall. In either case, the air that enters the chest cavity with each inspiration is trapped there; it cannot be expelled through the air passage or small hole in the chest wall.

A tension (pressure) thus is built up within the pleural space, which produces a collapse of the lung and a shift of the heart and the great vessels and trachea toward the unaffected side of the chest. This not only interferes with respiration but also disrupts circulatory function, because with increased intrathoracic pressure, venous return to the heart is compromised, causing decreased cardiac output and impairment of peripheral circulation. Diminished cardiac output leads to cardiac arrest. The clinical picture is one of air hunger, agitation, hypotension, tachycardia, profuse diaphoresis, and cyanosis.

- Relief of tension pneumothorax is considered an emergency measure.

Management. If a tension pneumothorax is suspected, the patient should immediately be given a high concentration of oxygen to treat the hypoxia. In an emergency situation, a tension pneumothorax can be converted quickly to a simple pneumothorax by insertion of a large-bore needle into the pleural space, which relieves the pressure and vents the intrathoracic air to the outside. Then a chest tube can be inserted and connected to suction to remove the remaining air and fluid and re-expand the lung.

If the lung expands and there is no continuing leakage from the lung, further drainage may be unnecessary. If the lung is still leaking, as evidenced by the reaccumulation of an inexhaustible volume of air during the thoracentesis, constant exit or removal of this air must be provided by a large-bore chest tube with water-seal drainage.

Penetrating Wounds of the Chest

Open Pneumothorax

Open pneumothorax implies an opening in the chest wall large enough to allow air to pass freely in and out of the thoracic cavity with each attempted respiration. Because the rush of air through the hole in the chest wall produces a sucking sound, such injuries are termed *sucking wounds* of the chest. In such patients, not only is the lung collapsed, but the structures of the mediastinum (heart and great vessels) are shifted toward the uninjured side with each inspiration and in the opposite direction with expiration. This is termed *mediastinal flutter*, and it produces serious circulatory embarrassment.

Management. Open pneumothorax calls for emergency interventions.

- Stopping the flow of air through the opening in the chest wall is a lifesaving measure.

In such an emergency, anything may be used that is large enough to fill the hole—a towel, a handkerchief, or the heel of the hand. If the patient is conscious, tell him to inhale and strain against a closed glottis. This action assists in the re-expansion of the lung and the ejection of the air from the thorax. In the hospital, the opening is plugged by sealing it with gauze impregnated with petrolatum. A pressure dressing is applied by circumferential strapping. Usually, a chest tube connected to water-seal drainage is inserted to permit exit of air and fluid. Antibiotics usually are prescribed to combat infection from contamination.

Stab Wounds

Stab wounds are a common cause of penetrating wounds of the chest, most of which are caused by knives and switchblades, and are frequently associated with alcohol or substance abuse. The appearance of the external wound may be very deceptive,

because pneumothorax, hemothorax, and cardiac tamponade along with severe and continuing hemorrhage can occur from any small wound, even one caused by an icepick.

Management. The objective of immediate management is to restore and maintain cardiopulmonary function. After an adequate airway is ensured and ventilation is corrected, the patient is examined for shock and intrathoracic and intra-abdominal injuries. The patient is undressed completely so that additional injuries will not be missed. There is a high risk for associated intra-abdominal injuries with stab wounds below the level of the fifth anterior intercostal space. Death can result from exsanguinating hemorrhage or intra-abdominal sepsis.

After the status of the peripheral pulses is assessed, a large-bore intravenous line is inserted. A diagnostic workup includes type and cross-match, chemistry profile, arterial blood gases, and an electrocardiogram. An indwelling catheter is inserted to monitor urinary volume and to collect a urine sample for laboratory study. A nasogastric tube is inserted to prevent aspiration, minimize leakage of abdominal contents, and decompress the gastrointestinal tract.

Shock is treated simultaneously with colloid solutions, crystalloids, or blood, as indicated by the condition of the patient. Chest radiographs are taken, and other diagnostic procedures are carried out (esophagogram, flat plate of the abdomen, arteriogram) as dictated by the needs of the patient.

A chest tube is inserted in the pleural space in most patients with penetrating wounds of the chest to achieve rapid and continuing re-expansion of the lungs. Frequently this will cause a complete evacuation of hemothorax and will decrease the incidence of clotted hemothorax. The chest tube allows early recognition of continuing intrathoracic bleeding, which will make surgical exploration necessary.

If the patient has a penetrating wound of the heart and great vessels, the esophagus, and the tracheobronchial tree, surgical intervention is required.

Pulmonary Contusion

Pulmonary contusion is damage to the lung parenchyma that results in hemorrhage and localized edema. It is associated with chest trauma when there is rapid compression and decompression of the chest wall.

Pathophysiology. The primary pathologic defect is the abnormal accumulation of fluid in the interstitial and intra-alveolar spaces. It is thought that injury to the lung parenchyma and its capillary network results in a serum protein and plasma leak. The extravascular serum protein exerts an osmotic pressure that enhances loss of fluid from the capillaries. Blood, edema, and cellular debris (from cellular response to injury) enter the lung and accumulate in the bronchioles and alveolar surface, where they interfere with the efficiency of gas exchange. There is an increase in pulmonary vascular resistance and pulmonary artery pressure. The patient experiences systemic hypoxia and carbon dioxide retention. Occasionally, a contused lung occurs on the other side of the point of body impact. This is called a *contrecoup contusion*.

Clinical Manifestations. Pulmonary contusion may be mild, moderate, or severe. The clinical manifestation will vary from tachypnea, tachycardia, pleuritic chest pain, hypoxemia, and blood-tinged secretions to more severe tachypnea, tachycardia, crackles, frank bleeding, severe hypoxemia, and respiratory acidosis. The efficiency of gas exchange is determined by arterial blood gas measurements. The chest films will show pulmonary infiltration.

Management. The goal of treatment includes maintenance of the airway, adequate oxygenation, and pain control. In mild cases of pulmonary contusion, ultrasonic mist nebulization is used to keep the secretions fluid. Postural drainage, physiotherapy, and sterile endotracheal suctioning are used to remove the secretions. Pain is managed by intercostal nerve blocks or by narcotics. Usually, antimicrobial therapy is administered, because a damaged lung is susceptible to infection. Oxygen by mask or cannula usually is given for 24 to 36 hours. Fluids are restricted because the injury is thought to be due to abnormal collection of fluid in the interstices of the lung.

If moderate lung contusion is encountered, in addition to the above symptoms, the patient will have a large amount of mucus, serum, and frank blood in the tracheobronchial tree. He coughs constantly but is unable to clear his secretions. This patient usually requires intubation with a cuffed endotracheal tube and is placed on a ventilator with low-concentration oxygen and PEEP to maintain the pressure and keep the lungs inflated. Diuretics may be given to reduce edema. A nasogastric tube is passed to relieve gastrointestinal distention. Metabolic acidosis is corrected with intravenous sodium bicarbonate. Frequent cultures of tracheobronchial secretions are obtained.

A patient with severe pulmonary contusion presents with the signs and symptoms of adult respiratory distress syndrome (ARDS), which include rapid respirations, tachycardia, cyanosis, agitation, combativeness, and continuous and productive coughing of mucoid, frothy, and bloody secretions. This patient is treated vigorously with endotracheal intubation and ventilatory support, plasma or albumin (to maintain normal oncotic pressure to prevent leakage from pulmonary capillaries), diuretics, fluid restriction, and perhaps the prophylactic administration of antimicrobials. Whole blood or fresh frozen plasma may be used to treat hypovolemia.

The complications of pulmonary contusion are infections, especially pneumonia in the contused segment, because the extravasation of fluid and blood into the alveolar and interstitial spaces is an excellent culture medium.

Cardiac Tamponade

Cardiac tamponade is the compression of the heart as a result of fluid within the pericardial sac. It usually is caused by blunt or penetrating trauma to the chest. (A penetrating wound of the heart is associated with a high mortality.) Cardiac tamponade also may follow diagnostic cardiac catheterization, angiographic procedures, and pacemaker insertion, which can produce perforations of the heart and great vessels. Pericardial effusion also may develop from metastases to the pericardium from malignant tumors of the breast and lung as well as from lymphomas and leukemias, uremia, tuberculosis, and high-dose radiation to the chest.

Pathophysiology. If the fluid formation is slow, the pericardium will distend without producing noticeable clinical symptoms until enough fluid develops to raise the intrapericardial pressure. A rapidly developing effusion interferes with ventricular filling and causes impairment of circulation. Thus, there is reduced cardiac output and insufficient venous return to the heart. Circulatory collapse can result.

Clinical Manifestations. The clinical manifestations depend on the speed of fluid accumulation. Important signs to watch for are a falling blood pressure, rising venous pressure (distended neck veins), and distant (muffled) heart sounds from impaired diastolic filling of the heart. Pulsus paradoxus (systolic blood pressure drops and fluctuates with respiration) may occur early in the development of cardiac tamponade. The patient may be anxious, confused, and restless and may have dyspnea, tachypnea, and precordial pain. The central venous pressure is elevated. However, the venous pressure may be low or normal if a large amount of blood has been lost as a result of associated injuries.

Management. The treatment of cardiac tamponade is thoracotomy for penetrating cardiac injuries where cardiorrhaphy (suturing the heart muscle) is performed to stop hemorrhage, relieve tamponade, and repair associated lacerations and lesions. (See the care of the patient undergoing heart surgery [Chap. 30] and of the patient undergoing chest surgery [Chap. 25].) Pericardiocentesis (needle aspiration of fluid from the pericardium, Chap. 29) may be performed to ''buy time'' before the patient is taken to surgery. This decompression of the pericardial sac permits effective heart action to be resumed.

Subcutaneous Emphysema

When the lung or the air passages are injured, air may enter the tissue planes and pass for some distance under the skin (*e.g.*, neck, chest). The tissues give a crackling sensation when palpated, and the subcutaneous air produces an alarming appearance as face, neck, body, and scrotum become misshapen by subcutaneous air. Fortunately, subcutaneous emphysema is of itself not a serious complication. The subcutaneous air is spontaneously absorbed if the underlying air leak is treated or stops spontaneously. Giving the patient inhalations of high concentrations of oxygen will promote the reabsorption of subcutaneous air by washing nitrogen from the blood and improving its diffusion from the subcutaneous tissues back into the circulation. In severe cases in which there is widespread subcutaneous emphysema, a tracheostomy is indicated to ensure patency of the airway.

The Clinical Problem of Aspiration

Aspiration (inhalation) of stomach contents is a serious complication that may cause death. It can occur when there is loss of protective airway reflexes, such as is seen in patients who are unconscious from drugs, alcohol, stroke, or cardiac arrest, or in instances when a nonfunctioning nasogastric tube allows the gastric contents to drain around the tube and cause silent aspiration.

Massive inhalation of gastric contents, if untreated, will, in a period of several hours, result in the clinical syndrome of tachycardia, dyspnea, cyanosis, and hypertension, followed by hypotension and finally death. The primary factors responsible for morbidity and mortality after aspiration of gastric contents are the volume of aspirated gastric contents and their character. A full stomach contains solid particles of food. If these are aspirated, the problem then becomes one of mechanical blockage of the airways and secondary infection. During periods of fasting, the stomach contains acidic gastric juice, which, if aspirated, may prove destructive to the alveoli and capillaries.

The presence of fecal contamination (more likely seen in intestinal obstruction) will increase the likelihood of mortality because the endotoxins produced by intestinal organisms may be absorbed systemically, or the thick proteinaceous material found in the intestinal contents may obstruct the airway, leading to atelectasis and secondary bacterial invasion.

Chemical pneumonitis may develop from aspiration and result in destruction of alveolar-capillary endothelial cells, with a consequent outpouring of protein-rich fluids into the interstitial and intra-alveolar spaces. This results in loss of surfactant, which in turn causes early closure of the airway. Finally, the impaired exchange of oxygen and carbon dioxide causes respiratory failure. Characteristics of aspiration include the following:

- Massive aspiration is usually fatal.
- Small, localized aspiration from regurgitation can cause pneumonia and respiratory distress.
- Silent regurgitation often occurs unobserved and may be more common than suspected.

Preventive Measures

When Reflexes Are Lacking.   Aspiration is likely to occur if the patient cannot adequately coordinate his protective glottic, laryngeal, and cough reflexes. This hazard is increased if the patient has a distended abdomen, is in a supine position, and has his upper extremities immobilized by intravenous infusions or hand restraints. When vomiting, a person can normally protect his airway by sitting up or turning on his side and coordinating his breathing, coughing, gag, and glottic reflexes. If these reflexes are active, an oral airway should not be inserted. If an airway is in place, it should be pulled out the moment the patient gags on it so as not to stimulate the pharyngeal gag reflex and promote vomiting and aspiration. Suctioning of oral secretions with a catheter should be performed with minimal pharyngeal stimulation yet at the same time be effective.

During Tube Feeding.   The patient who is receiving tube feedings is positioned upright during the feeding and for 30 minutes thereafter to allow the stomach to partially empty. Small volumes given under low pressure will help to prevent aspiration. Tube feedings must be given only when it is certain that the feeding tube is positioned correctly in the stomach.

Assessing for Delayed Emptying Time of Stomach.   A full stomach may cause aspiration because of increased intragastric or extragastric pressure. The following clinical situations cause delayed emptying time of the stomach and may contribute to aspiration: intestinal obstruction; increased gastric secretions during anxiety, stress, or pain; or abdominal distention because of ileus, ascites, peritonitis, drugs, severe illness, or vaginal delivery.

When a feeding tube is present, contents can be aspirated to determine the amount of the last feeding left in the stomach. If more than 50 ml is aspirated, there may be a problem with delayed emptying and the next feeding should be held.

After Prolonged Endotracheal Intubation.   Prolonged endotracheal intubation or tracheostomy can depress the laryngeal and glottic reflexes because of disuse. Patients with prolonged tracheostomies are encouraged to phonate and exercise their laryngeal muscles. The pharynx is suctioned before deflating the cuff to prevent aspiration of regurgitated material. It is important to remember that improperly administered IPPB treatments by mask can distend the stomach and promote aspiration.

Acute Respiratory Failure

Respiratory failure exists whenever the exchange of oxygen for carbon dioxide in the lungs cannot keep up with the rate of oxygen consumption and carbon dioxide production in the cells of the body. This results in a fall in arterial oxygen tension (hypoxemia) and a rise in arterial carbon dioxide tension (hypercapnia).

One must distinguish between acute respiratory failure and acute exacerbation of chronic respiratory failure. Acute respiratory failure is the respiratory failure appearing in the patient whose lung was structurally and functionally normal before the onset of the present illness. *Chronic respiratory failure* is the respiratory failure seen in patients with chronic lung diseases such as chronic bronchitis, emphysema, and black lung disease (coal miner's disease). These patients develop a tolerance to the gradually worsening hypoxia and hypercapnia. After acute respiratory failure, the lung usually returns to its original state. In chronic respiratory failure the structural damage is irreversible. The principles of management of these two conditions are different; this discussion will be confined to acute respiratory failure.

Causes of acute respiratory failure are numerous and may be subdivided into various categories. One major group includes those diseases in which respiratory failure results from inadequate ventilation: the lung itself remains structurally normal in the early stages. One of the most important causes of inadequate ventilation is upper airway obstruction. Its cause, diagnosis, and management are discussed on p. 530.

Central nervous system depression also will result in inadequate ventilation. The respiratory center, which controls every breath, lies in the lower part of the brain stem (pons and medulla). Drug overdose, anesthesia, head injury, stroke, brain tumors, encephalitis, meningitis, hypoxia, and hypercapnia are all capable of depressing the respiratory center. In these patients, respiration becomes slow and shallow. Respiratory arrest may occur in severe cases.

The impulses arising in the respiratory center travel through nerves that extend from the brain stem down the spinal cord to receptors in the muscles of respiration. Any disease of the nerves, spinal cord, muscles, or neuromuscular junction involved in respiration will seriously affect ventilation. Polyneuritis, myasthenia gravis, damage to the cervical segment of the spinal cord, large acute lesions of multiple sclerosis in the brain stem, and poliomyelitis are examples of such diseases.

Respiratory failure due to inadequate ventilation may occur in the immediate postoperative period, especially after major thoracic or upper abdominal surgery. The reasons for respiratory failure during this period are numerous. The effects of anesthetic drugs, analgesics, and sedatives (pentobarbital and morphine) are long-lasting. They depress respiration by their own effects or by enhancing the effects of narcotic analgesics. Pain in the thoracic and abdominal area interferes with deep breathing and coughing. Muscle relaxants frequently are used during anesthesia. Some patients may have difficulty in metabolizing or excreting these drugs, so that their effects last longer than usual, making patients weak in the postoperative period.

Use of small intravenous doses of morphine is recommended in the postanesthesia room, because they are short acting and easily titrated. Ventilation–perfusion abnormality also accounts for respiratory failure after major abdominal and thoracic operations.

Pleural effusion, hemothorax, and pneumothorax are conditions that interfere with ventilation by preventing expansion of the lung. They usually are produced by an underlying lung disease or pleural disease.

Trauma caused by motor vehicle accidents is a very common cause of acute respiratory failure. Accidents resulting in head injury, unconsciousness, and bleeding from the nose and mouth lead to upper airway obstruction and respiratory depression. Hemothorax, pneumothorax, and rib fractures may occur and may be responsible for inadequate ventilation. Flail chest also may occur and may lead to respiratory failure.

There are many acute diseases of the lung that may lead to acute respiratory failure. Of these diseases, pneumonia is perhaps the most common. It usually is caused by viral or bacterial activity. Chemical pneumonitis is pneumonia produced by the inhalation of irritant fumes or the aspiration of acidic gastric material. Bronchial asthma, atelectasis, pulmonary embolism, and pulmonary edema are some other conditions that can cause acute respiratory failure.

Adult Respiratory Distress Syndrome

Adult respiratory distress syndrome (ARDS), also known as noncardiogenic pulmonary edema, is a clinical syndrome characterized by a progressive decrease in arterial oxygen content occurring after a serious illness or injury. ARDS usually requires mechanical ventilation with a higher than normal airway pressure. There is a wide range of factors associated with the development of ARDS (see Table 26–3), including direct injury to the lungs (such as smoke inhalation) or indirect insult to the body (such as shock).

Pathophysiology.   ARDS occurs as a result of injury to the alveolar capillary membrane resulting in leakage of fluid into the alveolar interstitial spaces and alteration in the capillary bed (Fig. 26–4). There is a marked V/Q imbalance due to an impaired gas exchange and extensive shunting of blood in the lungs. The result is a decreased functional residual capacity, severe hypoxia, and hypocapnia.

Adult respiratory distress syndrome has been associated with a mortality rate of as high as 50% to 60%. The survival rate is somewhat improved when the cause can be determined, and early and aggressive treatment is implemented (especially the use of positive end-expiratory pressure).

Diagnostic Criteria

A diagnosis of ARDS may be made based on the following criteria:

- Acute respiratory failure
- Bilateral pulmonary infiltrates
- Hypoxemia (PaO_2 below 50 to 60 mm Hg) and inspired flow of oxygen (FIO_2) above 0.5 to 0.6.
- Pulmonary artery wedge pressure greater than 18 mm Hg.

Management

The management of ARDS includes the following:

1. Define and treat the cause.
2. Provide adequate ventilation.
3. Provide circulatory support.
4. Provide adequate fluid management.
5. Provide nutritional support.

Early diagnosis and treatment of the cause and prevention of infection are critical. Initially, the patient may require only supplemental oxygen. As the disease progresses, intubation and mechanical ventilation are instituted. The concentration of oxygen and ventilator settings are determined by the patient's status. PEEP is a critical part of the treatment of ARDS. PEEP increases FRC and reverses alveolar collapse, resulting in improved arterial oxygenation and a reduction in the V/Q imbalance. By using PEEP, a lower FIO_2 is required.

Systemic hypotension is not uncommon in ARDS. The cause frequently is related to hypovolemia secondary to leakage of fluid into the interstitial spaces. Hypovolemia should be carefully treated. Maintaining an adequate fluid balance without causing further overload is difficult. Intravenous crystalloid solutions are required with careful monitoring of pulmonary status.

TABLE 26–3.   *Factors Related to ARDS*

Aspiration (gastric secretions, drowning, hydrocarbons)

Drug ingestion and overdose

Hematologic disorders (disseminated intravascular coagulopathy, massive transfusions, cardiopulmonary bypass)

Prolonged inhalation of high concentrations of oxygen, smoke, or corrosive substances

Localized infection (bacterial, fungal, viral pneumonia)

Metabolic disorders (pancreatitis, uremia)

Shock (any cause)

Trauma (pulmonary contusion, multiple fractures, head injury)

Major surgery

Fat or air embolism

Systemic sepsis

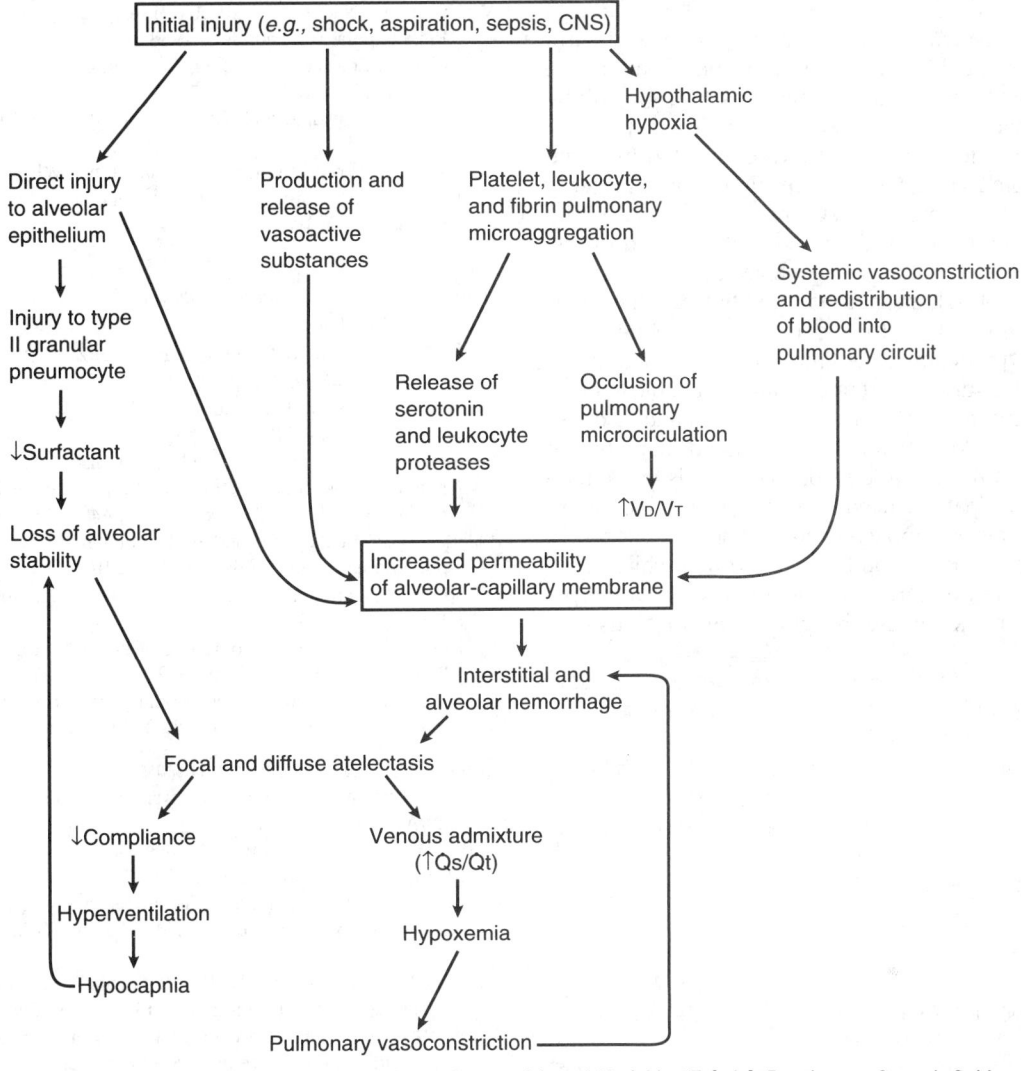

Figure 26–4. Pathogenesis of ARDS. (After Burton GG and Hodgkin JE [eds]. Respiratory Care: A Guide to Clinical Practice, 2nd ed. Philadelphia, JB Lippincott, 1984.)

Inotropic or vasopressor agents may be required. The Swan-Ganz readings are used to monitor the patient's fluid status.

The use of corticosteroids in the treatment of ARDS is controversial. Many believe that, in fact, their use may contribute to a deterioration in pulmonary function and the development of superinfections.

Adequate nutritional support is vital in the treatment of ARDS. Patients with ARDS require 35 to 45 kcal/kg a day to meet normal requirements. Enteral feeding is the first consideration; however, total parenteral nutrition also may be required.

Nursing Interventions

The patient with acute respiratory failure and ARDS is seriously ill and requires close monitoring because his condition could quickly change to a life-threatening situation. Most of the respiratory modalities discussed in Chapter 25 will be used in this situation (oxygen administration, mini-nebulizer therapy, chest physiotherapy, endotracheal intubation or tracheostomy, suctioning, tracheostomy care, and ventilator management).

Frequent assessment of the patient's status is necessary to evaluate the effectiveness of treatment.

In addition to implementing the medical plan of care, the nurse considers other needs of the patient. If the patient is not being mechanically ventilated, he is placed in semi-Fowler's or high-Fowler's position to allow maximum excursion of the thorax. He is supported in whatever position he feels most comfortable, using pillows, blankets, or an overbed table. If fluids are not restricted, fluid intake is encouraged to correct fluid loss that occurs during rapid breathing and to loosen secretions. The patient will be extremely anxious because of the hypoxemia and dyspnea. The nurse should reassure him of the ability and concern of the health care team, explain all procedures, and deliver care in a calm, patient manner. It is important to reduce the patient's anxiety because its manifestations prevent rest and increase oxygen expenditure. Rest is essential to conserve oxygen use, thereby reducing the oxygen need.

If the patient is on PEEP, there are several unique nursing considerations. PEEP is an unnatural pattern of breathing and will feel strange to the patient. He is reassured about his status and encouraged to work with the ventilator. If the PEEP level is not maintained, pancuronium (Pavulon) or another neuromuscular blocker may be administered. In this situation, the patient loses motor function but retains sensation. He will be paralyzed and unable to breathe, talk, or blink. The nurse must be sure the patient does not become disconnected from the ventilator. Neuromuscular blockers paralyze the respiratory muscles so the patient does not resist the ventilator and PEEP. This means that the patient will be apneic if removed or disconnected from the ventilator. Consequently, the nurse ensures that the patient is closely monitored at all times. When he is removed from the ventilator for suctioning or measurements, it is done quickly to minimize the time without ventilation. He also may experience discomfort or pain and be unable to communicate these sensations. The patient will appear unconscious, yet be awake and able to hear. He is reassured that what he is experiencing is a result of the medication and is temporary. The nurse must anticipate his needs regarding pain and comfort. The nurse checks his position to ensure that he is comfortable, and she talks *to* the patient and not *about* him while in his presence. Complete eye care is important because of the patient's inability to blink and the risk of corneal abrasions.

In summary, ARDS is a type of noncardiogenic pulmonary edema associated with a variety of clinical disorders, resulting in alveolar capillary membrane injury, causing leakage of fluid into the alveolar interstitial spaces and capillary bed. The morbidity and mortality rate in ARDS remains high despite advances in the understanding of the pathogenesis of the disease. Identification of ''at risk'' patients, early detection, and treatment are critical in improving patient outcomes.

Bibliography

Books

Baum GL and Wolinsky E. Textbook of Pulmonary Diseases, 4th ed, Vols 2 & 12. Boston, Little, Brown, 1989.

Braunwald E et al. Harrison's Principles of Internal Medicine. New York, McGraw-Hill, 1987.

Burton GA and Hodgkin JE. Respiratory Care: A Guide to Clinical Practice. Philadelphia, JB Lippincott, 1984.

Cox BG and Carr DT. Living with Lung Cancer: A Guide for Patients and their Families. Gainesville, Triad Publishing, 1987.

DiPiro JT et al. Pharmacotherapy: A Pathophysiologic Approach. New York, Elsevier, 1989.

Fincke MK and Lanros NE. Emergency Nursing: A Comprehensive Guide. Rockville, Aspen, 1986.

Fishman FP. Pulmonary Diseases and Disorders, 2nd ed, Vols 1–3. New York, McGraw-Hill, 1988.

Groenwald SL. Cancer Nursing: Principles and Practices. Boston, Jones & Bartlett, 1987.

Gurevich I. Infectious Diseases in Critical Care Nursing: Prevention and Precaution. Rockville, Aspen, 1989.

Hoeprich PD and Jordan MC. Infectious Disease, 4th ed. Philadelphia, JB Lippincott, 1989.

Holleb AI (ed). The American Cancer Society Cancer Book: Prevention, Detection, Diagnosis, Treatment, Rehabilitation, Cure. New York, Doubleday, 1986.

Kinney MR et al. AACN's Clinical Reference for Critical Care Nursing, 2nd ed. New York, McGraw-Hill, 1988.

Kitt S and Kaiser J. Emergency Nursing: A Physiologic and Clinical Perspective. Philadelphia, WB Saunders, 1990.

Mitchell RS et al (eds). Synopsis of Clinical Pulmonary Disease. St Louis, CV Mosby, 1989,

Morgan WKD and Seaton A. Occupational Lung Diseases, 2nd ed. Philadelphia, WB Saunders, 1984.

Murray JF and Nadel JA. Textbook of Respiratory Medicine, Vols 1 & 2. Philadelphia, WB Saunders, 1988.

Rea RE et al. Emergency Nursing Core Curriculum, 3rd ed. Philadelphia, WB Saunders, 1987.

Rowe JW and Besdine RW. Geriatric Medicine, 2nd ed. Boston, Little, Brown, 1988.

Roth JA et al. Thoracic Oncology. Philadelphia, WB Saunders, 1989.

Ziegfeld CR (ed). Core Curriculum for Oncology Nursing. Philadelphia, WB Saunders, 1987.

Journals

Asterisks indicate nursing research articles.

Pulmonary Infection

Bryan CS. Preventing pneumonia and influenza deaths in 1989–90. Consultant 1989 Nov; 29(11): 25–31.

Carden DL and Smith KJ. Pneumonias. Emerg Med Clin North Am 1989 May; 7(2): 255–278.

Griffiths MH et al. Diagnosis of pulmonary disease in human immunodeficiency virus infection: Role of transbronchial biopsy and bronchoalveolar lavage. Thorax 1989 Jul; 44(7): 554–558.

* Harkness GA, Bentley DW, and Roghmann KJ. Risk factors for nosocomial pneumonia in the elderly. Am J Med 1990 Oct; 89(4): 456–463.

Niederman MS. Pneumonia: The ongoing challenge. Emerg Med 1989 Apr 15; 21(7): 77–88.

Pennza PT. Aspiration pneumonia, necrotizing pneumonia and lung abscess. Emerg Med Clin North Am 1989 May; 7(2): 279–307.

Raju L. Community acquired pneumonia, today's organisms, today's treatment. Consultant 1988 Apr; 28(4): 49–57.

Chronic Obstructive Pulmonary Disease

* Gift AG. Clinical measurement of dyspnea. Dimens Crit Care Nurs 1989 Jul/Aug; 8(4): 210–216.

Harman EM. Status asthmaticus: Reduce risk factors and treat aggressively. Consultant 1989 May; 29(5): 129–135.

Hudson LD and Monti CM. Rationale and use of corticosteroids in chronic obstructive pulmonary disease. Med Clin North Am 1990 May; 74(3): 661–690.

* Janson–Bjerklie S and Shnell S. Effect of peak flow information on patterns of self-care in adult asthma. Heart Lung 1988 Sep; 17(5): 543–549.

Martin RJ. The sleep-related worsening of lower airways obstruction: Understanding and intervention. Med Clin North Am 1990 May; 74(3): 701–714.

McDonald AJ. Asthma. Emerg Med Clin North Am 1989 May; 7(2): 219–235.

Petty TL. Chronic obstructive pulmonary disease: Can we do better? Chest 1990 Feb Suppl; 97(2): 2S–5S.

* Renfroe KL. Effect of progressive relaxation of dyspnea and state anxiety in patients with chronic obstructive pulmonary disease. Heart Lung 1988 Jul; 17(4): 408–413.

Rosen RL and Bone RC. Treatment of acute exacerbations in chronic obstructive pulmonary disease. Med Clin North Am 1990 May; 74(3): 691–700.

Schneider SM. Chronic obstructive pulmonary disease. Emerg Med Clin North Am 1989 May; 7(2): 237–254.

Lung Cancer

Bragg DG. State-of-the-art assessment: Diagnostic imaging. Cancer 1989 Jul 1 Suppl; 64(1): 261–265.

Carr D. Lung cancer: Pitfalls and controversies in diagnosis and treatment. Consultant 1988 May; 28(5): 33–45.

Hulka BS. Cancer screening—Degrees of proof and practical application. Cancer 1988 Oct 15 Suppl; 62(8): 1776–1780.

Livingston R and Goodman GE. Small cell lung cancer. Curr Probl Cancer 1989 Jan/Feb; 7–54.

Trauma

Alexander MH. Mechanism and pattern of injury associated with use of seat belts. J Emerg Nurs 1988 Jul/Aug; 14(4): 214–216.

Carrero R and Wayne M. Chest trauma. Emerg Clin North Am 1989 May; 7(2): 389–418.

Coleman GM et al. Blunt chest trauma extrapericardial cardiac tamponade by mediastinal hematoma. Chest 1989 Apr; 95(4): 922–924.

Halpern JS. Mechanisms and patterns of trauma. J Emerg Nurs 1989 Sep/Oct; 15(5): 380–388.

Martin K. Reducing complications of thoracic gunshot wounds. Dimens Crit Care Nurs 1989 Sep/Oct; 8(5): 280–287.

Acute Respiratory Failure and ARDS

Bresler MJ and Steinback GL. The adult respiratory distress syndrome. Emerg Med Clin North Am 1989 May; 7(2): 419–430.

Hudson LD. The prediction and prevention of ARDS. Respir Care 1990 Feb; 35(2): 161–173.

Idell S. The deadly danger of ARDS. Emerg Med 1989 Apr 15; 21(7): 67–72.

Raffin TA. ARDS: Mechanisms and management. Hosp Pract 1987 Nov 15; 22(2): 65–80.

Root RK. The adult respiratory distress syndrome. West J Med 1989 Feb; 150(2): 187–194.

Pulmonary Vascular Disorders

Dunmire SM. Pulmonary embolism. Emerg Clin North Am 1989 May; 7(2): 339–354.

Manigle JE and Tenholder MF. Treatment for primary pulmonary hypertension: Back to the future. Chest 1989 Oct; 96(4): 900–905.

Pais SO and Tobin KD. Percutaneous insertion of the Greenfield filter. Am J Roentgenol 1989 May; 152(5): 933–938.

Schiff MJ. Finding and fighting pulmonary embolism. Emerg Med 1989 Apr 15; 21(7): 47–52.

Occupational Lung Diseases

Begin R et al. Lung function in silica-exposed worker: A relationship to disease severity assessed by CT scan. Chest 1988 Sep; 94(3): 539–545.

Dunn MM. Asbestos and the lung. Chest 1989 Jun; 95(6): 1304–1308.

Green F et al. Prevalence of silicosis at death in underground coal miners. Am J Indust Med 1989 Jun; 16(6): 605–615.

Mossman BT and Gee JB. Asbestos-related diseases. N Engl J Med 1989 Jun 19; 320(16): 1721–1730.

Miscellaneous

* Chulay M and Graeber GM. Efficacy of a hyperinflation and hyperoxygenation suctioning intervention. Heart Lung 1988 Jan; 17(1): 15–22.

Gothe B. Sleep apnea syndrome: An update. Respir Manag 1988 Mar/Apr; 18(2): 40–44.

* Henneman EA. Effect of nursing contact on the stress response of patients being weaned from mechanical ventilation. Heart Lung 1989 Sep; 18(5): 483–489.

* Kleiber C et al. Acute histologic changes in the tracheobronchial tree associated with different suction catheter insertion techniques. Heart Lung 1988 Jan; 17(1): 10–14.

* Lush MT et al. Dyspnea in the ventilator-assisted patient. Heart Lung 1988 Sep; 17(5): 528–535.

Martin LL. Obstructive sleep apnea: Preventing complications. Dimens Crit Care Nurs 1989 Mar/Apr; 8(2): 83–91.

* Preusser BA et al. Effects of two methods of preoxygenation on mean arterial pressure, cardiac out, peak airway pressure and post-suctioning hypoxemia. Heart Lung 1988 May; 17(3): 290–299.

* Roberts R et al. Diagnostic accuracy of fever as a measure of post-operative pulmonary complications. Heart Lung 1988 Mar; 17(2): 166–170.

* Rogge JA et al. Effectiveness of oxygen concentrations of less than 100% before and after endotracheal suction in patients with chronic obstructive pulmonary disease. Heart Lung 1989 Jan; 18(1): 64–70.

* Stone KS et al. Effects of lung hyperinflation on mean arterial pressure and post-suctioning hypoxemia. Heart Lung 1989 Jul; 18(4): 377–385.

* Stovsky B et al. Comparison of two types of communication methods used after cardiac surgery with patients with endotracheal tubes. Heart Lung 1988 May; 17(3): 281–289.

* Taggart JA et al. Airway pressures during closed system suctioning. Heart Lung 1988 Sep; 17(5): 536–542.

VuKick DL. Disease of the pleural space. Emerg Clin North Am 1989 May; 7(2): 309–324.

Wanner A. The role of mucus in chronic obstructive pulmonary disease. Chest 1990 Feb Suppl; 97(2): 11S–15S.

Waring NP. The late phase asthma response: The laboratory phenomenon that has become a hot clinical issue. Consultant 1988 Oct; 128(10): 123–133.

Nursing Research Profile for Unit 6

Respiratory Nursing

Overview

Most of the current respiratory nursing research centers on preventing detrimental sequelae to suctioning in intubated patients. The problems investigated ranged from postsuctioning hypoxemia to variances in mean arterial pressure and heart rate to tissue injury incurred by suction catheters. Many of those studies produced results easily incorporated into routine nursing practice.

Additionally, nurses are searching for methods to adequately assess dyspnea in patients and to assist patients with pulmonary disorders in coping with symptoms.

Dyspnea Management and Respiratory Muscle Exercise

▷ Janson-Bjerklie S and Shnell S. *Effect of peak flow information on patterns of self-care in adult asthma.* Heart Lung 1988 Sep; 17(5): 543–549.

This study investigated the influence of subjective and objective information on patients' selection of self-care strategies for management of asthma symptoms.

The design of this study was quasi-experimental with additional descriptive features. Twenty-eight patients (adults) with diagnosed asthma without other cardiopulmonary problems were recruited from the clinics of a large university medical center and placed in either the control or experimental group. Subjects were given logs in which to document the date and time of each symptom episode (a period of shortness of breath, chest tightness, or wheezing), to note the intensity of symptoms, and to record what they believed to be the precipitating factors and what strategies they used to control symptoms. The experimental group received mini Wright peak flowmeters to measure peak expiratory flow rates at the beginning and at the end of each episode. A visual analog scale (VAS) was used by all participants to rate the severity of their symptoms separately—dyspnea, wheezing, and chest tightness. This rating was performed for each episode and recorded in their logs.

All subjects experienced dyspnea, wheezing, and chest tightness and were able to differentiate and rate the intensity of each symptom. There were no significant differences in symptom scores between groups when compared by unpaired two-tailed *t* tests.

Precipitants of the recorded asthma symptom episodes were categorized into physical conditions, mechanical behaviors, emotions or moods, tense situations, allergens, environmental conditions, and physical activities. All categories of precipitants were recorded with equal frequency.

The mean number of relief strategies used by subjects from both groups during the study period was significantly less than the number of strategies reported by subjects in previous interviews as available methods of managing asthmatic symptoms. The number of strategies used by patients correlated significantly with high scores of dyspnea reported by patients. Use of prescribed medications was subjectively rated as the most efficacious of reported strategies. The control group rated most strategies as more efficacious than did the experimental group and used medication strategies significantly more often than the experimental group.

The results of this study indicate that when subjects have access to peak flow information, they use their medications less frequently. The peak flow information may have helped them use their medication more appropriately. However, they also used fewer other strategies. The authors also report that none of the patients in either group used their medications as originally prescribed.

Nursing Implications. The symptom of dyspnea, rather than other symptoms, led patients to use more strategies for relief. Health care providers need to be aware that patients are reliable sources of information about their degree of airflow obstruction. Additionally, the more strategies known by patients, the more strategies they use. Therefore, patients may benefit by being educated about a number of strategies to control symptoms. This study indicates that patients given peak flow information and appropriate education can adjust their medication regimens safely within prescribed guidelines. This study also indicates that physiologic feedback may facilitate self-care behaviors. Instructions to pay close attention to symptoms, such as dyspnea and chest tightness, and to correlate these with peak flow information, are vital.

▷ Lush MT et al. *Dyspnea in the ventilator-assisted patient.* Heart Lung 1988 Sep; 17(5): 528–535.

The authors' primary purposes were to document the occurrence of dyspnea in five patients receiving mechanical ventilation, to identify physiologic variables associated with dyspneic episodes, and to describe environmental factors associated with dyspnea. A secondary purpose was to establish the concurrent validity of two measures of dyspnea in patients with mechanical ventilation. Five alert and oriented patients with restrictive or obstructive pulmonary disease, who were receiving mechanical ventilation, participated in this study. At 4-hour intervals and at the complaint of dyspnea, patients quantified the severity of their dyspnea using a VAS and Modified Borg Scale (MBS). At each measurement, nurses observed concomitant physiologic and environmental variables for up to 30 minutes before the episode and took measures to relieve the dyspnea. A postextubation interview also was conducted.

All patients had episodes of dyspnea during the study. The level of dyspnea measured by the VAS for the five patients ranged from 0 to 95 mm on a scale of 0 to 100 mm. Selected physiologic variables readily observable and available at the bedside to nurses on a routine basis were correlated with severity of dyspnea as measured by the VAS. Few of the correlations were statistically significant. A moderate, positive statistically significant correlation was found between the number of environmental events and severity of dyspnea recorded on both the MBS and the VAS.

Each time dyspnea severity was measured, nurses recorded actions taken to control the symptoms. The most frequent actions taken by nurses were suctioning, changing the patient's position, and administering a breathing bag to the patient.

In the postextubation interview, most patients attributed the onset of dyspnea to nursing care activities such as suctioning, turning, weighing, and physical therapy exercises. The nurses' reports of supposed patient dyspnea were not necessarily supported by patients' ratings of dyspnea intensity.

Nursing Implications.   The number of conditions, events, and activities occurring simultaneously in the patient's environment may be related to the development of dyspnea. As this study indicated, a lack of congruence existed between nurses' and patients' perception of dyspnea. Consideration should be given to incorporating the VAS or MBS into nursing care to facilitate the routine evaluation of dyspnea. It is suggested that future studies examine the interactive effects of environmental events on the severity of dyspnea in patients undergoing mechanical ventilation.

▷ Renfroe KL. *Effect of progressive relaxation on dyspnea and state anxiety in patients with chronic obstructive pulmonary disease. Heart Lung* 1988 Jul; 17(4): 408–413.

Renfroe speculated that progressive muscle relaxation (PMR) training would have a positive effect on dyspnea and anxiety in patients with chronic obstructive pulmonary disease (COPD).

Twenty patients with diagnoses of COPD were randomly assigned to either the control or the experimental group. Criteria for inclusion in the study were (1) diagnosis of bronchial asthma, chronic bronchitis, emphysema, or all of these; (2) dyspnea on exertion; (3) absence of serious medical problems other than COPD; and (4) absence of acute disorders at the time of the study.

A VAS for dyspnea was used before and after each treatment session. Spielberger's State Anxiety Inventory, form Y-1, was also administered before and after each session. Forced expiratory volume (FEV) and forced vital capacity (FVC) were measured as indicators of pulmonary function before and after each session with a Wright portable spirometer. Heart and respiratory rates were measured for 1 full minute with a stopwatch.

After testing, each patient in the control group was es-

corted to a room equipped with lounge chairs and instructed to relax for 45 minutes in any way they wished. The experimental group was escorted to an identical room and instructed in the methods of PMR. The procedure recommended by Bernstein and Borkovec for tension-release in 16 muscle groups was followed. Each session lasted 45 minutes. Four weekly sessions in the clinical setting were conducted by the researcher. Patients were asked to practice the procedure once daily after the first session. A tape recording of the session was given to each patient for use at home.

After the 45-minute relaxation time, both groups were retested. A greater reduction in dyspnea and anxiety occurred during each session for patients in the PMR group than for patients in the control group. Additionally, respiratory and heart rate decreased significantly more in the PMR group from the beginning of the first session to the end of the fourth session.

Of the 20 patients who began the study, only 14 completed all four sessions. The 6 patients who did not complete the study did so for a variety of personal and medical reasons. Group membership of the study dropouts was not specified.

Nursing Implications.   This study supports the use of PMR to produce immediate reduction of dyspnea and anxiety for patients with COPD. Further, the data suggest that the two symptoms are probably related.

Progressive relaxation can be taught to patients in inpatient, outpatient, and home settings. The use of videotaped and audiotaped instructions could be provided as a patient teaching adjunct after a session of progressive relaxation training.

Endotracheal Suctioning

▷ Kleiber C, Krutzfield N, and Rose EF. *Acute histologic changes in the tracheobronchial tree associated with different suction catheter insertion techniques. Heart Lung* 1988 Jan; 17(1): 10–14.

The authors proposed to describe a safer method of deep endotracheal suctioning in the neonatal intensive care unit. Four groups of anesthetized, intubated kittens were involved in this study. Two groups were subjected to the insertion of a suction catheter to a calibrated or predetermined distance (0.5 cm beyond the end of the endotracheal tube) and withdrawal with or without the application of suction. The other two groups were subjected to the insertion of the catheter until resistance was met and withdrawal with or without the application of suction. A fifth group in which suction catheters were not introduced into the airway served as a control group.

The experimental groups had the following in common:

1. Each subject received the manually delivered breaths with a Hope II resuscitation bag before and after each suction catheter insertion to minimize hypoxemia.
2. Catheter insertions were performed three times per episode.
3. Sixteen episodes were completed with each subject, for a total of 48 suction catheter insertions per subject.
4. Episodes were spaced 10 minutes apart to allow for physiologic recovery from the suctioning events.
5. Catheters were size 6 Fr, 14 in long, sterile and vinyl, with two directly opposed side holes and a contoured open tip with 1-cm numeric markings.
6. The same experienced registered nurse performed all the suctioning episodes.

After these procedures, the animals were killed and autopsy was performed to examine the effects of the procedures on the mucosa of the trachea and bronchi. All the animals in the control group and the two groups in which the suction catheters were introduced to 0.5 cm beyond the end of the endotracheal tube had normal tissues. Nine of the 10 animals in the groups that had the suction catheter introduced to the point of resistance displayed focal areas of denudation of the epithelium of the mucosa with varying degrees of inflammation. The application of suction had no effect on the amount of tissue damage sustained.

Nursing Implications. The authors strongly suggest that catheter insertion should stop short of the carina. They suggest that, in addition to causing less tissue damage, this restriction may reduce the risk of a bacteremia caused by trauma to the bronchial epithelium during routine deep endotracheal suctioning.

Additionally, the authors caution practitioners to examine suction catheters and endotracheal tubes for the location and accuracy of markings.

Although one cannot generalize the results of these findings to human infants or adults, the authors suggest that caution be used in suction procedures. The findings also suggest the need for subsequent studies in humans.

▷ *Chulay M and Graeber GM. Efficacy of a hyperinflation and hyperoxygenation suctioning intervention. Heart Lung 1988 Jan; 17(1): 15–22.*

The authors proposed to describe the effects of five hyperinflation breaths with hyperoxygenation, administered before and after endotracheal tube suctioning, on arterial blood gas levels and cardiac dysrhythmias. The study used anesthetized paralyzed sheep (N = 27) in four different groups with protocols as follows:

Protocol 1. Sheep with normal lung function (N = 10) were studied. Suction alone was compared with mechanical delivery of the hyperinflation and hyperoxygenation intervention by means of a second ventilator.

Protocol 2. Sheep with abnormal lung function induced by the endotracheal instillation of hydrochloric and taurodeoxycholic acids (N = 7) were studied 3 hours after instillation. Suction alone was compared with mechanical delivery of the hyperinflation and hyperoxygen intervention using a second ventilator.

Protocol 3. Sheep with normal lung function (N = 5) were studied. Suction alone was compared with the manual delivery of the hyperinflation and hyperoxygenation intervention by means of two different models of manual resuscitation bags.

Protocol 4. Sheep with abnormal lung function induced by endotracheal instillation of hydrochloric and taurodeoxycholic acids (N = 5) were studied 3 hours after instillation. Suction alone was compared with manual delivery methods described in protocol 3.

The dependent variables in this study included arterial blood gas levels, heart rate, blood pressure, and electrocardiogram findings.

The animals in all groups had decreases in arterial oxygen tension (PaO_2) after endotracheal suction alone. The administration of five hyperinflation breaths with hyperoxygenation before and after endotracheal suctioning was effective in preventing PaO_2 decreases after suctioning in sheep with normal lung function when either a mechanical or a manual delivery technique was used. In sheep with abnormal lung function, the mechanical delivery technique was effective, but the manual delivery was not.

Only two animals had cardiac dysrhythmias during the study periods of any protocols. One animal (protocol 1) displayed frequent premature ventricular contractions during the aspiration of blood from a carotid artery catheter before the suctioning intervention. The other animal, also from protocol 1, experienced occasional premature atrial contractions throughout the study. There were no significant changes in heart rate or blood pressure during any of the suctioning interventions.

Nursing Implications. The findings suggest that the response to hyperinflation and hyperoxygenation differs in subjects with normal versus abnormal lung function as well as mechanical versus manual delivery techniques. Because of these differences, laboratory evaluation of endotracheal tube suctioning interventions should use abnormal lung function models rather than normal models to more closely approximate the critically ill population.

▷ *Preusser BA et al. Effects of two methods of preoxygenation on mean arterial pressure, cardiac output, peak airway pressure, and post-suctioning hypoxemia. Heart Lung 1988 May; 17(3): 290–299.*

The authors of this study proposed to determine which method of preoxygenation, manual resuscitation bag or ventilator, produced the least change in mean arterial pressure, cardiac output, and peak airway pressure and prevented post-suctioning hypoxemia during preoxygenation at two different lung inflation volumes.

An experimental research design was used in which the subjects served as their own controls. Ten patients scheduled to undergo coronary artery bypass surgery were included in the study. Three lung inflation breaths at fraction of inspired oxygen concentration (FIO_2) 1.0 were delivered at 12 and 14 ml/kg of lean body weight through ventilator or manual resuscitation bag, followed by 10 seconds of continuous endotracheal suctioning. This sequence was repeated once an hour for 4 consecutive hours.

The delivery of a preoxygenation breath, whether by manual resuscitation bag or ventilator, increased mean arterial pressure (MAP), cardiac output, and peak airway pressure (PAP). Volume also significantly affected these three variables. The manual resuscitation bag generated a significantly higher PAP than did the ventilator. The larger the volume in preoxygenation, the greater the increase in MAP and PAP irrespective of delivery method. Further, the cardiac output increased after the protocol with the manual resuscitation bag causing a greater increase than did the ventilator. Both methods effectively prevented postsuctioning hypoxemia. It was also found that the ventilator produced a peak PaO_2 that exceeded that produced by the resuscitation bag by 30%. In this study, the manual resuscitation bag caused a greater decline in pH and a greater increase in $PaCO_2$ than the ventilator at both preoxygenation volumes.

Nursing Implications. Based on study findings, it is recommended that nurses use smaller volumes delivered by means of a ventilator when preoxygenating before endotracheal suctioning.

If a manual resuscitation bag must be used, it is strongly recommended that the oxygen flowmeter be turned to flush, a bag with a large reservoir be used, and the bag be primed slowly using a two-handed compression followed by a slow refill. When possible, a test of the bag's FiO_2 with an oxygen analyzer should be performed. The patient should also receive preoxygenation breaths with smaller volumes synchronized with the patient's own respiratory efforts to minimize PAP. Finally, it is important to note the patient's MAP before the suctioning episode and to observe the patient, monitoring the mean arterial pressure, for at least 10 minutes after the procedure.

▷ Taggart JA, Dorinsky NL, and Sheahan JS. *Airway pressures during closed system suctioning.* Heart Lung 1988 Sep; 17(5): 536–542.

The authors proposed to delineate the airway pressures obtained during closed system suctioning (CSS) in an *in vitro* descriptive study involving the use of different ventilators as well as combinations of ventilator settings. Closed system suctioning is a method of removing secretions from the tracheobronchial tree of patients undergoing mechanical ventilation. Each ventilator was connected to a Vent Aid Training Test Lung and set at a ventilatory rate of 12/min and a tidal volume of 800 ml. CSS was performed at peak inspiratory flow rates of 25, 40, 50, and 60 L/min, at sensitivities of 0.5, 1.0, 2.0, and 3.0 cm H_2O, with and without positive end-expiratory pressure (PEEP) of 10 cm H_2O, and in modes of intermittent mandatory ventilation, assist control, and control.

With an *in vitro* lung model and the various combinations of ventilator types and settings, airway pressure was maintained above -10 cm H_2O during CSS in most situations. Two specific ventilator settings were associated with significant drops in airway pressure during CSS. First, the control mode of ventilation consistently produced peak negative pressures less than -10 cm H_2O. Second, when the Puritan-Bennett 7200 ventilator was set at a peak inspiratory flow rate of 25 L/min, the peak negative airway pressures dropped below -10 cm H_2O.

Nursing Implications. The findings of this study provide a framework to continue research in the clinical setting. The data suggest that the control mode of ventilation should be avoided in humans during CSS. In addition, peak inspiratory flow rates of greater than 25 L/min should be used with a Puritan-Bennett 7200 model ventilator. Future studies must also address ventilatory rate, because evidence suggests that CSS may produce dangerously low airway pressures when lower rates are used.

▷ Stone KS et al. *Effects of lung hyperinflation on mean arterial pressure and post-suctioning hypoxemia.* Heart Lung 1989 Jul; 18(4): 377–385.

The authors of this study proposed to determine the effect of five different lung hyperinflation volumes on the mean arterial pressure and postsuctioning hypoxemia.

Eight patients undergoing coronary artery bypass surgery were selected for the study. All patients (1) were intubated and placed on MA1 ventilators at 8 to 10 breaths/min at an FiO_2 of 40% without PEEP, (2) had arterial lines in place, and (3) were receiving IV lidocaine and nitroglycerine.

The five volumes examined in this study were based on the patient's lean body weight (LBW) and included the patient's prescribed tidal volume, 12 ml/kg LBW, 14 ml/kg LBW, 16 ml/kg LBW, and 18 ml/kg LBW.

The lung hyperinflation volumes were calculated and rounded to the nearest tenth. They were also calculated to accommodate for dead space.

The five volumes were randomly administered to each subject through a second primed MA1 ventilator. Control data regarding vital signs, MAP, and blood gases were gathered within 2 minutes before the experimental protocol was instituted. The patient received three consecutive lung hyperinflations at one of the randomly ordered volumes within a timed 15-second period. After the third hyperinflation, continuous suction was applied for 10 seconds. This sequence was repeated for a total of three times, then the patient was returned to the first ventilator. The study protocol was repeated each hour until all five volumes were randomly tested.

MAP was monitored continuously. Chest excursion was also measured as well as the electrocardiogram. Arterial blood gas samples were drawn after the suctioning at designated intervals.

The results of this study showed a statistically significant mean increase of 15 mm Hg in MAP over the three hyperinflation sequences. Results also showed a statistically significant change in MAP from one hyperinflation–suction sequence to the next. No statistically significant relationship was found between the five lung volumes and the change in MAP. The data indicated that these results were produced by the interaction of the lung hyperinflations and suctioning over time.

The greatest increase in PaO_2 occurred immediately after the suction pass. This increase was followed by a rapid decline at 30 seconds after suctioning that gradually returned to baseline.

With each increasing lung volume, there was a corresponding increase in PaO_2 immediately after the last suction pass. There was no statistically significant relationship between the five hyperinflation volumes and O_2 saturation.

Nursing Implications. A mean increase of 15 mm Hg in MAP for all five volumes tested can be clinically significant for patients after coronary artery bypass grafting surgery because these patients frequently have postoperative hypertension. These findings also have implications for patients with increased intracranial pressure.

A preliminary recommendation may be to limit the lung hyperinflation suction sequences to two per session.

In this study, all subjects had normal lung function. The study should be replicated in subjects with lung impairments.

Mechanical Ventilation: Communication Methods and Weaning

▷ Henneman EA. *Effect of nursing contact on the stress response of patients being weaned from mechanical ventilation.* Heart Lung 1989 Sep; 18(5): 483–489.

This prospective, randomized investigation was undertaken to determine the effect of direct nursing contact on the stress response of patients being weaned from mechanical ventilation. Twenty-six patients meeting the following criteria were placed in either the control or experimental group: (1) receiving mechanical ventilation for at least 24 hours, (2) being weaned by the T-piece method, (3) being weaned for the first time, (4) alert enough to follow simple commands, and (5) able to perceive verbal and tactile stimuli.

Before the initiation of weaning, both groups received the same physical and psychologic preparation from the nurse researcher. In the experimental group, the nurse stayed at the bedside, held the patient's hand, and talked with the patient throughout the weaning period. For the control group, the nurse stayed in the room but not in direct physical contact with the patient.

During the data collection period, the environment was strictly controlled with minimal interruptions. Heart rate, blood pressure, and respiratory rate measurements were collected at 5-minute intervals over a 25-minute period after the initiation of weaning.

No significant difference was found between the stress response of patients being weaned who received direct nursing care and those who did not. However, it is speculated that the nurse, by psychologically preparing the patient for weaning, being present during the process, and controlling the environment, effectively diminished the stress response for all patients in this study.

Nursing Implications. These findings suggest that touch and verbal interaction may not be stress reducing during efforts to wean patients from ventilators. Further study with a larger sample is indicated.

▷ *Stovsky B, Rudy E, and Dragonette P. Comparison of two types of communication methods used after cardiac surgery with patients with endotracheal tubes. Heart Lung 1988 May; 17(3): 281–289.*

Two types of communication techniques (planned and unplanned) were compared for effectiveness of communication in the early postoperative intubation period for patients undergoing cardiac surgery. The control group (N = 20) relied on the experience and creativity of the nurse providing the preoperative education and the postoperative care. The experimental group (N = 20) was instructed on the use of a communication board before surgery and used the board during the postoperative intubation period.

The research question addressed: Does a planned method of communication with a communication board increase patient satisfaction or nurse satisfaction as compared with an unplanned method using spontaneous communication techniques in the early postoperative intubation period with patients undergoing cardiac surgery?

The unplanned methods included (1) having the patient write, (2) having the patient use hand gestures such as pointing, (3) lip-reading, (4) asking the patient yes and no questions, and (5) trying to interpret nonverbal cues.

The planned communication consisted of the use of a picture board with words, termed a *communication board.* Four instruments were used in the study: an open-ended patient interview; a nurse bedside assessment tool; a patient and nurse satisfaction questionnaire; and a VAS on satisfaction with communication.

The results confirmed that the communication board group had increased satisfaction with communications during the intubation period as compared with the unplanned communication group. Nurses, on the other hand, reported no significant increase in satisfaction with communication while using the communication board.

These differences between patient and nurse perception of satisfactory and unsatisfactory communication only highlighted the necessity of seeking the patient's point of view.

Nursing Implications. On the basis of the results of the study, the authors made the following recommendations:

1. Patients undergoing mechanical ventilation after surgery should be instructed on specific communication techniques before surgery.

2. The communication techniques taught before surgery should be available to all patients who have endotracheal tubes after surgery.
3. A communication board should be considered a supplement to other methods of communication being used.
4. The communication methods most useful for individual patients should be identified and integrated into the written care plan.
5. Communication can be facilitated by providing the patient's eyeglasses, removing any ophthalmic ointment from the patient's eyes after surgery, and optimizing the patient's visual field.

Fever

▷ *Roberts R et al. Diagnostic accuracy of fever as a measure of post-operative pulmonary complications. Heart Lung 1988 Mar; 17(2): 166–170.*

The authors proposed to quantify the diagnostic accuracy of fever as a measure of postoperative pulmonary complications and to describe the sensitivity, specificity, and positive and negative predictive values of fever.

Assessments using fever and chest radiography were determined for 270 patients after elective intra-abdominal surgery in three hospitals with six practicing surgeons in a southern Ontario city. These patients were part of a large randomized controlled trial determining the effectiveness of different regimens of analgesia in averting postoperative pulmonary complications. As a methodologic substudy of this trial, the temperature for each patient was recorded every 4 hours for 4 days after surgery. The maximum daily temperature was noted.

The prevalence of postoperative atelectasis among 270 patients undergoing elective intra-abdominal surgery was 57%. The prevalence of fever was 40%. The sensitivity, specificity, positive and negative predictive values, and accuracy of fever within 48 hours after surgery in predicting atelectasis were calculated for this population with a disease prevalence of 57%.

A fever (temperature of 38°C or higher) during the first 48 hours after surgery correctly identified 47% of subjects having some degree of atelectasis as evidenced by chest radiograph on day 4. A normal temperature correctly placed 68% of those without atelectasis. Sixty-six percent of those with fevers had evidence of atelectasis (positive predictive value), and 49% of those without fevers were free of atelectasis (negative predictive value). The accuracy with which the presence or absence of fever predicted correctly those with and without atelectasis was 56%.

The specificity, or the proportion of patients without atelectasis who had normal temperatures, was high (over 80%) for each day. However, the sensitivity, or the proportion with atelectasis who had fevers was low (8% to 29%). Additionally, the diagnostic accuracy of fever was only about 50%.

Nursing Implications. Fever during the first 48 hours or any fever on days 1 to 4 after surgery is not an accurate diagnostic measure for radiologic evidence of atelectasis on day 4 after surgery. Neither the presence nor the absence of fever can ensure clinicians of a present or absent pathologic pulmonary process. The clinician's assessment might be more important than the finding of fever in determining the clinical need for more diagnostic measures. Further, the use of fever as a criterion for the eligibility of subjects or as an outcome measure in clinical research should be avoided as an invalid measure of pulmonary pathologic conditions.

unit 7

Cardiovascular, Circulatory, and Hematologic Function

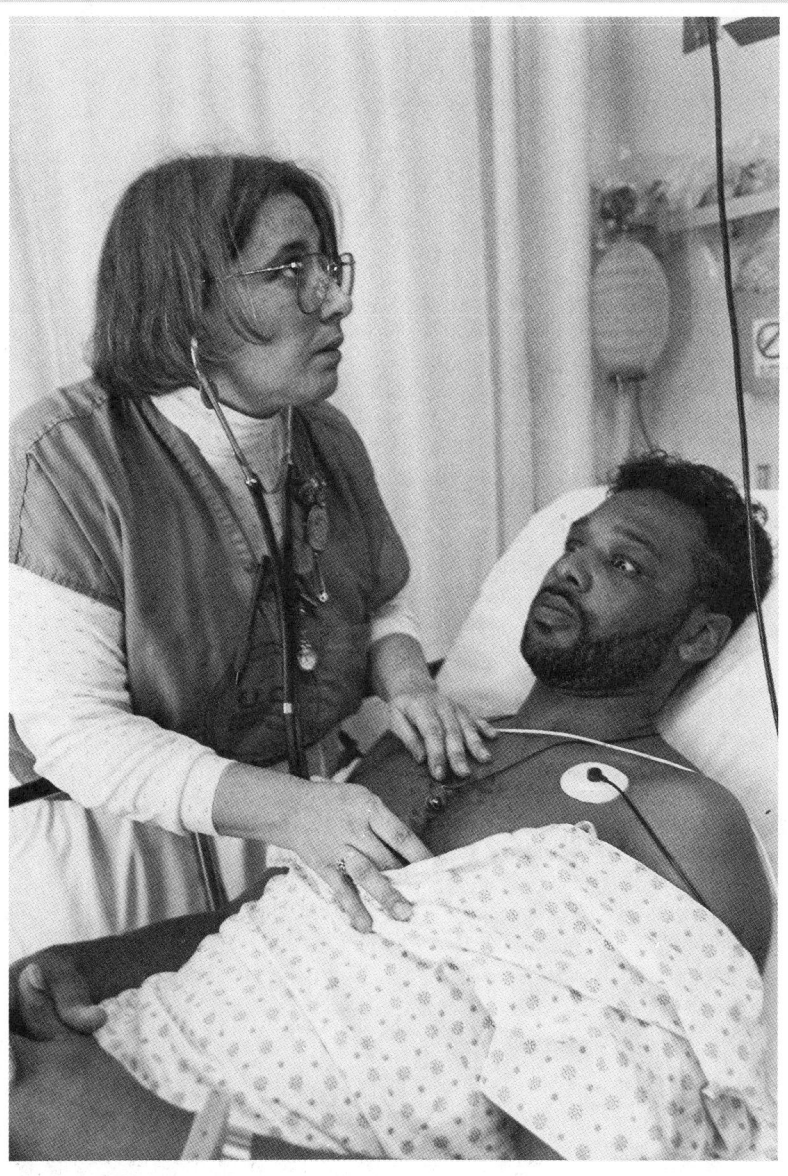

27

Assessment of Cardiovascular Function

Learning Objectives

On completion of this chapter, the learner will be able to:

1. Explain cardiac physiology in relation to cardiac anatomy and the normal conduction system of the heart
2. Incorporate assessment of cardiac risk factors into the health history and physical assessment of the cardiac patient
3. Use assessment parameters appropriate for determining the status of cardiovascular function
4. Correlate the components of the ECG with physiologic events of the heart
5. Use an ECG strip to determine heart rate
6. Determine the following information from an ECG strip: rate, presence or absence of P waves, PR interval, QRS interval, QT interval
7. Identify the clinical significance and related nursing implications of the various tests and procedures used for diagnostic assessment of cardiac function
8. Compare central venous pressure monitoring, pulmonary artery pressure monitoring, and systemic intra-arterial monitoring with regard to clinical usefulness and significance, nursing responsibilities, and possible complications

Nursing assessment of a patient with heart disease includes taking a history, performing a physical examination, and monitoring tests of cardiac functioning. Sound knowledge of cardiac anatomy, physiology, and pathophysiology is necessary for developing assessment skills, defining nursing diagnoses, planning nursing care, and understanding the purposes of diagnostic tests.

Overview of Cardiac Structure and Function

The heart is a hollow, muscular organ located in the center of the thorax, where it occupies the space between the lungs and rests on the diaphragm. It weighs approximately 300 g (10.6

oz), although heart weight and size are influenced by age, gender, body weight, frequency of physical exercise, and heart disease. The function of the heart is to pump blood to the tissues, supplying them with oxygen and other nutrients while removing carbon dioxide and other waste products of metabolism. There are actually two pumps within this organ, located on the right and left sides of the heart. The output of the right heart is distributed entirely to the lungs by the pulmonary artery, and the output of the left heart is distributed to the remainder of the body by the aorta. These two pumps eject blood simultaneously at approximately the same rate of output.

The pumping action of the heart is accomplished by the rhythmic contraction and relaxation of its muscular wall. During contraction of the muscle *(systole)*, the chambers of the heart become smaller as the blood is ejected. During relaxation of the muscles of the heart wall *(diastole)*, the heart chambers fill with blood in preparation for the subsequent ejection. A normal adult heart beats approximately 60 to 80 times per minute, ejects approximately 70 ml from either ventricle per beat, and has a total output of approximately 5 L/min.

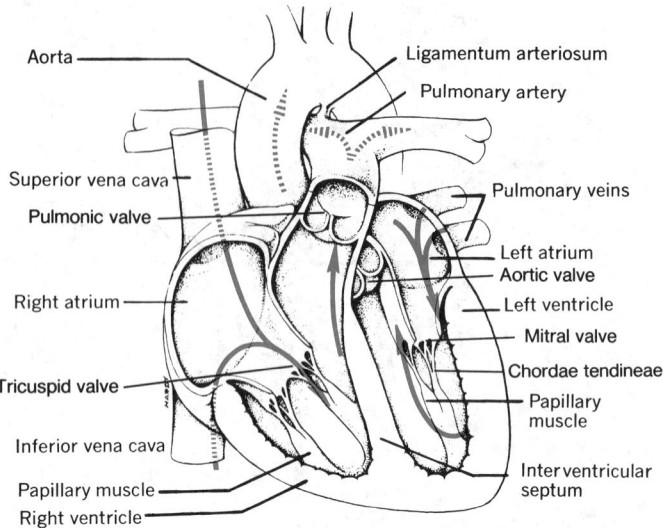

Figure 27–1.   Structure of the heart and course of blood flow through the heart chambers, as indicated by arrows. (Chaffee EE and Greisheimer EM. Basic Physiology and Anatomy. Philadelphia, JB Lippincott.)

Cardiac Anatomy

The area in the middle of the chest between the two lungs is called the *mediastinum*. The bulk of the mediastinal space is occupied by the heart, which is encased in a thin, fibrous sac called the *pericardium*.

The pericardium protects the surface of the heart but is not essential for its proper functioning. The space between the surface of the heart and the pericardial lining is filled with a very small amount of fluid, which lubricates the surface and reduces friction during cardiac muscle contraction.

Heart Chambers.   The right and left sides of the heart are each composed of two chambers, an *atrium* (pl. atria) and a *ventricle*. The common wall between the right and left chambers is called the *septum*. The ventricles are the chambers that eject blood into the arteries. The functions of the atria are to receive incoming blood from the veins and to act as temporary storage reservoirs for subsequent emptying into the ventricles. The relationship of the four chambers of the heart is shown in Figure 27–1.

The varying thicknesses of the atrial and ventricular walls relate to the workload required by each chamber. The atrial walls are thinner than those of the ventricles because of the lower-pressure work of the atria holding blood and channeling it to the ventricles. Because the left ventricle has the greater workload of the two bottom chambers, it is about 2½ times as thick as the right ventricle. The left ventricle ejects blood against the high systemic pressure, whereas the right ventricle ejects against the low pressure of the pulmonary vasculature.

Because of the rotation of the heart within the chest cavity, the right ventricle lies anteriorly (just beneath the sternum) and the left ventricle is situated posteriorly. The left ventricle is responsible for the apex beat or the *point of maximum impulse* (PMI), which is normally palpable in the left midclavicular line of the chest wall at the 5th intercostal space.

Cardiac Valves.   Cardiac valves permit blood to flow in only one direction through the heart. Valves, which are composed of thin leaflets of fibrous tissue, open and close passively in response to pressure changes and blood movement. There are two types of valves: *atrioventricular* and *semilunar*.

Atrioventricular Valves.   Valves separating the atria from the ventricles are termed atrioventricular valves. The *tricuspid valve*, so named because it its composed of three cusps, or leaflets, separates the right atrium from the right ventricle. The *mitral* or *bicuspid valve* (two cusps) lies between the left atrium and left ventricle (see Fig. 27–1).

Normally, when the ventricles contract, ventricular pressure tends to push the atrioventricular valve leaflets upward into the atrial cavity. If enough pressure were to be exerted on the valves, blood would be ejected backward from the ventricles to the atria. *Papillary muscles and chordae tendineae* (Fig. 27–1) are responsible for maintaining unidirectional blood flow through the atrioventricular valves. Papillary muscles are muscle bundles that are located on the sides of the ventricular walls. Chordae tendineae are fibrous bands extending from the papillary muscles to the edges of the valve leaflets, acting to tether the free edges of the valves to the ventricular wall. Contraction of the papillary muscles causes the chordae tendineae to become taut. This keeps the valve leaflets closed during systole, preventing backflow of blood. Papillary muscles and chordae tendineae are attached only to the mitral and tricuspid valves, and are notably absent from the semilunar valves.

Semilunar Valves.   Semilunar valves are situated between each ventricle and its corresponding artery. The valve between the right ventricle and the pulmonary artery is called the *pulmonic valve*; the valve between the left ventricle and the aorta is called the *aortic valve*. Both of the semilunar valves are normally composed of three cusps, which function properly without papillary muscles and chordae tendineae. There are no valves between the large veins and the atria.

Coronary Arteries.   The coronary arteries are the vessels that supply blood to the heart muscle, which has large metabolic requirements for oxygen and nutrients (Fig. 27–2). The heart

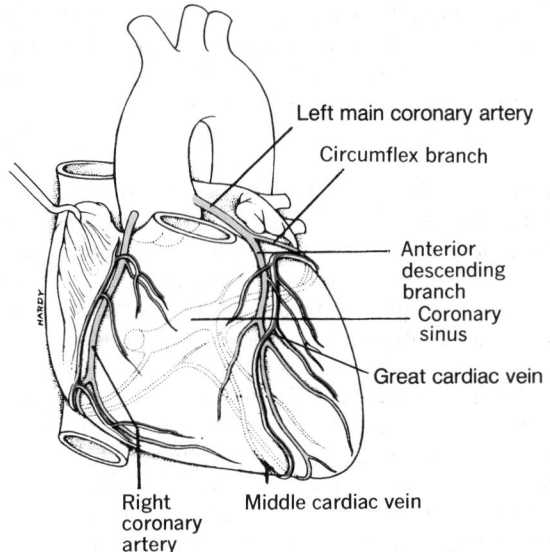

Figure 27–2. Diagram of the coronary arteries arising from the aorta and encircling the heart. Some of the coronary veins also are shown. (Chaffee EE and Greisheimer EM. Basic Physiology and Anatomy. Philadelphia, JB Lippincott.)

uses approximately 70% to 80% of the oxygen delivered through the coronary arteries; in contrast, other organs use, on the average, only one quarter of the oxygen delivered to them. The coronary arteries arise from the aorta near its origin at the left ventricle. The wall of the left side of the heart is supplied in large part through the left main coronary artery, which divides into several large branches that run down (left anterior descending coronary artery) and across the left side of the myocardium (circumflex artery). The right heart wall is supplied similarly from a separate right coronary artery. Unlike other arteries, the coronary arteries are perfused during diastole.

Cardiac Muscle. The specialized muscle tissue composing the wall of the heart is called cardiac muscle. Microscopically, cardiac muscle resembles striated (skeletal) muscle, which is under conscious control.

Functionally, however, heart muscle resembles smooth muscle because it is involuntary. The cardiac muscle fibers are arranged in an interconnected manner (called a *syncytium*) so that they can contract and relax in a coordinated manner. The sequential pattern of contraction and relaxation of individual muscle fibers ensures the rhythmic behavior of the heart muscle as a whole and enables it to function as a pump. The heart muscle itself is called the *myocardium*. The inner lining of the myocardium, which is in contact with the blood, is called the *endocardium*, and the outer layer of cells is called the *epicardium*.

Conduction System of the Heart

Cardiac muscle cells have an inherent rhythmicity, which is illustrated by the fact that a segment of myocardium removed from the rest of the heart will continue to contract rhythmically if maintained under the proper conditions. Sequential contrac-

tion of the atria and ventricles is necessary for the most effective blood flow, however. Orderly contraction occurs because the specialized cells of the conduction system methodically generate and conduct electrical impulses to myocardial cells.

The *sinoatrial* (SA) node, located at the junction of the superior vena cava and the right atrium, is the beginning of the conduction system and normally functions as the pacemaker for the entire myocardium (Fig. 27–3). The SA node initiates approximately 60 to 100 impulses per minute in a resting normal heart, but can change its rate in response to the needs of the body. The electrical signal initiated by the SA node is conducted along the myocardial cells of the atrium to the *atrioventricular* (AV) node. The AV node (located in the right atrial wall near the tricuspid valve) is another group of specialized muscle cells similar to the SA node, but with an intrinsic rate of about 40 to 60 impulses per minute. The AV node coordinates the incoming electrical impulses from the atria and, after a slight delay, relays an impulse to the ventricles. This impulse is conducted through a bundle of specialized muscle fibers (the *bundle of His*) that travel in the septum separating the left and right ventricles. The His bundle divides into right and left bundle branches, which terminate in fibers called *Purkinje fibers*. The right bundle fans out into the right ventricular muscle. The left bundle divides again into the left anterior and left posterior bundle branches, which fan out into the left ventricular muscle. Further spread of depolarization through the rest of the myocardium takes place by conduction through the muscle fibers themselves.

The heart rate is determined by the myocardial cells with the fastest intrinsic rate. Normally, the SA node is fastest. If the SA node malfunctions, the AV node generally takes over the pacemaker function of the heart. Should both the SA and AV nodes fail in their pacemaker function, the myocardium will continue to beat at a rate of less than 40 beats per minute, the intrinsic pacemaker rate of the ventricular myocardial cells.

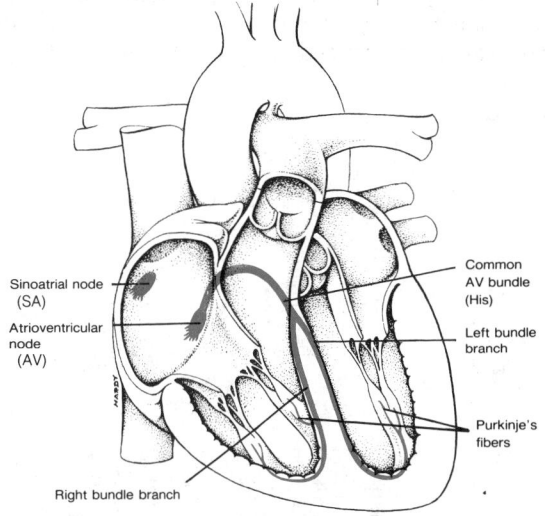

Figure 27–3. Conduction system. Diagram shows relationships of the sinoatrial node, the atrioventricular node, the common atrioventricular bundle and its branches. (Chaffee EE and Greisheimer EM. Basic Physiology and Anatomy. Philadelphia, JB Lippincott.)

Cardiac Physiology

Electrophysiologic Overview

Cardiac electrical activity is the result of movement of ions (charged particles such as sodium, potassium, and calcium) across the cell membrane. The electrical changes recorded within a single cell result in what is known as the cardiac action potential (Fig. 27–4).

In the resting state, cardiac muscle cells are polarized, which means an electrical difference exists between the negatively charged inside and the positively charged outside of the cell membrane. The cardiac cycle begins when an electrical impulse is released, beginning the phase of *depolarization.* The permeability of the cell membrane changes and ions move across it (see Fig. 27–4). With movement of ions into the cell, the inside of the cell becomes positive. Contraction of the muscle follows depolarization. A cardiac muscle cell is normally depolarized when a neighboring cell is depolarized (although it also can be depolarized by external electrical stimulation). Sufficient depolarization of a single specialized conduction system cell will therefore result in depolarization and contraction of the entire myocardium. *Repolarization* occurs as the cell returns to its baseline state (becomes more negative), and corresponds to relaxation of myocardial muscle.

After the rapid influx of sodium into the cell during depolarization, the permeability of the cell membrane to calcium is changed, allowing for uptake of calcium into the cell. The influx of calcium, occurring during the plateau phase of repolarization, is much slower than that of sodium and continues for a longer period. This interaction between changes in membrane voltage and muscle contraction is called *electromechanical coupling.*

Cardiac muscle, unlike skeletal or smooth muscle, has a prolonged refractory period during which it cannot be restimulated to contract. This protects the heart from sustained contraction (*tetany*), which would result in sudden cardiac death.

Normal electromechanical coupling and contraction of the heart are dependent on the composition of the interstitial fluid surrounding the heart muscle cells. The composition of this fluid is in turn influenced by the composition of the blood.

A change in blood calcium concentration therefore may alter contraction of the heart muscle fibers. A change in blood potassium concentration is also important, because potassium affects the normal electrical voltage of the cell.

Cardiac Hemodynamics

An important principle that determines the direction of blood flow is that fluid flows from a region of higher pressure to a region of lower pressure. The pressures that are responsible for blood flow in the normal circulation are generated by contraction of the ventricular muscle. When the muscle contracts, blood is forced from the ventricle into the aorta during the period when left ventricular pressure exceeds aortic pressure. When these two pressures become equal, the aortic valve closes and output from the left ventricle ceases. The blood that has entered the aorta increases the pressure in that vessel. This provides a pressure gradient to force blood progressively through the arteries and capillaries and into the veins. The blood returns to the right atrium because pressure in this chamber is lower than pressure in the veins. Similarly, a gradient of pressure is responsible for blood flow from the pulmonary artery through the lung and back to the left atrium. The pressure gradients within the pulmonary circulation are considerably lower than those in the systemic circulation because the resistance to flow in the pulmonary vessels is lower.

Cardiac Cycle.   Let us consider the pressure changes that occur in the chambers of the heart during the cardiac cycle, beginning with *diastole* when the ventricles are relaxed (Fig. 27–5). During diastole the atrioventricular valves are open, and blood returning from the veins flows into the atrium and then into the ventricle. Toward the end of this diastolic period, the atrial muscle contracts in response to a signal initiated by the SA node. The contraction raises the pressure inside the atrium and forces an increment of blood into the ventricle. This blood augments the volume of the ventricles by an additional 15% to 25%. At this point, the ventricles themselves begin to contract *(systole)* in response to propagation of the electrical impulse that began in the SA node some milliseconds previously. During systole, the pressure inside the ventricle rapidly rises, forcing the AV valves to close. The consequence of this action is that no further filling of the ventricle from the atrium can occur, and blood ejected from the ventricle cannot flow back to the atrium. The rapid rise of pressure inside the ventricles forces the pulmonic and aortic valves to open, and blood is ejected into the pulmonary artery and aorta, respectively. The exit of blood is at first rapid, and then, as the pressures in each ventricle and its corresponding artery approach equalization, the flow of blood gradually decreases. At the cessation of systole, the ventricular muscle relaxes and the pressure within the chamber rapidly decreases. This decrease in pressure creates a tendency for blood to flow back from the artery into the ventricle, which forces the semilunar valves to close. Simultaneously, as the pressure within the ventricle drops to below atrial pressure, the AV valves open, the ventricles begin to fill, and the entire sequence is repeated. It is important to note that the mechanical events related to filling and ejection by the heart are closely coupled to the corresponding electrical events that cause cardiac contraction and relaxation. When interpreting Figure 27–5, it is necessary to realize that the electrical events (ECG) precede the mechanical events (pressures). (See Analysis of the ECG, p. 631.)

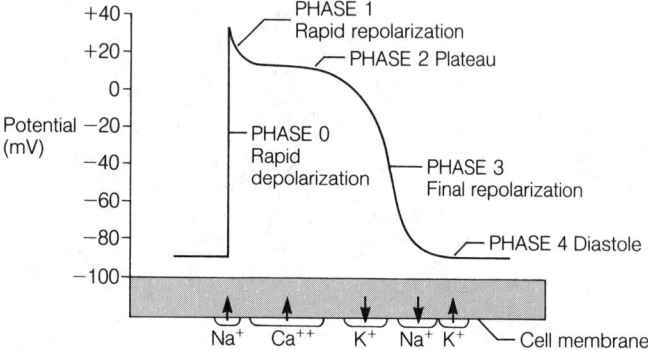

Figure 27–4.   Cardiac action potential. The arrows below the diagram indicate the approximate time and direction of movement of each ion influencing membrane potential. The phase of Ca^{++} moving out of the cell is not well-defined but is thought to occur during phase 4.

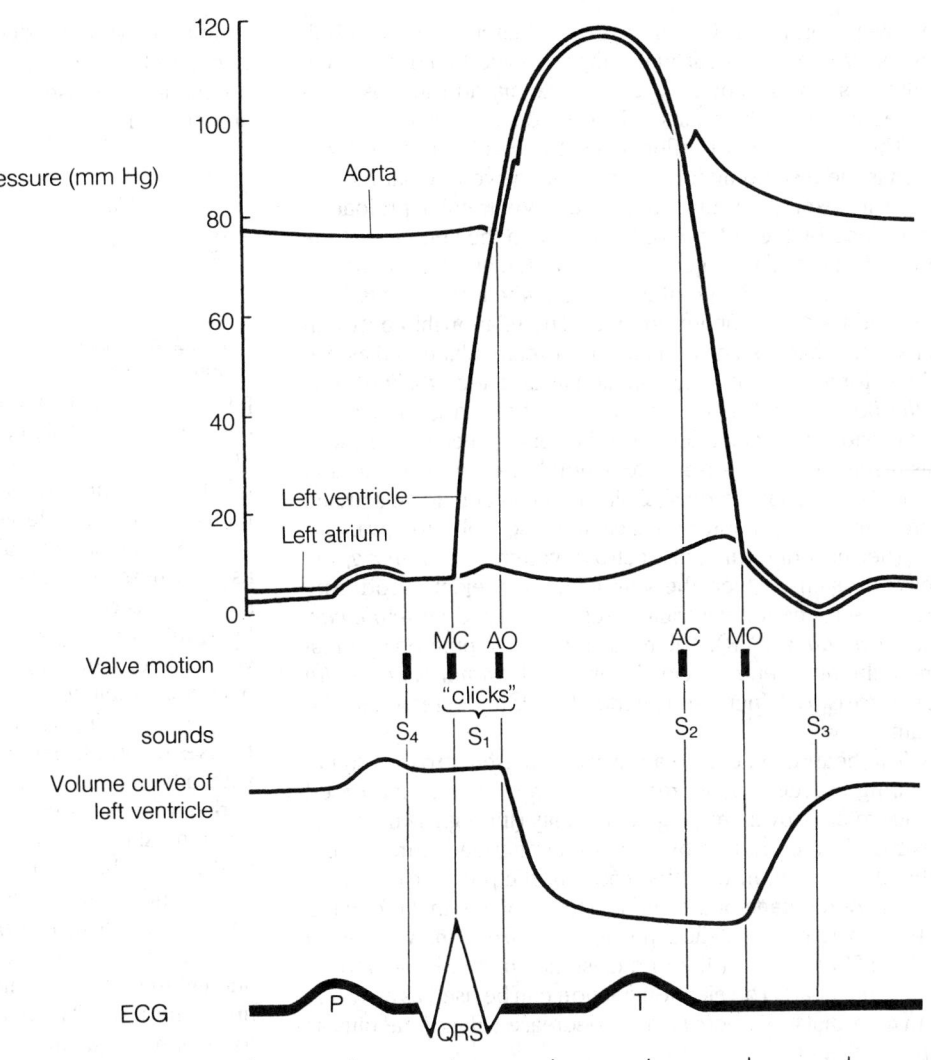

Figure 27–5. Events in the cardiac cycle. Three pressure curves are displayed: aortic, left ventricular, and left atrial. Electrocardiographic events precede the mechanical events. (See Analysis of ECG in this chapter.) Valve closure and opening are indicated, as is the relationship of the cardiac sounds to these events. (See Auscultation of the Heart in this chapter.)

The events just described lead to the repetitive rise and fall of pressures inside the ventricles. The maximum pressure reached is called *systolic pressure* and the minimum pressure *diastolic pressure*.

Cardiac Output

Cardiac output is the amount of blood pumped by the ventricles during a given period. The cardiac output of a typical adult is normally about 5 L/min but varies greatly, depending on the metabolic needs of the body. Cardiac output (CO) equals the stroke volume (SV) times the heart rate (HR).

$$CO = SV \times HR$$

Stroke volume is the amount of blood ejected per heartbeat. Cardiac output can be affected, therefore, by changes in either stroke volume or heart rate. The resting heart rate of an average adult is approximately 60 to 80 beats/min and the average stroke volume is about 70 ml/beat.

Control of Heart Rate. Because the function of the heart is to supply blood to all tissues of the body, its output must vary as the metabolic needs of the tissues themselves change. For example, during exercise the total cardiac output may in-

crease fourfold, to 20 L/min. This increase is normally accomplished by approximately doubling both the heart rate and the stroke volume. Changes in heart rate are accomplished by reflex controls mediated by the autonomic nervous system, including its sympathetic and parasympathetic divisions. The parasympathetic impulses, which travel to the heart through the vagus nerve, can slow the cardiac rate, whereas sympathetic impulses increase it. These effects on heart rate result from action on the SA node to either decrease or increase its rate of intrinsic depolarization. The balance between these two reflex control systems normally determines the heart rate. The heart rate is stimulated also by an increased level of circulating catecholamines (secreted by the adrenal gland) and by the presence of excess thyroid hormone, which produces a catecholamine-like effect.

Control of Stroke Volume. Stroke volume is primarily determined by three factors: (1) intrinsic contractility of the cardiac muscle, (2) the degree of stretch of the cardiac muscle before its contraction *(preload)*, and (3) the pressure against which the heart muscle has to eject blood during contraction *(afterload)*.

Intrinsic contractility is a term used to denote the force that can be generated by the contracting myocardium under any given condition. It is increased by circulating catecholamines, sympathetic neuronal activity, and certain drugs (such as digitalis). It is depressed by hypoxemia and acidosis. Increased contractility results in increased stroke volume.

The second factor influencing stroke volume is *preload,* which is the distending force stretching the ventricular muscle before its excitation and contraction. Ventricular preload is determined by the volume of blood within the ventricle at the end of diastole. The larger the preload, the greater will be the stroke volume, until a point is reached when the muscle is so stretched it can no longer contract. The relationship between increased stroke volume and increased ventricular end-diastolic volume for a given intrinsic contractility is called *Starling's law of the heart,* which is based on the fact that a greater initial length leads to a greater degree of shortening of cardiac muscle. This results from increased interaction between thick and thin filaments of the sarcomeres (similar to the interaction discussed more fully in the chapter on skeletal muscle physiology).

The third determinant of stroke volume is *afterload,* the pressure against which the ventricles must eject blood. The resistance to the left ventricle ejection is called *systemic vascular resistance* (SVR). The resistance by the pulmonary pressure to the right ventricle ejection is called *pulmonary vascular resistance* (PVR). Increased afterload leads to decreased stroke volume.

The heart can achieve a greatly increased stroke volume, as during exercise, by increasing preload (through increased venous return), by increasing contractility (through sympathetic nervous discharge), and by decreasing afterload (through peripheral vasodilation with decreased aortic pressure).

The percentage of the end-diastolic volume that is ejected with each stroke is called the *ejection fraction.* With each stroke, 55% to 75% of the end-diastolic volume is ejected by the normal heart. The ejection fraction can be used as an index of myocardial contractility; it is decreased if contractility is depressed.

Gerontologic Considerations

Atherosclerosis of the coronary arteries and the resultant effects on the heart have long been associated with the aging process. Recent investigations, however, show little evidence that age alone is the precipitating factor. Current evidence indicates that the cardiac changes once attributed to aging can be minimized by modifying life style and personal habits, that is, by following a low-sodium, low-fat diet, not smoking, and exercising regularly.

Studies have shown that the normal aging heart is able to provide an adequate cardiac output under ordinary circumstances, but may have limited functional ability to respond to situations that cause physical or emotional stress. In the elderly person who has decreased activity, the left ventricle may become smaller in response to the decreased workload demand. Aging also results in decreased elasticity and widening of the aorta, thickening and rigidity of the cardiac valves, and increased connective tissue in the SA and AV nodes and bundle branches. These changes lead to decreased myocardial contractility, increased left ventricular ejection time, and delayed conduction. Thus, stressful physical and emotional conditions, especially those that occur suddenly, may have adverse effects on the aged person. The heart is unable to respond to such

conditions with an adequate increase in rate, and more time is required for the heart rate to return to basal levels after even a minimal increase. In some patients, heart failure may be precipitated.

Health History

Nursing assessment for cardiac patients who are acutely ill requires a different initial health history than that for cardiac patients with stable or chronic problems. A patient experiencing an acute myocardial infarction requires immediate, and possibly life-saving, medical and nursing interventions—for example, relief of chest discomfort or prevention of dysrhythmias—rather than an extensive interview. For this patient, a few well-chosen questions about chest discomfort, associated symptoms (such as shortness of breath or palpitations), drug allergies, and smoking history are asked at the same time one is assessing heart rate, rhythm, and blood pressure and inserting an intravenous line. When the patient is more stable, a more extensive history is obtained.

When caring for an acutely ill cardiac patient, one first focuses on assessment of the heart and cardiac output. Patients with atherosclerotic coronary artery disease commonly experience chest discomfort (angina pectoris or myocardial infarction); shortness of breath, fatigue, and reduced urine output (left ventricular failure with decreased cardiac output); palpitations and dizziness (dysrhythmias due to ischemia, aneurysm, stress, or electrolyte imbalance); edema and weight gain (right ventricular failure); and postural hypotension with dizziness and light-headedness (intravascular volume depletion from diuretic therapy). Patients with valvular disease may have symptoms of heart failure, dysrhythmias, and chest discomfort.

When a patient is experiencing chest discomfort, questions to the patient should focus on differentiating a serious, life-threatening condition such as myocardial infarction from conditions that are less serious or that would be treated in a different manner. Not all chest discomfort is related to myocardial ischemia. Table 27–1 summarizes the characteristics and patterns of the more common cardiac and noncardiac causes of chest pain. There are some important points to remember, however, when evaluating chest discomfort:

- There is little correlation between the severity of the chest discomfort and the gravity of its cause. Some patients, such as the elderly or those with diabetes, may not experience pain with angina or myocardial infarction. Fatigue may be the predominant symptom.
- There is poor correlation between the location of chest discomfort and its source.
- The patient may have more than one clinical problem occurring simultaneously.
- In a patient with a history of atherosclerotic coronary artery disease, it is assumed that the chest discomfort is secondary to ischemia until proven otherwise.

To facilitate the gathering of subjective information for a cardiovascular health history, the patient is questioned as indicated below. It is important to individualize the questions for each patient, however, and to pursue areas where further clarification is necessary.

TABLE 27-1.   Assessment of Chest Pain

	Character, Location, and Radiation	Duration	Precipitating Events	Relieving Measures
ANGINA PECTORIS	Substernal or retrosternal pain spreading across chest. May radiate to inside of arm, neck, or jaws.	5–15 min	Usually related to exertion, emotion, eating, cold.	Rest, nitroglycerin, oxygen
MYOCARDIAL INFARCTION	Substernal pain or pain over precordium. May spread widely throughout chest. Painful disability of shoulders and hands may be present.	>15 min	Occurs spontaneously but may be sequelae of unstable angina.	Morphine sulfate, successful reperfusion of blocked coronary artery
PERICARDITIS	Sharp, severe substernal pain or pain to the left of sternum. May be felt in epigastrium and may be referred to neck, arms, and back.	Intermittent	Sudden onset. Pain increases with inspiration, swallowing, coughing, and rotation of trunk.	Sitting upright, analgesia, anti-inflammatory medications

(continued)

TABLE 27–1. *(Continued)*

	Character, Location and Radiation	*Duration*	*Precipitating Events*	*Relieving Measures*
PULMONARY PAIN	Pain arises from inferior portion of pleura. May be referred to costal margins or upper abdomen. Patient may be able to localize the pain.	30+ min	Often occurs spontaneously. Pain occurs or increases with inspiration.	Rest, time. Treatment of underlying cause, bronchodilators
ESOPHAGEAL PAIN (Hiatus hernia, reflux esophagitis or spasm)	Substernal pain. May be projected around chest to shoulders.	5–60 min	Recumbency, cold liquids, exercise. May occur spontaneously.	Food, antacid. Nitroglycerin relieves spasm
ANXIETY	Pain over left chest. May be variable. Does not radiate. Patient may complain of numbness and tingling of hands and mouth.	2–3 min	Stress, emotional tachypnea.	Removal of stimulus, relaxation

Breathing
- Are you ever short of breath?
- When do you become short of breath?
- How do you make your breathing better?
- What makes it worse?
- How long has shortness of breath been a problem?
- What activities are necessary for you to do that you are no longer able to do because of your breathing?
- Are you on any medication to improve your breathing?
- Does any medication you are taking affect your breathing?
- What time of day do you prefer to take your medication?

Circulation
- Describe the discomfort that you have in your chest.*
- Does the pain spread to your arms, neck, jaw, or back?
- Is there anything that seems to cause the pain?
- How long does the pain usually last?

* *Because patients do not always admit to having chest "pain," word equivalents of pain are used when eliciting the quality of discomfort. Common descriptions used by patients include strangling, constriction, tightness, aching, squeezing, pressing, heaviness, expanding sensation, choking in throat, indigestion, and burning.*

- What relieves the discomfort?
- Have you gained or lost any weight recently?
- Have you noticed any swelling of your hands, feet, or legs (or sacrum, if bedridden)?
- Do you ever feel dizzy or light-headed? Under what circumstances does this occur?
- Have you noticed any changes in your energy level? Fatigued?
- Do you ever feel as if your heart is racing, skipping beats, or pounding?
- Have you had problems with your blood pressure?
- Do you have headaches? What seems to cause them?
- Have you noticed that your hands or feet get unusually cold? When does this seem to happen?

Urination

- Is the amount of your urine output normal for you?
- Do you ever get up at night to use the bathroom? How many times? When did you notice the change?
- Do you take a diuretic? When do you take it?

Mentation

- Do you think as fast as you used to? As clearly?
- Do you laugh or cry more easily than before?
- When did you notice the change?
- Are you taking any medication that might affect your thinking?

When the patient's condition permits, other functional areas are also assessed.

Information obtained in the health history is needed to plan individualized care while the patient is hospitalized, to aid in discharge planning, and to provide appropriate teaching. Knowing how the patient perceives the effects of the disease process on activities of daily living will help to identify specific aims for cardiac rehabilitation or strategies for modifying certain activities. Because dietary modification (reduction of sodium, saturated fat, or caloric intake) probably will be prescribed, the history should include the following: food preferences (including cultural or ethnic), eating habits (canned or commercially prepared foods versus fresh foods, and restaurant cooking versus home cooking), who shops for groceries, and who prepares the meals. Knowledge of the patient's financial status assists the nurse in planning an affordable therapeutic regimen—one that includes, for example, economical options for healthy eating, exercise, and obtaining education through free community services. Refer to Chapter 6 for a more complete description of the health history.

Risk Factors in Coronary Artery Disease

The health history, as part of a cardiovascular assessment, needs to include questions about the patient's health promotion practices. Epidemiologic studies show that certain conditions or behaviors, called risk factors, are associated with a greater incidence of coronary artery disease. Risk factors are classified by the extent to which they can be modified by changing an element of life style or modifying personal behavior.

Nonmodifiable risk factors include the following:

- Positive family history
- Increasing age
- Gender (males at greater risk than females)
- Race (higher incidence in blacks than in whites)

Modifiable risk factors include the following:

- Hyperlipidemia
- Elevated blood pressure
- Cigarette smoking
- Elevated blood glucose (diabetes mellitus)
- Obesity
- Physical inactivity
- Stress
- Use of oral contraceptives

Assessment of these risk factors is an important and necessary part of cardiovascular assessment. Detailed discussion of these risk factors is presented in Chapter 28.

Effective patient teaching requires that the nurse have an adequate knowledge base supported by data from current research studies about risk factors. After effectively educating the patient about risk factors, the nurse assists the patient in setting realistic goals for modifying the risk factors. Although there is not complete agreement among health professionals about the effectiveness of modifying risk factors in patients with known coronary artery disease, it is generally accepted that making healthy changes (*e.g.*, reducing dietary fat intake and exercising regularly, promotes overall good health).

Physical Assessment

Assessment of physical findings is performed to confirm data obtained in the health history. Baseline information is obtained on admission. Until the examiner becomes skilled in physical assessment, the initial findings should be validated by an experienced clinician. For the acutely ill cardiac patient, physical examination is performed with routine vital signs (every 4 hours, or more frequently if indicated). Because nurses spend 24 hours a day with the patient, they are in the best position to identify any changes that may occur. Changes must be detected early, before serious complications develop. These changes are reported to the physician and noted in detail in the chart.

In addition to assessing the patient's appearance, a cardiac physical assessment should include an evaluation of the following:

- Effectiveness of the heart as a pump
- Filling volumes and pressures
- Cardiac output
- Compensatory mechanisms

Factors that reflect decreased contractility and efficiency of the heart as a pump are reduced pulse pressure, cardiac enlargement, and the presence of murmurs and gallop rhythms.

Filling volumes and pressures are estimated by the degree of jugular vein distention (JVD) and the presence or absence of congestion in the lungs, peripheral edema, and postural changes in blood pressure.

Cardiac output is reflected by heart rate, pulse pressure, peripheral vascular resistance, urine output, and central nervous system manifestations.

Examples of compensatory mechanisms that help maintain cardiac output are increased filling volumes and elevated heart rate. Note that findings on physical examination are correlated with data obtained from diagnostic procedures, such as invasive hemodynamic monitoring, which will be discussed later in this chapter.

The order of examination proceeds logically from head to toe, and with practice can be performed in about 10 minutes: (1) general appearance, (2) blood pressure, (3) pulse, (4) hands, (5) head and neck, (6) heart, (7) lungs, (8) abdomen, and (9) feet and legs.

General Appearance

The patient's level of distress is observed. Level of consciousness is noted and described. Appropriateness of thought content, reflecting the adequacy of cerebral perfusion, is particularly important to evaluate. Family members who are most familiar with the patient can be helpful in alerting the examiner to subtle behavioral changes. The nurse takes note of the patient's anxiety level and assesses the effects of the patient's anxiety on his cardiovascular status. The nurse attempts to put the anxious patient at ease throughout the examination.

Examination of Blood Pressure

Blood pressure is the pressure exerted on the walls of the arteries. It is affected by factors such as cardiac output, distensibility of the arteries, and the volume, velocity, and thickness (viscosity) of the blood. Blood pressure occurs as a cyclic phenomenon. The peak pressure occurs when the ventricles are contracting and is called *systolic pressure. Diastolic pressure* is the lowest pressure, which occurs when the ventricles are resting. Blood pressure usually is expressed as the ratio of the systolic pressure over the diastolic pressure, with normal adult values ranging from 100/60 to 140/90. The average normal blood pressure usually cited is 120/80.

The difference between the systolic and the diastolic pressures is called the *pulse pressure.* Normally, this amounts to approximately 40 mm Hg. An increase in blood pressure is called *hypertension;* a decrease is called *hypotension.* When only the systolic pressure is elevated *(systolic hypertension),* a widening of the pulse pressure results. This happens in atherosclerosis (hardening of the arteries) and in thyrotoxicosis. Elevation of the diastolic pressure is always associated with elevation of the systolic pressure. An increase in the diastolic pressure to 95 mm Hg gives rise to concern, particularly in younger patients; an increase in excess of 95 mm Hg in the diastolic pressure constitutes true hypertension and requires investigation and control.

Blood pressure can be measured directly or indirectly. The direct method requires the insertion of an arterial catheter into an artery, and is discussed later in this chapter. The indirect measurement is performed with a sphygmomanometer and a stethoscope. The sphygmomanometer consists of an inflatable cuff and a pressure gauge that communicates with the hollow portion of the cuff. The device is calibrated in such a manner that the pressure read on the manometer is comparable to the pressure in millimeters of mercury that is being transmitted to the brachial artery. The cuff is wrapped snugly and smoothly around the upper arm and is inflated by a bulb. Pressure on the cuff is increased until the radial or brachial pulse disappears. The disappearance of the pulse signifies that systolic blood pressure has been exceeded and the brachial artery is occluded. The cuff is then inflated 20 to 30 mm Hg above the point at which radial pulsation disappears. The cuff is slowly deflated,

and the reading is made either by auscultation or palpation. Auscultation enables a more accurate measurement of systolic and diastolic pressure.

To auscultate the blood pressure, the bell or diaphragm* of the stethoscope is placed over the brachial artery, just below the crease of the elbow (antecubital space), which is the point at which the brachial artery emerges from the two heads of the biceps muscle. The cuff is deflated by 2 to 3 mm Hg per second, while one listens for the onset of tapping sounds, which indicate the systolic blood pressure. These sounds, known as *Korotkoff sounds,* coincide with the heart beat, and will continue to emanate from the brachial artery until the pressure in the cuff has been reduced below diastolic pressure. At that point, the sound ceases. In actual practice, the sound more often becomes muffled (changes character) as diastolic pressure is reached and then disappears at approximately 10 mm Hg below normal diastolic pressure.

The disappearance of the sounds is closer to the true diastolic pressure. If there is greater than 10 mm Hg between the muffled sound and when it disappears, the blood pressure is recorded as a tripartite pressure, *e.g.,* 120/80/60, which implies that the sound became muffled at 80 mm Hg and disappeared at 60 mm Hg.

Sometimes, a temporary disappearance of sound occurs when auscultating the blood pressure. This is called an *auscultatory gap.* For example, Korotkoff sounds may be heard at 170 mm Hg, disappear at 150, return at 130, and disappear at 90. This patient has a 20-point auscultatory gap. It is common in patients with high blood pressure or severe aortic stenosis.

Palpation of blood pressure is similar to the procedure described above. When deflating the cuff, the radial or brachial pulse is palpated. The reading at which the pulse returns is the systolic pressure. Palpation is used when the blood pressure is difficult to hear, but with palpation the diastolic pressure cannot be accurately determined.

Accurate recording of the blood pressure depends on using a cuff that is the appropriate size for the patient. If the cuff is too large for the arm, as with a child, the pressure reading will be substantially below the true pressure. If the cuff is too small, as with using a standard adult cuff on obese persons, the pressure reading will be higher than the true pressure. The patient may appear to be hypertensive when the actual pressure is normal. Special cuffs are manufactured for various arm circumferences.

Initially, blood pressure is measured in both the right and the left arms. If a difference is found, the readings are reported to the physician and recorded. Subsequent measurements are taken on the arm with the higher pressure. If there is great difficulty in measuring the blood pressure in either arm, blood pressure also can be obtained in the lower extremities using an extra-wide cuff.

Several important details are summarized to ensure the accurate assessment of blood pressure:

- Cuff size must be appropriate for the patient.
- Cuff is firmly wrapped around the arm, and cuff bladder is centered over the brachial artery.
- Patient's arm should be at heart level.
- Initial recordings are made on both arms, and subsequent

---

* *The bell is better than the diaphragm in hearing the low-frequency Korotkoff sounds. In practice, however, the diaphragm is effective for blood pressure reading and is often used as well.*

measurements are taken on the arm with the higher pressure. Normally, in the absence of disease of the vasculature, there is no more than a difference of 5 mm Hg between arm pressures.

- Position of the patient and site of blood pressure measurement (*e.g.*, RA for right arm) are recorded.
- Palpation of the systolic pressure before auscultation helps to note an auscultatory gap more readily.
- The patient is instructed not to talk during blood pressure measurements. Researchers have found a significant increase in blood pressure and heart rate when subjects are talking.

Pulse Pressure.   Pulse pressure (difference between systolic and diastolic pressures) reflects stroke volume, ejection velocity, and systemic vascular resistance. Pulse pressure may serve as a noninvasive indicator of the patient's ability to maintain cardiac output. If the pulse pressure in the cardiac patient falls below 30 mm Hg, further assessment of the patient's cardiovascular status may be indicated.

Postural Blood Pressure Changes.   Postural (orthostatic) hypotension occurs when the blood pressure drops significantly after an upright posture is assumed; it usually is accompanied by dizziness, light-headedness, or syncope. Although there are many causes of postural hypotension, the three most commonly seen in the cardiac patient are intravascular volume depletion, inadequate vasoconstrictor mechanisms, and autonomic insufficiency. Postural changes in blood pressure, along with appropriate history, can help the clinician differentiate between these causes. The following points are considered when assessing postural blood pressure changes:

- Position the patient supine and as flat as symptoms permit for 10 minutes before the initial blood pressure and heart rate measurements.
- Always check supine measurements before checking upright measurements.
- Always record both heart rate and blood pressure and indicate the corresponding position (lying = ♂ ; sitting = ♀ ; standing = ♀)
- Do not remove the blood pressure cuff between position changes, but do check to see that it is still correctly placed.
- Assess postural blood pressure changes with the patient sitting on the edge of the bed with feet dangling and, if necessary, with the patient standing at the side of the bed.
- Wait 1 to 3 minutes after each postural change before recording blood pressure and heart rate.
- Be alert for any signs or symptoms of patient distress and, if necessary, return the patient to bed before test completion.
- Record any signs or symptoms that accompany the postural change.

Normal postural responses are increased heart rate of 15 to 20 beats above the resting rate (to offset reduced stroke volume and maintain cardiac output), up to a 15–mm Hg drop in systolic pressure, and a slight drop to an increase of 5 to 10 mm Hg in diastolic pressure.

Intravascular volume depletion should be suspected after diuretic therapy or bleeding when, in response to sitting or standing, the heart rate increases and *either* the systolic pressure decreases by 15 mm Hg *or* the diastolic blood pressure drops by 10 mm Hg. It is difficult to differentiate intravascular volume depletion from inadequate vasoconstrictor mechanisms by postural changes in vital signs alone. With intravascular volume

depletion, reflexes to maintain cardiac output (increased heart rate and peripheral vasoconstriction) function correctly but, because of lost volume, the blood pressure falls. With inadequate vasoconstrictor mechanisms, the heart rate again responds appropriately but, because of diminished peripheral vasoconstriction, the blood pressure drops. The following is an example of a postural blood pressure recording showing either intravascular volume depletion or inadequate vasoconstrictor mechanisms:

	Blood Pressure	*Heart Rate*
Lying down ♂	120/70	70
Sitting ♀	100/55	90
Standing ♀	98/52	94

In autonomic insufficiency, the heart rate is unable to increase to compensate for the gravitational effects of upright posture. Peripheral vasoconstriction may be absent or diminished. The presence of autonomic insufficiency does not rule out concurrent intravascular volume depletion. The following is an example of autonomic insufficiency as demonstrated by postural blood pressures changes:

	Blood Pressure	*Heart Rate*
Lying down ♂	150/90	60
Sitting ♀	100/60	60

Examination of the Pulse

In examining the pulse, the factors to be evaluated are rate, rhythm, quality, configuration of the pulse wave, and quality of the vessel itself.

Pulse Rate.   The normal pulse *rate* varies from a low of 50 in healthy, athletic, young adults to rates well in excess of 100 after exercise or during times of excitement. Anxiety frequently elevates the pulse rate during the physical examination. If the rate is higher than expected, it is appropriate to reassess it near the end of the physical examination, at a time when the examiner has established better rapport with the patient.

Pulse Rhythm.   Equally important in assessing the pulse is notation of the *rhythm*. Minor variations in the regularity of the pulse are normal. The pulse rate, particularly in young people, increases during inspiration and slows during expiration. This is called *sinus dysrhythmia*.

For the initial cardiac examination or if the pulse rhythm is irregular, the heart rate should be counted by auscultating the apical pulse for a full minute while simultaneously palpating the radial pulse. Two nurses may be necessary to accurately assess the apical pulse.

Any discrepancy between contractions heard and pulses felt is noted. Disturbances of rhythm (dysrhythmias) often result in a "pulse deficit," a difference between the apical rate (heart rate heard at the apex of the heart) and the peripheral rate. Pulse deficits commonly occur with atrial fibrillation, atrial flutter, premature ventricular contractions, and varying degrees of heart block. See Chapter 29 for a detailed discussion of these dysrhythmias.

An understanding of the complexity of dysrhythmias that may be encountered during the examination requires a sophisticated knowledge of cardiac electrophysiology, knowledge usually possessed by the nurse who specializes in cardiovascular nursing.

Pulse Quality.   The *quality*, or amplitude, of the pulse can be described as normal, diminished, or absent. Some authorities suggest a numerical classification based on a 0 to 4 scale:

>   0—absence of pulsation
>   +1—marked impairment of pulsation
>   +2—moderate impairment of pulsation
>   +3—slight impairment of pulsation
>   +4—normal pulsation

Numerical classification is quite subjective; thus, in written communication it is helpful to specify the scale range (*e.g.,* left radial +3/+4).

Pulse Configuration.   The configuration, or contour, of the pulse frequently conveys important information. In stenosis of the aortic valve, the pulse pressure is narrow and the pulse feels feeble. When insufficiency of the aortic valve is present, the rise of the pulse wave is abrupt and its fall is precipitous, a "collapsing" pulse. The true configuration of the pulse is best appreciated by palpating over the carotid artery rather than the distal radial artery, because the dramatic characteristics of the pulse wave may be distorted by transmission to smaller vessels.

Vessel Quality.   The condition of the vessel wall is also of concern, especially in older patients. Once rate and rhythm have been determined, the quality of the vessel is assessed by palpating along the radial artery and comparing it with normal vessels.

Does it appear to be thickened? Is it tortuous?

To assess peripheral circulation, all arterial pulses are located and evaluated. Arterial pulses are palpated at points where the arteries are near the skin surface and easily compressible against bones or firm musculature. Pulses are detected over the temporal, carotid, brachial, radial, femoral, popliteal, dorsalis pedis, and posterior tibial arteries. A reliable assessment of the pulses of the lower extremities depends on accurate identification of the artery location and careful technique (see Fig. 31–3). Firm finger pressure can easily obliterate the dorsalis pedis and posterior tibial pulses and confuse the examiner. Light palpation is essential. In approximately 10% of the population the dorsalis pedis arteries are not palpable. In such circumstances both are usually absent together, and the posterior tibial arteries alone provide adequate blood supply to the feet.

Hands

In the cardiac patient, the following are the most important findings to note when examining the upper extremities:

*   Peripheral cyanosis implies decreased flow rate of blood in the periphery, allowing more time for the hemoglobin molecule to become desaturated. This may occur normally with the peripheral vasoconstriction associated with a cold environment, or pathologically in conditions that reduce blood flow, for example, cardiogenic shock.

*   Pallor can denote anemia or an increased systemic vascular resistance.
*   Capillary refill time provides the basis for an estimate of the rate of peripheral blood flow. Normally, reperfusion occurs almost instantaneously. More sluggish reperfusion indicates a slower peripheral flow rate, for example, as in heart failure.
*   Hand temperature and moistness are controlled by the autonomic nervous system. Normally hands are warm and dry. Under stress, they may be cool and moist. In cardiogenic shock, hands become cold and clammy due to stimulation of the sympathetic nervous system and resulting vasoconstriction.
*   Edema decreases skin mobility.
*   Dehydration and aging reduce skin turgor.
*   Clubbing of the fingers and toes implies chronic hemoglobin desaturation, as in congenital heart disease.

Head and Neck

When examining the head as part of a cardiovascular assessment, one is concerned primarily with assessing the lips and earlobes for peripheral cyanosis. Peripheral cyanosis is a result of reduced blood flow to the periphery. More oxygen is extracted from the hemoglobin, resulting in a bluish color.

A gross estimate of right heart function can be made by observing the pulsations of the jugular veins of the neck. This enables estimation of central venous pressure, which reflects right atrial or right ventricular end-diastolic pressure (the pressure immediately preceding right ventricular contraction).

Jugular vein distention is caused by increased filling volume and pressure on the right side of the heart. Jugular vein pressure is measured as follows:

*   Begin with the patient supine, with the head of the examination table or bed elevated 15 to 30 degrees.
*   The patient's head is turned slightly away from the side of the neck that is being examined.
*   Identify the external jugular vein.
*   Locate the pulsations of the internal jugular vein. (Distinguish these pulsations from those of the adjacent carotid artery.)
*   Identify the highest point at which the internal jugular vein pulsations can be seen.
*   Using a centimeter ruler, measure the vertical distance between this point and the sternal angle (Fig. 27–6).
*   Record the distance in centimeters and indicate the angle at which the patient was lying (*e.g.,* "The internal jugular vein pulse is 5 cm above the sternal angle, with the head elevated to 30 degrees").
*   Measurements greater than 3 to 4 cm above the sternal angle are considered elevated.

When visualization of the internal jugular veins is difficult, observe the pulsations of the external jugular veins. These are more superficial and visible just above the clavicles adjacent to the sternocleidomastoid muscles. They are frequently distended while the patient lies supine on the examining table or bed. As the patient's head is elevated, the distention of the veins will disappear. The veins are not normally apparent if the head of the bed or examining table is elevated more than 30 degrees.

Obvious distention of the veins with the patient's head elevated 45 to 90 degrees indicates an abnormal increase in the volume of the venous system. This is associated with right-

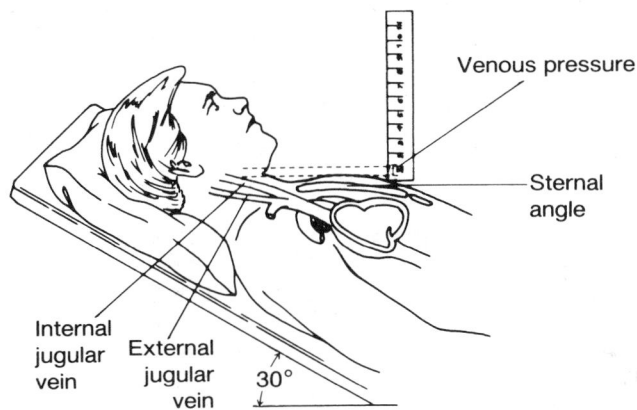

Figure 27–6. An assessment of jugular venous pressure. The highest point at which jugular vein pulsations can be seen is noted. The vertical distance between this point and the sternal angle is measured and recorded as centimeters above or below the sternal angle.

sided cardiac failure or, less commonly, with obstruction to flow in the superior vena cava, and although a rare event, acute massive pulmonary embolism.

Heart

The heart is examined indirectly by inspection, palpation, percussion, and auscultation of the chest wall. A systematic approach is the cornerstone of a thorough assessment. Examination of the chest wall is performed in the following six areas (Fig. 27–7).

1. *Aortic area* — second intercostal space* to the right of the sternum
2. *Pulmonary area* — second intercostal space to the left of the sternum
3. *Erb's point* — third intercostal space to the left of the sternum
4. *Right ventricular or tricuspid area* — fourth and fifth intercostal spaces to the left of the sternum
5. *Left ventricular or apical area* — fifth intercostal space to the left of the sternum
6. *Epigastric area* — below the xiphoid process

For the majority of the examination, the patient is supine, with head slightly elevated. The right-handed examiner is positioned at the right side of the patient and the left-handed examiner is at the left side.

Inspection and Palpation

In a systematic fashion, each area of the precordium is inspected and then palpated. Oblique lighting is used to assist the examiner in identifying subtle pulsation. There is a normal impulse that is discrete and well localized directly over the apex of the heart; it may be observed in young persons and in

---

* *Note: An accurate method of determining the correct intercostal space is to first locate the angle of Louis (see Fig. 27–7). This is done by locating the bony ridge near the top of the sternum at the junction of the body and the manubrium. From the angle of Louis, the second intercostal space is located by sliding one finger to the left or the right of the sternum. Subsequent intercostal spaces are located from this reference point by palpating down the rib cage.*

older persons who are thin. This is called the *apical impulse or point of maximal impulse* (PMI) and is normally located in the left fifth intercostal space in the mid-clavicular line.

The apical impulse can often be palpated. It normally is felt as a light pulsation, 1 to 2 cm in diameter. It is felt at the onset of the first heart sound and lasts only half of systole. The palm of the hand is used initially to locate the apical impulse, and the finger pads are used to describe its size and quality. If the apical impulse is broad and forceful, it is often referred to as a *left ventricular heave* or *lift*. It is so named because it appears to "lift" the hand from the chest wall during palpation.

- *Abnormal PMI.* Left ventricular enlargement from left ventricular failure is evident if the PMI is below the 5th intercostal space or lateral to the midclavicular line. Normally, the PMI is palpable in only one intercostal space. Palpation of the PMI in two or more adjacent intercostal spaces is indicative of left ventricular enlargement. If two distinctly separate areas with paradoxical movement are seen, a ventricular aneurysm should be suspected.

Murmurs, when they are exceptionally loud, also may be palpated and are felt by the palm of the hand as a "purring" sensation. This phenomenon is called a *thrill* and is always indicative of significant pathology within the heart. Thrills also may be palpated over vessels when there is significant substantial obstruction to blood flow, and will occur over the carotid arteries in the presence of narrowing (or stenosis) of the aortic valve.

Percussion

Normally, only the left border of the heart is detected by percussion. It extends from the sternum to the midclavicular line in the third to fifth intercostal space. The right border lies under the right margin of the sternum, but the sternum does not permit definition of the border. Enlargement of the heart to either the left of right usually can be noted. In many persons who have very thick chests, are obese, or have emphysema, the heart may lie sufficiently far beneath the thoracic surface so that not even its left border can be noted unless the heart is enlarged.

Unless the examiner detects a displaced apical impulse and suspects cardiac enlargement, percussion is omitted.

Auscultation

All areas identified in Figure 27–7, except the epigastric area, are auscultated. Events occurring at each of the four valves are uniquely reflected at specific locations on the chest wall. These locations do not correspond to the anatomic location of the valve within the chest. Rather, they are reflective of the patterns of radiation of heart sounds toward the chest wall. Sound in vessels through which blood is flowing is always reflected downstream. For example, events of the mitral valve are usually heard best in the fifth intercostal space at the midclavicular line. This is called the *mitral valve area*.

The examiner seeks to identify normal and abnormal heart sounds, which is a sophisticated and challenging process, but one with which the nurse can become familiar.

Heart Sounds: General Description. The normal heart sounds, S_1 and S_2, are produced primarily by closure of the heart valves. The time between S_1 and S_2 corresponds to systole. This is normally shorter than the time between S_2 and S_1 (diastole). As the heart rate increases, diastole shortens (Fig. 27–8). In normal physiology, the periods of systole and diastole are silent. Pathology of the ventricle, however, can give rise

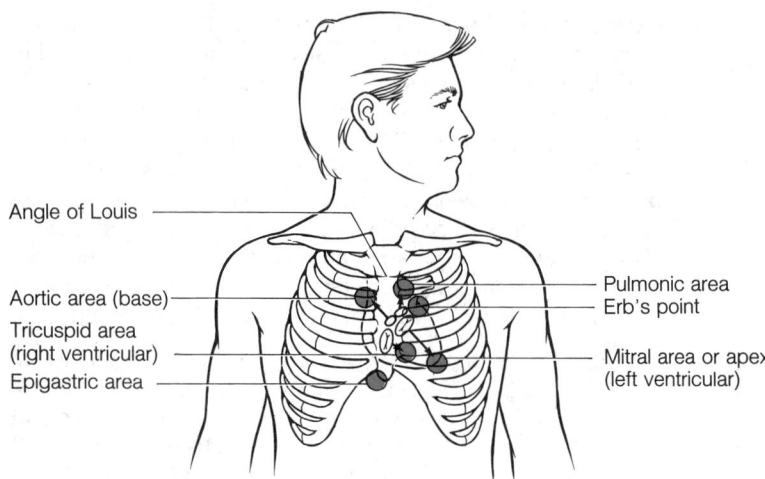

Angle of Louis

Aortic area (base)
Tricuspid area
(right ventricular)
Epigastric area

Pulmonic area
Erb's point

Mitral area or apex
(left ventricular)

Figure 27–7. Areas of the precordium to be assessed.

to transient sounds in systole and diastole that are called *gallops, snaps,* or *clicks.* Significant pathologic narrowing of the valve orifices at times when they should be open, or residual gapping of valves at times when they should be closed, gives rise to prolonged sounds that are called *murmurs.* A more detailed description of the various heart sounds follows below, and precedes a summary of the procedure for heart auscultation.

Normal Heart Sounds

First Heart Sound. The first heart sound (S_1) is created by the simultaneous closure of the mitral and tricuspid valves, although vibration of the myocardial wall also may contribute to this sound. Although heard over the entire precordium, it is heard best at the apex of the heart (mitral area). It is increased in intensity when the valve leaflets are made rigid by calcium in rheumatic heart disease and in any circumstance in which ventricular contraction intervenes at a time when the valve is caught wide open. The latter circumstance will occur, for example, when a premature ventricular contraction interrupts the normal cardiac cycle. The first heart sound varies in intensity from beat to beat when atrial contraction is not synchronous with ventricular contraction. This is because the valve may be fully or partially closed on one beat and quite widely patent on the subsequent one as a function of irregular atrial activity. The first heart sound is easily identifiable and serves as the point of reference for the remainder of the cardiac cycle (see Fig. 27–5).

Second Heart Sound. The second heart sound (S_2) is produced by the closure of the aortic and pulmonic valves. Although these two valves close almost simultaneously, the pulmonic valve usually lags slightly behind. Therefore, under certain circumstances, the two components of the second sound may be heard separately (split S_2). The splitting is more likely to be accentuated on inspiration and to disappear on expiration as a function of respiratory influence on right ventricular ejection (augmenting it on inspiration, inhibiting it on

expiration). S_2 is heard loudest at the base of the heart. The aortic component of the second sound is heard clearly in both the aortic and pulmonic areas, and is heard less clearly at the apex. The pulmonic component of the second sound, if present, may be heard only over the pulmonic area. Thus, one may hear a "single" second heart sound in the aortic area and a split second heart sound in the pulmonic area.

Gallop Sounds. Impedance to diastolic filling of the ventricle in certain disease states may give rise to transient vibrations in diastole that are much akin to, although usually softer than, the first and second heart sounds. Heart sounds then come in triplets and have the acoustical effect of a galloping horse; they are therefore called *gallops.* This may occur early in diastole, during the rapid-filling phase of the cardiac cycle, or later at the time of atrial contraction. A gallop sound occurring during rapid ventricular filling is called a *third heart sound* (S_3) and represents a normal finding in children and young adults (Fig. 27–9). Such a sound is heard in patients who have myocardial disease or in those who are in congestive heart failure and whose ventricles fail to eject all of their blood during systole. An S_3 gallop is heard best with the patient lying on the left side.

Gallop sounds heard during atrial contraction are called *fourth heart sounds* (S_4) (Fig. 27–10). An S_4 is often heard when the ventricle is hypertrophied and therefore resistant to filling. Such a circumstance may be associated with coronary artery disease, hypertension, or aortic stenosis. On rare occasions all four heart sounds are heard within a single cardiac cycle, giving rise to what is called a *quadruple rhythm.*

Gallop sounds are very low-frequency sounds and may only be heard with the bell of the stethoscope placed very lightly against the chest. They are heard best at the apex, although occasionally, when emanating from the right ventricle, they may be heard to the left of the sternum.

Snaps and Clicks. Stenosis of the mitral valve resulting from rheumatic heart disease gives rise to an unusual sound very early in diastole that is high-pitched and best heard along the

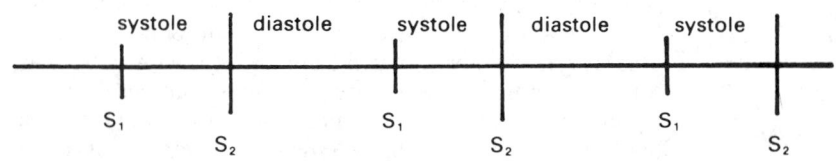

systole | diastole | systole | diastole | systole

S_1 S_1 S_1
    S_2 S_2 S_2

Figure 27–8. The normal heart sounds.

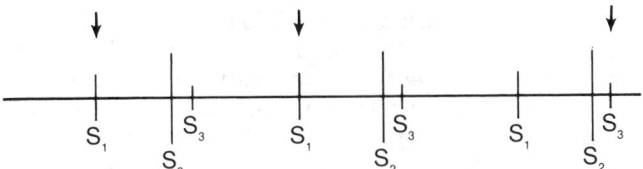

Figure 27-9. An S₃ gallop is heard immediately following the S₂.

left sternal border. The sound is caused by high pressure in the left atrium with abrupt displacement of a rigid mitral valve. The sound is called an *opening snap.* It occurs too long after the second sound to be mistaken for a split second sound and too early in diastole to be mistaken for a gallop. It almost always is associated with the murmur of mitral stenosis and is specific for the disease.

In an analogous manner, stenosis of the aortic valve gives rise to a short, high-pitched sound immediately after the first heart sound that is called an *ejection click.* This is due to very high pressure within the ventricle, displacing a rigid and calcified aortic valve.

Murmurs. Murmurs are created by the turbulent flow of blood. The causes of the turbulence may be a critically narrowed valve; a malfunctioning valve, which allows regurgitant blood flow; a congenital defect of the ventricular wall or between the aorta and the pulmonary artery; or an increased flow through a normal structure (*e.g.,* with fever, pregnancy, hyperthyroidism).

Murmurs are characterized and consequently identified by several characteristics, including *timing* in the cardiac cycle, *location* on the chest wall, *intensity, pitch, quality,* and *pattern of radiation.*

The *timing* of the murmur in the cardiac cycle is vital. First, the observer determines whether the murmur is occurring in systole or in diastole. Does it begin simultaneously with the first heart sound, or is there some delay between the sound and the beginning of a systolic murmur? Does the murmur run up to (or through) the second heart sound, or is there again delay between the end of the murmur and the occurrence of the second heart sound? Are diastolic murmurs continuous, or do they die out in mid- or late diastole?

Location of the murmur is critical. The diastolic murmur of *mitral stenosis* is heard only at the apex (mitral area) and may indeed be confined to only a few centimeters of the chest wall. The murmurs of *aortic and pulmonic stenosis,* although usually widely heard, are nevertheless heard best over their respective valve areas. The murmur of *aortic insufficiency* is heard best along the left sternal border, between the third and fourth interspace, while the patient is seated upright and leaning forward. (The murmur of aortic insufficiency may not be heard at all in the aortic area. This is because the "forward" direction of blood flow for regurgitation at the aortic valve is in the reverse direction.)

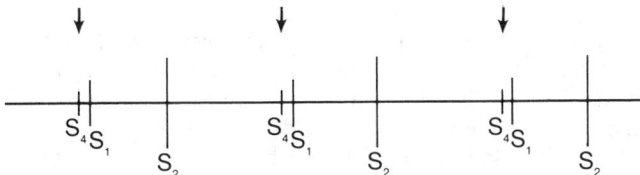

Figure 27-10. An S₄ gallop is heard immediately preceding the S₁.

The *intensity* of murmurs is conventionally graded from I through VI. It is sometimes difficult to hear a grade I murmur. A grade II cardiac murmur should be easily perceived. Murmurs of grades IV or louder are usually associated with thrills that may be palpated on the surface of the chest wall. A grade VI murmur often can be heard with the stethoscope off the chest. A murmur may vary in intensity from its inception to its conclusion. This is very characteristic of certain valvular disorders. The murmur of aortic stenosis, for example, begins sometime after the first heart sound, increases in intensity to midsystole, and then decreases in intensity, stopping before the second heart sound. The sound configuration is referred to as "diamond" in shape, and the murmur is referred to as an *ejection murmur* (Fig. 27-11). The midsystolic increase in intensity is characteristic of murmurs that result from ejection through either the aortic or the pulmonic valve. The murmur of mitral insufficiency and the murmur of a ventricular septal defect are, however, constant in intensity throughout systole. Moreover, they begin simultaneously with the first heart sound and end simultaneously with the second heart sound. They are referred to as *holosystolic* or *pansystolic murmurs.*

In the patient with coronary artery disease, the murmur most frequently heard is the holosystolic murmur (cardiac murmur that extends through systole) of mitral regurgitation. Backflow of blood from the left ventricle through the mitral valve occurs if the papillary muscles become ischemic and are no longer able to contract properly. This murmur is loudest at the apex, and may be heard with the diaphragm of the stethoscope.

The next important quality of a murmur is its *pitch.* The murmur of mitral stenosis is a low, rumbling sound, often heard only with the bell placed lightly on the chest wall. By contrast, the murmur of aortic insufficiency is a very high-pitched murmur, occasionally "whistling" in character, heard best with the diaphragm. Other murmurs, especially the murmur of aortic stenosis, contain the full spectrum of sound frequency, a characteristic that makes the murmur appear to be very harsh in quality.

The last feature of concern is *radiation* of the murmur. The murmur of mitral insufficiency, best heard at the apex (mitral area), radiates into the axilla. This, of course, reflects the "downstream" nature of its transmission. The murmur of

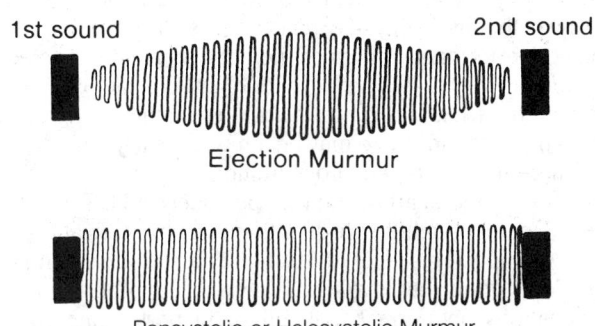

Figure 27-11. Differentiation between ejection murmurs generated at the pulmonic and aortic valves and pansystolic murmurs generated at the mitral and tricuspid valves. Ejection murmurs begin after the first sound, peak in midsystole, and generally end before the second sound. Pansystolic murmurs are of equivalent intensity throughout systole, beginning with the first sound and ending with the second sound.

aortic stenosis will, for similar reasons, radiate into the carotid arteries in the neck. The murmur of pulmonic stenosis, which may sound identical to that of aortic stenosis, will not radiate into the neck; rather, it may radiate into the left shoulder or into the back.

Friction Rub. In pericarditis, a harsh grating sound that can be heard in both systole and diastole is called a *friction rub*. It is caused by the abrasion of the pericardial surfaces during the cardiac cycle. This may be confused with a murmur; care should be taken to identify the sound when appropriate and to distinguish it from murmurs that may be heard in both systole and diastole. A pericardial friction rub can be heard best using the diaphragm of the stethoscope, with the patient sitting up and leaning forward.

Summary of the Procedure for Auscultation. For auscultation, the patient remains supine and the examining room is as quiet as possible. A stethoscope with a diaphragm and a bell is necessary for accurate auscultation of the heart.

Using the diaphragm, the examiner starts at the apical area and progresses upward along the left sternal border to the pulmonic and aortic areas. If desired, the examiner may choose to begin the examination at the aortic and pulmonic areas and progress downward to the apex of the heart. Initially, S_1 is identified and evaluated with respect to its intensity and splitting. Next, S_2 is identified and its intensity noted. After concentrating on S_1 and S_2, the examiner listens for extra sounds in systole and then in diastole. Sometimes it is useful to ask oneself the following questions: Do I hear snapping or clicking sounds? Do I hear any high-pitched blowing sounds? Is this sound in systole, or diastole, or both? The examiner again proceeds to "inch along" the designated areas of the precordium, listening carefully for these sounds. Finally, the patient is turned on the left side and the stethoscope is placed on the apical area, where an S_3 and a mitral murmur are more readily detected.

If an abnormality is heard, the entire chest surface is reexamined to determine the exact location of the sound and its radiation. It is important to reassure the patient who may be concerned about the prolonged examination. Once the characteristics of each phase of the cycle have been determined, the relationship of one to another and the synthesis of events within the cardiac cycle may be summarized.

Interpretation of Cardiac Sounds. The interpretation of cardiac sounds requires detailed knowledge of cardiac physiology and the pathophysiology of cardiac diseases. There are different levels of performance at which the nurse may be expected to function, however. The first level of function is simply the recognition that what one is hearing is not normal. There may be a third heart sound; there may be a murmur in systole or diastole; there may be a pericardial friction rub over the midsternum; the second heart sound may be widely split. These findings are to be brought to the attention of a physician and acted on accordingly. This level of function is useful in screening. It is the kind of activity involved in performing school physical examinations on normal children or in performing routine physical examinations of patients.

The second level of function involves pattern recognition. The nurse correctly observes the findings and is capable of recognizing the constellation of sounds and the diagnostic significance of common ones. This is the role in which the nurse practitioner has recently been placed.

At its most sophisticated level, cardiac diagnosis can be interpretive. Highly skilled nurses can differentiate among dysrhythmias and respond accordingly. They can determine the significance of the appearance and disappearance of gallops during treatment of patients who have had myocardial infarctions or who are in heart failure. This is the role that the coronary care nurse and the cardiovascular clinical nurse specialist assume. They function with a team of professionals for whom the fine details of cardiovascular diagnosis have become highly tuned, shared skills.

Lungs

Respiratory assessment is described in Chapter 24. Findings frequently exhibited by cardiac patients include the following:

- *Tachypnea.* Rapid, shallow breathing may be noted in patients who have heart failure or pain, or who are extremely anxious.
- *Cheyne–Stokes respirations.* Patients in severe left ventricular failure may exhibit Cheyne-Stokes breathing, which is a pattern of rapid respirations alternating with apnea. It is important to note the duration of the apnea.
- *Hemoptysis.* Pink, frothy sputum is indicative of acute pulmonary edema.
- *Cough.* A dry, hacking cough from irritation of small airways is common in patients with pulmonary congestion from heart failure.
- *Crackles.* Heart failure or atelectasis associated with bed rest, splinting from ischemic pain, or the effects of pain medication and sedatives, often results in the development of crackles. Typically, crackles are first noted at the bases (because of gravity's effect on fluid accumulation and decreased ventilation of basilar tissue) but may progress to all portions of the lung fields.
- *Wheezes.* Compression of the small airways by interstitial pulmonary edema may cause wheezing. Beta-blocking agents, such as propranolol, may precipitate airway narrowing, especially in patients with underlying pulmonary disease.

Abdomen

For the cardiac patient, two components of the abdominal examination are frequently performed.

- *Determination of liver size.* Liver engorgement occurs because of decreased venous return secondary to right ventricular failure. The liver will be enlarged, firm, nontender, and smooth. Hepatojugular reflux may be demonstrated by pressing firmly over the liver for 30 to 60 seconds and noting a 1-cm rise in jugular vein pressure.
- *Assessment of bladder distention.* Urine output is an important indicator of cardiac output. A patient who has not voided or who is unable to void is always assessed for bladder distention before initiating other measures. The suprapubic area is palpated for an oval-shaped mass and is percussed for dullness of a full bladder.

Feet and Legs

Many patients with heart disease have associated peripheral vascular disease, or peripheral edema secondary to right ventricular failure. Therefore, adequacy of peripheral arterial circulation and venous return should be assessed in all cardiac patients. In addition, thrombophlebitis is a complication associated with bed rest and requires careful monitoring. Refer to Chapter 31 for a complete description of these techniques.

Gerontologic Considerations

When performing a cardiovascular physical examination on an elderly client, a few considerations are noteworthy. In assessing peripheral pulses in an elderly patient, the arteries are palpated more readily because of increased hardness of the arteries and a loss of adjacent connective tissue. Palpation of the precordium in the elderly is affected by the changes in the shape of the chest. For example, a cardiac impulse may not be palpable in a patient with chronic obstructive pulmonary disease because of the increased anterior–posterior diameter of the chest. Kyphoscoliosis may dislocate the cardiac apex downward so that the diagnostic significance of palpating the PMI is obscured.

Systolic blood pressure increases with age, but diastolic blood pressure usually plateaus after 50 years. Conventionally, drug treatment for high blood pressure begins with a consistent systolic reading of 160 mm Hg or a diastolic reading of 95 mm Hg. For the elderly patient, however, many factors are considered before initiating medication therapy. Orthostatic hypotension may be present, reflecting a decreasing sensitivity of postural reflexes; the physician will consider this when prescribing medication therapy.

An S_4 is heard in about 90% of elderly patients, which is thought to be due to decreased compliance of the left ventricle. The S_2 is usually split. Murmurs are present in 60% or more of elderly patients. The most common murmur is a soft systolic ejection murmur due to sclerotic changes of the aortic leaflets.

In summary, a basic cardiac examination always includes an assessment of heart rate and rhythm, blood pressure, general appearance, and level of comfort and alertness. Blood pressure measurement is important for all patients, because hypertension is silent but exceedingly common in the population. If diagnosed early and adequately controlled, the potential risks of hypertension are significantly reduced.

Inspection of the anterior thorax is easily accomplished, and location of the PMI is noted. Percussion of the cardiac border is not essential for the nursing examination, and usually yields valuable information only when cardiac hypertrophy is present. The six principal areas are auscultated, and any variation from normal mandates further evaluation by a physician.

Diagnostic Tests and Procedures

Diagnostic tests and procedures are used to confirm data obtained by interview and examination. Some tests are easy to interpret, but others must be interpreted by expert clinicians. All require that basic explanations be given to patients. Some necessitate special orders before the test and special monitoring by the nurse after the procedure.

Laboratory Tests

Laboratory tests may be requested for a variety of reasons: to assist in the diagnosis of acute myocardial infarction (angina pectoris cannot be confirmed by either blood or urine studies); to measure abnormalities in blood chemistries that could affect the prognosis of a cardiac patient; to assess the degree of the inflammatory process; to screen for risk factors associated with the presence of atherosclerotic coronary artery disease; to determine baseline values before therapeutic intervention; to assess serum levels of medications; and to screen generally for any abnormalities. Laboratory studies relating specifically to the cardiac patient are summarized. Because many different methods of measurement are used, normal values may differ from one laboratory to the next.

Cardiac Enzymes

Plasma cardiac enzyme analysis is part of a diagnostic profile, including history, symptoms, and electrocardiogram, to diagnose acute myocardial infarction. Enzymes are released from cells when the cells are injured and their membranes rupture. Most enzymes are nonspecific in relation to the particular organ that has been damaged. Certain isoenzymes, however, come only from myocardial cells and are released when the cells are damaged by sustained hypoxia, resulting in infarction. The isoenzymes leak into the interstitial spaces of the myocardium and are carried into the general circulation by the lymph system and the coronary circulation, resulting in elevated blood levels. Because different enzymes are released into the blood at varying periods after myocardial infarction, it is crucial to evaluate the enzyme level in relation to the time of the onset of chest discomfort or other symptoms. Creatine kinase (CK) and its isoenzyme (CK-MB) are the most specific enzymes analyzed in the diagnosis of acute myocardial infarction, and they are the first enzymes to rise. Lactic dehydrogenase (LDH) and its isoenzymes also are analyzed for patients who have delayed seeking medical attention, because blood levels rise and peak later than CK (see Table 29–2 for the time course of cardiac enzymes).

Blood Chemistries

Serum Electrolytes.   Serum electrolytes can affect the prognosis of a patient with acute myocardial infarction or any cardiac condition. Serum sodium reflects relative water balance. Generally, hyponatremia indicates water excess and hypernatremia indicates water deficit. Calcium is necessary for blood coagulability and neuromuscular activity. Hypocalcemia and hypercalcemia can cause ECG changes and dysrhythmias.

Serum potassium is an indicator of renal function and may be decreased by diuretic agents that often are used to treat congestive heart failure. A decrease in potassium causes cardiac irritability and predisposes the patient receiving a digitalis preparation to digitalis toxicity and to the development of dysrhythmias. Elevated serum potassium has a myocardial depressant effect and a ventricular irritability effect. Hypokalemia and hyperkalemia each can lead to ventricular fibrillation or cardiac standstill.

Blood Urea Nitrogen.   Blood urea nitrogen (BUN) is an end product of protein metabolism and is excreted by the kidneys. In the cardiac patient, elevated BUN could reflect reduced renal perfusion (due to decreased cardiac output) or intravascular fluid volume depletion (due to diuretic therapy).

Glucose.   Serum glucose is important to measure because many cardiac patients also have diabetes mellitus. Serum glucose may be mildly elevated in stressful situations when mobilization of endogenous epinephrine results in conversion of liver glycogen to glucose.

Blood Lipids.   Total cholesterol, triglycerides, and lipoproteins are measured to evaluate a person's risk of developing atherosclerotic disease, especially if there is a positive family history of heart disease, or to diagnose a specific lipoprotein abnormality. Decreased levels of high-density lipoprotein (HDL) and elevated levels of low-density lipoprotein (LDL) increase the risk of atherosclerotic coronary artery disease. Although the total cholesterol value remains relatively constant over 24 hours, the measurement of a total lipid profile should be performed after a 12-hour fast. Prolonged stress may increase the total cholesterol.

Chest Radiography and Fluoroscopy

A chest radiograph usually is made to determine the size, contour, and position of the heart. It reveals cardiac and pericardial calcifications and demonstrates physiologic alterations in the pulmonary circulation. It does not aid in the diagnosis of acute myocardial infarction, but can confirm the presence of some complications (*e.g.,* congestive heart failure). Correct placement of cardiac catheters, such as pacemakers and pulmonary artery catheters, is also confirmed by chest radiograph.

Fluoroscopy provides visual observation of the heart on a luminescent x-ray screen. It shows cardiac and vascular pulsations and is useful in the assessment of unusual cardiac contours. Fluoroscopy is a useful tool for the placement and positioning of intravenous pacing electrodes and for guiding the catheter in cardiac catheterization.

Electrocardiography

The *electrocardiogram* (ECG) is a visual representation of the electrical activity of the heart as reflected from various angles to the skin surface.

The ECG is recorded as a tracing on a strip of paper or appears on the screen of an oscilloscope. To facilitate the interpretation of the ECG, data about the patient's age, sex, blood pressure, height, weight, symptoms, and medications (especially digitalis and antidysrhythmic drugs) should be noted on the ECG requisition. Electrocardiography is particularly useful in the evaluation of conditions that interfere with normal heart functions, such as disturbances of rate or rhythm, disorders of conduction, enlargement of heart chambers, presence of a myocardial infarction, and electrolyte imbalances.

The standard ECG consists of 12 leads. Information regarding the electrical activity of the heart is obtained by placing electrodes on the skin surface at standardized anatomic positions (Fig. 27–12). The various electrode positions that may be monitored are referred to as leads. For example, lead 1 measures the electrical activity between the left arm and the right arm. For a complete 12-lead ECG, the heart is viewed from each of 12 different anatomic positions.

Procedure for Obtaining an Electrocardiogram

To obtain a standard 12-lead ECG, electrodes are placed on the patient as shown in Figure 27–12. To ensure good contact between skin and electrode, the limb electrodes are placed on a flat surface just above the wrists and ankles, and electrode paste or an alcohol sponge is placed under each electrode.

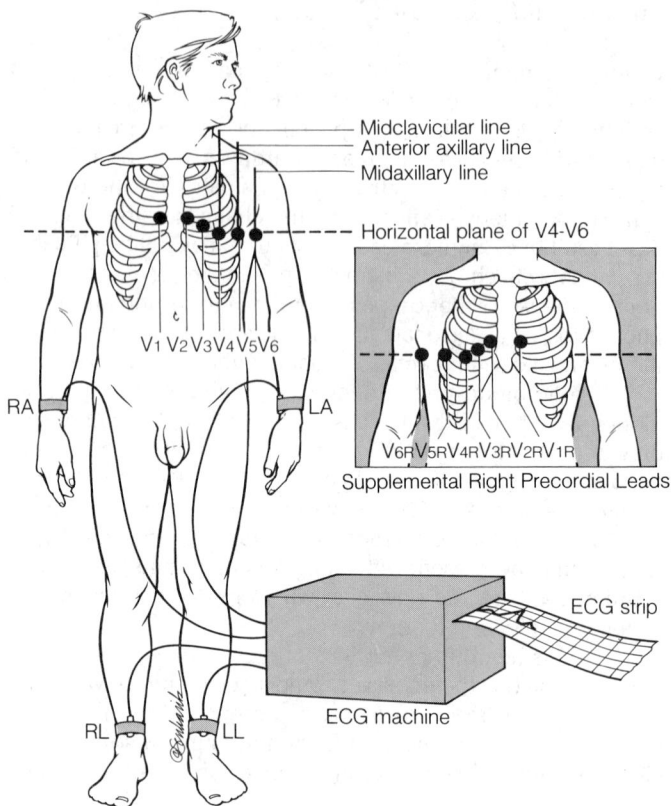

Figure 27–12.   ECG electrode placement. The standard left precordial leads are V_1: 4th intercostal space, R sternal border; V_2: 4th intercostal space, L sternal border; V_3: diagonally between V_2 and V_4; V_4: 5th intercostal space, L midclavicular line, V_5: same line as V_4, anterior axillary line; V_6: same line as V_4 and V_5, midaxillary line. The right precordial leads, placed across the right side of the chest, are the mirror opposite of the left leads.

The extremity straps are adjusted firmly to hold the electrodes in place. These straps should not pinch the patient's skin or be so tight as to decrease circulation distal to the strap.

With the four extremity straps in place, the first six leads can be recorded: lead I, II, and III, and AVR, AVL, and AVF. The six precordial or V leads are either held in place manually or attached by suction cups while recording.

With all electrodes attached, many ECG machines record all 12 leads automatically. Others may require manually selecting each lead on the machine or moving one chest electrode to each of the precordial lead positions. The arm and leg electrodes must be attached to the patient to obtain the V leads.

Each ECG should include the following identifying information:

1. Patient name and identification number
2. Location, date, and time of the recording
3. Patient age, sex, and cardiac medications
4. Race, body build (weight and height measurements), blood pressure, tentative clinical diagnosis, clinical status, and noncardiac medications such as phenothiazines
5. Any unusual position of the patient during the recording, or the presence of thoracic deformities, amputation, respiratory distress, or muscle tremor

Electrocardiographic Monitoring Variations

In performing an ECG, additional leads may be recorded to obtain more complete information. Right-sided precordial leads may be necessary (see Fig. 27–12) to better evaluate the right ventricle. An esophageal lead occasionally is used to evaluate the atria.

To have a patient's ECG continuously available for assessment, one of the 12 leads can be monitored on an oscilloscope. Two leads commonly used for continuous monitoring are lead II and a modification of V_1 (MCL_1) (Fig. 27–13). Lead II is selected when it is desirable to have accurate visualization of P waves. MCL_1 is selected when it is desirable to determine from which ventricle ectopic beats originate. The patient's rhythm is transmitted to the cardiac monitor either by direct contact of the electrode wires to the monitor or by telemetry. With telemetry, the ECG signals are transmitted as radiowaves from a battery-operated transmitter worn by the patient. Patients can walk around the unit while being monitored. Continuous ECG monitoring is part of the standard treatment regimen in critical care units, and is also frequently used on step-down and general units to detect dysrhythmias.

A few guidelines for electrode placement will ensure good conduction and a clear picture of the patient's rhythm on the monitor:

- Clean the skin surface with alcohol and gauze, before applying the electrodes. If the patient has much hair where the electrodes need to be placed, shave the area.
- Apply a little benzoin to the skin if the patient is diaphoretic and the electrodes are not adhering well.
- Change the electrodes at least every 24 hours, and examine the skin for irritation. Apply the electrodes to different locations each day.
- If the patient is sensitive to the electrodes, use hypoallergenic electrodes.

One lead of the ECG can be monitored by a small tape recorder (Holter recorder) and recorded on a continuous (1 to 24 hours) magnetic tape recording. The patient can then be monitored day or night to detect dysrhythmias or evidence of myocardial ischemia during activities of daily living. The tape recorder weighs approximately 2 pounds and can be car-

ried over the shoulder. The patient keeps a diary of activity, noting the time of any symptoms, experiences, or unusual activities performed. The tape recording is then examined (using a specialized instrument called a scanner), analyzed, and interpreted. Evidence obtained in this way is helpful in diagnosing dysrhythmias and myocardial ischemia and in evaluating therapy such as antidysrhythmic and antianginal drugs or pacemaker function.

For some patients considered at high risk for sudden cardiac death, a signal-averaged ECG is performed. This test is ordered separately from a standard ECG once the high-risk status has been identified. Signal averaging works by averaging about 150 to 300 QRS waveforms. The resulting averaged QRS complex is analyzed for certain characteristics that are likely to lead to lethal ventricular dysrhythmias. The recording is performed at the bedside and lasts about 15 minutes.

Another method of evaluating the ECG of a patient at home is by transtelephonic monitoring. The patient attaches a specific lead system and places a telephone mouthpiece over the transmitter box; the ECG is recorded and evaluated at another location. This method is often used for follow-up evaluation of permanent pacemakers.

Analysis of the ECG

When analyzed accurately, the ECG offers important information about the electrical activity of the myocardium. ECG waveforms are printed on graph paper. Time or rate is measured on the horizontal axis of the graph, and amplitude or voltage is measured on the vertical axis.

The ECG waveform represents the function of the heart's conduction system, which normally initiates and conducts the electrical activity.

Waves, Complexes, and Intervals. The ECG is composed of several waveforms, including the P wave, the QRS complex, the T wave, the ST segment, the PR interval, and possibly a U wave.

The *P wave* represents atrial muscle depolarization. It is normally 2.5 mm high or less and is 0.11 second or less in duration. The first negative deflection after the P wave is the Q wave, which is normally less than 0.03 second in duration and less than 25% of the R wave amplitude; the first positive

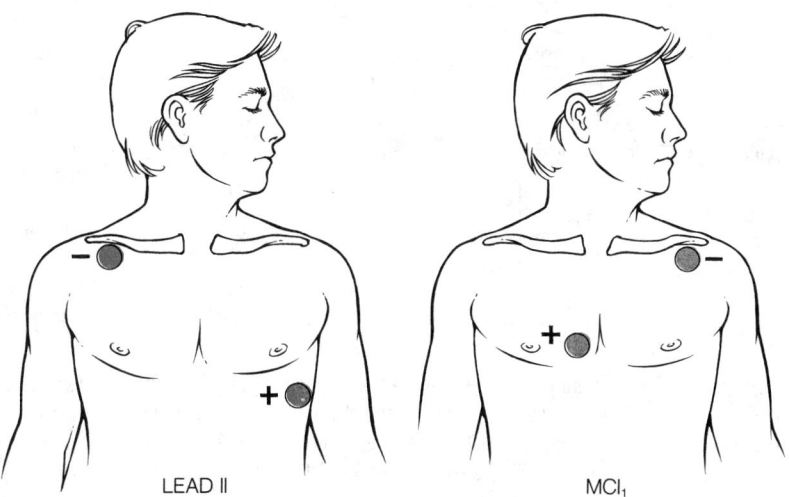

Figure 27–13. Two leads commonly used for continuous monitoring. Lead II—the negative electrode is placed on the right upper chest; the positive electrode is placed on the left lower chest. MCL_1—the negative electrode is placed on the left upper chest; the positive electrode is placed in the V_1 position. If a three-electrode system is used, the third electrode, which is the ground electrode, can be placed anywhere on the chest.

LEAD II MCl_1

deflection after the P wave is the *R wave;* and the *S wave* is the first negative deflection after the R wave (Fig. 27–14).

The *QRS complex* (beginning of Q wave, or R wave if there is no Q wave, to end of S wave) represents ventricular muscle depolarization. The QRS complex is normally 0.04 to 0.10 second in duration. When a wave is less than 5 mm vertically, small letters (q, r, s) are used; when a wave is larger than 5 mm vertically, capital letters (Q, R, S) are used. Not all QRS complexes have all three waveforms.

The *T wave* represents ventricular muscle repolarization. It follows the QRS complex and is usually of the same deflection as the QRS complex. If a *U wave* is seen, it will follow the T wave. The U wave is thought to represent repolarization of the Purkinje fibers but it sometimes is seen in patients with hypokalemia. If present, the U wave follows the T wave and is approximately the same size as the P wave. It may be mistaken for an extra P wave.

The *ST segment*, which represents early ventricular repolarization, lasts from the end of the S wave to the beginning of the T wave. It is normally isoelectric. It is analyzed for signs of ischemia.

The *PR interval* is measured from the beginning of the P wave to the beginning of the Q or R wave and represents the time required for atrial depolarization and the delay of the impulse in the AV node before ventricular depolarization. In adults, the PR interval normally ranges from 0.12 to 0.20 second in duration.

The QT interval, which represents the total time for ventricular depolarization and repolarization, is measured from the beginning of the Q wave, or R wave if no Q wave is present, to the end of the T wave. The QT interval varies with heart rate, is usually less than half the RR interval (measured from the beginning of one R wave to the beginning of the next R wave), and is usually 0.32 to 0.40 second in duration if the heart rate is 65 to 95.

Determination of Heart Rate From ECG.   Heart rate can be obtained from the ECG strip by several methods.

The graph paper on which the ECG is recorded is divided by light and dark vertical and horizontal lines at standard intervals (see Fig. 27–14). There are 300 large boxes in a 1-minute strip. Therefore, an easy and accurate method of determining heart rate with a regular rhythm is to count the number of large boxes between two R waves and divide the number into 300. If, for example, two large boxes are between two R waves, the heart rate is 150 (300 ÷ 2); if there are five large boxes, the heart rate is 60 (300 ÷ 5) (Fig. 27–15A).

An alternate but less accurate method for estimating heart rate, used when the rhythm is irregular, is to count the number of R-R intervals in 6 seconds and multiply that number by 10. The ECG paper is usually marked at 3-second intervals (15 large boxes, horizontally) by a vertical line at the top of the paper (see Fig. 27–15B). The RR intervals are counted rather than QRS complexes, because a computed heart rate based on the latter might be inaccurately high.

Abnormal Findings

Myocardial Ischemia and Injury.   Myocardial ischemia causes the T wave to be larger and inverted because of altered late repolarization. Possibly, the ischemic region remains depolarized, whereas adjacent areas have returned to the resting state. The change is seen in the leads closest to the involved surface of the heart. Ischemia also causes ST segment changes. If there is epicardial myocardial injury, the injured cells depolarize normally but repolarize more rapidly than do normal cells; thus, the ST segment is elevated. If the myocardial injury is on the endocardial surface, then the ST segment is depressed (1 mm or more) in the leads where the positive electrode faces the area of injury. With injury, the ST segment depression is horizontal or slopes downward and is 0.08 second in duration.

Myocardial Infarction.   Myocardial infarction (MI) is classified as either Q-wave or non–Q-wave. With Q-wave infarction, abnormal Q waves develop within 1 to 3 days, because of both the absence of depolarization current from necrotic tissue and opposing currents from other parts of the heart. An abnormal Q wave is 0.04 second or longer in duration and is, in depth, 25% of the R wave (provided the R wave itself exceeds 5 mm). Injury and ischemic changes are also present (Fig. 27–16). With non-Q-wave MI, the ST segment and T wave changes are not followed by a Q wave, but symptoms and cardiac enzyme analysis confirm the diagnosis.

During recovery from an MI, the ST segment often is first to return to normal (1 to 6 weeks). The T wave becomes large and symmetric for 24 hours, and then inverts within 1 to 3 days for 1 to 2 weeks. Q wave alterations are usually permanent. An old Q-wave MI is usually indicated by significant Q waves without ST segment and T wave changes.

Exercise Stress Testing

Exercise stress testing is a noninvasive means of assessing certain aspects of cardiac function. By evaluating cardiac action during physical stress, the heart's response to an increased demand for oxygen can be determined. The test is used for the following purposes: to assist in diagnosing the cause of

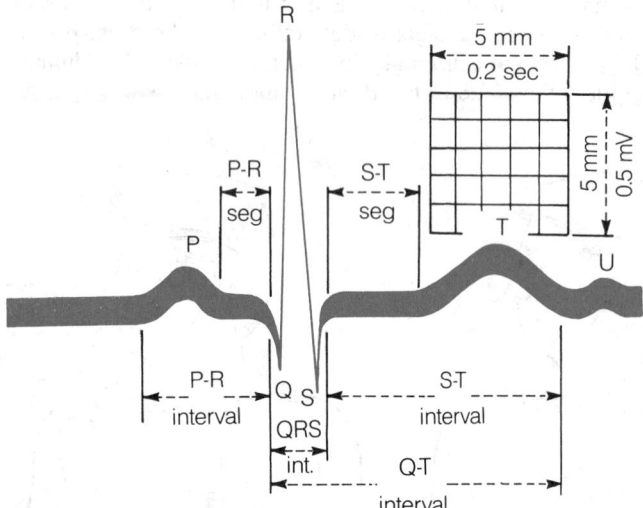

Figure 27–14. Commonly measured complex components. The PR interval is measured from the beginning of the P wave to the beginning of the QRS; the QRS is measured from the beginning of the Q wave to the end of the S wave; the QT interval is measured from the beginning of the Q wave to the end of the T wave.

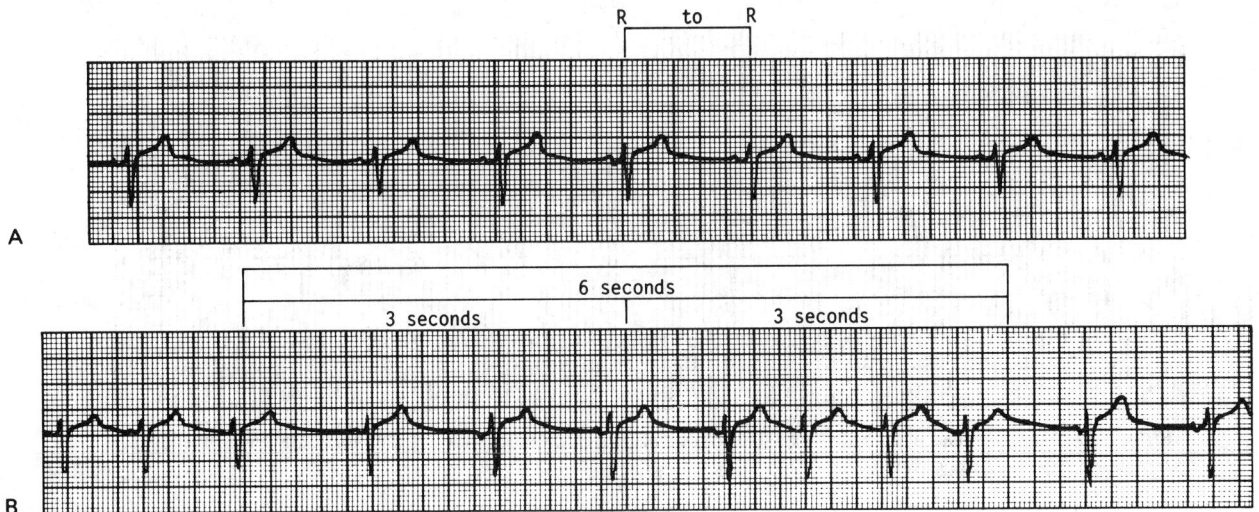

Figure 27–15. (**A**) Heart rate determination for a regular rhythm. There are five large boxes between two R waves. 300 divided by this number equals 60. The heart rate is approximately 60. (**B**) Heart rate determination if the rhythm is irregular. There are approximately seven RR intervals in 6 seconds. Seven times 10 equals 70. The heart rate is 70. (Underhill SL et al. Cardiac Nursing, 2nd ed. Philadelphia, JB Lippincott, 1989, p 314.)

chest pain, to screen for ischemic heart disease, to determine the functional capacity of the heart after an MI or after heart surgery, to assess the effectiveness of antianginal or antidysrhythmia drug therapy, to identify dysrhythmias that occur during physical exercise, and to aid in the development of a physical fitness program.

Exercise stress testing may be performed by having the patient walk on a treadmill, pedal a stationary bicycle, or climb a set of stairs. The patient is exercised by increasing walking speed and the incline of the treadmill or by increasing the load against which the bicycle is pedaled. ECG electrodes are applied to the patient, and tracings are made before, during, and after exercise testing (Fig. 27–17). Blood pressure, skin temperature, physical appearance, and the occurrence or worsening of chest pain are monitored closely during and after the test.

The test is continued until the patient's predetermined target heart rate is reached, but it is terminated early if the patient

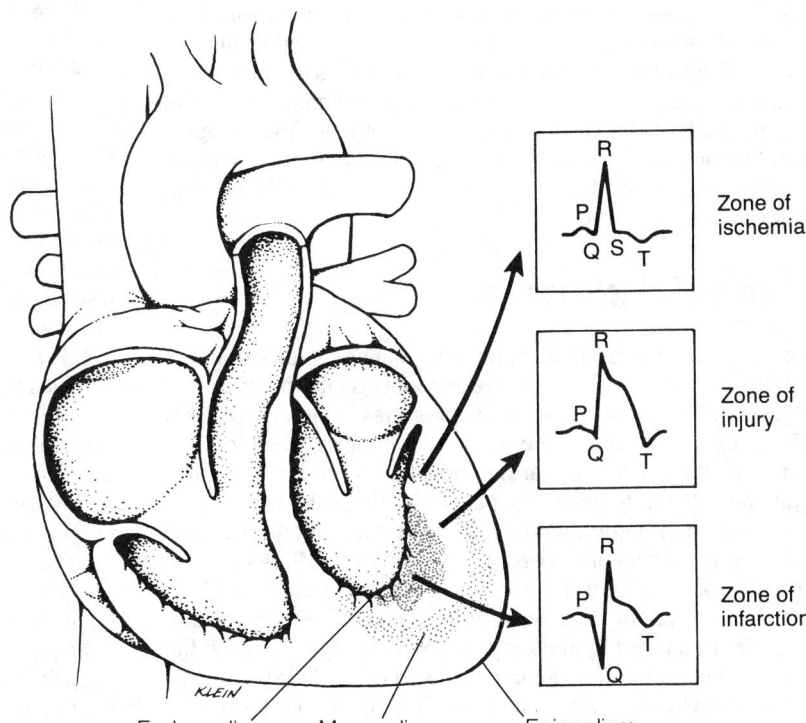

Figure 27–16. Effects of ischemia, injury, and infarction on ECG recording. Ischemia causes inversion of T wave because of altered repolarization. Cardiac muscle injury causes elevation of the ST segment. With Q-wave infarction, Q or QS waves develop because of the absence of depolarization current from the necrotic tissue and opposing currents from other parts of the heart.

Rest   Exercise

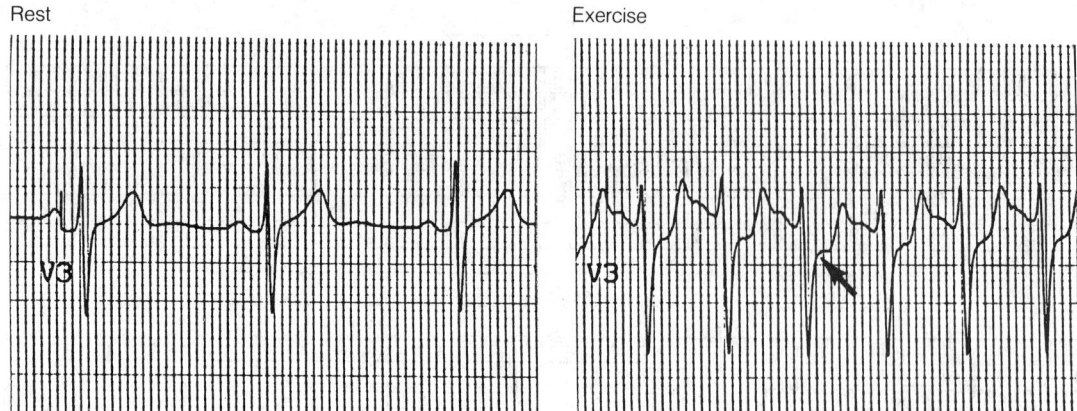

Figure 27-17.   One lead of a positive exercise stress test. The ECG demonstrates 4-mm horizontal ST-segment depression (*arrow*) during exercise.

experiences chest pain, extreme fatigue, drop in blood pressure or pulse rate, or other complications.

The patient is instructed to avoid smoking, eating, and drinking for 4 hours before the test and to wear comfortable shoes suitable for walking. Women are advised to wear a bra that provides adequate support. After the test the patient is instructed to rest for a period and to avoid stimulants, eating, or extreme temperature changes (*i.e.*, hot or cold showers, going out into the cold). Blood pressure and ECG are monitored for 10 to 15 minutes after completion of the test, or until they return to baseline.

Vectorcardiography

Vectorcardiography, which is similar to electrocardiography, presents a three-dimensional view of the electrical forces of the heart: horizontal or transverse, frontal, and left sagittal or lateral planes. This diagnostic modality amplifies understanding of the ECG and gives more accurate diagnostic information in certain areas of cardiac diagnosis (*e.g.*, ventricular hypertrophy, conduction disturbances, and myocardial infarction). The nurse assures the patient that the test is similar to an ECG and that it is safe and painless.

Cardiac Catheterization

Cardiac catheterization is an invasive diagnostic procedure in which one or more catheters are introduced into the heart and selected blood vessels to measure pressures in the various heart chambers and to determine oxygen saturation of the blood by sampling specimens. By far the most common use of cardiac catheterization is to assess the patency of the patient's coronary arteries and to determine the appropriate treatment, *e.g.*, percutaneous transluminal coronary angioplasty (PTCA) or coronary bypass surgery if atherosclerosis is present (see Chap. 30). During cardiac catheterization the patient's electrocardiogram is monitored by means of an oscilloscope. Because the introduction of the catheter into the heart can induce potentially fatal dysrhythmias, resuscitation equipment should be readily available when the procedure is being performed.

Angiography

Cardiac catheterization is usually performed with angiography, a technique of injecting contrast media into the vascular system to outline the heart and blood vessels. When a particular heart chamber or blood vessel is singled out for study, the procedure becomes *selective angiography*. Angiography makes use of *cineangiograms*, a series of rapidly changing films or movies on an intensified fluoroscopic screen that records the passage of the contrast media through the vascular site(s). The recording of the information allows for comparison of information over time.

Four of the more common sites for selective angiography are the aorta, the coronary arteries, and the right and left sides of the heart.

Aortography.   An aortogram is a form of angiography that outlines the lumen of the aorta and the major arteries arising from it. In *thoracic aortography*, contrast media are used to study the aortic arch and its major branches. The translumbar or retrograde brachial or femoral approach may be used.

Coronary Arteriography.   In coronary arteriography a radiopaque catheter is introduced into the right brachial or femoral artery and is passed into the ascending aorta and manipulated into the appropriate coronary artery under fluoroscopic control. Coronary arteriography is used to evaluate the degree of atherosclerosis and to determine the mode of treatment. It also is used to study suspected congenital anomalies of the coronary arteries.

Right-Heart Catheterization.   Right-heart catheterization involves passing a radiopaque catheter from an antecubital or femoral vein into the right atrium, right ventricle, and pulmonary vasculature. This is performed under direct visualization with a fluoroscope. Pressures within the right atrium are measured and recorded, and blood samples are removed for measurement of the hematocrit and oxygen saturation. The catheter is then passed through the tricuspid valve, and similar tests are performed on the blood within the right ventricle. Finally, the catheter is introduced into the pulmonary artery (through the pulmonic valve) and as far as possible beyond that point, where "capillary" samples are obtained and "capillary" pressures (also known as wedge pressures) are recorded. Then the catheter is withdrawn.

Right-heart catheterization is considered a relatively safe procedure. Potential complications, however, include cardiac dysrhythmias, venous spasm, infection of the cutdown site, cardiac perforation, and, rarely, cardiac arrest.

Left-Heart Catheterization. Left-heart catheterization usually is performed by retrograde catheterization of the left ventricle or by transseptal catheterization of the left atrium. In the retrograde technique, the catheter is inserted under direct vision into the right brachial artery (arteriotomy) and advanced under fluoroscopic control into the ascending aorta and into the left ventricle; or the catheter may be introduced percutaneously by puncture of the femoral artery.

In the transseptal approach, the catheter is passed from the right femoral vein (percutaneously or by saphenous vein cutdown) into the right atrium. A long needle is passed up through the catheter and is used to puncture the septum separating the right and left atria. The needle is withdrawn and the catheter is advanced under fluoroscopic control into the left ventricle. In both of these techniques the patient is monitored by electrocardiogram.

Left-heart catheterization is most often performed to evaluate the function of the left ventricular muscle and the mitral and aortic valves or the patency of the coronary arteries. It is used to evaluate patients before and after cardiac surgery. Usually, the right side of the heart is catheterized before the left side is catheterized. Potential complications include dysrhythmias, myocardial infarction, perforation of the heart or great vessels, and systemic embolization.

After the catheterization, the catheter is slowly withdrawn. With the brachial approach, the artery is repaired and the cutdown site is closed and bandaged. With the femoral puncture method, manual pressure is applied until the bleeding is stopped.

Nursing Interventions

Precatheterization nursing responsibilities include the following:

- Instruct the patient to fast, usually for 8 to 12 hours, before the procedure.
- Prepare the patient for the expected duration of the procedure; indicate that it will involve lying on a hard table for about 2 hours.
- Prepare the patient to experience certain sensations during the catheterization. Knowing what to expect can help the patient cope with the experience.

An occasional thudding sensation (palpitation) may be felt in the chest because of extra systoles that almost always occur, particularly when the catheter tip touches the myocardium. The patient may be asked to cough and deep breathe, especially after the dye injection. Coughing may help to disrupt a dysrhythmia and help to clear the dye from the arteries. Breathing deep and holding the breath helps to lower the diaphragm for better visualization of heart structures. The injection of contrast media into either side of the heart may produce a flushed feeling throughout the body and a feeling of micturition, which leaves in a minute or less.

- Encourage the patient to express fears and anxieties. Provide teaching and reassurance to reduce apprehension.
- Prepare the patient for the postcatheterization procedures.

Postcatheterization nursing interventions include the following:

- Observe the puncture (or cutdown) sites for bleeding or hematoma formation, and assess the peripheral pulses in the affected extremity (dorsalis pedis and posterior tibial pulses in the lower extremity, radial pulse in the upper extremity) every 15 minutes for 1 to 2 hours, and then every 1 to 2 hours until stable.
- Evaluate temperature and color of the affected extremity and any patient complaints of pain, numbness, or tingling sensations in the affected extremity to determine signs of arterial insufficiency. Report changes promptly.
- Observe for dysrhythmias by observing the cardiac monitor or by listening to the apical heart rate and evaluating the pulse for rhythm changes. A vasovagal reaction, consisting of bradycardia, hypotension, and nausea, can be precipitated by pain or a distended bladder, usually when a femoral site procedure has been performed. Prompt intervention is critical, which includes raising the feet and legs above the head, and administering intravenous fluids and sometimes intravenous atropine.
- If the procedure was performed percutaneously through the femoral artery, the patient will need to remain supine with the affected leg straight and the head elevated no more than 30 degrees for several hours. The patient is turned from side to side as needed for comfort. Analgesic medication is administered as prescribed for discomfort at the site.
- Report any complaint of chest discomfort immediately.
- Encourage fluids to increase urinary output and flush out the dye.
- Instruct the patient to ask for help in getting out of bed the first time after prolonged bed rest. Orthostatic hypotension may occur.

Echocardiography

Echocardiography is a noninvasive ultrasound test used to examine the size, shape, and motion of cardiac structures.

Three techniques for obtaining an echocardiogram are in use: M-mode, the unidimensional mode first introduced; two-dimensional or cross-sectional (Fig. 27–18); or Doppler. All three techniques involve the transmission of high-frequency sound waves into the heart through the chest wall and the recording of the return signals. The ultrasound is generated by a hand-held transducer (a device that converts one form of energy to another form of energy) applied to the front of the chest. The transducer picks up the echoes, converts them to electrical impulses, and transmits them to the echocardiography machine for display on an oscilloscope and for recording on a videotape. An ECG is recorded simultaneously to time events within the cardiac cycle. Echocardiography is a safe method that provides information similar in many respects to the data obtained with angiocardiography. It is especially useful in the diagnosis and differentiation of heart murmurs. An echocardiogram can show whether the heart is dilated, the walls or septum are thickened, or pericardial effusion is present. It has also been used to study the motion of prosthetic heart valves.

The patient should be assured that the test is safe and painless. He should know that he will be expected to change positions several times during the procedure, to breathe slowly, and periodically to hold his breath.

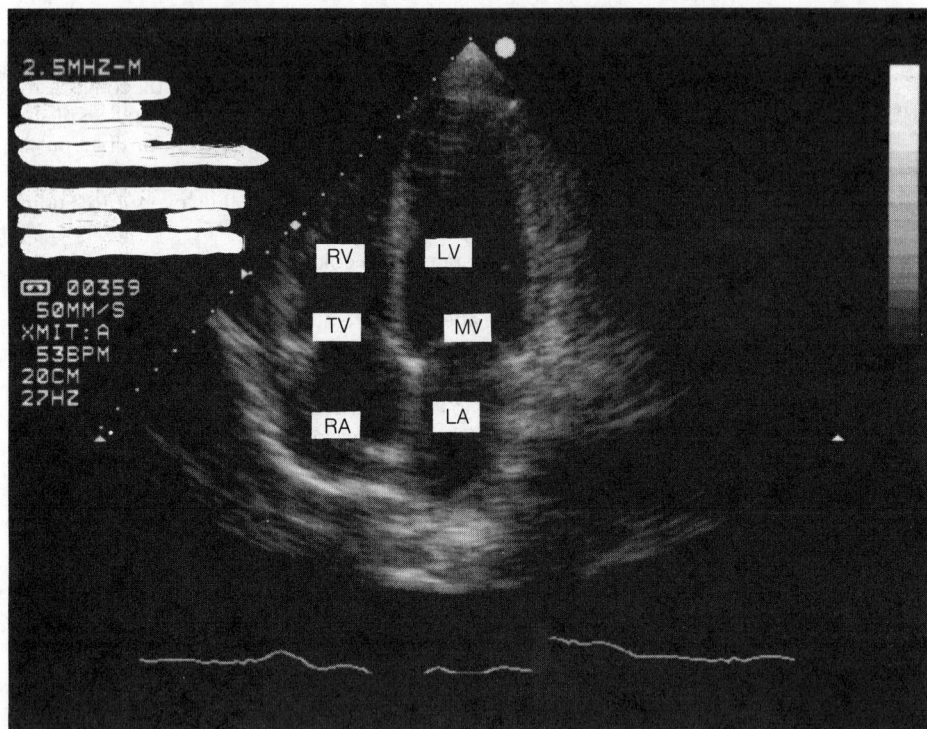

Figure 27–18. Two-dimensional echocardiographic view of the four chambers in a normal patient. (RV = right ventricle; LV = left ventricle; TV = tricuspid valve; MV = mitral valve; RA = right atrium; LA = left atrium.)

Phonocardiography

Phonocardiography is the graphic recording of heart sounds and pulse waves and their relation to time. It helps the observer to identify, accurately time, and differentiate among various sounds and murmurs. It is used to aid in the precise timing of cardiac events and in the diagnosis of valvular and other cardiac disorders.

Microphones containing miniature transducers are placed on the patient's chest at the apex and base of the heart. The transducers pick up heart sounds, amplify them, convert them to electrical impulses, and transmit them to a recorder, which produces a waveform graph of the sounds.

The patient is assured that the procedure is safe and painless. He is expected to remain still and quiet during the test except when asked to change positions, to breathe slowly, or to hold his breath.

Radioisotope Studies

Radioisotope studies are useful for detecting myocardial infarction and decreased myocardial blood flow, and for evaluating left ventricular function. The radioisotopes are injected intravenously, and scans are performed using a gamma scintillation camera.

Myocardial Infarction Imaging. Technetium pyrophosphate (^{99m}TC-PYP) is taken up in areas of the heart where there is damaged myocardial tissue, forming a *hot spot* on a scan made with a scintillation camera. Hot spots appear within 12 hours of infarction, are most evident 48 to 72 hours after infarction, and usually disappear within 1 week unless there is further myocardial damage.

The patient is assured that the scan involves less radiation exposure than a chest x-ray and is instructed to remain motionless during the scan.

Myocardial Blood Flow Evaluation. Thallium-201 is used to evaluate blood flow through vessels that are too small to visualize with coronary arteriography. Thallium concentrates in normal myocardial tissue but not in ischemic or necrotic tissues.

Often this test is paired with an exercise stress test to compare changes in myocardial perfusion immediately after exercise and at rest. One minute before the end of the exercise test, a dose of thallium-201 is injected in the intravenous line to allow for distribution to the heart before the exercise is completed. Images are taken immediately and repeated in 3 to 4 hours. Areas that do not show uptake of thallium are noted as "cold spots" and indicate lack of perfusion. "Cold spots" that disappear in the follow-up images indicate ischemia with exercise. Persistent "cold spots" indicate areas of infarction.

Although the most common thallium imaging is a one-dimensional view, a newer method with single photon emission tomography (SPECT) provides three-dimensional images. With SPECT, the camera moves around the patient in a 180- to 360-degree arc, to more precisely identify the areas of decreased myocardial perfusion.

The patient is assured that the thallium studies involve safe and acceptable radiation exposure, similar to other diagnostic x-rays.

Myocardial Wall Motion Scanning. The technique of gated cardiac blood pool scanning uses a computer to analyze left ventricular function. By determining the difference between the amount of the radioactive tracer ^{99m}Tc-PYP in the end-diastolic volume and the amount in the end-systolic volume, the ejection fraction can be calculated. This test can also be used to assess the differences in left ventricular function during rest and exercise.

In *multiple-gated acquisition* (MUGA) *scanning*, the scintillation camera records 14 to 64 points of one single cardiac cycle. The sequential pictures are studied to evaluate ventricular wall motion and to determine the ejection fraction.

The patient is assured that there is no known radiation danger, and he is instructed to remain motionless during the scan.

Positron Emission Tomography. Positron emission tomography (PET) is a newer scan providing information about myocardial perfusion and metabolism for patients with suspected or diagnosed coronary artery disease. Radioisotopes are administered by injection or inhalation and the radiation is then measured by the PET camera, which provides detailed three-dimensional images of the distribution. PET has limited accessibility and is more expensive than other tests like thallium. Because it provides more specific information, it is expected to become more widely available.

Hemodynamic Monitoring

Hemodynamic monitoring involves the use of invasive catheters placed in the vascular system of patients to closely monitor heart function, blood volume, and circulation. Patients requiring hemodynamic monitoring are usually critically ill and in an intensive care unit, although some stable patients on an intermediate care unit may have a central venous pressure catheter or an arterial catheter. The patient may have any number of underlying medical conditions, but the failure of the heart pump or a major circulation disturbance necessitates the invasive monitoring.

The specific monitoring catheters discussed below are central venous pressure (CVP), pulmonary artery pressure, and systemic arterial pressure catheters.

Central Venous Pressure Monitoring

CVP is the pressure within the right atrium and in the great veins within the thorax. It represents the filling pressure of the right ventricle and indicates the ability of the right side of the heart to manage a fluid load. It serves as a guide to fluid replacement in seriously ill patients and is a measure of effective circulating blood volume. Although CVP is one of several measurements obtained through a pulmonary artery catheter as described below, occasionally a patient on a general unit will have a catheter placed to measure CVP only.

CVP is a dynamic or changing measurement. The change in CVP correlated with the patient's clinical status is a more useful indication of adequacy of venous blood volume and alterations of cardiovascular function than is a single measurement of CVP. CVP reflects right ventricular function. Most right ventricular failure is secondary to left ventricular failure. Therefore, an elevated CVP can be a *late* sign of left ventricular failure. A lowered CVP indicates that the patient is hypovolemic, and this is verified when a rapid intravenous infusion causes the patient to improve. A rising CVP may be due to either hypervolemia or poor cardiac contractility.

The CVP site is prepared by shaving if necessary and cleansing with an antiseptic solution. A local anesthetic may be used. The catheter is threaded through the external jugular, antecubital, or femoral vein into the vena cava just above or within the right atrium. Once the CVP catheter is inserted, an-

tiseptic ointment and a dry, sterile dressing are applied. The dressing, intravenous fluid, manometer, and tubing are changed according to hospital policy and protocol. The usual intervals for changing the various components are: intravenous solution — every 24 hours; the line set-up — every 24 to 48 hours; the catheter insertion site dressing — every 24 to 72 hours.

CVP is measured by the height of a column of water in a manometer. When measuring CVP, it is crucial that the zero mark on the manometer be placed at a standard reference point, called the phlebostatic axis (Fig. 27–19). When this position is located, an ink mark is made on the chest to indicate the location. If the phlebostatic axis is used, CVP can be measured correctly with the patient supine at any backrest position up to 45 degrees. Normal CVP is 4 to 10 cm H_2O. The most common complications of CVP monitoring are infection and air embolism.

Pulmonary Artery Pressure Monitoring

The pulmonary artery (PA) catheter is an important assessment tool that is useful to effectively measure or calculate several right- and left-sided intracardiac pressures. Patients with pulmonary artery catheters are monitored only in critical care units and not on general medical-surgical nursing units.

Many models of PA catheters are currently used, varying in the number of lumina and the types of measurement capability. All types involve a balloon-tipped, flow-directed catheter inserted into a large vein (usually the subclavian or jugular veins) that leads into the superior vena cava and right atrium. The balloon is inflated, and the catheter is carried rapidly by the flow of blood through the tricuspid valve, into the right ventricle, through the pulmonic valve, and into a branch of the pulmonary artery. When the catheter reaches a small pulmonary artery, the balloon is deflated and the catheter is secured with sutures.

With the PA catheter correctly positioned, several parameters can be measured, including CVP or right atrial pressure, PA systolic and diastolic pressures, mean PA pressure, and pulmonary capillary wedge pressure. If certain thermodilution catheters are used, the cardiac output, systemic vascular resistance, pulmonary vascular resistance, and oxygen saturation can be measured or calculated. It is beyond the scope of this chapter to describe all the hemodynamic parameters in detail. The reader is referred to the bibliography for more detailed information about this aspect of critical care nursing. Some parameters are discussed below.

Pulmonary artery systolic and diastolic pressures are obtained with a transducer and blood pressure monitor. Normal pulmonary artery pressure is 25/9 mm Hg, with a mean pressure of 15 mm Hg. When the balloon is inflated, the catheter is "wedged" in the pulmonary artery. Pressures transmitted to the catheter reflect left ventricular end-diastolic pressure. At end-diastole, when the mitral valve is open, pulmonary artery wedge pressure is the same as the pressure in the left atrium and the left ventricle, *unless* the patient has mitral valve disease or pulmonary hypertension. Pulmonary artery wedge pressure is a mean pressure and is normally 4.5 to 13 mm Hg.

Catheter site care is essentially the same as that for a CVP catheter. The catheter flush solution is heparinized normal saline, delivered in small amounts using a pressure bag and flush device. See Chapter 29 for more specific guidelines for caring for a patient with a pulmonary artery catheter. As in measuring

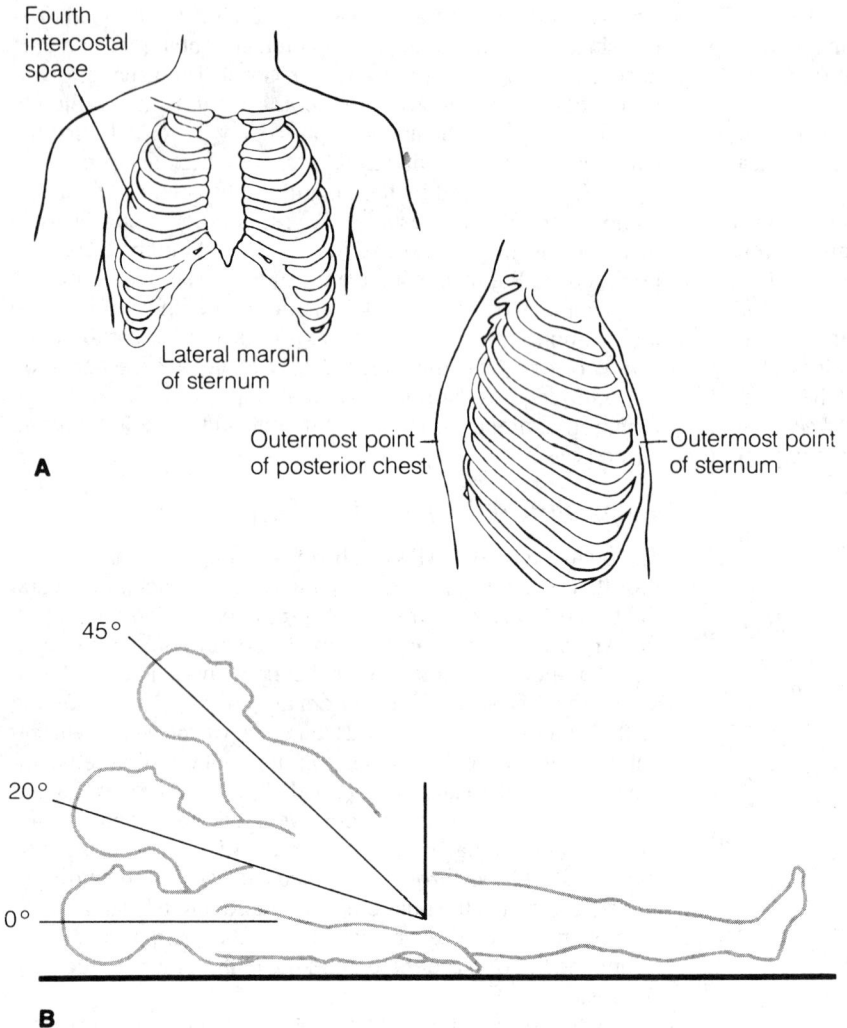

Figure 27–19. The phlebostatic axis and the phlebostatic level. (**A**) The phlebostatic axis is the crossing of two reference lines: (1) a line from the fourth intercostal space at the point where it joins the sternum, drawn out to the side of the body beneath the axilla; (2) a line midpoint between the anterior and posterior surfaces of the chest. (**B**) The phlebostatic level is a horizontal line through the phlebostatic axis. The transducer or the zero mark on the manometer must be level with this axis for accurate measurements. As the patient moves from the flat to erect positions, he moves his chest and therefore the reference level; the phlebostatic level stays horizontal through the same reference point. (After Shinn J et al: Heart Lung 8[2]:324.)

CVP, it is essential to place the transducer at the phlebostatic axis to ensure accurate readings. Measurement of cardiac output can also be obtained by using a pulmonary artery catheter. Complications of pulmonary artery monitoring include infection, pulmonary artery rupture, pulmonary thromboembolism, pulmonary infarction, catheter kinking, dysrhythmias, and air embolism.

Systemic Arterial Pressure Monitoring

Intra-arterial monitoring is used to obtain direct and continuous blood pressures in critically ill patients with severe high blood pressure or hypotension. Arterial catheters are also useful when obtaining arterial blood gases and serial blood samples. Intra-arterial monitoring is generally restricted to critical care units.

Once an arterial site is selected (radial, brachial, femoral, or dorsalis pedis), collateral circulation to the area must be confirmed before catheter placement. If no collateral circulation existed, and the cannulated artery became occluded, ischemia and infarction of the area distal to the cannulated site could occur. Collateral circulation can be checked by either the *Allen test* to evaluate the radial and ulnar arteries, or by using an ultrasonic *Doppler test* for any of the arteries. With the Allen test, the radial and ulnar arteries are simultaneously compressed, and the patient is asked to make a fist, causing

the hand to blanch. After the patient opens the fist, the pressure on the ulnar artery is released while maintaining pressure on the radial artery. The hand will turn pink if the ulnar artery is patent.

Site preparation and care are the same as for CVP catheters. The catheter flush solution is the same as for pulmonary artery catheters. A transducer is attached, and pressures are obtained in millimeters of mercury. Complications include local obstruction with distal ischemia, external hemorrhage, massive ecchymosis, dissection, air embolism, blood loss, pain, arteriospasm, and infection.

Chapter Summary

Assessment of cardiovascular function is a challenging process that requires knowledge of cardiac anatomy and physiology and the pathophysiology of cardiac diseases. This chapter has provided information basic to the subsequent chapters that describe the care of patients with cardiac disorders.

The extensiveness of the assessment of cardiovascular function varies depending on the setting, the acuity of the patient, and the situation. For the patient complaining of chest pain, the focus of the initial assessment is primarily to identify the cause of the pain and to determine the severity of the problem. If, however, a patient is admitted for an elective cardiac catheterization or is transferred to a general unit from a critical care unit, then a more extensive examination is important for assessing baseline changes.

A growing number of diagnostic tools are available for assessing cardiovascular function. For the most part, the nurse does not decide which tests to order. The nurse, however, must be knowledgeable about the methods to evaluate the resulting data. Most importantly, though, the nurse can be a strong advocate for patients by educating them about the tests and alleviating anxiety. The high technology can be overwhelming to patients. The more the nurse is equipped with a sound knowledge base about cardiovascular assessment, the more energy can be directed toward supporting patients through the process.

Bibliography

Books

Andreoli KG et al. Comprehensive Cardiac Care, 6th ed. St Louis, CV Mosby, 1987.

Bates B. A Guide to Physical Examination, 5th ed. Philadelphia, JB Lippincott, 1991.

Dubin D. Rapid Interpretation of EKG's, 4th ed. Tampa, Cover Publishing, 1989.

Ellestad MH. Stress Testing Principles and Practice, 3rd ed. Philadelphia, FA Davis, 1986.

Fowler NO. Noninvasive Diagnostic Methods in Cardiology. Philadelphia, FA Davis, 1983.

Grossman W. Cardiac Catheterization and Angiography. Philadelphia, Lea & Febiger, 1986.

Hurst JW et al. The Heart, 7th ed. New York, McGraw–Hill, 1990.

Malasanos L et al. Health Assessment, 4th ed. St Louis, CV Mosby, 1990.

Marriott HJL. Practical Electrocardiography, 8th ed. Baltimore, Williams & Wilkins, 1988.

Price MS and Fox JD. Hemodynamic Monitoring in Critical Care. Rockville, MD, Aspen Publishers, 1987.

Stein E and Delman AJ. Rapid Interpretation of Heart Sounds and Murmurs, 3rd ed. Philadelphia, Lea & Febiger, 1990.

Sweetwood H. Clinical Electrocardiography for Nurses, 2nd ed. Rockville, MD, Aspen Publishers, 1989.

Underhill SL et al. Cardiac Nursing, 2nd ed. Philadelphia, JB Lippincott, 1989.

Wingate S. Cardiac Nursing: A Clinical Management and Patient Care Resource. Rockville, MD, Aspen Publishers, 1991.

Journals

Asterisks indicate nursing research articles.

* Anderson KO and Masur FT. Psychologic preparation for cardiac catheterization. Heart Lung 1989 Mar; 18(2): 154–163.

Andrews LK. ECG rhythms made easier with algorithms. Am J Nurs 1989 Mar; 89(3): 365CC–371CC.

Barkett PA. Cardiac M.U.G.A. scan. Taking first-rate pictures of the heart. Nursing 1988 Oct; 18(10): 76–78.

Becker KL and Stevens SA. Get in touch and in tune with cardiac assessment. Part 1. Nursing 1988 Mar; 18(3): 51–55.

Bentley LJ. Radionuclide imaging techniques in the diagnosis and treatment of coronary heart disease. Focus Crit Care 1987 Dec; 14(6): 27–36.

Billiard SJ and Beattie S. A non-traditional approach to cardiac education: The use of cardiac catheterization films. Prog Cardiovasc Nurs 1990 Jan/Mar; 5(1): 21–25.

Billings JH. How to help cardiac patients reduce risk factors. Physician Sports Med 1989 Sep; 17(9): 71–83.

Caine R. Essentials of monitoring the electrocardiagram. Nurs Clin North Am 1987 Mar; 22(1): 77–87.

Calloway CK. Zeroing in on chest pain. Nursing 1990 Apr; 20(4): 44–45.

Caplan M and Ranieri C. What's his ECG telling you? A guide for nurses. RN 1989 Feb; 52(2): 42–52.

Charette AL. Bridging the gap between hemodynamics and monitoring. Crit Care Nurs Clin North Am 1989 Sep; 1(3): 539–546.

Ciaccio JM. Measurements of hemodynamics in side-lying positions: A review of the literature. Focus Crit Care 1990 Jun; 17(3): 250–254.

Clawson SP. Right ventricular infarction. Nursing 1990 Mar; 20(3): 34–39.

Criscitiello MG. Fine-tuning the cardiovascular exam. Patient Care 1990 Jun 15; 24(11): 51–62.

Decker S. Continuous EKG monitoring systems. Nurs Clin North Am 1987 Mar; 22(1): 1–13.

DeLeon AC. Fine-tuning the examination of the heart. Consultant 1989 Apr; 29(4): 51–54, 59–61.

Dennis JW and Greisler HP. Noninvasive cardiac monitoring. Nurs Clin North Am 1987 Mar; 22(1): 111–120.

Dennison RD. Understanding the four determinants of cardiac output. Nursing 1990 Jul; 20(7): 35–41.

* Freed CD et al. Blood pressure, heart rate, and heart rhythm changes in patients with heart disease during talking. Heart Lung 1989 Jan; 18(1): 17–22.

Gardner PE. Cardiac output. Theory, technique, and troubleshooting. Crit Care Nurs Clin North Am 1989 Sep; 1(3): 577–587.

Hill MN and Grim CM. How to take a precise blood pressure. Am J Nurs 1991 Feb; 91(2): 38–42.

Kennedy HL et al. Holter monitors: When and how. Patient Care 1989 Feb 15; 23(3): 90–94.

Kouvaras G et al. Q and non-Q wave myocardial infarction: Current views. Angiology 1988 Apr; 39(4): 333–340.

Kuecherer HF et al. Role of transesophageal echocardiography in diagnosis and management of cardiovascular disease. Cardiol Clin 1990 May; 8(2): 377–387.

Lansdowne LM. Signal-averaged electrocardiograms. Heart Lung 1990 Jul; 19(4): 329–336.

Lewis VC. Monitoring the patient with acute myocardial infarction. Nurs Clin North Am 1987 Mar; 22(1): 15–32.

Lough ME. Introduction to hemodynamic monitoring. Nurs Clin North Am 1987 Mar; 22(1): 89–110.

McConnell EA. Assessing groin pain after an arteriogram. Nursing 1990 Apr; 20(4): 86, 88.

Miracle VA. Get in touch and in tune with cardiac assessment. Part 2. Nursing 1988 Apr; 18(4): 41–47.

Moser DK et al. Noninvasive identification of patients at risk for ventricular tachycardia with the signal-averaged electrocardiogram. AACN Clin Issues Crit Care Nurs 1990 May; 1(1): 79–86.

Naggar CZ et al. Echocardiography: Clinical update. Hospital Med 1987 Aug; 23(8): 102–103, 106, 109–111.

Patterson RE et al. Cardiac imaging: Thallium and beyond. Patient Care 1990 May 15; 24(9): 24–43.

Perdue B. Cardiac catheterization—Before and after. Adv Clin Care 1990 Mar/Apr; 5(2): 16–18.

Reynolds T. Noninvasive hemodynamic assessment of intracardiac pressures and assessment of ventricular function with cardiac doppler. Crit Care Nurs Clin North Am 1989 Sep; 1(3): 629–634.

Roberts R. Enzymatic diagnosis of acute myocardial infarction. Chest 1988 Jan; 93(1): 3S–6S.

Schriner DK. Using hemodynamic waveforms to assess cardiopulmonary pathologies. Crit Care Nurs Clin North Am 1989 Sep; 1(3): 563–575.

Schweisguth D. Setting up a cardiac monitor—Without missing a beat. Nursing 1988 Nov; 18(11): 43–48.

Thompson VL. Chest pain: Your response to a classic warning. RN 1989 Apr; 52(4): 32–38.

Viall CD. Your complete guide to central venous catheters. Nursing 1990 Feb; 20(2): 34–42.

Walton J. Identification of patients at high risk for sudden cardiac death. Focus Crit Care 1987 Dec; 14(6): 70–75.

28

Management of Patients With Cardiac Disorders

Learning Objectives

On completion of this chapter, the learner will be able to:

1. Describe the relationship between coronary atherosclerosis, angina pectoris, and myocardial infarction
2. Develop teaching plans for patients with angina pectoris and myocardial infarction
3. Use the nursing process as a framework for care of patients with angina pectoris
4. Use the nursing process as a framework for care of patients with myocardial infarction
5. Compare the infectious diseases of the heart, their causes, pathologic changes, clinical manifestations, management, and prevention
6. Describe the nursing management of patients with pericarditis, with emphasis on prevention of complications
7. Distinguish between congestive, hypertrophic, and restrictive cardiomyopathies
8. Specify the significance of prophylactic antibiotic therapy for patients with rheumatic endocarditis, infective endocarditis, myocarditis, mitral prolapse, and mitral stenosis
9. Use the nursing process as a framework for care of patients with cardiomyopathy

Coronary Artery Disease

Coronary Atherosclerosis

The most common heart disorder in the United States is coronary atherosclerosis, a form of arteriosclerosis. This pathologic condition of the coronary arteries is characterized by an abnormal accumulation of lipid substances and fibrous tissue in the vessel wall that leads to changes in arterial structure and function and reduction of blood flow to the myocardium. Causes of atherosclerotic heart disease probably involve alterations in lipid metabolism, blood coagulation, and the biophysical and biochemical properties of the arterial walls.

Although there is disagreement among authorities with regard to the origin of lesions, there is agreement that atherosclerosis is a progressive disease and that its progress can be curtailed and in some cases reversed.

Pathophysiology. The functional lesion of atherosclerosis is called the *atheroma*. Atherosclerosis begins when the waxy cholesterol atheroma, which looks like pearly gray mounds of tissue, becomes deposited on the intima of the major arteries. These deposits interfere with the absorption of nutrients by the endothelial cells that compose the vessel lining, and obstruct blood flow by protruding into the lumen of the vessel (Fig. 28–1). The vascular endothelium in involved areas becomes necrotic and then scarred, further compromising the lumen and impeding the flow of blood. At sites such as these,

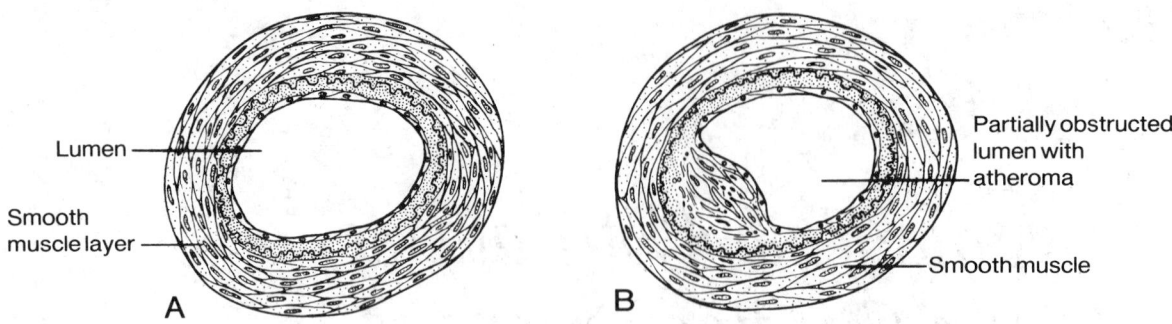

Figure 28–1. Cross-section of a normal and an atherosclerotic artery. (**A**) Cross-section of normal artery showing patent lumen. (**B**) Cross-section of artery showing atheroma and diminished patency of artery lumen.

where the lumen is narrowed and the wall rough, there is a great tendency for clots to form, which explains why intravascular coagulation, followed by thromboembolic disease, is among the most important complications of atherosclerosis.

Our knowledge of atherogenesis is limited. Several theories are proposed, but as yet none has been conclusively substantiated. Among suspected mechanisms are thrombus formation on the surface of the plaque, followed by fibrous organization of the thrombus, hemorrhage into a plaque, and continuing lipid accumulation. If the fibrous cap of the plaque ruptures, the lipid debris is swept into the bloodstream and obstruction of the arteries and capillaries distal to the ruptured plaque results.

The anatomic structure of the coronary arteries makes them particularly susceptible to the mechanisms of atherosclerosis (Fig. 28–2). They twist and turn as they supply the heart, thereby creating angles and nooks ripe for atheroma development.

Clinical Manifestations. Coronary atherosclerosis produces symptoms and complications as a result of the narrowing of the arterial lumen and obstruction of blood flow to the myocardium. This impediment to blood flow is progressive, and the inadequate blood supply (ischemia) that results deprives the muscle cells of the blood components they need for their

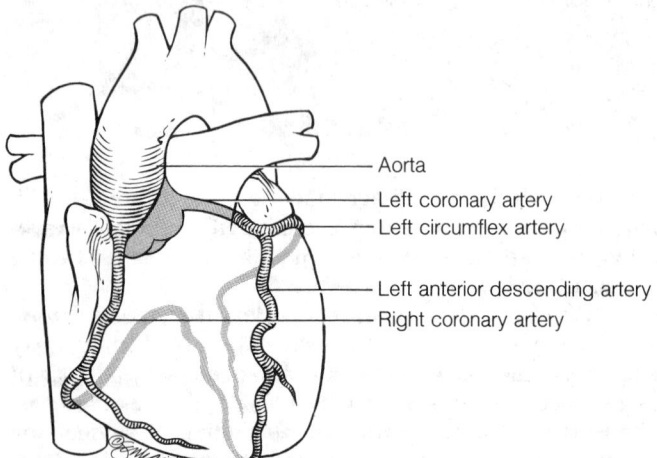

Figure 28–2. Angles of the coronary arteries. The many angles and curves of the coronary arteries contribute to the vessels' susceptibility to the development of atheromatous plaques. Arteries shown in color are behind the heart.

survival. Varying degrees of cell damage are produced by ischemia. The major manifestation of ischemia of the myocardium is chest pain. *Angina pectoris* refers to recurrent chest pain that is not accompanied by irreversible damage to myocardial cells. More severe ischemia with cell damage is termed *myocardial infarction.* Irreversibly damaged myocardium undergoes degeneration and is replaced by scar tissue. If the damage to the myocardium is extensive, the heart may eventually fail, that is, it may be unable to support the body's needs for blood by providing an adequate cardiac output.

Other clinical manifestations of coronary artery disease may be ECG changes, ventricular aneurysms, dysrhythmias, and sudden death.

Risk Factors and Prevention of Coronary Heart Disease

Epidemiologic studies show that there are conditions that may precede or accompany the onset of coronary heart disease. These conditions are called risk factors because the presence of one or more is believed to increase one's risk of developing coronary heart disease. A risk factor may be modifiable or nonmodifiable. A *modifiable risk factor* is one over which an individual may exercise control by changing a life style or personal habit; a *nonmodifiable risk factor* is a consequence of genetics over which an individual has no control (Chart 28–1). A risk factor may operate independently or in tandem with other risk factors. The more risk factors a person has, the greater is the likelihood of developing coronary artery disease. Persons at risk are advised to seek regular medical examinations and, where possible, to engage in a deliberate effort to reduce the number and extent of risks.

A major goal of risk factor identification and reduction is that of prevention of coronary heart disease. Prevention may be primary or secondary. Primary prevention involves measures taken before the development of symptoms of a disease process; secondary prevention involves those measures that may be taken to reduce the progress of or prevent the reoccurrence of a disease process.

Five modifiable risk factors—cigarette smoking, elevated blood pressure, hyperlipidemia, hyperglycemia, and certain behavior patterns—have received popular attention. Two of these risk factors cited as *major* causes of coronary artery disease (CAD) and its consequent complications are cigarette smoking and hypertension.

Chart 28–1
Risk Factors for Atherosclerosis

Nonmodifiable Risk Factors

Positive family history
Increasing age
Sex—Occurs three times more often in men than in women
Race—Higher incidence in blacks than in whites
Geography—Higher incidence in industrialized regions

Modifiable Risk Factors

Hyperlipidemia
Elevated blood pressure
Cigarette smoking
Elevated blood glucose (diabetes mellitus)
Obesity
Physical inactivity
Stress
Use of oral contraceptives
Personality traits such as highly competitive, aggressive, or
   ambitious

Cigarette Smoking. Cigarette smoking contributes to the development and severity of coronary artery disease in three ways. First, the inhalation of smoke increases the blood carbon monoxide (CO) level. Hemoglobin, the oxygen-carrying component of blood, combines more readily with CO than with O_2. Thus, the oxygen being supplied to the heart is severely limited, which makes the heart work harder to produce the same amount of energy. Second, nicotinic acid in tobacco products triggers the release of catecholamines, which cause arterial constriction. Blood flow and subsequent oxygenation are compromised. Third, cigarette smoking increases platelet adhesion, leading to a higher probability of thrombus formation. A person with increased risk for coronary heart disease is encouraged to stop smoking. The individual who successfully ceases to smoke reduces his risk of coronary heart disease by 50% within the first year of smoking cessation. The risk continues to decline as long as the individual refrains from smoking.

Elevated Blood Pressure. Elevated blood pressure is the most insidious of all risk factors because it is asymptomatic until hypertension is well advanced. An elevated blood pressure creates a very high pressure gradient against which the left ventricle must pump. The continued high pressure forces the myocardial oxygen demands to exceed the supply. This initiates the vicious cycle of pain associated with coronary artery disease.

Early detection of high blood pressure and compliance with a therapeutic regimen can prevent the serious consequences associated with untreated elevated blood pressure. Blood pressure is discussed in detail in Chapter 31.

Hyperlipidemia. The association of elevated blood lipids (fats) with coronary artery disease has been established through epidemiologic studies. *Lipids* are a mixed group of biochemical substances that may be manufactured by the body or derived from metabolism of ingested substances. An *endogenous lipid* is one produced by the normal metabolic functions of the body; an example of an endogenous lipid is sterol. An *exogenous lipid* is one derived from a source external to the body, such as a food that is high in fat.

Lipids have the common property of being more soluble in fat or organic solvents than in water. In the blood, the principal lipids are cholesterol and triglycerides; an elevation of one or both is referred to as hyperlipidemia. To render them

suitable for transport in the blood, the lipids are attached to a variety of proteins; the resulting product is called a lipoprotein. The presence of lipoproteins in the blood is *lipoproteinemia*.

The lipoproteins are described clinically by their respective densities. Each lipoprotein has a distinct function in the metabolism of exogenous and endogenous lipids. Some, such as LDL (low-density lipoprotein), are believed to play a role in the aggressiveness of the development of coronary heart disease (Chart 28–2). An excessive amount of lipoproteins in the blood is called *hyperlipoproteinemia*.

There are five types of hyperlipidemia. Table 28–1 describes the five types, the lipoprotein abnormality, and the potential clinical outcomes of elevated levels. Determining the underlying lipid abnormality by blood studies is essential before suggesting dietary control.

Hyperlipidemia may be primary or secondary. *Primary* hyperlipidemia is generally a hereditary disorder and is the rarest of the phenotypes. The *secondary* type occurs as a manifestation of numerous other diseases, including hypothyroidism, nephrotic syndrome, diabetes mellitus, and alcoholism. Therapy consists of treating the basic disorder.

For some individuals, the control of fat consumption is an important factor in preventive nutrition. Dietary fat may be regulated by changing the total amount or the type of fat in the diet, or both. Assisting the patient to modify dietary fat intake through effective counseling requires an understanding of the differences between saturated and polyunsaturated fatty acids, cholesterol, medium-chain triglycerides, and various other fractions, as well as of their functions in the human body.

No single diet or drug will be effective in all conditions in lowering the particular elevated lipid abnormality, but in most people with such an abnormality the level can be brought within the upper normal range.

For patients in whom diet alone cannot normalize the specific lipid, there are several medications that have a synergistic effect when taken with the prescribed diet. These agents are shown to be biochemically effective, in that elevated lipoprotein concentration tends to return toward normal, and manifestations of the abnormalities, such as xanthomas (yellow papules in the skin caused by lipid deposits), may disappear. Drug treatment also varies with the type of hyperlipidemia. The drugs used are usually grouped into two types: those that decrease

Chart 28–2
Composition, Sources, and Functions of Lipoproteins Present in Plasma

Lipoprotein	Composition		Source	Function	Linked to Coronary Heart Disease
High-density lipoproteins (HDL) (α-lipoproteins)	Protein Phospholipid Cholesterol Triglyceride	35%–60% 34%–44% 20%–28% 17%	Liver	Lowers LDL	No
Low-density lipoproteins (LDL) (β-lipoproteins)	Protein Phospholipid Cholesterol Triglyceride	20%–25% 25% 46% 14%	From breakdown of VLDL	Transports cholesterol from liver to periphery	Yes
Intermediate low-density lipoproteins (ILDL)	Intermediary between LDL and VLDL		Endogenous	Intermediate in transformation of VLDL to LDL	Yes
Very low-density lipoproteins (VLDL) (pre-β)	Protein Phospholipid Cholesterol Triglyceride	10% 20% 5% 65%	High dietary intake of CHO	Transports triglycerides from liver to periphery and serves as precursor to LDL	Yes
Chylomicrons	Protein Phospholipid Cholesterol Triglyceride	2% 6%–9% 2% 85%–95%	Dietary fat, exogenous	Removes cholesterol from liver	No

TABLE 28–1. *Primary Hyperlipidemias and Associated Clinical Features*

Phenotype	Dominant Lipids	Dominant Lipoproteins	Clinical Features of Elevated Levels
I (rare)	Triglycerides	Chylomicron	Xanthoma Enlarged liver Pancreatitis
II (common)			
A	Cholesterol	LDL	Premature atherosclerosis Xanthoma
B	Cholesterol Triglycerides	LDL	
III (uncommon)	Cholesterol Triglycerides	ILDL	Premature atherosclerosis Xanthoma
IV (uncommon)	Triglycerides	VLDL	Glucose intolerance Hyperuricemia Premature atherosclerosis
V (uncommon)	Triglycerides	Chylomicron VLDL	Xanthoma Enlarged liver Pancreatitis Glucose intolerance Hyperuricemia Premature atherosclerosis

LDL, low-density lipoprotein; ILDL, intermediate low-density lipoprotein; VLDL, very low-density lipoproteins.

lipoprotein synthesis, such as nicotinic acid and clofibrate, and those that increase lipoprotein breakdown (catabolism), such as cholestyramine, sitosterol, and D-thyroxine.

Harmful side effects can occur from the use of these drugs. Drug therapy is, therefore, reserved for the high-risk patient and is not regarded as a viable substitute for dietary modification. The usefulness of drugs in reversing coronary heart disease is still under investigation. It is, however, broadly accepted that preventive nutrition can have a significant impact on coronary heart disease.

Hyperglycemia. The relationship of elevated blood glucose and increased evidence of coronary heart disease is substantiated. Hyperglycemia fosters increased platelet aggregation, which can lead to thrombus formation. A high level of insulin (as is seen in some cases of adult onset diabetes) is said to cause damage to cells of the smooth muscle lining the vessels. The damaged vessel walls foster the growth of atheromas.

Other risk factors such as obesity and hypertension must be brought under control in addition to hyperglycemia. Control of hyperglycemia without modification of other risk factors does not reduce the risk of coronary heart disease.

Behavior Patterns of Coronary-Prone Persons. It is believed that stress and certain behaviors contribute to the pathogenesis of coronary (atherosclerotic) heart disease. Psychobiologic and epidemiologic studies have investigated behaviors that characterize people who are prone to coronary artery disease: competitive striving for achievement, exaggerated sense of time urgency, aggressiveness, and hostility. A person who manifests these behaviors is classified as type A coronary prone. It appears that, in addition to reducing other risk factors (smoking, dietary fats), such a person should take steps to alter life style and long-term habits.

The type A behavior pattern has been widely accepted as a risk factor for coronary heart disease. Contemporary research indicates that it may not be as significant as was once thought, but there is not yet conclusive evidence of its precise role.

Gerontologic Considerations

Atherosclerotic coronary artery disease is not a function of aging. Aging does, however, produce changes in the integrity of the lining of the walls of arteries (arteriosclerosis), thus impeding blood flow and tissue nutrition. These changes are often sufficient to diminish oxygenation and increase myocardial oxygen consumption (MVO_2). The result can be debilitating angina pectoris and eventually congestive heart failure.

In summary, the most commonly occurring form of heart disease today is coronary heart disease produced by atherosclerosis. The primary lesion of atherosclerosis is the atheroma. The coronary arteries, because of their anatomic structure, are particularly vulnerable to the development of atheroma. The two clinical entities caused by coronary atherosclerosis are angina pectoris and myocardial infarction.

Coronary heart disease is often preceded or accompanied by conditions that may increase one's likelihood of morbidity. These conditions are referred to as risk factors. They are considered nonmodifiable if they are beyond personal control, such as age. If they are amenable to personal control, such as smoking, they are considered to be modifiable. Risk factor identification and modification are major thrusts of coronary heart disease prevention and treatment.

Angina Pectoris

Definition, Etiology, and Pathophysiology

Angina pectoris is a clinical syndrome characterized by paroxysms of pain or a feeling of pressure in the anterior chest. The cause is considered to be insufficient coronary blood flow, resulting in inadequate oxygen supply of the myocardium; in other words, myocardial oxygen demands exceed supply.

Angina is usually caused by atherosclerotic heart disease, and almost invariably is associated with a significant obstruction of a major coronary artery. (The characteristics of the various types of angina are listed in Chart 28–3.)

A number of factors can produce anginal pain: (1) physical exertion can precipitate an attack by increasing myocardial oxygen demands; (2) exposure to cold can cause vasoconstriction and an elevated blood pressure, with increased oxygen demand; and (3) eating a heavy meal increases the blood flow to the mesenteric area for digestion, thus reducing the available blood supply to the heart. In a severely compromised heart, the shunting of blood for digestion can be sufficient to induce anginal pain. Stress or any emotion-provoking situation causing the release of adrenalin and increased blood pressure may accelerate the heart rate, thus increasing myocardial workload.

Identification of angina requires a careful history; effective treatment begins with patient teaching.

Clinical Manifestations

Ischemia of the heart muscle produces *pain,* varying in severity from upper substernal pressure to agonizing pain that is accompanied by severe apprehension and a feeling of impending death. The pain is usually felt deep in the chest behind the upper or middle third of the sternum (retrosternal). Although the pain frequently is localized, it may radiate to the neck, jaw, shoulders, and inner aspects of the upper extremities. The patient often experiences a tightness, a choking or strangling sensation that has a viselike, insistent quality. A feeling of weakness or numbness in the arms, wrists, and hands may accompany the pain. Along with the physical pain, the patient may also have a sense of impending death, an apprehension so characteristic of angina that if it occurs alone, as it sometimes does, it is sufficient for diagnosis. An important characteristic of anginal pain is that it subsides when the precipitating cause is removed.

Gerontologic Considerations

The elderly person who experiences angina may not exhibit the typical pain profile because of changes in neuroreceptors. Pain is often manifested in the elderly as weakness or fainting. When exposed to cold temperatures, elderly persons may experience anginal symptoms more quickly than younger persons because they have less subcutaneous fat to provide insulation. They should be encouraged to dress with extra clothing and advised to recognize feelings of weakness as an indication that they should rest or take prescribed medications.

Diagnostic Evaluation

The diagnosis of angina is often made by an evaluation of the clinical manifestations of pain and the patient's history. In certain types of angina, electrocardiogram (ECG) changes are

Chart 28–3
Types of Angina

Unstable Angina (Preinfarction Angina; Crescendo Angina)

Progressive increase in frequency, intensity, and duration of anginal attacks

Chronic Stable Angina

Predictable, consistent, occurs on exertion and is relieved by rest.

Nocturnal Angina

Pain occurs at night, usually during sleep; may be relieved by sitting upright.
Commonly due to left ventricular failure

Angina Decubitis

Angina while lying down

Intractable or Refractory Angina

Severe incapacitating angina

Prinzmetal's Angina (Variant: Resting)

Spontaneous type of anginal pain accompanied by ST-segment elevation in ECG
Thought to be due to coronary artery spasm
Associated with high risk of infarction

Silent Ischemia

Objective evidence of ischemia (such as stress test), but patient is asymptomatic

---

helpful in making a differential diagnosis of the angina. The patient's response to exertion or stress also may be tested by means of electrocardiographic monitoring while the patient exercises on a bicycle or treadmill.

Medical Management

The objectives of medical management of angina are to decrease the oxygen demands of the myocardium and to increase the oxygen supply. Medically these objectives are met through pharmacologic therapy and risk factor control. Surgically the objectives are met by revascularization of the blood supply to the myocardium, through coronary artery bypass surgery or percutaneous transluminal coronary angioplasty (PTCA), an interventional radiologic variant of surgery (see Chap. 30). Frequently a combination of medical and surgical therapies is employed.

Currently there are several new approaches being investigated to revascularize the myocardium. The application of intracoronary stents to enhance blood flow, the use of laser lights to vaporize plaques, and the use of percutaneous coronary endarterectomy to extract obstructions are three major achievements that hold great promise for the patient with coronary artery disease. Studies that compare the outcomes of one or all of the above with the well-established bypass surgery and PTCA are being conducted. The advances of science continue to offer relief of symptoms and retardation of the disease process for patients experiencing angina.

Pharmacologic Therapy: Nitroglycerin. The nitrates remain the mainstay of treatment for angina pectoris. Nitroglycerin is administered to reduce myocardial oxygen consumption, which decreases ischemia and relieves anginal pain. Nitroglycerin is a vasoactive drug that acts to dilate both the veins and the arteries and thus has an effect on the peripheral circulation. Dilation of the veins causes venous pooling of blood throughout the body. As a result, less blood is returned to the heart and there is a reduction in filling pressure (preload). Nitrates also

relax the systemic arteriolar bed and thus cause a fall in blood pressure (decreased afterload). These effects decrease myocardial oxygen requirements, bringing about a more favorable balance between supply and demand.

Nitroglycerin taken sublingually or in the buccal pouch alleviates the pain of ischemia within 3 minutes.

- The patient is instructed to keep the tongue still and to avoid swallowing saliva until the nitroglycerin tablet is dissolved. If the pain is severe, the tablet can be crushed between the teeth to hasten sublingual absorption.
- As a precaution, the patient should carry the medication with him at all times. Nitroglycerin is very unstable and is kept in a securely capped dark glass bottle. Nitroglycerin is not stored in metal or plastic pillboxes.
- Nitroglycerin is volatile and is inactivated by heat, moisture, air, light, and time. If the nitroglycerin is fresh, the patient will feel a burning sensation under the tongue and often a feeling of fullness or throbbing in the head. The nitroglycerin supply should be renewed every 6 months.
- Instead of using a fixed dosage, the patient regulates drug usage, taking the smallest dose that relieves pain. The drug should be taken in anticipation of any activity that may produce pain. Because nitroglycerin will increase the patient's tolerance for exercise and stress when taken prophylactically (*e.g.*, before exercise, stair-climbing, and sexual intercourse), it is best that it be taken *before* the pain develops.
- The patient should note how long it takes for the nitroglycerin to relieve the discomfort. If the pain is not relieved by nitroglycerin, an impending myocardial infarction may be suspected.

Side effects of nitroglycerin include flushing, throbbing headache, hypotension, and tachycardia. The use of long-acting nitrate preparations is controversial. Isosorbide dinitrate (Isordil) appears to be effective for up to 2 hours if taken sublingually, but has an uncertain effect if taken orally.

Topical Nitroglycerin Ointment.   Nitroglycerin is also available in a lanolin-petrolatum base. In this form it is applied to the skin to protect against anginal pain and promote its relief. It is especially useful when patients experience nocturnal angina or are involved in periods of extended activity (*e.g.*, golfing) because it has a prolonged effect of up to 24 hours. The dose is usually increased until headache or an excessive effect on blood pressure or heart rate occurs, and then is reduced to the largest dose that does not produce these side effects. Instructions for application accompany the various products. The user should be reminded to rotate the site of application to avoid skin irritation.

Beta-Adrenergic Blockers.   If the patient continues to have chest pain despite treatment with nitroglycerin and modification of life style, a beta-adrenergic blocking agent is recommended. Propranolol hydrochloride (Inderal) remains the drug of choice. This drug appears to reduce myocardial oxygen consumption by blocking the sympathetic impulses to the heart. The result is a reduction in heart rate, blood pressure, and myocardial contractility that establishes a more favorable balance between myocardial oxygen needs and the amount of oxygen available. This helps to control chest pain and allows the patient to work or exercise. Propranolol may be given with sublingual isosorbide dinitrate for anti-anginal and anti-ischemia prophylaxis. Propranolol is cleared by the liver at varying rates, depending on the individual patient. It is usually given at 6-hour intervals. Side effects include musculoskeletal weakness, hypotension, bradycardia, and mental depression.

When propranolol is started, blood pressure and heart rate should be monitored (while the patient is in an upright position) 2 hours after the medication has been administered. If the blood pressure drops significantly, a vasopressor may be needed. If severe bradycardia occurs, atropine is the antidote of choice. It is also important to remember that propranolol can precipitate congestive heart failure and asthma.

- The patient is cautioned not to stop taking propranolol abruptly, because there is evidence that angina may worsen and myocardial infarction may develop if this drug is abruptly discontinued.

Calcium Ion Antagonists/Channel Blockers.   The calcium channel blockers, or antagonists, possess properties that have profound effects on myocardial oxygen demands and supply, hence their value in the treatment of angina. Physiologically, the calcium ion performs at the cellular level to influence contraction of all types of muscle tissue and plays a role in the electrical stimulation of the heart.

Calcium ion antagonists/blockers increase myocardial oxygen supply by dilating the smooth muscle wall of the coronary arterioles, and decrease myocardial oxygen demands by reducing systemic arterial pressure and thus the workload of the left ventricle.

The three calcium ion antagonists/blockers most commonly used are nifedipine (Procardia), verapamil (Isoptin, Calan) and diltiazem (Cardizem). The vasodilating effects of these agents, particularly on the coronary circulation, have made them valuable in angina that results from coronary vasospasm (*Prinzmetal's angina*). Calcium blockers should be used with great caution in individuals with heart failure because they block the calcium that supports contractility. Hypotension may occur after intravenous (IV) administration. Other side effects that may occur are constipation, gastric distress, dizziness, or headache associated with dizziness.

Calcium ion antagonists/blockers are usually administered every 4 to 6 hours. Therapeutic doses vary from one person to another.

Risk Factor Control

Several other measures may be necessary to decrease the oxygen demands of the myocardium. It is important that the patient stop smoking, because smoking produces tachycardia and raises the blood pressure, thus increasing the work of the heart. Obese persons are advised to lose weight to reduce cardiac work.

Percutaneous Transluminal Coronary Angioplasty

Angina pectoris may persist for many years in a stable form with brief attacks. It is a serious disease, however. In the unstable stage, the episodes of chest pain become more frequent and intense, occurring without apparent provocation. When symptoms cannot be controlled despite an adequate trial of drug therapy, some form of revascularization is considered that can correct the basic problem by bringing a new blood supply to the ischemic myocardium (see p. 708).

Interventional radiology has made possible a procedure for the revascularization of the coronary arteries that is less invasive than bypass surgery. The procedure is referred to as *percutaneous transluminal coronary angioplasty*. A balloon-tipped catheter is inserted into the coronary artery and rapidly inflated and deflated. The purpose of this procedure is to compress the atheroma into the intimal lining of the artery, thereby increasing blood flow in the artery.

Patients eligible for this procedure have atherosclerotic disease, preferably noncalcified lesions, have had angina for less than 6 months, and are candidates for surgical revascularization. Lesions of the left main coronary artery are not suitable for PTCA because of the large amount of myocardial tissue at risk should total vessel occlusion occur. Patients with severely compromised left ventricular function are also ineligible for PTCA.

Myocardial infarction is a major complication of this procedure. For this reason it is recommended that this procedure be performed only if a cardiovascular surgical team is on standby.

▶ Nursing Process
The Patient With Angina Pectoris

▷ Assessment

In the hospital the nurse observes and records all facets of the patient's activities, with particular regard for those that have been found to precede and precipitate attacks of anginal pain. Appropriate questions may include:

> When do attacks tend to occur?
>> Following a meal?
>> After engaging in certain activities?
>> After physical activities in general?
>> After visits from members of the family or others?
> How does the patient describe the pain?

Is the onset of pain gradual or sudden?

How long does it last—seconds? minutes? hours?

Is the pain steady and persistent in quality?

Is the discomfort accompanied by other symptoms, such as excessive perspiration, light-headedness, nausea, palpitation, shortness of breath?

How many minutes after taking nitroglycerin does the pain last?

What is the mode of pain relief?

The answers to these questions form a basis for designing a logical program of prevention.

When sensing that an attack is imminent, a patient should cease all movement to reduce to a minimum the oxygen requirements of the ischemic myocardium. This is done with the hope that oxygen needs can be met by the limited blood oxygen supply available at the moment and the impending attack can thus be averted.

▷ Nursing Diagnoses

Based on the assessment data, major nursing diagnoses for the patient may include the following:

- Pain related to myocardial ischemia
- Anxiety related to fear of death
- Knowledge deficit about underlying nature of disease and methods for avoiding complications
- Potential noncompliance to therapeutic regimen related to nonacceptance of necessary life style changes

▷ Planning and Implementation

▷ *Goals:*   The major goals of the patient include prevention of pain, reduction of anxiety, awareness of the underlying nature of the disorder and understanding of the prescribed care, and adherence to the self-care program.

▷ Nursing Interventions

▷ *Prevention of Pain.*   The patient must understand the symptom complex and the need to avoid activities known to cause anginal pain, such as sudden exertion, exposure to cold, emotional excitement, and so forth. The patient must learn to change, modify, or adapt to these stresses.

There are patients whose attacks occur predominantly in the morning. For those patients a change in the schedule of daily activities is indicated. As a first step, the patient should plan to rise earlier each morning to shave, wash, and dress in a more leisurely fashion. Ideally, this unhurried pace should be maintained throughout the entire day, so that scheduled tasks and commitments are handled without haste or a sense of pressure. Any patient with angina pectoris should be instructed to initiate all movements with deliberation, avoid exposure to cold, avoid tobacco, eat regularly but lightly, and maintain weight within prescribed limits. Use of over-the-counter drugs should be discouraged, especially diet pills, nasal decongestants, or other drugs containing agents that will increase heart rate and blood pressure.

▷ *Reduction of Anxiety.*   This patient often has a strong fear of death. Staying with the patient is important as a step to minimize this fear. Nursing care is planned so that time away from the bedside is kept to a minimum, because this fear of death often is alleviated by the physical presence of another person. Essential information about the illness and explanation

of why it is important to follow prescribed directives are provided.

▷ *Understanding of the Illness and Strategies to Avoid Complications.*   The education of the patient with angina is designed to acquaint him with the basic nature of his illness and to furnish him with the facts he needs if he is to reorganize his living habits in a way that will reduce the frequency and severity of anginal attacks; delay the progress of the underlying disease, if possible; and help protect him from other complications. The factors outlined in Chart 28–4 are important in the education of the patient with angina pectoris.

▷ *Adherence to the Self-Care Program.*   The self-care program is prepared in collaboration with the patient and his significant other (see Chart 28–4). Activities should be planned so as to minimize the occurrence of episodes of angina. The patient should understand that any pain unrelieved by his usual methods should be treated at the closest emergency center.

▷ Evaluation

Expected Outcomes

1. Is relieved of pain (see Chart 28–4 on patient education)
2. Reduces anxiety
   a. Understands the illness and purpose of treatment
   b. Adheres to medical regimen
   c. Knows to seek medical assistance if pain persists or changes in quality
   d. Avoids being alone during painful episodes
3. Understands ways to avoid complications and demonstrates freedom from complications
   a. Describes the process of angina
   b. Explains reasons for measures to prevent complications
   c. Exhibits normal ECG and level of cardiac enzymes
   d. Is free of signs and symptoms of acute myocardial infarction
4. Adheres to self-care program
   a. Demonstrates an understanding of pharmacologic therapy
   b. Daily habits reflect modification of life style (see Chart 28–4)

In summary, the pain of angina pectoris results from an imbalance between the demand for and supply of oxygen to the myocardial tissue. The most typical form of angina is that which occurs on exertion. Most of the time, cessation of the exertion causes the pain to subside. The relief of angina is accomplished medically by using drug therapy such as nitrates and calcium ion antagonists/blockers. The patient who fails to gain relief from medications may be a candidate for revascularization of blood flow to the myocardium either by PTCA or coronary bypass surgery.

The nurse assists the patient in maximizing benefits from his medical therapies by thorough patient teaching. Evaluating the patient's responses to his therapeutic regimen through subjective and objective assessment offers the maximum opportunity for the patient to control his symptoms. Control of symptoms with medications and life-style changes can deter progress of the underlying disease and prevent complications.

Myocardial Infarction

Definition, Etiology, and Pathophysiology

Myocardial infarction refers to the process by which myocardial tissue is destroyed in regions of the heart that are deprived of

Chart 28–4
Patient Education for the Person With Angina

Goal: To improve the quality of life and promote health

Expected Outcomes

I. Patient reduces probability of an episode of anginal pain
  A. Uses moderation in all activities of life
    1. Participates in a regular daily program of activities that do not produce chest discomfort, shortness of breath, and undue fatigue
    2. Avoids exercises requiring sudden bursts of activity; avoids all isometric exercise
    3. Alternates activity with periods of rest. Some fatigue is normal and temporary
  B. Uses appropriate resources for support during emotionally stressful times, eg, counselor, nurse, clergy, physician
  C. Avoids overeating
    1. Eats smaller portions; may be necessary to eat frequently in smaller amounts to satisfy hunger
    2. Avoids excessive caffeine intake (coffee, cola drinks), which can increase the heart rate and produce angina
    3. Refrains from engaging in physical exercise for 2 hours after meals
  D. Does not use diet pills, nasal decongestants, or any over-the-counter medications that can increase the heart rate
  E. Stops smoking, as smoking increases the heart rate, blood pressure, and blood carbon monoxide levels
  F. Avoids cold weather, if possible; otherwise
    1. Wears scarf over nose/mouth during very cold weather to warm the air
    2. Walks more slowly in cold weather
    3. Dresses warmly in winter, including head, neck, and hand coverings

II. Patient manages an attack of anginal pain
  A. Carries nitroglycerin at all times
    1. Keeps nitroglycerin in a tightly capped, dark-colored glass bottle
    2. Discards the cotton filler/packing to allow prompt access to the pills
    3. Avoids opening the bottle unnecessarily
    4. Discards unused tablets after 5 months; obtains a fresh prescription
    5. When tablets are fresh, they cause a burning sensation when placed under the tongue
  B. Places nitroglycerin under the tongue at first sign of chest discomfort
    1. Does not swallow saliva until the tablet has dissolved
    2. Stops and rests until all pain subsides
    3. States the significance of using the upright position to potentiate the effects of nitroglycerin
    4. Usually, another nitroglycerin tablet may be taken in 3 to 5 minutes for two times. If the anginal discomfort is unrelieved by the usual number of nitroglycerin tablets, or if it recurs after a short interval, goes to the nearest emergency facility
  C. Takes nitroglycerin prophylactically to avoid pain that may occur with certain activities (stair-climbing, sexual intercourse)
  D. Is alert for the side effects of nitroglycerin: headache, flushing, dizziness

an adequate blood supply because of a reduced coronary blood flow. The cause of the reduced blood flow is either a critical narrowing of a coronary artery due to atherosclerosis or a complete occlusion of an artery due to embolus or thrombus. Decreased coronary blood flow may also result from shock and hemorrhage. In each case, there is a profound imbalance between myocardial oxygen supply and demand.

"Coronary occlusion," "heart attack," and "myocardial infarction" are all used synonymously, but the preferred term is *myocardial infarction* (MI). In the United States, well over a million of these attacks occur annually.

The pathophysiology of coronary heart disease and risk factors for it are discussed in the opening pages of this chapter.

Clinical Manifestations

The patient with myocardial infarction is usually male, over 40, and has atherosclerosis of the coronary vessels, often with arterial hypertension. Attacks also occur in women and in younger men in their early 30s or even 20s. Women who take oral contraceptives and also smoke are at very high risk. Overall, however, the rate of myocardial infarction is greater in men than in women at all ages.

Continuous chest pain, characterized by a sudden onset, usually over the lower sternal region and the upper abdomen, is the primary presenting symptom. The pain may increase steadily in severity until it becomes almost unbearable. It is a heavy, viselike pain, which may radiate to the shoulders and down the arms, usually the left arm. Unlike the pain of true angina, it begins spontaneously (not after effort, emotional upset, and the like), persists for hours or days, and is relieved neither by rest nor by nitroglycerin. In some cases the pain may radiate to the jaw and neck. The pain is often accompanied by shortness of breath; pallor; cold, clammy diaphoresis; dizziness or light-headedness; and nausea and vomiting.

The patient with diabetes mellitus may not experience severe pain with myocardial infarction. The neuropathy that accompanies diabetes can interfere with neuroreceptors, thus dulling the pain experience.

Gerontologic Considerations

The elderly patient may not experience the typical viselike pain associated with myocardial infarction because of the diminished responses of neurotransmitters that occur in the aging process. Often the pain is atypical, such as jaw pain, or fainting may be experienced.

The arteriosclerosis that accompanies aging may compromise tissue perfusion because of increased peripheral vascular resistance. Because elderly patients may have a well-established collateral circulation of the myocardium, they often are spared the lethal complications associated with myocardial infarction.

Diagnostic Evaluation

Diagnosis of myocardial infarction is generally based on history of the present illness, electrocardiogram, and serial serum enzymes. Prognosis depends on the severity of coronary artery obstruction and hence the extent of myocardial damage. Physical examination is always conducted but alone is insufficient to confirm the diagnosis.

Patient History.   The taking of a patient history occurs in two steps: (1) the history of the present illness and (2) the history of previous illnesses and family health history, particularly related to the incidence of heart disease in the family. Previous history often can provide valuable information about the patient's risk factors or coronary heart disease. The history of the present illness (*e.g.*, the onset and description of pain) is in many cases conclusive for the diagnosis of myocardial infarction.

The patient's history provides subjective data. The careful practitioner follows the history with interpretation of objective data offered by the ECG and serial enzyme studies.

The Electrocardiogram.   The ECG provides information about the electrophysiology of the heart. Through the use of serial readings, the physician is able to monitor the evolution and resolution of an MI. The location and relative size of the infarction also may be determined by ECG.

Although there are newer technologies that offer equivalent diagnostic data, the ECG remains the first diagnostic instrument of choice because of its bedside accessibility and its noninvasiveness.

Serum Enzymes and Isoenzymes.   Serial enzyme studies include the following:

Creatine Kinase and Its Isoenzymes.   Creatine kinase (CK, with its isoenzyme CK-MB) is regarded as the most sensitive and reliable indicator of all cardiac enzymes. There are three CK isoenzymes: CK-MM (skeletal muscle), CK-MB (heart muscle), and CK-BB (brain tissue). CK-MB is the cardiac-specific isoenzyme; that is, CK-MB is found only in cardiac cells and therefore rises only when there has been damage to these cells. CK-MB is the most specific index for the diagnosis of acute myocardial infarction. It is always increased in cases of severe angina pectoris, coronary insufficiency, and acute MI (AMI).

Lactic Dehydrogenase and Its Isoenzymes.   Lactic dehydrogenase (LDH) is not as reliable an indicator of acute myocardial damage as CK. Because it peaks later and is elevated longer than other cardiac enzymes, however, LDH is useful for diagnosis in patients who may have sustained AMI but have delayed admission to the hospital. There are five LDH isoenzymes, but only two (LDH_1 and LDH_2) are important in the diagnosis of AMI. Both LDH_1 and LDH_2 predominate in the heart, kidney, and brain, but normally the percentage of LDH_2 compared with LDH_1 is greater. When the percentage of LDH_1 exceeds that of LDH_2, the pattern is said to have "flipped," indicating AMI.

Table 28–2 shows the time courses of cardiac enzymes.

Medical Management

The goal of medical management is to minimize myocardial damage. Minimizing myocardial damage is accomplished by

TABLE 28–2.   *Time Course of Cardiac Enzymes Following Acute Myocardial Infarction*

Enzyme	Onset	Peak	Return to Normal
CK	3–6 hr	12–24 hr	3–5 days
CK-MB	2–4 hr	12–20 hr	48–72 hr
LDH	24 hr	48–72 hr	7–10 days
LDH_1	4 hr	48 hr	10 days
LDH_2	4 hr	48 hr	10 days

CK, creatine kinase; CK–MB, creatine kinase–MB isoenzyme; LDH, lactic dehydrogenase.

relieving pain, providing rest, and preventing complications such as lethal dysrhythmias and cardiogenic shock.

The most critical period for the patient with an MI is the first 2 to 3 days after the attack. The area of infarction can increase in size for several hours or days after the onset of the attack. Cardiogenic shock and ventricular fibrillation are common causes of sudden death during this period.

Thrombolytic Therapy.   The goal of management is to minimize myocardial damage and thus reduce the probability of complications. Important in reducing the size of the infarction is the administration of thrombolytic agents. The purpose of these drugs is to dissolve any thrombus that may have formed in a coronary artery, minimizing the occlusion and hence the infarction size. Critical to the effectiveness of these agents is the early administration of the drug after the onset of chest pain.

Three thrombolytic agents have proven to be valuable in thrombolysis: streptokinase, tissue-type plasminogen activator (t-PA), and anistreplase.

Streptokinase.   Streptokinase acts systemically on the body's hemostatic function. Although this medication has demonstrated effectiveness in clot lysis, the potential for systemic hemorrhage has made its use less than desirable. Streptokinase entails a risk of allergic reactions and has proven to be maximally effective only when injected directly into the coronary arteries. Intracoronary administration requires a cardiac catheterization facility, a highly skilled physician, and a cardiothoracic surgery standby team.

Tissue-Type Plasminogen Activator.   Tissue-type plasminogen activator, in contrast, has a specific action in the body's hemostatic function, so the risk of systemic bleeding is reduced. The enzyme t-PA is a naturally occurring enzyme, so allergic reactions are minimized. Finally, studies thus far indicate that intracoronary and intravenous administration of t-PA are equally effective.

Anistreplase.   Anistreplase, a clot-specific thrombolytic agent, parallels streptokinase and t-Pa in clinical effectiveness. Anistreplase is growing in acceptance because of its ease of administration and low cost.

These drugs are only effective if administered within 6 hours of the onset of chest pain, before transmural tissue necrosis occurs; the population of patients that this treatment benefits is thus limited. Coronary artery bypass surgery remains the viable alternative for revascularization of the myocardium in those persons for whom clot lysis is ineffective or contraindicated. (See Chap. 30 for a detailed discussion of bypass surgery.)

Nursing Implications of Thrombolytic Therapy

The nursing management of the patient receiving thrombolytic therapy is directed toward prevention and detection of the complications associated with administration of the drug and immediate intervention if complications occur.

The complications associated with streptokinase administration include systemic bleeding, dysrhythmias produced by coronary artery reperfusion, allergic reactions, and a recurrent thrombosis. Anxiety, which often accompanies the administration of a potentially dangerous drug, can be expected.

Before administration of streptokinase, the nurse conducts a baseline cardiovascular assessment and determines any contraindications to streptokinase therapy. During therapy, the patient's cardiac rhythm is assessed by ECG monitor so that if any new dysrhythmias are produced by reperfusion of a previously obstructed artery, early dysrhythmia management can be implemented. The potential for systemic bleeding can be minimized by monitoring coagulation study results, such as partial thromboplastin time (PTT). Patients who have had surgery in the recent past may not be candidates for this therapy because of the hazard of bleeding.

The complications associated with administration of t-PA are minimal compared with those associated with streptokinase. Tissue-type plasminogen activator acts directly on the clot and thus does not present the risk of systemic bleeding. Reperfusion dysrhythmias are as likely to occur as with streptokinase, thus necessitating monitoring of cardiac rhythm. The results of coagulation studies and the patient's response to concomitant anticoagulation therapy are monitored.

The nurse must remember at all times that thrombolytic therapy, whether streptokinase or t-PA, is superimposed on a patient who is experiencing or recovering from MI. Thus, the patient is continuously observed for complications of his primary illness.

Because of the aggressive nature of the therapies required to minimize myocardial damage, the patient suspected of having an MI is managed in a coronary or intensive care unit.

Intensive and coronary care units are equipped with continuous-monitoring equipment, which facilitates monitoring of dysrhythmias and other hemodynamic parameters. The patient is connected to a variety of monitoring devices. Nurses and physicians with special preparation and skills are assigned to care for these patients.

▶ Nursing Process
The Patient With Myocardial Infarction

▷ Assessment

One of the most important aspects of care of the patient with an MI is the nursing assessment. This serves to establish a baseline of information on the present status of the patient, so that any deviations may be noted immediately. The nursing assessment is orderly and inclusive and has as its objectives identification of the needs of the cardiac patient and determining their priority.

Systematic assessment of the patient includes a careful history, particularly as it relates to the description of symptoms: chest pain, dyspnea, palpitations, faintness (syncope), or sweating (diaphoresis). Each symptom must be evaluated with regard to time, duration, and precipitating and relieving factors.

In addition, a precise and complete physical assessment is critical to the observations for complications. A systematic method is used and should include the following:

1. *Level of consciousness.* The patient's orientation to time, place, and person is monitored closely. Often changes in sensorium are produced by medication therapies or impending cardiogenic shock. An altered sensorium can mean that the heart is not perfusing the cerebral circulation satisfactorily.
2. *Heart size.* The size of the heart may be assessed by identifying its location through palpation. The apical beat, often referred to as the point of maximal impulse (PMI), is normally found at the fifth intercostal space in the midclavicular line (Fig. 28–3). A shift of the heart to the left and downward may indicate left ventricular enlargement.
3. *Heart sounds.* Auscultation is used to identify the normal heart sounds. A stethoscope of good quality and proper fit is essential for the interpretation of heart sounds. The chest piece must have a bell to pick up low-pitched sounds and should have a diaphragm for the auscultation of high-pitched sounds. When using the bell of the stethoscope, it is applied to the skin lightly; when using the diaphragm, it is applied firmly.

The first heart sound (S_1), heard best over the apex of the heart and indicating the beginning of systole, should be identified first. The second sound (S_2), heard best at the base and indicating the beginning of diastole, is identified next (Fig. 28–4).

Abnormal sounds are noted. These include the third heart sound (S_3), known as ventricular gallop, and the fourth heart sound (S_4), known as an atrial or presystolic gallop. S_1 and S_2 together sound like the syllables "lub-dub." S_1 ("lub") is louder at the apex, and S_2 ("dub") is louder at the base. The S_3 sound follows closely after S_2 in a cadence similar to that of the word *Ken-tuck-y.* (S_1-S_2-S_3) The S_4 sound precedes the S_1 in the cadence of the word *Ten-nes-see* (S_4-S_1-S_2). Other sounds, that is, murmurs, created by blood flowing around an obstruction or flowing backward through an incompetent value, also are noted.

The nurse listens frequently after an MI for the development of an S_3. The sound of the S_3 is produced when the

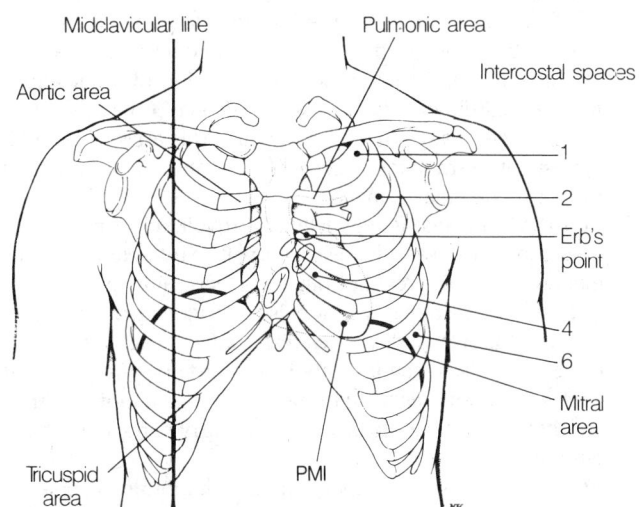

Figure 28–3. The apical beat, often referred to as the point of maximal impulse (PMI), is normally found at the fifth intercostal space in the midclavicular line.

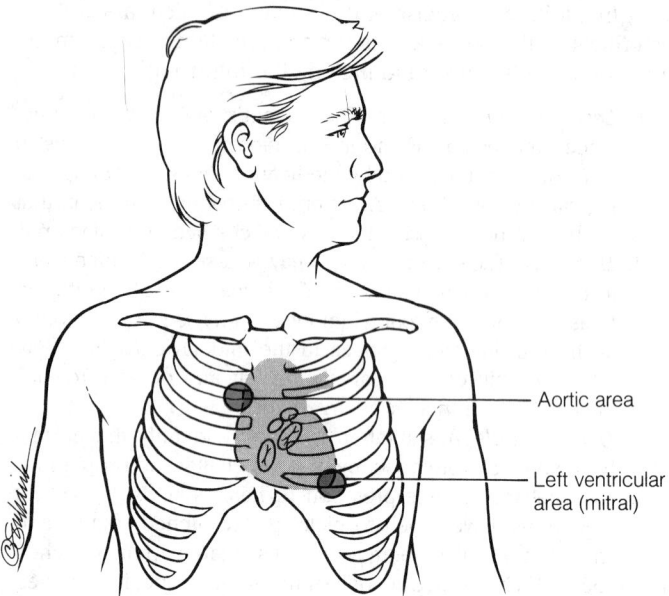

Figure 28–4. Preferred sites for auscultation of first and second heart sounds.

Aortic area

Left ventricular area (mitral)

blood in the ventricles hits against the noncompliant walls of a damaged myocardium. An S_3 can be an early sign of impending left ventricular failure. Early detection of an S_3 followed by aggressive medical management can prevent life-threatening pulmonary edema.

4. *Cardiac rhythm.* The incidence of dysrhythmias after an acute MI is approximately 90%. Early detection allows for initiation of antidysrhythmia medication therapy, which can prevent subsequent reduction in cardiac output, hypotension, reduction of perfusion to vital organs, and progression to lethal dysrhythmias. Although the interpretation of complex dysrhythmias is the responsibility of the critical care nurse, every nurse should be able to recognize normal sinus rhythm and deviations from the normal. It is also important to be familiar with the most commonly occurring dysrhythmias: premature ventricular contractions (PVCs), ventricular tachycardia, ventricular fibrillation, and bradydysrhythmias (see Chap. 29).

A cardiac monitor is used to continuously assess heart rate, rhythm, and conduction. These are documented at regular intervals and before the administration of medications that have cardiovascular effects. A 12-lead ECG is taken when any marked change in rhythm occurs. This assists in the diagnosis of dysrhythmias, conduction disturbances, and any further myocardial damage.

5. *Peripheral pulses.* Rate, rhythm, and volume of pulses are assessed. Cardiovascular disorders will be reflected here. For example, a rapid, regular, but weak pulse may indicate reduced cardiac output. A slow pulse may indicate heart block. An irregular pulse indicates cardiac dysrhythmias. Diminished or absent pulses may indicate that a thrombus from the left ventricle has embolized to the periphery. The femoral arteries are shown statistically to be a frequent site of peripheral arterial emboli.

6. *Fluid volume status.* Urinary output is important, especially in relation to intake. An early sign of cardiogenic shock is oliguria. The nurse observes for edema. In the patient who is on bed rest, the sacrum should be observed for edema.

7. *Pulse pressure.* Careful attention is given to pulse pressure measurements. Pulse pressure is the numeric difference between the systolic and diastolic pressures. A narrowing pulse pressure often is seen after an MI. Stroke volume may be inferred from the pulse pressure; that is, *stroke volume* is the amount of blood ejected with each ventricular contraction. Because effective ventricular contraction is a function of systole and diastole, the quantitative difference between these two hemodynamic parameters reflects the stroke volume.

8. *Bowel sounds.* An assessment of bowel motility is important in monitoring for mesenteric artery thrombosis. A reduction of blood supply will cause infarction of the bowel, a potentially fatal complication.

9. *Lung sounds.* Auscultation of the lung fields at frequent intervals is essential in assessing for signs of ventricular failure. Hearing an S_3 is almost predictable of crackles in the lung bases.

▷ Nursing Diagnoses

Based on the clinical manifestations, nursing history, and the diagnostic assessment data, the patient's major nursing diagnoses may include the following:

- Chest pain related to reduced coronary blood flow
- Potential ineffective breathing patterns related to fluid overload
- Potential altered tissue perfusion related to decreased cardiac output
- Anxiety related to fear of death
- Potential noncompliance with self-care program related to denial of diagnosis of MI

▷ Planning and Implementation

▷ *Goals:* The major goals of the patient include relief of chest pain, absence of respiratory difficulties, maintenance or attainment of adequate tissue perfusion, reduction of anxiety, and adherence to the self-care program.

▷ Nursing Interventions

▷ *Relief of Chest Pain.* The most expedient and appropriate method to relieve chest pain associated with MI is the intravenous administration of an analgesic agent, as prescribed by the physician. The drug of choice is morphine sulfate. Two important criteria are met by the administration of this drug intravenously rather than intramuscularly: a more rapid absorption is assured, and the serum enzyme levels are not falsely elevated as they would be by injection into a muscle. An additional benefit of morphine is the euphoric effect it produces, which is helpful in the management of anxiety. Morphine is also an effective preload and afterload reducer and thus serves to reduce myocardial workload. It accomplishes reduction of preload by causing vasodilation of the vascular smooth muscle, thus pooling the blood in the periphery. Arterial blood pressure is reduced concomitantly, which minimizes afterload. Because morphine is administered intravenously and takes effect rapidly, the nurse monitors the patient closely for hypotension, respiratory depression, and decreased mental acuity.

Administration of oxygen should occur in tandem with analgesia to assure maximum relief of pain. Inhalation of oxygen even in low doses raises the circulating level of oxygen and reduces pain associated with low levels of circulating oxygen.

Vigorous assessment of all vital signs should take place as long as the patient is experiencing pain. Physical rest, in bed with the backrest elevated or in a cardiac chair, will assist in decreasing chest discomfort and dyspnea. The head-up position is beneficial for the following reasons: (1) tidal volume is improved because there is reduced pressure from abdominal contents on the diaphragm, and thus oxygen exchange is improved; (2) drainage of the upper lobes of the lungs is improved; and (3) venous return to the heart is reduced (preload), which reduces the work of the heart.

▷ *Absence of Respiratory Difficulties.* Regular and vigorous assessment of respiratory function can help the nurse detect early signs of complications associated with the lungs. Scrupulous attention to fluid volume status will prevent overloading the heart and hence the lungs. Encouraging the patient to breathe deeply and change position frequently will prevent stagnation of fluid in the lung bases.

▷ *Maintenance or Attainment of Adequate Tissue Perfusion.* Keeping the patient on bed or chair rest is particularly helpful in reducing MVO_2. Checking skin temperature and peripheral pulses with frequency is important to the maintenance of adequate tissue perfusion. Oxygen may be administered to enrich the supply of circulating oxygen.

▷ *Reduction of Anxiety.* Developing a trusting and caring relationship with such patients is critical in reducing their anxiety. Frequent and private opportunities are provided for them to share their concerns and fears. An atmosphere of acceptance helps them to know that their feelings are both realistic and normal.

▷ *Compliance With a Self-Care Program.* The most effective way to increase the probability of compliance with a self-care regimen is adequate education about the disease process. Working with patients in the development of plans streamlined to meet their specific needs further enhances potential for compliance (Chart 28–5).

▷ **Evaluation**

Expected Outcomes
1. Patient experiences relief of pain
2. Shows no signs of respiratory difficulties
3. Maintains adequate tissue perfusion
4. Anxiety is reduced
5. Compliance with self-care program

Care of the patient with an uncomplicated MI is summarized in Nursing Care Plan 28–1.

(text continues on page 657)

Chart 28–5
Self-Care for the Patient With a Myocardial Infarction

A patient who has had an MI learns to regulate activity according to personal responses to each situation.

Goal: To extend and improve the quality of life

Expected Outcomes

I. Patient modifies activities during convalescence so that complete recovery is realized.
   A. Myocardial healing starts early but is not complete for varying periods, usually 6 to 8 weeks.
   B. A myocardial infarction usually requires some modification of life style; adaptation to a heart attack is an ongoing process.
      1. Avoids any activity that produces chest pain, dyspnea, or undue fatigue
      2. Avoids extremes of heat and cold and walking against the wind
      3. Loses weight, if indicated
      4. Stops smoking
      5. Alternates activity with rest periods. Some fatigue is normal and expected during convalescence.
      6. Uses personal strengths to compensate for limitations
      7. Develops regular eating patterns
         a. Avoids large meals and hurrying while eating
         b. Restricts caffeine-containing beverages, because caffeine can affect heart rate, rhythm, and blood pressure
         c. Complies with prescribed diet, modifying calories, fat, and sodium as prescribed
      8. Makes every effort to adhere to medical regimen, especially in taking medications
      9. Pursues activities that afford release of tension

II. Patient undertakes an *orderly* program of increasing activity and exercise for long-term rehabilitation.
   A. Engages in a regimen of physical conditioning with a gradual increase in activity levels
      1. Walks daily, increasing distance and time as prescribed
      2. Monitors pulse during physical activity until the maximum level of activity is attained
      3. Avoids activities that tense the muscles: isometric exercise, weight-lifting, any activity that requires sudden bursts of energy
      4. Avoids physical exercise immediately after a meal
      5. Shortens work hours when first returning to work
   B. Participates in a *daily* program of exercise that develops into a program of regular exercise for a lifetime

III. Manages occurrences of symptoms
      1. Reports to nearest emergency facility for chest pressure or pain not relieved in 15 minutes by nitroglycerin
      2. Contacts the physician when the following occur:
         a. Shortness of breath
         b. Fainting
         c. Slow or rapid heartbeat
         d. Swelling of feet and ankles

Nursing Care Plan 28–1

Care of the Patient With an Uncomplicated Myocardial Infarction

Nursing Interventions	Rationale	Expected Outcomes

Nursing Diagnosis: Chest pain related to reduced coronary blood flow

Goal: Relief of chest pain

1. Initially assess, document, and report to the physician the following:
 	
a. The patient's description of chest discomfort, including location, radiation, duration of pain, and factors that affect it
b. The effect of chest discomfort on cardiovascular hemodynamic perfusion—to the heart, to the brain, to the kidneys, and to the skin
	1. These data assist in determining the cause and effect of the chest discomfort and provide a baseline with which posttherapy symptoms can be compared.
	
	a. There are many conditions associated with chest discomfort. There are characteristic clinical findings of ischemic pain.
	b. Myocardial infarction decreases myocardial contractility and ventricular compliance, and may produce dysrhythmias. Cardiac output is reduced, resulting in reduced blood pressure and decreased organ perfusion. The heart rate may increase as a compensatory mechanism to maintain cardiac output.
		• Reports beginning relief of chest discomfort at once.
		• Appears comfortable:
		  Is restful
		  Respiratory rate, cardiac rate, and blood pressure return to prediscomfort level
		  Skin warm and dry
		• Adequate cardiac output as evidenced by:
		  Heart rate and rhythm
		  Blood pressure
		  Mentation
		  Urine output
		  Serum BUN and creatinine
		  Skin color, temperature, and moisture

2. Obtain a 12-lead ECG recording during pain, as prescribed, to determine extension of infarction.	2. An ECG during pain may be useful in the diagnosis of an extension of myocardial ischemia, injury, and infarction, and of variant angina.	
3. Administer oxygen as prescribed.	3. Oxygen therapy may increase the oxygen supply to the myocardium if actual oxygen saturation is less than normal.	
4. Administer narcotic or analgesic medications as prescribed and evaluate the patient's response continuously.	4. Narcotics are useful in alleviating chest discomfort, decreasing anxiety, and increasing sense of well-being. The side effects of these medications can be hazardous and the patient's status must be assessed.	
5. Ensure physical rest: use of the bedside commode with assistance; backrest elevated to comfort; full liquid diet as tolerated; arms supported during upper extremity activity; use of stool softener to prevent straining at stool. Visitor privileges are individualized, based on patient response. Provide a restful environment, and allay fears and anxiety by being supportive, calm, and competent.	5. Physical rest reduces myocardial oxygen consumption. Fear and anxiety precipitate the stress response; this results in increased levels of endogenous catecholamines, which increase myocardial oxygen consumption. Also, with increased epinephrine the pain threshold is decreased and pain increases the myocardial oxygen consumption.	
6. Promote the patient's physical comfort by providing individualized basic nursing care.	6. Physical comfort promotes the patient's sense of well-being and reduces anxiety.	

(continued)

Nursing Care Plan 28–1 *(Continued)*

Care of the Patient With an Uncomplicated Myocardial Infarction

Nursing Interventions	Rationale	Expected Outcomes

Nursing Diagnosis: Potential ineffective breathing pattern related to fluid overload

Goal: Absence of respiratory difficulties

1. Initially and every 4 hours, and with chest discomfort, assess, document, and report to the physician abnormal heart sounds (particularly S_3 and S_4 gallops and the holosystolic murmur of left ventricular papillary muscle dysfunction), abnormal breath sounds (particularly crackles), and patient intolerance to specific activities.	1. These data are useful in diagnosing left ventricular failure. Diastolic filling sounds (S_3-S_4 gallop) result from decreased left ventricular compliance associated with myocardial infarction. Papillary muscle dysfunction (from infarction of the papillary muscle) can result in mitral regurgitation and a reduction in stroke volume, leading to left ventricular failure. The presence of crackles (usually at the lung bases) may indicate pulmonary congestion from increased left heart pressures. The association of symptoms and activity can be used as a guide for activity prescription and a basis for patient teaching.	• Does not complain of shortness of breath, dyspnea on exertion, orthopnea, or paroxysmal nocturnal dyspnea.
		• Respiratory rate remains less than 20 breaths/min with physical activity and 16 breaths/min with rest.
		• Skin color is normal.
		• PaO_2 and $PaCO_2$ are within normal range.
		• Heart rate is less than 100 beats/min with blood pressure within patient's normal limits.
		• Chest film normal.
		• Patient reports relief of chest discomfort at once.
		• Appears comfortable:
		    Appears restful
		    Respiratory rate, cardiac rate, and blood pressure return to prediscomfort level.
		    Skin warm and dry

2. Promote the patient's physical comfort by providing individualized nursing care. Ensure physical rest.	2. Physical comfort promotes the patient's sense of well-being and reduces anxiety.	
3. Teach patient: a. To adhere to the diet prescribed (for example, explain low-sodium, low-calorie diet)	a. Low-sodium diet may reduce extracellular volume, thus reducing preload and afterload, and thus myocardial oxygen consumption. In the obese patient, weight reduction may decrease cardiac work and improve tidal volume.	
b. To adhere to activity prescription	b. The activity prescription is determined individually to maintain the heart rate and blood pressure within safe limits.	

Nursing Diagnosis: Potential inadequate tissue perfusion related to decreased cardiac output

Goal: Maintenance/attainment of adequate tissue perfusion

1. Initially and every 4 hours, and with chest discomfort, assess, document and report to the physician the following:
  a. Hypotension
  b. Tachycardia and other dysrhythmia
  c. Fatigability
  d. Mentation changes (use family input)
  e. Reduced urine output (less than 250 ml per 8 hours)
  f. Cool, moist, cyanotic extremities
	1. These data are useful in determining a low cardiac output state. An ECG with pain may be useful in the diagnosis of an extension of myocardial ischemia, injury, and infarction, and of variant angina.	• Blood pressure remains within the patient's normal range.
		• Ideally, normal sinus rhythm without dysrhythmia is maintained, or patient's baseline rhythm is maintained between 60 and 100 beats/min without further dysrhythmia.
		• No complaints of fatigue with prescribed activity
		• Remains fully alert and oriented and without personality change.

(continued)

Nursing Care Plan 28–1 (Continued)

Care of the Patient With an Uncomplicated Myocardial Infarction

Nursing Interventions	Rationale	Expected Outcomes

		• Appears comfortable
		  a. Appears restful
		  b. Respiratory rate, cardiac rate, and blood pressure return to prediscomfort level
		  c. Skin warm and dry
		• Urine output is greater than 40 ml/hr.
		• Extremities remain warm and dry with normal color.

2. Promote the patient's physical comfort and rest by providing individualized nursing care.	2. Physical comfort promotes the patient's sense of well-being and reduces anxiety. Rest reduces myocardial oxygen consumption.	

Nursing Diagnosis: Anxiety related to fear of death

Goal: Reduction of anxiety

Nursing Interventions	Rationale	Expected Outcomes
1. Assess, document, and report to the physician the patient's and family's level of anxiety and coping mechanisms.	1. These data provide information about the psychological well-being and a baseline so that post-therapy symptoms can be compared. Causes of anxiety are variable and individual, and may include acute illness, hospitalization, pain, disruption of activities of daily living at home and at work, changes in role and self-image due to chronic illness, and lack of financial support. Because anxious family members can transmit anxiety to the patient, the nurse must also reduce the family's fear and anxiety.	• Reports less anxiety. • Patient and family discuss their anxieties and fears about death. • Patient and family appear less anxious. • Appears restful, respiratory rate less than 16/min, heart rate less than 100/min without ectopic beats, blood pressure within patient's normal limits, skin warm and dry. • Participates actively in a progressive rehabilitation program. • Practices stress-reduction techniques
2. Assess the need for spiritual counseling and refer as appropriate.	2. If a patient finds support in a religion, religious counseling may assist in reducing anxiety and fear.	

3. Allow patient (and family) to express anxiety and fear:
  a. By showing a genuine interest and concern
  b. By facilitating communication (listening, reflecting, guiding)
  c. By answering questions
	3. Unresolved anxiety (the stress response) increases myocardial oxygen consumption.	

4. Use of flexible visiting hours allows the presence of a supportive family to assist in reducing the patient's level of anxiety.	4. The presence of supportive family members may reduce both patient's and family's anxiety.	
5. Encourage active participation in a hospital cardiac rehabilitation program.	5. Prescribed cardiac rehabilitation may help to eliminate fear of death, may reduce anxiety, and may enhance feelings of well-being.	

(continued)

Nursing Care Plan 28–1 *(Continued)*

Care of the Patient With an Uncomplicated Myocardial Infarction

Nursing Interventions	Rationale	Expected Outcomes
6. Teach stress reduction techniques.	6. Stress reduction may help to reduce myocardial oxygen consumption and may enhance feelings of well-being.	

Nursing Diagnosis: Potential noncompliance with self-care program related to denial of diagnosis of myocardial infarction

Goal: Complies with the home health-care program

(See Chart 28-5.)

(Adapted from Underhill SL et al. Cardiac Nursing. Philadelphia, JB Lippincott 1989.)

Cardiac Rehabilitation

Once an AMI has been diagnosed and the patient progresses to symptom-free status, an active rehabilitation program is provided.

The goals of rehabilitation for the patient with an MI are to extend and improve the quality of life. The immediate objectives are to return the patient as rapidly as possible to a normal or near-normal life style. These objectives are accomplished by training the patient for physical activity, educating both patient and family, and initiating psychosocial and vocational counseling when necessary.

Cardiac rehabilitation actually occurs in four phases. Phase 1 begins as soon as the acute episode of illness occurs, usually while the patient is still in the coronary care unit. Phase 2 occurs during the remainder of the hospitalization. During these stages, the nurse can assist the patient toward the realization of his goal of independence, even when he is on strict bed rest. This is achieved by directing his thinking toward the time when he will be active again. The goal here is not to change the patient's life style but to encourage necessary modifications. It is best to avoid focusing on what the patient cannot do. Instead, he is encouraged to develop short-term and long-range goals based on his needs. It is important to explain the nature of the disease, answer questions honestly, and reassure the patient that most persons return to a useful economic life and resume their usual activities. These positive approaches help to keep the patient from becoming a cardiac invalid.

Phase 3 begins with the patient's discharge to home and continues throughout his convalescence. The goal of phase 3 is to continue to restore the patient to activity levels that allow him to return to work or return to activities in which he participated before his illness. This phase is usually accomplished by enrolling the patient in a formal rehabilitation program that provides supervised incremental increases in activities and exercise. In lieu of a formal rehabilitation program, the physician may prescribe appropriate activities and exercises.

Phase 4 focuses on long-term conditioning and the maintenance of cardiovascular stability. The patient is usually very self-directed during this phase and does not require a supervised program. The goals of each phase build on the accomplishments of the previous phase.

Throughout all phases of rehabilitation the goals of activity and exercise tolerance are achieved through physical conditioning. Physical conditioning refers to the process of improving cardiac efficiency. Cardiac efficiency is achieved when work and activities of daily living can be performed at reduced heart rates and lower blood pressure. The outcome is that oxygen requirements of the heart are reduced, thus reducing cardiac workload.

Physical conditioning occurs in phase 1 with range of motion exercises for the arms. Phase 2 includes chair sitting, walking, and some stair climbing. Phase 3 may include walking more vigorously; finally, phase 4 may include jogging.

Physical conditioning is only conducted under the care of a physician. The patient is observed during activities for chest pain, dyspnea, weakness, fatigue, and an excessive increase in heart rate over his baseline rate. Should any of these signs or symptoms occur, the patient is cautioned to cease activity immediately and seek appropriate medical attention.

A complete discussion of cardiac rehabilitation is beyond the scope of this text; a rehabilitation text may be consulted for detailed explanations.

In summary, myocardial infarction refers to the process by which myocardial tissue is destroyed as a result of reduced coronary blood flow. The primary symptom is the sudden, unprovoked onset of severe viselike chest pain that may be accompanied by pallor, shortness of breath, or diaphoresis.

Medical diagnosis is made by evaluation of the patient's history, ECG, and serial serum enzymes. Of these three, the patient history is often sufficiently positive to confirm diagnosis. The goals of medical management are to minimize the damage to affected tissue, to preserve the integrity of the unaffected tissue, and to prevent lethal complications. Myocardial tissue preservation is accomplished by relieving pain, promoting rest to reduce myocardial work, and by administering thrombolytic therapy to enhance blood flow. In some cases revascularization through coronary artery bypass surgery is indicated. The intensive therapies required for the patient with an MI necessitate that the patient be in a critical care environment where continuous ECG monitoring can take place.

The patient experiencing an MI requires an intensive, orderly nursing assessment. Emphasis is placed on observation of physical signs associated with cardiovascular system competency such as heart rate and rhythm, urinary output, and level of consciousness.

Nursing interventions are directed at resolving altered comfort due to chest pain and then reducing anxiety. The patient is further assisted to recovery through a formalized cardiac rehabilitation program.

Infectious Diseases of the Heart

Rheumatic Endocarditis

Pathophysiology. The development of rheumatic endocarditis is directly attributed to rheumatic fever, a systemic disease caused by a group A streptococcal infection. Rheumatic fever affects all bony joints, producing a polyarthritis. The heart is also a target organ and is where the most serious damage occurs.

The heart damage and the joint lesions are not infectious in origin, in the sense that these tissues are not invaded and directly damaged by destructive organisms; rather, they represent a sensitivity phenomenon occurring in response to the *hemolytic streptococcus.* Blood leukocytes accumulate in the affected tissues and form nodules, which eventually are replaced by scars. The myocardium is certain to be involved in this inflammatory process; that is, *rheumatic myocarditis* develops, which temporarily weakens the contractile power of the heart. The pericardium likewise is affected; that is, *rheumatic pericarditis* also occurs during the acute illness. These myocardial and pericardial complications usually are without serious sequelae; conversely, the effects of *rheumatic endocarditis* are permanent and often crippling.

Rheumatic endocarditis anatomically manifests itself first by tiny translucent vegetations, which resemble beads about the size of the head of a pin, arranged in a row along the free margins of the valve flaps. These tiny beads look harmless enough and may disappear without injuring the valve flaps, but more often they have serious effects. They are the starting point of a process that gradually thickens the flaps, rendering them shorter and thicker than normal, which prevents them from closing the orifice of the valve perfectly. The result is leakage, a condition called *valvular regurgitation.* The most common site of valvular regurgitation is mitral regurgitation.

In other patients, the inflamed margins of the valve flaps become adherent, resulting in *valvular stenosis,* a narrowed or "stenotic" valvular orifice. A small percentage of patients with rheumatic fever become critically ill with intractable heart failure, serious dysrhythmias, and rheumatic pneumonia. These patients are treated in an intensive care unit.

Most patients recover with gratifying speed and their recovery ostensibly is complete. However, although free of symptoms, the patient is left with certain permanent residual effects that often lead gradually to progressive valvular deformities. The extent of cardiac damage, or even its existence, may not have been apparent in clinical examinations during the acute phase of the disease. Eventually, however, the heart murmurs that are characteristic of valvular stenosis, regurgitation, or both, become audible on auscultation and, in some patients, even detectable as "thrills" on palpation. The myocardium usually can compensate for these valvular defects very

well for a time, despite its increased burden. As long as it can do so, the patient remains in apparent good health. Sooner or later, however, it fails to compensate—and decompensation, when it occurs, is signaled by the manifestations of congestive heart failure, as described in Chapter 29.

Clinical Manifestations. The cardiac symptoms that appear will be dependent on which side of the heart is involved. The mitral valve is most often affected, producing the symptoms of left-sided heart failure: shortness of breath and crackles and wheezes in the lungs. See Chapter 29 for a discussion of left-sided versus right-sided failure. The severity of the symptoms depends on the size and location of the lesion.

The systemic symptoms that are present will be proportionate to the virulence of the invading organism. The identification of a new murmur in an individual with a systemic infection should be suspected as infectious endocarditis.

Management. The objectives of medical management are aggressive eradication of the causative organism and prevention of additional complications such as a thromboembolic event. Long-term antibiotic therapy is the treatment of choice. Penicillin administered parenterally remains the drug of choice.

The patient with rheumatic endocarditis, whose valve function is faulty but whose disease is quiescent, does not require therapy as long as the heart pumps effectively. Nevertheless, the danger exists of recurrent attacks of acute rheumatic fever, of bacterial endocarditis, of embolism from vegetations or mural thrombi in the heart, and of eventual cardiac failure. (The relationship between valvular disease and congestive failure and the treatment of heart failure are presented in Chap. 29.)

Prevention. The prevention of rheumatic endocarditis is accomplished through early and adequate treatment of streptococcal infections in all persons.

A first-line approach in preventing initial attacks of rheumatic endocarditis is to recognize streptococcal infections, treat them adequately, and control epidemics in the community. Every nurse should be familiar with the signs and symptoms of streptococcal pharyngitis (Chart 28–6).

- A throat culture is the only method by which accuracy of the diagnosis can be determined.

Susceptible patients may require long-term oral antibiotic therapy or, more commonly, be required to take prophylactic antibiotics before procedures that can potentiate invasion by a microorganism. Penicillin taken before dental checkups is an excellent example. The patient also must be reminded of less common procedures such as cystoscopy that may also require prophylaxis.

Infective Endocarditis

Pathophysiology. Infective endocarditis (bacterial endocarditis) is an infection of the valves and endothelial surface of the heart caused by direct invasion by bacteria or other organisms and leading to deformity of the valve leaflets. Causative microorganisms include bacteria (streptococci, enterococci, pneumococci, staphylococci,) fungi, rickettsiae, and *Streptococcus viridans.*

Infective endocarditis usually develops in patients who have a history of valvular heart disease. At great risk are patients with rheumatic heart disease or mitral valve prolapse and individuals who have had prosthetic valve surgery.

Chart 28-6
Signs and Symptoms of Streptococcal Pharyngitis

Rheumatic fever is a preventable disease. By eradication of rheumatic fever, the great cardiac crippler—*rheumatic heart disease*—would be virtually eliminated. Through the use of penicillin therapy in patients with streptococcal infections, almost all primary attacks of rheumatic fever can be prevented. A throat culture is the only method by which an accurate diagnosis can be determined. The signs and symptoms of streptococcal pharyngitis are the following:

- Fever (38.9° to 40°C, or 101° to 104°F)
- Chilliness
- Sore throat (sudden in onset)
- Diffuse redness of throat with exudate on oropharynx (may not appear until after the first day)
- Enlarged and tender lymph nodes
- Abdominal pain (more common in children)
- Acute sinusitis and acute otitis media (may be due to streptococcus)

Infective endocarditis often accompanies medical and surgical therapy. It is more common in older persons, probably because of decreased immunologic responses to infection, metabolic alterations arising from changes in the aging body, and increased instrumentation, especially in genitourinary disease. There is a high incidence of staphylococcal endocarditis among intravenous drug users, the disease occurring for the most part on normal valves.

Hospital-acquired endocarditis occurs most often in patients with debilitating disease, those with indwelling catheters, and those on prolonged intravenous or antibiotic therapy. Patients on immunosuppressive drugs or steroids may develop fungal endocarditis.

Clinical Manifestations. The onset of infective endocarditis usually is insidious. The signs and symptoms develop from toxicity of the infection, destruction of heart valves, and from embolization of fragments of vegetations.

The general manifestations, which may be mistaken for influenza, include vague complaints of malaise, anorexia, weight loss, cough, and back and joint pain. Fever is intermittent and may be absent in patients who are receiving antibiotics or corticosteroids or in those who are elderly or have congestive heart failure or renal failure. Splinter hemorrhages (linear and hemorrhagic streaks) may be noted under the fingernails and toenails, and petechiae may appear in the conjunctiva and mucous membranes. Hemorrhages with pale centers (Roth's spots) that may be seen in the fundi of the eyes are caused by emboli in the nerve fiber layer of the eye.

The cardiac manifestations include heart murmurs, which may be absent initially. Changing murmurs may be encountered and indicate valvular damage due to vegetations or to perforation of the valve or of the chordae tendinae. Heart enlargement or evidence of congestive heart failure is also seen.

The central nervous system manifestations include headache, transient cerebral ischemia, focal neurologic lesions, and strokes, which may be caused by emboli involving the cerebral arteries.

Embolization may be a presenting symptom, occurring at any time and involving other organ systems. The embolic phenomena may be manifested in the lung (recurrent pneumonia; pulmonary abscesses), kidney (hematuria; renal failure), spleen (left upper quadrant pain), heart (myocardial infarction), brain (stroke), or peripheral vessels.

Management. The objective of treatment is total eradication of the invading organism by adequate doses of an appropriate antimicrobial agent. The causative organism can be isolated through serial blood cultures. It is treated with a bactericidal agent or other appropriate medication, based on proven sensitivity to the causative agent. The antibiotic is usually administered parenterally in a continuous intravenous infusion for a period of 4 to 6 weeks. Bactericidal serum levels of the selected antibiotic are monitored by titering it against the causative organism. If the serum does not demonstrate bactericidal activity, increased dosages of the antibiotic are given or a different antibiotic is tried. There are numerous antimicrobial regimens currently in use, but penicillin is usually the drug of choice. Blood cultures are taken periodically to monitor the course of therapy.

Treatment with amphotericin B usually is required for the patient with fungal endocarditis.

After recovery from the infectious process, seriously damaged valves, as determined by severity of symptoms, may require replacement. The patient's temperature is monitored at regular intervals, because the course of fever is one indication of the effectiveness of treatment. Febrile reactions may occur also as a result of drug therapy, however. After adequate antimicrobial therapy is initiated, bacteria usually disappear. The patient should demonstrate an improved sense of well-being, better appetite, and decreased lethargy. During this time, patients require a great deal of psychosocial support, especially because they feel well but may find themselves confined to the hospital with restrictive IV therapy.

Complications. Even if the patient responds to the antimicrobial therapy, endocarditis can be very destructive to the heart and other organs. Congestive heart failure and cerebral vascular complications such as strokes may occur before, during, or after therapy. Valve stenosis or regurgitation, myocardial erosion, and mycotic aneurysms are some potential heart complications. Many other organ complications can result from septic or nonseptic emboli, immunologic responses, or hemodynamic deterioration.

Surgery. The advent of surgical valve replacement has favorably changed the prognosis of patients with severely damaged heart valves. Usually, valve excision and replacement are required for (1) patients who develop congestive heart failure as a result of aortic or mitral valve involvement in spite of adequate medical treatment; (2) patients who have more than one serious systemic embolic episode; and (3) persons with uncontrolled infection, recurrent infection, or fungal endocarditis. A large number of patients who have prosthetic valve endocarditis (infected prostheses) require valve replacement.

Prevention.   Infective endocarditis occurs most often in persons with structural abnormalities of the heart and great vessels, especially valvular heart disease. Any procedure that is associated with transient bacteremia may cause bacteria to lodge on damaged or abnormal valves. Persons at risk are patients with prosthetic cardiac valves, including bioprosthetic and homograft valves; previous bacterial endocarditis, even in the absence of heart disease; most congenital malformations; rheumatic and other acquired valvular dysfunction, even after valvular surgery; hypertrophic cardiomyopathy; and mitral valve prolapse with valvular regurgitation.

Antibiotic prophylaxis is recommended for persons at risk who undergo the following procedures and circumstances*:

Dental procedures known to induce gingival or mucosal bleeding, including professional cleaning
Tonsillectomy or adenoidectomy
Surgical operations that involve intestinal or respiratory mucosa
Bronchoscopy with a rigid bronchoscope
Sclerotherapy for esophageal varices
Esophageal dilatation
Gallbladder surgery
Cystoscopy
Urethral dilatation
Urethral catheterization if urinary tract infection is present
Urinary tract surgery if urinary tract infection is present
Prostatic surgery
Incision and drainage of infected tissue
Vaginal hysterectomy
Vaginal delivery in the presence of infection

Myocarditis

Pathophysiology.   Acute myocarditis is an inflammatory process involving the myocardium. The heart is a muscle; hence, its efficiency depends on the health of the individual muscle fibers. When the muscle fibers are healthy, the heart can function well in spite of severe valvular injuries; when the muscle fibers are damaged, life is in jeopardy.

Myocarditis usually results from an infectious process, particularly of viral, bacterial, mycotic, parasitic, protozoal, or spirochetal origin, or it may be produced by hypersensitivity states such as rheumatic fever. Therefore, myocarditis may be seen in patients with acute systemic infections, those receiving immunosuppressive therapy, or those with infective endocarditis.

Myocarditis can cause heart dilatation, mural thrombi, infiltration of circulating blood cells around the coronary vessels and between the muscle fibers, and degeneration of the muscle fibers themselves.

---

* A Statement for Health Professionals by the Committee on Rheumatic Fever, Endocarditis, and Kawasaki Disease of the Council on Cardiovascular Disease in the Young of the American Heart Association. JAMA 1990 Dec 12; 264(22):2919–2922

Clinical Manifestations.   The symptoms of acute myocarditis depend on the type of infection, the degree of myocardial damage, and the capacity of the myocardium to recover. Symptoms may be mild or absent. The patient may complain of fatigue and dyspnea, palpitations, and occasional precordial discomfort. Clinical examination may show cardiac enlargement, faint heart sounds, gallop rhythm, and a systolic murmur. A pericardial friction rub may be heard if the patient has associated pericarditis. Pulsus alternans (a pulse in which there is a regular alternation of weak and strong beats) may be present (see Chap. 27). Fever and tachycardia are frequently seen and symptoms of congestive heart failure may develop. Diagnosis can be confirmed by endomyocardial biopsy.

Management.   The patient is given specific treatment for the underlying cause, if it is known (*e.g.*, penicillin for hemolytic streptococci), and is placed on bed rest to decrease cardiac work, that is, to reduce the heart rate, stroke volume, blood pressure, and heart contractility. Bed rest also helps to decrease residual myocardial damage and the complications of myocarditis. The treatment is essentially the same as that used for congestive heart failure (see Chap. 29). The pulse, heart sounds, and temperature are evaluated to determine whether the disease is subsiding and whether congestive heart failure has occurred. If a dysrhythmia occurs, the patient should be placed in a unit with continuous cardiac monitoring so that personnel and equipment are readily available if a life-threatening dysrhythmia occurs.

When there is evidence of congestive heart failure, medication is administered to slow the heart rate and augment myocardial contractility.

- Patients with myocarditis are sensitive to digitalis. There must be continuing nursing surveillance to assess the patient for digitalis toxicity (evidenced by dysrhythmia, anorexia, nausea, vomiting, bradycardia, headache, malaise).

Elastic stockings and passive and active exercises should be used, because embolization from venous thrombosis and mural thrombi can occur.

Prevention.   The prevention of infectious diseases by means of appropriate immunizations and early treatment appears to be important in decreasing the incidence of myocarditis. After a bout of myocarditis, there is usually some residual heart enlargement. Physical activity is increased slowly, and the patient is instructed to report any symptoms that occur with increasing activity, such as a rapidly beating heart. Competitive sports and alcohol must be avoided.

Pericarditis

Definition and Etiology

Pericarditis refers to an inflammation of the pericardium, the membranous sac enveloping the heart. It may be a primary illness, or it may develop in the course of a variety of medical and surgical diseases. The following are some of the causes underlying or associated with pericarditis:

1. Idiopathic or nonspecific causes
2. Infection
   a. Bacterial (*e.g.*, streptococcus, staphylococcus, meningococcus, gonococcus)

  b. Viral (*e.g.*, coxsackie, influenza)
  c. Mycotic (fungal) (*e.g.*, rickettsia, parasite)
3. Disorders of connective tissue—systemic lupus erythematosus, rheumatic fever, rheumatoid arthritis, polyarteritis
4. Hypersensitivity states—immune reactions, drug reactions, serum sickness
5. Diseases of adjacent structures—myocardial infarction, dissecting aneurysm, pleural and pulmonary disease (pneumonia)
6. Neoplastic disease
  a. Secondary to metastasis from lung cancer, breast cancer
  b. Leukemia
  c. Primary (mesothelioma)
7. Radiation therapy
8. Trauma—chest injury, cardiac surgery, during cardiac catheterization, pacemaker implantation
9. Association with renal disorders (uremia)
10. Tuberculosis

Clinical Manifestations

The characteristic symptom of pericarditis is *pain* and the characteristic sign is a *friction rub*. Pain is almost always present in acute pericarditis and is most common over the precordium. The pain may be felt beneath the clavicle and in the neck and left scapular region. Pericardial pain is aggravated by breathing, turning in bed, and twisting the body; it is relieved by sitting up. In fact, the patient prefers to adopt a forward-leaning or a sitting posture. Dyspnea may occur as the result of pericardial compression of the heart's movements, which leads to a decreased cardiac output. The patient may appear extremely ill. Pericarditis *per se* often gives rise to no signs other than fever and the production of a friction rub.

Diagnostic Evaluation

Diagnosis is most often made on the presentation of signs and symptoms. The ECG may be helpful in confirming the diagnosis.

Management

The objectives of management are to determine the cause, to administer therapy for the specific cause (when known), and to be on the alert for *cardiac tamponade* (compression of the heart from fluid in the pericardial sac; see Chap. 30). The patient is placed on bed rest when cardiac output is impaired, until the fever, chest pain, and friction rub have disappeared.

Meperidine or morphine may be prescribed for pain relief during the acute phase. Salicylates relieve pain and hasten reabsorption of fluid in the patient with rheumatic pericarditis. Corticosteroids may be prescribed to control symptoms, hasten resolution of the inflammatory process in the pericardium, and prevent recurring pericardial effusion.

- Be alert to the possibility of cardiac tamponade. Use nursing assessment skills to anticipate and identify the triad of symptoms—falling arterial pressure, rising venous pressure, and distant heart sounds.

Patients with infections of the pericardium are treated with the antimicrobial agent of choice based on identification and sensitivity tests. The pericarditis of rheumatic fever may respond to penicillin. Isoniazid, ethambutol, rifampin, and streptomycin in various combinations are used in the treatment of tuberculosis that produces pericarditis. Amphotericin B is used in fungal pericarditis, and adrenal steroids are used in disseminated lupus erythematosus.

As the patient's condition improves, activity may be increased gradually. If pain, fever, or friction rub reappear, however, bed rest must be resumed.

▶ Nursing Process
The Patient With Pericarditis

▷ Assessment

Pain is the primary symptom of the patient with pericarditis. The pain of pericarditis is assessed by observation and by evaluation while having the patient vary positions in bed.

While observing the patient, the examiner tries to discover whether or not the pain is influenced by respiratory movements, with or without the actual passage of air; by flexion, extension, or rotation of the spine, including the neck; by movements of the shoulders and arms; by coughing; or by swallowing. Recognizing these relationships may be very helpful in establishing a diagnosis.

A pericardial friction rub occurs when the pericardial surfaces lose their lubricating fluid because of inflammation. The rub is audible on auscultation and is synchronous with the heartbeat. A pericardial friction rub is diagnostic of pericarditis and should be searched for diligently.

- The diaphragm of the stethoscope is placed tightly against the thorax; the left sternal edge in the fourth intercostal space, the site where the pericardium comes into contact with the left chest wall, is auscultated. A pericardial friction rub has a scratching or leathery sound. The rub is louder at the end of expiration and may be heard best while the patient is sitting.

If there is difficulty in distinguishing a pericardial friction rub from a pleural friction rub, the patient is asked to hold his breath. A pericardial friction rub will be continuous.

The patient's temperature is monitored frequently. Pericarditis will cause an abrupt onset of fever in a patient who has been afebrile.

▷ Nursing Diagnoses

Based on the assessment data, major nursing diagnoses of the patient may include the following:

- Pain related to inflammation of the pericardium
- Potential development of decreased cardiac output related to restriction of cardiac contraction

▷ Planning and Implementation

▷ *Goals:* The major goals of the patient may include relief of pain and maintenance or attainment of cardiac output.

▷ Nursing Interventions

▷ *Relief of Pain.* Relief of pain is achieved by having this patient remain on bed rest or chair rest, whichever is more comfortable. Because the posture the patient assumes to relieve the pain is that of sitting upright and leaning forward, chair rest may be more comfortable. As the chest pain and friction rub abate, activities of daily living may be resumed gradually.

If the patient is receiving medications for the pericarditis, such as analgesics, antibiotics, or corticosteroids, the patient's responses are monitored and recorded.

If chest pain and the friction rub recur, bed rest is resumed.

▷   *Maintenance/Attainment of Adequate Cardiac Output.*   If the patient does not respond to medical management, fluid may develop or accumulate between the pericardial linings or in the sac. This condition is called *pericardial effusion* (see Chap. 29). Fluid in the pericardial sac can cause constriction of the myocardium and interrupt its ability to pump. Thus, the cardiac output will decline with each contraction. Failure to identify the onset of this problem can lead to cardiac tamponade and the possibility of sudden death.

Early signs and symptoms of this event to observe for are those that indicate a falling arterial pressure. Usually the systolic pressure falls while the diastolic pressure remains stable; hence the pulse pressure narrows. Heart sounds may progress from being distant to being imperceptible. Neck vein distention and other signs of rising central venous pressure are observed. These signs and symptoms occur because, as the fluid-filled pericardial sac compresses the myocardium, blood continues to return to the heart from the periphery but cannot be pumped back into the circulation.

The physician must be notified immediately. The nurse should prepare for a pericardiocentesis (see Chap. 29). The nurse stays with the patient and continues to assess and record signs and symptoms until the physician arrives to prescribe more definitive therapy.

▷   Evaluation

Expected Outcomes
1. Patient is free of pain
   a. Performs activities of daily living comfortably
   b. Temperature returns to patient's normal range
   c. Pericardial friction rub is absent
2. Maintains or attains adequate cardiac output
   a. Blood pressure remains in patient's normal range
   b. Heart sounds are of good volume and can be auscultated
   c. Neck veins are not distended

Chronic Constrictive Pericarditis

Chronic constrictive pericarditis is a condition in which chronic inflammatory thickening of the pericardium compresses the heart and prevents it from expanding to normal size. The major hemodynamic deficit results from a restriction of ventricular filling.

Often the adherent pericardium becomes calcified. The heart action is greatly restricted by this tough, unyielding enclosure, and edema, ascites, and hepatic enlargement result. The fixation of the heart to the pericardium may produce a retraction of the chest wall with every beat.

Chronic restrictive pericarditis is caused by long-standing pyogenic infections, postviral infections, tuberculosis, or hemopericardium.

The signs and symptoms are predominantly those of congestive heart failure (see Chap. 29), but dyspnea on exertion is the most prominent symptom. Chronic atrial fibrillation is commonly present.

Surgical removal of the tough encasing pericardium (pericardiectomy) is the only treatment of any benefit. The objective of the operation is to release both ventricles from the constrictive and restrictive inflammation. (See Chap. 30 for care of the patient after cardiac surgery.)

In summary, the structure of the heart (see Chap. 27) renders it vulnerable to the toxic effects of the microorganisms that can invade the bloodstream. The organisms may be foreign, as in cases of infective endocarditis, or may be a result of an autoimmune response, as is suspected in collagen tissue–related diseases like rheumatic fever.

The responsible organism migrates to an area of heart tissue, attaches itself, and serves as a site for fibrin, bacteria, and platelet aggregation and ultimately scar tissue formation. The scarred tissue becomes thickened, stiffened, contracted, and deformed.

The degree of morbidity experienced by the patient is proportionate to the degree to which heart muscle mass is impaired. The symptomatology is also dependent on whether the right or left side of the heart is affected. Because infective heart disease is preventable, gaining knowledge about the causes and effects of infectious heart disease provides an opportunity for the nurse to play a pivotal role in the practice of prevention through teaching.

Acquired Valvular Diseases of the Heart

Mitral Valve Prolapse Syndrome

Pathophysiology.   The mitral valve prolapse syndrome is a dysfunction of the mitral valve leaflets that renders the mitral valve incompetent and results in valvular regurgitation. This syndrome may produce no symptoms or it may progress rapidly and result in sudden death. In recent years the syndrome has been diagnosed more frequently, ostensibly as a result of improved diagnostic methods.

Clinical Manifestations.   Many individuals have the syndrome but no symptoms. Often the symptoms are first identified during a physical examination of the heart, which discloses an extra heart sound referred to as a *mitral click*. The presence of a click indicates early valvular incompetence with disruption of normal blood flow. The mitral click may deteriorate into a murmur over time as the valve leaflets become progressively dysfunctional. Concomitant with the progression of the murmur may be signs and symptoms of heart failure as mitral regurgitation ensues.

Management.   Medical management is directed at controlling the associated symptoms. Some persons experience worrisome dysrhythmias and require antidysrhythmic agents. Others experience mild heart failure and require therapy (see Chap. 29 for a discussion of heart failure). In advanced stages, mitral valve replacement may be necessary.

It is important to educate patients with this syndrome about the need for prophylactic antibiotic therapy before undergoing invasive procedures that may introduce infectious agents systemically (*e.g.*, dental work, gastrourinary or gastrointestinal procedures, IV therapy). If in doubt about risk factors and the need for antibiotics, patients are advised to consult their physician.

Mitral Stenosis

Pathophysiology. Mitral stenosis is the progressive thickening and contracture of the mitral valve cusps, which causes narrowing of the orifice and progressive obstruction to blood flow.

Normally, three fingers should pass easily through this orifice, but in cases of marked stenosis a lead pencil will hardly fit through it. The left ventricle is not affected, but the left atrium has great difficulty in emptying itself through the narrow orifice into the ventricle. Therefore, it dilates and hypertrophies. Because no valve protects the pulmonary veins from a backward flow from this atrium, pulmonary circulation becomes markedly congested. As a result of the abnormally high pulmonary arterial pressure that must be maintained by the right ventricle, it is subjected to an excess strain and eventually fails.

Clinical Manifestations. Patients with mitral stenosis are likely to show progressive fatigue as a result of low cardiac output, hemoptysis, and dyspnea on exertion due to pulmonary venous hypertension, cough, and repeated respiratory infections.

The pulse is weak and often irregular because of atrial fibrillation caused by the atrium's dilation and hypertrophy. These render the atrium electrically unstable, resulting in a permanent atrial dysrhythmia. Diagnostic aids for the cardiologist are electrocardiography, echocardiography, and cardiac catheterization with angiography to verify the severity of the mitral stenosis.

Management. Antibiotic therapy is instituted to prevent recurrence of infections while congestive heart failure is treated with cardiotonics and diuretics. Surgical intervention consists of a valvotomy to rupture the fused commissures of the mitral valve or replacement of the mitral valve with a prosthetic valve (see Chap. 30). In some cases where surgery is contraindicated and medical therapy is failing, percutaneous transluminal valvuloplasty may offer some palliation of symptoms.

Mitral Insufficiency (Regurgitation)

Pathophysiology. Mitral insufficiency results when incompetence and distortion of the mitral valve prevent its free margins from coming into apposition during systole. The chordae tendinae may become shortened, preventing complete closure of the leaflets. Valvular movement is more restricted than in mitral stenosis. In about half of the patients, mitral regurgitation is caused by chronic rheumatic endocarditis.

Shortening or tearing of one or both of the mitral valve flaps prevents the perfect closure of the mitral orifice while the powerful left ventricle is forcing the blood into the aorta. Then, at each beat the left ventricle forces some of the blood back into the left atrium. Because this blood is added to the blood that is beginning to flow into this chamber from the lungs, the left atrium must dilate and hypertrophy. This backward flow of blood from the ventricle diminishes the volume of blood flowing from the lungs. As a result the lungs become congested, which adds an extra strain on the right ventricle. Therefore, the result of even slight mitral leak always involves both lungs and the right ventricle.

Clinical Manifestations. Palpitation of the heart, shortness of breath on exertion, and cough due to chronic passive pulmonary congestion are common symptoms. The pulse may be regular and of good volume, but frequently it becomes irregular as a result of either extrasystoles or atrial fibrillation, which may persist indefinitely.

Management. Management is the same as that for congestive heart failure. Surgical intervention consists of mitral valve replacement.

Aortic Valve Stenosis

Pathophysiology. Aortic valve stenosis is the narrowing of the orifice between the left ventricle and the aorta. In adults the stenosis may be congenital, or it may be a result of rheumatic endocarditis or cusp calcification of unknown cause. There is progressive narrowing of the valve orifice over a period of several years to several decades.

The leaflets of the aortic valve fuse and partially close the opening between the heart and the aorta. The left ventricle overcomes this obstruction to circulation by contracting more slowly but with greater energy than normal, forcibly squeezing the blood through the very small orifice. The heart's compensatory mechanisms begin to fail and clinical signs develop.

The obstruction to the aortic outflow tract places a pressure load on the left ventricle, which shows the strain by a thickening of the muscle wall. The heart muscle increases in size (hypertrophy) in response to all degrees of obstruction; heart failure occurs when obstruction is severe.

Clinical Manifestations. In moderate to severe cases of aortic stenosis, the patient first experiences exertional dyspnea, which is a manifestation of left ventricular decompensation with pulmonary congestion. Other signs are dizziness and fainting because of reduced volume of blood going to the brain. Angina pectoris is a frequent symptom that results from the increased oxygen demands imposed by the increased work of the left ventricle and by myocardial hypertrophy. Blood pressure can be low but is usually normal; often there is a low pulse pressure (30 mm Hg or less) because of diminished blood flow.

On physical examination, a loud, rough systolic murmur may be heard over the aortic area. The sound to listen for is a systolic crescendo–decrescendo murmur, which may radiate into the carotid arteries and to the apex of the left ventricle. The murmur is low-pitched, rough, rasping, and vibrating. If one rests a hand over the base of the heart, a vibration is felt that is the most intense of all cardiac thrills and resembles the purring of a cat. The purring is related to the turbulence caused by the blood flow across a narrowed valve orifice. The evidence of left ventricular hypertrophy may be seen on a 12-lead ECG.

Left-heart catheterization is necessary to accurately measure the severity of this valvular abnormality. Pressure tracings are taken from the left ventricle and the base of the aorta. The systolic pressure in the left ventricle is considerably higher than that in the aorta during systole.

Management. The singular definitive treatment for aortic stenosis is surgical replacement of the aortic valve. A significant risk of sudden death exists for those patients who are treated medically without surgical repair. The uncorrected condition can lead to irreversible heart failure that is intractable to medical therapies.

Aortic Insufficiency (Regurgitation)

Pathophysiology. Aortic insufficiency is caused by inflammatory lesions that deform the flaps of the aortic valve, preventing them from completely sealing the aortic orifice during diastole and thus allowing a backflow of blood from the aorta into the left ventricle. This valvular defect may result from endocarditis, congenital abnormalities, or diseases such as syphilis and dissecting aneurysm that cause dilation or tearing of the ascending aorta.

Because of the leak in the aortic valve during diastole, some of the blood in the aorta, always under high pressure, flows into the left ventricle, which must handle both the blood normally delivered by the left atrium into the ventricle through the mitral orifice and that returning from the aorta. The left ventricle dilates to accommodate this increased volume, hypertrophies to expel it, and does so with more than normal force, thus raising systolic blood pressure. The cardiovascular system tends to become accommodated through reflex vasodilation; the peripheral arterioles become relaxed, so peripheral resistance is lessened and diastolic pressure greatly lowered.

Clinical Manifestations. The disease develops insidiously, and the earliest manifestation is awareness of the increased force of the heartbeat. There may be marked arterial pulsations that are visible or palpable over the precordium. Arterial pulsation in the neck also will be marked. This is a result of the increased force and volume of the blood ejected from the hypertrophied left ventricle. Exertional dyspnea and easy fatigability follow. Signs and symptoms of left ventricular failure (orthopnea, paroxysmal nocturnal dyspnea) occur with moderate to severe regurgitation.

The pulse pressure (the difference between systolic and diastolic pressures) is considerably widened in these patients. One of the characteristic signs of the disease is the manner in which the pulse strikes the palpating finger with quick, sharp strokes and then suddenly collapses (water-hammer pulse). The nature of the pulse wave is quite unmistakable, because it rises rapidly to a peak and collapses quickly.

Diagnosis is made through ECG, echocardiogram, and cardiac catheterization.

Management. Aortic valve replacement is the treatment of choice, but the optimal time for valve replacement remains controversial. Surgery is recommended for any patient with left ventricular hypertrophy regardless of the presence or absence of other symptoms. If the patient has symptoms of congestive heart failure, medical management is recommended until surgery can be performed. (Management of the patient undergoing cardiac surgery is discussed in Chap. 30.)

In summary, the function of normal heart valves is to maintain the forward flow of blood from the atria to the ventricles and from the ventricles to the great vessels. Valvular damage may interfere with valvular function by stenosis (narrowing) of the valve or by impaired closure that allows backward leakage of blood (valvular insufficiency, regurgitation, or incompetence).

Acquired valvular heart disease often is a result of previous rheumatic endocarditis that has damaged one or more of the heart valves. The mitral valve is involved most frequently, followed by the aortic, tricuspid, and pulmonic valves. If the heart muscle remains strong, the circulatory apparatus can adjust itself efficiently even though a valve is badly injured. The details of such adjustment, called *compensatory changes*, include modifications in the rate and character of the heartbeat, changes in the blood, hypertrophy of the myocardium, and redistribution of the blood in the body. All of these changes minimize the consequences of the valve defect.

Cardiomyopathies

Definition, Etiology, and Pathophysiology

Myopathy is a disease of muscle. The cardiomyopathies are a group of diseases that affect the structure and function of the myocardium.

The cardiomyopathies are categorized by pathologic, physiologic, and clinical signs. They are defined as (1) dilated cardiomyopathy, or sometimes congestive cardiomyopathy; (2) hypertrophic cardiomyopathy; and (3) restrictive cardiomyopathy. Regardless of the category and the cause, these diseases lead to severe heart failure and often death.

Dilated or congestive cardiomyopathy is the most commonly occurring form of the cardiomyopathies. It is distinguished by a dilated and enlarged ventricular cavity along with decreasing muscle wall thickness, left atrial enlargement, and stasis of blood in the ventricle. Microscopic examination of the muscle tissue shows a diminishing of the contractile elements of the muscle fibers. Excessive chronic alcohol intake is often implicated in this type of cardiomyopathy.

Hypertrophic cardiomyopathy occurs less frequently and is most often associated with idiopathic hypertrophic subaortic stenosis (IHSS). In hypertrophic cardiomyopathies, the heart muscle actually increases in mass weight, especially along the septum. The septal size increase may produce obstruction to the flow of blood from the atria to the ventricles; hence, this category is divided further into obstructive and nonobstructive types. Nonobstructive hypertrophic cardiomyopathy is often linked to a hereditary etiology.

The last and least frequently occurring category is *restrictive cardiomyopathy*. This form is seen less frequently than all other forms and is characterized by an impairment of ventricular stretch and hence volume. Restrictive cardiomyopathy can be associated with amyloidosis and other such infiltrative diseases.

Regardless of the distinguishing features, the pathophysiology of cardiomyopathy is a series of progressive events that culminates in impaired pumping of the left ventricle. As the stroke volume becomes less and less, the sympathetic nervous system is stimulated, resulting in increased systemic vascular resistance. As in the pathophysiology of heart failure from any cause, the left ventricle enlarges to accommodate the demands and eventually fails. Failure of the right ventricle usually accompanies this process (Fig. 28–5).

Clinical Manifestations

The cardiomyopathies may occur at any age and affect both men and women. Most persons with cardiomyopathy present initially with signs and symptoms of heart failure. Dyspnea on exertion, paroxysmal nocturnal dyspnea (PND), cough, and easy fatigability are early symptoms. A physical examination usually indicates systemic venous congestion, jugular vein dis-

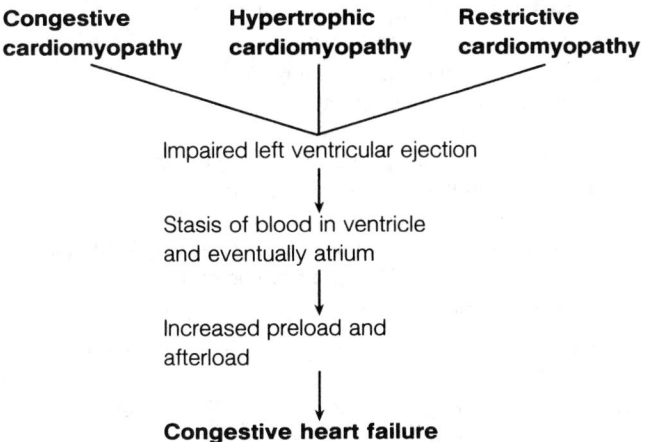

Figure 28–5. Cardiomyopathy and the development of congestive heart failure.

tention, pitting edema of dependent body parts, hepatic engorgement, and tachycardia.

Diagnostic Evaluation

Diagnosis of cardiomyopathy is usually made from findings disclosed by patient history and by ruling out other causes of the failure, such as myocardial infarction. There is no specific test that is best for diagnosing cardiomyopathy. The ECG will demonstrate changes consistent with left ventricular hypertrophy. The echocardiogram is probably one of the most helpful diagnostic tools in that the functioning of the left ventricle can be observed easily. Cardiac catheterization is sometimes used to rule out coronary artery disease as a causative factor.

Medical Management

Medical management is directed toward correcting the heart failure. When heart failure has progressed beyond being medically responsive, heart transplant is the patient's only hope for survival. In some cases ventricular assist devices are necessary to support the failing heart until a suitable donor becomes available (see Chap. 30).

▶ Nursing Process
The Patient With Cardiomyopathy

◊ Assessment

The nursing assessment for the patient with cardiomyopathy begins with a detailed history of the presenting signs and symptoms. Because of the chronic nature of this problem, a careful psychosocial history is also important. The patient's family support system should be identified very early and involved in the management of the patient.

The physical assessment should be directed toward signs and symptoms of congestive heart failure. A careful evaluation of fluid volume status, vital signs (including calculation of pulse pressure), and auscultation for an S_3 are all extremely important in a baseline assessment. The physician may want to place the patient on a cardiac monitor; however, once the diagnosis is

made or dysrhythmia is not a significant problem, the patient may not need to be monitored. The acuteness of the heart failure will determine whether or not the patient needs to be in a critical care unit.

◊ Nursing Diagnoses

Based on the assessment data, major nursing diagnoses for the patient may include the following:

- Potential ineffective breathing pattern related to myocardial failure
- Activity intolerance related to excessive fluid volume
- Anxiety related to the disease process
- Potential noncompliance with the self-care program

◊ Planning and Implementation

◊ *Goals:* The major goals of the patient include absence of respiratory difficulties, increased activity tolerance, reduction of anxiety, and compliance with the self-care program.

◊ Nursing Interventions

◊ *Absence of Respiratory Difficulties.* Because many of the patient's signs and symptoms are corrected by pharmacologic agents, attention to the timeliness of administration of prescribed medications is vitally important. Careful documentation of the patient's response is critical. Supporting respiratory exchange with oxygen by way of nasal prongs is also indicated.

The patient may be most comfortable if allowed to rest at the bedside in a chair. This position will be helpful in pooling venous blood in the periphery and reducing preload. Helping the patient to keep warm and to change position frequently will stimulate circulation and reduce the possibility of skin breakdown. Maintaining an environment free of dust, lint, flowers, and perfumes will also support easier respiratory exchange.

◊ *Increased Activity Tolerance.* Planning nursing care so that the patient participates frequently in activities of short duration is important. Allowing the patient to accomplish a goal, no matter how small, also will enhance his sense of well-being. For example, working with the patient to determine what part of the bath can be completed without aid, and then providing a period of rest before the nurse completes the bath, will help the patient conserve energy that is in short supply. Activities that deplete the patient's energy are avoided.

◊ *Reduction of Anxiety.* The patient is provided with appropriate information about his signs and symptoms. He is assisted to accomplish certain activities for himself. An atmosphere in which the patient feels free to verbalize his fears is provided, as is letting him know that his concerns are legitimate. If the patient is facing death or awaiting transplant surgery, he requires time to discuss his concerns. Spiritual, psychological, and emotional support may be indicated for the patient and his significant others.

◊ *Compliance With a Self-Care Program.* It is particularly important for the patient with cardiomyopathy to learn what self-care activities are necessary and how to perform them at home. An optimum health status is very desirable should the patient be a candidate for a heart transplant. Satisfactory improvement can be obtained by meticulous attention to a medication program, which usually consists of several different medications to maintain a state free of cardiac failure.

The nurse can be integral to the process as patients review life style and work to incorporate the above therapeutic activities with minimal intrusion. Helping patients to accept their disease status will facilitate their adherence to the self-care program at home.

Establishing trust is vital to the relationship with these chronically ill and debilitated patients. Providing realistic hope helps reduce their anxiety while awaiting a donor heart when transplant is an acceptable treatment modality.

When a patient can no longer be helped by any therapeutic technique, allowing the patient and significant others the freedom to begin the grieving process is vitally important.

▷ Evaluation

Expected Outcomes
1. Demonstrates improved respiratory function
   a. Respiratory rate is within normal limits
   b. Blood gases are normal
   c. Reports decreased dyspnea and increased comfort
   d. Uses oxygen therapy as prescribed
2. Increases activity tolerance
   a. Carries out activities of daily living (*e.g.*, brushes teeth, feeds self)
   b. Transfers self from chair to bed
   c. Reports increased tolerance to activity
3. Experiences reduction of anxiety
   a. Discusses prognosis freely
   b. Verbalizes fears and concerns
   c. Participates in support groups if appropriate
4. Complies with the program of self-care
   a. Takes medications according to prescribed schedule
   b. Modifies life style to accommodate activity limitations
   c. Identifies signs and symptoms to be reported to the health-care professional

In summary, cardiomyopathy is a disease of the heart muscle that affects myocardial structure and function. It is categorized by pathologic, physiologic, and clinical signs. Regardless of categorization, this disease results in severe heart failure and, if unamenable to treatment, it results in death.

The goal of medical management is to correct the heart failure. When the disease process becomes resistant to medical therapies, heart transplant is the patient's only hope for survival. In some cases ventricular assist devices are necessary to support the failing heart until a suitable donor becomes available.

The nurse is integral in supporting the patient with cardiomyopathy by encouraging an attitude of realistic hope. The intent is to foster compliant behavior. Compliance with medical therapies is critical to the well-being of the patient with cardiomyopathy.

Bibliography

Books/Pamphlets

Abels L. Critical Care Nursing. St Louis, CV Mosby, 1986.

Ahumada G. Cardiovascular Pathophysiology. New York, Oxford University Press, 1987.

An Older Person's Guide to Cardiovascular Health (pamphlet). American Heart Association, 1989.

Andreoli K et al. Comprehensive Cardiac Care. St Louis, CV Mosby, 1987.

Bates B. A Guide to Physical Examination. Philadelphia, JB Lippincott, 1991.

Brandenburg RO et al. Cardiology: Fundamentals and Practice. Chicago, Year Book Medical Publishers, 1987.

Braunwald E. Heart Disease: A Textbook of Cardiovascular Medicine. Philadelphia, WB Saunders, 1988.

Cheng T. The International Textbook of Cardiology. New York, Pergamon Press, 1986.

Chernow B. The Pharmacologic Approach to the Critically Ill Patient. Baltimore, Williams & Wilkins, 1988.

Cholesterol and Your Heart (pamphlet). American Heart Association, 1989.

Chung E. Principles of Cardiac Arrhythmias. Baltimore, Williams & Wilkins, 1989.

Chung EK. Manual of Acute Cardiac Disorders. Boston, Butterworths, 1988.

Coodley EL (ed). Geriatric Heart Disease, Littleton, MA, PSG Publishing, 1985.

Coronary Risk Factor Statement for the American Public (pamphlet). American Heart Association, 1987.

Dental Care for Adults With Heart Disease (pamphlet). American Heart Association, 1987.

Douglas MK and Shinn JA. Advances in Cardiovascular Nursing. Rockville, MD, Aspen Systems, 1985.

Eagle KA et al (eds). The Practice of Cardiology, Vols 1 and 2. Boston, Little, Brown, 1989.

Fozzard HA et al (eds). The Heart and Cardiovascular System. New York, Raven Press, 1986.

Harris R. Clinical Geriatric Cardiology. Philadelphia, JB Lippincott, 1986.

Heart Facts 1989 (pamphlet). American Heart Association, 1988.

Henning RJ and Grenvik A. Critical Care Cardiology. New York, Churchill Livingstone, 1989.

Hillis LD et al. Manual of Clinical Problems in Cardiology. Boston, Little, Brown, 1988.

Hojnacki LH and Halfman-Franey M. Handbook of Cardiac Rehabilitation for Nurses and Other Health Professionals. Englewood Cliffs, NJ, Prentice-Hall, 1985.

Holloway N. Nursing the Critically Ill Adult. Menlo Park, CA, Addison-Wesley, 1988.

Hunyor SN. Cardiovascular Drug Therapy. Baltimore, Williams & Wilkins, 1987.

Hurst JW (ed). The Heart. New York, McGraw-Hill, 1990.

Jillings CR. Cardiac Rehabilitation Nursing. Rockville, MD, Aspen, 1988.

Kern L. Cardiac Critical Care Nursing. Rockville, MD, Aspen, 1988.

Khan MG. Manual of Cardiac Drug Therapy. Philadelphia, WB Saunders, 1988.

King SB and Douglas SJ. Coronary Arteriography and Angioplasty. New York, McGraw-Hill, 1985.

Kinny M et al. AACN's Clinical Reference Manual. New York, McGraw-Hill, 1989.

Messerli FH. Cardiovascular Disease in the Elderly. Boston, Martinus Nijhoff, 1988.

Ornato JP. Cardiovascular Emergencies. New York, Churchill Livingstone, 1986.

Physician's Cholesterol Education Handbook (pamphlet). American Heart Association, 1988.

Price S and Wilson L. Pathophysiology—Clinical Concepts of Disease Process. New York, McGraw-Hill, 1986.

Sex and Heart Disease (pamphlet). American Heart Association, 1989.

Silber EN. Heart Disease. New York, Macmillan, 1987.

Smoking and Heart Disease (pamphlet). American Heart Association, 1989.

Sokolow M and McIlroy M. Clinical Cardiology. Los Altos, CA, Lange Medical Publications, 1986.

Suddarth DS. Lippincott Manual of Nursing Practice. Philadelphia, JB Lippincott, 1991.

Underhill SL et al. Cardiac Nursing. Philadelphia, JB Lippincott, 1989.

Understanding Angina (pamphlet). American Heart Association, 1989.

Warren JV and Lewis RP. Diagnostic Procedures in Cardiology. Chicago, Year Book Medical Publishers, 1985.

Wasserthel-Smoller S et al. Cardiovascular Health and Risk Management, Littleton, MA, PSG Publishing, 1989.

Webb WR and Kerstein MD. Cardiovascular Emergencies. Rockville, MD, Aspen, 1987.

Yee BH and Zorb SL. Cardiac Critical Care Nursing. Boston, Little, Brown, 1986.

Journals

Asterisks indicate nursing research articles.

Coronary Artery Disease

Becker DM et al. Cholesterol: Interpreting the new guidelines. Am J Nurs 1989 Dec; 89(12): 1622-1625.

Becker DM and Wilder LB. Nutritional and pharmacologic approaches to hypercholesterolemia. Cardiovasc Nurs 1987 May/Jun; 23(3): 12-16.

Braddy PK. Cardiac assessment tool. Crit Care Nurs 1989 Oct; 9(9):71-81.

Brenner ZR. Nursing elderly cardiac clients. Crit Care Nurs 1987 Mar/Apr; 7(2): 78-87.

Cohen J. Reducing cholesterol: Strategies for increasing patient awareness. Crit Care Nurs 1989 Mar; 9(3): 25-35.

Stoy DB. Controlling cholesterol with diet. Am J Nurs 1989 Dec; 89(12): 1625-1628.

Stoy DB. Controlling cholesterol with drugs. Am J Nurs 1989 Dec; 89(12): 1628-1631.

Stoy DB. Helping patients take cholesterol lowering drugs. Am J Nurs 1989 Dec; 89(12): 1631-1635.

* Thomas SA and Friedman E. Type A behavior and cardiovascular response during verbalization in cardiac patients. Nurs Res 1990 Jan/Feb; 39(1): 48-53.

Angina

Amsterdam E. Unstable angina: Ischemic chest pain that mimics MI. Consultant 1988 Apr; 28(4): 127-130.

Enger EL et al. Mechanisms of myocardial ischemia. J Cardiovasc Nurs 1989 Aug; 3(4): 1-15.

Hayward JM. Living with angina. Prof Nurs 1988 Oct; 4(1): 33–36.

Klein DM. Angina: Pathophysiology and the resulting signs and symptoms. Nursing 1988 Jul; 18(7): 44–46.

Maseri A. Clinical syndromes of angina pectoris. Hosp Prac 1989 Mar 15; 24(3): 65–69.

Miller C. Medications in angina. Focus Crit Care 1988 Jul/Aug; 15(4): 23–29.

Parker JO. Pharmacologic treatment of angina: Nitrate tolerance. Hosp Prac 1988 Nov 15; 23(11): 63–71.

Sakallaris B. Laser therapy for cardiovascular disease. Heart Lung 1987 Oct; 16(5): 506–518.

Schakenbach L. Prinzmetal's angina; Current perceptions and treatment. Crit Care Nurs 1987 Mar/Apr; 7(2): 90–99.

Shapiro W. Calcium channel blockers: Update on uses in ischemic heart disease. Consultant 1989 Aug; 29(8): 132–136.

Thompson VL. Chest pain: Your response to a classic warning. RN 1989 Apr; 52(4): 32–38.

Myocardial Infarction

Bauer W and Dracup K. Physiologic effects of back massage in patients with acute myocardial infarction. Focus Crit Care 1987 Nov; 14(6): 42–46.

Braun A. Drugs that dissolve clots. RN 1991 Jun; 54(6): 52–56.

Briones TL. Tissue-plasminogen activator: Nursing implications. Dimens Crit Care Nurs 1989 Jul/Aug; 8(4): 200–209.

* Cronin SN and Harrison B. Importance of nurse caring behaviors as perceived by patients after myocardial infarction. Heart Lung 1988 Aug; 17(4): 374–380.

Dillon J et al. Rapid initiation of thrombolytic therapy for acute MI. Crit Care Nurs 1989 Feb; 9(2): 55–61.

Finesilver C and Metzler DJ. Right ventricular infarction: The critically different MI. Am J Nurs 1991 Apr; 91(4): 32–36.

* Garding BS et al. Effectiveness of a program of information and support for myocardial infarction patients recovering at home. Heart Lung 1988 Jul/Aug; 17(4): 355–362.

Hilenberg C and Crowley C. Changes in family patterns after a myocardial infarction. Home Healthcare Nurs 1987 5(3): 26–32.

Kleven M. Comparison of thrombolytic agents: Mechanism of action, efficacy, and safety. Part 2. Heart Lung 1988 Nov/Dec; 17(6): 750–755.

Lewis V. Monitoring the patient with acute myocardial infarction. Nurs Clin North Am 1987 Mar; 22(1): 15–32.

Liddy Kg. Myocardial Infarction: Assessing the patient in the family setting. Home Healthcare Nurs 1989 7(3): 28–31.

Littrell K and Schumann LL. Promoting sleep for the patient with a myocardial infarction. Crit Care Nurs 1989 Mar; 9(3): 44–49.

Lowery BJ. Psychological stress, denial, and myocardial infarction. Image: Journal of Nursing Scholarship. 1991 Spring; 23(1): 51–55.

McGlashan R. Strategies for rebuilding self-esteem for the cardiac patient. Dimens Crit Care Nurs 1988 Jan/Feb; 7(1): 28–38.

Milligan KS. Tissue-type plasminogen activator: A new fibrinolytic agent. Heart Lung 1987 Jan/Feb; 16(1): 69–73.

Misinski M. Pathophysiology of acute myocardial infarction: A rationale for thrombolytic therapy. Part 2. Heart Lung 1988 Nov; 17(6): 743–750.

Moore HS. Preventing coronary artery reocclusion following t-PA. Crit Care Nurs 1990 Nov/Dec; 10(10): 52–58.

Mutnik A et al. Update on cardiac drugs: Inotropic and chronotropic agents. Nursing 1987 Oct; 17(10): 58–61.

Olson AR. What you should know about thrombolytic therapy. Nursing 1987 Dec; 17(12): 52–55.

* Raleigh E and Odtohan B. The effect of a cardiac teaching program on patient rehabilitation. Heart Lung 1987 May/Jun; 16(3): 311–317.

Rodriguez SW and Reed RL. Thrombolytic therapy for MI. Am J Nurs 1987 May; 87(5): 632–640.

Sipperly M. Expanding role of coronary angioplasty: Current implications, limitations and nursing considerations. Heart Lung 1989 Sep/Oct; 18(5): 507–513.

* Steele J and Ruzicki D. An evaluation of the effectiveness of cardiac teaching during hospitalization. Heart Lung 1987 May/Jun; 16(3): 306–310.

Vitello CJ. Thrombolytic therapy: Urokinase. J Cardiovasc Nurs 1987 Feb; 1(2): 59–64.

Infectious/Valvular Heart Disease

Bisno AL. Antimicrobial prophylaxis for infective endocarditis. Hosp Pract 1989 Mar 15; 24(3): 209–226.

Blaisdell MW et al. Percutaneous transluminal valvuloplasty. Crit Care Nurs 1989 Mar; 9(3): 62–68.

Grady K. Myocarditis: Review of a clinical enigma. Heart Lung 1989 Jul/Aug; 18(4): 347–353.

Mauie TJ. Infective endocarditis: A serious and changing disease. Crit Care Nurs 1987 Mar/Apr; 7(2): 31–46.

Ohler L et al. Aortic valvuloplasty: Medical and critical care nursing perspectives. Focus Crit Care 1989 Jul/Aug; 16(4): 275–287.

Owens-Jones S and Hopp L. Viral myocarditis. Focus Crit Care 1988 Jan/Feb; 15(1): 25–37.

Russell AC and Blake SM. Aortic valvuloplasty: Potential nursing diagnoses. Dimens Crit Care Nurs 1989 Mar/Apr; 8(2): 72–82.

Schactman M. A case study of atrial fibrillation and mitral stenosis. Focus Crit Care 1987 May; 14(3): 13–20.

Scrima D. Infective endocarditis: Nursing considerations. Crit Care Nurs 1987 Mar/Apr; 7(2): 47–56.

Serwer G. Acute rheumatic fever. Hosp Med 1989 Jan; 25(1): 25–42.

Utz S and Grass S. Mitral valve prolapse: Self-care needs, nursing diagnoses and interventions. Heart Lung 1987 Jan/Feb; 16(1): 77–83.

Cardiomyopathy

Casey P. Pathophysiology of dilated cardiomyopathy: Nursing implications. J Cardiovasc Nurs 1987 Nov; 2(1): 1–12.

Courtney–Jenkins A. The patient with hypertrophic cardiomyopathy. J Cardiovasc Nurs 1987 Nov; 2(1): 33–47.

Cragin P. Peripartum cardiomyopathy. Focus Crit Care 1988 Nov/Dec; 15(6): 39–44.

Geary CB. The patient with viral cardiomyopathy. J Cardiovasc Nurs 1987 Nov; 2(1): 48–52.

McHugh M. The patient with alcoholic cardiomyopathy. J Cardiovasc Nurs 1987 Nov; 2(1): 13–23.

Miracle V. Idiopathic hypertrophic subaortic stenosis. Crit Care Nurs 1988 Mar; 8(3): 102–111.

Purcell JA and Holder CK. Cardiomyopathy. Am J Nurs 1989 Jan; 89(1): 57–75.

Agencies
Governmental
National Heart, Lung, and Blood Institute
National Institutes of Health Building 31, Room 5A52, Bethesda, MD 20892

Voluntary
American Heart Association
7220 Greenville Ave, Dallas, TX 75231
Coronary Club
3659 Green Rd, Cleveland, OH 44122
Heartlife
PO Box 54305, Atlanta, GA 30308

29

Management of Patients With Complications of Cardiac Disorders

Learning Objectives

On completion of this chapter, the learner will be able to:

1. Determine the following information from an ECG strip: rate, presence or absence of P waves, PR interval, QRS interval, presence or absence of dysrhythmia, origin of dysrhythmia
2. Use the nursing process as a framework for care of patients with dysrhythmias
3. Compare the different types of pacemakers, their uses, nursing implications, and possible complications
4. Use the nursing process as a framework for care of patients with pacemakers
5. Compare the management of patients with cardiac failure with the management of patients with acute pulmonary edema
6. Use the nursing process as a framework of care for patients with cardiac failure
7. Demonstrate the techniques of cardiopulmonary resuscitation

Cardiac Complications: Overview

Complications of cardiac disorders are responsible for many deaths. The most common complications are dysrhythmias, acute pulmonary edema, cardiac failure, cardiogenic shock, thromboembolic episodes, and myocardial rupture. An important goal of medical and nursing management of patients with heart disease is the early identification of signs and symptoms that signal the onset of a complication.

Dysrhythmias are the most common complication of cardiac disease. They may vary in severity from a benign premature beat to a fatal ventricular fibrillation. Mobile intensive care units, new drug therapies, increasingly sophisticated

pacemakers, and automatic implantable defibrillators all have contributed to improvement in the control of compromising dysrhythmias.

Cardiac failure, which covers a spectrum of complications from acute pulmonary edema to cardiogenic shock, remains a leading cause of cardiac morbidity and mortality. The factor of greatest importance in cardiac failure is the extent of myocardial fiber damage. The severity of failure will be directly proportional to the extent of damaged muscle mass.

Although not as common today because of more aggressive activity programs for patients with heart disease, thromboembolic episodes still occur. The cerebral, renal, femoral, mesenteric, and pulmonary arteries are most often affected.

Myocardial rupture, too, is rare. It presents itself often

enough, however, that observing for signs and symptoms in the high-risk patient population is critical.

All complications of cardiac diseases can result in cardiac arrest. Cardiopulmonary resuscitation is the initial treatment of choice and is a skill that is essential for all health care workers.

The best defense in the reduction in number and severity of complications is nursing care that involves early recognition and reporting of cardinal signs and symptoms of the various complications.

Dysrhythmias

A dysrhythmia is a disorder of the heartbeat that includes a disturbance of rate, rhythm, or both. Dysrhythmias are derangements of the heart's conduction system and not of heart structure. Dysrhythmias are identified by analyzing electrocardiogram (ECG) waveforms. They are named according to the site of origin of the impulse and the mechanism of conduction involved. For example, a dysrhythmia that originates in the sinus node (SA node) and is slow in rate is called sinus bradycardia. There are four possible sites of origin of dysrhythmias, as indicated in Chart 29–1. Note also the possible altered conduction mechanisms that can occur.

Properties of Cardiac Muscle

The cardiac muscle possesses the physiologic properties of excitability, automaticity, conductivity, and contractility.

Excitability is the ability of a myocardial cell to respond to a stimulus; *automaticity* allows a cell to reach a threshold potential and generate an impulse without being stimulated by another source. *Conductivity* refers to the ability of the muscle to move an impulse from cell to cell. *Contractility* allows the muscle to shorten when stimulated.

When all of these properties are intact, the heart muscle is stimulated by impulses originating in the sinus node; hence, *the sinus node is referred to as the heart's pacemaker.* If disequilibrium occurs in one of the heart's basic properties, a dysrhythmia may result. The disequilibrium can be caused by normal activity such as exercise or by a pathologic occurrence such as a myocardial infarction. In myocardial infarction, because reduced oxygenation to the myocardium can increase excitability, the myocardium has an increased response to stimuli. This is an example of one of the most common causes of a dysrhythmia.

Normal Conduction Pathway. Once an impulse originates in the sinus node, a normal electrical pathway is followed. The impulse travels from the sinus node through the atria to the AV node or junction, which also includes the bundle of His. The impulse is delayed in time at the AV node to allow the ventricles to fill with blood. From the AV node the impulse travels very quickly through the bundle branches, terminating in the Purkinje fibers of the ventricular walls to initiate systole. The cycle then begins again. It is important to remember that an electrical stimulus is followed by a mechanical event of the heart (see Chap. 27).

Autonomic Nervous System. The heart is under the control of the automatic nervous system, which consists of sympathetic and parasympathetic fibers. The *sympathetic* system is also referred to as *adrenergic*, a word derived from the root word adrenalin. Thus, stimulation of the sympathetic system accelerates heart rate, raises blood pressure, and enhances the force of myocardial contraction. *Parasympathetic* stimulation, conversely, slows the heart rate, lowers blood pressure, and reduces the force of contraction.

Manipulation of the autonomic nervous system forms the foundation for much of the medication therapy in dysrhythmia control (*e.g.*, β-adrenergic blockers).

Dysrhythmias Originating in the Sinus Node

Sinus Bradycardia

Sinus bradycardia may be due to vagal stimulation, digitalis intoxication, increased intracranial pressure, or myocardial infarction (MI). It also is seen in highly trained athletes, in persons in severe pain, in persons on medication (propranolol, reserpine, methyldopa), in hypoendocrine states (myxedema, Addison's disease, panhypopituitarism), in anorexia nervosa, in hypothermia, and after surgical damage to the SA node.

The following are characteristics of this dysrhythmia (Fig. 29–1):

Rate: 40 to 60 beats per minute
P waves: Precede each QRS complex; PR interval normal
QRS complex: Usually normal

Chart 29–1
Identification of Dysrhythmias by Site of Origin

Sites of Origin	Mechanisms of Conduction
Sinus node	Bradycardia
Atria	Tachycardia
AV node or junction	Flutter
Ventricles	Fibrillation
	Premature beats
	Heart blocks

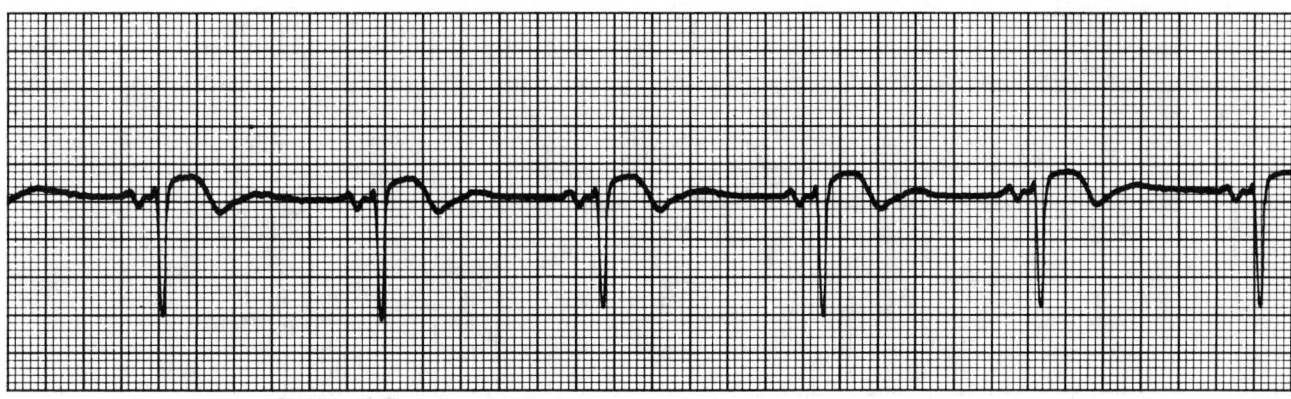

Figure 29–1.   Sinus bradycardia.

Conduction: Usually normal
Rhythm: Regular

All characteristics of sinus bradycardia are the same as those of normal sinus rhythm, except for the rate. If the slow heart rate is causing significant hemodynamic changes with resultant syncope, angina, or ectopic dysrhythmias, then treatment is directed toward increasing the heart rate. If the decrease in heart rate is due to vagal stimulation such as bearing down during defecation or vomiting, attempts are made to prevent further vagal stimulation. If the patient has digitalis intoxication, digitalis is withheld. The drug of choice in treating sinus bradycardia is atropine. Atropine blocks vagal stimulation, thus allowing a normal rate to occur.

Sinus Tachycardia

Sinus tachycardia may be caused by fever, acute blood loss, anemia, shock, exercise, congestive heart failure (CHF), pain, hypermetabolic states, anxiety, or sympathomimetic or parasympatholytic drugs. The ECG pattern is as follows (Fig. 29–2):

Rate: 100 to 180 beats per minute
P waves: Precede each QRS complex; may be buried in the preceding T wave; PR interval normal
QRS complex: Usually has a normal interval
Conduction: Usually normal
Rhythm: Regular

All aspects of sinus tachycardia are the same as those of normal sinus rhythm, except for the rate.

Carotid sinus pressure, applied to one side at a time, may be effective in slowing the rate temporarily, and thereby help to rule out other dysrhythmias. As heart rate increases, diastolic filling time decreases, resulting in reduced cardiac output and subsequent symptoms of syncope, fainting, and low blood pressure. If the rapid rate persists and the heart is unable to compensate for the decreased ventricular filling, the patient may develop acute pulmonary edema.

Treatment of sinus tachycardia is usually directed at abolishing the cause. Propranolol (Inderal) may be used if rapid reduction of rate is necessary. Propranolol blocks the effect of adrenergic fibers, thus slowing the rate.

Dysrhythmias Originating in the Atrial Muscle

Premature Atrial Contractions

Premature atrial contractions (PACs) may be due to atrial muscle irritability caused by caffeine, alcohol, nicotine, stretched atrial myocardium as in CHF, stress or anxiety, hypokalemia, atrial ischemia, injury, infarction, or hypermetabolic states.

Premature atrial contractions have the following characteristics (Fig. 29–3):

Rate: 60 to 100 beats per minute
P waves: Usually have a configuration different from that of the P waves that originate in the SA node. Another site in

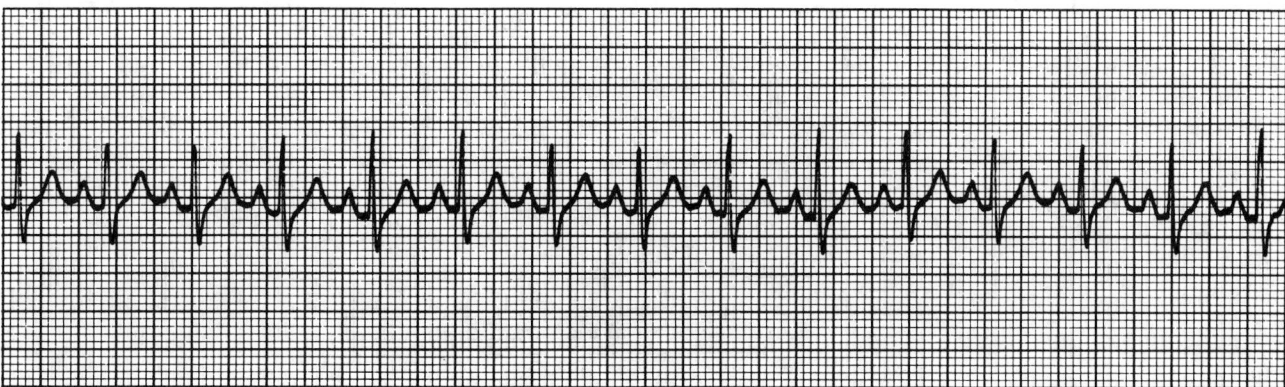

Figure 29–2.   Sinus tachycardia.

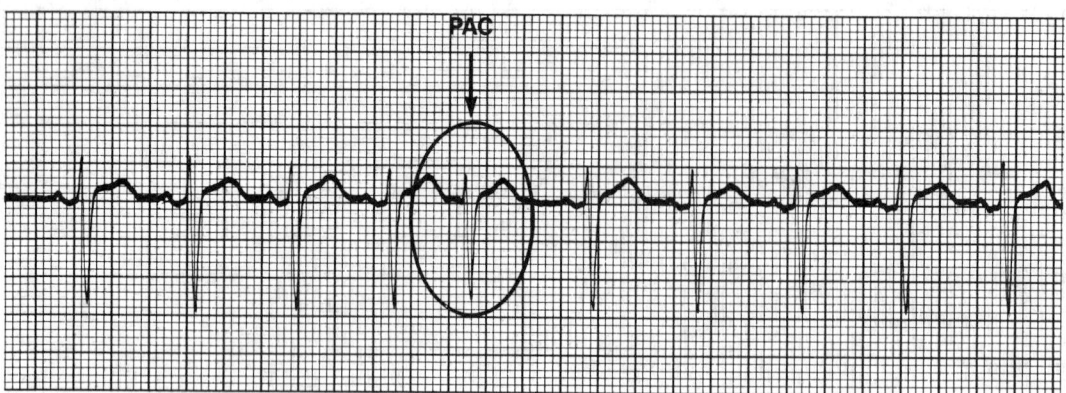

Figure 29–3. Premature atrial contraction.

the atria has become irritable (enhanced automaticity) and fires before the normal firing time of the SA node. PR interval may vary from the PR intervals of impulses originating in the SA node.

QRS complex: May be normal, aberrant, or absent. If the ventricles have completed their repolarization phase, they can respond to this early stimulus from the atria.

Conduction: Usually normal

Rhythm: Regular, except when the PACs occur. The P wave will be early in the cycle and usually will not have a complete compensatory pause. (Time between the preceding complex and the following complex is less than the time for two RR intervals.)

Premature atrial contractions are frequently seen in normal hearts. The patient may say that the heart "skipped a beat." A pulse deficit (the difference between apical and radial pulse rate) may exist. If PACs are infrequent, no treatment is necessary. If they are frequent (more than 6 per minute) or occur during atrial repolarization, this may herald more serious dysrhythmias such as atrial fibrillation. Again, treatment is directed toward the cause.

Paroxysmal Atrial Tachycardia

Paroxysmal atrial tachycardia (PAT) is characterized by abrupt onset and abrupt cessation. It may be triggered by emotions, tobacco, caffeine, fatigue, sympathomimetic drugs, or alcohol. Paroxysmal atrial tachycardia is not usually associated with organic heart disease. The rapid rate may produce angina due to decreased coronary artery filling. Cardiac output is reduced

and heart failure may occur. The patient frequently does not tolerate this rhythm for long periods.

Paroxysmal atrial tachycardia is characterized by the following (Fig. 29–4):

Rate: 150 to 250 beats per minute

P waves: Ectopic and distorted as compared with normal P wave; may be found in the preceding T wave; PR interval shortened (less than 0.12 second)

QRS complex: Usually normal, but may be distorted if aberrant conduction is present

Conduction: Usually normal

Rhythm: Regular

The patient may not be aware of PAT. Treatment is directed toward eliminating the cause and decreasing the heart rate. Morphine may slow the rate without further treatment. Carotid sinus pressure, applied to one side at a time, slows the rate or stops the attack and is usually more effective after digitalis or vasopressors. The use of vasopressors has a reflex effect on the carotid sinus by elevating the blood pressure and thus slowing the heart rate. Short-acting digitalis preparations may be used. Propranolol may be tried if digitalis is unsuccessful. Quinidine may be effective, or the calcium channel blocker verapamil (Calan) can be used. Cardioversion may be necessary if the patient does not tolerate the fast heart rate.

Atrial Flutter

Atrial flutter occurs when an atrial focus captures the heart rhythm and discharges impulses at a rate of between 250 and

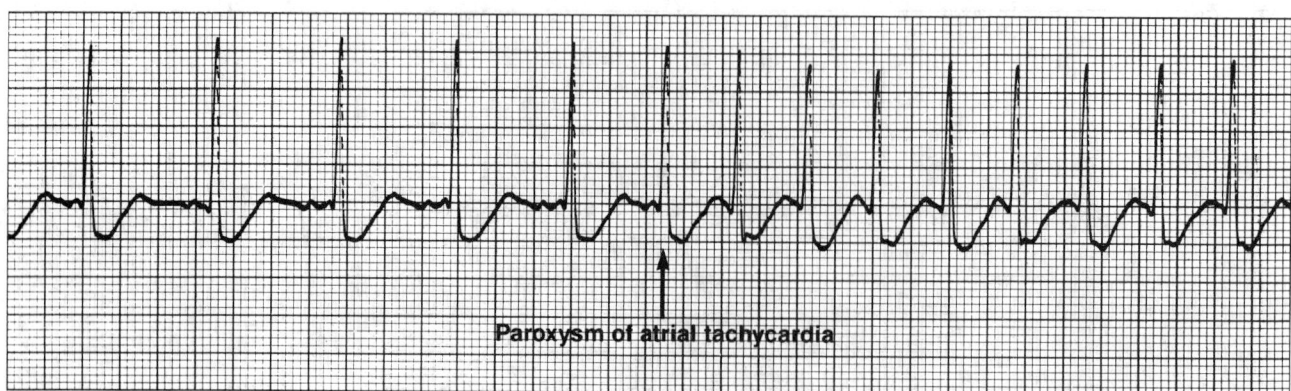

Figure 29–4. Paroxysmal atrial tachycardia.

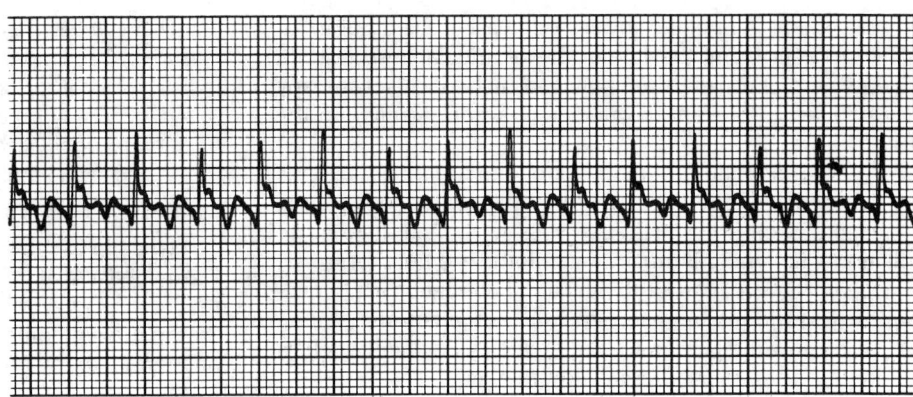

Figure 29–5. Atrial flutter. (Suddarth DS. Lippincott Manual of Nursing Practice, 5th ed. Philadelphia, JB Lippincott, 1991.)

400 times per minute. An important characteristic of the dysrhythmia is that a therapeutic block occurs at the AV node, which prevents some impulse transmission. Conduction of the impulse through the heart is otherwise normal, so the QRS complex is unaffected. This is an important feature of this dysrhythmia, as the 1:1 conduction of atrial impulses firing at 250 to 400 times per minute would result in ventricular fibrillation, a life-threatening dysrhythmia.

Atrial flutter is characterized by the following (Fig. 29–5):

Rate: Atrial rate between 250 and 400 beats per minute
Rhythm: Regular or irregular, depending on kind of block (*e.g.,* 2:1, 3:1, or a combination)
P wave: Not present; instead it is replaced by a saw-toothed pattern that is produced by the rapid firing of the atrial focus. These waves are referred to as *F* waves.
QRS complex: Normal configuration and normal conduction time
T wave: Present but may be obscured by flutter waves

The accepted treatment for atrial flutter is a digitalis preparation. This enhances the block at the AV node, thus slowing the rate. Quinidine also may be given to suppress the ectopic atrial focus. The concomitant use of digitalis and quinidine usually reverts the dysrhythmia to sinus rhythm. Other drug therapies that are useful are calcium channel and beta-adrenergic blockers.

If drug therapy is unsuccessful, atrial flutter often will respond to electrical cardioversion.

Atrial Fibrillation

Atrial fibrillation (disorganized and uncoordinated twitching of atrial musculature) is usually associated with atherosclerotic heart disease, valvular heart disease, CHF, thyrotoxicosis, cor pulmonale, or congenital heart disease.

Atrial fibrillation (Fig. 29–6) is characterized by the following:

Rate: An atrial rate of 350 to 600 beats per minute; ventricular response usually 120 to 200 beats per minute.
P waves: No discernible P waves; irregular undulation, termed fibrillatory or *f* waves, is seen; PR interval cannot be measured.
QRS complex: Usually normal.
Conduction: Usually normal through the ventricles. Characterized by an irregular ventricular response, because the AV node does not respond to the rapid atrial rate. Impulses that are transmitted cause the ventricles to respond irregularly.
Rhythm: Irregular and usually rapid, unless controlled. Irregularity of rhythm is due to concealed conduction within the AV node.

A rapid ventricular response reduces the time for ventricular filling and hence the stroke volume. The atrial kick, which is 25% to 30% of the cardiac output, is also lost. Congestive heart failure frequently follows. There is usually a *pulse deficit*, the numeric difference between apical and radial pulse rates.

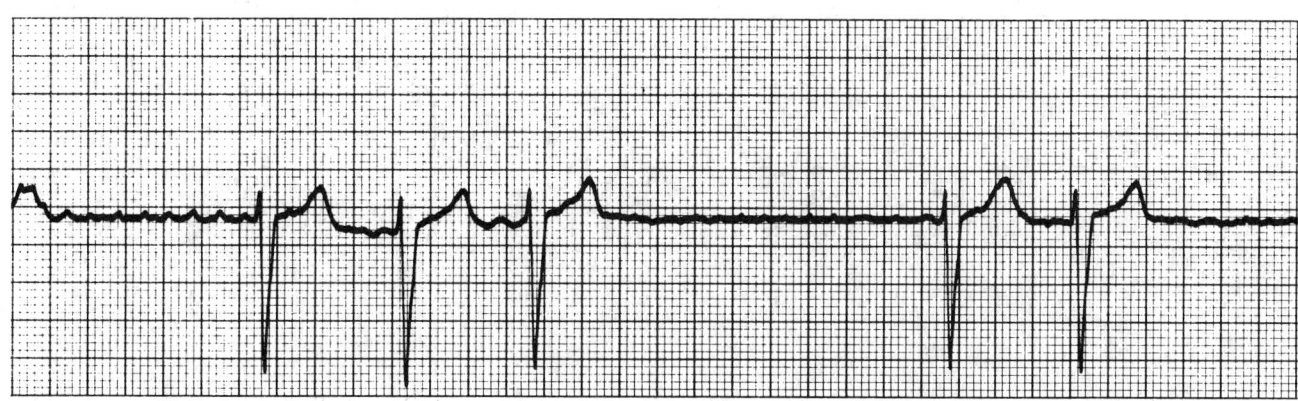

Figure 29–6. Atrial fibrillation.

Treatment is directed toward decreasing the atrial irritability and decreasing the rate of the ventricular response. In patients with chronic atrial fibrillation, anticoagulant therapy may be used to prevent thromboemboli from forming in the atria.

At times a mixture of atrial flutter and atrial fibrillation is seen, sometimes called atrial flutter-fibrillation or coarse atrial fibrillation. Such a dysrhythmia is best classified as atrial fibrillation when the criteria for atrial flutter are not met.

Medications of choice to treat atrial fibrillation are similar to those used in the treatment of PAT. A digitalis preparation is used to slow the heart rate, and an antidysrhythmic such as quinidine is used to suppress the dysrhythmia.

Dysrhythmias Originating in the Ventricular Muscle

Premature Ventricular Contractions

Premature ventricular contractions (PVCs) are the result of increased automaticity of the ventricular muscle cells. PVCs can be due to digitalis toxicity, hypoxia, hypokalemia, fever, acidosis, exercise, or increased circulating catecholamines.

Infrequent PVCs are not serious in themselves. Usually, the patient feels a palpitating sensation but has no other complaints. The concern, however, lies in the fact that these premature contractions may lead to more serious ventricular dysrhythmias.

In the patient with acute myocardial infarction (MI), PVCs are considered serious precursors of ventricular tachycardia and ventricular fibrillation when they (1) occur in increasing number, more than 6 per minute; (2) are multifocal or originate from several areas in the heart; (3) occur in pairs or triplets; and (4) occur in the vulnerable phase of conduction. The T wave represents the period when the heart is most likely to respond to any stray beat and be excited in a dysrhythmic manner. This phase of T-wave conduction is said to be the vulnerable phase.

Premature ventricular contractions (Fig. 29–7) have the following characteristics:

Rate: 60 to 100 beats per minute.
P waves: Will not be present because impulse originates in the ventricles.

QRS complex: Usually wide and bizarre. Usually longer than 0.10 second in duration. May have the same focus in the ventricle, or may have a wide variety of configurations if occurring from multiple foci in the ventricles.
Conduction: Occasionally retrograde through the junctional tissue and atria.
Rhythm: Irregular when the premature beat occurs.

To decrease the myocardial irritability, the cause must be determined and, if possible, corrected. An antidysrhythmic drug may be used for immediate and possibly long-term therapy. The drug most commonly used in acute care is lidocaine; for long-term therapy procainamide (Pronestyl) or quinidine may be effective.

Ventricular Bigeminy

Ventricular bigeminy is frequently associated with digitalis excess, coronary artery disease, acute MI, and CHF. The term *bigeminy* refers to a condition in which every other beat is premature.

Ventricular bigeminy (Fig. 29–8) has the following characteristics:

Rate: May occur at any heart rate, but rate is usually less than 90 beats per minute.
P waves: The same as described for PVCs; may be hidden within the QRS complex.
QRS complex: Every other beat is a PVC with a wide, bizarre QRS complex and a complete compensatory pause.
Conduction: The sinus beats are conducted from the sinus node in a normal fashion, but alternating PVCs start in the ventricles and may have retrograde conduction through the junctional tissue and atria.
Rhythm: Irregular.

If the ectopic beats occur every third beat, this is termed *trigeminy;* every fourth beat, *quadrigeminy.*

The treatment for ventricular bigeminy is the same as for PVCs. Because the underlying cause of ventricular bigeminy is frequently digitalis toxicity, this should be ruled out or treated if present. Ventricular bigeminy caused by digitalis toxicity is treated with phenytoin (Dilantin).

Ventricular Tachycardia

This dysrhythmia is caused by increased myocardial irritability, as are PVCs. It is usually associated with coronary artery disease

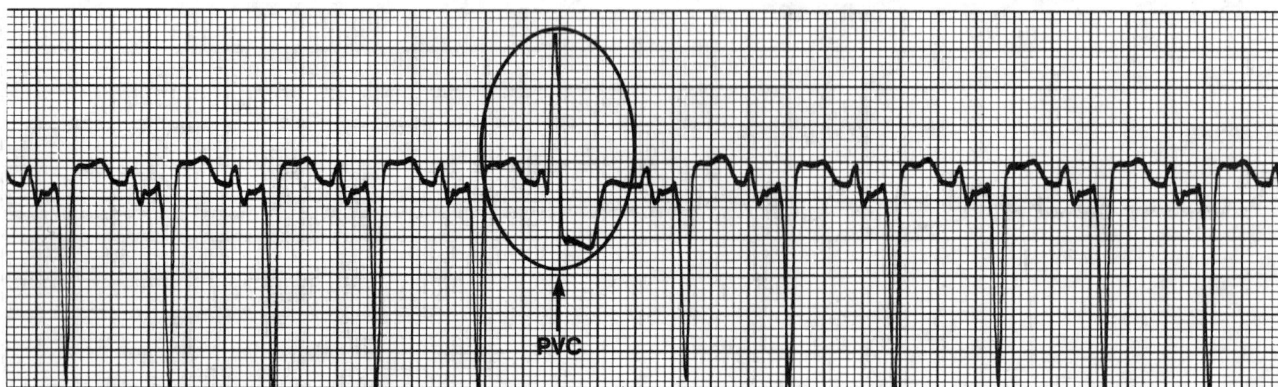

Figure 29–7. Premature ventricular contraction.

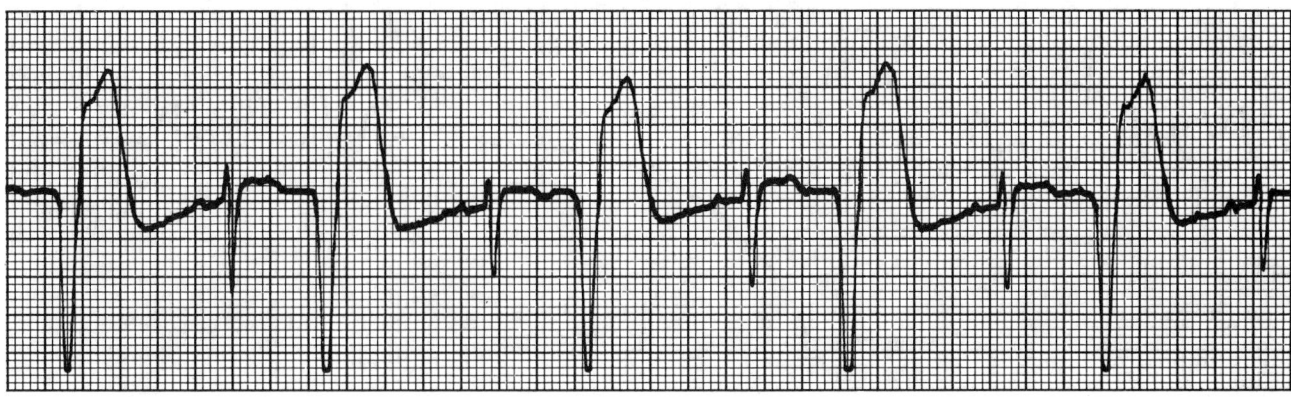

Figure 29–8. Ventricular bigeminy.

and may precede ventricular fibrillation. Ventricular tachycardia is extremely dangerous and should be considered an emergency. The patient is generally aware of this rapid rhythm and is quite anxious. Accelerated ventricular rhythm and ventricular tachycardia have the following characteristics (Fig. 29–9):

Rate: 150 to 200 beats per minute.
P waves: Usually buried in the QRS complex; if seen, they do not necessarily fall in the normal pattern with the QRS. The ventricular contractions are dissociated from the atrial contractions.
QRS complex: Have the same configurations as those of a PVC—wide and bizarre, with T waves in the opposite direction. A ventricular beat may fuse with a normal QRS, resulting in a fusion beat.
Conduction: Originates in the ventricle, with possible retrograde conduction to the junctional tissue and atria.
Rhythm: Usually regular, but irregular ventricular tachycardia is also seen.

The patient's tolerance or lack of tolerance for this rapid rhythm will dictate the therapy to be given. The cause of the myocardial irritability must be determined and corrected, if possible. Antidysrhythmic drugs may be used. Cardioversion may be indicated if the reduction in cardiac output is marked.

Ventricular Fibrillation

Ventricular fibrillation is rapid, ineffective quivering of the ventricles. With this dysrhythmia there is no audible heartbeat, no palpable pulse, and no respiration. This pattern is so grossly irregular it can hardly be mistaken for another type of dysrhythmia.

Ventricular fibrillation (Fig. 29–10) has the following characteristics:

Rate: Rapid, uncoordinated, ineffective.
P waves: Not seen.
QRS complex: Rapid, irregular undulation without specific pattern (multifocal). The ventricles have only a quivering motion.
Conduction: Foci are located in the ventricles, but so many foci are firing at one time that there is no organized conduction; no ventricular contractions occur.
Rhythm: Extremely irregular and uncoordinated, without specific pattern.

Immediate treatment is defibrillation.

Diagnosis

Electrophysiologic Studies. Electrophysiologic studies (EPSs) allow the physician to induce troubling dysrhythmias in a controlled environment. Catheters containing electrodes in the distal portion are placed within the heart. Stimulation of these electrode-containing catheters induces dysrhythmias. Once a dysrhythmia is induced, different medications are administered to determine which is the most effective in sup-

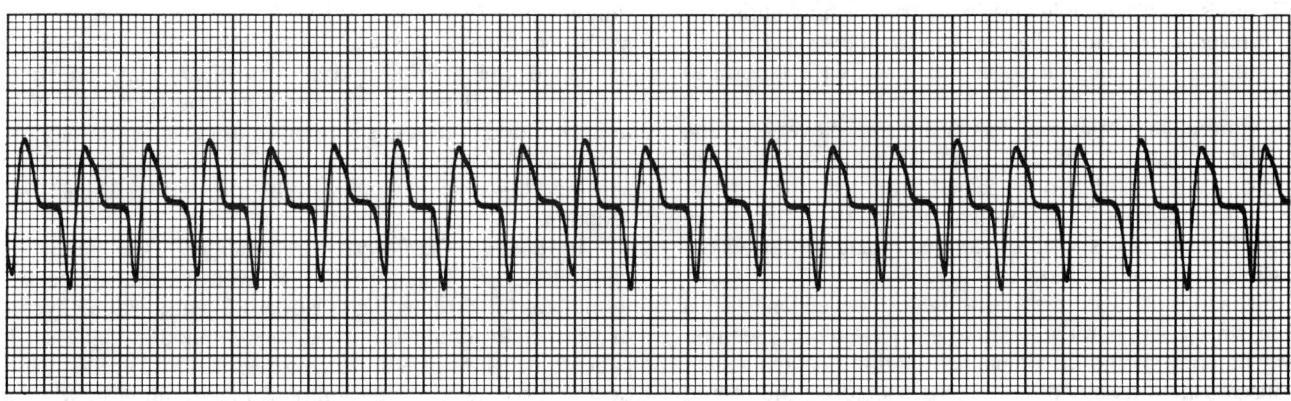

Figure 29–9. Ventricular tachycardia.

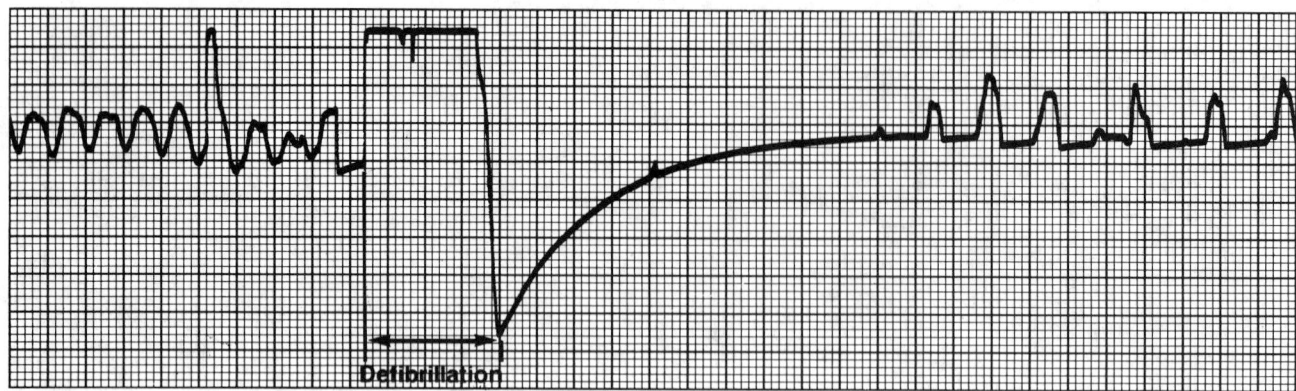

Figure 29–10. Ventricular fibrillation with defibrillation.

pressing the dysrhythmia. EPS is a new technology; the long-term benefit to the patient remains to be determined.

Electrocardiogram. The ECG pattern is analyzed for the presence of dysrhythmias.

Medical Management

Dysrhythmias are most commonly treated with medication therapy. In situations in which medications alone are not adequate, certain adjunctive mechanical therapies are available. The most common are elective cardioversion, defibrillation, and pacemakers.

Cardioversion

Cardioversion is the use of electricity to terminate dysrhythmias that have QRS complexes. It is usually an elective procedure. The patient is alert and informed consent is obtained. The patient is usually given diazepam (Valium) intravenously before cardioversion to promote anesthesia, and is usually intubated after being anesthetized. The amount of voltage used varies from 25 to 400 watt-seconds. Digoxin is usually withheld for 48 hours before cardioversion to prevent postcardioversion dysrhythmias.

The synchronizer is turned on. The defibrillator is synchronized with a cardiac monitor so that an electrical impulse is discharged during ventricular depolarization (the QRS complex). If not synchronized, the defibrillator could discharge during the vulnerable period (T wave), resulting in ventricular tachycardia or fibrillation.

There is no discernible QRS in ventricular fibrillation; the synchronizer is programmed to sense QRSs. If the synchronizer is left on, the machine will not fire as it waits to respond to a QRS.

If ventricular fibrillation occurs after cardioversion, the defibrillator must be recharged immediately, the synchronizer turned off, and defibrillation repeated. After use, the defibrillator must be turned off to prevent accidental discharge of the paddles. Oxygen flow should be stopped during cardioversion, if possible, to avoid the hazard of fire.

Indications of a successful response are conversion to sinus rhythm, strong peripheral pulses, and adequate blood pressure. Airway patency should be maintained, and the patient's state of consciousness assessed. Vital signs should be monitored and recorded until the patient is stabilized. ECG monitoring is required during and after cardioversion; therefore, these patients are in a critical care environment.

Defibrillation

Defibrillation is asynchronous cardioversion that is used in an emergency situation. Its use is usually confined to the treatment of ventricular fibrillation when there is no organized cardiac rhythm. Defibrillation completely depolarizes all the myocardial cells at once, allowing the sinus node to recapture its role as the pacemaker. The electrical voltage required to defibrillate the heart is much greater than that usually required for cardioversions. The following are some key points to remember in assisting with defibrillation or cardioversion:

- Use a good conducting agent between the skin and the paddles, such as saline pads or electrode paste.
- Position the paddles so as to create an effective arc (Fig. 29–11).
- Exert 20 to 25 pounds of pressure on each paddle to ensure good skin contact.
- Practice safety by being certain no one is touching the bed or patient when the paddles are discharged.
- In the case of ventricular fibrillation, cardiopulmonary resuscitation (CPR) is initiated and continued until mechanical defibrillation is available.

If defibrillation has been unsuccessful, cardiopulmonary resuscitation is resumed immediately. Epinephrine may be used if the pattern of ventricular fibrillation is fine; that is, no undulating waveform is discernible (Fig. 29–12). Epinephrine may make the fibrillation coarser and thus easier to convert with defibrillation (see Fig. 29–12). Sodium bicarbonate is prescribed to reverse the acidosis caused by lack of respiratory exchange. Epinephrine and sodium bicarbonate are incompatible when mixed together and must be administered separately. Blood pressure is supported using vasopressors. At no time during the resuscitation should the external cardiac massage and the assisted ventilation be stopped for longer than 5 seconds.

Implantable Cardioverter Defibrillator. The implantable cardioverter defibrillator (ICD) is a device that detects and terminates life-threatening episodes of ventricular tachycardia or ventricular fibrillation in patients deemed at high risk. The patients at high risk are those who have survived sudden cardiac death, who have sustained ventricular tachycardia, or who have syncope secondary to ventricular tachycardia. Many of these

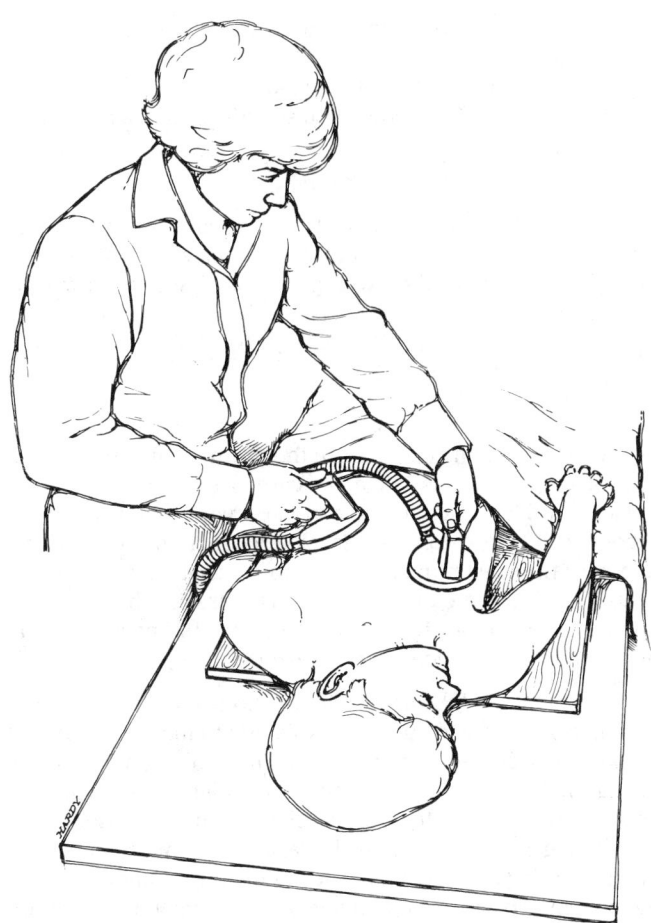

Figure 29–11. One method of paddle placement in cardioversion.

patients are unresponsive to medications or surgical ablation of irritable myocardial tissue. This is the population of patients most suitable for ICD.

The mechanical system consists of a pulse generator, two rate-sensing leads, and two leads through which electrical shock can be delivered directly to the myocardium (Fig. 29–13). This is an invasive device that is implanted by thoracotomy under surgical conditions. The rate-sensing leads are designed to respond to two criteria: a rate change and an altered length

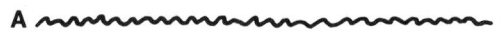

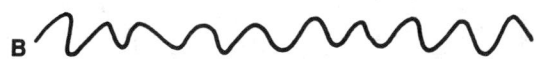

Figure 29–12. Very fine fibrillatory waves of ventricular fibrillation (**A**) can sometimes be coarsened into a more distinct fibrillatory pattern (**B**) by administration of epinephrine.

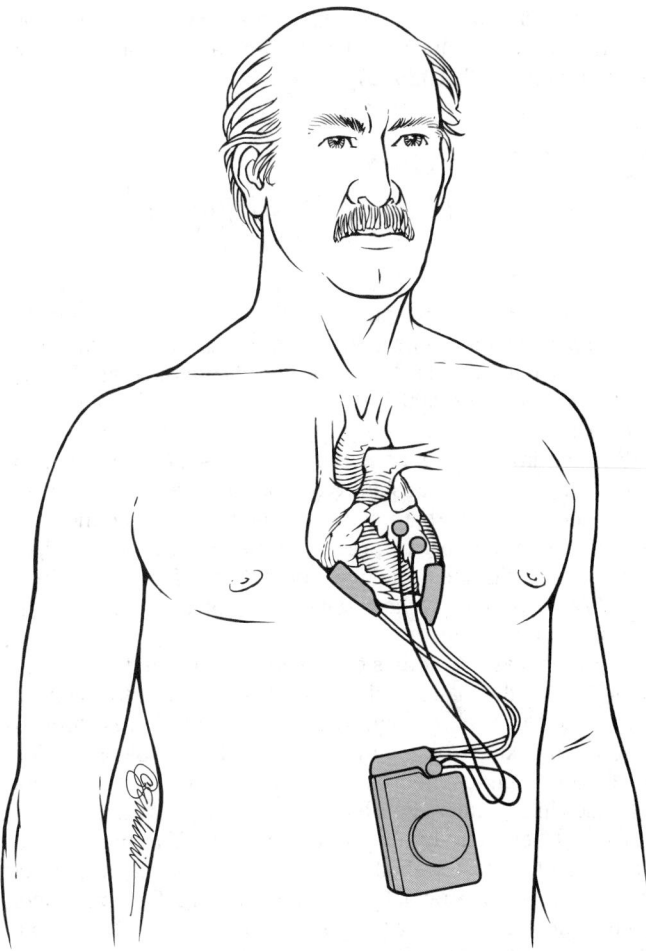

Figure 29–13. The implantable cardioverter-defibrillator mechanical system consists of a generator, two rate-sensing electrodes, and two epicardial patches.

of isoelectric line segments. When a dysrhythmia occurs, the rate sensors take 5 to 10 seconds to sense the dysrhythmia and another 5 to 7 seconds to charge the capacitors to deliver electrical shock to revert the rhythm. The device can deliver up to three shocks if necessary.

The use of the ICD does not eliminate the need for anti-dysrhythmic medication therapy. Medications are administered in conjunction with this technology.

The primary complications associated with the ICD are pulmonary in origin. The two most common complications are pulmonary dysfunctions secondary to the thoracotomy required for insertion of the ICD and surgical infections. There are lesser complications associated with the technical aspects of the equipment such as premature battery depletion or fractured leads. In spite of the possible complications, consensus among clinicians is that the benefit of this therapy to the patient exceeds the risks.

The nursing interventions for the patient with an ICD occur throughout three different phases, preoperative, postoperative, and predischarge. The first or preoperative phase may require management of acute episodes of life-threatening dysrhythmias in addition to providing the patient and family with explanations regarding the implantation of the ICD. The postoperative phase involves astute observation of the patient and his responses to his new technology. The predischarge phase involves more teaching and is vitally important to the patient's ability to live independently (Chart 29-2).

▶ Nursing Process
The Patient With a Dysrhythmia

▷ Assessment

The assessment of the patient with cardiac dysrhythmias is accomplished through patient history and physical and psychosocial assessments. A major focus of assessment is the dysrhythmia and the effect it is having on cardiac output (heart rate [HR] × stroke volume [SV]). When cardiac output is reduced, optimum oxygenation to the tissues and vital organs is diminished. This diminished oxygenation produces the signs associated with dysrhythmias. A patient history is conducted to determine the past or present existence of syncope, lightheadedness, dizziness, fatigue, chest discomfort, and palpitations. Any one or all of these signs can be present when cardiac output is decreasing.

Physical assessment is conducted to confirm the data obtained from the patient history and to observe for signs of diminished cardiac output. The nurse's attention is directed toward the skin, which can be pale and cool. Signs of fluid retention, such as neck vein distention and crackles and wheezes in the lungs are observed. The pulse is assessed apically and peripherally for rate and rhythm. The presence or absence of a pulse deficit is noted. The heart is auscultated for extra sounds, especially S_3 and S_4, which reflect a reduced compliance of the myocardium seen in reduced cardiac output. Blood pressure is measured and pulse pressure is determined. A declining pulse pressure indicates reduced cardiac output.

An isolated assessment may not disclose significant changes in cardiac output; therefore, the nurse compares multiple observations over time to recognize subtle changes.

▷ Nursing Diagnoses

Based on assessment data, major nursing diagnoses of the patient may include:

- Decreased cardiac output related to slow or rapid rate dysrhythmia
- Anxiety related to fear of the unknown
- Knowledge deficit about the disease and its treatment

▷ Planning and Implementation

▷ *Goals:* The major goals of the patient may include (1) maintenance of cardiac output, (2) minimization of anxiety, and (3) attainment of knowledge of the dysrhythmia and its treatment.

▷ Nursing Interventions

▷ *Maintenance of Cardiac Output.* Cardiac output is best protected by controlling episodes of the dysrhythmia. Administration of medications is managed carefully so that a constant serum blood level of the medication is maintained at all times. Frequent rhythm strips are analyzed to track the dysrhythmia and prevent its deterioration into a more malignant dysrhythmia, (*e.g.,* PVCs are aggressively managed before they become ventricular tachycardia). Rest is promoted for the patient so that myocardial oxygen needs are reduced.

▷ *Minimization of Anxiety.* The relationship between a dysrhythmia and cardiac output is explained to the patient so that he understands the rationale for his medical regimen. In particular, the relationship between myocardial oxygen demands and the subsequent effect on cardiac output is stressed.

During episodes of dysrhythmia, the nurse maintains a calm and reassuring attitude; this fosters a trusting relationship with the patient and assists in reducing anxiety. Small successes are shared with the patient so that his confidence in living with a dysrhythmia is promoted. For example, if a patient is having some dysrhythmia and a medication is administered that begins to lessen the number of ectopic beats, the nurse shares that information with the patient. The nursing goal is to maximize the patient's control and to make the unknown less threatening.

▷ *Attainment of Knowledge of the Dysrhythmia and Its Treatment.* In terms that the patient can understand and without unduly frightening the patient, information specific to his circumstances is explained. The importance of maintaining

---

Chart 29-2
Patient Education: The Patient With an Implantable Cardioverter Defibrillator

1. Avoid infection at the operative site.
   a. Observe incision site daily for redness, swelling, and heat.
   b. Avoid restrictive clothing that may produce friction over the wound site.
2. Avoid magnetic fields such as metal detection booths at airport security check points, MRIs, and microwaves.
   a. Magnetic fields can deactivate the ICD, negating any effect on a dysrhythmia.
3. Maintain a log to record shocks; record events that precipitate the sensation of shock. This provides important data for the physician to use in readjusting the medical regimen.
4. Avoid danger to self and others.
   a. The physician and patient together evaluate the appropriateness of driving.
   b. Adhere to appointments that are scheduled to test electronic performance of ICD.
   c. Call 911 for emergency assistance if you feel dizzy. Wear Medic-Alert identification that includes physician information.
5. Avoid frightening family or friends with unexpected shocks. Inform those closest to you that in the event they are touching you when a shock is delivered they may also feel the shock. It is especially important to warn sexual partners that this may occur.

therapeutic serum levels of antidysrhythmic medications is explained instead of a statement such as, always take your medications at a regular time each day.

Providing the patient with a plan of action for emergency needs is an effective means of increasing patient knowledge. Advising the patient to predetermine which hospital he would need to be taken to in the event of an emergency is strongly suggested.

◊ Evaluation

Expected Outcomes

1. Cardiac output is maintained
   a. Demonstrates minimal number of episodes of dysrhythmias
   b. Demonstrates blood pressure and pulse within normal parameters without wide variations
2. Anxiety is minimized
   a. Expresses a positive attitude about living with the dysrhythmia
   b. Expresses confidence in knowing what to do in case of an emergency
3. Attainment of knowledge of the dysrhythmia and its treatment
   a. Explains his dysrhythmia and its effect on cardiac output
   b. Articulates rationale for medication regimen and explains need for therapeutic serum level of the medication
   c. States actions to take in the event of an emergency

Conduction Abnormalities

First-Degree AV Block

First-degree AV block is usually associated with organic heart disease or may be due to the effect of digitalis. It is seen frequently in patients with inferior wall MIs.

First-degree heart block has the following characteristics (Fig. 29–14):

Rate: Variable, usually 60 to 100 beats per minute.
P waves: Precede each QRS complex. The PR interval is greater than 0.20 second in duration.
QRS complex: Follows each P wave; usually normal.
Conduction: Delayed conduction, usually anywhere between the junctional tissue and the Purkinje network, produces a prolonged PR interval. Ventricular conduction is usually normal.
Rhythm: Usually regular.

This dysrhythmia is important because it may lead to more serious forms of heart block. It is often a warning signal. Therefore, the patient should be monitored closely for any advancing block.

Second-Degree AV Block

Second-degree AV block is caused also by organic heart disease, an MI, or digitalis intoxication. This type of block results in a reduced heart rate and usually a reduced cardiac output (cardiac output = stroke volume × heart rate).

Second-degree heart block has the following characteristics (Fig. 29–15):

Rate: 30 to 55 beats per minute. The atrial rate may be two, three, or four times faster than the ventricular rate.
P waves: There are two, three, or four P waves for each QRS complex. The PR interval of the conducted beat is usually normal in duration.
QRS complex: Usually normal.
Conduction: One or more of the impulses are not conducted through the ventricles.
Rhythm: Usually slow and regular. When an irregularity is present, it is due to the fact that the block is varying from 2:1 to 3:1 or to some other combination.

Treatment is directed toward increasing the heart rate to maintain a normal cardiac output. Digitalis toxicity should be ruled out and myocardial depressant medications withheld.

Third-Degree AV Block

Third-degree AV block (complete heart block) is also associated with organic heart disease, digitalis toxicity, and MI. The heart rate may be markedly decreased, resulting in a decrease in perfusion to vital organs, such as the brain, heart, kidneys, lungs, and skin.

Complete block—third-degree AV block—has the following characteristics (Fig. 29–16):

Origin: Impulses originate in the SA node, but are not conducted to the Purkinje fibers. They are completely blocked. An escape rhythm from either the junctional or the ventricular area therefore takes over as the pacemaker.
Rate: Atrial rate, 60 to 100 beats per minute; ventricular rate, 40 to 60 beats per minute if the escape rhythm originated in the junction, 20 to 40 beats per minute if the escape rhythm originated in the ventricle.

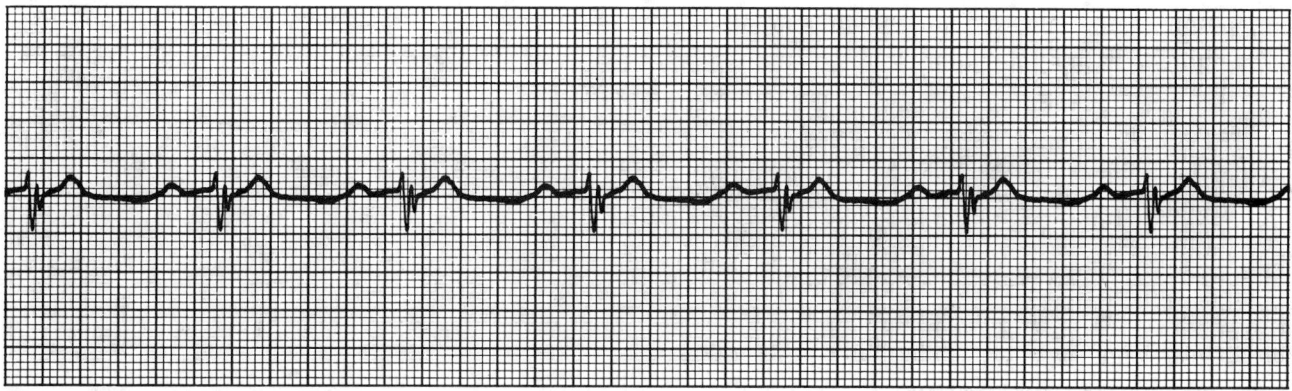

Figure 29–14. First-degree heart block.

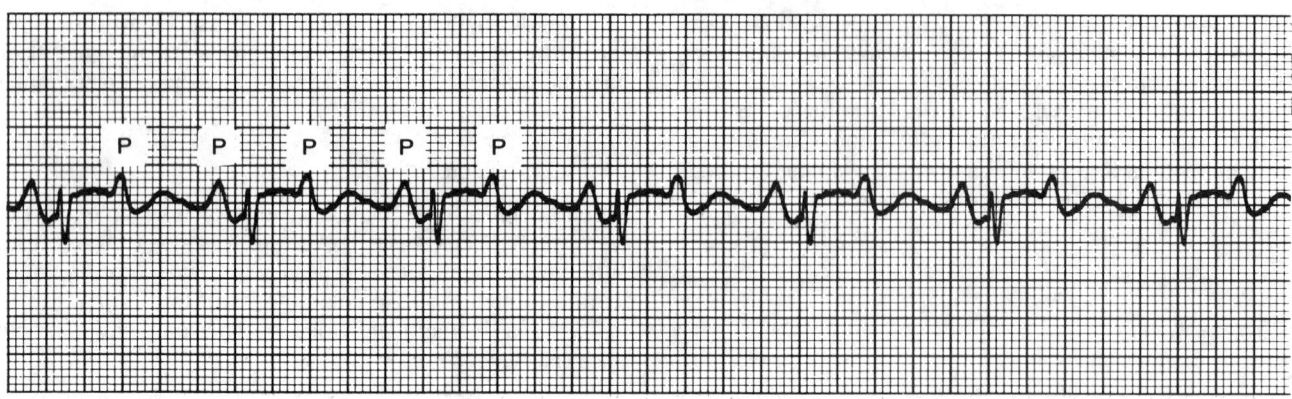

Figure 29–15. Second-degree heart block.

P waves: The P waves originating from the SA node are seen regularly throughout the rhythm, but they have no association with the QRS complexes.

QRS complex: If the escape rhythm originated in the junction, the QRS complexes have a normal supraventricular configuration, but have no association with the P waves. QRS complexes occur regularly. If the escape rhythm originated in the ventricle, the QRS complex is longer than 0.10 second in duration, and is usually broad and slurred. These QRS complexes have the same configuration as the QRS complex of a PVC.

Conduction: The SA node is firing, and P waves can be seen. They are all blocked and not conducted to the ventricles. Escape rhythms originating in the junction are usually conducted normally through the ventricles. Escape rhythms from the ventricles are ectopic with aberrant configuration.

Rhythm: Usually slow but regular.

Treatment is directed toward increasing perfusion to vital organs. The insertion of a temporary transvenous pacemaker is the acceptable treatment. A permanent pacemaker may be necessary if the block is persistent.

Ventricular Asystole

In ventricular asystole there are no QRS complexes. There is no heartbeat, no palpable pulse, and no respiration. Without immediate treatment, ventricular asystole is fatal.

Ventricular asystole (Fig. 29–17) has the following characteristics:

Rate: None.

P waves: May be visible, but they do not conduct through the AV node and ventricles.

QRS complex: None.

Conduction: Possibly, through the atria only.

Rhythm: None.

Cardiopulmonary resuscitation (CPR) is necessary to keep the patient alive. To decrease any vagal stimuli, atropine is administered intravenously. Epinephrine (intracardiac) should be administered and repeated at 5-minute intervals. Sodium bicarbonate may be given intravenously. Insertion of a transthoracic or transvenous pacemaker may be necessary.

Pacemaker Therapy

Definition and Indications for Use

A pacemaker is an electronic device that provides repetitive electrical stimuli to the heart muscle for the control of heart rate. It initiates and maintains the heart rate when the natural pacemakers of the heart are unable to do so. Pacemakers are generally used when a patient has a conduction disturbance or the forerunner of a conduction disturbance that causes failure of cardiac output. Pacemakers can be permanent or temporary. Permanent pacemakers are used most commonly for irreversible complete heart block; temporary pacemakers are used as adjunctive therapy to support patients who have had heart block after myocardial infarction or open-heart surgery. In some cases a pacemaker can also be used to control tachydysrhythmias that otherwise do not respond to medication therapy.

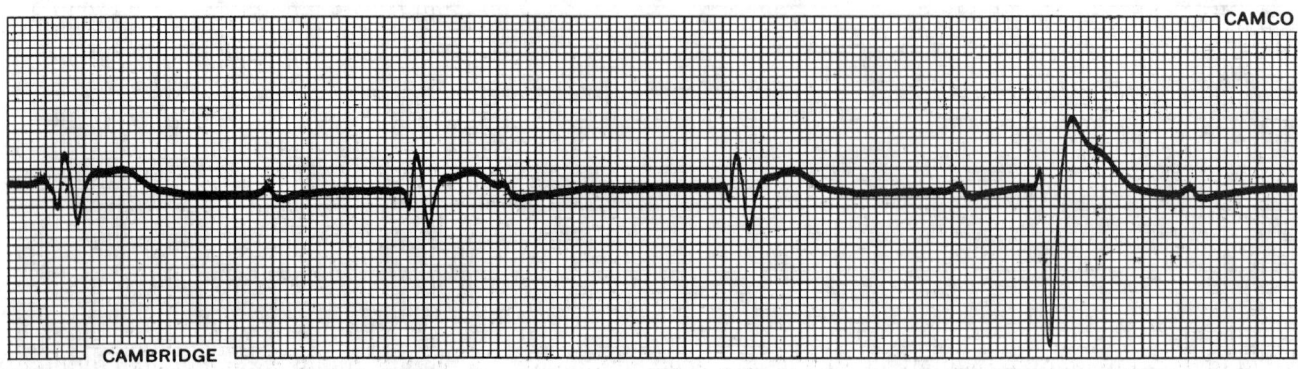

Figure 29–16. Third-degree heart block.

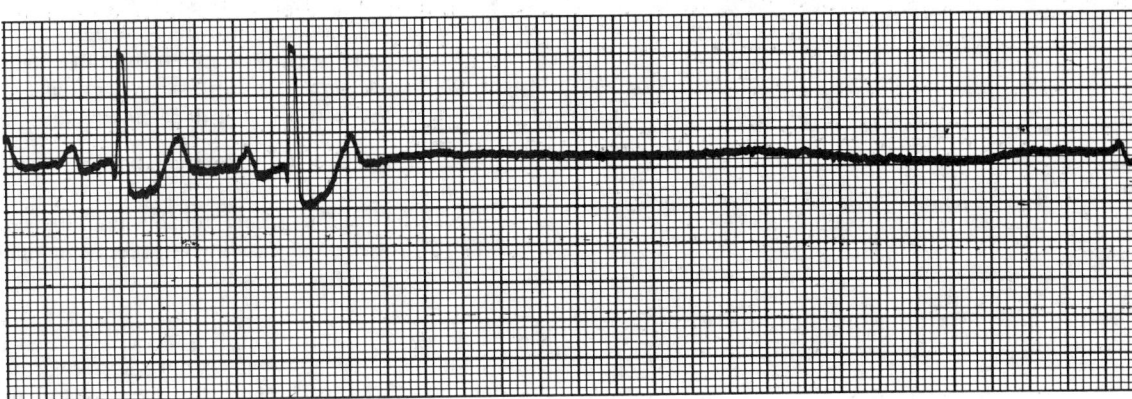

Figure 29–17. Ventricular asystole.

Pacemaker Design

Pacemakers consist of two component parts: (1) the electronic pulse generator, which contains the circuitry and batteries that generate the electrical stimulus; and (2) the pacemaker electrodes (also called leads or wires), which transmit the pacemaker impulses to the heart. The stimuli from the pacemaker travel through a flexible catheter electrode that is threaded through a vein into the right ventricle or introduced by direct penetration of the chest wall. The pulse generator is usually implanted in a subcutaneous pocket in the pectoral or axillary region; sometimes an abdominal site is selected.

Pacemaker generators are insulated to protect against body moisture and warmth. The pulse generator (or pacemaker) contains its own supply of power, which is provided by battery cells. The main power sources in current use are mercury-zinc batteries (lasting 3 to 4 years), lithium cell units (lasting up to 10 years), and a nuclear-powered pacemaker (^{238}plutonium source) that lasts 20 years to a lifetime. There are also pacemakers that can be recharged externally. Because pacemakers rely on batteries, battery exhaustion (with the exception of nuclear-powered and rechargeable batteries) is inevitable. Therefore, the generator that contains the batteries must be replaced periodically.

Types of Pacemakers

The most commonly used pacemaker is the *demand* (synchronous; noncompetitive) pacemaker, which is set for a specific rate and stimulates the heart when normal ventricular depolarization does not occur (Fig. 29–18). It functions only when the natural heart rate goes below a certain level. The *fixed rate* pacemaker (asynchronous; competitive) stimulates the ventricle at a preset constant rate that is independent of the patient's rhythm. It is used infrequently, usually in patients with complete and unvarying heart block.

Temporary Pacemaker Systems. Temporary pacing is usually an emergency procedure and permits the observation of the effects of pacing on heart function so that the optimum pacing rate for the patient can be selected before a permanent pacemaker is implanted. It is used in patients who have suffered myocardial infarction complicated by heart block, in patients with cardiac arrest with bradycardia and asystole, or in selected postoperative cardiac surgery patients. Temporary pacing may be done for hours, days, or weeks and is continued until the patient improves or a permanent pacemaker is implanted.

Temporary pacing may be carried out either by an endocardial (transvenous) approach or by the transthoracic approach to the myocardium. The transvenous electrode is passed under fluoroscopic guidance through any peripheral vein (antecubital, brachial, jugular, subclavian, femoral), and the catheter tip is positioned in the apex of the right ventricle. The most common complication occurring during pacemaker insertion is ventricular dysrhythmia. Cardiac perforation occurs rarely. A defibrillator should be immediately available.

Permanent Pacemaker Systems. For permanent pacing, the endocardial lead is passed transvenously into the right ventricle, and the pulse generator is implanted within the body underneath the skin below the right or left pectoral region or below the clavicle (Fig. 29–19). This is termed an endocardial

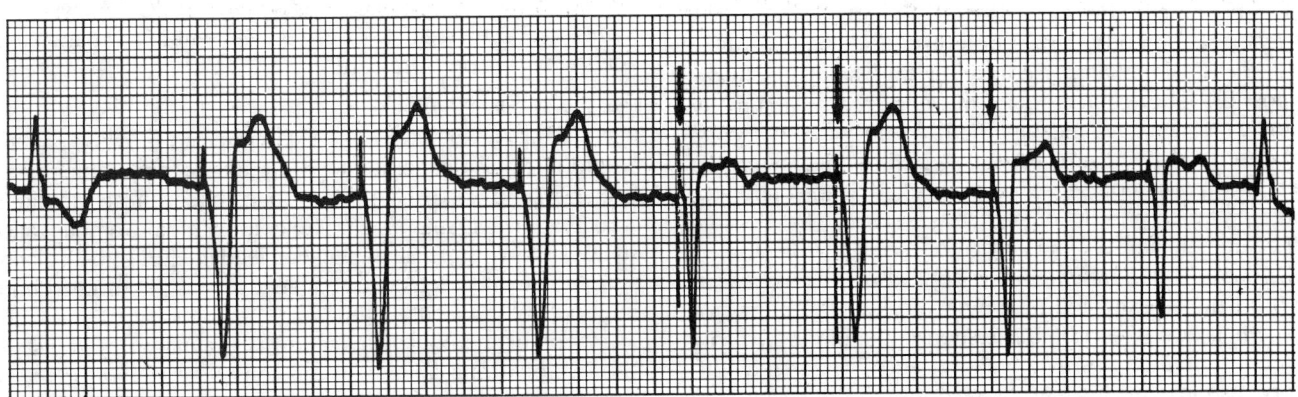

Figure 29–18. Synchronized pacemaker rhythm. Arrows indicate presence of sensed pacing spike.

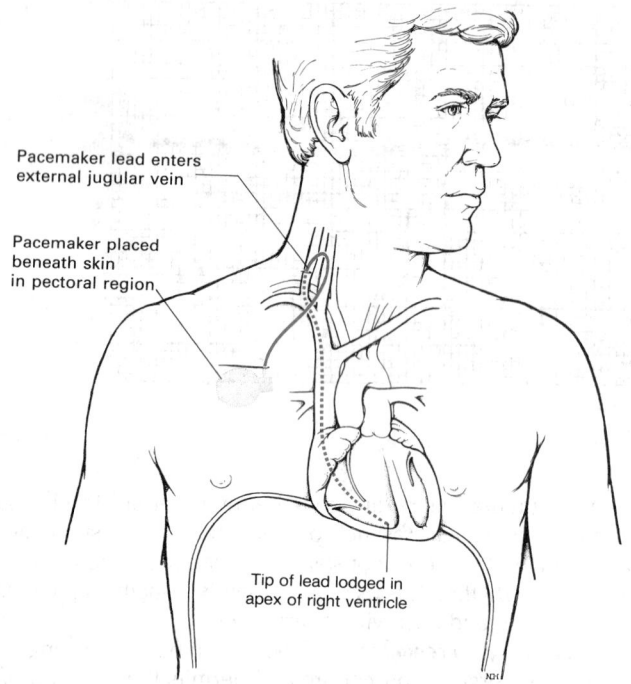

Pacemaker lead enters external jugular vein

Pacemaker placed beneath skin in pectoral region

Tip of lead lodged in apex of right ventricle

Figure 29-19. Implanted transvenous pacing electrode and pacemaker generator.

or transvenous implant. This procedure is usually performed under local anesthesia. Another method of permanent pacing is the implantation of the pulse generator in the abdominal wall. The electrode is passed transthoracically to the myocardium, where it is sutured in place. For this method, termed an *epicardial* or *myocardial implant,* a thoracotomy is required to provide access to the heart.

Atrioventricular Pacemakers (Physiologic Pacing). Pacemaker technology, through the development of AV pacemakers, has fostered the growth of safe and effective pacemaker therapy for many complex cardiac problems. AV pacemakers are considered highly desirable because they can be programmed to mimic the patient's own intrinsic cardiac function; hence they are referred to as *physiologic pacemakers.*

Because of the sophistication of these AV pacemakers, a universal code has been adopted to provide a means of safe communication about their function. The coding is referred to as the *ICHD code* because it is sanctioned by the Inter-Society Commission for Heart Disease. The complete code consists of five letters, but only three are used in common practice. The *first letter* of the code always describes the chamber being paced, that is, the chamber containing the pacing electrode. The possible letter characters for this code are A (atrium), V (ventricle), or D (dual, meaning both A and V). The *second letter* describes the chamber being sensed by the pacemaker generator. Information sensed is dispatched to the generator for interpretation and action by the generator. The possible letter characters here are once again A (atrium), V (ventricle), and D (dual). The *third letter* of the code always describes the type of response exhibited by the pacemaker. There are five characters used to describe this response, but of the five only two are in common use: I (inhibitory) and T (triggered). Inhibitory response means that the response of the pacemaker is controlled by the activity of the patient's own heart; that is,

the pacemaker will not function when the patient's heart beats. In contrast, triggered response means that the pacemaker will trigger a response based on intrinsic heart activity.

An example of an ICHD-coded pacemaker is DVI:

D —Both the atrium and the ventricle have a pacing electrode in place.
V —The pacemaker is sensing the activity of the ventricle only.
I —The pacemaker's stimulating effect is being inhibited by the activity of the patient's ventricle.

Complications

Complications associated with pacemakers relate to (1) their presence within the body, and (2) improper functioning. The following complications may arise from the presence of the pacemaker:

- Local infection (sepsis or hematoma formation) may occur at the site of venous cutdown or subcutaneous pacemaker placement.
- Dysrhythmias—ventricular ectopic activity may follow irritation of the ventricular wall by the electrode.
- Perforation of the myocardium or right ventricle by the catheter may occur.
- Abrupt loss of pacing caused by high ventricular threshold.

Pacemaker malfunction can arise from failure in one or more components of the pacing system. The majority of pulse generator failures are from depletion of the power supply (*i.e.,* battery failure). The patient should be informed that the battery cells are sealed in the pulse generator. When it is time for a battery change, a new incision is made over the old incision. The old pulse generator is removed, and the new unit is connected to the existing leads and reimplanted in the already existing pocket. This is usually performed under local anesthesia. Other complications include fracture (breakage) or dislocation of the electrodes and electronic failure.

Malfunction of the pacemaker can also occur with exposure to electromagnetic fields. Electromagnetic fields are produced by technologic equipment such as microwave ovens, magnetic resonance imaging (MRI) equipment, and the metal detectors now found at airport security check points. The patient is cautioned to avoid situations that threaten electromagnetic field exposure. The patient is advised to wear identification that will alert emergency health care personnel.

These complications are manifested by abrupt changes in heart rate and rhythm. Their visibility as symptoms will depend on the patient's level of dependency on the pacemaker. The diagnosis of these complications is made by ECG analysis. Manipulation of the electrodes or replacement of the pacemaker generator may be necessary.

Pacemaker Surveillance

Pacemaker clinics have been established to monitor patients and to test pulse generators for warnings of impending pacemaker system failure. Testing of pacemaker pulse amplitude and duration and analysis of pulse contour require amplification equipment. With special equipment, lead fracture and insulation disruption can be detected. A 12-lead ECG is performed during each patient visit to the clinic.

Another method of follow-up is evaluation by transtelephone monitoring of the transmission of the generator's pulse rate. By means of special equipment, the sound tone of the patient's pacemaker is transmitted over the telephone to a receiving system at a pacemaker clinic. The sounds are converted into an electronic signal and permanently recorded on an ECG strip. The pacemaker rate and other data concerning pacemaker function are obtained and evaluated by a cardiologist. This simplifies the diagnosis of a failing generator, provides reassurance, and improves the management of the person who is physically remote from pacemaker testing facilities.

Pacemaker Development

Activity Response Pacemaker. A pacemaker that will alter cardiac rate in response to changes in activity is being investigated. The preliminary designs depend on parameters such as physical activity, acid–base changes, and oxygen saturation, instead of depending on sinus node function. This pacemaker will be capable of improving cardiac output during exercise.

▶ Nursing Process
The Patient With a Pacemaker

▷ Assessment

After the insertion of either a temporary or a permanent pacemaker, the patient's heart rate and rhythm are monitored by electrocardiogram. The preset pacemaker rate is noted; the patient's heart rate may vary as much as five beats above or below the preset pacemaker rate. The new appearance or increasing frequency of dysrhythmia is observed and reported to the physician.

The incision site where the pulse generator is implanted (or the entry site for the pacing electrode if the pacemaker is temporary) is observed for bleeding, hematoma formation, or infection. Infection is a major threat to the patient who has received a new pacemaker. The insertion site is observed primarily for swelling, unusual tenderness, and increased heat. The patient may complain of continuous throbbing or pain. Any unusual drainage is reported to the physician.

All electrical equipment used in the vicinity of the patient is grounded. Improperly grounded equipment can generate leakage currents capable of producing ventricular fibrillation.

The nurse observes for potential sources of electrical hazards. No metal parts of the output terminal or pacemaker wires should be exposed. All such bare metal must be carefully covered with nonconductive tape to prevent accidental ventricular

fibrillation from stray currents. A biomedical engineer, electrician, or other qualified person should make certain that the patient is in an electrically safe environment.

▷ Complications

In the initial hours after the insertion of either a temporary or a permanent pacemaker, the most common complication is dislodgement of the pacing electrode. The identification of this complication is made by examination of the ECG pattern; the relationship between the pacing spike and the patient's QRS becomes asynchronous (Fig. 29–20).

The nurse can help to avoid this complication by minimizing the patient activities. If a temporary electrode is in place, the extremity is immobilized. The ECG is monitored very carefully for the presence of a pacing spike. Because of the importance of such monitoring, this patient is ideally in an intensive care unit.

Data about the model of pacemaker, date and time of its insertion, location of the pulse generator, stimulation threshold, and pacer rate should be noted on the patient's record. This information is important for solving any unusual dysrhythmia problem.

▷ Nursing Diagnoses

Based on assessment data, major nursing diagnoses of the patient may include the following:

- High risk for infection related to catheter or generator insertion
- Knowledge deficit regarding self-care program
- Potential for decrease in cardiac output related to pacemaker malfunction

▷ Planning and Implementation

▷ *Goals:* The major goals of the patient may include (1) absence of infection, (2) adherence to a self-care program, and (3) maintenance of pacemaker function.

▷ Nursing Interventions

▷ *Prevention of Infection.* The wound site is inspected daily for redness, edema, pain, or any unusual bleeding. The physician performs the initial dressing change and the nurse in-

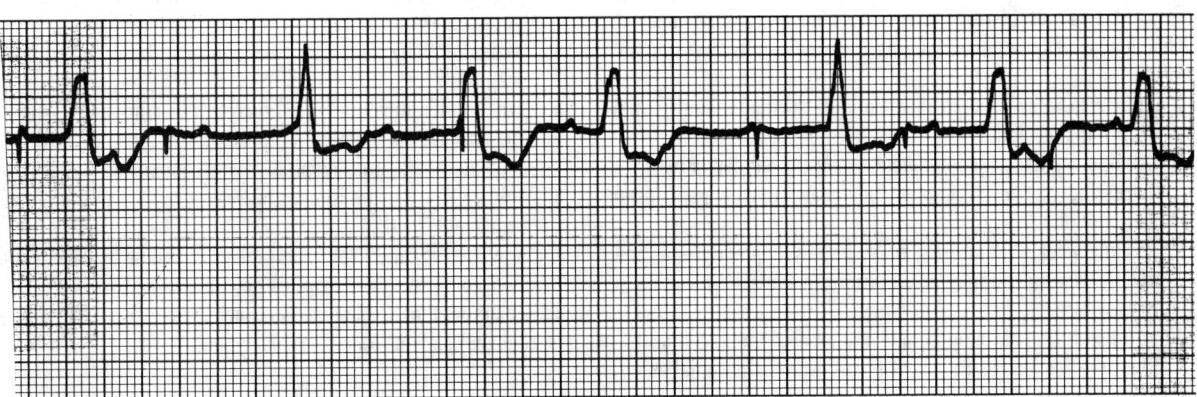

Figure 29–20. Loss of capture of pacemaker. Pacer discharges spike, but no mechanical activity follows.

spects and changes the dressing each day thereafter. Changes in the wound are reported to the physician.

▷ *Adherence to the Self-Care Program.* Because of the nature of the need for a pacemaker, most patients are very compliant with the home health-care program. See Chart 29–3 for details of patient education.

▷ *Maintenance of Pacemaker Function.* The patient follows a prescribed program of assessing and recording his pulse rate. See Chart 29–3 for additional details of maintenance of pacemaker function.

▷ Evaluation

Expected Outcomes

1. Free of infection
   a. Temperature normal
   b. WBCs within normal range (5,000 to 10,000/mm³)
   c. Exhibits no redness or swelling of pacemaker insertion site
2. Adheres to a self-care program
   a. Responds appropriately when queried about the signs and symptoms of infection
   b. Knows when to seek medical attention (as demonstrated in responses to signs and symptoms)
3. Maintains pacemaker function
   a. Measures and records pulse rate at regular intervals
   b. Experiences no abrupt changes in pulse rate or rhythm
   c. See Chart 29–3 for additional means of maintaining pacemaker function

In summary, cardiac dysrhythmias are the most common complications of cardiac disorders. Dysrhythmias may originate from disturbances in impulse formation or from conduction defects and may vary in severity from benign sinus dysrhythmia to life-threatening ventricular fibrillation. The effect that the dysrhythmia has on cardiac output determines the signs and symptoms that the patient will exhibit and the treatment that will be needed.

Dysrhythmias are diagnosed through ECG waveform analysis. An understanding of the properties of cardiac muscle and the heart's normal conduction system is fundamental to determining an accurate diagnosis.

Therapies for dysrhythmias include medications, pacemakers, and defibrillators. Mortality and morbidity from dysrhythmias are also being reduced by mobile intensive care units that permit immediate diagnosis and treatment of life-threatening dysrhythmias.

Acute Pulmonary Edema

Definition, Etiology, and Pathophysiology

Pulmonary edema is the abnormal accumulation of fluid in the lungs, either in the interstitial spaces or in the alveoli.

Pulmonary edema represents the ultimate stage of pulmonary congestion, in which fluid has leaked through the capillary walls and is permeating the airways, giving rise to dyspnea of dramatic severity. Pulmonary congestion occurs when the pulmonary vascular bed has received more blood from the right ventricle than the left can accommodate and remove. The slightest imbalance between inflow on the right side and outflow on the left side of the heart may have drastic consequences. For example, if with each heartbeat the right ventricle pumps out just one more drop of blood than the left, within the space of only 3 hours the pulmonary blood volume will have expanded 500 ml!

Noncardiac pulmonary edema has a wide variety of causes: toxic inhalants, drug overdose, and neurogenic pulmonary edema. Clinical management is directed toward reducing pulmonary blood flow and pulmonary arterial pressure.

The most common cause of pulmonary edema is cardiac

Chart 29–3
Patient Education: The Patient With a Pacemaker

1. Report to physician/pacemaker clinic periodically as prescribed, so that the rate of the pacemaker and its function can be checked. This is especially important during the first month after implantation.
   a. Adhere to weekly monitoring schedule during the first month after implantation.
   b. Check pulse daily. Report *immediately* any sudden slowing or increasing of the pulse rate. This may indicate pacemaker malfunction.
   c. Resume weekly monitoring when battery depletion is anticipated. (The time for reimplantation depends on the type of battery in use.)
2. Wear loose-fitting clothing around the area of the pacemaker.
   a. State the reason for the slight bulge over the pacemaker implant.
   b. Notify physician if the area becomes reddened or painful.
   c. Avoid trauma to the area of the pacemaker generator.

3. Study the manufacturer's instructions and become familiar with the pacemaker.
4. Physical activity does not usually have to be curtailed, with the exception of contact sports.
5. Carry an identification card/bracelet indicating physician's name, type and model number of pacemaker, manufacturer's name, pacemaker rate, and hospital where pacemaker was inserted.
6. Avoid close exposure to microwave ovens, MRI and other sources of magnetic fields.
7. Show identification card and request scanning by a hand scanner when going through weapons detector at airport.
8. Remember that hospitalization is necessary periodically for battery changes/pacemaker unit replacement.

disease—atherosclerotic, hypertensive, valvular, myopathic. Most patients with pulmonary edema have chronic heart disease of a type that imposes a strain on the left ventricle, such as arterial hypertension or aortic valve disease. The edema is particularly likely to arise from the damage to the heart muscle caused by acute MI. The development of pulmonary edema signifies that cardiac function has become grossly inadequate. There is an elevated left ventricular end-diastolic pressure and a rise in pulmonary venous pressure. This produces an increase in hydrostatic pressure, which results in transudation of fluid. Impaired lymphatic drainage contributes to the accumulation of fluid in the lung tissues.

The pulmonary capillaries, engorged with an excess of blood that the left ventricle is incapable of pumping, no longer are able to contain their contents. Fluid, first serous and later bloody, escapes into the adjacent alveoli through the communicating bronchioles and bronchi. It then mixes with air and, churned by respiratory agitation, is expelled from the mouth and nostrils. Because of the fluid buildup, the lungs become stiff and cannot expand, and air cannot enter. The result is severe hypoxia.

Death from pulmonary edema is by no means inevitable. If appropriate measures are taken promptly, attacks can be aborted and patients can survive this complication to benefit from measures directed against its recurrence. Fortunately, pulmonary edema usually does not develop precipitously but is preceded by the premonitory symptoms of pulmonary congestion.

Clinical Manifestations

The typical attack of pulmonary edema occurs at night after the patient has been lying down for a few hours. Recumbency increases the venous return to the heart and favors the resorption of edema fluid from the legs. The circulating blood becomes diluted, and its volume expands. The venous pressure rises and the right atrium fills with increasing rapidity. There is a corresponding increase in the right ventricular output, which eventually surpasses the output from the left ventricle. The pulmonary vessels become engorged with blood and proceed to leak. Meanwhile, the patient has become increasingly restless, anxious, and unable to sleep.

There is a sudden onset of breathlessness and a sense of suffocation. The patient's hands become cold and moist, the nail beds become cyanotic, and the skin color turns gray. In addition, the pulse is weak and rapid and the neck veins are distended. There is incessant coughing, which produces increasing quantities of mucoid sputum. As the pulmonary edema progresses, anxiety develops into near panic and the patient becomes confused, then stuporous. Breathing is noisy and moist, and the patient, nearly suffocated by the blood-tinged, frothy fluid now pouring into his bronchi and trachea, is literally drowning in his own secretions. The situation demands immediate action.

Diagnostic Evaluation

The diagnosis is made on evaluation of the clinical manifestations resulting from pulmonary congestion. A pulmonary artery catheter may be inserted to facilitate the monitoring of hemodynamic data (Chart 29-4) essential to the diagnosis and treatment.

Management

The goals of medical management for the patient with acute pulmonary edema are to reduce total circulating volume and to improve respiratory exchange. These goals are accomplished through a combination of oxygen and drug therapies and nursing support.

Oxygenation.   Oxygen is administered in concentrations adequate to relieve hypoxia and dyspnea.

If signs of hypoxemia persist, oxygen may be delivered by intermittent or continuous positive pressure. If respiratory failure occurs despite optimal management, endotracheal intubation and mechanical ventilation are required. The use of positive end expiratory pressure (PEEP) is effective in reducing venous return, lowering pulmonary capillary pressure, and improving oxygenation. Oxygenation is monitored by measurement of arterial blood gases.

Pharmacologic Therapy: Morphine.   Morphine is administered intravenously in small doses to reduce anxiety and dyspnea and to decrease peripheral resistance so that blood can be redistributed from the pulmonary circulation to the periphery. This action decreases pressure in the pulmonary capillaries and decreases transudation of fluid. The decrease in rate of respirations resulting from morphine is also beneficial.

- Morphine is not usually administered if pulmonary edema is caused by cerebral vascular accident or if chronic pulmonary disease or cardiogenic shock is present.
- The patient is observed for excessive respiratory depression; morphine antagonist (naloxone hydrochloride [Narcan]) is kept available.

Diuretics.   Either furosemide (Lasix) or ethacrynic acid (Edecrin) is administered intravenously to produce a rapid diuretic effect (Table 29-1). In addition, furosemide causes vasodilation and peripheral venous pooling, with a subsequent reduction in venous return that occurs even before the diuretic effect. Thus dyspnea is rapidly relieved and pulmonary congestion is decreased. Because a large volume of urine will be formed within minutes after administration of a potent diuretic, an indwelling catheter may be inserted.

- Falling blood pressure, increasing heart rate, and decreasing urinary output indicate that the total circulation is not tolerating diuresis.
- Patients with prostatic hyperplasia must be observed for signs of urinary retention.

Digitalis.   To improve the contractile force of the heart, thus increasing the output of the left ventricle, the patient may be given a rapid-acting digitalis preparation. The improved cardiac contractility will increase cardiac output, enhance diuresis, and reduce diastolic pressure. Thus pulmonary capillary pressure and the transudation of fluid into the alveoli will be reduced.

- Digitalis must be administered with extreme caution to patients with acute myocardial infarction, because these patients are sensitive to digitalis and may develop toxic dysrhythmias.
- The serum potassium level is measured at intervals because diuresis may have produced hypokalemia. The effect of digitalis in the presence of hypokalemia is enhanced, so digitalis toxicity may occur.
- If the patient has been on digitalis, the drug is usually with-

Chart 29–4
Guidelines: Hemodynamic Monitoring: Multilumen Pulmonary Artery Catheter

Nursing Action	Rationale/Amplification
Preparatory Phase	
1. Explain procedure to patient and family/significant other.	1. Tell the patient that it is normal to feel the catheter moving through the vein.
2. Check vital signs and apply ECG electrodes.	2. An initial assessment offers a baseline for comparison.
3. Place patient in a position of comfort; this is the baseline position.	3. Note the angle of elevation if patient cannot lie flat, as subsequent pressure readings are taken from this baseline position to ensure consistency.
4. Set up equipment according to manufacturer's directives:	4.
a. The pulmonary artery catheter requires a transducer, recording, amplifying, and flush systems.	a. Monitoring systems may vary greatly. The complexity of equipment requires an understanding of the equipment in use.
b. The pressure equipment is calibrated and flushed according to manufacturer's directives.	b. Flushing of the catheter system ensures patency and eliminates air bubbles.
c. The balloon is inflated with air or sterile water or saline to test for leakage (bubbles).	c. Testing is performed to ensure that the balloon is intact.
5. Shave and prepare the skin over insertion site.	5. Decreases risk of infection at insertion site.
Performance Phase (by the Physician)	
1. The pulmonary artery catheter is inserted through the internal jugular, subclavian, or any easily accessible vein by either percutaneous puncture or venotomy.	1. The internal jugular vein establishes a short route into the central venous system.
2. The catheter is advanced to the superior vena cava. Oscillations of the pressure waveforms will indicate when the tip of the catheter is within the heart. The patient may be asked to cough.	2. Catheter placement is determined by characteristic waveforms and changes. Coughing will produce deflections in the pressure tracing when the catheter tip is in the heart.
3. When the catheter is in the superior vena cava, it is inflated with air and advanced gently.	3. The amount of air to be used is indicated on the catheter.
4. The inflated balloon at the tip of the catheter will be guided by the flowing stream of blood through the right atrium and tricuspid valve into the right ventricle. From this position it finds its way into the main pulmonary artery, carried by blood flow. The catheter tip pressures are recorded continuously by specific pressure waveforms as the catheter advances through the various chambers of the heart.	4. Watch ECG monitor for signs of ventricular irritability as catheter enters the right ventricle. Report any signs of dysrhythmia to the physician.
5. The flowing blood will continue to direct the catheter more distally into the pulmonary tree. When the catheter reaches a pulmonary vessel that is approximately the same size or slightly smaller in diameter than the inflated balloon, it cannot be advanced any further. This is the wedge position, called pulmonary capillary wedge pressure (PCWP) or pulmonary artery wedge pressure (PAWP).	5. With the catheter in the wedge position, the balloon blocks the flow of blood from the right side of the heart toward the lungs. The resulting capillary wedge pressure is equal to the mean left atrial pressure.
6. The pressure is recorded with the balloon wedged in the pulmonary vascular bed. A mean capillary wedge pressure between 14 and 18 mm Hg appears to indicate optimal left ventricular function.	6. Wedge pressure reading provides information about the level of pulmonary congestion and is closely related to left atrial pressure and to left ventricular end-diastolic pressure (in the absence of mitral valve disease). This is a valuable measure of cardiac function. Filling pressures less than 8 to 10 mm Hg in an acutely injured heart are often associated with reduction in cardiac output, hypotension, and tachycardia. A pressure greater than 18 mm Hg indicates pulmonary congestion.
7. The balloon is deflated, causing the catheter to retract spontaneously into a larger pulmonary artery. This gives a continuous pulmonary artery systolic, diastolic, and mean pressure.	7. The normal systolic pulmonary range is 15 to 25 mm Hg, and the diastolic pulmonary pressure range is 8 to 12 mm Hg. The normal mean pulmonary artery pressure (average pressure in pulmonary artery throughout the entire cardiac cycle) ranges from 10 to 20 mm Hg.

(continued)

Chart 29-4 (Continued)

Nursing Action	Rationale/Amplification
Performance Phase (by the Physician)	
8. The catheter is sutured in place.	8. An antibiotic ointment may be placed around the site and covered with a sterile dressing.
9. The patency of the catheter is maintained with low-flow continuous irrigation.	9. A chest x-ray to confirm catheter position and as a baseline for future reference is obtained after Swan-Ganz catheter insertion.
To Obtain a Wedge Pressure Reading	
1. Close off the microdrip.	1. The transducer converts the pressure wave into an electronic wave that is displayed on a screen.
2. Inflate the balloon slowly until the contour of the pulmonary arterial pressure changes to that of pulmonary wedge pressure. As soon as a wedge pattern is observed, no more air is introduced. Do not introduce more air into balloon than specified.	2. *Caution: Do not allow catheter to remain in the wedge position when patient is unattended or when not directly making the measurement. Segmental lung infarction may occur if the catheter balloon is left inflated for long periods.*
3. Deflate the balloon as soon as the pressure reading is obtained.	
To Obtain a Central Venous Pressure Reading	
1. Turn the stopcock so that the CVP port is connected to the transducer.	1. Confirm the waveform to be that of the right atrium.
2. The pressure recorded is the central venous pressure.	2. Flush the tubing to ensure patency and return the stopcock to the continuous drip position.
Follow-Up Phase	
1. Inspect the insertion site daily. Observe for signs of infection, swelling, and bleeding.	1. A foreign body (catheter) in the vascular system increases the risk of sepsis.
2. Record data and time of dressing change and IV tubing change.	
3. If a peripheral vessel access site is used, assess the extremity for color, temperature, capillary filling, and sensation.	3. Ischemia (with possible loss of digits) may occur from inadequate arterial flow.
4. Evaluate pulse.	
5. Assess for complications: pulmonary embolism, dysrhythmias, heart block, damage to tricuspid valve, intracardiac knotting of catheter, thrombophlebitis, infection, balloon rupture, rupture of pulmonary artery.	
For Removal of the Catheter	
1. Be sure that the balloon is not inflated.	
2. The catheter is removed without excessive force of traction; pressure dressing is applied over the site.	2. This site should be checked periodically for bleeding.

held until the possibility of digitalis toxicity is ruled out (Chart 29-5).

Aminophylline. When the patient is wheezing and bronchospasm appears to play a significant role, aminophylline may be administered to relax bronchospasm.

- Aminophylline is administered by continuous intravenous drip in dosages based on body weight.

Positioning. Proper positioning can help reduce venous return to the heart.

- The patient is positioned upright, with legs and feet down, preferably with legs dangling over the side of the bed. This has the immediate effect of decreasing venous return, lowering the output of the right ventricle, and decreasing lung congestion (*e.g.*, reducing preload).
- If unable to sit with lower extremities dependent, the patient may be placed in an upright position in bed.

Rotating Tourniquets and Phlebotomy. The use of rotating tourniquets to mechanically reduce the volume of blood returning to the heart (preload) was once a first-line treatment for acute pulmonary edema. Tourniquets were applied to three of four extremities securely enough to impede venous return to the heart but not so tightly that they interfered with arterial flow to each extremity. To avoid the hazard of impaired oxygenation to an extremity, the tourniquets were rotated every 15 minutes in a clockwise pattern. The tourniquets were confining and disturbing to patients already struggling to breathe. In addition, the stagnation of blood in the extremities fostered the development of serious thromboembolic sequelae.

In recent years, the development of newer, more efficient pharmacologic agents in tandem with the ability to monitor fluid volume status via a multilumen pulmonary artery catheter (see Chart 29-4) has replaced the use of rotating tourniquets in most settings.

Phlebotomy, the removal of a specified volume of blood

TABLE 29–1.   *Commonly Used Diuretics*

Definition: Diuretics are agents that increase the rate of urine flow.
Action: Dependent on functionally active kidneys; most diuretics decrease the reabsorption of electrolytes (principally sodium) by the kidneys, promoting water loss as a secondary action. In the treatment of hypertension, the natriuretic (sodium excretion) effect is probably the action of importance. In edema states, the salt and water actions are both important.
Special Precaution: Some diuretics may produce electrolyte depletion, including potassium loss, which causes weakness and induces cardiac dysrhythmias. Vigorous diuresis can produce hypovolemia.
Dosage Determination: (1) Patient's daily weight; (2) clinical signs and symptoms; (3) state of renal function

Diuretic	Action	Nursing Implications
THIAZIDES AND RELATED DRUGS		
Chlorothiazide (Diuril) Hydrochlorothiazide (HydroDIURIL, Esidrix, Oretic) Methyclothiazide (Enduron) Polythiazide (Renese) Chlorthalidone (Hygroton) Quinethazone (Hydromox)	Increases renal excretion of sodium (natriuresis), potassium, chloride, bicarbonate (alkaline urine), with accompanying "osmotic" water loss Used principally in states of edema and hypertension Most widely used for prolonged administration	Monitor for electrolyte depletion: hyponatremia, hypokalemia, hypochloremic alkalosis Observe for signs and symptoms of electrolyte imbalance, dizziness, lightheadedness. Adverse reactions may occur, manifested by gastrointestinal, central nervous system, hematologic, and cardiovascular signs and symptoms. Supplementary potassium is usually prescribed with these diuretics.
POTASSIUM-SPARING DIURETICS		
Spironolactone (Aldactone)	Inhibits action of aldosterone in distal tubule and reduces reabsorption of sodium and chloride Gives gradual diuretic effect Used in treatment of cirrhosis and edema when other diuretics are toxic or ineffective	Monitor for electrolyte depletion. Usually used in combination with thiazide diuretic Observe for side effects—skin rash, gynecomastia.
Triamterene (Dyrenium)	Inhibits reabsorption of sodium ions in exchange for potassium and hydrogen ions in distal tubule	Usually used as an adjunct to thiazide therapy May cause elevation in blood uric acid Observe for nausea, vomiting, diarrhea, weakness, headache, and skin rash.
POTENT DIURETICS		
Furosemide (Lasix) Ethacrynic Acid (Edecrin)	Usually reserved for patients who do not respond to classical thiazide diuretics Blocks the reabsorption of sodium and water in proximal renal tubule and interferes with reabsorption of sodium in ascending limb of loop of Henle and in the most proximal portion of the distal tubule Associated with sodium, potassium, chloride, and hydrogen ion loss (acid urine) Has an almost immediate action (within 5 minutes) when given IV	Monitor for electrolyte depletion: may produce *profound diuresis* with hyponatremia, hypokalemia, hypochloremic alkalosis, and circulatory collapse. Potent and rapid acting Especially useful in acute pulmonary edema Observe for nausea, vomiting, diarrhea, skin rash, pruritus, blurring of vision, postural hypotension, vertigo, hearing loss. Furosemide is chemically related to sulfonamides; consider cross-allergies. Administer early in the day to avoid nocturia and consequent loss of sleep. Some patients may benefit from taking diuretics at bedtime to avoid paroxysmal nocturnal dyspnea.

for therapeutic reasons, was once used in severe cases of pulmonary edema. Although phlebotomy is a therapeutic technique for some hematologic conditions (*e.g.,* polycythemia vera), it is no longer an accepted standard of treatment for pulmonary edema.

Psychological Support.   Extreme fear and anxiety are car-

dinal features of pulmonary edema. These emotions, which are self-perpetuating, make the condition more severe. Reassuring the patient and providing skillful anticipatory nursing care are integral parts of the therapy. Because this patient experiences a sense of impending doom, it is essential that the nurse stay close. Touching the patient offers a sense of concrete

Chart 29-5
Digitalis and Cardiac Glycoside Preparations

Actions of Digitalis

Increases force of myocardial contractions
- Increases cardiac output by enhancing force of contraction of ventricle
- Slows heart rate
- Decreases heart size
- Decreases venous pressure
- Promotes diuresis
- Slows the ventricular rate in the setting of supraventricular dysrhythmias

Clinical Uses

- Congestive heart failure
- Atrial fibrillation; atrial flutter
- Supraventricular tachydysrhythmias
- Before cardiac surgery

Preparations

The choice of drug depends on the speed of onset desired, duration of action required, and individual patient response. The recommended dosage varies considerably.

Oral	Parenteral
Digitalis	Ouabain
Digoxin (Lanoxin)	Digoxin (Lanoxin)

Nursing Considerations and Actions

Special Precautions: The incidence of digitalis toxicity is high. Toxic effects do not always appear in a predictable manner.
- Monitor for toxic effects: dysrhythmias (most important toxic effect), anorexia, nausea, vomiting, bradycardia, headache, malaise.
- Assess clinical response of patient by relief of symptoms (dyspnea, orthopnea, crackles, hepatomegaly, peripheral edema).
- Elderly patients may tolerate digitalis therapy poorly; assess for bradycardia, impaired renal function.
- Monitor serum potassium levels in patients receiving digitalis, especially those receiving both digitalis and diuretics. There is a predisposition to dysrhythmias if a potassium imbalance is not detected and corrected.
- Assess for symptoms of electrolyte depletion in patients taking digitalis: lassitude, apathy, mental confusion, anorexia, decreasing urinary output, azotemia.
- The following factors may increase sensitivity to digitalis: myocardial infarction, myocarditis, potassium depletion, kidney or hepatic disease, diuretic therapy, diarrhea, loss of appetite, advancing age, hypoxia and hypercapnia in pulmonary disease, acidosis, alkalosis.
- Check apical rate before each dose. A rate of 60 or above with no dysrhythmias is desirable. Check with the physician regarding specific guidelines for each individual patient.

---

reality. Nursing care should be organized to maximize the nurse's presence at the bedside. The patient is given frequent simple, concise information about what is being done to treat the condition and what his responses to the treatment mean.

Prevention

Like most complications, pulmonary edema is easier to prevent than to treat. To recognize it in its early stages, when the presenting signs and symptoms are solely those of pulmonary congestion, the nurse auscultates the lung fields of patients with cardiac disease each day. A dry, hacking cough and the presence of a third heart sound (S_3) are often the earliest indicators of pulmonary congestion. The S_3 is best heard at the apex with the patient lying in the left lateral decubitus position.

In an early stage, the condition may be corrected by relatively simple measures. These include (1) placing the patient in an upright position with the feet and legs dependent, (2) eliminating overexertion and emotional stress to reduce the left ventricular load, and (3) administering morphine to reduce anxiety, dyspnea, and preload.

The long-range approach to the prevention of pulmonary edema must be directed at its precursor, pulmonary congestion. Measures to prevent congestive heart failure and the various facets of patient teaching are discussed in the next section.

In addition to these measures, the patient is advised to sleep with the head of the bed elevated on 25-cm (10-inch) blocks. It is especially important to use extreme caution when administering infusions and transfusions to cardiac patients and elderly persons.

- To prevent circulatory overload, which could precipitate acute pulmonary edema, intravenous fluids are administered at a slower rate, with the patient positioned upright in bed and under close nursing surveillance.
- Intravenous control devices are used to restrict the volume of fluid that can be delivered.

Surgical treatment may be necessary to eliminate or to minimize valvular defects that limit the flow of blood into or out of the left ventricle, because such defects impair the cardiac output and predispose the patient to the development of pulmonary congestion and edema.

Cardiac Failure
Definition, Etiology, and Pathophysiology

Cardiac failure, often referred to as congestive heart failure, is the inability of the heart to pump sufficient blood to meet the needs of the tissues for oxygen and nutrients. The term *congestive heart failure* is most commonly used when referring to left-sided and right-sided failure.

The underlying mechanism of cardiac failure involves impairment of the contractile properties of the heart, which leads to a lower-than-normal cardiac output. The concept of cardiac output is best explained by the equation $CO = HR \times SV$, where cardiac output (CO) is a function of heart rate (HR) times stroke volume (SV).

Heart rate is a function of the autonomic nervous system. When cardiac output falls, the sympathetic nervous system accelerates the heart rate to maintain adequate cardiac output. When this compensatory mechanism fails to maintain adequate tissue perfusion, the properties of stroke volume must adjust to maintain cardiac output.

However, in cardiac failure in which the primary problem is damaged and inhibited myocardial muscle fibers, stroke volume is impaired and normal cardiac output cannot be maintained. *Stroke volume*, the amount of blood pumped with each contraction, is dependent on three factors: preload, contractility, and afterload.

Preload is synonymous with Starling's Law of the Heart, in which the amount of blood filling the heart is directly proportional to pressure created by the length of the stretch of the myocardial fibers. *Contractility* refers to an alteration in the force of contraction that occurs at the cellular level and is related to changes in myocardial fiber length. *Afterload* refers to the amount of pressure the ventricle must create to pump blood across the pressure gradient created by the semilunar valves. In cardiac failure, any one or more of these three factors may be altered such that cardiac output is impaired. The relative ease of determining hemodynamic measurements through invasive monitoring procedures has greatly facilitated differential diagnosis and pharmacologic manipulation of the problem.

Cardiac failure most commonly occurs with disorders of cardiac muscle that result in decreased contractile properties of the heart. Common underlying conditions that lead to disordered muscle function include coronary atherosclerosis, arterial hypertension, and inflammatory or degenerative muscle disease.

Coronary atherosclerosis leads to myocardial dysfunction by interfering with the normal supply of blood to cardiac muscle. Hypoxia and acidosis (due to accumulation of lactic acid) result. Myocardial infarction (death of myocardial cells) frequently precedes the development of overt cardiac failure.

Systemic or pulmonary hypertension (increased afterload) increases the work requirement of the heart, and this in turn leads to hypertrophy of myocardial muscle fibers. This effect (*i.e.*, myocardial hypertrophy) can be considered a compensatory mechanism because it increases the contractility of the heart. For reasons that are not clear, however, the hypertrophied cardiac muscle does not function normally, and cardiac failure may eventually result.

Cardiac failure associated with inflammatory and degenerative diseases of the myocardium is due to direct damage to myocardial fibers, with a resultant decrease in contractility.

Cardiac failure may occur as a result of heart disease that only secondarily affects the myocardium. The mechanisms involved include impediment to flow of blood through the heart (*e.g.*, stenosis of a semilunar valve), inability of the heart to fill with blood (*e.g.*, pericardial tamponade, constrictive pericarditis, or stenosis of AV valves), or abnormal emptying of the heart (*e.g.*, insufficiency of AV valves). Sudden increase in afterload due to elevated systemic blood pressure ("malignant" hypertension) may result in cardiac failure in the absence of myocardial hypertrophy.

A number of systemic factors can contribute to the development and severity of cardiac failure. Increased metabolic rate (*e.g.*, fever, thyrotoxicosis), hypoxia, and anemia require an increased cardiac output to satisfy systemic oxygen demand. Hypoxia or anemia also may decrease the supply of oxygen to the myocardium. Acidosis (respiratory or metabolic) and electrolyte abnormalities may decrease myocardial contractility. Cardiac dysrhythmias, which may be present independently or secondary to cardiac failure, decrease the overall efficiency of myocardial function.

Clinical Manifestations

The dominant feature in cardiac failure is increased intravascular volume. Congestion of tissues results from increased arterial and venous pressures due to decreased cardiac output in the failing heart. Increased pulmonary venous pressure can lead to passage of fluid from pulmonary capillaries to the alveoli (pulmonary edema), manifested by cough and shortness of breath. Increased systemic venous pressure can result in generalized peripheral edema and weight gain.

The diminished cardiac output of cardiac failure has widespread manifestations because of diminished tissue and end-organ perfusion. Some commonly encountered effects related to low perfusion are dizziness, confusion, fatigue, exercise or heat intolerance, cool extremities, and oliguria. Renal perfusion pressure falls, which results in the release of renin from the kidney, which in turn leads to aldosterone secretion, sodium and fluid retention, and increased intravascular volume.

Left- and Right-Sided Cardiac Failure. The left and right ventricles can fail separately. Left ventricular failure most often precedes right ventricular failure. Pure left ventricular failure is synonymous with acute pulmonary edema. Because the outputs of the ventricles are coupled, failure of either ventricle may lead to decreased tissue perfusion. The congestive manifestations, however, may differ according to whether left or right ventricular failure exists.

Left-Sided Cardiac Failure. Pulmonary congestion predominates when the left ventricle fails, because the left ventricle is unable to adequately pump the blood coming to it from the lungs. The increased pressure in the pulmonary circulation causes fluid to be forced into the pulmonary tissues. The clinical manifestations that ensue include dyspnea, cough, fatigability, tachycardia with an S_3 heart sound, and anxiety and restlessness.

Dyspnea results from the accumulation of fluid in the alveoli, which impairs gas exchange. Dyspnea may occur even at rest or may be precipitated by minimal to moderate exertion. *Orthopnea*, difficulty in breathing when lying flat, may be present. The patient who experiences orthopnea will not lie flat, but instead will use pillows to prop himself up in bed or will sit in a chair, even to sleep. Some patients experience orthopnea only at night, a condition known as *paroxysmal nocturnal dyspnea* (PND). This occurs when the patient, who has been sitting for a long period with his feet and legs in a dependent position, returns to bed. After several hours the fluid that accumulated in the dependent extremities begins to be reabsorbed, and the impaired left ventricle is unable to adequately empty the increased volume. As a result, the pressure in the pulmonary circulation increases and causes further shifting of fluid into the alveoli.

The cough associated with left ventricular failure may be dry and nonproductive, but is most often moist. Large quantities of frothy sputum, which is sometimes blood-tinged, may be produced.

Fatigability results from the low cardiac output that deprives tissues of normal circulation and decreases the removal of catabolic waste products. It is also a result of the increased energy expended for breathing and the insomnia that results from respiratory distress and coughing.

Restlessness and anxiety result from the impaired oxygenation of tissues, the stress associated with respiratory difficulty, and the knowledge that the heart is not functioning properly. As anxiety increases, so does dyspnea, which in turn further enhances the anxiety, creating a vicious cycle.

Right-Sided Cardiac Failure. When the right ventricle fails, congestion of the viscera and the peripheral tissues predominates. This is because the right side of the heart is unable to adequately empty its blood volume and thus cannot accommodate all of the blood that normally returns to it from the venous circulation. The clinical manifestations that ensue include edema of the lower extremities (dependent edema), which is usually pitting edema, weight gain, hepatomegaly, distended neck veins, ascites, anorexia and nausea, nocturia, and weakness.

The dependent edema begins in the feet and ankles and can gradually progress up the legs and thighs and eventually into the external genitalia and lower trunk. Sacral edema is not uncommon for patients who are on bed rest, as the sacral area is dependent. *Pitting edema*, edema in which pits remain after even slight compression with the fingertips, is obvious only after retention of at least 4.5 kg (10 lb) of fluid.

Venous engorgement of the liver leads to hepatomegaly and tenderness in the right upper abdominal quadrant. As this process progresses, pressure within the portal vessels can become great enough to cause fluid to be forced into the abdominal cavity, a condition known as *ascites*. This collection of fluid in the abdominal cavity can cause pressure on the diaphragm and respiratory distress. Anorexia and nausea result from the venous engorgement and venous stasis within the abdominal organs.

Nocturia occurs because renal perfusion is promoted by periods of recumbency. Diuresis results, and is most common at night because cardiac output is improved with physical rest. The weakness that accompanies right-sided failure is due to the reduced cardiac output, impaired circulation, and inadequate removal of catabolic waste products from the tissues.

Diagnostic Evaluation

The diagnosis is made by evaluation of the clinical manifestations of pulmonary and systemic congestion. Of special importance in the determination of effective stroke volume is the use of the pulmonary artery catheter. This catheter may be inserted at the bedside. The catheter's technology has expanded to include a multilumen apparatus that allows for the measurement of more than one hemodynamic parameter via a single catheter. The catheter enters the right atrium through the superior vena cava. A balloon then is inflated, allowing the catheter to follow the blood flow through the tricuspid valve, through the right ventricle, through the pulmonic valve, and into the main pulmonary artery. Waveform and pressure readings are noted during insertion to identify location of the catheter within the heart. The balloon is deflated once the

catheter is in the pulmonary artery and properly secured (Fig. 29–21).

Actual measurements of preload, afterload, and cardiac output can be obtained. There are ports at various intervals along the catheter. One port lies at the level of the right atrium. Because preload is the amount of venous return to the heart and is therefore equal to the central venous pressure measurement, measuring the pressure at the proximal port yields an accurate preload and hence central venous pressure (CVP) measurement. The tip of the catheter rests in the pulmonary artery where left ventricular pressure measurements are made. The balloon is inflated and flows into a small pulmonary capillary, occluding or wedging the capillary. A pressure measurement is made that is the left ventricular end-diastolic pressure or afterload, the resistance against which the left ventricle must pump. Cardiac output is measured with a thermodilution lumen connected to a computer.

Measurements of the various pressures are made at intervals prescribed by the physician, and medication therapy is adjusted based on the readings.

The nursing management of the patient who has a hemodynamic catheter is highly specialized and is ideally conducted in an intensive care environment. The guidelines for managing a patient with a hemodynamic catheter are summarized in Chart 29–4.

Medical Management

The basic objectives in the treatment of patients with cardiac failure are the following:

1. To promote rest to reduce the workload on the heart
2. To increase the force and efficiency of myocardial contraction through the action of pharmacologic agents
3. To eliminate the excessive accumulation of body water by means of diuretic therapy, diet, and rest

Pharmacologic Therapy

Cardiac glycosides, diuretics, and vasodilators form the basis of the pharmacologic treatment of cardiac failure. Chart 29–5 summarizes the major cardiac glycosides, along with their actions and the nursing surveillance required when these medications are administered.

Digitalis. Digitalis increases the force of myocardial contraction and slows the heart rate. Several effects are produced: an increase in cardiac output; a decrease in venous pressure and blood volume; and an increase in diuresis, which relieves edema. The effect of a given dose of digitalis depends on the state of the myocardium, electrolyte and fluid balance, and renal and hepatic function.

A loading dose of digitalis may be administered to induce the full therapeutic effect of the drug. This is usually administered in the treatment of more severe forms of cardiac failure. Otherwise, the digitalis is started without a loading dose. A maintenance dose is administered and continued daily. In either case, the patient is observed closely and given a daily dose just adequate to replace the amount of drug that is metabolized or excreted, to maintain the digitalis effect without producing toxicity. The optimal dosage is the amount that relieves the patient's signs and symptoms of cardiac failure or slows the ventricular response therapeutically *without causing toxicity*. The patient is observed closely for relief of signs and symptoms:

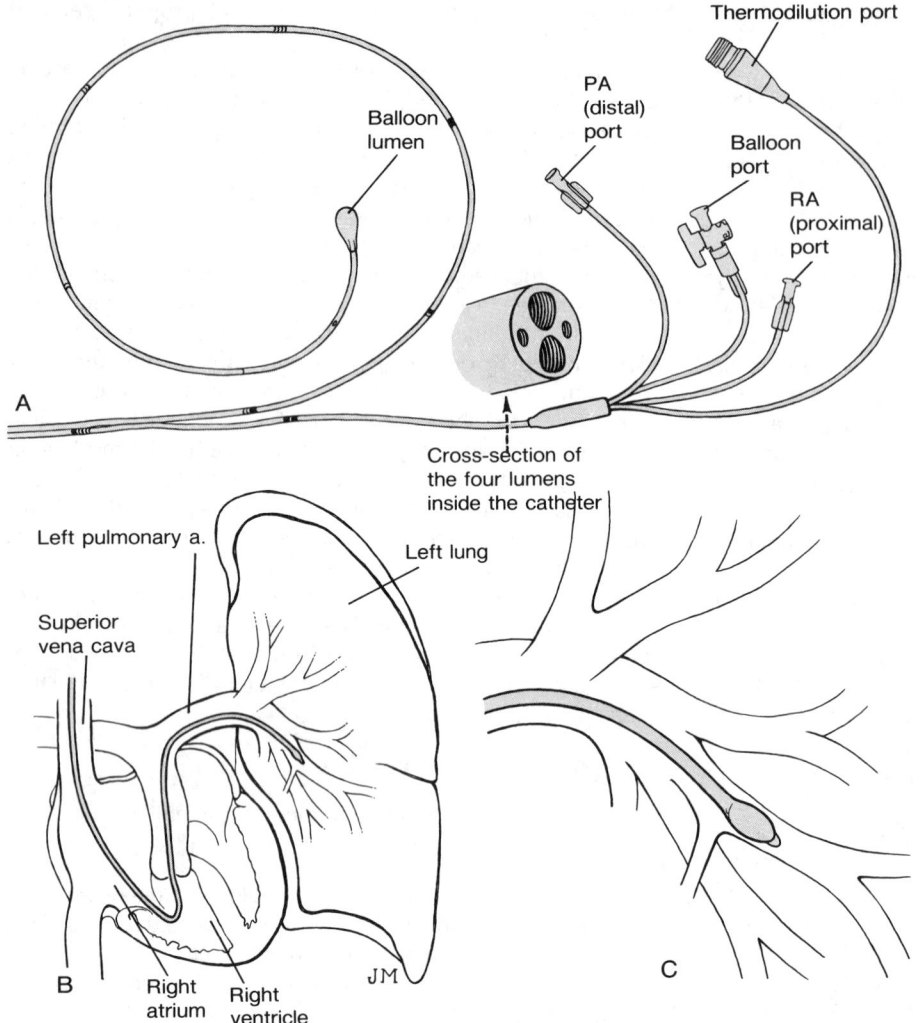

Figure 29–21. (**A**) The multilumen pulmonary artery catheter. (**B**) Location of the catheter within the heart. The catheter enters the right atrium via the superior vena cava. The balloon is then inflated, allowing the catheter to follow the blood flow through the tricuspid valve, through the right ventricle, through the pulmonic valve, and into the main pulmonary artery. Waveform and pressure readings are noted during insertion to identify location of the catheter within the heart. The balloon is deflated once the catheter is in the pulmonary artery and properly secured. (**C**) Pulmonary capillary wedge pressure (PWP). The catheter floats into a distal branch of the pulmonary artery when the balloon is inflated, and becomes "wedged." The wedged catheter occludes blood flow from behind, and the tip of the lumen records pressures in front of the catheter. The balloon is then deflated, allowing the catheter to float back into the main pulmonary artery. (Suddarth DS. The Lippincott Manual of Nursing Practice, 5th ed. Philadelphia, JB Lippincott, 1991.)

lessening dyspnea and orthopnea, decrease in crackles, and relief of peripheral edema.

Digitalis Toxicity.   Anorexia, nausea, and vomiting are early effects of digitalis toxicity. There may be alterations in the heart rhythm, bradycardia, premature ventricular contractions, ventricular bigeminy (coupling of normal and premature beat), and paroxysmal atrial tachycardia.

- The apical heart rate is taken before digitalis is administered. If there is excessive slowing of the heart rate or change in rhythm, the drug is withheld and the physician is notified. Frequently the physician withholds the digitalis preparation if the rate is 60 or less.
- If prescribed, the serum digitalis level is checked before administration of the drug.

Diuretic Therapy.   Diuretics are prescribed to promote the excretion of sodium and water through the kidneys. These medications may not be necessary if the patient responds to restricted activity, digitalis, and a low-sodium diet.

- When diuretics are prescribed they should be administered early in the morning so that the resultant diuresis does not interfere with the patient's nighttime rest.
- An intake and output record is kept, because the patient may lose a large volume of fluid after a single dose of a diuretic.

- As a basis for evaluating the effectiveness of therapy, a patient receiving diuretic medications is weighed daily at the same time. In addition, skin turgor is examined for evidences of edema or dehydration. The pulse rate is also monitored.

The dosage schedule is determined by the patient's daily weight, physical findings, and symptoms. Table 29–1 summarizes the diuretics in common use. Furosemide (Lasix) is a particularly useful diuretic in the treatment of heart failure because it dilates the venules, thereby increasing venous capacitance, which in turn reduces preload (venous return to the heart).

Diuretic Side Effects.   Prolonged diuretic therapy may produce *hyponatremia* (deficiency of sodium in the blood), which results in apprehension, weakness, fatigue, malaise, muscle cramps and twitching, and rapid, thready pulse.

Profuse and repeated diuresis can also lead to *hypokalemia* (potassium depletion). Signs are weak pulse, faint heart sounds, hypotension, muscle flabbiness, diminished tendon reflexes, and generalized weakness. Hypokalemia poses new problems for the cardiac patient, because among the complications of hypokalemia are marked weakening of cardiac contractions and the precipitation of digitalis toxicity in persons receiving digitalis, both of which increase the likelihood of dangerous dysrhythmias.

- Periodic assessment of the electrolytes will alert health team members to hypokalemia and hyponatremia.
- To lessen the risk of hypokalemia and its attendant complications, patients receiving diuretic medications may be given a potassium supplement (potassium chloride). Bananas, orange juice, dried prunes, raisins, apricots, dates, figs, peaches, and spinach are good dietary sources of potassium.

Other problems associated with diuretic administration are hyperuricemia, volume depletion, and hyperglycemia.

The elderly male patient requires ongoing nursing surveillance because the incidence of urethral obstruction due to prostatic hypertrophy is high in this age group. Signs of bladder distention should be observed for regularly by palpation over the bladder.

Vasodilator Therapy. Of particular significance in the management of cardiac failure are the vasoactive medications.

Vasodilator medications have been used to reduce impedance (resistance) to left ventricular ejection of blood. The drug action allows more complete ventricular emptying and increases venous capacity, so left ventricular filling pressure is reduced and a dramatic decrease in pulmonary congestion may be achieved rapidly.

Sodium nitroprusside may be given intravenously by means of carefully monitored infusions. The dosage is titrated to keep the arterial systolic pressure at the prescribed level, and the patient is monitored by measuring pulmonary artery pressures and cardiac output. Another commonly used vasodilator medication is nitroglycerin.

Providing Dietary Support

The rationale for dietary support is to provide a diet that will cause the heart the least possible work effort and muscular strain and maintain good nutritional status, taking into consideration the patient's likes, dislikes, and cultural food patterns.

Sodium Ion Manipulation. Restriction of sodium is indicated for the prevention, control, or elimination of edema, as in hypertension or cardiac failure. Sodium should be specified in describing the regimen rather than "low-salt" or "salt-free," and the quantity should be indicated in milligrams. Very often mistakes are made because of inconsistencies in the translation of salt to sodium. It is important to realize that salt is not 100% sodium. There are 393 mg, or approximately 400 mg, of sodium in 1 g (1000 mg) of salt.

Although the major source of sodium in the average American diet is salt, many types of natural foods contain varying amounts of sodium. Therefore, even if no salt is added in cooking and if salty foods are avoided, the daily diet may still contain approximately 1000 to 2000 mg of sodium.

Other sources of sodium can be found in some processed foods. Added food substances—such as sodium alginate, which improves texture; sodium benzoate, which acts as a preservative; or disodium phosphate, which improves cooking quality in certain foods—increase the sodium intake when included in the daily diet. Therefore, patients on low-sodium diets should be advised not to buy processed foods and to check labels carefully for such words as "salt" or "sodium," especially on canned foods. For diets that call for less than 1000 mg of sodium, low-sodium milk and bread and salt-free butter should be considered.

Patients on sodium-restricted diets also should be cautioned against using nonprescription medications, such as alkalizers, cough syrups, laxatives, sedatives, or salt substitutes,

because these products contain sodium or excessive amounts of potassium. Any over-the-counter medication of this type should not be purchased without first consulting the physician.

When diets are very restricted in both fat and sodium content, the patient may find the food unpalatable and may refuse to eat. A variety of flavorings such as lemon juice and herb seasonings may be used to improve the taste of the food and encourage the patient to accept the diet. Every effort should be made to take into account the patient's food preferences.

▶ Nursing Process
The Patient With Cardiac Failure

◇ Assessment

The focus of the nursing assessment for the patient with cardiac failure is directed toward observing for signs and symptoms of pulmonary and systemic fluid overload. All untoward signs are recorded and reported to the physician.

Respiratory. The lungs are auscultated at frequent intervals to determine the presence or absence of crackles and wheezes. Crackles are produced by the movement of air through fluid, and therefore, if present, are evidence that pulmonary congestion is developing. The rate and depth of respirations are also noted.

Cardiac. The heart is auscultated for the presence of an S_3 or S_4 heart sound. The presence of these signs may mean that the pump is beginning to fail and that there is increased blood volume remaining in the ventricle with each beat. The rate and rhythm are also noted. Rapid rates indicate that the ventricle has had less time to fill and there is therefore some stagnation of blood in the atria and eventually the pulmonary bed.

Sensorium/Level of Consciousness. As the intravascular volume increases, the circulating blood becomes dilute and its oxygen transport capacity is compromised. The brain tolerates inadequate oxygenation poorly, and the patient becomes confused.

Periphery. The dependent parts of the patient's body are assessed for edema. If the patient is sitting upright, the feet and lower legs are examined; if the patient is supine in bed, the sacrum and back are assessed for edema. Fingers and hands may also become edematous. In extreme cases of cardiac failure the patient may develop periorbital edema, in which the eyelids may be swollen shut.

The liver is examined for hepatojugular reflux (HJR). The patient is asked to breathe normally while manual pressure is applied over the liver for 30 to 60 seconds. If neck vein distention increases more than 1 cm, the test is positive for increased venous pressure.

Jugular vein distention (JVD) is assessed. This is performed by elevating the patient to a 45-degree angle. The distance between the angle of Louis and the level of jugular vein distension is estimated. (The *angle of Louis* is the junction between the body of the sternum and the manubrium.) A distance greater than 3 cm is said to be normal. Remember that this is an estimate and not an exact measurement.

Urinary Output. The patient may become oliguric or anuric. It is important to measure output frequently to develop a baseline to measure against in testing the efficacy of diuretic therapy. Intake and output records are rigorously maintained and the patient is weighed daily, at the same time and on the same scales.

▷ Nursing Diagnoses

Based on the assessment data, major nursing diagnoses for the patient may include the following:

- Activity intolerance related to fatigue and dyspnea secondary to decreased cardiac output
- Anxiety related to breathlessness and restlessness secondary to inadequate oxygenation
- Altered peripheral tissue perfusion related to venous stasis
- Potential knowledge deficit of self-care program related to nonacceptance of necessary life style changes

▷ Planning and Implementation

▷ *Goals:* The major goals of the patient may include promotion of rest, relief of anxiety, attainment of normal tissue perfusion, and knowledge of self-care program.

▷ Nursing Interventions

▷ *Promotion of Rest.* It is essential that the patient have both physical and emotional rest. Rest reduces the work of the heart, increases cardiac reserve, and reduces blood pressure. Periods of recumbency also promote diuresis by improving renal perfusion. Rest also decreases the work of the respiratory muscles and oxygen utilization. The heart rate is slowed, which prolongs the diastolic period of recovery and thus improves the efficiency of heart contraction.

▷ *Positioning.* The head of the bed may be elevated on 20- to 30-cm (8- to 10-in) blocks or the patient may be placed in a comfortable armchair. In this position the venous return to the heart (preload) and the lungs is reduced, pulmonary congestion is alleviated, and impingement of the liver on the diaphragm is minimized. The lower arms should be supported with pillows to eliminate the fatigue caused by the constant pull of their weight on the shoulder muscles. The orthopneic patient may sit on the side of the bed with feet supported on a chair, the head and arms resting on an over-the-bed table, and lumbosacral spine supported by a pillow. If pulmonary congestion is present, positioning the patient in an armchair is advantageous because this position favors the shift of fluid away from the lungs. Edema, which usually occurs in dependent parts of the body, shifts from the extremities to the sacral areas when the patient is confined to bed.

▷ *Relief of Anxiety.* Because of their inability to maintain adequate oxygenation, patients in cardiac failure are likely to be restless and anxious and feel overwhelmed by breathlessness. These symptoms tend to become exaggerated at night.

Raising the head of the bed and keeping a night light on are often helpful. The presence of a member of the family provides necessary reassurance to some persons. Oxygen may be administered during the acute stage to diminish the work of breathing and to increase the comfort of the patient. Small doses of morphine may be prescribed for extreme dyspnea, and chloral hydrate may be given as needed for sleep.

- The patient with hepatic congestion is unable to detoxify drugs with normal rapidity, and medications must be administered with caution. As a result of cerebral hypoxia with superim-

posed nitrogen retention, the patient may react unfavorably to sedative and hypnotic drugs, becoming confused and increasingly anxious in response to medication. Such a patient is restrained with caution; restraints are likely to be resisted, and resistance inevitably increases the cardiac load.

The patient who insists on getting out of bed at night can be seated comfortably in an armchair. As cerebral and systemic circulations improve, the quality of sleep will improve.

▷ *Avoiding Stress.* Rest is not possible in a highly anxious patient. Emotional stress produces vasoconstriction, elevates arterial pressure, and speeds the heart. Promoting physical comfort and avoiding situations that tend to promote anxiety and agitation may help the patient to relax. Rest is continued for a few days to a few weeks until the cardiac failure is controlled.

▷ *Attainment of Normal Tissue Perfusion.* The decreased tissue perfusion occurring in cardiac failure results from inadequate levels of circulating oxygen and stagnation of blood in the peripheral tissues. Moderate daily exercise will enhance the blood flow to peripheral tissues. Adequate oxygenation and appropriate diuresis will serve also to provide good tissue perfusion. Effective diuresis reduces hemodilution, thus providing more oxygen-carrying capacity to the vascular system.

Adequate rest is essential to the promotion of adequate tissue perfusion.

- There are dangers inherent in bed rest, such as pressure ulcers (especially in edematous patients), phlebothrombosis, and pulmonary embolism. Changes of position, deep breathing, elastic stockings, and leg exercises all help to improve muscle tone and at the same time aid venous return to the heart.

▷ *Knowledge About Self-Care.* The self-care program is prepared in cooperation with the patient and significant other (Chart 29–6). Activities of daily living should be planned to minimize breathlessness and fatigue. The patient should remember that intolerable breathlessness and fatigue associated with normal activities are reasons to seek medical attention.

▷ *Patient Education.* After cardiac failure is under control, the patient is encouraged to gradually resume the activities he was accustomed to before illness. The patient's earlier life style should be retained if possible. Some modifications in his habits, work, and interpersonal relationships usually have to be made. Any activity that produces symptoms must be curtailed or other adaptations made. The patient should be helped to identify his emotional stresses and to explore ways in which these may be resolved.

All too frequently patients keep returning to the clinic and hospital for recurring episodes of cardiac failure. Not only does this create psychological, sociologic, and financial problems, but the physiologic burden on the patient can be serious. Previously normal organs of the body may ultimately be damaged. Repeated attacks can lead to pulmonary fibrosis, liver cirrhosis, enlargement of the spleen and kidneys, and even brain damage due to insufficient oxygen during acute episodes.

Patient education, involvement, and cooperation are required to ensure that the patient will comply with his therapeutic regimen. Many of the recurrences of cardiac failure appear to be preventable. These include failure to follow the drug therapy properly, dietary indiscretions, inadequate medical follow-up,

Chart 29-6
Patient Education: Cardiac Failure

A patient with heart disease can learn to regulate his activity according to his individual response.

Goal: To deter progression of disease and the development of cardiac failure

The patient learns that to achieve these goals he will have to do the following:

I. Live within the limits of the cardiac reserve.
   A. Obtain adequate rest.
      1. Have a regular daily rest period.
      2. Shorten working hours if possible.
      3. Avoid emotional upsets.
   B. Accept the fact that taking digitalis and restricting sodium intake may be a permanent way of life.
      1. Take digitalis daily, exactly as prescribed.
         a. Avoid substituting another brand of digitalis for the one prescribed.
         b. Check own pulse rate daily.
         c. Have a check-off system to ensure that medicine(s) has been taken.
      2. Take diuretic as prescribed.
         a. Weigh at the same time daily to detect any tendency toward fluid accumulation.
         b. Report weight gain of more than 0.9 to 1.4 kg (2–3 pounds) in a few days.
         c. Know the signs and symptoms of potassium depletion; if taking oral potassium, keep a check-off system along with diuretic medication.
      3. Take vasodilator as prescribed.
         a. Learn to take own blood pressure at prescribed intervals.
         b. Know signs and symptoms of orthostatic hypotension and how to prevent it.
   C. Restrict sodium as directed.
      1. Consult the written diet plan and the list of permitted and restricted foods.
      2. Examine labels to ascertain sodium content (antacids, laxatives, cough remedies, and the like).
      3. Avoid using salt.
      4. Avoid excesses in eating and drinking.
   D. Review activity program.
      1. Increase walking and other activities gradually, provided that they do not cause fatigue and dyspnea.
      2. In general, continue at whatever activity level can be maintained without the appearance of symptoms.
      3. Avoid extremes of heat and cold, which increase the work of the heart. Air conditioning may be essential in a hot, humid environment.
      4. Keep regular appointments with physician or clinic.
II. Be alert for symptoms that may indicate recurring failure.
   A. Recall the symptoms experienced when illness began. Reappearance of previous symptoms may indicate a recurrence.
   B. Report immediately to the physician or clinic any of the following:
      1. Gain in weight
      2. Loss of appetite
      3. Shortness of breath on activity
      4. Swelling of ankles, feet, or abdomen
      5. Persistent cough
      6. Frequent urination at night

excessive physical activity, and failure to recognize recurring symptoms. A summary of what the patient should know is given in Chart 29–6.

The patient should be assisted to understand that cardiac failure can be controlled. Careful follow-up, maintenance of correct weight, sodium restriction, prevention of infection, avoidance of noxious agents such as coffee and tobacco, and avoidance of unregulated or excessive exercise all aid in preventing the onset of cardiac failure. In patients with valvular heart disease, surgical correction of the defect at the appropriate time may spare the heart and prevent failure.

▷ Evaluation

Expected Outcomes
1. Experiences reduced fatigue and dyspnea
   a. Obtains adequate physical and emotional rest
   b. Assumes positions that reduce fatigue and dyspnea
   c. Adheres to medication regimen
2. Experiences less anxiety
   a. Avoids situations that produce stress
   b. Sleeps comfortably at night
   c. Reports decreased stress and anxiety

3. Attains normal tissue perfusion
   a. Obtains adequate rest
   b. Performs activities that promote venous return: moderate daily exercise; active range of motion of extremities if immobile or in bed for long periods; wearing support stockings
   c. Skin warm and dry with normal color
   d. Exhibits no peripheral edema
4. Adheres to self-care regimen (see Chart 29–6, in which self-care activities are described)

Cardiogenic Shock

Cardiogenic shock (power failure), the end stage of left ventricular dysfunction, occurs when the left ventricle is extensively damaged. The heart muscle loses its contractile power, and the result is a marked reduction in cardiac output with inadequate tissue perfusion to the vital organs (heart, brain, kidneys). The degree of shock is proportional to the level of left ventricular dysfunction. Although cardiogenic shock is seen most commonly as a complication of MI, it also can occur with cardiac tamponade, pulmonary embolism, cardiomyopathy, and dysrhythmias.

Pathophysiology.   The signs and symptoms of cardiogenic shock reflect the circular nature of the pathophysiology of cardiac failure. The damage to the myocardium results in a decrease in cardiac output, which in turn reduces arterial blood pressure in the vital organs. Flow to the coronary arteries is reduced. This results in a decrease in the oxygen supply to the myocardium, which in turn increases ischemia and further reduces the heart's ability to pump. Thus, a vicious cycle is set in motion.

- The classic signs of cardiogenic shock are low blood pressure, rapid and weak pulse, cerebral hypoxia manifested by confusion and agitation, decreased urinary output, and cold, clammy skin.

Dysrhythmias are common and result from a decrease in oxygen to the myocardium. As in cardiac failure, the use of a pulmonary artery catheter to measure left ventricular pressure is important in assessing the severity of the problem and evaluating management. Continuing elevation of left ventricular end-diastolic pressure (LVEDP) accompanied by a fall in arterial blood pressure indicates the failure of the heart to function as an effective pump.

Medical Management.   There are many approaches to the treatment of cardiogenic shock. Any major dysrhythmias are corrected because they may have caused or contributed to the shock. If low intravascular volume is suggested or detected through pressure readings (*i.e.*, hypovolemia), the patient is treated by infusion of volume expanders. If hypoxia is present, oxygen is administered, often under positive pressure when regular flow is insufficient to meet tissue demands.

Medication therapy is selected and guided according to cardiac output and mean arterial blood pressure. One group of medications used is the catecholamines, which raise blood pressure and increase cardiac output. They tend to increase the workload of the heart, however, by increasing oxygen demand. Vasoactive medications such as sodium nitroprusside and nitroglycerin are effective medications that lower blood pressure and thus cardiac work. They cause arterial and venous dilation, thereby shunting much of the intravascular volume to the periphery and causing a reduction in preload and afterload. These vasoactive drugs are usually administered with dopamine, a vasopressor that assists in maintaining an adequate blood pressure.

Other therapeutic modalities employed in treating cardiogenic shock involve the use of circulatory assist devices. The most frequently used mechanical support system is the intra-aortic balloon pump (IABP). The IABP uses internal counterpulsation to augment the pumping action of the heart by the regular inflation and deflation of a balloon located in the descending thoracic aorta (Fig. 29–22). The device is connected to a control box that directs its activities by synchronization with the electrocardiogram. Hemodynamic monitoring is also essential to determine the patient's circulatory status during the use of the IABP. The balloon inflates during ventricular diastole and deflates during systole at a rate equal to the heart rate. The IABP augments diastole, which results in increased perfusion of the coronary arteries and myocardium and a decrease in left ventricular workload.

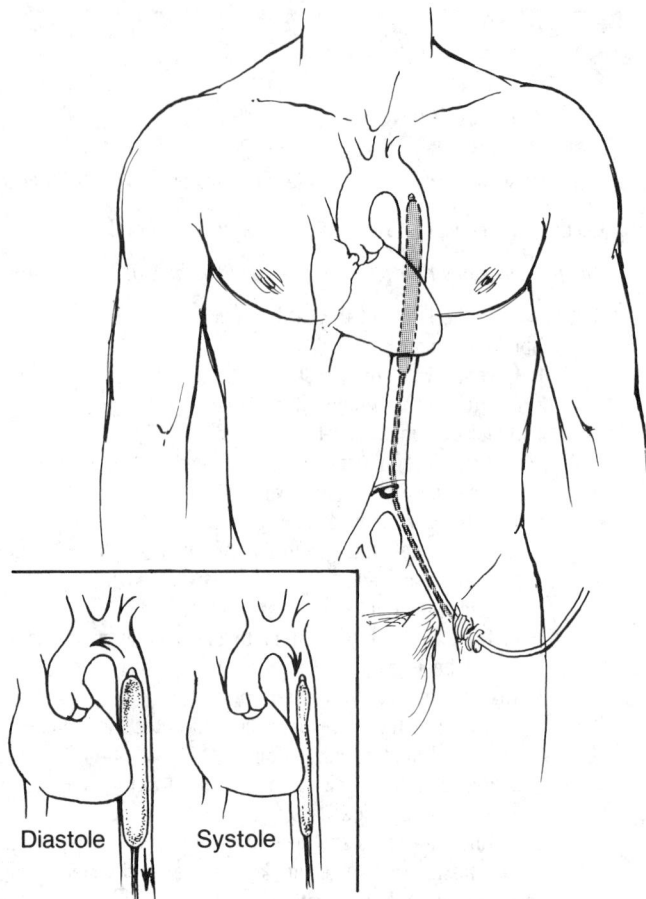

Diastole   Systole

Figure 29–22.   The intra-aortic balloon pump augments diastole, which results in increased perfusion of the coronary arteries and myocardium and a decrease in the left ventricular workload.

Nursing Implications.   The patient with cardiogenic shock requires constant nursing care and observation. Careful patient assessment, measurement of hemodynamic parameters, and recording of fluid intake and urinary output are essential. The patient must be closely monitored for dysrhythmias, which must be corrected immediately.

Because of the technology required for effective medical management in such cases, this patient is always treated in a critical care environment. Critical care nurses with highly developed skills are responsible for the nursing management. Every nurse, however, needs to understand the concepts of treatment modalities.

In summary, cardiac failure is a generic term that includes complications that are generally manifested by fluid volume overload resulting from cardiac decompensation. From pulmonary edema to cardiogenic shock, failure is a leading cause of morbidity and mortality in patients with heart disorders. The severity of symptoms of heart failure is directly proportional to the extent of cardiac muscle damage.

Damaged cardiac muscle impairs cardiac output primarily by disrupting stroke volume. Because stroke volume is a function of preload, afterload, and contractility, medical treatment is directed toward manipulating these parameters to improve cardiac output. Medication therapies are used to improve cardiac contraction and to reduce fluid volume overload.

Acute episodes of cardiac failure may be minimized through patient education. An important role for the nurse in managing the patient with failure is to provide education with regard to medications, diet, and weight control.

When cardiac failure progresses to the devastating state of cardiogenic shock, mortality rates increase significantly.

Thromboembolic Episodes

The decreased mobility of the patient and the impaired circulation that accompany cardiac diseases contribute to the development of intracardiac and intravascular thrombosis. As the patient increases activities, a thrombus may become detached (the detached thrombus is called an *embolus*) and may be carried to the brain, kidneys, intestines, or lungs.

The most common embolic episode is that of a pulmonary embolus. The symptoms of pulmonary embolism include chest pain, cyanosis, shortness of breath, rapid respirations, and hemoptysis. The pulmonary embolus may block the circulation to a part of the lung, producing an area of pulmonary infarction. The pain experienced is usually pleuritic—that is, it increases with respiration and may disappear when the patient holds a breath. Cardiac pain is continuous, however, and usually does not vary with respirations. The treatment of pulmonary embolism is discussed in Chapter 26.

Systemic embolism may occur from the left ventricle, and the resulting vascular occlusion may present as stroke or renal infarction; it may also compromise the blood supply to an extremity. The nurse must be aware of such possible complications and prepared to identify and report signs and symptoms.

Pericardial Effusion

Pathophysiology. Pericardial effusion refers to the escape of fluid into the pericardial sac. This may accompany pericarditis, advanced congestive heart failure, or cardiac surgery.

The characteristic sign of pericardial effusion is an extension of flatness on percussion across the anterior aspect of the chest wall. The patient may complain of a feeling of fullness within the chest or have substernal or ill-defined pain.

Normally, the pericardial sac contains less than 50 ml of fluid. Pericardial fluid may accumulate slowly without causing noticeable symptoms. A *rapidly* developing effusion, however, can stretch the pericardium to its maximum size and can cause decreased cardiac output and decreased venous return to the heart. The result is *cardiac tamponade* (compression of the heart) (Fig. 29–23).

Clinical Manifestations. Symptoms include a feeling of precordial oppression due to the stretching of the pericardial sac, shortness of breath, and a drop and fluctuation in blood pressure. Blood pressure is lowest on inspiration (*pulsus paradoxus*), at which point the pulse may not be perceptible. The venous pressure tends to rise, as evidenced by engorged neck veins.

The cardinal signs are falling arterial blood pressure, narrowing pulse pressure, rising venous pressure, and distant heart

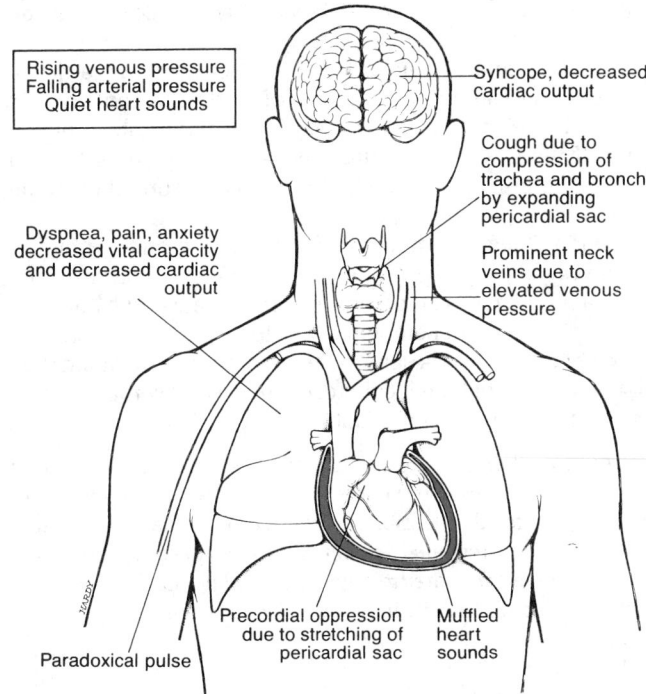

Figure 29–23. Assessment for cardiac tamponade due to pericardial effusion.

sounds. *This is a life-threatening situation, demanding immediate intervention.*

Diagnostic Evaluation. If the clinical manifestations are not immediately life threatening, the physician may choose to confirm the diagnosis by echocardiogram. Bedside assessment based on clinical signs and symptoms is usually diagnostic.

Management: Pericardial Aspiration (Pericardiocentesis). If the cardiac function becomes seriously impaired, a pericardial aspiration (puncture of the pericardial sac) is performed to remove fluid from the pericardial sac. The major goal for it is to prevent cardiac tamponade, which restricts normal heart action.

During the procedure the patient is monitored by ECG, and central venous pressure measurements are monitored. Emergency resuscitative equipment is readily available.

The head of the bed is elevated to a 45- to 60-degree angle, placing the heart in close proximity to the chest wall so that the needle can be inserted into the pericardial sac more easily. If not already in place, a peripheral intravenous device is inserted and a slow intravenous infusion is started in case it becomes necessary to administer emergency medications or blood products.

The pericardial aspiration needle is attached to a 50-ml syringe by a three-way stopcock. The V lead (precordial lead wire) of the ECG may be attached to the hub of the aspirating needle with alligator clips, because the monitoring of ECG oscillation is useful in determining whether or not the needle has contacted the myocardium. Contact is evidenced by an elevation of the ST segment or stimulation of premature ventricular contractions.

There are several possible sites for pericardial aspiration. The needle may be inserted in the angle between the left costal margin and the xiphoid, near the cardiac apex, to the left of the fifth or sixth interspace at the sternal margin, or on the right side of the fourth intercostal space. The needle is advanced slowly until fluid is obtained.

A fall in central venous pressure associated with a rise in blood pressure indicates that relief of cardiac tamponade has occurred. The patient almost always feels immediate improvement. If there is a substantial amount of pericardial fluid, a small catheter may be left in place to drain recurrent bleeding or effusion.

During the procedure, it is important to monitor drainage for the presence of bloody fluid. Pericardial blood does not clot readily, whereas blood obtained from inadvertent puncture of one of the heart chambers does clot.

Pericardial fluid is sent to the laboratory for examination for tumor cells, bacterial culture, chemical and serologic analysis, and differential cell count.

- After pericardiocentesis, care involves careful monitoring of the blood pressure, venous pressure, and heart sounds to evaluate for the possible recurrence of cardiac tamponade. If it recurs, repeated aspiration is necessary. Cardiac tamponade may require treatment by open pericardial drainage. The patient is ideally in an intensive care unit.

Myocardial Rupture

When a myocardial infarction, infectious process, pericardial disease, or other myocardial dysfunction weakens the cardiac muscle, the heart may rupture, leading to immediate death in most cases. Myocardial rupture, although fairly rare, can occur.

Death is caused by cardiac tamponade (the heart is bleeding into its pericardial sac). Pericardiocentesis and repair of the myocardium can be life-saving measures.

Cardiac Arrest

Cardiac arrest is defined as the sudden cessation of the heartbeat and effective circulation. All heart action may stop, or asynchronized muscular twitchings (ventricular fibrillation) may occur.

There is an immediate loss of consciousness and an absence of pulses and audible heart sounds. Dilation of the pupils of the eyes begins within 45 seconds. Convulsions may or may not occur.

- There is an interval of approximately 4 minutes between the cessation of circulation and the development of irreversible brain damage. The interval varies with the age of the patient. During this period, the diagnosis of cardiac arrest must be made and the circulation must be restored.
- *The most reliable sign of arrest is the absence of a carotid pulsation.* Valuable time should not be wasted taking the blood pressure or listening for the heartbeat.

Cardiopulmonary Resuscitation

Basic CPR consists of the following sequence: Airway, Breathing, and Circulation (Fig. 29–24). The resuscitation process consists of maintaining an open airway, providing artificial ventilation by means of rescue breathing, and providing artificial circulation by external cardiac compression.

The first step in CPR is to secure an airway. Any material is removed from the airway and the jaw is lifted forward. An oropharyngeal airway is inserted if available. The patient is ventilated with 12 breaths per minute using the bag and mask technique.

The next step after ventilation is external cardiac compression. This must be performed with the patient on a firm surface. The heel of one hand is placed on the lower half of the sternum, 3.8 cm (1½ in) from the tip of the xiphoid, and toward the patient's head. The other hand is placed on top of the first one. The fingers should not touch the chest wall. Using the body weight while keeping the elbows straight, quick, forceful compressions are applied to the lower sternum, 3.8 cm to 5 cm (1½ to 2 in) toward the spine. Regular compression and release are made 60 times per minute.

When two persons are available, the first person performs the cardiac compressions and the second ventilates the patient after five compressions. If only one person is available, the rate is two ventilations to every 15 cardiac compressions.

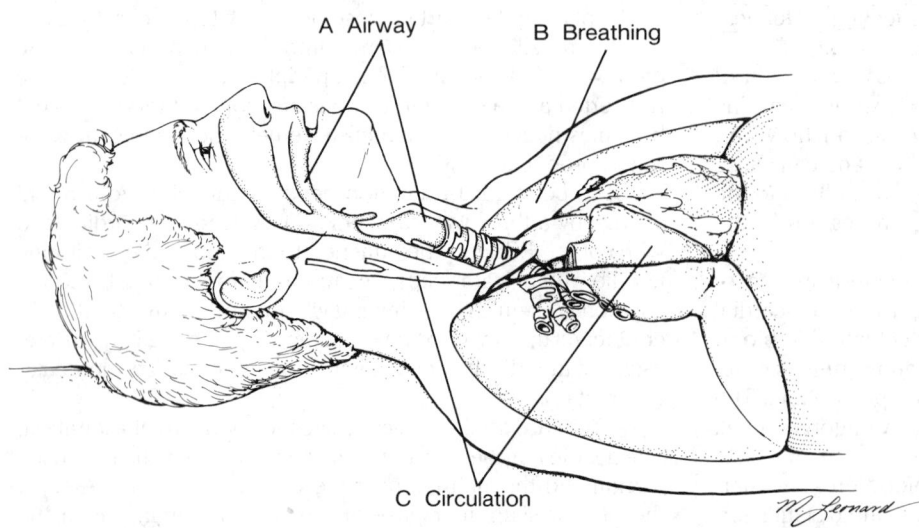

A Airway   B Breathing   C Circulation

Figure 29–24. The ABC's of basic life support.

TABLE 29–2. *Drug Therapy in Cardiopulmonary Resuscitation*

Drug	Objective	Side Effects and Comments
OXYGEN	To correct hypoxemia	No lung damage when used for less than 24 hours
LIDOCAINE	To suppress ventricular dysrhythmias. To raise the threshold for ventricular fibrillation (VF)	Myocardial and circulatory depression. CNS changes: drowsiness, disorientation, decreased hearing ability, paresthesias, muscle twitching, and agitation. Focal and grand mal seizures.
PROCAINAMIDE HYDROCHLORIDE	To suppress ventricular dysrhythmias when lidocaine is ineffective	Can cause ventricular asystole or fibrillation when administered IV.
ATROPINE	To accelerate cardiac rate by creating a positive chronotropic effect due to parasympatholytic action (reduces vagal tone) and by creating a positive dromotropic effect that accelerates AV conduction.	This increased heart rate may be deleterious in patients with acute MI. Atropine should be given to patients with acute MI only if the bradycardia results in hemodynamic changes.
EPINEPHRINE	To increase perfusion pressure during cardiac compressions To improve the myocardial contractile state To stimulate spontaneous contractions (eg, in asystole) To increase the vigor of VF	Epinephrine should not be added directly to a bicarbonate infusion, because catecholamines may be inactivated by alkaline solution.
SODIUM BICARBONATE (NaHCO₃)	To correct metabolic and respiratory acidosis	Because CO_2 production is increased, adequate ventilation is required. Excessive $NaHCO_3$ leads to metabolic alkalosis with displacement of oxyhemoglobin dissociation curve and consequent impairment of oxygen release to tissues. Hyperosmolality may also develop. Catecholamines and calcium salts should not be added to bicarbonate infusions because inactivation results. Because bicarbonate has a high pH, avoid mixing any drugs with it.

The decision to terminate resuscitation is based on medical considerations and will take into account the cerebral and cardiac status of the patient.

After successful resuscitation following cardiac arrest, the nurse should carefully monitor the situation because the patient is at great risk for another cardiac arrest. Continuation of ECG monitoring is essential, and any abnormalities of rhythm must be corrected. Electrolyte and acid–base balances must be established and maintained. Hemodynamic monitoring should be initiated if it was not previously instituted. Selected drugs are used during and after resuscitation (Table 29–2), and should be immediately available.

In summary, thromboembolic episodes, pericardial effusion, and myocardial rupture occur to a lesser extent than dysrhythmias or cardiac failure. Nonetheless, they can contribute significantly to morbidity and mortality when they do occur. It is incumbent on the nurse to be familiar with the warning signs and symptoms of these less common disorders to provide optimum care for patients with cardiac disease. Cardiopulmonary resuscitation is an immediate therapy that may be initiated for cardiac arrest. Evidence that an individual is breathless and pulseless is sufficient to warrant immediate resuscitation efforts.

Knowledge of cardiopulmonary resuscitation enhances the safety of both rescuer and rescuee.

Bibliography

Books

Abels L. Critical Care Nursing. St Louis, CV Mosby, 1986.

Ahumada G. Cardiovascular Pathophysiology. New York, Oxford University Press, 1987.

Andreoli K et al. Comprehensive Cardiac Care. St Louis, CV Mosby, 1987.

Brandenburg RO et al. Cardiology: Fundamentals and Practice. Chicago, Year Book Medical Publishers, 1987.

Braunwald E. Heart Disease: A Textbook of Cardiovascular Medicine. Philadelphia, WB Saunders, 1988.

Bustin D. Hemodynamic Monitoring for Critical Care. Norwalk, CT, Appleton–Century–Crofts, 1986.

Cardiopulmonary Resuscitation (CPR) (pamphlet). American Heart Association, 1986.

Cheng T. The International Textbook of Cardiology. New York, Pergamon Press, 1986.

Chernow B. The Pharmacologic Approach to the Critically Ill Patient. Baltimore, Williams & Wilkins, 1988.

Chung E. Principles of Cardiac Arrhythmias. Baltimore, Williams & Wilkins, 1989.

Chung E. Cardiac Emergency Care. Philadelphia, Lea & Febiger, 1985.

Chung E. Manual of Acute Cardiac Disorders. Boston, Butterworths, 1988.

Comerota AJ. Thrombolytic Therapy. New York, Grune & Stratton, 1988.

Conover MB. Understanding Electrocardiography. St Louis, CV Mosby, 1988.

Coodley EL (ed). Geriatric Heart Disease. Littleton, MA, PSG Publishing, 1985.

Daily ED and Schroeder JS. Techniques in Bedside Hemodynamic Monitoring. St Louis, CV Mosby, 1989.

Darovic GO. Hemodynamic Monitoring. Philadelphia, WB Saunders Company, 1987.

Douglas MK and Shinn JA. Advances in Cardiovascular Nursing. Rockville, MD, Aspen Systems, 1985.

Dunn MI and Lipman BS. Lipman–Massie Clinical Electrocardiography. Chicago, Year Book Medical Publishers, 1989.

Eagle KA et al (eds). The Practice of Cardiology, Vols 1 and 2. Boston, Little, Brown, 1989.

Edmonds JH. ECG STAT! Hospital Electrocardiography in Urgent Situations. Philadelphia, Lea & Febiger, 1988.

Facts About Congestive Heart Failure (pamphlet). American Heart Association, 1987.

Fozzard HA et al (eds). The Heart and Cardiovascular System. New York, Raven Press, 1986.

Frye SJ and Lounsbury P. Cardiac Rhythm Disorders: An Introduction Using the Nursing Process. Baltimore, Williams & Wilkins, 1988.

Grauer K and Curry WR. Clinical Electrocardiography: A Primary Care Approach. Oradell, NJ, Medical Economics, 1987.

Harris R. Clinical Geriatric Cardiology. Philadelphia, JB Lippincott, 1986.

Henning RJ and Grenvik A. Critical Care Cardiology. New York, Churchill Livingstone, 1989.

Hillis LD et al. Manual of Clinical Problems in Cardiology. Boston, Little, Brown, 1988.

Holloway N. Nursing the Critically Ill Adult. Menlo Park, CA, Addison-Wesley, 1988.

Hunyor SN. Cardiovascular Drug Therapy. Baltimore, Williams & Wilkins, 1987.

Hurst JW. The Heart. New York, McGraw-Hill, 1990.

Josephson ME. Sudden Cardiac Death. Philadelphia, FA Davis, 1985.

Julian DG and Wenger NK. Management of Heart Failure. Boston, Butterworths, 1986.

Kern L. Cardiac Critical Care Nursing. Rockville, MD, Aspen Systems, 1988.

Khan MG. Manual of Cardiac Drug Therapy. Philadelphia, WB Saunders, 1988.

Mandel WJ. Cardiac Arrhythmias: Their Mechanisms, Diagnosis, and Management. Philadelphia, JB Lippincott, 1987.

Marriott HJL. Practical Electrocardiography. Baltimore, Williams & Wilkins, 1988.

Marriott HL and Conover MR. Advanced Concepts in Arrhythmias. St Louis, CV Mosby, 1989.

Messerli F. Cardiovascular Disease in the Elderly. Boston, Martinus Nijhoff, 1988.

Norman AE. Rapid ECG Interpretation. New York, Macmillan, 1989.

Ornato JP. Cardiovascular Emergencies. New York, Churchill Livingstone, 1986.

Price S and Wilson L. Pathophysiology: Clinical Concepts of Disease Process. New York, McGraw-Hill, 1986.

Riegel B et al (eds). Dreifus' pacemaker therapy: An interprofessional approach. Philadelphia, FA Davis, 1986.

Silber EN. Heart Disease. New York, Macmillan, 1987.

Sokolow M and McIlroy M. Clinical Cardiology. Los Altos, CA, Lange Medical Publications, 1986.

Suddarth DS. Lippincott Manual of Nursing Practice. Philadelphia, JB Lippincott, 1991.

Underhill SL et al. Cardiac Nursing. Philadelphia, JB Lippincott, 1989.

Warren JV and Lewis RP. Diagnostic Procedures in Cardiology. Chicago, Year Book Medical Publishers, 1985.

Webb WR and Kerstein MD. Cardiovascular Emergencies. Rockville, MD, Aspen Sysems, 1987.

Yee BH and Zorb SL. Cardiac Critical Care Nursing. Boston, Little, Brown, 1986.

Journals

Asterisks indicate nursing research articles.

Dysrhythmias

Andrews LK. ECG rhythms made easier with algorithms. Am J Nurs 1989 Mar; 89(3): 365–369.

Andrews LK. Tracking electrical impulses. Am J Nurs 1989 Mar; 89(3): 370–371.

Arrhythmias. Med Times 1989 Jan; 117(1): 89–92.

Cheny R. Defibrillation. Crit Care Nurs Q 1988; 10(4): 9–15.

Conner RP. The Wenckebach phenomenon. Heart Lung 1987 Sep; 16(5): 506–518.

Conover M. A common arrhythmia. Crit Care Nurs 1988 May; 8(5): 112.

Cook JR and Nieminski K. Ventricular tachycardia. Crit Care Nurs 1988 Oct; 8(7): 15–17.

Crisp CB. Calcium channel blockers in emergency medicine. Emerg Care Q 1987 Aug; 3(2): 38–48.

Decker S. Continuous EKG monitoring systems. Nurs Clin North Am 1987 Mar; 22(1): 1–13.

*Dunnington CC et al. Patients with heart rhythm disturbances: Variables associated with increased psychologic stress. Heart Lung 1988 Jul/Aug; 17(4): 381–389.

Erickson SL. Wolff–Parkinson–White syndrome: A review and update. Crit Care Nurs 1989 May; 9(5): 28–35.

Geddes L. Monitoring the patient with conduction disturbances and blocks. Nurs Clin North Am 1987 Mar; 22(1): 33–47.

Lazarus M et al. Cardiac arrhythmias: Diagnosis and treatment. Crit Care Nurs 1988 Jul; 8(7): 57–65.

Lunger DG. Potassium supplementations: How and why? Focus Crit Care 1988 Oct; 15(5): 56–60.

Marden S and Chulay M. Esmolol HCL. Crit Care Nurs 1989 Nov/Dec; 9(10): 12–14.

Meola DR and Walker V. Responding quickly to tachydysrhythmias. Nursing 1987 Nov; 17(11): 34–41.

Mercer M The electrophysiology study: A nursing concern. Crit Care Nurs 1987 Mar/Apr; 7(2): 58–65.

Parker BM. Electrocardiography: Identifying diagnostic pitfalls. Consultant 1987 Aug; 27(8): 34–38.

Petrie JR. Distinguishing supraventricular aberrancies from ventricular ectopy. Focus Crit Care 1988 Jul; 15(4): 15–21.

Reyes A. Monitoring and treating life-threatening dysrhythmias. Nurs Clin North Am 1987 Mar; 22(1): 61–75.

Rhynsvurger J. Action stat! Third degree heart block. Nursing 1988 Oct; 18(10): 33.

Sargent RK. Advances in the treatment of ventricular dysrhythmias. Emerg Care Q 1987 Aug; 3(2): 18–26.

Schactman M. A case study of atrial fibrillation and mitral stenosis. Focus Crit Care 1987 May; 14(3): 13–20.

Stevens LL and Redd RM. Bedside electrophysiology study. Crit Care Nurs 1987 Jul/Aug; 7(4): 36–41.

Stevens L et al. Emergency catheter ablation of refractory ventricular tachycardia. Crit Car Nurs 1989 May; 9(5): 36–40.

Valle GA and Lemberg L. Electrolyte imbalances in cardiovascular disease: The forgotten factor. Heart Lung 1988 May; 17(3): 324–329.

Weller Dm and Noone J. Mechanisms of arrhythmias: Enhanced automaticity and reentry. Crit Care Nurs 1989 May; 9(5): 42–62.

Zimmaro DM. Catheter ablation of ventricular tachycardia and related nursing interventions. Crit Care Nurs 1987 Jul/Aug; 7(4): 20–29.

Pacemakers/Automatic Implantable Cardioverter Defibrillators

* Badger JM and Morris P. Observations of a support group for automatic implantable cardioverter-defibrillator recipients and their spouses. Heart Lung 1989 May; 18(3): 238–243.

Bayless WA. The elements of cardiac pacing. Crit Care Nurs 1988 Aug; 8(7): 31–41.

Catania SL. A simplified method for the interpretation of DDD pacemaker ECG's. Crit Care Nurs Q 1987; 9(4): 31–39.

Cooper D et al. Care of the patient with the automatic implantable defibrillator: A guide for nurses. Heart Lung 1987 Nov; 16(6) part 1: 640–648.

Featherston RG. Care of sudden cardiac death survivors: The aberrant cardiac patient. Heart Lung 1988 May; 17(3): 242–246.

Living with your pacemaker (pamphlet). American Heart Association, 1986.

Manolis AS et al. Automatic implantable cardioverter defibrillator. JAMA 1989 Sep 8; 262(10): 1362–1367.

McCrum AE and Tyndall A. Nursing care of patients with implantable defibrillators. Crit Care Nurs 1989 Sep; 9(9): 48–68.

Moser S et al. Caring for patients with implantable cardioverter-defibrillators. Crit Care Nurs 1988 Nov/Dec; 8(2): 52–65.

Nottingham A and Camp V. Remote cardiac monitoring nursing collaboration is the key. Dimens Crit Care Nurs 1987 May/Jun; 6(3): 176–178.

Persons CB. Transcutaneous pacing: Meeting the challenge. Focus Crit Care 1987 Feb; 14(1): 13–19.

Stevens L et al. Ventricular burst pacing. Crit Care Nurs 1989 Mar; 9(3): 38–43.

Stevens L and Buckingham T. Late potentials: A method for screening patients at risk for sudden cardiac death. Crit Care Nurs 1989 May; 9(5): 68–73.

Walton J. Identification of patients at high risk for sudden cardiac death. Focus Crit Care 1987 Nov/Dec; 14(6): 70–75.

Pulmonary Edema, Failure, Shock

Ardire L. IV NTG: Monitoring vital signs hourly versus every two hours. Crit Care Nurs 1990 Oct; 10(9): 52–56.

Bumann R and Speltz M. Decreased cardiac output: A nursing diagnosis. Dimens Crit Care Nurs 1989 Jan/Feb; 8(1): 6–15.

Contrades S. Altered cardiac output: An assessment tool. Dimens Crit Care Nurs 1987 Sep/Oct; 6(5): 274–282.

Jefferies PR and Whelan SK. Cardiogenic shock: Current management. Crit Care Nurs Q 1988; 11(1): 48–56.

Joseph DL and Bates S. Intra-aortic balloon pumping: How to stay on course. Am J Nurs 1990 Sep; 90(9): 42–47.

Lambert CE and Lambert V. Psychosocial impacts created by chronic illness. Nurs Clin North Am 1987 Sep; 22(3): 527–533.

Lough ME. Introduction to hemodynamic monitoring. Nurs Clin North Am 1987 Mar; 22(1): 89–110.

Masters S. Complications of pulmonary artery catheters. Crit Care Nurs 1989 Sep; 9(9): 82–91.

Moore J. Intravenous amrinone therapy at home for the patient with chronic congestive heart failure. Focus Crit Care 1988 Nov/Dec; 15(6): 32–37.

Mutnik A et al. Update on cardiac drugs: Inotropic and chronotropic agents. Nursing 1987 Oct; 17(10): 58–61.

Roberts S. Cardiogenic shock: Decreased coronary artery tissue perfusion. Dimens Crit Care Nurs 1988 Jul/Aug; 7(4): 196–208.

Schreiber TL et al. Management of myocardial infarction shock: Current status. Am Heart J 1989 Feb; 117(2): 435–443.

Schwertz D and Piano M. New inotropic drugs for treatment of congestive heart failure. Cardiovasc Nurs 1990 Mar/Apr; 26(2): 7–12.

Walter PJ (ed). Treatment of end-stage coronary artery disease. Adv Cardiol 1988; 36: 71–73.

Thromboembolism

Consensus Conference: Prevention of venous thrombosis and pulmonary emboli. JAMA 1986 Aug 8; 256(6): 744–749.

Daeschner SA. Action STAT! Pulmonary embolism. Nursing 1988 Sep; 18(9): 33.

Dickinson SP and Bury G. Pulmonary embolism—Anatomy of a crisis. Nursing 1989 Apr; 19(4): 34–42.

Gerdes L. Recognizing the multisystem effect of embolism. Nursing 1987 Dec; 17(12): 34–42.

Pericarditis/Rupture

Fraley MA. Differential diagnosis of chest pain. Physician Assist 1988 Jun; 12(6): 69, 73, 75.

Khan AH. Pericarditis: Diagnosis and treatment. Hosp Med 1987 Nov; 23(11): 43, 46, 48–50.

Kite JH. Cardiac and great vessel trauma: Assessment, pathophysiology and intervention. J Emerg Nurs 1987 Nov/Dec; 13(6): 346–351.

Mayberry-Toth B et al. Complications associated with acute myocardial infarction. Crit Care Nurs Q 1989 Sep; 12(2): 49–63.

Muirhead J. Constriction pericarditis: A review. Prog Cardiovasc Nurs 1988 Oct/Dec; 3(4): 122–127.

Truett L et al. Pericardial effusion with tamponade: Relief for the symptomatic patient. Dimens Oncol Nurs 1988 Fall; 2(3): 18–20.

Turk M. Acute pericarditis in the post-myocardial infarction patient. Crit Care Nurs Q 1989; 12(3): 34–38.

Unreliable enzymes in myocardial contusion. Emerg Med 1989 Mar 15; 21(5): 47–48.

Cardiac Arrest/Cardiopulmonary Resuscitation

Feeney–Stewart F. The sodium bicarbonate controversy. Dimens Crit Care Nurs 1990 Jan/Feb; 9(1): 22–28.

Jones S and Bagg A. L-E-A-D drugs for cardiac arrest. Nursing 1988 Jan; 18(1): 34–42.

Levy DB. Update on lidocaine. Emergency 1988 Sep; 20(9): 15–18.

Middaugh RE et al. Current considerations in respiratory and acid-base management during cardiopulmonary resuscitation. Crit Care Nurs Q 1988; 10(4): 25–33.

Standards for CPR and ECC. JAMA 1986 Jun 6; 255(21): 2915–2989.

Teplitz L. Clinical close-up on atropine. Nursing 1989 Nov; 19(11): 44–47.

Teplitz L. Clinical close-up on lidocaine. Nursing 1989 Sep; 19(9): 44–47.

Teplitz L. Clinical close-up on epinephrine. Nursing 1989 Oct; 19(10): 50–53.

Information/Resources

Agencies

Governmental

National Heart, Lung, and Blood Institute
National Institutes of Health Building 31, Room 5A52,
Bethesda, MD 20892

Voluntary

American Heart Association
7220 Greenville Ave, Dallas, TX 75231

Coronary Club
3659 Green Rd, Cleveland, OH 44122

Heartlife
PO Box 54305, Atlanta, GA 30308

30

Management of the Cardiac Surgery Patient

Learning Objectives

On completion of this chapter, the learner will be able to:

1. *Compare the various surgical procedures available for treatment of cardiac problems*
2. *Describe the significance of nursing assessment, patient teaching, and psychological support during preoperative preparation of the patient for cardiac surgery*
3. *Use the nursing process as a framework for the care of patients before cardiac surgery*
4. *Specify the critical nature of the components of postoperative management of the patient who has had cardiac surgery*
5. *Identify the possible complications after cardiac surgery, measures to prevent these complications, and assessment parameters appropriate for their identification*
6. *Use the nursing process as a framework for the care of patients after cardiac surgery*

Today, the patient with heart disease and related complications can be assisted to achieve a quality of life far greater than anticipated even as recently as a decade ago. Through sophisticated diagnostic modalities that allow for earlier and more accurate diagnosis, treatment can begin well before significant debilitation takes place. New treatment technologies and pharmacotherapeutics are being developed rapidly and with increasing safety of application and administration. Many of these have been discussed in the previous two chapters.

Perhaps no therapeutic intervention has contributed as much as cardiac surgery to the improved quality of life for the patient with heart disease.

The first successful cardiac surgery, closure of a right ventricular stab wound, was performed in 1895 by the Italian surgeon de Vecchi. In the United States the first such successful surgery, also a repair of a stab wound, was performed in 1902.

Valvular surgery followed in 1923 and 1925, closure of a patent ductus in 1937 and 1938, resection of a coarctation of the aorta in 1944, and the current era of coronary artery bypass grafting began in 1954.

The most revolutionary development in the advancement of cardiac surgery has been the evolution of the technique for cardiopulmonary bypass. It was first used successfully for humans in 1951. By 1989 over 250,000 procedures a year were being performed employing cardiopulmonary bypass (over 200,000 in North America). The majority of procedures are coronary artery bypass grafts (CABG) and valve repair or replacement.

Cardiac diseases may be circulatory (coronary artery disease, ascending aortic aneurysm), structural (valvular regurgitation/stenosis, atrial or ventricular septal defects, cardiomyopathy, traumatic) or conduction system disorders (bradycardias, lethal dysrhythmias). The causes of cardiac diseases may be classified as congenital, acquired, or idiopathic. The advances in diagnostics, medical management, surgical techniques, anesthesia techniques, and support systems such as cardiopulmonary bypass, critical care units, and rehabilitation programs have assisted in making surgery a viable treatment option for patients with cardiac disease. This chapter describes the surgical procedures and care of adults with acquired heart disease.

Cardiopulmonary Bypass

Many cardiac surgical procedures are possible because of cardiopulmonary bypass (extracorporeal circulation). The procedure provides a mechanical means of circulating and oxygenating blood for the body while "bypassing" the heart and lungs. The heart–lung machine allows for a bloodless surgical field while maintaining perfusion to the other body organs and tissues.

Cardiopulmonary bypass is accomplished by placement of a cannula in the right atrium, vena cava, or femoral vein to withdraw blood from the body. The cannula is connected to tubing filled with an isotonic crystalloid solution (usually 5% dextrose in Lactated Ringer's). Venous blood removed from the body by this cannula is filtered, oxygenated, cooled or warmed, and then returned to the body. The cannula returning

the oxygenated blood is usually in the ascending aorta, but may be in the femoral artery (Fig. 30–1).

Although cardiopulmonary bypass is a common technique in heart surgery, it is very complex. The patient requires anticoagulation with heparin to prevent thrombus formation and possible embolization that could occur when blood contacts the foreign surfaces of the cardiopulmonary bypass circuit and is pumped into the body by a mechanical pump (not the normal blood vessels and heart). After the patient is removed from the bypass machine, protamine sulfate is used to reverse the effects of heparin.

During the procedure hypothermia is maintained, usually 28° to 32°C (82.4° to 89.6°F). The blood is cooled during cardiopulmonary bypass and returned to the body. The cooled blood slows the body's basal metabolic rate, thereby decreasing the body's demand for oxygen. Cooled blood usually would have a higher viscosity, but the crystalloid solution used to prime the bypass tubing dilutes the blood. When the surgical procedure is completed, the blood is rewarmed as it passes through the cardiopulmonary bypass circuit. Urine output, blood pressures, arterial blood gases, electrolytes, coagulation studies, and the electrocardiogram all are used to monitor the patient's status during cardiopulmonary bypass.

There are still many things to learn about cardiopulmonary bypass. There are numerous types of bypass circuits and pumping mechanisms being used today. Attempts are being made to increase the time a patient may spend on the heart–lung machine. Researchers continue to refine cardiopulmonary bypass so that hemolysis, increased capillary membrane per-

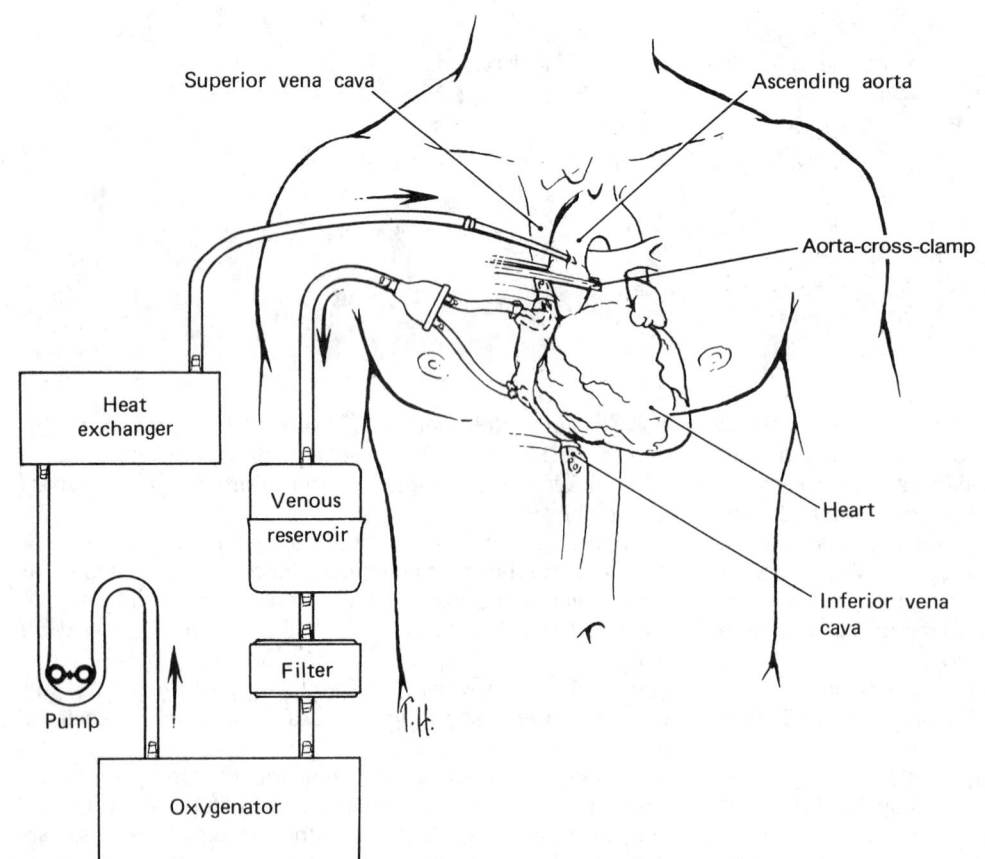

Figure 30–1. Schematic drawing of the cardiopulmonary bypass system.

meability, fluid and electrolyte shifts, tissue hypoxia/anoxia, thrombus/emboli formation, cardiac and vascular dissection, catecholamine and antidiuretic hormone (ADH) elevations, and the systemic inflammatory responses that complicate the procedure can be minimized or eliminated.

In summary, cardiopulmonary bypass maintains blood circulation and tissue perfusion while the patient has heart surgery. It oxygenates the blood and regulates temperature while providing the surgeon with a "bloodless" heart during surgery. Complications may result from coagulation alterations, high blood viscosity, fluid overload, oxygenation, and increased capillary permeability leading to edema.

Circulatory Cardiac Surgery

Percutaneous Transluminal Coronary Angioplasty

Coronary artery disease remains a major factor in the morbidity and mortality of Americans (see Chap. 28). Treatment categories have traditionally been clearly medical or surgical. Today, treatments that are invasive are not necessarily surgical. Technically, percutaneous transluminal coronary angioplasty (PTCA) is not a surgical procedure.

Patients who are considered candidates for PTCA are usually those who have lesions that occlude at least 70% of the internal lumen of a major coronary artery, placing a large amount of myocardium at risk for ischemia. These patients are ones whose conditions do not respond to medical treatments, and they should meet the criteria for coronary artery bypass surgery.

PTCA is attempted when the cardiologist believes that blood flow to the myocardium at risk for ischemia can be improved by the procedure. PTCAs are seldom attempted on patients with occlusions of the left main coronary artery that do not demonstrate collateral flow to the left anterior descending and circumflex arteries, patients with stenoses at the origin of the right coronary artery with the aorta, patients with coronary arteries that demonstrate an aneurysm proximal or distal to the stenosis, patients with diffusely diseased or more than 5-year-old saphenous vein grafts, or patients with questionable left ventricular function.

The cardiac catheterization laboratory is the procedure area used most frequently for PTCA. Patient care for PTCA is very similar to that for a cardiac catheterization. The patient's coronary arteries are examined by angiography, as they were during the diagnostic cardiac catheterization. The lesions are verified for location, extent, and calcification before a guidewire is passed into the artery beyond the lesion. A guide catheter is passed over the guidewire to the lesion. A balloon-tipped dilation catheter is then passed over the guidewire (through the guide catheter) and positioned over the lesion. When the balloon-tipped dilation catheter is properly positioned, pressurized air fills the balloon for an average of 30 to 60 seconds, cracking and possibly compressing the atherosclerotic lesion (Fig. 30–2). The coronary artery's media and adventitia are also stretched. Several inflations may be required to achieve the desired effect—usually defined as an increase in the artery's lumen of 20% or more. Other measures used to gauge the success of a PTCA are a residual stenosis of less

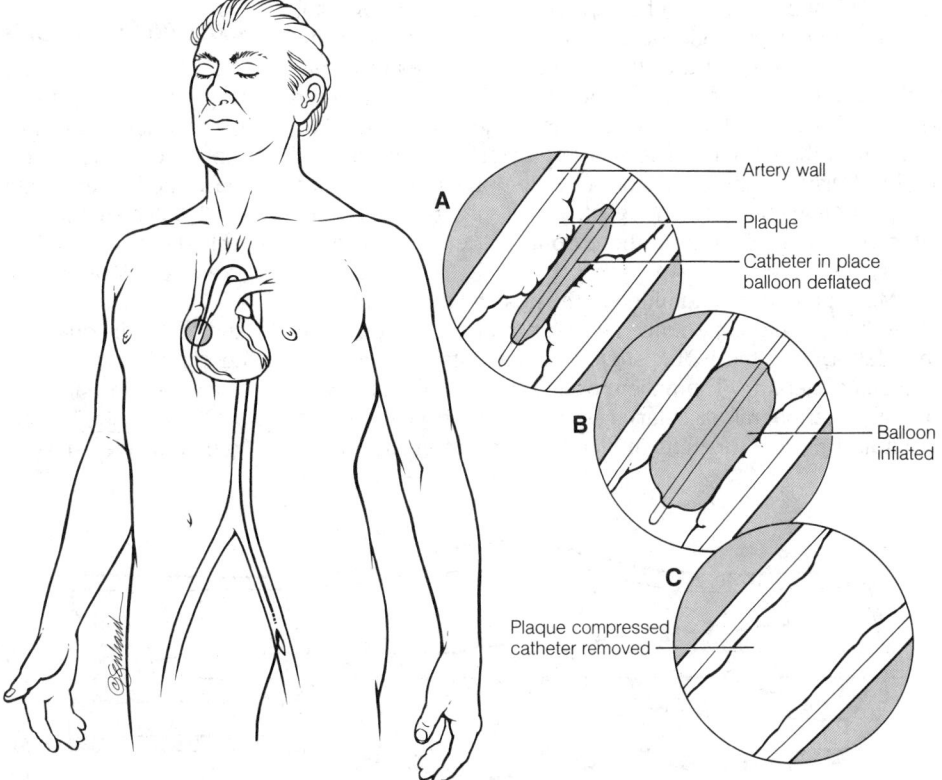

Figure 30–2. Percutaneous transluminal coronary angioplasty is a less invasive procedure than coronary artery bypass surgery in selected patients. (**A**) A balloon-tipped catheter is passed into the affected coronary artery and placed within the atherosclerotic lesion. (**B**) The balloon is then rapidly inflated and deflated with controlled pressure. (**C**) After the plaque is compressed, the catheter is removed, allowing improved blood flow for the vessel.

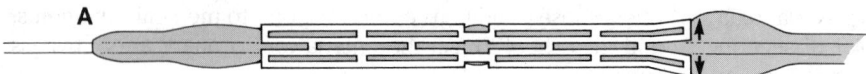

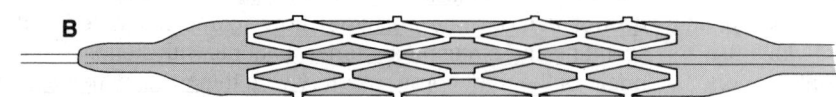

Figure 30–3. Schematic drawing of an intra-coronary artery stent: (**A**) closed, before balloon inflation; (**B**) open, after balloon inflation.

than 50% or less than 20 mm Hg difference in blood pressure from one side of the lesion to the other and no clinically obvious arterial trauma.

Complications during the PTCA procedure or the recovery period include dissection, abrupt closure, and spasm of the coronary artery. These may require emergency surgical treatment. For this reason, all PTCA candidates also must be coronary artery bypass candidates. A cardiac surgery operating room and surgical team are always on standby during a PTCA.

Three alternative procedures to emergency cardiac surgery are being examined. The first is redilation (PTCA). The second is redilation with an intravascular stent over the balloon. When the balloon is deflated the stent remains in the artery, holding the artery open (Fig. 30–3). Eventually endothelium covers the stent and it is incorporated into the vessel wall. The third alternative is the use of a laser. There are numerous types of lasers being used experimentally today. The theory is that the laser is able to "weld" the artery open or "melt" the plaque by the heat it generates.

The risks of emergency surgery also may be decreased by the use of a shunt catheter. It is sometimes possible to pass a shunt catheter through the reoccluded coronary artery (Fig. 30–4). This special catheter has numerous holes along its distal end. The openings begin before the coronary artery closure and continue to the end of the catheter. The holes proximal to the lesion permit arterial blood to flow into the catheter while the holes distal to the lesion permit the arterial blood to flow out of the catheter. The shunt catheter maintains a flow of blood distal to the occlusion while the patient is prepared for immediate, but not emergent, heart surgery. The shunt catheter is removed during the coronary artery bypass graft surgery.

Many patients are admitted to the hospital the day of their PTCA. Those who experience no complications go home the next day. During the PCTA procedure, patients receive large amounts of heparin. The patient often returns to the unit with the large peripheral vascular access cannula in place. He is monitored closely for signs of bleeding. The cannulas are re-

moved once the patient's clotting studies return to within 1.5 to 2 times the laboratory's normal values. Most patients receive intravenous heparin and nitroglycerine for a period after the procedure to prevent clot formation and arterial spasm. The patients are usually able to be weaned from the intravenous medications, resume self-care, and ambulate unassisted within 24 hours of the procedure.

In summary, PTCA is an invasive technique used to decrease the obstruction caused by atherosclerotic lesions in the coronary arteries. The procedure is often successful in decreasing the degree of coronary artery obstruction without development of complications; therefore, PTCA is an alternative to coronary artery bypass grafting. Because the procedure is not always successful and because some patients do develop complications, an open heart surgical suite and team are always on standby. As advances and improvements are made in PTCA, lesions that are longer, more numerous, and in more difficult locations are being treated. PTCAs are performed with and without the use of intracoronary stents, lasers, and shunt catheters.

Coronary Artery Revascularization

Coronary artery disease has been treated by some form of myocardial revascularization for approximately 30 years. Current coronary artery bypass graft (CABG) techniques have been performed for approximately 25 years. The most frequent CABG candidates are individuals with (1) angina that cannot be controlled by medical therapies, (2) unstable angina, (3) a positive exercise tolerance test and lesions that cannot be treated by PTCA, (4) a left main coronary artery lesion of more than 60%, and (5) individuals who have complications from or unsuccessful PTCAs.

The coronary arteries to be bypassed must have at least a 70% occlusive lesion (60% if it is the left main coronary artery) to be considered for CABG. The blood flow through an artery

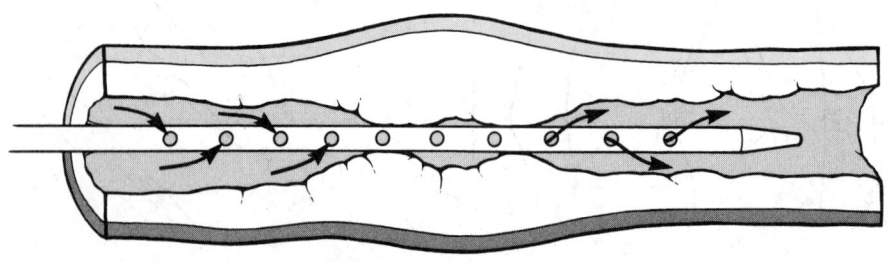

Figure 30–4. Schematic drawing of a shunt catheter.

with a lesion of less than 70% is enough to prevent adequate blood flow through the CABG. Thus, the CABG would clot, effectively negating the surgery performed.

Coronary artery bypass graft is performed under general anesthesia. A median sternotomy incision is made and the patient is placed on cardiopulmonary bypass. A blood vessel from another part of the body is grafted distal to the coronary artery lesion—"bypassing" the obstruction (Fig. 30–5). Cardiopulmonary bypass is discontinued and the incision is closed. The patient then is admitted to a critical care unit.

Initially the patient's care is focused on achieving or maintaining hemodynamic stability and recovery from general anesthesia. Within 48 hours the typical patient is transferred to a telemetry or surgical unit. The patient's care is focused on wound care, progressive activity, and diet; in addition, education about medications and risk factor modification is emphasized. Discharge from the hospital is usually 5 to 10 days after CABG. Patients can expect fewer symptoms from their coronary artery disease, with resulting increase in quality of life. CABG has not been shown to increase patients' life spans, however.

The most recent advances in the surgical procedure have been in the variety of blood vessels used to bypass the coronary artery lesion. The most common vessel has been the greater saphenous vein, followed by the lesser saphenous vein. Cephalic and basilic veins also have been used. The vein is removed from the leg (or arm) and grafted to the ascending aorta and to the coronary artery distal to the lesion. The saphenous veins are used in emergency CABG procedures be-cause they can be obtained by one surgical team while another team performs the chest surgery. One side effect of using a large vein is that the extremity from which it was taken often develops edema. The degree of edema is variable and may diminish over time. The saphenous veins develop symptomatic atherosclerotic changes approximately 5 to 10 years after CABG. The arm veins develop the same changes more quickly, approximately 3 to 6 years after the surgery.

The right and left internal mammary arteries had been used in the past, but the procedure of dissecting the artery from the chest wall required too much time under anesthesia and on the cardiopulmonary bypass machine. Advances in cardiopulmonary bypass and anesthesia have decreased the time required to begin the surgical procedures and have decreased the risks of longer surgical times, thus renewing interest in using arteries for CABGs. Because research had shown that arterial grafts did not develop atherosclerotic changes as quickly and maintained patency longer than vein grafts, use of the right and left internal mammary arteries regained popularity. The proximal end of the mammary artery is left intact. The distal end of the artery is dissected away from the chest wall. This distal end of the artery is then grafted to the coronary artery distal to the lesion.

The internal mammaries are not always long enough nor do they always have a sufficient diameter to be used for CABG. One side effect of the use of the internal mammary artery is ulnar nerve sensory damage, which can be temporary or permanent.

The gastroepiploic artery (located on the greater curvature

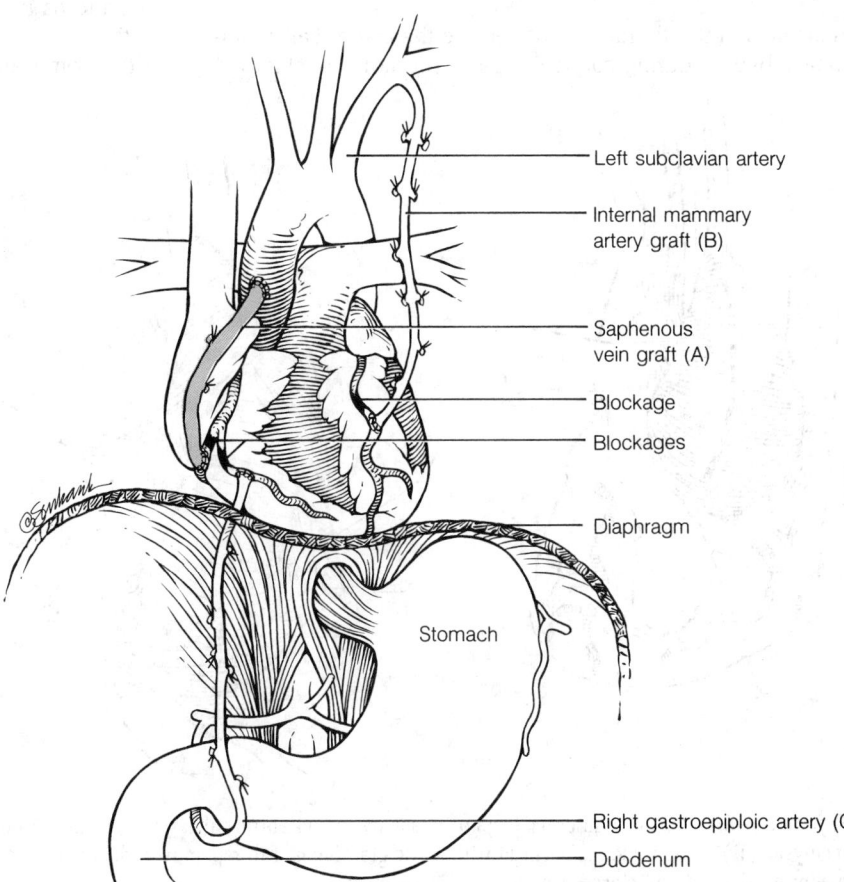

Figure 30–5. Schematic drawing of three coronary artery bypass grafts. One or more procedures may be performed. (**A**) Saphenous vein, the most frequently utilized bypass. (**B**) Left internal mammary artery, gaining in popularity because of its functional longevity. (**C**) Right gastroepiploic artery, rarely utilized because it has a more extensive blood supply to its wall and because of the risk of gastrointestinal tract contamination of the abdominal and/or mediastinal wound.

Left subclavian artery

Internal mammary artery graft (B)

Saphenous vein graft (A)

Blockage

Blockages

Diaphragm

Stomach

Right gastroepiploic artery (C)

Duodenum

of the stomach; see Fig. 30–5) also has been used for CABG. It has a much more extensive blood supply to its wall than the internal mammaries have, so it does not respond as well to use as a graft. Another disadvantage of the gastroepiploic artery is that the chest incision must be extended to the abdomen, thus exposing the patient to the additional risks of an abdominal incision and infection from gastrointestinal tract contamination of the surgical site.

Coronary artery bypass graft surgery may result in complications such as myocardial infarction, dysrhythmias, and hemorrhage. The patient's underlying coronary heart disease remains; so the patient may develop angina, exercise intolerance, or other symptoms experienced before CABG. Medications similar to those required preoperatively may need to be continued. The life style modifications recommended before surgery remain important, not just for the original pathology, but for the continued viability of the newly implanted grafts.

In summary, CABG is a major surgical intervention requiring the use of cardiopulmonary bypass. The internal mammary arteries have become the grafts of choice, although saphenous veins remain a commonly used alternative. The graft is anastomosed to the coronary artery distal to the lesion, increasing the flow of oxygenated blood to the distal myocardium. Patients must continue their diet, activity, and risk factor modifications and may need to continue medical management of their underlying disease to minimize symptoms and prolong the patency of their CABGs.

Ascending Aortic Aneurysm

Aneurysms of the thoracic aorta require the use of cardiopulmonary bypass during surgical repair. The aorta is clamped proximal and distal to the aneurysm. Care is taken to maintain blood flow to all of the aortic branches occluded by this procedure. The aneurysm is opened and a Dacron graft is sewn in place, extending beyond the ends of the aneurysm. The aorta then is closed over the graft. Attention is paid to preserving coronary artery blood flow.

The aneurysm also may involve the coronary artery sinuses and aortic valve. Surgical repair is similar, but the Dacron graft includes a prosthetic valve, and the coronary arteries must be anastomosed to the graft. Thus, the aortic valve is replaced as the aneurysm is repaired (Fig. 30–6).

The nursing care is primarily the same as for patients after open heart surgery. The patient is admitted to a critical care unit for at least 24 hours after surgery. Care focuses on the patient's recovery from anesthesia as well as assessing and maintaining tissue perfusion. The patient is transferred to a surgical unit once the blood pressure and neurovascular status are stable. Wound care, patient teaching regarding diet, activity, and medications, as well as assessing for signs of infection (redness, swelling, tenderness, drainage, temperature elevation or increased white blood cell count) continue through discharge.

Structural Cardiac Surgery

Valvuloplasty

The repair, rather than replacement, of a cardiac valve is referred to as *valvuloplasty*. The type of valvuloplasty depends on the cause of and type of valve dysfunction. Repair may be to the commissures between the leaflets (commissurotomy),

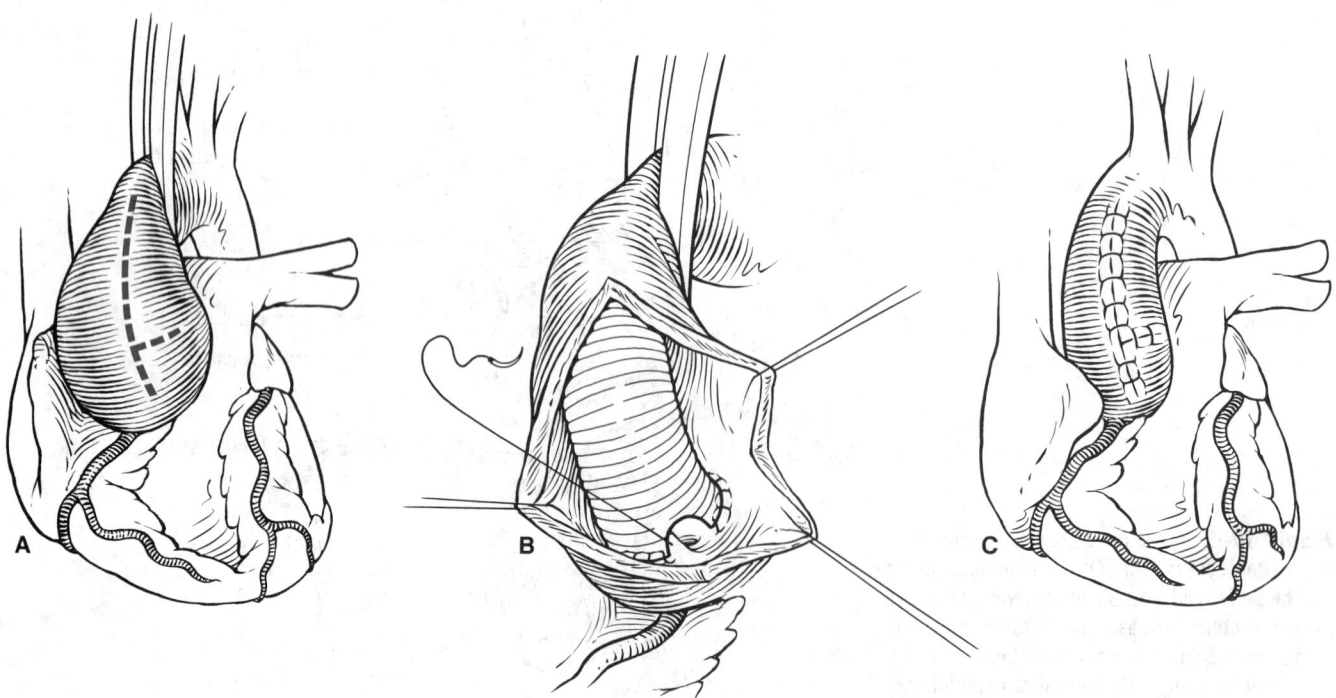

Figure 30–6. Repair of an ascending aortic aneurysm and aortic valve replacement: (**A**) incision into aortic aneurysm; (**B**) aortic value replacement with aortic graft implant to repair ascending aortic aneurysm; (**C**) aortic aneurysm trimmed and closed over graft.

to the annulus of the valve (annuloplasty), or to the leaflets and the chordae (chordoplasty). Most valvuloplasty procedures require general anesthesia and most also require cardiopulmonary bypass. Some procedures, however, can be performed in the cardiac catheterization laboratory; these procedures do not always require general anesthesia or cardiopulmonary bypass. A newly developed percutaneous, partial cardiopulmonary bypass technique is now used in some cardiac catheterization laboratories.

The patient is managed in a critical care unit for the first 24 to 72 hours postoperatively. Care focuses on hemodynamic stabilization and recovery from anesthesia. Most patients are then transferred to a telemetry or surgical unit for continued postsurgical care and teaching. Patients are discharged from the hospital in 2 to 10 days. In general, valves that have undergone valvuloplasty function longer than replacement valves and the patients do not require continuous anticoagulation.

Commissurotomy

The most common valvuloplasty procedure is the commissurotomy. Each valve has leaflets; the site where the leaflets meet each other is the commissure. The leaflets may adhere to one another, closing the commissure—*stenosis*. Less commonly the leaflets fuse in such a way that there is not only a stenosis, but the leaflets are also prevented from closing completely— *regurgitation* (the backward flow of blood). A commissurotomy is the procedure performed to separate the fused leaflets.

Closed commissurotomies do not require cardiopulmonary bypass. The patient is placed under general anesthesia, a midsternal incision is made, a small hole is cut into the heart, and the surgeon's finger or a dilator is used to break open the commissure. The valve is not directly visualized. This type of commissurotomy has been performed for mitral, aortic, tricuspid, and pulmonary valve disease.

Another procedure, balloon valvuloplasty (Fig. 30–7), has been beneficial for mitral valve stenosis in younger patients, as well as aortic valve stenosis in elderly patients and individuals with complex medical histories that place them at high risk for the complications of more extensive surgical procedures. Most commonly used for mitral and aortic valve stenosis, balloon valvuloplasty also has been used for tricuspid and pulmonic valve stenosis. The procedure is performed in the cardiac catheterization laboratory and may be performed with local anesthesia. Patients remain in the hospital 24 to 48 hours after the procedure.

The mitral procedure involves the passage of one or two catheters into the right atrium, through the atrial septum into the left atrium, across the mitral valve into the left ventricle, and out into the aorta. A guidewire is placed through each catheter and the original catheter is removed. A large balloon catheter is then placed over the guidewire and positioned with the balloon across the mitral valve. The balloon is then inflated with a dilute liquid angiographic solution. When two balloons are used, they are inflated simultaneously. The advantage of two balloons is that they are each smaller than the one large balloon often used, making smaller atrial septal defects. Also, as the balloons are inflated they usually do not completely occlude the mitral valve, thus permitting some forward flow of blood during the inflation period. All patients will experience some degree of mitral regurgitation after the procedure. Other possible complications include bleeding from the catheter insertion sites, emboli resulting in complications such as strokes,

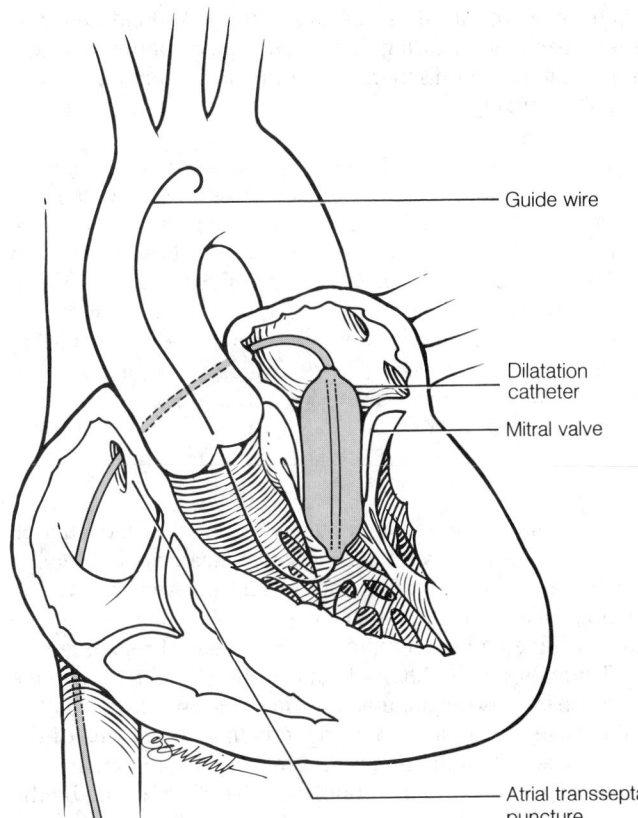

Figure 30–7. Balloon valvuloplasty: cross-sectional view of heart illustrating guide wire and dilatation catheter placed through an atrial transseptal puncture and across the mitral valve. The guide wire is extended out from the aortic valve into the aorta for catheter support.

and, rarely, left-to-right atrial shunts through an atrial septal defect caused by the procedure.

The aortic procedure also may be performed by passing the balloon or balloons through the atrial septum, but it is performed more commonly by introducing a catheter retrograde through the aorta, across the aortic valve, and into the left ventricle. Either the one-balloon or the two-balloon technique can be used for aortic stenosis. Unfortunately the dilation is not as effective as with the mitral valve, and the rate of restenosis is nearly 50% in the first 12 to 15 months after the procedure. Possible complications include aortic regurgitation, emboli, ventricular perforation, rupture of the aortic valve annulus, ventricular dysrhythmias, mitral valve damage, and bleeding from the catheter insertion sites.

Open commissurotomies are performed with direct visualization of the valve. The patient is under general anesthesia and a median sternotomy or left thoracic incision is made. The patient is placed on cardiopulmonary bypass, and an incision is made into the heart. A finger, scalpel, balloon, or dilator may be used to open the commissures. The added advantage of direct visualization of the valve is that thrombus may be noted and removed, calcifications seen, and if the valve has chordae/papillary muscles they also may be surgically repaired (see chordoplasty section of this chapter). The patient is admitted to a critical care unit after surgery. The care focuses on the patient's recovery from anesthesia and maintaining hemodynamic stability. The patient is usually transferred to a telemetry or surgical unit in 24 to 48 hours. Wound care and patient teaching regarding diet, activity, medications, and self-care continue until discharge from the hospital about 7 to 10 days after surgery.

In summary, repair of pathologies involving the commissures of a cardiac valve may be performed with few complications and low mortality. Closed and open procedures performed through a median sternotomy require hospital stays of 7 to 10 days. Percutaneous balloon commissurotomies require hospital stays of 1 to 2 days. Nursing care includes recovery from anesthetic and surgical procedures as well as preprocedure and postprocedure patient education. The greatest long-term success has been realized for mitral procedures. Aortic valves tend to restenose in 12 to 15 months. Tricuspid and pulmonic valve procedures are not frequently performed.

Annuloplasty

An annuloplasty is the repair of the valve annulus (the junction of the valve leaflets with the muscular heart wall). General anesthesia and cardiopulmonary bypass are required for all annuloplasties. The procedure narrows the diameter of the valve's orifice and is useful for the treatment of regurgitation.

There are two different annuloplasty techniques. One technique is to use an annuloplasty ring (Fig. 30–8). The leaflets of the valve are sutured to a ring, creating an annulus of the desired size. When the ring is in place, the tension created by the moving blood and the contracting heart are borne by the ring rather than by the valve or a suture line. Thus progressive regurgitation is prevented by the repair. The other technique involves tacking the valve leaflets to the atrium with sutures or taking "tucks" to tighten the annulus. The valve's leaflets and the suture lines are subjected to the direct forces of the blood and heart muscle movement, so the repair may degenerate more quickly than with the annuloplasty ring technique.

Leaflet Repair

Heart valve leaflets may be damaged by stretching out of shape, being shortened, or developing holes. The repair for elongated, ballooning, or other excess tissue leaflets is to remove the extra tissue. The elongated tissue may be folded over onto itself (tucked) and sutured—leaflet plication. A wedge of tissue may be cut from the middle of the leaflet and the gap sutured closed—leaflet resection (Fig. 30–9). Short leaflets are most often repaired by chordoplasty (see next section). Once the short chordae are released, the leaflets often "unfurl" and are able to resume their normal function of closing the valve during systole. A piece of pericardium may also be sutured to the leaflet. Most commonly the pericardial patch is used when it is necessary to repair holes in the leaflets.

Chordoplasty

Chordoplasty is the repair of the chordae tendineae. The mitral valve is involved with chordoplasty (as it has the chordae tendineae); seldom is chordoplasty required for the tricuspid valve. Regurgitation may be caused by stretched, torn, or shortened chordae tendineae. Stretched chordae tendineae can be shortened (Fig. 30–10), torn ones can be reattached to the leaflet, and shortened ones can be elongated. Regurgitation may also be caused by stretched papillary muscles, which can be shortened.

Valve Replacement

Prosthetic valve replacement began in the 1960s. When valvuloplasty is not a viable alternative, such as when the annulus or leaflets are immobilized by calcifications, valve replacement is performed. General anesthesia and cardiopulmonary bypass are used for all valve replacements. Most procedures are performed through a median sternotomy, although the mitral valve often is approached through a right thoracotomy incision.

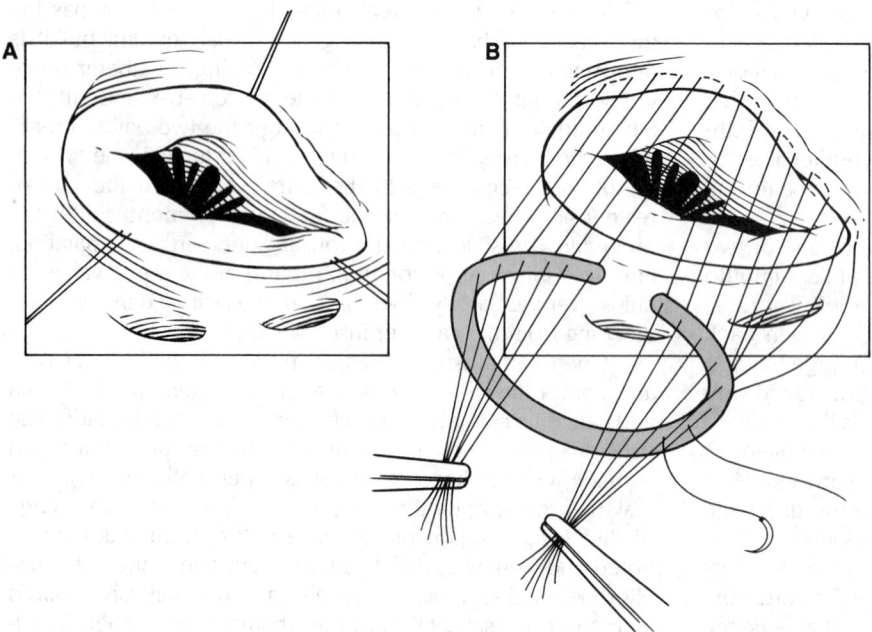
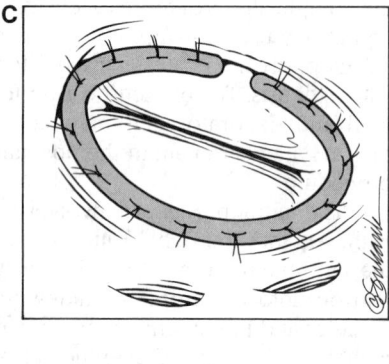

Figure 30–8. Annuloplasty ring insertion. (**A**) Mitral valve regurgitation; leaflets do not close. (**B**) Insertion of an annuloplasty ring. (**C**) Completed valvuloplasty; leaflets close.

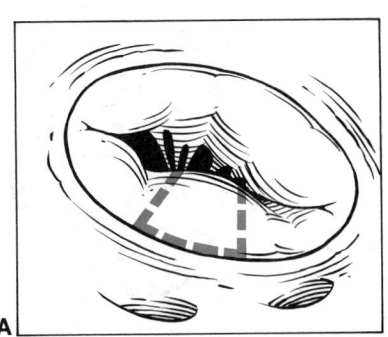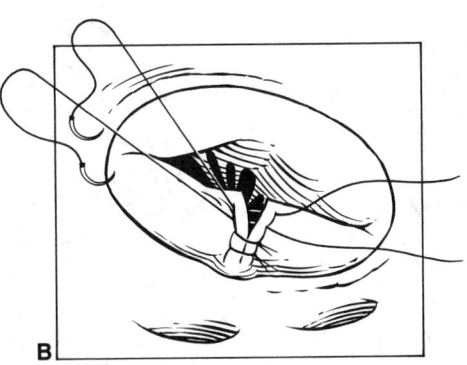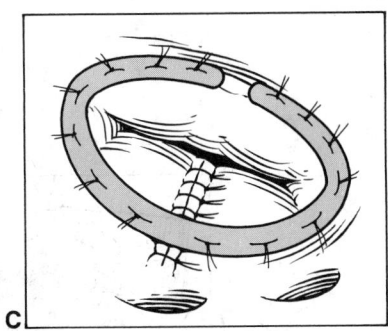

Figure 30-9. Valve leaflet resection and repair with a ring annuloplasty. (**A**) Mitral valve regurgitation; the section indicated by dashed lines will be excised. (**B**) Approximation of edges and suturing. (**C**) Completed valvuloplasty, leaflet repair, and annuloplasty ring.

Once the valve is visualized, the leaflets, and other valve structures such as chordae and papillary muscles, are removed. (There is some evidence to suggest that the posterior mitral valve leaflet, its chordae, and papillary muscles should be left *in situ* to maintain the shape and function of the left ventricle.) Sutures are placed around the annulus and then into the valve prosthesis. The replacement valve is slid down the suture into position and tied into place (Fig. 30–11). The incision is closed and the surgeon evaluates the function of the heart and quality of the prosthetic repair. The patient is weaned from cardiopulmonary bypass and surgery is completed. Complications unique to valve replacement are related to the sudden changes in intracardiac blood pressures; before surgery the heart gradually adjusted to the pathology, but the surgery abruptly "corrects" the way blood flows through the heart.

Three types of valve prostheses may be used—mechanical valves, xenografts, and homografts (Fig. 30–12). The mechanical valves are of the ball and cage or disc design. Mechanical valves are thought to be more durable than the other types of prosthetic valves and often are used for younger patients. Thromboemboli are significant complications associated with mechanical valves, so long-term anticoagulation with warfarin is required.

Xenografts are tissue valves (bioprostheses, heterografts); most are porcine but bovine valves may also be used. Their viability is 7 to 10 years. They are not thrombogenic, thus eliminating the need for long-term anticoagulation. They are used for women of childbearing age, as the potential complications of warfarin administration associated with menses and placental transfer to a fetus, as well as those associated with delivery of

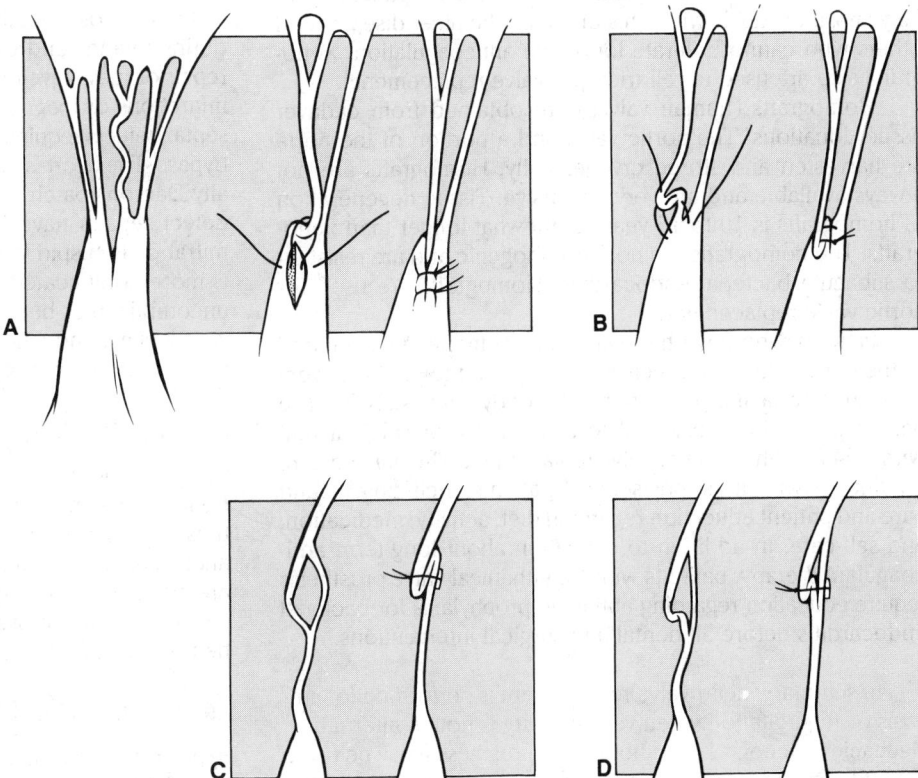

Figure 30-10. Chordoplasty to shorten elongated chordae. (**A**) Bury/trench technique. (**B–D**) Tucks that have been taken to shorten the chordae.

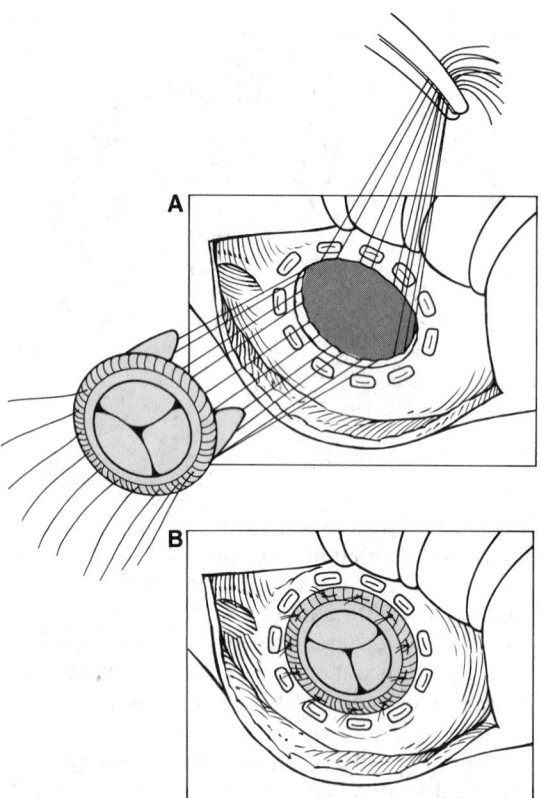

Figure 30–11. Illustration of a valve replacement. (**A**) Native valve excised and prosthetic valve inserted; (**B**) Completed valve replacement.

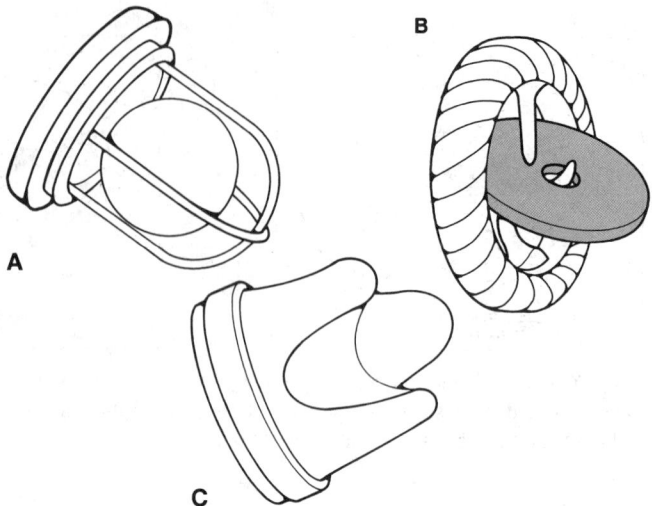

Figure 30–12. Common mechanical and biologic valve replacements. (**A**) Caged ball valve (Starr-Edwards/mechanical). (**B**) Tilting-disc valve (Medtronic-Hall/mechanical). (**C**) Porcine heterograft valve (Carpenter-Edwards/biologic).

a child, do not exist. Xenografts also are used for patients over 70 years, individuals with a history of peptic ulcer disease, and others who cannot tolerate long-term anticoagulation. Xenografts also are used for all tricuspid valve replacements.

Homografts (human valves) are obtained from cadaver tissue donations. The aortic valve and a portion of the aorta are harvested and stored cryogenically. Homografts are not always available and are very expensive. Tissue degeneration of homografts is 10 to 15 years, somewhat longer than xenografts. The homografts are not thrombogenic and are resistant to subacute bacterial endocarditis. Homografts are used for aortic valve replacement.

Patients who have had valve replacements are admitted to the critical care unit; their care is directed toward recovery from anesthesia and promotion of hemodynamic stability. The patient is usually transferred to a telemetry or surgical unit within 24 to 72 hours after valve replacement. The nursing care continues as for most postsurgical patients, including wound care and patient education regarding diet, activity, medication, and self-care. In addition to education about long-term anticoagulant therapy, patients with a mechanical valve prosthesis require education regarding antibiotic prophylaxis for bacterial endocarditis before all dental and surgical interventions.

In summary, heart valve replacement is performed for stenosis or regurgitation when valvuloplasty is not an alternative. Mechanical, xenograft, and homograft prostheses may be used. The sudden change in hemodynamics, as well as the procedure,

puts the patient at risk for many postoperative complications. These include bleeding, thromboembolism, infection, congestive heart failure, hypertension, dysrhythmias, hemolysis, and mechanical obstruction. Nursing care involves recovery from anesthesia, maintaining hemodynamic stability, and patient education.

Septal Repair

The atrial or ventricular septum may have an abnormal opening between the right and left sides of the heart: a septal defect. Although most septal defects are congenital and are repaired during infancy and childhood, adults may not have had early repair or may develop septal defects as a result of myocardial infarctions or diagnostic and treatment procedures. Repair of septal defects requires general anesthesia and cardiopulmonary bypass. The heart is opened and a pericardial or synthetic (usually Dacron) patch is used to close the opening. Atrial septal defect repairs have low morbidity and mortality. When the mitral or tricuspid valve is involved, however, the procedure is more complicated. Generally, ventricular septal repairs are uncomplicated, but the proximity of the defect to the intraventricular conduction system and the valves may make this repair more complex.

Left Ventricular Aneurysmectomy

Symptomatic left ventricular aneurysms may be surgically treated. The most common procedure, under general anesthesia and using cardiopulmonary bypass, is resection of the aneurysm. Less commonly, the aneurysm is plicated—folds are made of the aneurysm and sutured in place. Complications include ventricular dysrhythmias, heart failure, thromboemboli, hemorrhage, and infection.

Cardiomyopathy Surgery

Hypertrophic cardiomyopathies may impair outflow of blood from the left ventricle to the aorta. When the patient becomes symptomatic despite medical therapy and when a difference in pressure of 50 mm Hg or more exists between the left ventricle and the aorta, surgery is considered. The most common procedure is a myectomy (sometimes referred to as a myotomy–myectomy). Septal tissue approximately 1 cm wide and deep is cut from the enlarged septum below the aortic valve. The length of septum removed depends on the degree of obstruction caused by the hypertrophied muscle.

Instead of a septal myectomy, the left ventricle's outflow tract to the aortic valve may be opened by removing the mitral valve, chordae, and papillary muscles. The mitral valve then is replaced with a low-profile disc valve. The space taken up by the mitral valve is then much less and blood is able to move around the enlarged septum to the aortic valve in the area that the mitral valve previously occupied.

The primary complication of both procedures is dysrhythmia; in addition, the patient is at risk for the surgical complications described elsewhere in this chapter.

Transplantation

The first human-to-human heart transplant was performed in 1967. Since then transplant procedures, equipment, and medications have continued to improve. In 1983, cyclosporine became available for general use. Cyclosporine is an immunosuppressant that greatly decreases the body's ability to reject foreign proteins such as transplanted organs. Unfortunately cyclosporine also decreases the body's ability to resist infections, so a fine balance must be achieved between suppressing rejection and avoiding infection. Since the advent of cyclosporine in 1983, heart transplantation has become a therapeutic option for patients with end-stage heart disease.

Cardiomyopathy, ischemic heart disease, congenital heart disease, valvular disease, and rejection of previously transplanted hearts are the most common indications for transplantation. Candidates usually have severe symptoms uncontrolled by medical therapy, no other surgical options, and a prognosis of less than 12 months to live. Potential patients are screened by a multidisciplinary team before becoming candidates. The patient's age, pulmonary status, other chronic health conditions, infections, history of other transplants, compliance, and current health status are considered in the evaluation for transplantation.

When a donated heart becomes available, a computer generates a list of potential recipients on the basis of ABO blood group compatibility, sizes of donor and candidate, as well as the distance between the donor and potential recipient (distance is a variable because the transplanted heart's function is dependent on its being implanted within 4 hours of being harvested from the donor).

The most common surgical procedure is the orthotopic transplant (Fig. 30–13). A portion of the recipient's atria (with the vena cava and pulmonary veins) is left in place: the remainder of the candidate's heart is removed from the mediastinum. The donor heart, which usually has been preserved in ice, is prepared for implant by cutting away a small section of the atria that corresponds with the sections of the recipient's heart that were left in place. The donor heart is then implanted by suturing the donor atria to the residual atrial tissue of the recipient's native heart. The pulmonary artery and aorta are then anastomosed.

Less commonly the heterotopic technique is performed (Fig. 30–14). The donor heart is placed to the right and slightly

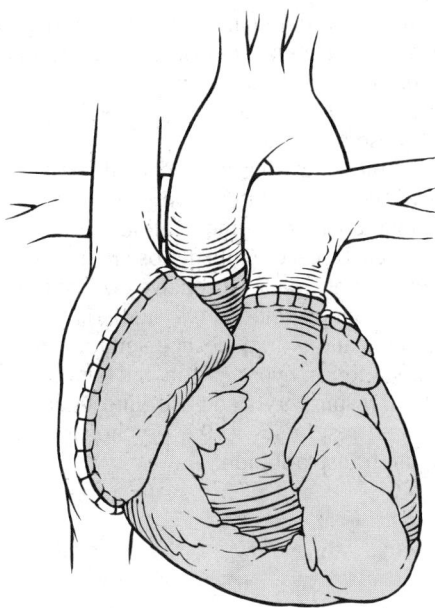

Figure 30–13. Orthotopic method of heart transplantation.

anterior to the recipient's heart; the recipient's heart is not removed. Initially it was thought that the original heart might provide some protection for the patient in the event that the transplanted heart was rejected. Although the protective effect has not necessarily been proven, other reasons for retaining the original heart have been identified: a small donor heart, a prolonged ischemic time for the donor heart, or a donor heart that may have been otherwise compromised but must be used in an emergency.

The transplanted heart does not have nerve connections with the recipient's body (denervated heart); thus the sympathetic and vagus nerves do not affect the transplanted heart. The resting rate of the transplanted heart is approximately 70 to 90 beats per minute, but will increase gradually if cate-

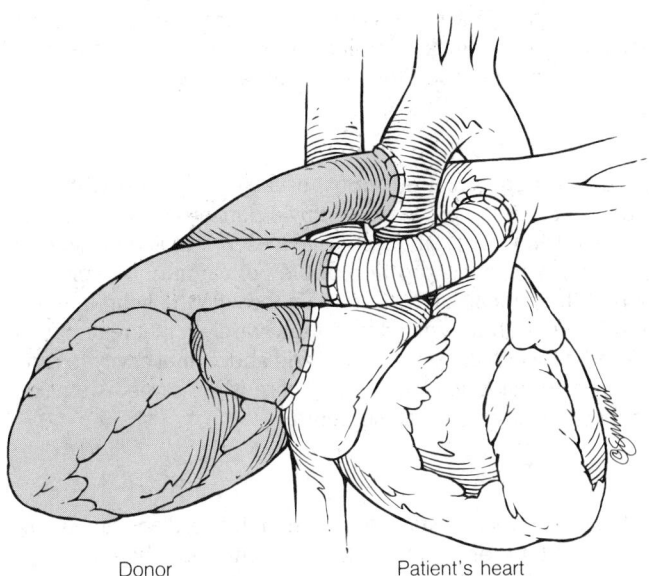

Donor   Patient's heart

Figure 30–14. Heterotopic method of heart transplantation.

cholamines are in the circulation. Patients must *gradually* increase and decrease their exercise (extended warm-up and cool-down periods), as 20 to 30 minutes may be required to achieve the desired heart rate. Atropine will not increase the heart rate of these patients.

Heart transplant patients are constantly balancing the risk of rejection with the risk of infection. They must comply with a complex regimen of diet, medications, activity, follow-up laboratory studies, biopsies (to diagnose rejection), and clinic visits. Most commonly, patients receive cyclosporine and corticosteroids to minimize rejection. In addition to rejection and infection, complications include accelerated arteriosclerosis of the coronary arteries, hypertension and hypotension, central nervous system, respiratory, and gastrointestinal disturbances, renal failure, and responses to the psychosocial stresses imposed by organ transplantation.

In summary, heart transplantation is a treatment option for some patients with end-stage cardiac disease. Cyclosporine and corticosteroids are the primary medications used today to suppress rejection of the transplanted heart. The medications must be carefully balanced to avoid making the patient susceptible to infection. Patients regain strength and obtain symptomatic relief from their disease, but must maintain lifelong compliance with a variety of diet, activity, medication, and follow-up regimens. The 1-year survival rate for heart transplant patients is approximately 80% to 90% and the 5-year survival rate is approximately 60% to 70%.

Tumor Excision

Tumors of the heart are quite rare. Primary tumors occur in less than 1% of the population; metastatic tumors have been reported to occur in 1.5% to 35% of oncology patients. Tumors may be a site for thrombus formation and therefore create a risk of embolism. Dysrhythmias may occur as the myocardium or conduction system is affected. Most cardiac tumors are benign. Surgical excision is performed only to prevent obstruction of a chamber or valve. Cardiopulmonary bypass is used, except for epicardial tumors, which can be excised without entering the heart and without stopping the heart from beating. The tumor location may necessitate valve replacement, myocardial patching, or pacemaker implantation. The nursing care is the same as that described for other cardiac surgery.

Pericardiotomy

Recurrent pericardial effusions, usually associated with neoplastic diseases, may be treated by a pericardiotomy (pericardial window). General anesthesia is used, but seldom cardiopulmonary bypass. A portion of the pericardium is excised to permit the pericardial fluid to drain through the lymphatic system into the abdominal cavity. More rarely, catheters may be placed between the pericardium and abdominal cavity to drain the pericardial fluid. The nursing care is the same as that described for other cardiac surgery.

Trauma Repair

Patients who receive surgical treatment for cardiac trauma have survived blunt force, gunshot, or stab injuries. The repairs are typically to the valves or septum in blunt force injuries, and to the ventricular and atrial walls in penetrating injuries. The wound is debrided and closed surgically when possible, but valve repair and replacement or patch grafts of the septum and atrial or ventricular walls may be required. The surgery is often emergent, so the risk of complications from the injury and surgery is high. The nursing care is the same as that described for other cardiac surgery.

Mechanical Assist Devices/Total Artificial Hearts

The use of cardiopulmonary bypass for cardiovascular surgery and the possibility of performing heart transplantation for end-stage cardiac disease have promoted the need for cardiac assist devices. Patients who cannot be weaned from cardiopulmonary bypass or patients who are in cardiogenic shock may benefit from a period of mechanical heart assistance. The most commonly used device is the intra-aortic balloon pump (IABP). The IABP decreases the work of the heart during contraction, but does not perform the actual work of the heart.

More complex devices that actually perform some or all of the pumping function for the heart also are being used. These more sophisticated ventricular assist devices can circulate as much, if not more, blood per minute as the patient's heart. Each ventricular assist device is used to support one ventricle. Today's most commonly used devices are centrifugal pumps. Many pneumatically driven devices are being used experimentally, and the clinical results are very encouraging (Fig. 30–15). Some ventricular assist devices can be combined with an oxygenator–extracorporeal membrane oxygenation (ECMO). The oxygenator–ventricular assist device combination is used for patients whose heart cannot pump blood through their lungs or their body.

Total artificial hearts are designed to replace both ventricles. The patient's heart must be removed to implant the total artificial heart. All of these devices are experimental. The Jarvik-7 had some short-term success, but the long-term results have been disappointing. Most total artificial heart researchers are hoping to develop a device that can be permanently implanted and that will eliminate the need for donated human heart transplantation for the treatment of end-stage cardiac disease.

Ventricular assist devices and total artificial hearts currently are being used as temporary treatments while the patient's own heart recovers or until a donor heart becomes available for transplant. Bleeding disorders, hemorrhage, thrombus, emboli, hemolysis, infection, and mechanical failure are some of the complications of ventricular assist devices and total artificial hearts. The nursing care for these patients focuses not only on assessing and minimizing these complications, but also must involve emotional support and education about the mechanical assist device.

Cardiac Conduction System Surgery

Antitachycardia Surgical Interventions

Atrial and ventricular tachycardias refractory to medications and not amenable to antitachycardia pacing may be treated by methods other than medications and pacemakers. These procedures usually are performed in the operating room under

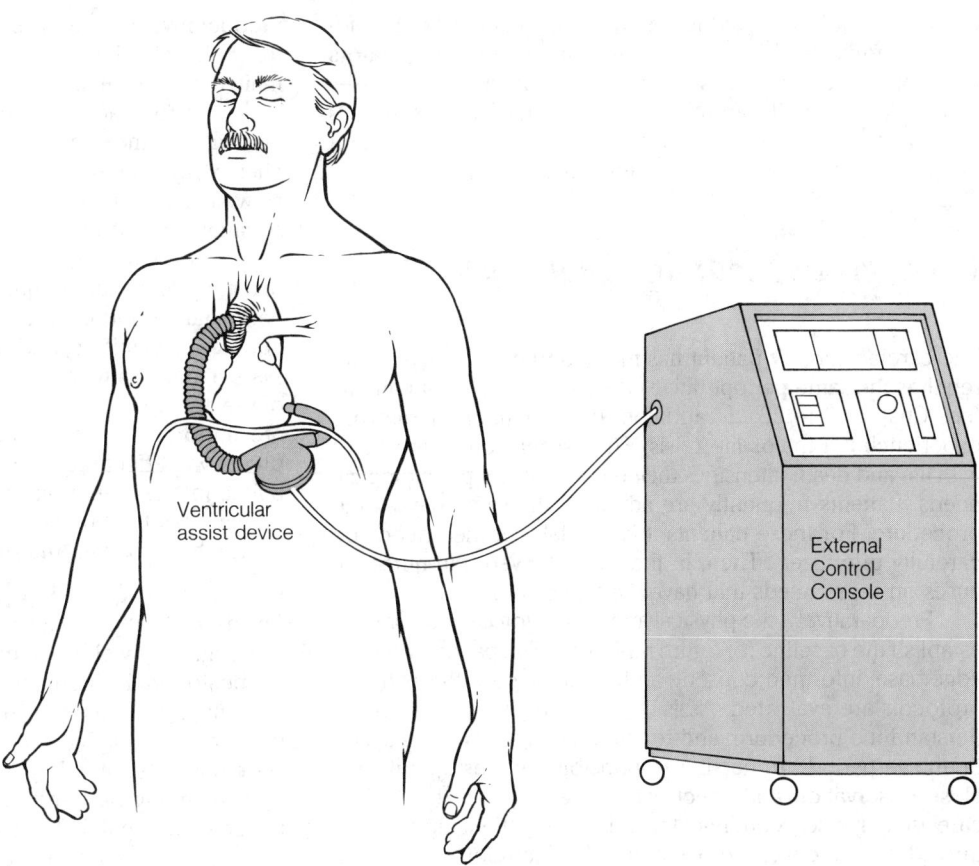

Figure 30–15. Left ventricular assist device.

general anesthesia. The first procedure is endocardial isolation. An incision is made into the endocardium separating the origin of the dysrhythmia from the surrounding endocardium. The edges of the incision are then sutured back together. The incision and its resulting scar tissue prevent the dysrhythmia from affecting the whole heart. A second surgical intervention is endocardial resection. The source of the dysrhythmia is identified and that area of the endocardium is peeled away. No reconstruction or repair is necessary. A third procedure is cryoablation. A special probe, cooled to a temperature of −60°C, is placed on the endocardium at the site of the dysrhythmia's origin for 2 minutes. The frozen area becomes a small scar and the origin of the dysrhythmia is eliminated. A fourth approach is electrical ablation. A catheter is placed at or near the origin of the dysrhythmia, and one to four shocks of 100 to 300 joules are administered through the catheter directly to the endocardium and surrounding tissue. The cardiac tissue is burned and scars, thus eliminating the source of the dysrhythmia. A fifth procedure has been used most recently—radiofrequency ablation. A special catheter is placed at or near the origin of the dysrhythmia. High-frequency sound waves are passed through the catheter, destroying the dysrhythmic tissue. The tissue damage is more specific to the dysrhythmic tissue with less trauma to the surrounding cardiac tissue than occurs with cryoablation or electrical ablation.

Cardioverter/defibrillators (implantable cardioverter defibrillator [ICD]) (Fig. 29–13) may be used in conjunction with the other surgical interventions previously described. The cardioverter/defibrillators are designed to terminate life-threatening dysrhythmias when they occur. Two leads are placed on or in the heart to sense the rhythm, and two electrodes are placed to cardiovert or defibrillate. The devices require a thoracotomy or subcostal incision for placement of some or all of the leads and defibrillation electrodes. The cardioverter/defibrillator is placed in a subcutaneous pocket in the left upper quadrant of the abdomen, and the lead and patch wires are connected to it. Each time the device detects a life-threatening dysrhythmia, it charges itself to 2 to 42 joules and then shocks the patient. Most devices have the capability of determining if the dysrhythmia is still present and can deliver two to six more shocks. If the dysrhythmia continues beyond that, the cardioverter/defibrillator will not shock the patient again until a normal rhythm has been reestablished.

The cardioverter/defibrillator is best suited for rapid ventricular tachydysrhythmias refractory to medication and documented as responsive to electrical cardioversion/defibrillation by electrophysiologic studies. Cardioverter/defibrillators are not suited for frequent dysrhythmias, because the patient would receive many shocks and the device would not last long (most devices can only cardiovert/defibrillate to a total of 100 to 200 times). It is recommended that family members and friends learn cardiopulmonary resuscitation (CPR) and know how to summon the emergency medical system. The risk to anyone touching the patient at the time of the shock is minimal, as the shocks are low energy and conduct (dissipate) through the patient's chest tissue before reaching the skin.

In summary, symptomatic tachydysrhythmias refractory to medications and antitachycardia pacemakers may be treated surgically. Surgical approaches include isolating, removing, or destroying the source of the dysrhythmia and implanting a device to terminate the dysrhythmia. Cardioverter/defibrillators used for sudden-death dysrhythmias, may be quite effective—however, the family and friends of sudden-death survivors should be encouraged to learn cardiopulmonary resuscitation and know how to use the emergency medical system.

Perioperative Nursing Management

The cardiac surgery patient has many of the same needs and requires the same perioperative care as other surgical patients (see Chaps. 20 to 22). In addition, the patient and family are experiencing a major life crisis. The association of the heart with life and death intensifies their emotional and psychological needs. Patients frequently are admitted the same day as the procedure. For these patients it is crucial that their needs be carefully prioritized. Then, in the time allowed, the nurse focuses on those needs that have the highest priority.

Preoperatively, the physical and psychological assessments establish the baseline for future reference. The patient's knowledge base, informed consent, and compliance with treatment protocols are evaluated. Assisting the patient to cope, to understand the procedure, and to maintain dignity during a safe operative period are nursing responsibilities. Postoperatively, close observation and specialized care begin in the critical care unit. Nurses continue to assist the patient and family through the recovery process on the step-down unit and through the rehabilitation phases until the patient and family are able to manage their own care.

Preoperative Nursing Management

The preoperative phase of cardiac surgery usually begins before hospitalization. Other disease conditions (diabetes, high blood pressure, chronic obstructive pulmonary disease, respiratory, endocrine, gastrointestinal [GI], genitourinary [GU], integumentary, and hematologic disorders) are treated and stabilized. Cardiac function is optimized; heart failure, dysrhythmias, and fluid and electrolyte imbalances are minimized. Sources of infection (dental, periodontal, integumentary, and GI infection) are investigated and treated.

Patients may be instructed to alter their medication regimen before surgery, such as tapering steroids and digoxin as well as decreasing or discontinuing anticoagulants. Medications for control of blood pressure, angina, diabetes, and dysrhythmia often are maintained until surgery. Maintaining activity patterns, a balanced diet, good sleep habits, and cessation of smoking are essential for minimizing the risks of surgery. Anxiety-reducing medications may be prescribed before surgery, to prevent the sympathetic responses of increased heart rate and blood pressure that may increase the patient's cardiac symptoms.

▶ Nursing Process
The Patient Awaiting Cardiac Surgery
▷ Assessment

Patients with nonacute heart disease may be admitted to the hospital the day before or the day of their surgery. Most of the preoperative evaluation is completed before the patient enters the hospital. Many surgeons' offices or hospitals will have mailed an information packet to the patient's home.

A history and physical examination are performed by nursing and medical personnel. The patient also may have a chest x-ray, electrocardiogram (ECG), and laboratory analyses as well as typing and cross-matching of blood. The health assessment focuses on obtaining baseline physiologic, psychological, and social information. The patient's and family's teaching needs are identified and addressed as necessary. Of particular importance is the patient's usual functional level, coping mechanisms, and support systems. The family support system and coping mechanisms, as well as the physical layout of the anticipated discharge environment, are assessed. These are important because the support of the family/significant others will affect the patient's postoperative course and rehabilitation. Discharge plans will be influenced by the life style demands of the home situation and the physical environment to which the patient returns after hospitalization.

▷ Health Assessment

The preoperative history and health assessment should be thorough and well documented because they provide a basis for postoperative comparison. A systematic assessment of all systems is performed, with emphasis on assessment of cardiovascular functioning. Functional status of the cardiovascular system is determined by reviewing the patient's symptomatology, including past and present experiences with chest pain, hypertension, palpitations, dyspnea, cyanosis, orthopnea, paroxysmal nocturnal dyspnea, peripheral edema, and intermittent claudication. Because alterations in cardiac output can affect renal, respiratory, gastrointestinal, integumentary, hematologic, and neurologic functioning, these systems also are assessed thoroughly. History of major illnesses, surgeries, and drug therapies, and use of drugs, alcohol, and tobacco are also explored. A complete physical examination is performed, with special emphasis on the following parameters:

- General appearance and behavior
- Vital signs
- Nutritional and fluid status, weight, and height
- Inspection and palpation of the heart, noting the point of maximal impulse (PMI), abnormal pulsations, thrills
- Auscultation of the heart, noting pulse rate, rhythm, and quality, S_3, S_4, snaps, clicks, murmurs, friction rub
- Jugular venous pressure
- Peripheral pulses
- Peripheral edema

▷ Psychosocial Assessment

The psychosocial assessment and the assessment of teaching–learning needs of the patient and family are as important as the physical examination. Anticipation of cardiac surgery is a source of great stress to the patient and family. They will be anxious and fearful and will have many unanswered questions. Their anxiety usually increases with the patient's admission to the hospital and the immediacy of surgery. An assessment of the level of anxiety is important. If it is low, this may indicate denial. If it is extremely high, it may interfere with the use of effective coping mechanisms and with preoperative teaching. Questions are asked to obtain the following information about both the patient and the family:

- The meaning of the surgery to the patient and family
- Coping mechanisms that are being used

- Measures used in the past to deal with stress
- Anticipated changes in life style
- Support systems in effect
- Fears regarding the present and the future
- Knowledge and understanding of the operative procedure, postoperative course, and long-term rehabilitation

Adequate time should be allowed for the patient and family to express their fears. The fears most often expressed are fear of the unknown, fear of pain, fear of body image change, and fear of dying.

Fear of the Unknown.   This fear is difficult to express. Lack of past experience with heart surgery does not provide sufficient detail to attach fears to any specific aspects. Instead of specific fears, which can be identified and for which coping mechanisms can be used, the patient and family often express a generalized dread.

Fear of Pain.   The patient may openly express a fear of pain and the inability to tolerate it, or may indirectly express this fear by asking many questions about pain, pain medications, and the process of recovering from anesthesia. The family may fear that they will be unable to cope with watching the patient experience pain.

Fear of Body Image Change.   Many patients have a fear of the scarring from surgery. This fear is frequently exaggerated because of lack of information. Patients may talk openly about this fear or express it indirectly through concern about continued love from others or excessive focus on postoperative pain.

Fear of Dying.   Some patients verbalize their fear of dying. Others only hint about their concern, such as questioning why they need to know about their surgery and postoperative course, asking for reassurance that someone will care for their family on the day of surgery, or becoming tearful around their family members or telling them to wait at home on the day of surgery. Likewise, family members who do not openly express their fear often will verbalize similar concerns.

During the assessment, the nurse determines how much the patient and family know about the impending surgery and the expected postoperative events. They are encouraged to ask questions and to indicate how much information they wish to have. Some patients prefer not to have detailed information, while others want to know as much as possible. Patients should be approached as unique individuals with their own specific learning needs, learning styles, and levels of understanding.

Patients requiring emergency heart surgery may have both cardiac catheterization and surgery within several hours of admission. The nurse will have little opportunity to assess and meet their emotional and teaching needs before surgery. As a result, they will need extra help postoperatively to adjust to the situation.

▷ Nursing Diagnoses

The nursing diagnoses for patients awaiting cardiac surgery will vary from patient to patient according to their cardiac disease process or abnormality and their symptomatology. The majority of patients will have a nursing diagnosis of decreased cardiac output (see Cardiac Failure in Chap. 29). In addition, preoperative nursing diagnoses for most patients will include the following:

- Fear related to the surgical procedure, its uncertain outcome, and the threat to well-being

- Knowledge deficit regarding the surgical procedure and the postoperative course

▷ Planning and Implementation

▷   *Goals:*   The major goals of the patient may include reduction of fear and learning about the surgical procedure and postoperative course.

▷ Nursing Interventions

During the preoperative phase of cardiac surgery, the nurse develops a plan of care that includes emotional support and teaching for the patient and family. Establishing rapport, answering questions, listening to fears and concerns, clarifying misconceptions, and providing information about what to expect are all interventions the nurse uses to prepare the patient and family emotionally for the surgery and for the postoperative events.

▷   *Reduction of Fear.*   The patient and family are allowed adequate time and repeated opportunities to express their fears. If there is fear of the unknown, other surgical experiences that the patient has had can be compared with the impending surgery. It is often helpful to describe to the patient the sensations that are expected. If the patient has already had a cardiac catheterization, the similarities and differences between that and the surgery may be compared. Also, the patient is encouraged to talk about any concerns related to previous experiences.

Discussion of the patient's fears about pain is initiated. A comparison between the pain experienced with cardiac surgery and other pain experiences is made. The preoperative sedation, the anesthetic, and the postoperative pain medications are described. The patient is reassured that the fear of pain is normal. It is explained that some pain will be experienced, but that the patient will be closely observed and that the use of medication, positioning, and relaxation will make the pain more tolerable.

Patients who have a fear of scarring from surgery are encouraged to discuss this. Misconceptions are corrected. It may be helpful to indicate that the health care team members will keep the patient informed about the healing process.

The patient and family are encouraged to talk about their fear of dying. They should be reassured that this fear is normal. For those who only hint about this concern despite efforts to encourage them to talk about their fear, coaching is helpful (*e.g.,* "Are you worrying about not making it through surgery? Most people who have heart surgery at least think about the possibility of dying."). Once the fear is expressed, the patient and family can be helped to explore their feelings.

By alleviating undue anxiety and fear, emotional preparation of the patient for surgery lessens the chance of preoperative problems, promotes smooth anesthesia induction, and enhances the patient's involvement postoperatively in care and recovery. In addition, preparation of the family for the events to come helps them to cope, to be supportive to the patient, and to participate in the postoperative and rehabilitative care.

▷   *Learning About the Surgical Procedure and Postoperative Course.*   Patient teaching is based on assessed learning needs. Teaching usually includes information about hospitalization, about the surgery (the preoperative care, the length of the surgery, what the patient will feel like, the visiting hours and procedures in the critical care unit), and about the recovery phase (length of hospitalization, when normal activities, such as housework, shopping, and work, can be resumed). Any changes made in medical therapy and preoperative preparations need to be explained and reinforced.

The patient is told that physical preparation usually involves several showers or scrubs with an antiseptic solution. Medication for sleep will be given the night before surgery and sedation just before surgery. Most cardiac surgical teams use prophylactic antibiotic therapy, and the antibiotics are started preoperatively.

If the preoperative hospitalization period is very short, teaching of the patient and family together may be most effective. The patient's anxiety increases with the admission process and the impending surgery. Unless the nurse has met the patient before the day of hospitalization, the time may be too short to establish a relationship that contributes to patient learning. Teaching of the patient and family together capitalizes on their established support relationship. Teaching in this phase should be directed primarily by the patient's and family's questions. Too much detail may only increase anxiety. The patient may be offered a tour of the intensive care unit, the postanesthesia recovery room, or both. (In some hospitals, the patient will initially go to the postanesthesia unit.) The patient recovering from anesthesia is reassured by having already seen and heard the environment and having met someone from the unit. The patient and family are informed about the equipment, tubes, and lines that will be present postoperatively and their purposes. They should know to expect several intravenous lines, chest tubes, and a urinary catheter. Explaining the purpose and the approximate time that these will be in place helps to reassure the patient. Most patients will remain intubated and on mechanical ventilation for 4 to 48 hours postoperatively. They need to be aware that this prevents them from talking, and they should be reassured that the staff are skilled in other ways to assess their needs.

The patient's questions about postoperative care and procedures should be answered. Deep breathing and coughing, using the incentive spirometer, and foot exercises are explained and practiced by the patient preoperatively. The family's questions at this time will focus primarily on the length of the surgery, who will discuss the results of the procedure with them and when this may occur, where to wait during the surgery, the visiting privileges in the intensive care unit, and how they can support the patient preoperatively and in the intensive care unit.

▷ Evaluation

Expected Outcomes

1. Experiences reduction of fear
   a. Identifies fears
   b. Discusses fears with family
   c. Uses past experiences as a focus for comparison
   d. Expresses positive attitude about outcome of surgery
   e. Expresses confidence in measures to be used to relieve pain
2. Acquires knowledge about the surgical procedure and postoperative course
   a. Identifies the purposes of the preoperative preparation procedure
   b. Tours the intensive care unit, if desired and appropriate
   c. Identifies limitations expected after surgery
   d. Discusses expected immediate postoperative environment, eg, tubes, machines, nursing surveillance

   e. Demonstrates expected activities after surgery (*e.g.*, deep breathing, coughing, foot exercises)

Intraoperative Nursing Management

Most of the surgical procedures previously described are performed through a median sternotomy incision. The patient is prepared for continuous monitoring: electrodes, indwelling catheters and probes are placed before the procedure to facilitate assessment of the patient's status and the need for changes in therapy. Intravenous lines will be inserted as needed for administration of fluids, medications, and blood products. In addition, the patient will be intubated and placed on mechanical ventilation.

Before the chest incision is closed, chest tubes are positioned to evacuate air and drainage from the mediastinum and the thorax. Epicardial pacemaker electrodes are implanted on the surface of the right atrium and the right ventricle. These epicardial electrodes can be used postoperatively to pace the heart or to monitor the heart for dysrhythmia differentiation with the atrial leads.

In addition to assistance with the surgical, anesthetic, and extracorporeal procedures, the surgical nurses are responsible for the comfort and safety of the patient. Some of their areas of intervention include emotional support of the patient and family, positioning, skin care, and wound care.

Possible intraoperative complications include dysrhythmias, hemorrhage, myocardial infarction, cerebral vascular accident, embolization, and organ failure secondary to shock, embolus, or adverse drug reactions. Astute intraoperative patient assessment is critical in preventing these complications and in detecting symptoms and initiating prompt therapy.

Postoperative Nursing Management

The immediate postoperative period for the patient who has undergone cardiac surgery presents many challenges to the health team. All efforts are made to facilitate the transition from the operating room to the intensive care unit or postanesthesia suite with a minimum of risk. Specific information about the operation and important factors about postoperative management are communicated by the surgical team and anesthesia personnel to the critical care nurse, who then assumes responsibility for the patient's care (Fig. 30–16).

▶ Nursing Process
The Patient Who Has Had Cardiac Surgery

▷ *Assessment*

When the patient is admitted to the critical care unit, and at least every 4 to 12 hours thereafter, a complete systematic assessment is performed to determine the postoperative status of the patient as compared with the preoperative baseline and anticipated changes since surgery. Assessment of the following parameters is performed:

* *Neurologic status*—level of responsiveness, pupil size and reaction to light, reflexes, movement of extremities, and hand grip strength

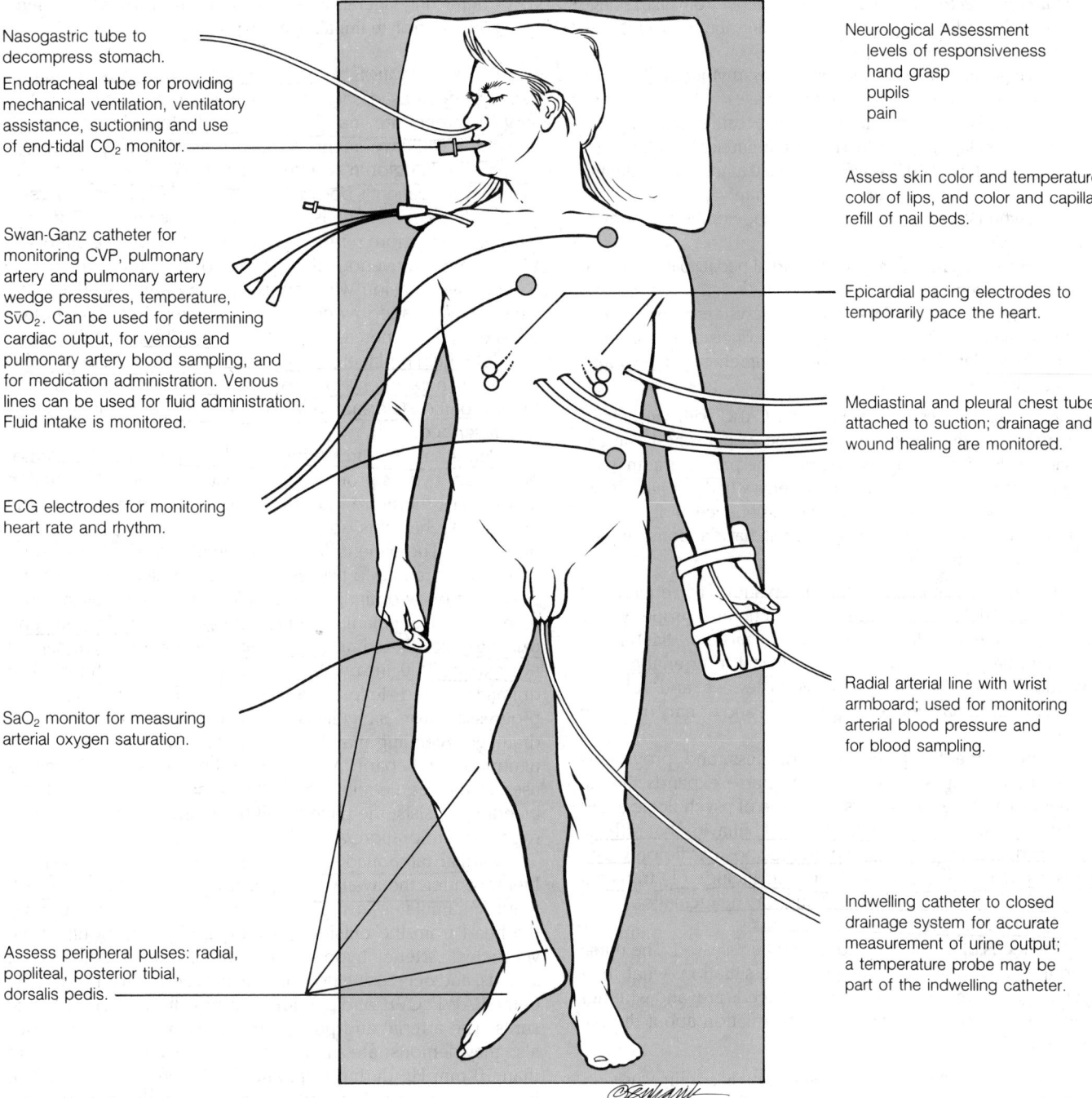

Nasogastric tube to decompress stomach.

Endotracheal tube for providing mechanical ventilation, ventilatory assistance, suctioning and use of end-tidal CO_2 monitor.

Swan-Ganz catheter for monitoring CVP, pulmonary artery and pulmonary artery wedge pressures, temperature, $S\bar{v}O_2$. Can be used for determining cardiac output, for venous and pulmonary artery blood sampling, and for medication administration. Venous lines can be used for fluid administration. Fluid intake is monitored.

ECG electrodes for monitoring heart rate and rhythm.

SaO_2 monitor for measuring arterial oxygen saturation.

Assess peripheral pulses: radial, popliteal, posterior tibial, dorsalis pedis.

Neurological Assessment
  levels of responsiveness
  hand grasp
  pupils
  pain

Assess skin color and temperature, color of lips, and color and capillary refill of nail beds.

Epicardial pacing electrodes to temporarily pace the heart.

Mediastinal and pleural chest tubes attached to suction; drainage and wound healing are monitored.

Radial arterial line with wrist armboard; used for monitoring arterial blood pressure and for blood sampling.

Indwelling catheter to closed drainage system for accurate measurement of urine output; a temperature probe may be part of the indwelling catheter.

Figure 30–16. Postoperative care of the cardiac surgical patient.

- *Cardiac status*—heart rate and rhythm, heart sounds, arterial blood pressure, central venous pressure (CVP), pulmonary artery pressure, pulmonary artery wedge pressure (PAWP), left atrial pressure (LAP), waveforms from the invasive blood pressure lines, cardiac output/index, systemic and pulmonary vascular resistance, pulmonary artery oxygen saturation ($S\bar{v}O_2$) if available, chest tube drainage, and pacemaker status and function
- *Respiratory status*—chest movement, breath sounds, venti-

lator settings (rate, tidal volume, oxygen concentration, mode [*e.g.,* IMV], positive end-expiratory pressure [PEEP], respiratory rate, ventilatory pressure, arterial oxygen saturation (SaO_2), end-tidal CO_2, chest tube drainage, arterial blood gases
- *Peripheral vascular status*—peripheral pulses; color of skin, nail beds, mucosa, lips and earlobes; skin temperature; edema; condition of dressings and invasive lines
- *Renal function*—urinary output, urine specific gravity and osmolarity

- *Fluid and electrolyte status*—intake; output from all drainage tubes; all cardiac output parameters, and the following indications of electrolyte imbalance:

  Hypokalemia: digitalis toxicity, dysrhythmias (U wave, AV block, flat or inverted T waves)

  Hyperkalemia: mental confusion, restlessness, nausea, weakness, paresthesias of extremities, dysrhythmias (tall, peaked T waves; increased amplitude; widening QRS complex; prolonged QT interval)

  Hyponatremia: weakness, fatigue, confusion, convulsions, coma

  Hypocalcemia: paresthesias, carpal pedal spasm, muscle cramps, tetany

  Hypercalcemia: digitalis toxicity, asystole

- *Pain*—nature, type, location, duration (incisional pain must be differentiated from anginal pain); apprehension; response to analgesics

- Note: Some patients who have had CABG with an internal mammary artery experience ulnar nerve paresthesia on the same side of the body as the graft. The paresthesia may be temporary or permanent. Also, patients who have had CABG with the gastroepiploic artery may experience an ileus for a longer period postoperatively and will have abdominal pain as well as chest pain.

Assessment also includes the observation of all equipment and tubes to determine if they are functioning properly: endotracheal tube, ventilator, end-tidal CO_2 monitor, SaO_2 monitor, pulmonary artery catheter, $S\bar{v}O_2$ monitor, arterial and intravenous lines, intravenous infusion devices and tubings, cardiac monitor, pacemaker, chest tubes, and urinary drainage system.

As the patient regains consciousness and progresses through the postoperative period, the nurse expands the assessment to include parameters indicative of psychological and emotional status. The patient may exhibit behavior that reflects denial or depression, or may experience postcardiotomy psychosis. Characteristic signs of psychosis include (1) transient perceptual illusions, (2) visual and auditory hallucinations, and (3) disorientation and paranoid delusions.

The needs of the family also should be assessed. The nurse ascertains how they are coping with the situation; what their psychological, emotional, and spiritual needs are; and whether or not they are receiving adequate information about the patient's condition.

Assessing for Complications. The patient is continuously assessed for indications of impending complications. The nurse and the physician function collaboratively to recognize early signs and symptoms of complications and to institute measures to reverse their progress.

Decreased Cardiac Output. A decrease in cardiac output is always a threat to the patient who has had cardiac surgery. It can be due to a variety of causes:

- Preload alterations—too little or too much blood volume returning to the heart because of hypovolemia, persistent bleeding, cardiac tamponade, or fluid overload
- Afterload alterations— arterioles and capillaries that are too constricted or too dilated because of alterations in body temperature or hypertension
- Heart rate alterations—too fast, too slow, or dysrhythmias

- Contractility alterations—cardiac failure, myocardial infarction, electrolyte imbalances, hypoxia

Preload Alterations. Hypovolemia is the most common cause of decreased cardiac output after cardiac surgery. The surgical procedure may have involved blood loss, although some of it will have been replaced to provide the patient with sufficient hemoglobin to carry oxygen to the tissues. As the hypothermic patient's body temperature rises, the blood vessels dilate and more volume is needed to fill the vessels. The capillary beds are more permeable as a result of cardiopulmonary bypass, and intravenous fluid is lost to the interstitial spaces. Arterial hypotension with low pulmonary artery wedge pressures (PAWP) and low central venous pressures (CVP) often are seen with an increased heart rate. The physician will usually prescribe fluid replacement with a colloid (albumin or protein) or starch (hetastarch), but packed red blood cells or a crystalloid solution (normal saline, lactated Ringer's solution) may be prescribed.

Persistent bleeding may cause hypovolemia. The cardiopulmonary bypass procedure may cause platelets to function abnormally, therefore blood may not clot normally. Also, the clotting mechanisms do not work well when a patient is hypothermic. The patient has experienced a surgical procedure that causes trauma to tissues and blood vessels that continue to ooze bloody drainage. In addition, the patient usually has received anticoagulants. Accurate measurement of wound and drainage tube bleeding is essential. Bloody drainage should not exceed 200 ml per hour for the first 4 to 6 hours. The drainage should decrease and stop within a few days, while progressing from sanguineous to serosanguineous and serous drainage. Bleeding may be treated with protamine sulfate to neutralize the heparin. Vitamin K and blood products may be used to replace deficiencies of the hematologic system. If the bleeding persists, the patient will be returned to the operating room for exploration; any bleeding sites are then controlled.

Cardiac tamponade also may decrease preload to the heart by preventing the available blood from getting into the heart. Fluid accumulates in the pericardial sac, which compresses the heart from the outside, preventing blood from filling the ventricles. Arterial hypotension, tachycardia, muffled heart sounds, and decreasing urine output are seen with an equalizing of the PAWP, CVP, and pulmonary artery diastolic (PAD) pressures. The arterial and pulmonary artery pressure waveforms also may demonstrate a pulsus paradoxus (a decrease of more than 10 mm Hg during inspiration). The chest tube drainage is usually decreased, suggesting that the drainage is trapped or clotted in the mediastinum. Efforts are made to assure that there are no kinks or obstructions in the tubing. The nurse may try to reestablish patency of the drainage system by milking the tubing (care must be taken not to strip the tubing, creating massive negative pressure within the chest, which may cause harm to the surgical repair or stimulate a dysrhythmia). A chest x-ray may show a widening mediastinum. Emergency medical management is required, which may include a pericardiocentesis (see Chap. 29).

Fluid overload is a less common problem for postcardiac surgery patients. High PAWP, CVP, and pulmonary artery diastolic pressures as well as crackles indicate fluid overload. Diuretics are usually prescribed and the rate of intravenous fluid administration is slowed. The patient may be placed on a fluid restriction. Alternative treatments are continuous arterial–venous hemofiltration, dialysis, and phlebotomy.

Afterload Alterations. Afterload is the force that the ventricle must overcome to move blood forward. Vascular resistance may be calculated to assess afterload and the effects of any vasoactive treatments. The patient's body temperature is the most common cause of alterations in afterload after cardiac surgery. With hypothermia, the blood vessels are constricted, increasing afterload. The treatment is to gradually rewarm the patient, although vasodilators may be required if the resistance is too great to wait for rewarming. Conversely, a fever or other hyperthermic condition dilates blood vessels, decreasing afterload. The treatment is to restore normothermia, but the patient may require vasopressor or volume support during a fever or if the vasodilation is severe.

Hypertension is another cause of increased afterload. Some patients will have a history of this condition and the nurse can anticipate treatment postoperatively. Other patients experience transient hypertension. Vasodilators (nitroglycerine, nitroprusside) may be used to treat hypertension. If hypertension was present before surgery, the patient is returned to the preoperative management regimen as soon as possible.

Heart Rate Alterations. Tachydysrhythmias should first be assessed to establish that they are not the result of preload or afterload alterations. If a tachydysrhythmia is the primary symptom, the heart rhythm is assessed and medications (*e.g.*, digoxin, quinidine, verapamil, esmolol, propranolol, lidocaine, procainamide, bretylium) are prescribed. Carotid massage may be performed by a physician to assist with diagnosing or treating the dysrhythmia. Cardioversion and defibrillation are alternatives for symptomatic tachydysrhythmias.

Bradycardias also may cause symptoms. Many postoperative patients will have temporary pacer wires that can be attached to a pulse generator (pacemaker) to stimulate the heart to beat at a faster rate. Less commonly, atropine, epinephrine, or isoproterenol may be used to increase the heart rate.

Dysrhythmias may or may not affect cardiac output. Those that do affect cardiac output are treated with medications, pacemakers, carotid massage, cardioversion, or defibrillation. The primary goal of treatment is to return the heart to a normal sinus rhythm. Some patients are unable to attain a normal sinus rhythm, so an alternate goal may be to establish a stable rhythm that produces a cardiac output sufficient for the patient.

Contractility Alterations. Cardiac failure results when the heart fails as a pump and the chambers cannot adequately empty (see Chap. 29). The nurse observes for and reports falling mean arterial pressure; rising PAWP, PAD, and CVP; increasing tachycardia; restlessness and agitation; peripheral cyanosis; venous distention; labored respirations; and edema. Medical management includes diuretics and digitalization.

Myocardial infarction may occur intraoperatively or postoperatively. A portion of the cardiac muscle dies; therefore contractility decreases. Until the infarcted area becomes edematous, the ventricular wall will move paradoxically during contractions, further decreasing cardiac output. Symptoms may be masked by the postoperative surgical discomfort or the anesthesia–analgesia regimen. Careful assessment of pain must be made to differentiate the type of pain the patient is experiencing. A myocardial infarction should be suspected if the mean blood pressure is low with normal preload. The systemic vascular resistance (afterload) and heart rate may be elevated to compensate for poor contractility. Serial ECGs and cardiac enzymes assist in making the diagnosis. Analgesics are prescribed in small amounts while the patient's blood pressure and respiratory rate are monitored (because vasodilation secondary to analgesics or decreasing pain may occur and compound the hypotension). Activity progression will depend on the patient's tolerance.

Hypoxia and electrolyte imbalances, such as hypokalemia (see the following section), decrease contractility of the cardiac muscle. Tachycardia and hypotension may be seen. The patient's ventricular stroke work index may be calculated to assist with assessment of contractility.

▷ *Altered Fluid and Electrolyte Balance.* Alterations in fluid and electrolyte balance may occur after cardiac surgery. Nursing assessment for these complications includes monitoring of intake and output, weight, PAWP, PAD, left atrial pressure and CVP readings, hematocrit levels, distention of neck veins, tissue edema, liver size, breath sounds (*i.e.*, fine crackles, wheezing), and electrolyte levels.

Changes in serum electrolytes are reported promptly so that treatment can be instituted. Especially important are dangerously high or low levels of potassium, sodium, and calcium.

Hypokalemia. *Hypokalemia* (low potassium) may be caused by inadequate intake, diuretics, vomiting, diarrhea, excessive nasogastric drainage, and stress due to surgery (increased aldosterone secretion produces decreased potassium-ion [K^+] and increased sodium-ion [Na^+] retention). The patient must be observed carefully when serum potassium rises or falls outside the normal level (K^+ = 3.5 to 5.0 mEq/L [3.5 to 5.0 mmol/L]). Some cardiac surgeons believe that it is important to maintain the K^+ level at 4.0 mEq/L (4.0 mmol/L) or higher to avoid dysrhythmias in the postoperative period. The following effects of low K^+ may be noted: digitalis toxicity, dysrhythmias, metabolic alkalosis, a weakened myocardium, and cardiac arrest. One possible specific ECG change is the presence of a U-wave that is more than 1 mm high. (A *U wave* is a positive deflection following the T wave.) Additional signs are AV block, flat or inverted T waves, and low voltage. When necessary, the physician prescribes intravenous potassium replacement.

Hyperkalemia. *Hyperkalemia* (high potassium) may be caused by increased intake, red cell breakdown caused by cardiopulmonary bypass or mechanical assist devices, acidosis, renal insufficiency, tissue necrosis, and adrenal cortical insufficiency. The following effects of high K^+ may be exhibited: mental confusion, restlessness, nausea, weakness, and paresthesias of the extremities. ECG changes specific for hyperkalemia are tall, peaked T waves, increased amplitude, a widening of the QRS complex, and a prolonged QT interval.

The physician may prescribe an ion exchange resin, sodium polystyrene sulfonate (Kayexalate), which binds the potassium in the GI tract and results in decreased serum potassium. Alternative treatments are intravenous (IV) sodium bicarbonate or IV insulin and glucose to temporarily drive the potassium back into the cells from the extracellular fluid.

Hypernatremia and Hyponatremia. Both *hypernatremia* (high sodium) and *hyponatremia* (low sodium) may occur after cardiac surgery; however, the latter is more common. Hyponatremia may result from a reduction of total body sodium or from an increase in water intake, which causes a dilution of body sodium. The patient must be observed for sodium values that vary from the normal ranges (*i.e.*, normal Na^+ = 135 to 145 mEq/L [135 to 145 mmol/L]). The nurse observes for symptoms of hyponatremia: weakness, fatigue, confusion, convulsions, and coma. When there is a true loss of sodium from the body, the physician prescribes sodium replacement. Diuretics are prescribed when reduction in sodium is due to increased water intake.

Hypocalcemia. *Hypocalcemia* (low calcium) can be caused by alkalosis, which reduces the amount of Ca^{++} in the extracellular fluid. Another cause may be transfusions of large amounts of citrated blood products—packed red blood cells or whole blood. (Most blood banks now use very little citrate to store blood as compared with the amounts used before 1985.) Citrate binds with calcium, reducing the amount of circulating ionized calcium.

The calcium level is monitored to determine if it is within normal limits (Ca^{++} = 8.8 to 10.3 mg/100 ml [2.20 to 2.58 mmol/L]). The nurse assesses the patient for symptoms of reduced calcium: numbness and tingling in the fingertips, toes, ears, and nose; carpal pedal spasm; and muscle cramps and tetany. Any symptoms of hypocalcemia are reported promptly so that the physician can institute calcium replacement immediately.

Hypercalcemia. *Hypercalcemia* (high calcium) can cause dysrhythmias that imitate those caused by digitalis toxicity. Calcium is known to potentiate, or enhance, the action of digitalis. Therefore, the nurse assesses the patient for signs of digitalis toxicity and reports these immediately so that the physician can institute treatment to prevent asystole and death.

Impaired Gas Exchange. Impaired gas exchange is another possible complication after cardiac surgery. All body tissues require an adequate supply of oxygen and nutrients for survival. To achieve this after surgery, an endotracheal tube with ventilator assistance may be used for 4 to 48 or more hours postoperatively. The assisted ventilation is continued until the patient's blood gas measurements are acceptable and the patient demonstrates the ability to breath independently. Patients who are stable after surgery may be extubated as early as 6 hours after surgery, which reduces their anxiety regarding their limited ability to communicate.

The patient is continuously assessed for indications of impaired gas exchange: restlessness, anxiety, cyanosis of mucous membranes and of peripheral tissues, tachycardia, and fighting the ventilator. Breath sounds are assessed frequently to detect fluid in the lungs, and to monitor lung expansion. Arterial blood gases are monitored.

▷ *Impaired Cerebral Circulation.* Brain function is dependent on a continuous supply of oxygenated blood. The brain does not have the capacity to store oxygen and must rely on adequate continuous perfusion by the heart. Thus it is important to observe the patient for any symptoms of hypoxia: restlessness, headache, confusion, dyspnea, hypotension, and cyanosis. Arterial blood gases, SaO_2, $S\bar{v}O_2$, and end-tidal CO_2 are assessed for decreased oxygen and increased carbon dioxide. An hourly assessment of the patient's neurologic status includes level of consciousness, response to verbal commands and painful stimuli, pupillary size and reaction to light, movement of extremities, hand grip strength, presence of pedal and popliteal pulses, and temperature and color of extremities. Any indication of a changing status is documented and any abnormal findings are reported to the surgeon immediately because they may signal the beginning of a complication in the postoperative period. Hypoperfusion or microemboli may produce central nervous system damage after cardiac surgery.

▷ Nursing Diagnoses

Based on the assessment data and the type of surgical procedure performed, major nursing diagnoses of the patient may include the following:

- Decreased cardiac output related to blood loss and compromised myocardial function
- Potential impaired gas exchange related to trauma of extensive chest surgery
- Potential alteration in fluid volume and electrolyte balance related to alteration in circulating blood volume
- Potential sensory–perceptual alterations related to sensory overload (critical care environment, surgical experience)
- Pain related to operative trauma and pleural irritation caused by chest tubes
- Potential alteration in tissue perfusion related to venous stasis, embolization, underlying atherosclerotic disease, effects of vasopressors, or coagulation problems
- Potential alteration in renal perfusion related to decreased cardiac output, hemolysis, or vasopressor drug therapy
- Potential hyperthermia related to infection or postpericardiotomy syndrome
- Knowledge deficit about self-care activities

▷ Planning and Implementation

▷ *Goals:* The major goals of the patient include restoration of cardiac output, adequate gas exchange, maintenance of fluid and electrolyte balance, reduction of symptoms of sensory overload, relief of pain, promotion of rest, maintenance of adequate tissue perfusion, maintenance of adequate renal perfusion, maintenance of normal body temperature, and learning self-care activities.

▷ Nursing Interventions

A typical postoperative nursing care plan for the cardiac surgery patient is presented in Nursing Care Plan 30–1.

▷ *Restoration of Cardiac Output.* Nursing management of the patient involves continuous observation of the patient's cardiac status and immediate notification of the surgeon of any changes that indicate decreased cardiac output. The nurse and the surgeon then work collaboratively to correct the problem.

In evaluating the patient's cardiac status, the nurse primarily determines the effectiveness of cardiac output through clinical observations and routine measurements: serial readings of blood pressure, heart rate, central venous pressure, arterial pressure, and left atrial or pulmonary artery pressure.

Renal function is related to cardiac function, as blood pressure and heart rate drive glomerular filtration; therefore, urinary output is measured and recorded. If urine output falls below 30 ml/hr, this may indicate a decrease in cardiac output.

(text continues on page 729)

Nursing Care Plan 30–1

Postoperative Nursing Care of the Cardiac Surgery Patient

Nursing Interventions	Rationale	Expected Outcomes

Nursing Diagnosis: Decreased cardiac output related to blood loss/volume status, vasoconstriction/vasodilation, tachycardia/brady-cardia/dysrhythmias, and compromised contractility (tamponade, electrolyte imbalances, anoxia, MI)

Goal: Restoration of cardiac output to maintain/attain desired life-style.

1. Monitor cardiovascular status. Serial readings of blood pressures (arterial, left atrial, pulmonary artery, pulmonary artery wedge pressure [PAWP], central venous pressure [CVP]), cardiac output/index, systemic and pulmonary vascular resistance, and cardiac rhythm and rate are obtained, recorded and correlated with the patient's condition.

   a. Assess arterial pressure every 15 minutes until stable, and as directed thereafter.

   b. Auscultate for heart sounds and rhythm.

   c. Assess all peripheral pulses (pedal, tibial, popliteal, femoral, radial, brachial, carotid).

   d. Measure left atrial pressure, pulmonary artery diastolic pressure (PAD), PAWP to determine left ventricular end-diastolic volume and to assess cardiac output (see Chart 29-4).

   e. Monitor PAWP, PAD, left atrial pressure, and CVP to assess blood volume, vascular tone, and pumping effectiveness of the heart. *Remember: Changes in values are more important than isolated readings;* mechanical ventilator may elevate CVP.

   f. Monitor ECG pattern for cardiac dysrhythmias (see Chap. 29 for discussion of dysrhythmias).

   g. Assess cardiac enzymes daily (if ordered).

1. Effectiveness of cardiac output is determined by hemodynamic monitoring.

   a. Blood pressure is one of the most important physiologic parameters to follow; vasoconstriction after cardiopulmonary bypass may make auscultatory blood pressure unobtainable.

   b. Auscultation provides evidence of cardiac tamponade (muffled distant heart sounds), pericarditis (precordial rub), dysrhythmias.

   c. Presence or absence and quality of pulses provide data about cardiac output as well as obstructive lesions.

   d. Rising pressures may indicate congestive heart failure or pulmonary edema.

   e. High PAWP, PAD, left atrial pressure, or CVP may result from hypervolemia, heart failure, cardiac tamponade; if blood pressure drop is due to low blood volume, PAWP, PAD, left atrial pressure, and CVP will show corresponding drop.

   f. Dysrhythmias may occur with coronary ischemia, hypoxia, alterations in serum potassium, edema, bleeding, acid–base or electrolyte disturbances, digitalis toxicity, cardiac failure. ST segment changes may indicate myocardial ischemia or coronary artery spasm. Pacemaker capture and antidys-rhythmic medication effects are used to maintain a heart rate and rhythm to support stable blood pressures.

   g. Elevations may indicate myocardial infarction.

The following parameters are within the patient's normal ranges:
- Arterial pressure
- Left atrial pressure
- PAWP
- Pulmonary artery pressures
- CVP
- Heart sounds
- Pulmonary and systemic vascular resistance
- Cardiac output and cardiac index
- Peripheral pulses
- Cardiac rate and rhythm
- Cardiac enzymes
- Urine output
- Skin and mucosal color
- Skin temperature

(continued)

Nursing Care Plan 30–1 *(Continued)*

Postoperative Nursing Care of the Cardiac Surgery Patient

Nursing Interventions	Rationale	Expected Outcomes
h. Measure urine output every ½ to 1 hour at first, then with vital signs.	h. Urine output less than 30 ml/hr indicates decreased cardiac output and decreased renal perfusion.	
i. Observe buccal mucosa, nail beds, lips, ear lobes, and extremities.	i. Duskiness and cyanosis may indicate decreased cardiac output.	
j. Assess skin; note temperature and color.	j. Cool moist skin indicates vasoconstriction and decreased cardiac output.	
2. Observe for persistent bleeding: steady, continuous drainage of blood; hypotension; low CVP; tachycardia. Prepare to administer blood products, IV solutions.	2. Bleeding can result from cardiac incision, tissue fragility, trauma to tissues, clotting defects.	• Less than 300 ml/hr of drainage through chest tubes during first 4 to 6 hours • Vital signs stable
3. Observe for cardiac tamponade: hypotension; rising PAWP, PAD, left atrial pressure, or CVP; muffled heart sounds; weak, thready pulse; neck vein distention; decreasing urinary output. Check for diminished amount of blood in chest drainage collection system. Prepare for pericardiocentesis (see Chap. 29). Assess for pulsus paradoxus.	3. Cardiac tamponade results from bleeding into the pericardial sac or accumulation of fluid in the sac, which compresses the heart and prevents adequate filling of the ventricles. Decrease in chest drainage may indicate fluid is accumulating in the pericardial sac.	• Vital signs stable • Chest tube drainage expected amount • CVP and left atrial pressures within normal limits • Urinary output within normal limits
4. Observe for cardiac failure: hypotension, rising PAWP, PAD, CVP, and left atrial pressure, tachycardia, restlessness, agitation, cyanosis, venous distention, dyspnea, ascites. Prepare to administer diuretics and digitalis.	4. Cardiac failure results from decreased pumping action of the heart; can cause deficient blood perfusion to vital organs.	• Vital signs stable • CVP and left atrial pressures within normal limits • Skin color normal • Respirations unlabored, clear breath sounds
5. Observe for myocardial infarction: ST segment elevations, T wave changes, decreased cardiac output in presence of normal circulating volume and filling pressures. Obtain serial ECGs and isoenzymes. Differentiate myocardial pain from incisional pain.	5. Symptoms may be masked by the patient's level of consciousness and pain medication.	• Vital signs stable • Pain limited to incision • ECG and isoenzymes negative for ischemic changes

Nursing Diagnosis: Potential impaired gas exchange related to trauma and extensive chest surgery

Goal: Adequate gas exchange

Nursing Interventions	Rationale	Expected Outcomes
Assess respiratory status and provide for adequate ventilation and tissue oxygenation.		
1. Maintain assist-controlled, or intermittent (synchronous if possible) ventilation.	1. Ventilatory support is used the first 4 to 48 hours to decrease work of the heart, to maintain effective ventilation, and to provide an airway in the event of cardiac arrest.	• Airway patent • ABGs within normal range • Endotracheal tube correctly placed, as evidenced by x-ray • Breath sounds clear
2. Monitor arterial blood gases, tidal volumes, peak inspiratory pressures, and extubation parameters.	2. ABGs and tidal volume indicate effectiveness of ventilator and changes that need to be made to improve gas exchange.	• Ventilator synchronous with respirations. • Breath sounds clear after suctioning. • Nail beds and mucous membranes pink.
3. Auscultate chest for breath sounds.	3. Crackles indicate pulmonary congestion;	• Mental acuity consistent with amount of sedatives and analgesics received.

(continued)

Nursing Care Plan 30–1 *(Continued)*

Postoperative Nursing Care of the Cardiac Surgery Patient

Nursing Interventions	Rationale	Expected Outcomes
	decreased or absent breath sounds indicate pneumothorax.	• Oriented to person; able to respond yes and no appropriately.
4. Sedate patient adequately, as prescribed, and monitor respiratory rate and depth if ventilations are not "controlled."	4. Sedation helps the patient to tolerate the endotracheal tube and to cope with ventilatory sensations; sedatives can depress respiratory rate and depth.	
5. Provide chest physiotherapy as prescribed.	5. Aids in preventing retention of secretions and atelectasis	
6. Promote coughing, deep breathing, and turning. Encourage use of incentive spirometer and compliance with breathing treatments. Teach incisional splinting with a "cough pillow" to decrease discomfort during deep breathing and coughing.	6. Aids in keeping airway patent, preventing atelectasis, and facilitating lung expansion	
7. Suction tracheobronchial secretions as needed, using strict aseptic technique.	7. Retention of secretions leads to hypoxia and possible cardiac arrest; retained secretions promote infection.	
8. See Chapter 25 for weaning process and endotracheal tube removal.		

Nursing Diagnosis: Potential alteration in fluid volume and electrolyte balance related to alternations in blood volume

Goal: Fluid and electrolyte balance

Nursing Interventions	Rationale	Expected Outcomes
1. Maintain fluid and electrolyte balance.	1. Adequate circulating blood volume is necessary for optimum cellular activity; metabolic acidosis and electrolyte imbalance can occur after use of cardiopulmonary bypass.	• Fluid intake and output balanced • Hemodynamic assessment parameters negative for fluid overload and dehydration • Exhibits normal blood pressure with position changes • Absence of dysrhythmia
a. Keep intake and output flow sheets; record urine volume every ½ to 2 hours while in critical care unit; then every 4 hours.	a. Provides a method to determine positive or negative fluid balance and fluid requirements	
b. Assess the following parameters: pulmonary artery pressures, left atrial pressures, blood pressure, CVP, pulmonary artery wedge pressure, weight, electrolyte levels, hematocrit, jugular vein pressure, tissue turgor, liver size, breath sounds, urinary output, and nasogastric tube drainage.	b. Provides information about state of hydration	
c. Measure postoperative chest drainage (should not exceed 300 ml/hr for first 4 to 6 hours); cessation of drainage may indicate kinked or blocked chest tube. Assure patency and integrity of the drainage system. Maintain autotransfusion system if in use.	c. Excessive blood loss from chest cavity can cause hypovolemia.	
2. Be alert to changes in serum electrolyte levels.	2. A specific concentration of electrolytes is necessary in both extracellular and intracellular body fluids to sustain life.	• Blood pH 7.35 to 7.45 • Serum potassium 3.5 to 5.0 mEq/L (3.5–5.0 mmol/L)

(continued)

Nursing Care Plan 30-1 (Continued)

Postoperative Nursing Care of the Cardiac Surgery Patient

Nursing Interventions	Rationale	Expected Outcomes
a. Hypokalemia (low potassium) *Effects:* dysrhythmias, digitalis toxicity, metabolic acidosis, weakened myocardium, cardiac arrest Observe for specific ECG changes. Administer IV potassium replacement as directed.	a. *Causes:* inadequate intake, diuretics, vomiting, excessive nasogastric drainage, stress from surgery	• Serum sodium 135 to 145 mEq/L (135–145 mmol/L) • Serum calcium 8.8 to 10.3 mg/100 ml (2.20–2.58 mmol/L)

b. Hyperkalemia (high potassium)
Effects: mental confusion, restlessness, nausea, weakness, paresthesias of extremities
   Be prepared to administer an ion-exchange resin (sodium polystyrene sulfonate [Kayexalate]), IV sodium bicarbonate or IV insulin and glucose.
	b. *Causes:* increased intake, hemolysis from cardiopulmonary bypass/mechanical assist devices, acidosis, renal insufficiency, tissue necrosis, adrenal cortical insufficiency.
	   The resin binds potassium and promotes intestinal excretion of it.
	   IV sodium bicarbonate drives potassium into the cells from extracellular fluid.
	   Insulin assists the cells with glucose absorption. The glucose provides the energy to activate the sodium/potassium pumps, which pull potassium into the cell while pumping sodium out.	

c. Hyponatremia (low sodium) *Effects:* weakness, fatigue, confusion, convulsions, coma Administer sodium or diuretics as directed.	c. *Causes:* reduction of total body sodium, or increased water intake causing dilution of sodium	
d. Hypocalcemia (low calcium) *Effects:* numbness and tingling in fingertips, toes, ears, nose; carpopedal spasm; muscle cramps; tetany Administer replacement therapy as directed.	d. *Causes:* alkalosis, multiple blood transfusions of citrated blood products	
e. Hypercalcemia (high calcium) *Effects:* dysrhythmias, digitalis toxicity, asystole Institute treatment as directed.	e. *Cause:* prolonged immobility	

Nursing Diagnosis: Potential sensory-perceptual alterations related to sensory overload

Goal: Reduction of symptoms of sensory overload; prevention of postcardiotomy syndrome

1. Use measures to prevent postcardiotomy syndrome: a. Explain all procedures and the need for patient cooperation. b. Plan nursing care to provide for periods of uninterrupted sleep with day-night pattern. c. Decrease sleep-preventing environmental stimuli as much as possible. d. Promote continuity of care from nurse to nurse.	1. Postcardiotomy syndrome may result from anxiety, sleep deprivation, increased sensory input, disorientation to night and day. Normally, sleep cycles are at least 50 minutes long. The first cycle may be as long as 90 to 120 minutes and then shorten during successive cycles. Sleep deprivation results when the sleep cycles are interrupted or there are not enough of them.	• Patient cooperates with procedures. • Sleeps for long, uninterrupted intervals • Oriented to person, place, time • Experiences no perceptual distortions, hallucinations, disorientation, delusions

(continued)

Nursing Care Plan 30-1 *(Continued)*

Postoperative Nursing Care of the Cardiac Surgery Patient

Nursing Interventions	Rationale	Expected Outcomes
e. Orient to time and place frequently. Encourage family to visit at regular times. f. Assess for medications that may contribute to delirium g. Teach relaxation techniques and diversions. h. Encourage self-care as much as tolerated to enhance self-control. Assess support systems and coping mechanisms 2. Observe for symptoms: perceptual distortions, hallucinations, disorientation, paranoid delusions.		

Nursing Diagnosis: Pain related to operative trauma and pleural irritation caused by chest tubes

Goal: Relief of pain

1. Record nature, type, location, and duration of pain. 2. Assist patient to differentiate between surgical pain and anginal pain. 3. Encourage routine pain medication dosing for the first 24 to 72 hours and observe for side effects of lethargy, hypotension, tachycardia, respiratory depression.	1. Pain and anxiety increase pulse rate, oxygen consumption, and cardiac workload. 2. Anginal pain requires immediate treatment. 3. Analgesia promotes rest, decreases oxygen consumption caused by pain, and aids patient in performing deep breathing and coughing exercises.	• States pain is decreasing in severity. • Reports absence of pain. • Restlessness decreased • Vital signs stable • Patient participates in deep breathing and coughing exercises. • Verbalizes fewer complaints of pain each day • Positions self; participates in care activities • Gradually increases activity

Nursing Diagnosis: Potential alteration in renal perfusion related to decreased cardiac output, hemolysis, or vasopressor drug therapy

Goal: Maintenance of adequate renal perfusion

1. Assess renal function: a. Measure urine output every ½ to 1 hour. b. Measure urine specific gravity c. Monitor and report lab results: BUN, serum creatinine, urine and serum electrolytes. 2. Prepare to administer rapid-acting diuretics or inotropic drugs (dopamine, dobutamine). 3. Prepare patient for peritoneal dialysis or hemodialysis if indicated.	1. Renal injury can be caused by deficient perfusion, hemolysis, low cardiac output, and use of vasopressor agents to increase blood pressure. a. Less than 20 ml/hr indicates decreased renal function. b. Indicates kidneys' ability to concentrate urine in renal tubules. c. Indicate kidneys' ability to excrete waste products 2. Promote renal function and increase cardiac output and renal blood flow	• Urine output consistent with fluid intake; greater than 20 ml/hr • Urine specific gravity 1.015 to 1.025 • BUN, creatinine, electrolytes within normal limits

(continued)

Nursing Care Plan 30-1 *(Continued)*

Postoperative Nursing Care of the Cardiac Surgery Patient

Nursing Interventions	Rationale	Expected Outcomes

Nursing Diagnosis: Potential hyperthermia related to infection or postpericardiotomy syndrome

Goal: Maintenance of normal body temperature

1. Assess temperature every hour.	1. Fever can indicate infectious process or postpericardiotomy syndrome.	• Normal body temperature
2. Use sterile technique when changing dressings, suctioning endotracheal tube; maintain closed system for all intravenous and arterial lines and for indwelling catheter.	2. Decreases chance of infection	• Incisions are free of infection and are healing • Absence of symptoms of postpericardiotomy syndrome
3. Observe for symptoms of postpericardiotomy syndrome: fever, malaise, pericardial effusion, pericardial friction rub, arthralgia.	3. Occurs in 10% to 40% of patients after cardiac surgery	
4. Administer anti-inflammatory agents as directed.	4. Relieve symptoms of inflammation (*e.g.*, warmth or feverish sensation, swelling, fullness, stiffness or aching sensation, and fatigue).	

Nursing Diagnosis: Knowledge deficit about self-care activities

Goal: Ability to perform self-care activities

1. Develop teaching plan for patient and family. Provide specific instructions for the following:
   • Diet
   • Activity progression
   • Exercise
   • Coughing, deep breathing, lung expansion exercises
   • Temperature monitoring
   • Medication regimen
   • Pulse taking
   • CPR, if appropriate for the family to learn
   • Entry to the emergency medical system
   • Need for Medic-Alert identification
	1. Each patient will have unique learning needs.	• Patient and family members explain and comply with all aspects of therapeutic regimen.
		• Patient and family member identify lifestyle changes necessitated by therapeutic regimen.
		• Has copy of discharge instructions.
		• Makes follow-up phone calls weekly
		• Keeps follow-up appointments with surgeon

2. Provide verbal and written instructions; provide several teaching sessions for reinforcement and answering questions.	2. Repetition promotes learning by allowing for clarification of misinformation. After cardiac surgery, patients have short-term memory difficulty; written information is helpful because it can be used as a resource even after discharge. The less familiar or greater the amount of the content the patient and family need to learn, the more time it will take to learn.	
3. Involve family in all teaching sessions	3. Family member responsible for home care is usually anxious and requires adequate time for learning.	
4. Provide information regarding follow-up phone call to surgeon or cardiologist and assigned liaison nurse; follow-up visit with surgeon in 4 to 6 weeks.	4. Arrangements for phone contacts with health-care personnel help to allay anxieties.	
5. Make appropriate referrals: Visiting Nurse service, community support groups, Mended Hearts Club.		

Urine specific gravity also is assessed (normal: 1.010 to 1.025), as is urine osmolality. Inadequate fluid volume may be manifested by low urinary output and a high specific gravity, whereas overhydration is exhibited by high urinary output with low specific gravity.

The growth and function of body cells depend on adequate cardiac output to provide a continuous supply of oxygenated blood to meet the changing demands of the organs and body systems. Because the buccal mucosa, nail beds, lips, and earlobes are sites with rich capillary beds, they should be observed for cyanosis or duskiness as possible signs of reduced heart action. Moist or dry skin may indicate either vasodilation or vasconstriction, respectively. Venous distention of the neck veins or of the dorsal surface of the hand raised to heart level may signal a changing demand or diminishing capacity of the heart. If cardiac output has fallen, the skin becomes cool, moist, and cyanotic or mottled.

Dysrhythmias, which may arise when poor perfusion of the heart exists, also serve as important indicators of cardiac function. The most common dysrhythmias encountered during the postoperative period are bradycardias, tachycardias, and ectopic beats. Continuous observation of the cardiac monitor for various dysrhythmias is an essential part of patient care and management.

Any indications of decreased cardiac output are reported promptly to the physician. These assessment data and further diagnostic tests are used by the physician to determine the cause of the problem. Once a diagnosis has been made, the physician and the nurse work collaboratively to restore cardiac output and prevent further complications. When indicated, the physician prescribes blood components, fluids, digitalis, diuretics, vasodilators or vasopressors. When further surgery is necessary, the patient and family are prepared for the procedure.

▷ *Adequate Gas Exchange.* To assure adequate gas exchange, the nurse assesses and maintains the patency of the endotracheal tube. The patient is suctioned when breath sounds demonstrate wheezes or coarse crackles (rhonchi). Suctioning may be performed with an in-line suction catheter; the nurse and respiratory therapist determine if the ventilator's fractional inspired oxygen (FiO_2) should be increased for three or more breaths before the patient is suctioned. Alternately, 100% oxygen is delivered to the patient by a manual resuscitation bag (Ambu) before and after suctioning to prevent hypoxia that can result from the suctioning procedure. Arterial blood gas determinations are compared with baseline data and reported to the physician promptly.

Because a patent airway is essential for O_2 and CO_2 exchange, the endotracheal tube must be secured to prevent it from slipping into the right mainstem bronchus and occluding the airway. Frequent change of position also provides for optimum pulmonary ventilation and perfusion by allowing the lungs to expand more fully. When the patient's condition stabilizes, body position is changed every 1 to 2 hours and the nurse listens to breath sounds to detect the presence of crackles, wheezes, and fluid in the lungs. Deep breathing and coughing also are encouraged to open the alveolar sacs and provide for increased perfusion. The patient should be taught and assisted to splint the surgical chest incision before and during coughing to minimize the discomfort.

The patient may be ready for extubation when gagging or "fighting/bucking" the ventilator is observed. Before extubation, the patient should have a cough/gag reflex; stable vital signs; be able to lift his head off the bed or give firm hand grasps; meet vital capacity, negative inspiratory force, and minute volume calculations for his size; and have acceptable arterial blood gases while breathing warmed humidified oxygen without the assistance of the ventilator. Extubation has been performed within these parameters without any adverse effects on the patient's condition or prognosis. During this time the nurse assists with the weaning process and, eventually, the removal of the tube.

▷ *Maintenance of Fluid and Electrolyte Balance.* To promote fluid and electrolyte balance, the nurse carefully assesses intake and output. Flow sheets are used to determine positive or negative fluid balance. All fluid intake is recorded, including intravenous fluids, flush solutions used in arterial and venous catheters and the nasogastric tube, and oral fluids. In addition, all output is recorded, including urine, nasogastric drainage, and chest drainage.

Hemodynamic parameters (blood pressure, pulmonary wedge and left atrial pressures, and CVP) are correlated with intake, output, and weight to determine the adequacy of hydration and cardiac output. Serum electrolytes are monitored and the patient is observed for signs of hypokalemia, hyperkalemia, hyponatremia, and hypocalcemia.

Any indications of dehydration, fluid overload, or electrolyte imbalance are reported promptly, and the physician and nurse work collaboratively to restore fluid and electrolyte balance. The patient's response to fluid and electrolyte replacements or restrictions is monitored closely.

▷ *Reduction of Symptoms of Sensory Overload.* Sensory overload is a common effect associated with the surgical experience and environmental factors in the critical care unit. *Postcardiotomy psychosis* may occur after cardiac surgery. The term refers to a group of abnormal behaviors that occur in varying intensity and duration in a large number of patients. In the early years of cardiac surgery this phenomenon occurred more frequently than it does today. At that time it was attributed to inadequate cerebral perfusion during surgery, microemboli, and the length of time that the patient remained on the cardiopulmonary bypass machine. Advances in surgical techniques have significantly decreased these factors. Today, when it occurs, it is thought to be due to anxiety, sleep deprivation, increased sensory input, and disorientation to night and day when the patient loses track of time. An important finding is that patients who do not or cannot express anxiety before surgery are more prone to develop psychosis in the postoperative period. Psychosis may appear after a brief lucid interval.

The nurse monitors the patient for signs of denial and provides an opportunity for emotional expression during the preoperative period. Careful explanations of all procedures and of the need for cooperation help to keep the patient oriented throughout the postoperative course. Continuity of care is desirable; a familiar face and a nursing staff with a consistent approach promote the delivery of quality nursing care. The use of a well-designed and individualized nursing care plan will provide guidelines to assist the nursing team in coordination of their efforts for the emotional well-being of the patient.

▷ *Relief of Pain.* Deep pain may not be reflected in the immediate area of injury but in a broader, more diffuse area. Patients who have had cardiac surgery experience pain caused by the interruption of intercostal nerves along the incision route and irritation of the pleura by the chest catheters. (Also, patients with internal mammary artery CABG report ulnar nerve paresthesias on the same side of their body as the graft.)

It is essential to observe and listen to the patient for verbal and nonverbal clues about pain. The nurse accurately records the nature, type, location, and duration of the pain. (Incisional pain must be differentiated from anginal pain.) The patient is encouraged to accept medication as often as it is prescribed to reduce the amount of pain. The patient should then be able to participate in deep breathing and coughing exercises and to progressively increase self-care.

Pain produces tension, which may stimulate the central nervous system to release adrenalin and thus constrict the arterioles. This can cause increased afterload and decreased cardiac output. Morphine sulfate alleviates anxiety and pain and induces sleep, which reduces metabolic rate and oxygen demands. After the administration of narcotics, any observations indicating relief of apprehension and pain are documented in the patient's record. The patient is observed for any respiratory depressant effects of the analgesic. If respiratory depression occurs, a narcotic antagonist (*e.g.*, naloxone [Narcan]) is used to counteract the effect.

▷ *Promotion of Rest.* Basic comfort measures used in conjunction with prescribed analgesics will potentiate the effects of the analgesics and promote rest. The patient is assisted in changing positions every 1 to 2 hours and is positioned in such a way that strain on the incisional line and chest tubes is avoided. Physical support of the incision during coughing and deep breathing helps to minimize pain. Nursing activities are scheduled as much as possible to provide undisturbed periods of rest. As the condition stabilizes and the patient is disturbed less frequently for monitoring and therapeutic procedures, rest periods can become extended.

▷ *Maintenance of Adequate Tissue Perfusion.* Peripheral pulses (pedal, tibial, popliteal, femoral, radial, brachial) are routinely palpated to assess for arterial obstruction. If a pulse is absent in any extremity, the cause may be prior catheterization of that extremity. The newly identified absence of any pulse is immediately reported to the physician.

After surgery, measures are taken to prevent venous stasis that can cause thrombus formation and subsequent embolization: (1) applying antiembolic stockings/elastic bandage wrap, (2) discouraging crossing of legs, (3) avoiding use of the knee gatch on the bed, (4) omitting pillows in the popliteal space, and (5) instituting passive exercises followed by active exercises to promote circulation and prevent loss of muscle tone.

Thrombus formation and resulting embolization also can result from injury to the intima of the blood vessels, dislodging of a clot from a damaged valve, loosening of mural thrombi, and coagulation problems. Air embolism may occur as a result of cardiopulmonary bypass. The usual embolic sites are the lungs, coronary arteries, mesentery, extremities, kidneys, spleen, and brain.

Symptoms of embolization, which vary according to site, should be observed for: (1) midabdominal or midback pain; (2) pain, cessation of pulses, blanching, numbness, or coldness in an extremity; (3) chest pain and respiratory distress with pulmonary embolus or myocardial infarction; and (4) one-sided weakness and pupillary changes, such as occur in cerebral vascular accident. All such symptoms are promptly reported to the physician.

▷ *Maintenance of Adequate Renal Perfusion.* Inadequate renal perfusion can occur as a complication of open-heart surgery. One possible cause is low cardiac output. In addition, trauma to blood cells during cardiopulmonary bypass can cause hemolysis of red blood cells. This leads to a buildup of toxic substances because the glomeruli are occluded by the debris of the damaged red cells. Use of vasopressor agents to increase blood pressure can lead also to reduction of the blood flow to the kidneys. Nursing management includes accurate measurement of urine output. An output of less than 20 ml/hour can indicate hypovolemia. Specific gravity tests should be carried out to determine the kidneys' ability to concentrate urine in the renal tubules. Rapid-acting diuretics or inotropic drugs (digitalis, isoproterenol) may be prescribed to increase cardiac output and renal blood flow. The nurse should be aware of the BUN and serum creatinine levels as well as urine and serum electrolytes. Abnormalities in these studies are reported promptly because it may be necessary to restrict fluids and limit the use of drugs that are normally excreted by the kidneys.

If efforts to maintain renal perfusion are not effective, the patient may require peritoneal dialysis or hemodialysis (see Chap. 42).

▷ *Maintenance of Normal Body Temperature.* Patients are usually hypothermic when admitted to the critical care unit from the cardiac surgical procedure. The patient must be gradually warmed to normothermia. This is accomplished partially by the patient's own basal metabolic processes and often with the assistance of warmed ventilator air, warm blankets, or heat lamps. While the patient is hypothermic, the clotting process is less efficient, the heart is prone to dysrhythmias, and oxygen does not readily transfer from the hemoglobin to the tissues. Because anesthesia suppresses the basal metabolism, oxygen supply usually meets the cellular demand.

After cardiac surgery the patient is at risk for developing elevated body temperature caused by infection or postpericardiotomy syndrome. The resultant increase in metabolic rate increases tissue oxygen demands and thus increases cardiac workload. Measures are taken to prevent this sequence of events or to halt it as soon as it is recognized.

Sites of infection include the lungs, urinary tract, incisions, and intravascular catheters. Meticulous care is used in preventing contamination at the sites of catheter and tube insertions. Sterile technique is used when changing dressings and when providing endotracheal tube care and catheter care. Clearance of pulmonary secretions is accomplished by frequent repositioning of the patient, chest physical therapy, and suctioning. A closed system is used to maintain all intravenous and arterial lines.

Postpericardiotomy syndrome occurs in approximately 10% to 40% of patients who undergo cardiac surgery. Its precise cause is unknown. A common factor appears to be trauma, with residual blood in the pericardial sac after surgery. The syndrome is characterized by fever, pericardial pain, pleural pain, dyspnea, pleural effusion and pericardial friction, and arthralgia. There may be a combination of these signs and symptoms. Leukocytosis is present, along with elevation of the sedimentation rate. These symptoms frequently appear after the patient is discharged from the hospital.

The syndrome must be differentiated from other postoperative complications (incisional pain, myocardial infarction, pulmonary embolus, bacterial endocarditis, pneumonia, or atelectasis). The treatment is dependent on the severity of the symptoms. Bed rest and anti-inflammatory agents, such as salicylates and steroids, lead to a dramatic improvement in symptoms.

▷ *Patient Teaching/Home Health Care.*   Depending on the type of surgery and postoperative progress, the patient may be discharged from the hospital as early as 5 to 10 days after surgery. Although the patient may be anxious to return home, usually both patient and family have apprehensions about this transition. The family often expresses the fear that they are not capable of caring for the patient at home. They often are concerned that complications will occur that they are unprepared to handle.

The nurse helps the patient and family to set realistic, achievable goals. A teaching plan that meets the patient's individual needs is developed with the patient and family. This is done several days before discharge to allow ample time for periodic review of the plan and answering of questions. Specific instructions are provided about diet; activity progression and exercise; coughing, deep breathing, and lung expansion exercises; weight and temperature monitoring; the medication regimen; and follow-up visits with the surgeon as well as the cardiologist or internist.

The nurse may find that some patients will have difficulty learning and retaining information after cardiac surgery. Studies have shown that many patients experience difficulties in cognitive function after cardiac surgery that have not been shown to occur after other types of major surgery. The patient may experience recent memory loss, short attention span, difficulty with simple math, poor handwriting, and visual disturbances. Patients who experience these difficulties often become frustrated when they try to begin resuming normal activities and learning how to care for themselves at home. The patient and family are reassured that the difficulty is temporary and will subside, usually in 6 to 8 weeks.

In the meantime, instructions are given to the patient at a much slower pace than normal, and a family member assumes responsibility for making sure that the prescribed regimen is followed. If necessary, arrangements are made for community nurse services to provide home care such as dressing changes, monitoring of vital signs, diet counseling, and support for the patient and family.

Patient education postoperatively does not end at the time of discharge. The patient is encouraged to maintain telephone contact with the surgeon, cardiologist, and nurse. This provides the patient and family with reassurance that questions can be answered and problems can be resolved when they arise. Many hospitals provide family support sessions that help family members to cope with their own stress related to the patient's home health care management. The patient is expected to have a follow-up visit with the surgeon 4 to 6 weeks after discharge.

Many patients and families benefit from supportive programs such as the postbypass rehabilitation programs offered by many medical centers. These programs provide exercise monitoring, instructions about diet and stress reduction, and support groups for patients and families. The American Heart Association sponsors the Mended Hearts Club, which provides information as well as an opportunity for families to share experiences.

▷ Evaluation

Expected Outcomes.   See Nursing Care Plan 30–1 for specific outcomes.

1. Achieves adequate cardiac output
2. Maintains adequate gas exchange
3. Maintains fluid and electrolyte balance
4. Experiences decreased symptoms of sensory overload; is reoriented to person, time, and place
5. Experiences relief of pain
6. Maintains adequate tissue perfusion
7. Achieves adequate rest
8. Maintains adequate renal perfusion
9. Maintains normal body temperature
10. Performs self-care activities

Chapter Summary

The cardiac surgery patient benefits from individualized, comprehensive nursing care that is directed toward meeting his physical and psychosocial needs within the context of his family/significant other support system. Preoperative assessment and education begin the course of care. The nursing diagnoses addressed during this period include fear and knowledge deficit. During the intraoperative period, safety, infection control, and prevention of complications become priorities. Postoperatively, nursing care focuses on physiologic needs, prevention of complications, and preparation of the patient and his family for discharge and self-care. Postoperative nursing diagnoses include decreased cardiac output, impaired gas exchange, alterations in fluid and electrolyte balance, sensory-perceptual alterations, pain, alteration in tissue perfusion and renal perfusion, hyperthermia, and knowledge deficit.

The nursing process provides a framework for meeting the needs of the patient and his family or significant others throughout the perioperative experience. Realistic, achievable goals are established in collaboration with the patient. The family members are assisted in supporting the patient's goals and progress toward self-care and discharge. Plans for follow-up care and referrals to support groups or programs are essential as the patient progresses from the hospital to his discharge residence.

Bibliography

Books

Braunwald E. Heart Disease: A Textbook of Cardiovascular Medicine, 3rd ed. Philadelphia, WB Saunders, 1988.

Clark DA. Coronary Angioplasty. New York, Alan R Liss, 1987.

Cohn LH et al. Decision Making in Cardiothoracic Surgery. Toronto, BC Decker, 1987.

Hudak CM et al. Critical Care Nursing, 5th ed. Philadelphia, JB Lippincott, 1990.

Hurst JW. The Heart, Arteries and Veins, 7th ed. New York, McGraw–Hill, 1990.

Reed CC and Stafford TB. Cardiopulmonary Bypass. The Woodlands, TX, Surgimedics/TMP, 1989.

Roberts AJ and Conti CR. Current Surgery of the Heart. Philadelphia, JB Lippincott, 1987.

Sigardson-Poor KM and Haggerty LM. Nursing Care of the Transplant Recipient. Philadelphia, WB Saunders, 1990.

Smith SL (Ed). Tissue and Organ Transplantation: Implications for Nursing Practice. St Louis, CV Mosby, 1990.

Sokolow M et al. Clinical Cardiology, 5th ed. Norwalk, CT, Appleton & Lange, 1990.

Journals

Asterisks indicate nursing research articles.

General

* Gortner SR et al. Improving recovery following cardiac surgery: A randomized clinical trial. J Adv Nurs 1988 Sep; 13(5): 649–661.

Goulart DT. Educating the cardiac surgery patient and family. J Cardiovasc Nurs 1989 May; 3(3): 1–9

Kronick–Mest C. Postpericardiotomy syndrome: Etiology, manifestations, and interventions. Heart Lung 1989 Mar; 18(2): 192–198.

* Ley SJ et al. Crystalloid versus colloid fluid therapy after cardiac surgery. Heart Lung 1990 Jan; 19(1): 31–40.

* Miller KM and Perry PA. Relaxation technique and postoperative pain in patients undergoing cardiac surgery. Heart Lung 1990 Mar; 19(2): 136–146.

Pierce WS et al. Cardiac surgery: A glimpse into the future. J Am Coll Cardiol 1989 Aug; 14(2): 265–175.

* Stovsky B et al. Comparison of two types of communication methods used after cardiac surgery with patients with endotracheal tubes. Heart Lung 1988 May; 17(3): 281–289.

Cardiopulmonary Bypass

Furst E. Cardiovascular technology. J Cardiovasc Nurs 1989 May; 3(3): 71–86.

Murkin JM. Pathophysiology of cardiopulmonary bypass. Can J Anaesth 1989 May; 36(3): S41–S44.

Percutaneous Transluminal Coronary Angioplasty

Goldberg S (ed). Coronary angioplasty. Cardiovasc Clin 1988; 19(2): 1–285.

Halfman–Franey M and Levine S. Intracoronary stents. Crit Care Nurs Clin North Am 1989 Jun; 1(2): 327–337.

Lynn–McHale DJ. Interventions for acute myocardial infarction: PTCA and CABGS. Crit Care Nurs Q 1989 Sep; 12(2): 38–48.

* Murphy MC et al. Education of patients undergoing coronary angioplasty: Factors affecting learning during a structured education program. Heart Lung 1989 Jan; 18(1): 36–45.

Sigwart U et al. Emergency stenting for acute occlusion after coronary balloon angioplasty. Circulation 1988 Nov; 78(5): 1121–1127.

Sipperly ME. Expanding role of coronary angioplasty: Current implications, limitations, and nursing considerations. Heart Lung 1989 Sep; 18(5): 507–513.

Coronary Artery Revascularization

Acinapura AJ et al. Internal mammary artery bypass grafting: Influence on recurrent angina and survival in 2100 patients. Ann Thorac Surg 1989 Aug; 48(2): 186–191.

* Allen JK et al. Factors related to functional status after coronary artery bypass surgery. Heart Lung 1990 Jul; 19(4): 337–343.

* Allen JK. Physical and psychosocial outcomes after coronary artery bypass surgery: Review of the literature. Heart Lung 1990 Jan; 19(1): 49–55.

* Artinian NT. Family member perceptions of a cardiac surgery event. Focus Crit Care 1989 Aug; (16)4: 301–308.

* Bartz C. An exploratory study of the coronary artery bypass graft surgery experience. Heart Lung 1988 Mar; 17(2): 179–183.

* Beckie T. A supportive-educative telephone program: Impact on knowledge and anxiety after coronary artery bypass graft surgery. Heart Lung 1989 Jan; 18(1): 46–55.

Calgar G. Future nursing: Coronary artery bypass with right gastroepiploic artery grafts. Cardiovasc Nurs 1988 Jul/Aug; 1(2): 8–9.

Foster ED and Kranc MAT. Alternative conduits for aortocoronary bypass grafting. Circulation [Suppl] 1989 Jun; 79(6): I-34-I-39.

Gersh BJ et al. Coronary bypass surgery in chronic stable angina. Circulation [Suppl] 1989 Jun; 79(6): I-46-I-57.

* Grady KL et al. Patient perception of cardiovascular surgical patient education. Heart Lung 1988 Jul; 17(4): 349–355.

Illes RW and Levitsky S. Review of invasive treatment of coronary artery disease. Surg Gynecol Obstet 1989 May; 168(5): 461–467.

* King KB and Parrinello KA. Patient perceptions of recovery from coronary artery bypass grafting after discharge from the hospital. Heart Lung 1988 Nov; 17(6): 708–715.

Lynn–McHale DJ. Interventions for acute myocardial infarction: PTCA and CABGS. Crit Care Nurs Q 1989 Sep; 12(2): 38–48.

McGoon DC (ed). Cardiac surgery. Cardiovasc Clin 1987; 17(3): 1–446.

* Mailis A et al. Chest wall pain after aortocoronary bypass surgery using internal mammary graft: A new pain syndrome? Heart Lung 1989 Nov; 18(6): 553–558.

Marker L. Coronary artery bypass. AORN 1989 Jun; 49(6): 1533–1548.

* Miller SP et al. Marital functioning after surgery. Heart Lung 1990 Jan; 19(1): 55–61.

* Newton KM and Killien MG. Patient and spouse learning needs during recovery from coronary artery bypass. Prog Cardiovasc Nurs 1988 Apr/Jun; 3(2): 62–69.

* Noll ML and Fountain RL. Effect of backrest position on mixed venous oxygen saturation in patients with mechanical ventilation after coronary artery bypass surgery. Heart Lung 1998 May; 19(3): 243–251.

* Norheim C. Family needs of patients having coronary artery bypass graft surgery during the intraoperative period. Heart Lung 1989 Nov; 18(6): 622–626.

* Penckofer S and Llewellyn J. Adherence to risk-factor instructions one year following coronary artery bypass surgery. J Cardiovasc Nurs 1989 May; 3(3): 10–24.

Pierce WS et al. Cardiac surgery: A glimpse into the future. J Am Coll Cardiol 1989 Aug; 14(2): 265–275.

* Shaw DK et al. Efficacy of shoulder range of motion exercises in hospitalized patients after coronary artery bypass graft surgery. Heart Lung 1989 Jul; 18(4): 364–369.

* Shively M. Effect of position change on mixed venous oxygen saturation in coronary artery bypass surgery patients. Heart Lung 1988 Jan; 17(1): 51–59.

* Stanley MJB and Frantz RA. Adjustment problems of spouses of patients undergoing coronary artery bypass graft surgery during early convalescence. Heart Lung 1988 Nov; 17(6 Part 1): 677–682.

Ascending Aortic Aneurysm

Sweeney MS et al. Cardiac surgical emergencies. Crit Care Clin 1989 Jul; 5(3): 659–678.

Valvuloplasty/Valve Replacement

Barden C et al. Balloon aortic valvuloplasty: Nursing care implications. Crit Care Nurs 1990 Jun; 10(6): 22–30, 86.

Blaisdell MW et al. Percutaneous transluminal valvuloplasty. Crit Care Nurs 1989 Mar; (9)3: 62–68.

Cooley DA. Technical problems in mitral valve repair and replacement. Ann Thorac Surg 1989 Sep; 48(3 Suppl): S91-2.

Cribier A and Letac B. Balloon catheter therapy and cardiac valvular disease. Annu Rev Med 1989; 40: 61–70.

Daily EK. Percutaneous balloon valvuloplasty in adult patients with valvular heart disease. Crit Care Nurs Clin North Am 1989 Jun; 1(2): 339–357.

* Finkelmeier BA et al. Implications of prosthetic valve implantation: An 8-year follow-up of patients with porcine bioprostheses. Heart Lung 1989 Nov; 18(6): 565–574.

Galloway AC et al. Current concepts of mitral valve reconstruction for mitral insufficiency. Circulation 1988 Nov; 78(5): 1087-1098.

Jones EL. Freehand homograft aortic valve replacement: The learning curve: A technical analysis of the first 31 patients. Ann Thorac Surg 1989 Jul; 48(1): 26-32.

Nichols L et al. Percutaneous aortic valvuloplasty procedure and implications for nursing. Heart Lung 1989 Jul; 18(4): 356-363.

Ohler L et al. Aortic valvuloplasty: Medical and critical care nursing perspectives. Focus Crit Care 1989 Aug; 16(4): 275-287.

Rahimtoola SH. Perspectives on valvular heart disease: An update. J Am Coll Cardiol 1989 Jul; 14(1): 1-23.

Russell AC and Blake SM. Aortic valvuloplasty: Potential nursing diagnoses. Dimens Crit Care Nurs 1989 Mar/Apr; 8(2): 72-82.

Safian RD et al. Improvement in symptoms and left ventricular performance after balloon aortic valvuloplasty in patients with aortic stenosis and depressed left ventricular ejection fraction. Circulation 1988 Nov; 78(5): 1181-1191.

* Tedesco C et al. Functional assessment of elderly patients after percutaneous aortic balloon valvuloplasty: New York Heart Association classification versus functional status questionnaire. Heart Lung 1990 Mar; 19(2): 118-125.

Ventricular Aneurysm

Magovern GJ et al. Surgical therapy for left ventricular aneurysms. Circulation 1989 Jun; 79(6): I-102-I-107.

Hypertrophic Cardiomyopathy

McIntosh CL and Maron BJ. Current operative treatment of obstructive hypertrophic cardiomyopathy. Circulation 1988 Sep; 78(3): 487-495.

Surgical treatment of hypertrophic obstructive cardiomyopathy. Lancet 1989 Feb 18; 1(8634): 358-360.

Transplantation

Copeland JG. Cardiac transplantation. Curr Probl Surg 1988 Sep; 25(9): 607-672.

Futterman LG. Cardiac transplantation: A comprehensive nursing perspective. Part 2. Heart Lung 1988 Nov; 17(1): 631-638.

Imperial FA et al. Cardiac transplantation. Crit Care Nurs Clin North Am 1989 Jun; 1(2): 399-415.

* Packa DR. Quality of life of adults after heart transplant. J Cardiovasc Nurs 1989 Feb; 3(2): 12-22.

Stevenson LW et al. Cardiac transplantation: Selection, immunosuppression and survival. West J Med 1988 Nov; 149(5): 572-582.

* Walden JA et al. Heart transplantation may not improve quality of life for patients with stable heart failure. Heat Lung 1989 Sep; 18(5): 497-506.

Tumor Excision

Larsson S et al. Atrial myxomas: Results of 25 years' experience and review of the literature. Surgery 1989 Jun; 105(6): 695-698.

McRae ME. Care plan for the patient undergoing intracardiac myxoma excision. Crit Care Nurs 1990 Oct; 10(9): 58-63.

Trauma Repair

Ivatury RR and Rohman M. The injured heart. Surg Clin North Am 1989 Feb; 69(1): 93-110.

Pevec WC et al. Blunt rupture of the myocardium. Ann Thorac Surg 1989 Jul; 48(1): 139-142.

Sweeney MS et al. Cardiac surgical emergencies. Crit Care Clin 1989 Jul; 5(3): 659-678.

Mechanical Assist Devices/Total Artificial Hearts

Berron K. Role of the ventricular assist device in acute myocardial infarction. Crit Care Nurs Q 1989 Sep; 12(2): 25-27.

Boley T et al. Last hope for the failing heart. Am J Nurs 1989 May; 89(5): 672-677.

Bolman RM et al. Circulatory support with a centrifugal pump as a bridge to transplantation. Ann Thorac Surg 1989 Jan; 47(1): 108-112.

Hill JD. Bridging to cardiac transplantation. Ann Thorac Surg 1989 Jan; 47(1):167-171.

Muneretto C et al. Total artificial heart: Survival and complications. Ann Thorac Surg 1989 Jan; 47(1): 151-157.

Portner PM et al. Implantable electrical left ventricular assist system: Bridge to transplantation and the future. Ann Thorac Surg 1989 Jan; 47(1): 142-150.

* Ruzevich SA et al. Nursing care of the patient with a pneumatic ventricular assist device. Heart Lung 1988 Jul; 17(4): 399-407.

Teplitz L. Patients with ventricular assist devices. Dimens Crit Care Nurs 1990 Mar/Apr; 9(2): 82-87.

Trafford AC and Gunter M. The left ventricular assist device. Nursing 1988 Nov; 18(11): 64B-64J.

Antitachycardia Surgical Interventions

* Badger JM and Morris PL. Observations of a support group for automatic implantable cardioverter-defibrillator recipients and their spouses. Heart Lung 1989 May; 18(3): 238-243.

Cox JL. Patient selection criteria and results of surgery for refractory ischemic ventricular tachycardia. Circulation 1989 Jun; 79(6 Suppl I): I-163-I-177.

Furst E. Automatic implantable cardioverter-defibrillator. J Cardiovasc Nurs 1988 Nov; 3(1): 77-81.

Hargrove WC and Miller JM. Risk stratification and management of patients with recurrent ventricular tachycardia and other malignant ventricular arrythmias. Circulation 1989 Jun; 79(6 Supp I): I-178-I-181.

Moser SA et al. Caring for patients with implantable cardioverter defibrillators. Crit Care Nurs 1988 Mar/Apr; 8(2): 52-65.

Teplitz L et al. Life after sudden death: The development of a support group for automatic implantable cardioverter-defibrillator patients. J Cardiovasc Nurs 1990 Feb; 4(2): 20-32.

Veseth-Rogers J. A practical approach to teaching the automatic cardioverter-defibrillator patient. J Cardiovasc Nurs 1990 Feb; 4(2): 7-19.

Vitello-Cicciu J. AICD implantation: Treatment for malignant ventricular dysrhytmias. J Cardiovasc Nurs 1988 Nov; 3(1): 82-87

Zipes DP. Cardiac electrophysiology: Promises and contributions. J Am Coll Cardiol 1989 May; 13(6): 1329-1349.

Information/Resources

Agencies

American Heart Association
7320 Greenville Ave, Dallas, TX 75231

International Society for Heart Transplantation, Thoracic and Cardiovascular Surgery
Newark Beth Israel Hospital, 201 Lyons Ave, Newark, NJ 07112

Mended Hearts
7320 Greenville Ave, Dallas, TX 75231

31

Assessment and Management of Patients With Vascular Disorders and Problems of Peripheral Circulation

Learning Objectives

On completion of this chapter, the learner will be able to:

1. Specify anatomic and physiologic factors that affect peripheral blood flow and tissue oxygenation

2. Use appropriate parameters for assessment of peripheral circulation

3. Use the nursing process as a framework of care for patients with circulatory insufficiency of the extremities

4. Compare the various diseases of the arteries, their causes, pathologic and physiologic changes, clinical manifestations, management, and prevention

5. Describe the "stepped care" approach to drug therapy for hypertension and the goals of health teaching for patients with hypertension

6. Use the nursing process as a framework of care for patients with hypertension

7. Describe the prevention and management of venous thrombosis

8. Compare the preventive management of venous insufficiency, leg ulcers, and varicose veins

9. Use the nursing process as a framework of care for patients with leg ulcers

10. Describe the relation between lymphangitis and lymphedema

Physiologic Overview

Adequate perfusion, which results in oxygenation and nutrition of body tissues, is dependent in part on a functionally intact cardiovascular system. Efficient pumping action of the heart, patent and responsive blood vessels, and an adequate circulating blood volume are essential for adequate blood flow. Nervous system activity, blood viscosity, and the metabolic needs of tissues influence the rate of blood flow, and hence the adequacy of blood flow.

The vascular system consists of two interdependent systems: the right heart pumps blood through the lungs to compose the pulmonary circulation, and the left heart pumps blood to all other body tissues to make up the systemic circulation. The blood vessels in both systems provide distensible channels for the transport of blood from the heart to the tissues and back to the heart. Cardiac ventricular contraction supplies the driving force for movement of blood through the vascular systems. *Arteries* distribute oxygenated blood from the left side of the heart to the tissues, whereas the *veins* convey deoxygenated blood from the tissues to the right side of the heart. *Capillary vessels*, located within the tissues, connect the arterial and venous systems and constitute the site of exchange of nutrients and metabolic wastes between the circulatory system and the tissues. *Arterioles* and *venules* immediately adjacent to the capillaries, together with the capillaries, compose the *microcirculation*. A schematic representation of the circulation is shown in Figure 31–1.

The *lymphatic system* complements the function of the circulatory system. Lymphatic vessels transport *lymph* (a fluid similar to plasma) and tissue fluids (containing smaller proteins, cells, and cellular debris) from the interstitial space to systemic veins.

Anatomy of the Vascular System

Arteries and Arterioles.   Arteries are thick-walled structures that carry blood from the heart to the tissues. The aorta, which has a diameter of approximately 25 mm (1 inch), gives rise to numerous branches, which in turn divide into smaller vessels, arteries and arterioles, that approach 4 mm (0.16 inch) in diameter by the time they reach the tissues. Within the tissues, the vessels divide further, diminishing to approximately 30 μm in diameter; these vessels are called arterioles.

The walls of the arteries and arterioles are composed of three layers: an inner endothelial cell layer called the *intima*, which is in contact with the blood; a middle layer called the *media*; and an outer layer called the *adventitia*. The intima provides a smooth surface for contact with the flowing blood.

The media makes up the major portion of the vessel wall in the aorta and other large arteries of the body. This layer is composed chiefly of elastic and connective tissue fibers that give the vessels considerable strength and allow them to constrict and dilate for the purpose of accommodating stroke volume and maintaining an even, steady flow of blood. The adventitia is a layer of connective tissue that anchors the vessel to its surroundings. There is much less elastic tissue in the smaller arteries and arterioles, and the media in these vessels is composed primarily of smooth muscle.

Smooth muscle controls vessel diameter by contraction and relaxation. Chemical, hormonal, and nervous system factors influence the activity of smooth muscle. Because arterioles can alter their diameter, thereby offering resistance to blood flow, they are often referred to as *resistance vessels*. Arterioles regulate the volume and pressure in the arterial system and rate of blood flow to the capillaries.

Because of the large amount of muscle, the wall of the arteries is relatively thick; it accounts for approximately 25%

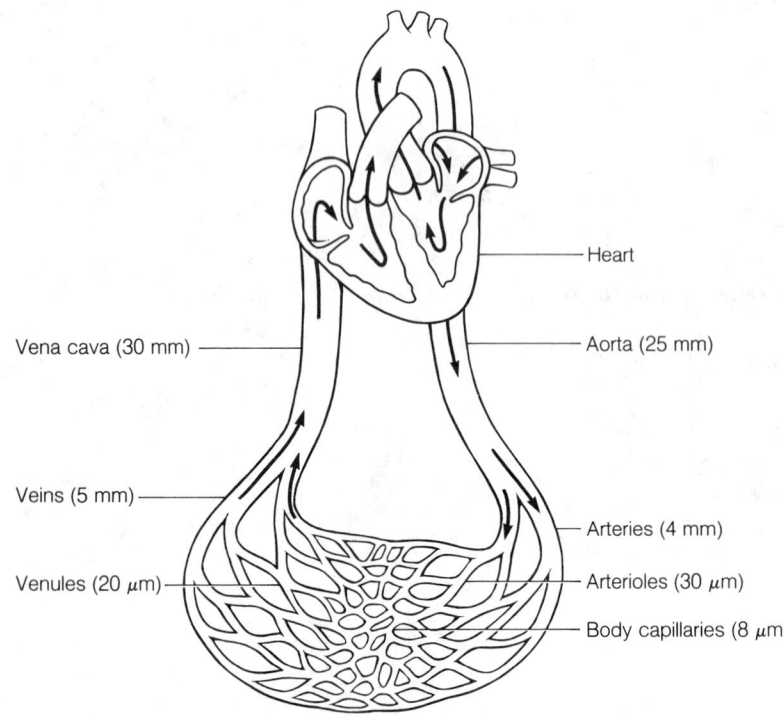

Vena cava (30 mm)

Veins (5 mm)

Venules (20 μm)

Heart

Aorta (25 mm)

Arteries (4 mm)

Arterioles (30 μm)

Body capillaries (8 μm)

Figure 31–1. Schematic drawing of systemic circulation. Oxygen-rich blood leaves the heart, goes through the aorta into the systemic arterial circulation until it reaches the capillaries, where the exchange of nutrients takes place. The deoxygenated blood returns to the heart by way of the venous system. Comparison of vessel size is demonstrated.

of the total diameter of the artery and approximately 67% of the total diameter of arterioles.

The intima and the inner third of the smooth muscle layer are in such close contact with the blood that the blood receives its nourishment from direct diffusion from the vessel. The adventitia and the outer media layers have a limited vascular system for nourishment. The muscle and adventitia of the arterial wall require their own blood supply to meet their metabolic needs.

Capillaries. Capillary walls lack smooth muscle and adventitia and are composed of a single layer of endothelial cells. This thin-walled structure permits rapid and efficient transport of nutrients to the cells and removal of metabolic wastes. The diameter of capillaries ranges from 5 to 10 μm, so red blood cells must alter their shape to pass through these vessels. Changes in capillary diameter are passive and are influenced by changes in the contractile state of precapillary and postcapillary vessels and in response to chemical stimuli. In some tissues a cuff of smooth muscle, called the precapillary sphincter, is located at the arteriolar end of the capillary and is responsible, along with the arteriole, for controlling capillary blood flow.

Some capillary beds, such as in the fingertips, contain *arteriovenous anastomoses*, through which blood passes directly from the arterial to the venous system. These vessels are believed to regulate heat exchange between the body and the external environment.

The distribution of capillaries throughout the tissues varies with the type of tissue. For example, skeletal tissue, which is metabolically active, has a more dense capillary network than does less active tissue such as cartilage.

Veins and Venules. Capillaries join together to form larger vessels called venules, which in turn join to form the veins. The venous system is therefore structurally analogous to the arterial system; venules correspond to arterioles, veins to arteries, and the vena cavae to the aorta. Analogous types of vessels in the arterial and venous systems have approximately the same diameters (see Fig. 31–1).

The walls of the veins, in contrast to those of the arteries, are thinner and considerably less muscular. The wall of the average vein amounts to only 10% of the vein diameter, in contrast to 25% in the artery. The wall of a vein, like that of an artery, is composed of three layers. These layers are not as well defined, however.

The thin, less muscular structure of the vein wall allows greater distensibility of these vessels. Greater distensibility and compliance permits the "storage" of large volumes of blood in the veins under low pressure. For this reason, veins are referred to as *capacitance vessels*. Approximately 75% of the total blood volume is contained in the veins. The sympathetic nervous system, which innervates the vein musculature, can stimulate venoconstriction, thereby reducing venous volume and increasing the general circulating blood volume.

Some veins, unlike arteries, are equipped with valves. In general, veins that transport blood against the force of gravity, as in the lower extremities, have one-way valves that interrupt the column of blood to prevent the distal reflux of blood as it is propelled toward the heart. Valves are composed of endothelial leaflets, the competency of which depends on the integrity of the vein wall.

Lymphatic Vessels. The lymphatics consist of a complex system of thin-walled vessels similar to the blood capillaries.

This network serves to collect lymph fluid from tissues and organs and to transport the fluid to the venous circulation. The lymphatics converge into two main trunks, the thoracic duct and the right lymphatic duct. These ducts empty into the junction of the subclavian and the internal jugular veins. The right lymphatic duct conveys lymph primarily from the right side of the head, neck, thorax, and upper arms. Peripheral lymphatics join larger lymph vessels and pass through regional lymph nodes before entering the venous circulation. The lymph nodes play an important role in the filtration of foreign particles.

The lymphatic vessels are permeable to large molecules and provide the only means whereby interstitial proteins can return to the venous system. With muscular contraction, lymph vessels become distorted to create spaces between the endothelial cells, which allow protein and particles to enter. Muscular contraction of the lymphatic walls and surrounding tissues aids in the propulsion of lymph toward venous drainage points.

Circulatory Needs of Tissues

The amount of blood flow needed by body tissues is constantly changing. The percentage of blood flow received by individual organs or tissues is determined by the rate of tissue metabolism, availability of oxygen, and the function of the tissues (Table 31–1). When metabolic requirements increase, blood vessels dilate to increase the flow of oxygen and nutrients to the tissues. When metabolic needs decrease, vessels constrict and blood flow to the tissues decreases. Metabolic demands of tissues increase with physical activity or exercise, local heat application, fever, and infection. Reduced metabolic requirements of tissues accompany rest or decreased physical activity, local cold application, and cooling of the body. Failure of blood vessels to dilate in response to the need for increased blood flow will result in tissue *ischemia* (deficient blood supply). The mechanism by which blood vessels dilate and constrict to adjust for metabolic changes assumes that a normal arterial pressure is maintained.

As blood passes through tissue capillaries, oxygen is removed and carbon dioxide added. The amount of oxygen extracted by each tissue is different. For example, heart muscle tends to extract about half the oxygen from arterial blood in one passage through its capillary bed, whereas in the kidneys only about 7% of the oxygen is removed as blood passes through these organs. The average amount of oxygen removed collectively by all of the body tissues is about 25%. This means that the blood in the vena cavae contains about 25% less oxygen than aortic blood. This is known as the *systemic arteriovenous oxygen difference*. It increases when the amount of oxygen delivered to the tissues is decreased relative to their metabolic needs. More detailed information about the blood flow and oxygen extraction as blood passes through capillary beds in various tissues is summarized in Table 31–1.

Blood Flow

Blood flow through the cardiovascular system always proceeds in the same direction: left heart to aorta, arteries, arterioles, capillaries, venules, veins, vena cavae, and finally to the right heart. The reason for this unidirectional flow is that a pressure difference exists between the arterial and venous systems. Because arterial pressure (approximately 100 mm Hg) is greater than venous pressure (approximately 4 mm Hg), and fluid al-

TABLE 31-1.   *Typical Values for Blood Flow and Oxygen Consumption for Various Human Organs*

Organ	Organ Weight (kg)	Blood Flow During Rest		Oxygen Usage During Rest	
		Organ Blood Flow (ml/min)	% Total Cardiac Output	Organ O$_2$ Usage (ml/min)	% Total O$_2$ Usage
Brain	1.4	750	14	45	18
Heart	0.3	250	5	25	10
Liver	1.5	1,300	23	75	30
GI tract	2.5	1,000			
Kidneys	0.3	1,200	22	15	6
Muscle	35.0	1,000	18	50	20
Skin	2.0	200	4	5	2
Remainder (*e.g.*, skeleton, bone marrow, fat, connective tissue)	27.0	800	14	35	14
TOTAL	70	6,500	100	250	100

(*Folkow B and Neil E. Circulation. New York, Oxford University Press.*)

ways flows from an area of high pressure to an area of low pressure, blood flows from the arterial to the venous system.

The pressure difference (ΔP) between the two ends of the vessel provides the impetus for the forward propulsion of blood. Impediments to blood flow offer the opposing force, which is known as resistance (R). Thus, the rate of blood flow is determined by dividing the pressure difference by the resistance:

$$\text{Flow} = \Delta P/R$$

From this equation it is clear that when resistance increases, a greater driving pressure is required to maintain the same degree of flow. Physiologically, an increase in driving pressure is accomplished by an increase in the force of contraction of the heart. If arterial resistance is chronically elevated, the heart muscle hypertrophies to sustain the greater contractile force.

In the majority of long smooth blood vessels, flow is laminar or streamlined, with blood in the center of the vessel moving slightly faster than the blood near the vessel walls. Laminar flow is silent. Laminar flow becomes turbulent with the increased rate of blood flow, with increased blood viscosity, with greater than normal vessel diameter, or when vessels have narrowed or constricted segments. Turbulent blood flow creates sounds that can be heard superficially with a stethoscope. The sound created by turbulent blood flow is called a *bruit*.

Blood Pressure.   See Chapter 27 for physiology and measurement of blood pressure.

Capillary Filtration and Reabsorption

Fluid exchange across the capillary wall is continuous. This fluid, which has the same composition as plasma without the proteins, forms the interstitial fluid. The equilibrium between hydrostatic and osmotic forces of the blood and interstitium, as well as capillary permeability, govern the amount and direction of fluid movement across the capillary. Hydrostatic force is a driving pressure that is generated by the blood pressure. Osmotic pressure is the pulling force that is created by plasma proteins. Normally, the hydrostatic pressure at the ar-

terial end of the capillary is relatively high, compared with that at the venous end. This high pressure at the arterial end of the capillaries tends to drive fluid out of the capillary and into the tissue space. Osmotic pressure tends to pull fluid back into the capillary from the tissue space, but this osmotic force cannot overcome the high hydrostatic pressure at the arterial end of the capillary. At the venous end of the capillary, however, the osmotic force predominates over the low hydrostatic pressure and there is a net reabsorption of fluid from the tissue space back into the capillary. Virtually all of the fluid that is filtered at the arterial end of the capillary bed is reabsorbed at the venous end, except for a very small amount. This excess filtered fluid enters the lymphatic circulation. These processes of filtration, reabsorption, and lymph formation aid in the maintenance of tissue fluid volume and in the removal of tissue waste and debris. Capillary permeability, under normal conditions, remains constant.

Under certain abnormal conditions, the fluid filtered out of the capillaries may greatly exceed the amounts reabsorbed and carried away by the lymphatics. This can result from damage to capillary walls and resulting increased permeability, obstruction of lymphatic drainage, elevation of venous pressure, or decrease in plasma protein osmotic force. The accumulation of fluid that results from these processes is known as *edema*.

Hemodynamic Resistance

The most important factor in the vascular system determining the resistance is the vessel radius. Small changes in vessel radius will lead to large changes in resistance. The predominant sites of change in caliber of blood vessels, and therefore in resistance, are the arterioles and the precapillary sphincter.

Peripheral vascular resistance is the opposition to blood flow provided by the blood vessels. Poiseuille's law provides the method by which resistance can be calculated.

$$R = \frac{8\eta L}{\pi r^4}$$

where

R = resistance
r = radius of the vessel
L = length of the vessel
η = viscosity of the blood
$8/\pi$ = a constant

This equation shows that the resistance is proportional to the viscosity of the blood and the length of the vessel, but inversely proportional to the fourth power of the vessel radius.

Blood viscosity and vessel length, under normal conditions, do not change significantly. Therefore, these factors do not usually play an important role in blood flow. A large increase in hematocrit, however, may increase blood viscosity and reduce capillary blood flow.

Peripheral Vascular Regulating Mechanisms

Because the metabolic needs of body tissues, even at rest, are continuously changing, an integrated and coordinated system of regulation is necessary so that blood flow to individual areas is maintained in proportion to the needs of that area. As might be expected, this regulatory mechanism is complex and consists of central nervous system influences, circulating hormones and chemicals, and independent activity of the arterial wall itself.

Sympathetic (adrenergic) nervous system activity, mediated by the hypothalamus, is the most important factor in regulating the caliber, and thus the blood flow, of peripheral blood vessels. All vessels are innervated by the sympathetic nervous system except the capillary and precapillary sphincters. Stimulation of the sympathetic nerves causes vasoconstriction. The neurotransmitter responsible for sympathetic vasoconstriction is norepinephrine. Sympathetic activation occurs in response to a number of physiologic and psychological stressors. Removal of sympathetic activity by medications or sympathectomy will result in vasodilation.

Other hormonal substances also affect peripheral vascular resistance. *Epinephrine*, released from the adrenal medulla, acts like norepinephrine in constricting peripheral blood vessels in most tissue beds. In low concentrations, however, epinephrine causes vasodilation in skeletal muscles, the heart, and the brain. *Angiotensin*, a potent substance formed from the interaction of renin (synthesized in the kidney) and a circulating serum protein, stimulates arterial constriction. Although the blood concentration of angiotensin is usually small, its profound vasoconstrictor effects become important in certain pathophysiologic states, such as congestive heart failure and hypovolemia.

Alterations in local blood flow are influenced by a number of circulating substances that have vasoactive properties. Potent vasodilator substances include histamine, bradykinin, prostaglandins, and certain muscle metabolites. A reduction in available oxygen and nutrients and changes in local *p*H also affect local blood flow. Serotonin, a substance liberated from platelets that aggregate at the site of vessel wall damage, constricts arterioles. The application of heat to parts of the body surface will cause local vasodilation, whereas the application of cold will cause vasoconstriction.

In summary, the delivery of adequate amounts of oxygen and nutrients to the cells and tissues depends on the integrity of several structural and functional systems. The peripheral vascular system provides the avenue for the delivery, and the metabolic demands of the cell dictate the utilization of the nutrients. Patent and intact arteries, capillaries, veins, and lymphatics constitute the structural elements of the vascular system. Cellular requirements, neuronal and hormonal control of the vessels, and the availability of oxygen and nutrients make up the functional components. When any of these elements are disrupted, the potential for tissue ischemia exists.

Pathophysiology of the Vascular System

Reduced blood flow through peripheral blood vessels characterizes all peripheral vascular diseases. The physiologic effects of altered blood flow depend on the extent to which tissue demands for oxygen and nutrients exceed their availability. If tissue needs are high, even modestly reduced blood flow may be inadequate to maintain tissue integrity, and tissues become *ischemic* (deficient in blood supply) and malnourished and ultimately die if adequate blood flow is not restored.

Heart Failure.   Inadequacy of peripheral blood flow occurs whenever the heart's pumping action becomes inefficient. Left-sided heart failure causes an accumulation of blood in the lungs and a reduction in forward flow or cardiac output, which results in inadequate arterial blood flow to the tissues. Right-sided heart failure causes systemic venous congestion and a reduction in forward flow (see Chap. 29).

Alterations in Blood and Lymphatic Vessels.   Intact, patent, and responsive blood vessels are necessary for adequate delivery of oxygen to tissues and removal of metabolic wastes. Arteries can become obstructed by atherosclerotic plaque, thrombus, or embolus. Damage and subsequent obstruction of arteries follow chemical or mechanical trauma, infections or inflammatory processes, vasospastic disorders, and congenital malformations. A sudden arterial occlusion causes profound and frequently irreversible tissue ischemia and tissue death. When arterial occlusions develop gradually, there is less risk for sudden tissue death because there is opportunity for the growth of new vessels to replace occluded ones (collateral circulation).

A reduction in venous blood flow can be caused by obstruction of the vein by a thrombus, incompetent venous valves, or a reduction in the effectiveness of the pumping action of surrounding muscles. Decrease in venous blood flow results in an increase in venous pressure, a subsequent rise in capillary hydrostatic pressure, a net filtration of fluid out of the capillaries into the interstitial space, and thus edema. Edematous tissues cannot receive adequate nutrition from the blood and consequently are more susceptible to breakdown or injury and to infection.

Obstruction of lymphatic vessels also results in edema. Lymphatics can become obstructed by tumor or by damage resulting from mechanical trauma or inflammatory processes.

Gerontologic Considerations.   The aging process produces changes in the walls of the blood vessels that affect the transportation of oxygen and nutrients to the tissues. The intima thickens as a result of cellular proliferation and fibrosis. Elastin fibers of the media become calcified, thin, and fragmented, and collagen accumulates in both the intima and the media.

These changes cause stiffening of the vessels, which results in increased peripheral resistance, impairment of blood flow, and increased left ventricular workload.

▶ Nursing Process
The Patient With Circulatory Insufficiency of the Extremities

▷ Assessment

Despite the variety of specific peripheral vascular diseases, all patients with these disorders experience ischemia (deficiency of blood supply to a body part) and therefore will have some of the same symptoms. The type and severity of symptoms present depends, in part, on the type, stage, and extent of the disease process as well as the speed with which the disorder develops. The distinguishing features of arterial and venous insufficiency are presented in Table 31–2.

▷ *Pain.*   A severe cramp-type pain in the extremities after activity or exercise is experienced by patients with peripheral arterial insufficiency. This pain, referred to as *intermittent claudication*, is due to the inability of the arterial system to provide adequate blood flow to the tissues in the face of increased demands for nutrients during exercise. As the tissues are forced to complete the energy cycle without the nutrients, muscle metabolites and lactic acid are produced. Pain is experienced as the metabolites aggravate the nerve endings of the surrounding tissue. Usually 75% of the vessel is obstructed before intermittent claudication is experienced. When the patient rests, and thereby decreases the metabolic needs of the muscles, the pain subsides. The progression of the vascular disease can be monitored by documenting the amount of exercise or the distance a patient can walk before pain is produced. Persistent pain in the extremities when the patient is resting indicates a severe degree of arterial insufficiency and a critical state of ischemia. This *rest pain* is often worse at night and may interfere with sleep.

The site of arterial disease can be deduced from the location of claudication. Calf pain may accompany reduced blood flow through the superficial femoral or popliteal artery, whereas pain in the hip or buttock may result from flow obstruction in the abdominal or common iliac artery.

▷ *Changes in Skin Appearance and Temperature.*   Adequate blood flow warms the extremities and gives them a rosy coloring. Inadequate blood flow results in cool and pale extremities. Further reduction of blood flow to these tissues, such as would occur with extremity elevation, results in an even whiter or more blanched appearance. A reddish blue discoloration of the extremities (*rubor*) may be observed within 20 seconds to 2 minutes after the extremity is dependent, and is indicative of severe peripheral arterial damage in which vessels are unable to constrict and remain dilated. *Cyanosis*, a bluish coloring of the skin, is manifested when the amount of oxygenated hemoglobin contained in the blood is reduced.

Additional adverse changes seen in the extremities as a result of chronically reduced nutrient supply include loss of hair, brittle nails, dry or scaling skin, atrophy, and ulcerations. Edema may be apparent either bilaterally or unilaterally. Gangrenous changes appear after prolonged severe ischemia and represent tissue necrosis.

TABLE 31–2.   *Clinical Manifestations of Peripheral Vascular Disease*

Arterial Insufficiency	*Venous Insufficiency*
ACUTE	
1. Asymmetric symptoms (affect only one leg)	1. Usually asymmetric symptoms
2. Severe, unrelenting pain	2. Sharp, deep muscle pain; may be relieved by elevation of extremity
3. Cold, pale extremity	3. Skin warm, red or red blue; with severe edema, skin cool and cyanotic
4. Diminished sensation	4. Pulses normal or diminished
5. Inability to move the extremity	5. Superficial veins full
6. Absence of pulses below the occlusion	6. Usually moderate to severe edema
7. No edema, initially	
CHRONIC	
1. Intermittent claudication, usually described as "cramps"; may progress to rest pain, usually described as "burning"	1. Discomfort described as aching, cramping, muscle fatigue; increased discomfort at end of day
2. Cool, pale extremity	2. Pigmentation, trophic changes, ulcers of lower legs and ankles
3. Diminished or absent distal pulses	3. Superficial veins prominent
4. Atrophy of skin, thickened nails, loss of hair	4. Edema moderate to severe
5. History of delayed wound healing	5. Paresthesias (burning, itching)
6. Reddish blue discoloration when extremity is dependent	6. Presence of ulcers around ankle
7. Presence of ulcers, superficial gangrene	

▷ *Pulses.* Determining the presence or absence, as well as the quality, of peripheral pulses is important in assessing the status of peripheral arterial circulation (Fig. 31-2). Absence of a pulse indicates that the site of obstruction is proximal to that location. Occlusive arterial disease impairs blood flow and can reduce or obliterate palpable pulsations in the extremities.

When pulses cannot be reliably palpated, it may be helpful to use a Doppler ultrasound device to detect peripheral flow (Fig. 31-3).

▷ *Gerontologic Considerations.* In the elderly person, the symptoms of peripheral vascular disease may be more pro-

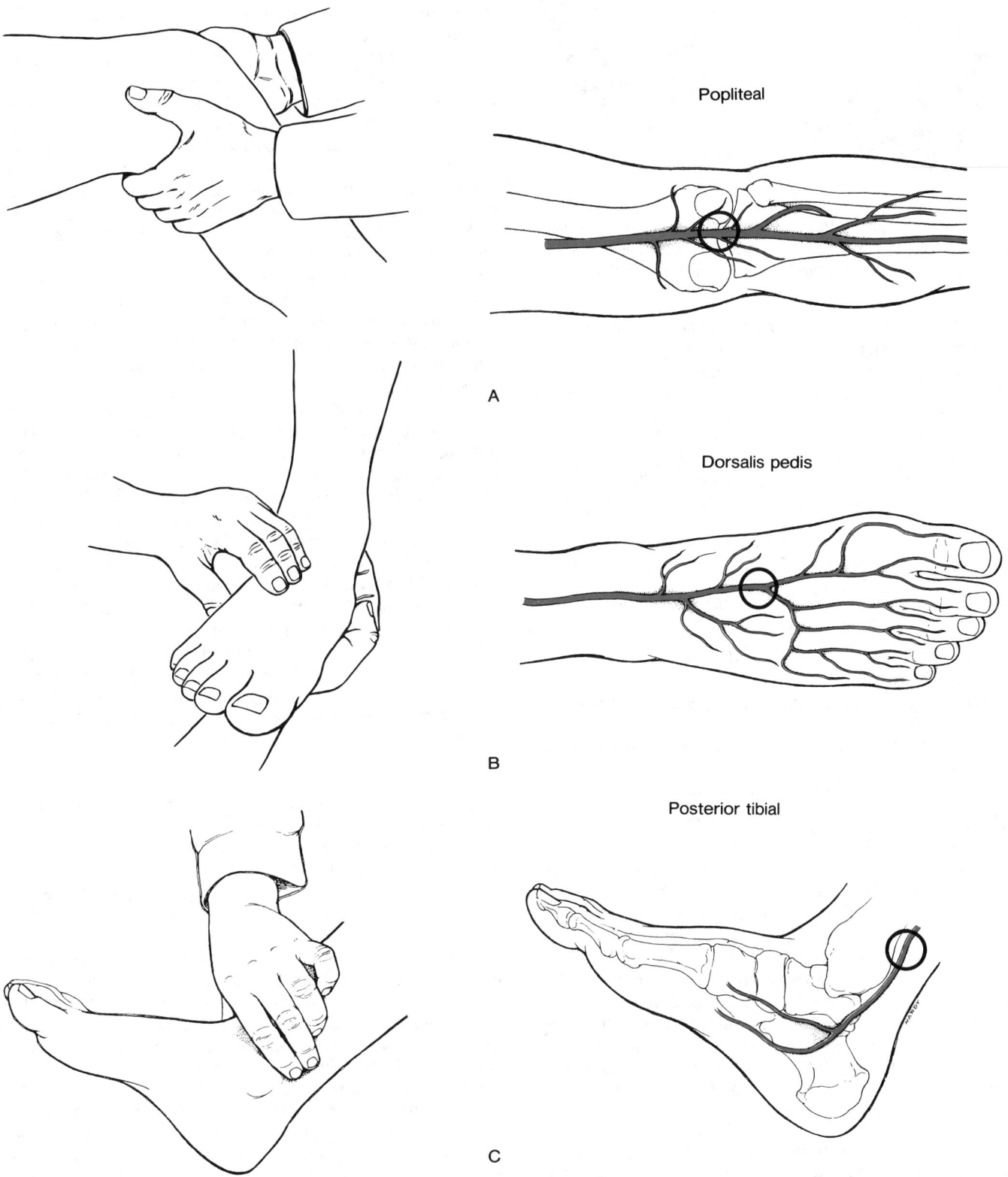

Figure 31-2. Assessing peripheral pulses. (**A**) Popliteal pulse. (**B**) Pedal pulse. (**C**) Posterior tibial pulse.

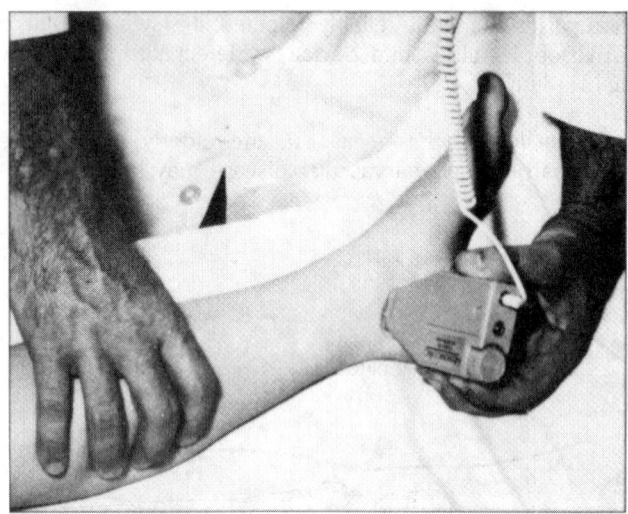

Figure 31–3. Doppler ultrasound transducer being used in screening for major deep-vein thrombosis. (Suddarth DS. The Lippincott Manual of Nursing Practice, 5th ed. Philadelphia, JB Lippincott, 1991.)

nounced than in the younger person because of the duration of the condition and the presence of coexisting chronic disease. Intermittent claudication may occur after walking only a few short blocks or after walking up a slight incline. Any prolonged pressure on the foot can cause pressure areas that become ulcerated, infected, and gangrenous. If chronic venous insufficiency is a problem, it also can lead to ulceration. The outcome of either arterial or venous insufficiency in the elderly person is increased impairment of mobility, activity, and independence.

◊ Nursing Diagnoses

Based on assessment data, major nursing diagnoses for the patient may include the following:

- Alteration in peripheral tissue perfusion related to compromised circulation
- Pain related to impaired ability of peripheral vessels to supply tissues with oxygen
- High risk for impairment of skin integrity related to compromised circulation
- Knowledge deficit regarding self-care activities

◊ Planning and Implementation

◊ **Goals:** The major goals of the patient may include increase in arterial blood supply to the extremities, decrease in venous congestion, promotion of vasodilation, prevention of vascular compression, relief of pain, attainment or maintenance of tissue integrity, and adherence to the self-care program.

Measures used by the patient and members of the health-care team to accomplish a single goal must be evaluated in terms of the positive as well as the negative effects they may have on the simultaneous achievement of other goals. A summary of the management of patients with peripheral vascular problems is presented in Nursing Care Plan 31–1.

◊ *Increase in Arterial Blood Supply to the Extremities and Decrease in Venous Congestion.* Arterial blood supply to a part can be enhanced when the part is placed below the level of the heart.

For the lower extremities, this can be accomplished by elevating the head of the bed on 15-cm (6-in) blocks or allowing the patient to assume a sitting position with the feet resting on the floor. Walking or other moderate or graded isometric exercises may be prescribed to promote blood flow by muscular exercise and thus to encourage the development of collateral circulation. Pain can serve as a guide in determining the amount of exercise a person should engage in. The onset of pain indicates that the tissues are not receiving adequate oxygen, signaling the patient to rest before continuing activity.

Active postural exercises, such as the *Buerger–Allen exercises*, may be prescribed for the patient with arterial insufficiency of the lower extremities. These exercises involve placing the extremities in three positions: elevation, dependency, and then at the horizontal position. The patient lies flat in bed with both legs elevated above the heart for 2 to 3 minutes. Then, sitting on the edge of the bed with the legs relaxed and dependent, the patient exercises the feet and toes (upward and downward, inward and outward) for about 3 minutes. Finally, the patient lies flat with the legs at the same level as the heart and covered for warmth for about 5 minutes. The times for each maneuver may vary, although the patient should attempt the series six times. Pain and dramatic color changes indicate the need for termination of the maneuver and rest. This routine may be repeated (Fig. 31–4) four times per day or as tolerated.

In patients with venous insufficiency, placing the lower extremities in a dependent position will only worsen the venous pooling associated with this condition. The pull of gravity impedes venous return to the heart and promotes venous stasis. Therefore, persons with venous insufficiency should elevate their legs above the level of the heart as much as possible. When upright, these patients should avoid standing still or sitting for prolonged periods. Walking aids venous return by the activation of the "muscle pump." In bed, patients with venous insufficiency should have the foot of the bed elevated on blocks.

Not all patients with peripheral vascular disease should exercise. Therefore, before recommending any program to patients, it is important to consult with the physician. Patients with leg ulcers, cellulitis, gangrene, or acute thrombotic occlusions require bed rest. These latter conditions can be made worse by activity.

◊ *Promotion of Vasodilation and Prevention of Vascular Compression.* Arterial dilation promotes increased blood flow to the extremities and is therefore a desirable goal in patients with peripheral arterial disease. In instances where the arteries are severely sclerosed, inelastic, or damaged, however, dilation is not possible. For this reason, measures to promote vasodilation, such as medications or surgery, may be only minimally effective.

Warmth promotes arterial flow by preventing chilling and thus the vasoconstriction associated with exposure to cold. Adequate clothing and warm environmental temperatures protect the patient from chilling. If chilling occurs, a warm bath or drink is helpful. When heat is applied directly to ischemic extremities, the temperature of the heat source should not exceed body temperature. Burn injuries can occur at lower temperatures in ischemic extremities than in normal limbs. In addition, excess heat may increase the metabolic rate of the extremities, and thus increase the need for oxygen until it cannot be met by the reduced arterial flow through the diseased

Nursing Care Plan 31–1

Care of the Patient With Peripheral Vascular Problems

Nursing Interventions	Rationale	Expected Outcomes

Nursing Diagnosis: Alteration in peripheral tissue perfusion related to compromised circulation

Goal: Increase in arterial blood supply to extremities

1. Lower the extremities below the level of the heart. 2. Encourage moderate amount of walking or graded extremity exercises. 3. Encourage active postural exercise (Buerger-Allen exercises).	1. Dependency of lower extremities enhances arterial blood supply. 2. Muscular exercise promotes blood flow and the development of collateral circulation. 3. With postural exercises, gravity alternately fills and empties the blood vessels.	• Extremities are warm to touch. • Has improved color of extremities • Experiences decreased muscle pain with exercise • Performs Buerger-Allen exercise series 6 times, 4 times per day or as tolerated

Goal: Decrease in venous congestion

1. Elevate extremities above heart level. 2. Discourage standing still or sitting for prolonged periods. 3. Encourage walking.	1. Elevation of extremities counteracts gravitational pull, promotes venous return, and prevents venous stasis. 2. Prolonged standing still or sitting promotes venous stasis. 3. Walking promotes venous return by activating the "muscle pump."	• Elevates lower extremities as prescribed • Decreased edema of extremities • Avoids prolonged standing still or sitting. • Gradually increases walking time daily

Goal: Promotion of vasodilation and prevention of vascular compression

1. Maintain warm temperature and avoid chilling. 2. Discourage smoking. 3. Counsel in ways to avoid emotional upsets; stress management. 4. Encourage avoidance of constrictive clothing and accessories (e.g., seat belts). 5. Encourage avoidance of leg crossing. 6. Administer vasodilator drugs and adrenergic blocking agents as prescribed, with appropriate nursing considerations.	1. Warmth promotes arterial flow by preventing the vasoconstriction effects of chilling. 2. Nicotine causes vasospasm, which impedes peripheral circulation. 3. Emotional stress causes peripheral vasoconstriction by stimulating the sympathetic nervous system. 4. Constrictive clothing and accessories impede circulation and promote venous stasis. 5. Leg crossing causes compression of vessels with subsequent impediment of circulation, resulting in venous stasis. 6. Vasodilators relax vascular smooth muscle; adrenergic blocking agents block the response to sympathetic nerve impulses or circulating catecholamines.	• Protects extremities from exposure to cold. • Does not smoke • Uses stress management program to minimize emotional upset • Avoids constricting clothing and appliances • Avoids leg crossing • Takes medication as prescribed

Nursing Diagnosis: Pain related to impaired ability of peripheral vessels to supply tissues with oxygen

Goal: Relief of pain

1. Promote increased circulation. 2. Administer analgesics as prescribed, with appropriate nursing considerations.	1. Enhancement of peripheral circulation increases the oxygen supplied to the muscle and decreases the accumulation of metabolites that cause muscle spasms. 2. Analgesics help to reduce pain and allow the patient to participate in activities and exercises that promote circulation.	• Uses measures to increase arterial blood supply to extremities. • Uses analgesics as prescribed.

(continued)

Nursing Care Plan 31–1 (Continued)

Care of the Patient With Peripheral Vascular Problems

Nursing Interventions	Rationale	Expected Outcomes

Nursing Diagnosis: High risk for impaired skin integrity related to compromised circulation

Goal: Attainment/maintenance of tissue integrity

1. Instruct in ways to avoid trauma to extremities.	1. Poorly nourished tissues are susceptible to trauma and bacterial invasion; healing of wounds is delayed or inhibited due to poor tissue perfusion.	• Inspects skin daily for evidence of traumatic injury • Avoids trauma and irritation to skin • Wears protective shoes • Adheres to meticulous hygienic regimen • Eats well-balanced diet that contains adequate protein and vitamins B and C
2. Encourage to wear protective shoes and padding for pressure areas.	2. Protective shoes and padding prevent foot injuries and blisters.	
3. Encourage meticulous hygiene: bathing with neutral soaps, applying lotions, carefully trimming nails.	3. Neutral soaps and lotions prevent drying and cracking of skin.	
4. Caution to avoid scratching or vigorous rubbing.	4. Scratching and rubbing can cause skin abrasions and bacterial invasion.	
5. Promote good nutrition: adequate intake of vitamins B and C and protein; control of obesity.	5. Good nutrition promotes healing and prevents tissue breakdown.	

Nursing Diagnosis: Knowledge deficit regarding self-care activities

Goal: Adherence to the self-care program

1. Include family/significant others in teaching program.	1–4. Adherence to the self-care program is enhanced when the patient receives support from family and from appropriate self-help groups and agencies.	• Practices frequent position changes as prescribed • Practices postural exercises as prescribed • Takes medications as prescribed • Avoids vasoconstrictors • Uses measures to prevent trauma • Uses stress management program • Accepts condition as chronic but amenable to therapies that will decrease symptomatology
2. Provide written instructions about foot and leg care.		
3. Help to secure properly fitting clothing, shoes, stockings.		
4. Refer to self-help groups as indicated: *e.g.*, Smoke-Enders, stress management.		

artery. Therefore, patients are instructed to test the temperature of bath water, hot water bottles, or heating pads before using them, or to avoid them altogether. Application of a heating pad to the abdomen can cause reflex vasodilation in the extremities and is safer than direct application of heat to affected extremities.

Nicotine causes vasospasm and can thereby dramatically reduce circulation to the extremities. Patients with arterial insufficiency who smoke must be fully informed of the circulatory consequences of this habit and encouraged to stop completely. Emotional upsets stimulate the sympathetic nervous system, which results in peripheral vasoconstriction. Although emotional stress is unavoidable, it can be minimized to some degree by environmental manipulation and a consistent stress management program. Emotionally charged or stressful situations should be avoided. Counseling services or relaxation training may be indicated for persons unable to cope effectively with situational stressors.

Constricting clothing and accessories such as garters, belts, girdles, and shoe laces will impede circulation to the extremities and promote venous stasis, and therefore should be avoided.

Leg crossing should be discouraged because it compresses vessels in the legs. The use of the bed knee gatch to elevate the legs causes further vascular compression and must be avoided.

Vasodilator medications and adrenergic blocking agents may be prescribed by a physician as adjunctive therapy. Vasodilators relax vascular smooth muscle, whereas adrenergic blocking agents block sympathetic response. Vasodilator therapy has not been proven to be successful, however, and may worsen tissue perfusion if systemic blood pressure becomes too low.

▷ *Relief of Pain.* Frequently, the pain associated with peripheral vascular disease is chronic and continuous. It limits activities, affects work and responsibilities, disturbs sleep, and alters one's sense of well-being. Because of this, patients are often depressed, irritable, and unable to exert the energy necessary to execute prescribed therapies. As a result it can be more difficult to alleviate pain, because the best means to do so is through the institution of measures that augment circulation. Analgesics can be helpful in reducing pain to the point

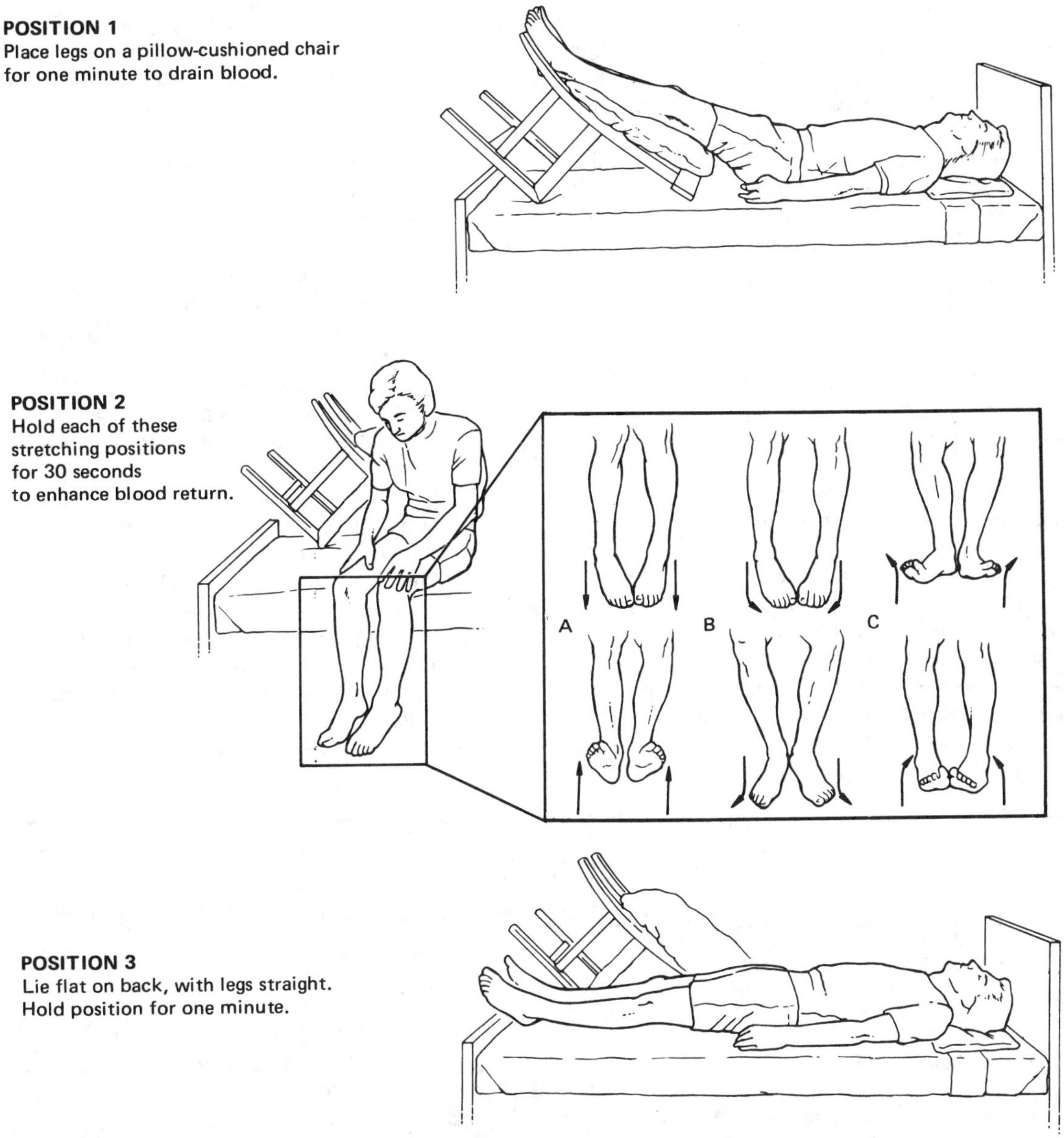

POSITION 1
Place legs on a pillow-cushioned chair
for one minute to drain blood.

POSITION 2
Hold each of these
stretching positions
for 30 seconds
to enhance blood return.

POSITION 3
Lie flat on back, with legs straight.
Hold position for one minute.

Figure 31–4. Buerger–Allen exercises. The exercise series is performed 6 times, 4 times a day. (Forshee T and Minckley B. Lumbar sympathectomy. RN; 39[2].)

where the patient may be more able to participate in the therapies that will increase circulation and ultimately relieve pain more effectively.

▷ *Maintenance of Tissue Integrity.*   Poorly nourished tissues are more susceptible to damage and infection. When lesions develop, healing may be delayed or inhibited because of the poor blood supply to the area. Infected, nonhealing ulcerations of the extremities can be debilitating and can require prolonged, often expensive hospitalization and treatments. Amputation of the extremity may eventually be necessary. Thus, measures to prevent these complications must be of high priority and vigorously implemented.

Trauma to the extremities must be avoided. Sturdy, well-fitting shoes or slippers should be worn when the patient ambulates to prevent foot injuries and blisters. The use of neutral soaps and body lotions prevents drying and cracking of skin. Scratching and vigorous rubbing can abrade skin and create a site for bacterial invasion; therefore feet should be patted dry. Stockings should be clean and dry. Fingernails and toenails should be carefully trimmed straight across after soaking in soap and warm water. If nails are thick and brittle and cannot be trimmed safely, a podiatrist should be consulted. Protective padding over corns and calluses will prevent breakdown and alleviate pressure. All signs of blisters, ingrown toenails, infection, or other problems should be reported to health-care professionals for treatment and follow-up. Persons with diminished vision may require assistance in periodically examining the lower extremities for trauma.

Good nutrition will promote healing and prevent tissue breakdown, and is thus included in the overall preventive program for persons with peripheral vascular disease. Vitamins B and C and adequate protein are necessary. Obesity strains the heart, increases venous congestion, and reduces circulation. A diet low in lipids may be indicated for patients with atherosclerosis. The physician and dietitian should be consulted.

▷ *Patient Education.* The self-care program should be planned with the patient so that those activities that will promote arterial and venous circulation, relieve pain, and promote tissue integrity will be acceptable to the patient. The patient and family should be helped to understand the reasons for each aspect of the program and the possible consequences of nonadherence. Care of the feet and legs is of prime importance in the prevention of trauma, ulceration, and gangrene. Detailed patient instruction in foot and leg care is provided in Chart 31–1.

▷ Evaluation

Expected Outcomes

1. Increases arterial blood supply to extremities
   a. Exhibits extremities warm to touch
   b. Has improved color of extremities (is free of rubor or cyanosis)
   c. Experiences decreased muscle pain with exercise
   d. Demonstrates palpable peripheral pulses
2. Decreases venous congestion
   a. Elevates lower extremities as prescribed
   b. Avoids prolonged standing still or sitting
   c. Has decreased edema in extremities
   d. Increases walking time
3. Promotes vasodilation; prevents vascular compression
   a. Protects extremities from exposure to cold
   b. Does not smoke
   c. Uses stress management program to minimize emotional upset
   d. Avoids constricting clothing and appliances (*e.g.*, tight seat belts)
   e. Avoids leg crossing
   f. Takes medication as prescribed
4. Is free of pain
   a. Uses measures to increase arterial blood supply to extremities
   b. Uses analgesics as prescribed
5. Attains or maintains tissue integrity
   a. Inspects skin daily for evidence of traumatic injury
   b. Avoids trauma and irritation to skin
   c. Wears protective shoes
   d. Adheres to meticulous hygienic regimen
   e. Eats well-balanced diet that contains adequate protein and vitamins B and C
   f. Consults podiatrist or primary physician for treatment of corns, blisters, trauma, and ingrown toenails.
6. Performs self-care activities
   a. Practices frequent position changes as prescribed by physician
   b. Practices postural exercises as prescribed by physician
   c. Takes medications as prescribed
   d. Avoids vasoconstrictors (*e.g.*, tight clothing, smoking, leg crossing)
   e. Uses measures to prevent trauma

Chart 31–1
Patient Education: Care of the Feet and Legs for the Person With A Peripheral Vascular Problem

Cleanliness

1. Wash feet at least once daily.
2. Use warm water and bland soap.
3. Dry feet thoroughly, especially between the toes. Blot and pat with a towel, but do not rub.

Warmth

1. Wear clean cotton hose, because they are comfortable and absorb moisture.
2. Prevent feet from getting cold; this reduces blood supply.
3. Avoid applying heat to the feet or legs unless approved by a physician or nurse.
4. Avoid swimming in cold water.
5. Avoid sunburn.

Safety

1. Protect feet by performing exercises on level ground.
2. Avoid walking in crowds.
3. Use care in cutting toenails.
   a. First soak feet for 10 minutes in warm water to soften nails.
   b. Cut nails straight across; avoid cutting nails close to flesh.
4. Do not go barefoot
5. Examine feet daily for trauma.
6. Consult podiatrist or primary physician for treatment of corns, blisters, trauma, and ingrown toenails.

Comfort Measures

1. Wear shoes that provide adequate toe room, have a good arch, and feel comfortable.
2. Apply powder if feet tend to become moist.
3. Apply a thin coating of lanolin if feet are dry and scaly.

Preventing Constriction of Blood Vessels

1. Avoid circular garters that cut off blood supply to legs and feet.
2. Do not cross legs at knees.
3. Place a pillow at foot end of bed under covers to prevent top bedding from exerting pressure on toes.
4. Apply lamb's wool between toes if they rub each other.

Exercise

Walk to stimulate circulation and promote tissue repair.

Medical Attention

1. Report redness, blistering, swelling, or pain.
2. Report athlete's foot, and peeling and itching between toes.
3. Do not use any medication on feet or legs unless prescribed by physician.

Smoking

Avoid tobacco in any form because it aggravates peripheral vascular conditions.

f. Participates in stress management program
g. Accepts condition as chronic but amenable to therapies that will decrease symptoms

Diseases of the Arteries

Arteriosclerosis and Atherosclerosis

Arteriosclerosis is the most common disease of the arteries; it literally means "hardening of the arteries." It is a diffuse process characterized by fibromuscular or endothelial thickening of the walls of small arteries and arterioles. Atherosclerosis refers to a generalized process characterized by focal changes in the intima of the large and medium-sized arteries. These changes consist of the accumulation of lipids, calcium, blood components, carbohydrates, and fibrous tissue (atheroma or plaque) on the intimal layer of the artery. Although the pathologic processes of arteriosclerosis and atherosclerosis differ, rarely does one occur without the other, and thus the terms are often used interchangeably. Because atherosclerosis is a generalized disease of the arteries, when it is present in the extremities it is usually present elsewhere in the body.

Pathophysiology and Etiology.   The most common direct results of atherosclerosis in arteries include narrowing (stenosis) of the lumen, obstruction by thrombosis, aneurysm development (abnormal dilatation of a blood vessel), ulceration, and rupture. Its indirect results are malnutrition and the subsequent fibrosis of the organs that the sclerotic arteries supply with blood. All actively functioning tissue cells require an abundant supply of nutrients and oxygen and are sensitive to any reduction in their supply. If such reductions are severe and permanent, these cells undergo ischemic necrosis (death of cells due to deficient blood flow) and are replaced by fibrous tissue, which requires much less nutrition.

Atherosclerosis primarily affects the main arteries throughout the entire arterial tree in varying degrees, usually in a patchy manner. Branch arteries are affected usually only at their bifurcations.

There have been many theories to explain why and how atherosclerosis develops. The primary lesion, the atheroma, is a focal area of a lipid plaque with a fibrous covering that slowly occludes the lumen of the vessel. No single theory has proven the pathogenesis; however, several parts of theories have been combined into the reaction-to-injury theory. According to this theory, vascular endothelial cell injury is due to prolonged hemodynamic forces, such as shearing stresses and turbulent flow, irradiation, chemicals, or chronic hyperlipidemia present in the arterial system. Injury to endothelium increases platelet and monocyte aggregation at the site of the injury. Smooth muscle cells migrate and proliferate, allowing a matrix of collagen and elastic fibers to form. It may be that there is not a single cause or mechanism for the development of atherosclerosis, but rather that multiple processes are involved.

Morphologically, atherosclerotic lesions are of two types: fatty streaks and fibrous plaque. Fatty streaks are yellow and smooth, protrude slightly into the lumen of the artery, and are composed of lipids and elongated smooth muscle cells.

These lesions have been found in the arteries of persons of all age groups, including infants. It is not clear whether fatty streaks predispose to the formation of fibrous plaques or if they are reversible. They do not usually cause clinical symptoms.

The *fibrous plaque* characteristic of atherosclerosis is composed of smooth muscle cells, collagen fibers, plasma components, and lipids. It is white to whitish-yellow and protrudes in varying degrees into the arterial lumen, at times completely obstructing it. These plaques are found predominantly in the abdominal aorta, coronary, popliteal, and internal carotid arteries. This plaque is believed to be an irreversible lesion (Fig. 31–5).

Gradual narrowing of the arterial lumen as the disease process progresses stimulates the development of collateral circulation (Fig. 31–6). This vascular "bypass" allows continued

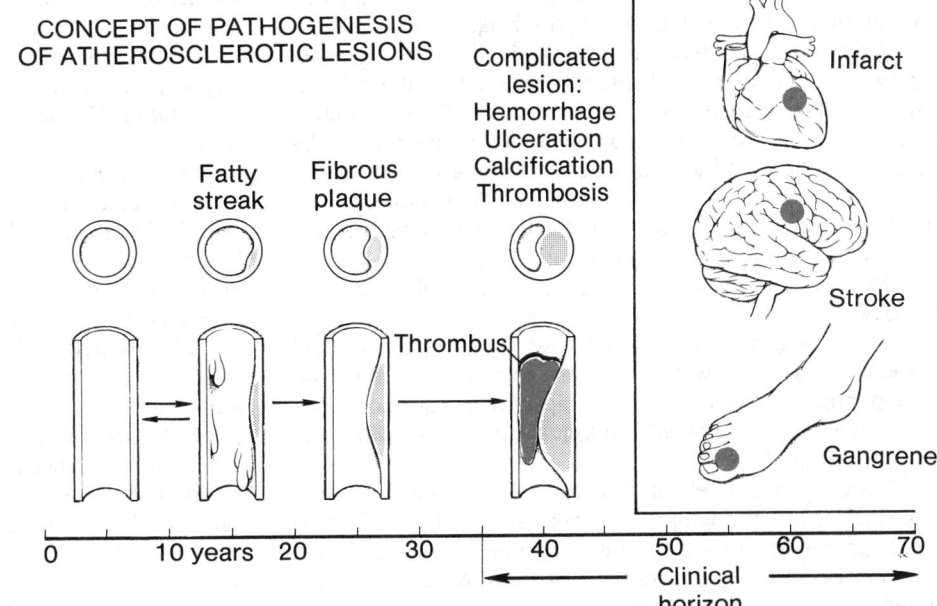

CONCEPT OF PATHOGENESIS OF ATHEROSCLEROTIC LESIONS

Figure 31–5. Schematic concept of the progression of atherosclerosis. Fatty streaks constitute one of the earliest lesions of atherosclerosis. Many fatty streaks regress, whereas others progress to fibrous plaques and eventually to atheromata. These may then become complicated by hemorrhage, ulceration, calcification, or thrombosis and may produce myocardial infarction. (Adapted from Hurst JW and Logue RB. The Heart. New York, McGraw-Hill.)

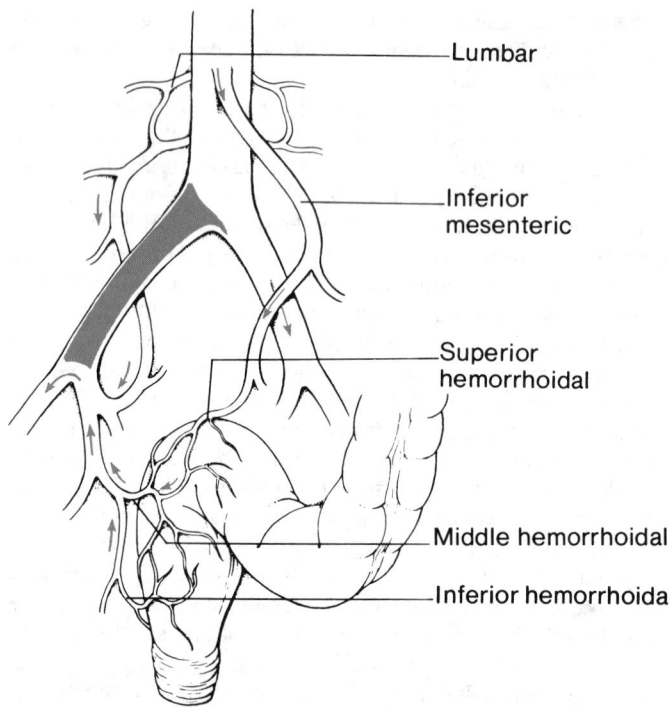

Lumbar

Inferior mesenteric

Superior hemorrhoidal

Middle hemorrhoidal

Inferior hemorrhoidal

Figure 31–6. Development of collateral channels in response to occlusion of the right common iliac artery and the terminal aortic bifurcation.

perfusion to the tissues beyond the arterial obstruction, but it is often inadequate to meet imposed metabolic demands, and ischemia results. The collateral vessels may or may not provide adequate perfusion to distal tissues.

Risk Factors.   Many factors are associated with the development of atherosclerosis. These factors have been determined from systematic observations of relationships between the development of atherosclerosis and certain characteristics. While it is not completely clear whether modification of these risk factors will prevent the development of cardiovascular disease, there is evidence that it may slow the disease process. Some risk factors, such as age or sex, cannot be modified. It is believed, however, that genetic factors can be influenced by alteration of other risk factors and therefore can be modified indirectly. These controllable risk factors include dietary factors, high blood pressure, diabetes, and smoking.

A diet high in fat has been strongly implicated in the causation of atherosclerosis. Approximately 39% of the calories Americans ingest are derived from fats. A complete explanation of the relationship between hyperlipidemia and cardiovascular disease can be found in Chapter 28. The American Heart Association recommends that, to reduce the risk of cardiovascular disease, persons should reduce the total amount of fat ingested in the diet, substitute unsaturated fats for saturated fats, and decrease the intake of cholesterol to no more than 300 mg per day.

Certain drugs are now being used to reduce blood lipid levels in conjunction with dietary modification. Among these are clofibrate, cholestyramine, colestipol, probucol, and niacin. Close supervision of patients on long-term therapy with these drugs is required.

Hypertension accelerates the rate of formation of atherosclerotic lesions in high-pressure vessels. The use of antihypertensive medication reduces the incidence of stroke. Diabetes also speeds up the atherosclerotic process by thickening the basement membranes of both the large and small vessels.

Smoking is identified as one of the strongest risk factors in the development of atherosclerotic lesions. Nicotine decreases blood flow to the extremities and increases heart rate and blood pressure by stimulating the sympathetic nervous system. Additionally, clot formation is enhanced by increased platelet aggregation. Carbon monoxide replaces oxygen from the hemoglobin, thus depriving the tissues of oxygen. The number of cigarettes smoked is directly related to the extent of the disease. Cessation of smoking is followed by a reduction of the risks. Many other factors such as obesity, stress, and lack of exercise have been identified as contributing to the disease process.

Although no single risk factor has been identified as the primary contributor to the development of atherosclerotic cardiovascular disease, it is clear that the greater the number of risk factors, the greater the likelihood of developing the disease. Therefore, the elimination of combined risk factors should be strongly emphasized.

Clinical Manifestations.   The clinical signs and symptoms resulting from the atherosclerotic process depend on the organ or tissue affected. Coronary atherosclerosis (heart disease), angina, and acute myocardial infarction are discussed in Chapter 28. Cerebrovascular disease, including transient cerebral ischemic attacks and stroke, is discussed in Chapter 56. Atherosclerosis of the aorta, including aneurysm, and atherosclerotic lesions of the extremities are discussed below.

Management.   The traditional management of atherosclerosis depends on risk factor modification, medication administration, and the nursing measures previously discussed. Recently, several surgical techniques have been shown to be important adjunctive therapies. Laser angioplasty is a technique whereby amplified light waves are transmitted by fiberoptic catheters. The laser beam heats the tip of a percutaneous catheter and vaporizes the atherosclerotic plaque. The rotational atherectomy device is a high-speed rotary cutter that removes lesions by abrading plaque. Although the technique is new, its results are encouraging because of the minimal damage to the normal endothelium and the low incidence of complications.

Gerontologic Considerations.   Atherosclerotic cardiovascular disease is found in 80% of the population over 65 years of age, and is the most common condition of the arterial system in the elderly. Risk factors are the same as for the general population.

Peripheral Arterial Occlusive Disease

Arterial insufficiency of the extremities is usually found in individuals over 50 years of age, most often in men, and predominantly in the lower extremities. The age of onset and severity are influenced by the type and number of atherosclerotic risk factors present. Obstructive lesions are predominantly confined to segments of the arterial system extending from the aorta, below the renal arteries, to the popliteal artery (Fig. 31–7).

Clinical Manifestations.   The hallmark of peripheral arterial insufficiency is *intermittent claudication*. This pain is insidious

and may be described as aching, cramping, tiredness, or weakness. *Rest pain* is persistent, aching, or boring and is usually present in the distal extremities. Elevation or horizontal placement of the extremity will aggravate the pain, whereas dependency of the extremity will reduce the pain. Some patients sleep with the affected leg hanging over the side of the bed in an attempt to relieve the pain.

A feeling of coldness or numbness in the extremities may accompany intermittent claudication and is a result of the reduced arterial flow. On examination, the extremities may be cool and exhibit pallor on elevation or a ruddy, cyanotic color when placed in a dependent position. Skin and nail changes, ulcerations, gangrene, and muscle atrophy may be evident. Bruits may be auscultated with a stethoscope (a *bruit* is the sound produced by turbulent flow of blood through an irregular, stenotic lumen or through a dilated [aneurysm] segment of the vessel). Peripheral pulses may be diminished or absent.

The examination of the peripheral pulses is an important part of the examination for arterial occlusive disease. Inequality of pulses between extremities or the absence of a normally palpable pulse is a reliable sign of occlusion. The femoral pulse

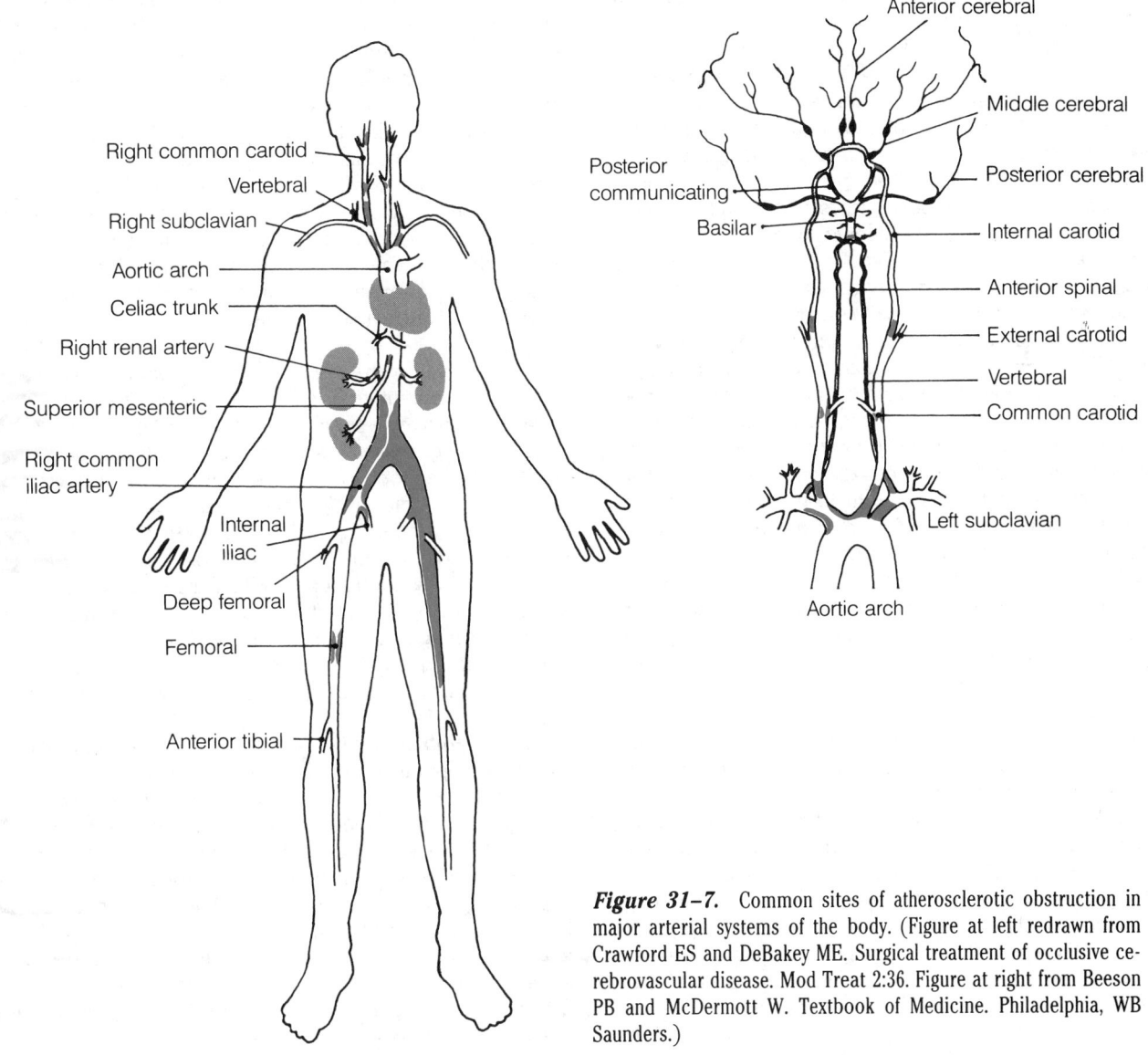

Figure 31–7.   Common sites of atherosclerotic obstruction in major arterial systems of the body. (Figure at left redrawn from Crawford ES and DeBakey ME. Surgical treatment of occlusive cerebrovascular disease. Mod Treat 2:36. Figure at right from Beeson PB and McDermott W. Textbook of Medicine. Philadelphia, WB Saunders.)

in the groin and the posterior tibial pulse behind the medial malleolus are most easily found. The popliteal pulse is sometimes difficult to palpate behind the knee in the obese patient, and the pedal artery varies in location on the dorsum of the foot and is normally absent in about 7% of the population.

Assessment.   The presence, anatomic location, and physiologic extent of arterial occlusive disease are determined by a careful history of the patient's symptoms and by physical examination. Observations of extremity color and temperature are made and pulses palpated. The nails may be thickened and opaque, and the skin shiny, atrophic, and dry with sparse hair growth. A comparative assessment is made of the two extremities.

Diagnostic Evaluation.   To determine the qualitative and quantitative aspects of the problem, Doppler ultrasonic flow studies can be performed.

The Doppler is an electronic stethoscope through which blood flow can be heard, even at times when pulses are not palpable. In addition, lower extremity blood pressure measurements can be obtained by coupling the Doppler with a standard pneumatic cuff. When comparing leg blood pressures with arm pressures, the patient with arterial occlusive disease of the lower extremities may demonstrate pressure in the legs lower than that in the arms.

Additional diagnostic tests for evaluating peripheral arterial occlusive disease include *oscillometry* to measure alterations in pulse volume at different levels of the extremity; an *exercise test* to determine the amount of activity possible before the onset of intermittent claudication; *plethysmography*, which monitors changes in pulse and leg size with each heartbeat; and a *lumbar sympathetic block*. This last test, used to evaluate peripheral circulation, involves injection of a local anesthetic into the lumbar epidural space to block the sympathetic nerves that go to the legs. Because the sympathetic nerves control the tension in the muscles of the blood vessels, a block of these nerves should produce vasodilation and increased temperature in the legs. Because atherosclerotic vessels are incapable of vasodilation; there is either no increase in temperature in the legs or only a slight increase. This test is often used to determine whether or not *sympathectomy* (interruption of afferent pathways in the sympathetic division of the autonomic nervous system) would be of benefit to the patient with impaired circulation of the legs. Sympathectomy eliminates vasospasm and improves peripheral blood supply.

Angiography may be used to confirm the diagnosis of occlusive arterial disease if surgery is considered. The procedure involves the injection of contrast medium directly into the vascular system and visualization of the vessels as the radiopaque material flows through them. In this manner, the location of vascular obstructions or aneurysms and the presence of collateral circulation can be demonstrated. Usually patients experience a temporary feeling of warmth as the contrast medium is injected. Local irritation at the injection site may occur. Infrequently, a patient may have an allergic reaction to the iodine contained in the contrast material. This reaction may appear immediately after the injection or may be delayed. Manifestations may include dyspnea, nausea and vomiting, sweating, tachycardia, and numbness of the extremities. Any such reaction is reported at once; treatment may include the administration of epinephrine (adrenalin), antihistamines, or steroids. In addition, there are risks of vessel injury and possibly stroke.

Digital subtraction angiography (DSA) is a radiologic visualization of arterial vessels using computer technology. Usually, angiography requires hospital admission from the day before the test until 24 hours after the test, and there are risks of severe complications after the procedure. With DSA, no hospitalization is necessary and the risks are fewer because entry into the arterial system is not necessary. By the use of an image-intensifier video system, vessels are displayed on a TV monitor. By computer, those images not required are subtracted so that the final intense image of the desired area is heightened.

Management.   The general care measures for patients with peripheral arterial disorders were described earlier in this chapter and are summarized in Chart 31–1. Generally, patients feel better on some type of exercise program. If this program is combined with weight reduction and the cessation of smoking, patients can often improve their activity limitations. Patients should not be promised that their symptoms will be relieved if they stop smoking. If claudication persists, they may lose their motivation not to smoke.

In some instances, *sympathectomy* may be beneficial to improve collateral circulation in patients with intermittent claudication. Excision of sympathetic ganglia will release arteriolar constriction and improve peripheral blood flow. In other patients, when intermittent claudication has become severe and disabling, or when the limb is at risk for amputation, vascular *grafting* or *endarterectomy* may be helpful. In the grafting procedure, either the diseased segment of artery is removed and a synthetic graft inserted in place of it, or the obstructed segment is left intact and instead "bypassed" by use of a graft. Material used for arterial bypass grafts may be synthetic (*e.g.,* Dacron, Teflon) or from autogenous veins (*e.g.,* saphenous vein). When an endarterectomy is performed, an incision is made into the artery and the atheromatous obstruction is "removed." The artery is then sutured closed to restore vascular integrity.

Percutaneous transluminal angioplasty (PTA) of arteries of the lower extremities is gaining acceptance as an alternative to vascular surgery, especially for those patients who are considered at high risk for surgical complications. Under local anesthesia, a balloon catheter is maneuvered across the area of stenosis or occlusion. The balloon is inflated and cracks the lesion, pushing it back up against the vessel wall. Complications from PTA include hematoma formation, embolus, arterial disection, and allergic reactions. Because surgery and general anesthesia are not required, the risks of morbidity are reduced, as are the length and cost of hospitalization. If reocclusion occurs, subsequent PTAs can be performed or, if that is not feasible, vascular surgery can be used to alleviate the obstruction.

Postoperative Nursing Management.   The primary objective in postoperative management of patients who have had these vascular procedures is to maintain adequate circulation through the arterial repair. Pulses of the affected extremities should be checked and recorded frequently and compared with those of the other extremity. Disappearance of a pulse may indicate thrombotic occlusion of the graft, so the surgeon is immediately notified. The color and temperature of the extremity are also monitored and any changes reported. An adequate circulating blood volume should be established and maintained. Continuous monitoring of urine output, central venous pressure, mental status, and pulse rate and volume will permit early recognition and treatment of fluid imbalances. Leg crossing and prolonged extremity dependency are avoided to prevent thrombosis. Leg elevation will reduce edema.

Thromboangiitis Obliterans (Buerger's Disease)

Buerger's disease is characterized by recurring inflammation of the intermediate and small arteries and veins of the lower and upper extremities, and results in thrombus formation and occlusion of the vessels. It is differentiated from other vessel diseases by its microscopic appearance. In contrast to atherosclerosis, Buerger's disease involves no lipid aggregates in the intimal coat, has more changes in the adventitia, results in a thrombosis that contains microabscesses, and does not cause vessel wall necrosis. Although this condition is different from atherosclerosis, in older patients atherosclerosis of the larger vessels may occur after involvement of the smaller vessels.

Etiology and Clinical Manifestations.   The cause of Buerger's disease is unknown. It occurs most often in men between the ages of 20 and 35, and it has been reported in all races in many areas of the world. There is considerable evidence that heavy smoking is either a causative or aggravating factor. Generally, the lower extremities are affected, but arteries in the upper extremities or viscera are also commonly involved. Superficial thrombophlebitis may be present. Arteriography confirms arterial occlusive disease.

Pain is the outstanding symptom of Buerger's disease. The patient complains of cramps in the feet (especially the instep) or legs after exercise (intermittent claudication), which are relieved by inactivity; often there is considerable burning pain that is aggravated by emotional disturbances, smoking, or chilling. Rest pain in the fingers and toes, a feeling of coldness, or a sensitivity to cold may be early symptoms. Various types of paresthesias may develop, and pulses may be diminished or absent.

As the disease progresses, definite redness or cyanosis of the part appears when it is dependent. Color changes may affect only one extremity or only certain digits or certain parts of a digit. Ulceration with gangrene may occur.

Management and Nursing Interventions.   The treatment of Buerger's disease is essentially the same as that for atherosclerotic peripheral vascular disease. The main objectives are to improve circulation to the extremities, prevent the spread of the disease, and protect the extremities from trauma and infection. The continuation of smoking is highly detrimental, and patients are advised to stop completely. Symptoms are often relieved by cessation of smoking.

Vasodilators are rarely prescribed because these drugs only cause dilation of healthy vessels; therefore, vasodilators may even divert blood away from the partially occluded vessels, which makes the situation worse. Regional sympathetic block or ganglionectomy may be useful in some instances to produce vasodilation and thereby increase blood flow.

Prognosis.   If gangrene of a toe develops as a result of arterial occlusive disease in the leg, it is unlikely that toe amputation or even a transmetatarsal amputation will succeed. Usually a below-knee amputation, or occasionally an above-knee amputation, is necessary. The indications for amputation are worsening gangrene, especially if moist; severe rest pain;

or sepsis secondary to gangrene. If any of these is present in a situation where bypass surgery is not feasible, amputation becomes necessary.

Aortic Diseases

The aorta is the main trunk of the arterial system and is divided into the ascending aorta (5 cm [2 inches] contained in the pericardium), the aortic arch (extending upward, backward, and downward), and the descending aorta. The entire aorta is designated as thoracic above the diaphragm and abdominal below the diaphragm.

Aortitis

Aortitis is inflammation of the aorta, particularly of the aortic arch. Two types are known to occur: Takayasu's disease and syphilitic aortitis. Takayasu's disease, or occlusive thromboaortopathy, is uncommon; syphilitic aortitis is almost never seen today.

Takayasu's Disease.   Takayasu's disease is a chronic inflammatory disease of the aortic arch and its branches seen primarily in young or middle-aged females. It results in ischemic symptoms affecting the upper extremity, brain, and eyes. In the early stages, it may respond to corticosteroids.

Syphilitic Aortitis.   Syphilitic aortitis usually begins before the age of 50. It starts at the root of the aorta and spreads in the form of a few discrete patches scattered over an otherwise normal intima. In most cases, the inflammatory process produces moderate dilation of the aorta, but it can produce more serious complications such as aortic insufficiency, aneurysm, or occlusion of the coronary ostia. Symptoms experienced by patients include sensations of substernal heaviness, viselike feelings of constriction of the chest, or attacks of agonizing pain. Sudden, short attacks of dyspnea may also occur.

In summary, atherosclerosis is a generalized disorder of the intimal layer of the arteries. Plaque, a lesion that consists of collagen fibers, lipids, and other blood components, accumulates on the intimal layer and obstructs the flow of oxygenated blood to distal tissues. These lesions may form in the coronary arteries, cerebrovascular system, aorta, or in the extremities. The clinical manifestations depend on the organ or tissues affected. At present the cause of atherosclerosis is unknown; however, several theories have been proposed. Both genetic and controllable risk factors have been determined.

Aortic Aneurysms

Classification of Aneurysms.   An aneurysm is a localized sac or dilatation of an artery formed at a weak point in the vessel wall (Fig. 31–8). Very small aneurysms due to local infection are designated *mycotic aneurysms*. An aneurysm that is somewhat larger but still limited in extent, projecting from one side of the vessel only, is called a *saccular aneurysm*. If an entire arterial segment becomes dilated, a *fusiform aneurysm* develops. Aneurysms are serious because rupture is always possible and can lead to hemorrhage and death.

The most common cause of aneurysm is atherosclerosis. Trauma to the wall of the artery, infection (pyogenic or syphilitic), and congenital defects of the artery wall also give rise to aneurysms, however.

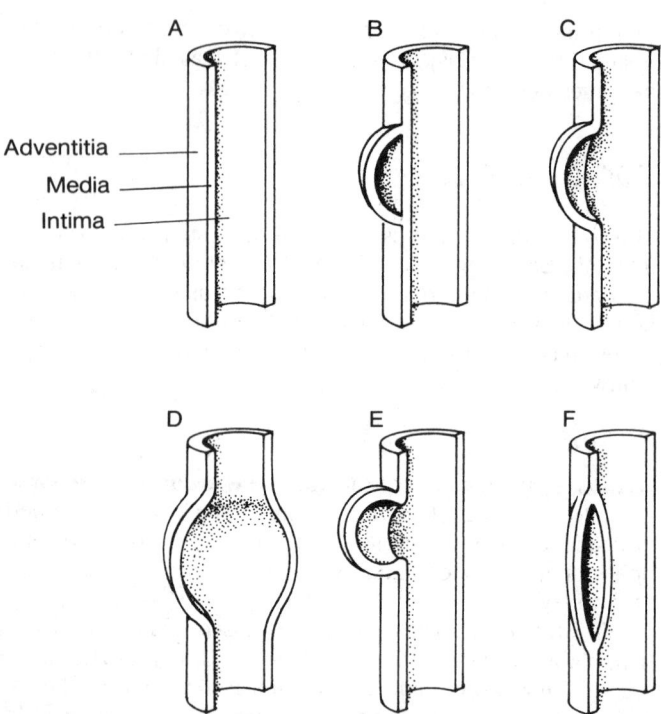

Figure 31–8.   Characteristics of arterial aneurysm. (**A**) Normal artery. (**B**) False aneurysm—actually a pulsating hematoma. The clot and connective tissue are outside the arterial wall. (**C**) True aneurysm. One, two, or all three layers may be involved. (**D**) Fusiform aneurysm—symmetrical, spindle-shaped expansion of entire circumference of involved vessel. (**E**) Saccular aneurysm—a bulbous protrusion of one side of the arterial wall. (**F**) Dissecting aneurysm—this usually is a hematoma that splits the layers of the arterial wall.

Aneurysm of the Thoracic Aorta

Approximately 85% of all cases of thoracic aortic aneurysm are caused by atherosclerosis. They occur most frequently in men between the ages of 40 and 70. The thoracic area is the most common site for the development of a dissecting aneurysm. About one third of patients with thoracic aneurysms die from rupture.

Clinical Manifestations.   Symptoms are variable and depend on how rapidly the aneurysm dilates and how the pulsating mass affects surrounding intrathoracic structures. Most are asymptomatic. In most cases *pain* is the most prominent symptom. It is usually constant and boring in character and may occur only when the person is lying in a supine position. Other conspicuous symptoms are *dyspnea*, the result of the pressure of the sac against the trachea, a main bronchus, or the lung itself; *cough*, frequently paroxysmal and with a brassy quality, *hoarseness*, stridor, weakness of the voice, or complete aphonia (manifestations of pressure against the left recurrent laryngeal nerve); and *dysphagia*, due to impingement on the esophagus.

Dilated superficial veins on the chest, the neck, or the arms, edematous areas on the chest wall, and cyanosis are often evident when large veins in the chest are compressed by the aneurysm. The pupils of the eyes may be unequal because of pressure against the cervical sympathetic chain. Diagnosis of a thoracic aortic aneurysm is principally by chest radiography and fluoroscopy.

Management.   Whether medical or surgical treatment is selected for thoracic aortic aneurysms depends on the type of aneurysm present. The goal of surgery is to remove the aneurysm and restore vascular continuity using a vascular graft (Fig. 31–9). Intensive monitoring is usually required after this type of surgery, and the patient is cared for in the critical care unit.

Medical management of the patient involves, in part, strict control of arterial blood pressure and a reduction in pulsatile aortic flow. Systolic pressure is maintained around 100 to 120 mm Hg with antihypertensive drugs (*e.g.*, reserpine, guanethidine). Pulsatile flow is reduced by medications that reduce cardiac contractility (*e.g.*, propranolol).

Abdominal Aortic Aneurysm

The most common cause of abdominal aortic aneurysm is atherosclerosis; syphilis is present in fewer than 1% of patients. Men are affected four times more often than women. The condition is more common among whites, and is most prevalent after the age of 60. Most of these aneurysms occur below the renal arteries. Untreated, the eventual outcome may be rupture and death.

Pathophysiology.   The factor common to all aneurysms is a damaged media in the vessel. This may be caused by congenital weakness, trauma, or disease process. Once an aneurysm develops, the tendency is toward an increase in size. Risk factors include genetic predisposition, smoking, and hypertension.

Clinical Manifestations and Diagnosis.   About two fifths of patients with abdominal aortic aneurysms have symptoms; the remainder are asymptomatic. Some patients complain that they can feel their "heart beating" in their abdomen when lying down. The most common symptom is intense *abdominal pain*, which may be persistent or intermittent and is often localized in the middle or lower abdomen to the left of the midline. The next most common symptom is *low back pain*, which is caused by pressure on the lumbar nerves. This is a serious symptom that usually signifies rapid expansion or impending rupture of the aneurysm. Less frequently, the patient complains of *feeling an abdominal mass* or *abdominal throbbing*. More than half of these patients exhibit hypertension. An interesting finding is the comparison of blood pressure readings of the thigh and arm. Ordinarily, the systolic blood pressure of the thigh exceeds that of the arm by 15 mm Hg or more. In about three quarters of patients with abdominal aortic aneurysm, the systolic pressure in the thigh is abnormally low in comparison to that in the arm.

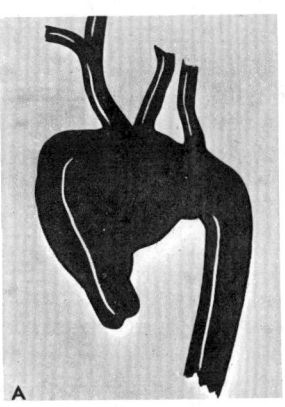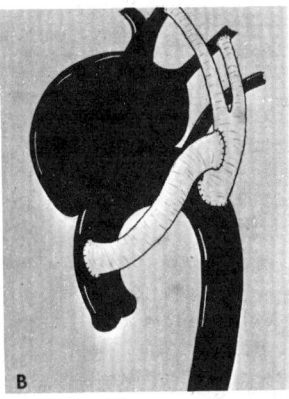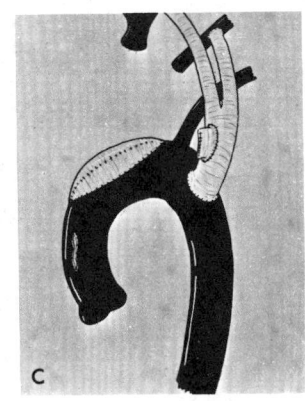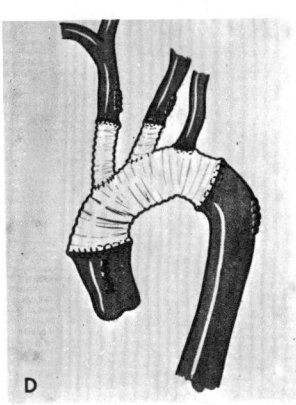

Figure 31–9. Surgical treatment of aortic aneurysm. (**A**) Location and extent of aortic aneurysm. (**B**) Method of treatment utilizing temporary bypass graft to maintain normal aortic circulation during excision of aneurysm. (**C**) Completed procedure with patch graft angioplasty to repair excised segment of aortic arch and conversion of temporary bypass graft to innominate and left common carotid arteries into the permanent graft. (**D**) Temporary bypass grafts used to maintain normal aortic circulation during excision and graft replacement of aneurysm have been completely removed, and aortic graft has been inserted. (DeBakey ME. Changing concepts in vascular surgery. J Cardiovasc Surg; 1:3–44.)

The most important diagnostic indication of this type of aneurysm is the presence of a pulsatile mass in the middle and upper abdomen. About 80% of abdominal aortic aneurysms can be palpated. A systolic bruit may be heard over the mass. Confirmation of the aneurysm by abdominal x-ray is possible if the aneurysm is calcified. An abdominal aortogram, ultrasonography, or DSA may also be used to define and confirm the presence of the aneurysm.

Management. The likelihood of rupture is significant in patients with an expanding or enlarging abdominal aneurysm. Consequently, surgery is the treatment of choice for abdominal aneurysms larger than 5 cm (2 in) in diameter or those that are enlarging. This involves resection of the aneurysm and insertion of a bypass (synthetic) graft (Fig. 31–10). Elective aneurysm repair, a major surgical procedure, has a reported mortality rate of 5%. The prognosis for a patient with a ruptured aneurysm is poor, and surgery is performed immediately.

Preoperatively, nursing assessment should be guided by the fact that the aneurysm might rupture, and by the recognition that the patient may have cardiovascular, cerebral, and pulmonary impairment secondary to atherosclerosis. Therefore, the functional capacity of all organ systems should be established. Medical therapies designed to stabilize physiologic function should be promptly implemented. Postoperative care requires intense monitoring of pulmonary, cardiovascular, renal, and neurologic status. Complications of surgery include arterial occlusion, graft hemorrhage and infection, ischemic colon, and impotence. After the acute recovery phase, an exercise schedule may be prescribed. Prolonged sitting should be avoided.

Indications of a rupturing abdominal aortic aneurysm include a constant intense back pain, falling blood pressure, decreasing red cell count and increasing white count, plus a soft abdomen. After a retroperitoneal rupture of an aneurysm, hematomas have been noticed in the scrotum, perineum, or penis. Signs of heart failure or loud bruit may suggest a rupture into the vena cava. Rupture into the peritoneal cavity is rapidly fatal. The overall surgical mortality rate with ruptured aneurysm is 50% to 75%.

Dissecting Aneurysm of the Aorta

Pathophysiology. Occasionally, an aorta diseased by arteriosclerosis develops an intimal tear due to a type of medial degeneration. This entity, which is often associated with poorly controlled hypertension, is three times more common in men than in women and occurs in the age group between 50 and 70 years. Dissecting aneurysms are extremely dangerous, resulting in death if untreated.

The intimal tear permits blood to dissect its way into the substance of the aortic wall. The result is the formation of a large hematoma in the arterial wall and the formation of a false channel between the intima and adventitia, which may extend for a considerable distance and produce severe and persistent pain. Death is usually caused by external rupture of the hematoma.

Clinical Manifestations and Assessment. The process of dissection leads to shearing and occlusion of the arteries branching from the aorta in the area involved by the process. The tear occurs most commonly in the region of the aortic arch, with the highest mortality associated with ascending aortic dissection. The dissection of the aorta may progress backward in the direction of the heart, obstructing the opening to the coronary arteries or producing hemopericardium (effusion of blood into the pericardial sac) or aortic insufficiency, or it may extend in the opposite direction, causing occlusion of the arteries supplying the gastrointestinal tract, the kidneys, the spinal cord, and even the legs.

The onset of symptoms is usually sudden. Severe and persistent pain, described as "tearing" or "ripping," may be reported in the anterior chest, epigastric area, back, or shoulders. Cardiovascular, neurologic, and gastrointestinal symptoms are responsible for other clinical manifestations, depending on the location and extensiveness of the dissection. The patient may manifest pallor, sweating, and tachycardia. Blood pressure may be elevated, unobtainable, or markedly different from one arm to the other. Because of the variable clinical picture associated with this condition, early diagnosis in often difficult.

Angiogram, computed tomography (CT) scan, ultrasound, and magnetic resonance imaging (MRI) aid in the diagnosis.

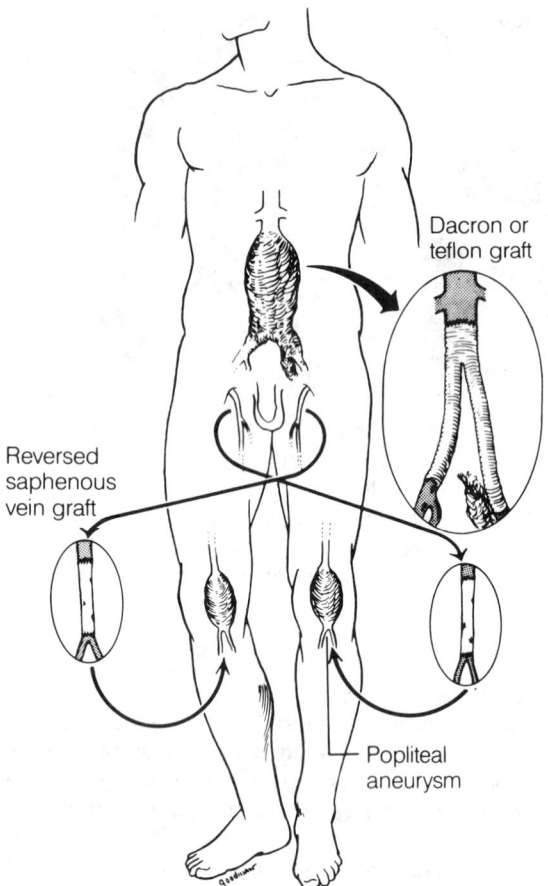

Figure 31–10. Surgical treatment of a large abdominal aneurysm involving the iliac arteries plus bilateral symptomatic popliteal aneurysms. Following resection, the abdominal aneurysm is replaced with a Teflon graft; the popliteal aneurysms are replaced by saphenous vein grafts, which appear to function much better at the flexion crease than the synthetic graft. (Hardy JD et al. Aneurysms of the popliteal artery. Surg Gynecol Obstet Mar; 140:402. By permission of Surgery, Gynecology & Obstetrics.)

Medical or surgical treatment of a dissecting aneurysm again depends on the type present and follows the general principles outlined for treatment of thoracic aortic aneurysms (see p. 754).

Other Aneurysms

Aneurysms may also arise in the peripheral vessels, most often as a result of atherosclerosis. These may involve such vessels as the renal artery, the subclavian artery, or (most frequently) the popliteal artery in the area of the knee. Such aneurysms may be bilateral.

The aneurysm produces a pulsating mass and a disturbance of peripheral circulation distal to it. Pain and swelling develop because of pressure on adjacent nerves and veins. Surgical repair of such aneurysms is now carried out with replacement grafts.

Gerontologic Considerations.   Most abdominal aneurysms occur between the age of 60 and 90 years. Aneurysm rupture is likely if there is coexistent hypertension or if the aneurysm is larger than 6 cm.

Arterial Embolism

Pathophysiology.   Arterial emboli arise most commonly from thrombi that develop in the chambers of the heart as a result of atrial fibrillation, myocardial infarction, infective endocarditis, or chronic congestive heart failure. These thrombi become detached and are carried from the left side of the heart into the arterial system, where they obstruct an artery that is smaller in size than the embolus. Emboli may also develop in advanced aortic atherosclerosis because of roughening or ulceration of the atheromatous plaques. The sequelae of arterial emboli depend primarily on the size of the embolus, the organ involved, and the state of the collateral vessels. The immediate effect is cessation of distal blood flow. The clot can progress above and below the obstruction. Secondary vasospasm can contribute to the ischemia. Fragmentation of the embolus can occur, resulting in occlusion of more distal vessels.

Emboli tend to lodge at arterial bifurcations and atherosclerotic narrowings. Cerebral, mesenteric, renal, and coronary arteries are often involved, in addition to the large arteries of the extremities.

Clinical Manifestations.   The symptoms of acute arterial embolism in extremities with poor collateral flow are acute, severe pain and a gradual loss of sensory and motor function. Pain may be aggravated by movement of and pressure on the extremity. Distal pulses are lost, and the extremity becomes pale, mottled, and numb. Superficial veins may be collapsed because of decreased blood flow to the extremity. A sharp line of color and temperature demarcation may occur distal to the site of the occlusion as a result of ischemia.

Management.   Medical management of an acute embolic occlusion includes intravenous anticoagulation with heparin, which will prevent propagation of the clot and thus reduce muscle necrosis. Thrombolytic agents such as streptokinase, urokinase, and tissue-type plasminogen activator (t-PA), are useful in hastening embolic lysis. Although the pharmacokinetics of these agents differ, the method of administration is similar. With radiographic visualization, a catheter is advanced to the clot into which the thrombolytic agent is infused. Thrombolytic therapy should not be used when there are known contraindications to therapy or when several additional hours of ischemia would necessitate amputation of the limb. Contraindications to thrombolytic therapy include active internal bleeding, stroke, recent major surgery, uncontrolled hypertension, and pregnancy. The treatment of choice in these instances is embolectomy.

Embolectomy involves incising the vessel and removing the clot. Before surgery, the patient remains on bed rest with the extremity level or slightly (15 degrees) dependent. The affected part is kept at room temperature and protected from trauma.

Postoperative Nursing Management.   During the postoperative period, every effort is made to encourage movement of the leg to stimulate circulation and prevent stasis. The nurse collaborates with the surgeon about the appropriate level of activity warranted based on the individual patient's condition. Anticoagulants may be continued for a time after surgery to prevent thrombosis of the affected artery and to diminish the development of thrombi at the initiating site. The nurse assesses the surgical wound frequently for evidence of hemorrhage, which can occur when anticoagulants are administered.

Arterial Thrombosis

Arterial thrombosis can also acutely occlude an artery. This slowly developing clot usually occurs at the site of damage of the arterial wall, which is most commonly due to atherosclerosis. Thrombi may also develop in an arterial aneurysm. The manifestations of an acute thrombolic arterial occlusion are similar to those described for embolic occlusion. However, treatment is made more difficult with a thrombus because the arterial occlusion has occurred in a degenerated vessel. This requires more extensive reconstructive surgery to restore flow than is required with an embolic event.

Raynaud's Disease

Raynaud's disease is a form of intermittent arteriolar vasoconstriction that results in coldness, pain, and pallor of the fingertips, toes, or tip of the nose. The cause is unknown, although many patients with the disease seem to have immunologic disorders. Recent studies indicate that the symptoms may be the result of a defect in basal heat production that eventually decreases the ability of cutaneous vessels to dilate. Episodes may be triggered by emotional factors or by unusual sensitivity to cold. The disease is most common in women between the ages of 16 and 40 years and is seen much more frequently in cold climates and during the winter months. The classic clinical picture reveals pallor brought on by the sudden vasoconstriction. Cyanosis follows as small amounts of blood enter the capillaries. Vasodilation then produces a red color. Thus the characteristic color change of Raynaud's phenomenon is described as white, blue, and red. The numbness, tingling, burning pain occurs as the color changes. The involvement tends to be bilateral and symmetric.

The term *Raynaud's phenomenon* is currently used to refer to localized, intermittent episodes of vasoconstriction of small arteries of the extremities, causing color and temperature changes. It is generally unilateral and affects only one or two digits. It is always associated with an underlying systemic disease. It may occur with scleroderma, systemic lupus erythematosus, rheumatoid arthritis, obstructive arterial disease, or trauma.

The prognosis for Raynaud's disease varies: some patients slowly improve, some grow slowly worse, and others show no change. Ulceration and gangrene are rare; however, chronic disease may cause atrophy of the skin and muscles.

Nursing Management. Avoidance of the particular stimuli that provoke vasoconstriction is the prime objective in controlling Raynaud's disease. An effort should be made to avoid situations that may upset the patient. Because concern over serious complications such as gangrene and amputation are certainly upsetting, the patient should be reassured that serious sequelae are not usual with Raynaud's disease. Smoking should be avoided.

Exposure to cold must be minimized. In areas where the fall and winter months are cold, the patient should remain indoors as much as possible and wear protective clothing when outdoors. Fabrics specially designed for cold climates (*e.g.*, Thinsulate) are recommended. Sharp objects should be handled carefully to avoid injuring the fingers. The physician may prescribe vasodilator and sympatholytic agents, such as reser-

pine or other rauwolfia derivatives, although their effectiveness is variable. The patient is cautioned about the postural hypotension that can result from these drugs and that this effect is increased by alcohol, exercise, and hot weather.

Interruption of the sympathetic nerves by removal of the sympathetic ganglia or division of their branches (*sympathectomy*) may afford some improvement in patients with Raynaud's disease.

Hypertension

Definition, Incidence, and Etiology

Hypertension can be defined arbitrarily as persistent levels of blood pressure in which the systolic pressure is above 140 mm Hg and the diastolic pressure is above 90 mm Hg. In the elderly population, hypertension is defined as systolic pressure above 160 mm Hg and diastolic pressure above 90 mm Hg. Hypertension is a major cause of heart failure, stroke, and kidney failure. It is called the "silent killer," because the person who has it is often symptom-free. The National Heart, Lung, and Blood Institute has estimated that half of persons with hypertension do not know they have it. Once it develops, a patient should have his blood pressure checked frequently because hypertension is a lifetime condition.

About 20% of the adult population develop hypertension; more than 90% of these have *essential* (primary) hypertension, which has no identifiable medical cause. The remainder develop elevations in blood pressure with specific cause (secondary hypertension), such as renovascular narrowing or parenchyma-renal disease, certain drugs, organ dysfunctions, tumors, and pregnancy.

Accompanying hypertension is the risk of premature morbidity and mortality, which increases as the systolic and diastolic pressures rise. The 1988 Report of the Joint National Committee on Detection, Evaluation, and Treatment of High Blood Pressure presented a recommended classification of blood pressure for persons aged 18 years and older (Table 31–3). This classification is helpful in establishing follow-up criteria when it is used with the knowledge that a diagnosis is based on the average of two or more readings on two or more occasions (Table 31–4).

Essential hypertension usually begins as a labile (intermittent) process in a person's late 30s to early 50s and gradually becomes "fixed." On occasion it appears abruptly and severely and takes an accelerated or "malignant" course that causes rapid deterioration of the patient's condition.

Emotional disturbances, obesity, excessive alcohol intake, and overstimulation with coffee, tobacco, and stimulatory drugs play a role, but the disease is strongly familial. It affects more women than men, but men, especially black men, are less able to tolerate the disease. The incidence increases with age in the United States, and the incidence for black Americans far exceeds that for white Americans.

Prolonged elevation of blood pressure eventually damages blood vessels throughout the body, most notably in the eyes, heart, kidneys, and brain, so that failing vision, coronary occlusion, renal failure, and strokes are the usual consequences of prolonged, uncontrolled hypertension. Cardiac muscle hy-

TABLE 31-3.   Classification of BP

Range, mm Hg	Category*
DIASTOLIC	
<85	Normal BP
85-89	High normal BP
90-104	Mild hypertension
105-114	Moderate hypertension
≥115	Severe hypertension
SYSTOLIC, WHEN DIASTOLIC BP IS <90	
<140	Normal BP
140-159	Borderline isolated systolic hypertension
≥160	Isolated systolic hypertension

* A classification of borderline isolated systolic hypertension (systolic BP 140 to 159 mm Hg) or isolated systolic hypertension (systolic BP ≥160 mm Hg) takes precedence over a classification of high normal BP (diastolic BP, 85 to 89 mm Hg) when both occur in the same person. A classification of high normal BP (diastolic BP 85 to 89 mm Hg) takes precedence over a classification of normal BP (systolic BP < 140 mm Hg) when both occur in the same person.
(The 1988 Report of The Joint National Committee on Detection, Evaluation, and Treatment of High Blood Pressure [NIH Publication No. 88-1088]. Arch Intern Med 1988 May; 148[5]:1024.)

pertrophies as the increased work of pumping against high pressure is sustained.

Increased peripheral resistance controlled at the arteriolar level is the basic cause for the elevated blood pressure, but the causes of increased resistance are poorly understood. Drug therapy is aimed at reducing peripheral resistance, to lower the blood pressure and lessen the stresses on the vascular system.

Pathophysiology of Essential Hypertension

The vasomotor center is situated in the medulla of the brain. Emanating from this vasomotor center are the sympathetic nervous system tracks, which go down the spinal cord and emerge from the spinal column at the sympathetic ganglia in the thorax and abdomen. Stimulation of the vasomotor center sets in motion impulses that travel down through the sympathetic nervous system to the sympathetic ganglia. At this point, the preganglionic neurons release acetylcholine, which stimulates the postganglionic nerve fibers in the blood vessel, where the release of norepinephrine results in constriction of the vessels. Numerous influences may affect the response of the blood vessel to these vasoconstrictor stimuli. Hypertensive persons are very sensitive to norepinephrine, although it is not known exactly why.

In the hypertensive patient, many factors moderate the vasomotor and vasoconstrictor responses, such as anxiety and fear.

Occurring concurrently with sympathetic nervous system stimulation of the blood vessels in response to emotional stimuli is stimulation of the adrenal gland. The adrenal medulla secretes epinephrine, which causes vasoconstriction. The adrenal cortex secretes cortisol and other steroids, which may enhance the vasoconstrictor response of the blood vessels. Vasoconstriction results in reduced blood flow to the kidney, causing the release of renin. Renin leads to the formation of angiotensin, a potent vasoconstrictor, which in turn stimulates secretion of aldosterone by the adrenal cortex. This hormone promotes sodium and water retention by the kidney tubules, causing an increase in intravascular volume. All of these factors tend to perpetuate the hypertensive state.

Gerontologic Considerations. Structural and functional changes in the peripheral vascular system are responsible for the changes in blood pressure that occur with age. Coupled with the age-related process of atherosclerosis, the loss of connective tissue elasticity, and a decrease in the relaxation of vascular smooth muscle, the ability of the vessels to distend and recoil is reduced. Consequently, the aorta and large arteries are less able to accommodate the ejected stroke volume, and a decrease in cardiac output and increase in peripheral resistance result.

The overall rise in prevalence of hypertension in those over 65 years of age is attributed to the increase in isolated systolic hypertension. The risk factors that are present in the general population continue into old age. These are approximately the same for elderly men and women.

Clinical Manifestations

Physical examination may reveal no abnormalities other than high blood pressure, but there may be changes in the retinae with hemorrhages, exudates (fluid accumulation), narrowed

TABLE 31-4.   Follow-Up Criteria for First-Occasion Measurement

Range (mm Hg)	Recommended Follow-Up*
DIASTOLIC	
<85	Recheck within 2 yr.
85-89	Recheck with 1 yr.
90-104	Confirm promptly (not to exceed 2 mo).
105-114	Evaluate or refer promptly to source of care (not to exceed 2 wk).
≥115	Evaluate or refer immediately to a source of care.
SYSTOLIC, WHEN DIASTOLIC BP IS <90	
<140	Recheck within 2 yr.
140-199	Confirm promptly (not to exceed 2 mo).
≥200	Evaluate or refer promptly to source of care (not to exceed 2 wk).

* If recommendations for follow-up of diastolic and systolic BPs are different for those aged 18 years or older, the shorter recommended time period supersedes and a referral supersedes a recheck recommendation.
(The 1988 Report of The Joint National Committee on Detection, Evaluation, and Treatment of High Blood Pressure [NIH Publication No. 88-1088]. Arch Intern Med 1988 May; 148[5]:1024.)

arterioles, and, in severe cases, papilledema (edema of the optic disc).

Persons with hypertension can be asymptomatic and remain so for many years. The appearance of symptoms usually indicates vascular damage, and specific manifestations are related to the organ systems served by the involved vessels. Coronary artery disease with angina is the most common sequela in hypertensive individuals. Left ventricular hypertrophy occurs in response to the increased workload placed on the ventricle as it contracts against higher systemic pressures. When the heart can no longer sustain the increased workload, left heart failure ensues. Pathologic changes in the kidneys may be manifested as nocturia and azotemia (increased blood urea nitrogen [BUN] and creatinine). Cerebral vascular involvement may produce a stroke or transient ischemic attack (TIA) manifested by temporary hemiplegia, blackouts, or alterations in vision. Cerebral infarctions account for 80% of the strokes and transient ischemic attacks in hypertensive persons.

Diagnostic Evaluation

A thorough history and physical examination are necessary. The retinae are examined, and laboratory studies are performed to assess target organ damage. Left ventricular hypertrophy (LVH) can be assessed by electrocardiogram; protein in the urine can be detected by urinalysis. Inability to concentrate the urine and an increase in the blood urea nitrogen may also be present. Special studies, such as renograms, intravenous pyelograms, renal arteriograms, split renal function studies, and the determination of renin levels, may also be performed to identify patients with renovascular disease. The presence of additional risk factors is assessed and evaluated.

Management

The objective of any treatment program selected for individual patients is to prevent associated morbidity and mortality by achieving and maintaining an arterial blood pressure below 140/90 mm Hg, whenever possible. The effectiveness of any program is determined by the degree of hypertension, complications, the cost of care, and perceived quality of life issues associated with the therapy.

Recent evidence demonstrates that nonpharmacologic approaches, including weight reduction; restriction of alcohol, sodium, and tobacco; exercise; and relaxation are definitive interventions that should be used in all antihypertensive therapy. When an individual with mild hypertension is at high risk (men, smokers), or where diastolic blood pressure is persistently elevated over 94 mm Hg, drug therapy should be initiated.

The step-care approach allows the practitioner to select the drug class that has the greatest effectiveness, fewest side effects, and best chance of acceptance by the patient (Fig. 31–11). Four classes of drugs are available as the first-line therapy, including thiazide diuretics, beta-blockers, calcium antagonists, and angiotensin-converting enzyme (ACE) inhibitors. When the patient with mild hypertension has been controlled for a year, the therapy can be stepped down or reduced.

In an attempt to promote compliance, complicated drug therapy schedules should be avoided. Table 31–5 describes the various pharmacologic agents used in the treatment of hypertension.

In summary, hypertension is defined as an elevation in blood pressure that exceeds 140/90 mm Hg when taken two or more times on two or more occasions. Although the exact cause of hypertension is unclear, it is known that there is an increase in vascular resistance at the arteriolar level. As resistance is sustained, vessels in the eyes, heart, kidney, and other organs are damaged. Eventually the left heart will thicken and hypertrophy in an attempt to supply the blood to the tissues.

Initially a hypertensive patient may not exhibit any overt manifestations of this disease; however, physical findings may reveal vascular or end-organ damage. Prevention of associated morbidity and mortality is the goal of all treatment programs. Reduction in blood pressure values can be accomplished by a combination of pharmacologic and nonpharmacologic approaches.

▶ Nursing Process
The Patient With Hypertension

◇ Assessment

Assessment of the patient with hypertension involves careful monitoring of the blood pressure at frequent intervals. The 1988 report of the Joint National Committee on Detection, Evaluation, and Treatment of High Blood Pressure has ex-

(text continues on page 764)

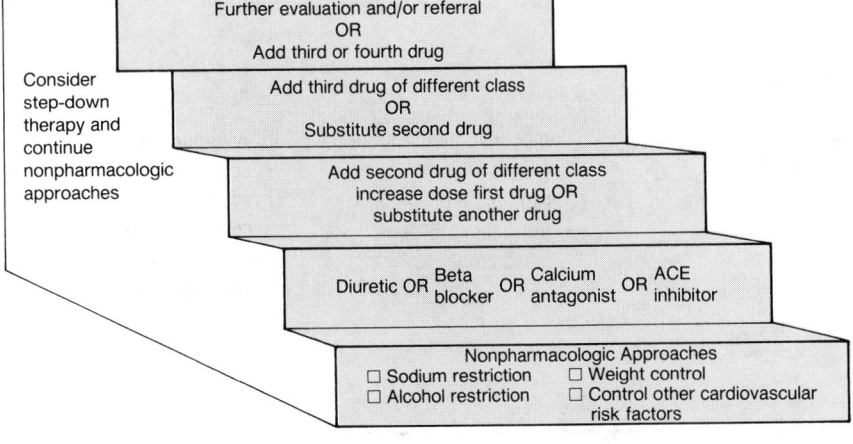

Figure 31–11. Individualized step-care therapy for hypertension. For some patients, nonpharmacologic therapy should be tried first. If blood pressure goal is not achieved, add pharmacologic therapy. Other patients may require pharmacologic therapy initially. In these instances, nonpharmacologic therapy may be helpful adjunct. ACE indicates angiotensin-converting enzyme; asterisk, drugs such as diuretics, β-blockers, calcium antagonists, ACE inhibitors, α-blockers, centrally acting α₂-agonists, rauwolfia serpentina, and vasodilators. (The 1988 Report of the Joint National Committee on Detection, Evaluation, and Treatment of High Blood Pressure [NIH Publication No. 88-1088]. Arch Intern Med 1988 May; 148[5]:1028.)

TABLE 31–5. *Medication Therapy for Hypertension*

Purpose: To maintain blood pressure within normal ranges by the simplest and safest means possible with the fewest side effects for each individual patient

Medication	Major Action	Advantages	Contraindications	Effects and Nursing Considerations
DIURETICS & RELATED DRUGS				
Thiazide Diuretics				
Chlorthalidone (Hygroton) Quinethazone (Hydromox) Chlorothiazide (Diuril) Hydrochlorothiazide (Esidrix; HydroDiuril)	Decrease of blood volume, renal blood flow, and cardiac output Depletion of extracellular fluid Negative sodium balance (from natriuresis), mild hypokalemia Directly affect vascular smooth muscle	Effective orally Effective during long-term administration Mild side effects Enhance other antihypertensive drugs Counter sodium retention effect of other antihypertensive drugs	Gout Known sensitivity to sulfonamide-derived drugs Severely impaired kidney function	Dry mouth, thirst, weakness, drowsiness, lethargy, muscle aches, muscular fatigue, tachycardia, GI disturbance Postural hypotension may be potentiated by alcohol, barbiturates, or narcotics Because thiazides cause sodium loss, patient is instructed to watch for postural hypotension in the summer. (Eating salted pretzels in hot weather may avert this.) Administer supplementary potassium. *Gerontologic Considerations:* Risk of postural hypotension is significant because of volume depletion; measure blood pressure in three positions.
Loop Diuretics				
Furosemide (Lasix) Ethacrynic acid (Edecrin)	Volume depletion Block reabsorption of sodium and water in kidney Antagonize action of aldosterone	Action rapid Potent To be used only when thiazides fail	Same as for thiazides	Volume depletion is rapid—profound diuresis Electrolyte depletion—replacement is required. Thirst, nausea, vomiting, skin rash, postural hypotension Sweet taste noted; oral and gastric burning *Gerontologic Considerations:* Same as thiazides
Potassium-Sparing Diuretics				
Spironolactone (Aldactone) Triamterene (Dyrenium)	Competitive inhibitors of aldosterone Act on distal tubule independently of aldosterone	Spironolactone is effective in treating hypertension accompanying primary aldosteronism. Both spironolactone and triamterene retain potassium.	Renal disease Azotemia Severe hepatic disease	Drowsiness, lethargy, headache—decrease the dosage. Diarrhea and other GI symptoms—administer drug after meals. Skin eruptions, urticaria

(continued)

TABLE 31–5. *(Continued)*

Medication	Major Action	Advantages	Contraindications	Effects and Nursing Considerations
DIURETICS & RELATED DRUGS *(continued)*				Mental confusion, ataxia— perhaps dosage needs to be reduced. Gynecomastia (not for triamterene)
ADRENERGIC INHIBITORS				
Reserpine (alkaloid of *Rauwolfia serpentina*)	Impairs synthesis and reuptake of norepinephrine	Slows pulse, which counteracts tachycardia of hydralazine	History of depression Psychosis Obesity Chronic sinusitis Peptic ulcer	May cause severe depression; report manifestations, as this may require that drug be omitted. Nasal stuffiness, which may require nasal vasoconstrictor Increases appetite— therefore, suggest stricter diet. Recurrence of peptic ulcer Administer with meals or milk. *Gerontologic Considerations:* Depression and postural hypotension common in elderly
Methyldopa (Aldomet)	Dopa-decarboxylase inhibitor; displaces norepinephrine from storage sites	Effective in patients not controlled with thiazide-reserpine (with or without hydralazine) Useful in patients with renal failure Does not decrease cardiac output or renal blood flow Does not induce oliguria	Liver disease	Drowsiness, dizziness Dry mouth; nasal stuffiness (troublesome at first but then tends to disappear) Hemolytic anemia (a hypersensitization reaction)—positive Coombs' test; may not indicate drug discontinuance *Gerontologic Considerations:* May produce mental and behavioral side effects in the elderly
Propranolol (Inderal)	Blocks the sympathetic nervous system (β-adrenergic receptors), especially the sympathetics to the heart, producing a slower heart rate and lowered blood pressure	Reduces pulse rate in patients with tachycardia and blood pressure elevation and is useful as an adjunctive drug with drugs that act at the neuroeffector site of the blood vessel	Bronchial asthma Allergic rhinitis Right ventricular failure due to pulmonary hypertension Congestive heart failure	Mental depression manifested by insomnia, lassitude, weakness, and fatigue Lightheadedness and occasional nausea, vomiting, and epigastric distress Blood dyscrasias such as agranulocytosis and thrombocytopenic purpura do occur, but are uncommon.

(continued)

TABLE 31–5.   *(Continued)*

Medication	Major Action	Advantages	Contraindications	Effects and Nursing Considerations
ADRENERGIC INHIBITORS (continued)				
				Gerontologic Considerations: Risk of toxicity is increased for elderly with decreased renal and liver function. Take blood pressure in three positions and observe for hypotension.
Prazosin hydrochloride (Minipress)	Peripheral vasodilator acting directly on the blood vessel; similar to hydralazine	Acts directly on the blood vessel and is an effective agent in patients with adverse reactions to hydralazine	Angina pectoris and coronary artery disease. Induces tachycardia if not preceded by administration of propranolol and a diuretic	Occasional vomiting and diarrhea, urinary frequency, and cardiovascular collapse, especially if given in addition to hydralazine without lowering the dose of the latter. Patients occasionally experience drowsiness, lack of energy, and weakness.
Clonidine hydrochloride (Catapres)	Exact mode of action not understood, but acts through the central nervous system, apparently through centrally mediated α-adrenergic stimulation in the brain, producing blood pressure reduction	Little or no orthostatic effect. Moderately potent, and sometimes is effective when other drugs fail to lower blood pressure	Severe coronary artery disease, pregnancy, children	Most common side effects are dry mouth, drowsiness, sedation, and occasional headaches and fatigue. Anorexia, malaise, and vomiting with mild disturbance of liver function have been reported. Skin rash, dreams and nightmares, insomnia, and anxiety have been reported but are not common.
Metoprolol (Lopressor)	Blocks access of norepinephrine to β_1-adrenergic receptors, especially in myocardium; decreases blood pressure by decreasing cardiac output and peripheral resistance	Rapid absorption	Cardiac failure Sinus bradycardia A-V conduction defects Diabetes mellitus	May cause bradycardia, congestive heart failure, intensification of heart block—take apical pulse before administration. May cause severe depression; report manifestations, as this may require that drug be omitted. Instruct patient to take radial pulse before each dose and report slow or irregular pulse to physician.
Nadolol (Corgard)	Blocks β-adrenergic receptors within the heart; reduces cardiac rate and output and	Can be used alone to treat hypertension, or in combination with a diuretic	Cardiac failure Sinus bradycardia Bronchial asthma COPD	May cause bradycardia; instruct patient to take pulse before each dose and report slow pulse to physician.

(continued)

TABLE 31–5.   *(Continued)*

Medication	Major Action	Advantages	Contraindications	Effects and Nursing Considerations
ADRENERGIC INHIBITORS *(continued)*				
	decreases myocardial automaticity; exact mode of action for decreasing standing and supine blood pressures unknown	Long half-life; once daily administration		May cause dizziness, sedation, behavioral changes, depression; caution patient to avoid driving and other dangerous activities until response is known.
Guanethidine (Ismelin)	Prevents release of sympathetic transmitter, norepinephrine. Is a depressant of adrenergic activity Depletes tissue stores Causes venous pooling, decreased venous return, and decreased cardiac output Decreases pulse rate, cardiac output, and renal blood flow	Potency	Pheochromocytoma, because greatly enhances pressor effect of catecholamines	Severe postural hypotension accentuated by alcohol, exercise, hot weather Warn against suddenly standing or standing for a long time. Diarrhea and nausea, nocturia Failure of ejaculation; counsel about possible sexual dysfunction. Fatigue and giddiness; blackout
VASODILATORS				
Hydralazine hydrochloride (Apresoline)	Decreases peripheral resistance but concurrently elevates cardiac output Acts directly on smooth muscle of blood vessels	Used as a third drug of choice when patient does not respond to thiazide-reserpine, thiazide-methyldopa, or thiazide-guanethidine	Angina or coronary disease Congestive heart failure Hypersensitivity	Headache, tachycardia, flushing, and dyspnea may occur—can be prevented by pretreating with reserpine. Peripheral edema may require diuretics. May produce lupus erythematosus-like syndrome
Minoxidil	Direct vasodilating action on arteriolar vessels, causing decreased peripheral vascular resistance; reduces systolic and diastolic pressures	Hypotensive effect more pronounced than hydralazine No effect on vasomotor reflexes; thus does not cause postural hypotension	Pheochromocytoma	Tachycardia, angina pectoris, ECG changes, edema; take blood pressure and apical pulse before administration; monitor I&O and daily weights.
ANGIOTENSIN-CONVERTING ENZYME INHIBITOR				
Captopril (Capoten)	Inhibits conversion of angiotensin I to angiotensin II Lowers total peripheral resistance	Fewer cardiovascular side effects Can be used with thiazide diuretic and digitalis Hypotension reversed by volume	Renal impairment	*Gerontologic Considerations:* Requires reduced dosages and loop diuretics with renal dysfunction
CALCIUM ANTAGONIST				
Diltiazem Hydrochloride (Cardizem)	Inhibits calcium ion influx Reduces cardiac afterload	Inhibits coronary artery spasm not controlled	Sick sinus syndrome; second or third	Do not discontinue suddenly

(continued)

TABLE 31–5.   *(Continued)*

Medication	Major Action	Advantages	Contraindications	Effects and Nursing Considerations
CALCIUM ANTAGONIST (continued)				
		by β-blockers or nitrates	degree AV block; hypotension; congestive heart failure	Observe for hypotension Report irregular heartbeat, dizziness, edema Instruct on regular dental care because of potential gingivitis
Nifedipine (Procardia: Adalat)	Inhibits calcium ion influx across membranes Vasodilating effects on coronary and peripheral arteriole Decreases cardiac work and energy consumption, increases delivery of oxygen to myocardium	Rapid action Effective oral or sublinqual No tendency to slow SA nodal activity or prolong AV node conduction	None	Administer on empty stomach Use with caution with diabetics Small frequent meals if complains of nausea Muscle cramps, joint stiffness, sexual difficulties disappear when dose decreased Report irregular heartbeat, constipation, shortness of breath, edema May cause dizziness
Verapamil (Calan, Isoptin)	Inhibits calcium ion influx Slows velocity of conduction of cardiac impulse	Effective antidysrhythmic Rapid IV onset Blocks SA and AV node channels	Sinus or AV node disease; severe heart failure Severe hypotension	Administer on empty stomach or before meal Do not discontinue suddenly Depression disappears when drug discontinued For headaches: reduce noise, monitor electrolytes Decrease dose for liver or renal failure *Gerontologic Considerations:* Requires reduced dose

panded its recommendations for the measurement of blood pressure. Conditions before measurement, equipment specifications, and techniques for measuring blood pressure are established so as to obtain a value that reflects the patient's usual status (Table 31–6). When the patient is placed on an antihypertensive drug therapy regimen, blood pressure readings are imperative to demonstrate the effectiveness of the drugs and to reveal decreases in pressure that would necessitate a change in the dosage of the drugs.

Physical examination also includes assessment of apical and peripheral pulses, their rate, rhythm, and character, to detect effects of the hypertension on the heart and the peripheral vessels. The patient is assessed for symptoms that would be indicative of multisystem sequelae of hypertension, such as nosebleeds, anginal pain, shortness of breath, alterations in vision, vertigo, headaches, or nocturia. A thorough assessment can yield valuable information about the extent of the effects of the hypertension throughout the body and any psychological factors related to the problem.

▷ Nursing Diagnoses

Based on the assessment data, nursing diagnoses for the patient may include the following:

- Knowledge deficit regarding the relation between the treatment regimen and control of the disease process
- Potential noncompliance to the self-care program related to negative side effects of prescribed therapy

▷ Planning and Implementation

▷ *Goals:* The major goals for the patient include understanding of the disease process and its treatment, and compliance with the self-care program.

TABLE 31-6. *Conditions, Equipment, and Techniques for Measuring Blood Pressure*

CONDITIONS BEFORE MEASUREMENT

No smoking or caffeine for 30 minutes.

Five minutes of quiet rest.

Patient seated with bare arm positioned at heart level and supported.

EQUIPMENT

For clinicians' use: mercury sphygmomanometer, recently calibrated aneroid manometer, or validated electronic device.

For patients' use (at home): automatic and semiautomatic devices using acoustic or oscillometric methods and digital display of readings.

Documented validity and reliability of all equipment types by manufacturer along with periodic calibration and maintenance.

Availability of several sizes of cuffs with appropriate one chosen so that rubber bladder encircles at least two thirds of arm (for children, bladder should encircle circumference of arm).

TECHNIQUES

Assessment based on average of at least two readings (if two readings differ by more than 5 mm Hg, additional readings are taken and used to calculate the average).

CONDITIONS AFTER MEASUREMENT

Inform patient of numeric BP value and need for periodic reassessment based on established follow-up criteria (wallet-sized cards designed for these purposes serve as useful reminders).

(Update on High Blood Pressure: Highlights from 1988 National Report. Nurs Prac 1988 Dec; 13[12]: 10.)

▷ **Nursing Interventions**

▷ *Patient Education to Avoid Progression of Vascular Changes.* The objective of treatment for hypertension is to lower the blood pressure to as close to normal levels as possible without introducing adverse effects. Adherence to therapy must be promoted in a cost-effective manner.

The treatment regimen consists of antihypertensive medications, dietary restrictions on sodium and fat, weight control, life-style changes, and follow-up health care at regular intervals. Because the therapeutic regimen becomes the responsibility of the patient, if able, or a significant other, counseling and education are imperative on an ongoing basis. Many patients benefit from hypertension clinics and support groups in which they can share their concerns with other patients and find the needed support for the life-style changes that accompany the therapy. The family should be involved in the educational and counseling programs so that they can support the patient's efforts to control hypertension.

Regular follow-up care is imperative so that the disease process can be assessed in terms of control or progression and treated accordingly. Symptoms of progression of the disease with involvement of other body systems must be detected early so that appropriate changes in the treatment regimen can be made.

▷ *Compliance With the Self-Care Program.* Noncompliance with the therapeutic program is a significant problem in people with hypertension. It is estimated that 50% discontinue their drug therapy within 1 year of its initiation, and that adequate blood pressure control is maintained in only 20%. Active participation of the patient in the program, including self-monitoring of blood pressure and diet, has been found to increase compliance by providing instant feedback and a greater sense of control.

A lot of energy is required of patients with hypertension to adhere to life-style, diet, and activity restrictions and to take regularly prescribed medications. The effort needed does not always seem reasonable, particularly when patients are symptom-free without medications but experience side effects with the medications. Much supervision, education, and encouragement are often needed with hypertensive persons to arrive at an acceptable plan for living with their hypertension and the treatment regimen. Compromises may have to be made on some aspects of the therapy to achieve success in higher-priority areas.

A thorough understanding of the disease process of hypertension as well as the impact of medication and health habits on this process is important. The concept of hypertension control rather than cure is important to explain. The temporary nature of medication side effects should be emphasized. Consultation with a dietitian may be useful in exploring the number of possible ways to modify salt and fat intake. Lists of low-salt foods and beverages should be provided. Salt substitutes are readily available and inexpensive. Beverages containing caffeine should be avoided. Alcohol may have synergistic effects with the medications, so the patient should be fully informed of this and encouraged to abstain from the use of alcohol. Because nicotine causes vasoconstriction, the use of tobacco should be discouraged. Support groups for control of weight, smoking, and stress may be beneficial for some patients. Others may need more support from family and friends.

Written information about the expected effects and side effects of medications is very useful in maintaining a safe self-administration program. When side effects do occur, patients need to know when and whom to contact. In addition, patients should be advised of the possibility of rebound hypertension with sudden discontinuation of antihypertensive medication, and of the possibility of sexual dysfunction related to the drugs.

The patient may be taught to measure blood pressure at home. Some authorities believe that this involves patients in their own care and emphasizes the fact that failing to take the medication can lead to a rise in blood pressure. It is difficult to convince many patients that the blood pressure is normally variable and does not stay fixed at one number.

Gerontologic Considerations. Compliance with the therapeutic program is even more difficult for the elderly person than for the general population. Drug therapy can be a significant problem because it must be continuous, it may require numerous doses daily, and it may be especially expensive for the person on a fixed income. Monotherapy, treatment with a single agent, may be appropriate in the elderly population. Special care must be taken to make sure that the patient understands the drug regimen and is able to read the instructions, and that provisions are made for having prescriptions refilled as needed. The elderly patient's family should always be included in the teaching program so that they can understand the patient's needs, support adherence to the therapeutic program, and know when to seek guidance from health professionals.

The patient and family should be especially cautioned that the antihypertensive drug therapy may cause problems of hypotension, which should be reported immediately. Because of their impaired cardiovascular reflexes, the elderly are often more sensitive than are younger persons to the volume depletion caused by diuretic therapy and by the sympathetic inhibition effect of adrenergic antagonists. In an attempt to prevent the postural hypotension that may ensue, the patient should be very careful to change positions slowly and to use supportive aids if necessary to prevent falls that could result from dizziness and syncope.

▷ Evaluation

Expected Outcomes

1. Maintains adequate tissue perfusion
   a. Maintains blood pressure within acceptable range with medication or diet therapy
   b. Gives no evidence of symptoms of angina, palpitations
   c. Reveals no electrocardiogram (ECG) changes indicative of left ventricular hypertrophy
   d. Has normal BUN and serum creatinine levels
   e. Exhibits no progression of retinal pathology
   f. Gives no evidence of symptoms of cerebral infarction, changes in mental status
   g. Peripheral pulses present
   h. Skin warm and dry
2. Complies with the self-care program
   a. Explains rationale for all aspects of the therapeutic regimen
   b. Includes family in decisions regarding changes in life style necessitated by the therapeutic regimen
   c. Adheres to the dietary regimen as prescribed: sodium, cholesterol, and calorie reduction
   d. Loses weight as prescribed
   e. Becomes involved in a regular program of exercise
   f. Takes own blood pressure daily (if appropriate)
   g. Takes medications as prescribed
   h. Reports side effects of medications to physician before altering or discontinuing medications
   i. Abstains from tobacco, caffeine, and alcohol
   j. Uses available community resources for stress management and reduction
   k. Explains rationale for continuance of therapeutic regimen, even though symptom free
   l. Keeps follow-up clinic or physician appointments

Hypertensive Emergencies

A hypertensive emergency exists when an elevated blood pressure must be lowered within 1 hour. These acute, life-threatening elevations in blood pressure require prompt treatment because of the serious end-organ damage that may occur. Hypertensive emergencies occur in patients whose hypertension has been poorly controlled or in whom medications have been abruptly discontinued. The presence of acute left ventricular failure or cerebral dysfunction indicates the need for immediate reduction in blood pressure.

The drugs of choice in hypertensive emergencies are those that have immediate effect. Intravenous nitroprusside has an immediate vasodilating action that is short-lived, and is thus widely used as the initial treatment in crisis. Other drugs used

for hypertensive emergencies include reserpine (Serpasil), methyldopa (Aldomet), phentolamine (Regitine), diazoxide (Hyperstat), and hydralazine (Apresoline). Most of these potent drugs are potentiated by diuretics. Extremely close monitoring of the patient's blood pressure and cardiovascular status is required during treatment with these medications. A precipitous drop in blood pressure can occur, and action must be taken immediately to prevent shock.

Vein Disorders

Venous Thrombosis, Thrombophlebitis, Phlebothrombosis, and Deep Vein Thrombosis

Although the above terms do not necessarily represent an identical pathology, for clinical purposes they are often used interchangeably.

Pathophysiology and Etiology

Although the exact cause of venous thrombosis remains unclear, three antecedent factors are believed to play a significant role in its development: stasis of blood, injury to the vessel wall, and altered blood coagulation. The presence of at least two factors appears to be necessary for thrombosis to occur.

Venous stasis occurs when blood flow is retarded, such as with heart failure or shock; when veins are dilated, such as after drug therapy; and when skeletal muscle contraction is reduced, as with immobility, extremity paralysis, or anesthesia. Bed rest has been shown to reduce blood flow in the legs at least 50%.

Disruption of the intimal lining of blood vessels creates a site for clot formation. Direct vessel trauma, such as after a fracture or dislocation, diseases of the veins, and chemical irritation of the vein from intravenous drugs or solutions, can all damage veins.

Increased coagulability of blood occurs most commonly in patients for whom anticoagulant medications have been abruptly withdrawn. Oral contraceptives and a number of blood dyscrasias can also lead to hypercoagulability.

Thrombophlebitis is inflammation of the walls of the veins, often accompanied by the formation of a clot. When a clot develops initially in the veins as a result of stasis or hypercoagulability, but without inflammation, the process is referred to as *phlebothrombosis*. Venous thrombosis can occur in any vein but is most frequent in the veins of the lower extremities. Both superficial and deep veins of the legs may be affected. Of the superficial veins, the saphenous vein is most frequently affected. Of the deep leg veins, the iliofemoral, popliteal, and small calf veins are most often involved.

Venous thrombi are composed of an aggregate of platelets attached to the vein wall and a tail-like appendage containing fibrin, white blood cells, and many red blood cells. The "tail" can grow larger or propagate in the direction of blood flow as successive layering of the clot constituents occurs. The danger associated with a propagating venous thrombosis is that parts of a clot can become detached and produce an embolic oc-

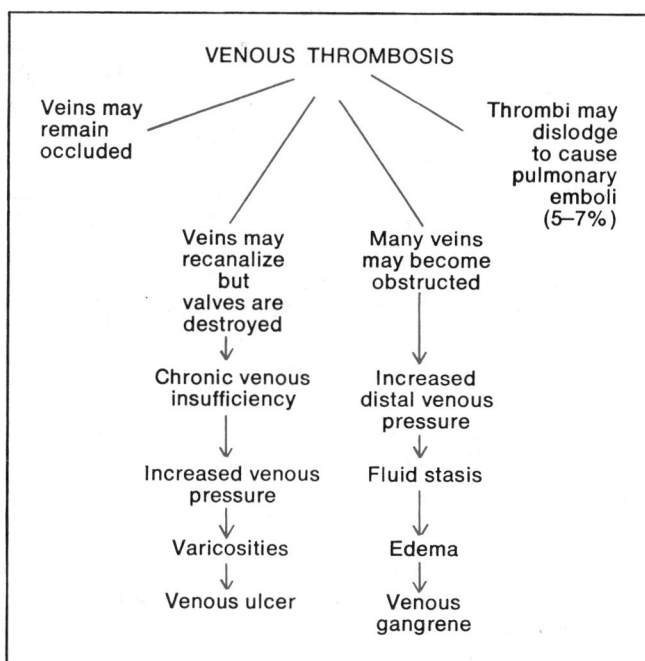

Figure 31-12. Complications of venous thrombosis. The seriousness of venous thrombosis is readily noted.

clusion of the pulmonary blood vessels. Fragmentation of the thrombus can occur spontaneously as the clot undergoes natural dissolution, or it can occur in association with elevation in venous pressure, such as occurs with sudden standing or muscular activity after prolonged inactivity. Other complications of venous thrombosis are described in Figure 31-12.

Clinical Manifestations

As many as 50% of all patients with venous thrombosis of the lower extremities have no symptoms. In others, symptoms are variable and not usually specific for thrombophlebitis. Despite this variability, however, the presence of clinical signs should always be investigated further.

Obstruction of the *deep* veins of the legs produces edema and swelling of the extremity because the outflow of venous blood is inhibited. The amount of swelling can be determined by measuring extremity circumference at various levels with a tape measure. One extremity is compared with the other at the same level for size differences. Bilateral swelling may be difficult to detect. The skin over the affected leg may become warmer, and superficial veins may become more prominent. Tenderness, which usually occurs later, is produced by inflammation of the vein wall and can be detected by gentle palpation of the extremity. *Homans' sign,* pain in the calf after sharp dorsiflexion of the foot, is not specific for deep venous thrombosis because it can be elicited in any painful condition of the calf. In some cases, signs of a pulmonary embolus are the first indication of a deep venous thrombosis.

Thrombosis of *superficial* veins produces pain or tenderness, redness, and warmth of the involved area. The risk of dislodgment and embolization of superficial venous thrombi is very low because the majority of them undergo spontaneous lysis; thus, this condition can be treated at home with rest, extremity elevation, analgesics, and possibly anti-inflammatory agents.

Nursing Assessment

Careful nursing assessment is invaluable in detecting early signs of venous disorders of the lower extremities. Patients with a history of varicose veins, hypercoagulation, neoplastic disease, cardiovascular disease, or recent major surgery or injury, and the obese, the elderly, and women taking oral contraceptives are in the high-risk group (Chart 31-2).

The following parameters are included in the nursing assessment:

- Question the patient about the presence of leg pain, heaviness, any functional impairment, or edema
- Inspect the legs from the groin to the feet, noting asymmetry and measuring and recording calf circumference. (One early indication of edema is engorgement of the concavity behind the medial malleolus.)
- Note any increase in temperature in the affected leg. (To determine temperature differences most effectively, cool hands in cold water, dry, and place them simultaneously on both of the patient's ankles and then on the calves.)
- To identify areas of tenderness and any thromboses (as evidenced by cordlike venous segments), palpate the leg carefully using three or four fingers, advancing the hands back and forth from the ankle to the knee and then to the groin.

Diagnostic Evaluation

Many noninvasive and invasive techniques are available to aid in verifying, defining, and localizing the presence of venous thrombosis. The noninvasive techniques of Doppler ultrasonography, impedence plethysmography, and duplex imaging rely on the thrombus to create abnormalities of venous flow.

Doppler ultrasonography involves the use of a Doppler probe placed over veins that are obstructed. The Doppler flow reading will be diminished in comparison with that for the opposite extremity, or absent. This method is relatively inexpensive, portable, simple, rapid, and noninvasive. Duplex venous imaging is able to obtain anatomic information, as well as to assess physiologic parameters.

Impedance plethysmography is used to measure changes in venous volume. A blood pressure cuff is applied to the patient's thigh and is inflated enough to impede venous flow (about 50 to 60 mm Hg) but not enough to impede arterial flow. Calf electrodes are used to measure electrical resistance that results from venous volume changes. In the presence of deep vein thrombosis, the increase in venous volume that nor-

---

Chart 31-2
Risk Factors for Thrombophlebitis

Bed rest—myocardial infarction, congestive heart failure, sepsis, traction
General surgery—in patients over 40 years of age
Leg trauma—especially fractures, casts
Previous venous insufficiency
Obesity
Oral contraceptives
Malignancy

mally results from blood trapped below the level of the cuff will be less than expected. False-positive results can be due to factors that cause vasoconstriction, increased venous pressure, decreased cardiac output, or external compression of the vein. False-negative results can be due to the existence of an old thrombus with subsequent development of adequate collateral circulation or to superficial phlebitis. The use of both Doppler ultrasonography and impedance plethysmography can significantly increase the accuracy of diagnosis.

Invasive techniques rely on the injection of contrast media into the venous system, which then bind with structural elements of the thrombus. ^{125}I-labeled fibrinogen and contrast phlebography are examples of these tests.

^{125}I-labeled fibrinogen scanning, a recently developed diagnostic procedure, has provided a sensitive method for early detection of venous thrombosis. The test relies on the fact that radioactive fibrinogen, when injected intravenously, will concentrate in the forming clot. The level of radioactivity can then be serially measured by an external counter, and the progression of the clot can be monitored. This test will not reveal thrombi that have already formed, however, nor thrombi in the groin or pelvic areas. A further drawback is the costliness of the test.

Contrast *phlebography* (venography) involves the injection of radiographic contrast media into the venous system through a dorsal foot vein. The diagnosis is based on the demonstration of an unfilled segment of vein in an otherwise completely filled vein with its connecting collaterals. Injection of the contrast media can cause a brief but painful vein inflammation. This test is generally accepted as the hallmark for diagnosis of venous thrombosis.

Preventive Measures

Venous thrombosis, thrombophlebitis, and deep vein thrombosis can often be prevented, especially if patients who are considered at high risk are identified and preventive measures are instituted without delay.

Elastic Stockings.   One approach to prophylaxis is the use of elastic stockings, which are usually prescribed for patients on a regimen of restricted activity, particularly those who are confined to bed. These stockings, by exerting a sustained, evenly distributed pressure over the entire surface of the calves, reduce the caliber of the superficial veins of the lower extremities, resulting in increased flow in the deeper veins. It is important to note that any type of stocking, including the elastic type, can be converted into a tourniquet if applied incorrectly (*i.e.*, rolled tightly at the top). In such instances, the stockings will produce stasis instead of preventing it. Elastic stockings are removed for a brief interval at least twice daily. While they are off, the skin is inspected for signs of irritation and the calves are examined for possible tenderness. Any skin changes or signs of tenderness are reported.

Intermittent pneumatic compression (IPC) devices can be used with the elastic stocking for the prevention of DVT. The IPC consists of an electric controller that is attached by air hoses to plastic leg sleeves. The leg sleeves are divided into compartments, which sequentially fill to apply pressure to the ankle, calf, and thigh at 35 to 55 mm Hg pressure. The IPC is capable of producing increases in blood velocity in excess of the elastic stockings. Nursing measures include ensuring that prescribed pressures are not exceeded and assessing for patient comfort.

Gerontologic Considerations.   Because of decreased strength and manual dexterity, elderly patients may be unable to apply elastic stockings properly. If such is the case, a family member should be taught how to assist the patient to apply the stockings so that they do not cause undue pressure on any part of the feet or legs.

Body Position and Exercise.   When the patient is on bed rest, the feet and lower legs should be elevated periodically above heart level. The superficial and tibial veins empty rapidly in this position and remain collapsed. Active and passive leg exercises, particularly those involving calf muscles, should be performed preoperatively and postoperatively to increase venous flow. Early ambulation is most effective in preventing venous stasis. Deep-breathing exercises are beneficial because they produce increased negative pressure in the thorax, which assists in emptying the large veins.

Management

The objectives of medical treatment are to prevent propagation of the thrombus and the inherent risk of pulmonary embolism and to prevent recurrent thromboemboli.

Therapeutic anticoagulation can accomplish both of these goals. Heparin, which is administered for 10 to 12 days by intermittent intravenous infusion or by continuous infusion, prevents the propagation of a clot and the development of new clots. Drug dosage is regulated by the partial thromboplastin time (PTT).

Four to 7 days before the heparin therapy is scheduled to be completed, an oral anticoagulant is started. The patient receives the oral anticoagulant for 3 months or longer for long-term prevention.

Unlike heparin, thrombolytic (fibrinolytic) therapy causes lysis and dissolution of a clot in 50% of patients. Therapy is given within the first 3 days after acute occlusion. Streptokinase, urokinase, and tissue-type plasminogen activator are from biologic sources and are about equal in thrombolytic activity. Advantages of lytic therapy include preservation of venous valves, and reduction of the incidence of postphlebitic syndrome and chronic venous insufficiency. There is, however, approximately a threefold greater incidence of bleeding with thrombolytic therapy than with heparin.

The patient's PTT, prothrombin time, hemoglobin, and hematocrit are monitored frequently. If bleeding occurs and cannot be stopped, the drug is discontinued. During and 24 hours after infusion, parenteral injections are withheld because the likelihood of bleeding from puncture sites is great.

Surgical Management.   Surgery for deep vein thrombosis is necessary when (1) anticoagulant or thrombolytic therapy is contraindicated; (2) the danger of pulmonary embolism is extreme; and (3) the venous drainage is so severely compromised that permanent extremity damage will probably result. A thrombectomy is the treatment of choice when surgery is necessary. A vena cava filter may be placed at the time of the thrombectomy, which will trap large emboli and prevent pulmonary emboli.

Nursing Management.   Bed rest, elevation of the affected extremity, elastic stockings, and analgesics for pain are adjuncts to therapy. Usually, bed rest is required for 5 to 7 days after a deep venous thrombosis. This is approximately the length of time necessary for the thrombus to adhere to the vein wall, thus preventing embolization. When the patient begins to ambulate, elastic stockings are used. Walking is superior to standing or sitting for long periods. Bed exercises, such as dorsiflexion of the foot against a foot board, are also recommended.

Warm, moist packs to the affected extremity reduce discomfort associated with deep venous thrombosis. Mild analgesics for pain control, as prescribed, provide additional relief. A summary of the management of thrombophlebitis is presented in Table 31–7.

In summary, venous disorders are characterized by stasis, hypercoagulability of the blood, and vessel wall injury. An inflammation of the vein wall can occur with the subsequent formation of a clot. Clots may occur anywhere, but are most commonly found in the veins of the lower extremities. Clinical findings are variable and may include edema, pain, and warmth. The goal of management is to resolve the current thrombus and prevent a recurrence. Resolution can be accomplished by anticoagulation or thrombolytic medications, or surgery. Prevention is dependent on identifying risk factors for the development of thrombus and educating the patient on appropriate interventions.

Anticoagulant Therapy for Thromboembolism

Anticoagulant therapy is the administration of a medication to delay the clotting time of blood, to prevent the formation of a thrombus in postoperative patients, and to forestall the extension of a thrombus once it has formed. Anticoagulants cannot dissolve a thrombus that has already formed.

Measures for the *prevention* or reduction of blood clotting within the vascular system are indicated in patients with thrombophlebitis, patients believed to have recurrent embolus formation, those with persistent leg edema secondary to heart failure, and the elderly person with a hip fracture who is likely to be immobilized for a considerable time. The usual treatment consists of the single or combined administration of heparin or coumarin derivatives, which reduce the normal activity of the clotting mechanism (Table 31–8).

Administration. *Continuous pump infusion* is the preferred method for administering heparin (provided there are appropriate facilities and adequate personnel for monitoring), because evidence suggests a lower incidence of hemorrhagic complications. Dosage is calculated on the basis of weight, and any possible bleeding tendencies are indicated by a pretreatment clotting profile. If renal insufficiency exists, lower doses are required. Periodic coagulation tests and hematocrit evaluations are obtained. Heparin is in the effective range when the PTT is 1½ times the control.

Intermittent intravenous injection is another means of administering heparin, in this instance as a dilute aqueous solution given every 4 hours. Administration may be facilitated by the use of a "heparin lock"—a small, butterfly-type scalp vein needle with an injection site at the end of the tubing (see Chap. 18).

Oral anticoagulants, such as Coumadin, are monitored by the prothrombin time. Because Coumadin has a lag period of 3 to 5 days, it is usually administered in conjunction with heparin until desired anticoagulation has been achieved (*i.e.*, when the prothrombin time is achieved at 1½ to 2 times the normal).

TABLE 31–7. *Comparison of Superficial and Deep Thrombophlebitis*

Superficial	*Deep*
CLINICAL MANIFESTATIONS	
Local swelling; bumpy and knotty	"Heaviness" on standing
Red, tender, local induration	Cramping leg pain
	Swelling:
	Calf vein thrombus—none
	Femoral vein thrombus—mild to moderate
	Ileofemoral vein thrombus—severe
	Positive Homans' sign
DIAGNOSTIC EVALUATION	
Venography—to rule out deep vein thrombosis	Blood flow studies to show inflow, filling, and emptying
	Venography—to determine presence of phlebitis, recanalization, extent of occlusion
MANAGEMENT	
Bed rest	Bed rest
Warm, moist compresses	Warm, moist compresses
Legs elevated; then elastic support after acute stage	Foot of bed elevated to 15 cm (6 in)
Heparin, intermittent or continuous	Surgery, possibly, to prevent embolic development
Acetaminophen for pain	
Antibiotics if necessary	
If deep veins are patent, superficial phlebitic veins may be removed.	

TABLE 31–8.   *Comparison of Heparin and Coumarin Derivatives*

Heparin Sodium	*Coumarin Derivatives*
PHYSIOLOGIC ACTION	
Interferes with clotting reaction at many points but primarily acts as an antagonist to thrombin and prevents conversion of fibrinogen to fibrin	Blocks the formation of prothrombin from vitamin K, a conversion that normally occurs in the liver
THERAPEUTIC ACTION	
Advantages	
Used for short-term therapy primarily (may also be used for long-term therapy)	Used for long-term therapy
Action is prompt and predictable.	Is given orally and provides efficient absorption from gastrointestinal tract
It can be used outside the body as well as inside: it may be used in certain dialysis procedures and in place of sodium citrate in donor blood.	Uniform strength of medication because of synthetic production
	Less expensive than heparin sodium
	Control factor better than with heparin sodium
	Sodium warfarin more completely absorbed than bishydroxycoumarin
Disadvantages	
Must be given parenterally, intravenously, or subcutaneously.	Prolonged lag period (2–3 days) before the appearance of its effect
A few patients have developed allergic reactions, and transient hair loss or osteoporosis has been reported (after several months of therapy).	Unpredictable duration of anticoagulant action (at times persisting up to 3 weeks)
ADMINISTRATION	
Test clotting and partial thromboplastin time (PTT) first.	Test prothrombin time first (see below).
PTTs are obtained every 4 to 6 hours, at which time repeat doses of heparin are given.	Warfarin: The average initial dose is 15 to 25 mg.
The object is to attain a PTT 1½ to 2½ times the normal control.	A second dose, somewhat smaller (10 mg), is prescribed on the following day.
Subcutaneous route–least recommended because of erratic absorption, possible puncture of vessels, and discomfort	Subsequent doses are adjusted on the basis of daily prothrombin levels.
The average therapeutic dose is 20,000 to 30,000 units daily either by *continuous infusion* with an infusion pump or in divided doses by *intermittent IV injection* every 4 to 6 hours.	Average dose is usually 5 mg/day
Prolonged therapy: May be given deep subcutaneously in lower abdomen. Use a fine, short, sharp needle (No. 25–27 gauge, 1.27 cm—1.60 cm [0.5–0.62 inches]).	Therapeutic level of hypoprothrombinemia may be reached in 3 to 5 days
Grasp roll of fat gently, and in dartlike fashion insert needle at right angle to the skin surface.	
After injection, do not rub site but firmly press site with an alcohol sponge.	
Each time use a new location on lower abdomen.	
Note: Intramuscular administration of heparin is avoided because of likelihood of local hematomas and tissue irritation.	
ACTION FOR ADVERSE EFFECTS	
Discontinue heparin.	Administer vitamin K preparations:
Protamine sulfate (acts as a base to neutralize acidic heparin)	*For mild bleeding control:*
Blood transfusion when hemorrhage occurs	Phytonadione tablets (oral use) (Mephyton) (vitamin K_1)
	For moderate to severe control:
	Phytonadione solution (Aqua-MEPHYTON) IV or IM. Transfusion may be required

Prothrombin time *is measured in seconds or percent of normal.*
Normal: *12.5 seconds or 100%.*
Desired Therapeutic Range: *25 to 30 seconds when the control is 12 seconds (approximately 1½–2½ times the control in seconds). When the prothrombin time is measured in percentage of normal, the desired therapeutic range is thought to be 20% to 30%.*

Precautions and Nursing Assessment. *The principal complication of anticoagulant therapy is the occurrence of spontaneous bleeding anywhere in the body.* Bleeding from the kidneys will be manifested by microscopic hematuria and is often the first sign of anticoagulant overdose. Bruises, nosebleeds, and bleeding gums are also early signs of bleeding. To promptly reverse the effects of heparin, the physician may prescribe intravenous injections of protamine sulfate. The reversal of the effects of coumarin derivatives is more difficult, but effective measures that the physician may prescribe include administering vitamin K and possibly fresh whole blood or plasma.

A further possible complication of heparin therapy is that of heparin-induced *thrombocytopenia* (decrease in platelets), which generally occurs 7 to 10 days after the treatment has been started. When this occurs it is a serious complication that results in thromboembolic manifestations, and the prognosis is extremely guarded. The thrombocytopenia is thought to be the result of an immunologic mechanism that causes aggregation of platelets. Prevention of this syndrome is dependent on regular monitoring of platelet counts and subsequent studies of platelet aggregation if thrombocytopenia becomes evident. The physician will discontinue heparin when this occurs and use protamine sulfate to reverse the heparin effects.

Oral anticoagulants interact with many other medications, and close monitoring of the patient's drug schedule is necessary. Drugs that potentiate oral anticoagulants include salicylates, anabolic steroids, chloral hydrate, glucagon, chloramphenicol, neomycin, quinidine, and phenylbutazone (Butazolidin.) Drugs that decrease the anticoagulant effect include phenytoin, barbiturates, diuretics, and estrogen. It is advisable to study drug interactions for patients taking specific oral anticoagulants.

Contraindications to anticoagulant therapy are summarized in Chart 31–3.

Patient Education About Oral Anticoagulants. The patient should be informed about the medication, its purpose, and the need to take the correct amount at the specific times prescribed, and should be aware that blood tests are scheduled periodically to determine whether a change in medication dosage is required. If the patient is unable or unwilling to cooperate with the therapeutic regimen, continuation of the drug therapy should be questioned. Specific teaching directives should include the following points:

- Take the anticoagulant tablet at the same time each day, usually between 8:00 and 9:00 AM.
- Wear or carry identification indicating what anticoagulant is being taken.
- Keep all appointments for blood tests.
- Because other medications affect the way the anticoagulant normally acts, do not take any of the following medications without the physician's consent: vitamins, cold medicines, antibiotics, aspirin, mineral oil, and anti-inflammatory drugs. The physician should be contacted before taking any over-the-counter drugs.
- Avoid alcohol since it may alter the body's response to an anticoagulant.
- Avoid food fads, crash diets, or marked changes in eating habits.
- Do not take Coumadin unless so directed by the physician.
- Do not stop taking Coumadin (when prescribed) unless so directed by the physician or nurse.

Chart 31–3
Contraindications to Anticoagulant Therapy

Lack of patient cooperation
Bleeding from the following systems:
    Gastrointestinal
    Genitourinary
    Respiratory
Hemorrhagic blood dyscrasias
Aneurysms
Severe trauma
Alcoholism
Compulsive drug use
Recent or impending surgery of:
    Eye
    Spinal cord
    Brain
Severe hepatic or renal disease
Recent cerebrovascular hemorrhage
Infections
Open ulcerative wounds
Occupations that involve a significant hazard of injury

- When seeking treatment from another physician, a dentist, or a podiatrist, indicate that an anticoagulant is being taken.
- Contact personal physician before dental extraction or elective surgery.
- If any of the following signs appear, report them immediately to the physician:
    Faintness, dizziness, or increased weakness
    Severe headaches or stomach pain
    Red or brown urine
    Any bleeding, such as cuts that do not stop bleeding
    Bruises that increase in size, nosebleeds, or unusual bleeding from any part of the body
    Red or black bowel movements
    Skin rash
- Avoid injury that can cause bleeding.
- Women should notify their physicians if they suspect that they are pregnant.

Chronic Venous Insufficiency

Pathophysiology and Clinical Manifestations

Venous insufficiency is a disease state resulting from the obstruction or reflux of venous valves in the legs. Both superficial and deep leg veins can be involved. The resulting venous hypertension can occur whenever there has been a prolonged increase in venous pressure, such as occurs with deep venous thrombosis.

Because the walls of veins are thinner and more elastic than walls of arteries, they distend readily when venous pressure is consistently high. In this state, leaflets of the venous valves are stretched and prevented from closing completely, thereby allowing a backflow or reflux of blood in the veins. Venography confirms the presence of obstruction and identifies the level of valvular incompetence.

When the deep veins in the legs have incompetent valves after a thrombus, *postphlebitic syndrome* may develop. This disorder is characterized by chronic venous stasis, resulting in edema, altered pigmentation, pain, stasis dermatitis, and stasis ulceration. Superficial veins may be dilated. The disorder is long-standing, difficult to treat, and often disabling.

Stasis ulcers develop as a result of the rupture of small skin veins and subsequent ulcerations. When these vessels rupture, red blood cells escape into surrounding tissues, and then degenerate and leave a brownish discoloration of the tissues. The pigmentation and ulcerations usually occur in the lower part of the extremity in the area of the medial malleolus of the ankle. The skin becomes dry, cracks, and itches. Subcutaneous tissues fibrose and atrophy. The risk of injury and infection of the extremities is increased.

Venous ulceration is the most serious complication of chronic venous insufficiency and can be associated with other conditions affecting the circulation of the lower extremities (Fig. 31–13). The potential complications and the principles of care, however, will be similar for all types.

Management and Patient Education

Management of the patient with venous insufficiency is directed at reducing venous stasis and preventing ulcerations. Measures that increase venous blood flow are antigravity activities and compression of superficial veins with elastic stockings.

Elevation of the legs decreases edema, promotes venous return, and provides symptomatic relief. Elevations should be performed frequently throughout the day (at least 30 minutes every 2 hours). At night, the patient should sleep with the foot of the bed elevated about 15 cm (6 inches). Prolonged sitting or standing still is detrimental, but walking should be encouraged. When sitting, the patient should avoid placing pressure on the popliteal spaces, such as occurs with leg crossing, or sitting with the legs dangling over the side of the bed. Constricting garments such as girdles or garters should be avoided.

Elastic compression of the legs reduces pooling of venous blood and enhances venous return to the heart. Thus, elastic hose are recommended for patients with venous insufficiency. The fit of the stocking is important. It should provide for a greater pressure at the foot and ankle, gradually declining to a lesser pressure at the knee or groin. If the top of the stocking

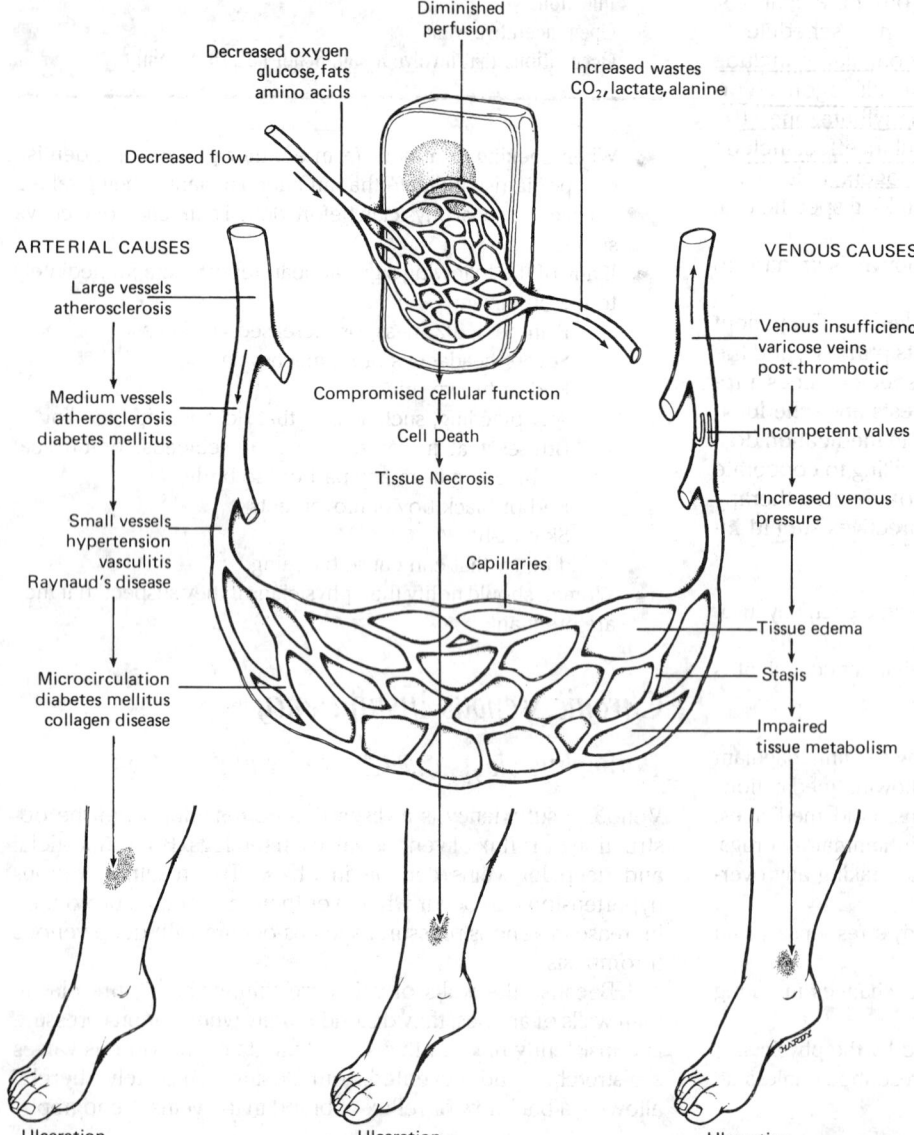

Figure 31–13. Pathophysiology of leg ulcers. Some of the conditions that cause diminished blood flow to peripheral tissue are indicated on the left. Oxygen and energy sources are further aggravated by capillary changes brought about by diabetes mellitus and collagen disease. Cellular function is compromised when insufficient oxygen and energy substrates are supplied. Tissue necrosis takes place and results in ulceration. A somewhat similar situation occurs when there is venous insufficiency brought about by a different hemodynamic pattern. Increased venous pressure reduces capillary flow. Edema and stasis result, impairing cellular metabolism and again leading to ulceration.

is too tight or twisting has occurred, a tourniquet effect is created, which worsens venous pooling. Stockings should be applied after a period of leg elevation, when the venous blood volume is at its lowest. The technique for putting on elastic hose is depicted in Figure 31–14.

Extremities with venous insufficiency are conscientiously protected from trauma. The skin is kept clean, dry, and soft. Signs of ulceration are immediately reported to the nurse or physician for treatment and follow-up.

Leg Ulcers

Definition and Etiology

A *leg ulcer* is an excavation of the skin surface that is produced by the sloughing of inflammatory necrotic tissue. The most frequent cause is vascular insufficiency, either venous or arteriolar. It is estimated that, of all leg ulcers, postphlebitic and varicose ulcers account for about 70%; the remaining 30%, such as those caused by burns, sickle cell anemia, and neurogenic disorders, are of nonvenous origin.

Pathophysiology

Inadequate exchange of oxygen and other nutrients in the tissue is the metabolic abnormality underlying the development of leg ulcers. When the cellular metabolism cannot maintain energy balance, cell death (necrosis) results. Alterations in blood vessels at the arterial, capillary, and venous levels may affect cellular processes and lead to the formation of ulcers (see Fig. 31–13).

Clinical Manifestations

The patient with a leg ulcer usually complains of aching, fatigue, heaviness, and swelling of the leg. The symptoms will vary depending on whether the problem is one that is arterial or venous in origin (see Table 31–2). The severity of the symptoms depends on the extent and duration of the vascular insufficiency. The ulcer itself appears as an open sore that is inflamed. Drainage may be present, or the area may be covered by a dark crust.

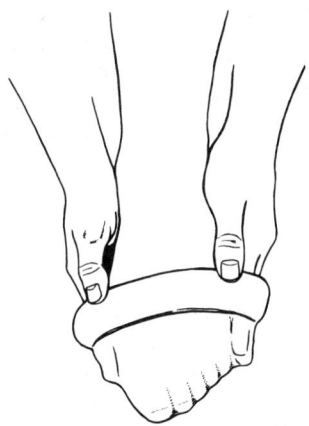

Figure 31–14. Method of applying a support stocking. A support stocking can be rolled, spread apart, and unrolled as the hands hold it in place—moving from foot to ankle and up the calf. Ideally, the stocking should be put on while the patient is in bed.

Diagnostic Evaluation

Because there are many causes of ulcers, it is important that an accurate causative diagnosis be made so that appropriate therapy can be prescribed. The history of the condition is important in determining the presence of venous or arterial insufficiency. The quality of all pulses of the lower extremities (femoral, popliteal, posterior tibial, and pedal) is carefully checked. More conclusive diagnostic aids are Doppler ultrasound studies, arteriography, and venography. Cultures of the ulcer drainage may be necessary to determine whether infection is the primary cause of the ulcer.

Management

Because most ulcers are infected and all ulcers have the potential for becoming infected, antibiotic therapy is prescribed when indicated by culture and sensitivity determinations. The route of administration prescribed is usually systemic because topical antibiotics have not proven to be effective for leg ulcers.

To promote healing, the wound is kept clean of drainage and necrotic tissue. This may be accomplished by flushing the area with normal saline; if that is unsuccessful, the physician may decide that debridement is necessary. Debridement can be performed using instruments to cut away devitalized tissue. It can also be done by applying isotonic saline dressings of fine mesh gauze to the ulcer bed. When dry, the dressing is removed along with the debris adhering to the gauze.

A variety of topical agents and soaps can be used in conjunction with washing and debridement therapies to promote healing of leg ulcers. The goals of treatment are to remove devitalized tissue and to keep the wound clean and moist while healing takes place. Adequate nutritional therapy must be maintained in the patient with venous ulcers for topical treatments to be successful.

Enzymatic debridement is preferred by some physicians, and enzyme ointments are used to treat the ulcer. The ointment is placed over the lesion but not over normal surrounding skin. The lesion and ointment are then covered with a saline-soaked sponge that has been thoroughly wrung out. A gauze dressing and a loose bandage are then applied. For the first 3 or 4 days the procedure is performed every 4 hours, and then every 8 hours. When pink granulating tissue develops, saline wet dressings are used.

Another method of treating ulcers involves the use of a debriding agent. Dextranomer (Debrisan) beads are small, highly porous, spherical beads (0.1 to 0.3 mm in diameter) that possess the ability to absorb wound secretions. Bacteria and products of tissue necrosis and protein degradation are actively suctioned into the bead layer. When the beads are completely saturated they take on a grayish yellow color, at which point their cleansing action stops. When the beads become saturated, they are removed and a fresh layer is applied.

Hyperbaric oxygen therapy may be considered in addition to topical therapy. The increase in the level of oxygen tension to 30 mm Hg increases fibroblast and collagen proliferation.

In patients where arterial insufficiency is the problem and the ulcer does not respond to antibiotics, cleansing, and debridement, more aggressive therapy may be necessary. Aortoiliac, aortofemoral, and femoropopliteal revascularization often are effective in correcting arterial insufficiency.

In summary, necrotic skin tissue of the leg, or a leg ulcer, is frequently caused by arterial or venous insufficiency. Vascular insufficiency does not allow for an adequate supply of oxygen and nutrients to the tissues. When cellular metabolic needs can no longer be satisfied, cellular death (necrosis) ensues. Manifestations are dependent on the type, duration, and extent of the insufficiency. Typically signs include an open sore, swelling of the extremity, and pain. Prevention of wound infection and the promotion of the healing process are the mainstays of treatment.

▶ Nursing Process
The Patient With Leg Ulcers

▷ Assessment

A careful nursing history and assessment of symptoms are important in determining venous or arterial insufficiency. The extent and type of pain are carefully assessed, as are the appearance and temperature of the skin of both lower extremities. The quality of all peripheral pulses is determined, and comparisons are made of the pulses bilaterally. The presence or absence of edema is determined. If the extremity is edematous, the degree of edema is determined. Any limitation of mobility and activity that results from the vascular insufficiency is determined. In addition, the patient's nutritional status is assessed and a history of the following conditions is obtained: diabetes, collagen disease, or varicose veins.

▷ Nursing Diagnoses

Based on the assessment data, major nursing diagnoses for the patient may include the following:

- Impairment of skin integrity related to vascular insufficiency
- Impaired physical mobility related to the activity restrictions of the therapeutic regimen and the presence of pain
- Altered nutrition, less than body requirements, related to increased need for nutrients that promote wound healing

▷ Planning and Implementation

▷ *Goals:*   The major goals of the patient may include restoration of skin integrity, improvement of physical mobility, and attainment of adequate nutrition.

The nursing challenge in caring for these patients is great, whether the patient is in the hospital or at home. The physical problem is often a long-term one that causes a substantial drain on the patient's physical, emotional, and economic resources.

▷ Nursing Interventions

▷ *Restoration of Skin Integrity.*   To promote wound healing, measures are used to keep the area clean. Cleansing requires very gentle handling, a mild soap, and lukewarm water. Strict aseptic technique is used to prevent contamination. Ointments and dressings are applied as prescribed.

Positioning of the legs depends on whether the cause of the ulcer is arterial or venous in origin. If there is arterial insufficiency, blood flow can be improved by elevating the head of the bed on 7.5- to 15-cm (3- to 6-in) blocks. This improved flow of blood increases oxygenation of the tissue and promotes healing. If there is venous insufficiency, resolution of dependent edema can be promoted by elevating the lower extremities. Decrease in the edema will allow for improved exchange of cellular nutrients and waste products in the area of the ulcer. Thus healing is promoted.

Avoidance of trauma to the lower extremities is imperative in promoting skin integrity. When the patient is ambulatory, all obstacles are moved from the path so that the patient's legs will not be bumped. When the patient is in bed, a bed cradle is used to relieve pressure from bed linens and to prevent anything from touching the legs. Heat in the form of heating pads, hot water bottles, or hot baths is avoided. Heat increases the oxygen demands and thus blood flow demands of the tissue, which in this case are already compromised.

▷ *Improvement of Physical Mobility.*   Generally, physical activity is restricted at first to promote healing. When infection has improved and healing has begun, ambulation will be resumed gradually and progressively. Activity aids arterial flow and venous return and is encouraged after the acute phase of the ulcer process.

Until full activity can be resumed, the patient is encouraged to move about when in bed, to turn from side to side frequently, and to exercise the upper extremities to maintain muscle tone and strength. Meanwhile, diversional activities that interest the patient are encouraged. Consultation with an occupational therapist may be helpful if the period of limited mobility and activity is prolonged.

If pain limits the patient's activity, analgesics are often prescribed by the physician. The pain of peripheral vascular disease is often chronic in nature, so non-narcotic analgesics are more desirable than narcotics because the problem of drug dependency is less. It is often desirable to administer the analgesic prior to scheduled activity periods to help the patient participate more comfortably in the activity.

▷ *Attainment of Adequate Nutrition.*   Nutritional deficiencies are determined from the patient's report of usual dietary intake. Alterations in the diet are made to remedy these deficiencies. In addition, a diet that is high in protein, vitamin C, and iron is encouraged in an attempt to promote the healing process.

Many patients with peripheral vascular disease are elderly. The caloric intake of these patients may need to be adjusted because of their decreased metabolic rate and decreased level of activity. Particular consideration should also be given to their iron intake, because many elderly people are anemic. Once a diet plan has been developed that meets the individual's nutritional needs, diet instruction is provided to the patient and family. The diet plan is designed to be compatible with the patient's and family's life style and preferences.

▷ Evaluation
Expected Outcomes

1. Skin integrity is restored
   a. Absence of inflammation
   b. Absence of drainage; negative culture report
   c. Uses measures to avoid trauma to the legs
   d. Uses prescribed position (head elevated or feet elevated) to promote circulation
2. Increases physical mobility
   a. Progresses gradually to optimum level of activity
   b. Reports that pain does not impede activity

3. Attains adequate nutrition
   a. Selects foods high in protein, vitamins, iron
   b. Discusses with family member dietary modifications that need to be made at home
   c. Plans, with family, a diet that is nutritionally sound

Varicose Veins

Incidence

Varicose veins (varicosities) are abnormally dilated, tortuous, superficial veins caused by incompetent venous valves (Fig. 31–15). Most commonly, this condition occurs in the lower extremities, the saphenous veins, or the lower trunk; however, it can occur elsewhere in the body (*e.g.*, esophageal varices; see Chap. 38).

It is estimated that varicose veins of the lower extremities affect one of five persons in the world. The condition is most common in women and in persons in occupations requiring prolonged standing, such as salespeople, barbers, beauticians, elevator operators, nurses, and dentists. A hereditary weakness of the vein wall may contribute to the development of varicosities, and it is not uncommon to see this condition occur in several members of the same family.

Pathophysiology and Manifestations

Varicose veins may be considered *primary* (without involvement of deep veins) or *secondary* (resulting from obstruction of deep veins). A reflux of venous blood in the veins results in venous stasis. If only the superficial veins are affected, the person may have no symptoms, but cosmetically the appearance of the dilated veins may be unappealing. If symptoms are present, they may take the form of dull aches, muscle cramps, and increased fatigue of muscles in the lower legs. Ankle edema and a feeling of heaviness of the legs may occur. Nocturnal cramps are a common symptom.

When deep venous obstruction results in varicose veins, patients may demonstrate the signs and symptoms of chronic venous insufficiency: edema, pain, pigmentation, and ulcerations. Susceptibility to injury and infection is increased.

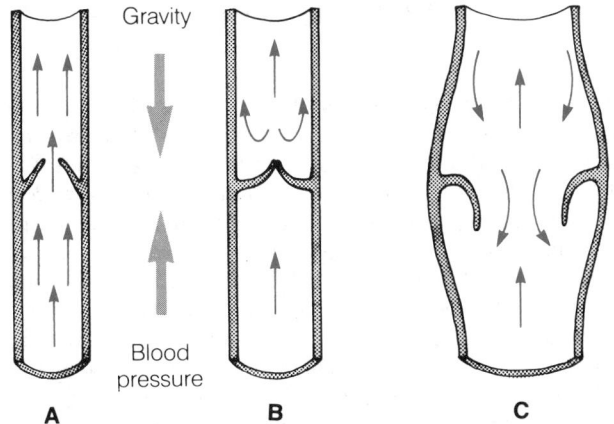

Figure 31–15. Competent valves showing blood flow patterns when the valve is open (**A**) and closed (**B**), allowing blood to flow against gravity. (**C**) With faulty, or incompetent, valves, the blood is unable to move toward the heart.

Diagnostic Evaluation

A common diagnostic test for varicose veins is the *Brodie–Trendelenburg test*. This test will demonstrate backward flow of blood through incompetent valves of the superficial veins and of the branches that communicate with the deep veins of the leg. With the patient lying down, the affected leg is elevated to empty the veins. A soft, rubber tourniquet is then applied around the upper thigh to occlude the veins, and the patient is asked to stand. If the valves of the communicating veins are incompetent, blood flows into the superficial veins from the deep veins. If, on release of the tourniquet, blood flows rapidly from above into the superficial veins, the inference is that the valves of the superficial veins are also incompetent. This test is used to determine the type of treatment to be recommended for the varicose veins.

The *Perthes' test* is a diagnostic procedure that easily indicates whether the deeper venous system and communicating veins are competent. A tourniquet is applied just below the knee and the patient is asked to walk. If the varicose veins disappear, the deep system and communicating vessels are competent. If the vessels do not empty and become even more distended on walking, incompetency or obstruction is inferred.

Additional diagnostic tests for the presence of varicose veins are the Doppler flow meter, phlebography, and plethysmography. The *Doppler flowmeter* can detect the retrograde flow of blood in superficial veins with incompetent valves after compression of the leg proximally. *Phlebography* involves the injection of radiographic contrast media into the leg veins so that vein anatomy can be visualized during various leg movements. *Plethysmography* allows measurement of changes in venous blood volume.

Prevention and Health Education

Activities that cause venous stasis should be avoided, such as wearing tight garters or a constricting panty girdle, crossing the legs at the thighs, and sitting or standing for long periods. Changing position frequently, elevating the legs when they are tired, and getting up to walk for several minutes of every hour promote circulation. The patient should be encouraged to walk 1 or 2 miles a day if there are no contraindications. Walking up the stairs rather than using the elevator or escalator is helpful in promoting circulation. Swimming is also good exercise for the legs.

Support hose or elastic stockings are useful. The overweight patient should be assisted in a weight-reduction plan.

Surgical Treatment

Surgery for varicose veins requires demonstrated patency of deep veins. Once this is established, *ligation* and division of the saphenous vein are accomplished under general anesthesia. The vein is ligated high in the groin where the saphenous vein meets the femoral vein. An incision is then made in the ankle, and a metal or plastic wire is passed the full length of the vein, "stripping" as it passes (Fig. 31–16). Pressure and elevation keep bleeding at a minimum during surgery.

Postoperative Nursing Management. Surgery can be performed at an outpatient setting, or patients can be admitted to the hospital on the day of surgery and discharged the following day. Bed rest is maintained for 24 hours, after which the patient begins walking every 2 hours for 5 to 10 minutes.

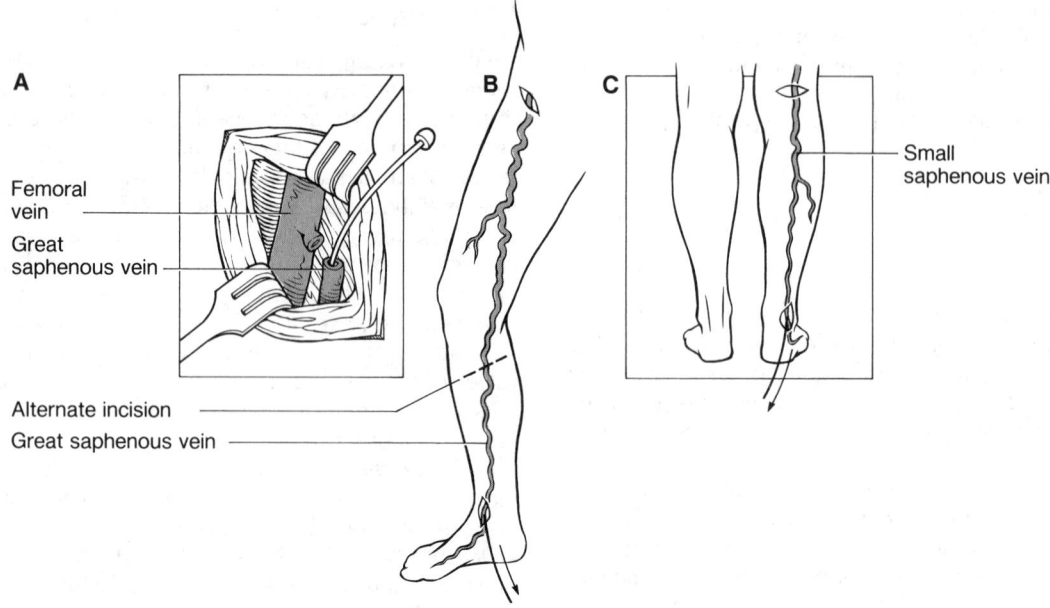

Figure 31–16. Ligation and stripping of the great and the small saphenous veins. (**A**) The tributaries of the saphenous vein have been ligated, and the saphenous vein has been ligated at the saphenofemoral junction. (**B**) Vein stripper has been inserted from the ankle superiorly to the groin. The vein is stripped from above downward. A number of alternate incisions may be needed to remove separate varicose masses. (**C**) The small saphenous vein is stripped from its junction with the popliteal vein to a point posterior to the lateral malleolus. (Rhoads et al. Surgery. Philadelphia, JB Lippincott.)

Elastic compression of the leg is maintained continuously for about 1 week after vein stripping. Exercise and movement of the legs and elevation of the foot of the bed are necessary. Standing still and sitting are contraindicated.

Analgesics may help patients move affected extremities more easily. The bandages are inspected for bleeding, particularly at the groin where the greatest risk of bleeding occurs. Sensations of "pins and needles" or hypersensitivity to touch in the involved extremity may indicate a temporary or permanent nerve injury resulting from surgery. The saphenous vein and saphenous nerve are in close proximity to each other in the leg.

Patients will require long-term elastic support of the leg after discharge from the hospital, and plans are made to provide adequate supplies. Exercises of the legs also will be necessary and the development of an individualized plan will require consultation with the patient and physician.

Sclerotherapy. In sclerotherapy, an irritating chemical, such as 0.5% sodium tetradecyl sulfate (Sotradecol), is injected into the vein, which irritates the venous endothelium and produces localized phlebitis and fibrosis, thereby obliterating the vein lumen. This treatment may be performed alone for small varicosities or may follow vein ligation or stripping. Sclerosing is a palliative, not curative, treatment. After injection of the sclerosing agent, elastic compression bandages are applied to the leg. These are worn for approximately 5 days. Compression stockings are then worn for an additional 5 weeks. Walking is important for maintenance of blood flow in the extremity and should be emphasized.

If the patient experiences a burning sensation in the injected leg for 1 or 2 days, a mild sedative and walking will relieve the problem. The bandage should be removed for the first time under the direction of the physician. Because bathing may be a problem during this time, a plastic bag may be placed over the bandaged leg and secured above the bandage to allow the patient to shower.

Sclerotherapy had declined in popularity in recent years because of the possible complications of thrombosis, injection site necrosis, vasospasm, hemolysis, and allergic reactions associated with stronger solutions. With the lower concentrations of sclerosing solutions available, however, sclerotherapy, with or without surgery, is regaining popularity.

The Lymphatic System

The lymphatic system consists of a set of vessels that spread throughout most of the body. These vessels start as lymph capillaries that drain tissue spaces of plasma that is not reabsorbed by the venular end of the capillaries. They unite to form the lymph vessels, which in turn pass through the lymph nodes and finally empty into the large thoracic duct that joins the jugular vein on the left side of the neck. *Lymph* is the fluid found in lymph vessels. *Tissue fluids* are found outside of vessels in the cellular interspaces. The lymphatic system of the abdominal cavity maintains a steady flow of digested fatty food (chyle) from the intestinal mucosa to the thoracic duct. In other parts of the body the lymphatic system's function is regional; the lymphatic vessels of the head, for example, empty into clusters of lymph nodes located in the neck, and those of the extremities into nodes in the axillae and the groin. The flow of lymph depends on the intrinsic contractions of the lymph vessels, the contraction of muscles, respiratory movements, and gravity.

Diagnosis by Lymphangiography

Radiologic visualization of the lymphatic system is possible after the injection of contrast media directly into lymphatic vessels in the hands and feet. This technique, *lymphangiography*, affords a means of detecting lymph node involvement by metastatic carcinoma, lymphoma, or infection in sites that are otherwise inaccessible to the examiner except by the direct surgical approach.

This procedure localizes a lymphatic vessel in each foot (or hand) by injecting Evans blue contrast media intradermally between the first and second digits. A blue lymphatic segment is identified, isolated, cannulated with a 25- to 30-gauge needle, and infused very slowly with contrast media containing iodine and oil. Appropriate x-ray pictures are taken at the conclusion of the injection, 24 hours later, and periodically thereafter, as indicated. The identified lymphomatous lymph nodes retain the contrast media for up to 1 year after the injection and any change in their size that may occur in response to radiation or chemotherapy can be measured and used as a criterion in determining therapeutic effect.

Lymphoscintigraphy is a reliable alternative to lymphangiography. A radioactive labeled colloid is injected subcutaneously in the second interdigital space. The limb is then exercised to facilitate the uptake of the media by the lymph system. Serial images then are completed at preset intervals. No adverse reactions are reported.

Lymphangitis and Lymphadenitis

Lymphangitis is an acute inflammation of the lymphatic channels. It arises most commonly from a focus of infection in an extremity. Usually, the infectious organism is the hemolytic streptococcus. The characteristic red streaks that extend up the arm or the leg from an infected wound outline the course of the lymphatics as they drain.

The lymph nodes located along the course of the lymphatic channels also become enlarged, red, and tender (*acute lymphadenitis*), and can become necrotic and form an abscess (*suppurative lymphadenitis*). The nodes involved most often are those in the groin, the axilla, or the cervical region.

Because these infections are nearly always caused by organisms that are sensitive to antibiotics, it is unusual to see abscess formation. Recurrent episodes of lymphangitis are often associated with progressive lymphedema.

After acute attacks, elastic support should be worn on the affected extremity for several months to prevent long-term edema.

Lymphedema and Elephantiasis

Lymphedemas are classified as primary (congenital malformations), or secondary (acquired obstruction). A swelling of tissues in the extremities occurs due to an increased quantity of lymph that results from an obstruction of lymphatics. It is especially marked when the extremity is in a dependent position. Initially the edema is soft, pitting, and relieved by treatment. As the condition progresses, the edema becomes firm, nonpitting, and unresponsive to treatment. The most common type is congenital lymphedema (lymphedema praecox), which is caused by hypoplasia of the lymphatic system of the lower extremity. This disorder is usually seen in women, and appears first between the ages of 15 and 25 years.

The obstruction may be in both the lymph nodes and the lymphatic vessels. At times it is seen in the arm, after a radical mastectomy for carcinoma, and in the leg in association with varicose veins or a chronic phlebitis. In the latter case, the lymphatic obstruction usually is due to a chronic lymphangitis. Lymphatic obstruction caused by a parasite (*Filaria*) is seen frequently in the tropics. When chronic swelling is present, there may be frequent bouts of acute infection characterized by high fever and chills and increased residual edema after the inflammation has resolved. These lead to chronic fibrosis, thickening of the subcutaneous tissues, and hypertrophy of the skin. This condition, in which chronic swelling of the extremity recedes only slightly with elevation, is referred to as *elephantiasis*.

Management

The goal of medical therapy is to reduce and control the edema and prevent infection. Strict bed rest with leg elevation may aid in mobilizing the fluids. Active and passive exercises assist in the movement of lymphatic fluid into the bloodstream. External compression devices milk the fluid proximally from the foot to the hip. When the patient is ambulatory, custom-fitted elastic stockings are worn.

In the initial therapy, furosemide (Lasix) is intermittently administered to prevent fluid overload. Diuretics have also been used palliatively for lymphedema in conjunction with elevation and elastic compression of the affected extremity. However, the use of diuretics is controversial.

If lymphangitis or cellulitis is present, antibiotic therapy is initiated. The patient is taught to inspect the skin for evidence of infection.

Surgical treatment of lymphedema is performed if the edema is severe and uncontrolled by medical therapy, if mobility is severely compromised, or if there is persistent infection. One surgical approach involves the excision of affected subcutaneous tissue and fascia, with skin grafting to cover the defect. Another procedure involves the transfer of superficial lymphatics into the deep lymphatic system by a buried dermal flap to provide a conduit for lymphatic drainage.

Postoperatively, the management of skin grafts and flaps is the same as when these therapies are used for other conditions. Prophylactic antibiotics may be prescribed for 5 to 7 days. Constant elevation of the affected extremity and observations for complications are essential. Complications can include flap necrosis, hematoma or abscess under the flap, and cellulitis.

In summary, disorders of the lymph system are generally considered to be treatable but not curable. The guiding principle for all therapy is the reduction of edema through increased muscular activity and enhanced venous return. This can be accomplished by a variety of therapies, including limb elevation, elastic support stockings, and external pneumatic compression devices.

Bibliography

Bates B. A Guide to Physical Examination, 5th ed. Philadelphia, JB Lippincott, 1991.

Berne R and Levy M. Physiology, 2nd ed. St Louis, CV Mosby, 1986.

Dossey BM et al. Essentials of Critical Care Nursing: Body, Mind, Spirit. Philadelphia, JB Lippincott, 1990.

Fahey VA. Vascular Nursing. Philadelphia, WB Saunders, 1988.

Guyton A. Textbook of Medical Physiology. Philadelphia, WB Saunders, 1986.

Hazzard WR et al. Principles of Geriatric Medicine and Gerontology, 2nd ed. New York, McGraw-Hill, 1990.

Jarrett F and Hirsch SA. Vascular Surgery of the Lower Extremity. St Louis, CV Mosby, 1985.

Lambert WC and Doty OB. Peripheral Vascular Surgery. Chicago, Year Book Medical Pub, 1987.

Page IH. Hypertensive Mechanisms. Orlando, Grune & Stratton, 1987.

Rakel RE (ed). Conn's Current Therapy. Philadelphia, WB Saunders, 1988.

Robbins S et al. Pathologic Basis of Disease, 4th ed. Philadelphia, WB Saunders, 1989.

Strandness DE (ed). Vascular Diseases: Current Research and Clinical Applications. Orlando, Grune & Stratton, 1987.

Journals

Asterisks indicate nursing research articles.

General

Berenson GS et al. Arterial wall injury and proteoglycan changes in atherosclerosis. Arch Pathol Lab Med 1988 Oct; 112(10): 1002–1009.

Eagan JS. Lasers: Applications in cardiovascular atherosclerotic disease. Crit Care Nurs Clin North Am 1989 Jun; 1(2): 311–326

* Foxall MJ et al. Comparative study of adjustment patterns of chronic obstructive pulmonary disease patients and peripheral vascular disease patients. Heart Lung 1987 Jul; 16(4): 354–363.

Kaplan NM. The deadly quartet: Upper-body obesity, glucose intolerance, hypertriglyceridemia, and hypertension. Arch Intern Med 1989 Jul; 149(7): 1514–1520.

Paul MC and Halfman–Franey M. Laser angioplasty in peripheral vascular disease. Crit Care Nurs 1990 May; 10(5): 65–77.

Stabile MJ and Warfield CA. The pain of peripheral vascular disease. Hosp Pract 1988 Mar; 23(3): 99–107.

Sweeney MS et al. Cardiac surgical emergencies. Crit Care Clin 1989 Jul; 5(3): 659–678.

Touhey JE et al. Hyperbaric oxygen therapy. Orthop Rev 1987 Nov; 16(11): 829–833.

Turner JA. Nursing interventions in patients with peripheral vascular disease. Nurs Clin North Am 1986 Jun; 21(2): 233–240.

Wagner MM. Pathophysiology related to peripheral vascular disease. Nurs Clin North Am 1986 Jun; 21(2): 195–205.

Wells I. Inferior vena cava filters and when to use them. Clin Radiol 1989 Jan; 40(1): 11–12.

Wills–Long SL et al. Hyperbaric oxygen therapy: Nursing opportunity. Dimen Crit Care Nurs 1989 May/Jun; 8(3): 176–182.

Young HL. Peripheral vascular disease: 1. Arterial disease of the lower limb. Br J Occup Ther 1989 Apr; 52(4): 127–129.

Young HL. Peripheral vascular disease: 2. Venous disorders of the lower limb. Br J Occup Ther 1989 Apr; 52(4): 130–132.

Anticoagulant and Thrombolytic Therapy

McCann RL and Sabiston DC. Current management of venous thromboembolic disease. Br J Surg 1989 Feb; 76(2): 113–114.

McConnell EA. APTT and PT: Two common-but-important coagulation studies. Nursing 1986 May; 16(5): 47–48.

Raskob GE et al. Anticoagulant therapy for venous thromboembolism. Prog Hemost Thromb 1989; 9: 1–27.

Sidorov J. Streptokinase v heparin for deep vein thrombosis. Arch Intern Med 1989 Aug; 149(8): 1841–1845.

Arterial Conditions

Bensen JL and Allastair MK. In situ artery bypass. AORN J 1987 Jan; 45(1): 40–55.

Bondy B. An overview of arterial disease. J Cardiovasc Nurs 1987 Feb; 1(2): 1–11.

Cardelli MB and Kleinsmith DM. Raynaud's phenomenon and disease. Med Clin North Am 1989 Sep; 73(5): 1127–1141.

Cheatle TR and Scurr JH. Abdominal aortic aneurysms: A review of current problems. Br J Surg 1989 Aug; 76(8): 826–829.

Cohle SD and Lie JT. Inflammatory aneurysm of the aorta, aortitis, and coronary arteritis. Arch Pathol Lab Med 1988 Nov; 112(11): 1121–1125.

Dixon MB. Acute aortic dissection. J Cardiovasc Nurs 1987 Feb; 1(2): 24–35.

Dixon MB and Nunnelee J. Arterial reconstruction for atherosclerotic occlusive disease. J Cardiovasc Nurs 1987 Feb; 1(2): 36–49.

Hotter AN. Preventing cardiovascular complications following AAA surgery. Dimen Crit Care Nurs 1987 Jan/Feb; 6(1): 10–18.

Hubner C. Exercise therapy and smoking cessation for intermittent claudication. J Cardiovasc Nurs 1987 Feb; 1(2): 50–58.

Olin JW. Thrombolytic therapy in the treatment of peripheral arterial occlusions. Ann Emerg Med 1988 Nov; 17(11): 1210–1214.

Paris BE et al. The prevalence and one-year outcome of limb arterial obstructive disease in a nursing home population. J Am Geriatr Soc 1988 Jul; 36(7): 607–612.

Reilly JM and Tilson MD. Incidence and etiology of abdominal aortic aneurysms. Surg Clin North Am 1989 Aug; 69(4): 705–711.

Stern PH. Occlusive vascular disease of lower limbs; diagnosis, amputation surgery and rehabilitation. Am J Phys Med Rehabil 1988 Aug; 67(4): 145–154.

Warbinek E and Wyness MA. Peripheral arterial occlusive disease. Part II: Nursing assessment and standard care plans. Cardiovasc Nurs 1986 Mar/Apr; 22(2): 6–10.

Zacca NM et al. Treatment of symptomatic peripheral atherosclerotic disease with a rotational atherectomy device. Am J Cardiol 1989 Jan; 63(1): 77–80.

Assessment and Diagnosis

Athanasoulis CA and Yucel EK. Venous reflux; Assessing the level of incompetence. Radiology 1990 Feb; 174(2): 326–327.

Bandyk DF. Perioperative imaging of aortic aneurysms. Surg Clin North Am 1989 Aug; 69(4): 721–735.

Bettman MA. Noninvasive and venographic diagnosis of deep vein thrombosis. Cardiovasc Intervent Radiol 1988 Nov; suppl: 515–520.

Comerota AJ et al. The diagnosis of acute deep venous thrombosis: Noninvasive and radioisoptic techniques. Ann Vasc Surg 1988 Oct; 2(4): 406–424.

Herman JA. Nursing assessment and nursing diagnosis in patients with peripheral vascular disease. Nurs Clin North Am 1986 Jun; 21(2): 219–231.

Hill MN and Grim CM. How to take a precise blood pressure. Am J Nurs 1991 Feb; 91(2): 38–42.

Massey JA. Diagnosis testing for peripheral vascular disease. Nurs Clin North Am 1986 Jun; 21(2): 207–218.

Moranoe JU and Raju S. Chronic venous insufficiency: Assessment with descending venography. Radiology 1990 Feb; 174(2): 441–444.

Wildus DM and Osterman FA. Evaluation and percutaneous management of atherosclerotic peripheral vascular disease. JAMA 1989 Jun; 261(21): 3146–3153.

Hypertension

Applegate WB. Hypertension in elderly patients. Ann Intern Med 1989 Jun; 110(11): 901–915.

Beare PG. Calcium channel blockers: Nursing care for hypertension. Crit Care Nurs 1989 Mar/Apr; 9(2): 37–44.

Black HR and Setaro JF. Monotherapy and beyond. Consultant 1989 Jan; 29(1): 88-91, 94, 99–100.

Black HR. Prescribing for compliance: The role of fixed-dose combinations. Consultant 1988 Jun; 28(6): 145-147, 150, 152.

Cressman MD and Vlasses PH. Recent issues in antihypertensive drug therapy. Med Clin North Am 1988 Mar; 772(2): 373–397.

Fontana SA. Update on high blood pressure: Highlights from the 1988 national report. Nurs Pract 1988 Dec; 13(12): 8, 10–12, 15, 18.

Frohlich ED. Calcium antagonist for initial therapy of hypertension. Heart Lung 1989 Jul; 18(4): 370–376.

Frohlich ED et al. Hypertensive cardiovascular disease. J Am Coll Cardiol 1987 Aug; 10(2): 57A–59A.

Graham DI. Morphologic changes during hypertension. Am J Cardiol 1989 Feb; 63(6): 6C–9C.

Greenberg G et al. The relationship between smoking and the response to antihypertensive treatment in mild hypertensives in the medical research council's trial of treatment. Int J Epidemiol 1987 Mar; 16(1): 25–30.

Hahn W, Brooks J, Hite R. Blood pressure norms for healthy young adults: Relation to sex, age, and reported parenteral hypertension. Res Nurs Health 1989 Feb; 12(1): 53–56.

Hill MN and Cunningham SL. The latest words for high BP. Am J Nurs 1989 Apr; 89(4): 504–508.

McGarry-Myers RJ and Franciosa JA. The role of new antihypertensive drugs. Chest 1988 Apr; 93(4): 868–869.

* Nakagawa-Kogan H et al. Self-management of hypertension: Predictors of success in diastolic blood pressure reduction. Res Nurs Health 1988 Apr; 11(2): 105–115.

* Powers MJ and Jalowiec A. Profile of the well-controlled hypertensive patient. Nurs Res 1987 Mar/Apr; 36(2): 106–110.

Rubenstein EB and Escalante C. Hypertensive crisis. Crit Care Clin 1989 Jul; 5(3): 477–495.

The 1988 Report of the Joint National Committee on Detection, Evaluation, and Treatment of High Blood Pressure. Arch Intern Med 1988 May; 148(5): 1023–1038.

Lymph Conditions

Gloviczki P et al. Noninvasive evaluation of the swollen extremity: Experiences with 190 lymphoscinitigraphic examinations. J Vasc Surg 1989 May; 9(5): 683–689.

Intenzo CM et al. Lymphedema of the lower extremities: Evaluation by microcolloidal imaging. Clin Nucl Med 1989 Feb; 142(2): 107–110.

Servelle M. Total superficial lymphangiectomy. AORN J 1988 Jun; 47(6): 1386–1387.

Wilson C and Bilodeau ML. Current management concepts for the patient with lymphedema. J Cardiovasc Nurs 1989 Nov; 4(1): 79–88.

Varicose Veins

Goldman MP and Fronek A. Anatomy and pathophysiology of varicose veins. J Dermatol Surg Oncol 1989 Feb; 15(2): 138–145.

de Groot WP. Treatment of varicose veins: Modern concepts and methods. J Dermatol Surg Oncol 1989 Feb; 15(2): 191–198.

Thompson NW. The diagnosis and treatment of varicose veins. NAPT J 1985 Jan/Feb; 17–23.

Venous Conditions

Inada K et al. Effects of intermittent pneumatic compression for prevention of postoperative deep vein thrombosis with special reference to fibrinolytic activity. Am J Surg 1988 Apr; 155(4): 602–605.

Lewis JD. The management of the limb in acute venous thrombosis. Blood Rev 1987 Mar; 1(4): 230–236.

Menzoian JO and Doyle JE. Venous insufficiency of the leg. Hosp Pract 1989 May; 24(5): 109–110, 113, 114, 116.

Nicolaides A et al. Progress in the investigation of chronic venous insufficiency. Ann Vasc Surg 1989 Jul; 3(3): 278–292.

Porteous MJ et al. Thigh length versus knee length stockings in the prevention of deep vein thrombosis. Br J Surg 1989 Mar; 76(3): 296–297.

Powers LR. Distal deep vein thrombosis. J Gen Intern Med 1988 May/Jun; 3(3): 288–293.

Reporting Standards in Venous Disease. J Vasc Surg 1988 Aug; 6(2): 172–181.

Scurr JH et al. Regimen for improved effectiveness of intermittent pneumatic compression in deep venous thrombosis prophylaxis. Surgery 1987 Nov; 102(5): 816–820.

Turpie AG et al. Prevention of deep vein thrombosis in potential neurosurgical patients. Arch Intern Med 1989 Mar; 149(3): 679–681.

Information/Resources

Agencies

Joint National Committee on Detection, Evaluation and Treatment of High Blood Pressure
National Heart, Lung and Blood Institute, Building 31, Room 4A05, Bethesda, MD 20892

National Heart, Lung and Blood Institute
Education Programs Information Center, 4733 Bethesda Ave, Suite 530, Bethesda MD 20814

32

Assessment and Management of Patients With Hematologic Disorders

Learning Objectives

On completion of this chapter, the learner will be able to:

1. Compare the hypoproliferative anemias to the hemolytic anemias
2. Use the nursing process as a framework for care of patients with anemia
3. Use the nursing process as a framework for care of patients with sickle cell anemia
4. Use the nursing process as a framework for care of patients with leukemia
5. Compare the leukemias, their incidence, physiologic alterations, clinical manifestations, management, and prognosis
6. Describe the stages of Hodgkin's disease in relation to extent of disease process, clinical manifestations, and therapeutic management
7. Differentiate between bleeding disorders that are vascular disorders, those that are platelet defects, and those that are clotting factor defects
8. Use the nursing process as a framework for care of patients with hemophilia
9. Describe the therapeutic usefulness of whole blood and each of its components
10. Develop a plan of care for the patient receiving a blood transfusion

Glossary

agranulocytosis—acute disease in which the white blood cell count decreases to extremely low levels and neutropenia is pronounced

aplasia—failure of an organ or tissue to develop normally

band cell—immature granulocyte

basophil—a granular leukocyte

ecchymosis—a blue-black macula that results from seepage of blood into skin or mucous membrane

eosinophil—a granular leukocyte

erythrocyte—red blood cell

erythropoiesis—the formation of red blood cells

(continued)

Glossary *(Continued)*

erythropoietin—*hormone that regulates red blood cell production*

glossitis—*inflammation of the tongue*

granulocyte—*granular leukocyte: polymorphonuclear leukocyte (neutrophil, basophil, or eosinophil)*

granulocytopenia—*abnormal reduction of granulocytes in the blood*

hematocrit—*fraction of the blood occupied by erythrocytes*

hematopoiesis—*production and development of blood cells*

hematopoietic—*blood producing*

hemoglobin—*iron-containing pigment of red blood cells*

hemolysis—*destruction of red blood cells with liberation of hemoglobin into the surrounding fluid*

histiocyte—*cell of loose connective tissue that shows phagocytic activity*

hyperplasia—*excessive proliferation of normal cells in normal tissue*

hypochromia—*blood possessing less than normal color and hemoglobin content*

leukocyte—*white blood cell*

leukopenia—*abnormal decrease of white blood cells*

lymphocyte—*a mononuclear leukocyte*

lysis—*disintegration or dissolution of cells*

macrocyte—*a large red blood cell*

macrophage—*cells of the reticuloendothelial system that have the ability to phagocytose particulate matter*

megaloblast—*abnormally large red blood cells*

microcyte—*a small red blood cell*

monocyte—*a mononuclear leukocyte*

mononuclear leukocyte—*agranulocyte (lymphocyte, monocyte)*

neutrophil—*a granular leukocyte*

normochromic—*normal color of cells*

normocytic—*normal size of cells*

oxyhemoglobin—*hemoglobin combined with oxygen*

pancytopenia—*reduction in all cellular elements of the blood*

petechiae—*small red or purple hemorrhagic spots on the skin*

phagocytosis—*the process of ingestion and digestion of bacteria and particles*

plasma—*liquid part of the blood*

platelet—*thrombocyte; cell fragment found in the blood that plays an important role in coagulation, hemostasis, and thrombus formation*

reticulocyte—*immature red blood cell*

reticuloendothelial system—*cells scattered throughout the body that have the ability to phagocytose particulate matter (bacteria, colloidal particles)*

serum—*the fluid portion of the blood that remains after coagulation*

spherocyte—*erythrocyte that assumes a spheroid shape*

thrombocyte—*platelet*

thrombocytopenia—*abnormal decrease in number of platelets*

Physiologic Overview

The hematologic system consists of the blood and the sites where blood is produced, including the bone marrow and lymph nodes. The blood is a specialized organ that differs from other organs in that it exists in a fluid state. The fluid consists of cellular components suspended in blood plasma. The blood cells are divided into *erythrocytes* (red blood cells, normally 5 million per mm³ of blood) and *leukocytes* (white blood cells, normally 5,000 to 10,000 per mm³ of blood). There are approximately 500 to 1000 erythrocytes for each leukocyte. Also suspended in the plasma are small, nonnucleated cell fragments called *platelets* (normally 150,000 to 450,000 platelets per mm³ of blood). These cellular components of blood normally make up 40% to 45% of the blood volume. The fraction of the blood occupied by erythrocytes is called the *hematocrit*. Blood appears as a thick, opaque, red fluid. Its color is imparted by the hemoglobin contained within the red blood cells.

The volume of blood in humans is approximately 7% to 10% of the normal body weight, which represents about 5 liters. The blood circulates through the vascular system and serves as a link between body organs, carrying oxygen absorbed from the lungs and nutrients absorbed from the gastrointestinal tract to the body cells for cellular metabolism.

The blood also carries waste products produced by cellular metabolism to the lungs, skin, liver, and kidneys for subsequent transformation and elimination from the body. It also carries hormones and antibodies to their sites of action or utilization.

To perform its functions, blood must remain in its normally fluid state. Because it is fluid, the danger always exists that trauma can lead to loss of blood from the vascular system. To prevent this, the blood has an intricate clotting mechanism that is activated when necessary to seal leaks in the blood vessels.

Excessive clotting is equally dangerous because it potentially obstructs blood flow to vital tissues. To prevent this complication, the body has a fibrinolytic mechanism that eventually dissolves the clots formed within blood vessels.

Bone Marrow

The bone marrow occupies the interior of spongy bones and the central cavity of the long bones of the skeleton. The marrow accounts for 4% to 5% of the total body weight and therefore is one of the larger organs of the body. The marrow can be either red or yellow. Red marrow is the site of active blood cell production and constitutes the major *hematopoietic* (blood-producing) organ. Yellow marrow, however, is composed mainly of fat and is not active in the production of blood elements. During childhood, the major portion of the marrow is red. As a person ages, a large portion of the marrow in the long bones is converted into yellow marrow, but it retains the potential for reversion to hematopoietic tissue if necessary. Red marrow in the adult is confined chiefly to the ribs, vertebral column, and other flat bones.

The marrow is a highly vascularized organ that consists of connective tissue containing free cells. The most primitive of this population of free cells are the stem cells, which are precursors of two different cell lines. The *myeloid line* includes erythrocytes, several types of leukocytes, and platelets. The *lymphoid line* differentiates into lymphocytes.

Erythrocytes

The normal red blood cell is a biconcave disc, its configuration resembling that of a soft ball compressed between two fingers. It has a diameter of about 8 μm but is a very flexible cell, so flexible that it is capable of passing easily through capillaries that may be as small as 4 μm in diameter. The volume of a red blood cell is about 90 μm^3. The red blood cell membrane is so thin that gases such as oxygen and carbon dioxide can easily diffuse across it. Mature red blood cells consist primarily of hemoglobin, which makes up 95% of the cell mass. These cells have no nuclei and have many fewer metabolic enzymes than do most other cells. The presence of a large amount of hemoglobin enables the cell to perform its principal function, the transport of oxygen between the lungs and tissues.

The oxygen-carrying pigment *hemoglobin* is a protein with a molecular weight of 64,000. The molecule is made up of four subunits, each containing a heme portion attached to a globin chain. Iron is present in the heme component of the molecule. An important property of the heme portion is its ability to bind to oxygen loosely and reversibly. When hemoglobin is combined with oxygen, it is called *oxyhemoglobin*. Oxyhemoglobin has a brighter red color than hemoglobin that does not contain oxygen (*reduced hemoglobin*), so arterial blood is brighter red than venous blood. Whole blood normally contains about 15 g of hemoglobin per 100 ml of blood (150 g/L), or 30 μg of hemoglobin per million erythrocytes.

Production of Erythrocytes (Erythropoiesis). Erythroblasts arise from the primitive stem cells in bone marrow. The erythroblast is a nucleated cell that in the process of maturing within the bone marrow accumulates hemoglobin and gradually loses its nucleus. At this stage, the cell is known as a *reticulocyte*. Further maturation into an erythrocyte entails the loss of dark staining material and a slight shrinkage in size. The mature erythrocyte is then released into the circulation. Under conditions of rapid *erythropoiesis*, reticulocytes and other immature cells may be released prematurely into the circulation.

Differentiation of the primitive multipotential stem cell of the marrow into an erythroblast is stimulated by *erythropoietin*, a substance produced primarily by the kidney. Under conditions of prolonged hypoxia, as in the case of persons living at high altitudes or after severe hemorrhage, erythropoietin levels are increased and red blood cell production is stimulated.

For normal erythrocyte production, the bone marrow requires iron, vitamin B$_{12}$, folic acid, pyridoxine (vitamin B$_6$), and other factors. If any of these factors is deficient during erythropoiesis, decreased red blood cell production and anemia result.

Iron Stores and Metabolism. Total body iron content in the average adult is approximately 3 g, most of which is present in hemoglobin or one of its breakdown products. Normally, about 0.5 to 1 mg of iron is absorbed per day from the intestinal tract to replace losses of iron in the feces. Additional amounts of iron, up to 2 mg per day, must be absorbed by the adult female to replace blood lost during menstruation. Iron deficiency in the adult (decreased total body iron content) generally indicates that blood has been lost from the body—for example, by hemorrhage or excessive menstruation.

The concentration of iron in blood is normally about 80 to 180 μg/dL (14 to 32 μmol/L) for men and 60 to 160 μg/dL (11 to 29 μmol/L) for women. With iron deficiency, bone marrow iron stores are rapidly depleted, hemoglobin synthesis is depressed, and the red blood cells produced by the marrow are small and low in hemoglobin.

Vitamin B$_{12}$ and Folic Acid Metabolism. Vitamin B$_{12}$ and folic acid are required for DNA synthesis in many tissues, but deficiencies of either of these vitamins have the greatest effect on erythropoiesis. Vitamin B$_{12}$ or folic acid deficiency is characterized by the production of abnormally large red blood cells called *megaloblasts*. Because these cells are abnormal, many are sequestered in the bone marrow and their rate of release is decreased. This condition results in megaloblastic anemia.

Both vitamin B$_{12}$ and the folic acid are derived from the diet. Vitamin B$_{12}$ combines with intrinsic factor produced in the stomach. The vitamin B$_{12}$–intrinsic factor complex is absorbed in the distal ileum. Folic acid is absorbed in the proximal small intestine.

Red Blood Cell Destruction. The average life span of a circulating red blood cell is 120 days. Aged red blood cells are removed from the blood by the reticuloendothelial system, particularly in the liver and the spleen. The reticuloendothelial cells produce a pigment called bilirubin from the hemoglobin that is released from the destroyed red blood cells. *Bilirubin* is a waste product that is excreted in the bile. The iron, freed from the hemoglobin during bilirubin formation, is carried in plasma bound to the protein called *transferrin* to the bone marrow, where it is reclaimed for production of new hemoglobin.

Function of Erythrocytes. The major function of the red blood cells is to transport oxygen from the lungs to the tissues. Erythrocytes are uniquely capable of performing this function because of their high concentration of hemoglobin. If hemoglobin were not present, the oxygen-carrying capacity of blood would be decreased by 99% and would not be sufficient to meet the metabolic needs of the body. An important property of hemoglobin is that it binds oxygen loosely and reversibly. As a result, oxygen readily binds to hemoglobin in the lungs, is carried as oxyhemoglobin in arterial blood, and readily dissociates from hemoglobin in the tissues. In venous blood, hemoglobin combines with hydrogen ions produced by cellular metabolism and thus buffers excess acid.

Leukocytes

Leukocytes are divided into two general categories, granulocytes and mononuclear cells (agranulocytes). In normal blood, the total leukocyte count is 5,000 to 10,000 cells per mm^3. Of these, approximately 60% are granulocytes and 40% are mononuclear cells. Leukocytes can be readily differentiated from erythrocytes by the presence of a nucleus, their larger size, and different staining properties.

Granulocytes. Granulocytes are defined by the presence of granules in their cytoplasm. The diameter of a granulocyte is generally two to three times that of an erythrocyte. Granulocytes are divided into three subgroups, which are characterized by their staining properties as seen on microscopic examination. *Eosinophils* have bright red granules in their cytoplasm, whereas the granules in *basophils* stain deep blue. The third, and by far the most numerous, cell in this series is the *neutrophil*, with granules that show a dull violet hue. The nucleus of the mature granulocyte generally has multiple lobes (usually two to four) connected by thin filaments of nuclear material. Because of their nuclear characteristics, these cells are called *polymorphonuclear* (PMN) leukocytes. The immature granulocyte has a single-lobed ovoid nucleus and is called a band cell. Ordinarily, band cells account for only a small percentage of circulating granulocytes, although their percentage can increase greatly under conditions in which the rate of production of PMN leukocytes is increased. The number of circulating granulocytes found in the healthy person is maintained relatively constant, but in the presence of infection large numbers of these cells are rapidly released into the circulation. Granulocyte production from the stem cell pool is thought to be controlled in a manner similar to the regulation of erythrocyte production by erythropoietin.

Mononuclear Leukocytes (Agranulocytes).   Mononuclear leukocytes (lymphocytes and monocytes) are white blood cells with a single-lobed nucleus and a granule-free cytoplasm. In normal adult blood, lymphocytes account for approximately 30% and monocytes approximately 5% of the total leukocytes. Mature *lymphocytes* are small cells with scanty cytoplasm. They are produced primarily in the lymph nodes and in the lymphoid tissue of the intestine, spleen, and thymus gland from precursor cells that originated as marrow stem cells. *Monocytes* are the largest of the blood leukocytes. They are produced by the bone marrow and give rise to tissue histiocytes, including Kupffer cells of the liver, peritoneal macrophages, alveolar macrophages, and other components of the reticuloendothelial system.

Function of the Leukocytes.   The function of the leukocytes is to protect the body from invasion by bacteria and other foreign entities. The major function of neutrophilic PMNs is to ingest foreign material (phagocytosis). Neutrophils arrive at the site within an hour of the onset of an inflammatory reaction and initiate phagocytosis, but are relatively short-lived. The influx of monocytes is later, but these cells continue their phagocytic activities for long periods.

The function of lymphocytes is primarily to produce substances that aid in the attack of foreign material. One group of lymphocytes (T lymphocytes) kills foreign cells directly or releases a variety of *lymphokines*, substances that enhance the activity of phagocytic cells. The other group of lymphocytes (B lymphocytes) produces antibodies, protein molecules that destroy foreign material by several mechanisms.

Eosinophils and basophils function as reservoirs of potent biologic materials such as histamine, serotonin, and heparin. Release of these compounds alters the blood supply to tissues, such as occurs during inflammation, and helps to mobilize body defense mechanisms. The increase in the number of eosinophils in allergic states indicates that these cells are involved in the hypersensitivity reaction.

Platelets

Platelets are small particles, 2 to 4 μm in diameter, that are present in the circulating blood plasma. Because they disintegrate quickly and easily, their number varies normally between 150,000 and 450,000 per mm^3 of blood, depending on the numbers that are produced, how they are used, and how quickly they are destroyed. They are formed from the fragmentation of giant cells of the bone marrow, called *megakaryocytes*. Platelet production is regulated by thrombopoietin.

Platelets play an essential role in the control of bleeding. When vascular injury occurs, platelets collect at the site. Substances released from platelet granules and other blood cells cause the platelets to adhere to each other and form a patch or plug, which temporarily stops bleeding. Additional substances released from platelets activate coagulation factors in the blood plasma.

Blood Coagulation

Blood coagulation is the process whereby the components of the liquid blood are transformed into a semisolid material called a *blood clot*. The blood clot is composed mainly of blood cells entrapped in a meshwork of fibrin. Fibrin is formed from proteins in the plasma as the result of a complex series of reactions.

Many factors are involved in the reaction cascade that forms fibrin. The clotting factors are listed in Table 32–1, and the extrinsic and intrinsic pathways for fibrin generation are shown diagrammatically in Figure 32–1. When tissue is injured, the extrinsic pathway is activated by the release from the tissue of a substance called thromboplastin. As the result of a series of reactions, prothrombin is converted to thrombin, which in turn catalyzes the conversion of fibrinogen to fibrin. Calcium (factor IV) is a necessary cofactor for many of these reactions. Clotting by the intrinsic pathway is activated when the collagen lining blood vessels is exposed. Clotting factors are then activated sequentially until, as with the extrinsic pathway, fibrin is ultimately formed. Although longer, this sequence is probably most often responsible for clotting *in vivo*. The intrinsic pathway is also responsible for initiating the clotting of blood that comes into contact with glass or other foreign surfaces, as when blood is withdrawn from the body into a test tube. It is for this reason that anticoagulants often must be used when drawing a specimen of blood for chemical or other tests. The anticoagulants usually used are either citrate, which binds the plasma calcium, or heparin, which prevents the conversion of prothrombin to thrombin. Citrate cannot be used as an anticoagulant *in vivo* because binding of plasma calcium would cause hypocalcemia and death. Heparin can be used clinically as an anticoagulant. Coumarins also are used clinically for their anticoagulant action of interfering with the production of several of the plasma-coagulating factors.

Clots that form in the body are eventually dissolved by the action of the fibrinolytic system, which consists of plasmin and other proteolytic enzymes. Through the action of this system, clots are dissolved as tissue is repaired, and the vascular system is returned to its normal baseline state.

Blood Plasma

After cellular elements are removed from blood, the remaining liquid portion is called blood plasma. It contains ions, proteins, and other substances. If plasma is allowed to clot, the remaining fluid is called *serum*. Serum has essentially the same composition as plasma, except that its fibrinogen and several of the clotting factors have been removed.

Plasma Proteins.   Plasma proteins consist primarily of albumin and globulins. The globulins in turn consist of alpha, beta, and gamma fractions derived by a laboratory test called *serum protein electrophoresis*. Each of these groups is made up of distinct proteins. The gamma globulins, which consist mainly of antibodies, are called *immunoglobulins*. These proteins are produced by the lymphocytes and plasma cells. Important proteins in the alpha and beta fractions are the transport globulins and the clotting factors, which are made in the liver. The transport globulins carry various substances in the bound

TABLE 32-1. *Clotting Factors*

Official Number	Synonym	Contemporary Version	
I	Fibrinogen	I	(Fibrinogen)
II	Prothrombin	II	(Prothrombin)
III	Tissue thromboplastin	III	(Tissue factor)
IV	Calcium	IV	(Calcium)
V	Labile	V	(Labile factor)
		VI	PF$_3$ (platelet coagulant activities)
		VI	PF$_4$
VII	Stable factor	VII	(Stable factor)
VIII	Antihemophilic factor	VIII	AHF (antihemophilic factor)
		VIII	VWF (von Willebrand factor)
		VIII	RAg (related antigen)
IX	Christmas factor	IX	(Christmas factor)
X	Stuart-Power factor	X	(Stuart-Power factor)
XI	Plasma thromboplastin (antecedent)	XI	(Plasma thromboplastin antecedent)
XII	Hageman factor	XII	HF (Hageman factor)
		XII	PK (Prekallikrein Fletcher)
		XII	HMWK (High-molecular-weight kininogen)
XIII	Fibrin-stabilizing factor	XIII	Fibrin-stabilizing factor

The Roman numerals and synonyms designating each clotting factor accepted by the International Committee on Blood Clotting Factors are located in the left-hand columns. Note the absence of factor VI. The version in the right-hand column incorporates more recently recognized clotting factors but is not officially recognized.
(Green D. General considerations of coagulation proteins. Ann Clin Lab Sci 8[2]:95–105.)

form around the circulation. For example, thyroid-binding globulin carries thyroxin, and transferrin carries iron. The clotting factors, including fibrinogen, remain in an inactive form in the blood plasma until activated by the clotting cascade.

Albumin is particularly important for the maintenance of fluid volume within the vascular system. Capillary walls are impermeable to albumin, so its presence in the plasma creates an osmotic force that keeps fluid within the vascular space. Albumin, which is produced by the liver, has the capacity to bind to a number of substances that are often present in plasma. In this way, it functions as a transport protein for metals, fatty acids, bilirubin, and drugs, among other substances.

Pathophysiology of the Hematologic System

Anemias. A frequent disorder of the hematologic system is a decrease in the number of circulating red blood cells. This condition, called *anemia,* can result from either underproduction of red blood cells by the bone marrow or increased destruction of circulating red blood cells. Underproduction of red blood cells can be due to a deficiency in cofactors for erythropoiesis, including folic acid, vitamin B$_{12}$, and iron. Red blood cell production may also be reduced if bone marrow is suppressed (by tumor or drugs) or is inadequately stimulated because of lack of erythropoietin, as occurs in chronic renal disease. Increased destruction of red blood cells may occur because of an overactive reticuloendothelial system (*e.g.,* hypersplenism) or because the bone marrow produces abnormal red blood cells (*e.g.,* sickle cell anemia). Because the red blood cell and its hemoglobin are important for the delivery of oxygen to tissues, anemias may result in tissue hypoxia.

Bleeding Disorders. Bleeding disorders can be attributed to deficiency in either platelets or clotting factors in the cir-

culating blood. Platelet function in the blood plasma can be reduced as the result of bone marrow insufficiency, increased splenic destruction, or abnormal circulating platelets. Deficiencies of clotting factors are usually due to underproduction of these factors by the liver. Hemophilia is a hereditary disorder that results from deficiency of clotting factors VIII and IX.

Manifestations of Blood Disorders. Problems commonly seen in patients with blood disorders are outlined in Chart 32–1.

Blood Study Procedures

Methods of Obtaining Blood

Venipuncture. Most routine hematologic studies are performed on venous blood, which is usually obtained from an antecubital vein. Occasionally, in very obese persons or those whose veins have been thrombosed by chemotherapy, it may be necessary to use one of the veins on the dorsum of the hand.

After a tourniquet has been applied around the upper arm, the arm and hand veins become prominent. The vein chosen for venipuncture should be straight not tortuous and should be well fixed in the subcutaneous tissue so that it does not roll away. The skin distal to the vein is stretched with one hand while the opposite hand is used to push the needle through the skin and then slowly into the vein. Blood is immediately placed in the collection tube appropriate for the particular test required. The tubes are color coded to specify what, if any, additive they contain. For some tests the blood is allowed to

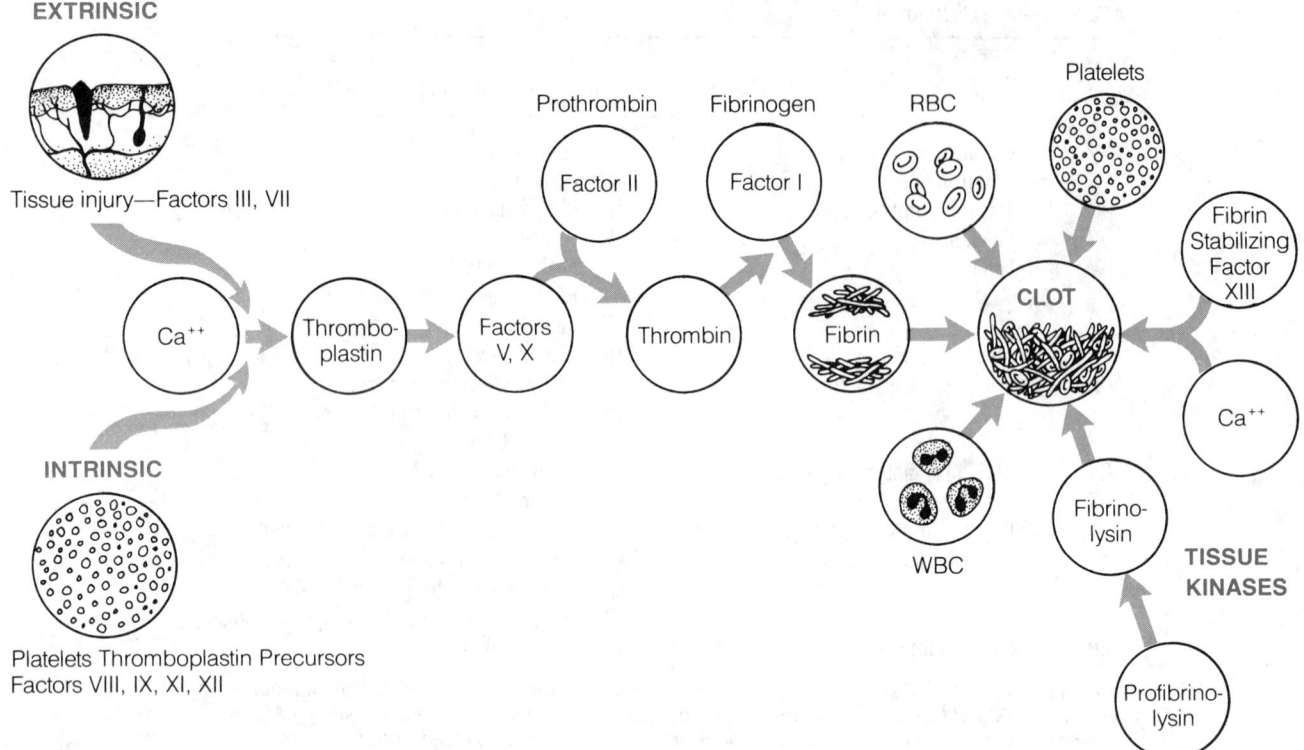

EXTRINSIC

Tissue injury—Factors III, VII

INTRINSIC

Platelets Thromboplastin Precursors
Factors VIII, IX, XI, XII

Prothrombin   Fibrinogen   RBC   Platelets

Factor II   Factor I

Ca^{++} Thrombo-plastin   Factors V, X   Thrombin   Fibrin   CLOT   Fibrin Stabilizing Factor XIII

Ca^{++}

WBC   Fibrino-lysin   **TISSUE KINASES**

Profibrino-lysin

Figure 32–1.   The blood-clotting mechanism. The schematic drawing represents the factors essential to change blood into a solid gel. The entire chain reaction in which fibrinogen (a plasma protein) is converted to fibrin (the clot) takes place at the site of vessel damage. (Adapted from Feller I and Archambeault C. Nursing the Burn Patient. Ann Arbor, The Institute for Burn Medicine.)

coagulate; for others it is kept fluid by the presence of an anticoagulant in the collection tube.

Finger Puncture.   The finger puncture method is used frequently for blood smears and counts. This method uses capillary blood, but for practical purposes the results are identical to those obtained with venous blood. Lancets of various shapes are available. These make a puncture of 1 to 2 mm. Best results are obtained if the patient's hand is warm and if the pulp of the index or middle finger is punctured. The skin should be cleaned with alcohol first and then carefully wiped dry with a lint-free sponge. If any alcohol remains, it will alter red cell morphology. The drops of blood obtained by this method can be gently touched to glass slides or cover slips, for peripheral smears. Capillary blood can also be drawn into calibrated red cell and white cell pipettes and into microhematocrit tubes.

The most common hematologic tests are described in Chart 32–2.

Bone Marrow Aspiration

Bone marrow is usually aspirated from the sternum or iliac crest in adults. Most patients need no more preparation than a careful explanation of the procedure, but for some very anxious patients, meperidine (Demerol) or a minor tranquilizer may be useful. It is always important for the physician or nurse to describe and explain the procedure as it is being performed and the sensations that will be experienced during the procedure. First, the skin area is cleansed as for any minor surgery. Then a small area is anesthetized with lidocaine (Xylocaine), through the skin and subcutaneous tissue to the periosteum of

the bone. The bone marrow needle is introduced with a stylet in place. When the needle is felt to go through the outer cortex of bone and enter the marrow cavity, the stylet is removed, a syringe is attached, and a small volume (0.5 ml) of blood and marrow is aspirated. The actual aspiration always causes brief pain, and the patient should be warned of this. Taking deep breaths or using relaxation techniques often helps.

If a bone marrow biopsy is necessary, it is best performed after the aspiration and with a special needle. Several types of needles are available, the procedure varying according to the type of needle used. Because these needles are large, the skin is punctured first with a surgical blade (no. 9 or 11) to make a 3- or 4-mm incision. Only the iliac bone is used for this procedure (Fig. 32–2), because the sternum is too thin.

The major hazard of these procedures is a slight risk of hemorrhage. This risk is increased if the patient's platelet count is low; therefore a platelet count is obtained before the procedure. After bone marrow aspiration, pressure is applied to the site for several minutes. After a biopsy, pressure is applied to the posterior iliac crest for 60 minutes by the combination of a pressure dressing and having the patient lie recumbent in bed. Most patients have no discomfort after a bone marrow aspiration, but the site of a biopsy may ache for a day or two.

In summary, the hematologic system is composed of the blood and the sites where blood is produced. This includes the bone marrow and lymph nodes. Blood is a tissue that circulates. It is composed of a straw-colored fluid, the plasma, in which are suspended the red and white blood cells and

Chart 32-1
Common Problems of Patients With Blood Disorders

Problem	Nursing Interventions
Fatigue and weakness	Plan nursing care to conserve the patient's strength and emotional energy. Provide frequent rest periods. Encourage ambulation and other activities as tolerated. Avoid disturbing activities, noise, and stress. Encourage optimal nutrition—high-protein and high-calorie foods and drinks.
Hemorrhagic tendencies	Keep the patient at rest during the bleeding episodes. Apply gentle pressure to the bleeding sites. Apply cold compresses to the bleeding sites when indicated. Do not disturb clots. Use small-gauge needles when administering medications by injection. Support the patient during transfusion therapy. Observe for symptoms of internal bleeding. Have a tracheostomy set available for the patient who is bleeding from the mouth or the throat.
Ulcerative lesions of the tongue, gums, or mucous membranes	Avoid irritating foods and beverages. Provide frequent oral hygiene with mild, cool mouthwash solutions. Use applicators or soft-bristled toothbrush. Keep the lips lubricated. Provide mouth care both before and after meals. Encourage regular visits to the dentist.
Dyspnea	Elevate the head of the bed. Use pillows to support the patient in the orthopneic position. Administer oxygen when indicated. Prevent unnecessary exertion. Avoid gas-forming foods.
Bone and joint pains	Relieve pressure of bedding by using a cradle. Administer either hot or cold compresses as prescribed. Administer analgesic as prescribed on a regular basis. Provide for joint immobilization when prescribed.
Fever	Provide cool sponges. Administer antipyretic (acetaminophen) drugs as prescribed. Encourage fluid intake unless contraindicated. Maintain a cool environmental temperature.
Pruritus or skin eruptions	Keep the patient's fingernails short. Use soap sparingly. Apply emollient lotions in skin care.
Anxiety of the patient and family	Explain the nature, the discomforts, and the limitations of activity associated with the diagnostic procedures and treatments. Encourage the patient and family to express their anxieties. Provide an atmosphere of acceptance and understanding. Promote the patient's relaxation and comfort. Consider the patient's individual preferences. Promote independence and self-care within the patient's limitations. Encourage the family to participate in the patient's care (as desired). Create a comfortable atmosphere for family visits with the patient.

Chart 32–2
Common Hematologic Laboratory Tests

Test	Definition
Complete blood count (CBC)	Includes enumeration of number of white cells, red cells, and platelets per cubic millimeter of venous blood, as well as a differential count, percentage of each type of nucleated cell in the blood, (e.g., percentage of polymorphonuclears, percentage of lymphocytes).
Reticulocyte count	Percentage of young (1–2 days old), nonnucleated erythrocytes in peripheral blood; they are recognized in special stains of blood smears as cells with lacy inclusions, which consist of RNA.
Hemoglobin electrophoresis	A drop of blood placed on a solid medium (paper, starch block, gel, or cellulose acetate) is exposed to a current of electricity while being bathed by a buffer solution. The different hemoglobins (e.g., A, A-2, F, S) travel at varying speeds, depending on their charge. At the end of the procedure, the paper or gel is stained, and the hemoglobins in each sample can be identified.
Sickling test	A drop of blood is mixed with a drop of a reducing agent (sodium metabisulfite). This substance deprives the red cells of oxygen and induces sickling if S hemoglobin is present. Sickling of red cells is observed under the microscope in 30 minutes if the blood was obtained from a person with either sickle trait or sickle cell anemia. Normal blood does not undergo any change.
Leukocyte alkaline phosphatase (LAP)	LAP is an enzyme present in high concentrations in granules of neutrophils. A special stain of peripheral blood smears is used to estimate the amount of LAP present per cell. The normal value is 20 to 130. Untreated chronic myelogenous leukemia patients have values of less than 20, and the test is useful to help diagnose CML. High values are seen in infection and steroid-induced leukocytosis.
Coombs' test	Determines the presence of immune globulin (hence, antibodies) on the surface of erythrocytes (direct Coombs' test) or in the plasma (indirect Coombs' test)
Bleeding time	A screening test for disorders of platelet function. It is the time taken for bleeding to cease after a standardized skin wound is produced, usually on the forearm. A prolonged time suggests an inherited or acquired platelet defect (e.g., von Willebrand's disease or aspirin ingestion).
Platelet aggregation	A measure of the time and completeness of the formation of platelet aggregates in a sample of plasma, after the addition of an agent such as epinephrine or ADP.
Prothrombin time	Measures the coagulant activity of the "extrinsic" system, including fibrinogen, prothrombin, and factors V, VII, and X. It is used to monitor therapy of coumarin derivatives, as well as to screen for liver disease.
Partial thromboplastin time	A screening test for deficiencies of all plasma coagulation factors except VII and XIII. It is usually considered abnormally prolonged if levels of factors are less than 30% of normal. It is often used to monitor heparin therapy.

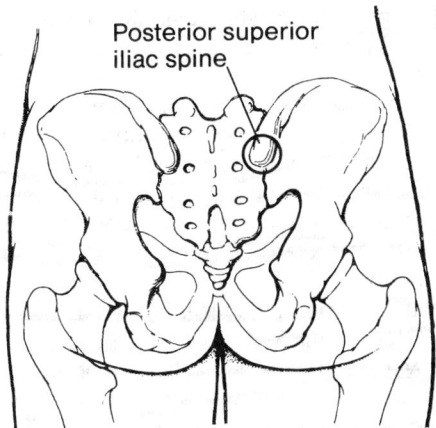

Figure 32–2. Site of bone marrow biopsy.

platelets. Through the vascular system, nutritive substances and oxygen needed for repair, growth, and metabolic actions are circulated to the body, and metabolic waste products, including carbon dioxide, are eliminated from the body. Blood has an intricate protective clotting mechanism that controls the excessive loss of blood from the body. Maintenance of the normal fluidity of the blood in the body is achieved through the fibrinolytic system.

Anemia

Definition and Etiology

Anemia is a laboratory term that indicates a low red cell count and a below-normal hemoglobin or hematocrit level. It is not a disease but rather reflects a disease state or altered body function. Physiologically, anemia exists when there is an insufficient amount of hemoglobin to deliver oxygen to the tissues.

There are many different kinds of anemias. Some are due to inadequate production of red blood cells, and others are due to premature or excessive destruction of red blood cells. The most common cause is blood loss, but other etiologic factors include deficits in iron and other nutrients, hereditary factors, and chronic diseases.

Pathophysiology

The appearance of anemia reflects either marrow failure or excessive red cell loss, or both. Marrow failure (*i.e.*, reduced erythropoiesis) may occur as a result of a nutritional deficiency, toxic exposure, tumor invasion, or, as in many instances, from causes unknown. Red cells may be lost through hemorrhage or hemolysis (destruction). In the latter case, the problem may be rooted in some red cell defect that is incompatible with normal red cell survival or explainable on the basis of some factor extrinsic to the red cell that promotes red cell destruction.

Red cell lysis (dissolution) occurs mainly within the phagocytic cells of the reticuloendothelial system, notably in the liver and spleen. As a byproduct of this process, bilirubin, formed within the phagocyte, enters the bloodstream. Any in-

crease in hemolysis is promptly reflected by an increase in plasma bilirubin. (This concentration normally is 1 mg/dl or less; levels above 1.5 mg/dl produce visible jaundice of the sclerae.)

If, as happens in certain specific hemolytic disorders, red cells are destroyed within the circulating bloodstream, hemoglobin itself appears in the plasma (*hemoglobinemia*). If the plasma concentration exceeds the capacity of the plasma haptoglobin to bind it all (*i.e.*, if the amount is more than about 100 mg/dl), this pigment diffuses through the renal glomeruli and into the urine (*hemoglobinuria*). Thus the presence or absence of hemoglobinemia and hemoglobinuria provides information about the location of abnormal blood destruction in a patient with hemolysis and can be a clue to the nature of the hemolytic process.

A conclusion as to whether the anemia in a particular patient is caused by hemolysis or by inadequate erythropoiesis usually can be reached on the basis of (1) the reticulocyte count in the circulating blood; (2) the degree to which young red cells are proliferating in the bone marrow and the manner in which they are maturing, as observed on biopsy; and (3) the presence or absence of hyperbilirubinemia and hemoglobinemia. Moreover, erythropoiesis can actually be quantified by measuring the rate at which injected radioactive iron is incorporated into circulating erythrocytes. The life span of the patient's red cells (therefore, the rate of hemolysis) can be measured by tagging a portion of these with radioactive chromium, reinjecting them, and following their disappearance from the circulating blood over the course of the ensuing days or weeks. Methods by which one particular type of marrow failure can be distinguished from another type, and one hemolytic disease from another, are specified in relation to each of these conditions discussed later in this chapter.

Gerontologic Considerations. Anemia is common in older persons and is the most common hematologic condition that affects the elderly, but studies indicate that the aging process does not cause changes in hematopoiesis. The cause is usually unexplained. Anemia is generally considered to be part of a pathologic process rather than a result of aging. Because the elderly person may be unable to respond adequately to the anemia with increased cardiac output or pulmonary ventilation, anemia in this population can have serious effects on cardiopulmonary function if not properly treated. Thus, it is particularly important to identify and treat the cause of the anemia rather than to consider it an inevitable consequence of aging.

Clinical Manifestations

Aside from the severity of the anemia, several factors affect the patient with anemia and tend to influence the severity and even the presence of symptoms: (1) the speed with which the anemia has developed, (2) its duration (*i.e.*, its chronicity), (3) the metabolic requirements of the particular patient, (4) the presence of other disorders or disabilities, and (5) special complications or concomitant features of the condition that produced the anemia.

The more rapidly an anemia develops, the more severe its symptoms. An otherwise normal person can tolerate as much as a 50% gradual reduction in hemoglobin, red count, or hematocrit without pronounced symptoms or significant incapacity, whereas the rapid loss of as little as 30% may precipitate profound vascular collapse in the same individual. A person who has been anemic for a very long time, with hemoglobin levels between 9 and 11 mg/dl (90 and 110 g/L), experiences few or no symptoms other than slight tachycardia on exertion. Exertional dyspnea is likely to occur below, but not above, 7.5 g/dl (75 g/L); weakness, only below 6 g/dl (60 g/L); dyspnea at rest, below 3 g/dl (30 g/L); and cardiac failure, only at the extremely low level of 2 to 2.5 g/dl (20 to 25 g/L).

Patients who customarily are very active are more likely to experience symptoms, and symptoms that are more pronounced, than a more sedentary person. A patient with hypothyroidism, who requires less than the usual amount of oxygen, may be completely asymptomatic, without tachycardia or increased cardiac output, at a hemoglobin level of 10 g/dl (100 g/L). Conversely, at any given level of anemia, patients with underlying heart disease are far more likely to experience angina or symptoms of congestive failure than someone without heart disease.

Finally, many anemic disorders are complicated by various other abnormalities that do not result from the anemia but are inherently associated with these particular diseases. These abnormalities may give rise to symptoms that completely overshadow those of the anemia, as is exemplified by the painful crises of sickle cell anemia (see p. 795).

Diagnostic Evaluation

A variety of hematologic studies are performed to determine the type and cause of the anemia. These include hemoglobin and hematocrit levels, red blood cell indices, white blood cell studies, serum iron level, measurement of total iron-binding capacity, folate level, vitamin B_{12} level, platelet count, bleeding time, prothrombin time, and partial thromboplastin time. Bone marrow aspiration and biopsy may be included. In addition, diagnostic studies are carried out to determine the presence of acute or chronic illness and the source of any chronic blood loss.

Management

Management of anemia is directed toward reversing the cause and replacing any blood that has been lost. The discussion below of each specific type of anemia includes its management.

▶ Nursing Process
The Patient With Anemia

▷ Assessment

The health history and physical examination are important when caring for a patient with anemia. They will reveal clues that may hasten the diagnostic process and alert the nurse to problems and concerns that often can be alleviated. Weakness, fatigue, and general malaise are common, as are pallor of the skin and mucous membranes. Jaundice may be present in patients with pernicious anemia or anemia that is hemolytic in nature. Dryness of the skin and hair and spooning (concave surface) of the nails are often seen in iron-deficiency anemia.

Cardiac status is carefully assessed. When the hemoglobin is low, the heart will attempt to compensate by pumping faster and harder in an effort to deliver more blood to hypoxic tissue. This increased cardiac workload results in such symptoms as tachycardia, palpitations, dyspnea, dizziness, orthopnea, and

exertional dyspnea. Congestive heart failure will eventually develop, as evidenced by cardiomegaly, hepatomegaly, and peripheral edema.

Neurologic examination is also important because of the effect of pernicious anemia on the central and peripheral nervous systems. The patient is assessed for peripheral numbness and paresthesias, ataxia, poor coordination, and confusion. Assessment of gastrointestinal function may disclose complaints of nausea, vomiting, diarrhea, anorexia, and glossitis (inflammation of the tongue).

The health history includes information about any medications the patient may be taking that could depress bone marrow activity or interfere with folate metabolism. The patient is also questioned about any loss of blood, as evidenced by blood in the stools, or, for women, excessive menstrual flow. Family history is important because certain anemias are inherited. A nutritional assessment may indicate deficiencies in essential nutrients such as iron, vitamin B_{12}, and folic acid.

▷ Nursing Diagnoses

Based on the assessment data, major nursing diagnoses for the patient may include the following:

- Activity intolerance related to weakness, fatigue, and general malaise
- Potential decreased cardiac output related to increased cardiac workload
- Altered nutrition, less than body requirements, related to inadequate intake of essential nutrients.

▷ Planning and Implementation

▷ *Goals:*   The major goals of the patient may include tolerance of normal activity, attainment or maintenance of normal cardiac output, and attainment or maintenance of adequate nutrition.

▷ Nursing Interventions

▷ *Tolerance of Normal Activity.*   Nursing care is planned to conserve the patient's strength and physical and emotional energy. Frequent rest periods are encouraged, and family support is elicited to promote a restful environment. A regular schedule of rest and sleep is imperative for restoring strength and activity tolerance. Ambulation and activities of daily living are encouraged as tolerated. As the anemia is treated and blood studies return to normal, the patient is encouraged to resume normal activities gradually. Activities that are found to cause undue fatigue are postponed until greater endurance becomes evident. Conditioning exercises may be used to increase endurance. Safety precautions are used to prevent falls resulting from poor coordination, paresthesias, and weakness.

▷ *Attainment and Maintenance of Normal Cardiac Output.*   With longstanding reduction of oxyhemoglobin, the heart may be less able to supply blood to hypoxic tissue. It will begin to enlarge, and cardiac output will decrease. Nursing measures are directed toward decreasing activities and stimuli that cause an increase in heart rate and increased cardiac output. The patient is encouraged to identify those situations that precipitate palpitations and dyspnea and to avoid them until the anemia is resolved. If dyspnea is a problem, measures such as elevation of the head of the bed and the use of pillows for support are used. Unnecessary exertion is avoided. Oxygen is administered when necessary. Vital signs are monitored frequently and the patient is observed for indications of fluid retention (*e.g.*, peripheral edema, decreased urinary output, and neck vein distention).

▷ *Attainment and Maintenance of Adequate Nutrition.*   Inadequate intake of essential nutrients, such as iron and folic acid, can cause some anemias. The symptoms associated with anemias, such as fatigue and anorexia, can in turn also interfere with nutrition. A well-balanced diet high in protein and high-calorie foods, fruits, and vegetables is encouraged. Spicy foods that can cause gastric irritation and foods that are gas producing are avoided. Dietary teaching sessions are planned for the patient; family members are included in these sessions because the diet plan should be acceptable to both the patient and the family. Dietary supplements (*e.g.*, vitamins, iron, folate) may prescribed by the physician.

▷ *Evaluation*

Expected Outcomes

1. Tolerates normal activity
   a. Follows a progressive plan of rest, activities, and exercises
   b. Paces activities according to energy level
2. Attains/maintains normal cardiac output
   a. Avoids activities that cause tachycardia, palpitations, dizziness, and dyspnea
   b. Uses rest and comfort measures to alleviate dyspnea
   c. Has normal vital signs
   d. Experiences no signs of fluid retention (*e.g.*, peripheral edema, decreased urinary output, neck vein distention)
3. Attains/maintains adequate nutrition
   a. Eats foods high in protein, calories, and vitamins
   b. Avoids foods that cause gastric irritation
   c. Develops a meal plan that promotes optimal nutrition

In summary, anemia is a reduction in the number of red cells or the amount of hemoglobin. It can be due to the following: blood loss, accelerated destruction by hemolysis, problems with production due to either a deficiency in the necessary building blocks (*e.g.*, iron, vitamin B$_{12}$, folic acid) or a structural problem in the marrow resulting from a tumor or lack of erythropoietin.

Classification of Anemias

There are several ways to classify the anemias. The physiologic approach is to determine whether the deficiency in red cells is due to a defect in production of red cells (*hypoproliferative anemia*) or to destruction of the red cells (*hemolytic anemia*).

In the hypoproliferative anemias, red cells usually survive normally, but the marrow is unable to produce adequate numbers of cells; thus, the reticulocyte count is depressed. This situation may be a result of marrow damage by drugs or chemicals (*e.g.*, chloramphenicol, benzene) or may be due to lack of erythropoietin (as in renal disease) or to lack of iron, vitamin B$_{12}$, or folic acid.

When hemolysis (dissolution of red blood cells with liberation of hemoglobin into surrounding fluid) is the major cause of anemia, the abnormality is usually within the red cell itself (as in sickle cell anemia or G-6-PD [glucose-6-phosphate dehydrogenase] deficiency), in the plasma (as in immune hemolytic anemias), or in the circulation (as in heart valve he-

molysis). With hemolytic anemias, the reticulocyte count is elevated and indirect bilirubin is high, often enough to cause clinical jaundice.

Hypoproliferative Anemias

Aplastic Anemia

Pathophysiology.   Aplastic anemia is anemia caused by a decrease in precursor cells in the bone marrow and replacement of the marrow with fat. The underlying cause of aplastic anemia remains unknown. It may be idiopathic, (*i.e.*, without apparent cause), may result from certain infections, or may be caused by drugs, chemicals, or radiation damage. Agents that regularly produce marrow aplasia in sufficient dosage include benzene and benzene derivatives; antitumor agents such as nitrogen mustard; the antimetabolites, including methotrexate and 6-mercaptopurine; and certain toxic materials, such as inorganic arsenic. Other agents occasionally responsible for aplasia or hypoplasia include certain antimicrobials, anticonvulsants, antithyroid drugs, oral hypoglycemic agents, antihistamines, analgesics, sedatives, phenothiazines, insecticides, and heavy metals. The most common offenders are the antimicrobials, chloramphenicol and the organic arsenicals, the anticonvulsants mephenytoin (Mesantoin) and trimethadione (Tridione), the anti-inflammatory analgesic drug phenylbutazone, sulfonamides, and gold compounds.

In many situations, aplastic anemia occurs when a drug or chemical is ingested in toxic amounts. However, in a small minority of persons, it develops after a drug has been taken in the recommended dosage. These latter cases may be considered a type of idiosyncratic drug reaction in persons who are highly susceptible for reasons as yet unknown. Provided that their exposure is terminated early (*i.e.*, on the first appearance of reticulocytopenia, anemia, granulocytopenia, or thrombocytopenia), a prompt and complete recovery may be anticipated. (Unfortunately, one cannot be so optimistic in the case of persons who have received chloramphenicol. Reactions to this drug may be completely unrelated to dosage; they may develop without premonitory changes in the hemogram long after the drug has been discontinued and can progress to a complete and fatal aplasia despite all available therapy.)

Whatever the offending agent, if exposure continues after signs of hypoplasia have appeared, bone marrow depression almost certainly progresses to the point of complete and irreversible failure—hence the importance of frequent complete blood counts for every patient receiving a drug or exposed regularly to any chemical that has been implicated in the production of aplastic anemia.

Diagnostic Evaluation.   Because the bone marrow is hypocellular, attempts at marrow aspiration frequently yield only a few drops of blood. A biopsy is usually necessary to demonstrate a severe decrease in normal marrow elements and replacement by fat. The abnormality is probably in the stem cell, the precursor for granulocytes, erythrocytes, and platelets. As a result, *pancytopenia* (deficiency in all of the cellular elements of the blood) occurs.

Clinical Manifestations.   The onset of aplastic anemia characteristically is a gradual one, marked by weakness, pallor, breathlessness on exertion, and other manifestations of anemia. Abnormal bleeding due to thrombocytopenia is a presenting symptom in about a third of the patients. When the granulocytic series is involved as well, the patient is likely to present with fever, acute pharyngitis, or some other form of sepsis, in addition to bleeding. Physical signs, except for pallor and skin hemorrhages, are unremarkable. The blood count is marked by variable degrees of pancytopenia. Red cells are *normocytic* and *normochromic*, that is, of normal size and color. Frequently, patients have no characteristic physical findings; adenopathy (enlargement of glands) and hepatosplenomegaly (liver and spleen enlargement) are lacking.

Management. As might be expected from a condition that affects all hematopoietic cells, aplastic anemia carries a very poor prognosis. Two methods of treatment are currently employed: (1) bone marrow transplantation and (2) administration of immunosuppressive therapy with antithymocyte globulin (ATG).

The goal of bone marrow transplantation is to provide the patient with an undamaged supply of functioning hematopoietic tissue. Successful transplantation requires the ability to match donor and recipient and to prevent complications during the recovery process. With the use of immunosuppressant cyclosporine, incidence of graft rejection is less than 10%.

The goal of immunosuppressive therapy with ATG is to remove the immunologic functions that prolong the aplasia and thus allow the patient's bone marrow to recover. ATG is given through a central venous catheter daily for 7 to 10 days. Patients who respond to the therapy usually do so within weeks to 3 months, but response may be as late as 6 months after treatment. Patients who have severe aplastic anemia and are treated early in the course of their disease have the best chance of responding to ATG. Trials with ATG and cyclosporine are in progress to see if the response rate can be improved further.

Supportive therapy plays a major role in the management of aplastic anemia. Any offending drug is discontinued. The patient is supported with transfusions of red cells and platelets as necessary to prevent symptoms. Eventually, such patients may develop antibodies to minor red cell antigens and to platelet antigens, so that transfusions no longer raise the counts sufficiently. Death is usually caused by hemorrhage or infection, although modern antibiotics, especially those active against gram-negative bacilli, have been a major advance for these patients. Patients with pronounced *leukopenia* (abnormal decrease of white blood cells) are protected from contact with people who have infections. Antibiotics should not be used prophylactically in neutropenic patients, because this favors the emergence of resistant bacteria and fungi.

Preventive Management. An extremely important area is prevention of drug-induced aplastic anemia. Because it is not possible to predict which patients will react adversely to a particular drug, potentially toxic medications should be used only when alternative therapies are not available. Blood cell counts must be carefully monitored in patients receiving potentially marrow-toxic drugs, such as chloramphenicol. Persons taking toxic drugs on a long-term basis should understand the need for periodic blood studies and know what symptoms to report.

Nursing Interventions. Patients with aplastic anemia are vulnerable to the effects of leukocyte, erythrocyte, and platelet deficiencies. They should be assessed carefully for signs of infection, tissue hypoxia, and bleeding. Any wound, abrasion, or ulcer of mucous membrane or skin is a potential site of infection and should be guarded against. Oral hygiene also is very important. Depending on the degree of weakness and fatigue, care should be planned to preserve the patient's energy. When thrombocytopenia is present, minor trauma, including subcutaneous and intramuscular (IM) injections, must be avoided. Regular atraumatic bowel movements are important, because hemorrhoids can develop and become infected or bleed.

Red Cell Aplasia

Red cell aplasia is an isolated anemia caused by lack of red cell formation in the marrow. This is a rare disorder in which only the erythroid cells are affected. The marrow is cellular, but the erythroid element is almost absent. There is a severe anemia without granulocytopenia or thrombocytopenia. The condition may be associated with tumors of the thymus or certain drugs, such as phenytoin (Dilantin), or it may arise during the course of a hemolytic anemia. Some patients produce an antibody to immature red cells that may be the cause of the disease. Treatment measures include red cell replacement, thymectomy, and administration of immunosuppressive drugs, such as corticosteroids and cyclosporine.

Myelophthisic Anemias

Myelophthisic anemias are a varied group of anemias that differ as to cause but are similar in that all show partial replacement of normal marrow space by abnormal tissue. This tissue may be fibrous (in myelofibrosis) or it may consist of plasma cells (in multiple myeloma) or metastatic carcinoma cells. A bone marrow biopsy is often necessary for the diagnosis. Pancytopenia is present, although it is usually less severe than in aplastic anemia, but there are also young marrow cells circulating, apparently because there is abnormal release from the damaged marrow. Myeloblasts and nucleated red cells are seen in small numbers. The treatment is that for the primary disease. Androgens occasionally improve the patient's condition.

Anemias in Renal Disease

There is a great deal of variability in degree of anemia seen in patients with end-stage renal disease, but in general, patients with a blood urea nitrogen (BUN) greater than 10 mg/dl are anemic. The symptoms of anemia are often the most disturbing of the patient's symptoms. The hematocrit usually falls to between 20% and 30%, although in rare cases it may fall below 15%. The red cells appear normal on peripheral smear.

This anemia is due to both a mild shortening of red cell survival and a deficiency of erythropoietin. Some erythropoietin is evidently produced outside the kidney, because some erythropoiesis does continue, even in anephric patients (those whose kidneys have been removed), and developing red cells can be seen in the bone marrow.

- Patients undergoing chronic hemodialysis lose blood into the dialyzer (artificial kidney) and may thus become iron deficient. Folic acid deficiency develops because this vitamin passes into the dialysate.
- Dialysis patients should be treated with iron and folic acid.
- The availability of recombinant erythropoietin has dramatically altered the management of anemia in end-stage renal disease. With this therapy, hematocrit levels can often be maintained at between 33% and 38%. Many patients report decreased

fatigue, increased energy levels, increased feelings of well-being, improved exercise tolerance, and better tolerance of dialysis treatments. In addition, this therapy has decreased the need for transfusion and its risks.

Anemias in Chronic Diseases

Many chronic inflammatory diseases are associated with anemia of a normochromic, normocytic type (red cells are normal in color and size). These include rheumatoid arthritis, lung abscesses, osteomyelitis, tuberculosis, and many malignancies. The anemia is usually mild and nonprogressive. It develops gradually over a period of 6 to 8 weeks and then stabilizes at hematocrit levels that are seldom below 25%. The hemoglobin rarely falls below 9 g/dl, and the bone marrow has normal cellularity with increased stores of iron. Erythropoietin levels are low, perhaps because of decreased production, and there is a block in the utilization of iron by erythroid cells. There is also a moderate shortening of red cell survival.

Most of these patients are comfortable and do not require treatment for the anemia. With successful treatment of the underlying disorder, the bone marrow iron is used to make red cells, and the hemoglobin rises.

Iron-Deficiency Anemia

Iron-deficiency anemia is a condition in which the total body iron content is decreased below a normal level. (Iron is needed for the synthesis of hemoglobin.) It is the most common type of anemia in all age groups.

Etiology. The common cause of iron deficiency in men and postmenopausal women is bleeding (*e.g.*, from ulcers, gastritis, or gastrointestinal tumors) or malabsorption, especially after gastric resection. The most common cause in premenopausal women is *menorrhagia* (excessive menstrual bleeding). Rarely, iron can be lost in the urine during intravascular hemolysis, as in paroxysmal nocturnal hemoglobinuria or heart valve hemolysis.

Clinical and Laboratory Manifestations. In persons who are iron deficient, the blood hemoglobin and the red blood cell count are reduced. The hemoglobin is reduced more than the red cell count, and for this reason the red cells tend to be small and relatively devoid of pigment, that is, *hypochromic*. Hypochromia is the hallmark of iron deficiency. The cause of this deficiency is the failure of the patient to ingest or absorb sufficient dietary iron to compensate for the iron requirements associated with body growth or for the loss of iron that attends bleeding, whether the bleeding is physiologic (*e.g.*, menstrual) or pathologic.

Patients with iron deficiency present primarily with the symptoms of anemia. If the deficiency is severe, they may also have a smooth, sore tongue; thin, spoon-shaped fingernails; and pica (a craving to eat unusual substances, such as clay, laundry starch, or ice). These symptoms subside after therapy.

The laboratory studies show a hemoglobin that is proportionately lower than the hematocrit and red count, because of the small, poorly hemoglobinized red cells (microcytosis and hypochromia). The serum iron concentration is low, the total iron-binding capacity is high, and the serum ferritin (a measure of the iron stores) is low. The white count is usually normal, and the platelet count is variable.

Management. It is always important to search for a cause of iron deficiency. It may be a sign of a curable gastrointestinal malignancy or of uterine fibroids or cancer. Except for pregnancy, when the cause is obvious, stool specimens should be tested for occult blood.

Several oral iron preparations are available for treatment: ferrous sulfate, gluconate, and fumarate. The least expensive and most effective preparation is ferrous sulfate. Tablets with enteric coating may be poorly absorbed and should be avoided. Usually, three or four doses a day are necessary. Although iron is absorbed best on an empty stomach, taking it with food is usually advised to minimize gastric distress. Patients may be better able to tolerate the therapy if the dose is started at 1 tablet daily and then raised. They should be warned that iron salts often change the stools to a darker color. Generally, the iron is continued for a year after the source of bleeding has been controlled. This allows for replenishing of the iron stores.

Nursing Interventions. Preventive education is important because iron-deficiency anemia is so common in menstruating and pregnant women. Food sources high in iron include organ and other meats, cooked white beans, leafy vegetables, raisins, and molasses. Taking iron-rich foods with a source of vitamin C enhances absorption.

The selection of a well-balanced diet is encouraged. Nutritional counseling is provided for those whose normal diet is less than adequate. Patients who have a history of fad diets are counseled that such diets often contain inadequate amounts of absorbable iron.

Iron therapy is usually continued for many months to replenish iron stores. In some cases, IM administration of iron (Imferon) may be prescribed; that is, when oral iron is not absorbed or is poorly tolerated or when iron is needed in large amounts. The injection causes some local pain and can stain the skin. A method for parenteral administration of iron preparations follows:

1. Discard needle used to draw medication into syringe; use new needle for injection to avoid tracking medication through subcutaneous tissue.
2. Allow a small amount of air into syringe.
3. Use a needle 5 cm (2 in) long—medication is injected deep into upper outer quadrant of buttock.
4. Retract skin over muscle *laterally* before inserting needle, to prevent leakage and staining of skin.
5. Inject solution slowly, followed by air in syringe; wait a few seconds before withdrawing needle. Do not massage the site.

Occasional febrile or allergic reactions are seen. Total iron replacement with a single intravenous injection is possible, but it can cause a severe anaphylactic reaction.

Patients with iron-deficiency anemia are encouraged to continue their iron therapy as long as it is prescribed, even though they may no longer be fatigued. If the iron supplement causes gastric distress, the patient is advised to take it with meals until the symptoms subside, and then to resume the between-meal schedule for maximum absorption. Because ferrous sulfate is likely to be deposited on the teeth and gums, the patient is advised to use frequent oral hygiene measures.

In summary, iron-deficiency anemia continues to be the most common anemia. The total body iron content is decreased below normal. In most adults it is associated with a history of bleeding or poor diet. The red cells appear microcytic and hypochromic. The patient presents with fatigue, irritability, numbness and tingling of the limbs, and soreness of the tongue.

Megaloblastic Anemias

The anemias caused by deficiencies of the vitamins B_{12} and folic acid show identical bone marrow and peripheral blood changes. This is because both vitamins are essential for normal DNA synthesis. In each case, *hyperplasia* (abnormal increase in the number of normal cells) of the marrow occurs, and the precursor erythroid and myeloid cells are large and bizarre; some are multinucleated. Many of these cells die within the marrow, however, so the mature cells, which leave the marrow, are decreased in number. Thus, a *pancytopenia* (deficiency of all cellular elements of the blood) develops. In a far advanced situation, the hemoglobin may be as low as 4 to 5 g/dl, the white blood count 2000 to 3000 per mm³, and the platelet count less than 50,000 per mm³. The red cells are large and the PMNs are hypersegmented.

Vitamin B_{12} Deficiency

Etiology.   A deficiency of vitamin B_{12} can occur in several ways. Inadequate dietary intake is very rare but can develop in strict vegetarians who consume no meat. Faulty absorption from the gastrointestinal tract is more common. An absence of intrinsic factor normally secreted by cells of the stomach is called *pernicious anemia*. This is primarily a disorder of elderly persons and has a familial tendency. The abnormality is in the gastric mucosa: the stomach wall becomes atrophic and fails to secrete intrinsic factor. This substance ordinarily binds with the dietary vitamin B_{12} and travels with it to the ileum, where the vitamin is absorbed. Without intrinsic factor, no orally administered B_{12} can enter the body. Even if adequate B_{12} and intrinsic factor are present, a deficiency can occur if disease involving the ileum or pancreas impairs absorption. Gastrectomy can also cause vitamin B_{12} deficiency.

Clinical Manifestations.   After the body stores of vitamin B_{12} are used up, patients begin to show signs of the anemia. They gradually become weak, listless, and pale. The hematologic effects of deficiency are accompanied by effects on other organ systems, particularly the gastrointestinal tract and nervous system. Patients with pernicious anemia develop a smooth, sore, red tongue and mild diarrhea. They may become confused, but more often have paresthesias in the extremities and difficulty keeping their balance because of damage to the spinal cord; they lose position sense. These symptoms are progressive, although the course may be marked by spontaneous partial remissions and exacerbations. Without treatment, patients die after several years, usually from congestive heart failure secondary to anemia.

Diagnostic Evaluation.   One means of determining the cause of vitamin B_{12} deficiency is the *Schilling test*. After fasting for 12 hours, the patient is given a small dose of radioactive B_{12} in water to drink, followed by a large, nonradioactive IM dose. When the oral vitamin is absorbed, it will be excreted in the urine; the IM dose helps to flush it into the urine. A 24-hour urine specimen is collected and measured for radioactivity. If very little has been excreted, the test is repeated several days later (the "second stage"), with a capsule of oral intrinsic factor added to the oral B_{12}. If the patient has pernicious anemia, this time much more radioactivity will be found in the 24-hour urine specimen. If the problem is due to an ileal or pancreatic defect, administration of digestive enzymes will increase absorption and subsequently increase urine radioactivity.

Management.   Vitamin B_{12} deficiency is treated by replacement. Strict vegetarians can prevent or treat deficiency with oral supplementation with vitamins or fortified soy milk. When, as is much more common, the deficiency is due to defective absorption or absence of intrinsic factor, replacement is by IM injections of vitamin B_{12}.

At first, B_{12} is given daily, but eventually most patients are managed with 100 μg IM monthly. This can produce dramatic recovery in desperately ill patients. The reticulocyte count rises within a week, and in several weeks the blood counts are all normal. The tongue improves in several days. The neurologic manifestations require more time for recovery; if there is severe neuropathy, paralysis, or incontinence, the patient may never recover fully.

- To prevent recurrence of the anemia, vitamin B_{12} therapy must be continued for the life of the patient who has had pernicious anemia or noncorrectable malabsorption.

Nursing Interventions.   These patients may need support during the diagnostic tests and nursing care for several aspects of their disease: anemia, congestive heart failure, neuropathy. When they are incontinent or paralyzed, care must be taken to prevent pressure ulcers and contracture deformities. The Schilling test can be useful only if the urine collections are complete; therefore, the nurse's assistance is essential. Patients must be taught about the chronicity of their disorder and the necessity for monthly injections even when they are asymptomatic. The gastric atrophy associated with pernicious anemia increases the risk of gastric carcinoma, so these patients need to understand that ongoing medical follow-up is important.

Folic Acid Deficiency

Folic acid is another vitamin that is necessary for normal red blood cell production. It is stored as different compounds, referred to as *folates*. The folate stores in the body are much smaller than those of vitamin B_{12}, so it is much more common to see dietary folate deficiency. This occurs in patients who rarely eat uncooked vegetables or fruits (*i.e.*, primarily elderly people living alone or persons with alcoholism). Alcohol increases folic acid requirements, and at the same time persons suffering from alcoholism usually have a diet that is deficient in the vitamin. Folic acid requirements are increased in chronic hemolytic anemias and in pregnancy, so these patients may develop the anemia while ingesting a normal diet.

- Patients on prolonged intravenous feeding or total parenteral nutrition may become folate deficient after several months, unless the vitamin is given intramuscularly. Some patients with diseases of the small bowel may not absorb it normally.

Clinical Manifestations and Laboratory Tests.   All of these patients have the characteristic findings of megaloblastic anemia along with a sore tongue. Symptoms of folic acid and vitamin B_{12} deficiencies are quite similar, and the two anemias may coexist. However, the neurologic manifestations of vitamin B_{12} do not occur with folic acid deficiency, and persist if B_{12} is not replaced. Therefore, careful distinction between the two anemias must be made. Serum levels of both vitamins can be measured.

Management.   Treatment is administration of a nutritious diet and 1 mg of folic acid a day. Folic acid is administered intramuscularly only in patients with malabsorption. With the exception of the vitamins given during pregnancy, most proprietary vitamin preparations do not contain folic acid, so it must be given as a separate tablet. When the hemoglobin returns to normal, the folic acid replacement can be stopped. However, persons suffering from alcoholism should continue receiving folic acid as long as they continue alcohol consumption.

In summary, megaloblastic anemias are caused by a lack of vitamin B_{12} or of folic acid. Both are required for normal DNA synthesis. Causes of vitamin B_{12} deficiency can be due to any of the following: dietary factors, gastric injury, lack of intrinsic factor, sprue, certain drugs (*e.g.*, neomycin, KCl), transport and utilization problems, increased demand (pregnancy, hyperthyroidism, certain neoplasms). Folic acid deficiency also occurs from decreased dietary intake, in malabsorption syndromes similar to those producing vitamin B_{12} deficiency, and through interference by drugs.

Hemolytic Anemias

In *hemolytic anemias*, the erythrocytes have a shortened life span. The bone marrow is usually able to compensate partially by producing new red cells at three or more times the normal rate. Consequently, all of these anemias share certain laboratory features: the reticulocyte count is elevated, the fraction of indirect bilirubin is increased, and the haptoglobin (a binding protein for free hemoglobin) is often low. The bone marrow is hypercellular, with erythroid proliferation. The only truly diagnostic test for hemolysis is the red cell survival study. This is usually necessary only for difficult diagnostic problems. About 20 to 30 ml of the patient's blood is removed, incubated with radioactive chromium-51, and then reinjected. The chromium-51 labels the red cells exclusively. After these cells have equilibrated with the circulating blood, small samples are taken at intervals over the next days and weeks, and the radioactivity is measured. A normal chromium-51 survival time is 28 to 35 days. Red cells of patients with severe hemolysis (such as sickle cell anemia) have survival times of 10 days or less.

Inherited Hemolytic Anemias

Hereditary Spherocytosis

Hereditary spherocytosis is a hemolytic anemia characterized by small, sphere-shaped red cells and splenomegaly (enlarged spleen). This is an uncommon disorder inherited in a dominant fashion.

Clinical Manifestations and Diagnostic Evaluation. An abnormality of the erythrocyte membrane causes cells to lose membrane as they pass through the spleen and to become spherical in shape. These spheres are relatively rigid and easily destroyed. The peripheral blood contains many of the characteristic small spherical cells, and the patient has an anemia that may be exacerbated during infections, even minor viral illnesses. In addition, the spleen is enlarged. The disorder is usually diagnosed in childhood, but may be missed until adult life because there are few symptoms.

Management. Surgical removal of the spleen (*splenectomy*) is the treatment. It does not change the erythrocyte defect but removes the site of membrane loss and hemolysis. After splenectomy (see p. 811), patients have normal hemoglobin levels, only slight shortening of red cell survival times, and few spherical cells in the peripheral smear. Patients have a normal life expectancy. The major complications prevented by splenectomy include (1) aplastic crises after infection, often with severe anemias; (2) nonhealing leg and ankle ulceration; and (3) gallstones.

Sickle Cell Anemia

Definition and Etiology. Sickle cell anemia is a severe hemolytic anemia resulting from a defective hemoglobin molecule and associated with attacks of pain. This disabling disease is found predominantly in Africans and in black Americans, but it also occurs in people from Mediterranean and Arab countries.

Pathophysiology. The defect is a single amino acid substitution in the β chain of hemoglobin. Because normal hemoglobin A contains two α and two β chains, there are two genes for synthesis of each chain. Persons with sickle cell trait have inherited only one abnormal gene, so their red cells can synthesize both normal β chains and β^s chains; thus, they have A and S hemoglobin. If two people with sickle trait marry, some of their children may inherit two abnormal genes and will then have only β^s chains and only S hemoglobin; these children have sickle cell anemia.

Clinical Manifestations. The sickle hemoglobin has the unfortunate property of acquiring a crystal-like formation when exposed to low oxygen tension. The oxygen in venous blood is low enough to cause this change; consequently, the cell containing S hemoglobin becomes deformed, rigid, and sickle-shaped when in the venous circulation (Fig. 32–3). These long, rigid cells can become lodged in small vessels and, when they pile up against each other, blood flow to a region or an organ may be slowed. When ischemia or infarction results, the patient may experience pain, swelling, and fever. Such a chain of events is presumed to explain the painful crises of this disease, but what triggers the chain or how to prevent it is not understood.

Symptoms are secondary to hemolysis and thrombosis. Patients are always anemic, with hemoglobin values in the 7 to 10 g/dl (70 to 100 g/L) range. Jaundice is characteristic and

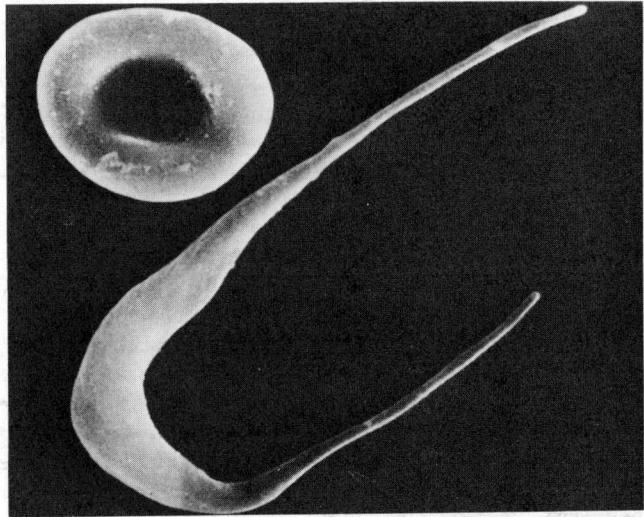

Figure 32–3. Photograph of a sickled cell and a normal red blood cell taken under the auspices of the Comprehensive Sickle Cell Center, University of Miami. (Photo by Dr. Bruce R. Cameron.)

is usually obvious in the sclerae. The bone marrow expands in childhood in a compensatory effort, sometimes leading to enlargement of the bones of the face and skull. The chronic anemia is associated with tachycardia, cardiac murmurs, and often cardiomegaly. Dysrhythmias and heart failure may occur in older patients.

Patients with sickle cell anemia may develop aplastic crises with infections and may have gallstones (due to increased hemolysis that leads to bilirubin stones) and leg ulcers. The ulcers may be chronic and painful and require skin grafting. These patients are unusually susceptible to infection, particularly pneumonias and osteomyelitis. Infection has been one of the most common causes of death.

All of the patient's tissues and organs are constantly vulnerable to microcirculatory interruptions by the sickling process, and therefore are susceptible to hypoxic damage or true ischemic necrosis at any time. Thrombotic episodes may result in minor pain in an extremity, in severe pain and swelling in a hand or knee, in chest pain due to pulmonary infarction, in pain simulating an acute abdominal crisis, or in the sudden appearance of a "stroke," with hemiplegia. These crises are completely unpredictable; they can occur monthly or very rarely and may last for hours, days, or weeks. Events that seem to precipitate crises include dehydration, fatigue, menstruation, intake of alcohol, emotional stress, and acidosis. Certain effects of infarction are permanent, such as hemiplegia, aseptic necrosis of the femoral head, and renal concentrating defects.

Diagnostic Evaluation.   The diagnosis can be made by hemoglobin electrophoresis or by "sickle prep," in which a drop of blood is mixed with sodium metabisulfite and observed under the microscope for sickling. Sickling in this test occurs whether the patient has sickle trait or sickle cell anemia; only electrophoresis can show the distinction. The patient with sickle trait has normal hemoglobin and hematocrit levels as well as a normal blood smear. In contrast, the patient with sickle cell anemia has a low hematocrit and sickled cells on smear.

Sickle Trait.   Patients with sickle trait are protected from crises because the hemoglobin A in their cells prevents the cells from sickling under ordinary circumstances. Such persons have no anemia and look and feel well. About 8% of black Americans have sickle trait.

Sickle Cell Anemia.   Patients with sickle cell anemia are usually diagnosed in childhood, because they are anemic in infancy and begin to have crises at 1 or 2 years of age. Many die in the first years of life, but antibiotics and patient and physician education about this disease have probably improved the outlook in the last 10 to 20 years, and some patients live into the sixth decade. All siblings of a patient with sickle cell anemia should be tested for the disease.

Management.   There is no specific treatment for the hemoglobin abnormality. The disease could be prevented only by intensive genetic counseling of the population at risk, a difficult and controversial task. Crises cannot now be prevented. Researchers are evaluating several chemicals with antisickling properties, but these are still in the investigational stage. Because infection seems to predispose to crises, all infections should be promptly treated or prevented when possible. Because dehydration and hypoxia promote sickling, patients are instructed to avoid high altitudes, anesthesia, or fluid loss. Because of the renal defect, these patients easily become dehydrated. Folic acid therapy is administered daily, because the marrow has an increased requirement.

When sickle crisis occurs, the mainstays of therapy are hydration and analgesia. Increased fluid intake helps to dilute the blood and reverse the agglutination of sickled cells within the small blood vessels. Patients and families can learn to handle minor crises at home but, if there is no relief after several hours, hospital admission may be necessary. The patients often have fever and leukocytosis with sickle cell crisis, so infection or appendicitis or cholecystitis may be suggested and must be ruled out. Intravenous fluids (3 to 5 L/day for adults) are essential. Narcotic analgesics are often necessary because of the severity of pain and should be given in adequate doses. They should never be used chronically, however, because of the risk of dependency. Relaxation techniques, breathing exercises, transcutaneous nerve stimulation, and whirlpool baths are helpful for some patients.

Transfusions are reserved for particular situations: (1) aplastic crisis, when the patient's hemoglobin falls rapidly; (2) severe painful crisis not responsive to any other therapy after several days; (3) as a preoperative measure to dilute the amount of sickled blood; and (4) sometimes during the latter half of pregnancy in an attempt to prevent crises.

▶ Nursing Process
The Patient With Sickle Cell Anemia

◁ Assessment

Because the sickling process can cause microcirculatory interruptions in any tissues and organs, with resultant hypoxia and ischemia, a careful assessment of all body systems is necessary. Particular emphasis is placed on assessing for pain, swelling, and fever. All joint areas are carefully examined for pain and swelling, as is the abdomen. A careful neurologic examination is important to elicit symptoms of cerebral hypoxia. The patient is also questioned about symptoms indicative of gallstones, such as food intolerances, epigastric distress, and pain in the right upper abdominal quadrant.

Because these patients are so susceptible to infections, they are assessed for the presence of any infectious process. Particular attention is given to examination of the chest and long bones and femoral head, as pneumonia and osteomyelitis are especially common. Leg ulcers, which may be infected, are sometimes present. Chronic anemia, another common problem associated with sickle cell anemia, is also considered during the physical examination.

Patients in crisis are questioned about factors that could have precipitated the crisis. They are asked to recall whether they have recently had symptoms of infection or dehydration or have been experiencing situations that promote fatigue or emotional stress. History of alcohol intake is also discussed. In addition, patients are asked to recall factors that seemed to precipitate previous crises and measures that they use to prevent crises. This information will provide guidelines for identifying and meeting their learning needs.

◁ Nursing Diagnoses

Based on the assessment data, major nursing diagnoses for the patient may include the following:

- Pain related to agglutination of sickled cells within blood vessels

- High risk for infection related to increased susceptibility as a factor of the disease process
- Knowledge deficit regarding prevention of crisis

▷ Planning and Implementation

A care plan for the patient with sickle cell crisis is presented in Nursing Care Plan 32–1.

The nurse can help the patient and family adjust to this chronic disease and understand the importance of hydration and prevention of infection. When leg ulcers are present, they require careful dressing and protection from trauma and wound contamination. If they fail to heal, skin grafting may be necessary. Cardiac disease is managed in the same way as for any patient who does not have sickle cell anemia. During crisis, the patient is kept quiet and allowed to rest undisturbed. Swollen extremities should not be exercised and pain should be relieved. Male patients may develop sudden, painful episodes of priapism (persistent penile erection) and need to know that it is common and has no long-term deleterious effects.

Other Hemoglobinopathies

C Hemoglobin.   C hemoglobin is less common among American blacks than S hemoglobin. Patients with the C trait are asymptomatic, and homozygous C disease is a mild hemolytic anemia with splenomegaly but no serious complications.

Thalassemia.   Thalassemia is a group of hereditary disorders associated with defective hemoglobin-chain synthesis. These anemias occur worldwide, but the highest prevalence is found in persons of Mediterranean, African, and Southeast Asian ancestry. The incidence is increasing in the United States with the influx of refugees from Southeast Asia. They are characterized by *hypochromia* (abnormal decrease in hemoglobin content of erythrocytes), *microcytosis* (smaller than normal erythrocytes), hemolysis, and variable degrees of anemia.

The thalassemias are classified into two major groups according to the affected globin chain of hemoglobin: α-thalassemias and β-thalassemias, which are associated with decreased or absent α-chain synthesis and β-chain synthesis, respectively. The α-thalassemias occur mainly in people from southeast Asia and Africa, and the β-thalassemias are most prevalent in Mediterranean populations. The α-thalassemias are milder than the β-forms and are often without symptoms. Patients with severe β-thalassemia will die within the first few years of life if untreated; if treated with regular transfusion therapy, they may survive into their 20s and 30s.

The β-thalassemias are classified according to their severity; minima, minor, intermedia, and major. Patients with *thalassemia minima* are asymptomatic; the majority of those with *thalassemia minor* are also without symptoms, although significant anemia that requires transfusion therapy may occur during pregnancy.

Thalassemia intermedia is more severe, with life expectancy of only about three or four decades. These patients often suffer from chronic fatigue, debilitating bone pain, cardiac disease, and hypersplenism. Because of an inadequate excretory pathway for iron, they often experience complications of iron overload (*e.g.*, hepatic fibrosis and cirrhosis), which is worsened by transfusion therapy.

Thalassemia major (Cooley's anemia) is characterized by severe anemia, marked hemolysis, and ineffective erythropoi-

esis. With early regular transfusion therapy, growth and development through childhood is facilitated. Organ dysfunction due to iron overload occurs. Regular chelation therapy with subcutaneous desferrioxamine has reduced the complications of iron overload and prolonged the life of these patients. The overall survival of patients receiving iron chelation continuously from the first few years of life is unknown, however.

Glucose-6-Phosphate Dehydrogenase Deficiency

The abnormality in this disorder is in G-6-PD, an enzyme within the red cell that is essential for membrane stability. A few patients have inherited an enzyme so defective that they have a chronic hemolytic anemia, but the most common type of defect results in hemolysis only when the red cells are stressed by certain situations, such as fever or the presence of certain drugs. The disorder came to the attention of researchers during World War II, when some soldiers developed hemolysis while taking primaquine, an antimalarial drug. Drugs that are hemolytic for G-6-PD–deficient persons are antimalarial drugs, sulfonamides, nitrofurantoin, the common coal tar analgesics (including aspirin), the thiazide diuretics, the oral hypoglycemic agents, chloramphenicol, para-aminosalicylic acid (PAS), vitamin K, and, for certain individuals subject to "favism," the fava bean. Blacks and persons of Greek or Italian origin are those primarily affected. The type of deficiency found in the Mediterranean population is more severe than that in the black population, resulting in greater hemolysis and sometimes in life-threatening anemias. All types are inherited as X-linked defects; thus, many more men are at risk than women. In the United States, about 15% of black men are affected.

Clinical Manifestations.   The patients are asymptomatic and have normal hemoglobin levels and reticulocyte counts most of the time. Several days after exposure to an offending drug, they may develop pallor, jaundice, and hemoglobinuria, and the reticulocyte count will rise. Special strains of the peripheral blood may then show *Heinz bodies* (degraded hemoglobin). Hemolysis continues for a week and then spontaneously the counts begin to improve because the new young red cells are resistant to lysis. In the Mediterranean type, this recovery does not occur.

Diagnostic Evaluation and Management.   The diagnosis is made by a screening test or a quantitative assay of G-6-PD. The treatment is removal of the drug. Transfusion is only necessary in the Mediterranean variety. The patient should be educated about the disease and given a list of drugs to avoid. These include sulfonamides, hypoglycemic agents, antimalarials, nitrofurantoin, phenacetin, aspirin (in high doses), and para-aminosalicylic acid.

In summary, hereditary hemolytic anemias are caused by membrane, metabolic, or hemoglobin defects of the red blood cell. Although there is extensive knowledge of the pathophysiology of these disorders, equivalent progress in therapy has not been matched.

Acquired Hemolytic Anemias

There are a variety of acquired hemolytic anemias, including paroxysmal nocturnal hemoglobinuria, immune hemolytic anemia, microangiopathic hemolytic anemia, heart valve hemolysis, and spur cell anemia, as well as those associated with

Nursing Care Plan 32–1

Care of the Patient With Sickle Cell Crisis

Nursing Interventions	Rationale	Expected Outcomes

Nursing Diagnosis: Pain related to agglutination of sickled cells within small blood vessels

Goal: Relief of pain

1. Assess severity and location of pain
Common sites of pain are
    Joints and extremities
    Chest
    Abdomen
2. Administer analgesics as prescribed.
 	
3. Encourage oral intake of fluids and administer IV fluids as prescribed; monitor intake and output.
4. Carefully position and support painful areas; encourage use of relaxation techniques and breathing exercises; apply moist heat to painful areas.
	1. Tissues and organs are susceptible to microcirculatory thrombosis with resulting hypoxic damage; hypoxia causes pain.
	
	2. Narcotic analgesics are necessary to relieve severe pain; avoid use of narcotics for chronic pain because of the possibility of dependency.
	3. Fluids promote hemodilution and reverse agglutination of sickled cells within small blood vessels.
	4. Joint pain can be minimized during a crisis by careful movement and with the use of moist heat; relaxation techniques and breathing exercises help the patient to focus attention away from the pain.
		• Verbalizes that pain is relieved after administration of analgesics
		• Moves body parts slowly and carefully to minimize pain
		• Increases fluid intake
		• Gradually experiences longer pain-free periods
		• Expresses interest in diversional activities

Nursing Diagnosis: High risk for infection related to increased susceptibility as a factor of the disease process

Goal: Prevention of infection

1. Assess for signs and symptoms of infection. Common sites of infection are
    Lungs
    Long bones; head of the femur
    Leg ulcers
2. Encourage early ambulation and pulmonary hygiene.
 	
3. Use aseptic technique when changing wound dressings.
4. Promote adequate nutrition and fluid intake
	1. The physiologic stress that results from infection often precipitates crises; resolution of infection at its onset can prevent or limit the duration of a crisis episode.
	2. Activity mobilizes pulmonary secretions; stagnant secretions are a prime medium for bacterial growth.
	3. Aseptic technique deters introduction of microorganisms into wound areas.
	4. Optimal nutrition and fluid balance promote tissue integrity.
		• Temperature normal
		• Breath sounds clear
		• WBCs within normal range (5,000–10,000/mm³)
		• Absence of pain of long bones
		• Cultures of wound drainage negative

Nursing Diagnosis: Knowledge deficit regarding prevention of crisis

Goal: Avoidance of situations that can precipitate crisis

1. Discuss factors that commonly precipitate crisis:
    Infection
    Dehydration
    Trauma
    Strenuous physical exertion
    Extreme fatigue
    Exposure to cold
    Hypoxia (e.g., high altitudes)
    Emotional stress
2. Discuss the chronic nature of the disease with patient and family; stress the importance of adequate hydration and avoidance of infection.
	1. Avoidance of situations that precipitate crisis can often increase the intervals between crisis attacks.
	
	2. Understanding of the chronicity of the disorder and the ability to minimize crises promotes adherence to the therapeutic regimen.
		• Patient identifies factors that can precipitate crisis
		• Identifies acceptable life-style changes necessary to prevent crisis
		• Elicits support of family in making changes in life style
		• Maintains adequate fluid intake
		• Identifies sources of infection that can be avoided
		• Identifies the need to seek prompt medical attention when infection occurs.

infections and hypersplenism. Table 32–2 identifies the causes, manifestations, and treatment of these anemias.

Immune Hemolytic Anemia

When antibodies combine with red cells they can be either *isoantibodies*, reacting with foreign cells, as in transfusion reactions or erythroblastosis fetalis, or *autoantibodies*, which react with the cells of the host. The immune hemolysis that results may be very severe. Antibodies coat the red cells, producing a positive Coombs's test. These cells are then removed by the spleen and the rest of the reticuloendothelial system. Many cells are destroyed, and others return to the circulation as spherocytes with reduced membrane and a shortened survival rate.

In *idiopathic autoimmune hemolytic states*, what induces the immune system to produce the antibodies is not known. The disease usually begins suddenly, often in persons over 40 years of age. In some cases, the hemolysis is associated with systemic disease (especially systemic lupus erythematosus, chronic lymphatic leukemia, or lymphoma). Other patients, with identical clinical features, can be shown to be producing antibodies to a drug (especially penicillin, cephalosporins, or quinidine). The antibodies or the drug–antibody complexes then attach to red cells, resulting in hemolysis. Patients taking large doses of methyldopa may develop antibodies to their own red cells; only a few of these patients have a significant hemolytic anemia.

Clinical Manifestations.   Presentation can be quite variable. A positive Coombs's test may be the only manifestation in mild cases. More often, signs of anemia are present. These include fatigue, dyspnea, palpitations, and jaundice. Occasionally, the anemia is so severe that the patient presents with overwhelming hemolysis and shock.

Management.   Any possibly offending medication should be discontinued. The treatment consists of high doses of corticosteroids until hemolysis decreases. When the hemoglobin has returned toward normal, usually after several weeks, the steroid dose can be lowered or, in some cases, discontinued entirely. In severe cases, blood transfusions may be required. Because the antibody may react with all possible donor cells, transfusion requires careful typing and slow, cautious administration.

Splenectomy removes a major site of red cell destruction; therefore, it may be performed if steroids do not produce a remission. If neither corticosteroid therapy nor splenectomy is successful, immunosuppressive drugs may be administered.

Polycythemia

Polycythemia refers to an increased concentration of red cells. It is a term used when the red cell count is greater than 6 million/mm^3 or the hemoglobin exceeds 18 g/dl. True polycythemia is present when the total body red cell mass is increased. "Relative" polycythemia occurs when the red cell mass is normal but the plasma volume is reduced; this may be produced by diuretic therapy or by unknown factors. Red cell mass can be measured accurately by an isotopic technique.

TABLE 32–2.   *Acquired Hemolytic Anemias*

Name	Cause	Manifestations and Treatment
Paroxysmal nocturnal hemoglobinuria	Unknown—sometimes occurs with aplastic anemia	Dark urine (hemoglobinuria), especially in morning Sometimes pancytopenia Multiple venous thrombosis No treatment known
Immune hemolytic anemia	Antibodies produced, sometimes secondary to drug (methyldopa [Aldomet], penicillin)	Jaundice, spherocytes Responds to steroids
Microangiopathic hemolytic anemia	RBC damaged during flow through abnormal small blood vessels, as in malignant hypertension	Fragmented RBC seen on smears Treat primary disease
Heart valve hemolysis	RBC damaged by regurgitant flow through incompetent valve prosthesis	Fragmented RBC Treatment: replace valve
Spur cell anemia	Severe liver disease, usually hypertension Increased lipid in RBC membrane	Spur-shaped RBC No treatment
Infections	Malaria, *Clostridum welchii*, especially after septic abortion	Hemoglobinuria possible Treat the infection
Hypersplenism	Large spleen from any cause: cirrhosis, lymphomas	Sometimes pancytopenia Treatment: splenectomy

Secondary Polycythemia

Secondary polycythemia is caused by excessive production of erythropoietin. This may occur in response to a hypoxic stimulus, as in chronic obstructive pulmonary disease or cyanotic heart disease, or in certain hemoglobinopathies in which the hemoglobin has an abnormally high affinity for oxygen (*e.g.,* hemoglobin$_{Chesapeake}$). In some cases of secondary polycythemia, the production of erythropoietin serves no purpose because there is no hypoxemia; this is the situation in a few patients with renal carcinoma, renal cysts, cerebellar hemangioblastoma, hepatoma, or uterine fibroids.

Management of secondary polycythemia involves treatment of the primary problem. If the cause cannot be corrected, *phlebotomy* (withdrawal of blood) may be necessary to reduce hypervolemia and hyperviscosity.

Polycythemia Vera

Polycythemia vera, or primary polycythemia, is a proliferative disorder in which all the marrow cells seem to have escaped from the normal control mechanisms. The bone marrow is intensely cellular, and in the peripheral blood the red count, white count, and platelets are often all elevated. Patients typically have a ruddy complexion and *hepatosplenomegaly* (enlarged liver and spleen). The symptoms are due to the increased blood volume (headache, dizziness, fatigue, and blurred vision) or to increased blood viscosity (angina, claudication, thrombophlebitis). Bleeding is also a complication, possibly because of the engorged capillaries. Another common and unexplained problem is pruritus.

Management

The objective of management is to reduce the high blood viscosity. Phlebotomy is an important part of therapy and can be performed repeatedly to keep the hemoglobin within normal range. Radioactive phosphorus or chemotherapeutic agents can be used to suppress marrow function but may increase the risk of leukemia. When the patient has an elevated uric acid level, allopurinol is used to prevent gouty attacks. Antihistamines may be administered to control pruritus.

In summary, polycythemia refers to an increase in red cell mass. In primary polycythemia vera there is a derangement of red blood cell reproduction. In secondary polycythemia a number of underlying conditions lead to increased erythropoietin levels. The response occurs because of decreased oxygen delivery.

Leukopenia and Agranulocytosis

Leukopenia is a condition in which the white cells number fewer than normal. Agranulocytosis is a potentially fatal condition in which there is almost complete absence of PMNs. A leukocyte count of fewer than 5000/mm³ or a granulocyte count of fewer than 2000/mm³ is abnormal and may be a signal of a generalized bone marrow disorder, such as megaloblastic anemia, aplasia, metastatic tumor, myelofibrosis, or acute leu-

kemia. Viral infections and overwhelming bacterial sepsis also can cause leukopenia. Most commonly, the cause is drug toxicity; phenothiazines are implicated frequently, and antithyroid drugs, sulfonamides, phenylbutazone, and chloramphenicol are also contributing factors. The patient is not symptomatic unless infection develops, which usually occurs when the granulocytes are fewer than 1000/mm³. Fever and severe sore throat with ulcerations are common complaints. Bacteremia may develop.

Management

Any possibly offending medications are withdrawn. If the granulocyte count is very low, the patient is protected from any obvious sources of infection. Cultures of all orifices and the blood are essential, and when fever occurs it is treated with broad-spectrum antibiotics until the specific organism is known. Good oral hygiene is helpful.

Hot saline irrigations of the throat are used to keep the throat clear of necrotic exudate. Comfort is provided by supplying an ice collar and whatever analgesic, antipyretic, and sedative drugs may be indicated. The goal of treatment, apart from eradicating the infection, is to eliminate, if possible, the factor responsible for the bone marrow depression. Spontaneous restoration of marrow function, except in the case of neoplastic diseases, often occurs in time, that is, within 2 or 3 weeks, if death from infection can be averted.

Hematopoietic Malignancies

Blood-forming tissues are characterized by rapid continuous turnover of cells. Normally, production of specialized blood cells from stem cell precursors is carefully regulated according to the body's needs. If homeostatic control of production is disrupted, neoplastic proliferation may result. A wide variety of hematopoietic malignancies can develop and they are often classified according to the cell line involved. *Leukemia*, literally "white blood," is a neoplastic proliferation of one particular cell (granulocytes, monocytes, lymphocytes, or megakaryocytes). The defect is believed to originate in the hematopoietic stem cell. The *lymphomas* are neoplasms of lymphoid tissue. Hodgkin's disease accounts for 40% of all lymphomas and is believed to result from defective T lymphocytes. Many other lymphomas are derived from B lymphocytes. Both Waldenström's macroglobulinemia and multiple myeloma are neoplasms affecting plasma cells produced by B lymphocytes.

Leukemia

The common feature of the leukemias is an unregulated proliferation or accumulation of white cells in the bone marrow, replacing normal marrow elements. There is also proliferation in the liver, spleen, and lymph nodes, and invasion of nonhematologic organs, such as the meninges, gastrointestinal tract, kidney, and skin. The leukemias are often classified according to the cell line involved, as either lymphocytic or myelocytic, and according to the maturity of the malignant cells, as either acute (immature cells) or chronic (differentiated cells).

The cause is unknown, but there is some evidence that genetic influence and viral pathogenesis may be involved. Bone marrow damage due to radiation exposure or chemicals (benzene) can cause leukemia.

Acute Myelogenous Leukemia

Acute myelogenous leukemia (AML) affects the hematopoietic stem cell that differentiates into all myeloid cells: monocytes, granulocytes (basophils, neutrophils, eosinophils), erythrocytes, and platelets. All age groups are affected; incidence rises with age. It is the most common nonlymphocytic leukemia.

Clinical Manifestations.   Most of the signs and symptoms evolve from insufficient production of normal blood cells. Vulnerability to infection results from granulocytopenia; weakness and fatigue occur due to anemia; and bleeding tendencies arise as a result of thrombocytopenia. The proliferation of leukemic cells within organs leads to a variety of additional symptoms: pain from enlarged liver or spleen; lymphadenopathy; headache or vomiting secondary to meningeal leukemia (most common in lymphocytic leukemia); and bone pain from expansion of marrow.

Onset is often insidious, with symptoms occurring over a period of 1 to 6 months. The peripheral blood will show a decrease in both erythrocyte and platelet counts. Although the total leukocyte count can be low, normal, or high, the percentage of normal cells is usually vastly decreased. A bone marrow specimen is diagnostic, disclosing an excess of immature blast cells. Auer rods present in the cytoplasm is diagnostic of AML.

Management.   Chemotherapy is the major form of therapy and in some instances results in remissions lasting a year or longer. Agents commonly used include daunorubicin hydrochloride (Cerubidine), cytarabine (Cytosar-U), and mercaptopurine (Purinethol). Supportive care consists of the administration of blood products and the prompt treatment of infections. When a tissue match with a close relative can be obtained, bone marrow transplantation is used to provide normal bone marrow after destruction of leukemic marrow by chemotherapy.

Prognosis.   Survival of treated patients averages only 1 year, with death usually a result of infection or hemorrhage. Untreated patients survive only about 2 to 5 months.

Chronic Myelogenous Leukemia

Chronic myelogenous leukemia (CML) is also believed to be a malignancy of myeloid stem cells. More normal cells are present than in the acute form, however, and therefore the disease is milder. A genetic abnormality termed the Philadelphia chromosome is found in 90% to 95% of patients. Uncommon before age 20, the incidence of CML rises with age.

Manifestations.   The clinical picture is similar to that of AML, but signs and symptoms are less severe. Many patients are without symptoms for years. Onset is typically insidious. Leukocytosis is always present, sometimes at extraordinary levels. Splenomegaly is common.

Management and Prognosis.   Therapies of choice are busulfan (Myleran) and hydroxyurea. Survival has been significantly improved with bone marrow transplantation. The final event in most patients is a transformation into an acute myelogenous leukemia that is usually resistant to all therapy.

Overall, patients live for 3 to 4 years. Death usually results from infection or hemorrhage. The nursing process is similar to that for acute leukemia (see p. 802).

Acute Lymphocytic Leukemia

Acute lymphocytic leukemia (ALL) is believed to be a malignant proliferation of lymphoblasts. It is most common in young children, males affected more than females, with a peak incidence at 4 years of age. After age 15, ALL is uncommon.

Manifestations.   Immature lymphocytes proliferate in marrow and peripheral tissue and crowd the development of normal cells. As a result of marrow proliferation of malignant cells, normal hematopoiesis is inhibited and leukopenia, anemia, and thrombocytopenia develop. Erythrocyte and platelet counts are low, and leukocyte counts may be either low or high but always include immature cells. Manifestations of leukemic cell infiltration into other organs are more common with ALL than with other forms of leukemia.

Management and Prognosis.   Therapy for this childhood leukemia has improved to the extent that approximately 60% of children survive at least 5 years. The major form of treatment is chemotherapy with combinations of vincristine, prednisone, daunorubicin, and asparaginase used for initial therapy and combinations of mercaptopurine, methotrexate, vincristine, and prednisone for maintenance. Irradiation of the craniospinal region and intrathecal injection of chemotherapeutic drugs help prevent central nervous system recurrence.

Chronic Lymphocytic Leukemia

A disease of elderly people, chronic lymphocytic leukemia (CLL) tends to be a mild disorder that primarily affects persons over age 40. It is more common in men than in women.

Clinical Manifestations.   Many patients are asymptomatic and are diagnosed during physical examination or treatment for another disease. Possible manifestations are those of anemia, infection, or enlargement of lymph nodes and abdominal organs. The erythrocyte and platelet counts may be normal or decreased. Lymphocytosis is always present.

Management and Prognosis.   If mild, CLL may require no treatment. When symptoms are severe, chemotherapy with steroids and chlorambucil (Leukeran) is often used. Highly variable in course, the average survival is 7 years.

Patients who no longer respond to therapy may be hospitalized for supportive care. They have often experienced remissions and exacerbations of the disease, and have known hope and despair. They are very tired and ill and require knowledgeable nursing assessment, support, and expert emotional and physical care. (See also section on patients with advanced carcinomas in Chap. 19.)

Gerontologic Considerations

Aging is accompanied by a gradual decline in the functioning of physiologic processes, among which is a reduction in the immune function, resulting in increased susceptibility to infections. Older patients also often delay reporting symptoms because of lack of knowledge, financial resources, or support systems. The complications of leukemia can be devastating to the already decreased reserves of the elderly. Comprehensive nursing care is critical in assisting the older patient to tolerate the side effects and treatment of the disease.

▶ Nursing Process
The Patient With Leukemia

◊ Assessment

Although the clinical picture will vary with the type of leukemia involved, the nursing history may reveal a range of signs and symptoms reported by the patient and noted during the physical examination. Included in the clinical manifestations may be weakness and fatigue, bleeding tendencies, petechiae and ecchymoses, pain, headache, vomiting, fever, and infection. Blood studies may show alterations of the white blood cells, anemia, and thrombocytopenia. Specific manifestations are identified under the discussion of each of the types of leukemia.

◊ Nursing Diagnoses

Based on the assessment data, nursing diagnoses for the patient may include the following:

- Ineffective coping related to the diagnosis and prognosis
- High risk for bleeding related to thrombocytopenia
- High risk for infection related to neutropenia
- Activity intolerance related to anemia
- Pain related to leukocytic infiltration of systemic tissues
- Altered nutrition, less than body requirements, related to gastrointestinal proliferative changes and toxic effects of chemotherapeutic agents
- Disturbance in body image related to alopecia

◊ Planning and Implementation

◊ *Goals:* The major goals of the patient may include ability to cope with the diagnosis and prognosis, absence of bleeding, absence of infection, tolerance of activity, attainment or maintenance of comfort, attainment or maintenance of adequate nutrition, and promotion of positive body image.

◊ Nursing Interventions

◊ *Ability to Cope With the Diagnosis and Prognosis.* Like other patients with malignant diseases, patients with leukemia are often depressed and frightened. A well-informed and sympathetic nurse can contribute immeasurably to their comfort by explaining procedures, anticipating side effects of drugs, and encouraging patients to participate in the therapeutic regimen. The therapy can become very complex, and too often patients feel that more is being done "to" them than "for" them. The nurse can be a sympathetic listener and help both patients and family mobilize defenses to cope with the emotional and physical stresses.

◊ *Prevention of Bleeding.* These patients should be approached in the same manner as those with aplastic anemia and should be assessed for thrombocytopenia, granulocytopenia, and anemia. The risk of bleeding correlates with the level of thrombocytopenia. In addition to having petechiae and ecchymoses, patients may develop major hemorrhages when their platelet counts drop below 20,000 per mm³ of blood. For undetermined reasons, fever or infection also increases the likelihood of bleeding. Any increase in petechiae and any melena, hematuria, or nosebleeds should be reported. Trauma and injections must be avoided, and acetaminophen, rather than aspirin, should be used for analgesia. Hormonal therapy may be prescribed to prevent menses. Hemorrhage is treated by bed rest and transfusions of red blood cells and platelets.

◊ *Prevention of Infection.* Because of the lack of mature and normal granulocytes, these patients are always threatened by infection, the major cause of death in leukemia. The likelihood of infection increases with the degree of neutropenia, so granulocyte counts under 100/ml of blood make the development of systemic infection highly probable. Immune dysfunction compounds the risk of infection. Patients must be systematically assessed for any evidence of infection.

It is essential to monitor the patient for the following signs and symptoms: temperature elevation, flushed appearance, chills, tachycardia, appearance of white patches in the mouth; redness, swelling, heat, or pain of eyes, ears, throat, skin, joints, abdomen, rectal and perineal areas; cough; changes in character or color of sputum, stool; and skin rash.

- The usual manifestations of infection are altered in patients with leukemia. Corticosteroid therapy may blunt the normal febrile and inflammatory responses to infection.

Some typical signs of infection, such as the appearance of exudates, are often not apparent and increase the need for careful observation. Frequent oral hygiene may decrease the likelihood of infection originating from the oral cavity. Because of the high risk of infection arising from intravenous cannulas, sterile gloves are worn to start infusions, daily site care should be provided, and the cannula should be changed every 48 hours. Rectal abscesses are not unusual, so it is important to ensure normal elimination and to avoid rectal thermometers, enemas, and rectal trauma. Vaginal tampons should be avoided. The urinary tract is another common site for infection. Catheterization should be avoided. When catheterization is essential, scrupulous asepsis during catheter insertion and maintenance is important.

◊ *Improvement of Activity Tolerance.* Anemia results from defective erythropoiesis, accelerated red cell destruction, and episodes of bleeding. If weak and easily fatigued, the patient may need assistance in choosing activity priorities and will need alternate rest and activity periods. Patients are also assessed for dyspnea, tachycardia, and other evidence of inadequate oxygen supply to vital organs.

◊ *Attainment/Maintenance of Comfort.* Infiltration of abnormal leukocytes into systemic tissues causes a variety of disabling symptoms. Pain is a common problem due to infiltration and enlargement of abdominal organs, lymph nodes, bones, and joints. Signs of central nervous system infiltration include headache, confusion, and other manifestations of meningeal irritation and increased intracranial pressure. Ongoing assessment of all body systems will help to identify these widespread effects so that care can be planned to decrease symptoms as they occur.

Careful positioning is helpful in preventing undue pain in the abdomen, lymph node areas, bones, and joints. Sudden movements are avoided and soft supports, such as pillows, are used to promote comfort. When necessary, analgesics are administered as prescribed to relieve pain. To avoid bleeding at puncture sites, small-gauge needles are used when analgesics are administered parenterally, and pressure is applied after injections.

The massive cell destruction resulting from chemotherapy increases uric acid levels and makes patients vulnerable to renal stone formation and renal colic. Therefore, patients require a high fluid intake to prevent crystallization of uric acid and subsequent stone formation.

▷ *Attainment or Maintenance of Adequate Nutrition.* Gastrointestinal problems may result from the infiltration of abnormal leukocytes into the abdominal organs as well as from the toxicity of the chemotherapeutic agents. Anorexia, nausea, vomiting, diarrhea, and mucosal lesions in the mouth are common. Because good nutrition is so important for cancer patients, careful timing of chemotherapeutic drug administration, prophylactic use of prescribed antiemetics, and the encouragement of foods and fluids that are the least irritating are essential. Frequent oral hygiene helps to prevent oral lesions and promotes appetite. Small, frequent feedings of foods and fluids that are high in protein and vitamins and that are palatable to the patient are often helpful in maintaining nutrition.

▷ *Promotion of Positive Body Image.* Because the hair is an important factor in a person's self-image, the occurrence of alopecia (hair loss) is usually traumatic. Patients are prepared for the occurrence of this problem and helped to express and resolve their feelings about it. It is often helpful for them to obtain a wig that they find aesthetically appealing before the hair loss occurs. Family members are encouraged to assist in selecting the wig. Involvement and support of the family are often invaluable in helping patients adjust to the problem.

▷ ## Evaluation

Expected Outcomes

1. Copes with diagnosis and prognosis
   a. Verbalizes feelings about prognosis to family/support system.
   b. Uses defense mechanisms appropriately
   c. Sets realistic goals
   d. Participates in the therapeutic regimen
2. Is free of bleeding
   a. Adheres to the therapeutic regimen
   b. Avoids situations that predispose to physical trauma (*e.g.*, razor and other sharp objects, forceful nose blowing, straining with stool, contact sports)
   c. Uses atraumatic measures of oral hygiene
   d. Monitors urine, stools, and vaginal discharge for evidences of bleeding
   e. Alerts health care personnel at first sign of bleeding
3. Is free of infection
   a. Attempts to maintain adequate nutritional intake
   b. Uses acceptable method of oral hygiene
   c. Describes signs and symptoms of infection and preventive measures
   d. Avoids persons with known infections
   e. Alerts health care personnel to first signs of infection
4. Experiences increased strength and endurance
   a. Explains causes for weakness and fatigue
   b. Spaces activities throughout the day
   c. Rests at specified intervals

d. Makes appropriate alterations in life style to accommodate decreased physical activity
   e. Shows progression in activity endurance from day to day
5. Attains or maintains comfort
   a. Identifies positions that promote comfort of the abdomen and extremities
   b. Positions self to relieve abdominal and extremity pain
   c. Rests with head of bed elevated to decrease headache
   d. Uses analgesics as prescribed
   e. Drinks adequate fluids to prevent renal stone formation
6. Attains or maintains adequate nutrition
   a. Identifies factors that precipitate gastrointestinal discomfort
   b. Uses antiemetics as prescribed to prevent nausea and vomiting
   c. Chooses foods that have the least chance of causing gastric irritation
   d. Attempts to increase intake of foods high in protein and vitamins
   e. Performs frequent oral hygiene
   f. Maintains/gains weight
7. Maintains positive body image
   a. Discusses feelings about alopecia
   b. Accepts help from nursing personnel and family in preparing for and coping with alopecia
   c. Obtains a wig that is appealing

In summary, the leukemias result from the malignant proliferation of the blood-forming cells. They are classified as acute or chronic and according to the cell type involved. Depending on the type of leukemia, the age of onset may vary from 2 to 80 years. The cause is not fully understood. Leukemic cells infiltrate the bone marrow, and normal hematopoiesis is impaired. Chemotherapy is the major form of therapy. Many of the complications of the disease arise not only from bone marrow failure but also from the cytotoxic effects of the treatment. Infection and bleeding may be life threatening. Prognosis varies according to the type of leukemia.

Nursing management includes careful assessment of actual and potential problems, education, and assisting both the patient and family to cope with the disease process.

Malignant Lymphomas

The lymphomas are neoplasms of the cells of lymphoid origin. They are often classified according to the degree of cell differentiation and the origin of the predominant malignant cell. These tumors usually start in lymph nodes, but can involve lymphoid tissue in the spleen, the gastrointestinal tract (for example, the wall of the stomach), the liver, or the bone marrow. They often spread to all of these areas and to extralymphatic tissues (lungs, kidneys, skin) by the time of death. The cause of these tumors is unknown.

Hodgkin's Disease

Hodgkin's disease, like other lymphomas, is a malignant disease of unknown origin that originates in the lymphatic system and involves predominantly the lymph nodes. It is somewhat more common in men and has two peaks of incidence: one in the early 20s and the other after age 50. Because many manifestations are similar to those occurring with infection, diagnostic studies are performed to rule out an infectious origin for the disease.

The malignant cell of Hodgkin's disease is the "Reed–Sternberg cell," a gigantic atypical tumor cell, morphologically unique and of uncertain lineage. It is the pathologic hallmark and essential diagnostic criterion for Hodgkin's disease.

Hodgkin's disease is customarily classified into subgroups based on pathologic criteria that reflect the grade of malignancy and suggest the prognosis. Lymphocyte predominance, for example, with fewest Reed-Sternberg cells and least disturbance of nodal architecture, carries a much more favorable prognosis than lymphocyte depletion, in which the lymph nodes are virtually replaced by tumor cells of the most primitive type. The majority of patients (those with conditions currently designated "nodular sclerosis" and "mixed cellularity") are in an intermediate position with respect to the density and destructiveness of tumor cells, therapeutic responsiveness, and overall outlook.

Clinical Manifestations

Hodgkin's disease usually begins as a painless enlargement of the lymph nodes on one side of the neck, which becomes increasingly conspicuous. For months, however, generalized pruritus may be the first and only symptom and later is often a most distressing one. The individual nodes remain firm and discrete (*i.e.*, they do not soften and do not fuse) and are seldom tender and painful. Soon the lymph nodes of other regions, usually the other side of the neck, also enlarge in the same manner. The mediastinal and retroperitoneal lymph nodes may also enlarge, causing severe pressure symptoms: pressure against the trachea results in dyspnea; pressure against the esophagus causes dysphagia; pressure on the nerves causes laryngeal paralysis and brachial, lumbar, or sacral neuralgias; pressure on the veins results in edema of one or both extremities and effusions into the pleura or peritoneum; and pressure on the bile duct causes obstructive jaundice. Later the spleen may become palpable, and the liver may enlarge. In some patients the first nodes to enlarge are those of one axilla or of one groin. Occasionally, the disease starts in mediastinal or peritoneal nodes and may remain limited to them. In still other cases the enlargement of the spleen is the only conspicuous lesion.

Eventually a progressive anemia develops. A leukocytosis often is observed with an abnormally high PMN count and an elevated eosinophil count. About half of the patients have a slight fever, with the temperature seldom rising above 38.3°C (101°F). Patients with mediastinal and abdominal involvement, however, present a remarkable intermittent fever. The temperature goes as high as 40.0°C (104°F) for periods of 3 to 14 days, returning to normal within a few weeks. Untreated, this disease is progressive in its course; the patient loses weight and becomes cachectic, infections develop, anemia becomes marked, *anasarca* (severe generalized edema) appears, the blood pressure falls, and death is likely in 1 to 3 years without treatment.

Diagnostic Evaluation

The diagnosis of Hodgkin's disease depends on the identification of characteristic histologic features in an excised lymph node. Once the diagnosis is confirmed, it is necessary to assess the total extent of tumor involvement and to define its distribution. In other words, the presence or absence of every tumor lesion inside and outside the lymphatic system and in organs and tissues is determined. This is a difficult, expensive, and uncertain undertaking but an extremely important one because these are the factors on which treatment is based.

Laboratory tests include a complete blood count, platelet count, sedimentation rate, and liver and renal function studies. A bone marrow biopsy and liver and spleen scans are performed to determine if there is involvement in these organs. Chest x-ray and bone scans of the pelvis, vertebrae, and long bones are performed to identify any involvement in these areas.

Management

Current concepts of treatment stem from the following observations and premises:

1. Hodgkin's disease spreads from its original location (usually a single node) by way of the lymphatic channels to contiguous lymph nodes, which in turn become the sites of tumor growth; it rarely skips lymph nodes en route to more distant sites of metastasis.
2. Hodgkin's disease rarely spreads beyond the lymphatic system to involve other organs and tissues until late in the disease.
3. Hodgkin's disease can be completely and permanently eradicated 95% of the time from any site that has received a radiation dose of 3500 to 4500 rad within the space of about 4 weeks. Megavoltage radiation techniques permit the delivery of such a dose to one or more entire lymph node chains.
4. Areas of the body in which the lymph node chains are located can tolerate doses of this magnitude without serious damage (as can the area of the spleen and the oronasopharynx, both of which may be involved in Hodgkin's disease), provided that vital structures such as the lungs, liver, gastrointestinal tract, kidneys, and bone marrow are protected by lead shields.

From the foregoing, it is postulated that Hodgkin's disease is potentially curable by radiotherapy, provided it has not extended beyond the lymph node chains, spleen, and oronasopharynx. Patients who do not have extension of the disease should have the benefit of "curative" radiotherapy in which doses large enough to destroy the tumors are delivered not only to obvious tumor nodes but to all adjacent nodes and lymph node chains as well. Conversely, any sign of spread beyond the treatable areas automatically disqualifies the Hodgkin's patient from such a program, in which case a combination of chemotherapy and palliative radiotherapy is indicated.

Staging of Hodgkin's Disease

For the sake of simplicity, uniformity, and convenience in categorizing patients with Hodgkin's disease with respect to the extent and activity of their disease and their eligibility for curative radiotherapy, the disease generally is classified, or "staged," as follows:

Stage I: Disease is limited to a single node and contiguous structures, or a single extralymphatic organ or site.

Stage II: Disease involves more than a single node or group of contiguous nodes, but is confined to one side of the diaphragm only.

Stage III: Disease is present both above and below the diaphragm and may include solitary involvement of the spleen, one extralymphatic site, or both.

Stage IV: Disease has disseminated diffusely to one or more extralymphatic sites with or without associated lymph node involvement.

Stages are further subdivided on the basis of the presence or absence of constitutional symptoms (*i.e.*, fever, night sweats, and unexplained weight loss). Patients without these symptoms are designated A and patients with them are designated B. The size or bulk of masses is also determined, as they may require separate therapy. Chemotherapy is often added for stage IIB and for stage IIIA. For stages IIIB and IV, combination chemotherapy is used, and radiation is generally reserved for the palliative treatment of local lesions that are especially destructive or painful. Currently patients diagnosed at stage IA or IIA have a 5-year survival rate of 90% and can essentially be considered cured. Survival rates decrease progressively with more advanced stages.

Nursing Interventions

Radiation therapy often requires many weeks of daily trips to the hospital. The dose to the tumor and adjacent lymph node areas is generally 4500 rad (45 grays).

Patients often develop esophagitis, anorexia, loss of taste, dry mouth, nausea and vomiting, diarrhea, skin reactions, and lethargy secondary to radiation therapy. Much ingenuity is needed to help patients cope with these unpleasant side effects. They should be encouraged to make a concerted effort to eat. Bland soft foods that they normally like are usually most palatable and are tolerated best when served at mild temperatures. Anesthetic throat lozenges may be helpful in relieving the mouth and throat discomfort that often interfere with eating. Decreased saliva increases the risk of dental caries and requires proper dental hygiene. The antiemetic that the physician prescribes should be administered during the peak times of nausea.

Skin reactions that give the appearance of sunburned or tanned skin are common. Patients are alerted that these are expected and that rubbing of the area and application of heat, cold, or lotions should be avoided. If the reaction is severe, the physician or nurse is to be notified.

The lethargy that accompanies radiation may cause patients to become discouraged about their progress. They are told that it is expected and that they must increase periods of rest and sleep to maintain a reasonable energy level. The family is encouraged to help patients in their attempts to rest. Diversional activities that require minimal energy expenditure may help to prevent boredom.

A commonly used chemotherapeutic regimen is a combination of nitrogen mustard, vincristine (Oncovin), prednisone, and procarbazine (MOPP). As for any patient receiving chemotherapy (see Chap. 19), support is necessary to help these patients tolerate the toxic effects, which include bone marrow depression, gastrointestinal disturbances, and alopecia. It often helps if patients are informed that the therapy will end at a specific time. This, along with the knowledge that there is a high likelihood of cure, often serves as an incentive for them to continue with the therapy. Helping patients to prepare for the alopecia by encouraging them to purchase a wig that is aesthetically acceptable to them before the problem occurs often averts some of the distress commonly associated with the loss of hair.

Patients with Hodgkin's disease are extremely vulnerable to infection, both as a result of radiation and chemotherapy and as a consequence of defective immune responses caused by the tumor. They are urged to report fever or any other signs of infection (skin redness, tenderness, lesions, cough) immediately so that treatment can be instituted. They are also apprised of the importance of avoiding contact with persons who are known to have infections.

Follow-up appointments with the physician are important for determining the effectiveness of the treatment and detection of complications. There is a high incidence of acute leukemia developing several years after treatment with radiation and chemotherapy. For this reason the patient and family are encouraged to keep all appointments.

Non-Hodgkin's Lymphomas

Non-Hodgkin's lymphomas are a more heterogenous group of disorders that can be defined as malignancies of the lymphoid tissue other than Hodgkin's disease. The cause is unknown; viral etiology has been suggested. There is an association with immunosuppressed states, (*e.g.*, acquired immunodeficiency syndrome [AIDS] and immunosuppressive therapy for organ transplant patients).

Manifestations are similar to those of Hodgkin's disease, but patients with these disorders are more likely to have generalized lymph node disease or extranodal disease when the disorder is first discovered. If the disease is localized, irradiation is the treatment of choice. If there is generalized involvement, combination chemotherapy is used. As with Hodgkin's disease, infection is a major problem. Central nervous system involvement is also common.

Mycosis Fungoides (Cutaneous T-Cell Lymphoma)

Mycosis fungoides is a relatively rare lymphoma of the skin that is found equally among blacks and whites, and is more common in men than women. It usually begins as a pruritic, red rash, and months or years later the skin becomes infiltrated with plaques and tumors of lymphoma. The specific lymphocyte involved is the T-cell lymphocyte. The body may be covered with mushroom-like growths varying in size from 1 cm to 5 cm (0.4 to 6 inches). Eventually, the malignant process reaches nodes, liver, spleen, and lungs. Patients are very uncomfortable with the itching and disfigurement of this disease. Treatment with nitrogen mustard (which may be used topically) or radiation can achieve palliation.

The patient with painful ulcerative lesions will require expert nursing care. A bed cradle may be used to remove the weight of bedding from painful skin lesions. Bacteriostatic ointment may be prescribed as a preventive measure against secondary infection and to protect open nerve endings from air exposure. Other aspects of management are similar to those for the patient with Hodgkin's disease.

Gerontologic Considerations

Non-Hodgkin's lymphoma is more common in the older adult and there appears to be an increased incidence of herpes zoster in these patients. Tissue in the elderly may be more sensitive to radiation and requires careful assessment for signs of complications.

In summary, the lymphomas are neoplasms that involve the cells of the immune system. They include Hodgkin's disease, which originates in lymphoid tissue, and non-Hodgkin's disease, which refers to all other malignant lymphomas not diagnosed as Hodgkin's disease. Mycosis fungoides is a T-cell lymphoma that affects the skin. The cause remains unknown and therapy consists mainly of chemotherapy and radiation. Prognosis for all lymphomas varies and primary complications resulting both from the disease and treatment include increased risk for infection, anemia, pain, and the possibility of developing a second malignancy. Careful assessment for disease progression and complications, education, and emotional support are essential components of nursing care.

Multiple Myeloma

Multiple myeloma is a malignant disease of plasma cells that infiltrate bone, lymph nodes, liver, spleen, and kidneys. It is not classified as a lymphoma. The malignant cell is the plasma cell, the neoplastic proliferation taking place mainly in the bone marrow.

Patients generally present with a normochromic, normocytic anemia, back pain, and sometimes leukopenia or thrombocytopenia due to bone marrow infiltration by malignant plasma cells. The diagnosis of myeloma can be made by aspiration or biopsy of the bone marrow. X-rays showing destructive lesions of many bones are suggestive but not diagnostic for this disease. The malignant plasma cells produce large quantities of abnormal globulins, which appear in the serum electrophoresis as a paraprotein "spike." Fragments of these globulins are excreted in urine as Bence Jones proteins.

Patients may be incapacitated by constant bone pain. The osteolytic lesions are often associated with hypercalcemia, and bone fractures are common, especially in the vertebrae or ribs. Median survival is between 2 to 5 years, with death usually resulting from infection or renal failure.

Management

Melphalan (Alkeran), cyclophosphamide, and steroids are the drugs used to decrease the tumor mass and relieve bone pain. They can prolong life from 1 year to 2 or 3 years. Radiation is very useful for palliation of bone pain and for reducing the size of extraskeletal plasma cell tumors. Good hydration is essential to prevent renal damage from precipitation of Bence Jones protein in the renal tubules, hypercalcemia, and hyperuricemia. Thus it is important to assess these patients for signs and symptoms of renal insufficiency. Allopurinol is used to prevent uric acid crystallization. When patients have severe pain they need narcotic analgesics and local radiation, and sometimes back braces to relieve pressure. Pathologic fractures are also possible. It is important to keep the patients as active as possible, because bed rest only increases the likelihood of hypercalcemia. Bacterial infections, especially pneumonia, are common in these patients, as they have impaired capacity for antibody production. Patients with multiple myeloma should not be put on fasting regimens for diagnostic tests because dehydrating procedures can precipitate acute renal failure.

Gerontologic Considerations. The incidence of multiple myeloma increases with age, rarely occurring before age 40. Because of the increasing older population, more patients are seeking treatment for this disease. Back pain should be closely investigated, as it often is a presenting complaint.

Bleeding Disorders

Pathophysiology

The body is normally protected against excessive and lethal blood loss by numerous complex and interrelated mechanisms. As indicated in Figure 32–1, hemostasis includes three phases. The first, the *vascular phase*, involves immediate vasoconstriction of injured vessels. This vessel spasm is sufficient to stop capillary bleeding. The second phase, or *platelet phase*, involves platelet aggregation at the site. These tiny cells are rapidly attracted to the damaged endothelium and form loose plugs. More platelets gather, and eventually these fuse and contract, forming stable plugs. The platelet plug effectively stops bleeding in small vessels such as venules, and provides temporary protection in larger injuries. Complete and permanent sealing of vascular wounds is accomplished through the clotting of the blood, which results in the production of an adherent gel-like mass that effectively controls most types of hemorrhage. This third phase, or *coagulation phase*, is initiated through either the intrinsic or the extrinsic pathway. A chain reaction occurs in which blood proteins are sequentially activated until factor Xa is formed. At this point, factor Xa interacts with factor V, calcium, and a platelet substance to convert prothrombin to thrombin. This is a very active enzyme that has several functions: one is to encourage further platelet aggregation; another is to convert fibrinogen to fibrin. Therefore, strands of fibrin begin to form in the vicinity of the platelet plug, reinforcing the plug and producing a larger clot. The fibrin clot is then further stabilized by the formation of bonds between the molecules, catalyzed by another plasma protein, factor XIII. The result is that the damaged vessel is sealed and blood flow in the area is slowed. Then, tissue repair of the vessel endothelium can proceed. Eventually, much of the fibrin clot will be lysed by another plasma protein system—the plasmin system, which produces fibrinolysis.

Abnormalities that predispose to hemorrhagic diseases can affect vessels, platelets, and any of the plasma coagulation factors, fibrin, or plasmin. Some patients can have defects at several sites simultaneously. Bleeding may be a manifestation of a primary coagulation defect (as in hemophilia), may occur secondary to another disease (as in cirrhosis, renal failure, or leukemia), or may be due to drugs (overdose of warfarin sodium).

Clinical Manifestations

The symptoms and signs of bleeding disorders vary, depending on the type of defect. A careful history can often give clues to the diagnosis. Abnormalities of the vascular system give rise to local bleeding, usually into the skin. Because platelets are primarily responsible for the cessation of bleeding from small vessels, patients with thrombocytopenia will have petechiae—small red or purple spots, often in clusters, seen on the skin and mucous membranes. Trauma results in excessive bruising but not large, uncontrolled hematomas. After cuts or skin puncture, bleeding stops promptly with local pressure and does not recur when pressure is released. In contrast, in hemophilia and abnormalities of other coagulation factors, the platelets function normally so that there are no petechial or superficial hemorrhages. Instead, deep bleeding occurs after minor trauma, such as intramuscular hematomas and hemorrhage into joint spaces. External bleeding recurs several hours after pressure is removed—as, for example, severe bleeding starting several hours after a tooth extraction.

Patients who have bleeding disorders or who have the potential for developing such disorders as a result of disease processes or therapeutic agents are observed carefully and frequently for bleeding. All drainage and excreta such as feces, urine, emesis, and gastric drainage are observed for occult as well as obvious blood. The skin is observed for petechiae and ecchymoses, and the nose and gums are assessed for bleeding. Abdominal, flank, or joint pain is promptly reported because it may be indicative of internal bleeding. In addition, the patient is closely observed for evidence of hypovolemia manifested by hypotension, tachycardia, pallor, cool clammy skin, altered responsiveness, and oliguria.

Vascular Disorders

Spontaneous rupture of small vessels that are defective or injured results in leakage of blood into the skin, and mucous membranes. The smallest hemorrhages, pinhead in size, are called *petechiae*. Larger lesions are termed *ecchymoses* or bruises. Platelet count and coagulation tests are usually normal.

Vascular dysfunction can be caused by a variety of mechanisms. Alterations in the connective tissue framework supporting blood vessels may explain the bleeding associated with vitamin C deficiency and adrenocortical hormone excess. Vascular injury also can result from systemic diseases such as diabetes mellitus or the action of bacterial toxins. A particularly important cause of vascular injury is immunologically mediated. As a consequence of drug reactions, bacterial infections, allergic disorders, or collagen-vascular diseases, vascular damage occurs. In general, bleeding from vascular disorders is mild.

Platelet Defects

The sudden onset of petechiae or excessive bruising or bleeding from the nose or gums should stimulate a search for a platelet defect. Deficiencies of platelet number, or thrombocytopenias, are most common, but there are also some rare disorders of platelet function in which the platelet count is normal but the clinical picture is identical to that in thrombocytopenia. The platelet function disorders can be diagnosed by special tests for platelet factor 3 and platelet adhesiveness and aggregation. An important functional platelet disorder is that induced by aspirin; even small amounts of aspirin prevent normal platelet aggregation, and the bleeding time is prolonged for several days after aspirin ingestion. Although this defect does not cause bleeding in most normal people, patients with another coagulation disorder (such as thrombocytopenia or hemophilia) can experience life-threatening hemorrhage after taking aspirin;

in addition, patients undergoing extensive surgery may experience bleeding postoperatively.

Thrombocytopenia

Thrombocytopenia is the most common cause of abnormal bleeding. It can result either from decreased production of platelets by the bone marrow or from increased peripheral destruction. Some of the causes are listed in Table 32–3. If the platelet deficiency is secondary to an underlying disease, this can usually be diagnosed from the examination of the patient or the bone marrow. When peripheral destruction is the cause of thrombocytopenia, the marrow shows increased megakaryocytes and normal platelet production. Bleeding and petechiae usually do not occur with platelet counts above 50,000/mm^3, although excessive bleeding can follow surgery.

When the platelet count drops below 20,000/mm^3, petechiae appear and there are nose bleeds, excessive menstrual bleeding, and hemorrhage after surgery or dental extractions. When the platelet count is less than 5000/mm^3, spontaneous fatal central nervous system hemorrhage or gastrointestinal hemorrhage can occur.

Management. The management for secondary thrombocytopenia is usually treatment of the underlying disease. If platelet production is impaired, platelet transfusions may raise platelet counts and stop bleeding or prevent intracranial hemorrhage. If excessive platelet destruction occurs, transfused platelets will also be destroyed and will not raise the count.

Idiopathic Thrombocytopenia Purpura

Idiopathic thrombocytopenia purpura (ITP) is a disease of all ages, but commonly affects children and young women. Although the precise cause remains unknown, viral infections sometimes precede the disease in children. Antiplatelet antibodies are produced, so platelet life span is markedly shortened. Occasionally, the antibodies can be demonstrated *in vitro*, but usually the diagnosis is made from the decreased platelet count and survival time and increased bleeding time. Other overt causes of thrombocytopenia must be excluded. Symptoms may begin suddenly, with petechiae, mucosal bleeding, and heavy menses in women. The platelet count is generally below 20,000/mm^3. Individuals with chronic ITP who are refractory to treatment are at increased risk for serious intracranial bleeding.

Management. Corticosteroids are the treatment of choice; the bleeding ceases in 1 to 2 days, and platelet counts rise in a week or so. About three fourths of patients respond to steroids, but many have a relapse when the drug is withdrawn. These patients, as well as those who do not respond to steroids, are treated with splenectomy. Splenectomy produces a lasting remission in 75% of patients, although transient recurrences of thrombocytopenia may occur months or years later. The rare patients who do not respond to splenectomy may be treated with the immunosuppressive drugs azathioprine or cyclosphosphamide. Patients are instructed to avoid all drugs that interfere with platelet function.

In summary, either quantitative or qualitative platelet defects can cause bleeding. Thrombocytopenia can be a result of decreased production, increased destruction, or increased utilization of platelets. Treatment is aimed at the underlying disease. ITP is thought to be mediated by autoantibodies that

TABLE 32–3.   *Thrombocytopenias*

Cause	Medical Management
FAILURE OF PRODUCTION	
Leukemia	Treat the leukemia.
Tumor invasion of marrow	
Aplastic anemia	Bone marrow transplant, androgens, antithymocyte globulin
Megaloblastic anemia	B_{12} or folic acid
Toxins	Discontinue toxin.
Drugs: heparin, chloramphenicol, cytotoxic drugs	Discontinue drug.
Infection, especially septicemia, viral infections, tuberculosis	Treat infection.
Alcohol	Discontinue alcohol.
INCREASED DESTRUCTION	
Due to antibodies	
Idiopathic thrombocytopenia purpura	Steroids, splenectomy
Lupus erythematosus	Steroids, immunosuppressive drugs
Malignant lymphoma	Steroids
Drugs: quinine, quinidine, digoxin, phenytoin, aspirin, sulfonamides, alcohol, gold	Discontinue drug.
Due to entrapment in large spleen	Splenectomy
Due to infections	Treat infection.
Bacteremia	
Postviral infections	
INCREASED UTILIZATION	
Disseminated intravascular coagulopathy	Heparin

shorten the life span of platelets. Corticosteroids, splenectomy, and immunosuppressive drugs are possible treatment modalities.

Clotting Factor Defects

Hemophilia

Definition and Etiology.   There are two hereditary bleeding disorders that are clinically indistinguishable, but that can be separated by laboratory tests—hemophilia A and hemophilia B. Hemophilia A is due to a deficiency of factor VIII clotting activity, whereas hemophilia B stems from a deficiency of factor IX. Factor VIII deficiency is about five times more common. Both types of hemophilia are inherited as X-linked traits, so almost all affected persons are males; their mothers and some of their sisters are carriers but are asymptomatic.

Clinical Manifestations.   The disease, which may be very severe, is manifested by large, spreading bruises and bleeding into muscles, joints, and soft tissues after even minimal trauma. Patients often note pain in a joint before swelling and limitation of motion are apparent. Recurrent joint hemorrhages can result in damage so severe that chronic pain or ankylosis (fixation) of the joint occurs. Many of the patients are crippled by the joint damage before they become adults. Spontaneous hematuria and gastrointestinal bleeding can occur. The disease

is recognized in early childhood, usually in the toddler age group.

Before factor VIII concentrates became available, many patients died of the complications before reaching adulthood. Some patients with hemophilia have a milder deficiency, having between 5% and 25% of the normal level of factor VIII or IX. These patients do not experience the painful and disabling muscle and joint hemorrhages, but bleed only after dental extractions or surgery. Nevertheless, such hemorrhages can prove fatal if the cause is not recognized quickly.

Management.   In the past, the only treatment was fresh frozen plasma, which had to be given in such large quantities that the patients became volume overloaded. Now factor VIII and IX concentrates are available to all blood banks. Patients are given concentrates when they are actively bleeding or as a prophylactic measure before dental extractions or surgery. Some families are taught how to administer the concentrate at home, at the first sign of bleeding.

A few patients eventually develop antibodies to the concentrates, so their factor levels cannot be elevated. Treatment of this problem is extremely difficult and often unsuccessful. Aminocaproic acid is an inhibitor of fibrinolytic enzymes. This drug can slow the dissolution of blood clots that do form, and it is sometimes used after oral surgery in patients with hemophilia.

In terms of general care, patients with hemophilia should never be given aspirin or IM injections. Dental hygiene is very important as a preventive measure, because dental extractions are so hazardous. Splints and other orthopedic devices may be very useful in patients who have suffered joint or muscle hemorrhages.

In recent years it has been found that patients with hemophilia are at high risk for developing AIDS as a result of the transfusions of blood and blood components that they previously received. To prevent this problem, people with AIDS and those at high risk for developing AIDS are no longer candidates for blood donation. In addition, all donated blood is now tested for the presence of antibodies to the AIDS virus. Commercial factor concentrates are heat-treated to reduce the possible transmission of infectious diseases.

▶ Nursing Process
The Patient With Hemophilia

▷ **Assessment**

Patients with hemophilia are carefully assessed for evidence of internal bleeding (abdominal, chest, or flank pain; hematuria; hematemesis, melena), muscle hematomas, and hemorrhage into joint spaces. Vital signs and hemodynamic pressure readings are assessed for indications of hypovolemia. All extremities and the torso are carefully examined for hematomas. All joints are assessed for swelling, limitation of mobility, and pain. Range of motion of the joints is performed slowly and carefully to avoid further damage. At the first indication of pain, joint motion is stopped. Patients are questioned about any limitations of activities and movement experienced in the past and any need they have had for assistive devices such as splints, a cane, or crutches.

If the patient has had recent surgery, the surgical site is frequently and carefully assessed for bleeding. Continuous monitoring of vital signs may be necessary until it is certain that excessive postoperative bleeding is not present.

All patients with hemophilia are questioned about how they and their family cope with their condition, measures that they use to prevent bleeding episodes, and any limitations that the condition imposes on their life style and daily activities. The patient who has frequent hospitalizations for bleeding episodes due to traumatic injury is carefully questioned about the factors that have led to these episodes. Such data are particularly helpful in determining the extent of the patient's acceptance of the condition and the need for patient and family education regarding measures to prevent unnecessary trauma.

▷ **Nursing Diagnoses**

Based on the assessment data, major nursing diagnoses for the patient may include the following:

- Pain related to joint hemorrhage and subsequent ankylosis
- Potential for decreased tissue perfusion related to bleeding
- Knowledge deficit regarding prevention of bleeding
- Ineffective coping related to the chronicity of the condition and its effects on life-style

▷ **Planning and Implementation**

▷ *Goals:* The major goals of the patient may include relief or minimization of pain, adequate tissue perfusion, use of measures to prevent bleeding, and coping with chronicity and altered life style.

▷ **Nursing Interventions**

▷ *Relief/Minimization of Pain.* Generally, analgesics are required to alleviate the pain associated with large muscle hematomas and joint hemorrhage. The physician usually prescribes oral non-narcotic analgesics when possible, because pain may be of long duration, and dependency on narcotics becomes a problem with chronic pain. It is often helpful to administer the analgesic before activities that are known to precipitate pain. This not only helps the patient to accomplish the activity, but also tends to decrease the amount of analgesic that the patient requires.

All efforts possible are taken to prevent or minimize pain due to activity. The patient is encouraged to move slowly and to prevent undue stress on involved joints. Many patients report that warm baths promote relaxation, improve mobility, and lessen pain. Heat is avoided during bleeding episodes, however, because it potentiates further bleeding.

Because joint pain restricts mobility, patients with excessive pain during activity may benefit from assistive devices. Splints, canes, or crutches are helpful in some cases in shifting body weight off joints that are particularly painful. Splints must be properly applied and crutches must be properly fitted to prevent undue pressure on body surfaces that could cause tissue trauma and bleeding.

▷ *Attainment or Maintenance of Adequate Tissue Perfusion.* The patient is assessed frequently for signs and symptoms of decreased tissue perfusion as evidenced by hypoxia to vital organs: restlessness, anxiety, confusion, pallor, cool clammy skin, chest pain, and decreased urinary output. Hypotension and tachycardia will occur as a result of volume depletion. The blood pressure, pulse, respiration, central venous pressure, and pulmonary artery pressure are monitored, as are the hemoglobin and hematocrit, coagulation and bleeding times, and platelet counts.

The patient is observed frequently for bleeding from the skin, mucous membranes, and wounds and for internal bleeding. During bleeding episodes, the patient is kept at rest and gentle pressure is applied to any external bleeding sites. Cold compresses are applied to bleeding sites when indicated.

Parenteral medications are administered with small-gauge needles to decrease trauma and the risk of bleeding. All possible efforts are made to protect the patient from trauma. The environment is kept free of obstacles that could cause falls, and the patient is turned and moved with care. Side rails are padded when necessary. Blood and blood components are administered as prescribed, and precautions are taken to avoid complications (see p. 815).

▷ *Use of Measures to Prevent Bleeding.* The patient and family are informed of the risk of bleeding and the necessary safety precautions to be taken. They are encouraged to alter the home environment as necessary to prevent physical trauma. Obstacles that could cause falls are removed. An electric razor is used for shaving and a soft toothbrush is used for oral hygiene. Forceful nose blowing and coughing and straining at stool are avoided. A stool softener is used if necessary. Aspirin and aspirin-containing drugs are to be avoided.

Physical activity is encouraged, but with proper safety

measures used. Noncontact sports such as swimming, hiking, and golf are acceptable activities, whereas contact sports are always to be avoided.

The necessity for regular checkups and laboratory studies is explained. With knowledge of the reasons for continued medical evaluation, the patient will be more likely to keep appointments.

▷   *Coping With Chronicity and Altered Life-Style.*   Patients with hemophilia often require assistance in coping with the condition because it is chronic, it places restrictions on their lives, and it is an inherited disorder that can be passed to future generations. From childhood, patients are helped to accept themselves and the disease and to identify the positive aspects of their lives. They are encouraged to be self-sufficient and to maintain independence by preventing unnecessary trauma that can cause acute bleeding episodes and temporarily interfere with normal activities. As they work through feelings about the condition and progress to acceptance of it, they will accept more and more responsibility for maintaining optimal health. They will cooperate with health care providers, keep regular medical and dental appointments, and strive toward a healthy, productive family life. Many patients benefit from the services of hemophilia care centers and support groups. These provide coordinated, ongoing care and the opportunity to interact with others who are faced with the same situation.

▷   ## Evaluation

Expected Outcomes
1. Experiences relief or minimization of pain
   a. Reports decrease in pain after taking analgesic
   b. Exhibits increased ability to tolerate joint motion
   c. Uses orthopedic aids (when necessary) to decrease pain
2. Maintains adequate tissue perfusion
   a. Vital signs and hemodynamic pressure readings remain normal
   b. Laboratory studies remain within normal ranges
   c. Experiences no active bleeding.
3. Uses measures to prevent bleeding
   a. Avoids physical trauma
   b. Alters home environment to increase safety
   c. Keeps appointments with health care professional
   d. Keeps appointments for laboratory studies
   e. Avoids contact sports
   f. Avoids aspirin and aspirin-containing drugs
   g. Wears Medic-Alert bracelet
4. Copes with chronicity and altered life style
   a. Identifies the positive aspects of present life
   b. Involves family members in decisions about the future and changes to be made in life style
   c. Strives toward independence
   d. Makes specific plans for continuation of health care

Von Willebrand's Disease

This is a common bleeding disorder, usually inherited as a dominant trait and affecting males and females equally. It is due to a mild deficiency of factor VIII (15% to 50% of normal) associated with an impairment of platelet function. The laboratory tests show normal platelet count, prolonged bleeding time, and slightly prolonged partial thromboplastin time. Pa-

tients commonly have nosebleeds, excessively heavy menses, bleeding from cuts, and postoperative bleeding. They do not suffer from massive soft tissue or joint hemorrhages. Both of the defects can be corrected either by the administration of cryoprecipitate, which contains factor VIII, fibrinogen, and factor XIII, or desmopressin (DDAVP), a synthetic vasopressin analogue.

In summary, hemophilia and von Willebrand's disease are the most common inherited clotting factor disorders. Hemophilia is a sex-linked recessive disorder that affects blood clotting. Factor VIII deficiency results in hemophilia A, whereas a low level or absence of factor IX results in less frequent hemophilia B. Both disorders are manifested by minimal or severe bleeding into muscles, joints, and soft tissues. Treatment consists of replacement therapy. Nursing management includes educating the patient and family about the disease process, prevention and management of bleeding episodes, and strategies for coping with chronic illness. Von Willebrand's disease is usually inherited as an autosomal dominant trait caused by a deficiency of factor VIII, part of which is necessary for normal platelet function. Severity may vary, and treatment consists of replacement therapy or desmopressin.

Hypoprothrombinemia

Prothrombin, as was previously noted, is essential for the clotting process. This protein is produced in the liver by a vitamin K–dependent chemical process. Vitamin K enters the body from food sources as well as from synthesis by bacteria that reside in the intestine. Normal prothrombin activity in the blood depends on adequate absorption of this vitamin from the gastrointestinal tract and on adequate liver function. Therefore, prothrombin deficiency may arise as a result of diarrhea, from a lack of bile in the gastrointestinal tract (necessary for absorption of fat-soluble vitamin K) due to biliary tract obstruction, from surgical removal or mucosal damage of a large part of the small intestine, from prolonged antibiotic therapy, or as the result of liver disease.

The principal manifestation of prothrombin deficiency, as observed in patients with hemophilia, is prolonged hemorrhage from blood vessels that are damaged by trauma or disease. This explains the characteristic occurrence of ecchymoses, hematuria, gastrointestinal bleeding, and postoperative hemorrhages.

Coumarin Toxicity.   The coumarins are drugs that often are employed to induce a partial depression of prothrombin activity, because the drugs interfere with the action of vitamin K in the liver. Therapy is usually calculated to prolong the prothrombin time by 1.5 to 2 times normal. In this range, thrombosis is inhibited and thrombophlebitis is prevented. If taken in excessive dosages, however, whether intentionally or mistakenly, or if certain other drugs that interfere with metabolism are administered simultaneously, the complete picture of prothrombin deficiency, with a severe hemorrhagic disorder, may be produced. Drugs that enhance coumarin-induced anticoagulation include phenylbutazone, indomethacin, phenytoin, and salicylates. Other drugs, such as barbiturates, decrease coumarin effects.

Management.   Hypoprothrombinemia, if due to vitamin K deficiency, responds to treatment with oral or parenteral administration of vitamin K. When corrective measures are urgently required, however, particularly in patients with liver disease or coumarin toxicity, fresh frozen plasma will promptly correct the deficit.

Liver Disease.   The liver produces all the plasma protein coagulation factors except factor VIII. Therefore, in severe hepatic disease of any sort, deficiencies in these factors may occur. The prothrombin time and partial thromboplastin time will both be prolonged. If the spleen is enlarged as well (as in cirrhosis), the platelet count also may be depressed. These patients frequently bruise easily and may have life-threatening hemorrhage from peptic ulcers or esophageal varices. Treatment includes fresh frozen plasma, cryoprecipitate, and platelets. Vitamin K does not improve the disorder.

Gerontologic Considerations.   The older patient is more likely to be taking several medications because of chronic illness. This can increase the possibility of an interaction with the coumarins. Frequent schedule or dose changes can be confusing to the elderly. Simple instructions should be written for the patient for later reference. Special emphasis is placed on helping the patient to recognize the need to avoid taking drugs that can have harmful interactions.

Disseminated Intravascular Coagulopathy

Occasionally, widespread clotting in small vessels of the body occurs, causing clotting factors and platelets to be used up. Thus, paradoxically, the patient presents with a bleeding disorder characterized by low fibrinogen, prolonged prothrombin time and partial thromboplastin time, thrombocytopenia, and elevated fibrin split products. Such patients may bleed from mucous membranes, venipuncture sites, and the gastrointestinal and urinary tracts. The bleeding can range from minimal occult internal bleeding to profuse hemorrhaging from all orifices. Patients may also develop organ necrosis, such as renal failure, due to fibrin deposition in small vessels. Many serious illnesses may predispose to DIC, including septicemia, premature separation of the placenta in a pregnant woman, metastatic malignancies, hemolytic transfusion reactions, massive tissue trauma, and shock. DIC should be suspected in any patient with a predisposing cause who develops purpura, a bleeding tendency, and signs of renal damage.

Serious hemorrhage requires replacement therapy: fluids, fresh frozen plasma, red cells, platelet concentrates, and, if indicated by very low fibrinogen level, cryoprecipitate. The best treatment is correction of the underlying disease, but in the meantime intravenous heparin may retard the coagulation process and permit normalization of clotting tests and a decrease in the hemorrhagic manifestations.

In summary, the most common acquired coagulation disorders are vitamin K deficiency, liver disease, and DIC. Vitamin K deficiency results in hypothrombinemia. Malabsorption, liver dysfunction, biliary obstruction, medications such as coumarin, or surgery can cause a decrease in vitamin K. Bleeding is dependent on the severity of the deficiency. Treatment in the form of replacement therapy or changes in medications depends on the underlying causative factor. DIC occurs secondary to another disease process. Overstimulation of the normal coagulation system leads to bleeding and thrombosis. Severity can be mild to acute, depending on the depletion of coagulation factors. Treatment is directed at the underlying disease.

Therapeutic Measures in Blood Disorders

Splenectomy

The surgical removal of the spleen is sometimes necessary after trauma to the abdomen. Because the spleen is very vascular, severe hemorrhage can result after splenic rupture. Under such circumstances, splenectomy becomes an emergency procedure.

Splenectomy is also often performed as a treatment for a number of hematologic disorders. An enlarged spleen may be the site of excessive destruction of blood cells; when this destruction is life threatening, the operation may prove palliative. This is the case in autoimmune hemolytic anemia or idiopathic thrombocytopenia purpura when these disorders do not respond to corticosteroids. Some patients with severe anemia due to inherited red cell defects (such as thalassemia or pyruvate kinase deficiency) may benefit from splenectomy. Patients with rheumatoid arthritis may develop splenomegaly that results in destruction of granulocytes and granulocytopenia; removal of the spleen may improve the blood count and reduce the tendency toward infection.

Splenectomy is often performed to relieve the pain and cytopenias caused by massive splenomegaly, which can occur in such diseases as myelofibrosis, chronic myelogenous leukemia, or Gaucher's disease (a rare chronic congenital disorder of lipid metabolism). Most patients with hereditary *spherocytosis* (spheroid shape of erythrocytes) are essentially cured of their hemolytic process by splenectomy.

When the spleen is large, the operation can be difficult, but generally there is a very low mortality. Morbidity may result from postoperative atelectasis, pneumonia, abdominal distention, and subphrenic abscess formation. Although young children are at the highest risk, all age groups are vulnerable to overwhelming lethal infections and should receive pneumococcal vaccine before surgery if possible. Patients are instructed to seek prompt medical attention when even relatively minor symptoms of infection occur. Patients with high platelet counts often are found to have even higher counts after splenectomy—greater than a million—and this can predispose the patient to serious thrombotic or hemorrhagic problems.

In summary, splenectomy may be necessary in cases of trauma, as a cure for certain diseases, or as palliative treatment. All asplenic patients are at increased risk for developing overwhelming sepsis. In addition to receiving pneumococcal vaccine, patients require education concerning the risks and treatment of any febrile illness.

Blood Transfusion
Blood Donation

Because blood and blood components are used so frequently, nearly all hospitals now have blood banks, and most large hospitals also have facilities for blood donation. Nurses employed in these departments screen prospective donors, perform the phlebotomies, and care for the health and safety of the donors.

Donor Interviewing

All prospective donors are examined and interviewed before the donation for their own protection and that of the recipients. The questioning must be tactful but complete, and an experienced interviewer will learn how to ask each question in several ways to obtain the most complete answers. Donors should appear to be in good health and should be free of any of the following disqualifying factors:

- A history of viral hepatitis, recently or at any time in the past, or a history of close contact with a hepatitis or dialysis patient within 6 months
- A history of receiving a blood transfusion or injection of any fraction of blood other than serum albumin or immune globulin within 6 months
- A history of untreated syphilis or malaria, because these can be transmitted by transfusion even years later. A person who has been free of symptoms and off therapy for 3 years after malaria may be a donor
- A history of evidence of drug abuse in which drugs were self injected, because intravenous drug users have a high hepatitis carrier rate and because of the risk of AIDS
- A history of possible exposure to the AIDS virus. A test for the presence of antibodies to AIDS virus in donated blood is now available. The population at risk includes those persons who engage in anal sex practices, persons with multiple sexual partners, intravenous drug users, sexual partners of individuals at risk for AIDS, and persons with hemophilia.
- A skin infection, because of the possibility of contamination of the phlebotomy needle
- A history of recent asthma, urticaria, or allergy to drugs, because hypersensitivity can be passively transferred to the recipient
- Pregnancy within 6 months, because of the nutritional demands of pregnancy on the mother
- A history of tooth extraction or oral surgery within 72 hours, because such procedures are frequently associated with transient bacteremia
- A history of recent tattoo, because of the higher risk of hepatitis
- A history of exposure to infectious disease within the past 3 weeks, because of the risk of transmission to the recipient
- Recent immunizations, because of the risk of transmitting live organisms (2-week waiting period for live, attenuated organisms; 1 month for rubella; 1 year for rabies)
- Presence of cancer, because of the lack of knowledge about transmission
- A history of whole blood donation within the past 56 days

Blood donors who pass this screen are then examined with regard to blood pressure, pulse, oral temperature, weight, and hemoglobin level. The last is often checked with a screening test that estimates only the hemoglobin. Persons under 17 and over 65 years of age are usually disqualified. Donors are expected to meet the following minimal requirements:

1. The body weight should exceed 50 kg (110 pounds) for a standard 450-ml donation. Donors weighing less than 50 kg (110 pounds) donate proportionately less blood.
2. The oral temperature should not exceed 37.5°C (99.6°F).
3. The pulse rate should be regular and between 50 and 100 beats per minute.
4. The systolic arterial pressure should be between 90 and 180 mm Hg, and the diastolic pressure between 50 and 100 mm Hg.
5. The hemoglobin level in the case of a woman should be at least 12.5 g/dl (125 g/L), and in the case of a man, 13.5 g/dl (135 g/L).

Phlebotomy

Phlebotomy consists of venipuncture and the withdrawal of blood. Universal precautions are used. Donors are placed in a semirecumbent position. The skin over the antecubital fossa is carefully cleansed with an iodine preparation. A tourniquet is applied, and venipuncture is performed. Withdrawal of 450 ml of blood takes less than 15 minutes. After removal of the needle, donors are asked to hold the involved arm straight up, and firm pressure is applied with sterile gauze for 2 or 3 minutes or until bleeding stops. A firm bandage is then applied. Donors are asked to remain recumbent until they feel able to sit up, usually 1 or 2 minutes. If weakness or faintness is experienced, they should rest for a longer period. After resting, they are given food and fluids in a reception area and asked to remain another 15 minutes. Donors should be instructed to leave the dressing on and avoid heavy lifting for several hours, to avoid smoking for 1 hour and alcoholic beverages for 3 hours, to increase fluid intake for 2 days, and to be sure to eat well-balanced meals for 2 weeks. The labels on the blood bag and tubes are checked carefully before and after donation to avoid any error that could prove fatal to a recipient.

Complications

Excessive bleeding at the site of venipuncture is sometimes due to a bleeding disorder in the donor, but more often is the result of a technical error: laceration of the vein, excessive tourniquet pressure, or failure to apply enough pressure after withdrawal of the needle.

Fainting is relatively common and may be related to emotional factors, vasovagal reaction, or prolonged fasting before donation. Because of the loss of blood volume, hypotension and syncope may occur when the donor assumes an erect position.

- A donor who appears pale or complains of faintness should immediately lie down or sit with head lowered below the knees. The nurse should observe the donor for another 30 minutes.

Anginal chest pain may be precipitated in patients with unsuspected coronary artery disease. *Convulsions* may occur in patients with epilepsy. Both angina and convulsions require further medical evaluation.

Blood and Blood Components

A unit of blood that has been drawn from a donor consists of approximately 450 ml of whole blood and 60 to 70 ml of preservative–anticoagulant. The latter serves as the anticoagulant and also provides the red cells with a sugar for metabolism. This blood can be maintained at 1° to 6°C in the blood bank for 21 to 35 days, depending on the type of preservative-anticoagulant used; after that time it is discarded if unused, because too many of the red cells are unable to survive *in vivo.* Whole blood stored more than 24 hours does not contain functional platelets or practical amounts of coagulation factors V and VIII.

Samples of the unit are always taken immediately after donation so that the blood can be typed and tested for the presence of syphilis, hepatitis, and antibodies. A test for the presence of AIDS antibodies in donated blood is now required. A label on the unit thereafter states the blood type and certifies that the unit is negative for syphilis serology, hepatitis B antigen, hepatitis C antibody, and AIDS antibodies.

Whole blood is a complex tissue with both cellular and many noncellular plasma components. Recently, it has been recognized that whole blood is necessary only in certain clinical situations; many times, component therapy can replace the particular deficiency without subjecting the patient to unnecessary risks, such as circulatory overload. In addition, the use for components is more economical because it makes it possible to meet the needs of more than one patient from a single blood donation. Many blood banks are able to separate whole blood into these fractions, and all of the components are available from the American Red Cross.

Whole Blood.   Whole blood may be used to treat acute, massive hemorrhage or hypovolemic shock due to hemorrhage. It is not indicated for the correction of anemia. Whenever possible, components should be used instead.

Packed Red Cells.   Red cells are separated from whole blood by centrifugation or sedimentation; most of the plasma is removed, leaving a hematocrit of approximately 80%. Packed red cells are indicated for transfusions in anemic patients, in surgical patients before and after operation, and in many cases of acute blood loss. The use of packed cells instead of whole blood reduces the volume load. Thus, this method is safer for patients with incipient congestive heart failure and reduces the incidence of transfusion reactions due to plasma factors.

Frozen Red Cells.   The method of freezing red cells allows storage for long periods—even years—but is expensive. Hence, frozen cells are used only under unusual circumstances, such as for patients with very rare blood types or with antibodies to the common minor antigens. Blood may also be stored for autotransfusion.

Platelets.   Patients with thrombocytopenia and hemorrhage often require transfusions of large numbers of platelets. Platelets taken from 4 to 8 units of blood are necessary to raise the count of a severely thrombocytopenic patient to a hemostatic level. Therefore, "platelet-rich plasma" with a small volume is used rather than whole blood. Several methods are available for harvesting fresh platelets: (1) Plasma can be removed after centrifugation of a unit of freshly collected whole blood; the plasma is then centrifuged again slowly to separate the platelets. Several such platelet "units" then can be pooled and given to the recipient, who thus receives platelets from several different donors. (2) A single donor can undergo *platelet apheresis,* in which blood is donated, the red cells are separated and returned to the donor immediately, and the plasma is spun down to obtain platelets in a volume of only 10 to 20 ml. In this way, multiple units can be donated.

Platelet concentrates are generally kept at room temperature with agitation and can be stored for 3 to 5 days. Each unit of platelets will raise the recipient's platelet count by about 10,000/mm³. For an adult with severe thrombocytopenia, 10 or more units of platelets may be needed daily. Even larger doses are needed for patients with fever or infection because these conditions decrease platelet effectiveness.

Single-donor platelet transfusions are especially valuable for patients who have received many transfusions and have developed antibodies to all except human leukocyte antigen (HLA) [transplantation antigen]–matched blood products.

Granulocytes.   Severely granulocytopenic patients with infection may benefit from transfusions of normal white cells. Large numbers of granulocytes less than 24 hours old must be administered. The donor's white cells are continuously removed as blood is drawn from one vein and returned through another vein. The process requires about 4 hours of donor time, and the donor must be anticoagulated during the procedure.

Plasma.   Whole plasma was originally used in the treatment of hypovolemic shock, but now, because plasma carries a risk of hepatitis equal to that of whole blood, other colloids (*e.g.,* albumin) or electrolyte solutions (*e.g.,* Ringer's lactate) are usually preferred. Plasma can be used to replace deficient coagulation factors in acquired or inherited bleeding disorders. Only fresh frozen plasma (which can be stored for 12 months) contains all the coagulation factors, including V and VIII. Fractions of plasma have now been prepared, however, that can replace all the factors except V in small-volume concentrates. Fresh frozen plasma may be administered to replace clotting factors in patients who are hemorrhaging and require massive transfusion with whole blood or packed red cells. It also is used to treat patients with severe liver disease.

Albumin.   Plasma albumin is a large protein molecule that usually stays within vessels and is a major contributor to plasma oncotic pressure. This material is used to expand the blood volume of patients in hypovolemic shock and to elevate the level of circulating albumin in patients with hypoalbuminemia. These preparations, in contrast to all other fractions of human blood, cellular or soluble, are subjected to heating at 60°C (140°F) for 10 hours, and therefore can be certified unequivocally as free of all viral contaminants, including the hepatitis virus. Whereas the risk of hepatitis transmission is an important consideration in connection with every other type of transfusion therapy (except immune globulin), this complication has not been reported with the use of albumin.

Cryoprecipitate.   Cryoprecipitate is a plasma derivative that is rich in factor VIII, fibrinogen, factor XIII, fibronectin, and von Willebrand factor. It is prepared by thawing one unit of fresh frozen plasma and removing all but 10 to 15 ml of plasma and the cold-insoluble globulins. The product is then refrozen and can be used for up to 1 year for the treatment of hemophilia A, von Willebrand's disease, DIC, and bleeding associated with renal disease.

Factor VIII Concentrate (Antihemophilic Factor).   A lyophilized (freeze-dried) concentrate of pooled fractionated human plasma that has been heat treated to reduce the transmission of hepatitis and human immunodeficiency virus (HIV) is used in the treatment of hemophilia A.

Factor IX Concentrate (Prothrombin Complex).   This commercial preparation is prepared by pooling, fractionating, and freeze-drying large volumes of plasma. Containing factors II, VII, IX, and X, it is used primarily for the treatment of patients with factor IX deficiency (hemophilia B or Christmas disease). It is also useful for the treatment of patients with congenital factor VII and X deficiencies. Heat treatment has reduced the risk of infectious disease transmission.

Transfusion Techniques

Administration of blood and blood components demands knowledge of correct techniques for administration and knowledge of possible complications. After verifying the physician's order and explaining the procedure to the patient, the nurse obtains the blood or blood component from the blood bank. Labels are carefully checked with another nurse. In accordance with Universal Precautions, gloves must be worn during all procedures involving possible contact with blood and other body fluids. Vital signs should be recorded before initiating the transfusion. Medications are *never* added to blood or blood products.

Whole blood or packed red cells generally are administered through a 19-gauge or larger needle into a large vein. Special tubing is used that contains a blood filter to screen out fibrin clots and other particulate matter. Certain electromechanical infusion pumps have been approved for controlled administration of blood and blood products. For the first 15 minutes, the transfusion is run very slowly, at about 2 ml/minute, and the patient is observed carefully for adverse effects. If no ill effects occur during this time, the flow rate is then increased unless the patient is at high risk for circulatory overload. Frequent observations of the patient continue throughout the transfusion. Major points to consider when administering blood components are listed in Table 32–4.

Assessment

Before initiating transfusion therapy, it is important to determine that the blood has been typed and cross-matched and that the

TABLE 32–4.   *Administration of Blood Components*

Product	Administration Technique	Major Complications
Packed red cells	Use Y-type infusion set, with 170-μm filter and make sure cells cover entire surface.	Transfusion reactions related to volume overload are less frequent than with whole blood.
	Administer 1 unit over 2–3 hours, do not exceed 4 hours.	Febrile nonhemolytic and allergic reactions.
	If necessary to help cells infuse, add 50–100 ml 0.9% NaCl.	Acute hemolytic reactions. Transfusion-transmitted diseases.
Platelets	Use component infusion set with minimum 170-μm filter. (Do not use small pore or leukocyte-depleting filters).	Febrile nonhemolytic and allergic reactions. Transfusion-transmitted diseases.
	Administer only with 0.9% NaCl.	
	Administer over 30–90 minutes, usually 4 units/hour (determined by volume tolerance).	
Granulocytes	Use Y-type infusion set with 170-μm filter. (Do not use leukocyte-depleting filter.)	Febrile, nonhemolytic, and allergic reactions. Leukoagglutinin reactions possible, leading to hypotension; anaphylaxis, and respiratory distress. Transfusion-transmitted diseases.
	Administer only with 0.9% NaCl.	
	Administer slowly over 1–2 hours (based on 200-ml volume).	
Plasma	Use blood component recipient set with 170-μm filter. (Do not use leukocyte-depleting filter.)	Risk of circulatory overload.
	Administer over 1–2 hours.	Risk of transfusion-transmitted diseases.
		Anaphylaxis (IgA-deficient recipients).
		Febrile and allergic reactions.
Albumin	Undiluted 25% albumin should be administered at 1 ml/min if patient is normovolemic.	Risk of circulatory overload.
	Use administration set supplied with product.	No risk of transfusion-transmitted diseases.
	Administer as rapidly as possible for patient in hypovolemic shock or at rate prescribed.	
Factor VIII concentrate	Reconstitute with sterile diluent provided. Use only plastic syringes.	Allergic and febrile reactions are common.
	Administer IV push through filtered needle or drip through component administration set.	Heat treatment has reduced risk of transfusion-transmitted diseases.
	Rate of administration dependent on patient's response.	
Factor IX complex	Reconstitute with sterile diluent provided.	Allergic and febrile reactions possible.
	Administer intravenously through a filter.	Heat treatment has reduced risk of transfusion-transmitted diseases.
	Rate of administration dependent on patient's response and product used.	
Cryoprecipitate	Infuse within 4 hours after preparation.	Febrile and allergic reactions.
	Use component infusion set with 170-μm filter.	Transfusion-transmitted diseases.
	Administer over 30–60 minutes.	

ABO group and Rh type on the blood containers are in accordance with the compatibility record. The blood also should be checked for the presence of gas bubbles and any abnormal color or cloudiness. Gas bubbles may indicate bacterial growth, and abnormal color or cloudiness may be a sign of hemolysis. The labels identifying the number and type of the donor blood and the recipient blood are noted. Patient identification is confirmed by asking for the patient's name and by checking the identification wrist band. At the same time, the patient's chart is checked for blood type and number. Temperature, pulse, respiration, and blood pressure are measured to provide a baseline for comparing vital signs at a later time.

After the blood transfusion is started, the patient is monitored closely for 15 to 30 minutes to detect signs of reaction or circulatory overload. Monitoring vital signs is carried out at regular intervals as indicated.

Complications and Nursing Management

Every patient who receives a blood transfusion is subject to the possible development of complications of transfusion therapy. Nursing management is directed toward the prevention of these complications and prompt initiation of measures to control any complications that occur. Transfusion complications include the following:

Circulatory overload
Febrile reaction
Allergic reaction
Septic reaction
Hemolytic reaction
Delayed hemolytic reaction
Diseases transmitted by the transfusion
    (*e.g.*, hepatitis, malaria, syphilis, AIDS)

Circulatory Overload.   In patients with normal blood volume (as in chronic anemia) or increased blood volume (as in renal failure or heart failure), the addition of whole blood or packed cells can precipitate pulmonary edema. Packed red cells are safer to use; if the rate of administration is sufficiently slow, circulatory overload may be prevented.

- The signs of circulatory overload include dyspnea, orthopnea, cyanosis, or sudden anxiety. If the transfusion is continued, severe dyspnea and coughing of pink, frothy sputum can occur. Neck vein distention, crackles at the base of the lungs, and rise in central venous pressure will occur.
- The patient is placed in an upright position with the feet in a dependent position, the blood is discontinued, and the physician is notified. The intravenous line is kept patent with a *very* slow infusion of normal saline to retain access to the vein in case intravenous medications are necessary. Phlebotomy or diuretics, oxygen, morphine, and aminophylline may be necessary if improvement does not occur rapidly.

Febrile Reaction.   Patients may develop a fever during transfusion because of the presence of bacterial pyrogens, sensitivity to leukocytes or platelets, hemolytic episodes, or unknown factors. Because of the widespread use of disposable transfusion equipment, bacterial pyrogens are rarely a cause. Infrequently, blood can be grossly contaminated with large numbers of microorganisms that survive in the 4°C (39.2°F) storage. If such blood is infused, the patient develops fever and shaking chills within 30 minutes, and shock soon follows.

Even when the cause of this reaction is recognized early (by Gram stain of the donor blood), mortality is high.

As soon as the reaction is recognized, the transfusion is discontinued and the intravenous line is kept open with normal saline. The physician and blood bank are notified and the blood container is returned to the blood bank. The patient's temperature is monitored 30 minutes after the chill and as indicated thereafter. Antipyretics are administered as prescribed.

Sensitivity to leukocyte or platelet antigens is much more common, especially in previously transfused patients or women who have borne children. The temperature rises during the administration of blood or shortly afterward and may be associated with chills and malaise. This type of reaction has a good prognosis; the treatment is an antipyretic. Subsequent transfusions should use leukocyte-poor blood.

Allergic Reaction.   Some patients may develop urticaria (hives) or generalized itching or, rarely, wheezing or anaphylaxis. The cause of these reactions is thought to be sensitivity to a plasma protein in the transfused blood, or passive transfer of antibodies from the donor that react with some antigen to which the recipient is exposed. The reactions are usually mild and respond to antihistamines. If urticaria is the only symptom, the transfusion can sometimes be continued at a slower rate. If the reaction is severe, parenteral epinephrine is used. Future reactions may be prevented by premedication with antihistamines.

Septic Reaction.   Septic reactions are severe reactions that result from transfusion of blood or components contaminated with bacteria. Preventive measures include administering blood within a 4-hour period before warm room temperatures promote bacterial growth, and inspecting blood or components for gas bubbles, clotting, or abnormal color before administration. If the transfusion is contaminated, the patient will respond with rapid onset of chills, high fever, vomiting, diarrhea, and marked hypotension. In such a case the transfusion is discontinued immediately and the intravenous line kept patent with normal saline. The physician and blood bank are notified, and the blood bag is returned to the blood bank. Blood cultures are obtained, and the patient is treated for septicemia with antibiotics, IV fluids, vasopressors, and steroids.

Hemolytic Reaction.   The most dangerous type of transfusion reaction occurs when the donor blood is incompatible with that of the recipient. Antibodies in the recipient's plasma rapidly combine with donor erythrocytes, and the cells are hemolyzed either in the circulation or in the reticuloendothelial system. The most rapid hemolysis occurs in ABO incompatibility (*e.g.*, if the donor is group A and the recipient is group O, and therefore has anti-A and anti-B antibodies). Rh incompatibility is often less severe.

- Symptoms consist of chills, low back pain, headache, nausea, or chest tightness, followed by fever and hypotension and vascular collapse. Severe reactions usually start within 10 minutes after the transfusion is begun. *Hemoglobinuria* (red urine) appears at the next voiding.
- The reaction must be recognized promptly and the transfusion discontinued immediately. Severity of complications is proportional to the volume of blood infused.

Treatment is directed toward correcting the hypotension and preventing the renal damage that can follow hemoglobinuria. The patient is supported with intravenous colloid and given mannitol as an osmotic diuretic to maintain adequate urine flow, glomerular filtration, and renal blood flow. An indwelling catheter may be necessary for accurate measurement of output. If, after 24 hours, urine flow cannot be maintained, mannitol is contraindicated because it can be assumed that acute tubular necrosis has occurred. The subsequent management will be that for the renal disorder and will include fluid restriction and possibly dialysis until spontaneous healing takes place.

Delayed Hemolytic Reaction.   Delayed hemolytic reactions usually occur at about 2 to 14 days and are recognized by fever, mild jaundice, a gradual fall in hemoglobin level, and a direct anti–human globulin test. Rarely is there hemoglobinuria, and generally these reactions are not dangerous. Recognition is important, however, because subsequent transfusions may cause an acute hemolytic reaction.

Diseases Transmitted by Blood Transfusion.   The following diseases are transmissible by blood transfusion.

Hepatitis.   Hepatitis is an important risk of transfusion therapy, both for whole blood and for most components (see previous discussion). Blood and blood products obtained from paid donors carry a higher risk than those from volunteer donors. Pooled blood products also constitute a significantly higher risk. Tests are used to detect hepatitis B virus, as well as hepatitis C (formerly non-A, non-B hepatitis). Hepatitis is further discussed in Chapter 38.

Malaria.   Malaria may be transmitted in blood donated by asymptomatic persons who have been exposed to the disease. Recipients develop high fever and headache several weeks after the transfusion.

Syphilis.   Syphilis is rarely transmitted now because of the serologic tests required on all units of blood and because the organism does not survive refrigeration.

Acquired Immunodeficiency Syndrome.   AIDS has been associated with transfusion of blood products. For this reason persons who engage in high risk behaviors (*i.e.*, sex with multiple partners, anal sex, intravenous drug use, sex with persons at risk for AIDS), and persons with signs and symptoms suggestive of the disease should not donate blood. All donated blood is now tested for the presence of antibodies to the AIDS virus.

Graft-Versus-Host Disease.   Engraftment of donor lymphocytes in immunocompromised recipients could result in graft-versus-host disease. Irradiating blood products inactivates donor lymphocytes.

Gerontologic Considerations.   The elderly patient who is receiving blood products is assessed for signs of circulatory overload. Rapid infusions of large volumes can result in congestive heart failure. Nursing care should include careful assessment of cardiac and pulmonary function and monitoring of fluid intake and output.

In summary, if it is suspected that a transfusion reaction is occurring because of any of the conditions mentioned previously, the nurse should stop the transfusion and notify the physician immediately. The following steps are taken so that a diagnosis may be made regarding the type and severity of the reaction:

- The transfusion set is disconnected, but the intravenous line is kept open with a saline solution in case intravenous medication should be needed rapidly.
- The *blood container and tubing are saved, not discarded.* They should be sent to the blood bank for repeat typing and culture.

- The patient's blood is drawn for plasma hemoglobin, culture, and retyping.
- A urine sample is collected as soon as possible and sent to the laboratory for a hemoglobin determination. Subsequent voidings of urine should be observed.
- The blood bank is notified that a suspected transfusion reaction has occurred.

Bone Marrow Transplantation

Bone marrow transplantation is an exciting addition to the therapeutic possibilities for hematologic disease. Bone marrow can be aspirated by needle from multiple sites of an anesthetized normal donor and easily transfused intravenously into the recipient. The marrow cells immediately travel to the marrow spaces that have been emptied by disease (*i.e.*, aplastic anemia) or by chemotherapy. The goal is for donor cells to proliferate in the marrow, releasing functional cells into the peripheral circulation. Complete marrow recovery may take 6 to 8 weeks.

The major barrier to the success of bone marrow transplantation is the antigenic difference between donor and recipient. Engraftment depends on the degree of tissue compatibility. Sources of donor cells are autologous or self; syngeneic (possessing identical genotypes) or a genetically identical twin; and allogeneic, where the donor is HLA compatible or histocompatible but may or may not be related to the recipient.

Recipients usually have pretransplant preparation. Depending on disease state and degree of immunologic compatibility, this preparation can consist of high-dose chemotherapy and sometimes total body irradiation to rid the marrow of malignant cells and suppress the immune system to avoid graft rejection. Many recipients succumb to graft-versus-host disease or severe infections while awaiting the recovery of the transplanted marrow. These complications increase with the age of the recipient. Patients over the age of 40 are usually not candidates for bone marrow transplantation. Methods of immunosuppression and supportive care have improved greatly over the last few years, however, and this is currently the best treatment for severe aplastic anemia. Bone marrow transplantation is also used to treat some forms of leukemia and thalassemia.

In summary, bone marrow transplantation is a therapeutic possibility for some patients with hematologic disorders, specifically severe aplastic anemia, some forms of leukemia, and thalassemia. Success depends on tissue compatibility and the patient's tolerance of immunosuppression. Research continues in this area; the goals are to overcome the complications of immunosuppression and to be able to offer bone marrow transplantation to more patients with hematologic disease.

Bibliography

Books

Babior BM and Stossel T. Hematology: A Pathophysiological Approach. New York, Churchill Livingstone, 1990.

Brain M and Carbone P. Current Therapy in Hematology–Oncology–3. Philadelphia, BC Decker, 1988.

Braunwald E et al (ed). Harrison's Principles of Internal Medicine. New York, McGraw–Hill, 1987.

Burns E. Clinical Management of Bleeding and Thrombosis. Boston Blackwell Scientific Publications, 1987.

Corriveau DM and Fritsona GA. Hemostasis and Thrombosis in the Clinical Laboratory. Philadelphia, JB Lippincott, 1988.

Fairbanks VF. Current Hematology and Oncology. Chicago, Yearbook Medical Publishers, 1988.

Goldberg K (ed). Nurse Review: Hematologic Problems. Springhouse, PA, Springhouse, 1990.

Mentzer WC (ed), Wagner GM. The Hereditary Hemolytic Anemias. New York, Churchill Livingstone, 1990.

Petz ZD and Swisher SN (ed). Clinical Practice of Transfusion Medicine. New York, Churchill Livingstone, 1989.

Powers LW. Diagnostic Hematology: Clinical and Technical Principles. St Louis, CV Mosby, 1989.

Rapaport S. Introduction to Hematology, Philadelphia, JB Lippincott, 1987.

Shahidi N (ed). Aplastic Anemia and Other Bone Marrow Failure Syndromes. New York, Springer–Verlag, 1990.

Turgeon M. Fundamentals of Immunohematology: Theory and Technique. Philadelphia, Lea & Febiger, 1989.

William WJ et al. Hematology. New York, McGraw-Hill, 1983.

Journals

Asterisks indicate nursing research articles.

General

Anderson GP. A fresh look at assessing the elderly. RN 1989 Jun; 52(6): 28–40.

Baldwin JG. True anemia: Incidence and significance in the elderly. Geriatrics 1989 Aug; 44(8): 33–36.

Brandt B. Nursing protocol for the patient with neutropenia. Oncol Nurs Forum 1988 Jan/Feb; 17(1 suppl): 9–15.

Chanarin I. How to diagnose (and not misdiagnose) pernicious anaemia. Blood Rev 1987 Dec; 1(4): 280–283.

Cattopadhyay B. Splenectomy, pneumococcal vaccination and antibiotic therapy. Br J Hosp Med 1989 Feb; 41(2): 172–174.

Farrant C. Multiple myeloma: Controlling pain, prolonging survival. RN 1987 Jan; 50(1): 38–42.

Gibson J. Autoimmune hemolytic anemia: Current concepts. Australian N Z J Med 1988 Jun; 18(4): 625–637.

Herring WB et al. When the hematocrit rises. Patient Care 1989 Aug; 23(13): 176–191.

Konradi D and Stockart P. A close-up look at leukemia. Nursing 1989 Jun; 19(6): 34–42.

Krause JR. The bone marrow in nutritional deficiencies. Hematol/Oncol Clin North Am 1988 Dec; 2(4): 557–566.

Maguire–Eisen M. Diagnoses and treatment of adult acute leukemia. Semin Oncol Nurs 1990 Feb; 6(1): 17–24.

May A and Choiseul M. Sickle cell anaemia and thalassemia: Symptoms, treatment and effects on lifestyle. Health Visitor 1988 Jul; 61(7): 212–215.

Morse M. Lymphoma: History, therapy and management of effects. J Assoc Pediatr Oncol Nurses 1989 Jan; 6(2): 19–20.

Ohee–Frempong K et al. Thalassemia syndromes: Recent advances. Hematol Oncol Clin North Am 1987 Sep; 1(3): 503–519.

Nibbon AC. Infection in the neutropenic patient. Semin Oncol Nurs 1990 Feb; 6(1): 50–60.

Pizzo PA. Combating infections in neutropenia patients. Hosp Pract 1989 Jul; 24(7): 93–110.

Rudolf VM. Oncology nursing protocols: A step toward autonomy. Oncol Nurs Forum 1989 Sep/Oct; 16(5): 643–647.

Scultz BM and Freedman M. Iron deficiency in the elderly. Baillieres Clin Haematol 1987 Jun; 1(2): 291–313.

Yardley J. Multiple myeloma. Nursing (Lond) 1989 Aug; 3(40): 4–7.

Walker CL. Stress and coping in siblings of childhood cancer patients. Nurs Res 1988 Jul/Aug; 37(4): 208–212.

Anemia

Beer J. Treatment of anaemia in chronic renal failure. Nurs Times 1988 Nov; 84(47): 55–57.

Dallman PR. Iron deficiency: Does it matter? J Intern Med 1989 Nov; 26(5): 367–372.

Farley PC and Foland J. Iron deficiency anemia: How to diagnose and correct. Post Grad Med 1990 Feb; 87(2): 89–101.

Frosberg JH. The anemias: Causes and courses of action. RN 1987 Jan; 52(1): 24–30.

Katsanes E and Ramsay NKC. Treatment of acquired severe aplastic anemia. Am J Pediatr Hematol Oncol 1989 Jan; 17(3): 360–367.

Marmont AM and Bacigaluo A. Aplastic anemia: Pathogenesis and treatment. Hematologica 1988 Apr; (73): 133–41.

Millman JA and Cerchio M. Caring for the aplastic patient at home: A practical guide. Caring 1988 Jan; 7(1): 28–41.

Patten E. Immunohematologic diseases. JAMA 1987 Nov; 258(20): 2945–2951.

Waterworth S. Management of anaemia. Nursing (Lond) 1989 Aug; 3(40): 12–15.

Wheby MS. Sizing up the seriousness of anemia. Emerg Med 1989 Aug; 21(14): 179–192.

Bleeding Disorders

Beris P and Mieschen P. Hematological complications of antiinfectious agents. Semin Hematol 1988 Apr; 25(2): 123–139.

Best Tests for Bleeding Disorders. Emerg Med 1989 Apr; 21(8): 150–161.

Coffin C. Potentially catastrophic bleeding disorders. Postgrad Med 1989 Sep 1; 86(3): 217–225.

Copplestone JA. Bleeding and coagulation disorders in the elderly. Baillieres Clin Haematol 1987 Jun; 1(2): 559–580.

Diethorn ML and Weld ZM. Physiologic mechanisms of hemostasis and fibrinolysis. Cardiovasc Nurs 1989 Nov; 4(1): 1–10.

Griffin JP. Be prepared for the bleeding patient. Nursing 1986 Jun; 16(6): 34–40.

Steed D et al. Surgery on the hemophiliac patient. AORN 1987 Jun; 45(6): 1412–1417.

Bone Marrow Transplantation

* Abramovitz L. Nurses' attitudes in caring for the pediatric bone marrow transplant patient. J Assoc Pediatr Oncol Nurses 1987 Jan; 4(1–2): 39.

Bater M. Preparing for bone marrow transplantation. Nursing Times 1989 Feb; 85(7): 46–47.

Buchsel P and Kelleher J. Bone marrow transplantation. Nurs Clin North Am 1989 Dec; 24(4): 907–934.

Ford R and Ballard B. Acute complications after bone marrow transplantation. Semin Oncol Nurs 1988 Feb; 4(1): 15–24.

Kelleher J and Jennings M. Nursing management of a marrow transplant unit: A framework for practice. Semin Oncol Nurs 1988 Feb; 4(1): 60–68.

Ramsay NK. Bone marrow transplantation. Transaction of the Association of Life Insurance Medical Directors of America 1988; 71: 162–173.

* Stutzer C. Work related stresses of pediatric bone marrow transplant nurses. J Pediatr Oncol Nurs 1989 Jul; 6(3): 70–78.

Wikle T et al. Bone marrow transplant today and tomorrow. Am J Nurs 1990 May; 90(5): 48–58.

Disseminated Intravascular Coagulation

Bick RL. Disseminated intravascular coagulation and related syndromes. Seminars Thromb Hemost 1988 Oct; 14(4): 299–338.

Carr ME. Disseminated intravascular coagulation: Pathogenesis, diagnosis, and therapy. J Emerg Med 1987 Jul/Aug; 5(4): 311–322.

Feinstein DI. Treatment of disseminated intravascular coagulation. Semin Thromb Hemost 1988 Oct; 14(4): 351–365.

Gregory SA et al. Hematologic emergencies. Med Clin North Am 1986 Sep; 70(5): 1129–1149.

Happ M. Life threatening hemorrhage in children with cancer. J Assoc Pediatr Oncol Nurses 1987 Jul; 4(3): 36–40.

Suchak BA and Barbon CB. Disseminated intravascular coagulation: A nursing challenge. Orthop Nurs 1989 Nov/Dec; 8(6): 61–9.

Young LM. DIC: The insidious killer. Crit Care Nurse 1990 Nov/Dec; 10(10): 26–33.

Sickle Cell Anemia

Davies SC and Brosovic M. The presentation, management and prophylaxis of sickle cell disease. Blood Rev 1989 Mar; 3(1): 29–44.

Galloway SJ and Harwood-Nuss AL. Sickle cell anemia—A review. J Emerg Med 1988 May/Jun; 6(3): 213–226.

Platt AF et al. The multidisciplinary management of pain in patients with sickle cell syndrome. J Acad Physician Assistants 1989 Mar/Apr; 2(2): 104–113.

Rivers R and Williamson N. Sickle cell anemia complex disease: Nursing challenge. RN 1990 Jun; 52(1): 24–29.

Smith JA. The natural history of sickle cell disease. Ann NY Acad Sci 1989 Jul; 565: 104–108.

Transfusion Therapy

Alter HJ et al. Detection of antibody to hepatitis C virus in prospectively followed transfusion recipients with acute and chronic non-A, non-B hepatitis. N Eng J Med 1989 Nov 30; 321: 1494–1500.

Blood transfusion: The state of the art. Emerg Med 1988 Nov; 20(20): 180–190.

Bonato J. Blood transfusions: Are they safe? Crit Care Nurs 1989 Jul/Aug; 9(7): 40–46.

Butler S. Current trends in autologous transfusion. RN 1989 Nov; 52(11): 44–55.

Hahn K. Monitoring a blood transfusion. Nursing 1989 Oct; 19(10): 20–21.

Kuo G et al. An assay for circulating anti-bodies to a major etiologic virus of human non-A, non-B hepatitis. Science 1989 Apr; 244: 362–364.

Litwack K. Practical points for transfusion therapy. J Post Anesthesia Nurs 1987 Nov; 11(4): 257–261.

Miller JA. Transfusion of blood and blood products. Prof Nurse 1989 Aug; 4(11): 560–565.

The latest protocols for blood transfusions. Committee on Transfusion Practices. American Association of Blood Banks. Nursing 1986 Oct; 16(10): 34–41.

Information/Resources

Government Agencies

National Heart, Lung and Blood Institute
National Institutes of Health, Building 31, Room 5A52, Bethesda, MD 29892

Voluntary Agencies

American Cancer Society
19 West 56 Street, New York, NY 10019

American Red Cross
1730 E Street NW, Washington, DC 20006

Leukemia Society of America
733 Third Avenue, New York, NY 10017

National Association for Sickle Cell Disease, Inc.
4221 Wilshire Boulevard, Suite 360, Los Angeles, CA 90010-3503

National Hemophilia Foundation
104 East 40th Street, Room 306, New York, NY 10016

Nursing Research Profile for Unit 7

Cardiovascular Nursing

Overview

In recent years, there have been increasing efforts among nursing researchers to study the needs of patients who have medical and surgical problems related to cardiovascular dysfunctions. Patient populations that have been studied most frequently are those who have experienced myocardial infarctions, those with hypertension, and those who have had cardiac surgery. Researchers have investigated the physiologic responses of these patients as well as the educational needs and coping abilities of patients and their families. Results of these studies have important nursing implications and indicate areas where further nursing research is needed.

Physiologic Assessment and Responses

▷ Byra-Cook CJ, Dracup KA, and Lazik AJ. Direct and indirect blood pressure in critical care patients. Nurs Res 1990 Sep/Oct; 39(5):285–288.

Various recommendations have been made about the methods to be used to auscultate blood pressure. Some authors have recommended use of the bell end of the stethoscope, some have recommended the diaphragm, and some have claimed that either listening device is accurate. In addition, some authors claim that the site of the antecubital fossa is most appropriate for blood pressure auscultation, while others claim that the area of the arm immediately superior to the internal medial condyle and medial to the biceps tendon (hereafter referred to as the upper arm) is the most appropriate site. This array of recommendations has resulted in inconsistent auscultation techniques in clinical practice. Thus, the purpose of this study was to determine whether the listening device and the site of auscultation affected the correlation between direct and indirect blood pressure readings. The assumption was made that direct blood pressure readings reflect the true value of the blood pressure.

A convenience sample of 50 critical care patients was studied. All subjects had indwelling radial arterial lines, audible Korotkoff sounds, arm circumferences of 25 to 35 cm, and regular sinus rhythms. Patients who were excluded were those with mechanical ventilators and intra-aortic balloon pumps and those who had trauma to or previous vascular surgery on the arm from which blood pressures were being assessed. Patients receiving vasoactive intravenous medications were excluded

if the dosage rate had been adjusted within 30 minutes of the pressure measurement.

Simultaneous blood pressure measurements were made in the same arm with use of the arterial line and auscultated readings. Three systolic and three diastolic pressure readings were obtained from each of the four auscultation techniques: bell/antecubital fossa, diaphragm/antecubital fossa, bell/upper arm, and diaphragm/upper arm. To obtain as close to simultaneous readings as possible, the auscultated readings started immediately after the direct arterial digital display changed. A 2-minute time period with the blood pressure cuff released from the arm elapsed between measurements.

The findings revealed positive correlations of systolic and diastolic blood pressure of each auscultation technique with direct measurements of systolic and diastolic pressures. However, auscultation with the diaphragm of the stethoscope over the brachial artery in the upper arm revealed the highest overall correlation between direct and indirect measurements for both systolic and diastolic pressures. Auscultation at this site with the diaphragm of the stethoscope also revealed the least mean difference between systolic and diastolic direct and indirect pressures overall.

Nursing Implications. (1) Further studies are required to confirm the findings of this study. However, in the critical care setting where small variations in blood pressure may be critical to appropriate therapeutic interventions, the nurse should be aware that differences in blood pressure readings may occur based on the technique by which blood pressures are auscultated. (2) To provide consistency of blood pressure measurements for patients, documentation should include the site and the method of measurement used. (3) Further studies are needed to identify additional factors (e.g., peripheral vascular disease, vasoactive medications) that may affect direct and indirect blood pressure measurements.

▷ Hahn W, Brooks J, and Hite R. Blood pressure norms for healthy young adults: Relation to sex, age, and reported parental hypertension. Res Nurs Health 1989 Feb; 12(1): 53–56.

The purpose of this study was to present normative blood pressure findings for white, healthy, normotensive young adults as a function of age, sex, and history of hypertension in one or both parents. Free blood pressure monitoring and health information were provided to students at a large midwestern university who participated in the study on a self-referral, walk-in basis. The 603 women and 919 men participating were between the ages of 18 and 22 years; were nonsmokers; were free of cancer, diabetes, kidney problems, heart disease, and stroke; and were not taking any medication with the exception of oral contraceptives. The subjects were asked to indicate if they had a positive family history for hypertension. Each person completed a questionnaire before having two sitting, resting blood pressure measurements taken on their right arms with an appropriate-size cuff. The average of the two measurements was used in the study analyses.

The findings showed that, among males, a parental history of hypertension (N = 306) was not related to the screening systolic or diastolic blood pressure. Additional analysis revealed a significant age effect, demonstrating that diastolic blood pressure increases with age for the age group studied. For women with histories of parental hypertension (N = 246), systolic blood pressure (mean, 107.4) and diastolic blood pressure (mean, 68.3) were higher than those for women without histories of parental hypertension (mean systolic, 105.5; mean diastolic, 66.6). Although these differences were slight, they were statistically significant. Women with two hypertensive parents had higher systolic blood pressures than did women with one hypertensive parent. Confounding the data collected for the female group was the use of oral contraceptives. Thirty-one percent of women with parental histories of hypertension were taking oral contraceptives as compared with 14% of the women without such parental histories.

Nursing Implications. (1) The report of parental hypertension by the normotensive young male and screening blood pressure measurements may be insufficient to detect normotensive males who are at risk for developing hypertension. (2) Diastolic blood pressure increases with age in healthy young men; thus, it is important to determine age when checking the blood pressure of young men. (3) The report of a parental history of hypertension by healthy young women is associated with higher levels of resting systolic and diastolic blood pressure; these higher levels may be associated with the use of oral contraceptives.

▷ *Thomas SA and Friedman E. Type of behavior and cardiovascular responses during verbalization in cardiac patients. Nurs Res 1990 Jan/Feb; 39(1):48–53.*

This study sought to determine whether physiologic mechanisms can be identified that link type A behavior patterns with an increased risk of coronary heart disease. Individuals described as having type A behavior patterns are believed to experience coronary heart disease more frequently than other individuals in the general population.

The study included two steps. First, patients were tested to determine their behavior pattern, type A versus type B. They were then monitored noninvasively for heart rate and blood pressure while reading quietly and then while verbalizing in a minimally stressful setting. The study population consisted of 111 cardiac patients (78 with a diagnosis of coronary heart disease and 33 with a diagnosis of hypertension) recruited from a cardiology clinic.

The objective data showed significant increases in blood pressure and heart rate in all subjects during verbalization. The study did not substantiate that patients with type A behavior patterns had any more adverse physiologic responses than any other patients in the study. The results of this study were consistent with previous studies. Responses under stressful circumstances were not measured.

Nursing Implications. (1) Rest and freedom from unnecessary verbalization are suggested for all patients experiencing coronary heart disease, regardless of behavior pattern. (2) Behavior pattern may not be a legitimate risk factor for developing coronary heart disease—further studies are needed. (3) Heart rate and blood pressure are sensitive indicators for measuring the body's response to verbal stimulation.

▷ *Freed CD et al. Blood pressure, heart rate, and heart rhythm changes in patients with heart disease during talking. Heart Lung 1989 Jan; 18(1):17–22.*

This study was designed with a twofold purpose: to determine the effects of low-affect (nonemotional) talking on blood pressure, heart rate, and cardiac rhythm of patients with coronary heart disease and to identify whether or not the response to talking is decreased by therapeutic doses of antihypertensive medications. The study population consisted of 37 adult volunteers who had been referred to a cardiac exercise laboratory for exercise ECG diagnostic examinations. All of the subjects had cardiac disease that had been documented by angiography. The study was conducted prior to the patients' exercise stress test procedures.

The study protocol consisted of a 6-minute period of time during which the subjects stood silently for 2 minutes, talked about their daily activities for 2 minutes, and then stood quietly again for 2 minutes. Blood pressure, heart rate, and heart rhythm were measured automatically and recorded each minute for the 6 consecutive minutes. Each subject was tested individually with only the experimenter present with the subject in the laboratory.

Systolic and diastolic blood pressures and heart rate were significantly higher while the patients were talking than while they stood silent. Larger blood pressure increases while talking were associated with higher resting blood pressure levels. Older patients manifested significantly greater systolic pressure increases during talking than did younger patients. For all patients, ventricular and atrial dysrhythmias were more frequent during talking than during quiet periods. Heart rate and blood pressure increases during talking were not blocked by therapeutic doses of antihypertensive medications. There were no significant differences related to sex.

Nursing Implications. (1) Changes in cardiovascular function during speech should be monitored for patients who have had myocardial infarction. This is particularly important relative to evidence that suggests a higher risk of sudden death among patients with cardiac disease who have ventricular ectopy. (2) Patients who have had myocardial infarctions should be taught to slow their rate of speech and to increase their periods of quiet relaxation during the recovery phase of their illness. (3) Careful consideration should be given to the interpersonal aspects of the lives of patients with cardiac disease.

Education and Support/Coping Needs

▷ *Anderson KO and Massur FT. Psychologic preparation for cardiac catheterization. Heart Lung 1989 Mar; 18(2):154–163.*

Cardiac catheterization, an invasive procedure that is known to be anxiety-producing, is performed on more than 500,000 patients yearly. Thus, it is important to identify ways to reduce or prevent anxiety in this group of patients. The purpose of this study was to identify the effectiveness of four psychologic preparatory strategies in reducing anxiety and enhancing adaptation during cardiac catheterization and to compare the effectiveness of these strategies to that of an attention placebo control intervention. The four psychologic preparatory strategies were as follows: sensory-procedural information, modeling, cognitive-behavioral coping skills, and modeling plus coping skills. Modeling was achieved through an audiovisual program that depicted a patient model who successfully underwent the steps of cardiac catheterization. The four experimental interventions and the control intervention were presented via audiovisual tapes.

The study population consisted of 60 patients who were undergoing their first cardiac catheterizations. The catheterizations were all performed by the same cardiologist. Each subject was randomly assigned to one of the four study interventions or to the control group. Prior to the intervention, the subjects completed a questionnaire that was designed to assess levels of anxiety, depression, and perceived ability to cope with the diagnostic procedure; they also completed an Adjective Check List (ACL) designed to measure depression, and the Palmar Sweat Index (PSI) was administered as a psychophysiologic indicator of anxiety. Following the interventions (provided one day precatheterization), the subjects completed a short test that measured retention of information about cardiac catheterization; the ACL and PSI were readministered. On the day of the catheterization, the subjects received no psychotropic medications. The cardiac catheterization nurse assessed the presence and intensity of anxiety-related behaviors as well as each patient's PSI before the cardiac catheterization. Immediately after this procedure, the nurse and the cardiologist (both of whom were blind to experimental conditions) rated the presence of anxiety-related behaviors and the extent to which the patient had followed instructions, moved around unnecessarily, and appeared anxious during the test. Each subject was asked to rate the levels of anxiety, depression, and coping ability experienced during the cardiac catheterization. Within 1 to 6 hours after the procedure, the subjects were again asked to rate the levels; in addition, the ACL and PSI were readministered, and the patients completed questionnaires about the information that they had received about the cardiac catheterization.

The findings of the study revealed that subjects who received the experimental interventions had lower levels of physiologic arousal during the cardiac catheterization and reported less anxiety after the procedure than did the subjects of the control group. Of the experimental preparatory strategies, the modeling strategy and the modeling plus coping skills strategies were the most effective. Subjects who received these two strategies demonstrated fewer anxiety-related behaviors and reported less anxiety and greater coping abilities.

Nursing Implications. (1) Psychologic preparation for cardiac catheterization is essential to decrease the anxiety that accompanies this invasive procedure. (2) The format and style of the preparatory information are important factors in positively influencing the patient's ability to cope with and adapt to the conditions of the catheterization. The use of a patient model (*i.e.*, a patient who has had a positive experience with the same procedure) is highly effective in decreasing anxiety and enhancing coping abilities.

▷ *Dunnington CS et al. Patients with heart rhythm disturbances: Variables associated with increased psychologic stress. Heart Lung 1988 Jul; 17(4):381–389.*

Patients experiencing and surviving malignant dysrhythmias (heart rhythm disturbances) are returned to the community following hospitalizations that involved numerous diagnostic studies and therapeutic procedures. This study examined the variables associated with psychologic distress following episodes of hospitalization for heart rhythm disturbances (HRD).

One hundred thirty-six patients with major HRDs (*i.e.*, ventricular tachycardia, fibrillation) unrelated to acute myocardial infarction were selected. Seventy-seven percent (N = 105) completed questionnaires designed to measure psychologic status, functional capacity, and occupational status.

Patients with HRDs demonstrated a high level of overall psychologic distress. This high level of distress was significantly correlated with long-term medication treatment, the need to modify work status, and advanced cardiac impairment. Patients who received long-term antidysrhythmic treatment had a higher distress level than did patients who received surgical treatment. Patients whose work status was curtailed had higher levels of distress than did patients who were allowed to continue work activity. Finally, patients who had a lower functional capacity were most distressed.

Nursing Implications. (1) Nurses must recognize the potential for psychologic distress in patients with heart rhythm disturbances. (2) Early involvement in a cardiac rehabilitation program may facilitate a sense of well-being because it focuses on what the patient can do as opposed to what he cannot do. (3) Individualization of support programs is imperative as patients leave the hospital to return to their family and community roles. (4) Vocational counseling may be appropriate for patients who must make job changes.

▷ *Garding BS, Kerr JC, and Bay K. Effectiveness of a program of information and support for myocardial infarction patients recovering at home. Heart Lung 1988 Jul; 17(4):355–362.*

This study addressed the important issue of patient education—specifically *when* information is best received by the patient. With the use of an experimental design for the study, 51 patients were randomly assigned to a control or experimental group. Predischarge teaching occurred for all participants, and they were then interviewed with a pretest based on the criterion measures of nursing care developed by Horn and Swain. The criteria included health knowledge and ability to perform self-care. The experimental group was followed postdischarge over 6 to 8 weeks by phone calls (at least three calls each) to clarify or reteach previously taught information. All study participants were then retested.

The results of the study substantiated higher post-test mean scores for the experimental group than for the control group in all content areas. The experimental group acquired a higher level of knowledge in the 6 to 8 weeks following discharge.

Nursing Implications. (1) Structured patient education programs may be minimally effective during hospitalization for acute illness. (2) Structured patient education programs may be more appropriate during the convalescent period. (3) Verbal communication and teaching via telephone can be considered reasonable supplements to traditional nurse–patient face-to-face teaching.

▷ *Nakagawa-Kogan H et al. Self-management of hypertension: Predictors of success in diastolic blood pressure reduction. Res Nurs Health 1988 Apr; 11(2):105–115.*

Thirty-four white, unmedicated, borderline hypertensive men were studied to determine which ones were most likely to succeed in self-management training. The purpose of the study was threefold: to test the effectiveness of self-management training for the acquisition of blood pressure self-regulation; to examine the cognitive/affective changes during self-management training; and to determine physiologic and psychologic entry characteristics that would be predictive of success in biofeedback training.

Borderline hypertensive subjects, ranging in age from 31

to 54 years (mean, 40 years), were accepted into the study if two of three diastolic blood pressure readings, taken on three separate days in a 2-week period of time, were between 90 and 105 mm Hg. The subjects completed a 90-item symptom checklist that was scored on nine subscales for psychologic distress. Self-management training consisted of 14 sessions of biofeedback, relaxation training, and cognitive/affective restructuring.

Subjects were classified into the success category, exit-normotensive, if the diastolic blood pressure was below 90 mm Hg at exit from the training program (N = 22). The remaining subjects were considered exit-hypertensive. Analysis of the symptoms checklist demonstrated that there were major reductions in all nine subscales of distress for both groups. Only the reduction on the anxiety subscale was statistically significant for the exit-normotensive group. The only subscale that was significantly reduced for the exit-hypertensive group was the hostility subscale. Comparison of the two groups showed that they began treatment at very different psychologic distress levels, with the exit-hypertensive group in more distress at entry than the exit-normotensive group. The physiologic parameters of the exit-normotensive group indicated reduced sympathetic arousal with an increase in heart rate and a decrease in systolic blood pressure.

Nursing Implications. (1) Cognitive/affective distress must be managed before self-management training can be used to control blood pressure. (2) High levels of distress limit the benefit of a short course of biofeedback training. (3) Psychologic distress in the form of anger and hostility is associated with elevated levels of systolic blood pressure. (4) Sympathetic activity influences cardiovascular activity in borderline hypertensive subjects.

▷ *Miller KM and Perry PA. Relaxation technique and postoperative pain in patients undergoing cardiac surgery. Heart Lung 1990 Mar; 19(2):136–146.*

The purpose of this study was to determine the effectiveness of a slow, deep-breathing relaxation technique in managing pain following coronary artery bypass graft surgery (CABG). A convenience sample of 29 subjects was studied. These patients ranged in age from 61 to 80 years, had not previously undergone CABG, did not have chronic pain or a diagnosis of cancer, and did not experience preoperative or postoperative complications.

Fifteen subjects were assigned to the experimental group; they received instructions for the slow, rhythmic, deep-breathing relaxation technique in addition to routine preoperative teaching and conversation. Fourteen subjects were assigned to the control group; they received only routine preoperative instructions and conversation. On the first postoperative day, the subjects completed two visual pain rating scales—a visual analog scale and a visual descriptor. In addition, the researchers collected chart information regarding blood pressure, heart rate, and respiratory rate.

Analysis of the data revealed significant decreases in blood pressure, heart rate, respiratory rate, and report of pain on the visual descriptor scale for the experimental group; there was either no change or an increase in each of the variables for the control group. No significant differences were found in the subjects' use of analgesics or visual analog scale scores. Most of the subjects in the experimental group reported that the relaxation technique was helpful in pain management and was simple to perform.

Nursing Implications. (1) Postoperative CABG pain reduction can be enhanced by supplementing analgesic medication with a slow, rhythmic, deep-breathing relaxation technique. (2) The relaxation technique is effective in decreasing blood pressure, heart rate, and respiratory rate after CABG. (3) Patients who learn the relaxation technique preoperatively find that it is simple to perform following CABG.

▷ *Penckofer S and Llewellyn J. Adherence to risk-factor instruction one year following coronary artery bypass surgery. J Cardiovasc Nurs 1989 May; 3(3):10–24.*

This study reports the results of follow-up data collected from patients 6 weeks and 1 year after elective CABG. The study was designed to measure the effectiveness of a structured discharge teaching guide used by nurses to educate patients and their families about the normal postoperative course that follows CABG and about risk factor modification. A convenience sample (N = 60) of two comparable groups was studied. One group received routine unstructured discharge teaching. The other group received structured teaching with the use of the written teaching guide. A test composed of 35 multiple-choice and true/false items was used to measure knowledge; an interview guide made up of both structured and open-ended questions was used to collect data about modification of the following risk factors: diet, exercise, smoking, obesity, and hypertension.

Before discharge, both groups demonstrated an increase in knowledge over the preteaching knowledge level. Six weeks after surgery, both groups reported an increase in adherence to risk factor modification instructions, with no differences between the groups. One year postsurgery there remained few significant differences between patients who received structured teaching and those who received routine unstructured teaching. Both groups reported improved well-being at 1 year, and most expressed satisfaction with the surgical outcomes. Most who were employed before surgery had returned to their previous jobs.

Nursing Implications. (1) Discharge teaching, whether structured or unstructured, appears to promote positive patient outcomes 1 year after CABG. (2) As the length of hospital stay following CABG decreases, there is a need to identify the information that is essential for patients to learn before discharge; this information should then be included in discharge instructions for all patients who have had CABG surgery. (3) Discharge information that cannot be taught prior to discharge can be presented to the patient and his family/significant others following discharge; for example, information about risk factor modification can be presented during the patient's follow-up visits to his health care provider.

▷ *Cronin SN and Harrison B. Importance of nurse caring behaviors as perceived by patients after myocardial infarction. Heart Lung 1988 July; 17(4):374–380.*

Caring is often defined as a foundational concept of nursing. Few studies have defined how caring behaviors are manifested in nursing practice. Cronin and Harrison studied 22 patients hospitalized with myocardial infarction in a coronary care unit to determine their perceptions of the caring behaviors of nurses. The subjects responded to open-ended questions and to the Caring Behaviors Assessment (CBA), an instrument designed to measure patients' perceptions of the degree to which nursing behaviors communicate caring.

The nursing behaviors that patients defined as being most indicative of caring were monitoring of patient condition (assessment) and demonstration of professional competence. The caring behaviors that ranked highest on the CBA were those that involved assistance with human needs (physical care). Teaching needs were also perceived as important. Less important to the patient were the qualitative, individualized aspects of care that nurses often espouse, such as visiting the patient when he is transferred to another unit or asking the patient how he would like to be addressed.

Nursing Implications. (1) Physical and safety needs are appropriately assigned the highest priority in planning care. (2) Nurses working in critical care units must be aware that patients view nurses' assessment activities and demonstration of clinical competence as caring behaviors.

▷ Badger JM *and* Morris PLP. *Observations of a support group for automatic implantable cardioverter-defibrillator recipients and their spouses. Heart Lung 1989 May; 18(3):238–243.*

The effectiveness of the implantable cardioverter-defibrillator has led to increasing numbers of individuals with this device implanted. Patients with this device have experienced a variety of symptoms of adjustment. The purpose of this study was to use group dynamics as a therapeutic intervention and then to determine the effects of the intervention on the patient and family.

Two groups of six patients each participated in the study. One group participated in an 8-week program that met once weekly; the other group did not meet and served as a contrast group. Each session had a defined agenda, and patients were accompanied by a family member. The patients were tested for the effect of therapy on role function and psychologic adjustment. They were tested before and after the 8-week program. For both areas tested, scores for the treatment group improved, although the scores were not statistically significant. The mean scores for the contrast group declined slightly.

Although the sample size is small and scientific rigor can be questioned, the study does demonstrate that there may be merit in group therapy sessions as a means of aiding adjustment to the implantable cardioverter-defibrillator.

Nursing Implications. Support groups for patients with implantable cardioverter-defibrillators may be helpful in promoting role function and psychologic adjustment to this therapeutic modality.

unit 8

Digestive and Gastrointestinal Function

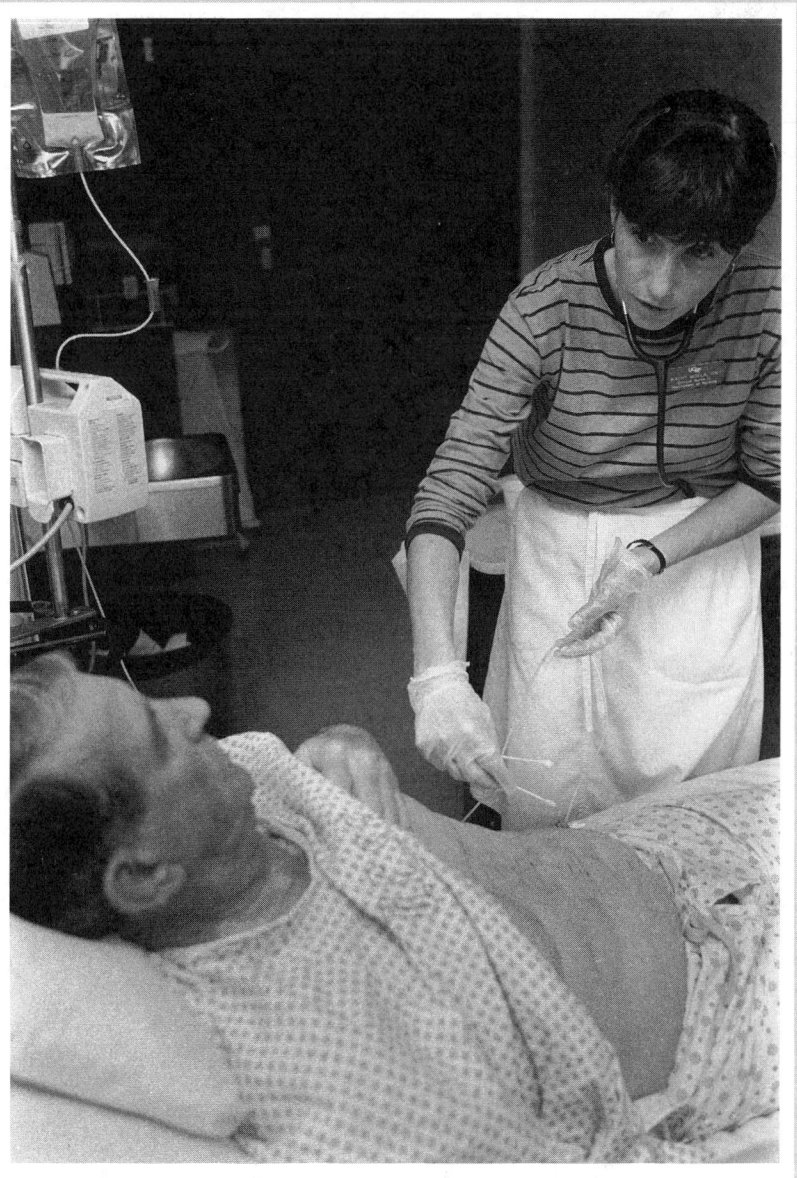

33

Assessment of Digestive and Gastrointestinal Function

Learning Objectives

On completion of this chapter, the learner will be able to:

1. Specify the mechanical and chemical processes involved in digestion and absorption of foods and elimination of waste products

2. Describe the patient preparation, teaching, and follow-up care appropriate for patients having diagnostic testing of the gastrointestinal tract

3. Use assessment parameters appropriate for determining the status of gastrointestinal function

Physiologic Overview

Anatomy of the Gastrointestinal Tract

The gastrointestinal tract is a tube that is continuous with the external environment at both ends. The pathway (23 to 26 feet in total length) extends from the mouth through the esophagus, stomach, and intestines to the anus. The *esophagus* is located in the mediastinum in the thoracic cavity, anterior to the spine and posterior to the trachea and heart. It is a collapsible tube about 25 cm (10 inches) in length that becomes distended when food passes through it.

The *stomach* is situated in the upper portion of the abdomen to the left of the midline, just under the left diaphragm. It is a distensible pouch with a capacity of approximately 1500 ml. The inlet to the stomach is called the *esophagogastric*

junction. It is surrounded by a ring of smooth muscle, called the lower esophageal sphincter (or cardiac sphincter), which, on contraction, closes the stomach from the esophagus. The outlet from the stomach is called the *pylorus.* Circular smooth muscle in the wall of the pylorus forms the *pyloric sphincter* and controls the size of the opening between the stomach and small intestine.

The *small intestine* is the longest segment of the gastrointestinal tract and accounts for about two thirds of the total length. It is folded back and forth on itself and occupies a major portion of the abdominal cavity. It is divided into three parts: an upper part, called the *duodenum;* the middle part, called the *jejunum;* and the lower part, called the *ileum.* The common bile duct, the conduit for both bile and pancreatic secretions, empties into the duodenum.

The junction between the small and large intestines usually lies in the right lower portion of the abdomen. It is in this area that the vermiform *appendix* is located. At the junction of the small and large intestines is the *ileocecal valve*, which functions in a similar fashion to the pyloric and esophageal sphincters. The *large intestine* consists of an *ascending* segment on the right side of the abdomen, a *transverse* segment that extends from right to left in the upper abdomen, and a *descending* segment on the left side of the abdomen. The terminal portion of the large intestine is the *rectum*, which is continuous with the *anus*. The anal outlet is surrounded by the external anal sphincter, which, unlike the other sphincters of the gastrointestinal tract, is composed of striated muscle and is under voluntary control (Fig. 33–1).

Blood Supply to the Gastrointestinal Tract

Because of its extended length, blood supply to the gastrointestinal tract is from arteries that originate along the entire length of the thoracic and abdominal aorta. Of particular importance are the vessels to the large and small intestines: the *superior* and *inferior mesenteric arteries*. These two arteries form small loops, or arcades, which encircle the intestine, supplying its wall with oxygen and nutrients (Fig. 33–2). Blood in the veins that drain the intestine is enriched by nutrients absorbed from the lumen of the gastrointestinal tract. These veins merge with others in the abdomen to form a large vessel called the *portal vein*, which carries the nutrient-rich blood to the liver. The blood flow to the entire gastrointestinal tract is about 20% of the total cardiac output, and it is significantly increased after eating.

Innervation

The gastrointestinal tract is innervated by both the sympathetic and parasympathetic parts of the *autonomic nervous system*. In general, sympathetic nerves exert an inhibitory effect on the gastrointestinal tract (except for the sphincters and blood vessels, which contract under the influence of the sympathetic nervous system). Parasympathetic nerve stimulation causes primary peristalsis to occur. The only portions of the tract under voluntary control are the upper esophagus and the external anal sphincter.

The Digestive Process

To perform their functions, all cells of the body require nutrients, which must be derived from the intake of food that contains protein, fat, carbohydrates, vitamins, and minerals, as well as cellulose fibers and other vegetable matter without nutritional value.

The primary digestive functions of the gastrointestinal tract are specifically related to providing these body needs:

- To break down food particles into their small constituent molecules for digestion
- To absorb the small molecules produced by digestion into the bloodstream
- To eliminate undigested and unabsorbed foodstuffs and other waste products from the body

As the food is being propelled through the gastrointestinal tract, it comes into contact with a wide variety of secretions that aid in digestion, absorption, and elimination of food particles (Fig. 33–3).

Oral Digestion

The process of digestion begins with the act of chewing, in which food is broken down into small particles that can be swallowed and mixed with digestive enzymes. The first secretion encountered is saliva, which is secreted in the mouth by the salivary glands at the rate of about 1.5 L daily. Saliva contains an enzyme, *ptyalin*, or salivary amylase, that helps in the digestion of starches (Table 33–1).

Eating or even the sight, smell, or thought of food can cause reflex salivation. The major function of saliva is to lubricate the food as it is chewed, thereby facilitating swallowing.

Swallowing

Swallowing, the initial act in the propulsion of food, is under voluntary control. It is regulated by a swallowing center in the medulla oblongata of the central nervous system. Voluntary efforts to initiate swallowing are ineffective unless there is something to swallow, such as air, saliva, or food. As the food is swallowed, the epiglottis moves to cover the tracheal opening and thus prevents aspiration of food into the lungs. Swallowing results in the propulsion of the bolus of food into the upper esophagus. The smooth muscle in the wall of the esophagus undergoes rhythmic contractions that move sequentially from top to bottom and help to propel the bolus of food from the upper esophagus toward the stomach. During this process of esophageal peristalsis, the lower esophageal sphincter, at the junction of the esophagus and the stomach, relaxes and permits the bolus of food to enter the stomach. Subsequently, the lower esophageal sphincter closes tightly to prevent reflux of stomach contents into the esophagus.

- When there is reflux of the acid contents of the stomach into the esophagus, an uncomfortable sensation occurs beneath the sternum. This sensation is commonly called *heartburn*.

Gastric Action

Within the stomach, food is exposed to gastric juice, the major characteristic of which is its very acid *p*H. The *p*H may be as low as 1 and is due to the secretion of *hydrochloric acid* by the glands of the stomach. The volume of gastric secretion is 2.5 L/day. The function of the highly acidic stomach secretion is to break down food into more absorbable components. The secretion of hydrochloric acid occurs in response to a meal.

- People who chronically secrete excessive amounts of gastric acid are susceptible to development of gastric and duodenal ulcers.

The gastric secretions also contain the enzyme *pepsin*, which is an important enzyme for the digestion of proteins.

Another component of gastric secretion is *intrinsic factor*. This compound is synthesized by cells of the stomach and combines with vitamin B_{12} in the diet, so that the vitamin can be absorbed in the ileum.

- In the absence of intrinsic factor, vitamin B_{12} cannot be absorbed, resulting in pernicious anemia.

Peristaltic contractions in the stomach propel its contents toward the pylorus. Large food particles cannot pass through the pyloric sphincter and are churned back into the body of

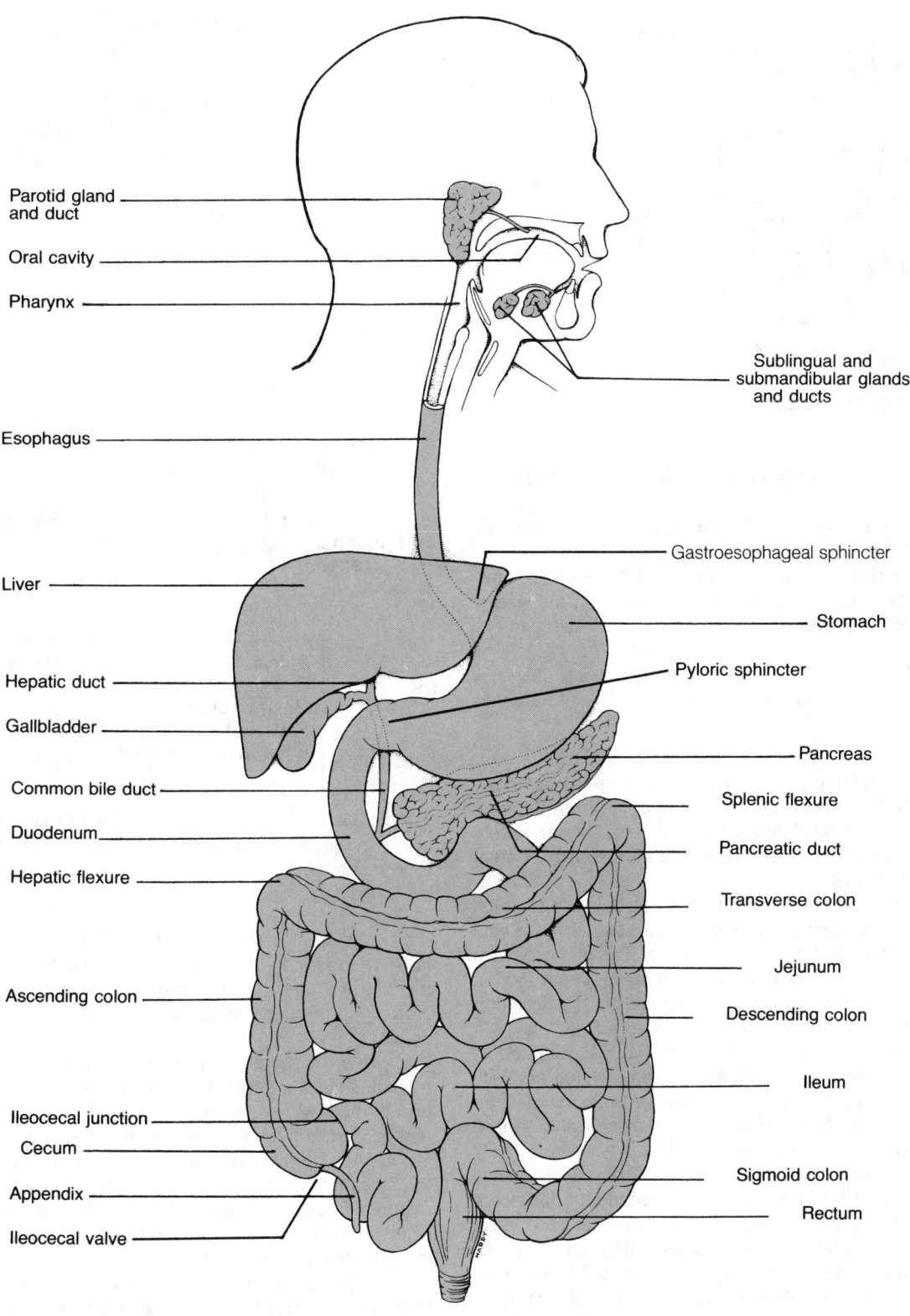

Parotid gland
and duct

Oral cavity

Pharynx

Sublingual and
submandibular glands
and ducts

Esophagus

Gastroesophageal sphincter

Liver

Stomach

Hepatic duct

Pyloric sphincter

Gallbladder

Pancreas

Common bile duct

Splenic flexure

Duodenum

Pancreatic duct

Hepatic flexure

Transverse colon

Jejunum

Ascending colon

Descending colon

Ileum

Ileocecal junction

Cecum

Sigmoid colon

Appendix

Rectum

Ileocecal valve

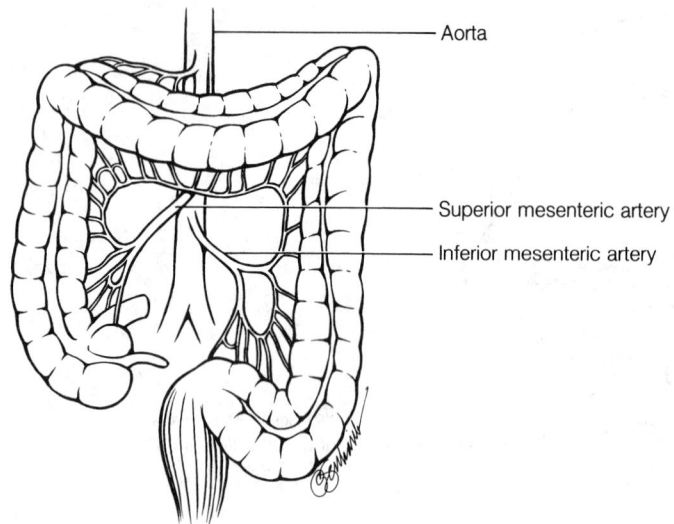

Figure 33–2. Anatomy and blood supply of the large intestine.

the stomach. In this way, food in the stomach is mechanically agitated and broken down into smaller particles.

Food remains in the stomach for a variable length of time, from a half hour to several hours, depending on the size of food particles, composition of the meal, and other factors. Peristalsis in the stomach and contractions of the pyloric sphincter allow the partially digested food to enter the small intestine at a rate that permits efficient absorption of nutrients.

Small Intestine Action

The remainder of the digestive process occurs primarily in the duodenum. Secretions in the duodenum come from the pancreas, the liver, and the glands in the wall of the intestine itself. The major characteristic of these secretions is their high content of digestive enzymes.

Pancreatic secretion has an alkaline *p*H, because of a high *bicarbonate* concentration. This serves to neutralize the acid entering the duodenum from the stomach. The pancreas also secretes digestive enzymes, including *trypsin*, which aids in the digestion of protein; *amylase*, which aids in the digestion of starch; and *lipase*, which aids in the digestion of fats.

Bile (secreted by the liver and stored in the gallbladder) contains *bile salts*, *cholesterol*, and *lecithin*, which emulsify the ingested fats and make them more accessible to digestion and absorption. The bile salts themselves are reabsorbed into the portal blood when they reach the ileum.

Secretions from the intestinal glands consist of mucus, which coats the cells and protects the duodenum from attack by hydrochloric acid; hormones; electrolytes; and enzymes. The total amount of intestinal secretions is approximately 1 L/ day of pancreatic juice, 0.5 L/day of bile, and 3 L/day from the glands of the small intestine. Intestinal peristalsis propels the contents of the small intestine toward the colon.

Gastrointestinal Regulatory Substances and Bacteria

Hormones

Three major hormones and two neuroregulators have been found to control the rate of secretion of the gastrointestinal

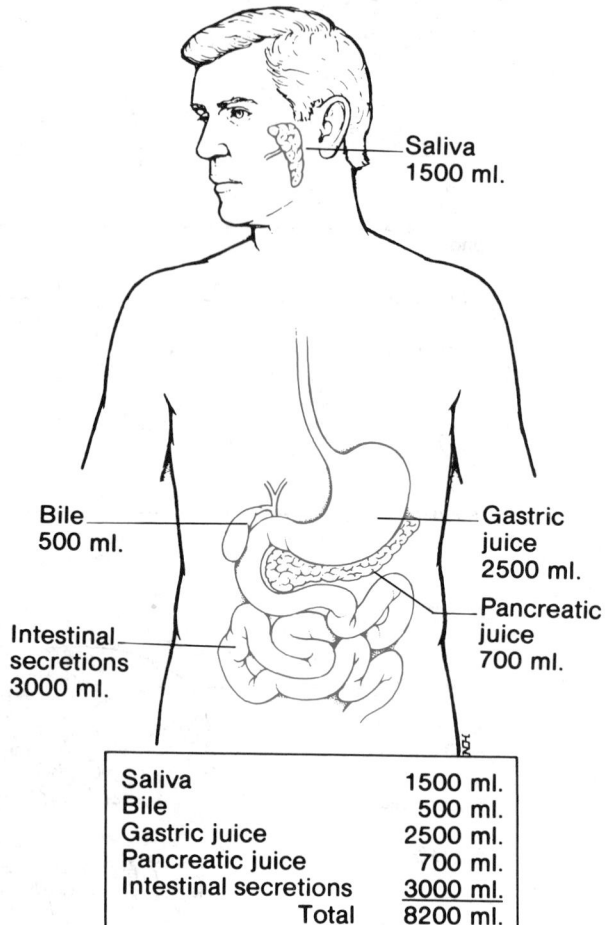

Figure 33–3. Total volume of digestive secretions produced in 24 hours. (Adapted from Bowen A. Intravenous alimentation in surgical patients. Mod Med.)

fluids and gastrointestinal motility (Table 33–2). Local regulators also play a role. *Acetylcholine* and *histamine* stimulate the gastric glands to increase the secretion of gastric acid. Norepinephrine and some prostaglandins inhibit gastric acid activity.

Gastrin is secreted by the cells of the stomach. It partially regulates the secretion of gastric acid and influences contraction of the lower esophageal and pyloric sphincters. The stimulus to gastrin release is distention of the stomach.

Secretin, secreted by the mucosa in the upper portion of the small intestine, stimulates the secretion of bicarbonate in pancreatic juice and inhibits the secretion of gastric acid. The stimulus to the release of secretin is acid entering the small intestine from the stomach.

Cholecystokinin-pancreozymin (CCK-PZ), also released from the cells in the upper small intestine, acts on both the gallbladder and the pancreas. It causes contraction of the gallbladder and release of digestive enzymes from the pancreas. The stimulus to the release of CCK-PZ is the presence of fatty acids and amino acids in the small intestine.

Bacteria

Bacteria are normal components of the contents of the gastrointestinal tract. Their presence is essential for normal gastrointestinal function. Few bacteria are present in the stomach

TABLE 33–1. *The Major Digestive Enzymes*

Name of Enzyme	Substrate	Products of Reaction	Source of Enzyme	Site of Action
ACTION OF ENZYMES THAT DIGEST CARBOHYDRATE				
Salivary amylase (ptyalin)	Starch (amylose) as in grains, potatoes, legumes	Dextrins, maltose, glucose	Secretions from parotid and submaxillary glands (saliva)	Mouth, if chewing is very thorough; some in fundus of stomach if mixing with acidic gastric juice is delayed
Pancreatic amylase (amylopsin)	Starch	α-Limit dextrins, maltose, glucose	Secretions from pancreas	Small intestine
	Dextrins	Maltose, glucose		
Disaccharidases	Disaccharides	Monosaccharides	Mucosal cells of small intestine (brush border)	Brush border of intestinal wall
Maltase	Maltose (in corn syrup, beer)	Glucose		
Isomaltase	Isomaltose	Glucose		
Sucrase	Sucrose (in table sugar; fruits)	Glucose and fructose		
Lactase	Lactose (in milk)	Glucose and galactose		
ACTION OF ENZYMES THAT DIGEST PROTEIN				
Pepsin (protease)	Protein	Large peptides	Chief cells of gastric mucosa (secreted as the inactive pro-enzyme pepsinogen*)	Stomach
Trypsin	Protein and polypeptides (Polypeptides are primarily from the partial digestion of protein.)	Polypeptides, dipeptides, amino acids	Pancreas (secreted as the inactive pro-enzymes trypsinogen, chymo-trypsinogen, and procarboxypeptidase*)	Lumen of the small intestine
Chymotrypsin				
Carboxypeptidase				
Aminopeptidase	Polypeptides	Smaller peptides, amino acids	Mucosal cells of small intestine	Brush border of small intestine
Dipeptidase	Dipeptides	Amino acids		
ACTION OF ENZYMES THAT DIGEST FAT (TRIGLYCERIDE)				
Pharyngeal lipase†	Triglycerides (in foods containing fat such as meat, butter, nuts, cheese)	Fatty acids, diglycerides, monoglycerides	Mucosa of pharynx	Fundus of stomach
Gastric lipase† (steapsin)	Short chain triglycerides (dairy fats)	Short-chain fatty acids, diglycerides, monoglycerides	Gastric mucosa	Stomach
Pancreatic lipase	Triglycerides, diglycerides	Diglycerides, monoglycerides, fatty acids (short, long, and medium chain)	Pancreas	Lumen of small intestine

* *Activation of pro-enzymes takes place in the lumen of the intestinal tract.*
† *Not essential for adequate digestion of fat.*
(Suitor CW and Crowley MF. Nutrition: Principles and Application in Health Promotion, 2nd ed. Philadelphia, JB Lippincott, 1984, p 219.)

TABLE 33–2.   *Gastrointestinal Regulatory Substances*

Substance	Stimulus for Production	Target Gland	Effect on Secretions	Effect on Motility
NEUROREGULATORS				
Acetylcholine	Sight, smell, chewing food, stomach distention	Gastric glands, other secretory glands, gastrointestinal muscle	Increased gastric acid	Generally increased; decreased sphincter tone
Norepinephrine	Stress, other various stimuli	Secretory glands, gastrointestinal muscle	Generally inhibitory	Generally decreased; increased sphincter tone
HORMONAL REGULATORS				
Gastrin	Myenteric reflexes caused by (1) distention of stomach with food; (2) secretagogues (partially digested protein; caffeine; other substances present in regular and decaffeinated coffee; alcohol; extractives)	Gastric glands	Increased secretion of gastric juice, which is rich in HCl	Increased motility of stomach, decreased time required for gastric emptying; Relaxation of ileocecal sphincter; Excitation of colon; Constriction of gastroesophageal sphincter
Cholecystokinin	Fat in duodenum	Gallbladder	Release of bile into duodenum	
		Pancreas	Increased production of enzyme-rich pancreatic secretions	
		Stomach	May inhibit gastric secretion somewhat	
Secretin	pH of chyme in duodenum below 4–5	Stomach	May inhibit gastric secretion somewhat	Inhibits stomach contractions
		Pancreas	Increased production of bicarbonate-rich pancreatic juice	
*Vasoactive intestinal peptide	Unclear	Pancreas	Increased pancreatic secretions	
		Stomach	Decreased gastric acid and pepsin produciton	Relaxation of stomach muscles
*Gastric inhibitory peptides (GIP)	Peptides, amino acids, fats, and glucose	Gastric glands	Decreased gastric acid production; Increased insulin production	Decreased gastric motility
*Motilin	Alkaline pH in duodenum	Stomach, intestines		Increased stomach and intestinal activity
LOCAL REGULATORS				
Histamine	Unclear; substances in food	Gastric glands	Increased gastric acid production	
* Prostaglandins (many types)	Possibly intestinal muscle contraction	Varied	Some (E_1, E_2, A) may inhibit gastric acid and pepsin secretion	PGE, PGF may cause contraction of longitudinal muscles

* *Specific physiologic roles not clear.*
(Suitor CW and Crowley MF. *Nutrition: Principles and Application in Health Promotion*, 2nd ed. Philadelphia, JB Lippincott, 1984, p 224.)

or upper small intestine, probably because they are killed by the acid secretions in the stomach. The bacterial population increases in the ileum, however, and becomes a major component of the contents of the large intestine. Here they assist in completing the breakdown of waste materials and bile salts.

Digestion and Absorption of Nutrients

Food, ingested in the form of fats, protein, and carbohydrates, is broken down into its constituent nutrients by the process of digestion.

Carbohydrates are broken down into disaccharides (*e.g.*, sucrose, maltose, and galactose) and monosaccharides (*e.g.*, glucose and fructose).

- Glucose is the major carbohydrate that the tissue cells use as fuel.

Proteins are broken down into amino acids and peptides. Ingested fats are emulsified into monoglycerides and fatty acids. Once the carbohydrates, proteins, and fats are broken down into smaller molecules, they can be more easily absorbed. Vitamins and minerals are not digested. They are absorbed essentially unchanged. Absorption takes place in the jejunum and is accomplished by both active transport and diffusion. Water and electrolytes from the diet and gastrointestinal secretions are absorbed by the gastrointestinal tract. Minimal amounts are excreted in the stool.

Colonic Action

Within 4 hours after eating, residual waste material (the consistency of gravy) passes into the terminal ileum and slowly passes into the proximal portion of the colon through the ileocecal valve.

This valve is normally closed and helps prevent colonic contents from refluxing back into the small intestine. With each peristaltic wave of the small intestine, the valve opens briefly and permits some of the contents to pass into the colon.

Weak peristaltic activity moves the colonic contents slowly, but intermittent strong peristaltic rushes propel the contents for considerable distances. When the contents reach and distend the rectum, an urge to defecate is experienced. When the next meal is eaten, hormones are again released that stimulate the gut. The first part of the waste materials from a meal reaches the rectum about 12 hours after eating. From the rectum to the anus, transport is much slower, and as much as one fourth of the waste materials from a meal may still be in the rectum 3 days after the meal was ingested. This slow transport of colonic contents allows efficient reabsorption of water and electrolytes.

Defecation

Distention of the rectum reflexively initiates contractions of its musculature and relaxation of the internal anal sphincter, which is ordinarily closed. The internal sphincter is controlled by the autonomic nervous system; the external sphincter is under the conscious control of the cerebral cortex. When the desire to defecate is felt, the external anal sphincter voluntarily relaxes,

permitting expulsion of colonic contents. Normally, the external anal sphincter is maintained in a state of tonic contraction. Thus, defecation is seen to be a spinal reflex that can be voluntarily inhibited by keeping the external anal sphincter closed. In this regard, it is similar to micturition. Contraction of abdominal muscles (straining) facilitates emptying of the colon.

The average frequency of defecation in humans is once daily, but the range is extremely variable. Changes in bowel habits may signify colonic disease. An increase in frequency of defecation is called *diarrhea*, whereas decreased frequency is called *constipation*.

The elderly are prone to constipation because of limited mobility and a decreased intake of fiber and foods that are hard to chew. A detailed explanation of gastrointestinal problems in the aged population is presented in Chapter 37.

Feces and Flatus

Feces consist of undigested foodstuffs, inorganic materials, water, and bacteria. Their composition is relatively unaffected by alterations of diet, because a large fraction of the fecal mass is of nondietary origin, derived from the gastrointestinal tract. This is why appreciable amounts of feces continue to be passed despite prolonged starvation. The brown color of the feces is due to breakdown of bile by the intestinal bacteria. Formation of chemicals, especially indole and skatole, by the intestinal bacteria are responsible in large part for the fecal odor.

The gastrointestinal tract normally contains approximately 150 ml of gas. Gas expelled from the upper gastrointestinal tract (belching) has its origin as swallowed air. Gas expelled from the lower gastrointestinal tract (flatulence) consists of swallowed air, as well as gas produced by bacteria in the colon. The gas in the colon contains methane, hydrogen sulfide, ammonia, and other gases. These gases can be absorbed into the portal circulation and are detoxified by the liver.

- Patients with liver disease are frequently treated with antibiotics to reduce the number of colonic bacteria and thereby inhibit the production of toxic gases.

In summary, with normal gastrointestinal functioning food passes through the component structures of the gastrointestinal tract, where it is digested, absorbed, and eliminated. Each component structure of the tract is specialized to assist in these functions. The overall goal of this process is to provide nutrients to the body's cells so that they can perform their functions effectively.

Diagnostic Tests and Procedures

Diagnostic assessment of the gastrointestinal tract includes the use of x-rays and ultrasound and the passage of various gastric and intestinal tubes. In general, the nurse has a supportive and educative role. Patients requiring such tests are frequently anxious, elderly, or debilitated. The preparation for many of these studies includes fasting and the use of laxatives or enemas, measures that are poorly tolerated by weakened patients and that have the potential to cause fluid and electrolyte imbalances. In addition, many of these tests require seemingly endless waiting, either for the tests to begin or to be completed, or for the results to be known.

Radiographic Diagnostic Tests

The entire gastrointestinal tract can be delineated by x-rays, after the introduction of barium sulfate or a similar radiopaque liquid as the contrast medium. This material, a tasteless, odorless, nongranular, and completely insoluble (hence, not absorbable) powder, is ingested in the form of a thick or thin aqueous suspension for purposes of upper gastrointestinal tract study *(upper GI series)*, and it is instilled rectally for visualization of the colon *(barium enema)*.

Upper Gastrointestinal Tract Study (Upper GI Series)

The upper GI series enables the examiner to detect or exclude any anatomic or functional derangement of the upper gastrointestinal organs or sphincters. It also aids in the diagnosis of ulcers, varices, tumors, regional enteritis, and malabsorption syndromes.

Patient Preparation

In preparation for a GI series, the patient may be asked to maintain a low-residue diet for 2 to 3 days before the test. The patient should receive nothing by mouth after midnight before the test. A laxative may be prescribed to clean out the intestinal tract. Because smoking can stimulate gastric motility, the patient is discouraged from smoking the morning before the examination.

Procedure

For purposes of examining the upper gastrointestinal tract, the patient is required to swallow barium under direct fluoroscopic examination.

As the contrast medium descends into the stomach, the position, patency, and caliber of the esophagus are visualized, enabling the examiner to detect or exclude any anatomic or functional derangement of that organ. An important observation can also be made in relation to the heart, namely, observing the presence or the absence of right atrial enlargement. An enlarged right atrium invariably impinges on the esophagus and is revealed by the resulting pressure defect in the esophagus. The appearance of the lower esophagus on radiographs after a swallow of thick barium suspension also allows for detection of esophageal varices, a manifestation of portal hypertension, as in cirrhosis of the liver.

Fluoroscopic examination next extends to the stomach, as its lumen fills with barium. The motility and the thickness of the gastric wall and the mucosal pattern are observed for evidence of spasms, ulcerations, malignant infiltrates, and other anatomic abnormalities, including pressure defects from without. The patency of the pyloric valve and the anatomy of the duodenum are also observed, with particular reference to possible ulceration of the mucosa, spasm of the wall, or displacement of the structure as a whole by a tumor in the adjacent area.

During the fluoroscopic examination, x-ray films are obtained to provide a permanent record of the findings. Additional films are taken at intervals, for as long as 24 hours thereafter, as a means of estimating the rate of gastric emptying and the degree of small bowel motility.

Double-Contrast Studies

The double-contrast method of examining the upper GI tract involves administering a thick barium suspension medium to outline the stomach and esophageal wall. Next, tablets that release carbon dioxide in the presence of water are given. The primary advantage of this technique is the finer detail that can be shown within the esophagus and stomach, permitting signs of early superficial neoplasms to be noted.

Continuous Infusion Method

A very detailed study of the small intestine involves the continuous infusion, through a duodenal tube, of 500 to 1000 ml of a thin barium sulfate suspension. This is carried out as a separate procedure. The barium fills the intestinal loops and is observed continuously by fluoroscope and filmed at frequent intervals as it progresses through the jejunum and the ileum.

Lower Gastrointestinal Tract Study (Barium Enema)

The purpose of a barium enema is to detect the presence of polyps, tumors, and other lesions of the large intestine and to demonstrate any abnormal anatomy or malfunction of the bowel.

Patient Preparation

The preparation of the patient includes those measures necessary to produce an empty and clean lower bowel. Usually, this includes a low-residue diet 1 to 3 days before the test, clear liquids the evening before, a laxative the evening before, taking nothing by mouth after midnight, and cleansing enemas until returns are clear.

- If the patient has active inflammatory disease of the colon, enemas are contraindicated. Active gastrointestinal bleeding may prohibit the use of laxatives and enemas. Barium enema is contraindicated in patients with suggested perforation or obstruction.

Procedure

In the x-ray department, the radiopaque substance is instilled rectally; it is viewed in the fluoroscope and then filmed. If the preparation of the patient has been adequate and the colon evacuated completely, the contour of the entire colon, including cecum and appendix (if patent), is clearly visible and the motility of each portion readily observed. The procedure takes about 15 minutes and is followed by an enema or laxative to facilitate barium removal.

Gastric Analysis/Gastric Acid Stimulation Test

Examination of the gastric juice offers a means of estimating the secretory activity of the gastric mucosa and of determining the presence, or the degree, of gastric retention in patients thought to have pyloric or duodenal obstruction.

- A diagnosis of pernicious anemia is excluded by the finding of acid.
- A diagnosis of gastric carcinoma may be established by the discovery of cancer cells in the gastric juice.

A small nasogastric tube with a catheter tip marked at various points from the distal end, is inserted through a nostril of the fasting patient. When the tube is at a point slightly less than 50 cm (21 in) distant, the tube should be within the stomach. Once in place, the tube is secured to the patient's cheek by means of a small strip of adhesive tape, and the patient is placed in a semireclining position. The entire stomach contents are aspirated by gentle suction into a syringe.

Histamine or betazole (Histalog) will be given subcutaneously to stimulate gastric secretions. The patient is told that he may experience a flushed feeling after the injection of this medication. Also, blood pressure and pulse are frequently monitored to detect hypotension. Emergency medications such as epinephrine and diphenhydramine (Benadryl) are available for use if required.

Gastric specimens are collected every 15 minutes for 1 hour. Specimens are labeled to indicate time before and after histamine injections. The acidity of the specimen is determined by means of an indicator, such as Töpfer's reagent, by indicator paper, or by a *p*H meter. Other examinations, in special instances, may include cytologic study by the Papanicolaou technique for the presence or absence of carcinoma cells. Enzyme analysis of the gastric juice may be indicated.

One of the most important items of information to be gained from gastric analysis relates to the ability of the mucosa to secrete hydrochloric acid:

- Patients with pernicious anemia secrete no acid under basal conditions or after stimulation.
- Patients with severe chronic atrophic gastritis secrete little or no acid. Some patients with gastric cancer secrete little or no acid.
- Patients with peptic ulcer invariably secrete some acid; patients with duodenal ulcers usually secrete an excess amount.

Upper Gastrointestinal Fiberoscopy/ Esophagogastroduodenoscopy

Fiberoscopy of the upper gastrointestinal tract allows for direct visualization of the gastric mucosa through a lighted endoscope (gastroscope). It is especially valuable when esophageal, gastric or duodenal abnormalities, inflammatory, neoplastic, or infectious processes are suspected (Fig. 33–4).

Fiberscopes are flexible scopes equipped with fiberoptic lenses. Colored photographs or motion pictures can be taken through them. Precautions must be taken to protect the scope, because the fiberoptic bundles may be broken if the scope is bent at an acute angle. Mouth guards are essential to prevent the patient from biting the scope.

An electronic video endoscope is available that is similar to the conventional fiberscope except that there is no viewing lens in the control section. The endoscope attaches directly to the video processor, which converts electronic signals to a television screen.

Fiberoptic gastroscopes are becoming more specialized. Side-viewing flexible scopes are now used to visualize the common bile, pancreatic, and hepatic ducts to evaluate jaundice, pancreatitis, tumors of the pancreas, common duct stones, and biliary tract disease. Common duct stones can even be retrieved using *endoscopic retrograde cholangiopancreatography*. Laser-compatible scopes are available. Laser therapy for gastrointestinal neoplasms is primarily palliative. It is used mainly to relieve obstruction, reduce tumor size, enlarge an obstructed lumen, and treat bleeding sites.

Patient Preparation

The patient is instructed to fast for 6 to 12 hours before the examination. Patient preparation includes spraying or gargling with a local anesthetic, along with the intravenous administration of diazepam (Valium) just before the scope is introduced. Atropine may be administered to reduce secretions. Glucagon may be given to relax smooth muscle. The patient is positioned on his left side to facilitate saliva drainage and easy access for the endoscopist.

Procedure

The pharynx is sprayed with tetracaine (Pontocaine) or a liquid gargle of ethyl aminobenzoate, after which the gastroscope is passed smoothly and slowly. The fiberoptic gastroscope is almost completely flexible and gives the physician an opportunity to view a large part of the gastric wall as well as the sphincters. The endoscope is then advanced into the duodenum for further examination. Biopsy forceps to obtain tissue specimens or cytology brushes to obtain cells for microscopic study also can be passed through the scope.

Follow-Up Care

After a gastroscopy the patient is instructed not to eat or drink until the gag reflex returns (in 1 to 2 hours); this is done to

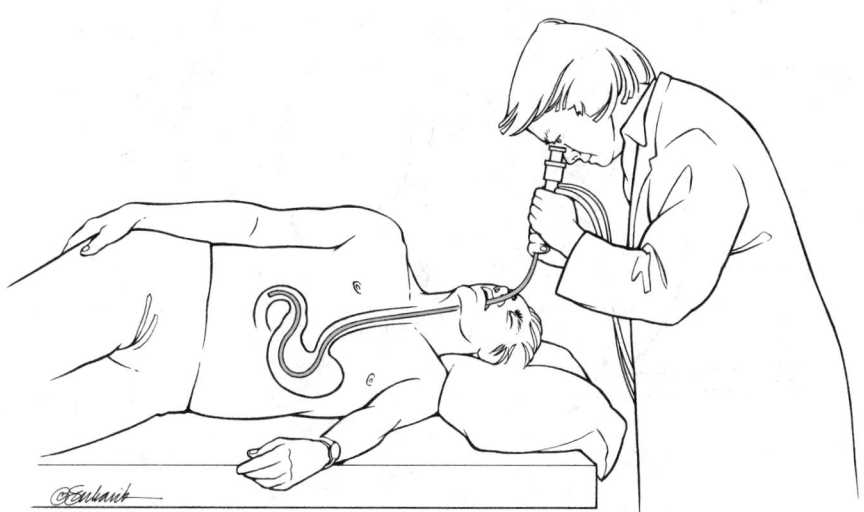

Figure 33–4. Patient undergoing gastroscopy.

prevent aspiration of food or fluids into the lungs. Postgastroscopy assessment by the nurse includes observation for signs of perforation, such as pain, unusual difficulty swallowing, and an elevated temperature. Minor throat discomfort can be relieved with lozenges, saline gargle, and oral analgesic medications after the gag reflex has returned.

Anoscopy, Proctoscopy, and Sigmoidoscopy

Procedures to view the lower bowel make use of instruments that use small beams of light that allow the lumen of the lower bowel to be viewed directly. The anoscope is used to examine the anal canal; proctoscopes and sigmoidoscopes are rigid scopes used to inspect the rectum and the sigmoid, respectively, for evidence of ulceration, tumors, polyps, or some other pathologic process.

The flexible sigmoidoscope permits examination of up to 40 to 50 cm (16 to 20 in) from the anus, more than the 25 cm (10 in) that can be seen with the rigid sigmoidoscope (Fig. 33–5) Rectal bleeding, a positive occult blood test, and anemia are indicators for a sigmoidoscopy even if the patient has a negative barium enema. Research has shown that the majority of carcinoid tumors begin in the terminal portion of the ileum. Repeated testing assures the detection of lesions in the early stages of malignancy and of precursor lesions (*i.e.*, polyps). Therefore, a flexible sigmoidoscopy should be performed at age 50, repeated in 1 year, and then performed every 3 years after that.

- Polyps and cancer lesions are found most commonly on the left side of the colon.

Patient Preparation

Such an examination requires that the lower bowel be clean; therefore, a warm tap-water enema or Fleet's enema is given until returns are clear. It may be necessary for the patient to take clear liquids the day before the examination. Generally, laxatives are not given.

Procedure for Rigid Scope Procedures

The patient assumes the knee–chest position, resting on his knees, feet extending over the edge of the bed or the examining table. With knees apart to give steady support, the patient leans over and rests the side of his face on the bed or the table, with his forearms on either side of the head and hands placed, one on top of the other, above the head. His back is now inclined at about a 45-degree angle, and he is in proper position for the introduction of an anoscope, proctoscope, or sigmoidoscope. Maximal convenience and comfort are provided by a table that has been especially designed for rectal endoscopy—the so-called proctoscopic table, which tilts the patient into the optimal position.

During a proctosigmoidoscopic examination, the patient is kept informed about the progress of the examination. He is informed that he will experience a feeling of pressure and will feel as though he is going to have a bowel movement. It is helpful to explain that this is from the pressure of the instrument and will last only a brief period. It may be necessary to attach suction equipment through the scope to remove any secretion, exudate, blood, or excreta that might be obstructing the area of observation. After each use, the collecting bottles and secretions must be disposed of safely. Disposable sigmoidoscopes are now available. Although they eliminate the need for cleaning, they must be disposed of safely.

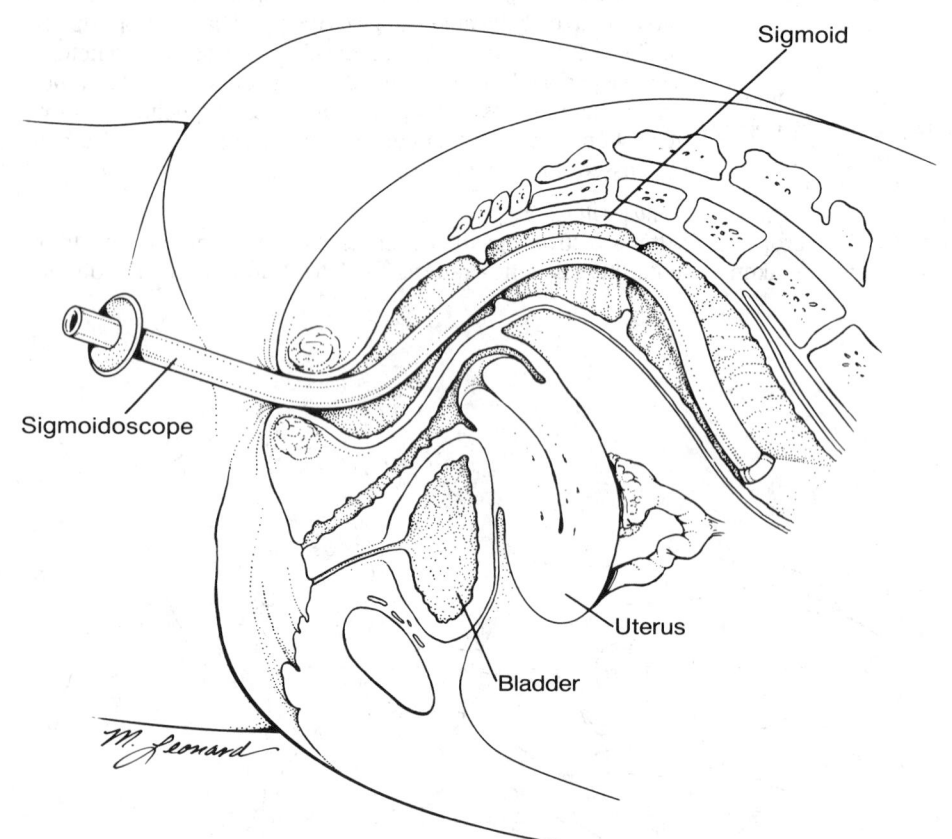

Figure 33–5. Sigmoidoscopy. Instrument is advanced past proximal sigmoid and then deflected into descending colon.

As part of the endoscopic examination, one or more small pieces of tissue may be removed for histologic study, a procedure referred to as a *biopsy*. This is performed with small biting forceps introduced through the instrument. Rectal and sigmoidal polyps, if present, may be removed by means of a wire snare, which is used to grasp the pedicle or stalk, and an electrocoagulating current, used to sever it and to prevent bleeding.

- It is extremely important that all tissue that is excised by the endoscopist be placed immediately in moist gauze or in an appropriate receptacle, labeled correctly and legibly, and then delivered without delay to the pathology laboratory for examination.

Procedure for Flexible Scope Procedures

The patient is placed in a comfortable position on his left side with his right leg bent and placed anteriorly. Biopsies and polypectomies can also be completed during this procedure. The same nursing implications apply as for the rigid scope procedures.

Fiberoptic Colonoscopy

Direct visual inspection of the colon is possible by means of a flexible fiberoptic colonoscope. This procedure is used as a diagnostic aid or for removal of foreign bodies, polyps, or tissue for biopsy (Fig. 33–6).

Patient Preparation

Success of the procedure depends on how well the colon is prepared. Therefore the intestinal tract is first emptied by limiting the patient's intake to liquids (perhaps for 1 to 3 days). Cleansing of the colon can be accomplished by one of two methods. The physician may order a laxative for 2 nights and a Fleet enema or saline enemas until clear the morning of the test. Currently, polyethylene glycol electrolyte lavage solutions (GoLYTELY, Colyte) are being used as effective intestinal lavages for cleansing the bowel. The patient is placed on a clear liquid diet starting at noon the day before the procedure. The lavage solutions are then ingested orally at intervals over the next 4 to 5 hours. The preparation is fast (rectal effluent is clear in about 4 hours) and tolerated fairly well by most patients.

Some side effects are nausea, fluid and electrolyte imbalance, and hypothermia (most patients are told to drink the preparation as cold as possible to make it more palatable.) The side effects are especially prominent among the elderly population.

- The patient is instructed not to take routine medications at the time of ingestion of the lavage solution, as they will not be digested. The use of lavage solutions is contraindicated in patients with intestinal obstructions.

Before the examination, a narcotic analgesic, usually meperidine (Demerol), may be administered. During the examination, diazepam (Valium) may be useful in relieving anxiety.

Procedure

Colonoscopy is performed with the patient lying on his left side with his legs drawn up. Discomfort may result from instilling air to open the colon or from insertion and movement of the scope. Biopsy forceps or a cytology brush may be passed through the scope to obtain specimens for histology and cytology exams. Complications are rare after this procedure, although perforation or hemorrhage is possible.

Follow-Up Care

The patient must be observed for signs and symptoms of bowel perforation (*e.g.*, rectal bleeding, abdominal pain/distention, or fever).

Colonoscopic Polypectomy

Colonoscopic polypectomy involves removal of a polyp through the use of cautery through a colonoscope. Many colon cancers begin with adenomatous polyps of the colon; therefore, the goal of colonoscopic polypectomy is early detection and pre-

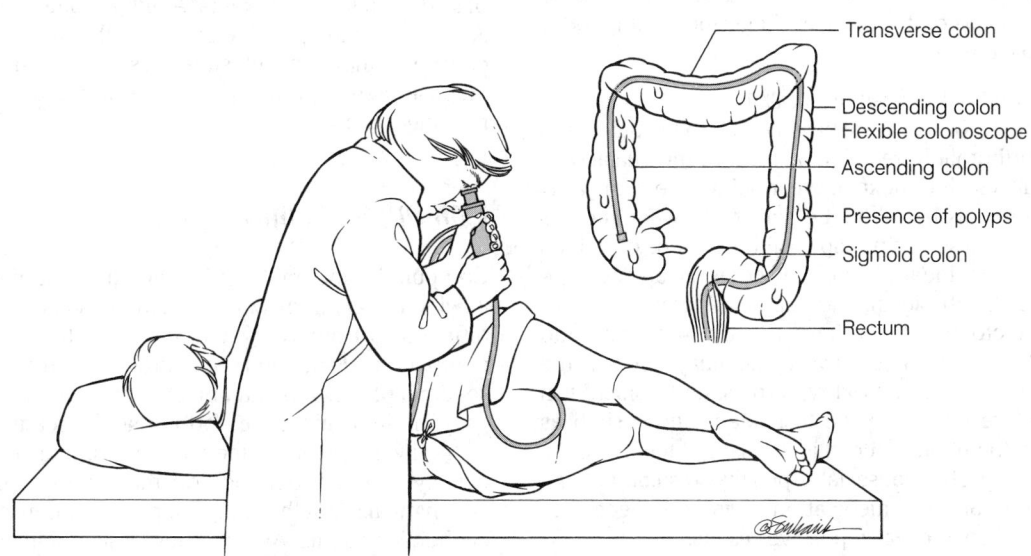

Figure 33–6. Colonoscopy. Flexible scope passes through rectum and sigmoid colon into the descending, transverse, and ascending colon.

vention of colorectal cancer. Resection and biopsy are performed to determine the cellular nature of the polyp, such as benign or malignant. All adenomatous colon polyps larger than 1.0 cm in diameter should be resected because malignancy is related to polyp size. All visible polyps must be removed.

Small Bowel Enteroscopy

A recent development is a small-caliber transnasal endoscope that will allow direct observation of the small intestine wall. Previously observation had been limited to the extreme proximal and distal portions using standard instruments. The examination is performed on an outpatient basis because it requires the tube to migrate with peristaltic movements through the bowel over several days.

Stool Examination

The basic examination of the stool includes an inspection of the specimen for its amount, consistency, and color, and a screening test for occult blood. Special tests indicated in specific cases may include tests for fecal urobilinogen, fat, nitrogen, parasites, food residues, and other substances.

Stool Color

The color of stools varies from light to dark brown. Various foods and medications affect stool color as follows: meat protein produces a dark brown coloration; spinach, a green hue; carrots and beets, red; cocoa, dark red or brown; senna, a yellowish hue; bismuth, iron, licorice, and charcoal, black; and barium, a milky white appearance.

- If shed in sufficient quantities into the upper gastrointestinal tract, blood produces a tarry black color (melena).
- Blood entering the lower portion of the gastrointestinal tract or passing rapidly through it will appear bright or dark red.
- Lower rectal or anal bleeding can be suspected if there is streaking of blood on the surface of the stool or if blood is noted on toilet tissue.

Tests for Occult Blood or to Confirm Melena

The most common stool tests are based on the benzidine, gum guaiac, or the orthotolidin reaction. A form of the guaiac test is the Hemoccult test. It is inexpensive, noninvasive, and easily performed at home. It should not be performed when there is hemorrhoidal bleeding. A dry paper slide is used, on which the stool specimen is smeared. The slide comes in an envelope that is mailed to the physician, and examined later.

There are factors that interfere with the sensitivity and specificity of the test. False-positive results may occur if the patient has eaten red meats, poultry, turnips, and horseradish immediately before or during the test. Medications such as iron, iodides, indomethacin, colchicine, salicylates, steroids, and vitamin C may also cause false-positive results. Careful assessment of diet and the medication regimen is necessary to eliminate the chance of false-positive results.

When stool tests are performed on an outpatient basis, patients are often instructed to restrict foods that cause false-positive results for 3 days before the test.

The American Cancer Society recommends annual fecal guaiac screening beginning at age 50. The screening test requires a 3-day serial stool testing.

Stool Consistency and Appearance

In various disorders the stool assumes a typical appearance:

- In *steatorrhea*, the stools are generally bulky, greasy, foamy, and foul in odor; stool color is gray, with a silvery sheen.
- With *biliary obstruction*, the stool becomes "acholic" and is light gray or clay colored, because of the absence of urobilin.
- In *chronic ulcerative colitis*, mucus or pus may be visible on gross inspection of the stool.
- *Constipation, obstipation*, or *fecal impaction* may result in the passage of small, dry, rocky-hard masses called *scybala*. This type of stool may traumatize the rectal mucosa sufficiently to cause bleeding, in which case the fecal masses are streaked with red blood.

Ultrasonography

Ultrasonography is a noninvasive diagnostic technique in which sound waves are passed into internal body structures; varying deflections of these sound waves are bounced back, much like a reflection. These, in turn, are displayed on an oscilloscope.

The chief advantage of the abdominal ultrasonography is the spatial reproduction of masses in transverse and longitudinal directions. The procedure is noninvasive, there are no noticeable side effects, and it is relatively inexpensive. This type of diagnostic procedure is useful in studying the liver, pancreas, spleen, gallbladder, and retroperitoneal tissues.

One disadvantage is that this technique cannot be used when a structure to be examined lies behind bony tissue, which prevents passage of sound waves to deeper structures. Also, gas in the abdomen or air in the lungs presents a problem, as ultrasound is not well transmitted through gas or air.

Endoscopic ultrasonography is a relatively new specialized enteroscopic procedure that will greatly aid in the diagnosis of gastrointestinal disorders. A high-frequency ultrasonic beam is added to the tip of the scope so that a transintestinal study can be completed. Intestinal gas, bone, and thick layers of adipose tissue that hamper conventional ultrasonography are no longer a problem.

Computed Tomography

Computed tomography (CT scanning) is a diagnostic method in which a very narrow x-ray beam is used to detect the density differences from very small cubes of tissue. These data are computerized and then reconstructed so that transverse cross-sections of the body can be shown on a television monitor.

The indications for abdominal CT scanning are diseases of the liver, spleen, kidney, pancreas, and pelvic organs. Adequacy of detail depends on the presence of fat, however, which means that this diagnostic tool is not useful for very thin, cachectic patients. Also, because a scanning time of 5 seconds is required, motion artifacts produced by heart beat and respiration cannot be avoided and the results are a less than clear picture. Finally, radiation doses are appreciable.

Magnetic Resonance Imaging

Magnetic resonance imaging (MRI) for gastroenterology is currently used to supplement, not replace, ultrasonography and CT. For MRI examination, the patient lies within a machine that reconstructs an image based on the magnetic field created between the machine and the structures it is studying.

- MRI is *definitely contraindicated* for patients with permanent pacemakers, because the magnetic field could cause pacer malfunction.

The entire procedure takes 30 to 90 minutes. There is no specific patient preparation except for abdominal or pelvic scans. Patients having MRI are instructed to avoid caffeine.

In summary, there are many diagnostic tools and procedures available to assist in assessment of the structure and function of the gastrointestinal tract. This discussion has provided specific information about these procedures including method, preparation, special instructions, and follow-up care.

Pathophysiologic and Psychological Considerations

Abnormalities of the gastrointestinal tract are numerous and exemplify every type of major pathology that can affect other organ systems. A composite view of the various types of gastrointestinal disorders that may occur is presented in Figure 33-7. Congenital, inflammatory, infectious, traumatic, and neoplastic lesions have been encountered in every portion, and at every site, along the length of the gastrointestinal tract. In common with many other organ systems, the GI tract is subject to circulatory disturbances, faulty nervous system control, and senescence.

Obstruction of the gastrointestinal tract is a common complication of the pathologic conditions identified in Figure 33-7. Various degrees of obstruction to the passage of intestinal contents in the gastrointestinal tract may result from tumors growing into the lumen, twisting or kinking of the intestine, infarction of tissue due to interruption of the blood supply, aspirated foreign bodies, or other reasons. As a consequence of obstruction, the force of the intestinal contractions is increased, the intestine becomes distended above the point of obstruction, and abdominal pain and bloating result. The peristaltic waves may actually reverse their direction, leading to vomiting. Excessive vomiting may result in the loss of large volumes of fluid from the body, causing dehydration, and loss of large amounts of hydrochloric acid, causing metabolic alkalosis. If the obstruction in the gastrointestinal tract occurs at, or below, the duodenum, biliary material will be in the vomitus, giving the characteristic green color. If the colon is obstructed, the ileocecal valve may become stretched and incompetent, colonic contents can reflux, and the patient may vomit fecal material.

Apart from the many organic diseases to which the gas-

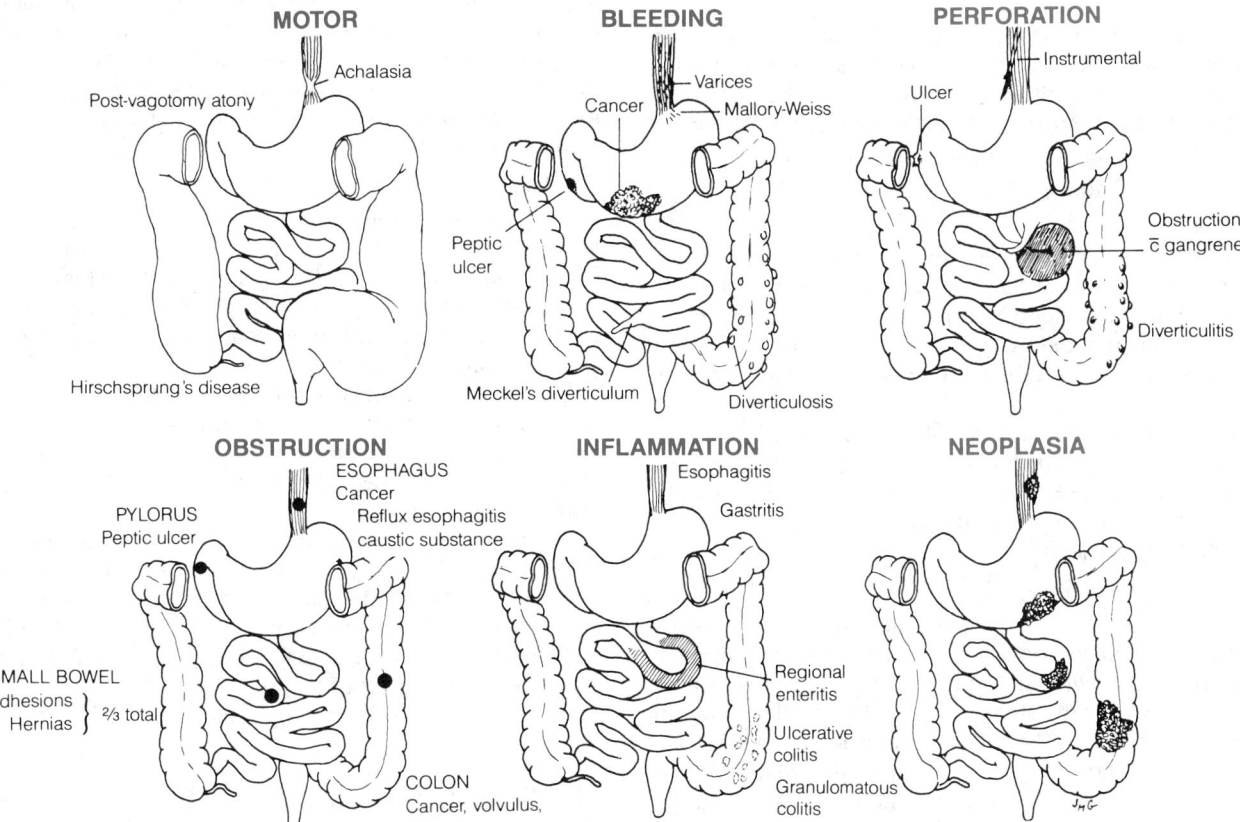

Figure 33-7. Pathophysiology of the gastrointestinal tract can be classified in many ways. The illustration vividly shows the many conditions that can occur under the six classifications. (Hardy JD. Rhoads Textbook of Surgery, 6th ed. Philadelphia, JB Lippincott, 1988.)

trointestinal tract is susceptible, there are many extrinsic factors—some related to disease, others not—that can interfere with its normal function and produce symptoms. Anxiety, for example, often finds its chief expression in indigestion, anorexia, or motor disturbances of the intestines, producing constipation or diarrhea. Students facing examinations or stressed executives facing major decisions may be susceptible to gastrointestinal disorders. Also, some psychological problems are thought to have a role in physical dysfunction. For example, personality factors are thought to have an influence in peptic ulcer disease.

In addition to the state of mental health, physical factors such as fatigue and an unbalanced or abruptly changed dietary intake can markedly affect the gastrointestinal tract. In both assessing the patient and instructing him, the nurse should realize that a combination of mental and physical factors affect the status of the gastrointestinal tract.

Nursing Assessment

The nurse performs a physical examination and takes a complete history. She focuses on symptoms common to gastrointestinal dysfunction. A sample assessment guide is found in Chart 33–1. Symptoms on which the assessment should focus include pain, indigestion, intestinal "gas," vomiting, hematemesis, diarrhea, and constipation.

Pain
Pain can be a major symptom of gastrointestinal disease. The character, duration, frequency, and time of the pain vary greatly, depending on the underlying cause, which affects the location and distribution of referred pain. Other factors, such as meals, rest, defecation, and vascular disorders, may directly affect pain.

Indigestion
Indigestion can result from disturbed nervous control of the stomach or from a disorder in the stomach or elsewhere in the body. Fatty foods tend to cause the most discomfort because they remain in the stomach longer than proteins or carbohydrates. Coarse vegetables and highly seasoned foods can also cause considerable distress.

Upper abdominal pain associated with eating is the most common complaint of patients with gastrointestinal dysfunction. The basis for the abdominal distress may be the patient's own gastric peristaltic movements. Bowel movements may or may not relieve the pain.

Intestinal "Gas" (Belching and Flatulence)
The accumulation of gas in the gastrointestinal tract may result in *belching*, the expulsion of gas from the stomach through the mouth, or *flatulence*, the expulsion of gas from the rectum.

Air that reaches the stomach is quickly expelled, but not necessarily by belching. Periodically, stomach gas moves into the lower esophagus (simple reflux) and then returns to the stomach because of a peristaltic contraction of the distal esophagus. Belching occurs when simple reflux is accompanied by contraction of the anterior abdominal muscles. At the first urge to belch, simply swallowing may interrupt the belch.

Usually, gases in the intestine pass into the colon and are released as flatus. Patients often complain of bloating, distention, or being "full of gas."

Vomiting
The involuntary act of vomiting is another major symptom of gastrointestinal disease. Vomiting is usually preceded by nausea, an unpleasant sensation suggesting that vomiting is imminent.

Hematemesis
Hematemesis is the vomiting of blood. When this happens soon after hemorrhage, the vomitus is bright red. If blood has been retained in the stomach, digestive processes change the hemoglobin to a brown pigment, which gives the vomitus a coffee-ground appearance.

Diarrhea
Diarrhea, which is defined as an abnormal increase in stool liquidity and in daily stool weight (volume), is a major abnormality of gastrointestinal function. A common mechanism for diarrhea is an increased rate of movement of the contents through the intestine and colon, so that inadequate time is available for absorption of the gastrointestinal secretions, resulting in an increased fluid content of the stool. Inflammation or other diseases of the colonic mucosa can also lead to diarrhea, as can infection from pathogens or parasites or overuse of cathartics. When these occur, water and electrolytes are not sufficiently reabsorbed and increased amounts of fluids or liquid reach the rectum, resulting in increased stool volume. *Steatorrhea*, defined as a large amount of fat in the stools, is commonly due to pancreatic disease. The decreased activity of pancreatic enzymes is responsible for decreased fat digestion. Disease of the biliary tract can also cause steatorrhea, because of the absence of bile salts. The consequences of diarrhea are loss of potassium, causing electrolyte imbalance; loss of bicarbonate, leading to acidosis; and loss of nutrients, leading to malnutrition.

Constipation
Constipation is the retention of or a delay in expulsion of fecal content from the rectum. In this situation, water is absorbed from the fecal matter, producing stools that are hard, dry, and of smaller volume than normal. A person is said to be constipated if he strains at stool more than 25% of the time or passes two or fewer stools per week.

A variety of factors can produce constipation, such as decreased food or fluid intake, or an intake of primarily low-residue foods; decreased exercise or activity patterns; atony of the aged bowel; neuroses; colon or rectal lesions; and intestinal obstructions.

In the elderly, constipation and impaction can result from a decrease in the sensation to defecate due to the decreased response of tactile and stretch receptors in the rectum and the anal canal; decreased exercise; and decreased intake of high-fiber foods because of chewing difficulties secondary to ill-fitting dentures or lack of teeth.

Nursing Interventions

Nursing interventions for the patient requiring gastrointestinal diagnostic assessment include the following:

Chart 33–1
Assessment of Gastrointestinal Functioning

General Nutritional Information

Patient name: _____
Current weight: _____ Ideal body weight: _____ Age: _____ Sex: _____
Height: _____ .
There has been a recent (weight gain, weight loss) _____ over _____ months of _____
pounds. At home, food is purchased by _____ and prepared by _____

Dietary record for past 72 hours: Food description and quantity

	Breakfast	Lunch	Dinner	Snack	Snack	Total Daily Calories
Day # 1						
Day # 2						
Day # 3						

Symptoms of Gastrointesinal Dysfunction

Is (able, unable) to chew food. Description of any disorder _____
Has recently experienced _____
  Anorexia, the lack of appetite for food.
  Dysphagia, difficulty with swallowing.
  Polyphagia, a voracious appetite or excessive eating.
  Odynophagia, pain on swallowing.
The above symptom has existed for _____ (days, weeks, months). It is aggravated by _____ and relieved
by _____
(Does, does not) experience indigestion. Foods that tend to cause the most discomfort are _____
Relief measures include _____
(Has, has not) experienced heartburn. Relief measures include _____
(Does, does not) experience pain. Pain can be described as _____ and of _____ duration. It occurs
(frequency) _____ It is aggravated by _____ and relieved by _____ It seems to be
localized in the _____ region.
It (does, does not) radiate to the _____
  Esophageal: Retrosternal; may radiate to back
  Gastric: Epigastric; may radiate to back, especially left subscapular
  Duodenal: Epigastric; may radiate to back, especially right subscapular
  Gallbladder: Right upper quadrant or epigastric; may radiate to back or right subscapular
  Pancreatic: Epigastric; may radiate to back or left lumbar
  Appendicular: Periumbilical, later to right lower quadrant
  Colonic: Hypogastrium, right or left lower quadrant
  Rectal: Pelvic area
Has recently experienced _____
  Vomiting, the forceful expulsion of gastric contents up through the esophagus.
  Retching, abdominal muscles contract in an attempt to expel contents.
  Hematemesis, the vomiting of blood that is bright red or "coffee ground" in appearance.
The above symptom has existed for _____ (days, weeks). It occurs _____ times per day.
Is aggravated by _____ and relieved by _____ Description of vomitus:
  Quantity _____ Odor _____ Color _____ Taste _____
  Presence of _____ (food particles, blood, mucus).
Has recently experienced _____ (diarrhea, constipation).
The above symptom has existed for _____ (days, weeks, months). It is aggravated by _____ and
relieved by _____ Description of stool: _____
  Content _____ Color _____ Consistency _____ Odor _____
Associated factors: Daily fluid intake _____ Exercise pattern _____
Intake of high fiber foods _____ Activity pattern _____
Presence of (bleeding, hemorrhoids).

- Providing general information about a balanced diet and the nutritional factors that can cause gastrointestinal disturbances. Specific information is provided after a diagnosis has been confirmed.
- Providing needed information about the test and the activities required of the patient; providing oral and written instructions
- Alleviating anxiety
- Assuring the patient that he will be helped to cope with his discomfort
- Encouraging family members, or others, to offer emotional support to the patient during the diagnostic testing

Bibliography

Books

Berk JE (ed). Bockus' Gastroenterology. Philadelphia, WB Saunders, 1985.

Elipoulos C. Gerontologic Nursing. 2nd ed. Philadelphia, JB Lippincott, 1987.

Fenoglio–Preiser et al. Gastrointestinal Pathology—An Atlas and Text. New York, Raven Press, 1989.

Given BA. Gastroenterology in Clinical Nursing. St Louis, CV Mosby, 1984.

Halevy J. Key Facts in Gastroenterology. New York, Plenum, 1986.

Kratzer GL and Demerest RJ. Office Management of Colon and Rectal Disease. Philadelphia, WB Saunders, 1985.

Misiewic JJ et al. Atlas of Clinical Gastroenterology. New York, Glaxo/Roche, 1985.

Porth CM. Pathophysiology: Concepts of Altered States. 3rd ed. Philadelphia, JB Lippincott, 1990.

Rossman I. Clinical Geriatrics. 3rd ed. Philadelphia, JB Lippincott, 1986.

Sivak M. Gastroenterologic Endoscopy. Philadelphia, WB Saunders, 1987.

Sleisenger M and Fordtan J. Gastrointestinal Disease—Pathology, Diagnosis, Management. 4th ed. Philadelphia, WB Saunders, 1988.

Williams SR. Nutrition and Diet Therapy. St Louis, Times Mirror/Mosby, 1989.

Journals

Archker E. Screening patients for colorectal cancer. Pract Gastroenterol 1989 Jan/Feb; 25(1): 37, 41–42.

Becker KL et al. Performing an in depth abdominal assessment. Nursing 1988 Jun; 19(6): 59–63.

Buchel E. Endoscopic ultrasonography. Endoscopic Review 1987 Mar/Apr; 4(2): 29–32.

Ciarleglio C. Gastric analysis: Old standby with a new purpose. SGA J 1988 Spring; 10(4): 202–204.

Ciarleglio C. Gastric analysis: Renaissance of an old technique. SGA J 1988 Fall; 11(2): 85–92.

Ciarleglio C. Gastric analysis Smart Chart. Gastroenterol Nurs 1989 Spring; 2(4):258.

Clarke B. Making sense of bowel prep for diagnostic procedures. Nursing Times 1989 Feb 1–7; 85(5): 46–47.

Coleman D. Anatomy and physiology of the small bowel. SGA J 1987 Spring; 10(1): 44–48.

Fiorenza V et al. Small intestinal motility: Normal and abnormal function. Am J Gastroenterol 1987 Nov; 98(11) : 1111–1114.

Fleisher M. Fecal occult blood screening tests. Endosc Rev 1987 May/Jun; 10(3): 31–39.

Groth K. Age related changes in the GI tract. Geriatr Nurs 1988 Sep/Oct; 9(5): 278–280.

Gruber M et al. The power of certainty. . . . Pattern recognition. AJN 1989 Apr; 89(4): 502–503.

Jacobs BB et al. Anatomy of the abdomen. Emergency Care Quarterly 1988 Feb; 3(4): 1–11.

Langfur F. Colonic lavage—Preparation for colonoscopy. Endosc Rev 1987 May/Jun; 10(3): 46–50.

Larson D Advanced anatomy and physiology of the colon. SGA J 1987 Fall; 10(2): 92–97.

Lencki BA. The esophagus. SGA J 1987 Fall; 10(2): 117–119.

Lewis BS and Waye JD. Small bowel enteroscopy in 1988: Pros and Cons. Am J Gastroenterol 1988 Aug; 99(8): 799–802.

Lind CD et al. Diagnosis: GI complaints in the geriatric patient. Part I. Hosp Med 1987 Oct; 23(10): 183–188, 193–4, 199.

Lind CD et al. Diagnosis: GI complaints in the geriatric patient. Part II. Hosp Med 1987 Nov; 23(11): 21–3, 27–9, 32.

Morazzo R et al. Colonoscopy complications. Endosc Rev 1988 Nov/Dec; 11(6): 9–29.

Nelson J and Castell D. Effects of aging on GI physiology. Pract Gastroenterol 1988 Nov/Dec; 24(6): 28–29, 32–35.

Newman FK et al. Magnetic resonance imaging: The latest in diagnostic technology. Nursing 1987 Jan; 17(1): 45–47.

Sekas G and Hutson W. Rectal exam by retroflexion maneuver during flexible sigmoidoscopy. Endoscopic Review 1987 May/Jun; 10(3): 29–31.

Smith CE. Assessing bowel sounds: More than just listening. Nursing 1988 Feb; 18(2): 42–43.

Smith CE. Investigating absent bowel sounds. Nursing 1987 Nov; 17(11): 73, 76–77.

Waye J. Colonoscopy, Why and How? Endosc Rev 1988 Nov/Dec; 11(6): 31–32.

Waye J. Expanding the uses of therapeutic endoscopy. Hosp Prac 1987 Aug 15; 22(8): 143–146, 151, 154.

Williams C. Preparing your patient for colonoscopy. Endosc Rev 1988 Nov/Dec; 11(6): 32–34.

34

Assessment and Management of Patients With Ingestive Problems and Upper Gastrointestinal Disorders

Learning Objectives

On completion of this chapter, the learner will be able to:

1. Use the nursing process as a framework for care of patients with conditions of the oral cavity
2. Describe the relationship of dental hygiene and dental problems to nutrition
3. Specify the nursing management of patients with abnormalities of the lips, gums, teeth, mouth, and salivary glands
4. Use the nursing process as a framework for care of patients with cancer of the oral cavity
5. Identify the physical and psychosocial long-term needs of patients with oral cancer
6. Use the nursing process as a framework for care of patients undergoing radical neck dissection.
7. Use the nursing process as a framework for care of patients with conditions of the esophagus
8. Describe the various conditions of the esophagus, their clinical manifestations, management, and rehabilitation

Because the process of ingestion begins with the mastication of food in the mouth, adequate nutrition is related to good dental health and the general condition of the mouth. Any discomfort or adverse condition in the oral cavity can have a deleterious effect on nutritional status. Changes in the oral cavity may influence the type and amount of food ingested as well as the degree to which food particles are properly mixed with salivary enzymes. Esophageal problems related to the apparently simple act of swallowing can also adversely affect food and fluid intake, thereby jeopardizing general health and well-being.

Given the close interrelationship between adequate nutritional intake and all of the structures of the upper gastrointestinal tract (lips, mouth, teeth, pharynx, esophagus), preventive health teaching should place heavy emphasis on helping people to prevent disorders associated with any of these structures.

▶ Nursing Process Overview
Patients With Conditions of the Oral Cavity

▷ Assessment

The principle nursing activities in the assessment phase include a health history to determine teaching and learning needs for preventive oral hygiene and to determine symptoms requiring medical evaluation.

The history includes questions about the patient's (1) normal brushing and flossing routine, (2) frequency of dental visits, (3) awareness of any lesions or irritated areas in the mouth, tongue, or throat, (4) need to wear dentures or partial plate, (5) recent history of sore throat or bloody sputum, (6) discomfort caused by certain foods, (7) daily food intake, and (8) use of alcohol and tobacco (including chewing tobacco).

Physical assessment includes inspection and palpation of both the internal and external structures of the mouth and throat. Removal of dentures and partial plates is necessary to ensure a thorough inspection of the gums. In general, the examination can be accomplished with the use of a bright light source (penlight) and a tongue depressor. Gloves are worn to palpate the tongue and any abnormalities.

The examination begins with inspection of the lips for moisture, hydration, color, texture, symmetry, and the presence of ulcerations or fissures. The lips should be moist, pink, and smooth and symmetric. The patient is instructed to open his mouth wide; a tongue blade is then inserted to expose the buccal mucosa for an assessment of color and lesions (Fig. 34–1A). Stensen's duct of each parotid gland is visible as a small red dot in the buccal mucosa next to the upper molars.

The gums are inspected for inflammation, bleeding, retraction, and discoloration. The odor of the breath is also noted. The hard palate is examined for color and shape. The dorsum of the tongue is inspected for texture, color, and lesions. A thin, white coat and large, vallate papillae in a V formation on the distal portion of the dorsum of the tongue are normal findings (see Fig. 34–1B). The patient is instructed to protrude his or her tongue and move it laterally. This provides the examiner with an opportunity to estimate the tongue's size as well as its symmetry and strength (assesses the integrity of the 12th cranial nerve [hypoglossal]). Further inspection of the ventral surface of the tongue and the floor of the mouth is accomplished by asking the patient to touch the tip of the tongue to the palate. Any lesions of the mucosa or any abnormalities involving the frenulum or superficial veins are noted. This is a common area for oral cancer, which presents as a white or red plaque, an indurated ulcer, or a warty growth.

A tongue blade is used to depress the tongue for adequate visualization of the pharynx. It is pressed firmly beyond the midpoint of the tongue. Proper placement avoids a gagging response and minimizes the patient's aversion to future oral examinations. The patient is told to tip his head back, open his mouth wide, take a deep breath, and say "ah." Often this will flatten the posterior tongue and briefly expose a full view of the anterior and posterior pillars, the tonsils, uvula, and posterior pharynx. These structures are inspected for color, symmetry, and evidence of exudate, ulceration, or enlargement. Normally, the uvula and soft palate rise symmetrically with a deep inspiration or "ah" and indicate an intact vagus nerve (10th cranial nerve).

A complete assessment of the oral cavity is essential, as many disorders such as cancer, diabetes, and immunosuppressive conditions from drug therapy or acquired immunodeficiency syndrome (AIDS) may be manifested by changes in the oral cavity.

▷ Nursing Diagnoses

Based on all the assessment data, major nursing diagnoses may include the following:

- Altered oral mucous membrane related to a pathologic condition, infection, or chemical/mechanical trauma (drugs, ill-fitting dentures)
- Altered nutrition, less than body requirements, related to in-

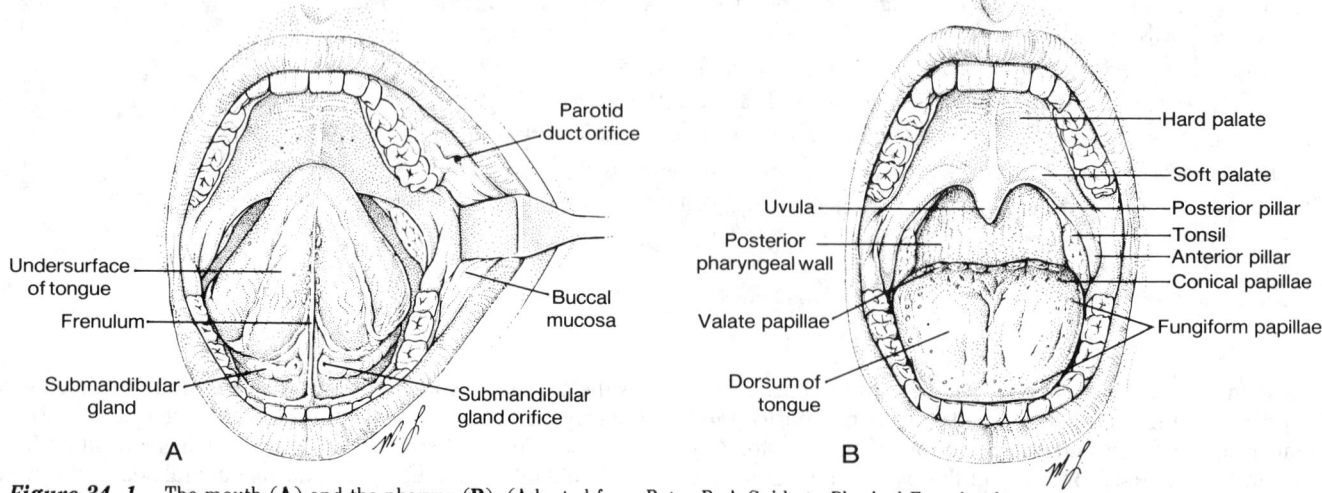

Figure 34–1.   The mouth (**A**) and the pharynx (**B**). (Adapted from Bates B. A Guide to Physical Examination and History Taking, 5th ed. Philadelphia, JB Lippincott, 1991.)

ability to ingest adequate nutrients secondary to oral/dental conditions.

- Disturbance in body image, related to a physical change in appearance subsequent to a disease condition or its treatment
- Pain related to oral lesion or treatment

◊ *Planning and Implementation*

◊ *Goals:* The major goals for the patient may include improvement in the condition of the oral mucous membrane, improvement in nutritional intake, attainment of a positive self-image, and attainment of comfort.

◊ *Nursing Interventions*

◊ *Mouth Care.* The nurse instructs the patient in the importance and techniques of preventive mouth care (Table 34–1). If a patient cannot tolerate brushing or flossing, an irrigating solution of 1 teaspoon of baking soda to 8 oz of warm water, or half-strength hydrogen peroxide is recommended (see Dudjak, 1987, in Nursing Research Profile for Unit 8). In the unconscious patient the nurse is responsible for oral hygiene (see Miller and Rubinstein, 1987, in Nursing Research Profile for Unit 8).

The cause of an oral mucus membrane disorder is identified by the physician so that it can be treated. The nurse monitors the intake of irritating substances. In the case of bacterial or fungal infections, the nurse administers the appropriate medication and instructs the patient in administration of medications for home care.

◊ *Nutritional Intake.* The patient's weight, age, and level of activity are recorded so an adequate daily calorie and nutritional intake can be estimated. A daily calorie count is maintained to determine the exact quantity of food and fluid ingested. The frequency and pattern of eating is recorded to determine if there are psychosocial factors as well as physiologic factors influencing ingestion. The nurse suggests that the patient avoid eating any foods that interfere with digestion. She recommends changes in the consistency of foods and the frequency of eating based on the disease condition and the patient's preferences. Consultation with a dietitian can be helpful. The goal is to help the patient attain and maintain a desirable body weight, healing of tissue, and sufficient energy.

◊ *Positive Self-Image.* If the patient has a disfiguring oral condition or has undergone disfiguring surgery, he may experience an alteration in self-image. The patient is encouraged to verbalize his perceived change in body appearance and realistically discuss actual changes or losses. The nurse offers support while the patient verbalizes his fears and negative feelings. The nurse encourages the patient to identify his reactions (withdrawal, depression, anger) and to describe himself and how he believes others see him so that he has a better understanding of his emotions. The nurse listens attentively and determines if the patient's needs are primarily psychosocial or cognitive-perceptual. This determination will help to individualize a plan of care. The patient's strengths and achievements are praised and his positive attributes reinforced.

The nurse should determine the patient's major anxieties concerning interpersonal relations at home and at work. The nurse then can recommend specific ways for the patient to interact with others and help him cope with his anxieties and fears. The nurse emphasizes that the patient's substance and worth are not diminished by a physical change in a body part.

The patient's progress in developing a positive self-esteem is recorded. The nurse should be alert to signs of grieving and should record emotional changes. Repeated opportunities are provided for listening, and the nurse should accept the patient's expressions of hostility. He is encouraged to relate his feelings in an atmosphere of acceptance.

◊ *Attainment of Comfort.* Oral lesions may be painful. The nurse instructs the patient in foods to avoid to minimize discomfort, such as spicy foods, hot foods, and hard foods (pretzels, nuts). The patient is also instructed in mouth care as above. It may be necessary to provide the patient with an analgesic such as viscous lidocaine (Xylocaine Viscous 2%) or narcotics as ordered by the physician.

◊ *Evaluation*

Expected Outcomes
1. Shows evidence of an intact oral mucous membrane
   a. Is free of pain/discomfort in the oral cavity
   b. No visible alteration in membrane integrity
   c. Identifies foods that are irritating (nuts, pretzels, spicy foods)
   d. States measures necessary for preventive mouth care
   e. Complies with medication regimen
2. Attains a desirable body weight
   a. Eats nutritionally balanced meals
   b. Keeps a daily record of calories
   c. Substitutes foods appropriately to maintain suggested caloric intake
   d. Maintains a recommended body weight plus or minus 2 to 3 kg (4 to 6 pounds)

TABLE 34–1. *Preventive Oral Hygiene*

1. Brush teeth using a soft toothbrush at least 2 times daily. Hold toothbrush at a 45-degree angle between brush and the gums and teeth. Gums and tongue surface should be brushed.
2. Floss at least once daily.
3. Use antiplaque mouth rinse.
4. Visit a dentist at least every 6 months, or when you have a chipped tooth, oral sore that persists longer than 2 weeks, or toothache.
5. Avoid alcohol and tobacco products, including smokeless tobacco.
6. Maintain adquate nutrition and avoid sweets.

3. Attains a positive self-image
   a. Freely discusses his body change
   b. Verbalizes anxieties
   c. Talks about himself as an important person
   d. Is able to accept change and modify his self-concept
   e. Speaks positively about his appearance
   f. Focuses energies away from self toward new identified goals
4. Attains an acceptable level of comfort
   a. Verbalizes that pain is absent or tolerable
   b. Avoids foods and liquids that cause discomfort
   c. Adheres to medication regimen

Conditions of the Oral Cavity

Abnormalities of the Lips, Gums, and Mouth

Many diseases are manifested as alterations in the oral cavity. This includes areas of the lips, mouth, or gums. Table 34–2 reviews abnormalities that may occur in these areas, as well as possible causes and nursing interventions.

Abnormalities of the Teeth

Dental Plaque and Caries

At least 95% of Americans sooner or later experience tooth decay. This is an erosive process that results from the action of bacteria on fermentable carbohydrates in the mouth, which in turn produces acids that dissolve tooth enamel. The extent of damage to the teeth depends on several factors, the most significant of which are (1) the presence of dental plaque; (2) the strength of the acids and the ability of the saliva to neutralize them; (3) the length of time the acids are in contact with the teeth; and (4) susceptibility of the teeth to decay. Dental plaque is a gluey, gelatin-like substance that adheres to the teeth. The initial action that causes damage to a tooth occurs under dental plaque.

Dental decay begins with a small hole, usually in a fissure or flaw of the enamel, or in an area that is hard to clean. Left unchecked, it penetrates the enamel into the dentin. Because the dentin is not as hard as the enamel, decay progresses somewhat more rapidly and in time reaches the pulp. When the blood, lymph vessels, and nerves are exposed, they become infected, and an abscess may form, either within the tooth or at the tip of the root. Soreness and pain usually accompany the abscess. As the infection increases, the patient's face may become swollen, and there may be pulsating pain. The dentist can determine by radiographs the extent of damage and the type of treatment needed. If treatment is not successful, it may be necessary to extract the tooth.

Preventive Management
Measures used in the prevention and control of dental caries include practicing effective mouth care, reducing the intake of sugars (refined carbohydrates), applying fluoride to the teeth or drinking fluoridated water, and the use of pit and fissure sealants.

Healthy teeth require conscientious and effective daily cleaning. The purpose of brushing is to mechanically break up the bacterial plaque that collects around teeth. See Table 34–1 for preventive oral hygiene.

The normal movement of the muscles of mastication and the normal flow of saliva also aid greatly in keeping the teeth clean. Because many ill patients do not eat and salivate normally, the natural cleaning process of the teeth is reduced. If a patient is unable to brush his teeth, which may occur in patients with cerebrovascular disease or those disabled by trauma, then it becomes a nursing responsibility. In any case, merely swabbing the patient's mouth and teeth with a swab is ineffective. The most effective method is mechanical cleansing. It is better to wipe the patient's teeth with a washcloth than to have him swish an antiseptic mouth wash several times and then emit it into the emesis basin. If the patient does not allow the nurse to use a toothbrush, a sponge swab immersed in a cleansing solution such as baking soda or half-strength hydrogen peroxide may be effective.

Lemon glycerin swabs, popular several years ago, are avoided because they are very drying to the patient's oral mucosa. Instead, the lips may be coated with a water-soluble gel to prevent drying.

Diet.   Dental caries may be prevented by decreasing the amount of sugar, especially between-meal snacks high in sugar. Alternative choices that are less cariogenic are fruits, vegetables, nuts, and possibly cheeses.

Fluoridation.   Fluoridation of public water supplies may decrease the amount of dental caries by 60%. Some areas of the country have natural fluoridation; other communities have mandated the addition of fluoride to public water supplies. Fluoridation may be attained through several other means, including vitamin preparations, application of a concentrated gel or solution by a dentist, addition of fluoride to home water supplies, or ingestion of sodium fluoride tablets or drops. To be most effective, fluoridation should take place between birth and 10 years of age.

Recent research has questioned the efficacy of fluoride and also suggests that the use of fluoride may be related to an increase in some types of cancer.

Pit and Fissure Sealants.   The occlusal surfaces of the teeth have pits and fissures that are areas prone to caries. Some dentists apply a special coating to fill and seal these areas from potential exposure to cariogenic processes.

Management
Treatment for dental caries includes fillings, extraction, dental implants, and dentures.

Fillings.   Carious areas in the teeth may be removed and the tooth refilled with a dental amalgam (alloy of several chemical elements). This procedure is performed by a dentist, often with the use of a local anesthetic.

Extraction.   Sometimes dental extraction is necessary if a tooth is defective or severely damaged. Extraction of one or several teeth is usually performed in the dental office. A local anesthetic is effective, and the procedure takes less than 30 minutes.

The patient may be admitted to a hospital for same-day surgery when all four molars are to be extracted at one time. Using endotracheal general anesthesia, the oral surgeon inserts a mouth retractor to provide exposure. Incisions are made laterally in the mandible to approach the impacted tooth. The jaw eventually regenerates bone that has been removed. Clo-

TABLE 34-2.   Abnormalities of the Lip, Mouth, and Gums

Condition	Signs and Symptoms	Possible Causes	Nursing Management
ABNORMALITIES OF THE LIP			
Actinic cheilitis	Irritation of lips associated with scaling, crusty, fissure. White overgrowth of horny layer of epidermis (hyperkeratosis).	Cumulative effect of exposure to sun. More frequently occuring in occupations with sun exposure such as farmers, and fair-skinned people. May lead to squamous cell cancer.	Teach patient importance of protecting lips from the sun by using protective ointment such as sun block. Instruct patient to have a periodic check-up by physician
Herpes simplex—cold sore or fever blister	Singular or clustered vesicles. May rupture.	Herpes simplex virus—an opportunistic infection. Frequently seen in immunosuppressed patients.	Acyclovir ointment or systemic administration as prescribed. Administer analgesics as prescribed. Avoid irritating foods.
Chancre	Reddened circumscribed lesion that ulcerates and becomes crusted.	Primary lesion of syphillis.	Cold soaks to lip for 20 minutes. Teach patient to avoid spicy food. Teach patient mouth care using half-strength hydrogen peroxide, or 1 teaspoon baking soda in 8 oz water.
Contact dermatitis	Red area or rash. Itching.	Allergic reaction to lipsticks, cosmetic ointments, or even toothpaste.	Instruct patient to avoid possible causes.
ABNORMALITIES OF THE MOUTH			
Leukoplakia (Fig. 34-2)	White patches, may by hyperkeratotic. Usually in buccal mucosa. Usually painless.	Less than 2% are malignant.	Instruct patient to see a physician if it persists longer than 2 weeks.
Hairy leukoplakia	White patches with rough hairlike projections. Typically found on lateral border of the tongue.	Smoking and use of tobacco. Seen often in persons who are HIV positive.	Instruct patient to see a physician if it persists longer than 2 weeks.
Lichen planus	White papules at the intersection of a network of interlacing lesions. Usually ulcerated and painful		Administer viscous lidocaine for pain. Instruct the patient to hold this in his mouth for 2–3 min. Apply triamcinolone (Kenalog) or Orabase after meals or at bedtime to assist with promotion of healing. Administer corticosteroids systemically or intralesionally, as prescribed. Instruct the patient in need for follow-up if condition is chronic.
Candidiasis—monilliases/thrush	Cheesy white plaque that looks like milk curds. When rubbed off, it leaves erythematous and often bleeding base.	*Candida ablicans* fungus. Predisposing factors include diabetes, antibiotic therapy, and immunosuppression.	Antifungal medications such as nystatin (Mycostatin), clotrimazole, or ketoconazole, as prescribed. These may be taken in pill form or as a suspension. When used as a suspension, the nurse teaches the patient to swish vigoroulsy for at least 1 minute and swallow.

(continued)

TABLE 34-2. *(Continued)*

Condition	Signs and Symptoms	Possible Causes	Nursing Management
Aphthous stomatitis—canker sore	Shallow ulcer with a white center and red border. Seen on the inner side of the lip and cheek. May also appear on the tongue. It begins with a burning or tingling sensation and slight swelling. Painful. Usually lasts 7–10 days and heals without a scar. Has a tendency to recur.	Unknown. It is associated with emotional or mental stress, fatigue, or hormonal factors.	Comfort measures such as a soft or bland diet. Antibiotics or steroids sometimes are helpful.
Leukoplakia buccalis—smoker's patch	This has two stages. Stage I has one or two thick pearly patches on the mucous membrane of the tongue or mouth. Over time the tongue and mouth become covered with a creamy thick white mucous membrane. They may slough, leaving a beefy red base.	Chronic irritation by carious, infected, poorly repaired teeth; tobacco; highly spiced foods; and occasionally due to syphilis.	Correction of the underlying cause will lead to disappearance.
Krythroplakia	Red patch on the oral mucous membrane.	Nonspecific inflammation. More frequently seen in the elderly.	
Kaposi's sarcoma	Appears first on the oral mucosa as a red, purple, or blue lesion. May be a singular lesion or multiple lesions. May be flat or raised.	HIV infection.	Instruct patient regarding side effects related to treatment such as surgery and radiation, or to use and side effects of medication.

ABNORMALITIES OF THE GUMS

Condition	Signs and Symptoms	Possible Causes	Nursing Management
Gingivitis	Painful, inflamed, swollen gums. Usually the gums bleed in response to light contact.	Poor oral hygiene—a collection of food debris, bacterial plaque, and calculus (tartar). The gums may also swell in response to normal processes such as puberty and pregnancy.	Teach patient proper oral hygiene (see Table 34-1).
Necrotizing gingivitis	Gray-white pseudomembranous ulcerations affecting the edges of the gums, mucosa of the mouth, tonsils, and pharynx. Foul breath. Painful, bleeding gums. Swallowing and talking are also painful.	Poor oral hygiene.	Instruct patient in proper oral hygiene (see Table 34-1).
Herpatic gingivostomatitis	Burning sensation with the appearance of small vesicles 24–48 hours later. Vesicles may rupture, forming sore shallow ulcers covered with a gray membrane.	Herpes simplex virus. This occurs most frequently in persons who are immunosuppressed. May occur in other infectious processes such as Streptococcal pneumonia, Meningococcal meningitis, and malaria.	Apply topical analgesics as prescribed. May need systemic narcotics if pain is severe. An antiviral agent such as systemic Acyclovir may be prescribed.
Peridontitis	Little discomfort at onset. May have bleeding, infection, gum recession, and loosening of teeth. Later in the disease the teeth may fall out.	Untreated gingivitis. Approximately 90% of persons over 40 are affected. Poor or inadequate dental hygiene and inadequate diet contribute to development.	Instruct patient in proper oral hygiene (see Table 34-1).

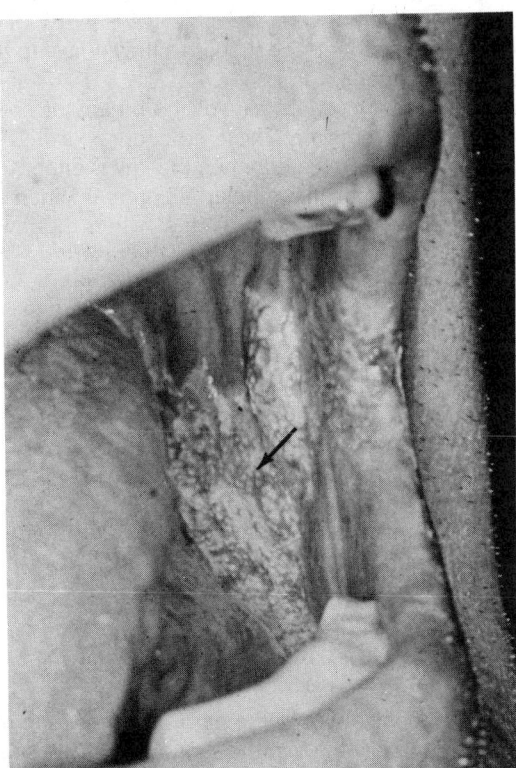

Figure 34–2. Leukoplakia. Note the white patches above and to the right of the teeth. (Lynch MA et al. Burket's Oral Medicine: Diagnosis and Treatment, 8th ed. Philadelphia, JB Lippincott, 1984.)

sure of the mucous membrane is accomplished with black silk sutures.

Tooth extraction is a simple procedure that usually has few complications. Elderly patients and patients taking anticoagulants may require special considerations. The elderly may have a chronic illness that makes it difficult for them to sit or recline in a dental chair for longer than 15 minutes. The dentist can keep the dental chair in the upright position and perform the procedure in spaced intervals. Patients taking an oral anticoagulant may be advised by the physician to withhold the medication and take oral vitamin K for 3 days before the dental procedure.

Nursing Interventions. After tooth extraction, oozing of blood may be apparent the first day. The patient is advised to rest and not rinse his mouth for the first 24 hours to lessen the likelihood of bleeding. If heavy bleeding occurs, he is told to place a clean, folded gauze pad directly on the bleeding spot and close his teeth tightly over the pad and apply pressure for about 30 minutes. He is advised to notify the dentist if there is prolonged or severe pain, swelling, or bleeding.

If impacted molars have been removed, the patient is advised to use ice packs to both sides of his face for 20-minute periods every hour for 24 hours to relieve swelling and soreness. Liquids are recommended for the first 24 hours. Most patients enjoy ice cream or milk shakes because they are filling, and the cool liquid soothes swollen tissues. A spouted container can be used if sucking from a straw is painful. The sutures are removed after the fifth day. Mouth rinsing or irrigations, usually with a salt water solution, are recommended for several days after tooth extraction. Brushing of the teeth is resumed when

the gums have healed. Prophylactic antibiotic treatment after extraction is often prescribed. These measures are taken because infection may be a complication. The patient is instructed to report any swelling or pain lasting longer than 1 week.

Dental Implants. Sometimes dental implants or transplantations are suggested if a patient has had multiple tooth extractions, or problems wearing dentures. Implants are metal replacements for teeth. The implant is stabilized in the bone structure of the gum.

Dentures. It is common practice for people to postpone indefinitely the final decision to obtain dentures, even though there is no possibility of having the few remaining teeth repaired. Hesitant patients are encouraged to pursue this health need by pointing out to them the positive aspects of obtaining dentures: improved appearance, better nutrition, and reduced likelihood of infection. The nurse should stress that when dentures are obtained, patience is required in learning to wear them effectively.

During the first 2 months of denture wear the patient is advised to

- Keep the dentures in place for 24 hours before the first adjustment so that any pressure areas or irritated tissue can be identified.
- Always put his dentures in place at least 6 hours before seeing the dentist for an adjustment.
- Be patient. It takes 6 to 8 weeks for gum tissue to adapt.
- Avoid large pieces of food, foods that irritate the gums (peanuts, celery, corn, seeds [as in fruits]), and foods that may get stuck between the gum tissue and the dentures, because the tissues are still swollen.
- Keep dentures clean and maintain healthy gum tissue by brushing twice a day with a soft toothbrush.

Pressure or irritation caused by dentures is reported to the dentist, who can make the proper adjustment. Uncorrected pressure areas may cause lesions.

Dentures require careful scrubbing, using a firm denture brush, mild soap and water, salt, and sodium bicarbonate. The addition of a drop of household chlorine acts as a deodorant and gives a fresher taste. Most dentists recommend that dentures be removed at night, scrubbed, and allowed to soak in a proprietary cleaner. When a patient is unable to clean his dentures, this becomes the responsibility of the nurse or family member.

Partial dentures should not be left in place for prolonged periods without being removed for a good cleaning. They are held in place with metal clasps that encircle the teeth. These clasps can be spread: using gentle force with two index fingers, one side and then the other can be loosened. When reapplied, the cleaned partial dentures usually can be pressed into place.

Many people prefer to have "immediate dentures." Usually, the back teeth are extracted first, which allows the tissues time to heal. Meanwhile, the artificial teeth are made and are ready for placement immediately after the front teeth have been extracted.

Dentoalveolar Abscess or Periapical Abscess

Periapical abscess, more commonly referred to as an abscessed tooth, results from a suppurative process involving the apical dental periosteum (fibrous membrane supporting the tooth structure) and the alveolar process in the periapical region (tissue surrounding the apex of the tooth where it is suspended in the tooth socket). It may appear in two forms. The acute form is usually secondary to a suppurative pulpitis that arises from an infection extending from dental caries. The infection of the dental pulp extends through the apical foramen of the tooth to form an abscess about the apex, its site of implantation in the alveolar bone. The abscess produces a dull, gnawing, continuous pain, often with a surrounding cellulitis and edema of the adjacent facial structures, and mobility of the involved tooth. The gum opposite the apex of the tooth is usually swollen on the cheek side, where the abscess is apt to point. Swelling and cellulitis of the facial structures may make it difficult to open the mouth. In well-developed abscesses there may be a systemic reaction, fever, and malaise.

Chronic dentoalveolar abscess is a slowly progressive infection with the same mode as the acute form. It differs from the acute form in that the process may progress to a fully formed abscess without the patient's knowing it. The infection eventually leads to a "blind dental abscess" that is really a periapical granuloma. It may enlarge to as much as 1 cm in diameter. It is often discovered on x-ray examination and is treated by extraction or root canal therapy, often with apicoectomy (excision of the apex of the tooth root).

Management

In the early stages of an infection, a dental surgeon may drill an opening into the pulp chamber to relieve tension and pain and to provide drainage. Usually, the infection has progressed to a periapical abscess. Drainage is provided by an incision through the gingivae down to the jaw bone. Foul pus escapes under pressure. This procedure is usually performed in the dental office. Occasionally the patient is admitted to the hospital for same-day surgery. After the inflammatory reaction has subsided, the tooth may have to be extracted or appropriate root canal therapy given.

Nursing Interventions

The nurse assesses the patient for bleeding after treatment. The patient is instructed to use a warm saline or water mouth rinse to keep the area clean. The nurse instructs the patient in the use of antibiotics and analgesics. The patient is also instructed to advance his diet from liquids to a soft diet as tolerated.

Malocclusion

Malocclusion is a faulty relationship between the teeth when the jaws are closed. Fifty percent of the population has some form of malocclusion. Correction of malocclusion requires several factors: an orthodontist who has special training, a patient who is motivated and cooperative, and adequate time. Most treatments begin when the patient has shed his last primary tooth and the last permanent successor has erupted, usually around 12 or 13 years of age.

Preventive orthodontics is started at age 5 if malocclusion is diagnosed early. Studies have shown the reduced need for teeth straightening in adolescence if preventive orthodontics is started with the primary teeth.

Management

To realign the teeth, the orthodontist gradually forces the teeth into a new location by the use of wires or plastic bands. Although the patient may object to the effect of these devices on his appearance, this psychological burden must be over-

come if good results are to be achieved in the future. In the final phase of treatment, a retaining device is worn for several hours each day to support the tissues as they adjust to the new alignment of the teeth.

Braces are also used as part of the means of correcting long or short jaw syndrome. These procedures, called *orthognathic surgery*, are performed when the jaw is either too long or too short for proper mandibular alignment. When the jaw is too long, bony material is extracted; when the jaw is too short, a bone graft or inert material may be inserted. The postoperative care of these patients is similar to that needed by patients with a fractured mandible (see pp. 858–859).

Nursing Interventions

It is essential that the patient keep his mouth meticulously clean. Encouragement is often necessary for the patient to persist in this most important part of the treatment. When an adolescent undergoing orthodontal correction is admitted to the hospital for some other problem, it may be necessary to remind him to continue wearing the retainer if it does not interfere with the problem requiring hospitalization.

Abnormalities of the Salivary Glands

The salivary glands consist of the parotid glands, one on each side of the face below the ear; the submaxillary and sublingual glands, both in the floor of the mouth; and the buccal gland, beneath the lips. About 1200 ml of saliva is produced daily. The glands' primary functions are lubrication, antibacterial protection, and digestion.

Parotitis

Parotitis (inflammation of the parotid gland) is the most common inflammatory condition of the salivary glands; however, infection can occur in the other glands as well. The essential lesion of mumps (epidemic parotitis) is an inflammation of the salivary gland (usually the parotid) and is primarily a pediatric communicable disease caused by viral infection.

Elderly, acutely ill, and debilitated people with decreased salivary flow due to general dehydration or medications are at high risk for developing parotitis. The infecting organisms travel from the mouth through the salivary duct.

The offending organism usually is *Staphylococcus aureus* (except in mumps). The onset of this complication is sudden, with an exacerbation of the fever and of the symptoms of the primary condition. The gland swells and becomes tense and tender. Pain is felt in the ear, and there is interference with swallowing. The swelling increases rapidly, and the overlying skin soon becomes red and shiny.

Nursing Interventions

Preventive mechanisms are essential. To prevent postoperative parotitis, patients are advised to have necessary dental work performed before surgery. In addition, optimal patient preparation includes maintaining an adequate nutritional and fluid intake along with good oral hygiene, and if possible discontinuing medications such as tranquilizers and diuretics that may cause a decrease in salivation. If parotitis occurs, antibiotic therapy is necessary. The nurse should also administer analgesics to control pain. If antibiotic therapy is not effective, incision and drainage (I & D) of the gland are necessary.

Sialadenitis

Sialadenitis (inflammation of the salivary glands) is caused by dehydration, radiation treatment, stress, or improper oral hygiene and is associated with infection with *Staphylococcus aureus, Streptococcus viridans,* or pneumococcus. Characteristics include pain, swelling, and a purulent discharge.

Management

Antibiotics are used to relieve acute symptoms. Massage, hydration, and steroids frequently cure the problem. Chronic sialadenitis, with uncontrolled pain, requires surgical excision of the gland and its duct.

Salivary Calculus (Sialolithiasis)

Salivary calculi (stones) occur in the submandibular gland. Sialograms (x-ray films taken with a radiopaque substance injected into the duct) may be required to demonstrate obstruction of the duct by stenosis. Salivary stones are formed mainly from calcium phosphate. If located within the gland, they are irregularly lobulated and vary in diameter from 3 to 30 mm. Stones in the duct are small and oval.

Calculi within the salivary gland cause no symptoms unless infection arises; but a calculus that obstructs the gland's duct causes sudden, local, and often colicky pain, which is suddenly relieved by a gush of saliva. This characteristic complaint can be elicited in a health history. When this condition exists, the gland is swollen and quite tender, the stone itself often is palpable, and its shadow may be seen on x-ray films.

The calculus can be extracted fairly easily from the duct in the mouth; sometimes enlarging the orifice permits the stone to pass spontaneously. It may be necessary to remove the gland surgically if there are repeated recurrences of symptoms and calculi in the gland itself.

Neoplasms

Although uncommon, neoplasms of almost any type may develop in the salivary gland. Tumors occur more frequently in the parotid gland. The incidence of salivary gland tumors is similar in men and women. Diagnosis is based on the history and physical examination and biopsy results.

Management

There is controversy regarding the best management of salivary gland tumors. Partial excision of the gland, along with all of the tumor and a wide margin, combined with careful dissection to preserve the vulnerable seventh cranial nerve (facial nerve), is the common procedure. For more involved tumors, it may not be possible to preserve the nerve when a parotidectomy is performed. If the tumor is malignant or mixed, radiation therapy may follow surgery. Chemotherapy may also be used followed by surgery. Local recurrences are common; the recurrent growth usually is more malignant than the original. It has also been observed that these patients have an increased incidence of second primary cancers.

Cancer of the Oral Cavity

Cancer of the oral cavity, which may occur in any part of the mouth or throat, is highly curable if discovered early. It is associated with the use of alcohol and tobacco. Many feel that the combination of alcohol and tobacco has a synergistic carcinogenic effect. Age is also a risk factor, with 75% of oral cancers occurring in persons over 60; but it is increasing in men under 30 because of the use of smokeless tobacco. It accounts for less that 2% of all cancer deaths in the United States. Men are afflicted twice as often as women; however, the incidence in women is increasing, possibly because of the increased use of tobacco and alcohol by women. The 5-year survival rate for cancer of the oral cavity and pharynx is 53% for whites and 31% for blacks. Of the 8150 annual deaths from oral cancer, the distribution by site is estimated as follows:

Lips	1% (100 cases)
Tongue	23% (1850 cases)
Mouth	29% (2400 cases)
Pharynx	47% (3800 cases)

The tumor seen with *cancer of the lip* is usually called an epithelioma. It occurs most frequently as a chronic ulcer on the lower lip in men. Basal cell carcinoma usually occurs on the upper lip and squamous cell carcinoma on the lower lip. Predisposing factors may be chronic irritation by a warm pipe stem or prolonged exposure to the sun and wind.

A typical lesion is a painless indurated ulcer with raised edges. Any wart or ulcer of the lip that does not heal in 2 weeks should be examined through biopsy.

Clinical Manifestations

Most oral cancers exhibit no symptoms in the early stages. The most frequent complaint of the patient is a painless sore or mass that will not heal. As the cancer progresses, the patient may complain of tenderness, difficulty in chewing, difficulty swallowing, difficulty speaking, coughing of blood-tinged sputum, or lumps in the area of the neck.

Diagnostic Evaluation

Diagnostic evaluation consists of an oral examination as well as assessment of cervical lymph nodes to evaluate for possible metastasis. Biopsies are performed on lesions suggestive of cancer. Suspicious lesions are those that have not healed in 2 weeks. Oral areas of high risk include the buccal mucosa and gingiva for persons who use snuff or smoke a cigar or pipe. For persons who smoke cigarettes and drink alcohol, high-risk areas include the floor of the mouth, ventrolateral tongue, and soft palate complex (the soft palate complex includes the soft palate, the anterior and posterior tonsillar area, uvula, and the area behind the molar and tongue junction).

Management

Management varies with the nature of the lesion, preference of the physician, and patient choice. Resectional surgery, radiation therapy, chemotherapy, or a combination of therapies may be effective.

In cancer of the lip, small lesions are usually excised liberally; larger lesions involving more than one third of the lip may be more appropriately treated by radiation therapy because of superior cosmetic results. The choice depends on the extent of the lesion, the skill of the surgeon or radiologist, and what is necessary to cure the patient while preserving the best appearance. For tumors larger than 4 cm there is a high recurrence rate.

Therapy for cancer of the tongue is usually aggressive, as the recurrence rate is high. For cancer of the lateral margin of the tongue, the two major treatments of choice are radiation therapy and surgery. It is often necessary to perform a hemiglossectomy (Fig. 34–3).

When cancer is present at the base of the tongue, surgical resection is more debilitating. Often radiation therapy may be the primary treatment. A combination of interstitial implants and external beam radiation may be employed. For larger lesions, external beam therapy alone is used.

Often cancer of the oral cavity has metastasized through the extensive lymphatic channel in the neck region (Fig. 34–4), thereby requiring a radical neck dissection (see p. 855).

▶ Nursing Process
The Patient With Cancer of the Oral Cavity

▷ Assessment

The principal nursing activities in the assessment phase include a careful nursing history (see p. 844). Particular attention is given to the patient's history of alcohol and tobacco use. The patient is also questioned regarding sores in the area of the oral cavity that have not healed for 2 weeks, and any lumps in the neck region.

Physical examination of the mouth is performed with careful description of any ulcerated areas. The neck is examined for enlarged lymph nodes (adenopathy).

▷ Nursing Diagnoses

Based on all the assessment data, the nursing diagnoses may include the following:

- Knowledge deficit about treatment plan and disease process
- Altered oral mucous membrane related to pathologic condition
- Alterated nutrition, less than body requirements, related to reduced intake of foods and fluids secondary to sensitive oral mucous membranes or decreased appetite
- Body image disturbance related to disfiguring appearance of an oral lesion or reconstructive surgery
- Fear of pain and social isolation and ineffective coping related to the diagnosis and prognosis of the disease process
- Impaired communication related to treatment or lesion.
- High risk for infection related to altered immunologic responses secondary to chemotherapy/irradiation
- Anticipatory grieving related to the diagnosis of cancer

▷ Planning and Implementation

▷ *Goals:*   The patient's major goals may include acquisition of knowledge about the treatment plan, maintenance of the integrity of the oral cavity, adequate intake of foods and fluids, attainment of a positive self-image and effective communication, acquisition of coping mechanisms, absence of infection, and acceptance of the diagnosis.

▷ Nursing Interventions

▷ *Patient Education.*   The nurse has the responsibility to make sure that the patient receives accurate information about his disease process if he wants the information. Some patients want to know everything about their diagnosis, and others want to know only what is necessary for them to manage their daily activities. The participation of family members or significant others is encouraged in any discussions.

The nurse must determine what the patient already knows and what he wants to know about the type of treatment recommended (chemotherapy, radiation therapy, surgery), the

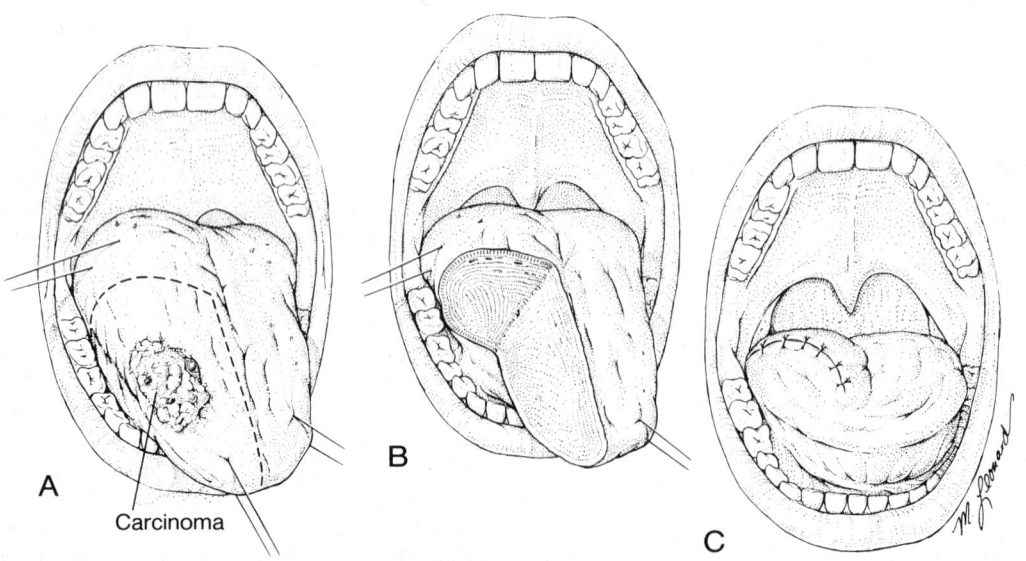

Figure 34–3.   (**A**) Surgery for cancer of the tongue. Small invasive cancer of the tongue. Tongue is extended and incision margins are outlined. (**B**) A deep resection provides for removal of a generous portion of nonmalignant tissue. (**C**) Sutured area results in a shallow margin that is less defined when the tongue is extended. (Adapted with permission from McQuarrie DG et al. Head and Neck Cancer. Chicago, Year Book Medical Publishers, 1986.)

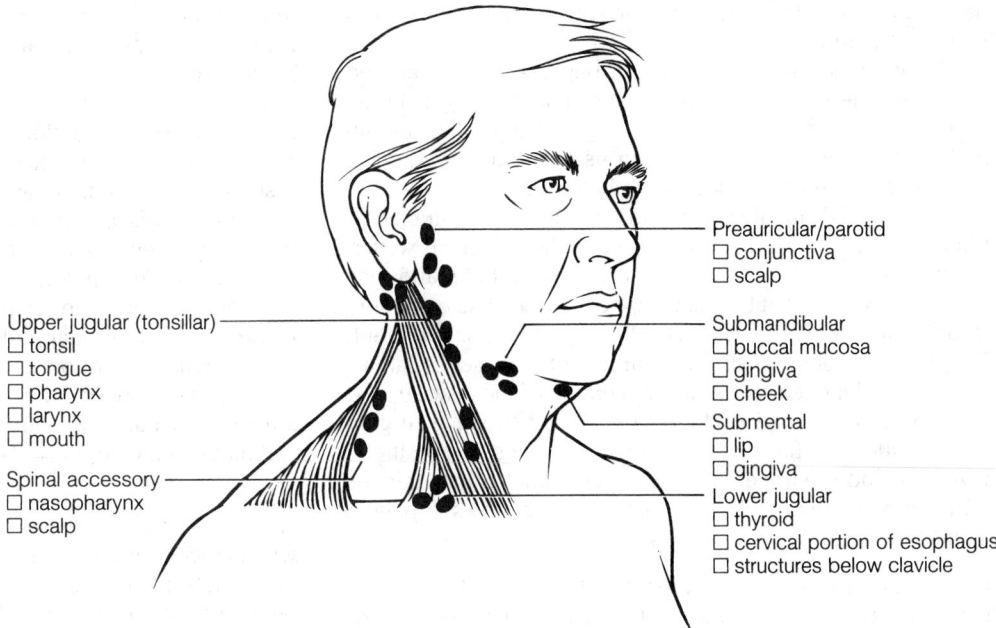

Upper jugular (tonsillar)
☐ tonsil
☐ tongue
☐ pharynx
☐ larynx
☐ mouth

Spinal accessory
☐ nasopharynx
☐ scalp

Preauricular/parotid
☐ conjunctiva
☐ scalp

Submandibular
☐ buccal mucosa
☐ gingiva
☐ cheek

Submental
☐ lip
☐ gingiva

Lower jugular
☐ thyroid
☐ cervical portion of esophagus
☐ structures below clavicle

Figure 34–4. Lymphatic drainage of the head and neck.

process involved, and the implications for his care. Information is presented at the patient's level of understanding and when he is relaxed, pain-free, and not distracted by visitors. Important facts are emphasized and repeated by the patient as necessary.

▷ *Mouth Care.* The nurse teaches the patient how to keep his mouth clean. Use of a soft toothbrush is recommended to minimize irritation of the gums. Flossing should be performed at least once a day to prevent the accumulation of food debris, which can aggravate sensitive tissues. If the patient cannot tolerate brushing or flossing, an irrigating solution of 1 teaspoon of baking soda to 8 ounces of warm water is recommended. Gentle lavage with a catheter inserted between the cheek and teeth loosens mucus and is refreshing. A power spray has the advantage of getting the solution into inaccessible areas. Commercial mouthwashes are not used because they contain alcohol, which can irritate the gums and dry the mouth.

Dryness of the mouth is a frequent sequela of oral cancer, particularly when the salivary glands have been exposed to radiation or major surgery. It is also noted in patients who are receiving psychopharmacologic agents or in those who are unable to close the mouth and therefore become mouth-breathers. To minimize this problem, the patient is advised to avoid dry, bulky, and irritating foods and fluids as well as alcohol and tobacco. He is also encouraged to increase intake of fluids, if not contraindicated. It may also be helpful to use a synthetic saliva.

Stomatitis or mucositis (breakdown of the oral mucosa) is often a side effect of chemotherapy or radiation therapy. Prophylactic mouth care is started when the patient begins receiving treatment; however, mucositis may become so severe that a break in treatment is necessary. If a patient receiving radiation therapy has poor dentition, it is often recommended that extraction of the teeth be performed before initiation of the treatment to the oral cavity to prevent infection.

With the unconscious patient, the nurse is wholly responsible for maintaining good oral hygiene. The use of a special mouth kit with all necessary applicator sticks, padded tongue

depressors, mouthwashes, and lubricants encourages frequent mouth attention. A water-soluble lip moisturizer is applied as needed to soothe dry and cracking lips.

▷ *Adequate Food and Fluid Intake.* Anorexia is a common problem in a patient with oral cancer because of the discomfort associated with eating. Soft or blenderized food may be helpful. Supplementary feedings (Sustacal, Ensure) help maintain an adequate protein and calorie intake. Weights are monitored and a daily nutritional assessment is performed to determine the quantity of food and fluid ingested. Consultation with a registered dietitian is helpful.

The desires as well as the nutritional needs of the patient should be taken into consideration. If he is not able to take anything by mouth, it may be necessary to provide nutrients parenterally or enterally to maintain fluid and electrolyte balance and to prevent starvation and negative nitrogen balance.

▷ *Coping Measures.* The patient requires patience and understanding. Quite naturally, he tends to withdraw from people, is self-conscious about mouth odors, and is sensitive about his appearance. The nurse is challenged to communicate with the patient, encourage his expression of fears and concerns, and offer him support and explanations as necessary. The immediate family needs to be aware of their supporting role and, in turn, should be informed of the plan of therapy for the patient and urged to participate in the plan of care.

A particular area of concern that interferes with communication, feeding, and swallowing is excessive salivation or drooling. The measures taken to control drooling depend on the cause, severity, and duration of the dysfunction. If the problem is moderate to severe but temporary, as may be the case after surgery, mechanical suction devices used with a soft catheter are effective. If drooling is mild, control may be obtained by training the patient to swallow more frequently, by providing emotional reassurance and support, and by using anticholinergic agents, such as those containing atropine or belladonna (Banthine, Robinul). For more severe drooling, it may be necessary to resort to plastic reconstructive surgery of the oral structures.

Mouth wipes, as well as a paper bag attached to the bed or the bedside stand to receive soiled tissues, always should be on hand. An effective way of holding dressings of the mouth or the lower jaw in place is by the use of a face mask. The strings can be tied at the top of the head.

The patient's family and friends should be encouraged to visit so that he is aware that others care about him. However, the patient may express a strong desire for solitude, and may be self-conscious about his appearance. The results of surgery or radiation concern him, especially the fear of disfigurement. The possibility of reconstructive surgery or prosthetics (an artificial part) depends on the site and extent of the disease, and needs to be explained to the patient. Reconstructive surgery may include skin flaps or grafts. Several types of prosthetic devices include an upper jaw device, a prosthetic that attaches to the upper teeth and extends back to replace the soft palate, or upper teeth.

▷ *Alleviation of Fear.*　The nurse has the patient describe his fears related to pain, isolation, altered life style, and loss of control. The description may provide a clue for managing the problem and developing a plan of care. The nurse assesses the patient's physical reactions to his fears. Common responses include muscle rigidity, fatigue, tachycardia, hypertension, dyspnea, and nausea.

The nurse can reduce fears in a number of ways. For example, the fear of pain can be managed by advising the patient that medication will be offered every 3 to 4 hours, and that if something more is needed the physician will be consulted to adjust the dosage or frequency. The nurse supports adaptive behaviors, encourages expressions of emotions, emphasizes the patient's abilities, and fosters positive self-esteem.

Distorted perceptions are corrected by providing accurate information. Control is fostered by encouraging the patient to participate in the treatment process. Support groups are recommended, and the nurse can offer to contact a representative from a support group to visit the patient.

The nurse should be receptive to the patient's expressions of potential loss. Behaviors associated with defense mechanisms such as projection, displacement, and rationalization need to be recognized. Many patients withdraw, cry easily, and experience a sense of hopelessness. Some of them progress through certain behaviors in anticipating death: denial, anger, depression, bargaining, resolution, and acceptance. The nurse's role is one of offering support. She projects an optimistic attitude, especially if the lesion has a high incidence of cure (90% for cancer of the lip). Visits by an appropriate counselor, social worker, or member of the clergy can be suggested.

▷ *Impaired Communication.*　For the patient undergoing radical surgical procedures for oral cancer, the potential for loss of verbal communication is high. Preoperatively the patient's ability to communicate in writing is assessed. He is provided with a magic slate or pen and paper to communicate postoperatively. If he is unable to write, a communication board with commonly used words or pictures is obtained preoperatively so that he may point to items he needs. A speech therapist is also involved postoperatively.

▷ *Infection Control.*　Thrombocytopenia and leukopenia, side effects of radiation and chemotherapy, weaken a patient's de-

fense mechanisms, making him more susceptible to infections. Anemia subsequent to malnutrition is also common. Laboratory results must be evaluated frequently, and the patient's temperature is checked every 6 to 8 hours for an elevation that may indicate an infection. Visitors who may transmit microorganisms are prohibited because the patient's immunologic system is depressed. Trauma to sensitive skin tissues is avoided to maintain skin integrity and prevent infection. Strict aseptic technique is necessary when changing dressings. Desquamation (shedding of the epidermis) is a reaction to radiation therapy that causes dryness and itching and can lead to a break in skin integrity and subsequent infection.

Adequate nutrition as discussed above is helpful in preventing infection. Signs of wound infection such as redness, swelling, drainage, or tenderness are reported to the physician. Antibiotics may be prescribed prophylactically.

▷ *Home Health Care.*　The posthospital objectives of patient care are similar to those during hospitalization. The patient who is recovering from treatment of a mouth condition needs to breathe, to obtain nourishment, to avoid infection, and to be alert for adverse signs. The patient, members of his family or the person responsible for his home care, the nurse, and whoever else may be involved, such as a speech therapist, dietitian, and psychologist, need to prepare an individualized plan of care. If suctioning the mouth or a tracheostomy tube is required, it is important to determine what equipment is needed and how to use it, as well as where it can be obtained. Consideration is given to the humidification and aeration of the room, as well as measures to control odors. Methods to prepare foods that are nutritious, properly seasoned, and of the right temperature can be explained. It may be more convenient for some patients to use commercial baby food than to prepare liquid and soft diets in a blender. If the patient is unable to take oral foods, instruction in the use of enteral or parenteral feedings is necessary. The use and care of prostheses must be understood. The importance of cleanliness with dressings and mouth care is reviewed. The person caring for the patient needs to know the signs of obstruction, hemorrhage, infection, depression, and withdrawal, as well as what to do about these problems. Follow-up visits to the clinic or physician are important to determine progression or regression and for the patient and caregiver to receive instructions about any modifications in medication or general care.

Over 90% of oral cancer recurrences appear within the first 18 months; therefore, meticulous inspection by the physician every 4 to 6 weeks is essential. Follow-up visits are indicated less frequently after 2 years but must be continued for life, because of the frequency of other primary carcinomas. One important part of continuing care is the elimination of alcohol consumption and smoking. Because of further extension of a malignancy by metastasis and necrosis, it may not be possible to halt the spread of disease. All efforts are then directed toward the comfort measures—physical, psychological, and spiritual. With the family's help these efforts may be continued in the hospital, a nursing home, a hospice setting, or the patient's own home.

▷ ## Evaluation

Expected Outcomes

1. Acquires information about disease process and course of treatment

a. Is motivated to learn about treatment and its implications and participates in the teaching sessions
b. Involves family members in teaching sessions as a means of support
2. Practices oral hygiene measures
   a. Brushes teeth and flosses daily; performs mouth care after each meal
   b. Inspects mouth routinely for the presence of lesions
   c. Avoids foods and fluids that irritate the gums or mouth
   d. Limits or avoids use of alcohol and tobacco (including smokeless tobacco)
   e. Uses lubricating agents for the mouth
   f. Exhibits no visible alteration in mucous membrane integrity
3. Maintains adequate intake of foods and fluids
   a. Eats soft, nonirritating foods several times a day
   b. Uses a modified eating utensil if necessary
   c. Maintains or gains weight
   d. Is hydrated
   e. Requests antiemetic agents as needed
   f. Adheres to enteral or parenteral feeding schedule
4. Evidences a positive self-image
   a. Interacts appropriately with family members
   b. Projects self-confidence
   c. Participates in social gatherings
   d. Discusses diagnosis and prognosis
   e. Verbally discusses emotional responses to the diagnosis
5. Reduces fears related to pain, isolation, and the inability to cope
   a. Accepts that pain will be managed if not eliminated
   b. Freely expresses fears and concerns
   c. Agrees to talk with a support group
   d. Communicates openly with family members and significant others
6. Communicates effectively with staff and family/friends
   a. Able to express needs verbally, with use of magic slate, pen and paper, or communication board
   b. Writes one positive thing about self each day
7. Is infection free
   a. Maintains normal laboratory values
   b. Is afebrile
   c. Maintains skin integrity
   d. Practices oral hygiene after every meal and at bedtime
   e. Avoids visitors with infectious conditions
   f. Eats a high-protein, high-carbohydrate diet

Gerontologic Considerations

Gerodontology is the branch of dentistry that deals with the elderly. About 50% of persons over 65 have lost all their teeth as a result of caries or periodontal disease. Although the goal in dentistry today is to retain the permanent teeth, that goal is not always possible for an aged person who has neglected caring for the teeth, and a partial or complete set of dentures may be necessary.

Tooth loss is not a normal aging process. Normal age-related changes in the oral mucosa include a drier and thinner epithelial skin layer and possibly a decrease in salivation. It is known that certain drugs frequently used in the elderly (such

as diuretics, drugs for Parkinson's disease, and some antihypertensives) will decrease salivary flow. There is a decrease in oral motor function (swallowing and chewing). Age is also a risk factor for development of oral cancer, as 75% of oral cancers occur in individuals over 60.

In summary, alterations in the oral cavity may be the result of a localized disease or a systemic disease that has oral manifestations. Several specific causes for these changes may include (1) neoplasms, (2) immunosuppression from drug therapy or human immunodeficiency virus (HIV) infection, (3) trauma, (4) diabetes, and (5) infectious lesions of bacterial, viral, or fungal origin. Treatment is dependent on the type, location, and extent of the oral condition.

Radical Neck Dissection

Malignancies of the head and neck, including cancers of the oral cavity, pharynx, and larynx, may be treated early by surgery, irradiation, or chemotherapy, with good results. These cancers (stages I and II) are in an area that can be easily seen, making early prognosis and treatment possible. Most observers agree that such patients do not die of recurrence at the site of the primary growth, but rather of metastasis to the cervical lymph nodes in the neck, which often takes place by way of the lymphatics before the primary lesion has been treated. Chemotherapy or radiation may be used in conjunction with radical neck dissection.

A radical neck dissection involves removal of all the tissue under the skin, from the ramus of the jaw down to the clavicle, and from the midline anteriorly back to the anterior border of the trapezius muscle posteriorly. This includes removal of the sternocleidomastoid muscle and other smaller muscles, as well as the jugular vein in the neck, because the lymphatic nodes are found widely distributed throughout these tissues (Fig. 34–5).

A *functional or modified neck dissection* involves only removal of the lymph nodes. Obviously, this approach appears a reasonable alternative to radical radiation therapy and is a preferred alternative to traditional neck dissection in the control of regional metastasis when neck disease is either occult or still confined to mobile lymph nodes.

▶ Nursing Process
The Patient Undergoing a Radical Neck Dissection

◊ Assessment

Preoperatively the patient is assessed for physical and psychological preparation for major surgery. He is also assessed for knowledge related to the preoperative and postoperative routines. Postoperatively the patient is assessed for complications such as altered respiratory status, wound infection, and hemorrhage. As healing occurs, the patient's range of motion of the neck is assessed.

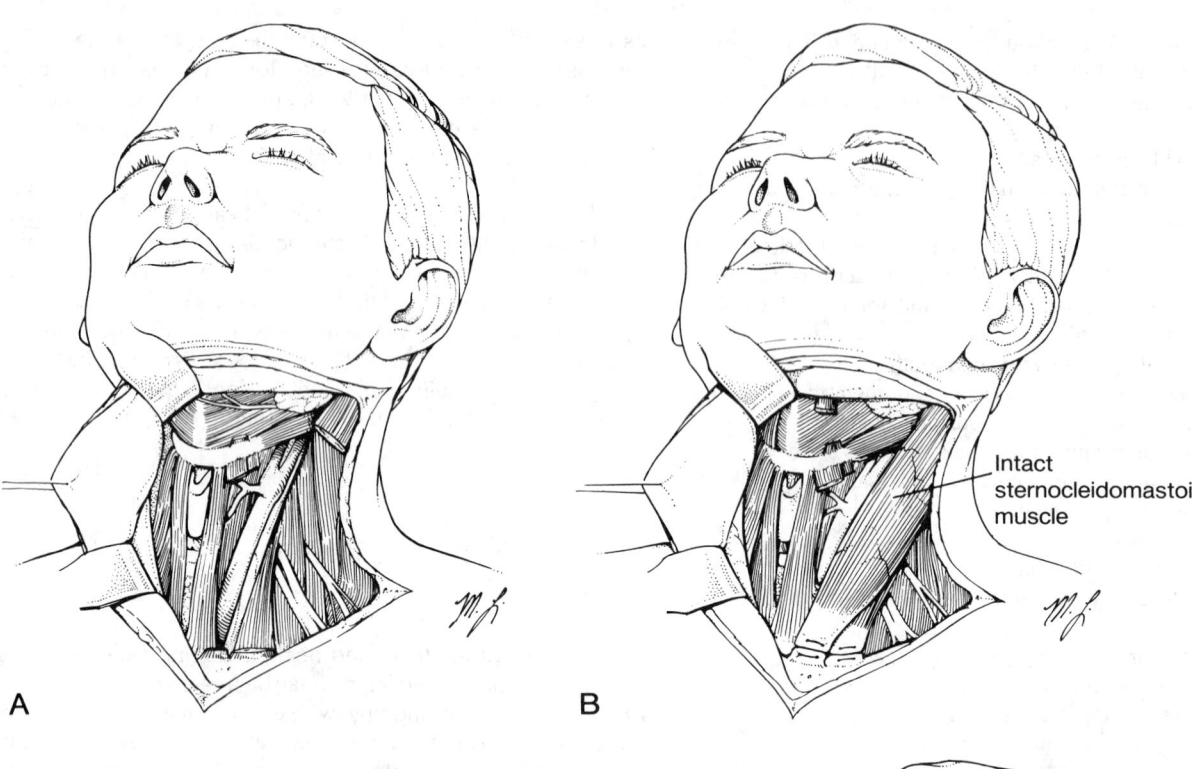

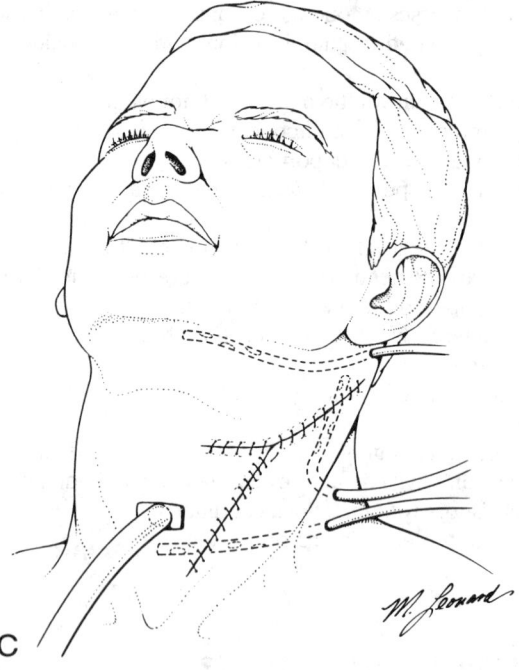

Intact
sternocleidomastoid
muscle

Figure 34–5. (**A**) A classic radical neck dissection in which the sternocleidomastoid and smaller muscles are removed. All tissue is removed, from the ramus of the jaw to the clavicle. The jugular vein has also been removed. The functional neck dissection (**B**) is similar but preserves the sternocleidomastoid muscle, internal jugular vein, and the spinal accessory nerve. The wound is closed (**C**), and portable suction drainage tubes are in place.

▷ Nursing Diagnoses

Based on all the assessment data, major nursing diagnoses may include the following:

- Knowledge deficit relative to preoperative and postoperative routine
- Ineffective airway clearance related to obstruction secondary to mucus, hemorrhage, or edema
- High risk for infection related to surgical intervention secondary to decreased nutritional status, or immunosuppression from chemotherapy/radiation therapy
- Altered nutrition, less than body requirements, related to disease process or treatment
- Ineffective coping related to diagnosis or prognosis
- Pain related to surgical incision and the presence of abnormal epithelial cells

  Potential Complications

- Hemorrhage
- Nerve injury

▷ Planning and Implementation

▷ *Goals:* The major goals for the patient may include participation in the treatment plan, maintenance of respiratory status, absence of infection, maintenance of adequate intake of food and fluids, effective coping strategies, attainment of comfort, absence of hemorrhage, and no long-term complications due to nerve injury.

▷ Nursing Interventions

▷ *Patient Education.*   Before the operation, the patient should be informed about the impending surgery, what is to be done in the operating room (amplification of the surgeon's explanation), and what the postoperative period will be like. At the same time, the patient is encouraged to express concerns about the upcoming surgery. During this exchange, the nurse has an opportunity to assess the patient's coping abilities, encourage questions, and develop a plan for offering assistance. A sense of mutual understanding and rapport will make the postoperative experience less troublesome for the patient. After the operation, any expressions of concern on the patient's part can guide the nurse in providing additional support. These intervention activities deliberately include supportive family members.

The general postoperative nursing intervention activities are similar to those described on pp. 860–862 for the patient who has had extensive neck surgery and therefore may have problems with breathing and swallowing. The specific postoperative physical nursing interventions for this patient include maintenance of a patent airway and continuous assessment of respiratory status; wound care and oral hygiene; nutritional needs; and observation for hemorrhage or nerve injury.

▷ *Airway Management.*   After the endotracheal tube or airway has been removed and the effects of the anesthesia have worn off, the patient may be placed in Fowler's position to facilitate breathing and promote comfort. This position also increases lymphatic and venous drainage, facilitates swallowing, and decreases venous pressure on the skin flaps.

Signs of respiratory distress, such as dyspnea, cyanosis, and changes in vital signs, are assessed because they may suggest edema, throat irritation from the endotracheal tube, hemorrhage, or inadequate drainage. Temperature is usually taken rectally.

In the immediate postoperative period, the nurse may be able to detect the presence of stridor (coarse, high-pitched sound on inspiration) by listening frequently at the trachea with a stethoscope. In this situation, the physician should be notified promptly.

Pneumonia may occur in the postoperative phase if pulmonary secretions are not removed. Coughing and deep breathing are encouraged to aid in the removal of secretions. The patient should assume a sitting position, with the nurse supporting his neck with her hands, so that he may be able to bring up excessive secretions. If this technique fails, the patient's respiratory tract may have to be suctioned. Care is exerted to protect the suture lines during suctioning. If a tracheostomy tube is in place, suctioning is performed through this tube using sterile technique. The patient may also be instructed to use the Yankeur suction (tonsil tip suction) to remove oral secretions.

▷ *Wound Care.*   With portable wound suction drainage, there is no need for pressure dressings because the skin flaps are drawn down tightly; 80 to 120 ml of serosanguineous secretions is usually drawn off by a portable suction unit the first day. This amount diminishes thereafter. If portable wound suction is not used, drains may be placed in the wound and pressure dressings applied to obliterate dead spaces and to provide immobilization. These pressure dressings may need to be reinforced from time to time. Dressings are observed for evidence of hemorrhage and constriction, which may affect respiration. The skin flap is assessed for color and temperature to determine viability. The flap should be pale and pink in color and warm to touch. The wound is also assessed for signs and symptoms of infection and these are reported to the physician. The patient is often placed on prophylactic antibiotics.

▷ *Nutritional Intake.*   Nutritional status is assessed preoperatively to decrease postoperative complications. Frequently nutrition is less than optimal because of inadequate intake. Therefore, the patient often requires parenteral supplements (total parenteral nutrition) preoperatively to attain a positive nitrogen balance. This may need to be continued for some time postoperatively if the patient is unable to take enough by mouth.

The patient may attain a positive nitrogen balance by taking supplemental substances such as Ensure, Sustacal, or Carnation Instant Breakfast (as a few examples) enterally either by mouth or by nasogastric feeding tube or gastrostomy. The need for supplements either parenterally or enterally is dependent on the patient's caloric intake versus his needs.

If the patient is able to take food by mouth, his ability to chew must be evaluated. The patient may require some diet modification, such as a soft, pureed, or liquid diet based on his chewing ability. Food preferences should also be discussed with the patient. Oral care before eating may enhance the patient's appetite.

▷ *Coping Measures.*   Preoperatively the patient is instructed in the planned surgery. The psychological postoperative nursing intervention is directed toward the support of a patient who has had a radical change in body image and who has major concerns regarding his prognosis. Such a patient also has difficulty in communication and is concerned about his continuing ability to breathe and swallow normally. Adjustment to the results of this surgery will take time, and the nurse enlists the support of family members in encouraging and reassuring the patient.

The person who has had extensive neck surgery often is sensitive about his appearance, either when the operative area is covered by bulky dressings or when an incision line is exposed, as with portable drainage. If the nurse conveys acceptance of the patient and his appearance and expresses a positive, optimistic attitude, the patient is more likely to be encouraged. In spite of the wide excision of tissue, the cosmetic and functional defects are less than might be expected. The patient also needs an opportunity to voice his concerns regarding the success of the surgery and his prognosis. Most patients are able to maintain and gain weight.

Alcohol and tobacco use are common in persons with cancer of the head and neck; therefore, the patient is encouraged to abstain from these substances. Alternative methods of coping need to be explored and introduced slowly.

▷ *Pain.*   Pain and the patient's fear of pain are potential complications of a radical neck dissection. Patients with head and neck cancer have often reported less pain than patients with other types of cancer (see Nicholsen, 1988, in Nursing Research Profile for Unit 8); however, the nurse should be aware that each person's pain experience is individual. The nurse should offer analgesics as ordered and assess the effectiveness of the analgesics.

◊ *Potential Complications*

◊ *Hemorrhage.*   Hemorrhage may occur from carotid artery rupture as a result of necrosis of the skin flap or damage to the artery itself from tumor or infection. The following measures are indicated to prevent or manage hemorrhage:

1. Assess vital signs. Tachycardia, tachypnea, and hypotension may indicate impending hypovolemic shock subsequent to hemorrhage.
2. Instruct the patient to avoid the Valsalva maneuver to prevent stress on the skin flap.
3. Report signs of impending rupture such as high epigastric pain or discomfort.
4. Observe dressings and wound drainage for excessive bleeding.
5. If hemorrhage occurs, stay with the patient and summon assistance. Hemorrhage requires the continuous application of pressure to the bleeding site or major associated vessel. Elevate the head of the patient's bed to maintain his airway and prevent aspiration. A controlled, calm manner will allay patient anxiety. A physician is notified immediately because vessel or ligature tear will require surgical intervention.

◊ *Nerve Injury.*   Complications due to nerve injury can occur if the cervical plexus or spinal accessory nerves are severed during surgery. Because lower facial paralysis may occur as a result of injury to the facial nerve, this is observed for and reported. Likewise, if the superior laryngeal nerve is damaged, the patient may have difficulty with swallowing liquids and food because of the partial lack of sensation of the glottis. Speech therapy may be indicated to assist with these complications. Excision of muscles and nerves results in weakness at the shoulder that can cause "shoulder drop," a forward curvature of the shoulder.

Many problems can be avoided with a conscientious exercise program. These exercises are usually begun when drains are removed and the neck incision is sufficiently healed. The purpose of the exercises depicted in Figure 34–6 is to promote maximum shoulder function and neck motion after surgery.

◊ *Home Care.*   The patient and family are instructed in the use of equipment for enteral or parenteral nutrition if the patient is unable to take food by mouth. Physical therapy and speech therapy also may be continued at home.

The patient is given information regarding support groups such as "I Can Cope" or "New Voice Club." The local chapter of the American Cancer Society may be helpful in providing information and equipment for the patient.

◊ *Evaluation*

Expected Outcomes

1. Acquires information about course of treatment
   a. Is motivated to learn preoperative and postoperative routines
   b. States preoperative and postoperative routines
   c. Involves family members in teaching sessions
2. Absence of respiratory distress
   a. Lungs are clear to auscultation
   b. States he is not short of breath
   c. Demonstrates ability to use suction effectively
3. Free of infection
   a. Maintains normal laboratory values
   b. Is afebrile
   c. Maintains skin integrity
   d. Practices oral hygiene after every meal and at bedtime
   e. Avoids visitors with infectious conditions
   f. Eats a high-protein, high-carbohydrate diet
4. Maintains adequate intake of foods and fluids
   a. Is compliant with altered route of feeding
   b. Is well hydrated
   c. Maintains or gains weight
5. Demonstrates ability to cope
   a. Is aware of diagnosis and understands prognosis
   b. Verbally discusses emotional responses to the diagnosis
   c. Attends support groups
6. Verbalizes comfort
   a. States he is comfortable
   b. States analgesic schedule

In summary, radical neck dissection is a surgical procedure that may be used in patients with head and neck cancer. The patient is instructed in the potential preoperative and postoperative complications. Often these patients require home care after hospitalization. See Nursing Care Plan 34–1 for details of nursing care.

Fracture of the Mandible: Jaw Repositioning and Reconstruction

Fractures of the mandible may consist of simple fractures without displacement, resulting from a blow on the chin. They also may be the result of planned surgical intervention, as in the correction of long or short jaw syndrome, or they may be very complicated, involving loss of tissue and bone from a severe accident. Mandibular fractures are usually closed fractures.

Management

In simple fractures, without loss of teeth, the lower jaw is immobilized by wiring it to the upper jaw. The wires are placed around the teeth in both the upper and lower jaw, on each side of the fracture line. The lower jaw is held tight against the upper jaw by cross-wires or rubber bands placed around the wires about the teeth. This simple form of fixation is used when there are teeth that can be used in the wire fixation. In other cases, in which teeth are missing or bone displacement has occurred, various other forms of fixation can be used. Some of these, such as metal arch bars, are applied in the mouth; other methods are more involved, requiring pins inserted into the bone, with fixation to a plaster head piece.

Nursing Interventions

Preoperatively the nurse must assure the patient that he will be able to breathe comfortably and to swallow. Immediately after surgery, the patient is placed on his side, with his head slightly elevated. The nasogastric suction tube inserted during surgery is connected to low-pressure suction to remove stomach contents and reduce the danger of aspiration. Antiemetic drugs are administered to prevent vomiting. If the patient vomits, the nurse must cut the wires to prevent aspiration. Surgery and rewiring will be repeated later.

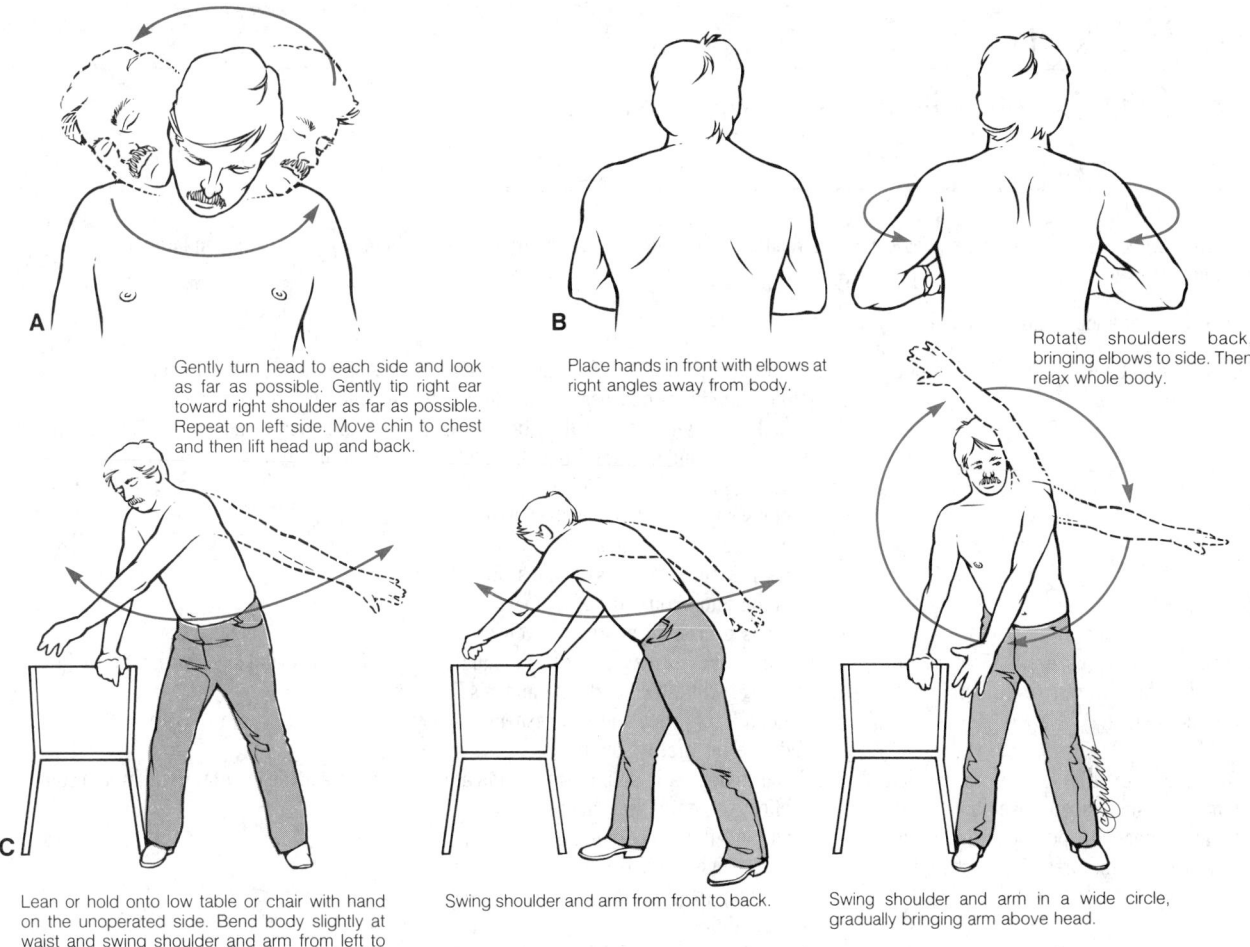

Gently turn head to each side and look as far as possible. Gently tip right ear toward right shoulder as far as possible. Repeat on left side. Move chin to chest and then lift head up and back.

Place hands in front with elbows at right angles away from body.

Rotate shoulders back, bringing elbows to side. Then relax whole body.

Lean or hold onto low table or chair with hand on the unoperated side. Bend body slightly at waist and swing shoulder and arm from left to right.

Swing shoulder and arm from front to back.

Swing shoulder and arm in a wide circle, gradually bringing arm above head.

Figure 34–6. Three rehabilitation exercises after head and neck surgery. The objective is to regain maximum shoulder function and neck motion after neck surgery. (Exercise for Radical Neck Surgery Patients. Head and Neck Service, Department of Surgery, Memorial Hospital, New York, New York.)

Clearing of the secretions of the nasopharyngeal area is performed with a small catheter inserted through the nasal orifice. The oral cavity can be aspirated by first inserting a tongue blade to move the cheek away from the teeth; the catheter is inserted in an area where there is a space between the teeth, where a tooth is missing, or in the space behind the third molar.

Constant attention by the nurse in the immediate postoperative period is necessary. As the patient regains consciousness, he needs to be reminded again that his jaw is wired but that he can breathe and swallow. As he emerges from anesthesia, his head is elevated. If an extraoral appliance is used to immobilize the mandible, the patient needs instruction for positioning himself so that he does not roll onto the device.

Careful attention to the hygiene of the mouth is essential, using warm alkaline mouthwashes at least every 2 hours, and after each feeding. In addition, the mouth is inspected at least once or twice daily to ensure thorough cleansing. A flashlight and a tongue blade to retract the cheeks are essential equipment. If permissible, a small, soft toothbrush can be used carefully. To prevent dry and cracking lips, a water-soluble lubricant is applied.

The diet must necessarily be liquid, but sufficient caloric and fluid intake can be given easily to these patients. They can be fed through a straw without much difficulty, and soft foods are given with a spoon. Water is given after each liquid feeding, followed by a mouthwash.

Usually, the patient is out of bed the first postoperative day and discharged in 2 to 3 days in the absence of other trauma. The wiring is usually removed in 6 to 8 weeks.

Patient Education and Home Health Care

The patient needs very specific guidelines for mouth care and feeding. He is reminded to see his physician for scheduled visits to make sure the fixation appliance is functioning properly. Any irritated areas are to be reported. A wire cutter is readily available and the patient and a family member are instructed about how to cut the wires in an emergency.

Conditions of the Esophagus

The esophagus is a mucus-lined, muscular tube that allows food to enter the stomach. It begins at the base of the pharynx

(text continues on page 862)

Nursing Care Plan 34–1

Care of the Patient Who Has Undergone Neck Dissection

Nursing Interventions	Rationale	Expected Outcomes

Nursing Diagnosis: Ineffective airway clearance related to obstruction secondary to edema, hemorrhage, or inadequate wound drainage

Goal: Maintenance of normal respiratory function

Nursing Interventions	Rationale	Expected Outcomes
1. Place the patient in high Fowler's position.	1. High Fowler's position facilitates expansion of the lungs because the diaphragm is pulled downward and the abdominal viscera are pulled away from the lungs. Breathing is promoted. This position also increases lymphatic and venous drainage, facilitates swallowing, and decreases venous pressure on the skin flaps. Regurgitation and aspiration of stomach contents is prevented postoperatively.	• Achieves a normal respiratory rate. • Breathes comfortably. • Avoids use of accessory muscles of respiration.
2. Monitor vital signs every 15 to 20 min initially, then every 1 to 2 hours for the first 24 hours.	2. Edema, hemorrhage, or inadequate drainage will alter heart rate and respirations. Tachypnea and restlessness may indicate respiratory distress.	• Maintains vital signs within normal range.
3. Auscultate breath sounds as needed. Place the stethoscope over the trachea in the immediate postoperative period to assess for the presence of stridor.	3. Abnormal breath sounds may indicate ineffective ventilation, decreased perfusion, and fluid accumulation. Stridor, a harsh, high-pitched sound primarily heard on inspiration, indicates airway obstruction.	• Shows evidence of normal breath sounds.
4. Encourage deep breathing and coughing. Place the patient in a sitting position and support the neck area with both hands.	4. Deep breathing before coughing promotes expansion of the airways and a more forceful cough. The coughing mechanism assists airway cilia with removal of secretions. Splinting the incision during coughing reduces strain and promotes the expulsion of secretions by allowing for deeper inspirations.	• Coughs effectively. • Maintains a patent airway.
5. Suction the airway as needed.	5. Suctioning mechanically clears the airway by removing secretions that the patient may be unable to cough up. Airway obstruction is prevented and coughing is stimulated. Atelectasis, caused by mucus blockage, is prevented.	• Breathes easier after suctioning.
6. Assess for hoarseness or dysphagia.	6. Edema subsequent to surgical trauma can cause pressure on the pharynx.	• Voice characteristics are unchanged. • Swallows without discomfort.

Nursing Diagnosis: High risk for infection related to improper wound healing

Goal: Absence of infection

Nursing Interventions	Rationale	Expected Outcomes
1. Instruct the patient in preoperative and postoperative oral hygiene using slightly alkaline solutions such as 8 oz of water mixed with 1 teaspoon of baking soda every 4 hours.	1. Oral care decreases oral bacteira, therefore decreasing the risk of bacterial infection postoperatively. Hydrogen peroxide *must not* be used, as it may break down fresh granulation tissue.	• Patient performs oral hygiene preoperatively and postoperatively every 4 hours. • Mouth remains clean.
2. Montior wound suction drainage.	2. Suction drainage negates the need for	• Wound drains less than 200 ml of sero-

(continued)

Nursing Care Plan 34–1 *(Continued)*

Care of the Patient Who Has Undergone Neck Dissection

Nursing Interventions	Rationale	Expected Outcomes
	pressure dressings because the skin flaps are pulled down tightly. Drainage should approximate 80 to 120 ml of serosanguineous secretions for the first 24 hours. Then the secretions should decrease daily. Continuous bloody drainage indicates small vessel oozing.	sanguineous drainage the first postoperative day. • No hematoma at skin graft.
3. Note drainage quantity and odor.	3. Purulent, malodorous drainage indicates an infection. Drainage greater than 300 ml in the first 24 hours is considered abnormal.	• Serosanguineous drainage is within normal limits.
4. Reinforce pressure dressing as needed.	4. If portable wound suction is not used, then pressure dressings are applied to obliterate dead spaces and provide immobilization. These are *reinforced,* not changed, as needed. Assess for any possible constrictions that would affect respirations.	
5. Use aseptic technique to cleanse skin around the drains; change the dressings on the second through fifth postoperative days.	5. Aseptic technique prevents wound contamination. Sterile saline effectively cleans the skin around the drains. A povidone-iodine solution, which is effective against a variety of microorganisms, can also be used as prescribed.	• Wound and surrounding skin remain clean and free of infection.
6. Assess condition of skin flap for viability every 4 hours after dressing is removed.	6. Cyanotic, cool, skin flap indicates possible necrosis.	• Flap will be pale pink in color and warm to touch. • Tissue will blanch to gentle touch.
7. Monitor vital signs. Assess for symptoms of infection: chills, diaphoresis, altered level of consciousness.	7. An elevated temperature, tachypnea, and tachycardia may indicate an infection.	• Is afebrile with normal respirations and a normal heart rate. • Is alert and aware of surroundings.

Nursing Diagnosis: Altered nutrition, less than body requirements, related to anorexia and dysphagia

Goal: Attainment of an optimal level of nutrition

1. Assess nutritional status preoperatively; consult with dietitian.	1. Poor nutrition preoperatively decreases wound healing and increases potential for infection.	• Patient does not have history of weight loss between 10% and 20%. If patient does have weight loss of 10% to 20%, supplements are given to maintain/increase weight and obtain positive nitrogen balance.
2. Administer tube feedings as prescribed.	2. A nasogastric tube may be in place for several days.	• Tolerates tube feedings.
3. Provide oral hygiene before and after meals.	3. Mouth hygiene enhances the appetite.	• Expresses a desire for food.

4. Assist with oral intake:
   a. Offer easily chewed foods; mash or blenderize if necessary.
   b. Suggest that the head be tilted to the unaffected side when swallowing.
   c. Inquire if privacy is desired when eating.
	4. Soft-textured foods facilitate swallowing. Passage of food may be tolerated better when pressure occurs on the side opposite the surgery. Self-feeding difficulties may cause embarrassment and interfere with digestion.	• Swallows food easily.
		• Is comfortable eating alone or with others.

(continued)

Nursing Care Plan 34–1 *(Continued)*

Care of the Patient Who Has Undergone Neck Dissection

Nursing Interventions	Rationale	Expected Outcomes

Nursing Diagnosis: Disturbance in self-concept and body image related to changes in appearance and alterations in communication

Goal: Attainment of a positive self-image

Nursing Interventions	Rationale	Expected Outcomes
1. Help the patient to communicate effectively. a. Provide materials for writing messages. b. Use communication board when appropriate. c. Make certain that the call bell is readily accessible. d. Develop nonverbal ways to communicate (*e.g.*, finger-tapping, sign language).	1. Temporary hoarseness is common after neck surgery. A tracheostomy is usually performed and verbal communication may not be possible. Communication with head movement may be impossible because of incisional pain.	• Recognizes that hoarseness is temporary. • Communicates nonverbally.
2. Encourage verbalization of fears: a. Provide time to listen. b. Project a positive, optimisitic attitude. c. Reinforce reality. d. Consult speech pathologist. e. Collaborate with family members to elicit their support and encouragement. f. Consult support groups such as New Voice Club through the American Cancer Society.	 a. Listening conveys acceptance and encourages further verbalization. b. An optimistic approach conveys interest and hope. c. Honesty will promote a trusting relationship. This includes confirming cosmetic and functional limitations. d. Speech pathologist may assist with other forms of communication such as esophageal speech or electrolarynx. e. Family members or significant others can provide valuable support to the patient.	• Willingly conveys fears and concerns. • Accepts prognosis with realistic limitations. • Patient develops alternative forms of communication (magic slate). • Accepts support as offered.
3. Observe for facial paralysis.	3. Injury to the facial nerve will cause lower facial paralysis.	• Absence of facial paralysis.
4. Observe for excessive drooling.	4. Damage to the hypoglossal nerve will result in excessive drooling and decreased ability to swallow.	• Absence of drooling and dysphagia.
5. Check for normal shoulder position and function.	5. Damage to the spinal accessory nerve will result in drooping of the shoulder. Rehabilitation exercises are begun when the incision is healed.	• Maintains normal shoulder functions.

and ends about 4 cm below the diaphragm. Its ability to transport food and fluid is facilitated by two sphincters: the pharyngoesophageal at the junction of the pharynx and the esophagus, and the gastroesophageal at the junction of the esophagus and the stomach. An incompetent gastroesophageal sphincter allows reflux (backward flow) of gastric contents.

Difficulty in swallowing (dysphagia) is the most common symptom of esophageal disease. This symptom may range from an uncomfortable feeling that a bolus of food is "caught" in the upper esophagus (before it eventually passes into the stomach) to acute pain on swallowing (odynophagia). Obstruction to the passage of food (solid and soft) and even liquids may be felt anywhere along the esophagus. Often the patient can indicate if the problem is located in the upper, middle, or lower third of the esophagus.

There are many pathologic conditions of the esophagus,

with the order of frequency beginning with achalasia (failure of the esophageal orifice of the stomach to relax) and progressing to diffuse spasm, diverticula, perforation, foreign bodies, chemical burns, hiatal hernias, benign tumors, and carcinoma. A discussion of these conditions is preceded by an overview of the nursing process for patients with esophageal disorders.

▶ Nursing Process Overview
Patients With Conditions of the Esophagus

◊ Assessment

The nurse elicits a complete health history. If an esophageal disorder is suspected, the nurse asks about the patient's appetite. Has it remained the same, increased, or decreased? Is there any discomfort with swallowing? If so, does it occur only with certain foods? Is it associated with pain? Does a change in position affect the discomfort? The patient is asked to describe the pain experience. Does anything aggravate it? Are there any other symptoms that occur regularly, such as regurgitation, nocturnal regurgitation, eructation (belching), heartburn, substernal pressure, a sensation that food is sticking in the throat, a feeling of early satiety, nausea, vomiting, or weight loss? Are the symptoms aggravated by emotional upset? If the patient admits to any of these complaints, the nurse questions the time of their occurrence; their relationship to eating; factors that relieve or aggravate them, such as position change, belching, antacids, or vomiting. This history also includes questions about the existence of past or present causative factors, such as infections and chemical, mechanical, or physical irritants. A history of alcohol and tobacco use is obtained. A review of daily intake of fruits and vegetables is elicited. The nurse determines if the patient appears emaciated and auscultates the patient's chest to determine if pulmonary complications exist.

◊ Nursing Diagnoses

Based on the assessment data, the nursing diagnoses may include the following:

- Altered nutrition, less than body requirements, related to difficulty with swallowing
- Pain, related to ingestion of an abrasive agent, a tumor, or frequent episodes of gastric reflux
- Knowledge deficit about the esophageal disorder, diagnostic studies, medical management, surgical intervention, and rehabilitation

◊ Planning and Implementation

◊ *Goals:* The major goals for the patient may include attainment of an adequate nutritional intake, relief of pain, and improvement in knowledge level.

◊ Nursing Interventions

◊ *Adequate Nutritional Intake.* The patient is encouraged to eat slowly and chew his food thoroughly to facilitate its passage to the stomach. Small, frequent feedings of bland food are recommended to promote digestion and prevent tissue irritation. Sometimes liquid swallowed with food will facilitate passage. An atmosphere for eating that will help stimulate the appetite should be provided. Irritants such as tobacco and alcohol should be avoided. A baseline weight is obtained and daily weights are recorded. The patient's intake of nutrients is assessed daily.

◊ *Relief of Pain.* Small, frequent feedings are recommended because large quantities of food overload the stomach and promote gastric reflux. The nurse suggests that very hot and cold beverages and spicy foods be avoided because they stimulate esophageal spasm and increase the secretion of hydrochloric acid. The patient is advised to avoid any activities that put strain on the thoracic area and increase pain. The patient should remain upright for 1 to 4 hours after each meal to prevent reflux by using gravity to decrease an elevated gastroesophageal pressure gradient. The head of the bed should be placed on 4- to 8-in (10- to 20-cm) blocks. Eating is discouraged before bedtime.

The patient is advised not to abuse over-the-counter antacids because excessive use can cause rebound acidity. Antacid use should be directed by a physician who can recommend the daily, safe quantity needed to neutralize gastric juices and prevent esophageal irritation. Histamine antagonists (Pepcid, Tagamet, Zantac) are administered as prescribed to decrease gastric acid irritation.

◊ *Patient Education.* The patient is prepared physically and psychologically for diagnostic tests, treatments, and possible surgical intervention. Reassurance and discussion about the procedures and their purposes are the principal nursing interventions. Some disorders of the esophagus evolve over time, whereas others are the result of trauma (*e.g.,* chemical burns or perforation). The emotional and physical preparation for treatment of the latter groups is more difficult because of the shortened time and the circumstances of the injury. Evaluation of treatment interventions must be ongoing; the patient is provided with sufficient information to participate in care and diagnostic efforts. If surgery is involved, immediate and long-term evaluation are similar to that of a patient undergoing thoracic surgery.

The goals of rehabilitation will depend on whether surgery or more conservative measures such as diet, positioning, and use of antacids were used in the treatment phase. If the condition is corrected, short-term evaluative measures may be sufficient. If an ongoing condition exists, the nurse must help the patient plan for needed physical and psychological adjustment and for follow-up care. Many elderly patients may experience ongoing conditions. These patients need support for realistic meal planning, use of medications, and participation in a full life. A multidisciplinary approach is helpful here, including the nutritionist, social worker, and family members.

◊ *Home Health Care.* Chronic esophageal conditions require an individualized approach to home management. There may be a need for special food preparation (blenderized foods; bland, soft diets) and increased frequency of eating (four to six small servings per day). The medication schedule is adjusted to the patient's daily activities as much as possible. Analgesics and antacids can be taken as needed every 3 to 4 hours.

Emergency conditions of the esophagus (perforation, chemical burns) usually happen in the home or away from medical help and require emergency management. The patient is treated for shock and respiratory distress and transported as quickly as possible to a medical facility. Specific emergency measures for chemical burns can be found on p. 867.

Foreign bodies in the esophagus do not pose an immediate threat to life unless pressure is exerted on the trachea, resulting in dyspnea or the cessation of respirations. Educating the public to prevent accidental swallowing of foreign bodies or corrosive agents is a major health issue. (See Chap. 63 for emergency resuscitation measures.)

Postoperative home health care focuses on nutritional support, management of pain, and respiratory function. Some patients are discharged from the hospital with total parenteral nutrition or enteral feeding by gastrostomy or jejunostomy tubes as a temporary measure. The patient and his family need specific instruction on the management of equipment and treatments. (See p. 885 for caring for a patient receiving total parenteral nutrition and p. 882 for the management of the patient with a gastrostomy. Postoperative nursing management for patients having thoracic or abdominal surgery can be found in Chaps. 22 and 25. Nursing management for a patient receiving radiation or chemotherapy is discussed in Chap. 19.)

▷ Evaluation

Expected Outcomes

1. Achieves an adequate nutritional intake
   a. Eats small, frequent meals
   b. Drinks water with small servings of food
   c. Avoids irritants (alcohol, tobacco, very hot beverages)
   d. Maintains desired weight
2. Is free of pain or able to control pain within an acceptable level
   a. Avoids large meals and irritating foods
   b. Takes antacids as prescribed
   c. Maintains the upright position after meals for 1 to 4 hours
   d. States that he has less eructation and chest pain
3. Increases knowledge level of esophageal condition, treatment, and prognosis
   a. States cause of condition
   b. Expresses rationale for medical or surgical management and diet/medication regimen
   c. Describes treatment program
   d. Practices preventive measures so accidental injuries are avoided

Achalasia

Achalasia is absent or ineffective peristalsis of the distal esophagus accompanied by failure of the esophageal sphincter to relax in response to swallowing. Narrowing of the esophagus just above the stomach results in a gradually increasing dilation of the esophagus in the upper chest. Achalasia may progress slowly. It is thought that there may be a familial incidence of achalasia.

Clinical Manifestations

The primary symptom of achalasia is that of difficulty in swallowing both liquids and solids. The patient has a sensation of food sticking in the lower portion of the esophagus. As the condition progresses, regurgitation of the food is common; this may occur spontaneously or may be brought about by the patient to relieve the discomfort that is produced by the prolonged distention of the esophagus by food that will not pass into the stomach. The patient may also complain of chest pain

and burning. Pain may not be associated with eating. There may be secondary pulmonary complications due to spillover of esophageal contents (aspiration pneumonia).

Diagnostic Evaluation

Radiologic studies show esophageal dilation above the narrowing at the gastroesophageal junction. Barium swallow and endoscopy may be used for diagnosis; however, the diagnosis is confirmed by manometry, which is the measurement of pressure in the esophagus. Manometry is performed by the radiologist or gastroenterologist.

Management

Two methods of management are recommended to treat the obstruction: forceful dilation (Fig. 34–7) and surgical separation of the muscle fibers (Fig. 34–8). Calcium channel-blockers have been used to decrease esophageal pressure and improve swallowing.

The conservative approach to treating early achalasia involves stretching the narrowed area of the esophagus. This is performed by passing a tube orally into the esophagus. A distensible bag (Mosher pneumatic) at the end of the tube is positioned and inflated. Vigorous dilation has a 75% success rate and a 3% incidence of perforation. The procedure can be painful; therefore, an analgesic or tranquilizer is administered before the treatment. The patient is monitored for perforation. Complaints of abdominal tenderness and fever may indicate that perforation has occurred (see later discussion on perforation).

A cardiomyotomy is the preferred surgical approach. A longitudinal incision about 12 cm in length is made through the muscularis of the esophagus extending about 1 cm into the gastric area. All muscle fibers are separated to relieve the lower esophageal stricture. While patients with a history of achalasia have a slightly higher incidence of esophageal cancer, long-term follow-up with esophagoscopy has not proved beneficial.

Diffuse Spasm

Diffuse spasm is a motor disorder of the esophagus characterized by dysphagia, odynophagia (painful swallowing), and chest pain similar to that of coronary artery spasm. Manometry indicates simultaneous contractions occurring irregularly. Radiographic studies show separated areas of spasm.

Conservative therapy includes administering sedatives and long-acting nitrates to relieve pain. Small, frequent feedings and a soft diet are usually recommended to decrease the esophageal pressure and irritation that lead to spasm. Pneumatic dilatation and esophageal myotomy may be necessary if pain becomes intolerable.

Diverticulum

A diverticulum is an outpouching of mucosa and submucosa that protrudes through a weak portion of the musculature (*pulsion* type). If there is a pulling outward of the esophageal wall from inflamed or scarred peribronchial lymph nodes, the term *traction diverticulum* is used. Diverticuli may occur in one of the three areas of the esophagus (1) pharyngoesophageal, (2) midesophageal, and (3) epiphrenic (Fig. 34–9).

Pharyngoesophageal Diverticulum

The most common type of diverticulum, which is found three times more frequently in men than in women, is pharyngo-

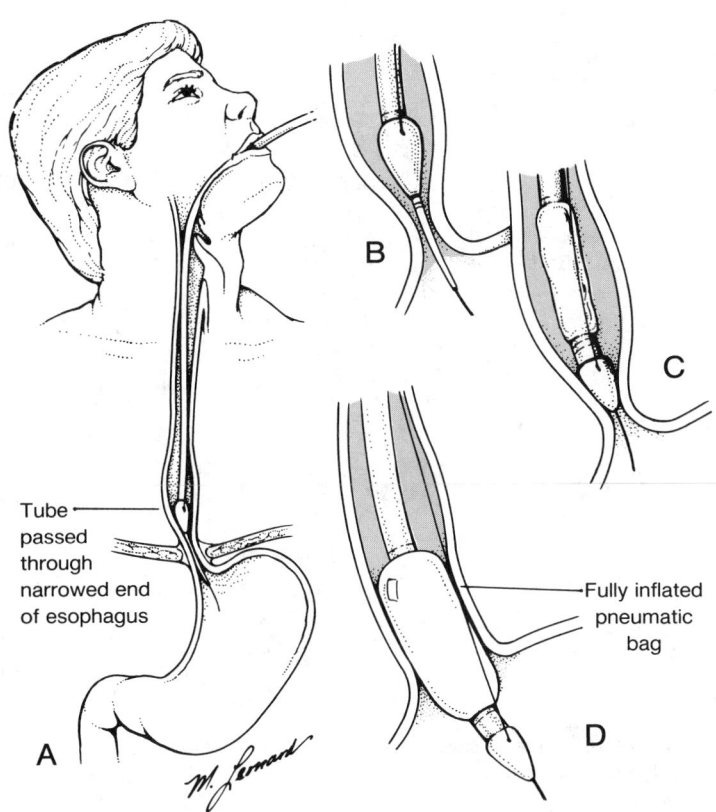

Figure 34–7. Treatment of achalasia by the conservative approach. (**A–C**) The dilator is passed, guided by a previously swallowed thread, into the upper stomach. (**D**) When the balloon is in proper position, it is distended by pressure sufficient to dilate the narrowed area of the esophagus.

esophageal pulsion diverticulum (Zenker's diverticulum), which occurs posteriorly through the cricopharyngeal muscle in the midline of the neck. It is usually seen in people over 60 years of age. The patient first notices difficulty in swallowing and a fullness in the neck. He may complain of belching, regurgitation of undigested food, and gurgling noises after eating. The diverticulum, or pouch, becomes filled with food or liquid. When the patient assumes a recumbent position, undigested food is regurgitated and may also cause coughing, because of irritation of the trachea. Halitosis and a sour taste in the mouth are also common, because of the decomposition of food retained in the diverticulum.

Diagnostic Evaluation and Management.   To determine the exact nature and location of a diverticulum, barium is ingested and x-ray films are taken. Esophagoscopy usually is contraindicated because of the danger of perforating the diverticulum, with resulting mediastinitis. The blind passing of a nasal tube should be avoided. The tube should be guided into the stomach

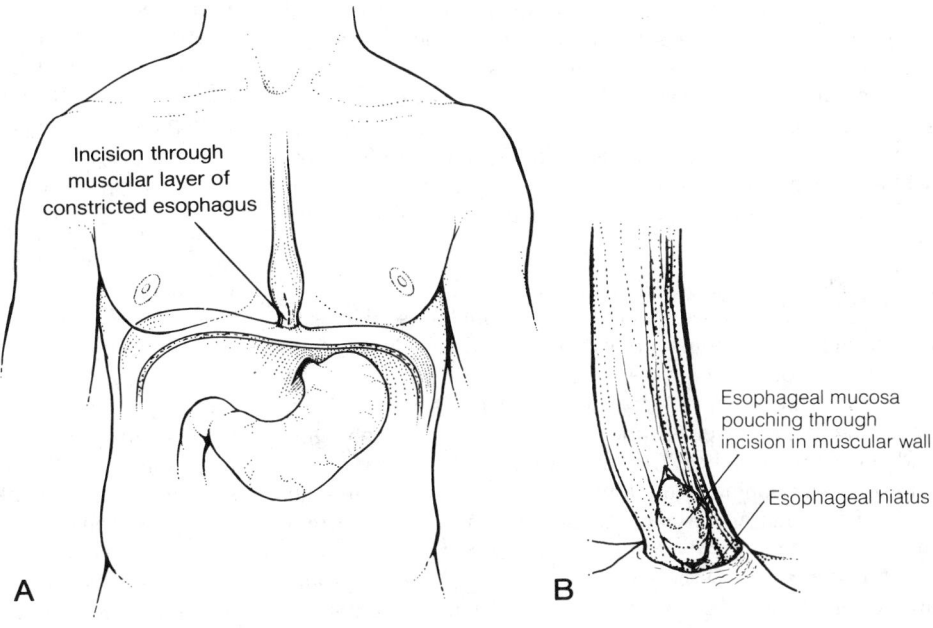

Figure 34–8. Treatment of achalasia: Major surgical approach. (**A**) The esophagus is approached from the front, on the left side. An incision is made through the muscularis of the esophagus. (**B**) The incision is of sufficient size to allow a pouching of the esophageal mucosa. Separation of the muscular fibers relieves the narrowing at the lower end of the esophagus and permits the patient to swallow normally again.

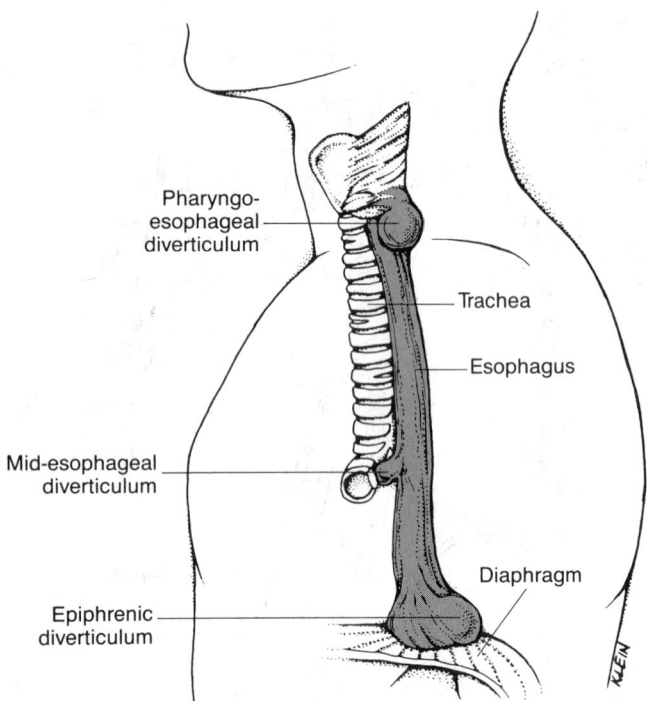

Figure 34-9. Possible sites for the occurrence of esophageal diverticula. The sites determine the location of the surgical incision to correct the problem.

under direct vision of a lighted scope. Because this patient often has a history of poor food and fluid intake, an evaluation of his nutritional state is performed to determine dietary needs.

Because the condition is progressive, the only means of cure is surgical removal of the diverticulum. Care is taken, surgically, to avoid undue trauma to the common carotid artery and internal jugular veins. The sac is dissected free and amputated flush with the esophageal wall. In addition to a diverticulectomy, a myotomy of the cricopharyngeal muscle is often performed, to relieve spasticity of the musculature, which otherwise seems to contribute to a continuation of the previous symptoms. Postoperatively, food and fluids are withheld until x-ray studies show no leakage at the surgical site. The diet is then begun with liquids and progressed as tolerated.

Nursing Interventions. When a patient has difficulty in swallowing, the diet is limited to foods that pass more easily. Blenderized meals supplemented with vitamins are often prescribed. The nurse arranges for the nutritionist to see the patient and his family to discuss plans for continuing this treatment at home.

Midesophageal and Epiphrenic Diverticula

The occurrence of diverticula in the midtubular esophagus is less common; symptoms are less acute, and usually the condition does not require surgery.

Epiphrenic diverticula are usually larger pulsion diverticula occurring in the lower esophagus just above the diaphragm, and occasionally higher. They are thought to be related to the improper functioning of the lower esophageal sphincter. One third of patients are asymptomatic, with the remaining two thirds complaining of dysphagia and chest pain.

Management. Surgery is indicated only if the symptoms are troublesome and growing progressively worse. A transtho-

racic (thoracotomy) approach is used; therefore preoperative and postoperative nursing management are similar to that for patients having thoracic surgery (see Chap. 25).

Nursing Interventions. After surgery the patient is fed through a nasogastric tube that usually is inserted at the time of operation. The feedings may include any liquid, but a careful record of their kind, amount, and character must be documented. After each feeding, the tube is flushed carefully with water. The wound also must be observed for evidence of leakage from the esophagus and a developing fistula.

If the operative risk is prohibitive, nursing management is similar to that advocated for the patient with a peptic ulcer: antacids, anticholinergics, and abstinence from coffee, alcohol, and smoking (see Chap. 36). In addition, reflux is avoided by (1) keeping the head of the bed elevated; (2) remaining upright for 2 hours in the postprandial period; (3) avoiding abdominal compression from garments and posture; (4) eating small meals; and (5) weight reduction, if overweight.

Perforation

The esophagus is not an uncommon site of injury. Perforation may result from stab or bullet wounds of the neck or chest, as well as from accidental puncture by a surgical instrument during examination or dilation. Spontaneous perforation of the esophagus has been known to occur during vomiting.

The patient experiences spontaneous pain followed by dysphagia. Infection, fever, leukocytosis, and severe hypotension may be noted. Hyperpnea and cervical tenderness are early signs of injury and crepitation. In some instances, signs of pneumothorax are observed. Radiographic examination and fluoroscopy can localize the site of the injury.

Management

Because of the high risk of infection, broad-spectrum antibiotic therapy is initiated. A nasogastric tube is passed, to provide suction and to reduce the amount of gastric juice that can reflux into the esophagus and mediastinum. Nothing is given by mouth, but nutritional needs are met by total parenteral nutrition. Surgery may be necessary to close the wound, and postoperative nutritional support then becomes a primary concern. Total parenteral nutrition is preferred to gastrostomy because the latter might cause reflux into the esophagus. Depending on the incisional site and nature of surgery, the postoperative nursing management will be similar to that for patients who have had thoracic or abdominal surgery.

Foreign Bodies

Swallowed foreign bodies (dentures, fishbones, pins) may injure the esophagus as well as obstruct its lumen. Pain and dysphagia may be present; dyspnea may occur as a result of pressure. Radiographic findings are useful in identifying the foreign body.

Usually, foreign bodies can be removed with the aid of the esophagoscope. When the foreign body is sharp (bobby pins, safety pins, needles, jacks, nails, and tacks), it may not be safe to allow the object to make its way slowly through the stomach and intestinal tract. A bar magnet, fastened to a cable, may be maneuvered into place with the aid of fluoroscopy and the object withdrawn. An indwelling catheter can be manipulated past the object, the balloon inflated, and the catheter and the foreign body removed. It is possible for a skilled esophagoscopist to remove open safety pins through the esophagoscope.

If an impacted bolus of food is lodged in the esophagus, the patient may be treated with a muscle relaxant such as Valium. This is sometimes sufficient to relax the esophageal muscle and allow the meat bolus to move through the esophagus. Another drug that may be used is glucagon injected intramuscularly. This medication also has a relaxing effect on the esophageal muscle. If these treatments are unsuccessful, an endoscopic procedure is performed to remove the impacting food.

Chemical Burns

The patient who accidentally or intentionally swallows a strong acid or base (such as lye) is emotionally distraught as well as in acute physical pain. An acute chemical burn of the esophagus is accompanied by severe burns of the lips, mouth, and pharynx, with pain on swallowing and, sometimes, difficulty in breathing, due either to edema of the throat or to a collection of mucus in the pharynx. The patient may be profoundly toxic, febrile, and in shock. The patient is treated immediately for shock, pain, and respiratory distress.

Management
Esophagoscopy and barium swallow are performed as soon as possible to determine the extent and severity of damage. The patient is kept NPO (nothing by mouth) and intravenous fluids are administered. A nasogastric tube may be placed by the physician.

The use of corticosteroid therapy, used to reduce inflammation and minimize subsequent scarring and stricture formation, is of questionable value. The value of prophylactic use of antibiotics for this patient has also been questioned; however, these treatments continue to be prescribed.

After the acute phase has subsided, the patient may require further treatment to prevent or manage strictures. Dilation using either peroral bougies or retrograde bougies (via a gastrostomy) may be sufficient treatment. For strictures that do not respond to dilation, surgical management is necessary. Reconstruction may be performed with an esophagectomy or colon interposition to replace the portion of esophagus removed.

Hiatal Hernia

The esophagus enters the abdomen through an opening in the diaphragm, and empties at its lower end into the upper part of the stomach. The opening in the diaphragm normally encircles the esophagus tightly; therefore, the stomach lies completely within the abdomen. In a condition known as *hiatus* (or *hiatal*) *hernia*, the opening in the diaphragm through which the esophagus passes becomes enlarged and part of the upper stomach tends to move up into the lower portion of the thorax. There are two types of hernias, type I and type II.

Type I. Type I or sliding hiatal hernias occur when the upper stomach and the gastroesophageal junction are displaced upward and slide in and out of the thorax. About 90% of patients with esophageal hiatal hernias have sliding hernias. Diagnosis is confirmed by radiographic studies and fluoroscopy (Fig. 34–10A).

Clinical Manifestations and Management. The patient may experience heartburn, regurgitation, and dysphagia. At least 50% of the patients are asymptomatic. Medical management includes frequent, small feedings that can pass easily through the esophagus. The patient is advised not to recline for 1 hour after eating to prevent reflux or movement of the hernia. The patient's bed is elevated at the head on 10- to 20-cm (4- to 8-inch) blocks to prevent movement of the hernia by gravity. Surgery is indicated in about 15% of patients.

Type II. The less frequent type II or rolling hernias occur when all or part of the stomach pushes through the diaphragm next to the gastroesophageal junction. Fewer than 10% of patients experience paraesophageal herniation, and many are

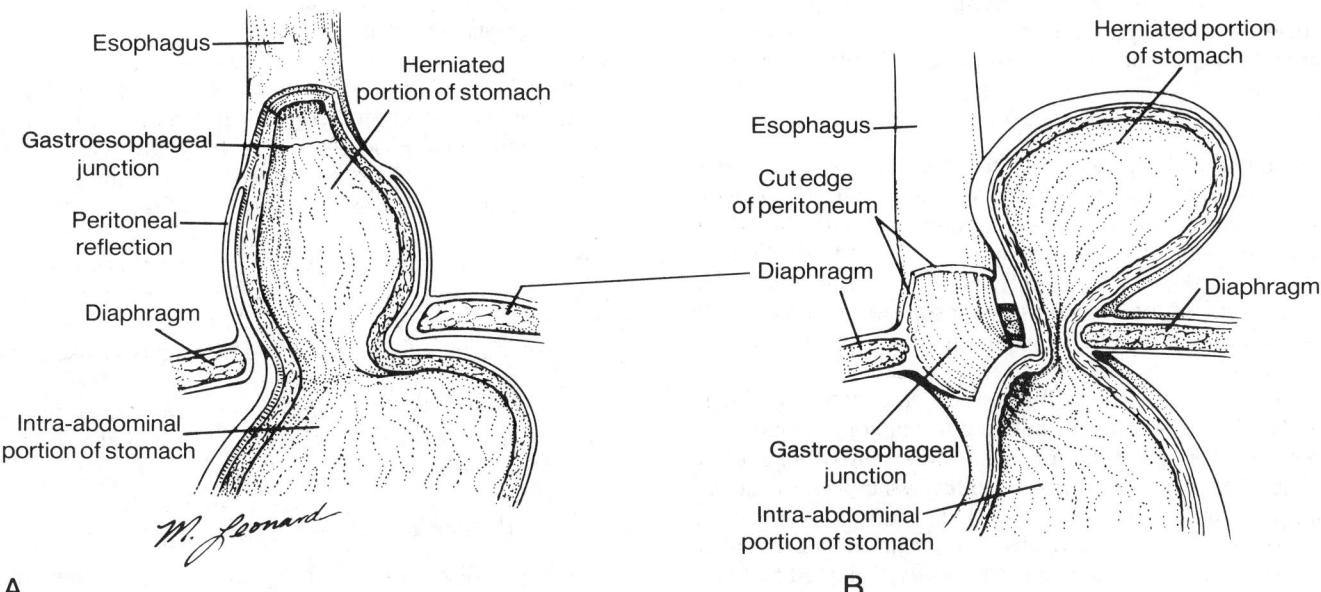

A   B

Figure 34–10. Sliding esophageal and paraesophageal hernias. (**A**) Sliding esophageal hernia. Upper stomach and cardioesophageal junction are moved upward and slide in and out of the thorax. (**B**) Paraesophageal hernia. All or part of the stomach pushes through the diaphragm next to the gastroesophageal junction.

asymptomatic. Reflux does not usually occur because the gastroesophageal sphincter is intact (see Fig. 34–10*B*).

Clinical Manifestations and Management.   The patient usually experiences a sense of fullness after eating. The complications of hemorrhage, obstruction, and strangulation can occur, so an anterior gastropexy (fixation of the prolapsed stomach in its normal position by suturing it to the abdominal wall) is the treatment of choice.

Esophageal Varices

Varices of the lower esophagus are a complication of cirrhosis of the liver and portal hypertension. This subject is discussed in Chapter 38.

Benign Tumors

Benign tumors may arise anywhere along the esophagus. The most common lesion is a leiomyoma, which can occlude the lumen of the esophagus. Most benign tumors are asymptomatic and are distinguished from cancerous growths by a biopsy. Small lesions are excised during esophagoscopy; thoracotomy may be necessary for intramural lesions.

Cancer of the Esophagus

In the United States, carcinoma of the esophagus occurs more than twice as often in men as in women. It is seen more frequently in blacks than in whites, and usually occurs in the fifth decade of life. Cancer of the esophagus has a much higher incidence in other parts of the world, including China and Northern Iran.

Chronic irritation is considered to be a risk factor for esophageal cancer. In the United States, cancer of the esophagus has been associated with ingestion of alcohol and the use of tobacco. In other parts of the world an association has been seen between esophageal cancer and the use of opium pipes, ingestion of excessively hot beverages, and nutritional deficiencies—especially lack of fruits and vegetables. It is thought that fruits and vegetables promote repair of irritated tissue.

Pathophysiology and Clinical Manifestations

Unfortunately, the patient may have an advanced ulcerated lesion of the esophagus before symptoms present. Malignancy, usually of the squamous cell epidermoid type, may spread beneath the esophageal mucosa, or it may spread directly into, through, and beyond the muscle layers into the lymphatics. In the latter stages, obstruction of the esophagus is noted, with possible perforation into the mediastinum and erosion into the great vessels.

When symptoms exist that are related to esophageal cancer, the disease is generally advanced. Symptoms include dysphagia, initially with solid foods and eventually with liquids; a feeling of a lump in the throat; painful swallowing; substernal pain or fullness; and, later, regurgitation of undigested food with foul breath and hiccoughs. The patient is first aware of intermittent and increasing difficulty in swallowing. At first only solid food gives trouble, but as the growth progresses and the obstruction becomes more complete, even liquids cannot pass into the stomach. Regurgitation of food and saliva occurs, hemorrhage may take place, and there is a progressive loss of

weight and strength due to starvation. Later symptoms include substernal pain, hiccough, respiratory difficulty, and foul breath. *The delay between onset of early symptoms and the time when the patient seeks medical advice is often 12 to 18 months.* Anyone with swallowing difficulties should be encouraged to see a physician immediately.

Diagnostic Evaluation

Diagnosis is confirmed in 95% of the cases by esophagoscopy with biopsy and brushings. Bronchoscopy usually is performed, especially in tumors of the middle and the upper third of the esophagus, to determine whether the trachea has been involved by the tumor and to help in determining whether the lesion can be removed. Mediastinoscopy is used to determine involvement of nodes and other mediastinal structures. Cancer of the lower end of the esophagus may be due to adenocarcinoma of the stomach extending upward into the esophagus.

Management

Treatment goals of esophageal cancer may be directed toward cure if found in an early stage; however, it is often found in late stages, making palliation the goal of therapy.

Treatment may include surgery, radiation, chemotherapy, or a combination of these modalities.

Surgery may be performed for cure or palliation based on the extent of the disease. Standard surgical management includes a total resection of the esophagus (esophagectomy) with removal of the tumor plus a wide tumor-free margin of the esophagus and lymph nodes in the area. The surgical approach may be through the thorax or the abdomen, depending on the location of the tumor. When tumors occur in the cervical or upper thoracic area, esophageal continuity may be maintained by interposition of a segment of the colon, use of a full thickness skin graft, or elevation of the stomach into the chest with implantation of the proximal end of the esophagus into the stomach. Tumors of the lower thoracic esophagus are more amenable to surgery than are tumors higher in the esophagus, and gastrointestinal tract integrity is maintained by implantation of the proximal esophagus into the stomach.

Surgical resection of the esophagus has a relatively high mortality rate because of infection, pulmonary complications, or anastomotic leak. Postoperatively, the patient has a nasogastric tube that should not be manipulated and the patient is kept NPO until radiographic studies confirm anastomotic integrity.

The use of radiation therapy either alone or in conjunction with surgery preoperatively or postoperatively may be the treatment of choice by some physicians. The use of chemotherapy combined with radiation and/or surgery is also being studied.

The ideal method of treating esophageal cancer has not yet been found; each patient is approached in a way that appears best for him.

Nursing Interventions

Intervention is directed toward improving the patient's nutritional and physical condition in preparation for surgery, radiation therapy, or chemotherapy. A weight-gaining program based on a high-caloric and high-protein diet, in liquid or soft form, is provided, if it can be managed by mouth. If not, total parenteral nutrition is initiated. Nutritional status is monitored throughout treatment.

The patient is educated about the nature of the postoperative equipment that will be used, including that required for closed chest drainage, nasogastric suction, parenteral fluid therapy, and perhaps gastric intubation. Immediate postoperative care is similar to that provided for patients undergoing thoracic surgery (see Chap. 25). After emergence from anesthesia, the patient is placed in semi-Fowler's position, and later Fowler's position, to assist in preventing reflux of gastric secretions. He is observed carefully for regurgitation and dyspnea. A common postoperative complication is aspiration pneumonia. Temperature is monitored to detect any elevation that may indicate seepage of fluid through the operative site into the mediastinum.

If a prosthetic tube has been inserted or an anastomosis has been performed, the patient will have a functioning continuum between the throat and the stomach. Immediately postoperatively the nasogastric tube should be marked for position and the physician notified if displacement occurs. The nurse does not attempt to reinsert a displaced nasogastric tube, as damage to the anastomosis may occur. The nasogastric tube is removed 5 to 7 days after surgery and a barium swallow is performed to evaluate for anastomotic leak before feeding the patient.

Once feeding begins the patient will need encouragement and patience as he begins to swallow small sips of water and, later, pureed small feedings. When he is able to increase food intake to a significant amount, parenteral fluids are discontinued. If a prosthetic tube (such as a pliable latex tube held open with fine wire coils) is used, it may easily become obstructed if food is not chewed sufficiently. After each meal, the patient is to remain upright for at least 2 hours to assist in movement of food. The nurse is challenged to encourage this patient to eat, since his appetite is usually poor. Family involvement and home-cooked favorite foods may help the patient to eat. If he complains of gastric distress, antacids may help. When radiation is part of the therapy, the patient's appetite is further depressed, and esophagitis may occur, causing the patient pain when he eats. Liquid supplements may be more easily tolerated.

Often, in either the preoperative or postoperative period, an obstructed or nearly obstructed esophagus causes difficulty with excess saliva, so that drooling becomes a problem. This is also a concern in an esophagostomy. In this situation, the use of small plastic bags fastened to the stoma are helpful in collecting secretions, or a wick-type piece of gauze may be placed at the corner of the mouth to direct secretions to a dressing or emesis basin. Of more concern is the possibility of aspiration of saliva into the tracheobronchial tree, with the danger of pneumonia.

When the patient is ready to go home, the family is instructed in how to give nutritional care, what to observe, how to handle signs of complications, how to keep the patient comfortable, and how to obtain needed physical and emotional support.

In summary, persons at risk for developing esophageal cancer include those who smoke cigarettes and drink alcohol, and the elderly. If the malignancy is detected early, removal is simplified and the continuity of the digestive system is easily maintained. The mortality rate among patients with cancer of the esophagus is high, however, because of three factors: (1) Usually, the patient is an older person, in whom the incidence of pulmonary and cardiovascular disorders is high. (2) Before significant symptoms occur, the tumor has already invaded surrounding structures. It is impossible to excise a liberal area of tissue because of the proximity of vital structures. (3) The malignancy tends to spread to nearby lymph nodes, and the unique relation of the esophagus to the heart and lungs makes these organs easily accessible to the extension of the tumor.

Bibliography

Books

Barton RE et al. The Dental Assistant. Philadelphia, Lea & Febiger, 1988.

Bates B. A Guide to Physical Examination and History Taking, 5th ed. Philadelphia, JB Lippincott, 1991.

DeVita VT, Hellman S, and Rosenberg SA (eds). Cancer. Principles and Practice of Oncology, 3rd ed. Philadelphia, JB Lippincott, 1989.

Groenwald S (ed). Cancer Nursing: Principles and Practices. Boston, Jones & Bartlett, 1990.

Jameson GG (ed). Surgery of the Esophagus. New York, Churchill Livingstone, 1988.

Skinner DB and Belsey RHR. Management of esophageal disease. Philadelphia, WB Saunders, 1988,

Taintor JF. The Oral Report. New York, Facts on File Publications, 1988.

Tenenbaum L. Cancer Chemotherapy. Philadelphia, WB Saunders, 1989.

Thawley SE et al. Comprehensive Management of Head and Neck Tumors. Philadelphia, WB Saunders, 1987.

Walsh J et al. Manual of Home Health Care Nursing. Philadelphia, JB Lippincott, 1987.

Journals

Asterisks indicate nursing research articles.

Conditions and Cancer of the Oral Cavity

Boring C et al. Cancer statistics 1991. CA 1991 Jan/Feb; 41(1): 19–36.

Brady LW and Davis LW. Treatment of head and neck cancer by radiation therapy. Semin Oncol 1988 Feb; 15(1): 29–38.

Bral M and Brownstein CN. Antimicrobial agents in the prevention and treatment of periodontal diseases. Dent Clin North Am 1988 Apr; 32(2): 217–241.

Conklin RJ and Blasberg B. Oral lichen planus. Dermatol Clin 1987 Oct; 5(4): 663–673.

Danielson KH. Oral care and older adults. J Gerontol Nurs 1988 Nov; 14(11): 6–10.

Dreyfuss AI et al. Cyclophosphamide, Doxorubicin, & CisPlat combination chemotherapy for advanced carcinoma of salivary gland origin. Cancer 1987 Dec 15; 60(12): 2869–2872.

* Dudjak LA. Mouth care for mucositis due to radiation therapy. Cancer Nurs 1987 Jun; 10(3): 131–140.

Freedman SD and Devine BA. A clean break: Postop oral care. Am J Nurs 1987 Apr; 87(4): 474–475.

Goodman T and Thomas C. Mandibular reconstruction. AORN 1988 Oct; 48(4): 678–688.

Green C. Orthodontics and temporomandibular disorders. Dent Clin North Am 1988 Apr; 32(3): 529–538.

Greenspan D and Greenspan JS. The oral clinical features of HIV infection. Gastroenterol Clin North Am 1988 Jul; 17(3): 535–543.

Hannon LM. Cancer of the oral cavity. Semin Oncol Nurs 1989 Aug; 5(3): 150–159.

Hutton KP and Rogers RS. Recurrent aphthous stomatitis. Dermatol Clin 1987 Oct; 5(4): 761–768.

Krolls SO and Smith WE. Sialolithiasis of the minor salivary glands. Ear Nose Throat J 1988 Apr; 67(4): 296–298.

Loughan DH and Smith LG. Infectious disorders of the parotid gland. N Engl J Med 1988 Apr; 85(4): 311–314.

McWalter GM et al. Draining facial sinus tracts of dental origin. Dental Sch Q 1987; 3(4): 1–4.

Mashberg A and Samit AM. Early detection, diagnosis and management of oral and oropharyngeal cancer. CA 1989 Mar/Apr; 39(2): 67–88.

* Miller R and Rubinstein L. Oral health care for hospitalized patients: The nurse's role. J Nurs Educ 1987 Nov; 26(9): 363–366.

Randle HW. White lesions of the mouth. Dermatol Clin 1987 Oct; 5(4): 641–650.

Ray TL. Oral candidiasis. Dermatol Clin 1987 Oct; 5(4): 651–662.

Schulmeister L. Join the fight against oral cancer. Nursing 1987 May; 17(5): 66–67.

Shaw JH. Causes and control of dental caries. N Engl J Med 1987 Oct 15; 317(16): 996–1004.

Suzuki JB. Diagnosis and classification of the peridontal diseases. Dent Clin North Am 1988 Apr; 32(2): 195–216.

Vogler WR et al. A randomized trial comparing Ketoconazole and Nystatin prophylactic therapy in neutropenic patients. Cancer Invest 1987 5(4): 267–273.

Wolfe R et al. Dental emergencies. Management by the primary care physician. Postgrad Med 1989 Feb 15; 85(3): 63–77.

Conditions and Cancer of the Head and Neck

Adams H et al. Oesophageal tears during pneumatic balloon dilitation for the treatment of achalasia. J Clin Radiol 1989 Jan; 40(1): 53–57.

Blitzer PH. Epidemiology of head and neck cancer. Semin Oncol 1988 Feb; 15(1): 2–9.

Breitbart W and Holland J. Psychosocial aspects of head and neck cancer. Semin Oncol 1988 Feb; 15(1): 29–38.

Dropkin MJ. Coping with disfigurement and dysfunction after head and neck cancer surgery: A conceptual framework. Semin Oncol Nurs 1989 Aug; 5(3): 213–219.

Ferguson MK et al. Early evaluation and therapy for caustic esophageal injury. Am J Surg 1989 Jan; 157(1): 116–120.

Foltz AT. Nutritional factors in the prevention of gastrointestinal cancer. Semin Oncol Nurs 1988 Nov; 4(4): 239–245.

Frank-Stromborg M. The epidemiology and primary prevention of gastric and esophageal cancer. Cancer Nurs 1989 Apr; 12(2): 53–64.

Frieling T et al. Family occurrence of achalasia and diffuse spasm of the oesophagus. Gut 1988 Nov; 29(11): 1595–1602.

Frogge MH. Future perspective and nursing issues in gastrointestinal cancer. Semin Oncol Nurs 1988 Nov; 4(4): 300–302.

Gelfand MD and Botoman VA. Esophageal motility disorders: A clinical overview. Am J Gastroenterol 1987 Mar; 82(3): 181–187.

Grant M et al. Nutrition management in the head and neck cancer patient. Semin Oncol Nurs 1989 Aug; 5(3): 195–204.

Harris LL and Smith S. Chemotherapy in head and neck cancer. Semin Oncol Nurs 1989 Aug; 5(3): 174–181.

Logemann JA. Swallowing and communication rehabilitation. Semin Oncol Nurs 1989 Aug; 5(3): 205–212.

Mahon S. Nursing interventions for the patient with a myocutaneous flap. Cancer Nurs 1987 Feb; 10(1): 21–31.

Martin LK. Management of the altered airway in the head and neck cancer patient. Semin Oncol Nurs 1989 Aug; 5(3): 182–190.

Medvec BR. Esophageal cancer: Treatment and nursing interventions. Semin Oncol Nurs 1988 Nov; 4(4): 246–256.

Mulder DG et al. Management of huge epiphrenic esophageal diverticula. Am J Surg 1989 Mar; 157(3): 303–307.

McCallum RW. The management of esophageal motility disorders. Hosp Pract 1988 Feb 15; 123(2): 239–250.

* Nicholsen BA et al. Assessment of pain in head and neck cancer patients using the McGill questionnaire. J Soc Otorhinolaryngol Head Neck Nurs 1988 Summer; 6(3): 8–12.

Schelper JR. Prevention, detection, and diagnosis of head and neck cancers. Semin Oncol Nurs 1989 Aug; 5(3): 139–149.

Schwartz SS and Yuska CM. Common patient care issues following surgery for head and neck cancer. Semin Oncol Nurs 1989 Aug; 5(3): 191–194.

Snow JB. Surgical management of head and neck cancer. Semin Oncol 1988 Feb; 15(1): 20–28.

Strohl RA. Radiation therapy for head and neck cancers. Semin Oncol Nurs 1989 Aug; 5(3): 166–173.

Agencies

American Association of Public Health Dentists
New York University Dental Center, 421 First Ave, New York, NY 10010
American Cancer Society
1599 Clifton Rd NE, Atlanta, GA 30329
American Dental Association
211 E Chicago Ave, Chicago, IL 60611
American Society of Geriatric Dentistry
1121 W Michigan St, Indianapolis, IN 46202

35

Gastrointestinal Intubation and Special Nutritional Management

Learning Objectives

On completion of this chapter, the learner will be able to:

1. Describe the purposes of gastrointestinal intubation and the care of patients with these therapies
2. Use the nursing process as a framework for care of the patient receiving a tube feeding
3. Explain the preoperative and postoperative care of the patient with a gastrostomy
4. Use the nursing process as a framework for care of the patient with a gastrostomy
5. Identify the purposes and uses of total parenteral nutrition
6. Use the nursing process as a framework for care of the patient receiving total parenteral nutrition
7. Specify the nursing measures that are used to prevent complications of total parenteral nutrition

Gastrointestinal Intubation

Gastrointestinal intubation is the insertion of a short or a long flexible rubber or plastic tube into the stomach or intestine by way of the mouth or nose to (1) decompress the stomach and remove gas and fluid, (2) diagnose gastrointestinal motility, (3) administer medications and feedings, (4) treat an obstruction or bleeding site, or (5) obtain gastric contents for analysis. Any solution administered through a tube is either poured through a syringe or delivered by drip regulated by gravity or by an electric pump. Aspiration (suctioning) to remove gas and fluids is accomplished by using a syringe, an electric suction machine, or a built-in wall suction outlet.

A variety of tubes are used for decompression, aspiration, irrigation, and for the control of bleeding from esophageal varices (Miller-Abbott, Cantor, Harris, Ewald, Levin, Moss, Salem sump, and Sengstaken-Blakemore) and for administra-

tion of feedings and medications (Levin, Moss, Dobhoff, Keo-feed, Flexiflo, Nutriflex, and Entriflex). The tubes differ in composition (rubber, polyurethane, silicone), length (90 cm to 3 m [36 inches to 10 feet]), size (6 to 18 Fr), purpose, and placement in the gastrointestinal tract (stomach, duodenum, jejunum).

Nasogastric Tubes

A nasogastric tube, or short tube, is introduced through the nose or the mouth into the stomach. Commonly used short tubes include the Levin tube, gastric sump tube, Nutriflex tube, Moss tube, and the Sengstaken-Blakemore esophageal-nasogastric tube, which are described below.

Levin Tube.   The Levin tube has a single lumen (No. 14 to 18 Fr) and is made of plastic or rubber with openings near its tip. The tube is used in adults to remove fluid and gas from the upper gastrointestinal tract, to obtain a specimen of gastric contents for laboratory studies, and to administer medications or feeding (gavage) directly into the gastrointestinal tract.

Circular markings at specific points on the tube serve as guides for insertion. A marking is made on the tube to indicate the midpoint (Fig. 35–1). The tube is advanced cautiously until this marking reaches the patient's nostril, indicating that the tube is in the stomach.

Placement may be checked further by aspirating gastric contents with a syringe and testing the *p*H of the aspirate. An x-ray film is the only sure way to verify the tube's location.

Gastric Sump Tube.   The gastric sump tube (Salem, VENTROL) is a radiopaque, clear-plastic, double-lumen nasogastric tube (Fig. 35–2). It is used to decompress the stomach and keep it empty. The inner, smaller tube vents the larger suction-

drainage tube to the atmosphere by means of an opening at the distal end of the tube. It is passed the same way as the Levin tube. It can protect gastric suture lines because, when used properly, the sump tube never allows the force of suction at the drainage openings, or outlets, to exceed 25 mm Hg, the level of capillary fragility. This action is controlled by a small vent tube (blue pigtail). Continuous suction is set at a low pressure of 30 mm Hg with the vent outlet kept open. If available suction is intermittent, rather than continuous, it may be set at 80 to 120 mm Hg. Because of its cyclic setting, by the time suction reaches the gastric mucosa it will be reduced to about 25 mm Hg.

To prevent reflux of gastric contents through the vent lumen (blue pigtail), the vent lumen is kept above the patient's midline; otherwise it will act as a siphon. Irrigation may be

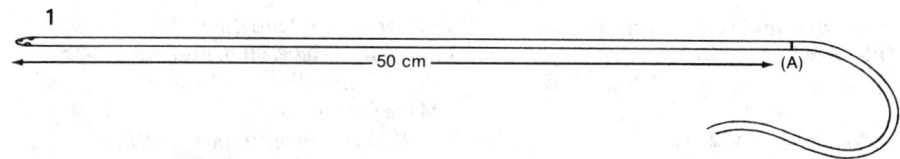

1. Mark the nasogastric tube at a point 50 cm. from the distal tip; call this point 'A'.

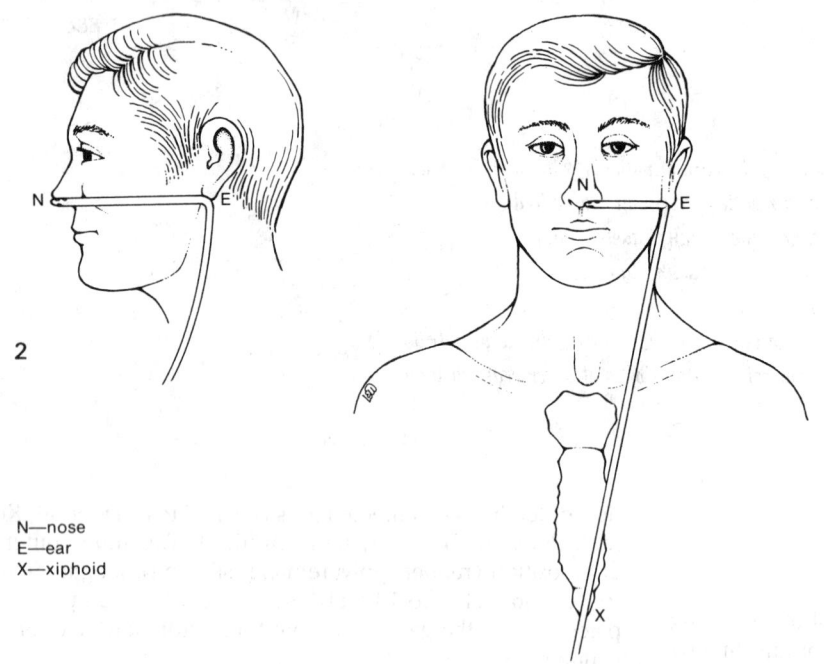

N—nose
E—ear
X—xiphoid

2. Have the patient sit in a neutral position with head facing forward. Place the distal tip of the tubing at the tip of the patient's nose (N); extend tube to the tragus (tip) of his ear (E), and then extend the tube straight down to the tip of his xiphoid (X). Mark this point 'B' on the tubing.

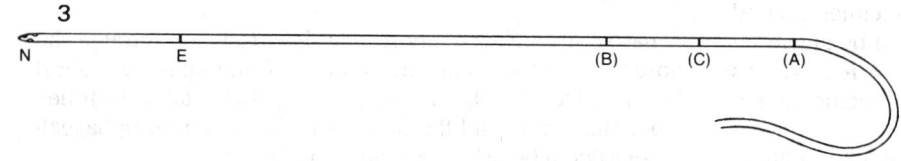

3. To locate point C on the tube, find the midpoint between points A and B. The nasogastric tube is passed to point C to ensure optimum placement in the stomach.

Figure 35–1.   Nasogastric intubation using the Levin tube (short tube) or the Salem sump tube. (Based on research reported in Hanson RL. Predictive criteria for length of nasogastric tube insertion for tube feeding. J Parenteral Enteral Nutr 3[3]:160–163.)

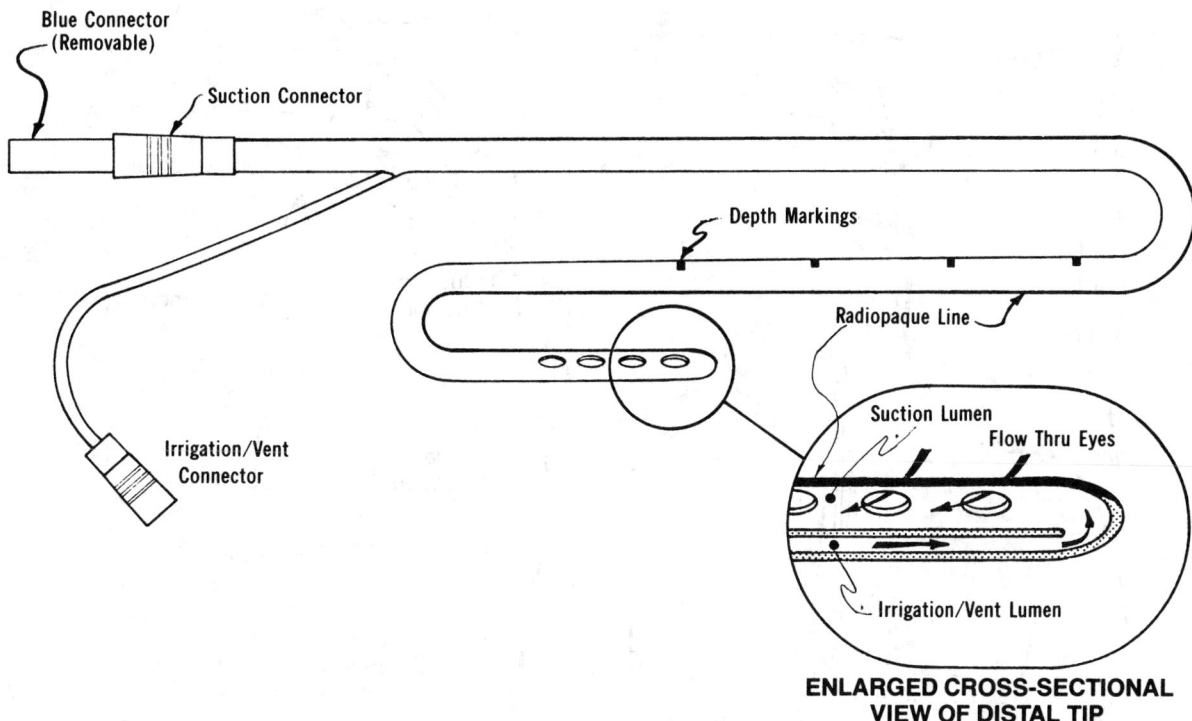

Figure 35–2. The VENTROL Levin (sump) tube. Note the enlarged version showing the direction of flow for suction and irrigation. (Courtesy of National Catheter Co, Argyle, NY.)

performed through either the main lumen or the vent lumen; if the vent lumen is used, irrigation is followed with injection of 10 ml of air, to clear the lumen.

Nutriflex Tube. The Nutriflex nasogastric feeding tube is 76 cm (30 in) long and has a mercury-weighted tip to facilitate insertion. It is coated with a Hydromer lubricant that is activated when moistened.

Moss Tube. The Moss nasoesophageal gastric decompression tube is 90 cm (35 inches) long and has a triple lumen (Fig. 35–3). It is anchored in the stomach by inflating the balloon. The decompression catheter provides for esophageal and gastric aspiration as well as lavage. The third lumen is an avenue for duodenal feedings.

Sengstaken-Blakemore (S-B) Tube. The S-B tube is used to treat bleeding esophageal varices (see Chap. 38 and Fig. 38–7). There are three lumina with two balloons. The balloons are checked for air leakage and proper inflation before insertion. One lumen is used to inflate a gastric balloon and the second one is used to inflate the esophageal balloon. The desired pressure in each balloon is 25 to 30 mm Hg. The tube should be clamped to secure set pressures. Frequent pressure checks should be made to guard against undetected air leaks in the system. The third lumen is used for gastric lavage to monitor bleeding. A pair of scissors is taped near the bedside so that if the patient develops respiratory distress the tube may be cut to deflate the balloons; the physician is notified.

In summary, short nasogastric tubes are used for decompression of the stomach, removal of gastric contents and feedings. Size, diameter and length vary depending on the indications for use and length of time needed. The S-B tube is used to control bleeding from esophageal varices.

Nasoenteric Tubes

A nasoenteric tube, or long tube, is introduced through the nose and passed through the esophagus and stomach into the intestinal tract. It is used to aspirate intestinal contents to prevent gas and fluid from distending the coils of intestine. This process is called *decompression*. Three major nasoenteric tubes that are used for aspiration and decompression are the Miller-Abbott tube, the Harris tube, and the Cantor tube. These tubes are used in the active treatment of obstruction of the small intestine. They are also used prophylactically, being inserted the night before an abdominal operation to prevent obstruction after the operation.

Because peristalsis is either absent or slowed for 24 to 48 hours after an operation, because of the effects of anesthesia and of visceral manipulation, nasogastric or nasoenteric suction is used for the following reasons:

- To evacuate fluids and flatus, so that vomiting is prevented and tension is reduced along the incision line
- To reduce edema, which can cause obstruction
- To enhance blood supply to the suture line, thereby providing nutrition to the site

Usually, the tubes are allowed to remain in place after the operation until peristalsis is resumed, as determined by the presence of bowel sounds.

Decompression Tubes

Miller-Abbott Tube. The Miller-Abbott tube is a double-lumen (No. 16 Fr) 3-m (10-foot) tube, one lumen of which is used to introduce mercury or to inflate the balloon at the end of the tube; the other lumen is used for aspiration. Before the

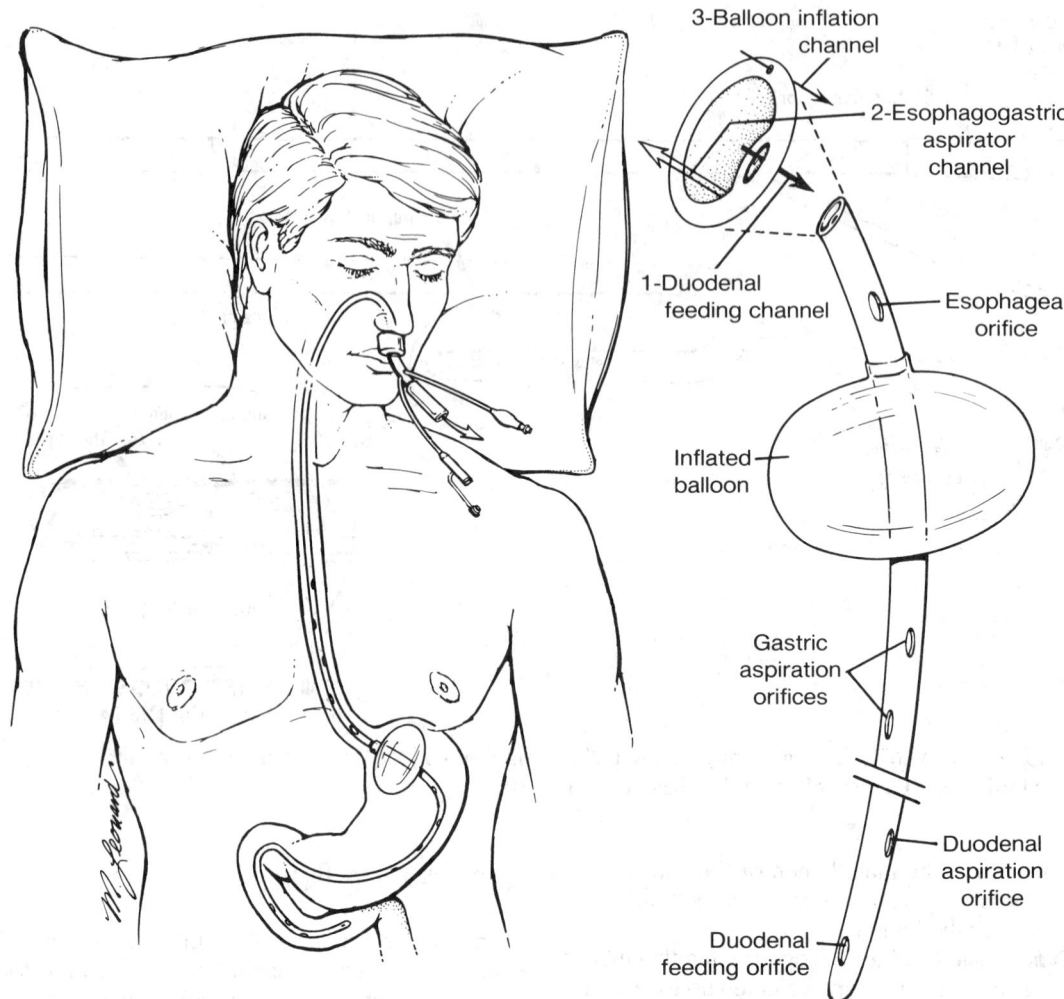

Figure 35–3. The Moss esophageal/duodenal decompression and feeding catheter. There are three channels: (1) the duodenal feeding channel; (2) the esophagogastric aspiration channel, which has additional openings into the proximal duodenum as well as the stomach and the distal esophagus; and (3) the balloon inflation channel.

tube is inserted, the balloon should be tested and its capacity measured; it is then deflated completely. The tube should be lubricated sparingly, and chilled well, before the tip is inserted through the patient's nose. Markings on the tube indicate the distance it has been passed.

Harris Tube.   The Harris tube is a single-lumen (14 Fr), mercury-weighted tube of about 1.8 m (6 feet). This tube has a metal tip that is lubricated and introduced into the nostril. The mercury-weighted bag follows. The weight of the mercury carries the bag by gravity. This tube is used solely for suction and irrigation. Usually, a Y-tube is attached to the end of the tube, so that the suction apparatus is attached to one side and an outlet with a clamp is available on the other side for irrigating purposes.

Cantor Tube.   The Cantor tube is 3 m (10 feet) long with a No. 18 Fr lumen. Its distinguishing feature is that it is larger than the other long tubes and has 4 or 5 ml of mercury in the bag at the extreme end of the rubber tubing. Before insertion, the bag is wrapped about the tube. After the tube is lubricated, it is passed through the nostril and advanced to the esophagus (Fig. 35–4). The patient is in a sitting position and is offered

sips of water to facilitate passage of the tube. Fluoroscopy is helpful in passing the tube into the duodenum.

In summary, long nasoenteric decompression tubes have single or double lumina and are used for decompression and gas and fluid removal. The tubes are used prophylactically before bowel surgery or to treat small bowel obstruction.

Feeding Tubes

Several nasoenteric tubes that are commonly used for feeding include the Keofeed, Nyphus/Nelson, Moss, and Dubbhoff tubes (Fig. 35–5). It usually takes 24 hours for the Dobhoff and the Keofeed tubes to pass through the stomach and into the intestines. Passage is facilitated by having the patient lie on his right side. The Nyhus/Nelson nasoenteral tube uses a twin-balloon design to provide both gastric decompression and jejunal feeding. Both the Nyhus/Nelson and the Moss tubes are inserted in the operating room and are used frequently for postoperative enteral feeding to avoid negative nitrogen balance, to enhance wound healing, and to promote gastric motility and peristalsis, therefore decreasing postoperative hospital

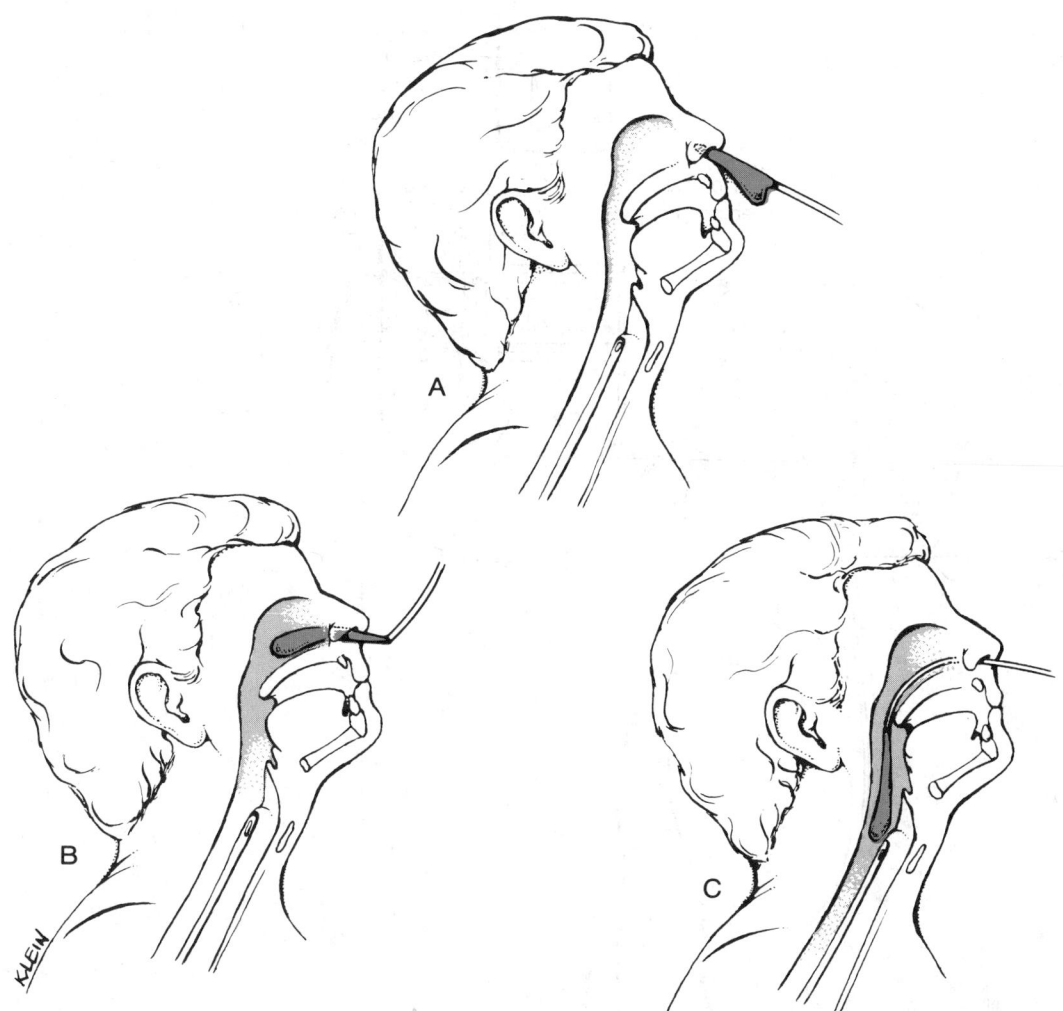

Figure 35–4. Passage of Cantor tube. (**A**) Tube with weighted mercury bag is introduced into the nostril. Note the natural tilt of the tubing. (**B**) After the mercury bag has entered the nostril, the catheter is tilted upward (head can also be tilted slightly upward) to facilitate gravity pull on the weighted bag. (**C**) The weight of the mercury pulls the bag downward. (Redrawn from Hardy JD. Rhoads Textbook of Surgery, 5th ed. Philadelphia, JB Lippincott.)

stay. Vivonex, a commercial tube feeding formula, is commonly used because it is in a partially digested form, allowing for rapid absorption by the intestine.

The polyurethane or silicone rubber feeding tubes have small diameters (6 to 8 Fr) and tungsten tips (rather than weighted mercury-filled bags), and some have a water-activated lubricant that makes it easier to place the tube and insert and remove the stylet. The various tubes come with instructions for ease of passage with or without a stylet. However, kinking of tubing may present a problem when a stylet is not used if the patient is uncooperative or unable to swallow. The stylet is used with caution with patients predisposed to esophageal punctures (elderly and frail with thin tissue). Essentially, such a tube is passed in the same way as a nasogastric tube, that is, with the patient in high Fowler's position. If this is not feasible, the patient is placed on his right side.

In summary, feeding tubes are used for total diet administration, supplementations, and for feedings postoperatively to promote positive nitrogen balance. They are useful for long-term therapy, as they are pliable and comfortable for the patient.

Nursing Interventions for Nasogastric and Nasoenteric Intubation

Nursing interventions are organized into the following areas:

- Instructing the patient about the purposes of the tube and the procedures required for insertion and advancement
- Inserting the nasogastric tube and assisting with the insertion of the nasoenteric tube
- Checking for placement of the nasogastric tube
- Advancing the nasoenteric tube
- Monitoring the patient
- Providing oral and nasal hygiene and care
- Assessing for possible complications
- Removing the tube

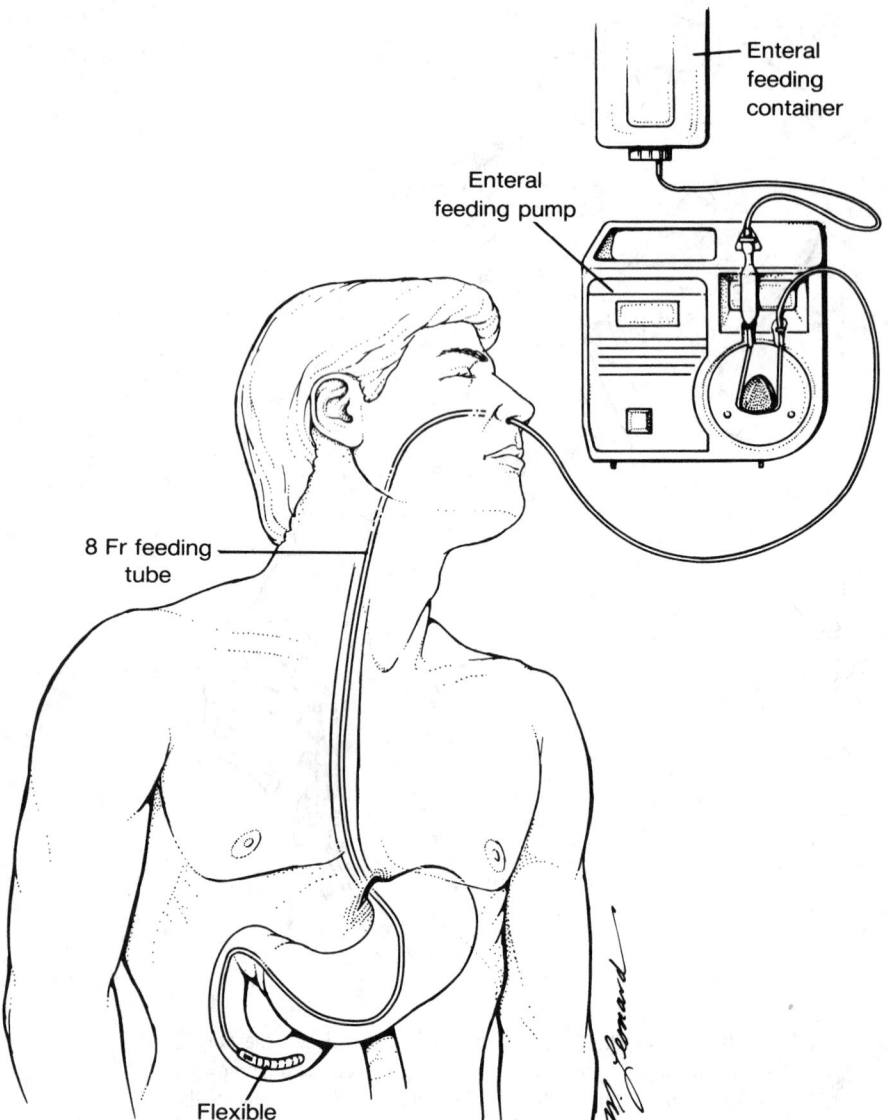

Figure 35–5. The enteral feeding tube (8 Fr) with a flexible weighted tip is readily passed into the stomach and through the pylorus into the duodenum or proximal jejunum.

Instruction

Before the patient is intubated, the nurse explains the purpose of the tube. This information may make the patient more cooperative and tolerant of an initially unpleasant procedure. The general activities related to the passage of the tube are then reviewed, including the fact that the patient may have to breathe through his mouth and that passage of the tube may cause him to gag until the tube has passed his gag reflex.

Insertion of the Tube

During insertion, the patient usually sits upright with a towel spread bib-fashion over his chest. Tissue wipes are made available. The patient is screened from other patients, and adequate light is provided. Occasionally, the physician will swab the nostril and spray the oropharynx with tetracaine (Pontocaine) to dull the nasal passage and the gag reflex and to make the procedure more tolerable. Gargling with a liquid anesthetic or holding ice chips in the mouth for a few minutes can have the same effect. Encouraging the patient to breathe through

his mouth or pant often helps, as does swallowing water, if permitted.

A polyurethane tube may need to be warmed to make it more pliable. The tube should be lubricated with a water-soluble substance (K-Y jelly) unless it has a dry coating called Hydromer, which, when moistened, provides lubrication for ease of insertion. After the tube is prepared, the patient is asked to tilt his head back so that the tube can be introduced through the nostril. The patient is encouraged to swallow as the tube is passed. When the tip is positioned in the stomach, the *nasogastric* tube is secured to the nose or cheek. (Fig. 35–6A) A recommended method is to apply tincture of benzoin to the skin where the nasogastric tube will be secured. The prepared area is covered with a strip of hypoallergenic tape or Op-site; then the tube is placed over the tape and secured with another piece of tape. The *nasoenteric* tube can be secured with tape to the malar eminence (use a slight U-shaped loop) or to the forehead (see Fig. 35–6B).

This technique secures the tube during patient movement. Nasoenteric tubes are *not* taped immediately, because it takes

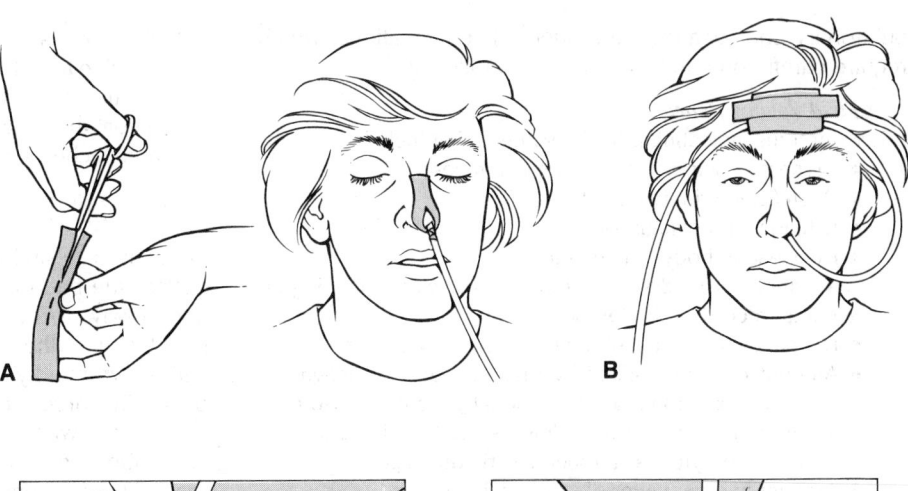

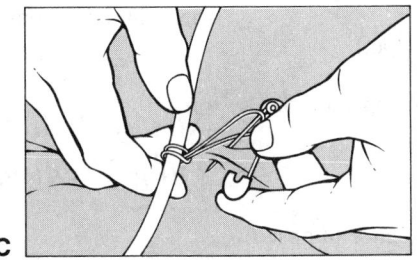
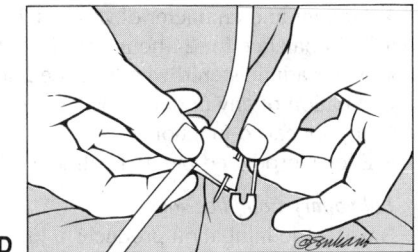

Figure 35–6. Securing nasogastric and nasoenteric tubes. (**A**) The *nasogastric* tube is secured to the nose with tape to prevent injury to the nasopharyngeal passages; the cheek may also be used. (**B**) Tape is placed on the forehead and the *nasoenteric* tube is taped to it, thereby allowing the Cantor tube to be advanced until desired placement is achieved. (**C** and **D**) Secure tubing to the patient's gown with either an elastic band or tape attached to a safety pin to prevent tension on the line during movement.

approximately 24 hours for these tubes to progress into the intestine.

Placement of the Nasogastric Tube

To ensure patient safety, it is important to confirm correct placement of the tube. Initially, this is often accomplished by x-ray. Subsequently, tube placement must be confirmed before instillation of liquids. In the past it has been recommended that this be performed by using a stethoscope to auscultate air insufflations through the tube. Recent studies, however, indicate that this ausculatory method is not accurate in differentiating between gastric and intestinal placement and gastric and respiratory placement. A more accurate method is to determine the pH of the tube aspirate. The pH of gastric aspirate is acidic (approximately 3); the pH of intestinal aspirate is approximately 6.5; and the pH of respiratory aspirate is more alkaline (7 or greater).

Advancement of the Nasoenteric Tube

After the tube has passed through the pyloric sphincter, it may be advanced 5 to 7.5 cm (2 to 3 in) every hour. So that gravity and peristalsis will aid in the passage of the tube, the patient is generally asked to lie on his right side for 2 hours, on his back for 2 hours, and then on his left side for 2 hours. Ambulation, if possible, also helps to advance the tube. If the tube is advanced too rapidly, it will curl and kink in the stomach.

Monitoring the Patient

The nasogastric tube is attached to straight drainage or intermittent low suction. If used for enteral nutrition, the end is wrapped in gauze and clamped closed or plugged between feedings. Confirmation of tube placement is essential before any fluids are instilled. Tube displacement may be caused by

tension on the tube (when the patient moves around in the bed or room), coughing, tracheal or nasotracheal suctioning, and airway intubation.

An accurate record is kept of all fluid intake, feedings, and irrigation. Normal saline is recommended for irrigations to avoid electrolyte loss through gastric drainage. The amount, color, and type of all drainage are recorded every 8 hours.

When double- or triple-lumen tubes are used, the individual lumina intended for aspiration, feeding, and balloon inflation are labeled. To avoid tension on the tube, the portion of the tube from the nose to the drainage unit is fixed in position, either with a safety pin or with adhesive-tape loops that are pinned to the patient's pajamas or gown. The tube must be looped loosely to prevent tension and dislodgment (see Fig. 35–6C, D).

Oral and Nasal Hygiene and Care

Regular and conscientious oral and nasal hygiene is a vital part of patient care, as the tube may be in place for several days. Moistened cotton-tipped swabs can be used to clean the nose. This can be followed by cleansing with water-soluble oil for lubrication. Frequent mouth attention is comforting. The nasal tape is changed every other day and nares are inspected for skin irritation. If the nasal and pharyngeal mucosa are excessively dry, steam or cool vapor inhalations may be beneficial. Throat lozenges, an ice collar, chewing gum (if permitted), and frequent movement also assist in relieving discomfort. These activities will keep the mucous membranes moist and will help prevent infection of the parotid glands.

Assessment for Possible Complications

Patients with nasogastric or nasoenteric intubation are susceptible to a variety of problems, including fluid volume deficit, pulmonary complications, and tube-related irritations, which require careful ongoing assessment, as follows:

Fluid Volume Deficit

1. Symptoms indicating a fluid volume deficit include
   - Dryness of skin and mucous membranes
   - Decreasing urinary output
   - Lethargy and exhaustion
   - Decrease in body temperature
2. Assessment of fluid volume deficit involves maintaining an accurate record of the following:
   - Drainage—amount, color, and type, every 8 hours
   - Amount of fluid instilled by irrigation of the nasogastric tube and the amount of water taken by mouth. An isotonic solution, such as normal saline, is used for irrigations to avoid electrolyte loss through gastric drainage
   - Amount and character of vomitus, if any
   - Fluid balance for 24 hours (intake versus output)
   - Water administered with tube feedings
   - Duration of any period in which the suction apparatus did not appear to function
   - Effects produced by the treatment

Pulmonary Complications

1. Nasogastric intubation produces a higher incidence of postoperative pulmonary complications by interfering with coughing and clearing of the pharynx.
2. The nurse assesses the lung fields regularly, through auscultation, to determine the presence of congestion. In addition, the patient is encouraged to cough and to take deep breaths regularly. The nurse also carefully confirms the proper placement of the tube before instilling any fluids.

Tube-Related Irritations

1. When providing oral hygiene, the nurse carefully inspects the mucous membranes for signs of irritation or excessive dryness. In addition, she palpates the area around the parotid glands to detect any soreness or lumps and any skin or mucous membrane irritation or necrosis.

2. The nostrils, oral mucosa, esophagus, and trachea are susceptible to irritation and necrosis. Visible areas are inspected frequently and the adequacy of hydration is assessed. In addition, the patient is assessed for the presence of esophagitis and tracheitis. Symptoms include sore throat and hoarseness.

Removal of Tube

When it is desirable to remove the tube, it is necessary to deflate the balloon if present and withdraw the tube, gently and slowly, for 15 to 20 cm (6 to 8 in), at intervals of 10 minutes, until the tip reaches the esophagus; the remainder is withdrawn rapidly from the nostril. If the tube does not come out easily, force should not be used—the physician is notified.

As it is withdrawn, the tube is concealed in a towel, because the sight of it may be unpleasant and cause the patient to vomit. After removal of the tube, oral hygiene is provided.

Nasogastric and Nasoenteric Tube Feedings

Tube feedings are given to meet nutritional requirements when oral intake is inadequate or not possible, as long as the gastrointestinal tract is functioning normally. Tube feedings are delivered to the stomach (nasogastric) or to the distal duodenum or proximal jejunum (nasoenteric) when it is necessary to bypass the esophagus and stomach. The numerous conditions requiring enteral nutrition are summarized in Table 35–1.

Liquid formulas are designed to improve nutritional intake by either oral or tube administration. Tube feedings have several advantages:

- Intraluminal delivery of nutrients preserves gastrointestinal integrity.

TABLE 35–1. *Conditions Requiring Enteral Nutrition*

Condition or Need	Cause
Preoperative preparation with elemental diet	
Gastrointestinal problems with elemental diet	Fistulas, short bowel syndrome, Crohn's disease, ulcerative colitis, nonspecific maldigestion or malabsorption
Cancer therapy	Radiation, chemotherapy
Convalescent care	Surgery, injury, severe illness
Coma, semiconsciousness*	Stroke, head injury, neurologic disorders
Hypermetabolic conditions	Burns, trauma, multiple fractures, sepsis
Alcoholism, chronic depression, anorexia nervosa*	Chronic illness, psychiatric or neurologic disorder
Debilitation*	Disease or injury
Maxillofacial or cervical surgery	Disease or injury
Oropharyngeal or esophageal paralysis*	Disease or injury
Mental retardation*	

* Some of these patients will be at risk for regurgitating or vomiting and aspirating administered formula. Accordingly, each case must be considered individually.
(Jensen T. Home enteral nutrition. Dietetic Currents, Ross Timesaver Jul/Aug; 9: 15–20.)

- Tube feedings preserve the normal sequence of intestinal and hepatic metabolism before nutrient delivery to the arterial circulation.
- The intestinal mucosa and liver are important in fat metabolism and are the only sites of lipoprotein synthesis.
- Normal insulin-glucagon ratios are maintained with the intestinal administration of carbohydrates.

Commercial formulas frequently present problems because the composition is "fixed." Some patients may not be able to tolerate certain ingredients, such as sodium, protein, or potassium. "Modular" diets are also prepared commercially, and the critical constituents of sodium, potassium, and fat can be added by the dietitian. Attention is given to including all essential minerals and vitamins. Total intake of calories, nutrients, and fluids are assessed when there is a reduction in total intake, or excessive dilution, of feedings.

Many patients do not tolerate tube feedings well, particularly those feedings administered by nasogastric intubation. Often a medium- or fine-bore Silastic tube is tolerated better than a plastic or rubber tube. The finer-bore tube, however, requires a finely dispersed formula to prevent the tube from clogging.

A wide variety of containers, feeding tubes and catheters, delivery systems, and pumps (Kangaroo 2, IMED-430, Dobhoff, Keofeed II, Flexiflo II) are available for use in tube or enteral feedings. The decision as to what to use is made after considering the most appropriate formula and delivery system for a given patient: nutrient sources, concentrations, osmolality, viscosity, and mineral content of a given formula, as well as the method and rate of administration, patient dexterity, available storage and refrigerator space, and cost of the formula and supportive equipment. Some commonly used commercial tube feedings include Ensure, Isocal, Sustacal, and Vivonex. Pulmocare is a specialized formula for patients with pulmonary disorders that is high in fat and low in carbohydrates. Its high density (1.5 calories/ml) is ideal for patients who require fluid restriction, and it is also designed to reduce carbon dioxide production. Some feedings are given as supplements, and others are provided to meet the patient's total nutritional needs. Nutritionists work closely with physicians and nurses in determining the best formula for the individual patient.

Osmosis and Osmolality

Solutions that are highly concentrated and foods that have certain characteristics can upset the normal water balance within the body. Fluid balance is maintained by the process of *osmosis*. It is accomplished within the body by moving water through membranes from a dilute solution of lower osmolality to a more concentrated one of higher osmolality until the solutions are nearly of equal osmolality. The osmolality of normal body fluids is approximately 300 mOsm/kg. The body attempts to keep the osmolality of the contents of the stomach and intestines at approximately this level.

Proteins are extremely large particles and therefore have little or no osmotic effect. Individual amino acids and carbohydrates are smaller particles, however, and therefore have greater osmotic effect. Fats are not water-soluble and do not form a solution in water; thus, they have no osmotic effect. Because electrolytes such as sodium and potassium are comparatively small particles, they have a great effect on osmolality, and consequently on tolerance.

Osmolality is an important consideration for patients being fed past the pylorus. When a concentrated solution of high osmolality is taken in large amounts, water will move to the stomach and intestines from fluid surrounding the organs and from the vascular compartment. The patient experiences a feeling of fullness, nausea, and diarrhea, which can bring about dehydration, resulting, in some cases, in hypotension and tachycardia. Collectively, these symptoms have been termed the *dumping syndrome*. This problem can generally be alleviated by starting the patient on a more dilute solution and by increasing the concentration over several days.

There is a wide range of tolerance among patients as to the effects of osmolality. Usually, debilitated patients are more sensitive to such disorders. Therefore, the nurse should be knowledgeable about the osmolality of formulas and should observe and prevent such disorders.

In summary, tube feeding solutions vary according to preparation, consistency, amount of calories and supplemental vitamins. The type chosen depends on the size and location of the tube, type of nutritional supplement (total versus partial), and convenience for the patient at home.

▶ Nursing Process
The Patient Receiving a Tube Feeding
▷ Assessment

The nurse participates in the assessment of patients with suspected nutritional problems. A preliminary assessment includes the family's need for information and should answer the following questions:

- What is the patient's nutritional status as judged by his current physical appearance; dietary history, including a history of food intolerance especially milk or lactose intolerance; and recent weight loss or gain?
- Are there any existing chronic illnesses or situations that will increase metabolic demands on the body?
- Is his fluid and electrolyte balance in order?
- Is his digestive tract functioning? Does it have good absorptive capacity?
- Are his kidneys and urinary system functioning normally?
- Are weight and fluid requirements met (*i.e.*, 30 to 40 ml/kg body weight)?
- What medications is he receiving and what other therapy is he receiving that may affect his digestive intake and digestive system?
- Does the dietary prescription fulfill his needs?

In addition, a more elaborate assessment is performed on those patients who may require extensive nutritional therapy. This is done by a team that includes the nurse, physician, and nutritionist. In addition to the history and physical examination and anthropometric measurements, nutritional assessment consists of recording any weight change, determining serum albumin and transferrin levels and total lymphocyte count, testing of delayed hypersensitivity reaction, and evaluating muscle function.

▷ Nursing Diagnoses

Based on all the assessment data, the major nursing diagnoses may include the following:

- Altered nutrition, less than body requirements, related to inadequate intake of nutrients
- Diarrhea related to the dumping syndrome
- Potential ineffective airway clearance related to aspiration of tube feeding
- High risk for fluid volume deficit related to hypertonic dehydration
- Potential ineffective individual coping related to the discomfort imposed by the presence of the nasogastric/nasoenteric tube

▷ **Planning and Implementation**

▷ *Goals:*   The major goals of the patient may include attainment and maintenance of nutritional balance, maintenance of a normal bowel pattern, maintenance of a patent airway, maintenance of adequate hydration, and improvement of individual coping.

▷ **Nursing Interventions**

▷ *Nutritional Balance.*   When preparing and administering a tube feeding, it is essential that all measures of cleanliness be observed. Temperature of the feeding, volume of the feeding, flow rate, and adequate fluid intake are also critically important.

The schedule determining the quantity and frequency of tube feedings is maintained. The nurse must therefore carefully monitor the rate of drip and avoid too rapid administration of fluids. Commonly used electrical pumps to control the rate and pressure of the delivery of viscous fluids are relatively heavy and must be attached to an intravenous (IV) pole. Several pumps that have been designed specifically for enteral tube feedings are lightweight and easy to handle, and require minimal instructions for use. Some examples are the Kangaroo Easy-Cap II (Cheeseborough-Pond); the Flexiflo II Portable Enteral Nutrition Pump (Ross Laboratories), which can be carried by using a nylon adjustable strap and can operate for 8 hours on a rechargeable battery; the Enteroport (Diatek), designed for continuous home feedings and available with a portable shoulder strap; the IMED 430 Enteral Delivery System (IMED); and the Flo Gard 2000 peristaltic pump (Travenol Laboratories).

Residual gastric content is checked before each feeding. (This solution is returned to the patient.) If the amount of aspirated gastric content is greater than 150 ml, the feeding is delayed and the patient's condition reassessed in 2 hours. If this occurs twice, the physician is notified.

Before and after each medication or administration of tube feeding and every 4 to 6 hours with continuous feedings, about 50 ml of water is administered to ensure patency and to decrease the chance of bacterial growth and crusting or occlusion of the tube. Some studies have reported water to be superior to cranberry juice in preventing tube occlusion. Medications may be given by single bolus, with flushing after each dose, depending on their preparation (Table 35-2).

When small-bore feeding tubes for continuous rates are irrigated, a 30-ml or larger syringe is used because pressure generated by smaller syringes can cause the tube to rupture. The bag and tubing are changed according to the agency's policy, usually every 24 to 48 hours, and fresh formulas are hung every 4 hours to reduce bacterial contamination.

Feedings are administered either by gravity (drip), bolus, or by continuous controlled pump that is either volumetric

TABLE 35-2.   *Medication Administered Via Feeding Tube*

Type	Preparation
Liquid	None
Simple compressed tablets	Crush and dissolve in water
Buccal or sublingual tablets	Give as intended
Enteric-coated tablets	Cannot be crushed; change in form is required

(ml/hour) or peristaltic (drops/hour). Gravity feedings are placed above the level of the stomach, and the speed of administration is determined by gravity. Bolus feedings are given in large volumes, 300 to 400 ml every 4 to 6 hours. Continuous feeding is the preferred method; allowing the feeding to be given in small set amounts over long periods reduces the risk of aspiration, distention, nausea, vomiting, and diarrhea.

Feedings are lactose free, with an osmolality of only 300 mOsm/kg; a feeding may be given undiluted and provides 1 calorie/ml. Feeding rates of about 100 to 150 ml/hr (2400 to 3600 calories/day) are effective in inducing positive nitrogen balance and progressive weight gain, without producing abdominal cramps and diarrhea. If the feeding is intermittent, 200 to 350 ml are given in 10 to 15 minutes.

Continuous monitoring of the tube-feeding regimen is necessary to determine its nutritional effectiveness. The following nursing interventions are implemented:

- Assess placement of tubing, position of patient, and flow rate
- Observe patient's ability to tolerate the formula (assess for feeling of fullness, bloating, urticaria, nausea, vomiting, diarrhea, and constipation)
- Check clinical responses, as noted in laboratory findings: blood urea nitrogen, hemoglobin, serum protein, and hematocrit
- Assess the patient's general condition by noting the appearance of the skin (turgor, dryness, color) and mucous membranes; urinary output; state of hydration; and weight gain or loss
- Observe for signs of dehydration (dry mucous membranes, thirst, decreased urine output)
- Record the actual formula intake by the patient
- Record incidents of vomiting and diarrhea or distention
- Note any changes in ability of the patient to communicate
- Report a urine glucose concentration of +3 or +4, decreased urinary output, sudden weight gain, and periorbital or dependent puffiness
- Hang fresh tube formula every 4 hours
- Change tube feeding container and line every 24 hours
- Assess residual volumes before each feeding or, in the case of continuous feedings, every 4 hours
- Monitor intake and output
- Weigh patient three times a week
- Consult dietician
- Assess for possible complications (Table 35-3)

▷ *Bowel Pattern.*   Patients receiving nasogastric or nasoenteric tube feedings frequently experience diarrhea (watery stools occurring three times in 24 hours). Pasty, unformed stool is expected with enteral therapy because many formulas have little or no residue. The dumping syndrome also leads to diar-

TABLE 35-3. *Complications of Enteral Therapy*

Complications	Cause
GASTROINTESTINAL	
Diarrhea	Hyperosmolar feedings
	Rapid infusion/bolus feedings
	Bacteria contamination of feedings
	Lactase deficiency
	Medications
	Decreased serum osmolarity level
	Food allergies
Nausea	Change in rate
	Offensive smell
	Hyperosmolar formula
	Inadequate gastric emptying
Gas/bloating/cramping	Air in tube
Dumping syndrome	Bolus feedings/rapid rate
	Cold formula
Atelectasis and possible pneumonia	Emesis and aspirated tube feeding
MECHANICAL	
Tube displacement	Excessive coughing/vomiting
	Tension on the tube/unsecured tube
	Tracheal suctioning
	Airway intubation
Tube obstruction	Inadequate flushing/formula
Residue	Inadequate crushing of medications
Nasopharyngeal irritation	Tube position
	Larger tubes
METABOLIC	
Dehydration and azotemia (excess urea in the blood)	Hyperosmolar feedings with insufficient fluid intake
Tube feeding syndrome	Excessive urea from high-protein mixture and formulas lacking fat
Electrolyte imbalances	Contents of formula and patient's medical diagnosis

rhea. To confirm that the dumping syndrome is causing the diarrhea, other possible causes must be ruled out: zinc deficiency (15 mg of zinc every 24 hours is recommended in the feeding to maintain a normal serum level of 50 to 150 μg/dl [7.65 to 22.95 μmol/L]), contaminated formula, malnutrition (a decrease in the intestinal absorptive area resulting from malnutrition can cause diarrhea), and drug therapy. Antibiotics such as clindamycin (Cleocin) and lincomycin (Lincocin), antidysrhythmic drugs (quinidine, propranolol [Inderal]), aminophylline (theophylline), and digitalis have been found to increase the frequency of the dumping syndrome in certain patients.

The dumping syndrome (discussed in Chap. 36) results from the rapid distention of the jejunum when hypertonic solutions are administered quickly (over 10 to 20 minutes). Foods high in carbohydrates and electrolytes draw extracellular fluid from the vascular system into the jejunum so that dilution and absorption can occur. The gastrointestinal symptoms (diarrhea,

nausea) associated with the dumping syndrome can be managed by

- Decreasing the instillation rate to provide time for carbohydrates and electrolytes to be diluted
- Administering the feedings at room temperature, because temperature extremes stimulate peristalsis
- Administering the feeding by continuous drip rather than bolus (if tolerated) to prevent sudden distention of the intestine
- Advising the patient to remain in semi-Fowler's position for 30 minutes after the feeding (this position prolongs transit time by decreasing the influence of gravity)
- Instilling the minimal amount of water needed to flush the tubing before and after a feeding because fluid given with a feeding increases transit time

▷ *Airway Management.* Airway obstruction occurs when stomach contents or enteral feedings are regurgitated and aspirated or when a nasogastric tube is improperly placed and feedings are instilled into the pharynx or the trachea. Nasoenteric tubes, especially those that provide for gastric and esophageal/duodenal decompression (Nyhus/Nelson, Moss), have helped decrease the frequency of regurgitation and aspiration.

To maintain a patent airway, the nurse must check tube placement before giving every feeding and always administer the feeding with the patient in the proper position to prevent regurgitation. To reduce the risk of reflux and pulmonary aspiration, the semi-Fowler's position is recommended for a nasogastric feeding; the patient's head should be elevated at least 30 degrees for a nasoenteric feeding. This position is maintained at least 30 minutes after completion of intermittent tube feedings; it is maintained at all times for patients receiving continuous tube feedings.

If aspiration is suspected, the feeding is stopped, and the pharynx and trachea are suctioned if necessary. The nurse notifies the physician.

▷ *Maintaining Adequate Hydration.* The hydration of the patient is monitored carefully because the patient often cannot communicate his need for water. Water is given every 4 to 6 hours and after feedings to prevent hypertonic dehydration. At the beginning of administration, the feeding is diluted to at least half-strength and not more than 50 to 100 ml is given at a time, or 40 to 60 ml/hr is given in continuous drip administration. This gradual administration helps the patient to develop tolerance, especially for hyperosmolar solutions. The following nursing measures are important:

- Observe for signs of dehydration (dry mucous membranes, thirst, decreased urine output).
- Administer water routinely and as needed
- Monitor intake and output

▷ *Promoting Coping Ability.* The psychosocial goal of nursing care is to provide support, encouragement, and a warm acceptance of the patient, while conveying hope that daily progressive improvement is possible. If the patient is having difficulty adjusting to the treatment, the nurse intervenes by

- Encouraging the patient when he adheres to the medical plan of care
- Encouraging self-care within the parameters of his activity level (making his bed, recording his daily weight and intake and output)
- Reinforcing an optimistic approach by identifying signs and symptoms that indicate progress (daily weight gain, electrolyte balance, absence of nausea and diarrhea)

▷ *Patient Education and Home Health Care.* Preparation for home care management of enteral feedings begins while the patient is hospitalized. The nurse teaches while administering the feedings so that the mechanics of the procedure are observed and reinforced. Before discharge, information is provided about the equipment, formula purchase and storage, and administration of the feedings (frequency, quantity, rate of instillation). Family members who will participate in the patient's home care are invited to all teaching sessions. Available printed information about the delivery equipment and formula is reviewed. The patient is encouraged to handle the equipment under the supervision of the nurse.

When the patient is at home, a visiting nurse will monitor his progress (weight, vital signs, activity level, electrolyte values)

and assess for any complications (dumping syndrome, nausea/vomiting, weight loss, lethargy, confusion, excessive thirst). The patient is encouraged to keep a diary in which he records times and amounts of feedings and any symptoms that occur. The nurse can review the diary during home visits.

▷ *Evaluation*

Expected Outcomes
1. Attains/maintains nutritional balance
   a. Has positive nitrogen balance
   b. Diagnostic studies within normal limits (*i.e.*, blood urea nitrogen [BUN], hemoglobin, hematocrit, serum protein)
   c. Attains or maintains hydration of body tissue
   d. Attains or maintains desired body weight
2. Is free from episodes of diarrhea
   a. Has fewer than three watery stools a day
   b. Does not have a bowel movement after a bolus feeding
   c. States he has no intestinal cramping
   d. Has normal bowel sounds
3. Maintains a patent airway
   a. Lungs clear to auscultation
   b. Normal heart rate and respirations
   c. Has a normal chest x-ray film
4. Attains or maintains hydration of body tissue
   a. Has a balanced intake and output every 24 hours
   b. Does not have dry skin or mucous membranes
   c. Has thirst needs met
5. Copes effectively with tube feeding regimen
   a. Asks to help with administering the feedings
   b. Participates in self-care activities
   c. Offers encouragement and support to others who are receiving tube feedings

Gastrostomy

A gastrostomy is an operation performed to create an opening into the stomach for the purpose of administering food and fluids. In some instances, a gastrostomy is used for prolonged nutrition, as in the elderly or debilitated patient. Gastrostomy is preferred to nasogastric feedings in the comatose patient because the gastroesophageal sphincter remains intact. Also, regurgitation may occur in nasogastric feedings but is less likely with a gastrostomy.

Several commonly employed feeding gastrostomies are the Stamm (temporary and permanent), Janeway (permanent), and percutaneous endoscopic gastrostomy (temporary). The Stamm and Janeway gastrostomies (Fig. 35–7) require either an upper abdominal midline incision or a left upper quadrant transverse incision. The Stamm procedure requires the use of concentric purse-string sutures to secure a tube to the anterior gastric wall. A stab wound exit is created in the left upper abdomen to provide for the gastrostomy. The Janeway procedure necessitates the creation of a tunnel (called a gastric tube) that is brought out through the abdomen to form a permanent stoma.

For the percutaneous endoscopic gastrostomy (PEG), a physician inserts a cannula into the stomach through an abdominal incision, using local anesthesia. The physician then

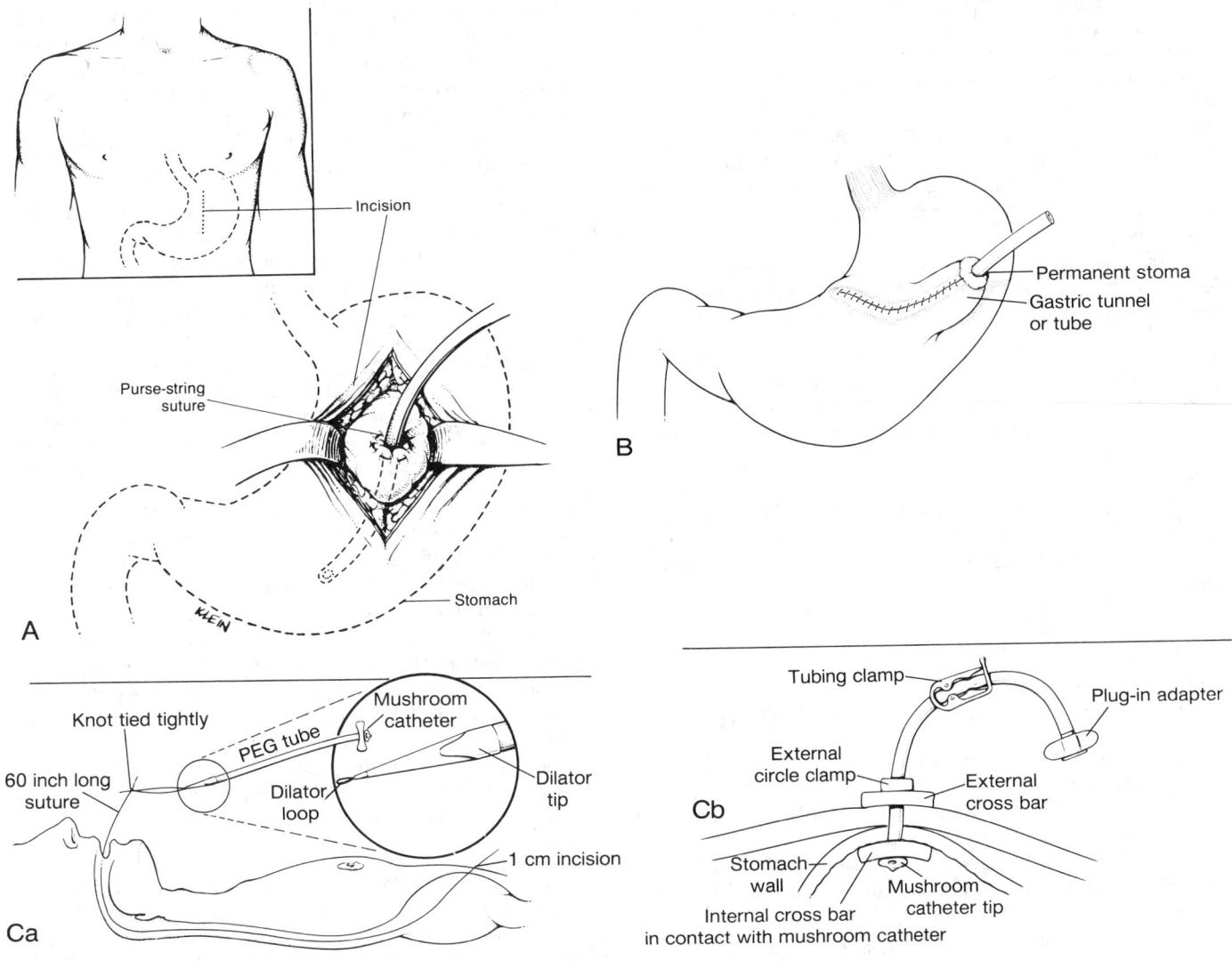

Figure 35–7. **(A)** Stamm gastrostomy, showing incision line and pursestring suture. **(B)** Janeway permanent gastrostomy. **(Ca)** Percutaneous endoscopic gastrostomy (PEG). **(Cb)** A close-up illustration of the abdomen, showing catheter fixation.

threads a nonabsorbable suture through the cannula. A second physician, looking through an endoscope, uses the endoscopic snare to grasp the end of the suture and guide it up through the patient's mouth. The suture is knotted to the dilator tip at the end of the PEG tube. The endoscopist then advances the dilator tip through the patient's mouth while the other physician pulls the suture through the cannula site. The attached PEG tube is guided down the esophagus, into the stomach and out through the abdominal incision. The mushroom catheter tip and internal crossbar secure the tube against the stomach wall. An external crossbar keeps the catheter in place. A tubing adaptor is in place between feedings and a clamp is used to close or open the tubing.

Patients with severe gastroesophageal reflux are at risk for aspiration pneumonia and therefore are not candidates for a gastrostomy. A jejunostomy is preferred, or jejunal feeding through a nasojejunal tube may be recommended.

In summary, a gastrostomy tube is for long-term use and total feeding supplementation. The risk of regurgitation is less frequent with this procedure than with nasogastric or nasoenteric feedings.

Nursing Process
The Patient With a Gastrostomy

Assessment

Preoperative
The focus of the preoperative assessment is on determining the patient's ability to understand the surgical experience and the manner in which he is dealing with the impending surgery. The ability to adjust to a change in body image and to participate in self-care is evaluated, along with the patient's and the family's psychological status. Is the patient depressed, angry, withdrawn, or optimistic? Will the family be supportive?

The purpose of the operative procedure is explained to the patient so that he will have a better understanding of his postoperative course. He needs to know that the purpose of this surgery is to bypass his esophagus and that liquid feedings will be administered directly into the stomach by means of a rubber or plastic tube or a prosthesis. If the prosthesis is to be permanent, the patient should be aware of it. Psychologically, this is often difficult for the patient to accept. When the procedure is being performed to relieve discomfort, prolonged vomiting, debilitation, and the inability to eat, however, it is more acceptable. Frequently a gastrostomy is performed on an elderly or a comatose patient who cannot tolerate nasogastric feedings.

The nurse evaluates the patient's skin condition and determines whether a delay in wound healing may be anticipated because of a systemic disorder (*e.g.*, diabetes mellitus, cancer).

▷ *Postoperative*

In the postoperative period the patient's fluid and nutritional needs are assessed to ensure proper food and fluid intake. The nurse checks the status of the tube and the wound for proper maintenance and any signs of infection. At the same time, the patient's reaction to the change in body image and his understanding of the methods for carrying out the feeding procedure are evaluated to determine the interventions needed to help him cope with the presence of the tube and to learn self-care measures.

▷ **Nursing Diagnoses**

Based on all the assessment data, the major nursing diagnoses in the postoperative period may include the following:

- Altered nutrition, less than body requirements, related to enteral feeding problems
- High risk for infection related to presence of wound and tube
- Impairment of skin integrity at tube site
- Ineffective coping related to the inability to eat normally
- Disturbance in self-concept/body image related to the presence of the tube
- Knowledge deficit about the feeding procedure

▷ **Planning and Implementation**

▷ *Goals:*   The major goals of the patient may include attainment of the desired level of nutrition, absence of infection, maintenance of skin integrity, improvement in coping methods, adjustment to changes in body image, and acquisition of sufficient knowledge about the tube feeding regimen.

▷ **Nursing Interventions**

▷ *Nutritional Needs.*   The first fluid nourishment is administered soon after surgery. This is usually tap water and 10% glucose. At first only 30 to 60 ml (1 to 2 oz) is given at a time, but the amount is gradually increased. By the second day, from 180 to 240 ml (6 to 8 oz) may be given at one time, provided it is tolerated and there is no leakage of fluid around the tube. Water and milk can be instilled after 24 hours for a permanent gastrostomy. High-calorie liquids are added gradually. In some settings, in the early postoperative period the nurse aspirates gastric secretions and reinstills them, after adding enough feeding to bring the volume to the desired total. By this method, gastric dilatation is avoided.

Blenderized foods are gradually added to clear liquids until a full diet is reached. Powdered feedings that are easily liquefied

are commercially available. A food blender can be used to liquefy a normal diet, which then can be fed through the tube. Blenderized tube feedings allow the patient to follow his usual diet pattern, which may prove to be psychologically more acceptable. In addition, good bowel function is promoted, as the fiber and residue are similar to that of a normal diet. Intake of milk is avoided in patients with lactase deficiency.

▷ *Tube Care and Infection Precautions.*   The tube can be held in place by a thin strip of adhesive that is first twisted about the tube and then firmly attached to the abdomen. A catheter plug or rubber-tipped hemostat may close the outlet of the tube immediately after a feeding to prevent leakage. A small dressing can be applied over the tube outlet; the tube can be coiled and held in place by Montgomery straps or a firm abdominal binder. This protects the skin surrounding the incision from the seepage of gastric acid contents and the spillage of feedings (Fig. 35–8). Thereafter, the dressing is changed every 2 or 3 days and the patient is taught how to do this for himself.

▷ *Skin Care.*   The skin surrounding a gastrostomy requires special care. It may become irritated because of the enzymatic action of gastric juices that leak around the tube. If untreated, the skin becomes macerated, red, raw, and painful. Daily washing with soap and water around the tube and the application of a bland ointment such as zinc oxide or petrolatum are protective measures. A long-term gastrostomy may require application of a stomahesive wafer to maintain the integrity of the skin around the tube, protect it from gastric secretions, and stabilize the entry site (Fig. 35–9).

Skin status is evaluated daily for signs of breakdown, irritation, or excoriation. The patient and family members should be encouraged to participate in this inspection and in hygiene activities.

▷ *Body Image Adjustment.*   The patient with a gastrostomy has experienced a major assault to his body image. Eating, which is a normal physiologic and social function, can no longer be taken for granted. The patient is also aware that gastrostomy as a therapeutic intervention is performed only in the presence of a major, chronic, or perhaps terminal illness. Calm discussion of the purposes and routines of gastrostomy feeding can help keep a gastrostomy from becoming an overwhelming situation. Talking with a person who has had a gastrostomy can also help the patient to accept the expected changes. Adjusting to a change in body image takes time and requires family support and acceptance. Evaluation of the existing family support sys-

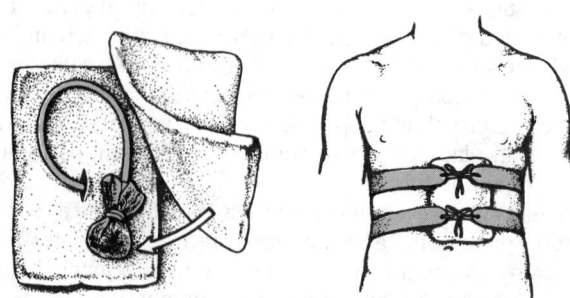

Figure 35–8.   Tube care. After a feeding, the opening of the tube is covered with a sterile gauze square held by a rubber band. The tubing is coiled on a dressing, covered, and secured with Montgomery straps.

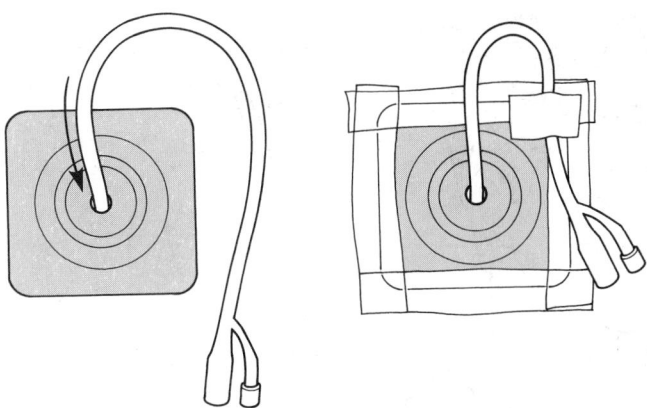

Figure 35–9. Securing a gastrostomy tube. (**Left**) Cut an opening in the stomahesive wafer the same shape as the exit site but one eighth larger. Then thread the gastrostomy tube through the hole and seal. (**Right**) Frame the wafer with tape; then tape the gastrostomy tube to the wafer to anchor and protect it.

tem is necessary. One family member may emerge as the primary support person who will become the major communicator between the patient and health care personnel.

▷ *Patient Education and Home Health Care.* The nurse assesses the patient's level of knowledge, interest in learning about the procedure, and ability to understand and apply the information. Detailed instructions about formula preparation and management of the tube feeding are provided. To facilitate self-care, the patient is instructed in posthospital care and encouraged to establish as normal a routine as possible. These goals are achieved through teaching about tube feedings and tube and skin care and through ongoing evaluation by questioning and return-demonstrations. The patient (and the caregiver in the home setting) must view himself as capable and responsible for care; know the method and frequency of administration of self-care activities; and have adequate supplies, including the physical, financial, and social resources to maintain care. In addition to individual teaching, the use of printed instruction is necessary as a reinforcement. Adequate provision of needed supervision and support must be arranged.

The demonstration begins by showing the patient how to check for residual gastric content before the feeding. The patient then learns how to determine the patency of the tube by administering water at room temperature before the feeding and after to clear the tube of food particles, which could decompose if allowed to remain in the tube. All feedings are given at room temperature or near body temperature.

For a bolus feeding, the patient is shown how to introduce the liquid into the catheter by using a funnel or the barrel of a syringe. The receptacle is tilted to allow air to escape while the liquid is initially being instilled. As the syringe or barrel fills with liquid, the feeding is allowed to flow into the stomach by gravity by holding the barrel or syringe perpendicular to the abdomen (Fig. 35–10). The rate of flow is regulated by raising or lowering the receptacle to no higher than 45 cm (18 in) above the abdominal wall.

With a bolus feeding, usually 300 to 500 ml is given for each meal and requires 10 or 15 minutes to complete. The amount is often determined by the patient's reaction. If he feels "full," it may be desirable to give smaller amounts more

frequently. *Keeping the head of the bed elevated for at least a half hour after feeding facilitates digestion and decreases the risk of aspiration.* Any obstruction requires that the feeding be stopped and the physician notified.

The tube is marked at skin level to provide the patient a baseline for comparison for later. The patient is advised to monitor the tube's length and notify his physician or home care nurse if the segment of the tube outside of the body becomes shorter or longer. The tube is flushed with 30 ml of water after each bolus or medication administration, and otherwise flushed daily to keep it patent. Care of the irrigation set involves daily cleaning with warm soapy water and rinsing after each use.

Some patients smell, taste, and chew small amounts of food before taking their tube feedings. This procedure stimulates the flow of salivary and gastric secretions and may give some sensation of normal eating. The chewed food is then deposited by the patient into a funnel attached to his gastrostomy tube and not swallowed.

A tube feeding may also be given by intermittent or continuous pressure by a feeding pump. Instruction in the use of the particular pump is provided. Most enteral feeding systems have built-in alarms that signal when the bag is empty, when the battery is low, or if an occlusion is present.

▷ **Evaluation**

Expected Outcomes

1. Achieves a balanced intake of nutrients
   a. Tolerates quantity and frequency of tube feedings
   b. Has 50 ml or less of residual gastric content before each feeding
   c. States he has no diarrhea
   d. Maintains or gains weight
   e. Has normal electrolyte values
2. Is free from infection and skin breakdown
   a. Is afebrile
   b. Has no drainage from the wound
   c. Demonstrates intact skin surrounding the incision
   d. Inspects incision twice a day
3. Is adjusting to the idea of change in body image
   a. Is able to discuss expected changes
   b. Verbalizes concerns
   c. Asks to speak with someone who has experienced this procedure
4. Is knowledgeable about the tube feeding regimen
   a. Helps prepare the prescribed formula or blenderized food
   b. Handles equipment competently
   c. Helps administer the feeding or does so independently
   d. Demonstrates how to maintain the patency of the tube
   e. Cleans the tubing as needed
   f. Keeps an accurate record of intake
   g. Is able to remove and reinsert the tube as needed for feedings

Total Parenteral Nutrition (Intravenous Hyperalimentation)

When a patient's intake of nutrients is significantly less than that required by the body to meet energy expenditures, a state

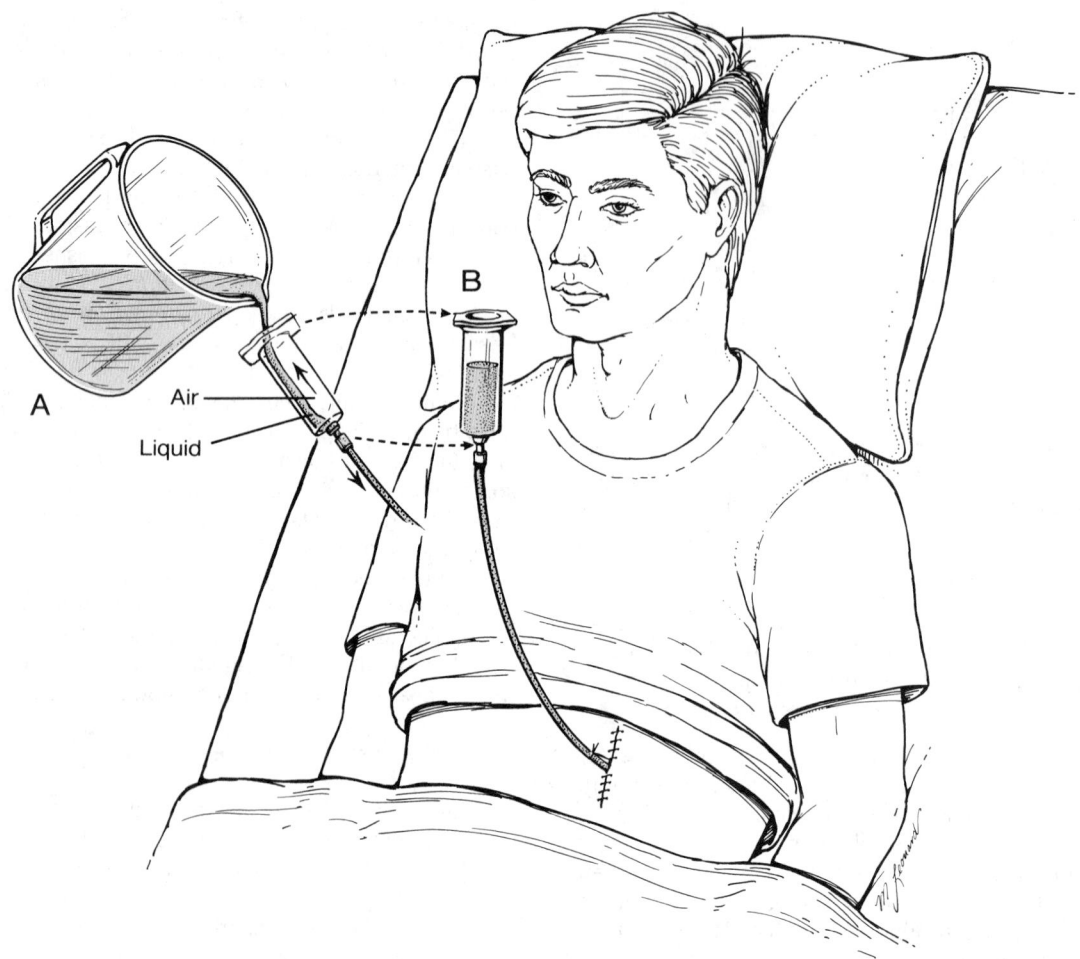

Figure 35–10.   Gastrostomy feeding by gravity. (**A**) Feeding is instilled at an angle so that air does not enter the stomach. (**B**) Syringe is raised perpendicular to stomach so feeding can enter by gravity.

of *negative nitrogen balance* results. This means that protein use is greater than protein intake. Total parenteral nutrition (TPN) is a method of supplying nutrients to the body. The goals of TPN are to attain improved nutritional status and weight gain and to improve healing ability.

Traditional intravenous feedings do not provide sufficient calories or nitrogen to meet the daily requirements of patients. In response, the body begins to convert protein to carbohydrates by the process of gluconeogenesis. TPN solutions, however, contain water, amino acids, glucose, vitamins, and electrolytes in a concentration that provides enough calories and nitrogen to meet the patient's daily nutritional needs. In general, TPN provides 30 to 35 kcal and 1.0 to 1.5 g/kg protein.

The average postoperative adult patient requires approximately 1500 calories a day to spare body protein. If this patient has conditions, such as fever, trauma, burns, or hypermetabolic disease, he may require up to 10,000 additional calories daily. The amount of volume necessary to provide these calories would surpass fluid tolerance and lead to pulmonary edema or congestive heart failure. To provide the required calories in small volume, it is necessary to increase the concentration and use a route of administration that will rapidly dilute incoming nutrients to the proper levels of body tolerance.

When hypertonic glucose is administered, it satisfies caloric requirements and allows amino acids to be released for protein synthesis, rather than being used for energy. Additional potassium is added to provide proper electrolyte balance and to transport glucose and amino acids across the cell membranes. To prevent deficiencies and fulfill requirements for tissue synthesis, other elements, such as calcium, phosphorus, magnesium, and sodium chloride, are added.

Patients who need TPN as well as additional intravenous solutions (chemotherapy, blood products, antibiotics) may be candidates for cyclic total parenteral nutrition. With cyclic total parenteral nutrition there is a set time during a 24-hour period when TPN is infused and a set time when it is not. This assures the patient that his nutritional and pharmacologic needs will be met. Ideally, cyclic TPN is infused over an 8- to 10-hour period during the night.

The pharmacist prepares the prescribed nutritional intravenous solutions. These are mixed, using strict aseptic precautions, under a filtered-air laminar flow hood. Basically, the solution consists of 25% glucose and synthetic amino acids (FreAmine); this provides the patient with 1000 calories and 6 g of nitrogen per liter. Electrolytes are added as determined by the serum electrolyte needs of the patient. Solutions delivered to the nursing unit are refrigerated until needed and then allowed to warm to room temperature. Commercial preparations (Amigen, Aminosol, FreAmine, Hyprotigen C, and others) are available and can be modified to meet individual needs.

Fat emulsions (Intralipid) can be administered simultaneously with TPN. Usually 500 ml of a 10% emulsion is administered over 6 hours, one to three times a week. Fat emulsions can provide up to 30% of the total daily calorie intake.

In summary, TPN is used to provide short- and long-term nutritional supplementation when the gastrointestinal tract cannot be used. Special monitoring of the patient's electrolytes, weight, glucose, and nutritional status is critical.

Clinical Indications

TPN is indicated for the following patients:

- Patients whose intake is insufficient to maintain an anabolic state (*e.g.*, those with severe burns, malnutrition, short-bowel syndrome)
- Patients unable to ingest food orally or by tube (*e.g.*, those with paralytic ileus, Crohn's disease with obstruction, post-radiation enteritis)
- Patients who refuse to ingest adequate nutrients (*e.g.*, those with anorexia nervosa, geriatric postoperative patients)
- Patients who should not be fed orally or by tube (*e.g.*, those with acute pancreatitis or high enterocutaneous fistula)
- Patients who need preoperative and postoperative nutritional support (*e.g.*, after bowel surgery)

Criteria that may be used to evaluate whether a patient should receive total parenteral nutrition include a 10% deficit in body weight; an inability to take oral food or fluids within 7 postoperative days; and hypercatabolic situations, such as major infection with fever.

Management

A nutritional support nurse, dietitian, or physician determines the patient's need for TPN by evaluating certain criteria: the degree of weight loss, the nitrogen balance, the amount of muscle loss and the total lean body mass, as well as the patient's inability to tolerate ingestion of food by the gastrointestinal tract. Ideally the nutritional support nurse, pharmacist, dietitian, and physician collaborate to determine the specific formula needed.

Partial parenteral nutrition is used to supplement oral intake when complete bowel rest is not indicated and nasogastric or nasoenteric suction is not required. Partial nutritional support is administered by peripheral vein because a less hypertonic solution is used. Dextrose concentrations above 10% should not be administered through peripheral veins because of the irritation that they cause to the intima of small veins. The usual length of therapy for partial parenteral nutrition is less than 2 weeks. Careful monitoring and conscientious care by experienced physicians and nurses can reduce the risk of many complications.

Method of Administration

Because TPN solutions have five or six times the solute concentration of blood (and exert an osmotic pressure of about 2000 mOsm/L), they are injurious to the intima of peripheral

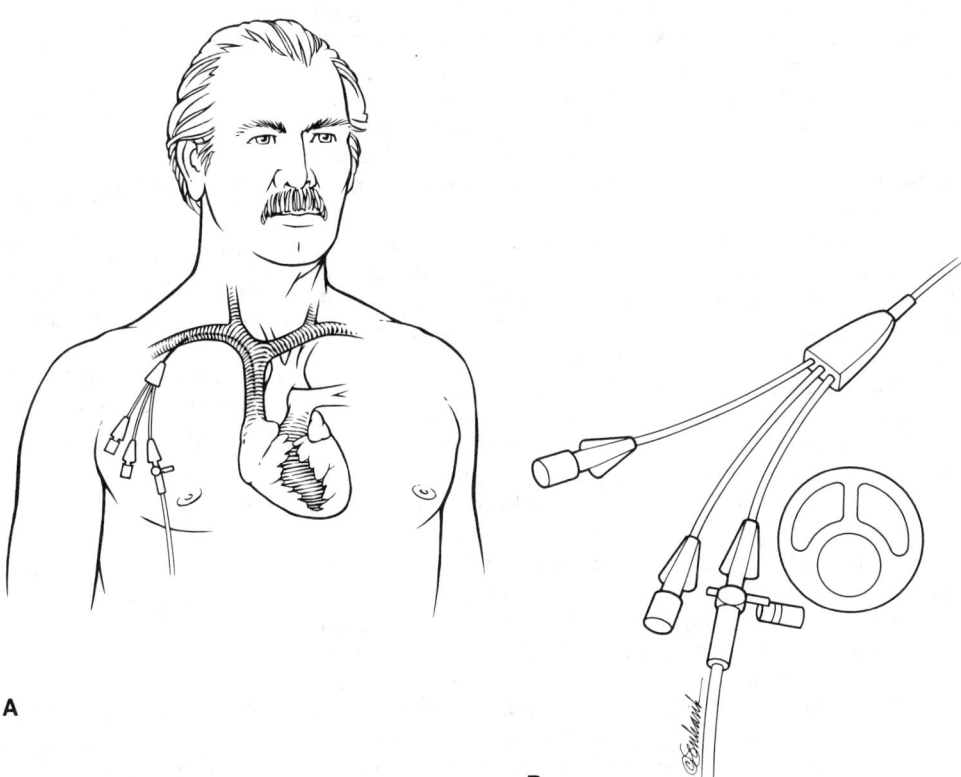

Figure 35–11. Subclavian triple lumen catheter used for total parenteral nutrition and other adjunct therapy. (**A**) The catheter is threaded through the subclavian vein and placed in the vena cava. (**B**) Each lumen is an avenue for solution administration; these are secured with Luer-Lok caps when not in use.

A

B

veins. Therefore, to prevent phlebitis and other venous complications, these solutions are administered into the circulatory system by means of a large-bore needle or catheter inserted into a high-flow large blood vessel (often the subclavian vein). Concentrated solutions are then diluted by the blood in this vessel, very rapidly, to isotonic levels.

Single-, double-, and triple-lumen catheters are available for subclavian lines. To ensure accessibility for short-term TPN therapy, it is recommended that a triple-lumen subclavian catheter is used that offers three ports of entry for various uses (Fig. 35–11). The distal lumen (16-gauge) is used to infuse blood and other viscous fluids. The 18-gauge middle lumen is reserved for TPN infusion. And the proximal port (18-gauge) is used for giving blood, medications and for drawing blood.

Catheters used for long-term therapy have single and double lumens; two types are the Hickman/Broviac catheter and the Groshong catheter. These catheters are inserted in the operating room. They are threaded under the skin (reduces risk of ascending infection) to the subclavian vein, and the distal end of the catheter is placed in the superior vena cava 2 to 3 cm above the junction with the right atrium (see Chart 19–4 and Fig. 19–4).

If a single-lumen catheter is used, various restrictions apply. Administering medications through the main catheter so they mix with the nutritional solution is not recommended because of the possibility of incompatibility of the medications with the nutritional solution (insulin is an exception). If drugs must be given, they should be infused through a peripheral IV line, not by piggyback at the TPN line. Transfusions of blood products also should not be given through the main line, as red cells may possibly coat the lumen of the catheter, thereby reducing the flow of nutritional solution.

Catheter Insertion

Patient Preparation.   The procedure is explained to the patient so that he realizes the importance of not touching the catheter insertion site and is aware that he will be able to be ambulatory during the extended time of therapy. For the insertion of the catheter, the patient is placed supine, in head-low position (to produce dilation of neck and shoulder vessels, which makes entry easier and prevents air embolus). The area is shaved, if necessary, and the skin prepared with acetone or ether to remove surface oils. Final skin preparation includes scrubbing with tincture of iodine or providone-iodine solution. The patient is instructed to turn his head facing the side opposite from the site of venipuncture; he is to remain motionless while the catheter is inserted and the wound dressed, so as to afford maximum accuracy in the placement of the tube.

Insertion of the Catheter.   The preferred route is by way of the subclavian vein, which leads into the superior vena cava. An alternate route is the internal jugular to the superior vena cava. An indwelling catheter is a constant source of potential infection, and it is recommended that the site be changed every 4 weeks.

Sterile drapes are applied to the upper chest. The patient may wear a face mask to prevent the spread of mircoorganisms.

Procaine or lidocaine is injected into the skin and underlying tissues for local anesthesia. The target area is the inferior border at the midpoint of the clavicle (see Fig. 35–11A). A large-bore needle on a syringe is inserted and moved parallel to and beneath the clavicle until it enters the vein. The syringe is then detached and a radiopaque catheter is inserted through the needle into the vein. When the catheter is positioned, the needle is withdrawn and the catheter attached to the intravenous tubing. Until the syringe is detached from the needle and the catheter inserted, the patient may be asked to perform the Valsalva maneuver. (To do this, he is instructed to take a deep breath, hold it, and bear down with his mouth closed. Compression of the abdomen may also accomplish the maneuver.) The Valsalva maneuver is performed to produce a positive phase in central venous pressure to lessen the possibility of air being drawn into the circulatory system (air embolism). The physician sutures the catheter to the skin to avoid accidental dislodgment.

The catheter insertion site is swabbed with a germicide solution, and antibiotic ointment is applied directly to the insertion site. A gauze or transparent dressing is applied using strict sterile technique.

The position of the tip of the catheter is checked at this point with x-ray to confirm its location and to rule out a pneumothorax before the TPN solution is administered. Once the catheter position is confirmed, the prescribed solution is started by connecting the catheter to the IV administration set. Initial rate of infusion is usually set at 50 ml/hr and gradually increased to maintenance rate or predetermined dose (100 to 125 ml/hr).

Each lumen is secured with Luer-Lok caps and labeled according to location (proximal, middle, distal). To ensure patency, the physician may prescribe that all lumina be flushed with a diluted heparin flush initially and twice a day when not in use, after each intermittent infusion, after blood drawing, and whenever an infusion is disconnected. Blood is not aspirated from TPN tubing for blood studies unless it is a lifesaving measure. Force is *never* used to irrigate the catheter. If resistance is met, the physician is notified; he may try to dissolve the clot with urokinase. If attempts to clear the lumen do not work, the lumen is labeled as "clotted off."

In summary, TPN requires close monitoring of the patient for complications. Consistent care provided to the catheter site and daily monitoring of the patient's lab values will ensure safe solution administration.

Discontinuance of Total Parenteral Nutrition

TPN is discontinued gradually to allow for adjustment to decreased levels of glucose. After the administration of hypertonic solution, isotonic glucose is administered for several hours to protect against rebound hypoglycemia. Oral carbohydrates will shorten tapering time. Specific symptoms of rebound hypoglycemia include weakness, faintness, sweating, shakiness, feeling cold, confusion, and increased heart rate.

▶ Nursing Process
The Patient Receiving Total Parenteral Nutrition

◊ Assessment

The nurse assists in identifying a patient who may be a candidate for TPN. Indicators to observe for include any significant weight loss (10% or more of weight when healthy), a decrease in oral food intake for more than 1 week, any significant sign of protein loss (serum albumin levels below 3.2 g/dl [32 g/L], muscle wasting, decreased tissue healing, or abnormal urea nitrogen excretion), and persistent vomiting and diarrhea. The nurse carefully monitors the patient's hydration, electrolyte balance, and calorie intake.

During TPN therapy the nurse monitors body weight, intake and output, blood glucose levels, serum electrolytes, and the complete blood count for any abnormalities. A number of major complications can occur with TPN. See Table 35–4 for a list of potential complications and associated nursing interventions.

▷ Nursing Diagnoses

Based on all the assessment data, the major nursing diagnoses may include the following:

- Altered nutrition, less than body requirements, related to inadequate intake of nutrients
- High risk for infection related to contamination of the catheter site or integrity of the line
- Fluid volume excess related to altered infusion rate
- High risk for fluid volume deficit related to an altered infusion rate
- High risk for activity intolerance related to fear of dislodgment or occlusion of the catheter

▷ Planning and Implementation

▷ *Goals:*   The major goals for the patient may include attainment of an optimal level of nutrition, absence of infection, maintenance of adequate fluid volume, and achievement of an optimal level of activity within individual limitations.

▷ Nursing Interventions

▷ *Optimal Nutrition.*   A continuous, uniform infusion of TPN solution over a 24-hour period is desired. In some cases, however (*e.g.,* home care patients), cyclic parenteral nutrition may be appropriate. This allows patients to receive optimal amounts of calories and electrolytes while receiving other needed intravenous agents through the same line. A set number of hours per day is provided for the TPN.

The patient is weighed three times a week at the same time of the day under the same conditions, for accurate comparison. Under the TPN regimen (without additional energy expenditure), a satisfactory weight gain is usually achieved. Accurate intake and output records and fluid balances are kept. A caloric count is kept of any oral nutrients. Trace elements (copper, zinc, chromium, manganese, and selenium) are included in TPN solutions but may need to be individualized for each patient. The TPN solutions are evaluated and ordered daily by the physician according to laboratory values and patient tolerance.

▷ *Absence of Infection.*   Total parenteral nutrition solutions are ideal culture media for bacterial and fungal growth, and central venous catheters provide a port of entry. Dressings are changed aseptically, usually three times a week and as needed. *Candida albicans* is the most common infectious organism. Others include *Staphylococcus aureus, S. epidermidis,* and *Klebsiella pneumoniae.*

The patient is placed in low Fowler's position for a dressing change. The nurse and patient may reduce the possibility of airborne contamination by wearing masks. Old dressings are removed carefully to prevent the catheter from becoming dis-

lodged. The area is checked for leakage, kinked catheter, and skin reactions such as inflammation, redness, swelling, tenderness, or purulent drainage. Using sterile gloves, the nurse cleanses the area with acetone, followed by tincture of iodine or thimerosal (Merthiolate), with the aid of a sponge holder and 3 × 3-inch gauze pledgets. Cleaning begins from the center and moves outward. Alcohol may be used in the same manner to remove iodine. Antibiotic ointment is applied to the insertion site if prescribed, and the site is covered with a small dressing, slit to fit around the catheter. A gauze pad or transparent dressing is centered over the area. When the intravenous tubing extension is changed, it is replaced rapidly to prevent buildup of organisms along the lumen of the inner tubing. The union of the catheter and tubing is then covered and secured with adhesive tape to prevent separation and exposure to air. Mainline intravenous tubing and filters are changed every 24 hours, and all connections are taped securely to avoid break in the integrity of the system. The tubing is labeled with date, time, and initials when changed.

If the patient has a draining wound, such as a tracheostomy, in the nearby area, additional precautions are taken to keep the wound dry by applying transparent plastic operating-room adhesive drape over the dressings, to ensure waterproofing. Hypoallergenic adhesive tape can be used if the patient complains of itching from conventional tape. The dressing change is recorded, and the condition of the area and the patient's reaction are reported.

▷ *Maintenance of Adequate Fluid Volume Balance.*   An infusion pump is recommended for TPN. Rates are set at a designated rate of milliliters per hour. The rate is checked every half hour to 1 hour; an alarm signals a problem. The infusion rate cannot be increased or decreased to compensate for fluids that are infusing too quickly or too slowly. If the IV runs out, a bag of 10% dextrose and water is hung until the next TPN bag is available from the pharmacy.

If the rate is too rapid, hyperosmolar diuresis occurs (excess sugar will be excreted), which if severe enough may cause intractable seizures, coma, and death. Symptoms of rapid hypertonic fluid intake include headache, nausea, fever, chills, and increasing lassitude. If the flow rate is too slow, the patient does not get the maximum benefit of calories and nitrogen.

Intake and output are recorded every 8 hours so that fluid imbalance can be readily detected. The patient is weighed three times a week; he should not show a weight loss or a great weight gain. The nurse assesses for signs of dehydration (thirst, decreased skin turgor, lowered central venous pressure reading) and reports any findings to the physician immediately. It is essential to monitor blood glucose status because hyperglycemia can cause diuresis and excessive fluid loss.

▷ *Optimal Level of Activity.*   Activities and ambulation are encouraged when the patient is physically capable. With a plastic catheter in the subclavian vein, the patient has freedom to move his extremities and should be encouraged to maintain good muscle tone. The teaching and exercise program initiated in the occupational and physical therapy departments should be reinforced.

▷ *Patient Education and Home Health Care.*   Successful home parenteral nutrition requires teaching the patient and his family specialized skills by means of an intensive training program and follow-up supervision in the home. This must be done through a team effort. The financial costs of such programs

TABLE 35-4.   *Potential Complications of Total Parenteral Nutrition*

Complication	Cause	Nursing Action
Sepsis	Separation of tubing and contamination	Tape all tubing connection sites
		Never interrupt the mainline or piggyback other lines.
	Separation of dressings	Reinforce or change quickly, using aseptic technique.
	Contaminated solution	Discard.
	Infection at insertion site of catheter	Notify physician. Monitor vital signs every 4 hours.
		Catheter site changed every 4 weeks.
Air embolism	Disconnected tubing	Tape all tubing connection sites initially
		Replace tubing immediately and notify physician
	Cap missing from port	Replace cap and notify physician.
	Blocked segment of vascular system	Turn patient on his left side and place in the head-low position. Notify physician
Clotted catheter line	Inadequate or infrequent heparin flushes.	Administer heparin flush in unused lines twice a day
	Disruption of infusion	Monitor infusion rate hourly and inspect the integrity of the line
Catheter displacement	Excessive movement, possibly with a nonsecured catheter	Stop the infusion and notify the physician.
Hyperglycemia	Glucose intolerance	Monitor glucose levels (blood and urine)
		Observe for stupor, confusion, lethargy.
		Notify physician; insulin is added to the TPN solution as prescribed
Fluid overload	Fluid infusing rapidly	Decrease infusion rate.
		Monitor vital signs.
		Notify physician.
		Treat respiratory distress by sitting patient upright and administering oxygen as needed, if prescribed.
Pneumothorax	Improper catheter placement and inadvertent puncture of the pleura	Place in Fowler's position.
		Offer reassurance.
		Monitor vital signs.
		Be prepared for respiratory arrest.
		Prepare for thoracentesis or chest tube insertion.
Rebound hypoglycemia	TPN feedings are stopped	Monitor for symptoms (weakness, tremors, diaphoresis, headache, hunger, and apprehension); if occurs, notify physician.
		Wean patient off TPN gradually.

are less than those incurred in a hospital. Initiation of a home program may be the only way the patient can be discharged. Ability to learn, availability of family interest and support, adequate finances, and the physical plan of the home are factors that must be assessed when the decision for home TPN is made. Institutions sponsoring home TPN programs have developed teaching brochures for every aspect of the treatment, including catheter and dressing care, use of an infusion pump, fat emulsions, and instillation of heparin flushes.

A home care teaching program prepares the patient to manage his specific form of TPN. He is taught how to store his solutions, set up his infusion, flush the line with heparin, change his dressings, and troubleshoot for complications. The most frequent complication is infection. The nurse emphasizes handwashing and strict asepsis in handling equipment, changing the dressing, and preparing the solution.

Mechanical problems usually arise from technical complications found within the infusion pump or catheter site. The patient is taught how to troubleshoot for catheter problems (leakage, loose cap, tear in the tubing, blood clot) and is given a list of directions explaining what to do for each problem. Malfunctioning pumps can usually be replaced in 24 hours. The patient is given a list of symptoms indicative of metabolic complications (neuropathies, mentation changes, diarrhea, nausea, skin changes, urine output) and directed to contact his home health care nurse or physician if he thinks he is experiencing a complication. The patient is asked to have weekly serum chemistry and hematology monitoring and to have the glucose level of his urine checked daily.

The nurse should be aware that the average patient will need about 2 weeks of instruction and reinforcement. Additional time will be needed from a nutritional support nurse or pharmacist for the patient who is going to mix his own solution at home instead of using a premixed solution supplied by an outside vendor.

The psychosocial aspects of home parenteral nutrition are just as significant as the physiologic and technical concerns. These patients must cope with the loss of eating and the changes in life style brought by sleep disturbances (frequent urination during infusions, usually two to three times during the night). Major psychosocial reactions include depression, anger, withdrawal, anxiety, and altered self-image. A successful home parenteral nutrition program depends on motivation, emotional stability, and technical competence.

▷ Evaluation

Expected Outcomes
1. Attains/maintains nutritional balance
   a. Attains/maintains positive nitrogen balance
   b. Has results of specific diagnostic studies within normal limits (BUN, serum protein, hemoglobin, hematocrit)
   c. Attains or maintains desired body weight
   d. Attains or maintains hydration of body tissue
2. Is infection free
   a. Is afebrile
   b. Has no purulent drainage from the catheter insertion site
   c. States that the catheter site is not tender or painful
   d. IV line integrity is maintained
3. Is hydrated
   a. Has good skin turgor
   b. Maintains a balanced daily intake and output
   c. Maintains current weight or gains 1 to 2 pounds weekly until ideal body weight is achieved
4. Achieves an optimal level of activity within self-limitations
   a. Performs isometric and isotonic exercises as directed
   b. Participates in exercise program recommended by physician and physiotherapists
   c. Ambulates freely according to his abilities and the physician's direction

In summary, goals for patients receiving TPN include attainment of optimal nutrition and absence of the complications of infection, fluid volume excess, and activity limitation. On-going assessment is directed toward monitoring the patient's response to the therapy: weight, intake and output, laboratory values, signs of infection at the site of the IV catheter, and level of mobility and activity. The physician's order for the TPN solution is changed as appropriate to meet the patient's individual needs.

Some patients receive parenteral nutrition at home. These patients and their families/significant others must be motivated and able to learn the skills necessary for successful management of the therapy in the home setting. Follow-up supervision by health care personnel is essential to assure that the patient's care is satisfactory and that his physical and psychosocial needs are met.

Bibliography

Books
Alpers D et al. Manual of Nutritional Therapeutics. Boston, Little, Brown, 1988.
Cerra FB. Pocket Manual of Surgical Nutrition. St Louis, CV Mosby, 1984.
Deitel M (ed). Nutrition in Clinical Surgery. Baltimore, Williams & Wilkins, 1985.
Dixon JA (ed). Surgical Application of Lasers, 2nd ed. Chicago, Year Book Medical Publishers, 1987.
Eastwood GL. Core Textbook of Gastroenterology. Philadelphia, JB Lippincott, 1984.
Hardy JD et al (eds). Hardy's Textbook of Surgery. Philadelphia, JB Lippincott, 1988.
Hermann JB and Wertheimer MD. Case Studies in General Surgery. Baltimore, Williams & Wilkins, 1988.
Hudak CM et al. Critical Care Nursing. A Holistic Approach. Philadelphia, JB Lippincott, 1989.
Nyhus LN and Wastell C. Surgery of the Stomach and Duodenum, 4th ed. Boston, Little, Brown, 1986.
Rombeau JL and Caldwell MD (eds). Clinical Nutrition, Vol I. Enteral and Tube Feeding. Philadelphia, WB Saunders, 1984.
Sabiston DC (ed). Textbook of Surgery: The Biological Basis of Modern Surgical Practice. Philadelphia, WB Saunders, 1986.
Schwartz S et al (eds). Principles of Surgery, 5th ed. New York, McGraw-Hill, 1989.
Williams SR. Nutrition and Diet Therapy. St Louis, Times Mirror/Mosby, 1989.

Journals
Asterisks indicate nursing research articles.

Nasogastric and Nasoenteric Intubation and Feeding
Andrassy RJ. Preserving the gut mucosal barrier and enhancing immune response. Contemp Surg 1988 Feb; 32(2-A): 1–7.
* Anliker AW. Bacterial contamination of continuous-infusion enteral feedings. Nutr Supp Serv 1988 Jul; 8(7): 11–12, 32.
Breach CL and Saldanha LG. Tube feeding complications, Part I: Gastrointestinal. Nutr Supp Serv 1988 Mar; 8(3): 15–16, 19.
Breach CL and Saldanha LG. Tube feeding complications. Part II: Mechanical. Nutr Supp Serv 1988 May; 8(5): 28, 32.
Breach CL and Saldanha LG. Tube feeding complications, Part III: Metabolic. Nutr Supp Serv 1988 Jun; 8(6): 16, 19.
Cerrato PL. Fast action for tube-fed patient's diarrhea. RN 1988 Mar; 51(3): 89–90.
Creighton H. Legal implications of removal of feeding tubes. Nurs Manage 1987 Mar; 18(3): 20, 22, 24.
Davis PD et al. A tube-feeding monitoring flow sheet. Nutr Supp Serv 1988 Jul; 8(7): 21–23.
Eisenberg P. Enteral nutrition: Indications, formulas, and delivery techniques, Nurs Clin North Am 1989 Jun; 24(2): 315–338.
* Eisenberg P et al. Characteristics of patients who remove their nasal feeding tube. Clin Nurse Spec 1987 Mar; 1(3): 94–98.

Fagerman KE and Lysen LK. Enteral feeding tubes: A comparison and history. Nutr Supp Serv 1987 Sep; 7(9): 10–14.

Farley J. About enteral tube nutrition, Nursing 1988 Aug; 18(8): 82.

Farley JM. Current trends in enteral feedings. Crit Care Nurse 1988 Apr; 8(4): 23–28.

Flynn KT et al. Enteral tube feeding: Indications, practices and outcomes. Image: J Nurs Scholarship 1987 Spring; 19(1): 16–19.

Freedman J. Speaking out on nasogastric feedings. Geriatr Nurs 1987 Jan/Feb; 8(1): 7.

Guiness R. How to use the new small-bore feeding tubes. Nursing 1986 Apr; 16(4): 51–56.

Hanson RL. Predictive criteria for length of nasogastric tube insertion for tube feeding. J Parenter Enteral Nutr 1979 May/Jun; 3(3): 160–163.

Hard choices: Ethical issues in nutritional support. Nutr Supp Serv 1987 Feb; 7(2): 19–21.

Hatchett–Cohen L. Nasoduodenal tube feeding. Geriatr Nurs 1988 Feb; 9(2): 88–91.

Heaphey L. Home nutritional support: Current consumer concerns. Nutr Supp Serv 1988 Apr; 8(4): 24.

Herfindal TE et al. Survey of home nutritional support patients. J Parenter Enteral Nutr 1989 May/Jun; 13(3): 255–261.

Herrmann ME et al. Subjective distress during continuous enteral alimentation: Superiority of silicone rubber over polyurethane. J Parenter Enteral Nutr 1989 May/Jun: 13(3): 281–285.

Holmes S. Dietetics artificial feeding. Nursing Times 1987 Aug; 83(31): 49–54.

Horbal–Shuster M and Irwin M. Keeping enteral nutrition on track. Am J Nurs 1987 Apr; 87(4): 523–524.

* Huddleston K et al. MIC or Foley: Comparing gastrostomy tubes. MCN 1989 Jan/Feb; 14(1): 20–23.

Jensen T. Home enteral nutrition. Dietetic Current Ross Timesaver 1982 Jul/Aug; 9: 15–20.

Jones S. Simpler and safer tube-feeding techniques. RN 1984 Oct; 47(10): 40–47.

Krachenfels MM. Update on tube-feeding formulas. Home Healthcare Nurse 1987 Mar; 5(3): 47–50.

McCarthy MS. Early postoperative jejunal feedings with gastric decompression: Implications for nursing practice. Nutr Supp Serv 1988 Sep; 8(9): 8–9.

McLaren M. Home tube feedings: Gastrointestinal complications. Home Healthcare Nurse 1987 Mar; 5(3): 41–42.

* Metheny N. Measures to test placement of nasogastric feeding tubes: A review. Nurs Res 1988 Nov/Dec; 37(6): 324–329.

* Metheny N et al. Effectiveness of the auscultatory method in predicting feeding tube location. Nurs Research 1990 Sep/Oct; 1990; 39(5): 262–267.

* Metheny N et al. Effect of feeding tube properties and three irrigants on clogging rates. Nurs Res 1988 May/Jun; 37(3): 165–169.

* Metheny NA et al. Aspiration pneumonia in patients fed through nasoenteral tubes. Heart Lung 1986 May; 15(3): 256–261.

Moore MC. Do you still believe these myths about tube feedings? RN 1987; 50(5): 51–54.

Padilla GV et al. Subjective distress of nasogastric tube feeding. J Parenter Enteral Nutr 1979 Feb; 13(2): 53–57.

* Pritchard V. Tube feeding-related pneumonias. J Gerontol Nurs 1988 Jul; 14(7): 32–36.

Sanders S. Nursing home problems in tube feeding the geriatric patient. Nutr Supp Serv 1987 Jul; 7(7): 21–22.

Schwartz DB and Darrow AK. Hypoalbuminemia-induced diarrhea in the enterally alimented patient. Nutr Clin Pract 1988 Dec; 12(6): 235–237.

Shronts EP. Enteral formulas update. Nutr Supp Serv 1988 Apr; 8(4): 16.

Stavropoulos MN et al. Long term enteral nutrition for management of gastric outlet obstruction following acid digestion. Nutr Clin Pract 1988 Aug; 3(4): 148–149.

Steinborn PA. Home enteral nutrition. Caring 1988 Sep; 12(9): 20–23.

Strong RM et al. Enteral tube feedings utilizing a pH sensor enteral feeding tube. Nutr Supp Serv 1988 Aug; 8(8): 11, 24–25.

Winkler HR. Home enteral nutrition in practice. Nutr Supp Serv 1987 Dec; 7(12): 27–29.

* Wilson MF and Haynes–Johnson V. Cranberry juice or water? A comparison of feeding-tube irrigant. Nutr Supp Serv 1987 Jul; 7(7): 23–24.

Williams PJ. How do you keep medicines from clogging feeding tubes? Am J Nurs 1989 Feb; 89(2): 181–182.

Winston D. Advances in gastroenterology and nutrition. Nutr Supp Serv 1988 May; 8(5): 7, 10.

Winston DH. Treatment of severe malnutrition in anorexia nervosa with enteral tube feedings. Nutr Supp Serv 1987 Jun; 7(6): 24–25.

Gastrostomies

Alltop SA. Teaching for discharge: Gastrostomy tubes. RN 1988 Nov; 51(11): 42–46.

Bruckstein DC. Percutaneous endoscopic gastrostomy. Geriatr Nurs 1988 Mar/Apr; 9(2): 92–93.

Hogan K and Rensselaer LV. An improved method of anchoring a gastrostomy tube. Nutr Supp Serv 1988 Mar; 8(3): 12–14.

Irwin M. Managing leaking gastrostomy sites. Am J Nurs 1988 Mar; 88(3): 359–360.

McGee L. Feeding gastrostomy: Nursing care. Part 2. J Enterostom Ther 1967 Sep/Oct; 14(5): 201–211.

Starkey JF et al. Taking care of percutaneous endoscopic gastrostomy. Am J Nurs 1988 Jan; 88(1): 42–45.

Total Parenteral Nutrition

Camp LD. Care of the Groshong catheter. Oncology Nursing Forum 1988 Nov/Dec; 15(6): 745–748.

Johndrow PD. Making your patient and his family feel at home with TPN. Nursing 1988 Oct; 18(10): 65–69.

Klass K. Trouble-shooting central line complications. Nursing 1987 Nov; 17(11): 58–61.

Lee B. Total parenteral nutrition. Nurs Times 1987 Jan; 83(1): 33–35.

Lee B. Total parenteral nutrition. Nurs Times 1987 Aug; 83(31): 58–59.

Morris LL. Critical care's most versatile tool. RN 1988 May; 51(5): 42–46.

* Petrosino B et al. Infection rates in central venous catheter dressings. Oncol Nurs Forum 1988 Nov/Dec; 15(6): 709–717.

Reilly JJ et al. Economic impact of malnutrition: A model system for hospitalized patients. J Parenter Enteral Nutr 1988 Apr; 12(4): 371–376.

Scott WL. Complications associated with central venous catheters. Chest 1988 Dec; 94(6): 1221–1224.

Sohl L et al. Working with triple-lumen central venous catheters. Nursing 1988 Jul; 18(7): 50–55.

Szwanek M et al. Trace elements and parenteral nutrition. Nutr Supp Serv 1987 Aug; 7(8) 8–13.

Yamanaka H et al. Preoperative nutritional assessment to predict postoperative complications in gastric cancer patients. J Parenter Enteral Nutr 1989 May/Jun; 13(3): 286–291.

Ziegenbein RC. Focused review criteria for central parenteral nutrition. Nutr Clin Pract 1989 Feb; 4(1): 24–30.

Information/Resources

Agencies

Society of Gastrointestinal Assistants, Inc.
   1070 Sibley Towers, Rochester, NY 14604
American Cancer Society
   90 Park Ave, New York, NY 10016
American Institute of Nutrition
   9650 Rockville Pike, Bethesda, MD 20014
American Society for Gastrointestinal Endoscopy
   PO Box 1565, 13 Elm St, Manchester, MA 01944
Nutrition Institute of America
   200 W 86th St, New York, NY 10024

36

Management of Patients With Gastric and Duodenal Disorders

Learning Objectives

On completion of this chapter, the learner will be able to:

1. Compare acute gastritis, chronic gastritis, and peptic ulcer
2. Use the nursing process as a framework for care of patients with gastritis
3. Use the nursing process as a framework for care of patients with peptic ulcer
4. Describe the dietary, pharmacologic, and surgical treatment of peptic ulcer
5. Describe the nursing management of patients who undergo surgical procedures for treatment of obesity
6. Use the nursing process as a framework for care of patients with gastric cancer
7. Use the nursing process as a framework for care of patients undergoing gastric surgery.
8. Identify the complications of gastric surgery and their prevention and management
9. Describe the home health care needs of the patient who has had gastric surgery

Gastritis

Acute Gastritis

Gastritis (inflammation of the stomach mucosa) is most often due to a dietary indiscretion. The person eats too much or too rapidly or eats food that is noxious because it is too highly seasoned or is infected. Other causes of acute gastritis include alcohol, aspirin, uremia, or radiation therapy. Gastritis also may be the first sign of an acute systemic infection.

Pathophysiology and Clinical Manifestations.   The gastric mucous membrane becomes edematous and hyperemic and undergoes superficial erosion; it secretes a scanty amount of gastric juice, containing very little acid but much mucus. Superficial ulceration may occur and can lead to hemorrhage. The patient may have an uncomfortable feeling in his abdomen, with headache, lassitude, nausea, and anorexia, often accompanied by vomiting and hiccuping. Some patients, however, are asymptomatic.

The gastric mucosa is capable of repairing itself after a bout of gastritis. Occasionally, hemorrhage may require surgical intervention. If the irritating food is not vomited but reaches the bowel, colic and diarrhea may result. As a rule, the patient is well in about a day, although he may not have much appetite for the next 2 or 3 days.

Chronic Gastritis

Inflammation of the stomach that exists for a prolonged period can be caused by either benign or malignant ulcers of the stomach, by cirrhosis complicated by portal hypertension, and by uremia (the breakdown in the gastric mucosa is believed to be caused by the excess of urea in the blood or possibly by bacteria).

Pathophysiology.   Chronic gastritis may be classified as type A or type B. Type A disease results from parietal cell changes leading to atrophy and cellular infiltration. It is associated with autoimmune diseases such as pernicious anemia. It occurs in the fundus or body of the stomach.

Type B gastritis affects the antrum (lower end of the stomach near the duodenum). It has recently been associated with the presence of the bacilli *Campylobacter pylori*. It may also be associated with dietary factors such as hot drinks or spices; use of drugs; alcohol; smoking; or reflux of intestinal contents into the stomach.

Clinical Manifestations.   Type A gastritis is essentially asymptomatic except for symptoms of vitamin B_{12} deficiency (see Chap. 32). In type B gastritis, the patient may complain of anorexia (poor appetite), heartburn after eating, belching, sour taste in the mouth, or nausea and vomiting.

Diagnostic Evaluation.   Type A gastritis is associated with achlorhydria or hypochlorhydria (absence or low levels of hydrochloric acid), whereas type B gastritis is associated with hyperchlorhydria. Diagnosis is determined by gastroscopy, upper gastrointestinal x-ray series, and histologic examination.

Corrosive Gastritis

A more severe form of acute gastritis is caused by the ingestion of strong acids or alkalies. The mucosa may become gangrenous or perforate. Scarring can occur, resulting in pyloric obstruction.

Management of Gastritis

For *acute gastritis*, management consists of permitting the patient to ingest nothing by mouth until symptoms subside. When the patient is able to take nourishment by mouth, a bland diet, perhaps supplemented by alkalies, is provided. If the symptoms persist, parenteral administration of fluids may become necessary. If bleeding is present, management is similar to the procedures used for upper gastrointestinal tract hemorrhage (see p. 903).

For *chronic gastritis*, management is directed toward diet modification, rest, stress reduction, and pharmacotherapy. There is no reliable cure for *C. pylori*. The bacteria may be suppressed by the use of bismuth salt preparations such as Pepto-Bismol. Patients with type A gastritis usually have evidence of malabsorption of vitamin B_{12} caused by the presence of antibodies against intrinsic factor.

For *corrosive gastritis*, immediate treatment consists of diluting and neutralizing the offending substance.

- To neutralize acids, common antacids (*e.g.*, aluminum hydroxide) are used; to neutralize an alkali, diluted lemon juice or diluted vinegar is used.
- If corrosion is extensive or severe, emetics and lavage are avoided because of the danger of perforation.

Therapy thereafter is supportive, including nasogastric intubation, analgesics and sedatives, antacids, intravenous fluids, and electrolytes. It may be necessary to evaluate the patient by fiberoptic endoscopy. Emergency surgery may be required to remove gangrenous or perforated tissue. Gastrojejunostomy or gastric resection may be necessary to treat pyloric obstruction.

▶ Nursing Process
The Patient With Gastritis
▷ Assessment

During the history, the nurse asks about the patient's presenting signs and symptoms. Does the patient experience heartburn, indigestion, nausea, or vomiting? Do the symptoms occur at any specific time of the day, before or after meals, after ingesting spicy or irritating foods, or after the ingestion of certain drugs or alcohol? Are the symptoms related to anxiety, stress, allergies, eating or drinking too much, or eating too quickly? How are the symptoms relieved? Is there any history of previous gastric disease or surgery? A diet history plus a 72-hour diet recall is helpful. A history is important to identify whether known dietary excesses or other indiscretions are associated with the current symptoms, whether others in the patient's environment have similar symptoms, whether the patient is vomiting blood, and whether any known caustic element has been swallowed.

The nurse performs a complete physical assessment. Signs to note include abdominal tenderness, dehydration (altered skin turgor, dry mucous membranes), and evidence of any systemic disorder that might be responsible for the symptoms of gastritis (chronic uremia, cirrhosis). The length of time that the current symptoms last and any methods used by the patient to treat his symptoms, and their effects, should also be identified.

▷ Nursing Diagnoses

Based on all the assessment data, the patient's major nursing diagnoses may include the following:

- Anxiety related to treatment
- Altered nutrition, less than body requirements, related to inadequate intake of nutrients
- High risk for fluid volume deficit related to insufficient fluid intake and excessive fluid loss subsequent to vomiting
- Knowledge deficit about dietary management
- Pain related to irritated stomach mucosa

▷ Planning and Implementation

▷ *Goals:*   The major goals of the patient may include reduction of anxiety, reduced intake of irritating foods and adequate intake of nutrients, maintenance of fluid balance, increased awareness of dietary management, and relief of pain.

▷ Nursing Interventions

▷ *Reduction of Anxiety.* For corrosive gastritis, emergency measures are carried out as quickly as possible. Supportive therapy is offered to the patient and family during treatment and after the ingested acid or alkali has been neutralized or diluted. The patient may need to be prepared for additional diagnostic studies (endoscopy) or surgery. Anxiety about the pain and treatment modalities is usually present as well as fear of permanent damage to the esophagus. A calm approach is used by the nurse, and questions are answered as completely as possible. All procedures and treatments are explained according to the patient's interest and level of understanding.

▷ *Nutritional Measures.* For *acute gastritis*, physical and emotional support is provided and the patient is helped to deal with his symptoms, which may include nausea, vomiting, heartburn, and fatigue. Foods and fluids are not permitted by mouth for hours or days until the acute symptoms subside. Intravenous therapy may be necessary and is monitored, and serum electrolyte values are evaluated daily. When the symptoms subside, ice chips followed by clear liquids are offered. Small, frequent, bland meals are introduced as soon as possible to provide oral nutrition, decrease the need for intravenous therapy, and minimize irritation to the gastric mucosa. As food is introduced, any symptoms suggesting a repeat episode of gastritis are evaluated and reported to the physician. The intake of caffeinated beverages is discouraged because caffeine is a central nervous system stimulant that increases gastric activity and pepsin secretion. Cigarette smoking is discouraged because nicotine reduces the secretion of pancreatic bicarbonate and thus inhibits the neutralization of gastric acid in the duodenum. Nicotine also increases parasympathetic stimulation, which increases muscular activity in the bowel and can lead to nausea and vomiting.

▷ *Fluid Balance.* Daily intake and output are monitored to detect early signs of dehydration (minimal urine output of 30 ml/hr, minimal intake of 1.5 L/day). If food and fluids are withheld, 3 liters of intravenous fluids daily is prescribed. Fluid intake plus caloric value is measured (1 liter 5% dextrose in water = 170 calories of carbohydrate). Electrolyte values (sodium, potassium, chloride) are assessed every 24 hours to detect early indicators of fluid imbalance.

The nurse must always be alert for any indicators of hemorrhagic gastritis (hematemesis, tachycardia, hypotension). If these occur, the physician is alerted, vital signs are monitored as the patient's condition warrants, and the guidelines for managing upper gastrointestinal tract bleeding are followed (see below).

▷ *Patient Education.* The patient's knowledge about gastritis is evaluated so that a teaching plan can be individualized. A bland diet is prescribed that takes into account daily caloric needs, food preferences, and the desired frequency of eating.

The patient is given a list of substances to avoid (*e.g.*, caffeine, nicotine, spicy foods, irritating or highly seasoned foods, alcohol). Antacids, bismuth salts, sedatives, or anticholinergics are administered as prescribed. Patients with pernicious anemia are given instructions regarding the need for long-term vitamin B_{12} injections.

▷ *Relief of Pain.* The patient is instructed to avoid foods and beverages that may be irritating to the gastric mucosa (see above). The nurse assesses the patient's level of pain and attainment of comfort through the use of medications and avoidance of irritating substances.

▷ Evaluation

Expected Outcomes

1. Exhibits less anxiety
   a. Reports less anxiety
   b. States how anxiety increases symptoms
2. Eats fewer irritating foods
   a. Eliminates caffeinated beverages from diet
   b. Avoids spicy foods and seasonings (pepper)
   c. Chooses nonirritating seasonings for foods (mint, parsley)
   d. Avoids alcoholic beverages.
3. Maintains fluid balance
   a. Drinks 6 to 8 glasses of water daily
   b. Tolerates intravenous therapy of at least 3 L daily
   c. Has a urinary output of about 1.5 L daily
   d. Displays adequate skin turgor
   e. Increases oral intake of fluids and foods as symptoms decrease
4. Adheres to dietary regimen
   a. Repeats dietary restrictions to the nurse
   b. Selects nonirritating foods and beverages
   c. Modifies caloric intake to individual preferences
   d. Takes medications as prescribed
5. Experiences less pain
   a. Avoids irritating foods and beverages
   b. Takes prescribed medications as scheduled
   c. Reports relief of pain

In summary, gastritis, or irritation of the stomach mucosa, may be divided into acute and chronic forms. Acute gastritis results from ingestion of irritating substances and usually subsides in a few days. Chronic gastritis is divided into two types, A and B. Type A is associated with pernicious anemia and is usually treated with vitamin B_{12}. Type B gastritis has recently been associated with the bacilli *C. pylori*, which is suppressed with the use of bismuth salts such as PeptoBismol. Avoidance of alcohol and irritating foods is usually helpful.

Upper Gastrointestinal Tract Bleeding

Gastritis and hemorrhage from peptic ulcer are the two most common causes of upper gastrointestinal tract bleeding. *Hematemesis* refers to the vomiting of blood. The vomited blood can be bright red or have a "coffee ground" appearance (hemoglobin changes to methemoglobin in the stomach). The passage of dark, tarry stools (melena) indicates upper gastrointestinal tract bleeding. Management depends on the amount of blood lost and the rate of bleeding.

Management. Management of upper gastrointestinal tract bleeding consists of (1) quickly determining the amount of blood lost and the rate of bleeding, (2) rapidly correcting the blood loss, (3) stopping the bleeding with water or saline lavage, (4) stabilizing the patient, and (5) diagnosing and treating the cause. Specific medical and nursing interventions for upper gastrointestinal tract bleeding are discussed in the section Complications of Peptic Ulcers.

Once the patient has been stabilized, endoscopy is performed to determine the cause and precise site of bleeding. Endoscopy is about 80% effective in identifying the bleeding site. If the diagnosis is inconclusive, then upper gastrointestinal x-ray films can provide more information.

Rebleeding occurs in about 25% of patients and warrants surgical intervention. The patient is carefully monitored so that indicators of bleeding can be quickly detected. These signs include decreased central venous pressure, tachycardia, tachypnea, hypotension, mental confusion, thirst, and oliguria.

Peptic Ulcer

A peptic ulcer is an excavation formed in the mucosal wall of the stomach, the pylorus, the duodenum, or the esophagus (Fig. 36–1). A peptic ulcer is frequently referred to as a gastric, duodenal, or esophageal ulcer, depending on its location. It is caused by the erosion of a circumscribed area of mucous membrane. This erosion may extend as deeply as the muscle layers or through the muscle to the peritoneum. Peptic ulcers are more likely to be in the duodenum than in the stomach. As a rule, they occur singly, but there may be a number of them present at one time. Chronic gastric ulcers tend to occur in the lesser curvature of the stomach, near the pylorus. See Table 36–1 for a comparison of the features of gastric and duodenal ulcers.

Etiology and Incidence

The etiology of peptic ulcer is poorly understood. It is known that peptic ulcers occur only in the areas of the gastrointestinal tract that are exposed to hydrochloric acid and pepsin. The disease occurs with the greatest frequency between the ages of 40 and 60 years, but is relatively uncommon in women of childbearing age, although it has been observed in childhood and even in infancy. More men than women are affected (3: 1), although there is some evidence that the incidence in women is increasing. After menopause, the incidence of peptic ulcer in women is almost equal to that in men. Peptic ulcers in the body of the stomach can occur without excessive acid secretion; therefore, an attempt should be made to differentiate gastric from duodenal ulcers.

It is estimated that 5% to 15% of the population in the United States have ulcers, but only about half of these are recognized. Duodenal ulcer was first recognized around 1900, and the incidence increased until the 1950s. Since then there has been a steady decrease in the United States, but the reason is unclear. The incidence has declined by 50% over the past 20 years. Duodenal ulcers are 5 to 10 times more common than gastric ulcers.

Predisposition

Attempts continue to be made to delineate the "ulcer personality." Psychoanalysts claim that an ulcer results from repression of strong dependency needs. Others claim that occupational stress, with no opportunity to express hostility, is another strong factor. Ulcers seem to develop in persons who are emotionally tense, but whether this is the cause or the effect of the condition is uncertain. Familial tendency also appears as a significant predisposing factor; three times as many ulcer patients have relatives with the same diagnosis. A further hereditary link is noted in the finding that persons in blood group O are 35% more susceptible than persons with type A, B, or AB blood. Other predisposing factors associated with peptic ulcer include emotional stress, eating hurriedly and irregularly, and smoking excessively. Rarely, ulcers are due to excessive amounts of the hormone gastrin, produced by tumors (gastrinomas—Zollinger–Ellison syndrome). There is also the possibility that gastric ulcers may be associated with bacterial infection such as *C. pylori*.

Pathophysiology

Peptic ulcer occurs mainly in the gastroduodenal mucosa because this tissue is unable to withstand the digestive action of gastric acid and pepsin. The erosion is due to an increase in concentration or activity of acid-pepsin or to a decrease in the normal resistance of the mucosa. A damaged mucosa is unable to secrete enough mucus to act as a barrier against hydrochloric acid.

Gastric secretion occurs in three phases: (1) cephalic, (2) gastric, and (3) intestinal. Because these phases are interactive and not independent of one another, a disturbance in any one phase may be ulcerogenic.

Cephalic (Psychic) Phase. The first phase is initiated by stimuli such as the sight, smell, or taste of food, acting on cerebral cortical receptors that, in turn, stimulate the vagal nerves. Essentially, an unappetizing meal has little effect on gastric secretion, whereas a more tasty, appealing meal evokes a high secretion. This accounts for the traditional emphasis on serving a bland meal to the peptic ulcer patient. Today many gastroenterologists agree that the bland diet has no significant effect on gastric acidity or ulcer healing. Excessive vagal activity during the night, however, when the stomach is empty, is a significant irritant.

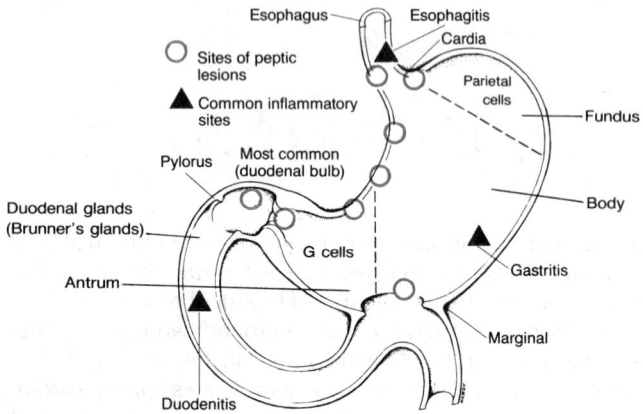

Figure 36–1. Peptic lesions may occur in the esophagus (esophagitis), stomach (gastritis), or duodenum (duodenitis). Note peptic ulcer sites and common inflammatory sites. Hydrochloric acid is formed by parietal cells in the fundus; gastrin is secreted by G cells in the antrum. The duodenal glands secrete an alkaline mucus solution.

TABLE 36-1. *Comparison of Duodenal and Gastric Ulcer*

Chronic Duodenal Ulcer	*Chronic Gastric Ulcer*
AGE	
30–60	Usually 50 and over
SEX	
Male-female: 3:1	Male-female: 2:1
BLOOD GROUP	
Most frequently—O	No differentiation
GENERAL NOURISHMENT	
Usually well nourished	Often malnourished
ACID PRODUCTION: STOMACH	
Hypersecretion	Normal—hyposecretion
PAIN	
2–3 hours after a meal; nighttime: often awakened between 1 and 2 AM	Occurs ½ to 1 hour after a meal; nighttime: rarely; relieved by vomiting
Ingestion of food relieves pain	Ingestion of food does not help; sometimes pain is increased
VOMITING	
Uncommon	Common
HEMORRHAGE	
Melena more common than hematemesis	Hematemesis more common than melena
MALIGNANCY POSSIBILITY	
Never	Perhaps in less than 10%
ASSOCIATED WITH USE OF NONSTEROIDAL ANTI-INFLAMMATORY DRUGS	
No	Yes

Gastric Phase. The gastric phase of gastric secretion is mediated by the hormone *gastrin*. Gastrin, which can be measured by a radioimmunoassay, enters the bloodstream from the antrum and is carried to glands in the fundus and body of the stomach; here it stimulates the production of gastric juice. Gastrin activity may be greater in patients with pyloric stenosis. The antrum of the patient with gastric ulcer contains less gastrin than that of the patient with a duodenal ulcer. After partial gastrectomy or gastrojejunostomy, if part of the antrum is left in place but no longer is in contact with the acid-secreting portion of the stomach, the antrum continues to release gastrin, because acid no longer bathes the mucosa to inhibit gastrin release. Excess gastrin in the blood can lead to marginal ulcers. Excessive gastrin is also present in Zollinger–Ellison syndrome.

Intestinal Phase. During the intestinal phase, a hormone, secretin, is secreted when hydrochloric acid enters the duodenum. Secretin, in turn, stimulates bicarbonate secretion from the pancreas, which neutralizes the acid. Secretin also inhibits the gastric phase of gastric secretion.

Gastric Mucosal Barrier. In humans, gastric secretion is a mixture of mucopolysaccharides and mucoproteins secreted continuously by the mucosal glands. This mucus adsorbs pepsin and protects it against acid. Hydrochloric acid is secreted continuously, but secretions increase because of neurogenic and hormonal mechanisms that are initiated by gastric and intestinal stimuli. If hydrochloric acid were not buffered and neutralized, and if the outer layer of mucosa did not offer protection, hydrochloric acid, along with pepsin, would destroy the stomach. Hydrochloric acid comes into contact with only a small portion of the gastric mucosal surface; it diffuses into it with amazing slowness. This impenetrability of the mucosa is called the *gastric mucosal barrier*. It is the chief defense of the stomach against being digested by its secretions. Other factors that influence mucosal resistance are blood supply, acid–base balance, integrity of the mucosal cells, and epithelial regeneration.

Therefore, a person is likely to develop a peptic ulcer from one of two causes: (1) hypersecretion of acid-pepsin, and (2) a weakened gastric mucosal barrier. Anything that decreases the production of gastric mucus or damages gastric mucosa is ulcerogenic; salicylates and other nonsteroidal anti-inflammatory drugs, alcohol, and anti-inflammatory drugs fall into this category.

Clinical Manifestations

Symptoms of duodenal ulcer (the most common form of peptic ulcer) may last for a few days, weeks, or months and may even disappear only to reappear, often without an identifiable cause. Exacerbations seem to occur in the spring or fall, but even this pattern is inconsistent. Many persons have symptomless ulcers, and in 20% to 30%, perforation or hemorrhage may occur without any preceding manifestations.

Pain.   As a rule, the patient with duodenal ulcer complains of dull, gnawing pain; or a burning sensation in the midepigastrium or in the back. It is believed that the pain occurs when the increased acid content of the stomach and duodenum erodes the lesion and stimulates the exposed nerve endings. Another theory suggests that contact of the lesion with acid stimulates a local reflex mechanism that initiates contraction of the adjacent smooth muscle.

Pain is usually relieved by eating, as food neutralizes the acid, or by taking alkali; however, once the stomach has emptied or the alkali wears off, the pain returns. Sharply localized tenderness can be elicited by gentle pressure on the epigastrium at or slightly to the right of the midline. Some relief is obtained by local pressure on the epigastrium.

Pyrosis (Hypersialorrhea, Heartburn).   Some patients experience a burning sensation in the esophagus and stomach, which moves up to the mouth, occasionally with sour eructation. Eructation, or burping, is common when the patient's stomach is empty.

Vomiting.   Although rare in uncomplicated duodenal ulcer, vomiting may be a symptom of peptic ulcer. It is due to gastric outlet obstruction caused by either muscular spasm of the pylorus or mechanical obstruction. The latter may be due to scarring or to acute swelling of the inflamed mucous membrane adjacent to the acute ulcer. Vomiting may or may not be preceded by nausea; usually it follows a bout of severe pain, which is relieved by ejection of the acid gastric contents. The vomitus may contain food particles from the previous day.

Constipation and Bleeding.   Constipation may be apparent in the patient with duodenal ulcer, probably as a result of diet and medications.

- About 20% of patients who bleed from an acute duodenal ulcer have had no previous digestive complaints, but they develop symptoms thereafter.

Diagnostic Evaluation

A physical examination may reveal pain, epigastric tenderness, or abdominal distention. Bowel sounds may be absent. A barium study of the upper gastrointestinal tract may show an ulcer; however, endoscopy is the preferred diagnostic procedure.

Upper gastrointestinal endoscopy is used to identify inflammatory changes, ulcers, and lesions. Endoscopy permits direct visualization of the duodenal mucosa and is used to augment radiographic studies. Endoscopy has been found to detect 20% of those lesions not evident in x-ray studies because of the size or location of the lesion. Stools may be collected daily until the laboratory reports are negative for occult blood. Gastric secretory studies are of value in diagnosing achlorhydria (the absence of hydrochloric acid in gastric juices) and Zollinger-Ellison syndrome. Pain that is relieved by ingesting food or antacids and the absence of pain on arising are also highly suggestive of duodenal ulcer.

A breath test has been developed that detects *C. pylori*. Although this bacterium is present in many patients with peptic ulcer disease and gastritis, no causative relationship has been proven.

Management

From the beginning, once the diagnosis is established, the patient is informed that he can learn how to keep his problem under control, but he may expect remissions and recurrences.

Control of Gastric Secretions.   Gastric acidity can be managed with appropriate sedation and neutralization of the gastric juice at frequent and regular intervals with drugs, nonirritating foods, and antacids.

Drugs that block the acid-secreting action of histamine (H_2 blockers), such as ranitidine, cimetidine, or famotidine, or drugs that produce an acid-resistant barrier over the ulcer, such as sucralfate, have been shown to be effective in healing duodenal ulcers. Antispasmodics may be given to reduce pylorospasm and intestinal motility. Anticholinergic agents may be prescribed to inhibit gastric secretion. Hospitalization, if required at all, can be limited to a few days, unless bleeding, obstruction, perforation, or severe nocturnal pain is present.

Rest and Stress Reduction.   Reducing environmental stress is a difficult task requiring physical and mental interventions on the patient's part and aid and cooperation of family members and significant others. The patient may need help in identifying situations that are stressful or exhausting. A rushed life style and an irregular schedule may aggravate symptoms and interfere with regular meals taken in relaxed settings and with regular administration of medications. In addition to suggestions for stress reduction, the patient also may benefit from suggestions about regular rest periods during the day, at least during the acute phase of the disease.

Smoking.   Studies have shown that smoking decreases the secretion of bicarbonate from the pancreas into the duodenum. Therefore, the acidity to the duodenum is higher when one smokes. Research indicates that continuation of cigarette smoking may significantly inhibit ulcer repair.

Diet.   Because there is little evidence to support the theory that bland diets are more beneficial than regular meals, patients have been encouraged to eat whatever agrees with them. There are, however, a few precautions to consider in the early stages of healing. The goal of the diet for patients with peptic ulcers is to avoid oversecretion and hypermotility in the gastrointestinal tract. These can be minimized by avoiding extremes of temperature and overstimulation by meat extracts, alcohol, and coffee, (including decaffeinated coffee, which also stimulates acid secretion). In addition, an effort is made to neutralize acid by eating three regular meals a day. Small, frequent feedings are not necessary as long as antacids or a histamine blocker is taken.

Diet compatibility becomes an individual matter. If the patient tolerates a particular food, he may eat it. If it produces pain, he should avoid it. Milk and cream are no longer considered central to therapy. In fact, diets rich in milk and cream are potentially harmful, because they are potent acid stimuli and over a long period they increase serum lipids, a contributing factor in producing atherosclerosis.

H_2 Receptor Antagonists.   Histamine has two receptors for its action. H_1 receptor is located on bronchial and nasal mucosa, cardiac tissue, and blood vessels; H_2 receptor is found primarily in the parietal cells in the stomach, in uterine and bronchial muscle, and in T lymphocytes. Even though H_2 receptors are distributed in body tissue, only gastric receptors appear to be affected by H_2 receptor antagonists. Common antihistamines block the action of H_1 receptors but have no effect on H_2 receptors in the stomach. H_2 receptor antagonists, cimetidine, ranitidine, and famotidine, have a dramatic effect on lowering acid secretion in the stomach. High doses of these drugs reduce secretion to almost unmeasurable levels.

Cimetidine (Tagamet) is given orally with each meal and at bedtime. A 300-mg tablet can inhibit acid secretion by greater than 90% for about 5 hours. It also inhibits the body's secretory response to gastrin, acetylcholine, and histamine. Cimetidine relieves ulcer pain and thus decreases the need for antacids. Although research has shown that liquid antacids used appropriately are as effective as cimetidine, most patients prefer to take tablets than a liquid preparation throughout the day. Short-term treatment with cimetidine has resulted in complete ulcer healing, but low-dose maintenance therapy may be needed to prevent recurrence. Side effects may include changes in liver function studies, gynecomastia, confusion in older patients, and drug interactions (especially with warfarin anticoagulants, Valium and theophylline).

Ranitidine (Zantac) is another H_2 antagonist that is given in a tablet form twice a day. Studies have shown this drug to be more effective than cimetidine, and it causes fewer side effects than cimetidine. Side effects that have been noted include dizziness, constipation, gynecomastia, and depression. Depression usually begins in 6 to 8 weeks. It takes several weeks for the depression to lift after the drug has been stopped.

Famotidine (Pepcid) is an H_2 receptor antagonist that is taken once a day, usually at bedtime. Trial clinical studies have shown rapid ulcer healing in 4 to 8 weeks for about 85% of those treated. Thereafter a reduced dosage is recommended for maintenance therapy. Famotidine's absorption rate is not significantly affected by antacids, which can be given at the same time. Studies on elderly patients have shown no significant changes in pharmacodynamics. Table 36–2 gives a listing of the recommended dosage and scheduling of these drugs.

Antacids. Antacids continue to be a mainstay of peptic ulcer treatment even though they are not capable of maintaining a *p*H of 3.5 or above (necessary for pepsinogen inactivity) for

TABLE 36–2. *Drug Therapy for Duodenal Ulcer Disease*

Drug Class/ Drug	Dosage/Duration
ANTACIDS (various)	30 ml 1 and 3 hours after meals and at bedtime for 4 weeks or longer
H_2-RECEPTOR ANTAGONISTS	
Cimetidine	300 mg qid for 4–6 wk (alternative schedules: 400 mg bid and 800 mg once a day)
	To prevent recurrence: 400 mg/day at bedtime
Ranitidine	150 mg bid for 4–6 wk (alternative schedule: 300 mg once a day)
	To prevent recurrence: 150 mg/day at bedtime
Famotidine	40 mg once a day for 4–6 wk
	Maintenance therapy: 20 mg/day at bedtime
CYTOPROTECTIVE AGENTS	
Sucralfate	1 g qid or 2 g bid

(Reprinted with permission from Koch MJ. How to detect and heal lesions and relieve pain. Consultant 1987 May; 27[5]: 21–24.)

longer than 45 minutes. The objective is to select the antacid that provides the safest and longest period of acid neutralization. Usually, antacids leave the stomach rapidly, so that frequent doses are required. Recommended dosages should not be exceeded because systemic alkalosis or rebound hyperacidity can occur.

Sodium bicarbonate is probably the best neutralizer of acid contents in the stomach but is *not* recommended because it is emptied from the stomach too rapidly and over time can easily lead to alkalosis.

Antacids can be divided into those that contain magnesium, magnesium and aluminum, or aluminum alone. Those that contain magnesium tend to cause diarrhea, and those that contain aluminum cause constipation. Antacids that contain calcium are not recommended because calcium produces an increase in serum gastrin and in acid secretion.

In the past, concern about sodium content determined selection of antacid type; however, recently producers of antacids have decreased the sodium content in all antacids. All antacids have been found to be more effective if given in the liquid form.

Antacid intake is scheduled to correspond to the delay in gastric emptying. A recommended schedule is 1 to 2 tablespoons (15 to 30 ml), 1 to 3 hours after each meal and at bedtime. The effectiveness of antacid therapy can be prolonged if antacids are taken 1 hour after meals because this is when there is peak acid output. Antacids usually have a short duration and need to be taken again in 2 hours. For convenience, some people use the tablet form. Patients are advised to read the package directions and consult their physician for dosage schedule. If the patient is awakened at night with epigastric pain, he notes the time, and thereafter may set his alarm clock for an hour earlier to take the antacid.

Anticholinergics. Anticholinergics block acetylcholine, which is a major stimulant of acid secretion. Their effectiveness is limited because undesirable side effects may occur at therapeutic doses. Therefore, they are only prescribed for those patients who suffer from severe, persistent nocturnal pain, and they are rarely recommended for long-term use. Anticholinergics decrease gastric motor activity and thus allow an antacid to remain in the stomach longer. They are occasionally used at nighttime with a double dose of antacid for persistent night pain.

Side effects of anticholinergic drugs include dryness of the mouth and throat; excessive thirst; difficulty in swallowing; flushed, dry skin; rapid pulse and respiration; dilated pupils; and emotional excitement.

- Because of these side effects, anticholinergic medications are contraindicated in several conditions including glaucoma, tachycardia, dysrhythmias, pyloric obstruction, ulcerative colitis, paralytic ileus, and urinary retention.

Other Drugs. Sucralfate (Carafate) is a locally acting drug that has also been shown to have anti-ulcer properties. Sucralfate forms complexes with proteinaceous exudates, such as albumin and fibrinogen, in the ulcer crater, producing an adherent barrier over the ulcer. This barrier is acid resistant, as opposed to acid reducing. The result is that acid is prevented from passing through to the ulcer, but the acid is not appreciably neutralized. Sucralfate is only minimally absorbed from the gastrointestinal tract and does not depend on systemic activity for its anti-ulcer effects.

Duration of Treatment.   The patient should adhere to the drug program to ensure complete healing of the ulcer. Because most patients become free of symptoms in a week, it becomes a nursing goal to stress the importance of following the prescribed regimen so that the breakdown of the healing process and the return of chronic ulcer symptoms are averted. Rest, sedatives, and tranquilizers add to the patient's comfort and are used as needed. Maintenance dosages of H_2 receptor antagonists are usually recommended for 1 year.

After the first week, the purpose of using antacids changes from that of relieving symptoms to preventing symptoms. The best plan appears to be to have the patient eat regular meals.

From the sixth or seventh week to 6 months, antacid is taken about an hour after meals and at bedtime. Thereafter, antacid therapy is usually halted. If the person experiences a stressful situation or has not been careful with his diet and symptoms recur, he may resume antacid therapy until he is free of symptoms. The patient is advised to stop smoking entirely. Methods to stop smoking and relieve stress are encouraged.

Surgical Intervention.   With the advent of H_2 receptor antagonists, surgical intervention for peptic ulcers is less common. Surgery is recommended for patients with intractable ulcers, life-threatening hemorrhage, perforation, or obstruction. Surgical procedures include vagotomy, vagotomy with pyloroplasty, or Billroth I or II. See p. 912, Nursing Process: The Patient Undergoing Gastric Surgery.

Prognosis

Recurrence of an ulcer is possible and may occur within 2 years in about one third of all patients, although this incidence may be reduced with prophylactic use of the H_2 receptor antagonists. The likelihood of recurrence is reduced if the person avoids smoking, tea, coffee and cola (including decaffeinated), alcohol, and ulcerogenic drugs (such as anti-inflammatory agents).

▶ Nursing Process
The Patient With a Peptic Ulcer

▷ Assessment

The history serves as an important base for diagnosis. The patient is asked to describe the pain and methods that he uses to relieve it (food, antacids). Peptic ulcer pain is usually described as "burning" or "gnawing" and occurs about 2 hours after a meal. It frequently awakens the patient between midnight and 3:00 AM. The patient will usually state that the pain is relieved by taking antacids or foods or by vomiting. The patient is asked if he has vomited. Is emesis bright red or coffee ground? Has he had blood in his stools? During the history the nurse asks the patient to list his usual food intake for a 72-hour period and to include his food habits (speed of eating, regularity of meals, preference for spicy foods, use of seasonings, use of caffeinated beverages). The patient's level of tension or nervousness is assessed. Does he smoke cigarettes and how many? How does he express anger? How does he describe his work and family life? Is there occupational stress or problems within his family? Is there a family history of ulcer disease?

Vital signs are assessed for indicators of anemia (tachycardia, hypotension), and the stool is examined for occult blood. A physical examination is performed, and the abdomen is palpated for localized tenderness.

▷ Nursing Diagnoses

Based on all the assessment data, the patient's nursing diagnoses may include the following:

* Pain, related to the effect of gastric acid secretion on damaged tissue
* Anxiety related to coping with an acute disease
* Knowledge deficit about prevention of symptoms and management of the condition

▷ Planning and Implementation

▷ *Goals:*   The major goals of the patient may include relief of pain, reduction of anxiety, and acquisition of knowledge about prevention and management.

▷ Nursing Interventions

▷ *Relief of Pain.*   Pain relief can be attained by administering prescribed medications (antacids, anticholinergics, histamine antagonists). Aspirin and foods and beverages that contain caffeine (cola, tea, coffee, chocolate) are avoided. Regularly spaced meals are encouraged in a relaxed atmosphere. The patient is encouraged to learn relaxation techniques to help him cope with stress and pain and to stop smoking. See Nursing Care Plan 36–1, Care of The Patient With Peptic Ulcer Disease.

▷ *Reduction of Anxiety.*   The nurse should assess what the patient knows and wants to know about his disease. His level of anxiety is evaluated. Patients with peptic ulcers are usually anxious, but their anxiety is not always obvious. This attempt at coping frequently aggravates their disease process. Information is provided at the patient's level of learning, and his questions are answered. The patient is allowed to express his fears openly and without criticism. Diagnostic tests are explained, and medications are administered on schedule. These patients are frequently time oriented, and any schedule deviation or disruption can cause anxiety and increase gastric secretion. The nurse emphasizes that nurses are nearby if there is a problem. The nurse interacts with the patient in a relaxing manner and helps him to identify stressors and learn effective coping techniques and relaxation methods. The nurse encourages the participation of the patient's family in his care and emotional support if this is feasible.

▷ *Patient Education and Home Health Care.*   To deal successfully with ulcer disease, the patient must understand his situation and those factors that will help or aggravate his condition. Areas that need consideration and perhaps modification, along with evaluative questions, are the following:

1. *Medication:* Does the patient know what medications are to be taken at home, including name, dosage, frequency, and possible side effects? Does the patient know what drugs to avoid?
2. *Diet:* Does the patient know what particular foods tend to upset him? Does the patient know that coffee, tea, colas, and alcohol have acid-producing potential? Does he know to avoid overeating? Does he understand the importance of regular meals taken in a relaxed setting?

Nursing Care Plan 36–1

Care of the Patient With Peptic Ulcer Disease

Nursing Interventions	Rationale	Expected Outcomes

Nursing Diagnosis: Knowledge deficit regarding the prevention of symptoms and management of the condition

Goal: Acquisition of knowledge about prevention and management

1. Assess the patient's level of knowledge and "readiness to learn."	1. Attending to learning is dependent on the patient's physical condition, level of anxiety, and mental readiness.	• Expresses an interest in learning how to manage his disease.
2. Teach necessary information: a. Use words at the level of learner. b. Choose a time when the patient is rested and interested. c. Limit teaching sessions to 30 minutes or less.	2. Individualization of the teaching plan promotes learning.	• Participates in teaching sessions. • Asks questions.
3. Reassure the patient that the disease can be managed.	3. Knowledge can have a positive influence on behavior modification.	• States a desire to be responsible for self-care.

Nursing Diagnosis: Pain, related to irritated mucosa and muscle spasms

Goal: Relief of pain

1. Administer drug therapy as prescribed: a. Antacids b. Histamine antagonists c. Anticholinergics	1. Pharmacotherapy helps reduce pain as follows: a. Antacids neutralize acidity of gastric secretions. b. Histamine antagonists interfere with the secretion of gastric acid. c. Anticholinergics inhibit the release of gastric acid.	• Takes medications as prescribed. • Experiences less pain with drug therapy.
2. Recommend avoidance of ulcerogenic over-the-counter drugs.	2. Drugs that contain salicylates are irritating to the gastric mucosa.	• Substitutes acetaminophen (Tylenol) for aspirin. • Avoids over-the-counter drugs that contain acetylsalicylic acid (Contac, Alka-Seltzer)
3. Advise patient to avoid foods/beverages that are irritating to the stomach lining: caffeine and alcohol.	3. Foods/beverages that contain caffeine stimulate the secretion of hydrochloric acid.	• Complies with recommended restrictions.
4. Instruct patient to increase intake of water.	4. Water is considered a good antacid.	• Drinks 6 to 8 glasses of water daily.
5. Instruct patient to eat slowly and chew small pieces of food.	5. The greater the size of food particles, the greater the secretion of hydrochloric acid.	• Eats smaller amounts of food at one time and chews food slowly.
6. Advise patient to space meals and snacks at regular intervals.	6. Regularly scheduled meals help keep food particles in the stomach, which helps to neutralize the acidity of gastric secretions.	• Adheres to a schedule of regularly spaced meals and snacks.
7. Advise patient to stop smoking	7. Smoking increases the possibility of recurrence of ulcer	• Patient stops smoking

Nursing Diagnosis: Anxiety related to the fear of coping with an acute disease

Goal: Reduction of anxiety

1. Encourage the patient to express concerns and fears and ask questions as needed.	1. Open communication fosters a trusting relationship, which helps reduce anxiety and stress.	• Expresses fears and concerns.

(continued)

Nursing Care Plan 36–1 (Continued)

Care of the Patient With Peptic Ulcer Disease

Nursing Interventions	Rationale	Expected Outcomes
2. Explain the reasons for adhering to a planned treatment schedule: a. Pharmacotherapy b. Diet restriction c. Modified activity levels d. Reduction or cessation of smoking	2. Knowledge reduces the anxiety found with "fear of the unknown." Knowledge can have a positive influence on behavior modification.	• Understands rationale for various treatments and restrictions. • Modifies behavior appropriately.
3. Assist the patient identify anxiety-producing situations.	3. Stressors need to be identified before they can be managed.	• Identifies anxiety-producing situations.
4. Teach stress-reducing exercises: meditation, distraction, and imagery.	4. Decreased anxiety decreases hydrochloric acid secretion.	• Uses relaxation measures appropriately.

Nursing Diagnosis: Altered nutrition, less than body requirements, related to pain associated with eating

Goal: Attainment of an optimal level of nutrition

1. Recommend nonirritating foods and beverages.	1. Nonirritating foods reduce epigastric pain.	• Avoids irritating foods and beverages.
2. Suggest that meals be eaten at regularly scheduled times, avoid snacks before bedtime	2. Regular meals help neutralize gastric secretions, snacks before bedtime increase acid secretion from stomach.	• Eats meals and snacks at regularly scheduled intervals.
3. Encourage eating meals in a relaxed atmosphere.	3. A relaxed atmosphere is less anxiety producing. Decreasing anxiety helps decrease the secretion of hydrochloric acid.	• Chooses a relaxed atmosphere for meals.

3. *Smoking:* Does the patient know that smoking may interfere with ulcer healing? Is he aware of programs to assist with smoking cessation?

4. *Rest and stress reduction:* Is the patient aware of sources of stress in family and work environments? Has this illness or other situations produced symptoms of stress or poor coping in the family or work setting? Is the patient aware that smoking probably increases the irritation to his ulcer? Can the patient identify rest periods during the day? Can the patient plan for added periods of rest or relaxation after unavoidable periods of stress? Does the patient need extended psychological counseling?

5. *Awareness of complications:* Is the patient alert to signs and symptoms of complications that should be reported?
   - *Hemorrhage:* cool skin, confusion, increased heart rate, labored breathing, blood in the stool
   - *Perforation:* severe abdominal pain, rigid and tender abdomen, vomiting, elevated temperature, increased heart rate
   - *Pyloric obstruction:* nausea, vomiting, distended abdomen, abdominal pain
   - *Intractability:* persistent pain and discomfort related to stress, food intake, or drug regimen

6. *Follow-up care:* Does the patient realize that follow-up supervision is necessary for about 1 year? Does he realize that his ulcer could recur? Does he know to seek medical assistance if symptoms recur?

◊ Evaluation

Expected Outcomes

1. Experiences no pain
   a. Is free of pain between meals
   b. Uses antacids as prescribed
   c. Adheres to medication regimen
   d. Avoids foods and fluids that cause pain
   e. Eats meals at regular times
   f. Experiences no side effects of antacids (diarrhea or constipation)
2. Experiences less anxiety
   a. Identifies situations that produce stress
   b. Identifies life-style adjustments necessary to reduce stress
   c. Involves family in decisions regarding life-style adjustments
   d. Alters life style as appropriate
   e. Uses sedatives and tranquilizers as prescribed
   f. Experiences no side effects of sedatives and tranquilizers
3. Complies with therapeutic regimen
   a. Avoids irritating foods and beverages
   b. Eats regularly scheduled meals
   c. Eats slowly and in a relaxed atmosphere
   d. Takes prescribed medications as scheduled
   e. Uses coping mechanisms to deal with stress

Complications of Peptic Ulcers

There are four major complications of peptic ulcer: hemorrhage, perforation, pyloric obstruction, and intractable ulcer.

Hemorrhage

Manifested by hematemesis, melena, or both, hemorrhage is the *most common complication* of peptic ulcer. Hemorrhage occurs in 10% to 20% of patients with ulcers and has a mortality rate of 30% to 40%. The most frequent site is the distal portion of the duodenum. When the hemorrhage is of large proportions (2000 to 3000 ml), most of the blood is vomited. The patient may become almost exsanguinated, and rapid correction of blood loss will be required to save his life. When the hemorrhage is small, much or all of the blood may be passed in the stools, which will appear tarry black because of the digested hemoglobin.

Assessment. The nurse assesses the patient for early symptoms of faintness or dizziness; nausea may precede or accompany bleeding. Dyspepsia may not be present. Vital signs are evaluated for tachycardia, hypotension, and tachypnea. The hemoglobin and hematocrit are analyzed. The stool is tested for gross or occult blood, and 24-hour urinary output is recorded to detect anuria or oliguria.

Management. Because bleeding can be fatal, the cause and severity of the hemorrhage are quickly identified and the blood loss is treated to prevent hypovolemic shock.

- Preparations are made for a peripheral intravenous line for infusion of saline and blood and possibly a central line for infusion of fluids as well as for measurement of central venous pressure. Blood component therapy is initiated if there are signs of tachycardia, sweating, and coldness of the extremities.
- The hemoglobin and hematocrit are monitored to detect bleeding.
- An indwelling urinary catheter is inserted to monitor urinary output.
- Nasogastric intubation is used to distinguish fresh blood from "coffee ground" material and to administer saline for lavage (clot removal, vasoconstriction of superficial vessels). The normal saline solution may be taken by mouth and the fluid withdrawn through the tube by suction. This removes acid, prevents nausea and vomiting, and provides a means of monitoring further bleeding. The *p*H of gastric secretions may be checked hourly through the nasogastric tube and antacids administered for a *p*H less than 4.
- Oxygen therapy may be instituted.
- The patient is placed in the recumbent position to prevent hypovolemic shock.
- Vital signs are monitored as warranted by the patient's condition.
- Hypovolemic shock is treated as described in Chap. 22.

If bleeding cannot be managed by the measures just described, then the following may be performed:

1. Endoscopic therapy: Control of bleeding may be accomplished by using several endoscopic therapies such as coagulation by laser, heat probes, or injection techniques (injection of drugs to control the bleeding, such as epinephrine).

A combination of these therapies may be employed. There is much debate regarding how soon endoscopy should be performed. Some believe endoscopy should be performed within the first 24 hours after hemorrhage has been stabilized. Others believe endoscopy can be performed during acute bleeding, as long as visualization is possible.

2. Intra-arterial vasopressin infusions, by pump, directly into a bleeding artery: A repeat arteriogram is needed to evaluate the efficacy of treatment.

3. Selective embolization: Emboli of autologous blood clots with or without Gelfoam (absorbable gelatin sponge), or a mixture of the patient's own blood or blood products are forced through a catheter to a point above the bleeding lesion. This procedure is done by a radiologist.

Surgical Treatment. If bleeding recurs in 48 hours after medical therapy has begun, or if more than 6 units of blood are required in 24 hours to maintain blood volume, the patient is likely to be scheduled for surgery. Some physicians recommend surgical intervention if a patient with peptic ulcer hemorrhages three times.

Other determining factors for surgery are the patient's age (if he is over 60, massive hemorrhaging is three times more likely to be fatal), a history of chronic duodenal ulcer, and a coincidental gastric ulcer.

The area of the ulcer is removed, or the bleeding vessels are ligated. In many patients a procedure is included that is aimed at controlling the underlying causes of the ulcer (*e.g.,* vagotomy and pylorectomy, or gastrectomy).

Perforation. Perforation of a peptic ulcer may occur unexpectedly, without much evidence of preceding indigestion. Perforation into the peritoneal cavity is an abdominal catastrophe and an indication that surgery is required.

Signs and symptoms to note include the following:

- Sudden, severe upper abdominal pain (persisting and increasing in intensity)
- Pain, which may be referred to the shoulders, especially the right shoulder, because of irritation of the phrenic nerve in the diaphragm
- Vomiting and collapse (fainting)
- Extremely tender and rigid (boardlike) abdomen
- Shock

Immediate surgical intervention is indicated, because chemical peritonitis develops within a few hours after perforation and is followed by a bacterial peritonitis. Therefore, the perforation must be closed as quickly as possible. In a few patients, it may be deemed safe and advisable that surgery be performed for the ulcer disease, in addition to the perforation being sutured.

Postoperatively, the stomach contents are drained by means of a nasogastric tube. The nurse monitors fluid and electrolyte balance and assesses the patient for peritonitis or localized infection (increased temperature, abdominal pain, paralytic ileus, increased or absent bowel sounds, abdominal distention). Antibiotic therapy is given parenterally as prescribed.

Pyloric Obstruction

Pyloric obstruction occurs when the area distal to the pyloric sphincter becomes scarred and stenosed from spasm or edema or from scar tissue that is formed when the ulcer alternately heals and breaks down. The patient has symptoms of nausea and vomiting, constipation, epigastric fullness, anorexia, and (later) weight loss.

In treating the patient, the first consideration is the insertion of a nasogastric tube to decompress the stomach. At the same time, attempts are made to confirm that obstruction is the cause of discomfort. This is done by checking the amount of fluid aspirated from the nasogastric tube. A residual of over 200 ml is strongly suggestive of obstruction. Some physicians also use the load test, which involves infusing 750 ml of normal saline through the nasogastric tube into the mid-antrum of the stomach. The patient is rotated, to permit normal gastric emptying; 20 minutes later, aspiration is performed, and if more than 400 ml is retrieved, obstruction is confirmed.

Before surgery is undertaken, decompression continues and extracellular fluid volume and electrolyte and metabolic derangements are corrected. Conscientious daily fluid monitoring is continued. With supportive measures, the patient's condition may improve. It may be feasible to repeat the load test; if negative, medical treatment continues. If positive, surgery, in the form of a vagotomy and antrectomy, may be required. If the patient is severely malnourished, total parenteral nutrition may be used.

Intractable Ulcer

An intractable ulcer is one that continues to give problems and is resistant to all forms of treatment. It is the most common, persistent problem seen with peptic ulcer disease and the most common reason given by patients for choosing surgery.

A careful patient history includes a thorough review of dietary and drug habits, which could disclose long-term use of caffeine-containing drinks or aspirin-containing medications. The entire gastrointestinal tract is carefully assessed to determine other possible problems, such as hiatus hernia, gallbladder disease, or diverticulitis.

The patient and family are informed of the fact that surgery is no guarantee that an ulcer is cured. Possible postoperative sequelae, such as intolerance to dairy products and sweet foods, are also discussed.

Surgical Approaches

Surgery for ulcer disease is performed when medical therapy has not been successful or when complications arise, such as hemorrhage, perforation, or pyloric obstruction. Patients requiring ulcer surgery may have had a long illness, be discouraged, have interruptions in their work role, and experience pressures in their family life. Various types of surgical procedures may be used in treating peptic ulcer disease (Table 36-3).

- *Subtotal gastrectomy* is removal of one third of the stomach. The remaining segment is anastomosed to the duodenum or the jejunum.
- *Antrectomy* involves removing the antral (lower) portion of the stomach (which contains the G cells that secrete gastrin) as well as a small portion of the duodenum and pylorus. The remaining segment is anastomosed to the duodenum (Billroth

I) or the jejunum (Billroth II) (Fig. 36-2). An antrectomy may also be performed in conjunction with a truncal vagotomy.
- *Vagotomy*, severing of the vagus nerves, may be performed to reduce gastric acid secretion.
  - *Truncal vagotomy*, severing of the right and left vagus nerves as they enter the stomach at the distal part of the esophagus, is the type of vagotomy most commonly used to decrease acid secretion and reduce gastric and intestinal motility.
  - *Selective vagotomy* involves severing vagal innervation to the stomach but maintaining the innervation to the rest of the abdomen.
  - *Parietal cell vagotomy* involves severing only those vagus nerves that innervate the parietal cell mass in the upper portion of the stomach. Antrum innervation remains intact, decreasing the need for a pyloroplasty.
- *Pyloroplasty* is a drainage operation in which a longitudinal incision is made into the pylorus and transversely sutured closed to enlarge the outlet and relax the muscle (see Fig. 36-2). A pyloroplasty usually accompanies truncal and selective vagotomies, which produce delayed gastric emptying.

Nursing Interventions

Preoperative nursing care for the patient undergoing surgery for peptic ulcer disease includes the following:

- *Preparing the patient for diagnostic tests:* The patient undergoes laboratory analyses, x-ray series, and a general physical examination before surgery. The nurse prepares the patient for each of these diagnostic measures by explaining their nature and significance.
- *Attending to the patient's fluid and nutritional needs:* The nutritional and fluid needs of the patient are of major importance. In those patients with pyloric obstruction, there usually is prolonged vomiting, with resultant weight and fluid loss. Every effort is made to restore an adequate nutritional level and to maintain an optimal fluid and electrolyte balance.
- *Clearing and emptying the gastrointestinal tract:* Nasogastric suction often is required to empty the stomach, especially in patients with pyloric obstruction. The tube is inserted before the operation and left in place for operative and postoperative use.

  It is important that the colon be empty when the patient goes to surgery; this is ensured by an enema the day before surgery. If gastrointestinal films have been made shortly before the day of surgery, enemas are given to completely remove the barium that may remain in the colon.
- *Limiting fluid intake:* The patient's oral intake is usually limited to fluids during the 24-hour period before surgery.

Postoperative care is the same as that for gastric surgery. (See pp. 912–914, Nursing Process: The Patient Undergoing Gastric Surgery, as well as pp. 907–909, Nursing Care Plan 36-2, Care of the Patient Undergoing a Gastric Resection.)

In summary, peptic ulcers, gastric ulcers, and esophageal ulcers are more frequently seen in persons under stress or in persons who smoke or drink alcohol in excess. There is also some indication that gastric ulcers and perhaps duodenal ulcers are associated with the bacilli *C. pylori.*

Treatment involves use of H_2 receptor antagonists and

TABLE 36–3. *Gastric Operations for Peptic Ulcers*

Operation	Description	Mortality	Recurrence	Advantages	Sequelae
Vagotomy with drainage: pyloroplasty or gastroenterostomy	Vagotomy may by truncal or selective (preserving hepatic, celiac, and pancreatic branches)	Under 1%	12%	Fairly simple surgical procedure Clinical results: 75%—excellent 10%—fair 10%—poor	Some patients experience problems of fullness after eating (33%), dumping syndrome (10%), diarrhea (10%), and gastritis (90%)
Vagotomy with antrectomy	Resection of vagus nerves and removal of antrum	3.9%	3.3%	Marginal ulceration rate lowest	In some patients, fullness after eating, dumping syndrome, diarrhea, anemia, malabsorption
Subtotal gastrectomy Billroth I (gastroduodenostomy; anastomosis after resection)	Removal of distal third of stomach; anastomosis with duodenum	2%	10%	Restores normal continuity	Dumping syndrome, anemia, malabsorption, and weight loss Billroth I has a 4% marginal ulceration rate.
Billroth II (gastrojejunostomy; anastomosis after resection)	Removal of distal segment of stomach and antrum: anastomosis with jejunum		1%–3%		Billroth II has a 2% marginal ulceration rate.
Proximal (parietal cell) gastric vagotomy without drainage	Denervation of acid-secreting parietal cells but preserving vagal innervation to gastric antrum and extragastric abdominal viscera	Under 1%	1%–9%	No dumping syndrome, reflex gastritis, or diarrhea No need for antibiotics, because gastrointestinal tract is not open	Appears to be a safe procedure; needs long-term assessment

antacids. The use of cytoprotective drugs has been recently approved. When the patient is experiencing life-threatening hemorrhage, perforation, obstruction, or is not responding to medications, surgical intervention may be warranted.

Zollinger–Ellison Syndrome (Gastrinoma)

Zollinger–Ellison syndrome is suspected when a patient presents with several peptic ulcers. It is identified by the following findings: hypersecretion of gastric juice, multiple duodenal ulcers (second and third portions of the duodenum), an increase in parietal cell mass, hypertrophied duodenal glands, and gastrinomas (islet cell tumors) in the pancreas. The gastrinomas may also be found in the duodenum and stomach. The incidence of malignancy is high.

The huge amounts of secreted hydrochloric acid almost have the effect of the stomach's trying to digest itself. The serum gastrin level is increased. In Zollinger–Ellison syndrome, secretin stimulates gastrin secretion rather than inhibits it. Steatorrhea (unabsorbed fat in the stool) may be evident, because excessive gastric acid inactivates lipase in the intestine, thereby precipitating bile salts and decreasing fat digestion. The result is steatorrhea and diarrhea. Gastrin also decreases water and salt absorption, which in turn leads to diarrhea.

Management. Hypersecretion of acid may be controlled with high doses of H_2 receptor antagonists such as cimetidine, ranitidine, and famotidine. Patients may require twice the normal dose, and dosages usually need to be increased with prolonged use. H_2 receptor antagonists may be used in conjunction with an anticholinergic agent. The drug omeprazole, which inhibits the gastric acid pump, also may be used.

Surgical treatment may be helpful for patients not responding to medications. Total gastrectomy or parietal-cell vagotomy are the recommended surgical procedures. Twenty percent of patients are found to have metastasis at the time of surgery.

Nursing Assessment. The patient is assessed for fluid and electrolyte imbalances secondary to diarrhea and possible hypercalcemia. The nurse prepares the patient for diagnostic tests.

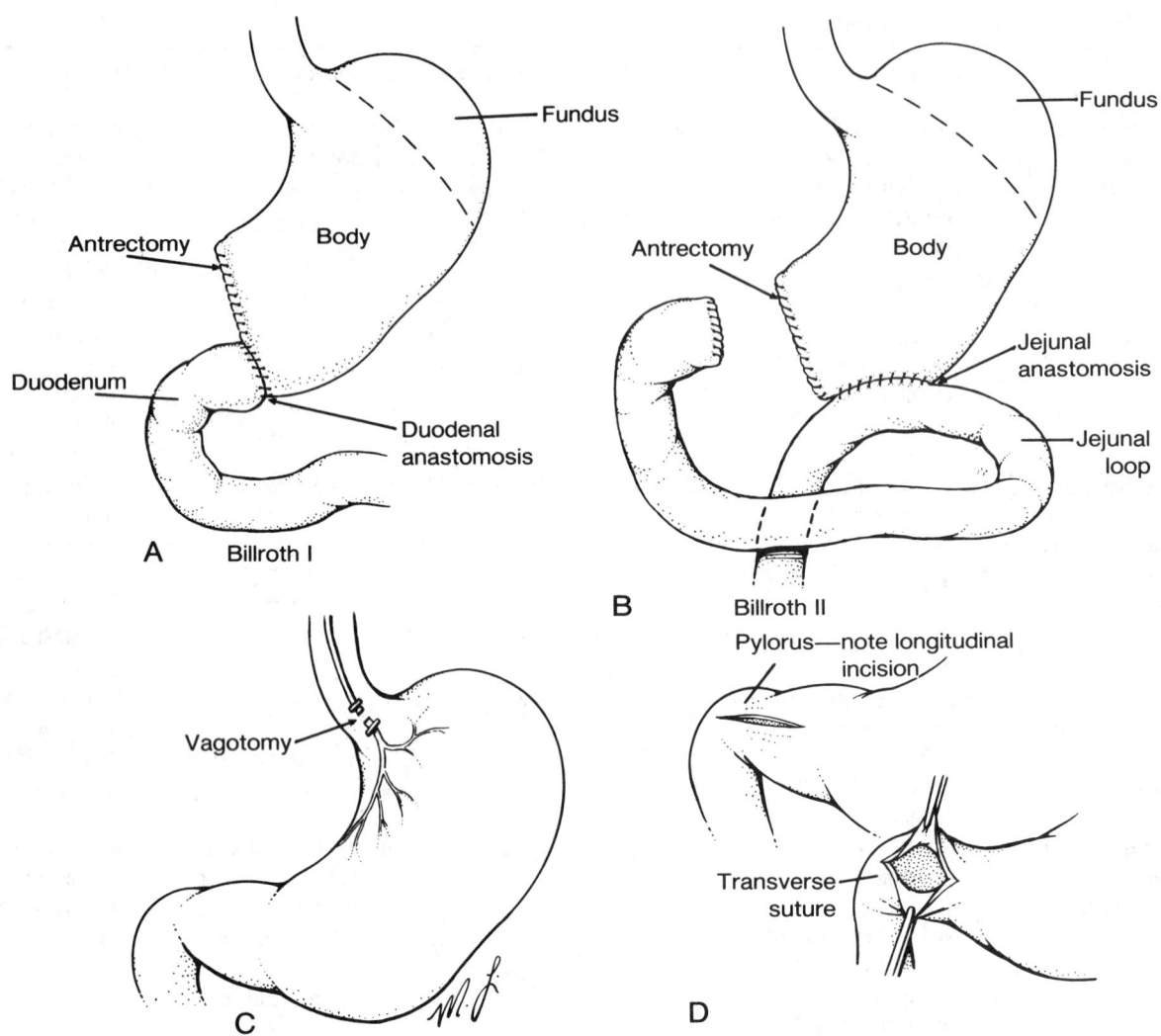

Figure 36–2. Surgical procedures for ulcer disease. (**A**) Antrectomy with anastomosis to the duodenum (Billroth I). (**B**) Antrectomy with anastomosis to the jejunum (Billroth II). (**C**) Severing of the vagus nerves (vagotomy). (**D**) A longitudinal incision into the pylorus followed by a transverse suture to enlarge the opening (pyloroplasty).

After diagnosis is confirmed, the nurse instructs the patient in the need to comply with the medication regimen and follow-up care. For patients requiring surgery, see Nursing Care Plan 36–2.

Stress Ulcer

Stress ulcer is the term given to acute mucosal ulceration of the duodenal or gastric area that occurs following physiologically disturbing conditions.

Pathophysiology and Etiology.   Stressful conditions such as burns, shock, severe sepsis, and multiple organ trauma can initiate the development of stress ulcers. Fiberoptic endoscopy within 24 hours of injury shows shallow erosions of the stomach wall; by 72 hours, multiple gastric erosions are observed. As the stressful condition continues, the ulcers spread. When the

patient recovers, the lesions are reversed. This pattern is typical of stress ulceration.

Differences of opinion exist as to the actual causation of mucosal ulceration. Usually, it is preceded by shock; this leads to a decrease in gastric mucosal blood flow and to a reflux of duodenal contents into the stomach. In addition, large quantities of pepsin are released. The combination of ischemia, acid, and pepsin creates an ideal climate to produce ulceration. Stress ulcers should be distinguished from Cushing's ulcers and Curling's ulcers. Cushing's ulcers are common in patients with trauma to the brain. They may occur in the esophagus, stomach, or duodenum and are usually deeper and more penetrating than stress ulcers. Curling's ulcer, another type of gastric ulcer, is frequently observed about 72 hours after extensive burns.

Management.   Antacids are the basis of treatment. If the patient is acutely ill, antacids may be given through the nasogastric tube. Frequent gastric aspiration is performed to check *p*H, in an attempt to get it to, or above, 3.5. Antacid therapy

Nursing Care Plan 36–2

Care of the Patient Undergoing a Gastric Resection

Nursing Interventions	Rationale	Expected Outcomes

PREOPERATIVE

Nursing Diagnosis: Knowledge deficit regarding the surgical procedure and postoperative course

Goal: Attainment of information about the procedure and postoperative course

Nursing Interventions	Rationale	Expected Outcomes
1. Make certain the patient understands what type of surgery he is to have.	1. Preoperative knowledge helps the patient understand the reasons for postoperative procedures.	• Improves adherence to treatment regimen.
2. Advise the patient that he will be placed in a modified Fowler's position after recovery from anesthesia.	2. Modified Fowler's position promotes comfort and drainage of the stomach.	
3. Advise the patient that he will be asked to breathe deeply and cough, postoperatively.	3. Coughing and deep breathing will prevent pulmonary complications.	• Avoids shallow breathing associated with incisional pain.
4. Advise the patient that he will have a nasogastric tube in place postoperatively and fluids will be withheld until peristalsis returns.	4. The nasogastric tube provides for gastric drainage that may contain some blood for the first 12 hours.	• Tolerates discomfort of nasogastric tube.
5. Inform the patient that he will be receiving parenteral fluids. Oral fluids will be withheld until the nasogastric tube is removed and peristalisis returns.	5. Parenteral fluids meet fluid and nutritional needs and compensate for fluids lost in drainage and vomitus.	• Accepts fluid restriction by mouth.
6. Inform the patient that bland foods are added gradually.	6. Small increments of food and fluid (120 ml between meals) are initiated to determine the patient's tolerance.	• Adheres to dietary regimen.
7. Inform the patient that he will be assisted to ambulate on the first postoperative day.	7. Early ambulation prevents venous stasis and phlebothrombosis.	• Is willing to ambulate as soon as possible.
8. Inform the patient that wound dressings may have drainage. Excessive drainage or bright red blood will be reported immediately.	8. Serosanguineous drainage is expected postoperatively, especially if tubes are left in the wound.	• Understands that dressings will have drainage and will be reinforced.

POSTOPERATIVE

Nursing Diagnosis: Pain related to the surgical incision

Goal: Relief of pain

Nursing Interventions	Rationale	Expected Outcomes
1. Promote frequent turning for comfort and for the prevention of pulmonary and vascular complications.	1. Inactivity encourages the pooling of pulmonary secretions.	• Cooperates with pulmonary routine.
2. Administer analgesics or narcotics as prescribed.	2. Pain control results from selective depression of the central nervous system.	• Requests pain medication as needed.
3. Withhold oral fluids until prescribed.	3. Sealing of the suture line is enhanced if patient is NPO.	• Remains NPO.
4. Use gastric suction to remove liquids, blood, and gas from stomach.	4. Promotes healing of suture line. Prevents unnecessary distention and pain.	

(continued)

Nursing Care Plan 36–2 (Continued)

Care of the Patient Undergoing a Gastric Resection

Nursing Interventions	Rationale	Expected Outcomes

Nursing Diagnosis: High risk for fluid volume deficit, related to shock or hemorrhage

Goal: Experiences no fluid volume deficit

Nursing Interventions	Rationale	Expected Outcomes

1. Assess patient for signs of shock:
  a. Evaluate drainage from dressing and drainage bottle.
  b. Evaluate blood pressure, pulse, and respiratory rate.
  c. Administer blood and fluids as prescribed.
  d. Instruct patient regarding symptoms to report.
	1. Decreased circulating blood volume can lead to hypovolemic shock.	• Alerts nurse to any dizziness, increased heart rate, confusion, excessive fatigue, or clammy skin.

2. Be alert to signs of hemorrhage:
  a. Observe gastric aspirate in drainage bottle for evidence of blood.
  b. Observe the suture line for bleeding.
  c. Evaluate blood pressure, pulse, and respiratory rate.
  d. Prepare patient for blood transfusion, and initiate therapy as prescribed.
  e. If bleeding continues, prepare patient for surgical intervention.
	2. Hemorrhage can lead to hypovolemic shock and death.	• Alerts nurse to any signs of bleeding.

Nursing Diagnosis: Altered nutrition, less than body requirements, related to the surgical procedure

Goal: Attainment of optimum nutrition

Nursing Interventions	Rationale	Expected Outcomes
1. Administer intravenous fluids as prescribed.	1. Intravenous fluids help prevent shock and maintain fluid and electrolyte balance.	• Cooperates with intravenous therapy.
2. Administer oral fluids as prescribed when audible bowel sounds are present	2. Positive bowel sounds indicate peristalsis is present.	
3. Increase fluids according to patient's tolerance.	3. Maintain fluid balance.	• Accepts fluids as tolerated.
4. Keep patient on bland diet with vitamin supplements as indicated by his condition.	4. Bland foods are less irritating to gastric mucosa.	• Adheres to diet therapy.
5. Maintain supplementary iron and vitamin therapy as prescribed.	5. Iron and vitamin therapy is necessary to supplement postoperative diet to promote tissue repair and prevent anemia.	• Takes iron and vitamin supplements as prescribed.
6. Discourage foods that may initiate development of dumping syndrome; encourage moderate amount of fat, low carbohydrates.	6. Decreased hypertonicity of intestinal contents prevents the osmotic pull of extracellular fluid into the intestinal area.	• Adheres to diet therapy.

Nursing Diagnosis: High risk for infection related to surgical incision.

Goal: Free of infection

Nursing Interventions	Rationale	Expected Outcomes
1. Assess wound for signs and symptoms of infection such as redness, swelling, tenderness, purulent drainage; fever. Report signs and symptoms if present.	1. Wound should be clean; some serosanguinous drainage may occur the first 24 hours and then subside.	• Absence of signs and symptoms of infection

(continued)

▶ Nursing Care Plan 36–2 *(Continued)*

Care of the Patient Undergoing a Gastric Resection

Nursing Interventions	Rationale	Expected Outcomes
2. Assess abdomen for signs of peritonitis—tenderness, rigidity, distention.	2. Peritonitis may occur secondary to gastric surgery.	• Absence of symptoms of peritonitis.
3. Administer prophylactic antibiotics as prescribed.	3. Antibiotics are frequently administered to the patient following abdominal surgery to prevent infection.	• No reaction to antibiotics.

Nursing Diagnosis: Potential noncompliance with the therapeutic regimen related to denial

Goal: Adherence to therapeutic regimen

1. Help patient to modify his environmental stresses.	1. Stress increases the secretion of hydrochloric acid, which irritates a compromised/damaged stomach mucosa.	• Uses stress reduction methods (biofeedback, imagery, distraction).
2. Encourage patient to remain under medical supervision.	2. Periodic hematologic studies are necessary to monitor for anemia. A complete physical examination may yield data about possible metastasis.	• Sees physician every 6 to 12 months as scheduled.
3. Arrange for some person or agency to help the patient cope: home health worker, clergyman, psychologist, nurse practitioner.	3. Long-term coping may require a support system.	• Seeks help when needed.

can also inhibit the activity of the proteolytic enzyme, pepsin. Stress ulcers are treated aggressively with cimetidine therapy in addition to antacids. Other methods of management of upper gastrointestinal tract hemorrhage are discussed on p. 903.

Morbid Obesity

Morbid obesity is a term applied to people who are twice their ideal body weight. Management consists of placing the person on a reducing diet, implementing behavioral modification, and encouraging enrollment in a weight loss clinic. Some physicians recommend acupuncture and hypnosis. When conservative measures have been tried for more than 3 to 5 years and have failed, a surgical procedure may be performed.

Surgical Management

Maxillomandibular Fixation. In maxillomandibular fixation, the person's jaws are wired to prevent the mouth from opening more than a fraction. The object is to restrict the patient's oral intake of fluids. Weight loss with this method is slow, and most patients regain their weight.

Intragastric Balloon. The intragastric balloon is a soft polyurethane sac that is inserted into the stomach, where its presence reduces the space available for food. The patient is sedated for the procedure, and the balloon, which is about the size of a small juice can, is inserted into the stomach by means of an endoscope. Although the exact mechanism of action is not known, it is believed that the balloon stimulates gastric nerve fibers that induce satiety. Patients feel full and eat smaller meals. The balloon is meant to supplement diet management and behavior modification. It must be removed after 4 months and is reinserted if needed. A major concern with this method of treatment is the danger that the balloon may break, necessitating removal by endoscope to prevent it from passing through the duodenum.

Jejunoileal Bypass. Jejunoileal bypass is the anastomosis of the proximal jejunum to the terminal ileum. It is preferred only for those patients weighing more than 500 pounds and only as a temporary measure. It is usually followed by gastric bypass or gastroplasty when the patient has lost sufficient weight to be considered a good surgical candidate. Jejunoileal bypass is associated with a high incidence of metabolic complications (hepatic cirrhosis, renal stones, hypoproteinemia) and is therefore not recommended for long-term management of morbid obesity.

Gastric Bypass and Vertical Banded Gastroplasty. Gastric bypass and vertical banded gastroplasty are the current gastric restrictive operations of choice. In gastric bypass surgery, the proximal segment of the stomach is transected to form a small pouch with a small gastroenterostomy stoma. The Roux-en-Y gastric bypass is the recommended procedure for long-term weight loss. In the Roux-en-Y bypass, a horizontal row of staples creates a stomach pouch with a 1-cm stoma that is anastomosed with a portion of distal jejunum, creating a gastroenterostomy. The transected proximal portion of the jejunum is anastomosed to the distal jejunum (Fig. 36–3).

In vertical banded gastroplasty, a double row of staples is

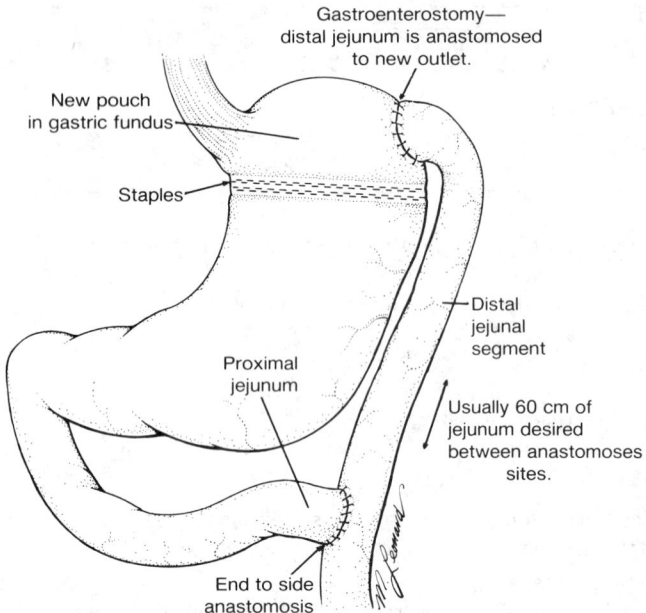

Figure 36–3. Gastric bypass with Roux-en-Y. A horizontal row of staples creates a pouch with a capacity of 50 ml or less. The proximal jejunum is transected and the distal end anastomosed to the new pouch. The proximal segment is anastomosed to the jejunum.

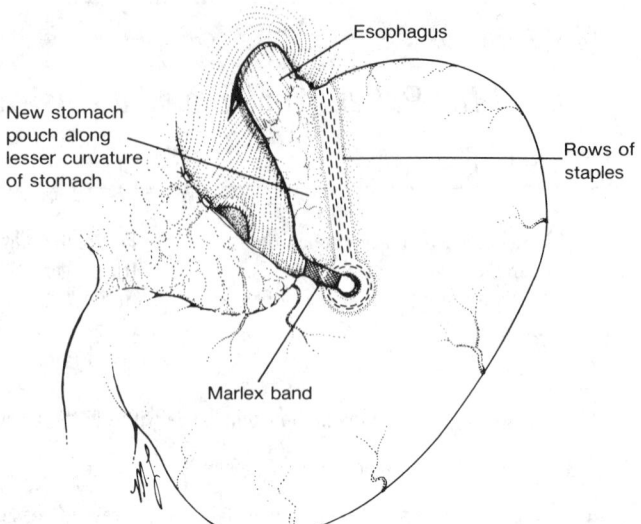

Figure 36–4. Vertical banded gastroplasty. A vertical row of staples along the lesser curvature of the stomach creates a new, smaller stomach pouch.

applied vertically along the lesser curvature of the stomach, beginning at the angle of His. A small stoma is created at the end of the staples by adding a circle of staples or a band of polypropylene mesh or silicone tubing (Fig. 36–4).

Nursing Interventions. General postoperative nursing care is similar to that for any patient experiencing gastric resection (see Nursing Care Plan 36–2). Patients are usually discharged in 1 week with detailed dietary instruction. Patients are usually given six small feedings consisting of a total of 600 to 800 calories. Fluid intake is encouraged to prevent dehydration. Patients are instructed to report any excessive thirst or concentrated urine to their physician. Outpatient visits are scheduled monthly.

Psychosocial considerations are essential for these patients. All efforts are directed toward helping them modify their eating behaviors and cope with their body image change. Noncompliance usually results in patients eating too much or too fast. If this happens, vomiting and painful esophageal distention may occur.

Postoperative complications may occur in the immediate postoperative period and include peritonitis, stomal obstruction, stomal ulcers, atelectasis and pneumonia, thromboembolism, and metabolic sequelae resulting from prolonged vomiting and diarrhea.

Gastric Cancer

Cancer of the stomach continues to decrease in the United States, (there has been a 60% decline during the past 40 years). It is still a serious problem, however, accounting for 13,700 deaths annually, mostly in people over the age of 40, and occasionally in younger people. Most stomach cancers occur in the pylorus or antrum of the stomach and are adenocarcinomas. The incidence of gastric cancer is much greater in Japan, which has led to mass screening for earlier diagnosis in that country. Diet appears to be a significant factor. A diet high in smoked foods and lacking in fruits and vegetables may increase the risk of gastric cancer. Other factors related to the incidence of gastric cancer include chronic inflammation of the stomach, pernicious anemia, achlorhydria, and possibly heredity. The prognosis is poor, as most patients have metastasis at the time of diagnosis.

Clinical Manifestations

The early symptoms of gastric cancer are often indefinite, because most of these tumors begin on the lesser curvature, where they cause little disturbance to gastric functions. In the early stages of gastric cancer, symptoms may be absent or indefinite. Some studies have shown that early symptoms may resemble those of patients with benign ulcers such as pain relieved with antacids. Symptoms of progressive disease may include indigestion, anorexia, dyspepsia, weight loss, abdominal pain, constipation, anemia, and nausea and vomiting.

Diagnostic Evaluation

Physical examination is usually not helpful, as most gastric tumors are not palpable. X-ray examination by upper GI and double-contrast barium swallow followed by endoscopy for biopsy and cytologic washings are the usual diagnostic studies. Because metastasis frequently occurs before warning signs are experienced, computed tomography (CT) scan, bone scan, and liver scan are valuable in determining the extent of the problem. Dyspepsia of more than 4 weeks' duration in any person over age 40 calls for complete x-ray examination of the gastrointestinal tract.

Management

There is no successful treatment of gastric carcinoma except removal of the tumor. If the tumor can be removed while it is still localized to the stomach, the patient can be cured. If the tumor has spread beyond the area that can be excised surgically, cure cannot be effected. In many of these patients, however, effective palliation, to prevent symptoms such as obstruction, may be obtained by resection of the tumor (see pp. 912–914, Nursing Process: The Patient Undergoing Gastric Surgery). If a *radical subtotal gastrectomy* has been performed, the stump of the stomach is anastomosed to the jejunum, as in the gastrectomy for ulcer. When *total gastrectomy* is performed, gastrointestinal continuity is restored by an anastomosis between the ends of the esophagus and jejunum. Palliative, rather than radical, surgery is performed if there is metastasis to other vital organs, such as the liver.

For patients in whom surgical treatment does not offer cure, treatment with chemotherapy may offer further control of the disease or palliation. Frequently used drugs include a combination of 5-fluorouracil (5FU), Adriamycin, and mitomycin-C. Radiation has little success in gastric cancer.

▶ # Nursing Process
The Patient With Gastric Cancer

▷ ## Assessment

The nurse elicits a history of diet from the patient such as high intake of smoked or cured foods and low intake of fruits and vegetables. Has the patient lost weight; how much?

Does the patient smoke cigarettes? If so, how many a day? How long has he been smoking? Does he notice any stomach discomfort during or after smoking? Does he drink alcohol? If so, how much?

The nurse asks the patient if there is a family history of cancer. If so, are immediate family members or close or distant relatives affected? This information is helpful when determining possible support systems. What is the patient's marital status? Is there someone who is going to provide emotional and financial support?

During the physical examination it may be possible to palpate a mass. Other organs are examined for tenderness or masses. Pain is usually a late symptom.

▷ ## Nursing Diagnoses

Based on all the assessment data, the patient's major nursing diagnoses may include the following:

- Anxiety related to anticipating the surgical procedure
- Altered nutrition, less than body requirements, related to anorexia
- Pain, related to the presence of abnormal epithelial cells
- Anticipatory grieving related to the diagnosis of cancer
- Knowledge deficit regarding self-care activities

▷ ## Planning and Implementation

▷ *Goals:* The major goals of the patient may include reduction of anxiety, attainment of optimum nutrition, relief of pain, and adjustment to the diagnosis and to anticipated life style changes.

▷ ## Nursing Interventions

▷ *Reducing Anxiety.* A relaxed, nonthreatening atmosphere is provided so that the patient can express his fears, concerns,

and possibly anger with the diagnosis and prognosis. The nurse encourages the family to listen or ventilate as appropriate. The nurse offers assurance and supports positive coping measures. She advises the patient about any procedures and treatments so that he knows what to expect and suggests that he discuss his feelings with a member of the clergy if desired.

▷ *Promoting Optimal Nutrition.* Small frequent feedings of nonirritating foods are encouraged to decrease gastric irritation. Food supplements should be high in vitamins A and C and iron so that tissue repair is facilitated. If a total gastrectomy is to be performed, then parenteral vitamin B_{12} will need to be administered indefinitely. The nurse monitors the rate and frequency of intravenous therapy. The nurse records intake, output, and daily weights to make sure the patient is maintaining or gaining weight. Signs of dehydration (thirst, dry mucous membranes, poor skin turgor, tachycardia) are assessed and results of daily laboratory studies are reviewed to note any metabolic abnormalities (sodium, potassium, glucose, blood urea nitrogen). Antiemetics are administered as prescribed.

▷ *Relief of Pain.* Analgesics are administered as prescribed. A continuous drip infusion may be necessary for severe pain. The frequency, intensity, and duration of the pain is assessed to determine the effectiveness of the analgesic being administered. The nurse works with the patient to help him manage his pain (*e.g.*, position changes, decreased environmental stimuli, restricted visiting). Nonpharmacologic methods for pain relief such as imagery, distraction, relaxation tapes, backrubs, and massage are suggested, and periods of rest and relaxation are encouraged.

▷ *Psychosocial Support.* The nurse helps the patient express his fears and concerns about his diagnosis. The patient is allowed the freedom to grieve in his own way. His questions are answered honestly, and he is encouraged to participate in his treatment decisions. Some patients mourn the loss of a body part and perceive their surgery as a type of mutilation. Some express disbelief and need reality reinforcement. Privacy should be provided during periods of crying if the patient wants to be alone.

The nurse offers emotional support and involves family members and significant others whenever possible. She must be aware of mood swings and defense mechanisms (denial, rationalization, displacement, regression) and reassure the patient and family members that emotional responses are normal and expected. Professional services are provided if necessary, including those of clergy, psychiatric clinical nurse specialists, psychologists, social workers, and psychiatrists. The nurse projects an empathetic approach and spends time with the patient. Most patients will begin to participate in self-care activities when they have acknowledged their loss.

▷ *Patient Education and Home Health Care.* The patient is advised that it may take 6 months before regular meals can be eaten after a partial resection. Small, frequent feedings are given initially, or he will be fed through a tube; intravenous hyperalimentation may be necessary. With any enteral feeding, the possibility of the dumping syndrome exists, so it must be explained and ways to manage it reviewed.

The patient is told that it may take 3 months before normal activities can be resumed. Daily periods of rest are necessary, and he will have to visit his physician frequently after he is discharged. Changes in life style will be affected by chemotherapy and radiation therapy. The patient needs to know what to expect: length of treatments, expected reactions (nausea, vomiting, anorexia, fatigue), and need for transportation to and from the treatments. Psychological counseling may be necessary for some.

Nutritional counseling is started in the hospital and reinforced at home. Any tube feeding procedure is supervised by a visiting nurse, who teaches the patient and family members how to use the equipment and formulas and how to detect complications. (See pp. 878–882 to review management of tube feedings.) The patient learns to record his daily intake, output, and weight and is taught how to cope with pain, nausea, vomiting, and bloating. He is made aware of those complications that require medical attention, such as bleeding (overt or covert hematemesis, melena), obstruction, perforation, or any symptoms that become consistently worse.

The nurse teaches the patient how to care for his incision and how to examine the wound for signs of infection (malodorous drainage, pain, heat, inflammation, swelling). Any chemotherapy regimen is explained. The patient as well as his family need to know what kind of care will be needed during and after treatments.

▷ Evaluation

Expected Outcomes

1. Experiences less anxiety
   a. Expresses his fears and concerns about surgery
   b. Seeks emotional support
   c. Discusses feelings about surgery with family
   d. Discusses the surgical procedure and postoperative course
2. Attains optimum nutrition
   a. Eats small, frequent meals
   b. Eats foods high in iron and vitamins A and C
   c. Maintains recommended weight
3. Experiences less pain
   a. Takes prescribed medications as scheduled
   b. Rests periodically during the day
   c. Uses relaxation techniques
4. Adjusts to diagnosis
   a. Freely expresses his fears and concerns
   b. Seeks emotional support from family members
   c. Discusses his prognosis
5. Performs self-care activities and adjusts to life style changes
   a. Resumes normal activities within 3 months
   b. Alternates periods of rest and activity
   c. Tolerates three regular meals daily within 6 months after surgery
   d. Manages tube feelings
   e. Adjusts to intravenous hyperalimentation
   f. Adheres to chemotherapy or radiation regimen
   g. Keeps follow-up clinic or physician appointments

In summary, although relatively rare in the United States, cancer of the stomach is of epidemic proportions in certain areas of the world, including portions of Japan. There is a high suspicion that cancer of the stomach is linked to dietary factors. It is usually diagnosed in an advanced stage, making prognosis poor.

Gastric Surgery

Gastric surgery may be performed on patients with peptic ulcers who have life-threatening hemorrhage, obstruction, perforation, or do not respond to medication. It also may be indicated for patients with gastric cancer or trauma. Operative procedures may include a partial gastrectomy (removal of the stomach) or total gastrectomy with either end-to-end or end-to-side esophagojejunostomy anastamosis.

▶ Nursing Process
The Patient Undergoing Gastric Surgery

▷ Assessment

Preoperatively, the patient is assessed for knowledge of preoperative and postoperative surgical routines. The patient's and family's knowledge of the rationale for surgery is assessed. Also preoperatively, the nutritional status is assessed: Has the patient lost weight? How much? Over how long? Does the patient have nausea and vomiting? Has the patient had hematemesis? The patient is assessed for presence of bowel sounds. Palpation of the abdomen is performed to determine if masses can be felt or if there is tenderness.

Postoperatively, the patient is assessed for complications secondary to the surgical intervention such as hemorrhage, infection, abdominal distention, or decreased nutritional status. (See Nursing Process: Caring for The Postoperative Patient in Chap. 22, and The Patient Undergoing Thoracic Surgery in Chap. 25 for the patient who has had a total gastrectomy, as the chest cavity may be entered).

▷ Nursing Diagnoses

Based on all the assessment data, the patient's major nursing diagnoses may include the following:

1. Anxiety related to surgical intervention
2. Knowledge deficit about surgical procedures and postoperative course
3. Altered nutrition, less than body requirements
4. Pain related to surgical incision
5. Knowledge deficit regarding home care

The following potential problems are treated collaboratively by the physician and nurse:

1. Hemorrhage
2. Shock
3. Pulmonary complications
4. Dumping syndrome
5. Steatorrhea
6. Vitamin B_{12} deficiency
7. Gastritis and esophagitis

▷ Planning and Implementation

▷ *Goals:* The major goals of the patient may include reduction of anxiety, knowledge and understanding about the surgical procedure and postoperative course, attainment of optimum nutrition, relief of pain, ability to care for self at home, and absence of complications.

▷ Nursing Interventions

▷ *Reducing Anxiety.* An important part of the preoperative nursing care involves allaying the patient's fears and anxieties about the impending surgery and its implications. The nurse encourages the patient to express his feelings and answers his questions. If the patient is experiencing hemorrhage, perforation, or acute obstruction, adequate psychological preparation of the patient may not be possible. In this event, the nurse caring for the patient postoperatively should anticipate his concerns, fears, and questions. For all postoperative patients the nurse should be available for support and further explanations.

▷ *Increasing Knowledge.* It is also necessary to explain the routine preoperative and postoperative activities to the patient such as preoperative medications, nasogastric intubation, intravenous fluids, abdominal dressings, and pulmonary care. These procedures will need to be reinforced postoperatively—especially if the patient had emergency surgery.

▷ *Maintaining Adequate Nutrition.* The patient should be evaluated preoperatively for nutritional status. Many patients with gastric cancer are malnourished and may require preoperative enteral or more frequently total parenteral nutrition (see p. 885). Postoperatively, parenteral nutrition may be continued to provide caloric needs as well as provide fluids lost in drainage and vomitus.

After the return of bowel sounds and removal of the nasogastric tube, fluids may be given, followed by food in small portions. Bland foods are gradually added until the patient is able to eat six small meals a day and drink 120 ml of fluid between meals. The key to increasing the dietary content is to offer food and fluids gradually as tolerated and to recognize that each person's tolerance is different.

Dysphagia may be noticed in those patients who have had truncal vagotomy, which causes trauma to the lower esophagus. If regurgitation occurs in patients who have had gastric surgery, the patient may be eating too much or too fast. It also may indicate that edema along the suture line is preventing fluids and food from moving into the intestinal tract. If gastric retention does occur, it may be necessary to reinstate nasogastric suction; pressure must be low to avoid disruption of the suture line.

With regard to long-term management of these patients, weight loss is a common problem because the patient experiences early fullness that curbs his appetite. Anorexia may also be due to the dumping syndrome (see below) which occurs in about one fifth of patients after partial gastrectomy.

The following teaching points are emphasized:

- Fluids should be taken before or between meals rather than with meals
- Smaller but more frequent meals should be eaten
- Meal composition should be more dry than liquid
- Foods with small molecule carbohydrates, such as sucrose and glucose, should be avoided; fat may be consumed to tolerable levels

- It may be advisable to supplement the diet with vitamins and medium chain triglycerides

Other dietary deficiencies the nurse should be aware of include (1) malabsorption of organic iron, which may require supplementation with oral or parenteral iron, and (2) low serum level of vitamin B_{12}, which may require supplementation by the intramuscular route.

▷ *Relief of Pain.* The patient is given analgesics postoperatively as prescribed by the physician to maintain an acceptable level of comfort. Care must be taken to maintain the patient's ability to adequately perform pulmonary care activities (deep breathing and coughing) and to ambulate. The nurse assesses the effectiveness of analgesic intervention. Positioning the patient in a modified Fowler's position promotes comfort as well as allows for easy drainage of the stomach in the patient with a partial gastrectomy.

The function of the nasogastric tube is maintained to prevent distention and resultant pain. The amount of nasogastric drainage from the patient following a total gastrectomy will normally be small.

▷ *Home Health Care.* Patient teaching is based on assessment of the patient's physical and psychological readiness to return to his home and the community. (If the patient has gastric cancer, goals may be for maintenance and palliation.) The patient and family will benefit from a team approach to discharge care. The team members include the community nurse, physician, nutritionist, and the social worker. Written instructions about meals, activities, medications, and follow-up care are indicated.

▷ Collaborative Interventions

▷ *Hemorrhage.* Hemorrhage is occasionally a complication after gastric surgery. The patient exhibits the usual signs (see Chap. 22), and may vomit bright red blood in considerable amounts. Nasogastric drainage should be assessed for the type and amount of drainage; some bloody drainage for the first 12 hours is expected, but excessive bleeding should be reported. The abdominal dressing should also be assessed for bleeding.

Because this experience is likely to be upsetting to the patient and family, the nurse should remain calm and reassure the patient. Emergency measures are performed, such as nasogastric lavage and administration of blood and blood products.

▷ *Shock.* Shock has been mentioned as a complication, especially in very ill patients. The restoration of normal temperature and the administration of fluids are the prophylactic measures necessary. For symptoms and treatment of shock, see Chap. 22.

▷ *Pulmonary Complications.* Pulmonary complications frequently follow upper abdominal incisions because of the tendency for shallow respirations. Therefore, the nurse uses foresight and initiates appropriate preventive measures to promote optimum oxygen–carbon dioxide exchange and adequate circulation such as coughing, deep breathing, and ambulation. Auscultation of the patient's lungs is performed every 4 hours.

▷ *Dumping Syndrome.* The term *dumping syndrome* designates an unpleasant set of vasomotor and gastrointestinal symptoms that occur after meals in 10% to 50% of patients who have had gastrointestinal surgery or a form of vagotomy.

Clinical Manifestations. Early symptoms may include a sensation of fullness, weakness, faintness, dizziness, palpitations, diaphoresis, cramping pains, and diarrhea. Later, there is a rapid elevation of blood glucose, followed by a compensatory reaction of insulin secretion. This results in a reactive hypoglycemia, which also is unpleasant for the patient. Symptoms that may occur 10 to 90 minutes after eating are vasomotor and are manifested by pallor, perspiration, palpitations, headache, and feelings of warmth, dizziness, and even drowsiness.

Pathophysiology. The pathophysiology underlying this syndrome is not completely understood, but there may be several causes for its occurrence. One is the mechanical result of surgery in which a small gastric remnant connects into the jejunum through a large opening. Foods that are high in carbohydrates and electrolytes have to be diluted in the jejunum before absorption can take place; yet the passage of food from the stomach remnant into the jejunum is too rapid. The ingestion of fluid at mealtime is another factor that causes the stomach contents to empty rapidly into the jejunum. The symptoms that occur are probably a result of rapid distention of the jejunal loop anastomosed to the stomach. The hypertonic intestinal contents draw extracellular fluid from the circulating blood volume into the jejunum to dilute the high concentration of electrolytes and sugars.

Nursing Interventions. In anticipation of the possibility of the patient's experiencing the dumping syndrome, nursing intervention is directed toward proper dietary instruction.

- The patient should be positioned in a semirecumbent position during mealtime. After the meal, he should lie down for 20 to 30 minutes to delay stomach emptying.
- Fluids are discouraged with meals, but may be given up to an hour before mealtime or 1 hour after mealtime.
- Fat may be given to tolerance, but carbohydrate intake should be kept low (sucrose and glucose are avoided).
- Antispasmodics, as prescribed, also may aid in delaying the emptying of the stomach.

Surgery is resorted to only if absolutely necessary (less than 1% of patients).

▷ *Steatorrhea.* Steatorrhea (unabsorbed fat in the stool) is partially the result of rapid gastric emptying, which prevents adequate mixing with pancreatic and biliary secretions. In mild cases, steatorrhea can be controlled by reducing the intake of fat and administering an antimotility drug.

▷ *Vitamin B$_{12}$ Deficiency.* Total gastrectomy brings to a complete halt the production of "intrinsic factor," the gastric secretion that is required for the absorption of vitamin B$_{12}$ from the gastrointestinal tract. Therefore, unless this vitamin is supplied by parenteral injection throughout life, the patient inevitably suffers from vitamin B$_{12}$ deficiency, which leads in time to a condition identical to that of a patient with pernicious anemia in relapse. All of the manifestations of pernicious anemia, including macrocytic anemia and combined system disease, may be expected to develop within a period of 5 years or less, to progress in severity thereafter, and, in the absence of therapy, to prove fatal. This complication is avoided by the regular monthly intramuscular injection of 100 to 200 μg of vitamin B$_{12}$, a regimen that should be started without delay after gastrectomy.

▷ *Gastritis and Esophagitis.* With the removal of the pylorus, which acts as a barrier to the reflux of duodenal contents, bile reflux gastritis and esophagitis may occur. This is manifested by burning epigastric pain and the vomiting of bile material. Eating or vomiting does not relieve the situation. Binding agents such as cholestyramine, (Questran), aluminum hydroxide gel, or metoclopramide hydrochloride (Reglan) have been used with some success.

▷ Evaluation

Expected Outcomes

1. Experiences less anxiety
   a. States understanding of surgical procedure
   b. Expresses his fears and concerns about surgery
   c. Seeks emotional support via appropriate channels
2. Expresses knowledge regarding postoperative course
   a. Discusses the surgical procedure and postoperative course
   b. Discusses feelings about surgery with family
3. Attains optimum nutrition
   a. Maintains a reasonable weight
   b. Explains the rationale for feeding schedule
   c. Is compliant with vitamin supplementation
   d. Does not experience nausea and vomiting
4. Attains optimal level of comfort
   a. Verbalizes sufficient pain control
5. Is compliant with home care needs
   a. States need for supplemental vitamins
   b. States dietary restrictions
   c. Is aware of home care agencies available
6. Exhibits absence of complications
   a. Maintains stable vital signs
   b. Exhibits no hemorrhage
   c. Deep breathes and coughs every 2 to 4 hours
   d. Lungs are clear to auscultation
   e. Ambulates first or second postoperative day
   f. Maintains weight
   g. Is compliant with medication regimen

In summary, the patient undergoing gastric surgery requires explanation of preoperative and postoperative procedures. Surgery may be performed for emergency situations such as hemorrhage, perforation, and obstruction, or for patients not responding to medication for ulcer treatment, as well as for patients with trauma or gastric cancer. Each patient must be considered as an individual with individualized needs. Nursing Care Plan 36–2 summarizes the nursing care that these patients may require.

Bibliography

Books

Bates B. A Guide to Physical Examination and History Taking, 5th ed. Philadelphia, JB Lippincott, 1991.

DeVita VT, Hellman S, and Rosenberg SA (eds). Principles and Practice of Oncology, 3rd ed. Philadelphia, JB Lippincott, 1989.

Gitnick G et al. Principles and Practices of Gastroenterology and Hepatology. New York, Elsevier, 1988.

Groenwald S (ed). Cancer Nursing: Principles and Practices. Boston, Jones & Bartlett, 1990.

Margulis AR and Burhemn HJ. Alimentary Tract Radiology, 4th ed. St Louis, CV Mosby, 1989.

Sleisenger MH and Fordran JS. Gastrointestinal Diseases: Pathophysiology, Diagnosis, Management. Philadelphia, WB Saunders, 1989.

Walsh J et al. Manual of Home Health Care Nursing. Philadelphia, JB Lippincott, 1987.

Journals

Asterisks indicate nursing research articles.

Peptic Ulcers and Gastritis

Carson JL and Strom BL. The gastrointestinal side effects of the nonsteroidal anti-inflammatory drugs. J Clin Pharmacol 1988 Jun; 28(6): 554–559.

Ganz RA. Smoking, life stresses, and personality disorders in ulcer patients. Gastroenterooology 1987 Jul; 93(1): 221–222.

Hornick RB. Peptic ulcer disease: A bacterial infection? N Engl J Med 1987 Jun; 316(25): 1598–1600.

Koch MJ. How to detect and heal lesions and relieve pain. Consultant 1987 May; 27(5): 21–24.

Konopad E and Noseworthy T. Stress ulceration: A serious complication in critically ill patients. Heart Lung 1988 Jul; 17(4): 339–347.

Matthewson K et al. Which peptic ulcer patients bleed. Gut 1988 Jan; 29(1): 70–74.

McNulty CA. Campylobacter-associated gastritis. Practitioner 1987 Feb; 231(424): 176–178.

Michaletz PA and Graham DY. Gastritis. Postgrad Med 1988 Feb; 83(3): 98–106.

Miller TA. Emergencies in acid-peptic disease. Gastroenterol Clin North Am 1988 Jun; 17(2): 303–315

Wyatt J and Dixon MF. Chronic gastritis: A pathogenetic approach. J Pathol 1988 Feb; 154(2): 113–124.

Gastrointestinal Bleeding

Christensen J et al. Incidence of perforated and bleeding peptic ulcers before and after the introduction of H_2 receptor antagonists. Ann Surg 1988 Jan; 207(1): 4–6.

Eastwood GL. Upper GI bleeding: Differential diagnosis and management. Hosp Med 1987 Feb; 23(2): 57–63.

Eastwood GL. Upper GI bleeding: Differential diagnosis and management. Hosp Med 1987 Mar; 23(3): 44–52.

Farley J. Myths and facts about gastrointestinal bleeding. Nursing 1988 Mar; 18(3):25.

Patras AZ et al. Managing GI bleeding. It takes a two-tract mind. Nursing 1988 Apr; 18(4): 68–75.

Morbid Obesity

Borkin JS et al. The effects of morbid obesity and the Garren–Edwards gastric bubble on solid phase gastric emptying. Clin J Gastroenterol 1988 Dec; 83(12): 1364–1367.

*Bufalino J et al. Surgery for morbid obesity: The patient's experience. Appl Nurs Res 1989 Feb; 2(1): 16–22.

Council of Scientific Affairs. Treatment of obesity in adults. JAMA 1988 Nov 4: 260(17): 2547–2551.

Kennedy–Caldwell C. The morbidly obese surgical patient. Crit Care Nurse 1987 Sep/Oct; 7(5): 87–89.

Gastric Cancer

Boring et al. Cancer statistics 1991. CA 1991 Jan/Feb; 41(1): 19–36.

Feickert DM et al. Gastrectomy for stomach carcinoma. AORN 1988 Jun; 47(6): 1395–1406.

Frank–Stromborg M. The epidemiology and primary prevention of gastric and esophageal cancer. Cancer Nurs 1989 Apr; 12(2): 53–64.

Foltz AT. Nutritional factors in the prevention of gastrointestinal cancer. Semin Oncol Nurs 1988 Nov; 4(4): 239–245.

Frogge MH. Future perspectives and nursing issues in gastrointestinal cancer. Semin Oncol Nurs 1988 Nov; 4(4): 300–302.

Treat J et al. Therapy of advanced gastric carcinoma. Am J Clin Oncol 1989 Apr; 12(2): 162–168

Wong JF. Stomach cancer. Semin Oncol Nurs 1988 Nov; 4(4): 257–264.

Zollinger–Ellison Syndrome

Maton PN et al. Medical management of patients with Zollinger–Ellison syndrome who have had a previous gastric surgery: A prospective study. Gastroenterology 1988 Feb; 94(3): 294–299.

Wolfe MM and Jensen RT. Zollinger–Ellison syndrome. Current concepts in diagnosis and management. N Engl J Med 1987 Nov; 317(19): 1200–1209.

Therapy

Boey J. Proximal gastric vagotomy. The preferred operation for perforations in acute duodenal ulcer. Ann Surg 1988 Aug; 208(2): 169–174.

Critchlow JF. Comparative efficacy of parenteral histimine (H_2)-antagonists in acid suppression for the prevention of stress ulceration. Ann Surg 1987 Dec; 83(6A): 23–28.

Feickert DM. Gastric surgery: Your cruicial pre- and postop role. RN 1987 Jan; 50(1): 24–35.

Gustavsson S and Kelly A. Total gastrectomy for benign disease. Surg Clin North Am 1987 Jun; 67(3): 539–550.

Haglund U et al. Esophageal and jejunal motor function after total gastrectomy and Roux-Y esophagojejunostomy. Am J Surg 1989 Mar; 157(3): 308–311.

Smout AJ et al. Gastric emptying and postprandial symptoms after Billroth II resection. Surgery 1987 Jan; 101(1): 27–34.

Sontag SJ. Current status of maintenance therapy in peptic ulcer diseases. Am J Gastroenterol 1988 Jun; 83(6): 607–617.

Texter EC. A critical look at the clinical use of antacids in acid-peptic disease and gastric acid rebound. Am J Gastroenterol 1989 Feb; 84(2): 97–108.

Information/Resources

Agencies

American Cancer Society
  1599 Clifton Rd, NE, Atlanta, GA 30329
American Digestive Disease Society
  420 Lexington Ave, New York, NY 10017
American Gastroenterological Association
  6900 Grove Rd, Thorofare, NJ 08086
National Interagency Council on Smoking and Health
  419 Park Ave South, New York, NY 10016

37

Management of Patients With Intestinal and Rectal Disorders

Learning Objectives

On completion of this chapter, the learner will be able to:

1. Specify the health care teaching needs of patients with constipation and those with diarrhea
2. Use the nursing process as a framework for care of patients with constipation and patients with diarrhea
3. Compare the primary malabsorption conditions with regard to their pathophysiology, clinical manifestations, and management
4. Use the nursing process as a framework for care of patients with appendicitis and those with diverticulitis
5. Compare Crohn's disease and ulcerative colitis with regard to their pathophysiology, clinical manifestations, diagnostic evaluation, and medical, surgical, and nursing management
6. Use the nursing process as a framework for care of the patient with a chronic inflammatory bowel disease
7. Describe the responsibilities of the nurse in meeting the needs of the patient with an intestinal ostomy
8. Use the nursing process as a framework for care of the patient with cancer of the colon or rectum
9. Describe the various types of intestinal obstruction and their management
10. Use the nursing process as a framework for care of the patient with an anorectal condition

Gastrointestinal (GI) diseases constitute a major health problem, afflicting more than 34 million Americans. About 20 million of them have a chronic disorder and about 2 million are permanently disabled. Gastrointestinal diseases account for 200,000 absences from work daily and for men are the leading cause of time lost from work. About $100 million is paid annually in benefits to veterans who receive payments for service-connected disabilities due to digestive conditions. The greatest cost, however, is in the number of lives lost annually (200,000).

These gastrointestinal diseases are significant because the majority of the digestive process occurs on the intestinal surface and in the intestinal cell. Absorption also occurs here. The types of diseases and disorders that affect the lower GI tract are many and varied. Two problems that occur frequently with many of these diseases and disorders are constipation and diarrhea. These two problems are also commonly seen in the elderly. In all age groups, a fast-paced life-style, high levels of stress, irregular eating habits, insufficient intake of fiber and water, and lack of daily exercise contribute to these problems. Laxatives are among the most popular over-the-counter medications purchased in the United States today, and laxative abuse is becoming a serious problem in the aged population. Nurses can have an impact on the chronicity of these problems by identifying behavior patterns that put patients at risk, by educating the public about prevention and management, and by helping those afflicted improve their condition and prevent complications.

Constipation

Constipation refers to an abnormal infrequency of defecation, and also to abnormal hardening of stools that makes their passage difficult and sometimes painful.

Most individuals have at least one bowel movement a day. The range of normal, however, extends from three movements per day to three or fewer per week. In persons who are constipated, defecation is irregular and is complicated by hardened stools. Some constipated persons occasionally have a diarrhea of liquid stools as a result of the irritation caused by the presence in the colon of hard, dry fecal masses. Such stools contain a good deal of mucus, secreted by glands in the colon in response to these irritating masses. In severe constipation, the rectum may become impacted, that is, filled with masses of hard feces that must be softened by instillations of oil before they can be washed out by an enema.

Constipation can be caused by certain medications (tranquilizers, anticholinergics, narcotics, antacids with aluminum), rectal/anal disorders (hemorrhoids, fissures), obstruction (cancer of the bowel), metabolic and neurologic conditions (diabetes mellitus, multiple sclerosis), endocrine conditions (hypothyroidism, pheochromocytoma), lead poisoning, and connective tissue disorders (scleroderma, lupus erythematosus). Other diseases of the colon commonly associated with constipation are irritable bowel syndrome and diverticular disease.

Causative factors include weakness, immobility, debility, fatigue, and inability to increase intra-abdominal pressure to facilitate the passage of stools, such as occurs with emphysema.

Many people develop constipation because they are busy and cannot or will not take the time to defecate. In the United States constipation is also seen as a result of dietary habits (low consumption of fiber), lack of regular exercise, and a stress-filled life.

Constipation also can result from the chronic use of laxatives, which eventually override the bowel's sensitivity to the need to eliminate. Chronic laxative use is a major health concern in the United States.

The inability to pass a hard stool can also occur with acute processes such as appendicitis. Laxatives given in this instance may produce perforation of the inflamed appendix. In general, a cathartic should not be given while the patient has fever, nausea, or pain merely because the bowels fail to move. A cathartic should never be prescribed in the presence of inflammatory bowel disease.

Gerontologic Considerations. Elderly persons report problems with constipation five times more frequently than younger people. A number of factors contribute to this increased frequency. Persons who have loose-fitting dentures or have lost their teeth have difficulty chewing and frequently choose soft, processed foods that are low in fiber. Convenience foods, also low in fiber, are popular for those who have lost interest in eating. Some older people reduce their fluid intake if they are not eating regular meals; decreased fluid intake decreases bulk and makes passage of stool more difficult. Lack of exercise and prolonged bed rest also contribute to constipation by decreasing abdominal muscle tone.

Sometimes older persons imagine that they are constipated because they do not have a daily bowel movement and have misconceptions about what is and is not normal.

Pathophysiology. The pathophysiology of constipation is poorly understood. It is believed, however, to be related to interference with one of three major functions of the colon: mucosal transport (mucosal secretions facilitate movement of colon contents), myoelectric activity (mixing of the rectal mass and propulsive actions), or the processes involved in defecation. The urge to defecate is normally stimulated by rectal distention, which initiates a series of four actions: stimulation of the inhibitory rectoanal reflex, relaxation of the internal sphincter muscle, relaxation of the external sphincter muscle and muscles in the pelvic region, and increased intra-abdominal pressure. Interference in any of these four processes can thus lead to nonorganic or idiopathic constipation.

When the urge to defecate is ignored, the rectal mucous membrane and musculature become insensitive to the presence of fecal masses, and consequently a stronger stimulus is required to produce the necessary peristaltic rush for defecation. The initial effect of this fecal retention is to produce irritability of the colon, which at this stage frequently goes into spasm, especially after meals, giving rise to colicky midabdominal or low abdominal pains. After several years of this process, the colon loses muscular tone; it is essentially unresponsive to normal stimuli. At this point, the patient may be said to have *atonic constipation*, whereas in the earlier stage the condition is sometimes referred to as *spastic constipation*, although neither type should be regarded as a separate entity. Atony of the bowel also occurs with aging, and this can be complicated with constant use of laxatives.

Clinical Manifestations. Clinical manifestations include abdominal distention, *borborygmus* (intestinal rumbling), pain and pressure, decreased appetite, headache, fatigue, indigestion, a sensation of incomplete emptying, straining at stool, and the elimination of small-volume, hard, dry stool.

Diagnostic Evaluation.   Diagnosis of constipation is based on a complete physical examination, a barium enema, a sigmoidoscopy, and stool testing for occult blood. These tests are completed to determine whether this symptom is due to spasm or narrowing of the bowel. Anorectal pressure studies may be performed to determine malfunction of the muscle and sphincter. Idiopathic constipation is diagnosed after an organic cause is eliminated.

Management.   Treatment should be aimed at the underlying cause of constipation. Management includes discontinuing abusive laxative use, recommending the inclusion of fiber in the diet, prescribing an exercise routine to strengthen abdominal muscles, and patterning behaviors related to establishing a normal bowel movement (responding to reflexes, "heeding the call," setting a daily defecation time, drinking warm water with a meal). The daily addition to the diet of 6 to 12 teaspoonfuls of unprocessed bran is recommended, especially for the treatment of constipation in the elderly. A high-residue diet induces rapid movement through the colon and a large, soft stool.

If laxative use is necessary, one of the following may be prescribed: bulk-forming agents, saline/osmotic agents, lubricants, stimulants, or fecal softeners. The physiologic action and patient teaching related to these laxatives are described in Table 37–1. Enemas and rectal suppositories are not rec-

TABLE 37–1.   *Laxatives: Classification, Agent, Action, and Patient Education*

Classification	Sample Agent	Action	Patient Education
Bulk-Forming	Psyllium hydrophilic muciloid (Metamucil)	Polysaccharides and cellulose derivatives mix with intestinal fluids, swell, and stimulate peristalsis.	Take with 8 ounces of water and follow with 8 ounces of water. Do not take dry. Report abdominal distention or unusual amount of flatulence.
Saline/Osmotic Agent	Magnesium hydroxide (Milk of Magnesia)	Nonabsorbable magnesium ions alter stool consistency by drawing water into the intestines by osmosis; peristalsis is stimulated. Action occurs within 2 hours.	The liquid preparation is more effective than the tablet form. Only short-term use is recommended because of toxicity (CNS or neuromuscular depession, electrolyte imbalance). Magnesium laxatives should not be taken by patients with renal insufficiency.
Lubricant	Mineral oil	Nonabsorbable hydrocarbons soften fecal matter by lubricating the intestinal mucosa. The passage of stool is facilitated. Action occurs within 6–8 hours.	Do not take with meals because mineral oils may impair the absorption of fat-soluble vitamins and delay gastric emptying. Swallow carefully because drops of oil that gain access to the pharynx may produce a lipid pneumonia.
Stimulant	Bisacodyl (Dulcolax)	Irritates the colon epithelium by stimulating sensory nerve endings and increasing mucosal secretions. Action occurs within 6–8 hours.	Catharsis may cause fluid and electrolyte imbalance, especially in the elderly. Tablets should be swallowed, not crushed or chewed. Avoid milk or antacids within 1 hour of taking the drug because the enteric coating may dissolve prematurely.
Fecal Softener	Dioctyl sodium sulfosuccinate (Colace)	Hydrates the stool by its surfactant action on the colonic epithelium (increases the wetting efficiency of intestinal water). Aqueous and fatty substances are mixed. The medication does not exert a laxative action.	Can be used safely by patients who should avoid straining (cardiac patients, patients with anorectal disorders)

ommended for constipation and should be reserved for the treatment of impaction or for bowel preparation for surgery or diagnostic procedures. If long-term laxative use is absolutely necessary, the physician may prescribe a bulk-forming agent in combination with an osmotic laxative.

▶ Nursing Process
The Patient With Constipation

▷ Assessment

When talking with patients about their bowel habits, it is important to keep in mind that some may be embarrassed to discuss such a personal body function. Tact and respect for the patient are generally appreciated. Questions of a more personal matter may be placed later in the history after rapport has been established.

Health History
- Onset and duration of constipation
- Life style (exercise, nutrition, stress)
- Occupation
- Past elimination pattern
- Current elimination pattern
- Laxative/enema use
- Current drug therapy
- Past medical history
- Description of color, odor, consistency of stool
- Presence of any of the following:
    Rectal pressure/fullness
    Abdominal pain
    Straining at defecation
    Watery diarrhea
    Flatulence

Physical Assessment
- Auscultation of abdomen for bowel sounds
- Characteristics of bowel sounds—infrequent, absent, high-pitched, gurgling
- Palpation for distention—absent, slight, moderate, severe
- Inspection of perianal area for hemorrhoids, fissures, and signs of irritation

▷ Nursing Diagnoses

Based on all the assessment data, the patient's major nursing diagnoses may include the following:

- Constipation or fecal impaction related to health habits
- Knowledge deficit about health maintenance practices to prevent constipation
- Anxiety related to concern about irregular elimination pattern

▷ Planning and Implementation

▷ *Goals:*   The major goals of the patient may include restoration/maintenance of a regular pattern of normal bowel elimination, adequate intake of fluids and roughage foods, understanding of methods for avoiding constipation, and relief of anxiety.

▷ Nursing Interventions

▷ *Maintenance of Elimination.*   The maintenance of elimination is basic to the care of every patient. The effort entailed in defecation is considerable. With the use of a bedpan, the muscular strain is inevitably greater; when constipation is also present, the performance of this function can be extremely fatiguing if not altogether exhausting. This is a serious consideration in the management of patients with congestive heart failure, those who have suffered a recent myocardial infarction and are susceptible to cardiac rupture, and those with arterial hypertension.

To facilitate elimination, the patient is assisted to assume the normal position for defecation. The semi-squatting position maximizes the use of the abdominal muscles and the force of gravity. Hospitalized patients who cannot use the bathroom experience less strain if assisted to a bedside commode, or if they are seated on a bedpan at the side of the bed with feet supported on a chair. If the patient cannot sit up, a small support should be placed under the lumbosacral curve to minimize strain and increase comfort while using the bedpan.

▷ *Patient Education and Home Health Care.*   Most of the patient's goals can be achieved through a thorough teaching program that presents information about the causes of constipation and the dietary practices and exercise activity that can promote healthy bowel habits.

In functional constipation, the role of the nurse is to assist with the reeducation of the patient. The physiology of defecation should be explained carefully, with particular emphasis on the importance of heeding promptly the urge to defecate. The patient is instructed to have a regular time for defecation, preferably after a meal. Thinking about the act of defecation (*i.e.*, "autosuggestion") may be an aid in initiating the reflex. A small footstool to promote flexion of the hips ensures an optimal posture during defecation.

The patient must know what constitutes a normal diet and should be aware of the similarities and differences between the prescribed diet and the normal diet. In general, a high-residue, high-fiber diet is prescribed for atonic constipation; a bland or low-residue diet is indicated for the patient with an irritable colon. For the elderly, the addition of 2 g of bran to cereal daily can markedly increase the number of spontaneous bowel movements and decrease the use of cathartics, stool softeners, and enemas.

The nurse recommends frequent ambulation and abdominal muscle toning exercises to promote defecation. Abdominal toning exercises consist of contracting abdominal muscles four times daily, doing sit-ups with knees flexed and heels on the floor, and doing straight leg lifts while in a lying position. A patient confined to bed is encouraged to perform range-of-motion exercises, turn frequently from side to side and lie prone (if not contraindicated) for 30 minutes every 4 hours. These exercises increase abdominal muscle tone, which helps propel colon contents.

▷ *Reduction of Anxiety.*   Patients who worry about having a *daily* bowel movement need reassurance. It is helpful to carefully explain that some healthy persons have a bowel movement three times daily while others do so only two or three times a week. Knowing that some of the food eaten may normally remain in the intestinal tract 48 hours after ingestion will help the patient to understand and accept the fact that a daily bowel evacuation is not always necessary. The use of laxatives should be discontinued. If the feces remain in the rectum too long and become dehydrated and hardened, the patient may be instructed to instill 60 to 90 ml (2 to 3 oz) of warm oil into the rectum at bedtime to soften the feces. A small enema of physiologic saline the next morning should help in removal of the softened feces.

If a laxative regimen has been prescribed, the patient should be made aware of the consequences of laxative dependency and possible fecal impaction. Preventive measures include the gradual tapering off of laxative use; sufficient fluid and fiber intake; an adequate exercise program; and modification of contributory life-style factors (*e.g.*, ignoring the urge to defecate, stress).

Evaluation

Expected Outcomes
1. Establishes a regular pattern of bowel elimination
   a. Includes a time for defecation as part of daily routine
   b. Participates in a regular exercise program
   c. Avoids laxative abuse
   d. Drinks 2 to 3 liters of water daily
   e. Includes foods high in bulk in the diet (fresh fruits, bran, nuts, whole grain breads and cereals, cooked fruits and vegetables)
   f. Reports soft, formed stool every day or every 2 to 3 days
2. Demonstrates understanding of measures appropriate for preventing constipation
   a. Identifies measures that promote defecation
   b. Explains importance for fluids and foods high in bulk.
   c. Performs abdominal muscle toning exercises
3. Experiences less anxiety about bowel function
   a. Identifies measures that can be used to prevent or relieve constipation
   b. Alters life-style to promote normal bowel function.
   c. Avoids use of laxatives unless prescribed.

Complications of Constipation

Valsalva Maneuver.   Straining at stool has a striking effect on the arterial blood pressure (*Valsalva maneuver*). During the period of active straining, the flow of venous blood in the chest is temporarily impeded because of an increase in intrathoracic pressure that tends to collapse the large veins in the chest. The atria and the ventricles receive less blood, and consequently less is delivered by the systolic contractions of the left ventricle; the cardiac output is decreased, and there is a transient drop in arterial pressure. Almost immediately after this period of hypotension, a rise in arterial pressure occurs; the pressure is elevated momentarily to a point far exceeding the original level (the "rebound" phenomenon). In patients with arterial hypertension, this compensatory reaction may be exaggerated greatly, and the peaks of pressure attained may be dangerously high—sufficient, indeed, to rupture a major artery in the brain or elsewhere.

Fecal Impaction.   Fecal impaction refers to an accumulated mass of dry feces that cannot be expelled. The mass may be palpable on digital examination, may cause pressure on the colon mucosa that results in ulcer formation, and may cause the frequent seepage of liquid stools. Treatment consists of mineral oil and saline enemas and manual extraction of the stool.

Megacolon.   Megacolon refers to a dilated and atonic colon caused by a fecal mass that obstructs the passage of colon contents. Symptoms include constipation, liquid fecal incontinence, and abdominal distention. The obstruction, which is diagnosed on radiographic examination, can lead to perforation and an emergency colectomy.

Cathartic Colon.   Cathartic colon refers to mucosal atrophy of the colon with muscle thickening and fibrosis subsequent to the chronic use of laxatives. Symptoms include hypokalemia, metabolic alkalosis, malabsorption, and liquid fecal seepage. Treatment is directed at relieving the symptoms.

Diarrhea

Diarrhea is a condition in which there is an unusual frequency of bowel movements (more than 3/day), as well as changes in the amount (more than 200 g/day), and the consistency (increased stool liquidity). It is usually associated with urgency, perianal discomfort, incontinence, or a combination of these. Three factors determine its severity: intestinal secretions, altered mucosal absorption, and increased motility.

Diarrhea can be classified as *large volume*, *small volume*, or *infectious*. Depending on the quantity of daily unformed stools, it can also be described as mild (1 to 3 unformed stools/24 hours), moderate (3 to 6 unformed stools/24 hours), or severe (more than 6 unformed stools/24 hours with associated symptoms, fever, or blood in stool).

Disease processes that are associated with diarrhea are irritable bowel syndrome, ulcerative colitis, carbohydrate malabsorption, anal sphincter deficit, Zollinger–Ellison syndrome, intestinal obstruction/ileus, viral infection, and bacterial infection.

Pathophysiology.   *Acute*, or *large-volume*, *diarrhea* is caused by an increased secretion of water and electrolytes by the intestinal mucosa. This occurs because water is pulled into the intestines by the osmotic pressure of nonabsorbed particles or because intestinal secretions are increased. *Small-volume diarrhea* is caused by increased peristaltic action of the intestines and is usually due to inflammatory bowel disease (ulcerative colitis, Crohn's disease). *Infectious diarrhea*, which is caused by an infectious agent, results in an acute increase in the water content of feces due to increased mucosal cell secretion of water. Peristaltic action is also increased. Common infectious agents are *Shigella*, *Escherichia coli*, and *Campylobacter jejuni*. The most common intestinal irritants are the products of certain bacteria present either in the intestine or in the food before it was eaten. In the case of the enteric pathogens, the organisms causing bacillary dysentery, bacterial growth with release of the irritating toxins takes place in the intestine. Conversely, many cases of food poisoning are due to the ingestion of food that is contaminated and already contains the toxin. *Staphylococcus aureus*, for example, if given an opportunity to multiply in food, produces a toxin that is extremely irritating to the intestinal tract.

Preventive Health Measures.   Precautions include ensuring that proper storage and refrigeration facilities are available and are used for the handling of all fresh fruits and meats. Meat products should be cooked thoroughly and either consumed promptly or refrigerated immediately. Milk and milk products should be refrigerated and protected from contamination. Food items that are particularly likely to cause infection because they provide the best environment for bacterial growth, include custards and cream fillings. Such materials should be cooked thoroughly and then refrigerated immediately.

Proper cleaning, especially in the kitchen, is obviously very important in the prevention of epidemic diarrhea. All materials used in the preparation and the serving of food must be cleaned rigorously and kept in immaculate condition. All food handlers should receive detailed instructions in hygienic principles and practices and, on the development of any illness that is potentially infectious, should be relieved of their duties immediately.

Clinical Manifestations.   In acute cases the stools are grayish brown, foul smelling, and filled with undigested particles of food and mucus. The patient complains of abdominal cramps, distention, intestinal rumbling (borborygmus), anorexia, and thirst. Painful straining (tenesmus) of the anus may occur with each defecation.

The diarrhea in food poisoning is explosive in onset, develops within a very few hours after the toxic meal, and, except in severe cases, subsides within 1 or 2 days—as soon as the toxin is excreted and the inflammatory response decreases. There is little or no fever, and usually the only associated symptoms are those directly attributable to the diarrhea, namely, dehydration and weakness.

Dysentery resulting from the growth of gastrointestinal pathogens within the gastrointestinal tract, however, develops with a more gradual onset and persists for several days or weeks.

Diagnostic Evaluation.   Patients with diarrhea in whom the diagnosis is not evident should have a complete blood count (CBC), chemical profile, urinalysis, and a routine stool examination as well as a stool exam for infectious or parasitic organisms. Proctosigmoidoscopy and barium enema may also be necessary.

Management.   Primary medical management is directed at controlling or curing the underlying disease. Certain drugs, (*e.g.*, prednisone) may reduce the severity of the diarrhea and the disease. Sometimes there is specific therapy for the underlying process.

For mild diarrhea, oral fluids are immediately increased and an oral glucose and electrolyte solution may be prescribed to rehydrate the patient. For moderate diarrhea, nonspecific drugs such as diphenoxylate (Lomotil) and loperamide (Imodium) are also prescribed to decrease motility for diarrhea of a noninfectious source. Antimicrobial agents are prescribed when an infectious agent has been identified or when the diarrhea is severe.

Intravenous therapy may be necessary for rapid hydration, especially for the very young or the elderly.

Gerontologic Considerations.   Older persons can quickly become dehydrated and hypokalemic from episodes of diarrhea. Accurate intake and output records are kept to determine fluid loss. All output is measured, including liquid stools. Urinary output of less than 30 ml/hour for 2 to 3 consecutive hours is reported to the physician. Hypokalemia is manifested by muscle weakness, paresthesia, hypotension, anorexia, and drowsiness. A potassium level below 3.0 mEq/L is reported to the physician,

because decreased potassium causes cardiac dysrhythmias that can lead to death (atrial and ventricular tachycardia, ventricular fibrillation, and premature ventricular contractions). The older person taking digitalis must be aware of the signs of hypokalemia, because low levels of potassium potentiate the action of digitalis, which can lead to digitalis toxicity.

Older persons need ready access to a bathroom because they may not be able to control elimination fully. They may need help with ambulation if a mobility problem exists.

The older person's skin is very sensitive because of decreased turgor and reduced subcutaneous fat layers. Enzymes from diarrheal stool are irritating and can cause excoriation. The patient is instructed and assisted if necessary to keep the anal area dry and clean. Washing with a mild soap is recommended. The area is patted dry and petrolatum can be applied after stool passage to serve as a protective barrier.

▶ Nursing Process
The Patient With Diarrhea

▷ Assessment

Health History
- Onset and pattern of diarrhea
- Presence of any of the following:
    Abdominal pain
    Cramping
    Urgency
    Watery stools
    Greasy stools
    Mucus or pus in the stool
- Current drug therapy
- Daily dietary intake
- Past medical history (any chronic disease)
- Allergies
- Recent exposure to acute illness
- Recent travel to another geographic area

Physical Assessment
- Auscultation of abdomen for bowel sounds
- Characteristic bowel sounds—frequent, borborygmus
- Palpation for distention and tenderness
- Inspection of the stool—consistency, color, and odor
- Inspection of skin and mucous membranes for dehydration
- Auscultation for postural hypotension, tachycardia
- Daily weight and intake and output

Watery stools are characteristic of small-bowel disease, whereas loose, semisolid stools are associated more often with disorders of the colon. Voluminous, greasy stools suggest intestinal malabsorption, and the presence of mucus and pus in the stools denotes inflammatory enteritis or colitis. Oil droplets on the toilet water are almost always diagnostic of pancreatic insufficiency. Nocturnal diarrhea may be a manifestation of diabetic neuropathy.

▷ Nursing Diagnoses

Based on all the assessment data, the patient's major nursing diagnoses may include the following:

- Diarrhea related to infection, ingestion of irritating foods, or disorder of the bowel.
- High risk for fluid volume deficit related to frequent passage of stools and insufficient fluid intake
- Anxiety related to frequent, uncontrolled elimination
- High risk for impaired skin integrity related to the passage of frequent, loose stools
- High risk for transmission of infection

▷ Planning and Implementation

▷ *Goals:* The major goals of the patient may include cessation of diarrhea, avoidance of fluid volume deficit, reduction of anxiety, maintenance of skin integrity, and prevention of spread of infection.

▷ Nursing Interventions

▷ *Measures to Control Diarrhea.* During an episode of acute diarrhea, the patient is encouraged to rest in bed and take liquids and foods that are low in bulk until the acute period subsides. When food intake is tolerated, the nurse recommends a bland diet. Caffeine intake is limited because caffeine stimulates intestinal motility. Milk may be restricted for several days because transient lactase deficiency may be seen in some forms of acute diarrhea. Antidiarrheal drugs such as diphenoxylate (Lomotil) are administered as prescribed.

▷ *Maintaining Fluid Balance.* Fluid balance is difficult to maintain during an acute episode of diarrhea because the rapid propulsion of feces through the intestines decreases water absorption; output exceeds intake. The nurse assesses for dehydration (decreased skin turgor, tachycardia, decreased pulse volume, decreased serum sodium, thirst) and keeps an accurate record of intake and output. The patient is weighed daily. The nurse encourages oral fluid replacement in the form of water, juices, bouillon, and commercial preparations such as Gatorade. Parenteral fluids are administered as ordered.

▷ *Reducing Anxiety.* An opportunity is provided for the patient to express fears/worry about being embarrassed by lack of control over bowel elimination. This fear of embarrassment is often a major concern.

The patient is assisted to identify irritating foods and stressors that precipitate an episode of diarrhea. Elimination or reduction of these factors helps control defecation. The patient is encouraged to be sensitive to body clues that warn of impending urgency (abdominal cramping, hyperactive bowel sounds). Special absorbent underwear, that will protect clothes if there is accidental fecal discharge, may be helpful.

An understanding, tolerant, and relaxed demeanor is essential. The patient's efforts to use coping mechanisms are supported and encouraged. Antianxiety medications are administered as prescribed.

▷ *Skin Care.* The perianal area becomes excoriated because diarrheal stool contains digestive enzymes that cause local irritation. The nurse instructs the patient to follow a perianal care routine such as the following: wipe or pat the area dry after defecation, cleanse with a mild soap and warm water, pat dry immediately with cotton balls, and apply lotion or ointment as a skin barrier.

▷ *Precautionary Infection Measures.* All patients with diarrhea should be treated as potentially infectious until they are proven otherwise. If the diarrhea is of an infectious origin, the nurse should determine whether there is any diarrhea among the family and neighbors. Proper precautions must be taken to prevent the spread of the disease through contamination of hands, clothing, bed linens, and other objects with feces or vomitus.

The nurse tries to determine if there is a causal relationship between episodes of diarrhea and food intake. If a food contaminant is suggested, food is tested by bacteriologic cultures. Food that is not contaminated can still act as an irritant to the patient's gastrointestinal tract.

▷ Evaluation

Expected Outcomes

1. Avoids irritating foods
   a. Identifies foods that act as irritants
   b. Eliminates irritating foods from diet
   c. Reports a decrease in number and frequency of daily stools
   d. Reports formed stools
2. Maintains fluid and electrolyte balance
   a. Takes sufficient fluids orally
   b. Tolerates parenteral fluid and electrolyte replacement
   c. States absence of fatigue and muscle weakness
   d. Is alert and oriented
   e. Displays moist mucous membranes and normal tissue turgor
   f. Has a balanced intake and output
   g. Has normal urine specific gravity
3. Experiences less anxiety
   a. Verbalizes concerns and fears
   b. States symptoms that signal an impending attack
   c. Uses coping mechanisms effectively
   d. Wears special absorbent underwear that protects clothing from soiling if needed
4. Maintains skin integrity
   a. Keeps area clean after defecation
   b. Uses lotion or ointment as a skin barrier

In summary, two problems that occur frequently with intestinal and rectal disorders are constipation and diarrhea. Patients with constipation, abnormal infrequency in defecation, and patients with diarrhea, unusual frequency of defecation, require nursing intervention directed toward the following goals: maintenance of fluid and electrolyte balance, relief of discomfort and anxiety, and restoration of normal bowel pattern.

Conditions of Malabsorption

Digestion is the process whereby nutrients are reduced to appropriate form for intestinal absorption. Intestinal absorption transports nutrients across the mucosa to the portal blood system.

Along with nutrients, the intestinal tract is the recipient of a large volume of fluid and electrolytes. Of about 1500 ml of liquid ingested daily, plus about 7000 ml from the gastrointestinal tract (salivary, gastric, biliary, pancreatic, and intestinal sources), all but 500 ml is absorbed proximal to the ileocecal valve. Thus, the intestine continually shifts the volume and composition of its contents to fulfill its major function of absorption.

Interruptions in the complex digestive process may occur anywhere to cause malabsorption, the inability of the digestive system to absorb one or more of the major nutrients—carbohydrates, fats, and proteins. Malabsorption occurs when the digestive process has been altered by:

- The inability of nutrients to be readily catabolized and transported (gastric resection, Zollinger–Ellison syndrome, pancreatic insufficiency)
- The decreased absorption of nutrients by the intestinal mucosa (jejunal diverticula, ileal dysfunction)
- A combination of causes (parasitic diseases, Whipple's disease, celiac disease)

In addition to these causes, certain inflammatory bowel disorders, such as ulcerative colitis and regional enteritis (Crohn's disease), cause increased protein breakdown (catabolism) in the small intestine, with resulting loss of protein into the lumen of the intestine (protein-losing enteropathy).

Pathophysiology.   Three primary malabsorption diseases are (1) tropical sprue, (2) adult celiac disease (nontropical sprue, gluten-induced celiac disease), and (3) lactose intolerance. Tropical sprue and adult celiac disease are similar in clinical manifestations and pathologic changes, but differ in their geographic incidence and causes, and also respond to different treatments. In adult celiac disease, protein malabsorption is frequently seen as an allergic reaction to gluten, which is found in wheat, rye, oats, and barley. Gluten causes the mucosal villi to atrophy, thus restricting their absorptive abilities. Lactose intolerance occurs when there is a deficiency of lactase, a digestive enzyme that breaks down milk sugar (the disaccharide lactose). The resulting high concentration of lactose in the intestines causes an osmotic retention of water, which results in abdominal cramping, nausea, and possibly diarrhea.

Clinical Manifestations.   The hallmarks of the malabsorption syndrome, of whatever cause, are diarrhea or frequent loose, bulky, foul stools that have increased fat content and are often grayish in color; associated weakness, weight loss, and lack of well-being are often present. The chief result of malabsorption is malnutrition, manifested by weight loss.

Patients with the malabsorption syndrome, if untreated, become weak and emaciated because of starvation. Failure to absorb the fat-soluble vitamins A, D, and K causes these patients to develop a corresponding avitaminosis. Manifestations of abnormal bleeding are likely to appear as a result of vitamin K deficiency and hypoprothrombinemia (see p. 810). Anemia develops, which is of the macrocytic type characteristic of folic acid deficiency (see p. 794). Impaired absorption of calcium may be responsible for gradual demineralization of the skeleton. Moreover, calcium deficiency may lead to extreme neuromuscular hyperirritability, including attacks of hypocalcemic tetany.

See Table 37–2 for the clinical and pathophysiologic aspects of malabsorption and maldigestion diseases.

Management.   Diagnostic studies are helpful in determining the disorder responsible for the malabsorption syndrome (Table 37–3). Dietary considerations are preeminent in the

treatment of adult celiac disease and lactose intolerance. In celiac disease, the elimination of gluten from the patient's diet is followed by striking clinical improvement. The diarrhea ceases and nutritional status is restored to normal. This remission may be expected to last only as long as the patient remains on a gluten-free diet. Unfortunately, the total exclusion of gluten is difficult to accomplish, because it is incorporated into many foods as a binder and filler. It is contained in almost every bakery product, "wheat-free" or otherwise, and is an ingredient of other foodstuffs as well, including some brands of ice cream.

The treatment for lactose intolerance consists of removing lactose-containing foods from the diet (*e.g.*, milk, ice cream). Soy milk products can be substituted. Most adults can digest fermented milk products such as cheese and yogurt. These products supply a vital need for calcium, and their use is encouraged.

The factors primarily responsible for the onset and the progression of tropical sprue have not as yet been clarified. Of greatest benefit in this condition is the administration of folic acid, which usually is prescribed for a period of 4 to 6 months after remission has occurred. Broad-spectrum antibiotics are equally important. The beneficial effects of folic acid in patients with tropical sprue appear with such regularity and on occasion are so striking as to suggest that this particular malabsorption syndrome may be attributable to, as well as productive of, folic acid deficiency.

Acute Inflammatory Intestinal Disorders

Acute inflammatory intestinal disorders such as appendicitis and peritonitis may at first have similar clinical manifestations: abdominal pain and tenderness, nausea and vomiting, anorexia, a low-grade temperature, tachycardia, and leukocytosis. Diagnosis is based on a complete history and physical examination. Surgery is the treatment of choice. Common nursing goals are relief of pain, prevention of fluid volume deficit, reduction in anxiety, elimination of infection due to the potential/actual disruption of the gastrointestinal tract, maintenance of skin integrity, and attainment of optimum nutrition.

Appendicitis

The appendix is a small, fingerlike appendage about 10 cm (4 in) long, attached to the cecum just below the ileocecal valve. No definite function can be assigned to it in humans. The appendix fills with food and empties as regularly as does the cecum, of which it is a part. It empties inefficiently, however, and its lumen is small, so that it is prone to become obstructed and is particularly vulnerable to infection (appendicitis).

Appendicitis is the most common cause of acute inflammation in the right lower quadrant of the abdominal cavity. About 7% of the population will have appendicitis at some time in their lives; males are affected more than females, and teenagers more than adults. It occurs most frequently between the ages of 10 and 30.

The disease is more prevalent in countries in which people

TABLE 37-2. *Pathophysiologic and Clinical Aspects of Diseases of Malabsorption and Maldigestion*

Diseases/Disorders	Physiologic Pathology	Clinical Features
Gastric resection with gastrojejunostomy	Decreased pancreatic stimulation because of duodenal bypass; poor mixing of food, bile, pancreatic enzymes; decreased intrinsic factor, bacterial stasis in afferent loop	Weight loss, moderate steatorrhea, anemia (combination of iron deficiency, vitamin B_{12} malabsorption, folate deficiency)
Pancreatic insufficiency (chronic pancreatitis, pancreatic carcinoma, pancreatic resection, cystic fibrosis)	Reduced intraluminal pancreatic enzyme activity, with maldigestion of lipid and protein	History of abdominal pain followed by weight loss; marked steatorrhea, azotorrhea; also frequent glucose intolerance (70% in pancreatic insufficiency)
Ileal dysfunction (resection or disease)	Loss of ileal absorbing surface leads to reduced bile-salt pool size and reduced vitamin B_{12} absorption; bile in colon inhibits fluid absorption.	Diarrhea, weight loss with steatorrhea, especially when greater than 100 cm resection, decreased vitamin B_{12} absorption
Stasis syndromes (surgical strictures, blind loops, enteric fistulas, multiple jejunal diverticula, scleroderma)	Overgrowth of intraluminal intestinal bacteria, especially anaerobic organisms, to greater than 10^6/ml, results in deconjugation of bile salts, leading to decreased effective bile-salt pool size, also bacterial utilization of vitamin B_{12}.	Weight loss, steatorrhea; low vitamin B_{12} absorption, may have low D-xylose absorption
Zollinger-Ellison syndrome	Hyperacidity in duodenum inactivates pancreatic enzymes.	Ulcer diathesis, steatorrhea
Lactose intolerance	Deficiency of intestinal lactase results in high concentration of intraluminal lactose with osmotic diarrhea.	Affects 80% of U.S. black persons and probably all other noncaucasian races; varied degrees of diarrhea and cramps after ingestion of lactose-containing foods; positive lactose tolerance test, decreased intestinal lactase
Celiac disease (gluten enteropathy)	Toxic response to a gluten fraction by surface epithelium results in destruction of absorbing surface.	Weight loss, diarrhea, bloating, anemia (low iron, folate), osteomalacia, steatorrhea, azotorrhea, low D-xylose absorption; folate and iron malabsorption; diagnostic biopsy change
Tropical sprue	Unknown toxic factor results in mucosal inflammation, partial villous atrophy.	Weight loss, diarrhea, anemia (low folate, vitamin B_{12}); steatorrhea; low D-xylose absorption, low vitamin B_{12} absorption; typical but nonspecific biopsy change
Whipple's disease	Bacterial invasion of intestinal mucosa	Arthritis, hyperpigmentation, lymphadenopathy, serous effusions, fever, weight loss; steatorrhea, azotorrhea, diagnostic biopsy change
Certain parasitic diseases (giardiasis, stronglyoidiasis, coccidiosis, capillariasis)	Damage to, or invasion of, surface mucosa	Diarrhea, weight loss; steatorrhea; organism may be seen on jejunal biopsy or recovered in stool
Immunoglobulinopathy	Decreased local gut defenses, lymphoid hyperplasia, lymphopenia	Frequent association with *Giardia*: hypogammaglobulinemia or isolated IgA deficiency; diagnostic or typical biopsy changes

(Halsted JA. The Laboratory In Clinical Medicine, Philadelphia, WB Saunders.)

consume a diet low in fiber and high in refined carbohydrates. In the United States, about 200,000 appendectomies are performed annually for acute appendicitis.

Pathophysiology. The appendix becomes inflamed and edematous because of either kinking or an occlusion, possibly caused by a fecalith (hardened mass of stool), tumor, or foreign body. The inflammatory process increases intraluminal pressure, initiating a progressively severe generalized or upper abdominal pain that, within a few hours, becomes localized in the right lower quadrant of the abdomen. Eventually, the inflamed appendix fills with pus and then is likely to perforate. Just how much tenderness there will be, how much muscle

TABLE 37–3.   *Suggested Diagnostic Studies for Disorders Resulting in Malabsorption*

Diagnostic Study	Test Result With Malabsorption Syndrome
Hemoglobin and hematocrit	Decreased if anemia is present.
Mean corpuscular volume	Decreased values are found with malabsorption of vitamin B_{12}.
Serum carotene level	Decreased values are associated with steatorrhea and fat malabsorption syndrome.
Upper GI series	Abnormal findings with malabsorption syndrome may include thickening of the intestinal mucosa, a change in fecal transit time, or narrowed mucosa of the terminal ileum.
Sudan stain for fecal fat	Abnormally large numbers of fat droplets can help to distinguish malabsorption from maldigestion.
A 72-hour stool collection for fat	A diet containing 80 g of fat must be ingested for 2 days before and during the test. Stool fat greater than 5 g/24 hr indicates a fat digestion disorder.
D-Xylose absorption test	Urine excretion over 5 hours after the ingestion of 5 g of D-xylose should be 5 g of xylose. Decreased excretion is indicative of malabsorption or enterogenous steatorrhea (fatty stools caused by a disease of the small intestines).

(Adapted from Eastwood GL. Core Textbook of Gastroenterology. Philadelphia, JB Lippincott.)

spasm, and whether or not there is constipation or diarrhea depend not so much on the severity of the appendiceal infection as on the location of the appendix. If the appendix curls around behind the cecum (*retrocecal* appendix), pain and tenderness may be felt in the lumbar region; if its tip is in the pelvis, these signs may be elicited only on rectal examination. Pain on defecation suggests that its tip is against the rectum; pain on micturition suggests that it is near the bladder or impinges on the ureter.

Clinical Manifestations.   The lower quadrant pain is usually accompanied by a low-grade fever, nausea, and often vomiting. At *McBurney's point* (Fig. 37–1), located halfway between the umbilicus and the anterior spine of the ilium, local tenderness is noted when pressure is applied and there is some rigidity of the lower portion of the right rectus muscle. A moderate leukocytosis is often present. Loss of appetite is common. If the appendix has ruptured, the pain becomes more diffuse; abdominal distention develops as a result of paralytic ileus, and the patient's condition worsens.

Complications.   The major complication of appendicitis is perforation. Appendiceal perforation leads to peritonitis or abscess formation. The incidence of perforation is 10% to 32%. The incidence is higher in young children and the elderly. Per-

foration generally occurs at any time after 24 hours of onset of pain. Symptoms include fever of 37.7°C (100°F) or greater, toxic appearance, and continued abdominal pain or tenderness.

Diagnostic Evaluation.   Diagnosis is based on a complete physical examination and a CBC.

On physical examination, common findings include slight muscular rigidity, normal bowel sounds, and local and *rebound tenderness* (production or intensification of pain when pressure is released). Early palpation of the abdomen shows diffuse tenderness around the umbilicus and midepigastrium. As the condition progresses, pain shifts to the lower right quadrant. If the patient coughs or the anterior abdominal wall is percussed, pain is enhanced. *Rovsing's sign* may be elicited by palpating the left lower quadrant (Fig. 37–1), which, paradoxically, causes pain to be felt by the patient in the right lower quadrant.

The more severe the pain, the more the patient will guard and protect the abdomen and the greater will be muscular rigidity. A posture of right hip flexion is a protective maneuver used by the patient, suggesting irritation of the psoas muscle (*positive psoas sign*) by the inflamed appendix. Radiologic signs in about 50% of the patients show right lower quadrant density or localized air-flow levels.

The patient has a low-grade temperature and a leukocyte count greater than 10,000/mm³. The neutrophil count is frequently elevated above 75%. In about 10% of those with acute appendicitis, however, leukocyte and differential cell counts are normal.

Management.   Surgery is indicated if appendicitis is suggested, unless there is good evidence that perforation has occurred recently and that generalized peritonitis has developed. If the question of surgery is undecided, a narcotic analgesic is withheld, even in the face of moderate pain, because it may mask the patient's symptoms. After the decision regarding surgery has been made, the patient may be given medication for pain.

The nurse assists in preparing the patient for surgery. An intravenous infusion is used to promote adequate renal function and replace existing fluid loss. Aspirin may be prescribed to lower the elevated temperature. Antibiotic therapy is often instituted as a preventive measure against infection. If there is evidence or likelihood of paralytic ileus, a nasogastric tube may be inserted. The patient is asked to void, and the prescribed preoperative medications are given. Usually, an enema is not given.

The patient who has been suffering from acute abdominal pain may view the operation as a means of relief. This acceptance of surgery makes the anesthetic and postanesthetic course a relatively easy one. The operation may be performed under general or spinal anesthesia.

Immediately on recovery from the anesthesia, the patient is placed in the Fowler's position. A narcotic analgesic, usually morphine sulfate, is given at intervals of 3 or 4 hours. Oral fluids are usually given when they can be tolerated unless the patient has been dehydrated, in which case they are given intravenously. Food may be given as desired on the day of operation, if the patient's condition permits.

For the uncomplicated appendectomy, the patient can be discharged on the day of surgery if the temperature is within normal limits and there is no undue discomfort in the operative area. The sutures are removed from the incision between the fifth and seventh days, in the physician's office. An appendec-

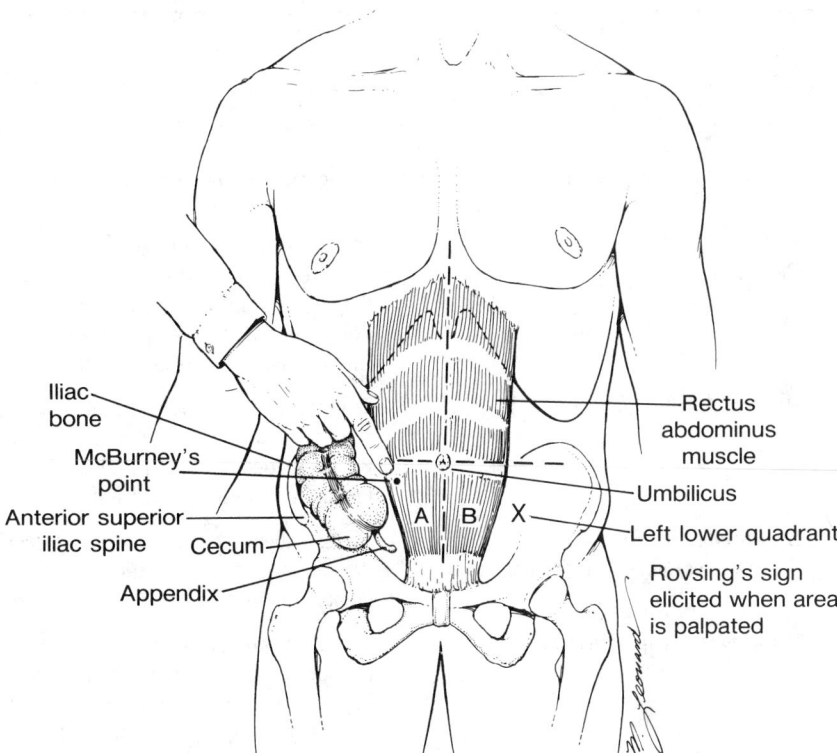

Figure 37–1. McBurney's point. When the appendix is inflamed, tenderness can be noted in the right lower quadrant at McBurney's point (**A**), which is between the umbilicus and the anterior superior iliac spine. Rovsing's sign occurs when pain is felt in the right lower quadrant after the left lower quadrant has been palpated (**B**).

tomy is usually an emergency procedure, however, and frequently complications such as perforation are present.

If there is a possibility of peritonitis, a drain is left in place at the area of incision. Patients are monitored carefully for signs of intestinal obstruction and secondary hemorrhage. Secondary abscesses may form in the pelvis, under the diaphragm, or in the liver. These cause an elevation of temperature and pulse rate, with an increase in the leukocyte count. A fecal fistula, with discharge of feces through the drainage tract, may occur after the drainage of an appendiceal abscess. Any sign of feces on the dressing is brought to the attention of the surgeon.

Other potential complications after treatment are identified in Chart 37–1.

Peritonitis

Peritonitis is inflammation of the peritonium—the membranous coat lining the abdominal cavity and covering the viscera. Usually it is a result of bacterial infection, the organisms coming from disease of the gastrointestinal tract or, in women, the internal reproductive organs (Fig. 37–2). Secondary peritonitis comes from external sources by injury, or by extension of inflammation from an extraperitoneal organ, such as the kidney. The most common bacteria implicated are *E. coli*, *Klebsiella*, *Proteus*, and *Pseudomonas*. *Inflammation* and *ileus* are the direct effects of the infection. Other common causes of peritonitis are appendicitis, perforated ulcers, diverticulitis, and bowel perforation. Peritonitis may be associated with abdominal trauma, operative procedures, and peritoneal dialysis.

Pathophysiology. Peritonitis is caused by leakage of contents from abdominal organs into the abdominal cavity, usually as a result of inflammation, infection, ischemia, trauma, or tu-

mor perforation, or, in the case of peritoneal dialysis, through the inadvertent introduction of contaminated fluid. Edema of tissues results, and in a short while exudation develops. Fluid in the peritoneal cavity becomes turbid with increasing amounts of protein, white cells, cellular debris, and blood. The immediate response of the intestinal tract is hypermotility, soon followed by paralytic ileus, with an accumulation of air and fluid in the bowel.

Clinical Manifestations. Symptoms depend on the location and extent of the inflammation, which are determined by the infection causing the peritonitis. At first a diffuse type of pain is felt. This tends to become constant, localized, and more intense near the site of the process. It is usually aggravated by movement. The affected area of the abdomen becomes extremely tender, and the muscles become rigid. Rebound tenderness and ileus may be present. Usually, nausea and vomiting occur and peristalsis is diminished. The temperature and pulse rate increase, and there is almost always an elevation of the leukocyte count. Shock may result from hypovolemia or septicemia. The early clinical manifestations of peritonitis frequently are the symptoms of the disorder causing the condition.

Management. Fluid, colloid, and electrolyte replacement is the major focus of medical management. Hypovolemia occurs because massive amounts of fluids and electrolytes move from the intestinal lumen into the peritoneal cavity and deplete the vascular space. This in turn decreases renal perfusion. In addition, the fluid in the abdominal cavity can impair ventilation by causing pressure on the diaphragm. Several liters of an isotonic solution are prescribed.

Intestinal intubation and suction assist in relieving abdominal distention and in promoting intestinal function. Oxygen therapy by nasal cannula or mask will promote ventilatory function, but occasionally airway intubation and ventilatory assistance may be required.

Chart 37–1
Potential Complications Following Appendectomy

Prompt recognition by the nurse and effective management of treatment can prevent prolonged disability for the patient.

Complication	Nursing Assessment and Interventions
Peritonitis	Observe for abdominal tenderness, fever, vomiting, abdominal rigidity, and tachycardia. Employ constant nasogastric suction. Correct dehydration as prescribed. Give antibiotic agents as prescribed.
Pelvic or lumbar abscess	Evaluate for anorexia, chills, fever, and diaphoresis. Observe for diarrhea, which may indicate pelvic abscess. Prepare patient for rectal examination. Prepare patient for operative drainage procedure.
Subphrenic abscess (abscess under the diaphragm)	Assess patient for chills, fever, and diaphoresis. Prepare for x-ray examination. Prepare for surgical drainage of abscess.
Ileus (paralytic and mechanical)	Assess for bowel sounds. Employ nasogastric intubation and suction. Replace fluids and electrolytes by intravenous route as prescribed. Prepare for surgery, if diagnosis of mechanical ileus is established.

If the cause of the peritonitis is removed at an early stage, the inflammation subsides and the patient recovers. Frequently, however, the inflammation is not localized and the whole abdominal cavity becomes involved.

Because sepsis is the major cause of death from peritonitis, massive antibiotic therapy is usually initiated early in the treatment. Cultures of peritoneal fluid are taken and, until the laboratory reports are available, large doses of a broad-spectrum antibiotic are given intravenously. When laboratory results are completed, the organism-specific antibiotic therapy is initiated.

Eventually, unless the cause of peritonitis is eliminated, the patient may succumb to intestinal obstruction. This is brought about by small bowel adhesions and even local abscess formation. If these can be localized, surgical drainage is effective.

Surgical objectives include removing the infected material and correcting the cause. Surgical treatment is directed toward excision (appendix), resection with or without anastomosis (intestine), repair (perforation), and drainage (abscess). With extensive sepsis, the creation of an ostomy may be necessary.

Nursing Interventions. Accurate assessment of pain is important. A description of the nature of the pain, its location in the abdomen, and any shifts in location may help ascertain the source of difficulty.

Accurate recording of all intake and output assists in calculating fluid replacement. In addition, determination of central venous pressure (see p. 637) may be helpful. A rise in pressure levels to 15 cm H_2O or higher may indicate circulatory overload.

Drains are frequently inserted during the operation, and it is essential that the nurse observe and record the character of the drainage. Care must be taken in moving and turning the patient to prevent the drains from being dislodged accidentally.

Signs that the peritonitis is subsiding include a decrease in temperature and pulse rate, softening of the abdomen, return of peristaltic sounds, passing of flatus, and bowel movements. Foods and fluids (taken by mouth) will be gradually increased and parenteral fluids reduced.

Two of the most common complications that must be observed for are wound evisceration and abscess formation. Any suggestion from the patient that an area of the abdomen is tender or painful or "feels as if something just gave way" must be reported. The sudden occurrence of serosanguineous wound drainage strongly suggests wound dehiscence (see Chap. 22).

Diverticular Disorders

A *diverticulum* is an outpouching or herniation of the mucous membrane lining of the bowel through a defect in the muscle layer. Diverticula, in fact, may occur anywhere along the course of the gastrointestinal tract, from the esophagus to the rectum.

Diverticulosis exists when multiple diverticula are present without inflammation or symptoms. *Diverticulitis* results when food and bacteria retained in a diverticulum produce infection and inflammation that can impede drainage and lead to perforation or abscess formation. Diverticulitis is found in approximately 10% of the United States population, but is more common in those over 60 years. Its incidence is approximately 60% in those over 80 years of age. A congenital predisposition is likely when the disorder is present in those under 40 years of age. A low intake of dietary fiber is considered a major cause of the disease.

It has been estimated that approximately 20% of patients with diverticulosis experience diverticulitis at some point. Diverticulitis is most common in the sigmoid colon (95%). It may

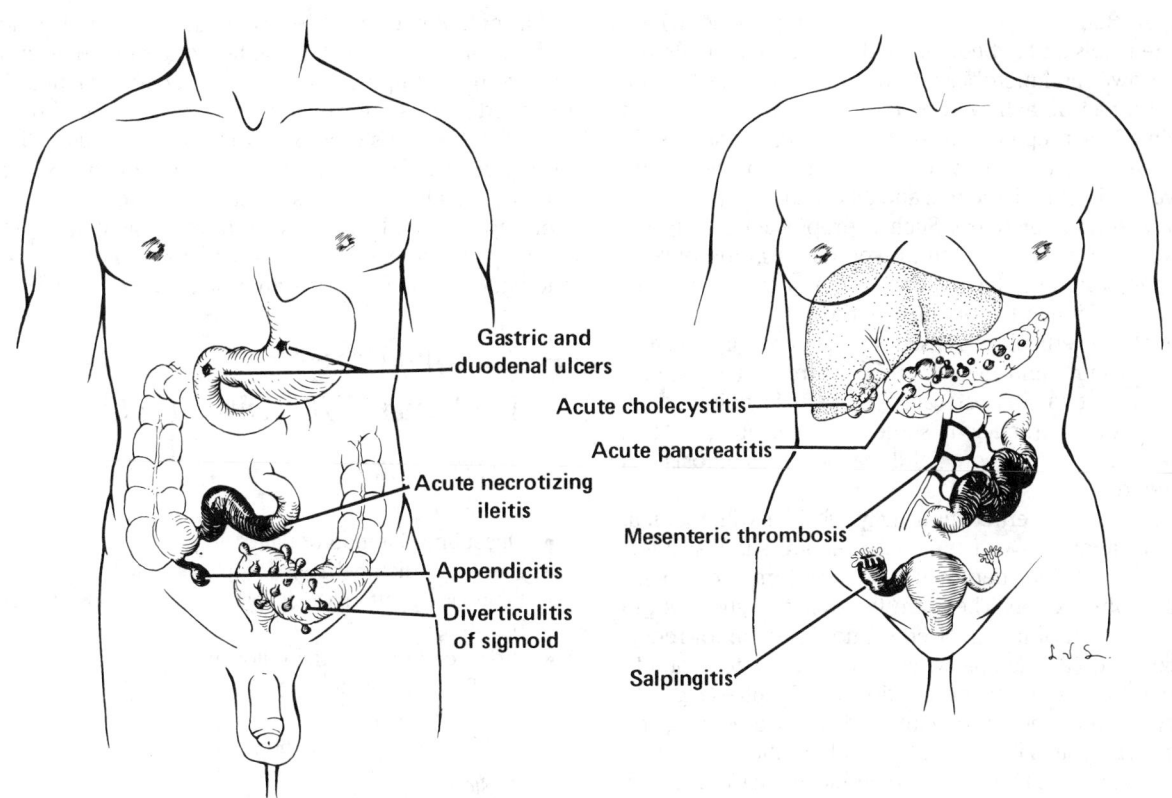

Figure 37–2.   Common primary causes of peritonitis. (Way LW [ed]. Current Surgical Diagnosis and Treatment, 9th ed. Los Altos, CA, Lange Medical Publishers, 1991.)

occur in acute attacks or may persist as a long-continued, smoldering infection.

Pathophysiology.   A diverticulum forms when the mucosa and submucosal layers of the colon herniate through the muscular wall because of high intraluminal pressure (thickened muscle layers occlude the lumen), low volume in the colon (fiber-deficient contents), and decreased muscle strength in the colon wall (muscular hypertrophy from hardened fecal masses). A diverticulum can become obstructed and then inflamed if the obstruction continues. The inflammation tends to spread to the surrounding bowel wall, giving rise to irritability and spasticity of the colon. An abscess may develop, leading to peritonitis, and erosion of the blood vessels (arterial) may produce bleeding.

Clinical Manifestations.   Constipation from spastic colon syndrome often precedes the development of diverticulosis by many years. Other signs of diverticulosis are bowel irregularity and diarrhea. A moderately severe acute diverticulitis has as its most common symptom crampy pain in the left lower quadrant of the abdomen, and a low-grade fever. After local inflammation of the diverticula, there may be a narrowing of the large bowel with fibrotic stricture, leading to cramps, narrow stools, and increased constipation. With the development of granulation tissue, occult bleeding may occur, producing iron-deficiency anemia. In addition, weakness and fatigue are evident. If an abscess develops, there is tenderness, a palpable mass, fever, and leukocytosis. If an inflamed diverticulum perforates, abdominal pain results that is localized over the involved segment—usually the sigmoid; local abscess or peritonitis results. With the development of peritonitis, the symptoms of rigidity, abdominal pain, loss of bowel sounds, and shock develop.

Uninflamed or slightly inflamed diverticula may erode areas adjacent to arterial branches, thus causing massive rectal bleeding.

Gerontologic Considerations.   The incidence of diverticular disease increases with age. There are structural changes in the circular muscle layers of the colon as well as cellular hypertrophy. The elderly may not notice abdominal pain until infection occurs. They may delay reporting symptoms because they fear surgery or are afraid that they may have cancer.

Although blood in the stool is a common sign of diverticular disease in the elderly, it is frequently overlooked because a person fails to examine the stool or cannot see changes because of diminished vision.

Diagnostic Evaluation.   Diverticulosis may be diagnosed from radiographic studies that show narrowing of the colon and thickened muscle layers.

A history generally elicits the two main presenting symptoms of diverticulitis: pain in the lower left quadrant and a marked change in bowel habits (diarrhea or constipation). Diagnosis is made on the basis of sigmoidoscopy (direct visualization), colonoscopy, and x-ray findings with a barium enema (after inflammation has subsided). A computed tomography (CT) scan can reveal abscesses.

Management.   In *diverticulosis*, a high-fiber diet is prescribed to prevent constipation. In *diverticulitis*, the bowel is rested by withholding oral fluids, administering intravenous fluids, and instituting nasogastric suctioning. Broad-spectrum antibiotics and analgesics are prescribed. Oral intake is increased as symptoms subside. A low-fiber diet may be necessary until signs of infection decrease.

For spastic pain, antispasmodics such as propantheline

bromide (Pro-Banthine) and oxyphencyclimine (Daricon) are taken before meals and at bedtime. Sedatives and tranquilizers, as well as bowel antimicrobials, also may be required. Stool normalization can be achieved by the use of one or more of the following: bulk preparations, such as Metamucil; stool softeners, such as dioctyl sodium sulfosuccinate (Colace); instillation of warm oil into the rectum; and an evacuant suppository, such as bisacodyl (Dulcolax). Such a prophylactic plan will reduce the bacterial flora of the bowel, diminish the bulk of the stool, and soften the fecal mass, so that it traverses more easily the area of inflammatory obstruction.

Surgery for diverticulosis is usually necessary only if severe hemorrhage occurs, and even then is controversial because studies show that in 50% of cases, surgery is followed by a recurrence of diverticula. If surgery is indicated, a total colectomy with an ileorectal/ileoanal anastomosis is recommended.

Although acute diverticulitis usually subsides with medical management, about 25% of the cases require surgical intervention for perforation, peritonitis, abscess formation, hemorrhage, and obstruction. There are two types of surgery: (1) one-stage resection of the involved sigmoid section for recurrent attacks, and (2) multiple-staged procedures for complications, such as obstruction, perforation, and fistulae (Fig. 37–3). Surgery is preceded by barium studies. In preparing the patient for surgery, it is important to avoid irritating the colon, which is already sensitive and susceptible to perforation. A mild saline laxative and carefully administered cleansing enemas may be sufficient.

The type of surgery performed varies with the operative findings. When possible, the area of diverticulitis is resected and the remaining bowel joined end to end (primary resection and end-to-end anastomosis). A two-stage resection may be performed, in which the diseased colon is resected, as in a one-stage operation, but no anastomosis is performed and both ends of the bowel are brought out onto the abdomen as stomas. The "double-barrel" colostomy is then anastomosed in a later procedure. In some patients such an operation may appear impossible or inadvisable, in which case a colostomy is performed in the right transverse colon. Diverting the fecal flow from the area of diverticulitis allows the inflammatory process to subside, and a later operation to remove the part of the colon containing the diverticulitis is performed, followed by an anastomosis. When this method of treatment is chosen, the colostomy is temporary; after the area of diverticulitis has been removed and the intestinal continuity established by the anastomosis, the colostomy is closed. This is thus a three-stage procedure. A colostomy on the right side of the transverse colon drains liquid or mushy feces and requires that a bag be worn constantly. Irrigations are rarely indicated in this type of colostomy. The patient may take baths or showers, using soap and water to cleanse the skin around the colostomy stoma.

▶ Nursing Process
The Patient With Diverticulitis

▷ Assessment

Health History
- Onset and duration of pain
- Review of dietary habits for low fiber intake
- Elimination pattern (constipation with periods of diarrhea with bleeding)
- Presence of any of the following:
  Straining at stool
  Tenesmus
  Bloated feeling in abdomen

Physical Assessment
- Auscultation for bowel sounds
- Characteristics of bowel sounds
- Palpation for left lower quadrant pain or tenderness
- Palpation of sigmoid as a firm mass
- Inspection of stool for pus, mucus, and blood
- Elevation of temperature and pulse rate
- Laboratory findings of elevated white blood cell count and sedimentation rate

▷ Nursing Diagnoses

Based on all the assessment data, the patient's major nursing diagnoses may include the following:

- Constipation related to narrowing of the colon secondary to thickened muscular segments and strictures

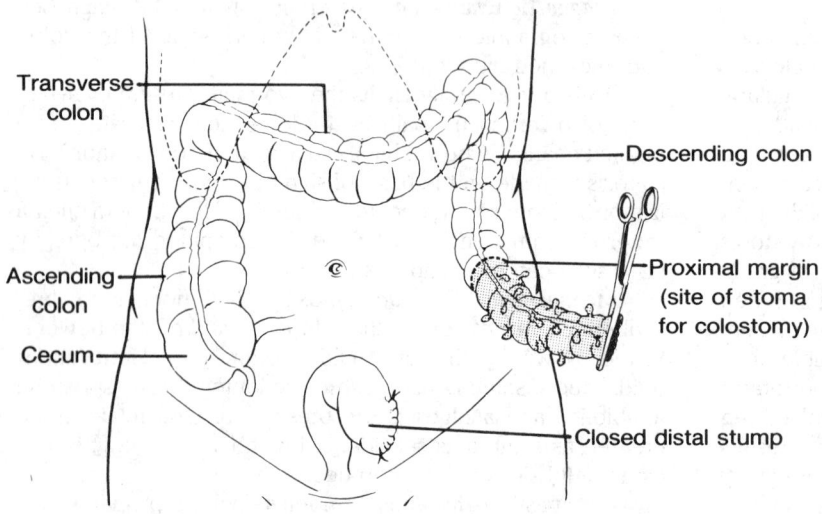

Figure 37–3. The Hartmann procedure for diverticulitis. Primary resection for diverticulitis of the colon. The affected segment (shaded) has been divided at its distal end. If primary anastomosis is to be done, the proximal margin (dotted line) is transected, and the bowel is anastomosed end-to-end. If a two-stage procedure will be used, a colostomy is formed at the proximal margin, and the distal stump is oversewn (Hartmann procedure, as shown), or exteriorized as a mucous fistula. The second stage consists of colostomy takedown and anastomosis. (Way LW [ed]. Current Surgical Diagnosis and Treatment. 9th ed. Los Altos, CA, Lange Medical Publishers, 1991.)

- Pain related to inflammation and infection
- Altered gastrointestinal tissue perfusion related to infection secondary to abscess formation, perforation, and peritonitis

◊ *Planning and Implementation*

◊ *Goals:* The major goals of the patient may include attainment of normal elimination, reduction in pain, and improvement in gastrointestinal tissue perfusion.

◊ *Nursing Interventions*

◊ *Maintenance of Normal Elimination Patterns.* A fluid intake of 2 to 3 L/day (within limits of the patient's cardiac reserve), is recommended. Foods that are soft but have increased fiber, such as peas and prunes, are suggested to promote defecation. For uncomplicated diverticular disease, unprocessed bran, soups, salads, and cereals are added. An individualized exercise program is encouraged to improve abdominal muscle tone. The patient's daily routine is reviewed to establish a schedule for meals and a set time for defecation. The patient is assisted to identify undesirable habits that may have been used to suppress the urge to defecate. The daily intake of bulk laxatives such as Metamucil, which helps to propel feces through the colon, is encouraged. Stool softeners are administered as prescribed to decrease straining at stool, which in turn decreases intestinal pressure. Oil-retention enemas may be prescribed to soften the stool and decrease inflammation.

◊ *Pain Relief.* Analgesics and antispasmodic drugs are administered as prescribed. A low-fiber diet is recommended until the inflammation subsides. The intensity, duration, and location of pain are recorded to determine severity and progression or remission of the inflammatory process. Pain is felt in the left lower quadrant and can be referred to the back. Any abdominal rigidity, which may indicate perforation and peritonitis, is reported promptly.

◊ *Preventing Complications.* The major nursing focus is prevention through identification of persons at risk and management of those suffering from diverticular disease. The nurse encourages fluid intake to promote hydration to maintain normal stool consistency and prevent straining. During acute inflammation, however, oral foods and fluids may be restricted, in which case intravenous fluids are prescribed to prevent dehydration.

If food is tolerated while infection is present, a low-fiber diet is prescribed and the nurse advises the patient about dietary management. The nurse assesses for indicators of perforation: a tender, rigid abdomen; an elevated while blood cell count; an elevated sedimentation rate; the presence or absence of pain; increased temperature; tachycardia, and hypotension. Perforation constitutes a surgical emergency.

The patient should understand the nature of the problem and recognize that the objective is to rest the intestinal tract. Heretofore, diverticulosis of the colon was considered relatively harmless, but, because of the potential for developing complex problems, prevention is now given major emphasis.

◊ *Evaluation*

Expected Outcomes
1. Attains a normal pattern of elimination
   a. Reports less abdominal cramping and pain
   b. Reports the passage, without pain, of soft, formed stool

   c. Adds unprocessed bran to foods
   d. Drinks at least 10 glasses of fluid a day (if fluid intake is tolerated)
   e. Exercises daily
2. Experiences less pain
   a. Requests analgesics as needed
   b. Adheres to a low-fiber diet
3. Achieves normal gastrointestinal tissue perfusion
   a. Complies with food restrictions
   b. Remains on bed rest
   c. Is afebrile
   d. Has a soft, nontender abdomen with normal bowel sounds

Meckel's Diverticulum

Meckel's diverticulum is a congenital abnormality consisting of a blind tube, comparable to the appendix, that usually opens into the distal ileum near the ileocecal valve. A portion of this duct persists as a diverticulum in approximately 2% of the population. It is more common in men than in women.

The importance of Meckel's diverticulum lies in the fact that its mucosal lining may become inflamed and may lead to intestinal obstruction, or it may perforate, causing peritonitis.

The most common symptoms of a diseased Meckel's diverticulum are abdominal pain, typically umbilical in location, or the passage of stools containing blood. The blood is a dark crimson color. (A slowly bleeding gastric or upper intestinal lesion is tarry black; a colonic hemorrhage usually produces bright red bleeding). The treatment is surgical excision of the diverticulum.

In summary, appendicitis, peritonitis, and diverticulitis are acute inflammatory disorders manifested by many of the same signs and symptoms. Each, however, involves different infectious pathophysiology. Nursing goals for patients with these disorders are similar—relief of pain, maintenance of fluid and electrolyte balance, reduction of anxiety, and prevention of complications.

Chronic Inflammatory Bowel Disease

The term *inflammatory bowel disease* is used to designate two chronic inflammatory gastrointestinal disorders: regional enteritis (Crohn's disease, granulomatous colitis) and ulcerative colitis. The incidence of inflammatory bowel disease in the United States is estimated to be between 4% and 10%, with 25,000 new cases occurring annually. The disease is seen more frequently in whites and most frequently in the Jewish population. A familial history is found in 20% to 40% of patients.

The current belief is that regional enteritis and ulcerative colitis are separate entities with similar etiologies. Both are characterized by exacerbations and remissions. A specific chromosomal abnormality has not been identified. Each disease may be triggered by environmental agents such as pesticides, food additives, tobacco, and radiation. An immunologic influence has been suggested because of studies that show abnormalities in humoral and cell-mediated immunity in people with these disorders. Lymphocytotoxic antibodies have been found in patients with inflammatory bowel disease, but more definitive research is needed to link immunologic and environmental factors.

A psychological factor has also been suggested. Many individuals with ulcerative colitis are found to be dependent, passive, immature, perfectionist, and anxious to please. Coping behaviors are often inappropriate and can include withdrawal, denial, and repression. Some people have a decreased level of tolerance for the pain and discomfort associated with intestinal cramping and diarrhea. Some clinicians suggest that the personality traits are the cause—not the result—of the disease symptoms, but more clinical research is needed to establish a causal relationship. See Table 37–4 for a comparison of regional enteritis and ulcerative colitis.

TABLE 37–4.   *Comparison of Regional Enteritis and Ulcerative Colitis*

	Regional Enteritis	**Ulcerative Colitis**
HISTORY	Prolonged, variable course	Exacerbations, remissions
PATHOLOGY		
Early	Transmural thickening	Mucosal ulceration
Late	Deep, penetrating granulomas	Mucosal minute ulceration
CLINICAL MANIFESTATIONS		
Location	Ileum, right colon (usually)	Rectum, left colon
Bleeding	Usually not, but may occur	Common—severe
Perianal involvement	Common	Rare—mild
Fistulas	Common	Rare
Rectal involvement	About 20%	Almost 100%
Diarrhea	Less severe	Severe
DIAGNOSTIC STUDIES		
X-ray films	Regional, discontinuous lesions	Diffuse involvement
	Narrowing of colon	No narrowing of colon
	Mucosal edema	No mucosal edema
	Stenosis, fistulas	Stenosis, rare; no fistulas
Sigmoidoscopy	May be unremarkable unless accompanied by perianal fistulas	Abnormal inflamed mucosa
Colonoscopy	Distinct ulcerations separated by relatively normal mucosa in right colon	Friable mucosa with pseudopolyps or ulcers in left colon
THERAPEUTIC MANAGEMENT		
	Steroids, sulfonamides (Sulfasalazine [Azulfidine])	Steroids, sulfonamides; Azulfidine is useful in preventing recurrence
	Total parenteral nutrition	
	Partial or complete colectomy, with ileostomy or anastomosis	Proctocolectomy, with ileostomy
	Rectum can be preserved in some patients.	Rectum can be preserved in only a few patients "cured" by colectomy.
	Recurrence common	
Systemic complications	Small bowel obstruction	Toxic megacolon
		Malignant neoplasms
	Right-sided hydronephrosis	Pyelonephritis
	Nephrolithiasis	Same
	Cholelithiasis	Cholangiocarcinoma
	Arthritis	Same
	Retinitis, iritis	Same
	Erythema nodosum	Same

Regional Enteritis (Crohn's Disease)

Pathophysiology.   Regional enteritis commonly occurs in adolescents or young adults, but can appear at any time of life. The most common areas in which it is found are the distal ileum and colon. It can occur anywhere along the alimentary canal, however, from the mouth to the anus. This inflammatory disease process extends through all layers of the bowel wall. This is a subacute and chronic inflammation that extends through the intestinal mucosa. This transmural involvement accounts for the formation of fistulas, fissures, and abscesses. The lesions are characteristically discontinuous or separated by normal tissue. Granulomas occur in half of the cases. In advanced cases the intestinal mucosa has a "cobblestone" appearance. As the disease advances, the intestinal lumen narrows, causing obstruction.

Clinical Manifestations.   With regional enteritis, the onset of symptoms is usually insidious, but abdominal pain, diarrhea, and weight loss are prominent, and are unrelieved by defecation. Diarrhea is present in 90% of patients. Scar tissue and formation of granulomas interfere with the ability of the intestine to transport products of the upper intestinal digestion through the constricted lumen, resulting in crampy abdominal pains. Because intestinal peristalsis is stimulated by the eating of food, the crampy pains occur after meals. To avoid these bouts of crampy pain, the patient avoids food or takes it only in amounts and types inadequate for normal nutritional requirements, so that weight loss, malnutrition, and secondary or macrocytic anemia occur. In addition, ulcers form in the lining membrane of the intestine and other inflammatory changes take place, resulting in a constant irritating discharge that is emptied into the colon from the weeping, swollen intestine. This causes a chronic diarrhea. The end result is a very uncomfortable person who is thin and emaciated from inadequate food intake and constant fluid loss. In some patients, the inflamed intestine may perforate and form intra-abdominal and anal abscesses. Melena may occur, along with malabsorption syndrome. Fever and leukocytosis occur. Abscesses, fistulas, and fissures are common.

Diagnostic Evaluation.   The most conclusive diagnostic aid is a barium study of the upper gastrointestinal tract that shows the classic "string sign" on x-ray of the terminal ileum, indicating the constriction of a segment of intestine.

A proctosigmoidoscopic examination is usually performed initially to establish whether there is an inflammatory process in the rectosigmoid area. If this area is normal, the diagnosis of ulcerative colitis is ruled out.

A stool examination may be positive for occult blood and steatorrhea. Leukocytosis and an elevated sedimentation rate may be present. Bowel sounds are hyperactive over the right lower quadrant.

Ulcerative Colitis

Pathophysiology.   Ulcerative colitis is a recurrent ulcerative and inflammatory disease of the colon and rectum, with rare involvement of the distal ileum. It is a serious disease, accompanied by systemic complications and a high mortality rate. Eventually 10% to 15% of the patients develop carcinoma of the colon. Ulcerative colitis affects the superficial mucosa of the colon and is characterized by multiple ulcerations, diffuse inflammations, and desquamation of the colonic epithelium, with alternating periods of exacerbation and remission. The lesions are continuous and ultimately spread throughout the large intestine. Eventually the bowel narrows, shortens, and thickens because of muscular hypertrophy and the deposition of fat.

Clinical Manifestations.   The predominant symptoms of ulcerative colitis are diarrhea, abdominal pain, intermittent tenesmus, and rectal bleeding. In addition, anorexia, weight loss, fever, vomiting, and dehydration may be evident, as well as cramping and the feeling of an urgent need to defecate. The patient may report passing 10 to 20 liquid stools daily. Hypocalcemia and anemia frequently develop. Rebound tenderness may occur in the right lower quadrant.

Diagnostic Evaluation.   In the diagnosis of chronic ulcerative colitis, careful stool examination is performed to rule out dysentery caused by the common intestinal organisms, especially *Entamoeba histolytica* infection. The stool is positive for blood. Leukocytosis, anemia, and bone marrow depression are common. Other indicators include a loss of plasma proteins due to liver dysfunction, electrolyte imbalance, thrombocytosis due to the inflammatory process, and decreased serum iron levels secondary to blood loss. Sigmoidoscopy and barium enema are of value in distinguishing this condition from other diseases of the colon with similar symptoms.

- In acute ulcerative colitis, cathartics are contraindicated when the patient is being prepared for barium enema because they may cause severe exacerbation of the condition, which may lead to megacolon (excessive dilatation of the colon), perforation, and death. If the patient is required to have this diagnostic test, a liquid diet for a few days before the x-ray and a gentle tap water enema on the day of examination may be prescribed.

Medical Management of Inflammatory Bowel Disorders

Medical treatment for both regional enteritis and ulcerative colitis is aimed at reducing inflammation, suppressing inappropriate immune responses, and providing rest for a diseased bowel, so that healing may take place.

Low-residue, high-protein diets with supplemental vitamin therapy and iron replacement are effective in meeting nutritional needs. Fluid and electrolyte imbalance due to dehydration caused by diarrhea is corrected by intravenous therapy. Any foods that exacerbate diarrhea should be avoided. Milk may contribute to diarrhea if lactose intolerance is present. In addition, cold foods are to be avoided, along with smoking, because both increase intestinal motility. Total parenteral nutrition may be indicated.

Sedative and antidiarrheal/antiperistaltic medications are used to reduce to a minimum the colonic peristalsis to rest the inflamed bowel. They are continued until the patient's stools approach normal frequency and consistency. Sulfonamides such as sulfasalazine (Azulfidine) or sulfisoxazole (Gantrisin) are often effective for mild or moderate inflammation. Antibiotics are used for secondary infections, particularly for purulent complications such as abscesses, perforation, and peritonitis. Azulfidine is helpful in preventing recurrences.

Adrenocorticotropic hormone (ACTH) and corticosteroids

are most effective early in the course of the acute inflammatory phase rather than in the chronic phase. When steroids are reduced or stopped, the symptoms of disease are likely to return. If steroids are continued, adverse sequelae such as hypertension, fluid retention, cataracts, hirsutism, and adrenal suppression may develop.

Psychotherapy is aimed at determining what factors distress the patient, dealing with these factors, and attempting to resolve conflicts so that they no longer aggravate the patient.

Surgical Management of Inflammatory Bowel Disorders

When conservative measures fail to relieve the severe symptoms of inflammatory bowel disease, surgery may be recommended.

If a lesion can be delineated in regional enteritis (obstruction, abscess, fistula, stricture), it is resected (excised, removed), and the remaining portions of the bowel are anastomosed (joined together). Loss of 50% of the small bowel can usually be tolerated. The surgical procedures of choice are the following:

- Total colectomy (excision of the entire colon) with ileostomy (surgical creation of an opening into the ileum, usually by means of an ileal stoma on the abdominal wall)
- Segmental colectomy (removal of a segment of the colon) with anastomosis (joining of the remaining portions of the colon)
- Subtotal colectomy (removal of nearly all of the colon) with ileorectal anastomosis (joining of the ileum and rectum)

The rate of recurrence after surgery is 20% to 40% in the first 5 years. Patients under 25 years of age have the highest recurrence rate.

Approximately 15% to 20% of the patients with ulcerative colitis require surgical intervention. Indications for surgery include lack of improvement and continued deterioration, profuse bleeding, perforation, stricture formation, and indications that carcinoma has developed. The operation of choice is a total colectomy and ileostomy; any procedure more limited will prove to be of only temporary benefit in most patients. A proctocolectomy (complete excision of colon, rectum, and anus) is recommended when the rectum is severely involved.

In the 1970s, a surgical procedure was introduced that combined proctocolectomy with a continent ileal reservoir (*Kock's pouch*). This procedure eliminates the need for an external fecal collection bag. Approximately 30 cm of the distal ileum is reconstructed to form a reservoir with a nipple valve that is created by intussusception of a portion of the terminal ileal loop (Fig. 37–4*A*). Gastrointestinal effluent can be stored in the pouch for several hours and is then removed by means of a catheter inserted through the nipple valve. The major problem with the Kock pouch is malfunction of the nipple valve, which is seen in 20% to 40% of the patients.

A new surgical procedure is being performed for chronic ulcerative colitis and familial polyposis that eliminates the permanent ileostomy, establishes an ileal reservoir, and retains anal sphincter control of elimination. The procedure involves an ileoanal anastomosis performed in conjunction with a total abdominal colectomy and a mucosal proctectomy (see Fig. 37–4*F*). A temporary diverting-loop ileostomy is constructed at the time of surgery and closed about 3 months later. With ileoanal anastomosis, the diseased colon and rectum are removed, voluntary defecation is maintained, and anal continence is preserved. The ileal reservoir decreases the number of bowel movements by 50%, from approximately 14 to 20 per day to 7 to 10 per day. Nighttime elimination is gradually reduced to one bowel movement. Complications of the ileoanal anastomosis include perianal skin excoriation from leakage of fecal contents, stricture formation at the anastomosis site, and small bowel obstruction.

▶ Nursing Process
The Patient With a Chronic Inflammatory Bowel Disease

▷ Assessment

Health History
- Onset and duration of abdominal pain
- Presence of any of the following:
    Diarrhea
    Tenesmus
    Nausea
    Anorexia
    Weight loss
- Relationship of symptoms to stress or dietary indiscretions
- Family history of inflammatory bowel disease
- Allergies, especially to milk/lactose
- Dietary pattern, including amounts of alcohol, caffeine, and nicotine used daily/weekly
- Depression, anxiety
- Sleep disturbances

Physical Assessment
- Auscultation for bowel sounds, noting characteristics
- Palpation for distention, tenderness, pain
- Inspection for rectal bleeding

With regional enteritis, pain is usually localized in the right lower quadrant where hyperactive bowel sounds can be heard because of borborygmus and increased peristalsis. Abdominal tenderness is noted on palpation. The most prominent symptom is intermittent pain associated with diarrhea that does not decrease with defecation. Pain in the periumbilical region usually indicates involvement of the terminal ileum. With ulcerative colitis, the abdomen may be distended and rebound tenderness present. Rectal bleeding is a dominant sign.

▷ Nursing Diagnoses

Based on all the assessment data, the patient's major nursing diagnoses may include the following:

- Diarrhea related to the inflammatory process
- Abdominal pain and cramping, related to increased peristalsis
- Fluid volume and electrolyte deficits related to anorexia, nausea, and diarrhea
- Altered nutrition, less than body requirements, related to anorexia secondary to diarrhea
- Activity intolerance related to fatigue
- Anxiety related to impending surgery
- Ineffective individual coping related to repeated episodes of diarrhea

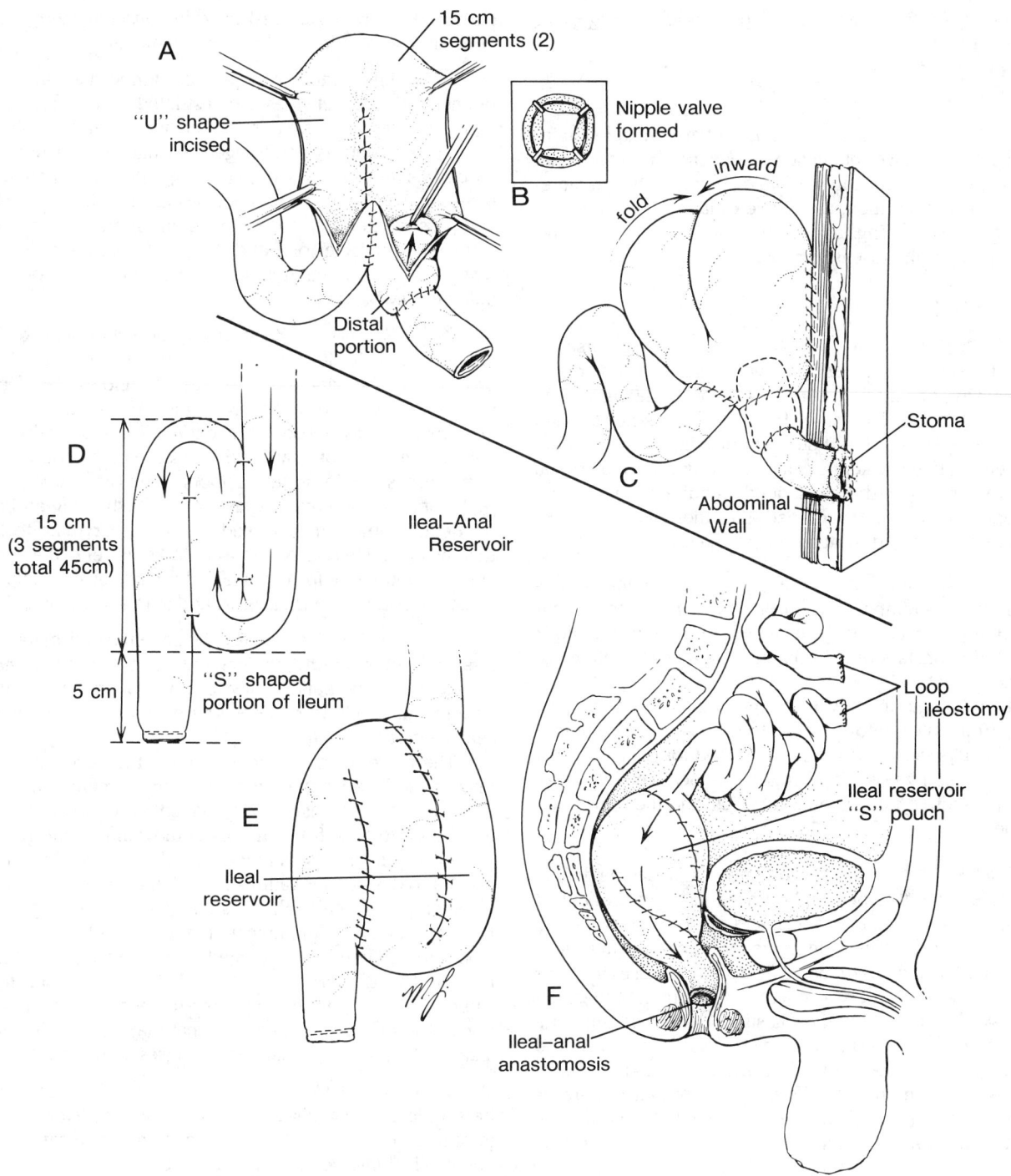

Figure 37–4. An ileal reservoir for the Kock pouch and for an ileoanal anastomosis.

For the Kock pouch: (**A**) A 30-cm portion of the ileum is sutured together to form a U shape. It is then excised open and the distal portion is pulled back into the ileum (similar to an intussusception). (**B**) A nipple valve is formed by suturing the pulled-back portion of the intestine to itself. (**C**) The top of the ileum is folded onto itself and a stoma is formed from the distal portion.

For the ileoanal anastomosis: (**D**) A 50-cm portion of the distal ileum is aligned in an S shape. (**E**) The bowel is opened along the antimesenteric surface and then adjacent walls are anastomosed to create a reservoir. (**F**) A mucosal proctectomy precedes anastomosis of the ileal reservoir. A temporary loop ileostomy diverts effluent discharge for several months.

- Knowledge deficit concerning the process and management of the disease

▷ Planning and Implementation

▷ *Goals:* The major goals of the patient may include attainment of normal bowel elimination, reduction in abdominal pain and cramping, prevention of fluid volume deficit, maintenance of optimal nutrition, avoidance of fatigue, reduction of anxiety, effective coping, and acquisition of knowledge and understanding of the disease process.

▷ Nursing Interventions

▷ *Maintenance of Normal Elimination Patterns.* The nurse ascertains if there is a relationship between diarrhea and certain foods, activity, or emotional stress. Any precipitating factors are reported, as well as stool frequency, consistency, and amount. Ready access to a bathroom or bedpan is provided, and the environment is kept clean and odor free. Antidiarrheal agents are administered as prescribed, and the frequency and consistency of stools are recorded after therapy has started. Bed rest is encouraged to decrease peristalsis.

▷ *Pain Relief.* The character of the pain is documented as dull, burning, or cramplike. Its onset is relevant: Does it occur before or after meals, during the night, or before elimination? Is the pattern constant or intermittent? Is it relieved with medications?

Anticholinergic medications are administered as prescribed, 30 minutes before a meal to decrease intestinal motility, and analgesics are given as prescribed for pain. Pain can also be reduced by position changes, the local application of heat (as prescribed), diversional activities, and the prevention of fatigue.

▷ *Maintenance of Fluid Intake.* To detect fluid volume deficit, an accurate record of oral and intravenous fluids is kept as well as a record of output (urine, liquid stool, vomitus, wound or fistula drainage). Daily weights are monitored because they indicate rapid fluid gains or losses. The nurse assesses for signs of fluid volume deficit: dry skin and mucous membranes, decreased skin turgor, oliguria, exhaustion, decreased temperature, increased hematocrit, elevated urine specific gravity, and hypotension. Oral intake of fluids is encouraged, and intravenous flow rate is monitored. Measures to decrease diarrhea are initiated: dietary restrictions, stress reduction, and administration of antidiarrheal agents.

▷ *Nutritional Measures.* Total parenteral nutrition (TPN) is used when the symptoms of inflammatory bowel disease are severe. With TPN, the nurse maintains an accurate record of fluid intake and output as well as the patient's daily weight. The patient should gain 0.5 kg daily during therapy. The urine is tested for glucose, acetone, and specific gravity daily when TPN is being used. Elemental feedings that are high in protein and low in fat and residue are instituted after TPN therapy because they are digested primarily in the jejunum, do not stimulate intestinal secretions, and allow the bowel to rest. Intolerance is noted if the patient exhibits nausea, vomiting, diarrhea, or abdominal distention.

If oral foods are tolerated, small, frequent feedings are given to avoid overdistending the stomach and stimulating

peristalsis. Activities are restricted to conserve energy, reduce peristalsis, and reduce calorie requirements.

▷ *Rest.* Intermittent rest periods during the day are recommended and activities are restricted to conserve energy and reduce the metabolic rate. Activity within the limit of the patient's capacity is encouraged, so that he will not regard himself as an invalid. Bed rest is suggested for a patient who is febrile, has frequent diarrheal stools, or is bleeding. Active and passive exercises are encouraged for anyone on bed rest to maintain muscle tone and prevent thromboembolic complications. Activity restrictions are evaluated and modified on a day-to-day basis.

▷ *Reducing Anxiety.* Rapport can be established by being attentive and displaying a calm, confident manner. Time is provided for the patient to ask questions and express feelings. Careful listening and sensitivity to nonverbal indicators of anxiety (restlessness, tense facial expressions) are helpful. The patient may be emotionally labile because of the consequences of the disease, so information about impending surgery should be tailored to the patient's level of understanding and desire for detail. Some persons need to know everything to lessen their anxiety, whereas others want to know very little. Pictures and illustrations help to explain the surgical procedure and assist the patient to visualize what a stoma looks like.

▷ *Coping Measures.* Because the patient feels isolated, helpless, and out of control, understanding and emotional support are essential. The patient may respond to stress with infantile or demanding behavior, perfectionism, anger, denial, and social self-isolation.

The nurse needs to recognize that the patient's behavior may be affected by innumerable factors unrelated to inherent emotional characteristics. Any patient who is suffering from the discomforts of frequent bowel movements and rectal soreness is anxious, discouraged, and depressed. Thus, it is important to develop a relationship with the patient that supports his attempts to deal with the stresses that have plagued him. It is important to communicate that his complaints are understood: the patient is encouraged to talk and ventilate his feelings, and to discuss any matters that are disturbing to him. Attention is directed to the patient rather than to his intestinal tract. Stress reduction measures that may be used include relaxation techniques, breathing exercises, and biofeedback.

▷ *Patient Education and Home Health Care.* The patient's understanding of the disease process and need for additional information about medical management (medications, diet) and surgical interventions are assessed.

Information about nutritional management is provided. A bland, low-residue, high-protein, high-calorie, and high-vitamin diet relieves symptoms and decreases diarrhea. The rationale for the use of steroids, anti-inflammatory agents, antibacterial and antidiarrheal drugs, and antispasmodics is provided. The importance of taking medications as prescribed and not abruptly discontinuing them is emphasized (especially the steroid agents, which can cause serious medical problems if suddenly stopped).

If surgery is required, the nurse explains the procedure and the preoperative and postoperative care. Ileostomy care is reviewed if necessary. See Nursing Care Plan 37-1 for the patient with an intestinal ostomy.

(text continues on page 940)

Nursing Care Plan 37-1

Care of the Patient With an Intestinal Ostomy

Nursing Interventions	Rationale	Expected Outcomes

Nursing Diagnosis: Knowledge deficit of the surgical procedure and preoperative preparation

Goal: Understands the surgical process and the necessary preoperative preparations

Nursing Interventions	Rationale	Expected Outcomes
1. Ascertain if the patient has had a previous surgical experience and ask for recollections of positive and negative impressions.	1. Fear of a repeated negative experience increases anxiety. Talking about the experience with a nurse helps clarify misconceptions and helps the patient ventilate any repressed emotions. Positive experiences are reinforced.	• Expresses anxieties and fears about the surgical process • Projects a positive attitude toward the surgical procedure • Repeats in own words information supplied by the surgeon • Identifies normal anatomy and physiology of gastrointestinal tract and how it will be altered. Can point to expected location of abdominal wound and stoma. Describes stoma appearance and size • Adheres to "bowel prep" regimen of antimicrobials or mechanical cleansing • Tolerates the presence of nasogastric/nasoenteric tube
2. Determine what information the surgeon provided and whether it was understood. Clarify and elaborate as necessary. Know whether the stoma is permanent or temporary. Be aware of the patient's prognosis if carcinoma exists.	2. Clarification prevents misunderstandings and alleviates anxiety. A positive affect may be more difficult to project if the ostomy is permanent or the prognosis poor.	
3. Use pictures or drawings to illustrate the location and appearance of the wounds (abdominal, perineal) and the stoma if the patient is interested and receptive.	3. Knowledge, for some, alleviates anxiety because they have decreased their fear of the unknown. Others choose not to know because it makes them more anxious.	
4. Explain that oral/parenteral antimicrobials will be administered to cleanse the bowel preoperatively. Mechanical cleansing may also be required.	4. Antimicrobials and mechanical cleansing will reduce intestinal bacterial flora.	
5. Assist the patient during nasogastric/nasoenteric intubation. Measure drainage from the tube.	5. Nasoenteral intubation is used for decompression and drainage of gastrointestinal contents before surgery.	

Nursing Diagnosis: Disturbance in self-concept related to altered body image

Goal: Attainment of a positive self-concept

Nursing Interventions	Rationale	Expected Outcomes
1. Encourage the patient to verbalize feelings about the stoma.	1. Free expression of feelings allows the patient the opportunity to verbalize and identify concerns. Expressed concerns can be therapeutically addressed by health care team members.	• Freely expresses concerns • Accepts support • Seeks help as needed • States is willing to talk with an ostomate
2. Offer to be present when the stoma is first viewed and touched.	2. Anxiety can be reduced if questions are immediately answered.	
3. Suggest that the spouse or significant other view the stoma.		
4. Offer counseling, if desired.		
5. Arrange for a visit with an ostomate.	5. Ostomates provide an empathetic approach because they can share mutual feelings, and offer support.	

(continued)

➤ Nursing Care Plan 37–1 (Continued)

Care of the Patient With an Intestinal Ostomy

Nursing Interventions	Rationale	Expected Outcomes

Nursing Diagnosis: Anxiety related to the loss of bowel control

Goal: Reduction of anxiety

1. Provide information about expected bowel function:
  a. Characteristics of effluent
  b. Frequency of discharge
2. Teach the patient how to prepare the pouch for an adequate fit.
  a. Choose the drainage pouch that will provide a secure fit around the stoma. Measure the stoma size with a measuring guide provided by the ostomy manufacturer and compare with the opening on the pouch. About 3-mm (⅛-in) clearance should be provided around the stoma.
  b. Remove any plastic covering that protects the pouch adhesive. *Note:* The pouch is applied by pressing the adhesive for 30 seconds to the skin or skin barrier.
3. Demonstrate how to change the pouch before leakage occurs. Be aware that the elderly person may have diminished vision and difficulty handling equipment.
4. Demonstrate how to irrigate the colostomy (usually on the 4th–5th day.) Recommend that irrigating be done on a regular time, depending on the type of colostomy.
	1. Emotional adjustment is facilitated if adequate information is provided at the level of the learner.
	
	  a. The pouch opening should be larger than the stoma for an adequate fit. Available brands come in different sizes to fit the stoma. Adjustments can be made if necessary.
	
	  b. The pouch is ready to apply directly to the skin or skin protector.
	
	3. Manipulation of the appliance is a learned motor skill that requires practice and positive encouragement.
		• Expresses interest in learning about expected bowel function
		• Handles equipment correctly.
		• Changes the pouch unassisted
		• Irrigates colostomy successfully
		• Progresses toward a regular schedule of elimination

Nursing Diagnosis: High risk for impaired skin integrity related to irritation of the peristomal skin by the effluent

Goal: Attainment of skin integrity

1. Provide information about signs/symptoms of irritated or inflamed skin. Use pictures if possible. 2. Teach patient how to gently cleanse the peristomal skin 3. Demonstrate how to apply a skin barrier (powder, gel, paste, wafer). 4. Demonstrate how to remove the pouch.	1. Peristomal skin should be slightly pink without abrasions and similar to that of the entire abdomen. 2. Mild friction with warm water and a gentle soap cleanses the skin and minimizes irritation and possible abrasions. Patting the skin dry prevents tissue trauma. 3. Skin barriers protect the peristomal skin from enzymes and bacteria. 4. Gently separate adhesive from the skin to avoid irritation. Never pull!	• Describes appearance of healthy skin • Correctly cleanses the skin • Successfully applies a skin barrier • Gently removes the drainage pouch without skin damage • Demonstrates intact skin around the colostomy stoma

(continued)

Nursing Care Plan 37-1 *(Continued)*

Care of the Patient With an Intestinal Ostomy

Nursing Interventions	Rationale	Expected Outcomes

Nursing Diagnosis: Potential alteration in nutrition, less than body requirements, related to avoidance of foods that may cause gastrointestinal discomfort

Goal: Achievement of an optimal nutritional intake

1. Conduct a complete nutritional assessment to identify any foods that may increase peristalsis by irritating the bowel.	1. Patients react differently to certain foods because of individual sensitivity.	• Modifies diet to avoid offensive foods yet maintains a balanced nutritional intake
2. Advise the patient to avoid food products with a cellulose or hemicellulose base (nuts, seeds).	2. Cellulose food products are the nondigestable residue of plant foods. They hold water, provide bulk, and stimulate elimination.	• Avoids foods such as peanuts • Modifies intake of certain fruits
3. Recommend moderation in intake of certain irritating fruits such as prunes, grapes, and bananas.	3. These fruits tend to increase the quantity of effluent.	

Nursing Diagnosis: Sexual dysfunction related to altered body image

Goal: Attainment of satisfactory sexual performance

1. Encourage the patient to verbalize his fears. The sexual partner is welcomed to participate in the discussion.	1. Expressed needs help the therapist develop a plan of care.	• Expresses fears and concerns • Discusses alternative sexual positions • Accepts services of a professional counselor
2. Recommend alternative sexual positions.	2. Avoid patient embarassment with the visual appearance of the stoma. Avoid peristomal skin irritation secondary to friction.	
3. Seek assistance from a sexual therapist or psychiatric clinical specialist.	3. Some patients need professional sexual counseling.	

Nursing Diagnosis: High risk for fluid volume deficit related to anorexia and vomiting

Goal: Attainment of fluid balance

1. Estimate fluid intake and output:
   a. Strict intake and output
	1. Provides indication of fluid balance.
	   a. An early indicator of fluid imbalance is a daily, significant difference between intake and output. The average person ingests (food, fluids) and loses (urine, feces, lungs) about 3 liters of fluid every 24 hours.
		• Maintains fluid balance
		• Maintains normal serum and urinary values for sodium and potassium
		• Normal skin turgor
		• Surface of tongue is pink with a moist mucous membrane

b. Daily weights	b. A gain/loss of 1 liter of fluid is reflected in a body weight change of 2.2 pounds.	
2. Assess serum and urinary values of sodium and potassium.	2. Sodium is the major electrolyte regulating water balance. Vomiting results in decreased urinary and serum sodium levels. Urinary sodium values, in contrast to serum values, reflect early, sensitive	

(continued)

Nursing Care Plan 37–1 (Continued)

Care of the Patient With an Intestinal Ostomy

Nursing Interventions	Rationale	Expected Outcomes
	changes in sodium balance. Sodium works in conjunction with potassium, which is also decreased with vomiting. A significant deficiency in potassium is associated with a decrease in intracellular potassium bicarbonate, which leads to acidosis and compensatory hyperventilation.	
3. Observe and record skin turgor and the appearance of the tongue.	3. Adequate hydration is reflected by the skin's ability to return to its normal shape after being grasped between the fingers. *Note:* In the older person, it is normal for the return to be delayed. Changes in the mucous membrane covering of the tongue are an accurate and early indicator of hydration status.	

Patients who are being medically managed at home need to understand that their disease can be controlled and that they can lead a healthy life between exacerbations. Control implies management based on an understanding of inflammatory bowel disease and its treatment.

During a flare-up, patients are encouraged to rest as needed and modify activities according to energy levels. If possible they should limit activities to one floor in the house. Patients are advised to limit tasks (*e.g.*, housekeeping chores) that impose strain on the lower abdominal muscles. Patients should sleep in a room close to the bathroom because of frequent diarrheal stools (10 to 20 a day). Quick access to a toilet helps alleviate the worry of embarrassment if an accident occurs. Room deodorizers help control odors.

Patients in the home setting need information about their medications (drug name, dosage, side effects, frequency of administration) and need to take them on schedule. Medication reminders are helpful (containers that separate pills according to day and time, daily checklists).

Dietary modifications can control but not cure the disease. A low-residue, high-protein, high-calorie diet is recommended, especially during an acute phase. Patients are encouraged to keep a record of those foods that irritate the bowel and to eliminate them from their diet.

The prolonged nature of the disease often causes a strain on family life and financial resources. Family support is vital; however, some family members experience resentment, guilt, fatigue, and an inability to continue coping with the emotional demands of the illness as well as with the physical demands of caring for another.

Some persons will not socialize for fear of being embarrassed. Many prefer to eat alone. Because they have lost control over elimination they believe that they have lost control over other aspects of their life. They need time to ventilate their fears and frustrations.

▷ Evaluation

Expected Outcomes

1. Reports a decrease in the frequency of diarrheal stools
   a. Recognizes a causal relationship between certain foods, activity, or stress, and elimination
   b. Complies with activity restrictions; maintains bed rest
   c. Takes medications as prescribed
2. Experiences less pain
   a. Uses diversional activities to decrease anxiety and pain
   b. Takes anticholinergics before meals
   c. Takes analgesics as needed and as prescribed
3. Maintains fluid volume balance
   a. Drinks 1 to 2 liters oral fluids daily
   b. Has a normal body temperature
   c. Displays adequate skin turgor and moist mucous membranes
4. Attains optimal nutrition
   a. Tolerates small, frequent feedings without diarrhea
   b. Complies with total parenteral nutrition therapy
   c. Accepts elemental feedings if necessary
5. Avoids episodes of fatigue
   a. Rests periodically during the day
   b. Adheres to bed rest restrictions
   c. Performs exercises as needed
6. Feels less anxious
   a. Discusses fears and worries
   b. Describes the surgical procedure in own words
   c. Handles equipment with ease and skill
   d. Speaks willingly with an ostomate

7. Copes successfully with diagnosis
   a. Ventilates feelings freely
   b. Socializes with family members and friends
   c. Uses appropriate stress-reduction behaviors
8. Acquires an understanding of the disease process
   a. Modifies diet appropriately to decrease diarrhea
   b. Adheres to medication regimen
   c. Describes possible surgical interventions

In summary, regional enteritis and ulcerative colitis are chronic inflammatory disorders with resultant changes in the physiologic function of the area of the intestine/colon involved. Initially, both conditions are generally treated medically, but may eventually require surgical intervention.

Nursing care for patients with regional enteritis and ulcerative colitis are similar, with goals directed toward relief of anxiety and pain, attainment and maintenance of fluid, electrolyte, and nutritional balance, and ability to cope with the effects of the illness. Patients who require surgery (*e.g.*, ileostomy) need preoperative education and emotional support to prepare for the surgery.

Nursing Considerations for the Patient Requiring an Ileostomy

Preoperative Nursing Interventions

A period of preparation, with intensive fluid, blood, and protein replacement, is necessary before surgery is attempted. Antibiotics may be prescribed. If the patient has been taking steroids, then steroids will be continued during the surgical phase. The patient is assessed for adrenal insufficiency by observing and recording pulse, blood pressure, urinary output, general appearance, and reactions.

Usually, the patient is given a low-residue diet offered in frequent small feedings. All other preoperative measures are similar to those for general abdominal surgery. The abdomen is marked for the proper placement of the stoma by the surgeon or the ostomy nurse. Care is taken to see that the ostomy stoma is conveniently placed.

Information about an ileostomy is presented to the patient by means of literature, models, and discussion. The patient must have a thorough understanding of the surgery and what to expect postoperatively. Teaching before surgery will relate to managing the drains from the outlet, the nature of drainage, and the need for nasogastric intubation, parenteral fluids, and perineal packing and care.

Postoperative Nursing Interventions

General abdominal surgery wound care is required. As soon as the operation is completed, a temporary plastic bag with an adhesive facing is placed over the ileostomy and firmly pressed onto surrounding skin. The opening of the small intestine on the abdomen continuously discharges the liquid contents of the small intestine, because the stoma does not have a controlling sphincter. The contents draining from the ileostomy drain into the plastic bag and are thus kept from coming into contact with skin. They are collected and measured as the bag becomes full. After the ileostomy has had a chance to heal, a permanent appliance is obtained and held in place on the skin with a special cement. The stomal size should be rechecked in 3 weeks, when the edema has subsided. The final size and type of appliance may be selected in 3 months, after the patient's weight has stabilized and the stoma shrinks to a stable shape.

Because these patients lose much fluid and food in the early postoperative period, an accurate record of fluid intake, urinary output, and fecal discharge is necessary to help gauge the fluid needs of the patient. Fluids and a low-residue, high-calorie diet are encouraged.

Nasogastric suction is also a part of immediate postoperative care, with the tube requiring frequent irrigation, as prescribed. The purpose of nasogastric suction is to facilitate healing and to relieve pressure on the suture line by preventing a buildup of gastric contents. The patient receives parenteral fluids for 4 to 5 days. Thereafter, sips of clear liquids are offered, and the diet progresses gradually. Nausea and abdominal distention are observed as signs of an obstruction. Should they occur, the physician is notified.

As with other patients undergoing abdominal surgery, early ambulation is encouraged. Prescribed pain medications are administered as required.

By the end of the first week, rectal packing is removed. Because this procedure may be uncomfortable, the patient may be given a sedative an hour before it is performed. After the packing is removed, the perineum is irrigated two to three times daily until full healing takes place.

Psychosocial Considerations

The patient understandably may think that everyone is aware of the ileostomy, and may view the stoma as mutilative in comparison with other abdominal incisions that heal and are hidden. Because there is loss of a body part and a major change in anatomy, the ileostomy patient often goes through the various phases of grieving: shock, disbelief, denial, rejection, anger, and restitution. Nursing support through these phases is important, and understanding of the patient's emotional outlook in each instance should determine the nurse's approach. For example, teaching may be of no avail until the patient has reached the stage of restitution. Concern over body image may lead to questions related to family relationships, sexual function, and the ability to become pregnant and to deliver a baby normally.

Finally, such patients need to know that someone understands and cares about them. A calm, nonjudgmental attitude exhibited by the nurse will aid in gaining the patient's confidence, so important to therapy and preoperative preparation. It is important to recognize the dependency needs of these patients.

Such patients probably are challenging to the nurse. Their prolonged illness can make them irritable, anxious, and depressed. The nurse can coordinate patient care through nursing conferences attended by consultants such as the physician, psychologist, psychiatrist, social worker, enterostomal therapist, and dietitian. The team approach lends support in approaching a complex nursing problem.

Conversely, an operation establishing an ileostomy can

produce dramatic positive changes in patients who have suffered from colitis for several years. Once the continuous discomfort of the disease has decreased and patients learn how to take care of an ileostomy, they develop a more positive outlook. But until they progress to this phase, an empathetic and tolerant approach by the nurse will play an important part in recovery.

The support of other ostomates is also a help. A nonprofit health service agency that is dedicated to the rehabilitation of ostomates is the United Ostomy Association (36 Executive Park, Irvine, CA 92714). This organization gives patients useful information about living with an ostomy through an educational program of literature, lectures, and exhibits. Local associations provide visiting services by qualified members who provide hope, as well as rehabilitation services, to new ostomy patients. Hospitals in the region may have an enterostomal therapy nurse on the staff; this is a valuable resource person for the ileostomy patient.

Rehabilitation and Patient Education After an Ileostomy

There are certain rehabilitation problems unique to the ileostomy patient, one of which is irregularity of bowel evacuation. The patient with an ileostomy cannot establish regular bowel habits because the contents of the ileum are fluid and are discharging continuously. Therefore, the patient must wear a pouch day and night. The pouch is regarded, then, as an intestinal prosthesis.

Several days after the operation, the ileostomy diameter is carefully measured with a stoma-measuring card (various apertures indicate different sizes). Disposable pouches may be ordered to fit the stoma or the pouches may be cut down to size as necessary. The patient can carry on normal activities without fear of leakage or odor.

The location and length of the stoma are significant in the management of the ileostomy by the patient. The surgeon places the stoma as close to the midline as possible and in a position where even an obese patient with a protruding abdomen can care for it easily. Usually, the ileostomy stoma is about 2.5 cm (1 in) long, which makes it convenient for the attachment of an appliance.

The ileostomy may be noisy at first because of edema caused by slight obstruction of tissues. Eventually it will become quieter. A low-fiber diet is followed at first, with strained fruits and vegetables. These foods are important for vitamins A and C. Later there are few dietary restrictions, except for avoiding foods that are high in fiber or hard-to-digest kernels, such as celery, popcorn, corn, poppy seeds or caraway seeds, and coconut. Fluids may be a problem during the summer, when they are lost during perspiration as well as through the ileostomy. Drinks such as Gatorade are helpful in maintaining electrolyte balance. If the effluent (fecal discharge) is too watery, fibrous foods (such as whole grain cereals, fresh fruit skins, beans, corn, and nuts) are restricted.

If the effluent is excessively dry, salt intake is increased. An increased intake of water or fluid will not increase the effluent because excess water is excreted in the urine.

Another possible problem is skin excoriation around the stoma. The ileostomy drainage contains enzymes that rapidly excoriate the skin. If irritation and yeast growth are present, nystatin powder (Mycostatin) is dusted lightly on the peristomal skin.

A regular schedule for changing the pouch before leakage occurs is established. In teaching the patient to use and care for his pouch, a procedure similar to that in Chart 37-2 should be established. The amount of time that a person can keep the appliance sealed to the body depends on the location of the stoma and on body structure. Usually, the normal wearing time is 5 to 7 days. The appliance is emptied every 4 to 6 hours, or at the same time the patient empties his bladder. An emptying spout at the bottom of the appliance is closed with a special clip made for this purpose. Most pouches used at this time are disposable and odorproof. Foods such as spinach and parsley act as deodorizers in the intestinal tract; foods that cause odors include cabbage, onions, and fish. Bismuth subcarbonate tablets prescribed by the physician and taken by mouth three or four times a day are effective in reducing odor. Some physicians prescribe a stool thickener, such as diphenoxylate (Lomotil) (by mouth), to assist in odor control.

A continent ileostomy may have been created instead of the traditional ileostomy. A nipple valve is constructed at the outlet to facilitate drainage. The patient must be taught the procedure for drainage of the pouch (Chart 37-3).

When discharge is thick, water can be injected through the catheter to loosen and soften it. Effluent consistency is affected by food intake. At first drainage is only 60 to 80 ml, but as time goes on it will increase significantly. The pouch will stretch, eventually accommodating 500 to 1000 ml. The gauge to determine the frequency of the need for drainage is the sensation of pressure in the pouch.

Patient Education and Home Health Care. The spouse and family should be familiar with the adjustment that will be necessary when the patient returns home. They need to know why it is necessary for the ileostomate to occupy the bathroom for 10 minutes at certain times of the day, and why certain equipment is needed. Their understanding is necessary to reduce tension—a relaxed patient tends to have fewer problems.

Psychosocial needs of the patient are stressed. For the patient who has a continent ileostomy, knowing that it will not be necessary to wear an ileostomy bag is often sufficient encouragement for the patient to master control over the pouch.

A successful cover for the stoma for home use consists of a dressing that is absorbent on one side and plasticized on the other. (High-quality disposable diapers can be cut into 7.5 × 7.5-cm [3 × 3-in] squares; these make an ideal dressing.) The dressing is held in place with tape. To reduce skin excoriation, the tape is placed differently with each application so that it does not contact the same area of skin each time.

A water-soluble lubricant, rather than petrolatum, should be used. The latter has a tendency to clog the catheter and is difficult to wash from it.

The position to assume in the bathroom is one of individual preference and convenience. The patient may sit on the toilet seat, stand in front of the toilet, or sit on a chair in front of the toilet. It is suggested that an adapter and a length of tubing be available to attach to the catheter, so that effluent does not splatter but drains easily into the toilet bowl.

Experimentation is encouraged when there are problems with drainage. If the catheter meets resistance when attempts

Chart 37–2
Guidelines for Changing an Ileostomy Appliance

Changing an ileostomy appliance is necessary to prevent leakage (the bag is usually changed every 2 to 4 days), to allow for examination of the skin around the stoma, and to assist in controlling odor if this becomes a problem. The appliance should be changed at any time that the patient complains of burning or itching under the disc or pain in the area of the stoma; routine changes should be performed early in the morning before breakfast or 2 to 4 hours after a meal, when the bowel is least active.

Procedure

Nursing Action	Rationale/Amplification
1. Promote patient comfort and involvement in the procedure.	Providing a relaxed atmosphere and adequate explanations help the patient to become an active participant in the procedure.
A. Have the patient assume a relaxed position. Provide privacy.	
B. Explain details of the procedure.	
C. Expose the ileostomy area; remove the ileostomy belt (if worn).	
2. Remove the appliance.	
A. Have the patient sit on the toilet or on a chair facing the toilet. If the patient prefers to stand, have him face the toilet.	These positions facilitate disposal or drainage.
B. The appliance (pouch) can be removed by gently pushing the skin away from the adhesive.	
3. Cleanse the skin.	
A. Wash the skin gently with a soft cloth moistened with tepid water and mild soap, the patient may prefer to bathe before putting on a clean appliance.	The patient may shower with or without the pouch. Micropore or waterproof tape applied to the sides of the faceplate will keep it secure while bathing.
B. Rinse and dry the skin thoroughly after cleansing.	Moisture or soap residue will interfere with appliance adhesion.
4. Apply appliance (when there is *no* skin irritation):	
A. An appropriate skin barrier is applied to the peristomal skin before the pouch is applied.	Many pouches have a built-in skin barrier.
B. Remove cover from adherent surface of disc of disposable plastic pouch and apply directly to the skin.	The skin should be thoroughly dried before applying the pouch.
C. Press firmly in place for 30 seconds to insure adherence.	
5. Apply appliance (when there is skin irritation):	
A. Cleanse the skin thoroughly but gently; pat dry.	To remove debris.
B. Apply Kenalog spray; blot excess moisture with a cotton pledget and dust lightly with nystatin (Mycostatin) powder.	The steroid preparation (Kenalog) helps to decrease inflammation. The antifungal (nystatin) treats those types of infections that are common around stomas. A prescription is required for both medications.
(1) An alternate effective measure is to apply a wafer of Stomahesive (Squibb), which is available in 10×10-cm (4×4-in) and 20×20-cm (8×8-in) pieces. The stomal opening should be cut the same size as the stoma; use a cutting guide (supplied with Stomahesive). The wafer is applied directly to the skin.	Stomahesive is a substance that facilitates healing of excoriated skin. It adheres well even to moist, irritated skin.
(2) A second alternative is to moisten a karaya gum washer and apply when it is tacky. If the skin is moist, karaya powder may be applied first and any excess dusted off gently.	Karaya also facilitates skin healing. Tackiness promotes adherence.
C. The pouch is then applied to the treated skin.	This will allow skin to heal while the appliance is in place.
6. Check the pouch bottom for closure; use the rubber band or clip provided.	Proper closure controls leakage.

Chart 37-3
Guidelines for Draining a Continent Ileostomy (Koch Pouch)

A *continent ileostomy* is the surgical creation of a pouch of small intestine that can serve as an internal receptacle for fecal discharge; a nipple valve is constructed at the outlet. Postoperatively, a catheter extends from the stoma and is attached to a closed drainage suction system. To assure patency of the catheter, usually every 3 hours 10 to 20 ml of normal saline is instilled gently into the pouch; return flow is not aspirated but is allowed to drain by gravity.

After approximately 2 weeks, when the healing process has progressed to the point at which the catheter is removed from the stoma, the patient is taught to drain the pouch. The equipment required includes a catheter, tissues, water-soluble lubricant, gauze squares, a syringe, irrigating solution in a bowl, and an emesis or receiving basin.

The following procedure is used to drain the pouch; the patient is assisted to participate in this procedure so that he can learn to perform it unassisted.

Nursing Action	Rationale/Amplification
1. Lubricate the catheter and gently insert it about 5 cm (2 in), at which some resistance may be felt at the valve or "nipple."	When gentle pressure is used, the catheter usually will enter the pouch.
2. If there is much resistance, fill a syringe with 20 ml of air or water and inject it through the catheter, while still exerting some pressure on the catheter.	This will permit the catheter to enter the pouch.
3. Place the other end of the catheter in a drainage basin held below the level of the stoma. Later this process can be carried out at the toilet with drainage delivered into the toilet bowl.	Gravity facilitates drainage. Drainage may include flatus as well as effluent.
4. After drainage, the catheter is removed and the area around the stoma is gently washed with warm water. Pat dry and apply an absorbent pad over the stoma. Fasten the pad with hypoallergenic tape.	The entire procedure requires about 5 to 10 minutes; at first it is performed every 3 hours. The time between procedures is gradually lengthened to three times daily.

are made to insert it, the patient is encouraged to relax before draining the pouch and to be sure to lubricate the catheter well. It may be easier for the patient to lie down when the catheter is inserted and then stand up for drainage purposes.

Skin care, odor reduction, diet, and activities are similar to those recommended for other ostomy patients.

Complications

Minor complications occur in about 40% of patients who have an ileostomy; less than 20% of the complications require surgical intervention. *Peristomal skin irritation*, the most common complication of an ileostomy, is due to leakage of effluent. An ill-fitting pouch is frequently the cause. The pouch is adjusted by the nurse or an enterostomal therapist and skin barriers are applied. *Diarrhea*, manifested by very irritating effluent that rapidly fills the pouch (every hour or sooner), can quickly lead to dehydration and electrolyte losses. Supplemental water, sodium, and potassium are given to prevent hypovolemia and hypokalemia. Antidiarrheal agents are administered. *Stenosis* is caused by circular scar tissue formation at the stoma site. The scar tissue is surgically released. *Urinary calculi* occur in about 10% of ileostomy patients because of dehydration secondary to decreased fluid intake. Intense lower abdominal pain that radiates to the legs, hematuria, and signs of dehydration alert the nurse to strain all urine. Sometimes small stones are passed during urination; otherwise treatment is necessary to crush or remove the calculi. *Cholelithiasis* (formation of gall-

stones) due to cholesterol occurs three times more frequently than in the general population because of changes in the absorption of bile acids that occurs preoperatively. Spasm of the gallbladder causes severe upper right abdominal pain that can radiate to the back and right shoulder. *Ileitis* is usually seen with a recurrence of inflammatory bowel disease.

Intestinal Obstruction

Intestinal obstruction exists when there is any pathologic impediment to the normal flow of intestinal contents through the intestinal tract. This flow can be impeded by two types of processes:

1. *Mechanical*—there is an intraluminal obstruction or mural obstruction from pressure on the intestinal walls. Examples are intussusception, polypoid tumors, stenosis, strictures, adhesions, hernias, and abscesses.
2. *Paralytic*—the intestinal musculature is unable to propel the contents along the bowel. Examples are amyloidosis, muscular dystrophy, endocrine disorders like diabetes mellitus, or neurologic diseases like Parkinson's disease. It also can be residual from surgical operations.

The obstruction can be partial or complete. Its seriousness depends on the region of bowel that is affected, the degree to which the lumen is occluded, and, especially, the degree to which the blood circulation in the bowel wall is disturbed.

Adhesions are the most common cause of small bowel obstruction (60% incidence), followed by hernias and neoplasms. Other causes include intussusception, volvulus, and paralytic ileus.

Adhesions

After abdominal operations, there are many areas within the abdomen that may not be completely healed, and loops of intestine may become adherent to these areas. Such inflammatory adhesions usually are only temporary and of no particular importance. Occasionally, however, these adhesions may produce a kinking of an intestinal loop, which causes obstruction of the intestinal flow. This obstruction usually appears on the third or fourth day after operation, when peristalsis is normally resumed and when food and fluids are being given to the patient for the first time.

Intussusception

Intussusception is a condition in which one part of the intestine slips into another part located below it, much as a telescope is shortened by pushing one section into the next. This occurs through peristalsis. The point at which intussusception develops most commonly is at or near the ileocecal valve. The telescoping, or *invagination*, also may start at the point of attachment of a tumor in the colon and become engaged by a peristaltic wave and propelled along the colon, dragging into the lumen that portion of the wall to which its pedicle is attached (Fig. 37–5A.)

Volvulus

A volvulus (see Fig. 37–5B) is a life-threatening obstruction in which the bowel is twisted on itself and the intestinal lumen is obstructed both proximally and distally. The accumulation of gas and fluid in the trapped bowel and compromised vascular supply lead to necrosis, perforation, and peritonitis.

Paralytic Ileus

A paralytic ileus is a paralysis of peristaltic movement due to the effect of trauma or toxins on the nerves that regulate intestinal movement. Functional paralytic ileus after abdominal surgery may last 12 to 36 hours. Because of this, food and fluids are withheld until normal peristalsis returns, as indicated by bowel sounds (heard with the stethoscope) or the passing of flatus. Paralytic ileus also may occur after back injuries, after operation on the kidney, and frequently with peritonitis.

The lack of peristalsis results in a distention of the intestine with gas produced by decomposition of the intestinal contents or by swallowing of air. Few or no peristaltic sounds can be heard, and the patient may be extremely uncomfortable, if not in marked pain.

Abdominal Hernias

An abdominal hernia is a protrusion of an abdominal organ (commonly the small intestine) through an opening in the abdominal wall. Most hernias result from congenital or acquired weakness of the abdominal wall, coupled with sustained increased intra-abdominal pressure from coughing or straining,

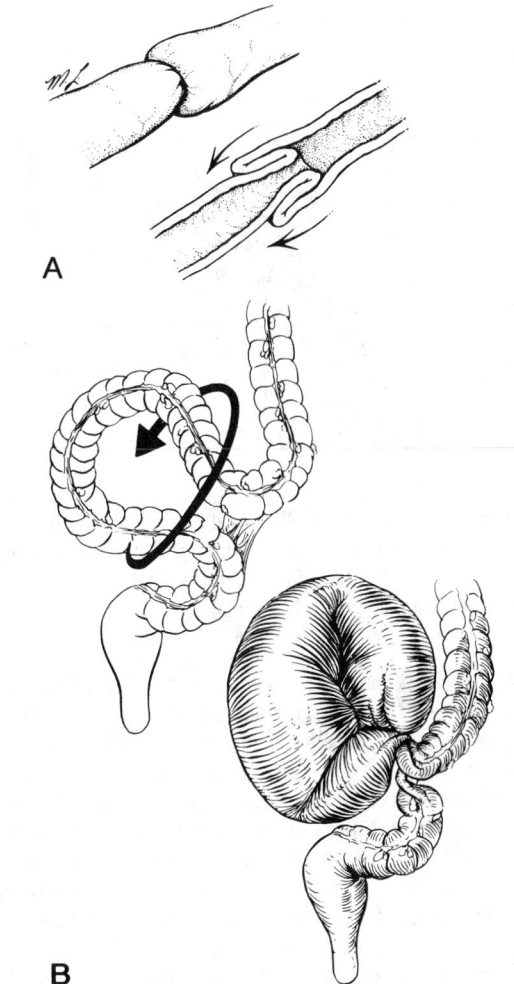

A

B

Figure 37–5. Two courses of intestinal obstruction. (**A**) Intussusception. Note invagination or shortening of colon by the movement of one segment of bowel into another. (**B**) Volvulus of the sigmoid colon. The twist is counterclockwise in most cases of sigmoid volvulus. Note the edematous bowel. (*B:* Way LW [ed]. Current Surgical Diagnosis and Treatment, 9th ed. Los Altos, CA, Lange Medical Publishers, 1991.)

or from an enlarging lesion within the abdomen. Once the hernia occurs, it has a tendency to increase in size.

The hernial sac is formed by an outpouching of the peritoneum and may contain the large or small intestine, the omentum, and occasionally the bladder. When the hernia is initially formed, the sac is filled only when the patient is standing up; the contents return to the abdominal cavity as soon as the patient lies down. There are several types of hernias.

Indirect inguinal hernia is the most common type of hernia (It is due to a weakness of the abdominal wall at the point through which the spermatic cord emerges in the male, and the round ligament in the female). Through this opening the hernia extends down the inguinal canal and often into the scrotum or the labia (Fig. 37–6). It is common in the male, and it may appear at any age.

Direct inguinal hernia passes through the posterior inguinal wall. It also is more common in males. It is more difficult to repair than indirect inguinal hernia, and often recurs after surgery. It is believed to be hereditary or related to a defect in the synthesis of collagen.

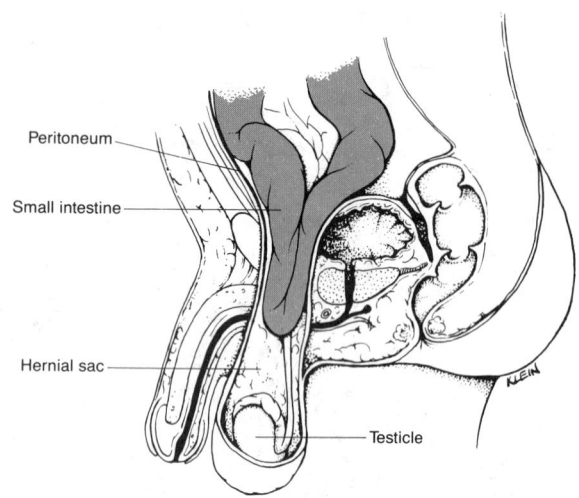

Figure 37-6. Inguinal hernia. Note that the sac of the hernia is a continuation of the peritoneum of the abdomen and that the hernial contents are intestine, omentum, or other abdominal contents that pass through the hernial opening into the hernial sac.

Umbilical hernia results from failure of the umbilical orifice to close. It is most common in obese women and in children, as a protrusion at the umbilicus. This hernia is also seen with increased intra-abdominal pressure in cirrhosis and ascites.

Ventral or incisional hernias occur because of a weakness in the abdominal wall. They are due most frequently to previous operations in which drainage was necessary, complete closure of the tissues being impossible. Weakened by infection, only a slight bulge results at first, but this increases gradually in size until a definite hernial sac is produced.

Femoral hernia appears below the inguinal (Poupart's) ligament (*i.e.,* below the groin) as a round bulge. It is more frequent in women because of changes during pregnancy.

The major complication of an abdominal hernia is intestinal obstruction. For this reason, surgical repair is performed before any further complications can occur.

A hernia is referred to as *reducible* when the protruding mass can be placed back into the abdominal cavity. This can occur naturally when the patient lies down, or it may require manual reduction (the mass is pushed back into the cavity). As time goes on, adhesions form between the sac and its contents, so that the hernia becomes *irreducible* or *incarcerated*. Such a hernia is one that cannot be reduced and in which the intestinal flow may be obstructed completely.

In a *strangulated hernia*, not only are the contents irreducible, but the blood and intestinal flow through the intestine in the hernia ceases completely. This condition develops when the loop of intestine in the sac becomes twisted or swollen and a constriction is produced at the neck of the sac. The result then is an acute intestinal obstruction, with the added danger of gangrene of the bowel. The symptoms are pain at the site of strangulation, followed by colicky abdominal pain, vomiting, and swelling of the hernial sac.

Mechanical Reduction.   Very often patients can reduce their own hernias. To keep the mass from protruding when a standing position is assumed, a *truss* (a pad made of firm material that is placed externally over the hernia and held in place with a belt) may be worn. Most authorities agree that a truss creates more problems than it can solve. Skin irritation and

lesions may result from constant rubbing. When improperly fitted, it may cause strangulation of the hernia. A truss may be recommended, however, (1) for infants, when there is need to wait for a weight gain before surgery or for remission of another problem, such as bronchitis; (2) for adults who have an underlying problem that needs to be resolved first; or (3) when a patient has worn a truss for years, is terrified of the hospital, and will not part with the truss. In this last instance, the proper fitting of the truss must be done by a qualified person. The Valsalva maneuver can also be used to check for the effectiveness of the truss. Daily bathing and the use of corn starch powder can lessen the possibility of skin irritation. Usually the truss is worn directly over the hernia and not over clothing, which could cause slipping. It must be emphasized that *a truss does not cure a hernia*; it simply prevents the abdominal contents from entering the hernial sac.

The hernia should always be repaired by surgery; otherwise, it is in continual danger of strangulation. When strangulation occurs, surgery becomes imperative and is attended invariably by considerable risk.

The surgical procedure involves removal of the hernial sac after it has been dissected free from surrounding structures, the contents have been replaced in the abdominal cavity, and its neck has been ligated. The muscle and the fascial layers then are sutured together firmly over the hernial orifice to prevent a recurrence. The incidence of recurrence is 5% to 25%. When the tissues are not sufficiently strong, reinforcement can be obtained by overlaying the suture line with synthetic sutures or mesh, which is also sutured in place (*hernioplasty*). The presence of the mesh stimulates more than the usual amount of fibroblastic activity and thereby enhances the strength of the repair. When strangulation has occurred, the operation is complicated by intestinal obstruction and injury to the bowel.

Preoperative Nursing Interventions.   Most patients undergoing a *herniorrhaphy* (surgical repair of a hernia) are in good physical condition and have elected to have the surgery. They may be prompted by the knowledge that an unrepaired hernia can become a serious emergency, or that the condition can cause difficulty in securing employment. The patient may come into the hospital the morning of surgery or the night before, or the procedure can be performed in a surgical clinic/center. In emergency conditions of strangulated or incarcerated hernia, the nurse prepares the patient as in any other acute surgical problem.

Assessment includes determining whether the patient has an upper respiratory infection, chronic cough from excessive smoking, or sneezing due to an allergy. It may be necessary to postpone the operation, because coughing or sneezing could weaken the postoperative wound, thereby negating the purpose of surgery.

Postoperative Nursing Interventions.   The patient is allowed out of bed several hours after surgery. Young, healthy patients without other diseases are often discharged on the day of surgery. After local or spinal anesthesia, diet is determined by the desires of the patient. When general anesthesia is used, fluid and food are restricted until peristalsis returns.

Urinary retention is common in the postoperative period. If the patient gets out of bed to void within several hours after surgery, however, there usually is no difficulty. In any case, it is necessary to prevent bladder distention; this may require catheterization if other nursing measures fail.

The patient who coughs or sneezes after the operation is

instructed to splint the incision site with one hand, both to lessen the pain and to protect the incision site from the increased intra-abdominal pressure caused by the coughing and sneezing.

After repair of an inguinal hernia, swelling of the scrotum may occur. Because this is extremely painful, the patient is reluctant to move. Elevating the scrotum on a rolled towel and applying small ice bags intermittently are helpful. A narcotic may be prescribed for pain, and antibiotics may be prescribed to prevent epididymitis. A suspensory bandage or a scrotal support may be applied for support and comfort.

Infection that interferes with healing occurs occasionally. Soreness in the operative region and temperature elevation may suggest such a problem. Systemic antibiotics or local wound treatment with heat application, followed by incision and drainage, may be required.

For more extensive hernia repair, such as may be required after umbilical or large incisional hernia, nasogastric suction may be used to prevent distention, vomiting, and straining. Stool softeners are prescribed to prevent straining during defecation.

Patient Education and Home Health Care Considerations. Hospitalized patients may go home the day after herniorrhaphy or may stay 3 to 5 days or longer, depending on their age and medical condition. Many patients have same-day surgery with local anesthesia. The patient at home needs to know that pain and scrotal swelling will be present after surgery for 24 to 48 hours. Local applications of ice, elevation of the scrotum, use of a scrotal support, and pain medication should relieve the pain. The patient is instructed to report severe pain to the physician.

Some surgeons permit patients to do whatever they wish if they agree not to engage in painful activity, thereby preventing injury to the incision. Most, however, recommend limited activities for 5 to 7 days, and restriction of heavy lifting for 4 to 6 weeks. The use of correct body mechanics at all times is encouraged.

The patient is advised to report any drainage from the incision to the physician. Straining during defecation is avoided by diet modification, bulk cathartics, or stool softeners, and a daily fluid intake of 2000 ml. Pain or difficulty with urination is reported to the physician.

Evaluation. Short-term evaluation of nursing interventions can be carried out through an assessment of the return of peristalsis, adequate urinary output, decrease in scrotal swelling, absence of infection, relief of pain, and avoidance of straining with defecation. Long-term evaluation can be carried out through an assessment of the patient's understanding of the restrictions established.

Small Bowel Obstruction

Pathophysiology. Proximal to the intestinal obstruction, there is an accumulation of intestinal contents, fluid, and gas. In the small intestine, distention reduces the absorption of fluids and stimulates gastric secretion. As a result, fluids and electrolytes are lost. With increasing distention, pressure within the intestinal lumen causes a decrease in venous and arteriolar capillary pressure. This, in turn, causes edema, congestion, necrosis, and eventual rupture or perforation of the intestinal wall.

Reflux vomiting may also occur from the abdominal distention. With vomiting, there is a loss of hydrogen ions and potassium from the stomach, producing hypochloremia, hypokalemia, and metabolic alkalosis. Then dehydration and acidosis develop because of water loss and sodium loss. When there are acute fluid losses, hypovolemic shock may occur.

Clinical Manifestations. The initial symptom is usually pain that is wavelike in character. The patient may pass blood and mucus, but no fecal matter and no flatus. Vomiting occurs. This pattern is often characteristic. If the obstruction is complete, the peristaltic waves become extremely vigorous and assume a reverse direction, the intestinal contents being propelled toward the mouth instead of toward the rectum. If the obstruction is in the ileum, fecal vomiting takes place. First, the patient vomits the stomach contents, then the bile-stained contents of the duodenum and the jejunum, and finally, with each paroxysm of pain, the darker, fecal-like contents of the ileum. Soon, because of the loss of water, sodium, and chlorides in the vomitus, the unmistakable signs of dehydration become evident. The patient complains of intense thirst, drowsiness, generalized malaise, and aching. The tongue and the mucous membranes become parched; the face acquires a pinched appearance. The abdomen becomes distended, the lower the obstruction in the gastrointestinal tract, the more marked is the distention. If the situation is allowed to continue uncorrected, shock appears, due to dehydration and loss of plasma volume. The patient is prostrated; the pulse becomes increasingly weak and rapid; the temperature and the blood pressure are lowered; the skin is pale, cold, and clammy. With strangulation, the patient experiences severe abdominal pain and tenderness, high fever with leukocytosis, and symptoms of shock.

Diagnostic Evaluation. Diagnosis is based on presentation of symptoms as identified above and also radiologic studies. The abdominal radiograph will show abnormal quantities of gas in the bowel. Laboratory studies, (*i.e.*, electrolyte studies and complete blood count) will reveal a picture of dehydration and loss of plasma volume, and possibly infection.

Management. Decompression of the bowel through a nasoenteral tube is successful in the majority of cases. When the bowel is completely obstructed, the possibility of strangulation warrants surgical intervention. While awaiting the surgical procedure, intravenous therapy is used to replace the depleted water, sodium, chloride, and potassium.

The surgical treatment of intestinal obstruction depends largely on the cause of the obstruction. In the most common causes of obstruction, such as strangulated hernia and obstruction by adhesions, the operation consists of repair of the hernia or division of the adhesion to which the intestine is attached. In some hernias, the strangulated portion of bowel may be removed and an anastomosis performed. The complexity of the operation for intestinal obstruction depends on the duration of the obstruction and the condition of the intestine found at operation.

Large Bowel Obstruction

About 15% of intestinal obstructions occur in the large bowel, and most are found in the sigmoid. The most common causes are carcinoma, diverticulitis, inflammatory bowel disorders, and benign tumors.

Pathophysiology. Obstruction at the ileocecal valve produces changes similar to those in small bowel obstruction. Obstruction in the colon can lead to severe distention and perforation unless some gas and fluid can flow back through the ileum (incompetent valve). Large bowel obstruction, even if complete, is also comparatively undramatic if the blood supply to the colon is not disturbed. If the blood supply is cut off, however, intestinal strangulation and necrosis (tissue death) occur, and the patient's life is in jeopardy. In the large intestine, dehydration occurs more slowly than in the small intestine because the colon is able to absorb its fluid contents and can distend to a size considerably beyond its normal full capacity.

Clinical Manifestations. Large bowel obstruction differs clinically from the small bowel type in that the symptoms develop and progress relatively slowly. In patients with obstruction in the sigmoid or the rectum, constipation may be the only symptom for days. Eventually, the abdomen becomes markedly distended, loops of large bowel become visibly outlined through the abdominal wall, and the patient suffers from crampy lower abdominal pain. Finally, fecal vomiting develops. The terminal features are essentially those of ileum obstruction.

Radiographic studies show a distended colon. Barium studies are contraindicated.

Management. The usual treatment is surgical resection, with the formation of a colostomy or ileostomy in right colon obstruction and perforation. Sometimes an ileoanal anastomosis is performed. A *cecostomy* (insertion of a tube into the lumen of the cecum) may be performed for those patients who are poor surgical risks and urgently need relief from the obstruction. The procedure provides an outlet for releasing gas and a small amount of drainage.

In summary, bowel obstruction may result from a pathophysiologic problem in the small or large intestine. Symptoms of pain and abdominal distention are similar in both situations. Diagnosis must be based on radiologic findings. The treatments vary from decompression of the bowel to surgical resection.

Cancer of the Large Intestine: Colon and Rectum

Tumors of the small intestine are rare; conversely, tumors of the colon are relatively common. In fact, cancer of the colon and rectum is now one of the most common types of internal cancer in men in the United States. It is estimated that 147,000 new cases of colorectal cancer (76,000 in women and 71,000 in men) are diagnosed in this country each year. Colon cancer affects more than twice as many people as rectal cancer.

The incidence increases with age (most patients are over age 50), and is higher in persons with a family history of colon cancer and those with ulcerative colitis. The distribution of cancer sites throughout the colon can be seen in Figure 37–7. Changes in the percentage distribution have been recorded recently. The incidence of cancer in the sigmoid and rectal areas has decreased, whereas the incidence in the ascending and descending colon has increased.

Of the more than 147,000 people diagnosed annually, about half that number die annually—although almost three

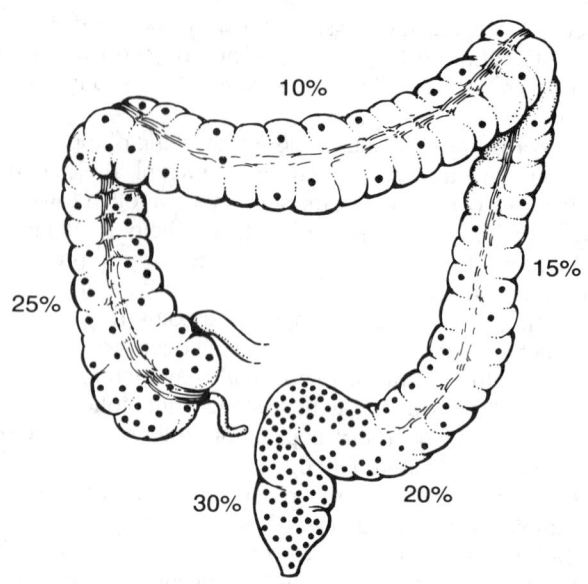

Figure 37–7. Distribution of cancer of the colon and rectum. (After Way LW [ed]. Current Surgical Diagnosis and Treatment, 9th ed. Los Altos, CA, Lange Medical Publishers, 1991.)

out of four patients could be saved by early diagnosis and prompt treatment. The low 5-year survival rate of 40% to 50% is due primarily to late diagnosis. Most people are asymptomatic for long periods and seek medical help only when they notice a change in bowel habits or rectal bleeding. Risk factors are listed in Chart 37–4.

Pathophysiology. Cancer of the colon and rectum always arises from the epithelium lining of the intestine. Like other types of cancer, the cancer cells invade and destroy normal tissues and extend into surrounding structures. Cancer cells may break away from the primary tumor and spread to other parts of the body (most often to the liver.) Persons with a history of inflammatory bowel disease or polyps are at high risk. The effects produced depend largely on the location of the cancer.

Clinical Manifestations. Most colorectal cancers are detected only after symptoms have appeared. The chief symptoms are changes in bowel habits (the most common presenting symptom), the passage of blood in the stools (second most common symptom), mucus, rectal/abdominal pain, persistent narrowing of stool, tenesmus, and the feeling of incomplete emptying after bowel movements. Symptoms may also include unexplained anemia, weight loss, and fatigue. A suddenly developing obstruction may be the first symptom of cancer involving the colon anywhere between the cecum and the sigmoid, for in this region, where the bowel contents are liquid, a slowly developing obstruction will not become evident until the lumen is practically closed. Cancer of the sigmoid and the rectum causes earlier symptoms of partial obstruction, with constipation alternating with diarrhea, lower abdominal crampy pains, and distention.

- Any patient with a history of unexplained change in bowel habit, with changes in the shape of the stool, or with passage of blood in the stools should be studied carefully to rule out cancer of the large bowel.

Gerontologic Considerations. The incidence of carcinoma of the colon and rectum increases with age. These cancers are

Chart 37–4
Risk Factors for Cancer of the Colon

Age—over 40
Blood in stool
History of rectal polyps
Presence of adenomatous polyps or villous adenomas.
Family history of colon cancer or familial polyposis
History of chronic inflammatory bowel disease
Diet—high in fat, protein, beef, and low in fiber

considered the most common malignancies in old age except for prostatic cancer in men. The presentation of symptoms is often insidious. Fatigue is almost always present, due primarily to iron-deficiency anemia. The symptoms most commonly reported by the elderly are abdominal pain, obstruction, tenesmus, and rectal bleeding.

Colonic carcinoma in the elderly has been closely associated with dietary carcinogens. Lack of fiber is a major causative agent because fecal transit time is prolonged, which in turn prolongs exposure to possible carcinogens. Excess fat is believed to alter bacterial flora and convert steroids into compounds that have carcinogenic properties.

Diagnostic Evaluation. Along with the abdominal and rectal examination, the most important diagnostic procedures for cancer of the colon are fecal occult blood testing, barium enema, proctosigmoidoscopy, and colonoscopy. As many as 60% of colorectal cancer cases can be identified by sigmoid-

oscopy with biopsy or cytology smears. For people 50 years of age and older, sigmoidoscopy is recommended every 2 years.

The level of carcinoembryonic antigen (CEA) found in colon cancer tissue was previously believed to be a highly reliable indicator in diagnosing colon cancer. Recent studies, however, show that CEA levels are only 30% to 40% accurate as a basis for diagnosis, although they are reliable in predicting prognosis. With complete tumor excision, the elevated levels of CEA should return to normal within 48 hours. Elevations of CEA at a later date suggest recurrence.

Guiac-based tests for fecal occult blood are still the most widely accepted diagnostic at-home test. A quantitative assay known as the *Hemo Quant test*, which detects *heme* (the iron-containing nonprotein portion of the hemoglobin molecule) that is altered during fecal transit, is also used. Results are reported as milligrams of hemoglobin per gram of stool.

Surgical Management

Surgery is the primary treatment for most colon cancers. *In situ* cancers are removable through the colonoscope. Bowel resection is indicated for stage I, II, and III colon cancers. The type of surgery depends on the location and size of the tumor. When the tumor can be removed, the involved colon is excised for some distance on each side of the growth to remove the tumor and the area of its lymphatic spread (Fig. 37–8). This is called a partial colectomy, or hemicolectomy. The intestine is rejoined by an end-to-end anastomosis of the colon.

Immediate reconnection may not always be possible because of the presence of infection. A temporary colostomy is

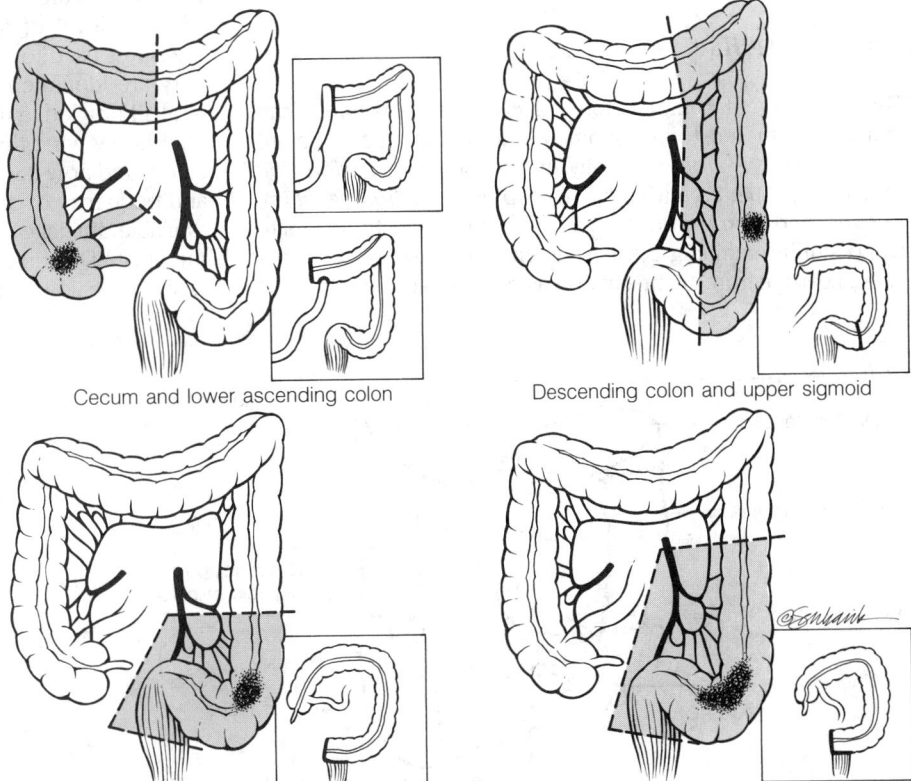

Cecum and lower ascending colon

Descending colon and upper sigmoid

Low sigmoid and upper rectum

Rectal

Figure 37–8. Examples of areas where cancer can occur, what area is removed, and (in the very small diagrams) how the anastomosis is done. (Adapted from American Cancer Society.)

then performed, creating an opening called a stoma for the elimination of wastes. The location of the tumor and amount of invasion into surrounding tissues dictates the placement of the colostomy (Fig. 37–9). Surgery is sometimes recommended for stage IV colon cancer. The goal of this procedure is palliative. In the event that the tumor has spread and involves surrounding vital structures, it is considered to be inoperable.

Surgery is also the primary treatment for most rectal cancers. Again, the type of surgical procedure will vary depending on the size and site of the tumor. An attempt is always made to preserve the anal sphincter so that a permanent colostomy is not needed. Wide removal of the tumor with anastomosis is sometimes possible. When the growth in the rectum or sigmoid is inoperable, especially when symptoms of partial or complete obstruction are present, a permanent colostomy must be formed. When the growth is situated low in the sigmoid or rectum, the growth is removed through a perineal incision. The procedure is called abdominoperineal resection. A permanent colostomy is formed (Fig. 37–10).

Medical Management

Several other forms of treatment for colon and rectal cancer are becoming a popular mode of adjunctive treatment. Radiation therapy is now being used preoperatively, intraoperatively, and postoperatively to shrink the tumor, to achieve better results from the surgery, and to reduce the risk of reccurence. For inoperative tumors, radiation is being used to give significant relief from the symptoms. Intracavity and implantable radiation devices are used. Benefit may be obtained when chemotherapy is used in conjunction with surgery. Immunotherapy is presently being studied in clinical trials.

Complications

The incidence of complications for colostomies is about half that seen with ileostomies. Some common complications are *prolapse of the stoma* (usually due to obesity), *perforation* (due to improper stoma irrigation), *stoma retraction, fecal impaction*, and *skin irritation*. Leakage from an anastomotic site can occur if remaining bowel segments are diseased or weakened. Leakage from an intestinal anastomosis causes abdominal

distention and rigidity, temperature elevation, and signs of shock. Surgical repair is necessary.

Pulmonary complications are always a concern with abdominal surgery. Patients over 50 years of age are considered to be at high risk, especially if they are or have been receiving antibiotics or sedatives, or are being maintained on bed rest for a prolonged period. Two primary pulmonary complications are pneumonia and atelectasis. These can be prevented by frequent movement (turning the patient from side to side every 2 hours), deep abdominal breathing, coughing, and early ambulation.

See Chart 37–5 for a list of potential complications to observe for after intestinal surgery.

Nursing Considerations for the Patient Requiring a Colostomy

Preoperative Nursing Interventions

Psychosocial Support

A patient diagnosed with cancer of the colon or rectum may require a permanent colostomy and may grieve about the diagnosis and the impending surgery. Emotional reactions and the family's ability to provide support are assessed. Patients undergoing surgery for a temporary colostomy may express fears and concerns similar to those of a person with a permanent stoma. A temporary colostomy can become permanent for a patient whose condition deteriorates and who cannot tolerate additional surgery. Coping behaviors and verbalization of concerns are encouraged.

The level of anxiety (mild, moderate, severe) and any measures used to cope with the diagnosis and impending surgery are identified. Questions are asked to ascertain the patient's knowledge about the surgical procedure. Does the patient know what the stoma will look like, where it will be located, and how it will function? Is the patient aware of the type and frequency of drainage that are expected? Has he seen the available drainage pouches? Has he spoken to an enterostomal therapist? Does he know anyone who has a stoma? Does he wish to speak with an ostomate (a person with a ostomy)? All

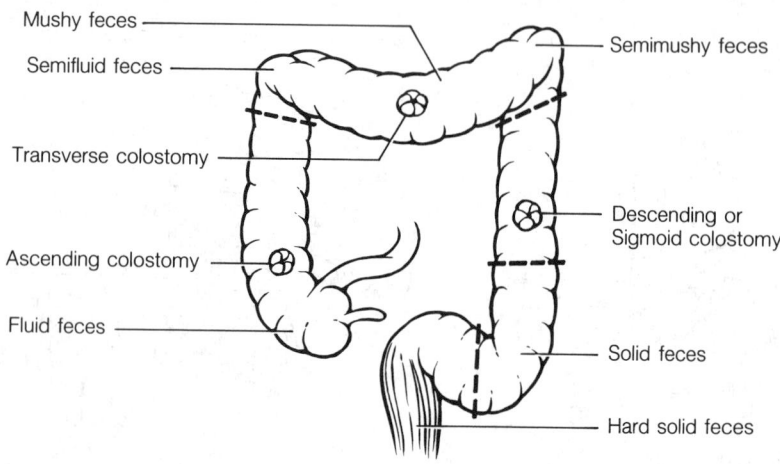

Figure 37–9. A diagrammatic representation of the placement of permanent colostomies and the nature of the discharge at these sites.

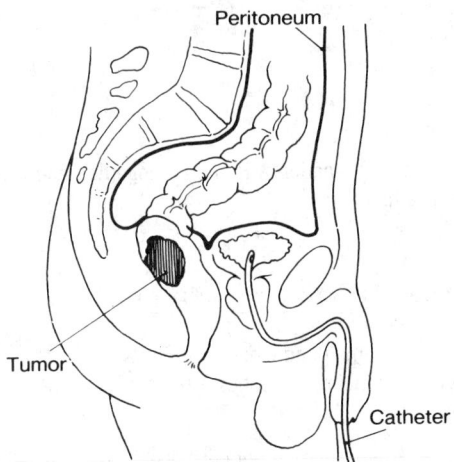

1. Presurgical patient. Note tumor in rectum.

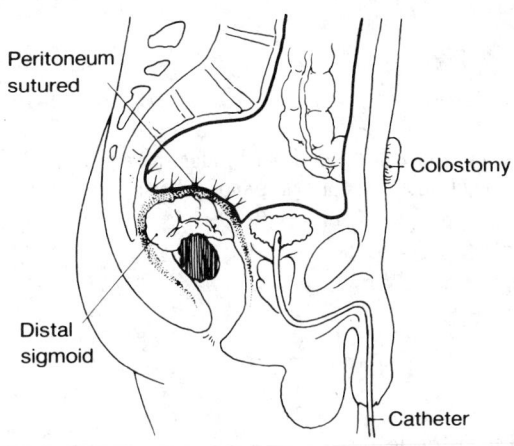

2. At operation, sigmoid is removed and colostomy established. The distal bowel has been dissected free to a point below pelvic peritoneum, which is sutured over the closed end of the distal sigmoid and rectum.

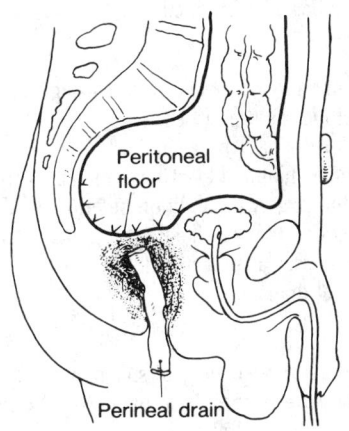

3. Perineal resection includes removal of the rectum and free portion of the sigmoid from below. A drain is inserted in this void.

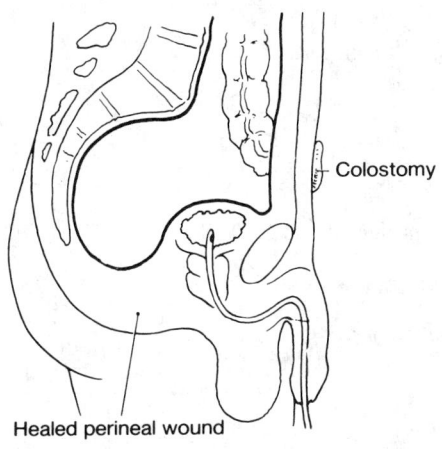

4. The final result after healing. Note healed perineal wound and the permanent colostomy.

Figure 37–10. Abdominoperineal resection for carcinoma of rectum.

members of the health team, the enterostomal therapy nurse, and the family should be available for assistance and support.

Speaking with a person who is successfully managing a colostomy is often helpful. The United Ostomy Association is a nonprofit agency that gives patients useful information on living with an ostomy, through an educational program of literature, lectures, and exhibits. Visiting services by qualified members and rehabilitation services for new ostomy patients are provided by national organizations (see p. 963).

Anticipated changes in body image and life style are profoundly disturbing, and patients may need empathetic support in trying to adjust to them. Because the stoma is located on the abdomen, the patient may think that everyone will be aware of the ostomy. The nurse can help reduce this apprehension by presenting factual information about the surgical procedure and the creation and management of the ostomy. If the patient is receptive, diagrams, photographs, and appliances may be used to explain and clarify. Because the patient is experiencing emotional stress, the nurse may need to repeat some of the

information. Time should be provided for the patient to ask questions. The nurse's acceptance and understanding of the patient's concerns and feelings convey a caring, competent attitude that promotes confidence and cooperation.

Preparation for Surgery

Usually, a high-calorie, low-residue diet is given for several days before surgery, if time and the patient's condition permit. If an emergency does not exist, prescribed intestinal antimicrobials, such as kanamycin, erythromycin, and neomycin, are given by mouth for several days to reduce the bacterial content of the colon and to soften and decrease the bulk of the contents of the colon. In addition, mechanical cleansing of the bowel may be accomplished by laxatives, enemas, or colonic irrigations.

Careful attention is given to reports of pain, which are assessed and described as to their nature, location, and duration. The nurse records fluid losses such as occur with vomiting and diarrhea. This will aid in regulating the fluid intake

Chart 37-5
Summary of Potential Complications After Surgery of the Intestines

Anticipation of and vigilance for complications have first priority in caring for postoperative patients. Prompt recognition and management of these complications can prevent prolonged disability and, in some instances, death.

Complication	Nursing Assessment and Interventions
Paralytic ileus	Initiate or continue nasogastric intubation. Prepare patient for x-ray study. Ensure adequate fluid and electrolyte replacement. Administer prescribed antibiotics if patient has symptoms of peritonitis.
Mechanical obstruction	Evaluate patient for intermittent colicky pain, nausea, and vomiting.
Intraperitoneal infection and abdominal wound infection	Assess for evidence of constant or generalized abdominal pain, rapid pulse, and elevation of temperature. Prepare for tube decompression of bowel. Administer fluids and electrolytes by IV route as prescribed. Administer antibiotics as prescribed
Intra-abdominal septic conditions	
Peritonitis	Evaluate patient for nausea, hiccups, chills, spiking fever, tachycardia. Administer antibiotics as prescribed. Prepare patient for drainage procedure. Institute intravenous fluid and electrolyte therapy as prescribed. Prepare patient for surgery if condition deteriorates.
Abscess formation	Administer antibiotics as prescribed. Apply warm compresses as prescribed. Prepare for surgical drainage.
Wound complications	
Infection	Monitor temperature for evidences of spiking fever. Observe for redness, tenderness, and pain around wound. Assist in establishing local draiange. Obtain specimen of drainage material for culture and sensitivity studies.
Wound disruption	Observe for sudden appearance of profuse serous drainage from wound. Cover wound area with sterile towels held in place with binder. Prepare patient immediately for surgery.
Anastomotic complications	
Dehiscence of anastomosis Fistulas	Prepare patient for surgery. Assist in bowel decompression. Administer parenteral fluids as prescribed to correct fluid and electrolyte defects.

and maintaining adequate fluid balance. If the hemoglobin is below 12 g, blood transfusions may be prescribed because anemia is common. Preoperative nasogastric intubation may be indicated and minimizes postoperative distention. An indwelling catheter is inserted as prescribed to ensure that the bladder is empty during surgery. This will aid in keeping postoperative perineal dressings dry. The abdomen and perineum are prepared for surgery.

Postoperative Nursing Interventions

Postoperative nursing care for patients undergoing a colostomy is similar to nursing care for any abdominal surgery patient (see Chap. 22). The patient is monitored for signs of the complications discussed earlier in this section (p. 950). These include leakage from an anastomotic site, prolapse of the stoma, perforation, stoma retraction, fecal impaction, and skin irritation, as well as pulmonary complications associated with abdominal surgery. Patients experiencing a colostomy are helped out of bed on the first postoperative day and encouraged to care for the colostomy from the first irrigation. The return to normal diet is rapid, and every effort is made to encourage them to live as they did before the operation.

Gerontologic Considerations

Elderly patients may have some degree of decreased vision and impaired hearing, as well as difficulty with skills that require fine motor coordination. Therefore, it may be helpful for the patient to handle the ostomy equipment preoperatively and simulate cleaning the peristomal skin and irrigating the stoma.

Accidents resulting from falls occur frequently among the elderly. It is important to determine whether the patient can walk unassisted to the bathroom.

Skin care is a major concern for the elderly ostomate because of skin changes that occur with aging. The epithelial and subcutaneous fatty layers become thin and skin is easily irritated. To prevent breakdown, special attention is paid to skin cleansing and the proper fit of an appliance. Arteriosclerosis causes decreased blood flow to the wound and stoma site. As a result, transport of nutrients is delayed, and healing takes longer.

Some patients experience delayed elimination after irrigation because of decreased peristalsis and reduced mucus production. Most require 6 months before they feel comfortable with their ostomy care.

Care of the Colostomy

Colostomy function will begin 3 to 6 days postoperatively. The nurse manages the colostomy until the patient begins to learn to care for it himself. Skin care must be taught as well as application and management of the drainage pouch and irrigation.

Skin Care

The effluent discharge will vary with the type of ostomy. The stool is soft and mushy but irritating to the skin with a transverse colostomy, and fairly solid and slightly irritating with a descending or sigmoid colostomy. The patient is advised to protect the peristomal skin by frequently washing the area with a mild soap, applying a protective skin barrier around the stoma, and securely attaching the drainage pouch. Nystatin powder (Mycostatin) can be dusted lightly on the peristomal skin if irritation or yeast growth is present.

The skin is cleaned gently with a moist, soft cloth and a mild soap. Any excess skin barrier is removed. Soap acts as a mild abrasive agent to remove enzyme residue from fecal spillage. During the time the skin is being cleansed, a gauze dressing may cover the stoma or a vaginal tampon can be inserted gently to absorb excess drainage. The patient may be permitted to bathe or shower before putting on the clean appliance. Micropore tape applied to the sides of the pouch will keep it secure during bathing. The skin is patted completely dry with a gauze pad; rubbing the area is avoided. A skin barrier (wafer, paste, powder) is used around the stoma to protect the skin from fecal drainage.

Application of the Drainage Pouch

The stoma is measured to determine the correct size for the pouch. The pouch opening should be about 0.3 cm (⅛ inch) larger than the stoma. The skin is cleansed according to the above procedure. A peristomal skin barrier is applied. The backing from the adherent surface of the pouch is removed and the bag is pressed down over the stoma for 30 seconds. Mild skin irritation may require dusting the skin with Karaya powder or stomahesive powder before attaching the pouch.

Management of the Drainage Pouch

Colostomy bags may be worn immediately after irrigation; then a change to a simple dressing may be effective. Patients can choose from a wide variety of pouches, depending on their individual needs. Most pouches are disposable and odor resistant. Commercially prepared deodorizers are available for use.

As a rule, colostomy bags are not necessary. As soon as the patient has learned a routine for evacuation, bags may be dispensed with and a closed ostomy pouch or a simple dressing of disposable tissue (often covered with plastic wrap) is used, held in place by an elastic belt or girdle. Except for the escape of gas and a slight amount of mucus, nothing comes from the colostomy opening between irrigations; therefore, a colostomy bag is unnecessary.

Removal of the Appliance

The drainage appliance is changed when it is one-third to one-fourth full so that the weight of its contents does not cause the pouch to separate from the adhesive disc and spill the contents. The patient assumes a comfortable sitting or standing position and *gently* pushes the skin down from the faceplate while pulling the pouch up and away from the stoma. Gentle pressure prevents traumatizing the skin as well as preventing the spillage of any liquid fecal contents.

Irrigation of the Colostomy

The stoma on the abdomen does not have voluntary muscular control and may empty at irregular intervals. Regulation is achieved either by irrigation or by allowing the bowel to evacuate naturally without irrigations. The choice often depends on the individual and the nature of the colostomy. The type and frequency of effluent vary according to the type of colostomy (see Fig. 37–9).

The purpose of irrigating a colostomy is to empty the colon of gas, mucus, and feces so that the patient can go about social and business activities without fear of fecal drainage. By irrigating the stoma at a *regular* time, there is less gas and retention of irrigating fluids.

The time of irrigation should be consistent with the schedule the person will follow after leaving the hospital. Refer to Chart 37–6 for the irrigating procedure and Figure 37–11 for the equipment.

Care of the Perineal Wound

If the malignancy has been removed by the perineal route, the wound is observed carefully for signs of hemorrhage. This

Chart 37–6
Guidelines for Irrigating a Colostomy

Irrigation of a colostomy is performed for the purposes of emptying the colon of feces, gas, or mucus, cleansing the lower intestinal tract, and establishing a regular pattern of evacuation so that normal life activities may be pursued. A suitable time for the irrigation is selected, preferably after a meal, so that this time is compatible with the patient's posthospital pattern of activity. Irrigation should be performed at the same time each day.

Before the procedure the patient sits on a chair in front of the toilet or on the toilet itself. An irrigating reservoir with 500 to 1500 ml lukewarm tap water is hung 45 to 50 cm (18 to 20 in) above the stoma (shoulder height when the patient is seated). Dressings or pouch are removed. The following procedure is used; the patient is assisted to participate in the procedure so that he can learn to perform it unassisted.

Nursing Action	Rationale/Amplification
1. Apply an irrigating sleeve or sheath to the stoma. Place the end in the commode (see Fig. 37–11).	This helps to control odor and splashing and allows feces and water to flow directly into the commode.
2. Allow some of the solution to flow through the tubing and catheter/cone.	Air bubbles in the setup are released so that air is not introduced into the colon, which would cause crampy pain.
3. Lubricate the catheter/cone and gently insert it into the stoma. Insert the catheter no more than 8 cm (3 in). Hold the shield/cone gently, but firmly, against the stoma to prevent backflow of water.	These steps are necessary to prevent intestinal perforation.
4. If the catheter does not advance easily, allow water to flow slowly while advancing catheter. *Never force the catheter!*	A slow rate of flow helps to relax the bowel and facilitates passage of the catheter.
5. Allow the fluid to enter the colon slowly. If cramping occurs, clamp off the tubing and allow the patient to rest before progressing. Water should flow in over a 5- to 10-minute period.	Painful cramps are usually caused by too rapid a flow or by too much solution. 500 ml is usually sufficient for initial postoperative irrigation. Volume may be increased with subsequent irrigations to 1000 or 1500 ml as needed by the patient for effective results.
6. Hold the shield/cone in place 10 seconds after the water has been instilled; then gently remove it.	
7. Allow 10 to 15 minutes for most of the return; then dry the bottom of the sleeve/sheath and attach it to the top, or apply the appropriate clamp to the bottom of the sleeve.	Most of the water, feces, and flatus will be expelled in 10 to 15 minutes.
8. Leave the sleeve/sheath in place about 20 minutes while the patient gets up and moves around.	Ambulation stimulates peristalsis and completion of the irrigation return.
9. Cleanse the area with a mild soap and water; pat the area dry.	Cleanliness and dryness will provide the patient with hours of comfort.
10. Replace the colostomy dressing or pouch.	The patient should use a pouch until the colostomy is sufficiently controlled.

wound may contain a drain or packing that is removed gradually, so that by about the seventh day all drains are out. There may be sloughing bits of tissue for the following week or 10 days. This process is hastened by the mechanical irrigation of the wound or with sitz baths.

This may be done two or three times a day, and then gradually less frequently. The condition of the perineal wound, any bleeding, infection, or necrosis are recorded and reported. During the procedure it is important to protect the bed with an extra waterproof sheet and absorbent pads, and it may be well to plan the irrigation so that it can be performed before the patient receives morning care.

Changing the patient's position from one side to the other every 2 to 4 hours is desirable, because not only is it uncomfortable to lie in a dorsal recumbent position, but such a position may also interfere with healing by causing wound separation.

An indwelling catheter remains in place for several days

to prevent urinary retention and pressure on the perineal area. Continuing assessment of the patient's urinary status is maintained to detect infection and assist in monitoring hydration.

Patient Education and Home Health Care

The spouse and family should be familiar with the adjustment that will be necessary when the patient returns home. They need to be encouraged to verbalize their concerns. Their understanding is necessary to reduce tension; a relaxed patient tends to have fewer problems.

Before the patient's discharge from the hospital, an individualized routine for stoma care and irrigation is reviewed with the patient and family. Supplemental literature is helpful, because those involved may have questions when the patient is back in the home setting. Someone in the family should

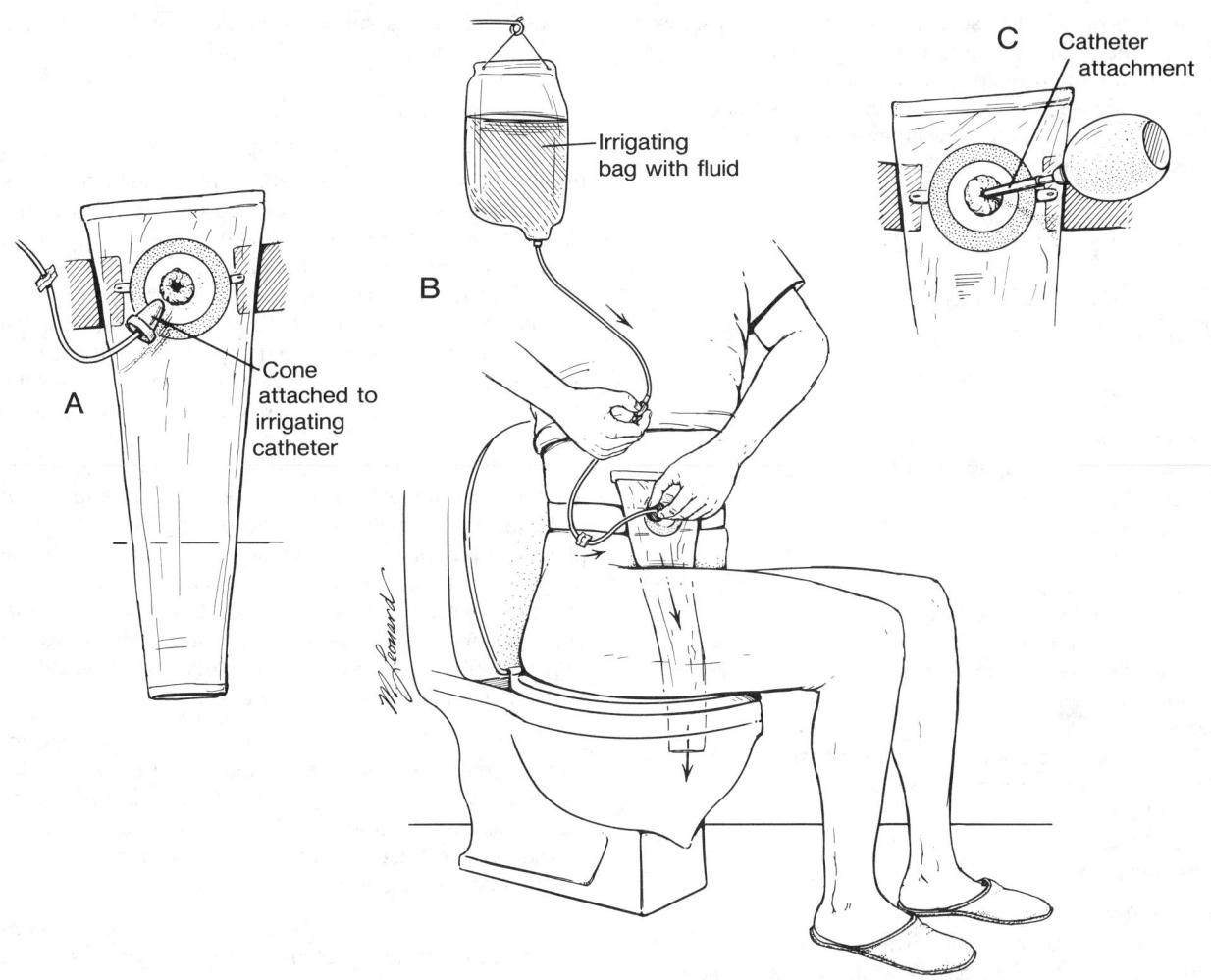

Figure 37–11. Colostomy irrigation. (**A**) Irrigating catheter has a cone attachment to prevent injury to stomal tissue. (**B**) Irrigating fluid is instilled with sleeve in place. Drainage contents empty into toilet. (**C**) The bulb syringe method can be used to stimulate fecal drainage. Note that a portion of the hard nozzle is removed and a catheter attached to minimize stomal irritation.

assume responsibility for purchasing the equipment and supplies that will be needed at home. Many patients benefit from referral to a visiting nurse agency or from the services of the local chapter of The American Cancer Society.

Nutritional Status

In general, the patient is reminded that good health practices will promote feelings of well-being and positive adjustment to the colostomy. The diet is individualized as long as it is well balanced and does not cause diarrhea or constipation.

A complete nutritional assessment is performed. Foods that cause excessive odor and gas are avoided. These include foods in the cabbage family, eggs, fish, beans, and cellulose products such as peanuts. It is important to determine if the elimination of food is causing any nutritional deficiencies. Nonirritating foods are substituted for those that are restricted so that deficiencies are corrected. The patient is advised to experiment with an irritating food several times before restricting it, because the reaction may be an initial sensitivity that will decrease with use.

Hydration status is assessed (skin turgor, mucous membranes, intake and output, weight) and signs of dehydration are reported. If the patient has problems with diarrhea, the frequency of diarrheal stools is noted, along with the occurrence of abdominal cramping, urgency, and hyperactive bowel sounds. The patient is assisted to identify any foods or fluids that may be causing diarrhea, such as fruits, high-fiber foods, soda, coffee, tea, or carbonated beverages. The use of paregoric, bismuth subgallate, bismuth subcarbonate, or diphenoxylate with atropine (Lomotil) will control the diarrhea. For constipation, prune or apple juice or a mild laxative is effective.

Sexual Activity

The patient is encouraged to discuss plans to return to usual sexual activity. Some patients may initiate questions about sexual activity directly or give indirect clues about their fears. Some may view the surgery as mutilating and a threat to their sexuality; some fear impotence. Others may express worry about odor or leakage from the pouch during sexual activity. Alternative sexual positions are recommended as well as alternative methods of stimulation to satisfy sexual drives. The nurse assesses the patient's needs and attempts to identify specific concerns. If the nurse is uncomfortable with this, or if the patient's concerns seem complex, the nurse should seek assistance from an appropriate source, such as the enterostomal therapy nurse, sex counselor, or clinical specialist.

▶ Nursing Process
The Patient With Cancer of the Colon or Rectum

▷ Assessment

Health History
- Presence of abdominal pain
- Characteristics of pain:
     Location
     Frequency
     Duration
     Associated with food intake
- Past elimination pattern
- Present elimination pattern—exact changes
- Current drug therapy
- Past medical history
- Description of color, odor, consistency of stool
- Presence of blood or mucus in stool
- Weight loss
- Dietary habits, including alcohol use
- Unusual fatigue

Physical Assessment
- Auscultation of abdomen for bowel sounds
- Palpation for areas of tenderness, distention, solid masses
- Inspection of stool for blood

▷ Nursing Diagnoses

Based on all the assessment data, the patient's major nursing diagnoses may include the following:

Preoperative
- Anxiety related to impending surgery and the diagnosis of cancer
- Pain related to tissue compression secondary to obstruction
- Altered nutrition, less than body requirements, related to nausea and anorexia
- High risk for fluid volume deficit related to vomiting and dehydration

Postoperative
- High risk for infection related to possible contamination of the abdominal cavity during the surgical procedure
- Knowledge deficit concerning the diagnosis, the surgical procedure, and self-care after discharge
- Impaired skin integrity related to the surgical incisions (abdominal and perianal) and the formation of a stoma

▷ Planning and Implementation

▷ *Goals:*   The major goals of the patient may include reduction in anxiety, reduction/alleviation of pain, attainment of an optimal level of nutrition, maintenance of fluid and electrolyte balance, prevention of infection, acquisition of information

about the diagnosis, surgical procedure, and self-care after discharge, and maintenance of optimal tissue healing.

▷ Nursing Interventions

▷ *Reducing Anxiety*   The patient's level of anxiety (mild, moderate, severe) is assessed. Coping mechanisms used to deal with stress are identified. Supportive efforts include: provision for privacy if desired, relaxation exercises, biofeedback; time is set aside to sit with the patient who wishes to ventilate, cry, or ask questions. A member of the clergy is contacted if desired. A time for the family to meet with the physicians and nurses if the patient wishes to discuss the treatment/prognosis with them is arranged. A meeting with an enterostomal therapist may be useful. An ostomate is asked to visit if the patient desires this.

A relaxed and empathetic attitude is projected. Questions are answered honestly. All tests and procedures are explained at the level of the patient's understanding. Any information the physician has provided is clarified, if necessary. Sometimes anxiety is relieved if the patient knows what physical preparation is necessary preoperatively and what to expect postoperatively. Some patients appreciate seeing pictures or drawings, whereas others would prefer not to know details. The patient's needs and desires for information are assessed.

▷ *Pain Reduction/Alleviation.*   Analgesics are administered as prescribed. The environment is made conducive to relaxation by dimming the lights, turning off the television or radio, and restricting visitors and telephone calls. Additional comfort measures are offered: position changes, a back rub, distraction, and relaxation techniques.

▷ *Nutritional Measures.*   If the patient's condition permits, a diet high in calories, protein, and carbohydrates and low in residue is given preoperatively for several days to provide adequate nutrition and decrease excessive peristalsis, to minimize cramping. A full-liquid diet may be prescribed 24 hours before surgery to decrease bulk. Total parenteral nutrition is required for some patients to replace depleted nutrients, vitamins, and minerals. Daily weights are recorded and the physician is notified if the patient continues to lose weight while receiving parenteral nutrition.

Anemia is common. If the hemoglobin falls below 12 g (1.86 mmol/L), blood transfusions may be prescribed by the physician. When administering a blood transfusion, normal safety guidelines and agency policy regarding safety are followed. The patient is monitored for indicators of an allergic reaction (rash, flushing, hives, chills, dyspnea, vomiting, tachycardia); the transfusion is stopped if a reaction appears.

▷ *Maintenance of Fluid and Electrolyte Balance.*   Intake and output, including vomitus, are measured and recorded, to provide an accurate record of fluid balance. The patient's intake of oral food and fluids is restricted to prevent vomiting. If vomiting is expected, antiemetics are administered as prescribed. Full or clear liquids may be tolerated, or the patient may be allowed nothing by mouth. A nasogastric tube will be inserted preoperatively to drain accumulated fluids and prevent abdominal distention. An indwelling catheter may be inserted to allow for monitoring of hourly output. An output of less than 30 ml/hr is reported to the physician.

Intravenous administration of fluids and electrolytes is monitored. Serum electrolytes are monitored to detect hypokalemia and hyponatremia, which occur with gastrointestinal fluid loss. Vital signs are assessed to detect hypovolemia: tachycardia, hypotension, and decreased pulse volume. Hydration status is assessed, and decreased skin turgor, dry mucous membranes, concentrated urine, and increased urine specific gravity are reported.

▷ *Prevention of Infection.* Antibiotics such as kanamycin sulfate (Kantrex), erythromycin (Erythrocin), and neomycin sulfate are administered as prescribed to reduce intestinal bacteria in preparation for bowel surgery. These are administered by mouth to reduce the bacterial content of the colon and to soften and decrease the bulk of the contents of the colon. In addition, the bowel can be cleansed by laxatives, enemas, or colonic irrigations.

▷ *Preoperative Patient Education.* The patient's present knowledge about the diagnosis, prognosis, surgical procedure, and expected level of functioning postoperatively is assessed. Learning ability and interest are identified. Information that is needed, how it should be presented, when the patient would be most receptive, and who should be present during the instruction are determined. The patient is encouraged to participate in the learning process. A time and location conducive to learning are chosen. Repetition and praise are used to reinforce learning.

Information that the patient needs about the physical preparation for surgery, the expected appearance and care of the wound postoperatively, the technique of ostomy care, dietary restrictions, pain control, and medication management are included in the teaching plan. (See Nursing Care Plan 37–1 for the patient with an intestinal ostomy.)

▷ *Wound Care.* The abdominal wound is examined frequently during the first 24 hours to make sure that it is healing without complications (infection, dehiscence, hemorrhage, excessive edema). Dressings are changed as needed to prevent infection. The patient is shown how to splint the abdominal incision during coughing and deep breathing to lessen tension on the edges of the incision. Temperature, pulse rate, and respirations are monitored for elevations that may indicate an infectious process. A temperature higher than 38.3°C (101°F) is reported to the physician.

The stoma is examined for swelling (slight edema due to surgical manipulation is normal), color (a healthy stoma should be pink), discharge (a small amount of oozing is normal), and bleeding (an abnormal sign). The peristomal skin is cleansed gently and patted dry to prevent irritation. Perineal wound care is described on p. 953.

▷ *Patient Education and Home Health Care.* Discharge planning requires the combined efforts of the physician, nurse, enterostomal therapist, social worker, and dietitian. Patients being discharged are given specific information, individualized to their needs, about ostomy care and complications to observe for: obstruction, infection, stoma stenosis, retraction or prolapse, and peristomal skin irritation. Dietary instructions are essential to help patients identify and eliminate irritating foods that can cause diarrhea or constipation. Patients are given a list of the medications prescribed for them, with information on the action, purpose, and possible side effects of each. A system for remembering when to take the medication is developed with the patient.

Treatments (irrigations, wound cleansing) and dressing

changes are reviewed, and the family is encouraged to participate. Patients need very specific directions about when to call the physician. They need to know exactly what complications require prompt attention (bleeding, abdominal distention and rigidity, diarrhea, and the "dumping syndrome"—see p. 913). Patients are directed to weigh themselves weekly and notify the physician if they experience continued or abrupt weight loss of 1 to 2 pounds per week. If radiation therapy is necessary, the possible side effects of anorexia, vomiting, diarrhea, and exhaustion are reviewed.

▷ **Evaluation**

Expected Outcomes

1. Experiences less anxiety
   a. Verbalizes concerns and fears freely
   b. Uses coping measures to deal with stress
   c. Shares feelings/concerns with family members
   d. Meets with support persons (clergy, social worker, ostomate)
2. Experiences less pain
   a. Requests analgesics as needed
   b. Uses diversional activities successfully
   c. Reports absence of pain
3. Achieves an optimal level of nutrition
   a. Eats a low-residue, high-protein, high-calorie diet
   b. Reports less abdominal cramping
   c. Tolerates parenteral nutrition therapy
4. Achieves fluid balance
   a. Restricts oral intake of foods and fluids when nauseated
   b. Urinates about 1.5 L/24 hr
   c. Denies paresthesia, dizziness, unusual fatigue (signs of hypokalemia), excessive thirst
   d. Denies dry, itchy, or scaly skin
   e. Maintains recommended weight
5. Avoids infection
   a. Takes oral antibiotics
   b. Cooperates with bowel cleansing
   c. Is afebrile
6. Acquires information about the diagnosis, surgical procedure, and self-care after discharge
   a. Discusses the diagnosis, surgical procedure, and postoperative self-care
   b. Asks specific questions
   c. Relates concerns and fears
   d. Participates actively in the learning process (listens attentively, clarifies procedures, restates important concepts, answers questions correctly)
   e. Communicates individual needs for self-care after discharge
   f. Understands technique of ostomy care
7. Maintains clean incision, stoma, and perineal wound
   a. Describes the appearance of incision site accurately
   b. States that there is some pain in the incisional area, but that it is relieved by analgesics
   c. Discusses the appearance of the stoma as raised and pink, with minimal edema
   d. Describes peristomal skin as normal color and without irritation
   e. Assists the nurse with dressing changes
   f. Begins to clean the stoma and peristomal skin whenever necessary

g. Cooperates with perineal wound irrigations
h. Splints incisional area with hand when coughing and taking deep breaths
i. Is afebrile

In summary, colorectal cancer causes an abnormality in the physiologic functioning of the lower gastrointestinal tract and therefore changes in bowel habits. Surgery is the primary treatment and may result in a colostomy. Preoperative and postoperative nursing care are directed toward psychosocial support and patient and family education related to the care of the colostomy.

Polyps of the Colon and Rectum

A polyp is a mass of tissue that protrudes into the lumen of the bowel and can be found anywhere in the intestinal tract and rectum. Polyps can be classified into two groups: neoplastic (adenomas and carcinomas) and non-neoplastic (mucosal and hyperplastic). Adenomatous polyps (benign epithelial growths) are common in the western world. They occur more frequently in the large intestine than in the small intestine. Although the vast majority of them do not develop into invasive neoplasms, their presence must be identified and closely followed. Polyps occur in 10% to 60% of the population; occurrence is most frequent in the fifth decade of life.

Clinical manifestations depend on the size of the polyp and the amount of pressure it exerts on intestinal tissue. The most common symptom is rectal bleeding. Lower abdominal pain may also occur. If the polyp is large enough, symptoms of obstruction will be present.

The diagnosis is based on history and digital rectal exam, barium enema studies, sigmoidoscopy, or colonoscopy. Once they are identified, polyps are removed through a colonoscope by the use of special equipment (*i.e.*, biopsy forceps and snares). Microscopic exam of the polyp then identifies the type of polyp, and the physician determines whether surgery is indicated. The principle reason for performing a colonic polypectomy is because of the possibility that malignancy is already present or may develop.

Diseases of the Anorectum

Patients with anorectal disorders seek medical care primarily because of pain and rectal bleeding. Other frequent complaints are protrusion of hemorrhoids, anal discharge, itching, swelling, anal tenderness, stenosis, and ulceration. Constipation occurs because defecation is delayed because of pain.

Rectal Examination and Patient Preparation

Visual inspection (anoscopy) and digital examination of the anus and the rectum are indispensable for detecting and identifying lesions involving these structures. Moreover, rectal ex-

amination is extremely useful in diagnosing or excluding many intra-abdominal and pelvic conditions, including appendicitis; diverticulitis; salpingitis; tumors of the ovary, uterus, and colon; and prostatic lesions of various types.

Rectal examinations may be performed with the patient in the knee–chest or Sims's lateral position, or on a special proctoscopic table. Whatever position is used, the patient is informed of the procedure and how it is to be performed, and is draped so that only the rectal area is exposed.

Anorectal Abscess

Anorectal abscess is an infection in the pararectal spaces. Persons with regional enteritis and other immunodeficient states such as AIDS are particularly susceptible to these infections. Many of these abscesses will result in fistulas.

Clinical Manifestations and Management.   An abscess may occur in a variety of spaces in and around the rectum. Often it contains a quantity of foul-smelling pus and is painful. If the abscess is superficial, swelling, redness, and tenderness are observed. A deeper abscess may result in toxic symptoms and even lower abdominal pain, as well as fever. More than half of rectal abscesses will result in fistulas.

Palliative therapy consists of sitz baths and analgesics. Prompt surgical treatment is the treatment of choice, however. This consists of incision and drainage. When deeper infection exists, with the possibility of a fistula, it is necessary to remove the fistulous tract. This may be done initially, or it may require a second operation. Often no packing is used; if it is used, usually the wound is lined with petrolatum gauze. Later, when it is necessary to remove the packing, soaking it first with saline solution is helpful.

These wounds are allowed to heal by granulation. Bowel movements should be formed, rather than liquid or soft. Cathartics or mineral oil are not usually used.

Anal Fistula

An anal fistula is a tiny, tubular, fibrous tract that extends into the anal canal from an opening located beside the anus (Fig. 37–12*A*). Fistulas usually result from an infection. They may also develop from trauma, fissures, or regional enteritis.

Clinical Manifestations.   Pus or stool may leak constantly from the cutaneous opening. Other symptoms are passage of flatus or feces from the vagina and pruritis. Untreated fistulas may cause systemic infection with related symptoms.

Treatment.   Surgery is always recommended because few fistulas heal spontaneously. A *fistulectomy* (excision of the fistulous tract) is the recommended surgical procedure. Three or four hours before the operation, the perineum is shaved and the lower bowel evacuated thoroughly with several prescribed enemas. The last enema should return clear and should be evacuated entirely.

The patient usually is placed in the lithotomy position, and the sinus tract is identified by inserting a probe into it or by injecting the tract with methylene blue solution. The fistula is dissected out or laid open by an incision from its rectal opening to its outlet. The wound is packed with gauze.

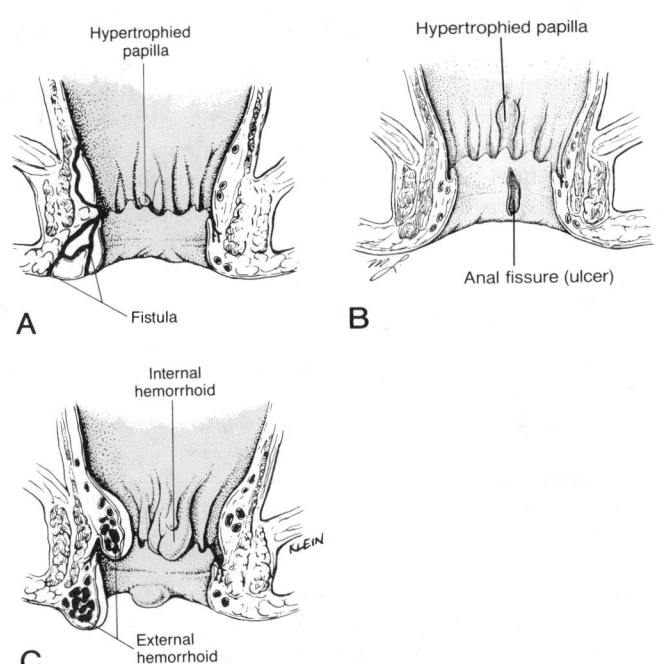

Figure 37–12. Various types of anal lesions. (**A**) Fistula. (**B**) Fissure. (**C**) External and internal hemorrhoids.

Anal Fissure

An anal fissure is a longitudinal tear in the anal canal (see Fig. 37–12*B*). Fissures are usually caused by trauma from passing a large firm stool or persistent tightening of the anal canal secondary to stress and anxiety (leading to constipation). Other causes include childbirth, trauma, and cathartic abuse. The most pronounced symptom is extreme pain during defecation.

Clinical Manifestations and Management. Fissures are characterized by painful defecation, burning, and bleeding. Most of these fissures will heal if treated by conservative measures. These measures include stool softeners and bulk agents, an increase in water intake, sitz baths, and emollient suppositories. A suppository combining an anesthetic with a steroid is comforting. Anal dilation under anesthesia may be required.

If fissures do not respond to conservative treatment, surgery is indicated. Several types of operations may be performed: in some cases, the anal sphincter is dilated and the fissure is excised; in others, a part of the external sphincter is divided. This produces a paralysis of the external sphincter, with consequent relief of spasm, and permits the ulcer to heal. When there is a large, overhanging sentinel hemorrhoid, excision of the ulcer and of the hemorrhoid is performed.

Hemorrhoids

Hemorrhoids are hyperplastic areas of vascular tissue in the anal canal. They are very common. By the age of 50, 50% of people have hemorrhoids to some extent. Pregnancy is known to initiate or aggravate the symptoms of hemorrhoids. Hemorrhoids are classified into two types. Those occurring above the internal sphincter are called *internal hemorrhoids*, and those appearing outside the external sphincter are called *external hemorrhoids* (see Fig. 37–12*C*). They cause itching, pain, and are the most common cause of bright red bleeding with defecation. Internal hemorrhoids prolapse frequently through the sphincter and cause considerable discomfort.

Clinical Manifestations and Management. External hemorrhoids are associated with severe pain due to inflammation and edema caused by thrombosis. Internal hemorrhoids are not usually painful until they bleed or prolapse with enlargement. Hemorrhoid symptoms and discomfort can be relieved by good personal hygiene and by avoiding excessive straining during defecation. A high-residue diet that contains fruit and bran may be all the treatment that is necessary; failing this, a hydrophilic laxative may help. Sitz baths, ointments, and suppositories containing anesthetics, astringents (witch hazel), and bed rest are measures that allow the engorgement to subside. There are several types of nonoperative treatments for hemorrhoids. Infrared photocoagulation and bipolar diathermy are new techniques that can be used to afix the mucosa to the underlying muscle. Injection of sclerosing solutions is also effective for small, bleeding hemorrhoids.

A conservative surgical treatment of internal hemorrhoids is the rubber-band ligation treatment. As the hemorrhoid is visualized through the anoscope, its proximal portion above the mucocutaneous lines is grasped with an instrument, and a small rubber band is slipped over it. Tissue distal to the rubber band becomes necrotic after several days and is removed. Because of fibrosis, lower anal mucosa is drawn up and adheres to the underlying muscle. Although this treatment has been satisfactory in some patients, it has proven painful in others and may cause some secondary hemorrhage. This method has been known to cause perianal sepsis.

Cryosurgical hemorrhoidectomy involves freezing the tissues of the hemorrhoid for a sufficient time to cause necrosis. Although it is painless, it is not popular because the discharge is very foul-smelling and wound healing is prolonged.

Excision of an external hemorrhoidal tag can be performed with laser therapy. The treatment is usually performed in the physician's office and is quick and relatively painless.

The methods of treating hemorrhoids just described are not effective for advanced thrombosed veins, which must be treated by more extensive surgery.

Hemorrhoidectomy, or surgical excision, can be performed to remove all of the redundant tissue involved in the process. The operation usually involves digital dilatation of the rectal sphincter and removal of the hemorrhoids by the use of a clamp and cautery or by ligation and excision. After completion of the operative procedures, a small tube, often covered with petrolatum gauze, may be inserted through the sphincter to permit the escape of flatus and also of blood, if there should be any bleeding. Instead of the tube, some surgeons place pieces of Gelfoam or Oxycel gauze over the anal wounds. Dressings, in such cases, are held in place by a T-binder.

Patient Education and Home Health Care. Stool softeners are usually prescribed for several days to prevent pain and discomfort during elimination. Local cooling astringents such as witch hazel help reduce discomfort. The physician usually recommends aspirin or acetaminophen for pain. Normal bowel elimination without pain should occur within a week (see Nursing Process: The Patient With an Anorectal Condition).

Pilonidal Sinus (Cyst)

A pilonidal sinus or cyst is found in the intergluteal cleft on the posterior surface of the lower sacrum (Fig. 37–13). It is thought by some to be formed by an infolding of epithelial tissue beneath the skin, which may communicate with the skin surface through one or several small sinus openings. Hair frequently is seen protruding from these openings, and this gives the cyst its name—*pilonidal*—a nest of hair. The cysts rarely give symptoms until adolescence or early adult life, when infection produces an irritating drainage or an abscess. This area is easily irritated by perspiration and friction.

Management.   In the early stages of the inflammation, the infection may be controlled by antibiotic therapy. Once an abscess has formed, as in cases of a hair-containing sinus, surgery is indicated. When an abscess is present, incision and drainage are performed. In patients with hair-containing sinuses without marked inflammatory reaction, surgery is also necessary to remove hair and debris, potential sources of irritation and infection. The entire cyst and the secondary sinus tracts are excised. In many patients the resulting defect may be sutured, but in some the defect may be so large that it cannot be closed entirely, and it is allowed to heal by granulation. Extensive excisions are no longer considered necessary.

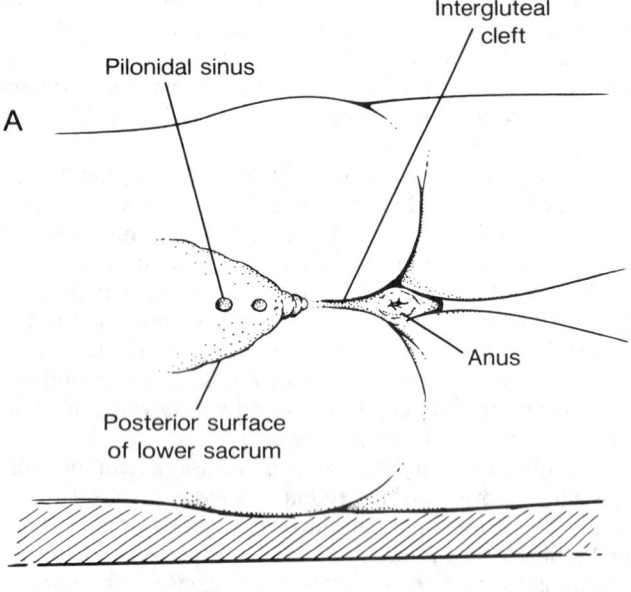

Figure 37–13.   (**A**) Pilonidal sinus on lower sacrum about 5 cm (2 in) above the anus in the intergluteal cleft. (**B**) Note hair particles emerging from sinus tract. Localized indentations of the skin (pits) can occur near the sinus openings.

Nursing Interventions.   In those patients with abscess, hot, moist applications are used frequently. After excision of the cyst, the care is that of any superficial wound. Shaving of hair around the wound is recommended to avoid recurrence. For the first few days, the patient often is more comfortable lying on his abdomen or side with a pillow between the legs. Most patients are allowed out of bed soon after surgery, and their postoperative care is managed at home.

▶ Nursing Process
The Patient With an Anorectal Condition

▷ Assessment

Health History
- Presence of bleeding
- Description of bleeding—amount, color
- Presence of pain
- Characteristics of pain—during evacuation, length of pain, associated abdominal pain
- Presence of discharge—mucoid, purulent, bloody
- Diet history—fiber intake
- Elimination pattern
- Laxative use
- Occupation—requirement of prolonged standing or sitting

Physical Assessment
- Inspection of the perianal area of hemorrhoids, fissures, drainage of pus or feces, signs of irritation
- Inspection of stool for blood or mucus

▷ Nursing Diagnoses

Based on all the assessment data, the patient's major nursing diagnoses may include the following:

- Constipation related to ignoring the urge to defecate because of pain during elimination
- Anxiety related to impending surgery and embarrassment
- Pain, related to irritation, pressure, and sensitivity in the rectal/anal area secondary to anorectal disease and sphincter spasms postoperatively
- Altered urinary elimination related to postoperative fear of pain
- High risk for injury, hemorrhage, related to the surgical incision
- Potential noncompliance with the therapeutic regimen

▷ Planning and Implementation

▷ *Goals:*   The major goals of the patient may include attainment of adequate elimination, reduction in anxiety, relief of pain, promotion of urinary elimination, prevention of hemorrhage, and compliance with the therapeutic regimen.

▷ Nursing Interventions

▷ *Measures for Relief of Constipation.*   The intake of at least 2000 ml of water daily is encouraged to provide adequate hydration. High-fiber foods are recommended to promote bulk in the stool and facilitate easy passage through the rectum. Bulk laxatives such as Metamucil and stool softeners are administered as prescribed. The patient is advised to set aside a time for defecation and to heed the urge to defecate. Relaxation exercises may be helpful before defecation to relax the abdominal perineal muscles that may be constricted or in spasm because of anticipated pain with elimination.

▷ *Reducing Anxiety.* Patients facing rectal surgery may be upset and irritable because of discomfort, pain, and embarrassment. Specific psychosocial needs are identified and the plan of care is individualized. Privacy is provided by limiting visitors, if agreeable to the patient. The patient's privacy is maintained when giving care. Soiled dressings are removed from the room promptly to prevent unpleasant odors. Room deodorizers may be needed if dressings are foul-smelling.

▷ *Relieving Pain.* During the first 24 hours after rectal surgery, there may be painful spasms of the sphincter and perineal muscles. Therefore, control of pain is a prime consideration. The patient is encouraged to assume positions of comfort (bed rest with prolapsed internal hemorrhoids, avoidance of walking with an abscess). Ice and analgesic ointments may decrease pain. Warm compresses may promote circulation and soothe irritated tissues. Sitz baths, three or four times a day, will relieve soreness and pain by relaxing sphincter spasm. After 24 hours have elapsed, topical anesthetic agents may be beneficial for relief of local irritation and soreness.

Wet dressings saturated with equal parts of cold water and witch hazel help relieve edema. When wet compresses are being used continuously, petrolatum should be applied around the anal area to prevent skin maceration. The patient is instructed to assume a prone position at intervals, because this position promotes dependent drainage of edema fluid.

Medications may include suppositories that contain anesthetics, astringents, antiseptics, tranquilizers, and antiemetics. Patients will be more compliant, and less apprehensive and uncomfortable, if the suppository is inserted properly. The most effective position for the patient to assume while the suppository is being inserted is sidelying, with the uppermost leg flexed. The suppository is unwrapped; the buttocks are spread apart with one hand and the suppository is inserted with the other. If the suppository was stored in the refrigerator (to prevent melting), it may be warmed to room temperature to lessen irritation of rectal mucosa. Water-soluble suppositories may be lubricated with water or lubricating jelly; however, cocoa butter suppositories are self-lubricating.

▷ *Promoting Urinary Elimination.* Voiding may be a problem, because of a reflex spasm of the sphincter at the outlet of the bladder and a certain amount of muscle-guarding from apprehension and pain. All methods to encourage voluntary micturition (increasing fluid intake, listening to running water, dripping water over the urinary meatus) should be tried before resorting to catheterization. After rectal operations, patients are usually allowed out of bed to void.

▷ *Preventing Hemorrhage.* The operative site is examined for rectal bleeding. The patient is assessed for systemic indicators of excessive bleeding (tachycardia, hypotension, restlessness, thirst). After hemorrhoidectomy, hemorrhage may occur from the veins that were cut. If a tube has been inserted through the sphincter after operation, evidence of bleeding should be apparent on the dressings. If bleeding is obvious, direct pressure is applied to the area and the physician is notified.

▷ *Patient Education and Home Health Care.* The patient should keep the perianal area as clean as possible. This is accomplished by gentle cleansing with warm water and drying with absorbent cotton wipes. The patient is instructed to avoid rubbing the area with toilet tissue.

The patient prevents constipation by responding quickly to the urge to defecate. Over-the-counter laxatives should be avoided. Diet is modified to increase fluids and fiber. The patient is encouraged to ambulate as soon as possible.

When it is time for discharge from the hospital, the patient should know how to take sitz baths and how to test the temperature of the water. Sitz baths may be given in a bathtub three or four times a day, or a plastic sitz bath unit (usually sold in a drugstore) can be used.

The patient is informed about the prescribed diet, made aware of the significance of proper eating habits, and told what laxatives can be taken safely and why exercise is important. The surgeon usually outlines a schedule in detail to cover the daily routine. This is reviewed with the patient by the nurse.

▷ Evaluation

Expected Outcomes

1. Attains a normal pattern of elimination
   a. Sets aside a time for defecation, usually after a meal or at bedtime
   b. "Heeds the call" and takes the time to sit on the toilet and try to defecate
   c. Uses relaxation exercises as needed
   d. Increases fluid intake to 2 L/24 hr
   e. Adds high-fiber foods to diet
   f. Reports passage of soft, formed stools
   g. Reports less abdominal discomfort
2. Projects less anxiety
   a. Discusses fears and concerns
   b. Describes surgical procedure
   c. Describes postoperative recovery procedures
   d. Communicates privacy needs
3. Experiences less pain
   a. Modifies body position and activities to minimize pain and discomfort
   b. Applies heat/cold to rectal/anal area
   c. Takes sitz baths four times a day
   d. Changes dressing frequently; requests assistance if needed
   e. Reports less pain
4. Achieves voluntary micturition
   a. Voids without difficulty
   b. Is free of urinary pain/discomfort
5. Is free of any bleeding problems
   a. Has a clean incision
   b. Exhibits normal vital signs
   c. Is free of hemorrhage
6. Adheres to a therapeutic regimen
   a. Keeps perianal area dry
   b. Eats bulk-forming foods
   c. Has soft, formed stools on a regular basis
   d. Ambulates as soon as possible

In summary, diseases of the anorectum cause similar signs and symptoms even though the pathophysiologic basis differs with each disease entity. Nursing interventions in each case are directed toward assisting the patient to obtain normal elimination patterns, experience less pain and anxiety, and avoid complications.

Bibliography

Books

Allan RN et al. Inflammatory Bowel Diseases. New York, Churchill Livingstone, 1990.

Bolt RJ et al. The Digestive System. New York, John Wiley & Sons, 1983.

Brandt L. Gastrointestinal Disorders of the Elderly. New York, Raven Press, 1984

Chopra S and May R. Pathophysiology of Gastrointestinal Diseases. Boston, Little, Brown, 1989

Cohen S. Clinical Gastroenterology: A Problem Solving Approach. New York, John Wiley & Sons, 1983.

Corman ML. Colon and Rectal Surgery, 2nd ed. Philadelphia, JB Lippincott, 1989.

Danzi JT. Idiopathic Inflammatory Bowel Disease: Current Clinical Practice. Philadelphia, WB Saunders, 1987.

Donovan MI and Girton SE. Cancer Care Nursing. Norwalk, CT, Appleton–Century–Crofts, 1984.

Eastwood GI. Core Textbook of Gastroenterology. Philadelphia, JB Lippincott, 1984.

Eliopoulus C. Gerontologic Nursing, 2nd ed. Philadelphia, JB Lippincott, 1987.

Fenoglio–Preiser et al. Gastrointestinal Pathology: An Atlas and Text. New York, Raven Press, 1989.

Ferrari BT et al. Complications of Colon and Rectal Surgery. Philadelphia, WB Saunders, 1985.

Gitnick G. Handbook of GI Emergencies, 2nd ed. New York, Elsevier, 1987.

Given B and Simmons S. Gastroenterology in Clinical Nursing. St Louis, CV Mosby, 1984.

Hamilton H. Gastrointestinal Disorders (Nurses Clinical Library). Springhouse, PA, Springhouse, 1985.

Kirsner J and Shorter R. Diseases of the Colon, Rectum, and Anal Canal. Baltimore, Williams & Wilkins, 1988.

Kirsner J and Shorter R. Inflammatory Bowel Disease, 3rd ed. Philadelphia, Lea & Febiger, 1988.

Misiewicz JJ et al. Atlas of Clinical Gastroenterology. New York, Glaxo/Roche, 1985.

Price AL. Ileostomy Care: Stoma Care and Management Techniques. Springfield, IL, Charles C Thomas, 1984.

Shackelford RT and Zuidema GD. Surgery of the Alimentary Tract. Philadelphia, WB Saunders, 1986.

Sivak M. Gastroenterologic Endoscopy. Philadelphia, WB Saunders, 1987.

Sleisenger MH and Fordtran JS. Gastrointestinal Disease: Pathophysiology, Diagnosis, and Management. Philadelphia, WB Saunders, 1988.

Spiro HM. Clinical Gastroenterology. New York, Macmillan, 1983.

Spratt JS. Neoplasms of the Colon, Rectum, and Anus. Philadelphia, WB Saunders, 1984.

Steiner P et al. A Sourcebook for Living With Inflammatory Bowel Disease. Nat'l Foundation for Ileitis and Colitis, 1985.

Way LW. Current Surgical Diagnosis and Treatment. Los Altos, CA, Lange Medical Publishers, 1991.

Welch CE et al. Manual of Lower Gastrointestinal Surgery. New York, Springer–Verlag, 1986.

Journals

Asterisks indicate nursing research articles.

General

Birkett DH. Hemorhoids: Diagnosis and treatment options. Hosp Pract 1988 Jan 30; 23(1): 99–102, 105+.

Bitterman RN. Nonspecific abdominal pain. Emerg Med 1989 Mar 30; 21(6): 63, 67–68.

Kelly M. Adjusting to ileostomy. Nurs Times 1987 Aug 19–25; 83(33): 29–31.

Koster TJ. Sounding out appendicitis. Emerg Med 1988 Feb 15; 20(3): 133–136.

Lanardhanan R et al. Cecal volvulus: Decompression. Am J Gastroenterol 1987 Sep; 88(9): 912–914.

Morrissey K and Cohan A. Colonoscopic decompression for non-obstructive colonic dilatation. Curr Concepts Gastroenterol 1989; 13(2): 7–13.

Palmer RC. Diverticular disease: Dietary and other measures that help control these lesions. Consultant 1988 May; 28(5): 75–82.

Shabsin H. Behavioral considerations in evaluating and treating chronic GI pain. Endosc Rev 1988 May/Jun; 11(3): 67–72.

Waye JD et al. Small colon polyps. Am J Gastroenterol 1988 Feb; 88(2): 120–122.

Constipation and Diarrhea

Basch A. Changes in elimination associated with cancer. Semin Oncol Nurs 1987 Nov; 3(4): 287–292.

Bayless TM. Chronic diarrhea: Newly appreciated syndromes. Hosp Pract 1989 Jan 15; 24(1): 117–131.

Beck ML. Imodium. SGA J 1988 Fall; 11(2): 112–113.

MacLeod J. Fecal incontinence: A practical program of management. Endosc Rev 1988 Nov/Dec; 11(6): 45–59.

* McMillan SC. Validity and reliability of the constipation assessment scale. Cancer Nurs 1989 Jun; 12(3): 183–188.

McShane RE. Constipation: Impact of etiological factors. J Gerontol Nur 1988 Apr; 14(4): 31–34, 46–47.

Ogorek C and Reynolds J. Chronic constipation: Diagnosis and treatment. Endos Rev 1987 Nov/Dec; 4(6): 47–53.

Vargas J. Sorting out the causes of vomiting and diarrhea. Emerg Med 1988 Feb 15; 20(3): 138–148.

Bowel Obstruction

Cobert BL. Obstruction of the small and large bowel. Hosp Med 1989 Aug; 23(8): 77–89.

Dalzell T. Acute intestinal obstruction. Nurs Times 1989 Jan 11; 85(1): 59–61.

Johnson J. Colonoscopy and diseases of the large bowel. Endosc Rev 1989 Jul/Aug; 12(4): 29–34.

Ricci E et al. Endoscopic management of colonic stenosis. Endosc Rev 1989 May/Jun; 12(3): 8–25.

Webb W. Endoscopic therapy of colonic strictures, volvulus, and pseudo-obstruction. Endosc Rev 1989 Jul/Aug; 12(4): 41–44.

Postsurgical Malabsorptions

Dowling H. Short bowel syndrome. Endosc Rev 1988 Jul/Aug; 12(4): 47–57.

McConnell EA. Fluid and electrolyte concerns in intestinal surgical procedures. Nurs Clin North Am 1987 Dec; 22(4): 853–860.

Colon, Rectal, and Anal Disorders

Fazio VW. Anorectal disorders. Gastroenterol Clin North Am 1987 Mar; 16(1): 1–198.

Harbick SV. Colorectal cancer. SGA J 1988 Spring; 10(4): 208–210.

Kretchevsky D. Epidemiology of colon cancer. Endosc Rev 1987; 4(3): 12–20.

Luk GD. Colorectal cancer. Gastroenterol Clin North Am 1988 Dec; 17(4): 1–200.

Owen D. Premalignant lesions of the GI tract. Endosc Rev 1987 May/Jun 4(3): 18–30.

Patterson BH et al. Food choices and cancer guidelines. Am J Public Health 1988 Mar; 78(3): 282–286.

Inflammatory Bowel Disease

Bennett P. Psychological aspects of physical illness: IBD (Part I). Nurs Times 1987 Nov 18–24; 83(46): 51–53.

Black M. Crohn's disease, pathophysiology, diagnosis, and management. Gastroenterol Nurs 1989 Spring; 2(4): 259–262.

Clause RE et al. Inflammatory bowel disease: A systematic approach to diagnosis and management. Physician Assist 1988 Jul; 12(7): 43–45, 49+.

Farraye FA et al. Inflammatory bowel disease: Advances in management of ulcerative colitis and Crohn's disease. Consultant 1988 Oct; 28(10): 39–43, 46–47.

Feuenstein IM. Radiologic evaluation of IBD: CT and Ultrasonography. Appl Radiol 1987 Nov; 16(11): 160–162.

Ginsberg A. Management of inflammatory bowel disease. Gastroenterol Clin North Am 1989 Mar; 18(1): 1–198.

Ginsberg A. New treatment for inflammatory bowel disease. Endosc Rev 1987 Jul/Aug; 4(4): 25–27.

Greenstein AJ. The surgery for Crohn's disease. Surg Clin North Am 1987 Jun; 67(3): 573–596.

Hennesy K. Nutritional support and gastrointestinal disease. Nurs Clin North Am 1989 Jun; 24(2): 373–382.

Kinash RG. Inflammatory bowel disease: Implications for the patient, challenges for nurses. Rehabil Nurs 1987 Dec; 34(12): 82–89.

Lubat E and Balthazar EJ. Current role of CAT Scan in IBD. Am J Gastroenterol 1988 Feb; 89(2): 107–113.

Nold HJ. Complications of inflammatory bowel disease. Hosp Pract 1987 Nov 30; 22(11): 65–75.

Prasad ML. Surgical options for the patient with inflammatory bowel disease. SGA J 1988 Winter; 10(3): 141–144.

Sirlin SM et al. Inflammatory bowel disease. Physician Assist 1988 Mar; 12(3): 24–25, 29–32, 34.

Smith L. Surgery for inflammatory bowel disease. Endosc Rev 1987 Jul/Aug; 4(4): 34–38.

Swartz M. Beyond the scope: A nursing view of the extraintestinal manifestations of inflammatory bowel disease. Gastroenterol Nurs 1989 Summer; 1(1): 3–9.

Information/Resources

Agencies

American Cancer Society
1599 Clifton Rd NE, Atlanta, GA 30329
International Association for Enterostomal Therapy
2081 Business Circle Dr, Suite 290, Irvine, CA 92715
National Foundation for Ileitis and Colitis
444 Park Ave S, New York, NY 10016
United Ostomy Association
36 Executive Park, Irvine, CA 92714

Nursing Research Profile for Unit 8

Digestive and Gastrointestinal Problems

Overview

Recent nursing research studies relative to gastrointestinal conditions and therapeutic modalities have provided information that is useful in clinical practice. A variety of topics have been studied. The focus of these studies has been on identifying those nursing measures that serve to promote health and prevent complications that cause discomfort or prolong disability.

The following research studies are examples of the research that has been conducted in the areas of oral hygiene and tube-feeding procedures. Although the subect populations were in some cases small and generalization of the findings is not always feasible, the nursing implications warrant consideration and further study.

Oral Hygiene

▷ Miller R and Rubinstein L. Oral health care for hospitalized patients: The nurse's role. J Nurs Ed 1987 Nov; 26(9): 362–366.

The researchers designed this study for the purpose of determining whether senior nursing students had sufficient knowledge about the oral health care needs of hospitalized patients. A 12-item open- and closed-ended, self-administered questionnaire was designed and used to obtain data from senior nursing students in two university programs, one diploma program, and one community college program. The questions measured knowledge regarding plaque, dental diseases, and daily oral health care and opinions about the nurse's role in providing oral health care for hospitalized patients. One hundred sixty-four questionnaires were returned, a response rate of 75.2%.

The results of the study showed that the majority of students who were surveyed demonstrated basic knowledge about plaque, gingival disease, plaque removal aids, and denture care. In addition, 85% identified the nurse as the health care member most appropriate to assist patients with daily oral hygiene. However, less than half the students felt that they were able to recognize the signs of periodontal disease, and few students

(11%) identified the necessity for controlling bacterial plaque for immunosuppressed patients.

Nursing Implications. (1) Nurses have a need for more knowledge about oral hygiene care for hospitalized patients. (2) Nurses assume significant responsibility for assisting hospitalized patients with oral health care.

▷ Dudjak LA. Mouth care for mucositis due to radiation therapy. Cancer Nurs 1987 Jun; 10(3):131–140.

Advances in the treatment of cancer with chemotherapy, radiation therapy, and immunotherapy have improved cure rates and extended life spans. However, these therapies have destructive effects on normal tissue. The tissue alterations and functional changes of the oral cavity that result from radiation treatment of patients with cancer of the head and neck are of great significance and concern. The researchers identified a need to establish a protocol for the control and treatment of oral mucositis that results from radiation therapy.

The purpose of this study was to determine the effects of two oral care protocols (half-strength hydrogen peroxide and a solution of baking soda and water) on the physical condition of the oral mucosa and on the perception of comfort for patients receiving radiation therapy to the head and neck. The study population consisted of 15 patients who were prescribed a minimum of 5000 rad to the oral cavity. The subjects were randomly assigned to one of two mouth care protocols; the protocols differed only with regard to the agent used (half-strength hydrogen peroxide versus a solution of baking soda and water). An Oral Examination Guide that measures the physical condition of the mouth and an Oral Perception Guide that assesses perception of comfort were used to collect data initially and at the completion and 1 month after completion of radiation therapy.

Findings of the study revealed no significant difference in physical condition of the mouth in the subjects assigned to the two different protocols. However, there was a significant difference in the level of comfort between the two groups; subjects using the half-strength hydrogen peroxide protocol indicated higher levels of comfort. Both groups had the same rate of oral infection, which was lower than that suggested in the literature. It was concluded that systematic performance of oral care may be more effective than the specific oral agent used in decreasing the destructive effects of radiation on the oral mucosa.

Nursing Implications. (1) Patient and family education

should focus on the potential value of an oral care regimen. (2) Consistency of reinforcement and encouragement about compliance with the oral care regimen are important nursing strategies; family members should be involved in providing this reinforcement and encouragement.

Tube Feeding

▷ **Metheny N et al. Effectiveness of the ausculatory method in predicting feeding tube location. Nurs Res 1990 Sep/Oct; 39(5):262–267.**

Nutrients are often provided to patients through nasogastric or nasointestinal feeding tubes. To ensure patient safety, confirmation of correct placement of these tubes initially and prior to each feeding has long been recommended. Auscultation of air inserted into the tube is one of the most common procedures used for this purpose.

The purpose of this study was twofold: to determine the extent to which sounds produced by air insufflations through feeding tubes can be used to predict where in the gastrointestinal tract (esophagus, stomach, or proximal small intestine) the tube's ports end and to determine the extent to which air insufflations through feeding tubes can be used to differentiate between gastric and respiratory placement of tubes.

This subject population consisted of 85 acutely ill adults who had either a small-bore nasogastric or a nasointestinal feeding tube. Following x-ray verification of tube position, sounds generated by a series of air insufflations through the tubes were tape-recorded. One hundred fifteen recordings of sound sequences were obtained. The tapes were played for five skilled clinicians who independently recorded their impressions of the sounds.

The findings of the study revealed that the ausculatory method is not effective in specifying the location of a feeding tube in the gastrointestinal tract. Only 34.4% of the responses to the taped sounds were correct.

During the study there were three subjects with feeding tubes inadvertently placed in the respiratory tract. Air insufflations through two of these tubes were clearly audible; in addition, sounds were transmitted from the lung or pleural space throughout the upper abdomen.

Nursing Implications. (1) The ausculatory method should not be relied upon to differentiate between tube placement in the stomach and tube placement in the small intestine. (2) Likewise, the ausculatory method is not reliable in differentiating between gastric and respiratory placement of a tube. (3) Determination of the *p*H of feeding tube aspirates is recommended for differentiation between gastric and intestinal placement of a tube and gastric and respiratory placement.

▷ **Anliker AW. Bacterial contamination of continuous-infusion enteral feedings. Nutri Supp Serv 1988 Jul; 8(7):11–12, 32.**

Enteral feedings administered by continuous-drip are used for many patients in hospitals, extended care facilities, and home settings. Because the feeding solution remains at room temperature for long periods of time, it is susceptible to bacterial contamination, which can result in gastroenteritis.

The researchers investigated the bacterial growth over time of continuous-drip-administration enteral feeding sets. It was hypothesized that the number of bacterial colonies cultured from the feeding sets would increase over time.

A convenience sample of 10 patients who received a continuous-drip enteral feeding for a minimum of 72 hours was studied. Cultures of the nutrient solutions were obtained from the tubing at 0, 24, 48, and 72 hours after the tubing was initially hung. Eighty percent of the subjects had positive culture results during the 72-hour period; 13 different organisms were cultured.

The findings revealed that there was no significant difference between the colony count means of 0 and 24 hours, 24 and 48 hours, and 48 and 72 hours. However, a significant difference existed between the 0- and 48-hour intervals, the 0- and 72-hour intervals, and the 24- and 72-hour intervals.

Nursing Implications. It is suggested that continuous-drip feeding sets can be safely left in place for 48 hours. However, replication of the study with larger sample sizes is necessary to confirm the findings.

▷ **Wilson MF and Haynes-Johnson V. Cranberry juice or water? A comparison of feeding-tube irrigants. Nutri Supp Serv 1987 Jul; 7(7):23–24.**

One of the most common mechanical complications associated with enteral feeding tubes is tube lumen obstruction. The subsequent need to irrigate the tube and to replace it if irrigation is unsuccessful results in increased costs of supplies and physical and emotional trauma to the patient related to tube reinsertion.

The purpose of this study was to compare the effectiveness of cranberry juice and water in maintaining the patency of Dobbhoff feeding tubes. The subject population consisted of 30 patients who were receiving continuous pump infusions of Osmolite liquid nutrition through newly inserted Dobbhoff feeding tubes that had been inserted via the nasal passage. The subjects were randomly assigned to receive either 30 ml of water or 30 ml of cranberry juice every 4 hours.

The study results revealed that tubes irrigated with water had a significantly lower incidence of occlusion than those irrigated with cranberry juice. None of the tubes irrigated with water became occluded, as compared with 73.3% of the tubes irrigated with cranberry juice.

Nursing Implications. (1) Water can be considered an effective, inexpensive irrigant for maintaining patency in Dobbhoff feeding tubes inserted via the nasal passage and used for continuous pump infusions of Osmolite. (2) Follow-up studies should be conducted with other commonly used nutrient solutions.

▷ **Metheny N, Eisenberg P, and McSweeney M. Effect of feeding tube properties and three irrigants on clogging rates. Nurs Res 1988 May/Jun; 37(3):165–169.**

The purpose of this study was twofold: to examine the effects of the feeding tube properties of material and diameter on the incidence of tube clogging and to compare the efficacy of cranberry juice, water, and Coca-Cola as irrigants in preventing tube clogging.

One hundred and eight feeding tubes were studied over three consecutive 12-hour periods. Half the tubes were made of polyurethane and half were silicone; each tube type group was equally divided among external diameters of 8, 10, and 12 Fr. Each tube was connected to gravity-flow feeding sets containing the same isotonic enteral solution. The flow rate was adjusted to the same rate for all tubes. Rates were not readjusted until the scheduled (every 4 hours) irrigations were completed. One third of the tubes were irrigated with cranberry juice, one third with water, and one third with Coca-Cola.

The findings revealed that the polyurethane material was superior to silicone and that Coca-Cola and water were consistently superior to cranberry juice as irrigants; the tube diameter had no significant effect on the incidence of tube clogging.

Nursing Implications. (1) Feeding tubes that are least likely to result in tube clogging are recommended; polyurethane tubes are superior to silicone tubes. (2) Because thicker formulas may require tubes with larger diameters, it is reasonable to select either 10 or 12 Fr tubes for gastric feeding use. (3) Choosing a tube that is least likely to clog is more cost-effective than replacing a less expensive tube that tends to clog more easily.

▷ Eisenberg P, Spies M, and Metheny NA. *Characteristics of patients who remove their nasal feeding tube. Clin Nurse Spec* 1987 Mar; 1(3):94–98.

Nurses caring for patients who are receiving enteral feeding are often concerned that the patients will remove the feeding tubes. Displacement of the tube results in interruption of nutritional intake as well as the need to replace the tube, which results in increased costs and possible complications for the patient.

The researchers conducted a 6-month prospective study for the purposes of identifying and quantifying risk factors for patients who discontinue their tubes. The study population consisted of 109 patients who received enteral nutrition from the placement of a total of 213 nasoenteral tubes. Forty-one percent of the subjects removed their tubes at least once. Restlessness and disorientation were significant factors in these subjects. Patients with the primary diagnosis of cerebrovascular accident, head trauma, and sepsis who demonstrated disorientation and restlessness were significantly more likely to remove their tubes than were patients with other diagnoses who were also disoriented and restless.

Nursing Implications. (1) Patients with feeding tubes must be assessed to determine if they are at risk for removing their tubes. (2) Devices to prevent removal of tubes must be used for at-risk patients; nasal anchoring devices and wrist restraints are useful; frequent reassessment is imperative. (3) Patients' families should be involved in efforts directed toward preventing patients from removing feeding tubes.

unit *9*

Metabolic and Endocrine Function

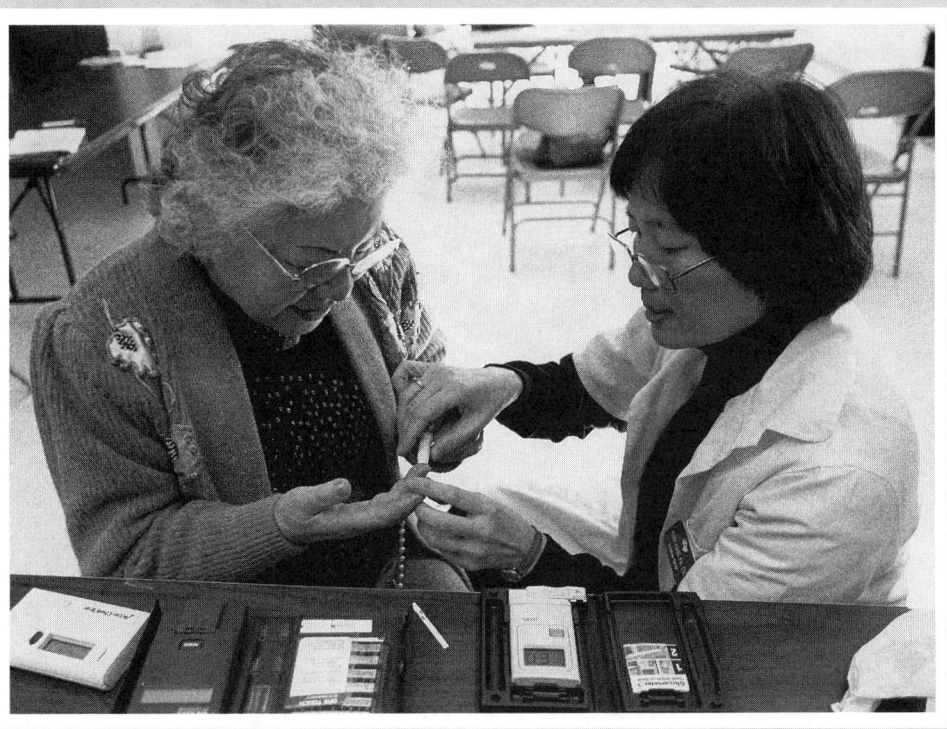

38

Assessment and Management of Patients With Hepatic and Biliary Disorders

Learning Objectives

On completion of this chapter, the learner will be able to:

1. Identify the metabolic functions of the liver and the alterations in these functions that occur with liver disease

2. Explain liver function tests and clinical manifestations of liver dysfunction in relation to the pathophysiologic alterations of the liver

3. Relate jaundice, portal hypertension, ascites, nutritional deficiencies, and hepatic coma to the pathophysiologic alterations of the liver

4. Compare the various types of hepatitis and their causes, prevention, clinical manifestations, management, prognosis, and home health care needs

5. Use the nursing process as a framework for care of the patient with cirrhosis of the liver

6. Describe the medical and nursing management of patients with esophageal varices

7. Compare the nonsurgical and surgical management of patients with cancer of the liver

8. Describe the postoperative nursing care of the patient undergoing liver transplantation

9. Compare approaches to management of cholelithiasis

10. Use the nursing process as a framework for care of patients with cholelithiasis and those undergoing cholecystectomy

Physiologic Overview

The liver, the largest gland of the body, can be considered a chemical factory that manufactures, stores, alters, and excretes a large number of substances involved in metabolism. The location of the liver is essential in this function, because it receives nutrient-rich blood directly from the gastrointestinal tract and then either stores or transforms these nutrients into chemicals that are used elsewhere in the body for metabolic needs. The liver is especially important in the regulation of glucose and protein metabolism. The liver manufactures and secretes bile, which has a major role in the digestion and absorption of fats in the gastrointestinal tract. It functions as an organ of excretion by removing waste products from the bloodstream and secreting them into the bile. The bile produced by the liver is stored temporarily in the gallbladder until it is needed for the process of digestion, at which time the gallbladder empties and bile enters the intestine.

Anatomy

The liver is located behind the ribs in the upper right portion of the abdominal cavity. It weighs about 1500 g and is divided into four lobes. Each lobe is surrounded by a thin layer of connective tissue, which extends into the lobe itself and divides the liver mass into small units, called *lobules*. A schematic diagram of the liver and its anatomic relationships is shown in Figure 38–1.

The circulation of the blood into and out of the liver is of major importance in its function. The blood that perfuses the liver is derived from two sources. Approximately 75% of the blood supply comes from the portal vein, which drains the gastrointestinal tract and is rich in nutrients. The remainder of the blood supply enters by way of the hepatic artery and is rich in oxygen. Terminal branches of these two blood supplies join to form common capillary beds, which constitute the sinusoids of the liver. Liver cells (hepatocytes) are thus bathed by a mixture of venous and arterial blood. The sinusoids empty into a venule that occupies the center of each liver lobule and is called the *central vein*. The central veins join to form the hepatic vein, which constitutes the venous drainage from the liver and empties into the inferior vena cava, close to the diaphragm. Thus there are two sources of blood flowing into the liver but there is only one exit pathway.

In addition to hepatocytes, phagocytic cells belonging to the reticuloendothelial system are present in the liver. Other organs that contain reticuloendothelial cells are the spleen, bone marrow, lymph nodes, and lungs. In the liver, these cells are called *Kupffer cells*. Their main function is to engulf particulate matter (such as bacteria) that enters the liver through the portal blood.

The smallest bile ducts, called *canaliculi*, are located between the lobules of the liver. These canaliculi receive secretions from the hepatocytes and carry them to larger bile ducts, which eventually form the *hepatic duct*. The hepatic duct from the liver and the cystic duct from the gallbladder join to form the *common bile duct*, which empties into the small intestine. The flow of bile into the intestine is controlled by the sphincter of Oddi, located at the junction where the common bile duct enters the duodenum.

The gallbladder, a pear-shaped, hollow, saclike organ, 7.5 to 10 cm (3 to 4 inches) long, lies in a shallow depression on the inferior surface of the liver, to which it is attached by loose connective tissue. The capacity of the gallbladder is 30 to 50 ml of bile. Its wall is composed largely of smooth muscle. The gallbladder is connected to the common bile duct by the cystic duct.

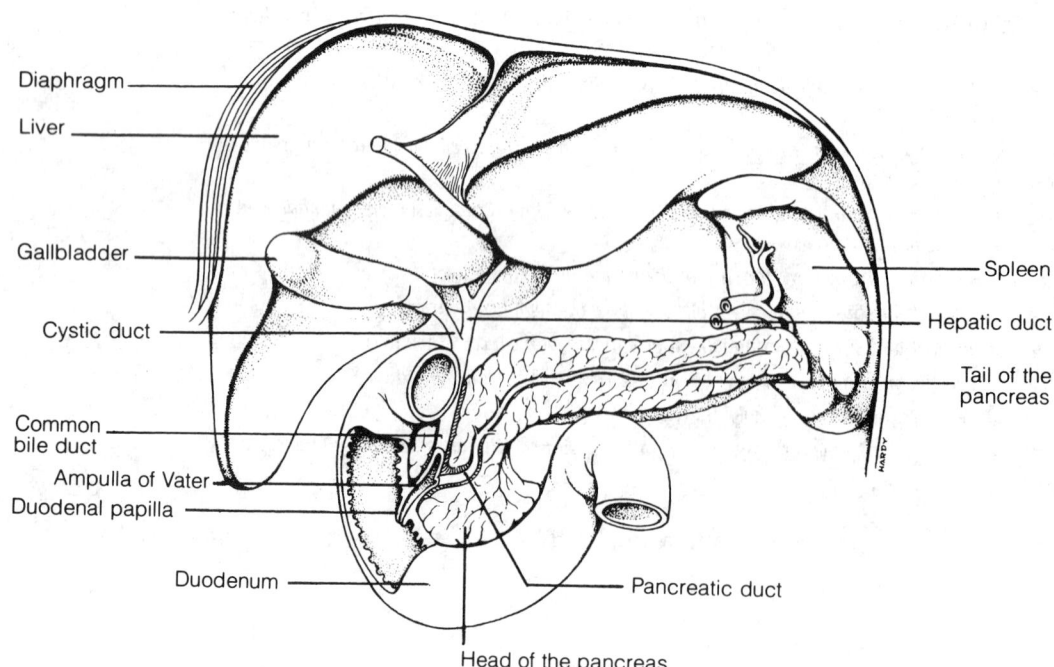

Figure 38–1. Liver and biliary system. (Chaffee EE and Greisheimer EM. Basic Physiology and Anatomy. 4th ed. Philadelphia, JB Lippincott.)

Metabolic Functions of the Liver

The liver plays a major role in the regulation of blood glucose concentration. After a meal, glucose is taken up from the portal venous blood by the liver and converted into glycogen, which is stored in the hepatocytes. Subsequently, the glycogen is converted back to glucose and released as needed into the bloodstream to maintain normal levels of blood glucose. Additional glucose can be synthesized by the liver through a process called *gluconeogenesis*. For this process, the liver uses amino acids from protein breakdown or lactate produced by exercising muscles.

Use of amino acids for gluconeogenesis results in the formation of ammonia as a by-product. The liver converts this metabolically generated ammonia into urea. Ammonia produced by bacteria in the intestines is also removed from portal blood for urea synthesis. In this way, the liver converts ammonia, a potential toxin, into urea, a harmless compound that can be excreted in the urine.

The liver also plays an important role in protein metabolism. It synthesizes almost all of the plasma proteins (except τ-globulin), including albumin, α- and β-globulins, blood-clotting factors, specific transport proteins, and most of the plasma lipoproteins. Vitamin K is required by the liver for synthesis of prothrombin and some of the other clotting factors. Amino acids serve as the building blocks for protein synthesis.

The liver is also active in fat metabolism. Fatty acids can be broken down for the production of energy and production of ketone bodies (acetoacetic acid, β-hydroxybutyric acid, and acetone). Ketone bodies are small compounds that can enter the bloodstream and provide a source of energy for muscles and other tissues. Breakdown of fatty acids into ketone bodies occurs predominantly when the availability of glucose for metabolism is limited, as during starvation or in diabetic patients. Fatty acids and their metabolic products are also used for the synthesis of cholesterol, lecithin, lipoproteins, and other complex lipids. Under some conditions, lipids may accumulate in the hepatocytes and result in the abnormal condition called fatty liver.

Vitamins A, B_{12}, D, and several of the B complex vitamins are stored in large amounts in the liver. Certain metals, such as iron and copper, are also stored within the liver. Because the liver is rich in these substances, liver extracts have been used for therapy of a wide range of nutritional disorders.

Drug Metabolism

Many drugs, such as barbiturates and amphetamines, are metabolized by the liver. Metabolism generally results in loss of activity of the drug, although in some cases activation may occur. One of the important pathways for drug metabolism involves conjugation (binding) of the drug with a variety of compounds, such as glucuronic or acetic acid, to form more soluble substances. The conjugated products may be excreted in the feces or urine, similar to bilirubin excretion.

Bile

Bile is continuously formed by the hepatocytes and collected in the canaliculi and bile ducts. It is composed mainly of water and electrolytes, such as sodium, potassium, calcium, chloride, and bicarbonate, and also contains significant amounts of lecithin, fatty acids, cholesterol, bilirubin, and bile salts. Bile is collected and stored in the gallbladder and is emptied into the intestine when needed for digestion. The functions of bile are excretory, as in the excretion of bilirubin, and as an aid to digestion through the emulsification of fats by bile salts.

Bile Salts. Bile salts are synthesized by the hepatocytes from cholesterol. After conjugation with amino acids (taurine and glycine), they are excreted into the bile. The bile salts, together with cholesterol and lecithin, are required for emulsification of fats in the intestine. This process is necessary for efficient digestion and absorption. Bile salts are then reabsorbed, primarily in the distal ileum, into portal blood for return to the liver and are again excreted into the bile. This pathway from hepatocytes to bile to intestine and back to the hepatocytes is called the *enterohepatic circulation*. Because of the enterohepatic circulation, only a small fraction of the bile salts that enter the intestine is excreted in the feces. This decreases the demand for active synthesis of bile salts by the liver cells.

Bilirubin Excretion

Bilirubin is a pigment derived from the breakdown of hemoglobin by cells of the reticuloendothelial system, including the Kupffer cells of the liver. Hepatocytes remove bilirubin from the blood and chemically modify it through conjugation to glucuronic acid, which makes the bilirubin more soluble in aqueous solutions. The conjugated bilirubin is secreted by the hepatocytes into the adjacent bile canaliculi and is eventually carried in the bile into the duodenum. In the small intestine, bilirubin is converted into urobilinogen, which is in part excreted in the feces and in part absorbed through the intestinal mucosa into the portal blood. Much of this reabsorbed urobilinogen is removed by the hepatocytes and is secreted into the bile once again (enterohepatic circulation). Some of the urobilinogen enters the systemic circulation and is excreted by the kidneys in the urine. Elimination of bilirubin in the bile represents the major route of excretion for this compound. The bilirubin concentration in the blood may be increased in the presence of liver disease, when the flow of bile is impeded (*e.g.*, with gallstones in the bile ducts), or with excessive destruction of red blood cells. With bile duct obstruction, bilirubin does not enter the intestine and, as a consequence, urobilinogen will be absent from the urine.

Gallbladder

The gallbladder functions as a storage depot for bile. Between meals, when the sphincter of Oddi is closed, bile produced by the hepatocytes enters the gallbladder. During storage, a large portion of the water in bile is absorbed through the walls of the gallbladder, so that gallbladder bile is five to ten times more concentrated than that originally secreted by the liver. When food enters the duodenum, the gallbladder contracts, and the sphincter of Oddi relaxes, allowing the bile to enter the intestine. This response is mediated by secretion of the hormone cholecystokinin-pancreozymin (CCK-PZ) from the intestinal wall.

Pathophysiology

Liver dysfunction results from damage to the liver parenchymal cells, either directly, from primary liver diseases, or indirectly, due to obstruction to bile flow or to derangements of hepatic circulation.

Disease processes that lead to hepatocellular dysfunction may be caused by infectious agents, such as bacteria and viruses, and by anoxia, metabolic disorders, toxins and drugs, nutritional deficiencies, and states of hypersensitivity. Probably the most common cause of parenchymal damage is malnutrition, especially in alcoholism. The response of the parenchymal cells is much the same for most noxious agents: replacement of glycogen by lipids, producing fatty infiltration, with or without cell death or necrosis. This is commonly associated with inflammatory cell infiltration and growth of fibrous tissue. Cell regeneration can occur if the disease process is not too toxic to the cells. The end result of chronic parenchymal disease is the shrunken, fibrotic liver seen in cirrhosis.

Hepatocellular dysfunction is manifested by alteration of the metabolic and excretory functions of the liver. Serum bilirubin concentration rises, leading to *jaundice* (yellowing of the skin mucous membranes, sclerae, and other tissues); this results from intrahepatic obstruction of bile channels. Abnormalities of carbohydrate, fat, and protein metabolism occur with liver dysfunction. Abnormal protein metabolism results in decreased serum albumin concentration and edema. Ammonia, a by-product of metabolism, is absorbed from the gastrointestinal tract but is not converted to urea by the damaged liver cells. An increased serum ammonia level may produce signs of central nervous system impairment.

The vascular architecture of the liver may be disturbed, causing increased portal vein blood pressure, which results in leakage of fluid into the peritoneal cavity, or ascites, and esophageal varices. The lack of normal production of various blood-clotting factors can lead to bleeding from any site, but the patient is particularly prone to gastrointestinal bleeding.

Many endocrine abnormalities also occur with liver dysfunction as a result of the inability of the liver to metabolize hormones normally, including androgens or sex hormones. Although the exact mechanisms for their appearance are not well established, gynecomastia, amenorrhea, testicular atrophy, and other disturbances of sexual function and sex characteristics are thought to result from failure of the damaged liver to normally inactivate estrogens.

Acute liver damage may cause acute liver failure, may be completely reversible, or may progress to chronic liver disease. The end result of chronic liver damage is cirrhosis, characterized by replacement of parenchymal cells with fibrotic tissue. Liver failure occurs when the liver is unable to carry out its excretory functions, and metabolic functions of the liver are inadequate to meet the needs of the body. Hepatic coma results when liver dysfunction is so severe that the liver is unable to remove ammonia, an end product of protein metabolism from the bloodstream. This accumulates in the circulation and nervous system, producing severe, life-threatening manifestations.

Gerontologic Considerations

The most common change in the liver in the elderly is a decrease in the size and weight of the liver accompanied by a decrease in total hepatic blood flow. In general, however, these decreases are in proportion to the decreases in body size and weight seen in normal aging. Results of liver function tests do not normally change in the elderly; abnormal results in an elderly patient indicate abnormal liver function and are not the result of the aging process itself.

The immune system is altered in the aged, and a less responsive immune system may be responsible for the increased incidence and severity of hepatitis B in the elderly and the increased incidence of liver abscesses secondary to decreased phagocytosis by the Kupffer cells.

Drug metabolism by the liver appears to be decreased in the elderly, but such changes are usually also accompanied by changes in intestinal absorption, renal excretion, and altered body distribution of some drugs secondary to changes in fat deposition. These alterations necessitate careful administration and monitoring of all medications with reduction of dosage to prevent drug toxicity.

Diagnostic Evaluation of Hepatic Function

Liver Function Tests.   Over 70% of the parenchyma of the liver may be damaged before liver function tests become abnormal. Function is generally measured in terms of serum enzyme activity (*e.g.*, alkaline phosphatase, transaminases, lactic dehydrogenase), and serum concentrations of proteins, bilirubin, ammonia, clotting factors, and lipids. Several of these tests may be helpful for assessment of patients with liver disease; however, the nature and extent of hepatic dysfunction cannot be determined by these tests alone. Many other disorders can influence their results; therefore, the tests are not sensitive indicators of liver dysfunction. A list of the commonly used liver function tests is shown in Table 38–1.

Other Diagnostic Tests.   Ultrasonography, computed tomography (CT) scanning, and magnetic resonance imaging (MRI) have been useful in identifying normal structures and abnormalities of the liver and biliary tree.

Examination of the Liver.   The liver may be palpable in the right upper quadrant. A palpable liver presents as a firm, sharp ridge with a smooth surface (Fig. 38–2). The size of the liver is estimated by percussion of the liver's upper and lower borders. When the liver is not palpable, but tenderness is suspected, tapping the lower right thorax briskly may elicit tenderness. The patient's response is then compared by performing a similar maneuver on the left lower thorax.

If the liver is palpable, the examiner notes and records its size, consistency, whether it is tender, and whether its outline is regular or irregular. If the liver is enlarged, the degree to which it descends below the right costal margin is recorded to provide some indication of its size. The examiner determines if the liver edge is sharp and smooth or blunt and if the enlarged liver is nodular or smooth. The liver of a patient with cirrhosis is small and hard, while the liver of a patient with acute hepatitis is quite soft and the edge is easily moved by the hand. Tenderness of the liver implies recent acute enlargement with consequent stretching of the liver capsule. The absence of tenderness may imply that the enlargement is of long-standing duration. The liver of a patient with viral hepatitis is tender, and that of a patient with alcoholic hepatitis is not. Enlargement of the liver is an abnormal finding requiring further evaluation.

Liver Biopsy.   A procedure that greatly facilitates the diagnosis of most hepatic disorders is the liver biopsy (*i.e.*, the sampling of liver tissue by needle aspiration for the purpose

TABLE 38–1. *Liver Function Studies*

Test	Normal	Clinical Functions
PIGMENT STUDIES		
Serum bilirubin, direct	0–0.3 mg/dl (0–5.1 μmol/L)	These studies measure the ability of liver to conjugate and excrete bilirubin. Results are abnormal in liver and biliary tract disease and are associated with jaundice clinically.
Serum bilirubin, total	0–0.9 mg/dl (1.7–20.5 μmol/L)	
Urine bilirubin	0 (0)	
Urine urobilinogen	0.05–2.5 mg/24 hr (0.09–4.23 μmol/24 hr)	
Fecal urobilinogen (infrequently used)	40–200 mg/24 hr (0.068–0.34 mmol/24 hr)	
PROTEIN STUDIES		
Total serum protein	7.0–7.5 g/dl (70–75 g/L)	Proteins are manufactured by the liver. Their levels may be affected in a variety of liver impairments.
Serum albumin	3.5–5.5 g/dl (35–55 g/L)	
Serum globulin	1.5–3.0 g/dl (15–30 g/L)	
Serum protein electrophoresis	3.2–5.6 g/dl (32–56 g/L)	Albumin Cirrhosis
Albumin		Chronic hepatitis
α_1-Globulin	0.1–0.4 g/dl (1–4 g/L)	Edema, ascites)
α_2-Globulin	0.4–1.2 g/dl (4–12 g/L)	Globulin Cirrhosis
β-Globulin	0.5–1.1 g/dl (5–11 g/L)	Liver disease
γ-Globulin	0.5–1.6 g/dl (5–16 g/L)	Chronic obstructive jaundice
		Viral hepatitis
Albumin/globulin (A/G) ratio	A > G or 1.5:1–2.5:1	A/G ratio is reversed in chronic liver disease (decreased albumin and increased globulin).
PROTHROMBIN TIME		
Response of prothrombin time to vitamin K	100% return to normal	Prothrombin time may be prolonged in liver disease. It will not return to normal with vitamin K in severe liver cell damage.
SERUM ALKALINE PHOSPHATASE	Varies with method: 2–5 Bodansky units 20–90 IU/L at 30° (20–90 U/L at 30°)	Serum alkaline phosphatase is manufactured in bones, liver, kidneys, and intestine and excreted through biliary tract. In absence of bone disease, it is a sensitive measure of biliary tract obstruction.
SERUM TRANSAMINASE STUDIES		
SGOT or AST	10–40 units (4.8–19 U/L)	The studies are based on release of enzymes from damaged liver cells. These enzymes are elevated in liver cell damage.
SGPT or ALT	5–35 units (2.4–17 U/L)	
LDH	165–400 units (80–192 U/L)	
BLOOD AMMONIA	20–120 μg/dl (11.1–67.0 μmol/L)	Liver converts ammonia to urea. Ammonia level rises in liver failure.
CHOLESTEROL		
Ester	150–250 mg/dl (3.90–6.50 mmol/L) 60% of total (fraction of total cholesterol: 0.60)	Cholesterol levels are elevated in biliary obstruction and decreased in parenchymal liver disease.

Additional Studies	Clinical Functions
RADIOLOGIC STUDIES	
Barium study of esophagus	For varices, which indicate increased portal pressure
Plain film of abdomen	To determine gross liver size
Liver scan with radio-tagged iodinated rose bengal, gold, or technetium	To show size and shape of liver; to show replacement of liver tissue with scars, cysts, or tumor
Cholecystogram and cholangiogram	For gallbladder and bile duct visualization
Celiac axis arteriography	For liver and pancreas visualization
Splenoportogram (splenic portal venography)	To determine adequacy of portal blood flow

(continued)

TABLE 38–1. *(Continued)*

Additional Studies	Clinical Functions
PERITONEOSCOPY OR LAPAROSCOPY	Direct visualization of anterior surface of liver, gallbladder, and mesentery through a trocar
LIVER BIOPSY	To determine anatomic changes in liver tissue
MEASUREMENT OF PORTAL PRESSURE	Elevated in cirrhosis of the liver
ESOPHAGOSCOPY/ENDOSCOPY	To search for esophageal varices and abnormalities
ELECTROENCEPHALOGRAM	Abnormal in hepatic coma and impending hepatic coma
ULTRASONOGRAPHY	To show size of abdominal organs and presence of masses
COMPUTED TOMOGRAPHY (CT SCAN)	To detect hepatic neoplasms; diagnose cysts, abscesses, and hematomas; and distinguish between obstructive and nonobstructive jaundice
ANGIOGRAPHY	Visualizes hepatic circulation and detects presence and nature of hepatic masses
MAGNETIC RESONANCE IMAGING (MRI)	To detect hepatic neoplasms; diagnose cysts, abscesses, and hematomas

of histologic study). Nursing responsibilities in relation to liver biopsy are summarized in Chart 38–1. A graphic presentation is found in Figure 38–3.

Clinical Manifestations of Hepatic Dysfunction

The complications of liver disease are numerous and varied. In many instances their ultimate effects are incapacitating or lethal; their presence is ominous, and their treatment is often difficult.

Among the most frequent and important of these complications are the following:

• Jaundice, resulting from increased bilirubin concentration in the blood
• Portal hypertension and ascites, resulting from circulatory changes within the diseased liver and producing severe gastrointestinal hemorrhages and excessive sodium and fluid retention.
• Nutritional deficiencies, attributable to the inability of the

malfunctioning liver cells to metabolize certain vitamins, and responsible for impaired functioning of the central and peripheral nervous systems and for abnormal bleeding tendencies
• Hepatic coma, reflecting accumulation of ammonia in the serum because of impaired protein metabolism by the diseased liver.

Nursing care of the patient with impaired liver function is summarized in Nursing Care Plan 38–1.

Jaundice

When, for any reason, the bilirubin concentration in the blood becomes abnormally increased, all the body tissue, including the sclerae and the skin, becomes yellow-tinged or greenish yellow. This condition is called *jaundice*. Jaundice becomes clinically evident when the serum bilirubin level exceeds 2 to 2.5 mg/dl (SI: 34–43 µmol/L). Increased serum bilirubin levels and jaundice may result from impairment of hepatic uptake, conjugation of bilirubin, or excretion of bilirubin into the biliary system. There are several types of jaundice: (1) hemolytic, (2) hepatocellular, (3) obstructive, and (4) jaundice due to hered-

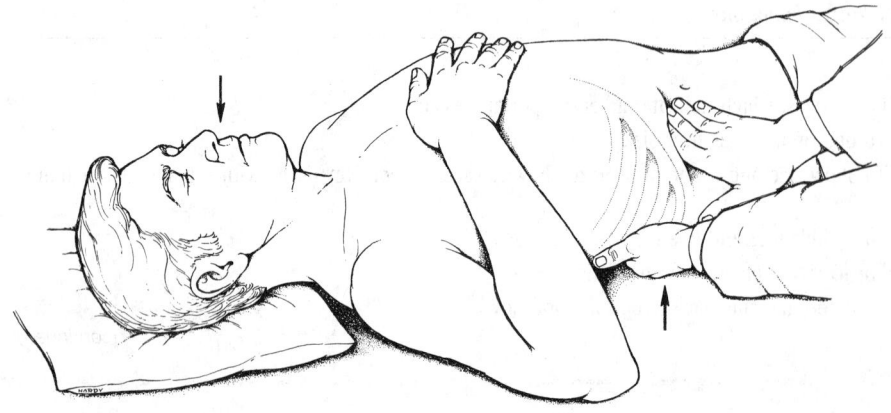

Figure 38–2. Technique for palpation of the liver. As the patient inhales, a palpable liver edge descends to meet the index finger of the right hand. At the height of inspiration, the examiner releases the pressure of the right hand slightly and tries to feel the liver edge "slip" under the fingertips.

Chart 38–1
Liver Biopsy and the Role of the Nurse

Nursing Activities	Rationale
Preprocedure	
1. Ascertain that coagulation tests (prothrombin time, PTT, and platelet count) have been requested, completed, and reported and that compatible donor blood is available.	Many patients with liver disease have clotting defects and are prone to bleed abnormally.
2. Check for signed consent.	
3. Measure and record the patient's pulse, respirations, and arterial pressure immediately before biopsy.	Prebiopsy values provide a basis on which to compare the patient's vital signs and evaluate his status after the procedure.
4. Describe to the patient in advance:	Explanations serve to allay his fears and ensure his cooperation.
• Steps of the procedure	
• Sensations expected	
• After-effects anticipated	
• Restrictions of activity and monitoring procedures to follow	
During Procedure	
5. Give support to the patient during the procedure.	The presence of a supportive nurse enhances comfort and promotes a sense of security.
6. Expose the right side of the patient's upper abdomen (right hypochondriac).	The skin at the site of penetration will be cleansed and infiltrated with local anesthetic.
7. Instruct the patient to inhale and exhale deeply several times, finally to exhale, and to hold his breath at the end of expiration (see Fig. 39–3).	Holding the breath immobilizes the chest wall and the diaphragm; penetration of the diaphragm thereby is avoided, and the risk of lacerating the liver is minimized.
• The physician promptly introduces the biopsy needle by way of the transthoracic (intercostal) or transabdominal (subcostal) route, penetrates the liver, aspirates, and withdraws. The entire procedure is completed within 5 to 10 seconds.	
8. Instruct the patient to resume breathing.	
Postprocedure	
9. Immediately after the biopsy, assist the patient to turn onto his right side; place a pillow under his costal margin, and caution him to remain in this position, recumbent and immobile, for several hours.	In this position, the liver capsule at the site of penetration is compressed against the chest wall, and the escape of blood or bile through the perforation is impeded.
10. Measure and record the patient's pulse, respiratory rate and his blood pressure at 10- to 20-minute intervals for the prescribed period, or until their values are stable, and his condition is satisfactory. Be alert to and report promptly any increase in pulse rate or any decrease in arterial pressure, any complant of pain, or manifestations of apprehension.	These signs may indicate the presence and the progress of hepatic bleeding, severe hemorrhage, or bile peritonitis, the most frequent complications of liver biopsy.

itary hyperbilirubinemia. Hepatocellular and obstructive jaundice are the two types commonly associated with liver disease.

Hemolytic Jaundice. Hemolytic jaundice is the result of an increased destruction of the red blood cells, the effect of which is to flood the plasma with bilirubin so rapidly that the liver, although functioning normally, cannot excrete the bilirubin as quickly as it is formed. This type of jaundice is encountered in patients with hemolytic transfusion reactions and other hemolytic disorders. The bilirubin in the blood of these patients is predominantly of the unconjugated, or "free," type. Fecal and urine urobilinogen are increased; conversely, the urine is free of bilirubin. Patients with this type of jaundice, unless their hyperbilirubinemia is extreme, do not experience symptoms or complications as a result of the jaundice *per se.*

Very prolonged jaundice, however, even if mild, predisposes to the formation of "pigment stones" in the gallbladder, and extremely severe jaundice (*e.g.*, in patients with levels of free bilirubin above 20 to 25 mg/dl) poses definite risk of possible brain stem damage.

Hepatocellular Jaundice. Hepatocellular jaundice is caused by the inability of diseased liver cells to clear normal amounts of bilirubin from the blood. The cellular damage may be from infection, such as in hepatitis A, hepatitis B, hepatitis C (from virus-infected blood transfusion), or yellow fever virus, or from drug or chemical toxicity (*e.g.*, carbon tetrachloride, chloroform, phosphorus, arsenicals, certain psychotherapeutic drugs, or ethanol).

Cirrhosis of the liver is a form of hepatocellular disease

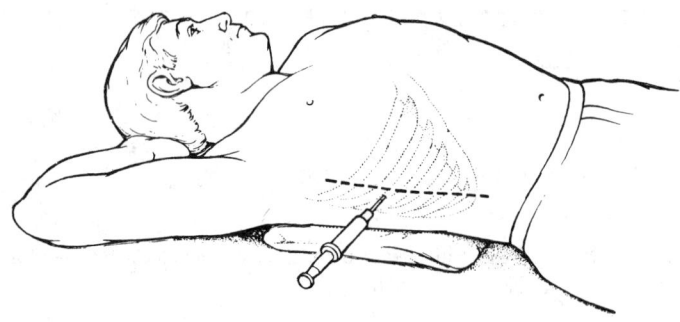

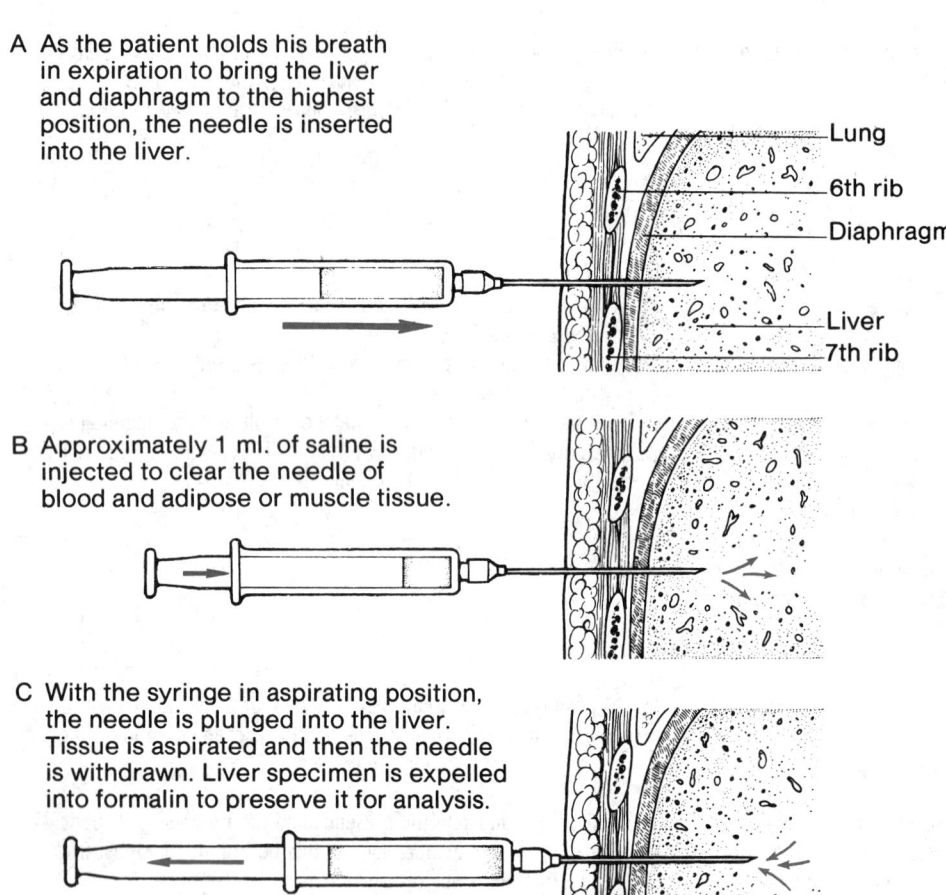

A As the patient holds his breath in expiration to bring the liver and diaphragm to the highest position, the needle is inserted into the liver.

B Approximately 1 ml. of saline is injected to clear the needle of blood and adipose or muscle tissue.

C With the syringe in aspirating position, the needle is plunged into the liver. Tissue is aspirated and then the needle is withdrawn. Liver specimen is expelled into formalin to preserve it for analysis.

Figure 38–3. Technique of liver biopsy.

that may produce jaundice. It is usually associated with excessive alcohol intake; however, it may also be a late result of liver cell necrosis caused by viral infection. In prolonged obstructive jaundice, cell damage eventually develops, so that both types appear together.

Clinical Manifestations.   Patients with hepatocellular jaundice may be mildly or severely ill, with lack of appetite, nausea, loss of vigor and strength, and possible weight loss. In some instances of hepatocellular disease, obvious jaundice may not be apparent. The serum bilirubin concentration and urine urobilinogen level may be elevated, however. In addition, levels of serum glutamic oxaloacetic transaminase (SGOT) and serum glutamic pyruvic transaminase (SGPT)* may be increased, in-

dicating cellular necrosis. At onset there may be complaints of headache, chills, and fever, if the cause is infectious. Depending on the cause and extent of the liver cell damage, hepatocellular jaundice may or may not be completely reversible.

Obstructive Jaundice.   Obstructive jaundice of the extrahepatic type may be caused by the bile duct's being occluded by a gallstone, by an inflammatory process, by a tumor, or by pressure from an enlarged organ. The obstruction may also involve the small bile ducts within the liver substance (*i.e.,* intrahepatic obstruction), caused, for example, by pressure on these channels from inflammatory swelling of the liver or by an inflammatory exudate within the ducts themselves. Intrahepatic obstruction due to stasis and inspissation (thickening) of bile within the canaliculi is an occasional occurrence, following the ingestion of certain drugs, which accordingly are referred to as "cholestatic" agents. These include phenothi-

---

* Aspartate aminotransferase (AST) and alanine aminotransferase (ALT) may be used alternatively in place of SGOT and SGPT, respectively.

Nursing Care Plan 38-1

Care of the Patient With Impaired Liver Function

Nursing Interventions	Rationale	Expected Outcomes

Nursing Diagnosis: Activity intolerance related to fatigue, lethargy, and malaise

Goal: Increased activity tolerance

1. Assess level of activity tolerance and degree of fatigue, lethargy, and malaise.	1. Provides baseline for further assessment and criteria for assessment of effectiveness of interventions.	• Exhibits increased interest in activities and events.
2. Assist with activities and hygiene when fatigued.	2. Promotes some exercise and hygiene within patient's level of tolerance.	• Participates in activities and gradually increases exercise within physical limits.
3. Encourage rest when fatigued or when abdominal pain or discomfort occurs.	3. Conserves energy and protects the liver.	• Reports increased strength and well-being.
4. Assist with selection of desired activities and exercise.	4. Stimulates patient's interest in activities of interest to him.	• Reports absence of abdominal pain and discomfort.

Nursing Diagnosis: Altered nutrition related to abdominal distention and discomfort and anorexia

Goal: Improved nutritional status

1. Assess dietary intake and nutritional status through diet history and diary, daily weight measurements, laboratory data, and anthropometric assessment.	1. Identifies deficits in nutritional intake and adequacy of nutritional state.	• Exhibits improved nutritional status by increased weight (without fluid retention), improved laboratory data and anthropometric measurements.
2. Provide diet high in carbohydrates with protein intake consistent with liver function.	2. Provides calories for energy, "sparing" protein for healing.	• States rationale for dietary modifications.
3. Elevate the head of the bed during patient's meals.	3. Reduces discomfort from abdominal distention and decreases sense of fullness produced by pressure of abdominal contents and ascites on the stomach.	• Identifies foods high in carbohydrates and within protein requirements (high in cirrhosis and hepatitis, low in hepatic failure).
4. Provide oral hygiene before meals and pleasant environment for meals at meal time.	4. Promotes positive environment and increased appetite.	• Reports improved appetite.

Nursing Diagnosis: Impaired skin integrity related to jaundice and edema

Goal: Improved skin integrity

1. Assess degree of discomfort related to pruritus and edema experienced by patient.	1. Assists in determining appropriate strategies.	• Exhibits intact skin without redness, excoriation, or breakdown.
2. Note and record degree of jaundice and extent of edema.	2. Provides baseline for detecting changes and evaluating effectiveness of interventions.	• Reports relief of pruritus.
3. Keep patient's fingernails short and smooth.	3. Prevents skin excoriation and infection from scratching.	• Exhibits no skin excoriation from scratching.
4. Provide frequent skin care avoiding use of soaps and alcohol-based lotions.	4. Removes waste products deposited in skin while preventing dryness of skin.	• Uses nondrying soaps and lotions. States rationale for use of nondrying soaps and lotions.
5. Massage bony prominences and turn frequently.	5. Minimizes prolonged pressure on bony prominences susceptible to breakdown and promotes mobilization of edema.	• Turns self periodically. Exhibits reduced edema of dependent parts of the body.

(continued)

Nursing Care Plan 38–1 (Continued)

Care of the Patient With Impaired Liver Function

Nursing Interventions	Rationale	Expected Outcomes

Nursing Diagnosis: High risk for injury related to altered clotting mechanisms and altered level of consciousness

Goal: Reduced risk of injury

1. Assess level of consciousness and cognitive level.	1. Assists in predicting patient's ability to protect self and comply with required self-protective actions; may detect deterioration of hepatic function.	• Is oriented to time, place, and person. • Exhibits no ecchymoses (bruises), cuts, or hematoma. • Exhibits no hallucinations, and demonstrates no efforts to get up unassisted or to leave hospital.
2. Provide safe environment (pad side rails, remove obstacles in room, prevent falls).	2. Minimizes falls and accidents and damage if falls occur.	
3. Provide frequent surveillance to orient patient and minimize use of restraints.	3. Protects patient from harm while stimulating and orienting patient; minimizes use of restraints, which may disturb patient further.	

Nursing Diagnosis: Body image disturbance related to changes in appearance, sexual dysfunction, and role function

Goal: Improvement of body image and self-esteem

1. Assess changes in appearance and the meaning these changes have for patient and family.	1. Provides information for assessing impact of changes in appearance, sexual function, and role on the patient and his significant other.	• Verbalizes concerns related to changes in appearance, life, and life-style. • Shares concerns with significant others. • Identifies past coping strategies that have been effective.
2. Encourage patient to verbalize his reactions and feelings about these changes.	2. Enables patient to identify and express concerns; encourages patient and significant others to share these concerns.	• Uses past effective coping strategies to deal with changes in appearance, life, and life-style.
3. Assess patient's and significant others' previous coping strategies.	3. Permits encouragement of those coping strategies that are familiar to patient and have been effective in the past.	• Maintains good grooming and hygiene. • Identifies short-term goals and strategies to achieve them.
4. Assist and encourage patient to maximize appearance and explore alternatives to previous sexual and role functions.	4. Encourages patient not to abandon those roles and functions that may return with appropriate treatment while encouraging exploration of alternatives.	• Exercises an active role in decision making about self and care. • Identifies resources that are not harmful. • Verbalizes that some of previous life-style practices have been harmful.
5. Assist patient in identifying short-term goals.	5. Accomplishing these goals serves as positive reinforcement and increases self-esteem.	• Uses healthy expressions of frustration, anger, and so forth.
6. Encourage and assist patient in decision-making about care.	6. Promotes patient's taking control of life and improves sense of well-being and self-esteem.	
7. Identify with patient resources to provide additional support (counselor, clergy).	7. Assists patient in identifying resources and accepting assistance from others when indicated.	
8. Assist patient in identifying previous practices that may have been harmful to self (alcohol and drug abuse).	8. Recognition and admission of the harmful effects of these practices is necessary for identifying a more healthy life-style.	

azines, antithyroid medications, sulfonylureas, tricyclic antidepressants, and nitrofurantoin.

Clinical Manifestations. Whether the obstruction is intrahepatic or extrahepatic, and whatever its cause may be, if bile cannot flow normally into the intestine, but is backed up into the liver substance, it is reabsorbed into the blood and carried throughout the entire body, staining the skin, the mucous membranes, and the sclerae. It is excreted in the urine, which becomes deep orange and foamy. Because of the decreased amount of bile in the intestinal tract, the stools become light or clay-colored. The skin may itch intensely, requiring repeated starch or oil baths. Dyspepsia, and especially an intolerance to fatty foods, may develop temporarily, due to impairment of fat digestion in the absence of intestinal bile. Here the SGOT and SGPT levels rise only moderately, but the bilirubin and alkaline phosphatase levels are elevated.

Hereditary Hyperbilirubinemia.   Increased serum bilirubin levels (hyperbilirubinemia) due to several inherited disorders can also produce jaundice. *Gilbert's syndrome* is a familial disorder that is due to a diminution of glucuronyl transferase and an increased unconjugated bilirubin level that causes jaundice. Although serum bilirubin levels are increased, liver histology and liver function test results are normal, and there is no hemolysis. Other conditions that are probably caused by inborn errors of biliary metabolism include *Dubin–Johnson syndrome* (chronic idiopathic jaundice, with pigment in the liver) and *Rotor's syndrome* (chronic familial conjugated hyperbilirubinemia without pigment in the liver); "benign" cholestatic jaundice of pregnancy, with retention of conjugated bilirubin, probably secondary to unusual sensitivity to the hormones of pregnancy; and probably also benign recurrent intrahepatic cholestasis.

Portal Hypertension and Ascites

Obstruction to blood flow through the damaged liver results in increased blood pressure (*portal hypertension*) throughout the portal venous system. Although portal hypertension is commonly associated with hepatic cirrhosis, it can also occur with noncirrhotic liver disease.

There are two major sequelae of portal hypertension:

1. The formation of esophageal, gastric, and hemorrhoidal varicosities (*varices*) occurs because of the elevated pressures transmitted to all of the veins that drain into the portal system. These varicosities are prone to rupture and often are the source of massive hemorrhages from the upper gastrointestinal tract and the rectum (see p. 999). The likelihood of bleeding is increased by the blood clotting abnormalities frequently present in patients with cirrhosis.
2. The second important manifestation of portal hypertension is accumulation of fluid (*ascites*) in the abdominal cavity. As ascites develops, intravascular volume tends to fall and renin is released by the kidneys. This results in secretion of increased quantities of the hormone aldosterone by the adrenal glands, which in turn causes the kidneys to retain sodium and water in an attempt to return intravascular volume to normal. Unfortunately, if portal hypertension continues, fluid retention will contribute to the formation of even more ascites as the albumin in the ascitic fluid creates an osmotic gradient and pulls more fluid into the peritoneal cavity.

Assessment

The presence and extent of ascites can be determined by percussion of the abdomen. When fluid has accumulated in the peritoneal cavity, the flanks will bulge when the patient assumes a supine position. The presence of fluid accumulation can be confirmed either by percussing for shifting dullness (Fig. 38-4A, B) or by detecting a fluid wave (Fig. 38-4C). A fluid wave is likely to be found only when there is a large amount of fluid present. Daily measurement and recording of abdominal girth and body weight are carried out to assess the progression of ascites and its response to treatment. The roles of dietary modification, drug therapy, paracentesis, and shunting in controlling ascites are discussed below.

Controlling Fluid Retention and Ascites

Nutritional Control.   The goal of treatment for the patient with ascites is a negative sodium balance to reduce fluid retention. Table salt, salty foods, salted butter and margarine, and all ordinary canned and frozen foods (those foods that are not specifically prepared for low-sodium/salt diets) should be avoided. The taste of unsalted foods can be improved by using salt substitutes, such as lemon juice, oregano, and thyme. Commercial substitutes need to be cleared with the physician; for example, those containing ammonia could precipitate hepatic coma. Liberal use should be made of powdered, low-sodium milk and milk products. If fluid accumulation is not controlled on this regimen, the salt restriction must be more stringent, with the daily sodium allowance reduced to 200 mg, and diuretics administered.

Diuretics.   Another method of reducing edema and ascites is to induce diuresis. This involves the reduction of sodium intake to 9 to 22 mEq (200 to 500 mg) daily; restriction of fluids, if the serum sodium concentration is low; and administration of oral diuretics such as furosemide (Lasix) or ethacrynic acid (Edecrin). These diuretics are used cautiously, because with long-term use they may induce severe sodium depletion (hyponatremia). Spironolactone (Aldactone), an aldosterone-blocking agent, also may be administered to supplement the action of these diuretics and to help prevent undue potassium loss. Ammonium chloride and acetazolamide (Diamox) are contraindicated because of the possibility of precipitating hepatic coma. Daily weight loss should not exceed 0.227 kg (or less than ½ lb) daily.

Diuretic therapy is carefully monitored by the nurse to detect possible complications: fluid and electrolyte disturbances and encephalopathy. Possible fluid and electrolyte problems include hypovolemia, hypokalemia, hyponatremia, and hypochloremic alkalosis. Encephalopathy may be precipitated by dehydration and hypovolemia. Additionally, when potassium stores are depleted, the amount of ammonia in the systemic circulation increases, which may cause impaired cerebral functioning and encephalopathy. Careful assessment and documentation of intake and output, abdominal girth, and daily weight are undertaken to assess fluid status. Serum ammonia and electrolyte levels are monitored to assess electrolyte balance, response to therapy, and risk of encephalopathy.

Skin integrity will be affected if skin care is not adequate. Pressure over bony prominences and edematous tissue must be relieved by frequently changing body position, or possibly by using an alternating-pressure mattress. Lower extremities may have to be elevated and support hose applied. Salt-poor albumin may be given intravenously to temporarily elevate the serum albumin level, which increases serum osmotic pressure. This helps reduce edema by causing the ascitic fluid to be drawn back into the bloodstream and ultimately eliminated by the kidneys.

Paracentesis

Paracentesis is the removal of fluid (ascites) from the peritoneal cavity through a small surgical incision or puncture made through the abdominal wall. Once considered a routine form of treatment for ascites, paracentesis is now primarily for di-

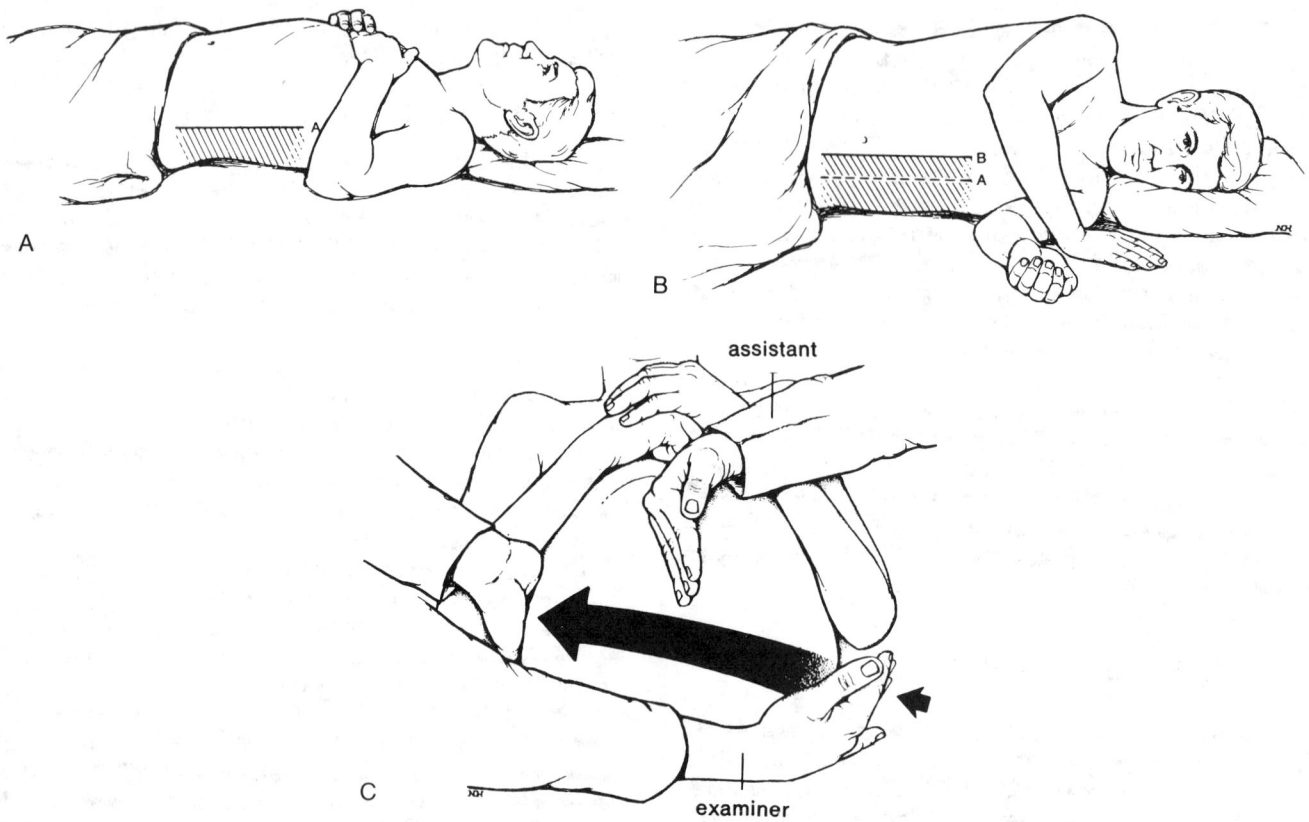

Figure 38–4. Assessing for ascites. (**A**) To percuss for shifting dullness, each flank is percussed with the patient in a supine position. If fluid is present, dullness is noted at each flank. The most medial limits of the dullness should be marked as indicated in **A.** The patient should then be shifted to his side. (**B**) Note what happens to the area of dullness if fluid is present. (**C**) To detect the presence of a fluid wave, the examiner places one hand alongside each flank. A second person then places a hand, ulnar side down, along the patient's midline, and applies light pressure. The examiner then strikes one flank sharply with one hand, while the other hand remains in place to detect any signs of a fluid impulse. The assistant's hand dampens any wave impulses traveling through the abdominal wall. (Copyright 1974, American Journal of Nursing Company. Reproduced with permission from American Journal of Nursing 1974, Sep; 74[9].)

agnostic examination of ascitic fluid, for treatment of massive ascites resistant to other therapy and causing severe problems to the patient, and as a prelude to other procedures, including radiography, peritoneal dialysis, ascites reinfusion, or surgery.

If paracentesis is warranted (Fig. 38–5), the aspiration is limited to the slow removal of 2 to 3 liters, to relieve acute symptoms. Removing large amounts of fluid may cause hypotension, oliguria, and hyponatremia. If fluid in excess of this amount is removed, ascitic fluid tends to form again, drawing fluid from extracellular tissue throughout the body.

Nursing Interventions.   The nurse prepares the patient for paracentesis by providing the necessary information, instructions, and reassurance.

- The patient is instructed to void as completely as possible just before paracentesis, to reduce the risk of inadvertent puncture of the bladder.

Sterile equipment and appropriate collection receptacles are made ready. Preparatory to the procedure, the patient is placed in the upright position on the edge of the bed or in a chair, fully supported, with his feet resting on a stool. One arm is fitted with a sphygmomanometer cuff. The trocar is intro-

duced with aseptic technique through a puncture wound in the midline below the umbilicus, and the fluid is removed through a drainage tube into a container.

During the procedure the nurse helps the patient to maintain the proper posture.

- The patient is monitored closely for evidence of vascular collapse, such as the appearance of pallor, increase in pulse rate, or decline in blood pressure. Blood pressure readings are recorded at frequent intervals from the beginning of the procedure.

When the procedure is concluded, the patient is placed in a comfortable position. The amount of fluid collected is measured, described, and recorded; and samples of the fluid, properly labeled, are sent to appropriate laboratories for examination of the cellular sediment, its specific gravity, protein concentration, and bacterial content.

Shunts

Attempts have been made to treat ascites through reinfusion of ascitic fluid into the general circulation; however, there is

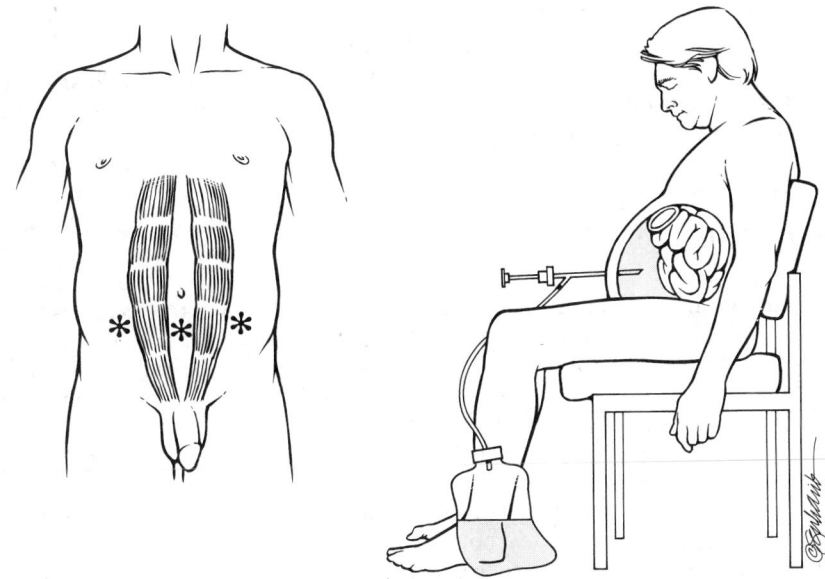

Figure 38–5. The patient undergoing paracentesis.

risk of infection from such treatment. In addition, this treatment is temporary, and reaccumulation of ascites occurs within 2 months in more than 70% of patients.

The insertion of a LeVeen or peritoneovenous shunt has been successful in reducing ascites and maintaining intravascular protein and fluid volume by "shunting" or redirecting the ascitic fluid from the peritoneal cavity into the systemic circulation (Fig. 38–6). In this method, a perforated silicon tube is directed through a small transverse abdominal incision into the peritoneal cavity. The proximal end of the tube is attached to a valve; from the valve another tube emerges and is threaded subcutaneously to the superior vena cava. The valve is normally closed, but opens when the pressure in the peritoneal cavity rises 3 cm H_2O above the pressure of the intrathoracic vena cava, which is located in the thorax. When the valve opens, the ascitic fluid flows into the superior vena cava. When pressure falls, the valve closes.

In the postoperative period, the patient is observed closely and the hematocrit is measured every 4 hours to monitor vascular volume expansion and hemodilution that may result from the inflow of ascitic fluid. Excessive hemodilution may be interrupted by placing the patient in a sitting position, which reduces the difference between the pressures of the peritoneal cavity and intrathoracic pressure, closing the valve and temporarily stopping the drainage of ascitic fluid to the vena cava. A diuretic such as furosemide may be prescribed to avoid the possibility of pulmonary edema. Laboratory studies include careful monitoring of the coagulation profile, because reabsorption of substances in the ascitic fluid may inhibit clotting and lead to bleeding. Body weight, abdominal girth, and urinary output are recorded every 2 hours. Ordinarily, the hematocrit falls, abdominal girth decreases, weight drops, and urinary output rises. Reversal of these changes may indicate that the shunt is no longer patent and that the ascitic fluid is reaccumulating.

After the relief of ascites, fluid and sodium intake will depend on the cardiac status and presence of peripheral edema. These patients require continued care and monitoring, for even though the ascites may be cleared, the underlying liver disorder is not reversed by the insertion of a peritoneovenous shunt.

Factors limiting the use of peritoneovenous shunt procedures include a significant rate of bacterial infection and coagulation disorders. Complications of peritoneovenous shunting (obstruction of the valve, thrombosis of the superior vena cava) may result in reaccumulation of ascites. As a result, portosystemic shunt procedures (described on p. 1003) have been performed in an effort to manage intractable ascites. Although

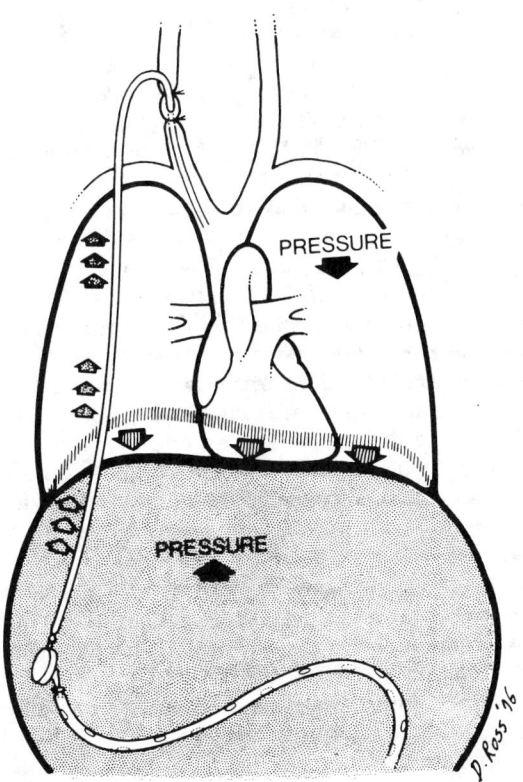

Figure 38–6. Peritoneojugular shunt for reducing ascites. The valve lies in the lower right side extraperitoneally, and a perforated collecting tube extends into the peritoneal cavity. (Schiff L [ed]. Diseases of the Liver, 6th ed. Philadelphia, JB Lippincott, 1987.)

these procedures have been shown to control ascites, they are often accompanied by significant risk of encephalopathy. The incidence of encephalopathy has been reported as higher in patients treated for ascites than for esophageal varices, suggesting that the risk may be increased in patients with intractable ascites.

Nutritional Deficiencies

Another group of complications that is common to patients with severe chronic liver disease of all types is caused by inadequate intake of proper vitamins. Among the specific deficiency states that occur on this basis are (1) vitamin A deficiency, beriberi, polyneuritis, and Wernicke-Korsakoff psychosis, all attributable to a deficiency of thiamine; (2) skin and mucous membrane lesions characteristic of riboflavin deficiency; (3) pyridoxine deficiency, (4) hypoprothrombinemia (see p. 810), characterized by spontaneous bleeding and ecchymoses, due to vitamin K deficiency; (5) the hemorrhagic lesions of scurvy (*i.e.*, vitamin C deficiency); and (6) the macrocytic anemia of folic acid deficiency.

- The threat of these avitaminoses provides the rationale for supplementing the diet of every patient with chronic liver disease (especially when alcoholism is involved) with ample quantities of vitamins A, B complex, C, K, and folic acid.

Hepatic Coma

Hepatic coma, one of the dreaded complications of liver disease, occurs with profound liver failure and results from the accumulation of ammonia and other identified toxic metabolites in the blood. Ammonia accumulates because damaged liver cells fail to detoxify and convert to urea the ammonia that is constantly entering the bloodstream as a result of its absorption from the gastrointestinal tract and its liberation from kidney and muscle cells. The increased ammonia concentration in the blood causes brain dysfunction and damage, resulting in hepatic encephalopathy and hepatic coma.

Assessment and Clinical Manifestations. The earliest symptoms of hepatic coma include minor mental changes and motor disturbances. The patient appears to be slightly confused and experiences alterations in mood. He becomes unkempt in appearance and experiences altered sleep patterns. He tends to sleep during the day and to experience restlessness and insomnia at night. As hepatic coma progresses, he may be difficult to awaken. He may exhibit *asterixis* (flapping tremor of the hands). Simple tasks, such as handwriting, become difficult. A sample of handwriting, taken daily, may provide graphic evidence of progression or reversal of hepatic coma. In the early stages of hepatic coma, the patient's reflexes are hyperactive; with deepening of coma these reflexes disappear and the extremities may become flaccid.

The electroencephalogram (EEG) shows generalized slowing and an increase in amplitude of brain waves. Except for the triphasic waves, all of the other manifestations noted are also observable in other conditions. Occasionally, *fetor hepaticus*, a characteristic breath odor like freshly mowed grass, acetone, or old wine, may be noticed. In a more advanced stage there are gross disturbances of consciousness

and the patient is completely disoriented with respect to time and place. With further progression of the disorder, he lapses into frank coma and may have convulsions. Approximately 35% of all patients with cirrhosis of the liver die in hepatic coma.

Aggravating and Precipitating Factors. Circumstances that increase blood ammonia content tend to aggravate or precipitate hepatic coma. The largest source of blood ammonia is the enzymatic and bacterial digestion of dietary and blood proteins in the gastrointestinal tract. Ammonia from these sources is *increased* as a result of gastrointestinal (GI) bleeding (*i.e.*, bleeding esophageal varices or chronic GI bleeding), a high-protein diet, bacterial growth in the small and large intestines, and uremia. The ingestion of ammonium salts will also increase the blood ammonia level. In the presence of alkalosis or hypokalemia, increased amounts of ammonia are absorbed from the gastrointestinal tract and from the renal tubular fluid. Conversely, serum ammonia is *decreased* by elimination of protein from the diet and by the administration of antibiotics, such as neomycin sulfate, that reduce the number of intestinal bacteria capable of converting urea to ammonia.

Other factors unrelated to increased blood ammonia that may induce hepatic coma in susceptible patients include excessive diuresis, dehydration, infections, surgery, fever, and consciousness-altering drugs, such as sedatives, tranquilizers, and narcotics. Table 38–2 presents the stages of hepatic coma, common signs and symptoms and potential nursing diagnoses for each stage.

Management

Principles of management of hepatic coma include the following:

- The patient with impending hepatic coma is observed frequently, to assess neurologic status. A daily record is kept of handwriting and performance in arithmetic to monitor mental status.
- Fluid intake and output and body weight are recorded each day.
- Vital signs are measured and recorded every 4 hours.
- Evidence suggesting pulmonary or other infection is assessed frequently and reported promptly if observed.
- Serum ammonia level is monitored daily.
- If signs of impending hepatic coma occur, the patient's protein intake is reduced sharply or eliminated altogether, for a time.
- To reduce ammonia absorption from the gastrointestinal tract, a high-cleansing enema may be prescribed.
- In addition, an antibiotic drug such as neomycin is given as an intestinal antiseptic.
- Electrolyte status is carefully monitored and corrected if abnormal.
- Sedative and analgesic drugs, if prescribed at all, are administered to this patient in very conservative doses and under very close observation.

Lactulose (Cephulac) is administered to reduce blood ammonia; it probably acts by a combination of mechanisms that promote the excretion of ammonia in the stool: (1) ammonia is kept in the ionized state, resulting in a fall in colon pH—this reverses the normal passage of ammonia from the colon to the blood; (2) catharsis takes place, which decreases the ammonia absorbed from the colon; and (3) the fecal flora

TABLE 38-2. *Stages of Hepatic Encephalopathy and Possible Nursing Diagnoses**

Stage	Clinical Symptoms	Clinical Signs and EEG Changes	Selected Potential Nursing Diagnoses
1	Normal level of consciousness with periods of lethargy and euphoria; reversal of day–night sleep patterns	Asterixis; impaired writing and ability to draw line figures. Normal EEG	Activity intolerance Self-care deficit Sleep pattern disturbances
2	Increased drowsiness; disorientation; inappropriate behavior; mood swings; agitation	Asterixis; fetor hepaticus. Abnormal EEG with generalized slowing	Impaired social interaction Altered role performance High risk for injury
3	Stuporous; difficult to arouse; sleeping most of time; marked confusion; incoherent speech	Asterixis; increased deep tendon reflexes; rigidity of extremities. EEG markedly abnormal.	Altered nutrition Impaired mobility Impaired communication
4	Comatose; may not respond to painful stimuli	Absence of asterixis; absence of deep tendon reflexes; flaccidity of extremities. EEG markedly abnormal.	High risk for aspiration Impaired gas exchange Impaired tissue integrity

* Nursing diagnoses are likely to progress so that most nursing diagnoses present at earlier stages will occur during later stages as well.

are changed to organisms that do not produce ammonia from urea.

Two or three soft stools per day are desirable; this indicates that lactulose is performing as intended. Watery diarrheal stools, however, indicate drug overdose. Possible side effects include intestinal bloating and cramps, which usually disappear in a week. To overcome the sweet taste to which some patients object, lactulose can be diluted with fruit juice. The patient is closely monitored for hypokalemia and dehydration. Other laxatives are not given during lactulose administration because their effects would disturb dosage regulation. Lactulose enemas have also been used effectively in acute hepatic encephalopathy for patients who are comatose or in whom oral administration is contraindicated or impossible.

Other Manifestations of Liver Dysfunction

Many patients with liver dysfunction develop generalized edema due to hypoalbuminemia that results from decreased hepatic production of serum albumin. The production of blood clotting factors by the liver is also reduced, leading to an increased incidence of bruising, nosebleeds, bleeding from wounds, and, as described above, gastrointestinal bleeding. Decreased production of several clotting factors may be due, in part, to deficient absorption of vitamin K from the gastrointestinal tract. This probably is caused by the inability of liver cells to use vitamin K to make prothrombin. Absorption of the other fat-soluble vitamins (vitamins A, D, and E) as well as dietary fats may also be impaired, because of decreased secretion of bile salts into the intestine.

Abnormalities of glucose metabolism also occur; the blood glucose level may be abnormally high shortly after a meal (*i.e.*, a diabetic-type glucose tolerance test result), but hypoglycemia may occur during fasting because of decreased hepatic glycogen reserves and decreased gluconeogenesis.

- Because of decreased ability to metabolize drugs, usual drug dosages must be reduced for the patient with liver failure.

Decreased metabolism of estrogens by the damaged liver can lead to gynecomastia, testicular atrophy, loss of pubic hair in the male, and menstrual irregularities in the female, as well as spider angiomata and reddened palms ("liver palms"). Splenomegaly (enlarged spleen) with possible hypersplenism occurs commonly as a manifestation of portal hypertension. Patients with liver dysfunction due to biliary obstruction commonly develop severe itching (pruritus) due to retention of bile salts.

Hepatic Disorders

Viral Hepatitis

The increasing incidence of viral hepatitis is a growing public health concern. The disease is important because of its ease of transmission, morbidity, and the prolonged loss of time from school or employment that it can cause.

It is estimated that 60% to 90% of cases of viral hepatitis go unreported. The occurrence of subclinical cases, failure to recognize mild cases, and misdiagnosis are thought to contribute to the underreporting. Although approximately 50% of adults in the United States have antibodies against hepatitis A virus, many are unable to recall an earlier episode or the occurrence of the symptoms of hepatitis.

Breakthroughs in better understanding of viral hepatitis in the past have been due to recognition in 1968, by Blumberg, that Australian (Au) antigen was a specific immunologic marker for hepatitis B infection. This led to a series of new designations, and Australian antigen now is referred to as hepatitis B surface antigen: HB_sAg. More recently, a specific antigen for hepatitis A has been identified (HA Ag). Also, tests have been developed to detect anti-HAV, anti-HB_s, and anti-HB_c antibodies, as well as the e-antigen and anti–e-antibody associated with hepatitis B. This means that diagnostic tests, including complement fixation, immune adherence, and radioimmunoassay, are available for recognizing hepatitis A and hepatitis B. The existence of one or more agents capable of producing hepatitis C (non-A, non-B hepatitis) has also been recognized.

A guide to the terminology associated with viral hepatitis is provided in Chart 38-2.

Nursing Implications.   The nurse is especially concerned with four major problem areas of viral hepatitis: (1) the care of the patient with hepatitis; (2) the increased risks in hemodialysis units and in intravenous drug users; (3) the fact that many people who have the disease are asymptomatic, which may present serious epidemiologic problems; and (4) the apparent health needs of the community that are required for its elimination. The last category includes the following considerations:

- Proper community and home sanitation
- Conscientious individual hygiene at all times
- Safe practices for preparing and dispensing food
- Effective health supervision in schools, dormitories, extended care facilities, barracks, and camps
- Continuous health education programs
- Reporting of every case of viral hepatitis to the local health department

For a comparison of the many aspects of the major forms of viral hepatitis, see Table 38-3.

Hepatitis A Virus

Hepatitis A, formerly designated infectious hepatitis, is caused by an RNA virus of the enterovirus family. The mode of transmission of this disease is the fecal–oral route, primarily through the ingestion of food or liquids infected by the virus. The virus has been found in the stool of infected patients before the onset of symptoms and during the first few days of illness. Typically, a young adult acquires the infection at school and brings it home, where haphazard sanitary habits spread it through the family. It is more prevalent in underdeveloped countries or in instances of overcrowding and poor sanitation. An infected food handler can spread the disease, and people can contract it by consuming water or shellfish from sewage-contaminated waters. It is rarely, if ever, transmitted by blood transfusions.

The incubation period is estimated to be from 1 to 7 weeks, with an average of 30 days. The course of the illness may be prolonged, lasting from 4 to 8 weeks. It generally lasts longer and is more severe in those over the age of 40.

Chart 38-2
Hepatitis Glossary

Hepatitis A

HAV	Hepatitis A virus; etiologic agent of hepatitis A, (formerly infectious hepatitis).
Anti-HAV	Antibody to hepatitis A virus; appears in serum soon after onset of symptoms; disappears after 3–12 months.
IgM anti-HAV	IgM antibody to HAV; indicates recent infection with HAV; positive up to 6 months after infection.

Hepatitis B

HBV	Hepatitis B virus; etiologic agent of hepatitis B (formerly serum hepatitis)
HB$_s$Ag	Hepatitis B surface antigen (Australian antigen); indicates acute or chronic hepatitis B or carrier state; indicates infectious state
Anti-HB$_s$	Antibody to hepatitis B surface antigen; indicates prior exposure and immunity to hepatitis; may indicate passive antibody from HBIG or immune response from hepatitis B vaccine
HB$_e$Ag	Hepatitis B e-antigen; present in serum early in course; indicates highly infectious stage of hepatitis B; persistence in serum indicates progression to chronic hepatitis.
Anti-HB$_e$	Antibody to hepatitis B e-antigen; suggests low titer of HBV
HB$_c$Ag	Hepatitis B core antigen; found in liver cells; not easily detected in serum
Anti-HB$_c$	Antibody to hepatitis B core antigen; most sensitive indicator of hepatitis B; appears late in the acute phase of the disease; indicates infection of HBV at some time in the past
IgM anti-HB$_c$	IgM antibody to HB$_c$Ag; present for up to 6 months after HBV infection.

Hepatitis C

HCV	Hepatitis C virus (formerly non-A, non-B virus); may be more than one virus

Hepatitis D

HDV	Hepatitis D virus (delta agent); etiologic agent of hepatitis D; HBV is required for replication
HDAg	Hepatitis delta antigen; detectable in early acute HDV infection
Anti-HDV	Antibody to HDV; indicates past or present infection with HDV

TABLE 38–3.   *Comparison of Types of Viral Hepatitis*

	Hepatitis A	*Hepatitis B*	*Hepatitis C*	*Hepatitis D*
Other Names	HAV, Type A hepatitis, infectious or epidemic hepatitis; IH virus	HBV, Type B hepatitis, serum hepatitis, SH virus, Dane particle	Non-A, non-B hepatitis	Delta virus or agent
EPIDEMIOLOGY				
Cause	Hepatitis A virus	Hepatitis B virus	Hepatitis C virus; may be more than 1 virus	Hepatitis D virus
Method of transmission	Fecal–oral route; poor sanitation Person to person Waterborne, foodborne—shellfish Rarely, if at all, by blood transfusion	Parenterally, or by intimate contact with carriers or those with acute disease; male homosexuals. Vertical transmission from mothers to infants Contaminated instruments, syringes, needles; renal dialysis*	Transfusion of blood and blood products Personnel in renal transplant and dialysis units Parenteral drug abusers Institutions with long-term residents*	Same as hepatitis B Requires hepatitis B surface antigen for replication; therefore follows pattern similar to that of hepatitis B
Source of virus/antigen	Blood, feces, saliva	Blood, saliva, semen, vaginal secretions	Appears to be blood-borne	
Distribution by age	Young adults (15–29) and middle-aged who have escaped childhood infection	Affects all ages, but mostly young adults	Same as HBV	
Incubation period	3–5 weeks; average: 30 days	2–5 months; average: 90 days	Variable: 14–115 days; average: 50 days	
Occurrence	Worldwide	Worldwide	Worldwide Accounts for 20% of sporadic cases	
Antibody	Anti-HAV Present in convalescent sera and immune serum globulin (ISG)	Anti-HB$_c$ (core antigen) Anti-HB$_s$ (surface antigen)		
Immunity	Homologous	Homologous		
Severity	Most anicteric and asymptomatic	More severe than HAV	Wide spectrum of severity, resembling HAV or HBV; often prolonged illness—months May progress to chronic hepatitis*	Increased incidence of fulminant hepatitis May progress to chronic active hepatitis and cirrhosis.
NATURE OF ILLNESS				
Signs and symptoms	May occur with or without symptoms: flulike illness Preicteric phase: Headache, malaise, fatigue, anorexia, lassitude, fever Icteric phase: Dark urine, scleral icterus, jaundice, liver tenderness, and perhaps enlargement	May occur without symptoms 1000 IU/L-serum transaminase level May develop antibodies to virus Similar to HAV, but more severe Fever and respiratory symptoms rare, but may have arthralgias, rash	Similar to HBV Less severe and anicteric	Similar to hepatitis B

(continued)

TABLE 38–3. *Comparison of Types of Viral Hepatitis* (Continued)

	Hepatitis A	*Hepatitis B*	*Hepatitis C*	*Hepatitis D*
Diagnosis and method	Elevated serum transaminase Complement fixation rate Radioimmunoassay	HB_sAg, HB_eAg, anti-HB_c, in absence of anti-HB_s (obtainable as a panel) in serum Elevated serum transaminase Radioimmunoassay— hemagglutination		Anti-delta antibodies in the presence of HB_sAg
Severity	Usually mild Fatality rate 0%–1%	Variable, may be severe Fatality rate varies: 1%–10%	Frequent occurrence of chronic carrier state and chronic liver disease	Similar to hepatitis, but greater likelihood of chronic active hepatitis and cirrhosis
Specific treatment	Adequate fluids, rest, nutrition	Same as HAV In research: vaccine antiviral chemotherapy to eliminate chronic HBV carrier state (being tested)	In investigation: alpha-interferon	In investigation: alpha-interferon
PREVENTION	Good sanitation Proper personal hygiene Effective sterilization procedures Careful screening of food handlers Immune globulin given within a few days of exposure	Specific hepatitis B immune globulin (HBIG), probably useful after exposure by ingestion, inoculation, or splash involving hepatitis B surface antigen (HB_sAg) Hepatitis B vaccine recommended for preexposure immunization of those at high risk Screening of blood donors	Screening of blood donors	Avoid exposure to hepatitis B

* Recent intensive research suggests probably the same for HBV and hepatitis C.

The virus is present only briefly in the serum; by the time jaundice occurs, the patient is likely to be noninfectious.

Assessment and Clinical Manifestations.   Many patients are anicteric (without jaundice) and symptomless. When symptoms appear, they are of a mild, flulike upper respiratory tract infection, with low-grade fever. Anorexia is an early symptom and is often severe. It is thought to result from release of a toxin by the damaged liver or by failure of the damaged liver cells to detoxify an abnormal product. Later, jaundice and dark urine may become apparent. Indigestion is present, in varying degrees, marked by vague epigastric distress, nausea, heartburn, and flatulence. The patient may also develop a strong aversion to the taste of cigarettes or the presence of cigarette smoke and other strong odors. These symptoms tend to clear as soon as the jaundice reaches its peak—perhaps 10 days after its initial appearance. The liver and the spleen are often moderately enlarged for a few days after onset; otherwise, apart from jaundice, there are few physical signs to be elicited.

Although symptoms may be very mild in children, adults are more likely to be symptomatic, the symptoms more severe, and the course of the disease prolonged.

Management.   Bed rest during the acute stage and a diet that is both acceptable and nutritious are part of the treatment and nursing care. During the period of anorexia, the patient should receive frequent small feedings, supplemented, if nec-

essary, by intravenous infusions of glucose. Because this patient would rather not look at food or eat, gentle persistence and ingenuity may be required to stimulate his appetite. Optimal food and fluid levels are necessary to counteract weight loss and prolonged recovery. Even before the icteric phase, however, many patients recover their appetites and thereafter need no reminders to maintain a good diet.

The patient's sense of well-being as well as laboratory test results are generally appropriate guides to bed rest and restriction of physical activity. Gradual but progressive ambulation seems to hasten recovery, provided the patient rests after activity and does not participate in activities to the point of fatigue.

Patient Education and Home Health Care.   The patient is usually managed at home unless symptoms are particularly severe. Therefore, the patient and family need to be assisted to cope with the incapacitation and fatigue that are common problems in hepatitis and to be aware of the indications to seek additional health care if the symptoms persist or worsen. Additionally, the patient and family need specific guidelines about diet, rest, follow-up blood work, as well as sanitation and hygiene measures, particularly handwashing, to prevent spread of the disease to other family members.

Prognosis.   Recovery from hepatitis type A is the rule; a rare case progresses to acute liver necrosis or fulminant hepatitis, terminating in cirrhosis of the liver, or death. Hepatitis

A confers immunity against itself; however, the person may contract other forms of hepatitis. The mortality rate of hepatitis A is approximately 0.5%. No carrier state exists, and no chronic hepatitis is associated with hepatitis A.

Control and Prevention. Ways to reduce the risk of contracting hepatitis A include:

- Good personal hygiene, stressing careful handwashing (after bowel movement and before eating)
- Environmental sanitation—safe food and water supply, as well as effective sewage disposal
- Administration of immune globulin: Type A hepatitis can be prevented by the administration of globulin intramuscularly during the period of incubation, if this treatment is instituted within 2 weeks of exposure. This bolsters the persons's own antibody production and provides 6 to 8 weeks of passive immunity. Immune globulin may suppress overt symptoms of the disease; the resulting subclinical case of hepatitis A would produce active immunity to subsequent attacks of the virus. Although rare, systemic reactions to immune globulin may occur. (Caution is required when anyone who has previously had angioedema, hives, or other allergic reactions is treated with any human immune globulin. Epinephrine should be available for use in systemic or anaphylactic reactions.)
- Preexposure prohylaxis is recommended for international travelers to developing countries and settings with poor or uncertain sanitation conditions.
- Immune globulin is also recommended for household members and sexual contacts of persons with hepatitis A.

Hepatitis B Virus

Hepatitis B virus is a double-shelled particle containing DNA. This particle is composed of the following:

HB$_c$Ag—hepatitis B core antigen (antigenic material in an inner core)
HB$_s$Ag—hepatitis B surface antigen (antigenic material in an outer coat)
HB$_e$Ag—an independent protein circulating in the blood

Each antigen elicits its specific antibody:

anti-HB$_c$—persists during the acute phase of illness; may indicate continuing hepatitis B virus in the liver
anti-HB$_s$—detected during late convalescence; usually indicates recovery and development of immunity
anti-HB$_e$—usually signifies reduced infectivity

HB$_s$Ag can be detected transiently circulating in the blood in 80% to 90% of infected patients. HB$_c$Ag cannot be detected in blood. HB$_s$Ag may be noted in the blood for months and years, which suggests that these patients may be asymptomatic carriers, if HB$_e$Ag is absent. If it is present, these patients may have chronic hepatitis and may be more infectious.

From the community health point of view, about 15% of American adults are positive for anti-HB$_s$, which indicates that they have had hepatitis B. Anti-HB$_s$ may be positive in as many as two thirds of IV drug users.

Unlike hepatitis A, which is transmitted primarily by the fecal–oral route, hepatitis B is transmitted primarily through blood (percutaneous and permucosal routes). The virus has been found in blood, saliva, semen, and vaginal secretions and can be transmitted through mucous membranes and breaks in the skin. Hepatitis B has a long incubation period. It replicates in the liver and remains in the serum for relatively long periods, allowing transmission of the virus. Therefore, those at risk of developing hepatitis B include the general surgeon, clinical laboratory worker, dentist, nurse, and respiratory therapist. Staff and patients in hemodialysis and oncology units and homosexually active males and IV drug users are also at increased risk. Mandatory screening of blood donors for HB$_s$Ag has greatly reduced the occurrence of hepatitis B after blood transfusion.

Assessment and Clinical Manifestations. Clinically, the disease closely resembles hepatitis A. The incubation period, however, is much longer (between 2 and 5 months). The mortality is appreciable, ranging from 1% to 10%, depending on the infective dose and the condition of the patient. Symptoms and signs of hepatitis B may be insidious and variable. Fever and respiratory symptoms are rare: some patients have arthralgias and rashes. The patient may lose his appetite and experience dyspepsia, abdominal pain, generalized aching, malaise, and weakness. Jaundice may or may not be evident. If jaundice occurs, it is accompanied by light-colored stools and dark urine. The patient's liver may be tender and enlarged to 12 to 14 cm vertically. The spleen is enlarged and palpable in a small number of patients; the posterior cervical lymph nodes may also be enlarged.

Gerontologic Considerations. The elderly patient who contracts hepatitis B has a serious risk of severe liver cell necrosis or fulminant hepatic failure, particularly if other illnesses are present. The patient is seriously ill and the prognosis is poor.

Management. Recent clinical trials with alpha-interferon have shown that early treatment with daily subcutaneous injections of 5 million units of alpha-interferon for 4 months induces remission of hepatitis B in over one third of patients and eliminates hepatitis B surface antigen (indicates carrier state) in 10% of patients. Although these results are very promising, it must be noted that interferon is ineffective in a sizable number of patients, must be given by daily injection, and is not without side effects. These may include influenza-like symptoms and fatigue. Long-term follow-up is required to determine if the effects of interferon are sustained and if this therapy ultimately decreases the incidence of hepatocellular carcinoma in patients with hepatitis B.

Regardless of other treatment, bed rest is usually recommended until the symptoms of hepatitis have subsided. Subsequently, the patient's activities are restricted until the hepatic enlargement and the elevation of the level of serum bilirubin and liver enzymes have disappeared. Adequate nutrition should be maintained; proteins are restricted when the ability of the liver to metabolize protein by-products is impaired, as demonstrated by symptoms. Other therapeutic measures employed to control the dyspeptic symptoms and general malaise include the use of antacids, belladonna, and antiemetics. However, all medications should be avoided if emesis is a problem. This patient should be hospitalized and treated with fluid therapy. Because of the mode of transmission, the patient is evaluated for other blood-borne diseases.

Convalescence may be prolonged, with complete symptomatic recovery sometimes requiring 3 to 4 months or longer. During this stage, gradual restoration of physical activity is permitted and encouraged, after complete clearing of the jaundice.

Psychosocial considerations are identified by the nurse, particularly the effects of isolation and separation from family and friends during the acute and infective stages. Special planning is required to minimize alterations in sensory perception. The family is included in planning to decrease the fears and anxieties of the patient and family about the spread of the disease.

Patient Education and Home Health Care.   Because of the prolonged period of convalescence, the patient and family must be prepared for home care. Provision for adequate rest and nutrition must be ensured before the patient's discharge. Those family members and friends who have had intimate contact with the patient should be informed about the risks of contracting hepatitis B, and arrangements should be made for them to receive hepatitis B vaccine or hepatitis B immune globulin. Those at risk must be aware of early signs of hepatitis B and of ways to reduce risk to themselves. Follow-up home visits by a community health nurse are indicated to assess the patient's progress and answer family members' questions about transmission of the disease. A home visit also permits evaluation of the understanding of the patient and family about the importance of adequate rest and nutrition. Because of the risk of transmission through sexual intercourse, use of strategies to prevent exchange of body fluids is advised; these include abstinence or the use of condoms.

Prognosis.   Mortality of hepatitis B has been reported to be as high as 10%. Another 10% of patients who have hepatitis B progress to a carrier state or develop chronic hepatitis. It remains the chief cause of cirrhosis and hepatocellular carcinoma worldwide.

Control and Prevention.   The goals are (1) to interrupt the chain of transmission, (2) to protect those people at high risk through the use of hepatitis B vaccine, and (3) to use passive immunization for unprotected people exposed to hepatitis B virus.

Continued screening of potential blood donors for the presence of HB$_s$Ag will further decrease the risk of transmission by blood transfusion. A reduction in the number of people acquiring hepatitis B could occur if paid blood donors could be replaced by an all-volunteer donor population. The use of disposable syringes, needles, and lancets reduces the risk of spreading this infection from one patient to another during the collection of blood samples or the administration of parenteral therapy. Good personal hygiene practices are fundamental to infection control. In the clinical laboratory, work areas should be disinfected daily. Gloves are worn when handling all blood and body fluids as well as HB$_s$Ag-positive specimens. Eating is prohibited in the laboratory.

Administering medication by individual-dose ampules is essential. Where IV drug users share the same needles, serious outbreaks of hepatitis have occurred.

Hepatitis B Vaccine.   Active immunization is recommended for individuals at high risk for hepatitis B. Two forms of hepatitis B vaccine are available. One form is prepared from plasma of humans chronically infected with HBV. Although enthusiasm for vaccination for hepatitis B has been dampened because of the association of acquired immunodeficiency syndrome (AIDS) and HBV and concern about possible transmission of human immunodeficiency virus (HIV) infection, numerous studies have shown no evidence that AIDS can be transmitted by HBV vaccine. All viruses, including HIV, are killed during the preparation of the vaccine. A yeast-recombinant hepatitis B vaccine (Recombivax HB) has been developed recently. Its response is similar to plasma-derived vaccine,

TABLE 38–4.   *Persons at Increased Risk for Hepatitis B*

Health care workers with frequent exposure to blood, blood products, or other body fluids, including
but not limited to
  Hemodialysis staff
  Oncology/chemotherapy nurses
  Others at risk for needlesticks
  Operating room staff
  Respiratory therapists
  Dentists
Hemodialysis patients
Homosexually active men
Users of illicit intravenous drugs
Household and sexual contacts of carriers of HBV
Travelers to settings with poor or uncertain sanitary conditions
Heterosexuals with multiple sexual partners
Recipients of blood products (ie, clotting factor concentrate)

but with a lower antibody titer; therefore, booster doses may be required. The duration of protection and recommendation for booster doses has not yet been established.

Both forms of the hepatitis B vaccine are given in three doses, the second and third doses 1 and 6 months after the first dose. Hepatitis B vaccination should be given to adults in the deltoid muscle, as administration in the gluteal region may result in suboptimal response. Persons at high risk, including nurses and other health care personnel exposed to blood or blood products, should receive active immunization. (See Table 38–4 for a list of other persons at risk for HBV who should receive hepatitis B vaccine.) Health care workers who have had frequent contact with blood are screened for anti-HBs to determine if immunity is already present from previous exposure. Studies have shown that the vaccine produces active immunity to HBV in 90% of healthy persons. It does not provide protection to those already exposed to HBV and provides no protection against hepatitis A or hepatitis C. Side effects of immunization are infrequent. Soreness and redness at the injection site are the most common postinjection complaints.

Hepatitis B Immune Globulin.   Hepatitis B immune globulin, or HBIG, is indicated for persons exposed to HBV who have never had hepatitis B and have never received hepatitis B vaccine. Specific indications for postexposure vaccine with HBIG include: (1) accidental exposure to HB$_s$Ag-positive blood through percutaneous (needle-stick) or transmucosal (splashes in contact with mucous membranes) routes, (2) sexual contact with persons who are positive for HB$_s$Ag, and (3) perinatal exposure. HBIG, which provides passive immunity, is prepared from plasma selected for high titers of anti-HBs. Again, there has been no evidence that HIV infection can be transmitted by HBIG.

Both active and passive immunization are recommended for persons exposed to hepatitis B through sexual contact or through percutaneous or transmucosal routes. If HBIG and hepatitis B vaccine are administered at the same time, separate sites and separate syringes should be used.

Hepatitis C (Non-A, Non-B Hepatitis)

A significant proportion of cases of viral hepatitis are neither hepatitis A, hepatitis B, nor hepatitis D; as a result they are classified as hepatitis C (formerly non-A, non-B hepatitis or NANB hepatitis). This form of hepatitis can be caused by at least three different viruses. In the United States, over 90% of cases are a result of blood transfusion, and hepatitis C is the primary form of hepatitis associated with transfusions. Individuals at special risk for hepatitis C include children receiving frequent transfusions or those who require large volumes of blood. Hepatitis is more likely from commercial or paid blood donors than from volunteer donors. Hepatitis C occurs not only in patients after blood transfusions and among IV drug users but also in personnel associated with renal dialysis units and in residents in homes for the mentally retarded; it also is transmitted through sexual intercourse.

The incubation period is variable, reflecting the variety of causative agents. Symptoms of post-transfusion hepatitis C usually occur at 6 to 7 weeks after transfusion. The clinical course of acute hepatitis C is similar to that of hepatitis B; symptoms are usually mild. A chronic carrier state occurs frequently, however, and significant chronic liver disease often occurs after hepatitis C. There is an increased risk of cirrhosis or liver cancer after hepatitis C. Long-term, low-dose interferon therapy has been effective in preliminary trials in some patients with hepatitis C.

A method of screening blood transfusions for hepatitis C was approved in 1990 and is likely to lead to substantial reduction in cases of hepatitis associated with blood transfusions.

Hepatitis D

Hepatitis D (delta agent) occurs in some cases of hepatitis B. Because the virus requires hepatitis B surface antigen for its replication, only individuals with hepatitis B are at risk for hepatitis D. Anti-delta antibodies in the presence of HB_sAg on testing confirm the diagnosis. It is also common in persons who are IV drug users, hemodialysis patients, and recipients of multiple blood transfusions. The symptoms of hepatitis D are similar to those of hepatitis B except that patients are more likely to have fulminant hepatitis and to progress to chronic active hepatitis and cirrhosis. Treatment is similar to that of other forms of hepatitis, although interferon as a specific treatment for hepatitis D is under investigation.

Toxic Hepatitis and Drug-Induced Hepatitis

Certain chemicals have poisonous effects on the liver and when taken by mouth or injected parenterally produce acute liver cell necrosis, or *toxic hepatitis*. The chemicals most commonly implicated in this disease are carbon tetrachloride, phosphorus, chloroform, and gold compounds. These are true hepatotoxins.

Many drugs may induce hepatitis but are sensitizing rather than toxic. The result, *drug-induced hepatitis*, is similar to acute viral hepatitis; however, parenchymal destruction tends to be more extensive. Some examples of drugs that can lead to hepatitis are isoniazid, halothane, acetaminophen, and certain antibiotics, antimetabolites, and anesthetic agents.

Clinical Manifestations and Management.   Toxic hepatitis resembles viral hepatitis in onset. Obtaining a history of exposure to hepatotoxic chemicals, drugs, or other agents assists in earlier initiation of treatment and removal of the offending agent. Anorexia, nausea, and vomiting are the usual symptoms; jaundice and hepatomegaly are noted on physical assessment.

Symptoms are more intense for the more severely poisoned patient.

Recovery from acute toxic hepatitis is rapid if the hepatotoxin is identified early and removed or if exposure to the agent has been limited. Recovery, however, is unlikely if there is a prolonged period between exposure and onset of symptoms. There are no effective antidotes. The fever rises; the patient becomes deeply toxic and prostrated. Vomiting may be persistent, with the vomitus containing blood. Clotting abnormalities may be severe, and hemorrhages may appear under the skin. The severe gastrointestinal symptoms may lead to vascular collapse. Delirium, coma, and convulsions develop, and within a few days the patient usually dies of fulminant hepatic failure (see section that follows).

Short of liver transplantation, few treatment options are available. Therapy is directed toward restoring and maintaining fluid and electrolyte balance, blood replacement, and provision of comfort and supportive measures. A few patients recover from acute toxic hepatitis only to develop chronic liver disease.

In the event that the liver heals, there may be scarring, followed by postnecrotic cirrhosis. Manifestations of sensitivity to a drug may occur on the first day of its use or not until several months later, depending on the drug. Usually, the onset is abrupt, with chills, fever, rash, pruritus, arthralgia, anorexia, and nausea. Later, there may be jaundice and dark urine and an enlarged and tender liver. When the offending drug is withdrawn, symptoms may gradually subside. Reactions may be severe, however, and even fatal, even though the drug is stopped. If fever, rash, or pruritus occurs from any medication, its use should be stopped immediately.

Concern has been expressed regarding the effect on the liver of halothane (Fluothane), a commonly used nonexplosive inhalation anesthetic. Because halothane may cause serious, and sometimes fatal, liver damage, its use is contraindicated in (1) patients with known liver disease; (2) repeated instances, particularly in patients who have had a fever of unknown cause after the first administration of halothane; and (3) patients with evidence of prior sensitization. Such sensitization would have been in evidence during the second postoperative week, with such manifestations as fever, rash, eosinophilia, arthralgia, or jaundice.

Fulminant Hepatic Failure

Fulminant hepatic failure is characterized by the development of hepatic encephalopathy within 8 weeks of the onset of disease in a patient without prior evidence of hepatic dysfunction. It is characterized by dramatic and rapid clinical deterioration caused by massive hepatocellular injury and necrosis. Mortality is extremely high (60% to 85%), despite intensive treatment.

Viral hepatitis is the most common cause of fulminant hepatic failure; other causes include toxic drugs (*i.e.*, acetaminophen) and chemicals (*i.e.*, carbon tetrachloride), metabolic disturbances (Wilson's disease), and structural changes (Budd–Chiari syndrome).

The presence of jaundice and profound anorexia may be the initial reason for the patient to seek health care. Fulminant hepatic failure is often accompanied by coagulation defects, renal failure and electrolyte disturbances, infection, hypoglycemia, encephalopathy, and cerebral edema.

Treatment modalities have included blood or plasma exchanges, charcoal hemoperfusion, and corticosteroids. Despite these treatment modalities, however, mortality remains high. Consequently, liver transplantation has become the treatment of choice for persons with fulminant hepatic failure. Liver transplantation is discussed on p. 1006.

Hepatic Cirrhosis

Cirrhosis of the liver refers to scarring of the liver. Three kinds are generally considered:

1. *Laennec's portal cirrhosis* (alcoholic, nutritional), in which the scar tissue characteristically surrounds the portal areas. This is most frequently due to chronic alcoholism and is the most common type of cirrhosis.
2. *Postnecrotic cirrhosis*, in which there are broad bands of scar tissue, as a late result of a previous acute viral hepatitis.
3. *Biliary cirrhosis*, in which there is pericholangitic, perilobular scarring. This type usually is the result of chronic biliary obstruction and infection (cholangitis); its incidence is considerably lower than that of Laennec's and postnecrotic cirrhosis.

The portion of the liver chiefly involved consists of the portal and the periportal spaces, where the bile canaliculi of each lobule communicate to form the liver bile ducts. These areas become the site of inflammation, and the bile ducts become occluded with inspissated (thickened) bile and pus. An attempt is made by the liver to form new bile channels; hence, there is an overgrowth of tissue made up largely of disconnected, newly formed bile ducts and surrounded by scar tissue. Clinical manifestations of this disease include intermittent jaundice and fever. Initially the liver is enlarged, hard, and irregular; eventually it becomes atrophic. The treatment is the same as that for any form of chronic liver insufficiency.

Pathophysiology

Although several factors have been implicated in the etiology of cirrhosis, alcohol consumption is considered the major causative factor. Cirrhosis occurs with greatest frequency among alcoholics. Although nutritional deficiency with reduced protein intake contributes to liver destruction in cirrhosis, excessive alcohol intake is the major causative factor in fatty liver and its consequences. Cirrhosis, however, is also observed among people who do not consume alcohol, and it has been observed in those with a high alcohol intake despite a normal diet.

Some people appear to be more susceptible than others to this disease, whether they are alcoholics or malnourished or not. Other factors may play a role, including exposure to certain chemicals (carbon tetrachloride, chlorinated naphthalene, arsenic, or phosphorus) or infectious schistosomiasis. Twice as many men as women are affected, and the majority of patients are between 40 and 60 years of age.

Laennec's cirrhosis is a disease characterized by episodes of necrosis involving the liver cells, sometimes occurring repeatedly throughout the course of the disease. The destroyed liver cells are gradually replaced by scar tissue; eventually the amount of scar tissue exceeds that of the functioning liver tissue. Islands of residual normal tissue and regenerating liver tissue may project from the constricted areas, giving the cirrhotic liver its characteristic hobnail appearance. The disease usually

has a particularly insidious onset and a very protracted course, occasionally proceeding over a period of 30 or more years.

Clinical Manifestations

Early in the course of cirrhosis, the liver tends to be large and its cells loaded with fat. The liver is firm and has a sharp edge noticeable on palpation. Abdominal pain may be present because of recent, rapid enlargement of the liver, producing tension on the fibrous covering of the liver (Glisson's capsule). Later in the course of the disease, the liver decreases in size as scar tissue contracts the liver tissue. The liver edge, if palpable, is nodular.

The late manifestations are due partly to chronic failure of liver function and partly to obstruction of the portal circulation. Practically all the blood from the digestive organs is collected in the portal veins and carried to the liver. Because a cirrhotic liver does not allow the blood free passage, it is backed up into the spleen and the gastrointestinal tract, with the result that these organs become the seat of chronic passive congestion; that is, they are stagnant with blood and thus cannot function properly. Such patients are likely to have chronic dyspepsia (indigestion) and constipation or diarrhea. There is gradual weight loss. Fluid rich in protein may accumulate in the peritoneal cavity, producing ascites. This can be demonstrated through percussion for shifting dullness or a fluid wave (see Fig. 38–4). Splenomegaly may also be present. Spider telangiectases, or dilated superficial arterioles resembling bluish-red spiders, are frequently observed on inspection of the face and trunk.

The obstruction to blood flow through the liver resulting from the fibrotic changes also results in the formation of collateral blood vessels in the gastrointestinal system and shunting of blood from the portal vessels into blood vessels with lower pressures. As a result, the patient with cirrhosis will often have prominent, distended abdominal blood vessels, which are visible on abdominal inspection (caput medusae), and distended blood vessels throughout the gastrointestinal tract. The esophagus, stomach, and lower rectum are common sites of collateral blood vessels. These distended blood vessels form varices or hemorrhoids, depending on their location. Because these vessels were not intended to carry the high pressure and volume of blood imposed by cirrhosis, they may rupture and bleed. Therefore, assessment must include observation for occult and frank bleeding from the gastrointestinal tract. Approximately 25% of patients develop small hematemesis; others have profuse hemorrhage from the stomach and esophageal varices.

Other late symptoms of cirrhosis are attributable to chronic failure of liver function. The concentration of plasma albumin is reduced, predisposing to the formation of edema. Overproduction of aldosterone occurs, causing sodium and water retention and potassium excretion. Because of inadequate formation, use, and storage of certain vitamins (notably vitamins A, C, and K), signs of their deficiency frequently are encountered, particularly hemorrhagic phenomena associated with vitamin K deficiency. Chronic gastritis and impaired gastrointestinal function, together with inadequate dietary intake and impaired liver function, account for the anemia often associated with this disease. The anemia and the patient's poor nutritional status and poor state of health result in severe fatigue, which interferes with the ability to carry out routine daily activities.

Additional clinical manifestations include deterioration of

mental function with impending hepatic encephalopathy and hepatic coma. Therefore, neurologic assessment is indicated and includes the patient's general behavior, cognitive abilities, orientation to time and place, and speech patterns.

In addition to noting the occurrence of clinical manifestations, the nurse obtains accurate information about the patient's dietary and alcohol intake. It is also important to document exposure to toxic agents encountered during work or recreation. Any potentially hepatotoxic medications or drugs taken by the patient or exposure to general anesthetic agents are documented and reported.

Diagnostic Evaluation

The extent of liver disease and the type of treatment are determined after studying the laboratory findings. Because the functions of the liver are complex, there are many diagnostic tests that may provide information about its function (see Table 38–1). The patient needs to know why these tests are being performed, why they are important, and how to cooperate. In severe parenchymal liver dysfunction, the serum albumin level tends to decrease, and the serum globulin level rises. Enzyme tests indicate liver cell damage: serum alkaline phosphatase, SGOT, and SGPT levels increase, and the serum cholinesterase level may decrease. Bilirubin tests are performed to measure bile excretion or bile retention. Photolaparoscopy, in conjunction with biopsy, permits direct visualization of the liver.

Ultrasound scanning will measure the difference in density of parenchymal cells and scar tissue. Computed tomography (CT scan) and radioisotopic liver scans give information about liver size and hepatic blood flow and obstruction.

Management

The management of the patient with cirrhosis is usually based on the patient's presenting symptoms. For example, antacids are prescribed to decrease gastric distress and minimize the possibility of gastrointestinal bleeding. Vitamins and nutritional supplements promote healing of damaged liver cells and improve the patient's general nutritional status. Potassium-sparing diuretics (*e.g.*, spironolactone) may be indicated to decrease ascites, if present, and minimize fluid and electrolyte changes common with other diuretic agents. The physician also strongly encourages the patient to avoid further alcohol use, a recommendation that is reinforced in a nonjudgmental way by the nurse. Although the fibrosis of the cirrhotic liver cannot be reversed, its progression may be halted or slowed by such measures.

Preliminary studies indicate that colchicine, an anti-inflammatory drug used to treat the symptoms of gout, may increase the length of survival in patients with mild to moderate cirrhosis.

▶ Nursing Process
The Patient With Hepatic Cirrhosis

◊ Assessment

Nursing assessment focuses on history of precipitating factors, particularly long-term alcohol abuse, as well as changes in the patient's physical and mental status. The patient's past and current patterns of alcohol use (duration and amount) are assessed and documented. Mental status is assessed through interview and other interaction with the patient; orientation to person, place, and time is noted. The patient's ability to carry on a job or household activities provides some information about physical and mental status. Additionally, the patient's relationship with family, friends, and coworkers may give some indication about incapacitation secondary to alcohol abuse and cirrhosis. Abdominal distention and bloating, gastrointestinal bleeding, bruising, and weight changes are noted.

◊ Nursing Diagnoses

Based on all the assessment data, the patient's major nursing diagnoses may include the following:

- Activity intolerance related to fatigue, general debility, muscle wasting, and discomfort
- Altered nutrition related to chronic gastritis, decreased gastrointestinal motility, and anorexia
- Impaired skin integrity related to edema, jaundice, and compromised immunologic status
- High risk for injury related to altered clotting mechanisms and portal hypertension
- Altered thought processes related to deterioration of liver function and increased serum ammonia level

◊ Planning and Implementation

◊ *Goals:*   The goals of the patient may include independence in activities, improvement of nutritional status, improvement of skin integrity, decreased potential for injury, and improvement of mental status.

◊ Nursing Interventions

To assist in accomplishing these goals, the major objectives of therapy are (1) to promote rest to reduce the demands on the dysfunctional liver, (2) to meet the patient's nutritional needs, (3) to prevent further threats to skin integrity, (4) to minimize risk of bleeding, and (5) to minimize metabolic derangements and limit those factors causing further deterioration of mental function.

◊ *Rest.*   The patient with active liver disease requires rest and other supportive measures to permit the liver to reestablish its functional ability. The patient's weight and the volume of his fluid intake and output are measured and recorded daily. His position in bed is adjusted for maximal respiratory efficiency, which is especially important if ascites is marked, as it interferes with adequate thoracic excursion. Oxygen therapy may be required in liver failure to oxygenate the damaged cells and prevent further cell destruction.

Rest reduces the demands on the liver and increases the liver's blood supply. Because the patient is more susceptible to infection, efforts to prevent respiratory, circulatory, and vascular disturbances need to be initiated. These measures may help prevent such problems as pneumonia, thrombophlebitis, and pressure ulcers. When the patient's nutritional status improves and the patient gains strength, he is encouraged to increase his activity gradually. Activity and mild exercise, as well as rest, are planned.

◊ *Improved Nutritional Status.*   The patient with cirrhosis who has no ascites or edema and exhibits no signs of impending coma should receive a nutritious, high-protein diet supplemented by vitamins of the B complex and others as indicated (including vitamins A, C, and K and folic acid). Because proper nutrition is so important, every effort must be made to encourage the patient to eat. This is as important as any medication. Often small, frequent meals are tolerated better than three large meals because of the abdominal pressure exerted by ascites.

Patient preferences are considered. Patients with prolonged or severe anorexia, or those who are vomiting or eating poorly for any reason, may receive nutrients by nasogastric tube or total parenteral nutrition (TPN).

Patients with fatty stools (steatorrhea) should receive water-soluble forms of fat-soluble vitamins—A, D, and E (Aquasol A, D, and E). Folic acid and iron are prescribed to prevent anemia. If the patient shows signs of impending or advancing coma, a low-protein diet should be given temporarily; too much high-protein food such as meats may produce portal-systemic encephalopathy (PSE), and too little may cause negative nitrogen balance and wasting. Suggested protein foods are dairy products (eggs, skim milk), cereal (wheat germ, white rice), and fish. A high-caloric intake should be maintained, and supplementary vitamins and minerals should be provided (*e.g.*, oral potassium, if the serum potassium is normal or low and if renal function is normal). As soon as the patient's condition permits, the protein intake should be restored to normal, or above. Diet therapy is determined on an individualized basis.

▷ *Skin Care.*   Careful skin care is provided because of the presence of subcutaneous edema, the immobility of the patient, jaundice, and increased susceptibility to skin breakdown and infection. Frequent position changes are necessary to prevent pressure ulcers. Irritating soaps and use of adhesive tape are avoided to prevent trauma to the skin. Lotion may be soothing to irritated skin; measures are taken to minimize the patient's scratching of the skin.

▷ *Prevention of Bleeding.*   Because of decreased production of prothrombin and the diseased liver's decreased synthesis of substances necessary for blood coagulation, hemorrhage is possible. Precautionary measures include protecting the patient with padded side rails, applying pressure to any injection site, and avoiding injury from sharp objects. The nurse should observe for melena and check stools for blood as signs of possible internal bleeding. Vital signs also are monitored regularly. Precautions are taken to minimize rupture of esophageal varices by avoiding further increases in portal pressure. Dietary modification and appropriate use of stool softeners may assist in preventing straining during defecation. The patient is monitored closely for gastrointestinal bleeding; equipment (Sengstaken-Blakemore tube), intravenous fluids, and medications needed to treat hemorrhage from esophageal varices are kept readily available (see pp. 1000–1001).

▷ *Improved Mental Function.*   Portal-systemic encephalopathy (PSE) is a possible neurologic syndrome that includes deteriorating mental status and dementia as well as physical signs such as abnormal voluntary and involuntary movements. It has occurred in patients after shunting and in those with advanced cirrhosis. PSE is mainly caused by ammonia and its effect on cerebral metabolism. Many factors predispose the patient with cirrhosis to PSE; some are unforeseeable, but many are avoidable. The nurse is in a position to observe early evidence of

this condition and promote early treatment. The nurse also uses strategies to orient the patient to reality.

▷ *Patient Education and Home Health Care.*   During hospitalization, the patient is prepared for discharge by the nurse and other health care providers through dietary instruction. Of greatest importance is the exclusion of alcohol from the diet. The patient may need referral to Alcoholics Anonymous, psychiatric care, or support from a trusted clergy person.

Sodium restriction will continue for a considerable time, if not permanently. If this diet is to be followed correctly, the patient will require written instructions, teaching, reinforcement, and support from the staff as well as the family members.

The success of treatment depends on convincing the patient of the need to adhere completely to the therapeutic plan. This includes rest; probably a change in life style; an adequate, well-balanced diet; and the elimination of alcohol. The patient and family are also instructed about the symptoms of impending encephalopathy and the possibility of bleeding tendencies and easy susceptibility to infection. Recovery is neither rapid nor easy; there are frequent setbacks and apparent lack of improvement. Many patients find it difficult to refrain from using alcohol for comfort or escape. The understanding nurse can play a significant role in offering support and encouragement to this patient. Referral of the patient to a community health nurse who visits the patient in the home after discharge may assist the patient in dealing with the transition from hospital to home, where use of alcohol may have been an important part of the patient's normal home life. The community health nurse is able to observe the patient's progress at home and the manner in which he and his family cope with the elimination of alcohol and the dietary restrictions. Additionally, the nurse is able to reinforce previous teaching and answer questions that may not have occurred to the patient or family until the patient is back home and trying to reestablish new patterns of eating, drinking, and life-style.

▷ *Summary.*   For an overall view of the nursing management of the patient with cirrhosis, refer to Nursing Care Plan 38–2.

▷ Evaluation

Expected Outcomes
1. Demonstrates ability to participate in activities
    a. Plans activities and exercises to allow alternating periods of rest and activity
    b. Reports increased strength and well-being
    c. Displays increased weight gain without increased edema and ascites formation
    d. Participates in hygienic care
2. Increases nutritional intake
    a. Demonstrates intake of appropriate nutrients and avoidance of alcohol as reflected by diet log
    b. Gains weight without increased edema and ascites formation
    c. Reports decrease in gastrointestinal disturbances and anorexia
    d. Identifies foods and fluids that are nutritious and allowed on diet
    e. Identifies foods restricted from diet
    f. Adheres to vitamin therapy regimen

(text continues on page 999)

Nursing Care Plan 38–2

Care of the Patient With Cirrhosis

Nursing Interventions	Rationale	Expected Outcomes

Nursing Diagnosis: Activity intolerance related to fatigue and weight loss

Goal: Increased energy and increased participation in activities

1. Offer high-protein, high-caloric diet.	1. Provides calories for energy and protein for healing.	• Reports increased strength and well-being.
2. Give supplementary vitamins (A, B-complex, C, and K).	2. Provides additional nutrients.	• Plans activities to allow ample periods of rest.
3. Encourage alternating periods of rest and exercise.	3. Conserves patient's energy while encouraging exercise within patient's tolerance.	• Increases activity and exercise as strength increases.
4. Encourage and assist with gradually increasing periods of exercise.	4. Improves general well-being and self-esteem.	• Gains weight without increased edema or ascites formation.
		• Demonstrates adequate intake of nutrients and excludes alcohol from diet.

Nursing Diagnosis: Altered body temperature: hyperthermia related to inflammatory process of cirrhosis

Goal: Maintenance of normal body temperature

1. Record temperature regularly.	1. Provides baseline to detect fever and to evaluate interventions.	• Reports normal temperature and absence of chills or sweating.
2. Encourage fluid intake.	2. Corrects fluid loss from perspiration and fever and increases patient's level of comfort.	• Demonstrates adequate intake of fluids.
3. Apply cool sponges or icebag for elevated temperature.	3. Promotes reduction of fever by conduction and evaporation and increases patient's comfort.	
4. Administer antibiotics as prescribed.	4. Promotes appropriate serum concentration of antibiotics to treat infection.	
5. Avoid exposure to infections.	5. Minimizes risk of further infection and further increases in body temperature and metabolic rate.	
6. Keep patient at rest while temperature is elevated.	6. Reduces metabolic rate.	

Nursing Diagnosis: Impaired skin integrity related to edema formation

Goal: Improved skin integrity and protection of edematous tissue

1. Restrict sodium as prescribed.	1. Minimizes edema formation.	• Exhibits normal turgor of skin of extremities and trunk.
2. Give careful attention and care to the skin.	2. Edematous skin and tissue has compromised nutrient supply and is very vulnerable to pressure and trauma.	• Exhibits absence of skin breakdown.
3. Turn and change position of patient frequently.	3. Minimizes prolonged pressure and promotes mobilization of edema.	• Exhibits normal tissue without evidence of redness, discoloration, or increased warmth over bony prominences.
4. Weigh patient daily and record intake and output.	4. Permits best estimate of fluid status and monitoring of fluid retention and loss from tissues.	• Changes position frequently.
5. Carry out passive range of motion exercises; elevate edematous extremities.	5. Promotes mobilization of edema.	
6. Provide small foam, rubber supports under heels, malleoli, and other bony prominences.	6. Protects bony prominences and minimizes trauma *if used correctly.*	

(continued)

Nursing Care Plan 38–2 (Continued)

Care of the Patient With Cirrhosis

Nursing Interventions	Rationale	Expected Outcomes

Nursing Diagnosis: Impaired skin integrity related to jaundice and compromised immunologic status

Goal: Improved skin integrity and minimization of skin irritation

1. Note and record degree of jaundice of skin and sclerae.	1. Provides baseline for detecting changes and evaluating interventions.	Demonstrates improved skin integrity:
2. Provide frequent skin care, bathing without soap, and massage with emollient lotions.	2. Prevents dryness of skin and minimizes pruritus.	• Exhibits intact skin without evidence of breakdown or infection.
3. Keep patient's fingernails short.	3. Prevents skin excoriation from scratching.	• Reports absence of pruritus. • Demonstrates decreasing jaundice of skin and sclerae. • Uses emollients and avoids soaps in daily hygiene.

Nursing Diagnosis: Altered nutrition, less than body requirements, related to anorexia and gastrointestinal disturbances

Goal: Improved nutritional status

1. Encourage patient to eat meals and supplementary feedings.	1. Encouragement is essential for the patient with anorexia and gastrointestinal discomfort.	Increased intake of nutritious diet: • Demonstrates intake of sufficient high-protein, high-caloric meals.
2. Offer frequent, small feedings.	2. Small meals are frequently easier for the anorexic patient to tolerate.	• Identifies food and fluid that are nutritious and permitted on diet.
3. Provide attractive meals and an aesthetically pleasing setting at meal time.	3. Promotes appetite and sense of well-being.	• Gains weight without increased edema or ascites formation.
4. Eliminate alcohol.	4. Eliminates "empty calories" and avoids the gastric irritation produced by alcohol.	• Identifies the rationale for small, frequent meals.
5. Provide oral hygiene before meals.	5. Reduces unpleasant taste and stimulates appetite.	• Reports increased appetite and well-being. • Excludes alcohol from diet.
6. Apply an ice collar for nausea.	6. May reduce incidence of nausea.	• Participates in oral hygiene measures before meals and to counteract nausea.
7. Administer medications prescribed for nausea, vomiting, diarrhea, or constipation.	7. Reduces gastrointestinal symptoms and discomforts that decrease the appetite and interest in food.	• Takes medications for gastrointestinal disorders as prescribed.
8. Encourage increased fluid intake and exercise if the patient reports constipation.	8. Promotes normal bowel pattern and reduces abdominal discomfort and distention.	• Reports normal gastrointestinal function with regular bowel function.
9. Observe for evidence of gastrointestinal bleeding.	9. Detects serious gastrointestinal complications.	• Identifies reportable symptoms of abnormal gastrointestinal function: melena, gross bleeding.

Nursing Diagnosis: High risk for injury related to portal hypertension, altered clotting mechanisms, and impaired detoxification of drugs.

Goal: Decreased risk of injury

1. Observe each stool for color, consistency, and amount.	1. Permits detection of bleeding in gastrointestinal tract.	• Exhibits absence of frank bleeding from gastrointestinal tract.
2. Be alert for symptoms of anxiety, epigastric fullness, weakness, and restlessness.	2. May indicate early signs of bleeding and shock.	• Exhibits absence of restlessness, epigastric fullness, and other indicators of hemorrhage and shock.
3. Test each stool and emesis for occult blood.	3. Detects early evidence of bleeding.	• Exhibits negative results of test for occult gastrointestinal bleeding.
4. Observe for hemorrhagic manifestations: ecchymosis, epistaxis, petechiae, and bleeding gums.	4. Indicates altered clotting mechanisms.	• Is free of ecchymotic areas or hematoma formation. • Exhibits normal vital signs.

(continued)

> ## Nursing Care Plan 38-2 *(Continued)*

Care of the Patient With Cirrhosis

Nursing Interventions	Rationale	Expected Outcomes
5. Record vital signs at frequent intervals.	5. Provides baseline and evidence of hypovolemia, shock.	• Maintains rest and remains quiet if active bleeding occurs.
6. Keep patient quiet and limit activity.	6. Minimizes risk of bleeding and straining.	• Identifies rationale for blood transfusions and measures to treat bleeding.
7. Assist physician in passage of tube for esophageal balloon tamponade.	7. Promotes nontraumatic insertion of tube in anxious and combative patient for immediate treatment of bleeding.	• Uses measures to prevent trauma (*e.g.,* uses soft toothbrush, blows nose gently, avoids bumps and falls, avoids straining during defecation).
8. Observe during blood transfusions.	8. Permits detection of transfusion reactions (risk is increased with multiple blood transfusions needed for active bleeding from esophageal varices).	• Experiences no side effects of medications.
9. Measure and record nature, time, and amount of vomitus.	9. Assists in evaluating extent of bleeding and blood loss.	• Takes all medications as prescribed.
10. Maintain patient in fasting state, if indicated.	10. Reduces risk of aspiration of gastric contents and minimizes risk of further trauma to esophagus and stomach by preventing vomiting.	• Identifies rationale for precautions with use of all medications.
11. Administer vitamin K as prescribed.	11. Promotes clotting by providing fat-soluble vitamin necessary for clotting mechanism.	
12. Stay in constant attendance during episodes of bleeding.	12. Reassures anxious patient and permits monitoring and detection of further needs of the patient.	
13. Offer cold liquids by mouth when bleeding stops (if prescribed).	13. Minimizes risk of further bleeding by promoting vasoconstriction of esophageal and gastric blood vessels.	

14. Institute measures to prevent trauma:
  a. Maintain safe environment.
 	
  b. Encourage *gentle* blowing of nose.
 	
  c. Provide soft toothbrush and avoid use of toothpicks.
  d. Encourage intake of foods with high content of vitamin C.
  e. Apply cold compresses where indicated.
  f. Record location of bleeding sites.
 	
  g. Use small-gauge needles for injections.
	14. Promotes safety of patient.
	  a. Minimizes risk of trauma and bleeding by avoiding falls and cuts, etc.
	  b. Reduces risk of nosebleed (epistaxis) secondary to trauma and decreased clotting.
	  c. Prevents trauma to oral mucosa while promoting good oral hygiene.
	  d. Promotes healing.
	
	  e. Minimizes bleeding into tissues by promoting local vasoconstriction.
	  f. Permits detection of new bleeding sites and monitoring of previous sites of bleeding.
	  g. Minimizes oozing and blood loss from repeated injections.	

15. Administer medications carefully; monitor for side effects.	15. Reduces risk of side effects secondary to damaged liver's inability to detoxify (metabolize) drugs and medications normally.	

Nursing Diagnosis: Pain and discomfort related to enlarged tender liver and ascites

Goal: Increased level of comfort

1. Maintain bed rest when patient experiences abdominal discomfort.	1. Reduces metabolic demands and protects the liver.	• Maintains bed rest and decreases activity in presence of pain.

(continued)

Nursing Care Plan 38-2 (Continued)

Care of the Patient With Cirrhosis

Nursing Interventions	Rationale	Expected Outcomes
2. Administer antispasmodics and sedatives as prescribed.	2. Reduces irritability of the gastrointestinal tract and decreases abdominal pain and discomfort.	• Takes antispasmodics and sedatives as indicated and as prescribed.
3. Observe, record, and report presence and character of pain and discomfort.	3. Provides baseline to detect further deterioration of status and to evaluate interventions.	• Reports decreased pain and abdominal discomfort.
4. Reduce sodium and fluid intake if prescribed.	4. Minimizes further formation of ascites.	• Reports pain and discomfort if present.
		• Reduces sodium and fluid intake to prescribed levels if indicated to treat ascites.
		• Obtains pain relief.
		• Exhibits decreased abdominal girth and appropriate weight changes.

Nursing Diagnosis: Fluid volume excess related to ascites and edema formation

Goal: Restoration of normal fluid volume

1. Restrict sodium and fluid intake if prescribed.	1. Minimizes formation of ascites and edema.	• Consumes diet low in sodium and within prescribed fluid restriction.
2. Administer diuretics, potassium, and protein supplements as prescribed.	2. Promotes excretion of fluid through the kidneys and maintenance of normal fluid and electrolyte balance.	• Takes diuretics, potassium, and protein supplements as indicated without experiencing side effects.
3. Record intake and output.	3. Assesses effectiveness of treatment and adequacy of fluid intake.	• Exhibits increased urine output.
4. Measure and record abdominal girth daily.	4. Monitors changes in ascites formation and accumulation.	• Exhibits decreasing abdominal girth.
5. Explain rationale for sodium and fluid restriction.	5. Promotes patient's understanding of restriction and cooperation with it.	• Identifies rationale for sodium and fluid restriction.

Nursing Diagnosis: Altered thought processes related to deterioration of liver function and increased serum ammonia level

Goal: Improved mental status

1. Restrict dietary protein as prescribed.	1. Reduces source of ammonia (protein foods).	Demonstrates improved mental status:
2. Give frequent small feeding of carbohydrates.	2. Promotes adequate carbohydrate for energy requirements and "spares" protein from breakdown for energy.	• Exhibits serum ammonia level within normal limits.
3. Protect from infection.	3. Minimizes risk of further increase in metabolic requirements.	• Is oriented to time, place, and person.
4. Keep environment warm and draft-free.	4. Minimizes shivering, which would increase metabolic requirements.	• Reports normal sleep patterns.
5. Pad the side-rails of the bed.	5. Provides protection for the patient in the event that hepatic coma and seizure activity occur.	• Demonstrates an interest in events and activities around him.
6. Limit visitors.	6. Minimizes patient's activity and metabolic requirements.	• Demonstrates normal attention span.
7. Provide careful nursing surveillance to ensure patient's safety.	7. Provides close monitoring of new symptoms and minimizes trauma to the confused patient.	• Follows and participates in conversations appropriately.
8. Avoid narcotics and barbiturates.	8. Prevents masking of symptoms of hepatic coma and prevents drug overdose secondary to reduced ability of the damaged liver to metabolize narcotics and barbiturates.	• Reports urinary and fecal continence.
		• Experiences no seizures.

(continued)

► ## Nursing Care Plan 38-2 (Continued)

Care of the Patient With Cirrhosis

Nursing Interventions	Rationale	Expected Outcomes
9. Arouse at intervals.	9. Provides stimulation to the patient and opportunity for observing the patient's level of consciousness.	

Nursing Diagnosis: Ineffective breathing pattern related to ascites and restriction of thoracic excursion secondary to ascites, abdominal distention, and fluid in the thoracic cavity

Goal: Improved respiratory status

Nursing Interventions	Rationale	Expected Outcomes
1. Elevate head of bed.	1. Reduces abdominal pressure on the diaphragm and permits fuller thoracic excursion and lung expansion.	Experiences improved respiratory status: • Reports decreased shortness of breath.
2. Conserve patient's strength.	2. Reduces patient metabolic and oxygen requirements.	• Reports increased strength and sense of well-being.
3. Change position at intervals.	3. Promotes expansion and oxygenation of all areas of the lungs.	• Exhibits respiratory rate (12–18 min) with no adventitious sounds.
4. Assist patient during paracentesis or thoracentesis.	4. Paracentesis and thoracentesis (performed to remove fluid from the thoracic cavity) may be frightening to the patient. Helps obtain patient's cooperation with the procedure, minimizing discomfort and risks.	• Exhibits full thoracic excursion without shallow respirations. • Exhibits normal blood gases. • Experiences absence of confusion or cyanosis.
a. Support and maintain position during procedure.		
b. Record both the amount and the character of fluid aspirated.	b. Provides record of fluid removed and indication of severity of limitation of lung expansion by fluid.	
c. Observe for evidence of coughing, increasing dyspnea, or pulse rate.	c. Indicates irritation of the pleural space and evidence of ventilatory function compromised by pneumothorax or hemothorax (air or blood accumulating in pleural space).	

g. Describes the rationale for small, frequent meals
h. Excludes alcohol from diet
3. Demonstrates improved skin integrity
   a. Shows intact skin without evidence of breakdown or infection
   b. Achieves decreased edema in extremities and trunk
   c. Demonstrates normal turgor of skin of extremities and trunk
   d. Changes position frequently
   e. Inspects bony prominences daily
   f. Avoids trauma to skin
   g. Reports decreased or absent pruritus
   h. Uses lotions to decrease pruritus
4. Experiences decreased risk of bleeding
   a. Is free of ecchymotic areas or hematoma formation
   b. Reports absence of frank bleeding from gastrointestinal tract (*e.g.*, absence of melena and hematemesis)
   c. Reports negative results of test for occult gastrointestinal bleeding
   d. Uses measures to prevent trauma (*e.g.*, uses soft tooth-

brush, blows nose gently, arranges furniture to prevent bumps and falls, avoids straining during defecation)
5. Demonstrates improved mental function
   a. Has serum ammonia level within normal limits
   b. Is oriented to time, place, and person
   c. Demonstrates normal attention span (*e.g.*, is able to complete reading of desired articles, books; is able to watch television with interest)
   d. Converses with family and health care team members appropriately
   e. Reports urinary and fecal continence
   f. Identifies early, reportable signs of impaired thought processes

Bleeding Esophageal Varices

Bleeding or hemorrhage from esophageal varices occurs in approximately one third of patients with cirrhosis and varices.

The mortality rate resulting from the first bleeding episode is 45% to 50%; it is one of the major causes of death in patients with cirrhosis.

Pathophysiology and Clinical Manifestations

Esophageal varices are dilated tortuous veins usually found in the submucosa of the lower esophagus; however, they may develop higher in the esophagus or extend into the stomach. Such a condition nearly always is caused by portal hypertension, which, in turn, is due to obstruction of the portal venous circulation within the cirrhotic liver (see p. 381). Because of increased obstruction of the portal vein, venous blood from the intestinal tract and spleen seeks an outlet through collateral circulation (new pathways of return to the right atrium). The effect is increased strain, particularly on the vessels in the submucosal layer of the lower esophagus and upper part of the stomach. These collateral vessels are not very elastic but rather are tortuous and fragile and bleed easily. Other less common causes of varices are abnormalities of the circulation in the splenic vein or superior vena cava and hepatic venothrombosis.

Bleeding esophageal varices are life threatening and can result in hemorrhagic shock, producing decreased cerebral, hepatic, and renal perfusion. In turn, there will be an increased nitrogen load from bleeding into the gastrointestinal tract and an increased serum ammonia level, which increase the risk of encephalopathy. Bleeding esophageal varices should be suspected in the presence of hematemesis and melena, especially in the patient who has abused alcohol. Usually, the dilated veins cause no symptoms unless the portal pressure increases sharply and the mucosa or supporting structures become thin. Then massive hemorrhage takes place. Factors that contribute to hemorrhage are muscular strain from lifting heavy objects, straining at stool, sneezing, coughing or vomiting, esophagitis, or irritation of vessels by poorly chewed foods or irritating fluids. Salicylates and any drug that erodes esophageal mucosa or interferes with cell replication also may contribute to bleeding.

Assessment

The patient's history and physical examination will assist in identifying the cause of the bleeding. Immediate endoscopy is indicated to identify the cause and site of bleeding; at least 30% of patients suspected of bleeding from esophageal varices bleed from other sources (gastritis, ulcers). Barium swallow, ultrasound, CT scan, and angiography are also used to identify the source of the bleeding. Neurologic assessment will assist in identifying possible hepatic encephalopathy resulting from the breakdown of blood in the gastrointestinal tract and a rising serum ammonia level. Manifestations range from drowsiness to coma. Portal hypertension may be suggested if dilated abdominal veins and rectal hemorrhoids are detected. Also apparent may be a palpable enlarged spleen (splenomegaly) and ascites. Laboratory tests that may be required are various liver function tests, such as serum transaminase, bilirubin, alkaline phosphatase, and serum proteins.

Nursing support before and during examination by endoscopy to identify the site of bleeding can be effective in relieving a stressful experience. Careful monitoring can detect early signs of cardiac dysrhythmias, perforation, and hemorrhage. After the examination, fluids are not given until the gag reflex returns. Lozenges and gargles may be used to relieve throat discomfort if the patient's condition permits and he is able to participate in his care. If the patient is actively bleeding, oral intake will not be permitted and the patient will be prepared for further diagnostic and therapeutic procedures.

Portal vein pressure can be measured in the operating room by introducing a needle into the spleen; a manometer reading above 20 ml saline is abnormal. Combined umbilical-portal and hepatic vein catheterization is the most practical method for measuring portal pressure and at the same time permits radiologic study of the hepatic vascular bed. Blood flow studies also may be performed, which assists in determining cardiac output.

Splenoportography involves serial or segmental x-ray films to detect extensive collateral circulation in esophageal vessels, which would be indicative of varices. Other tests are hepato-portography and celiac angiography. These are usually performed in the operating room or radiology department.

Overall nursing assessment includes monitoring of the patient's physical condition and evaluation of his emotional reactions to the bleeding episode. Vital signs are monitored and recorded, and the patient's nutritional status is assessed.

Bleeding from esophageal varices can quickly lead to hemorrhagic shock and should be considered an emergency.

Management

The patient with bleeding varices is critically ill, requiring aggressive medical care and expert nursing care (Chart 38–3). Assessment requires that the extent of bleeding be evaluated and vital signs monitored continuously when hematemesis and melena are present. Signs of potential hypovolemia are noted, such as cold clammy skin, tachycardia, a drop in blood pressure, decreased urine output, restlessness, and increased or shallow peripheral pulses. Blood volume is monitored by means of a central venous pressure or arterial catheter. Oxygen is required to prevent hypoxia and to maintain adequate blood oxygenation.

Because patients with bleeding esophageal varices are subject to electrolyte imbalance, intravenous fluids and volume expanders are provided to restore fluid volume and replace electrolytes. Blood transfusion also may be needed. Urinary output is carefully monitored; an indwelling catheter may be inserted.

Nonsurgical Management. Nonsurgical treatment is preferable because of the high mortality of emergency surgery for control of bleeding esophageal varices and because of the poor physical condition of the patient with severe liver dysfunction.

Pharmacologic Therapy. Vasopressin (Pitressin) may be the initial mode of therapy because of its constriction of the splanchnic arterial bed and resulting decrease in portal pressure. It may be given intravenously or by intra-arterial infusion. Either method requires monitoring by the nurse. Gastric aspiration and vital signs offer indices of the effectiveness of vasopressin. Electrolyte evaluation and monitoring of fluid intake and output are necessary, as hyponatremia may occur and vasopressin may have an antidiuretic effect.

Coronary artery disease in this patient would be a contraindication to the use of vasopressin, because coronary vasoconstriction is a side effect that may precipitate myocardial infarction.

The combination of vasopressin and nitroglycerin (ad-

Chart 38–3
Management Modalities and Nursing Care for the Patient With Bleeding Esophageal Varices

Treatment Modality*	Action	Nursing Priorities
Nonsurgical Modalities		
Pharmacologic agents		
Vasopressin (Pitressin)	Reduces portal pressure by constricting splanchnic arteries	Observe response to therapy. Monitor for side-effects. (*Vasopressin*: angina. Nitroglycerin may be prescribed to prevent or treat angina.
Propranolol (Inderal)	Reduces portal pressure by β-adrenergic blocking action	*Propranolol*: decreased pulse and blood pressure, impaired cardiovascular response to hemorrhage.)
Somatostatin		Administer medication as prescribed. Support patient during treatment.
Balloon tamponade	Exerts pressure directly to bleeding sites in esophagus and stomach	Monitor closely to prevent accidental removal or displacement of tube, subsequent airway obstruction, and aspiration. Explain procedure to patient briefly to obtain cooperation with insertion and maintenance of esophageal-tamponade tube and reduce patient's fear of the procedure. Provide frequent oral hygiene. Report the onset of chest pain.
Iced saline lavage	Produces vasoconstriction of the esophageal and gastric blood vessels	Ensure patency of the nasogastric tube to prevent aspiration. Observe gastric aspirate for blood and cessation of bleeding. Protect the patient from chilling.
Injection sclerotherapy	Promotes thrombosis and sclerosis of bleeding sites by injection of sclerosing agent into the esophageal varices	Observe for aspiration, perforation of the esophagus, and recurrence of bleeding following treatment.
Surgical Modalities		
Portal-systemic shunts	Reduces portal hypertension by diverting blood flow away from obstructed portal system	Observe for development of portal systemic encephalopathy (altered mental status, neurologic dysfunction), hepatic failure, and rebleeding. Requires intensive, expert nursing care for prolonged period. Provide post-thoracotomy care.
Surgical ligation of varices	Ties off blood vessels at the site of bleeding	Observe for rebleeding.
Esophageal transection and devascularization	Separates bleeding site from portal system	Observe for rebleeding.

* Several modalities may be used concurrently or in sequence.

ministered by intravenous, sublingual, or transdermal routes) has been effective in reducing or preventing the side effects (constriction of coronary vessels and angina) caused by vasopressin alone.

Somatostatin has been reported to be more effective than vasopressin in decreasing bleeding from esophageal varices

without the vasoconstrictive effects of vasopressin. Propranolol, a β-blocking agent that decreases portal pressure, has been shown to prevent bleeding from esophageal varices in some patients; however, it is recommended that it be used only in combination with other treatment modalities such as sclerotherapy or balloon tamponade. Further studies of these drugs are necessary to evaluate their use in treatment and prevention of bleeding episodes.

Balloon Tamponade. To control the hemorrhage in certain patients, pressure is exerted on the cardia (upper orifice of the stomach) and against the bleeding varices by a double-balloon tamponade (Sengstaken–Blakemore tube) (Fig. 38–7). The three openings in the tube are for specific purposes: gastric aspiration, inflation of the gastric balloon, and inflation of the esophageal balloon.

The balloon in the stomach is inflated, and the tube is pulled gently to exert a force against the cardia. Irrigation of the tubing is performed to detect bleeding; if returns are clear, the esophageal balloon is not inflated. If bleeding continues, the esophageal balloon is inflated. The desired pressure in both balloons is 25 to 30 mm Hg, as measured by the manometer. After the balloon is inflated, there is a possibility of injury or rupture of the esophagus. Constant nursing surveillance is necessary at this time. Traction may be placed on the tube. A nasogastric tube may be inserted through the other nares to

aspirate esophagopharyngeal secretions if a three-lumen tube is used. This is not necessary with the four-lumen tube (Fig. 38–7C) because a fourth lumen provides a direct route for esophageal aspiration. Confirmation of the position of the tube and balloons by x-ray is recommended.

A cathartic such as magnesium sulfate may be administered through the tube to eliminate blood in the gastrointestinal tract; otherwise, ammonia absorption could occur, which may lead to hepatic coma and death. Thereafter, neomycin is administered to reduce intestinal bacterial flora, which are a source of ammonia-forming enzymes.

Gastric suction is provided by connecting the proper catheter outlet to suction. The tubing is irrigated hourly, and drainage will indicate whether bleeding has been controlled. Iced saline lavage or irrigation may be used in the gastric balloon to constrict the gastric vessels. In such instances, the nurse will anticipate possible chilling of the patient and provide comfort measures. The pressures on the tubes and traction are released periodically, as prescribed. Balloon tamponade is

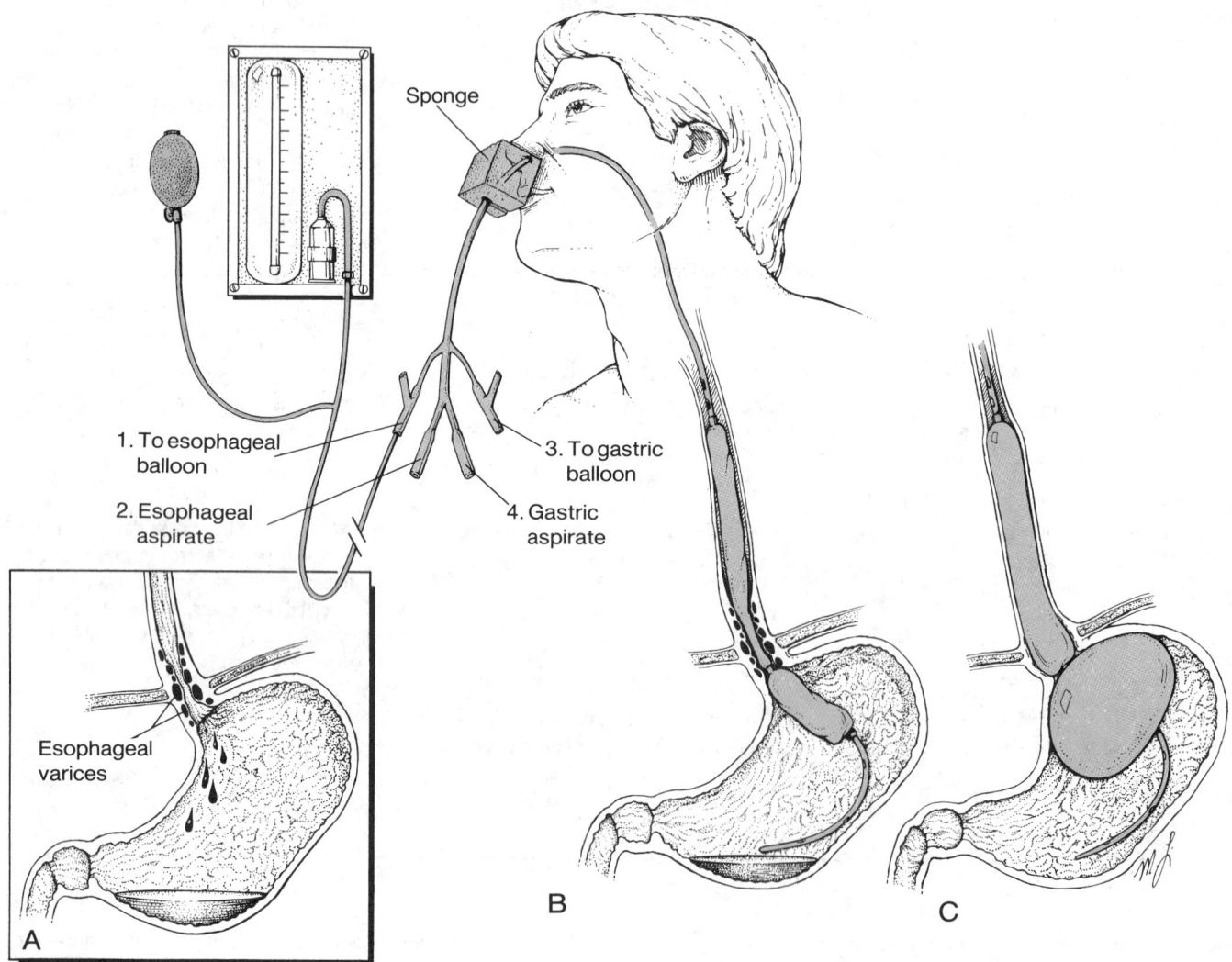

Figure 38–7. Esophageal balloon tamponade to treat bleeding esophageal varices. (**A**) Dilated, bleeding esophageal veins (varices) of the lower esophagus. (**B**) A four-lumen esophageal tamponade tube with balloons (uninflated) in place. (**C**) Compression of bleeding esophageal varices by inflated esophageal and gastric balloons. The gastric and esophageal outlets permit aspiration of secretions.

continued for several days and then cautiously released, followed by removal of the tube if no bleeding recurs.

Although this method has been fairly successful, it is important to note some inherent dangers. If the tube is left in place or inflated too long or at too high a pressure, ulceration and necrosis of the mucosa of the stomach or esophagus may occur. If the tube suddenly ruptures, the result is disastrous—airway obstruction and aspiration of gastric contents into the lungs. Using a new, tested tube may minimize this risk. Asphyxiation is another problem, caused by accidental pulling of the tube and inflated balloon into the oropharynx. These potential dangers suggest the need for intensive and expert care. A confused or restless patient with this tube in place and balloons inflated should not be left alone because of these risks.

Aspiration of blood and secretions is frequently associated with the use of balloon tamponade, especially in the stuporous or comatose patient. Endotracheal intubation before insertion of the tube protects the airway and minimizes the risk of aspiration.

The balloon may be deflated at intervals if prescribed to prevent erosion and necrosis of the mucosa of the stomach and esophagus and to determine if bleeding has ceased.

Nursing comfort measures include frequent mouth and nasal care. For secretions that accumulate in the mouth, tissues should be within easy reach of the patient. Oral suction may be necessary in some patients for removal of oral secretions. The patient who has experienced esophageal hemorrhage is usually anxious and frightened. The patient is less anxious if he knows that the nurse is nearby and will respond immediately to his call. The experience of having the tube inserted is uncomfortable and never pleasant. Explanations during the procedure and while the tube is in place may be reassuring to the patient.

Although use of balloon tamponade effectively stops the bleeding in most (90%) patients, bleeding recurs in the majority of patients, necessitating other treatment modalities. Once the balloons are deflated or the tube is removed, the patient must be assessed frequently because of the high risk of recurrent bleeding.

Injection Sclerotherapy. In injection sclerotherapy (Fig. 38–8), a sclerosing agent is injected through a fiberoptic endoscope into the bleeding esophageal varices to promote thrombosis and eventual sclerosis. Although controlled studies have not demonstrated conclusively that injection sclerotherapy is superior to other treatments or improves long-term survival, the procedure has been used successfully to treat gastrointestinal hemorrhage. In addition, it has been used to treat esophageal varices before bleeding has occurred; however, its use as a prophylactic measure is controversial because of the inability to predict which third of those patients with esophageal varices will experience bleeding. After treatment, the patient must be observed for bleeding, perforation of the esophagus, aspiration pneumonia, and esophageal stricture. Antacids may be given after the procedure to counteract the effects of peptic reflux.

Repeated courses of sclerotherapy may be needed to obliterate all the varices. The patient and family need to be aware of the importance of these additional treatments and continued long-term follow up even though the patient may not be actively bleeding.

Other Measures. Bleeding is also treated by sedation and complete rest of the esophagus; therefore, parenteral feedings are initiated. Straining and vomiting must be prevented. Gastric

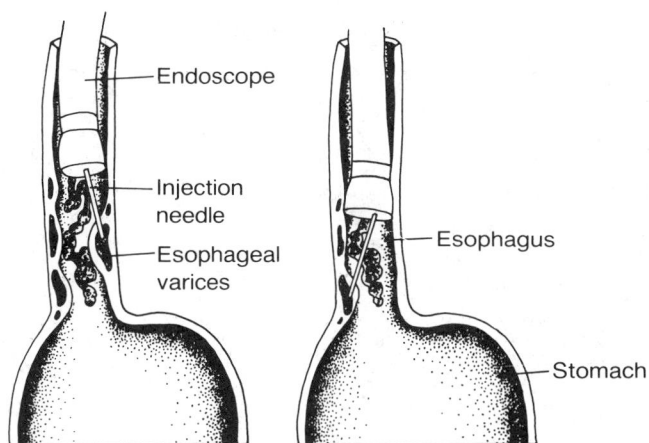

Figure 38–8. Injection sclerotherapy. Injection of sclerosing agent into esophageal varices through an endoscope.

suction usually is employed to keep the stomach as empty as possible. The patient often complains of severe thirst, which may be relieved by frequent oral hygiene and moist sponges to the lips. The nurse keeps close surveillance on the patient's blood pressure. Vitamin K therapy and multiple blood transfusions often are indicated. A quiet environment and calm reassurance will help to relieve the patient's anxiety.

Surgical Management. Surgical procedures that may be employed for esophageal varices are direct surgical ligation of varices, portacaval and splenorenal venous shunt operations, and esophageal transection with devascularization.

Surgical Bypass Procedures. The most common procedure is to create an anastomosis between the portal vein and the inferior vena cava—a *portacaval anastomosis* (Fig. 38–9). When portal blood is shunted into the vena cava, the pressure in the portal system is decreased, and consequently the danger of hemorrhage from esophageal and gastric varices is reduced. When the portal vein cannot be used because of thrombosis, or for other reasons, a shunt may be made between the splenic vein and the left renal vein (*splenorenal shunt*) after splenectomy. Some surgeons prefer this shunt to the portacaval shunt, even when the portal vein can be used.

A *mesocaval* shunt is a third type of bypass procedure, in which the inferior vena cava is severed and the proximal end of the vena cava is anastomosed to the side of the superior mesenteric vein.

These operations are extensive procedures and are not always successful, because of secondary clotting in the veins used for the shunt. Nevertheless, a shunt is the only method by which a lowering of pressure in the portal system may be effected. Because hemorrhages from the esophageal varices are often fatal, many of these relatively poor-risk patients must be subjected to these attempts to save their lives.

Devascularization and Transection. Devascularization and staple-gun transection operations to separate the bleeding site from the high-pressure portal system have been used in emergency management of variceal bleeding. The lower end of the esophagus is reached through a small gastrostomy incision; the staple gun permits reanastomosis of the transected ends of the esophagus. Controlled studies of this procedure are necessary to determine if it is a potential alternative to other therapies.

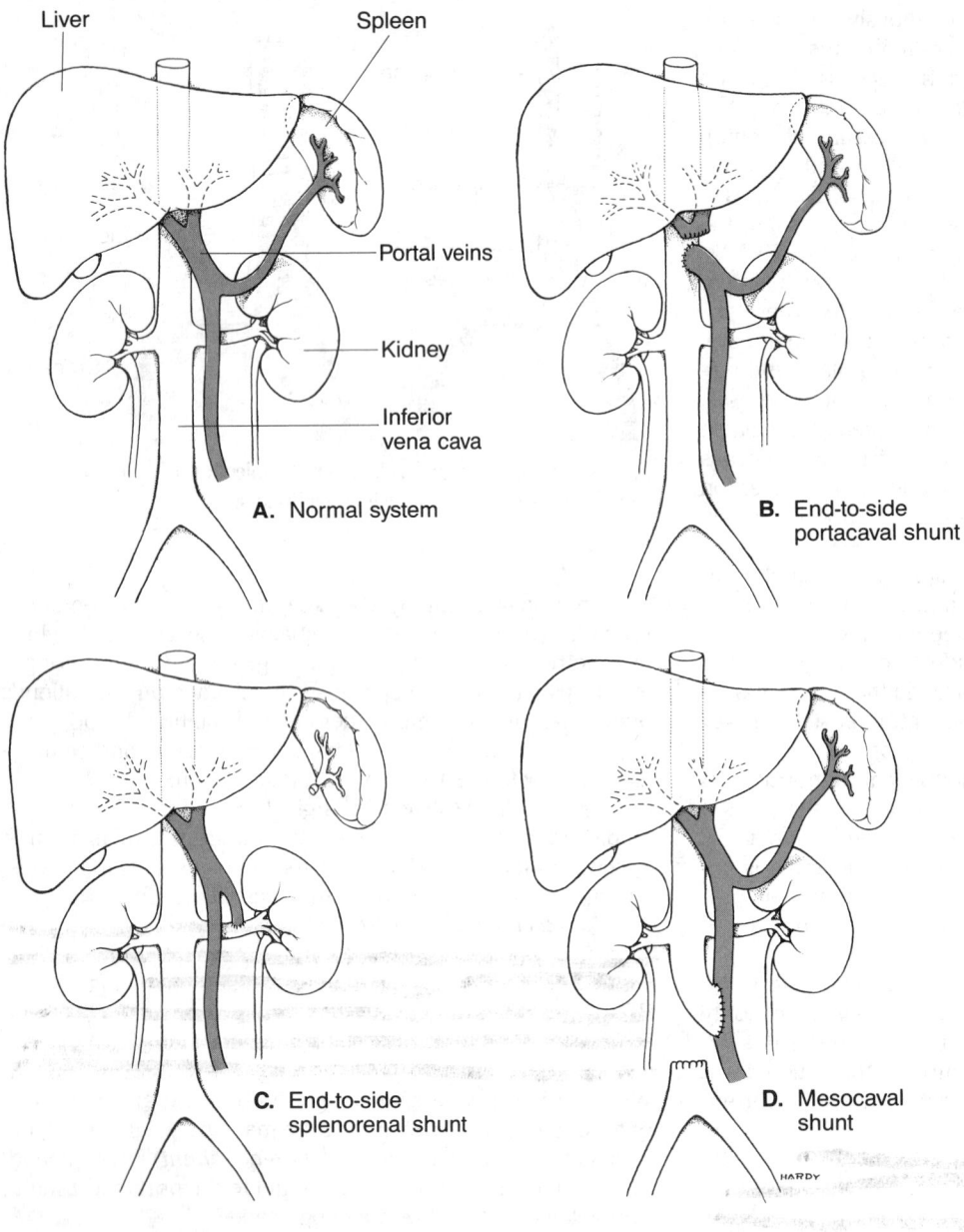

Liver   Spleen

Portal veins

Kidney

Inferior
vena cava

A. Normal system

B. End-to-side
portacaval shunt

C. End-to-side
splenorenal shunt

D. Mesocaval
shunt

Figure 38–9. Normal portal system
and examples of portal-systemic shunts.

Postoperative Nursing Interventions. Bleeding anywhere in the body is anxiety provoking, resulting in a crisis situation for the patient and his family. If the patient is an alcoholic, delirium secondary to alcohol withdrawal can further complicate the situation. The nurse provides support and pertinent explanations regarding medical and nursing interventions. Monitoring the patient closely will help in detecting and managing complications.

Postoperative care is similar to that for any abdominal operation, but complications may arise, including hypovolemic or hemorrhagic shock, hepatic encephalopathy, electrolyte imbalance, metabolic and respiratory alkalosis, alcohol withdrawal syndrome, and seizures. The surgical procedures do not alter the course of the progressive liver disease, and bleeding may recur as new collateral vessels develop.

Management modalities and nursing care of the patient with bleeding esophageal varices are summarized in Chart 38–3.

Cancer of the Liver

Hepatic tumors generally are cancerous. It has been only in recent years that benign liver tumors have gained any significance, as their incidence has increased with the use of oral contraceptives.

As for cancerous tumors, few cancers originate in the liver. Those that are primary tumors ordinarily occur in patients with cirrhosis, especially of the postnecrotic type. Such a *hepatoma* is usually nonresectable because of rapid extension and metastasis elsewhere. *Cholangiocarcinoma* is a primary malignant tumor, usually arising in normal liver. If found early, cure may be possible, but the likelihood of early detection is small.

In addition, cirrhosis, hepatitis B, and exposure to certain chemical toxins (*e.g.*, vinyl chloride, arsenic) have been implicated in the etiology of primary cancer of the liver. Cigarette smoking has also been identified as a risk factor, especially when combined with alcohol use. Other substances that have been implicated include aflatoxins or carcinogens in herbal medicines, and nitrosamines.

Metastases from other primary sites are found in the liver in about one half of all late cancer cases. Malignant tumors are likely to reach the liver eventually by way of the portal system, the lymphatic channels, or by direct extension from an abdominal tumor. Moreover, the liver apparently is an ideal place for these malignant cells to thrive. Often the first evidence of cancer in an abdominal organ is the appearance of liver metastases, and, unless exploratory operation or autopsy is performed, the primary tumor may never be discovered.

The early manifestations of malignant disease of the liver include signs and symptoms of any cancer that interferes with nutrition; these include recent loss of weight, loss of strength, anorexia, and anemia. Abdominal pain may be present and accompanied by rapid enlargement of the liver, which on palpation presents an irregular surface. Jaundice is present only if the larger bile ducts are occluded by the pressure of malignant nodules in the hilum of the liver. Ascites occurs if such nodules obstruct the portal veins or if tumor tissue is seeded in the peritoneal cavity.

The diagnosis of cancer of the liver is made on the basis of clinical signs and symptoms, history and physical examination, and results of laboratory and radiologic findings. Increased serum levels of bilirubin, alkaline phosphatase, glutamic oxaloacetic transaminase (SGOT), and lactic dehydrogenase (LDH) may occur. Leukocytosis (increased white blood cells, erythrocytosis [increased red blood cells], hypercalcemia, hypoglycemia, and hypocholesterolemia may also be seen on laboratory assessment. The serum level of alphafetoprotein (which serves as a tumor marker) is abnormally elevated in 30% to 40% of patients with liver cancer.

Many patients have metastases from the primary liver tumor to other sites by the time diagnosis is made; metastases occur primarily to the lung, but may also occur to regional lymph nodes, adrenals, bone, kidneys, heart, pancreas, and stomach.

Nonsurgical Management

Radiation therapy and chemotherapy have been used in the treatment of malignant disease of the liver with varying degrees of success. Although these therapies may prolong survival and improve the patient's quality of life by reducing pain and discomfort, the major effect remains palliative.

Radiation Therapy. Pain and discomfort have been effectively reduced in 70% to 90% of patients with radiation therapy; anorexia, weakness, and fever also have been reduced. Liver function tests may improve temporarily. Other methods of delivering radiation include (1) intravenous injection of antibodies to tumor-associated antigens tagged with radioactive isotopes and (2) percutaneous placement of a high-intensity source for interstitial radiation therapy. Their purpose is to deliver radiation directly to the tumor cells. Radiation therapy combined with chemotherapy has also been attempted, with no additional benefit demonstrated.

Chemotherapy. Chemotherapy has been used to improve the patient's quality of life and prolong survival; it also may be used as adjuvant therapy after surgical resection of hepatic tumors. Systemic chemotherapy and regional infusion chemotherapy are two methods used to administer antineoplastic agents to patients with primary and metastatic hepatic tumors.

An implantable pump has been used to deliver a high concentration of chemotherapy to the liver through the hepatic artery. This method provides a reliable, controlled, and continuous infusion of drug that can be carried out in the patient's home.

Patient Education and Home Health Care. The patient and family are instructed to assess and report complications and side effects of the drug. Therefore, they need to be well informed about its actions and desired and undesirable effects. They are instructed by the nurse about the importance of follow-up visits to permit frequent checks on the response of the patient and the tumor to chemotherapy, the condition of the site of the pump insertion, and the occurrence of toxic effects. The patient is encouraged to resume routine activities as soon as possible, but warned to avoid contact sports and other activities that may damage the pump.

Percutaneous Biliary Drainage. Percutaneous biliary or transhepatic drainage is used to bypass biliary ducts obstructed by liver, pancreatic, or bile duct tumors in patients with inoperable tumors or in those considered poor surgical risks. Under fluoroscopy, a catheter is inserted through the abdominal wall, past the obstruction into the duodenum. Such procedures are used to reestablish biliary drainage, relieve pressure and pain from buildup of bile behind the obstruction, and decrease pruritus and jaundice. As a result, the patient is more comfortable and quality of life and survival are improved. For several days after its insertion, the catheter is opened to external drainage. The bile is observed closely for amount, color, and the presence of blood and debris.

Complications of percutaneous biliary drainage include sepsis, leakage of bile, hemorrhage, and reobstruction of the biliary system by debris in the catheter or from encroaching tumor. Therefore, the patient is observed for fever and chills, bile drainage around the catheter, changes in vital signs, and evidence of biliary obstruction, including increased pain or pressure, pruritus, and recurrence of jaundice.

Patient Education and Home Health Care. The patient and his family often fear that the catheter will be dislodged. They need reassurance and instruction to reduce their fear that the catheter will fall out easily. Additionally, the patient and family require verbal and written instruction as well as demonstration of catheter care. They are instructed in techniques to keep the catheter site clean and dry and to assess the catheter and its insertion site. Irrigation of the catheter with sterile normal saline or water may be prescribed to keep the catheter patent and free of debris. The patient and his caregivers are taught proper technique to avoid introducing bacteria into the biliary system or catheter during irrigation. They are instructed not to aspirate or draw back on the syringe during irrigation to prevent entry of irritating duodenal contents into the biliary tree or catheter. The patient and his caregivers are also instructed about the signs of complications and are encouraged to notify the nurse or physician if problems or questions occur.

Other Nonsurgical Treatment Modalities. Hyperthermia has been used as a treatment modality for hepatic metastases. Heat has been directed to tumors through several methods to cause necrosis of the tumors while sparing normal tissue. Freezing hepatic tumor cells by *cryosurgery* and use of *laser surgery* are in the early stages of development as treatment modalities. *Immunotherapy* is another treatment modality currently under investigation. In this therapy, lymphocytes with antitumor reactivity are administered to the patient with a hepatic tumor. Regression of the tumor, the desired outcome, has been demonstrated in patients with metastatic cancer in whom standard treatment has failed. These newer modes of therapy require further study before their benefits and side effects are known.

Surgical Management

Successful hepatic lobectomy for cancer can be performed when the primary hepatic tumor is localized or when, in the case of metastasis, the primary site can be completely excised and the metastasis is limited. Metastases to the liver, however, are rarely limited or solitary. Capitalizing on the regenerative capacity of the liver cells, some surgeons have successfully removed 90% of the liver. The presence of cirrhosis limits the ability of the liver to regenerate.

Preoperative Evaluation and Preparation. As the patient is being prepared for surgery, his nutritional, fluid, emotional, and physical needs are evaluated and addressed. Support, explanation, and encouragement are provided to help him prepare physically and psychologically for the surgery. Meanwhile, he may be undergoing extensive and exhausting diagnostic studies. It may be necessary to prepare the intestinal tract by way of cathartics, colonic irrigation, and intestinal antibiotics to minimize the possibility of ammonium accumulation and to anticipate the possibility of incision into the intestines at surgery. Specific studies may include liver scan, liver biopsy, cholangiography, selective hepatic angiography, percutaneous needle biopsy, peritoneoscopy, laparoscopy, ultrasound and CT scans, and blood tests, particularly determinations of serum alkaline phosphatase and serum glutamic oxaloacetic acid levels.

Surgical Intervention. If it is necessary to restrict blood flow from the hepatic artery and portal vein beyond 15 minutes (under normothermic conditions, 15-minute occlusion is permissible), it is likely that hypothermia will be used. Most surgeons prefer the anatomic (surgical) division of the lobes. Here the liver is divided into a right and a left lobe by a lobar fissure that is almost in line with the gallbladder bed and the inferior vena cava on the visceral surface. According to this division, the branching of hepatic vessels and the portal vein lend themselves to a more even segmentation. A right-liver lobectomy according to the surgical division is less extensive than it would be in the functional division.

For a right-liver lobectomy or an extended right lobectomy (including medial left lobe), a thoracoabdominal incision is used. An extensive abdominal incision is made for a left lobectomy.

Postoperative Nursing Interventions. There are potential problems related to cardiopulmonary involvement, vascular complications, and respiratory and liver dysfunction. Metabolic abnormalities require careful attention. A constant infusion of 10% glucose may be required in the first 48 hours to prevent a precipitous fall in blood sugar, resulting from decreased gluconeogenesis. Protein synthesis and lipid metabolism are also altered, necessitating infusions of albumin. Extensive blood loss may occur, and, as a result, the patient will receive infusions of blood and intravenous fluids. The patient requires constant close monitoring and care for the first 2 or 3 days, as described for abdominal and thoracic postsurgical nursing care (see Chap. 22). Early ambulation is encouraged. Liver regeneration is rapid; in one patient who had a 90% resection of the liver, a normal liver mass was restored in 6 months.

Liver Transplantation to Treat Liver Tumors. Removal of the liver and its replacement by a healthy donor organ has been successful. Recurrence of the primary liver malignancy after transplantation, however, has been reported to be 80% to 85%. Therefore, it has been recommended that the patient be treated with systemic chemotherapy or radiation therapy along with liver transplantation.

Liver Transplantation

Liver transplantation is used to treat life-threatening end-stage liver disease for which no other form of treatment is available. The results of liver transplantation have improved remarkably with the use of cyclosporine. This immunosuppressive agent, used in combination with corticosteroids, has contributed to the current 1-year success rate of 80%. Despite this success, liver transplantation is not a routine procedure and may be accompanied by complications related to the lengthy surgical procedure, immunosuppressive therapy, infection, and technical difficulties encountered in reconstruction of blood vessels and the biliary tract. Additionally, long-standing systemic problems resulting from the patient's primary liver disease may complicate the patient's preoperative and postoperative course. Previous surgery of the abdomen, including procedures to treat complications of advanced liver disease (i.e., shunt procedures used to treat portal hypertension and esophageal varices), increase the complexity of the transplantation procedure.

The indications for liver transplantation are not as limited today as a result of use of veno-venous bypass, advances in immunosuppressive therapy, and improvements in biliary tract reconstruction. General indications for liver transplantation include irreversible advanced chronic liver disease, fulminant hepatic failure, metabolic liver diseases, and hepatic malignancies, where resection for cure requires complete removal of the liver. Examples of disorders that are indications for liver transplantation include hepatocellular liver disease (e.g., viral hepatitis, drug- and alcohol-induced liver disease, and Wilson's disease) and cholestatic diseases (e.g., primary biliary cirrhosis, sclerosis cholangitis, and biliary atresia). Liver transplantation is now recognized as an established therapeutic modality rather than as an experimental procedure to treat these disorders. As a result, centers where liver transplantation is performed are proliferating. Patients requiring transplantation are often referred from distant hospitals to these sites. To prepare the potential patient and his family for liver transplantation, nurses in all settings require an understanding of the process and the procedure of liver transplantation.

Orthotopic liver transplantation involves total removal of the diseased liver and its replacement with a healthy liver. Removal of the patient's liver leaves a space for the new liver and permits anatomic reconstruction of the hepatic vasculature and biliary tract as close to normal as possible. The patient being considered for liver transplantation frequently has many systemic problems that influence preoperative and postoperative care. Because success of transplantation is more difficult when the patient has developed severe gastrointestinal bleeding and advanced hepatic coma, efforts are made to perform the procedure before this stage.

Preoperative Nursing Interventions. Once it is evident that a patient has irreversible severe liver dysfunction, he may be considered a potential candidate for transplantation. The patient will undergo extensive diagnostic evaluation to determine if he is a suitable candidate for transplantation. The patient and his family are given full explanations about the procedure and about the chances of success of transplantation and its risks, including the side effects of long-term immunosuppression. The need for close follow-up and lifelong compliance with the therapeutic regimen, including immunosuppression, is explained to the patient and his family. Once the patient is accepted as a suitable candidate for transplantation, his name is placed on a waiting list at the transplant center; patient information is entered into the United Network Organ Sharing (UNOS) computer system so that candidates may be identified and matched when appropriate organs become available. Because a liver becomes available for transplantation only with the death of another individual, usually healthy except for severe brain injury and brain death, the patient and his family undergo a stressful waiting period. The nurse is often the major source of support for the patient and family during this period. The patient must be accessible at all times in case an appropriate liver becomes available. During this time the patient's liver function may deteriorate further and he may experience other complications from the primary liver disease. Because of the current shortage of donor organs, patients sometimes die awaiting transplantation.

Malnutrition, massive ascites, and fluid and electrolyte disturbances are treated before surgery to increase the patient's chances of a successful outcome. If the patient's liver dysfunction has a very rapid onset, as in fulminant hepatic failure, there is little time or opportunity for the patient to consider and weigh options and their consequences; often this patient has developed coma, and the decision to proceed with transplantation is made by the patient's family.

The nurse coordinator is an integral member of the transplant team who plays an important role in the evaluation of the patient for liver transplantation. She serves as a patient and family advocate and assumes the important role of link between the patient and the other members of the transplant team. Additionally, the nurse serves as a resource to other nurses and health care team members involved in evaluation and care of the patient undergoing this procedure.

Surgical Procedure

The donor liver is freed from other structures; the bile is flushed from the gallbladder to prevent damage to the walls of the biliary tract; and the liver is perfused with a preservation solution, and cooled. Before placing the donor liver in the recipient, it is flushed with cold lactated Ringer's solution to remove potassium and air bubbles. Anastomoses of the blood vessels and bile duct between the donor and the recipient's liver are performed. Biliary reconstruction is performed with an end-to-end anastomosis of the donor and recipient common bile ducts; a stented T-tube is inserted to permit external drainage of bile. If an end-to-end anastomosis is not possible because of diseased or absent bile ducts, an end-to-side anastomosis will be made between the common bile duct of the graft and a loop (Roux-en-Y portion) of jejunum; in this case, bile drainage will be internal and a T-tube will not be inserted. Liver transplantation is a long procedure partly because the patient with liver failure often has portal hypertension and subsequently many venous collateral vessels that must be ligated. Blood loss during the surgical procedure may be extensive. If the patient has adhesions from previous abdominal surgery, lysis of adhesions is often necessary. If a shunt procedure was performed previously, it must be surgically reversed to permit adequate portal venous blood supply to the new liver.

Postoperative Nursing Interventions.   The patient is maintained in an environment as free from bacteria, viruses, and fungi as possible because immunosuppressive drugs reduce the body's natural defenses. In the immediate postoperative period, the patient is monitored continuously for cardiovascular, pulmonary, renal, neurologic, and metabolic function. Mean arterial and pulmonary artery pressures are monitored continuously. Cardiac output, central venous pressure, pulmonary capillary wedge pressure, arterial and mixed venous blood gases, urine output, heart rate, and blood pressure are used to evaluate the patient's hemodynamic status and intravascular fluid volume. Liver function tests, electrolyte levels, the coagulation profile, chest x-ray, cardiogram, and fluid output including urine, bile, and drainage from chest tubes and Jackson Pratt tubes are monitored closely. Because the liver is responsible for storage of glycogen and synthesis of protein and clotting factors, monitoring and replacement of these substances in the immediate postoperative period are essential.

Because of the likelihood of atelectasis and an altered ventilation–perfusion ratio due to insult to the diaphragm during the surgical procedure, prolonged anesthesia, immobility, postoperative pain, and the presence of chest tubes, the patient will have an endotracheal tube in place and require mechanical ventilation during the initial postoperative period. Suctioning is performed as required and sterile humidification is provided.

The postoperative complication rate is high and is related primarily to technical complications or infection. Immediate postoperative complications may include bleeding, infection, rejection, and impaired biliary drainage. Disruption, infection, or obstruction of biliary anastomosis may occur. Bleeding is common in the postoperative period and may result from coagulopathy, portal hypertension, and fibrinolysis caused by ischemic injury to the donor liver. Hypotension may occur in this phase secondary to blood loss. Administration of platelets, fresh frozen plasma, and other blood products may be necessary. Hypertension is more common; however, its cause is uncertain. This is treated if blood pressure elevation is significant or sustained.

Infection is the leading cause of death after liver transplantation. Pulmonary and fungal infections are common; susceptibility to infection is increased by immunosuppression needed to prevent rejection. Therefore, precautions must be taken to prevent nosocomial infections by strict asepsis when manipulating arterial, urinary, bile, and other drainage systems, obtaining specimens, and changing dressings.

A transplanted liver is perceived by the immune system as a foreign antigen. It triggers an immune response, leading to the activation of T lymphocytes that attack and destroy the transplanted liver. Cyclosporine is used to prevent this response and rejection of the transplanted liver. It inhibits the activation of immunocompetent T lymphocytes to prevent the production of effector T cells. Although the 1- and 5-year survival rates have increased dramatically since the advent of cyclosporine, it is not without major side effects. Nephrotoxicity is the major side effect of cyclosporine; this problem seems to be dose related, and renal dysfunction can be reversed if the dose of cyclosporine is appropriately decreased. Liver biopsy and ultrasound may be required to investigate suspected episodes of rejection. Corticosteroids, azathioprine, anti-lymphocytic globulin, and monoclonal antibody OKT3 are other agents in use in transplantation. Clinical trials of newer immunosuppressive agents continue; FK506 is a new immonosuppressive agent that appears to have fewer side effects than cyclosporine.

Retransplantation is usually attempted if failure of the transplanted liver occurs. The success rate of retransplantation does not approach that of the initial transplantation, however.

Patient Education and Home Care Considerations. Teaching the patient and family about long-term measures to promote health is an important function of the nurse. The patient and his family must understand the reasons for required continuous adherence to the therapeutic regimen, with special emphasis on the methods of administration, rationale, and side effects of the prescribed immunosuppressive agents. The patient is given written as well as verbal instructions about how and when to take the medications and is instructed to take steps to be sure that an adequate supply of medication is available so that he does not run out of the medication or skip a dose. He is instructed about the signs and symptoms that are indications of problems requiring consultation with the transplant team. The patient with a T-tube in place will be instructed in care of the tube.

The importance of follow-up blood work and visits to the transplant team is emphasized. Cyclosporine trough levels will be obtained along with other blood tests that indicate the function of the liver and kidneys. During the first months, the patient is likely to require blood work two to three times a week. As his condition stabilizes, blood work and visits to the transplant team will be scheduled less frequently. The importance of routine ophthalmology examinations is emphasized because of the increased incidence of cataracts and glaucoma with long-term steroid therapy. Regular oral hygiene and follow-up dental care, with administration of prophylactic antibiotics before dental treatments, are recommended because of the immunosuppression.

The patient is advised that while a successful transplantation will not return him to normal, it does increase his chances for survival and a more normal life than he had before transplantation, if rejection and infection can be prevented. Many patients have lived successful and productive lives after liver transplantation. Several women have had normal pregnancies and delivered normal infants after liver transplantation.

Liver Abscesses

Whenever an infection develops anywhere along the gastrointestinal tract, there is danger that the infecting organisms may reach the liver through the biliary system, portal venous system, or hepatic arterial or lymphatic systems. Most bacteria are promptly destroyed, but occasionally some gain a foothold. The bacterial toxins destroy the neighboring liver cells, and the necrotic tissue produced serves as a protective wall for the organisms. Meanwhile, leukocytes migrate into the infected area. The result is an abscess cavity full of a liquid containing living and dead leukocytes, liquefied liver cells, and bacteria. Pyogenic abscesses of this type may be either single or multiple and small.

The clinical picture is one of sepsis with few or no localizing signs. The temperature is elevated and may be accompanied by chills. The patient may complain of dull abdominal pain and tenderness in the right upper quadrant of the abdomen. Hepatomegaly, jaundice, and anemia may develop. The result is a life-threatening disease. In the past, mortality was 100% because of the vague clinical symptoms, inadequate diagnostic tools, and inadequate surgical drainage of the abscess. With the aid of a CT scan and a liver scan for early diagnosis, and surgical drainage of the abscess, mortality has been greatly reduced.

Treatment includes intravenous antibiotic therapy; the specific antibiotic used in treatment depends on the organism identified. *Entamoeba histolytica* is the most common cause of liver abscess. In certain geographic areas, gram-negative bacilli have been implicated with increased frequency. Continuous supportive care is indicated because of the serious condition of the patient.

In summary, the liver is a highly complex organ in terms of structure and function. Therefore, when dysfunction of the liver occurs, systemic problems ranging from mild flulike symptoms to gastrointestinal hemorrhage and hepatic coma are possible. Patients with liver dysfunction are often chronically ill; however, acute fulminating liver disease may occur. Management of liver disease today ranges from symptomatic treatment of symptoms such as ascites, jaundice, and GI bleeding to replacement of a severely damaged liver through transplantation. Nursing care of the patient with chronic liver dysfunction may include assisting a patient with cirrhosis to cope with chronic or long-term symptoms and promoting healthy life styles. Nursing management of the patient with acute liver disease and liver failure may focus on relieving the systemic effects of the dysfunction, assessment, and early intervention for life-threatening symptoms such as GI hemorrhage, and assisting with recovery from liver transplantation.

Liver failure is the fourth leading cause of death in the United States, and disease of the liver is responsible for considerable disability. Many liver disorders are preventable; therefore, education regarding use of alcohol, drugs, and other health promotion strategies is an important aspect of the nurse's role in health promotion and prevention of liver disease.

Biliary Conditions

Several disorders affect the biliary system and interfere with normal drainage of bile into the duodenum. These disorders include carcinoma that obstructs the biliary tree and infection of the biliary system. Gallbladder disease with gallstones, however, is the most common disorder of the biliary system. Although not all occurrences of gallbladder infection (*cholecystitis*) are related to gallstones (*cholelithiasis*), 95% of patients with acute cholecystitis have gallstones. Most of the 15 million Americans with gallstones have no pain, however, and are unaware of the presence of stones. For a guide to the terminology associated with biliary disorders and procedures, see Chart 38-4.

Chart 38–4
Terminology—Biliary Disorders and Procedures

Cholecystitis—inflammation of the gallbladder
Cholelithiasis—the presence of calculi in the gallbladder
Cholecystectomy—removal of the gallbladder
Cholecystostomy—opening and drainage of the gallbladder
Choledochotomy—opening into the common duct
Choledocholithiasis—stones in the common duct
Choledocholithotomy—incision of common bile duct for removal of stones
Choledochoduodenostomy—anastomosis of common duct to duodenum
Choledochojejunostomy—anastomosis of common duct to jejunum
Lithotripsy—disintegration of gallstones by shock waves
Laparoscopic cholecystectomy—removal of gallbladder through endoscopic procedure
Laser cholecystectomy—removal of gallbladder using laser rather than scalpel and traditional surgical instruments

---

Cholecystitis

The gallbladder may be the site of an acute infection (cholecystitis) that causes acute pain, tenderness, and rigidity of the upper right abdomen, associated with nausea and vomiting and the usual signs of an acute inflammation. This condition is referred to as *acute cholecystitis*. If the gallbladder is found to be filled with pus, there is an *empyema* of the gallbladder.

Ninety percent of patients with acute cholecystitis have *calculous cholecystitis*; that is, a gallbladder stone obstructs bile outflow. Bile remaining in the gallbladder initiates a chemical reaction; autolysis and edema occur; and the blood vessels in the gallbladder are compressed, compromising its vascular supply. Consequently, gangrene of the gallbladder with perforation results. Bacteria play a minor role in acute cholecystitis. Bacterial invasion may occur *after* breakdown of local defense mechanisms.

Acalculous cholecystitis describes acute gallbladder inflammation in the absence of obstruction by gallstones. Acalculous cholecystitis occurs after major surgical procedures, severe trauma, or burns. It is speculated that it results from alterations in fluids and electrolytes and in regional blood flow in the visceral circulation. Its occurrence with major procedures or trauma makes its diagnosis difficult.

Cholelithiasis

Cholelithiasis (calculi, or gallstones) usually form in the gallbladder from the solid constituents of bile and vary greatly in size, shape, and composition (Fig. 38–10).

Gallstones are uncommon in children and young adults but become increasingly prevalent after age 40. The incidence of cholelithiasis increases thereafter to such an extent that it has been estimated that by the age of 75, one of every three people will have gallstones.

Pathophysiology

There are two major types of gallstones: those composed predominantly of pigment and those composed primarily of cho-

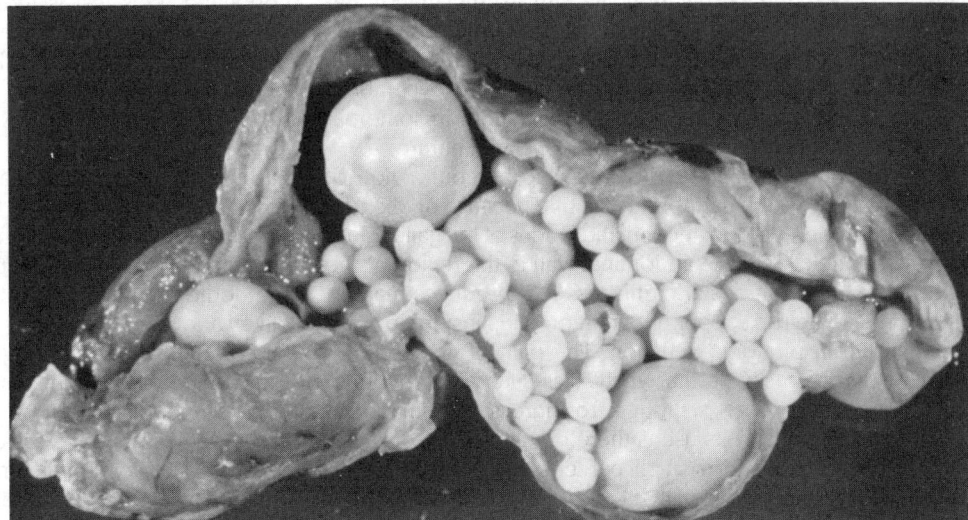

Figure 38–10. Multiple gallstones in a gallbladder. (Courtesy of National Institute of Diabetes and Digestive and Kidney Diseases.)

lesterol. Pigment stones probably form when unconjugated pigments in the bile precipitate to form stones. The risk of developing such stones is increased in patients with cirrhosis, hemolysis, and infections of the biliary tree. These stones cannot be dissolved and must be removed surgically.

Cholesterol stones account for most gallbladder disease in the United States. Cholesterol, a normal constituent of bile, is insoluble in water. Its solubility depends on bile acids and lecithin (phospholipids) in bile. In gallstone-prone patients, there is decreased bile acid synthesis and increased cholesterol synthesis in the liver, resulting in a bile supersaturated with cholesterol, which precipitates out of the bile to form stones. The cholesterol-saturated bile predisposes to the formation of gallstones and acts as an irritant, producing inflammatory changes in the gallbladder.

Four times more women than men develop cholesterol stones and gallbladder disease; they are usually over 40 years of age, multiparous, and obese. The incidence of stone formation is increased in users of oral contraceptives, estrogens, and clofibrate, which are known to increase biliary cholesterol saturation. The incidence of stone formation increases with age as a result of increased hepatic secretion of cholesterol and decreased bile acid synthesis. In addition, there is increased risk because of malabsorption of bile salts in patients with gastrointestinal disease or T-tube fistula or in those who have had ileal resection or bypass.

Clinical Manifestations

Gallstones may be silent, producing no pain and only mild gastrointestinal symptoms. Such stones may be detected incidentally during surgery or evaluation for nonrelated problems.

The patient with gallbladder disease due to gallstones may develop two types of symptoms: those due to disease of the gallbladder itself and those due to obstruction of the bile passages by a gallstone. The symptoms may be acute or chronic. Epigastric distress, such as fullness, abdominal distention, and vague pain in the right upper quadrant of the abdomen, may occur. This distress may follow a meal high in fried or fatty foods.

If a gallstone obstructs the cystic duct, the gallbladder becomes distended and eventually infected. The patient develops a fever and may have a palpable abdominal mass. The patient may experience biliary colic with excruciating upper right abdominal pain that radiates to the back or right shoulder, is usually associated with nausea and vomiting, and is noticeable several hours after a heavy meal. The patient moves about restlessly, unable to find a comfortable position. In some patients the pain is constant rather than colicky in nature.

Such a bout of biliary colic is caused by contraction of the gallbladder, which cannot release bile because of obstruction by the stone. When distended, the fundus of the gallbladder comes in contact with the abdominal wall in the region of the right ninth and tenth costal cartilages. This produces marked tenderness in the right upper quadrant on deep inspiration and prevents full inspiratory excursion. The pain of acute cholecystitis may be so severe that analgesics such as meperidine are required. Morphine is thought to increase spasm of the sphincter of Oddi, and its use is therefore avoided.

Jaundice occurs in a small percentage of patients with gallbladder disease and usually occurs with obstruction of the common bile duct. Obstruction of the flow of bile into the duodenum results in the following characteristic symptoms: the bile, no longer carried to the duodenum, is absorbed by the blood, giving the skin and mucous membrane a yellow color. This is frequently accompanied by marked itching of the skin.

The excretion of the bile pigments by the kidneys gives the urine a very dark color. The feces, no longer colored with bile pigments, are grayish, like putty, and usually described as "clay-colored."

Obstruction of bile flow also interferes with absorption of the fat-soluble vitamins A, D, E, and K. Therefore, the patient may exhibit deficiencies of these vitamins if biliary obstruction has been prolonged. Vitamin K deficiency will interfere with normal blood clotting.

If the gallstone is dislodged and no longer obstructs the cystic duct, the gallbladder drains and the inflammatory process subsides after a relatively short time. If the gallstone continues to obstruct the duct, abscess, necrosis, and perforation with generalized peritonitis may result.

Diagnostic Evaluation

Abdominal Radiograph.   An abdominal radiograph may be obtained if gallbladder disease is suggested and to exclude other causes of symptoms. Only 15% to 20% of gallstones are sufficiently calcified to be visible on such films, however.

Ultrasonography.   Ultrasonography has replaced oral cholecystography as the diagnostic procedure of choice because it is rapid and accurate and can be used in patients with liver dysfunction and jaundice. Additionally, it does not expose patients to ionizing radiation. The procedure is most accurate if the patient fasts overnight so that the gallbladder is distended. The use of ultrasound is based on reflected sound waves. Ultrasonography can detect calculi in the gallbladder or a dilated common bile duct. It is reported to detect gallstones with 95% accuracy.

Radionuclide Imaging or Cholescintography.   Cholescintigraphy is used successfully in diagnosis of acute cholecystitis. In this procedure a radioactive agent is administered intravenously. It is then taken up by the hepatocytes and rapidly excreted through the biliary system. The biliary tract is then scanned, and images of the gallbladder and biliary tree are obtained. This test is more expensive than ultrasonography, takes longer to perform, exposes the patient to radiation, and cannot detect gallstones. Its use may be limited to those cases in which ultrasonography is not conclusive.

Cholecystography.   Although it has been replaced by ultrasonography as the test of choice, cholecystography is still used if ultrasound equipment is not available or if the ultrasound results are inconclusive. Oral cholangiography may be performed to detect gallstones and to assess the ability of the gallbladder to fill, concentrate its contents, contract, and empty. An iodide-containing contrast medium that is excreted by the liver and concentrated in the gallbladder is administered to the patient. The normal gallbladder fills with this radiopaque substance. If gallstones are present, they appear as shadows on the radiograph.

Medications given as contrast media include iopanoic acid (Telepaque), iodipamide meglumine (Cholografin), and sodium ipodate (Oragrafin). These preparations are given in oral doses,

10 to 12 hours before x-ray study. The patient is permitted nothing by mouth after administration of the contrast medium, to prevent contraction and emptying of the gallbladder.

The patient is questioned about allergies to iodine or seafood. If no allergy is identified, the patient receives the oral form of the contrast medium the evening before the radiographs are obtained. A radiograph of the right upper abdomen is obtained. If the gallbladder is found to fill and empty normally and to contain no stones, it is concluded that no gallbladder disease is present. If gallbladder disease is present, the gallbladder may not be visualized because of obstruction by gallstones. A repeat of the oral cholecystogram with a second dose of the contrast medium may be necessary if the gallbladder is not visualized on the first attempt. Cholecystography in the obviously jaundiced patient is not useful because the liver cannot excrete the radiopaque dye into the gallbladder in a jaundiced patient. Oral cholecystogram is likely to continue to be used as part of the evaluation of patients who have been treated with gallstone dissolution therapy or lithotripsy.

Endoscopic Retrograde Cholangiopancreatography. Endoscopic retrograde cholangiopancreatography (ERCP) permits direct visualization of structures once available only during laparotomy. It involves insertion of a flexible fiberoptic endoscope into the esophagus to the descending duodenum (Fig. 38–11). The common bile duct and pancreatic duct are cannulated and contrast material is injected into the ducts, permitting visualization and evaluation of the biliary tree. ERCP also permits direct visualization of these structures and access to the distal common bile duct to retrieve a retained gallstone.

Nursing Interventions. The procedure requires a cooperative patient to permit insertion of the endoscope without damage to the gastrointestinal tract structures, including the biliary

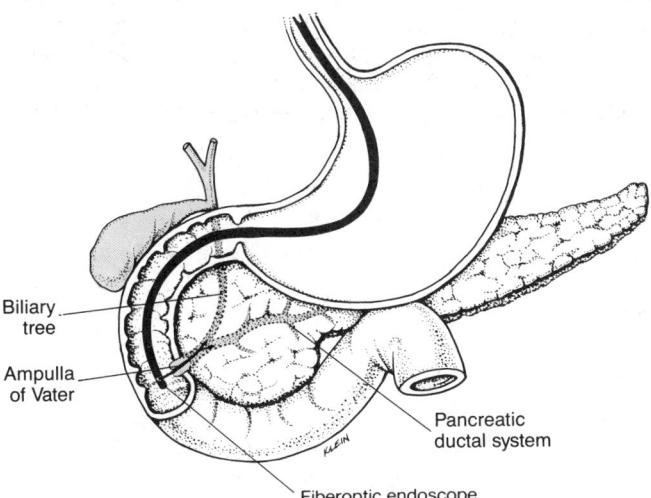

Biliary tree

Ampulla of Vater

Pancreatic ductal system

Fiberoptic endoscope

Figure 38–11. Endoscopic retrograde cholangiopancreatography (ERCP). By means of a side-viewing fiberoptic duodenoscope, the ampulla of Vater is catheterized and the biliary tree injected with contrast material. The pancreatic ductal system is also assessed, if indicated. This procedure is of special value in ampullary or periampullary neoplasms, which may be simultaneously visualized and a biopsy performed. Acute pancreatitis is a contraindication. (Redrawn from Misra PS and Bank S. Gallbladder disease: Guide to diagnosis. Hosp Med.)

tree. Before the procedure, the patient is given an explanation of the procedure and his role in it. Sedation is administered immediately before the procedure. During ERCP, the nurse monitors intravenous fluids, administers medications, and positions the patient. After the procedure, the nurse monitors the patient's condition, observing vital signs and checking for signs of perforation or infection. The nurse also monitors the patient for side effects of any medications received during the procedure and return of the patient's gag reflex after the use of local anesthetics.

Percutaneous Transhepatic Cholangiography. Percutaneous transhepatic cholangiography (PTC) involves the injection of dye directly into the biliary tree. Because of the relatively large concentration of dye that is introduced into the biliary system, all components of the system, including the hepatic ducts within the liver, the entire length of the common bile duct, the cystic duct, and the gallbladder, are clearly outlined.

This procedure can be carried out even in the presence of liver dysfunction and jaundice. It is useful in distinguishing jaundice caused by liver disease (hepatocellular jaundice) from that due to biliary obstruction; for investigating the gastrointestinal symptoms of patients whose gallbladders have been removed; for locating stones within the bile ducts; and in diagnosing cancer involving the biliary system.

Procedure. The patient, who is fasting and well sedated, lies supine on the x-ray table. The injection site, which is usually in the midclavicular line immediately beneath the right costal margin, is disinfected and anesthetized with lidocaine (Xylocaine). A small incision is made at this point and a thin, flexible needle ("skinny" needle) with stylet is inserted cephalad, posteriorly at a 45-degree angle and parallel to the midline. When the needle has penetrated to a depth of approximately 10 cm (4 in), the stylet is removed and replaced by a plastic connector tube with a 50-ml syringe attached. Gentle suction is applied while the needle is slowly withdrawn, until bile appears in the syringe. As much bile as possible is withdrawn, a radiopaque dye is injected, and an x-ray film obtained.

Before the needle is removed, as much dye and bile as possible are aspirated to forestall subsequent leakage into the needle tract and eventually into the peritoneal cavity, to minimize the risk of bile peritonitis.

Nursing Interventions. Although the complication rate after this procedure is low, the patient must be observed closely for symptoms of bleeding, peritonitis, and septicemia. Pain and indicators of these complications should be reported immediately. Antibiotics should be administered as prescribed to minimize the risk of sepsis and septic shock.

Nonsurgical Management

The major objectives of medical therapy are to reduce the incidence of acute attacks of gallbladder pain and cholecystitis by supportive and dietary management, and, if possible, to remove the cause of cholecystitis by pharmacotherapy, endoscopic procedures, or surgical intervention.

Supportive and Dietary Management. Approximately 80% of the patients with acute gallbladder inflammation achieve a remission with rest, intravenous fluids, nasogastric suction, analgesia, and antibiotics. Unless the patient's condition deteriorates, surgical intervention is delayed until the patient's acute symptoms subside and complete evaluation can be carried out.

The diet immediately after an attack is usually limited to low-fat liquids. Powdered supplements high in protein and carbohydrate can be stirred into skim milk. The following may then be added as tolerated: cooked fruits, rice or tapioca, lean meats, mashed potatoes, non–gas-forming vegetables, bread, coffee, or tea. Eggs, cream, pork, fried foods, cheese and rich dressings, gas-forming vegetables, and alcohol are avoided. The patient needs to be reminded that fatty foods may bring on an attack.

Dietary management may be the major mode of therapy in those patients who have experienced only dietary intolerance to fatty foods and vague gastrointestinal symptoms.

Pharmacotherapy. Chenodeoxycholic acid (chenodiol or CDCA) has been effective in dissolving about 60% of radiolucent gallstones composed primarily of cholesterol. The mechanism of action is the inhibition of liver synthesis and secretion of cholesterol, thereby desaturating bile. Existing stones can be decreased in size, small ones dissolved, and new stones prevented from forming. The therapy is most effective if the stones are small. The effective dose of chenodiol depends on body weight. Chenodiol is generally indicated for those patients who refuse surgery or for whom it is considered too risky.

Certain other medications, such as estrogens, oral contraceptives, clofibrate, and dietary cholesterol, may adversely affect the results of treatment with chenodeoxycholic acid. If the patient is taking these medications, the physician should be made aware of this.

Recurrence of stones has been reported in 20% to 50% of patients after chenodeoxycholic acid is terminated; therefore, a low dose of this drug may be continued to prevent recurrence. Patients' adherence to this mode of therapy requires further study and follow-up.

If acute symptoms of cholecystitis continue or recur, pharmacotherapy is inappropriate as a substitute for more definitive treatment, and surgical intervention or lithotripsy is indicated.

Long-term follow-up and monitoring of the patient's liver enzymes are indicated. The patient is instructed to report adverse side effects of medications and the recurrence of symptoms of cholecystitis.

Ursodeoxycholic acid (UDCA), another drug with similar effects, is also used to dissolve gallstones. UDCA has fewer side effects than chenodiol and can be given in smaller doses to achieve the same effect.

Nonsurgical Removal of Gallstones. Methods of treating gallstones by infusion of solvents into the gallbladder are under investigation. One method involves infusion of a solvent through a tube or catheter inserted percutaneously directly into the gallbladder. Other procedures have involved infusion of the solvent (mono-octanoin or methyl tertiary butyl ether [MTBE]) through a tube or drain inserted through a T-tube tract to dissolve stones not removed at the time of surgery, through an ERCP endoscope, or through a transnasal biliary catheter. In this last procedure, the catheter is introduced through the mouth and inserted into the common bile duct. The upper end of the tube is then rerouted from the mouth to the nose and left in place. This enables the patient to eat and drink normally while passage of stones is monitored or chemical solvents are infused to dissolve the stones.

Several nonsurgical methods are used to remove stones that were not removed at the time of cholecystectomy or have become lodged in the common bile duct. A catheter and instrument with a basket attached are threaded through the T-tube tract or fistula formed at the time of T-tube insertion; the basket is used to retrieve and remove the stone lodged in the common bile duct. A second procedure is use of the ERCP endoscope. After the endoscope is inserted, a cutting instrument is passed through the endoscope into the ampulla of Vater of the common bile duct. It may be used to cut the submucosal fibers, or papilla, of the sphincter of Oddi, enlarging the opening, which may allow the lodged stone to pass spontaneously into the duodenum. Another instrument with a small basket or balloon at its tip may be inserted through the endoscope to retrieve the stone (Fig. 38–12). Although complications after this procedure are rare, the patient must be observed closely for bleeding, perforation, and the development of pancreatitis. This procedure is particularly useful in the diagnosis and treatment of patients presenting with symptoms after biliary tract surgery, for those patients with intact gall-

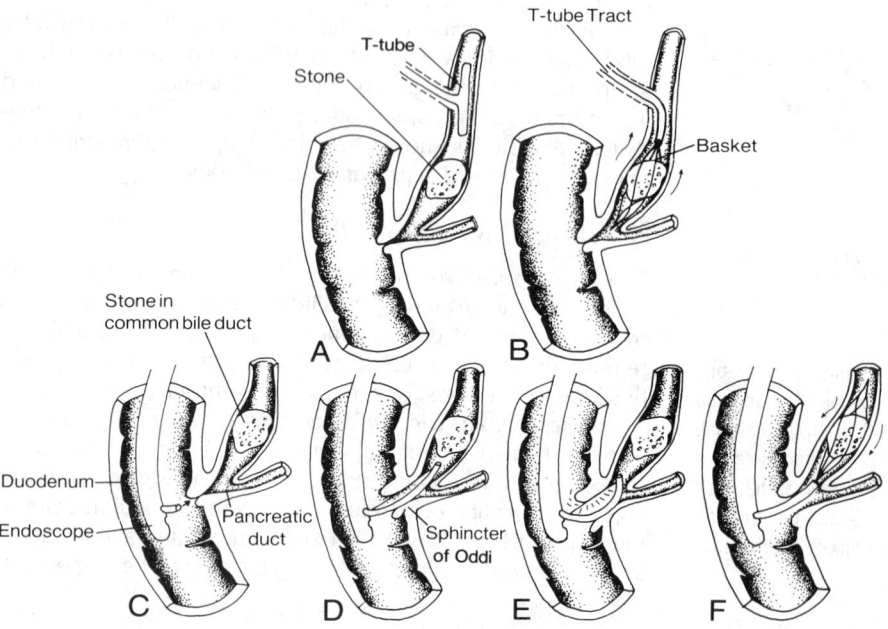

Figure 38–12. Removal of gallstone. (**A**) Use of T-tube tract for removal of retained stone. (**B**) Removal of stone with basket attached to catheter threaded through T-tube tract. (**C**) ERCP endoscope inserted into duodenum. (**D**) Papillotome inserted into common bile duct. (**E**) Enlarging opening of sphincter of Oddi. (**F**) Retrieval and removal of stone with basket inserted through endoscope.

bladders, and for patients in whom surgery is particularly hazardous.

Extracorporeal Shock-Wave Lithotripsy. Extracorporeal shock wave therapy (lithotripsy or ESWL) has been successfully used for nonsurgical fragmentation of gallstones. The word lithotripsy is derived from *lithos,* meaning stone, and *tripsis,* meaning rubbing or friction. This noninvasive procedure uses repeated shock waves directed at the gallstone located in the gallbladder or common bile duct to fragment the stones. Shock waves are generated in a liquid medium by an electric spark, piezoelectric, or electromagnetic discharges. The energy is transmitted to the body through a water bath or fluid-filled bag (Fig. 38–13A). The converging shock waves are directed to the stones to be fragmented; because of differences in impedance among tissues, little shock-wave energy is absorbed before

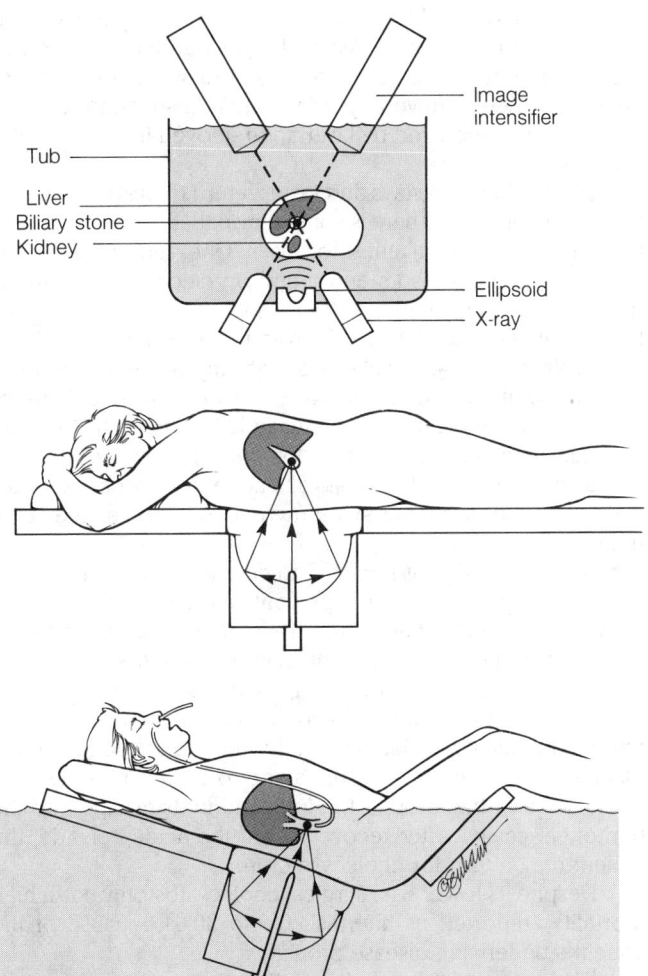

Figure 38–13. (**A**) Schematic illustration of extracorpreal shock wave therapy. The gallbladder stone is localized by imaging. Shock waves are generated in the ellipsoid reflector and transmitted through the water to the stone. (**B**) Positioning of the patient for treatment of stones located in the gallbladder. The fluid-filled bag is recessed in the table; the fluid-filled bag transmits the shock waves from the generator to the patient's skin. (**C**) Positioning of the patient for treatment of stones located in the common bile duct. The patient is partially immersed in a water bath. A nasobiliary tube is used to introduce contrast material to permit visualization and localization of the stone and to decompress the biliary tree.

reaching the stone, and thus minimal tissue damage to surrounding tissue is expected if those tissues with large air contents or solid tissue (lung, GI tract, bone) are avoided.

After the stones are gradually broken up, the stone fragments pass from the gallbladder or common bile duct spontaneously, are removed by endoscopy, or are dissolved with oral bile acid or solvents. Because the procedure requires no incision and no hospitalization, patients may be admitted overnight or may be treated as outpatients; most return to their usual routines within 48 hours of treatment.

If the lithotriptor uses high total shock wave energy, a general, spinal, or epidural anesthetic is administered to the patient. If the lithotriptor uses low total shock wave energy, the treatment can be administered without anesthesia; however, more shocks must be used with this equipment before stones are fragmented.

The patient with gallbladder stones is placed in a prone position over the shock wave generator (see Fig. 38–13B). A fluid-filled cushion is placed between the patient and the lithotriptor. If treatment is for bile duct stones, the patient may be partially immersed in a water bath (see Fig. 38–13C); a nasobiliary catheter or other biliary catheter is inserted to permit introduction of radiocontrast material into the biliary tree and to decompress the bile duct during the treatment. Ultrasound is used to visualize the stones. The shock waves are timed with the electrocardiogram to reduce the risk of dysrhythmias.

Side effects of lithotripsy used to treat gallstones have included cutaneous petechiae (14%) and gross hematuria (3%), probably caused by microscopic injury to the right kidney from passage of shock waves through it. More serious side effects, such as pancreatitis or bile duct obstruction, are possible, but their incidence is small. The patient is monitored after the procedure for the occurrence of these symptoms. Because discharge may occur soon after completion of the treatment, the patient must be adequately prepared for discharge and self-care. Teaching includes information about the symptoms that should be reported. If oral bile salts are prescribed, the patient is instructed about the importance of compliance and follow-up.

Intracorporeal Lithotripsy. With intracorporeal lithotripsy, stones in the gallbladder or common bile duct may be fragmented by ultrasound, pulsed laser, or hydraulic lithotripsy applied through an endoscope directly to the stones. The stone fragments or debris are then removed by irrigation and aspiration. The procedure may be followed by removal of the gallbladder through an incision or by laparoscopy. If the gallbladder is not removed, a drain may be inserted for 7 days.

These nonsurgical methods of removing stones are expected to decrease the need for surgery, reduce the length of hospital stay, and enable patients to return to their normal activities more quickly than they could if they had undergone traditional cholecystecomy for surgical removal of the stones.

Surgical Management

Surgical treatment of gallbladder disease and gallstones is carried out for the relief of long-continued symptoms, for the removal of the cause of biliary colic, and for treatment of acute cholecystitis. Surgery may be elective when the patient's symptoms have subsided or may be performed as an emergency procedure if the patient's condition necessitates it.

Preoperative Management. In addition to x-ray studies of the gallbladder, chest x-rays, electrocardiogram, and liver function tests (see Table 38–1) may be performed. Vitamin K may be administered if the patient's prothrombin level is low. Blood component therapy may be given before surgery.

Nutritional requirements are considered; if the patient is not eating properly, it may be necessary to provide intravenous glucose with protein hydrolysate supplements to aid wound healing and help prevent liver damage.

Preparation for a gallbladder operation is similar to that for any upper abdominal laparotomy. Instruction and explanation are given before surgery with regard to turning and deep breathing. Because the abdominal incision is high, the patient is often reluctant to move and turn; pneumonia and atelectasis are possible postoperative complications that are often avoided by breathing deeply and by turning. Because drainage tubes are usually required after surgery, the patient should be informed of this, so that he knows what to expect. The patient should also be informed about the likelihood of a nasogastric tube and suction during the immediate postoperative period.

Surgical Intervention and Drainage Systems. Patients usually are placed on the operating table with the upper abdomen raised somewhat by an air pillow or sandbag to make the biliary area more accessible.

Cholecystectomy. Cholecystectomy is one of the most frequent surgical procedures, with over 600,000 performed each year in the United States. In this operation, the gallbladder is removed after ligation of the cystic duct and artery. The operation is performed in most cases of acute and chronic cholecystitis. A drain (Penrose) is placed in the gallbladder and brought out through a stab wound for drainage of blood, serosanguineous fluids, and bile into absorbent dressings.

Minicholecystectomy. Minicholecystectomy is a surgical procedure in which the gallbladder is removed through a 4-cm incision. If needed, the surgical incision is extended to remove large gallbladder stones. Drains may or may not be used with minicholecystectomy. Cost savings resulting from patients' shorter hospital stays have been identified as major reasons for pursuing this type of procedure. There has been debate about the use of this procedure because it limits exposure to all the involved biliary strictures.

Laparoscopic Cholecystectomy. Laparoscopic (or endoscopic) cholecystectomy is performed through a small incision or puncture made through the abdominal wall in the umbilicus. The laparoscopic cholecystectomy procedure includes insufflation of the abdominal cavity with carbon dioxide (pneumoperitoneum) to assist in insertion of the endoscope and aid the physician in visualization of the abdominal structures. A fiberoptic endoscope is inserted through the small umbilical incision. Several additional punctures or small incisions are made in the abdominal wall to introduce other surgical instruments into the operative site. The surgeon is able to visualize the biliary system through the endoscope; a camera attached to the endoscope permits transmission and visualization of the intra-abdominal site to a television monitor.

The patient is prepared physically and psychologically for the possibility of a traditional abdominal surgical procedure if problems are encountered during the endoscopic procedure. Although an open abdominal procedure has only occasionally been necessary, the patient is given general anesthesia and informed that an open abdominal procedure may be necessary. The advantage of this procedure is that the patient does not experience the paralytic ileus that occurs with open abdominal surgery and the patient experiences less postoperative abdominal pain. The patient is usually discharged from the hospital within 1 to 2 days of surgery and is able to resume full activity and employment within a week of the surgery. It has been recommended that laparoscopic cholecystectomy be used only for nonacute cholecystitis and performed only in those centers where the surgeon and operating team are skilled in laparoscopic techniques.

Laser Cholecystectomy. Use of a laser rather than traditional surgical instruments (*e.g.*, scissors, scalpel, etc.) has been reported with open abdominal cholecystectomy and laparoscopic cholecystectomy. The laser scalpel is used to accomplish dissection of the gallbladder. With laparoscopic laser cholecystectomy, several ports (small punctures) are necessary to allow access of instruments to grasp and remove the gallbladder and for visualization by fiberoptic endoscopy. The gallbladder is drained and irrigated; stones in the gallbladder may be fragmented by intracorporeal lithotripsy. The stone fragments or debris are then removed by irrigation and aspiration, and the gallbladder is dissected by laser and removed through the endoscope.

Shorter hospital stays and faster return to previous activity have been reported. There is continuing debate, however, about the safety and effectiveness of laser. One author states that dissection using scissors and aided by electrocoagulation is quicker, safer, cheaper, and less complicated than the use of laser to dissect the gallbladder from the liver bed.

Choledochostomy. In choledochostomy, an incision is made into the common duct for removal of stones. After the stones have been evacuated, a tube usually is inserted into the duct for drainage of bile until edema subsides. This tube is connected to gravity drainage tubing. The gallbladder also contains stones and, as a rule, a cholecystectomy is performed at the same time.

Surgical Cholecystostomy. Cholecystostomy is performed when the patient's condition prevents more extensive surgery or when an acute inflammatory reaction obscures the biliary system. The gallbladder is surgically opened, the stones and the bile or the pus are removed, and a drainage tube is secured with a purse-string suture. As soon as the patient is returned to bed, the nurse should connect this tube to a drainage bottle placed at the side of the bed. Failure to do this may result in the leakage of bile around the tube and in its escape into the peritoneal cavity. After recovery from the acute episode, the patient may return for cholecystectomy.

Despite its lower risk, surgical cholecystostomy has a high mortality (reported as high as 20% to 30%) because of the patient's underlying disease process.

Percutaneous Cholecystostomy. Percutaneous cholecystostomy has been used in the treatment and diagnosis of acute cholecystitis in patients who are poor risks for any surgical procedure or for general anesthesia. These may include patients with sepsis or severe cardiac, renal, pulmonary or liver failure. Under local anesthesia, a fine needle is inserted through the abdominal wall and liver edge into the gallbladder under the guidance of ultrasound or CT scan. Bile is aspirated to ensure adequate placement of the needle, and a catheter is inserted into the gallbladder to decompress the biliary tract. Almost immediate relief of pain and resolution of signs and symptoms of sepsis and cholecystitis have been reported with this procedure. Antibiotics are administered before, during, and after the procedure.

Gerontologic Considerations. Surgical intervention for disease of the biliary tract is the most common operative procedure performed in the elderly. Although the incidence of gallstones increases with age, the symptoms experienced by the elderly patient may not be the typical picture of fever, pain, chills, and jaundice. Biliary tract disease in the elderly may be accompanied or preceded by symptoms of septic shock: oliguria, hypotension, mental changes, tachycardia, and tachypnea.

Although surgery in the elderly presents risk because of preexisting associated diseases, the mortality from serious complications from biliary tract disease itself is also high. The risk of mortality and morbidity is increased in the elderly patient who undergoes emergency surgery for life-threatening disease of the biliary tract. Despite associated or preoperative medical illness in the elderly, elective cholecystectomy is usually well tolerated and can be carried out with low risk if expert assessment and care are provided before, during, and after the surgical procedure.

Because of recent changes in the health care system, there has been a decrease in the number of elective surgical procedures, including cholecystectomies, performed. As a result, patients requiring the procedure are seen in the later stages of disease. Simultaneously, patients undergoing surgery are increasingly over 60 years of age and are presenting with complicated acute cholecystitis. The higher risk of complications and shorter hospital stays make it essential that older patients and their family members receive specific information about signs and symptoms of complications and measures to prevent them.

▶ Nursing Process
The Patient Undergoing Surgery for Gallbladder Disease

◊ Assessment

The health history and examination focus on the occurrence of abdominal pain and discomfort as well as those factors that tend to precipitate discomfort. The presence of abdominal pain several hours after eating a meal high in fats is noted. The history and examination also include information about respiratory status, as the high abdominal incision required during surgery may interfere with full respiratory excursion. A history of smoking or previous respiratory problems is noted. Shallow respirations, a persistent or ineffective cough, and the presence of adventitious breath sounds are noted. Nutritional status is evaluated through dietary history, general examination, and laboratory results.

◊ Nursing Diagnoses

Based on all the assessment data, the major nursing diagnoses for the patient with gallbladder disease and undergoing surgery may include the following:

- Pain and discomfort related to obstruction of the biliary system and inflammation and distention of the gallbladder

- Impaired gas exchange related to the high abdominal surgical incision
- Impaired skin integrity related to altered biliary drainage after surgical intervention
- Altered nutrition related to inadequate bile secretion.
- Knowledge deficit about self-care activities after discharge.

◊ Planning and Implementation

◊ **Goals:** The patient's goals include relief of pain, absence of respiratory complications, absence of complications of altered biliary drainage related to surgical intervention, improved nutritional intake, and understanding of self-care routines.

◊ Nursing Interventions

◊ *Postoperative Nursing Interventions.* As soon as the patient has recovered from anesthesia, he is placed in low Fowler's position. Fluids may be given intravenously, and nasogastric suction (tube probably inserted immediately before surgery) may be instituted to relieve abdominal distention. Water and other fluids may be given in about 24 hours, and a soft diet started later, after bowel sounds return.

◊ *Relief of Pain.* The location of the subcostal incision is likely to cause the patient to avoid turning and moving and to splint the operative site by taking shallow breaths to prevent pain. Because full aeration of the lungs and gradually increased activity are necessary to prevent postoperative complications, analgesics should be given as prescribed and the patient assisted to turn, cough, breathe deeply, and ambulate as indicated. Use of a pillow or binder over the incision may reduce the amount of pain during these maneuvers.

◊ *Improvement of Respiratory Status.* These patients are especially prone to pulmonary complications, as are all patients with upper abdominal incisions. Thus, they should be taught to take deep breaths every hour to expand the lungs fully and prevent atelectasis. Early ambulation prevents pulmonary complications as well as other complications, such as thrombophlebitis. Pulmonary complications are more likely to occur in the elderly and the obese patient.

◊ *Biliary Drainage and Skin Care.* As previously mentioned, in patients who have undergone a cholecystostomy or choledochostomy, the drainage tubes must be connected immediately to a drainage receptacle. In addition, tubing should be fastened to the dressings or to the bottom sheet, with enough leeway for the patient to move without dislodging or kinking it. Because a drainage receptacle remains attached when the patient is ambulating, the collecting bag may be placed in a bathrobe pocket or fastened so that it is below the waist or common duct level. If a Penrose drain is used, as it is for cholecystectomy, the dressings are changed as required. Montgomery straps are helpful in maintaining a comfortable dressing.

After these surgical procedures, the patient is observed for indications of infection, leakage of bile into the peritoneal cavity, and obstruction of bile drainage. If bile is not draining properly, an obstruction is probably causing bile to be forced back into the liver and bloodstream. Because jaundice may result, the nurse should be particularly observant of the color of the patient's sclerae. The nurse should also note and report right upper quadrant abdominal pain, nausea and vomiting, bile drainage around the T-tube, clay-colored stools, and a change in vital signs.

Bile may continue to drain from the drainage tract in considerable quantities for a time, necessitating frequent changes of the outer dressings and protection of the skin from irritation. Skin pastes of zinc oxide, aluminum, or petrolatum prevent the bile from literally digesting the skin.

To prevent total loss of bile, the drainage tube or collecting receptacle may be elevated above the level of the abdomen, so that the bile drains externally only if pressure develops in the duct system. The bile collected is measured every 24 hours; the amount, color, and character of the drainage are documented. After several days of drainage, the tubes may be clamped for an hour before and after each meal, with the purpose being to deliver bile to the duodenum to aid in digestion. Within 7 to 14 days, the drainage tubes are removed from the gallbladder or common bile duct.

In all patients with biliary drainage, the stools should be observed daily and their color recorded. Specimens of both urine and stool may be sent to the laboratory for examination for bile pigments. In this way, it is possible to determine that the bile pigment is disappearing from the blood and is draining again into the duodenum. A careful record of fluid intake and output is kept and totaled for each 24 hours.

▷ *Improvement of Nutritional Status.* The diet of these patients may be low in fats and high in carbohydrates and proteins immediately after surgery. At the time of hospital discharge, there are usually no special dietary instructions, other than to maintain a nutritious diet and avoid excessive fats. Fat restriction usually is lifted in 4 to 6 weeks when biliary ducts dilate to accommodate the volume of bile once held by the gallbladder and when the ampulla of Vater again functions effectively. After this, when one eats fat, adequate bile will be released into the digestive tract to emulsify the fats and allow their digestion. Before this, fats would not be digested completely or adequately in some persons, and flatulence might occur. However, one purpose of gallbladder surgery is ultimately to allow for a normal diet.

▷ *Patient Education and Home Health Care.* Because the patient may be discharged from the hospital while the drainage system is still in place, the patient and family will need instructions about its management. They must be instructed in proper care of the drainage tube and should know to report to the physician promptly changes in the amount or characteristics of drainage. Assistance in securing the appropriate dressings will reduce the patient's anxiety about going home with the drain or tube still in place.

The patient should be instructed about which medications are required (vitamins, anticholinergics, and antispasmodics) and their actions. He also should be aware of symptoms that are reportable to his physician—jaundice, dark urine, pale-colored stools, pruritus, or signs of inflammation and infection, such as pain or fever.

Some patients note "looseness of the bowels," consisting of one to three bowel movements a day—the result of a continual trickle of bile through the choledochoduodenal junction after cholecystectomy. Usually, such frequency diminishes over a period of a few weeks to several months. Follow-up visits are essential for this patient.

▷ Evaluation

Expected Outcomes

1. Achieves relief of pain
   a. Reports decrease in pain of cholecystitis and cholelithiasis, and absence of postoperative incisional pain
   b. Splints abdominal incision to decrease pain
   c. Avoids foods that cause pain
   d. Uses postoperative analgesia as prescribed
   e. Uses appropriate preventive activities when pain-free postoperatively (*e.g.*, turns, coughs, breathes deeply, ambulates).
2. Is free of respiratory complications.
   a. Is free of temperature elevation, cough, and increased respiratory rate
   b. Demonstrates full respiratory excursion with deep inspiration and expiration
   c. Coughs effectively, using pillow to splint abdominal incision
   d. Uses postoperative analgesia as prescribed
   e. Exercises as prescribed (*e.g.*, turns, ambulates)
3. Exhibits normal skin integrity around biliary drainage site
   a. Is free of fever, abdominal pain, change in vital signs, or bile around drainage tube
   b. Exhibits or reports gradual decrease in bile drainage
   c. Reports skin, mucous membranes, stool, and urine to be of normal color
   d. Demonstrates proper management of catheter; identifies reportable complications (*e.g.*, redness or purulent drainage at site)
   e. Demonstrates that skin around T-tube or drainage tube is intact and free of excoriation
   f. Identifies signs and symptoms of biliary obstruction to be noted and reported
   g. Has serum bilirubin level within normal range
4. Obtains relief of dietary intolerance
   a. Maintains adequate dietary intake
   b. Avoids foods that cause gastrointestinal symptoms
   c. Reports decreased incidence or absence of nausea, vomiting, diarrhea, flatulence, and abdominal discomfort

In summary, the presence of gallstones is common in adults in the United States. Symptoms resulting from gallbladder disease are one of the most common reasons for hospitalization. Despite recent advances in treatment modalities, surgery of the gallbladder remains one of the most frequent surgical procedures performed. Newer treatment modalities have enabled many patients to forego surgery by electing nonsurgical therapies to treat their gallstones; however, long-term results of these therapies are not yet known. Same-day surgery and early discharge programs have enabled some patients undergoing elective cholecystectomy to return home within 24 hours of surgery. Shorter hospital stays make it essential that patients and their families receive instructions about signs and symptoms of complications after surgical and nonsurgical management of gallstones, as well as measures to prevent them.

The frequency of elective gallbladder surgery has decreased in the last decade. Subsequently, many patients are seen during the later stages of disease with complicated acute cholecystitis, and their symptoms are often severe. These may include severe pain, gastrointestinal symptoms, fluid and electrolyte disturbances, and sepsis. Emergency surgery may be required. Many patients with acute cholecystitis undergoing emergency surgery are elderly and at increased risk for postoperative complications.

Bibliography

Books

Bengmark S. Progress in Surgery of the Liver, Pancreatitis, and Biliary System. Boston, Nijhoff, 1988.

Hodgson WJB. Liver Tumors: Multidisciplinary Management. St Louis, Warren H Green, 1988.

Sigardson–Poor KM and Haggerty LM. Nursing Care of the Transplant Recipient. Philadelphia, WB Saunders, 1990.

Thompson R. Lecture Notes on the Liver. Oxford, Blackwell Scientific Publications, 1985.

US Department of Health and Human Services. Sixth Special Report to the US Congress on Alcohol and Health. Washington, DC, Public Health Service. National Institute on Alcohol Abuse and Alcoholism, 1987.

Wanebo HJ (ed). Hepatic and Biliary Cancer. New York, Marcel Dekker, 1987.

Journals

Liver

General

Adinaro D. Liver failure and pancreatitis: Fluid and electrolyte concerns. Nurs Clin North Am 1987 Dec; 22(4): 843–852.

Bannister P et al. Sex hormone changes in chronic liver disease: A matched study of alcoholic versus non-alcoholic liver disease. Q J Med 1987 Apr; 63(240): 305–313.

Burnett DA. Rational uses of hepatic imaging modalities. Semin Liver Dis 1989 Feb; 9(1): 1–6.

Hirayama T. A large-scale cohort study on risk factors for primary liver cancer, with special reference to the role of cigarette smoking. Cancer Chemother Pharmacol 1988; 23(Suppl): S114–S117.

Kemeny N and Schneider A. Regional treatment of hepatic metastases and hepatocellular carcinoma. Curr Probl Cancer 1989 Jul/Aug; 13(4): 203–283.

Oberfield RA et al. Liver cancer. CA 1989 Jul/Aug; 39(4): 206–218.

O'Mary SS. Liver cancer: Primary and metastatic disease. Semin Oncol Nurs 1988 Nov; 4(4): 265–273.

Rikkers LF. Current status of the management of patients with portal hypertension. Surg Annu 1988; 20: 179–200.

Rustgi A, Saini S, and Schapiro BH. Hepatic imaging and advanced endoscopic techniques. Med Clin North Am 1989 Jul; 73(4): 895–909.

Williams NN and Daly JM. Current trends in management of hepatic metastases. Surg Annu 1989 21: 215–235.

Hepatitis

Balistreri WF. Viral hepatitis. Pediatr Clin North Am 1988 Jun; 35(3): 637–669.

Bruckstein AH. Immunoprophylaxis of viral hepatitis. Postgrad Med 1988 Jul; 84(1): 85–88, 91–92, 94.

Conrad ME and Lemon SM. Prevention of endemic icteric viral hepatitis by administration of immune serum gamma globulin. J Infect Dis 1987 Jul; 156(1): 56–63.

Hoffnagle JH and Jones EA. Therapy of chronic viral hepatitis: Past, present, and future. Semin Liver Dis 1989 Nov; 9(4): 231–234.

Hoffnagle JH. Chronic hepatitis B. N Engl J Med 1990 Aug 2; 323(5): 337–339.

Lange R. Viral hepatitis and international travel. Am Fam Pract 1987 Jul; 36(1): 179–184.

Lisanti P and Talotta D. Hepatitis D: Yet another reason to get your HBV vaccine. Am J Nurs 1990 Apr; 90(4): 29–30.

McLean AA, Monahan GR, and Finkelstein DM. Prevalence of hepatitis B serologic markers in community hospital personnel. Am J Public Health 1987 Aug; 77(8): 998–999.

Perrillo RP et al. A randomized controlled trial of interferon alfa-2b alone and after prednisone withdrawal for the treatment of chronic hepatitis B. N Engl J Med 1990 Aug 2; 323(5): 295–301.

Peters M. Mechanisms of action of interferons. Semin Liver Dis 1989 Nov; 9(4): 235–239.

Renault PF and Hoofnagle JH. Side effects of alpha interferon. Semin Liver Dis 1989 Nov; 9(4): 273–277.

Schiff E. Immunoprophylaxis of viral hepatitis: A practical guide. Am J Gastroenterol 1987; Apr; 82(4): 287–291.

Seeff LB and Dienstag JL. Transfusion-associated non-A, non-B hepatitis. Where do we go from here? (Editorial). Gastroenterology 1988 Aug; 95(2): 530–533.

Smith LG and Perez G. Viral hepatitis. The alphabet game. Postgrad Med 1988 Oct; 84(5): 179–184, 186.

Cirrhosis

Boyer JL and Ransohoff DF. Is colchicine effective therapy for cirrhosis? N Engl J Med 1988 June 30; 318(26): 1751–1752.

Franco D et al. Should portosystemic shunt be reconsidered in the treatment of intractable ascites in cirrhosis? Arch Surg 1988 Aug; 123(8): 987–991.

Kaplan MM. Medical treatment of primary biliary cirrhosis. Semin Liver Dis 1989 May; 9(2): 138–143.

Kershenobich D et al. Colchicine in the treatment of cirrhosis of the liver. N Engl J Med 1988 June 30; 318(26): 1709–1713.

Mackay IR and Gershwin ME. Primary biliary cirrhosis: Current knowledge, perspectives, and future directions. Semin Liver Dis 1989 May; 9(2): 149–157.

Stanley MM et al. Peritoneovenous shunting as compared with medical treatment in patients with alcoholic cirrhosis and massive ascites. N Eng J Med 1989 Dec 14; 321(24): 1632–1638.

Test your knowledge of medical/surgical nursing. Part 3. (Assess your readiness to care for a patient with cirrhosis). Nursing 1989 Dec; 72–75.

Tzakis AG et al. Liver transplantation for primary biliary cirrhosis. Semin Liver Dis 1989 May; 9(2): 144–157.

Williams GD. Trends in alcohol-related morbidity and mortality Public Health Rep 1988 Nov/Dec; 103(6): 592–597.

Fulminant Hepatic Failure

Brems JJ et al. Fulminant hepatic failure: The role of liver transplantation as primary therapy. Am J Surg 1987 Jul; 154(1): 137–141.

O'Grady JG et al. Controlled trials of charcoal hemoperfusion and prognostic factors in fulminant hepatic failure. Gastroenterology 1988 May; 94(5): 1186–1192.

Russell GJ, Fitzgerald JF, and Clark JH. Fulminant hepatic failure. J Pediatr 1987 Sep; 111(3): 313–319.

Schafer DF and Shaw BW Jr. Fulminant hepatic failure and orthotopic liver transplantation. Semin Liver Dis 1989 Aug; 9(3): 189–194.

Esophageal Varices

Burns SM and Martin MJ. VP/NTG therapy in the patient with variceal bleeding. Crit Care Nurs 1990 Oct; 10(9): 42–49.

Burroughs AK. The management of bleeding due to portal hypertension. Part 1. The management of acute bleeding episodes. Q J Med 1988 Jun; 67(254): 447–458.

Feneyrou B et al. Initial control of bleeding from esophageal varices with the Sengstaken–Blakemore Tube. Experience in 82 patients. Am J Surg 1988 Mar; 155(3): 509–511.

Fleig WE and Strange EF. Esophageal varices: Current therapy in 1989. Endoscopy 1989 Mar; 21(2): 89–86.

Garden OJ et al. Propranolol in the prevention of recurrent variceal hemorrhage in cirrhotic patients. A controlled trial. Gastroenterology 1990 Jan; 98: 185–190.

Hosking SW et al. Management of bleeding varices in the elderly. Br Med J 1989 Jan 21; 298(6667): 152–153.

O'Connor KW et al. Comparison of three nonsurgical treatments for bleeding esophageal varices. Gastroenterology 1989 Mar; 96(3): 899–906.

Panés J et al. Efficacy of balloon tamponade in treatment of bleeding gastric and esophageal varices. Dig Dis Sci 1988 Apr; 33(4): 454–459.

Peck SN and Griffith DJ. Reducing portal hypertension and variceal bleeding. Dimens Crit Care Nurs 1988 Sep/Oct; 7(5): 269–278.

Pierce JD, Wilkerson E, and Griffiths SA. Acute esophageal bleeding and endoscopic injection sclerotherapy. Crit Care Nurs 1990 Oct; 10(9): 67–72.

Pinto HC et al. Long-term prognosis of patients with cirrhosis of the liver and upper gastrointestinal bleeding. Am J Gastroenterol 1989 Oct; 84(10): 1239–1243.

Sarin SK. Endoscopic sclerotherapy for esophago-gastric varices: A critical reappraisal. Aust N Z J Med 1989 Apr; 19(2): 162–171.

Tabibian N. Sclerotherapy for esophageal varices. Am Fam Physician 1988 Jun; 37(6): 147–152.

Terblanche J. The surgeon's role in the management of portal hypertension. Ann Surg 1989 Apr; 209(4): 381–395

Terblanche J, Burroughs AK, and Hobbs, KEF. Controversies in the management of bleeding esophageal varices. Part 1. N Engl J Med 1989 May 25; 320(21): 1393–1398.

Terblanche J, Burroughs AK, and Hobbs, KEF. Controversies in the management of bleeding esophageal varices. Part 2. N Engl J Med 1989 Jun 1; 320(22): 1469–1475.

Terblanche J, Kahn D, and Bornman PC. Long-term injection sclerotherapy treatment for esophageal varices. Ann Surg 1989 Dec; 210(6): 725–731.

Zeppa R et al. Portal hypertension. A fifteen year perspective. Am J Surg 1988 Jan; 155(1): 6–9.

Liver Transplantation

Beckermann S and Galloway S. Elective resection of the liver: Nursing care. Crit Care Nurs 1989 Nov/Dec; 9(10): 40–42, 44, 46–48.

Buckels JAC. Liver transplantation in acute fulminant hepatic failure. Transplantation Proc 1987 Oct; 19(5): 4365–4366.

Donovan JP et al. Preoperative evaluation, preparation, and timing of orthotopic liver transplantation in the adult. Semin Liver Dis 1989 Aug; 9(3): 168–175.

Gruppi LA, Killen AR, and Rodriguez W. Liver transplantation: Key nursing diagnoses. Dimens Crit Care Nurs 1990 Sep/Oct; 9(5): 272–279.

Gruppi LA et al. Launching a multidisciplinary staff development program for liver transplantation. Nurs Connect 1990 Sep; 3(2): 55–60.

Kirby RM et al. Orthotopic liver transplantation: Postoperative complications and their management. Br J Surg 1987 Jan; 74(1): 3–11.

Kozlowski LM. Case study in identification and maintenance of an organ donor. Heart Lung 1988 Jul; 17(4): 366–371.

Miller HD. Liver transplantation: Postoperative ICU care. Crit Care Nurs 1988 Sep; 8(6): 19–21, 24–31.

Omery A and Caswell D. A nursing perspective of the ethical issues surrounding liver transplantation. Heart Lung 1988 Nov; 17(6, Part 1): 626–631.

Pezze JL. RATG: Implications for nursing care in organ transplantation. Crit Care Nurs 1990 Oct; 10(9): 18–24.

Shaw BW et al. Postoperative care after liver transplantation. Semin Liver Dis 1989 Aug; 9(3): 202–230

Sheets L. Liver transplantation. Nurs Clin North Am 1989 Dec; 24(4): 881–889.

Smith SL. Liver transplantation: Implications for critical care nursing. Heart Lung 1985 Nov; 14(6): 617–627.

Spisso J, Clark B, and Wallace T. The postoperative liver transplant patient. Crit Care Nurs 1988 Jan/Feb; 8(1): 53–58.

Starzl TE et al. Orthotopic liver transplantation for alcoholic cirrhosis. JAMA 1988 Nov 4; 260(17): 2542–2544.

Starzl TE and Demetris AJ. Liver transplantation: A 31-year perspective, Part I. Curr Probl Surg 1990 Feb; 27(2): 55–115.

Starzl TE and Demetris AJ. Liver transplantation: A 31-year perspective, Part II. Curr Probl Surg 1990 Mar; 27(3): 123–178.

Starzl TE and Demetris AJ. Liver transplantation: A 31-year perspective, Part III. Curr Probl Surg 1990 Apr; 27(4): 187–240.

Van Thiel DH, Makowka L, and Starzl TE. Liver transplantation: Where it's been and where it's going. Gastroenterol Clin North Am 1988 Mar; 17(1): 1–18.

Vargo RL and Rudy EB. Infection as a complication of liver transplant. Crit Care Nurs 1989 Apr; 9(4): 52–62.

Whiteman K et al. Liver transplantation. Am J Nurs 1990 Jun; 90(6): 68–72.

Wood RP et al. A review of liver transplantation for gastroenterologists. Am J Gastroenterol 1987 Jul; 82(7): 593–606.

Wood RP et al. Complications requiring operative intervention after orthotopic liver transplantation. Am J Surg 1988 Dec; 156(6): 513–518.

Gallbladder Disease

American College of Physicians, Health and Policy Committee. How to study the gallbladder (Position Paper). Ann Intern Med 1988 Nov 1; 109(9): 752–754.

Aranha GV, Kruss D, and Greenlee HB. Therapeutic options for biliary tract disease in advanced cirrhosis. Am J Surg 1988 Mar; 155(3): 374–377.

Burnett D et al. Use of external shock-wave lithotripsy and adjuvant ursodiol for treatment of radiolucent gallstones. A national multicenter study. Dig Dis Sci 1989 Jul; 34(7): 1011–1015.

Carter DC. Pancreatitis and the biliary tree: The continuing problem. Am J Surg 1988 Jan; 155(1): 10–17.

Cass AS. Extracorporeal shock wave lithotripsy for gall stones. How effective is it? Postgrad Med 1989 Feb 15; 85(3):111, 112, 117–120, 122.

Chapman WC, Stephens WH, and Williams LF Jr. Principles of biliary extracorporeal lithotripsy. Technical considerations and clinical implications. Am J Surg 1989 Sep; 158(3): 179–191.

Cuschieri A. The laparoscopic revolution–Walk carefully before we run (editorial). J R Coll Surg Edinb 1989 Dec; 34(6): 295.

Cuschieri A, Berci G, and McSherry CK. Laparoscopic cholecystectomy (editorial). Am J Surg 1990 Mar; 159(3): 273.

Delikaris PG. Choledochoduodenostomy. Surg Annu 1989; 21: 181–199.

Diettrich NA, Cacippo JC, and Davis RP. The vanishing elective cholecystectomy: Trends and their consequences. Arch Surg 1988 Jul; 123(7): 810–814.

Dubois F et al. Coelioscopic cholecystectomy: Preliminary report of 36 cases. Ann Surg 1990 Jan; 211(1): 60–62.

Fitzgibbons RJ et al. Alternatives to conventional surgical therapy for calculous biliary tract disease. Surg Annu 1989; 21: 237–262.

Frimberger E. Operative laparoscopy: Colecystotomy. Endoscopy 1989 Dec; 21(Suppl I): 367–372

Goco IR and Chambers LG. Dollars and cents: Minicholecystectomy and early discharge. South Med J 1988 Feb; 81(2): 162–163.

Gutman H et al. Changing trends in surgery for benign gallbladder disease. Am J Gastroenterol 1988 May; 83(5): 545–548.

Heinerman PM, Boeckl O, and Pimpl W. Selective ERCP and preoperative stone removal in bile duct surgery. Ann Surg 1989 Mar; 209(3): 267–271.

Hwang MH et al. Transcholecystic endoscopic choledocholithotripsy: Successful management of retained common bile duct stone. Endoscopy 1987 Jan; 19(1): 24–27.

Inui K et al. Nonsurgical treatment of cholecystolithiasis with percutaneous transhepatic cholecystoscopy. Am J Gastroenterol 1988 Oct; 83(10): 1124–1127.

Jurf JB, Clements L, and Llorente J. Cholecystectomy made easier. Am J Nurs 1990 Dec; 90(12): 38–39.

Klimberg S, Hawkins I, and Vogel SB. Percutaneous cholecystostomy for acute cholecystitic in high-risk patients. Am J Surg 1987 Jan; 153(1): 125–129.

Lancaster S and Bears–Marshall D. Gallstone lithotripsy. Am J Nurs 1988 Dec; 88(12): 1629–1630.

Lauritsen KB et al. Cholescintigraphy and ultrasonography in patients suspected of having acute cholecystitis. Scand J Gastroenterol 1988 Jan; 23(1): 42–46.

Lee PH, Hopkins TB, and Howard PJ. Percutaneous cholecystolithotomy. Urology 1989 Jan; 33(1): 37–39.

Lewis RT et al. Simple elective cholecystectomy: To drain or not. Am J Surg 1990 Feb; 159(2): 241–245.

Margiotta SJ et al. Cholecystectomy in the elderly. Am J Surg 1988 Dec; 156(6): 509–512.

Martin KI and Doubilet P. How to image the gallbladder in suspected cholecystitis. Ann Intern Med 1988 Nov 1; 109(9): 722–729.

McGahan JP. A new catheter design for percutaneous cholecystotomy. Radiology 1988 Jan; 166(1 pt 1): 49–52.

Moody FG et al. Lithotripsy for bile duct stones. Am J Surg 1989 Sep; 158(3): 241–247.

Neoptolemos JP et al. ERCP findings and the role of endoscopic sphincterotomy in acute gallstone pancreatitis. Br J Surg 1988 Oct; 75(10): 954–960.

Perissat J, Collett DR, and Bellard R. Gallstones: Laparoscopic treatment, intracorporeal lithotripsy followed by cholecystostomy or cholecystectomy—A personal technique. Endoscopy 1989 Dec; 21(Suppl I): 373–374.

Rhodes M et al. Cholesystokinin (CCK) provocation test: Long-term follow-up after cholecystectomy. Br J Surg 1988 Oct; 75(10): 951–953.

Richter JM and Weinstein DF. Extracorporeal shock-wave lithotripsy of common bile duct stones. Gastroenterology 1989 Jan; 96(1): 252–254.

Sackman M et al. Shock-wave lithotripsy of gallbladder stones. The first 175 patients. N Engl J Med 1988 Feb 18; 318(7): 393–397.

Sauerbruch T. Gallstone lithotripsy by extracorporeal shock waves. Am J Surg 1989 Sep; 158(3): 188–191.

Sharp KW. Acute cholecystitis. Surg Clin North Am 1988 Apr; 68(2): 269–279.

Shively EH et al. Operative cholangiography. Am J Surg 1990 Apr; 159(4): 380–384.

Siegman–Igra Y et al. Septicemia from biliary tract infection. Arch Surg 1988 Mar; 123(3): 366–368.

Sivak MV Jr. Endoscopic management of bile duct stones. Am J Surg 1989 Sep; 159(3): 228–240.

Smith N and Max MH. Gallbladder surgery in patients over 60: Is there an increased risk? South Med J 1987 Apr; 80(4): 472–474.

Stahlgren LH. Biliary lithotripsy. Am J Surg 1988 Sep; 156(Part 2): 5B–8B.

Sullivan WA Jr. Treatment of acute cholecystitis. Selection of the optimum approach. Postgrad Med 1987 Jan; 81(1): 191–198.

Teplick SK et al. Percutaneous cholecystostomy in patients at high risk. Treatment of acute acalculous cholecystitis. Postgrad Med 1987 Jan; 81(1): 209–211, 214.

Vanderpool D et al. Cholecystectomy. South Med J 1989 Apr; 82(4): 450–452.

Vogelzang RL and Nemcek AA Jr. Percutaneous cholecystostomy: Diagnostic and therapeutic efficacy. Radiology 1988 Jul; 168(1): 29–34.

Wenk H et al. Percutaneous transphepatic cholecysto-lithotripsy (PTCL). Endoscopy 1989; 21(5): 221–222.

Information/Resources

Agencies

American Liver Foundation
    998 Pompton Ave, Cedar Grove, NJ 07009
National Institute on Alcohol Abuse and Alcoholism
    Rockville, MD 20857
Alcoholics Anonymous World Service (AA)
    PO Box 459 Grand Central Station, New York, NY 10163
National Council on Alcoholism, Inc
    12 W 21st St, New York, NY 10010

39

Assessment and Management of Patients With Diabetes Mellitus

Chapter Outline

Learning Objectives

On completion of this chapter, the learner will be able to:

1. Differentiate between type I and type II diabetes
2. Describe etiologic factors associated with diabetes
3. Relate the clinical manifestations of diabetes to the associated pathophysiologic alterations
4. Identify the diagnostic and clinical significance of blood glucose tests
5. Explain the dietary modifications used for management of persons with diabetes
6. Describe the relationship between diet, exercise, and medication (i.e., insulin or oral hypoglycemic agents) for persons with diabetes
7. Develop a plan for teaching insulin self-administration
8. Identify the role of oral hypoglycemic agents in diabetic therapy
9. Differentiate between hypoglycemia and diabetic ketoacidosis, and hyperosmolar nonketotic syndrome
10. Describe management strategies for a person with diabetes to use during "sick days"
11. Describe the major macrovascular, microvascular and neuropathic complications of diabetes and the self-care behaviors important in their prevention
12. Identify the teaching aids and community support groups that are available for persons with diabetes
13. Use the nursing process as a framework for care of the patient with diabetes

Definition

Diabetes mellitus is a heterogeneous group of disorders characterized by an elevation in the level of glucose in the blood. There is normally a certain amount of glucose circulating in the blood that is derived from ingested food and from the formation of glucose by the liver. Insulin, a hormone produced by the pancreas, controls the blood glucose level by regulating the production and storage of glucose.

In diabetes there may be a decrease in the body's ability to respond to insulin and/or a decrease or absence of insulin produced by the pancreas. This leads to abnormalities in the metabolism of carbohydrates, proteins, and fats. The resulting hyperglycemia may lead to acute metabolic complications such as diabetic ketoacidosis and hyperosmolar nonketotic syndrome. Long-term hyperglycemia may contribute to chronic microvascular complications (kidney and eye disease) and neuropathic complications. Diabetes is also associated with an increased occurrence of macrovascular diseases, including myocardial infarction, strokes, and peripheral vascular disease.

Types of Diabetes

There are several different types of diabetes mellitus; they may differ in cause, clinical course, and treatment. The major classifications of diabetes are as follows:

- Type I: Insulin-dependent diabetes mellitus (IDDM)
- Type II: Non–insulin-dependent diabetes mellitus (NIDDM)
- Diabetes mellitus associated with other conditions or syndromes
- Gestational diabetes mellitus (GDM)

About 5% to 10% of people with diabetes have type I, insulin-dependent diabetes. In this form of diabetes, inadequate amounts of insulin are produced by the pancreas, resulting in the need for insulin injections to control the blood glucose. This type is characterized by a sudden onset usually before the age of 30 years.

About 90% to 95% of people with diabetes have type II, non–insulin-dependent diabetes. Type II diabetes results from a decrease in the sensitivity of the cells to insulin (called insulin resistance) and a decrease in the amount of insulin produced. Type II diabetes is first treated with diet alone. If elevated glucose levels persist, diet is supplemented with oral hypoglycemic agents. In some individuals with type II diabetes, oral agents will not control hyperglycemia, and insulin injections will be required. In addition, during periods of acute physiologic stress (such as illness or surgery), individuals who usually control their type II diabetes with diet and oral agents may require insulin injections. Type II diabetes occurs most frequently in people who are over 30 years of age and obese.

Diabetes complications may develop in any person with type I or type II diabetes—not just in patients who take insulin. Some persons with type II diabetes who are treated with oral medications may have the impression that they do not really have diabetes or that they simply have "borderline" diabetes. They may feel that, compared with diabetic patients who require insulin injections, their diabetes is not a "serious" problem. It is important for the nurse to emphasize to them that if they have had glucose levels diagnostic for diabetes and require oral medications to control blood glucose, they actually have diabetes and not a borderline problem with sugar. ("Borderline" diabetes is currently classified as impaired glucose tolerance and refers to a condition in which glucose levels fall between normal and those levels considered diagnostic for diabetes [see p. 1026].)

Table 39-1 summarizes the major classifications of diabetes, current terminology, old labels, and major clinical characteristics. It is important to recognize that this classification system is dynamic rather than static in two ways. First, as research findings become available, it appears that there are many differences among individuals within each category. Second, with time, patients may move from one category to another. For example, a woman with gestational diabetes may, after delivery, move into the non–insulin-dependent (type II) category. These types also differ in their etiology, clinical course, and management.

Epidemiology

Diabetes mellitus is a chronic disease of major importance in the United States today, currently affecting an estimated 11 million people. According to the National Diabetes Data Group of the National Institutes of Health, 5.8 million of the 11 million cases have been diagnosed; the remainder are undiagnosed. About 500,000 new cases of diabetes are diagnosed yearly.

Diabetes is especially prevalent in the elderly. Among people over 65 years of age, 8.6% have type II diabetes. This figure includes 15% of the nursing home population. Hispanic, black, and some Native American populations have a higher rate of diabetes than the white population. In American Indian populations, such as the Pima Indians, 20% to 50% of the adults have diabetes.

Diabetes is the leading cause of new blindness (among 25- to 74-year-olds) and nontraumatic amputations in the United States. Twenty-five percent of patients on dialysis have diabetes. Diabetes is the third leading cause of death by disease, mostly because of the high rate of coronary artery disease among people with diabetes.

The economic cost of diabetes continues to rise because of increasing medical costs and an aging population. Costs directly related to diabetes are conservatively estimated at $20 billion annually, including direct medical care expenses and indirect costs due to disability and premature death.

Hospitalization rates are 2.4 times greater for adults and 5.3 times greater for children with diabetes than for the general population. The rate of hospitalization increases for the elderly with diabetes. Half of all persons with diabetes who are over 65 are hospitalized each year. Severe and life-threatening complications often contribute to increased rates of hospitalization for patients with diabetes.

TABLE 39-1. *Classification of Diabetes Mellitus and Related Glucose Intolerances*

Current Classification	Previous Classifications	Clinical Characteristics
Type I: Insulin-dependent diabetes mellitus (IDDM) (5%–10% of all diabetes)	Juvenile diabetes Juvenile-onset diabetes Ketosis-prone diabetes Brittle diabetes	Onset any age, but usually young Usually thin at diagnosis Etiology includes genetic, immunologic, and/or environmental factors (*e.g.,* virus) Often have islet cell antibodies Often have antibodies to insulin even before insulin treatment Little or no endogenous insulin Need insulin to preserve life Ketosis-prone when insulin absent Acute complication of hyperglycemia: diabetic ketoacidosis
Type II: Non–insulin-dependent diabetes (NIDDM) (90%–95% of all diabetes: obese—80% of type II; nonobese—20% of type I)	Adult-onset diabetes Maturity-onset diabetes Ketosis-resistant diabetes Stable diabetes	Onset any age, usually over 30 Usually obese at diagnosis Etiology includes obesity, heredity, and/or environmental factors No islet cell antibodies Decrease in endogenous insulin Majority can control blood glucose through weight loss if obese Oral hypoglycemic agents may improve blood glucose levels if dietary modification alone is unsuccessful May need insulin on a short- or long-term basis to prevent hyperglycemia Ketosis rare, except in stress or infection Acute complication: hyperosmolar nonketotic syndrome
Diabetes mellitus associated with other conditions or syndromes	Secondary diabetes	Accompanied by conditions known or suspected to cause the disease: pancreatic diseases; hormonal abnormalities; drugs such as glucocorticoids and estrogen-containing preparations Depending on the ability of the pancreas to produce insulin, the patient may require treatment with oral agents or insulin.
Gestational diabetes	Gestational diabetes	Onset is during pregnancy, usually in the second or third trimester Due to hormones secreted by the placenta, which inhibit the action of insulin Above-normal risk of perinatal complications, especially macrosomia (abnormally large babies) Treat with diet and, if needed, insulin to strictly maintain normal blood glucose levels Occurs in about 2%–5% of all pregnancies Glucose intolerance transitory but may recur: • In subsequent pregnancies • 30%–40% will develop overt diabetes (usually type II) within 5–10 years (especially if obese) Risk factors include: obesity, age over 30 years, family history of diabetes, previous large babies (over 9 lb)

(continued)

TABLE 39-1. *(Continued)*

Current Classification	Previous Classifications	Clinical Characteristics
		Screening tests (glucose challenge test) should be performed on ALL pregnant women between 24 and 28 weeks' gestation
Impaired glucose tolerance	Borderline diabetes	Blood glucose levels between normal and that of diabetes
	Latent diabetes	25% eventually develop diabetes
	Chemical diabetes	Above-normal susceptibility to atherosclerotic disease
	Subclinical diabetes	Renal and retinal complications usually not significant
	Asymptomatic diabetes	May be obese or nonobese; obese should reduce weight
		Should be screened for diabetes periodically
Previous abnormality of glucose tolerance (PrevAGT)	Latent diabetes Prediabetes	Current normal glucose metabolism
		Previous history of hyperglycemia (*e.g.,* during pregnancy or illness)
		Periodic blood glucose screening after age 40 if there is a family history of diabetes or if symptomatic
		Encourage ideal body weight
Potential abnormality of glucose tolerance (PotAGT)	Prediabetes	No history of glucose intolerance
		Increased risk of diabetes if:
		• Positive family history
		• Obesity
		• Mothers of babies over 9 pounds at birth
		• Members of certain Native American Indian tribes with high prevalence of diabetes (*e.g.,* Pima)
		Screening and weight advice as in PrevAGT

Pathophysiology and Clinical Manifestations

Normal Physiology

Insulin is secreted by the *beta* cells, which are one of four types of cells in the islets of Langerhans in the pancreas. Insulin is considered to be an anabolic, or storage, hormone. When a meal is eaten, insulin secretion increases and moves glucose from the circulation into muscle, liver, and fat cells. In those cells, insulin has the following effects:

- Stimulates storage of glucose in the liver and muscle (in the form of glycogen)
- Enhances storage of dietary fat in adipose tissue
- Accelerates transport of amino acids (derived from dietary protein) into cells

Insulin also inhibits the breakdown of stored glucose, protein, and fat.

During "fasting" periods (between meals and overnight), there is a lower, but continuous, release of insulin. This is accompanied by an increased release of another pancreatic hormone called glucagon (which is secreted by the *alpha* cells of the islets of Langerhans). The net effect of the balance between insulin and glucagon levels is to maintain a constant level of glucose in the blood through release of glucose from the liver.

Initially, the liver produces glucose through the breakdown of glycogen (*glycogenolysis*). After 8 to 12 hours without food, new glucose is formed by the liver from noncarbohydrate substances, including amino acids (*gluconeogenesis*).

Pathophysiology of Diabetes

Type I Diabetes. In type I diabetes there is a marked deficiency in the production of insulin by the pancreatic beta cells. Fasting hyperglycemia occurs as a result of unchecked glucose production by the liver. In addition, glucose derived from food eaten cannot be stored but instead remains in the bloodstream and contributes to postprandial (after meal) hyperglycemia.

If the concentration of glucose in the blood is sufficiently high, the kidneys may not reabsorb all of the filtered glucose; the glucose then appears in the urine (*glucosuria*). When excess glucose is excreted in the urine, it is accompanied by excessive fluid and electrolyte loss. This is called *osmotic diuresis*. As a result of the excess loss of fluid, the patient experiences increased urination (*polyuria*) and increased thirst (*polydipsia*).

Insulin deficiency also impairs the metabolism of proteins and fats, leading to weight loss. Patients may experience an increased appetite (*polyphagia*) because of the decreased storage of calories. Other symptoms include fatigue and weakness.

As the insulin deficiency progresses, the processes that are usually inhibited by insulin occur unrestrained. Thus, glycogenolysis (breakdown of stored glucose) and, more significantly, gluconeogenesis (production of new glucose from amino acids and other substrates) contribute further to hyperglycemia. In addition, the breakdown of fat occurs, resulting in an increased production of ketone bodies, which are the by-products of fat breakdown. *Ketone bodies* are acids that disturb the acid–base balance of the body when they accumulate in excess amounts. The resulting diabetic ketoacidosis (DKA) may cause signs and symptoms such as abdominal pain, nausea, vomiting, hyperventilation, fruity odor of the breath, and, if left untreated, altered level of consciousness, coma, and even death.

The onset of type I diabetes usually occurs abruptly and before the age of 30. Initiation of insulin treatment along with fluid and electrolytes as needed for DKA rapidly improves the metabolic abnormalities and resolves symptoms of hyperglycemia and DKA. Diet and exercise with frequent monitoring of blood glucose levels are also important components of therapy.

Type II Diabetes.   In type II diabetes there are two main problems related to insulin: insulin resistance and impaired insulin secretion. Insulin resistance refers to a decreased sensitivity of the tissues to insulin. Normally, insulin binds to special receptors on cell surfaces. As a result of insulin binding to these receptors, a series of reactions involved in glucose metabolism occurs within the cell. The insulin resistance of type II diabetes is associated with a decrease in these intracellular reactions. The insulin thus becomes less effective at stimulating glucose uptake by the tissues.

In order to overcome insulin resistance and to prevent the buildup of glucose in the blood, there must be an increase in the amount of insulin secreted. This occurs in impaired glucose tolerance in which a normal or slightly elevated glucose level is maintained only through excess secretion of insulin. However, if the beta cells are unable to keep up with the increased demand for insulin, the glucose level rises and type II diabetes develops.

Despite the impaired insulin secretion that is characteristic of type II diabetes, there is enough insulin present to prevent the breakdown of fat and the accompanying production of ketone bodies. Therefore, DKA does not occur in type II diabetes. Uncontrolled type II diabetes may, however, lead to another acute problem called hyperosmolar nonketotic syndrome (see p. 1052).

Type II diabetes occurs most commonly in people over 30 years of age who are obese. Because it is associated with a slow (over years), progressive glucose intolerance, the onset of type II diabetes may go undetected for many years. If symptoms are experienced, they are frequently mild and may include fatigue, irritability, polyuria, polydipsia, skin wounds that heal poorly, vaginal infections, or blurred vision (if glucose levels are very high).

For most patients (approximately 75%), type II diabetes is detected incidentally (*e.g.*, when routine laboratory tests are performed). One consequence of diabetes going undetected for many years is that long-term diabetes complications (*e.g.*, eye disease, peripheral neuropathy, peripheral vascular disease) may have developed before the actual diagnosis of diabetes is made.

Because insulin resistance is associated with obesity, the primary treatment of type II diabetes is weight loss. Exercise is also important in enhancing the effectiveness of insulin. Oral hypoglycemic agents may be added if diet and exercise are not successful in controlling blood glucose levels. If the use of maximum doses of oral agents fails to reduce glucose levels to satisfactory levels, insulin is used. Some patients require insulin on an ongoing basis, while a few may require insulin on a temporary basis during periods of acute physiologic stress, such as illness or surgery.

Complications of Diabetes.   The complications associated with both types of diabetes are classified as acute or chronic complications. Acute complications result from an imbalance in the treatment regimen. They include:

- Hypoglycemia (low blood sugar), which is also called insulin reaction or insulin shock
- Hyperglycemia (high blood sugar), which, if uncontrolled, may lead to diabetic ketoacidosis (DKA) in type I diabetes or hyperosmolar nonketotic syndrome (HNKS) in type II diabetes

If not treated appropriately, the acute complications may lead to coma or even death.

The chronic complications of type I and type II diabetes generally occur 10 to 15 years after the onset of diabetes. There are three main types of chronic complications:

- Macrovascular (large vessel) disease—affecting coronary, peripheral vascular, and cerebrovascular circulations
- Microvascular (small vessel) disease—affecting the eyes (retinopathy) and kidneys (nephropathy)
- Neuropathic diseases—affecting sensorimotor and autonomic nerves and contributing to such problems as impotence and foot ulcers

Controlling blood glucose levels is important in delaying, or possibly avoiding, the onset of microvascular and neuropathic complications. For macrovascular complications, nephropathy, and probably retinopathy, blood pressure control is also important. Chart 39-1 presents an overview of the complications of diabetes.

Etiology

Type I Diabetes

Type I diabetes is characterized by destruction of the pancreatic beta cells. Currently it is thought that a combination of genetic, immunologic, and possibly environmental (*e.g.*, viral) factors contribute to beta cell destruction.

Genetic Factors.   People do not inherit type I diabetes itself; rather, they inherit a genetic predisposition, or tendency, toward developing type I diabetes. This genetic tendency has been found in people with certain HLA (human leukocyte antigen) types. HLA refers to a cluster of genes responsible for transplantation antigens and other immune processes. Ninety-five percent of white patients with type I diabetes exhibit specific HLA types (DR3 and/or DR4). The risk of developing type I diabetes is increased three to five times in people who have one of these two HLA types. The presence of both DR3 and DR4 HLA types confers a 10- to 20-fold increased risk of developing type I diabetes (as compared with the general population).

Chart 39–1
Complications of Diabetes

Acute Complications

1. Hypoglycemia (low blood glucose). Also known as: hypoglycemic reaction, insulin reaction, insulin shock
2. Hyperglycemia (high blood glucose). May lead to:
   - Diabetic ketoacidosis in type I diabetes
   - Hyperosmolar, nonketotic syndrome in type II diabetes

Long-Term (Chronic) Complications

1. Macrovascular Disease
   a. Coronary artery disease (leading to myocardial infarction)
   b. Cerebrovascular disease (leading to stroke)
   c. Peripheral vascular disease*
2. Microvascular Disease
   a. Retinopathy (eye disease)
   b. Nephropathy (kidney disease)
3. Neuropathy (nerve damage)
   a. Sensorimotor neuropathy (affecting the extremities)*
   b. Autonomic neuropathy (affecting gastrointestinal, cardiovascular, genitourinary functioning)

* Contributes to the development of foot ulcers and the high incidence of amputations in diabetes.

Immunologic Factors. In type I diabetes there is evidence of an autoimmune response. This is an abnormal response in which antibodies are directed against normal tissues of the body, responding to these tissues as if they are foreign. Autoantibodies against islet cells and against endogenous (internal) insulin have been detected in people at the time of diagnosis and even several years prior to the development of clinical signs of type I diabetes. Currently, research is being conducted to evaluate the effect of immunosuppressive agents on progression of disease in persons with newly diagnosed type I diabetes or persons with prediabetes (those with detectable antibodies but no clinical symptoms of diabetes).

Environmental Factors. There are ongoing investigations into possible external factors that may initiate destruction of the beta cell. For example, it has been proposed that certain viruses or toxins may precipitate the autoimmune process that leads to beta cell destruction.

The interaction of genetic, immunologic, and environmental factors in the etiology of type I diabetes is the subject of continuing research. While the events that lead to beta cell destruction are not fully understood, it is generally accepted that a genetic susceptibility is a common underlying factor in the development of type I diabetes.

Type II Diabetes

The exact mechanisms that lead to insulin resistance and impaired insulin secretion in type II diabetes are unknown at this time. Genetic factors are thought to play a role in the development of insulin resistance. In addition, there are certain risk factors that are known to be associated with the development of type II diabetes. These include:

- Age (insulin resistance tends to occur with age over 65)
- Obesity
- Family history
- Ethnic group (in the United States, there is a higher chance of type II diabetes developing in Hispanic and certain American Indian populations, and, to a lesser degree, in the black population)

Diagnostic Evaluation

The presence of abnormally high blood glucose levels is the criterion on which the diagnosis of diabetes should be based. Fasting plasma glucose levels above 140 mg/dl (SI: 7.8 mmol/L) or random plasma glucose levels over 200 mg/dl (SI: 11.1 mmol/L) on more than one occasion suggests a diagnosis of diabetes. If fasting glucose levels are normal or nearly normal, the diagnosis must be based on a glucose tolerance test.

Glucose Tolerance Test. Currently, the oral glucose tolerance test (OGTT) is more sensitive than the intravenous glucose tolerance test (IVGTT), which is used only in special circumstances (*e.g.*, for the patient who has had gastric surgery). The OGTT is carried out through administration of a simple carbohydrate solution.

The patient ingests high-carbohydrate (150 to 300 g) meals for 3 days preceding the test. After an overnight fast, a blood sample is drawn. Then a 75-g carbohydrate load, usually in the form of a carbonated sugar beverage (Glucola), is given to the patient. The patient is instructed to sit quietly during the test and to avoid exercise, smoking, coffee, and any other oral intake except water.

The World Health Organization (WHO) recommends that blood samples be drawn 2 hours after glucose ingestion. Recommendations from the National Diabetes Data Group include also drawing blood samples at 30 and 60 minutes after glucose ingestion. See Chart 39-2 for specific WHO diagnostic criteria for diabetes mellitus.

Several factors affect the OGTT, including the method of analysis, source of the specimen (whole blood, plasma, or serum, capillary or venous blood), diet, activity level, amount of bed rest, presence of chronic disease, medication, and amount of the glucose load. In the elderly, diet, activity level, and medications present particular problems in interpreting the test results.

Dietary preparation for the test is very important because food intake may affect test results. It may be necessary to give written instructions to the patient to ensure the required intake of carbohydrate. If the diet is normal and the person's weight is stable, 150 gm per day are usually sufficient.

Medications that affect glucose tolerance should be discontinued, if possible, for about 3 days before the test. Four commonly prescribed medications affect the OGTT: diuretics (usually thiazides), glucocorticoids, synthetic estrogens, and phenytoin (Dilantin). Other interfering agents include high doses of nicotinic acid, ethanol, and the chronic ingestion of salicylates and monoamine oxidase inhibitors (especially hydrazine derivatives).

Special circumstances that affect the OGTT are pregnancy, gastric surgery, and advanced age. There is a special modification of the diagnostic criteria for the pregnant patient. In patients who have had gastric surgery, the IVGTT is necessary because an oral glucose load passes quickly into the small intestine, leading to a rapid absorption of glucose and therefore to glucose levels that are abnormal.

Gerontologic Considerations.   Elevated blood glucose levels appear to be age-related and occur in both men and women throughout the world. Elevation of blood glucose appears in the fifth decade of life and increases in frequency with advancing age. When elderly people with overt diabetes are excluded from the statistics, about 10% to 30% of elderly people have age-related hyperglycemia.

The question then arises whether age-related hyperglycemia is part of the normal aging process and benign, or whether it is pathologic and requires therapeutic intervention. Several studies have suggested that the hyperglycemia is pathologic because it leads to macrovascular complications.

The cause of age-related changes in carbohydrate metabolism is still not resolved. Apparently, delayed absorption from the gastrointestinal tract is not a factor. Other possibilities include poor diet, physical inactivity, a decrease in the lean body mass in which ingested carbohydrate may be stored, altered insulin secretion, and insulin resistance.

Management

The main goal of the treatment of diabetes is to try to normalize insulin activity and blood glucose levels in an attempt to reduce the development of the vascular and neuropathic complications. The therapeutic goal within each type of diabetes is to lower blood glucose levels as much as possible without seriously disrupting the patient's usual activity patterns.

There are five components of management for diabetes:

Diet
Exercise
Monitoring
Medication (as needed)
Education

Treatment is variable throughout the course of the disease because of changes in life-style and physical and emotional status as well as advances in therapy resulting from research. Therefore, the management of diabetes involves constant assessment and modification of the treatment plan by health professionals as well as daily adjustments in therapy by the patient himself. Although the health care team directs the treatment, it is the patient who is faced with the daily charge of managing the intricacies of a complex therapeutic regimen. For this reason, patient and family education is seen as an essential component of diabetes treatment—equal in importance to other components of the treatment regimen.

Chart 39-2
World Health Organization Diagnostic Criteria for Diabetes Mellitus in Nonpregnant Adults

On at least two occasions:
1. *Random* plasma glucose >200 mg/dl (11.1 mmol/L)
or

2. *Fasting* plasma glucose >140 mg/dl (7.8 mmol/L)
or

3. *2-hour sample* during 75-g OGTT (Oral Glucose Tolerance Test) >200 mg/dl (11.1 mmol/L)

(World Health Organization. Diabetes mellitus. Report of a WHO study group. Tech Report Series No. 727, 1985.)

Dietary Management

General Principles.   Diet and weight control constitute the foundation of diabetes management. Nutritional management of the patient with diabetes is geared toward the following goals:

1. Provision of all the essential food constituents (*e.g.,* vitamins, minerals)
2. Achievement and maintenance of ideal weight
3. Meeting energy needs
4. Prevention of wide daily variations in blood glucose levels and achieve blood glucose levels as close to normal as is safe and practical
5. Decrease of blood lipid levels, if elevated

For patients who require insulin to help control blood glucose levels, maintaining as much consistency as possible in the amount of calories and carbohydrates eaten at different meal times is important for control of blood glucose. In addition, consistency in the approximate time intervals between meals, with the addition of snacks, if necessary, helps in the prevention of hypoglycemic reactions and in overall blood glucose control.

For obese patients (especially those with type II diabetes), weight loss is the key to the treatment of diabetes. For obese patients in general, weight loss is the major preventive factor for the development of diabetes. Obesity is associated with an increased resistance to insulin and is one of the main etiologic factors associated with type II diabetes. Some obese type II diabetic patients who require insulin or oral agents for control of blood glucose may be able to significantly reduce or completely eliminate the need for medication through weight loss. Even as small a weight loss as 10% of total weight can significantly improve blood glucose levels. For obese diabetic patients who do not take insulin, consistency of meal content or timing is not as critical. Rather, the major focus is on decreasing the overall number of calories eaten.

Long-term adherence to the meal plan is one of the most challenging aspects of diabetes management. For obese patients it may be more realistic to only moderately restrict calories. For those who have lost weight, maintaining the weight loss is often difficult. In order to assist these patients in incorporating new dietary habits into their life-styles, participation in behavioral therapy, group support, and ongoing nutrition counseling is encouraged.

For all diabetic patients, the meal plan must take into consideration the patient's food likes and dislikes, life-style, usual eating times, and ethnic and cultural background. For patients using intensive insulin therapy regimens, there may be a greater flexibility in the timing and content of meals provided the patient can safely alter the insulin dose as needed (see p. 1035).

Calorie Intake

Calorie Requirements.   The first step in preparing the meal plan is to determine the patient's basic calorie requirements, taking into consideration age, sex, body weight, and degree of activity. There are several methods of assessing calorie needs. A simple method, for instance, in most weight-maintenance diets is to multiply ideal weight by 28 cal/kg. For weight reduction, a 15 to 20 cal/kg of the patient's ideal weight is suitable.

For most people, long-term reduction diets can be achieved with caloric levels between 1000 and 1200 calories. The calorie requirement can be raised to a maintenance level when the patient achieves the desired weight.

The most important objective in the dietary treatment of diabetes is control of total calorie intake to attain or maintain ideal weight. Success of this measure alone is often associated with reversal of the hyperglycemia in type II diabetic patients. In a young patient with type I diabetes, priority should be given to providing a diet with enough calories to maintain normal growth and development. Some patients may be underweight at the onset of type I diabetes because of rapid weight loss from severe hyperglycemia. The goal with these patients may initially be to provide a higher calorie diet to regain lost weight.

Calorie Distribution.   In addition to a recommended number of daily calories, the diabetic meal plan also focuses on the percentage of calories to come from carbohydrate, protein, and fats. There are two main types of carbohydrates—complex and simple. Starches such as bread, cereal, rice, and pasta are complex carbohydrates; fruit and sugars are examples of simple carbohydrates. In general, carbohydrate foods have the greatest effect on blood glucose levels because they are more quickly digested than other foods and are converted into glucose rapidly. Several decades ago it was recommended that diabetic diets contain more calories from protein and fat foods than from carbohydrates in order to reduce post-meal increases in blood glucose levels. However, more recently it has been found that complex carbohydrates are absorbed more gradually from the gastrointestinal tract and cause less of a blood glucose rise than initially thought. In addition, diets that contained fewer calories from carbohydrates contained increased calories from fats—a problem in trying to reduce the cardiovascular disease commonly associated with diabetes.

The caloric distribution recommended at present is higher in carbohydrates than in fat and protein. However, research into the appropriateness of a higher carbohydrate diet in patients with decreased glucose tolerance is ongoing, and recommendations may be changed accordingly. Currently, the American Diabetes and American Dietetic Associations recommend that for all levels of caloric intake, 50% to 60% of calories be derived from carbohydrates, 20% to 30% from fat, and the remaining 12% to 20% from protein. These recommendations are also consistent with those of the American Heart Association and American Cancer Society.

Carbohydrates.   A high intake of carbohydrates—especially simple sugars—is typical in the American diet. The goal of the diabetic diet is to emphasize the intake of complex carbohydrates (especially those higher in fiber), such as breads, cereals, pastas, and beans. However, because certain nutritious foods such as milk and fruit contain simple sugars (lactose and fructose), encouraging complete avoidance of simple sugars is inappropriate. In addition, the use of moderate amounts of sucrose (table sugar) is gaining wider acceptance provided the patient can maintain adequate blood glucose levels, blood lipid levels (including all types of cholesterol and triglycerides), and weight control. For some patients, a more liberal use of simple carbohydrates can be a major factor in promoting adherence to a meal plan.

Fat.   The recommendations regarding fat content of the diabetic diet include both reduction in the total percentage of calories from fat sources and limitation of the amount of saturated fats (10% of total calories). In addition, limitation of total intake of dietary cholesterol is recommended. These recommendations may help in the reduction of risk factors, such as elevated serum cholesterol levels, which are associated with the development of coronary heart disease, the leading cause of death and debility among diabetic patients.

Protein. The meal plan may include the use of some non-animal sources of protein in order to help in the reduction of saturated fat and cholesterol intake. In addition, recommendations for the amount of protein intake may be reduced in patients with early signs of developing renal disease.

Fiber. The use of fiber in diabetes has received increasing attention in the past 10 years as researchers study the effects on diabetes of a high-carbohydrate, high-fiber diet. This type of diet plays a role in lowering total cholesterol and LDL (low-density lipoprotein) cholesterol in the blood. Increasing fiber in the diet may also improve blood glucose levels, leading to a decrease in the need for exogenous insulin.

There are two classifications of dietary fibers: soluble and insoluble. Soluble fiber—in foods such as legumes, oats, and some fruits—plays more of a role in lowering blood glucose and lipid levels than does insoluble fiber.

The mechanism of action of soluble fiber is thought to be related to the formation of a gel in the gastrointestinal tract. This gel slows the emptying of the stomach and the movement of food through the upper digestive tract. The potential glucose-lowering effect of fiber may be due to the slower rate of glucose absorption from food that contains soluble fiber.

Insoluble fiber is found in whole-grain breads and cereals and in some vegetables. This type of fiber plays more of a role in increasing stool bulk and preventing constipation. Both insoluble and soluble fibers increase satiety, which is helpful for weight loss.

One risk involved in suddenly increasing fiber intake is that it may require adjusting the dosage of insulin or oral agents medications to prevent hypoglycemia. Other problems may include abdominal fullness, nausea, diarrhea, increased flatulence, and constipation if fluid intake is inadequate. If fiber is added to or increased in the meal plan, it should be done gradually and in consultation with a dietitian. The 1986 Exchange Lists for Meal Planning is an excellent guide for increasing fiber intake. Food choices within the vegetable, fruit, and starch/bread exchanges are highlighted in the lists.

Research continues into the role of dietary fiber. It appears that adding more fiber to the meal plan is beneficial. However, further research will help to determine how fiber works, which fibers are best, and the amount of fiber that is optimal for blood glucose and lipid control.

Alcohol. The ingestion of alcohol by diabetic patients need not be completely restricted. It is important, however, for patients and health care professionals to be aware of the potential adverse effects of alcohol specific to diabetes.

In general, the same precautions regarding the use of alcohol by the general public should be applied to patients with diabetes. Moderation in the amount of alcohol consumed is recommended. The main danger with the use of alcohol by a diabetic patient is hypoglycemia. This is especially true for patients who take insulin. Alcohol may decrease the normal physiologic reactions in the body that produce glucose (gluconeogenesis). Thus, if a diabetic patient takes alcohol on an empty stomach, there is an increased likelihood of hypogly-

cemia developing. In addition, excessive alcohol intake may impair a person's ability to recognize and appropriately treat hypoglycemia and to follow a prescribed meal plan in order to prevent hypoglycemia.

For the person with type II diabetes treated with oral agents, a potential side effect of alcohol consumption is a disulfiram (Antabuse) type of reaction. Depending upon the amount of alcohol consumed, the person taking chlorpropamide (Diabinese) may experience facial flushing, warmth, headache, nausea, vomiting, sweating, and/or thirst within minutes of consuming alcohol. This reaction seems to be less common with other oral agents.

In addition to these immediate potential untoward effects, alcohol consumption may also lead to excessive weight gain (because of the high caloric content of alcohol), hyperlipidemia, and (especially if mixed drinks and liqueurs are consumed) elevated glucose levels.

Patient teaching regarding alcohol intake must emphasize moderation in the amount of alcohol consumed; lower calorie or less sweet drinks such as "light" beer or dry wine, and the intake of food along with alcohol are advised. For type II diabetic patients especially, incorporating the calories from alcohol into the overall meal plan is important for weight control.

Food Classification Systems

In order to teach diet principles and to help patients in meal planning, several systems have been developed in which foods are organized into groups. The general concept is that foods are separated into groups that possess common characteristics, such as number of calories, composition of foods (*i.e.*, amount of protein, fat, and/or carbohydrate in the food), or effect on blood glucose levels.

Exchange Lists. A common tool in use is the Exchange Lists for Meal Planning. There are six main exchange lists: bread/starch, vegetable, milk, meat, fruit, and fat. Foods included on one list (in the amounts specified) contain equal numbers of calories and are approximately equal in grams of protein, fat, and carbohydrate.

Patients are given meal plans (tailored to their individual needs and preferences) based on a recommended number of food choices from each exchange list. Foods within one list may be interchanged with one another, thus facilitating the patient's ability to choose a variety of foods to eat while maintaining as much consistency as possible in the nutrient content of foods eaten. Table 39-2 presents three sample lunch menus that are interchangeable in terms of carbohydrate, protein, and fat content.

During recent years there has been an expansion in information available regarding food exchanges. Information on combination foods such as pizza, chili, and chow mein is now readily available in the exchange list information from the American Diabetes and American Dietetic Associations. In addition, exchanges for a variety of foods, including convenience packaged foods, dessert foods, and snack foods, are published in various books and publications. Some of the food manufacturing companies publish exchange lists that describe their products.

The 1986 exchange list emphasizes a high-carbohydrate, high-fiber diet and reflects the order in which foods are usually considered in meal planning. High-fiber foods and those with

TABLE 39–2. *Sample Menus Based on the Exchange Lists*

Exchanges	Sample Lunch #1	Sample Lunch #2	Sample Lunch #3
2 starch	2 slices bread	Hamburger bun	1 cup cooked pasta
3 meat	2 oz sliced turkey and 1 oz lowfat cheese	3 oz lean beef patty	3 oz boiled shrimp
1 vegetable	Lettuce, tomato, onion	Green salad	½ cup plum tomatoes
1 fat	1 tsp mayonnaise	1 tbsp salad dressing	1 tsp olive oil
1 fruit	1 medium apple	1¼ cup watermelon	1¼ cup fresh strawberries
"Free" items (optional)	Iced tea	Diet soda	Ice water with lemon
	Mustard, pickle, hot pepper	1 tbsp catsup, pickle, onions	Garlic, basil

a high sodium content are identified to aid in diet planning for patients on special diabetic diets that are high in fiber and low in sodium.

Basic Four Food Groups. For patients who need a simplified meal plan, "balanced" meals are encouraged with foods from a modified grouping of the "basic four" food groups. These groups include the bread/cereal group, the milk/cheese group, the meat/fish/poultry/bean group, and the fruit and vegetable group. For the diabetic diet, the fruit and vegetable groups must be separated because of the very different effect of these two types of foods on blood glucose levels. This system may not provide the same consistency in intake as the exchange lists, but it will discourage meal planning that emphasizes one type of food that may increase blood glucose levels while totally eliminating another type of food.

Another similar approach might be simply to teach patients about which foods contain carbohydrate (*i.e.*, starch and simple sugars), protein, and fat. Menu planning should include meals with all three types of foods—emphasizing complex carbohydrates (starches) and limiting simple sugars and fat.

Calorie Counting. Meal planning approaches for use with type II (non–insulin-requiring) obese patients may emphasize food choices based on numbers of calories. In these patients it may be less critical for meals to be consistent in the exact percentage of calories derived from the various nutrients (carbohydrates, proteins, and fats). Rather, assuring overall limits on the number of calories consumed is emphasized.

Glycemic Index. One of the main goals of diet therapy in diabetes is to avoid sharp, rapid increases in blood glucose levels after food is eaten. Some patients, therefore, in the past were taught to avoid or limit the intake of foods that were assumed to cause the greatest increases in post-meal glucose levels.

It had long been thought that simple carbohydrates have a greater impact on post-meal blood glucose than complex carbohydrates. Recent research, however, has suggested that some complex carbohydrates may act more like the simple carbohydrates. In addition, it has been found that certain foods that are equal in carbohydrate content may have very different effects on the blood glucose level.

The term *glycemic index* is used to describe how much a given food raises the blood glucose level as compared with an equivalent amount of glucose. In general, some of the research studies have found that root vegetables such as carrots and potatoes have a higher glycemic index than other complex and simple carbohydrates, such as pasta, legumes, and fructose.

These studies, however, were sometimes based on the glucose response to eating a fairly large amount of just one type of food. Therefore, the glycemic index cannot be used to predict the effect of a particular food when eaten in a normal mixed diet.

More recent research has found a very complex set of factors that may affect the glycemic index of food. These factors include:

- Protein, fat, and fiber content of the meal
- Form in which the carbohydrate is ingested (*e.g.*, raw versus cooked)
- Content and time of previous meal
- Rate of meal intake
- Variations in the digestive, absorptive, and metabolic processes of the person ingesting the food

Studies of the glycemic index have raised many questions regarding the traditional approach to diabetic meal planning. For example, questions are raised regarding the equivalency of foods on the same exchange list. Foods on one list may be equivalent in terms of the amount of carbohydrate but may not be equivalent in their effect on blood glucose. Similarly, foods on one list may have different glycemic effects depending upon how they are prepared.

Despite the necessity for further research on the glycemic index, there are general guidelines that can be used in making dietary recommendations:

- Combining starch foods with protein- and fat-containing foods tends to slow down their absorption and lower the glycemic response
- Eating foods that are raw and whole, in general, will result in a lower glycemic response than eating chopped, pureed, or cooked foods
- When adding foods with simple sugars to the diet, a lower glycemic response may result if they are eaten with other more slowly absorbed foods

Patients can create their own glycemic index by monitoring their blood glucose level after ingesting a particular food. This can help patients improve their blood glucose levels through individualized manipulation of the diet. Many patients who use frequent monitoring of blood glucose levels can use this information to adjust their insulin doses for variations in food intake.

Sweeteners and Food Labels. The use of sweeteners is acceptable for patients with diabetes, especially if it assists in overall dietary adherence. Moderation in the amount of sweetener used is encouraged to avoid potential adverse effects.

There are two main types of sweeteners: nutritive and non-nutritive. The nutritive sweeteners contain calories, while the non-nutritive sweeteners have few or no calories in the amounts normally used.

Nutritive sweeteners
- Include fructose (fruit sugar), sorbitol, xylitol
- Are not calorie-free
- Provide calories in amounts similar to those in sucrose (table sugar)
- Cause less elevation in blood sugar levels than sucrose
- Are often used in "sugar-free" foods
- May have a laxative effect (sorbitol)

Non-nutritive sweeteners
- Have minimal or no calories
- Are used in products and are also available for table use
- Produce minimal or no elevation in blood sugar levels
- Saccharin—no calories
- Aspartame—packaged with dextrose, 4 calories/packet, loses sweetness with heat
- Acesulfame K—packaged with dextrose, 1 calorie/packet

Food Labeling. Foods that are labeled "sugarless" or "sugar-free" may still provide calories equal to those of the equivalent non–sugar-free products if made with nutritive sweeteners. Thus, for weight loss, these products may not always be useful. In addition, patients must not consider them "free" foods to be eaten in unlimited quantity because they may cause elevations in blood glucose levels.

Foods that are labeled "dietetic" are not necessarily reduced-calorie foods. They may be lower in sodium or have other special dietary uses. Patients must realize that foods labeled "dietetic" may still contain significant amounts of sugar or fat.

Patients must also be taught to read labels of "health" foods—especially snacks—because they often contain sugar products such as honey, brown sugar, and corn syrup. In addition, these "health" snacks frequently contain saturated vegetable fats (such as coconut or palm oil), hydrogenated vegetable fats, or animal fats, which may be contraindicated in the patient with elevated blood lipids.

Health Teaching About Diet

The clinical dietitian uses various educational tools, teaching materials, and approaches to meal planning. Initial education will address the importance of consistency in eating habits, the relationship of food and insulin, and the provision of an individualized meal plan. Follow-up education will then focus on more in-depth management skills, such as restaurant eating, reading food labels, and adjusting the meal plan for exercise, illness, and special occasions. The nurse plays an important role in communicating pertinent information to the dietitian and reinforcing the patient's understanding.

For some patients, learning to use the exchange system may be too difficult. This may be related to limitations in what the patient is intellectually capable of understanding and retaining. It may also be related to emotional issues, such as difficulty accepting the diagnosis of diabetes or feelings of deprivation and undue restriction in eating. It is important to simplify information as much as possible and to provide many opportunities for practice and repetition of information. In addition, it should be emphasized that using the exchange system (or any food classification system) provides a new way of thinking about food rather than a completely new way of eating.

Exercise

Exercise is extremely important in the management of diabetes because of its effects on lowering blood glucose and reducing cardiovascular risk factors. Exercise lowers blood glucose by increasing the uptake of glucose by body muscles and improving insulin utilization. It also improves circulation and muscle tone. These effects are useful in diabetes in relation to losing weight, easing stress, and maintaining a feeling of well-being. Exercise also alters blood lipids—increasing levels of high-density lipoproteins (HDL) and decreasing total cholesterol and triglyceride levels. This is especially important to the person with diabetes because of the increased risk of cardiovascular disease.

However, patients with blood glucose levels over 250 mg/dl (14 mmol/L) who have ketones in their urine should not begin exercising until the urine ketone test is negative and the blood glucose level is lower. Exercising with elevated blood glucose levels will cause increased secretions of glucagon, growth hormone, and catecholamines. The liver will then release more glucose, resulting in an increase in blood glucose. Exercise should not be performed until blood glucose levels are under 250 mg/dl (14 mmol/L).

Initially, the insulin-requiring patient should be taught to eat a 15-gm carbohydrate snack (a fruit exchange) or a snack of complex carbohydrate with a protein before engaging in moderate exercise, in order to prevent unexpected hypoglycemia. The exact amount of food needed varies from person to person and should be determined with the use of blood glucose monitoring results. Some patients find that they do not require a pre-exercise snack if they exercise within 1 to 2 hours after a meal. Other patients may require extra food regardless of the timing of exercise. If extra food is required, it need not be deducted from the regular meal plan.

Another potential problem for patients who take insulin is hypoglycemia that occurs many hours *after* exercise. To avoid postexercise hypoglycemia, especially after strenuous exercise, the patient may need to eat a snack at the end of the exercise session. In addition, it may be necessary to have the patient reduce the dosage of insulin that is peaking at the time of exercise.

Patients participating in extended periods of exercise should test blood glucose before, during, and after the exercise period, and they should eat carbohydrate snacks as needed to maintain blood glucose levels. Other participants or observers should be aware that the person exercising has diabetes, and they should know what assistance to give if severe hypoglycemia occurs.

In obese persons with type II diabetes, exercise in addition to dietary management both improves glucose metabolism and enhances loss of body fat. Exercise coupled with weight loss improves insulin sensitivity and may decrease the need for insulin or oral agents. Eventually, the patient's glucose tolerance may return to normal. The type II diabetic patient who is not taking insulin or an oral agent may not need extra food before exercise.

Persons with diabetes should be taught to exercise at the same time (preferably when blood glucose levels are at their peak) and in the same amount each day. Regular daily exercise, rather than sporadic exercise, should be encouraged. Exercise recommendations must be altered as necessary for patients with diabetic complications such as retinopathy, autonomic neuropathy, sensorimotor neuropathy, and cardiovascular disease. Increased blood pressure associated with exercise may aggravate diabetic retinopathy and increase the risk of a hemorrhage into the vitreous or retina. In patients with ischemic heart disease, there is a risk of triggering angina or a myocardial infarction. Avoidance of trauma to the lower extremities is especially important in the patient with numbness related to neuropathy.

In general, a slow, gradual increase in the length of the exercise period is encouraged. For many patients, walking is a safe and beneficial form of exercise that requires no special equipment (except for proper shoes) and can be performed anywhere.

If the patient is over 30 years of age and has two or more of the risk factors for heart disease, an exercise stress test is recommended. Risk factors for heart disease include hypertension, obesity, high cholesterol levels, abnormal resting electrocardiogram, sedentary life-style, smoking, and a family history of heart disease. In general, persons with diabetes should discuss an exercise program with their physician.

Gerontologic Considerations

Physical activity that is consistent and realistic is beneficial to the elderly person with diabetes. Advantages include a decrease in hyperglycemia, a general sense of well-being, and the utilization of ingested calories, resulting in weight reduction. Because there is an increased incidence of cardiovascular problems in the elderly, a pattern of slow, consistent exercise should be planned that does not exceed the patient's physical capacity. Physical impairment from other chronic diseases must also be considered.

Monitoring of Glucose and Ketones

Self-Monitoring of Blood Glucose

The 1980s were a time of rapid advancements in the technology available for glucose monitoring. The development of methods for self-monitoring of blood glucose (SMBG) is seen as the greatest breakthrough in diabetes management since the discovery of insulin.

With the use of frequent SMBG results, people with diabetes are now able to adjust the treatment regimen to obtain optimal blood glucose control. This allows for detection and prevention of hypo- and hyperglycemia and plays a crucial role in normalizing blood glucose levels, which will possibly reduce long-term diabetic complications.

Procedure. There are various methods available for SMBG. Most of them involve obtaining a drop of blood from the fingertip, applying the blood to a special reagent strip, and allowing the blood to stay on the strip for a specific amount of time (usually between 45 and 60 seconds, as specified by the manufacturer). For some of the products, the blood is then wiped off the strip (using cotton or tissue per manufacturer

specifications). The reagent pad of the strip changes color and can then be matched to a color chart on the product package (Fig. 39-1) or is inserted into a meter that gives a digital readout of the blood glucose value.

Several newer blood glucose monitors are available that have eliminated the step of blood removal from the strip. The strip is placed in the meter first, before blood is applied to it. Once the blood is placed on the strip, it remains there for the duration of the test. The meter automatically displays the blood glucose level after a short period of time (under 1 minute). One of the newest products uses a glucose sensor cartridge (instead of strips) onto which the blood is placed. These new types of meters tend to give blood glucose results in a shorter period of time, and most of them have automatic timers that do not need to be activated by the user.

Meters have also been developed that can be used by patients with visual impairments. They have audio components that assist the patient in performing the test and obtaining the result.

Advantages and Disadvantages of SMBG Systems.   It is very important that the method used by patients be appropriately matched to their skill level. Factors affecting SMBG performance include: visual deficits, fine motor coordination, intellectual capability, comfort with technology, willingness, and cost.

Visual methods are the least expensive and require less equipment. However, they require the ability to distinguish colors and to be exact in timing the procedures.

Meters in general are more expensive (at least initially), but they eliminate the subjective aspect of trying to match colors visually.

Meters that require removal of blood from the reagent strip have more steps that must be performed in an exact sequence. However, they allow for double-checking the results through visual reading of the strips. The newer generation of meters that do not require removal of blood from the strip generally have simpler techniques for usage. However, most of them do not provide a backup method for visually checking the meter results. Figure 39-2 illustrates two systems available for glucose monitoring.

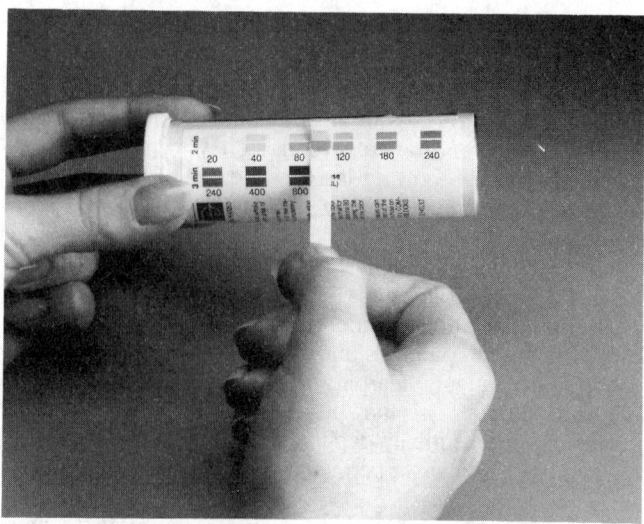

Figure 39–1.   With this product, the user visually compares the color on the reagent strip to a chart.

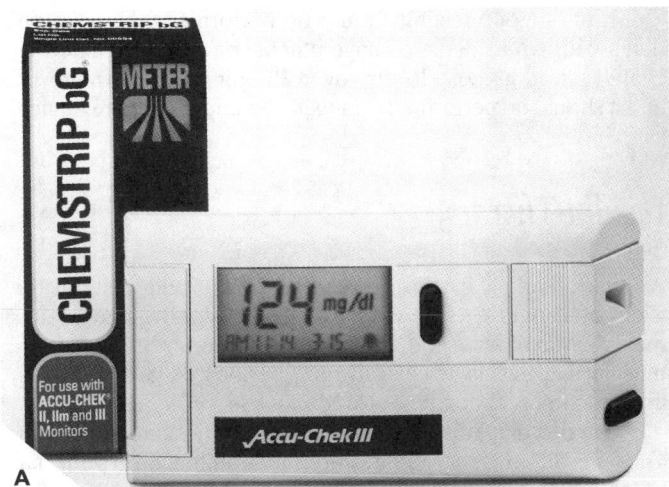
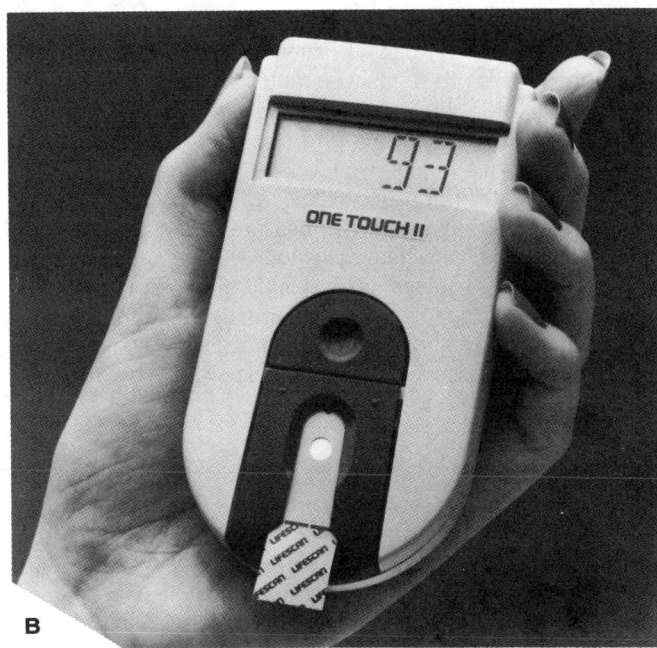

Figure 39–2. Examples of two blood glucose monitors. (**A**) The Accu-Chek III meter allows for double checking results through visual reading. (There is also a new nonwipe version of this meter called Accu-Chek Easy, not shown.) (**B**) The One Touch II is one example of a meter that does not require removal of blood from the strip. (*A*: Courtesy of Boehringer Manheim Corp, Indianapolis. *B*: Courtesy of Lifescan, Inc, a Johnson and Johnson Company.)

A potential hazard of all methods of SMBG is that the patient may obtain and report erroneous blood glucose values as a result of using incorrect techniques. Some common sources of error include:

- Improper application of blood (*e.g.*, drop too small)
- Improper timing
- Improper blood removal (*e.g.*, wiping too hard or too lightly or not using recommended material for wiping)
- Improper cleaning and maintenance of meters (*e.g.*, allowing dust and/or blood to accumulate on the optic window)

The nurse plays an important role in providing initial education in SMBG techniques. Equally important is evaluating the techniques of patients who are "experienced" in self-monitoring. Patients should be discouraged from purchasing SMBG products from stores or catalogs that do not provide direct education. Every 6 to 12 months, patients should conduct a comparison of their meter with a simultaneous laboratory-measured blood glucose level in their physician's office.

Candidates for SMBG. Blood glucose monitoring is a useful procedure for all people with diabetes. It is a cornerstone of treatment for any intensive insulin therapy regimen (including two to four injections per day or insulin pumps) and for managing pregnancy complicated by diabetes. It is also highly recommended for patients with:

- Unstable diabetes
- A tendency for severe ketosis or hypoglycemia
- Hypoglycemia without warning symptoms
- Abnormal renal glucose thresholds

For patients not taking insulin, SMBG is helpful for monitoring the effectiveness of exercise, diet, and oral agents. It can also help to motivate patients to continue with treatment. For type II diabetic patients, SMBG should also be recommended during periods of suspected hyperglycemia (*e.g.*, illness) or hypoglycemia (*e.g.*, unusual increased activity levels).

Frequency of SMBG. For most insulin-requiring patients, testing two to four times per day is recommended (usually before meals and at bedtime). For patients who take insulin prior to each meal, testing at least three times per day is required for safely determining each insulin dose. Patients not on insulin may be instructed to check blood glucose levels a minimum of two to three times per week.

For all patients, testing is recommended if possible whenever hypoglycemia or hyperglycemia is suspected.

Using Results of SMBG. The tendency to discontinue SMBG may be seen in patients who were never instructed on how to utilize the results for altering their treatment regimen. Instructions will vary according to the patient's understanding and the physician's philosophy of diabetes management. At the very least, patients should be given parameters for calling the physician. Patients using intensive insulin therapy regimens may be given sophisticated algorithms (rules) for changing the insulin doses based on patterns of values greater or less than the target range.

Glycosylated Hemoglobin

This is a blood test that reflects average blood glucose levels over a period of approximately 2 to 3 months. When blood glucose levels are elevated, a glucose molecule attaches itself to hemoglobin in a red blood cell. The longer the glucose in the blood remains above normal, the more glycosylated hemoglobins form. This complex (the hemoglobin attached to the glucose) is permanent and lasts for the life of the red blood cell, approximately 120 days. If near-normal blood glucose levels are maintained, with only occasional rises in blood glucose, the overall value will not be greatly elevated. However, if the blood glucose values are consistently high, then the test result will also be elevated. If patients report mostly normal results on records of self-glucose monitoring but the glycosylated hemoglobin is high, there may be errors in the methods used for glucose monitoring, errors in recording results, or frequent elevations in glucose levels at times during the day when the patient is not usually checking the blood.

There are various tests that measure the same thing but have different names, including hemoglobin A_{1C} and hemoglobin A_1. The normal values differ slightly from test to test and from laboratory to laboratory and normally range from 4% to 8%. Values within the normal range indicate consistently near-normal blood glucose levels, a goal made easier by patients' self-monitoring of blood glucose levels.

Urine Testing for Glucose

Prior to the availability of SMBG methods, urine glucose testing was the only method available for day-to-day monitoring of diabetes. It currently has limited use in diabetes management.

The general procedure involves applying urine to a reagent strip or tablet and matching colors on the strip with a color chart. The results are expressed as a percentage (*e.g.*, 1/10%, 1/4%, 2%) or on a scale of 1+ to 4+. (The percentage reading method is preferred because this scale is consistent from method to method).

There are several disadvantages to urine testing, including:

- Results do not reflect the blood glucose level at the time of the test
- It is impossible to detect hypoglycemia because a "negative" urine glucose result may occur when blood glucose ranges from zero to 180 mg/dl (10 mmol/L) or higher
- Patients may have a false sense of being in "good" control when results are always negative
- Various medications (*e.g.*, aspirin, vitamin C, some antibiotics) may interfere with test results
- In the elderly and in patients with kidney disease, the renal threshold (*i.e.*, the level of blood glucose at which glucose starts to appear in the urine) is increased; thus, falsely negative readings may occur at dangerously elevated glucose levels

The advantages of urine glucose testing are that it is less expensive than SMBG and it is not invasive.

Urine glucose testing is sometimes used in combination with SMBG to detect extreme hyperglycemia at times when blood glucose testing is not being performed. Otherwise, urine glucose testing should be limited to patients who cannot or will not perform blood glucose testing.

Urine Testing for Ketones

Ketones (or ketone bodies) in the urine signal that control of type I diabetes is deteriorating. When there is almost no effective insulin available, the body starts to break down stored fat for energy. Ketone bodies are by-products of this fat breakdown, and they accumulate in the blood and urine. The only method available for self-testing of ketone bodies by patients is urine testing.

The most commonly used method to detect ketonuria is to use a urine "dipstick" (Ketostix or Chemstrip uK), which measures one type of ketone body. The reagent pad on the strip turns a purplish color when ketones are present. (Note: one of the ketone bodies is called "acetone," and this term is

frequently used interchangeably with the term "ketones.") There are also strips available that measure both glucose and ketones (Keto-Diastix or Chemstrip uGK). Large amounts of ketones may depress the color development of the glucose test area.

Urine ketone testing should be performed whenever patients with type I diabetes have glucosuria or unexplained elevated blood glucose levels (over 250 mg/dl or 14 mmol/L), and it should be performed during illness and during pregnancy.

Insulin Therapy

As stated earlier, insulin is secreted by the beta cells of the islets of Langerhans. It works to lower blood glucose after meals by facilitating the uptake and utilization of glucose by muscle, fat, and liver cells. During periods of fasting, insulin inhibits the breakdown of stored glucose, protein, and fat.

In type I diabetes, the body fails to produce enough insulin. Thus, insulin must be administered indefinitely. In type II diabetes, insulin may be necessary on a long-term basis to control glucose levels if diet and oral agents have failed. In addition, some patients whose type II diabetes is usually controlled by diet alone or by diet and an oral agent may require insulin temporarily during illness, infection, pregnancy, surgery, or some other stressful event.

Frequently, insulin injections are taken two times per day (or even more) in order to control post-meal and overnight increases in blood glucose. Because the insulin dose required by the individual patient is determined by the level of glucose in the blood, accurate monitoring of blood glucose levels is essential. Self-monitoring of blood glucose levels has become the cornerstone of insulin therapy because of its role in evaluating the effectiveness of the insulin dosage and promoting better control of blood glucose levels.

Insulin Preparations. A number of insulin preparations are available. They vary according to four main characteristics: time course of action, concentration, species (source), and manufacturer.

Time Course. Insulins may be grouped into three main categories based on the onset, peak, and duration of action.

Short-Acting Insulins Include:
- Regular insulin (marked "R" on the bottle)
- Semilente insulin ("SL")

The onset of regular insulin action is ½ to 1 hour; peak, 2 to 4 hours; duration, 6 to 8 hours. Another name for regular insulin is crystalline zinc insulin (CZI). Semilente insulin has a slightly longer time course of action: onset, 1 to 2 hours; peak, 4 to 6 hours; and duration, 8 to 12 hours.

Both insulins are clear in appearance and are usually administered 20 to 30 minutes before a meal, either alone or in combination with a longer-acting insulin.

Intermediate-Acting Insulins Include:
- NPH insulin (neutral protamine Hagedorn)
- Lente insulin ("L")

The onset is 3 to 4 hours; peak, 8 to 16 hours; duration, 20 to 24 hours.

Both insulins are similar in their time course of action and are white and milky in appearance. If NPH or Lente insulin is taken alone, it is not critical that it be taken a half hour before the meal. It is important, however, for the patient to have eaten some food around the time of the onset and peak of these insulins.

Long-acting insulin is sometimes referred to as "peakless" insulin because it tends to have a long, slow, sustained action rather than sharp, definite peaks in action. Available long-acting insulin is:

- Ultralente insulin (UL)

The onset is 6 to 8 hours; peak, 14 to 20 hours; duration, greater than 32 hours.

(Note: the nurse may find that different sources list differing numbers of hours for the onset, peak, and duration of action of the three main types of insulin. The nurse should focus on which meals—and snacks—are being "covered" by which insulin doses. In general, the short-acting insulins are expected to cover meals immediately following the injection; the intermediate-acting insulins are expected to cover subsequent meals; and the long-acting insulins provide a relatively constant level of insulin and control primarily the fasting glucose level.)

Concentration. The most common concentration of insulin used in the United States is U-100. This means that there are 100 units of insulin per 1 cubic centimeter. Thus, a syringe that holds 100 units of U-100 insulin is a 1-ml (cc) syringe. If a syringe holds 50 units of U-100 insulin, it is a ½-ml, U-100 syringe.

Years ago, U-40 and U-80 insulins were also widely available in the United States, but U-80 insulin is no longer available and U-40 is used infrequently today.

Species (Source). In the past, all insulins were derived from the pancreases of cows (beef insulin) and pigs (pork insulin). In the last several years, "human insulins" have become widely available. They are produced in two ways—either converting pork insulin into human insulin by substituting one amino acid for another in order to achieve the same amino acid sequence found in human insulin, or using recombinant DNA technology to produce human insulin.

Manufacturer. The two manufacturers of insulin in the United States are the Lilly and Novo Nordisk companies. The insulins made by the different companies are usually interchangeable, provided the concentration (*e.g.*, U-100), species (*e.g.*, human), and type (*e.g.*, NPH) of insulin are the same.

Human insulins made by the different companies are given different brand names:

- Lilly human insulins = "Humulin"
- Novo Nordisk human insulins = "Novolin"

Therefore, a patient taking 20 units of human NPH insulin may be using either Humulin N or Novolin N. A more complete list of the available insulins appears in Table 39-3.

Insulin Regimens. Insulin regimens vary from one to four injections per day. Usually there is a combination of a short-acting insulin and a longer-acting insulin. The normally functioning pancreas continuously secretes small amounts of insulin during the day and night. In addition, whenever there is a rise in blood glucose after ingestion of food, there is a rapid burst of insulin secretion in proportion to the glucose-raising effect of the food. The goal of all but the simplest, one-injection insulin regimen is to mimic this normal pattern of insulin secretion as closely as possible. In general, the more complex the regimen, the greater the possibility of normalizing the blood glucose levels—especially for the patient with variations in eating and activity patterns. Table 39-4 describes several different insulin regimens and the advantages and disadvantages of each one.

Patients can be taught to use the results of self–blood glucose testing in order to vary the insulin doses. This allows patients more flexibility in the timing and content of meals and exercise periods. However, complex insulin regimens require a strong level of commitment, intensive education, and close follow-up by the health care team. In addition, patients aiming for normal blood glucose levels run the risk of more hypoglycemic reactions.

The type of regimen used by any particular patient will vary according to a number of factors. For example, patient knowledge, willingness, goals, health status, and finances may all affect decisions regarding insulin treatment. In addition, the physician's philosophy about blood glucose control and the availability of equipment and support staff may influence decisions regarding insulin therapy.

There are two general approaches to insulin therapy. One is to simplify the insulin regimen as much as possible with the aim of avoiding the acute complications of diabetes (*i.e.*, hypoglycemia and symptomatic hyperglycemia). With this type of simplified regimen (*e.g.*, one to two injections per day), patients may frequently have blood glucose levels well above normal. This approach would be appropriate for the terminally ill, the frail elderly with limited self-care abilities, or any patient who is completely unwilling or unable to engage in self-management activities that are part of a more complex insulin regimen.

The second approach is to use a more complex insulin regimen (two to four injections per day) in order to achieve as good blood glucose control as is safe and practical. Some diabetologists believe that maintaining blood glucose levels as close to normal as possible may prevent or slow the progression of long-term diabetic complications. Another reason for using a more complex insulin regimen is to allow patients more flexibility to change their insulin doses from day to day in accordance with changes in their eating and activity patterns and as needed for variations in the prevailing glucose level.

It is very important for patients to be involved in the decision regarding which insulin regimen to use. Patients need to compare the potential benefits of different regimens with the potential costs (such as time involved, number of injections or fingersticks for glucose testing, amount of record keeping, etc.). There are no set guidelines as to which insulin regimen should be used for which patients. It must not be assumed that an elderly patient or a patient with visual impairment should automatically be given a simplified regimen. Likewise, it must not be assumed that all young people will want to be involved in a complex treatment regimen.

Nurses play an important role in educating patients about the availability of different approaches to insulin therapy. Nurses should refer patients to diabetes specialists or diabetes education centers for further training and education in the various insulin treatment regimens.

Health Teaching—Insulin Injection. Insulin injections are administered into the subcutaneous tissue with the use of special insulin syringes. A variety of syringes and injection-aid devices are available. Charts 39-3 and 39-4 summarize important factors to include in teaching patients about insulin.

TABLE 39–3. Insulin Preparations Available in the United States

Manufacturer	Product	Species Source	Type
RAPID-ACTING			
Lilly	Iletin I	Beef/pork	Regular
Lilly	Iletin II	Beef or pork	Regular
Lilly	Humulin Regular	Human	Regular
Novo Nordisk	Regular	Pork	Regular
Novo Nordisk	Purified Pork Regular	Pork	Regular
Novo Nordisk	Novolin R	Human	Regular
Lilly	Iletin I Semilente	Beef/pork	Semilente
Novo Nordisk	Semilente	Beef	Semilente
Novo Nordisk	Purified Pork S	Pork	Semilente
INTERMEDIATE-ACTING			
Lilly	Iletin I NPH	Beef/pork	NPH
Lilly	Iletin II NPH	Beef or pork	NPH
Lilly	Humulin NPH	Human	NPH
Novo Nordisk	NPH	Beef	NPH
Novo Nordisk	Purified Pork N	Pork	NPH
Novo Nordisk	Novolin N	Human	NPH
Lilly	Iletin I Lente	Beef/pork	Lente
Lilly	Iletin II Lente	Beef or pork	Lente
Lilly	Humulin L	Human	Lente
Novo Nordisk	Lente	Beef	Lente
Novo Nordisk	Purified Pork L	Pork	Lente
Novo Nordisk	Novolin L	Human	Lente
LONG-ACTING			
Lilly	Iletin I Ultralente	Beef/pork	Ultralente
Lilly	Humulin U	Human	Ultralente
Novo Nordisk	Ultralente	Beef	Ultralente
Novo Nordisk	Purified Beef U	Beef	Ultralente
MIXED			
Lilly	Humulin 70/30	Human	70% NPH/30% Reg
Novo Nordisk	Novolin 70/30	Human	70% NPH/30% Reg

Equipment

Insulin. Short-acting insulins are clear in appearance, and longer-acting insulins are cloudy and white. The longer-acting insulins must be mixed (gently inverted or rolled in the hands) before use.

Some sources specify that insulin bottles in use be refrigerated, while others simply suggest that insulin be kept at room temperature. There is agreement that extremes of temperature are to be avoided; thus, insulin should not be allowed to freeze and should not be kept in direct sunlight or in a hot car. Before injection, it is recommended that insulin be at room temperature (which may require rolling it in the hands or removing it from a refrigerator for a period of time prior to the injection).

Insulin bottles should also be checked for *flocculation*, which is a frosted, whitish coating inside the bottle of inter- mediate- or long-acting insulins. This occurs most commonly with human insulins that are not refrigerated. If a frosted, adherent coating is present, the insulin is inactivated and should not be used.

Syringes. Syringes must be matched with the insulin concentration (*e.g.*, U-100). Currently, three sizes of U-100 insulin syringes are available:

- 1-ml (cc) syringes—hold 100 units
- ½-ml syringes—hold 50 units
- ³/₁₀-ml syringes—hold 30 units

The needle length (approximately ½ inch) is similar with all types of syringes, and the needle is usually between 27 and 29 gauge. The smaller syringes are marked in 1-unit increments

Chart 39–3
Teaching Insulin Administration

Equipment

Insulin
1. Identifies information on label of insulin bottle
   - Type (*e.g.*, NPH, regular, 70/30)
   - Species (human, beef, pork)
   - Manufacturer (Lilly, Novo Nordisk)
   - Concentration (*e.g.*, U-100)
   - Expiration date
2. Checks appearance of insulin
   - Clear or milky white
   - Checks for flocculation (clumping, frosted appearance)
3. Identifies where to purchase and store insulin
   - Indicates approximately how long bottle will last (1000 units per bottle U-100 insulin)
   - Indicates how long opened bottles can be used

Syringes
1. Identifies concentration (U-100) marking on syringe
2. Identifies size of syringe (*e.g.*, 100-unit, 50-unit, 30-unit)
3. Describes appropriate disposal of used syringe

Preparation and Administration of Insulin Injection

1. Draws up correct amount and type of insulin
2. Properly mixes two insulins if necessary
3. Cleanses skin, inserts needle, and injects insulin
4. Describes site rotation
   - Demonstrates injection with all anatomic areas to be used
   - Describes pattern for rotation, such as using abdomen only or using certain areas at the same time of day
   - Describes system for remembering site locations, such as horizontal pattern across the abdomen as if drawing a dotted line

Knowledge of Insulin Action

1. Lists prescription
   - Type and dosage of insulin
   - Timing of insulin injections
2. Describes approximate time course of insulin action
   - Identifies long- and short-acting insulins by name
   - States approximate time delay until onset of insulin action
   - Identifies need to delay food until 15–30 minutes after the injection (indicated when injecting regular insulin)
   - Knows that longer time delays are safe when blood glucose level is high and time delays may need to be shortened when blood glucose level is low

Incorporation of Insulin Injections Into Daily Schedule

1. Recites proper order of pre-meal diabetes activities
   - May use mnemonic device such as the word "tie," which helps the patient remember the order of activities ("t" = test [blood glucose], "i" = insulin injection, "e" = eat)
   - Describes daily schedule, such as test, insulin, eat, before breakfast and dinner; test and eat, before lunch and bedtime
2. Describes information regarding hypoglycemia
   - Symptoms: shakiness, sweating, nervousness, hunger, weakness
   - Causes: too much insulin, too much exercise, not enough food
   - Treatment: 10–15 g of simple carbohydrate, such as 2–3 glucose tablets, 1 tube glucose gel, ½–1 cup juice
   - After initial treatment, follow with snack including starch and protein, such as cheese and crackers, milk and crackers, half sandwich
3. Describes information regarding prevention of hypoglycemia
   - Avoid delays in meal timing
   - Eat a meal or snack approximately every 4–5 hours (while awake)
   - Do not skip meals
   - Increase food intake before exercise
   - Check blood glucose regularly
   - Change insulin doses only with medical supervision
   - Carry a form of fast-acting sugar at all times
   - Wear a medical ID bracelet
   - Teach family, friends, coworkers about signs and treatment of hypoglycemia
   - Have family, roommates, traveling companions learn to use injectable glucagon for severe hypoglycemic reactions
4. Regular follow-up for evaluation of diabetes control
   - Keeps written record of blood glucose, insulin doses, hypoglycemic reactions, variations in diet
   - Keeps all appointments with health professionals
   - Sees physician regularly (usually 2–4 times per year)
   - States how to contact physician in case of emergency
   - States when to call physician to report variations in blood glucose levels

and may be easier to use for patients with visual deficits or patients taking very small doses of insulin. Some of the 1-ml syringes are marked in 2-unit increments.

Preparing the Injection

Mixing Insulins. When a short- and longer-acting insulin are to be given simultaneously, they are usually mixed together in the same syringe.

There is some question as to whether the two insulins are stable if the mixture is kept in the syringe for more than 5 to 15 minutes. This may depend on the ratio of the insulins as well as the time between mixing and injecting. Some research studies have suggested that when mixing regular insulin with the long-acting insulin, there is a binding reaction that slows the action of the regular insulin. This may also occur to a lesser

(text continues on page 1040)

TABLE 39-4. Insulin Regimens

Schematic Representation	Description	Advantages	Disadvantages
Normal pancreas (graph: μU/ml, 0 to 100; x-axis BR LU DI SN BR)	Insulin release increases when blood glucose levels rise and continues at a low steady rate between meals		
One injection per day (graph: Insulin effect; REG, NPH; x-axis BR LU DI SN BR)	Before breakfast: • NPH* or • NPH with regular	Simple regimen	Difficult to control fasting blood glucose if effects of NPH do not last Afternoon hypoglycemia may result from attempts to control fasting glucose level by increasing NPH dose
Two injections per day (graph: Insulin effect; REG, NPH, REG, NPH; x-axis BR LU DI SN BR)	Before breakfast and dinner: • NPH or • NPH with regular or • Premixed (N and R) insulin	Simplest regimen that attempts to mimic normal pancreas	Need relatively fixed schedule of meals and exercise Cannot independently adjust NPH or regular if premixed insulin is used

Three or four injections per day

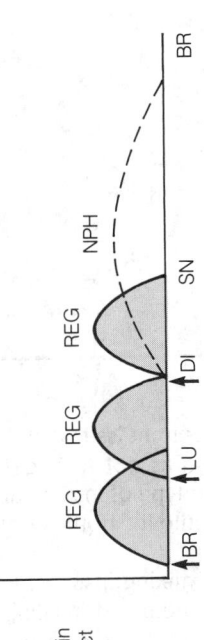

Regular before each meal with:
- NPH at dinner or
- NPH at bedtime or
- Ultralente one or two times per day

More closely mimics normal pancreas than two-injection regimen

Decide each premeal dose of regular insulin independently

More flexibility with meals and exercise

Requires more injections than other regimens

Requires multiple blood glucose tests on a daily basis

Requires intensive education and follow-up

Insulin pump

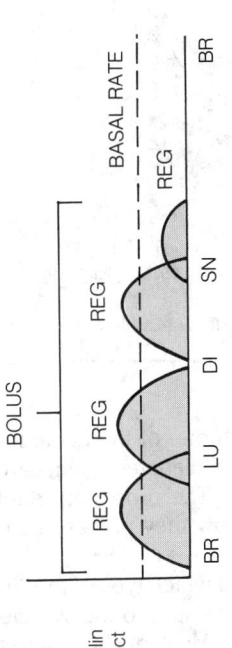

Uses ONLY regular insulin infused at continuous, low rate called *basal rate* (commonly 0.5–1.5 units/hour) and pre-meal *bolus doses* activated by pump wearer

Most closely mimics normal pancreas

Decreases unpredictable peaks of intermediate- and long-acting insulins

Increases meal and exercise flexibility

Requires intensive training and frequent follow-up

Potential for mechanical problems

Requires multiple blood glucose tests on a daily basis

Potential increase in expenses (depending upon insurance coverage)

*Where NPH appears, Lente insulin may also be used (however, the rate of absorption of regular insulin may be decreased when mixed with Lente preparations).
BR, breakfast; LU, lunch; DI, dinner; SN, snack; ↑ indicates insulin injection.*

1039

Chart 39-4
Self-Injection of Insulin

1. Cleanse the skin with alcohol where the injection is to be made. Wait (5–10 seconds) for the alcohol to dry completely.

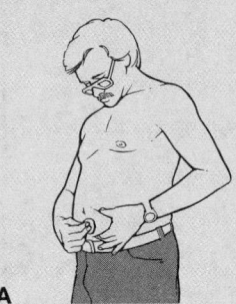

A

2. With one hand, stabilize the skin by spreading it or pinching up a large area.

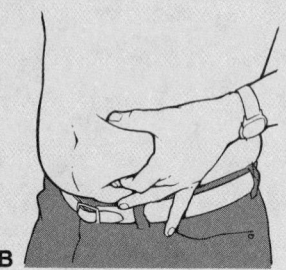

B

3. Pick up syringe with the other hand and hold it as you would a pencil. Insert needle straight into the skin.*

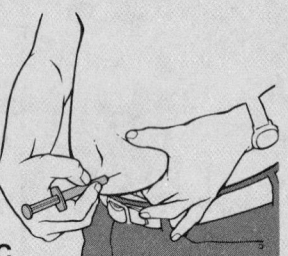

C

4. To inject the insulin, push the plunger all the way in.†

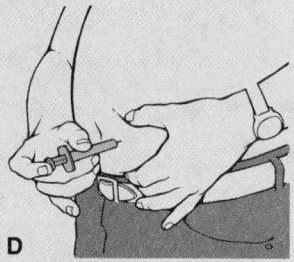

D

5. Pull needle straight out of skin. Press alcohol swab or cotton ball over injection site for several seconds.

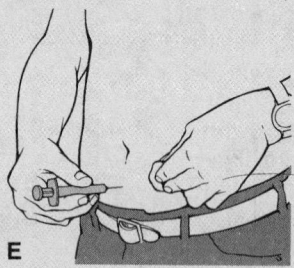

E

6. Use disposable syringe only once and discard into hard plastic container (with a tight-fitting top) such as an empty bleach or detergent container.‡

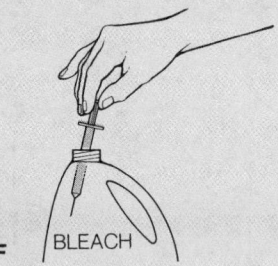

F   BLEACH

* Some patients may be taught to insert the needle at a 45-degree angle.
† Some patients may be taught to pull back slightly on the plunger to check for blood in the syringe before pushing the plunger.
‡ Some studies suggest that it may be safe to reuse disposable syringes.

degree when mixing regular insulin with one of the Lente insulins. Patients are advised to consult their diabetes health care professionals for advice on this matter. The most important issue is that patients be consistent in how they prepare their insulin injections from day to day.

There are varying opinions regarding which type of insulin (short- or longer-acting) should be drawn up into the syringe first when they are going to be mixed. Most of the printed materials from the drug companies recommend drawing up the regular insulin first. The most important issues are that the patient be consistent in technique so as not to accidentally draw up the wrong dose or the wrong type of insulin, and that patients not inject one type of insulin into the bottle containing a different type of insulin.

For patients who have difficulty mixing insulins, two options are available. They may use a premixed insulin, which contains 70% NPH and 30% regular insulin in one bottle, or they may have prefilled syringes prepared.

Two brands of premixed insulins currently available in the United States are Novolin 70/30 (Novo Nordisk) and Humulin 70/30 (Lilly). Mixed insulins with other ratios, such as 80% NPH with 20% regular insulin, may soon be available in the United States. The appropriate initial dosage of premixed insulin must be calculated so that the ratio of NPH to regular insulin most closely approximates the separate doses needed.

For patients who are able to inject insulin but have difficulty drawing up a single or mixed dose, syringes can be prefilled with the help of home health nurses and/or family and neighbors living close by. A 3-week supply of insulin syringes may be prepared and kept in the refrigerator.

Withdrawing Insulin. Most (if not all) of the printed materials available on insulin dose preparation instruct patients to inject air into the bottle of insulin equivalent to the number of units of insulin to be withdrawn. The rationale behind this is to prevent the formation of a vacuum inside the bottle, which would make it difficult to withdraw the proper amount of insulin.

Some nurses specializing in diabetes have found that some patients (who have been taking insulin for many years) have stopped injecting air prior to withdrawing the insulin. These patients found that the extra step was not necessary for accurately drawing up the insulin doses. An interesting research study conducted in England called into question the necessity of teaching patients to inject air into the bottles. Approximately one-third of the patients (and most of the nurses) questioned in this study did not routinely inject air. In addition, 52 patients were asked to draw up insulin without injecting air first. Most of the patients reported that it was easier to withdraw the insulin by eliminating the step and reported no difficulty in preparing the proper insulin dose (Lockwood et al, 1988).

Elimination of this step (or alteration of this practice, *e.g.,* injecting a syringe full of air into the vial once per week) facilitates the teaching process for some patients learning to draw up insulin for the first time. Some patients become confused with the sequence of steps involved in injecting air into two separate bottles in two different amounts prior to drawing up a mixed dose. For the elderly, simplification of the procedure for preparing insulin injections may have a major impact on maintaining independence in daily living.

As with other variations in insulin injection technique, the most important factor is that the patient maintain consistency in the procedure and that nurses be flexible when teaching new patients or assessing the skills of patients experienced with insulin injections.

Administering the Injection

Site Selection and Rotation. The four main areas for injection are the abdomen, arms (posterior surface), thighs (anterior surface), and hips (Fig. 39-3). Insulin is absorbed faster when injected into certain areas. Speed of absorption is greatest in the abdomen and decreases progressively in the arm, thigh, and hip.

Systematic rotation of injection sites is recommended to prevent localized changes in fatty tissue. In addition, to promote consistency in insulin absorption, patients should be encouraged to use all available injection sites within one area rather than randomly rotating sites from area to area. For example, some patients almost exclusively use the abdominal area, administering each injection ½ to 1 inch away from the previous injection. Another approach to rotation is to always use the

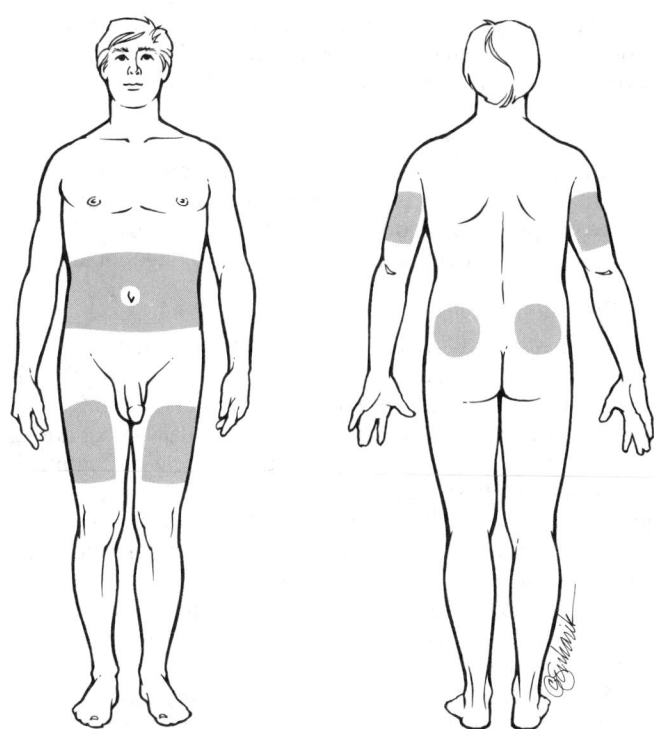

Figure 39-3. Suggested areas for insulin injection.

same area at the same time of day. For example, patients may inject morning doses into the abdomen and evening doses into the arms or legs.

A few general principles apply to all rotation patterns. First, patients should try not to use the same *site* more than once in 2 to 3 weeks. In addition, if the patient is planning to exercise, insulin should not be injected into the limb that will be exercised, because inconsistent insulin absorption may result.

In the past, patients were taught to rotate injections from one area to the next (*e.g.,* injecting once in the right arm, then once in the right abdomen, then once in the right thigh). Patients who still use this system must be taught to use the same area for injection in a more consistent fashion.

Needle Insertion. There are varying approaches to insertion of the needle for insulin injections. These include spreading versus bunching the skin; using a 45-degree versus a 90-degree angle; and aspirating versus not aspirating prior to injecting the insulin.

The technique used for holding the skin and inserting the needle must ensure that the insulin is injected into the subcutaneous tissue. Injection that is too deep (*e.g.,* intramuscular) or too shallow may affect the rate of absorption of the insulin.

Aspiration involves inserting the needle and then pulling back on the plunger to check for blood being drawn into the syringe. If no blood is seen, the plunger is then pushed in to inject the insulin. If blood is seen, the insulin is not given at that site in order to avoid giving the injection directly into a blood vessel.

The necessity of aspiration with self-injection of insulin is being questioned. The usefulness of this procedure with a very small gauge needle is being further investigated. In addition, many patients who have been using insulin for an extended period of time have eliminated this step from their insulin injection routine with no apparent adverse effects.

For some patients, aspiration is a difficult and unsafe procedure. Patients with visual impairments or deficits in fine motor coordination may accidentally withdraw all or some of the needle during this procedure. Aspiration is virtually impossible for the patient limited to the use of one hand (*e.g.,* a stroke patient). In addition, patients who use injection-aid devices into which the syringe is loaded are not able to visualize the syringe during the injection. Patients using insulin "pen" devices do not have the ability to pull back on the plunger at all.

Problems With Insulin

Local Allergic Reactions.   A local allergic reaction in the form of redness, swelling, tenderness, and induration or a 2- to 4-cm wheal may appear at the site of injection 1 to 2 hours after the injection is given. These reactions usually occur during the beginning stages of therapy and disappear with continued use of insulin. These allergic reactions are becoming less frequent because of the increased purity of insulins. The physician may prescribe an antihistamine to be taken 1 hour before the injection if such a local reaction occurs.

Occasionally, if alcohol is not allowed to dry on the skin before injection, it is carried into the tissues. This results in a localized reddened area.

Systemic Allergic Reactions.   Systemic allergic reactions to insulin are rare. First, there is an immediate local skin reaction that gradually spreads into generalized urticaria. The treatment is desensitization, with small doses of insulin given in gradually increasing amounts. These rare reactions are occasionally associated with generalized edema or anaphylaxis.

Insulin Lipodystrophy.   *Lipodystrophy* refers to a localized disturbance of fat metabolism, in the form of either lipoatrophy or lipohypertrophy, occurring at the site of insulin injections. *Lipoatrophy* is loss of subcutaneous fat and appears as slight dimpling or more serious pitting of subcutaneous fat. The use of U-100 insulin, which is 99% pure, has almost eliminated this disfiguring complication. Lipoatrophy is treated by injection of purified insulin into the periphery of the lipoatrophic area.

Lipohypertrophy is the development of fibrofatty masses at the injection site and is caused by the repeated use of an injection site. If insulin is injected into scarred areas, the absorption may be delayed. This is one reason why rotation of injection sites is so important. The patient should avoid injecting insulin into these areas until the hypertrophy disappears.

Insulin Resistance.   Most patients at one time or another have some degree of insulin resistance. This may occur for various reasons, the most common being obesity, which can be overcome by weight loss.

Clinical insulin resistance has been defined as a daily insulin requirement of 200 units or more. In most diabetic patients taking insulin, immune antibodies develop and bind the insulin, thereby decreasing the insulin available for use. All animal insulins, as well as human insulins to a lesser degree, cause antibody production in humans.

Very few of these patients develop high levels of antibodies. Many of these patients give a history of insulin therapy interrupted for several months or more. Treatment consists of administering a purer insulin preparation, and occasionally prednisone may be needed to block the production of antibodies. This may be followed by a gradual reduction in insulin requirement. Therefore, patients need to monitor themselves for hypoglycemia.

Alternative Methods of Insulin Delivery.   In the 1980s, intensive insulin therapy regimens became more widely used. Patients started taking three or four doses of insulin per day in an attempt to more closely approximate normal insulin release. Several devices were created in at attempt to simplify the procedures involved in drawing up and injecting insulin multiple times daily.

Injection Ports.   These devices are subcutaneous access ports that are inserted into the subcutaneous tissue by the patient and remain in place for up to 3 days. The Button Infuser has a 27-gauge needle attached to a resealable injection port. A newer device called the Insuflon has a flexible Teflon catheter with an injection port attached. Similar to an IV catheter, there is an introducer needle that is removed once the catheter is in place. Patients tape the device in place and then give their insulin injections through the resealable port rather than puncturing their skin multiple times daily.

Insulin Pens.   These devices use small (200-unit) prefilled insulin cartridges that are loaded into a penlike holder. A disposable needle is attached to the device for insulin injection. Insulin is delivered by dialing in a dose and/or pushing a button for every 1- or 2-unit increment given. People using these devices still need to insert the needle for each injection; however, they do not need to carry insulin bottles or to draw up insulin before each injection. These devices are most useful for patients who need to inject only one type of insulin at a time (*e.g.,* premeal regular three times a day and bedtime NPH) or who can use the premixed 70% NPH/30% regular insulins.

Jet Injectors.   As an alternative to needle injections, jet injection devices deliver insulin through the skin under pressure in an extremely fine stream. These devices are more expensive than other alternative devices mentioned above and require thorough training and supervision when first used. In addition, patients should be cautioned that absorption rates, peak insulin activity, and insulin levels may be different when switching to a jet injector. (Insulin given by jet injector usually works faster.)

Insulin Pumps.   These are small, externally worn devices that closely mimic the functioning of the normal pancreas. Insulin pumps contain a 3-ml syringe that is attached to a long (42-inch), thin, narrow-lumen tube with a needle or Teflon catheter attached to the end (Figs. 39-4 and 39-5). The patient inserts the needle or Teflon catheter into the subcutaneous tissue (usually on the abdomen) and secures it with tape or a transparent dressing. The needle or Teflon catheter is changed at least every 3 days. The pump is then worn either on a belt or in a pocket. Some women keep the pump tucked into the front or side of the bra or wear it on a garter belt on the thigh.

The pump uses only regular insulin, which is delivered in two different ways. First, there is a continuous "basal rate" of insulin that infuses typically at a rate of 0.5 to 2.0 units/hr. Then, prior to each meal, the patient activates the pump (through a series of button pushes) to deliver a "bolus" dose of insulin. The patient can decide on the amount of insulin bolus to infuse based on blood glucose levels and anticipated food intake and activity level.

There has been debate in the diabetes literature as to whether insulin pumps offer better control of blood glucose than other multiple-dose regimens (*e.g.,* three or four injections per day). One advantage of insulin pumps is that patients do not have to use intermediate- or long-acting insulins, which may have unpredictable peaks of action and may therefore

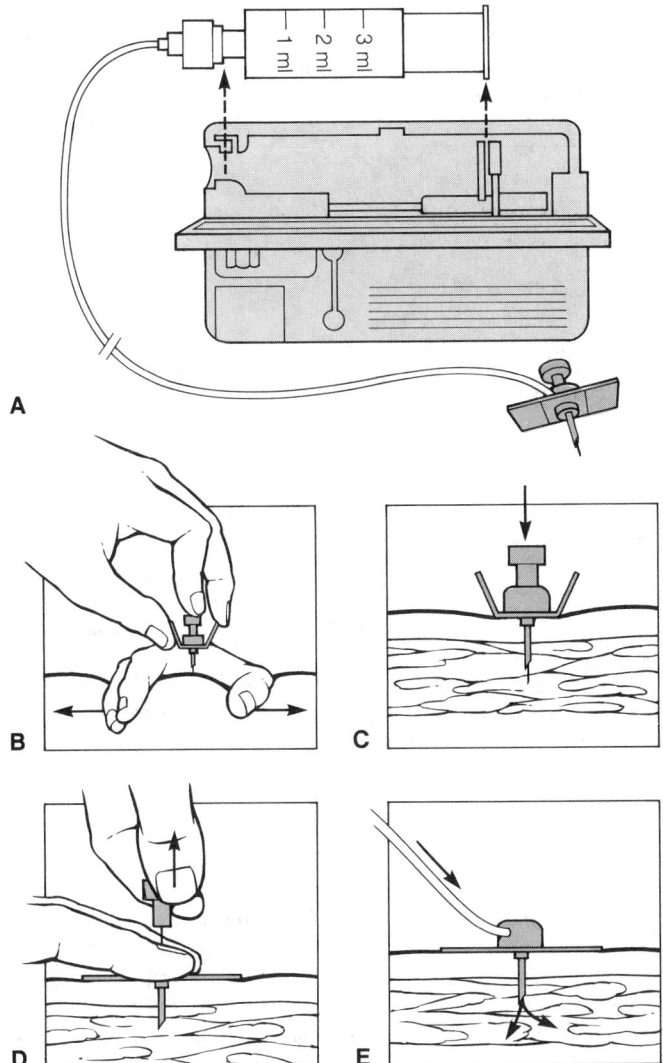

Figure 39-4. (**A**) Diagram of an insulin pump showing syringe in place inside pump and connection of pump via tubing to needle site. (**B–E**) Actual insertion site before, during, and after the needle and catheter have been inserted.

cause unexpected swings in blood glucose. Some of the other advantages of insulin pumps include increased flexibility in life-style (in terms of timing and amount of meals, exercise, and travel) and, for some patients, improved blood glucose control.

A disadvantage of insulin pumps is that unexpected disruptions in the flow of insulin from the pump may occur if the tubing or needle becomes occluded, if the supply of insulin runs out, or if the battery is depleted. Another disadvantage is the potential for infection at needle insertion sites. Hypoglycemia may occur with insulin pump therapy; however, this is usually related to the lowered blood glucose levels many patients achieve rather than to a specific problem with the pump itself. In addition, some patients may find that having to wear the pump virtually 24 hours per day is an inconvenience. (It can easily be disconnected, per patient preference, for limited periods of time [*e.g.*, for showering, exercise, sexual activity].)

Many insurance policies cover the cost of pump therapy; if it is not covered, the extra expense of the pump and associated supplies may be a deterrent for some patients.

Insulin pump candidates must be willing to check blood glucose levels multiple times daily while on pump therapy. In addition, they must be psychologically stable and open about having diabetes, because the insulin pump is often a visible sign to others and a constant reminder to the patient that he has diabetes. Most important, patients using insulin pumps must have extensive education in the use of the insulin pump and in self-management of blood glucose and insulin doses. They must work closely with a team of health care professionals who are experienced in insulin pump therapy.

Research Into Alternative Insulin Delivery.   Research into mechanical delivery of insulin has involved implantable insulin pumps that can be externally programmed according to blood glucose testing. Clinical trials with these devices are currently in progress. In addition, there is research into the development of implantable devices that both measure the blood glucose and deliver insulin as needed.

Transplantation.   Transplantation of the whole pancreas or a segment of the pancreas is being performed on a limited population (mostly diabetic patients receiving kidney transplantations simultaneously). One main issue regarding pancreatic transplantation is weighing the risks of antirejection medications against the advantages of pancreas transplantation. Another approach under investigation is the implantation of insulin-producing pancreatic islet cells. This latter approach involves a less extensive surgical procedure and a potentially lower incidence of immunogenic problems.

Oral Hypoglycemic Agents

Oral hypoglycemic agents may be effective for type II diabetic patients who cannot be treated by diet alone. See Table 39-5 for a list of these agents.

In the United States, the oral hypoglycemic agents available are the sulfonylureas. They are thought to exert their primary

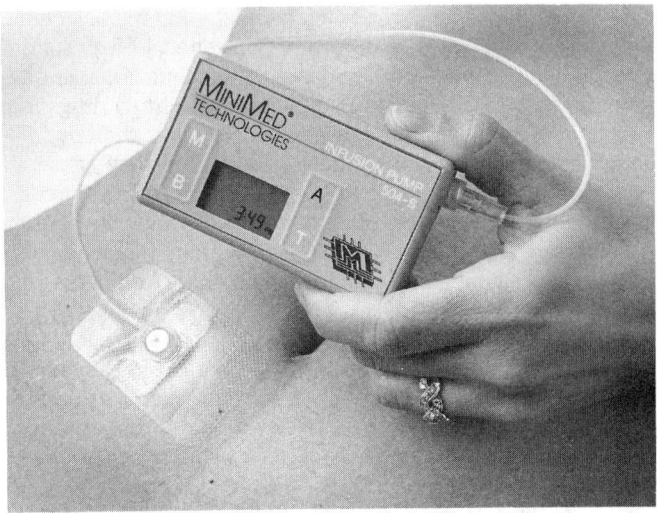

Figure 39-5.   MiniMed insulin pump. (Courtesy of MiniMed Technologies, Sylmar, CA.)

TABLE 39–5.   *Oral Hypoglycemic Agents Used in the United States*

Generic Name (Trade Name)	Tablet Size (mg)	Usual Daily Dose Range (mg)	Maximum Dose (mg)	Duration of Action (hr)
FIRST-GENERATION COMPOUND				
Tolbutamide (Orinase)	250, 500	500–2000 (divided)	3000	6–12
Chlorpropamide (Diabinese)	100, 250	100–500 (single)	750	60
Acetohexamide (Dymelor)	250, 500	250–1500 (single or divided)	1500	12–24
Tolazamide (Tolinase)	100, 250, 500	100–750 (single or divided)	1000	12–24
SECOND-GENERATION COMPOUND				
Glyburide (Micronase, Diabeta)	1.25, 2.5, 5	2.5–10 (single or divided)	20	12–24
Glipizide (Glucotrol)	5, 10	5–25 (single or divided)	40	10–24

(Davidson MB. Update on therapy of diabetes mellitus: Diet, sulfonylurea agents and insulin. Mt Sinai J Med 1987 Mar; 54[3]:201.)

action by directly stimulating the pancreas to secrete insulin. Therefore, a functioning pancreas is necessary for these agents to be effective, and they cannot be used in the treatment of patients who have type I diabetes and are prone to ketoacidosis. An additional important action of oral agents, unrelated to a direct pancreatic effect, is to improve insulin action at the cellular level. They may also directly decrease glucose production by the liver, although this action is controversial.

The sulfonylureas can be divided into short- intermediate- and long-acting agents with varying duration of action. The most common side effects of these drugs include gastrointestinal symptoms and dermatologic reactions. Hypoglycemia may occur when an excessive dose of a sulfonylurea is used or when meals are omitted or food intake is decreased. Because of the prolonged hypoglycemic effects of oral agents (especially chlorpropamide), some patients need to be hospitalized for treatment of oral agent–induced hypoglycemia. Another side effect of chlorpropamide is a disulfiram (Antabuse)–type reaction when alcohol is ingested (see section on alcohol for more information).

Some drugs may directly interact with oral hypoglycemic agents, potentiating their hypoglycemic effects (*e.g.*, sulfonamides, chloramphenicol, clofibrate, phenylbutazone, and bisohydroxycoumarin). In addition, there are certain drugs that may independently affect blood glucose levels, thereby indirectly interfering with oral agents. Drugs that may cause an elevation of glucose levels include potassium-losing diuretics, glucocorticoids, estrogen compounds, and diphenylhydantoin (Dilantin). Drugs that may cause hypoglycemia include salicylates, propranolol, MAO (monoamine oxidase) inhibitors, and pentamidine.

It is important for patients to realize that oral agents are prescribed as an addition to (and not as a substitution for) other treatment modalities such as diet and exercise. Oral hypoglycemic drugs may need to be abandoned temporarily in favor of insulin if the patient develops hyperglycemia due to infection, trauma, or surgery.

If, as time goes on, a patient's blood glucose values that were once responsive to oral hypoglycemic agents are no longer responsive to these agents, the patient is then treated with insulin. This is referred to as a *secondary failure*. A *primary failure* occurs when the blood glucose level remains high a month after initial drug use.

Using a combination of oral agents with insulin has been proposed as a treatment for some patients with type II diabetes. However, the effectiveness of this approach has not yet been proved.

Education

Diabetes mellitus is a chronic illness requiring a lifetime of special self-management behaviors. Because diet, physical activity, and physical and emotional stress can affect diabetic control, patients must learn to balance a multitude of factors. Not only must patients learn daily self-care skills for avoidance of acute decreases or increases in blood glucose, but they must also incorporate into their life-style many preventive behaviors for avoidance of long-term diabetic complications. An appreciation for the knowledge and skills that diabetic patients must acquire can help the nurse in providing effective patient education and counseling.

Approaches to Teaching.   Changes in the health care delivery system as a whole have had a major impact on diabetes education and training. Patients with new-onset diabetes are having much shorter hospital stays or may even be managed completely on an outpatient basis. In recent years there has been a proliferation of outpatient diabetes education and training programs with increasing support of third-party reimbursement. Nonetheless, *for some patients, exposure to diabetes teaching during the course of a hospitalization may be the only opportunity the patient has for learning skills of self-management and avoidance of diabetic complications.*

At many hospitals there are nurses who specialize in diabetes education and management. However, because of the large number of diabetic patients that are admitted to every unit of a hospital, the staff nurse plays a vital role in identifying diabetic patients, assessing self-care skills, providing basic education, reinforcing teaching provided by the specialist, and referring patients for follow-up after discharge.

Organizing Information.   There are various schemes for organizing and prioritizing the vast amount of information that must be taught to diabetic patients. In addition, many hospitals and outpatient diabetes centers have devised written guidelines, care plans, and documentation forms (often based on guidelines from the American Diabetes Association) that may be used to document and evaluate diabetes teaching.

A general approach to organizing diabetes education is to divide information and skills into two main types:

1. Basic, initial, or "survival" skills and information
2. In-depth ("advanced") or continuing education

Survival Skills.   This information must be taught to any patient with newly diagnosed type I diabetes or any type II diabetic patient starting on insulin for the first time. This basic survival information is literally that which the patient must know in order to "survive" (*i.e.*, avoid severe hypoglycemic or acute hyperglycemic complications) after discharge. Categories of survival information include:

1. Simple pathophysiology
   a. Basic definition of diabetes (having high blood sugars)
   b. Normal blood sugar ranges
   c. Effect of insulin and exercise (decrease sugar)
   d. Effect of food and stress, including illness and infections (increase sugars)
   e. Basic treatment approaches
2. Treatment modalities
   a. Insulin administration
   b. Basic diet information (*e.g.*, food groups and timing of meals)
   c. Monitoring of blood glucose, urine ketones
3. Recognition, treatment, and prevention of acute complications
   a. Hypoglycemia
   b. Hyperglycemia
4. Pragmatic information
   a. Where to buy and store insulin, syringes, glucose-monitoring supplies
   b. When and how to reach the physician

Newly diagnosed type II diabetic patients also need to learn some of this basic information. Most of the emphasis is initially placed on diet teaching. For patients started on oral hypoglycemic agents, it is also very important to teach about hypoglycemia. If the diabetes has gone undetected for many years, the patient may already be experiencing some of the chronic diabetic complications. Thus, for some patients with newly diagnosed type II diabetes, the basic diabetes teaching must include information on preventive skills such as foot care and eye care (*i.e.*, planning yearly examinations by the ophthalmologist and understanding that retinopathy is largely asymptomatic until the advanced stages). It is important for patients to realize that once they master the basic skills and information, further diabetes education must be pursued. Acquiring in-depth and advanced diabetes knowledge occurs throughout the patient's lifetime both informally (through experience and sharing of information with other people with diabetes) and formally (through programs of continuing education).

In-Depth/Continuing Education.   This involves teaching more detailed information related to survival skills (such as learning to vary diet and insulin and preparing for travel) as well as learning preventive measures for the avoidance of long-term diabetic complications. These include:

- Foot care
- Eye care
- General hygiene (*e.g.*, skin care, oral hygiene)
- Risk factor management (control of blood pressure and blood lipids, normalizing blood glucose levels)

More advanced continuing education may include the use of alternative methods for insulin delivery (*e.g.*, the insulin pump and learning sophisticated algorithms or rules for evaluating and adjusting insulin doses). For example, patients can be taught to increase or decrease insulin doses based on a several-day pattern of blood glucose levels.

The amount of "advanced" diabetes education to be provided will depend upon patient interest and ability. However, learning preventive measures (especially foot care and eye care) is mandatory and vitally important for reducing the occurrence of amputations and blindness in the diabetic population.

Timing of Teaching.   Before initiating diabetes education, it is important to assess the patient's (and family's) readiness to learn. When patients are first diagnosed with diabetes (or first told of their need for insulin), they go through various stages of the grieving process. These stages may include shock and denial, depression, negotiation, anger, and acceptance. The amount of time it takes for patients and family members to work through the grieving process will vary from patient to patient. They may experience feelings of helplessness, guilt, and altered body image, loss of self-esteem, and concern about the future. The nurse must assess the patient's coping strategies and reassure patients and families that feelings of depression and shock are normal.

Asking the patient and family about their major concerns or fears is an important way to learn about any misinformation that may be unnecessarily contributing to feelings of anxiety. Some common misconceptions regarding diabetes and its treatment are listed in Chart 39-5. Simple, direct information should be provided to dispel misconceptions. More in-depth information can be provided once survival skills are mastered.

After dispelling misconceptions or answering questions that concern the patient the most, the nurse must use a firm, but caring, approach to focus attention on concrete survival skills. Because of the immediacy of needing to learn multiple new skills, initiating teaching as soon as possible after diagnosis is crucial. For patients who are in the hospital, there is not usually the luxury of waiting until the patient feels ready to learn. Early discharge necessitates initiation of survival skill education as early as possible in the hospital stay. Early teaching allows the patient ample opportunity to practice skills with supervision of the nurse prior to discharge. Follow-up by home health nurses is often necessary for reinforcement of survival skills.

Teaching Methods.   Maintaining flexibility in teaching approaches is important. Teaching skills and information in a "logical" sequence is not always the most helpful for patients. For example, many patients are focused on their fear of the injection. Before they learn how to draw up, purchase, store, and mix insulins, they should be taught to insert the needle and inject insulin (or practice with saline). Furthermore, numerous demonstrations by the nurse or practice injections (*e.g.*, using an orange) before the patient (or family) gives the first injection may actually increase the patient's anxiety and fear of self-injection.

Chart 39–5
Misconceptions Related to Diabetes and Its Treatment

Misconception	Nurse's Response
Diabetes is caused by eating too much sugar.	Once diabetes develops, eating too much sugar can cause the glucose level to rise. However, the reason that diabetes develops initially is that there is a decrease in the amount of insulin in the body or a decrease in the ability of insulin to control the blood glucose level. These problems are *not* caused by eating too much sugar.
	In type I diabetes, in which the pancreatic beta cells produce little or no insulin, various factors contribute to beta-cell damage, including genetics, a defect in the immune system, and/or an external factor (such as a virus).
	In type II diabetes, the body is resistant to the effect of insulin. The amount of insulin released by the beta cells is not enough to overcome this insulin resistance, and hyperglycemia results. Insulin resistance and decreased insulin release are *not* caused by eating too much sugar. Two factors that do contribute to the development of type II diabetes are being obese and having a family history of diabetes.
Sugar is found only in dessert foods.	There are several different types of sugars (simple carbohydrates) that increase blood glucose levels. Dessert foods often contain sucrose, one type of sugar. Many other packaged foods (such as flavored yogurt, cereals, canned beans, sauces, salad dressing, "health food bars") also contain some form of sugar. Patients should be instructed to check labels for sources of sugar such as corn syrup, dextrose, brown sugar, honey.
	Fruit and fruit juices also contain sugar. Even if the juice is labeled "unsweetened" or "no sugar added," there is still natural fruit sugar in the product, which causes elevations in the glucose level.
The only diet change needed in the treatment of diabetes is to stop eating sugar.	First, it is important for the patient to realize that it is not feasible (nor is it advisable) to remove *all* sources of sugar from the diet. There are nutritious foods (such as fruit) that contain some form of sugar and that should be included in the meal plan. In addition, recent research has shown that increasing the amount of simple sugars (including table sugar) allowed in the diabetic meal plan may not adversely affect glucose levels.
	For patients requiring insulin, the meal plan includes limiting concentrated sweets as well as maintaining consistency in time intervals between meals. In addition, patients need to learn to adjust the insulin dose if there are variations in the amount of food eaten or in the carbohydrate content of meals.
	For patients on oral hypoglycemic agents, it is important to avoid skipping meals and to limit intake of sugars. If the patient is obese, the meal plan emphasizes limiting total calories, which is best achieved by decreasing the fat content of meals.
Once insulin injections are started (for treatment of type II diabetes) they can never be discontinued.	During periods of acute stress (such as illness, infection, or surgery) or when receiving certain medications that cause elevations in blood glucose, some patients with type II diabetes will require insulin. If the diabetes had previously been well controlled with diet alone or diet with oral hypoglycemic agents, the patient should be able to resume previous methods for control of diabetes when the stress is resolved.
	In addition, insulin is sometimes used to control blood glucose levels in obese type II diabetic patients who have been unsuccessful at weight loss. If the patient is able to lose weight after insulin therapy is initiated, the insulin doses may be tapered and the patient may be able to switch to diet and exercise alone or with oral hypoglycemic agents for control of blood glucose.
	(For patients with type I diabetes, insulin is needed on an ongoing basis. For thin patients with type II diabetes, once insulin has to be started, it is usually required permanently).
If increasing doses of insulin are needed to control the blood glucose, the diabetes must be getting "worse."	Explain to the patient that, unlike other medications that are given in standard doses, there is not a standard dose of insulin that is effective for all patients. Rather, the dose must be adjusted according to blood glucose test results. If the initial insulin dose prescribed for

(continued)

Chart 39-5 *(Continued)*

Misconception	*Nurse's Response*
	the patient does not adequately decrease the glucose level, the patient may assume that he has a "bad" case of diabetes or that the diabetes is getting worse. It is important to instruct patients that many different factors may affect the ability of insulin to lower the glucose, including obesity, puberty, pregnancy, illness, and certain medications.
	In addition, to avoid hypoglycemia, physicians frequently initiate insulin therapy with smaller dosages than will eventually be needed. The doses are then increased in small increments until blood glucose levels are in the desired range.
Insulin causes blindness (or other diabetic complications).	When patients have a diabetic acquaintance in whom the initiation of insulin therapy happened to coincide with the onset of diabetic complications, the patient may view insulin as the cause of complications such as blindness or amputation. In these situations, the acquaintance probably had type II diabetes that was no longer controllable with diet and oral hypoglycemic agents. It must be explained to the patient that factors such as elevated blood glucose and elevated blood pressure levels (and not insulin therapy) contribute to some of the diabetic complications. Furthermore, emphasize that insulin is a natural hormone that is present in every person's body, helps control blood glucose levels, and definitely does not cause long-term complications of diabetes.
Insulin must be injected directly into the vein.	When patients first learn that one area used for insulin injections is the arm, they may envision inserting the needle directly into a vein in the antecubital area, as in blood withdrawal. The patient must be reassured that insulin is injected into the fat tissue on the *back* of the arm (or on the abdomen, thigh, or hip) and that the needle is much shorter than that used for venipuncture.
There is extreme danger in injecting insulin if there are any air bubbles in the syringe.	Patients may have a fear of dying if air bubbles are injected with a syringe. (This may be related to the misconception that insulin is injected directly into the vein.) Reassure patients that the main danger in having air bubbles in the insulin syringe is that the amount of insulin being injected is less than the required dosage. It is often difficult to remove every small "champagne" bubble from the syringe. Thus, the patient should be reassured that injection of insulin when these bubbles are present will not cause any harm.
Urine and blood glucose testing are interchangeable (*i.e.*, they provide the same information).	Explain to the patient that directly testing the blood is the most accurate method of measuring the glucose level. The *urine* glucose test, which measures the amount of glucose that has "spilled" into the urine since the bladder was last emptied, is only an indirect way of determining the glucose level in the *blood.* The kidneys will not allow sugar to spill into the urine until the blood glucose reaches a level about 180 to 200 mg/dl (10–11.1 mmol/L). Therefore, the urine will test negative for glucose when the *blood* glucose is at any level between 0 and 200 mg/dl. Hypoglycemia cannot be detected with urine testing, nor can the blood glucose level be strictly controlled.
Blood glucose levels remain the same throughout the day.	Explain to patients that there is normally a variation in blood glucose levels—with the lowest levels before meals and the highest levels 1 to 2 hours after eating. The goal of the diabetes treatment plan is to minimize wide swings in glucose levels, not to eliminate the normal variations.

(Pearce MA, Rosenberg CS, and Davidson MB. Patient education. In Davidson MB [ed]. Diabetes Mellitus: Diagnosis and Treatment, 3rd ed. New York, Churchill Livingstone, 1991.)

For most patients, once they have actually performed the part of the skill they feared the most, they are much more prepared to hear and comprehend other related information. (If the patient then wants to use a pillow or orange to practice a skill already tried, that would be appropriate). Thus, having the patient self-inject first or having the patient perform a fingerstick for glucose monitoring first may enhance his ability to then learn how to draw up the insulin or operate the glucose monitor.

Various tools can be used to aid in teaching. Many of the companies that manufacture products for diabetes self-care also provide booklets and videotapes to assist in patient teaching. It is important to use a variety of written handouts that are matched to the patient's ability (including different languages, low-literacy information, information with large print) to reinforce teaching. Patients can be encouraged to stay current with diabetes care through participation in activities sponsored by local hospitals and diabetes organizations. In addition, there are many diabetes magazines geared toward the patient with diabetes that provide information on all aspects of diabetes management.

Ample opportunity should be provided for the patient and family for repetition and supervised practice of skills (including self-injection, self-testing, meal selection, verbalization of symptoms, and treatment of hypoglycemia). Once skills have been mastered, participation in ongoing support groups may assist patients in incorporating new habits and maintaining adherence to the treatment regimen.

Teaching the "Experienced" Diabetic Patient. For patients who have had diabetes for many years, assessment of survival skills is important. Some research studies have found that up to 50% of patients may make errors in self-care skills. Assessment of these patients must include *observation* of skills, not just asking patients to describe self-care behaviors. In addition, it is imperative that these patients be fully aware of preventive measures related to foot care, eye care, and risk factor management.

If patients are experiencing long-term diabetic complications for the first time, they may go through the grieving process again. Some of these patients may experience a renewed interest in diabetes self-care in the hope of delaying further complications. Other patients may be overwhelmed by feelings of guilt and depression. The nurse must encourage the patient to discuss feelings and fears related to complications and to provide appropriate information regarding diabetic complications. Again, participation in support groups may assist the patient and family in coping with changes in life-style that occur with the onset of diabetic complications.

Promoting Adherence. Patients who are having difficulty adhering to the diabetes treatment plan must be approached with a sense of caring and understanding. The use of "scare" tactics (such as threats of blindness or amputation if the patient does not adhere to the treatment plan) or making the patient feel guilty is not productive and may interfere with establishing a trusting relationship with the patient. Using judgmental terminology, such as asking the patient if he has "cheated" on his diet, only promotes feelings of guilt and low self-esteem.

If problems exist with glucose control or with the development of preventable complications, it is important to distinguish between nonadherence, knowledge deficit, and a self-care deficit. It should not be assumed that problems with diabetes management are related to nonadherence. The patient may simply have forgotten or never learned certain information. The problem may be correctable simply through providing complete information and assuring patient comprehension of information.

If knowledge deficit is not the problem, certain physical or emotional factors may be impairing the patient's ability to perform self-care skills. For example, decreased visual acuity may impair the patient's ability to accurately administer insulin, measure blood glucose, or inspect skin and feet. In addition, decreased joint mobility (especially in the elderly) impairs the ability to inspect the bottom of the feet. Emotional factors such as continual denial of the diagnosis or depression may impair the patient's ability to carry out multiple daily self-care measures.

It is also important to assess the patient for signs of infection or emotional stress that may lead to elevated blood glucose levels despite adherence to the treatment regimen.

The following approaches by the nurse are helpful for promoting adherence:

1. Deal with any underlying factors (*e.g.*, knowledge deficit, self-care deficit, illness) that may affect diabetic control
2. Simplify the treatment regimen if it is too difficult for the patient to follow
3. Adjust the treatment regimen to meet patient requests (*e.g.*, adjust diet or insulin schedule to allow for increased flexibility in meal content or timing)
4. Establish a specific plan or contract with the patient with simple, measurable goals
5. Provide positive reinforcement of self-care behaviors performed instead of focusing on behaviors that were neglected (*e.g.*, praise a patient for blood glucose testing that was performed instead of focusing on the number of "missed" tests)
6. Help the patient to identify personal motivating factors rather than focusing on wanting to please the doctor or nurse
7. Encourage pursuit of life goals and interests; discourage undue focus on diabetes

Acute Complications of Diabetes

There are three major acute complications of diabetes related to short-term imbalances in blood glucose: hypoglycemia, diabetic ketoacidosis (DKA), and hyperosmolar nonketotic syndrome (HNKS) (also known as hyperosmolar hyperglycemic nonketotic coma—HHNKC).

Hypoglycemia (Insulin Reactions)

Hypoglycemia (abnormally low blood glucose level) occurs when the blood glucose falls below 50 to 60 mg/dl (2.7 to 3.3 mmol/L). It can be caused by too much insulin or oral hypoglycemic agents, too little food, or excessive physical activity. Hypoglycemia may occur at any time of the day or night. It often occurs before meals, especially if meals are delayed or snacks are omitted. For example, midmorning hypoglycemia may occur when the morning regular insulin is peaking, while hypoglycemia that occurs in the late afternoon coincides with the peak of the morning NPH or Lente insulin. Middle-of-the-night hypoglycemia may occur because of peaking evening NPH or Lente insulins, especially in patients who have not eaten a bedtime snack.

Symptoms. The symptoms of hypoglycemia may be grouped into two categories: adrenergic symptoms and central nervous system symptoms.

In mild hypoglycemia, as the blood glucose level falls, the sympathetic nervous system is stimulated. The surge of adrenalin causes symptoms such as sweating, tremor, tachycardia, palpitation, nervousness, and hunger.

In moderate hypoglycemia, the fall in blood glucose level deprives the brain cells of needed fuel for functioning. Signs of impaired function of the central nervous system may include inability to concentrate, headache, lightheadedness, confusion, memory lapses, numbness of the lips and tongue, slurred speech, incoordination, emotional changes, irrational behavior, double vision, and drowsiness. Any combination of these symptoms (in addition to adrenergic symptoms) may occur with moderate hypoglycemia.

In severe hypoglycemia, central nervous system function is so impaired that the patient needs the assistance of another person for treatment of hypoglycemia. Symptoms may include disoriented behavior, seizures, difficulty arousing from sleep, or loss of consciousness.

Hypoglycemic symptoms may occur suddenly and unexpectedly. The combination of symptoms varies considerably from person to person. To some degree, this may be related to the actual level to which the blood glucose drops or to the rate at which it is dropping. For example, patients who usually have blood glucose in the hyperglycemic range (*e.g.*, in the 200s or greater) may feel hypoglycemic (adrenergic) symptoms when their blood glucose quickly drops to 120 mg/dl (6.6 mmol/L) or less. Conversely, patients who frequently have glucose in the low range of normal may be asymptomatic when the blood glucose slowly falls under 50 mg/dl (2.7 mmol/L).

Another factor contributing to altered hypoglycemic symptoms is a decreased hormonal (adrenergic) response to hypoglycemia. This occurs in some patients who have had diabetes for many years. It may be related to one of the chronic diabetic complications—autonomic neuropathy (see section on hypoglycemic unawareness). As the blood glucose falls, the normal surge in adrenalin does not occur. The patient does not feel the usual adrenergic symptoms, such as sweating and shakiness. The hypoglycemia may not be detected until moderate or severe central nervous system impairment occurs. It is imperative that these patients perform self-monitoring of blood glucose on a frequent regular basis, especially before driving or engaging in other potentially dangerous activities.

Treatment.　Immediate treatment must be given when hypoglycemia occurs. The usual recommendation is for 10 to 15 g of a fast-acting sugar orally:

  2–4 commercially prepared glucose tablets
  4–6 oz of fruit juice or regular soda
  6–10 Life Savers or other hard candies
  2–3 tsp of sugar or honey

(It is not necessary to add sugar to juice, even if it is labeled as "unsweetened" juice. The fruit sugar in juice contains enough simple carbohydrate to sufficiently raise the blood glucose level. Adding table sugar to juice may cause a sharp increase in the blood glucose, and the patient may experience hyperglycemia for hours after treatment.)

If the symptoms persist more than 10 to 15 minutes after initial treatment, the treatment is repeated. Once the symptoms resolve, a snack containing protein and starch (such as milk or cheese and crackers) is recommended unless the patient plans on eating a regular meal or snack within 30 to 60 minutes.

It is important for diabetic patients (especially those on insulin) to carry some form of simple sugar with them at all times. There are many different commercially prepared glucose tablets and gels that patients may find convenient to carry. If the patient experiences a hypoglycemic reaction and does not have any of the recommended emergency foods available, any available food (preferably a simple carbohydrate food) should be consumed.

Patients are to be discouraged from eating high-calorie, high-fat dessert foods (such as cookies, cakes, donuts, ice cream) to treat hypoglycemia. The high fat content of these foods may slow the absorption of the glucose, and the hypoglycemic symptoms may not be resolved as quickly as they are with the intake of simple carbohydrates. The patient may subsequently eat more of the foods when symptoms do not resolve rapidly. This in turn may cause very high levels of blood glucose for several hours after the reaction and may also contribute to weight gain.

Patients who feel unduly restricted by their meal plan may view hypoglycemic episodes as a time to "reward" themselves with desserts. It may be more prudent to teach these patients to incorporate occasional desserts into the meal plan. This may make it easier for them to limit their treatment of hypoglycemic episodes to simple (low-calorie) carbohydrates such as juice or glucose tablets.

Treatment of Severe Hypoglycemia.　For patients who are unconscious, are unable to swallow, or refuse treatment, an injection of glucagon 1 mg can be administered either subcutaneously or intramuscularly. Glucagon is a hormone produced by the alpha cells of the pancreas that stimulates the liver to release glucose (through the breakdown of glycogen, the stored glucose). It is packaged as a powder in 1-mg vials and must be mixed with a diluent before being injected. After injection of glucagon, it may take up to 20 minutes for the patient to regain consciousness. A simple sugar followed by a snack should be given to the patient upon awakening to prevent recurrence of hypoglycemia, because the duration of the action of glucagon is brief. Some patients experience nausea following the administration of glucagon. The patient should be instructed to notify the physician after severe hypoglycemia has occurred.

Glucagon is sold by prescription only and should be part of the emergency supplies kept available by persons with diabetes who require insulin. Family members, neighbors, or co-workers should be instructed in the use of glucagon. This is especially true for patients who receive little or no warning of hypoglycemic episodes.

In the hospital, patients who are unconscious or unable to swallow may be treated with 25 to 50 ml of 50% dextrose in water ("D-50"), which is administered intravenously. The effect is usually seen within minutes. Patients may complain of a headache and of pain at the IV site. Assuring patency of the intravenous line used for injection of 50% dextrose is important; hypertonic solutions such as 50% dextrose are very irritating to the vein.

Prevention and Patient Education.　Hypoglycemia is prevented by following a regular pattern for eating, administering insulin, and exercising. Between-meal and bedtime snacks may be needed to counteract the maximum insulin effect. In general, the patient should cover the time of peak activity of insulin by eating a snack and by taking additional food when engaging in an increased level of physical activity. Routine blood glucose tests are performed so that changing insulin requirements may be anticipated and adjusted.

Because unexpected hypoglycemia may occur, all patients treated with insulin should wear an identification bracelet or tag indicating that they have diabetes.

Patients and family members must be instructed on the various potential symptoms of hypoglycemia. Family members especially must be made aware that any subtle (but unusual) change in behavior may be an indication that hypoglycemia is occurring. They should be taught to encourage and even insist that the person with diabetes check his blood glucose if hypoglycemia is suspected. Some patients (when hypoglycemic) become very resistant to testing or eating and become angry at family members trying to treat the hypoglycemia. Family members must be taught to persevere and to understand that the hypoglycemia can cause irrational and unintentional behavior.

Some patients with autonomic neuropathy or those taking propranolol for the treatment of hypertension or cardiac dysrhythmias may not experience the typical symptoms of hypoglycemia. It is very important for these patients to perform blood glucose tests on a frequent and regular basis.

Type II diabetic patients who take oral hypoglycemic agents may also develop hypoglycemia (especially those taking chlorpropamide, which is a long-lasting oral hypoglycemic agent).

Gerontologic Considerations.   In the elderly, hypoglycemia is a particular concern for many reasons:

Elderly people frequently live alone and may not recognize the symptoms of hypoglycemia

With decreasing renal function, it takes a longer time to clear oral hypoglycemic agents, which are excreted primarily by the kidneys

Skipping meals may occur because of decreased appetite or financial limitations on meal planning

Decreased visual acuity may lead to errors in insulin administration

Diabetic Ketoacidosis

Pathophysiology.   Diabetic ketoacidosis (DKA) is caused by an absence or markedly inadequate amount of insulin. This results in disorders in the metabolism of carbohydrate, protein, and fat. The three main clinical features of DKA are:

Dehydration
Electrolyte loss
Acidosis

When insulin is lacking, the amount of glucose entering the cells is reduced. In addition, there is unrestrained production of glucose by the liver. Both of these factors lead to hyperglycemia. In an attempt to rid the body of the excess glucose, the kidneys excrete the glucose along with water and electrolytes (such as sodium and potassium). This osmotic diuresis, which is characterized by excessive urination (polyuria), leads to *dehydration* and marked *electrolyte loss*. Patients with severe DKA may lose an average of 6.5 liters of water and up to 400 to 500 mEq each of sodium, potassium, and chloride over a 24-hour period.

Another effect of insulin deficiency is the breakdown of fat (lipolysis) into free fatty acids and glycerol. The free fatty acids are converted into ketone bodies by the liver. In DKA there is an excess production of ketone bodies because of the lack of insulin that would normally prevent this from occurring. Ketone bodies are acids, and when they accumulate in the circulation they lead to metabolic *acidosis*.

Signs and Symptoms.   The signs and symptoms of DKA are outlined in Figure 39-6. The hyperglycemia of DKA leads to polyuria and polydipsia (increased thirst). In addition, patients may experience blurred vision, weakness, and headache. Patients with marked intravascular volume depletion may have

orthostatic hypotension (drop in systolic blood pressure of 20 mm Hg or more upon standing). Volume depletion may also lead to frank hypotension with a weak, rapid pulse.

The ketosis and acidosis characteristic of DKA lead to gastrointestinal symptoms such as anorexia, nausea, vomiting, and abdominal pain. The abdominal pain and physical findings on examination can be so severe that it appears that there is an intraabdominal process occurring that will require surgery. Patients may have acetone breath (a fruity odor), which occurs with elevated levels of ketone bodies. In addition, hyperventilation (with very deep, but not labored, respirations) may occur. These *Kussmaul respirations* represent the body's attempt to decrease the acidosis, counteracting the effect of the ketone buildup.

Mental status changes in DKA vary widely from patient to patient. Patients may be alert, lethargic, or comatose, most likely depending upon the plasma *osmolarity* (concentration of osmotically active particles).

Laboratory Values.   Blood glucose levels may vary from 300 to 800 mg/dl (16.6 to 44.4 mmol/L). Some patients may have even lower glucose values, while others may have values as high as 1000 mg/dl (55.5 mmol/L) or more (usually depending upon the degree of dehydration). *It is important for the nurse to realize that the severity of DKA is not necessarily related to the blood glucose level.* Some patients may have severe acidosis with blood glucose levels in the high 100- to low 200-mg/dl (5.5 to 11.1 mmol/L) range, while others may have no evidence of DKA despite blood glucose levels of 400 to 500 mg/dl (22.2 to 27.7 mmol/L).

Evidence of ketoacidosis is reflected in low serum bicarbonate (0 to 15 mEq/L) and low *p*H (6.8 to 7.3) values. A low pCO_2 level (10 to 30 mm Hg) reflects the respiratory compensation (Kussmaul respirations) for the metabolic acidosis. Accumulation of ketone bodies (which precipitates the acidosis) is reflected in blood and urine ketone measurements.

Sodium and potassium levels may be low, normal, or high, depending upon the amount of water loss (dehydration). It is important to remember that despite the plasma concentration there has been a marked total body depletion of these (and other) electrolytes. Ultimately, these electrolytes will need to be replaced.

Elevated levels of creatinine, blood urea nitrogen (BUN), hemoglobin, and hematocrit may also be seen with dehydration. After rehydration, continued elevation in the serum creatinine and BUN levels will be present in the patient with underlying renal insufficiency.

Causes.   Three main causes of DKA are:

- A decreased or missed dose of insulin
- An illness or infection
- The initial manifestation of undiagnosed and untreated diabetes

A decrease in insulin may result from an insufficient dosage of insulin being prescribed or from an insufficient dosage of insulin being administered by the patient. Erroneous decreases in insulin dosage may be made by patients who are ill and who assume that if they are eating less or if they are vomiting, they must decrease their insulin doses. (Because illness [especially infections] may cause increased blood glucose levels, patients do not need to decrease doses to account for decreased food intake when ill and may even need to increase insulin.)

Other potential causes of decreased insulin include patient

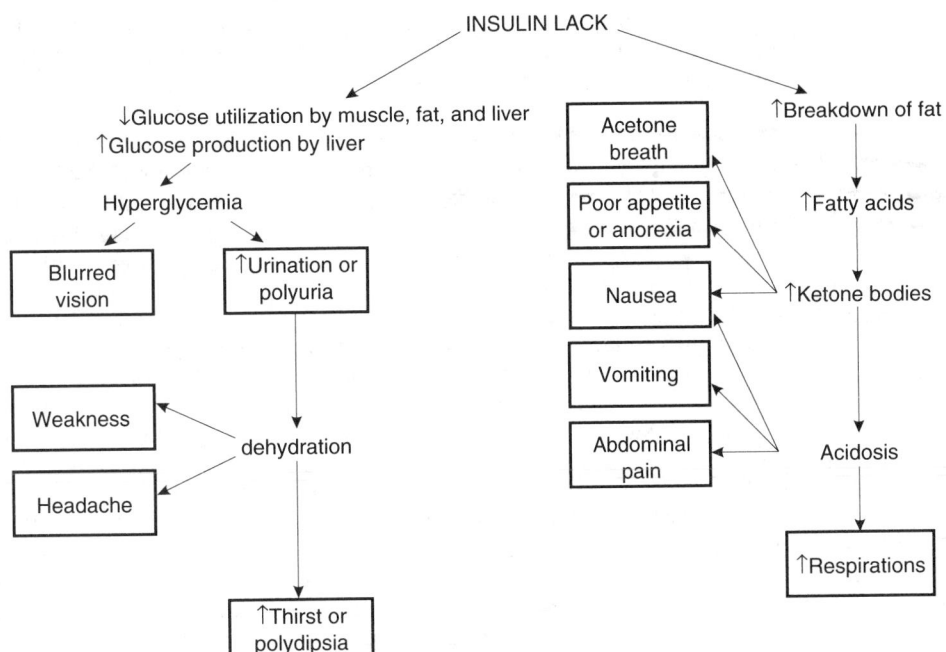

Figure 39-6. Abnormal metabolism that causes signs and symptoms of diabetic ketoacidosis: ↑, increased; ↓, decreased. (Pearce MA, Rosenberg CS, and Davidson MD. Patient education. In Davidson MB [ed]. Diabetes Mellitus: Diagnosis and Treatment, 3rd ed. New York, Churchill Livingstone, 1991.)

error in drawing up or injecting insulin (especially in patients with visual impairments); intentional skipping of insulin doses (especially in adolescents with diabetes who are having difficulty coping with diabetes or other aspects of their lives); or equipment problems (*e.g.,* occlusion of insulin pump tubing).

Illness and infections are associated with insulin resistance. In response to physical (and emotional) stresses, there is an increase in the level of "stress" hormones—glucagon, epinephrine, norepinephrine, cortisol, and growth hormone. These hormones promote glucose production by the liver and interfere with glucose utilization by muscle and fat tissue, counteracting the effect of insulin. If insulin levels are not increased during times of illness and infection, hyperglycemia may progress to DKA.

Treatment.   Treatment of DKA is aimed at correction of the three main problems: dehydration, electrolyte loss, and acidosis.

Dehydration.   Rehydration is important for maintaining tissue perfusion. In addition, fluid replacement enhances the excretion of excess glucose by the kidneys. Patients may need up to 6 to 10 liters of intravenous fluid to replace fluid loss caused by polyuria, hyperventilation, diarrhea, and vomiting.

Initially, 0.9% normal saline is administered at a very high rate—usually 0.5 to 1 L/hr for 2 to 3 hours. Hypotonic normal saline (0.45%) may be used for patients with hypertension or hypernatremia or those at risk for congestive heart failure. After the first few hours, 0.45% normal saline is the fluid of choice for continued rehydration, provided the blood pressure is stable and the sodium level is not low. Moderate to high rates of infusion (200 to 500 ml/hr) may continue for several more hours.

Monitoring fluid volume status involves frequent measurement of vital signs (including checking for orthostatic changes in blood pressure and heart rate), lung assessment, and monitoring intake and output. Initial urine output will lag behind intravenous fluid intake as dehydration is corrected. Plasma expanders may be necessary for correction of severe hypo-

tension that does not respond to intravenous fluid treatment. Monitoring for signs of fluid overload is especially important for the older patient or patients at risk for congestive heart failure.

Electrolyte Loss.   The major electrolyte of concern during treatment of DKA is potassium. Although the initial plasma concentration of potassium may be low, normal, or even high, there is a major loss of potassium from body stores. Furthermore, the level of potassium will drop during the course of treatment of DKA and therefore must be monitored frequently.

Some of the factors related to treatment of DKA that reduce the serum potassium concentration include:

Rehydration leading to increased plasma volume and subsequent decreases in the concentration of serum potassium

Rehydration leading to increased urinary excretion of potassium

Insulin administration enhancing the movement of potassium from the extracellular fluid into the cells

Cautious but timely replacement of potassium is vital for the avoidance of severe cardiac dysrhythmias that may occur with hypokalemia. Up to 40 mEq/hr (added to IV fluids) may be required for several hours. Because the potassium level will drop during treatment of DKA, *potassium must be infused even if the plasma concentration of potassium is normal.* Then, as DKA is resolving, the rate of potassium replacement will be decreased. For safe infusion of potassium, the nurse should check that:

There are no signs of *hyper*kalemia on the ECG (tall, peaked T waves)

The laboratory values of potassium are normal or low

The patient is urinating (*i.e.,* not experiencing renal shutdown)

Frequent (every 2 to 4 hours initially) ECG readings and laboratory measurements of potassium are necessary during the first 8 hours of treatment. Potassium replacement is withheld only if hyperkalemia is present or if the patient is not urinating.

However, because the potassium level may drop quickly as a result of rehydration and insulin treatment, potassium replacement must be initiated as soon as potassium levels drop to normal.

Acidosis. The accumulation of ketone bodies (acids) is the result of fat breakdown. The acidosis that occurs in DKA is reversed with insulin. Insulin inhibits the fat breakdown, thereby stopping the buildup of acids.

Insulin is usually infused intravenously at a slow, continuous rate (*e.g.*, 5 units per hour). Hourly blood glucose values must be measured. Dextrose is added to IV fluids (*e.g.*, D_5NS or $D_5.45NS$) when blood glucose levels reach 250 to 300 mg/dl (13.8 to 16.6 mmol/L) to avoid too rapid a drop in the blood glucose level.

Various intravenous mixtures of regular insulin may be used. The nurse must convert hourly rates of insulin infusion (frequently ordered as "units per hour") to IV drip rates. For example, if 100 units of regular insulin are mixed in 500 ml of 0.9NS, then 1 unit of insulin equals 5 ml. Thus, an initial insulin infusion rate of 5 units per hour would equal 25 ml/hr. It is best to infuse the insulin separately from the rehydration solutions to allow for frequent changes in rate and content of rehydration solutions.

When mixing the insulin drip, it is important to flush the insulin solution through the entire IV infusion set and to discard the first 50 ml of fluid. Insulin molecules adhere to the glass and plastic of IV infusion sets; thus, the initial fluid may contain a decreased concentration of insulin.

It is imperative that the IV insulin be infused *continuously* until subcutaneous administration of insulin is resumed. Any interruption in insulin administration may result in the reaccumulation of ketone bodies and worsening acidosis. Even if blood glucose levels are dropping to normal, the insulin drip must not be turned off. Rather, the rate or concentration of the dextrose infusion should be increased.

It is important to remember that blood glucose levels are usually corrected before the acidosis is corrected. Thus, IV insulin may be continued for 12 to 24 hours, until the serum bicarbonate improves (to at least 15 to 18 mEq/L) and until the patient can eat. Normalized blood glucose levels are *not* an indication that the acidosis has resolved.

In general, bicarbonate infusion for correction of severe acidosis is avoided during treatment of DKA because it precipitates further, sudden (and potentially fatal) decreases in serum potassium levels. Continuous insulin infusion is usually sufficient for reversing the acidosis of DKA.

Prevention and Education. For prevention of DKA related to illness, patients must be taught "sick day rules" for managing their diabetes when ill (Chart 39-6). The most important issue is to teach patients not to eliminate insulin doses when nausea and vomiting occur. Rather, they should take their usual insulin dose (or previously prescribed special "sick day" doses) and then attempt to consume frequent small portions of carbohydrates (including foods usually avoided, such as juices, regular sodas, and Jell-O). Drinking fluids every hour—including broth—is important for avoidance of dehydration. Blood glucose and urine ketones must be checked every 3 to 4 hours.

If the patient is unable to take fluids without vomiting, or if elevated glucose or ketone levels persist, the physician must be contacted. Patients are taught to plan ahead and have foods available for use on sick days. In addition, a supply of urine test strips (for ketone testing) and blood glucose test strips should be available. Patients must know how to contact their physician 24 hours a day.

Diabetes self-management skills (including insulin administration and blood glucose testing) should be assessed to ensure that accidental error in insulin administration or blood glucose testing did not occur. Psychologic counseling is recommended for patients and family members if intentional alteration in insulin dosing was the cause of the DKA.

Hyperosmolar Nonketotic Syndrome

Pathophysiology and Clinical Manifestations. Hyperosmolar nonketotic syndrome (HNKS) is a situation in which hyperglycemia and hyperosmolarity predominate, with alterations of the sensorium (sense of awareness). At the same time, ketosis is minimal or absent. The basic biochemical defect is lack of effective insulin. The patient's persistent hyperglycemia causes osmotic diuresis, resulting in losses of water and electrolytes. To maintain osmotic equilibrium, water shifts from the intracellular fluid space to the extracellular fluid space.

Chart 39-6
Guidelines to Follow During Periods of Illness ("Sick Day Rules")

- Take insulin or oral hypoglycemic agents as usual.
- Test blood glucose and (for type I diabetic patients) test urine ketones every 3 to 4 hours.
- Report elevated glucose levels (greater than 300 mg/dl, 16.6 mmol/L, or as otherwise specified) or urine ketones to the physician.
- Insulin-requiring patients may need supplemental doses of regular insulin every 3 to 4 hours.
- If usual meal plan cannot be followed, substitute soft foods (*e.g.*, ⅓ cup regular gelatin, 1 cup cream soup, ½ cup custard, 3 squares graham crackers) six to eight times per day.
- If vomiting, diarrhea, or fever persists, take liquids (*e.g.*, ½ cup regular cola or orange juice, ½ cup broth, 1 cup Gatorade) every ½ to 1 hour to prevent dehydration and to provide calories.
- Report nausea, vomiting, and diarrhea to the physician because extreme fluid loss may be dangerous.
- For patients with type I diabetes, inability to retain oral fluids may warrant hospitalization to avoid diabetic ketoacidosis and possibly coma.

With glucosuria and dehydration, hypernatremia and increased osmolarity occur.

One major difference between HNKS and DKA is that ketosis and acidosis do not occur in HNKS. Differences in the amount of insulin present in each condition are thought to be partially responsible for this. In DKA there is virtually no insulin present; thus, breakdown of stored glucose, protein, and fat occurs (the latter leading to production of ketone bodies and subsequent ketoacidosis). In HNKS, the level of insulin is not as low. While there is not enough insulin to prevent hyperglycemia (and subsequent osmotic diuresis), the small amount of insulin present is enough to prevent fat breakdown. Patients with HNKS do not experience the gastrointestinal symptoms related to ketosis that cause the patient with DKA to seek medical attention. Often, patients developing HNKS tolerate polyuria and polydipsia for weeks, and only when neurologic changes occur or when an underlying illness worsens do they (or more often family or staff at an extended care facility) seek medical attention. Thus, the hyperglycemia and dehydration are more severe in HNKS secondary to delays in treatment.

The clinical picture of HNKS is one of hypotension, profound dehydration (dry mucous membranes, poor skin turgor), tachycardia, and variable neurologic signs (*e.g.*, alteration of sensorium, seizures, hemiparesis). This is a serious condition with a mortality rate ranging from 5% to 30%, usually related to an underlying illness.

Causes. This condition occurs most frequently in older people (50 to 70 years) who have had no previous history of diabetes or only mild type II diabetes. The acute development of the condition can be traced to some precipitating event, such as an acute illness (pneumonia, myocardial infarction, stroke), ingestion of drugs known to provoke insulin insufficiency (thiazide diuretics, propranolol), or therapeutic procedures (peritoneal dialysis/hemodialysis, hyperalimentation). There is a history of days to weeks of polyuria, with inadequate fluid intake.

Management. The overall approach to the treatment of HNKS is similar to that of DKA: fluids, electrolytes, and insulin. Because of the increased age of the typical patient with HNKS, close monitoring of volume and electrolyte status may be needed for prevention of congestive heart failure and cardiac dysrhythmias. Fluid treatment is started with 0.9% or 0.45% normal saline depending upon the sodium level and severity of volume depletion. Central venous or arterial pressure monitoring may be necessary to guide fluid replacement. Potassium is added to replacement fluids when urinary output is adequate and is guided by continuous EKG monitoring and frequent laboratory determinations of potassium.

Extremely elevated blood glucose levels will drop as the patient is rehydrated. Insulin plays a less crucial role in the treatment of HNKS because it is not needed for reversal of acidosis, as in DKA. Nonetheless, insulin is usually given at a continuous low rate to treat hyperglycemia, and dextrose is added to replacement fluids (as in DKA) when the glucose level reaches the 250- to 300-mg/dl range (13.8 to 16.6 mmol/L).

Other therapeutic modalities are determined by the underlying illness of the patient and the results of continuing clinical and laboratory evaluation. Treatment is continued until metabolic abnormalities are corrected and neurologic symptoms clear. It may take as many as 3 to 5 days for neurologic symptoms to resolve; thus, treatment of HNKS usually continues well beyond the time when metabolic abnormalities are resolved.

After recovery from HNKS, many patients can control diabetes with diet alone or diet with oral hypoglycemic agents. Insulin may not be needed once the acute hyperglycemic complication is resolved.

Morning Hyperglycemia

An elevated blood glucose level on arising in the morning may be due to an insufficient level of insulin, to the dawn phenomenon, or to the Somogyi effect. The dawn phenomenon is characterized by a relatively normal blood glucose level until approximately 3 AM, when blood glucose levels begin to rise. The phenomenon is thought to result from nocturnal surges in growth hormone secretion that create a greater need for insulin in the early morning hours in patients with type I diabetes. It must be distinguished from insulin waning or the Somogyi effect (nocturnal hypoglycemia followed by rebound hyperglycemia).

It is often difficult to tell from the patient's history which of these causes is responsible for morning hyperglycemia. In order to determine the cause, the patient must be awakened once or twice during the night to test blood glucose levels. Testing the blood glucose level at bedtime, at 3 AM, and upon awakening will provide information that can be used in making an insulin adjustment to avoid morning hyperglycemia caused by the dawn phenomenon. Table 39-6 summarizes the differences between insulin waning, the dawn phenomenon, and the Somogyi effect.

▶ Nursing Process
The Patient With Newly Diagnosed Diabetes Mellitus

▷ Assessment

Nursing history and physical assessment focus on the signs and symptoms of prolonged hyperglycemia and on physical, social, and emotional factors that may affect the patient's ability to learn and perform diabetes self-care activities.

The patient is interviewed and asked for a description of symptoms that preceded the diagnosis of diabetes, such as polyuria, polydipsia, polyphagia, skin dryness, blurred vision, weight loss, vaginal itching, and nonhealing ulcers. The blood glucose and, for patients with type I diabetes, urine ketone levels are measured.

Patients with type I diabetes are assessed for signs of DKA, including ketonuria, Kussmaul respirations, orthostatic hypotension, and lethargy. The patient is questioned regarding symptoms of DKA, such as nausea, vomiting, and abdominal pain. Laboratory values are monitored for signs of metabolic acidosis, such as decreased *p*H and decreased bicarbonate, and for signs of electrolyte imbalance.

Patients with type II diabetes are assessed for signs of HNKS, including hypotension, altered sensorium, seizures, and decreased skin turgor. Laboratory values are monitored for signs of hyperosmolarity and electrolyte imbalance.

(*Note:* If the patient exhibits signs and symptoms of DKA or HNKS, nursing care first focuses on treatment of these acute

TABLE 39-6. *Causes of Morning Hyperglycemia*

Characteristic	Treatment
INSULIN WANING Progressive rise in blood glucose from bedtime to morning	Increase evening (pre-dinner or bedtime) dose of intermediate- or long-acting insulin or institute a dose of insulin before the evening meal if one is not already in use.
DAWN PHENOMENON Relatively normal blood glucose until about 3 AM, when the level begins to rise	Change time of injection of evening intermediate-acting insulin from dinner time to bedtime.
SOMOGYI EFFECT Normal or elevated blood glucose at bedtime, a decrease at 2-3 AM to hypoglycemic levels, and a subsequent increase caused by the production of counter-regulatory hormones	Decrease evening (pre-dinner or bedtime) dose of intermediate-acting insulin and/or increase bedtime snack.

complications as outlined in previous sections. Once these complications are resolving, nursing care then focuses on long-term management of diabetes as discussed in this section.)

The patient is assessed for physical factors that may impair his ability to learn or perform self-care skills, such as:

- Visual deficits (have the patient read numbers or words on the insulin syringe, menu, newspaper, and/or written teaching materials)
- Deficits in motor coordination (observe patient eating or performing other tasks or have patient practice handling syringe or finger-lancing device)
- Neurologic deficits (*e.g.*, due to stroke) (from history in chart; assess for aphasia or decreased ability to follow simple commands)

The nurse evaluates the patient's social situation for factors that may influence the diabetes treatment and education plan, such as:

- Decreased literacy (assess this while assessing for visual deficits by having patient read from teaching materials)
- Limited financial resources/lack of health insurance
- Presence or absence of family support
- Typical daily schedule (ask patient about timing and number of usual daily meals, work and exercise schedule, plans for travel)

The patient's emotional status is assessed through observation of general demeanor (*e.g.*, withdrawn, anxious) and body language (*e.g.*, avoids eye contact). The patient is asked what his major concern is or what he fears most about diabetes (this allows for assessment of any misconceptions or misinformation regarding diabetes). Coping skills are assessed by asking the patient how he has dealt with difficult situations in the past.

▷ Nursing Diagnoses

Based on the assessment data, the patient's major nursing diagnoses may include the following:

- High risk for fluid volume deficit related to polyuria and dehydration
- Altered nutrition related to imbalance of insulin, food, and physical activity
- Knowledge deficit about diabetes self-care skills/information
- Potential self-care deficit related to physical impairments or social factors
- Anxiety related to loss of control, fear of inability to manage diabetes, misinformation related to diabetes, fear of diabetes complications

▷ Planning and Implementation

▷ *Goals:* The major goals of the patient may include attainment of fluid and electrolyte balance, optimal control of blood glucose, regaining weight lost, ability to perform basic (survival) diabetes skills and self-care activities, and reduction in anxiety.

Nursing Interventions

▷ *Maintenance of Fluid and Electrolyte Balance.* Intake and output are measured. Intravenous fluids and electrolytes are administered as ordered, and oral fluid intake is encouraged. Laboratory measurements of serum electrolytes (especially sodium and potassium) are monitored. The patient's vital signs are monitored to detect signs of dehydration: tachycardia, orthostatic hypotension.

▷ *Correction of Metabolic Abnormalities.* Bedside glucose monitoring is performed (usually before meals and at bedtime). Insulin is administered as ordered. Juice or glucose tablets are used for treatment of hypoglycemia. Supplemental insulin doses are given (not more often than every 3 to 4 hours) as ordered for hyperglycemia. The patient is encouraged to eat full meals and snacks as ordered per diabetic diet. Arrangements are made with the dietitian for extra snacks before increased physical activity. It is important for the nurse to ensure that insulin orders are altered as needed for delays in eating due to diagnostic and other procedures.

▷ *Patient Education.*   The patient is taught survival skills, including simple pathophysiology; treatment modalities (insulin administration, monitoring of blood glucose and—for type I diabetes—urine ketones, diet); recognition, treatment, and prevention of acute complications (hypoglycemia and hyperglycemia); and pragmatic information (where to obtain supplies, when to call physician). If the patient has any signs of long-term diabetes complications at the time of diagnosis of diabetes, teaching about appropriate preventive behaviors (*e.g.*, foot care or eye care) should be included.

▷ *Specialized Patient Education and Home Health Care.*   Special equipment is used for instruction on diabetes survival skills, such as a magnifying glass for insulin preparation or an injection aid device for insulin injection. Low-literacy information is used as needed. The family is instructed to assist in diabetes management (*e.g.*, to prefill syringes, to monitor blood glucose). The diabetes specialist is consulted regarding various blood glucose monitors and other equipment for use with patients with physical impairments. Follow-up education is arranged with a home health nurse or an outpatient diabetes education center. The patient is assisted in identifying community resources for education and supplies as needed; consideration is given to financial limitations or physical limitations (such as centers for the visually impaired). Other members of the health care team are informed about variations in the timing of meals and the work schedule (*e.g.*, if patient works at night or in the evenings and sleeps during the day) so that the diabetes treatment regimen can be adjusted accordingly.

▷ *Reducing Anxiety.*   The nurse provides emotional support and sets aside time to sit with the patient who wishes to ventilate, cry, or ask questions about this new diagnosis. Any misconceptions the patient or family may have regarding diabetes are dispelled (see Chart 39-5). The patient and family are assisted to focus on learning self-care behaviors. The patient is encouraged to perform the skills that he fears most, and he must be reassured that once a skill such as self-injection or puncturing a finger for glucose monitoring is performed for the first time, anxiety will be relieved. The patient is given much positive reinforcement for the self-care behaviors he has attempted, even if the technique has not yet been completely mastered.

▷ Evaluation

Expected Outcomes

1. Achieves fluid and electrolyte balance
   a. Demonstrates intake and output balance
   b. Exhibits electrolyte values that are within normal limits
   c. Vital signs remain stable with resolution of orthostatic hypotension and tachycardia.

2. Achieves metabolic balance
   a. Avoids extremes of glucose levels (hypoglycemia or hyperglycemia)
   b. Demonstrates rapid resolution of hypoglycemic episodes
   c. Avoids further weight loss and begins to approach desired weight
3. Demonstrates/verbalizes diabetes survival skills, including:

Simple Pathophysiology

a. Defines diabetes as a condition in which high blood glucose is present
b. States normal blood glucose range
c. Identifies factors that cause the blood glucose level to fall (insulin, exercise)
d. Identifies factors that cause the blood glucose level to rise (food, illness and infections)
e. Describes the major treatment modalities—diet, exercise, monitoring, medication, education

Treatment Modalities (Insulin, Diet, Monitoring, Education)

a. Demonstrates proper technique for drawing up and injecting insulin (including mixing two types of insulin if necessary)
b. Verbalizes insulin injection rotation plan
c. Verbalizes understanding of classification of food groups (depending upon system used)
d. Verbalizes appropriate schedule for eating snacks and meals
e. Orders appropriate foods on menus and identifies foods that may be substituted for one another on the meal plan
f. Demonstrates proper technique for monitoring blood glucose, including using finger-lancing device; obtaining large, hanging drop of blood; applying blood properly to strip; removing blood from strip at appropriate time interval (if necessary); obtaining value of blood glucose; and recording blood glucose value. If meter is used, patient is able to calibrate and clean meter, change batteries, and identify alarms and warnings on meter.
g. Demonstrates proper technique for disposing of needles used for blood glucose monitoring and insulin injections (*e.g.*, discarding needles into hard plastic container such as empty bleach or detergent container)
h. Demonstrates proper technique for urine ketone testing (for patients with type I diabetes) and verbalizes appropriate times to check for ketones—when ill or when glucose test results are repeatedly and unexplainably over 250 to 300 mg/dl (13.8 to 16.6 mmol/L)
i. Identifies community, outpatient resources for obtaining further diabetes education

Acute Complications (Hypoglycemia and Hyperglycemia)

a. Verbalizes symptoms of hypoglycemia (shakiness, sweating, headache, hunger, numbness or tingling of lips or fingers, weakness, fatigue, difficulty concentrating, change of mood) and dangers of untreated hypoglycemia (seizures and coma)
b. Identifies appropriate treatment of hypoglycemia, including 10 to 15 gm of simple carbohydrate (*e.g.*, 2 to 4 glucose tablets, 4 to 6 oz of juice or soda, 2 to 3 tsp of sugar, or 6 to 10 Lifesavers) followed by a snack of protein and

carbohydrate, such as cheese and crackers or milk, or by a regularly scheduled meal
c. Identifies potential causes of hypoglycemia—too much insulin, delayed or decreased food intake, increased physical activity
d. Verbalizes preventive behaviors, such as frequent monitoring of blood glucose when daily schedule is changed, taking snack before exercise. Verbalizes importance of wearing medical identification and carrying a source of simple carbohydrate *at all times*.
e. Verbalizes symptoms of prolonged hyperglycemia—increased thirst and urination
f. Verbalizes rules for sick-day management (Chart 39-6)

Pragmatic Information
a. Verbalizes where to purchase and store insulin, syringes, and glucose-monitoring supplies
b. Identifies appropriate circumstances for calling the physician, including when ill, when glucose levels are repeatedly over a certain level (per physician guidelines), or when skin wounds fail to heal
c. Identifies name and phone number to reach physician or other member of health care team 24 hours per day

Long-Term Complications of Diabetes

There has been a steady decline in deaths of diabetic patients due to ketoacidosis and infection but an alarming rise in deaths due to cardiovascular and renal complications. Long-term complications are becoming more common as more persons live longer with their diabetes.

The long-term complications of diabetes can affect almost every organ system of the body. The general categories of chronic diabetic complications are:

Macrovascular disease
Microvascular disease
Neuropathy

The specific causes and pathogenesis of each type of complication are still being investigated. It appears, however, that increased levels of blood glucose may play a role in neuropathic disease, microvascular complications, and risk factors contributing to macrovascular complications. Hypertension may also be a major contributing factor, especially in macrovascular and microvascular diseases.

Long-term complications are seen in both type I and type II diabetes, usually not occurring within the first 5 to 10 years of the diagnosis. Renal (microvascular) disease is more prevalent among type I diabetic patients, while cardiovascular (macrovascular) complications are more prevalent among older type II diabetic patients.

Macrovascular Complications

Atherosclerotic changes in the larger blood vessels commonly occur in diabetes. These atherosclerotic changes are similar to those seen in nondiabetic patients except that they tend to occur at an earlier age and with greater frequency in diabetic

patients. Depending upon the location of the atherosclerotic lesions, different types of macrovascular diseases may result.

Coronary Artery Disease. Atherosclerotic changes in the coronary arteries lead to an increased occurrence of myocardial infarctions in persons with diabetes (twice as frequent in diabetic men and three times as frequent in diabetic women). In diabetes there is an increased likelihood of complications resulting from the myocardial infarction and of a second myocardial infarction occurring. Some studies suggest that coronary artery disease may account for 50% to 60% of all deaths in patients with diabetes.

One unique feature of coronary artery disease in patients with diabetes is that the typical ischemic symptoms may be absent. Thus, patients may not experience the early warning signs of decreased coronary blood flow and may have "silent" myocardial infarctions in which chest pain or other typical symptoms are not experienced. These "silent" myocardial infarctions may be discovered only as changes on the electrocardiogram. This lack of ischemic symptoms may be secondary to autonomic neuropathy.

Cerebral Vascular Disease. Atherosclerotic changes in cerebral blood vessels or the formation of an embolus elsewhere in the vasculature that then lodges in a cerebral blood vessel can lead to the occurrence of transient ischemic attacks and strokes. Cerebrovascular disease in diabetic patients is similar to that of nondiabetic patients except that people with diabetes may have twice the risk of developing cerebrovascular disease, and studies suggest that there may be a greater likelihood of death due to cerebrovascular disease in diabetes. In addition, recovery from a stroke may be impaired in patients who have elevated blood glucose levels at the time of diagnosis and immediately following a cerebrovascular accident.

Symptoms of cerebrovascular disease may be quite similar to those of the acute diabetic complications (HNKS or hypoglycemia). These may include dizziness, decreased vision, slurred speech, and weakness. It is very important that patients reporting these types of symptoms be assessed for blood glucose levels (and treated as indicated for blood glucose abnormalities) prior to the initiation of extensive diagnostic testing for cerebrovascular disease.

Peripheral Vascular Disease. Atherosclerotic changes in the large blood vessels of the lower extremities are responsible for the increased (two to three times higher than in nondiabetic persons) incidence of occlusive peripheral arterial disease in diabetic patients. Signs and symptoms of peripheral vascular disease may include diminished peripheral pulses and intermittent claudication (pain in the buttock, thigh, and/or calf during walking). It is the severe form of arterial occlusive disease in the lower extremities that is largely responsible for the increased incidence of gangrene and amputation in diabetic patients.

Neuropathy and impairments in wound healing also play a role in diabetic foot disease (see next sections).

Role of Diabetes in Macrovascular Diseases. Diabetes researchers continue to investigate the relationship between diabetes and macrovascular diseases. The atherosclerotic changes that occur in the blood vessels of diabetic patients are no different from those that occur in the nondiabetic population. While diabetic patients are more likely to develop macrovascular diseases, there is no clear-cut explanation for why they are more prone to develop atherosclerotic changes than their nondiabetic counterparts. The main feature unique to diabetes is an elevated level of blood glucose. However, a direct link has not been found between hyperglycemia and atherosclerosis.

There are certain risk factors that are associated with accelerated atherosclerosis. These include elevated blood lipids, hypertension, cigarette smoking, obesity, lack of exercise, and family history. These risk factors appear to play equal roles in the development of macrovascular diseases in both the diabetic and nondiabetic population. While certain risk factors may be more common among diabetic patients (*e.g.*, obesity, increased triglyceride levels, hypertension), there continues to be a higher rate of macrovascular diseases among diabetic patients as compared to nondiabetic patients possessing the same risk factors. Thus, diabetes itself is seen as an independent risk factor for the development of accelerated atherosclerosis.

Other potential factors that may play a role in diabetes-related atherosclerosis are the subject of debate among diabetes researchers. These include platelet and clotting-factor abnormalities, decreased flexibility of red blood cells, decreased oxygen release, changes in the arterial wall related to hyperglycemia, and possibly hyperinsulinemia.

Treatment and Prevention of Macrovascular Diseases. At present, prevention and treatment of the commonly accepted risk factors for atherosclerosis are recommended. Diet is important in the management of obesity, hypertension, and hyperlipidemia. In addition, the use of medications for control of hypertension and hyperlipidemia may be indicated. There is some evidence that increased triglyceride levels may improve with the control of blood glucose levels.

Regular exercise is important; however, there may be certain limitations that need to be considered. The presence of intermittent claudication may limit the patient's ability to exercise. These patients need to be given recommendations for slowly increasing the amount of exercise so as to increase blood flow to the lower extremities, thereby increasing exercise tolerance. In addition, pentoxifylline (Trental) may be prescribed for relief of pain from claudication. This medication improves blood flow to ischemic areas through its effect on red blood cell flexibility, platelet adhesiveness, and blood viscosity.

As mentioned earlier (see section on exercise), the presence of other diabetic complications (*e.g.*, neuropathy, retinopathy) may limit the types of exercises that can be performed. Exercise is timed to promote lowering of post-meal hyperglycemia while avoiding hypoglycemia at peak times of insulin action.

Risk factor management is an important aspect of diabetes treatment. For patients on insulin, attention is often focused exclusively on blood glucose levels and adjustment of insulin doses. It is important to teach patients that risk factor management is an equally important part of diabetic treatment and must not be forgotten, even by patients who successfully maintain strict blood glucose control.

When macrovascular complications do occur, treatment is the same as with nondiabetic patients. In addition, it is important to pay attention to blood glucose control. Physiologic stress that accompanies illnesses such as strokes and myocardial infarctions, as well as the stress of surgical procedures, may cause an increase in blood glucose levels. Appropriate adjustment of medications is important. For some type II diabetic patients there may be a need to switch from oral hypoglycemic medications to insulin.

The ability to perform diabetes self-care skills may be adversely affected in patients who have experienced a stroke and who have a deficit in upper extremity function. The use of special equipment for assistance in blood glucose monitoring and insulin administration may be indicated.

Microvascular Complications

While macrovascular atherosclerotic changes are seen in both diabetic and nondiabetic patients, the microvascular changes are unique to diabetes. Diabetic microvascular disease (or microangiopathy) is characterized by capillary basement membrane thickening. The basement membrane surrounds the endothelial cells of the capillary. Researchers postulate that increased blood glucose levels through a series of biochemical responses lead to a thickening of the basement membrane to several times its normal thickness.

Two places where impaired capillary function may have devastating effects are the microcirculation of the retina of the eye and the kidney. The resulting diabetic retinopathy is the leading cause of blindness in people between 20 and 74 years of age in the United States. Similarly, about one in every four individuals starting dialysis has diabetic nephropathy.

Diabetic Retinopathy

The eye pathology referred to as diabetic retinopathy is caused by changes in the small blood vessels in the retina of the eye (Fig. 39-7). The retina is the area of the eye that receives images and sends information about the images to the brain. It is richly supplied with blood vessels of all kinds—small arteries and veins, arterioles, venules, and capillaries.

There are three main stages of retinopathy: nonproliferative (background) retinopathy, preproliferative retinopathy, and proliferative retinopathy. The majority of diabetic patients develop some degree of background retinopathy within 5 to 15 years of the diagnosis of diabetes. A very small percentage of these patients go on to develop the more serious proliferative stage or the condition called *macular edema*, in which visual impairment is common.

Nonproliferative (Background) Retinopathy. Some of the pathologic capillary changes involved in this early stage of retinopathy include thickening of the basement membrane, increased capillary permeability, and capillary occlusions. Examination of the retina may reveal microaneurysms (''outpouching'' of the capillary walls), leakage of fluid/serum (''exudates'') through the microaneurysms and weakened capillary walls, and small intraretinal hemorrhages.

As many as 90% of diabetic patients (with poorly controlled blood glucose) may develop clinical evidence of background retinopathy. In these patients, the only indication that retinopathy is present may be a scattering of microaneurysms seen on ophthalmologic examination. The majority of these patients will have no visual impairments at this stage and have little risk of developing blindness in the future.

One problem that can lead to visual impairments at this stage of retinopathy is *macular edema*. When capillary leakage or hemorrhage occurs, one result may be retinal edema around the areas of capillary damage. If this leakage occurs around the macula (the part of the retina on which images in the center of the visual field are focused), visual distortion and loss of

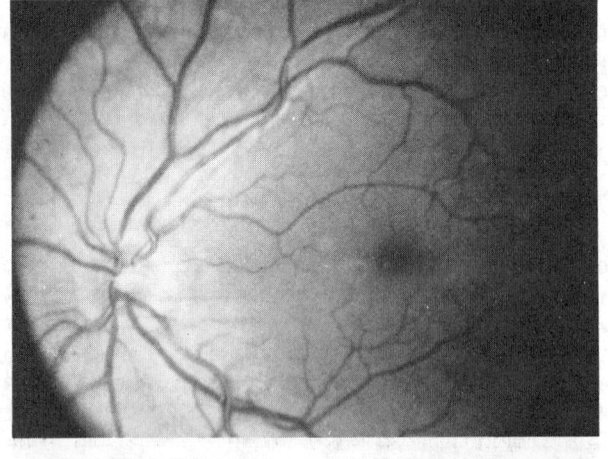

A

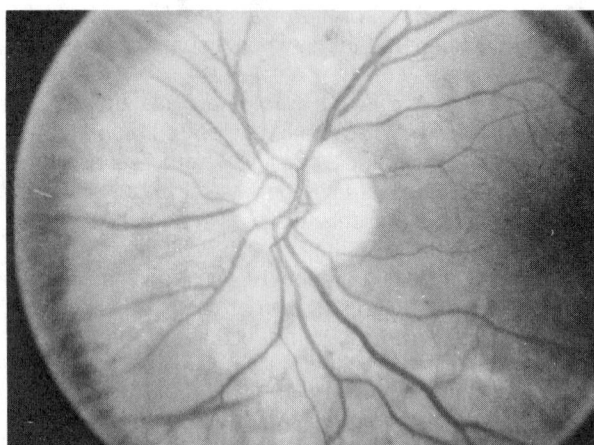

B

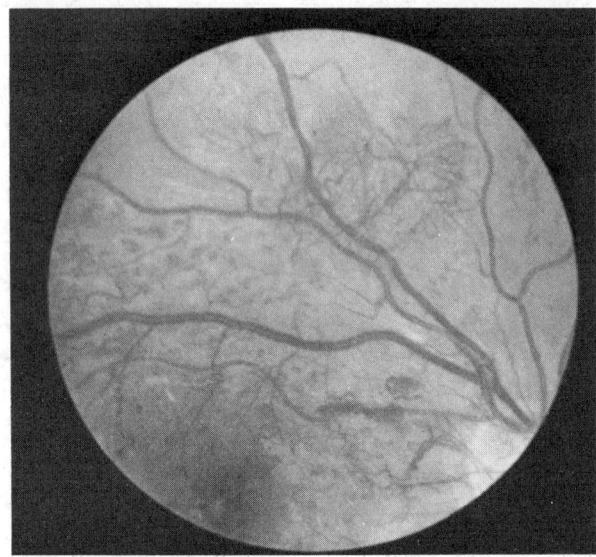

C

Figure 39–7. Diabetic retinopathy. (**A**) In the fundus photograph of a normal eye, the light circular area to the left, over which a number of blood vessels converge, is the optic disc, where the optic nerve meets the back of the eye. To the right of the optic disc is a smaller, dark spot on the photograph, the macula. The macula is the part of the retina on which images in the center of a person's visual field are focused. This part of the retina has a high concentration of light-sensitive cells, called *cones,* which provide sharp, clear color vision in bright light. (**B**) The fundus photograph of a patient with diabetic retinopathy shows neovascularization—growth of a fine network of abnormal new vessels—directly on the optic disc. Small dots on the photograph are microaneurysms, while larger blotches are hemorrhages. One example of a hemorrhage in this photo is an almost horizontal streak on the lower left. (**C**) This fundus photograph showing severe diabetic retinopathy reveals widespread neovascularization, microaneurysms, and hemorrhaging. (Photo courtesy of National Eye Institute.)

central vision may occur. Peripheral vision may not be affected. The prevalence of macular edema in people with type I and type II diabetes is approximately 10%.

Preproliferative Retinopathy. This advanced form of background retinopathy is considered a precursor to the more serious proliferative retinopathy. Epidemiologic evidence suggests that 10% to 50% of patients with preproliferative retinopathy will develop proliferative retinopathy within a short time (maybe as little as 1 year).

In the preproliferative stage there are signs of capillary closure and of a retinal response to decreased perfusion. Beaded veins, clusters of blot hemorrhages, and areas of localized ischemia (called soft exudates or "cotton wool spots") may be seen.

In response to the decreased delivery of oxygen and nutrients to the retina, there may be a budding of new blood vessels. It is thought that in the preproliferative stage, dilated, tortuous capillaries within the retina represent early stages of new vessel formation. If these new vessels leak, they may contribute to the development of macular edema.

As with background retinopathy, if visual changes occur during the preproliferative stage, they are usually due to macular edema.

Proliferative Retinopathy. The greatest threat to vision occurs in this advanced stage of retinopathy. The term proliferative refers to the growth of new blood vessels in and around the retina. Whereas the preproliferative stage might involve growth of new vessels within the retina itself, in the proliferative stage new vessels may extend out into the vitreous space (toward the front of the eye). These new vessels are very fragile, with thin, leaky walls, and they are prone to hemorrhaging.

The visual loss associated with proliferative retinopathy is due to vitreous hemorrhage or retinal detachment. The vitreous is normally clear, allowing light to be transmitted to the retina. When there is a hemorrhage, the vitreous becomes clouded and cannot transmit light; the result is loss of vision. Another consequence of vitreous hemorrhaging is that resorption of the blood in the vitreous leads to the formation of fibrous scar tissue. This scar tissue may place traction on the retina, resulting in retinal detachment and subsequent visual loss.

Patients may have a fairly significant degree of proliferative retinopathy and may even have some hemorrhaging without major visual changes. It is important, however, if they report any symptoms indicative of hemorrhaging, such as "floaters" or "cobwebs" in the visual field, or if they report sudden visual changes, that they be referred immediately for an ophthalmologic evaluation and possible laser treatment.

Diagnostic Evaluation. Diagnosis is by direct visualization with an ophthalmoscope or with a technique known as fluorescein angiography. Fluorescein angiography can document

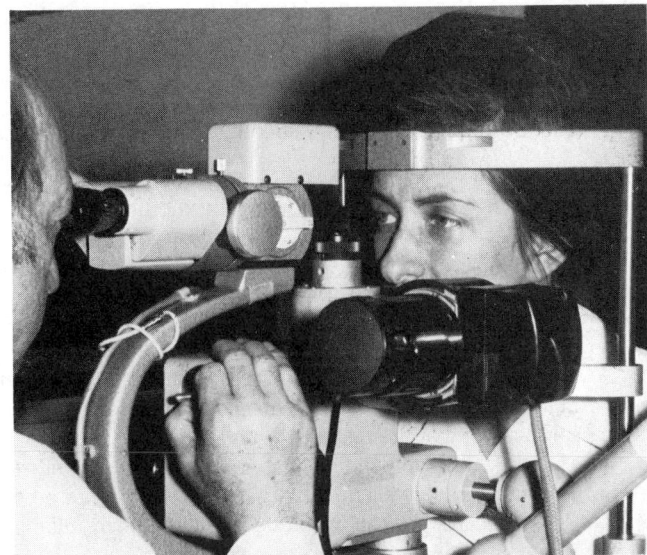

A

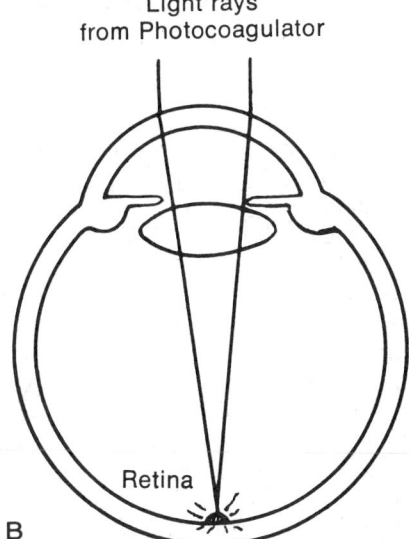

Light rays
from Photocoagulator

Retina

B

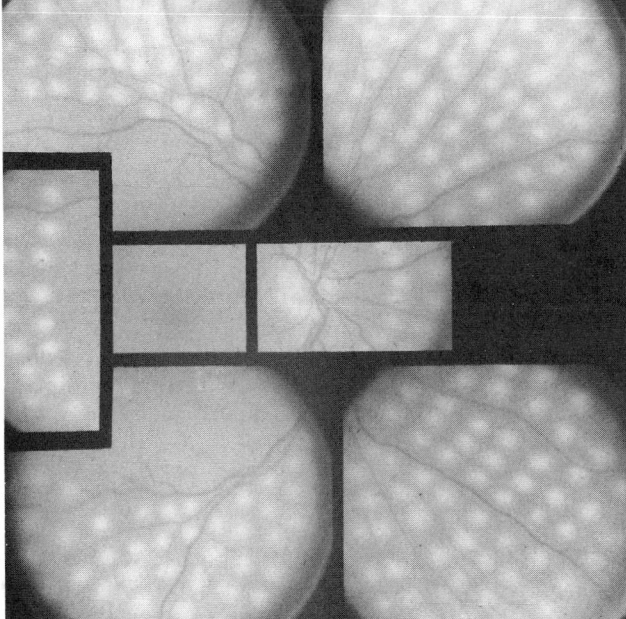

C

Figure 39–8. Photocoagulation. (**A**) The photograph shows a person receiving treatment with the argon laser, which generates a fine but intense blue–green beam of light. In this therapy the intense beam of light is directed into the eye and focused on a tiny spot in the retina. (**B**) Principle underlying photocoagulation. The intense beam of light acts in much the same way as the sun's rays focused through a magnifying glass produce a small burn on a leaf. (**C**) Fundus photograph of the right eye demonstrating fresh panretinal argonlaser photocoagulation burns that have been delivered in a grid-like fashion sparing the macular area. (*A:* Courtesy of Dr. Arnall Patz, Wilmer Eye Institute, Johns Hopkins Hospital, Baltimore, Maryland. *B:* American Association of Workers for the Blind, Inc, Blindness Annual. *C:* Klein R. Management of eye diseases in the insulin-dependent diabetic patient. Primary Care Clin 1983; 10[4]:686.)

the type and activity of the retinopathy. It is a technique in which a dye is injected into an arm vein. The dye is carried to various parts of the body through the blood, but especially through the vessels of the retina of the eye. This technique allows the ophthalmologist, using special instruments, to see the retinal vessels in bright detail and gives useful information that cannot be obtained with just an ophthalmoscope. Photographs of the fundus of the eye are taken through a series of filters that excite and record the fluorescence of the dye. The dye is bound to the blood proteins and first appears in the choroid and then in the arterial branches of the retina. Areas of leakage from the vessels and areas of neovascularization (new vessel formation) are stained with fluorescein.

Side effects of this diagnostic procedure performed in an outpatient setting may include:

• Nausea during the dye injection
• A yellowish, fluorescent discoloration of the skin and urine that may last 12 to 24 hours
• An occasional allergic reaction, usually hives or itching

However, it is generally a safe diagnostic procedure. Patient preparation includes explaining the following:

• The sequence of the steps of the procedure
• The fact that the procedure is painless
• The potential side effects
• The type of information the technique can provide
• That the flash of the camera may be slightly uncomfortable for a short period of time

Management

Photocoagulation ("Laser"). The main treatment of diabetic retinopathy is argon-laser photocoagulation (Fig. 39-8). The laser treatment destroys leaking blood vessels and areas of neovascularization. Recent national studies of diabetic retinopathy have identified certain characteristics (in terms of retinal changes) that represent increased risks for hemorrhaging. In these patients, a procedure called *panretinal photocoagulation* may significantly reduce the rate of progression to blindness. Panretinal photocoagulation involves the systematic application of multiple (more than 1000) laser burns throughout the retina (except in the macular region). This stops the widespread growth of new vessels and hemorrhaging of damaged vessels.

The role of "mild" panretinal photocoagulation (with one-third to one-half as many laser burns) in the early stages of proliferative retinopathy or in patients with preproliferative changes is being investigated.

For macular edema, "focal" photocoagulation is used to apply smaller laser burns to specific areas of microaneurysms in the macular region. Recent studies have shown that this may reduce the rate of visual loss from macular edema by 50%.

Photocoagulation treatments are usually performed on an outpatient basis, and most patients can return to their usual activities by the next day. For some patients, limitations may be placed on activities involving weight-bearing or bearing down. For most patients, the treatment does not cause intense pain, although they may report varying degrees of discomfort. Usually an anesthetic eye drop is all that is needed during the treatment. A small percentage of patients may experience slight visual loss, loss of peripheral vision, or impairments in adaptation to the dark. For most patients, however, the risk of slight visual changes from the laser treatment itself is much less than the potential for loss of vision from progression of retinopathy.

Vitrectomy.   When a major hemorrhage into the vitreous occurs, the vitreous fluid becomes mixed with blood and prevents light from passing through the eye, which can cause blindness. A vitrectomy is a surgical procedure in which vitreous humor filled with blood or fibrous tissue is removed with a special drill-like instrument and replaced with saline or another liquid.

A vitrectomy is performed on patients who already have a visual loss and in whom the vitreous hemorrhage has not cleared on its own after 6 months. The purpose is to restore useful vision; recovery to near-normal vision is not usually expected.

Other (Medical) Treatments.   Studies continue into other ways to slow the progression of diabetic retinopathy. These include:

- Control of hypertension
- Control of blood glucose
- Cessation of smoking

Other Ophthalmologic Complications.   Diabetic retinopathy is not the only complication of diabetes that can affect the vision. Cataracts, hypo- and hyperglycemia, neuropathy, and glaucoma may also affect vision.

- *Cataracts:* Opacity of the lens of the eye; cataracts occur at an earlier age in patients with diabetes.
- *Lens changes:* The lens of the eye can swell when blood glucose levels are elevated. For some patients, visual changes related to lens swelling may be the first symptoms of diabetes. It may take up to 2 months of blood glucose control before hyperglycemic swelling subsides and vision stabilizes. Therefore, patients are advised not to change eyeglass prescriptions during the 2 months following discovery of hyperglycemia.
- *Hypoglycemia:* Temporary visual disturbances such as blurring and double vision may occur during episodes of hypoglycemia. These symptoms should subside after blood glucose levels return to normal.
- *Extraocular muscle palsy:* This may occur as a result of di-

abetic neuropathy. The involvement of various cranial nerves responsible for ocular movements may lead to double vision. This usually resolves spontaneously.
- *Glaucoma:* Glaucoma may occur with slightly higher frequency in the diabetic population.

Health Teaching

In all forms of therapy for retinopathy, something is destroyed in the process of saving vision. The facts must be presented to the patient and family as honestly as possible. The course of the retinopathy will be long and stressful. In counseling the patient, it is important to stress:

- That the appearance of retinopathy can be expected after many years of diabetes, and its appearance does not necessarily mean that the diabetes is on a downhill course
- That the odds for maintaining vision are in the patient's favor
- That frequent eye examinations are the best way to preserve vision, because they allow for the detection of any retinopathy

Some additional points to keep in mind when the patient with diabetes has some type of visual impairment are the following:

- Visual impairment can be a shock to anyone. A person's response to vision loss depends on personality, self-concept, and coping mechanisms.
- As in any loss, blindness and its acceptance by the patient will occur in stages; some patients may learn to accept blindness in a rather short period of time, while others may never accept it.
- Although retinopathy occurs bilaterally, the severity may differ in the two eyes.
- Many of the chronic complications of diabetes occur simultaneously. For example, a blind diabetic patient may also have peripheral neuropathy and may experience impairment of manual dexterity and tactile sensation.

Nephropathy

People with diabetes account for about 25% of patients with end-stage renal disease requiring dialysis or transplantation each year in the United States. Persons with diabetes have a 20% to 40% chance of developing renal disease.

People with type I diabetes frequently show initial signs of renal disease after 15 to 20 years, while patients with type II diabetes develop renal disease within 10 years of the diagnosis of diabetes. Many of these patients with type II diabetes may have had diabetes for many years before it was diagnosed and treated.

To date, there is no reliable method to predict whether a person will develop renal disease. Studies are currently in progress to determine the effect of blood glucose control on the prevention or delay of nephropathy. Controlling blood pressure is the only intervention currently known to slow the progression of established renal disease.

Pathology.   New evidence suggests that soon after the onset of diabetes, increased filtering by the kidneys occurs. The molecular makeup of the basement membrane of the kidney capillaries (*glomeruli*) is structured to serve as a selective filter. Over a period of years, the basement membrane thickens as a result of chronic high blood glucose levels. Not only is the amount of basement membrane increased, but the proportion of the various glycoproteins is altered so that the molecular architecture of the membrane is changed. The membrane is thicker as well as more permeable, and blood proteins are lost in the urine.

Soon after the development of diabetes, and especially if the blood glucose levels are elevated, the kidney's filtration mechanism is stressed. As a result, the pressure in the blood vessels of the kidney increases. It is thought that the elevated pressure serves as the stimulus for the development of nephropathy. Various medications and diets are being tested to prevent these complications.

Diagnostic Evaluation. One of the most important blood proteins that begins leaking in the urine is albumin. Small amounts may leak undetected for years. Early microalbuminuria may be discovered in a 24-hour urine sample. In patients with microalbuminuria, more than 85% will eventually develop clinical nephropathy. However, if microalbuminuria is not present, fewer than 5% will develop nephropathy. Carefully designed low-protein diets appear to reverse early leakage of small amounts of protein from the kidney.

When a urine dipstick test reads consistently positive for significant amounts of albumin, the patient is tested for serum creatinine and blood urea nitrogen levels. At this point in the development of renal disease, diagnostic testing for cardiac or other systemic problems may also be required. Some of the tests involve injection of special dyes that are not easily cleared by the damaged kidney. Therefore, the value of the diagnostic test must be weighed against the potential risks.

People (both diabetic and nondiabetic) who are in the early stages of renal disease frequently develop hypertension. However, essential hypertension occurs in up to 50% of all people with diabetes (for unknown reasons); thus, it should not be assumed that someone with diabetes who has hypertension also has renal disease. Other diagnostic criteria must also be present.

Clinical Manifestations. Most of the signs and symptoms of renal dysfunction in the person with diabetes are similar to those seen in patients without diabetes. (See Chap. 42 for the management of patients with renal disorders.) Additionally, as renal failure progresses, the catabolism (breakdown) of both exogenous and endogenous insulin decreases, and frequent hypoglycemic episodes may result. Insulin needs change as a result of changes in the catabolism of insulin and also as a result of changes in diet related to the treatment of nephropathy. The stress of renal disease affects self-esteem, family relationships, marital relations, and virtually all aspects of daily life. As renal function decreases, the patient frequently experiences multiple-system failure (*e.g.*, declining visual acuity, impotence, foot ulcerations, congestive heart failure, and nocturnal diarrhea).

Prevention and Management. In addition to achieving and maintaining near-normal blood glucose levels, management for all patients with diabetes should include careful attention to the following:

- Control of hypertension (the use of angiotensin-converting enzyme inhibitors for control of hypertension may also decrease early proteinuria)
- Prevention and/or vigorous treatment of urinary tract infections
- Avoidance of nephrotoxic substances
- Adjustment of medications as renal function changes

- A diet low in sodium
- A diet low in protein (especially in the early stages of nephropathy)

In renal failure, two types of treatment are available: dialysis (hemodialysis or peritoneal dialysis) and transplantation from a relative or a cadaver.

Hemodialysis for the patient with diabetes is similar to that for patients without the disease (see Chap. 42). Because hemodialysis creates additional stress on patients with cardiovascular disease, it may not be indicated in certain patients. In addition, it is extremely intrusive into a patient's life.

Both *continuous ambulatory peritoneal dialysis* (CAPD) and *intermittent peritoneal dialysis* are being used by an increasing number of patients with diabetes, mainly because of the independence they allow to patients. In addition, insulin can be mixed into the dialysate, which may result in better blood glucose control and end the need for insulin injections. However, these patients may require more insulin because the dialysate contains glucose. A major risk of peritoneal dialysis is infection and peritonitis.

Renal disease is frequently accompanied by advancing retinopathy that may require laser treatments and surgery. Severe hypertension also worsens eye disease because of the additional stress it places on the blood vessels. Patients being treated by hemodialysis who require eye surgery may be switched to peritoneal dialysis and have their hypertension aggressively controlled for several weeks before surgery. The rationale for this change is that hemodialysis requires anticoagulants that can increase the risk of bleeding after the operation, and peritoneal dialysis minimizes pressure changes in the eyes.

In recent years, the success rate for kidney transplantation in patients with diabetes has improved. In medical centers performing large numbers of transplants, the chances are 75% to 80% that the transplanted kidney will continue to function in the patient with diabetes for at least 5 years. Like the original kidneys, transplanted kidneys in patients with diabetes can eventually be damaged if blood glucose levels are consistently high following the transplantation. Therefore, monitoring blood glucose levels frequently and adjusting insulin levels in diabetic patients with transplanted kidneys are essential for long-term success.

The mortality rate for diabetic patients undergoing dialysis is higher than that in nondiabetic patients undergoing dialysis and is closely related to the severity of cardiovascular problems.

The Neuropathies of Diabetes

Neuropathy in diabetes refers to a group of diseases that affect all types of nerves, including peripheral (sensorimotor), autonomic, and spinal nerves. The disorders appear to be clinically diverse and depend on the location of the affected nerve cells.

The prevalence increases with the age of the patient and the duration of the disease and may be as high as 50% in patients who have had diabetes for 25 years. Elevated blood glucose levels over a period of years have been implicated in the etiology of neuropathy.

The pathogenesis of neuropathy in diabetes may be due to either a vascular or a metabolic mechanism or both, but their relative contributions have not yet been determined. Capillary basement membrane thickening and capillary closure may be present. In addition, there may be demyelinization of the nerves, which is thought to be related to hyperglycemia. Nerve conduction is disrupted when there are aberrations of the myelin sheaths.

The two most common types of diabetic neuropathy are sensorimotor polyneuropathy and autonomic neuropathy. Cranial mononeuropathies, for example affecting the oculomotor nerve, also occur in diabetes, especially among the elderly. (See section on eye disorders in diabetes.)

Clinical Manifestations of Sensorimotor Polyneuropathy. This type of neuropathy is also called *peripheral neuropathy*. It most commonly affects the distal portions of the nerves and especially the lower extremities. It affects both sides of the body in a symmetrical fashion and may progressively spread in a proximal direction.

Initial symptoms include paresthesias (prickling, tingling, or heightened sensation) and burning sensations (especially at night). As the neuropathy progresses, the feet become numb. In addition, there is a decrease in proprioception (awareness of posture and movement of the body and of position and weight of objects in relation to the body), and a decrease in the sensation of light touch may lead to an unsteady gait. Decreased sensations of pain and temperature place patients with neuropathy at increased risk for injury and undetected foot infections.

On physical examination, a decrease in deep tendon reflexes and vibratory sensation is found. For some patients who have few or no symptoms of neuropathy, these physical findings may be the only indication that neuropathic changes are taking place. For patients with signs or symptoms of neuropathy, it is important to rule out other possible neuropathies, including alcoholic or vitamin-deficiency neuropathies.

Management of Sensorimotor Polyneuropathy. There have been some reports of improvement in symptoms with strict control of blood glucose. There is ongoing research into the role of blood glucose control in halting the progression of neuropathy or in preventing neuropathy altogether.

For some patients, neuropathic pain spontaneously resolves within 6 months. For other patients, pain persists for many years. Various approaches to pain management can be tried. These include analgesics (preferably non-narcotic); tricyclic antidepressants, phenytoin or carbamazepine (anticonvulsants); mexiletine (an antidysrhythmic); or transcutaneous electrical nerve stimulation (TENS).

Experiments continue with a group of drugs called aldose reductase inhibitors, which may block the damaging effects of hyperglycemia. There is also a new topical medication, capsaicin (Axscain), which has been shown in preliminary reports to decrease lower extremity neuropathic pain. Further investigations into the role of this topical medication in neuropathy continue.

Clinical Manifestations of Autonomic Neuropathy. Involvement of the autonomic nervous system covers a broad range of dysfunctions affecting almost every organ system of the body. Treatment of the autonomic neuropathy will depend on which organ system is affected. Generally, treatment of specific problems will be the same as it would be for similar problems in the nondiabetic population. Six main effects of autonomic neuropathy are described here.

Cardiovascular. Three manifestations of autonomic neu-ropathy are a fixed, slightly tachycardiac heart rate; orthostatic hypotension; and "silent," or painless, myocardial infarctions.

Gastrointestinal. Delayed gastric emptying may occur with the typical symptoms of early satiety, bloating, nausea, and vomiting. In addition, there may be unexplained wide swings in blood glucose levels related to inconsistent absorption of the glucose from ingested foods. "Diabetic" constipation or diarrhea (especially nocturnal diarrhea) is also associated with gastrointestinal autonomic neuropathy.

Urinary. Urinary retention, a decreased sensation of bladder fullness, and other urinary symptoms of neurogenic bladder result from autonomic neuropathy. Patients with a neurogenic bladder are predisposed to developing urinary tract infections. This is especially true in patients with poorly controlled diabetes because hyperglycemia impairs resistance to infection.

Adrenal Gland/"Hypoglycemic Unawareness." Autonomic neuropathy of the adrenal medulla is responsible for diminished or absent adrenergic symptoms of hypoglycemia. Patients may report that they no longer feel the typical shakiness, sweating, nervousness, and palpitations associated with hypoglycemia. Strict blood glucose control is *not* recommended for these patients. Their inability to detect and appropriately treat these warning signs of hypoglycemia puts them at risk for developing dangerously low blood glucose levels.

Sudomotor Neuropathy. This neuropathic condition refers to a decrease or absence of sweating ("anhidrosis") of the extremities with a compensatory increase in upper body sweating. The dryness of the feet increases the risk for development of foot ulcers.

Sexual Dysfunction. Sexual dysfunction, especially impotence in men, is one of the most well-known and feared complications of diabetes. The effects of autonomic neuropathy on female sexual functioning are not well documented. Reduced vaginal lubrication has been mentioned as a possible neuropathic effect; however, research studies to support this and other potential female sexual dysfunctions are lacking.

Impotence, the difficulty or inability of the penis to become rigid and sustain an erection, occurs with greater frequency in diabetic men than in nondiabetic men of the same age. It is important for the nurse and patient to realize, however, that in diabetic men neuropathy is *not* the only cause of impotence. Medications such as antihypertensives, psychologic factors, and other medical conditions (*e.g.*, vascular insufficiency) that may affect nondiabetic men also play a role in impotence in diabetic men.

A thorough evaluation of possible factors affecting erectile dysfunction is extremely important. Treatment of potential underlying causes, such as changing antihypertensive medications or providing sexual or marital counseling, must take place prior to more extensive, invasive treatments such as surgical penile implants.

Many patients may be embarrassed to discuss sexual issues. A sensitive and straightforward approach to obtaining a sexual history is important. Some patients may be unaware that sexual dysfunction commonly occurs for medical reasons and may simply assume it is due to increasing age or stress. Conversely, psychogenic impotence may result from undue worry or misinformation about diabetes-related impotence. Providing correct information about various causes of impotence in diabetes is important.

The role of hyperglycemia and vascular disease in impotence is not clearly defined. Poorly controlled blood glucose, pain, and other symptoms related to diabetic complications may contribute to an overall feeling of malaise and weakness. These symptoms may contribute to decreased interest in sexual relations. In autonomic neuropathy, libido, the ability to ejaculate, and the sensation of orgasm are usually *not* diminished.

Treatment of Impotence. In recent years, several nonsurgical options have been developed for impotence due to diabetic autonomic neuropathy. There are external vacuum erection aid devices that manually draw blood into the penis. The erection is maintained through the use of a constrictor band, which is placed around the base of the penis. It is important for patients to realize that ejaculation may still occur even with the band in place and that contraception should be used if indicated.

Another nonsurgical treatment for impotence is self-injection of a vasodilating medication, such as papaverine. The patient injects the medication into the corpus cavernosum of the penis, causing an erection.

Surgical approaches include insertion of penile implants such as an inflatable penile prosthesis, which can be activated by the patient when erection is desired.

Retrograde Ejaculation. Some men with autonomic neuropathy have normal erectile function and are able to experience orgasm but do not ejaculate. Retrograde ejaculation occurs, in which seminal fluid is propelled backward through the posterior urethra and into the urinary bladder. Examination of the urine confirms the diagnosis because of the large number of active sperm present. Fertility counseling is necessary for couples attempting conception.

Foot and Leg Problems in Diabetes

Fifty to 75% of lower extremity amputations are performed on people with diabetes. As many as 50% of these amputations are thought to be preventable, provided patients are taught preventive foot care measures and practice preventive foot care on a daily basis.

Three diabetic complications contribute to the increased risk of foot infections. They are:

Neuropathy: Sensory neuropathy leads to loss of pain and pressure sensation, and autonomic neuropathy leads to increased dryness and fissuring of the skin (secondary to decreased sweating).

Peripheral vascular disease: Poor circulation of the lower extremities contributes to poor wound healing and the development of gangrene.

Immunocompromise: Hyperglycemia impairs the ability of specialized leukocytes to destroy bacteria. Thus, in poorly controlled diabetes there is a lowered resistance to certain infections.

The typical sequence of events in the development of a diabetic foot ulcer begins with a soft-tissue injury of the foot, formation of a fissure between the toes or in an area of dry skin, or formation of a callus. Injuries are not felt by the patient with an insensitive foot and may be thermal (*e.g.*, from using heating pads, walking barefoot on hot concrete, or testing bath water with the foot), chemical (*e.g.*, burning the foot while using caustic agents on calluses, corns, or bunions), or traumatic (*e.g.*, injuring skin while cutting nails, walking with an undetected foreign object in the shoe, or wearing ill-fitting shoes and socks).

If the patient is not in the habit of thoroughly inspecting both feet on a daily basis, the injury or fissure may go unnoticed until a serious infection has developed. Drainage, swelling, redness (from cellulitis) of the leg, or gangrene may be the first sign of foot problems that the patient notices.

Treatment of foot ulcers involves bed rest, antibiotics, and debridement. In addition, controlling glucose levels that tend to increase when infections occur is important for promoting wound healing. In patients with peripheral vascular disease, foot ulcers may not heal because of the decreased ability of oxygen, nutrients, and antibiotics to reach the injured tissue. Amputation may be necessary to prevent further spread of infection.

Foot assessment and foot care instruction are most important when dealing with patients who are at high risk for developing foot infections. Some of the high-risk characteristics include:

- Duration of diabetes over 10 years
- Age over 40 years
- History of smoking
- Decreased peripheral pulses
- Decreased sensation
- Anatomic deformities or pressure areas (such as bunions and calluses)
- History of previous foot ulcers or amputation

Foot Care. Preventive foot care includes properly bathing, drying, and lubricating feet (care must be taken not to allow moisture to accumulate from water or lotion between the toes). Feet must be inspected on a daily basis for any redness, blisters, fissures, calluses, or ulcerations. For patients who have a visual impairment or have decreased joint mobility (especially the elderly), use of a mirror for inspection of the bottom of the feet or instruction of a family member in foot inspection may be necessary. The interior surfaces of shoes should be inspected for any rough spots or foreign objects. Visual and manual (with the hand) inspection on a daily basis is important. Feet should be examined on a regular basis by a podiatrist, physician, or nurse. Patients with pressure areas, such as calluses, or patients with thick toenails should see the podiatrist routinely for shaving of calluses and trimming of nails.

Patients should be taught to wear well-fitting, closed-toe shoes. Podiatrists can provide patients with inserts to remove pressure from pressure points on the foot. New shoes should be broken in slowly (*i.e.*, worn for 1 to 2 hours initially with gradual increases in the length of time worn) to avoid blister formation. High-risk behaviors should be avoided, such as walking barefoot, using heating pads on the feet, wearing open-toed shoes, and shaving calluses. Toenails should be trimmed straight across without rounding the corners. If patients have visual deficits or thickened toenails, a podiatrist should cut the nails.

Patients should be counseled on reducing risk factors, such as smoking and elevated blood lipids, that contribute to peripheral vascular disease. Blood glucose control is important for avoiding decreased resistance to infections and for avoiding diabetic neuropathy.

Special Issues in Diabetes

The Patient With Diabetes Undergoing Surgery

During periods of physiologic stress, such as surgery, blood glucose levels tend to rise as a result of an increase in the level of stress hormones (epinephrine, norepinephrine, glucagon, cortisol, and growth hormone). If hyperglycemia is not adequately controlled during surgery, the resulting osmotic diuresis may lead to excessive loss of fluids and electrolytes. Type I diabetic patients also risk developing ketoacidosis during periods of stress.

Hypoglycemia is also a concern in diabetic patients undergoing surgery. This is especially a concern during the preoperative period if surgery is delayed beyond the morning in a patient who received a morning injection of intermediate-acting insulin.

There are various approaches to the management of glucose control during the perioperative period. Frequent capillary glucose monitoring of the diabetic patient is vitally important throughout the pre- and postoperative periods, regardless of the method used for glucose control.

For patients who usually take insulin, one-half to two-thirds of the usual morning dose (either intermediate-acting insulin alone or both short- and intermediate-acting insulins) may be administered subcutaneously in the morning before surgery. The remainder is then administered after surgery. Another approach with subcutaneous insulin is to divide the total number of units of insulin taken daily into four equal doses of regular insulin. This is then administered at 6-hour intervals.

The use of intravenous insulin and dextrose has become more widespread with the increased availability of meters for intraoperative glucose monitoring. The morning of surgery, all subcutaneous insulin doses are usually withheld (unless the blood glucose level is elevated, for example, above 200 mg/dl [11.1 mmol/L], in which case a small dose of subcutaneous regular insulin may be ordered).

Blood glucose is controlled during surgery with the intravenous infusion of regular insulin, which is balanced by an infusion of dextrose. The insulin and dextrose infusion rates are adjusted according to frequent (hourly) capillary glucose determinations. Postoperatively, the insulin infusion may be continued until the patient is able to eat. If intravenous insulin is discontinued, subcutaneous regular insulin may be administered at set intervals (every 4 to 6 hours), or intermediate-acting insulin may be administered every 12 hours with supplemental regular insulin as necessary until the patient is eating and the usual pattern of insulin dosing is resumed.

The nurse taking care of a diabetic patient who is receiving intravenous insulin must carefully monitor the insulin infusion rate and blood glucose levels. Intravenous insulin has a much shorter duration of action than subcutaneous insulin. Thus, if the infusion is interrupted or discontinued, hyperglycemia will result within a few hours. The nurse must ensure that subcutaneous insulin is administered either immediately before or by 1 hour after the intravenous insulin infusion is discontinued.

Type II diabetic patients who do not usually take insulin may require insulin during the perioperative period to control blood glucose elevations. Patients who are taking chlorpropamide, a long-acting oral hypoglycemic agent, may be instructed to discontinue the oral agent 1 day before surgery. Some of these patients may resume their usual regimen of diet and oral agent during the recovery period. Other patients (who are probably not well controlled with diet and an oral hypoglycemic agent before surgery) will need to continue with insulin injections after discharge.

For type II diabetic patients who are undergoing minor surgery but who do not normally take insulin, glucose levels may remain stable provided no dextrose is infused during the surgery. Postoperatively, they may require small doses of regular insulin until the usual diet and oral agent are resumed.

During the postoperative period, diabetic patients must also be closely monitored for cardiovascular complications because of the increased prevalence of atherosclerosis in patients with diabetes, wound infections, and skin breakdown (especially in the patient with decreased pain sensation in the extremities due to neuropathy). Maintaining adequate nutrition and blood glucose control promotes wound healing.

Management of Hospitalized Diabetic Patients

At any one point in time, 10% to 20% of general medical–surgical patients in the hospital have diabetes. This number may increase as the elderly make up a greater proportion of the population. While some hospitals may have a specialized diabetic/metabolic unit, typically diabetic patients are admitted to all units of the hospital.

Often diabetes is not the primary medical diagnosis, yet problems with the control of diabetes frequently result from changes in the patient's normal routine or from illness or surgery. Some of the main issues pertinent to nursing care of the hospitalized diabetic patient are presented in the following section.

Self-Care Issues. All patients admitted to the hospital must relinquish control of most aspects of daily care to the hospital staff. For the diabetic patient who is actively involved in diabetes self-management (especially insulin dose adjustment), relinquishing control over meal timing, insulin timing, and insulin dosage may be particularly difficult. The patient may fear hypoglycemia and express much concern over possible delays in receiving attention from the nurse when hypoglycemic symptoms are experienced.

It is important for the nurse to acknowledge the patient's concerns and to involve the patient as much as possible in the plan of care. If the patient disagrees with certain aspects of the nursing or medical care related to diabetes, the nurse must communicate this to other members of the health care team and, where appropriate, make changes in the plan to meet patient needs.

Hyperglycemia During Hospitalization. Hyperglycemia may occur in the hospitalized patient as a result of the original illness that led to the need for hospitalization. In addition, a number of other factors may contribute to hyperglycemia, such as:

- Changes in the usual treatment regimen (*e.g.*, increased food, decreased insulin, decreased activity)
- Medications (*e.g.*, glucocorticoids such as prednisone, which are used in the treatment of a variety of inflammatory disorders)
- Intravenous dextrose, which may be part of the maintenance fluids or may be used for intravenous administration of antibiotics and other medications
- Overly vigorous treatment of hypoglycemia
- Mismatched timing of meals and insulin (*e.g.*, post-meal hyperglycemia may occur if insulin is given immediately before or even after meals)

Nursing action to correct some of these factors is important for the avoidance of unnecessary hyperglycemia. Assessment of the patient's usual home routine is important. The nurse should try to approximate as much as possible the home schedule of insulin, meals, and activities. Monitoring blood glucose levels and obtaining orders for extra doses of insulin (at times when insulin is usually taken by the patient) are important nursing functions.

- *Insulin doses must not be withheld when blood glucose levels are normal.*

Regular insulin is usually needed to avoid post-meal hyperglycemia (even in the patient with normal pre-meal glucose levels), and NPH insulin will not peak until many hours after the dose is given. Intravenous antibiotics should be mixed in normal saline (if possible) to avoid excess infusion of dextrose (especially in the patient who is eating). It is important to avoid overly vigorous treatment of hypoglycemia, which may lead to hyperglycemia. Treatment of hypoglycemia should be based on the established hospital protocol (usually 10 to 15 gm of carbohydrate in the form of juice, glucose tablets, or, if necessary, ½ to 1 ampule of 50% dextrose given intravenously). Adding extra sugar to the juice is unnecessary. If the initial treatment does not adequately increase the glucose level, the same treatment may be repeated.

Common Causes of Hypoglycemia. Hypoglycemia in a hospitalized patient is usually the result of too much insulin or delays in eating. Specific examples include:

- Overuse of "sliding scale" regular insulin, particularly as a supplement to regularly scheduled, twice-daily short- and intermediate-acting insulins
- Lack of dosage change when dietary intake is changed (*e.g.*, in patient taking nothing by mouth)
- Overly vigorous treatment of hyperglycemia (*e.g.*, giving too frequent successive doses of regular insulin before the time of peak insulin activity is reached) so that there is an accumulated effect

Nurses must assess the pattern of glucose values and avoid giving doses of insulin that repeatedly lead to hypoglycemia. Successive doses of subcutaneous regular insulin should be given no more frequently than every 3 to 4 hours. For patients receiving NPH or Lente insulin before breakfast and dinner, the nurse must use caution in administering supplemental doses of regular insulin at lunch and bedtime. Hypoglycemia may occur when two insulins peak at similar times (*e.g.*, morning NPH peaks with lunchtime regular insulin and may lead to late

afternoon hypoglycemia, while dinnertime NPH peaks with bedtime regular insulin and may lead to nocturnal hypoglycemia). To avoid hypoglycemic reactions due to delayed food intake, the nurse should arrange for a snack to be given to the patient if meals are going to be delayed because of procedures, physical therapy, or other activities.

Common Alterations in Diet

NPO (*Nothing by Mouth*). For the patient who must have nothing by mouth in preparation for a procedure, the nurse must ensure that the usual insulin dosage has been changed. These changes may include eliminating the regular insulin and giving a decreased amount (*e.g.*, half of the usual dose) of intermediate-acting NPH or Lente insulin. Another approach is to use frequent (every 3 to 4 hours) dosing of regular insulin only. Intravenous dextrose may be ordered to provide calories and to avoid the development of hypoglycemia.

It is important to remember that even when no food is taken, glucose levels may rise as a result of hepatic glucose production, especially in type I and lean type II diabetic patients. Furthermore, in type I diabetic patients, complete elimination of the insulin dose may lead to the development of diabetic ketoacidosis. Thus, administering insulin to the type I diabetic patient who is receiving nothing by mouth is an important nursing action.

For type II diabetic patients taking insulin, DKA does not develop when insulin doses are eliminated because the patient's own pancreas produces some insulin. Thus, skipping the insulin dose altogether when the patient has type II diabetes (and is *not* receiving intravenous dextrose) may be safe.

For patients who receive nothing by mouth for extended periods of time, glucose testing and insulin administration should be performed at regular intervals, usually 2 to 4 times per day. Insulin regimens for the patient who is fasting for an extended period may include NPH insulin every 12 hours (with regular insulin added to the NPH depending on the results of glucose testing) or regular insulin only every 4 to 6 hours. These patients should receive dextrose infusions to provide some calories and limit ketosis.

Clear Liquid Diet. When the diet is advanced to include clear liquids, the diabetic patient will be receiving more simple carbohydrate foods, such as juice and Jell-O, than are usually included in the diabetic diet. It is important for hospitalized patients to maintain their nutritional status as much as possible to promote healing. Thus, the use of reduced-calorie substitutes such as diet soda or diet Jell-O would not be appropriate when the only source of calories is clear liquids. Simple carbohydrates, when eaten alone, cause a rapid rise in glucose levels; thus, it is important to try to match peak times of insulin with peaks in glucose. If a patient was receiving insulin at regular intervals while receiving nothing by mouth, the scheduled times for glucose tests and insulin injections must be changed to match meal times.

Enteral Tube Feedings. Solutions used for tube feedings in patients with nasogastric tubes or other feeding tubes contain more simple carbohydrates and less protein and fat than the typical diabetic diet. This results in increased levels of glucose. It is important that insulin doses be administered at regular intervals (*e.g.*, NPH every 12 hours or regular insulin every 4 to 6 hours) when tube feedings are given at a continuous rate. If insulin is administered at routine (pre-breakfast and pre-dinner) times, hypoglycemia during the day may result from patients receiving more insulin without more calories, while hyperglycemia may occur during the night when feedings continue but insulin action wanes.

A common cause of hypoglycemia in patients receiving continuous tube feedings and insulin is inadvertent or purposeful discontinuation of the feeding. The nurse must discuss with the medical team any plans for temporarily discontinuing the tube feeding (*e.g.*, when the patient is away from the unit). Planning ahead may allow alterations to be made in the insulin dose, or it may allow for intravenous dextrose to be initiated. In addition, if problems with the tube feeding develop unexpectedly (*e.g.*, the patient pulls out the tube, the tube clogs, or the feeding is discontinued when residual gastric contents are found), the nurse must notify the physician, assess glucose levels more frequently, and administer intravenous dextrose if indicated.

Total Parenteral Nutrition (TPN). The diabetic patient receiving TPN may receive both intravenous insulin (added to the TPN container) and subcutaneous intermediate-acting and/or short-acting insulins. Similar to the patient receiving continuous nasogastric tube feedings, the blood glucose monitoring and insulin administration should be performed at regular intervals if the TPN infuses continuously. If the TPN is infused over a limited number of hours, subcutaneous insulin should be administered such that peak times of insulin action coincide with times of TPN infusion.

Hygiene. The nurse caring for a hospitalized diabetic patient must focus attention on oral hygiene and skin care. Because diabetic patients commonly develop periodontal disease, it is important for the nurse to assist patients with daily dental care. The patient should also be assisted in keeping skin clean and dry—especially in areas of contact between two skin surfaces (such as groin, axilla, and, in obese women, under the breasts), where chafing and fungal infections tend to occur.

For the bedridden diabetic patient, nursing care must emphasize the prevention of skin breakdown at pressure points. The heels are particularly susceptible to breakdown because of loss of sensation of pain and pressure associated with sensory neuropathy.

Feet should be cleaned, dried, lubricated (except in the area between the toes), and inspected frequently. If the patient is in the supine position, pressure on the heels can be alleviated by elevating the lower legs on a pillow with the heels hanging over the edge of the pillow. When the patient is seated in a chair, the feet should be positioned so that pressure is not placed on the heels. If the patient has a foot ulcer, it is important to perform preventive foot care of the unaffected foot as well as to carry out special care of the infected foot.

As always, every opportunity should be taken to teach the patient about diabetes self-management, including daily oral, skin, and foot care. Female diabetic patients should also be instructed about measures for the avoidance of vaginal infections, which occur more frequently when blood glucose levels are elevated. Patients often take their cues from the nurse and will realize the importance of daily personal hygiene if this is emphasized during the course of their hospitalization.

Stress

As mentioned earlier, physiologic stresses, such as infections and surgery, contribute to hyperglycemia and may precipitate DKA or HNKS. Emotional stress may have a negative impact on diabetic control as well. An increase in "stress" hormones leads to an increase in glucose levels, especially when the intake of food and insulin remains unchanged. In addition, during periods of emotional stress, the person with diabetes may alter the usual pattern of meals, exercise, and medication. This contributes to hyperglycemia or even hypoglycemia (*e.g.*, in the patient on insulin or oral hypoglycemic agents who stops eating in response to stress).

People who have diabetes must be made aware of the potential deterioration in diabetic control that can accompany emotional stress. They must be encouraged to try to adhere to the diabetes treatment plan as much as possible during times of stress. In addition, learning strategies for minimizing stress and coping with stress when it does occur are an important aspect of diabetes education.

Gerontologic Considerations

People with diabetes are living longer; therefore, both type I and type II diabetes are seen more frequently in the elderly population. Regardless of the type or duration of diabetes, the goals of diabetes treatment may need to be altered when caring for the elderly. The focus is on quality-of-life issues, such as maintaining independent functioning and promoting general well-being. While striving for strict blood glucose control may not be safe or appropriate, prolonged symptomatic hyperglycemia should be avoided.

Some elderly patients will not be able to manage a detailed diabetes treatment plan. However, it must not be assumed that all patients over a certain age can adhere only to the simplest regimen. Although the goal may be simply to avoid hypoglycemia and symptomatic hyperglycemia, certain patients may prefer more complex regimens that allow more flexibility in meals and daily schedule. As with all people with diabetes, individualization of the treatment plan with frequent follow-up by the health care team is important.

Some of the barriers to learning and self-care that may be seen in the elderly include decreased vision, hearing loss, memory deficits, decreased mobility and fine motor coordination, increased tremors, depression and loneliness, decreased financial resources, and limitations related to other medical illnesses.

Assessing patients for these barriers as well as discussing any misconceptions or folk beliefs regarding the cause and treatment of diabetes is important in setting up a diabetes treatment plan and educational activities. Presenting brief, simplified instructions with ample opportunity for practice of skills is important. The use of special devices such as a magnifier for the insulin syringe, an insulin pen, or a mirror for foot inspection is helpful. If necessary, family members and other community resources are called upon to assist with basic diabetes survival skills. If possible, it is preferable to teach patients and/or family members to test *blood* glucose at home, because urine glucose tests are usually less accurate in the elderly as a result of increased renal threshold and increased frequency of renal and urinary problems. Frequent evaluation of self-care skills (insulin administration, blood glucose monitoring, foot care, diet planning) is essential, especially in patients with deteriorating vision and memory.

Dietary adherence is difficult for some elderly patients because of decreased appetite, poor dentition, and decreased physical and financial ability to prepare meals. In addition, patients may be unwilling to change long-standing dietary habits. Altering the meal plan in order to incorporate these eating habits or other limitations may be necessary.

Careful monitoring for diabetes complications must not be neglected in the elderly. Hypoglycemia is especially dangerous because it may go undetected and result in falls. Dehydration is a concern in patients who have chronically elevated blood glucose levels. Assessment for long-term complications—especially eye and foot problems—is important. Avoiding blindness and amputation through early detection and treatment of retinopathy and foot ulcers may mean the difference between institutionalization and continued independent living for the elderly person with diabetes. Changes seen in the elderly person with diabetes are summarized in Chart 39-7.

▶ Nursing Process
The Patient With Diabetes as a Secondary Diagnosis

People with diabetes frequently seek medical attention for problems not directly related to blood glucose control. However, during the course of treatment of the primary medical diagnosis, the blood glucose control may worsen. In addition, the only opportunity for some diabetic patients to update their knowledge in diabetes self-care and prevention of complications is during the time of hospitalization. Therefore, it is important for the nurse taking care of the diabetic patient to focus attention on diabetes, regardless of the primary problem. Furthermore, control of blood glucose levels is important because hyperglycemia impairs resistance to certain infections and may contribute to impaired wound healing.

▷ Assessment

Assessment of the diabetic patient with a primary problem such as cardiac disease, renal disease, cerebrovascular disease, peripheral vascular disease, surgery, or any other type of illness is the same as that for a nondiabetic patient and is described in other chapters. In addition to nursing assessment for the primary problem, assessment of the diabetic patient must also focus on hypo- and hyperglycemia, skin breakdown, and diabetes self-care skills, including survival skills and measures for prevention of long-term complications.

The patient is assessed for hypo- and hyperglycemia with frequent capillary glucose monitoring (usually ordered before meals and at bedtime) and with monitoring for signs and symptoms of hypoglycemia or prolonged hyperglycemia (including DKA or HNKS) as described in previous sections.

Careful assessment of the skin, especially at pressure points and on the lower extremities, is important. The skin is assessed for dryness, cracks, skin breakdown, and redness. The patient is questioned regarding a history of neuropathy and symptoms of neuropathy, such as tingling and pain or numbness of the feet. Deep tendon reflexes are assessed.

Assessment of diabetes self-care skills is performed as early as possible in order to determine if the patient will require further diabetes teaching. The nurse *observes* the patient preparing and injecting the insulin, monitoring blood glucose, and performing foot care. (Simply questioning the patient about these skills without actually observing him perform the skills is not sufficient.) Knowledge about diet can be assessed with the help of the dietitian through direct questioning and review of patient choices on the menu. The patient is questioned regarding signs, treatment, and prevention of hypoglycemia and hyperglycemia. The patient's knowledge of risk factors for macrovascular disease, including hypertension, increased lipids, and smoking, is assessed. The patient is questioned regarding the date of the last eye examination (including dilation of the pupil).

▷ Nursing Diagnoses

Based on the assessment data, the patient's major nursing diagnoses may include the following:

Chart 39–7
Changes in the Elderly That May Affect Diabetes

Sensory Changes

- Decreased vision
- Decreased smell
- Taste changes
- Decreased proprioception

Gastrointestinal Changes

- Dental problems
- Appetite changes
- Delayed gastric emptying
- Decreased bowel motility

Activity/Exercise Pattern Changes
- More sedentary

Renal Function Changes

- Decreased function
- Decreased drug clearance

Affective/Cognitive Changes

- Medications/meals omitted or taken erratically

Socioeconomic Factors

- Fad diets
- Loneliness/living alone
- Lack of money

Chronic Diseases

- Hypertension
- Arthritis
- Neoplasms
- Acute/chronic infections

Potential Drug Interactions

- Use of another person's medications
- Consulting multiple physicians for different illnesses
- Alcohol

- Altered nutrition related to increase in stress hormones (due to primary medical problem) and imbalances in insulin, food, and physical activity
- High risk for impaired skin integrity related to immobility and lack of sensation (due to neuropathy)
- Potential knowledge deficit about diabetes self-care skills (due to lack of basic diabetes education or lack of continuing in-depth diabetes education)

▷ *Planning and Implementation*

▷ *Goals:*   The major goals of the patient may include attainment of optimal control of blood glucose, maintenance of skin integrity, and ability to perform basic diabetes self-care skills as well as preventive care for the avoidance of long-term diabetes complications.

▷ *Nursing Interventions*

▷ *Maintenance of Optimal Blood Glucose Control.*   Blood glucose is monitored and insulin is administered as ordered. It is important for the nurse to ensure that insulin orders are altered as needed for changes in the patient's schedule or eating pattern. Treatment is given for hypoglycemia (with oral glucose) or hyperglycemia (with supplemental regular insulin not more often than every 3 to 4 hours). Blood glucose records are assessed for patterns of hypoglycemia and hyperglycemia at the same time of day, and findings are reported to the physician for alteration in insulin orders. In the patient with prolonged elevated blood glucose levels, laboratory values and the patient's physical condition are monitored for signs of DKA or HNKS.

▷ *Skin Care.*   The skin is assessed daily for dryness or breaks in skin. The feet are cleaned with warm water and soap. Excessive soaking of the feet is avoided. The feet are dried thoroughly, especially between the toes, and lotion is applied to the entire foot except between the toes. For bedridden patients (especially those with a history of neuropathy), the heels are elevated off the bed with a pillow placed under the lower legs and the heels resting over the edge of the pillow. Dermal ulcers are treated as indicated and prescribed. The nurse promotes optimal blood glucose control in patients with skin breakdown.

▷ *Patient Education.*   The nurse requests that the patient give repeated return demonstrations of skills that were not performed correctly during the initial assessment. The patient is taught self-care activities for the prevention of long-term complications, including foot care, eye care, and risk factor management.

▷ *Evaluation*

Expected Outcomes

1. Achieves optimal control of blood glucose
   a. Avoids extremes of hypoglycemia and hyperglycemia
   b. Hypoglycemic episodes are rapidly resolved
2. Maintains skin integrity
   a. Skin remains smooth without dryness and cracking
   b. Avoids ulcers due to pressure and neuropathy
3. Demonstrates/verbalizes diabetes survival skills and preventive care

Treatment Modalities
   a. Demonstrates proper technique for administering insulin and checking blood glucose

b. Demonstrates appropriate knowledge of diet through proper menu selections and identification of pattern used for selection of foods at home
   c. Verbalizes appropriate signs, treatment, and prevention of hypo- and hyperglycemia

Demonstrates Proper Foot Care
   a. Inspects feet (using mirror if necessary to see bottom of foot), including inspection for cracks between toes
   b. Washes feet with warm water and soap; dries feet thoroughly
   c. Applies lotion to entire foot except between toes
   d. Verbalizes behaviors that decrease the risk of foot ulcers, including:
   - Wearing shoes at all times
   - Using hand or elbow, *not foot,* to test bath water
   - Avoiding use of heating pad on feet
   - Wearing cotton socks
   - Avoiding constrictive shoes
   - Wearing new shoes for brief periods of time
   - Avoiding home remedies for treatment of corns and calluses
   - Having feet examined at every appointment with the physician
   - Consulting a podiatrist for regular nail hygiene if necessary

Verbalizes Measures and Information Regarding Prevention of Eye Disease
   a. Necessity of *yearly* eye examinations by an ophthalmologist (starting at 5 years after diagnosis for type I diabetes or the year of diagnosis for type II diabetes)
   b. Relates that retinopathy usually causes *no* change in vision until serious damage to the retina has occurred
   c. Relates that early laser treatment along with good control of blood glucose and blood pressure may prevent visual loss from retinopathy
   d. Identifies hypoglycemia and hyperglycemia as two causes of (temporary) blurred vision

Verbalizes Measures for Controlling Macrovascular Risk Factors
   a. Smoking cessation
   b. Dietary limitation of fats and cholesterol
   c. Control of hypertension
   d. Exercise

Chapter Summary

Diabetes mellitus is a group of disorders characterized by abnormalities in the metabolism of carbohydrate, protein, and fat. These abnormalities are related to a lack of insulin or a decrease in the amount of insulin produced by the pancreas. In addition to the metabolic disorders, there are many vascular and neurologic complications associated with diabetes mellitus that may contribute to such problems as blindness, renal failure, amputation, and an increased rate of strokes and heart attacks.

   Treatment of diabetes involves diet management, monitoring glucose levels in blood and sometimes urine, monitoring urinary ketones in patients with type I diabetes, exercise, and medications such as oral hypoglycemic agents and insulin. Major advances in treatment modalities over the last decade have allowed diabetic patients to achieve near-normal blood glucose levels and to have more flexibility in life-style. The most important aspect of diabetes treatment is education. Nurses play a vital role in providing patients and their families with the tools and knowledge necessary for successful management of diabetes. Patients must learn skills for the daily management of diabetes, the avoidance and treatment of acute complications such as hypoglycemia and hyperglycemia, and the avoidance of long-term complications. In addition, nurses play an important role in promoting psychosocial well-being in patients and families who are dealing with this chronic illness.

Bibliography

Books

Biermann J and Toohey B. The Diabetic's Book. Los Angeles, J Tarcher, 1990.

Biermann J and Toohey B. The Diabetic's Total Health Book. Los Angeles, J Tarcher, 1988.

Davidson M. Diabetes Mellitus: Diagnosis and Treatment, 3rd ed. New York, John Wiley & Sons, 1990.

Guthrie D (ed). Diabetes Education: A Core Curriculum for Health Professionals. Chicago, American Association of Diabetes Educators, 1988.

Jensen N and Moore M (eds). Learning to Live Well with Diabetes, 2nd ed. Minnetonka, MN, Diabetes Center, Inc, 1987.

Jovanovic L, Biermann J, and Toohey B. The Diabetic Woman. Los Angeles, J. Tarcher, 1987.

Krall L and Beaser R. Joslin Diabetes Manual, 12th ed. Philadelphia, Lea & Febiger, 1989.

Lebovitz H (ed). Physician's Guide to Non-Insulin-Dependent (Type II) Diabetes: Diagnosis and Treatment, 2nd ed. Alexandria, VA, American Diabetes Association, 1988.

Monk A et al. Managing Type II Diabetes. Wayzata, MN, DCI Publishing, 1988.

Olson O. Diagnosis and Management of Diabetes Mellitus, 2nd ed. New York, Raven Press, 1988.

Peterson C and Jovanovic L. The Diabetes Self-Care Method, 2nd ed. New York, Simon & Schuster, 1991.

Redman BK. The Process of Patient Education, 6th ed. St Louis, CV Mosby, 1988.

Sperling M (ed). Physician's Guide to Insulin-Dependent (Type I) Diabetes: Diagnosis and Treatment. Alexandria, VA, American Diabetes Association, 1988.

Position Statements/Consensus Statements

American Association of Diabetes Educators. Effective utilization of blood glucose monitoring: Position statement. The Diabetes Educator 1989 Sep/Oct; 15:(5):461.

American Association of Diabetes Educators. Prevention of transmission of blood-borne infectious agents during blood glucose monitoring: Position statement. The Diabetes Educator 1988 Sep/Oct; 14(5):425.

American Diabetes Association. Office guide to diagnosis and classification of diabetes mellitus and other categories of glucose intolerance: Position statement. Diabetes Care 1991 Mar; 14(Suppl 2):3–4.

American Diabetes Association. Gestational diabetes mellitus: Position statement. Diabetes Care 1991 Mar; 14(Suppl 2):5–6.

American Diabetes Association. Screening for diabetes: Position statement. Diabetes Care 1991 Mar; 14(Suppl 2):7–9.

American Diabetes Association. Standards of medical care for patients with diabetes mellitus: Position statement. Diabetes Care 1991 Mar; 14(Suppl 2):10–13.

American Diabetes Association. Prevention of type I diabetes mellitus: Position statement. Diabetes Care 1991 Mar; 14(Suppl 2):14–15.

American Diabetes Association. Eye care guidelines for patients with diabetes mellitus: Position statement. Diabetes Care 1991 Mar; 14(Suppl 2):16–17.

American Diabetes Association. Foot care in patients with diabetes mellitus: Position statement. Diabetes Care 1991 Mar; 14(Suppl 2):18–19.

American Diabetes Association. Nutritional recommendations and principles for individuals with diabetes mellitus: Position statement. Diabetes Care 1991 Mar; 14(Suppl 2):20–21.

American Diabetes Association. Use of noncaloric sweeteners: Position statement. Diabetes Care 1991 Mar; 14(Suppl 2):28–29.

American Diabetes Association. Insulin administration: Position statement. Diabetes Care 1991 Mar; 14(Suppl 2):30–33.

American Diabetes Association. Continuous subcutaneous insulin infusion: Position statement. Diabetes Care 1991 Mar; 14(Suppl 2): 34–35.

American Diabetes Association. Diabetes mellitus and exercise: Position statement. Diabetes Care 1991 Mar; 14(Suppl 2):36–37.

American Diabetes Association. Bedside blood glucose monitoring in hospitals: Position statement. Diabetes Care 1991 Mar; 14(Suppl 2):38.

American Diabetes Association. Urine glucose and ketone determinations: Position statement. Diabetes Care 1991 Mar; 14(Suppl 2):39–40.

American Diabetes Association. Concurrent care: Position statement. Diabetes Care 1991 Mar; 14(Suppl 2):41.

American Diabetes Association. Hospital admission guidelines for diabetes mellitus: Position statement. Diabetes Care 1991 Mar; 14(Suppl 2): 42–43.

American Diabetes Association. Third-party reimbursement for outpatient diabetes education and counseling: Position statement. Diabetes Care 1991 Mar; 14(Suppl 2):44.

American Diabetes Association. Management of diabetes in correctional institutions: Position statement. Diabetes Care 1991 Mar; 14(Suppl 2):45.

American Diabetes Association. Responsible use of animals in research: Position statement. Diabetes Care 1991 Mar; 14(Suppl 2):46.

American Diabetes Association. Hypoglycemia and employment/licensure: Position statement. Diabetes Care 1991 Mar; 14(Suppl 2):47.

American Diabetes Association. Food labeling: Position statement. Diabetes Care 1991 Mar; 14(Suppl 2):48.

American Diabetes Association. Jet injectors: Technical review. Diabetes Care 1991 Mar; 14(Suppl 2):50.

American Diabetes Association. Exercise and NIDDM: Position statement. Diabetes Care 1991 Mar; 14(Suppl 2):52–56.

American Diabetes Association. Self-monitoring of blood glucose: Consensus statement. Diabetes Care 1991 Mar; 14(Suppl 2):57–62.

American Diabetes Association. Diabetic neuropathy: Consensus statement. Diabetes Care 1991 Mar; 14(Suppl 2):63–68.

American Diabetes Association. Role of cardiovascular risk factors in prevention and treatment of macrovascular disease in diabetes. Diabetes Care 1991 Mar; 14(Suppl 2):69–75.

American Diabetes Association. National standards for diabetes patient education and American Diabetes Association review criteria. Diabetes Care 1991 Mar; 14(Suppl 2):76–81.

Journals
Asterisks indicate nursing research articles

General

Anderson R. The challenge of translating scientific knowledge into improved diabetes care in the 1990s. Diabetes Care 1991 May; 14(5):418–421.

Armstrong N. Coping with diabetes mellitus: A full-time job. Nurs Clin North Am 1987 Sep; 22:559–568.

Birk R. Feelings and emotions: Their role in diabetes care. Caring 1988 Nov; 7(11):46–48.

Bohannon J. Diabetes in the elderly. Postgrad Med 1988 Oct; 84(5):283–295.

Brosseau J. (Diabetes in) Native Americans. Diabetes Forecast 1988 Sep; 41(9):42–45.

Cameron K and Gregor F. Chronic illness and compliance. J Adv Nurs 1987 Nov; 12(6):671–676.

Carr P. When overcompliance means trouble. Nursing 1990 Mar; 20(3):65–66.

Harris J. Impaired glucose tolerance in the U.S. population. Diabetes Care 1989 Jul/Aug; 12(7):464–474.

Harris M. Hypercholesterolemia in diabetes and glucose intolerance in the U.S. population. Diabetes Care 1991 May; 14(5):366–374.

Jewler D. (Diabetes in) Americans of Latin descent. Diabetes Forecast 1988 Sep; 41(9):27–32.

Lipson L et al. (Diabetes in) Black Americans. Diabetes Forecast 1988 Sep; 41(9):34–38.

Lipson L and Kato-Palmer S. (Diabetes in) Asian Americans. Diabetes Forecast 1988 Sep; 41(9):48–51.

* Lundman B, Asplund K, and Norberg A. Living with diabetes: Perceptions of well-being. Res Nurs Health 1990 Aug; 13(4):255–262.

Mayou R, Bryant B, Turner R. Quality of life in non-insulin-dependent diabetes and a comparison with insulin-dependent diabetes. J Psychosom Res 1990; 34(1):1–11.

Morrow L and Halter J. Diabetes mellitus in the older adult. Geriatrics 1988 Dec; 43(Suppl):57–65.

National Diabetes Data Group. Classification and diagnosis of diabetes mellitus and other categories of glucose intolerance. Diabetes 1979 Dec; 28(12):1039–1057.

Skyler JS. Insulin dependent diabetes mellitus. Postgrad Med 1987 May 1; 81(6):163–174.

Songer T et al. Health, life and automobile insurance characteristics in adults with IDDM. Diabetes Care 1991 Apr; 14(4):318–324.

Stern M. Kelly West lecture: Primary prevention of type II diabetes mellitus. Diabetes Care 1991 May; 14(5):399–410.

World Health Organization. Diabetes mellitus. Report of a WHO study group. Tech Report Series No. 727, 1985.

Zimmet PZ. Primary prevention of diabetes mellitus. Diabetes Care 1988 Mar; 11(3):258–262.

Management

Abraira C and Derler J. Large variations is sucrose in constant carbohydrate diets in type II diabetes. Am J Med 1988 Feb; 84(2):193–200.

Anderson J and Campbell R. Mixing insulins in 1990. Diabetes Educator 1990 Sep/Oct; 16(5):380–386.

Anderson J and Geil P. New perspectives in nutrition management of diabetes mellitus. Am J Med 1988 Nov; 85(Suppl 5A):159–165.

* Beaulieu J. Nursing diagnoses co-occurring in adults with insulin-dependent diabetes mellitus. Classif Nurs Diagn Proc Eighth Conf 1989; 199–205.

Bingham P and Riddle M. Combined insulin–sulfonylurea treatment of type II diabetes. Diabetes Educator 1989 Sep/Oct; 15(5):450–455.

Clouse R and Sandrock M. Intensive nutritional support. Diabetes Spectrum 1989 Sep/Oct; 2(5):329–334.

Crapo P. Use of alternative sweeteners in diabetic diet. Diabetes Care 1988 Feb; 11(2):174–182.

Dunning D. Safe travel tips for the diabetic patient. RN 1989 Apr; 52(4):51–55.

* Edelstein J and Linn M. Locus of control and the control of diabetes. Diabetes Educator 1987 Jan/Feb; 13(1):51–54.

Farkas-Hirsch R and Levandoski L. Implementation of continuous subcutaneous insulin infusion (insulin pump) therapy: An overview. Diabetes Educator 1988 Sept; 14(5):401–406.

* Germain C and Nemchik R. Diabetes self-management and hospitalization. Image: Journal of Nursing Scholarship 1988 Summer; 20(2):74–78.

Gohdes D. Diet therapy of minority patients with diabetes. Diabetes Care 1988 Feb; 11(2):189–191.

Graham C. Exercise and aging: implications for persons with diabetes. Diabetes Educator 1991 May/Jun; 17(3):189–195.

Hamera E et al. Self-regulation in individuals with type II diabetes. Nurs Res 1988 Nov/Dec; 37(6):363–367.

Horton E. Role and management of exercise in diabetes mellitus. Diabetes Care 1988 Feb; 11(2):201–211.

Huzar J and Cerrato P. Diabetes now: The role of diet and drugs. RN 1989 Apr; 52(4):46–50.

Jovanovic–Peterson L, et al. Identifying sources of error in self-monitoring of blood glucose. Diabetes Care 1988 Nov/Dec; 11(10):791–794.

* Keith K and Pieper B. Perioperative blood glucose levels: a study to determine the effect of surgery. AORN J 1989 Jul; 50(1):103–110.

Kittler P and Sucher K. Diet counseling in a multicultural society. Diabetes Educator 1990 Mar/Apr; 16(2):127–132.

* Krug L, Haire-Joshu D, and Heady S. Exercise habits and exercise relapse in persons with non-insulin dependent diabetes mellitus. Diabetes Educator 1991 May/Jun; 17(3):185–188.

Lockwood D, Trand M, and Mather H. Is injecting air into insulin bottles necessary? Br Med J 1988 Nov; 297(6659):1315–1316.

Marynuik M and Cox J. The role of diet in reducing the risks of hyperlipidemia. Diabetes Educator 1988 Sep/Oct; 14(5):435–437.

* McCarthy J, Sink P, and Covarrubias B. Reevaluation of single-use insulin syringes. Diabetes Care 1988 Nov/Dec; 11(10):817–818.

Paige M and Heins J. Nutritional management of diabetic patients during intensive insulin therapy. Diabetes Educator 1989 Nov; 14(6):505–509.

Pendleton L, House W, and Parker L. Physicians' and patients' views of problems of compliance with diabetes regimens. Public Health Rep 1987 Jan/Feb; 102(1):21–26.

* Poteet G, Reinert B, and Ptak H. Outcome of multiple usage of disposable syringes in the insulin-requiring diabetic. Nurs Res 1987 Nov/Dec; 36(6):350–352.

Robertson C. When an insulin-dependent diabetic must be NPO. Nursing 1986 Jun; 16(6):30–31.

Robertson C. The new challenges of insulin therapy. RN 1989 May; 52(5):34–38.

Rosenberg C. Current status of insulin pumps. Mt Sinai J Med 1987 Mar; 54(3):217–220.

Sawicki P et al. Color discrimination and accuracy of blood glucose self-monitoring in type I diabetic patients. Diabetes Care 1991 Feb; 14(2):135–137.

Skyler J. Intensive insulin therapy: A personal and historical perspective. Diabetes Educator 1989 Jan/Feb; 15(1):33–39.

Smith L and Casso M. Exercise and the intensively treated IDDM patient. Diabetes Educator 1988 Nov/Dec; 14(6):510–515.

Smithgall J. Parenteral nutrition in diabetes mellitus. Diabetes Educator 1987 Winter; 13(1):41–46.

Steil C. Insulin storage. Diabetes Educator 1988 Nov/Dec; 6(14):564–565.

Strock E et al. Managing diabetes in the home: A model approach. Caring 1988 Feb; 7(2):50–56.

Trevelyan J. The reluctant patient. Nurs Times 1990 Jan 24–30; 86(4):68, 71–72.

Tomky D. Tapping the full power of insulin pumps. RN 1989 Jun; 52(6):46–48.

Tomky D. Diabetes now: A three-pronged approach to monitoring. RN 1989 Mar; 52(3):24–30.

* Wakefield B et al. Does contamination affect the reliability and validity of bisected Chemstrip bGs? West J Nurs Res 1989 June; 11(3):328–333.

Wylie-Rosett J. Evaluation of protein in dietary management of diabetes mellitus. Diabetes Care 1988 Feb; 11(2):143–148.

Wylie-Rosett J, Swenscionis C, Stern J. Nutritional and behavioral strategies for the obese individual with diabetes. Top Clin Nutr 1988 Oct; 3(4):9–19.

Patient and Family Education

* Anderson R et al. The diabetes care and education provided by nurses working in physicians' offices. Diabetes Educator 1988 Nov; 14(6):532–536.

Bartlett E. The stepped approach to patient education. Diabetes Educator 1988 Mar/Apr; 14(2):130–135.

Cleary M. Aiding the person who is visually impaired from diabetes. Diabetes Educator 1985 Winter; 10(4):12–23.

Donohue–Porter P. Diabetes now: Patient education makes all the difference. RN 1989 Nov; 52(11):56–64.

Fox B. Geriatric patient education: Issues and answers. J Contin Educ Nurs 1988 Jul/Aug; 19(4):169–173.

Funnel M. Role of diabetes educator for older adults. Diabetes Care 1990 Feb; 13(Suppl 2):60–65.

Funnell M et al. Empowerment: An idea whose time has come in diabetes education. Diabetes Educator 1991 Jan/Feb; 17(1):37–41.

Hahn K. Teaching patients to administer insulin. Nursing 1990 Apr; 20(4): 70.

Harris R et al. Development of the diabetes health belief scale. Diabetes Educator 1987 Summer; 13(3):292–297.

Herget M and Williams A. New aids for low-vision diabetics. Am J Nurs 1989 Oct; 89(10):1319–1322.

Hurxthal K. Quick! Teach this patient about insulin. Am J Nurs 1988 Aug; 88(8):1097–1100.

Istre SM: The art and science of successful teaching. Diabetes Educator 1989 Jan/Feb; 15(1):67–75.

Jackson M and Broussard B. Cultural challenges in nutrition education among American Indians. Diabetes Educator 1987 Winter; 13(1):47–50.

Rubin R, Peyrot M, and Saudek C. Differential effect of diabetes education on self-regulation and life-style behaviors. Diabetes Care 1991 Apr; 14(4):335–337.

Smith J et al. Survey of computer programs for diabetes management and education. Diabetes Educator 1988 Sep/Oct; 14(5):412–415.

Tabak E. The relationship of information exchange during medical visits to patient satisfaction: A review. Diabetes Educator 1987 Winter; 13(1):36–40.

* Teza S, Davis W, and Hiss R. Patient knowledge compared with national guidelines for diabetes care. Diabetes Educator 1988 May/June; 14(3): 207–211.

Westberg J and Jason H. Building a helpful relationship: The foundation of effective patient education. Diabetes Educator 1986 Fall; 12(4): 374–378.

Complications

Ai E and Ferris F. The early treatment of diabetic retinopathy. Diabetes Educator 1988 Sep/Oct; 14(5):421–424.

Bamburger D, Days G, and Gerding D. Osteomyelitis in the feet of diabetes patients: Long-term results, prognostic factors, and the role of antimicrobial and surgical therapy. Am J Med 1987 Oct; 83(4):653–660.

Bild DE et al. Lower-extremity amputation in people with diabetes: Epidemiology and prevention. Diabetes Care 1989 Jan; 12(1):24–31.

Broadstone V et al. Diabetic peripheral neuropathy. Part I: Sensorimotor neuropathy. Diabetes Educator 1987 Winter; 13(1):30–35.

Cyrus J et al. Diabetic peripheral neuropathy. Part II: Autonomic neuropathies. Diabetes Educator 1987 Spring; 13(2):111–115.

The DCCT Research Group. Are continuing studies of metabolic control and microvascular complications in IDDM justified? The diabetes control and complications trial (DCCT). N Engl J Med 1988 Jan; 318(4):246–250.

* D'Eramo G and Fain J. Adult foot care perceptions and practices. Practical Diabetology 1988 Nov/Dec; 7(6):1–2.

Dills S et al. Coping with neuropathy, the forgotten complication. Diabetes Educator 1987 Spring; 13(2):148–151.

Fritz ME. Periodontal disease and diabetes. Clin Diabetes 1989 Sept/Oct; 7(5):77, 80–84.

Funnel M and McNitt P. Autonomic neuropathy: Diabetics' hidden foe. Am J Nurs 1986 Mar; 86(3):266–270.

Graham C and Lasko–McCarthey P. Exercise options for persons with diabetic complications. Diabetes Educator 1990 May/Jun; 16(3):212–220.

Hahn K. The many signs of renal failure. Nursing 1987 Aug; 17(8):34–42.

Haire-Joshu D. Smoking, cessation, and the diabetes health care team. Diabetes Educator 1991 Jan/Feb; 17(1):54–65.

Havlin C and Cryer P. Hypoglycemia: The limiting factor in the management of insulin-dependent diabetes mellitus. Diabetes Educator 1988 Sep/Oct; 14(5):407–411.

Hoops S. Renal and retinal complications in insulin-dependent diabetes mellitus: The art of changing the outcome. Diabetes Educator 1990 May/Jun; 16(3):221–231.

Hultman J and Mohr R. Evaluation and treatment of diabetic foot problems. Mt Sinai J Med 1987 Mar; 54(3):253–260.

Huzar J. Diabetes now: Preventing acute complications. RN 1989 Aug; 52(8):34–40.

Jerums G et al. Spectrum of proteinuria in type I and type II diabetes. Diabetes Care 1987 Jul/Aug; 10(4):419–427.

Kaiser F and Korenman S. Impotence in diabetic men. Am J Med 1988 Nov; 85(5A):147–152.

Katzin L. Chronic illness and sexuality. Am J Nurs 1990 Jan; 90(1):54–59.

Leese D. Diabetic cranial mononeuropathies: A patient's perspective. Diabetes Educator 1988 Nov; 14(6):527–531.

Maliszewiski M, Dennis C, and Decoste K. Prevention, detection, and treatment of diabetic eye disease: An overview and demonstration project. Diabetes Educator 1988 Sep/Oct; 14(5):416–420.

Miller R and Evans W. Nurse and patient: Allies preventing amputation. RN 1988 Jul; 51(7):38–44.

Mueller MJ et al. Insensitivity, limited joint mobility, and plantar ulcers in patients with diabetes mellitus. Phys Ther 1989 Jun; 69(6):453–459, (response to commentary) 461–462.

Narins B and Narins R. Clinical features and health-care costs of diabetic nephropathy. Diabetes Care 1988 Nov/Dec; 11(10):933–939.

Nawoczenski D et al. The neuropathic foot—A management scheme: A case report. Phys Ther 1989 Apr; 69(4):287–291.

* Nylin K. Diabetic patients facing long-term complications: coping with uncertainty. J Adv Nurs 1990 Sep; 15(9):1021–1029.

Ramsey P. Hyperglycemia at dawn. Am J Nurs 1987 Nov; 87(3):1424–1426.

Ratner R and Whitehouse F. Motor vehicles, hypoglycemia, and diabetic drivers. Diabetes Care 1989 Mar; 12(3):217–222.

Robertson C. Caring for the diabetic with PAD (peripheral arterial disease). RN 1988 Jul; 51(7):42–44.

Robertson C. Coping with chronic complications. RN 1989 Sep; 52(9):34–43.

Rosenberg C. Wound healing in the patient with diabetes mellitus. Nurs Clin North Am 1990 Mar; 25(1):247–261.

Rosenthal J. Timely recognition of diabetic retinopathy. Emerg Med 1989 Jun 15; 21(11):87–90.

Schreiner–Engel P. Diagnosing and treating the sexual problems of diabetic women. Clin Diabetes 1988 Nov/Dec; 121:126–136.

Sabo C and Michael S. Managing D.K.A. and preventing a recurrence. Nursing 1989 Feb; 19(2):50–56.

Selby J et al. The natural history and epidemiology of diabetic nephropathy. Implications for prevention and control. JAMA 1990 Apr 11; 263(14): 1954–1959.

Tuck M. Treatment of hypertensive diabetic patients. Diabetes Care 1988 Nov/Dec; 11(10):828–832.

Viberti G. Recent advances in understanding mechanisms and natural history of diabetic renal disease. Diabetes Care 1988 Nov/Dec; 11(Suppl 1):3–9.

Vinicor F. Atherosclerosis and DM. Diabetes Spectrum 1988 Nov/Dec; 5: 319–323.

Watkins P. Editorial: Diabetic autonomic neuropathy. JAMA 1990 Apr 12; 322(15):1078–1079.

The Working Group on Hypertension in Diabetes. Statement on hypertension in diabetes mellitus. Final report. Arch Intern Med 1987 May; 147(5):830.

Wulsin L et al. Psychosocial aspects of diabetic retinopathy. Diabetes Care 1987 May/Jun; 10(3):367–373.

Investigational Therapies

Editorial: Transplant or insulin. Lancet 1990 June 9; 335(8702):1371–1372.

Becker S. The risks and rewards of pancreatic transplant. RN 1989 Jul; 52(7):54–57.

Herold K and Rubenstein A. Immunosuppression for insulin-dependent diabetes. N Engl J Med 1988 Mar 17; 318(11):701–703.

Marks J and Skyler J. Clinical review: Immunotherapy of type I diabetes mellitus. J Clin Endocrinol Metab 1991 Jan; 72(1):3–9.

Selam J and Charles M. Devices for insulin administration. Diabetes Care 1990 Sep; 13(9):955–979.

Soon-Shiong P and Lanza R. Pancreas and islet-cell transplant. Potential cure for diabetes mellitus. Postgrad Med 1990 Jun; 87(8):133–134, 139–140.

Sutherland D. Coming of age for pancreas transplantation. West J Med 1989 Mar; 150(3):314–318.

Diabetes Series

American Diabetes Association. 1991 Buyer's guide to diabetes products. Diabetes Forecast 1990 Oct; 43(10):34–74.

Davidson M and Braunstein G (eds). Diabetes mellitus: Recent developments in treatment. Mt Sinai J Med 1987 Mar; 54(3):195–271.

Laxton C (ed). Diabetes and home care. Caring 1988 Nov; 7(2):3–67.

Rizza R and Greene D (eds). Diabetes mellitus. Med Clin North Am 1988 Nov; 72(6):1271–1607.

Information/Resources

Agencies

American Association of Diabetes Educators
500 North Michigan Ave Suite 1400, Chicago, IL 60611 (312) 661-1700

American Diabetes Association
1660 Duke St, Alexandria, VA 22313 (703) 549-1500

American Dietetic Association
430 North Michigan Ave, Chicago, IL 60611 (312) 280-5000

American Foundation for the Blind
15 West 16th St, New York, NY 10011 (212) 620-2000

Juvenile Diabetes Foundation
432 Park Ave S, New York, NY 10016 (212) 889-7575

Medic Alert Foundation International
2323 Colorado St, Turlock CA 95381-1009 (209) 668-3333

National Library Services for the Blind and Physically Handicapped
1291 Taylor St, NW Washington, DC 20542 (202) 287-5100

Journals for Patients

Diabetes '90, Subscription Department, American Diabetes Association, 1660 Duke St, Alexandria, VA 22314

Diabetes Forecast, American Diabetes Association, Membership Center, PO Box 2055, Harlan, IA 51593–0238

Diabetes in the News, Ames Center for Diabetes Education, Miles Inc, PO Box 3105, Elkhart, IN 46515

Diabetes Self-Management, PO Box 51125, Boulder, CO 80321-1125

Health-O-Gram, SugarFree Center, 13725 Burbank Blvd, Van Nuys, CA 91401

Living Well With Diabetes, Diabetes Center, 13911 Ridgedale Dr, Suite 250, Minnetonka, MN 55343

40

Assessment and Management of Patients With Endocrine Disorders

Learning Objectives

On completion of this chapter, the learner will be able to:

1. Specify the functions and hormones secreted by each of the endocrine glands
2. Identify the diagnostic tests used to determine alterations in function of each of the endocrine glands
3. Compare hypothyroidism and hyperthyroidism: their causes, clinical manifestations, management, and nursing interventions
4. Construct a nursing care plan for the patient undergoing thyroidectomy
5. Compare hyperparathyroidism and hypoparathyroidism: their causes, clinical manifestations, management, and nursing interventions
6. Compare Addison's disease to Cushing's syndrome: their causes, clinical manifestations, management, and nursing interventions
7. Use the nursing process as a framework for care of patients with adrenal insufficiency
8. Use the nursing process as a framework for care of patients with Cushing's syndrome
9. Specify the teaching needs of patients requiring corticosteroid therapy
10. Differentiate between acute and chronic pancreatitis
11. Use the nursing process as a framework for care of patients with acute pancreatitis
12. Identify the limitations of surgical treatment of tumors of the pancreas

Physiologic Overview

Endocrine glands, which secrete their products directly into the bloodstream, are clearly differentiated from exocrine glands, such as sweat glands, which secrete through ducts onto epithelial surfaces. The chemical substances secreted by the endocrine glands are called *hormones*. Hormones help to regulate organ function in concert with the nervous system. This dual regulatory system, in which rapid action by the nervous system is balanced by slower hormonal action, permits precise control of body functions in response to varied changes within and outside the body.

There are steroid hormones, such as hydrocortisone; peptide or protein hormones, such as insulin; and amine hormones, such as epinephrine. These different classes of hormones act on the target tissues by different mechanisms, as discussed below. A schematic diagram of the important endocrine glands is shown in Figure 40-1. Table 40-1 lists the important hormones, their target tissue, and some of their properties.

Certain anatomic features are common to the endocrine glands. The glands are composed of secretory cells arranged in minute clusters (acini). No ducts are present, but the glands have a rich blood supply, so that the chemicals they produce can rapidly enter the bloodstream.

The concentration in the bloodstream of most hormones is maintained at a relatively constant level. If the hormone concentration rises, further production of that hormone is inhibited. When the hormone concentration falls, the rate of production of that hormone increases. This mechanism for regulation of hormone concentration in the bloodstream is called *feedback control*. The principle of feedback control is important in the regulation of many biologic processes.

Mechanism of Hormone Action.   Hormones can alter the function of the target tissue by interacting with chemical receptors located either on the cell membrane or in the interior of the cell. Peptide and protein hormones interact with receptor sites on the cell surface, which results in the stimulation of the intracellular enzyme adenyl cyclase. This in turn results in increased production of cyclic 3′,5′-adenosine monophosphate (cyclic AMP). The cyclic AMP inside the cell alters enzyme activity. Thus, cyclic AMP is the "second messenger" that links the peptide hormone at the cell surface to a change in the intracellular environment. Some of the protein and peptide hormones may also act by changing membrane permeability. These hormones act relatively rapidly, within seconds or minutes. The mechanism of action for amine hormones is similar to that for peptide hormones.

Because of their smaller size and higher lipid solubility, steroid hormones penetrate the cell membranes and interact

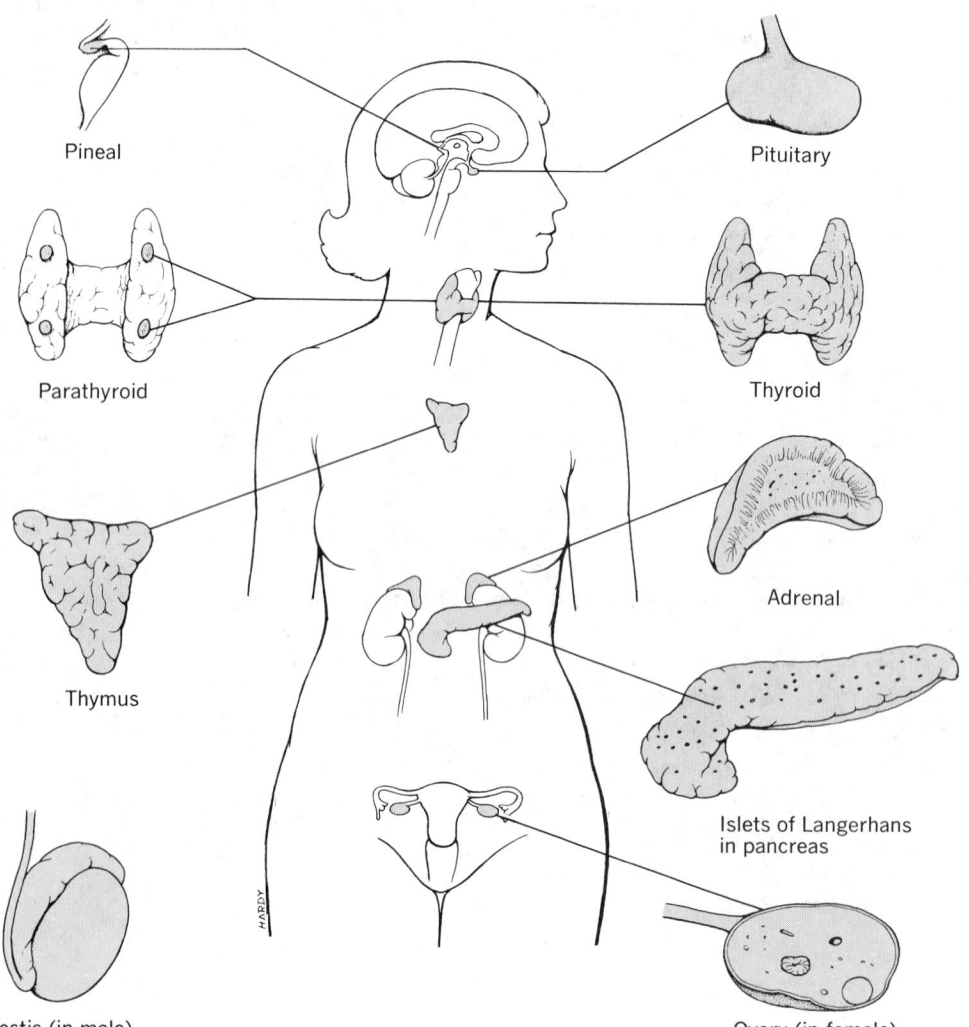

Pineal

Pituitary

Parathyroid

Thyroid

Thymus

Adrenal

Islets of Langerhans in pancreas

Testis (in male)

Ovary (in female)

Figure 40-1.   General location of the major endocrine glands. (Chaffee EE and Greisheimer EM. Basic Physiology and Anatomy, 4th ed. Philadelphia, JB Lippincott.)

with intracellular receptors. This steroid-receptor complex modifies cell metabolism and formation of messenger ribonucleic acid (RNA) from deoxyribonucleic acid (DNA). The messenger RNA then stimulates protein synthesis within the cell. Steroid hormones, because they exert their action by the modification of protein synthesis, require several hours in order to exert their effects.

The Pituitary Gland

The pituitary gland, or the hypophysis, has been referred to as the master gland of the endocrine system. It secretes hormones that, in turn, control the secretion of hormones by other endocrine glands. The pituitary itself is controlled in large part by the hypothalamus, an adjacent area of the brain.

The pituitary gland is a round structure about 1.27 cm (½ inch) in diameter located on the inferior aspect of the brain and connected to the hypothalamus by the pituitary stalk. The pituitary gland is divided into anterior, intermediate, and posterior lobes.

The important hormones secreted by the *posterior* lobe of the pituitary gland are *vasopressin* (antidiuretic hormone [ADH]) and *oxytocin*. These hormones are synthesized in the hypothalamus and travel down the nerve cells that connect the hypothalamus to the posterior pituitary gland, where they are stored. Vasopressin secretion is stimulated by an increase in the osmolality of the blood or by a decrease in blood pressure. The primary function of vasopressin is to control the excretion of water by the kidney. Oxytocin secretion is stimulated during pregnancy and at the time of childbirth. The primary functions of oxytocin are to facilitate milk ejection during lactation and to increase the force of uterine contractions during labor and delivery. Exogenous oxytocin is used therapeutically to initiate labor.

The important hormones of the *anterior* pituitary gland are follicle-stimulating hormone (FSH), luteinizing hormone (LH), prolactin, adrenocorticotropic hormone (ACTH), thyroid-stimulating hormone (TSH), and growth hormone. The secretion of each of these major hormones is controlled by releasing factors (RF) that are secreted by the hypothalamus. These releasing factors reach the anterior pituitary by way of the bloodstream in a special circulation called the pituitary portal blood system.

The hormones released by the anterior pituitary enter the general circulation and are transported to their target organs. TSH, ACTH, FSH, and LH have as their main function the release of hormones from other endocrine glands. Prolactin acts on the breast to stimulate milk production. Growth hormone has widespread effects on many target tissues and is discussed below. The other trophic hormones will be discussed in conjunction with their target organs.

Growth Hormone. Growth hormone, also referred to as somatotropin, is a protein hormone that increases protein synthesis in many tissues, increases the breakdown of fatty acids in adipose tissue, and increases the glucose level in the blood. These actions of somatotropin are essential for normal growth, although other hormones, such as thyroid hormone and insulin, are required as well. The secretion of growth hormone is increased by stress, exercise, and low blood glucose. The half-time of growth hormone activity in the blood is 20 to 30 minutes. It is largely inactivated in the liver. If secretion of growth hormone is insufficient during childhood, generalized limited growth and dwarfism result. Conversely, oversecretion during childhood results in gigantism, with a person reaching 7 or even 8 feet in height. Excess growth hormone in adults results in deformities of bone and soft tissue and enlargement of viscera but no increase in height. This condition is known as acromegaly.

Abnormal Pituitary Function. Abnormalities of pituitary function are caused by oversecretion or undersecretion of any of the hormones produced or released by the gland. Abnormalities of the anterior and posterior portions of the gland may occur independently. Oversecretion (hypersecretion) most commonly involves ACTH or growth hormone, resulting in the conditions known as Cushing's disease or acromegaly, respectively. Undersecretion (hyposecretion) commonly involves all of the anterior pituitary hormones and is termed *panhypopituitarism*. In this condition, the thyroid gland, the adrenal cortex, and the gonads atrophy because of loss of the trophic hormones. The most common disorder related to posterior lobe dysfunction is diabetes insipidus, a condition in which abnormally large volumes of dilute urine are excreted as a result of deficient production of vasopressin.

The Thyroid Gland

The thyroid gland is a butterfly-shaped organ located in the lower neck anterior to the trachea. It consists of two lateral lobes connected by an isthmus. The gland is approximately 5 cm long and 3 cm wide and weighs about 30 g. The blood flow to the thyroid, per gram of gland tissue, is very high (about 5 ml/min/g of thyroid), approximately five times the blood flow to the liver. This reflects the high metabolic activity of the thyroid gland. The thyroid gland produces three different hormones: *thyroxine* (T_4) and *triiodothyronine* (T_3), which are referred to collectively as thyroid hormone, and *calcitonin*.

Thyroid Hormone. Two separate hormones produced by the thyroid gland make up thyroid hormone: thyroxine and triiodothyronine. These hormones are amino acids that have the unique property of containing iodine molecules bound to the amino acid structure. T_4 contains four iodine atoms in each molecule, while T_3 contains only three. These hormones are synthesized and stored bound to a glycoprotein called thyroglobulin in the cells of the thyroid gland until needed for release into the bloodstream.

Iodine Uptake and Metabolism. Iodine is essential to the thyroid gland for synthesis of its hormones. In fact, the major use of iodine in the body is by the thyroid, and the major derangement in iodine deficiency is alteration of thyroid function. Iodide is ingested in the diet and absorbed into the blood in the gastrointestinal tract. The thyroid gland is extremely efficient in taking up iodide from the blood and concentrating it within the cells. There, iodide ions are converted to iodine molecules, which react with tyrosine (an amino acid) to form the thyroid hormones.

Regulation of Thyroid Function. The secretion of thyrotropin, or thyroid-stimulating hormone (TSH), by the pituitary gland controls the rate of thyroid hormone release. In turn, the release of TSH is determined by the level of thyroid hormones in the blood. If thyroid hormone concentration in the blood decreases, release of TSH increases, which causes increased output of T_3 and T_4. This is an example of feedback control. Thyrotropin-releasing hormone (TRH), secreted by the hypothalamus, exerts a modulating influence on the release of

TABLE 40–1. *Endocrine System in Summary*

Endocrine Gland and Hormone	Principal Site of Action	Principal Processes Affected
PITUITARY GLAND		
Anterior Lobe		
Growth hormone (somatotropin)	General	Growth of bones, muscles, and other organs
Thyrotropin	Thyroid	Growth and secretory activity of thyroid gland
Adrenocorticotropin	Adrenal cortex	Growth and secretory activity of adrenal cortex
Follicle-stimulating	Ovaries	Development of follicles and secretion of estrogen
	Testes	Development of seminiferous tubules, spermatogenesis
Luteinizing or interstitial cell stimulating	Ovaries	Ovulation, formation of corpus luteum, secretion of progesterone
	Testes	Secretion of testosterone
Prolactin or lactogenic (luteotropin)	Mammary glands and ovaries	Secretion of milk; maintenance of corpus luteum
Melanocyte-stimulating	Skin	Pigmentation (?)
Posterior Lobe		
Antidiuretic (vasopressin)	Kidney	Reabsorption of water; water balance
	Arterioles	Blood pressure (?)
Oxytocin	Uterus	Contraction
	Breast	Expression of milk
PINEAL GLAND		
Melatonin	Gonads (?)	Sexual maturation (?)
THYROID GLAND		
Thyroxine and triiodothyronine	General	Metabolic rate; growth and development; intermediate metabolism
Thyrocalcitonin	Bone	Inhibits bone resorption; lowers blood level of calcium
PARATHYROID GLANDS		
Parathormone	Bone, kidney, intestine	Promotes bone resorption; increases absorption of calcium; raises blood calcium level
ADRENAL GLANDS		
Cortex		
Mineralocorticoids (*e.g.,* aldosterone)	Kidney	Reabsorption of sodium; elimination of potassium
Glucocorticoids (*e.g.,* cortisol)	General	Metabolism of carbohydrate, protein, and fat; response to stress; anti-inflammatory
Sex hormones	General (?)	Preadolescent growth spurt (?)
Medulla		
Epinephrine	Cardiac muscle, smooth muscle, glands	Emergency functions: same as stimulation of sympathetic nervous system
Norepinephrine	Organs innervated by sympathetic nervous system	Chemical transmitter substance; increases peripheral resistance
ISLET CELLS OF PANCREAS		
Insulin	General	Lowers blood sugar; utilization and storage of carbohydrate; decreased gluconeogenesis
Glucagon	Liver	Raises blood glucose; glycogenolysis
Somatostatin	General	Lowers blood glucose by interfering with release of growth hormone and glucagon
TESTES		
Testosterone	General	Development of secondary sex characteristics
	Reproductive organs	Development and maintenance; normal function

(continued)

TABLE 40-1. *(Continued)*

Endocrine Gland and Hormone	Principal Site of Action	Principal Processes Affected
OVARIES		
Estrogens	General	Development of secondary sex characteristics
	Mammary glands	Development of duct system
	Reproductive organs	Maturation and normal cyclic function
Progesterone	Mammary glands	Development of secretory tissue
	Uterus	Preparation for implantation; maintenance of pregnancy
GASTROINTESTINAL TRACT		
Gastrin	Stomach	Production of gastric juice
Enterogastrone	Stomach	Inhibits secretion and motility
Secretin	Liver and pancreas	Production of bile; production of watery pancreatic juice (rich in $NaHCO_3$)
Pancreozymin	Pancreas	Production of pancreatic juice rich in enzymes
Cholecystokinin	Gallbladder	Contraction and emptying

(Adapted from Chaffee EE, and Lytle IM. Basic Physiology and Anatomy, 4th ed. Philadelphia, JB Lippincott.)

TSH from the pituitary. Environmental factors, such as a fall in temperature, may lead to increased secretion of TRH and thereby result in elevated secretion of thyroid hormones. Figure 40-2 shows the hypothalamic–pituitary–thyroid axis, which regulates thyroid hormone production.

Function of Thyroid Hormones. The primary function of the thyroid hormones T_3 and T_4 is to control the cellular metabolic activity. These hormones serve as a general pacemaker by accelerating metabolic processes. The effects on the metabolic rate are frequently produced by increasing the level of specific enzymes that contribute to oxygen consumption and altering the responsiveness of tissues to other hormones. The thyroid hormones influence cell replication and are important in brain development. The presence of adequate thyroid hormone is also necessary for normal growth. The thyroid hormones, through their widespread effects on cellular metabolism, influence every major organ system.

Calcitonin. Calcitonin, or thyrocalcitonin, is another important hormone secreted by the thyroid gland. Its secretion is not controlled by TSH. It is secreted by the thyroid gland in response to high plasma levels of calcium, and it reduces the plasma level by increasing calcium deposition in bone.

Abnormalities of Thyroid Function. Inadequate secretion of thyroid hormone during fetal and neonatal development will result in stunted physical and mental growth (cretinism) due to general depression of body metabolic activity. In the adult, hypothyroidism (myxedema) is manifested by lethargy, slow mentation, and generalized slowing of body functions. Oversecretion of thyroid hormones (hyperthyroidism) is manifested by a greatly increased metabolic rate. Many of the other characteristics of hyperthyroid patients result from the increased response to circulating catecholamines (epinephrine and norepinephrine). Hypothyroidism and hyperthyroidism are discussed in detail in a later section of this chapter. Oversecretion of thyroid hormones is usually associated with an enlarged thyroid gland (goiter). Goiter also commonly occurs in the presence of iodide deficiency. In this latter condition, lack of iodide results in low levels of circulating thyroid hormones, which causes increased release of TSH; the elevated TSH causes overproduction of thyroglobulin and hypertrophy of the thyroid gland. *Euthyroid* refers to thyroid hormone production that is within normal limits.

The Adrenal Glands

There are two adrenal glands in the human, each attached to the upper portion of a kidney. Each adrenal gland is, in reality, two endocrine glands. The adrenal medulla at the center of

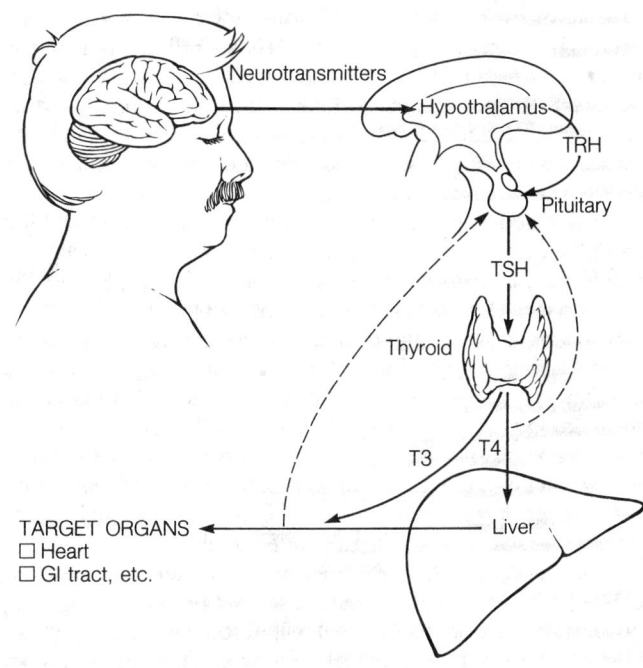

Figure 40-2. Hypothalamic-pituitary-thyroid axis. Thyroid-releasing hormone (TRH) from the hypothalamus stimulates the pituitary gland to secrete thyroid-stimulating hormone (TSH). TSH stimulates thyroid hormone (T_3 and T_4) production by the thyroid gland. High circulating levels of T_3 and T_4 inhibit further TSH secretion and thyroid hormone production through a negative feedback mechanism (*dashed lines*).

the gland secretes catecholamines, while the outer portion of the gland, the adrenal cortex, secretes corticosteroids.

Adrenal Medulla.   The adrenal medulla functions as part of the autonomic nervous system. Stimulation of preganglionic sympathetic nerve fibers, which travel directly to the cells of the adrenal medulla, causes release of the catecholamine hormones epinephrine and norepinephrine. About 90% of the secretion of the human adrenal medulla is epinephrine (also called adrenalin). Catecholamines regulate metabolic pathways to promote catabolism of stored fuels to meet caloric needs from endogenous sources. The major effects of epinephrine release are involved in preparation to meet a challenge (fight-or-flight response). Secretion of epinephrine causes decreased blood flow to tissues that are not needed in emergency situations, such as the gastrointestinal tract, and causes increased blood flow to those tissues that are important for effective fight or flight, such as cardiac and skeletal muscle. Catecholamines also induce release of free fatty acids, increase the basal metabolic rate, and elevate the level of blood glucose.

Adrenal Cortex.   The three kinds of steroid hormones produced by the adrenal cortex are glucocorticoids, the prototype of which is hydrocortisone; mineralocorticoids, mainly aldosterone; and sex hormones, mainly androgens (male sex hormones).

Glucocorticoids.   The glucocorticoids are given their name because they have an important influence on glucose metabolism; increased hydrocortisone secretion results in elevated blood glucose levels. However, the glucocorticoids have major effects on the metabolism of almost all organs of the body. Glucocorticoids are secreted from the adrenal cortex in response to the release of ACTH from the anterior lobe of the pituitary gland. This system represents an example of negative feedback. The presence of glucocorticoids in the blood inhibits the release of corticotropin-releasing factor (CRF) from the hypothalamus and also inhibits ACTH secretion from the pituitary. The resultant decrease in ACTH secretion causes diminished release of glucocorticoids from the adrenal cortex. A functioning adrenal cortex is necessary for life, although survival is possible by appropriate replacement with exogenous adrenocortical hormones.

The glucocorticoids are frequently administered to inhibit the inflammatory response to tissue injury and suppress allergic manifestations. Side effects of glucocorticoids include possible development of diabetes, osteoporosis, peptic ulcer, increased protein breakdown resulting in muscle wasting and poor wound healing, and redistribution of body fat. The presence of large amounts of exogenously administered glucocorticoids in the blood inhibits release of ACTH and endogenous glucocorticoids. Because of this, the adrenal cortex can atrophy. If exogenous glucocorticoid administration is suddenly discontinued, adrenal insufficiency results because of the inability of the atrophied cortex to respond adequately.

Mineralocorticoids.   Mineralocorticoids exert their major effects on electrolyte metabolism. They act principally on renal tubular and gastrointestinal epithelium to cause increased sodium ion absorption in exchange for excretion of potassium or hydrogen ions. Aldosterone secretion is only minimally influenced by ACTH. It is primarily secreted in response to the presence of angiotensin II in the bloodstream. Angiotensin II is a substance that elevates the blood pressure by constricting arterioles. Its concentration is increased when renin is released from the kidney in response to decreased perfusion pressure.

The resultant increased aldosterone levels promote sodium reabsorption by the kidney and the gastrointestinal tract, which tends to restore blood pressure to normal. The release of aldosterone is also increased by hyperkalemia. Aldosterone is the primary hormone for the long-term regulation of sodium balance.

Adrenal Sex Hormones (Androgens).   Androgens, the third major type of steroid hormones produced by the adrenal cortex, exert effects similar to those of male sex hormones. The adrenal gland may also secrete small amounts of some estrogens, or female sex hormones. Secretion of adrenal androgens is controlled by ACTH. When secreted in normal amounts, the adrenal androgens probably have little effect, but when secreted excessively, in certain inborn enzyme deficiencies, masculinization may result. This is termed the *adrenogenital syndrome.*

The Parathyroid Gland

The parathyroid glands, normally four in number, are situated in the neck, embedded in the posterior aspect of the thyroid gland. These small glands are easily overlooked and can be removed accidentally at the time of thyroid surgery. Inadvertent surgical removal is the most common cause of hypoparathyroidism.

Parathormone, the protein hormone from the parathyroid glands, regulates calcium and phosphorus metabolism. Increased secretion of parathormone results in increased calcium absorption from the kidney, the intestine, and bones, thereby raising the blood calcium level. Some actions of this hormone are increased by the presence of vitamin D. Parathormone also tends to lower the blood phosphorus level. Excess parathormone can result in markedly elevated levels of serum calcium, a potentially life-threatening situation. When the product of serum calcium and serum phosphorus (calcium $\times$ phosphorus) becomes high, calcium phosphate may precipitate in various organs of the body and cause tissue calcification.

The output of parathormone is regulated by the serum level of ionized calcium. Increased serum calcium results in decreased parathormone secretion, forming a feedback system.

The Pancreas

The pancreas, located in the upper abdomen, has both exocrine (digestive enzymes) and endocrine gland function. In contrast to endocrine glands, an exocrine gland is one whose secretions travel through a duct to their site of utilization and are not secreted into the bloodstream.

Exocrine Pancreas.   The secretions of the exocrine portion of the pancreas are collected in the pancreatic duct, which joins the common bile duct and enters the duodenum at the ampulla of Vater. Surrounding the ampulla is the sphincter of Oddi, which partially controls the rate at which the secretions from both the pancreas and the gallbladder enter the duodenum.

The secretions of the exocrine pancreas are digestive enzymes high in protein content and an electrolyte-rich fluid. The secretions are very alkaline because of their high concentration of sodium bicarbonate and are capable of neutralizing the highly acid gastric juice that enters the duodenum. The enzyme secretions include *amylase*, which aids in the digestion of carbohydrates; *trypsin*, which aids in the digestion of proteins; and *lipase*, which aids in the digestion of fats. Other enzymes that promote the breakdown of more complex foodstuffs are also secreted.

The secretion of these exocrine pancreatic juices is stimulated by hormones originating in the gastrointestinal tract. *Secretin* is the major stimulus for increased bicarbonate secretion from the pancreas, while the major stimulus for digestive enzyme secretion is the hormone *cholecystokinin-pancreozymin* (CCK-PZ). The vagus nerve also influences exocrine pancreatic secretion.

Endocrine Pancreas.   The islets of Langerhans, the endocrine part of the pancreas, are collections of cells embedded in the pancreatic tissue. They are composed of alpha, beta, and delta cells. The hormone produced by the beta cells is called *insulin;* the alpha cells secrete *glucagon*, and the delta cells secrete *somatostatin*. A major action of insulin is to lower blood glucose by permitting entry of the glucose into the cells of the liver, muscle, and other tissues, where it is either stored as glycogen or burned for energy. Insulin also promotes the storage of fat in adipose tissue and the synthesis of proteins in various body tissues. In the absence of insulin, glucose is not able to enter the cells and is excreted in the urine. This condition, called diabetes mellitus, can be diagnosed by high levels of glucose in the blood and urine. In diabetes mellitus, stored fats and protein are used for energy instead of glucose, with consequent loss of body mass. The rate of insulin secretion from the pancreas is normally regulated by the level of glucose in the blood. The effects of glucagon (opposite to those of insulin) are chiefly to raise the blood glucose by converting glycogen to glucose in the liver. Glucagon is secreted by the pancreas in response to a fall in the level of blood glucose. Somatostatin exerts a hypoglycemic effect by interfering with release of growth hormone from the pituitary and glucagon from the pancreas, both of which tend to raise blood glucose levels.

Endocrine Control of Carbohydrate Metabolism.   Glucose for body energy needs is derived by metabolism of ingested carbohydrates and also from proteins by the process of gluconeogenesis. Glucose can be stored temporarily in the liver, muscles, and other tissues in the form of glycogen. The endocrine system controls the level of blood glucose by regulating the rate at which glucose is synthesized, stored, and moved to and from the bloodstream. Through the action of hormones, blood glucose is normally maintained at approximately 100 mg/dl (5.5 mmol/L) of blood. Insulin is the primary hormone that leads to a lowering of the blood glucose level. Hormones that act to raise the blood glucose level are glucagon, epinephrine, adrenocorticosteroids, growth hormone, and thyroid hormone.

The Thyroid Gland

Assessment: Tests of Thyroid Function

Several tests are available and may be necessary to give a complete and accurate picture of thyroid function. In addition, clinical signs and symptoms are evaluated and provide useful information about the function of the thyroid gland.

The stimulating effect of the thyroid gland is exerted through the production and distribution of two hormones: thyroxine (T_4), which maintains body metabolism in a steady state, and triiodothyronine (T_3), which is approximately five times as potent as T_4 and has a more rapid metabolic action. Measurement of the levels of thyroid hormones in the blood is used to assess thyroid function.

Serum T_4.   The test most commonly used is the determination of serum T_4 by radioimmunoassay or competitive binding techniques. The range of T_4 in serum is normally between 4.5 and 11.5 μg/dl (58.5 to 150 nmol/L); T_4 is bound mainly to thyroxine-binding globulin (TBG) and prealbumin; T_3 is bound less firmly. T_4 is normally bound to proteins. Any factor that alters these binding proteins also changes the T_4 levels. Serious systemic illnesses, medications (*i.e.*, oral contraceptives, steroids, phenytoin, salicylates), and protein-wasting as a result of nephrosis and use of androgens may interfere with accurate test results.

Serum T_3.   The serum T_3 test measures free and bound, or total, serum content of T_3. Its secretion occurs in response to TSH secretion, as does that of T_4. Although T_3 and T_4 serum levels generally increase or decrease together, T_3 levels appear to be more accurate indicators of hyperthyroidism, which causes a greater rise in T_3 than T_4 levels. The normal range for serum T_3 is 70 to 220 ng/dl (1.15 to 3.10 nmol/L).

Resin T_3 Uptake.   The resin T_3 uptake test uses a reagent of radioactive T_3 to measure thyroid hormone levels in the serum by determining the amount of hormone bound to TBG and the number of available binding sites. Normally, TBG is not fully saturated with thyroid hormone, and additional binding sites are available to combine with radioiodine-labeled T_3 added to the patient's blood specimen. Measurement of the number of free binding sites, therefore, provides an index to the amount of thyroid hormone already present in the patient's circulation. The normal T_3 uptake value is 25% to 35% (relative uptake fraction: 0.25 to 0.35), which indicates that approximately one-third of the available sites of TBG are occupied by thyroid hormone. If the number of free or unoccupied binding sites is low, as in hyperthyroidism, the T_3 uptake is greater than 35% (0.35). If the number of available sites is high, as occurs in hypothyroidism, the test results are less than 25% (0.25).

T_3 uptake is useful in the evaluation of thyroid hormone levels in patients who have received diagnostic or therapeutic doses of iodine. The test results may be altered by the use of estrogens, androgens, salicylates, phenytoin, anticoagulants, or steroids.

Tests of Thyroid-Stimulating Hormone.   The secretion of T_3 and T_4 by the thyroid gland is under the control of TSH (thyrotropin) from the anterior pituitary gland. Measurement of serum TSH concentration is valuable in the diagnosis and management of thyroid disorders and in differentiation between disorders due to disease of the thyroid gland itself and disorders due to disease of the pituitary or hypothalamus.

TSH Radioimmunoassay.   The level of TSH in the serum can be measured by radioimmunoassay. It is increased in patients with primary hypothyroidism. Immunoradiometric assay with labeled monoclonal antibody to TSH is a recently developed technique with increased specificity and sensitivity in the measurement of TSH.

Thyrotropin-Releasing Hormone Test.   The TRH stimulation test provides a direct means of testing pituitary reserve for TSH and is useful when T_3 and T_4 test results are inconclusive. The patient fasts overnight. Just before and 30 minutes after intravenous administration of TRH, blood samples are drawn for

TSH levels. In hypothyroidism due to primary disease of the thyroid gland, there is an increased serum TSH level; in hypothyroidism due to disease of the pituitary or hypothalamus, there is an absent or delayed response to TRH. Prior to the test, the patient is warned that the intravenous administration of TRH may cause temporary facial flushing, nausea, or a desire to urinate.

Thyroglobulin. Thyroglobulin, a precursor for T_3 and T_4, can be measured reliably in the serum by radioimmunoassay. Those factors that increase or decrease thyroid gland activity and the secretion of T_3 and T_4 have a similar effect on thyroglobulin synthesis and secretion. Thyroglobulin levels are increased in thyroid carcinoma, hyperthyroidism, and subacute thyroiditis. They may be high in normal physiologic conditions such as pregnancy. They may be increased or decreased by medications or by diagnostic and therapeutic procedures that temporarily increase the serum levels of thyroglobulin. Measuring the thyroglobulin level is useful in the follow-up and management of patients with thyroid carcinoma and metastatic thyroid disease.

Radioactive Iodine Uptake. The radioactive iodine uptake test measures the rate of iodine uptake by the thyroid gland. The patient is given a tracer dose of ^{131}I, and a count is made over the thyroid with use of a scintillation counter, which detects and counts the gamma rays released from the breakdown of ^{131}I in the thyroid. Thyroid activity divided by the amount of administered activity (expressed as a percentage) is the uptake value. It is a simple test and provides reliable results. It is affected by the patient's intake of iodide or thyroid hormone; therefore, a careful preliminary clinical history is essential in evaluating results. Normal values vary from one geographic region to another and with the intake of iodine. Patients with hyperthyroidism accumulate a high proportion of the ^{131}I (in some patients up to 90%), whereas patients with hypothyroidism exhibit a very low uptake. This test is also used to determine what dose of ^{131}I should be given to treat a patient with hyperthyroidism.

Thyroid Scan, Radioscan, or Scintiscan. Similar to the radioactive iodine uptake test, in a thyroid scan a highly focused scintillation detector moves back and forth across the area to be studied in a series of parallel tracks that move progressively downward. At the same time, a printing device records a mark whenever a predetermined number of counts has been received. This produces a visual representation of the localization of radioactivity in the area being scanned. Although ^{131}I has been the most commonly used isotope, ^{125}I and ^{99m}Tc (sodium pertechnetate) are also being used because of their physical and biochemical properties, which allow a lower radiation dose to be given to the patient.

Scanning is helpful in determining location, size, shape, and anatomic function of the thyroid gland, particularly when thyroid tissue is substernal or large. Identification of areas of increased function ("hot" areas) or decreased function ("cold" areas) can assist in diagnosis. Although most areas of decreased function are not malignancies, lack of function increases the likelihood of malignancy, particularly if only one nonfunctioning area is present. Scanning of the entire body, to obtain the total body profile, may be carried out in a search for a functioning thyroid metastasis.

Protein-Bound Iodine. Protein-bound iodine is a conjugated molecule formed when T_4 becomes attached to certain plasma protein components. Thyroid function may be assessed in relation to the concentration of protein-bound iodine in the blood. In this test, serum proteins are precipitated, washed, and then measured for iodine content. Normal values range from 4 to 8 $\mu g/dl$ (0.32 to 0.63 $\mu mol/L$) of plasma. Values above 8 $\mu g/dl$ indicate thyroid overactivity; conversely, concentrations below 4 $\mu g/dl$ are considered evidence of hypothyroidism. Unreliable results that may occur if the patient has taken medications containing iodine have decreased the use of this test.

Nursing Implications of Thyroid Tests. When a patient is scheduled for thyroid tests, it is necessary to determine if he has taken medications or drugs that contain iodine, because these will alter the results of some of the scheduled tests. Iodide-containing medications include contrast media and those used in the treatment of thyroid disorders. Other less obvious sources of iodine are topical antiseptics, multivitamin preparations and food supplements frequently found in health food stores, cough syrups, and amiodarone, an antidysrhythmic agent. Other medications that may affect thyroid function test values are estrogens, salicylates, amphetamines, chemotherapeutic agents, antibiotics, steroids, and mercurial diuretics. The patient should be questioned about the use of these medications, and their use should be noted on the laboratory requisition for thyroid function tests. See Table 40-2 for a partial list of agents that may interfere with accurate testing of thyroid gland function.

Examination of the Thyroid Gland

The thyroid gland is inspected and palpated routinely on all patients. The identification of specific anatomic landmarks is required to ensure an accurate assessment. The lower neck region between the sternocleidomastoid muscles is inspected for anterior swelling or asymmetry. The patient is instructed to extend his neck slightly and swallow. Thyroid tissue rises normally with swallowing. The thyroid is then palpated for size, shape, consistency, symmetry, and the presence of tenderness.

The examiner may perform this portion of the examination from an anterior or a posterior position. For the beginning examiner, the thyroid is most effectively palpated from a position behind the patient, with both hands encircling the patient's neck (Fig. 40-3). The thumbs are rested on the nape of the patient's neck, while the index and middle fingers palpate for the thyroid isthmus and the anterior surfaces of the lateral lobes. When palpable, the isthmus is perceived as firm and of a rubber-band consistency. The left lobe is examined by po-

TABLE 40-2. *Partial List of Drugs That May Alter Thyroid Test Results*

Estrogens	Opiates
Sulfonylureas	Androgens
Glucocorticoids	Salicylates
Iodine	Lithium
Propranolol	Amiodarone
Cimetidine	Clofibrate
5-Fluorouracil	Furosemide
Diphenylhydantoin	Diazepam
Heparin	Danazol
Chloral hydrate	Dopamine antagonists
X-ray contrast agents	Propylthiouracil

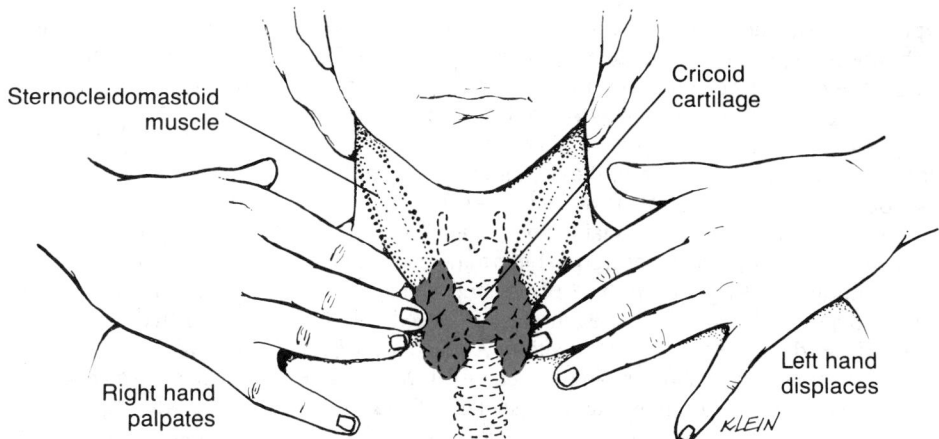

Figure 40–3. Technique of palpation of the thyroid gland. The isthmus of the thyroid may be felt in the midline, approximately 1 cm below the cricoid cartilage. The gland is felt laterally beneath the insertion of the sternocleidomastoid muscle.

sitioning the patient with his neck flexed slightly forward and to the left. The thyroid cartilage is then displaced to the left with the fingers of the right hand. This maneuver displaces the left lobe deep into the sternocleidomastoid muscle, where it can be more easily palpated. The left lobe is then palpated by placing the left thumb deep into the posterior area of the sternocleidomastoid muscle, while the index and middle fingers exert opposite pressure in the anterior portion of the muscle. Having the patient swallow during the maneuver may assist the examiner to locate the thyroid as it ascends in the neck. The procedure is reversed for an examination of the right lobe. The isthmus is the only portion of the thyroid that is normally palpable. If a patient has a very thin neck, occasionally two thin, smooth, nontender lobes may also be palpable.

If the thyroid gland is enlarged on palpation, auscultation over both lobes with the diaphragm of the stethoscope is performed. Auscultation will identify the localized audible vibration of a bruit. This is an abnormal finding indicative of increased blood flow through the thyroid gland and necessitates referral to a physician. The presence of tenderness, enlargement, or nodularity within the thyroid also requires additional evaluation by a physician.

Hypothyroidism and Myxedema

Hypothyroidism is a condition in which there is a slow progression of thyroid hypofunction, followed by symptoms indicating thyroid failure. It results from suboptimal levels of thyroid hormone. More than 95% of patients with hypothyroidism have *primary* dysfunction of the thyroid gland itself. When the thyroid dysfunction is due to failure of the pituitary gland, it is known as *secondary hypothyroidism;* when failure of the hypothalamus is the underlying cause, the term *tertiary hypothyroidism* is used. When thyroid deficiency is present at birth, the condition is known as *cretinism.* In such instances, the mother may also suffer from thyroid deficiency.

The most common cause of hypothyroidism in adults is autoimmune thyroiditis (Hashimoto's thyroiditis), in which the immune system attacks the thyroid gland. Symptoms of hyperthyroidism (see p. 1083) may later be followed by those of hypothyroidism and myxedema. Hypothyroidism also commonly occurs in patients with previous hyperthyroidism who have been treated with radioiodine, surgery, or antithyroid drugs. It occurs most frequently in older women.

Clinical Manifestations

Early symptoms of hypothyroidism are nonspecific, but extreme fatigue makes it difficult for the person to complete a full day's work or participate in usual activities. Complaints of hair loss, brittle nails, and dry skin are common, and numbness and tingling of the fingers may occur. On occasion, the voice may become husky, and the patient may complain of hoarseness. Menstrual disturbances such as menorrhagia or amenorrhea occur, in addition to loss of libido.

With more severe hypothyroidism, the temperature and pulse rate become subnormal. The patient usually begins to gain weight even without an increase in food intake. (Severely hypothyroid patients, however, may be cachectic.) The skin becomes thickened because of an accumulation of mucopolysaccharides in the subcutaneous tissues (the origin of the term *myxedema*). The hair thins and falls out; the face becomes expressionless and masklike. The patient often complains of being cold even in a warm environment.

At first the patient may be irritable and may complain of fatigue, but as the condition progresses, the emotional responses are subdued. The mental process becomes dulled, and the patient appears apathetic. Speech is slow, the tongue enlarges, and hands and feet increase in size. The patient frequently complains of constipation. Deafness also may occur. The advanced myxedematous state may produce personality changes.

Myxedema affects women five times more frequently than men and occurs most often between 30 and 60 years of age. It is not without its complications, because there is an associated tendency to the rapid development of atherosclerosis, with all its consequences. The patient with advanced myxedema is hypothermic and abnormally sensitive to sedatives, opiates, and anesthetic agents. Therefore, these drugs are given only with extreme caution.

Patients with unrecognized hypothyroidism who are undergoing surgery are at increased risk for intraoperative hypotension and postoperative congestive heart failure and altered mental status.

Management

The prime objective is to restore a normal metabolic state by replacing the missing hormone. Synthetic levothyroxine (Synthroid or Levothroid) is the preferred preparation for treating hypothyroidism and suppressing nontoxic goiters. The dosage for hormone replacement is based on the patient's serum TSH concentration. Desiccated thyroid is used less frequently because it often results in transient elevated serum concentrations of T_3, with occasional symptoms of hyperthyroidism. If replacement therapy is adequate, the symptoms of myxedema disappear and normal metabolic activity is resumed.

The treatment consists of maintaining vital functions. Arterial blood gases may be measured to determine carbon dioxide retention and to guide the use of assisted ventilation to combat hypoventilation. Fluids are administered cautiously because of the danger of water intoxication. Application of external heat (*i.e.*, heating pads) is avoided because it will increase oxygen requirements and may lead to vascular collapse. If hypoglycemia is evident, concentrated glucose may be given to provide glucose without precipitating fluid overload. Thyroid hormone (usually Synthroid) is given intravenously until consciousness is restored if myxedema has progressed to myxedema coma. Then the patient is continued on oral thyroid hormone therapy. Because of an associated adrenocortical insufficiency, steroid therapy may be initiated.

Precautionary Concerns

- Myocardial ischemia or infarction may occur in response to therapy in patients with myxedema.

Any patient who has been myxedematous for a long period of time is almost certain to have elevated serum cholesterol levels, atherosclerosis, and coronary artery disease. As long as metabolism is subnormal and the tissues, including the myocardium, require relatively little oxygen, a reduction in blood supply is tolerated without overt symptoms of coronary artery disease. However, when thyroid hormone is given, the oxygen demand increases but oxygen delivery cannot be increased unless, or until, the atherosclerosis improves. This will occur very slowly, if at all. The signal that the oxygen needs of the myocardium exceed its blood supply is angina pectoris. Angina or dysrhythmias may occur when thyroid replacement is initiated, because thyroid hormones enhance the cardiovascular effects of catecholamines.

The nurse must be alert for signs of angina, especially during the early phase of treatment, and if detected, it must be reported and treated at once in order to avoid a fatal myocardial infarction. Obviously, the administration of thyroid hormone must be discontinued immediately, and later, when it can be resumed safely, thyroid hormone replacement should be given cautiously at a lower level of dosage and under the close observation of the physician and the nurse.

Elderly arteriosclerotic patients may also become confused and agitated if their metabolic rates are raised too quickly in myxedema.

Marked clinical improvement follows the administration of hormone replacement; such medication must be continued for life, even though signs of myxedema disappear over a 3- to 12-week period.

Precautions must be taken during the course of therapy because of the interaction of thyroid hormones with other drugs. Thyroid hormones may increase blood glucose levels, which may necessitate adjustment in doses of insulin or oral hypoglycemic agents. The effects of thyroid hormone may be increased by phenytoin and tricyclic antidepressants. Thyroid hormones may also increase the pharmacologic effects of dig-

italis glycosides, anticoagulants, and indomethacin, requiring careful observation and assessment by the nurse for side effects of these drugs.

- Severe untreated hypothyroidism is characterized by an increased susceptibility to all hypnotic and sedative drugs.

These drugs, even in small doses, may induce profound somnolence, lasting far longer than anticipated. Moreover, they are likely to cause respiratory depression, which could easily be fatal because of the decreased respiratory reserve and alveolar hypoventilation that occur in myxedema.

With this in mind, the dosage of any such drug is most conservative (*e.g.*, no more than a half or one-third the dosage ordinarily employed in patients of similar age and weight with normal thyroid function). Sedative and hypnotic agents are not used unless the indications are very specific. If they are given, the nurse must monitor the patient closely for signs of impending narcosis (stupor-like condition) or respiratory failure.

Nursing Management

The patient with hypothyroidism experiences decreased energy and moderate to severe lethargy. As a result, he is at risk for the complications of immobility. His ability to exercise and participate in activities is further limited by the changes in cardiovascular and pulmonary status resulting from the myxedematous state. A major role of the nurse is to support the patient by assisting with care and hygiene while encouraging him to participate in activities within his tolerance to prevent complications of immobility. The patient's vital signs and cognitive level are monitored closely during diagnostic workup and initiation of treatment to detect (1) deterioration of his physical and mental status, (2) symptoms indicating that an increased metabolic rate resulting from treatment exceeds the ability of the cardiovascular and pulmonary systems to respond, and (3) continued limitations or complications of myxedema.

- Medications are administered to the patient with hypothyroidism very cautiously because of his altered metabolism and excretion and his already depressed metabolic rate and respiratory status.

The patient often experiences chilling and extreme intolerance to cold even if the room temperature feels comfortable or hot to others. Extra clothing and blankets are provided, and the patient is protected from drafts. Although he may ask for a heating pad or electric blanket to decrease chilling and discomfort, these measures are avoided because of the risk of causing peripheral vasodilation, further loss of body heat, and vascular collapse. Additionally, the patient could be burned by using these items without being aware of it because of delayed responses and decreased mental status.

The patient and his family are often very concerned about the changes they have observed as a result of the hypothyroid state. It is often reassuring to the patient and family to be informed that many of the symptoms will disappear as treatment becomes effective. The patient is instructed to continue to use medications as prescribed even after symptoms improve. Dietary instruction is provided to promote weight loss once medication has been initiated and to promote return of normal bowel patterns. Because of the decreased mentation that occurs with hypothyroidism, it is important that a family member also be informed and instructed about treatment goals, medication schedules, and side effects that are to be reported to the physician. Additionally, these instructions and guidelines are provided in writing for the patient, family, and community health nurse to refer to once the patient returns home.

The patient with moderate to severe hypothyroidism may experience severe emotional reactions to his altered physical state. Changes in appearance and body image and the frequent delay in diagnosis of the disorder because of the nonspecific, early symptoms may produce negative reactions by family members and friends. The patient may have been labeled by family and friends as mentally unstable, uncooperative, or unwilling to take proper care of himself. As hypothyroidism is treated successfully and symptoms subside, he may experience depression and guilt as a result of the progression and severity of symptoms that occurred. The patient and family are informed that the symptoms and inability to recognize them are common occurrences and part of the disorder itself. The patient and family may require assistance and counseling to deal with the emotional concerns and reactions that occur.

Patient Education and Home Health Care.   The patient with hypothyroidism and myxedema, usually an older woman, is in need of considerable follow-up, teaching, and health care. Prior to hospital discharge, arrangements are made to ensure that the patient returns to an environment that will promote adherence to the prescribed treatment plan. The patient will require encouragement and assistance in the daily administration of medications. Assistance in devising a schedule or record ensures accurate and complete administration of medications. The importance of continued thyroid hormone replacement is reinforced, and the patient and family members are instructed about the signs of over- and undermedication. A weekly visit from the community health nurse is arranged to assess the patient's physical and cognitive status and ability to cope with the recent changes.

Gerontologic Considerations.   Most patients with primary hypothyroidism are 40 to 70 years of age and present with long-standing mild to moderate hypothyroidism. The higher prevalence of hypothyroidism in the elderly may be related to alterations in immune function with age. The signs and symptoms of hypothyroidism are often atypical in the elderly; the elderly patient may have few or no symptoms until the dysfunction is severe. Depression, apathy, or decreased mobility or activity may be the major initial symptom. In all patients with hypothyroidism, the effects of analgesics, sedatives, and anesthetic agents are prolonged; particular caution is necessary in administration of these agents to the elderly because of concurrent changes in liver and renal function.

In the elderly patient with mild-to-moderate hypothyroidism, thyroid hormone replacement must be started with low doses and increased gradually to prevent serious cardiovascular and neurologic side effects. Angina, for example, may occur because of rapid thyroid replacement in the presence of coronary disease secondary to the hypothyroid state. Congestive heart failure and tachydysrhythmias may worsen during the transition from the hypothyroid state to the normal metabolic state. Dementia may become more apparent during early thyroid hormone replacement in the elderly patient.

Myxedema and myxedema coma generally occur exclusively in patients over 50 years of age. The high mortality of myxedema mandates immediate intravenous administration of high doses of thyroid hormone as well as supportive care.

Nursing care of the patient with hypothyroidism/myxedema is summarized in Nursing Care Plan 40-1.

Hyperthyroidism (Graves' Disease)

Hyperthyroidism constitutes a well-defined disease entity, commonly designated as *Graves' disease* or *exophthalmic goiter*. Its etiology is unknown, but the excessive output of thyroid hormones is thought to be due to abnormal stimulation of the thyroid gland by circulating immunoglobulins. Long-acting thyroid stimulator (LATS) is found in significant concentration in the serum of many of these patients and may be related to a defect in the patient's immune surveillance system. The disorder, which affects women five times more frequently than men and peaks in incidence in the third and fourth decades, may appear after an emotional shock, stress, or an infection, but the exact significance of these relationships is not understood.

Clinical Manifestations

Patients with well-developed hyperthyroidism exhibit a characteristic group of symptoms and signs (sometimes referred to as *thyrotoxicosis*). Their presenting symptom is often nervousness. They are often emotionally hyperexcitable, irritable, and apprehensive; they cannot sit quietly; they suffer from palpitations; and their pulse is abnormally rapid at rest as well as on exertion. They tolerate heat poorly and perspire unusually freely; the skin is flushed continuously, with a characteristic salmon color, and is likely to be warm, soft, and moist. A fine tremor of the hands may be observed. Patients may exhibit exophthalmos (bulging eyes), which produces a startled facial expression.

Other important symptoms include an increased appetite and dietary intake, progressive loss of weight, abnormal muscular fatigability and weakness, amenorrhea, and changes in bowel function, with constipation or diarrhea. The pulse rate of these patients ranges constantly between 90 and 160 beats/min; the systolic, but characteristically not diastolic, blood pressure is elevated; atrial fibrillation may occur; and cardiac decompensation in the form of congestive heart failure is common, especially in elderly patients.

The thyroid gland invariably is enlarged to some extent. It is soft and may pulsate; a thrill often can be felt and a bruit is heard over the thyroid arteries, which are signs of greatly increased blood flow through the organ.

In advanced cases, the diagnosis is made on the basis of the symptoms and the tests described previously: an increase in serum T_4 and an increased ^{131}I uptake by the thyroid, in excess of 50%.

The course of the disease may be mild, characterized by remissions and exacerbations and terminating with spontaneous recovery in the course of a few months or years. On the other hand, it may progress relentlessly, with the untreated person becoming emaciated, intensely nervous, delirious, even disoriented, and the heart eventually fails.

Symptoms of hyperthyroidism may occur with release of excessive amounts of thyroid hormone as a result of inflammation following irradiation of the thyroid or destruction of thyroid tissue by tumor. Such symptoms may also occur with

(text continues on page 1086)

Nursing Care Plan 40–1

Care of the Patient With Hypothyroidism/Myxedema

Nursing Interventions	Rationale	Expected Outcomes

MILD TO MODERATE MYXEDEMA

Nursing Diagnosis: Activity intolerance related to fatigue and depressed cognitive process

Goal: Increased participation in activities and increased independence

1. Promote independence in self-care activities.
  a. Space activities to promote rest and exercise as tolerated.
  b. Assist with self-care activities when patient is fatigued.
  c. Provide stimulation through conversation and nonstressful activities.
  d. Monitor patient's response to increasing activities.
	a. Encourages activities while allowing time for adequate rest.
	  b. Permits patient to participate to the extent possible in self-care activities.
	  c. Promotes interest without overly stressing the patient.
	  d. Guards against over- and underexertion by the patient.
		• Participates in self-care activities.
		• Reports decreased level of fatigue.
		• Displays interest and awareness in environment.
		• Participates in activities and events in environment.
		• Participates in family events and activities.
		• Reports no chest pain, increased fatigue, or breathlessness with increased level of activity.

Nursing Diagnosis: Altered body temperature

Goal: Maintenance of normal body temperature

1. Provide extra layer of clothing or extra blanket. 2. Avoid and discourage use of external heat source (*e.g.*, heating pads, electric or warming blankets) 3. Monitor patient's body temperature and report decreases from patient's baseline value. 4. Protect from exposure to cold and drafts.	1. Minimizes heat loss. 2. Reduces risk of peripheral vasodilatation and vascular collapse. 3. Detects decreased body temperature and onset of myxedema coma. 4. Increases patient's level of comfort and decreases further heat loss.	• Experiences relief of discomfort and cold intolerance. • Maintains baseline body temperature. • Reports adequate feeling of warmth and lack of chilling. • Uses extra layer of clothing or extra blanket. • Explains rationale for avoiding external heat source.

Nursing Diagnosis: Constipation related to depressed gastrointestinal function

Goal: Return of normal bowel function

1. Encourage increased fluid intake within limits of fluid restriction. 2. Provide foods high in fiber. 3. Instruct patient about foods with high water content. 4. Monitor bowel function. 5. Encourage increased mobility within patient's exercise tolerance. 6. Encourage patient to use laxatives and enemas sparingly.	1. Promotes passage of soft stools. 2. Increases bulk of stools and more frequent bowel movements. 3. Provides rationale for patient to increase fluid intake. 4. Permits detection of constipation and return to normal bowel pattern. 5. Promotes evacuation of the bowel. 6. Minimizes patient's dependence on laxatives and enemas and encourages normal pattern of bowel evacuation.	• Attains return of normal bowel function. • Reports normal bowel function. • Identifies and consumes foods high in fiber. • Drinks recommended amount of fluid each day. • Participates in gradually increasing exercises. • Uses laxatives as prescribed and avoids excessive dependence on laxatives and enemas.

(continued)

Nursing Care Plan 40–1 *(Continued)*

Care of the Patient With Hypothyroidism/Myxedema

Nursing Interventions	Rationale	Expected Outcomes

MILD TO MODERATE MYXEDEMA *(Continued)*

Nursing Diagnosis: Knowledge deficit about the therapeutic regimen for lifelong thyroid replacement therapy

Goal: Knowledge and acceptance of the prescribed therapeutic regimen

1. Explain rationale for thyroid hormone replacement	1. Provides rationale for patient to use thyroid hormone replacement as prescribed.	• Describes therapeutic regimen correctly.
2. Describe effects of medication to patient.	2. Provides encouragement to patient by identifying improved physical status and well-being that will occur with thyroid hormone therapy.	• Explains rationale for thyroid hormone replacement. • Identifies positive outcomes of thyroid hormone replacement.
3. Assist patient to develop schedule and checklist to ensure self-administration of thyroid replacement.	3. Increases assurance that medication will be taken as prescribed.	• Administers medication to self as prescribed. • Identifies adverse side effects that should be reported promptly to physician: recurrence of symptoms of hypothyroidism and occurrence of symptoms of hyperthyroidism.
4. Describe signs and symptoms of over- and underdose of medication.	4. Serves as check for patient to determine if therapeutic goals are met.	

SEVERE MYXEDEMA

Nursing Diagnosis: Ineffective breathing pattern related to depressed ventilation

Goal: Improved respiratory status and maintenance of normal breathing pattern

1. Monitor respiratory rate, depth, and pattern.	1. Identifies patient's baseline to monitor further changes and evaluate effectiveness of interventions.	• Shows improved respiratory status and maintenance of normal breathing pattern. • Demonstrates normal respiratory rate, depth, and pattern.
2. Encourage deep breathing and coughing.	2. Prevents atelectasis and promotes adequate ventilation.	• Takes deep breaths and coughs when encouraged.
3. Administer medications (hypnotics and sedatives) with caution.	3. Myxedema patients are *very* susceptible to respiratory depression because of use of hypnotics and sedatives.	• Demonstrates normal breath sounds without adventitious sounds on auscultation.
4. Maintain patent airway through suction and ventilatory support if indicated (see Chap. 22 for care of patients with ventilator).	4. Use of an artificial airway and ventilatory support may be necessary with respiratory depression.	• Explains rationale for cautious use of medications. • Cooperates with suction procedure and ventilator when necessary.

Nursing Diagnosis: Altered thought processes related to depressed metabolism and altered cardiovascular and respiratory status

Goal: Improved thought processes

1. Orient patient to time, place, date, and events around him.	1. Provides reality orientation to patient.	• Shows improved cognitive functioning. • Identifies time, place, date, and events correctly.
2. Provide stimulation through conversation and nonthreatening activities.	2. Provides stimulation within patient's level of tolerance for stress.	• Responds when stimulated.
3. Explain to patient and family that change in cognitive and mental functioning is a result of disease process.	3. Reassures patient and family about the cause of the cognitive changes and that a positive outcome is possible with appropriate treatment.	• Responds spontaneously as treatment becomes effective. • Interacts spontaneously with family and environment.
4. Monitor cognitive and mental processes and response of these to medication and other therapy.	4. Permits evaluation of the effectiveness of treatment	• Explains that change in mental and cognitive processes is a result of disease process. • Takes medications as prescribed to prevent decrease in cognitive processes.

excessive administration of thyroid hormone for treatment of hypothyroidism.

Management

As yet, no treatment for hyperthyroidism has been discovered that combats its basic cause. However, reduction of thyroid hyperactivity provides effective symptomatic relief and removes the principal source of its most important complications. Management will depend on the etiology of the hyperthyroidism.

Three forms of treatment are available for treating hyperthyroidism and controlling excessive thyroid activity: (1) pharmacotherapy, employing antithyroid drugs that interfere with the synthesis of thyroid hormones and other agents that control manifestations of hyperthyroidism; (2) irradiation, involving the administration of the radioisotope ^{131}I or ^{125}I for destructive effects on the thyroid gland; and (3) surgery, with removal of most of the thyroid gland.

Pharmacotherapy.   The objective of pharmacotherapy is to inhibit one or more stages in hormone synthesis or hormone release; another goal may be to reduce the amount of thyroid tissue, with resulting decreased thyroid hormone production.

Antithyroid drugs effectively block the utilization of iodine by interfering with the iodination of thyrosine and the coupling of iodothyrosines in the synthesis of thyroid hormones. This prevents the synthesis of thyroid hormone. The most commonly used medications are propylthiouracil (Propacil, PTU) or methimazole (Tapazole), until the patient is euthyroid (*i.e*, neither hyperthyroid nor hypothyroid). These drugs block extrathyroidal conversion of T_4 to T_3. Because antithyroid drugs do not interfere with release or activity of previously formed thyroid hormones, it may take several weeks for relief of symptoms, at which time the maintenance dose is established, followed by a gradual withdrawal of the medication over the next several months.

Therapy is determined on the basis of clinical criteria, including changes in pulse rate, pulse pressure, body weight, size of the goiter, and results of laboratory studies of thyroid function. Toxic complications of antithyroid drugs are relatively uncommon; nevertheless, periodic examinations cannot be neglected, in view of the possibility that drug sensitization, followed by fever, rash, urticaria, or even agranulocytosis and thrombocytopenia, may develop. With any sign of infection, especially pharyngitis and fever or the occurrence of mouth ulcers, the patient is advised to stop the medication, notify the physician immediately, and have hematologic studies performed. Rash, arthralgias, and fever occur in 5% of patients. Agranulocytosis is the most serious toxic side effect and occurs in 1 in every 200 patients. Its incidence is higher in those patients over 40 years of age who are treated with high doses of methimazole. It generally occurs within the first 3 months of therapy.

Patients on antithyroid drugs are instructed not to use decongestants for nasal stuffiness because they are poorly tolerated. Antithyroid drugs are contraindicated in late pregnancy because they may produce goiter and cretinism in the fetus.

Thyroid hormone may occasionally be given with antithyroid drugs to put the thyroid gland at rest. In this approach, hypothyroidism from excess antithyroid drug is avoided, as is stimulation of the thyroid gland by TSH. Thyroid hormone is available as desiccated thyroid, thyroglobulin (Proloid), and levothyroxine sodium (Synthroid). These are slow-acting preparations that take about 10 days to achieve their full effect.

Liothyronine sodium (Cytomel) has a more rapid onset and lasts a short time.

Adjunctive Therapy.   Iodine or iodide compounds, once the only therapy available for patients with hyperthyroidism, are no longer used as the sole method of treatment. Such compounds decrease the release of thyroid hormones from the thyroid gland and reduce the vascularity and size of the thyroid. Compounds such as potassium iodide, Lugol's solution, and saturated solution of potassium iodide (SSKI) are used in combination with antithyroid agents or β-adrenergic blockers to prepare the patient with hyperthyroidism for surgery. These drugs reduce the activity of the thyroid hormone and the vascularity of the thyroid gland, making the surgical procedure safer.

Solutions of iodine and iodide compounds are more palatable in milk or fruit juice and are administered through a straw to prevent staining of the teeth. These compounds reduce the metabolic rate more rapidly than antithyroid drugs, but their action does not last as long.

- Patients receiving these drugs should be observed for the development of goiter and should be cautioned against use of over-the-counter medications that contain iodides and can increase the response to iodide therapy. Cough medications, expectorants, bronchodilators, and salt substitutes may contain iodide and should be avoided by the patient receiving iodide therapy.

Beta-adrenergic blocking agents may be used to control the sympathetic nervous system effects that occur in hyperthyroidism. For example, propranolol is useful in controlling nervousness, tachycardia, tremor, anxiety, and heat intolerance.

Radioactive Iodine.   The goal of treatment with radioactive iodine (^{131}I) is to destroy the overactive thyroid cells. Almost all the iodine that enters and is retained in the body becomes concentrated in the thyroid gland. Therefore, radioactive isotope of iodine will be concentrated in the thyroid gland, where it will destroy thyroid cells without jeopardizing other radiosensitive tissues. Over a period of weeks or months, those thyroid cells exposed to the radioactive iodine will be destroyed, resulting in reduction of the hyperthyroid state and eventually hypothyroidism.

Prior to treatment with radioactive iodine, the patient receives antithyroid drugs for 6 to 18 months. Following return of thyroid hormone production to normal levels, radiation or surgical therapy can be undertaken safely.

The patient is instructed as to what to expect of this tasteless, colorless radioiodine, which is administered by the physician. If the patient is hospitalized during administration of ^{131}I, radiation safety precautions identified by the hospital's radiation safety committee should be followed. Following treatment with ^{131}I, the patient is discharged and usually followed closely until the euthyroid state is reached.

A single dose of the drug is given by mouth, based on 80 to 160 μCi/gm of estimated thyroid weight. The patient is observed for signs of thyroid storm (see p. 1089). Seventy percent to eighty-five percent of patients are cured by one dose of ^{131}I. An additional 10% to 20% require two doses; rarely is a third dose necessary.

In 3 to 4 weeks, symptoms of hyperthyroidism subside. Because the incidence of hypothyroidism following this form of treatment is very high (*i.e.*, over 90% at 10 years), close supervision is required by periodic visits to the physician to evaluate thyroid function. Thyroid hormone replacement will be necessary.

Radioactive iodine has been used in toxic adenomas or multinodular goiter and in most varieties of thyrotoxicosis (rarely permanently successful) and is preferred for the treatment of patients beyond the childbearing years with diffuse toxic goiter. It is contraindicated in pregnancy and in nursing mothers because radioiodine crosses the placenta and is secreted in breast milk.

Those caring for the patient need to give reassurance, because patients often fear such medications as radioactive drugs, which require special supervision.

Surgical Intervention. The surgical removal of about five-sixths of the thyroid tissue (subtotal thyroidectomy) practically assures a prolonged remission in most patients with exophthalmic goiter. Before surgery, the patient is given propylthiouracil until signs of hyperthyroidism have disappeared. Iodine (Lugol's solution or potassium iodide) is prescribed to reduce the size and the vascularity of the goiter.

- Patients receiving iodine medication must be monitored for evidence of iodine toxicity (iodism), the appearance of which is the signal for immediate withdrawal of the drug. Symptoms of iodism include swelling of the buccal mucosa, excessive salivation, coryza, and skin eruptions.

Thyroidectomy for treatment of hyperthyroidism usually is scheduled soon after the patient's basal metabolic rate has been reduced to normal. Management of the patient undergoing thyroidectomy is discussed on p. 1091.

Relapse Rate and Risk of Hyperthyroidism Following Treatment. None of the treatments for thyrotoxicosis is without side effects, and all three forms of treatment (*i.e.*, antithyroid drugs, surgery, and radioactive iodine therapy) share the same complications: relapse or recurrent hyperthyroidism and permanent hypothyroidism. The rate of relapse is increased in patients who initially had very severe disease, a long history of dysfunction, ocular and cardiac symptoms, large goiter, and relapse after previous treatment. Although reports of rate of relapse and the occurrence of hypothyroidism vary among studies, relapse with antithyroid drugs is approximately 45% 1 year following completion of therapy and almost 75% 5 years later. Discontinuation of antithyroid drugs before therapy is complete usually results in relapse within 6 months in the majority of patients. The relapse rate following radioactive iodine therapy approaches 26% at 1 year; hypothyroidism occurs in almost 28% of patients at 1 year and in 90% to 100% by 5 years. The incidence of relapse with subtotal thyroidectomy is 19% at 18 months; an incidence of hypothyroidism of 25% has been reported at 18 months after surgery. The risk of these complications illustrates the necessity for long-term follow-up of patients undergoing treatment of hyperthyroidism.

Gerontologic Considerations

Patients over age 60 account for 10% to 20% of the cases of thyrotoxicosis. Although some older patients develop typical signs and symptoms of thyrotoxicosis, in most, an atypical picture is present. The major symptoms of the elderly patient with hyperthyroidism may be depression and apathy, often accompanied by significant weight loss. In addition, the patient may report cardiovascular symptoms and difficulty climbing stairs or rising from a chair because of muscle weakness. The elderly patient may experience a single manifestation such as atrial fibrillation, anorexia, or weight loss. These general symptoms may mask the underlying thyroid disease. Spontaneous remission of hyperthyroidism is rare in the elderly. Measurement of T_4 and T_3 uptake is indicated in elderly patients with unexplained physical or mental deterioration.

The use of ^{131}I is generally recommended for treatment of thyrotoxicosis in the elderly rather than surgery unless an enlarged thyroid gland is pressing on the airway. However, the hypermetabolic state of thyrotoxicosis must be controlled by antithyroid drugs before ^{131}I is used because radiation may precipitate thyroid storm by increasing the release of hormone from the thyroid gland. Thyroid storm, if it occurs, has a mortality rate of 10% in the elderly.

The use of β-blockers may be indicated to decrease the cardiovascular and neurologic signs and symptoms of thyrotoxicosis. However, these agents must be used with extreme caution to minimize adverse effects on cardiac function that may produce congestive heart failure. If antithyroid agents are used, the patient must be monitored closely because the elderly patient is more likely to develop granulocytopenia.

The dosage of other medications to treat other chronic illnesses in the elderly patient may need modification because of the altered rate of metabolism in hyperthyroidism.

▶ **Nursing Process**
The Patient With Hyperthyroidism

▷ **Assessment**

The health history and examination focus on the occurrence of symptoms related to accelerated or exaggerated metabolism. These include the patient's and family's report of irritability and increased emotional reaction. It is also important to determine the impact that these changes have had on the patient's interaction with family, friends, and co-workers. The history includes other stressors and the patient's ability to cope with stress. Nutritional status and the presence of symptoms are assessed. The occurrence of symptoms related to excessive output of the nervous system and changes in vision and the appearance of the eyes are noted.

▷ **Nursing Diagnoses**

Based on all the assessment data, the major nursing diagnoses of the patient with hyperthyroidism include the following:

- Altered nutrition related to exaggerated metabolic rate, excessive appetite, and increased gastrointestinal activity
- Ineffective coping related to irritability, hyperexcitability, apprehension, and emotional instability
- Disturbance in self-esteem related to changes in appearance, excessive appetite, and weight loss
- Altered body temperature

▷ **Planning and Implementation**

▷ *Goals:* The patient's goals may be improved nutritional status, improved coping ability, improved self-esteem, and maintenance of normal body temperature.

▷ **Nursing Interventions**

▷ *Improvement of Nutritional Status.* Hyperthyroidism affects all body systems, including the gastrointestinal system. The patient's appetite is increased but may be satisfied by several well-balanced meals of small size, even up to six meals a day. Foods and fluids are selected to replace fluid lost through diarrhea and diaphoresis and to control diarrhea that results from increased peristalsis. Rapid movement of food through the gastrointestinal tract may result in nutritional imbalance and further weight loss. In order to reduce diarrhea, highly seasoned foods and stimulants such as coffee, tea, cola, and alcohol are discouraged. High-calorie, high-protein foods are encouraged. A quiet atmosphere during mealtime may aid digestion. The patient's weight and dietary intake are recorded to monitor nutritional status.

▷ *Coping Measures.*   The patient with hyperthyroidism needs assurance that the emotional reactions he is experiencing are a result of the disorder and that with effective treatment those symptoms will be controlled. Because of the negative effect that these symptoms have on interaction and communication of the patient with family and friends, they too need reassurance that these symptoms are expected to disappear with treatment. It is important to use a calm, unhurried approach with the patient. Additionally, stressful experiences are minimized; therefore, the patient is not placed in a hospital room with very ill or talkative patients. The environment is kept quiet and uncluttered. Noises, such as loud music, conversation, and equipment alarms, are minimized. Relaxing activities are encouraged if they do not overstimulate the patient.

If thyroidectomy is planned, the patient is likely to be apprehensive and anxious about the surgery. The patient is informed that while surgery is planned, treatment is necessary to prepare the patient and the thyroid gland for surgical treatment. The patient is assisted by the nurse to take the medications as prescribed and to develop a plan to encourage adherence to the therapeutic regimen. The patient's hyperexcitability and shortened attention span may necessitate repetition of this information and written instructions.

▷ *Improved Self-Esteem.*   The hyperthyroid patient is likely to experience changes in appearance, appetite, and weight that are beyond his control. These factors, along with the patient's recognition that he is not coping well with his family, environment, and illness, may result in loss of self-esteem. The nurse conveys to the patient an understanding of his concern about these problems and expresses willingness to assist him to deal with them. The patient is informed that these changes are a result of the dysfunction of the thyroid gland and are in fact out of his control. If changes in appearance are very disturbing to the patient, mirrors may be removed from the room so that the patient is not constantly reminded of his changed appearance. In addition, family members and personnel are reminded to avoid bringing these changes to the patient's attention. The nurse explains to the patient that most of these changes are expected to disappear after effective treatment. If the patient experiences eye changes secondary to hyperthyroidism, eye care and protection may become necessary. The patient may need instructions about correct instillation of eye drops or ointment prescribed to soothe the eyes and protect the exposed cornea.

The patient may be embarrassed by the very large meals that he consumes as a result of his greatly increased metabolic rate. Therefore, the nurse arranges the setting so that the patient eats alone if desired and avoids commenting on the large dietary intake of the patient, while at the same time making sure that the patient receives sufficient food.

▷ *Maintenance of Normal Body Temperature.*   The patient with hyperthyroidism frequently finds a normal room temperature uncomfortably warm because of his exaggerated metabolic rate and heat production. The nurse provides a cool, comfortable environment for the patient and provides fresh bedding and gown as needed. Giving cool baths, providing cool or cold fluids, and monitoring body temperature are important in providing relief. The reason for the patient's discomfort and the importance of providing a cool environment are explained to the family and staff.

▷ *Patient Education and Home Health Care.*   The patient with hyperthyroidism is instructed how and when to take prescribed medication. Additionally, he needs to know how the medication regimen fits in with the broader therapeutic plan. Because of the patient's hyperexcitability and decreased attention span, a written plan is provided for the patient to use at home. The type and amount of information given to the patient are individualized because of the resulting stress and possible emotional reactions by the patient. The patient and family members receive verbal and written information about the desired effects as well as possible side effects of the medications. The patient is instructed by the nurse about which adverse effects should be reported to the physician. The importance of long-term follow-up is stressed because of the possibility of hypothyroidism following thyroidectomy or treatment with antithyroid drugs or [131]I.

If the patient is expected to have a total or subtotal thyroidectomy, he is informed about what to expect. This information, however, will be repeated to the patient as the time of surgery approaches. The patient is also instructed to avoid those situations that have the potential to stimulate the life-threatening occurrence of thyroid storm.

▷ Evaluation

Expected Outcomes

1. Improves nutritional status.
   a. Reports adequate dietary intake and decreased feelings of hunger.
   b. Reports stabilization of weight.
   c. Identifies high-calorie, high-protein foods.
   d. Explains reasons for increased appetite.
   e. Identifies foods to be avoided on diet.
   f. Avoids use of alcohol and other stimulants.
   g. Reports decreased episodes of diarrhea.
   h. Demonstrates normal skin turgor and normal fluid balance.
2. Demonstrates effective coping methods in dealing with family, friends, and co-workers.
   a. Reports more effective conversation and interaction with family, friends, and co-workers.
   b. Explains reasons for irritability and emotional instability.
   c. Identifies situations, events, and people that are stress-producing.
   d. Avoids stressful situations, events, and people.
   e. Participates in relaxing, nonstressful activities.
   f. Explains to family and friends reasons for irritability and expectation that behavior will change when treatment takes effect.

g. Identifies expected goals/outcomes of surgery or other treatment.

h. Explains reason for delay in surgery and identifies own role during waiting period.

i. Takes medications as prescribed in preparation for surgery or other treatment.

3. Achieves increased self-esteem.

a. Verbalizes feelings about self and illness.

b. Describes feelings of frustration and loss of control to others.

c. Describes reasons for increased appetite.

d. Discusses events in environment rather than concentrating on changes in own appearance.

e. Dresses in attractive clothes that do not emphasize changes in physical appearance.

4. Maintains normal body temperature.

a. Reports relief of discomfort and a more comfortable environment.

b. Uses clothing or bedding that is cool and comfortable.

c. Notifies staff when fresh clothing or bedding is needed.

d. Reports normal body temperature.

e. Drinks cool fluids within fluid allowance.

f. Uses air conditioner or fan if indicated.

g. Avoids hot, uncomfortable environments.

Thyroid Storm (Thyrotoxic Crisis)

Thyroid storm (thyrotoxic crisis) is a form of severe hyperthyroidism, usually of abrupt onset and characterized by high fever (hyperpyrexia), extreme tachycardia, and altered mental state, which frequently appears as delirium. Thyroid storm is a life-threatening condition and is usually precipitated by stress such as injury, infection, nonthyroid surgery, thyroidectomy, tooth extraction, insulin reaction, diabetic acidosis, pregnancy, digitalis intoxication, abrupt withdrawal of antithyroid drugs, or vigorous palpation of the thyroid. These factors will precipitate thyroid storm in the partially controlled or completely untreated hyperthyroid patient. Patients who are maintained in a euthyroid state through the proper adjustment of an antithyroid drug may experience stressful conditions uneventfully and without thyrotoxic crisis.

Although thyroid crisis may be difficult to identify, the following signs are suggestive: (1) tachycardia (over 130 beats/min), (2) temperature above 37.7°C (100°F), (3) exaggerated symptoms of hyperthyroidism, and (4) disturbances of a major system, for example, gastrointestinal (weight loss, diarrhea, abdominal pain), neurologic (psychosis, somnolence, coma), or cardiovascular (edema, chest pain, dyspnea, palpitations).

Untreated thyroid storm is almost always fatal, but with proper treatment the mortality rate can be reduced substantially.

Management. The immediate objective is to reduce body temperature and heart rate and prevent vascular collapse. Measures to reduce the temperature include a hypothermia mattress or blanket, ice packs, a cool environment, and hydrocortisone.

- Salicylates are not used because they displace thyroid hormone from binding proteins and worsen the hypermetabolism.

Humidified oxygen is administered to improve tissue oxygenation and meet the high metabolic demands. Intravenous fluids containing dextrose are administered to replace liver glycogen stores that have been decreased in the hyperthyroid patient. Propylthiouracil (PTU) or methimazole is given to impede formation of thyroid hormone and block conversion of T_4 to T_3, the more active form of thyroid hormone. Hydrocortisone is prescribed to treat shock or adrenal insufficiency. Iodine is administered to decrease output of T_4 from the thyroid gland. For cardiac problems such as atrial fibrillation, dysrhythmias, and congestive heart failure, sympatholytic agents may be given. Propranolol in combination with digitalis has been effective in reducing severe cardiac symptoms.

- The patient with thyroid storms or crisis is critically ill and requires astute observation and aggressive and supportive nursing care during and after the acute stage of illness. Care of the patient with hyperthyroidism is the basis of nursing management of the critically ill patient with thyroid storm or crisis.

Thyroiditis

Subacute or granulomatous thyroiditis (deQuervain's thyroiditis), an inflammatory disorder of the thyroid gland that predominantly affects women in their 50s, presents as a painful swelling in the anterior neck that lasts 1 or 2 months and then disappears spontaneously without residual effect. There is evidence that this disorder may be due to a viral infection. The thyroid enlarges symmetrically and occasionally is painful. The overlying skin is often reddened and warm. Swallowing may be difficult and uncomfortable. Irritability, nervousness, insomnia, and weight loss—manifestations of hyperthyroidism—are common, and many patients experience chills and fever as well.

Another form of thyroiditis occurs in the postpartum period and is thought to be an autoimmune reaction.

The purpose of treatment is to control the inflammation. In general, acetylsalicylic acid (aspirin) controls the symptoms of inflammation in mild cases but should be avoided if symptoms of hyperthyroidism occur, because it displaces thyroid hormone from its binding sites and increases the amount of circulating hormone. Beta blocking agents may be used to control symptoms of hyperthyroidism; antithyroid agents, which block the synthesis of T_4 and T_3, are *not* effective in thyroiditis because the associated thyrotoxicosis results from the release of stored thyroid hormones rather than from their increased synthesis. In more severe cases, glucocorticoids may be effective but do not usually affect the underlying cause.

Chronic Thyroiditis (Hashimoto's Thyroiditis). Chronic thyroiditis, which occurs most frequently in women 30 to 50 years of age, has been termed *Hashimoto's disease,* depending on the histologic appearance of the inflamed gland. In contrast to acute thyroiditis, the chronic forms are usually not accompanied by pain, pressure symptoms, or fever, and thyroid activity is usually normal or low, rather than increased.

There is evidence that cell-mediated immunity plays a significant role in the pathogenesis of thyroiditis. A genetic predisposition also seems to be significant in its etiology. If untreated, the disease runs a slow, progressive course, leading eventually to hypothyroidism.

The objective of treatment is to reduce the size of the thyroid gland and prevent myxedema. Thyroid hormone therapy is prescribed to reduce thyroid activity and the production of thyroglobulin. If hypothyroid symptoms are present, thyroid hormone is given. Surgery may be required if pressure symptoms persist.

Thyroid Tumors

Tumors of the thyroid gland are classified on the basis of being benign or malignant, as well as on the presence or absence of associated thyrotoxicosis and the diffuse or irregular quality of the glandular enlargement. If the enlargement is sufficient to cause a visible swelling in the neck, the tumor is referred to as a *goiter*.

All grades of goiter are encountered, from those that are barely visible to those producing disfigurement. Some are symmetrical and diffuse, others nodular. Some are accompanied by hyperthyroidism, in which case they are described as *toxic;* others are associated with a euthyroid state and are called *nontoxic* goiters.

Endemic (Iodine-Deficient) Goiter. The most common type of goiter, encountered chiefly in geographic regions where the natural supply of iodine is deficient (*e.g.*, the Great Lakes areas of the United States), is the so-called simple or colloid goiter. Aside from being caused by an iodine deficiency, simple goiter may also be caused by an intake of large quantities of goitrogenic substances in patients with unusually susceptible glands. These substances include excessive amounts of iodine or lithium, which is currently used in the treatment of manic-depressive states.

Simple goiter represents a compensatory hypertrophy of the thyroid gland, presumably due to stimulation by the pituitary gland. The pituitary gland produces a hormone controlling thyroid growth, and this production increases if there is subnormal thyroid activity, as when insufficient iodine is available for production of the thyroid hormone. Such goiters usually cause no symptoms except for the swelling in the neck, which may result in tracheal compression when excessive.

Management. Many goiters of this type recede after iodine imbalance is corrected. Supplementary iodine such as saturated solution of potassium iodide (SSKI) is prescribed in order to depress the pituitary's thyroid-stimulating activity.

When surgery is recommended, postoperative complications can be minimized when certain criteria exist: (1) a relatively young person without the complications of concurrent medical illnesses, such as diabetes, heart disease, drug allergies; (2) a preoperative euthyroid state resulting from treatment with antithyroid drugs; (3) preoperative iodide administration to reduce the size and vascularity of the goiter; and (4) a surgical team experienced in thyroid surgery.

Patient Education. Simple or endemic goiter can be prevented by providing children in iodine-poor districts with iodine compounds. If the mean iodine intake is less than 40 μg/day, the thyroid gland hypertrophies. The World Health Organization recommends that salt be iodized to a concentration of one part in 100,000, which is adequate for the prevention of endemic goiter. In the United States, salt is iodized to one part in 10,000. The introduction of iodized salt has been the single most effective means of preventing goiter in susceptible populations.

Nodular Goiter. Certain thyroid glands are nodular because of the presence of one or several areas of *hyperplasia* (overgrowth) that appear to develop under conditions similar to those responsible for the colloid or simple goiter. No symptoms may arise as a result of this condition, but, not uncommonly, these nodules slowly increase in size, with some descending into the thorax, where they cause local pressure symptoms. Some nodules become malignant and some become associated with a hyperthyroid state. Thus, many nodular thyroids eventually require surgical intervention.

Thyroid Cancer

Cancer of the thyroid is much less prevalent than other forms of cancer. According to the American Cancer Society, approximately 1000 patients die annually of this malignancy. The most common type is *papillary adenocarcinoma*, which accounts for over half of thyroid malignancies. This neoplasm starts in childhood or early adult life, remains localized, and eventually metastasizes along the lymphatics and lymph nodes if untreated. It appears as an asymptomatic nodule in a normal gland. If papillary adenocarcinoma occurs in the elderly, it is generally more aggressive, as are other types of thyroid cancer when they occur in the elderly. The risk of malignancy increases with family history of thyroid cancer.

An association exists between external radiation of the head, neck, or chest in infancy and childhood and subsequent development of thyroid carcinoma. Between 1940 and 1960, radiation therapy was occasionally used to shrink enlarged tonsillar and adenoid tissue, to treat acne, or to reduce an enlarged thymus.

For people exposed to external radiation in childhood, there appears to be a continuing increase in thyroid cancer 5 to 40 years after irradiation. Consequently, people who underwent such treatment should consult a physician, request an isotope thyroid scan as part of the evaluation, follow recommended treatment of abnormalities of the gland, and continue with annual checkups if all is normal.

Follicular adenocarcinoma appears in later life, usually over age 40, and accounts for 20% to 25% of thyroid neoplasms. It is encapsulated and feels elastic or rubbery on palpation. This tumor eventually spreads by hematogenous routes to bone, liver, and lung. The prognosis is not as favorable as for papillary adenocarcinoma.

Lesions that are single and hard and fixed on palpation or associated with cervical lymphadenopathy suggest malignancy.

Other types of cancer are *medullary* (5%), which presents as solid, hard nodular tumors, and *anaplastic* (5%), which is hard, irregular masses that grow quickly and may be painful and tender. Almost 50% of anaplastic thyroid carcinomas are found in patients over 60 years of age. These tumors have an exceedingly poor prognosis.

Diagnostic Evaluation. The tests of thyroid function may be helpful in the evaluation of thyroid nodules and masses. However, their results are rarely conclusive.

Needle biopsy of the thyroid gland is used as an outpatient procedure to make a diagnosis of thyroid cancer and to differentiate cancerous thyroid nodules from noncancerous ones. The procedure is safe and usually requires only a local anesthetic. However, patients who undergo the procedure are followed closely because cancerous tissues may be missed during the procedure. Additional diagnostic studies include ultrasound, thyroid scans, and thyroid suppression tests.

Management. The treatment of choice of thyroid carcinoma is surgical removal. Total or near-total thyroidectomy is performed when possible.

Modified neck dissection is performed if there is lymph node involvement. Following surgery, ablation procedures are carried out with ^{131}I to eradicate residual thyroid tissue if the tumor is radiosensitive. Radioactive iodine also maximizes the chance of discovering thyroid metastasis at a later date if total body scans are carried out.

Following surgery, thyroid hormone is administered in suppressive doses to lower the levels of TSH to a euthyroid state.

Patient Education. Postoperatively, the patient will require instructions about the need to take exogenous thyroid hormone to prevent the occurrence of hypothyroidism. Later follow-up includes clinical assessment for recurrence of nodules or masses in the neck and signs of hoarseness, dysphagia, or dyspnea. Chest x-ray films are performed as recommended. Total body scans are advised annually for the first 3 postoperative years and less frequently thereafter. Prior to planned total body scans, thyroid hormones are stopped for about a month preceding the tests.

T_4, TSH, serum calcium, and phosphorus levels are monitored to determine if the thyroid hormone supplementation is adequate and to note whether calcium balance is maintained.

Although local and systemic reactions to radiation may occur and may include neutropenia or thrombocytopenia (see p. 807), these complications are rare when ^{131}I is used. Surgery combined with radioiodine produces a higher survival rate than does surgery alone.

Thyroidectomy

Partial or complete thyroidectomy may be carried out as primary treatment of thyroid carcinoma, hyperthyroidism, or hyperparathyroidism. The type and extent of the surgery depend on the diagnosis, goal of surgery, and prognosis.

Preoperative Management. Before undergoing surgery for treatment of hyperthyroidism (see p. 1086), the patient will be treated with appropriate drug therapy to return his thyroid hormone levels and metabolic rate to normal and to reduce the risk of thyroid storm and hemorrhage during the postoperative period. One important approach in the preoperative period is to gain the confidence of the patient and lessen his anxiety. Some forms of occupational therapy are recommended if they are quieting and relaxing.

The patient with hyperthyroidism often comes from a home made tense by his restlessness, irritability, and nervousness. It is necessary to protect the patient from such tension and stress in order to avoid precipitating thyroid storm. If there is evidence of increased stress when family or friends visit, it may be advisable to limit visiting privileges during the preoperative period.

Nutritional intake is regulated to include adequate carbohydrate and protein foods. A high daily caloric intake is necessary because of the increased metabolic activity and rapid depletion of glycogen reserves. Supplementary vitamins, particularly thiamine and ascorbic acid, are provided. Tea, coffee, cola, and other stimulants are avoided.

If the patient is to undergo diagnostic testing prior to surgery, he is informed of the purpose of the test and the preoperative preparations in order to reduce anxiety. In addition, special efforts are made to ensure a good night's rest preceding surgery.

Preoperative teaching includes demonstrating to the patient how to support his neck with his hands after surgery to prevent stress on the incision; that is, raising his elbows and placing his hands behind his neck will provide support and put much less strain and tension on the neck muscles and the surgical incision.

Postoperative Management. The patient is moved and turned carefully so as to support the head and avoid tension on the sutures. The most comfortable position is the semi-Fowler's position with the head elevated and supported by pillows. Narcotics are administered as prescribed for pain. The patient may receive humidified oxygen to facilitate breathing. The nurse should anticipate apprehension in the patient and inform him that oxygen will assist his breathing and provide humidity. Intravenous fluids will be administered during the immediate postoperative period; water may be given by mouth as soon as nausea ceases. Usually, there is a little difficulty in swallowing; initially, cold fluids and ice may be taken better than other fluids. Often patients prefer a soft diet to a liquid diet in the immediate postoperative period.

The surgical dressings should be checked periodically and reinforced when necessary. It is important to remember that when the patient is in the dorsal position, the sides and the back of the neck as well as the anterior dressing are to be observed for bleeding. In addition to monitoring the pulse and the blood pressure for any indication of internal bleeding, it is also important to be on the alert for complaints of sensation of pressure or fullness at the incision site. Such symptoms may indicate hemorrhage subcutaneously and should be reported.

Occasionally, difficulty in respiration occurs as a result of edema of the glottis or an injury to the recurrent laryngeal nerve. This complication requires that an airway be inserted. Therefore, a tracheostomy set is kept at the patient's bedside at all times, and the surgeon is summoned at the first indication of respiratory distress.

The patient is advised to talk as little as possible, but when he does speak, the nurse should note any voice changes that might indicate injury to the recurrent laryngeal nerve, which lies just behind the thyroid next to the trachea.

An over-bed table may be used to provide easy access to those materials and items that are needed frequently, such as paper tissues, water pitcher and glass, and a small emesis basin. These are kept within easy reach so that the patient will not need to turn his head in search of them. It is also convenient to use this table when vapor-mist inhalations are given for the relief of excessive mucus secretions.

The patient usually is permitted out of bed as soon as he feels able, and he is provided his choice of diet. A well-balanced, high-calorie diet is prescribed to promote weight gain. Sutures or skin clips usually are removed on the second day. The patient is usually ready for discharge from the hospital the day of surgery or soon afterward if the postoperative course is uncomplicated.

Complications. Hemorrhage, edema of the glottis, and injury to the recurrent laryngeal nerve are complications that have been reviewed previously. Occasionally, in thyroid operations, the parathyroid glands may be injured or removed, producing a disturbance of the calcium metabolism of the body. As the blood calcium level falls, hyperirritability of the nerves, with spasms of the hands and feet and muscular twitchings, occurs. This group of symptoms is termed *tetany,* and its appearance should be reported at once because laryngospasm, although rare, may occur and obstruct the patient's airway. Tetany of this type is usually treated by the intravenous administration of calcium gluconate. This calcium abnormality may be temporary following thyroidectomy.

Patient Education and Home Health Care. The necessity for rest, relaxation, and nutrition is explained to both the patient and his family. Specific instructions are given regarding follow-up visits to the physician or the clinic, which are important for monitoring the patient's thyroid status. The patient should be permitted to resume his former activities and responsibilities completely once he has recovered from surgery.

Responsibilities and factors relating to the home environment that produce emotional tension often have been implicated as precipitating causes of thyrotoxicosis. The patient's hospitalization affords an opportunity to evaluate these factors and possibly alter the environmental situation.

Prevention of Radiation-Induced Thyroid Damage and Cancer

The thyroid gland has a very efficient mechanism to remove iodine from the bloodstream and concentrate or "trap" it for subsequent synthesis of thyroid hormone. The effectiveness of this mechanism to concentrate iodide is reflected in a concentration of iodide 20 to 40 times the concentration of iodide in the plasma. If milk and other food sources become contaminated with radioactivity as a result of a nuclear detonation or a nuclear power plant accident, the radioactive iodide would become concentrated in the thyroid gland at this very high concentration, irradiate the thyroid gland, and increase the risk of thyroid gland cancer. Therefore, in communities exposed to increased radioactivity, attempts have been made to block the uptake of radioactive iodide by flooding or saturating the thyroid gland with nonradioactive iodide. Saturated solutions of potassium iodide (SSKI) or other iodide preparations administered as soon as possible after exposure occurs almost completely inhibit thyroid absorption of the radioactive iodide and promote rapid excretion of any that is absorbed.

The Parathyroid Glands

Hyperparathyroidism

Hyperparathyroidism, which is due to overproduction of parathyroid hormone by the parathyroid glands, is characterized by bone calcification and the development of renal stones containing calcium. Primary hyperparathyroidism occurs two to four times more often in women than in men and is most frequently seen in patients over 70 years of age. Secondary hyperparathyroidism with similar manifestations occurs in patients with chronic renal failure and so-called renal rickets as a result of phosphorus retention, increased stimulation of the parathyroid glands, and increased parathyroid hormone secretion.

Clinical Manifestations and Diagnosis. The patient may have no symptoms or may experience signs and symptoms resulting from involvement of several body systems. He may develop apathy, fatigue, muscular weakness, nausea, vomiting, constipation, and cardiac dysrhythmias, all attributable to an increased concentration of calcium in the blood. Psychologic manifestations may vary from emotional irritability and neurosis to psychoses due to the direct effect of calcium on the brain and nervous system. An increase in calcium produces an increase in the excitation potential of nerve and muscle tissue. Occasionally, the patient may be misdiagnosed as "psychoneurotic."

The formation of stones in one or both kidneys, related to the increased urinary excretion of calcium and phosphorus, is one of the important complications of hyperparathyroidism and occurs in 55% of patients with primary hyperparathyroidism. Renal damage results from the precipitation of calcium phosphate in the renal pelvis and parenchyma, resulting in renal calculi (kidney stones), obstruction, pyelonephritis, and uremia.

Musculoskeletal symptoms accompanying hyperparathyroidism may result from demineralization of the bones or bone tumors, composed of benign giant cells resulting from overgrowth of osteoclasts. The patient may develop skeletal pain and tenderness, especially of the back and joints; pain on weight-bearing; pathologic fractures; deformities; and shortening of body stature.

The incidence of peptic ulcer and pancreatitis is increased with hyperparathyroidism and may be responsible for many of the gastrointestinal symptoms that occur.

The diagnosis of primary hyperparathyroidism is established on the basis of increased serum calcium levels and an elevated level of parathormone. Radioimmunoassays for parathormone are very sensitive and differentiate primary hyperparathyroidism from other causes of hypercalcemia in more than 90% of patients with elevated serum calcium levels. An elevated serum calcium level is a nonspecific finding because serum levels may be altered by diet, medications, and renal and bone changes. Bone changes may be detected on x-ray films in advanced cases of the disease. Ultrasound, MRI, thallium scan, and fine-needle biopsy have been used to evaluate the function of the parathyroids and to localize parathyroid cysts, adenomas, or hyperplasia.

Management. The insidious onset and chronic nature of hyperparathyroidism, and its diverse and often vague symptoms, may result in depression and frustration of the patient. The family may have considered the patient's illness to be psychosomatic. An awareness of the course of the disorder and an understanding approach by the nurse may help the patient and family to deal with their reactions and feelings.

The treatment of primary hyperparathyroidism is the surgical removal of abnormal parathyroid tissue. In the preoperative period it must be recognized that kidney involvement is possible, because these patients are subject to renal calculi. A fluid intake of 2000 ml or more is encouraged to help prevent calculus formation. Cranberry juice is suggested because there is evidence that it may lower urinary *p*H. It can be added to juices and ginger ale for variety. Because of the possibility of stone formation, urine is strained and any evidence of calculi is saved for laboratory analysis. The patient is observed for other manifestations of renal calculi, such as abdominal pain and hematuria. Thiazide diuretics should not be used in the patient with hyperparathyroidism because they decrease the renal excretion of calcium and cause further elevations in serum calcium levels.

Mobility of the patient, with walking or use of a rocking chair, is encouraged as much as possible because bones subjected to normal stress give up less calcium. Bed rest, on the other hand, increases calcium excretion and predisposes the patient to formation of renal calculi.

Oral phosphate lowers the serum calcium level in some patients. Long-term use is not recommended because of ectopic calcium phosphate deposits in soft tissues.

Nutritional needs are met, but foods high in calcium and phosphorus, such as milk and milk products, are limited. If the patient has a coexisting peptic ulcer, specifically prescribed antacids and protein feedings will be necessary. Because anorexia is common, efforts are made to encourage the patient's appetite. Prune juice, stool softeners, and physical activity, along with increased fluid intake, help to offset constipation, which is a common postoperative problem for this patient.

The nursing management of the patient undergoing parathyroidectomy is essentially the same as that for a thyroidectomy patient (see p. 1091). Although not all parathyroid tissue will be removed during surgery in an effort to maintain control of calcium–phosphorus balance, the patient must be monitored closely to detect symptoms of tetany, which may be an early postoperative complication. Most patients quickly regain function of the remaining parathyroid tissue and experience only mild, transient postoperative hypocalcemia. In patients with significant bone disease or bone changes, a more prolonged period of hypocalcemia should be anticipated.

Hypercalcemic Crisis. Acute hypercalcemic crisis can occur in hyperparathyroidism. This occurs with extreme elevation of serum calcium levels. Serum calcium levels higher than 15 mg/dl (3.7 mmol/L) result in neurologic, cardiovascular, and renal symptoms that can be life-threatening. Treatment includes rehydration with large volumes of intravenous fluids, diuretic agents to promote renal excretion of excess calcium, and phosphate therapy to correct hypophosphatemia and decrease serum calcium levels by promoting calcium deposit in bone and decreasing gastrointestinal absorption of calcium. Cytotoxic agents, calcitonin, and dialysis may be used in emergency situations to decrease serum calcium levels quickly. The patient in acute hypercalcemic crisis requires close monitoring for complications, deterioration of his condition, and reversal of serum calcium levels.

A combination of calcitonin and glucocorticoids has been administered in emergencies to reduce the serum calcium level by increasing calcium deposition in bone.

The patient requires expert assessment and care to minimize complications and reverse the life-threatening hypercalcemia. Medications are administered with care, and attention is given to fluid balance to promote return of normal fluid and electrolyte balance in this patent. Supportive measures are necessary for the patient and family.

Hypoparathyroidism

The most common cause of hypoparathyroidism is inadequate secretion of parathyroid hormone following interruption of the blood supply or surgical removal of parathyroid gland tissue during thyroidectomy, parathyroidectomy, or radical neck dissection. Atrophy of the parathyroid glands of unknown etiology is a less common cause of hypoparathyroidism.

Pathophysiology. Symptoms of hypoparathyroidism are due to a deficiency of parathormone that results in an elevation of blood phosphate (hyperphosphatemia) and a decrease in the concentration of blood calcium (hypocalcemia). Hypocalcemia results because in the absence of parathormone there is decreased intestinal absorption of dietary calcium and decreased resorption of calcium from bone and through the renal tubules. Decreased renal excretion of phosphate causes hypophosphaturia, and low serum calcium levels result in hypocalciuria.

Clinical Manifestations. Hypocalcemia causes irritability of the neuromuscular system and contributes to the chief symptom of hypoparathyroidism, *tetany*—a general muscular hypertonia, with tremor and spasmodic or uncoordinated contractions occurring with or without efforts to make voluntary movements. In latent tetany there is numbness, tingling, and cramps in the extremities, with the patient complaining of stiffness in the hands and feet. In overt tetany the signs include bronchospasm, laryngeal spasm, carpopedal spasm (flexion of the elbows and wrists and extension of the carpophalangeal joints; see Fig. 18-6), dysphagia, photophobia, cardiac dysrhythmias, and convulsions. Other symptoms include anxiety, irritability, depression, and even delirium.

Diagnostic Evaluation. Latent tetany is suggested by a positive Trousseau's sign or a positive Chvostek's sign. *Trousseau's sign* is positive when carpopedal spasm is induced by occluding the blood flow to the arm for 3 minutes with use of a blood pressure cuff. *Chvostek's sign* is positive when a sharp tapping over the facial nerve just in front of the parotid gland and anterior to the ear causes the mouth, nose, and eye to twitch.

The diagnosis is often difficult because of vague symptoms of aches and pains. Therefore, laboratory studies are especially helpful. Tetany develops at serum calcium levels of 5 to 6 mg/dl (1.2 to 1.5 mmol/L) or lower. Serum phosphate levels are increased, and x-ray studies of bone show increased density. Calcification is detected on x-ray films of subcutaneous or paraspinal basal ganglia of the brain.

Management. The objective of therapy is to raise the serum calcium level to 9 to 10 mg/dl (2.2 to 2.5 mmol/L) and to eliminate the symptoms of hypoparathyroidism and hypocalcemia. When hypocalcemia and tetany occur following a thyroidectomy, the immediate treatment is to administer calcium gluconate intravenously. If this does not decrease neuromuscular irritability and seizure activity immediately, sedatives such as pentobarbital may be administered.

Parenteral parathormone can be administered to treat acute hypoparathyroidism with tetany. However, the high incidence of allergic reactions to injections of parathormone limits its use to acute episodes of hypocalcemia. The patient receiving parathormone is monitored closely for changes in serum calcium levels and allergic reactions.

Because of neuromuscular irritability, the patient with hypocalcemia and tetany requires an environment that is free of noise, sudden drafts, bright lights, or sudden movement.

Tracheostomy or mechanical ventilation may become necessary, along with bronchodilating medications, if the patient develops respiratory distress.

Nursing management of the patient with possible acute hypoparathyroidism includes the following actions:

- The attention of the nurse in the care of postoperative patients having thyroidectomy, parathyroidectomy, and radical neck dissection is directed toward anticipating signs of tetany, convulsions, and respiratory difficulties.
- Calcium gluconate is kept at the bedside with equipment necessary for intravenous administration. If the patient has cardiac problems, is subject to dysrhythmias, or is receiving digitalis, then calcium gluconate is administered slowly and cautiously.
- Calcium and digitalis increase systolic contraction, and, furthermore, they potentiate each other. This may produce potentially fatal dysrhythmias. Consequently, the cardiac patient requires continuous cardiac monitoring and careful assessment.

Therapy for the patient with chronic hypoparathyroidism is determined after serum calcium levels are obtained. The prescribed diet is high in calcium and low in phosphorus. Although milk, milk products, and egg yolk are high in calcium, they are restricted because they also contain high levels of phosphorus. Spinach is also avoided because it contains oxalate, which would form insoluble calcium substances. Oral tablets of calcium salts, such as calcium gluconate, may supplement the diet. Aluminum hydroxide gel or aluminum carbonate (Gelusil, Amphojel) is also given after meals to bind phosphate and promote its excretion through the gastrointestinal tract.

Variable dosages of a vitamin D preparation—dihydrotachysterol (AT 10 or Hytakerol) or ergocalciferol (vitamin D_2) or cholecalciferol (vitamin D_3)—are usually required and enhance calcium absorption from the gastrointestinal tract.

An important aspect of nursing care is teaching about medications and diet therapy. The patient needs to know the reason for a high calcium and low phosphate intake and the symptoms of hypocalcemia and hypercalcemia so that he immediately contacts his physician if these symptoms occur.

The Adrenal Gland

Pheochromocytoma

A pheochromocytoma is a tumor that usually is benign and originates from the chromaffin cells of the adrenal medulla. In 80% to 90% of patients, the tumor arises in the medulla; in the remaining patients it occurs in the extra-adrenal chromaffin tissue located in or near the aorta, ovaries, spleen, or other organs. Pheochromocytoma occurs at any age, but its peak incidence is between ages 25 and 50. It affects men and women equally. Because of the high incidence of pheochromocytoma in family members, the patient's family should also be screened for this tumor. Ten percent of the tumors are bilateral and 10% are malignant.

Although uncommon, pheochromocytoma is the cause of high blood pressure in 0.1% to 0.5% of patients with hypertension. It is one form of hypertension that is usually cured by surgery; without detection and treatment, it is usually fatal.

Pheochromocytoma may occur in the familial form as part of multiple endocrine neoplasia, Type II (MEN-II); therefore, it should be considered a possibility in patients with medullary thyroid carcinoma and parathyroid hyperplasia or tumor.

Clinical Manifestations.   Functioning tumors of the adrenal medulla cause hypertension and other cardiovascular disturbances. The nature and severity depend on the relative proportions of epinephrine and norepinephrine secretion.

The hypertension may be intermittent or persistent. However, only 50% of patients with pheochromocytoma have sustained or persistent hypertension. If the hypertension is of the sustained type, it may be difficult to distinguish from so-called essential hypertension. In addition to hypertension, the symptoms are essentially the same as those encountered after the administration of epinephrine in large doses, namely, tachycardia or palpitations, excessive perspiration, tremor, headache, flushing, and anxiety. Hyperglycemia may result from conversion of liver and muscle glycogen to glucose by epinephrine secretion; insulin may be required to maintain normal blood glucose levels.

The clinical picture in the paroxysmal form of pheochromocytoma usually is characterized by acute, unpredictable attacks, lasting seconds or several hours, during which the patient is extremely anxious, tremulous, and weak. The patient may experience headache, vertigo, blurring of vision, tinnitus, air hunger, and dyspnea. Other symptoms include polyuria, nausea, vomiting, diarrhea, abdominal pain, and a feeling of impending doom. Palpitations and tachycardia are common.

Blood pressures as high as 350/200 mm Hg have been recorded. Such blood pressure elevations are dangerous and may precipitate life-threatening complications, including cardiac dysrhythmias, dissecting aneurysm, stroke, and acute renal failure. Postural hypotension occurs in 70% of untreated cases of pheochromocytoma.

Diagnostic Evaluation.   The diagnosis of pheochromocytoma is suspected if signs of sympathetic nervous system overactivity occur in association with marked elevation of blood pressure. However, determination of the catecholamines in urine and blood offers the most direct and conclusive test for overactivity of the adrenal medulla.

Total plasma catecholamine (norepinephrine and epinephrine) concentration is measured with the patient supine and at rest for 30 minutes. To prevent elevation of catecholamine levels by the stress of venipuncture, a butterfly needle, scalp vein needle, or venous catheter may be inserted 30 minutes before the blood specimen is obtained. Factors that may elevate catecholamine levels must be controlled in order to obtain valid results; these factors include consumption of coffee or tea, use of tobacco, emotional and physical stress, and use of many prescription and over-the-counter medications (*i.e.*, amphetamines, nose drops or sprays, decongestants, and bronchodilators). Normal plasma values of epinephrine are 100 pg/ml (SI: 590 pmol/L); normal values of norepinephrine are generally less than 100 to 550 pg/ml (SI: 590 to 3240 pmol/L). Values of epinephrine greater than 400 pg/ml (SI: 2180 pmol/L) or norepinephrine values greater than 2000 pg/ml (SI: 11,800 pmol/L) are considered diagnostic of pheochromocytoma; values that fall between normal values and those diagnostic of pheochromocytoma indicate the need for further testing.

Measurement of metabolites of catecholamines in the urine is useful in diagnosis. Urinary metanephrine is the most diagnostic urine test of adrenal medulla function. A 24-hour specimen of urine may be collected for determination of vanillylmandelic acid (VMA), a metabolite of catecholamines; foods and medications (*e.g.*, coffee, tea, bananas, chocolate, vanilla, aspirin) that alter the test results must be eliminated to assure accuracy of the test. Urine collected over a 2- or 3-hour period after an attack of hypertension can be assayed for catecholamine content.

Provocative tests and most suppression tests have been eliminated from the evaluation of the patient with suspected pheochromocytoma because of the occurrence of false-positive and false-negative test results and because of the risks of hypertensive and hypotensive episodes that may occur.

If the results of plasma and urine tests of catecholamines are inconclusive, a clonidine suppression test may be performed. Clonidine (Catapres) is a centrally acting, antiadrenergic drug that suppresses the release of neurogenically mediated catecholamines. The suppression test is based on the principle that catecholamine levels are normally increased through the activity of the sympathetic nervous system; in pheochromocytoma, increased catecholamines result from diffusion of excess catecholamines into the circulation, bypassing normal storage and release mechanisms. Therefore, in pheochromocytoma, clonidine will not suppress release of catecholamines. The results of the test are considered normal if 2 to 3 hours after a single oral dose of clonidine the total plasma catecholamine value decreases at least 40% from the patient's baseline and the absolute value falls below 500 pg/ml. Patients with pheochromocytoma exhibit no change in catecholamine levels.

Diagnostic tests may also be carried out to localize the pheochromocytoma and to determine if more than one tumor is present. Computed tomography, magnetic resonance imaging (MRI), ultrasonography, intravenous pyelography, and aortography or arteriography may be performed. However, these procedures are carried out only after the patient is prepared with blocking agents to prevent hypertensive attacks.

A new procedure using ^{131}I-metaiodobenzylguanidine (MIBG) is used to determine the location of the pheochromocytoma and detect metastatic sites outside the adrenal gland. MIBG is a radioactive compound that is taken up by adrenergic cells. It has been helpful in identifying tumors not detected by other tests or procedures. MIBG scintigraphy is a noninvasive, safe procedure that will increase the accuracy of diagnosis of adrenal tumors.

Other diagnostic studies may focus on evaluation of function of other endocrine glands because of the association of pheochromocytoma in some patients with other endocrine tumors.

Management. During an episode or attack of hypertension, tachycardia, anxiety, and the other symptoms of pheochromocytoma, the patient is placed on bed rest with the head of the bed elevated to promote an orthostatic decrease in blood pressure. The patient may be moved to the intensive care unit to permit close monitoring of electrocardiographic changes and careful administration of α-adrenergic blocking agents such as phentolamine (Regitine) or smooth muscle relaxants (sodium nitroprusside [Nipride]) to quickly lower the blood pressure. Phenoxybenzamine (Dibenzyline) is a long-acting α-blocker that may be used after the patient's blood pressure is stable to begin preparation of the patient for surgery.

The treatment of pheochromocytoma is surgical removal of the tumor, usually with adrenalectomy. Bilateral adrenalectomy may be necessary if tumors of both adrenal glands are present. Preliminary patient preparation includes effective control of blood pressure and blood volumes. Usually, this is carried out over 10 days to 2 weeks. Phentolamine or phenoxybenzamine (Dibenzyline) may be used safely without causing undue hypotension. These agents inhibit the effects of catecholamines but do not alter their synthesis or degradation. β-Adrenergic blocking agents may be used in patients with cardiac dysrhythmias or in those not responsive to α-adrenergic blocking drugs. α-Adrenergic and β-adrenergic blocking agents must be used with caution, because patients with pheochromocytoma may have increased sensitivity to them. Still another group of drugs that may be used preoperatively are catecholamine synthesis inhibitors such as α-methyl-*p*-tyrosine (metyrosine). These are occasionally used when the effects of catecholamines are not reduced by adrenergic blocking agents.

Manipulation of the tumor during surgical excision may cause release of stored epinephrine and norepinephrine with marked increases in blood pressure and changes in heart rate. Therefore, use of sodium nitroprusside and α-adrenergic blocking agents may be required during and after surgery. Exploration of other possible sites of tumor is frequently undertaken to ensure removal of all tumor. As a result, the patient is subject to the stress and effects of a long surgical procedure, which may increase the risk of hypertension postoperatively.

Corticosteroid replacement is required if bilateral adrenalectomy has been necessary. Corticosteroids may also be necessary for the first few days or weeks after removal of a single adrenal gland. Intravenous administration of corticosteroids (methylprednisolone sodium succinate [Solu-Medrol]) may begin the evening before surgery and continue during the early postoperative period to prevent adrenal insufficiency. Oral preparations of corticosteroids (prednisone) will be prescribed after the acute stress of surgery diminishes.

The patient will be monitored for several days in the intensive care unit with special attention given to electrocardiographic changes, arterial pressures, fluid and electrolyte balance, and blood glucose levels. Several intravenous lines will be inserted for administration of fluids and medications. Hypotension and hypoglycemia may occur in the postoperative period because of the sudden withdrawal of excessive amounts of catecholamines. Therefore, careful attention is directed toward monitoring and treating these changes.

Hypertension usually disappears with treatment. However, it can persist or recur if the blood vessels have been damaged by severe and prolonged hypertension or if all pheochromocytoma tissue has not been removed.

Several days after surgery, urine and plasma levels of catecholamines and their metabolites are measured to determine whether surgery has been successful. When levels have returned to normal, the patient may be discharged. Thereafter, periodic checkups are required, especially in young patients or in patients whose families have a history of pheochromocytoma. Pre- and postoperative nursing care is summarized in Nursing Care Plan 40-2.

Patient Education and Home Health Care. The patient who has undergone surgery to treat pheochromocytoma has experienced a stressful preoperative and postoperative course and may remain fearful of repeated attacks. Although it is usually expected that all pheochromocytoma tissue has been removed, there is a possibility that other sites were undetected and that attacks may recur. The patient is scheduled for periodic follow-up appointments to observe for return of normal blood pressure and serum and urine levels of catecholamines. He may be required to collect urine specimens for 24 hours before follow-

Nursing Care Plan 40-2

Care of the Patient With Pheochromocytoma

Nursing Interventions	Rationale	Expected Outcomes

PREOPERATIVELY AND DURING ACUTE ATTACKS

Nursing Diagnosis: Anxiety and fear related to excessive amount of circulating catecholamines and resulting symptoms

Goal: Relief of fear and anxiety

Nursing Interventions	Rationale	Expected Outcomes
1. Remain with patient during acute episode/attack. Be calm in approach.	1. Remaining with patient will help decrease his fear and level of panic.	• Reports decreased level of fear and anxiety.
2. Reassure patient that attack will end and that assistance to treat problem will be provided.	2. Fear and anxiety may further stimulate production of adrenal medulla hormones and increase blood pressure.	• Expresses hope and expectation that problem will be handled effectively by health care team.
3. Decrease external stimulation.	3. Quiet environment will stimulate patient less than a hurried one.	• Rests comfortably and quietly in intensive care unit.
4. Explain all procedures and events but in a factual, brief way.	4. Procedures and events will be less frightening if the patient understands their purpose and the expected outcomes.	• Explains rationale for procedures and events. • Exhibits no further increase in blood pressure, heart rate, or other symptoms.

Potential Complication: Recurrence of attacks due to excessive circulating catecholamines

Goal: Reduction of factors that have the potential to precipitate attacks

Nursing Interventions	Rationale	Expected Outcomes
1. Explain to patient activities that may precipitate attacks: a. Palpation of tumor b. Anxiety c. Vigorous exercise d. Trauma e. Exerting pressure on tumor f. Lying in certain positions (differs with each patient)	1. Certain activities may cause stimulation of the tumor and produce release of excess catecholamines.	• Identifies events and activities to be avoided to reduce the risk of further attacks. • Explains rationale for avoiding events and activities that increase risk of further attacks. • Does not permit palpation of tumor by all health care team members. • Identifies foods that increase risk of attacks.
2. Caution patient to avoid certain foods (beer, red wines, aged cheese, yogurt) and drugs (i.e., antitussive agents [cough syrup], MAO inhibitors, isoproterenol, amphetamines).	2. Certain foods and drugs may precipitate an attack by direct effects on the tumor, causing release of catecholamines.	• Consumes no foods that increase the risk of attacks. • Explains rationale for avoiding foods that may precipitate attacks. • Experiences no attacks.
3. Monitor patient's response to stressful events.	3. Surgical removal of one or both adrenal glands makes the patient more susceptible to stress and less able to respond to stressors.	• Identifies side effects of corticosteroids and ways to minimize side effects and complications.
4. Instruct patient how and when to administer own corticosteroids, if indicated (see p. 1105 for care of patient on long-term steroid therapy).	4. Lifetime replacement of corticosteroids will be necessary if a bilateral adrenalectomy was performed.	

(continued)

Nursing Care Plan 40-2 (Continued)

Care of the Patient With Pheochromocytoma

Nursing Interventions	Rationale	Expected Outcomes
POSTOPERATIVELY		
See Chapter 22 for care of the postoperative patient.		
Potential Complications: Rapid changes in blood pressure, fluid and electrolyte imbalances, pain, surgical stress		
Goal: Reduction of risk of postoperative complications		
1. Monitor blood pressure and fluid and electrolyte status.	1. Manipulation of the tumor during surgery and sudden withdrawal of catecholamines postoperatively make the patient susceptible to rapid changes in blood pressure and fluid and electrolyte balance.	• Exhibits normal fluid and electrolyte status. • Reports pain relief and comfort. • Exhibits normal response to stress. • Maintains normal blood pressure and pulse rate.
2. Administer pain medication to assure patient of adequate pain relief.	2. Postoperative pain and surgical stress increase the risk of postoperative complications (changes in blood pressure, fluid imbalance).	• Exhibits appropriate psychologic response to stressful events. • Explains rationale for steroid replacement. • Takes medication as prescribed.

up visits to the clinic or physician's office and is given verbal and written instructions about the procedure. If long-term steroid replacement is necessary, the patient is given instructions on the correct schedule to follow (see p. 1105 for care of patients on long-term steroid therapy). A visit from a community health nurse may be arranged to assure the patient that he is adhering to the medication schedule correctly and to assist him in dealing with problems that may result from long-term steroid use.

Disorders of the Adrenal Cortex

The adrenal cortex is necessary for life. Adrenocortical secretions make it possible for the body to adapt to stress of all kinds. How well one adapts to stress varies from person to person. Without the adrenal cortex, severe stress will cause peripheral circulatory failure, shock, and prostration. Life would be maintained only with nutritional, electrolyte, and fluid replacement and replacement of adrenocortical hormones.

Adrenocortical hormones are classified into three groups: mineralocorticoids, glucocorticoids, and sex hormones. *Mineralocorticoids* are concerned with sodium and water retention and potassium excretion. Examples are aldosterone and desoxycorticosterone, a natural precursor of aldosterone. *Glucocorticoids* are concerned with metabolic effects, including carbohydrate metabolism. Examples are cortisol and corticosterone. Glucocorticoids enhance the metabolic breakdown of body proteins and fat to provide a source of energy during periods of fasting. They antagonize the action of insulin, enhance protein catabolism, and inhibit protein synthesis. They affect defense mechanisms of the body and influence emotional functioning either directly or indirectly. They also suppress inflammation and inhibit scar tissue formation. In adrenal insufficiency, patients may be depressed or anxious, whereas with excessive replacement they tend to become euphoric. The *sex hormones* secreted by the adrenal cortex are androgens and estrogens.

Disorders of the adrenal cortex develop as a result of hyposecretion or hypersecretion of the adrenocortical hormones. Adrenal insufficiency may result from disease, atrophy, hemorrhage, or surgical removal of the adrenal gland or glands.

Chronic Primary Adrenocortical Insufficiency (Addison's Disease)

Pathophysiology. Addison's disease, caused by a deficiency of cortical hormones, results when the adrenal cortex is surgically removed with bilateral adrenalectomy or is destroyed, often as a result of idiopathic atrophy or infections such as tuberculosis or histoplasmosis. Inadequate secretion of ACTH from the pituitary gland results in adrenal insufficiency because of decreased stimulation of the adrenal cortex. The symptoms of adrenocortical insufficiency may also result from the sudden cessation of exogenous adrenocortical hormonal therapy, which suppresses the body's normal response to stress and interferes with normal feedback mechanisms.

Clinical Manifestations. Addison's disease has a characteristic clinical picture. The chief clinical manifestations include muscular weakness, anorexia, gastrointestinal symptoms, fatigue, emaciation, dark pigmentation of the skin, hypotension, low blood glucose, low serum sodium, and high serum potassium. In severe cases the disturbance of sodium and potassium metabolism may be marked by depletion of the sodium and water and severe, chronic dehydration.

As the disease progresses, with acute hypotension developing as a result of hypocorticism, the patient develops adsonian crisis, which is a medical emergency marked by cyanosis, fever, and the classic signs of shock: pallor, apprehension, rapid and weak pulse, rapid respirations, and low blood pressure. In addition, the patient may complain of headache, nausea, abdominal pain, and diarrhea and show signs of confusion and restlessness. Even slight overexertion, exposure to cold, acute infections, or a decrease in salt intake may lead to circulatory collapse. The stress of surgery or dehydration resulting from preparation for diagnostic tests or surgery may precipitate an addisonian or hypotensive crisis.

Diagnostic Evaluation.   Although the clinical manifestations presented appear specific, the onset of Addison's disease usually occurs with nonspecific symptoms. The diagnosis of Addison's disease is confirmed by laboratory test results. Suggestive laboratory findings include a decrease in the concentrations of blood glucose and sodium (hypoglycemia and hyponatremia), an increased concentration of serum potassium (hyperkalemia), and an increased white blood cell count (leukocytosis).

The definitive diagnosis is confirmed by low levels of adrenocortical hormones in the blood or urine. Serum cortisol levels are decreased in adrenal insufficiency. If the adrenal cortex is destroyed, baseline values are low and ACTH injection fails to cause the normal rise in plasma cortisol and urinary 17-hydroxycorticosteroids. If the adrenal gland is normal but not stimulated properly by the pituitary, a normal response to repeated dosages of exogenous ACTH is seen, but no response follows the administration of metyrapone, which stimulates endogenous ACTH.

Management.   Immediate treatment is directed toward combating shock: restoring blood circulation, administering fluids, monitoring vital signs, and placing the patient in a recumbent position with legs elevated. Hydrocortisone (Solu-Cortef) is given intravenously and followed with 5% dextrose in normal saline. Vasopressor amines may be required if hypotension persists.

Antibiotics may be prescribed if infection has precipitated adrenal crisis in a patient with chronic adrenal insufficiency. Additionally, the patient will be examined closely to determine other factors or illnesses that led to the acute episode.

Oral intake may be initiated as soon as tolerated by the patient. Gradually, intravenous fluids are decreased as oral fluids are accepted.

If the adrenal gland does not regain function, the patient will require life-long replacement of corticosteroids and mineralocorticoids to prevent recurrence of adrenal insufficiency and to prevent addisonian crisis in times of stress and illness. Additionally, the patient will probably be required to supplement his dietary intake with added salt during times of gastrointestinal losses of fluids through vomiting and diarrhea.

▶ Nursing Process
The Patient With Adrenal Insufficiency

▷ Assessment

The health history and examination focus on the presence of symptoms of fluid imbalance and on the patient's level of stress. The blood pressure and pulse rate are observed as the patient moves from a lying to a standing position to detect inadequate fluid volume. Additionally, the patient's skin color and turgor are assessed for changes related to chronic adrenal insufficiency and decreased fluid volume. A history of weight changes, the presence of muscle weakness, and the level of fatigue are obtained. The patient and family members are asked about the onset of illness or increased stress that may have precipitated the acute crisis.

▷ Nursing Diagnoses

Based on all the assessment data, the major nursing diagnoses of the patient with adrenal insufficiency include the following:

- Fluid volume deficit related to inadequate fluid intake and to fluid loss secondary to inadequate adrenal hormone secretion
- Activity intolerance related to inadequate production of adrenal hormones
- Knowledge deficit about the need for hormone replacement and dietary modification

▷ Planning and Implementation

▷   *Goals:*   The patient's goals may include improved fluid balance, improved response to activity and decreased stress in life, and increased knowledge about the need for hormone replacement and dietary modifications.

▷ Nursing Interventions

▷   *Fluid Balance Measures.*   Weight changes are recorded daily because they provide information about the adequacy of the patient's fluid and hormone replacement. Additionally, the patient's skin turgor and mucous membranes are assessed to provide information about fluid balance. The patient is instructed to report increased thirst, which may indicate impending fluid imbalance. Frequent monitoring of lying, sitting, and standing blood pressures also provides a useful indicator of fluid balance. A decrease of systolic pressure (20 mm Hg or more) may be indicative of depletion of fluid volume, especially if accompanied by symptoms.

The patient is encouraged to consume foods and fluids that will assist in restoring and maintaining fluid and electrolyte balance. With the assistance of the dietitian, the nurse can provide guidance to the patient to select foods high in sodium during gastrointestinal disturbances and very hot weather.

In collaboration with the physician, the nurse assists the patient in learning to administer hormone replacement as prescribed and to modify the dosage during illness and other stressful occasions. The patient is provided written and verbal instructions about the administration of mineralocorticoid (Florinef) and/or glucocorticoid (prednisone) as prescribed (see p. 1105 for care of patient on corticosteroid therapy).

▷   *Improved Activity Tolerance.*   Until the patient's condition is stabilized, precautions are taken to avoid unnecessary activity and events that might be stressful and could precipitate another hypotensive episode. Attempts are made to detect signs of infection or the presence of other stressors that may have triggered the crisis in the first place. Even minor events or stressors that ordinarily would go unnoticed may be excessive in the presence of adrenal insufficiency. During the acute crisis, a quiet, nonstressful environment is maintained. All activities (*e.g.,* bathing, turning) are carried out *for* the patient. All procedures are explained to the patient in order to reduce fear and anxiety. The nurse explains to the family the rationale for minimizing stress during the acute crisis and the measures for helping the patient reduce or avoid stress.

▷   *Patient Education.*   Because of the need for life-long replacement of adrenal cortex hormones to prevent adrenal insufficiency and acute adrenal crises with vascular collapse, the patient and family members receive explicit verbal and written instructions about the rationale for replacement therapy and proper dosage. Additionally, they receive instructions from the nurse and physician about how to balance the drug dosage and increase salt intake in times of illness and other stressful situations. The patient and family are frequently provided with a syringe and a vial of injectable steroid, such as Solu-Cortef, for use in emergencies, and they need careful instruction about how and when to use it. The patient is advised to inform other health care providers, such as dentists, that he is receiving steroids, to wear a Medic Alert bracelet, and to have information about his need for steroids with him at all times.

The patient and family need to know the signs of excessive or insufficient hormone replacement. The development of edema may signify *too high* a dose of hormone; postural hypotension (fall in systolic blood pressure, lightheadedness, and dizziness on standing) frequently signifies *too low* a dose.

The patient is also instructed about modifications in diet that are helpful in maintaining fluid and electrolyte balance. During illness and very hot weather, the patient should increase foods high in sodium to counteract increased sodium loss. Adequate fluids are also encouraged to maintain normal fluid balance. The patient is encouraged to weigh himself daily to detect any significant changes in weight that may indicate fluid loss or retention due to too much or too little hormone or a recurrence of adrenal insufficiency with changes in stress level.

◊ *Home Health Care.* Although most patients are able to return to job and family responsibilities soon after hospital discharge, others are unable to do so because of concurrent illnesses or incomplete recovery from the episode of adrenal insufficiency. In these circumstances, it is useful for the nurse to make a referral to the community health nurse who will visit the patient at home, assess recovery, monitor hormone replacement, and assess stress in the home. Additionally, the nurse will have the opportunity to assess the knowledge the patient and family have about drug therapy and dietary modifications. A home visit also provides the opportunity to assess the patient's plans for follow-up visits to the clinic or physician's office.

◊ *Evaluation*

Expected Outcomes

1. Achieves improved fluid balance.
   a. Exhibits normal skin turgor and moist mucous membranes.
   b. Reports stable weight and no excessive thirst.
   c. Reports absence of symptoms of postural hypotension (lightheadedness, dizziness, fainting on rising).
   d. Explains rationale for increasing salt and fluid intake in times of illness, increased stress, and very hot weather.
   e. Identifies foods high in sodium.
   f. Consumes high-sodium foods during illness, in very hot weather, and in times of increased stress.
   g. Seeks health care when illness or stress level exceeds the ability of patient to manage it.
2. Improves response to stress and decreases stress level.
   a. Reports normal daily stresses without development of symptoms of adrenal crisis.
   b. Identifies sources of excessive stress and ways to avoid them.
3. Increases knowledge about the need for hormone replacement and dietary modifications.

   a. Explains rationale for hormone replacement.
   b. Identifies consequences of inadequate hormone replacement.
   c. Demonstrates proper technique of administering injectable hormone for use in emergencies.
   d. Explains how to modify hormone dosage and diet to meet changing needs during illness, stress, and hot weather.
   e. Wears Medic Alert bracelet and carries medical information with him at all times.
   f. Designs schedule to ensure adherence to required medication therapy.
   g. Takes medication as prescribed.
   h. Identifies signs and symptoms of overdosage and underdosage of hormone.
   i. Exhibits absence of signs and symptoms of overdosage and underdosage of hormone.

Cushing's Syndrome

Cushing's syndrome is the opposite of Addison's disease, with its clinical characteristics reflecting excessive, rather than deficient, adrenocortical activity. The syndrome may result from excessive administration of cortisone or ACTH or from hyperplasia of the adrenal cortex.

Pathophysiology. The basic lesion responsible for Cushing's syndrome may be a tumor of the pituitary gland that produces ACTH and stimulates the adrenal cortex to increase its hormone secretion despite adequate amounts being produced. Primary hyperplasia of the adrenal glands in the absence of a pituitary tumor is less common. Administration of cortisone or ACTH may also produce Cushing's syndrome. Regardless of the cause, the normal feedback mechanisms that control the function of the adrenal cortex become ineffective, and the usual diurnal pattern of cortisol is lost. The signs and symptoms of Cushing's syndrome are primarily a result of unregulated secretion of glucocorticoids and androgens (sex hormones), although there may also be altered mineralocorticoid secretion.

Clinical Manifestations. When overproduction of the adrenal cortical hormone occurs, growth arrest, obesity, and musculoskeletal changes occur.

The classic picture of Cushing's syndrome in the adult shows a characteristic central type obesity, with a fatty "buffalo hump" in the neck and supraclavicular areas, a heavy trunk, and relatively thin extremities (Fig. 40-4). The skin is thinned, fragile, and easily traumatized; ecchymoses and striae develop. The patient complains of weakness and lassitude. Sleep is disturbed because of altered diurnal secretion of cortisol. Excessive protein catabolism occurs, producing muscle wasting and osteoporosis. Kyphosis, backache, and compression fractures of the vertebrae may result. Retention of sodium and water occurs as a result of increased mineralocorticoid activity, contributing to the hypertension and congestive heart failure commonly seen in Cushing's syndrome.

The patient develops a "moon-faced" appearance and may experience increased oiliness of the skin and acne. There is increased susceptibility to infection. Hyperglycemia or overt diabetes may develop. The patient may also report weight gain, slow healing of minor cuts, and bruises.

In females of all ages, virilization may occur as a result of excess androgens. Virilization is characterized by the appearance of masculine traits and the recession of feminine traits.

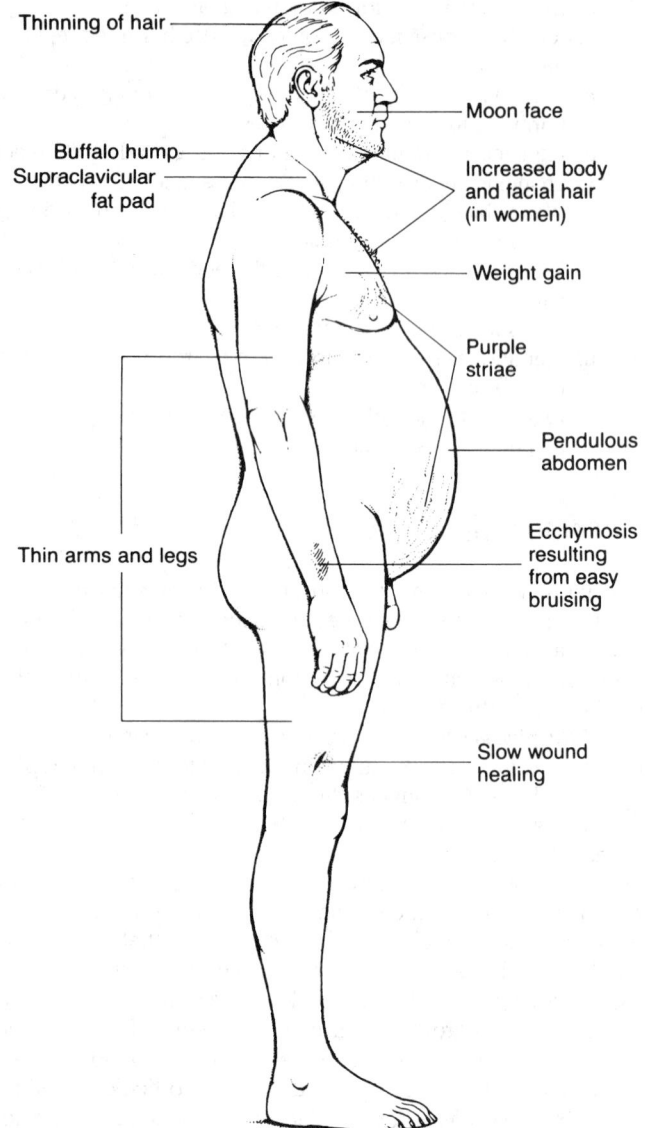

Figure 40–4.   Features of Cushing's syndrome invariably include truncal obesity, thin extremities, moon face, buffalo hump, and supraclavicular fullness. Broad purple striae appear at stretch points, such as the abdomen, hips, and shoulders. Body and facial hair is increased, and thinning of scalp hair may be noted only if androgens are increased.

There is an excessive growth of hair on the face (hirsutism), the breasts atrophy, menses cease, the clitoris enlarges, and the patient's voice deepens. Libido is lost in males and females.

Changes occur in mood and mental activity; a psychosis may develop on occasion. Distress and depression are common and are increased by the magnitude of the physical changes that occur with this syndrome. If Cushing's syndrome is a consequence of pituitary tumor, visual disturbances may occur because of pressure of the growing tumor on the optic chiasm.

Diagnostic Evaluation.   Indicators of this syndrome include an increase in serum sodium and blood glucose levels and a decreased serum concentration of potassium, a reduction in the number of blood eosinophils, and a disappearance of lymphoid tissue. Measurements of plasma and urinary cortisol levels are obtained. Several blood samples may be collected to determine if the normal diurnal variation in plasma levels is present. This variation is frequently abolished in adrenal dys-

function. If several blood samples are required, it is essential that they be collected at the times specified and that the time of collection be noted on the requisition slip.

A 24-hour urinary free cortisol level provides the most accurate test of adrenal function. Radioimmunoassay of plasma ACTH is useful in identifying the cause of Cushing's syndrome. Diagnostic studies may also include 24-hour urine collection for levels of 17-hydroxycorticosteroids and 17-ketosteroids, the urinary metabolites of cortisol and androgens. In Cushing's syndrome, these levels and plasma cortisol levels are elevated.

A low-dose dexamethasone suppression test may be performed, in which a low dose of dexamethasone, a potent synthetic glucocorticoid, is administered and plasma cortisol and urine 17-hydroxycorticosteroid levels are obtained. In patients with normal adrenal function, even low doses of the glucocorticoid will produce decreased cortisol and 17-hydroxycorticosteroid levels. This test is complex and requires administration of the drug every 6 hours for 48 hours and collection of plasma and 24-hour urine specimens. Hospitalization is therefore often necessary for completion of this test.

The corticotropin-releasing factor (CRF) stimulation test is useful in distinguishing pituitary tumors from ectopic sites of ACTH production as the cause of Cushing's syndrome. Several of these tests are likely to be performed to screen the symptomatic patient for Cushing's syndrome and to confirm the results of other tests.

A CT scan or MRI may be performed to localize adrenal tissue and detect tumors of the adrenal gland.

Management.   Because the majority of cases of Cushing's syndrome are due to pituitary tumors rather than tumors of the adrenal cortex, treatment is usually directed at the pituitary gland. Surgical removal of the tumor (transsphenoidal hypophysectomy) is the primary treatment of choice and has a very high rate of success (90%) when performed by a skilled neurosurgeon. Implantation of needles containing radioactive isotopes into the pituitary gland has also been successful. Adrenalectomy (see p. 1102) is the treatment of choice in patients with primary adrenal hypertrophy.

Postoperatively, symptoms of adrenal insufficiency may begin to appear 12 to 48 hours after surgery because of reduction of the high levels of circulating adrenal hormones. Temporary replacement therapy with hydrocortisone may be necessary for several months until the adrenal glands begin to respond normally to the body's needs. If both adrenal glands have been removed (bilateral adrenalectomy), lifetime replacement of adrenal cortex hormones will be necessary.

If the Cushing's syndrome is a result of externally administered (exogenous) corticosteroids, an attempt will be made to reduce or taper the drug dose to the minimum level adequate to treat the underlying disease process (*e.g.*, autoimmune and allergic diseases and rejection of transplanted organs). Frequently, alternate-day therapy decreases the symptoms of Cushing's syndrome and allows recovery of the adrenal glands' responsiveness to ACTH.

▶ Nursing Process
The Patient With Cushing's Syndrome

▷ **Assessment**

The health history and examination focus on the effects on the body of high concentrations of adrenal cortex hormones and on the inability of the adrenal cortex to respond to changes in cortisol and aldosterone levels. The history includes information about the patient's level of activity and ability to carry out routine and self-care activities. The patient's skin is observed and assessed for trauma, infection, breakdown, bruising, and edema. Changes in physical appearance are noted, and the patient's responses to these changes are elicited. Throughout the interview and examination, the nurse assesses the patient's mental function, including mood, responses to questions, awareness of his environment, and level of depression.

◊ Nursing Diagnoses

Based on all the assessment data, the major nursing diagnoses of the patient with Cushing's syndrome include the following:

- Self-care deficit related to weakness, fatigue, muscle wasting, and altered sleep patterns
- Impaired skin integrity related to edema, impaired healing, and thin and fragile skin
- High risk for injury and infection related to altered protein metabolism and inflammatory response
- Body image disturbance related to altered physical appearance, impaired sexual functioning, and decrease in activity level
- Altered thought processes related to mood swings, irritability, and depression

◊ Planning and Implementation

◊ *Goals:* The patient's major goals include increased ability to carry out self-care activities, improved skin integrity, decreased risk of injury and infection, improved body image, and improved mental function.

◊ Nursing Interventions

◊ *Rest and Activity.* Weakness, fatigue, and muscle wasting make it difficult for the patient with Cushing's syndrome to carry out normal activities. Yet moderate activity should be encouraged to prevent complications of immobility and promote increased self-esteem. Insomnia often contributes to the patient's fatigue. Rest periods are planned and spaced throughout the day. Efforts are made to promote a relaxing, quiet environment for rest and sleep.

◊ *Skin Care.* Meticulous skin care is necessary to avoid traumatizing the patient's fragile skin. Use of adhesive tape is avoided because it can irritate the skin and tear the fragile skin when the tape is removed. The skin and bony prominences are assessed frequently, and the patient is encouraged and assisted to change positions frequently to prevent skin breakdown.

◊ *Decreased Risk of Injury and Infection.* A protective environment must be established to prevent falls, fractures, and other injuries to bones and soft tissues. The patient who is very weak may require assistance in ambulating to prevent falls or bumping into sharp corners of furniture. Unnecessary exposure to visitors, staff, or patients with infections is avoided. The patient is assessed frequently for subtle signs of infection because the anti-inflammatory effects of glucocorticoids may mask the common signs of inflammation and infection. Foods high in protein, calcium, and vitamin D are recommended to minimize muscle wasting and osteoporosis.

◊ *Improved Body Image.* If removal of the cause of Cushing's syndrome is possible and is carried out, the major physical changes will disappear in time. However, the patient may benefit from discussion of the impact the changes have had on self-concept and relationships with others. The weight gain and edema seen with Cushing's syndrome may be modified by a low-carbohydrate, low-sodium diet. A high-protein intake may reduce some of the other bothersome symptoms.

◊ *Improved Thought Processes.* Explanations to the patient and family members about the cause of emotional instability are important in helping them cope with the mood swings, irritability, and depression that may occur. Psychotic behavior may occur in a few patients and should be reported. The patient and family members are encouraged to verbalize their feelings.

Additionally, the patient is prepared for adrenalectomy if indicated, and postoperative care (see below). Peptic ulcer and diabetes mellitus are common in the patient with Cushing's syndrome; therefore, management includes assessment of stools for blood and testing of urine for glucosuria and appropriate intervention if indicated.

◊ Evaluation

Expected Outcomes

1. Increases participation in self-care activities.
   a. Plans activities and exercises to allow alternating periods of rest and activity.
   b. Participates in hygienic care.
   c. Reports improved well-being.
   d. Sleeps soundly at night and during planned rest periods.
   e. Is free of complications of immobility.
2. Attains/maintains skin integrity.
   a. Has intact skin, without evidence of breakdown or infection.
   b. Shows evidence of decreased edema in extremities and trunk.
   c. Avoids trauma to skin.
   d. Changes position frequently.
   e. Inspects bony prominences daily.
3. Decreases risk of injury and infection.
   a. Is free of fractures or soft-tissue injuries.
   b. Is free of ecchymotic areas.
   c. Uses measures to prevent trauma (*e.g.*, seeks assistance when necessary, arranges rugs and furniture to prevent falls and bumps).
   d. Avoids people with cold or flu symptoms.
   e. Experiences no temperature elevation, redness, pain, or other signs of infection and inflammation.
   f. Explains rationale for foods high in protein, calcium, and vitamin D.
   g. Selects and eats foods high in protein, calcium and vitamin D.
4. Achieves improved body image.
   a. Uses makeup appropriately and selects clothes that enhance appearance.
   b. Socializes with others.
   c. Uses good grooming (*e.g.*, skin care, hair care).
   d. Is not gaining weight.
   e. Adheres to diet (*e.g.*, consumes high-protein, low-carbohydrate, low-sodium diet).
   f. Verbalizes feelings about changes in appearance, sexual function, and activity level.

g. States that physical changes are a result of excessive corticosteroids.

5. Exhibits improved mental functioning.
   a. Identifies excessive corticosteroid level as the reason for mood changes.
   b. Verbalizes feelings to nurse and to family.
   c. Participates in family activities.
   d. Notifies nurse, physician, and family if feelings become overwhelming.

Primary Aldosteronism

The principal action of aldosterone is to conserve body sodium. Under the influence of this hormone, the kidneys excrete less sodium and more potassium and hydrogen.

Excessive production of aldosterone, which occurs in some patients with functioning tumors of the adrenal gland, causes a distinctive pattern of biochemical changes and a corresponding set of clinical manifestations that are diagnostic of this condition. Such patients exhibit a profound decline in the blood levels of potassium (hypokalemia) and hydrogen ions (alkalosis), as demonstrated by an increase in *p*H and carbon dioxide combining power. The serum sodium level is normal or elevated depending on the amount of water reabsorbed with the sodium. Hypertension is usually present, although aldosteronism is the primary cause of only 3% of cases of hypertension.

Hypokalemia is responsible for the variable muscle weakness in patients with aldosteronism, as well as an inability on the part of the kidneys to acidify or concentrate the urine. Accordingly, the urine volume is excessive, leading to reports of polyuria. Serum, by contrast, becomes abnormally concentrated, contributing to excessive thirst (polydipsia) and arterial hypertension. A secondary increase in blood volume and possible direct effects of aldosterone on nerve receptors such as the carotid sinus are other factors producing the hypertension. Hypokalemic alkalosis may decrease the plasma-ionized calcium level and predispose the patient to tetany and paresthesias. Trousseau's and Chvostek's signs can be used to assess neuromuscular irritability before overt paresthesia and tetany occur (see p. 1093).

Diagnostic studies reveal, in addition to a high or normal serum sodium level and low serum potassium level, high serum aldosterone levels and low serum renin levels. The measurement of aldosterone excretion rate following salt loading by IV infusions of saline for 3 days or the addition of 10 to 12 g of sodium chloride to the patient's diet for 5 to 7 days is a useful diagnostic test for primary aldosteronism.

Treatment of primary aldosteronism usually involves surgical removal of the adrenal tumor through adrenalectomy.

Adrenalectomy

Adrenalectomy is the treatment of choice in primary Cushing's syndrome and aldosteronism. In addition, it is also used in the treatment of adrenal tumors and for malignancy of the breast and prostate gland.

For Adrenal Tumors.   All of the endocrine disturbances associated with a hypersecreting tumor of the adrenal cortex or medulla can be relieved completely, and the patient im-

proved dramatically, by surgical removal of the involved gland. Adrenalectomy is performed through an incision in the loin or the abdomen. In general, the postoperative care resembles that given for any abdominal operation. Following surgery for adrenal cortical tumors, the patient is susceptible to fluctuations in adrenocortical hormones and may require administration of corticosteroids, fluids, and other agents to maintain blood pressure and prevent acute complications. Attention is also directed toward maintenance of a normal serum glucose level with insulin and appropriate intravenous fluids and dietary modifications.

Nursing management in the postoperative period includes frequent assessment of vital signs so that early indications of hemorrhage and possible adrenal crisis may be detected and treated. Stressful situations can be avoided by explaining the treatment, promoting comfort measures, establishing priorities of care, and providing rest periods.

For Malignancy of Breasts or Prostate.   Certain malignancies, notably those of the breast and the prostate, are affected by the hormones produced by endocrine glands. Thus, ovarian hormones are known to have an effect on carcinoma of the breast and hormones of the testes on carcinoma of the prostate. In some patients, the hormones are still present even after suppression of endocrine stimulation, and they have been found to arise from adrenal glands. For this reason, bilateral adrenalectomy may be performed in an effort to control recurrent carcinoma of the breast or the prostate. The adrenals are approached either transabdominally or through the posterior bed of the 12th rib.

Postoperatively, adrenocortical hormones must be administered in appropriate dosage to overcome the sudden reduction of those hormones by the surgical procedure. The dosage of adrenocortical hormone may be reduced gradually as the body adjusts itself to its new level of hormone production.

Corticosteroid Therapy

Corticosteroids are used extensively for adrenal insufficiency and are also widely used in suppressing inflammation and autoimmune reactions, controlling allergic reactions, and reducing the rejection process in transplantation. Commonly used steroid preparations are listed in Table 40-3. Their *anti-inflammatory* and *antiallergy* actions make corticosteroids effective in treating rheumatic or connective tissue diseases such as rheumatoid arthritis and systemic lupus erythematosus. High doses seem to permit patients to tolerate high degrees of stress. Such *antistress* action may be due to the ability of corticosteroids to aid circulating vasopressor substances in keeping the blood pressure elevated, or it may be due to other effects, such as the maintenance of the plasma glucose level.

Although the synthetic steroids are safer for some patients because of relative freedom from mineralocorticoid activity, most natural and synthetic corticosteroids produce similar kinds of side effects. The size of the dose required to bring about desired anti-inflammatory and antiallergy effects also causes metabolic effects, pituitary and adrenal gland suppression, and changes in the function of the central nervous system. Such changes may be disabling and even dangerous.

In view of these possible side effects, it is obvious that while adrenocorticosteroids are highly effective therapeutically, they may also be very dangerous. Dosages of these medications

TABLE 40-3. *Commonly Used Steroid Preparations*

Generic Names	Trade Names
GLUCOCORTICOIDS	
Hydrocortisone	Cortisol, Hydrocortone, Cortef, Compound F
Cortisone	Cortone, Cortogen, Compound E
Dexamethasone	Decadron, Hexadrol, Dexameth, Deronil, Delalone, Dexasone, 9α-fluoro-16α-methylpredisolone
Prednisone	Meticorten, Deltasone, 1,2-dehydrocortisone, Orasone
Prednisolone	Meticortelone, 1,2-dehydrocortisol
Methylprednisolone	Medrol, Solu-medrol
Triamcinolone	Aristocort, Kenacort, Kenalog, Cenocort, Azmacort, Aristospan
Beclomethasone	Beconase, Beclovent, Vanceril, Vancenase, Propaderm
Betamethasone	Celestone, Betameth, Betnesol
MINERALOCORTICOIDS	
Desoxycorticosterone or desoxycorticosterone acetate	Percorten, Cortate, DOCA
Fludrocortisone	Florinef, F-Cortef, 9α-fluorohydrocortisone
Aldosterone	Electrocortin, Aldocorten

are frequently altered to allow high concentrations when absolutely necessary and then tapered in an attempt to avoid undesirable effects. This requires that patients be closely observed for side effects and that the dose be reduced when high doses are no longer required. Suppression of the adrenal cortex may persist up to a year after a course of corticosteroids of only 2 weeks' duration.

Therapeutic Effects and Complications of Corticosteroid Therapy

The dosage of corticosteroids is determined by the nature and chronicity of the illness as well as by any other medical problem the patient has. Rheumatoid arthritis and bronchial asthma are chronic disorders that corticosteroids do not cure; however, these drugs may be useful when other measures do not provide adequate control of symptoms. In such a situation, the adverse effects of steroids are weighed against the current problems of the patient. These drugs may be used for a period of time but then should be gradually reduced as the patient's symptoms subside. The nurse plays an important role in providing encouragement and understanding during the times the patient may experience recurrence of symptoms and apprehension about these while taking smaller doses.

Acute flare-ups and crises are treated with large doses of corticosteroids, as in emergency treatment for bronchial obstruction in status asthmaticus and shock from septicemia caused by gram-negative bacteria. Other measures, such as anti-infective agents or medications are also used with corticosteroids to treat shock and other major symptoms.

At times corticosteroids are continued past the acute flare-up stage for the purpose of combating possible complications that are deemed worse than the side effects of steroids. Systemic lupus erythematosus is an example of such a condition.

A different problem exists when corticosteroids are used in treating eye infections. Outer eye infection can be treated by topical application of eye drops, because these do not cause systemic toxicity. However, long-term application may cause an increase in intraocular pressure, which may lead to glaucoma in some patients. In other patients, prolonged use of steroids may lead to cataract formation.

Topical administration of steroids in the form of creams, ointments, lotions, and aerosols is especially effective in many dermatologic disorders. It may be more effective in some conditions to use occlusive dressings around the affected part so that maximum absorption of the drug is achieved. Steroid penetration and absorption are also increased if the drug is applied when the skin is hydrated or moist (*e.g.*, immediately after bathing). Absorption of topical steroids varies with body location. For example, absorption is greater through the layers of skin on the scalp, face, and genital area than on the forearm, and as a result these sites are more susceptible to the side effects of the drug than other sites. The recent availability of over-the-counter topical steroids increases the risk of side effects of steroids in patients who are unaware of the potential risks of these drugs or use them indiscriminately. Excessive use of these agents, especially on large surface areas of inflamed skin, can lead to decreased therapeutic effects and increased side effects.

Major Side Effects of Corticosteroid Therapy

Adverse effects are more likely to occur when steroid therapy is used for long periods of time. In general, such effects are classified as follows:

Metabolic Effects.   Changes in the metabolism may occur following large doses of glucocorticoids or mineralocorticoids. Excessive glucocorticoid activity (hypercorticism) causes clinical manifestations of Cushing's syndrome (see p. 1099), including the characteristic rounding of the face and an abnormal distribution of body fat.

Because of changes in the metabolism of carbohydrate, protein, and fat, certain other complications may occur. For example, some patients may develop peptic ulcer, diabetes mellitus, or osteoporosis. Therefore, preventive actions or supportive therapy is required to minimize the threat of these other conditions. For example, it is necessary for the patient with a history of peptic ulcer to continue with antacids and perhaps antispasmodic medications, at the same time recognizing that peptic ulcer pain may not be present as a warning sign during the administration of corticosteroids. For the patient with diabetes, oral hypoglycemic agents should be continued or insulin dosages adjusted as needed. For the patient with osteoporosis, it is helpful to adhere to a high-protein diet and to take calcium salt and vitamin D supplement, observing for possible hypercalciuria. Special efforts are made to prevent an injury that may result in a fracture.

Infection may spread with minimal symptoms because of suppression of the immune system and the inflammatory process. Viral and fungal infections are general contraindications for steroid use because of the difficulty in treating these conditions.

Endocrine Effects. Prolonged steroid therapy has a tendency to suppress certain functions of the anterior portion of the pituitary gland. Hence, growth in children may be halted following long-term treatment with steroids because of adrenal atrophy and suppression of the pituitary's release of ACTH. Although this effect may not be apparent under ordinary circumstances, it is obvious during times of unusual stress. During these periods, acute adrenal insufficiency may occur, requiring massive doses of corticosteroids to prevent adrenal collapse.

Central Nervous System Effects. Euphoria and mood changes result from the action of corticosteroids on the central nervous system. Because such a reaction often creates psychologic dependency on steroids, the patient may resist being removed from these drugs. With prolonged use of corticosteroids, the patient may experience mood swings that include excitement, restlessness, depression, and sleeplessness. Nursing support and understanding are required as the patient experiences these changes. Any tendency to emotional, psychologic, or psychotic difficulties needs to be brought to the attention of the physician before steroids are prescribed. Table 40-4 lists some of the common side effects of corticosteroid therapy.

Chart 40-1 provides an overview of the management of the patient on steroid therapy.

Dosage Schedule

Attempts have been made to determine the best time to administer pharmacologic doses of steroids. Once the patient's symptoms have been controlled on a 6-hour or 8-hour program, a once-daily or every-other-day schedule may be implemented. In keeping with the natural secretion of cortisol, the best time of the day for the total steroid dose is in the early morning from 7 to 8 AM. Large-dose therapy at 8 AM, when the gland is most active, produces maximal suppression of the gland. A large 8 AM dosage is more physiologic, because it allows the body to escape effects of the steroids from 4 PM to 6 AM, when serum levels are normally low, hence minimizing cushingoid effects. If symptoms of the disease being treated are successfully suppressed, alternate-day therapy is helpful in reducing pituitary–adrenal suppression in patients requiring prolonged

TABLE 40-4. *Potential Side Effects of Glucocorticoid Therapy*

OPHTHALMIC	*SKELETAL*
Cataracts	Osteoporosis
Glaucoma	Spontaneous fractures
	Aseptic necrosis of femur
CARDIOVASCULAR	Vertebral compression fractures
Hypertension	
Congestive heart failure	*GASTROINTESTINAL*
	Peptic ulcer
ENDOCRINE/METABOLIC	Pancreatitis
Truncal obesity	
Moon face	*MUSCULAR*
Buffalo hump	Myopathy
Sodium retention	Muscle weakness
Hypokalemia	
Metabolic alkalosis	*DERMATOLOGIC*
Hyperglycemia	Thinning of skin
Menstrual irregularities	Petechiae
Impotence	Ecchymoses
Negative nitrogen balance	Striae
Altered calcium metabolism	Acne
Adrenal suppression	
	PSYCHIATRIC
IMMUNE FUNCTION	Mood alterations
Decreased inflammatory responses	Psychoses
Impaired wound healing	
Increased susceptibility to infections	

therapy. Taking the total steroid dose every other day presents some problems in that patients complain of discomfort on the second day. It may be necessary for the nurse to explain to the patient that this regimen may be necessary to minimize side effects and suppression of adrenal function.

Tapering of Steroids. Corticosteroid dosages are reduced gradually (tapered) to allow normal adrenal function to return and to prevent steroid-induced adrenal insufficiency. Up to 1 year or more after use of corticosteroids, the patient is at risk of adrenal insufficiency in times of stress. For example, if surgery for any reason is necessary, the patient is likely to require intravenous steroids during and after surgery to prevent the occurrence of acute adrenal crisis.

The Pituitary Gland

Hypopituitarism

Hypopituitarism is pituitary insufficiency resulting from destruction of the anterior lobe of the pituitary gland. *Panhypopituitarism* (Simmonds' disease) is total absence of all pituitary secretions and is rare. Postpartum pituitary necrosis (Sheehan's syndrome) is another uncommon cause of failure of the anterior pituitary. It is more likely to occur in women with severe blood loss, hypovolemia, and hypotension at the time of delivery.

Chart 40–1
Side Effects and Implications of Steroid Therapy

Side Effects	Nursing Management	Possible Medical Management
Cardiovascular system effects: Hypertension Thromboembolic complications Arteritis	Report to physician. Continue assessment of patient.	Reduce dose of steroids.
Infection and masking of signs of inflammation	Assess for atypical indicators of infection. Report to physician. Limit visitors and prevent exposure to infection if possible. Promote cleanliness.	Prescribe antimicrobial agents.
Eye complications: Glaucoma Corneal lesions	Report to physician.	Refer to ophthalmologist.
Adrenal insufficiency as manifested by peripheral circulatory collapse (orthostatic hypotension)	Report to physician. Remain with patient. Decrease sources of stress. Assist with administration of fluids and steroids.	Prescribe hydrocortisone and intravenous normal saline; prescribe oral corticosteroid when patient's condition is stable.
Musculoskeletal effects	Encourage diet high in calcium and vitamin D. Use caution in moving and ambulating patient. Avoid trauma and falls.	Prescribe synthetic estrogens or androgens. Prescribe calcium supplement and oral preparations of vitamin D.
Moon face (Cushing's syndrome) Weight gain and edema Potassium loss	Suggest caloric restriction. Suggest sodium restriction. Report symptoms to physician. Suggest foods high in potassium.	Consider a different steroid medication. Prescribe diuretics. Prescribe potassium supplement.
Acne Increased urinary frequency and nocturia	Suggest frequent washing. Assess for urinary tract infection and glycosuria.	Prescribe topical medications. Evaluate for diabetes mellitus and order urinalysis and urine culture and sensitivity if indicated.

Counseling of Patients on Long-Term Steroid Therapy

1. Recognize that steroids are valuable and useful medications, but if taken longer than 2 weeks certain side effects may be noticed.
2. Side effects that are to be reported to the physician include dizziness when rising from chair or bed (postural hypotension indicative of adrenal insufficiency), nausea, vomiting, thirst, abdominal pain, pain of any type, feelings of depression or nervousness, and development of an infection.
3. Other side effects may include weight gain (may be due to water retention or increased food intake), acne, headaches, fatigue, and increased urinary frequency.
4. If the patient experiences trauma (fall, motor vehicle accident) or significant stress, adrenal failure may be precipitated; a Medic-Alert tag/bracelet must be worn to identify drug therapy in case of injury or crisis. The patient and family may be instructed in emergency administration of hydrocortisone injection.
5. Adequate medication must be kept on hand so that the patient does not run out of the prescribed corticosteroid.

Hypopituitarism is also a complication of radiation therapy to the head and neck area. The total destruction of the pituitary gland by trauma, tumor, or vascular lesion removes all stimuli that are normally received by the thyroid, the gonads, and the adrenal glands. The resulting endocrinopathy is characterized by extreme weight loss, emaciation, atrophy of all endocrine glands and organs, hair loss, impotence, amenorrhea, hypometabolism, and hypoglycemia. Coma and death will ensue without replacement of the missing hormones.

Pituitary Tumors

Tumors of the pituitary gland are three principal types, representing an overgrowth of (1) eosinophilic cells, (2) basophilic cells, or (3) chromophobic cells (*i.e.*, cells with no affinity for either eosinophilic or basophilic stains).

Eosinophilic tumors, if they develop early enough in life, result in gigantism. The person thus affected may be over 7 feet tall and large in all proportions, yet so weak and lethargic that he can hardly stand. If the disorder begins during adult life, the excessive skeletal growth occurs only in the feet, the hands, the superciliary ridges, the molar eminences, the nose, and the chin, giving rise to the clinical picture called *acromegaly.* Enlargement, moreover, is not confined to the skeleton but involves every tissue and organ of the body. Many of these patients suffer from severe headaches and visual disturbances because the tumors exert pressure on the optic nerves. Assessment of central vision and visual fields may reveal loss of color discrimination, diplopia (double vision), or blindness of a portion of a field of vision. Decalcification of the skeleton, muscular weakness, and endocrine disturbances, similar to those occurring in patients with hyperthyroidism, also are associated with tumors of this type.

Basophilic tumors give rise to *Cushing's syndrome* (see p. 1099) with features largely attributable to hyperadrenalism, including masculinization and amenorrhea in females, truncal obesity, hypertension, osteoporosis, and polycythemia.

Chromophobic tumors, which constitute 90% of pituitary tumors, produce no hormones but destroy the rest of the pituitary gland, causing hypopituitarism. Patients with this disease are inclined to be obese and somnolent, exhibiting fine, scanty hair; dry, soft skin; pasty complexion; and small bones. They also experience headaches, loss of libido, and visual defects progressing to blindness. Other symptoms include polyuria, polyphagia, a lowering of the basal metabolic rate, and a subnormal body temperature.

Management of Acromegaly or Pituitary Tumors. Surgical removal of the pituitary tumor through a transsphenoidal approach is considered the treatment of choice (described below). In cases where surgery is not possible, treatment has included radiation therapy and the use of bromocriptine and somatostatin analogue. Bromocriptine, a dopamine agonist, and somatostatin analogue (SMS 201-995) inhibit growth hormone production or release. Marked improvement of symptoms has been reported.

Hypophysectomy

Hypophysectomy, or removal of the pituitary gland, may be performed for several reasons, including treatment of primary tumors of the pituitary gland. In diabetic retinopathy, it is used to halt the progress of hemorrhagic retinopathy and avoid blindness. Hypophysectomy may also be performed as a palliative measure to relieve bone pain secondary to metastasis of malignant lesions of the breast and prostate. Pituitary hormones influence the growth of the normal breast and stimulate the function of the ovaries and the adrenal glands. Hypophysectomy removes the hormonal influences of these glands and reduces stimuli to the continued growth of the neoplasm.

There are several methods of pituitary ablation (removal). It can be performed surgically through the transfrontal, subcranial, or oronasal–transsphenoidal approaches. The pituitary can also be destroyed by irradiation or cryosurgery. (See Chap. 56 for the transsphenoidal approach to the removal of a pituitary tumor and for the nursing management of a patient undergoing cranial surgery.)

The absence of the pituitary gland alters the function of many parts of the body. Menstruation ceases and infertility occurs after total or nearly total ablation of the pituitary gland. Replacement therapy with adrenal steroids (hydrocortisone) and thyroid hormone may be necessary.

Diabetes Insipidus

Diabetes insipidus is a disorder of the posterior lobe of the pituitary gland due to a deficiency of vasopressin, the antidiuretic hormone (ADH). It is characterized by great thirst (polydipsia) and large volumes of dilute urine. It may be secondary to head trauma, brain tumor, or surgical ablation or irradiation of the pituitary gland. Without the action of vasopressin on the distal nephron of the kidney, an enormous daily output of very dilute, waterlike urine with a specific gravity of 1.001 to 1.005 occurs. The urine contains no abnormal substances, such as glucose and albumin. Because of the intense thirst, the patient tends to drink 4 to 40 liters of fluid daily, with a special craving for cold water.

In the hereditary form of diabetes insipidus, the primary symptoms may begin at birth. When it occurs in adults, the polyuria may have an insidious onset, although sometimes it occurs suddenly and may be related to an injury.

The disease cannot be controlled by limiting the intake of fluids, because loss of high volumes of urine continues even without fluid replacement. Attempts to restrict fluids cause the patient to experience an insatiable craving for fluid and to develop hypernatremia and severe dehydration.

Diagnostic Evaluation. The fluid deprivation test is carried out, in which fluids are withheld for 8 to 12 hours or until 3% of the body weight is lost. The patient is weighed frequently during the time fluid is withheld. Plasma and urine osmolality studies are performed at the beginning and end of the test. The inability to increase specific gravity and osmolality of the urine is characteristic of diabetes insipidus. The patient with diabetes insipidus will continue to excrete large volumes of urine with low specific gravity and will experience weight loss, rising serum osmolality, and elevated serum sodium levels. The patient's condition needs to be assessed frequently during the test, and the test is terminated if the patient develops problems such as tachycardia, excessive weight loss, or hypotension.

Management. The objectives of therapy are (1) to assure adequate fluid replacement, (2) to replace vasopressin (which is usually a long-term therapeutic program), and (3) to search for and correct the underlying intracranial pathology.

Desmopressin (DDAVP), synthetic vasopressin without the vascular effects of natural ADH, is particularly valuable because it has a longer duration of action and fewer adverse effects than other preparations previously used to treat the disease. It is administered intranasally with the patient sniffing the solution into his nose through a flexible calibrated plastic tube. Two administrations daily appear to control the symptoms.

Another form of therapy is the intramuscular administration of ADH, vasopressin tannate in oil, which is given every 24 to 96 hours. The effect is a reduction in urinary volume for 24 to 96 hours. The vial of medication should be warmed or shaken vigorously prior to administration. The injection is given in the evening so that maximum results are obtained during sleep. Abdominal cramps are a side effect of this drug. Rotation of injection sites is necessary to prevent lipodystrophy.

The drug lypressin (Diapid) is absorbed through the nasal mucosa into the blood and is another method of administering vasopressin. Its duration may be too short for patients with severe disease. The patient should be observed for chronic rhinopharyngitis if this modality of treatment is used.

Clofibrate, a hypolipidemic agent, has been found to have an antidiuretic effect on patients with diabetes insipidus who have some residual hypothalamic vasopressin. Chlorpropamide (Diabinese) and thiazide diuretics are also used in mild forms of the disease, because they potentiate the action of vasopressin. The patient receiving chlorpropamide should be warned of the possibility of hypoglycemic reactions.

The patient will require encouragement and support if he is undergoing studies of a possible cranial lesion. The patient and family members are instructed about follow-up care and emergency measures. The patient is also advised to wear a Medic Alert bracelet and to carry information about this disorder and his medications with him at all times. Caution must be used with administration of vasopressin if coronary artery disease is present because it causes vasoconstriction.

Syndrome of Inappropriate Antidiuretic Hormone Secretion

The syndrome of inappropriate antidiuretic hormone secretion (SIADH) refers to excessive ADH secretion from the pituitary gland even in the face of subnormal serum osmolality. Patients with this disorder cannot excrete a dilute urine. They retain fluids and develop a sodium deficiency (dilutional hyponatremia). SIADH is often of nonendocrine origin. That is, the syndrome may occur in patients with bronchogenic carcinoma in which malignant lung cells synthesize and release ADH. SIADH has also occurred with severe pneumonia, pneumothorax, and other disorders of the lungs in addition to malignant tumors that affect other organs.

Disorders of the central nervous system, such as head injury, brain surgery or tumor, or meningitis, are thought to produce SIADH by direct stimulation of the pituitary gland. Some drugs (vincristine, phenothiazines, tricyclic antidepressants, and others) have been implicated in SIADH; they either directly stimulate the pituitary gland or increase the sensitivity of renal tubules to circulating ADH.

This syndrome is generally managed by eliminating the underlying cause if possible and restricting the patient's fluid intake. Because retained water is slowly excreted through the kidneys, the extracellular fluid volume contracts and the serum sodium concentration gradually increases toward normal. Diuretics may be used along with fluid restriction if severe hyponatremia is present.

Close monitoring of fluid intake and output, daily weight, urine and blood chemistries, and neurologic status is indicated for the patient at risk for SIADH. Supportive measures and explanations of procedures and treatments assist the patient to deal with this disorder.

In summary, the endocrine glands secrete substances known as hormones directly into the circulation. The hormones work with the nervous system to regulate organ function. The concentration of the hormones in the bloodstream is normally maintained at a relatively constant level through feedback mechanisms. That is, when the concentration of a hormone is reduced, the production or secretion of the hormone is stimulated until the normal concentration of the hormone is restored. When the hormone level rises in the bloodstream, its production or secretion is reduced until a normal concentration is once again achieved. The disorders of the endocrine glands generally result from overproduction (*hyper-*) or underproduction (*hypo-*) of hormones. Because of the widespread action of the hormones, dysfunction of one of the endocrine glands results in major disturbances throughout the body. Hypofunction of the endocrine glands is generally treated with replacement of the specific hormone that is affected. Hyperfunction is usually treated by removal of part or all of the gland that is overproducing the hormones.

The Pancreas

The pancreas has both endocrine and exocrine functions, and these functions are interrelated. The major exocrine function is to facilitate digestion through secretion of enzymes into the proximal duodenum. Secretin and cholecystokinin-pancreozymin (CCK-PZ) are hormones from the gastrointestinal tract that aid in the digestion of food substances by control of secretions of the pancreas. Additionally, neural factors also influence pancreatic enzyme secretion. Considerable dysfunction of the pancreas must occur before enzyme secretion decreases and protein and fat digestion becomes impaired. Pancreatic enzyme secretion is normally 1000 to 4000 ml/day, with the amount depending on the quantity and type of food intake.

Gerontologic Considerations. There is little change in the size of the pancreas with age. There is, however, an increase in fibrous material and some fatty deposition in the normal pancreas in patients over age 70. Additionally, there may be some slight focal changes of arteriosclerosis with age. Studies have suggested a decreased pancreatic secretion rate (decreased lipase, amylase, and trypsin) and bicarbonate output in older patients. There may be some impairment of normal fat absorption with increasing age, possibly due to delayed gastric emptying and pancreatic insufficiency. Decreased calcium absorption may also occur. These changes require care in interpreting diagnostic tests in the normal elderly person and in providing dietary counseling.

Pancreatitis

Pancreatitis (inflammation of the pancreas) is a serious disorder of the pancreas that can assume several forms. *Acute pancreatitis,* in which the structure and function of the pancreas usually return to normal after the acute attack, occurs most frequently as a result of gallstones. *Chronic pancreatitis* is characterized by permanent abnormalities of pancreatic function and is usually a result of long-term alcohol use. Patients with long-standing, undiagnosed chronic pancreatitis may develop acute episodes of pancreatitis, making the clinical picture less clear.

Several classification systems have been used to categorize the various stages and forms of pancreatitis. One classification system describes acute pancreatitis on the basis of findings on laparotomy or autopsy. These include interstitial (edematous) and hemorrhagic (acute necrotizing) pancreatitis. The 1984

International Symposium on Classification of Pancreatitis categorizes the disease as acute or chronic pancreatitis, with obstructive chronic pancreatitis added as a type of chronic pancreatitis.

Several theories exist about the cause and mechanism of pancreatitis, which is generally described as the autodigestion of the pancreas. Generally, these theories state that obstruction of the pancreatic duct is present and is accompanied by hypersecretion of the exocrine enzymes of the pancreas. These enzymes enter the bile duct, where they are activated and, together with bile, back up (reflux) into the pancreatic duct, causing pancreatitis.

Acute Pancreatitis

Pathophysiology and Etiology.   Acute pancreatitis or inflammation of the pancreas is brought about by the digestion of this organ by the very enzymes it produces, principally trypsin. Eighty percent of patients with acute pancreatitis have biliary tract disease; however, only 5% of patients with gallstones develop pancreatitis. Gallstones enter the common bile duct and lodge at the ampulla of Vater, obstructing the flow of pancreatic juice or causing a reflux of bile from the common bile duct into the pancreatic duct, thus activating the powerful enzymes within the pancreas. Normally, these remain in an inactive form until the pancreatic juice reaches the lumen of the duodenum. Spasm and edema of the ampulla of Vater, resulting from duodenitis, can probably produce pancreatitis.

Long-term alcohol use is a common cause of acute episodes of pancreatitis, but the patient usually has had undiagnosed chronic pancreatitis before the first episode of acute pancreatitis occurs. Other less common causes of pancreatitis include bacterial or viral infection, with pancreatitis a complication of mumps virus. Blunt abdominal trauma, peptic ulcer disease, ischemic vascular disease, hyperlipidemia, hypercalcemia, and the use of corticosteroids, thiazide diuretics, and oral contraceptives have been associated with an increased incidence of pancreatitis. Acute pancreatitis may follow surgery on or near the pancreas or after instrumentation of the pancreatic duct. In addition, there is a small incidence of hereditary pancreatitis.

Mortality of acute pancreatitis is high (10%) because of shock, anoxia, hypotension, or fluid and electrolyte imbalances. Attacks of acute pancreatitis may result in complete recovery, may recur without permanent damage, or may progress to chronic pancreatitis. The patient admitted to the hospital with a diagnosis of pancreatitis is acutely ill and requires expert nursing and medical care.

Classification.   Pancreatitis ranges in severity from a relatively mild, self-limiting disorder to a rapidly fatal disease that does not respond to any treatment. Edema and inflammation confined to the pancreas are the major events in the more mild form of pancreatitis, which is termed *interstitial* or *edematous pancreatitis*. Although this is considered the more mild form of pancreatitis, the patient is acutely ill and at risk of developing shock, fluid and electrolyte disturbances, and sepsis.

Acute hemorrhagic pancreatitis represents a more advanced form of acute interstitial pancreatitis. Enzymatic digestion of the gland is more widespread and complete. The tissue becomes necrotic, and the damage extends to the vasculature,

so that blood escapes into the substance of the pancreas and into the retroperitoneal tissues. Late complications consist of pancreatic cysts or abscesses. The mortality rate of acute hemorrhagic pancreatitis is 30%.

Clinical Manifestations.   Severe abdominal pain is the major symptom of pancreatitis that brings the patient to medical care. Abdominal pain and tenderness, along with back pain, result from irritation and edema of the inflamed pancreas that stimulate the nerve endings. Increased tension on the pancreatic capsule and obstruction of the pancreatic ducts also contribute to the pain. Typically, the pain occurs in the midepigastrium. Pain is frequently acute in onset, occurring 24 to 48 hours after a very heavy meal or alcohol ingestion, and it may be diffuse and difficult to locate. It is generally more severe after meals and is unrelieved by antacids. Pain may be accompanied by abdominal distention, a poorly defined palpable abdominal mass, and decreased peristalsis.

The patient appears acutely ill. Abdominal guarding is present. A rigid or boardlike abdomen may occur and is generally an ominous sign. The abdomen may, however, remain soft in the absence of peritonitis. Ecchymosis (bruising) in the flank or around the umbilicus may indicate severe, hemorrhagic pancreatitis.

Nausea and vomiting are common in acute pancreatitis. The vomitus is usually gastric in origin but may also be bile-stained. Fever, jaundice, mental confusion, and agitation may also occur.

Hypotension is typical and reflects hypovolemia and shock due to loss of large amounts of protein-rich fluid into the tissues and peritoneal cavity. The patient may develop tachycardia, cyanosis, and cold, clammy skin in addition to hypotension. Acute renal failure is common.

Respiratory distress and hypoxia are common, and the patient may develop diffuse pulmonary infiltrates, dyspnea, tachypnea, and abnormal blood gas values. Myocardial depression, hypocalcemia, hyperglycemia, and disseminated intravascular coagulation may also occur with acute pancreatitis.

The diagnosis of acute pancreatitis is based on a history of abdominal pain, the presence of known risk factors, physical examination findings, and selected diagnostic findings.

Diagnostic Evaluation.   Serum amylase is the most important aid in diagnosing acute pancreatitis. Peak levels are reached in 24 hours, with a rapid fall to normal levels within 48 to 72 hours. Urinary amylase levels also become elevated and remain elevated longer than serum amylase levels. The white blood cell count is usually elevated; hypocalcemia is present in many patients and appears to be correlated with the severity of pancreatitis. Transient hyperglycemia and glucosuria and elevated serum bilirubin levels occur in some patients with acute pancreatitis.

X-ray films of the abdomen and chest are obtained to differentiate pancreatitis from other disorders that may cause similar symptoms and to detect the development of pleural effusions. Sonograms and tomograms (CT scans) are used to identify an increase in the diameter of the pancreas and to detect pancreatic cysts or pseudocysts.

Usually the stools of patients suffering with pancreatic disease are bulky, pale, and foul smelling. Fat content varies between 50% and 90% in pancreatic disease; normally, the fat content is 20%.

Management. Management of the patient with acute pancreatitis is symptomatic and is directed toward preventing or treating complications. All oral intake is withheld to inhibit pancreatic stimulation and secretion of pancreatic enzymes. Although there is some controversy about the use of total parenteral nutrition (TPN) in acute pancreatitis because of the possibility that it may stimulate pancreatic secretion, it is usually an important part of therapy, particularly in debilitated patients. Nasogastric suction may be used to relieve nausea and vomiting, to decrease painful abdominal distention and paralytic ileus, and to remove hydrochloric acid so that it does not enter the duodenum and stimulate the pancreas. Cimetidine (Tagamet) is also used to decrease hydrochloric acid secretion.

Adequate pain medication is essential during the course of acute pancreatitis to provide sufficient pain relief and minimize the patient's restlessness, which may stimulate pancreatic secretion further.

Adequate correction of fluid and blood loss and low albumin levels is necessary to maintain fluid volume and prevent renal failure. The patient is usually acutely ill and is monitored in the intensive care unit. Antibiotics are frequently administered to control infection; insulin may be required if significant hyperglycemia occurs. Peritoneal lavage has been effective in severe pancreatitis or if ascites is significant.

Aggressive respiratory care is indicated because of the increased likelihood of elevation of the diaphragm, pulmonary infiltrates and effusion, and atelectasis. Hypoxemia occurs in a significant number of patients with acute pancreatitis even without abnormalities present on x-ray. Respiratory care may range from close monitoring of arterial blood gases to use of humidified oxygen to intubation and use of a ventilator.

Placement of biliary drains (for external drainage) and stents (indwelling tubes) in the pancreatic duct through endoscopy has been performed recently with some success. This treatment reestablishes drainage of the pancreas without surgery and has resulted in decreased pain and increased weight gain.

Antacids may be used when the acute episode of pancreatitis begins to resolve. Oral feedings that are low in fat and protein content are initiated very gradually. Caffeine and alcohol are eliminated from the diet. If the episode of pancreatitis occurred during treatment with thiazide diuretics, glucocorticoids, or oral contraceptives, these medications are discontinued. Follow-up of the patient may include ultrasound, x-ray studies, or endoscopic retrograde cholangiopancreatography (ERCP) to determine if the pancreatitis is resolving and to assess for abscesses and pseudocysts. ERCP may also be used to identify the cause of acute pancreatitis if it is in question and for endoscopic sphincterotomy and removal of gallstones from the common bile duct.

Research is currently under way to identify agents that would prevent the increased capillary permeability and edema that occur with acute pancreatitis.

Gerontologic Considerations. Acute pancreatitis affects people of all ages; however, the mortality from acute pancreatitis increases with advancing age. In addition, the pattern of complications changes with age. Younger patients tend to develop local complications, while the incidence of multiple organ failure increases with age, possibly as a result of progressive decreases in physiologic function of major organs with increasing age. Close observation of major organ function (*i.e.*, lungs, kidneys) is indicated and aggressive treatment is necessary to reduce mortality from acute pancreatitis in the elderly.

▶ Nursing Process
The Patient With Acute Pancreatitis

◇ Assessment

The health history focuses on the presence and character of the patient's abdominal pain and discomfort. The presence of pain, its location, its relationship to eating and to alcohol consumption, and the effect of the patient's efforts to obtain pain relief are noted. The patient's nutritional and fluid status and history of gallbladder attacks and alcohol use are assessed. A history of gastrointestinal problems, including nausea, vomiting, diarrhea, and passage of stools containing fat, is elicited. The abdomen is assessed for pain, tenderness, guarding, and bowel sounds; the presence of a boardlike or soft abdomen is noted. Respiratory status, respiratory rate and pattern, and breath sounds are assessed. Normal and adventitious breath sounds and abnormal findings on chest percussion, including dullness at the bases of the lungs and abnormal tactile fremitus (see Chap. 24, p. 506), are documented.

◇ Nursing Diagnoses

Based on all the assessment data, the major nursing diagnoses of the patient with acute pancreatitis include the following:

- Severe pain related to inflammation, edema, distention of the pancreas, and peritoneal irritation
- Altered fluid and nutritional status related to vomiting, inadequate fluid intake, fever and diaphoresis, and fluid shifts
- Ineffective breathing pattern related to severe pain, pulmonary infiltrates, pleural effusion, and atelectasis

◇ Planning and Implementation

◇ *Goals:* The major goals for the patient include relief of pain and discomfort, improved fluid and nutritional status, and improved respiratory function.

◇ Nursing Interventions

◇ *Relief of Pain and Discomfort.* Because the pathologic process responsible for pain is autodigestion of the pancreas, the objectives of therapy are to relieve pain and to decrease secretion of the enzymes of the pancreas. The pain of acute pancreatitis is often very severe, necessitating the liberal use of analgesics. Meperidine (Demerol) is the drug of choice; morphine sulfate is avoided because it causes spasm of the sphincter of Oddi. Oral feedings are withheld to decrease the formation and secretion of secretin. The patient is maintained on parenteral fluids and electrolytes to restore and maintain fluid balance. Nasogastric suction is used to remove gastric secretions and to relieve abdominal distention. The nurse provides frequent oral hygiene and care to decrease discomfort from the nasogastric tube and relieve dryness of the mouth; dryness of the mucous membranes will be increased if the patient is receiving anticholinergic drugs to decrease pancreatic secretions.

The acutely ill patient will be maintained on bed rest to decrease the metabolic rate and reduce the secretion of pancreatic and gastric enzymes. If the patient experiences increasing severity of pain, this is reported to the physician, because the patient may be experiencing hemorrhage of the pancreas, or the dose of analgesic may be inadequate.

The patient with acute pancreatitis often has a clouded sensorium because of severe pain, fluid and electrolyte disturbances, and hypoxemia. Therefore, he will require frequent and repeated but simple explanations about the need for withholding fluid intake and about maintenance of gastric suction and bed rest.

▷ *Fluid Balance and Nutritional Status.* Nausea, vomiting, gastric suction, movement of fluid from the vascular compartment to the peritoneal cavity, and diaphoresis and fever increase the patient's need for fluid and electrolyte replacement. Intravenous fluids will be administered and may be accompanied by transfusion of blood and albumin to maintain the patient's blood volume and to prevent or treat shock. The patient's fluid and electrolyte status is assessed by noting skin turgor and moistness of mucous membranes. The patient is weighed daily, and fluid intake and output are carefully measured, including urine output, nasogastric secretions, and diarrhea. The nurse observes the patient for the presence of ascites and measures abdominal girth if ascites is suspected.

During the attack of acute pancreatitis, the patient will not be permitted food and oral fluid intake; however, it is important for the nurse to assess the patient's nutritional status and to note any events that alter the patient's fluid and nutritional needs. These signs include increased body temperature, restlessness and increased physical activity, and fluid and nutrient loss through diarrhea. Frequent assessment of the patient is indicated and emergency medications are kept readily available because of the risk of circulatory collapse and shock. Decreased blood pressure and reduced urine output are reported promptly because they may indicate hypovolemia and shock or renal failure.

As the patient's acute symptoms subside, oral feedings are reintroduced gradually. Between acute attacks, the patient receives a diet high in carbohydrates and low in fat and proteins. Heavy meals are avoided, as are alcoholic beverages.

▷ *Improved Breathing Pattern.* The patient is maintained in a semi-Fowler's position to decrease pressure on the diaphragm by a distended abdomen and to increase respiratory expansion. Frequent changes of position are necessary to prevent atelectasis and pooling of respiratory secretions. Anticholinergic medications, if given to decrease gastric and pancreatic secretions, also dry the secretions of the respiratory tract, predisposing the patient to obstruction and infection. Pulmonary assessment is essential to observe for any changes in respiratory status. The patient is instructed in techniques of coughing and deep breathing to improve respiratory function.

▷ *Patient Education and Home Health Care.* The patient who has experienced and survived an episode of acute pancreatitis has been acutely ill. He will require a prolonged period of time to regain strength and return to his previous level of activity. Because of the severity of the acute illness, the patient may not recall many of the facts and explanations given during the acute phase. As a result, this patient often requires repetition and reinforcement of information and instructions. If acute pancreatitis is a result of biliary tract disease such as gallstones and gallbladder disease, the patient requires reinforcement about the need for a low-fat diet and avoidance of heavy meals. If the pancreatitis is a result of alcohol abuse, the patient needs to be reminded of the importance of eliminating *all* alcohol. When the acute attack has subsided and he returns to his previous environment, he may be inclined to return to his previous habits. Specific information about resources and support groups that may be of assistance in avoiding alcohol in the future is provided to the patient and his family. Referral to Alcoholics Anonymous or other appropriate support groups is essential.

A referral to the community health nurse is often indicated to permit the nurse to assess the patient's home situation, reinforce instructions about fluid and nutrition intake and avoidance of alcohol, and permit the patient and family members to discuss their questions and concerns.

A summary of nursing management of the patient with acute pancreatitis is provided in Nursing Care Plan 40-3.

▷ **Evaluation**

Expected Outcomes

1. Experiences relief of pain and discomfort.
   a. Reports relief of pain and discomfort.
   b. Explains rationale for nasogastric tube and suction.
   c. Uses analgesics as prescribed, without overuse.
   d. Participates in oral hygiene measures.
   e. Maintains bed rest as prescribed.
   f. Uses anticholinergics appropriately if prescribed.
   g. Avoids alcohol to decrease abdominal pain.
2. Achieves improved fluid and nutritional balance.
   a. Demonstrates normal skin turgor and moist mucous membranes.
   b. Reports stabilization of weight.
   c. Demonstrates no increase in abdominal girth.
   d. Reports decrease in number of episodes of diarrhea.
   e. Identifies and consumes high-carbohydrate, low-protein foods.
   f. Explains rationale for eliminating alcohol intake.
   g. Maintains adequate fluid intake within prescribed guidelines.
3. Experiences improved respiratory function.
   a. Maintains semi-Fowler's position when in bed.
   b. Changes position in bed frequently.
   c. Coughs and takes deep breaths at least every hour.
   d. Demonstrates normal respiratory rate and pattern and full lung expansion.
   e. Demonstrates normal breath sounds and absence of adventitious breath sounds.
   f. Drinks at least 8 glasses of nonalcoholic fluids per day (if within fluid allowance) to liquefy pulmonary secretions.
   g. Demonstrates normal body temperature and absence of indications of respiratory infection.

Chronic Pancreatitis

Chronic pancreatitis is an inflammatory disease characterized by progressive anatomic and functional destruction of the pancreas. As cells are replaced by fibrous tissue with repeated attacks of pancreatitis, pressure within the pancreas increases. The end result is mechanical obstruction of the pancreatic and common bile ducts and the duodenum. Additionally, there is atrophy of the epithelium of the ducts, inflammation, and destruction of the secreting cells of the pancreas.

Alcohol consumption in Western societies and malnutrition worldwide are the major causes of chronic pancreatitis. In alcoholism, the incidence of pancreatitis is 50 times the rate in the nondrinking population. Chronic consumption of alcohol produces hypersecretion of protein in pancreatic secretions. The result is protein plugs and calculi within the pancreatic ducts. There is also evidence that alcohol has a direct toxic effect on the cells of the pancreas. Damage to these cells is more likely to occur and to be more severe in patients whose diets are poor in protein content and either very high or very low in fat. The incidence of chronic pancreatitis is increased in adult men and is characterized by recurring attacks of severe upper abdominal and back pain, accompanied by vomiting. Attacks often are so painful that narcotics, even in large doses, do not provide relief. As the disease progresses, recurring attacks of pain will be more severe, more frequent, and of longer duration. Some patients complain of continuous severe pain; others have a dull, nagging constant pain. The risk of addiction to opiates is increased in pancreatitis because of the chronic nature and severity of the pain.

Weight loss is a major problem in chronic pancreatitis; over 75% of patients experience significant weight loss usually due to decreased dietary intake secondary to anorexia or fear that eating will precipitate another attack. Malabsorption occurs late in the disease when as little as 10% of pancreatic function remains. As a result, the digestion of foodstuffs, especially proteins and fats, is disrupted. The stools become frequent, frothy, and foul-smelling because of the impairment of fat digestion, which results in stool with a high fat content. This condition is referred to as *steatorrhea*. As the disease progresses, calcification of the gland may occur and calcium stones may form within the ducts.

Diagnostic Evaluation. Endoscopic retrograde cholangiopancreatography (ERCP) is the most useful study in the diagnosis of chronic pancreatitis. It provides detail about the anatomy of the pancreas and of the pancreatic and biliary ducts. It is also helpful in obtaining tissue for analysis and in differentiating pancreatitis from other conditions such as carcinoma. A CT scan or ultrasonography is helpful to detect the presence of pancreatic cyst formation. A glucose tolerance test evaluates pancreatic islet cell function, information necessary for making decisions about surgical resection of the pancreas. An abnormal glucose tolerance test indicative of diabetes may be present. In contrast to the patient with acute pancreatitis, serum amylase levels and the white blood cell count may not be grossly abnormal.

Management. The management of chronic pancreatitis depends on its probable cause in each patient. Nonsurgical approaches may be indicated for the patient who refuses surgery, is a poor surgical risk, or whose disease and symptoms do not warrant surgical intervention. Treatment is directed toward prevention and management of acute attacks, the relief of pain and discomfort, and management of exocrine and endocrine insufficiency of pancreatitis. Treatment and prevention of abdominal pain and discomfort are similar to those used in acute pancreatitis; however, the focus is usually on the use of nonopiate methods to prevent or treat pain. The physician as well as the nurse and dietitian emphasize to the patient and family the importance of avoiding alcohol and other foods that the patient has found tend to produce abdominal pain and discomfort. The fact that no other treatment is likely to relieve pain if the patient continues to consume alcohol is stressed to the patient.

Diabetes mellitus resulting from dysfunction of the pancreatic islet cells is treated with diet, insulin, or oral hypoglycemic agents. The hazard of severe hypoglycemia with alcohol use is stressed to the patient and family members. Pancreatic enzyme replacement is indicated in the patient with malabsorption and steatorrhea.

Surgery is generally carried out to relieve abdominal pain and discomfort, to restore drainage of pancreatic secretions, and to reduce the frequency of acute attacks of pancreatitis. The surgical procedure to be performed depends on the anatomic and functional abnormalities of the pancreas, including the location of disease within the pancreas, the presence of diabetes, exocrine insufficiency, biliary stenosis, and pseudocysts of the pancreas. Other factors taken into consideration in determining if surgery is to be performed and what procedure is indicated include continued use of alcohol and the ability of the patient to manage the endocrine or exocrine changes that are expected from surgical alterations.

Pancreaticojejunostomy with a side-to-side anastomosis or joining of the pancreatic duct to the jejunum allows drainage of the pancreatic secretions into the jejunum. Pain relief occurs by 6 months in over 80% of the patients who undergo this procedure, but pain returns in a substantial number of these patients as the disease itself progresses. Patients who undergo surgery may experience increased weight gain and improved nutritional status; this may result from reduction in pain associated with eating rather than from correction of malabsorption. A variety of other surgical procedures are performed for different degrees and types of disease, ranging from revision of the sphincter of the ampulla of Vater, to internal drainage of a pancreatic cyst into the stomach, to wide resection or removal of the pancreas. Attempts have been made to preserve the endocrine function of the pancreas by autotransplantation or implantation of the patient's pancreatic islet cells. Testing and refinement of this procedure continue in an effort to improve the results. Morbidity and mortality following these surgical procedures are high because of the poor physical condition of the patient prior to surgery and the concomitant occurrence of cirrhosis.

Despite these operative procedures, the patient is likely to continue having pain and digestive difficulties from the pancreatitis unless he abstains completely from the use of alcohol.

Pancreatic Cysts

As a result of the local necrosis that occurs at the time of acute pancreatitis, collections of fluid may form in the vicinity of the pancreas. These become walled off by fibrous tissue and are called pancreatic cysts. They are the most common type of pancreatic cysts; other types develop as a result of congenital anomalies or secondary to chronic pancreatitis or trauma to the pancreas.

Diagnosis of pancreatic cysts is made by ultrasound, CT scan, and ERCP. ERCP may be used to define the anatomy of the pancreas and to evaluate the patency of pancreatic drainage. Pancreatic cysts may attain considerable size. Because of their location behind the posterior peritoneum, when they en-

(text continues on page 1114)

Nursing Care Plan 40-3

Care of the Patient With Acute Pancreatitis

Nursing Interventions	Rationale	Expected Outcomes

Nursing Diagnosis: Severe pain and discomfort related to edema, distention of the pancreas, and peritoneal irritation

Goal: Relief of pain and discomfort

1. Administer meperidine (Demerol) frequently, as prescribed, based on patient's level of pain and discomfort.	1. Meperidine acts by depressing the central nervous system and thereby increasing the patient's pain threshold. Morphine is not usually given because it has a tendency to produce spasm of the sphincter of Oddi.	• Reports relief of pain. • Moves and turns without increasing pain and discomfort. • Rests comfortably and sleeps for increasing periods of time. • Reports less frequent episodes of pain, discomfort, and cramping.
2. Assess pain level before and after administration of analgesic.	2. Assessment and control of pain are important because restlessness increases body metabolism, which stimulates the secretion of pancreatic and gastric enzymes.	
3. Report unrelieved pain or increasing intensity of pain.	3. Pain may increase pancreatic enzymes and may also indicate pancreatic hemorrhage.	
4. Assist the patient to assume positions of comfort; turn and reposition q2h.	4. Frequent turning relieves pressure and aids in preventing pulmonary and vascular complications.	

Goal: Reduction of stimulation of the pancreas

1. Give anticholinergic drugs as prescribed.	1. Anticholinergic drugs reduce gastric and pancreatic secretion.	• Reports relief of pain, discomfort, and abdominal cramping.
2. Withhold oral intake.	2. Pancreatic secretion is increased by food and fluid intake.	• Takes no fluid and food during acute phase.
3. Maintain the patient on bed rest.	3. Bed rest decreases body metabolism and thus reduces pancreatic and gastric secretions.	• Maintains bed rest.

4. Use continuous nasogastric suction.
  a. Measure gastric secretions at specified intervals.
  b. Observe and record color and viscosity of gastric secretions.
  c. Ensure that the nasogastric tube is patent to permit free drainage.
	4. Nasogastric suction removes gastric contents and prevents gastric secretions from entering the duodenum and stimulating the secretin mechanism. Decompression of the intestines (if intestinal intubation is used) also assists in relieving respiratory distress.	• Explains rationale for fluid and dietary restrictions and use of nasogastric drainage.

Goal: Relief of discomfort associated with nasogastric drainage

1. Use water-soluble lubricant around external nares.	1. Prevents irritation.	• Exhibits intact skin and tissue of nares at site of nasogastric tube insertion.
2. Turn patient at intervals; avoid pressure or tension on NG tube	2. Relieves pressure of tube on esophageal and gastric mucosa.	• Reports no pain or irritation of nares or oropharynx.
3. Give oral hygiene and gargling solutions without alcohol.	3. Relieves dryness and irritation of oropharynx.	• Exhibits moist, clean mucous membranes of mouth and nasopharynx.
4. Explain rationale for use of nasogastric drainage.	4. Assists patient to cope with the drainage, nasogastric tube, and suction.	• States that thirst is relieved by oral hygiene. • Restates rationale for nasogastric tube and suction.

(continued)

Nursing Care Plan 40-3 *(Continued)*

Care of the Patient With Acute Pancreatitis

Nursing Interventions	Rationale	Expected Outcomes

Nursing Diagnosis: Fluid volume deficit related to vomiting, decreased fluid intake, fever and diaphoresis, and fluid shifts

Goal: Improvement in fluid and electrolyte status

Nursing Interventions	Rationale	Expected Outcomes
1. Assess fluid and electrolyte status (skin turgor, mucous membranes, urine output, vital signs).	1. The amount and type of fluid and electrolyte replacement are determined by the status of the blood pressure, the laboratory evaluations of serum electrolyte and blood urea nitrogen levels, the urinary volume, and the assessment of the patient's condition.	• Exhibits moist mucous membranes and normal skin turgor.
		• Exhibits normal blood pressure without evidence of postural (orthostatic) hypotension.
		• Excretes adequate urine output.
		• Exhibits normal, not excessive, thirst.
2. Assess sources of fluid and electrolyte loss (vomiting, diarrhea, nasogastric drainage, excessive diaphoresis).	2. Electrolyte losses occur from nasogastric suctioning, severe diaphoresis, emesis, and as a result of the patient's being in a fasting state.	• Maintains normal pulse and respiratory rate.
		• Remains alert and responsive.
3. Combat shock if present.	3. Extensive acute pancreatitis may cause peripheral vascular collapse and shock. Blood and plasma may be lost into the abdominal cavity, and, therefore, there is a decreased blood and plasma volume. The toxins from the bacteria of a necrotic pancreas may cause shock.	• Exhibits normal arterial pressures and blood gases.
a. Administer corticosteroids as prescribed to those who do not respond to conventional treatment.		• Exhibits normal electrolyte levels.
b. Evaluate the amount of urinary output. Attempt to maintain this at 50 ml/hr.		• Exhibits no signs or symptoms of calcium deficit (*e.g.*, tetany, carpopedal spasm).
4. Administer intravenous electrolytes (sodium, potassium, chloride) as prescribed.	4. Patients with hemorrhagic pancreatitis lose large amounts of blood and plasma, which decreases effective circulation and blood volume.	• Exhibits no additional losses of fluids and electrolytes through vomiting, diarrhea, or diaphoresis.
5. Administer plasma, albumin, and blood as prescribed.	5. Replacement with blood, plasma or albumin, assists in ensuring effective circulating blood volume.	• Reports stabilization of weight.
		• Demonstrates no increase in abdominal girth.
6. Keep a supply of intravenous calcium gluconate readily available.	6. May be prescribed to prevent or treat tetany.	• Demonstrates no fluid wave on palpation of the abdomen.
7. Assess abdomen for ascites formation:	7. During acute pancreatitis, plasma may be lost into the abdominal cavity, which diminishes the blood volume.	
a. Measure abdominal girth daily.		
b. Weigh patient daily.		
c. Palpate abdomen for fluid wave (p. 982).		

Nursing Diagnosis: Altered nutrition: Less than body requirements related to inadequate dietary intake, impaired pancreatic secretions, increased nutritional needs secondary to acute illness, and increased body temperature

Goal: Improvement in nutritional status

Nursing Interventions	Rationale	Expected Outcomes
1. Assess current nutritional status and increased metabolic requirements.	1. Alteration in pancreatic secretions interferes with normal digestive processes. Acute illness, infection, and fever increase metabolic needs.	• Maintains normal body weight.
		• Demonstrates no additional weight loss.
		• Maintains normal serum glucose levels.
2. Monitor serum glucose levels and give insulin as prescribed.	2. Impairment of endocrine function of the pancreas leads to increased serum glucose levels.	• Reports decreasing episodes of vomiting and diarrhea.
		• Reports return of normal stool characteristics and bowel pattern.
3. Administer intravenous fluid and electrolytes and parenteral nutrition as prescribed.	3. Parenteral administration of fluids, electrolytes, and nutrients is essential to provide fluids, calories, electrolytes, and nutrients when oral intake is prohibited.	• Consumes foods high in carbohydrate, low in fat and protein.
		• Explains rationale for high-carbohydrate, low-fat, low-protein diet.

(continued)

Nursing Care Plan 40–3 (Continued)

Care of the Patient With Acute Pancreatitis

Nursing Interventions	Rationale	Expected Outcomes
4. Provide high-carbohydrate, low-protein, low-fat diet when tolerated.	4. These foods increase caloric intake without stimulating pancreatic secretions beyond the ability of the pancreas to respond.	• Eliminates alcohol from diet. • Explains rationale for limiting coffee intake and avoiding spicy foods.
5. Instruct patient to eliminate alcohol.	5. Alcohol intake produces further damage to pancreas and precipitates attacks of acute pancreatitis.	
6. Counsel patient to avoid excessive use of coffee and spicy foods.	6. Coffee and spicy foods increase pancreatic and gastric secretions.	

Nursing Diagnosis: Ineffective breathing pattern related to splinting from severe pain, pulmonary infiltrates, pleural effusion, and atelectasis

Goal: Improvement in respiratory function

1. Assess respiratory status (rate, pattern, breath sounds).	1. Acute pancreatitis produces retroperitoneal edema, elevation of the diaphragm, pleural effusion, and inadequate lung ventilation. Intra-abdominal infection and labored breathing increase the body's metabolic demands, which further decreases pulmonary reserve and leads to respiratory failure.	• Demonstrates normal respiratory rate and pattern and full lung expansion. • Demonstrates normal breath sounds and absence of adventitious breath sounds. • Demonstrates normal arterial blood gases. • Maintains semi-Fowler's position when in bed. • Changes position in bed frequently. • Coughs and takes deep breaths at least every hour. • Demonstrates normal body temperature. • Exhibits no signs or symptoms of respiratory infection or impairment. • Is alert and responsive to environment.
2. Maintain semi-Fowler's position	2. Decreases pressure on diaphragm and allows greater lung expansion.	
3. Instruct and encourage patient to take deep breaths and to cough every hour.	3. Taking deep breaths and coughing will clear the airways and reduce atelectasis.	
4. Assist patient to turn and change position every 2 hours.	4. Changing position frequently assists aeration and drainage of all lobes of the lungs.	

5. Reduce the excessive metabolism of the body.
    a. Administer antibiotics as prescribed.
    b. Place patient in an air-conditioned room.
    c. Administer nasal oxygen as required for hypoxia.
    d. Use a hypothermia blanket if necessary.
	5. Pancreatitis produces a severe peritoneal and retroperitoneal reaction that causes fever, tachycardia, and accelerated respirations. Placing the patient in an air-conditioned room and supporting him with oxygen therapy decrease the workload of the respiratory system and the tissue utilization of oxygen. Reduction of fever and pulse rate decreases the metabolic demands on the body.	

large, they impinge on and displace the stomach or the colon, which are adjacent. Eventually, through pressure or secondary infection, they produce symptoms, requiring that they be drained.

Management.   Drainage into the gastrointestinal tract or through the skin surface of the abdominal wall may be established. In the latter instance, the drainage is likely to be profuse and destructive to tissue because of the enzyme contents. Hence, steps must be taken to protect the skin in areas adjacent

to the drainage site to prevent excoriation. Ointments protect the skin, provided that they are applied before excoriation takes place. Another method involves the constant aspiration of digestive juice from the drainage tract by means of a suction apparatus, so that skin contact with the digestive enzymes is avoided. This method demands expert nursing attention to be sure that the suction tube does not become dislodged from the drainage tract and that the entire apparatus functions properly without interruption.

Consultation with an enterostomal therapist is advised to identify appropriate strategies to maintain drainage while protecting the patient's skin.

When chronic pancreatitis develops in association with gallbladder disease, efforts are made to relieve the obstruction by surgically exploring the common duct and removing the stones; usually, the gallbladder is removed at the same time. In addition, an attempt is made to improve the drainage of the common bile duct and the pancreatic duct by dividing the sphincter of Oddi, a muscle that is located at the ampulla of Vater (this operation is known as a *sphincterotomy*). Nursing management after such an operation is the same as that indicated for all patients undergoing biliary tract surgery. A T tube usually is placed in the common bile duct, requiring a drainage system to collect the bile after the operation.

Pancreatic Tumors

Carcinoma of the Pancreas

The incidence of pancreatic cancer has been steadily increasing for the past 20 to 30 years, especially in nonwhite males. It is the fourth leading cause of cancer deaths in the United States and occurs most frequently in the sixth and seventh decades of life. Exposure to industrial chemicals or toxins in the environment, a high-fat diet, and cigarette smoking are associated with an increased incidence of pancreatic cancer, although their role in the etiology is unclear. The risk of pancreatic cancer is increased in persons with hereditary pancreatitis.

Cancer may arise in any portion of the pancreas (in the head, the body, or the tail), producing clinical manifestations that vary, depending on the location of the lesion and whether or not functioning, insulin-secreting pancreatic islet cells are involved. Tumors that originate in the head of the pancreas, the most common location, give rise to a distinctive clinical picture. Functioning islet cell tumors, whether benign (adenoma) or malignant (carcinoma), are responsible for the syndrome of hyperinsulinism (see p. 1119). With these exceptions, the symptoms are nonspecific, and patients usually do not seek medical attention until late in the course of their illness; 80% to 85% of patients have advanced, unresectable disease when the tumor is first detected.

Clinical Manifestations.   Anorexia, weight loss, abdominal pain, or jaundice may be the initial symptom and may develop only when the disease is far advanced. Other signs include rapid, profound, and progressive weight loss as well as vague upper or midabdominal pain or discomfort that is unrelated to any gastrointestinal function and difficult to describe. Such discomfort radiates as a boring pain in the midback and is unrelated to posture or activity. Patients with pancreatic carcinoma often find that they get some relief from pain by sitting hunched forward; pain is often accentuated by lying supine. Pain is often progressive and severe, requiring the use of narcotic analgesics. It is often more severe at night. The formation of ascites is common.

A very important sign, when present, is the onset of symptoms of insulin deficiency: glucosuria, hyperglycemia, and abnormal glucose tolerance. Diabetes may be an early sign of carcinoma of the pancreas. Meals often aggravate epigastric pain, which usually occurs weeks before the appearance of

jaundice and pruritus. A gastrointestinal x-ray series may demonstrate deformities in adjacent viscera caused by the impinging pancreatic mass. Ultrasonography, CT scanning, and ERCP are useful in establishing the diagnosis.

Percutaneous fine-needle aspiration biopsy of the pancreas is used to diagnose pancreatic tumors and to confirm the diagnosis in patients whose tumors are not resectable, eliminating the stress and postoperative pain of ineffective surgery. In candidates for surgery, a preoperative diagnosis of the tumor is helpful in planning the surgical procedure. In this procedure, a needle is inserted through the anterior abdominal wall into the pancreatic mass under the guidance of CT scan, ultrasound, ERCP, or other imaging techniques. The aspirated material is examined for malignant cells.

Another procedure, a percutaneous transhepatic cholangiography (PTC), may be performed to identify obstructions of the biliary tract by a pancreatic tumor. Research is currently under way to identify tumor markers that would aid in diagnosing patients with pancreatic tumors.

Management.   Therapy usually is limited to palliative measures. Definitive surgical treatment (*i.e.,* total excision of the lesion) often is not feasible because of the extensive growth when the lesion is finally diagnosed and the probable widespread metastases—especially to the liver, lungs, and bones.

The surgical procedure is usually extensive if carried out to remove resectable localized tumors. Although pancreatic tumors may be resistant to standard radiation therapy, the patient may be treated with radiation and chemotherapy. Pain management and attention to nutritional requirements are important nursing measures to improve the patient's level of comfort. A full-length foam-rubber pad placed under the patient has proved beneficial and protects the bony prominences from pressure.

Tumors of the Head of the Pancreas

Assessment.   Tumors in this region of the pancreas cause obstruction of the common bile duct where it passes through the head of the pancreas to join the pancreatic duct and empty at the ampulla of Vater into the duodenum. Obstruction to the flow of bile produces jaundice, clay-colored stools, and dark urine.

Malabsorption of nutrients and fat-soluble vitamins may result from the obstruction and from the absence of bile from the gastrointestinal tract. Some degree of abdominal discomfort or pain and pruritus may be noted. Nonspecific symptoms such as anorexia, weight loss, and malaise may be present. If these signs and symptoms are present, cancer of this part of the pancreas is suspected.

The jaundice of this disease must be differentiated from the jaundice due to a biliary obstruction caused by a gallstone in the common duct, which usually is intermittent and appears typically in obese patients, most often women, who have had previous symptoms of gallbladder disease. The tumors producing the obstruction may arise from the pancreas, from the common bile duct, or from the ampulla of Vater.

Management.   When these patients come to the hospital, they are in such a poor nutritional and physical state that a fairly long period of preparation is necessary before operation can be attempted. Various liver and pancreatic function studies are carried out, vitamin K is given to restore the blood prothrombin activity, and a diet high in protein is often given with pancreatic enzymes. TPN may be administered. Blood transfusions frequently are used as well.

Following conventional blood and x-ray studies, more sophisticated diagnostic aids may be used, including duodenography, angiography by hepatic or celiac artery catheterization, pancreatic scanning, percutaneous transhepatic cholangiography, ERCP, and percutaneous needle biopsy of the pancreas. Laparotomy with biopsy of the pancreas may be performed to aid diagnosis.

Surgical Management. A biliary-enteric shunt may be performed to relieve the jaundice and, perhaps, provide time for a thorough diagnostic evaluation. Pancreatoduodenectomy (Whipple's procedure), which involves removal of the gallbladder, distal portion of the stomach, duodenum, and head of the pancreas, and anastomosis of the remaining pancreas, stomach, and common duct to the jejunum, is the operation of choice for potentially curable cancer of the head of the pancreas (Fig. 40-5*A, B*). The result is removal of the tumor, allowing flow of bile into the jejunum. When excision of the tumor cannot be performed, the jaundice may be relieved by diverting the bile flow into the jejunum by anastomosing the jejunum to the gallbladder, a procedure known as cholecystojejunostomy (Fig. 40-5*C*). (Whipple's resection has also been carried out to relieve the pain of chronic pancreatitis.)

Nursing Management. Extensive preoperative preparation is indicated and includes adequate hydration and nutrition, correction of prothrombin deficiency with vitamin K, and treatment of anemia to minimize postoperative complications.

The postoperative management of patients who have undergone a pancreatoduodenectomy or Whipple's procedure is similar to the management of patients following extensive gastrointestinal and biliary surgery. The psychosocial considerations, however, are more specific and must be properly approached by the nurse. In view of the fact that the patient has undergone major and risky surgery and is severely ill, he may experience anxiety and depression that will affect his response to therapy.

The mortality rate following this procedure has decreased recently because of advances in methods of nutritional support and improved techniques of surgical anastomosis. Preoperatively and postoperatively, the challenge for the nurse is to promote patient comfort, prevent complications, and assist the patient in returning to and maintaining as normal and comfortable a life as possible.

Hemorrhage, vascular collapse, and hepatorenal failure remain the major complications of this extensive surgical procedure. The patient will be monitored closely in the intensive care unit following surgery, have multiple intravenous and arterial lines in place for fluid and blood replacement as well as for monitoring arterial pressures, and be on a mechanical ventilator in the immediate postoperative period. Careful attention is given to changes in the patient's vital signs, arterial blood gases and pressures, laboratory values, and urine output. Although the patient's physiologic status is the focus of the physician and nurse in the immediate postoperative period, his psychologic and emotional state must be considered along with that of his family. The immediate and long-term outcome of this extensive surgical resection is uncertain, and the patient and family require emotional support and understanding in the critical and stressful preoperative and postoperative periods.

See Nursing Care Plan 40-4 (pp. 1117–1119) for care of

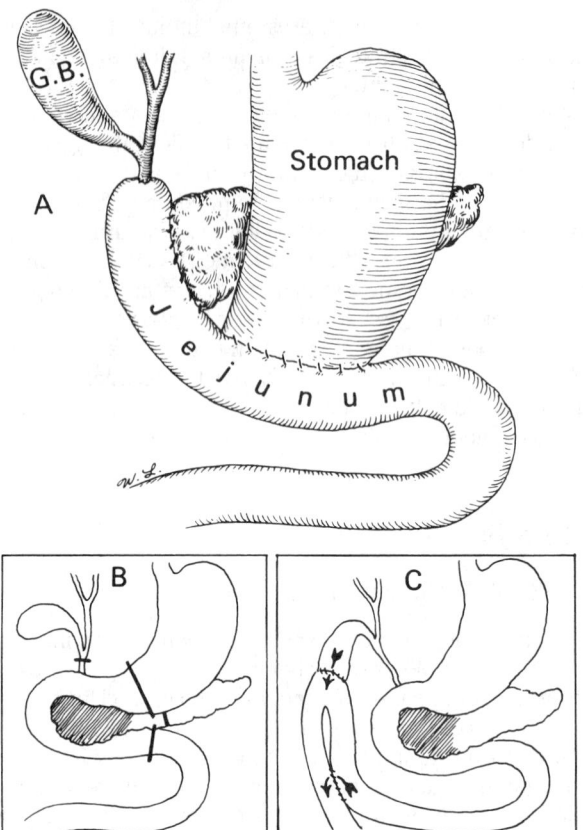

Figure 40–5. Pancreatoduodenectomy (Whipple's procedure or resection). (**A**) End result of resection of the carcinoma of the head of the pancreas or the ampulla of Vater. The common duct is sutured to the end of the jejunum, and the remaining portion of the pancreas and the end of the stomach are sutured to the side of the jejunum. (**B**) Lines indicate removal of head of pancreas, duodenum, adjacent stomach, and distal segment of common bile duct. (**C**) Cholecystojejunostomy is an alternative procedure if a tumor of the head of the pancreas is inoperable. Bile flows into the intestine through the anastomosis of the jejunum and gallbladder.

the patient following pancreatoduodenectomy (Whipple's procedure).

Pancreatic Islet Tumors

The pancreas contains the islets (islands) of Langerhans—small nests of cells that secrete directly into the bloodstream and, therefore, are part of the endocrine system. The secretion, insulin, is essential for metabolism of glucose. Diabetes mellitus (see Chap. 39) is the result of deficient secretion of insulin.

At least two types of tumors of the pancreatic islet cells are known: those that secrete insulin and those in which insulin secretion is not increased, known as "nonfunctioning" islet cell cancer.

Tumors of the islet cells frequently produce hypersecretion of insulin and an excessive rate of metabolism of glucose. Hypoglycemia, the resulting fall in serum glucose level, produces symptoms of weakness, mental confusion, and even convul-

(text continues on page 1119)

Nursing Care Plan 40–4

Care of the Patient Following Pancreatoduodenectomy (Whipple's Procedure)

Nursing Interventions	Rationale	Expected Outcomes

Nursing Diagnosis: Pain and discomfort related to extensive surgical incision and presence of nasogastric tube

Goal: Relief of pain and discomfort

1. Assess pain frequently before and after administration of analgesics.	1. Increasing pain may indicate occurrence of complications (pancreatitis, peritonitis, perforation of organ, or leakage of anastomosis).	• Reports decreasing pain and discomfort. • Experiences no increase in severity or frequency of pain. • Takes pain medication as prescribed.
2. Administer pain medication frequently, as prescribed.	2. Previous use of pain medications for past persistent pain may alter patient's response to pain medications and necessitate larger doses.	• Turns frequently with assistance to positions of comfort. • Rests comfortably without pain and discomfort.
3. Assist patient to assume position of comfort.	3. Position changes relieve pressure areas and decrease pressure and stress on suture lines.	• Exhibits intact, nonirritated skin and tissue of nares at site of nasogastric tube insertion.
4. Use water-soluble lubricant around external nares.	4. Lubricates the tissues and decreases friction at site of nasogastric tube insertion.	• Reports no pain or irritation of nasopharynx, oropharynx, or nares. • Exhibits moist, clean mucous membranes of mouth and nasopharynx.
5. Provide oral hygiene and gargling solutions.	5. Relieves dryness and irritation of oropharynx.	• Reports no excessive thirst.
6. Explain reasons for nasogastric tube and drainage.	6. Information may increase the patient's ability to cope with nasogastric tube and drainage.	• States rationale for nasogastric tube and suction.

Nursing Diagnosis: Ineffective breathing pattern related to extensive surgical incisions, immobility, prolonged anesthesia

Goal: Improvement of respiratory function

1. Assess patient's respiratory status:
  a. Dependence on mechanical ventilator
  b. Respiratory rate and pattern
  c. Thoracic excursion
  d. Breath sounds and adventitious sounds
	1. Splinting from extensive surgical incisions, prolonged immobility, and anesthesia frequently produce ineffective respiratory patterns and retained pulmonary secretions.	• Exhibits respiratory rate of 12 to 18/min with adequate thoracic excursion.
		• Breathes effectively without the mechanical ventilator.
		• Exhibits normal breath sounds without adventitious sounds.

2. Aspirate pulmonary secretions from the endotracheal tube or tracheostomy tube, as indicated.	2. Retained secretions interfere with adequate oxygen–carbon dioxide exchange.	• Takes deep breaths and coughs hourly while splinting abdominal incisions. • Coughs productively clear or white sputum.
3. Encourage and assist patient to cough and take deep breaths every hour.	3. Coughing and deep breathing aid in removal of pulmonary secretions and prevent atelectasis.	• Changes position frequently. • Exhibits normal body temperature and absence of respiratory infection.
4. Assist patient to change positions every hour.	4. Frequent changes of position will assist drainage of all lobes of the lungs.	

Nursing Diagnosis: Altered nutrition: Less than body requirements related to inadequate nutrition prior to surgery, increased metabolic demands secondary to extensive surgery, tissue repair, and altered gastrointestinal function

Goal: Improved nutritional state

1. Assess and report changes in factors affecting nutritional needs and status:
  a. Increased body temperature
  b. Increased gastrointestinal drainage and fluid loss
	1. Fever, increased gastrointestinal drainage, infection, and increased level of stress increase metabolic and nutritional needs.	• Maintains or increases body weight without edema formation.
		• Demonstrates no increase in metabolic rate and nutritional requirements:
		  Exhibits normal body temperature.

(continued)

Nursing Care Plan 40–4 (Continued)

Care of the Patient Following Pancreatoduodenectomy (Whipple's Procedure)

Nursing Interventions	Rationale	Expected Outcomes
c. Signs of infection d. Stress level 2. Administer parenteral fluids, electrolytes, and nutrients as prescribed. 3. Examine skin and tissue for breakdown and fistula formation. 4. Monitor serum glucose level and observe for symptoms of hyperglycemia and hypolgycemia. 5. Provide a high-carbohydrate, high-protein, high-vitamin diet as prescribed when oral intake is tolerated. 6. Administer pancreatic enzymes (Pancrease or Viokase) with meals if prescribed.	2. Parenteral administration of fluids, electrolytes, and nutrients is essential for healing when oral intake is prohibited. 3. The likelihood of breakdown of tissue increases with malnutrition and in turn increases need for nutrients. 4. The insulin-secreting islets of Langerhans of the pancreas may be impaired or may be removed during surgery, increasing the risk of hypoglycemia or hyperglycemia. 5. A high-carbohydrate, high-protein, high-vitamin diet is necessary to meet increased nutritional needs, prevent loss of muscle mass, promote healing of surgical incisions, and maintain weight. 6. Surgical resection of the pancreas may result in inadequate pancreatic enzymes, leading to malabsorption and further malnutrition.	Experiences no excessive gastrointestinal losses of fluid or nutrients. Demonstrates absence of signs of infection and inflammation. Exhibits decreasing levels of stress. • Exhibits rapid healing of incisions and no fistula formation. • Exhibits intact skin without evidence of breakdown. • Exhibits normal serum glucose levels. • Consumes foods high in carbohydrates, proteins, and vitamins. • Reports enhanced appetite. • Explains rationale for foods high in carbohydrates, proteins, and vitamins. • Identifies foods high in carbohydrates, proteins, and vitamins. • Takes pancreatic enzymes with meals as prescribed. • Reports decreasing episodes of diarrhea and steatorrhea. • Explains rationale for use of pancreatic enzymes with meals.

Nursing Diagnosis: Impaired skin and tissue integrity

Goal: Improvement of skin and tissue integrity

1. Avoid pressure on anastomoses and sutures:
  a. Irrigate nasogastric tube and other drainage tubes *gently* and *only* if prescribed.
 	
  b. Assess for adequate drainage from T tube, nasogastric tube, and any other drainage systems.
  c. Prevent kinking of tubing.
 	
2. Withhold oral intake until gastrointestinal function returns and diet and fluids are prescribed.
 	
3. Assess bowel sounds and abdomen for distention.
4. Inspect surgical incisions for inflammation, infection, and abscess formation.
	a. Ensures patency of drainage tubes but avoids increased intraluminal pressure and disruption of anastomosis and suture lines.
	  b. Ensures patency of drainage tubes.
	
	  c. Prevents buildup of intraluminal pressure and pressure on anastomosis.
	2. Too early intake of foods and fluid may cause abdominal distention and vomiting, increasing the risk of disrupting surgical anastomoses.
	3. Provides data about gastrointestinal function and early intestinal obstruction.
	4. Poor nutritional state and extensive surgery increase susceptibility to poor wound healing and increased skin and tissue breakdown.
		• Exhibits expected type and amount of drainage from T tube, nasogastric tube, and other drainage tubes.
		• Exhibits no untoward effects after irrigation of drainage tubes, if irrigation is needed.
		• Demonstrates return of normal bowel sounds.
		• Exhibits no abdominal distention.
		• Passes flatus.
		• Reports no nausea or vomiting.
		• Exhibits clean surgical incision without signs of inflammation, infection, or abscess formation.
		• Exhibits normal body temperature.
		• Exhibits pink, intact skin without signs of breakdown, irritation, or excoriation.
		• Demonstrates no purulent drainage or leakage of gastrointestinal secretions to skin surface.

(continued)

Nursing Care Plan 40-4 (Continued)

Care of the Patient Following Pancreatoduodenectomy (Whipple's Procedure)

Nursing Interventions	Rationale	Expected Outcomes
5. Inspect skin for breakdown, irritation, and excoriation.	5. Leakage of gastrointestinal drainage may cause digestion and excoriation of skin.	• Reports no increased pressure or pain at surgical incisions or sites of drainage tubes.
6. Maintain aseptic technique in handling wound dressings and drainage and all secretions.	6. Minimizes the risk of infection in susceptible patient.	
7. Apply paste or salve to skin at sites of drainage.	7. Protects skin from further excoriation and damage.	

sions. These may be relieved almost immediately by oral or intravenous administration of glucose. The 5-hour glucose tolerance test is helpful in diagnosing insulinoma, the tumor of the pancreatic islet cells that produces excessive insulin, and in distinguishing it from the more common functional hypoglycemia.

Once the diagnosis of a tumor of the islet cells has been made, surgical treatment with removal of the tumor usually is recommended. The tumors may be benign adenomas or they may be malignant. Complete removal usually results in a dramatic cure. In some patients, such symptoms may not be produced by an actual tumor of the islet cells but by a simple hypertrophy of this tissue. In such cases a partial *pancreatectomy*—removal of the tail and part of the body of the pancreas—is performed.

Management. In preparing these patients for surgery, the nurse must be alert for symptoms of hypoglycemia and be ready to administer glucose, should they appear. After operation, the nursing management is the same as that following any upper abdominal operation, with special emphasis on observation of serum glucose levels.

Hyperinsulinism

Hyperinsulinism results from the overproduction of insulin by the pancreatic islets. Symptoms resemble those of excessive doses of insulin and are attributable to the same mechanism— an abnormal reduction in blood glucose levels. Clinically, it is characterized by episodes during which the patient experiences unusual hunger, nervousness, sweating, headache, and faintness; in severe cases, convulsive seizures and episodes of unconsciousness may occur. The findings at operation or on postmortem examination may indicate hyperplasia (overgrowth) of the islets of Langerhans or a benign or malignant tumor involving the islets and capable of producing large amounts of insulin (see preceding discussion). Occasionally, tumors of nonpancreatic origin produce an insulin-like material that can cause hypoglycemia. This condition occasionally is responsible for convulsions coinciding with decreases in the blood glucose to levels that are inadequate to sustain normal brain function (*i.e.*, below 30 mg/dl [1.6 mmol/L]).

All of the symptoms that accompany spontaneous hypoglycemia are relieved by the oral or parenteral administration of glucose. Surgical removal of the hyperplastic or neoplastic tissue from the pancreas offers the only successful method of treatment. About 15% of patients with spontaneous or functional hypoglycemia eventually develop diabetes mellitus.

Ulcerogenic (Zollinger-Ellison) Tumors

Some tumors of the islets of Langerhans are associated with a hypersecretion of gastric acid that produces ulcers in the stomach, the duodenum, and even the jejunum. The hypersecretion is so great that even after partial gastric resection enough acid to produce further ulceration may remain. When a marked tendency to develop gastric and duodenal ulcers is noted, an ulcerogenic tumor of the islets of Langerhans is suspected.

These tumors, which may be benign or malignant, are treated, when possible, by excision. Frequently, however, because of extension beyond the pancreas, removal is not possible. In many patients, a total gastrectomy may be necessary to reduce the secretion of gastric acid sufficiently to prevent further ulceration.

In summary, the pancreas has both endocrine and exocrine functions. Pancreatitis and cancer of the pancreas are the most common disorders of the pancreas other than diabetes mellitus, which results from an inadequate insulin supply. The patient who experiences acute or chronic pancreatitis or cancer of the pancreas may be malnourished and suffering from acute or chronic abdominal pain. The patient often undergoes extensive diagnostic studies to determine the specific etiology of the symptoms and dysfunction and to assist in determining appropriate treatment. Treatment may be surgical or nonsurgical, depending on the etiology; nursing care is directed toward reducing the patient's acute or chronic symptoms, assisting him to cope with the diagnostic and treatment regimens, and promoting a healthy life-style and supportive environment.

Bibliography

Books

Baumel H and Deixonne B (eds). Exocrine Pancreatic Cancer. New York, Springer–Verlag, 1987.

Becker KL (ed). Principles and Practice of Endocrinology and Metabolism. Philadelphia, JB Lippincott, 1990.

Burch WM. Endocrinology for the House Officer. Baltimore, Williams & Wilkins, 1988.

Howard JM, Jordan GL Jr, and Reber HA. Surgical Diseases of the Pancreas. Philadelphia, Lea & Febiger, 1987.

Ingbar SH and Braverman LE (eds). Werner's The Thyroid: A Fundamental Clinical Text, 5th ed. Philadelphia, JB Lippincott, 1986.

Malfertheiner P and Ditschuneit H. Diagnostic Procedures in Pancreatic Disease. New York, Springer–Verlag, 1986.

Malseed RT and Harrigan GS. Textbook of Pharmacology and Nursing Care. Using the Nursing Process. Philadelphia, JB Lippincott, 1989.

National Cancer Institute. Cancer of the Pancreas. Research Report. U.S. Department of Health and Human Services, National Institutes of Health, Washington, DC, October 1987.

Riccabona G. Thyroid Cancer: Its Epidemiology, Clinical Features, and Treatment. New York, Springer–Verlag, 1987.

Toledo–Pereyra LH (ed). Pancreas Transplantation. Boston, Kluwer Academic Publishers, 1988.

Toledo–Pereyra LH. The Pancreas: Principles of Medical–Surgical Practice. New York, John Wiley & Sons, 1985.

Wilson JD and Foster DW (eds). Williams' Textbook of Endocrinology, 7th ed. Philadelphia, WB Saunders, 1985.

Journals
General

Aron DC. Endocrine complications of the acquired immunodeficiency syndrome. Arch Intern Med 1989 Feb; 149(2):330–333.

Beall GN. Immunologic aspects of endocrine diseases. JAMA 1987 Nov 27; 258(20):2952–2956.

Bravo EL. Clinical aspects of endocrine hypertension. Med Clin North Am 1987 Sep; 71(5):907–920.

Goldmann DR. Surgery in patients with endocrine dysfunction. Med Clin North Am 1987 May; 71(3):499–509.

Hague WM. Prescribing in pregnancy: Treatment of endocrine diseases. Br Med J 1987 Jan 31; 294(6567):297–300.

Hobbie WL and Schwartz CL. Endocrine late effects among survivors of cancer. Semin Oncol Nurs 1989 Feb; 5(1):14–21.

Lancaster LE. Renal and endocrine regulation of water and electrolyte balance. Nurs Clin North Am 1987 Dec; 22(4):761–772.

Lobo A et al. Emotional disturbances in endocrine patients: Validity of the scaled version of the General Health Questionnaire (GHQ-28). Br J Psychiatry 1988 Jun; 152:807–812.

Truhan AP and Ahmed AR. Corticosteroids: A review with emphasis on complications of prolonged systemic therapy. Ann Allergy 1989 May; 62(5):375–391.

Disorders of the Thyroid

Bethune JE. Interpretation of thyroid function tests. Dis Mon 1989 Aug; 25(8):546–595.

Brabant A et al. The role of glucocorticoids in the regulation of thyrotropin. Acta Endocrinol (Copenh) 1989 Jul; 121(1):95–100.

Connor CS et al. Radioiodine therapy for differentiated thyroid carcinoma. Am J Surg 1988 Dec; 156(6):519–521.

Dall'Aglio E et al. Graves' disease and thyroxine-binding globulin deficiency. Arch Intern Med 1988 Jun; 148(6):1445–1446.

Faber J et al. Pituitary–thyroid axis in critical illness. J Clin Endocrinol Metab 1987 Aug; 65(2):315–320.

Gavin LA. The diagnostic dilemmas of hyperthyroxinemia and hypothyroxinemia. Adv Intern Med 1988; 33:185–204.

Greenspan FS (ed). Thyroid diseases. Med Clin North Am 1991 Jan; 75(1):1–234.

Jackson JA, Verdonk CA, and Spiekerman AM. Euthyroid hyperthyroxinemia and inappropriate secretion of thyrotropin. Arch Intern Med 1987 Jul; 147(7):1311–1313.

Lervang H-H, Pryds O, and Østergaard Kristensen HP. Thyroid dysfunction after delivery. Acta Med Scand 1987; 222(4):369–374.

Levin RM. Editorial: Thyrotoxicosis in the elderly. J Am Geriatr Soc 1987 Jun; 35(6):587–589.

Mathewson MK. Thyroid disorder. Crit Care Nurs 1987 Jan/Feb; 7(1):74–85.

Mechlis S et al. Amiodarone-induced thyroid gland dysfunction. Am J Cardiol 1987 Apr 1; 59(8):833–835.

Melliere D, Etienne G, and Becquemin J-P. Operation for hyperthyroidism: Methods and rationale. Am J Surg 1988 Mar; 155(3):395–399.

Mier A et al. Reversible respiratory muscle weakness in hyperthyroidism. Am Rev Respir Dis 1989 Feb; 139(2):529–533.

O'Neil JR. Thyroid crisis. Nursing 1987 Nov; 17(11):33.

Reeve TS. Surgical treatment for thyrotoxicosis. Br J Surg 1988 Sep; 75(9):833–834.

Reid DJ. Hyperthyroidism and hypothyroidism complicating the treatment of thyrotoxicosis. Br J Surg 1987 Nov; 74(11):1060–1062.

Sakiyama R. Common thyroid disorders. Am Fam Physician 1988 Jul; 38(1):227–238.

Scott MA. Admission thyroid function testing in elderly patients. Aust N Z J Med 1986 Oct; 16(5):699–702.

Thomas R and Reid RL. Thyroid disease and reproductive dysfunction: A review. Obstet Gynecol 1987 Nov; 70(5):789–798.

Whiteside–Yim C and MacAdams MR. Thyroid disorders: The general internist's approach. Postgrad Med 1987 Apr; 81(5):231–235, 238–240, 245.

Yeomans AC. Assessment and management of hypothyroidism. Nurse Pract 1990 Nov 15(11):8–15.

Disorders of the Parathyroid Glands

Chambers JK. Metabolic bone disorders: Imbalances of calcium and phosphorus. Nurs Clin North Am 1987 Dec; 22(4):861–872.

Favus LH et al. Recurrent parathyroid cystic disease. Am Fam Physician 1989 Jul; 40(1):119–122.

Fitzpatrick LA and Bilezikian JP. Acute primary hyperparathyroidism. Am J Med 1987 Feb; 82(2):275–282.

McCance DR et al. Parathyroid carcinoma: A review. J R Soc Med 1987 Aug; 80(8):505–509.

Mondal BK, Biswas RL, and Mondal KN. Primary hyperparathyroidism. Br J Clin Pract 1988 Nov; 42(11):475–477.

Nikkilä MT, Saaristo JJ, and Koivula TA. Clinical and biochemical features in primary hyperparathyroidism. Surgery 1989 Feb; 105(2 pt 1):148–153.

Peck WW et al. Hyperparathyroidism: Comparison of MR imaging with radionuclide scanning. Radiology 1987 May; 163(2):415–420.

Randal SB et al. Parathyroid variants: US evaluation. Radiology 1987 Oct; 165(1):191–194.

Disorders of the Adrenal Medulla

Angermeier KW and Montie JE. Perioperative complications of adrenal surgery. Urol Clin North Am 1989 Aug; 16(3):597–606.

Cooper MB et al. Phaeochromocytoma in the elderly: A poorly recognised entity? Br Med J 1986 Dec 6; 293(6560):1474–1475.

Girard M and Deluca SA. Pheochromocytoma. Am Fam Physician 1989 May; 39(5):139–142.

Greene JP and Guay AT. New perspectives in pheochromocytoma. Urol Clin North Am 1989 Aug; 16(3):487–503.

Hull CJ. Phaeochromocytoma: Diagnosis, preoperative preparation and anaesthetic management. Br J Anaesth 1986 Dec; 58(12):1453–1468.

Jovenich JJ. Anesthesia in adrenal surgery. Urol Clin North Am 1989 Aug; 16(3):583–587.

MacDougall IC et al. Overnight clonidine suppression test in the diagnosis and exclusion of pheochromocytoma. Am J Med 1988 Jun; 84(6):993–1000.

Malone MN et al. Preoperative and surgical management of pheochromocytoma. Urol Clin North Am 1989 Aug; 16(3):567–582.

Samaan NA, Hickey RC, and Shutts PE. Diagnosis, localization, and management of pheochromocytoma. Cancer 1988 Dec 1; 62(11):2451–2460.

Stenström G, Ernest I, and Tisell LE. Long-term results in 64 patients operated upon for pheochromocytoma. Acta Med Scand 1988; 223(4):345–352.

Telenius–Berg M et al. Catecholamine release after physical exercise: A new provocative test for early diagnosis of pheochromocytoma in multiple endocrine neoplasia type 2. Acta Med Scand 1987; 222(4):351–359.

Young MJ et al. Biochemical tests for pheochromocytoma: Strategies in hypertensive patients. J Gen Intern Med 1989 Jul/Aug; 4(4):273–276.

Disorders of the Adrenal Cortex

Avgerinos PC et al. The corticotropin-releasing hormone test in the postoperative evaluation of patients with Cushing's syndrome. J Clin Endocrinol Metab 1987 Nov; 65(5):906–913.

Bloom LS and Libertino JA. Surgical management of Cushing's syndrome. Urol Clin North Am 1989 Aug; 16(3):547–565.

Chandler WF et al. Surgical treatment of Cushing's disease. J Neurosurg 1987 Feb; 66(2):204–212.

Freidberg SR. Transsphenoidal pituitary surgery in the treatment of patients with Cushing's disease. Urol Clin North Am 1989 Aug; 16(3):589–595.

Fuhrman SA. Appropriate laboratory testing in the screening and work-up of Cushing's syndrome. Am J Clin Pathol 1988 Sep; 90(3):345–350.

Guilhaume B et al. Transsphenoidal pituitary surgery for the treatment of Cushing's disease: Results in 64 patients and long-term follow-up studies. J Clin Endocrinol Metab 1988 May; 66(5):1056–1064.

Mampalam TJ, Tyrrell JB, and Wilson CB. Transsphenoidal microsurgery for Cushing disease: A report of 216 cases. Ann Intern Med 1988 Sep 15; 109(6):487–493.

Melby JC. Therapy of Cushing disease: A consensus for pituitary microsurgery. Ann Intern Med 1988 Sep 15; 109(6):445–446.

Nieman LK et al. The ovine corticotropin-releasing hormone (CRH) stimulation test is superior to the human CRH stimulation test for the diagnosis of Cushing's disease. J Clin Endocrinol Metab 1989 Jul; 69(1):165–169.

Perry RR et al. Primary adrenal causes of Cushing's syndrome. Ann Surg 1989 Jul; 210(1):59–68.

Sandler LM et al. Long-term follow-up of patients with Cushing's disease treated by interstitial irradiation. J Clin Endocrinol Metab 1987 Sep; 65(3):441–447.

Schira MG. Steroid-dependent states and adrenal insufficiency: Fluid and electrolyte disturbances. Nurs Clin North Am 1987 Dec; 22(4):837–841.

Sheeler LR. Cushing's syndrome. Urol Clin North Am 1989 Aug; 16(3):447–445.

Disorders of the Pituitary Gland

Barkan AL. Case report: Pituitary atrophy in patients with Sheehan's syndrome. Am J Med Sci 1989 Jul; 298(1):38–40.

Barkan AL et al. Treatment of acromegaly with the long-acting somatostatin analog SMS 201-995. J Clin Endocrinol Metab 1988 Jan; 66(1):16–23.

Bloom SR. Acromegaly. Am J Med 1987 May 29; 82(Suppl 5B):88–91.

Cobb WE and Jackson IMD. Short-term recovery of visual field loss in acromegaly during treatment with a long-acting somatostatin analogue. Am J Med 1989 Apr; 86(4):496–498.

Diamond T, Nery L, and Posen S. Spinal and peripheral bone mineral densities in acromegaly: The effects of excess growth hormone and hypogonadism. Ann Intern Med 1989 Oct 1; 111(1):567–573.

Germon K. Fluid and electrolyte problems associated with diabetes insipidus and syndrome of inappropriate antidiuretic hormone. Nurs Clin North Am 1987 Dec; 22(4):785–796.

Impallomeni M et al. Investigation of anterior pituitary function in elderly in-patients over the age of 75. Q J Med 1987 Jun; 63(242):505–515.

Lam KSL et al. Long-term effects of megavoltage radiotherapy in acromegaly. Aust N Z J Med 1989 Jun; 19(3):202–206.

Melmed S and Fagin JA. Acromegaly update—Etiology, diagnosis and management. West J Med 1987 Mar; 146(3):328–336.

Oelkers W. Hyponatremia and inappropriate secretion of vasopressin (antidiuretic hormone) in patients with hypopituitarism. N Engl J Med 1989 Aug 24; 321(8):492–496.

Poe CM and Taylor LM. Syndrome of inappropriate antidiuretic hormone: Assessment and nursing implications. Oncol Nurs Forum 1989 May/Jun; 16(3):373–381.

Roberts DM. Sheehan's syndrome. Am Fam Physician 1988 Jan; 37(1):223–227.

Ross DA and Wilson CB. Results of transsphenoidal microsurgery for growth hormone-secreting pituitary adenoma in a series of 214 patients. J Neurosurg 1988 Jun; 68(6):854–867.

Schultz PN. Hypopituitarism in patients with a history of irradiation to the head and neck area: Diagnoses and implications for nursing. Oncol Nurs Forum 1989 Nov/Dec; 16(6):823–826.

Sukegawa I et al. Urinary growth hormone (GH) measurements are useful for evaluating endogenous GH secretion. J Clin Endocrinol Metab 1988 Jun; 66(6):1119–1123.

Tulandi T, Yusuf N, and Posner BI. Diabetes insipidus: A postpartum complication. Obstet Gynecol 1987 Sep; 70(3 pt 2):492–495.

van't Verlaat JW et al. Transsphenoidal microsurgery as primary treatment in 25 acromegalic patients: Results and follow-up. Acta Endocrinol (Copenh) 1988 Feb; 117(2):154–158.

Wang C et al. Comparison of the effectiveness of 2-hourly *versus* 8-hourly subcutaneous injections of a somatostatin analog (SMS 201–995) in the treatment of acromegaly. J Clin Endocrinol Metab 1989 Sep; 69(3):670–677.

Pancreatitis

Adinaro D. Liver failure and pancreatitis: Fluid and electrolyte concerns. Nurs Clin North Am 1987 Dec; 22(4):843–852.

Bourliere M and Sarles H. Pancreatic cysts and pseudocysts associated with acute and chronic pancreatitis. Dig Dis Sci 1989 Mar; 34(3):343–348.

Carter DC. Pancreatitis and the biliary tree: The continuing problem. Am J Surg 1988 Jan; 155(1):10–17.

DiMagno EP. Early diagnosis of chronic pancreatitis and pancreatic cancer. Med Clin North Am 1988 Sep; 72(5):979–992.

Ebbehøj N et al. Pancreaticogastrostomy for chronic pancreatitis. Am J Surg 1989 Mar; 157(3):315–317.

Fan ST et al. Influence of age on the mortality from acute pancreatitis. Br J Surg 1988 May; 75(5):463–466.

Grendell JH and Egan J. Acute pancreatitis (medical staff conference). West J Med 1987 May; 146(5):598–602.

Hayakawa T et al. Chronic alcoholism and evolution of pain and prognosis in chronic pancreatitis. Dig Dis Sci 1989 Jan; 34(1):33–38.

Jeffres C. Complications of acute pancreatitis. Crit Care Nurs 1989 Apr; 9(4):38–44, 46, 48.

Kiviluoto T et al. Pseudocysts in chronic pancreatitis. Arch Surg 1989 Feb; 124(2):240–243.

Kozarek RA et al. Endoscopic placement of pancreatic stents and drains in the management of pancreatitis. Ann Surg 1989 Mar; 209(3):261–266.

Nealon WH, Townsend CM, and Thompson JC. Operative drainage of the pancreatic duct delays functional impairment in patients with chronic pancreatitis: A prospective analysis. Ann Surg 1988 Sep; 208(3):321–326.

Nealon WH, Townsend CM, and Thompson JC. Preoperative endoscopic retrograde cholangiopancreatography (ERCP) in patients with pancreatic pseudocyst associated with resolving acute and chronic pancreatitis. Ann Surg 1989 May; 209(5):532–537.

Neoptolemos JP et al. Acute cholangitis in association with acute pancreatitis: Incidence, clinical features and outcome in relation to ERCP and endoscopic sphincterotomy. Br J Surg 1987 Dec; 74(12):1103–1106.

Neoptolemos JP et al. ERCP findings and the role of endoscopic sphincterotomy in acute gallstone pancreatitis. Br J Surg 1988 Oct; 75(10): 954–960.

Pitchumoni CS, Agarwal N, and Jain NK. Systemic complications of acute pancreatitis. Am J Gastroenterol 1988 Jun; 83(6):597–606.

Potts JR III. Acute pancreatitis. Surg Clin North Am 1988 Apr; 68(2):281–299.

Robertson JFR and Imrie CW. Acute pancreatitis associated with carcinoma of the ampulla of Vater. Br J Surg 1987 May; 74(5):395–397.

Sax HC et al. Early total parenteral nutrition in acute pancreatitis: Lack of beneficial effects. Am J Surg 1987 Jan; 153(1):117–124.

Spross JA. Pancreatic cancer: Nursing challenges. Semin Oncol Nurs 1988 Nov; 4(4):274–284.

Stahl TJ et al. Partial biliary obstruction caused by chronic pancreatitis: An appraisal of indications for surgical biliary drainage. Ann Surg 1988 Jan; 207(1):26–32.

Stone WM. Chronic pancreatitis: Results of Whipple's resection and total pancreatectomy. Arch Surg 1988 Jul; 123(7):815–819.

Thompson JS et al. Postoperative pancreatitis. Surg Gynecol Obstet 1988 Oct; 167(5):377–380.

Thompson SR et al. Epidemiology and outcome of acute pancreatitis. Br J Surg 1987 May; 74(5):398–401.

Tollison AA. Danger signs: Rebound tenderness. Nursing 1988 Feb; 18(2): 78–79.

Venu RP et al. Idiopathic recurrent pancreatitis: An approach to diagnosis and treatment. Dig Dis Sci 1989 Jan; 34(1):56–60.

Warshaw AL and Schapiro RH. Pancreas divisum and pancreatitis. Surg Annu 1988; 20:101–120.

Walhout MF. Insulinoma: Diagnosis and treatment. Crit Care Nurs 1990 Oct; 10(9):26–35.

Worsing H. Exocrine pancreatic substitution: Facts and controversies. Scand J Gastroenterol 1986; 126(Suppl):49–54.

Nursing Research Profile for Unit 9

Nursing Care of Patients With Diabetes

Overview

Nursing research in the area of diabetes covers a variety of topics. Most of the studies deal with promoting self-care abilities in patients with diabetes. Some of the research focuses on pragmatic issues such as cost-saving recommendations made by nurses, including reusing insulin syringes and halving reagent strips used for glucose monitoring. Nurse investigators have also focused on the knowledge base of diabetic patients and on evaluating methods for meeting standards of diabetes education set forth by national organizations. Research into patients' assessment of the status of their diabetes has revealed that their interpretations of symptoms do not always coincide with information taught regarding symptoms.

The emotional aspects of diabetes and coping patterns in diabetic patients and families are the focus of nursing research as well as research published in the psychologic and medical literature. As with other chronic illnesses, research into the patient's perception of susceptibility to disease complications and of the benefits of certain self-care actions is conducted to guide nurses in designing effective programs for educating diabetic patients and promoting long-term adherence to treatment regimens.

Nursing research related to hospitalized diabetic patients covers topics such as (inpatient) blood glucose management, patient responses to hospitalization, and knowledge of nurses about diabetes in the hospital setting.

▷ Poteet GW, Reinert B, and Ptak HE. *Outcome of multiple usage of disposable syringes in the insulin-requiring diabetic.* Nurs Res 1987 Nov/Dec; 36(6): 350–352.

The study focused on reuse of disposable insulin syringes by diabetic patients. A sample of 166 diabetic patients completed a questionnaire regarding their current insulin injection practices. Seventy-four (44.6%) of the subjects reported multiple usage of the disposable syringes. Sixty-seven (90.5%) of these subjects reused their syringes 2 to 4 times; the remainder reused them 5 to 20 times. Patients who reused their syringes tended to be older, to have lower income, and to require a greater number of injections per day.

Forty-four of the 74 subjects who reported reusing disposable syringes were randomly selected for further study. These 44 subjects, all of whom required more than one injection of insulin per day, were asked not to alter their usual injection routine and to save one of their syringes for collection after the final injection of the day. Syringes from these subjects were collected and cultured for bacterial growth. Forty (91%) of the syringes showed no bacterial growth, and the four remaining syringes showed normal skin flora growth.

While a few of the patients in this study did report redness at the injections sites (4% of reusers and 14% of nonreusers), infections did not occur in the subjects who reused syringes. The authors postulate that skin redness, which was more common in subjects who used syringes only once, may be related to skin preparation technique.

Nursing Implications. This study confirms the findings of several other studies that reported safe syringe reuse. The authors nonetheless caution against changing counseling practices before further studies have been conducted with a larger sample size, with bacterial cultures being taken at the point at which syringes would routinely be discarded, and with further investigation of the possible causes of redness at injection sites. Although it is generally accepted that many diabetic patients in the community reuse their syringes without apparent harm, most institutional policies prohibit this practice. Nurses who are questioned by patients regarding reuse of syringes must follow institutional guidelines for patient teaching. However, the nurse may also inform patients that syringe reuse is a subject of study, and they may want to share the results of studies that have been published so that patients can make informed decisions about their own practice.

▷ McCarthy JA, Sink PF, and Covarrubias BM. *Reevaluation of single-use insulin syringes.* Diabetes Care 1988 Nov/Dec; 11(10): 817–818.

In this study, various methods for reusing insulin syringes were tested. The subjects included 25 persons with diabetes who were taking two injections per day using human insulins. There were four protocols of syringe reuse and one protocol of single use of the syringe that each subject performed for 12-day periods. The first protocol to be used was randomly assigned to each subject, as was the order in which the other four protocols would be used. Syringe reuse protocols included using the syringe four times with the following measures:

- Wipe the needle with alcohol, cap it, and keep the syringe in a refrigerator after each use.
- Wipe the needle with alcohol, cap it, and keep the syringe at room temperature after each use.
- Cap the needle and keep the syringe in a refrigerator after each use.
- Cap the needle and keep the syringe at room temperature after each use.

Injection sites were monitored by the subjects for signs of infection for 72 hours after the injection. Signs of infection included redness, swelling, warmth, and tenderness. Subjects were to call the researchers immediately to report any signs of infection. Plans would then be made to have the subject seen by a physician and to culture any draining from the site.

The results of the study showed that no subjects reported signs of infection with any of the protocols. The authors suggest that syringe reuse (for at least four injections) may be safe under a variety of conditions of care of the syringe.

Nursing Implications. If nurses are questioned by patients about reuse of insulin syringes, the results of this study could be shared with patients with a description of the various methods of storing the syringe between uses.

▷ **Wakefield B et al. Does contamination affect the reliability and validity of bisected Chemstrip bGs?** West J Nurs Res 1989 Jun; 11(3): 328–333.

This study investigated the safety of the practice of cutting in half reagent strips used for visual determinations of blood glucose. The authors sought to determine if this procedure, which is recommended by some nurses as a cost-saving measure, affects the reliability and validity of blood glucose results. The study evaluated two potential factors that may adversely affect strip interpretations: contamination of strips through contact with skin or nonsterile cutting utensils, and availability of less (half) of the usual color pad for visual interpretation of blood glucose values.

Capillary blood was obtained from 56 subjects. Blood from each subject was applied to five chemstrips, each of which was subjected to one of five conditions: whole strips used according to manufacturer instructions; whole strips contaminated by having the subject squeeze the reagent pad between the unwashed thumb and finger for 5 seconds; strips cut in half by use of sterile equipment; strips cut in half by use of scissors cleaned with soap and water; and strips cut in half with uncleaned scissors. The blood glucose tests were performed by one of two RNs who read all of the strips visually. In addition, whole strips were interpreted by the Accu-Chek meter. The subjects included RN students (nondiabetic) and diabetic patients so that a range of blood glucose levels would be available for interpretation.

The range of mean blood glucose readings from the various strip conditions was small (151.0 to 161.8 mg/dl). While there was a statistically significant difference in readings between the Accu-Chek (mean, 151 mg/dl) and visual readings of the nurses (mean, 160 mg/dl), this difference is not clinically significant. The study results revealed that nurses' interpretations of chemstrips were not markedly affected by cutting the strips in half or by contaminating the strips.

Nursing Implications. Although this study supports the safety of cutting strips in half as a cost-saving measure, the authors point out that further research is needed to determine whether these conditions affect patients' ability to interpret strip values. Additional studies are needed to determine the effect of precutting the strips well in advance of their use. Nurses must avoid making recommendations to patients that have not been set forth by the product manufacturer. However, nurses may share with patients the results of research studies such as this one so that patients can make informed decisions regarding the splitting of reagent strips.

▷ **Teza SL, Davis WK, and Hiss RG. Patient knowledge compared with national guidelines for diabetes care.** Diabetes Educator 1988 May/Jun; 14(3): 207–211.

The study by Teza and co-workers examined the level of patient knowledge of diabetes as compared to national standards set forth by the American Diabetes Association and the American Association of Diabetes Educators. The sample consisted of 428 patients randomly selected from 61 primary care physician practices in 8 communities. Subjects represented an age range of 16 to 85 years and were divided into three main categories based on type and management of diabetes: insulin-dependent diabetes mellitus (IDDM), non–insulin-dependent diabetes mellitus (NIDDM) using insulin, and NIDDM not using insulin. Among the three groups, the average duration of diabetes was 19.6 years (IDDM), 13.3 years (NIDDM using insulin), and 7.9 years (NIDDM not using insulin).

The subjects were given a written examination covering issues in diabetes care, including diet, insulin, exercise, oral hypoglycemic agents, hypoglycemia, ketoacidosis, and care of the lower extremities.

Study results revealed that subjects with IDDM had the highest overall score (71% correct), subjects with NIDDM using insulin had 57% correct, and subjects with NIDDM not using insulin had 52% correct. Four content areas in which subjects for all three groups scored the lowest were rationale behind the meal plan, classification of food examples into food groups, diet management when ill, and care of minor injuries to feet and lower extremities.

The authors suggest that the emphasis placed on patient education by the national diabetes groups during the 1980s has not necessarily produced the desired outcomes in communities where diabetes management is coordinated by general practitioners. Furthermore, the authors postulate that the better performance found among patients on insulin may be reflective of an attitude among health care professionals and patients that NIDDM is a less serious disease than IDDM and that it requires less daily care and patient knowledge than IDDM.

The differences in examination scores of each group of patients led the authors to comment on the importance of dividing the diabetic population into separate groups when preparing educational programs or proposing research projects to analyze patient knowledge.

Nursing Implications. The poor test performance of patients with long-standing diabetes, especially in areas of diet, sick day management, and foot care, emphasizes the important role nurses have in assessing the self-care practices of all diabetic patients. This study supports the notion that diabetes education is an ongoing process and that it must not be assumed that patients who have had diabetes for many years have gained knowledge beyond the initial survival skills taught at diagnosis.

▷ *Hamera E et al. Self-regulation in individuals with type II diabetes. Nurs Res 1988 Nov/Dec; 37(6): 363–367.*

In this study, Hamera and co-workers examine methods used by individuals with diabetes for obtaining feedback regarding the effects of the treatment regimen. A model of self-regulation of diabetes was proposed in which individuals with diabetes use symptoms as a measure of blood glucose levels and take actions based on symptom relief. The purpose of this study was to determine the effect of symptom association and action taking on diabetes control.

The study sample included 173 subjects with type II diabetes ranging in age from 27 to 83 years. Subjects had diabetes for an average of 9.9 years, and all of the subjects reported having received some type of diabetes education. Treatment of diabetes included oral agents (46.8% of subjects), insulin (42.8%), and diet alone (10.4%). Eighty-five percent of subjects reported monitoring blood glucose, and 6.9% reported testing urine.

The subjects were interviewed to determine whether they monitor symptoms and whether they take action in response to symptoms. Subjects were asked questions about the symptom or group of symptoms that they viewed as the best indicator of high blood glucose and low blood glucose. They were questioned regarding their confidence in the accuracy of these symptoms, what actions they took when they experienced these symptoms, and whether they felt that these actions modified blood glucose and relieved symptoms.

Results of the study revealed that most of the subjects (85%) associated symptoms with high or low blood glucose and that there was a wide variety of symptoms reported, some of which were consistent with symptoms typically described in the literature and others that were not consistent with typically described symptoms. Just over half of the subjects believed that the symptoms accurately reflected the blood glucose level, although most subjects did not objectively measure the accuracy of symptoms by self-monitoring of blood glucose.

Seventy-six percent of the subjects took action when experiencing symptoms they associated with high blood glucose (*e.g.,* watched diet, took a nap, drank a noncaloric beverage, or ate or drank a high-calorie food or beverage), and 88% took action when experiencing symptoms associated with low blood glucose (*e.g.,* ate a high-calorie food, took a nap).

The level of formal diabetes education, frequency of self-monitoring of blood glucose, and duration of diabetes were not related to use of this self-regulatory process. Two factors that were associated with use of the self-regulatory process were gender and insulin use. Women and subjects using insulin were more likely to associate symptoms with high or low blood glucose and to take action to relieve symptoms. Level of diabetes control (as measured by glycosylated hemoglobin) was not related to self-regulation.

The authors suggest that lack of correlation of this self-regulation process with diabetic control may be related to the fact that subjects may be interpreting symptoms inaccurately, subjects are not objectively measuring blood glucose levels when symptoms occur, and some of the actions taken (*i.e,* taking a nap) would have no effect on, or may even worsen, blood glucose levels.

Nursing Implications. This study illustrates the important role of ongoing blood glucose monitoring in diabetes. Nurses who work with patients who feel that they can determine blood glucose levels based on symptoms should encourage these patients to continue to monitor blood glucose, especially to verify symptoms of low or high blood glucose, which usually lead the patient to take action. In addition, the inappropriate responses of some of the subjects to perceived high and low blood glucose levels emphasizes the importance of ongoing diabetes assessment and education, even many years after the diagnosis of diabetes.

▷ *Edelstein J and Linn MW. Locus of control and the control of diabetes. Diabetes Educator 1987; 13(1): 51–54.*

In this study, Edelstein and Linn examined the relation between the personality characteristic of locus of control (LOC) and metabolic control among a group of diabetic men. LOC refers to a person's perception of the relation between his own behavior and outcomes resulting from that behavior. Regarding health care behaviors, it has been assumed that patients with an internal LOC expect health outcomes to be related to their own behavior and may be more inclined toward preventive self-care behaviors. Conversely, it has been assumed that patients with an external LOC relate outcomes to external forces, may be less self-directed in health care behaviors, and need more of a directive approach from the health care provider. However, the authors discuss a number of conflicting research findings in the area of LOC and illness outcomes in which patients with an external LOC were more inclined to take favorable health actions.

The sample in this study consisted of 120 diabetic men using insulin. The subjects had an average age of 51 years, and the average duration of diabetes was 12 years. All of the subjects received diabetes follow-up at the same clinic and had been exposed to the same educational program. The subjects were seen every 6 months for 3 years and were given a battery of psychologic, stress, and physiologic tests. The psychologic tests included completion of Rotter's 23-item Locus of Control Scale, in which higher scores indicated a more external orientation. Physiologic testing for metabolic control included glycosylated hemoglobin A$_1$C, blood glucose, triglyceride, and cholesterol tests.

The authors found that in general an external personality orientation was associated with better control of diabetes at the subsequent visit. One possible explanation for this is that externally oriented patients may be more receptive to instructions from others. For internally oriented diabetic patients, the unpredictable nature of the course of the disease may lead them to stop complying with certain behaviors if they do not believe that these behaviors positively affect outcomes.

One limitation of this study was that the authors found that LOC was not as good a predictor of metabolic control in patients with poorly controlled diabetes.

Nursing Implications. Despite conflicting results reported in the literature regarding LOC and patient adherence to treatment regimens, this study points out that health care programs may best serve patients if a number of different approaches are used in helping patients learn self-care behaviors and skills for coping with chronic disease. Further studies are needed to explore LOC and health outcomes and to examine changes in internal versus external orientation in the same patient over time.

▷ Keith KS and Pieper B. *Perioperative blood glucose levels: A study to determine the effect of surgery.* AORN J 1989 July; 50(1):103–110.

The purpose of this study was to examine changes in the blood glucose levels of IDDM, NIDDM, and nondiabetic patients undergoing surgery. The sample consisted of 36 patients (13 with IDDM, 11 with NIDDM, and 12 nondiabetics) with a median age of 52.6 years who were undergoing one of eight surgical procedures, the three most common of which were cholecystectomy, cataract extraction, and abdominal hysterectomy. The types of anesthesia used included general (61%), spinal (11%), and local (28%). Capillary blood glucose levels were measured with a glucose meter at least five times: the morning of surgery, in the preoperative holding room, 15 minutes after the start of surgery, every hour during the surgery, and 15 minutes after admission to the postanesthesia care unit.

The results revealed a significant difference in preoperative blood glucose levels between the diabetic and nondiabetic patients. Mean morning blood glucose values for the nondiabetic, IDDM, and NIDDM patients were 107, 177, and 190 mg/dl, respectively. During the intraoperative and postoperative periods, however, there was no significant difference in blood glucose values in the three groups. For all three groups (including the nondiabetic patients), blood glucose levels increased during the intraoperative period regardless of the treatment used to control blood glucose. Mean peak blood glucose levels at 75 minutes into surgery for nondiabetic, IDDM, and NIDDM patients were 276, 245, and 295 mg/dl, respectively. These values decreased to the 160 to 200 mg/dl range by the time the patients reached the postanesthesia care unit. Analysis of results by type of anesthesia did not yield significant differences in blood glucose levels, although the numbers of patients receiving spinal and local anesthesia were small.

Nursing Implications. The authors pointed out that two potential problems associated with elevated blood glucose levels are impaired wound healing and fluid and electrolyte imbalance due to osmotic diuresis. They further suggest that to prevent osmotic diuresis, the goal should be to keep blood glucose levels below the renal threshold for glucose, which is approximately 180 mg/dl. The results of this study point out that more vigorous treatment with insulin is needed, especially in patients who continue to have elevated blood glucose levels in the immediate postoperative period. Further investigation into the possible effects of elevated blood glucose in the nondiabetic surgical patient is warranted.

Nurses play an important role in monitoring blood glucose values, especially in the operating room where use of a blood glucose meter may eliminate the need for additional personnel and movement required to take blood specimens to the laboratory.

▷ Germain CP and Nemchik RM. *Diabetes self-management and hospitalization.* Image: J Nurs Scholarship 1988 Summer; 20(2): 74–78.

Germain and Nemchik examined the beliefs and experiences of diabetic patients regarding self-management of diabetes during hospitalization. A convenience sample of 73 persons with diabetes completed a questionnaire addressing their current diabetes self-care regimen; beliefs and desires regarding self-care during hospitalization; experiences during hospitalization; and concerns regarding future hospitalizations. Fifty-one (71%) of the subjects reported on a recent hospitalization. Most of the hospitalizations were not clearly linked to diabetes problems. For most of the subjects, diabetes care activities were carried out by hospital staff. The four self-care activities reported most frequently by subjects who did participate in diabetes management included diet selection, insulin injection, urine testing, and treatment of hypoglycemia.

Most subjects responded positively to questions that asked if diabetic patients should be allowed to continue self-management in the hospital. Another question asked subjects to describe the worst occurrences regarding their diabetes care while hospitalized. Two responses were (1) receiving the wrong type or dosage of insulin and (2) not being listened to by staff and physicians. Concerns regarding future hospitalizations included fear of insulin reactions without access to food, worries about timing and dosage of medication, and doubts regarding knowledge of the hospital staff.

Nursing Implications. This study points out the importance of assessing patient desires for participation in diabetes self-care and of establishing hospital policies that allow for self-care when desired. Allowing self-preparation and self-administration of insulin and having appropriate food available for treatment of hypoglycemia may help to decrease the occurrence of preventable hypoglycemia and hyperglycemia in hospitalized diabetic patients. This study also illustrates the importance of ensuring that the hospital staff who deal with diabetic patients have updated knowledge on diabetes care. This will help to promote a sense of confidence in diabetic patients, especially when self-care abilities are temporarily impaired. Furthermore, promoting diabetes self-care during hospitalization will give nurses ample opportunity for assessment of patient skills and provision of diabetes teaching as needed.

▷ Drass JA et al. *Perceived and actual level of knowledge of diabetes mellitus among nurses.* Diabetes Care 1989 May; 12(5): 351–356.

The adequacy of staff nurse knowledge of diabetes and the ability of staff nurses at a large research/teaching hospital to assess their own level of diabetes knowledge were investigated by Drass and co-workers. A sample of 184 staff nurses from a variety of clinical areas completed three questionnaires. A basic demographic data sheet collected information such as years in nursing, education, and presence of diabetes in self or family. A diabetes self-report tool was designed by the investigators to assess the staff nurses' perception of their own knowledge of diabetes. A third questionnaire was a diabetes knowledge test, with 45 multiple-choice questions used to assess the level of basic diabetes knowledge. Categories of content areas covered by the test included etiology of diabetes, treatment modalities, acute and chronic complications, hygiene, surgery, and stress.

The mean percent of questions answered correctly by subjects was 64% of the questions that tested knowledge about diabetes. Common content areas that were answered incorrectly included treatment of hypoglycemia, duration of action of oral hypoglycemic agents, blood glucose monitoring, and etiology of IDDM. Staff nurses who scored higher on the diabetes self-report tool achieved a lower score on the knowledge test. This inverse correlation indicates that the more staff nurses perceived that they were knowledgeable about diabetes, the less they actually knew. Additionally, nurses who had been in nursing for many years and nurses who had not attended an inservice lecture on diabetes within the past 6 months tended to score lower on the knowledge test. One interesting finding was that nurses who had diabetes or who had family members with diabetes tended to score lower on the diabetes self-report tool. In general, it appeared that the more involved the nurses were with diabetes, the more they realized that there is much new information to learn about diabetes.

Nursing Implications.   The authors suggest that the combination of rapid technologic advances in diabetes management and lack of exposure to information regarding diabetes in nurses who have been out of school for a period of years leads to a lack of knowledge of diabetes and a lack of awareness of their knowledge deficit. In many hospitals, the staff nurse is expected to participate in initial and continuing diabetes education of patients. Participation of nurses, especially those who have not recently been exposed to new diabetes information in continuing education classes, is important. Not only will this improve the nurses' knowledge level, it may also contribute to an increase in patient knowledge and self-care abilities.

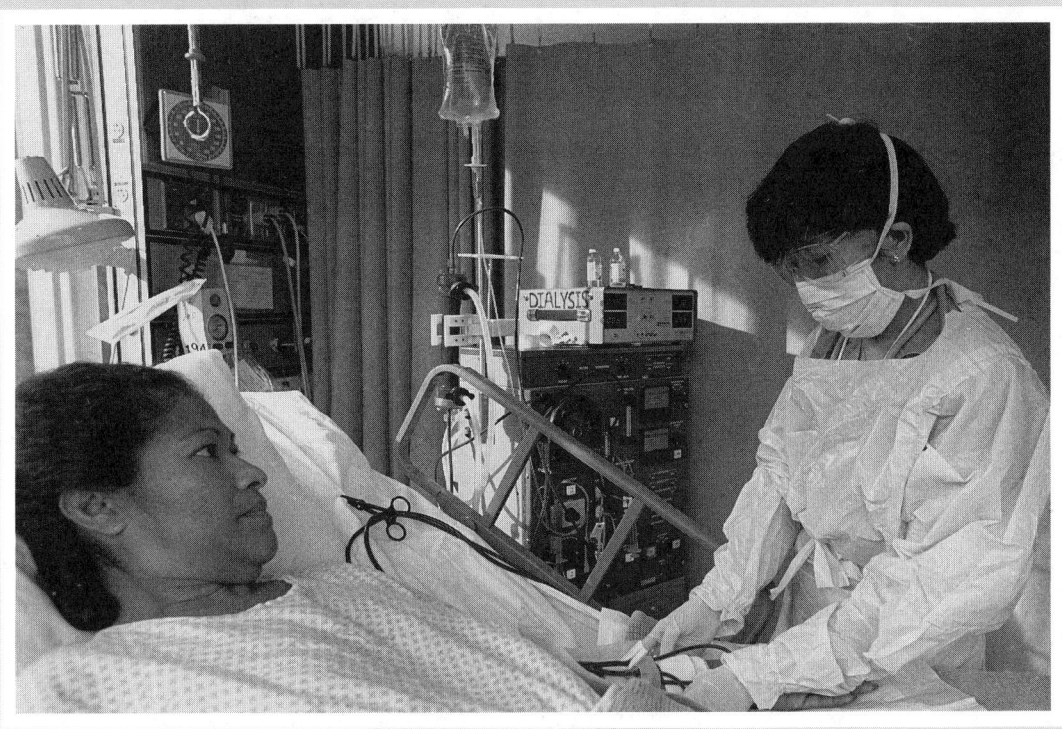

41

Assessment of Urinary and Renal Function

Learning Objectives

On completion of this chapter, the learner will be able to:

1. Describe the role of the kidney in the regulation of fluid, electrolyte, and acid–base balance
2. Use assessment parameters for determining the status of renal and urinary function
3. Describe diagnostic tests used to determine renal and urinary function
4. Develop a nursing care plan for patients undergoing assessment of the urinary/renal system

Physiologic Overview

The kidneys, ureters, bladder, and urethra compose the urinary system. The kidneys' main functions are regulation of the fluid and electrolyte composition of the body fluids and removal of metabolic end products from the blood. The urine that is formed as a result of these processes is transported from the kidneys through the ureters to the urinary bladder, where it is temporarily stored. During the act of urination (micturition), the bladder contracts and the urine is excreted from the body through the urethra. Although fluid and electrolytes can be lost by other routes, such as in perspiration or feces, it is the kidneys that precisely regulate the internal environment of the body. The renal excretory function is necessary for maintenance of life. However, unlike the cardiovascular and respiratory systems, complete malfunction of the kidneys may not cause death for several days. Dialysis (the "artificial kidney") and other treat-ment modalities can be used as substitutes for certain functions of the kidneys.

An important feature of the urinary system is its ability to adapt to wide variations in fluid load based on individual habits and patterns. Basically, the kidneys must be able to excrete dietary and metabolic waste products that are not eliminated by other organs. This usually amounts to 1 to 2 liters of water per day, 6 to 8 g of salt (sodium chloride) per day, 6 to 8 g of potassium chloride per day, and 70 mg of acid equivalents per day. In addition, protein is ingested and metabolized by the body into urea and other waste products that must also be excreted in the urine.

Anatomy of the Urinary System

The kidneys are paired organs, each weighing approximately 125 g, located in a position lateral to the bodies of the lower thoracic vertebrae, a few centimeters to the right and left of the midline. They are surrounded by a thin, fibrous tissue known

1131

as the capsule. Anteriorly, the kidneys are separated from the abdominal cavity and its contents by layers of peritoneum. Posteriorly, they are shielded by the lower thoracic wall. Blood is supplied to each kidney through the renal artery and is drained through the renal vein. The renal arteries arise from the abdominal aorta, and the renal veins carry blood back into the inferior vena cava. The kidneys can efficiently clear the blood of waste materials, in part because blood flow through the kidneys is great and represents 25% of cardiac output.

Urine is formed within the functional units of the kidneys, known as *nephrons*. The urine formed within these nephrons passes into collecting ducts, the tubules, that join to form the pelvis of each kidney. Each kidney pelvis gives rise to a ureter. The ureter is a long tube with a wall composed largely of smooth muscle. It connects each kidney to the bladder and functions as a conduit for urine.

The urinary bladder is a hollow organ that is situated anteriorly just behind the pubic bone. It acts as a temporary storage reservoir for the urine. The walls of the bladder consist largely of smooth muscle called the detrusor muscle. Contraction of this muscle is mainly responsible for emptying the bladder during urination. The urethra arises from the bladder; it passes through the penis in the male and opens just anterior to the vagina in the female. In the male, the prostate gland, which lies just below the bladder neck, surrounds the urethra posteriorly and laterally. A short distance from its origin, the urethra is encircled by a small bundle of muscle fibers called the external urinary sphincter. This sphincter is the major site for control of the initiation of urination.

The Nephron.   The kidney is divided into an outer portion called the cortex and an inner portion known as the medulla (Fig. 41-1). In the human, each kidney is composed of approximately 1 million nephrons. The nephron, considered the functional unit of the kidney, consists of a glomerulus and a tubule (Fig. 41-2). The glomerulus, the beginning of the nephron, is composed of tufts of capillaries that are supplied with blood by an afferent arteriole and drained by an efferent ar-

teriole. The latter is a thick-walled muscular vessel that helps to maintain a high pressure in the glomerular capillaries. Like capillaries in general, the walls of the glomerular capillaries are composed of a layer of endothelial cells and a basement membrane. Epithelial cells that form the beginning of the tubule are located on one side of the basement membrane. The tubule itself is divided into three parts: a proximal tubule, the loop of Henle, and a distal tubule. The distal tubules coalesce to form collecting ducts. The ducts pass through the renal cortex and the medulla to empty into the pelvis of the kidney.

Function of the Nephron.   The process of urine formation begins as blood flows through the glomerulus. Fluid is filtered through the walls of the glomerular capillary tufts into the proximal tubule. Under normal conditions, approximately 20% of the plasma passing through the glomerulus is filtered into the nephron, amounting to about 180 liters of filtrate per day. The filtrate, very similar to blood plasma without its proteins, consists essentially of water, electrolytes, and other small molecules. Within the tubule and collecting ducts, some of these substances are selectively reabsorbed into the blood. Other substances are secreted into the filtrate as it travels down the tubule. The urine is the remaining fluid (along with its contents) that reaches the pelvis of the kidney. Some substances, such as glucose, are normally completely reabsorbed in the tubule and do not appear in the urine. The processes of reabsorption and secretion in the tubule frequently involve active transport and require the utilization of metabolic energy. The amount of various substances normally filtered by the glomerulus, reabsorbed by the tubules, and excreted in the urine is shown in Table 41-1.

Urine Composition

The kidney functions as the main excretory organ of the body. It disposes of end products of the body's metabolism as well as ingested nutrients. In the normal person, the amounts of these materials excreted per day are exactly equal to the

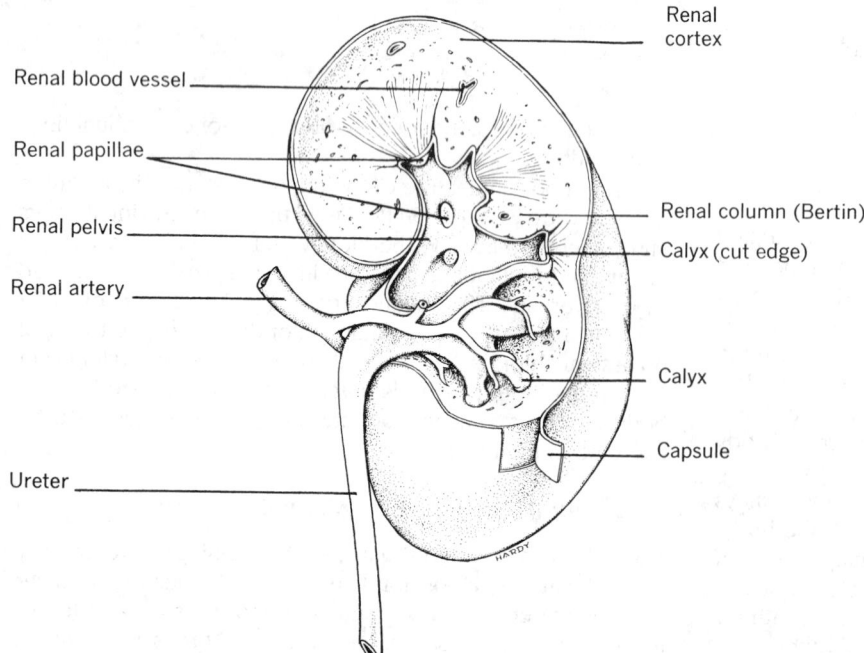

Renal cortex

Renal blood vessel

Renal papillae

Renal pelvis

Renal artery

Ureter

Renal column (Bertin)

Calyx (cut edge)

Calyx

Capsule

Figure 41–1.   Diagram of internal structure of kidney, showing relations of renal pelvis and calyces to pyramids in medullary region. (Chaffee EE and Greisheimer EM. Basic Physiology and Anatomy, 3rd ed. Philadelphia, JB Lippincott.)

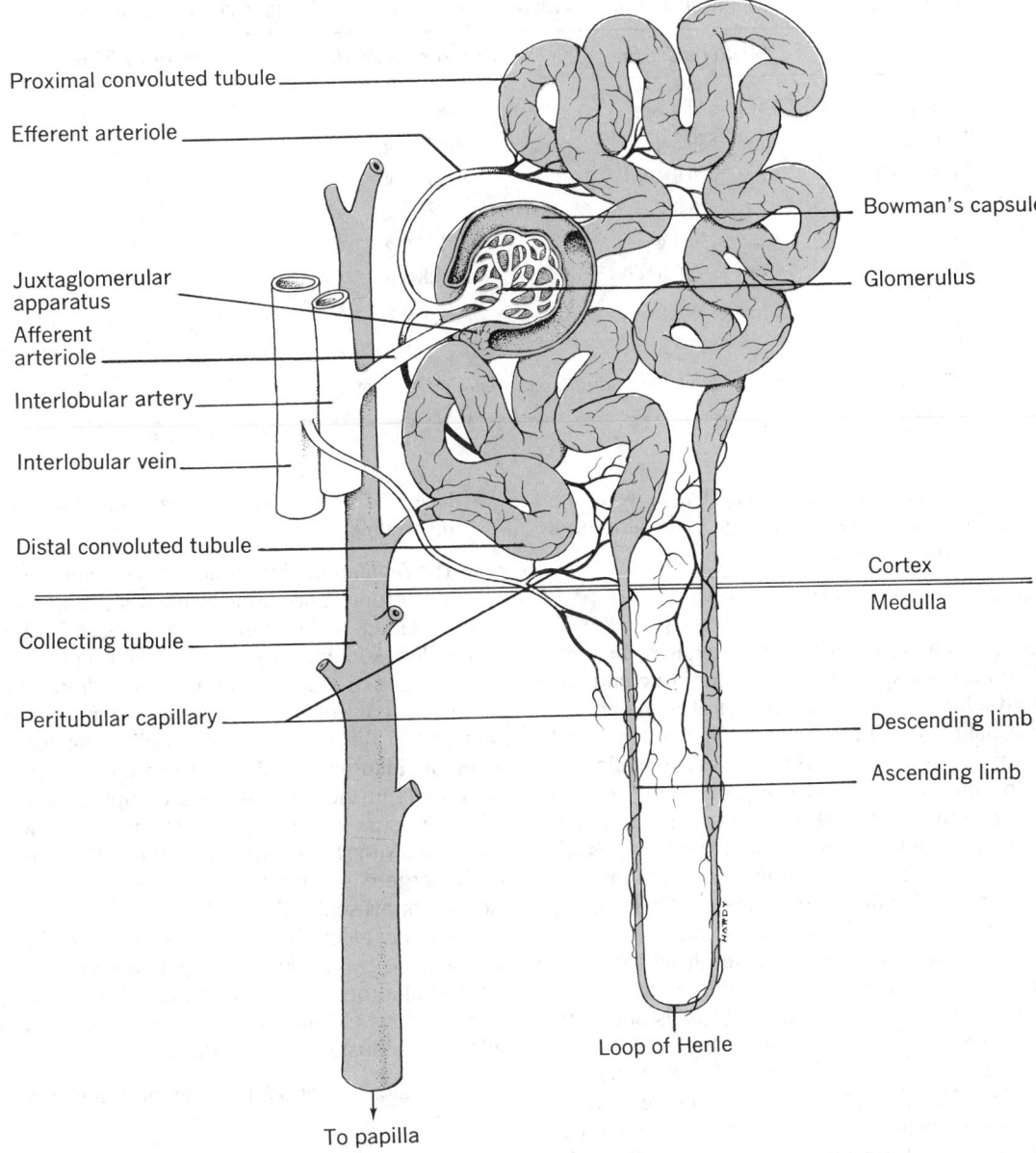

Proximal convoluted tubule

Efferent arteriole

Bowman's capsule

Glomerulus

Juxtaglomerular apparatus

Afferent arteriole

Interlobular artery

Interlobular vein

Distal convoluted tubule

Cortex

Medulla

Collecting tubule

Peritubular capillary

Descending limb

Ascending limb

Loop of Henle

To papilla

Figure 41–2. A nephron and its blood supply. The collecting tubule receives urine from neighboring nephron units. Note that the loop of Henle dips into the medullary layer of the kidney. (Chaffee EE and Greisheimer EM. Basic Physiology and Anatomy, 3rd ed. Philadelphia, JB Lippincott.)

amounts ingested and formed, so that over a period of time there is no net change in the total body composition.

Urine is composed primarily of water. A normal person ingests approximately 1 to 2 liters of water per day, and normally all but 400 to 500 ml of this fluid intake is excreted in the urine. The remainder is lost from the skin, from the lungs during breathing, and in the feces. Electrolytes, including sodium, potassium, chloride, bicarbonate, and other less abundant ions, are also excreted by the kidneys. The average American diet contains about 6 to 8 g each of sodium chloride (salt) and potassium chloride per day, and nearly all of this is excreted in the urine.

The third group of substances appearing in the urine is made up of the end products of protein metabolism. The major end product is urea, of which about 25 g is produced and excreted per day. Other products of protein metabolism that

must be excreted are creatinine, phosphates, and sulfates. Uric acid, formed as a product of nucleic acid metabolism, is also eliminated in the urine.

It is important to recognize that some substances that are present in high concentrations in the blood are ordinarily completely reabsorbed by active transport in the renal tubule. Amino acids and glucose, for example, are usually filtered at the glomerulus and reabsorbed so that none of either is excreted in the urine. Glucose, however, will appear in the urine if its blood level is so high that its concentration in the glomerular filtrate exceeds the capacity of the tubules to reabsorb it. Normally, the glucose is completely reabsorbed when its concentration in the blood is less than 200 mg/dl (11 mmol/L). In diabetes, where the blood glucose levels exceed the kidney's reabsorption capacity, glucose will appear in the urine. Protein is also not normally found in the urine. These molecules are not filtered

TABLE 41-1.   *Filtration, Reabsorption, and Excretion of Certain Normal Constituents of Plasma*

	Filtered 24 Hr	*Reabsorbed 24 Hr*	*Excreted 24 Hr**
Sodium	540.0 g	537.0 g	3.3 g
Chloride	630.0 g	625.0 g	5.3 g
Bicarbonate	300.0 g	300.0 g	0.3 g
Potassium	28.0 g	24.0 g	3.9 g
Glucose	140.0 g	140.0 g	0.0 g
Urea	53.0 g	28.0 g	25.0 g
Creatinine	1.4 g	0.0 g	1.4 g
Uric acid	8.5 g	7.7 g	0.8 g

* *These are typical normal values. Wide variation is found, depending on diet.*

at the glomerulus because of their large size. The appearance of protein in the urine usually signifies damage to the glomeruli that causes them to become "leaky."

Regulation of Acid Excretion

The catabolism or breakdown of proteins involves the production of acid compounds, in particular phosphoric and sulfuric acids. In addition, a certain amount of acid material is ingested daily. Unlike CO_2, these are nonvolatile acids and cannot be eliminated by the lung. Because accumulation of these acids in the blood would lower its pH, (more acidic) and inhibit cell function, they must be excreted in the urine. A person whose kidney function is normal excretes approximately 70 mEq of acid each day. The kidney is able to excrete some of this acid directly into the urine to the extent of lowering its pH to 4.5, 1000 times more acidic than blood.

More acid usually needs to be eliminated from the body than can be excreted directly as free acid in the urine. This is accomplished by the renal excretion of acid that is bound to chemical buffers. The acid (H^+) is secreted by the renal tubular cells into the filtrate, where it is buffered chiefly by phosphate ions and ammonia (NH_3). Phosphate is present in the glomerular filtrate, and ammonia is produced by the cells of the renal tubules and secreted into the tubular fluid. Through the buffering process, the kidney is able to excrete large quantities of acid in a bound form without further lowering the pH of the urine.

Regulation of Electrolyte Excretion

The amount of electrolytes and water that must be excreted by the kidney each day varies greatly, depending on the amounts ingested. The 180 liters of filtrate formed by the glomeruli each day contain about 1100 g of sodium chloride. All but 2 liters of water and 6 to 8 g of sodium chloride are normally reabsorbed by the kidneys. Water from the filtrate follows the reabsorbed sodium in order to maintain osmotic balance. The remaining water, sodium chloride, other electrolytes, and waste products are then excreted as urine. Thus, more than 99% of the water and sodium filtered at the glomerulus is reabsorbed into the blood by the time the urine leaves the body. By regulating the amount of sodium (and therefore water) reabsorbed, the kidney can regulate the volume of body fluids.

- If sodium is excreted in excess of the amount ingested, the patient will become dehydrated.

- If less sodium is excreted than is ingested, the patient will retain fluid.

The regulation of the amount of sodium excreted depends on aldosterone, a hormone synthesized and released from the adrenal gland. In the presence of increased aldosterone in the blood, less sodium is excreted in the urine.

Release of aldosterone from the adrenal gland is largely under the control of angiotensin, a peptide hormone manufactured in the liver and activated in the lung. Angiotensin levels are in turn controlled by renin, a hormone that is released from cells in the kidneys. This complex system is activated when pressure in the renal arterioles falls below normal levels, as occurs with shock and dehydration. The effect of activation of this system is to increase the retention of water and expansion of intravascular fluid volume.

Another electrolyte whose concentration in the body fluids is regulated by the kidney is potassium, the most abundant intracellular ion. The excretion of potassium by the kidney is increased by elevated aldosterone levels, in contrast to the effects of aldosterone on sodium excretion.

- Retention of potassium is the most life-threatening effect of renal failure.

Regulation of Water Excretion

Regulation of the amount of water excreted is also an important function of the kidney. With a large water or fluid intake, a large volume of dilute urine must be excreted. Conversely, with a low fluid intake, the urine that is excreted must be concentrated. The relative degree of dilution or concentration of the urine can be measured in terms of its *osmolality*. This term refers to the amount of solid material (electrolytes and other molecules) dissolved in the urine. The filtrate in the glomerular capillary normally has the same osmolality as the blood, with a value of approximately 300 mOsm/L (300 mmol/L). As the filtrate passes through the tubules and collecting ducts, the osmolality may vary from 50 to 1200 mOsm/L, reflecting the maximal diluting and concentrating abilities of the kidney.

The osmolality of the urine specimen can be measured. *Osmolality* reflects the number of particles of solute in a unit of solution, unlike *specific gravity*, which is less precise and reflects both the quantity and the nature of particles. Therefore, protein, glucose, and intravenous contrast medium affect specific gravity more than osmolality. Osmolality is measured when a precise assessment of the concentrating and diluting abilities of the kidneys is needed. Normal urine osmolality is 500 to 800 mOsm/L. Normal specific gravity is 1.015 to 1.025 (when fluid intake is normal).

Regulation of water excretion and urine concentration is carried out in the tubule by varying the amount of water that is reabsorbed in relation to electrolyte reabsorption. The glomerular filtrate has essentially the same electrolyte composition as the blood plasma without the proteins. The amount of water that is reabsorbed is under the control of antidiuretic hormone (ADH or vasopressin). ADH is a hormone that is secreted by the posterior part of the pituitary gland in response to changes in osmolality of the blood. With decreased water intake, blood osmolality tends to rise and stimulate ADH release. ADH then acts on the kidney in order to cause increased reabsorption of water, thereby returning the osmolality of the blood toward normal. With excess water intake, the secretion of ADH by the pituitary is suppressed and, therefore, less water is reabsorbed by the kidney tubule. This latter situation leads to increased urine volume (*diuresis*).

- Loss of the ability to concentrate and dilute the urine is the most common early manifestation of kidney disease. A dilute urine of fixed specific gravity (approximately 1.010) or fixed osmolality (approximately 300 mOsm/L) is excreted.

Renal Clearance

The test most commonly used to evaluate how well the kidney performs its excretory function is termed *clearance*. Clearance of a substance A is shown by the following equation: clearance equals (the urine concentration of A) times (the urine volume in a given time) divided by the plasma concentration of A.

Clearance =

$$\frac{(\text{urine concentration of A}) \times (\text{urine volume in a given time})}{\text{plasma concentration of A}}$$

For example, if the arterial plasma concentration of a substance is 0.1 mg/ml, the urine concentration of the same substance is 50 mg/ml, and the urine volume is 1.0 ml/min, the clearance of that substance according to the above equation is 500 ml/min. This means that 500 ml of blood are completely cleared of that substance in one minute. In the body, few substances are actually completely cleared from the blood during a single pass through the kidney. In the example given above, if the blood is cleared of only 50% of the substance, urine concentration of the substance would be 25 mg/ml and the calculated renal clearance would be 250 ml/min. It is possible to measure the renal clearance of any substance, but the one that has proved particularly useful is the creatinine clearance. *Creatinine* is an endogenous waste product of skeletal muscle that is excreted by glomerular filtration and is not appreciably reabsorbed or secreted by the renal tubules. Therefore, creatinine clearance is a good measure of the glomerular filtration rate (GFR). The normal adult GFR is about 100 to 120 ml/min (1.67 to 2.00 ml/sec).

Storage of Urine and Voiding

Urine formed by the kidney is transported from the renal pelvis through the ureters and into the bladder. This movement is facilitated by peristaltic waves occurring about one to five times per minute and generated by the smooth muscle in the ureter wall. Urine flows into the bladder sporadically, propelled by peristaltic contractions. There are no sphincters between the bladder and the ureters, although reflux of urine from the bladder in normal subjects is prevented by the unidirectional nature of the peristaltic waves and because each ureter enters the bladder at an oblique angle. However, with overdistention of the bladder due to disease, the elevated pressure in the bladder can be transmitted back through the ureters, leading to ureteral distention and possible reflux or back-up of urine. This can lead to kidney infection (pyelonephritis) and damage from the elevated pressure (hydronephrosis).

The pressure in the bladder is normally very low, even as the urine accumulates, because the bladder's smooth muscle adapts to the increased stretch as the bladder is slowly filled. The first sensations of bladder filling ordinarily occur when about 100 to 150 ml of urine are present in the bladder. In most cases, there is a desire to void when the bladder contains approximately 200 to 300 ml. With 400 ml, a marked feeling of fullness is usually present.

Voiding of urine is controlled by contraction of the *external urethral sphincter*. This muscle is under voluntary control and is innervated by nerves from the sacral area of the spinal cord. Voluntary control is a learned behavior that is not present at birth. When there is a desire to urinate, the external urethral sphincter is relaxed, and the *detrusor muscle* (bladder smooth muscle) contracts and expels the urine from the bladder through the urethra. The pressure generated in the bladder during urination (micturition) is approximately 50 to 150 cm of water. Urine remaining in the urethra drains by gravity in the female and is expelled by voluntary muscle contractions in the male.

The contraction of the detrusor muscle is regulated by a reflex involving the parasympathetic nervous system. The reflex is integrated in the sacral portion of the spinal tract. The sympathetic nervous system plays no essential part in micturition but does prevent semen from entering the bladder during ejaculation. If the pelvic nerves to the bladder and sphincter are destroyed, voluntary control and reflex urination are abolished and the bladder becomes overdistended with urine. If the spinal pathways from the brain to the urinary system are destroyed (for example, after a spinal cord transection), reflex contraction of the bladder is maintained but voluntary control over the process is lost. In both of these types of loss of innervation, the muscle of the bladder can contract and expel urine but the contractions are generally insufficient to empty the bladder completely, and *residual urine* (urine left in the bladder after voiding) remains.

Catheterization—passage of a catheter through the urethra into the bladder—can be used to assess bladder function by permitting measurement of the volume of residual urine. Normally this is no more than 50 ml. However, catheterization is avoided whenever possible (and strict asepsis is used whenever it is necessary) because it increases the risk of infection. Another test for bladder dysfunction is to measure the pressure in the bladder after instillation of various volumes of saline. This latter procedure is called a *cystometrogram*.

Overview of Renal Pathophysiology

Diseases of the kidney can be classified according to the segment of the nephron that is primarily affected. Glomerulonephritis and the various forms of the nephrotic syndrome primarily affect the renal glomerulus. Vascular diseases, infections, and toxins primarily affect the renal tubule, although some degree of glomerular dysfunction may coexist. Obstruction of the outflow of urine due to calculi (stones), protein, or other material in the collecting ducts or ureters may eventually lead to damage throughout the nephron. When the degree of kidney damage is severe, renal failure occurs and may result in *uremic syndrome.*

Glomerular Disorders

Nephritic Syndrome. The nephritic syndrome occurs in response to a group of diseases in which inflammation of the glomerulus (glomerulonephritis) is predominant. The major manifestations are hematuria, proteinuria, sodium and fluid retention, hypertension, and occasionally oliguria. These abnormalities are due to damage to the glomerular capillaries that permits leakage of red blood cells into the tubular lumen. Glomerulonephritis most commonly results from immune reactions. Common causes are the reaction to some streptococcal infections, predominantly in children, and the autoimmune diseases such as Goodpasture's syndrome and lupus erythematosus. Glomerulonephritis may resolve completely, although in some patients renal failure may result.

Nephrotic Syndrome. The nephrotic syndrome results from a group of glomerular diseases associated with increased permeability of the glomerulus to proteins. Frequently there are no alterations of kidney structure observable by light microscopy. The primary manifestation of the disease is the loss of plasma proteins, particularly albumin, in the urine. Although the liver is capable of increasing its production of albumin, it is unable to keep up with the daily loss of albumin through the kidney; thus, hypoalbuminemia results. The resultant decreased oncotic pressure leads to generalized edema as fluid moves from the vascular system into the extracellular fluid spaces. A decreased circulating blood volume activates the renin–angiotensin system, leading to retention of sodium and further edema. Patients with nephrotic syndrome also exhibit an elevated lipid concentration in their blood (*hyperlipidemia*), the cause of which is not known. The nephrotic syndrome can occur with almost any intrinsic renal disease or systemic disease that affects the glomerulus.

Renal Failure

The following description of renal failure is presented in this chapter to provide an overview of the multiplicity and complexity of abnormalities and problems that can result from renal disease. A complete description of acute and chronic renal failure is presented in Chapter 43.

Renal failure is present when the excretion of water, electrolytes, and metabolic waste products is insufficient because of kidney damage that prevents the kidneys from maintaining the normal internal environment of the body. Acute renal failure has a sudden onset and is frequently reversible. Chronic renal failure usually develops gradually but can also occur as a consequence of an acute episode. One normal kidney is generally sufficient for maintenance of fluid and electrolyte balance and elimination of metabolic end products, so renal failure requires bilateral kidney damage. The signs and symptoms of renal failure are in large part a result of altered fluid and electrolyte

balance of the body. The diagnosis is generally made by the finding of *azotemia*, defined as elevation of nitrogenous waste products in the blood. *Uremic syndrome*, or *uremia*, characterized by the signs and symptoms resulting from accumulation of these waste products, occurs when the condition is severe.

Pathogenesis of Renal Failure. Decreased excretion of metabolic waste products can occur as a result of decreased blood flow to the kidney (prerenal), acute obstruction of the flow of urine from the kidney (postrenal), or damage to the kidney itself (intrarenal).

- Decreased renal blood flow can occur with hypotension, congestive heart failure, dehydration, or thrombosis of renal arteries. An acute decrease in renal blood flow may lead to secondary renal damage and renal failure. Decreased excretion of waste products due to decreased renal blood flow in the absence of kidney damage is called *prerenal azotemia.*

- Decreased urine output due to complete urinary obstruction can occur in patients who have an enlarged prostate, stones (calculi) in the ureters or urethra, or infiltrating tumors. Secondary damage to the kidneys and renal failure will result if the obstruction is not relieved promptly. This is termed *obstructive* or *postrenal* failure.

- Acute renal failure due to direct injury to the kidney results from acute vasculitis, acute glomerulonephritis, severe ("malignant") hypertension, or, more commonly, acute damage to the renal tubules (acute tubular necrosis, ATN). The clinical conditions that may result in acute tubular necrosis include hypotension (shock), exposure to nephrotoxic chemicals, disintegration of blood components (intravascular hemolysis) leading to a buildup of hemoglobin in the urine (due to transfusion reactions, extensive burns, or infusion of water intravenously), and crushing injuries that damage muscle tissue. These injuries cause a release of myoglobin, which is carried to the kidneys and excreted in the urine (myoglobinuria). These are *intrarenal* causes of renal failure.

Chronic renal failure may follow acute renal failure (if not reversed) or it may result from the same causes as acute renal failure; in addition, it may result from infection of the kidneys, nephrosclerosis, diabetic nephropathy, collagen diseases, and other chronic, progressive kidney diseases.

Uremic Syndrome (Uremia)

Uremic syndrome, or *uremia*, is a term used to designate the manifestations of chronic renal dysfunction that leads to an accumulation in the blood of substances normally excreted in the urine. Uremia is a generalized condition that affects all organ systems of the body.

Fluids and Electrolytes. The fluid and electrolyte abnormalities that occur in renal failure are the result of a decreased number of functioning nephrons. The basic pathophysiologic alteration in the kidney is a decreased glomerular filtration rate (GFR) due to a reduced number of filtering glomeruli, leading to decreased clearance of substances that depend on filtration for their excretion. Decreased GFR can be diagnosed by a decreased creatinine clearance. As creatinine clearance decreases, serum creatinine increases. Because of creatinine's constant production, it is a specific and sensitive indicator of kidney disease. The blood urea nitrogen (BUN) also increases with kidney damage, but its level is also affected by protein intake and tissue breakdown.

In addition to decreased GFR, a decrease in the number of functioning nephrons results in decreased ability of the tubules to modify the glomerular filtrate prior to its excretion as urine. As a result, the urine resembles plasma, having a fixed specific gravity or osmolality. This inability to concentrate or dilute the urine prevents appropriate responses by the kidneys to changes in the daily intake of water and electrolytes. Decreased intake of fluid or salt can lead to dehydration or sodium depletion; excess salt or water intake may cause water intoxication or sodium overload. Decreased tubular function also results in an inability of the kidney to excrete increased loads of potassium (K^+) and acid (H^+). With advanced renal disease, the normal production of H^+ by body metabolism or release of K^+ from damaged cells of the body can result in acidosis or hyperkalemia. Decreased excretion of acid results primarily from the inability of the tubules to secrete ammonia (NH_3) and to reabsorb sodium bicarbonate ($NaHCO_3$). There may also be decreased excretion of phosphates and organic acids. Decreased excretion of potassium results from an inability of the tubules to secrete this ion into the urine. In addition, the excretion of drugs may be markedly altered, necessitating adjustment of their usual dosages.

Calcium Metabolism and Bone Changes. Disorders of calcium metabolism with secondary bone changes are among the major manifestations of uremia. The primary finding is usually a decreased serum calcium concentration. Several mechanisms have a role in the development of hypocalcemia. Calcium levels are dependent on the amount of phosphorus present. (Calcium and phosphorus levels have a reciprocal relationship; that is, when one rises, the other decreases.) Thus, a decreased excretion of phosphorus in the urine and an elevation of the serum phosphorus level cause a decrease in the amount of free calcium in the body. Additionally, there is decreased conversion of vitamin D to its active form by the damaged kidneys, leading to diminished absorption of calcium from the gastrointestinal tract.

Decreased serum calcium secondarily stimulates the parathyroid glands to produce increased parathormone, resulting in secondary *hyperparathyroidism*, which is characterized by demineralization of bone and formation of bone cysts. The bone changes are worsened by decreased deposition of calcium due to decreased active vitamin D and increased resorption of calcium due to chronic acidosis. The demineralization of bone leads to frequent fractures and bone pain. The term *renal osteodystrophy* is frequently used to designate the complex bone changes that occur with uremia.

Anemia. Anemia, another common manifestation of uremia, is generally caused by a decreased rate of production of erythrocytes or red blood cells (RBCs) by the bone marrow and increased rates of destruction of RBCs. Decreased erythropoiesis (the formation of RBCs) is related to a decreased rate of production of erythropoietin by the kidneys. In this form of anemia, the RBCs in the peripheral blood generally appear to be of normal size and of normal hemoglobin concentration (normocytic, normochromic anemia). Blood loss due to bleeding from the gastrointestinal tract or other sites may contribute to the anemia.

Cardiovascular Manifestations. Hypertension, frequently associated with chronic renal failure, may be either the cause or the result of renal damage. Primary hypertension leads to kidney damage as a result of atherosclerosis of the renal vasculature manifested by nephrosclerosis. Secondary hyperten-

sion occurs as a result of increased renin production by the diseased kidney, leading to generalized vasoconstriction as well as salt retention, which leads to fluid retention and an expansion of the vascular volume.

- Patients with impaired renal function are prone to volume overload because they are unable to compensate for acute increases in water and salt intake.
- Chronic congestive heart failure with pulmonary and peripheral edema frequently occurs as a consequence of hypertensive cardiac disease complicated by the effects of fluid overload and anemia.
- Congestive heart failure results in decreased renal blood flow with elevation of BUN out of proportion to the degree of kidney damage.

Other Manifestations of Uremia. Among the diverse manifestations of uremia are gastrointestinal symptoms, including anorexia, nausea, vomiting, and hiccups, and neuromuscular symptoms, including mental clouding, inability to concentrate, drowsiness, lethargy, twitching, convulsions, and tetany related to the low serum calcium. Dermatologic symptoms, including severe itching (pruritus), are common. Uremic frost, the deposit of urea on the skin by perspiration, is uncommon today because of early treatment of uremia. Patients with uremia also have altered cellular immunity, with decreased delayed hypersensitivity and increased susceptibility to infection probably related to a decreased ability of leukocytes to kill bacteria.

The precise mechanisms for many of these diverse manifestations have not been identified. However, retention of products normally excreted in the urine, such as ammonia, phenols, and other organic and inorganic compounds, is the probable cause.

Course of Renal Failure

The basic mechanisms underlying the pathophysiologic changes of acute and chronic renal failure are similar. However, their clinical presentations are markedly different. There are two phases of acute renal failure: the oliguric phase and the diuretic phase.

Oliguric Phase. Acute renal failure occurs because of sudden insults to the kidney that result in a decreased rate of urine formation. This is called the *oliguric phase* of acute renal failure.

- During the oliguric phase, the potential life-threatening complications are related to fluid and electrolyte retention, (in particular, hyperkalemia and acidosis).

Diuretic Phase. If the original insult is removed and permanent damage has not yet occurred, the recovery process begins with a gradually increasing glomerular filtration rate. At this stage, the renal tubular cells may still be unable to reabsorb the water and electrolytes in the increasing volume of glomerular filtrate. As a result, the volume of urine rises above normal, resulting in the *diuretic* phase of acute renal failure.

- During the diuretic phase, the potential life-threatening complications are dehydration and electrolyte depletion.

Complete recovery from renal failure may require several months or up to a year. Some patients with acute renal failure will not recover normal renal function despite removal of the initial insult and will develop chronic renal failure. More commonly, however, chronic renal failure develops insidiously over time. The disease is frequently not discovered until the patient develops symptoms related to fluid and electrolyte abnormalities. At this stage, kidney function has generally decreased by more than 50% and the creatinine concentration in the blood has risen above normal. The nursing care of patients with renal failure is discussed in Chapter 43.

Assessment of Urinary Function

Clinical Manifestations of Urinary Dysfunction

The following signs and symptoms are suggestive of urinary tract disease: pain, changes in voiding, and gastrointestinal symptoms.

Pain

Genitourinary pain is not always present in renal disease but is generally seen in the more acute conditions. Pain of renal disease is usually caused by obstruction and subsequent sudden distention of the renal capsule. Its severity is related to how quickly the distention develops.

Kidney pain may be felt as a dull ache in the costovertebral angle (the area formed by the rib cage and vertebral column) and may extend to the umbilicus. Ureteral pain produces pain in the back that radiates to the abdomen, upper thigh, testis, or labium. Pain in the flank (the region between the ribs and ilium), radiating to the lower abdomen or epigastrium and often associated with nausea, vomiting, and paralytic ileus, may indicate renal colic. Bladder pain (low abdominal pain or pain over the suprapubic area) can be due to an overdistended bladder or bladder infection. Urgency, tenesmus (painful straining), and terminal dysuria (pain at the end of voiding) are usually present. Pain at the urethral meatus occurs with irritation of the bladder neck or urethra due to infection (urethritis), trauma, or a foreign body in the lower urinary tract.

Severe pain in the scrotal region results from inflammation and edema of the epididymis or testicle or from torsion of the testicle, while perineal and rectal fullness and pain signal acute prostatitis or prostatic abscess. Back and leg pain may be due to metastasis of cancer of the prostate to the pelvic bones. Pain in the penile shaft may originate from urethral problems, while pain in the glans penis is usually due to prostatitis.

Changes in Voiding (Micturition)

Voiding or micturition is normally a painless function occurring five to six times daily and occasionally once at night. The average person forms and voids 1200 to 1500 ml of urine in 24 hours. This amount is modified by fluid intake, sweating, outside temperature, vomiting, or diarrhea.

Urinary frequency is voiding that occurs more often than usual when compared with the patient's usual pattern or the generally accepted norm of once every 3 to 6 hours. It may result from a variety of conditions: infection, diseases of the urinary tract, metabolic disease, hypertension, and certain medications such as diuretics.

Urgency (strong desire to void) may be due to inflammatory lesions in the bladder, prostate, or urethra; acute bacterial infections or chronic prostatitis in men; or chronic posterior urethrotrigonitis (inflammation of the urethra and trigone of the bladder) in women.

Burning on urination is seen in patients with urethral irritation or bladder infection. Urethritis frequently causes burning during the act of voiding, whereas cystitis may produce burning both during and after urination.

Dysuria (painful or difficult voiding) stems from a wide variety of pathologic conditions.

Hesitancy (undue delay and difficulty in initiating voiding) may indicate compression of the urethra, neurogenic bladder, or outlet obstruction.

Nocturia (excessive urination at night) suggests decreased renal concentrating ability, heart failure, diabetes mellitus, or incomplete bladder emptying.

Urinary incontinence (involuntary loss of urine) may result from injury of the external urinary sphincter, acquired neurogenic disease, or severe urgency from infection.

Stress incontinence (intermittent leakage of urine due to sudden strain) results from weakness of the sphincteric mechanism.

Enuresis (involuntary voiding during sleep) is physiologic to the age of 3 years. After that time, it may be functional or symptomatic of obstructive disease of the lower urinary tract.

Polyuria (a large volume of urine voided in a given time) may be due to diabetes mellitus, diabetes insipidus, chronic renal disease, diuretics, or excessive fluid intake.

Oliguria (a small volume of urine; output between 100 and 500 ml/24 hr) and *anuria* (absence of urine in the bladder; output less than 100 ml/24 hours) indicate a serious renal dysfunction requiring immediate medical intervention. These conditions may result from such causes as shock, trauma, incompatible blood transfusion, and drug toxicity. Complete absence of urine (absolute anuria) is usually indicative of complete obstruction of the urinary tract.

Hematuria (red blood cells in the urine) is considered a serious sign because it may indicate cancer of the genitourinary tract, acute glomerulonephritis, or renal tuberculosis. The color of bloody urine depends on the pH of the urine and the amount of blood present; acid urine is a dark, smoky color, while alkaline urine is red. Hematuria may also be due to systemic causes such as blood dyscrasias (abnormalities of clotting), anticoagulant therapy, neoplasms, trauma, and extreme exercise.

Proteinuria (albuminuria) (abnormal amounts of protein in the urine) is characteristically seen in all forms of acute and chronic renal disease. Normal urine does not contain persistent protein in significant quantities.

Gastrointestinal Symptoms

Gastrointestinal symptoms may occur with urologic conditions because the gastrointestinal and urinary tracts have common autonomic and sensory innervation and because of renointestinal reflexes. The anatomic relation of the right kidney to the colon, duodenum, head of the pancreas, common bile duct, liver, and gallbladder may cause gastrointestinal disturbances. The proximity of the left kidney to the colon (splenic flexure), stomach, pancreas, and spleen may also result in intestinal symptoms. These may include nausea, vomiting, diarrhea, abdominal discomfort, and paralytic ileus. Appendicitis also may be accompanied by urinary symptoms.

Health History

When obtaining a health history, it is essential that the nurse use language and terms understandable to the patient and be aware of the patient's embarrassment or discomfort in discussing genitourinary functions and symptoms. The patient may "forget" or deny symptoms because of anxiety or embarrassment. The following information related to urinary function is sought:

- What is the patient's chief health concern or reason for seeking health care?
- Is pain present?
    - Location? Character? Radiation? Duration? Related to voiding? What brings it on? What relieves it?
- Has the patient had fever? Chills? Passage of stones?
- Are there any disorders of voiding?
    - Dysuria? When does it occur? Initial or terminal dysuria? Hesitancy? Straining? Pain during or after urination? Changes in color of urine? Diminished urine output? Incontinence? Stress incontinence? Urgency incontinence?
    - Any history of hematuria?
- Is nocturia present or absent? Date of onset?
- What is the past history in relation to urinary problems?
- Is there a family history of renal disease?
- Is there a history of urinary infections?
- Has the patient ever been hospitalized with urinary tract infection?
    - Before the age of 12?
    - Cystoscopy? Indwelling catheter? Kidney x-ray procedures?
- Is the patient at risk for urinary tract infections?
- Does the patient have diabetes mellitus? Hypertension? Allergies?
- What are the patient's present and past occupations? (Any exposure to occupational hazards relevant to the urinary tract, *e.g.,* chemicals, plastics, pitch, tar, or rubber?)
- Has the patient been exposed to any environmental toxins?
- What is the patient's smoking history?
- What childhood diseases did the patient have?
- Did enuresis extend beyond the usual age (past 3 years of age)?
- Any history of genital lesions or sexually transmitted diseases?
- For the female patient:
    - Number of children? Their ages? Forceps deliveries? Catheterized? When? Why?
    - Any signs of vaginal discharge? Vaginal/vulvar itch or irritation?
- Is the patient receiving any prescription or over-the-counter medications that may affect urinary or renal function? Have any medications been prescribed for treatment of renal or urinary problems?

The nurse not only elicits information about the patient's physical complaints but also assesses psychosocial status and educational needs. The nurse evaluates the patient's anxiety, perceived threats to body image, support systems, and sociocultural patterns. By putting together the information gathered during the initial and subsequent nursing assessments, the nurse finds valuable clues regarding misunderstandings, lack of knowledge, and needs for patient teaching.

Physical Assessment

Because renal dysfunction affects all body systems, a general assessment is indicated (see specific discussions in following sections). Additionally, the assessment focuses on the urinary tract specifically.

By direct palpation it is sometimes possible to determine the size and mobility of the kidneys.

- With the patient in a supine position, the examiner places one hand under the patient's back so that her fingers are clear of the lower ribs. The other hand (palm down) is placed anterior to the kidney, with the fingers just above the level of the umbilicus.
- The patient is instructed to inhale deeply and the examiner's anterior hand is pushed forward.

It may be possible to feel the smooth, rounded lower pole of the kidney between the hands; the right kidney is felt more easily than the left kidney because it is somewhat lower than the left one.

Renal disease may produce tenderness over the costovertebral angle, which lies where the twelfth or bottom rib joins the spine. Auscultation of the upper quadrants of the abdomen is performed to assess for *bruits* (vascular sounds that might indicate stenosis of the renal arteries).

In a rectal examination in the male, the prostate gland may be palpated digitally as a part of the study of urinary difficulty that occurs when there is hyperplasia of the prostate in older men (see Chap. 49).

The inguinal area is examined for enlarged nodes, an inguinal or femoral hernia, and a varicocele. In women, the vulva, urethra, and vagina are examined.

During the physical assessment, the patient is assessed for edema, which would indicate fluid retention; the face and dependent parts of the body are specifically assessed.

Diagnostic Evaluation

Urinalysis

Urinalysis may provide important clinical information. Although its routine use on admission and in preoperative screening of patients undergoing elective surgery has become controversial recently because of few positive findings, it remains a routine test in most clinical settings. Urine examination includes evaluation of the following:

1. Urine color and clarity
2. Urine odor
3. Measurement of urine acidity and specific gravity
4. Tests for the presence of protein, glucose, and ketone bodies in the urine (proteinuria, glucosuria, and ketonuria, respectively)
5. Microscopic examination of the urine sediment after centri-

TABLE 41–2. *Indications for Diagnostic Admission Urinalysis*

HISTORY OF FOLLOWING SYMPTOMS
Dysuria	Frequency
Hesitancy	Urethral discharge
Flank pain	

HISTORY OF DISORDERS THAT CAN AFFECT RENAL FUNCTION
Renal disease	Diabetes mellitus
Collagen vascular disease	Exposure to nephrotoxins

PHYSICAL ASSESSMENT FINDINGS
Fever of unknown origin	Tenderness of costovertebral angle
Generalized edema	Prostate gland abnormalities
Jaundice	

(Adapted from Aken BV et al. Efficacy of routine admission urinalysis. Am J Med 1987 Apr; 82[4]:719–722.)

fuging for the detection of red blood cells (hematuria), white blood cells, casts (cylindruria), crystals (crystalluria), pus (pyuria), and bacteria (bacteriuria)

Indications for admission urinalysis, if it is not a procedure routinely carried out, are presented in Table 41-2. Dipstick urinalysis tests provide a rapid method of screening symptomatic patients for certain constituents, including hemoglobin, ketones, protein, and the presence of leukocytes (pyuria). Numerous additional tests are applicable in special situations.

Collection of Urine Samples

All urine tests are ideally performed on fresh specimens, preferably the first voiding of the day because this specimen is most concentrated and more likely to reveal abnormalities. Random specimens are satisfactory for most analyses, provided that they have been collected in clean containers and have been adequately protected against bacterial contamination and chemical deterioration. All specimens should be refrigerated

as soon as they are obtained. If left standing at room temperature, the urine becomes alkaline because of contamination of urea-splitting bacteria from the environment. Microscopic examination should be performed within a half hour of collection; delay allows dissolution of cellular elements and bacterial overgrowth in nonsterile specimens. Urine cultures should be processed immediately. If this is not possible, they should be stored at 4°C (39°F).

- Urine specimens should be collected from the patient by means of the clean-catch midstream technique, with use of a wide-mouthed container (see Fig. 41-3).

24-Hour Urine Collection

Many quantitative analytic tests are carried out on specimens of urine collected over a 24-hour period. The procedure is as follows:

The patient is instructed to empty the bladder at a specified time (such as 8:00 AM). This urine is discarded. All urine voided during the next 24 hours is collected. The last specimen is collected and saved 24 hours after the collection began (*i.e.*, 8:00 AM).

The patient's bladder should be empty when the test starts and empty when it ends. The urine is collected in a clean container. Depending on the test to be performed, a preservative may be added or the urine may need to be refrigerated. Discarding even one specimen voided during the test period invalidates the test. A successful collection requires complete understanding and cooperation on the part of the patient and of all unit personnel concerned with the patient's care.

Clean-Catch Midstream Urine Specimens

Urine specimens voided in the usual manner are practically useless for bacteriologic study because of inevitable contamination by organisms residing in the vicinity of the urethral meatus. Such contamination can be avoided by catheterizing the urinary bladder. However, catheterization is no longer recommended routinely to obtain urine specimens except for specific indications because of the risk of infection. Reliable bacteriologic studies are possible without catheterization, with use of the clean-catch midstream technique.

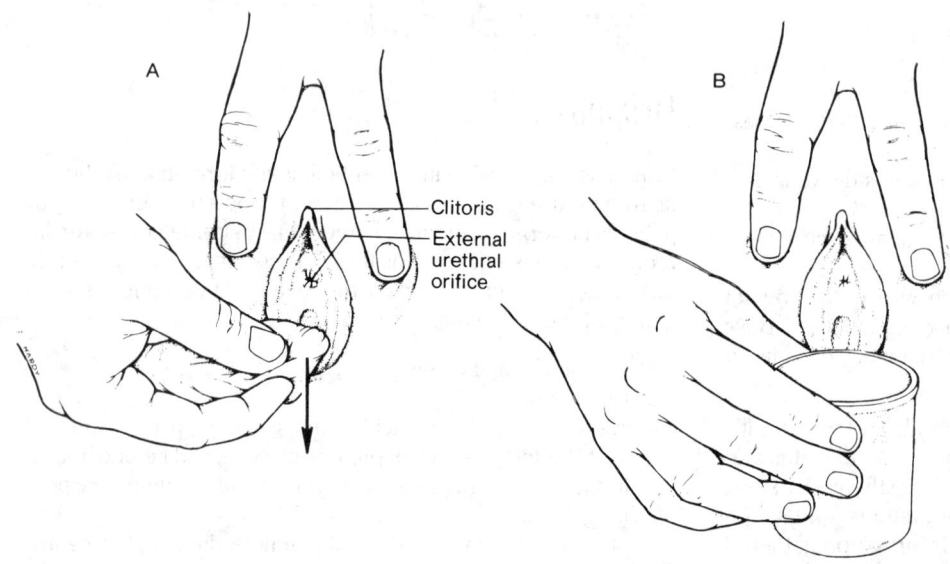

Figure 41–3. A clean-catch midstream urine specimen in the female. (**A**) The patient is instructed to hold the labia apart and wash from high up front toward the back with gauze soaked in soap. (**B**) The collection cup is held so that it does not touch the body, and the sample is obtained only while the patient is voiding with the labia held apart.

Instructions to the Male Patient

- Expose the glans and cleanse the area around the meatus with soap. Remove all soap with water-soaked pledgets.
- Do not collect the first portion of the voiding; discard it.
- Collect the next portion by voiding into a sterile wide-mouthed bottle or large-caliber tube that is protected by a sterile closure.
- Do not collect the last few drops of urine because prostatic secretions may be introduced into the urine at the end of the urinary stream.

Instructions to the Female Patient

- Separate the labia to expose the urethral orifice (see Fig. 41-3).
- Cleanse around the urinary meatus with sponges soaked in liquid soap.
- Wipe the perineum from the front to the back.
- Remove all soap with water-soaked pledgets, wiping from front to back.
- Keep the labia separated and void forcibly, but do not collect the first portion of the voiding. (The distal portion of the urethral orifice is colonized by bacteria; the initial voiding washes away the urethral contaminants.)
- Collect the midstream portion of the urinary flow, making sure that the container does not come in contact with the genitalia.

Renal Function Tests

Renal function tests are used to evaluate the severity of kidney disease and to follow the patient's clinical progress. These tests also provide information about the kidneys' effectiveness in carrying out their excretory function. Results of function tests may be within normal limits until renal function is reduced to less than 50% of normal. Renal function can be assessed most accurately if several tests are performed and their results analyzed together. Table 41-3 lists the more common tests of renal function. Because of the important role of the kidneys in maintaining fluid and electrolyte balance, serum electrolyte levels also are assessed.

Ultrasound

Ultrasound (ultrasonic scan) uses sound waves that are passed into the body. Organs in the urinary system create characteristic ultrasonic images. Abnormalities such as masses, malformations, or obstructions can be identified. Ultrasound is a noninvasive technique, and no special patient preparation is required. Because of its sensitivity, ultrasound has replaced many other diagnostic procedures as the initial diagnostic procedure.

TABLE 41-3.   Tests of Renal Function

Test	Purpose/Rationale	Test Protocol
RENAL CONCENTRATION TEST		
Specific gravity Osmolality of urine	Tests the ability to concentrate solutes in the urine. Concentration ability is lost early in kidney disease; hence, this test shows early defects in renal function.	Fluids may be withheld for 12 to 24 hours to assess the concentrating ability of the tubules under controlled conditions. Specific gravity measurements of urine are taken at specific times to determine urine concentration.
CREATININE CLEARANCE* (ENDOGENOUS CREATININE CLEARANCE) TEST		
	Provides an approximation of rate of glomerular filtration Measures volume of blood cleared of creatinine in 1 minute Most sensitive indication of early renal disease Useful to follow progress of patient's renal status	All urine is collected over 24-hour period. Draw one sample of blood within the 24-hour period.
SERUM CREATININE TEST		
	A test of renal function reflecting the balance between production and filtration by renal glomerulus Most sensitive measure of renal function	Test is performed on blood serum.
SERUM UREA NITROGEN (BLOOD UREA NITROGEN [BUN]) TEST		
	Serves as index of renal excretory capacity Serum urea nitrogen is dependent on the body's urea production and on urine flow. (Urea is the nitrogenous end product of protein metabolism.) Affected by protein intake, tissue breakdown	Test is performed on blood serum.

* Clearance is the amount of blood cleansed of a constituent per unit of time.

X-Ray and Other Imaging Studies

Kidney, Ureter, and Bladder X-Ray.   An x-ray of the abdomen or KUB (kidney, ureters, and bladder) may be performed to delineate the size, shape, and position of the kidneys and to reveal any abnormalities, such as calculi (stones) in the kidneys or urinary tract, hydronephrosis, cysts, tumors, or kidney displacement by abnormalities in the surrounding tissues.

Computed Tomography and Magnetic Resonance Imaging. Computed tomography (CT or CAT scan) and magnetic resonance imaging (MRI) are noninvasive techniques that provide excellent cross-sectional views of the kidney and urinary tract. They provide information about the extension of invasive lesions of the kidney. No special patient preparation is needed.

Infusion Drip Pyelography.   Infusion drip pyelography is an intravenous infusion of a large volume of dilute solution of contrast material to produce opacification of the renal parenchyma and complete filling of the urinary tract. This method of examination is useful when regular urographic techniques fail to show the drainage structures satisfactorily (*e.g.*, in a patient with an elevated blood urea nitrogen) or when prolonged opacification of the drainage structures is desired so that *tomograms* (body section radiography) can be made. Films are obtained at specified intervals after the start of the infusion to examine the filled and distended collecting system. The patient preparation is the same as for excretory urography (see below), except that fluids are not restricted.

Excretory Urography (Intravenous Urogram or Intravenous Pyelogram).   An excretory urogram or intravenous pyelogram (IVP) permits visualization of the kidneys, ureter, and bladder. A radiopaque contrast medium is administered intravenously and is cleared from the bloodstream and concentrated by the kidneys. A *nephrotomogram* may be carried out as part of the study to visualize different layers of the kidney and the diffuse structures within each layer and to differentiate solid masses or lesions from cysts in the kidneys or urinary tract.

Excretory urography is conducted as part of the initial assessment of any suspected urologic problem, especially in the diagnosis of lesions in the kidneys and ureters. It also provides a rough estimate of renal function. After the contrast material (sodium diatrizoate or meglumine diatrizoate) is administered intravenously, multiple films are taken serially to visualize drainage structures.

Patient Preparation.   The patient may be prepared for the procedure as follows:

1. The patient's history should be obtained to check for any indications of allergies that might cause an adverse reaction to the contrast material. The physician and the radiologist are notified of allergy (especially to iodine or shellfish) or suspicion of allergy so that appropriate measures are taken to prevent serious allergic reactions. The suspected allergy is also noted prominently in the patient's record.
2. A laxative may be prescribed the night before the scheduled examination to eliminate feces and gas from the intestinal tract.
3. Liquids may be restricted 8 to 10 hours before the test to promote a concentrated urine. However, elderly patients with marginal renal reserve or function, patients with multiple myeloma, and those with uncontrolled diabetes mellitus may not tolerate dehydration. With the approval of the physician, the nurse may give such patients water to drink during the hours before the test. The patient should not be overhydrated,

because this may dilute the contrast material and thus cause inadequate visualization.
4. The procedure itself and the sensations produced by injection of the contrast medium and during the procedure (*e.g.*, a temporary feeling of warmth and flushing of the face) are described to the patient.

If the patient has a history of allergies, a test dose of the contrast material may be injected intradermally. If no skin reaction occurs in 15 minutes, the regular intravenous test dose of contrast material is administered. Although rare, as with the administration of any intravenous drug, an anaphylactic reaction may occur. (This reaction may occur even if the skin sensitivity test has been negative.)

- All IV urogram rooms should have emergency drugs (epinephrine, corticosteroids, vasopressors), as well as oxygen, tracheostomy, and other equipment, ready for immediate therapy in case an anaphylactic reaction occurs.

Retrograde Pyelography.   In retrograde pyelography, ureteral catheters are passed up through the ureters into the renal pelvis by means of cystoscopy. A contrast material is then introduced into the catheters by gravity or syringe. Retrograde pyelography is usually performed if intravenous urography provides inadequate visualization of the collecting systems. It is being used less frequently because of improved techniques in excretory urography.

Cystogram.   A catheter is inserted into the bladder and contrast material is instilled to outline the bladder wall and to aid in evaluation of *vesicoureteral reflux* (backflow of urine from the bladder into one or both ureters). Cystograms are also taken in conjunction with simultaneous pressure recordings inside the bladder.

Cystourethrogram.   A cystourethrogram provides visualization of the urethra and bladder either by retrograde injection of the contrast material into the urethra and bladder or by x-ray films taken while the patient excretes the contrast material. The *voiding cystourethrogram* is described on p. 1144.

Renal Angiography.   This procedure permits visualization of the renal arteries. A needle is used to pierce the femoral (or axillary) artery, and a catheter is threaded up through the femoral and iliac arteries into the aorta or renal artery. Contrast material is injected to opacify the renal arterial supply. Angiography enables evaluation of blood flow dynamics, demonstrates abnormal vasculature, and helps to differentiate renal cysts from renal tumors.

Nursing Interventions.   Before the procedure, a laxative may be prescribed to eliminate fecal material and gas from the colon so that unobstructed x-rays can be obtained. The proposed injection sites (groin for femoral approach or axilla for axillary approach) are shaved. The peripheral pulse sites (radial, femoral, dorsalis pedis) are marked for easy access in postprocedural assessment. The patient is informed that a feeling of heat may be sensed briefly along the course of the vessel when the contrast material is injected.

Following the procedure, the vital signs are monitored until stable. If the axillary artery was the site of the injection, the blood pressure is taken on the opposite arm. The puncture site is examined for swelling and hematoma formation. The peripheral pulses are palpated. The color and temperature of the involved extremity are noted and compared with those of the uninvolved extremity. Cold compresses may be applied to the puncture site to decrease edema and pain.

Endourology (Urologic Endoscopic Procedures)

The Cystoscopic Examination

The cystoscopic examination (*cystoscopy* or *"cysto"*) is a method of direct visualization of the urethra and bladder. The cystoscope, which is inserted through the urethra into the bladder, has a self-contained optical lens system that provides a magnified, illuminated view of the bladder. The cystoscope is manipulated to allow complete visualization of the urethra and bladder as well as the ureteral orifices and prostatic urethra. Small ureteral catheters can be passed through the cystoscope, allowing assessment of the ureter and the pelvis of the kidney. The cystoscope also permits the urologist to obtain a urine specimen from each kidney to evaluate its function. Cup forceps can be inserted through the cystoscope for biopsy. Calculi may be removed from the urethra, bladder, and ureter via cystoscopy.

The endoscope is passed under direct vision. After inspection of the urethra, the bladder is inspected. Sterile irrigating solution is instilled to distend the bladder and wash away blood clots, thereby allowing better visualization (Fig. 41-4). The use of a high-intensity light and interchangeable lenses allows excellent visualization and permits still and motion pictures to be taken of these structures.

Prior to the procedure, a sedative may be administered. A local topical anesthetic is instilled into the urethra by the urologist before the cystoscope is inserted. Intravenous diazepam (Valium) in combination with topical urethral anesthesia may be administered. Alternatively, spinal or general anesthesia may be used.

Nursing Interventions.   As with any diagnostic procedure, the nurse describes the examination and procedure in order to inform the patient and allay fears. Additional preprocedure preparation may include having the patient drink one or two glasses of water before going to the radiology department.

Postprocedure management is directed at relieving any possible discomfort resulting from the examination. Some burning upon voiding, blood-tinged urine, and urinary frequency from trauma to the mucous membrane may occur after cystoscopic examination. Moist heat to the lower abdomen or warm sitz baths are helpful in relieving pain and promoting muscle relaxation. Occasionally, following cystoscopic examination the patient with obstructive pathology may experience urinary retention as a result of edema caused by the instrumentation. The patient with prostatic hyperplasia is carefully monitored for urinary retention. Warm sitz baths and relaxant medications are helpful for relieving retention, but an indwelling catheter may be required.

The patient who has undergone instrumentation of the urinary tract (*i.e.*, cystoscopy) is monitored for signs and symptoms of urinary tract infection.

Renal and Ureteral Brush Biopsy

Brush biopsy techniques provide specific information when abnormal x-ray findings for the ureter or renal pelvis raise uncertainty as to whether the defect is a tumor, a stone, a blood clot, or an artifact. First, a cystoscopic examination is conducted. Then a ureteral catheter is introduced, followed by a biopsy brush that is passed through the catheter. The suspected lesion is brushed back and forth in order to obtain cells and surface tissue fragments for histologic analysis.

Following the procedure, intravenous fluids may be administered to help clear the kidneys and prevent clot formation. Urine may contain blood (usually clearing in 24 to 48 hours) from oozing at the brushing site. Postoperative renal colic occasionally occurs and responds to analgesics.

Renal Endoscopy (Nephroscopy)

Renal endoscopy (nephroscopy) is the introduction of a fiberscope into the pelvis of the kidney, through an incision (pyelotomy) or percutaneously, to view the interior of the renal pelvis, remove calculi, biopsy small lesions, and aid in the diagnosis of renal hematuria and selected renal tumors.

Needle Biopsy of the Kidney

Needle biopsy of the kidney is performed by percutaneous needle biopsy through renal tissue or by open biopsy through a small flank incision. It is useful in evaluating the course of renal disease and in obtaining specimens for electron and immunofluorescent microscopy, particularly for glomerular disease. Before the biopsy is carried out, coagulation studies are conducted to identify any risk for postbiopsy bleeding.

The patient may be placed on a fasting regimen 6 to 8 hours before the test. An intravenous line is established. A urine specimen is obtained and saved for comparison with the postbiopsy specimen. The patient is informed that it will be necessary to hold his breath (to prevent movement of the kidney) during insertion of the renal biopsy needle.

The sedated patient is placed in a prone position with a sandbag under the abdomen. A local anesthetic agent is infiltrated into the skin at the biopsy site. The biopsy needle is introduced just inside the renal capsule of the outer quadrant of the kidney. The location of the needle may be confirmed by fluoroscopy or by ultrasound, in which a special probe is used. Open biopsy may also be carried out, through a small flank incision.

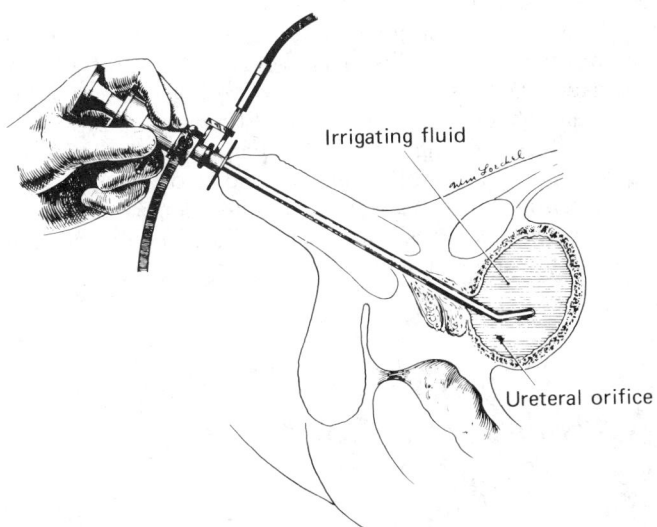

Figure 41-4.   Cystoscopic examination. A cystoscope is introduced into the bladder of the male. The upper cord is an electric line for the light at the distal end of the cystoscope. The lower tubing leads from a reservoir of sterile irrigating fluid that is used to inflate the bladder.

Postbiopsy Nursing Management. After the specimen is obtained, pressure is applied to the biopsy site. The patient may be kept in a prone position immediately following biopsy and on bed rest for 24 hours to minimize risk of bleeding.

The nurse observes for hematuria, which may appear soon after biopsy. The kidney is a highly vascular organ, and approximately one fourth of the entire cardiac output circulates through it in about 1 minute. The passage of the biopsy needle punctures the kidney capsule, and bleeding can occur in the perirenal space. Usually, the bleeding subsides on its own, but a large amount of blood can accumulate in this space in a short period of time without noticeable signs until cardiovascular collapse is evident.

- To detect early signs of bleeding, it is important that the vital signs be monitored every 5 to 15 minutes for the first hour and then with decreasing frequency as indicated.
- Signs and symptoms suggestive of bleeding include a rise or fall in blood pressure, anorexia, vomiting, and the development of a dull, aching discomfort in the abdomen.
- Any symptoms of backache, shoulder pain, or dysuria are reported to the physician.

Flank pain may occur but usually represents bleeding into the muscle rather than around the kidney. Colicky pain similar to that of ureteral colic may develop when a clot is present in the ureter and may cause excruciating, sharp flank pain that radiates to the groin.

All urine voided by the patient is scrutinized for evidence of bleeding and compared with the prebiopsy specimen and subsequent voiding samples. If bleeding persists, as indicated by an enlarging hematoma, palpating or manipulating the abdomen is avoided. A hematocrit and hemoglobin study is performed within 8 hours to assess for anemia. Usually, the fluid intake is maintained at 3000 ml daily unless the patient has renal insufficiency. If bleeding occurs, the patient is prepared for blood transfusion and surgical intervention for control of hemorrhage, which may necessitate surgical drainage or rarely nephrectomy (removal of kidney).

Patient Education. Delayed hemorrhage can occur several days after biopsy. Therefore, the patient is instructed to avoid strenuous activity and sports, and heavy lifting for at least 2 weeks. The physician or clinic is to be notified if any of the following occurs: flank pain, hematuria, lightheadedness and fainting, rapid pulse, or any other signs and symptoms of bleeding.

Radioisotope Studies

Radioisotope studies are noninvasive procedures that do not interfere with normal physiologic processes and require no specific patient preparation. Radiopharmaceuticals (^{99}Tc-labeled compound or ^{131}I-hippurate) are injected intravenously. Studies are obtained with a scintillation camera placed posterior to the kidney, with the patient in a supine, prone, or sitting position. The resultant image (called a *scan*) indicates the distribution of the radiopharmaceutical within the kidney.

The *Tc scan* provides information about kidney perfusion and is useful when renal function is poor. The *hippurate scan* provides information about kidney function.

Urodynamic Measurements

Urodynamic measurements provide physiologic and structural tests to evaluate bladder and urethral function by measuring the (1) rate of urine flow, (2) bladder pressures during voiding and at rest, (3) internal urethral resistance, and (4) bladder contraction and relaxation. Abdominal, bladder, and detrusor pressures, sphincter activity, bladder innervation, muscle tone, and sacral reflex are assessed.

The following are the urodynamic measurements most frequently performed.

Uroflowmetry (flow rate) is the record of the volume of urine passing through the urethra per time unit (ml/sec).

A *cystometrogram* is a graphic recording of the pressures in the bladder (intravesical) at various phases of filling and emptying of the urinary bladder to assess its function. During the procedure, the amount of fluid instilled into the bladder and voided, as well as the patient's sensations of bladder fullness and urge to void, are recorded. These are then compared with the pressures measured in the bladder during bladder filling and voiding. The patient is first asked to void, and the physician observes the time it takes to initiate voiding; the size, force, and continuity of the urinary stream; and the degree of straining and hesitancy. A retention catheter is passed through the urethra and into the bladder. The residual volume is measured and the catheter left in place. The urethral catheter is connected to a water manometer, and sterile solution is allowed to flow into the bladder, usually at the rate of 1 ml/sec. The patient informs the examiner when the first desire to void is felt, and again when the bladder feels full. The degree of bladder filling at these points is recorded. The pressures above the zero level at the symphysis pubis are measured, and the pressures and volumes within the bladder are plotted and recorded.

The *urethral pressure profile* measures urethral resistance along the length of the urethra. Gas and fluid are instilled through a catheter that is withdrawn while the pressures along the urethral wall are obtained.

A *cystourethrogram* permits visualization of the urethra and bladder either by retrograde injection or by voiding of contrast material.

In a *voiding cystourethrogram,* the bladder is filled with contrast medium, and the patient voids while rapid spot films are taken. The presence or absence of vesicoureteral reflux or congenital abnormalities in the lower urinary tract can be demonstrated. The voiding cystourethrogram is also used to investigate difficulty in bladder emptying and incontinence.

Electromyography involves the placement of electrodes in the pelvic floor/musculature or anal sphincter to evaluate neuromuscular function of the lower tract.

Nursing Care of Patients Undergoing Assessment of the Urinary/ Renal System

All patients, regardless of the extent or type of urinary tract dysfunction, undergo tests to assess the function of the urinary

Nursing Care Plan 41-1

Care of the Patient Undergoing Assessment for Urinary/Renal Dysfunction

Nursing Interventions	Rationale	Expected Outcomes

Nursing Diagnosis: Knowledge deficit about procedures and diagnostic tests

Goal: Patient acquires knowledge and understanding of the procedure and tests and expected behaviors

Nursing Interventions	Rationale	Expected Outcomes
1. Assess patient's current level of understanding of planned tests and procedures.	1. Provides basis for further explanations and teaching and gives indication of patient's perception of procedures.	• States rationale for planned diagnostic procedures and tasks and behaviors expected during the procedures.
2. Provide factual description of tests in language and terms the patient understands.	2. Understanding what is expected enhances patient's compliance and cooperation.	• Complies with urine collection, fluid modifications, or other procedures required for diagnostic evaluation.
3. Assess patient's understanding of test results following their completion.	3. Apprehension may interfere with patient's ability to understand information and results provided by physician and other health care providers.	• Restates in own words results of diagnostic assessment. • Asks for clarification of terms and procedures.
4. Reinforce information provided to patient about test results and implications for follow-up care.	4. Provides opportunity for patient to clarify points and anticipate follow-up care.	• Explains rationale for follow-up care. • Participates in follow-up care.

Nursing Diagnosis: Pain and discomfort related to infection, edema, obstruction, or bleeding along urinary tract or invasive diagnostic tests

Goal: Relief of pain and discomfort

Nursing Interventions	Rationale	Expected Outcomes

1. Assess level of pain and discomfort.
  a. Dysuria
  b. Burning on urination
  c. Abdominal pain and discomfort
  d. Flank pain
  e. Bladder spasm
	1. Provides baseline for evaluating success of interventions and progression of dysfunction.	• Reports decreasing levels of pain and discomfort.
		• Uses sitz bath as indicated.
		• Consumes increased fluid intake if indicated.

2. Encourage fluid intake (unless contraindicated).	2. Promotes dilute urine and flushing of lower urinary tract.	• Reports absence of local symptoms (urgency, frequency, dysuria, and burning on urination).
3. Encourage warm sitz baths.	3. Relieves local discomfort and promotes relaxation.	• States ability to start and stop urinary stream without discomfort. • Identifies signs and symptoms to be reported to health care provider.
4. Report increased pain to physician.	4. May indicate progression of dysfunction, recurrence of dysfunction, or untoward signs (*e.g.*, bleeding, calculi).	• Takes medications as prescribed • Does not delay in emptying bladder • Uses appropriate hygienic practices:
5. Administer analgesics and antispasmodics for pain and spasm as prescribed.	5. May be prescribed for pain and spasm.	Avoids use of bubble bath Uses appropriate hygiene after bowel movements
6. Assess voiding patterns and practices of hygiene and provide instructions about recommended voiding patterns and hygienic practices.	6. Delayed emptying of the bladder and some poor practices of hygiene contribute to discomfort and pain secondary to renal or urinary tract dysfunction.	

Nursing Diagnosis: Fear related to (1) potential alteration in renal function and body part and (2) embarrassment secondary to discussion of urinary function and invasion of genitalia

Goal: Reduced fear

Nursing Interventions	Rationale	Expected Outcomes
1. Assess patient's level of fear and apprehension.	1. A high level of fear or apprehension can interfere with learning and cooperation.	• Appears relaxed with low level of fear and apprehension.

(continued)

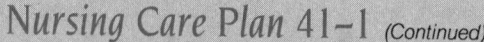

Nursing Care Plan 41–1 *(Continued)*

Care of the Patient Undergoing Assessment for Urinary/Renal Dysfunction

Nursing Interventions	Rationale	Expected Outcomes
2. Explain all procedures and tests to patient.	2. Knowledge about what is expected helps to reduce fear and apprehension.	• States rationale for tests and procedures in a calm, relaxed manner
3. Provide privacy and respect patient's modesty by closing doors and keeping patient covered and clothed. Keep urinal and bedpan covered and out of sight.	3. Communicates that you are aware of and accept patient's need for privacy and modesty.	• Maintains usual privacy and modesty • Discusses own urinary tract dysfunction in correct terminology without overt indications of embarrassment or discomfort
4. Use correct terminology in factual manner when questioning patient about urinary tract dysfunction.	4. Conveys that nurse is comfortable discussing patient's urinary dysfunction and symptoms with patient.	• Is able to relate fears and concerns • Shows correct understanding of procedures and possible outcomes
5. Assess patient's fears about perceived changes associated with tests and other procedures.	5. May reveal unfounded fears and misperceptions that can be alleviated by correct understanding.	
6. Instruct patient in relaxation exercises	6. May promote relaxation and assist the patient in coping with uncertainty about outcomes.	

tract. Even those who have had these tests repeatedly in the past experience fear and apprehension about the procedures and the results. Additionally, they frequently feel discomfort and embarrassment about a previously private and personal function: voiding. Although this is a function that health care providers deal with frequently in the course of providing care, it is important to remember that it is not so routine to patients.

Nursing Diagnoses

Potential nursing diagnoses for these patients include the following:

- Knowledge deficit about the procedures and diagnostic tests
- Pain and discomfort related to renal infection, edema, obstruction, or bleeding along the urinary tract or invasive diagnostic procedures
- Fear related to possible diagnoses of serious illness and alteration in renal function
- Fear related to embarrassment secondary to discussion of urinary function and invasion of genitalia

Planning, Implementation, and Evaluation

The goals, nursing interventions, rationales for interventions, and expected outcomes are discussed in more detail in Nursing Care Plan 41-1, Care of the Patient Undergoing Assessment for Urinary/Renal Dysfunction.

Gerontologic Considerations

Renal and urinary tract function change with age. After age 40, there is a progressive decline in the glomerular filtration rate to approximately 50% of normal by age 70. Tubular function, including reabsorption and concentrating ability, is re-

duced also with increasing age. Although renal function usually remains adequate despite these changes, renal reserve is decreased and may reduce the kidneys' ability to respond effectively to drastic or sudden physiologic changes. At the same time, changes in other body systems often alter the patient's response to illness, resulting in signs and symptoms of illness or infection that are atypical or different from those that commonly occur in younger patients.

Structural or functional abnormalities that occur with aging may prevent complete emptying of the bladder and increase the risk of urinary tract infection, the most common cause of sepsis in patients over 65 years of age. In addition to changes in renal function, there are changes in function of the ureters, bladder, and urethra with aging. The likelihood of prostatic enlargement in the elderly male patient makes assessment of urinary patterns extremely important, because undetected urethral obstruction can result in renal failure and urinary tract infections in elderly men. Elderly women often have incomplete emptying of the bladder and urinary stasis.

The increased occurrence of chronic illness in the elderly and the increased use of prescription drugs and over-the-counter drugs indicate the need for a complete health history to identify predisposing conditions, the use of medications, or interactions of several medications that could compromise renal function further. Preparation of the elderly patient for diagnostic tests must be managed carefully to prevent dehydration that might precipitate renal failure in a patient with marginal renal reserve. Limitations in mobility often imposed on elderly patients may affect the patient's ability to void adequately or to consume adequate fluids. Patients may limit their own fluid intake to minimize the frequency of voiding or the risk of incontinence; teaching the patient and family about the dangers of an inadequate fluid intake is an important role of the nurse caring for the elderly patient.

Chapter Summary

Normal function of the urinary tract is essential for excretion of metabolic end products and maintenance of normal fluid, electrolyte, and acid–base balance. Any disorder of the kidneys and lower urinary tract has the potential to cause systemic manifestations. Evaluation of the patient with such disorders may focus on the specific structures of the lower urinary tract or may be directed toward the effects of the disorder on electrolyte concentrations in the blood. Diagnostic evaluation may require extensive tests and procedures. Because voiding is a function usually carried out in private and the urinary tract is closely associated with the genitalia and sexual function, the patient may be uncomfortable and embarrassed about discussing symptoms and may be hesitant to ask questions about tests, procedures, test results, and kidney and bladder function. The patient's concerns should be anticipated and validated; these concerns and the family's concerns are answered in a matter-of-fact but sensitive manner to minimize their embarrassment and discomfort.

Bibliography

Books

Bates B. A Guide to Physical Examination and History Taking. Philadelphia, JB Lippincott, 1991.

Brenner BM, Coe FL, and Rector FC Jr. Clinical Nephrology. Philadelphia, WB Saunders, 1987.

Catto ORD. Pregnancy and Renal Disorders. Dordrecht, Kluwer Academic Publishers, 1988.

DeWardener HE. The Kidney: An Outline of Normal and Abnormal Function, 5th ed. New York; Churchill Livingstone, 1985.

Fischbach F. A Manual of Laboratory Diagnostic Tests, 3rd ed. Philadelphia, JB Lippincott, 1988.

Guzzetta CE et al. Clinical Assessment Tools for Use With Nursing Diagnoses. St Louis, CV Mosby, 1989.

Hanno PM and Wein AJ. A Clinical Manual of Urology. Englewood Cliffs, NJ, Appleton–Century–Crofts, 1987.

Kunin CM. Detection, Prevention and Management of Urinary Tract Infections. Philadelphia, Lea & Febiger, 1987.

Massry SG and Glassock RJ. Textbook of Nephrology, 2nd ed. Baltimore, Williams & Wilkins, 1989.

Rose BD and Black RM. Manual of Clinical Problems in Nephrology. Boston, Little, Brown, 1988.

Schrier RW and Gottshalk CW (eds). Diseases of the Kidney. Boston, Little, Brown, 1988.

Toledo-Pereyra LH (ed.) Kidney Transplantation. Philadelphia, FA Davis, 1988.

Journals

Aken BV et al. Efficacy of the routine admission urinalysis. Am J Med 1987 Apr; 82(4):719–722.

Baer CL. Assessing flank pain. Nursing 1989 Oct; 19(10):75–79.

Becker KL and Stevens SA. Performing in-depth abdominal assessment. Nursing 1988 Jun; 18(6):59–64.

Campbell JPM and Gunn AA. Plain abdominal radiographs and acute abdominal pain. Br J Surg 1988 Jun; 75(6):554–556.

Del Mar C and Badger P. The place of routine urine testing on admission to hospital. Med J Aust 1989 Aug 7; 151(7):151–153.

Fairley KF and Birch DF. Detection of bladder bacteriuria in patients with acute urinary symptoms. J Infect Dis 1989 Feb; 159(2):226–231.

Garrett VE et al. Bladder emptying assessment in stroke patients. Arch Phys Med Rehabil 1989 Jan; 70(1):41–43.

Kahn RI. Outpatient endourologic procedures. Urol Clin North Am 1987 Feb; 14(1):77–89.

Kanel KT. The intravenous pyelogram in acute pyelonephritis. Arch Intern Med 1988 Oct; 148(19):2144–2148.

Kee JL and Hayes ER. Assessment of patient laboratory data in the acutely ill. Nurs Clin North Am 1990 Dec; 25(4):751–759.

Kellogg JA et al. Clinical relevance of culture versus screens for the detection of microbial pathogens in urine specimens. Am J Med 1987 Oct; 83(4):739–745.

Kiel DP and Moskowitz MA. The urinalysis: A critical appraisal. Med Clin North Am 1987 Jul; 71(4):607–624.

Lawrence VA, Gafni A, and Gross M. The unproven utility of the preoperative urinalysis: Economic evaluation. J Clin Epidemiol 1989; 42(12):1185–1192.

Mainprize TC and Drutz HP. Accuracy of total bladder volume and residual urine measurements: Comparison between real-time ultrasonography and catheterization. Am J Obstet Gynecol 1989 Apr; 160(4):1013–1016.

Needham CA. Rapid detection methods in microbiology: Are they right for your office? Med Clin North Am 1987 Jun; 71(4):591–605.

Pfaller M et al. The usefulness of screening tests for pyuria in combination with culture in the diagnosis of urinary tract infection. Diagn Microbiol Infect Dis 1987 Mar; 6(3):207–209.

Stark JL. A quick guide to urinary tract assessment. Nursing 1988 Jul; 18(7):56–58.

Striegel J, Michael AF, and Chavers BM. Asymptomatic proteinuria. Postgrad Med 1988 Jun; 83(8):287–290, 293, 294.

Walter FG and Knopp RK. Urine sampling in ambulatory women: Midstream clean-catch versus catheterization. Ann Emerg Med 1989 Feb; 18(2):166–172.

Woolhandler S et al. Dipstick urinalysis screening of asymptomatic adults for urinary tract disorders. JAMA 1989 Sep 1; 262(9):1215–1219.

42

Management of Patients With Urinary and Renal Dysfunction

Learning Objectives

On completion of this chapter, the learner will be able to:

1. Describe the sequence of events leading to urinary tract infection in a patient with an indwelling urinary catheter

2. Outline the principles of management of a patient with an indwelling urinary catheter

3. Compare and contrast urinary retention and urinary incontinence: their causes, clinical manifestations, complications, and management

4. Use the nursing process as a framework for the care of patients with urinary retention

5. Discuss strategies for the management of urinary incontinence in the elderly patient

6. Compare and contrast hemodialysis and peritoneal dialysis: underlying principles, procedures, complications, and nursing considerations

7. Describe nursing management of the hospitalized dialysis patient

8. Use the nursing process as a framework for care of patients undergoing kidney surgery

Psychosocial Considerations

Conditions of the genitourinary tract may generate emotional stresses and feelings of embarrassment when the external genitalia are examined and treated or urinary function is discussed. Problems of incontinence may cause distress, disgust, and feelings of helplessness. Many patients are constantly uneasy about the possibility of an "accident"; occasionally a patient appears indifferent.

Surgical procedures affecting the male reproductive organs can pose a threat to the sexuality of the patient, no matter what his age. Although many men may hide their fears of impotency by blaming "prostate trouble," many sexual problems of males (such as difficulty in achieving erection and premature ejaculation) are psychologic in origin and related to a variety of causes—fear, guilt, aversion to partner, and fatigue. Because of such fears and feelings, a male patient may react with anger and hostility to those caring for him, or he may turn his anger inward, resulting in more than the usual amount of pain. Patients with urinary infections may become depressed when they undergo prolonged periods of treatment. Anxiety in any stressful situation can produce urinary frequency and urgency.

Patients with urologic disorders, like any other patients, need to be respected as individuals and understood. They want their questions answered, fears allayed, and discomfort relieved. Additionally, their modesty and privacy need to be maintained. They require reassurance, support, and acceptance from the nurse.

Fluid and Electrolyte Imbalance

A major problem for patients with renal disorders is fluid and electrolyte imbalance. The nurse must be skilled in observing and documenting the clinical condition of the patient. The patient with a urologic disorder has a fluid intake–output chart for recording all fluid intake, whether by ingestion or by parenteral administration. The volume of urine and other output and the patient's weight are monitored and recorded. These records are essential in determining the patient's fluid allowance.

The nurse is alert to manifestations of body fluid disturbances (see Chap. 18). For example, the following signs and symptoms may occur in patients with renal disease:

1. Acute weight gain (in excess of 5%), edema, moist crackles in lungs, puffy eyelids, and shortness of breath—could indicate fluid volume excess.
2. Acute weight loss (in excess of 5%), a drop in body temperature, dryness of skin and mucous membranes, longitudinal wrinkles or furrows of tongue, and oliguria or anuria—could indicate fluid volume deficit.
3. Abdominal cramps, apprehension, convulsions, fingerprinting on sternum, and oliguria or anuria—could indicate sodium deficit.
4. Dry, sticky mucous membranes, flushed skin, oliguria or anuria, thirst, and rough and dry tongue—could indicate sodium excess.
5. Anorexia, abdominal distention, silent intestinal ileus, weakness, and soft, flabby muscles—could indicate potassium deficit.
6. Diarrhea, intestinal colic, irritability, and nausea—could indicate potassium excess.
7. Abdominal cramps, carpopedal spasm, muscle cramps, tetany, and tingling of ends of fingers—could indicate calcium deficit.
8. Deep bone pain, flank pain, and muscle hypotonicity—could indicate calcium excess.
9. Deep, rapid breathing (Kussmaul), shortness of breath on exertion, stupor, and weakness—could indicate primary base bicarbonate deficit.
10. Depressed respiration, muscle hypertonicity, and tetany—could indicate primary base bicarbonate excess.
11. Chronic weight loss, emotional depression, pallor, fatigue, and soft, flabby muscles—could indicate protein deficit.
12. Positive Chvostek's sign, convulsions, disorientation, hyperactive deep reflexes, and tremor—could indicate magnesium deficit.

The nurse needs a thorough understanding of the patient's gains and losses of body fluids, and she shares this information with other members of the health care team. When administering and monitoring intravenous therapy, the nurse adjusts the flow rate in accordance with the physician's prescription and the patient's fluid requirements. Repeated blood samples are obtained for evaluation of electrolyte balance. The nurse

explains the purpose of the studies and prepares the patient for venipuncture.

Maintaining Adequate Urinary Drainage

For the patient with urologic disease, as for any other person, urinary excretion of waste materials is necessary for life. The composition of the body fluids is determined not so much by what the patient ingests as by what the kidneys retain. In health, the kidneys are very efficient, excreting the substances that are not needed and retaining those that are. In the patient with a urologic disorder or one with marginal kidney function, care must be taken to assure adequacy of urinary drainage and preservation of kidney function.

When artificial drainage of the urinary system becomes necessary, catheters may be inserted directly into the bladder, the ureter, or the kidney pelvis. Catheters are available in various sizes, shapes, and lengths and may have one or more openings placed in various positions near the tip. A catheter may be constructed of hard or soft rubber, woven fabric, silicone, metal, glass, or plastic. The tip may be open or closed and have a mushroom shape, such as the Pezzer catheter; have a winged shape, such as the Malecot catheter; or simply be round and blunt. The type of catheter chosen depends on its purpose.

Catheterization

Principles of Management

There are times when insertion of a catheter is lifesaving, as is the case when the urinary tract is obstructed or the patient is unable to void. At other times, catheterization may be necessary to determine the amount of residual urine in the bladder after the patient has voided, to bypass an obstruction that blocks the flow of urine, to provide postoperative drainage following bladder, vaginal, or prostate surgery, or to provide a means to monitor hourly urinary output in critically ill patients.

- A patient should be catheterized only if absolutely necessary because catheterization commonly leads to urinary tract infection.

Urinary tract infections are responsible for over a third of all hospital-acquired infections. Most of these (at least 80%) follow instrumentation of the urinary tract, usually catheterization. The pathogens responsible for catheter-associated urinary tract infections include *Escherichia coli*, *Klebsiella*, *Proteus*, *Pseudomonas*, *Enterobacter*, *Serratia*, and *Candida*. Many of these are part of the patient's endogenous bowel flora or are acquired through cross-contamination by patients or hospital personnel or through exposure to nonsterile equipment.

Catheters impede most of the natural defenses of the lower urinary tract by obstructing the periurethral ducts, irritating the bladder mucosa, and providing an artificial route of entry for organisms to enter the bladder. When catheters are used, microorganisms may gain access to the urinary tract by three main pathways: (1) by introduction from the urethra into the bladder at the time of catheterization; (2) from the thin film of urethral fluid outside of the catheter at the catheter–mucosa interface; and (3) by migration to the bladder along the internal lumen of the catheter after contamination (most common).

To safeguard the patient, the following points of care are essential in urethral catheter management:

- Strict surgical asepsis is employed.
- The urethra is adequately cleansed.
- The catheter should be smaller than the external urinary meatus to minimize trauma and allow secretions to drain out alongside the catheter.
- The catheter is well lubricated with an appropriate antimicrobial lubricant.
- The catheter is inserted gently and skillfully.
- The catheter is removed as soon as possible.

Figure 42-1 summarizes the sequence of events that often follows long-term use of an indwelling urinary catheter in the elderly patient leading to infection and leakage of urine.

Nursing Care of the Patient With an Indwelling Catheter and a Closed Urinary Drainage System. When an indwelling catheter is necessary, a closed drainage system—one designed to minimize or prevent disconnection of the tubing and risk of contamination—is essential. Such a system may consist of an indwelling catheter, a connecting tube, and a collecting bag emptied by a drainage valve; it may consist of a triple-lumen indwelling urethral catheter attached to a closed sterile drainage system. The three-way catheter allows urinary drainage through one channel, inflation of the retention balloon with water or air through the second channel, and continuous irrigation of the bladder with antibacterial solution through the third channel.

▶ ## Nursing Process

The Patient With an Indwelling Catheter and a Closed Urinary Drainage System

▷ ### Assessment

The patient with an indwelling catheter is observed for signs and symptoms of urinary tract infection: cloudy urine, hematuria, fever, chills, anorexia, and malaise. The area around the urethral orifice is observed for drainage and excoriation. Urine cultures provide the most accurate means for assessment of infection. The color, odor, and volume of urine are also monitored.

Nursing assessment includes observation of the drainage system to ensure that the system provides adequate drainage of urine. The catheter itself is observed to make sure that it is properly anchored to prevent pressure on the urethra at the penoscrotal junction in the male patient, and tension and traction on the bladder in both male and female patients. An accurate record of the patient's fluid intake and urine output provides additional information about the adequacy of renal function and urinary drainage.

Additionally, patients at risk for urinary tract infection from catheterization are identified; these include persons who are elderly, debilitated, chronically ill, immunosuppressed, or diabetic. The patient's understanding of the purpose of catheterization is also assessed. Because of the increased risk of

infection and subsequent septicemia, assessment for signs and symptoms of bacteriuria, infection, and sepsis is essential.

The elderly patient who has an indwelling urinary catheter for management of incontinence may not exhibit the usual or typical signs and symptoms of infection. Therefore, any subtle change in the patient's physical condition or mental status must be considered a possible indication of infection.

▷ ### Nursing Diagnoses

Based on the assessment data, the patient's major nursing diagnoses may include the following:

- High risk for infection of the urinary tract related to contamination of the urinary tract
- High risk for impaired tissue integrity (urethra and bladder) related to catheterization

▷ *Goals:* The major goals for the patient may include absence of urinary tract infection and absence of trauma to the urethra and bladder.

▷ ### Nursing Interventions

▷ *Infection Control.* Certain principles of care are essential when managing a closed urinary drainage system.

- Strict asepsis is necessary during insertion of the catheter.
- A preassembled and sterile closed urinary drainage system is necessary and should not be disconnected before, during, or after insertion of the catheter.
- To prevent contamination of a closed system, the tubing is *never* disconnected. No part of the collection bag or drainage tube should ever be contaminated.
- The bag is never raised above the level of the patient's bladder because this will cause flow of contaminated urine by gravity into the patient's bladder from the bag.
- Urine should not be allowed to collect in the tubing because a free flow of urine must be maintained to prevent infection. Improper drainage occurs when the tubing is kinked or twisted, allowing pools of urine to collect in the loops of the tubing.
- The drainage bag must not touch the floor. The bag and collecting tubing are changed if contamination occurs, if the urine flow becomes obstructed, or if the tubing junctions start to leak at the connections.
- The bag is emptied at least every 8 hours through the drainage valve, and more frequently if there is a large volume of urine, to lessen the risk of bacterial proliferation.
- Care is taken to see that the drainage tube (valve/spout) is not contaminated. A receptacle in which to empty the bag is provided for each patient.
- Irrigation of the catheter is *not* carried out routinely.
- The catheter is *never* disconnected from the tubing to obtain urine samples, irrigate the catheter, or ambulate or transport the patient.
- Inadvertent handling or manipulation of the catheter by the patient or staff is avoided.
- Hand washing is *mandatory* before and after handling of the catheter, tubing, and drainage bag.

The catheter is a foreign body in the urethra and produces a reaction in the urethral mucosa with some urethral discharge. However, meatal care during catheterization is discouraged,

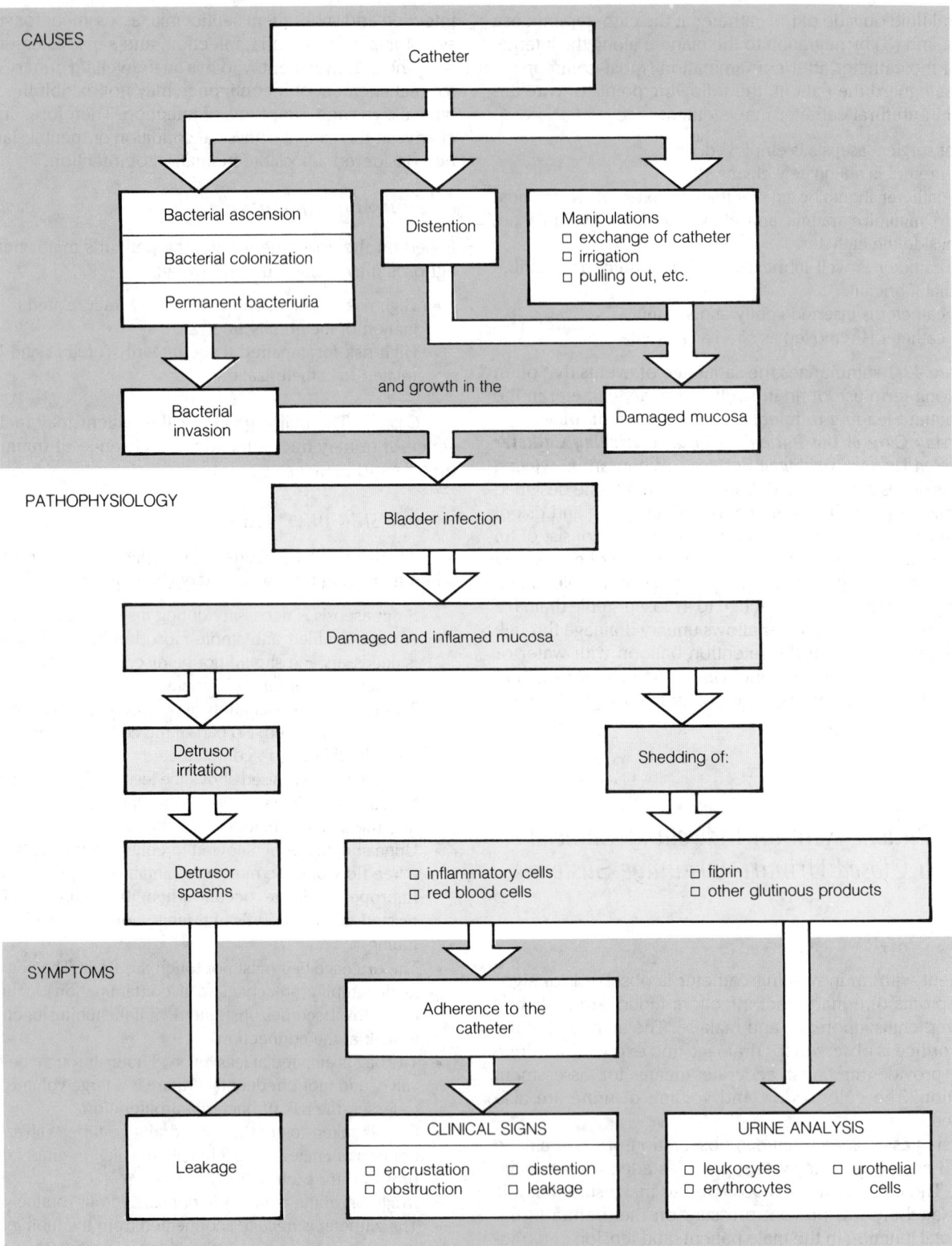

Figure 42–1. Pathophysiology and symptoms of bladder infection in long-term catheterized elderly. (Redrawn from Seiler WO and Stahelin HB. Practical management of catheter-associated UTIs. Geriatrics 1988 Aug; 43[8]: 44.)

because catheter manipulation, including that involved in cleansing, results in increased rates of infection. Gentle washing with soap during the daily bath is warranted to cleanse and to remove obvious encrustations from the external catheter surface. The catheter is anchored as securely as possible to prevent to-and-fro movement in the urethra. Drainage and encrustation occur at the exit of any tube. Encrustation arising from urinary salts may serve as a nucleus for stone formation. There appears to be significantly less crust formation when silicone catheters are used.

A liberal fluid intake and an increased urine output must be assured to mechanically flush the catheter and to dilute urinary constituents that might form encrustations. (The intake must be within limits of the patient's cardiac reserve.) Keeping the urine acidic helps to prevent tube obstruction and encrustation of urinary sand and calculus deposits. Ascorbic acid or potassium acid phosphate may be prescribed to acidify the urine.

Measures must be taken to prevent cross-contamination because many urinary tract infections are due to extrinsically acquired organisms transmitted by cross-contamination. Patients at risk are women, elderly debilitated patients, and those who are critically ill.

- There must be renewed emphasis on *hand washing* between patients and before and after handling any part of the catheter or drainage system.
- Patients with indwelling urinary catheters should not be in the same room with other catheterized patients or those who are severely disabled. Only one patient with an indwelling catheter should be assigned to a room to minimize the risk of cross-contamination.

Urine cultures are obtained as prescribed or indicated in monitoring for infection; many catheters have an aspiration (puncture) port from which a specimen can be obtained. With an indwelling urinary catheter in place, bacterial colonization (bacteriuria) will occur within 2 weeks in half the patients and in almost all patients within 4 to 6 weeks of catheter insertion, even if recommendations for infection control and catheter care are carefully followed. Controversy exists about the usefulness of culture and the treatment of bacteriuria in patients with indwelling catheters who are asymptomatic because bacteriuria is inevitable and overtreatment may lead to resistant strains of bacteria.

▷ *Minimizing Trauma.* A catheter of the appropriate size is used to minimize trauma to the urethra during its insertion. The catheter is lubricated adequately so that it can be inserted easily and gently. It is inserted far enough into the bladder to prevent trauma to the urethral tissues when the retention balloon of the catheter is inflated. Manipulation of the catheter is most often the cause of damage to the bladder mucosa in the catheterized patient. Infection then inevitably occurs when urine invades the damaged mucosa. The catheter is secured properly to prevent it from moving, causing traction on the urethra, or being accidentally removed. Care is taken to ensure that any patient who is confused does not accidentally remove the catheter with the retention balloon still inflated, because such an action would cause bleeding and considerable trauma to the urethra.

In the male patient, the catheter is taped laterally to the thigh or to the abdomen (Fig. 42-2) to prevent pressure on the

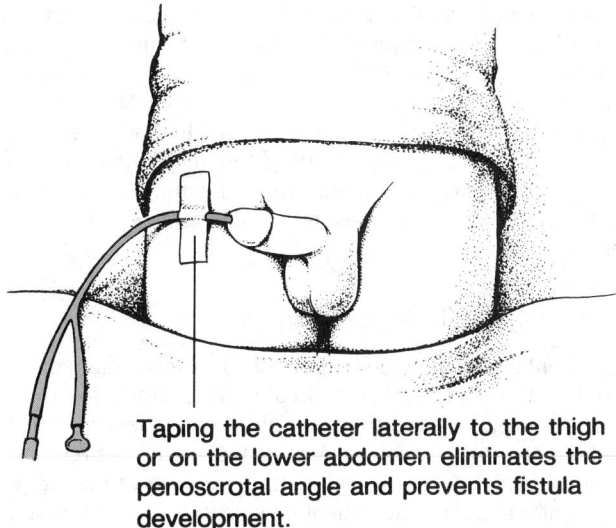

Taping the catheter laterally to the thigh or on the lower abdomen eliminates the penoscrotal angle and prevents fistula development.

Figure 42–2. For the male patient, the catheter is taped to the thigh or to the abdomen.

urethra at the penoscrotal junction, which can eventually lead to the formation of a urethrocutaneous fistula.

In the female patient, the drainage tubing attached to the catheter is taped to the thigh to prevent tension and traction on the bladder.

▷ Evaluation

Expected Outcomes

1. Free of urinary tract infection
   a. Excretes urine that is clear and yellow or amber, with a specific gravity of 1.015 to 1.025
   b. Has a urine culture negative for microorganisms
   c. Has a normal temperature
   d. Demonstrates adequate fluid intake and urine output
   e. Does not have excessive drainage or excoriation around the urethral orifice
   f. Maintains position of the drainage bag below the level of the bladder when in bed, sitting, or ambulating
2. Is free of trauma to urethra and bladder
   a. Reports absence of pain or discomfort in urethra or bladder
   b. Demonstrates no blood in urine or irritation of urethra
   c. Maintains proper anchoring of the catheter to prevent movement and accidental removal of the catheter
   d. Avoids kinking or twisting of the catheter or drainage tubing
   e. Is free of pain or discomfort on voiding following catheter removal
   f. Eliminates 200 to 400 ml of urine with each voiding following catheter removal
   g. Shows no signs of urinary incontinence

In summary, although indwelling urinary catheters are commonplace in health care settings, they must be considered and treated as potential sites of urinary tract infection and major factors in sepsis, morbidity, and mortality. Meticulous technique is essential in management of an indwelling urinary catheter to prevent contamination, bacteriuria, and urinary tract infection. The nurse caring for the elderly patient with an indwelling catheter must take into consideration the nonspecific and often atypical signs and symptoms of urinary tract infection that occur in the elderly. Careful assessment is essential to detect the subtle signs and symptoms of urinary tract infection in the elderly patient and the indicators of sepsis and septic shock in this population in order to reduce the morbidity and mortality resulting from the use of urinary catheters. Instructions to the patient, family, and other care providers may reduce the incidence of complications of this mode of management. When possible, alternatives to this mode of treatment must be considered.

Intermittent Self-Catheterization

Intermittent self-catheterization provides periodic drainage of urine from the bladder. It is the treatment of choice following spinal cord injury and other neurologic disorders in which bladder emptying is impaired. Aseptic techniques are required during the patient's in-hospital training because of the risk of cross-contamination. The patient may use a "clean" (nonsterile) technique at home, where the risk of cross-contamination is reduced. Self-catheterization promotes independence, results in few complications, and permits more normal sexual relations. The objectives are to decrease the morbidity associated with the long-term use of an indwelling catheter and to achieve catheter-free status if possible.

Teaching emphasizes the importance of frequent catheterization and the emptying of the bladder at the prescribed time irrespective of the circumstances. (If the bladder becomes overdistended, blood flow through the bladder wall is decreased and the risk of infection is increased.)

The female patient requires a mirror to help locate the urinary meatus. She is taught to catheterize herself by inserting a catheter 7.5 cm (3 in) into the urethra in a downward and backward direction. The male patient is taught to lubricate the catheter and retract the foreskin of the penis with one hand while grasping the penis and holding it at a right angle to the body. (This maneuver straightens the urethra and makes it easier to insert the catheter.) The catheter is inserted 15 to 25 cm (6 to 10 in) until the urine begins to flow. After the catheter is removed, it is washed in soapy water, rinsed, and wrapped in a paper towel, plastic bag, or case. A patient following this routine should be seen by a urologist at regular intervals for assessment of urinary function and the occurrence of complications.

If the patient is unable to perform intermittent self-catheterization, frequently a family member is taught to carry out the procedure at regular intervals during the day.

Suprapubic Bladder Drainage

Suprapubic bladder aspiration is a method of establishing drainage from the bladder by inserting a catheter or tube into the bladder through a suprapubic ("above the pubis") incision or puncture. It is used as a temporary measure to divert the flow of urine from the urethra when the urethral route is impassable (because of injuries, strictures, prostatic obstruction), after gynecologic operations when bladder dysfunction is likely to occur (vaginal hysterectomy, vaginal repair surgery), and after pelvic fractures.

To facilitate insertion of the suprapubic catheter, the patient is placed in a supine position and the bladder is distended by administration of oral or intravenous fluids or by instillation of sterile saline into the bladder via a urethral catheter. These measures make it easier to locate the bladder.

The suprapubic area is surgically prepared and the puncture site located approximately 5 cm above the symphysis pubis. The bladder may be entered through an incision in the bladder or through a puncture made by a small trocar. The catheter or suprapubic drainage tube is threaded into the bladder and secured with sutures or tape (Fig. 42-3). The area around the catheter is covered with a sterile dressing. The catheter is connected to a sterile closed drainage system, and the tubing is secured to prevent tension on the catheter.

Suprapubic bladder drainage may be maintained continuously for several weeks. If the patient's ability to void is to be tested, the catheter is clamped for 4 hours, during which time the patient attempts to void. After the patient voids, the catheter is unclamped and the residual urine is measured. Usually, if the amount of residual urine is less than 100 ml on two separate occasions (morning and evening), the catheter is removed. However, if the patient complains of pain or discomfort, the suprapubic catheter is usually left in place until he is able to void successfully.

Patients with suprapubic drainage are usually able to void sooner after surgery than those with urethral catheters. Suprapubic drainage may be more comfortable than an indwelling catheter. It also provides greater patient mobility, allows measurement of residual volume without urethral instrumentation, and presents less of a risk for bladder infection. The suprapubic catheter is removed when it is no longer necessary, and a sterile dressing is placed over the site.

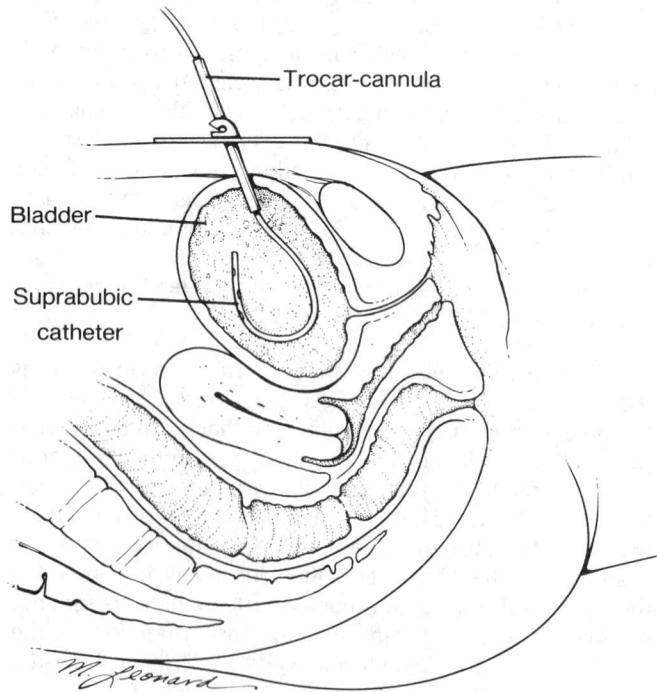

Figure 42-3. Suprapubic bladder drainage. A trocar-cannula is used to puncture the abdominal and bladder walls. The catheter is threaded through the trocar cannula, which is then removed, leaving the catheter in place. The catheter is secured by tape or sutures to prevent accidental removal.

Alterations in Voiding Patterns

Urinary Retention

Urinary retention (both acute and chronic) refers to the inability to urinate despite the patient's urge or desire to do so. Chronic retention will often lead to overflow incontinence (due to pressure of retained urine in the bladder) or residual urine. *Residual urine* refers to urine that remains in the bladder after voiding.

Retention may occur in any postoperative patient, particularly in those who have undergone surgery on the perineal or anal regions that resulted in reflex spasm of the sphincters. It may also occur in the acutely ill, the elderly, or the bedridden. Urinary retention may be due to anxiety, prostatic enlargement, urethral pathology (infection, tumor, calculus), trauma, neurogenic bladder dysfunction, and other conditions. Some medications cause urinary retention, including anticholinergics–antispasmodics, such as atropine; antidepressant–antipsychotic agents, such as phenothiazine; antihistamine preparations, such as pseudoephedrine hydrochloride (Sudafed); β-adrenergic blockers, such as propranolol; and antihypertensive agents, such as hydralazine.

Urinary retention may lead to infection, which may develop as a result of overdistention of the bladder, compromised blood supply to the bladder wall, and proliferation of bacteria. Impaired renal function may also occur, particularly if obstruction of the urinary tract is present.

Management. Measures are instituted to prevent overdistention of the bladder and to treat infection or obstruction. Many problems, however, can be prevented by careful nursing assessment and appropriate nursing interventions.

▶ ## Nursing Process
The Patient With Urinary Retention

▷ ### Assessment

The signs and symptoms of urinary retention may easily be overlooked unless the nurse consciously assesses for them.

- What are the time and volume of the last voiding?
- Is the patient passing small amounts of urine frequently?
- Is the patient dribbling?
- Is the patient complaining of pain or discomfort in the lower abdomen? (Discomfort may be relatively mild if the bladder distends slowly.)
- Is there a rounded swelling arising out of the pelvis (could indicate retention)?
- Is there dullness on percussion in the suprapubic region (may indicate a full bladder)?
- Are there other indicators of urinary retention, such as restlessness and agitation.?

▷ ### Nursing Diagnoses

Based on the assessment data, nursing diagnoses for the patient may include the following:

- Urinary retention related to pain, tension, lack of privacy, or unfamiliar surroundings and position for voiding
- Pain and discomfort related to bladder distention

▷ *Goals:* The patient's major goals may be return of normal voiding patterns and relief of discomfort.

▷ ### Nursing Interventions

▷ *Promoting Urinary Elimination.* Nursing measures to encourage voiding include providing privacy, assisting the patient to the bathroom or commode in order to provide a more natural setting for voiding, or allowing the male patient to stand beside the bed while using the urinal (because most men find this position more comfortable and natural for urination). Additional measures include providing warmth to relax the sphincters (*i.e.,* sitz baths, warm compresses to the perineum, showers), giving the patient hot tea to drink, and offering psychologic reassurance and support.

Following surgical procedures, the prescribed analgesic should be administered because pain in the incisional area can make voiding difficult. When the patient cannot void, careful catheterization is used to prevent overdistention of the bladder. In the case of prostatic obstruction, attempts at catheterization (by the urologist) may not be successful, requiring that a suprapubic catheter be inserted.

▷ *Relief of Pain and Discomfort.* Relief of urinary retention generally brings relief of abdominal distention, pain, and discomfort. Treatment of the cause (*i.e.,* obstruction) usually relieves the patient's fear that the problem will recur.

▷ ### Evaluation

Expected Outcomes
1. Demonstrates normal voiding patterns
   a. Voids 300 to 400 ml of urine every 3 hours
   b. Exhibits no abdominal distention
   c. Is free of sensation of bladder fullness
2. Experiences relief of pain and discomfort
   a. Reports no abdominal or bladder pain and discomfort
   b. Uses appropriate measures to prevent recurrence of urinary retention and bladder discomfort

Urinary Incontinence

Urinary incontinence is the involuntary or uncontrolled loss of urine from the bladder. If urinary incontinence results from an inflammatory condition (cystitis), it will probably be temporary in nature. However, if it results from a serious neurologic condition (paraplegia), it is likely to be a permanent problem.

Over 10 million adults in the United States suffer from urinary incontinence. It affects persons from all age groups but is particularly common in the elderly. It has been reported that over half of all nursing home residents have urinary incontinence. Although urinary incontinence is *not* a normal consequence of aging, age-related changes in the urinary tract predispose the older person to incontinence. Age, gender, and number of previous deliveries are established risk factors and explain, in part, the increased incidence in women. Other suggested risk factors include urinary tract infection, menopause, genitourinary surgery, chronic illness, and various medications.

Rashes, pressure ulcers, skin and urinary tract infections, and restrictions of activity are consequences of urinary incontinence. The costs of care for patients with urinary incontinence are estimated to be over $10.3 billion annually. The psychosocial costs of urinary incontinence are enormous; embarrassment, loss of self-esteem, and social isolation are common outcomes. Urinary incontinence in the elderly often leads to their institutionalization.

Stress incontinence is the involuntary loss of urine through an intact urethra as a result of a sudden increase in intraabdominal pressure. It is seen mostly in women and is often due to obstetric injury, lesions of the bladder neck, extrinsic pelvic disease, fistulas, detrusor dysfunction, and a variety of other conditions. In addition, it may result from congenital conditions (extrophy of the bladder, ectopic ureter).

Urge incontinence occurs when the patient senses the urge to void but is unable to inhibit voiding long enough to reach the toilet. In many cases, uninhibited contraction of the bladder is also a concomitant factor; this may occur in the patient with neurologic dysfunction that impairs inhibition of bladder contraction, or in the patient with local symptoms of irritation due to urinary tract infection or bladder tumors.

Overflow incontinence is characterized by frequent, sometimes almost constant, loss of urine from the bladder. The bladder cannot empty normally and becomes overdistended. Despite frequent urine loss, the bladder never empties. It may be caused by neurologic abnormalities (*i.e.,* spinal cord lesions) or by factors that obstruct the outflow of urine (*i.e.,* medications, tumors, strictures, and prostatic hyperplasia). Neurogenic bladder is discussed separately in the next section.

Functional incontinence refers to those instances in which the function of the lower urinary tract is intact but other factors, such as severe cognitive impairment, make it difficult for the patient to identify the need to void (*i.e.,* Alzheimer's dementia) or physical impairments make it difficult or impossible for the patient to reach the toilet in time for voiding.

Mixed forms of urinary incontinence, which include characteristics of those just described, may also occur. Additionally, urinary incontinence can be a result of the interaction of many factors. Only with appropriate recognition of the problem, assessment, and referral for diagnostic evaluation and treatment can the outcome of incontinence be determined. *All* persons with incontinence should be considered for evaluation and treatment.

Treatment for urinary incontinence depends on the underlying causative factors. However, before appropriate treatment can be initiated, the presence of the problem must be identified and the possibility of successful treatment recognized. If nurses and other health care workers accept incontinence as an inevitable part of aging and illness or consider it irreversible and untreatable at any age, it cannot be successfully treated. Collaborative, multidisciplinary efforts are often essential in the assessment and effective treatment of urinary incontinence.

Successful management depends on the nature of urinary incontinence and on the causative factors. Urinary incontinence may be transient or reversible; once the underlying cause is successfully treated, the patient's voiding pattern reverts to normal. Those causes that are reversible and often transient can be recalled by the acronym *DIAPPERS.* These causes include the following: *d*elirium, *i*nfection of the urinary tract, *a*trophic vaginitis or urethritis, *p*harmacologic agents (anticholinergics, sedatives, alcohol, analgesics, diuretics, muscle relaxants, adrenergic agents), *p*sychologic factors (depression, regression), *e*ndocrine disorders, *r*estricted activity, *r*etention of urine, and *s*tool impaction. Once these are successfully treated, the patient's voiding pattern often reverts to normal.

Once the presence of incontinence is recognized, a thorough history is necessary. This will include a detailed description of the problem and a history of medication use. Voiding history, voiding log or diary, and bedside tests (*i.e.,* postvoiding residual urine volume, stress maneuvers) may be used to aid in determining the type of urinary incontinence. A more extensive urodynamic diagnostic evaluation may be performed.

Depending on the results of the evaluation, nursing management and/or medical management may be indicated. Nursing measures that are often effective may be simple measures that include assuring an environment that promotes toileting; placing the call light, bedpan or urinal within easy reach; leaving a light on in the patient's darkened room; and helping the patient to select clothing that facilitates quick dressing and undressing to use the toilet. Other measures the nurse may use to treat urinary incontinence include instructing and encouraging the patient in the use of pelvic floor (Kegel) exercises, initiation of a program of prompted voiding or habit retraining, and increasing the patient's fluid intake to prevent constipation and stool impaction, which are frequent factors in urinary incontinence in the sedentary patient. Bladder training (discussed on p. 241), which may involve the use of biofeedback or behavioral strategies, has also been reported to be successful.

Surgical correction may be indicated for stress incontinence. There is a wide range of surgical procedures: vaginal repair, abdominal suspension of the bladder, and elevation of the bladder neck. A modified artificial sphincter that uses a silicone-rubber balloon as a self-regulating pressure mechanism is being used to close the urethra. Another method of controlling stress incontinence is the application of electronic stimulation to the pelvic floor by means of a miniature pulse generator with electrodes mounted on an intra-anal plug.

For other types of incontinence, those nursing measures described above are often more appropriate.

Neurogenic Bladder

Neurogenic bladder refers to a bladder disturbance that results from a lesion of the nervous system. It may be caused by spinal cord injury or tumor, certain neurologic diseases (multiple sclerosis), congenital anomalies (spina bifida, myelomeningocele), infection, and certain systemic disorders (diabetes mellitus). There are two types of neurogenic bladders: (1) *spastic* or *hypertonic* bladder, characterized by automatic, reflex, or uncontrolled expulsion of urine from the bladder with incomplete emptying, and (2) *flaccid* bladder, with loss of sensation of bladder fullness and thus overfilling and distention of the bladder.

The major complication of neurogenic bladder is infection that results from stasis of urine and subsequent catheterization. Hypertrophy of the bladder walls also results, ultimately leading to *vesicoureteral reflux* (backing up of urine from the bladder to the ureters) and *hydronephrosis* (dilation of the internal structures of the kidney by increased pressure of the backed-up urine). *Urolithiasis* (stones in the urinary tract) may develop from urinary stasis and infection and from demineralization of bone due to prolonged bed rest. Renal failure is the major cause of death of patients with neurologic impairment of the bladder.

Nursing Interventions

The care of the patient with neurogenic bladder is a major challenge to the health care team. There are several long-term objectives appropriate for all types of neurogenic bladders: (1) to prevent overdistention of the bladder, (2) to empty the bladder regularly and completely, (3) to maintain urine sterility with no stone formation, and (4) to maintain adequate bladder capacity without vesicoureteral reflux.

The immediate management of the patient with a neurogenic bladder consists of catheterizing the patient intermittently or inserting a three-way catheter with closed drainage to avoid overdistention. In intermittent catheterization, the bladder is catheterized at designated intervals (4, 6, or 8 hours) with a small-diameter catheter. This intermittent emptying approximates physiologic bladder function and avoids complications usually encountered with an indwelling catheter. An hourly fluid intake and output record is maintained to assess the patient's voiding patterns.

If continuous catheterization and drainage are used in a male patient, the catheter is taped laterally to the thigh or to the abdomen to avoid the sharp angulation of the catheter and prevent pressure at the penoscrotal angle (see Fig. 42-2).

With the use of either intermittent or continuous catheterization, a liberal fluid intake is encouraged to reduce the urinary bacterial count, reduce stasis, decrease the concentration of calcium in the urine, and minimize the precipitation of urinary crystals and subsequent stone formation. The patient is kept as mobile as possible, through early ambulation if feasible, or through use of a wheelchair or tilt table. A diet low in calcium is recommended to prevent calculi.

The problems of patients with neurogenic bladder disease vary considerably from patient to patient. It may be difficult initially to assess what the long-term rehabilitation potential and eventual urologic disability may be.

Diagnostic Evaluation

As soon as the patient's condition permits, evaluation studies are performed to assess for bladder and bladder neck problems. The initial studies provide a baseline against which later changes can be measured. Serial studies of BUN, creatinine clearance, and serum creatinine are performed to determine the status of renal function. A cystogram determines the presence of vesicoureteral reflux. A urethrogram may be performed to detect the presence of urethral complications. Pressure and flow studies and an IV urogram are also performed. A cystoscopic examination may be performed to assess loss of muscle fibers and elastic tissues and to provide an opportunity for biopsy if necessary.

Spastic Bladder

The spastic (reflex, automatic, or hypertonic) bladder disorder is caused by any lesion of the cord above the voiding reflex arc (upper motor neuron lesion). The result is a loss of conscious sensation and cerebral motor control. There is reduced bladder capacity and marked hypertrophy of the bladder wall. As a result, the bladder empties on reflex, with minimal or no controlling influence to regulate its activity.

The objective of the bladder program is to develop effective spontaneous reflex voiding, which is accomplished in the following manner:

- The patient drinks a measured amount of fluid from 8 AM to 10 PM; no fluids (except sips) are taken after 10 PM to avoid bladder overdistention.
- At a specific time(s), the patient attempts to void by applying pressure over the bladder, by tapping the abdomen, or by stretching the anal sphincter with a finger to trigger the bladder.
- Immediately following the voiding attempt, the patient is catheterized to determine the amount of residual urine.
- The volumes of urine voided and catheterized are measured.
- The bladder is palpated at repeated intervals to determine whether distention of the bladder occurs.
- The patient without usual sensation is instructed to be alert for any signs that indicate a full bladder, such as perspiration, coldness of hands or feet, and feelings of anxiety.
- The intervals between catheterizations are lengthened and the patient's program progresses as the volume of residual urine decreases. Catheterization is usually discontinued when the volume of residual urine is at an acceptable level.

Flaccid Bladder

The flaccid (atonic, nonreflex, or autonomous) neurogenic bladder is caused by a lower motor neuron lesion, most commonly due to trauma. This form of neurogenic bladder has increasingly been recognized as a problem in patients with diabetes mellitus. The bladder continues to fill and becomes greatly distended. The bladder muscle does not contract forcefully at any time. Sensory loss may accompany a flaccid bladder, so the patient feels no discomfort. Overdistention causes damage to the bladder musculature, infection due to stagnant urine, and damage to the kidneys as a result of pressure from the urine.

A patient with a flaccid bladder may be placed on the type of bladder routine outlined above under Spastic Bladder. A 2-hour voiding schedule is established to prevent overdistention. Parasympathomimetic drugs (bethanechol [Urecholine]) may help to increase the contraction of the detrusor muscle. This approach may be very effective, especially for a hypotonic bladder in which there is no significant obstruction of the bladder outlet.

Patients can also be taught to perform self-catheterization at intervals until spontaneous complete emptying of the bladder is achieved. Although intermittent catheterization may have to be carried out for a prolonged period of time, it is a safe and successful method of managing patients who have neurogenic bladders.

Sometimes it is not possible for the patient to achieve reflex bladder control or self-catheterization. The male patient then may use an external (condom catheter) collecting device if the bladder empties well and no residual urine remains. The female patient may need to wear pads or waterproof pants. However, these strategies should be resorted to only after thorough evaluation and attempts at other modes of management. Surgical intervention may be carried out to correct bladder neck contractures or vesicoureteral reflux or to perform some type of urinary diversion procedure (see Chap. 43).

In summary, urinary incontinence is a problem that is expected to increase in incidence as the population ages. A key to the management of urinary incontinence is the recognition that many causes of incontinence are transient and reversible. In many cases, recognition that incontinence exists is a major step in assessment and treatment. In order for appropriate treatment to be initiated, nurses and other health care workers must consider urinary incontinence to be treatable and reversible rather than an inevitable part of illness and aging. Collaborative, multidisciplinary efforts are essential in the assessment and effective treatment of urinary incontinence. Many strategies directed toward urinary incontinence are medically directed; however, even more strategies are under the direction of the nurse, who must be sensitive to the problem and committed to effective treatment of this problem.

Dialysis

Dialysis is a process used to remove fluid and waste products from the body when the kidneys are unable to do so because of impaired function or when toxins or poisons must be removed immediately to prevent permanent or life-threatening damage. In dialysis, solute molecules diffuse through a semipermeable membrane, passing from the side of higher concentration to that of lower concentration. Fluids pass through the semipermeable membrane by means of osmosis or ultrafiltration (application of external pressure to the membrane).

The purposes of dialysis are to maintain the life and well-being of the patient until kidney function is restored and to remove unwanted substances from the blood if renal function does not return. Methods of therapy include *hemodialysis*, *hemofiltration*, and *peritoneal dialysis*.

Dialysis is used in renal failure to remove toxic substances and body wastes normally excreted by healthy kidneys and in the management of patients with intractable (not responsive to treatment) edema, hepatic coma, hyperkalemia, hypercalcemia, hypertension, and uremia. The main indications for *acute dialysis* are a high and rising level of serum potassium, fluid overload or impending pulmonary edema, increasing acidosis, pericarditis, and severe confusion. It may also be used to remove certain drugs or other toxins (poisoning or drug overdose).

The indications for initiating *chronic or maintenance dialysis* in chronic renal failure (end-stage renal disease) include the occurrence of uremic signs and symptoms: nausea and vomiting, severe anorexia, increasing lethargy, mental confusion, elevated serum potassium level, fluid overload not responsive to diuretics and fluid restriction, and a general lack of well-being. In addition, the occurrence of a pericardial friction rub is an urgent indication for dialysis in the patient with chronic renal failure. The decision to initiate dialysis is one that should be reached after thoughtful discussion between the patient, family, and physician. The nurse can assist the patient and family by answering their questions, clarifying information, and supporting their decision.

Hemodialysis

It is estimated that more than 100,000 patients currently receive hemodialysis. Hemodialysis is a process used for patients who are acutely ill and require short-term dialysis (days to weeks) or for patients with end-stage renal disease (ESRD) who require long-term therapy. A synthetic, semipermeable membrane replaces the renal glomeruli and tubules and acts as the filter for the impaired kidneys.

For patients with chronic renal failure, hemodialysis provides reasonable rehabilitation and life expectancy. However, hemodialysis does not cure or reverse renal disease and is not able to compensate for losses of the kidneys' endocrine or metabolic activities. These patients must undergo dialysis treatment for the rest of their lives (usually three times a week for at least 3 to 4 hours per treatment) or until they receive a successful kidney transplant. Patients are placed on chronic dialysis when they require dialysis therapy for survival and for control of uremic symptoms.

The requirements for hemodialysis for a patient with end-stage renal failure are: (1) access to the patient's circulation, (2) a dialyzer with a semipermeable membrane (the artificial kidney), and (3) an appropriate dialysate bath.

Access to the Patient's Circulation

Access to the patient's circulation for long-term hemodialysis is achieved through subclavian catheterization or a more permanent vascular access. A double-lumen or multi-lumen catheter is inserted into a subclavian vein. Although this method of vascular access is not without risks (*i.e.*, vascular injury such as hematoma, pneumothorax, infection, thrombosis of the subclavian vein, and inadequate flow), it can often be used for several weeks.

Fistula.   The fistula is created surgically by connecting or joining (anastomosis) an artery to a vein, either side to side or end to side. The fistula takes 4 to 6 weeks to "mature" before it is ready for use. This gives time for healing to take place and for the venous segment of the fistula to dilate in order to accommodate two large-bore (14- or 16-gauge) needles. The needles are inserted into the vessel to obtain blood flow adequate to pass through the dialyzer. The arterial segment of the fistula is used for arterial flow and the venous segment for retransfusion of the dialyzed blood.

Graft.   A graft is created by suturing a piece of bovine artery or vein, Gore-Tex material (heterograft), or saphenous vein graft into the patient's own vessel. This is carried out to provide an available segment in which to place the needles for dialysis. Usually, the graft is created when the patient's own vessels are not suitable to be used for a fistula. Grafts are usually placed in the forearm, upper arm, or upper thigh. Patients with compromised vascular systems, such as those with diabetes, often need to have a graft in order to have hemodialysis.

Other Means of Access.   Catheters inserted into the femoral blood vessels may be used for patients who require emergency hemodialysis but have no vascular access available (fistula, graft). A Scribner shunt (AV or arteriovenous shunt) may be created for short-term use for hemodialysis. With the shunt, tubing is anchored in an artery and an adjacent vein; between treatments, the two sides of the tubing are joined together in an arc. When dialysis is performed, a connector between the arterial and venous tubing is removed and the tubing is connected to the dialysis machine. The use of such shunts is uncommon today, but they have been used for hemofiltration (described on p. 1160).

Underlying Principles of Hemodialysis

The objectives of hemodialysis are to extract toxic nitrogenous substances from the blood and to remove excess water. The composition of the blood is altered by exposing the blood to a modified salt solution, or dialysate, separated from the blood by a semipermeable membrane. Heparin is added to the blood to prevent clotting. The blood passes, by means of a pump, to the semipermeable membrane, and the dialysate bath flows on the other side of the membrane. The toxins and wastes in the blood are removed by *diffusion,* moving from an area of greater concentration in the blood to an area of lesser concentration in the dialysate. The dialysate is composed of all the important electrolytes in their ideal extracellular concentrations. The electrolyte level in the blood can be brought under control by proper adjustment of the dialysate bath. (Small pores in the semipermeable membrane do not allow the loss of red blood cells and proteins.)

Excess water is removed from the blood by *osmosis.* The removal of water can be controlled by creating a desired pressure gradient (*ultrafiltration*). The body's buffer system is maintained by the addition of acetate, which diffuses from the dialysate to the patient's blood and metabolizes to form bicarbonate. Purified blood is returned to the body through the patient's vein. By the end of the dialysis treatment, many waste products have been removed, electrolyte and water balance has been restored, and the buffer system has been replenished.

During dialysis, the patient, the dialyzer, and the dialysate bath require constant monitoring to detect the numerous complications that can arise (*e.g.,* air embolism, inadequate or excessive ultrafiltration, blood leaks, contamination, and shunt or fistula complications). The nurse in the dialysis unit has an important role in monitoring and supporting the patient and in carrying out a continuing program of patient assessment and education.

There have been many continuing developments in dialyzers and technology for the treatment of end-stage renal disease, but most dialyzers conform to one of the following types: the coil dialyzer, the flat plate dialyzer, and the hollow fiber artificial kidney.

Management of the Patient on Long-Term Hemodialysis

An optimum dietary program is important for patients on hemodialysis because of the effects of uremia (wasting, poor dietary intake, the reduced palatability of the restricted diet, the loss of nutrients during dialysis, and any concurrent illnesses).

With the effective use of hemodialysis, the patient's dietary intake can be improved. However, the diet usually involves some adjustment or restriction of protein, sodium, potassium, or fluid intake. Protein intake must be of high biologic quality and of complete amino acid composition (eggs, meat, milk, fish) to prevent poor protein utilization and to maintain positive nitrogen balance and replace amino acids lost during dialysis. If many water-soluble nutrients and metabolites have been removed from the tissues as a result of the effects of dialysis, the patient may require additional vitamins and minerals. After dialysis procedures are initiated, the patient's clinical condition usually improves, and there is usually a diminished need for stringent dietary restrictions.

Many drugs are excreted wholly or in part by the kidneys. Patients requiring drug therapy (cardiac glycosides, antibiotics, antidysrhythmic agents, antihypertensive agents) are monitored closely to ensure that blood and tissue levels of these drugs are maintained without toxic accumulation. This type of information is kept in mind when the patient asks, "Is it all right to take this medicine for a headache?" It is also important to keep in mind that some medications are removed from the blood during dialysis, requiring adjustment of the dosage by the physician.

Complications

Although hemodialysis can prolong life indefinitely, it does not alter the natural course of the underlying kidney disease, nor does it completely replace kidney function or control uremic symptoms. The patient is subject to a number of problems and complications. The leading cause of death among patients undergoing chronic hemodialysis is arteriosclerotic cardiovascular disease. Disturbances of lipid metabolism (*hypertriglyceridemia*) appear to be accentuated by hemodialysis. Congestive heart failure, coronary heart disease and anginal pain, stroke, and peripheral vascular insufficiency may incapacitate the patient. Anemia and fatigue contribute to diminished physical and emotional well-being, lack of energy and drive, and loss of interest. Gastric ulcers and other gastrointestinal problems occur from the physiologic stress of chronic illness, medication, and related problems. Disturbed calcium metabolism leads to renal osteodystrophy that produces bone pain and fractures. Other problems include fluid overload associated with congestive heart failure, malnutrition, and disequilibrium syndrome from rapid fluid and electrolyte changes.

Patients with virtually no renal function have been maintained for a number of years by hemodialysis. For some, a successful kidney transplant would eliminate the need for chronic, long-term hemodialysis treatment. Despite these limitations of dialysis, many patients have been able to return to productive, satisfying lives. Pregnancy and delivery of healthy babies have even been reported in a few dialysis patients.

Although the costs of dialysis for all patients are now reimbursed by Medicare, limitations in work ability imposed by illness and dialysis result in concerns about finances for patients and their families.

Psychosocial Considerations

Persons undergoing long-term hemodialysis are concerned with very real problems. Generally, their medical status is unpredictable and their lives are disrupted; they often have financial problems, difficulty in holding a job, waning sexual desires and impotence, depression from living the life of a chronically ill person, and fear of dying. Younger persons worry about marriage, having children, and the burden that they bring to their families. A regimented life-style necessitated by the frequent dialysis treatments and restrictions in food and fluid intake is often demoralizing to the patient and family.

Dialysis imposes an altered life-style on the family. The amount of time required for dialysis decreases social activities and can create conflict, frustration, guilt, and depression in the family. Frequently, family and friends regard the patient as a "marginal person" with a limited life expectancy. It may be difficult for the patient, spouse, and family to express anger and negative feelings.

The nurse can support the family by letting them know that feelings of anger and distress are normal emotional reactions in this situation. It also helps to provide verbal and written instructions and to inform them of resources that are available for assistance and support. The family should be involved in treatment and decision making.

The patient should be given the opportunity to express any feelings of anger and concern over the limitations imposed by the disease and treatment, as well as possible financial problems, job insecurity, pain, and discomfort. If anger is not expressed, it may be directed inward and lead to depression, despair, and attempts at suicide; the incidence of suicide is increased in dialysis patients. If the anger is projected outward to other people, it may destroy an already threatened family relationship. The patient needs a close relationship with someone to turn to in times of stress and discouragement. Some patients will use denial to deal with the overwhelming array of medical problems (*e.g.*, infections, hypertension, anemia, neuropathy). The nurse can help by supporting the patient in coping with these ever-present problems and fears.

Home Hemodialysis

For selected patients, hemodialysis is carried out in the home. However, not all people are candidates because this procedure requires a highly motivated patient who is willing to take responsibility for the dialysis procedure and is able to adjust each treatment to meet the body's changing needs.

The patient with kidney failure and the family member who will serve as helper must undergo a training program to learn how to prepare, operate, and disassemble the dialysis machine; maintain and clean the equipment; administer medications (heparin) into the machine lines; and handle emergency problems (hemodialysis coil rupture, shock, convulsions). The home is surveyed to see if electrical outlets and plumbing facilities are adequate. The emphasis is on the patient's assuming primary responsibility for the treatment and a more normal life-style.

When financial assistance became available for long-term dialysis, most patients elected to have their dialysis performed in outpatient centers (satellite or limited-care dialysis centers) rather than in the home.

High-Flux Dialysis

High-flux dialysis is a new development in dialysis that increases the clearance of small- and middle-molecular-weight molecules and large volumes of fluid through high blood flow rates through the dialyzer, increased dialysate flow, and a high permeability membrane with a large surface area. This new development is expected to increase the efficiency of dialysis while shortening the duration of treatments. However, it is not suitable for all patients; those patients whose physical condition is unstable are unlikely to be candidates for high-flux dialysis because of the rapid removal of fluid.

Continuous Arteriovenous Hemofiltration

Hemofiltration or *continuous arteriovenous hemofiltration* (CAVH) is another system for temporarily replacing kidney function. It is used at the bedside in the intensive care unit for patients with fluid overload secondary to oliguric (low urinary output) renal failure or those patients whose kidneys are unable to handle their acute high metabolic or nutritional needs. The blood is circulated through a small-volume, low-resistance filter by the patient's own arterial pressure rather than that of the blood pump used in hemodialysis (Fig. 42-4). Blood flows from an artery (via an arteriovenous shunt or arterial catheter) to a hemofilter. Here excess fluids, electrolytes, and nitrogenous waste products are removed by ultrafiltration. The blood then returns to the patient's circulation via the venous arm of the arteriovenous shunt or a venous catheter. The ultrafiltrate resulting from filtration of the blood contains unwanted solutes and fluid. The ultrafiltrate is discarded. Intravenous fluids may be administered to replace fluid removed by the procedure. The process of hemofiltration is continuous and slow, making it particularly suitable for patients with unstable cardiovascular systems.

Continuous Arteriovenous Hemodialysis

Continuous arteriovenous hemodialysis (CAVHD) shares many of the characteristics of CAVH but offers the advantage of a concentration gradient to facilitate more rapid clearance of urea. This is accomplished by the circulation of dialysate on one side of a semipermeable membrane. The blood flow through the system depends on the patient's arterial pressure, as it does in CAVH; a blood pump is not used as it is in standard hemodialysis.

Major advantages of CAVH and CAVHD are that they do not produce rapid fluid shifts, they do not require dialysis machines or dialysis personnel to carry out the procedures, and they can be initiated quickly in hospitals without dialysis facilities. Access to the vascular system for these procedures may be through a previously established internal fistula (as used for hemodialysis), through an externally placed access (such as a Scribner shunt), or by cannulation of the femoral or radial blood vessels.

Peritoneal Dialysis

In peritoneal dialysis, the surface of the peritoneum, which amounts to approximately 22,000 cm^2, acts as the diffusing surface. An appropriate sterile dialyzing fluid (dialysate) is introduced into the peritoneal cavity at intervals. Urea and creatinine, both metabolic end products normally excreted by the kidneys, are removed (cleared) from the blood during peritoneal dialysis. Urea is cleared at a rate of 15 to 20 ml/min, while creatinine is removed more slowly.

With the development of nonirritating silicone catheters and improvements in commercial dialyzing solution, peritoneal dialysis has become easier to perform. In addition to the indications previously mentioned, peritoneal dialysis has been used to treat peritonitis (inflammation of the peritoneum) by adding antibiotics to the dialysate, which comes in direct contact with the infected site during dialysis. It is also occasionally used as a means of lavage in abdominal trauma and acute pancreatitis. Peritoneal dialysis can be carried out a few days after abdominal surgery.

It usually takes 36 to 48 hours to achieve with peritoneal dialysis what hemodialysis accomplishes in 6 to 8 hours. Peritoneal dialysis can be intermittent (several times per week, each 6 to 48 hours) or continuous.

Because of the development of a surgically implantable Silastic catheter for permanent access to the peritoneal cavity, automated closed-cycle peritoneal dialysis machines, and

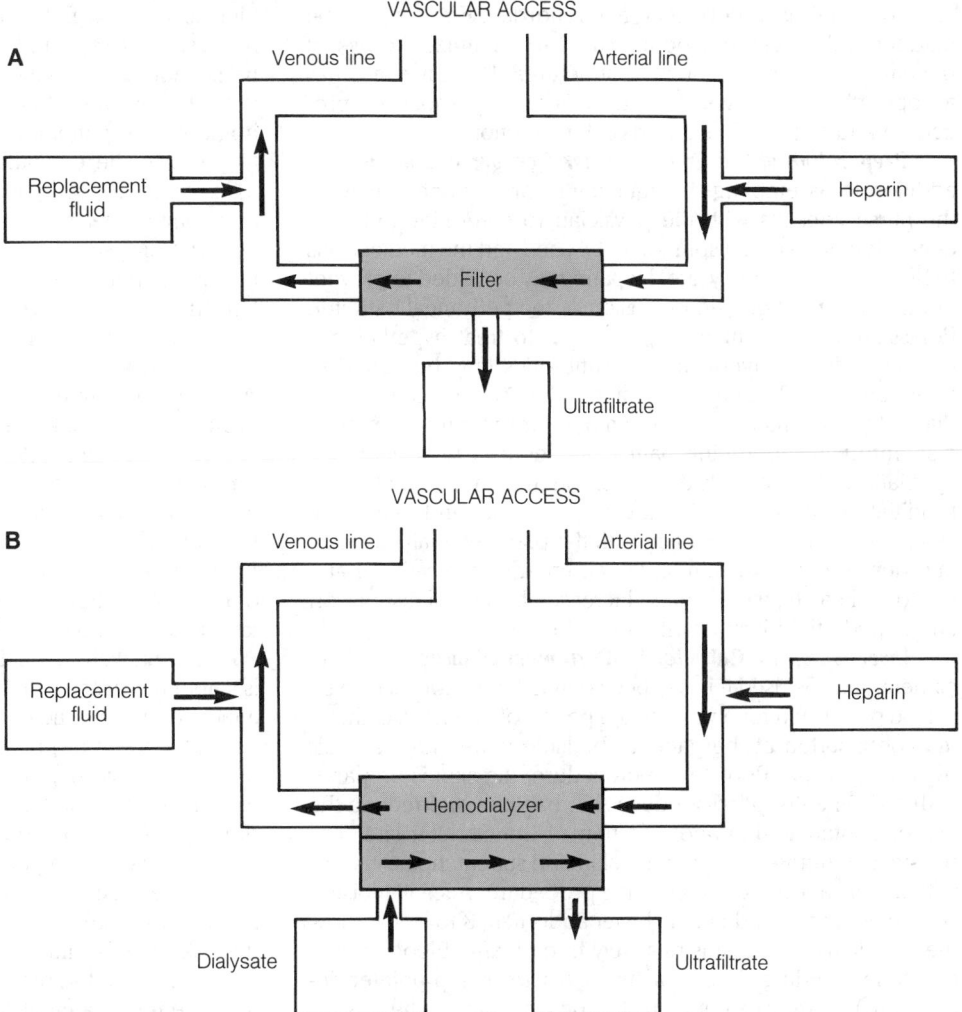

Figure 42–4. Schematic representation of (**A**) continuous arteriovenous hemofiltration (CAVH) and (**B**) continuous arteriovenous hemodialysis (CAVHD). (Redrawn from Nahman NS and Middendorf DF. Continuous arteriovenous hemofiltration. Med Clin North Am 1990 Jul; 74[4]:977.)

plastic bags to hold the dialysate, this procedure is carried out in the home for long-term therapy of patients with chronic renal failure.

Although there are variations in the scheduling of dialysis treatments with the different forms of peritoneal dialysis, the underlying principles are the same.

Principles of Peritoneal Dialysis. One to 3 liters (usually 2 liters) of sterile dialyzing solution (dialysate) is infused through an abdominal catheter into the peritoneal cavity. The solution flows into the cavity by gravity. The fluid comes in close contact with the blood vessels of the peritoneal cavity, which serves as the dialyzing membrane. Toxic wastes and excess fluid move from the patient's circulation by diffusion and osmosis into the peritoneal cavity during the *dwell* or *equilibration time,* the period in which the fluid remains in the abdominal cavity before it is drained. At the end of the dwell time, the solution is drained from the abdominal cavity by siphon and gravity and discarded. A new container of fluid is added and infused. An exchange (infusion, dwell time, and drainage) may range from less than an hour (as may be indicated in acutely ill patients) to many hours (overnight or throughout the day, as in continuous ambulatory peritoneal dialysis or continuous cycling peritoneal dialysis).

Goals and Indications for Peritoneal Dialysis. The goals of this method of treatment are to assist in the removal of toxic substances and metabolic wastes, to reestablish normal fluid balance by removing excessive fluid, and to restore electrolyte balance. Peritoneal dialysis may be the treatment of choice for patients with renal failure who are unable or unwilling to undergo hemodialysis or renal transplantation. Patients who are susceptible to the rapid fluid, electrolyte, and metabolic changes that occur during hemodialysis experience fewer of these problems with the slower rate of peritoneal dialysis. Therefore, patients with diabetes or cardiovascular disease, many older patients, and those who may be at risk for side effects of systemic use of heparin would be likely candidates for peritoneal dialysis to treat their renal failure. Additionally, severe hypertension, congestive heart failure, and pulmonary edema not responsive to usual treatment regimens have been successfully treated with peritoneal dialysis.

Preparation of the Patient for Peritoneal Dialysis. The patient about to undergo peritoneal dialysis may be acutely ill, thus requiring short-term treatment to correct severe disturbances in fluid and electrolyte status, or may be undergoing one of many treatments, as in continuous peritoneal dialysis to treat chronic renal failure. Therefore, the nurse's preparation of the patient and family for peritoneal dialysis is dependent on the patient's physical and psychologic status, level of alertness, previous experience with dialysis, and understanding of and familiarity with the procedure.

The procedure is explained to the patient and a signed consent in obtained. Baseline vital signs, weight, and serum

1162   UNIT 10: Urinary and Renal Function

electrolyte levels are obtained and recorded. Emptying of the bladder and bowel may be indicated to minimize the risk of puncture of internal organs and structures. The nurse also has an opportunity to assess the patient's anxiety about the procedure and to provide support and instruction.

Preparation of the Equipment for Peritoneal Dialysis. In addition to assembling the equipment for peritoneal dialysis, the nurse consults with the physician to determine the concentration of dialyzing solution to be used and the medications to be added to the dialysate. Heparin may be added to prevent fibrin clot formation and occlusion of the peritoneal catheter. Potassium chloride may be prescribed to treat hyperkalemia without inducing hypokalemia. Antibiotics may be added to treat peritonitis. Prior to the addition of these medications, the dialysate is warmed to body temperature to prevent patient discomfort and abdominal pain and to increase urea clearance by dilation of the vessels of the peritoneum. Immediately prior to initiation of dialysis, the administration set and tubing are assembled. The tubing is filled with the prepared dialysate fluid in order to reduce the amount of air entering the catheter and peritoneal cavity, which could increase abdominal discomfort and impede fluid instillation and drainage.

Insertion of the Catheter for Peritoneal Dialysis. A stylet catheter may be used if it is expected that the peritoneal dialysis will be performed for a very limited period of time. The catheter may be inserted at the patient's bedside under strict asepsis by the physician. Prior to the procedure, the skin is prepared with a local antiseptic to reduce skin bacteria and reduce the risk of contamination and infection of the catheter site. The physician infiltrates the patient's skin and subcutaneous tissues with a local anesthetic prior to the procedure. A small incision or stab wound is made in the lower abdomen, 3 to 5 cm below the umbilicus; this area is relatively free of large blood vessels and little bleeding should occur. A *trocar* (sharp pointed instrument) is used to puncture the peritoneum as the patient tightens the abdominal muscles by raising his head. The catheter is threaded through the trocar and positioned. Dialysis fluid that has been previously prepared is infused into the peritoneal cavity, pushing the *omentum* (peritoneal lining extending from the abdominal organs) away from the catheter. A pursestring suture may be used to secure the catheter in place.

The dialyzing solution is allowed to flow freely into the peritoneal cavity. Five to ten minutes are usually required for infusion of 2 liters of fluid. The fluid is allowed to remain in the peritoneal cavity for the prescribed dwell or equilibration time to allow diffusion and osmosis to occur. Diffusion of small molecules such as urea and creatinine takes place maximally in the first 5 to 10 minutes of the dwell time. At the end of the dwell time, the drainage tube is unclamped and the peritoneal cavity is drained by siphon and gravity through a closed system. Drainage is normally completed in 10 to 30 minutes, and the drained fluid is normally colorless or straw-colored. It should not be cloudy; bloody drainage should not appear after the first few exchanges. Guidelines for care of the patient during peritoneal dialysis are included in Chart 42-1.

Continuous Ambulatory Peritoneal Dialysis

Continuous ambulatory peritoneal dialysis (CAPD) is a form of dialysis used for many patients with end-stage renal disease. Traditional peritoneal dialysis requires skilled nurses and tech-

nicians to perform the procedure. Treatments are intermittent, necessitating repeated sessions usually lasting from 6 to 48 hours, during which the patient is immobile. In contrast, CAPD is continuous and usually self-administered. It is performed at home by the patient. Sometimes a family member is trained to perform the exchanges for the patient. The technique is adjusted to the patient's physiologic requirements for dialysis and ability to learn the procedure.

The dialysate is delivered from flexible plastic containers through a permanent peritoneal catheter. A catheter of the type developed by Tenckhoff is implanted in the abdomen surgically. This catheter has one or two Dacron cuffs. Growth of tissue around the cuff provides a bacteria-resistant seal. A subcutaneous tunnel (5 to 10 cm in length) provides further protection against bacterial infection (Fig. 42-5).

After the dialysate is infused into the peritoneal cavity through the catheter, the bag is folded and tucked underneath the clothing during the dwell or equilibration time. This provides the patient with some freedom and reduces the number of connections and disconnections necessary at the catheter end of the tubing, thereby reducing the accompanying risk of contamination and peritonitis.

Alternatively, a Y-set system of tubing is used. The catheter is capped off after dialysate fluid is infused. After tubing is attached to the catheter and a fresh bag of dialysate is attached, a small amount of fluid is flushed from the fresh solution bag to the drainage bag. Dialysate is then drained from the peritoneal cavity to the drainage bag. Following completion of drainage, fresh solution is infused into the peritoneal cavity. This permits washing out of any contaminants introduced during connection of the bags; these contaminants are infused into the drainage bag rather than the peritoneal cavity, reducing the risk of peritonitis.

To reduce the risk of peritonitis, meticulous care is taken to prevent contamination of the catheter, fluid, or tubing and accidental disconnection of the catheter from the tubing. The catheter is protected from manipulation and the catheter entry site is meticulously cared for according to a set protocol.

The success of CAPD depends upon the maintenance of the permanent catheter placed in the peritoneal cavity. Catheter problems that can arise include one-way obstruction, dislodgment from the pelvis, omental wrapping, dialysate leak, exit-site infection, fibrin-clot formation, and bacterial/fungal contamination.

Principles. CAPD works on the same principles involved in other forms of peritoneal dialysis: diffusion and osmosis. However, because CAPD is a continuous treatment, a steady state of blood values of the nitrogenous waste products results. The precise blood levels depend on the residual kidney function, on the daily dialysate volume, and, of course, on the rate of production of the waste products. There are less extreme fluctuations in the serum chemistries on CAPD, because the dialysis is constantly in progress. The serum electrolytes usually stay in the normal range.

The longer length of time that the dialysate stays in the peritoneal cavity has a positive effect on the clearance of middle-sized molecules. It is thought that these middle molecules may be significant uremic toxins. Their clearance is greatly enhanced by CAPD. Low-molecular-weight substances, such as urea, diffuse more rapidly than middle-sized molecules in dialysis, but they are removed more slowly during CAPD than during hemodialysis.

Chart 42–1
Guidelines for Nursing Care of the Patient During Intermittent Peritoneal Dialysis

Nursing Action	Rationale
I. Promote patient comfort during procedure.	
A. Provide physical comfort measures.	The dialysis period is lengthy, and the patient becomes fatigued.
1. Provide frequent back care and massage of pressure areas.	
2. Assist patient to turn from side to side.	
3. Elevate head of bed at intervals.	
4. Allow patient to sit in chair for brief periods if condition permits (only with surgically implanted catheter, with trocar, patient is on strict bed rest).	
B. Keep patient informed of progress and results.	Being informed helps the patient to cope and cooperate with the lengthy procedure.
1. Reinforce teaching about the procedure and its goals.	
2. Give patient information about progress (*e.g.,* fluid loss, weight loss, return of electrolyte balance).	
C. Provide care of the whole patient.	Focus on the dialysis procedure, rather than on the patient, threatens the patient's psychologic well-being and may result in failure to detect physiologic and emotional problems.
1. Provide physiologic and psychologic care throughout procedure, remembering patient's predialysis needs, reactions, concerns, and health problems.	
2. Keep family informed about the patient's status and progress.	
II. Maintain peritoneal dialysis fluid infusion and drainage.	
A. If the fluid is not draining properly, move the patient from side to side to facilitate the removal of peritoneal drainage. The head of the bed may also be elevated. *Never push in the catheter.* Assess the patency of the catheter. Check for closed clamp, kinked tubing, or air lock.	If the drainage stops, or slows to a drip before the dialyzing fluid has been adequately drained, this may indicate that the catheter tip is buried in the omentum. Turning the patient may be helpful (or it may be necessary for the physician to reposition the catheter). Pushing in the catheter is contraindicated because it introduces bacteria into the peritoneal cavity.
B. Use strict aseptic technique when adding exchanges or emptying drainage containers.	Minimizes risk of infection.
C. Monitor blood pressure and pulse every 15 minutes during the first exchange, and every hour thereafter. Monitor the heart rhythm for signs of dysrhythmia.	A drop in blood pressure may indicate excessive fluid loss due to the glucose concentrations of the dialyzing solutions. Changes in vital signs may indicate impending shock or overhydration.
D. Monitor the patient's temperature every 4 hours (especially after catheter removal).	An infection may become evident after dialysis has been discontinued.
E. The procedure is repeated until the blood chemistry levels improve. The usual time is 36 to 48 hours; the patient will receive 24 to 48 exchanges (the number dependent on patient's condition). In acute conditions, catheters are usually removed within 48 to 72 hours. A new trocar is inserted for the next treatment.	The duration of the dialysis depends on the severity of the condition and on the size and weight of the patient.
III. Monitor changes in fluid and electrolyte status, weight changes, vital signs, and intake and output records.	
A. Maintain an exact record of the patient's fluid balance during the treatment.	Complications (dehydration, circulatory collapse, hypotension, shock, and death) may occur if the patient loses too much fluid through peritoneal drainage. Large fluid losses around the catheter may be missed unless the dressings are checked carefully.
1. Calculate the status of the patient's loss or gain of fluid at the end of each exchange; check dressing for leakage, and weigh on gram scale if leakage is significant.	
2. The fluid balance should be about even or should show *slight* fluid loss or gain, depending on the patient's fluid status.	
3. Assure that the record includes the following:	
a. Exact time of beginning and end of each exchange; starting and finishing time of drainage	
b. Amount and type of solution infused and drained	

(continued)

Chart 42–1 *(Continued)*

Nursing Action	*Rationale*
c. Fluid balance (cumulative) d. Number of exchanges e. Medications added to dialyzing solution f. Pre- and postdialysis weight, plus daily weight g. Level of responsiveness at beginning, throughout, and at end of treatment h. Assessment of vital signs and patient's condition	
IV. Monitor for complications.	

A. Peritonitis
  1. Observe for nausea and vomiting, anorexia, abdominal pain, tenderness, rigidity, and cloudy dialysate drainage.
  2. Send specimen of dialysate for WBC and cultures.
	Peritonitis is the most common complication. Antibiotics may be added to the dialysate or administered systemically.

B. Bleeding
  1. Observe catheter site and drainage for bleeding.
  2. Monitor vital signs.
  3. Monitor serum hemoglobin and hematocrit.
	A small amount of bleeding around a newly inserted catheter is not significant if it does not persist. During the first few exchanges, blood-tinged fluid from subcutaneous bleeding is not uncommon. Small amounts of heparin may be added to inflow solution to prevent the catheter from becoming obstructed or occluded. A hematocrit of the drainage fluid may be obtained to assess the amount of bleeding.

C. Respiratory difficulty
  1. Slow the inflow rate.
  2. Make sure tubing is not kinked and is draining properly.
  3. Prevent air from entering the peritoneal cavity by keeping the drip chamber of the tubing three-fourths full of fluid.
  4. Elevate head of bed; encourage coughing and breathing exercises.
  5. Turn patient from side to side.
	Respiratory difficulty is caused by pressure from the fluid in the peritoneal cavity and the upward displacement of the diaphragm, producing shallow respirations.
	In severe respiratory difficulty, the fluid from the peritoneal cavity should be drained immediately and the physician notified.

D. Abdominal pain Encourage patient to move about.	Pain may be caused by the dialyzing solution's not being at body temperature, incomplete drainage of the solution, chemical irritation, irritation by the catheter, peritonitis, or air pressing on the diaphragm and causing referred shoulder pain.

E. Leakage
  1. Change the dressings frequently around the trocar; use care not to dislodge the catheter.
  2. Use sterile, plastic drapes to prevent contamination.
	Leakage around the catheter predisposes to peritonitis.

F. Constipation
  1. Assist patient to move about.
  2. Provide high-fiber foods and fluid within dietary restrictions.
	Inactivity, decreased nutrition, phosphate binders, and the presence of fluid in the abdomen tend to cause constipation.

G. Low serum albumin
  1. Monitor serum protein levels.
  2. Assess for edema, hypotension, weight changes.
	Small amounts of albumin are lost with each exchange, resulting in a lowered serum albumin. Edema may occur with possible hypotension.

The removal of excess water during peritoneal dialysis is achieved by the addition of hypertonic glucose to the dialysate, creating an osmotic gradient. Glucose solutions of 1.5%, 2.5%, and 4.25% are available in several sizes, from 500 ml to 3000 ml, thus allowing the dialysate selection to fit the patient's tolerance, size, and physiologic needs.

An exchange is performed usually four times a day and the fluid is changed four times a day. This technique is continuous, 24 hours a day, 7 days a week. The patient performs the exchanges at intervals spread throughout the day (*e.g.*, at 8 AM, noon, 5 PM, and 10 PM) and sleeps during the night. Each exchange usually takes 30 to 60 minutes or longer to perform; its duration depends on the length of the prescribed dwell time. This consists of a 5- or 10-minute period of infusion, a 20-minute drain period, and a 10-minute, 30-minute, or longer dwell time.

Indications.   CAPD is the treatment of choice for most patients who want to perform their own dialysis at home. CAPD is indicated for those patients on maintenance or chronic hemodialysis who have problems with their present treatment

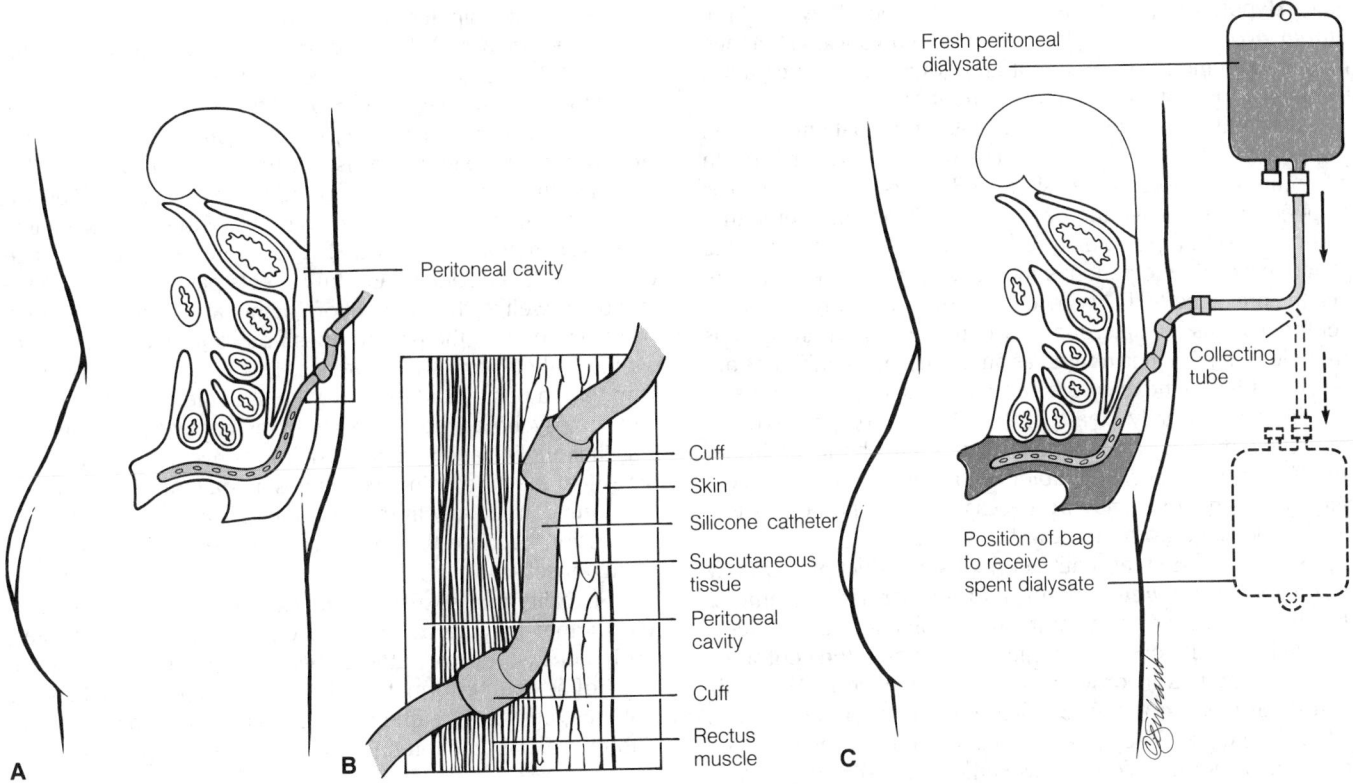

Figure 42–5. Continuous ambulatory peritoneal dialysis. (**A**) The peritoneal catheter is implanted through the abdominal wall. (**B**) Dacron cuffs and a subcutaneous tunnel provide protection against bacterial infection. (**C**) Dialysate fluid flows by gravity to the peritoneal catheter into the peritoneal cavity. Following equilibration, the fluid is removed by siphon and gravity and discarded.

modality, such as vascular access dysfunction or failure, excessive thirst, severe hypertension, postdialysis headaches, and severe anemia requiring frequent transfusion.

Patients awaiting a kidney transplant can be safely maintained on CAPD. Diabetic persons with end-stage renal disease may be a group for whom CAPD is an *absolute* indication. The excellent control of hypertension, the control of uremia, and the satisfactory control of glycemia by intraperitoneal administration of insulin may arrest the diabetic complications.

Older patients generally do well on CAPD if family or community supports are available. Patients who are able to take an active part in their treatment, want more freedom, and are motivated and willing to carry out the required treatment also do well on CAPD. The patient's family support system, as well as his ability to perform CAPD, is considered when the mode of treatment is selected.

Patients choose CAPD to gain freedom from a machine, to have control over their daily activities, to avoid dietary restrictions, to have greater fluid intake, to elevate the serum hematocrit, to have blood pressure under greater control, to have freedom from venipuncture, and, hopefully, to gain a general overall feeling of well-being. Almost half of all new end-stage renal disease patients are choosing CAPD for their form of therapy. The number of patients receiving CAPD is expected to continue to increase.

Contraindications. Contraindications for CAPD include poor clearance of solutes due to adhesions from previous operations or to systemic inflammatory disease. Another contraindication is recurrent chronic backache with preexisting disc disease (which could be aggravated by the continuous pressure of dialysis fluid in the abdomen). The presence of a colostomy, ileostomy, nephrostomy, or ileal conduit may increase the risk of peritonitis. Patients receiving immunosuppressive treatment have increased complications because of poor healing of the catheter exit site.

Patients with arthritis or poor hand strength may require assistance in performing the exchange. Blind or partially blind patients and those with other physical limitations have been instructed to perform CAPD successfully.

Complications

CAPD is not without complications. Most complications are minor in nature, but several, if left unattended, can have serious consequences for the patient.

Peritonitis. Peritonitis is the most common complication and also the most serious; it occurs in 60% to 80% of patients on peritoneal dialysis. Most peritonitis episodes are due to accidental contamination caused by *Staphylococcus epidermidis*. These episodes result in mild symptoms and have a good prognosis; however, peritonitis due to *Staphylococcus aureus* produces a higher morbidity rate, has a more serious prognosis, and runs a longer course. Gram-negative organisms may originate in the bowel, particularly when there is more than one organism in the peritoneal fluid and when the organisms are anaerobic. Indications of peritonitis include cloudiness of the peritoneal dialysis effluent (drainage) and diffuse abdominal pain. Hypotension and other signs of shock may occur if *Staphylococcus aureus* is the responsible organism. Drainage fluid is examined for cell count and gram stain and cultured to identify the organism and guide treatment.

Peritonitis is treated in the hospital if the patient is too ill to perform his own exchanges. The patient is usually put on intermittent peritoneal dialysis for 48 hours or more or it is stopped entirely while the patient is receiving parenteral antibiotic therapy. Stopping dialysis for several days also promotes phagocytosis by the patient's macrophages; there is evidence that the presence of dialysate in the peritoneal cavity may hamper the response of macrophages to infection. If the symptoms are mild, the patient is treated as an outpatient. Antibiotics are usually added to the dialysate and also taken orally for 10 days. The infection usually clears in 2 to 4 days. To preserve the patient's remaining renal function, care must be taken in determining the dosage of antibiotics that may be nephrotoxic. Surgical intervention may be necessary if the peritonitis is a result of leakage from the bowel.

With a persistent catheter exit-site infection (usually *Staphylococcus aureus*), removal of the permanent catheter may be necessary to prevent the development of peritonitis.

Patients with fungal peritonitis need to have the peritoneal catheter removed in order to clear the infection. Peritonitis with three positive peritoneal fluid cultures also necessitates catheter removal. The patient is maintained on hemodialysis for about 1 month before a new catheter is inserted.

Regardless of the organism responsible, the patient with peritonitis loses large amounts of protein through the peritoneum; acute malnutrition and delayed healing may result. Therefore, attention must be given to assessment and prompt treatment of these infections.

Leakage. Leakage of dialysate through the incision/insertion site may be noted immediately after catheter insertion. Usually, the leak stops spontaneously if dialysis is withheld for several days to give the incision and exit site enough time to heal. During this period, it is important to reduce factors that might delay healing, such as undue abdominal muscle activity and straining during bowel movement.

Late leaks can occur spontaneously months or years after catheter placement. They may be leaks through the exit site or into the abdominal wall.

Bleeding. A bloody effluent (drainage) may be observed occasionally, especially in young, menstruating females. In most cases, no cause can be found for the bleeding. Catheter displacement from the pelvis has occasionally been associated with the bleeding. Some patients have had bloody effluent following an enema or from minor trauma. Invariably, bleeding stops after a day or two and requires no specific intervention. More frequent exchanges during this time may be necessary to prevent obstruction of the catheter by blood clots.

Other Complications. Other complications include abdominal hernias, probably resulting from the continuously increased intra-abdominal pressure. The types of hernias that have developed include incisional, inguinal, diaphragmatic, and umbilical hernias. The persistently raised intra-abdominal pressure also aggravates symptoms of hiatal hernia and hemorrhoids.

Hypertriglyceridemia is frequently found in patients on CAPD, suggesting that this therapy may accelerate atherogenesis. Cardiovascular disease remains a major cause of death in this population of patients.

Low back pain and anorexia due to the presence of fluid in the abdomen and the constant sweet taste related to absorption of glucose may also occur with CAPD.

Altered Body Image and Sexuality. Although CAPD has given end-stage renal disease patients more freedom and control over their treatment, it is not without its problems. The patients often experience an altered body image because of the abdominal catheter and the presence of the bag and tubing. Waist size increases from 1 to 2 in (or more) with the presence of fluid in the abdomen, and this affects patients' clothing selection as well as their feeling of "being fat." Body image may be so altered that the patient does not want to look at or care for the catheter for days or weeks. Talking with other patients who have a positive attitude may help. Some patients seem to have no psychologic problems with the catheter; they think of it as their lifeline and as a life-sustaining device. Patients sometimes feel they are doing exchanges all day long and have no free time, particularly in the beginning. They may experience depression because they feel overwhelmed with the responsibility of self-care.

Sexuality and sexual activity can be altered; the patient and partner may be reluctant to engage in sexual activities, partly because of the catheter being psychologically "in the way" of sexual performance. The presence of the 2 liters of dialysate, peritoneal catheter, and drainage bag may interfere with the sexual function and body image of these patients.

Patient Education and Home Health Care

Patients are taught to perform CAPD once they are medically stable. They may be taught as inpatients or outpatients. The training usually takes 5 days to 2 weeks.

During the training period, patients are taught basic anatomy and physiology about the kidney, the disease process, the exchange procedure, possible complications and the appropriate way to respond to these problems, the measurement of vital signs, catheter care, proper hand washing techniques, and, most important, when and whom to call with a problem. Because of the consequences of peritonitis, the patient and family are thoroughly instructed about indicators of peritonitis, preventive measures, and early treatment strategies.

The dietitian and social worker meet with the patient and the family during the training period and at intervals thereafter. Information and instruction about diet are provided. Although the diet of CAPD patients can be liberal, some recommendations are necessary. Because of protein loss with continuous peritoneal dialysis, patients are instructed to eat a high-protein, well-balanced diet. They are also encouraged to increase their fiber intake daily to help prevent constipation. Often patients gain from 3 to 5 pounds within a month of initiation of CAPD, so they may be asked to limit their carbohydrate intake so they do not gain an excessive amount of weight. Potassium, sodium, and fluid restrictions are not usually needed.

Patients usually lose about 2 liters of fluid over and above the 8 liters of dialysate infused into the abdomen during a 24-hour period, allowing a normal fluid intake even in an anephric patient (a patient without kidneys).

Patients are taught according to their own learning ability and learning level, and only as much at one time as they can handle without feeling uncomfortable or highly stressed. Follow-up care during phone calls and visits to the outpatient department as well as continuing home care assist patients in the transition to the home and to the role of active participants in their own health care. Patients often depend on being able to check with the nurses to see if they are making the right choices as to dialysate or control of blood pressure, or simply to discuss a problem. They are seen by the CAPD team as outpatients once a month or more if needed. The patient's exchange procedure is evaluated at that time to see that strict aseptic technique is being used. The patient's administration tubing is changed by the CAPD nurses every 4 to 8 weeks. Infrequent tubing changes decrease the chance of possible contamination. Blood chemistries are followed closely to make certain the therapy is adequate for the patient.

CAPD is not for everyone with end-stage renal disease, but it is a viable form of therapy for those patients who not only want to do self-care but experience a feeling of independence from a machine and its accompanying rigid schedule. If patients are willing to do the exchange as taught, and are able to fit the therapy into their own routines, they can live relatively normal lives and feel a measure of accomplishment and success with CAPD. Often patients relate that they feel better on CAPD, have more energy, and feel more like they did before they had renal failure.

It would be wrong to encourage all patients to seek CAPD. Instead, patients should be helped to find the therapy most suitable for their particular life-style and with which they can best reach an optimal state of well-being.

Continuous Cycler Peritoneal Dialysis

Continuous cycler peritoneal dialysis (CCPD) is a combination of overnight intermittent peritoneal dialysis with a prolonged dwell during the day.

The patient is connected to a cycler machine every evening and receives three to five 2-liter exchanges during the night; in the morning, the patient caps off the catheter after infusing 1 to 2 liters of fresh dialysate. This dialysate stays in the abdominal cavity until the patient's reattachment to the cycler machine at bedtime. The patient is able to sleep because the machine is very quiet, and extra-long tubing from the machine allows the patient to move and turn normally during sleep.

This technique decreases the infection rate because of fewer opportunities for contamination with bag changes and tubing disconnections and permits the patient to be free of exchanges throughout the day, making it possible to work more freely and carry out activities of daily living.

Care of the Hospitalized Dialysis Patient

The patient who receives hemodialysis or peritoneal dialysis may be hospitalized for treatment of complications related to the underlying renal abnormality or the dialysis treatment itself. In addition, the patient may experience problems not related to renal dysfunction or its treatment. When the hemodialysis patient is hospitalized for any reason, care must be taken to protect the vascular access from damage. Therefore, the vascular access is assessed for patency, and precautions are taken to ensure that the extremity with the vascular access is not used for blood pressure measurements or obtaining blood specimens. The CAPD patient is usually well versed in care of

the catheter exit site; however, it is important to use the patient's hospitalization to assess his adherence to recommended catheter care and to correct any misperceptions or deviations from appropriate technique. The medications prescribed for all dialysis patients must be closely monitored to avoid those that are toxic to the kidneys; dosage must be monitored and perhaps altered to prevent either toxic effects on the kidney or overdosage because of impaired renal excretion. Care must be taken to listen to and evaluate all problems and symptoms reported by the patient without attributing them broadly to renal failure or to the fact that the patient is on dialysis.

After the patient has been receiving dialysis for a while, he may begin to reevaluate his status, the treatment modality, his satisfaction with life, and the impact of these on his family. Opportunity must be provided for the patient to verbalize feelings and reactions and to explore possible options. It is not uncommon for a patient to consider discontinuing dialysis treatment. His feelings and reactions must be taken seriously, and opportunity must be provided for discussion of them with the dialysis team as well as with a psychologist, psychiatrist, psychiatric nurse, or trusted friend or member of the clergy. The decision of the patient to begin dialysis does not require that he continue dialysis. The patient's informed decision, after thoughtful deliberation, should be respected.

In summary, dialysis has become almost commonplace in the management of patients with renal failure. However, to patients and their families, the need for and dependence on dialysis for survival are often devastating. The patient and family faced with dialysis usually require extensive counseling and education; this need often occurs when they are confronted with the realization that renal failure is a life-threatening illness. Although techniques of dialysis are of paramount importance in the nursing management of the patient's disorder, the ability of the patient and his family to deal with the illness and its treatment is also important if the patient is to understand and cope with the complex treatment. A sympathetic nurse who understands the importance of the technologic aspects of dialysis and the psychologic impact of treatment is often critical to the adjustment of the patient and his family to treatment.

The Patient Undergoing Kidney Surgery

A patient may undergo surgery of the kidney to remove obstructions (tumors or calculi), to insert a tube for drainage of the kidney (nephrostomy, ureterostomy), or to remove the kidney itself to treat unilateral kidney disease, to treat renal carcinoma, or as part of management of the patient undergoing renal transplantation.

Preoperative Considerations

Operations on the kidney are attempted only after a period of evaluation and preparation to ensure that renal function is as good as possible. Fluids are encouraged to promote increased excretion of waste products before surgery, unless contraindicated because of preexisting renal or cardiac dysfunction. If kidney infection is present preoperatively, a wide-spectrum antimicrobial agent may be given to avoid the hazards of bacteremia. Coagulation studies (prothrombin time, partial thromboplastin time, platelet count) may be indicated if the patient has a history of bruising and bleeding. The general preoperative preparation is similar to that described in Chapter 20.

Patients facing kidney surgery are often apprehensive. They may enter the hospital with pain, fever, and hematuria. Thus, the nurse encourages the patient to recognize and express any feelings of anxiety. Confidence is reinforced by establishing a relationship of trust and by providing expert care. Patients faced with the prospect of losing a kidney may think that they will be dependent on dialysis for the rest of their lives. However, normal function may be maintained by a single healthy kidney.

Perioperative Concerns

The operative incisions for renal surgery include flank, intercostal, lumbodorsal, and transverse abdominal or thoracoabdominal incisions (Fig. 42-6). The difficulties in renal surgery are related to difficulty in access to the kidney. Plans are made at this time for managing altered urinary drainage and drainage systems.

Postoperative Management

Because the kidney is such a vascular organ, hemorrhage and shock are the chief complications following renal surgery. Fluid and blood replacement is frequently indicated in the immediate postoperative period to prevent or treat intraoperative blood loss.

Abdominal distention and paralytic ileus are fairly common following operations on the kidney and ureter and are thought to be due to a reflex paralysis of intestinal peristalsis and to manipulation of the colon or duodenum during surgery. Abdominal distention is relieved by decompression via a nasogastric tube. (See p. 445 for treatment of paralytic ileus.) Oral fluids are permitted when auscultation reveals active bowel sounds or the passage of flatus is noted.

If infection occurs, antibiotics are given as necessary on the basis of culture identification of the causative organism. The toxic manifestations of these agents must be kept in mind when assessing the patient and evaluating his renal function. Therapy with low doses of heparin may be initiated postoperatively; subcutaneous administration of heparin has been shown to prevent thromboembolism in urologic patients.

Management may also include insertion of a nephrostomy or other drainage tube and the use of ureteral stents. See p. 1169 for a description of these devices and nursing implications.

Management of Drainage Tubes

Almost all patients undergoing kidney and urologic surgery and many patients with other kidney and urologic disturbances

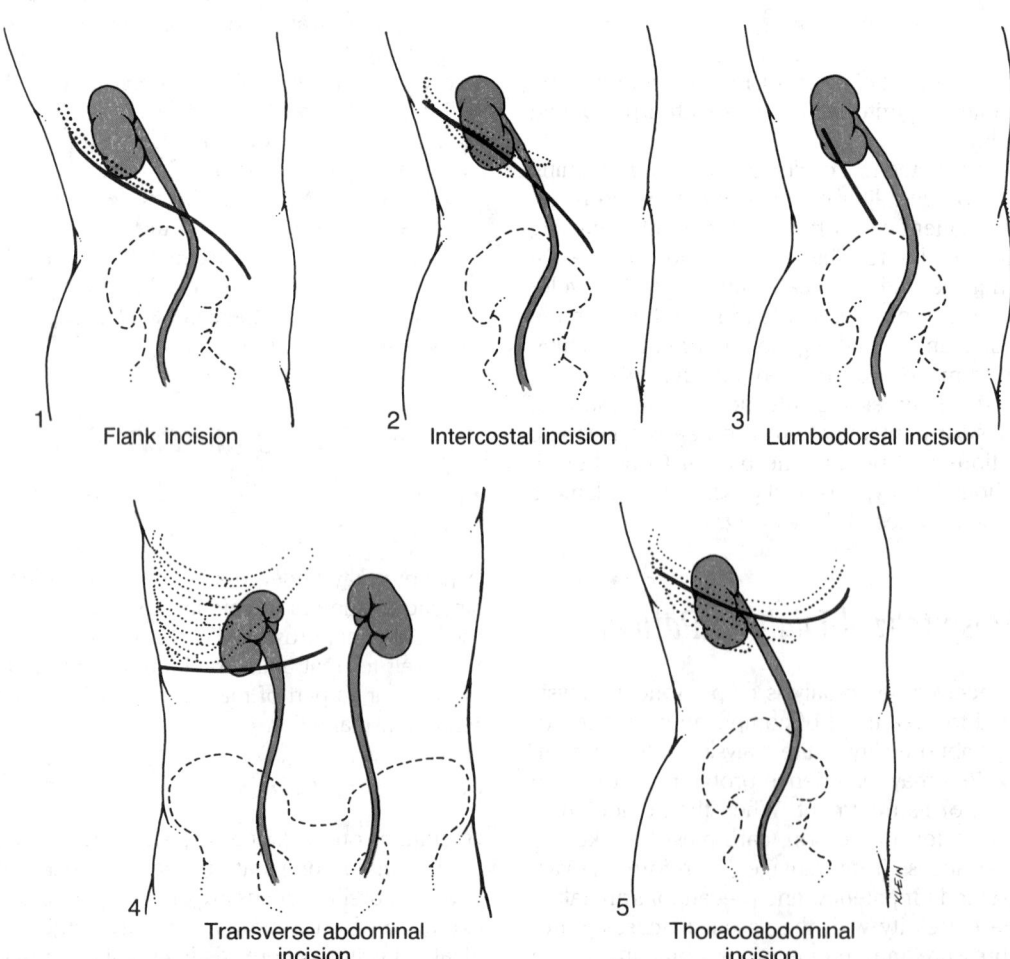

1 Flank incision

2 Intercostal incision

3 Lumbodorsal incision

4 Transverse abdominal
incision

5 Thoracoabdominal
incision

Figure 42-6. Standard incisions for urologic surgical procedures.

have drains, tubes, or catheters in place. Following operations such as nephrostomy, pyelotomy, and ureterotomy, drainage tubes may be placed directly in the kidney, pelvis, or ureter in order to divert or drain the urine and keep the wound dry. All catheters and tubes must remain functioning (*e.g.*, draining) to prevent obstruction by blood clots, which can cause infection. Pain similar to renal colic is caused by the passage of blood clots down the ureter.

Nephrostomy Drainage. A nephrostomy tube is inserted directly into the kidney for temporary or permanent urinary diversion either percutaneously or through a surgical incision. This may be accomplished by a single tube or by a self-retaining U-loop or circular nephrostomy tube (see p. 1208). The purposes of nephrostomy drainage are to provide drainage from the kidney after surgery, conserve and permit physiologic restoration of renal tissue traumatized by obstruction, and provide drainage when the ureter is no longer draining. The nephrostomy tube is attached to closed drainage system or to a urostomy appliance.

Percutaneous nephrostomy is the insertion of a tube through the skin into the pelvis of the kidney. It is performed to provide external drainage of urine from an obstructed ureter, to provide a route for insertion of a ureteral stent (see following discussion), to dissolve renal calculi, to dilate strictures, to close fistulas, to administer drugs, to allow insertion of a brush biopsy instrument and nephroscope, and to perform selected surgical procedures.

The skin site is prepared and anesthetized, and the patient is asked to inhale and hold his breath while a spinal needle is advanced into the renal pelvis. Urine is aspirated for culture, and contrast material may be injected into the pyelocalyceal system. An angiographic catheter guide wire is introduced through the needle to the kidney. The needle is withdrawn and the tract dilated by the passage of tubes or guidewires. The nephrostomy tube is introduced and positioned within the kidney or ureter, fixed by skin sutures, and connected to a closed drainage system.

The patient and tubing are observed for signs of bleeding (immediate or delayed), urinary stones or debris, fistula formation, and infection.

- Assess for bleeding at the nephrostomy site (main complication).
- Assure unobstructed drainage of the nephrostomy tube/catheter. Obstruction of the tube produces pain, trauma, pressure and stress on the suture lines, and infection. If the tube is dislodged inadvertently, it must be immediately replaced by the surgeon because the nephrostomy opening will contract, making it difficult to reinsert the tube.
- A *nephrostomy tube is never clamped*, because such an action will precipitate acute pyelonephritis.
- The nephrostomy tube is rarely irrigated. If necessary, irrigation may be performed by the surgeon.

If irrigation is necessary, only 10 ml of warm, sterile saline is used for irrigation because of the small size of the renal pelvis and the risk of mechanical damage to the kidney or infection from pyelorenal backflow. Fluid intake is encouraged to produce good mechanical flushing and to dilute urinary particles that cause calculus formation. The urine is kept acidic to prevent tube encrustation by urinary sediments. If the patient has a nephrostomy tube in each kidney, output for each catheter is measured and recorded separately. The catheters may be

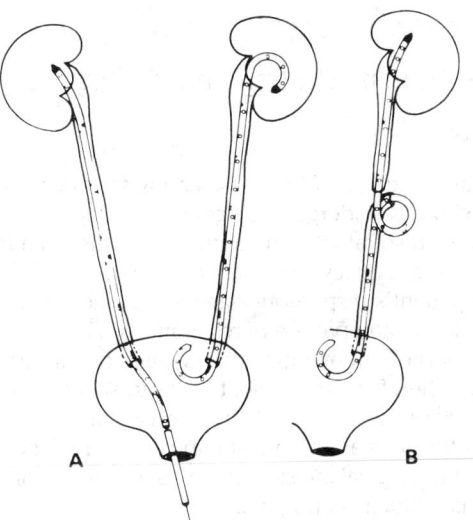

Figure 42–7. Ureteral stents. (**A**) Retrograde passage of ureteral stent. The Double-J ureteral stent is shaped to resist migration. The proximal J hooks into the lower calix or renal pelvis, and the distal J curves into the bladder. (**B**) Open surgical placement of double-J stent prior to an ureteral anastomosis. (Courtesy of Medical Engineering Corporation, Racine, WI.)

attached to leg collection bags when the patient becomes ambulatory.

Ureteral Stents

A ureteral stent is a tubular device designed for placement within the ureter to maintain ureteral flow in patients with ureteral obstruction (from edema, stricture, fibrosis, advanced malignancy), to restore kidney function, to divert urine, to promote healing, and to maintain the caliber/patency of the ureter after surgery (Fig. 42-7).

The stent, usually of soft, flexible silicone, may be temporary or permanent. It may be inserted through a cytoscope or nephrostomy tube or by open operation. Complications include infection, inflammation secondary to the presence of a foreign body in the genitourinary tract, tube encrustation, bleeding or clot obstruction within the stent, and dislodgment of the stent.

Newer stent designs avoid some of these problems. The double-J ureteral stent has a J-shaped curve molded into each end, which prevents upward or downward migration. This stent can be used in place of a nephrostomy or pyelostomy for short- or long-term urinary drainage. The double-pigtail ureteral stent has a pigtail coil at each end of the stent, which permits placement of the upper coil (pigtail) in the renal pelvis, with the lower coil at the ureteral orifice. The coils prevent the stent from moving and allow free body movement.

The nursing interventions are to monitor for bleeding, observe and measure output, assess for purulent drainage at the insertion site or in the drainage bag, and monitor for stent dislodgment, which is denoted by colicky pain and a decrease in urine output.

An indwelling stent usually induces local ureteral reaction, including mucosal edema, which can cause temporary obstruction of the ureter.

► Nursing Process
The Patient Undergoing Kidney Surgery
◊ Assessment

Immediate concerns of the nurse caring for the postoperative patient who has undergone surgery of the kidney include assessment of respiratory and circulatory status, pain level, and patency and adequacy of urinary drainage.

The patient's respiratory status is assessed by monitoring the rate, depth, and pattern of respirations. The location of the surgical incision frequently causes pain on inspiration and coughing. Therefore, the patient tends to splint the chest wall and respirations tend to be shallow. Auscultation is performed to assess for normal and adventitious breath sounds. The location of the surgical incision provides a guide for anticipating respiratory problems and pain.

The vital signs and arterial or central venous pressure are monitored. Skin color and temperature and urine output will also provide information about the adequacy of circulatory status. The surgical incision and drainage tubes are observed frequently to aid in the detection of unexpected blood loss and hemorrhage.

Pain is a major problem for the patient postoperatively because of the site of the surgical incision and the position assumed on the operating table to permit adequate access to the kidney. The location and severity of pain are assessed before and after administration of analgesics. Abdominal distention, which increases the patient's level of discomfort, is also noted.

The patient's urinary output and drainage from tubes inserted during surgery are monitored for amount, color, and type of output and drainage. Decreased or absent drainage is reported promptly to the physician, because it may indicate obstruction that could cause pain, infection, and disruption of the suture lines.

◊ Nursing Diagnoses

Based on the history and assessment data and the type of surgical procedure performed, major nursing diagnoses for the patient include the following:

- High risk for ineffective airway clearance related to the location of the surgical incision
- High risk for altered cardiac output related to blood loss
- Pain and discomfort related to the location of the surgical incision, the position assumed on the operating table during surgery, and abdominal distention
- Alteration in patterns of urinary elimination related to urinary drainage

◊ Planning and Implementation

◊ *Goals:* The major goals for the patient may include maintenance of effective airway clearance, maintenance of cardiac output, relief of pain and discomfort, and maintenance of urinary elimination.

◊ Nursing Interventions

◊ *Maintaining Airway Clearance.* The surgical approaches to the kidney predispose the patient to respiratory complications and paralytic ileus. Also, with a subcostal or posterior incision, the patient may have severe pain on breathing and coughing.

If the pleura has been opened, pneumothorax may be a problem. The incision is generally close to the diaphragm and, with a substernal incision, the nerves may be stretched and bruised.

Adequate use of analgesic medications is necessary to relieve pain so that the patient is able to take deep breaths and cough. If the analgesia is administered at regular, frequent intervals, the patient will be able to perform deep-breathing and coughing exercises more effectively. The incentive spirometer may be used to help maximize lung inflation. The patient is encouraged to cough after each deep breath to loosen secretions. Relief of abdominal distention will promote fuller respiratory effort and thoracic excursion.

◊ *Maintaining Cardiac Output.* Bleeding, hemorrhage, hypovolemia, and shock are the major complications of kidney surgery. The nurse's role is to observe for these complications, to report their signs and symptoms, and to administer prescribed parenteral fluids and blood if complications occur. Monitoring of the patient's vital signs, skin condition, urinary drainage system, and surgical incision is necessary to detect evidence of decreased circulating blood and fluid volume and cardiac output.

◊ *Relieving Pain.* In addition to the incisional pain, the patient may experience pain and discomfort from distention of the renal capsule (tumor, blood clot), ischemia (from occlusion of blood vessels), and stretching of the intrarenal blood vessels. Adequate pain relief is necessary to permit the patient to take deep breaths, cough, turn, and move about. The patient also frequently experiences muscular aches and pains resulting from the position assumed on the operating table, which places anatomic and physiologic stresses on the body. Massage, moist heat, and analgesic medications provide relief.

◊ *Promoting Urinary Elimination.* Attention to the patient's urinary output and drainage is essential to preserve and protect the patient's remaining kidney function. Therefore, adequate drainage is critical to prevent obstruction and infection. The output from each urinary drainage tube is recorded separately; very accurate output measurements are essential in monitoring renal function and the patency of the urinary drainage system. Strict asepsis is used during manipulation of the drainage catheter and tube. Hand washing is mandatory before and after touching any parts of the system. Use of closed drainage systems is essential to avoid contamination of the system and infection. The patient's urinary drainage is monitored closely for changes in volume, color, odor, and constituents. Urinalysis and urine cultures are indicated to follow the patient's progress. Care is taken to be sure that the collection bag is suspended below the patient's bladder to prevent reflux of urine into the urinary tract. However, the bag is kept off the floor to prevent contamination. Most urinary drainage systems do not require routine irrigation. If irrigation is necessary and prescribed, however, it should be performed carefully, with the use of sterile solution, with minimal pressure, consistent with the physician's instructions, and with strict asepsis without interruption of the closed drainage system.

◊ *Patient Education and Home Care.* If the patient is to be discharged from the hospital with the drainage system in place, measures are taken to be sure that both patient and family understand the importance of maintaining the system correctly and preventing infection. Verbal and written instructions and

(text continues on page 1173)

Nursing Care Plan 42–1

Care for the Patient Undergoing Surgery of the Kidney

Nursing Interventions	Rationale	Expected Outcomes

Nursing Diagnosis: High risk for ineffective airway clearance related to pain of high abdominal or flank incision, abdominal discomfort, and immobility

Goal: Adequate airway clearance

Nursing Interventions	Rationale	Expected Outcomes
1. Administer analgesics as prescribed.	1. Pain relief enables patient to take deep breaths and cough	• Takes deep breaths and coughs adequately when encouraged and assisted
2. Splint patient's incision with hands or pillow to assist patient in coughing.	2. Splints incision and promotes adequate cough and prevention of atelectasis	• Exhibits respiratory rate of 12–18/min • Exhibits normal breath sounds without adventitious sounds
3. Assist patient to change positions frequently.	3. Promotes drainage and inflation of all lobes of the lungs	• Exhibits full thoracic excursion without shallow respirations
4. Encourage use of incentive spirometer or blow bottles if indicated or prescribed.	4. Encourages adequate deep breaths	• Uses incentive spirometer or blow bottles with encouragement
5. Assist with and encourage early ambulation.	5. Mobilizes pulmonary secretions	• Splints own incision while taking deep breaths and coughing • Reports progressively less pain and discomfort with coughing and deep breaths • Exhibits normal blood gases and chest x-ray • Exhibits normal body temperature with no signs of atelectasis or pneumonia on assessment

Nursing Diagnosis: Pain and discomfort related to surgical incision, positioning, and stretching of muscles during kidney surgery

Goal: Relief of pain and discomfort

Nursing Interventions	Rationale	Expected Outcomes
1. Assess patient's level of pain.	1. Provides baseline for later assessment of pain-relief strategies	• Reports relief of severe pain and discomfort
2. Administer analgesics as prescribed.	2. Promotes pain relief	• Takes analgesia as prescribed
3. Apply moist heat and massage to areas with muscular aches and discomfort.	3. Promotes relaxation and relief of muscle pain and discomfort	• States rationale for use of moist heat and massage
4. Splint patient's incision with hands or pillow during movement or deep breathing and coughing exercises.	4. Minimizes sensation of pulling or tension on incision and provides sense of support to the patient	• Exercises aching muscles within recommendations • Gradually increases physical activity and exercise
5. Assist and encourage early ambulation.	5. Promotes resumption of muscle activity exercise	• Uses distraction, relaxation exercises, and imagery for pain relief • Exhibits absence of behavioral manifestations of pain and discomfort (*e.g.*, restlessness, perspiration, verbal expressions of pain) • Participates in deep-breathing and coughing exercises

Nursing Diagnosis: Fear and anxiety related to diagnosis, outcome of surgery, and alteration in urinary function

Goal: Reduction of fear and anxiety

Nursing Interventions	Rationale	Expected Outcomes
1. Assess patient's anxiety and fear levels prior to surgery if possible.	1. Provides a baseline for postoperative assessment	• Verbalizes reactions and feelings to staff
2. Assess patient's knowledge about pro-	2. Provides a basis for further teaching	• Shares reactions and feelings with spouse or significant other

(continued)

Nursing Care Plan 42-1 (Continued)

Care for the Patient Undergoing Surgery of the Kidney

Nursing Interventions	Rationale	Expected Outcomes
cedure and expected surgical outcome preoperatively.		• Grieves appropriately for self and for changes in role and function
3. Evaluate the meaning alterations have for patient and spouse or significant other.	3. Enables understanding of patient's reactions/responses to expected and unexpected results of surgery	• Identifies information needed to promote own adaptation and coping
4. Encourage patient to verbalize reactions, feelings, and fears.	4. Verbalization of responses is often necessary for patient's understanding of them and ultimate resolution.	• Participates in activities and events going on around immediate environment
5. Encourage patient to share feelings with spouse or significant other.	5. Enables patient and spouse to receive mutual support and reduces sense of isolation from each other	• Accepts visit from support person or participates in support group
6. Offer and arrange for visit from member of support group (e.g., ostomy group, if indicated).	6. Provides support from another person who has encountered the same or a similar surgical procedure and an example of how others have coped with the alteration	• Identifies support person from own experience and peer group

Nursing Diagnosis: Altered patterns of urinary elimination related to urinary drainage

Goal: Maintenance of urinary elimination

Nursing Interventions	Rationale	Expected Outcomes
1. Assess urinary drainage system immediately.	1. Provides basis for further assessment and action	• Exhibits adequate urinary output and patent drainage system
2. Assess adequacy of urinary output and patency of drainage system.	2. Provides baseline	• Exhibits urine output consistent with fluid intake
3. Use asepsis and hand washing when providing care and manipulating drainage system.	3. Prevents or reduces risk of contamination of urinary drainage system	• Demonstrates normal laboratory values: BUN, creatinine, and urine specific gravity
4. Maintain closed urinary drainage system.	4. Reduces risk of bacterial contamination and infection	• Exhibits sterile urine on urine culture
5. If irrigation of the drainage system is necessary, use gloves and sterile irrigating solution, and a closed drainage and irrigation system.	5. Permits irrigation when necessary while maintaining closed drainage system, minimizing risk of infection	• Exhibits clear, dilute urine without debris or encrustation in the drainage system
		• States rationale for avoiding manipulation of catheter, drainage or irrigation system
6. If irrigation is necessary and prescribed, it is carried out gently with sterile saline and the prescribed amount of irrigating fluid.	6. Maintains patency of the catheter or drainage system and prevents sudden increases in pressure in the urinary tract that may cause trauma, pressure on sutures or urinary tract structures, and pain	• Exhibits normal placement of urinary stent or ureteral catheters until removed by physician
		• Maintains closed urinary drainage system
		• Exhibits normal body temperature without signs or symptoms of urinary tract infection
7. Assist patient in turning and moving in bed and when ambulating to prevent displacement or accidental removal of urinary stent or ureteral catheters if in place.	7. Prevents trauma from accidental displacement of urinary stent or ureteral catheter, necessitating repeated instrumentation of the urinary tract (e.g., cytoscopy) to replace them	• Cleans urinary meatus and catheter with soap and water
		• Consumes adequate fluid intake (6–8 glasses of water or more per day unless contraindicated)
8. Observe urine color, volume, odor, and constituents.	8. Provides information about adequacy of urine output, condition and patency of drainage system, and debris in urine	• Urinary drainage system remains in place until removed or discontinued by physician
		• Maintains urinary drainage system without infection or obstruction
9. Minimize trauma and manipulation of catheter, drainage system, and urethra.	9. Reduces risk of contamination of drainage system and eliminates site of bacterial invasion	• Maintains urinary diversion as instructed

(continued)

> ## Nursing Care Plan 42-1 *(Continued)*
>
> ## Care for the Patient Undergoing Surgery of the Kidney

Nursing Interventions	Rationale	Expected Outcomes
		• Maintains self-care so that environment is odor-free
10. Clean meatus gently with soap during bath.	10. Removes debris and encrustations without causing trauma or contamination of urethra	• States rationale for close follow-up and maintains recommended schedule of appointments with health care providers
11. Anchor drainage tube.	11. Prevents movement or slipping of drainage tube, minimizing trauma and contamination of urethra or catheter	
12. Maintain adequate fluid intake.	12. Promotes adequate urinary output and prevents urinary stasis	
13. Assist with and encourage early ambulation while ensuring placement of urinary drainage system.	13. Minimizes cardiovascular and pulmonary complications while preventing loss, dislodging, or disruption of drainage system	
14. If patient is to be discharged with urinary drainage system (catheter) in place or a urinary diversion, instruct patient and family member in care.	14. Knowledge and understanding of the drainage system or urinary diversion are essential to prevent infection and other complications	

guidelines are provided to the patient prior to discharge. Specific indications that necessitate notifying the nurse or physician are identified.

Arrangements are made to have the patient visited at home by the visiting nurse. The specific instructions and guidelines given to the patient are shared with the visiting nurse prior to the home visit. She will assess the patient's ability to carry out the instructions and guidelines in the home and answer questions the patient or family may have about the procedure. Additionally, the nurse assesses the patient for infection and obstruction of the urinary tract, encourages an adequate fluid intake, and assesses the patient's compliance with recommendations. She reviews with the patient and family those signs, symptoms, problems, and questions that should be referred to the physician or other primary health care provider.

Specific nursing interventions for the patient undergoing kidney surgery are presented in Nursing Care Plan 42-1.

Evaluation

Expected Outcomes

1. Achieves effective airway clearance
   a. Exhibits clear and normal breath sounds
   b. Demonstrates normal respiratory rate and unrestricted thoracic excursion
   c. Performs deep-breathing exercises and coughs every 2 hours
   d. Uses the incentive spirometer as directed
   e. Demonstrates normal temperature and vital signs
2. Maintains cardiac output
   a. Demonstrates normal vital signs and arterial and central venous pressures
   b. Exhibits normal skin turgor, temperature, and color
   c. Demonstrates no additional losses of blood or fluid

   d. Exhibits absence of signs and symptoms of shock and hypovolemia (*e.g.*, decreased urine output, restlessness, rapid pulse)
3. Experiences reduced pain and discomfort
   a. Reports progressive decrease in pain
   b. Requires analgesics at less frequent intervals
   c. Turns, coughs, and takes deep breaths as suggested
   d. Ambulates progressively
   e. Uses moist heat and massage to reduce muscular aches
4. Maintains urinary elimination
   a. Demonstrates unobstructed urine flow from drainage tubes
   b. Exhibits normal fluid and electrolyte balance (normal skin turgor, serum electrolytes within normal range, absence of symptoms of imbalances)
   c. Reports no increase in pain, tenderness, or pressure at drainage site
   d. Exhibits cautious handling of own drainage system
   e. Washes hands before and after handling drainage system and handles it only when necessary
   f. States rationale for use and maintenance of a closed drainage system
   g. Identifies signs and symptoms that should be reported to the health care provider
   h. Exhibits absence of signs of infection (such as fever and pain)

In summary, surgery of the kidney may be performed to remove an obstruction, to reestablish drainage of the urinary tract, or to remove the kidney itself. The patient undergoing surgery of the kidney is often uncomfortable preoperatively, apprehensive about the surgical procedure, and fearful about the outcome. Postoperatively, the patient experiences pain and discomfort because of the location of the surgical incision and the positions necessary during surgery to provide adequate access to the surgical field. Major responsibilities of the nurse in the postoperative period include provision of adequate analgesia to relieve the patient's pain and make him comfortable so that he is able to take measures to prevent respiratory complications. Maintenance and monitoring of the urinary drainage system are crucial to prevent deterioration of kidney function and to assist in maintenance and replacement of fluids. The nurse also prepares the patient who is to go home with a drainage system in place to manage the system safely.

Chapter Summary

Treatment modalities used in the management of patients with renal and urinary tract disorders relieve symptoms, improve the patient's well-being, and prolong life. However, these treatment modalities do not duplicate kidney and urinary function, may not cure the disorder, and often present the patient with myriad other unexpected problems. The patient is subject to many side effects and complications of treatment. The treatment methods may consume considerable time, effort, and physical and emotional energy. The patient must adjust to new and different ways of managing functions considered basic to life. Social and economic well-being may be negatively affected by the disorder itself or by the demands imposed by the often "high-tech" treatment methods that are necessary. Stress and uncertainty are common in the patient and his family. The nurse caring for the patient treated with any of these modalities requires an understanding of their physical, social, psychologic, and economic impact on the patient and his family. The patient and his family will require assistance to master the skills needed for successful management and assistance in developing strategies to cope with the changes that result.

Bibliography

Books

Brenner BM, Coe FL, Rector FC Jr. Clinical Nephrology. Philadelphia, WB Saunders, 1987.

Catto ORD. Pregnancy and Renal Disorders. Dordrecht, Kluwer Academic Publishers, 1988.

DeWardener HE. The Kidney: An Outline of Normal and Abnormal Function, 5 ed. New York: Churchill Livingstone, 1985.

Gingell C and Abrams P (eds). Controversies and Innovations in Urologic Surgery. New York, Springer–Verlag, 1988.

Hanno PM and Wein AJ. A Clinical Manual of Urology. Englewood Cliffs, NJ, Appleton–Century–Crofts, 1987.

Kunin CM. Detection, Prevention and Management of Urinary Tract Infections. Philadelphia, Lea & Febiger, 1987.

Massry SG and Glassrock RJ. Textbook of Nephrology, 2nd ed. Baltimore, Williams & Wilkins, 1989.

Nolph KD. Peritoneal Dialysis, 3rd ed. Norwell, MA, Kluwer Academic, 1989.

Pak CYC. Renal Stone Disease: Pathogenesis, Prevention and Treatment. Boston, Nijhoff, 1987.

Riehle RA Jr. Principles of Extracorporeal Shock Wave Lithotripsy. New York: Churchill Livingstone, 1987.

Rose BD and Black RM. Manual of Clinical Problems in Nephrology. Boston, Little, Brown, 1988.

Schrier RW and Gottshalk CW (eds). Diseases of the Kidney. Boston: Little, Brown, 1988.

Journals
Asterisks indicate nursing research articles.

General

Chambers JK. Fluid and electrolyte problems in renal and urologic disorders. Nurs Clin North Am 1987 Dec; 22(4):815–826.

Chambers JK. Metabolic bone disorders. Imbalances of calcium and phosphorus. Nurs Clin North Am 1987 Dec; 22(4):861–872.

Chenevey B. Overview of fluids and electrolytes. Nurs Clin North Am 1987 Dec; 22(4):749–759.

Lancaster LE. Renal and endocrine regulation of water and electrolyte balance. Nurs Clin North Am 1987 Dec; 22(4):761–772.

Urinary Catheters

Brettman LR. Nosocomial infection risks associated with short-term and long-term inpatient care. Urology 1988 Sep; 32(3):21–23.

* Bristol S et al. The mythical danger of rapid urinary drainage. Am J Nurs 1989 Mar; 89(3):344–345.

* Dodds P and Hans AL. Distended urinary bladder drainage practices among hospital nurses. Appl Nurs Res 1990 May; 3(2):68–72.

Jaff MR and Paganini EP. Meeting the challenge of geriatric UTIs. Geriatrics 1989 Dec; 44(12):60–62, 65, 69.

Ouslander JG, Greengold B, and Chen S. Complications of chronic indwelling urinary catheters among male nursing home patients: A prospective study. J Urol 1987 Nov; 138(5):1191–1195.

Ouslander JG, Greengold B, and Chen S. External catheter use and urinary tract infections among incontinent male nursing home patients. J Am Geriatr Soc 1987 Dec; 35(12):1063–1070.

* Roe BH. Study of information given by nurses for catheter care to patients and their carers. J Adv Nurs 1989 Mar; 14(3):203–210.

* Roe BH. Use of bladder washouts: A study of nurses' recommendations. J Adv Nurs 1989 Mar; 14(3):494–500.

Seiler WO and Stähelin HB. Practical management of catheter-associated UTIs. Geriatrics 1988 Aug; 43(8):43–50.

* Watson R. A nursing trial of urinary sheath systems on male hospitalized patients. J Adv Nurs 1989 Jun; 14(6):217–225.

Zilkoski MW, Smucker DR, and Mayhew HE. Urinary tract infections in elderly patients. Postgrad Med 1988 Sep 1; 84(3):191–198.

Urinary Incontinence

Abdellah FG. Incontinence: Implications for health policy. Nurs Clin North Am 1988 Mar; 23(1):291–297.

* Brink CA et al. A digital test for pelvic muscle strength in older women with urinary incontinence. Nurs Res 1989 Jul/Aug; 38(4):196–199.

Cella M. The nursing costs of urinary incontinence in a nursing home population. Nurs Clin North Am 1988 Mar; 23(1):159–168.

* Creason NS et al. Prompted voiding therapy for urinary incontinence in aged female nursing home residents. J Adv Nurs 1989 Feb; 14(2): 120–126.

Jirovec MM, Brink CA, and Wells TJ. Nursing assessments in the inpatient geriatric population. Nurs Clin North Am 1988 Mar; 23(1):219–230.

McCormick KA, Scheve AAS, and Leahy E. Nursing management of urinary incontinence in geriatric inpatients. Nurs Clin North Am 1988 Mar; 23(1):231–264.

Morishita L. Nursing evaluation and treatment of geriatric outpatients with urinary incontinence: Geriatric day hospital model. A case study. Nurs Clin North Am 1988 Mar; 23(1):189–206.

National Institutes of Health Consensus Development Conference Statement. Urinary incontinence in adults. 1988 Oct 3–5; 7(5):1–114.

Newman DK et al. Restoring urinary continence. Am J Nurs 1991 Jan; 91(1):28–34.

Palmer MH. Incontinence: The magnitude of the problem. Nurs Clin North Am 1988 Mar; 23(1):139–157.

Palmer MH. Urinary incontinence. Nurs Clin North Am 1990 Dec; 25(4): 919–934.

Petrilli CO, Traughber B, and Schnelle JF. Behavioral management in the inpatient geriatric population. Nurs Clin North Am 1988 Mar; 23(1): 265–277.

Smith DAJ. Continence restoration in the homebound patient. Nurs Clin North Am 1988 Mar; 23(1):207–218.

* Whippo CC and Creason NS. Bacteriuria and urinary incontinence in aged female nursing home residents. J Adv Nurs 1989 Mar; 14(3): 217–225.

Wyman JF. Nursing assessment of the incontinent geriatric outpatient population. Nurs Clin North Am 1988 Mar; 23(1):169–187.

Dialysis (General)

Cloonan CC, Gatrell CB, Cushner HM. Emergencies in continuous dialysis patients: Diagnosis and management. Am J Emerg Med 1990 Mar; 8(2):134–138.

Frank DI. Psychosocial assessment of renal dialysis patients. ANNA J 1988 Aug; 15(4):207–210, 232.

Gibson S. Renal replacement therapy, I. Practitioner 1989 Nov 22; 233(1479):1535–1537.

Jones KR. Policy and research in end-stage renal disease. Image: J Nurs Scholarship 1987 Fall; 19(3):126–129.

Lewis SL. Alteration of host defense mechanisms in chronic dialysis patients. ANNA J 1990 Apr; 17(2):170–180.

Mailloux LU et al. Predictors of survival in patients undergoing dialysis. Am J Med 1988 May; 84(5):855–862.

Martino AN. Rehabilitation: How can more dialysis and transplant patients be fully rehabilitated? Transplant Proc 1987 Apr; 19(2 Suppl 2):107–110.

* Nyamathi A. Coping responses of spouses of MI patients and of hemodialysis patients as measured by the Jalowiec coping scale. J Cardiovasc Nurs 1987 Nov; 2(1):67–74.

* O'Brien ME. Compliance behavior and long-term maintenance dialysis. AM J Kidney Dis 1990 Mar; 15(3):209–214.

Port FK. Mortality and causes of death in patients with end-stage renal failure. Am J Kidney Dis 1990 Mar; 15(3):215–217.

Redrow M et al. Dialysis in the management of pregnant patients with renal insufficiency. Medicine 1988 Jun; 67(4):199–208.

Snyder TE. An exercise program for dialysis patients. Am J Nurs 1989 Mar; 89(3):362–364.

Hemodialysis, Continuous Arteriovenous Ultrafiltration, and Continuous Arteriovenous Hemodialysis

Betts DK and Crotty GD. Response to illness and compliance of long-term hemodialysis patients. ANNA J 1988 Apr; 15(2):96–99.

Chmielewsli C, Zellers L, and Eyer J. Continuous arteriovenous hemofiltration in the patient with hepatorenal syndrome: A case study. Crit Care Nurse Clin North Am 1990 Mar; 2(1):115–121.

Jameson MD and Wiegmann TB. Principles, uses and complications of hemodialysis. Med Clin North Am 1990 Jul; 74(4):945–960.

* Jones LC and Pruett SG. Self-care activities and processes used by hemodialysis patients. ANNA J 1988 Apr; 13(2):73–79.

Lawyer LA and Valasco A. Continuous arteriovenous hemodialysis in the ICU. Crit Care Nurs 1989 Jan; 9(1):29–41.

Lievaart A and Voerman HJ. Nursing management of continuous arteriovenous hemodialysis. Heart Lung 1991 Mar; 20(2):152–158.

Nahman NS Jr and Middendorf DF. Continuous arteriovenous hemofiltration. Med Clin North Am 1990 Jul; 74(4):975–984.

Paradiso C. Hemofiltration: An alternative to dialysis. Heart Lung 1989 May; 18(3):282–290.

Price CA. Continuous arteriovenous ultrafiltration: A monitoring guide for ICU nurses. Crit Care Nurs 1989 Jan; 9(1):12–19.

Peritoneal Dialysis

Cairns HS et al. Treatment of resistant CAPD peritonitis by temporary discontinuation of peritoneal dialysis. Clin Nephrol 1989 Jul; 32(1):27–30.

Carbone V. Continuous ambulatory peritoneal dialysis procedures. Crit Care Nurs 1987 Jul/Aug; 7(4):74–80.

Covalesky R. . . . About peritoneal dialysis. Nursing 1990 Apr; 20(4):91.

Goodenough GK, Lutz LJ, and Gregory MC. Home-based renal dialysis. Am Fam Physician 1988 Feb; 37(2):203–214.

Khanna R and Nolph KD. The physiology of peritoneal dialysis. Am J Nephrol 1989; 9(6):504–512.

Maher JF and Maher AT. Continuous ambulatory peritoneal dialysis. Am Fam Physician 1989 Nov; 40(5):187–192.

Nolph KD, Lindblad AS, and Novak JW. Continuous ambulatory peritoneal dialysis. N Engl J Med 1988 Jun 16; 318(24):1595–1600.

Saklayen MG. CAPD peritonitis: Incidence, pathogens, diagnosis, and management. Med Clin North Am 1990 Jul; 74(4):997–1010.

Steiner RW and Jalasz NA. Abdominal catastrophes and other unusual events in continuous ambulatory peritoneal dialysis patients. Am J Kidney Dis 1990 Jan; 15(1):1–7.

Strangio L. Peritoneal dialysis made easy. Nursing 1988 Jan; 18(1):43–46.

Twardowski ZJ. Peritoneal dialysis: Current technology and techniques. Postgrad Med 1989 Apr; 85(5):161–164, 167, 170, 173, 174, 181, 182.

Renal Surgery

Applegeet CJ. Nursing aspects of outpatient surgery. Urol Clin North Am 1987 Feb; 14(1):21–25.

Cass AS. Nephrectomy: A review of the surgical approaches. Today's OR Nurse 1990 Jun; 12(6):16–21.

Mackety CJ. Lasers in urology. Nurs Clin North Am 1990 Sep; 25(3):697–709.

McDonald HP Jr. Office ambulatory surgery in urology. Urol Clin North Am 1987 Feb; 14(1):27–30.

Cassady JF Jr. Regional anesthesia for urologic procedures. Urol Clin North Am 1987 Feb; 14(1):43–50.

Wetchler BV. Outpatient general and spinal anesthesia. Urol Clin North Am 1987 Feb; 14(1):31–42.

Information/Resources

Agencies

American Society for Artificial Internal Organs
  P.O. Box C Boca Raton, FL 33429 (407) 391-8589
American Association of Kidney Patients
  1 Davis Blvd., Suite LL1, Tampa, FL 33606 (813) 251-0725
National Institute of Diabetes and Digestive and Kidney Diseases
  National Institutes of Health, Bethesda, MD 20892
National Kidney Foundation
  30 East 33rd St., New York, NY 10016 (212) 889-2210

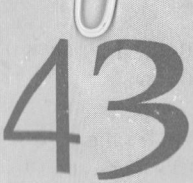

43

Management of Patients With Urinary and Renal Disorders

Learning Objectives

On completion of this chapter, the learner will be able to:

1. Identify factors contributing to urinary tract infections

2. Develop a teaching plan for the patient with urinary tract infection

3. Compare and contrast pyelonephritis, glomerulonephritis, and the nephrotic syndrome: causes, pathophysiologic changes, clinical manifestations, and management

4. Describe causes of acute renal failure and chronic renal failure

5. Use the nursing process as a framework for the care of patients with acute renal failure

6. Use the nursing process as a framework for the care of patients with chronic renal failure

7. Develop a postoperative nursing care plan and teaching plan for the patient undergoing kidney transplantation

8. Describe modalities for management of renal calculi (kidney stones)

9. Develop a teaching plan for the patient undergoing treatment for renal calculi (kidney stones)

10. Formulate preoperative and postoperative nursing diagnoses for the patient undergoing surgery for urinary diversion

11. Describe interstitial cystitis and its physical and psychologic impact on the patient

Disorders of the urinary tract and kidneys range from those that are usually easily treated infections to life-threatening disorders necessitating organ replacement or long-term treatment with dialysis. Recent advances in pharmacotherapeutics and technology have improved the diagnostic and treatment possibilities for these disorders. Additionally, those disorders that once required surgical intervention and prolonged recuperation can be treated today with noninvasive, nonsurgical techniques.

Infections of the Urinary Tract

Overview of Urinary Tract Infections

Urinary tract infections (UTIs) are caused by the presence of pathogenic microorganisms in the urinary tract, with or without signs and symptoms. Infection may occur at any site within the urinary tract and may affect the bladder (cystitis), urethra (urethritis), prostate (prostatitis), or kidney (pyelonephritis). The normal urinary tract is sterile except near the urethral orifice. General risk factors for UTI include inability or failure to empty the bladder completely, decreased natural host defenses, and instrumentation of the urinary tract, including catheterization. Diabetes, pregnancy, and neurologic disorders also increase the risk of UTI because they result in incomplete emptying of the bladder and stasis of urine.

Bacteriuria refers to the presence of bacteria in the urine. Infections in any part of the urinary tract may persist for months or even years without symptoms. Although uncommon, gram-negative sepsis and death may result. Two percent of all patients admitted to the hospital acquire urinary tract infections during their hospital stay, accounting for 500,000 hospital-acquired urinary tract infections each year. One percent, or 5000, of these become life-threatening. In at least 80% of hospital-acquired urinary tract infections, instrumentation of the urinary tract or catheterization is the precipitating cause. The incidence of infection in patients with indwelling urinary catheters rises dramatically after 2 days. Urinary tract infections may be categorized as *uncomplicated* (usually seen in young, healthy women), *complicated* (usually seen in men; usually the result of a structural or functional urinary abnormality in men or women), or *recurrent* (characterized by symptomatic episodes of infection alternating with symptom-free periods).

Factors Contributing to Urinary Tract Infections

The sterility of the bladder is maintained through several mechanisms: the physical barrier of the urethra, urine flow, various antibacterial enzymes and antibodies, and anti-adherence effects mediated by the mucosal cells of the bladder. When bladder function is normal, even large numbers of bacteria are normally quickly and effectively eliminated from the bladder through the combined effects of these mechanisms. For infection to occur, bacteria must gain access to the bladder, attach to and colonize the epithelium of the urinary tract to avoid being washed out with voiding, evade host defense mechanisms, and initiate inflammation. The majority of urinary tract infections result from fecal organisms that ascend from the perineum to the urethra and the bladder, adhering to the mucosal surfaces. An anti-adherence factor, glycosaminoglycan (GAG), normally exerts a nonspecific protective effect against various bacteria. The GAG molecule attracts water molecules, and a water barrier is formed that serves as a defensive layer between the bladder and the urine. GAG may be impaired by certain agents (cyclamate, saccharin, aspartame, and tryptophan metabolites). Research is under way to identify agents that may enhance anti-adherence activity. Another substance, Tamm-Horsfall protein, coats the bladder epithelial cells, is found in urine, and acts as a defense mechanism. Inflammation, abrasion of the urethral mucosa, incomplete emptying of the bladder, altered metabolic states (diabetes, pregnancy, gout),

and immunosuppression increase the risk of UTI by interfering with these normal mechanisms.

Urethrovesical reflux refers to the reflux (flowing back) of urine from the bladder into the urethra. It is caused by an increase in intrabladder pressure with coughing and sneezing, which may force the urine out of the bladder into the urethra. When the pressure returns to normal, the urine flows back into the bladder, bringing into the bladder the bacteria from the anterior portions of the urethra. Urethrovesical reflux is also caused by dysfunction of the bladder neck or urethra. The urethrovesical angle and urethral closure pressure may be altered with menopause, increasing the incidence of infection in postmenopausal women.

Ureterovesical or *vesicoureteral reflux* refers to the flowing back of urine from the bladder into one or both ureters. Normally, the ureterovesical junction prevents urine from traveling back into the ureter, particularly at the time of voiding. When the ureterovesical valve is impaired because of congenital causes or ureteral abnormalities, the bacteria may reach the kidneys and eventually destroy the kidneys.

Fecal contamination of the urethral meatus is a common route of entry of bacteria into the urinary tract. *Sexual intercourse* plays a role in the ascent of organisms from the perineum into the bladder in women. *Instrumentation of the urinary tract* (with catheterization or cystoscopic examinations) is also a major factor in urinary tract infections. *Stasis of urine* in the bladder may lead to infection, which may ultimately spread through the entire urinary system. Any *obstruction* to urinary flow increases the urinary tract's susceptibility to infection. Common causes of urinary tract obstruction are congenital anomalies, urethral strictures, contracture of the bladder neck, bladder tumors, calculi (stones) in the ureters or kidneys, compression of the ureters, and neurologic abnormalities. Infections may spread to the urinary tract by way of the blood (hematogenous spread) or the lymphatic system (lymphogenous spread). Common causes of UTI are summarized in Figure 43-1.

Six million patients are treated yearly for urinary tract infections; those affected are primarily women. Because the significance and treatment of UTI differ considerably in women and men, UTIs in women and men are discussed separately.

Urinary Tract Infections in Women.   The incidence of UTI is much higher in women than men because of obvious differences in anatomy. One of every five women in the United States develops a UTI sometime during her lifetime; 3% of these women experience recurrent disease. Discomfort and inconvenience secondary to UTI account for 6 to 7 million visits to the physician's office per year. Over 250,000 cases of acute pyelonephritis occur in the United States each year. Although most (90%) of episodes of UTI in women are simple, uncomplicated infections, such infections during pregnancy must be treated promptly even in the absence of symptoms because there is an increased risk of acute pyelonephritis and premature delivery.

Women are more prone to develop bladder infections because of the short female urethra and its anatomic proximity to the vagina, periurethral glands, and rectum. The organisms most frequently responsible for UTIs in women are those normally found in the gastrointestinal tract: *Escherichia coli* (80%) and *Staphylococcus saprophyticus* (11%). Other organisms responsible for urinary tract infections include *Proteus mirabilis;* one or more species of *Klebsiella, Enterobacter,* and

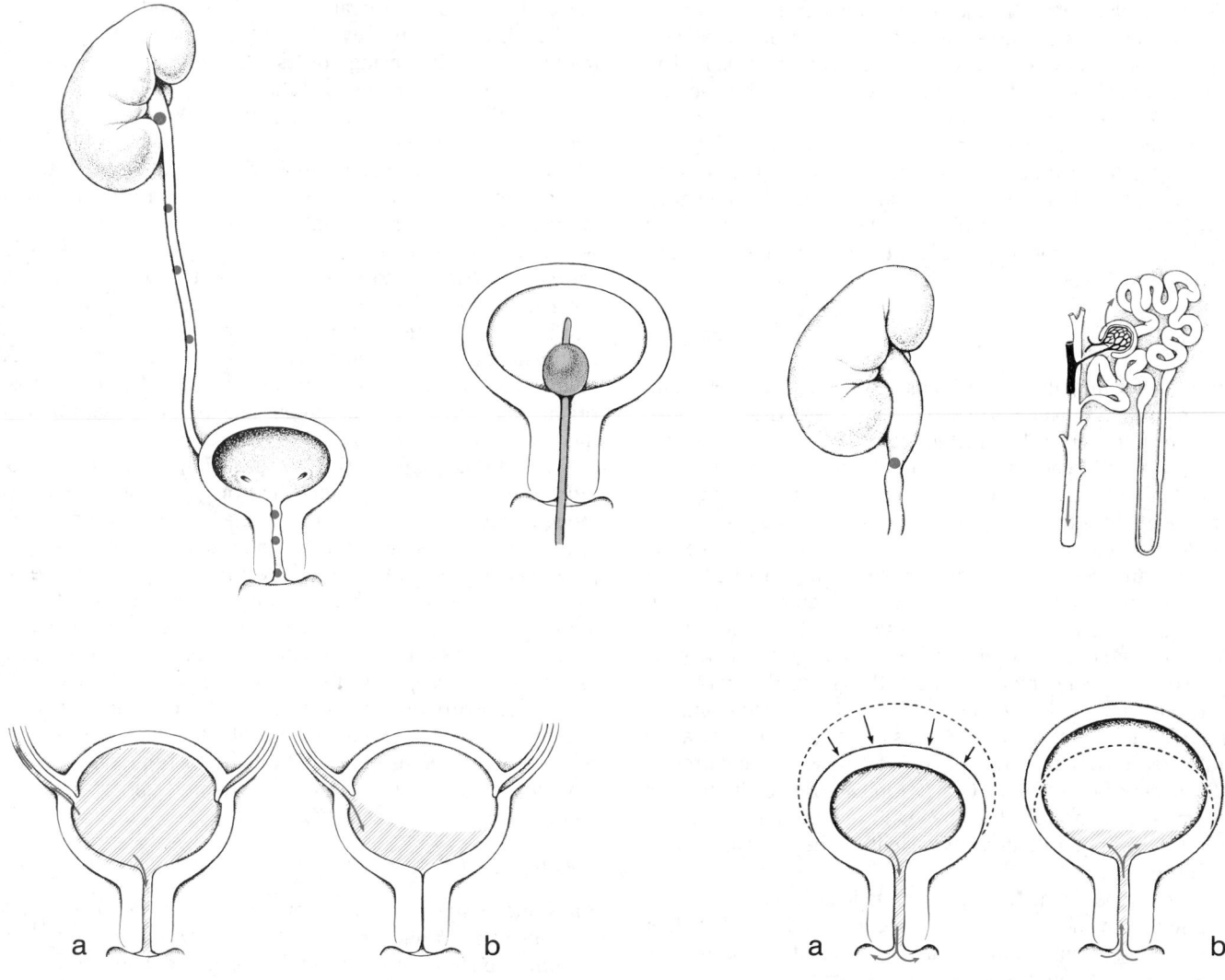

With failure of the ureterovesical valve action, urine moves up the ureters during voiding (*a*) and flows into the bladder when voiding has stopped (*b*). This prevents complete emptying of the bladder, stasis, and contamination of the ureters with bacteria-laden urine.

With coughing and straining, the bladder pressure rises, which may force urine from the bladder into the urethera (*a*). When bladder pressure returns to normal, the urine flows back to the bladder (*b*), which introduces bacteria from the urethra to the bladder.

Figure 43–1. Causes of urinary tract and kidney infections.

Pseudomonas; and the various enterococci. Bacterial colonization of the vaginal introitus with these fecal flora has been identified as an early initial event in UTI. Subsequently, flora colonize the urethra and then ascend to the bladder, where adhesion of microorganisms to the urothelium (the epithelium of the urinary tract) occurs. Adherence of bacteria tends to be higher during the early, estrogen-dependent phase of the menstrual cycle, with hysterectomy, and with aging, suggesting that hormonal status has a role. Additionally, atrophy of the urethral epithelium with aging may reduce the force of the urinary stream and therefore may reduce the effectiveness of the washing out of bacteria with voiding. Most women with uncomplicated urinary tract infections respond to a single course of treatment with an appropriate antimicrobial agent.

Urinary Tract Infections in Men.   Urinary tract infections in men result from ascending infection from the urethra, just as they do in women. However, the length of the urethra, its distance from the rectum in men, and the bactericidal properties of prostatic fluid generally protect men from urinary tract infections. As a result, urinary tract infections in men are much less frequent, and when they do occur, they usually indicate a functional or structural abnormality of the genitourinary tract. As a result, UTIs in men are generally considered "complicated." It has been recommended that men who experience even a single episode of UTI should undergo a urologic workup and be examined for urinary obstruction, prostatic infection, renal stones, or systemic disease. *Escherichia coli* is responsible for 75% of infections in men. Many other gram-negative bacteria, particularly *Proteus* species, are responsible for the remaining infections. Recurrent infections in men are usually relapses; that is, they are caused by the same organism. The cause may be failure of the treatment to eradicate the bacteria or the presence of structural or functional abnormalities of the urinary tract; bacteriuria is unlikely to be eradicated until the cause is treated. Urinary tract infections in men generally do not respond to short-term (3 to 4 days) therapy; such short-term therapy is likely to result in relapsing, recurrent urinary tract infections. Complicated UTIs in men often require treatment of 4 to 6 weeks.

Gerontologic Considerations

Urinary tract infection is the most common cause of acute bacterial sepsis in patients over 65 years of age. Gram-negative sepsis resulting from UTI in the elderly is associated with a mortality rate exceeding 50%. Structural abnormalities and neurogenic bladder secondary to strokes or autonomic neuropathy of diabetes may prevent complete emptying of the bladder and lead to an increased risk of UTI. When indwelling catheters are used to treat these problems, the risk of UTI rises dramatically, because the presence of a catheter in the bladder causes increased adherence of bacteria to the bladder wall. The incidence of bacteriuria increases with age and disability, with women affected more frequently than men. Elderly women often have incomplete emptying of the bladder and urinary stasis. Postmenopausal women are susceptible to colonization and increased adherence of bacteria to the vagina and urethra in the absence of estrogen. Oral or topical estrogen is effective in some postmenopausal women with recurrent cystitis to restore the glycogen content of vaginal epithelial cells and an acidic *p*H.

The antibacterial activity of prostatic secretions that protects men from bacterial colonization of the urethra and bladder decreases with aging. Although urinary tract infections are rare in men, the prevalence in men over 65 years of age approaches that of women in the same age group. The dramatic rise in UTI in men as they get older is due largely to prostatic hyperplasia or carcinoma, strictures of the urethra, and neuropathic bladder. Renal calculi, the use of indwelling urinary catheters, and debilitating illness are other contributing factors. The use of catheterization or cystoscopy in the evaluation or treatment may contribute further to UTI. Bacteriuria is more common in men with confusion or dementia and those with bowel or bladder incontinence. Chronic bacterial prostatitis should be suspected in the elderly patient with relapsing urinary tract infections because it is the most common cause of such infections. Transurethral resection (TUR) of the prostate gland may help to reduce its incidence. Infected prostatic calculi (stones) are another cause of urinary tract infections in elderly men; continuous suppressive antimicrobial therapy or surgical treatment may be necessary to treat these infections.

Nursing home patients are a major reservoir of pathogens resistant to many antibiotics because of the high incidence of chronic illness in that population, the frequent use of antimicrobial drugs, the high number and close proximity of patients with indwelling urinary catheters, and the presence of infected pressure ulcers. Immobility and related incomplete bladder emptying may be a factor in UTI in nursing home patients. UTI is more likely to occur with the use of a bedpan than with use of a commode or toilet. Diligence in hand washing, careful perineal care, and separation of catheterized patients from others with catheters may decrease the incidence of urinary tract infections in nursing homes.

The organisms responsible for urinary tract infections in the institutionalized elderly may differ from those found in patients residing in the community; this is thought to be due in part to the frequent use of antibiotics by patients in nursing homes. *Escherichia coli* is the most common organism seen in the elderly in the community or hospital. However, patients with indwelling catheters are more likely to be infected with *Proteus, Klebsiella, Pseudomonas,* or enterococci. Patients in nursing homes may require 7 to 10 days of medication for the treatment to be effective. Controversy exists about the need for treatment of asymptomatic bacteriuria in the institutionalized elderly patient because of the possibility that antibiotic-resistant organisms produced by treatment may be of greater threat to the patient if sepsis occurs.

The recognition of UTI and sepsis in the elderly is made more difficult by the frequent lack of typical symptoms. Although frequency, urgency, and dysuria may occur, nonspecific symptoms such as altered sensorium, lethargy, anorexia, hyperventilation, and a low-grade fever may be the only clues to the presence of a UTI. The probability of frequent reinfection increases with advancing age. Treatment must be initiated as soon as infection is detected because of the high mortality associated with sepsis in the elderly. Age-related changes in intestinal absorption of medications and decreased renal function and hepatic flow may necessitate alterations in the antimicrobial regimen used to treat urinary tract infections in the elderly. Renal function must be monitored and the dose of medications altered accordingly.

Clinical Manifestations

Signs and symptoms of UTI cover a broad range. Frequently, the patient is asymptomatic and is found to have bacteria in the urine (bacteriuria) while undergoing a routine physical examination. Signs and symptoms of lower UTI (cystitis) include frequent pain and burning on urination, sometimes accompanied by spasms in the region of the bladder and suprapubic area. Hematuria and back pain may also be present. Signs and symptoms of upper UTI (pyelonephritis) include fever, chills, flank pain, and painful urination. Upon physical examination, there is pain and tenderness in the area of the costovertebral angle (CVA). If extensive damage to the kidneys has occurred, manifestations of renal failure may be present and may include nausea, vomiting, pruritus, weight loss, edema, and shortness of breath.

Diagnostic Evaluation

Urinary tract infection is diagnosed by the presence of bacteria in the urine. A colony count of at least 100,000 colonies per milliliter of urine on a clean-catch midstream or catheterized specimen has been considered the major criterion for the presence of infection. However, UTI and subsequent sepsis have occurred with lower bacterial colony counts. Approximately one-third of women with symptoms of acute infections will have negative midstream urine cultures and may go untreated if 100,000 CFU (colony-forming units)/ml is used as the criterion for infection. The presence of *any* bacteria in specimens obtained by suprapubic needle aspiration of the urinary bladder or catheterization is considered indicative of infection. Microscopic hematuria is present in approximately 50% of patients with acute infection. White blood cells are also detected in urinary tract infections; a large number of these cells may be associated with upper rather than lower UTI. Urine cultures may be obtained to identify the specific organism present. However, because of the high probability that the organism in young women with a first or occasional UTI is *Escherichia coli,* cultures are often omitted. It has been suggested that urinalysis and urine cultures are indicated only for patients with persistent or recurrent symptoms, or for neutropenic patients, renal transplant patients, or patients who have indwelling urinary catheters. Specific indications for urine cultures are identified in Table 43-1.

Acute urethritis due to sexually transmitted organisms (*i.e.,* *Chlamydia trachomatis, Neisseria gonorrhoeae,* and herpes simplex) or acute vaginitis infections (caused by *Trichomonas* or *Candida*) may be responsible for symptoms similar to those of UTI, requiring evaluation to distinguish between them. Dysuria that occurs when the urine flows over the perineum is generally associated with vaginitis rather than UTI. Urine cultures are usually performed in men with infections of the urinary tract because of the likelihood of structural or functional abnormalities as the cause. A culture of prostatic fluid or urine voided after massage of the prostate gland may be obtained.

In persons at high risk for complicated or recurring infection, diagnostic studies such as intravenous pyelography (IVP) and cystography may be carried out following treatment to determine if the infection is secondary to abnormalities of the urinary tract. An excretory urogram or ultrasonic evaluation, cystoscopy, and urodynamic studies may be indicated to identify the cause of recurrent infection that is resistant to treatment. IVP, retrograde cystography or cystoscopy, and ultrasonography may be used to determine if calculi, a renal mass or abscess, hydronephrosis, or prostatic hypertrophy is a factor in the infection.

Cystitis (Lower Urinary Tract Infection)

Cystitis is an inflammation of the urinary bladder that is most often caused by an ascending infection from the urethra. It may be caused by urine flowing back from the urethra into the bladder (urethrovesical reflux), fecal contamination, or the use of a catheter or cystoscope. (Interstitial cystitis, a noninfectious, inflammatory disorder of the bladder characterized by symptoms similar to those of lower urinary tract infection, is discussed on p. 1215.)

Cystitis occurs more often in women than men. The distal portion of the urethra is frequently colonized with bacteria

TABLE 43-1. *Indications for Urine Cultures in Patients With Symptoms of Urinary Tract Infections (UTIs)*

Complicated or unusual features

History of UTI in the past 3 weeks (suggests relapse)

Persistence of symptoms for 7 days or more

Recent hospitalization or catheterization (suggests nosocomial infection)

Pregnancy

following colonization of the vaginal introitus. A defect of the mucosa of the urethra, vagina, or external genitalia may allow organisms to adhere and colonize at periurethral sites and to invade the bladder. Acute cystitis in women is usually caused by *Escherichia coli* and often follows sexual intercourse. The onset of sexual activity is associated with an increased frequency of urinary tract infections in women, particularly in women who fail to void after intercourse; voiding may wash bacteria from the bladder. Infection is also associated with diaphragm–spermicide contraception. Diaphragm–spermicide use may cause a partial urethral obstruction and serve as a foreign body. Additionally, it has been shown to alter the vaginal flora, which may be a factor in colonization of the vagina by *Escherichia coli* and alterations in bacterial attachment to the epithelial cells of the urinary tract. Cystitis in men is secondary to some other factor (*i.e.,* infected prostate, epididymitis, or bladder stones). Consequently, men will undergo a diagnostic workup after the first episode of cystitis to identify and treat the cause.

The patient with cystitis experiences urgency, frequency, burning and pain on urination, nocturia, and pain or spasm in the region of the bladder and suprapubic area. Pyuria (white blood cells in the urine), bacteria, and often red blood cells (hematuria) are found on examination of the urine. Office culturing kits provide general qualitative information about the bacterial colony count and identify the organism as grampositive or gram-negative.

Management

The ideal treatment for UTI is an antibacterial agent that effectively eradicates bacteria from the urinary tract with minimal effects on fecal and vaginal flora, thereby minimizing the incidence of vaginal yeast infections. (Yeast vaginitis occurs in as many as 25% of patients treated with antimicrobial agents that affect vaginal flora and often causes more symptoms and is more difficult and more costly to treat than the original UTI.) Additionally, the drug should be low in cost and should produce few side effects and low resistance. Because the organism in initial, uncomplicated urinary tract infections in women is most likely *Escherichia coli* or other fecal flora, the drug should also be effective against these organisms. Nitrofurantoin generally meets these requirements; nausea, the major gastrointestinal side effect, can be minimized by the administration of nitrofurantoin macrocrystals (Macrodantin) with meals. Other medications that have been used effectively for uncomplicated lower urinary tract infections include sulfisoxazole (Gantrisin) and trimethoprim-sulfamethoxazole (TMP/SMZ, Bactrim or Septra). Drugs such as ampicillin and amoxicillin increase the likelihood of drug-resistant organisms. Various treatment regimens have been used successfully to treat uncomplicated lower urinary tract infections in women; these include single-dose administration, short-course (3 to 4 days) medication regimens, or 7- to 10-day courses. Regardless of the regimen prescribed, the patient is instructed to take *all* the doses prescribed, even if relief of symptoms occurs promptly. Longer medication courses are indicated for men, pregnant women, and women with pyelonephritis and with other types of complicated urinary tract infections.

Recurrence. Although treatment of UTI for 3 days is usually adequate in women, recurrence of infection occurs in about 20% of women treated for uncomplicated UTI. Repeated infections at close intervals suggest persistence (same organism); this is relatively rare in women and if it occurs it is a cause for referral to a urologist to investigate and correct abnormalities. It may also occasionally occur if initial treatment was inadequate or administered for too short a period of time. Recurrent infections in men are usually due to persistence of the same organism; further evaluation and treatment are indicated.

Reinfection of the female patient with new bacteria is more common than persistence of the initial bacteria. If the diagnostic evaluation reveals no structural abnormalities in the urinary tract, the woman with recurrent urinary tract infections may be instructed to begin treatment on her own whenever symptoms occur and to contact the health care provider only with persistence of symptoms or the occurrence of fever. This patient is instructed in the use of dip-slide culture devices to detect the presence of bacteria.

Long-term use of antimicrobial agents decreases the risk of reinfection and may be indicated in patients with recurrent infections. If recurrence is caused by persistent bacteria from preceding infections, the causative factor (*i.e.*, stone, abscess), if one is present, must be treated. Following treatment and sterilization of the urine, low-dose preventive therapy (nitrofurantoin macrocrystals) each night at bedtime is often used.

With recurrence after completion of antimicrobials, another short course (3 to 4 days) of full-dose antimicrobial therapy followed by a regular bedtime dose of antimicrobials may be prescribed. If there is no recurrence, medication is taken every other night for 6 to 7 months. Other options include a dose of an antimicrobial agent following sexual intercourse, a dose of the antimicrobial at bedtime, or a dose of the prescribed antimicrobial every other night or three times per week.

► Nursing Process
The Patient With Lower Urinary Tract Infection

◊ Assessment

A history of urinary signs and symptoms is obtained from the patient with a suspected urinary tract infection. The presence of pain, frequency, urgency, and hesitancy and changes in urine are assessed, documented, and reported. The patient's usual pattern of voiding is assessed to detect factors that may predispose the patient to urinary tract infection. Infrequent emptying of the bladder, the association of symptoms of urinary tract infection with sexual intercourse, contraceptive practices, and personal hygiene are assessed. The patient's knowledge about prescribed antimicrobial medications and preventive health care measures is also assessed. Additionally, the patient's urine is checked for volume, color, concentration, cloudiness, and odor, all of which are altered by bacteria in the urinary tract.

◊ Nursing Diagnoses

Based on the assessment data, the nursing diagnoses may include the following:

- Pain and discomfort related to inflammation and infection of the urethra, bladder, and other urinary tract structures

- Knowledge deficit regarding factors predisposing to infection and recurrence, detection and prevention of recurrence, and pharmacologic therapy

◊ Planning and Implementation

◊ *Goals:*   The patient's major goals may include relief of pain and discomfort and increased knowledge of preventive measures and treatment modalities.

◊ Nursing Interventions

◊ *Relieving Pain and Discomfort.*   Dysuria, frequency, hesitancy, urgency, and other types of discomfort associated with urinary tract infection are frequently relieved quickly once antimicrobial therapy is initiated. Antispasmodic drugs may be useful in relieving bladder irritability and pain. Aspirin, heat to the perineum, and hot tub baths help relieve urgency, discomfort, and spasm. The patient is encouraged to drink liberal amounts of fluids to promote renal blood flow and to flush the bacteria from the urinary tract. However, fluids that may be irritating to the bladder (*e.g.*, coffee, tea, colas) are avoided. Frequent voiding (every 2 to 3 hours) is encouraged to empty the bladder completely, because this can significantly lower urine bacterial counts, reduce urinary stasis, and prevent reinfection.

◊ *Patient Education and Home Health Care.*   Women who have repeated urinary tract infections should receive detailed instructions on the following points:

1. Reduce concentrations of pathogens at the vaginal introitus by hygienic measures:
   a. Shower rather than bathe in a tub, because bacteria in the bath water may enter the urethra.
   b. Cleanse around the perineum and urethral meatus after each bowel movement.
2. Drink liberal amounts of fluid during the day to flush out bacteria.
3. Void every 2 to 3 hours during the day and completely empty the bladder. This prevents overdistention of the bladder and compromised blood supply to the bladder wall, which predispose the patient to urinary tract infection.
4. If sexual intercourse is the initiating event for development of bacteriuria:
   a. Void immediately after sexual intercourse.
   b. Take the prescribed single dose of an oral antimicrobial agent following sexual intercourse.
5. If bacteria continue to appear in the urine, long-term antimicrobial therapy may be required to prevent colonization of the periurethral area and recurrence of infection. The medication should be taken after emptying the bladder just before going to bed to ensure adequate concentration of the drug during the overnight period.
6. If prescribed, monitor and test the urine for bacteria with dip-slides (Microstix) as follows:
   a. Wash around the urethral meatus several times, using different washcloths.
   b. Collect a midstream urine specimen.
   c. Remove a slide from its container, dip it into the urine sample, and return it to the container.
   d. Incubate the slide at room temperature according to product directions.

e. Read the results by comparing the slide with the colony density chart that comes with the product.

f. Initiate therapy as prescribed and complete the full prescribed course of medication.

g. Notify health care provider if fever occurs or if signs and symptoms persist.

7. See health care provider regularly for follow-up, recurrence of symptoms, infections nonresponsive to treatment, or further involvement of the urinary tract.

▷ Evaluation

Expected Outcomes

1. Experiences relief of pain, urgency, dysuria, and fever.
   a. Reports absence of pain, urgency, dysuria, hesitancy on voiding.
   b. Takes antimicrobial agent as prescribed.
   c. Takes analgesics and hot tub baths for discomfort.
   d. Drinks 8 to 10 glasses of fluids daily.
   e. Voids every 2 to 3 hours.
   f. Voids urine that is clear and free from odor.
2. Increases knowledge of preventive measures and prescribed treatment modalities.
   a. States rationale for using shower rather than tub for daily hygiene.
   b. Uses appropriate cleansing action following each bowel movement.
   c. States rationale for appropriate cleansing method following each bowel movement.
   d. Voids frequently during day and at bedtime to prevent overdistention of bladder.
   e. Voids immediately after sexual intercourse.
   f. Takes oral antimicrobial agents as prescribed following sexual intercourse.
   g. Takes entire course of antimicrobial agent as prescribed.
   h. Demonstrates correct use of dipslides to monitor for urinary tract infection.
   i. Reports recurrence of symptoms to health care provider.
   j. Adheres to follow-up schedule as recommended by health care provider.
   k. Reports symptoms of further involvement of the urinary tract.

Pyelonephritis (Upper Urinary Tract Infection)

Pyelonephritis is a bacterial infection of the renal pelvis, tubules, and interstitial tissue of one or both kidneys. Bacteria may gain access to the bladder via the urethra and ascend to the kidney or may reach the kidney through the bloodstream. Pyelonephritis is frequently secondary to ureterovesical reflux, in which an incompetent ureterovesical valve allows the urine to back up (reflux) into the ureters, usually at the time of voiding (see Fig. 43-1). Urinary tract obstruction (which increases the susceptibility of the kidneys to infection) and renal diseases are among other causes. Pyelonephritis may be acute or chronic.

Acute pyelonephritis is an active infection that presents with chills and fever, flank pain, costovertebral angle tenderness, leukocytosis, bacteria and white blood cells in the urine, and frequently symptoms of lower urinary tract involvement, such as dysuria and frequency. Upper urinary tract infection is associated with antibody coating of the bacteria in the urine. (Antibodies coat the bacteria in the renal medulla; when the bacteria are excreted in the urine, the immunofluorescent test can detect the antibody coating.)

There are areas of inflammation in the kidney with interstitial infiltrations of inflammatory cells that in time may produce tubular destruction and abscess formation. Low-grade interstitial inflammation may result in atrophy and destruction of tubules and the glomeruli. Eventually, when pyelonephritis becomes chronic, the kidneys become scarred, contracted, and nonfunctioning.

Diagnostic Evaluation and Management.   An intravenous urogram and other diagnostic tests may be performed to locate any obstruction in the urinary tract. The relief of obstruction is essential to save the kidney from destruction. The treatment is essentially the same as that for cystitis, although the course of treatment is likely to be longer. Urine culture and sensitivity tests are obtained because the choice of antimicrobial agent is determined by the causative organism. Medication should produce sustained antibacterial concentration of the drugs in the renal parenchyma. The antimicrobial drug must be given for a period long enough to prevent reseeding of residual foci of infection.

A possible problem in treatment is a chronic or recurring infection persisting for months or years without symptoms. After the initial antimicrobial regimen, the patient is maintained on continuous antimicrobial treatment until there is no evidence of infection, all causative factors have been treated or controlled, and kidney function is stabilized. The patient is monitored with serum creatinine determinations and blood counts for the duration of the long-term therapy.

Chronic Pyelonephritis

Repeated bouts of acute pyelonephritis may lead to chronic pyelonephritis (chronic interstitial nephritis). However, recent evidence suggests that chronic pyelonephritis is less frequently a cause of chronic renal failure than previously thought.

The patient with chronic pyelonephritis usually has no symptoms of infection unless an acute exacerbation occurs. Noticeable signs may include fatigue, headache, poor appetite, polyuria, excessive thirst, and weight loss. Persistent and recurring infection may produce progressive scarring of the kidney with ultimate kidney failure.

Complications of chronic pyelonephritis include end-stage renal disease (from progressive loss of nephrons secondary to chronic inflammation and scarring), hypertension, and formation of kidney stones (from chronic infection with urea-splitting organisms, resulting in stone formation).

Diagnostic Evaluation and Management.   The extent of the disease is assessed by intravenous urogram and measurements of BUN, creatinine levels, and creatinine clearance. Eradication of bacteria from the urine is undertaken if present. The choice of an antimicrobial is based on culture identification of the pathogen. If the urine cannot be made bacteria-free, nitrofurantoin or a combination of sulfamethoxazole and trimethoprim may be used to suppress bacterial growth. Hypertension and chronic renal failure are the major complications of chronic pyelonephritis. Compromised renal function alters the excretion of antimicrobial agents and necessitates careful monitoring of renal function; this is particularly important if the medications are potentially toxic to the kidneys.

Perinephric Abscess

Perinephric abscess is an abscess in the fatty tissue of the kidney that may arise secondary to an infection of the kidney or as a hematogenous (spread through the bloodstream) infection originating elsewhere in the body. It may be secondary to a staphylococcal infection of the kidney or to the spread of infection from adjacent areas, such as from diverticulitis or appendicitis. The symptoms often are acute in onset, with chills, fever, leukocytosis, and other signs of suppuration. Locally, there is flank or abdominal tenderness or pain. The patient usually appears seriously ill.

Management. The treatment consists of administration of the appropriate antimicrobial agent and incision and drainage of the abscess. Drains are usually inserted and left in the perinephric space until all significant drainage has ceased. Because the drainage often is profuse, frequent changes of the outer dressings may be necessary. As in the treatment of an abscess in any site, the patient is monitored for sepsis, fluid intake and output, and general response to treatment.

Carbuncle of the Kidney

Carbuncle of the kidney is an infection of hematogenous origin that is caused usually by *Staphylococcus*. It usually follows a cutaneous boil or carbuncle and is characterized by fever, malaise, and dull pain in the region of the kidney. This type of infection, if recognized, usually subsides with chemotherapy and penicillin. Recently, carbuncles of the kidney from gramnegative bacteria have increased in incidence.

Tuberculosis of the Kidney and Genitourinary Tract

Pathophysiology and Clinical Manifestations. Tuberculosis of the kidney and urinary tract is caused by the organism *Mycobacterium tuberculosis* and usually spreads from the lungs by way of the bloodstream to the kidneys and to other organs of the genitourinary tract. At first the symptoms are mild; there is usually a slight afternoon fever and a loss of weight and appetite. The process of tuberculosis generally starts in one of the renal pyramids; ulceration into the kidney pelvis follows. The organisms are carried down with the urine into the bladder so that the bladder is likely to become infected.

Tuberculosis of the lower genitourinary tract is always secondary to renal tuberculosis, with the infection having disseminated downward. In the male, the prostate and epididymis may become infected.

Tuberculosis of the urinary bladder is an extension of tuberculosis of a kidney. This disease gives rise to several small ulcers, the majority of them near the trigone of the bladder. The symptoms of bladder tuberculosis are those of cystitis in general but with an unusual degree of bladder irritability because of the location of the lesions. Suggestive early symptoms of this disease are an increased urinary output that contains considerable pus and yet is acid in reaction (in nearly all other pyurias the urine is alkaline) and hematuria (either microscopic or gross). The features of pain, dysuria, and urinary frequency, when they occur, are due to bladder infection. Signs of bladder irritability (frequency, nocturia) are a later manifestation of the disease.

Management. A search for tuberculosis elsewhere in the body is conducted when tuberculosis of the kidney or urinary tract is found. Inquiry is made to determine if the patient has had known exposure to tuberculosis. Three or more clean-voided first morning urine specimens are obtained for culture for *M. tuberculosis*.

The objective of treatment is to eradicate the offending organism. Combinations of ethambutol, isoniazid, and rifampin are used to delay the emergence of resistant organisms. Shorter-course chemotherapy (4 months) has been effective in eradicating the organism and in penetrating renal tissue. Because renal tuberculosis is a manifestation of a systemic disease, all measures to promote the general health of the person are used. Surgical intervention may be necessary to prevent obstructive problems and to remove an extensively diseased kidney. The patient is counseled about the need for follow-up examinations (urine cultures, excretory urograms) usually for a period of a year.

Treatment will need to be reinstituted if a relapse occurs and the tubercle bacilli again invade the genitourinary tract. Ureteral stenosis or bladder contractures are complications that may develop during the healing process.

In summary, UTIs range from uncomplicated infections that result from contamination of the urethra and bladder with sexual intercourse to complicated infections that require careful follow-up and long-term therapy to prevent damage to the kidneys and renal dysfunction. The elderly patient is at particular risk of urinary tract infection; in this segment of the population, UTI may lead to life-threatening sepsis. Nursing care for the patient with UTI focuses on identification and assessment of those factors that increase the patient's risk of infection and education about strategies to reduce those risks. Although many of the clinical manifestations of uncomplicated UTI are not life-threatening, they are often uncomfortable and distressing to the patient, requiring assistance and understanding on the part of the nurse.

Acute Glomerulonephritis

Acute glomerulonephritis refers to a group of kidney diseases in which there is an inflammatory reaction in the glomeruli. It is not an infection of the kidney *per se* but rather the result of untoward side effects of the defense mechanism of the body. In most types of glomerulonephritis, IgG, the major immunoglobulin (antibody) found in the serum of humans, can be detected in the glomerular capillary walls. As a result of an antigen–antibody reaction, aggregates of molecules (complexes) are formed and circulate throughout the body. Some of these complexes lodge in the glomeruli, the filtering bed of the kidney, and induce an inflammatory response.

In most cases, the stimulus of the reaction is group A streptococcal infection of the throat, which ordinarily precedes the onset of glomerulonephritis by an interval of 2 to 3 weeks. The streptococcal product, acting as an antigen, stimulates circulating antibodies and results in deposit of the complexes in the glomeruli, producing injury to the kidney. Glomerulonephritis may also follow scarlet fever and impetigo (infection of the skin) and acute viral infections (upper respiratory infections, mumps, varicella, Epstein–Barr, hepatitis B, and HIV infections). The many forms of glomerulonephritis include proliferative, membranous, membranoproliferative, focal proliferative, and rapidly progressive. The pathology of these various types of glomerulonephritis has yet to be defined satisfactorily.

Pathophysiology.   Cellular proliferation (increased production of endothelial cells lining the glomerulus), infiltration of the glomerulus by leukocytes, and thickening of the glomerular filtration membrane or basement membrane result in scarring and loss of filtering surface. In acute glomerulonephritis, the kidneys become large, swollen, and congested. All the renal tissues—glomeruli, tubules, and blood vessels—are affected in all forms of glomerulonephritis, but in each form the tissues are involved to varying degrees. In some patients, antigens outside the body (bacteria, viruses) initiate the process, resulting in the complexes being deposited in the glomeruli. In other patients, the membrane tissue of the kidney becomes altered by disease and serves as the inciting antigen. With electron-microscopy and immunofluorescent identification of the immune mechanism, the nature of the lesion can be studied.

Clinical Manifestations.   The disease may be so mild that it is discovered inadvertently through a routine urinalysis, or the history may reveal a preceding episode of pharyngitis or tonsillitis with fever. In the more severe form of the disease, the patient presents with headache, malaise, facial edema, and flank pain. Mild to severe hypertension is seen, and tenderness over the costovertebral angle (CVA) is common. (The costovertebral angles, used as landmarks, are the angles formed on each side of the body by the bottom rib of the rib cage and the vertebral column.)

Acute glomerulonephritis is predominantly a disease of youth. Some poststreptococcal cases that develop later are acute exacerbations of a glomerulonephritis that is already present but undetected. Viral forms of glomerulonephritis occur across the age spectrum.

Diagnostic Evaluation.   The urine is scanty and often bloody; there may even be *no* urine (anuria) for 1 or more days, although this is rare. Usually, early in the disease, the patient voids 50 to 200 ml daily of a cola-colored urine, with an elevated specific gravity (specific gravity may be low if the renal concentrating ability is impaired) and a thick sediment of red blood cells, leukocytes, and all kinds of casts. (RBC casts indicate glomerular injury.) The urine contains large amounts of protein. A large percentage of patients have an increased antistreptolysin O titer as a result of a reaction to the streptococcal organism. Usually, there are rising values of BUN and serum creatinine. The patient may be anemic because of loss of the red blood cells in the urine and changes in the hematopoietic mechanism of the body.

Serial determinations of antistreptolysin O (ASO) or anti-Dnase B (ADB) titers are often elevated in poststreptococcal glomerulonephritis. Serum complement levels may be decreased but generally return to normal within 2 to 8 weeks. Renal biopsy may be obtained to aid in diagnosis.

As the patient improves, the amount of urine increases, while the urinary protein and urinary sediment diminish. Usually, more than 90% of children recover. The percentage of recovery for adults is not well established but is probably about 70%. Some patients become severely uremic within weeks and re-

quire dialysis for survival. Others, after a period of apparent recovery, insidiously develop chronic glomerulonephritis.

Management.   The goals of management are to protect the patient's poorly functioning kidneys and to treat complications promptly. If residual streptococcal infection is suspected, penicillin is prescribed. Bed rest is encouraged during the acute phase until the urine clears and the BUN, creatinine, and blood pressure return to normal. Rest also facilitates diuresis. The urine of the patient may serve as a guide to the duration of bed rest, because excessive activity may increase proteinuria and hematuria.

Dietary protein is restricted when renal insufficiency and nitrogen retention (elevated BUN) develop. Sodium is restricted when hypertension, edema, and congestive heart failure are present. Diuretics and antihypertensive agents may be prescribed to control hypertension. Carbohydrates are given liberally to provide energy and reduce the catabolism of protein.

Fluids are given according to the patient's fluid losses and daily body weight. Insensible fluid loss through respiration and feces (500 to 1000 ml) is considered in estimating fluid loss. The intake and output are measured and recorded. Usually, diuresis begins 1 to 2 weeks after the onset of symptoms. Edema decreases and hypertension lessens. However, proteinuria and microscopic hematuria may persist for many months. In some patients, the disease may progress to chronic glomerulonephritis. Complications include hypertensive encephalopathy, congestive heart failure, and pulmonary edema. Hypertensive encephalopathy is considered a medical emergency, and therapy is directed toward reducing the blood pressure without impairing renal function.

In rapid progressive glomerulonephritis, plasma exchange (plasmapheresis) and treatment with steroids and cytotoxic drugs have been used to reduce the inflammatory response. In this form of glomerulonephritis, the risk of progression to end-stage renal disease is high without aggressive treatment. Dialysis is occasionally necessary in acute glomerulonephritis if manifestations of uremia are severe.

Patient Education and Home Health Care.   Instructions to the patient include explanations and scheduling for follow-up evaluations of (1) blood pressure, (2) urinalysis for protein, and (3) blood for BUN and creatinine studies to determine if there is exacerbation of disease activity. The patient is instructed to notify the physician if symptoms of renal failure occur (*e.g.*, fatigue, nausea, vomiting, diminishing urinary output). Any infection must be treated promptly. A referral to the community health nurse may be indicated for those patients who live alone to provide an opportunity for careful assessment of the patient's progress and to detect the onset of early symptoms of renal insufficiency. Blood pressure is monitored, and serum and urine specimens may be obtained to detect changes in renal function. If steroids or cytotoxic drugs are prescribed, verbal and written instructions about dosage, desired actions, side effects, and precautions to be followed are provided to the patient and his family.

Chronic Glomerulonephritis

Pathophysiology.   Chronic glomerulonephritis may have its onset as acute glomerulonephritis or may represent a milder type of antigen–antibody reaction, one so mild that it is overlooked. After repeated occurrences of these reactions, the kidneys are reduced to as little as one-fifth their normal size, consisting largely of fibrous tissue. The cortex shrinks to a layer of 1 to 2 mm in thickness or less. Bands of scar tissue distort the remaining cortex, making the surface of the kidney rough and irregular. Many glomeruli and their tubules become scarred, and the branches of the renal artery are thickened. The result is severe glomerular damage that results in chronic glomerulonephritis, a common cause of chronic renal failure.

Clinical Manifestations.   The symptoms of chronic glomerulonephritis are variable. Some patients with severe disease have no symptoms at all for a long time. They may discover their condition as the result of a blood test or when their blood pressure is found to be elevated. The diagnosis may be suggested during a routine eye examination when vascular changes or retinal hemorrhages are found. The first indication of disease may be a sudden, severe nosebleed, a stroke, or a convulsion. Many patients merely notice that their feet are slightly swollen at night. The majority of patients also have such general symptoms as loss of weight and strength, increasing irritability, and nocturia. Headaches, dizziness, and digestive disturbances are common.

Physical examination may reveal a poorly nourished patient with a yellow-gray pigmentation of the skin and periorbital and peripheral (dependent) edema. Blood pressure may be normal or severely elevated. Retinal findings include hemorrhage, exudate, narrowed tortuous arterioles, and papilledema. Mucous membranes are pale because of anemia.

As chronic glomerulonephritis progresses, the patient develops the following signs and symptoms of renal insufficiency and chronic renal failure. The neck veins may be distended as a result of fluid overload. Cardiomegaly, a gallop rhythm, and other signs of congestive heart failure may be present. Crackles can be heard in the lungs. Peripheral neuropathy with depressed deep tendon reflexes and neurosensory changes occurs late in the illness. When frank uremia occurs, the patient becomes confused and his attention span will be limited. An additional late finding includes evidence of pericarditis with a pericardial friction rub and pulsus paradoxus (an exaggerated drop in blood pressure or weakening of pulse amplitude with inspiration secondary to impaired cardiac flow during inspiration).

A number of laboratory abnormalities occur. Urinalysis reveals a fixed specific gravity of 1.010, variable proteinuria, and urine sediment changes. As glomerular filtration becomes depressed, hyperkalemia and decreased serum bicarbonate (metabolic acidosis) develop. Fatal hypermagnesemia may develop if magnesium-containing antacids are given to patients with renal failure. Anemia secondary to decreased erythropoiesis (production of red blood cells) and shortened red cell survival time, hypoalbuminemia with edema secondary to protein loss through the damaged renal glomeruli, and depressed serum calcium and increased serum phosphorus values occur as renal failure progresses. Impaired nerve conduction velocity develops in about 50% of patients once the glomerular filtration rate falls below 50 ml/min as a result of rising levels of waste products in the tissues and nervous system and electrolyte abnormalities. Chest films may show cardiac enlargement and pulmonary edema. The electrocardiogram may be normal but may also reflect hypertension with left ventricular hypertrophy and electrolyte disturbances, such as hyperkalemia and spiked T waves.

Management.   The treatment of the ambulatory patient is guided by the patient's symptoms. Therefore, if hypertension is present, treatment is directed toward readjusting the diet and fluid intake in an effort to maintain as normal a metabolic state as possible. Protein intake (of high biologic value) is adjusted according to the response of the patient, with adequate calories to prevent the use of protein for energy. If there is a urinary tract infection, a possible factor in producing further renal damage, treatment is initiated.

If severe edema develops, the patient is placed on bed rest and the head of the bed is elevated to promote comfort and diuresis. Weight is monitored daily, and diuretics are used to reduce fluid overload. Sodium intake and fluid intake are adjusted according to the ability of the patient's kidneys to excrete water and sodium.

Initiation of dialysis is considered early in the course of the disease to keep the patient in optimal physical condition, prevent fluid and electrolyte imbalances, and minimize the risk of complications of renal failure. The course of dialysis is smoother if treatment is initiated before the patient develops significant complications.

Nursing Interventions.   The nurse has a major role in explaining to the patient and family what is occurring. Additionally, the nurse gives emotional support throughout the course of the disease and treatment by providing opportunities for the patient and family to verbalize their concerns and have their questions answered and their options discussed.

The nurse observes the patient for changes in fluid and electrolyte status and for signs of deterioration of renal function. Changes in fluid and electrolyte status and in cardiac and neurologic status are reported promptly to the physician. If dialysis is initiated, the patient and family will require considerable assistance and support in dealing with the need for this therapy and its long-term implications. See Chapter 42 for a discussion of dialysis and pp. 1197–1199 for a discussion of kidney transplantation.

Nephrotic Syndrome

The nephrotic syndrome is a clinical disorder characterized by (1) a marked increase in protein in the urine (proteinuria), (2) a decrease in albumin in the blood (hypoalbuminemia), (3) edema, and (4) excess cholesterol in the blood (hypercholesterolemia). It is seen in any condition that seriously damages the glomerular capillary membrane. Although generally considered a disorder of childhood, nephrotic syndrome does occur in adults, including the elderly. Causes include chronic glomerulonephritis, diabetes mellitus with intercapillary glomerulosclerosis, amyloidosis of the kidney, systemic lupus erythematosus, and renal vein thrombosis. The pathophysiology of nephrotic syndrome is discussed on p. 1136.

Clinical Manifestations.   There is a slow onset of fluid retention that progresses to pitting edema. The patient loses protein in the urine, leading to depletion of body proteins. In addition, the blood cholesterol level is high. The diagnosis is based on assessment of the patient's signs and symptoms, physical examination, renal function tests, measurements of 24-hour urine protein, and serum electrolyte evaluations. Urinalysis shows microscopic hematuria, urinary casts, and other abnormalities. Needle biopsy of the kidney may be performed for histologic examination of renal tissue to confirm the diagnosis. Morbidity is increased with nephrotic syndrome because of infection, a hypercoagulable state, and accelerated atherogenesis. Those patients who have heavy proteinuria *and* elevated serum creatinine levels are at increased risk of progressing to end-stage renal disease.

Management.   The objective of management is to preserve renal function. It may be necessary to keep the patient on bed rest for a few days to promote diuresis to reduce the edema. A high-protein diet is given to replenish wasted tissues and restore body proteins. If the edema is severe, the patient is placed on a low-sodium diet. Diuretics are prescribed for the patient with severe edema, and adrenocorticosteroids (prednisone) may be used to reduce proteinuria. Cyclosporine may be prescribed in steroid-resistant nephrotic syndrome.

Nursing Interventions.   In the early stages, the nursing management is similar to that of the patient with acute glomerulonephritis, but as the disease worsens, management is similar to that of the patient with chronic renal failure (see pp. 1193–1196).

The patient who is receiving steroids or cyclosporine requires instructions about the medications and about the signs and symptoms that warrant reporting to the physician. Additionally, assistance with selecting a high-protein diet while restricting cholesterol may be necessary.

Nephrosclerosis

Nephrosclerosis is hardening, or sclerosis, of the arteries of the kidney and is usually seen in association with hypertension. It is the renal manifestation of generalized arteriosclerosis. There are two forms: malignant and benign. Malignant nephrosclerosis is thought to be a generalized vascular disease that starts in the kidney and finally involves the entire vascular tree. Patients with the malignant type progress rapidly through the stages of proteinuria, increasing hypertension, failing renal function, and retinal vessel changes. They usually die within several months. The factor responsible for death may be uremia, congestive heart failure due to hypertensive heart disease, or a cerebrovascular accident. It occurs most commonly during the third to the fifth decade of life.

Patients who develop benign nephrosclerosis are found in older age-groups. These patients rarely complain of renal symptoms, although for years the urine has a low and fixed specific gravity and contains a small amount of protein and an occasional hyaline or granular cast. Only late in the disease does renal insufficiency appear.

Hydronephrosis

Hydronephrosis due to obstruction of urinary flow is dilatation of the pelvis and calyces of one or both kidneys with resulting thinning of the renal parenchyma. Obstruction to the normal flow of urine causes the urine to back up, resulting in increased pressure in the kidney. If the obstruction is in the urethra or the bladder, the back-pressure affects both kidneys, but if the obstruction is in one of the ureters because of a stone or kink, only one kidney is damaged.

Partial or intermittent obstruction may be caused by a renal stone that has formed in the renal pelvis but has dropped into the ureter and blocked it. Or the obstruction may be due to a tumor pressing on the ureter or to bands of scar tissue resulting from an abscess or inflammation near the ureter that pinches it. The disorder may be due to an odd angle of the ureter as it leaves the renal pelvis or to an unusual position of the kidney, favoring a ureteral twist or kink. In elderly males, the most common cause is urethral obstruction at the bladder outlet caused by an enlarged prostate.

Whatever the cause, as the urine accumulates in the renal pelvis, it distends the pelvis and its calyces. In time, atrophy of the kidney results. As one kidney undergoes gradual destruction, the contralateral kidney gradually enlarges (compensatory hypertrophy). Ultimately, there is impairment of renal function.

Clinical Manifestations.   The patient may be asymptomatic if the onset is gradual. Acute obstruction may produce aching in the flank and back. If infection is present, dysuria, chills, fever, tenderness, and pyuria may occur. There may be bleeding from the affected kidney and hematuria. If both kidneys are affected, signs and symptoms of chronic renal failure may occur.

Management.   The goals of management are to identify and correct the cause of the obstruction, to treat infection, and to restore and conserve renal function.

To relieve the obstruction, the urine may have to be diverted by nephrostomy (see Chap. 42) or other types of diversion. The infection is treated with antimicrobials because residual urine in the calyces produces infection and pyelonephritis. The patient is prepared for surgical removal of obstructive lesions (calculus, tumor, obstruction of the ureter). If one kidney is severely damaged and its function is destroyed, nephrectomy (removal of the kidney) may be performed.

Renal Failure

Renal failure results when the kidneys are unable to remove the body's metabolic wastes or perform their regulatory functions. The substances normally eliminated in the urine accumulate in the body fluids as a result of impaired renal excretion and lead to a disruption in endocrine and metabolic functions as well as fluid, electrolyte, and acid–base disturbances. Renal failure is a systemic disease and is a final common pathway of many different kidney and urinary tract diseases. Each year an estimated 42,000 Americans die of irreversible kidney failure.

Acute Renal Failure

Pathophysiology

Acute renal failure is a sudden and almost complete loss of kidney function caused by failure of the renal circulation or by glomerular or tubular dysfunction. It is manifested by sudden oliguria (less than 500 ml of urine per day), high urinary output, or anuria (less than 50 ml of urine per day). Regardless of the volume of urine excreted, the patient with acute renal failure experiences rising serum creatinine and blood urea nitrogen (BUN) levels and retention of other metabolic waste products normally excreted by the kidneys. Any condition that causes reduction in renal blood flow, such as volume depletion, hypotension, or shock, leads to a reduction in glomerular filtration, renal ischemia, and tubular damage. Renal failure may also result from the adverse effects of burns, crushing injuries, and infection as well as from nephrotoxic agents that cause acute tubular necrosis and temporary cessation of renal function. With burns and crush injuries, myoglobin (a protein released from muscle when injury occurs) and hemoglobin are liberated, causing renal toxicity, ischemia, or both. Severe transfusion reactions may also cause renal failure because the hemoglobin, released through hemolysis, filters through the kidney glomeruli and becomes concentrated in the kidney tubules to such a degree that precipitation occurs, interfering with the excretion of urine. After these events, the kidneys become swollen and edematous, and the epithelial cells in the tubules may undergo necrosis (Chart 43-1).

Although the exact pathogenesis of acute renal failure and oliguria is not always known, various possible mechanisms have been suggested. In many instances, there is a clear-cut underlying disease, mechanical obstruction of the urinary tract by calculi or tumor, or renal artery obstruction. Another causative factor in acute renal failure is the use of nonsteroidal anti-inflammatory agents, especially in the elderly. These agents interfere with prostaglandins that normally protect renal blood flow, and their use impairs this protective mechanism, leading to hypoperfusion of the kidneys.

Some of the factors that lead to acute renal failure may be reversible if identified and treated promptly, before kidney function is impaired. This is true of the following conditions that reduce blood flow to the kidney and impair kidney function: (1) hypovolemia; (2) hypotension; (3) reduced cardiac output and congestive heart failure; (4) obstruction of the kidney or lower urinary tract by tumor, blood clot, or kidney stone; and (5) bilateral obstruction of the renal arteries or veins. If treated and corrected before the kidneys are permanently damaged, the increased BUN, oliguria, and other signs associated with these conditions may be reversed.

There are three clinical phases of acute renal failure: the period of oliguria, a period of diuresis, and a period of recovery. The *period of oliguria* (urinary volume less than 400 to 600 ml/24 hr) is accompanied by a rise in the serum concentration of the elements usually excreted by the kidneys (urea, creatinine, uric acid, organic acids, and the intracellular cations—potassium and magnesium). The oliguric phase lasts approximately 10 days.

In some patients there can be a decrease in renal function with increasing nitrogen retention, yet the patient is actually excreting 2 or more liters of urine daily. This is the so-called high-output failure or nonoliguric form of renal failure and occurs predominantly after nephrotoxic antibiotics are administered to the patient; it may occur with burns, traumatic injury, and halogenated anesthesia.

In the second phase, the *period of diuresis,* the patient experiences a gradually increasing urinary output, which signals that glomerular filtration has started to recover. Although the

Chart 43-1
Causes of Acute Renal Failure

Prerenal

Hypovolemia
   Hemorrhage
   Dehydration
Ischemia
   Cross-clamping of the aorta
   Surgery of the aorta or renal vessels
   Extensive surgery in the elderly
Septicemia
   Septic shock

Intrarenal

Prolonged renal ischemia
"Pigment nephropathy"
   Hemoglobinuria (transfusion reactions, hemolytic anemia)
   Myoglobinuria (crush injury, burns, massive tissue injury)
Exposure to nephrotoxic agents
   Aminoglycoside antibiotics (gentamicin, kanamycin)
   Heavy metals (lead, mercury)
   Solvents and chemicals (arsenic, ethylene glycol, carbon tetrachloride)
   Nonsteroidal anti-inflammatory drugs (NSAIDs)
   Radiopaque contrast media
Acute glomerulonephritis
Acute pyelonephritis

Postrenal

Urinary tract obstruction
   Calculi
   Tumors
   Prostatic hypertrophy
   Strictures

volume of urinary output may reach normal or elevated levels, renal function may be markedly abnormal in the diuretic phase. Therefore, expert medical and nursing management is still required.

The *period of recovery* signals the improvement of renal function and may take from 3 to 12 months. Usually, there is a permanent partial reduction in the glomerular filtration rate and the ability to concentrate urine.

Clinical Manifestations

Almost every system of the body is affected when there is failure of the normal renal regulatory mechanisms. The patient appears critically ill and is lethargic with persistent nausea, vomiting, and diarrhea. The skin and mucous membranes are dry from dehydration, and the breath may have the odor of urine. Central nervous system manifestations include drowsiness, headache, muscle twitching, and convulsions. The urinary output is scanty, may be bloody, and has a low specific gravity (1.010 compared with 1.025 normally). There is a steady daily rise in the serum creatinine value, with the rate of rise dependent on the degree of catabolism (breakdown of protein).

A patient with renal disease in which the glomerular filtration rate is reduced is unable to excrete potassium. Protein catabolism results in the release of cellular potassium into the body fluids, causing severe hyperkalemia (high serum K^+ levels). Hyperkalemia may lead to dysrhythmias and cardiac arrest. Sources of potassium include normal tissue catabolism; dietary intake; blood anywhere outside the vascular system, such as in the gastrointestinal tract; or blood transfusion and other sources (intravenous infusions, potassium penicillin, and extracellular shift in response to metabolic acidosis).

There may be large losses of sodium from the gastrointestinal tract from diarrhea and vomiting. Patients with acute oliguria cannot eliminate the daily metabolic load produced by the normal metabolic processes. This is reflected by a fall in the blood carbon dioxide combining power and blood *p*H. Thus, progressive acidosis accompanies renal failure. There may be an increase in serum phosphate concentrations, and serum calcium levels may be low in response to decreased absorption of calcium from the intestine and in association with an elevation of serum phosphate levels.

Anemia inevitably accompanies acute renal failure from blood loss due to uremic gastrointestinal lesions, reduced red cell life span, and reduced erythropoietin production.

Prevention and Health Maintenance

A careful history is indicated to determine if the patient has been taking potentially nephrotoxic antimicrobial agents or has been exposed to environmental toxins. The kidneys are especially susceptible to the adverse effects of drugs because they receive such a large blood flow (25% of the cardiac output at rest) and are a major excretory pathway for antimicrobial drugs. The nephrons are exposed to high concentrations of antimicrobials as a result of glomerular filtration and tubular secretion and reabsorption and thus are more likely to suffer toxic effects of drugs. Therefore, in patients taking potentially nephrotoxic drugs (aminoglycosides, gentamicin, tobramycin, colistimethate, polymyxin B, amphotericin B, vancomycin, amikacin, capreomycin, cyclosporine), renal function should be monitored by evaluating BUN and serum creatinine levels within 24 hours of initiation of drug therapy and at least twice a week while the patient is receiving therapy. Any agent that reduces renal blood flow (*i.e.*, chronic analgesic use) may cause renal deterioration. Chronic analgesic use, particularly with nonsteroidal anti-inflammatory drugs (NSAIDs), causes interstitial nephritis and papillary necrosis. Patients with congestive heart failure or cirrhosis with ascites are at particular risk for NSAID-induced renal failure. Age, existing renal diseases, and the administration of several nephrotoxic agents simultaneously increase the risk of kidney damage.

Other precautionary measures taken to avoid renal complications include the following:

- Adequate hydration procedures are initiated before, during, and after operative measures.
- Shock, in any clinical situation, is prevented or treated promptly with blood and fluid replacement.
- Critically ill patients are monitored by measuring central venous pressure and hourly urinary output to detect the onset of renal failure as early as possible.
- Hypertension is treated promptly.

- Patients undergoing intensive diagnostic studies requiring fluid restriction (*e.g.*, barium enema, intravenous pyelogram), especially elderly patients who may not have adequate renal reserve, should be adequately hydrated to prevent dehydration.
- All precautions are taken to ensure that the correct person receives the appropriate blood in order to avoid severe transfusion reactions, which can precipitate renal complications.
- Infections, which may produce progressive renal damage, are controlled and avoided.
- Special attention is paid to draining wounds, burns, and other causes of sepsis and to septicemia.
- Meticulous care is given to patients with indwelling catheters to prevent ascending infections. Catheters are removed as soon as possible.
- Adequate hydration for patients with neoplastic disorders, patients with disorders of metabolism (*i.e.*, gout), or those receiving chemotherapy is provided.

Management

The kidney has a remarkable ability to recover from insult. Therefore, the objective of treatment of acute renal failure is to restore normal chemical balance and prevent complications so that repair of renal tissue and restoration of renal function can take place. A search is made to identify, treat, and eliminate any possible cause.

Dialysis may be initiated to prevent serious complications of uremia, such as hyperkalemia (potassium intoxication), pericarditis, and seizures. Dialysis corrects many biochemical abnormalities; allows for liberalization of fluid, protein, and sodium intake; diminishes bleeding tendencies; and may help wound healing. Hemodialysis, hemofiltration, or peritoneal dialysis may be carried out. These forms of dialysis are discussed in Chapter 42, which presents treatment modalities for patients with renal dysfunction.

Fluid and electrolyte imbalances are a major problem in acute renal failure; hyperkalemia is the most life-threatening of these disturbances. Thus, monitoring for hyperkalemia includes monitoring serum electrolyte levels (potassium value above 6.0 mEq/L; SI: 6.0 mmol/L), eletrocardiographic assessment (peaked T waves), and the patient's clinical status. The elevated potassium levels may be reduced by administering ion exchange resins (sodium polystyrene sulfonate [Kayexalate]) orally or by retention enema. The drug's action depends on the ability to move resin through the intestinal tract. Sorbitol induces water loss in the gastrointestinal tract and may be given orally or as an enema with Kayexalate. The patient is assessed for the development of fecal impaction. If a retention enema is given (the colon is the major site for potassium exchange), a rectal catheter with a balloon may be prescribed to facilitate retention if necessary. The patient should retain the resin 30 to 45 minutes to promote potassium removal.

- A patient with a high and rising level of serum potassium requires immediate peritoneal dialysis, hemodialysis, or hemofiltration.
- Intravenous glucose and insulin or calcium gluconate may be used as an emergency and temporary measure to treat hyperkalemia.
- Sodium bicarbonate may be given to promote an elevation of plasma *p*H. Sodium bicarbonate increases the *p*H, which causes potassium to move into the cell, and the result is low-

ering of the patient's serum potassium level. This is short-term therapy and is used with other long-term measures, such as dietary restriction and dialysis.

- All external sources of potassium are eliminated or reduced.

Management of fluid balance is based on daily body weight, serial measurements of central venous pressure, serum and urine concentrations, fluid losses, blood pressure, and the clinical status of the patient. A flow chart may be used to record pertinent information to indicate the degree to which the patient's condition is improving or deteriorating. The parenteral and oral intake and the output of urine, gastric drainage, stools, wound drainage, and perspiration are calculated and are used as the basis for fluid replacement. The fluid lost through the skin and lungs and produced through the normal metabolic processes is also considered in fluid management.

The patient is weighed daily and can be expected to lose 0.2 to 0.5 kg (½ to 1 lb) daily if he is in negative nitrogen balance (*i.e.*, receiving caloric intake that is less than his caloric requirement). This weight loss represents tissue breakdown. If the patient does not lose weight or develops hypertension, fluid retention should be suspected. Fluid excesses can be evaluated by the clinical findings of dyspnea, tachycardia, and distended neck veins. The lungs are auscultated for signs of moist crackles (rales). Because pulmonary edema may be caused by excessive administration of parenteral fluids, the development of generalized edema is assessed by examining the presacral and pretibial areas several times daily. Sodium losses are estimated (by evaluating serum and urine sodium levels) and corrected.

Adequate blood flow to the kidneys in some patients may be restored by intravenous fluids and medications. Mannitol, furosemide, or ethacrynic acid may be prescribed to initiate a diuresis and prevent or minimize subsequent renal failure. If acute renal failure is caused by hypovolemia secondary to hypoproteinemia, an infusion of albumin may be prescribed. Shock and infection, if present, are treated.

When severe acidosis is present, the arterial blood gases must be monitored and appropriate ventilatory measures instituted if respiratory problems develop. The patient may require sodium bicarbonate therapy or dialysis.

The patient's elevated serum phosphate concentration may be controlled with phosphate-binding agents (aluminum hydroxide); these help prevent a continuing rise in serum phosphate levels by decreasing absorption of phosphate from the intestinal tract.

Dietary proteins are limited to approximately 1 g/kg during the oliguric phase to minimize protein breakdown and to prevent accumulation of toxic end products. Caloric requirements are met with high-carbohydrate feedings, because carbohydrates have a protein-sparing effect (in a high-carbohydrate diet, protein is not used for meeting energy requirements but is "spared" for growth and tissue healing). Foods and fluids containing potassium and phosphorus (bananas, citrus fruits and juices, coffee) are restricted. Potassium intake is usually restricted to 40 to 60 mEq/day, and sodium is usually restricted to 2 g/day. The patient may require total parenteral nutrition (see Chap. 35).

The oliguric phase of acute renal failure may last from 10 to 20 days and is followed by the diuretic phase, at which time urinary output begins to increase, signaling that glomerular filtration is taking place. Blood chemistry evaluations are made to determine the amounts of sodium, potassium, and water

needed for replacement along with assessment for overhydration or underhydration.

After the diuretic phase, the patient is placed on a high-protein, high-calorie diet and is encouraged to resume activities gradually, because muscle weakness will be present from excessive catabolism.

Nursing Interventions

The nurse has an important role in management of the patient with acute renal failure. In addition to directing attention to the patient's primary disorder, which may be a factor in the development of acute renal failure, the nurse monitors the patient for complications, participates in emergency treatment of fluid and electrolyte imbalances, assesses the patient's progress and response to treatment, and provides physical and emotional support. Additionally, the nurse keeps the patient's family informed about the patient's condition, assists them in understanding the treatments, and provides psychologic support. Although the development of acute renal failure may be the most life-threatening problem, the nurse must continue to include in the plan of care those nursing measures indicated for the patient's primary disorder (*e.g.*, burns, shock, trauma, obstruction of the urinary tract).

The serious fluid and electrolyte imbalances that can occur with acute renal failure require the nurse to closely monitor the patient's serum electrolyte levels and physical indicators of these complications during all phases of the disorder. Additionally, parenteral fluids, all oral intake, and all medications are screened carefully to ensure that hidden sources of potassium are not inadvertently administered or consumed. The patient's cardiac function and musculoskeletal status are monitored closely for changes suggestive of hyperkalemia. The patient's fluid status is monitored by careful attention to fluid intake, urine output, changes in body weight, the presence of edema, distention of the jugular veins, alterations in heart sounds and breath sounds, and increasing difficulty in breathing. Indicators of deterioration of fluid and electrolyte status are reported immediately to the physician, and preparation is made for emergency treatment, including the use of glucose and insulin, calcium gluconate, or cation-exchange resins (Kayexalate) to treat hyperkalemia, and the initiation of hemodialysis, peritoneal dialysis, or hemofiltration to correct fluid and electrolyte disturbances.

The nurse also directs attention to reducing the patient's metabolic rate during the acute stage of renal failure to reduce catabolism and the subsequent release of potassium and accumulation of endogenous waste products (urea and creatinine). Bed rest may be indicated to reduce exertion and the metabolic rate during the most acute stage of the disorder. Fever and infection, both of which increase metabolic rate and catabolism, are prevented or treated promptly. Attention is given to pulmonary function, and the patient is assisted to turn, cough, and take deep breaths frequently to prevent atelectasis and respiratory infection. Drowsiness and lethargy may prevent the patient from moving and turning without encouragement and assistance. Asepsis is essential with invasive lines and catheters to minimize the risk of infection and increased metabolism. An indwelling catheter is avoided if possible because of the high risk of urinary tract infection.

Skin care is an important part of nursing intervention because the patient's skin may be dry or susceptible to breakdown as a result of edema. Additionally, excoriation and itching of the skin may result from the deposit of irritating toxins in the patient's tissues. Massaging bony prominences, turning the patient frequently, and bathing with cool water are frequently comforting and prevent skin breakdown.

The patient with acute renal failure will require treatment with hemodialysis, peritoneal dialysis, or hemofiltration to prevent serious complications; the length of time that these treatments will be necessary varies with the cause and extent of damage to the kidneys. The patient and family will need assistance, explanation, and support during this time. The purpose and rationale of the treatments will be explained to the patient and family by the physician. However, their high levels of anxiety and fear may necessitate repeated explanation and clarification by the nurse. The family members may initially be afraid to touch and talk to the patient during the procedure but should be encouraged and assisted to do so. Although many of the nurse's functions will be devoted to the technical aspects of the procedure, the psychologic needs and concerns of the patient and family cannot be ignored. Continued assessment of the patient for complications of acute renal failure and of its precipitating cause is essential.

Chronic Renal Failure (End-Stage Renal Disease)

Chronic renal failure or end-stage renal disease (ESRD) is a progressive, irreversible deterioration in renal function in which the body's ability to maintain metabolic and fluid and electrolyte balance fails, resulting in uremia (a syndrome resulting from an excess of urea and other nitrogenous wastes in the blood). It may be caused by chronic glomerulonephritis; pyelonephritis; uncontrolled hypertension; hereditary lesions, such as in polycystic kidney disease; vascular disorders; obstruction of the urinary tract; renal disease secondary to systemic disease (diabetes); infections; drugs; or toxic agents. Environmental and occupational agents that have been implicated in chronic renal failure include lead, cadmium, mercury, and chromium. Dialysis or kidney transplantation eventually becomes necessary to maintain life.

Pathophysiology. As renal function declines, the end products of protein metabolism, which are normally excreted in urine, accumulate in the blood. There are imbalances in the body chemistry and in the cardiovascular, hematologic, gastrointestinal, neurologic, and skeletal systems. Skin and reproductive changes are also seen.

The patient tends to retain sodium and water, increasing the risk of edema formation, congestive heart failure, hypertension, and, occasionally, ascites. Hypertension may also result from activation of the renin–angiotensin axis and the concomitant increased aldosterone secretion.

Other patients have a tendency to lose salt, and they run the risk of hypotension and hypovolemia. Episodes of vomiting and diarrhea may produce sodium and water depletion, which worsens the uremic state. Metabolic acidosis occurs as a result of the reduced ability of the kidney to excrete hydrogen ions, produce ammonia, and conserve bicarbonate.

The body's serum calcium and phosphate levels are reciprocal; as one rises, the other decreases. With decreased filtration through the kidney's glomerulus, there is an increase in the serum phosphate level and a reciprocal or corresponding decrease in the serum calcium level. Secretion of parathormone increases in response to this decreased calcium level. However, in renal failure, the body does not respond normally to the increased secretion of parathormone, and, as a result, calcium leaves the bone, often producing bone changes and bone disease. Uremic bone disease (renal osteodystrophy) develops from changes in calcium, phosphate, and parathormone balance. Also, the active metabolite of vitamin D (1,25-dihydroxycholecalciferol) normally manufactured by the kidney decreases with the progression of renal disease. In other patients, the calcification process in the bone may fail, resulting in osteomalacia. The serum magnesium level may rise because of the inability of the kidney to excrete magnesium.

Anemia develops as a result of inadequate erythropoietin production, the shortened life span of red blood cells, nutritional deficiencies, and the uremic patient's tendency to bleed, particularly from the gastrointestinal tract. Erythropoietin, a substance normally produced by the kidney, stimulates bone marrow to produce red blood cells. In renal failure, erthyropoietin production decreases and profound anemia results, producing fatigue, angina, and shortness of breath.

Neurologic complications of renal failure may occur as a result of renal failure itself, severe hypertension, an electrolyte imbalance, water intoxication, and drug effects. Such manifestations include altered mental function, changes in personality and behavior, convulsions, and coma.

A decrease in libido, impotence, and amenorrhea may occur; however, pregnancy in the patient with chronic renal failure is possible. Skin changes include pruritus (in part from calcium/phosphate imbalance), which adds to the patient's distress.

The rate of decline in renal function and progression of chronic renal failure is related to the underlying disorder, to the urinary excretion of protein, and to the presence of hypertension. The chronic renal failure of those patients who excrete significant amounts of protein or have elevated blood pressure tends to progress more rapidly than that of patients without these conditions.

Clinical Manifestations

Although at times the onset of chronic renal failure is sudden, in the majority of patients it begins with one or more symptoms—fatigue and lethargy, headache, general weakness, gastrointestinal symptoms (anorexia, nausea, vomiting, diarrhea), bleeding tendencies, and mental confusion. There is decreased salivary flow, thirst, a metallic taste in the mouth, loss of smell and taste, and parotitis or stomatitis. If active treatment is begun early, the symptoms may disappear. Otherwise, these symptoms become more marked, and others appear as the metabolic abnormalities of uremia affect virtually every body system.

The patient gradually becomes more and more drowsy; the respirations become Kussmaul in character; and a deep coma develops, often with convulsions, which may occur as muscle twitchings or severe spasms (myoclonic jerks) quite similar to those of epilepsy. A white, powdery substance, "uremic frost," composed chiefly of urates, appears on the skin. Unless treatment is initiated, death soon follows.

Management

The goal of management is to retain kidney function and maintain homeostasis for as long as possible. All factors that contribute to the problem and those that are reversible (*e.g.*, obstruction) are identified and treated.

With the deterioration of renal function, dietary intervention is necessary with careful regulation of protein intake, fluid intake to balance fluid losses, sodium intake to balance sodium losses, and some restriction of potassium. At the same time, adequate calorie intake and vitamin supplementation must be ensured. There is some restriction of protein because urea, creatinine, uric acid, and organic acids—the breakdown products of dietary and tissue proteins—will accumulate rapidly in the blood when there is impaired renal clearance (the ability to remove or "clear" these substances from the blood). The allowed protein must be of high biologic value: dairy products, eggs, meats. High-biologic-value proteins are those that are complete proteins and supply the essential amino acids that are necessary for growth and cell repair. Usually, the fluid allowance is 500 to 600 ml of fluid more than the 24-hour urine output.

Sodium and potassium allowance is determined by concentrations of these electrolytes in the serum and urine. If a patient has a tendency to lose sodium, appropriate supplementation is given. Hyperphosphatemia and hypocalcemia have in the past been treated with aluminum-based antacids that bind dietary phosphorus in the gastrointestinal tract. However, concern about the potential long-term toxicity of aluminum and the association of high aluminum levels with neurologic symptoms and osteomalacia have led some physicians to prescribe calcium carbonate in place of high doses of aluminum-based antacids. This medication also binds dietary phosphorus in the intestinal tract and permits the use of smaller doses of antacids. Both calcium carbonate and phosphorus-binding antacids must be given with food to be effective.

Calories are supplied by carbohydrates and fat to prevent wasting. Vitamin supplementation is necessary because a protein-restricted diet does not give the necessary complement of vitamins. (Also, the patient on dialysis may lose water-soluble vitamins from the blood during the dialysis treatment.)

Hypertension is managed by intravascular volume control and a variety of antihypertensive medications. The metabolic acidosis of chronic renal failure usually produces no symptoms and requires no treatment; however, sodium bicarbonate supplements or dialysis may be needed to correct the acidosis.

The patient is observed for early evidence of neurologic abnormalities. These may vary from slight twitching to headache or delirium. The patient is protected from injury during involuntary movements; thus, it is advisable to pad the side rails of the bed. The onset of seizures is recorded along with their type, duration, and general effect on the patient. The physician is notified immediately. Intravenous diazepam (Valium) or phenytoin (Dilantin) is usually given to control seizures. (The nursing management of the patient having seizures is discussed in Chap. 57.) Heart failure, infection, and volume depletion may also require treatment.

Management of anemia has benefited from the recent availability of recombinant human erythropoietin (Epogen). The patient with chronic renal failure who has a low hematocrit (less than 30%) usually experiences significant symptoms of the anemia and is a candidate for this therapy. Hematocrit levels are used to assess the patient's response to therapy. The goal of therapy is to obtain and maintain a hematocrit of 33% to 38%, which generally results in alleviation of the patient's symptoms of anemia. A rise in the level of the hematocrit may take 2 to 6 weeks to occur. Therapy is administered either intravenously or subcutaneously three times a week. Side effects of recombinant erythropoietin include aggravation of hypertension, due to hemodynamic changes as the anemia is corrected, and increased platelets, which may increase the blood's clotting tendency. Adjustment of heparin may be necessary to prevent clotting of the dialysis lines during hemodialysis treatments. Following initiation of therapy, the patient's hematocrit is monitored frequently. Serum iron and transferrin levels are monitored to assess iron stores. Because adequate stores of iron are necessary for an adequate response to erythropoietin, supplementary iron may be prescribed. The patient's blood pressure and serum potassium levels are monitored to detect hypertension and rising serum potassium levels, which may occur with therapy and the increasing red cell mass. The occurrence of hypertension requires initiation or adjustment of the patient's antihypertensive therapy. Hypertension that cannot be controlled is a contraindication for recombinant erythropoietin therapy. The patient may experience flulike symptoms with initiation of therapy; these tend to subside with repeated doses. Patients who have received recombinant erythropoietin therapy have reported decreased levels of fatigue, an increased feeling of well-being, better tolerance of dialysis, higher energy levels, and improved exercise tolerance. Additionally, this therapy has decreased the need for transfusion and its risks (infectious disease, antibody formation, and iron overload).

The patient with increasing symptoms of chronic renal failure is referred to a dialysis and transplantation center early in the course of progressive renal disease. Dialysis is usually initiated when the patient cannot maintain a reasonable lifestyle with conservative treatment. The details of dialysis treatment can be found in Chapter 42.

Nursing Interventions

The patient with chronic renal failure requires astute nursing care to avoid the complications of reduced renal function and the stresses and anxieties of dealing with a life-threatening illness.

Potential nursing diagnoses for these patients include the following:

- Fluid volume excess and electrolyte imbalance related to decreased urine output and dietary and fluid restrictions
- Altered nutrition: less than body requirements related to anorexia, gastrointestinal discomfort, and dietary restrictions
- Knowledge deficit regarding condition and treatment regimen
- Activity intolerance related to fatigue
- Self-esteem disturbance related to dependency and role changes

Nursing care is directed toward assessing fluid and electrolyte status and identifying potential sources of imbalance, implementing a dietary program to ensure proper nutritional intake within the limits of the treatment regimen, providing explanations and information to the patient and family concerning the consequences of reduced renal function and the need to follow the protocols prescribed by the physician, and promoting positive feelings by encouraging increased self-care and greater independence. Specific interventions, along with rationale and evaluation criteria, are presented in more detail in Nursing Care Plan 43-1 for a patient with chronic renal failure.

Gerontologic Considerations

Changes in the Elderly. Changes in kidney function with normal aging increase the susceptibility of the elderly to kidney

(text continues on page 1196)

Nursing Care Plan 43–1

Care of the Patient With Chronic Renal Failure

Nursing Interventions	Rationale	Evaluation

Nursing Diagnosis: Fluid volume excess and electrolyte imbalance related to decreased urine output and dietary and fluid restrictions

Goal: Maintenance of fluid and electrolyte balance

Nursing Interventions	Rationale	Evaluation

1. Assess fluid and electrolyte status:
  a. Serum electrolyte levels
  b. Daily weight changes
  c. Precise intake and output balance
  d. Skin turgor and presence of edema
  e. Distention of neck veins
  f. Blood pressure and pulse rate and rhythm
  g. Signs of calcium imbalance (Chvostek's and Trousseau's signs)
  h. Respiratory rate and effort
2. Identify potential sources of fluids:
  a. Medications
  b. Foods
  c. Intravenous fluids used to administer antibiotics
  d. Oral fluids used to ingest oral medication
3. Explain to patient and family rationale for restrictions of certain foods and fluids.
4. Assist patient and family in identifying hidden sources of restricted electrolytes.
5. Administer antacids as prescribed.
 	
6. Avoid use of magnesium-based antacids and other medications with magnesium.
7. Provide foods and fluids within dietary restrictions.
8. Assist patient to cope with the discomforts resulting from restrictions.
  a. Provide or encourage frequent oral hygiene.
  b. Encourage use of distraction.
	1. Assessment provides baseline and continuing data base for monitoring changes and evaluating interventions for disturbances in fluid balance, sodium balance, and potassium and calcium balance.
	
	2. Unrecognized sources of excessive fluid, sodium, potassium, and phosphate may be uncovered.
	
	3. Understanding promotes patient and family cooperation with necessary food and fluid restrictions.
	4. Independence and involvement of patient and family in maintaining fluid and dietary restrictions are encouraged.
	5. Antacids promote binding of phosphate in intestinal tract and normal calcium and phosphorus levels.
	6. Magnesium toxicity is avoided.
	
	7. Adequate dietary intake and fluid and electrolyte balance are promoted.
	8. Increasing patient comfort promotes compliance with dietary restrictions.
	  a. Oral hygiene minimizes dry oral mucous membranes.
	  b. Focus on food and fluid restrictions is reduced.
		• Exhibits normal or acceptable serum electrolyte levels.
		• Demonstrates no rapid weight increases or decreases.
		• Maintains dietary and fluid intake within restrictions.
		• Exhibits normal skin turgor without evidence of edema.
		• Exhibits normal blood pressure.
		• Exhibits regular pulse rhythm.
		• Exhibits no distention of neck veins.
		• Reports no difficulty breathing or shortness of breath.
		• Demonstrates absence of Chvostek's and Trousseau's signs.
		• States rationale for dietary restrictions and limited fluid intake.
		• Reads labels of prepared foods and correctly identifies foods to be avoided.
		• Takes antacids as prescribed, avoiding those antacids that contain magnesium.
		• States rationale for use of antacids as prescribed.
		• States rationale for avoiding magnesium-containing antacids.
		• Uses oral hygiene frequently.
		• Reports decreased dryness of oral mucous membranes.
		• Reports decreased thirst.
		• Exhibits interest in activities not related to food or fluid.

Nursing Diagnosis: Altered nutrition: less than body requirements, related to anorexia, gastrointestinal discomfort, and dietary restrictions

Goal: Maintenance of adequate nutritional intake

Nursing Interventions	Rationale	Evaluation

1. Assess nutritional status:
  a. Weight changes
  b. Anthropometric measures
  c. Laboratory values
	1. Baseline data are provided for monitoring changes and evaluating interventions.	• Identifies foods within dietary restrictions that are appealing.
		• Consumes high biologic value proteins.
		• Consumes foods high in calories within other dietary allowances.

(continued)

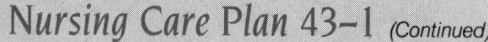

Nursing Care Plan 43–1 *(Continued)*

Care of the Patient With Chronic Renal Failure

Nursing Interventions	Rationale	Evaluation
2. Assess patient's nutritional dietary patterns: a. Diet history b. Food preferences c. Calorie counts	2. Past and present dietary patterns can be considered in planning meals.	• Reports increased appetite at mealtime. • Takes antacids on a schedule that does not produce a feeling of fullness before meals.
3. Assess for factors contributing to altered nutritional intake: a. Anorexia b. Nausea and vomiting c. Unpalatable diet d. Depression e. Lack of understanding of dietary restrictions f. Stomatitis	3. Information about other factors that may be altered or eliminated to promote adequate dietary intake is provided.	• Explains in own words the rationale for dietary restrictions and the relationship of dietary restrictions to urea and creatinine levels. • Consults written lists of acceptable foods when selecting foods. • Identifies ways of increasing food's palatability without using sodium or potassium.
4. Provide patient's food preferences within dietary restrictions.	4. Increased dietary intake is encouraged.	• Identifies foods that are prohibited on diet and rationale for their exclusion.
5. Promote intake of high biologic value protein foods: eggs, dairy products, meat.	5. Complete proteins are provided for positive nitrogen balance necessary for growth and tissue healing within protein restriction.	• States rationale for dietary changes when dialysis is initiated. • Uses oral hygiene before each meal.
6. Encourage high-calorie, low-protein, low-sodium, and low-potassium snacks between meals.	6. This diet eliminates/reduces sources of restricted foods and provides calories for energy while sparing protein for growth and tissue healing.	• Reports increased appetite in more pleasant surroundings. • Exhibits no rapid increases or decreases in weight.
7. Alter schedule of medications so that they are not administered immediately before meals.	7. Ingestion of medications immediately before meals may produce anorexia or a feeling of fullness that may interfere with dietary intake. (Antacids given to bind phosphate in the intestinal tract and reduce the serum phosphate level frequently produce a feeling of fullness.)	• Demonstrates normal skin turgor without edema; healing; and acceptable plasma protein and albumin levels.
8. Explain rationale for dietary restrictions and their relationship to kidney dysfunction and increased urea and creatinine levels.	8. Promotes patient understanding of relationships between diet and urea and creatinine levels to disturbed kidney function.	
9. Provide written lists of foods allowed and suggestions for improving their taste without the use of sodium or potassium.	9. Lists provide a positive approach to dietary restrictions and a reference for the patient and his family to use when at home.	
10. Provide written lists of foods that are to be used in limited amounts or avoided entirely.	10. Lists include those foods that must be avoided to prevent serious electrolyte and nutritional problems.	
11. Explain changes in diet and more liberal dietary intake if dialysis is initiated.	11. Frequent dialysis removes waste products (*e.g.*, urea, creatinine); protein is removed by peritoneal dialysis and hemodialysis.	
12. Provide oral hygiene before meals.	12. Oral hygiene temporarily improves the patient's sense of taste by eliminating waste products and moistens mucous membranes.	
13. Provide pleasant surroundings at mealtime.	13. Unpleasant factors that contribute to patient's anorexia are eliminated.	

(continued)

Nursing Care Plan 43-1 (Continued)

Care of the Patient With Chronic Renal Failure

Nursing Interventions	Rationale	Evaluation
14. Weigh patient daily.	14. Nutritional status can be monitored.	
15. Assess for evidence of inadequate protein intake: a. Edema formation b. Delayed healing c. Decreased serum albumin levels	15. Inadequate protein intake can lead to decreased albumin and other plasma proteins, edema formation, and delay in healing.	

Nursing Diagnosis: Knowledge deficit regarding condition and treatment regimen

Goal: Increased knowledge about condition and related treatment

1. Assess knowledge and understanding of cause of renal failure, consequences of renal failure, and its treatment: a. Cause of patients's renal failure b. Meaning of renal failure c. Understanding of renal function d. Relationship of fluid and dietary restrictions to renal failure e. Rationale for substitute for kidney function (hemodialysis, peritoneal dialysis, kidney transplantation)	1. Baseline information is provided for further explanations and teaching.	• Verbalizes relationship of cause of renal failure and consequences. • States relationship of renal failure and need of substitute for renal function in own words. • Explains fluid and dietary restrictions as they relate to failure of kidneys' regulatory functions. • Asks questions about treatment options, indicating readiness to learn. • Verbalizes plans to continue as normal a life as possible. • Uses written information and instructions to clarify questions and seek additional information.
2. Provide explanations of renal function and consequences of renal failure at patient's level of understanding in language understood by patient and guided by patient's level of readiness.	2. Patient can learn about renal failure and its treatment as he becomes ready to understand and accept the diagnosis and its consequences.	
3. Assist patient to identify ways to incorporate changes and treatment into life.	3. Patient can see that his life does not have to change completely or revolve around his disease and its treatment.	
4. Provide verbal and written information and instructions as appropriate about: a. Renal function and failure b. Fluid and electrolyte restrictions c. Dietary restrictions d. Medication schedule e. Reportable problems, signs and symptoms f. Follow-up schedule g. Community resources h. Treatment options	4. Patient has information that he can refer to for further clarification during hospital stay and at home.	

Nursing Diagnosis: Activity intolerance related to fatigue

Goal: Participation in activity within tolerance

1. Assess factors contributing to fatigue: a. Anemia b. Fluid and electrolyte imbalances c. Accumulation of end products of metabolism (*e.g.*, urea and creatinine) d. Depression	1. Indications of severity of fatigue are provided.	• Participates in increasing levels of exercise and activity. • Reports increased energy and sense of well-being. • Alternates rest and activity. • Participates in selected self-care activities.

(continued)

Nursing Care Plan 43–1 (Continued)

Care of the Patient With Chronic Renal Failure

Nursing Interventions	Rationale	Evaluation
2. Promote independence in self-care activities within patient's activity tolerance.	2. Mild/moderate activity and improved self-esteem are promoted.	• Identifies activities and events of importance to him.
3. Encourage alternating activity with rest.	3. Activity and exercise within limits are promoted and adequate rest encouraged.	
4. Assist with self-care activities when fatigued.	4. Adequate hygiene and opportunity for rest are promoted.	
5. Assist patient to determine which activities are of most value to him.	5. Patient can use energy to participate in those activities and events of most importance to him.	

Nursing Diagnosis: Self-esteem disturbance related to dependency and role changes

Goal: Improved self-concept

1. Assess patient's (and family's) responses and reactions to illness and its treatment.	1. Data are provided about problems encountered by patient and family in coping with changes in life and life-style.	• Identifies previously used coping styles that have been effective
2. Assess relationship of patient and significant family members.	2. Strengths and supports of patient and family are identified.	• Identifies previously used coping styles that are no longer possible because of renal failure and its treatment (e.g., alcohol and drug use; extreme physical exertion)
3. Assess usual coping patterns of patient and family members.	3. Coping patterns that may have been effective may be potentially destructive in view of restrictions imposed by renal failure and its treatment.	• Patient and family identify and verbalize their responses and feelings in reaction to renal failure and the necessary changes in their life and life-style.
4. Encourage patient and family to express concerns and reactions to changes produced by renal failure and its treatment: a. Role changes b. Changes in life-style c. Changes in occupation d. Sexual changes e. Dependence on health care team f. Altered food and fluid patterns g. Lack of energy	4. Patient can identify concerns and steps necessary to deal with them.	• Seeks professional counseling, if necessary, to cope with changes resulting from renal failure and its treatment. • Seeks information from nurse and other health care providers about treatment options. • Identifies own strengths and those of supportive family members when considering treatment options.
5. Assist patient and family in seeking professional counseling to deal with severe reactions if necessary.	5. Additional source of support and strength to deal with complex reactions and feelings is provided.	• Takes active role in decision making about treatment options.
6. Provide realistic descriptions of treatment options (hemodialysis, peritoneal dialysis, transplantation) to patient and family.	6. The patient and family have the data to assist in making decisions about treatment options in a positive, future-oriented manner.	

dysfunction and renal failure. Alterations in renal blood flow, glomerular filtration, and renal clearance increase the risk of drug-associated changes in renal function. Precautions are indicated with the administration of all medications because of the frequent use of multiple prescription and over-the-counter drugs and the risk of side effects. The incidence of systemic diseases such as atherosclerosis, hypertension, cardiac failure, diabetes, and malignancy increases with advancing age, predisposing the elderly to renal disease associated with these

disorders. Fluid and electrolyte balance in the elderly is usually maintained in normal circumstances. However, with age, the kidney is less able to respond to acute fluid and electrolyte changes. Therefore, acute problems need to be prevented if possible or recognized and treated quickly to avoid kidney damage. Precautions are warranted when the elderly patient must undergo extensive diagnostic tests, or when new medications (e.g., diuretics) are added, to prevent dehydration, which can compromise marginal renal function and lead to acute renal failure. The elderly patient may develop nonspecific and atypical signs of disturbed renal function and fluid and electrolyte imbalances. Recognition of these problems is further hampered by their association with previously existing disorders and the misconception that they are normal changes of aging.

Acute Renal Failure in the Elderly. The incidence of acute renal failure is increasing in older, hospitalized patients. Approximately 50% of those patients who develop acute renal failure during hospitalization for a medical or surgical problem are over 60 years of age. In the past, acute renal failure was predominantly caused by hypotension due to dehydration and electrolyte imbalance. More recently, acute tubular necrosis due to shock and the use of nephrotoxic drugs has been the most common cause of acute renal failure in the elderly. Exposure of the patient with pre-existing renal insufficiency to radiocontrast material during diagnostic studies is a major cause of renal failure in the elderly. Multiple myeloma and diabetes mellitus increase the risk of contrast-induced renal failure in the patient with pre-existing renal dysfunction because of precipitation of cellular debris in the kidney, which is exaggerated by fluid restriction imposed for many diagnostic tests. Multiple prescriptions and the increased use of over-the-counter drugs increase the risk of drug-induced renal damage. Suppression of thirst, enforced bed rest, the use of restraints, and confusion all contribute to the older patient's failure to consume adequate fluids and his subsequent dehydration, thus compromising the already decreased renal function.

Chronic Renal Failure in the Elderly. Rapidly progressive glomerulonephritis, membranous glomerulonephritis, and nephrosclerosis have been identified as the most common biopsy-proven causes of chronic renal failure in the elderly. Clinically derived figures indicate that glomerulonephritis, interstitial nephritis, renovascular disease, and urinary tract obstruction are the most common causes of chronic renal failure in the elderly. Renal failure associated with multiple myeloma is a common cause of chronic renal failure in the elderly. It is frequently associated with dehydration and hypercalcemia or the use of nonsteroidal anti-inflammatory drugs. Primary hypertensive disease and urinary tract obstruction as causative factors tend to increase in incidence with aging, while diabetes and cystic renal disease become less common as the cause of end-stage renal disease with advancing age.

Clinical Manifestations. The signs and symptoms of renal disease in the elderly are often nonspecific; the occurrence of symptoms of other disorders (congestive heart failure, dementia) can mask the symptoms of renal disease and delay or prevent diagnosis and treatment. Nephrotic syndrome is common as a manifestation of renal disease in the older patient.

Management of the Older Patient With Renal Failure. Hemodialysis and peritoneal dialysis have been used effectively in the treatment of elderly patients. Although there is no single age limitation for renal transplantation, concomitant disorders (*i.e.*, coronary artery disease, peripheral vascular disease) have made it less common as a form of treatment for the elderly. The outcome has been shown to be comparable to that of younger patients. Some elderly patients elect not to participate in these management strategies. Conservative management (nutritional therapy and other less conventional treatment modalities) may be considered in those patients who are not suitable for or elect not to participate in dialysis or transplantation.

Kidney Transplantation

Because of the patient's improved satisfaction with life and more normal life-style following transplantation, it has become the treatment of choice for the majority of patients with end-stage renal disease. Kidney transplantation involves transplanting a kidney from a living donor or human cadaver to a recipient who has end-stage renal disease. Most patients have been on dialysis for months or years prior to transplantation. The patient with irreversible end-stage renal disease is evaluated as a candidate for possible kidney transplantation.

The patient's kidneys, which are nonfunctioning, may or may not be removed, and dialysis may be instituted until a kidney from a suitable donor is obtained. Kidney transplants from well-matched living donors who are related to the patient (those with compatible ABO and HLA antigens) are more successful than those from cadaver donors. The transplanted kidney is placed in the patient's iliac fossa anterior to the crest of the ilium. The ureter of the newly transplanted kidney is transplanted into the bladder or anastomosed to the ureter of the recipient (Fig. 43-2).

Preoperative Management

The preoperative goal of management is to bring the patient's metabolic state to a level as close to normal as possible. Tissue typing is performed to determine compatibility of the tissues and cells of the donor and recipient. Antibody screening is also performed. Immunosuppressive drugs (azathioprine [Imuran], prednisone, and cyclosporine) are given to suppress the body's immunologic defense mechanism and prevent later rejection of the transplanted kidney. Hemodialysis may be performed the day before the scheduled transplant. The patient must be free of infection at the time of renal transplantation because of immunosuppression and the risk of spread of infection. Therefore, the patient is evaluated and treated for gingival disease and dental caries. The lower urinary tract is studied to assess bladder neck function and to detect ureteral reflux.

Nursing Interventions. The nursing aspects of preoperative management are similar to those for patients undergoing renal and vascular surgery. The patient may have experienced considerable discouragement, depression, and anxiety while on dialysis awaiting a cadaver kidney. The patient who receives a kidney from a living related donor may be concerned about the donor and experience other emotional reactions. Helping the patient to deal with these concerns is part of the nurse's role in preoperative management.

Postoperative Management

The goal of care is to maintain homeostasis until the transplanted kidney is functioning well. The major limiting factor of this procedure is the body's immunologic response, which may lead to rejection and destruction of the transplanted kidney. The survival of a transplanted kidney depends on the success of techniques that suppress this normal immunologic reaction. The risks of immunosuppression must be weighed against the effects of rejection. In order to overcome or minimize the body's defense mechanism, immunosuppressive drugs such as azathioprine (Imuran), corticosteroids (predni-

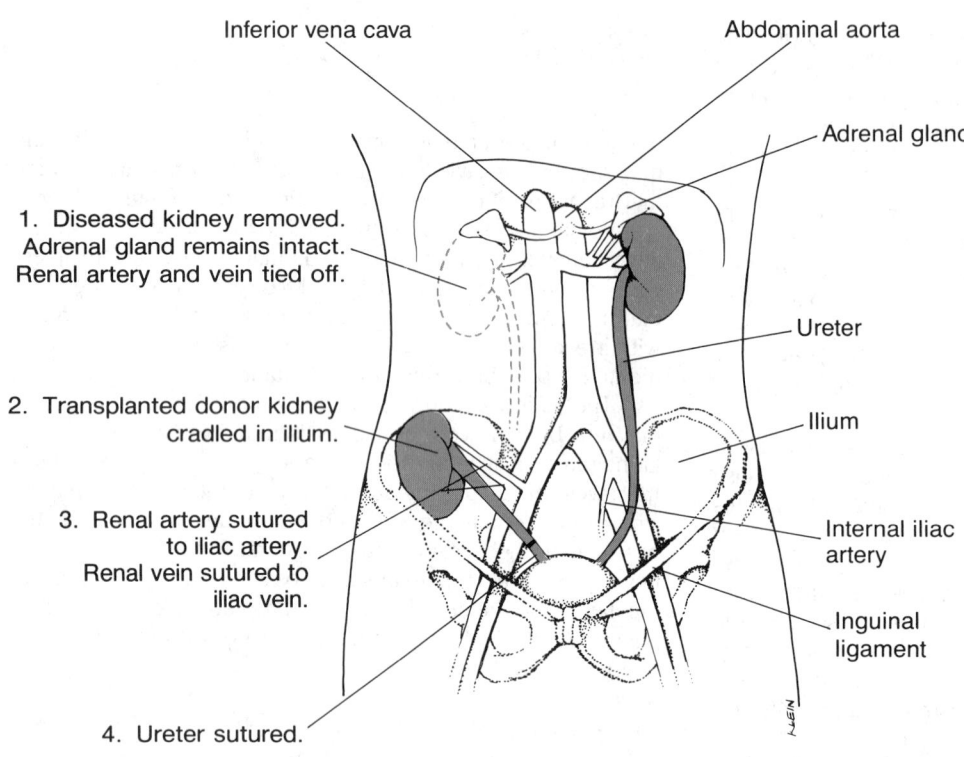

1. Diseased kidney removed. Adrenal gland remains intact. Renal artery and vein tied off.

2. Transplanted donor kidney cradled in ilium.

3. Renal artery sutured to iliac artery. Renal vein sutured to iliac vein.

4. Ureter sutured.

Inferior vena cava

Abdominal aorta

Adrenal gland

Ureter

Ilium

Internal iliac artery

Inguinal ligament

Figure 43–2. Renal transplantations (**1**) The diseased kidneys may be removed and the renal artery and vein are tied off. (**2**) The transplanted kidney is placed in the iliac fossa. (**3**) The renal artery of the donated kidney is sutured to the iliac artery, and the renal vein is sutured to the iliac vein. (**4**) The donated kidney's ureter is sutured to the bladder or to the patient's ureter.

sone), and cyclosporine are given. Plasmaleukapheresis (PLP), lymph drainage, antilymphocytic globulin (ALG), and cyclophosphamide are other methods of immunosuppression that are used less commonly. The doses are gradually tapered over a period of several weeks, depending on the patient's immunologic response to the transplant. This therapy is continued indefinitely. The use of monoclonal antibodies (*i.e.*, OKT3 and IL-2R) for immunosuppression is currently under investigation.

Renal graft rejection and failure may occur early (24 to 72 hours), within a few days (3 to 14 days), or later (after 3 weeks). Ultrasound may be used to detect enlargement of the kidney, while renal biopsy and radiographic techniques are used to evaluate a failing renal transplant. When severe rejection occurs or when excessive immunosuppression is required to maintain the kidney, the transplanted kidney is removed and the patient is returned to dialysis.

Postoperative Nursing Interventions

Assessing for Rejection and Infection.   Following a kidney transplant, the patient is assessed for signs and symptoms of threatened graft rejection: oliguria, edema, fever, increasing blood pressure, apprehension, weight gain, and swelling or tenderness over the graft. Results of blood chemistry tests and leukocyte and platelet counts are monitored closely, because immunosuppression depresses the formation of leukocytes and platelets.

The patient is closely monitored for infection because the kidney recipient is susceptible to faulty healing and infection due to immunosuppressive therapy and complications of renal failure.

- A distinction must be made between infection and rejection because impaired renal function and fever are evidence of both infection and rejection, and treatment differs.

Immunosuppressive drugs make the transplant patient more vulnerable to opportunistic infections (candidiasis, cytomegalic viral disease, *Pneumocystis carinii* pneumonia) and infection with other relatively nonpathogenic viruses, fungi, and protozoa, which can be a major hazard. The patient is protected from exposure to hospital staff, visitors, and other patients who have active infections. Careful hand washing is imperative; face masks may be worn by hospital staff and visitors to reduce the risk of transmitting infectious agents while the patient is receiving high doses of immunosuppressive drugs. Septicemia (bacteremia or fungemia) in renal transplant patients is responsible for a significant number of the deaths.

- Clinical manifestations of septicemia include shaking chills, fever, rapid heartbeat and respirations (tachycardia and tachypnea), and either an increase or a decrease in white blood cells (leukocytosis or leukopenia).

The portal of entry for infection may be the urinary tract, the lung, the operative site, and other sources. Urine cultures are performed frequently in view of the high incidence of bacteriuria during both the early and the late stages of transplant. Any type of wound drainage should be viewed as a potential source of infection because drainage is an excellent culture medium for bacteria. Catheter and drain tips may be cultured on removal by cutting off the tip of the catheter or drain (using aseptic technique) and placing it in a sterile container for laboratory culture.

Monitoring Urinary Function.   The vascular access for hemodialysis is monitored to ensure patency and to evaluate for evidence of infection. Following a successful renal transplant, the vascular access usually clots. This may result from improved coagulation with the return of renal function. Hemodialysis may be necessary postoperatively to maintain homeostasis until the transplanted kidney is functioning well.

A kidney from a living related donor usually begins to function immediately after grafting and may produce large quantities of dilute urine. A cadaver kidney may or may not undergo tubular necrosis and may not function for 2 or 3 weeks. The kidney may produce amounts of urine varying from extremes of no urine to large volumes of urine. During this stage, the patient may experience significant changes in fluid and electrolyte status; therefore, careful monitoring is indicated. The output from the urinary catheter (connected to a closed drainage system) is measured every 30 minutes to an hour. After the catheter is removed, the patient is instructed to void frequently to avoid stressing the bladder suture line. Intravenous fluids are administered in accordance with urine volume and serum electrolyte levels and as prescribed by the physician.

Other Possible Complications. Gastrointestinal ulceration and steroid-induced bleeding may occur. Fungal colonization of the gastrointestinal tract (especially the mouth) and urinary bladder may occur secondary to steroid and antibiotic administration. Cardiovascular disease is emerging as an important cause of death following transplantation, due in part to the increasing age of transplantation patients. An additional problem is possible tumor growth, because patients on long-term immunosuppressive therapy have been found to develop malignancies more frequently than the general population. This requires understanding and the expert management of emotional crises by all concerned with the person's care.

Psychologic Considerations. The rejection of a transplanted kidney remains a matter of concern to the patient, the patient's family, and the supporting health care team for many months. The fears of kidney rejection and the complications of immunosuppressive therapy (Cushing's syndrome, diabetes, capillary fragility, osteoporosis, glaucoma, cataracts, acne) place tremendous psychologic stresses on the patient. Anxiety and uncertainty about the future and difficult post-transplant adjustment are often sources of stress for the patient and his family.

Patient Education and Home Health Care. The patient is advised that follow-up care after transplantation is a lifelong necessity. He receives individual and written instructions concerning diet, medication, fluids, daily weight, daily measurement of urine, management of intake and output, prevention of infection, and resumption of activity and avoidance of contact sports in which the transplanted kidney may be injured.

The nurse works closely with the patient and family to ensure their understanding of the need for continuing the immunosuppressive drug as prescribed. Additionally, the patient and family are instructed to assess for and report signs of rejection of the transplanted kidney, signs of infection, or significant side effects of the immunosuppressive drugs. These include decrease in urinary output; weight gain; malaise; fever; respiratory distress; tenderness over the graft; anxiety; depression; changes in eating, drinking, or other habit patterns; and changes in blood pressure readings. The National Association of Kidney Patients is a nonprofit organization that serves the needs of those with kidney disease. It has many helpful suggestions for patients and family members learning to cope with dialysis and transplantation.

Organ Donation. An inadequate number of available organs remains the greatest limitation to the successful treatment of patients with end-stage renal disease. For those interested in donating a kidney, the National Kidney Foundation* will provide written information describing the organ donation

---

* *See bibliography at end of chapter for address.*

program and a card specifying the organ to be donated in the event of death. The card is signed by the donor and two witnesses and is to be carried by the donor at all times. Procurement of an adequate number of kidneys for potential recipients is still a major problem; however, many states have legislation that requires physicians to ask relatives of deceased patients with potential cadaver kidneys if they would consider donation. Nurses are often called on by family members to explain or clarify donation and the possible outcomes.

In summary, the patient with renal failure experiences changes that affect every organ and system of the body and often alter the patient's work, recreation, home, and family life. The patient who requires dialysis or transplantation usually undergoes considerable physiologic and psychologic stress during the long course of illness and treatment. Although dialysis reduces the patient's symptoms and improves his physical status, he still has end-stage renal disease that requires frequent, often exhausting treatments for survival. Transplantation is considered by many patients to be the last hope of a normal or near-normal life. The patient facing or recovering from transplantation often has a number of complex medical complications and concomitant nursing diagnoses that require a high degree of clinical knowledge and skill on the part of the nurse. The nurse caring for the patient with renal failure or transplantation must also have those skills necessary for assessing the psychologic status of the patient and family as the patient and family adjust to new complex treatments and setbacks.

Urolithiasis

Urolithiasis refers to the presence of stones (calculi) in the urinary system. Stones are formed in the urinary tract by the deposit of crystalline substances (calcium oxalate, calcium phosphate, uric acid) excreted in the urine. They may be found anywhere from the kidney to the bladder and vary in size from minute granular deposits, called sand or gravel, to bladder stones the size of an orange. The different sites of calculus formation in the urinary tract are shown in Figure 43-3.

Certain factors favor the formation of stones, including infection, urinary stasis, and periods of immobility (produces slowing of renal drainage and altered calcium metabolism). Hypercalcemia (high concentration of blood calcium compounds) and hypercalciuria (large amounts of calcium in the urine) may be caused by hyperparathyroidism, renal tubular acidosis, excessive intake of vitamin D, excessive intake of milk and alkali, and certain myeloproliferative diseases (leukemia, polycythemia vera, multiple myeloma), which produce an unusual proliferation of blood cells derived from bone marrow. These factors promote increased calcium concentrations in blood and urine, causing precipitation of calcium and formation of stones. Struvite calculi, or infection stones, are likely to occur when urease, a bacterial enzyme, is present in the urine. Some stones are caused by an excessive excretion of uric acid, the end product of purine metabolism. Urinary stone formation may also occur with inflammatory bowel disease and in those with an ileostomy or bowel resection, particularly of the small bowel, because these persons absorb more oxalate.

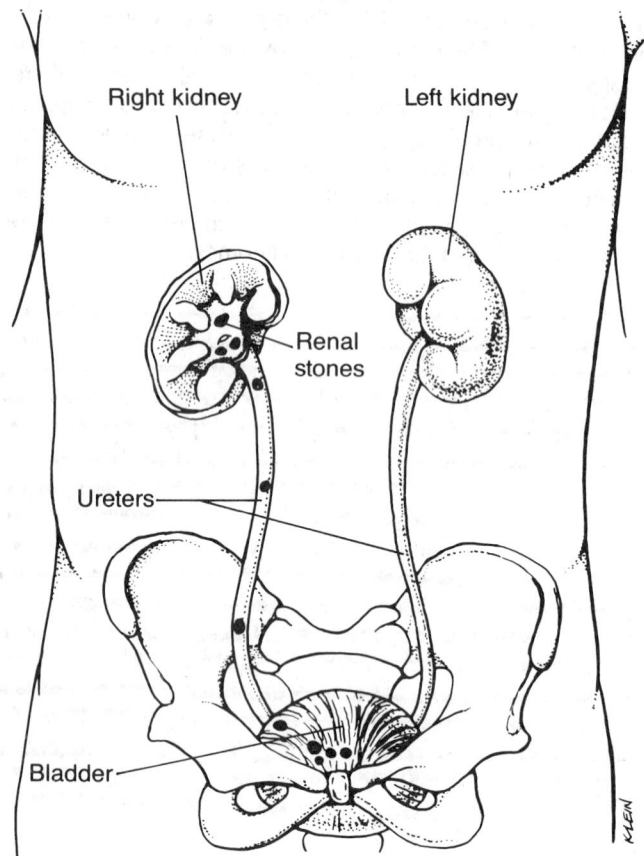

Right kidney

Left kidney

Renal stones

Ureters

Bladder

Figure 43–3. Various sites of calculous disease of the urinary tract (urolithiasis).

Vitamin A deficiency may be another cause. In many patients, however, no cause may be found.

The problem occurs predominantly in the third to fifth decades and affects men more than women. Persons who have had two stones tend to have recurrences. The majority of stones contain calcium or magnesium in combination with phosphorus or oxalate. Most stones are radiopaque and can be detected by roentgenography.

Clinical Manifestations

The clinical manifestations of stones in the urinary tract depend on the presence of obstruction, infection, and edema. When the stones block the flow of urine, obstruction develops, and the constant irritation of the stone may be followed by a secondary infection that causes pyelonephritis and cystitis with chills, fever, and dysuria. Some stones cause few if any symptoms while slowly destroying the functional units (nephrons) of the kidney; others cause excruciating pain and discomfort. Stones in the renal pelvis may be associated with intense, deep ache in the loin (part of the back between the thorax and pelvis) and with voiding of increased amounts of urine containing blood and white blood cells (pyuria). The stone produces an increase in hydrostatic pressure and distends the renal pelvis and proximal ureter. Thus, painful afferent sensations are initiated. Pain originating in the renal area radiates anteriorly and downward toward the bladder in the female and toward the testis in the male. If the pain suddenly becomes acute, the loin exquisitely tender, and nausea and vomiting

appear, the patient is having an attack of *renal colic*. Diarrhea and abdominal discomfort may accompany the attack. These gastrointestinal symptoms are due to renointestinal reflexes and the anatomic proximity of the kidneys to the stomach, pancreas, and large intestines.

When stones lodge in the ureter, acute, excruciating, colicky pain is experienced, radiating down the thigh and to the genitalia. The pain usually occurs in waves. There is usually a frequent desire to void, but very little urine is passed, and it usually contains blood because of the abrasive action of the stone. This group of symptoms is called *ureteral colic*. In general, the patient will spontaneously pass stones 0.5 to 1 cm in diameter. Those over 1 cm in diameter usually must be removed or broken up so that they can be removed or passed spontaneously. When stones lodge in the bladder, they usually produce symptoms of irritation and may be associated with urinary tract infection and hematuria. If the stone obstructs the bladder neck, there will be urinary retention.

Diagnostic Evaluation

The diagnosis is confirmed by intravenous urography or retrograde pyelography. Blood chemistries and a 24-hour urine test for measurement of calcium, uric acid, creatinine, sodium, *p*H, and total volume are part of the diagnostic workup. A dietary and drug history and family history of renal stones are obtained to identify factors predisposing the patient to the formation of stones.

Management

The basic goals underlying the management of the patient's disease are to eradicate the stone, to determine the stone type, to prevent nephron destruction, to control infection, and to relieve any obstruction that may be present. Infection and back-pressure of obstructed urine can destroy the renal parenchyma.

The immediate objective of treatment of renal or ureteral colic is to relieve the pain until its cause can be eliminated; morphine or meperidine is administered to prevent shock and syncope that may result from the excruciating pain. Hot baths or moist heat to the flank areas may also be useful. Unless the patient is vomiting, fluids are encouraged, because this treatment tends to increase the hydrostatic pressure behind the stone and thus assists it in its downward passage. A high round-the-clock fluid intake reduces the concentration of urinary crystalloids and ensures a high urinary output. A high fluid intake also reduces the specific gravity of the urine.

Cystoscopic examination and passage of a small ureteral catheter to dislodge the obstructive stone (when possible) immediately relieves back-pressure on the kidney and alleviates the intense pain.

When stones are recovered, chemical analysis is carried out to determine their composition. For example, calcium oxalate or calcium phosphate stones usually indicate disorders of oxalate or calcium metabolism, while urate stones suggest a disturbance in uric acid metabolism. Struvite stones (infection stones) account for 15% to 20% of urinary calculi. Specific antibacterial agents are administered if infection is present.

Diet and Drug Therapy. Diet therapy is most effective when stones are caused by metabolic abnormalities resulting in increased excretion of stone constituents (hypercalciuria) or altered physiochemical properties of the urine (urine acidity). Most stones contain calcium combined with phosphate or other substances. For these patients, the diet selected is moderately reduced in calcium and phosphorus content (Chart 43-2). The urine is acidified. Sometimes stones will cease enlarging simply by ensuring an adequate fluid intake and limiting certain foods in the diet that make up the main ingredient of the stone (*e.g.,* calcium).

Sodium cellulose phosphate has been reported to be effective in preventing calcium stones. It binds calcium from food in the intestinal tract, reducing the amount of calcium absorbed into the circulation. If increased parathormone production (resulting in increased serum calcium levels in blood and urine) is a factor in the formation of stones, thiazide therapy may be beneficial in reducing the calcium loss in the urine and lowering the elevated parathormone levels.

Patients who develop phosphatic calculi may be prescribed a diet low in phosphorus (see Chart 43-2). To offset excess phosphorus, aluminum hydroxide gel often is prescribed because it combines with the excess phosphorus, causing it to be excreted through the intestinal tract rather than in the urinary system.

For uric acid stones, the patient is placed on a low-purine diet to reduce the output of uric acid in the urine. Foods high in purine (shellfish and organ meats) are avoided, and other proteins may be limited. Allopurinol (Zyloprim) may be given to reduce serum and urinary uric acid excretion. The urine is alkalinized. For cystine stones, a low-protein diet is prescribed, the urine is alkalinized, and penicillamine is administered to reduce the amount of cystine in the urine.

For oxalate stones, a dilute urine is maintained and the intake of oxalate is limited. This means avoiding green, leafy vegetables, beans, celery, beets, rhubarb, chocolate, tea, coffee, and peanuts.

If the stone is not passed spontaneously or complications occur, treatment modalities may include extracorporeal shock wave therapy, percutaneous stone removal, or ureteroscopy.

Extracorporeal Shock Wave Lithotripsy. Extracorporeal shock wave lithotripsy (ESWL; Fig. 43-4) is a nonsurgical procedure used to break up stones in the calyx of the kidney. After the stones are reduced to small fragments the size of grains of sand, the remnants of the stones are passed in the urine through the lower urinary tract and voided.

In ESWL, or lithotripsy, a high-energy amplitude of pressure, or shock wave, is generated by the abrupt release of energy and transmitted through water and soft tissues. When the shock wave encounters a substance of different intensity (a kidney stone), a compression wave causes the surface of the stone to fragment. Repeated shock waves focused on the stone eventually reduce it to many small pieces that may be passed from the upper portion of the urinary tract spontaneously. The need for anesthesia for the procedure depends on the type of lithotriptor used, which determines the number and intensity of shock waves delivered. The shock waves are timed with the patient's electrocardiogram to prevent cardiac dysrhythmias. Multiple shocks are necessary, with their number depending on the size of the kidney stone to be fragmented. Although the shock waves usually do not damage other tissue,

---

Chart 43-2
Calcium- and Phosphorus-Restricted Diet Plan*

Foods Used

Milk: Limited to 1 cup (½ pint) a day. Cream may be substituted for part of the milk.

Cheese: Pot or cottage cheese only; limited to 2 oz.

Fats: As desired.

Eggs: Limited to 1 a day; egg whites as desired.

Meat, fish, fowl: Limited to 4 oz daily of beef, lamb, pork, veal, chicken, turkey, fish. See those to be avoided.

Soups and broths: All; cream soups made with milk allowance only.

Vegetables: At least 3 servings besides potato. One or 2 servings of deep-green or deep-yellow vegetables to be included daily. See list of those to be avoided.

Fruits: All except rhubarb. Include citrus fruit daily.

Breads, cereals, pastas: White, enriched bread, rolls, and crackers except those made from self-rising white flour; farina (not enriched); cornflakes; corn meal; hominy grits; rice; Rice Krispies; Puffed Rice; macaroni; spaghetti; noodles.

Desserts: Fruit pies, fruit cobblers, fruit ices, gelatin, puddings made with allowed milk and egg, angel food cake. (Do not use packaged mixes.)

Beverages: Coffee, Postum, Sanka, tea, gingerale.

Condiments: Sugar, jellies, honey, salt, pepper, spices.

Foods to Be Avoided

Cheese: All except pot or cottage cheese.

Meats, fish, fowl: Brains, heart, liver, kidney, sweetbreads, game (pheasant, rabbit, deer, grouse), sardines, fish roe.

Vegetables: Beet greens, chard, collards, mustard greens, spinach, turnip greens, dried beans, peas, lentils, soybeans.

Fruits: Rhubarb.

Breads, cereals, pastas: Whole-grain breads, cereals, and crackers; rye bread; all breads made with self-rising flour; oatmeal; brown and wild rice; bran; Bran Flakes; wheat germ; all dry cereals except those allowed.

Desserts: All except those allowed.

Beverages: Carbonated soft drinks, cocoa.

Miscellaneous: Nuts, peanut butter, chocolate, cocoa, condiments with a calcium or a phosphate base (read labels).

* This diet will contain 500 to 700 mg of calcium and from 1000 to 1200 mg of phosphorus.
(Anderson L et al. Nutrition in Health and Disease, 17th ed. Philadelphia, JB Lippincott.)

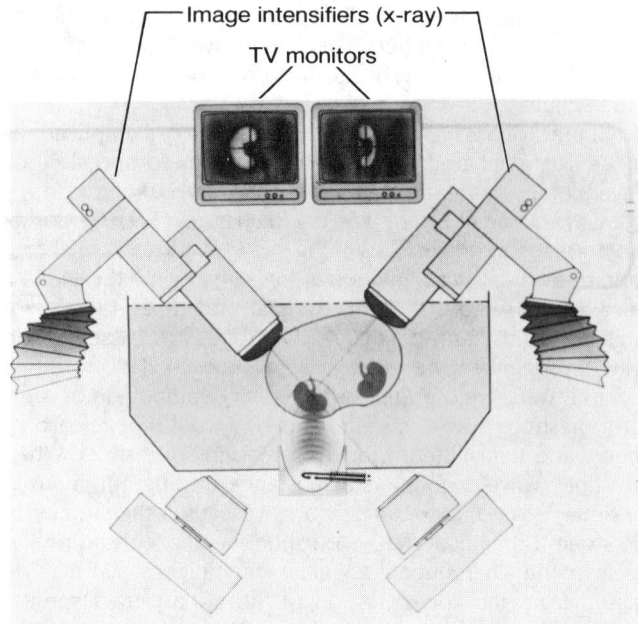

A

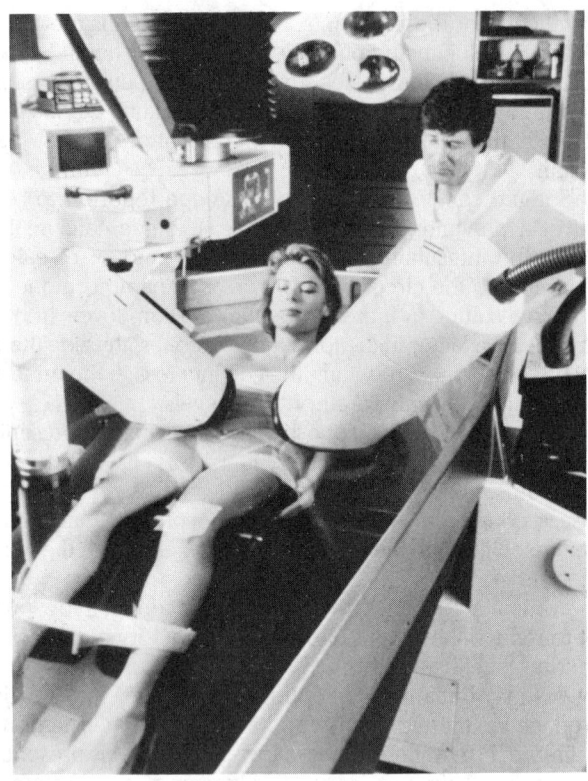

B

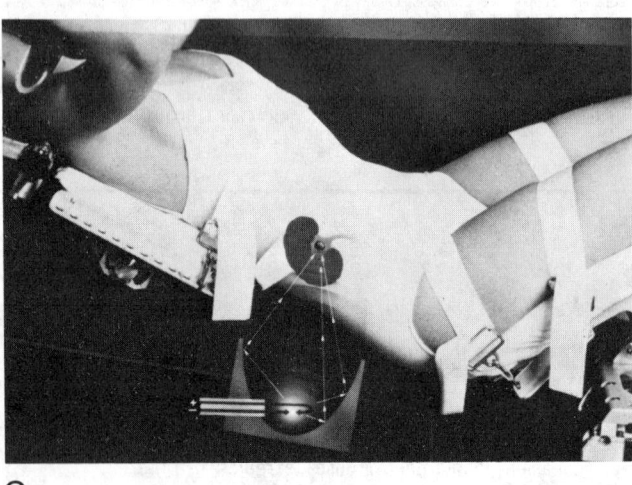

C

Figure 43–4.   Extracorporeal shock wave lithotripsy (ESWL). (**A**) Schematic diagram of the lithotripter directed toward a stone located in a patient's kidney (seen in cross-section). The patient is positioned to ensure precise three-dimensional localization of the kidney stone using fluoroscopy to visualize the stone on the TV monitors. (**B**) Patient positioned in the water bath for treatment. (With second-generation lithotripters, a fluid-filled bag may be used. The patient is positioned over the bag; submersion into a water bath is not necessary.) (**C**) Shock waves are directed at the kidney stone. (Courtesy of Dornier Medical Systems, Inc.)

discomfort from the multiple shocks may occur. Additionally, the patient is observed for damage to lung tissue as well as obstruction and infection resulting from blockage of the urinary tract by stone fragments. All urine is strained following the procedure; voided gravel or sand is sent to the laboratory for chemical analysis. The patient is encouraged to increase his fluid intake to assist in the passage of stone fragments, which may occur for 6 weeks to several months after the procedure.

Although lithotripsy is a costly treatment, it has decreased hospital stay and expenses by reducing the amount of time required by the patient to recover, because an invasive surgical procedure to remove the kidney stone is avoided. ESWL has also been used effectively on an outpatient basis; in this case, the patient and his family are instructed about signs and symptoms that indicate the occurrence of complications. The patient is followed closely to ensure that treatment has been effective and that no complications, such as obstruction, infection, renal hematoma, or hypertension, have developed. Several treatments may be necessary to ensure disintegration of stones.

Endourologic Methods of Stone Removal.   The field of endourology integrates the skills of the radiologist and urologist to extract renal calculi without major surgery. A percutaneous nephrostomy (or percutaneous nephrolithotomy) is performed (see Chap. 42), and a nephroscope is introduced through the dilated percutaneous tract into the renal parenchyma. Depending on its size, the stone may be extracted with forceps or by a stone basket, or an ultrasound probe is introduced through the nephrostomy tube and ultrasonic waves are used to pulverize the stone. Small stone fragments and stone dust are irrigated and suctioned out of the collecting system. Larger stones may be further reduced by ultrasonic disintegration and then removed with forceps or a stone basket. In a similar method, an electrical discharge is used to create a hydraulic shock wave to break up the stone (electrohydraulic lithotripsy).

A probe is passed through the cystoscope, and the tip of the lithotriptor is placed near the stone. The strength of the discharge and pulse frequency can be varied. This procedure is performed under topical anesthesia.

After stone extraction, the percutaneous nephrostomy tube is left in place for a time to ensure that the ureter is not obstructed by edema or blood clots. The most common complications are hemorrhage, infection, and urinary extravasation. Only a very small skin incision is required to remove the stone, a short hospital stay is required, and postoperative morbidity is minimal. After tube removal, the nephrostomy tract closes spontaneously.

Ureteroscopy. Ureteroscopy involves visualization and access to the ureter by insertion of instruments through a ureteroscope via cystoscopy. Stones can be removed or stones can be fragmented with the use of laser, electrohydraulic lithotripsy, or ultrasound and then removed. A stent may be inserted and left in place for 48 hours or more after the procedure to maintain patency of the ureter. Hospital stays are generally very short, and some patients can be successfully treated as outpatients.

Stone Dissolution. Infusions of chemolytic solutions (*e.g.*, alkylating agents, acidifying agents) for the purpose of stone dissolution may be performed as an alternative treatment for patients who are poor risks for other therapy, who refuse other methods, or who have easily dissolved (struvite) stones. Usually, a percutaneous nephrostomy is performed, and the warm irrigating solution is allowed to flow continuously onto the stone. The irrigating solution leaves the renal collecting system via the ureter or the nephrostomy tube. The pressure inside the renal pelvis is monitored during the procedure.

Several of these treatment modalities may be used in combination to ensure successful removal of the stones.

Surgical Removal. Once the major mode of therapy for the treatment of renal stones, surgical removal today is considered appropriate treatment for only 1% to 2% of patients. Surgical intervention is indicated if the stone does not respond to other forms of treatment. Surgery is also performed to correct any anatomic abnormalities within the kidney to improve urinary drainage.

If the stone is in the kidney, the operation performed may be a *nephrolithotomy* (incision into the kidney with removal of the stone) or a *nephrectomy*, if the kidney is nonfunctional secondary to infection or hydronephrosis. Stones in the kidney pelvis are removed by a *pyelolithotomy*, those in the ureter by *ureterolithotomy*, and those in the bladder by *cystotomy*. Sometimes an instrument is inserted through the urethra into the bladder, and the stone is crushed in the jaws of this instrument. Such an operation is called a *cystolitholapaxy*. The postoperative nursing management following kidney surgery is discussed in Chapter 42.

▶ **Nursing Process**
The Patient With Renal Stones

▷ **Assessment**

The patient with suspected renal stones is assessed for pain and discomfort. The severity and location of pain are assessed along with the area of radiation of the pain. The patient is also assessed for the presence of associated symptoms, such as nausea, vomiting, diarrhea, and abdominal distention. Additionally, the nursing assessment includes observations for signs of urinary tract infection (chills, fever, dysuria, frequency, and hesitancy) and obstruction (frequent urination of small amounts, oliguria, or anuria). The urine is observed for the presence of blood and strained for stones or gravel.

The history focuses on factors that predispose the patient to urinary tract stones or that may have precipitated the current episode of renal or ureteral colic. Factors that predispose the patient to stone formation may include family history of stones, the presence of cancer or bone marrow disorders or the use of chemotherapeutic agents, inflammatory bowel disease, or a diet high in calcium or purines. Factors that may precipitate stone formation in the patient predisposed to renal calculi include episodes of dehydration, prolonged immobilization, and infection. The patient's knowledge about renal stones and measures to prevent their occurrence or recurrence is also assessed.

▷ **Nursing Diagnoses**

Based on the assessment data, the nursing diagnoses of the patient with renal stones may include the following:

- Pain and discomfort related to inflammation, obstruction, and abrasion of the urinary tract
- High risk for infection and obstruction related to blockage of the urinary track by a stone or edema
- Knowledge deficit regarding prevention of recurrence of renal stones

▷ **Planning and Implementation**

▷ *Goals:* The patient's major goals may include relief of pain and discomfort, prevention of infection and obstruction, and prevention of recurrence of renal stones.

▷ **Nursing Interventions**

▷ *Relieving Pain.* Immediate relief of severe pain from renal or ureteral colic is promoted through the use of narcotic analgesics as prescribed. Intravenous or intramuscular administration may be prescribed to provide rapid relief and prevent shock from developing as a result of the excruciating pain. Moist heat to the flank may also be prescribed and may provide some relief. The patient is encouraged and assisted to assume a position of comfort. If the patient obtains some pain relief by ambulating, he is assisted to do so. The patient's pain is monitored closely, and increases in severity are reported promptly to the physician so that relief can be provided and additional treatment initiated. The patient is prepared for other treatment (*e.g.*, lithotripsy, percutaneous stone removal, ureteroscopy, or surgery) if severe pain is unrelieved and the stone is not passed spontaneously.

▷ *Preventing Infection and Obstruction.* The patient with suspected renal stones is at risk of infection and obstruction of the urinary tract. He is instructed to report decreased urine volume and bloody or cloudy urine. The total urine output and patterns of voiding are monitored. Increased fluid intake is encouraged to prevent dehydration and increase hydrostatic pressure within the urinary tract to promote passage of the stone. If the patient is unable to take adequate fluids orally, intravenous fluids will be prescribed. The patient is assisted with walking because ambulation may help to move the stone through the urinary tract.

The nursing care of patients with calculi requires constant observation to detect the spontaneous passage of a stone. All urine is strained through gauze, because uric acid stones may crumble. Any blood clots passed in the urine should be crushed and the sides of the urinal and bedpan inspected for clinging stones.

▷ *Patient Education and Home Health Care.* Because it is known that urinary calculi may recur after the first stone forms, the patient is encouraged to follow a regimen to avoid further stone formation. One facet of prevention is to *maintain a high fluid intake,* because stones form more readily in a concentrated urine. A patient who has shown a tendency to form stones should drink enough to excrete 3000 to 4000 ml of urine every 24 hours, should adhere to the prescribed diet, and should avoid sudden increases in environmental temperatures, which may cause a fall in urinary volume. Occupations and sports that produce excessive sweating can lead to severe temporary dehydration; therefore, fluid intake should be increased. Sufficient fluids should be taken in the evening to prevent urine from becoming too concentrated at night. Urine cultures may be performed every 1 to 2 months the first year and periodically thereafter. Recurrent urinary infection is treated vigorously.

Because prolonged immobilization slows renal drainage and alters calcium metabolism, increased mobility is to be encouraged whenever possible. In addition, excessive ingestion of vitamins (especially vitamin D) and minerals is discouraged.

If the patient has undergone lithotripsy, percutaneous stone removal, ureteroscopy, or other surgical procedures for stone removal, he is instructed about the signs and symptoms of complications that warrant that the physician be notified. The importance of follow-up to assess kidney function and to ensure the successful eradication or removal of all kidney stones is emphasized to the patient and his family.

If medications are prescribed for the prevention of stone formation, the actions and importance of the medications are explained to the patient. Additionally, detailed information about foods to be included and excluded is provided verbally and in writing. The patient may be instructed to monitor his urinary pH; he will be instructed by the nurse about the procedures of determining the pH and interpreting the results. Because of the high risk of recurrence, the patient with renal stones is taught the signs and symptoms of stone formation, obstruction, and infection. He is directed to report these to the physician promptly.

▷ *Evaluation*

Expected Outcomes

1. Experiences relief of pain.
   a. Reports decreased pain and discomfort.
   b. Assumes a position of comfort.
   c. Ambulates progressively with assistance.
   d. Requests analgesia as prescribed.
   e. Uses moist heat to flank area and hot baths to relieve discomfort.
   f. Exhibits no signs of pain-induced shock or syncope.

2. Exhibits no indications of urinary tract infection or obstruction.
   a. Voids clear urine without red blood cells.
   b. Voids 200 to 400 ml of urine per voiding.
   c. Reports absence of dysuria, frequency, and hesitancy.
   d. Exhibits normal body temperature.
   e. Reports no chills.

3. Exhibits increased knowledge of health behaviors to prevent recurrence.
   a. Consumes high fluid intake (10 to 12 glasses of fluid per day).
   b. Voids dilute urine that is clear in color and free of blood.
   c. Identifies actions to take to avoid dehydration.
   d. Avoids prolonged periods of immobilization and activity if possible.
   e. Consumes diet prescribed to reduce dietary factors predisposing to stone formation.
   f. Avoids foods high in calcium, phosphorus, oxalate, or purine.
   g. Identifies symptoms to be reported to health care provider (fever, chills, flank pain, hematuria).
   h. Monitors urinary pH as directed.
   i. Takes prescribed medication as directed to reduce stone formation.
   j. Notifies health care provider of signs and symptoms of complications following stone removal or fragmentation procedures.

In summary, the introduction of new technology and new methods of treatment for kidney stones increases the importance of the nurse's role in patient education, counseling, and follow-up. Many of the new modes of therapy are performed on an outpatient basis or involve very short hospital stays. Therefore, patients and their families need appropriate instruction and education about possible complications, including methods to assess for complications, strategies to take to treat or minimize complications, and situations that require follow-up by the physician or nurse.

Renal Trauma

Various types of injuries of the flank, back, or upper abdomen may result in bruising, lacerations, or rupture of the kidney or pedicle injury. The kidneys are protected by the musculature of the back posteriorly and by a cushion of abdominal wall and viscera anteriorly. They are highly mobile and are "fixed" only at the renal pedicle. With traumatic injury, the kidney can be thrust against the lower ribs, resulting in contusion and rupture. Rib fractures occurring with renal displacement or a fracture of the transverse process of the upper lumbar vertebrae may be associated with renal contusion or laceration. Injuries may be blunt (auto and motorcycle accidents, falls, athletic injuries) or penetrating (gunshot wounds, stabbings). Failure to wear seat belts contributes to the incidence of renal trauma in motor vehicle accidents (MVAs). Renal trauma is frequently associated with other injuries.

The most common renal injuries are contusions, laceration, rupture, and renal pedicle injuries or small internal laceration of the kidney. The kidneys receive half of the blood flow from the abdominal aorta; therefore, even a fairly small renal laceration can produce massive bleeding.

Clinical Manifestations.   The clinical manifestations include pain, renal colic (due to clots/fragments obstructing the collecting system), hematuria, flank mass, ecchymoses, and lacerations or wounds of the lateral abdomen and flank. Signs and symptoms of hypovolemia and shock are likely with significant hemorrhage.

Management.   The goals of management are to control hemorrhage, pain, and infection; to preserve and restore renal function; and to maintain urinary drainage.

Hematuria is the most common manifestation of renal trauma; therefore, the appearance of blood in the urine following an injury suggests the possibility of renal injury. There is no relationship between the degree of hematuria and the degree of injury. Hematuria may be absent or detectable only on microscopic examination. Therefore, all urine is saved and sent to the laboratory for analysis to detect the presence of red blood cells and to follow the course of bleeding. The time the urine is voided and the volume are recorded. Hematocrit and hemoglobin levels are monitored closely; decreasing values indicate hemorrhage.

The patient is monitored for oliguria and signs of hemorrhagic shock, because a pedicle injury or shattered kidney can lead to rapid exsanguination (lethal blood loss). An expanding hematoma may cause rupture of the kidney capsule. To detect the presence of hematoma, the area around the lower ribs, upper lumbar vertebrae, flank, and abdomen is palpated for tenderness. A palpable flank or abdominal mass with local tenderness, swelling, and ecchymosis suggests renal hemorrhage or extravasation. The area of the original mass can be outlined with a marking pencil so that the observer can evaluate the area for change. Severe flank or costovertebral pain may signal a pedicle injury, which can cause ischemic necrosis of the kidney. Renal trauma is often associated with other injuries to the abdominal organs (liver, colon, small intestines); therefore, the patient is assessed for skin abrasions, lacerations, and entry and exit wounds of the upper abdomen and lower thorax, because these may be associated with renal injury. Up to 80% of patients with renal trauma have associated injuries of other internal organs.

Renal trauma may be classified on the basis of the mechanism of injury (blunt versus penetrating injuries), the anatomic location, or the severity of the injury. *Minor* renal trauma includes contusions, hematomas, and some lacerations of the cortex of the kidney. *Major* renal injuries include major lacerations with rupture of the capsule of the kidney. *Critical* renal trauma involves multiple and severe lacerations of the kidney with injury to the vascular supply of the kidney.

In minor injuries to the kidney, healing may take place with conservative measures. The patient is kept on bed rest until hematuria clears. Intravenous infusions may be necessary, because retroperitoneal bleeding may produce a reflex paralytic ileus.

Antimicrobial drugs may be prescribed to prevent infection from perirenal hematoma or urinoma (a cyst containing urine). Patients with retroperitoneal hematomas may develop a low-grade fever as absorption of the clot takes place.

The patient should be evaluated frequently during the first few days following injury in order to detect flank and abdominal pain, muscle spasm, and swelling over the flank.

- Any *sudden* change in the patient's condition may indicate hemorrhage and require surgical intervention. The vital signs are monitored to detect evidence of bleeding. Narcotic analgesia is avoided because this may mask accompanying abdominal symptoms.
- The patient is prepared for surgical exploration if increasing pulse rate, hypotension, and impending shock occur.

Critical renal injuries and most penetrating injuries require surgical exploration because of the high incidence of involvement of other organ systems and the serious complications that may result if these injuries are untreated. The damaged kidney may have to be removed (nephrectomy), although on occasion it is possible to repair it. Patients with major renal injuries may be treated conservatively (bed rest, no surgery) or through surgical intervention, depending on the patient's condition and the nature of the injury.

Early postoperative complications (within 6 months) include rebleeding, abscess, sepsis, urine extravasation, and fistula formation.

Patient Education and Home Health Care.   Follow-up care includes monitoring the blood pressure to detect hypertension that may occur on a renovascular basis. Other complications include stone formation, infection, cysts, vascular aneurysms, and loss of renal function. Activity is usually restricted for 1 month following trauma to minimize the incidence of delayed or secondary bleeding. The patient is instructed about what changes should be reported to the physician. Guidelines for increasing activity gradually are also provided.

Bladder Injuries

Injury to the bladder may occur with pelvic fractures and multiple trauma or from a blow to the lower abdomen when the bladder is full. Blunt trauma may result in contusion (an ecchymosis or large discolored bruise resulting from escape of blood into the tissues and involving a segment of the bladder wall) or in rupture of the bladder, extraperitoneally, intraperitoneally, or a combination of both. Complications from these injuries (hemorrhage, shock, sepsis, and extravasation of blood into the tissues) must be treated promptly.

A retrograde urethrogram is performed first to evaluate for urethral injury. The patient is catheterized *after* the urethrogram is performed to minimize the risk of urethral disruption and extensive, long-term complications.

Management.   Treatment for traumatic rupture of the bladder involves immediate surgical exploration and repair of the laceration, with suprapubic drainage of the bladder and the perivesical space (around the bladder) along with insertion of an indwelling urethral catheter.

In addition to the usual postoperative care following urologic surgery, the drainage systems (suprapubic, indwelling urethral catheter, and perivesical drains) are closely monitored to ensure adequate drainage until healing takes place. The patient with a ruptured bladder may have gross bleeding for several days after repair. Complications of urethral injuries include stricture, incontinence, and impotence.

Renal Cysts

Cysts of the kidney may be multiple (polycystic) or single. Polycystic disease of the adult is inherited as an autosomal dominant trait and usually involves both kidneys. The patient presents with abdominal or lumbar pain, hematuria, hypertension, palpable renal masses, and recurrent urinary tract infections. Renal insufficiency and failure usually develop in the terminal stages. Polycystic renal disease is also associated with cystic diseases of other organs (liver, pancreas, spleen) and aneurysms of the cerebral arteries. It is characteristically seen in midlife.

Management.   Because there is no specific treatment for polycystic renal disease, care of the patient is directed toward relief of pain, symptoms, and complications. Hypertension and urinary tract infections are treated aggressively. Dialysis is indicated when signs of renal insufficiency and failure occur. Genetic counseling is part of patient education, because polycystic kidney disease is a hereditary disease. The patient is advised to avoid sports and occupations that present a risk of trauma to the kidney.

Simple cysts of the kidney usually occur unilaterally and differ clinically and pathophysiologically from polycystic kidney disease. The cyst may be drained percutaneously.

Congenital Anomalies

Congenital anomalies of the kidney are not uncommon. Occasionally there is fusion of the two kidneys, forming what is called a *horseshoe kidney*. One kidney may be small and deformed and often is nonfunctioning. Not infrequently there may be a double ureter or congenital stricture of the ureter. The treatment of these anomalies is necessary only if they cause symptoms, but it is important to determine that the other kidney is present and functioning before surgery is undertaken.

Renal Tumors

Cancer of the kidney accounts for 2% of all cancers in adults in the United States; it affects almost twice as many men as women. Risk factors include tobacco use, occupational exposure to industrial chemicals, obesity, and dialysis (the incidence of renal cysts and renal tumors is increased in patients on long-term dialysis). Renal tumors may arise from the renal capsule, parenchyma (renal cell carcinomas), connective tissue (sarcomas), or fatty tissue, or they may be neurogenic or vascular. Almost 90% of all tumors are adenocarcinomas. These tumors may metastasize early to the lungs, bone, liver, brain, and contralateral kidney. One-fourth to one-half of patients will have metastatic disease at the time of diagnosis.

Clinical Manifestations

Many renal tumors produce no symptoms and are discovered on a routine physical examination as a palpable abdominal mass. The classic triad, occurring late in the course of the disease, is blood in the urine (hematuria), pain, and a mass in the flank. *The usual sign that first calls attention to the tumor is painless hematuria,* which may be either intermittent and microscopic or continuous and gross. There may be a dull pain in the back from back-pressure produced by compression of the ureter, extension of the tumor into the perirenal area, or hemorrhage into the substance of the kidney. Colicky pains occur if a clot or mass of tumor cells passes down the ureter. Symptoms from metastasis may be the first manifestation of renal tumor and include unexplained weight loss, increasing weakness, and anemia.

The diagnosis of a renal tumor may require intravenous urography, cystoscopic examination, nephrotomograms, renal angiograms, ultrasonography, or computed tomography (CT scan). These tests may be exhausting for a patient already debilitated by the systemic effects of a tumor, for the elderly patient, and for one anxious about the diagnosis and outcome. The nurse assists the patient physically and psychologically in preparation for these procedures and monitors him carefully for signs of dehydration and exhaustion.

Management

The goal of management is to eradicate the tumor before metastasis occurs. A radical nephrectomy is the preferred treatment if the tumor can be removed. This includes removal of the kidney (and tumor), adrenal gland, surrounding perinephric fat and Gerota's fascia, and lymph nodes. Radiation therapy, hormonal therapy, or chemotherapy may be used along with surgery. Immunotherapy may be helpful.

Renal Artery Embolization.   In patients with metastatic renal carcinoma, embolization of the renal artery is performed to occlude the blood supply to the tumor and thus cause the death of tumor cells. Several days after completion of angiographic studies, a catheter is advanced into the renal artery, and embolizing materials (Gelfoam, autologous blood clot, steel coils) are injected into the artery and carried with the arterial blood flow to mechanically occlude the tumor vessels. This decreases the local blood supply, making removal of the kidney (nephrectomy) easier, and theoretically stimulates an immune response. This is based on the concept that infarction of the renal cell carcinoma will release tumor-associated antigens that will enhance the patient's response to metastatic lesions. The procedure may also reduce the number of tumor cells entering the venous circulation during surgical manipulation.

Following renal artery embolization and tumor infarction, a characteristic symptom complex labeled "postinfarction syndrome" occurs, lasting 2 to 3 days. The patient has pain localized to the flank and abdomen, an elevated temperature, and gastrointestinal complaints. Pain is treated with parenteral analgesics, while aspirin controls the fever; antiemetics, restriction of oral intake, and maintenance with intravenous fluids are used to treat the gastrointestinal complaints.

Biologic Therapy.   Success in treating renal tumors with biologic response modifiers has recently been reported. Patients may be treated with interleukin-2 (IL-2), a protein that regulates cell growth. This may be used alone or in combination with lymphokine-activated killer (LAK) cells, which are white blood cells that have been stimulated by IL-2 to increase their ability to kill cancer cells. Interferon, another biologic response modifier, is also under investigation as a mode of therapy for treating advanced renal cancer.

Nursing Interventions

The patient with a renal tumor may undergo extensive diagnostic and therapeutic procedures, including surgery, radiation therapy, and chemotherapy. Following surgery, the patient usually has catheters and drains in place to maintain a patent urinary tract, to remove drainage, and to permit very accurate measurement of urine output. Because of the location of the surgical incision and the position of the patient during the surgical procedure, pain and muscle soreness are common. The patient requires frequent analgesia during the postoperative period and assistance with turning. He is encouraged to turn, cough, and take deep breaths to prevent atelectasis and other pulmonary complications. The patient and his family require assistance and support to cope with the diagnosis and uncertainties about outcome. (See Chap. 42 for postoperative care of the patient undergoing renal surgery and Chap. 19 for care of the oncology patient.)

Follow-up care is essential to detect signs of metastases as well as to reassure the patient and family about the patient's continued well-being. The patient who has had surgery for renal carcinoma should have a yearly physical examination and x-ray of the chest throughout life, because late metastases are not uncommon. All subsequent symptoms should be evaluated with possible metastases in mind.

Cancer of the Bladder

Cancer of the urinary bladder is seen more frequently in persons from age 50 onward and affects men more than women (3:1). Statistics indicate that these tumors make up approximately 2% of all cancers in the body and are on the increase. The most common type is transitional cell cancer.

Risk factors for cancer of the bladder include cigarette smoking and carcinogens in the work environment, such as dyes, rubber, leather, ink, or paint. There may be a relationship between coffee drinking and bladder cancer. Chronic schistosomiasis (parasitic infection that irritates the bladder) is also a risk factor. Cancers arising from the prostate, colon, and rectum in males and from the lower gynecologic tract in females may metastasize to the bladder.

Clinical Manifestations. These tumors usually arise at the base of the bladder and involve the ureteral orifices and bladder neck. *Gross, painless hematuria* is the most common symptom of cancer of the bladder. Infection of the urinary tract is a common complication, producing frequency, urgency, and dysuria. However, any alteration in voiding or change in the urine may indicate cancer of the bladder. Pelvic or back pain may occur with metastasis.

The diagnostic evaluation may include excretory urography, computed tomography (CT scan), ultrasonography, cystoscopy, and bimanual examination under anesthesia. Biopsies of the tumor and adjacent mucosa are the definitive diagnostic procedures.

Transitional cell carcinomas and carcinomas *in situ* shed recognizable cancer cells. Cytologic examination of fresh urine and saline bladder washings provide information about the patient's prognosis, especially for those at high risk for recurrence of primary bladder tumors.

Management. Treatment of bladder cancer depends on the grade of the tumor (based on the degree of cellular differentiation), the stage of tumor growth (the degree of local invasion and the presence or absence of metastasis), and the multicentricity (having many centers) of the tumor. The patient's age and physical, mental, and emotional status are considered in determining treatment modalities.

Transurethral resection or fulguration may be performed for simple papillomas (benign epithelial tumors). These procedures eradicate the tumors through surgical incision or electrical current with the use of instruments inserted through the urethra. One of the greatest challenges is the management of superficial bladder cancers, because there are usually widespread abnormalities in the bladder mucosa. The entire lining of the urinary tract, or urothelium, is at risk, because carcinomatous changes are found not only in the mucosa of the bladder but also in that of the renal pelvis, ureter, and urethra. Recurrences are a serious problem; approximately 60% of superficial bladder tumors recur after transurethral resection or fulguration. Persons with benign papillomas should be followed with cytology and cystoscopy periodically for the rest of their lives because aggressive malignancies may develop from these tumors.

Chemotherapy with use of a combination of methotrexate, vinblastine, doxorubicin (Adriamycin), and cisplatin (M-VAC) has been effective in producing partial remission of transitional cell carcinoma of the bladder in some patients with advanced disease. Clinical trials are under way to evaluate the use of M-VAC with surgery and radiation therapy.

Topical chemotherapy (intravesical chemotherapy or instillation of antineoplastic agents into the bladder resulting in contact of the agent with the bladder wall) is considered when there is high risk of recurrence, when cancer *in situ* is present, or when tumor resection has been incomplete. Topical chemotherapy delivers a high concentration of drug (thiotepa, doxorubicin, 5-fluorouracil) to the tumor to promote tumor destruction. Fluid intake may be limited during instillation of the drug to prevent the need to void during the procedure, which takes approximately 2 hours. At the conclusion, the patient is encouraged to void and to drink liberal amounts of fluid to flush the drug from the bladder.

The tumor may be irradiated preoperatively to reduce microextension of the neoplasm and viability of tumor cells, thus reducing the chances that the cancer may recur in the immediate area or spread through the circulatory or lymphatic systems. Radiation therapy is also used in combination with surgery or to control the disease in the patient with an inoperable tumor.

A simple cystectomy (removal of the bladder) or a radical cystectomy is performed for invasive or multifocal bladder cancer. Radical cystectomy in the male involves removal of the bladder, prostate, and seminal vesicles and immediate adjacent perivesical tissues. In the female, radical cystectomy involves removal of the bladder, lower ureter, uterus, tubes, ovaries, anterior vagina, and urethra. It may or may not include a pelvic lymphadenectomy (removal of lymph nodes). Removal of the bladder requires a urinary diversion procedure (see below).

The transitional cell variety of bladder cancer responds poorly to chemotherapy. Cisplatin, doxorubicin, and cyclophosphamide have been administered in various doses and schedules and appear most effective.

Bladder cancer may also be treated by direct infusion of the cytotoxic agent through the arterial supply of the involved organ. Thus, a higher concentration of the chemotherapeutic agent can be achieved with reduction of its systemic toxic effects. For more advanced bladder cancer or for patients with intractable hematuria (especially following radiation therapy), a large water-filled balloon placed within the bladder produces tumor necrosis by reducing the blood supply of the bladder wall (hydrostatic therapy). The instillation of formalin, phenol, or silver nitrate has achieved relief of hematuria and strangury (slow and painful discharge of urine) in some patients.

Urinary Diversion

Urinary diversion refers to a means of diverting the urine away from the bladder so that it exits via a new route, usually through an opening in the skin (stoma). This is performed primarily when a large or invasive bladder tumor requires removal of the entire bladder. Urinary diversion has also been used in the management of pelvic malignancy, birth defects, strictures and trauma to ureters and urethra, neurogenic bladder, chronic infection causing severe ureteral and renal damage, and intractable interstitial cystitis.

There is controversy concerning the best means of establishing permanent diversion of the urinary tract. Additionally, new techniques are frequently introduced in an effort to improve patient outcomes. The age of the patient, condition of the bladder, body build, degree of obesity, degree of ureteral dilation, state of renal function, and the patient's acceptance of the results of the procedure and his learning ability are all taken into consideration in determining the appropriate surgical procedure.

Long-term acceptance of urinary diversion by the patient depends to a large degree on the location or position of the stoma, a water-tight seal of the drainage pouch/bag to the skin, and his ability to manage the pouch and drainage apparatus. Therefore, attention must be given to these considerations to promote a positive outcome.

There are two categories of urinary diversion: *ureteroenterocutaneous diversions* (a portion of the intestines is used to create a new reservoir for urine) and *cutaneous diversions* (a diversion in which urine drains through an opening created in the abdominal wall and skin).

The most common methods of urinary diversion are listed below:

Ureteroenterocutaneous Diversions
1. *Conventional conduit:* transplanting the ureters to an isolated section of the terminal ileum, (*ileal conduit*) and bringing one end to the abdominal wall (Fig. 43-5A). The ureter may also be transplanted into the transverse sigmoid colon (colon conduit) or proximal jejunum (jejunal conduit).
2. *Continent ileal urinary reservoir (Kock pouch):* transplanting the ureters to an isolated segment of ileum (pouch) with a nipple-like one-way valve; urine is drained by catheter (Fig. 43-6).
3. *Ureterosigmoidostomy:* introducing the ureters into the sig-

moid, thereby allowing urine to flow through the colon and out of the rectum (see Fig. 43-5B).

Cutaneous Urinary Diversions
4. *Cutaneous ureterostomy:* bringing the detached ureter through the abdominal wall and attaching it to an opening in the skin (see Fig. 43-5C).
5. *Vesicostomy:* suturing the bladder to the abdominal wall and creating an opening (stoma) through the abdominal and bladder walls for urinary drainage (see Fig. 43-5D).
6. *Nephrostomy:* inserting a catheter into the renal pelvis via an incision into the flank or by percutaneous catheter placement into the kidney (see Fig. 43-5E).

Ileal Conduit Urinary Diversion (Ileal Loop)

In an ileal conduit, the urine is diverted by implanting the ureter into a loop of ileum that is led out through the abdominal wall. This loop of ileum is a simple conduit (passageway) for urine from the ureters to the surface. A loop of the sigmoid colon may also be used. An ileostomy bag is used to collect the urine. The resected (cut) ends of the remaining intestine are anastomosed (connected) to provide an intact bowel.

Stents, usually made of thin, pliable tubing, are placed in the ureters to prevent occlusion secondary to postsurgical edema. They may be left in place 5 to 15 days postoperatively. To compensate for the space of the removed bladder, Jackson Pratt tubes or other types of drains are inserted to prevent the accumulation of fluid that occurs.

After surgery, a skin barrier and a transparent, disposable urinary drainage bag are applied around the conduit and connected to drainage. A custom-cut appliance is used until the edema subsides and the stoma shrinks to normal size. The clear bag allows the stoma to be visualized and the patency of the stent and the urinary output to be better monitored. The ileal bag drains urine constantly (not feces). The appliance (bag) usually remains in place as long as it is watertight; it is changed when necessary to prevent leakage of urine.

Nursing Interventions. In the immediate postoperative period, urine volumes are checked hourly, because an output below 30 ml/hr may indicate an obstruction in the ileal conduit with possible backflow or leakage from the ureteroileal anastomosis. A catheter may be inserted through the urinary conduit if prescribed to check for possible stasis or residual urine from a constricted stoma.

The stoma is inspected frequently for bleeding. Minimal bleeding may be seen and implies good blood supply. A change in color of the stoma from a normal pink to red color to a dark purplish color suggests that the vascular supply may be compromised. If cyanosis and compromised blood supply persist, surgical intervention is likely.

The stoma is not sensitive to touch, but the skin around the stoma becomes very sensitive if it becomes irritated by urine or by the appliance. The skin is inspected for (1) signs of irritation and bleeding of the stomal mucosa; (2) alkaline encrustation with skin irritation around the stoma (from alkaline urine coming in contact with exposed skin); and (3) wound infections.

Moisture in bed linens or clothing or the odor of urine around the patient should alert the nursing personnel to the possibility of leakage from the appliance, the presence of an infection, or a problem in hygienic management. Because se-

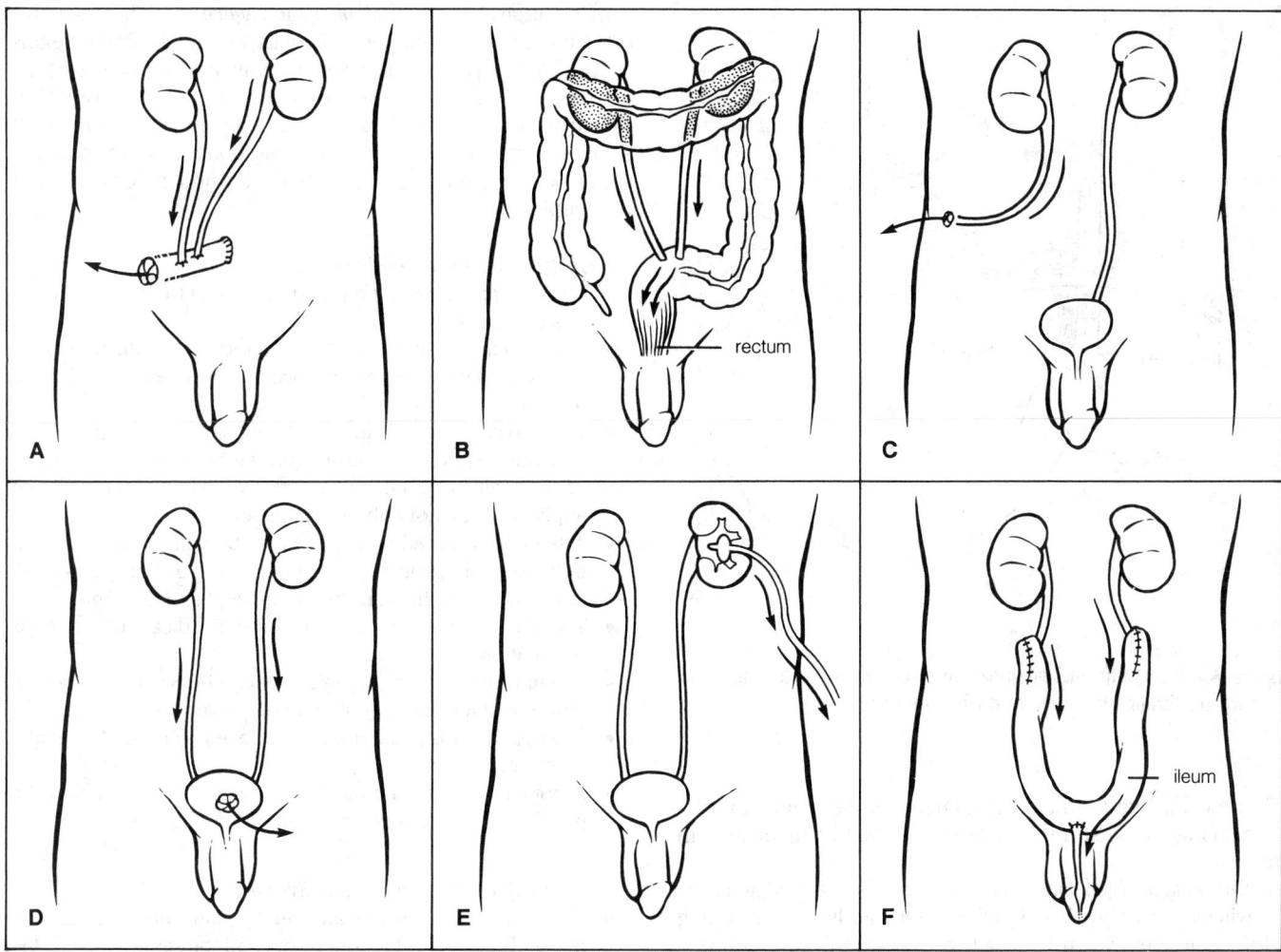

Figure 43–5. Methods of urinary diversion. (**A**) Ileal conduit. (**B**) Ureterosigmoidostomy. (**C**) Cutaneous ureterostomy. (**D**) Vesicostomy. (**E**) Nephrostomy. (**F**) Camey Procedure.

vere alkaline encrustation can accumulate rapidly around the stoma, the urine *p*H is kept below 6.5. Urine *p*H can be determined by testing the urine draining from the stoma, not from the collecting appliance. A properly fitted appliance is essential to prevent exposure of the peristomal skin (skin around the stoma) to urine. If the urine is foul smelling, the stoma is catheterized, if prescribed, in order to obtain a specimen for culture and sensitivity or to determine if the stoma is patent and draining properly and to detect the presence of residual urine. Scarring of the stoma can interfere with urine drainage.

A high-fluid diet is encouraged in order to flush the ileal conduit and decrease the accumulation of mucus. The patient may excrete a fairly large amount of mucus mixed with urine as a result of the use of a mucous membrane for formation of the conduit. To relieve anxiety, the patient is reassured that this is a normal occurrence following an ileal conduit.

Complications. Complications following this method of urinary diversion include wound infection or wound dehiscence, urinary leakage, ureteral obstruction, hyperchloremic acidosis, small bowel obstruction, and stomal gangrene. Delayed complications include ureteral obstruction, contraction or narrowing of the stoma (stomal stenosis), pyelonephritis, and renal calculi.

Patient Education and Home Care

Appliance Selection. The urinary appliance may consist of one or two pieces and may be disposable (usually used once and discarded) or reusable. The choice of appliance is determined by the location of the stoma and the patient's normal activity, body build, and economic resources. A reusable appliance has a faceplate that is attached to the skin surface with cement or adhesive. Either reusable pouches or disposable pouches may be used with the reusable faceplate. Disposable appliances are discarded after each use. They have the advantage of having a surface that is already prepared and of being lightweight and easy to conceal. A skin barrier must be used to protect the skin from excoriation due to exposure to the urine. See Figure 43-7 for examples of appliances.

Determining the Stoma Size. As the postoperative edema subsides, the stoma opening is recalibrated every 3 to 6 weeks for the first few months postoperatively. The correct appliance size is determined by measuring the widest part of the stoma with a ruler. The permanent appliance should be no more than

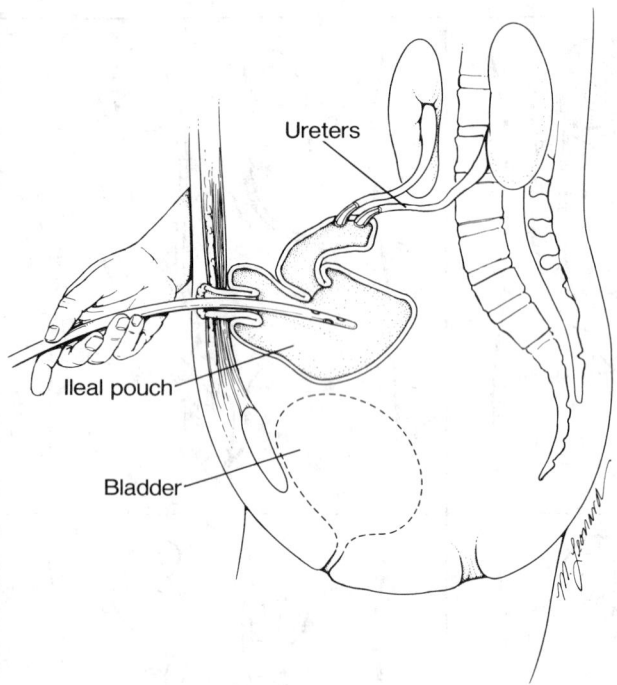

Figure 43–6. Continent ileal urinary reservoir (Kock pouch). Insertion of a catheter through the valve to drain stored urine.

1.6 mm (⅛ in) larger than the diameter of the stoma and the same shape as the stoma to prevent contact of the skin with drainage.

Changing the Appliance. The appliance is changed at a time that will be most convenient to the patient. Early in the morning before fluids are taken is usually a convenient time because the urine output is reduced. The collecting appliance usually lasts 3 to 5 days before leakage occurs.

Instructions for Application of the Appliance. The objective is to change the system before it leaks, but definitely if it begins to leak. A variety of appliances are available; regardless of the type of appliance used, a skin barrier is essential to protect the skin from irritation and excoriation. To maintain peristomal skin integrity, a skin barrier or leaking pouch is never patched with tape to prevent accumulation of urine under the skin barrier or faceplate.

Instructions for a Reusable System
- The new appliance is prepared according to the manufacturer's directions.
- The opening of the faceplate is tailored to the patient's stoma.
- The edge of the faceplate is moistened with water or adhesive remover.
- The peristomal skin is cleansed with a small amount of soap and warm water. It is thoroughly rinsed and dried; if a film of soap remains on the skin or the skin is not dried well, the appliance may not adhere adequately.
- A tampon or rolled gauze pad may be gently placed on top of the stomal opening (not inserted into the stoma) to absorb urine and keep the skin dry during appliance change.
- The skin surrounding the stoma is inspected carefully for signs of irritation.
- A skin protector wipe or seal ring can be used prior to centering the faceplate opening directly over the stoma.
- The appliance is positioned and applied with firm but gentle pressure.
- A pouch cover can be used or cornstarch applied under the pouch to prevent perspiration and skin irritation.

Instructions for a Disposable System
- The stoma is measured and an opening made in the skin barrier ⅛ in larger than the stoma and the same shape as the stoma.
- The old system is removed.

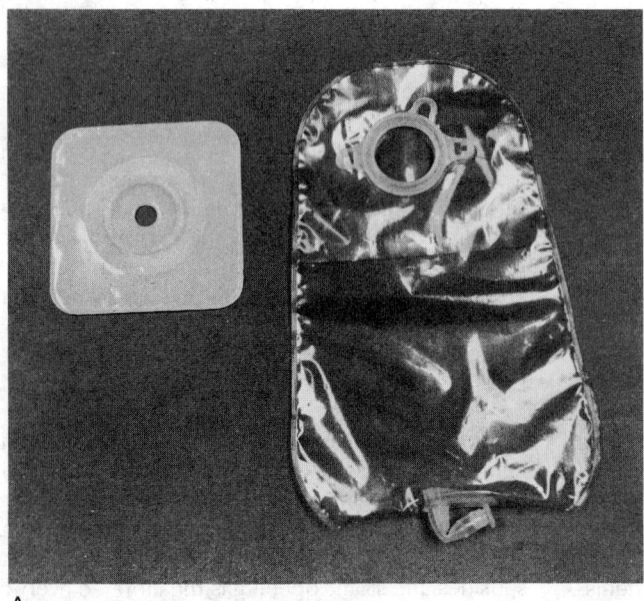 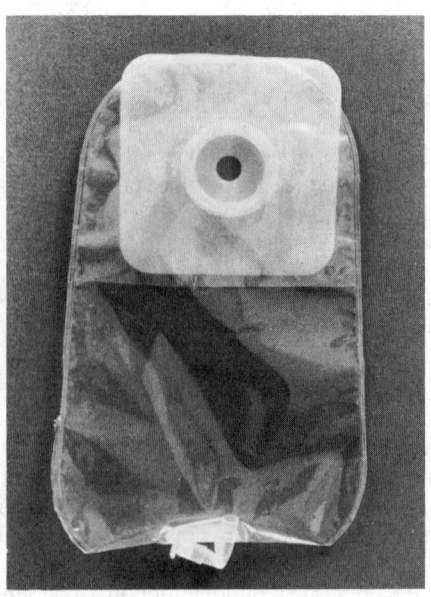

A   B

Figure 43–7. Skin-protective barrier used with urostomy pouch. (**A**) Squibb Stomahesive wafer (*left*) and Sur-Fit urostomy pouch (*right*). (**B**) Stomahesive wafer with pouch attached.

- The skin is cleansed with warm water and dried thoroughly.
- The peristomal skin is assessed for irritation.
- A tampon or rolled gauze pad may be gently placed on top of the stomal opening (not inserted into the stoma) to absorb urine and keep the skin dry during appliance change.
- The paper backing is removed from the skin barrier.
- The opening is centered over the stoma and applied with firm but gentle pressure to attain a watertight seal.
- If a two-piece system is used, the pouch is snapped onto the flanged wafer that adheres to the abdomen.
- The drainage tap/spout at the bottom of the pouch is closed.
- A pouch cover can be used or cornstarch applied under the pouch to prevent perspiration and skin irritation.
- Hypoallergenic tape is applied in a picture-frame effect around the skin barrier/wafer.

Because the degree to which the stoma protrudes is not the same in all patients, there are various accessories and custom-made appliances to solve individual problems.

Odor Control.   The patient should be advised to avoid foods that give the urine a strong odor: asparagus, cheese, and eggs. A few drops of liquid deodorizer or diluted white vinegar may be introduced through the drain spout into the bottom of the pouch with a syringe or eyedropper. Taking ascorbic acid by mouth helps acidify the urine and suppress urine odor. Also, the patient should be reminded that the pouch will develop an odor if it is worn too long and not cared for properly.

Managing the Ostomy Appliance.   The pouch is emptied via a drain valve when it is one-third full, because the weight of the urine will cause it to separate from the skin. Some patients prefer wearing a leg bag attached with an adaptor to the drainage apparatus. To promote uninterrupted sleep, a collecting bottle and tubing (one unit) are snapped onto an adaptor that connects to the ileal appliance. A small amount of urine is left in the bag when the adaptor is attached to prevent the bag from collapsing against itself. The tubing may be threaded down the pajama leg to prevent kinking. The collecting bottle and tubing are rinsed daily with cool water and once a week with a 3:1 solution of water and white vinegar.

Cleaning and Deodorizing the Appliance.   Usually the reusable appliance is rinsed in warm water and soaked in a 3:1 solution of water and white vinegar or a commercial deodorizing solution for 30 minutes. It is rinsed with tepid water and air dried away from direct sunlight. (Hot water and exposure to direct sunlight will dry out the pouch and increase the incidence of cracking.) After drying, the appliance may be powdered with cornstarch and stored. Two appliances are necessary—one to be worn while the other is air drying.

The patient is encouraged to contact the local ostomy association for visits, reassurance, and practical information.*

Continent Ileal Urinary Reservoir (Kock Pouch)

The continent ileal urinary reservoir is another type of urinary diversion created for patients whose bladder is removed or can no longer function (neurogenic bladder). In this procedure, a segment of the small intestine is surgically isolated from the intestine and serves for storage of urine (Fig. 43-6). The ureters are implanted in the isolated segment and an opening is created connecting the new "bladder" to the abdominal wall. To pre-

vent leakage of urine, a nipple-like valve is created by intussuscepting (telescoping) the intestine. To drain the stored urine, a catheter is inserted through the nipple valve and urine is drained at prescribed intervals. The advantage of this urinary diversion is that the valve prevents leakage of urine and the drainage of urine is under the control of the patient. The reservoir must be drained at regular intervals by a catheter to prevent absorption of metabolic waste products from the urine, reflux of urine to the ureters, and urinary tract infections.

Ureterosigmoidostomy

Ureterosigmoidostomy is an implantation of the ureters into the sigmoid colon. It is usually performed for the patient who has had extensive pelvic radiation, previous small bowel resection, or coexisting small bowel disease. In addition to the usual preoperative regimen, the patient may be placed on a liquid diet for several days preoperatively to reduce residue in the colon. Antimicrobial agents (neomycin, kanamycin) are administered for bowel disinfection. Ureterosigmoidostomy requires a competent anal sphincter, adequate renal function, and active renal peristalsis. The degree of anal sphincter control may be determined by assessing the patient's ability to retain enemas.

The patient is informed that, following surgery, voiding will occur from the rectum for the rest of his life and that an adjustment in life-style will be necessary because of urinary frequency (as often as every 2 hours); drainage will have a consistency equivalent to a watery diarrhea. There will be some degree of nocturia. Activities will have to be planned around the frequent need to urinate, which in turn may affect the patient's social life. However, the patient has the advantage of urinary control without having to wear an external appliance.

Postoperatively, a catheter is placed in the rectum to drain the urine and prevent reflux of urine into the ureters and kidneys. The tube is taped to the buttocks and special skin care is given around the anus to prevent excoriation. Irrigations of the rectal tube may be prescribed, but force should not be used because of the danger of introducing bacteria into the newly implanted ureters.

In this operation, larger areas of the bowel mucosa are exposed to urine and electrolyte reabsorption; as a result, electrolyte imbalance and acidosis may occur. Potassium and magnesium imbalances may occur from the presence of urine in the bowel, which simulates diarrhea. Fluid and electrolyte balance is maintained in the immediate postoperative period by closely monitoring the patient's serum electrolyte levels and administering appropriate intravenous infusions. Acidosis may be prevented by placing the patient on a low-chloride diet supplemented with sodium potassium citrate. The patient should be instructed never to wait longer than 2 to 3 hours before emptying urine from the intestine in order to keep rectal pressure low and to minimize the absorption of urinary constituents from the colon. It is essential to teach the patient about the symptoms of urinary tract infection: fever, flank pain, and frequency.

After the rectal catheter is removed, the patient learns to control the anal sphincter through special sphincteric exercises. At first, urination is frequent. With reassurance and encouragement and the passage of time, the patient will gain greater control and will learn to differentiate between the need to void and the need to defecate.

---

* See bibliography at end of chapter for address.

Pyelonephritis (upper urinary tract infection due to reflux of bacteria from the colon) is fairly common. Long-term antimicrobial therapy may be prescribed to prevent infection.

Specific dietary instructions include avoidance of gasforming foods, because flatus can cause stress incontinence and offensive odors. Other ways to avoid gas are to avoid chewing gum, smoking, and any other activity that involves swallowing air. Salt intake may be restricted to prevent hyperchloremic acidosis. Potassium intake is increased through foods and medication because potassium may be lost in acidosis. A late complication is adenocarcinoma of the sigmoid colon, possibly due to the exposure of colonic mucosa to urine, leading to cellular changes.

Cutaneous Ureterostomy

A cutaneous ureterostomy is accomplished by bringing the detached ureters through the abdominal wall and attaching them to an opening in the skin. This procedure is used for selected patients with ureteral obstruction (advanced pelvic cancer); for poor-risk patients, because it requires less extensive surgery than other urinary diversion procedures; and for patients who have had previous abdominal radiation.

A urinary appliance is fitted immediately following surgery. The management of the patient with a cutaneous ureterostomy is very similar to the care of the patient with an ileal conduit (see p. 1208), although the stomas are usually flush with the skin or retracted.

Cystostomy

An infrequently used method of urinary diversion is the suprapubic cystostomy. A special catheter is usually inserted under local anesthesia through the abdomen into the bladder through either an incision in the lower abdominal wall or a puncture made by a trocar. Generally, a cystostomy is performed on the patient with an obstruction below the bladder (prostatic obstruction) when it is not possible to insert a urethral catheter. A cystostomy may be temporary (until corrective surgery can be performed) or permanent.

The patient with a cystostomy requires liberal amounts of fluid to prevent encrustation around the catheter. Other problems encountered include the formation of bladder stones, acute and chronic infections, and problems in collecting urine. The advice and assistance of an enterostomal therapist is needed in choosing the most suitable urine collection bag and educating and assisting the patient in its use.

Other Urinary Diversion Procedures

There are frequent variations on these procedures and innovations in surgical procedures in an effort to identify and perfect procedures that will improve patient outcomes and reduce the incidence of postoperative problems. These include cecal, patched cecal, Mainz reservoirs, and Indiana pouches. These techniques involve isolation of part of the large intestine to create a reservoir for urine and creation of an abdominal stoma. Another surgical procedure, the Camey procedure (Fig. 43-5*F*), uses a portion of the ileum as a bladder substitute. In this procedure, the isolated ileum serves as the reservoir for urine; it is anastomosed directly to the portion of the remaining urethra following cystectomy. This procedure permits emptying of the bladder through the urethra.

General Management of Patients Undergoing Urinary Diversion Procedures

Preoperative Management

A careful preoperative assessment of cardiopulmonary function is performed because patients undergoing cystectomy (excision of the urinary bladder) are usually older people who may not fare well in a lengthy complex procedure. As part of preoperative management, the bowel is cleansed to minimize fecal stasis, to decompress the bowel, and to minimize postoperative ileus; a low-residue diet is prescribed; and antimicrobial drugs are administered to reduce pathogenic flora in the bowel and to reduce the risk of infection and sepsis. Adequate preoperative hydration is imperative to ensure urine flow during surgery and to prevent hypovolemia during the prolonged operative procedure. The patient undergoing a urinary diversion procedure for cancer may have severe problems with malnutrition because of increased tumor mass, radiation enteritis, and decreased food intake. Enteral or total parenteral nutrition can be used to support the patient, minimize toxicity, promote healing, and improve response to treatment. The risk of skin problems is increased in the patient who has received preoperative radiation therapy.

Postoperative Management

Postoperative management focuses on maintaining urinary function, preventing postoperative complications (respiratory complications, fluid and electrolyte imbalances), and promoting patient comfort. Catheters or drainage systems are observed and urine output is monitored carefully. A nasogastric tube is inserted during surgery for decompression of the gastrointestinal tract and to relieve pressure on the intestinal anastomosis. It is usually kept in place for several days following surgery. As soon as bowel function resumes, as manifested by bowel sounds, the passage of flatus, and a soft abdomen, the patient is given fluids by mouth. Until that time, fluids and electrolytes are administered intravenously. The patient is assisted to ambulate as soon as possible.

Because of the complexity of the surgery, the usual reasons (cancer, trauma) for urinary diversion procedures, and the frequently less-than-optimal nutritional status, complications are not unusual. These may include the usual postoperative complications (atelectasis, fluid and electrolyte imbalances, etc.) as well as breakdown of the anastomoses, sepsis, fistula formation, fecal or urine leakage, and skin irritation. If these occur, the patient will remain hospitalized for an extended length of time and will probably require total parenteral nutrition, gastrointestinal decompression via nasogastric suction, and further surgery. The goals of management will be to establish drainage, to provide adequate nutrition for healing to occur, and to prevent sepsis.

Nursing Interventions

The role of the nurse in the immediate postoperative phase is to assess the patient for complications and prevent their occurrence. The catheters and urinary collection receptacle inserted or applied during surgery are monitored closely. Urine volume, patency of the drainage system, and color of drainage are noted. A sudden decrease in urine volume or increase in drainage is reported promptly to the physician because this may indicate obstruction of the urinary tract, inadequate blood volume, or bleeding. Analgesia is administered as prescribed to promote patient comfort and permit the patient to turn, cough, and take deep breaths without excessive pain and discomfort. The nursing care indicated for this patient includes measures for the patient undergoing intestinal surgery (see Chap. 37) and surgery of the urinary tract (see Chap. 42). The remainder of the postoperative management and the nursing care related to the physical needs of the patient are covered under the previous discussions of the specific urinary diversion procedures.

◆ Nursing Process
The Patient Undergoing a Urinary Diversion Surgical Procedure

▷ Assessment

The patient admitted to the hospital for a urinary diversion surgical procedure is assessed thoroughly. The assessment focuses on the patient's and the family's understanding of the procedure and the changes in physical structure and function that will result from the surgery. The patient's self-concept and self-esteem are also assessed in addition to his usual way of coping with stress and loss. The patient's mental status, hand dexterity and coordination, and preferred method of learning are noted because these will influence his ability to participate in self-care postoperatively.

▷ Nursing Diagnoses

Based on the assessment data, the nursing diagnoses for the patient undergoing urinary diversion surgery may include the following:

Preoperative Diagnoses
- Anxiety related to anticipated losses associated with the surgical procedure
- Knowledge deficit about outcomes of the surgical procedure

Postoperative Diagnoses
- Knowledge deficit about management of urinary function
- High risk for self-esteem disturbance related to altered body image
- Ineffective individual coping related to fear of the diagnosis and the impact of surgery
- Potential for sexual dysfunction related to after-effects of surgery and self-consciousness about stoma
- High risk for impaired skin integrity related to problems in managing appliance

▷ Planning and Implementation

Preoperative Goals: The patient's major goals may include relief of anxiety and increased knowledge about expected outcomes of the surgery.

Postoperative Goals: The patient's major goals may include increased knowledge about management of urinary function, increased self-esteem, appropriate coping mechanisms to accept and deal with altered urinary function and sexuality, and maintenance of peristomal skin integrity.

▷ Nursing Interventions
▷ Preoperative

▷ *Relieving Anxiety.*   The threat of bladder removal and cancer creates fear related to losses—loss of love, body image, and security. In addition to problems in adapting to an external appliance, a stoma, and a scar, the patient must also adapt to alterations in toileting habits, and the male patient must also adapt to sexual impotency. (A penile implant is considered if the patient is a candidate for the procedure.) Women face the fear of loss of appearance because of changed body image. A supportive approach is needed that includes physical and psychosocial support. It involves taking a personal interest in the patient, assessing the patient's concept and perception of self and the manner in which he responds to stress and loss, and helping him to maintain his usual life-style and independence with as few modifications as possible. The patient is encouraged to express his fears and anxiety. A visitor from the Ostomy Visitation Program of the American Cancer Society can give emotional support and make adaptation easier both before and after surgery.

▷ *Patient Education.*   An enterostomal therapist is invaluable for preoperative teaching. Explanations of the surgical procedure and the reasons for wearing a collection device postoperatively are given to the patient and the family. The stoma site is planned preoperatively with the patient standing, sitting, and lying in order to locate the stoma away from bony prominences, skin creases, and fat folds. *The patient must be able to see and comfortably reach the site for ease of self-care.* The optimum site is marked with indelible ink for intraoperative location. It may be helpful to have the patient practice wearing the appliance partially filled with water before surgery.

▷ Postoperative

▷ *Patient Education.*   A major postoperative objective is to assist the patient to achieve the highest level of independence and self-care possible. The primary nurse or enterostomal therapist, if available, works closely with the patient and family to instruct and assist them in all phases of management of the ostomy. The patient is encouraged to participate in decisions regarding the type of collecting appliance and the time of day to change the appliance. The patient is assisted and encouraged to look at and touch the stoma early so that he overcomes his fears.

The patient and family are instructed about the signs and symptoms to be reported to the physician and about problems that they can handle themselves. Information and increased responsibility for self-care are provided according to the patient's physical recovery from surgery and his ability to accept and acquire the knowledge and skill needed for independence. Verbal and written instructions are provided, and the patient is given the opportunity to practice and demonstrate his skill in the management of his urinary drainage.

▷ *Increased Self-Esteem.*   In addition to alterations in urinary drainage, the patient with a urinary diversion also experiences loss or fear of loss of relationships with others, altered sexuality and sexual function, dependence, and changes in life-style. The patient's ability to cope with these potential changes depends to some degree on his body image and self-esteem before the surgery and the support and reaction of others around him. The nurse can assist the patient to improve his self-concept by providing him with the skills and confidence to be independent in the management of his altered urinary drainage. Additionally, acceptance of his feelings and reactions as he adjusts to alteration of the previously private and routine act of voiding may assist him in accepting these changes.

▷ *Improved Sexuality.* The patient who experiences altered sexual function as a result of the surgical procedure may mourn this loss and its meaning to him and his partner. Encouraging the patient and partner to share their feelings about this loss with each other and acknowledging the importance of sexual function and expression may assist the patient and spouse to seek sexual counseling if necessary and to explore alternative ways of expressing sexuality. A visit from another ''ostomate'' who is functioning fully in society and family life may also assist the patient and family in recognizing that full recovery is possible.

▷ *Maintenance of Peristomal Skin Integrity.* Strategies to promote skin integrity begin with reducing and controlling those factors that increase the patient's risk of poor nutrition and poor healing. Meticulous skin care and management of the drainage system are provided by the nurse until the patient is able to manage them and is comfortable doing so. Adequate supplies and complete instruction are necessary to enable the patient and a family member to develop competence and confidence in their skills. Written and verbal instructions are provided, and the patient is encouraged to contact the nurse or physician for follow-up questions. Follow-up phone calls from the nurse to the patient and family after the patient's discharge may provide added support. Follow-up visits and reinforcement of correct skin care and appliance management techniques also promote skin integrity. Specific techniques for management of the appliance are described on pp. 1210–1211.

▷ Evaluation

Expected Outcomes

Preoperative

1. Experiences reduced anxiety.
   a. Verbalizes fears and anxieties about surgery and its outcomes.
   b. Grieves about alterations openly as appropriate.
   c. Shares fears, anxieties, and concerns with partner.
   d. Accepts visit from Ostomy Visitation Program.
   e. Reports reduction in level of anxiety.
   f. Exhibits interest in other activities and events.
2. Increases knowledge about expected outcomes of surgery.
   a. States purpose and expected outcomes of surgical procedure.
   b. Describes anticipated alterations in urinary drainage in own words.
   c. Asks primary nurse or enterostomal therapist relevant questions related to postoperative course.
   d. Assists primary nurse, enterostomal therapist, or surgeon in identifying appropriate site for stoma.

Postoperative

1. Increases knowledge about management of urinary function.
   a. Participates in management of urinary drainage system.

   b. Verbalizes own preferences and opinions in making decisions about care and management.
   c. Describes anatomic alteration due to surgery.
   d. Describes and uses recommended skin care measures.
   e. Revises daily routine to accommodate urostomy (urinary drainage) management.
   f. Identifies potential problems and measures to handle them.
   g. Identifies reportable signs and symptoms.
   h. Asks questions relevant to care at home.
   i. Identifies health care professional and other support persons to contact following discharge for questions and concerns about management of urinary function.
2. Exhibits improved self-concept.
   a. Verbalizes acceptance of urinary diversion, stoma, and appliance.
   b. Demonstrates increasing independence in self-care.
   c. Verbalizes plans to resume normal activities of daily living and return to usual life-style.
   d. Identifies alternative ways of sexual expression (if impotent).
   e. Verbalizes acceptance of support and assistance from family members and health care providers.
   f. Exhibits proper hygiene and grooming.
   g. Accepts visit from ''ostomate.''
   h. Volunteers to visit other patients about to undergo urinary diversion surgery.
3. Improves sexuality.
   a. Verbalizes concerns about possible alterations in sexuality and sexual function.
   b. Verbalizes interest in alternative methods of sexual expression.
   c. Discusses sexual concerns with partner and appropriate counselor.
   d. Seeks sexual counseling if appropriate.
   e. Engages in mutually satisfying activities with partner.
4. Maintains skin integrity.
   a. Demonstrates intact peristomal skin.
   b. Reports no pain or discomfort of peristomal area.
   c. Verbalizes actions to take if skin excoriation occurs.
   d. Demonstrates skill in managing drainage system and appliance.

In summary, the patient who undergoes urinary diversion requires expert medical and nursing care to reduce the occurrence of preventable complications and to assess and intervene when other problems occur. The patient undergoing these procedures is often concerned about not only the alteration in normal voiding and his body image but also the disorder (*e.g.*, cancer) that has necessitated the surgical procedure. Patience, understanding, and sensitivity to the implications of this major change in body function are important characteristics of the nurse who is going to be effective in assisting the patient and family to learn the management techniques needed for complete rehabilitation. The nurse must work effectively with other health care providers (*e.g.*, enterostomal therapist, discharge planning nurse, visiting nurse) to identify and appropriately utilize those services that will assist the patient in adjusting to a modified life-style.

Interstitial Cystitis

Interstitial cystitis is a relatively common disorder in older women; it may occur in men but does so with much less frequency. There are between 20,000 and 90,000 diagnosed cases in the United States, but it is estimated that there are four to five times that number undiagnosed. It is characterized by severe irritable voiding symptoms and a markedly diminished bladder capacity. Symptoms may include urinary frequency, nocturia, urgency, suprapubic pressure, and pain with bladder filling; the pain may occur in the abdomen or perineum or radiate to the groin. These symptoms are often partially or completely relieved by emptying of the bladder. The findings on biopsy suggest an inflammatory or autoimmune basis for this condition, although specific chemical mediators have not been identified. The reason the disease is localized to the bladder is unknown. Suggested causes include penetration of urinary irritants into the urothelium or suburothelial tissues due to a defect in the barrier between the urine and bladder wall mucosa.

The urine contains both red and white blood cells even though it is *uninfected* and cytology is benign. An increased number of mast cells in the urine is suggestive of interstitial cystitis. The presence of Hunner's ulcers (superficial erosions of the bladder wall) is considered diagnostic; however, these do not occur in all women. Interstitial cystitis is a diagnosis made by the process of exclusion because there are no definitive diagnostic criteria. As a result, several years may pass before a definitive diagnosis is made. The median age of onset is between ages 40 and 50; its duration is 7 to 10 years. Symptoms increase in severity over the first few years, then stabilize and fluctuate. Interstitial cystitis is a progressive disease if not treated, and early diagnosis may improve the response to treatment. It is a chronic and disabling condition of the bladder; the picture of the patient with interstitial cystitis is often one of chronic pain syndrome. The pain and frequency may hamper the patient's ability to work or participate in social activities; nocturia may lead to chronic sleep deprivation. The lack of more specific diagnostic criteria does not mean that this is a psychologically based disease; rather, it is a physical disorder with psychologic consequences. Many patients have difficulty in coping with the lack of a diagnosis, the inability of health care professionals to provide an explanation for their symptoms, the persistence of symptoms, and the lack of empathy from health care providers.

Diagnostic Process

The diagnosis of interstitial cystitis is made by eliminating other causes of these symptoms and on the basis of history, symptoms, signs, cystoscopy, urodynamic studies, histology, and laboratory tests. A micturition chart or diary with recordings of the frequency of voiding and the volume of each voiding over at least 48 to 72 hours may aid in the diagnostic process. Biopsy and radiographic studies such as urography, cystography, skeletal and pelvic x-ray films, ultrasound, and CT scan are of value to exclude other conditions that could cause similar symptoms. The only abnormal x-ray finding characteristic of interstitial cystitis is a small bladder; however, this is not com-

monly present. Urinalysis, culture, residual volume, and flow rate are usually normal in patients with interstitial cystitis.

Interstitial cystitis is characterized by mucosal glomerulations of the bladder wall seen on cystoscopic examination. Glomerulations are pinpoint petechial hemorrhages that develop throughout the bladder. These areas often coalesce to become hemorrhagic spots on the bladder mucosa that bleed when the bladder is distended under general anesthesia (an important diagnostic criterion). Unlike other causes of painful bladder syndrome, interstitial cystitis may progress to contraction of the bladder with diminished bladder volume. Cystoscopy is performed and fluid is instilled in the bladder to 80 cm of water pressure for 1 minute with the patient under anesthesia. The bladder is distended to its maximum capacity and the fluid is then drained; in most patients, few abnormalities are encountered during this first filling. However, as soon as bladder capacity is reached and the irrigating fluid is drained, the last portion of the fluid drained is usually blood-tinged. Fissures and scars of the bladder mucosa tend to split as the bladder capacity is reached, thus producing the characteristic appearance of a Hunner ulcer. Re-examination reveals glomerulations and often splotchy hemorrhages throughout the bladder, although their distribution may be patchy. This picture is a late manifestation of interstitial cystitis. The cystoscopic picture does not necessarily correlate with severity of symptoms or response to therapy.

Treatment

Treatment strategies have included the use of tricyclic antidepressants that may decrease the excitability of smooth muscle in the bladder through their central and peripheral anticholinergic actions. Treatment has ranged from destruction of ulcers with laser photoirradiation, to bladder instillation of a variety of agents (*i.e.,* silver nitrate, neomycin, chlorpactin), to bladder removal and urinary diversion. There have been reports that urinary diversion may give total relief even though the bladder remains in place. Intractable pain and severe bladder contracture with incontinence are the most common indications for surgery.

Investigations are under way to identify treatments that will relieve symptoms. Agents currently undergoing clinical trial include subcutaneous heparin (stabilizes mast cells; antagonizes histamine, bradykinin, and prostaglandin E; and inhibits the complement system and action of inflammatory agents); dimethyl sulfoxide (DMSO; has anti-inflammatory, immunologic, analgesic, and bacteriostatic properties); and other agents (sodium pentosanpolysulfate) to correct defects in the protective layer of the bladder mucosa. Bladder instillation of various compounds has been used to try to provide relief. TENS (transcutaneous electrical nerve stimulation) has been used in some patients to relieve symptoms.

Nursing Interventions

The patient who presents with the symptoms of interstitial cystitis has often experienced symptoms for a prolonged period of time and has usually been unable to participate in normal activities and carry out normal activities of daily living because of these symptoms. Because the diagnosis of interstitial cystitis is not made readily, the patient may have previously encountered health care providers who doubted the existence of the reported symptoms. The patient has usually been treated by a number of health care providers, often with little relief of symptoms. Consequently, the patient may be depressed and anxious. Additionally, the patient may be distrustful and skeptical of proposed treatments, particularly if these have been tried before and have been unsuccessful. Therefore, it is crucial that the nurse convey to the patient that she believes the symptoms exist and appreciates their severity and their effect on life-style. The nurse provides explanations about diagnostic tests and treatment modalities. The nurse also assesses the effectiveness of the patient's ability to cope with this disorder and provides psychologic support.

Urethral Conditions

Caruncle

A caruncle is a small, red, extremely vascular polyplike growth situated just within, and protruding from, the external urethral meatus of women. On rare occasions it causes no subjective symptoms. However, it may be acutely sensitive, causing increased frequency of urination, which is exquisitely painful, and a local burning pain exaggerated by exertion. Local excision of the caruncle will relieve the symptoms.

Urethritis

Urethritis, inflammation of the urethra, is usually an ascending infection and may be classified as gonorrheal (see Chap. 62) or nongonorrheal. However, both conditions may be present in the same patient.

Gonorrheal Urethritis.   Gonorrheal urethritis is caused by *Neisseria gonorrhoeae* and is transmitted by sexual contact. In the male, inflammation of the meatal orifice occurs with burning on urination. A purulent urethral discharge appears 3 to 14 days (or longer) after sexual exposure. However, the disease may be asymptomatic. In the female, a urethral discharge is not always present and the disease also is often essentially asymptomatic. Therefore, gonorrhea in the female is frequently not diagnosed and reported. In the male, the infection involves the tissues around the urethra, causing periurethritis, prostatitis, epididymitis, and urethral stricture. Sterility may occur as a result of vasoepididymal obstruction. Treatment of gonorrhea is discussed and patient education information is provided in Chapter 62.

Nongonorrheal Urethritis.   Urethritis not associated with *Neisseria gonorrhoeae* is usually caused by *Chlamydia trachomatis* or *Ureaplasma urealyticum*. If the male patient is symptomatic, he will complain of mild to severe dysuria and a scanty to moderate urethral discharge. Nongonorrheal urethritis requires prompt antimicrobial treatment with tetracycline or doxycycline, or in those patients who do not respond or are allergic to the tetracyclines, erythromycin may be substituted. Follow-up care is necessary to make certain that a cure is achieved. All persons who are sexual partners of patients with nongonorrheal urethritis must be examined for sexually transmitted disease and treated.

Urethral Strictures

A urethral stricture is a narrowing of the lumen of the urethra due to scar tissue and contraction. Strictures result from urethral injury (caused by insertion of surgical instruments during transurethral surgery, indwelling catheters, or cystoscopic procedures), straddle injuries and automobile accidents, untreated gonorrheal urethritis, and congenital abnormalities.

The force and size of the urinary stream is diminished and symptoms of urinary infection and retention occur. Stricture causes urine to back up, resulting in cystitis, prostatitis, and pyelonephritis. An important element of prevention is to treat all urethral infections promptly. Prolonged urethral catheter drainage is to be avoided and utmost care should be taken in any type of instrumentation involving the urethra, including catheterization.

Management.   The treatment may be palliative (gradual dilatation of the narrowed area with metal sounds or bougies) or surgery under direct vision (internal urethrotomy). If the stricture has become so small as to prevent the passage of a catheter, the urologist uses several small filiform bougies in search of the opening. When one bougie passes beyond the stricture into the bladder, it is fixed in place, and urine will drain from the bladder. The stricture then can be dilated to a larger size by the passage of a larger sound (a dilating instrument) following behind the filiform as a guide. Following dilatation, hot sitz baths and non-narcotic analgesics are administered to control the pain. Antimicrobials are prescribed for several days after dilatation to minimize the infectious reaction, thus reducing discomfort.

Surgical excision or urethroplasty may be necessary for severe cases. A suprapubic cystostomy may be necessary in some patients. The postoperative treatment for cystostomy is described on p. 1212.

Chapter Summary

Disorders of the urinary tract and kidneys have the potential to alter the function of many body systems as well as fluid and electrolyte and acid–base balance. The resulting changes in normal function include both physiologic complications and psychologic responses to physiologic changes. The nurse caring for the patient with disorders of the urinary tract and kidneys must have an understanding of the complex functions of the kidneys and lower urinary tract; an understanding of fluid and electrolyte imbalances that may occur secondary to urinary tract and renal dysfunction is essential. Although disorders may be limited to uncomplicated urinary tract infections that are usually easily treated, the nurse has an important role in patient education to assure compliance with therapy and follow-up if indicated. When renal dysfunction or urinary tract disorders necessitate complex treatments such as dialysis, transplantation, lithotripsy, or urinary diversion, the nurse is responsible not only for major aspects of patient teaching but also for many high-technology aspects of care. As patients who undergo such treatments are hospitalized for shorter periods of time, home care considerations take on increasing importance to assure continuity of quality care, preservation of remaining renal function, and patient recovery.

Bibliography

Books

Brenner BM, Coe FL, and Rector FC Jr. Clinical Nephrology. Philadelphia, WB Saunders, 1987.

Catto GRD. Clinical Transplantation: Current Practice and Future Prospects. Lancaster, England, MTP Press Limited, 1987.

Cerilli GJ. Organ Transplantation and Replacement. Philadelphia, JB Lippincott, 1988.

Gingell C and Abrams P (ed). Controversies and Innovations in Urologic Surgery. New York, Springer-Verlag, 1988.

Hanno PM and Wein AJ. A Clinical Manual of Urology. Englewood Cliffs, NJ, Appleton-Century-Crofts, 1987.

Kunin CM. Detection, Prevention and Management of Urinary Tract Infections. Philadelphia, Lea & Febiger, 1987.

Massry SG and Glassrock RJ. Textbook of Nephrology, 2nd ed. Baltimore, Williams & Wilkins, 1989.

Nolph KD. Peritoneal Dialysis, 3rd ed. Norwell, MA, Kluwer Academic, 1989.

Pak CYC. Renal Stone Disease: Pathogenesis, Prevention and Treatment. Boston, Nijhoff, 1987.

Riehle RA Jr. Principles of Extracorporeal Shock Wave Lithotripsy. New York, Churchill Livingstone, 1987.

Rose BD and Black RM. Manual of Clinical Problems in Nephrology. Boston, Little, Brown & Co, 1988.

Sigardson-Poor KM and Haggerty LM. Nursing Care of the Transplant Recipient. Philadelphia, WB Saunders, 1990.

Smith PH. Combination Therapy in Urological Malignancy. New York, Springer-Verlag, 1989.

Smith SL (ed). Tissue and Organ Transplantation: Implications for Nursing Practice. St Louis, CV Mosby, 1990.

Journals

Asterisks indicate nursing research articles.

General

Chambers JK. Fluid and electrolyte problems in renal and urologic disorders. Nurs Clin North Am 1987 Dec; 22(4):815-826.

Chenevey B. Overview of fluids and electrolytes. Nurs Clin North Am 1987 Dec; 22(4):749-759.

Lancaster LE. Renal and endocrine regulation of water and electrolyte balance. Nurs Clin North Am 1987 Dec; 22(4):761-772.

Faubert PF and Porush JG. Managing hypertension in chronic renal disease. Geriatrics 1987 Jan; 42(1):49-58.

Innerarity SA. Electrolyte emergencies in the critically ill renal patient. Crit Care Nurs Clin North Am 1990 Mar; 2(1):89-99.

Pearlstein G. Renal system compliations in HIV infection. Crit Care Nurs Clin North Am 1990 Mar; 2(1):79-87.

Urinary Tract Infections

Andriole VT. Urinary tract infections: Recent developments. J Infect Dis 1987 Dec; 156(6):865-869.

Asher EF, Oliver BG, and Fry DE. Urinary tract infections in the surgical patient. Am Surg 1988 Jul; 54(7):466-469.

Boscia JA et al. Therapy vs no therapy for bacteriuria in elderly ambulatory nonhospitalized women. JAMA 1987 Feb 27; 257(8):1067-1071.

Brettman LR. Nosocomial infection: Risks associated with short-term and long-term inpatient care. Urology 1988 Sep; 32(Suppl 3):21-23.

Brettman LR. Pathogenesis of urinary tract infections: Host susceptibility and bacterial virulence factors. Urology 1988 Sep; 32(Suppl 3):9-11.

Breitenbucher RB. UTI: Managing the most common nursing home infection. Geriatrics 1990 May; 45(5):68-75.

Brooks D. UTI: A practical approach to management. Practitioner 1989 May 22; 233(1469):762-764.

Cook DJ, Achong MR, and Dobranowski J. Emphysematous pyelonephritis.

Complicated urinary tract infection in diabetes. Diabetes Care 1989 Mar; 12(3):229-232.

Dolan JG, Bordley DR, and Polito R. Initial management of serious urinary tract infection: Epidemiologic guidelines. J Gen Intern Med 1989 May/Jun; 4(3):190-194.

Fihn SD. Behavioral aspects of urinary tract infection. Urology 1988 Sep; 32(Suppl 3):16-18.

Foxman B. Recurring urinary tract infection: Incidence and risk factors. Am J Public Health 1990 Mar; 80(3):331-333.

Gleckman RA and Czachor JS. Managing diabetes-related infections in the elderly. Geriatrics 1989 Aug; 44(8):37-39, 44-46.

Jaff MR and Paganini EP. Meeting the challenge of geriatric UTIs. Geriatrics 1989 Dec; 44(12):60-65, 69.

Johnson JR and Stamm WE. Urinary tract infections in women: Diagnosis and treatment. Ann Intern Med 1989 Dec 1; 111(11):906-917.

Jones P, Jones SL, and Katz J. A randomized trial to improve compliance in urinary tract infection patients in the emergency department. Ann Emerg Med 1990 Jan; 19(1):16-20.

Josephson S et al. *Gardnerella vaginalis* in the urinary tract: Incidence and significance in a hospital population. Obstet Gynecol 1988 Feb; 71(2):245-250.

Karafin LJ and Coll ME. Lower urinary tract disorders in the postmenopausal woman. Med Clin North Am 1987 Jan; 71(1):111-121.

Kaye D (ed). Urinary tract infections. Med Clin North Am 1991 Mar; 75(2): 241-513.

Krieger JN. Urinary tract infections in women: Causes, classification, and differential diagnosis. Urology 1990 Jan; 35(Suppl 1):4-7.

Leibovici L et al. A clinical model for diagnosis of urinary tract infection in young women. Arch Intern Med 1989 Sep; 149(9):2048-2050.

Lipsky BA. Urinary tract infections in men. Epidemiology, pathophysiology, diagnosis, and treatment. Ann Internal Med 1989 Jan 15; 110(2): 138-150.

McNeeley SG Jr. Treatment of urinary tract infections during pregnancy. Clin Obstet Gynecol 1988 Jun; 32(2):480-487.

Meares EM Jr. Urinary tract infections in the male patient. Urology 1988 Sep; 32(Suppl 3):19-20.

Mott PD and Barker WH. Treatment decisions for infections occurring in nursing home residents. J Am Geriatr Soc 1988 Sep; 36(9):820-824.

Nicolle LE et al. Localization of urinary tract infection in elderly, institutionalized women with asymptomatic bacteriuria. J Infect Dis 1988 Jan; 157(1):65-70.

Platt R. Adverse consequences of asymptomatic urinary tract infections in adults. Am J Med 1987 Jun 26; 82(Suppl 6B):47-52.

Rudman D et al. Clinical correlates of bacteremia in a Veterans Administration extended care facility. J Am Geriatr Soc 1988 Aug; 36(8): 726-732.

Safrin S, Siegel D, Black D. Pyelonephritis in adult women: Inpatient versus outpatient therapy. Am J Med 1988 Dec; 85(6):793-798.

Saviteer SM, Samsa GP, Rutala WA. Nosocomial infections in the elderly. Am J Med 1988 Apr; 84(4):661-668.

Schaeffer AJ. Recurrent urinary tract infection in the female patient. Urology 1988 Sep; 32(Suppl 3):12-15.

Seiler WO and Stähelin HB. Practical management of catheter-associated UTIs. Geriatrics 1988 Aug; 43(8):43-50.

Smith JW. Southwestern Internal Medicine Conference: Prognosis in pyelonephritis: Promise or progress. Am J Med Sci 1989 Jan; 297(1):53-62.

Stamey TA. Recurrent urinary tract infections in female patients: An overview of management and treatment. Rev Infect Dis 1987 Mar/Apr; 9(Suppl 2):S195-S210.

Stamm WE et al. Urinary tract infections: From pathogenesis to treatment. J Infect Dis 1989 Mar; 159(3):400-406.

Stover SL et al. Urinary tract infection in spinal cord injury. Arch Phys Med Rehabil 1989 Jan; 70(1):47-54.

* Whippo CC and Creason NS. Bacteriuria and urinary incontinence in aged female nursing home residents. J Adv Nurs 1989 Mar; 14(3): 217-225.

Wilhelm MP and Edson RS. Antimicrobial agents in urinary tract infections. Mayo Clin Proc 1987 Nov; 62(11):1025–1031.

Zilkowski MW, Smucker DR, and Mayhew HE. Urinary tract infections in elderly patients. Postgrad Med 1988 Sep 1; 84(3):191–194, 197–199, 201, 202, 205, 206.

Zilkowski MW. Urinary tract infections in the elderly. Am Fam Physician 1989 May; 39(5):125–134.

Disorders of the Kidney

Bernard DB. The nephrotic syndrome: A clinical approach. Hosp Pract 1990 Sep 15; 25(9):86–88, 93–102.

Cameron JS. Treatment of primary glomerulonephritis using immunosuppressive agents. Am J Nephrol 1989; 9(Suppl 1):33–40.

Couser WG. Rapidly progressive glomerulonephritis: Classification, pathogenetic mechanisms, and therapy. Am J Kidney Dis 1988 Jun; 11(6):449–464.

FitzSimmons SC et al. Kidney disease of diabetes mellitus: NIDDK initiatives for the comprehensive study of its natural history, pathogenesis, and prevention. Am J Kidney Dis 1989 Jan; 13(1):7–10.

Goyer RA. Environmentally related diseases of the urinary tract. Med Clin North Am 1990 Mar; 74(2):377–389.

Jennette JC and Falk RJ. Diagnosis and management of glomerulonephritis and vasculitis presenting as acute renal failure. Med Clin North Am 1990 Jul; 74(4):893–908.

Johnson DL. Nephrotic syndrome: A nursing care plan based on current pathophysiologic concepts. Heart Lung 1989 Jan; 18(1):85–93.

Keller F et al. Long-term treatment and prognosis of rapidly progressive glomerulonephritis. Clin Nephrol 1989; 39(4):192–197.

Murphy PJ, Wright G, and Rai GS. Nephrotic syndrome in the elderly. J Am Geriatr Soc 1987 Feb; 35(2):170–173.

Packham DK et al. Primary glomerulonephritis and pregnancy. Q J Med 1989 Jun; 71(266):537–553.

Paller MS. Drug-induced nephropathies. Med Clin North Am 1990 Jul; 74(4):909–917.

Reddi AS and Camerini–Davalos RA. Diabetic nephropathy. An update. Arch Intern Med 1990 Jan; 150(1):31–43.

Rosenfeld JA. Renal disease and pregnancy. Am Fam Physician 1989 Apr; 39(4):209–212.

Whelton PK and Klag MJ. Hypertension as a risk factor for renal disease. Hypertension 1989 May; 13(5pt2):I19–I27.

Williams W. Poststreptococcal glomerulonephritis: How important is it as a cause of chronic renal failure? Transplant Proc 1987 Apr; 19(2):97–100.

Zarconi J and Smith MC. Glomerulonephritis. Bacterial, viral, and other infectious causes. Postgrad Med 1988 Jul; 84(1):239–251.

Acute Renal Failure

Baer CL. Acute renal failure. Recognizing and reversing its deadly course. Nursing 1990 Jun; 20(6):34–40.

Burke JF Jr. and Francos GC. Surgery in the patient with acute or chronic renal failure. Med Clin North Am 1987 May; 71(3):489–497.

Finn WF. Diagnosis and management of acute tubular necrosis. Med Clin North Am 1990 Jul; 74(4):873–891.

Harper J. Rhabdomyolysis and myoglobinuric renal failure. Crit Care Nurs 1990 Mar; 10(3):32–36.

Martinez–Maldonado M and Kumjian DA. Acute renal failure due to urinary tract obstruction. Med Clin North Am 1990 Jul; 74(4):919–932.

Miller CA and Evans D. CNS manifestations of acute renal failure. Crit Care Nurs 1987 May/Jun; 7(3):94–95.

Norris MKG. Acute tubular necrosis: Preventing complications. Dimens Crit Care Nurs 1989 Jan/Feb; 8(1):16–26.

Chronic Renal Failure

Ad Hoc Committee for the National Kidney Foundation. Statement on the clinical use of recombinant erythropoietin in anemia of end-stage renal disease. Am J Kidney Dis 1989 Sep; 14(3):163–169.

Anderson S and Brenner BM. Progressive renal disease. A disorder of adaptation. Q J Med 1989 Mar; 70(263):185–189.

Asrat T and Nageotte MP. Renal failure in pregnancy. Semin Perinatol 1990 Feb; 14(1):59–67.

Beaman M et al. Changing pattern of acute renal failure. Q J Med 1987 Jan; 62(237):15–23.

Berg J. Assessing for pericarditis in the end-stage renal disease patient. Dimens Crit Care Nurs 1990 Sep/Oct; 9(5):266–271.

* Betts DK and Crotty GD. Response to illness and compliance of long-term hemodialysis patients. ANNA J 1988 Apr; 15(2):96–99.

Chambers JK. Metabolic bone disorders. Imbalances of calcium and phosphorus. Nurs Clin North Am 1987 Dec; 22(4):861–872.

Dillard P. Nursing care of the black renal patient—The role, challenge and reward. Transplant Proc 1987 Apr; 19(2):118–120.

Erlich L. Use of EPOGEN for treatment of anemia associated with chronic renal failure. Crit Care Nurse Clin North Am 1990 Mar; 2(1):101–113.

Eschbach JW. The anemia of chronic renal failure: Pathophysiology and the effects of recombinant erythropoietin. Kidney Int 1989 Jan; 35(1):134–148.

Eschbach JW et al. Treatment of the anemia of progressive renal failure with recombinant human erythropoietin. N Engl J Med 1989 Jul 20; 321(3):158–163.

Eschbach JW and Adamson JW. Guidelines for recombinant human erythropoietin therapy. Am J Kidney Dis 1989 Aug; 14(2 Suppl 1):2–8.

Food and Drug Administration. Epoetin alfa approved for anemia treatment. JAMA 1989 Jul 14; 262(2):184.

Gehm L and Propp DA. Pulmonary edema in the renal failure patient. Am J Emerg Med 1989 May; 7(3):336–339.

Glück Z and Nolph KD. Ascites associated with end-stage renal disease. Am J Kidney Dis 1987 Jul; 10(1):9–18.

Hahn K. The many signs of renal failure. Nursing 1987 Aug; 17(8):34–41.

Hall PM. Can progression of renal disease be prevented? Postgrad Med 1989 Jul; 86(1):113–115, 120.

Jones KR. Policy and research in end-stage renal disease. Image: J Nurs Scholar 1987 Fall; 19(3):126–129.

Julius M et al. Independence in activities of daily living for end-stage renal disease patients: Biomedical and demographic correlates. Am J Kidney Dis 1989 Jan; 13(1):61–69.

Kleeman CR. Metabolic coma. Kidney Int 1989 Dec; 36(6):1142–1158.

Levin ML. The elderly patient with advanced renal failure. Hosp Pract 1989 Mar 30; 24(3A):35–44.

Lim VS. Reproductive function in patients with renal insufficiency. Am J Kidney Dis 1987 Apr; 9(4):363–367.

Miller LR et al. Acquired renal cystic disease in end-stage renal disease: An autopsy study of 155 cases. Am J Nephrol 1989; 9(4):322–328.

* Moore MN. Development of a sleep–awake instrument for use in a chronic renal population. ANNA J 1989 Feb; 16(1):15–19.

* Nyamathi A. Coping responses or spouses of MI patients and of hemodialsis patients as measured by Jalowied coping scale. J Cardiovasc Nurs 1987 Nov; 2(1):67–74.

* O'Brien ME. Compliance behavior and long-term maintenance dialysis. Am J Kidney Dis 1990 Mar; 15(3):209–214.

Oldenburg B, McDonald GJ, and Perkins RJ. Prediction of quality of life in a cohort of end-stage renal disease patients. J Clin Epidemiol 1988; 41(6):555–564.

Plawecki HM, Brewer S, and Plawecki JA. Chronic renal failure. J Gerontol Nurs 1987 Dec; 13(12):14–17.

Rostand SG et al. Renal insufficiency in treated essential hypertension. N Engl J Med 1989 Mar 16; 320(11):684–688.

Roy AT et al. Renal failure in older people. J Am Geriatr Soc 1990 Mar; 38(3):239–253.

Sacks CR, Peterson RA, and Kimmel PL. Perception of illness and depression in chronic renal disease. Am J Kidney Dis 1990 Jan; 15(1):31–39.

Sasak C and Giordano E. Case management of the anemic patient. Epoetin alfa: Focus on patient teaching. ANNA J 1990 Apr; 17(2):188–190.

Schwartz AB et al. Erythropoietin for the anemia of chronic renal failure. Am Fam Pract 1988 Jun; 37(6):211–215.

Sekkarie MA et al. Recovery from end-stage renal disease. Am J Kidney Dis 1990 Jan; 15(1):61–65.

Stenvinkel P, Alvestrand A, and Bergström J. Factors influencing progression in patients with chronic renal failure. J Intern Med 1989 Sep; 226(3): 183–188.

Tzamaloukas AH. Diagnosis and management of bone disorders in chronic renal failure and dialyzed patients. Med Clin North Am 1990 Jul; 74(4):961–974.

Kidney Transplantation

Bass M. Infection in renal transplantation: The first six months. Crit Care Nurs Clin North Am 1990 Mar; 2(1):133–138.

Briggs JD. Renal transplantation. Q J Med 1989 Jul; 72(267):589–597.

Cunningham N and Smith SL. Postoperative care of the renal transplant patient. Crit Care Nurs 1990 Oct; 10(9):74–80.

Fedric TN. Immunosuppressive therapy in renal transplantation. Crit Care Nurs Clin North Am 1990 Mar 2(1):123–131.

Gaudier FL et al. Pregnancy after renal transplantation. Surg Gynecol Obstet 1988 Dec; 167(6):533–543.

Harasyko C. Kidney transplantation. Nurs Clin North Am 1989 Dec; 24(4): 851–863.

Holechek MJ, Burrell-Diggs D, and Navarro MO. Renal transplantation: An option for end-stage renal disease patients. Crit Care Nurs 1991 Feb; 13(4):62–71.

Luke RG. Hypertension in renal transplant recipients. Kidney Int 1987 Apr; 31(4):1024–1037.

Mathew TH. Recurrence of disease following renal transplantation. Am J Kidney Dis 1988 Aug; 12(2):85–96.

Renshaw DC. Sex and the renal transplant patient. Clin Ther 1987; 10(1): 2–7.

Shah B et al. Current experience with renal transplantation in older patients. Am J Kidney Dis 1988 Dec; 12(6):516–523.

Surman OS. Psychiatric aspects of organ transplantation. Am J Psychiatry 1989 Aug; 146(8):972–982.

* Sutton TD and Murphy SP. Stressors and patterns of coping in renal transplant patients. Nurs Res 1989 Jan/Feb; 38(1):46–49.

Yoshimura N and Oka T. Medical and surgical complications of renal transplantation: Diagnosis and management. Med Clin North Am 1990 Jul; 74(4):1025–1037.

Renal Calculi

Atala A and Steinbock GS. Extracorporeal shock-wave lithotripsy of renal calculi. Am J Surg 1989 Mar; 157(3):350–358.

Cass AS. Extracorporeal shock wave lithotripsy. How does it work? Who are candidates for it? Postgrad Med 1988 May 1; 83(6):185–190, 192.

Dickinson IK et al. Combination of percutaneous surgery and extracorporeal shockwave lithotripsy for the treatment of large renal calculi. Br J Urol 1986; 58(6):581–584.

Kramolowsky EV, Quinlan SM, and Loening SA. Extracorporeal shock wave lithotripsy for the treatment of urinary calculi in the elderly. J Am Geriatr Soc 1987 Mar; 35(3):251–254.

Newman DM et al. Extracorporeal shock-wave lithotripsy. Urol Clin North Am 1987 Feb; 14(1):63–71.

Roth RA and Beckmann CF. Complications of extracorporeal shock-wave lithotripsy and percutaneous nephrolithotomy. Urol Clin North Am 1988 May; 15(2):155–166.

Segura JW. Surgical management of urinary calculi. Semin Nephrol 1990 Jan; 10(1):53–63.

Smith LH. The pathophysiology and medical treatment of urolithiasis. Semin Nephrol 1990 Jan; 10(1):31–52.

Tillotson SL and DeLuca SA. Complications of extracorporeal shock wave lithotripsy. Am Fam Physician 1988 Dec; 38(6):161–163.

Willscher MK et al. Safety and efficacy of electrohydraulic lithotripsy by ureteroscopy. J Urol 1988 Nov; 140(5):957, 958.

Wilson WT and Preminger GM. Extracorporeal shock wave lithotripsy. An update. Urol Clin North Am 1990 Feb; 17(1):231–242.

Renal Trauma

Cass AS et al. Deaths from urologic injury due to external trauma. J Trauma 1987 Mar; 27(3):319–321.

Cass AS and Luxenberg M. Management of extraperitoneal ruptures of bladder caused by external trauma. Urology 1989 Aug; 33(3):179–183.

Gasparis L and Noone J. Managing emergencies. Renal genitourinary emergencies. Nursing 1989 Mar; 19(3):96–100.

Smith MF. Renal trauma: Adult and pediatric considerations. Crit Care Clin North Am 1990 Mar 2(1):67–77.

Sommers MS. Blunt renal trauma. Crit Care Nurs 1990 Mar; 10(3):38–48.

Weiskittel P and Sommers MS. The patient with lower urinary tract trauma. Crit Care Nurs 1989 Jan; 9(1):53–65.

Whitehorne M, Cacciola R, Quinn ME. Multiple trauma: Survival after the golden hour. J Adv Med Surg Nurs 1989 Dec; 2(1):27–39.

Tumors of the Urinary Tract and Urinary Diversion

Broadwell DC. Peristomal skin integrity. Nurs Clin North Am 1987 Jun; 22(2):321–332.

Erickson PJ. Ostomies: The art of pouching. Nurs Clin North Am 1987 Jun; 22(2):311–320.

Fowler JE Jr. Continent urinary reservoirs. Surg Annu 1988; 2:201–225.

Killeen KP and Libertino JA. Management of bowel and urinary tract complications after urinary diversion. Urol Clin North Am 1988 May; 15(2): 183–194.

Lange MP et al. Management of multiple enterocutaneous fistulas. Heart Lung 1989 Jul; 18(4):386–390.

Lieskovsky G, Skinner DG, and Boyd SD. Complications of the Kock pouch. Urol Clin North Am 1988 May; 15(2):195–205.

National Cancer Institute. U.S. Department of Health and Human Services. National Institutes of Health. What you need to know about bladder cancer. NIH Pub. No. 90-1559. Washington, DC, 1989.

National Cancer Institute. U.S. Department of Health and Human Services. National Institutes of Health. Adult kidney cancer and Wilms' tumor. NIH Pub. No. 90-2342. Washington, DC, 1989.

Petillo MH. The patient with a urinary stoma: Nursing management and patient education. Nurs Clin North Am 1987 Jun; 22(2):263–279.

Rolstad BS. Innovative surgical procedures and stoma care in the future. Nurs Clin North Am 1987 Jun; 22(2):341–356.

Sagalowsky AI. Technique of the continent ileal bladder: Camey procedure. Urol Clin North Am 1987 Aug; 14(3):643–651.

Schover LR. Sexuality and fertility in urologic cancer patients. Cancer 1987 Aug; 60(Suppl 1):553–558.

Shipes E. Psychosocial issues: The person with an ostomy. Nurs Clin North Am 1987 Jun; 22(2):291–302.

Shipes E. Sexual function following ostomy surgery. Nurs Clin North Am 1987 Jun; 22(2):303–310.

Interstitial Cystitis

Albers DD and Geyer JR. Long-term results of cystolysis (supratrigonal denervation) of the bladder for intractable interstitial cystitis. J Urol 1988 Jun; 139(6):1205, 1206.

Fall M. Transcutaneous electrical nerve stimulation in interstitial cystitis. Update on clinical experience. Urology 1987 Apr; 29(4 Suppl):40–42.

Fowler JE Jr. et al. Interstitial cystitis is associated with intraurothelial Tamm-Horsfall protein. J Urol 1988 Dec; 140(6):1385–1389.

Gillenwater JY and Wein AJ. Summary of the National Institute of Arthritis, Diabetes, Digestive and Kidney Diseases Workshop on Interstitial Cystitis. National Institutes of Health, Bethesda, MD, Aug 28–29, 1987. J Urol 1988 Jul; 140(1):203–206.

Hanno PM and Wein AJ. Editorial: Interstitial cystitis. J Urol 1987 Sep; 138(3):595, 596.

Hanno PM, Buehler J, and Wein AJ. Use of amitriptyline in the treatment of interstitial cystitis. J Urol 1989 Apr; 141(4):846–848.

Hanno PM et al. Diagnosis of interstitial cystitis. J Urol 1990 Feb; 143(2): 278–281.

Holm-Bentzen M et al. Painful bladder disease: Clinical and pathoanatomical differences in 115 patients. J Urol 1987 Sep; 138(3):500–502.

Holm-Bentzen M et al. A prospective double-blind clinically controlled multicenter trial of sodium pentosanpolysulfate in the treatment of interstitial cystitis and related painful bladder disease. J Urol 1987 Sep; 138(3):503–507.

Messing EM. The diagnosis of interstitial cystitis. Urology 1987 Apr; 29(4 Suppl):4–7.

Painful bladder diseases: Interstitial or abacterial cystitis? Lancet 1988 Feb 13; 1(8581):337–338.

Parsons CL and Mulholland SG. Successful therapy of interstitial cystitis with pentosanpolysulfate. J Urol 1987 Sep; 138(3):513–516.

Perez–Marrero R, Emerson LE, and Feltis JT. A controlled study of dimethyl sulfoxide in interstitial cystitis. J Urol 1988 Jul; 140(1):36–39.

Perez–Marrero R, Emerson LE, and Juma S. Urodynamic studies in interstitial cystitis. Urology 1987 Apr; 29(4 Suppl):27–30.

Steinkohl WB and Leach GE. Urodynamic findings in interstitial cystitis. Urology 1989 Dec; 34(6):399–401.

Information/Resources

Agencies

American Cancer Society
  1599 Clifton Rd. NE, Atlanta, GA 30329, (404) 320-3333

Cancer Information Service
  1-800-4-CANCER

American Society for Artificial Internal Organs
  PO Box C, Boca Raton, FL 33429, (407) 391-8589

International Association for Enterostomal Therapy
  2081 Business Center Dr., Suite 290, Irvine, CA 92715, (714) 476-0268

Interstitial Cystitis Association
  PO Box 1553, Madison Square Garden Station, New York, NY 10159, (212) 979-6057

American Association of Kidney Patients
  1 Davis Blvd., Suite LL1, Tampa, FL 33606, (813) 251-0725

National Institute of Diabetes and Digestive and Kidney Diseases
  National Institutes of Health, Bethesda, MD 20892

National Kidney Foundation
  30 East 33rd St., New York, NY 10016, (212) 889-2210

United Ostomy Association
  36 Executive Park, Suite 120, Irvine, CA 92714-6744, (714) 660-8624

Nursing Research Profile for Unit 10

Urinary and Renal Nursing

Overview

A few of the topics that have recently received increased attention by nurse researchers have included urinary incontinence, aspects of management of indwelling urinary catheters, and stress and coping related to dialysis and transplantation.

An important area for research is that of urinary incontinence. Studies reported here focus on assessment of the patient with urinary incontinence and strategies to reduce the incidence of urinary incontinence.

Indwelling urinary catheters remain a concern for the nurse; further study is needed to identify nursing interventions related to management of urinary catheters and drainage systems and problems experienced by patients discharged to their homes with catheters in place.

Stressors associated with hemodialysis and renal transplantation and psychologic reactions to those stressors remain an area of considerable interest to nurse researchers. Fewer studies have focused on stressors related to peritoneal dialysis. As technologic advances continue and move into the home and long-term care setting, nursing research must keep pace with their impact on patients and families, and their psychologic and physical implications.

Further research related to physiologic and psychologic reactions to urinary diversions and nursing interventions related to these procedures is needed. Research related to recurrent urinary tract infection and interstitial cystitis is urgently needed because of the physiologic, psychologic, and economic costs of these disorders.

Urinary Incontinence

▷ Brink CA *et al.* A *digital test for pelvic muscle strength in older women with urinary incontinence*. Nurs Res 1989 Jul/Aug; 38(4):196–199.

Because of the high incidence of stress urinary incontinence and its association with pelvic muscle weakness, a clinically useful objective means of assessing pelvic muscle strength is needed. This study describes test–retest and inter-rater reliability and validity of a digital test of pelvic muscle strength

in older women with urinary incontinence. The pelvic muscle rating scale tested in this study assessed vaginal and pelvic muscle contraction when the examiner's gloved fingers were inserted 4 to 6 cm into the vaginal canal. A seven-point scale ranging from 0 to 4 (0, 0.3, 0.5, 1, 2, 3, 4) was used to rate the strength of the pressure exerted with pelvic muscle contraction, alteration of the vertical plane of the examiner's fingers, and duration of the contraction.

The sample included 338 noninstitutionalized women with urinary incontinence. Their ages ranged from 55 to 90 years; mean age was 67.5 years (SD = 8.9). Stress incontinence was the most common type of urinary incontinence in the sample; symptoms of stress incontinence were described by the majority of subjects. Pelvic muscle strength was rated by nurse practitioners trained by the researchers to conduct the assessment and to use the seven-point rating scale. Additionally, a perinometer (a measurement instrument) was used to assess pelvic muscle strength, specifically first maximal sustained contraction, mean strength of six 10-second held contractions, and the mean of five rapid unsustained contractions of the pelvic muscles. The perinometer was used to assess criterion validity of the rating scale.

Test–retest reliability was assessed by correlating scores obtained twice on 228 subjects with an interval of 4 to 6 weeks between examinations; significant correlations of the measures were reported. Inter-rater reliability was obtained by correlating scores obtained by two examiners who examined the same patient on the same day; correlations of the scores were significant. Significant correlations were also obtained when ratings were correlated with measures of pelvic muscle strength of 298 subjects obtained by perinometer, supporting the validity of the digital rating scale. Additional analyses indicated that women who reported inability to stop the urinary stream in the midst of urination and those who reported a large amount of urine loss with episodes of incontinence were associated with scores indicative of weaker pelvic muscles.

Nursing Implications. The findings of this study demonstrate sufficient reliability and validity of a digital rating scale of pelvic muscle strength to warrant further testing in studies of women with urinary incontinence. A valid, reliable measure to assess pelvic muscle strength is an important step in determining factors responsible for urinary incontinence, in selecting strategies to assist women who are incontinent, and in evaluating the effectiveness of those strategies.

> Creason NS et al. Prompted voiding therapy for urinary
> incontinence in aged female nursing home residents. J Adv
> Nurs 1989 Feb; 14(2):120–126.

This study compared the effect of prompted voiding and socialization on incontinence in 85 elderly female nursing home residents. Patients included in the sample were residents of one of four nursing homes, were 65 years of age or older, were incontinent of urine 2 weeks or longer, and had no indwelling catheter in place. The first group (N = 30) received prompted voiding; subjects in a second group (N = 27) received socialization; and subjects in a third group (N = 28) constituted the control group.

Subjects in the *prompted voiding group* were checked every waking hour by nursing assistants and asked about the need to void. They were assisted to the bathroom if necessary. Wetness/dryness checks were conducted hourly. The *socialization group* received a 2- to 3-minute hourly social contact with no mention of voiding made by the staff. Assistance to the bathroom was given if the desire to void was expressed by the patient; wet/dry checks were made hourly. The *control group* received usual care provided in the nursing home; wet/dry checks consistent with the routine of the specific nursing home were conducted, usually ever 2 to 3 hours. Data collected from subjects in each group included assessment of cognitive function with the Mini-Mental Status Examination (MMS) and assessment of functional capacities with the Katz Index of Activities of Daily Living (KADL) assessment. Episodes of incontinence were recorded for later analysis; data from the wet/dry checks were graphed for all three groups to visualize patterns. If patterns were detected after 2 weeks, the experimental treatments were implemented based on subjects' voiding patterns; if no patterns were detected, hourly checks and treatments continued as initially assigned.

The sample included 85 subjects whose ages ranged from 65 to 99 years; the mean age was 87 years. Sixty-five percent (N = 55) of the subjects were at the lowest level of cognitive function; 16% (N = 14) were at the next level; and 19% (N = 16) were in a normal range of cognitive function. KADL scores indicate that the overwhelming majority of patients had significant or extreme functional limitations requiring assistance with bathing, dressing, and toileting.

Because randomization of subjects to groups was not possible, the authors examined similarities of the experimental and control groups prior to application of the experimental treatments. The control group and prompted voiding group were similar on the variables of interest, but the socialization group was more functional, more continent, younger, and had a higher level of cognition compared with the other two groups prior to initiation of treatment.

Age, decreased cognitive status, and impaired functional status were all found to be related to incontinence. The older the resident and the more severe the loss of cognitive or functional status, the more severe the incontinence. Analysis of the proportion of incontinence episodes (number of times found incontinent/number of times checked) at the end of the first 5 weeks of intervention revealed that by the fifth week the prompted voiding group was more similar to the socialization

group than to the control group (which received no intervention other than usual care).

Nursing Implications. Although this study is hampered with methodologic flaws inherent in this type of study, as discussed by the researchers, it does demonstrate that prompted voiding can be effective in decreasing episodes of incontinence. Prompted voiding may also be effective in reducing costs associated with frequent changes of linen and skin excoriation secondary to incontinence and in maintaining or restoring a patient's dignity and self-esteem.

> Whippo CC and Creason NS. Bacteriuria and urinary
> incontinence in aged female nursing home residents.
> J Adv Nurs 1989 Mar; 14(3):217–225.

Urinary incontinence has been identified as a symptom of urinary tract infection (UTI). However, preexisting incontinence in elderly patients makes it difficult to determine how important this is as an indicator of UTI. The aim of this study was to identify factors associated with bacteriuria in women known to be incontinent of urine who were residents of a nursing home.

Sixty-five female nursing home residents with urinary incontinence constituted the sample; the mean age was 85 years (range, 64 to 97 years). Clean-catch midstream urine specimens collected under controlled conditions were analyzed by the laboratory; urine culture was performed if the urine screen was positive for bacteria. Subjects were then divided into three groups by urine bacteria counts: (1) those with negative urine screens, (2) those with bacteria counts greater than 100,000/ml of urine, and (3) those with bacteria counts less than 100,000/ml of urine. Data collected on subjects grouped into these three categories included: frequency of episodes of urinary incontinence, frequency of physical symptoms commonly associated with UTI (*i.e.*, urgency, dysuria, urinary frequency, tachycardia, fever, and hematuria), and abnormal physical examination findings found to be associated with urinary incontinence. The MMS and the KADL were used to assess cognitive function and functional abilities, respectively.

Results indicate that the classic symptoms of pain and burning are all but absent in all groups. A high incidence of abnormal findings on physical examination was found. No differences were found among the three groups in the following symptoms: nocturia, daytime frequency of urination, difficulty initiating urination, straining to start urination, and inability to wait for 5 minutes to void after feeling the urge to urinate. Although there were some differences in some physical symptoms across groups (*i.e.*, urge to void and inability to hold urine once the urge to void was felt), group differences were not in the predicted direction. There was a tendency for patients with reduced cognitive function to be more likely to have UTI, although the statistical level fell just short of significance. There was a relationship between level of independence as measured by KADL and incidence of UTI; the higher the level of independence, the less the likelihood that UTI would be present.

Nursing Implications. The findings of this study support the notion that UTIs in the elderly may not be accompanied by the usual signs and symptoms of UTI. Careful physical and cognitive assessment of patients must be undertaken because differences in cognitive function and level of independence may account for the failure to recognize and report symptoms of UTI and the inability to act on them.

Catheter Care

▷ Roe BH. *Study of information given by nurses for catheter care to patients and their carers.* J Adv Nurs 1989 Mar; 14(3):203–210.

The purpose of this study was to determine what information about catheter care is provided by hospital and district nurses to community-based patients with indwelling urethral catheters. A sample of 46 district nurses and 60 hospital nurses were interviewed about information and instruction they gave to patients with indwelling urinary catheters. A semi-structured interview schedule and topic checklist were used to guide the interview. The information included: recommendations regarding type of catheter, frequency of catheter changes, meatal cleansing, urinary drainage system, frequency of bag change, use of bladder washouts, hand hygiene, and nurses' opinions about catheters. Each item of advice about catheter and catheter care reported by each nurse was scored; the highest score possible was 19. Data about nurses' level of education and work setting (hospital versus district) were obtained.

The median checklist scores among nurses by work setting and educational preparation ranged from a low of 3.39 to a high of 5.60 on the 19-item scale. The range of individual nurses was from 0 (indicating that no information was given) to 12. No significant differences in scores were found among nurses of different educational levels. Significant differences were found according to nurses' work setting; scores indicated that district nurses reported giving more information and instruction than did hospital nurses. Results also indicated considerable variation among nurses in their opinions about the type, size, and length of catheter that should be used, and there were differences in opinion about frequency of catheter change and recommendations regarding meatal cleansing. None of these opinions differed by educational level; differences in opinion about type of catheter (silicone versus silicone-coated) existed by work setting.

Nursing Implications. The scores on the checklists reported by hospital nurses and district nurses regarding their instructions to patients and their caregivers indicate that often little or incomplete information about catheter management is given. Additionally, the information that is reportedly given to patients and their caregivers is inconsistent; many of the instructions given are not consistent with information provided in the literature. Although the use of indwelling catheters has decreased, there are occasions when such a catheter is indicated. In those circumstances, the patient who is to go home with a catheter in place and his caregivers must receive comprehensive information about catheter care. The nurse preparing the patient and caregiver for home care needs to collaborate as well with the nurse who visits the patient at home to provide consistent instructions and assistance with catheter care to assure comfort and freedom from complications.

Hemodialysis and Kidney Transplantation

▷ Jones LC and Pruett SG. *Self-care activities and processes used by hemodialysis patients.* ANNA J 1986 Apr; 13(2):73–79.

The authors theorized that hemodialysis patients use self-care activities to deal with the stressors commonly attributed to hemodialysis treatment. The purpose of the study was to explore those self-care activities used by hemodialysis patients to deal with hemodialysis-related stressors. Twenty-five hemodialysis patients constituted the sample. The sample included 24 male and 1 female patient. The patients' ages ranged from 31 to 70 years (mean age, 47 years), and the duration of treatment with hemodialysis ranged from 15 to 139 months (mean duration of hemodialysis treatment, 58.4 months). Semistructured interviews were used to obtain data about patients' ways of dealing with treatment-related stressors. The stressors used in this study were identified from previously published research. Qualitative analysis was used to analyze data obtained through the interviews.

Self-care activity responses related to the treatment regimen were categorized and tabulated for each stressor. Data were analyzed to identify recurrent themes and concepts related to self-care activities. The authors describe self-care activities as specific acts initiated by individual patients and self-care processes as responses that serve as adaptive mechanisms in performing self-care. Four patterns of self-care processes were identified and defined: (1) *equalizing,* the process of weighing, judging, and shifting competing demands for time, energy, finances, desires, and requirements; (2) *substituting,* the process of replacing and exchanging desires and activities; (3) *withdrawing,* the process of moving away from events, people, and ideas; and (4) *guarding,* the process of maintaining vigilance over the body and delivery of care. Different subjects used different self-care responses to cope with the same stressor. For example, one patient reported eating restricted foods just before treatment when the negative effect of the food item would be moderated by treatment soon after its ingestion (equalizing); another avoids thinking about restricted foods (withdrawing); and a third substitutes other food items for those that are restricted (substituting).

Nursing Implications. The exploratory nature of this study precludes implications for clinical practice but does suggest the need for individual assessment of patients' strategies for dealing with stressors related to hemodialysis. Patients tend to develop strategies such as equalizing or substituting to deal with specific physiologic stressors, such as fluid imbalance and dietary restrictions. They require accurate information about the consequences of their judgments and actions to be able to make safe, informed judgments. The inclusion of only one female patient in the study further limits the generalizability of the findings.

▷ Betts DK and Crotty GD. *Response to illness and compliance of long-term hemodialysis patients.* ANNA J 1988 Apr; 15(2):96–99.

The overall purpose of this study was to examine relationships between responses to illness and level of compliance in long-term hemodialysis patients. The study specifically assessed (1) the relationship between response to illness and serum potassium and serum phosphorus levels and between-dialysis weight gain and (2) the relationship of these three physiologic measurements.

Forty-six stable patients who had been receiving long-term hemodialysis treatments for at least 2 years completed the study. Subjects were interviewed with the Response to Illness Questionnaire (RIQ), a 34-item questionnaire that assesses the various meanings that an illness may have for a patient and the patient's cognitive, affective, and behavioral responses to it.

Subjects were presented statements about their illness and asked to indicate their agreement or disagreement on a four-point Likert-type scale ranging from 0 (the most negative response) to 3 (the most positive response). The range of possible total scores was 0 to 102.

Demographic data including age, length of time on dialysis, and ethnicity were obtained. Between-dialysis weight gain and serum potassium and phosphorus levels were obtained. Patients were weighed before each dialysis treatment and at the conclusion of each treatment. For this study, compliance was defined as a weight gain of 0 to 4 pounds between dialysis treatments, serum potassium levels between 3.5 and 5.5 mEq/L, and serum phosphorus levels between 3.5 and 5 mg/100 ml.

Results. The mean RIQ score of 73.9 indicates an overall positive response to illness. While the majority (71.7%) of patients stayed within designated acceptable limits for potassium levels, only 23.9% stayed within acceptable limits for phosphorus levels and 6.5% stayed within limits for weight gain. There were no significant relationships between response to illness as measured by the RIQ and any of the physiologic measurements. Age was significantly correlated with the subjects' responses to illness and with between-dialysis weight gain. The older the subject, the more positive the response to illness. Older subjects also gained less weight between dialysis treatments than younger subjects in the sample.

The results of this study suggest that the feelings of hemodialysis patients about their illness, as measured by the RIQ, have little bearing on adherence to treatment, as measured by between-treatment weight gain and serum potassium and phosphorus levels. The authors suggest that other variables may have greater influence on patients' adherence to the fluid and dietary restrictions that are part of the hemodialysis regimen.

Nursing Implications. The extent of patients' adherence to the treatment regimen differs considerably from patient to patient and from one aspect of the treatment regimen to another. Difficulty in adhering to the prescribed treatment regimens must be assessed on an individual or case-by-case basis. Factors influencing adherence to restrictions must be explored with the patient. Adherence to one restriction or recommendation cannot be considered an indication of adherence to all restrictions or recommendations.

▷ O'Brien ME. *Compliance behavior and long-term maintenance dialysis. Am J Kidney Dis 1990 Mar; 15(3): 209–214.*

The purpose of this longitudinal study was to examine the relationships between social support and compliance behavior in long-term maintenance hemodialysis patients. A second aim was to evaluate changes in compliance behavior over time as patients moved from the stages of early to long-term coping with end-stage renal disease and hemodialysis treatment.

Social support was conceptualized as being related to the caring and expectations of significant others about the patient's treatment-associated behavior. Compliance was defined as adherence to the total therapeutic regimen prescribed for an individual dialysis patient. At time 1, 12 to 18 months following initiation of hemodialysis, the sample consisted of 126 subjects. At time 2, 3 years later, the sample consisted of 63 subjects from the original sample. At time 3, another 3 years later, there were 33 subjects remaining in the sample. The relationship between social support and compliance behavior was assessed

at all three points. Changes in social support and compliance behavior over time were assessed at time 2 and time 3.

The Primary Support System Scale and Secondary Support System Scale were used to assess primary (family and kin) and secondary (professional caregivers) social support. Patient compliance behavior was assessed by the Hemodialysis Regimen Compliance Schedule. Sociodemographic data were also obtained. Qualitative data were collected at time 3 with a Dialysis Patient Focused Interview Guide, which included items that focused on family and caregiver support and expectations regarding the patient's compliance with various aspects of the therapeutic regimen and the patient's attitudes toward and behavior involving compliance with dialysis treatment.

Results. The findings of the study indicate that social support by family members and professional caregivers is strongly related to compliance with the hemodialysis regimen early in its course. In lower socioeconomic groups, support from professional caregivers is more closely related to compliance than is that of the family. Long-term compliance changed over time; some patients became more compliant with the therapeutic regimen from time 1 to time 2, while others became less compliant.

When patients who survived to be interviewed at time 2 and time 3 were compared to those who died early in the course of the study, it was found that those who died earliest (between time 1 and time 2) had the highest compliance. Those who survived to time 3 had the lowest level of compliance. Analysis of the qualitative data suggested that survivors learned on their own what their own limits were and that they would take steps to stay within those limits.

Nursing Implications. Reasoned compliance, that is, compliance based on the patient's own experiences of what his safe limits are, may be more conducive to survival than rigid or ritual compliance with strict behavioral prescriptions. In order for a patient to develop an understanding and appreciation of his own limits, he needs complete and accurate information about the cause-and-effect relationship between actions and their consequences. A realistic, individualized approach to teaching the hemodialysis patient about treatment and its consequences may allow the patient some flexibility, better adjustment, and longer survival.

▷ Sutton TD and Murphy SP. *Stressors and patterns of coping in renal transplant patients. Nurs Res 1989 Jan/Feb; 38(1):46–49.*

The purposes of this study were (1) to determine the incidence and severity of selected stressors and the coping strategies used by a group of postoperative renal transplant patients and (2) to explore the influence of time on stress and coping patterns of renal transplant patients. Forty patients who had received a renal transplant less than 4 years previously constituted the sample. The 35-item End-Stage Renal Disease (ESRD) stressor scale, modified for use with transplant patients, was administered to the subjects. Ten additional items specific to transplantations, such as fear of transplant rejection and feelings toward the organ donor, were added. The severity of each of the 45 stressors was rated by subjects on a five-point Likert scale from not at all (0) to a great deal (5).

The Jalowiec coping scale was used to assess coping behaviors of transplant patients. Demographic data were also obtained; these included age, sex, marital status, and race, and illness-related information (*i.e.*, pretransplant treatment modalities, type of transplant, time since transplantation, other major health problems, and current medications).

Forty patients who had received a kidney transplant within the last 4 years constituted the sample. They were approached and asked to participate in the study during routine post-transplant appointments for follow-up care. The mean total severity score for the stressor scale was 74.1 ± 24.8, with scores ranging from 45 to 149 (the highest possible score was 175). The five stressors rated as most stressful were: cost, fear of rejection, weight gain, uncertainty regarding future, and limitation of physical activities. There were no significant correlations between stressor scores and any demographic characteristics.

To examine changes over time, the patients were categorized by time since transplant into two groups: those whose transplant was 0 to 23 months ago and those who received their transplant 24 to 48 months ago. Patients who had received their transplant 24 to 48 months ago had higher stress scores than patients who had received a transplant more recently. Subjects who received their transplant more recently rated cost as the most stressful item; subjects who had received their transplant 24 to 48 months ago rated fear of kidney rejection as most stressful. Although there were differences in rankings of severity of some items by the two groups, the rankings were generally similar.

The mean total coping score was 102.3 ± 15.5, with a range of 69 to 129 (the highest possible score was 200). No significant correlations were found between total coping scores and any demographic characteristics. Subscores for problem-oriented coping and affective-oriented coping were calculated. The mean score on the problem-oriented coping subscale was significantly higher than the mean affective-oriented coping score. Higher scores on the affective-oriented coping subscale were associated with having a diagnosis of diabetes and being on insulin. Total stressor scores were not correlated with total coping scores or problem-oriented coping scores. There was a positive correlation between total stressor scores and affective-oriented coping.

Nursing Implications.   Stressors persist up to 4 years after transplantation. Cost and fear of rejection remain of major concern to patients. Patients' questions and concerns about the function of the transplant should be taken seriously. Although the author's contention that stressors change over time would be better measured with a longitudinal study, there is some suggestion that stressors early in the post-transplantation course are different from those later in the course. During the early post-transplantation phase, patients may feel that they have more control over successful outcomes. Later in the post-transplant course, when transplant function may decrease, they may perceive that they have less control. Therefore, providing patients with accurate information and options (when possible) may provide more of a sense of control and may reduce their stress level.

Bibliography

Other Related Research Studies

Dodds P and Hans AL. Distended urinary bladder drainage practices among hospital nurses. Appl Nurs Res 1990 May; 3(2):68–72.

Moore MN. Development of a sleep–awake instrument for use in a chronic renal population. ANNA J 1989 Feb; 16(1):15–19.

Nyamathi A. Coping responses of spouses of MI patients and of hemodialysis patients as measured by the Jalowiec coping scale. J Cardiovasc Nurs 1987 Nov; 2(1):67–74.

Roe BH. Use of bladder washouts: A study of nurses' recommendations. J Adv Nurs 1989 Jun; 14(6):494–500.

Watson R. A nursing trial of urinary sheath systems on male hospitalized patients. J Adv Nurs 1989 Jun; 14(6):467–470.

unit 11
Reproductive Function

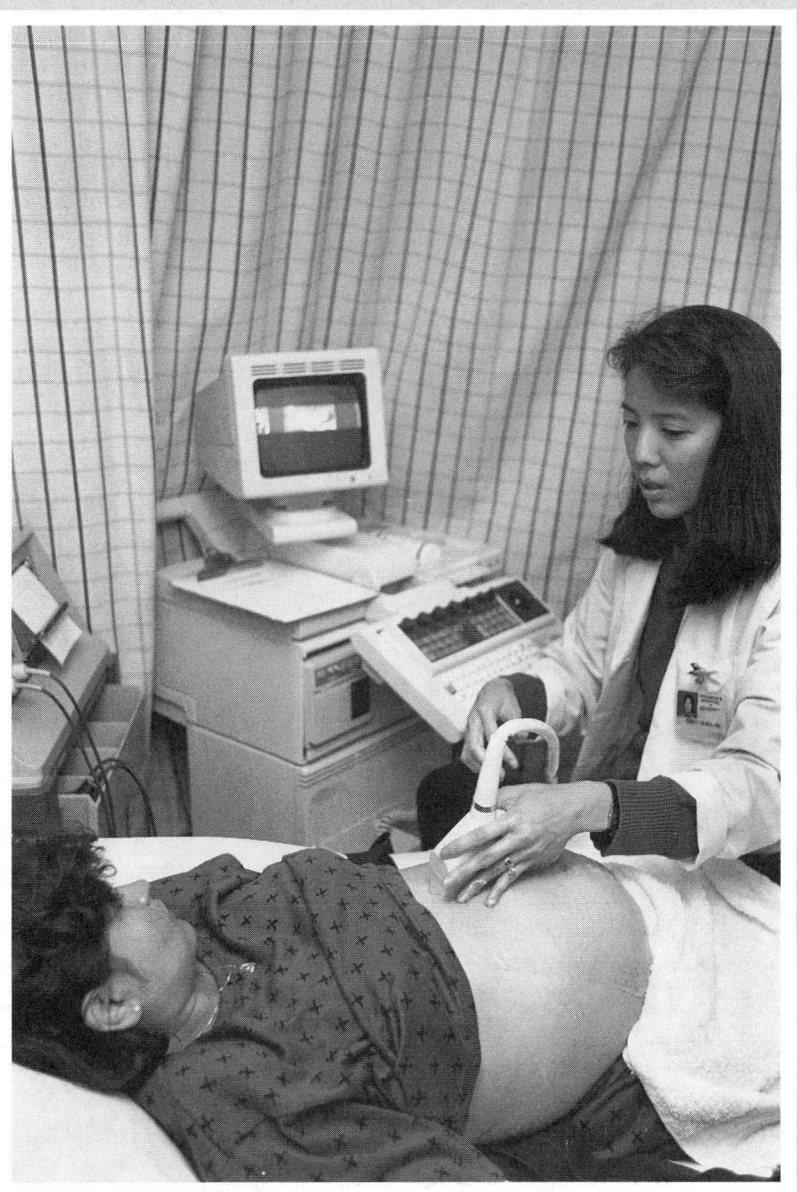

44

Management of Problems Related to Female Physiologic Processes

Learning Objectives

On completion of this chapter, the learner will be able to:

1. Describe diagnostic examinations and tests used to determine alteration in functioning of the female reproductive organs and the nurse's role during these procedures
2. Describe uses of vaginal and vulvar irrigations and vaginal creams and principles that guide their use
3. Describe the physiology of menstruation and the related physical changes and psychosocial considerations
4. Use the nursing process as a framework for care of patients with premenstrual syndrome
5. Specify factors that cause disturbances of menstruation and the related nursing implications
6. Develop a teaching plan for women experiencing menopause
7. Describe methods of contraception and implications for health care and education for each method
8. Describe the nursing management of the patient having an abortion
9. Specify the causes and management of infertility
10. Use the nursing process as a framework for the care of patients with tubal ectopic pregnancies
11. Describe indicators of domestic violence and abuse of women and strategies for the nurse caring for a woman who is a victim of abuse

Physiologic Overview

The female reproductive system consists of two ovaries, two fallopian (uterine) tubes, a uterus, and a vagina. The *vulva* is the region of the external genitalia; it includes two thick folds of tissue called the *labia majora* and two smaller lips of delicate tissue called the *labia minora*, which lie within the labia majora. The upper portions of the labia minora unite to form a partial covering for the *clitoris*, a highly sensitive organ composed of erectile tissue. Between the labia minora, below and posterior to the clitoris, is the urinary meatus, the external opening of

the female urethra, which measures a little more than 3 cm in length (1.5 inches). Below this orifice is a larger opening, the vaginal orifice (Fig. 44–1). On each side of the vaginal orifice is a *vestibular (Bartholin's) gland*, which is a bean-sized structure that empties its mucous secretion by way of a small duct. The orifice of the duct is found within the labia minora, external to the hymen. The tissue between the external genitalia and the anus is called the fourchette. All of the tissue that makes up the female external genitalia is called the perineum.

The *vagina* is the canal lined with mucous membrane that is 7.5 to 10 cm (3 or 4 inches) long and extends downward and forward from the uterus to the vulva. Anterior to it are the

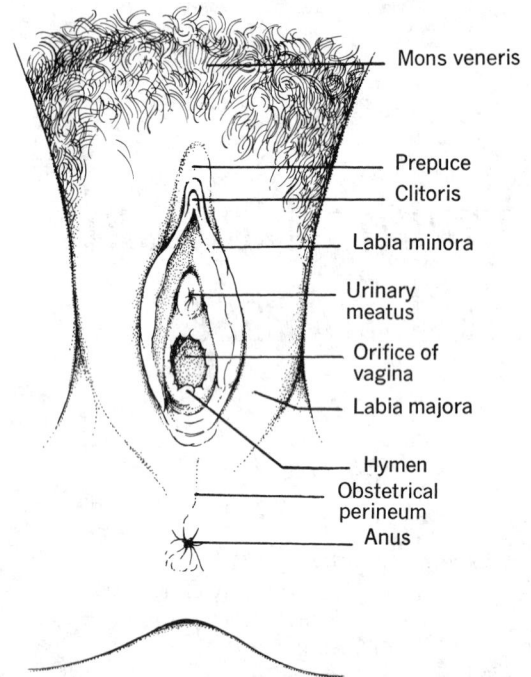

Figure 44–1. External female genitalia. (Chaffee EE and Greisheimer EM. Basic Physiology and Anatomy. Philadelphia, JB Lippincott.)

bladder and the urethra, and below it lies the rectum. The anterior and posterior walls of the vagina normally lie in contact with one another. The upper part of the vagina, the *fornix*, surrounds the *cervix* (the neck of the uterus).

The *uterus* is a pear-shaped muscular organ that is about 7.5 cm (3 inches) long and about 5 cm (2 inches) wide at its upper part. Its walls are about 1.25 cm (0.5 inch) thick. The

size of this organ may vary depending on parity (number of children).

A young woman who has not completed a pregnancy to the stage of fetal viability (*nullipara*) frequently has a smaller uterus than one who has completed two or more pregnancies to the stage of fetal viability (*multipara*).

The uterus is divided into a narrow neck, or cervix, that projects into the vagina and a larger upper part, the *fundus* or body, which is covered posteriorly and partly anteriorly by peritoneum. The uterus lies posterior to the bladder and is held in position in the pelvic cavity by several ligaments. The *round ligaments* extend anteriorly and laterally to the internal inguinal ring and down the inguinal canal, where they blend with the tissues of the labia majora. The *broad ligaments* are folds of peritoneum extending from the lateral pelvic walls and enveloping the fallopian tubes. The uterosacral ligaments extend posteriorly to the sacrum, and the uterovesical ligaments pass anteriorly. The inner portion of the fundus is triangular. It narrows to a small canal in the cervix that has a constriction at each end, referred to as the external and internal ossa. The upper lateral parts of the uterus are called the *cornua*. From here the oviducts or fallopian tubes extend outward, with their lumina continuous internally with the uterine cavity.

The *ovaries* lie behind the broad ligaments, behind and below the tubes. They are oval bodies about 3 cm (1.2 inches) in length, which contain thousands of tiny egg cells or ova. The ovaries and the fallopian tubes are called the *adnexa* (Fig. 44–2).

The ovary, which normally contains 30,000 to 40,000 ova, remains quiescent in early life. At the time of puberty (usually between the 12th and 14th years), however, the ova begin to ripen or mature, enlarging as a type of cyst known as a *graafian follicle*. The cyst enlarges during the follicular phase until it reaches the surface of the ovary, where rupture occurs, and the ovum is discharged into the peritoneal cavity. This periodic

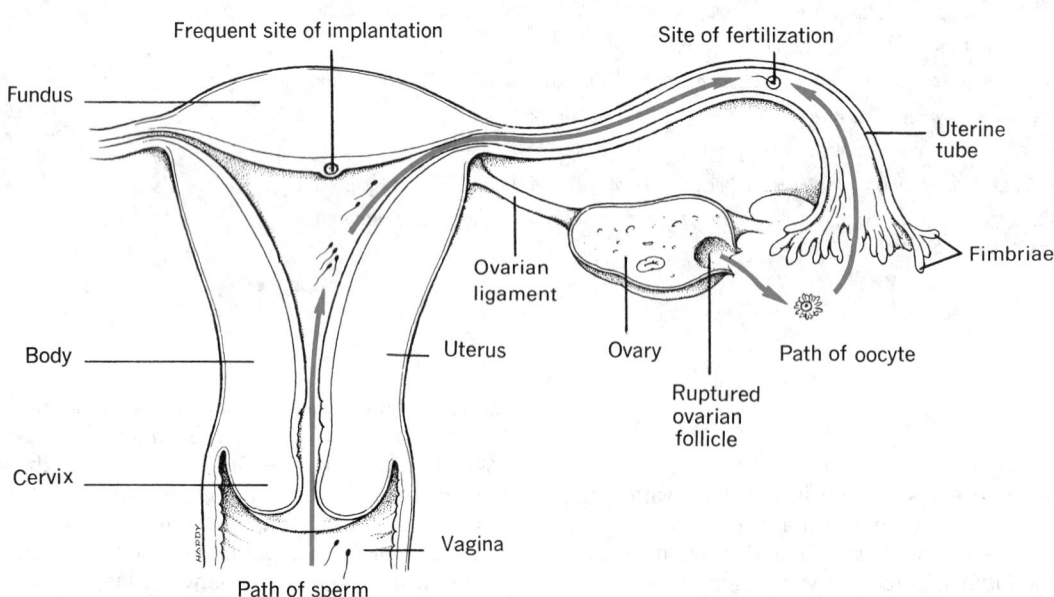

Figure 44–2. Schematic drawing of female reproductive organs, showing path of oocyte from ovary into fallopian tube, path of spermatozoa, and the usual site of fertilization. (Chaffee EE and Greisheimer EM. Basic Physiology and Anatomy. Philadelphia, JB Lippincott.)

discharge of matured ova is referred to as *ovulation* when the menstrual cycle enters the luteal phase. The ovum usually finds its way into the fallopian tube, where it is carried to the uterus. If it meets a spermatozoon, the male reproductive cell, a union occurs and *conception* takes place. After the discharge of the ovum, the cells of the graafian follicle undergo a rapid change. Gradually they become yellow (*corpus luteum*) and produce a secretion that has the function of preparing the uterus for the reception of the fertilized ovum.

If conception does not occur, the ovum disintegrates and the mucous membrane lining the uterus (*endometrium*), which has become thickened and congested, becomes hemorrhagic. The upper layer of lining cells and the blood that appears in the uterine cavity are discharged through the cervix and the vagina. This flow of blood (*menstruation*) mixes with mucus and cells and occurs approximately every 28 days during the sexual life of females, although normal ovulatory cycles can vary from 21 to 42 days. The period of flow usually lasts from 4 to 5 days, during which time 50 to 60 ml of blood is lost. After the cessation of the menstrual flow, the endometrium proliferates and thickens from estrogenic stimulation, ovulation recurs, and the cycle begins again. Ovulation usually occurs midway between menstrual periods.

Between the ages of 45 and 52 years (average age is 51.3 years), the menstrual flow ceases in most women. This period, called the *menopause* (change of life, climacteric), is associated with atrophy of the breasts and genital organs and sometimes with emotional and vascular changes and losses in bone density.

Health Maintenance

Over the past two decades, increased attention has focused on women's health problems and health maintenance, probably due in part to women's increased interest and concern about their own health care. Biologic as well as psychosocial changes that have a direct bearing on the health of women continue to be studied from conception to death.

As women have moved into the labor market, they have faced changes in life style, such as new family patterns, multiple roles, and competition; exposure to environmental hazards and stress; and greater participation in damaging health practices (*e.g.,* drug use). Greater responsibility for one's personal health (self-care) is being assessed. Physical exercise and competitive sports that once were considered nonfeminine are now popular. Stress-related illnesses have increased, and programs to control stress are common.

Delaying the time of having children until well after a career is established is a common practice. The use of oral contraceptives and intrauterine devices (IUDs) is popular, as is the use of the diaphragm and other barrier methods of contraceptives. Recent problems traced to certain IUDs dampened the enthusiasm for this form of contraception. Newly developed IUDs are a safer option for appropriate candidates.

Nurses are becoming more knowledgeable about preventive care for women, particularly with regard to their unique needs. The nurse encourages female clients to determine their own goals and behaviors. This can be facilitated by assessing health and illness manifestations; offering intervention strategies; and providing support, counseling, and ongoing monitoring as women move toward their health goals.

Hygienic Features: Client/Patient Education

The nurse is in a key position to teach and to advise girls and women about the principles of good health and personal hygiene, especially principles dealing with feminine hygiene related to those parts of the female body concerned with reproduction. The reproductive system in a healthy individual, like any other part of the anatomy, functions well if nutrition, exercise, rest, and elimination are adequate. Aside from teaching female patients about these general aspects of care, the nurse should provide instruction about sexually transmitted diseases (STDs) and preconceptional, prenatal, and postnatal care.

Concepts of feminine hygiene vary greatly with different cultures. What may be considered appropriate care for a European woman may be viewed differently by an American or Japanese woman. In some societies, an emphasis on cleanliness and neatness may be considered unnecessary, whereas in others climate and local customs may affect the habits practiced. Even members of the same family may have different opinions about personal habits.

Nurses need to understand the variations in attitudes and practices of hygiene and their relation to sexual function. Because many methods of feminine hygiene are empirical, it is necessary to apply common sense. Douching of the vagina has been passed down from certain old cultures as a traditional practice of feminine hygiene. Modern studies of vaginal physiology, however, show no health benefit from douching; indeed, many douches that were once considered to be necessary may irritate the vaginal mucosa or reduce the normal mechanisms of resistance to infection.

Contrary to popular opinion, genital odor infrequently arises from the vagina but is often of external origin, arising from the interaction of oil secreted by the vulvar skin with surface bacteria. Occasionally, old menstrual blood or seminal fluid ejaculated in coitus produces some vaginal odor. A simple, low-pressure, warm water irrigation or, at most, a douche of a solution of 30 ml of white vinegar to a liter of water is appropriate. Significant malodor from the vagina can result from a retained tampon or another foreign body or vaginitis, which requires examination and treatment.

Assessment

Health History

The nurse is in a unique position to teach patients about the normal physiologic processes of menstruation and menopause. Many difficulties encountered by a young girl or middle-aged woman usually can be corrected easily; if allowed to go untreated, they may cause damage.

- Danger signals that every woman should report to a health care professional are spotting, irregular or excessive bleeding, or any bleeding after menopause.

Persistent painful menstruation, leukorrhea, and urinary disturbances should be investigated. Many of these early signs can be corrected simply and permanently. An annual breast and pelvic examination is important for all women who are more than 18 years old or who are sexually active, regardless of age.

The gynecologic patient often requires understanding because of the emotional as well as physical considerations that govern the situation. A woman may resent any reference to her genitourinary system, feeling that she is suspected of questionable social or sexual habits.

Psychic factors may also present during the menopausal period. The loss of reproductive capacity may cause disappointment if the woman has had no children. For a woman with a grown family, it may mean that she feels she is no longer useful, or more positively, may result in feelings of sexual and personal freedom. Circumstances affect the responses of each patient and must be considered on an individual basis.

Because gynecologic conditions often are of such a personal and private nature, the nurse is expected to respect the confidentiality of the patient. This information is shared only with those directly involved in professional patient care, as is true with all patient information. Nursing ethics and legal liability demand confidentiality.

Domestic Violence and Abuse of Women

Nurses who care for women must be aware of the prevalence of violence toward women in our society. Six million women are victims of domestic violence each year; therefore, many battered women are encountered in nursing practice. Abuse can be physical, emotional-psychological, or can involve threats or damage to her children, pets, or property. Male violence seems to be related to issues of power and control, and maintaining the traditional role of men as heads of households. Abuse involves fear of one partner by another, and control by threats, insults, or physical abuse.

Nurses are in a unique position to bring problems of abuse to light. By being well informed on this subject, alert to problems related to abuse, and knowledgeable about the kinds of questions that might elicit information from women concerning abuse in their lives, nurses can offer intervention for a problem that would otherwise go undetected. Many women are not comfortable admitting that they are involved in an abusive relationship. Many see it as their fault; that is, if they were better wives, this would not be happening. They are sometimes embarrassed to admit that their husbands or partners are hurting them. If they are not directly questioned by health professionals about abuse, women may not admit the cause of their health problem or injuries, or the reason they are seeking health care. Direct questioning is an important part of health assessment of all women by nurses. Simply asking a woman if anyone is hurting her, if she has ever been hurt by a male partner, or if she is ever afraid of her partner may open the door for a woman to share her problems.

Asking these questions in more than one way is helpful. Any time a diagnosis of abuse goes undetected during a health care encounter, the opportunity to intervene has been lost and the violence continues. Assessment for risk of abuse must be done with the woman alone. Asking her about her husband's or partner's behavior in his presence or within his hearing could endanger the patient and obviously is not conducive to disclosure and intervention.

Nurses may question why women stay in violent and abusive situations. Many reasons exist, and none of them are related to masochism or pleasure in being persecuted. Women stay to keep their family together, because they hope the batterer will change, because of lack of financial resources, fear of homelessness, and often because they have been threatened with death if they leave. They stay despite the violence not because of it.

There are no specific signs or symptoms of battering victimhood. Nurses may see vague symptoms, such as injuries that do not fit a description of the incident, such as a bruise on the side of the upper arm from ''walking into a door,'' suicide attempts, drug and alcohol abuse, frequent emergency department visits, vague pelvic pain, and depression.

Violence is not a one-time occurrence in a relationship. It usually continues and escalates in severity over time. This is an important point to emphasize when a woman states that her partner has hurt her but has promised to change. Batterers can change but not without extensive counseling and motivation.

Familiarity with local services is important. Once nurses ask about domestic violence, they must be prepared to offer appropriate referral information. Once they have assured the patient that she is not alone, and state the belief that no one deserves to be hurt or hit, proper documentation and referrals are appropriate.

The National Coalition Against Domestic Violence has information on local shelters in all states and is listed at the end of this chapter. Nurses can also call local shelters for pamphlets describing their services to place in waiting rooms, rest rooms, and pamphlet racks. Every health care setting where women receive health care should have a pamphlet rack with information about abuse and appropriate resources and services. Some nurses have found that by leaving literature on domestic violence in the rest room, patients are more comfortable looking at it than they would be in a waiting room with other patients.

Optimal nursing care involves considering every woman a possible victim of abuse, assessing all women by questioning, and looking for clues and signs that may be indicative of abuse. Once abuse is identified, an empathetic demeanor conveying the belief that violence is not acceptable, along with information on local shelters and emergency hot lines can help a woman determine what is best for her. Even if she decides to return to her partner, intervention by identifying and documenting the abuse and providing information about resources to the woman may help the next time violence occurs.

Pelvic Examination

The pelvic examination is a facet of physical assessment that may be performed by the nurse. Competency can be attained with proper training and clinical supervision.

Although several positions may be used for the pelvic examination, the supine lithotomy position is used most frequently. Another technique employs the lithotomy position in which the woman assumes a semisitting stance. This position offers several advantages: (1) it is more comfortable; (2) it allows better eye contact between patient and examiner; (3) it provides an easier means for the examiner to carry out the bimanual examination; and (4) it enables the woman to use a mirror to see her anatomy, note the presence of any lesions, and learn methods for certain types of contraceptive techniques.

If the examiner is required to perform the pelvic assessment in the hospital on a patient who is too ill, disabled, or neurologically impaired to be placed on a table equipped with stirrups, the Simms' position may be used. In the Simm's position, the patient lies on her left side, with her left arm behind her and her right leg bent at a 90-degree angle. The right labia may be retracted for adequate access to the vagina.

The patient is instructed to void before the pelvic examination for her own comfort and for ease of examination. A urine specimen is obtained if urine tests are part of the total assessment.

The patient is then placed on the table with her legs in stirrups; she is encouraged to relax so that her buttocks are positioned at the edge of the examination table and her thighs are spread as widely apart as possible. The patient is appropriately draped to avoid embarrassment. The following equipment is necessary: good light source, vaginal speculum, unsterile gloves, lubricant, spatula, cytobrush or cotton-tipped applicators, glass slides, fixative solution or spray, and appropriate material for occult blood screening.

When the patient is prepared, the labia majora and minora are examined. The epidermal tissue of the labia majora, with its hair follicles characteristic of skin, fades to the pink mucous membrane of the vaginal introitus. In the nulliparous woman, the labia minora should come together at the opening of the vagina. In women who have borne children, the labia minora may gape, and vaginal tissue may protrude. The patient is asked to "bear down." Trauma to the anterior vaginal wall during childbirth may have resulted in incompetency of musculature, so that a bulge representing bladder intrusion into the submucosa of the anterior vaginal wall may be seen. This is called a *cystocele*. Childbirth trauma also may have affected the posterior vaginal wall, so that a bulge representing the cavity of the rectum may protrude, presenting as a *rectocele*. The cervix or the uterus itself may descend under pressure through the vaginal canal and present itself at the introitus. This is termed *prolapse* of the uterus.

The introitus should be free of superficial mucosal lesions. The labia minora may be separated by the fingers of the gloved hand and the lower part of the vagina palpated. In virginal women, a *hymen* of variable thickness may be felt circumferentially within 1 or 2 cm of the vaginal opening. The hymenal ring usually permits the insertion of two fingers but occasionally is sufficiently restricting so that only one finger may enter the vagina. Rarely, the hymen totally occludes the vaginal entrance. In nonvirginal women, a rim of scar tissue representing the remnants of the hymenal ring may be felt circumferentially around the vagina near its opening. The greater vestibular glands (Bartholin's glands) lie between the labia minora and the remnants of the hymenal ring. These glands frequently become infected in gonococcal disease. Patients may occasionally present with an abscess of one of these glands that can become uncomfortable and may need incision and drainage.

Speculum Examination

Assorted sizes of the bivalved speculum are available in metal and plastic, both of which are warmed with hot water or a heating pad to make insertion less uncomfortable. The speculum is not lubricated, because lubrication with commercial jellies may interfere with cervical cytology. Two setscrews may be seen on the metal speculum. One is along the handle and holds the two valves of the speculum together; this one is tightened. The setscrew that holds the thumbrest in place is loosened. The speculum is grasped in the right hand, with the thumb against the back of the thumbrest to keep the tips of the valves closed.

The speculum is rotated slightly counterclockwise and the vaginal orifice is held open by the thumb and the forefinger of the gloved left hand by some examiners. Other practitioners find that straight insertion of a speculum with downward pressure on the vagina is more comfortable for the patient (Fig. 44-3).

The speculum is gently inserted into the posterior portion of the introitus and slowly advanced to the top of the vagina. The tip of the speculum may then be elevated and the speculum rotated to a transverse position. The speculum is then slowly opened to show the cervix of the uterus. The cervix having been brought into view, the setscrew of the thumbrest may be tightened to hold the speculum open.

If any purulent material appears at the cervical os, it is cultured with a sterile cotton-tipped applicator and immediately placed in an appropriate medium for transfer to a laboratory. In high-risk populations, routine cultures for gonococcus and chlamydia are advocated in light of the high incidence of both diseases and because of the high risk for pelvic infection and tubal damage and infertility from these infections.

The cervix is inspected. In nulliparous women, the cervical os is 2 to 3 mm in diameter and smooth. Women who have borne children may have a laceration, usually transverse, frequently giving the cervical os a "fishmouth" appearance. Moreover, epithelium from the endocervical canal may have grown out onto the surface of the cervix, appearing as beefy red surface epithelium circumferentially arranged around the os.

Malignant changes may not be obviously differentiated from the remainder of the cervical mucosa. The presence of endocervical epithelium around the cervical os can lead to chronic infection and discharge from the orifice. Small cysts may appear on the surface of the cervix under these circumstances. These are usually bluish or white and are termed *nabothian cysts*. A polyp of endocervical mucosa may protrude through the os and appears dark red. These can cause irregular bleeding, are rarely malignant, and are usually removed easily in an office or clinic setting. A carcinoma may appear as a cauliflower-like growth. It is friable and bleeds easily when traumatized. Blueness of the cervix is a sign of early pregnancy (Chadwick's sign).

From 1940 to 1970, diethylstilbestrol (DES) was given orally to women experiencing bleeding in pregnancy to avoid miscarriage. Although this drug was effective in many cases, it has been associated with abnormalities of the genital tract in females and males. One of every thousand women exposed to DES *in utero* may develop vaginal or cervical clear cell adenocarcinoma. All women born during this period should be

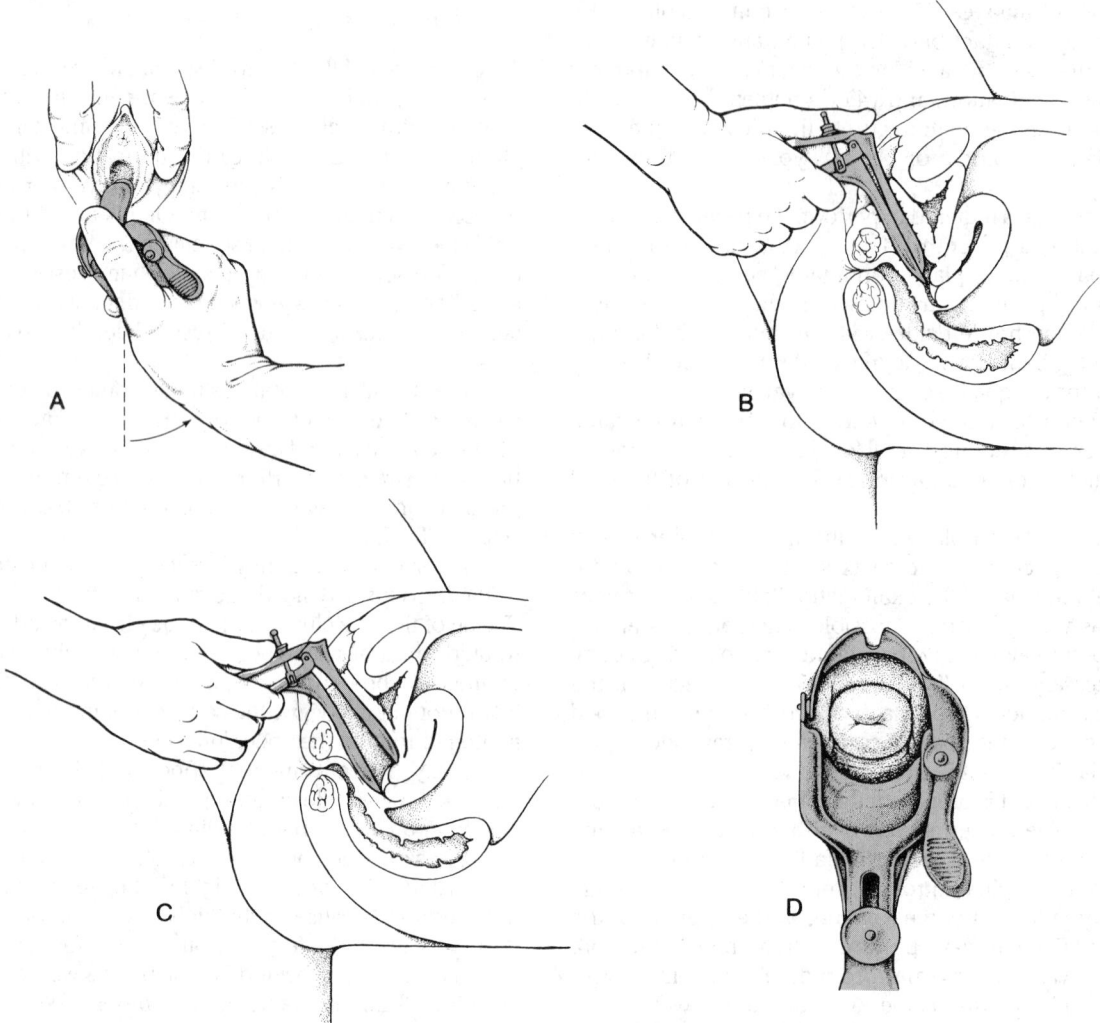

Figure 44–3. Technique for speculum examination of the vagina and cervix. (**A**) The labia are spread apart with a gloved left hand, while the speculum is grasped in the right hand and turned counterclockwise before being inserted into the vagina. (**B**) The closed speculum is inserted into the vagina. (**C and D**) The blades of the speculum are then spread apart to reveal the cervical os.

questioned about this possibility. Occasionally, the cervices of these women have a hooded appearance (a peaked aspect superiorly or a ridge of tissue surrounding them) and are evaluated by colposcopy when identified.

The vagina is examined as the speculum is withdrawn. It is smooth in young girls and becomes more thickened after puberty, with many rugae and much redundancy in the epithelium. Vaginal discharge may be present. Discharge due to bacteria is yellow and has a purulent appearance. Discharge due to *Trichomonas* is thin and watery, often yellow, and occasionally frothy and malodorous. Discharge due to *Candida* is thick and white and may have a cheesy appearance. The menopausal vagina thins because of less estrogen, and rugae often are no longer present.

Bimanual Examination

The examiner assumes a standing position for the bimanual examination. This examination is performed with the forefinger

and middle finger of the gloved and lubricated hand (Fig. 44-4). These fingers are placed in the vaginal orifice, while the other fingers are held tightly out of the way, with the thumb completely adducted. The fingers are advanced vertically along the vaginal canal, and the vaginal wall is palpated. Firmness of any part of the vaginal wall may represent old scar tissue from childbirth trauma. Such tissue may be tender. Anterior tenderness or burning may represent urethritis associated with a urinary tract infection (UTI).

The cervix is palpated and assessed for its consistency, mobility, size, and position. The normal cervix is uniformly firm but not hard. Softening of the cervix and elongation of the cervical canal are seen in early pregnancy. Hardness may reflect invasion by neoplasia. The cervix and uterus are normally freely movable.

Pain on movement of the cervix is called a positive *chandelier sign* and is usually indicative of a pelvic infection. Fixation of the uterus in the pelvis may be a sign of endometriosis or malignancy. The body of the uterus is normally twice the di-

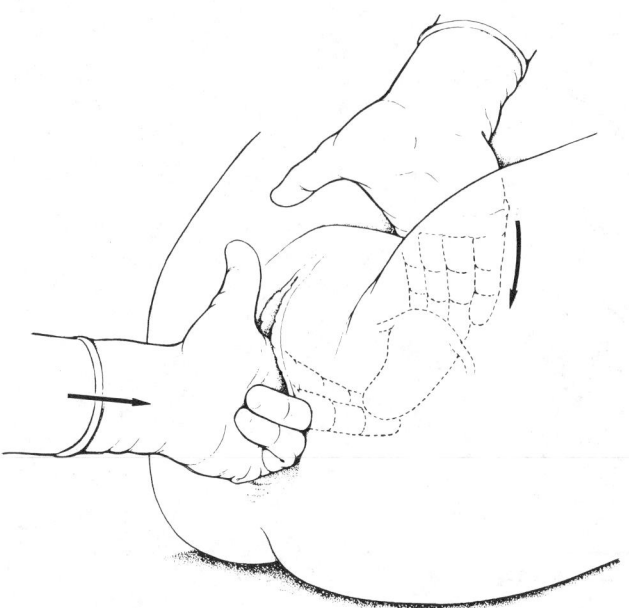

Figure 44-4. Technique for the bimanual examination of the pelvis in women.

ameter and twice the length of the cervix, curving anteriorly toward the abdominal wall. One of five women has a retroflexed uterus, which curves posteriorly toward the sacrum.

The opposite hand is now placed halfway between the umbilicus and the pubis and is pressed firmly toward the vagina. If the uterus is in an appropriate position, movement of the abdominal wall causes the body of the uterus to descend, and the pear-shaped organ becomes freely movable between the abdominal examining hand and the examining fingers of the pelvic examining hand.

An accurate impression can be gained of the size, mobility, and regularity of the contour of the uterus. Nurse practitioners, nurse midwives, and physicians obtain this skill after performing many examinations with supervision.

The right and left parametria are now palpated. The fallopian tubes and ovaries are contained within these structures. The fingers of the pelvic hand are moved first to one side, then to the other, while the abdominal hand is moved correspondingly to either side of the abdomen and downward. The adnexa are trapped between the two examining hands and are palpated for an obvious mass, tenderness of adnexal tissue, and mobility of the parametrial contents.

It is common for the ovaries to be slightly tender. Patients need to be reassured that slight discomfort is normal. Bimanual palpation of the vagina and cul-de-sac is accomplished by placing the index finger in the vagina and the middle finger in the rectum. A gentle movement of these fingers toward each other compresses the posterior vaginal wall and the anterior rectal wall and assists the examiner in identifying the integrity of these structures. This procedure may give the patient the sensation of having a bowel movement. The examiner reassures the patient that although she has the urge to defecate, she is not in fact doing so.

To prevent cross-contamination between the vaginal and rectal orifices, the examiner changes gloves between these examinations. Explanation throughout the examination is reassuring and educational.

Diagnostic Evaluation

Tests Performed During the Gynecologic Examination

Cytologic Test for Cancer (Papanicolaou Smear)

This cytologic test is done to detect cervical cancer. Vaginal secretions are aspirated or scraped from the cervical os and transferred to a glass slide (Fig. 44-5) and "fixed" immediately by immersing in or spraying with a fixative. The patient should be instructed not to douche before this examination, because cellular material can be washed away. The Papanicolaou (Pap) smear should be done during a nonmenstrual phase of the cycle because the presence of blood interferes with an accurate interpretation.

The finding of an abnormal smear (with the exception of class V) does not mean that the patient has cancer but points out that colposcopy-directed biopsies are indicated. Mild inflammation or atypias are usually repeated in 3 to 6 months. Patients are usually apprehensive, as most women assume that an abnormal Pap smear means cancer.

The pathologist examines and interprets the cytologic smear. The classification for cytologic findings as suggested by Papanicolaou is as follows:

Class I: Absence of atypical or abnormal cells
Class II: Atypical cytology, usually cervical inflammation but no evidence of malignancy
Class III: Cytology suggestive of, but not conclusive for, malignancy
Class IV: Cytology strongly suggestive of malignancy
Class V: Cytology conclusive for malignancy

Newer classifications are descriptive and omit numbers; terms used in these systems to describe findings include normal; inflammation; atypia (not typical); koilocytosis (a change in cells affected by human papillomavirus); mild, moderate, or severe dysplasia; and invasive carcinoma.

New terminology includes the following categories: *Low-grade squamous intraepithelial lesion* (LGSIL) is equivalent to cervical intraepithelial neoplasia (CIN) types I and II. *High-grade squamous intraepithelial lesion* (HGSIL) is equivalent to CIN type III or the equivalent of carcinoma *in situ*. These new terms are seen on Pap smear findings and encompass all precursors to invasive carcinoma of the cervix. These diagnostic terms are currently being implemented and are described more fully in Table 44-1.

Cervical Biopsy

The type and extent of biopsy of the cervix vary according to the abnormality or to the results of an abnormal Pap smear. When a lesion is clearly visible or can be seen with a magnifying instrument called a *colposcope*, one or more punch biopsies may be performed as an office procedure without anesthesia, because the cervix is less sensitive to cutting procedures than is the vagina. All suspicious Pap smears (*i.e.*, persistent inflammation or dysplasia) are followed by a colposcopy. If biopsy specimens during this examination show premalignant cells or CIN, usually cryotherapy or a cone biopsy (biopsy excision of an inverted cone of tissue from the cervix) is needed.

If a cone biopsy is necessary for high-grade squamous intraepithelial lesion or carcinoma *in situ*, the patient is advised to rest for 24 hours after this surgical procedure and to leave

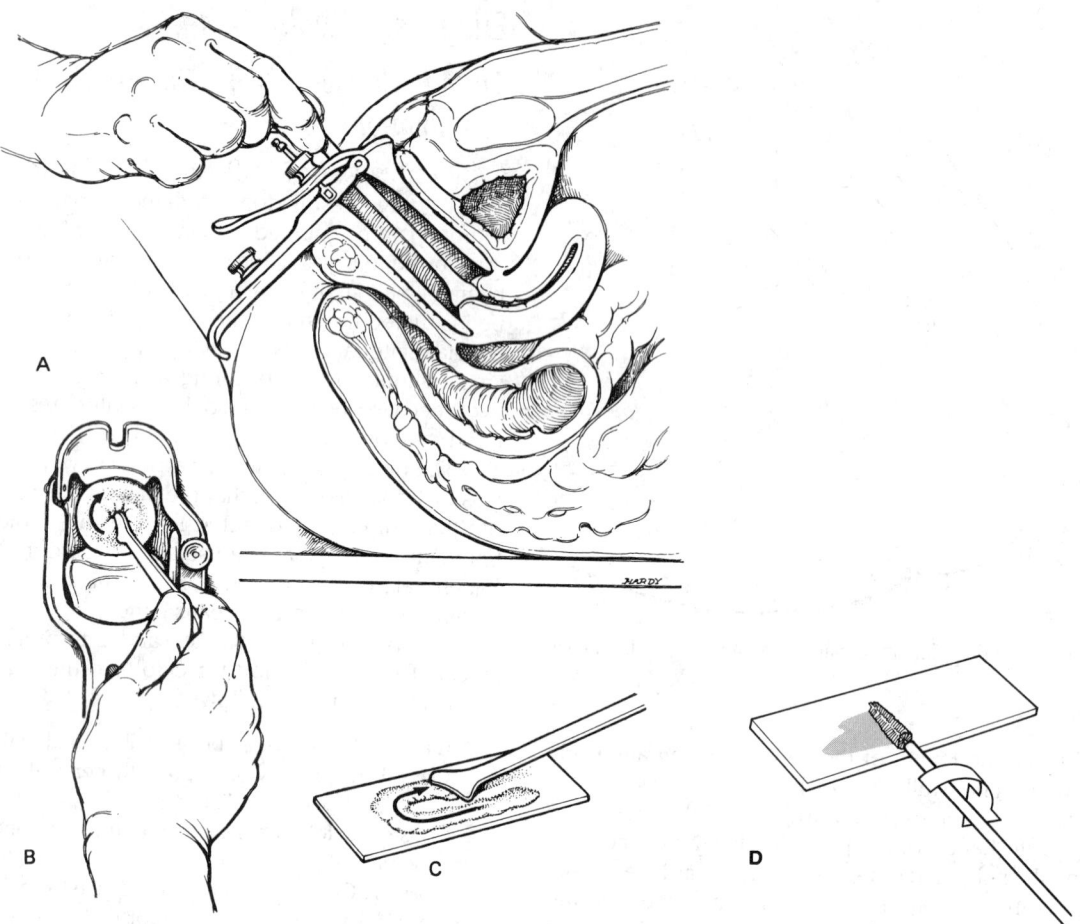

Figure 44–5. Method of using a wooden Ayre spatula to obtain cervical secretions for cytology. (**A**) Speculum in place and the Ayre spatula in position at the cervical os. (**B**) The tip of the spatula is placed in the cervical os and the spatula rotated 360 degrees, firmly but nontraumatically. (**C**) Cellular material clinging to the spatula is then smeared smoothly on a glass slide, which is promptly placed in a fixative solution. (**D**) Cytobrush is rotated in the cervical os and rolled onto a glass slide.

any packing in place until the physician removes it, usually the following day. Any excess bleeding should be reported to the patient's care provider. Guidelines regarding sexual activity, bathing, and other activities postoperatively are provided by the physician. Condoms are recommended after biopsy because of exposure of tissues and increased risk of HIV infection with exposure to the virus.

Endometrial (Aspiration) Smears and Biopsy

A smear obtained directly from the endometrium provides an accurate method of cytologic diagnosis of the endometrium. There are many ways of obtaining endometrial tissue for cytologic analysis. Evaluation can be made of endometrial secretions, cells, or lavage solutions introduced into the endometrial cavity.

Endometrial biopsy is performed during the gynecologic pelvic examination as an outpatient procedure. It usually can be performed without anesthesia; however, a paracervical block is effective if required. A uterine sound, a measuring device, is inserted into the uterus, followed by a thin, hollow curette. Suction also may be used for retrieving endometrial tissue for laboratory analysis. This procedure is probably the most accurate outpatient method for evaluating endometrial cancer

and is usually indicated in cases of irregular bleeding, infertility, and in some women on estrogen replacement therapy.

Schiller's Test

With the patient in the lithotomy position (cervix exposed by speculum), a long cotton-tipped applicator is used to paint the cervix with aqueous iodine solution. The appearance of a mahogany-brown color covering the entire surface indicates a reaction between the iodine and the glycogen of normal cells. Such a reaction is considered negative. If the cervix is abnormal, immature cells are present and tissues are not stained brown, indicating that the test is positive. The absence of staining directs attention to the sites requiring additional study (*i.e.,* biopsy), such as those related to cancer, scars, erosion, and zones of nonmalignant leukoplakia.

Dilatation and Curettage

In a dilatation and curettage (D&C), the cervical canal is widened with a dilator and the uterine endometrium is scraped with a curette. The purpose of the procedure is to secure endometrial or endocervical tissue for cytologic examination, to

TABLE 44-1.   *Comparison of Five Classifications of the Pap Smear*

Interpretation of Result	Numerical System	Dysplasia Cytologic Classification	Cervical Intraepithelial Neoplasia Classification	Dyskariosis Classification	Bethesda Classification
Negative	Class I	Negative; squamous metaplasia	No designation	Negative	Negative
	Class II	Atypical squamous metaplasia			Atypical Squamous cells
Suspicious		Mild dysplasia	CIN I	Borderline	Low-grade squamous intraepithelial lesion*
	Class III	Moderate dysplasia	CIN II	Mild Moderate	
Probable	Class IV	Severe dysplasia Carcinoma *in situ*	CIN III	Severe	High-grade squamous intraepithelial lesion*
Positive	Class V	←----------------------------- Invasive carcinoma ----------------------------→			

* The Bethesda working group (1989) suggests that "these two new terms encompass the spectrum of terms currently used to delineate the squamous cell precursors to invasive squamous carcinoma, including the grades of CIN, the degrees of dysplasia, and carcinoma in situ."
(Fullerton JT and Barger MK. Papanicolaou smear: An update on classification and management. J Am Acad Nurse Pract 1989 Jul/Sep; 1[3]:87.)

control abnormal uterine bleeding, and as a therapeutic measure for incomplete abortion.

Because this procedure is usually carried out under anesthesia and requires surgical asepsis, it is performed in the operating room. Many gynecologists perform D&Cs under local anesthesia, supplemented with diazepam (Valium), midazolam (Versed), or meperidine (Demerol). Explanations as well as psychological and physical preparations are given by the nurse. The patient has a right to know what the procedure will involve (usually explained by her gynecologist) and what to expect in the way of postoperative discomfort, drainage, or limitations. Many physicians do not require that the perineum be shaved, but voiding and evacuation of the intestinal tract by a small enema are usually desired.

In the operating room, the patient is placed in the lithotomy position, the cervix is dilated with an instrument, and scrapings of the endometrium are obtained by means of a curette. Tissue for biopsy also may be obtained with an electric needle or a punch biopsy forceps. A cone of tissue may be obtained with a cautery or scalpel if indicated. Packing is placed in the cervical and vaginal canal, and a sterile perineal pad is placed over the perineum. A sanitary belt is used to hold the pad in place, or a self-adhesive pad is used. When the pad must be changed while the packing is still in place (usually 24 hours), it is replaced with a sterile pad. Evidence of excessive bleeding is reported. After the surgical procedure, the patient remains in bed for the remainder of the day, although she may get up to go to the bathroom. No restrictions are placed on dietary intake. If pelvic discomfort or low back pain occurs, mild analgesics usually suffice. The physician indicates when sexual intercourse may be safely resumed. Most physicians advise no vaginal penetration for 2 weeks to reduce the risk of infection and bleeding.

Endoscopic Examinations

Laparoscopy (Pelvic Peritoneoscopy)
A laparoscopy is the insertion of a scope (diameter about 10 mm) into the peritoneal cavity through a 2-cm (¾-inch) subumbilical incision (Fig. 44-6), to allow visualization of the pelvic

structures. Indications for laparoscopy are diagnostic (*i.e.*, in cases of pelvic pain when no cause can be found). It is also possible to perform minor operative procedures, such as tubal sterilization, ovarian biopsy, and lysis of peritubal adhesions, by means of laparoscopy. A D&C precedes this procedure, not only because it affords additional information but also because a surgical instrument (intrauterine sound or cannula) may be positioned to permit manipulation of the uterus during laparoscopy, affording better visualization.

A better view of the pelvis, lower abdomen, and visceral contents is also facilitated by the injection of a prescribed amount of carbon dioxide intraperitoneally into the cavity (insufflation). This separates the intestines from the pelvic organs. The tubes may be electrocoagulated, and a segment removed for histologic verification. After the purpose of the laparoscopy has been accomplished, the scope is withdrawn and carbon dioxide is allowed to escape through the outer cannula. The skin incision is closed with sutures or a small clip and covered with a bandage.

The patient is carefully observed for several hours to detect any untoward signs indicating bleeding, injury, or burns from the coagulator. These complications rarely occur, however. Laparoscopy is a cost-effective outpatient procedure.

Hysteroscopy
Hysteroscopy (transcervical intrauterine endoscopy) allows direct visualization of all parts of the uterine cavity by means of a lighted optical instrument. The procedure is best performed about 5 days after completion of menstruation (estrogenic phase of the menstrual cycle). The vagina and vulva are cleansed, and a pericervical anesthetic block is performed. The instrument used for the procedure, a *hysteroscope*, is passed into the cervical canal and advanced under direct vision 1 or 2 cm; uterine-distending fluid (saline or 5% dextrose) is infused through the instrument to dilate the uterine cavity and to provide better visualization.

Hysteroscopy is most commonly indicated as an adjunct to a D&C in cases of infertility, unexplained bleeding, retained IUD, and recurrent early pregnancy loss. This procedure is

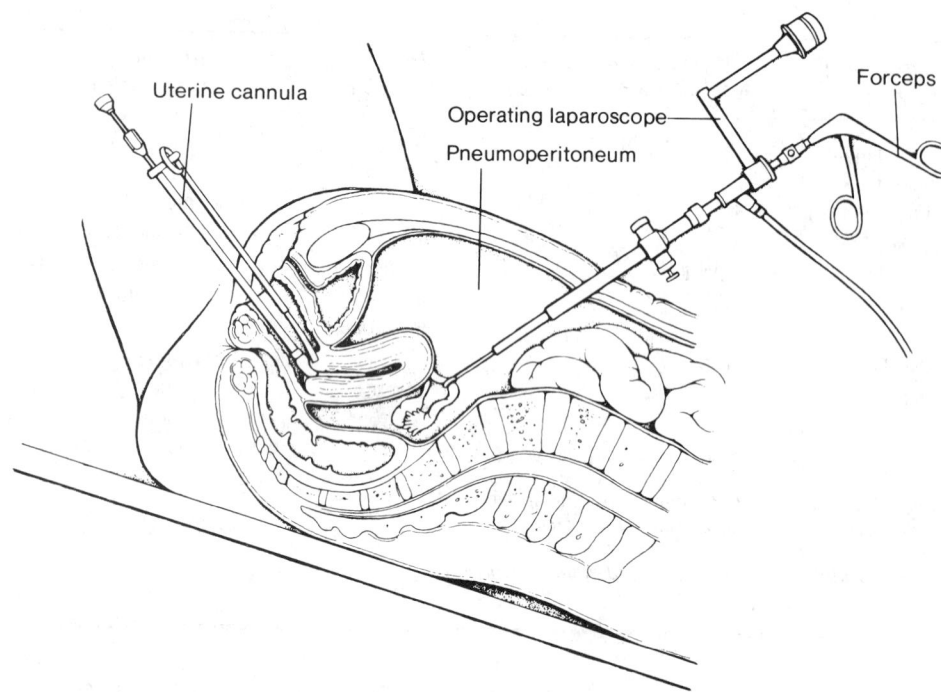

Figure 44–6. Laparoscopy. The laparoscope (**right**) is inserted through a small incision in the abdomen. A forceps is inserted through the scope to grasp the uterine tube. To improve the view, a uterine cannula (**left**) is inserted into the vagina to push the uterus upward. Insufflation of gas creates an air pocket (pneumoperitoneum), and the pelvis is elevated (note the angle), which forces the intestines higher in the abdomen.

contraindicated in patients with cervical or endometrial carcinoma or acute pelvic inflammation.

Colposcopy and Colpomicroscopy

The *colposcope* (magnification from 10 to 25 times) and *colpomicroscope* (magnification to 400 times) are optical instruments designed to permit three-dimensional views of stained or unstained cervical epithelium *in situ*. These instruments permit visualization of suspicious areas, but biopsy of the tissue and other diagnostic methods are required for accurate diagnosis. Nurse colposcopists (nurses with specific training) and gynecologists require special training in this diagnostic technique.

Radiographic Diagnostic Procedures

Many radiologic procedures are helpful in diagnosing pelvic conditions. Ordinary x-ray films, barium enemas, gastrointestinal x-ray series, intravenous urography, and cystography are just a few examples. Other diagnostic procedures include hysterosalpingogram, computed tomography, and radioisotope scanning.

Hysterosalpingogram (Uterotubogram)

A uterotubogram is an x-ray study of the uterus and the fallopian tubes after the injection of a contrast medium. The diagnostic procedure is performed to study sterility problems, to evaluate tubal patency, and to determine the presence of any abnormal condition in the uterine cavity.

The patient is placed in the lithotomy position, and the cervix is exposed with a bivalved speculum. A cannula is inserted into the cervix, and contrast medium is injected into the uterine cavity and the tubes. X-ray films are taken to show the path and the distribution of the contrast materials.

In preparation for a hysterosalpingogram, the intestinal tract is prepared by a cathartic and an enema so that gas shadows do not distort the x-ray films. An analgesic is prescribed for comfort, as some patients experience nausea, vomiting,

cramps, and faintness. After the test, it may be advisable for the patient to apply a perineal pad for several hours, because the radiopaque medium may stain clothing.

Computed Tomography

Computed tomographic (CT) scanning has several advantages over ultrasound (described later), even though it involves radiation exposure and is more costly. It is more effective with obese patients or a patient with a distended bowel or stomach. A CT scan also can demonstrate the presence of cancer and its extension into retroperitoneal lymph nodes and skeletal involvement, although it is of limited value in diagnosing other gynecologic abnormalities.

Angiography and Radioisotope Scanning

The procedures of angiography and radioisotope scanning are also used as required. Because the uterus and adnexa are in proximity to the kidneys, ureter, and bladder, urologic diagnostic aids, such as the KUB (kidney, ureter, and bladder) and pyelogram, are frequently used.

Other Diagnostic Aids

Ultrasonography

Ultrasonography employs a simple procedure based on transmission of sound waves similar to the sonar detection used in submarines. Diagnostic ultrasonic scanning equipment uses pulsed ultrasound waves of a frequency exceeding 20,000 Hz (formerly cycles per second); the pelvis and abdomen are scanned in linear fashion. The transducer, which is placed in contact with the abdomen or into the vagina, converts mechanical energy into electrical impulses, which in turn are amplified and recorded on an oscilloscope screen. A photograph or video is taken of the patterns. The entire procedure takes about 10 minutes, involves no ionizing radiation, and is not uncomfortable, aside from a full bladder, which is necessary for good visualization during an abdominal scan. (A vaginal sonogram does not require a full bladder.) The findings of this test, in combination with other diagnostic tools, provide useful adjuncts to the physical examination, particularly in the obstetric patient or the obese patient in whom pelvic examination may have been unsatisfactory.

Magnetic Resonance Imaging

Magnetic resonance imaging produces patterns that are more delicate and definitive than other radiographic processes. Its chief advantage is absence of radiation. It is more costly, however, and generally less available.

In summary, the patient who undergoes gynecologic examination and gynecologic diagnostic testing as part of routine preventive health care, or in response to disturbances in normal function, may be uncomfortable, anxious, or embarrassed by these procedures. Misinformation and misconceptions about reproductive and gynecologic functions may occur because of reluctance of the patient to ask questions of the health care provider. The nurse can use the opportunity of gynecologic examination and testing to answer questions, allay the patient's fears, and promote regular gynecologic health care practices.

Nursing Interventions for Patients With Gynecologic Conditions

A variety of local treatments may be prescribed to treat gynecologic conditions; these include douches, irrigations, and vaginal jellies. *Douches* are therapeutic measures used in the treatment of patients with gynecologic diseases. They are used both before and after surgery and are of two types: vulvar and vaginal. *Vaginal irrigations* are used therapeutically to cleanse or disinfect the vagina and adjacent parts, both before and after surgery. They also serve to soothe inflamed tissues. Occasionally, warm or cold douches are indicated in the treatment of oozing of vaginal discharge.

The patient is placed on the bedpan in the dorsal position with the knees apart and the labia separated. Undue exposure of the patient is prevented, and the bed is protected by placing an absorbent pad under the bedpan. Commonly used solutions include sterile water, normal saline, and antiseptic solutions.

Douches should be given at a temperature of 43.3°C (100°F) or as prescribed. The container holding the prescribed solution is raised not more than 60 cm (2 feet) above the level of the patient's hips. The nurse then puts on examination gloves, and separating the labia with the thumb and the forefinger of the left hand, cleans the vaginal orifice and inserts the douche nozzle gently into the vagina for a distance of 5 cm (2 inches), with the tip directed toward the hollow of the sacrum. The clamp then is removed from the tube, and the solution is allowed to flow. Pressure should be avoided to prevent fluid from refluxing through the uterus, which can result in ascending transmission of bacteria to the uterine cavity and tubes. The solution can be allowed to flow intermittently until at least 1 liter of solution has been used.

The treatment should not be done hastily if therapeutic benefits are to be achieved; it should take from 20 to 30 minutes. After the solution has been instilled, the nozzle may be removed and the patient should be asked to strain as if trying

to have a bowel movement. This act tends to expel any fluid remaining in the vagina. Then the bedpan is removed, and the perineum is dried with cotton. The patient is instructed to remain recumbent for at least an hour after a warm douche.

After the douche has been completed, the apparatus is cleansed and sterilized (if not disposable), including the bedpan. When douching is performed at home, the patient usually lies in the bathtub and follows the same practices just described.

Vulvar irrigations are indicated chiefly after operations on the perineum. They should be given after each urination or bowel movement in an effort to keep the incision free from infection. The patient is prepared for a vulvar irrigation in the same manner as for a vaginal douche. Warm, sterile water then is poured gently over the vulva from a sterile container. The area is dried with sterile gauze or cotton, and a sterile dressing or pad is applied and held in place with a T-binder, or a self-adhesive pad is used.

Vaginal antiseptic jellies are another form of medication that the patient can apply herself by means of an applicator. Creams or jellies can be used before and after surgery and in many instances are substituted for therapeutic and cleansing douches. It may be necessary for the patient to wear a perineal pad after application of medication.

Menstruation

Physiologic Overview

The *gonads* are the organs that produce either the egg cells (ova) or the sperm cells of an organism. In the female, the gonads are called *ovaries* and are located in the pelvis on either side of the uterus. In the male, the gonads are the *testes* and are contained within the scrotum. In addition to their reproductive function, the gonads are important endocrine glands.

Ovarian Hormones

The ovaries produce steroid hormones, predominantly *estrogens* and *progesterone*. Several different estrogens are produced by the ovarian follicle, which consists of the developing ovum and its surrounding cells. The most potent of the ovarian estrogens is *estradiol*. Estrogens are responsible for the development and maintenance of the female reproductive organs and the secondary sex characteristics associated with the adult female. Estrogens have an important role in breast development and in the cyclic changes of the uterus that occur monthly.

Progesterone is also important in regulating the changes that occur in the uterus during the menstrual cycle. It is secreted by the *corpus luteum*, which consists of the ovarian follicle after the ovum has been released. Progesterone is the most important hormone for conditioning the lining of the uterus (endometrium) in preparation for implantation of the fertilized ovum. If pregnancy occurs, the secretion of progesterone becomes largely a function of the placenta. This secretion is important for the maintenance of normal pregnancy. In addition, progesterone, working in concert with estrogen, prepares the breast for production and secretion of milk.

Androgens are also produced by the ovaries, but only in small amounts, and play a complex role in the early development of the follicle. Their other functions in the female are still under investigation.

Regulation of Ovarian Hormone Secretion

Follicle-stimulating hormone (FSH) secreted by the pituitary is primarily responsible for stimulating estrogen secretion. *Luteinizing hormone* (LH) is primarily responsible for stimulating the production of progesterone. Feedback mechanisms in part regulate FSH and LH secretion. Increased estrogen levels in the blood inhibit FSH secretion but promote LH secretion. Elevated progesterone levels inhibit LH secretion. In addition gonadotropin-releasing hormone (GnRH) from the hypothalamus affects the rate of gonadotropin (FSH and LH) release.

Menstrual Cycle

In the female, secretion of ovarian hormones follows a cyclic pattern that results in changes of the uterine endometrium (the inner lining of the uterus) and in menstruation (Fig. 44-7). At the beginning of the cycle (just after menstruation), FSH output is increased and estrogen secretion is stimulated. This causes the endometrium to thicken and become more vascular (proliferative phase). Near the middle portion of the cycle, LH output increases and progesterone secretion is stimulated. It is at this time that ovulation occurs. Under the combined stimulus of estrogen and progesterone, the endometrium reaches its peak of thickening and vascularization (secretory phase). If the ovum has been fertilized, estrogen and progesterone levels remain high and the complex hormonal changes of pregnancy follow. If fertilization has not occurred, the output of FSH and LH diminishes; secretion of estrogen and progesterone falls rapidly; and the vascularized, thickened endometrium is sloughed, with resultant vaginal bleeding (menstruation). The cycle then begins again.

Psychosocial Considerations

The girl between the ages of 10 and 14 who is approaching the *menarche*, or onset of menstruation, should be instructed about this normal process. Psychologically, it is more healthy to refer to this event as "my period" rather than as "being sick" or "having the curse." With adequate nutrition, rest, and exercise, most women feel little discomfort. Some girls do experience breast tenderness and a feeling of fullness a day or two before the onset of menstruation. There may be a greater tendency of fatigue and some discomfort of the lower back, legs, and pelvis on the first day; temperament and mood changes may be apparent. Slight deviations from the usual healthy pattern of daily living are considered normal, but signs of excessive deviations may require investigation. The perineal pad is a widely used method of disposing of menstrual discharge; deodorant pads are available, but some women are allergic or sensitive to the deodorants that are used, so their use is discouraged. Tampons are also used extensively; usually, there is no significant evidence of untoward effects from their use, providing there is not difficulty in inserting them. Tampons should not be worn for more than 4 hours to prevent toxic shock syndrome (discussed more fully in Chap. 45). Should the "tail" string break and difficulty be encountered in removing the tampon, the woman's physician or nurse practitioner should be consulted.

As was mentioned earlier, menstruation may be handled differently in different cultures. Some women believe that it is detrimental to change a pad or tampon too frequently; they believe that by allowing this discharge to accumulate, an increased flow is stimulated, which is considered desirable. For the nurse to insist that a pad be changed before the time the patient believes proper may cause conflict. These differences must be carefully reconciled so that proper understanding develops.

Other psychosocial aspects may need to be considered, such as belief in the vulnerability of women to illness during menstruation. Many believe it is detrimental to swim, take a shower, receive a "permanent wave," get teeth filled, or eat certain foods during one's period. Some young women erroneously believe that they are unable to conceive at this time, so they use no contraception. Such myths need to be recognized and corrected. Many other examples of misunderstanding could be listed; however, the objective is to alert the nurse to these unexpressed, deep-rooted beliefs. Aspects of gynecologic problems cannot always be expressed easily. The nurse needs to convey confidence, as well as offer sound advice, to set up an exchange of communication.

Premenstrual Syndrome

Premenstrual syndrome (PMS) is a combination of symptoms experienced by some women before the onset of each menstrual cycle. The cause is unknown, but several theories suggest estrogen excess or progesterone deficit in the luteal phase. Major symptoms include headache, fatigue, low back pain, engorged or painful breasts, and a feeling of abdominal fullness. General irritability may include mood swings, fear of losing control, binge eating, and crying spells. Symptoms vary widely from one woman to another and from one cycle to the next in the same person. A generally stressful life appears related to the intensity of physical symptoms. Women report moderate to severe life disruption, even affecting interpersonal relationships among family members. PMS can be a factor in reduced productivity, work-related accidents, and absenteeism.

The *timing* of the above symptoms helps in determining the diagnosis. Symptoms recur regularly at the same phase of each menstrual cycle and, in the same cycle, are usually followed by a symptom-free phase once the menstrual flow has started.

Management

There is no single treatment or known cure for PMS. Women are encouraged to chart their own symptoms, which can help in learning to anticipate symptoms and when they occur. Some physicians prescribe pain relievers, diuretics, and natural and synthetic progesterones. Long-term risks of progesterone use are unknown. Prostaglandin inhibitors (*e.g.*, ibuprofen and anaprox) are also used.

▶ Nursing Process
The Patient With Premenstrual Syndrome

▷ Assessment

The nurse should establish a rapport with the patient while obtaining a health history, which should note when symptoms began and their intensity. The nurse determines whether the onset is related to a major hormonal change, such as after use of oral contraceptives, a pregnancy, tubal ligation, or after a period of amenorrhea, although it is unclear how these changes

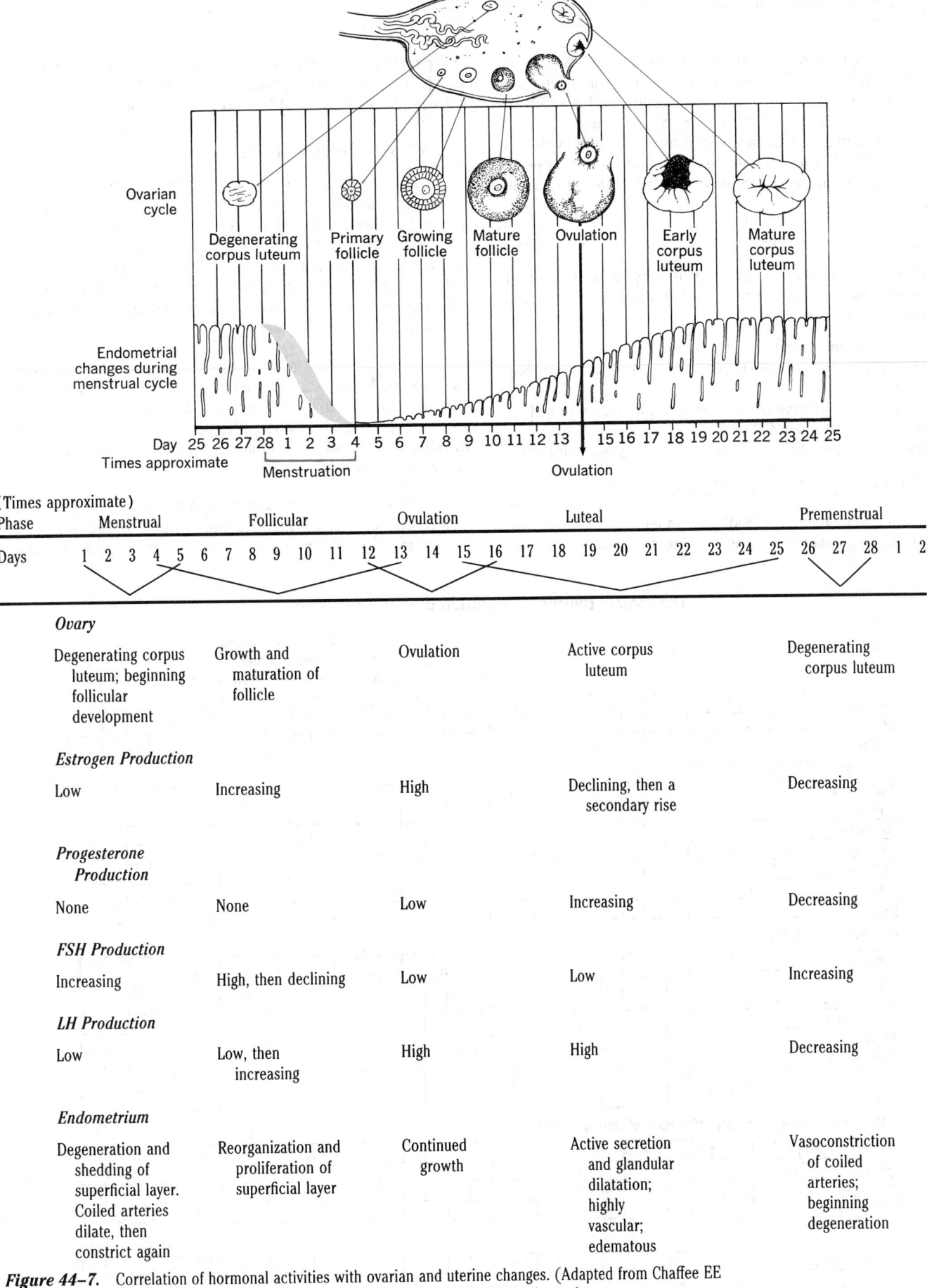

Figure 44-7. Correlation of hormonal activities with ovarian and uterine changes. (Adapted from Chaffee EE and Greisheimer EM. Basic Physiology and Anatomy, 3rd ed. Philadelphia, JB Lippincott.)

might affect symptoms. In addition to obtaining a record of symptoms and times of occurrence, the nurse can offer guidance in developing a chart showing the timing and intensity of symptoms, as shown in Figure 44-8. Such a record, to be meaningful, is maintained over a minimum of three cycles. A nutritional history is also elicited to determine dietary excesses of salt, alcohol, and caffeine, or a diet that is insufficient in essential nutrients.

◊ Nursing Diagnoses

Based on the health and nutritional history as well as other assessment data, the major nursing diagnoses for the patient may include the following:

- Anxiety related to the effects of PMS
- Ineffective coping of both patient and family related to effects of PMS
- High risk for violence directed at family members or self related to symptoms of PMS
- Knowledge deficit about causes and management of PMS

◊ Planning and Implementation

◊ *Goals:* The major goals of the patient may include reduction of anxiety (mood swings, crying, binge eating, fear of losing control), ability to cope with usual interpersonal relations with family and at work, absence of violent reactions, improved knowledge regarding PMS and use of control measures.

◊ Nursing Interventions

◊ *Reducing Anxiety.* General support and counseling are provided. The patient is asked to participate in her care by keeping a chart of her symptoms (see Fig. 44-8); she is encouraged to plan activities around the troublesome times. Her partner and children are included in discussing her problem, if desired. Sharing this information can lead to mutual understanding and lessened tension for the patient. Analgesics or tranquilizers may be prescribed.

◊ *Coping Measures.* Positive coping measures are facilitated. Partners can be advised to assist by offering support, increased involvement with child care, and seeking marital counseling if problems get out of control. The patient can try to plan her working time to accommodate the days she will be less productive because of PMS.

◊ *Reducing Stress.* Stress reduction through exercise, meditation, imagery, or creative activities should be encouraged. The nurse is attentive and understanding because this provides

Diagnostic Diary A: Evaluation of PMS Symptoms

NAME _____

YEAR _____

Grading of Symptoms:
0—No Symptoms   2—Moderate Symptoms
1—Mild Symptoms   3—Severe Symptoms (i.e., Disabling)

DAY OF CYCLE	1	2	3	4	5	6	7	8	9	10	11	12	13	14	15	16	17	18	19	20	21	22	23	24	25	26	27	28	29	30	31
DATE																															
MENSES																															

PSYCHOLOGICAL SYMPTOMS

Depression																															
Anxiety																															
Irritability																															
Lethargy																															
Insomnia																															
Forgetfulness																															
Confusion																															

PHYSICAL SYMPTOMS

Swelling																															
Breast Tenderness																															
Abdominal bloating																															
Palpitations																															
Weight gain																															
Constipation																															
Headache																															
Rhinitis																															

PAIN SYMPTOMS (Usually NOT associated with PMS)

Menstrual cramps																															
Painful intercourse																															
Pelvic pain																															
Backache																															

Morning weight (lb)																															

Figure 44–8. Diagnostic diary for evaluation of PMS symptoms. (Chihal HJ. Premenstrual Syndrome: A Clinic Manual, 2nd ed. Dallas, Essential Medical Information Systems, 1990, pp 80–81.)

relief to the patient; it is helpful to the patient to know that others recognize and understand what she is experiencing.

◊   *Patient Education.*   The nurse can suggest that the patient keep a 3-month record of symptoms and consult with a health care professional in determining the specific diagnosis. She is encouraged to follow the recommendations for additional testing to rule out other possible causes of the symptoms.

The patient should assume responsibility for following a dietary plan or eating small meals and eliminating or restricting sugar, salt, alcohol, caffeine, and nicotine. Supplements of vitamin B_6, calcium, and magnesium may be prescribed. Exercise and relaxation each day are encouraged, and the importance of participating in various health promotion strategies such as weight reduction if applicable is emphasized. Perhaps flexible work schedules can be arranged to accommodate the troublesome period each month. Enrolling in a PMS group that meets to discuss mutual problems can also be helpful. Such groups provide support and have a tendency to make problems more bearable when others have the same or worse symptoms. The findings of nurse researchers working with partners of patients with PMS are discussed in the Research Profile. Premenstrual syndrome seems to be self-limiting, and no treatment has been proved effective.

Any suggestion of suicidal tendencies must be evaluated by psychiatric consult immediately. Probability of child abuse must be reported.

◊   **Evaluation**

Expected Outcomes

1. Patient experiences reduction in anxiety
   a. Verbalizes awareness of the nature of the problem
   b. Relates that her new support system (health care personnel) has reduced her concerns
2. Demonstrates adequate coping mechanisms
   a. Keeps a monthly calendar of her symptoms
   b. Schedules activities around her "problem times"
   c. Reports greater comfort and reduced stress
3. Follows dietary practices that improve behavior
   a. Reduces intake of refined sugar and salt
   b. Increases intake of magnesium-rich foods (whole grains, nuts, green vegetables)
   c. Avoids caffeine, cigarettes, and alcohol
   d. Takes vitamin B_6 (pyridoxine) as prescribed

Dysmenorrhea

Primary dysmenorrhea is painful menstruation with no identifiable pelvic pathology. It usually occurs within a few years after the menarche and appears to be related to the establishment of ovulatory cycles. It is a common condition, occurring in more than half of menstruating women. Painful cramps are the result of excessive production of prostaglandins, which causes increased uterine hypercontractility and arteriolar vasospasm. Psychological factors such as anxiety and tension may also contribute to dysmenorrhea. As the woman grows older, pain tends to decrease; it often completely resolves after childbirth.

In *secondary dysmenorrhea,* a pelvic pathologic process is confirmed, such as endometriosis, tumor, or pelvic inflammatory disease (PID). These conditions are discussed in Chapter 45.

Assessment and Clinical Manifestations

In primary dysmenorrhea, the symptoms are mild cramps that may begin 12 to 24 hours before the onset of flow and become more acute with the flow, lasting an additional 12 to 24 hours. The pain is crampy, is located in the lower midabdomen and may radiate to the lower back and upper thighs, and may be associated with chills, nausea, vomiting, headache, and irritability. Occasionally, diarrhea occurs. In secondary dysmenorrhea, patients are usually older and pain is not always limited to the time of menses and first day of flow.

A complete physical examination is performed to rule out possible abnormalities, such as strictures of the cervix or vagina or an imperforate hymen, as well as other conditions, such as endometriosis, PID, adenomyosis, and fibroid uterus. A hysterosalpingogram, ultrasound examination, or laparoscopy may be required to identify organic causes.

Management and Nursing Interventions

In primary dysmenorrhea, the reason for the discomfort is explained, and the patient is assured that menstruation is a normal function of the reproductive tract. If the patient is a young girl and is accompanied by her mother, the mother may also need reassurance. Many daughters are conditioned to expect dysmenorrhea because their mothers experienced it. The pain, which is real, can be treated once worry and concern over its possible significance are dispelled through accurate understanding. Symptoms subside in a few years or with normal sexual function and childbearing.

More specific methods of affording relief are as follows. The patient is encouraged to carry on her usual activities, because mind-occupying functions and physical exercise provide a neurophysiologic basis for relief. Taking analgesics before cramps start, in anticipation of discomfort, is advised. Aspirin, a mild prostaglandin inhibitor, may be taken at recommended doses every 4 hours. If necessary, antiemetics, antispasmodics, and mild tranquilizers may be prescribed by the physician. Prostaglandins have been cited as causing dysmenorrhea, so prostaglandin antagonists are helpful (ibuprofen [Motrin], naproxen [Naprosyn], mefenamic acid [Ponstel], naproxen [Anaprox]). If one inhibitor does not provide relief, the patient is advised to try another. Usually these medications are well tolerated, but some women experience gastrointestinal side effects. Contraindications include allergy, peptic ulcer history, sensitivity to aspirin-like medications, asthma, and pregnancy. Low-dose oral contraceptives often provide relief in over 90% of patients.

Management of secondary dysmenorrhea is directed to treating the underlying cause (*e.g.,* endometriosis, PID).

Amenorrhea (Absence of Menstrual Flow)

Primary amenorrhea (delayed menarche) refers to those instances when a young woman over age 16 has not yet begun to menstruate but otherwise shows evidence of sexual maturation or by age 14 in the absence of secondary sexual characteristics. This may be of considerable concern to the person as well as to her mother but is more than likely due to minor variations in body build, heredity, and environment, as well as to physical, mental, and emotional development.

The understanding nurse provides an opportunity for the girl to express her concerns and anxiety about this problem, because she may feel that she is not like her peers. A complete physical examination, careful history, and simple laboratory studies assist in excluding physiologic disorders, metabolic or endocrine difficulties, and other systemic diseases. Treatment is directed toward correction of any abnormalities.

Secondary amenorrhea (no menses for the length of three cycles or 6 months) occurs after a normal menarche and during pregnancy and lactation. In the adolescent, the most common cause is a minor emotional upset related to being away from home, attending college, tension from school work, or interpersonal problems. Because the second most common cause is pregnancy, this possibility should always be investigated.

Secondary nutritional disturbances may also be apparent, such as weight loss or weight gain. On occasion there may be a pituitary or thyroid dysfunction that may be treated successfully by appropriate measures. Consultation with a physician is necessary.

Abnormal Uterine Bleeding

Menorrhagia

Menorrhagia is excessive bleeding at the time of the regular menstrual flow. In early life, it may be due to endocrine disturbances, but with increase in duration of the menstrual periods in later life, it is usually due to inflammatory disturbances, tumors of the uterus, or hormonal imbalance. Emotional disturbance may also affect bleeding.

A woman with menorrhagia is encouraged to see her gynecologist and describe the nature of the excessive bleeding. Although difficult to measure, an estimate might be given in terms of numbers of pads or tampons, their type and absorbency and number saturated per hour.

Metrorrhagia

Metrorrhagia is the appearance of blood from the uterus between regular menstrual periods. It may be a symptom of disease, possibly cancer or benign tumors of the uterus; therefore, it merits early diagnosis and treatment. Metrorrhagia is probably the most significant form of menstrual dysfunction and warrants further investigation, usually by D&C. Any bleeding 1 year after cessation of menses mandates medical evaluation, and malignancy must be considered until proved otherwise.

Perimenopause

Perimenopause is the period extending from the first signs of menopause, usually hot flashes, to beyond the complete cessation of menses (1 year beyond). *Menopause* is described as the physiologic cessation of menses associated with failing ovarian function. It is often diagnosed in retrospect when a year has passed with no menses . The *climacteric* period is the transition period in the life of a woman during which the reproductive function gradually diminishes and is lost. *Postmenopause* is the period about 1 year past the cessation of menses and beyond.

Physiologic Overview

The menopausal period of a woman's life marks the end of her active reproductive life. It usually occurs between the ages of 49 and 52, but it may occur in some women as early as 42 or as late as 55. Median age is 51. Menstruation then ceases, and as a result of the complete cessation of activity on the part of the ovaries, the reproductive organs and the mammary glands may begin to atrophy. No more ova mature; therefore, no ovarian hormones are produced. A similar situation occurs earlier if the ovaries are removed or are destroyed by irradiation, producing an artificial menopause.

Menopause is not a pathologic phenomenon; in addition to estrogen deficiency, there are multifaceted psychological and physiologic changes, including neuroendocrinologic, biochemical, and metabolic changes related to the aging process.

Clinical Manifestations

Usually, symptoms of menopause can be classified according to cause, as arising from endocrine changes due to a lack of estrogen or psychological changes. The process starts gradually and is recognized by the change in menstruation. The monthly flow becomes smaller in amount, then irregular, and finally ceases. Often, the time between periods becomes longer—there may be a lapse of several months between them. Any prolonged menstrual flow or bleeding between periods should be reported promptly to the physician.

Hot or warm flashes and night sweats are reported by some women and are directly attributable to hormonal changes. The hot flash is a symptom denoting vasomotor instability. Flashes may be mild, moderate, and severe, varying from a warm feeling, often fleeting, that is barely noticed to an extremely hot feeling accompanied by profuse sweating that is uncomfortable. The latter may require the woman to seek relief by fanning or showering.

Physical manifestations may include atrophic changes, skin dryness, weight gain, decreased stature, and osteoporosis. Although the entire genitourinary system is affected by reduced estrogens, changes in the vulvovaginal area are most apparent. There is a thinning of hair (mons veneris) and a gradual shrinkage of the labia. Vaginal secretions diminish, and dyspareunia (painful intercourse) may be experienced. This can be avoided by added lubrication, such as K-Y Jelly, Replens, Surgilube, or contraceptive foam. The vaginal *p*H rises, predisposing to bacterial infections (vaginitis). Itching and burning of vulvar tissues may be noted.

Psychological Manifestations

Symptoms of a more psychological type may occur before or during these changes in the monthly periods (*e.g.*, dizziness, weakness, nervousness, insomnia, headaches, and inability to concentrate). This often is the time in a woman's life when children have grown up and left home; thus, she may no longer feel needed. This realization, added to an acute awareness of the aging process, can have an effect on symptoms expressed. Fear of growing old may trigger feelings of depression. These feelings may be more of a problem for women who have not worked outside the home. For those who are involved with interesting and meaningful work, such reactions occur less frequently. Many woman have mild symptoms, and some have none.

Management

Most patients respond to a program of education, reassurance, modification of their living habits, and an improved regimen of health.

Occasionally, mild sedatives and tranquilizers are necessary to control nervousness and to counteract depression, which is not unusual at this time, although these symptoms may be due to factors other than hormonal change. If routine problems become too difficult to handle, counseling can be helpful.

Persistent and severe hot flashes require treatment by estrogen therapy given on a cyclic basis. The dosage is regulated by the physician according to a desired schedule, such as taking the medication for the first 25 days of each month. A progestational agent is usually added for the last 13 days of estrogen administration.

Continued use of estrogen therapy to prevent widespread degenerative changes, including physical aging, is still controversial. Most authorities are conservative and prescribe estrogen replacement on an individual basis for acute estrogen deprivation or annoying signs of estrogen deficiency, such as atrophic vaginitis, hot flashes, or osteoporosis. Restraint in prescribing estrogens for all menopausal women arose from concern that protracted treatment would induce neoplastic changes in estrogen-sensitive aging tissue. Some of these changes are offset by the addition of progesterone.

Nursing Interventions

Measures should be taken to promote the woman's general health. The nurse can explain to the patient that the cessation of the menses is a physiologic function that is rarely accompanied by extreme nervous symptoms and illness.

The current expected life span after menopause for the average woman is 30 to 35 years, and it encompasses as many years as the childbearing phase of her life. The menopause is not a complete change of life. The normal sexual urges remain, and women retain their usual reaction to sex long after menopause. There is nothing abnormal about the change of life, and nothing unusual about the continuation of satisfying sexual relations afterward. Many women enjoy better health after the menopause than they have had for years. This is especially true with persons who have suffered with dysmenorrhea.

Patient Education

The following factors are stressed in patient teaching:

- The climacteric period is normal and self-limiting.
- Overfatigue and environmental problems exaggerate the symptoms.
- A nutritious diet and weight control will improve physical condition.
- An exercise program in keeping with the patient's needs promotes vitality.
- Interest and participation in outside activities help to reduce anxiety and tension.
- Changes are expected in former support networks: departure of children, aging and dependent parents, death of loved ones.
- This is an excellent time for intellectual growth and the stimulation of new ideas and experiences.
- Menopause does not mean a termination of the patient's sex life.
- An annual physical examination is essential to the maintenance of continuing good health.

For the handling or prevention of physical annoyances, the following instructions to the patient may be helpful:

- For itching or burning vulvar areas, seek evaluation and if appropriate, a prescription for a cortisone or hormonal cream.

- To prevent dyspareunia (pain with sexual intercourse), use a water-soluble lubricant, such as K-Y Jelly, Replens, or contraceptive foam.
- Improve perineal muscle tone and bladder control by practicing Kegel's exercises daily:
  When lying on the back with a pillow under the knees, contract the perineal muscles as though stopping urination; hold for 5 seconds and release. Repeat 10 times for 3 or 4 times a day. This also can be done while sitting or standing.
- Use bland skin cream and lotions to prevent drying, itching, and cracking skin.
- Avoid bubble baths, as most ingredients are drying to the skin.
- Pay increased attention to good grooming, including attractive color coordination of clothes, make-up, and hair-styling to give a needed lift when it is most needed.
- Join a weight-reduction support group such as *Weight Watchers* or a similar support group if weight is a problem. There is a tendency to gain weight, particularly around the hips, thighs, and abdomen.
- Observe a proper level of calcium intake because calcium requirements increase after menopause. Milk and calcium supplements may be helpful in slowing the progress of osteoporosis (see Chap. 61 for discussion of this condition).

The individual woman's evaluation of herself and her worth, now and in the future, certainly affects her emotional reaction to this change in her life.

Gerontologic Considerations

Frequent examinations can help in preventing problems of the reproductive tract in the aging female. Often, older women do not have regular gynecologic examinations; many who have delivered their children at home have never had a pelvic examination. Some regard it as an embarrassing and unpleasant procedure. The role of the nurse in emphasizing an annual pelvic examination for all women is of major health teaching significance. The nurse, nurse practitioner, or nurse midwife can make the examination a time for education and reassurance, rather than an embarrassment.

With aging, the vulva loses hair and subcutaneous fat, accompanied by general tissue atrophy. As a result, the woman is easily susceptible to irritation and infection. Pruritus is a common symptom. Physiologic changes include diminished vaginal lubrication and elasticity.

The primary change is the absence of responsive follicles in the ovary. This results in the reduction of estrogen secretion and concomitant changes in androgen production. Estrogen deficiency directly affects the ovaries, endometrium, vaginal epithelium, and skin, which is known to possess estrogen receptors. Clinical effects are dyspareunia and increased susceptibility to vaginal trauma and urinary tract infection (UTI). Frequent sexual activity helps to maintain the elasticity of the vagina. Six to eight glasses of water per day with vitamin C (500 mg) may lessen the incidence of UTI.

With relaxing pelvic musculature, prolapse of the uterus can occur. Appropriate evaluation and surgical repair can provide relief if the patient is a candidate for surgery. When surgery is indicated, it must be recognized that more time is needed for the healing and repair of tissues. In addition, concern needs to be given to the psychosocial aspects of care. Support resources are essential in achieving the desired outcomes of self-sufficiency in the woman.

The incidence of cancer is increased in the aging person. Gerontologic implications are presented in Chapter 12. Sexual changes are discussed in Chapter 17.

Contraception

Control of human reproduction has been practiced for various reasons since ancient times. Many methods exist, and their acceptance has fluctuated. An ideal method has not been developed; all have advantages and disadvantages. Most methods apply to women. Research has addressed male methods of contraception, but for varying reasons few seem close to marketable, although several are being explored.

Family planning refers to limiting or spacing the number of children born. In preventing unwanted or unplanned births, the means described below are available:

Natural planning—using any natural means of pregnancy prevention to the exclusion of chemical or mechanical means

Contraception—a means of temporarily avoiding pregnancy

Sterilization—a means of permanently preventing pregnancy

In the United States, sterilization is the most prevalent method of contraception of women who have completed their childbearing. Oral contraceptives are the most prevalent method in women who have not begun or completed childbearing.

Patient Education.   Much has been written about family planning and the availability and use of contraceptive devices. The nurse is in a strong position to help patients understand the options available. Religious groups have made clear their teaching and dogma regarding birth control, and these beliefs need to be respected and understood as couples make their own decisions. Research is changing the methods used in fertility control, and more acceptable and longer-lasting types are sought.

Natural Methods

The advantages of natural methods of contraception include the following: (1) they are not hazardous to a person's health; (2) they are inexpensive; and (3) they are approved by some religions. The disadvantages are that they require discipline by the couple and periods of abstinence. Also, unless the patient is well educated in the sympto-thermal method of ovulatory timing, this is less effective than other methods. Courses are available in the sympto-thermal method at Catholic hospitals and some family planning clinics. *Abstinence* or *celibacy* is the only completely effective means of preventing pregnancy.

Coitus interruptus is the withdrawal of the penis from the vagina before ejaculation, which requires strong willpower. The uncertainty and unreliability of this method are due to the presence of many sperm in the pre-ejaculatory fluid.

Rhythm Method.   The rhythm method of contraception can be difficult to use because it is based on the woman's ability to determine her time of ovulation and on the avoidance of intercourse during the fertile period. The fertile phase (which requires sexual abstinence) is estimated to occur about 14 days before menstruation, although it may occur between the 10th and 17th days. It is assumed that spermatozoa can fertilize an ovum up to 72 hours after intercourse and that the ovum can be fertilized for about 24 hours after it leaves the ovary. Studies show that of 100 women practicing the rhythm method, up to 40 conceive during a year.

According to some researchers, if a woman carefully determines her "safe period," based on precise recording of her menstrual dates for at least 1 year and follows a carefully worked out formula, she may achieve 80% protection. It requires a long period of abstinence during each cycle, however. These prerequisites require more time and control than many women have. New methods of detecting ovulation (*e.g.,* ovulimeter) have improved statistics.

To increase the effectiveness of the rhythm method, the woman is encouraged to:

- Keep a daily chart recording the nature of cervical mucus; and vaginal wetness; this changes as the menstrual cycle progresses
- Measure her temperature at waking (temperature rises for a few days after ovulation)
- Estimate when ovulation will occur based on past experience
- Take a course in this method with her partner

A group of researchers has discovered how to predict ovulation. The presence of the enzyme *guaiacol peroxidase* in cervical mucus signals ovulation 6 days beforehand and controls viscosity. Sperm can get through the cervical canal *only* when mucus is watery (ovulation time) and an egg is present.

Test kits are available over the counter and are easily understandable and reliable but can be expensive. Ovulation prediction kits are more effective for planning conception than for avoiding it.

Oral Steroids/Oral Contraceptives

Physiologic Basis.   Oral synthetic steroid preparations of estrogen and progesterone tend to block the stimulation of the ovary by the central nervous system by preventing the release of FSH from the anterior pituitary. In the absence of FSH, a follicle does not ripen and ovulation does not take place. This is the mechanism of action of oral contraceptives. Progestin (a synthetic form of progesterone) suppresses the LH surge, preventing ovulation. It also renders cervical mucus impenetrable to sperm. Synthetic estrogens and progestins vary in potency as well as androgenic and anabolic activity.

There are two kinds of therapy: "combined" and "progestin only." The difference lies in the dosage of progestin and the presence of estrogen. In combination pills, estrogen and progesterone are present in every pill. Most women taking oral contraceptives take this type. Progestins interfere with cervical mucus production and prevent the uterine endometrium from fully developing to receive the fertilized ovum, resulting in a lighter than normal menstrual flow after pills are taken for 21 days and then stopped for 7 days. The flow is withdrawal bleeding from stopping hormones, as a normal period occurs only with ovulation. Combined pills now include biphasics, which contain a constant amount of estrogen with an increase in the progestin on day 10, and triphasics, which provide low doses of estrogen that vary, along with varying levels of progesterone during the 21-day cycle. The intent of this variation is to provide an effective contraceptive that mimics the normal cycle and has enough progesterone to prevent ovulation and spotting.

To initiate pill usage, depending on package instructions, one pill is taken on the Sunday after a period starts, or on the first day of a period, or on the fifth day. Pills are taken for 21 days followed by 7 hormone-free days. Some packages include sugar pills for 7 days that are hormone-free. Some women find it easier to stay in the habit of taking one pill every day, and some prefer 7 days without pills. After 7 days off or 7 sugar pills, a new package is started.

In a small percentage of patients, side effects may be noted, such as nausea, depression, headache, weight gain, leg cramps, and breast soreness. Usually, these symptoms disappear after 3 or 4 months. Because such symptoms are sometimes related to sodium and water retention caused by estrogen, a smaller dose of the hormone or a different hormonal combination, along with salt reduction in the diet, may alleviate the problem.

Other problems encountered are the occurrence of thromboembolic disorders, more rapid growth of uterine fibroids, and jaundice, although these are infrequent. Therefore, these drugs should not be used by women who have had thromboembolic disorders, uterine fibroids, or liver or gall bladder disease. Noted also is an increased incidence of heart attacks in smokers over the age of 35 who are on the pill. Occasionally, neuro-ocular complications arise, but a cause-and-effect relationship has not been established. Should visual disturbances occur, the drug should be discontinued and another method of birth control used.

Women with infrequent periods usually are advised to use another method of contraception. If they use oral contraceptives, it may take a while for their ovaries to resume functioning after they discontinue pill use. With respect to how soon fertility returns after use of oral contraceptives, resumption of normal menses is delayed 2 to 3 months in approximately 20% of users. Most obstetricians recommend that the woman use a barrier method for 3 months after stopping the pill before becoming pregnant. To date, studies have not found a link between the pill and breast cancer. Studies have shown that the pill lessens the incidence of benign breast disease, cancer of the uterus, cancer of the ovaries, and pelvic infection.

"Mini" pills contain a progestin only and are less protective against pregnancy. Forty percent of women have ovulatory cycles on this pill. These pills are helpful for women who have had estrogen-related side effects on combination pills (*i.e.,* headaches, hypertension, leg pain, chloasma, weight gain, or nausea). They also can be used in those who are over 35 (nonsmokers) or those with varicose veins.

Some obstetricians recommend this pill for lactating women who need a hormonal method of contraception. Spotting during the pill cycle and lack of withdrawal bleeding during the 7 days off occur frequently if timing is not regular, that is, one pill every 24 hours.

Patients who take oral contraceptives seem to be at higher risk for contracting chlamydia, a common sexually transmitted disease (STD). This is an important point for nurses to emphasize when teaching patients about their use. They may be safe from pregnancy, but if they have multiple partners, chlamydial infection and other STDs, including HIV infection, are a risk.

It is generally accepted that no definite long-term undesirable effects after prolonged use of oral contraceptives have been observed. Fetal anomalies do not appear to be a concern, and normal reproductive tract function and fertility are restored (although somewhat delayed, as was indicated above) after discontinuance of the oral contraceptive. Meanwhile, research and experimentation continue toward the development of a single monthly pill or injection that would be safe as well as effective. The risk factors of oral contraceptives are listed in Chart 44-1.

Contraindications include hypertension, congenital hyperlipidemia, liver disease, cholestatic jaundice, amenorrhea, cigarette smoking (more than half a pack per day), acute phase of mononucleosis, and sickle cell disease. Oral contraceptives at present are recommended for young women, and use by low-risk nonsmokers can be extended until 35 to 40 years of age. A new combination pill containing a progestin and only 20 μg of estrogen, as opposed to most pills, which contain 35 μg of estrogen, is now being used in nonsmoking, low-risk women up to the time of menopause. Some gynecologists allow patients with migraine headaches to take oral contraceptives as long as headaches do not worsen with their use. Some diabetologists allow their patients to use the pill with careful glucose monitoring. Leiomyomas (fibroid tumors) of the uterus can enlarge with pill use, so patients with this condition are advised of this risk and then monitored carefully or taken off the pill and offered other methods.

Mechanical Barriers

Diaphragm.   The diaphragm is an effective contraceptive device. It is a round flexible spring (50 to 90 mm in diameter) that is covered with a domelike latex rubber cup. A spermicidal jelly or cream is used to coat the concavity of the diaphragm before it is inserted deep into the vagina. The combination of a diaphragm and spermicide prevents spermatozoa from entering the cervical canal. The diaphragm presents no discomfort when fitted properly and inserted correctly, because it is lodged against the back wall of the vagina and anteriorly against the edge of the pubic bone. Because women vary in size, diaphragms are designed to fit the client; therefore, it is necessary for the woman to be fitted for the proper size by a physician or a nurse practitioner. At this time, the woman is instructed in its use and care. A return demonstration ensures that the diaphragm is inserted correctly to cover the cervix and upper vagina.

Each time the diaphragm is used, it must be examined carefully by holding it up to a bright light and making sure it

---

Chart 44-1
Absolute Contraindications to the Use of Oral Contraceptives

Known, suspected, or history of estrogen-dependent neoplasia
Known, suspected, or history of cancer of the breast
Thrombophlebitis or thromboembolic disease, or history of
Cerebrovascular or coronary artery disease, or history of
Abnormal uterine bleeding from an unknown cause
Known or suspected pregnancy
Benign or malignant liver tumor

has no pinpoint holes, cracks, or tears. Contraceptive jelly or cream is applied in a prescribed manner to the dome of the diaphragm; if it is applied more than 6 hours before intercourse, it must be reapplied. The diaphragm is then positioned to cover the cervix completely. The diaphragm is left in place at least 6 hours after coitus. On removal it is cleansed thoroughly with mild soap and water, rinsed, and dried before it is stored in its original container.

Cervical Cap.   The cervical cap is much smaller (22 to 35 mm) than the diaphragm and covers only the cervix; it is used with a spermicide. If the woman knows how to insert a diaphragm, it is not difficult to apply a cervical cap. The chief advantage is that the cap may be left in place for 2 days.

Some research has shown that the cap, although convenient, may cause cervical irritation, so most clinicians obtain a Pap smear before fitting a cap and repeat it after 3 months of use.

Sponge and Spermicide.   A more recent contraceptive is a sponge made of urethane and a spermicide (nonoxynol-9) that is marketed under the trade name of Today. It is inserted into the vaginal tract, fits loosely over the cervix, and may be left in place up to 24 hours. A polyester loop attached to the sponge permits its retrieval. It is available without prescription and appears, according to some tests, to be as effective as the diaphragm.

In actual practice, it seems less effective than the diaphragm, possibly because it is not fitted individually. It also has been found to cause occasional sensitivity reactions and to come apart on removal. Despite these disadvantages, it is easily available, inexpensive, and is more effective than no contraceptive at all.

Condom.   The condom is an impermeable snug-fitting rubber or plastic cover applied to the erect penis before it enters the vaginal canal. The penis with condom in place is to be removed from the vagina while still erect to prevent leakage of ejaculate.

The condom is an effective method when used with contraceptive foam. The latex condom is also a barrier to the transmission of STDs, especially gonorrhea, infection with chlamydia, and human immunodeficiency virus (HIV). It is the *only* barrier method recommended for reducing risk of HIV infection. Women need to know that they have a right to insist that a partner use a condom and a right to refuse to have sex without its use.

Intrauterine Device

An intrauterine device (IUD) is a plastic device of varying shapes, usually 2.5 × 2 cm (1 × ¾ inches), that is inserted by a gynecologist through the cervix into the endometrial cavity to prevent pregnancy. The method by which an IUD prevents contraception is thought to be due to a local inflammatory reaction caused by the presence of a foreign body in the uterus. The inflammatory reaction appears to be toxic to spermatozoa and blastocytes. One type of IUD, the Progestasert-T, releases progestin and is replaced each year. The progestin may decrease cramping during menses, but this type of IUD has a slightly higher pregnancy rate than copper-bearing IUDs. Another IUD available is the Paraguard, a copper-bearing IUD that is effective for 6 years.

The advantages of this method are that it is effective over a long time, appears to have no systemic effects, and reduces the factor of patient error. The disadvantages are that such a device may cause excessive bleeding, become displaced, perforate the cervix and uterus, and may cause infection. There is also the risk of pregnancy-related complications, such as spontaneous or septic abortion, and ectopic pregnancy. This method is contraindicated in nulliparous women, women with multiple partners, women with heavy or crampy periods, or those with a history of ectopic pregnancy or pelvic infection. IUDs do *not* reduce risk of STDs.

Implant Contraceptive

The Norplant System is a reversible, 5-year, low-dose progestin-only contraceptive consisting of six soft Silastic capsules that are placed subdermally in a woman's upper arm. By slowly releasing levonorgestrel over the 5 years that the device is effective, it seems to provide effective contraception. The average annual pregnancy rate over 5 years is less than 1%. Recently approved by the Food and Drug Administration (FDA) for use in the United States, this method of contraception has been used by about 500,000 women in other countries. Contraindications to the use of this method are acute liver disease or liver tumors, unexplained vaginal bleeding, breast cancer, or a history of thrombophlebitis or pulmonary embolism.

Insertion takes place under aseptic conditions in an outpatient setting such as an office or clinic. A small incision is made in the upper arm under local anesthesia. The Norplant capsules should be inserted within the first 7 days of the menstrual cycle to avoid the possibility of a preexisting pregnancy. The contraceptive effect occurs within 24 hours. The device can be removed at any time but is effective for 5 years. Both insertion and removal usually take about 15 minutes. The most common side effect with this method is irregular bleeding.

Information included in patient teaching about this method includes:

1. Little or no discomfort is experienced on insertion.
2. The Norplant System is not visible but is palpable on the inside of the upper arm if pressure is applied to that area.
3. Irregular bleeding may occur.
4. If pregnancy is desired, previous fertility levels should resume shortly after removal.
5. The risk of ectopic pregnancy in Norplant users is the same as those using no method or those with an IUD in place. Any abdominal pain should be reported to the patient's care provider immediately.
6. The risks of smoking in combination with the use of this method are unknown. Women should be advised not to smoke.

Interception (Postcoital Conception Control)

A properly timed administration of an adequate dosage of estrogen after intercourse prevents pregnancy. Such a "morning after" pill is not applicable for use in long-term contraception but is of real value in emergency situations such as rape, defective or torn condom or diaphragm, or other "accidental" intercourse. It has been used for more than 8 years in care provided after rape.

Such medication given immediately after fertilization and before the occurrence of implantation is effective. Usually, the therapy is continued over 5 days using DES. Nausea can be minimized by taking the medication with meals and with an antiemetic drug. Other side effects, such as breast soreness and irregular bleeding, may occur but are transient. Ovral, an oral contraceptive containing norgestrel, is used also as a "morning after" method. Two tablets are taken within 12 to 24 hours of sexual intercourse and two tablets are taken 12 hours later. Any patient using this method should be advised that there is a 1.6% failure rate and should also be counseled about other methods of contraception. The effect of morning-after contraception is related to luteal phase dysfunction, producing an endometrium that is out of phase.

Postcoital IUD insertion has also been used with copper-bearing IUDs. This method may not be appropriate in post-rape situations or if other contraindications mentioned above exist.

Permanent Conception Control

Sterilization is becoming increasingly common and in fact is the preferred method of contraception for couples who no longer desire to have children. Sterilization is most often achieved by tubal ligation in the female and by vasectomy in the male. Ligations may be reversible; however, they are still considered a permanent means of sterilization. Hysterectomy or oophorectomy, performed for other reasons, also results in sterility.

Tubal Sterilization. Tubal sterilization (ligation or electrocoagulation of uterine tubes) terminates a woman's ability to have children without affecting her ovulatory or menstrual function. Various surgical techniques have been developed using the abdominal or vaginal approach.

Laparoscopy is the most common method of tubal ligation in the United States. The surgeon performs a *laparotomy* (an abdominal incision) and locates the fallopian tubes. The tubes then are occluded using clips or sutures. Another possible technique is to resect a segment of the tube. This operation may be done during other abdominal surgery or cesarean section, provided informed consent has been obtained.

Tubal ligation is most often performed through a *mini-laparotomy* (small abdominal incision). The surgeon places an instrument into the vagina and moves the uterus and tubes up against the abdominal wall, where access is gained through the small incision to ligate the tube.

Sterilization also can be done through a *colpotomy* (incision of the vagina). A culdoscope is inserted into the vagina and through a colpotomy incision. The fimbriated fallopian tube is then ligated and excised or occluded by tantalum clips. With the clips, however, there is the possibility that sterilization can be reversed at some point in the future. The advantage of this method is the absence of an abdominal scar and less intraperitoneal insufflation (injection of gas, as is done with an abdominal laparoscope), but because of an increased incidence of postoperative infection, this method is used infrequently.

Patient Education. Usually before sterilization is done, an IUD, if present, is removed. If the patient is receiving an oral contraceptive, it is usually continued up to the time of the procedure. Postoperatively there is some abdominal soreness for a few days. The patient is instructed to report any of the following: bleeding, pain that continues or increases, and elevated temperature. For 2 weeks, she is to avoid intercourse and strenuous exercises or lifting.

Vasectomy. A vasectomy is the ligation and transection of a section of the vas deferens in the male, with or without removal of a segment of the vas. The severed ends are occluded with ligatures or clips, or the lumen of each vas is coagulated. A bilateral vasectomy may be done as a sterilization procedure, as it interrupts the transportation of the sperm. (The spermatozoa, which are manufactured in the testes, are unable to travel up the vas deferens because of surgical interruption.)

Seminal fluid is mostly manufactured in the seminal vesicles and prostate gland, which are unaffected by vasectomy. Thus, there will be no noticeable decrease in the amount of ejaculated fluid, except that it contains no spermatozoa. Because the sperm cells have no exit, they are reabsorbed into the body. The procedure has no effect on sexual potency, erection, ejaculation, or production of male hormones.

Two behavioral responses seem to be common after vasectomy. Persons who were anxious about intercourse because of fear of pregnancy due to contraceptive failure often report a decrease in anxiety and an increase in spontaneous sexual arousal. Some men adopt stereotyped masculine behavior, supposedly to allay concerns that the surgery has decreased their masculinity. Concise and factual preoperative discussion may minimize or prevent the latter behavior. Findings of some studies suggest that vasectomy can lead to autoimmune disorders, in that antibodies that agglutinate the patient's own spermatozoa may form and persist for many years after the procedure. An increased incidence of autoimmune disorders after vasectomy has not been clinically proved, and no pathology has been linked to antibody formation.

The patient is advised that he will be sterile but that potency will not be altered after a bilateral vasectomy. The procedure does not prevent STD. On rare occasions, a spontaneous reanastomosis of the vas deferens occurs, which may result in pregnancy of the partner. A legal consent form must be obtained before the procedure is performed.

Complications of vasectomy include scrotal ecchymoses and swelling, superficial wound infection, vasitis (inflammation of the vas deferens), epididymitis or epididymo-orchitis, hematomas, and sperm granuloma. A *sperm granuloma* is an inflammatory response to the collection of sperm in the scrotum due to leakage from the severed end of the proximal vas. This can initiate recanalization of the vas, possibly resulting in pregnancy of the partner.

For a comparison of vasectomy and female sterilization, see Chart 44-2.

Patient Education. Ice bags are applied intermittently to the scrotum for several hours after surgery to reduce swelling and relieve discomfort. The patient is advised to wear cotton jockey-type briefs for added comfort and support. He may become greatly concerned about the discoloration of the scrotal skin and superficial swelling. This occurs frequently after vasectomy and responds to sitz baths.

Sexual intercourse may be resumed as desired by the patient, although he should be informed that he will still be fertile for a varying time after vasectomy, until the spermatozoa that are stored distal to the point of interruption of the vas have been evacuated.

Contraceptives should be used until the patient is declared infertile. This declaration is made by examination of ejaculate. Some physicians examine a specimen 4 weeks after the vasectomy to determine sterility; others use two consecutive specimens 1 month apart, and still others consider a patient sterile after 36 ejaculations.

Chart 44–2
Sterilization Methods

Vasectomy

Advantages

Safe—slight morbidity
Almost no mortality
Simple
Inexpensive in comparison with female sterilization
Brief—20-minute procedure

Disadvantages

Not effective until sperm in reproductive system are ejaculated.
Complications: bleeding, swelling, infection

Failure Rate
0%–5.3%

Reversibility
5%–90%

Anesthesia
Local

Recovery Time
1–5 days

Laparoscopic Tubal Sterilization

Advantages

Low rate of complications
Short recovery
Minimal morbidity
Leaves small scar
Brief—20-minute procedure

Disadvantages

Infrequent complications can be serious.
Some women note crampier menses after sterilization

Failure Rate
0%–2%

Reversibility
10%–90%

Anesthesia
Usually general

Recovery Time
0–5 days

(Adapted from Hatcher R et al. Contraceptive Technology, 1990–1992, 15th ed. Irvington, NY, Irvington Publishers, 1990.)

Vasovasostomy (Sterilization Reversal). Microsurgical techniques are being used for vasectomy reversal (vasovasostomy), which restores patency to the vas deferens.

Many men will have sperm in their ejaculate after a reversal, but only 29% to 85% are able to impregnate a partner.

Banking of Sperm. Storage of fertile semen in a sperm bank *before* a vasectomy is a possibility should unforeseen life events cause a desire in the patient to father a child. The success rate in achieving pregnancy with frozen sperm is uncertain. Legal problems have become an issue with this method and will probably continue to be an issue in the future.

Investigational Conception Control

Researchers recognize that the perfect method of conception control (barring abstention or sterilization), does not exist; every method has some risk. Research and testing of types of contraception control have decreased considerably because of the cost of testing and the risk of liability. The following are under investigation:

Vaginal rings may be available that also release progestin. Placed around the cervix, vaginal rings may be effective for 3 months, are removed during coitus, and require careful vaginal hygiene.

RU-486 (Mifepristone) is a progesterone antagonist that prevents implantation and leads to menses. Administered by mouth within 10 days of an expected period, it produces a medical abortion in most patients. Prolonged bleeding may be one side effect. If combined with a prostaglandin suppository, it causes an abortion in up to 95% of patients up to 5 weeks after conception. Other uses for this drug may include treatment of breast cancer, endometriosis, and ectopic pregnancy.

Abortion

Interruption of pregnancy or expulsion of the contents of the pregnant uterus before the fetus is viable is called *abortion*.

The fetus is usually considered to be viable any time after the sixth month of gestation. The aborted fetus weighs less than 1000 g. Above this weight, the fetus is usually viable and the term *premature labor* is used.

Spontaneous Abortion

It is estimated that 1 of every 5 to 10 conceptions results in spontaneous abortion. Most of these occur because of an abnormality in the fetus, so abortion is nature's way of rejecting a defective conception. Other causes may be due to systemic diseases, hormonal imbalance, or anatomic abnormalities. This type of abortion is commonly called a miscarriage. If the patient is experiencing bleeding and cramping, a threatened abortion is diagnosed, as abortion is usually imminent. Spontaneous abortion occurs most commonly in the second or third month of gestation, probably because of a defective ovum and subsequent developmental defects of the fetus and placenta.

There are various kinds of spontaneous abortion, depending on the nature of the process (threatened, inevitable, incomplete, and complete). Uterine bleeding and pain (uterine contractions) are suggestive of an abortion in a woman of childbearing age. In such a *threatened abortion*, the cervix does not dilate; with bed rest and conservative treatment, it may be prevented. If it cannot be prevented, an *inevitable abortion* is imminent. If some of the tissue, but not all, is passed, the abortion is referred to as *incomplete*; however, if the fetus and all related tissue are expressed (removed), the abortion is *complete*.

Habitual Abortion

Habitual abortion is successive, repeated spontaneous abortions of unknown cause. As many as 60% may be due to chromosomal anomalies. After two consecutive abortions, most patients are referred for genetic counseling and testing. Ultraconservative measures are employed in an attempt to save the pregnancy, such as complete bed rest, administration of progesterone to support the endometrium and occasionally thyroid extract therapy and counseling.

In the condition known as *incompetent cervical os*, the cervix dilates painlessly in the second trimester of pregnancy, resulting in a spontaneous abortion. A surgical procedure called the *Shirodkar* or *cervical cerclage* is designed to prevent the cervix from dilating prematurely. A pursestring suture is placed around the cervix at the level of the internal os. Bed rest is often ordered with this procedure. It is most important that the patient and nurses caring for her, including those in community health agencies, be informed that such a suture is in place. Two to 3 weeks before term or the onset of labor, the suture is cut. Delivery is usually by cesarean section.

Management of Patients Undergoing Spontaneous Abortion. Signs of a threatening abortion are vaginal bleeding and abdominal cramps. The woman is encouraged to see a physician, who will probably recommend bed rest, sexual abstinence, light diet, and no straining on defecation. If infection is suspected, antibiotics may be prescribed.

Nursing Interventions

All tissue passed vaginally is saved for examination by the physician. In the hospital, all personnel caring for the patient are alerted to save the contents of the bedpan for possible placental or fetal tissue. If there is much bleeding, the patient may require transfusions and fluid replacement. An estimate of the amount of bleeding can be determined by recording the number of perineal pads and the nature of saturation per 24 hours. For an incomplete abortion, oxytocin may be prescribed to contract the patient's fundus before a dilatation and evacuation (D&E) or suctioning of the uterus. A patient with such an evacuation of retained secretions requires the same nursing care as a person having a D&C (see p. 1236).

Because patients experience loss of a pregnancy, *caring* is an important aspect of nursing. The response of the woman who desperately wants a baby is different from that of the woman who does not want to be pregnant but may be frightened of the possible consequences of an abortion. The nurse must not overlook the fact that in many instances, particularly for the woman having a spontaneous abortion, there is a grieving period that must be handled. Such grieving may be delayed or unresolved, resulting in other problems until the grief reaction has been worked out. There are many reasons for delayed grief reaction: friends may not have known the woman was pregnant; the woman may not have seen the lost fetus and can only imagine the sex, size, and so forth of the person who never developed; there is no burial service; those who know about the abortion (family, friends, caregivers) encourage denial and rarely encourage crying and talking about the loss.

In any event, providing opportunities for the patient to talk and vent her emotions not only helps her but also provides clues for the nurse in planning more specific care. Those persons closest to the woman are encouraged to hug her and allow her to talk and cry. If grief is unresolved, it may manifest itself by persistent vivid memories of the events surrounding the time of loss, persistent sadness or anger, and frequent flooding of emotion when recalling the loss. Pathologic grief may require the assistance of a therapist skilled in grief work.

Elective Abortion

A voluntary termination of pregnancy is called an elective abortion and should be performed by skilled medical personnel. In 1973, the Supreme Court ruled that decisions about abortion rest between a woman and her physician in the first trimester. The ruling stated that during the second trimester, the state may regulate practice in the interest of women's health, and during the final weeks of pregnancy the state may choose to protect the life of the fetus, except when necessary to preserve the life or health of the woman.

In July of 1989, the Supreme Court upheld a Missouri law prohibiting the use of public facilities for abortion. More recent court decisions have restricted access and returned power to the states.

Legal abortions may be carried out in the following ways, usually in an outpatient setting.

Dilatation and Evacuation or Suction Curettage

The cervix is dilated manually with instrumentation or by use of a laminaria, and a uterine aspirator is introduced. Suction is applied and tissue is removed from the uterus. This method is not used by some if the pregnancy has advanced beyond 12 weeks. More recently, some clinics have extended the period to 16 weeks and even beyond.

Hypertonic Saline Injection

A small amount of amniotic fluid is removed and replaced by hypertonic saline. Serious hazards can occur, including cardiovascular collapse, cerebral and pulmonary edema, renal failure if intravenous injection occurs, and disseminated intravascular coagulopathy (DIC). Augmentation with oxytocin speeds this process. This method is not used frequently.

Prostaglandins

These substances can be introduced into the amniotic fluid or by vaginal suppository or intramuscular injection in later pregnancy. Strong uterine contractions ensue, usually resulting in abortion. This method avoids the DIC associated with saline abortions mentioned above. Gastrointestinal symptoms (*i.e.*, nausea, vomiting, diarrhea, and abdominal cramping) and fever can occur.

Laminaria

An age-old method of cervical dilatation has been revived in medical practice. Laminaria tents are made from a species of seaweed that grows in cold ocean waters. They are shaped into tampon-shaped forms with a string on one end. When placed in a moist environment, the tent, which is highly hygroscopic, swells to three to five times its original diameter, causing dilatation. The greatest amount of swelling occurs in 4 or 5 hours; however, additional dilatation may occur over the next few hours.

Advantages over mechanical dilators include less trauma and more acceptance and tolerance by patients. Disadvantages include some discomfort and slight cramping. This method also requires one visit for the insertion and then a return visit 4 to 6 hours later. There is also a risk of low-grade endometritis (inflammation of the endometrium), even though the laminaria is sterilized by radiation or gas. Removal is occasionally difficult, and slippage into the uterus has occurred.

An alternative is Lamicel, a synthetic polyethylene sponge impregnated with magnesium sulfate and compressed into a rod. It works more rapidly than *Laminaria* tents.

Hysterotomy

A hysterotomy is a miniature cesarean section. This operation is infrequently used as a method for termination of pregnancy.

Septic Abortion

When unskilled attempts to end a pregnancy are made, the methods usually include administering large amounts of drugs (effects are toxic and never really evacuate the uterus) or performing a curettage, with an associated high risk of rupture of the uterus, hemorrhage, or infection.

Although this has been a major problem in the past, with the dissemination of birth control information and the liberalization of abortion laws, a decline in septic abortion has occurred.

If a woman who has had a simple, uncomplicated septic abortion receives proper medical attention early enough, with treatment using broad-spectrum antibiotics, the prognosis is excellent. Fluid and blood component replacement is required before careful attempts are made to evacuate the uterus.

For the treatment of septic abortion complicated by impending shock, see the discussions of shock (Chap. 22) and PID (Chap. 45).

Management of the Patient Undergoing Elective Abortion.
Before the procedure, fears, feelings and options are explored with the patient by a nurse or counselor trained in pregnancy counseling. After ascertaining the patient's choice (*i.e.*, continuation of pregnancy and parenthood, continuation of pregnancy followed by adoption, or termination of the pregnancy by abortion), a pelvic examination is performed to determine uterine size. Laboratory studies before an abortion must include a pregnancy test to confirm the pregnancy, hematocrit to rule out anemia, an Rh determination, and an STD screen. A patient with anemia may need blood component replacement; an Rh-negative patient may require Rhogam to prevent isoimmunization; and all patients should be screened for STD before the procedure to prevent possible infection.

A variety of methods are available to postpone or prevent pregnancy and are reviewed with the patient. Their effectiveness is dependent on the method used and the extent to which the correct instructions for use are followed by the couple. The woman who uses any method of birth control should be assessed for her understanding of the method and its potential side effects and her satisfaction and the satisfaction of her partner with the method. The patient needs to continue her regular health examinations, including gynecologic examinations and Pap smears. The nurse is in an ideal position to assess

the patient's understanding and to provide health teaching related to reproductive issues and women's health care. An increasingly important issue to be included in teaching related to contraceptive use is the need for barrier methods (*i.e.*, condoms) along with those contraceptive methods that do not provide protection against transmission of HIV infection. Chart 44-3 summarizes information provided to women after elective abortion.

Infertility

Infertility usually refers to a couple's failure to achieve a pregnancy after 1 year of unprotected intercourse. *Primary* infertility refers to a couple who have never had a child. *Secondary* infertility means that at least one conception has occurred but currently the couple is unable to achieve a pregnancy. In the United States, infertility is a major medical and social problem affecting 10% to 15% of North American couples. Both partners are urged to seek health care for complete examinations and evaluation if they desire children.

Etiology

Possible causative uterine factors of infertility include displacement, tumors, congenital anomalies, and inflammation. For an ovum to become fertilized, the vagina, fallopian tubes, cervix, and uterus must be patent and the mucosal secretions must be receptive to the sperm. Semen is alkaline, as is cervical secretion; normal vaginal secretion is acid. Often, more than one factor may be responsible for the problem. Such tests may require the services of a gynecologist, urologist, endocrinologist, or internist.

Diagnostic Evaluation

Careful evaluation includes not only anatomic and endocrinologic investigation but also consideration of psychosocial factors. A complete history, physical examination, and laboratory studies are performed on both partners to rule out such causative factors as previous STD, anomalies, injuries, tuberculosis, mumps, orchitis, and psychosocial disorders.

Other factors can include impaired sperm production, endometriosis, DES, or antisperm antibodies. Legal abortions are not a factor in the ability to conceive, unless they are complicated by a postprocedure infection.

Five types of factors are considered basic to infertility: for the woman, (1) ovarian, (2) tubal, (3) cervical, or (4) uterine conditions; and for the man, (5) seminal conditions. A composite estimate of the relative frequency of causes of the infertility follows:

Unexplained—28%
Sperm problem—21%
Ovulatory failure—18%
Tubal damage—14%
Endometriosis—6%
Coital problems—5%
Cervical mucus—3%
Other male problems—2%*

---

* From Speroff L et al. Clinical Gynecologic Endocrinology and Infertility, 4th ed. Baltimore, Williams & Wilkins, 1989, p 518.

Chart 44-3
For Your Information: Post-Abortion Care

1. Someone needs to accompany you to have your abortion and to drive you home.
2. Normal activities may be resumed as soon as you feel able.
3. You may be given some medication (Methergine or Ergotrate) to take, which will help your uterus return to its normal size. It is important to take this medication as directed. Because this medication makes your uterus contract, some uterine cramping is normal and to be expected. You also may be given some antibiotics to prevent infection.
4. To prevent infection, do not have intercourse or insert anything into your vagina for 2 to 3 weeks. Other forms of sexual activity or orgasm will not be harmful. Douching, tub bathing, swimming, and tampons are not allowed for the same length of time.
5. Bleeding will probably stop after 3 to 4 days but may last up to 3 weeks. Some patients have no bleeding. If you are saturating two sanitary pads per hour or have a fever, call your health care provider immediately.
6. You will have a normal period in 4 to 6 weeks.
7. A follow-up examination 2 weeks after the procedure is important to ensure that your body has returned to normal and that no infection has occurred. This appointment is a time to discuss feelings that you may be having and a time to discuss a method of contraception.
8. If you have chosen birth control pills as your method of contraception, start your pills on the Sunday after the abortion procedure. Otherwise, use contraceptive foam and condoms together, to prevent another pregnancy.
9. Notify your nurse practitioner or physician if you have any of the following symptoms:
   Fever (38°C or 100.4°F or above)
   Abdominal pain or cramps (severe or increasing)
   Abdominal tenderness with pressure, coughing, or walking
   Bleeding that is heavy or lasts for more than 3 weeks
   Foul-smelling vaginal discharge
   Rash, hives, asthma (possible reaction to medication)
   No period after 6 weeks

(Adapted from Hawkins J et al. Protocols for Nurse Practitioners in Gynecologic Settings. Tiresias Press, 1988; and Hatcher R et al. Contraceptive Technology, 1990–1992. 15th ed. Irvington, NY, Irvington Publishers, 1990.)

Ovarian Factor.   Tests are performed to determine whether there is regular ovulation and a progestational endometrium adequate for implantation. This includes keeping a basal body temperature chart for at least four cycles, taking an endometrial biopsy, and performing other tests for ovulation and progesterone production.

Tubal Factor (Tubal Insufflation or Rubin's Test).   To determine tubal patency, carbon dioxide is introduced through a sterile cannula into the uterus and the fallopian tubes, and then into the peritoneal cavity. By listening with a stethoscope on the abdomen, the physician may hear gas swishing into the abdomen, indicating that the tubes are patent. Another positive indication of tubal patency is the feeling by the patient of referred pain under the scapula or shoulder on the side of the patent tube. This suggests that the gas is under the diaphragm, exerting pressure on the phrenic nerve. If normal patency is present, there is a rise in pressure of 80 to 120 mm Hg, with a sudden drop to 50 to 70 mm Hg as gas passes into the peritoneal cavity. If the gas pressure gauge reaches 200 mm Hg, the test is considered negative, indicating an occlusion.

Hysterosalpingography (see p. 1238) is a radiographic study that is useful to rule out uterine or tubal abnormalities.

Laparoscopy (see p. 1237) permits direct visualization of tubes and adnexa and can assist in the diagnosis of conditions that may inferfere with fertility (*i.e.,* endometriosis).

Cervical Factor.   Cervical mucus can be examined to determine whether proper changes occur at ovulation that are favorable to sperm penetration, survival, and growth.

A postcoital cervical mucus test (Sims-Huhner test) is performed between 2 and 8 hours after intercourse. Intercourse and ejaculation are avoided for 24 to 48 hours before the test. The physician aspirates cervical secretions, using a medicine dropper or special cannula. The woman has been instructed not to bathe or douche between coitus and the examination; a perineal pad may be worn until she is placed in a lithotomy position in the examination room. Aspirated material is placed on a slide and examined under the microscope for presence and viability of sperm cells.

Uterine Factor.   Fibroids, polyps, and congenital malformations are possible problems in this category. Their presence may be determined by pelvic examination or by hysterosalpingography.

Seminal Factor.   After 2 to 3 days of sexual abstinence, the sperm specimen is collected in a clean, dry glass container, kept at or below room temperature; and examined within 1 hour for volume, sperm motility, morphology, and cell count.

Two to 6 milliliters of watery alkaline semen is normal; a normal count is 60 to 100 million per milliliter, although the incidence of impregnation is lessened only when the count is below 20 million per milliliter.

Miscellaneous Factors.   Miscellaneous factors, including immunologic factors, are being investigated. Some cases of recurrent early pregnancy loss or recurrent abortion are due to an abnormal maternal response to antigens on fetal or placental tissues. Some women have been treated with infusions of their partner's lymphocytes with some success, but this treatment remains experimental, and long-term effects are unknown.

Management

Sterility may be difficult to treat, because it often is due to a combination of several factors. Statistics show that many couples undergoing study conceive without the cause of infertility coming to light; likewise, although some couples undergo all tests, the cause of the problem may remain undiscovered. Between these extremes, many problems, simple as well as complex, can be discovered and corrected.

Therapy may require surgery to correct a malfunction or anomaly, hormonal supplements, attention to proper timing, and recognition and correction of psychological or emotional factors.

Reproductive Technologies

Numerous technologies have been developed to help in the reproduction process and to assist in the basic right of procreativity. Mechanisms already exist under U.S. law to foster safe medical procedures while safeguarding the integrity of the participants. Institutional review boards and procedures for informed consent are two such mechanisms.

Artificial Insemination.   Artificial insemination is the deposition or introduction of semen into the female genital tract by artificial means. If the sperm cannot penetrate the cervical canal normally, consideration may be given to *artificial insemination*, using the husband's semen (AIH). In the event of azoospermia (lack of sperm in the semen), semen from carefully selected donors may be used (AID).

Indications for using artificial insemination are (1) inability of the man to deposit semen in the vagina, which may be due to premature ejaculation, pronounced hypospadias, or dyspareunia (painful intercourse experienced by the woman); and (2) inability of semen to be transported from the vagina to the uterine cavity; this is usually due to faulty chemical conditions, such as may be produced with an abnormal cervical discharge. Another indication for artificial insemination is the desire of a single woman to have a child.

Husband's Semen.   Certain conditions need to be established before semen is transferred to the vagina. The woman must have no abnormalities of the genital system, the tubes must be patent, and ova must be available. In the man, sperm need to be normal in shape, amount, motility, and endurance. The time of ovulation in the woman should be determined as accurately as possible, so that the 2 or 3 days during which fertilization is possible each month can be used. Fertilization seldom occurs from a single insemination. Usually, insemination is attempted between the 10th and 17th days of the cycle; three different attempts may be made during one cycle. Semen is collected in a wide-mouth, 2-ounce jar after masturbation. Withdrawal and use of condoms are considered unsatisfactory by many infertility specialists because of loss of or effect on sperm.

Donor's Semen.   A donor may be used when the sperm of the woman's partner is defective or absent, or when, for hereditary reasons, it is feared that an undesirable disease may be transmitted. Safeguards need to be set up to prevent legal, ethical, emotional, and religious problems. Written consent may protect all parties involved, including the woman, the donor, and the resulting child.

The donor is selected on the basis of close resemblance to the husband, both physically and intellectually; there should be no family history of epilepsy, diabetes, or known genetic defects, and a negative test result for syphilis and HIV should be obtained. Preferably, precautions should be taken so that the donor is not known to the recipient, and vice versa.

Insemination Procedure.   The recipient is placed in the lithotomy position on the examining table, a speculum is inserted, and the vagina and cervix are swabbed clean with a cotton-tipped applicator. Semen is drawn into a sterile syringe, and a cannula is attached. The semen is then directed to the external os. If this is contraindicated, the semen may be inserted directly into the uterus (intrauterine insemination). In this procedure, the sperm are washed before insertion to remove biochemicals. This is indicated when mucus is inadequate, when antibodies are present, or when sperm count is low. After the careful withdrawal of the syringe, the patient is to lie flat on the examining table for a half hour. Thereafter, there are no restrictions on the activities of the woman.

The success rate for artificial insemination varies. About three to six inseminations are required over a 2- to 4-month period. Because this procedure is opposed by the Roman Catholic Church, this method should be discussed with patients, who may then choose to consult their spiritual advisor.

In Vitro Fertilization.   *In vitro* fertilization (IVF) is accomplished by first stimulating the ovary to produce multiple eggs or ova, usually with Pergonal or Clomid, because pregnancy success rates are greater with more than one early embryo. At the appropriate time, discerned by hormonal measurement and ultrasound, the ova are recovered by transvaginal ultrasound retrieval. Sperm and egg are coincubated for up to 36 hours and embryos are transferred approximately 48 to 80 hours after retrieval. Implantation should occur in 2 to 3 days. Gamete intrafallopian transfer (GIFT) is a variation of IVF in which oocytes are removed and drawn into a catheter with sperm and then inserted into the fallopian tube, where fertilization occurs. Success rates vary from 20% to 30%.

The most common indications for the above procedures are irreparable tubal damage, endometriosis, immunologic problems, unexplained infertility, inadequate sperm, and DES exposure.

Although IVF produced mixed reactions at first, it is now accepted as a standard form of infertility treatment, with more than 200 programs in the United States.

Nursing research shows that couples attempting this method of conception need education and support from medical professionals caring for them to cope with the anxiety involved; pertinent research is discussed in the research profile at the end of this unit.

All nurses should be aware of RESOLVE, an organization that provides invaluable information and group support for infertile patients. This nonprofit self-help group was originated by a nurse who had experienced the problem herself. The literature on infertility that is produced by this group is an important resource for patients and professionals. Most areas across the country have local support groups. More information can be obtained by writing to RESOLVE, Inc. (see address at end of chapter).

In summary, infertility, the inability to conceive a pregnancy after a year or more of regular sexual relations without contraception, or the inability to carry a pregnancy to a live birth, affects about 15% of the U.S. population.

Factors are related to abnormalities of the female reproductive system, allergic reaction to sperm, endometriosis, abnormalities of the male reproductive tract, inadequate sperm production, endocrine abnormalities, sexual dysfunction, or genetic abnormality.

After a thorough history and physical examination, assessment follows a careful diagnostic protocol. One of the roles that nurses in this field fulfill is that of an educator; education helps to lessen the anxiety and emotional difficulty the couple experiences during the diagnostic period. After factors affecting infertility are determined, patients may undergo various treatments, including ovulation induction, artificial insemination, or *in vitro* fertilization. The nurse's role in these treatments is specialized, and certification in this specific area is possible. Counseling, education, emotional support and assistance, research, and clinical responsibilities are all part of the nurse's role in this sensitive and unique field.

Ectopic Pregnancy

Ectopic pregnancy occurs when the fertilized ovum does not reach the cavity of the uterus but becomes implanted on any tissue other than the lining of the uterine cavity, such as the fallopian tube or, occasionally, in the ovary or the abdomen, or even the cervix of the uterus (Fig. 44-9).

As the fertilized ovum increases in size, the tube becomes more and more distended, until finally, 4 to 6 weeks after conception, rupture takes place, and the ovum is discharged into the abdominal cavity.

Etiology and Incidence

The highest incidence of ectopic implantation occurs in women from 35 to 44 years of age, when about 1 in 50 pregnancies is ectopic. Precipitating factors include salpingitis, endometri-osis, PID, chemotherapy for pelvic tuberculosis, congenital anomalies of the tubes, spasm of the tubes with muscular insufficiency altering tubal function, previous pelvic or abdominal surgery, an IUD, progestin-only contraceptives, DES exposure, or the history of a previous tubal pregnancy. Increasing occurrence is due to the rise of STDs such as gonorrhea and those caused by chlamydia; improved antibiotic therapy to treat PID, which may prevent total tubal closure; and the late onset of childbearing by an increased number of women. Unfortunately, 50% of those with one ectopic pregnancy do not produce a living child, and 20% have a repeat occurrence.

Clinical Manifestations

Delay in menstruation from 1 to 2 weeks followed by slight bleeding (spotting) may suggest the problem of an ectopic pregnancy. Some form of menstrual bleeding occurs in more than half of ectopic pregnancies, so most physicians and patients do not immediately suspect a tubal pregnancy. Symptoms may begin with vague soreness on the affected side, probably due to uterine contractions and distention of the tube; frequently the patient experiences sharp, colicky pain at times.

When tubal rupture occurs, there is agonizing pain, dizziness, faintness, and some nausea and vomiting (see Fig. 44-9 for nursing assessment). These symptoms are related to peritoneal reaction to blood escaping from the tube. Air hunger and symptoms of shock indicate that the patient is desperately ill; all the signs of hemorrhage—rapid, thready pulse; subnormal temperature; restlessness; pallor, sweating—are in evidence. Later the pain becomes generalized in the abdomen and radiates to the shoulder and neck because of intraperitoneal accumulation of blood that causes an irritation of the diaphragm. During vaginal examination, the surgeon may feel a large mass of clotted blood that has collected in the pelvis behind the uterus or a tender adnexal mass.

Occasionally, the clinical picture makes the diagnosis relatively simple; however, when it is questionable, other aids are

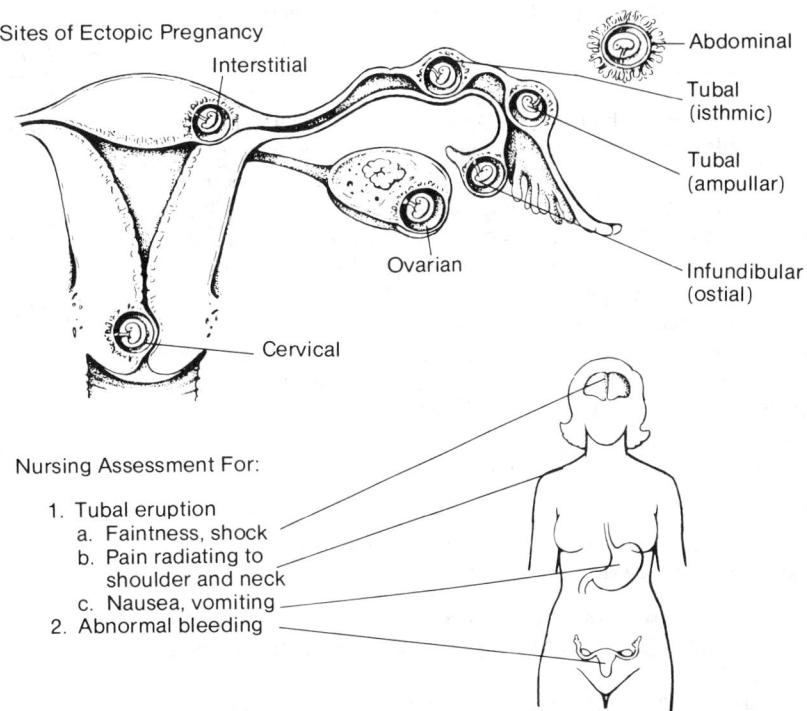

Sites of Ectopic Pregnancy

Interstitial

Abdominal

Tubal (isthmic)

Tubal (ampullar)

Ovarian

Infundibular (ostial)

Cervical

Nursing Assessment For:

1. Tubal eruption
   a. Faintness, shock
   b. Pain radiating to shoulder and neck
   c. Nausea, vomiting
2. Abnormal bleeding

Figure 44-9. Ectopic pregnancy. The various possible sites for ectopic pregnancy are shown in the upper diagram of the uterus and uterine tube.

of value. Ultrasound often can be effective in differentiating between an intrauterine and ectopic pregnancy. Laparoscopy is most often used because the physician can visually note an unruptured tubal pregnancy, thereby circumventing the risk to the patient of a tubal rupture. A beta-subunit blood test to detect the presence of human chorionic gonadotropin, a hormone secreted by the trophoblast soon after conception, is an essential part of the diagnosis. This value increases twofold every 72 hours in a normal pregnancy. If this level is greater than 6500 units without an intrauterine sac visible on ultrasound, an ectopic pregnancy is likely.

Management
The goal of treatment is the surgical removal of the ectopic pregnancy, because it is a life-threatening problem.

When the operation is performed early, practically all patients recover rapidly; if tubular rupture occurs, the mortality increases. The type of surgery is determined by the size and extent of local tubal damage; surgery ranges from conservative to more extensive. Conservative surgery would include "milking" an ectopic pregnancy from the tube. A resection of the involved tube the with end-to-end anastomosis may be effective. Some surgeons today perform a salpingostomy, which involves opening and evacuating the tube and controlling bleeding. The tube may be left open or sutured closed. More radical surgery includes salpingectomy or salpingo-oophorectomy. Depending on the amount of blood lost, blood transfusions and treatment for shock may be necessary preoperatively and during the surgery.

Prognosis
The pregnancy rate after treatment is enhanced; the expectancy of another ectopic pregnancy or miscarriage is five to six times greater than for a woman who has not had an ectopic pregnancy.

▶ Nursing Process
The Patient With an Ectopic Pregnancy

◊ Assessment
The health history includes the menstrual pattern and any (even slight) bleeding since conception. The patient's description of pains and their location is elicited. Did she experience any sharp, colicky pains? The nurse notes whether pain eventually radiates to the shoulder and neck, which may be due to pressure on the diaphragm. Signs and symptoms of rupture are more prominent and suggest hemorrhage and shock.

The meaning of a tubal pregnancy to the patient should be assessed, if possible, noting its psychological impact, how she is coping with the problem, and evidence of grief. Vital signs, level of consciousness, and nature and amount of vaginal bleeding are monitored.

◊ Nursing Diagnoses
Based on the assessment data, the patient's major nursing diagnoses may include the following:

- Pain related to the progression of the tubal pregnancy
- Grieving related to the loss of pregnancy and effect on future pregnancies
- Knowledge deficit of treatment and impact on future pregnancies

Potential complications of ectopic pregnancy are hemorrhage and shock. Careful assessment is essential to detect the development of these serious problems.

◊ Planning and Implementation
◊ *Goals:* The major goals of the patient may include relief of pain, acceptance and resolution of grief and pregnancy loss, and achievement of understanding of the unnatural pregnancy, its treatment, and its outcome. In addition, early detection of complications is a goal.

◊ Nursing Interventions
◊ *Relief of Pain.* After determining location of pain, the nurse uses measures to relieve discomfort by position changes, distraction, and relaxation techniques. She provides emotional support by listening and correcting misconceptions. Analgesics are administered if prescribed. If the patient is to have surgery, preanesthetic medications also provide pain relief.

◊ *Grief Support.* The loss of early pregnancy may or may not be expressed verbally by the patient and her partner. The impact may not be fully realized or even accepted until much later. The nurse should be available to listen and provide support. The patient's partner should share in this obvious loss and sad time. Other professionals such as a psychotherapist or clergy can be consulted if required.

◊ *Patient Education.* With rapid changes, confusion may occur in the early hospital experience of the patient. Life-threatening symptoms resulting from possible hemorrhage and shock must be addressed and treated first. At this time the patient's attention is focused on a crisis and not on learning. Therefore, it may be later that the patient is in a position to learn and ask questions about what has happened and why certain diagnostic measures and interventions were performed. Treatments are explained as they are presented and understood by the patient. The patient's partner is included when possible. After recovery from the postoperative discomforts, the time may be more appropriate to address any questions and problems, such as the effect of this aborted pregnancy on future pregnancies.

◊ *Assessment of Complications.* Continuous monitoring of vital signs, level of consciousness, amount of bleeding, and intake and output provides information about the possibility of hemorrhage and the need to prepare for intravenous therapy. Bed rest is indicated. Laboratory results relative to hematocrit and hemoglobin, as well as blood gases, are noted. Significant deviations in these laboratory values are reported to the physician, and the patient is prepared for the possibility of surgery.

◊ Evaluation
Expected Outcomes
1. Exhibits no signs of hemorrhage and shock
   a. Has lessened amounts of discharge (vaginal pad)
   b. Has normal skin color and turgor
   c. Has stable vital signs
2. Patient experiences a lessening of pain and discomfort
3. Begins to accept pregnancy loss and expresses grief
   a. Expresses sorrow over loss
   b. Expresses the future hope for another child
4. Acquires knowledge about tubal pregnancy and its resolution
   a. Demonstrates an understanding of the causes of tubal pregnancy

b. Describes the need for careful health assessment during any future pregnancy
5. Experiences no complications
   a. Exhibits normal vital signs
   b. Exhibits no signs of bleeding
   c. Urine output is adequate

In summary, the woman who experiences a tubal ectopic pregnancy often experiences manifestations of pain, physiologic shock due to hemorrhage, and grief simultaneously. In addition to providing high-quality physical care to the patient, the nurse also must be sensitive to the sense of loss and grief that often occurs with loss of a tubal pregnancy. The patient may also express feelings of self-blame and concern for her future childbearing capacity. The patient's partner may also experience these concerns and reactions, and therefore should be included in the plan of care.

Chapter Summary

An important role of the nurse is promotion of positive practices and behaviors related to women's health. This includes providing the woman with information about the importance of regular gynecologic examinations for promotion of health and early detection of problems, assessing for problems related to gynecologic and reproductive function and discussing questions or concerns related to sexual function and sexuality. Providing an open, nonjudgmental environment is critical if the woman is to feel comfortable discussing these personal issues. The nurse must convey to the patient understanding and sensitivity about these issues and must be knowledgeable about their impact on the woman and her partner.

The patient who experiences a disorder related to the reproductive system is often distressed, anxious, and embarrassed because of the personal or private nature of reproduction and sexuality. The woman who experiences such disorders requires quality nursing care and understanding and sensitivity to the patient's psychological reactions.

Bibliography

Books

Barger M (ed). Protocols for Gynecologic and Obstetric Health Care. Orlando, Grune & Stratton, 1988.

Campbell J and Humphreys J. Nursing Care of Victims of Family Violence. Reston, VA, Reston Publishing, 1984.

Cefalo R and Moos M-K. Preconceptional Health Promotion: A Practical Guide. Rickville, MD, Aspen Systems, 1988.

Chihal H. Premenstrual Syndrome: A Clinic Manual, 2nd ed. Dallas, Essential Medical Information Systems, 1990

Cunningham F et al. Obstetrics, 18th ed. Norwalk, CT, Appleton & Lange, 1989

Dickey R. Managing Contraceptive Pill Patients, 6th ed. Durant, OK, Creative Infomatics, 1990.

Doress P and Siegal D. The Midlife and Older Women Book Project, New York, Touchstone, 1987.

Emans S and Goldstein D. Pediatric and Adolescent Gynecology. Boston, Little, Brown & Co, 1990.

Fogel C and Lauver D. Sexual Health Promotion. Philadelphia, WB Saunders, 1990.

Gillis C et al. Toward a science of family nursing. Menlo Park, CA, Addison-Wesley, 1989.

Hatcher R et al. Contraceptive Technology, 1990–1992, 15th ed. Irvington, NY, Irvington Publishers, 1990.

Hawkins J et al. Protocols for Nurse Practitioners in Gynecologic Settings, 2nd ed. New York, Tiresias Press, 1988.

Hollingsworth D and Resnik R. Medical Counseling Before Pregnancy. New York, Churchill Livingstone, 1988

Hoole A et al. Patient Care Guidelines for Nurse Practitioners. Boston, Little, Brown & Co, 1988.

Jensen M and Bobak I. Maternity and Gynecologic Care: The Nurse and The Family, 4th ed. St Louis, CV Mosby, 1989.

Lichtman R and Papera S. Gynecology: Well-Woman Care. Norwalk, CT, Appleton & Lange, 1990.

Menning B. Infertility: A Guide for the Childless Couple. New Jersey, Prentice-Hall, 1988.

Moore K (ed). Public Health Policy Implications of Abortion: A Government Relations Handbook for Health Professionals. ACOG, 1990.

Niswander K (ed). Manual of Obstetrics, 3rd ed. Boston, Little, Brown & Co, 1988

Overall C. Ethics and Human Reproduction: A Feminist Analysis. Boston, Allen & Unwin, 1987.

Pernoll M and Benson R. Current Obstetric and Gynecologic Diagnosis and Treatment, 7th ed. Norwalk CT, Appleton & Lange, 1991.

Precis 3: An Update in Obstetrics and Gynecology. American College of Obstetricians and Gynecologists, Washington, DC, 1986.

Raff V and Friesner A. Quick Reference to Maternity Nursing. Rockville, MD, Aspen Systems, 1989.

Salzer LP. Infertility: How Couples Can Cope. Boston, GK Hall, 1986.

Shapiro C. Infertility and Pregnancy Loss: A Guide for Helping Professionals. San Francisco, Jossey-Bass, 1988.

Speroff L et al. Clinical Gynecologic Endocrinology and Infertility, 4th ed. Baltimore, Williams & Wilkins, 1989.

Stewart F et al. Understanding Your Body. Toronto, Bantam, 1987.

Journals

Asterisks indicate nursing research articles.

General Articles

Andrist L. Taking a sexual history and educating clients about safe sex. Nurs Clin North Am 1988 Dec; 23(4):959–973.

Brundage J and Pacholski C. Guiding Young Women's Health. NAACOG's Clin Iss Perinatal Health 1991; 2(2):271–277.

Edelman D. Diethylstilbestrol exposure and risk of clear cell carcinoma. Int J Fertil 1989 Jul/Aug; 34(4):251–255.

Gimpelson R. Office hysteroscopy: Indications and limitations. Female Patient 1989 May; 14(5):14–24.

Home Study Program on Well Women Gynecology. J Nurse Midwifery 1990 Nov/Dec; 35(6):339–384.

Jennings C. Corner on issues: Raising consciousness about women's health issues. J Am Acad Nurse Pract 1991 Apr/Jun; 3(2):92–94.

Maximovich A. Minimal endometriosis: When to treat. Fam Pract 1989 Jul; 14(7):51–58.

McBride A. Mental health effects of women's multiple roles. Image: Journal of Nursing Scholarship 1988 Spring; 20(1):41–47.

Modica M and Timor-Tritsch I. Transvaginal sonography provides a sharper view into the pelvis. JOGNN 1988 Mar/Apr; 17(2):89–95.

Schnarch D. Inhibited sexual desire: Diagnostic and treatment strategies. Female Patient 1989; 14(4):83–88.

Sheahan S. Identifying female sexual dysfunctions. Nurse Pract 1989 Feb; 14(2):25–34.

Smith M and Heaton D. Health concerns of lesbian women. Female Patient 1989 Jul; 14(7):43–74.

Shattuck J. Pelvic inflammatory disease: Education for maintaining fertility. Nurs Clin North Am 1988 Dec; 23(4):899–906.

Premenstrual Syndrome

Beckley F. The essential role of nurses in PMS management. OB/Gyn Nurs Pt Counsel 1991 Winter; 3(1):6–7.

Budhoff P. Use of prostaglandin inhibitors in the treatment of PMS. Clin Obstet Gynecol 1987 Jun; 30(2):453–464.

Cerrato P. Dietary help for PMS patients. RN 1988 Jan; 51(1):69–71.

Chisley J and Levy K. The media construct a menstrual monster: A content analysis of PMS articles in the popular press. Women Health 1990 Feb; 16(2):89–104.

Cortese J and Brown M. Coping responses of men whose partners experience premenstrual symptomatology. JOGNN 1989 Sep/Oct; 18(5): 405–412.

Freeman E et al. Effects of medical history factors on symptom severity in women meeting criteria for premenstrual syndrome. Obstet Gynecol 1988 Aug; 72(2):236–239.

Keye W. General evaluation of premenstrual symptoms. Clin Obstet Gynecol 1987 Jun; 30(2):396–407.

Magos A and Studd J. A simple method for the diagnosis of premenstrual syndrome by use of a self-assessment disk. Am J Obstet Gynecol 1988 May; 158(5):1024–1028.

Robinson G. Premenstrual syndrome: Current knowledge and management. Can Med Assoc J 1989 Mar 15; 140(6):605–611.

Rubinow D and Schmidt J. Models for the development and expression of symptoms in premenstrual syndrome. Psychiatr Clin North Am 1989 Mar; 12(1):53–68.

Walton J and Youngkin E. The effect of a support group on self-esteem of women with premenstrual syndrome. JOGNN 1987 May/Jun; 16(3): 174–178.

Winter E et al. Dispelling myths: A study of PMS and relationship satisfaction. Nurse Pract 1991 May; 16(3):34–45.

Woods N. Premenstrual symptoms: Another look. Public Health Rep [Suppl] 1987 Jul/Aug; 106–112.

Diagnostic Evaluation

Beal M. Understanding cervical cytology. Nurse Pract 1987 Mar; 12(3): 15–22.

Enterline E and Leonardo J. Condylomata accuminata. Nurse Pract 1989 Apr; 14(8):8–16.

McQuiston C. The relationship of risk factors for cervical cancer and HPV in college women. Nurse Pract 1989 Apr; 14(4):18–26.

Nelson J et al. Cervical intra-epithelial neoplasia (dysplasia and carcinoma in situ) and early invasive cervical carcinoma. CA 1989 May; 39(3): 157–178.

Piver M. Preventing deaths from cervical cancer: The Papanicolaou smear controversy. Female Patient 1988 Oct; 13(10):19–37.

Menstruation

Connell A. Abnormal uterine bleeding. Nurse Pract 1989 Apr; 14(4):44–57.

* Heitkemper M et al. Gastrointestinal symptoms and bowel patterns across the menstrual cycle in dysmenorrhea. Nurs Res 1988 Mar/Apr; 37(2): 108–113.

* Heitkemper M et al. GI symptoms, function and psychophysiological arousal in dysmenorrheic women. Nurs Res 1991 Jan/Feb; 40(1):20–26.

Kelly J and Hatfield S. Menstrual irregularities and bone loss in female athletes. Fam Pract 1989; 17(7):35–39.

Murata J. Abnormal genital bleeding and secondary amenorrhea: Common gynecological problems. JOGNN 1990 Jan/Feb; 19(1):26–36.

Moghissi K. Secondary amenorrhea: Treatment decisions. Female Patient 1989 Feb; 14(2):95–98.

Treybig M. Primary dysmenorrhea or endometriosis. Nurse Pract 1989 May; 14(5):8–18.

Menopause and Postmenopause

Ausenhus M. Osteoporosis: Prevention during the adolescent and young adult years. Nurse Pract 1988 Sep; 13(9):42–48.

Denny M et al. Gynecological health needs of elderly women. J Gerontol Nurs 1989 Jan; 15(1):33–38.

* Dickson GL. The metalanguage of menopause research. Image: Journal of Nursing Scholarship 1990 Fall; 22(3):168–173.

* Dickson G. A feminist poststructuralist analysis of the knowledge of menopause. Adv Nurs Sci 1990 Mar; 12(3):15–31.

Miller P. New hope for osteoporosis. Female Patient 1990 Jan; 15(1):49–61.

Notelovitz M. Women and the climacteric: Ensuring physical and mental wellness. Clin Nurs Pract 1989 Summer; 7(2):6–11.

Piziak V. Osteoporosis: What can be done. Female Patient 1989 Feb; 14(2): 57–68.

Resnick N and Greenspan S. "Senile" osteoporosis reconsidered. JAMA 1989 Feb 17; 261(7):1025–1029.

Conception Control

Breckholdt M et al. Oral contraception in disease states. Am J Obstet Gynecol 1990 Dec; 163(6 pt 2):2213–2216.

Brokaw A et al. Fitting the cervical cap. Nurse Pract 1988 Jul; 13(7):49–55.

Connell E. Barrier contraceptives: Their time has returned. Female Patient 1989 May; 14(5):66–75.

Connell E. Contraceptive advances. Part 1. Hormonal methods. Female Patient 1989 Dec; 14(12):29–36.

Duchin S et al. Oral contraceptives: Risks, benefits and guidelines. Patient Care 1989 Mar; 23(6):89–111.

Durant RH et al. Contraceptive behavior among sexually active Hispanic adolescents. J Adolesc Health Care 1990 Nov; 11(6):490–496.

Franklin M. Recently approved and experimental methods of contraception. J Nurse Midwifery 1990 Nov/Dec; 35(6):365–376.

Grimes D. IUD insertion: A clinical refresher. Female Patient 1989 Feb; 14(2):51–54.

* Hughes C and Torre C. Predicting effective contraceptive behavior in college females. Nurse Pract 1987 Sep; 12(9):44–54.

Jarrett M et al. The contraceptive needs of midlife women. Nurse Pract 1990 Dec; 15(12):34–39.

Kjersgaard A. Male or female sterilization: A comparative study. Fertil Steril 1989 Mar; 51(3):439–445.

Lethbridge D. The use of breastfeeding as a contraceptive. JOGNN 1989; 18(1):31–37.

* Loucks A. A comparison of satisfaction with types of diaphragms among women in a college population. JOGNN 1989; 18(3):194–200.

* Norris A. Cognitive analysis of contraceptive behavior. Image: Journal of Nursing Scholarship 1988 Fall; 20(3):135–139.

North B. Age appropriate contraceptive counseling for women. Med Aspects Hum Sexuality 1989; 23(7):22–28.

Rosenfield A. RU 486 and the politics of reproduction. Female Patient 1989 Feb; 14(2):69–74.

Sonenstein F et al. Sexual activity, condom use and AIDS awareness among adolescent males. Fam Plann Perspect 1989; 21(4):152–158.

Infertility

Bernstein J et al. Psychological status of previously infertile couples after a successful pregnancy. JOGNN 1988 Nov/Dec; 17(6):404–408.

* Blenner JL. Passage through infertility treatment: A state theory. Image: Journal of Nursing Scholarship 1990 Fall; 22(3):153–158.

Davis D and Dearman C. Coping strategies of infertile women. JOGNN 1991 May/Jun; 20(3):221–228.

Hirsch A and Hirsch S. The effect of infertility on marriage and self concept. JOGNN 1989 Jan/Feb; 18:13–20.

Kempers R (ed). The infertile woman. Obstet Gynecol Clin North Am 1987 Dec; 14(4):1–XXX.

* Milne B. Couples experiences with in vitro fertilization. JOGNN 1988 Sep/Oct; 17(5):347–351.

* Olshansky E. Responses to high tech infertility treatment. Image: Journal of Nursing Scholarship 1988 Fall; 20(3):128–131.

Ory S. Keeping up to date on donor insemination. Contemp Obstet Gynecol 1989; 33(3):88–112.

Owens S. Gamete intra-fallopian transfer. JOGNN 1989 Mar/Apr; 18(2): 93–97.

Update on infertility: A symposium. J Reprod Med 1989 Feb; 34(2):117–155.

Pregnancy Preparation

Chez R. Identifying maternal/fetal risks before pregnancy. Med Aspects Human Sexuality 1991 Apr; 25(4):66–71.

Jimenez S. Starting a preconception class. Childbirth Educ 1989; 8(4):46–49.

Why it's important to help patients prepare for pregnancy: A symposium. Contemp Obstet Gynecol 1989; 33(6):64–85.

Abortion

Atrash H et al. Legal abortion in the U.S.: Trends and mortality. Contemp Obstet Gynecol 1990 Feb; 35(2):58–69.

Franco K et al. Psychological profile of dysphoric women post-abortion. JAMWA 1989; 44(4):113–115.

Kissling F. The abortion debate: Moving forward. Conscience 1991 Jan/Feb; 12(2):1–3.

Llewellyn S and Pytches R. An investigation of anxiety following termination of pregnancy. J Adv Nurs 1988 Jul; 13(4):468–471.

* Wells N. Management of pain during abortion. J Adv Nurs 1989 Jan; 14(1):56–62.

Ectopic Pregnancy

Barber H. Ectopic pregnancy: A diagnostic challenge. Female Patient 1989 Apr; 14(4):113.

Davis K et al. Ectopic pregnancy: What to do during the 20 day window. J Reprod Med 1989 Feb; 34(2):162–166.

Battered Women

Bachman G. Childhood sexual abuse and the consequences in adult women. Obstet Gynecol 1988 Apr; 71(4):631–642.

* Campbell J. A test of two explanatory models of women's responses to battering. Nurs Res 1989 Jan/Feb; 38(1):18–23.

Campbell J and Alford P. The dark consequences of marital rape. Am J Nurs 1989 Jul; 89(7):946–949.

Chez R. Woman battering. Am J Obstet Gynecol 1988; 158(1):1–4.

Helton A. Battering during pregnancy. Am J Nurs 1986; 86(8):910–913.

* Weingourt R. Wife rape in a sample of psychiatric patients. Image: Journal of Nursing Scholarship 1990 Fall; 22(3):144–147.

Information/Resources

Agencies

American College of Obstetricians and Gynecologists
    600 Maryland Avenue SW, Washington, DC 20024-2588

American Infertility Society
    2131 Magnolia Ave Suite 201, Birmingham, AL 35256

Association for Voluntary Sterilization
    708 Third Ave, New York, NY 10017

National Abortion Rights Action League
    825 15th St NW, Washington, DC 2005

National Coalition Against Domestic Violence
    PO Box 15127, Washington, DC 2003-0127

Nurses Association of the American College of Obstetricians and Gynecologists
    409 12th Street SW, Washington, DC 20024-2191

Planned Parenthood Federation of America
    810 Seventh Ave, New York, NY 10019

Resolve, Inc.
    P.O. Box 474, Belmont, MA 02178

45

Management of Patients With Disorders of the Female Reproductive System

Chapter Outline

Learning Objectives

On completion of this chapter, the learner will be able to:

1. Compare the various types of vaginal infections and the risk factors associated with each type

2. Develop an educational program for the patient with vaginal infection

3. Use the nursing process as a framework for the care of the patient with a vulvovaginal infection

4. Use the nursing process as a framework for the care of the patient with genital herpesvirus infection

5. Describe nursing implications for prevention and management of toxic shock syndrome and the rationale for each intervention

6. Use the nursing process as a framework for the care of the patient with toxic shock syndrome

7. Compare the malignant disorders of the female reproductive tract

8. Use the nursing process as a framework for the care of the patient undergoing hysterectomy

9. Describe indications for vulvectomy and the preoperative and postoperative nursing interventions

10. Use the nursing process as a framework for the care of the patient undergoing vulvectomy

11. Compare nursing interventions indicated for the patient undergoing radiation therapy and chemotherapy for malignancy of the female reproductive tract

Infections of the Female Reproductive System

Vulvovaginal Infections

Overview and Prevention

The vagina is protected against infection by its normally low pH (3.5 to 4.5), which is maintained by the actions of Döderlein's bacilli (a part of the normal vaginal flora) and the hormone estrogen. The risk of infection is greater if the woman's resistance is lowered, the pH is altered, and the number of invading organisms is increased.

Vulvovaginal disorders are common problems in women. The nurse has a key role in providing information that will assist in preventing and treating many of these conditions. Young girls and women need to understand female anatomy, proper personal hygiene, and the advantages of absorbent cotton underwear.

The epithelium of the vagina is highly responsive to estrogen, which induces the formation of glycogen. The breakdown of glycogen into lactic acid produces a low vaginal pH. When estrogen decreases, such as during lactation and menopause, there is a decrease in glycogen. In adolescents or young women who take oral contraceptives, the normal vaginal flora and glycogen formation are reduced. Compounding the problem, many in this age group develop acne for which tetracycline is prescribed; this drug further destroys the normal vaginal flora, which are needed to maintain the lower pH that inhibits the growth of most organisms. With reduction in glycogen formation, infections are common and require careful diagnosis for proper treatment to be prescribed.

As the vaginal epithelium matures during the reproductive years, other causative factors initiate infections, such as sexual intercourse with an infected partner, poor feminine hygiene, and the wearing of tight, nonabsorbent, and heat-retaining clothing.

During the perimenopausal period, when estrogen production ceases, the vaginal labia and tissue may become atrophied and fragile, making the area more susceptible to injury and infection.

Risk factors for vulvovaginal infections are summarized in Chart 45-1.

Vulvitis, Leukorrhea, and Nonspecific Vaginitis

Vulvitis, an inflammation of the vulva, usually occurs in conjunction with other or systemic disorders, such as a dermatologic problem, poor hygiene, or sexually transmitted disease (STD), or it may be secondary to a specific vaginitis.

Vaginitis, an inflammation of the vagina, occurs when candida, *Trichomonas*, or bacterial vaginosis, previously called *Gardnerella* vaginalis and nonspecific bacterial vaginitis, invade the vagina. The normal whitish vaginal discharge (known as *leukorrhea*), which occurs in slight amounts during ovulation or just before menarche or the onset of menstruation, becomes more profuse when vaginitis occurs. Often vaginitis is accompanied by urethritis because of the proximity of the urethra to the vagina. The discharge may cause itching, redness, burning, and edema, which may be aggravated by voiding and defecation.

Treatment for vaginitis may be directed toward enhancing the natural flora of the vagina. This can be accomplished by a weak acid douche, 15 ml of vinegar to 1 liter of warm water (1 tablespoon of white vinegar to 1 quart of warm water), to restore acidity.

Disadvantages of douching are the potential introduction of bacteria upward and further erosion of the natural flora. If patients are instructed to douche, they must be advised to use low pressure. Whether using disposable bottles or reusable irrigating equipment, douches must always be introduced with minimal pressure. If disposable bottles are evacuated with force, or if irrigating equipment is used by holding it at an elevated level, bacteria may be forced upward into the cervix and may possibly infect the pelvis. Patients are instructed to douche, if necessary, in a supine position, using minimal pressure.

Once a diagnosis has been made, local intravaginal applications of appropriate medication may be dispensed from a tube with an applicator. The applicator is inserted into the vagina, and medication is expressed in the desired amount. Hydrocortisone vulvar ointment or cream may be applied locally, as prescribed, for symptomatic relief of itching or irritation.

Specific Vaginal Infections

Specific vaginal infections include candidiasis, bacterial vaginosis, and trichomoniasis (Table 45-1). Chlamydial infections usually affect the cervix.

Chart 45-1
Risk Factors for Vulvovaginal Infections

Premenarche	Allergies
Pregnancy	Oral contraceptives
Perimenopause	Broad-spectrum antibiotics
Poor personal hygiene	Diabetes mellitus
Tight undergarments	Low estrogen levels
Synthetic clothing	Intercourse with infected partner
Frequent douching	Oral–genital contact (yeast can inhabit the mouth and intestinal tract)

TABLE 45–1. *Vaginal Infections*

Condition	Cause	Clinical Manifestations	Management Goals
Candidiasis	*Candida albicans, glabrata,* or *tropicalis*	Inflammation of vaginal epithelium producing itching, reddish irritation White, cheeselike discharge clinging to epithelium	Eradicate the fungus by administration of an antifungal agent. Frequently used brand names of vaginal creams and suppositories are Monistat, Femstat, Terazol, and Gyne-Lotrimin Review other causative factors (*i.e.,* antibiotic therapy, nylon underwear, tight clothing, pregnancy, oral contraceptives) Determine whether diabetes is present in those with recurrent monilia
Gardnerella-associated bacterial vaginosis or nonspecific vaginitis	*Gardnerella vaginalis* and vaginal anaerobes	Usually no edema or erythema of vulva or vagina. Grayish white to yellow-white discharge clinging to external vulva and vaginal walls	Administer metronidazole, with instructions about avoiding alcohol while taking this medication If infection is recurrent, treat partner
Trichomonas vaginalis vaginitis (STD)	*Trichomonas vaginalis*	Inflammation of vaginal epithelium, producing burning and itching Frothy yellowish white or yellowish brown vaginal discharge	Remove exudate, relieve inflammation, restore acidity, and reestablish normal bacterial flora: oral metronidazole for patient and partner
Bartholinitis (infection of greater vestibular gland)	*Escherichia coli* *Trichomonas vaginalis* *Staphylococcus* *Streptococcus* Gonococcus	Erythema around vestibular gland Swelling and edema Development of vestibular gland abscess	Drain the abscess; provide antibiotic therapy; excise gland of patients with chronic bartholinitis
Cervicitis: acute and chronic	Chlamydia Gonorrhea *Streptococcus* Many pathogenic bacteria	Profuse purulent vaginal discharge Backache Urinary frequency and urgency	Determine the cause: perform cytologic examination of cervical smear and appropriate cultures Eradicate the gonococcus, if present: penicillin (as directed) or spectinomycin or tetracycline, if patient is allergic to penicillin Tetracycline, Vibramycin to eradicate chlamydia Eradicate other causes: cervical cauterization.
Atrophic vaginitis	Lack of estrogen; glycogen deficient	Discharge and irritation with alkaline *p*H of vaginal secretions	Provide estrogen therapy for vaginal epithelialization; provide topical vaginal estrogen therapy; improve nutrition if necessary; relieve dryness through use of Replens

Candidiasis

Candidiasis is a fungal infection caused by *Candida albicans.* This organism is frequently a normal inhabitant of the mouth, throat, large intestine, and vagina; it propagates in areas that are moist and warm, such as in mucous membranes and folds of tissue. *C. albicans* is also found in patients who have been on penicillin, cephalosporin, or tetracycline therapy and other antibiotics, because these medications alter natural protective organisms usually present in the vaginal tract. Clinical infection may occur during pregnancy, with a systemic condition such as diabetes mellitus, or when the patient is taking steroids or oral contraceptives. Other varieties have also been implicated as causative organisms.

Clinical manifestations are a vaginal discharge that causes intense pruritus; is irritating, watery, and tenacious; and may contain white, cheesy particles. A burning sensation may follow urination, especially if there is excoriation from scratching. Symptoms are often more severe just before menstruation, but are more refractory (less yielding to treatment) during pregnancy. Diagnosis is made by identifying the spores on a wet potassium hydroxide slide.

Management. The goal is to eliminate this infection. Assessment of the patient includes identifying any underlying factors that may contribute to the overgrowth of candidal organisms, such as pregnancy, diabetes, or use of estrogenic or oral contraceptive medications.

Preferred medications are antifungal agents such as miconazole, nystatin (Mycostatin), and clotrimazole cream; these agents may be applied internally by applicator into the vagina at bedtime for 7 nights or longer if the problem is chronic. The cream may be applied to the vulvar area for pruritus. Treatment is continued even through a menstrual cycle. Medications are most effective in a three-dose regimen or a 7-night course of treatment.

Vaginal creams effective in eliminating candidiasis or yeast infections are available without a prescription. However, patients are cautioned to use these creams only if they are certain of the diagnosis. If they are uncertain or if they have not obtained relief, they are instructed to seek health care.

Bacterial Vaginosis

Bacterial vaginosis has also been called *Gardnerella*, nonspecific, and bacterial vaginitis. It is characterized by vaginal odor that patients usually describe as fishlike. It is usually accompanied by a heavier than normal discharge and seems to be particularly noticeable after sexual intercourse. It can occur throughout the menstrual cycle and does not produce any local discomfort or pain. The discharge is gray to yellowish white. The odor can be detected readily when a drop of potassium hydroxide is added to a sample of vaginal mucus on a glass slide. Under the microscope, vaginal cells are coated with bacteria and are described as "clue cells." The *p*H of the discharge is usually above 4.7.

Management.   Metronidazole given twice a day for 1 week is effective. If patients are unable to take this medication, ampicillin or amoxicillin is used. Some practitioners treat the woman's sexual partners if the infection recurs, whereas others treat partners with an initial infection and with recurrences.

Trichomoniasis

Trichomonas vaginalis is a flagellated protozoan that causes a common sexually transmitted vaginitis. The male may be an asymptomatic carrier who harbors the organism in his urogenital tract and transmits the infection to his female partner.

Clinical manifestations include a vaginal discharge that is thin (sometimes frothy), yellow to yellow-brown, malodorous, and very irritating. An accompanying vulvitis may result, with intense vulvovaginal burning and itching. In some women, the problem tends to become chronic. It is diagnosed by microscopic detection of the pear-shaped, mobile, flagellate organisms. On inspection with a speculum, tissue may reveal vaginal erythema with multiple small petechiae ("strawberry spots"), which also can be seen on the cervix.

Management.   The most effective treatment for trichomoniasis is metronidazole (Flagyl). Both partners are treated with either a one-time loading dose or a smaller dose three times a day for 1 week. The one-time dose is more convenient, and compliance tends to be greater. The week-long treatment has occasionally been noted to be more effective. Some patients complain of an unpleasant but temporary metallic taste when taking metronidazole. Nausea and vomiting, as well as a hot, flushed feeling occur when this medication is taken in combination with an alcoholic beverage. In view of these possible side effects, the patient should be strongly advised not to drink alcohol while taking the drug.

In addition, intercourse is avoided unless a condom is used. For those who have uncomfortable side effects from metronidazole, antitrichomonal suppositories are available (*e.g.*, Vagisec Plus). Relief may be experienced, but not a complete cure. Metronidazole therapy is contraindicated in patients

with some blood dyscrasias or central nervous system diseases, women who are breast-feeding their infants, and those in the first trimester of pregnancy. Flagyl has been found to cause diminished white blood cell production. It is not prescribed without examination, and many practitioners will not prescribe Flagyl more than once within a year without first obtaining a complete blood count. Both trichomonas and bacterial vaginosis have been implicated in the occurrence of premature labor if they are not detected and treated during pregnancy.

Chlamydial Infections

Sexually transmitted infection with *Chlamydia trachomatis*, a bacterium, is on the increase (see Chap. 62). Clinical manifestations in women resemble those of gonorrhea (cervicitis and mucopurulent discharge). In males, urethritis and epididymitis are noted. Chlamydia affects the genitourinary tract and can cause dysuria. The condition also may be asymptomatic. Diagnosis can be confirmed by direct smear or culture.

The Centers for Disease Control recommends treatment with tetracycline, doxycycline, or erythromycin usually for 1 week at prescribed doses. Pregnant women are cautioned not to take tetracycline because of potential adverse effects on the fetus. Results of treatment are usually good if it is begun early enough. Possible complications from delayed treatment are tubal disease, pelvic inflammatory disease (PID), and infertility.

Gerontologic Considerations

A common postmenopausal occurrence is atrophy of the vaginal mucosa, which then becomes more prone to infection by pyogenic bacteria—*atrophic vaginitis*. An annoying leukorrhea (vaginal discharge) causes itching and burning. Management is similar to that for nonspecific bacterial vaginitis. In addition, estrogenic hormones, either taken orally or applied locally as an ointment, are effective in restoring epithelium.

◗ Nursing Process
The Patient With a Vulvovaginal Infection

◊ ### Assessment

The woman with a vulvovaginal problem should be examined soon after the onset of symptoms. As part of the preparation she is instructed not to douche, since this would alter the appearance of the vaginal mucosa and vulvar surfaces. The area is observed for erythema, edema, excoriation, and discharge. Each of the organisms producing infections appears to have its own characteristic discharge and effect (see Table 45-1). The patient is asked if there has been an increase in the amount of secretions and how she would describe any sensations, such as odor, itching, or burning. Dysuria often occurs as a result of local irritation of the urinary meatus.

Factors that may be involved should be assessed: (1) physical and chemical factors, such as increased perspiration plus decreased evaporation (from tight or synthetic clothing), antiperspirants, perfumes and powders, soaps, bubble bath, a soiled perineal area, contraceptive sponges, or suppositories and feminine hygiene products, (2) psychogenic factors; and (3) medical conditions or endocrine factors such as a predisposition for vulvar involvement in the diabetic, geriatric, or chronically ill patient. The medications the patient has been taking are noted, as some hormones and antibiotics, for example, may have altered the vaginal flora, resulting in an overgrowth of *C. albicans.*

The nurse may prepare a vaginal smear (wet mount) to assist in diagnosing the nature of the infection. A common method is for the examiner to collect vaginal secretions with a cotton-tipped applicator and place the secretions on separate glass slides. A drop of saline is added to one slide, and a drop of 10% potassium hydroxide is added to another slide. Under a microscope, if *Gardnerella* or bacterial vaginitis is present, the slide with normal saline added shows epithelial cells dotted with bacteria referred to as clue cells. If trichomonas is present, small motile cells are seen. In the presence of yeast, the potassium hydroxide slide reveals the characteristics that are typical of monilia.

▷ Nursing Diagnoses

Based on the nursing assessment and other data, the patient's major nursing diagnoses may include the following:

- Pain and discomfort related to burning or itching from the infectious process
- High risk for reinfection or spread of infection
- Knowledge deficit about proper hygiene and preventive measures

▷ Planning and Implementation

▷ *Goals:* The major goals of the patient may include relief of pain and discomfort; prevention of reinfection, complications, and infection of sexual partner; and acquisition of knowledge about methods for preventing vulvovaginal infections and managing self-care.

▷ Nursing Interventions

▷ *Relief of Discomfort and Pain.* Vulvovaginal conditions are treated on an outpatient basis, unless the patient has other medical problems. Tact and gentleness are important. Psychosocial comfort is also significant because many women express embarrassment and even guilt that the infection may have been acquired from a sex partner. In some instances, treatment plans may include the partner.

The nurse's role is to reinforce instructions for warm perineal irrigations that can provide comfort and also cleanse the infected area if indicated. Irrigations are also occasionally recommended after each voiding and defecation. A sitz bath may be taken in a bathtub or with the use of a small disposable unit that fits over the toilet seat. If chafing of the upper thighs is present, a dusting of cornstarch powder may alleviate the discomfort.

Generally, sexual intercourse is discouraged until a cure is achieved. Use of a condom is suggested to prevent reinfection and irritation of sensitive tissues. If dyspareunia is experienced, the woman is counseled about other ways of showing affection and achieving sexual satisfaction.

▷ *Prevention of Reinfection or Spread of Infection.* One of the basic goals of preventing reinfection is to reduce tissue irritation due to scratching or wearing tight clothing. The area is to be kept clean by daily bathing and adequate cleansing after voiding and defecation.

In postmenopausal patients, the level of naturally secreted estrogen decreases. Vaginal mucosal cells and vulvar skin lose glycogen. Vaginal acidity declines, and the atrophic tissues become more fragile and susceptible to trauma and infection. Therefore, gentleness and proper lubricating ointments are essential.

In teaching the patient how to use medications such as suppositories and applicators to dispense cream or ointment, the nurse may demonstrate by using a model of the pelvis. The importance of handwashing is stressed before and after administration of each medication. To prevent loss of medication from the vagina, the patient should lie down for 30 minutes after insertion. If there is some medication seepage, a perineal pad is worn to prevent soilage of clothing. When certain drugs are prescribed, the nurse can instruct the patient about appropriate precautions. For example, tetracycline, if prescribed for infection with chlamydia, is taken 1 to 2 hours after meals and not with dairy products, iron, or other mineral-containing substances. In addition, sunlight exposure should be avoided when this medication is taken. In general, long-term use of antibiotics should be avoided to prevent candidiasis, which can result when normal flora are destroyed by the antibiotics.

▷ *Patient Education and Self-Care.* In addition to reviewing ways of preventing reinfection, the nurse assesses the individual learning needs of the patient relative to the immediate problem. The patient needs to know the characteristics of a normal versus abnormal discharge. Questions often arise about douching. Normally, douching is unnecessary, because daily bathing and proper cleaning after voiding and defecation keep the perineal area clean. Many patients are misinformed about the presumed necessity for douching or using feminine hygiene products. Douching has a tendency to eliminate normal flora; this tends to reduce the woman's ability to ward off infection. Repeated douching may result in vaginal epithelial breakdown and chemical irritation. Douching may be recommended and prescribed, however, to reduce unpleasant, abnormal odors, to remove excessive discharge, to change the *p*H (such as vinegar douches), and to serve as an antiseptic irrigating solution. The procedure is reviewed with the patient, as is the care and cleaning of equipment so that it is properly disinfected.

After douching, and whenever necessary, the woman should keep the perineum dry; a hair dryer turned on low is an effective aid. She is advised to wear loose-fitting cotton underwear, not tight-fitting synthetic, nonabsorbent, heat-retaining garments (pantyhose, tight pants or slacks). It is suggested that the woman also avoid wearing damp swimsuits for long periods.

Sexual intercourse should be avoided until cure is achieved. If pain during intercourse (dyspareunia) is no longer a problem, a condom may be used and efforts made not to further injure the vaginal tissue. The use of water-soluble lubricant (K-Y Jelly) decreases excoriation. If infection recurs, it may be necessary to repeat the treatment regimen and to treat the partner.

▷ Evaluation

Expected Outcomes

1. Experiences reduced pain and discomfort
   a. Cleans the perineum as prescribed
   b. Reports that itching is relieved
   c. Has normal vital signs
   d. Urine output is within normal limits

2. Is free from infection
   a. Has no signs of inflammation, pruritus, odor, or dysuria
   b. Notes vaginal discharge appears normal (thin, clear, non-frothy)
   c. Reports that her partner is free from infection
3. Participates in self-care
   a. Takes medication as prescribed
   b. Wears absorbent underwear
   c. Avoids unprotected sexual intercourse
   d. Douches only as prescribed

Human Papillomavirus

Human papillomavirus (HPV) infection causes an STD that most commonly results in small, warty growths on the vulva, labia, cervix, vaginal walls or rectum. Some strains (numbers 16, 18, and 31) of the virus are associated with cervical cancer. Treatment is necessary to eradicate these growths, although a few resolve spontaneously. Treatment modalities include trichloroacetic acid and cautery or laser treatment.

Patients should have Pap smears every 6 months for several years after this diagnosis because of the propensity of this virus to cause dysplasia. Male partners should be evaluated by a urologist, because HPV lesions may be difficult to visualize. If a partner has a small lesion that is invisible to him, intercourse may result in reinfection of his treated partner. Urologists may use a colposcope or an application of acetic acid, followed by magnified inspection.

Herpesvirus Type 2 Infection (Herpes Genitalis, Herpes Simplex Virus)

Herpes genitalis is a viral infection that causes herpetic (blisters) lesions on the cervix, vagina, and external genitalia; it is an STD but also may be transmitted asexually from wet surfaces or by self-transmission (*i.e.*, touching a cold sore and then touching the genital area).

This form of herpes is of major concern to health care providers and consumers because of the increasing prevalence of the disease (400,000 to 500,000 new cases each year). Not only is the infection painful, it also can recur.

There is no cure at present. The condition requires accurate diagnosis, effective care, and specific measures to prevent possible complications.

Etiology and Pathophysiology.   Of the known herpesviruses, six affect humans: (1) herpes simplex type 1 (HSV-1), usually causing "cold sores" of lips; (2) herpes simplex type 2 (HSV-2); (3) varicella zoster; (4) Epstein–Barr virus; (5) cytomegalovirus; and (6) human B-lymphotropic virus (HBLV). HSV-2 appears to be the causative virus in over 80% of genital and perineal lesions; about 20% are HSV-1.

There is considerable overlap between HSV-1 and HSV-2, which are clinically indistinguishable. Close human contact via mouth, oropharynx, mucosal surface, vagina, and cervix seems necessary to acquire the infection. Other susceptible sites are skin lacerations and conjunctivae. Usually the virus is killed at room temperature by drying. When virus replication diminishes, the virus ascends the peripheral sensory nerves and remains inactive in the nerve ganglia. Another outbreak occurs when the host is subjected to stressors, such as fatigue, illness, dental work, stress, or sunburn. In pregnant women with active herpes, babies delivered vaginally may become infected with the virus. There is a high risk of significant fetal morbidity and mortality if this occurs. Cesarean section is performed if an outbreak occurs near the time of delivery.

Clinical Manifestations.   Itching and pain accompany the process as the area becomes red and edematous. The vesicular state may appear as a pimple, which later coalesces, ulcerates, and encrusts. In the female, the labia is the usual primary site, and then possibly the cervix, vagina, and perianal skin. The male is affected on the glans penis, foreskin, and penile shaft. Flulike symptoms may occur 3 or 4 days after the appearance of lesions. Inguinal lymphadenopathy, temperature elevation, malaise, headache, myalgia, and dysuria are noted. In the female, a purulent discharge may develop from a secondary bacterial infection. Pain is evident during the first week and then decreases. The lesions disappear in about 2 weeks unless they become secondarily infected.

Complications arise from extragenital spread, such as to the buttocks or upper thighs and even to the eyes as a result of touching them with hands that have not been washed. Other potential problems are aseptic meningitis, and severe psychologic stress related to the diagnosis.

Management.   There is no cure for HSV-2 infection, but treatment is aimed at relieving the symptoms. The goals are to prevent the spread of infection, to make the patient comfortable, to decrease potential health risks, and to be supportive and initiate a counseling and education program. Acyclovir (Zovirax), an antiviral agent that can alter the course of the infection, is available for topical, oral, and intravenous use. In general, acyclovir may reduce the duration of the infection and is effective in treating recurrences. Resistance and long-term side effects do not seem to be major problems. Recurrences tend to be much milder than the initial episode. Symptoms include mild perineal burning and itching.

▶ Nursing Process
The Patient With a Genital Herpesvirus Infection

▷ Assessment

The health history, physical and pelvic examination, plus collaboration with other health care personnel taking care of this patient establish the nature of the infectious condition.

▷ Nursing Diagnoses

Based on all the assessment data, the patient's major nursing diagnoses may include the following:

- Pain related to the presence of genital lesions
- High risk for reinfection or spread of infection
- Anxiety and distress related to embarrassment over the presence of the disease
- Knowledge deficit about the disease process and about methods of avoiding spread and preventing recurrences.

▷ Planning and Implementation

▷ *Goals:*   The major goals of the patient may include relief of pain and discomfort, control of infection and its spread, relief of anxiety, and knowledge of and adherence to the treatment regimen and self-care.

◊ Nursing Interventions

◊ *Relief of Pain.* The local lesions are to be kept clean, and proper hygienic practices are advocated. Small ice packs may be applied intermittently to painful areas to bring relief. Clothing should be clean, loose, soft, and absorbent. Tepid sitz baths are comforting and cleansing. Aspirin and other analgesics are effective in controlling pain. Occlusive ointments and powders are to be avoided because they prevent the lesions from drying, which in turn helps to kill the virus.

If there is considerable pain and malaise, bed rest may be required. It is necessary to assess the fluid intake of the patient, the presence of bladder distention, and the frequency of voiding. Adequate fluid intake is encouraged; voiding is assisted by pouring warm water over the vulva. Such measures help in preventing urinary retention and infection. Oral acyclovir is taken as prescribed, and side effects such as rash, headache, insomnia, acne, sore throat, muscle cramps, and lymphadenopathy are monitored but are unlikely. Rest and an appropriate diet are recommended. An indwelling urinary catheter may be necessary in severe cases of urethritis or dysuria. Voiding in a sitz bath or through an empty toilet tissue tube may lessen discomfort, as both methods keep undiluted urine from contact with the lesions.

◊ *Control of Infection.* Because herpesvirus can spread from the discharge of lesions, efforts are made to keep these areas dry. Cautious use of a hair dryer turned on low and cool is comforting and drying. Acyclovir ointment as prescribed may be applied locally to the lesions four or five times daily to control the spread of infection and to hasten healing. For general methods of preventing the spread of the infection, see the recommendations mentioned in the next section on self-care instruction. Acyclovir taken four or five times a day for a week may be prescribed.

◊ *Patient Education.* The problems of genital herpes are both physical and psychological. Usually, the patient experiences a great deal of stress on learning the diagnosis, and this in itself aggravates the problem. Therefore, when counseling the patient, the nurse should review the causes of the condition and the manner in which it progresses. The client's questions are encouraged because such questions indicate a receptive time to learn. The highly individual nature of the disease, its widespread incidence, the prevention of complications, and promising research findings are discussed. The nurse can reassure the patient that in a few weeks she will be able to function normally both socially and sexually. Self-care measures for the person with genital herpes are listed in Chart 45-2.

◊ Evaluation

Expected Outcomes

1. Experiences minimal pain and discomfort
   a. Takes aspirin/analgesic/acyclovir as prescribed
   b. Rests and conserves energy
   c. Uses warm sitz baths
   d. Wears clean, loose, cotton clothing
   e. Abstains from sexual activity while symptomatic
   f. Develops a plan for relaxation and stress reduction
2. Keeps infection under control
   a. Practices proper hygienic techniques
   b. Washes hands after going to the bathroom/cleansing perineum to avoid transmitting the virus to other areas, especially the eyes
   c. Avoids use of occlusive ointments
3. Acquires knowledge about genital herpes
   a. Defines the limitations of social and sexual practices as the condition permits
   b. Describes intent to follow proper health habits and to control stress
   c. Indicates a willingness to arrange for follow-up care if necessary

Chart 45-2
Patient Education and Self-Care for Genital Herpes

- Herpes is transmitted mainly by direct contact; abstinence is required for a brief period.
- Control of the condition will not require a major life-style change. Intercourse is avoided during treatment, but hand-holding and kissing are permissible.
- Women can be reassured that they can have children; their obstetricians need to know that they have the condition so they can be monitored appropriately.
- Conscientious hygienic practices of cleanliness (hand washing, perineal cleanliness) must be practiced. The patient should wear loose, comfortable clothing, eat a balanced diet, and get adequate rest and relaxation.
- Lesions should be washed gently with mild soap and running water and lightly dried
- Prolonged exposure to the sun should be avoided, as it seems to cause recurrences (and skin cancer).
- Occlusive ointments, strong perfumed soaps, or bubble bath should be avoided.
- Medications must be taken as prescribed; follow-up appointments with health care personnel should be kept, and recurrences, which are not as severe as the initial episode, reported.
- The patient is encouraged to join a group to share solutions and experiences and hear about newer treatments. Information can be obtained from HELP (Herpetics Engaged in Living Productively), 260 Sheridan Avenue, Palo Alto, CA 94306.
- Usually precautions are unnecessary in the absence of active lesions.
- Lesions away from the mouth or perineum can be covered with a dressing and an impermeable cover during intercourse; such lesions are infrequent.
- For a partner with no history of genital herpes, a condom should be used.

Toxic Shock Syndrome

Toxic shock syndrome (TSS), a condition first identified in the late 1970s, is caused by the bacterium *Staphylococcus aureus* and usually occurs in women under age 30 who are menstruating and using tampons (particularly highly absorbent tampons). Its incidence is 6 to 7 per 100,000 menstruating women. Its peak incidence occurred in 1980.

TSST-1, a protein toxin released by some strains of *S. aureus*, probably enters the bloodstream by reflux from the uterus to the tubes or through surface abrasions on the vaginal wall.

TSS also has occurred in nonmenstruating women and in men and has been associated with such conditions as cellulitis, surgical wound infections, subcutaneous abscesses, and conditions requiring nasal packing.

Clinical Manifestations.   In an otherwise healthy person, the onset of TSS occurs with a sudden fever (up to 38.9°C [102°F]), vomiting, diarrhea, myalgia, hypotension, chills, headache, palmar erythema, and signs suggesting the onset of septic shock. A red, macular rash similar to a sunburn often develops. In some patients, this rash makes its first appearance on the torso, and in others, it first appears on the hands (palms and fingers) and feet (soles and toes); it then may desquamate in 7 to 10 days. Myalgia and dizziness are common.

Urine output is decreased and the urea nitrogen level becomes elevated; such urinary dysfunction may initiate disorientation because of fluid deficit and toxins. Respiratory distress has been reported as a result of pulmonary edema.

If adult respiratory distress syndrome (ARDS) occurs, the outlook becomes grave. Inflammation of mucous membranes also may occur. Blood studies indicate leukocytosis and elevated bilirubin, urea nitrogen, and creatine values.

Two to 3% of patients with TSS die of complications.

Diagnostic Evaluation.   Blood and urine cultures are taken, along with throat cultures when appropriate. Vaginal and possibly cervical specimens also are evaluated.

Management.   The patient is placed on bed rest, and the treatment plan is directed primarily at controlling the infection with antibiotics and restoration of circulating blood volume.

If there is respiratory distress, oxygen therapy is instituted; if signs of acidosis appear, sodium bicarbonate is given. Calcium is prescribed for hypocalcemia.

Swan-Ganz catheters, intravenous dopamine, and military antishock trousers (MAST) may be used to assist in management of shock.

The entire treatment plan is adjusted according to the individual patient's condition, which may vary from mild to very acute. Certainly not overlooked are the patient's emotional and psychological concerns.

▶ Nursing Process
The Patient With Toxic Shock Syndrome

◊ Assessment

The nursing history is directed toward determining whether the patient has used tampons recently, what kind she used, how long she retained a single tampon before changing it, and whether she noted any problems when inserting the tampon, which may have injured the vaginal tissue. Sometimes, rough edges on the plastic or cardboard applicator can scratch or injure the mucosa when the tampon is inserted. The injured or broken tissue becomes an open avenue through which organisms invade the bloodstream.

◊ Nursing Diagnoses

Based on the nursing assessment and other data, the patient's major nursing diagnoses may include the following:

- Anxiety related to the severity and suddenness of the symptoms
- Fluid volume deficit related to vomiting and diarrhea
- Knowledge deficit about the use of tampons and personal hygiene

◊ Planning and Implementation

◊   *Goals:*   The major goals of the patient may include reduction of anxiety and emotional stress, absence of vomiting and diarrhea, absence of complications, and acquisition of relevant knowledge.

◊ Nursing Interventions

The nursing interventions follow the goals according to priority of needs. Emotional support and reassurance often reduce anxiety and apprehension. Close monitoring and documentation of vital signs and blood gases provide valuable indices regarding the patient's physical status. The nurse notes skin changes as well as fluid intake and loss, inasmuch as these data assist in evaluating hydration and kidney function. The patient is often critically ill and is cared for in the intensive care unit where constant monitoring and immediate response to complications are possible.

Cultures of all body excretions and of the nose, throat, vagina, and cervix are taken. The results of these studies assist the physician in prescribing appropriate antibiotic therapy.

Disseminated intravascular coagulopathy (DIC) has been observed in patients with TSS; therefore, it is essential for the nurse to be observant for hematomas; petechiae; oozing from needle puncture sites; cyanosis; and coolness of the nose, fingertips, and toes. Management of the patient with shock and DIC is described in Chapters 22 and 19, respectively.

◊   *Patient Education and Home Health Care.*   Because the use of tampons during menstruation has been linked with TSS, it is recommended that superabsorbent tampons not be used. If tampons are preferred, tampons should be changed frequently (every 4 hours). Tampons should be inserted carefully to avoid abrasions (applicators with rough edges should not be used). If a diaphragm is used, it should not be left in place longer than 6 hours. Use of tampons is discouraged if the patient has had TSS, as is use of the diaphragm or sponge during menses or in the first 3 months postpartum.

The risk of developing TSS is increased at any time a woman is bleeding vaginally, that is, during menses and postpartum.

◊ Evaluation

Expected Outcomes

1. Exhibits reduced anxiety and emotional stress
2. Is free of fluid loss and imbalance
   a. Notes absence of vomiting and diarrhea
   b. Takes adequate fluids and food

3. Exhibits absence of complications
   a. Is free of purulent discharge
   b. Has normal arterial blood gases and coagulation studies
   c. Is free of infection
4. Demonstrates awareness of self-care measures
   a. Understands the role of diet and exercise through recovery and beyond in prevention of recurrence
   b. Avoids the use of tampons after a diagnosis of TSS

Endocervicitis/Cervicitis

Endocervicitis is an inflammation of the mucosa and the glands of the cervix. It is a fairly common problem that may occur when organisms gain access to the cervical glands after intercourse, abortion, intrauterine manipulation, or delivery. It is an infection that, if untreated, may extend into the uterus, fallopian tubes, and pelvic cavity. In most patients, the inflammation is caused by ordinary pyogenic organisms, but gonorrheal and chlamydial infection of the glands can occur.

Inflammation can cause erosion of the cervical tissue, resulting in spotting or bleeding. The chief symptom is leukorrheal discharge, at times associated with sacral backache, low abdominal pain, and urinary and menstrual disturbances.

Chlamydia is frequently the bacterium causing mucopurulent cervicitis. It is estimated that between 3 and 10 million cases occur each year in the United States. It is most commonly found in young sexually active patients with more than one partner and is transmitted through sexual intercourse. It can cause pelvic infections and sterility. Chlamydial infections of the cervix are often asymptomatic, but cervical discharge, dyspareunia, dysuria, and bleeding may occur. Other complications include conjunctivitis and perihepatitis. In pregnancy, stillbirth, neonatal death, and premature labor may occur. Chlamydial infection and gonorrhea often coexist. As many as 25% of females who have chlamydial infections also have gonorrhea. Treatment is aimed at eradication of both organisms, usually with amoxicillin followed by tetracycline.

Management.   Treatment should be preventive as well as curative. Prevention of gonorrhea and chlamydial infection by condom and spermicidal use, and avoidance of partners who are unknown or who have a penile drip or discharge, reduce the incidence of endocervicitis and STDs. If chlamydia is the cause, tetracycline or doxycycline is prescribed.

Chronic cervicitis is sometimes associated with abnormal Pap smear and cervical biopsy results. If a cone biopsy is necessary, it is performed under general anesthesia. The tip of an electric instrument is inserted into the external os and rotated to cut and coagulate a cone of tissue. Packing is usually required and is removed by the physician. If cauterization or cryotherapy is necessary, these office procedures are explained to the patient. The patient is also alerted to the fact that a heavy, malodorous discharge is to be expected for up to 3 weeks because of sloughing of cervical tissue after these procedures. A follow-up visit in 2 to 3 weeks is important to check the cervical healing and to check for possible stenosis, which may require dilatation. The patient is instructed to report any heavy bleeding.

The loop electrosurgical excision procedure (LEEP) is a new method to remove abnormal cervical tissue found on colposcopic examination after an abnormal Pap smear. It is performed as an outpatient procedure and removes a button-shaped piece of tissue with relatively little discomfort and few complications.

Pelvic Infection (Pelvic Inflammatory Disease)

Pelvic infection is an inflammatory condition of the pelvic cavity that may involve the fallopian tubes (salpingitis), ovaries (oophoritis), pelvic peritoneum, or pelvic vascular system. Infection may be acute, subacute, recurrent, or chronic and may be localized or widespread. It is usually bacterial but also may be caused by a virus, fungus, or parasite.

Etiology.   Pathogenic organisms usually enter the body through the vagina, pass through the cervical canal and into the uterus, and under various conditions may proceed to one or both fallopian tubes and ovaries and into the pelvis. In bacterial infections that occur after childbirth or abortion, and in some intrauterine device–related infections, pathogens are disseminated directly through the tissues that support the uterus by way of the lymphatics and blood vessels (Fig. 45-1A). The increased blood supply required by the placenta provides more pathways for infection. These postpartal and postabortion infections tend to be unilateral.

In gonorrheal infections, the gonococci pass through the cervical canal and into the uterus, where the environment, especially during menstruation, allows them to multiply rapidly and spread to the fallopian tubes and into the pelvis (see Fig. 45-1B). The infection is usually bilateral. In rare instances, some diseases (*e.g.,* tuberculosis) gain access to the reproductive organs by way of the bloodstream from the lungs (see Fig. 45-1C).

One of the most frequent causes of salpingitis is a chlamydia infection, possibly accompanied by gonorrhea. Chlamydial infection involves the cervix and then extends upward, infecting the fallopian tubes or the uterus.

Clinical Manifestations.   The onset of pelvic infection is usually manifested by vaginal discharge, lower abdominal pelvic pain, and tenderness that occurs after the menses. The type of discharge varies with the infecting organism. It is usually heavy and purulent with gonorrhea or staphylococcal infection; with streptococcal infection, the discharge tends to be thinner and more mucoid. Systemic symptoms include fever, general malaise, anorexia, nausea, headache, and possibly vomiting. On pelvic examination, intense tenderness may be noted. Symptoms may be acute and severe or low grade and subtle. The patient is placed on broad-spectrum antibiotic therapy. Women with mild to moderately severe infections are usually treated as outpatients. Patients who are acutely ill, however, may require hospitalization.

In the hospital, intensive therapy includes bed rest, intravenous fluids to correct dehydration and acidosis, and intravenous antibiotic therapy. If abdominal distention or ileus is present, nasogastric intubation and suction are initiated. Careful monitoring of vital signs and symptoms assists in evaluating the status of the infection. Treatment of sexual partners is necessary to prevent reinfection.

Complications.   Pelvic or generalized peritonitis may develop, as may abscess formation, strictures, and obstruction of the fallopian tubes. Obstruction may result in an ectopic pregnancy in the future if a fertilized egg is unable to pass the stricture. Or, scar tissue may occlude the tubes, resulting in sterility. Adhesions are a common development that eventually may require removal of the uterus, tubes, and ovaries. Other complications include bacteremia with septic shock and thrombophlebitis with possible embolization.

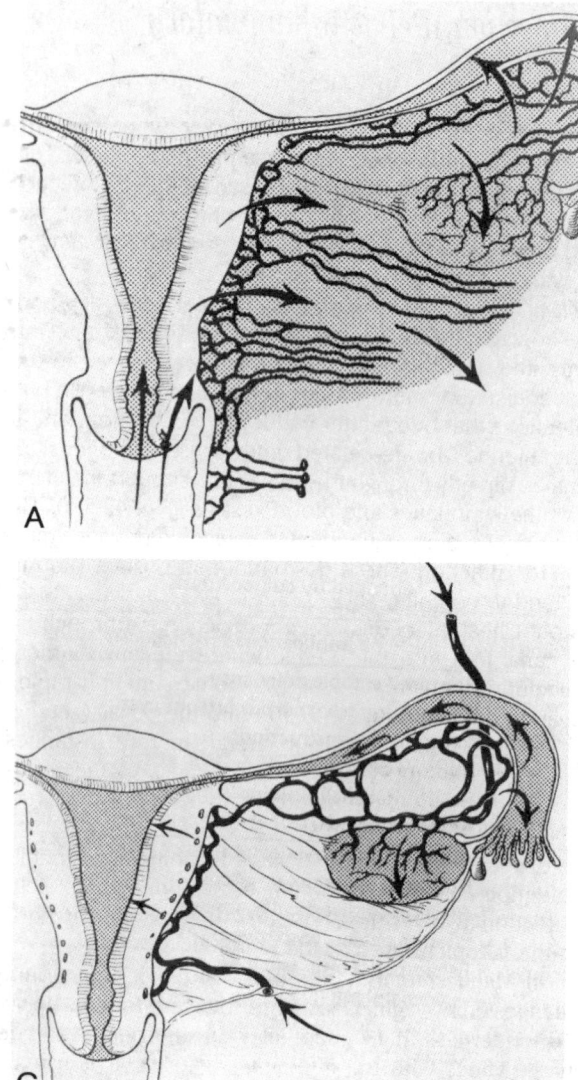

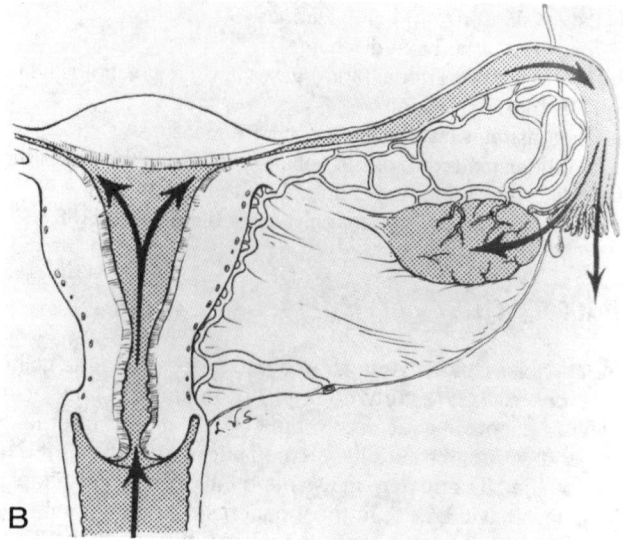

Figure 45–1. Proposed pathways of dissemination of microorganisms in pelvic infections. (**A**) Direct spread of bacterial infection other than gonorrhea (through the lymphatics). (**B**) Direct spread of gonorrhea. (**C**) Hematogenous spread of bacterial infection (*e.g.*, tuberculosis). (Pernoll M and Benson R [eds]. Current Obstetric and Gynecologic Diagnosis and Treatment, 7th ed. Norwalk, CT, Appleton & Lange, 1991.)

Nursing Interventions

Infection may be distressing, both physically and emotionally. The patient may feel well one day and experience vague symptoms and discomfort the next. She may suffer from constipation and menstrual difficulties.

The hospitalized patient is maintained on bed rest and is usually placed in semi-Fowler's position to facilitate dependent drainage. For comfort, heat (heating pad) can be applied to the abdomen externally and warm douches may be prescribed to improve local circulation. In addition, the patient is supported nutritionally and with selective antibiotic therapy as prescribed. Catheterization and the use of tampons are avoided to prevent the spread of the infection.

Proper recording of vital signs and the nature and amount of vaginal discharge are necessary as a guide to therapy.

The dissemination of infection to others can be controlled in many ways:

- Perineal pads are handled carefully with an instrument or gloves, and the soiled pad is disposed of according to hospital guidelines.
- Hands are washed carefully with a germicidal soap.

- All items that come in contact with the patient (utensils, bedpans, toilet seats, and linens) are properly disinfected by the correct procedure for controlling the specific organisms responsible for the infection.

The patient must be informed of the need for these precautions and encouraged to take part in procedures to prevent contamination of others as well as to protect herself from reinfection.

If reinfection or spread of infection occurs, symptoms may include abdominal pain, nausea and vomiting, fever, malaise, malodorous purulent vaginal discharge, and leukocytosis.

Patient Education and Home Health Care. Patient teaching consists of explaining how pelvic infections occur and how they can be controlled and avoided.

Guidelines and instructions provided to the patient include:

- Be aware that organisms can gain entrance to the reproductive area during sexual intercourse or after pelvic surgery, abortion, and childbirth.
- Realize that some users of intrauterine devices may be more susceptible to infections, particularly those with multiple partners.

- Follow proper perineal care, especially wiping from front to back.
- Do not douche frequently because this practice reduces natural flora that can combat infecting organisms.
- Wear clean, cotton, loose-fitting undergarments.
- Consult with a health care provider if unusual vaginal discharge or odor is noted.
- Avoid tampons if they have caused problems.
- Do not wear pads or tampons longer than 4 hours.
- Remember to remove a diaphragm after using it for 6 hours.
- Maintain optimal health practices with proper nutrition, exercise, weight control, and relaxation.
- Visit a gynecologist at least once a year.
- Before intercourse, insist on a partner's wearing a condom if there is any question of infection.

If a partner is not well known, or has had another partner recently, condoms are preventive. All patients who have had PID need information about the signs and symptoms of ectopic pregnancy (pain, abnormal bleeding, faintness, dizziness, and shoulder pain [see Chap. 44]).

HIV Infection and AIDS

Any discussion of vulvovaginal disorders must include the diagnosis of human immunodeficiency virus (HIV) and AIDS, described in Chapter 48.

Women with HIV accounted for almost 12% of reported HIV cases in 1990, compared with 8% in 1987. Most are in the reproductive age group, and more than 70% are black or Hispanic. Over half are IV drug users, whereas the other half have been exposed through sexual contact with HIV-infected partners.

The preexistence of any genital ulcers or lesions increases the risk of infection (*i.e.*, a herpetic lesion or syphilitic chancre could provide a portal of entry). Syphilis seems to accelerate in HIV-positive patients, proceeding directly from primary to tertiary in some patients. Chlamydia is associated with a higher rate of HIV, possibly related to inflammatory changes of the cervix, providing entry sites. HIV-positive women have a higher rate of human papillomavirus and also seem to develop larger and more painful herpes lesions with more recurrences, probably related to immunosuppression from their disease. Acyclovir is appropriate for such patients. Candidiasis is frequent in this population, and oral candidiasis may be a sign of rapid advancement of the disease.

Women with HIV must be counseled about contraception and safer sex. Because there is a 25% to 50% chance of perinatal transmission, decisions to conceive or to use contraception must be made with adequate education and care. For those who choose to avoid conception, condoms and a spermicidal agent or a condom with oral contraceptives are good choices. Risk of transmission of the virus to or from a partner will be reduced with either choice, along with protection from unwanted pregnancies.

In summary, although most infections of the female reproductive tract are not life threatening, they often cause pain, discomfort, fear, and embarrassment. The occurrence of symptoms may raise anxiety about the significance of their occurrence and fear of life-threatening disorders (*i.e.*, AIDS). The patient who acquires a vaginal infection may develop mistrust of her sexual partners, and her intimate relationships may be threatened.

The patient with a vulvovaginal infection often requires assistance to obtain relieve of symptoms and instruction about self-care measures, safer sexual practices, and hygiene measures. Additionally, she may require assistance in dealing with the psychological reactions (*i.e.*, distrust, anger, depression) that may occur in response to acquiring a vaginal infection. She also needs adequate information about the possible effects of the infection on the risk of acquiring STDs and on future childbearing. Patients who have experienced toxic shock syndrome and those who use tampons or contraceptive sponges need instruction about safe use of these products.

Structural Disorders

Fistulas of the Vagina

A fistula is an abnormal, winding opening between two internal hollow organs or between an internal hollow organ and the exterior of the body. The name of the fistula indicates the two areas that are connected abnormally; a *ureterovaginal fistula* is an opening between the ureter and vagina; a *vesicovaginal fistula*, an opening between the bladder and the vagina; and a *rectovaginal fistula*, an opening between the rectum and the vagina (Fig. 45-2).

Etiology.   Fistulas may occur congenitally; in adults, however, breakdown often occurs because of tissue damage resulting from injury sustained during surgery, delivery, radiation therapy, or disease processes such as carcinoma.

Clinical Manifestations.   The immediate problem becomes one of infection and resulting excoriation. For example, the patient who has a vesicovaginal fistula has a continuous trickling of urine into the vagina. With a rectovaginal fistula, there is fecal incontinence, and flatus is discharged through the vagina. When such a discharge combines with a leukorrhea, a malodorous condition develops that is difficult to control.

Methylene blue dye can be used to delineate the course of the fistula. In vesicovaginal fistula, the dye is instilled into the bladder and appears in the vagina. After a negative methylene blue test, indigo carmine is injected intravenously; if the dye appears in the vagina, a ureterovaginal fistula is indicated. Cystoscopy is often used to determine the exact location.

Management.   The goal is to eliminate the fistula, thereby also controlling infection and excoriation. Frequently, a fistula will heal without surgical intervention. Otherwise surgery is indicated. Usually the vaginal approach is used for vesicovaginal and urethrovaginal fistulas. The abdominal approach is used for fistulas higher in the abdomen. Fistulas that are difficult to repair or very large may require urinary or fecal diversion.

Because fistulas often are related to obstetric or surgical trauma, if these occur without the previously mentioned history of trauma, the health care provider should consider Crohn's disease or lymphogranuloma venereum (LGV) as a possible cause.

Nursing Interventions.   Nursing measures are planned to relieve discomfort, prevent infection, and improve the patient's self-perception and self-care abilities.

Healing of the tissues is promoted by proper nutrition with an increase in intake of vitamin C and protein, by local clean-

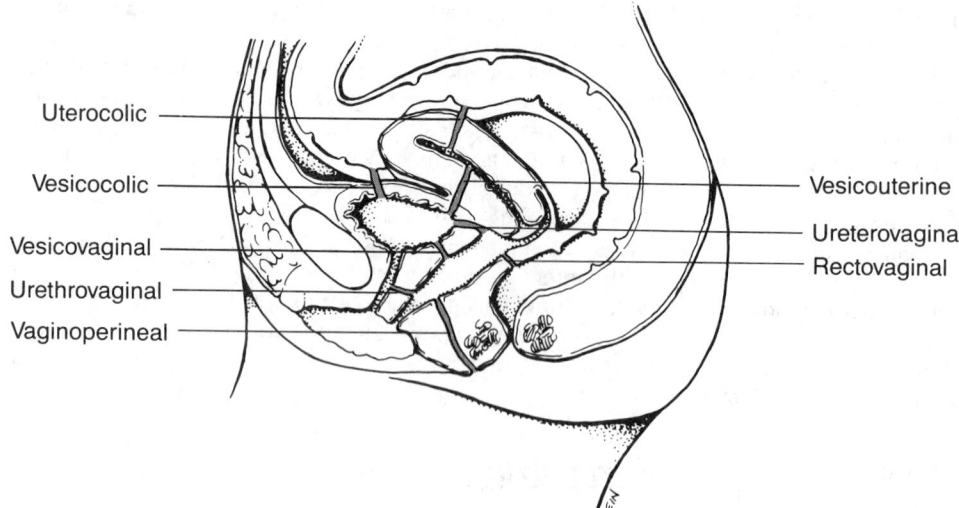

Figure 45–2. Common sites for fistulas: *Uterocolic*—uterus and colon. *Vesicocolic*—bladder and colon. *Vesicovaginal*—bladder and vagina. *Urethrovaginal*—urethra and vagina. *Vaginoperineal*—vagina and perineal area. *Vesicouterine*—bladder and uterus. *Ureterovaginal*—ureter and vagina. *Rectovaginal*—rectum and vagina.

liness through douching and enemas, by rest, and by taking prescribed intestinal antibiotics. A rectovaginal fistula will heal faster if the patient is placed on a low-residue diet and if proper drainage of affected tissues is initiated.

If the person is older, more rest is required than in most postoperative patients because of a higher incidence of debilitation and the delicate as well as sensitive nature of the tissues. Warm perineal irrigations and controlled heat-lamp treatments are effective in stimulating the healing process.

For the patient who has had repair of a vesicovaginal fistula, an indwelling catheter is usually inserted. Drainage from the catheter is observed carefully, and care is taken to ensure that the catheter is functioning properly. If the catheter becomes clogged, urine may collect in the bladder, causing pressure that may damage the repaired tissue. If prescribed, bladder irrigation and vaginal irrigations are performed gently, with minimal pressure.

Effective measures to assist the woman whose fistula cannot be repaired must be planned on an individual basis. Cleanliness, frequent sitz baths, and deodorizing douches are required, as well as the use of perineal pads and protective undergarments. Particular attention to skin care is necessary to prevent excoriation. Bland creams or a light dusting of cornstarch may be soothing. Attention to the social and psychological needs of this patient are essential components of effective care.

Despite the best surgical intervention, fistulas may recur. Preoperative treatment of any existing vaginitis is important to successful surgery. Usually, observation for 2 years is needed to evaluate successful intervention.

Cystocele, Rectocele, Enterocele, and Lacerations of the Perineum

Cystocele is a downward displacement of the bladder toward the vaginal orifice (Fig. 45-3). Occasionally it is caused by tissue weakness, but most often it is a result of injuries received during childbirth. The condition appears some years later when genital atrophy associated with aging takes place.

Rectocele and lacerations of the perineum may occur as injuries to the muscles and the tissues of the pelvic floor and may happen at the time of childbirth. Because of tears in muscles below the vagina, the rectum may pouch upward, pushing the posterior wall of the vagina in front of it. This condition is termed a rectocele. At times, the lacerations may extend to such a degree as to sever completely the fibers of the anal sphincter (complete tear). An enterocele is a protrusion of intestinal wall into the vagina.

Clinical Manifestations.   A cystocele occurs as a bulging downward of the anterior vaginal wall that causes a sense of pelvic pressure, fatigue, and often such urinary symptoms as incontinence, frequency, and urgency. Back pain (dragging and strain type) and pelvic pain are experienced.

The symptoms of rectocele are similar to those of cystocele, with one exception—instead of urinary symptoms, the patient experiences constipation and incontinence of gas and feces when complete tears have occurred.

Management.   Perineal exercises are prescribed and help to strengthen the weakened muscles. These are more effective in the early stages of a cystocele. If surgery is contraindicated, or refused, a pessary may be used. Such a device may be prescribed for mild problems.

A *pessary* is a device inserted in the upper vagina and positioned to assist in keeping on organ, such as the bladder, uterus, or intestine, in proper alignment. It is usually shaped as a ring or doughnut and is made of a variety of materials, such as rubber or plastic. The size and type of pessary are selected and fitted by the gynecologist. The patient can be taught to remove the pessary at bedtime and to reinsert it in the morning. If it remains in place and is not removed by the patient, she should have it removed, checked, and cleaned by the physician or nurse practitioner at prescribed intervals. At this time, tissues need to be inspected for pressure points or signs of irritation. Normally, there is no pain, discomfort, or discharge with its use. Douching may be recommended if there is a discharge.

Surgical Management.   The treatment of cystocele is surgical, the operation for the repair of the anterior vaginal wall being termed *anterior colporrhaphy*. The operation for the repair of rectocele and lacerations of the perineum is called a *perineorrhaphy* or a *posterior colporrhaphy*.

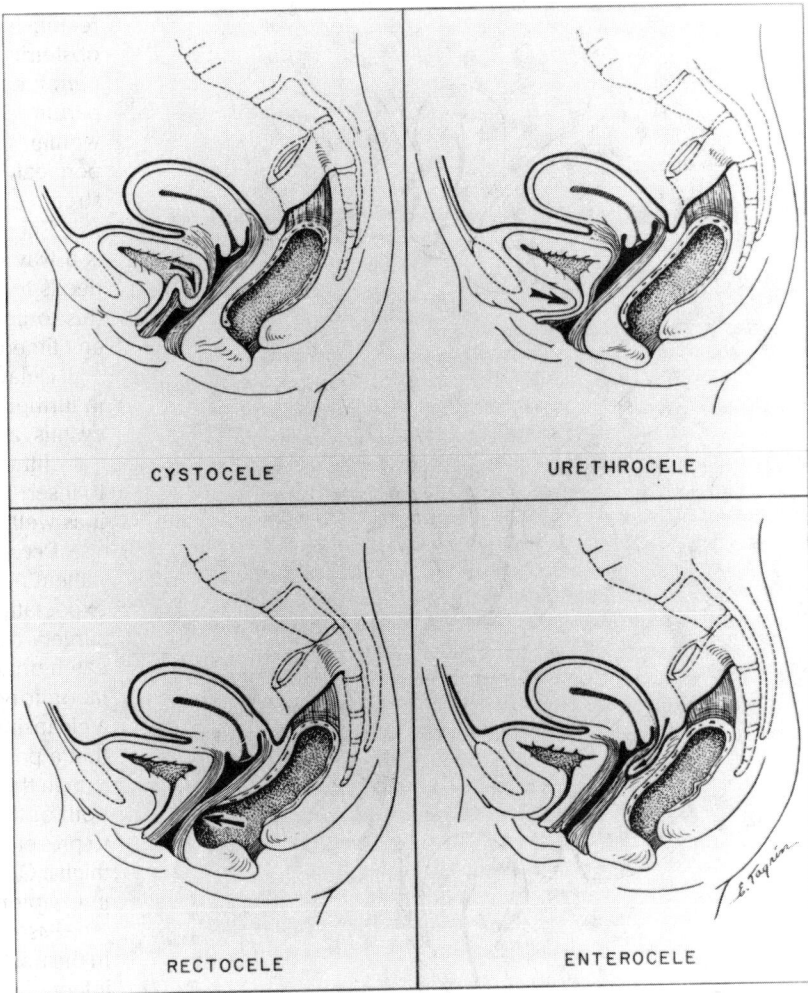

Figure 45–3. Diagrammatic representation of the four most common types of pelvic floor relaxation: cystocele, urethrocele, rectocele, and enterocele. Arrows depict sites of maximum protrusion. (Kistner RW. Gynecology: Principles and Practice, 4th ed. Chicago, Year Book Medical Publishers, 1986.)

Displacements of the Uterus

Most commonly, the uterus lies with the cervix at right angles to the long axis of the vagina and with the body of the uterus inclined slightly forward. However, it is freely movable, because of the requirements of pregnancy. The strain of pregnancy, the formation of adhesions, or a weakening of its natural supports or individual variations may produce changes in the normal position of the uterus that usually cause no severe problems to the patient but may give rise to troublesome symptoms.

Backward Displacements. Backward displacements (*retroversion* and *retroflexion*) of the uterus (Fig. 45-4) may give rise to such symptoms as backache or a sense of pelvic pressure. Most retrograde displacements are asymptomatic.

Asymptomatic retroversion of the uterus occurs in approximately 20% of women and is a variant of normal. Such women may have more discomfort in the lower back rather than in the abdominal area during labor.

Prolapse and Procidentia. Because of the weakening of the supports of the uterus, most often brought about by childbirth, the uterus may work its way down the vaginal canal (prolapse) and even appear outside the vaginal orifice (procidentia) (Fig. 45-5).

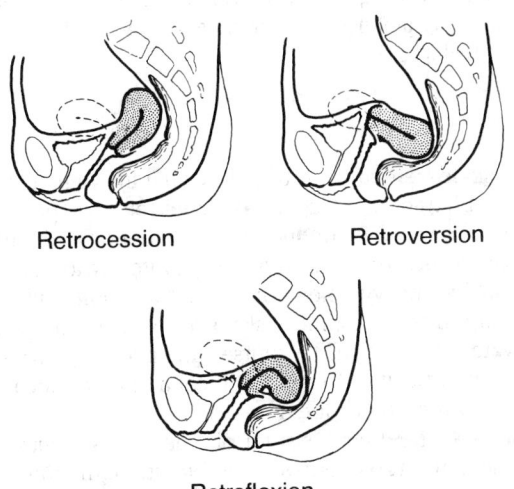

Figure 45–4. Retrodisplacements of the uterus. The dotted line indicates the normal position of the uterus. In *retrocession*, the uterus tilts posteriorly. In *retroversion*, the uterus turns posteriorly as a whole unit. In *retroflexion*, the fundus bends posteriorly above the cervical end. (Hardy JD. Hardy's Textbook of Surgery, 2nd ed. Philadelphia, JB Lippincott, 1988.)

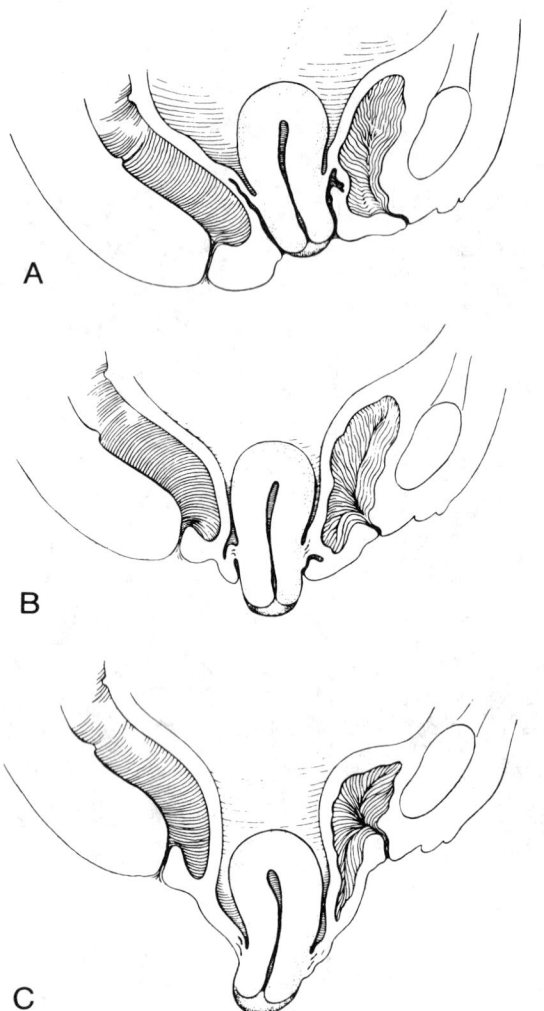

Figure 45–5. Prolapse of the uterus and the vagina. (**A**) First-degree prolapse—cervix comes down to introitus. (**B**) Second-degree prolapse—cervix protrudes through introitus. (**C**) Third-degree prolapse—total procidentia: uterus protrudes through introitus. (Adapted from Gray LA. Postgrad Med 30:209.)

In its descent, the uterus pulls with it the vaginal walls and even the bladder and the rectum. Symptoms are pressure plus urinary symptoms (incontinence and retention) from displacement of the bladder, which are aggravated when the woman coughs, lifts a heavy object, or stands for a long while. Normal activities are troublesome tasks; even walking up stairs may aggravate the problem. The nurse can encourage women who have such difficulties to seek medical attention, because time will not correct the problem.

The best treatment is surgical. The uterus is sutured back into place, and repair is performed to strengthen and tighten muscle bands. In postmenopausal women, the uterus may be removed (hysterectomy). For elderly women or those who are too ill to withstand the strain of surgery, pessaries may be the treatment of choice.

Nursing Interventions

Patient Education and Home Health Care. Many of the problems related to relaxation of the pelvic muscles (cystocele,

rectocele, uterine prolapse) might have been prevented. During obstetric care, early visits to the nurse midwife or obstetrician permit early detection of potential problems. During the postpartum period, perineal exercises can be taught so that the woman develops the ability to tighten and relax gluteal and perineal floor muscles. Learning to start and stop the urinary stream also enhances perineal muscle tone.

Encouraging the patient to start and stop the urinary stream is a way of teaching her how to isolate the muscles that she needs to strengthen. After isolating the muscle while voiding, this toning exercise (Kegel's exercises) can be performed at any time during the day.

Delays in obtaining evaluation and treatment may result in further complications such as infection, cervical ulceration, cystitis, and hemorrhoids.

If the patient is to have a pessary, she needs to know how to insert it, how long it may remain in place, and how to clean it as well as reinsert it.

Preoperative Nursing Management. Before surgery, the patient needs to know the extent of the proposed surgery, the expectations for the postoperative period, and the effect of surgery on future sexual functions. Often, a midstream clean-catch urine specimen is required. The specimen is sent to the laboratory immediately. For a rectocele repair, a cathartic and a cleansing enema may be prescribed. Some surgeons request that a perineal shave be completed.

In the operating room, special attention is given to placing both of the patient's legs in and out of stirrups simultaneously to prevent muscular strain and excess pressure on the legs and thighs. Other preoperative details are similar to those described in Chapter 20.

Postoperative Nursing Management and Rehabilitation. In the postoperative period, the immediate goals are to prevent infection and pressure on the suture line. This will require perineal care and may preclude the use of dressings. The patient is always urged to void within a few hours after operations for cystocele and complete tear. If the patient does not void within this period, feels uncomfortable, or has pain in the region of the bladder after 6 hours, catheterization is performed. Some physicians prefer to leave an indwelling catheter in place for 2 to 4 days. There are various other methods of bladder care, as described in Chapter 42.

After each urination or bowel movement, the perineum is irrigated with warm sterile saline (see p. 1239) and the area blotted dry with sterile cotton.

There are several methods used in caring for the sutures. In one method, the sutures are left alone until healing occurs (*i.e.*, for 5 to 10 days). Thereafter, daily vaginal douches of sterile saline are given during the period of convalescence. In another method—the wet method—small douches of sterile saline are given twice daily, beginning on the day after operation and continuing throughout convalescence.

A heat lamp or hair dryer may be used to help dry the area and enhance the healing process. Commercially available sprays containing a combination of antiseptic and anesthetic solutions are soothing and effective. An ice pack applied locally may relieve discomfort. For effective relief of this type, a plastic bag can be filled with ice chips. However, the weight of the bag must rest on the bed and not on the patient.

The routine postoperative care is much like that for an abdominal operation. The patient is placed in bed, with the head and the knees elevated slightly. A liquid diet is given on the first day, and then a full diet is begun as soon as desired.

After an operation for a complete perineal laceration (through the rectal sphincter), special care and attention are required. The bladder is emptied by catheterization to prevent strain on sutures.

Throughout the convalescence of all patients who have had surgical repairs, stool-softening agents are given each night after the patient is permitted a soft diet.

Patient Education and Home Health Care.   Predischarge instructions include information pertaining to douching, the use of mild laxatives, the amount of exercise recommended, and the need to avoid lifting heavy objects or standing for prolonged periods. The patient is reminded to return to the gynecologist for a follow-up visit and to check with the physician regarding safe resumption of sexual intercourse.

In particular, the patient is instructed to report any pelvic pain, observation of unusual discharge, inability to care for personal hygiene, and bleeding from the vagina. She is advised to continue with perineal exercises, which are recommended to assist in strengthening muscles. The patient is instructed as follows: tense the perineal muscles by pressing the buttocks together; hold this position; relax. This exercise, done 10 to 20 times each hour, can be performed while the person is sitting or standing.

In summary, structural disorders of the female reproductive tract may affect the vagina, uterus, or bladder. These disorders are commonly attributed to aging or the trauma of childbirth; long-standing consequences may be vaginal discharge, infection, and excoriation. Symptoms of urinary tract involvement or gastrointestinal symptoms may occur. Their severity may range from occasional, mild symptoms to those that are severe and disruptive of normal activities, thus requiring surgical intervention. Kegel exercises may strengthen the muscles of the pelvic floor and decrease the incidence of some structural disorders that can occur after childbirth and accompanying aging.

Benign Tumors and Conditions

Vulvar Cysts

A cyst of the greater vestibular gland is a cystic dilation of the duct of the Bartholin's gland resulting from obstruction. This is the most common of vulvar tumors and is located in the posterior third of the vulva, near the vestibule. A simple cyst may be asymptomatic. Infection may be due to the gonococcus organism, *Escherichia coli*, or *Staphylococcus aureus* and can cause an abscess with or without inguinal adenopathy. The best treatment is incision and drainage, plus antibiotics.

If a cyst is asymptomatic, treatment is unnecessary. Often, moist heat or sitz baths will result in drainage and resolution.

Vulvar Dystropy

Vulvar dystrophy, also called leukoplakia and lichen sclerosus, is a condition causing dry, thickened skin on the vulva or slightly raised whitish papules or macules. Symptoms usually consist of varying degrees of itching, but some patients have no symptoms. A small percentage of patients with cancer of the vulva

have an associated dystrophy. Biopsy and careful follow-up are the usual approach. If malignant cells are detected on biopsy, a simple vulvectomy is usually performed. If the biopsy is negative for malignancy, testosterone, estrogen, or cortisone creams are prescribed, depending on the type of dystrophy, to keep symptoms at a minimum.

Ovarian Cysts

Pathophysiology.   The ovary is a frequent site for the development of cysts. These may be simply pathologic enlargements of normal ovarian constituents, the graafian follicle, or corpus luteum, or they may arise from abnormal growth of the ovarian epithelium.

Dermoid cysts are tumors that are believed to arise from parts of the ovum that disappear normally as ripening (maturation) takes place. Because their origin is undefined, all that can be said is that they are tumors made up of undifferentiated embryonal cells. They grow slowly and are found during surgery to contain a thick, yellow, sebaceous material arising from a skin lining. Hair, teeth, bone, brain, eyes, and many other tissues often are found in a rudimentary state within these cysts.

Clinically, cysts are manifested by their obvious presence as an ovarian mass. There may be lower abdominal pain that may be acute or chronic. Rupture may occur and simulate a variety of acute abdominal emergencies, such as appendicitis or ectopic pregnancy. Larger cysts may produce abdominal swelling and pressure on adjacent abdominal organs.

The treatment of ovarian cysts is usually surgical. If cysts are less than 5 cm in diameter and appear to be fluid filled or physiologic, in a young, healthy patient, oral contraceptives are frequently used to attempt suppression of ovarian activity and resolution of the cyst. Ninety-eight percent of tumors that occur in women aged 29 and younger are benign. At 50 years of age, only 50% are benign. The postoperative nursing care after surgical removal of an ovarian cyst is similar to that for abdominal surgery, with one exception. The marked decrease in intra-abdominal pressure incidental to the removal of a large cyst often leads to considerable abdominal distention. This complication may be prevented to some extent by the application of a snug-fitting abdominal binder.

Benign Tumors of the Uterus: Leiomyomas (Fibroids, Myomas, and Fibromyomas)

Myomatous or fibroid tumors of the uterus are almost always benign (99.5%) and arise from the muscle tissue of the uterus. They are common, occurring in about 20% of white women and 40% to 50% of black women. They develop slowly between the ages of 25 and 40 years and often become large in size after this period. There are instances in which such a tumor causes no symptoms. The most common symptom is abnormal vaginal bleeding. Other symptoms are due to pressure on the surrounding organs—pain, backache, constipation, and urinary symptoms. In addition, such tumors often cause metrorrhagia and even sterility.

Management.   The treatment of uterine fibroids depends to a large extent on their size and location. The patient with minor symptoms is observed closely. If she plans to have children, treatment is as conservative as possible. As a rule, large tumors that produce pressure symptoms should be removed. Usually, the uterus is removed (hysterectomy), and the ovaries are preserved, if possible. If the tumor is small, it may be removed (myomectomy); the wound in the uterus is then closed. Laser is being used also for treatment of fibroids.

Fibroids shrink and disappear during menopause without the stimulation of estrogen. Experimental drugs that induce medical menopause have been seen to be helpful in tumor shrinkage (*e.g.*, Lupron).

The nursing process for a patient having a hysterectomy is on pp. 1280–1281.

Endometriosis

Endometriosis is a benign lesion in which cells similar to those lining the uterus are found growing aberrantly in the pelvic cavity outside the uterus. It is a puzzling disease because symptoms vary and may be misleading. Extensive endometriosis may cause few symptoms, whereas an isolated lesion may produce many symptoms.

Pathophysiology.   In order of frequency, pelvic endometriosis attacks the ovary, ureterosacral ligaments, cul-de-sac, rectovaginal septum, uterovesical peritoneum, cervix, outside surface of the uterus, umbilicus, laparotomy scars, hernial sacs, and appendix. The misplaced endometrium responds to ovarian hormonal stimulation and is indeed dependent on this stimulation. When the uterus goes through the process of menstruation, this ectopic tissue bleeds—mostly into areas having no outlet—which then causes pain and adhesions. These lesions are typically small, puckered, and brown or blue-black, indicating concealed bleeding. If the endometrial tissue is within an ovarian cyst, there is no outlet for the bleeding and the formation is referred to as a *pseudocyst* (chocolate cyst).

Incidence.   The diagnosis of endometriosis has increased in recent years because of the availability of laparoscopy. Before the use of the laparoscope, major surgery was necessary before a diagnosis could be made. There is a high incidence among patients who marry later, bear children later, and have fewer children. In countries such as India, where tradition favors early marriage and early childbearing, endometriosis is rare.

It is characteristically found in the young, nulliparous woman aged 25 to 35. A similar condition affecting the uterine lining in older, multiparous patients is referred to as adenomyosis. At present, these two conditions, which at one time were thought to be related, are now considered separate entities, although symptoms may be similar and both conditions may be present.

There appears to be a predisposition to endometriosis; it is more common in women whose close female relatives have this condition.

Etiology.   The more popular theories regarding the origin of endometrial lesions are the transplantation theory and the metaplasia theory. The transplantation theory suggests that a backflow of menses (retrograde menstruation) causes endometrial tissue to be transported to ectopic sites through the uterine tubes. Transplantation can also occur during surgery if endometrial tissue is transferred inadvertently by way of instruments. Endometrial tissue can be spread also by lymphatic or venous channels. The metaplasia theory relates to retained remnants of embryonic epithelial tissue, which during the growth process may be transformed into endometrial tissue

by means of outside stimuli. The real cause of endometriosis may be a combination of factors.

Clinical Manifestations and Diagnostic Evaluation.   Symptoms vary with the location of endometrial tissue. Usually the chief symptom is a type of dysmenorrhea, unlike typical uterine cramps. The patient complains of a deep-seated aching in the lower abdomen, vagina, posterior pelvis, and back that occurs 1 or 2 days before the menstrual cycle and lasts 2 or 3 days. Some patients, however, have no pain. Abnormal uterine bleeding and dyspareunia (painful intercourse) also may be evident in sexually active women.

Excess prostaglandin release from the cells that are shed may contribute to nausea and diarrhea. Infertility is another possible effect.

A health history, including the menstrual pattern, is necessary to elicit specific symptoms. On bimanual pelvic examination, fixed tender nodules may be detected and the uterus may be restricted in motility, indicating the presence of adhesions. Laparoscopy confirms the diagnosis.

Management.   Treatment depends on the nature of the symptoms, desire for pregnancy, and the extent of the disease. If the woman is asymptomatic, observation every 6 months may be all that is required. Other therapy for varying degrees of symptoms may be palliation, hormone administration, or surgery. Palliative efforts include analgesics, prostaglandin inhibitors, and pregnancy; the latter will alleviate symptoms because of amenorrhea during gestation.

Hormonal therapy, in which oral contraceptives are given for 6 to 9 months, will suppress menstruation and relieve menstrual pain (dysmenorrhea). There may be side effects, however, such as fluid retention, nausea, weight gain, vaginal discharge, or other complications related to oral contraceptive use. If these side effects are troublesome, this form of therapy is discontinued or changed to a different formulation.

Another type of hormonal therapy involves the use of a synthetic androgen, danazol (Danocrine), which causes atrophy of the endometrium and subsequent amenorrhea. The drug inhibits the release of gonadotropin with minimal overt sex hormone stimulation. This medication is expensive and may cause troublesome side effects such as fatigue, depression, weight gain, oily skin, decreased breast size, mild acne, hot flashes, and atrophy of the vagina.

Most women continue treatment despite side effects, and symptoms improve for 80% to 90% of women with mild to moderate endometriosis. This drug is contraindicated in pregnancy, while breast-feeding, and in those patients with a history of abnormal vaginal bleeding, liver, heart, or kidney disease.

A gonadotropin-releasing hormone (GnRH) agonist or GnRH blocker called Synarel results in decreased estrogen production and subsequent amenorrhea. It is administered by nasal spray twice a day for 6 months. Side effects are related to low estrogen levels (*e.g.*, hot flashes and vaginal dryness). This effective medication reduces the discomfort of endometriosis and is helpful in patients who are trying to conceive but are hindered by this condition.

If conservative measures are not helpful, surgery may be necessary. The procedure selected will depend on the individual patient's needs. A laparoscopy may be performed during which it may be feasible to fulgurate (cut with high-frequency current) endometrial implants and to lyse (cut) adhesions. Laser surgery is another option made possible by laparoscopy. Lasers are used to vaporize the endometrial implants or to coagulate the implant, thereby destroying it.

Depending on circumstances, other surgical procedures may be used, including laparotomy, uterine suspension, abdominal hysterectomy, bilateral salpingo-oophorectomy, and appendectomy.

Prognosis. In mild to moderate endometriosis, the use of hormonal or surgical treatment relieves pain and enhances the chance of pregnancy. For women over age 35 or those willing to sacrifice reproductive capability, definitive surgery (total hysterectomy) provides another alternative.

Nursing Interventions. The health history and physical examination concentrate on identifying the specific symptoms, determining when and how long they have been bothersome, and on the woman's reproductive desires. This information is most helpful in contributing to the treatment plan.

Patient goals include relief of pain, relief of dysmenorrhea and dyspareunia, and avoidance of infertility. Nursing interventions will include assessment of pain and evaluation of the techniques and prescribed medications that provide relief. Explanations of the various diagnostic procedures often alleviate anxiety.

Emotional support is provided to the woman and her partner who desire pregnancy and childbearing. As the treatment plan progresses, it may become apparent that pregnancy is not easily possible. The psychosocial impact of this realization on the couple must be respected and addressed.

Alternatives such as *in vitro* fertilization (IVF) or adoption are discussed at an appropriate time and referrals offered.

The nurse's role in patient education is to dispel myths, such as a causative relationship between the use of tampons and endometriosis, and to encourage investigation of dysmenorrhea or abnormal bleeding patterns. The Endometriosis Association (listed at the end of this chapter) is a good resource for patients seeking further information and support.

Adenomyosis. In this condition, the tissue that lines the endometrium invades the uterine wall; the incidence is highest in women from 40 to 50 years of age. Symptoms are hypermenorrhea (excessive and prolonged bleeding), acquired dysmenorrhea, polymenorrhea (abnormally frequent bleeding), and premenstrual staining. On physical examination, the uterus is felt to be enlarged, firm, and tender. Treatment depends on the severity of bleeding and pain; hysterectomy offers greater relief than more conservative forms of therapy, and is currently the treatment of choice.

Malignant Conditions

Malignant tumors of the female reproductive system (excluding breast cancer) are estimated to be the cause of over 23,500 deaths in the United States each year. It is expected that 13,500 new cases of invasive cancer of the cervix will be detected, and this diagnosis will result in 6000 deaths. These estimates do not include *in situ* cancers. About 33,000 new cases of uterine cancer are estimated and 4000 deaths are predicted to occur yearly. For ovarian cancer, 20,500 new cases will be diagnosed and 12,400 deaths will be due to this disease. Four thousand nine hundred other genital cancers will be diagnosed and 1100 deaths will be due to this diagnosis annually (Cancer Facts and Figures, 1990—American Cancer Society).

Although some cancers are difficult to detect or prevent, yearly pelvic examinations with Pap smear are painless and relatively inexpensive methods of early detection. Health professionals can encourage women to follow this health practice by making examinations a pleasant, educational, supportive opportunity for their patients. It has been suggested that Pap smears become a routine requirement during pre-employment, pre-admission, or insurance physicals. If more women realized that this test does not have to be uncomfortable or embarrassing, early detection rates would undoubtedly improve. An increase in the number of women having this simple, painless test will save lives that otherwise would be claimed by cancer.

Cancer of the Cervix

There are two main types of primary uterine cancer—carcinoma of the cervix, which is predominantly epidermoid cancer, and carcinoma of the endometrium (corpus and body of the uterus).

Cancer of the cervix is less common than it used to be because of early detection by Pap smear. Invasive cervical cancer over the last 40 years has decreased from 45 per 100,000 to 15 per 100,000, but it is still the third most common reproductive cancer in women, excluding breast cancer. It occurs most commonly between 30 and 45 years of age, but can occur as early as 18 years of age. Sexual activity has a relationship to the incidence of cancer of the cervix; before age 25, it is more prevalent in those who have had multiple sexual partners and several early pregnancies. Studies tend toward the conclusion that this type of cancer is an STD.

Risk factors, aside from early age at first intercourse, early childbearing, and multiple partners, include exposure to HPV, smoking, and exposure to diethylstilbesterol (DES) *in utero*. Most cervical malignancies are squamous cell cancers. Adenocarcinoma is less common.

Diagnosis may follow an abnormal Pap smear with dysplasia or persistent atypical smears, followed by a biopsy identifying cervical intraepithelial neoplasia (CIN) or a high-grade squamous intraepithelial lesion (HGSIL). It may be detected when a patient complains of discharge or irregular bleeding, but it is most often asymptomatic.

Leukorrhea may be the only abnormal symptom. The discharge increases gradually in amount and becomes watery and, finally, dark and foul smelling because of necrosis and infection of the tumor mass. The bleeding occurs at irregular intervals, between periods (metrorrhagia) or after menopause. It may be very slight, just enough to spot the undergarments, and it is noted usually after some form of mild trauma (intercourse, douching, or defecation). As the disease continues, the bleeding may become constant and may increase in amount.

Chronic infections of the cervix seem to play a significant part in the development of cervical cancer. Such pathology becomes evident as a large reddish growth or a deep, ulcerating crater before any symptoms appear.

As the cancer advances, the tissues outside the cervix may be invaded, including the lymph glands anterior to the sacrum. In one third of patients with invasive cervical cancer, the disease involves the fundus. The nerves in this region become involved, producing excruciating pain in the back and the legs that is relieved only by large doses of narcotics. The final picture, when untreated, is one of extreme emaciation and anemia, often with fever due to secondary infection and abscesses in the ulcerating mass.

Diagnostic Evaluation. A valuable tool for the physician is the clinical staging of a disease. By estimating the extent of the disease, treatment can be planned more specifically and prognosis reasonably predicted. The International Classification adopted by the International Federation of Gynecology and Obstetrics (Table 45-2) is most widely used; the TNM (tumor, nodes, and metastases) classification is also used in describing malignancies (see Chart 19-2, p. 349). In this system, T refers to extent of primary tumor, N to lymph node involvement, and M to extent of metastasis.

Signs and symptoms are evaluated, and x-ray and laboratory studies plus special examinations such as punch biopsy and colposcopy are done. Depending on the stage, other tests may be used, including dilatation and curettage (D&C), computed tomography, lymphangiography, and possibly magnetic resonance imaging, intravenous pyelography (IVP), and barium x-ray studies.

Management.   When precursor lesions such as low-grade squamous intraepithelial lesions (LGSIL) or HGSIL are found by colposcopy and biopsy, conservative nonsurgical removal is possible. Cryotherapy (freezing with nitrous oxide refrigerant) or laser therapy is effective. Conization (removal of a cone-shaped portion of the cervix) is performed when biopsy demonstrates CIN III or HGSIL, equivalent to carcinoma *in situ.*

CIN I and II are consistent with mild to moderate dysplasia or LGSIL (the new Bethesda classification).

CIN III or HGSIL is consistent with severe dysplasia and carcinoma *in situ.* (For clarification of these terminology changes, see Table 44-1, which describes changes in Pap smear terminology in recent years. The Bethesda classification is the most current.) Table 45-3 describes other terms that are used in cytologic descriptions. Table 45-4 describes proper technique for obtaining a cervical specimen for cytologic examination.

If preinvasive cervical cancer occurs when a woman has completed childbearing, a simple hysterectomy will probably be recommended. Frequent subsequent periodic examinations are performed to check for recurrence. For invasive cervical cancer, radiation or radical hysterectomy or both may be methods of treatment. The method selected depends on the stage of the lesion (see Table 45-2) and on the judgment and skill of the physician. Radical surgery is advocated by some authorities, especially when a patient is unable to withstand the effects of radiation or has a radiation-resistant cancer. Surgical procedures commonly carried out include the following:

Total hysterectomy—removal of the uterus, cervix, and ovaries.
Radical hysterectomy (Wertheim)—an abdominal incision is made, and the uterus, adnexa, proximal vagina, and bilateral lymph nodes are removed en masse.
Radical vaginal hysterectomy (Schauta)—a vaginal approach is used to remove the uterus, adnexa, and proximal vagina. (*Note:* "Radical" used before each of the above procedures means that an extensive area of the paravaginal, paracervical, parametrial, and uterosacral tissues is removed with the uterus.)

TABLE 45-2.   *International Classification of Carcinoma of the Uterine Cervix*

Stage of Lesion	Area	Description
Stage 0	Carcinoma *in situ*	Cancer limited to epithelial layer; no evidence of invasion
Stage I	Carcinoma strictly confined to cervix	Size is not a criterion
Stage IA		Microinvasive
Stage IB		Clinically obvious stage I
Stage II	Vaginal cancer	Lesion has spread beyond cervix to involve vagina (not lower third) or paracervical region on one or both sides
Stage IIA		Vaginal extension only
Stage IIB		Paracervical extension with or without vaginal involvement
Stage III	Cancer involves lower third of vagina or has extended to one or both pelvic walls	Unequivocal palpable lymph node disease on the pelvic wall
		IV pyelogram shows one or both ureters obstructed by the tumor
Stage IIIA		Extends to lower third of vagina only
Stage IIIB		Isolated carcinomatous metastases are palpable on the pelvic wall
Stage IV	Bladder extension	Evidence that carcinoma involves the bladder seen in cystoscopic examination or by presence of vesicovaginal fistula
	Rectal extension	Carcinoma spreads outside true pelvis to other organs
	Distant spread	

TABLE 45-3. *Other Descriptive Terms Used in Cervical Cytology*

Atypical squamous metaplasia
Metaplastic squamous cells that contain nuclear features of active inflammation.

Chronic cervicitis
Inflammatory exudate associated with epithelial changes.

Dyskeratocytes
Mature, squamous cells with dense and refringent cytoplasm indicative of human papilloma virus.
May be falsely read as dysplasia.

Giant cells
Large multinucleated cells that may be indicative of herpes.

Koilocytotic atypia (warty atypia)
Hollow squamous cells indicative of human papilloma virus.

Parakeratosis
Indicative of estrogen-deficient states.

Regeneration and Repair
Features of inflammation and repair seen in squamous and columnar cells.

(Fullerton JT and Barger MK. Papanicolaou smear: An update on classification and management. J Am Acad Nurse Pract 1989 Jul/Sep; 1[3]:87.)

Bilateral pelvic lymphadenectomy—Removal of the common iliac, external iliac, hypogastric, and obturator lymphatics and nodes.
Pelvic exenteration—removal of the pelvic organs, including bladder or rectum and pelvic lymph nodes.
Salpingo-oophorectomy—removal of uterine tube and ovary.

Follow-up by gynecologic oncologists is imperative.

Cancer of the Endometrium

Cancer of the endometrium (fundus or corpus) of the uterus has increased in incidence partly because people are living longer and there is more accurate reporting. The major emphasis for the nurse is to encourage all women over the age of 18 to have annual checkups, including a gynecologic examination. After breast, colorectal, and lung malignancies, endometrial cancer is the fourth most common cancer in women and the most common pelvic neoplasm. Treatment consists of total hysterectomy and bilateral salpingo-oophorectomy. Depending on the stage, intracavitary radiation or external pelvic irradiation may be part of the treatment preoperatively or postoperatively.

About half of all women with postmenopausal bleeding have cancer of the uterus. The median age is 61, and most

TABLE 45-4. *Method for Obtaining an Optimal Pap Smear*

Technique	Rationale
1. Do not obtain a Pap smear in the presence of menses or frank bleeding (exception: high suspicion of neoplasia).	Blood obscures a proper reading of cells.
2. If performing more than one test (*e.g.,* Pap and GC), obtain the Pap smear first.	This will maintain the integrity of the superficial layer of cells that will be sampled.
3. Label frosted end of slide with pencil.	Ink rubs off glass.
4. After speculum insertion; gently remove mucus and blood that may interfere with visualization or cytology.	If not removed, this material may be obtained instead of cervical cells.
5. Insert a saline-moistened cotton-tipped applicator or cytobrush* 2–3 cm into endocervical canal. Rotate 180–360 degrees and roll out onto a slide.	This obtains endocervical cells and may sample squamocolumnar junction in the cervical canal. Saline prevents absorption of cells into the cotton, thus increasing the yield transferred to the slide.
6. Place longer end of the Ayre spatula† in cervical canal and firmly scrape the exocervix in a full circle.	This technique will obtain a sampling of exocervix and squamocolumnar junction. (If transformation zone is far out from the os, it may be necessary to move the spatula away from the os.)
7. Obtain a vaginal pool sample from the posterior vaginal fornix. (Optional unless a suspicious lesion is present.)	This sample may reveal endometrial or vaginal wall cancer. Women over age 45 are at increased risk for endometrial cancer, and these cells might be shed into the posterior fornix.
8. For women who have had a hysterectomy, obtain a sample from the vaginal cuff.	This sampling may detect residual vaginal wall cancer.
9. Do not rub, repeat, or overlap strokes on the slide.	Avoids breaking or destroying cells.
10. Immediately fix slide with cytologic fixative, unscented hairspray, or place in a jar of 95% alcohol.	Exposure to air or light causes distortion of cells.

* *Some care providers recommend use of the spatula before the use of the cytobrush to obtain a better sample, as the cytobrush often causes slight bleeding. The spatula obtains cells at the squamocolumnar junction, whereas the brush or swab collects endocervical cells. Both components are necessary for an adequate sampling.*
† *An Ayre spatula is a small wooden spatula with a forked end that is universally available in gynecologic settings in the United States.*
(Fullerton JT and Barger MK. Papanicolaou smear: An update on classification and management. J Am Acad Nurse Pract 1989 Jul/Sep; 1[3]:86.)

patients are at least 55 years old. Obese women have a slightly higher risk, as they have increased levels of estrone from excess weight. This is due to conversion of androstenedione to estrone in body fat. This exposes the uterus to unopposed estrogen.

Unopposed estrogen given in replacement therapy is also a risk factor. Currently, progesterone is added to offset this risk, but in the past some women have been treated with estrogen alone and are at increased risk. Other risk factors include nulliparity and late menopause (*i.e.*, after age 52). This cancer is more common in white women and in women who have diabetes. Most uterine cancers are adenocarcinomas and originate in the lining of the uterus. Treatment is based on stage of disease but almost always begins with a total abdominal hysterectomy (TAH) along with bilateral salpingo-oophorectomy (BSO).

Hysterectomy

A total hysterectomy involves the removal of the uterus, including the cervix. This procedure is performed for many conditions, including dysfunctional uterine bleeding; endometriosis; malignant and nonmalignant growths on the uterus, cervix, and adnexa; problems of pelvic relaxation and prolapse; and irreparable injury to the uterus. Malignant conditions require a total abdominal hysterectomy and bilateral salpingo-oophorectomy.

▶ Nursing Process
The Patient Undergoing a Hysterectomy

◊ Assessment

The health history and physical and pelvic examination plus a review of the laboratory studies enable the nurse to establish a broad picture of the patient's problems. Additional questions will include psychosocial implications, as a hysterectomy in most instances affects very personal and deep-seated experiences and relationships. If the hysterectomy is performed because of a malignancy, anxiety related to cancer and death adds to the stress of this procedure.

◊ Nursing Diagnoses

Based on all the assessment data, the patient's major nursing diagnoses may include the following:

- Anxiety related to the diagnosis of cancer, fear of pain, perceived loss of femininity, and disfigurement
- Body image disturbance related to altered sexuality, fertility, and relationships with family and partner
- Pain related to surgery and other adjuvant therapy.
- Knowledge deficit of the perioperative aspects of hysterectomy and self-care

◊ Planning and Implementation

◊ *Goals:*   The major goals of the patient may include relief of anxiety, acceptance of self as altered, absence of pain or discomfort, and increased knowledge of self-care requirements.

◊ Nursing Interventions

◊ *Relief of Anxiety.*   Anxiety in the woman undergoing a hysterectomy stems from a number of variables: unfamiliar environment, effects of surgery on body image and reproductive ability, fear of pain and other discomforts, and sensitivity and possibly feelings of embarrassment about exposure of the genital area in the perioperative period. Conflicts between medical treatment and religious beliefs may be troubling. It is necessary for the nurse to determine the meaning of this experience to the patient, and it is also necessary for the patient to verbalize her feelings to someone who understands and can help.

The nurse identifies the patient's strengths that will produce a positive effect. Through the preoperative period, explanations are given relative to the phases of physical preparation.

◊ *Preoperative Preparation.*   The physical preparation differs little from the details described for the preparation of a patient undergoing a laparotomy. The lower half of the abdomen and the pubic and perineal regions usually are carefully shaved and cleansed with soap and water (some operating rooms do not require shaving). The intestinal tract and the bladder are empty before the patient is taken to the operating room. This is important to prevent contamination and accidental injury to the bladder or intestinal tract. An enema and antiseptic douche are usually prescribed the evening before surgery to be followed by sedation for a restful night. Preoperative medications given the morning of surgery will help the patient relax.

◊ *Improved Body Image.*   The nursing assessment reveals how the woman feels about having a hysterectomy. It is a personal experience that is affected by the nature of the diagnosis, significant others who may be involved (family, partner), religious beliefs, and prognosis. Concerns may surface, such as the inability to have children, loss of femininity, and questions about the impact on sexual relationships and satisfaction. The patient needs to be reassured that she will still have a vagina and that sexual intercourse can be experienced after a temporary period of abstinence postoperatively while the tissues heal.

Education includes the information that sexual satisfaction and orgasm arise from clitoral stimulation rather than the presence or absence of a uterus. Most women note some change in sexual feelings after hysterectomy, but they vary in intensity. In some cases, the vagina is shortened by surgery, and this may affect some sexual feelings or comfort.

Moreover, when hormonal balances are upset, as often occurs in disturbances of the reproductive system, the patient may exhibit depression and heightened emotional sensitivity to people and situations. Each patient must be understood in the light of such factors and approached and evaluated individually. This understanding must be shared by the family as well as the health care providers. The nurse who exhibits interest, concern, and willingness to listen to the patient's fears will add immeasurably to the patient's progress throughout the surgical experience. Because the decision to have a hysterectomy rests with the patient, her decision must be respected and supported.

◊ *Relief of Pain.*   A hysterectomy may be performed by way of an abdominal incision or by a vaginal route. The surgeon makes this decision based on the diagnosis and size of the uterus. The vaginal hysterectomy usually allows earlier ambulation. An abdominal incision is used in cases of malignancy and when the uterus is enlarged. Pain and abdominal discomfort are not uncommon. Analgesics are administered as prescribed to relieve pain and promote daily ambulation.

To combat the discomfort of abdominal distention, a nasogastric tube may be inserted before the patient leaves the operating room, especially if excessive handling of viscera has taken place. If a large tumor was present, its excision could cause edema because of the sudden release of pressure. In the postoperative period, fluids and food may be restricted for 1 or 2 days. If there is abdominal flatus, a rectal tube may be prescribed, as well as heat to the abdomen. When peristalsis, begins, as determined by abdominal auscultation, the patient is served additional fluids and a soft diet. Ambulation facilitates the return of normal peristalsis.

◊ *Postoperative Care.*   The principles of general postoperative care for abdominal surgery apply. Particular attention is given to peripheral circulation, such as noting presence of varicosities and promoting circulation with leg exercises and antiembolic stockings. Major risks are infection and hemorrhage. In addition, because of the proximity of the surgical intervention to the bladder, problems of voiding may occur, particularly after a vaginal hysterectomy.

Edema or nerve trauma may cause temporary atony, and an indwelling catheter may be used. If no catheter is in place, catheterization may be necessary if the patient has not voided after 8 hours. If the catheter is in place, it is usually removed shortly after ambulation. During surgery, the handling of the bowel may cause ileus and interfere with bowel functioning.

◊ *Patient Education and Home Health Care.*   Information is provided to the patient according to her needs and desires. It is important for her to know what limitations or restrictions, if any, may be expected. Menstruation will no longer occur; symptoms of menopause will not result if the ovaries are intact, but if they have been removed, hormonal replacement may be considered. Although a hysterectomy has been minimizingly described by some as "simply a bit more than an appendectomy," it does cause some reduced strength and fatigue for a few weeks. This is to be expected and should gradually improve.

The patient should resume activities gradually; however, this does not mean sitting for long periods because this may cause pooling of the blood in the pelvis and the risk of thromboembolism. Showers are preferable to tub bathing to reduce the possibility of infection and to avoid the dangers of injury from stepping in and out of the tub. The patient is advised to avoid straining, lifting, sexual intercourse, or driving until these activities are permitted by the physician. Vaginal discharge, foul odor, excessive amount of bleeding, and an elevated temperature are reported to a health care professional promptly.

The nurse will reinforce information given to the patient by the physician regarding the resumption of sexual intercourse. Other methods of sexual expression and other less strenuous coital positions may be suggested.

◊ *Evaluation*

Expected Outcomes

1. Experiences decreased anxiety
   a. Asks specific questions regarding the effects of surgery on menstruation, procreation, sexual relations, and cancer
   b. Discusses the surgical procedure and postoperative course

2. Accepts herself as she is now
   a. Includes her partner in planning her convalescence
   b. Verbalizes understanding of her disorder and projected solution
   c. Takes time and care with her appearance
   d. Shares her plans with the nurse regarding her first 2 weeks at home
   e. Displays no depression or sadness
3. Experiences minimal pain and discomfort
   a. Reports relief of abdominal pain and discomfort
   b. Ambulates without pain
4. Exhibits absence of complications
   a. Is afebrile for 24 hours before discharge
   b. Has stable vital signs
   c. Ambulates early
   d. Notes absence of calf pain, redness, tenderness, or swelling in extremities
   e. Reports no urinary problems or abdominal distention
5. Confirms her acquisition of knowledge and understanding of self-care
   a. Practices deep breathing, turning, and leg exercises as taught
   b. Increases activity and ambulation daily
   c. Reports adequate fluid intake and adequate urinary output
   d. Alternates periods of rest with activity
   e. Identifies what symptoms to report
   f. Describes purposes of prescribed hormonal replacement
   g. Repeats instructions and identifies side effects to be reported
   h. Keeps follow-up clinic/office appointments
   i. Understands that some women note decreased sexual satisfaction after hysterectomy; others note no change

Cancer of the Vulva

Primary cancer of the vulva represents 3% to 4% of all gynecologic malignancies and is seen mostly in postmenopausal women. More whites than nonwhites are afflicted. Epidermoid cancer is the most common type. Intraepithelial cancer includes squamous cell carcinoma *in situ* and extramammary Paget's disease. Less common are Bartholin's gland cancer, basal cell carcinoma, and malignant melanoma. Little is known of the cause of this condition.

The median age for cancer *in situ* is 44 years, whereas the median age for invasive cancer of the vulva is 61 years. Numbers are higher in women with hypertension, obesity, and diabetes. Less radical approaches than vulvectomy, discussed below, are being used.

Clinical Manifestations and Diagnostic Evaluation.   Long-standing pruritus is the most common symptom of vulvar cancer. Bleeding, foul-smelling discharge, and pain also may be present, and are usually signs of advanced disease. Early lesions appear as a chronic dermatitis; later a lump may be noted that continues to grow and becomes a hard, ulcerated, cauliflower-like growth. Biopsy is the chief means of diagnosing vulvar cancer.

- A biopsy should be performed on any vulvar lesion that is persistent or ulcerated or does not heal quickly with proper therapy.

The nurse is in a unique position to encourage a woman

with these manifestations to seek health care, because this is one of the most curable of all malignant conditions; it is visible and accessible and grows relatively slowly. It begins on the skin surface and is easily noticed as a small ulcer that becomes irritated, itchy, or increases in size. Possible increased risk may be related to chronic vulvar irritation and vulvar dystrophy.

Management. Vulvar carcinomas, depending on their extent, may be treated by wide excision, laser vaporization, chemotherapy creams (*i.e.*, 5-fluorouracil), or radiation.

The primary treatment for vulvar malignancy is a wide excision. Radiation is used for unresectable tumors. Laser treatment is an option for *in situ* lesions. If a widespread area is involved, a vulvectomy may be the treatment of choice.

Vulvectomy is most often reserved for women who are over 60 years of age with premalignant lesions or recurrent carcinoma *in situ* lesions, atypical hyperplasias, extensive disease, or dystrophic lesions. Regional lymphadenectomy is also performed at the time of vulvectomy in invasive disease. Chemotherapy and immunotherapy have been used as adjunctive measures.

► Nursing Process
The Patient Undergoing a Vulvectomy

◊ Assessment

In addition to the findings on physical and pelvic examination, the health history is a valuable tool because it is at this time that rapport on a one-to-one basis can be developed between nurse and patient. The reason the patient has sought health counsel is apparent. What needs to be tactfully determined is the reason for any delay if any delay in seeking health care occurred. Was it modesty, economics, denial, or simply neglect? How will this affect her future care and needs? Health habits are ascertained, and receptability for learning is evaluated. Psychosocial factors are also assessed. Preoperative preparation and psychological encouragement are also begun at this time.

◊ Nursing Diagnoses

Based on all the assessment and other data, the patient's major nursing diagnoses may include the following:

- Anxiety related to the diagnosis and aftermath of surgery
- Alteration in skin integrity related to wound drainage
- High risk for infection related to proximity of excretory function
- Pain related to surgical incision and subsequent wound care
- Sexual dysfunction related to change in body part and functioning—vulvectomy
- Self-care deficit related to lack of understanding of perineal care and general health status

◊ Planning and Implementation

◊ *Goals:*   The major goals of the patient may include acceptance of and preparation for surgical intervention, avoidance of infection and postsurgical complications, recovery of optimal sexual function, and ability to perform adequate and appropriate self-care.

◊ Nursing Interventions

◊ Preoperative

◊ *Relieving Anxiety.*   The patient must be allowed time to talk and ask questions. Fear of mutilation and loss of function is lessened when a woman of childbearing age learns that the possibility of having sexual relations is good and that pregnancy is possible after a simple vulvectomy. The nurse must know what the physician has told the patient in this regard.

◊ *Physical Preparation.*   In addition to the nursing care described in Chapter 20 regarding physical and psychological preparation, wide preparation of the skin may include cleansing the lower abdomen, inguinal areas, upper thighs, and vulva with a detergent germicide for several days before the surgical procedure. The extent of surgery is dependent on the extent of the spread; more extensive lesions require deep pelvic node dissection. Antibiotic and heparin prophylaxis may be prescribed preoperatively and continued postoperatively because of risk of infection and pulmonary emboli.

◊ Postoperative

◊ *Wound Care.*   When the patient returns from the operating room, perineal dressings are more likely to remain in place and be comfortable if a T-binder is used. Groin wounds may be exposed or covered with simple dressings. Pressure dressings may be placed over the wounds to aid in preventing the accumulation of lymph and serum. Many surgeons insert plastic tubes or drains through stab wounds in each inguinal area with attachment to portable suction. This arrangement facilitates apposition of tissue flaps and prevents accumulation of serum.

The wound is cleansed daily with warm normal saline irrigations or other antiseptic solutions as prescribed. After a *gentle* cleansing, a warm-water spray is pleasant and nontraumatizing and enhances circulation. The wound should be exposed to the air at frequent intervals to decrease moisture and maceration of the incision site. While sutures are in place, dry heat from a heating lamp or hair dryer may be prescribed.

◊ *Comfort Measures.*   Because sutures may be taut because of the surgeon's attempt to approximate tissues, comfortable positioning is required. Perhaps a low Fowler's position, or occasionally a pillow placed under the knees, will relieve tension on the incision. When placed on her side, it is more comfortable for the patient and reduces tension on the wound to have a pillow placed between her legs and against the lumbar region.

An air mattress or "egg crate" pad or mattress can assist in distributing weight and relieving pressure points. Moving from one position to another requires time and patience on the part of both patient and nurse. An overbed trapeze bar helps the patient to move herself. Ambulation may be attempted on the second day.

Analgesics are administered as required for comfort. Because primary healing rarely occurs, débridement is usually performed to provide satisfactory conditions for healing by secondary intention. Because the healing process is slow and the nature of the surgery is often distressing to the patient, she is likely to be discouraged. The nurse must be aware of the patient's uneasiness about being unduly exposed when visitors arrive or someone enters the room. She will tend to be sensitive and apologetic about odors. Thus, cleanliness, deodorant sprays, immediate removal of soiled dressings, and adequate ventilation contribute to a more pleasant environment.

◊ *Prevention of Infection.* A low-residue diet will prevent straining on defecation and wound contamination. Of particular concern is urethral and catheter care, inasmuch as an indwelling catheter is usually in place. The incidence of infection is high, which emphasizes the need for the meticulous care using principles of asepsis. Sitz baths are discouraged after a vulvectomy because of the risk of infection.

◊ *Patient Education and Home Health Care.* The patient is encouraged to share her concerns as she recovers and begins to assume increasing responsibility for her care. As she participates in changing her dressings and cleansing herself, she can use a mirror to see the perineal area. By commenting on how well the tissues are healing, and that they are looking more and more normal, the nurse will be able to provide reassurance and encouragement.

The nurse explains the need for the patient to share her concerns with her sexual partner. She can relay her daily progress to him. Activities are gradually increased and words of encouragement mean a great deal.

Posthospital care requires giving complete instructions to a family member who will assist in caring for this patient at home or to the community nurse who will be visiting her. Gradual resumption of physical and social activities is encouraged. The cure rate of properly treated vulvar carcinoma is 50% to 60%. In the absence of lymph node metastasis, the cure rate is approximately 85% to 90%.

A radical vulvectomy is often extensive and may require a second admission and operation for skin grafting. This is determined on an individual basis.

◊ ## Evaluation

Expected Outcomes
1. Adjusts to the surgical experience
   a. Uses available resources in coping with and alleviating emotional stress
   b. Asks questions related to postoperative expectations
   c. Demonstrates willingness to discuss alternate methods for expressing love and affection
2. Avoids infection and postoperative complications
   a. Is free of any signs and symptoms of infection: normal vital signs
   b. Begins to move with a minimum of discomfort
   c. Maintains cleanliness of the site following micturition or defecation
3. Assumes appropriate self-care
   a. Participates more each day in caring for her dressing changes
   b. Uses the mirror to check progress in wound healing
   c. Irrigates the wound for comfort and to stimulate healing

Cancer of the Vagina

Cancer of the vagina usually occurs as a result of metastasis from choriocarcinoma or from cancer of the cervix or adjacent organs, such as from the uterus, vulva, bladder, or rectum. Primary cancer of the vagina is uncommon.

Risk factors include previous cervical malignancy, *in utero* exposure to DES, previous vaginal or vulvar cancer, previous radiation therapy, history of HPV, or history of pessary use.

Any patient with previous cervical cancer should be examined regularly for vaginal lesions.

Before 1970, cancer of the vagina was considered to be a condition that occurred predominantly in the postmenopausal woman. In the 1970s, it was shown that maternal ingestion of DES affected female offspring who were exposed *in utero.* Benign genital tract abnormalities have occurred in some of these young women. Adenosis of the vagina may also occur.

The risk of clear cell tumor with DES exposure is 0.14 to 1.4 in 1000 women. Colposcopy is usually indicated for all women exposed to this drug. If adenosis or a significant cervical lesion is found, follow-up is individualized but essential.

Vaginal pessaries, used to provide support for prolapse in those not appropriate for surgical repair, have been found to be related to vaginal cancer if not cared for properly (*i.e.,* cleansed and checked by a health professional on a regular basis), since they can be a source of irritation.

Symptoms of cancer of the vagina are spontaneous bleeding, vaginal discharge, pain, and urinary and or rectal symptoms. Inguinal adenopathy (enlargement of lymph nodes in the inguinal region) is rare.

Laser treatment is becoming a more frequently used option in early vaginal and vulvar cancer. Surgery and radiation therapy are other methods of treatment used, depending on the extent of the disease.

Nursing Interventions. Encouraging close cooperation with health care personnel is the prime target of nursing intervention with young women who were exposed to DES *in utero.* They are at an age when sexuality in all its ramifications, including pregnancy, is of significance. Emotional support for mothers and daughters is important. For young women who have had vaginal reconstructive surgery, specific vaginal dilating procedures may be initiated. Water-soluble lubricants are helpful in reducing dyspareunia. If a possible malignancy develops that requires treatment, all aspects and effects of radiation therapy, chemotherapy, or surgery need to be explored on an individual basis.

Nurses can provide education to patients about early detection of vaginal and vulvar cancer by reporting unusual discharge or bleeding to their health care provider. Patients are also instructed in genital self-examination during a routine gynecologic examination. With a mirror, the patient can be shown what constitutes normal female anatomy and informed about changes that should be reported—lesions, sores, lumps, and persistent itching. The patient can be taught to perform this self-screening procedure at the same time as her monthly breast self-examination.

Cancer of the Fallopian Tubes

Malignancies of the fallopian tube are the least common type of genital cancer and are very rare. Symptoms can include a profuse, watery discharge and a colicky lower abdominal pain or abnormal vaginal bleeding. An enlarged tube may be found on examination. Surgery followed by radiation therapy is the usual treatment.

Cancer of the Ovary

Ovarian cancer is a frustrating disease to patients and health care providers because its silent onset and lack of warning symptoms usually result in advanced disease by the time of diagnosis. It is difficult to diagnose and is unique in that it may give rise to many primary cancers and may be the site of metastases from other cancers. It carries an annual mortality rate of 12,000 deaths and is the fourth most prevalent cause of cancer deaths in women, exceeded only by breast, colon, and lung malignancies. The peak incidence is in the fifth decade, with most cases occurring between 45 and 65 years of age. Its incidence is highest in industrialized countries, except for Japan, where its incidence is low.

A woman with ovarian cancer has a threefold to fourfold increased risk of breast cancer and women with breast cancer have an increased risk of ovarian cancer. No definitive causative factors have been determined, but oral contraceptives provide a protective effect. Heredity may play a part, and many physicians advocate biannual pelvic examinations for women with one or two relatives with ovarian cancer. Despite careful examination, these tumors are usually deep in the pelvis and difficult to detect. No early screening mechanism exists at present, although tumor markers are being explored. At present, tumor-associated antigens are more helpful in follow-up after diagnosis and treatment, but are not helpful for early screening.

Risk factors may include: a high-fat diet, smoking, alcohol, use of talcum powder perineally, a history of breast, colon, or endometrial cancer, and a family history of breast or ovarian cancer. Nulliparity, infertility, and anovulation are included as risks. The overall 5-year survival rate is 37%. This low survival rate is related to difficulty in diagnosis and unknown cause.

Clinical Manifestations.   Symptoms can include irregular menses, increasing premenstrual tension, menorrhagia with breast tenderness, early menopause, abdominal discomfort, dyspepsia, pelvic pressure, and urinary frequency. These symptoms can often be vague, but any woman with gastrointestinal symptoms without a known diagnosis must be evaluated with this diagnosis in mind. Flatulence, fullness after a light meal, and increasing abdominal girth are significant symptoms.

Diagnosis.   Any enlarged ovary must be investigated. Pelvic examination will not detect early ovarian cancer, and pelvic imaging techniques are not always definitive. Seventy-five percent of ovarian cancers have metastasized outside the ovary by the time the diagnosis is made, and 60% have spread beyond the pelvis.

There are many different cell types of ovarian cancer but epithelial tumors constitute 90%. Germ cell tumors and stromal tumors make up the other 10%.

Management.   Surgical removal is the goal of treatment. Preoperative workup can include barium enema, proctosignoidoscopy, upper GI series, chest radiograph, and IVP. Because of the high morbidity and mortality, staging of the tumor is important to direct treatment accordingly. Staging is described in Table 45-5. A total abdominal hysterectomy with bilateral salpingo-oophorectomy and omentectomy is the usual operative choice for early disease. Radiation therapy and chemotherapy using cisplatin, alkeran, and other agents, immu-

TABLE 45-5. *Stages of Cancer of the Ovary*

I—Growth limited to the ovaries
II—Growth involves one or both ovaries with pelvic extension
III—Growth involves one or both ovaries with metastases outside the pelvis or positive retroperitoneal or inguinal nodes.
IV—Growth involves one or both ovaries with distant metastases

nostimulants (*i.e.*, interferon), and intraperitoneal radioisotopes are all used, depending on staging. Hormonal regulation with tamoxifen, an antihormonal agent, may be effective. Because ovarian cancer often results in small metastatic implants in the pelvis, the pelvis and abdomen are often irradiated by a moving strip technique. The abdomen is divided into 2.5-cm strips and treated sequentially to lessen incidence of side effects.

After adjunct therapies, a second-look laparatomy may be performed to evaluate results of treatment with multiple biopsies of internal organs. Occasionally, catheters are left in place if radioactive agents are to be used postoperatively. Chemotherapy is the most common form of treatment in advanced disease.

Nursing Management.   The combination of two major clues, a long history of ovarian dysfunction and vague, undiagnosed persistent gastrointestinal symptoms, should alert the nurse to the possibility of early ovarian malignancy. Usually, ovarian malignancy is extensive at the time of diagnosis. After assessment and evaluation of other data, nursing measures will include those related to the various treatment modalities of surgery, radiation, chemotherapy, and palliation. Emotional support, comfort measures, plus attentiveness and caring are meaningful aids to this patient and her family.

Radiation Therapy

Radiation therapy plays an important role in the treatment of gynecologic malignancy (see Chap. 19, p. 351). In the treatment of squamous cell carcinoma of the cervix, it is frequently the procedure of choice, depending on the stage.

In the management of uterine and ovarian cancers, radiation is usually employed as an adjunct to surgery. In the definitive treatment of cervical disease by radiation, a combination of external pelvic radiation and internal intracavitary radiation may be used. Only in the earliest microinvasive carcinomas of the cervix is internal (intracavitary) radiation used alone. Cure rates of 85% or greater can be expected with cervical cancer that is limited to the cervix alone. As the disease extends into the parametrium, the cure rate drops to about 65%. Once the disease extends to the pelvic sidewalls, however, perhaps only one third of the patients will be cured, although many more will benefit from the palliative effects of radiation as a result of the reduction in tumor bulk and the control of infection, pain, and bleeding.

External pelvic irradiation delivered by supervoltage or megavoltage equipment usually extends over 4 to 6 weeks. Thereafter, intracavitary radiation is performed. This sequence may be reversed, depending on anatomic considerations. The cervix and uterus lend themselves naturally to internal irradiation because they act as a receptacle for radioactive sources. Isotopes of radium and cesium are used for intracavitary irradiation.

Intraoperative radiation is a technique that allows radiation to be applied directly to the affected area during surgery.

Intraoperative radiation therapy uses an electron beam directed to the operative site. This direct-view irradiation may be used when para-aortic nodes are positive for neoplasm or for unresectable or partially resectable neoplasms. Benefits are accurate beam direction, precisely limiting the radiation to the tumor only, and the ability during treatment to block sensitive organs from radiation. This new method is usually combined with external beam radiation preoperatively or postoperatively. It may be used after a cone biopsy or after hysterectomy.

External Beam Therapy. Betatrons, linear accelerators, and cobalt-60 units are capable of delivering high doses of radiation deep within the pelvis to the site of the tumor. Radiation side effects are cumulative and tend to appear as the total dose exceeds the body's natural capacity to repair the radiation effect. Radiation enteritis, resulting in diarrhea and abdominal cramping, and radiation cystitis, manifested by frequency, urgency, and dysuria, may occur; this is a natural manifestation of the normal tissues' response to the radiation therapy program. The radiation therapist and nurse inform the patient in advance of these possible side effects and employ a variety of measures to modify their impact when they occur. These measures include dietary control (by restricting the amount of fiber, roughage, and lactose), and the use of antispasmodic drugs.

The patient may be placed on a low-residue diet to prevent frequent bowel movements and to avoid blockage of a possibly stenosed gastrointestinal tract.

The following guidelines may be helpful:

- Limit dairy products to two servings daily.
- Avoid raw fruits, beans, peas, and popcorn.
- Eat white or refined breads and cereals only.
- Eat ground or well-cooked, tender meats, eggs, and cheese.
- Eat juices without pulp, canned fruit, and cooked vegetables.

Evaluation of the physical, emotional, and learning needs of the patient and needs of the family are part of the nursing assessment before and during treatment. Information overload, along with anxiety that impairs learning, must be anticipated.

On occasion, severe reactions will require that treatment be suspended briefly until the normal tissues repair themselves.

Internal (Intracavitary) Irradiation. In the operating room, an examination is performed under anesthesia, after which specially prepared applicators are inserted into the endometrial cavity and vagina. These devices are not loaded with radioactive material until the patient has returned to her room. X-ray films are obtained to determine the precise relationship of the applicator to the normal pelvic anatomy and to the tumor. Only when this study is completed does the radiation therapist load the applicators with predetermined amounts of radioactive material. This is called *afterloading* and allows for precise control of the radiation exposure received by the patient, with minimal exposure of the physician and nursing and health care personnel. A patient undergoing internal radiation treatment is placed in a private room until the application is completed. Adjacent rooms may also need to be evacuated. A lead shield is placed at the doorway to the patient's room.

Various applicators have been developed for intracavitary treatment. Some are inserted into the endometrial cavity and endocervical canal as multiple small irradiators (*e.g.,* Heyman's capsules). Others consist of a central tube (tandem or intrauterine "stem") placed through the dilated endocervical canal into the uterine cavity, which remains in fixed relationship with irradiators placed in the upper vagina on each side of the cervix (vaginal ovoids) (Fig. 45-6).

At the time of insertion of the applicator, an indwelling bladder catheter is inserted. The applicator is secured in place with vaginal packing. The objective of the internal treatment is to maintain the distribution of internal radiation at a fixed dosage throughout the application. Such applications usually last 24 to 72 hours, depending on dose calculations made by the radiation physicist.

Nursing Management During Intracavitary Radiation Therapy

The radioactive elements used in intracavitary therapy are radium and cesium. Cesium has a long half-life and no gaseous by-products. During the treatment, diligent nursing care must be given. The patient is carefully observed and attended, although the nursing staff must try to reduce as much as possible the radiation exposure to themselves and should use the principles of time, distance, and shielding to protect themselves from excessive exposure:

- Minimize amount of time near a radioactive source.
- Maximize distance from radioactive source.
- Use required shielding to keep exposure at a minimum.

Nurses who are or may be pregnant should not be involved in the immediate care of such patients. Visits to the patient should not be aimless; nurse–patient contacts provide a good opportunity for the patient to talk about her anxiety and fear. To minimize radiation exposure, the nurse may stay at the foot of the bed or at the entrance to the room.

During the treatment, the patient is on absolute bed rest. She may move from side to side with her back supported by a pillow, and the head of the bed may be raised to 45 degrees. The patient should be encouraged to practice deep-breathing

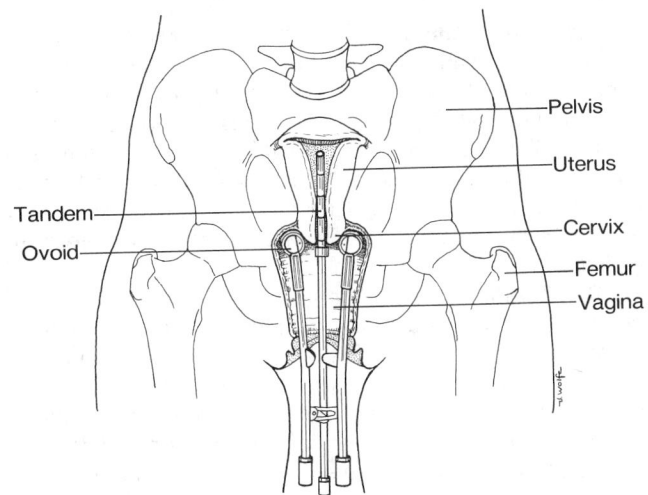

Figure 45–6. Placement of tandem and ovoids for internal radiation therapy. (Copyright 1987 J. Wolfe.)

and coughing exercises and to flex and extend the feet to stretch the calf muscles to promote venous return. Back care is much appreciated by the patient, but adequate care is given within the minimum amount of time at the bedside.

Usually, the patient is on a low-residue diet to prevent frequent bowel movements. One is less concerned here with dislodging the applicator than with the social and physical discomforts that the patient may experience. The nurse should inspect the catheter frequently to make sure that it is draining properly. The chief hazard of improper drainage is that the bladder may become distended and its walls exposed to radiation. Although perineal care is omitted at this time, any profuse discharge should be reported immediately to the radiation therapist or gynecologic surgeon.

The patient is observed for evidence of temperature elevation, nausea, and vomiting. These symptoms should be reported, because they may indicate infection or perforation. Finally, the radiation therapist takes steps to secure the internal applicator in place. Nursing personnel need not be preoccupied with the fear that the applicator will be prematurely extruded. However, one should check from time to time to see that the applicator or the radioactive sources have not been dislodged. Should this happen, the Radiation Safety Department is notified immediately. Radioactive sources should never be grasped with the hand or fingers.

The Radiation Safety Department will give specific safety precautions to those who will be in contact with the patient, including care providers and family. Nurses caring for the patient will receive directives regarding time and distance related to care provision. Other instructions vary but may include the following:

1. Film badges or pocket ion chambers are worn to monitor exposure.
2. Rubber gloves are needed to dispose of any soiled matter that may be contaminated.
3. Specific laundry and housekeeping directions will be provided.
4. The patient will be restricted to her room and not allowed visitors who are or may be pregnant or who are younger than 18 years of age.
5. A discharge survey is usually performed by Radiation Safety personnel before the patient leaves the room to ensure that all sources of radiation have been removed.

Applicator Removal.   The radiation therapist calculates precisely the radiation dose delivered. At the end of the prescribed period, the nurse may be requested to assist the physician in removing the applicator. Because the sources are "afterloaded," they can be removed by the physician in the same manner as they were inserted. This does not require local or general anesthesia and is performed in the patient's room. Medication with a mild sedative may be required before the applicator is removed.

Post-Treatment Care.   Progressive ambulation is recommended after the period of enforced bed rest. Diet may be offered as tolerated. The patient may shower as soon as she wishes. Patients should be instructed not to douche after removal of the applicator. Because the cervix has been dilated, any chance of bacterial contamination should be minimized.

Nurses caring for patients undergoing radiation therapy assess any possible misconceptions about this mode of treatment that the patient and family may have both before and after treatment. The oncology clinical nurse specialist may be

consulted for information and assistance with problem solving, if necessary. Resources for further clinical and patient information are listed at the end of Chapter 19.

In summary, malignancy may develop in any of the organs of the female reproductive tract. Although early detection of cancer has increased as a result of adherence to the recommendations of the American Cancer Society for breast self-examinations, gynecologic examinations, and mammograms, many women do not follow these recommendations, or ignore or deny the appearance of symptoms. The nurse who provides care for women during hospitalization, in a clinic, long-term care facility, or the home has the opportunity to teach and counsel women about practices that will protect them from undetected malignancy.

The patient who is diagnosed with malignancy of the female reproductive system often is anxious and fearful about the diagnosis, and its implications for her well-being and the well-being of her family. She often has realistic fears about her treatment options and their potential effects on her survival as well as her ability to care for her family and to carry on her usual activities. The nurse who is sensitive to the impact of the diagnosis of malignancy of the reproductive system and knowledgeable about the treatment options and their potential benefits and side effects is better able to provide quality care to the patient.

Chapter Summary

As they care for women and their health problems, nurses must maintain a high level of professional curiosity about research results and current protocols regarding changes in approach to disease treatment and prevention as they care for women and their health problems. Constant changes, improvements, and new modes of treatment must be considered in any nursing care plan.

Awareness of those at risk for cervical, uterine, and ovarian cancer provides a starting point for patient education programs. Individual patient counseling includes warning signs, symptoms, and methods of prevention. Pelvic infections, possibly related to chlamydial infection and other STDs, may cause disability and pain. The threat of infertility and the complexity of treatment for this entity deserve every preventive method of education that nurses treating women can develop. The current epidemic of HPV or genital warts with its propensity for causing premalignant cervical changes is again a challenge for nurses, who have the ability to make a difference through patient education. The emotional trauma of herpes simplex requires nursing intervention, reassurance, and education about what this viral entity means for the patient's future.

Because a large part of future patient care will involve geriatric populations, awareness of teaching methods, disease states, and manifestations are of paramount importance to all nurses. Gynecologic health of older women is often ignored, but some nurses have initiated changes in this area and others can continue current programs and improve on them.

Sensitivity to fears of death and mutilation are considered in care planning and in response to patient behavior. Women who have assisted friends or relatives through radiation or chemotherapy may have preconceived notions about outcomes that need to be explored.

Provision of adequate access to care for the homeless, financially restricted, HIV infected, prevention ignorant, young, old, abused, or any woman is a challenge for today's nurse.

Bibliography

Books

Ashwanden P et al. Oncology Nursing: Advances, Treatments and Trends into the 21st Century. Rockville, MD, Aspen Systems, 1990.

DeVita V et al. Cancer: Principles and Practice of Oncology, 3rd ed. Philadelphia, JB Lippincott, 1989.

DeVita V et al. AIDS, 2nd ed. Philadelphia, JB Lippincott, 1989.

Dunnihoo D. Fundamentals of Gynecology and Obstetrics. Philadelphia, JB Lippincott, 1990.

Emans J and Goldstein D. Pediatric and Adolescent Gynecology, 3rd ed. Boston, Little, Brown, 1990.

Fogel C and Lauver D. Sexual Health Promotion. Philadelphia, WB Saunders, 1990.

Glass R. Office Gynecology, 3rd ed. Baltimore, Williams & Wilkins, 1988.

Groenwald S. Cancer Nursing: Principles and Practice. Boston, Jones & Bartlett, 1987.

Jones H and Jones G. Novak's Textbook of Gynecology, 11th ed. Baltimore, Williams & Wilkins, 1988.

Lichtman R and Papera S. Gynecology Well-Woman Care. Norwalk, CT, Appleton and Lange, 1990.

Newcomer V and Young E. Geriatric Dermatology. New York, Igaku-Shoin, 1989.

Nichols D and Randall C. Vaginal Surgery, 3rd ed. Baltimore, Williams & Wilkins, 1989.

Nori D and Hilaris B. Radiation Therapy of Gynecological Cancer. New York, Alan R Liss, 1987.

Pernoll M and Benson R (eds). Current Obstetric and Gynecologic Diagnosis and Treatment. Norwalk, CT, Appleton & Lange, 1987.

Precis III: An Update in Obstetrics and Gynecology. Washington, DC, American College of Obstetrics and Gynecology, 1986.

Quilligan E and Zuspan F (eds). Current Therapy in Obstetrics and Gynecology 3. Philadelphia, WB Saunders, 1990.

Recurrent Vulvovaginal Candidiasis: A Continuing Education Program for Nurse Practitioners. Palo Alto, CA, Syntex-NAACOG, 1989.

Stewart F et al. Understanding Your Body: Every Woman's Guide to Gynecology and Health. Toronto, Bantam, 1987.

Veronesi U (ed). Surgical Oncology: A European Handbook. Berlin, Springer-Verlag, 1989.

Wang C (ed). Clinical Radiation Oncology. Littleton, MA, PSG, 1988.

Wittes R (ed). Manual of Oncologic Therapeutics. Philadelphia, JB Lippincott, 1989/1990.

Ziegfeld C (ed). Core Curriculum for Oncology Nursing. Philadelphia, WB Saunders, 1987.

Journals

Asterisks indicate nursing research articles.

General

Centers for Disease Control: 1989 Sexually transmitted diseases treatment guidelines. MMWR 1989; 38(S-8):1–43.

Chacko M et al. Vaginal douching in teenagers attending a family planning clinic. J Adolesc Health Care 1989 Mar; 10(3):217–219.

Foley S. Preventive gynecologic nursing in an inpatient setting. J Obstet Gynecol Neonatal Nurs 1987 May-Jun; 16(3):160–166.

Lawhead R. Vulvar self-examination: What your patient should know. Female Patient 1990 Jan; 15(1):33–38.

Lichtman R. Perimenopausal hormone replacement therapy: Review of the literature. J Nurse Midwifery 1991 Jan/Feb; 36(1):30–48.

Nussbaum M et al. Attitudes vs performance in providing gynecologic care to adolescents by pediatricians. J Adolesc Health Care 1989 Mar; 10(3):203–208.

Gerontological Considerations

Blesch K and Prohaska T. Cervical cancer screening in older women: Issues and interventions. Cancer Nurs 1991 Jun; 14(3):141–147.

Coopland A. Geriatric urogynecology. Obstet Gynecol Clin North Am 1989 Dec; 16(4):931–937.

Denny M and Koren M. Gynecological health needs of elderly women. J Gerontol Nurs 1989; 15(1):33–38.

* Dickson G. A feminist poststructuralist analysis of the knowledge of menopause. Adv Nurs Sci 1990 Mar; 12(3):15–31.

McKay M. Genital dermatoses in geriatric dermatology. In: Newcomer V and Young E. Geriatric Dermatology. New York, Igaku-Shoin, 1989, pp 477–492.

Morrison BD and Robbins L. Sexual assessment and the aging female. Nurs Pract 1989 Dec;14(12):35–45.

Vulvovaginal Infections

Burnhill M. Clinician's guide to counseling patients with chronic vaginitis. Contemp Obstet Gynecol 1990 Jan:35(1);37–44.

Eschenbach D. Bacterial vaginosis: Emphasis on upper genital tract complications. Obstet Gynecol Clin North Am. 1989 Sept 16(3):593–610.

Gietyl K. Role of the nurse practitioner in the management of vaginitis. Am J Obstet Gynecol 1988 Apr; 158(4):1009–1011.

Hammill H. Some unusual causes of vaginitis (excluding trichomonas, bacterial vaginosis and candida albicans). Obstet Gynecol Clin North Am 1989 Sep; 16(3): 337–345.

Hammill H. Normal vaginal flora in relation to vaginitis. Obstet Gynecol Clin North Am 1989 Jun; 16(2):329–336.

Landers D. The treatment of vaginitis: Trichomonas, yeast and bacterial vaginosis. Clin Obstet Gynecol 1988 Jun; 31(2):473–479.

Pelosi M and Apuzzio J. Vaginitis: Update on diagnosis and treatment. Female Patient 1989 May; 14(5):84–98.

Secor RMC. Bacterial vaginosis: A comprehensive review. Nurs Clin North Am 1988 Dec; 23(4):865–875.

Sobel JD. Bacterial vaginosis: Assessment and treatment. Med Aspects Hum Sexuality 1990 Jun; (6):42–46.

Wolner-Hanssen P et al. Clinical manifestations of vaginal trichomoniasis. JAMA 1989 Jan; 261(4):571–576.

Herpes Simplex Type 2

Breslin E. Genital herpes simplex. Nurs Clin North Am 1988 Dec; 23(4): 907–915.

Brock B et al. Frequency of asymptomatic shedding of herpes simplex virus in women with genital herpes. JAMA 1990 Jan; 19; 263(3):418–420.

Cohen P and Young A. Herpes simplex: Update on diagnosis and management of genital herpes infection. Med Aspects Hum Sexuality 1988 Mar; 22(3):93–100.

Davies K. Genital herpes: An overview. JOGNN 1990 Sep/Oct; 19(5):401–406.

Lafferty W. Genital herpes: Recommendations for comprehensive care. Postgrad Med 1988 Feb; 83(2):157–165.

Landy H and Grossman J. Herpes simplex virus. Obstet Gynecol Clin North Am 1989 Sep; 16(3):495–515.

Peng T and Johnson T. HSV in the pregnant patient. Female Patient 1989 Aug; 14(8):27–41.

Endometriosis

Corfman R and Grainger D. Endometriosis: Associated infertility and treatment options. J Reprod Med 1989 Feb; 34(2):135–141.

Filer R and Wu C. Coitus during menses: Its effect on endometriosis and pelvic inflammatory disease. J Reprod Med 1989 Nov; 34(11):887–890.

Lomano J. Fiberoptic laser laparoscopy in the treatment of pelvic endometriosis. Laser Nurs 1989 Winter; 3(4):9–11.

Rock J (ed). Endometriosis. Obstet Gynecol Clin North Am 1989 Mar; 16(1).

Treybig M. Primary dysmenorrhea or endometriosis. Nurs Pract 1989 May; 14(5):8–18.

Pelvic Inflammatory Disease

Apuzzio J and Pelosi M. The "new salpingitis": Subtle symptoms, aggressive management. Female Patient 1989 Nov; 14(11):25–35.

Moscicki A. HPV infection in teenage girls. Med Aspects Hum Sexuality 1990 Jul; 24(7):2227.

Pastorek J. Pelvic inflammatory disease and tubo-ovarian abscess. Obstet Gynecol Clin North Am 1989 Jun; 16(2):347–361.

Pokorny S. Pelvic inflammatory disease: An epidemic among American teenagers. Female Patient 1989 Aug; 14(8):42–44.

Shattuck J. Pelvic inflammatory disease: Education for maintaining fertility. Nurs Clin North Am 1988 Dec; 23(4):899–906.

Wardell D. Ectopic pregnancy: A growing concern. J Am Acad Nurs Pract 1989 Oct/Dec; 1(4):119–125.

Condyloma Acuminata: Human Papillomavirus

Carlone J (ed). Human papillomavirus: A growing epidemic. Nurs Pract Forum 1990 Jun; 1(1):10–62.

Deitch K. Symptoms of chronic vaginal infection and microscopic condyloma in women. JOGNN 1990 Mar/Apr; 19(2):133–138.

Enterline J and Leonardo J. Condylomata accuminata. Nurs Pract 1989 Apr; 14(4):8–16.

Koutsky L and Wolner-Hanssen P. Genital papillomavirus infection. Obstet Gynecol Clin North Am 1989 Sep; 16(3):541–564.

Lehr S and Lee M. The psychosocial and sexual trauma of a genital HPV infection. Nurs Pract Forum 1990 Jun; 1(1):25–30.

Lucas V. Human papillomavirus: A potentially carcinogenic STD. Nurs Clin North Am 1988 Dec; 23(4):917–935.

McQuiston C. The relationship of risk factors for cervical cancer and HPV in college women. Nurs Pract 1989 Apr; 14(4):18–26.

Nettina S and Kauffman F. Diagnosis and management of sexually transmitted genital lesions. Nurs Pract 1990 Jan; 15(1):20–39.

Toole K et al. Cervical dysplasia and condyloma as risks for carcinoma: Two case studies. Am J Maternal Child Nurs 1990 May/Jun; 15(3):170–175.

Walker J et al. Human papillomavirus genotype as a prognostic indicator in carcinoma of the uterine cervix. Obstet Gynecol 1989 Nov; 74(5):781–785.

Endocervicitis: Chlamydia

Bachman G. Psychosexual aspects of hysterectomy. Womens Health Iss 1990 Fall; 1(1):41–49.

Bourcier K and Seidler A. Chlamydia and condylomata acuminata: An update for the nurse practitioner. J Obstet Gynecol Neonatal Nurs 1987 Jan-Feb; 16(1):17–22.

Brown H. Recognizing common STD's in adolescents. Contemp Obstet Gynecol 1989 Mar; 33(3):47–62.

Cohen I. *Chlamydia trachomatis* in the perinatal period. Contemp Obstet Gynecol 1989 Jun; 33(6):22–34.

Dulaney P et al. A comprehensive education and support program for women experiencing hysterectomies. JOGNN 1990 Jul/Aug; 19(4):319–325.

Loucks A. Chlamydia: An unheralded epidemic. Am J Nurs 1987 Jul; 87(7):920–922.

Paavonen J et al. Randomized treatment of mucopurulent cervicitis with doxycycline or amoxicillin. Am J Obstet Gynecol 1989 Jul; 161(11):128–135.

Whelan M. Nursing management of the patient with *Chlamydia trachomatis* infection. Nurs Clin North Am 1988 Dec; 23(4): 877–883.

Woolard D et al. Screening for *Chlamydia trachomatis* at a university health service. J Obstet Gynecol Neonatal Nurs 1989, Mar/Apr; 18(2):145–149.

Hysterectomy

Cohen S et al. Another look at psychologic complications of hysterectomy. Image: Journal of Nursing Scholarship 1989 Spr; 21(1):51–53.

Hysterectomy and its alternatives. Consum Rep 1990 Sep; 55(9):603–607.

Patient guide: Hysterectomy. Female Patient 1990 Jan; 15(1):62–63.

Sloan D. The expendable organ. Female Patient 1989 Jun; 14(6):35–37.

AIDS In Women

Anderson J. Gynecologic manifestations of AIDS and HIV. Female Patient 1989 Sep; 14(9): 57–68.

Fiumara N. Human immunodeficiency virus infection and syphilis. J Am Acad Dermatol 1989 Jul; 21(1): 141–142.

Gee G. AIDS: Context of care. Semin Oncol Nurs 1989 Nov; 5(4):244–248.

* Jacob J. Self-assessed learning needs of oncology nurses caring for individuals with HIV related disorders: A national survey. Cancer Nurs 1990 Aug; 13(4):246–255.

Me first! Medical manifestations of HIV in women. New Jersey Women and AIDS Network, 5 Elm Row, New Brunswick, NJ 08901.

Moroso G and Holman S. Counseling and testing women for HIV. NAACOG's Clinical Issues in Perinatal and Women's Health Nursing 1990; 1(1):10–19.

Redfield R and Burke D. HIV infection: The clinical picture. Sci Am 1988 Oct; 259(4):90–98.

Ryan J. Clinicians and HIV infections. Nurs Pract 1989 Sep; 14(10):4040–4046.

Sinclair B. Epidemiology and transmission of infection by human immunodeficiency virus. NAACOG's Clinical Issues in Perinatal and Women's Health Nursing 1990; 1(1):1–9.

Wenstrom K and Gall S. HIV infection in women. Obstet Gynecol Clin North Am 1989 Sep; 16(3):627–643.

Wofsy C. Women and acquired immunodeficiency syndrome. West J Med 1988 Dec; 149(6):687–690.

Reproductive Malignancy

Berek J (Mod). Monoclonal antibodies role in combating gyn malignancies. Contemp Obstet Gynecol 1990 Feb; 35(2):109–120.

* Christman N. Uncertainty and adjustment during radiotherapy. Nurs Res 1990 Jan/Feb; 39(1):17–20.

Coughman SM and Russo G. Cutaneous signs of internal cancer. Patient Care 1989 Jan 30; 23(2):28–41.

Dattoli M et al. Analysis of multiple prognostic factors in patients with stage 1b cervical cancer: Age as a major determinant. Int J Radiat Oncol Biol Phys 1989 Jul; 17(1):41–47.

Feldman J. Ovarian failure and cancer treatment: Incidence and interventions for the premenopausal woman. Oncol Nurs Forum 1989 May; 16(5):651–657.

Fullerton J and Barger M. Papanicolaou smear: An update on classification and management. J Am Acad Nurs Pract 1989 Jul/Sep; 1(3):84–90.

Gribbin M. Could you detect these oncological crises? RN 1990 Jun; 53(6): 36–42.

Harbeck S. Intraoperative radiation therapy. Oncol Nursing Forum 1988; 15(2):143–147.

Holloway R et al. Monitoring the course of cervical cancer with the squamous cell carcinoma serum radioimmunoassay. Obstet Gynecol 1989 Dec; 74(6):944–949.

Kwikkel H. Treating CIN: Laser vaporization or cryotherapy. Contemp Obstet Gynecol 1989 Mar; 33(3):29–44.

* Mishel M and Sorenson D. Uncertainty in gynecological cancer: A test of mediating functions of mastery and coping. Nurs Res 1991 May/Jun; 40(3):167–171.

Pearcy R et al. The value of pre-operative intracavitary radiotherapy in patients treated by radical hysterectomy and pelvic lymphadenectomy for invasive carcinoma of the cervix. Clin Radiol 1988 Jan; 39(1):95–98.

* Picard H. Fatigue in cancer patients: A descriptive study. Cancer Nurs 1991 Feb; 14(1):13–19.

Qian H et al. Smoking and reproductive cancer: A report from China. Female Patient 1989 Jun; 14(6):42–51.

Rubin M and Lauver D. Assessment and management of cervical intraepithelial neoplasia. Nurs Pract 1990, Oct; 15(10):23–31.

Schover L et al. Sexual dysfunction and treatment for early stage cervical cancer. Cancer 1989 Jan; 63(1):204–212.

Shy K et al. Papanicolaou smear screening interval and risk of cervical cancer. Obstet Gynecol 1989 Dec; 74(6):838–843.

Slattery M et al. Cigarette smoking and exposure to passive smoke are risk factors for cervical cancer. JAMA 1989 Mar; 261(11):1593–1633.

Strohl R. The nursing role in radiation oncology: Symptom management of acute and chronic reactions. Oncol Nursing Forum 1988; 15(4): 429–434.

Wilczynski S, et al. Adenocarcinoma of the cervix associated with human papillomavirus. Cancer 1988 Oct; 62(7):1331–1336.

Woodward J. The triple C approach to the detection of cervical cancer. Nurs Pract Forum 1990 Jun; 1(1):31–39.

Ovarian Cancer

Heintz A et al. The treatment of advanced ovarian carcinoma: Clinical variables associated with prognosis. Gynecol Oncol 1988 Jul; 30(3): 347–358.

Koonings P et al. Relative frequency of primary ovarian neoplasms: A ten-year review. Obstet Gynecol 1989 Dec; 74(6):921–925.

McGowan L. Ovarian cancer after hysterectomy. Obstet Gynecol 1987 Mar; 69(3):386–389.

Vaginal and Vulvar Cancer

Baggish M et al. Quantitative evaluation of the skin and accessory appendages in vulvar carcinoma in situ. Obstet Gynecol 1989 Aug; 74(2): 169–173.

Chamorro T. Cancer of the vulva and vagina. Semin Oncol Nurs 1990 Aug; 6(3):198–205.

Edelman D. Diethylstilbestrol exposure and the risk of clear cell cervical and vaginal adenocarcinoma. Int J Fertil 1989 Apr; 34(4):251–255.

Uterine Cancer

Boyd M. Endometrial cancer. Can J Surg 1989 Mar; 32(2):89–92.

Dunton C. Treatment of early invasive (1A) and advanced stage (IIB-IVA)

cervical carcinoma. Am J Gynecol Health 1990 Nov/Dec; 4(6):192–194.

Feldman J. Ovarian failure and cancer treatment: Incidence and intervention for the premenopausal woman. Oncol Nurs Forum 1989 May; 16(5): 651–657.

Gilman C. Management of early-stage endometrial carcinoma. Am Fam Physician 1987 Apr; 35(4):103–112.

Greven K et al. Analysis of failure patterns in stage III endometrial carcinoma and therapeutic implications. Int J Radiat Oncol Biol Phys 1989 Jul; 17(1):35–39.

Hricak H et al. Endometrial carcinoma staging by MR imaging. Radiology 1987 Feb; 162(2):297–305.

Hubbard J et al. Cancer of the endometrium. Semin Oncol Nurs 1990 Aug; 6(3):206–213.

Kuten A et al. Results of radiotherapy in recurrent endometrial carcinoma: A retrospective analysis of 51 patients. Int J Radiat Oncol Biol Phys 1989 Jul; 17(1):29–34.

Lewandowski G and Delgado G. Postoperative adjuvant external beam radiotherapy in surgical stage I endometrial carcinoma. Cancer 1989 Oct; 64(7):1414–1417.

Rostad ME. The radical vulvectomy patient: Preventing complications. Dimens Crit Care Nurs 1988 Sep/Oct; 7(5):289–294.

Schulz M and Shen J. Treatment of stage I endometrial carcinoma. J Reprod Med 1989 Feb; 34(2):167–172.

Agencies

American Cancer Society
777 Third Avenue, New York, NY 10017

Herpetics Engaged in Living Productively (HELP)
260 Sheridan Avenue, Palo Alto, CA 94306

46

Assessment and Management of Patients With Breast Disorders

Learning Objectives

On completion of this chapter, the learner will be able to:

1. Develop a teaching plan for self-examination of the breast for the hospitalized patient and for consumer groups
2. Describe diagnostic tests used to detect breast disorders
3. Use the nursing process as a framework for care of the patient with cancer of the breast
4. Compare the therapeutic usefulness of chemotherapy, surgery, and radiation in treating cancer of the breast
5. Describe the physical, psychosocial, and rehabilitative needs of the patient who has had a mastectomy

Anatomic Overview

Breasts of males and females are the same until puberty, when estrogen and other hormones initiate breast development in women. This usually occurs about the age of 10 and continues until about age 16, although the range is wide and can vary from 9 to 18 years of age. Stages of development of the breast are described as Tanner stages 1 through 5 after the physician who initiated classification of adolescent breast changes. Stage 1 describes a prepubertal breast. Stage 2 is breast budding, the first sign of puberty in a female. Stage 3 involves further enlargement of breast tissue and the areola, and stage 4 occurs when the nipple and areola form a secondary mound on top of breast tissue. Stage 5 is a larger breast with a single contour.

Figure 46-1 shows the anatomy of the breast when de-velopment is completed. The breast contains glandular (parenchyma) and ductal tissue along with fibrous tissue that binds the lobes together and fatty tissue in and between the lobes. These paired mammary glands are located between the second and sixth ribs over the pectoralis major muscle from the sternum to the midaxillary line and extend into the axillae, an area of breast tissue called the *tail of Spence*. Cooper's ligaments, which are fascial bands, support the breast on the chest wall.

Each breast consists of 12 to 20 cone-shaped lobes that are made up of lobules. Lobules are clusters of acini, small structures ending in a duct. All of the ducts in each lobule empty into an ampulla, which then opens onto the nipple after narrowing. Eighty-five percent of breast tissue is fat.

Psychosocial Implications

In Western culture, the breast is considered a significant component of feminine beauty. A woman's reaction to any actual

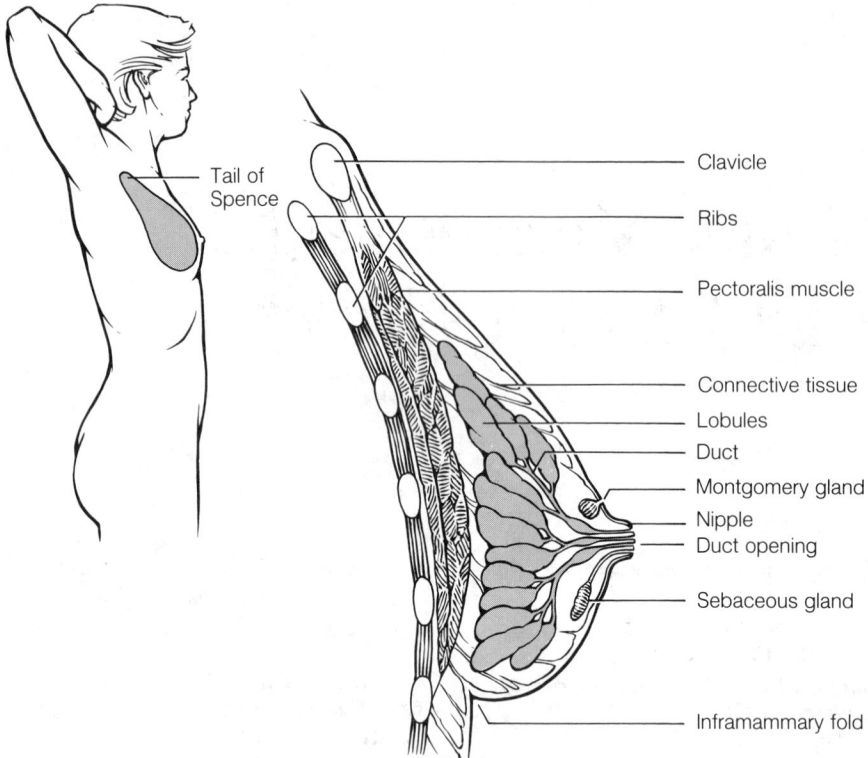

Tail of Spence

Clavicle

Ribs

Pectoralis muscle

Connective tissue

Lobules

Duct

Montgomery gland

Nipple

Duct opening

Sebaceous gland

Inframammary fold

Figure 46–1. Anatomy of the breast.

or suspected disease may include fear of disfigurement, fear of loss of sexual attractiveness, and fear of death. These fears may be major impediments to evaluation of a breast problem.

All health care providers, aware of these implications, should encourage women to examine their own breasts and teach them to recognize early signs of changes that may indicate problems. The nurse plays a pivotal role in preventive education. Almost all settings lend themselves to teaching, disseminating information, and encouraging appropriate care for prevention, detection, and treatment of breast problems.

Incidence of Breast Disease

Although most disorders of the female breast are benign, the breast is estimated to be the site of 28% of all cancers in women in the United States and is estimated by the National Cancer Institute to cause 18% of all cancer deaths. Death from cancer of the breast is exceeded only by lung cancer.

Benign breast disease also occurs frequently in women and arouses a great deal of anxiety. Because of the variations in breast tissue that occur during the menstrual cycle, pregnancy, and menopause, normal changes must often be distinguished from those that may be pathologic. Most women notice increased tenderness and lumpiness prior to their menstrual period; therefore, breast self-examination (BSE) is encouraged after menses when less fluid retention is present. Many women have grainy-textured breast tissue, but these areas are usually less nodular after menses. Benign lesions include, among others, fibrocystic changes, fibroadenomas, and cysts.

Assessment: Breast Examination

Female Breast

Examination of the female breast is conducted during any general physical or gynecologic examination or whenever the patient presents with suspicion, complaint, or fear of breast disease. A professional breast examination is recommended at least every 3 years for women aged 20 to 40, and then annually. A complete and thorough breast examination including instruction in BSE takes at least 5 minutes or more.

Inspection. Examination begins with inspection. The patient disrobes to the waist and is seated in a comfortable position facing the examiner. The breasts are inspected for size and symmetry. A slight difference in size is common and is generally a normal finding. The skin is inspected for color, thickening or edema, and venous pattern. Erythema may indicate local inflammation or superficial lymphatic invasion by a neoplasm. An increased venous pattern can signal increased blood supply demanded by a tumor. Edema and pitting of the skin caused by blocked lymph drainage from a possible neoplasm can give the skin an orange-peel appearance (*peau d'orange*), a classic sign of advanced breast malignancy.

Nipples, though variable in each patient, are normally similar in size and shape. A slight inversion of one or both nipples is not uncommon and is a significant finding only when of recent origin. Ulceration, rashes, or nipple discharge requires evaluation. To elicit a dimpling or retraction that may otherwise go undetected, the examiner instructs the patient to raise both arms overhead. This maneuver normally elevates both breasts equally. Next, the patient is instructed to place her hands at her waist and push in. These movements, causing contraction of the pectoral muscles, do not normally alter the breast contour or nipple direction. Any dimpling or retraction during these position changes is suggestive of a potential malignancy. The clavicular and axillary regions are inspected and palpated for swelling, discoloration, lesions, or enlarged lymph nodes.

Palpation. Palpation of the axillary and clavicular areas is easily performed with the patient in a sitting position. For examination of axillary lymph nodes, the patient's arm is gently abducted from the thorax by the examiner's hand. The patient's left forearm is grasped gently and supported with the examiner's left hand. The right hand is then free to palpate the axilla, noting the presence or absence of nodes that may be lying against the thoracic wall. The flat parts of the fingertips are used to gently palpate the areas of the central, lateral, subscapular, and pectoral nodes. Normally, these lymph nodes are not palpable. If enlarged, their size, location, mobility, consistency, and tenderness are noted. The patient is then assisted to a supine position. Before breast palpation, the shoulder is elevated by a small pillow to balance the breast on the chest wall. Failure to do this allows the breast tissue to fall laterally, and a breast mass may be missed in this thickened tissue.

Light palpation in a systematic fashion includes the entire surface of the breast, including the axillary tail. The examiner may choose to proceed in a clockwise direction following imaginary concentric circles from the outer limits of the breast toward the nipple. Other acceptable methods are to palpate from each number on the face of the clock toward the nipple in a clockwise fashion or along imaginary vertical lines on the breast.

During palpation, the consistency of the tissue and the presence of tenderness or masses are noted. If a mass is detected, it is described by its location (*i.e.,* left breast, 2 cm from the nipple at the 2 o'clock position). Size, shape, consistency, border delineation, and mobility are included in the description. Lastly, the areola around the nipple is gently compressed to determine the presence or absence of breast discharge or secretion.

The breast tissue of the adolescent is usually firm and lobular, while the postmenopausal woman is more likely to have breast tissue that feels thinner and more granular. During pregnancy and lactation, the breasts are firmer and larger, and lobules are more distinct. Areolae usually darken during pregnancy because of hormonal changes. Cysts are often found in menstruating women and are usually well defined and freely movable. Premenstrually, cysts may be larger and more tender. Malignancies, on the other hand, tend to be hard, poorly defined, fixed to the skin or underlying tissue, and often nontender. Any abnormalities detected during inspection and palpation require evaluation by a physician.

Male Breast

Examination of the male breast and axillae is not to be overlooked. The nipple and areola are inspected for masses, lesions, or discharge. The areola is palpated for masses. Gynecomastia (overdeveloped mammary glands in the male) is differentiated from the soft, fatty enlargement of obesity by the firm enlargement of glandular tissue beneath and immediately surrounding the areola. The same procedure for inspection and palpation of the female axillae is employed during an assessment of the male axillae.

One percent of all patients with carcinoma of the breast are male. Although most of this chapter emphasizes treatment of female patients, treatment of breast cancer in males is similar. Most cancers in men are found at a later stage, possibly because men are not as conscious about breast lumps as are women.

Self-Examination of the Breast

Because many breast cancers are detected by women themselves, top priority must be given to teaching all women how and when to examine their breasts. It is estimated that only a minority of women (25% to 30%) perform BSE each month. Even among women who perform BSE, there are often delays in seeking medical attention. The reasons for this continue to be the subject of research; fear is a major factor. Economic factors, lack of education, reluctance to act if no pain is involved, psychologic factors, and modesty may all enter into delay and denial.

The nurse is in a unique position to inform and educate all women about the benefits of regular BSE and early detection. Several nursing strategies that may increase motivation to perform BSE have been identified. A personal commitment to this practice on the part of the nurse is one of these strategies. Films about BSE can be obtained from local chapters of the American Cancer Society. Methods are described more fully in Figure 46-2. The BSE in-hospital program from the National Cancer Institute in Bethesda, Maryland, offers information and teaching aids for nurses in hospitals to teach patients about BSE and breast cancer.

The optimal time for BSE is between the fifth and eighth day of the menstrual cycle, counting the first day of menses as day one. If a woman is postmenopausal, she is encouraged to examine her breasts on the first day of every month to encourage regularity and routine.

All patients who have had a mastectomy are carefully instructed in BSE of the remaining breast. The incision site is also palpated to detect any nodularity, which may indicate recurrence of disease.

Diagnostic Techniques

Mammography

Mammography is a breast imaging modality that does not require the injection of a contrast medium but can detect nonpalpable lesions. The procedure takes about 20 minutes and is performed in an x-ray department of a hospital or in a private radiology office. Two views are taken of each breast: a craniocaudal view and a mediolateral view. For these views, the breast is compressed from top to bottom and side to side. Fleeting discomfort may be experienced because maximum compression aids proper visualization.

Mammography may diagnose breast cancer before it is clinically palpable (*i.e.,* smaller than 1 cm). This test does have limitations and is not foolproof. A false-negative rate of 5% to 10% applies.

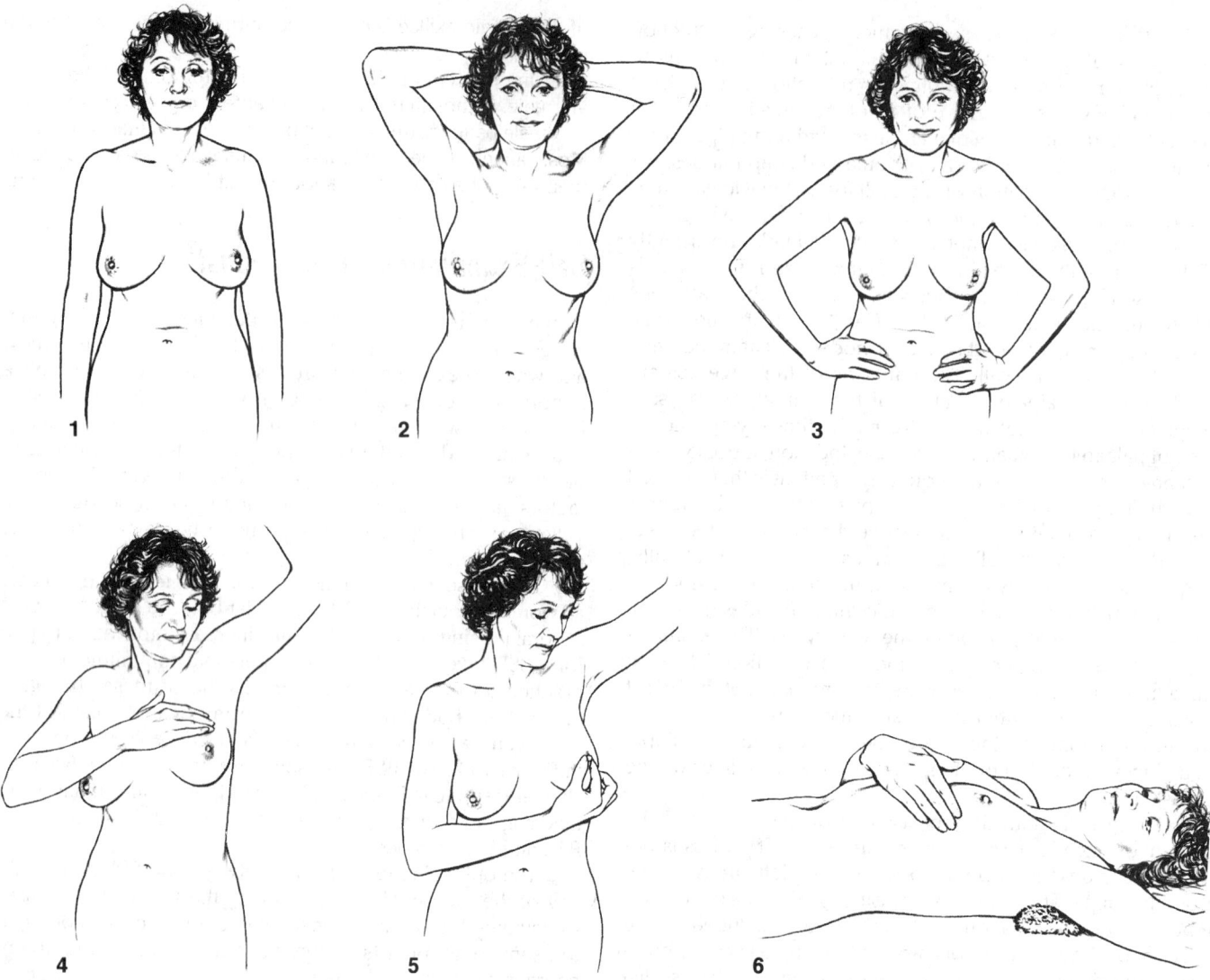

Figure 46-2. Breast self-examination (BSE). (**1**) Stand before a mirror. Check both breasts for anything unusual. Look for a discharge from the nipples, puckering, dimpling, or scaling of the skin. The next two steps are done to check for any change in the shape or contour of your breasts. As you do them, you should be able to feel your chest muscles tighten. (**2**) Watching closely in the mirror, clasp your hands behind your head and press your hands forward. (**3**) Next, press your hands firmly on your hips and bow slightly toward the mirror as you pull your shoulders and elbows forward. Some women do the next part of the exam in the shower. Your fingers will glide easily over soapy skin, so you can concentrate on feeling for changes inside the breast. (**4**) Raise your left arm. Use three or four fingers of your right hand to feel your left breast firmly, carefully, and thoroughly. Beginning at the outer edge, press the flat part of your fingers in small circles, moving the circles slowly around the breast. Gradually work toward the nipple. Be sure to cover the whole breast. Pay special attention to the area between the breast and the underarm, including the underarm area itself. Feel for any unusual lump or mass under the skin. (**5**) Gently squeeze the nipple and look for a discharge. (If you have any discharge during the month—whether or not it is during BSE—see your doctor.) Repeat the exam on your right breast. (**6**) Steps 4 and 5 should be repeated lying down. Lie flat on your back, with your left arm over your head and a pillow or folded towel under your left shoulder. This position flattens the breast and makes it easier to check. Use the same circular motion described above. Repeat on your right breast. (What you need to know about breast cancer. U.S. Department of Health and Human Services, Public Health Service, National Institutes of Health, Bethesda, MD, 1989.)

Galactography, injection of less than 1 ml of radiopaque material through a cannula into a ductal opening on the areola followed by a mammogram, is performed when the patient has a bloody nipple discharge or when a solitary dilated duct is noted on mammography. These symptoms may be indicative of a benign lesion or a cancerous one. This procedure is usually not painful because the dilated duct is already slightly enlarged. If pain is experienced, the dye has usually been inserted into the wrong duct.

Patients scheduled for a mammogram may raise the issue of exposure to radiation. Although the radiation is approximately equivalent to an hour in the sun, patients would have to have many mammograms in a year to increase their risk of cancer. The benefits of this test outweigh the risks.

A baseline or first mammogram is recommended for all women between 35 and 40 years of age. From 40 to 50 years of age, a mammogram every 1 to 2 years is advised by the American Cancer Society. After 50 years of age, annual testing is recommended.

Thermography and Xeroradiography

Thermography is a technique that measures surface temperature of breast tissue. It was previously hoped that this modality would provide a technique of breast screening not involving radiation. While it is still used occasionally, it is not a reliable diagnostic tool at present.

Xeroradiography is similar to a mammogram, but results are portrayed with a bas-relief effect. A selenium-coated plate is subjected to an electrical charge, the x-ray exposure is made, and then a special development process reveals soft tissue of the breast, including skin. This diagnostic test is used less frequently than mammography.

Ultrasound

A transducer is used to focus a beam of high-frequency sound waves through the skin and into the breast. The echo of the sound waves varies with the density of the underlying tissue. The echo is then displayed on a screen. This technique is 95% to 99% accurate in diagnosing cysts but is not definitive in ruling out malignancy.

Fine-Needle Aspiration and Surgical Biopsy

Biopsy of the breast, which involves obtaining tissue specimens for examination, can be performed on an outpatient basis. The procedure may be performed with or without a local anesthetic. After the injection of a local anesthetic (if used), a fine needle is directed into the site to be sampled. Suction is applied to a syringe, and tissue or fluid is drawn into the needle. This material is spread on a slide and sent to the laboratory. Many lesions can be accurately diagnosed by this method.

Other biopsies are performed in the operating room under general or local anesthesia. The entire lesion is generally removed and a frozen section and pathologic examination are performed. If cancer is diagnosed, the tissue is also tested for estrogen and progesterone receptor status. Hormonal therapy may be used in patients who test positive for these receptors (described on p. 1303) once the definitive surgical procedure has been performed. Needle localization is used when minute pinpoint calcifications, indicating a potential malignancy, are noted. A small needle is inserted, usually painlessly, followed by another mammogram to ensure that the needle designates the area to undergo biopsy. A small guide wire remains after needle withdrawal to ensure a precise diagnostic biopsy.

In summary, although breast examinations and diagnostic studies of the breast are recommended in an effort to detect problems early in their course, many women are anxious as well as uncomfortable during these procedures. The nurse who discusses them with the patient in a sensitive, routine manner may assist the patient in becoming more comfortable during these procedures. During contact with *every* patient, male or female, the nurse who encourages BSE is promoting preventive health behaviors.

When a problem is detected and the patient requires more extensive diagnostic testing or surgery to correct or treat a disorder of the breast, the nurse must consider the physical and psychologic impact of breast disorders on the patient. Providing accurate information about the procedures and tests and giving emotional support often help to alleviate some of the patient's distress.

Conditions Affecting the Nipple

Fissure. A fissure is a longitudinal ulcer that tends to develop in breast-feeding women. Constantly irritated by infant sucking, a raw area can become painful and infected; bleeding can also occur. Prevention is important. Daily washing with water, massage with lanolin, and exposure to air are helpful. Breast-feeding can be continued with a nipple shield, if necessary. If the fissure is severe or extremely painful, the woman is advised to stop breast-feeding; a breast pump can be used until breast-feeding can be resumed. Persistent ulceration requires further diagnostic and therapeutic approaches.

Bleeding or Bloody Discharge From the Nipple. At times, a bloody discharge may seep from the nipple. Often it is produced when pressure is placed on one area at the edge of the areola. Although a bloody discharge can be a sign of malignancy, it is most commonly due to a wartlike, benign epithelial tumor or papilloma growing in one of the larger collecting ducts just at the edge of the areola, or in an area of cystic disease. Bleeding occurs with any trauma, and the blood collects in the duct until it is pressed out at the nipple. Treatment includes excision of the duct with the papilloma. This lesion is usually benign, but histologic evaluation is necessary upon removal to rule out malignancy.

Paget's Disease of the Breast. Paget's disease of the breast is seen most frequently in women over age 45 and is usually unilateral. The cause of this condition is unknown but often begins as a mild eczema-like condition that may spread over the areola and onto the breast. The first symptom may be mild burning or itching. Ulceration or erosion may develop. In the more advanced stages, retraction of the nipple may occur. Any areolar lesion that has not cleared after a few weeks of treatment by simple cleansing and protective measures must be biopsied to rule out this condition. A mastectomy follows this diagnosis because of its malignant nature. If involvement is limited to the areola, the chance of metastasis to axillary nodes is about 5%, but if a mass is present, the prospect for cure by surgery is reduced.

Breast Infections

Mastitis. Lactational mastitis, or inflammation or infection of breast tissue, may occur at any time while breast-feeding. It may result from the transfer of microorganisms to the breast by the hands of the patient or those of personnel caring for her. A breast-fed infant with an oral, eye, or skin infection may be a source of infection. Mastitis may be caused by bloodborne organisms. An infection of the ducts results, causing stagnation of milk in one or more lobules. The breast texture becomes tough or doughy, and the patient complains of dull pain in the region affected. A nipple that is discharging purulent material, serum, or blood requires investigation.

Treatment consists of antibiotics and local heat. Lactation can continue and a breast pump may be used. A broad-spectrum antibiotic may be prescribed for 7 to 10 days. The patient should wear a snug bra and follow careful personal hygiene. Adequate rest and hydration are important aspects of management.

Lactational Abscess. A breast abscess may develop as a sequela of an acute mastitis, although it can occur in women who are not breast-feeding an infant. The area affected becomes very tender and red. Purulent matter can often be expressed from the nipple. Breast-feeding is often discontinued if an abscess occurs, but many surgeons advocate continuation if the patient concurs. Firm breast support is provided and antibiotics are prescribed. Incision and drainage may be necessary if the abscess fails to respond to conservative treatment. Warm, wet compresses may hasten resolution.

Benign Cysts and Tumors of the Breast

Fibrocystic Breast Changes. Fibrocystic changes of the breast may be referred to as mammary dysplasia or chronic cystic mastitis. Many women develop multiple cysts, usually due to an overgrowth of fibrous tissue in ductal areas. This condition occurs most commonly from 30 to 50 years of age, and although the cause is unknown, dependency on estrogen seems to be a factor, because the cysts usually disappear after menopause. Cystic areas often fluctuate in size, depending on the menstrual cycle. They are usually larger premenses and smaller postmenses because of premenstrual fluid retention. They may be painless or may become very tender premenstrually. Occasionally, shooting pains may be felt. A supportive bra, decreased salt and caffeine intake, and supplementation with vitamin E may be helpful; however, some women note no change with this regimen. Some women report that these symptoms increase with stress and caffeine consumption.

Many cysts can be aspirated with or without local anesthesia; however, some cystic breast tissue does not consist of aspiratable cysts but lumpy, grainy breast tissue. Biopsy is occasionally necessary to differentiate cystic changes from a true mass. If a biopsy specimen of a fibrocystic mass shows atypical hyperplasia, the patient has an increased risk for development of breast cancer.

If pain and tenderness are severe, danazol (Danocrine) may be prescribed; this drug has an antiestrogenic effect and therefore decreases breast pain and nodularity. Danazol is used only in severe cases because of its potential side effects: flushing, vaginitis, and androgenic changes (virilization).

Mild analgesics can be suggested. Occasionally, mild diuretics are prescribed. A low-salt diet and the elimination of methylxanthines (coffee, tea, cola, and theophylline) may be helpful. Symptoms usually subside with menopause.

Breast Discharge

In patients who are not lactating, breast discharge can be related to many causes. Carcinoma, papilloma, pituitary adeno-

mas, cystic breasts, and many medications can result in discharge of fluid from the nipple. Oral contraceptives, pregnancy, estrogen replacement therapy, chlorpromazine-type drugs, frequent breast stimulation, or suckling may be contributory. Some athletic women may develop breast discharge due to the movement of breast tissue while running or during aerobic exercises. Breast discharge should be evaluated by the patient's health care provider but is often not cause for alarm.

Other Conditions

Fat necrosis is a rare condition of the breast that is indistinguishable from carcinoma. The entire mass is usually excised.

Gigantomastia or *macromastia* (overly large breasts) is a problem for some women. Weight loss and various medications have been used with little effect. Reduction mammoplasty is an elective procedure for the patient who is physically or emotionally distressed; this procedure is discussed later in the chapter.

Fibroadenomas are firm, round, movable, benign tumors of the breast, usually occurring in the late teens to late thirties. They are nontender and are usually removed for diagnostic certainty.

Cystosarcoma phylloides is a type of fibroadenoma that tends to grow rapidly. It is rarely malignant and is surgically excised. If it is malignant, mastectomy follows. (Variations in breast masses are described in Table 46-1.)

Lipomas are small, fatty tumors that are benign. They may resemble malignancy because they can be firm and poorly encapsulated. Biopsy may be required.

In summary, although the breast disorders just described are rarely life-threatening, they are often uncomfortable and distressing; their presence and detection may be mistaken by the patient as an indication of more serious disorders. Understanding by the nurse about the possible impact of these disorders on the patient is important in helping the patient understand their significance and the strategies that are necessary to deal with them.

Malignant Breast Disease and Breast Cancer

One of every nine women in the United States will develop breast cancer. This staggering statistic forces nurses to look at this diagnosis with prevention, education, and care in mind. The incidence of breast cancer is increasing while mortality rates remain about the same. This disease entity may occur at any age after the onset of menses but is far more common over the age of 40.

Incidence

The incidence of breast cancer has continued to increase at the rate of 1% per year since the early 1970s, while the mortality rate has changed little. It is hoped that early diagnosis and treatment will make a difference in these numbers. Worldwide,

TABLE 46-1. *Variations in Breast Masses*

The most common breast masses are due to fibrocystic changes, fibroadenomas, or malignancy. Biopsy is often needed for confirmation, but the following characteristics are diagnostic clues.

	Fibrocystic Changes	*Fibroadenomas*	*Malignancy*
(Illustrations show how the lump may feel, because it is usually not visible.)			
Age	20 years to menopause	Puberty to menopause	20–90 years; most common, 40–80 years
Number	Single or multiple	Usually single	Usually single
Shape	Round	Round, disc, or lobular	Irregular
Consistency	Soft to firm	Usually firm	Firm or hard
Mobility	Mobile	Mobile	May be fixed
Tenderness	Often tender	Nontender	Usually nontender
Retraction signs	Absent	Absent	May be present

(Adapted from Bates B. A Guide to Physical Examination. Philadelphia, JB Lippincott, 1991.)

breast cancer is diagnosed in over 1 million women annually. According to the American Cancer Society, 175,000 new cases of breast cancer will be diagnosed in 1991. Estimated deaths are 44,500 for the same year. Mortality continues to increase with age except during menopause, when there is a slight decrease in incidence; the reason for this is unknown. A low incidence is noted in women who have had an early menopause brought on by an oophorectomy. Racial differences have been noted; black and Oriental women seem to have lower rates than white women. Japanese women have a very low rate, but Japanese women who immigrate to the United States and adopt a Western culture have an increased rate; therefore, diet or environment may be a risk factor.

Risk Factors

Risk factors include:

1. A history of breast cancer (8% to 17% of women develop breast cancer in their other breast)
2. Daughters or sisters of women with breast cancer (risk is increased two to three times, and if the malignancy occurred prior to menopause, the risk is increased further)
3. Nulliparity (risk is increased in women without children)
4. Women having their first child after age 30 (risk is greater than that of nulliparous women)
5. Prolonged exposure to hormonal stimulation (*i.e.,* women who had early menarche prior to age 12 and late menopause after age 50 may be at increased risk). (This factor may be related to exposure to estrogen, without the presence of progesterone. This may be a time when another co-factor, possibly environmental, may provide an opportunity for neoplastic

development. Oral contraceptives and estrogen replacement therapy do not seem to increase risk.)
6. History of high exposure levels of ionization (previous x-ray treatment or exposure to nuclear fallout)
7. Malignancies of the uterus, ovary, or colon
8. High fat intake, obesity, and alcohol intake. A slightly increased risk is found in women who are moderate drinkers. In countries where wine is consumed regularly (*e.g.,* France and Italy), the rate is slightly higher. Some research findings suggest that young women who drink alcohol are more vulnerable to this effect in later years.
9. History of atypical hyperplasia, either lobular or ductal on biopsy
10. Female gender (most women have no discernible risk factors but are at risk because of gender, so all women must be evaluated carefully)

Clinical Manifestations

The symptoms of the disease are insidious. A nontender lump, which may be movable, develops in the breast, usually in the upper outer quadrant, more often on the left than on the right. Ninety percent are found by women themselves or their partners. Pain is usually absent, except in the later stages. Few women are first made aware of a problem by a well-localized discomfort that may be described as burning, stinging, or aching. Some women have no symptoms and no palpable lump but have an abnormal mammogram. Eventually in advanced cases, without detection and treatment, a dimpling or peau d'orange (orange-peel skin) appearance of the skin may be observed, which is due to swelling produced by obstruction of lymphatic circulation in the dermal layer. On examination in the mirror, the patient may note asymmetry and an elevation of the affected breast. Nipple retraction may be evident. Later, the breast becomes more or less fixed on the chest wall. Ulceration and metastasis follow. Diagnosis is made by maintaining a high index of suspicion, taking a thorough history, and performing a careful examination and a mammographic study. If findings are suspicious, an excisional biopsy of the area is performed.

Whether biopsy is performed with a fine needle or by excision, an adequate sample is essential. If the tissue proves to be positive for carcinoma, additional studies are performed. These include a complete profile, including liver studies, CEA (carcinoembryonic antigen), a nonspecific marker found in the blood that increases if metastasis occurs, bone scan, and chest radiography, and liver scan. The purpose of these studies is to rule out metastasis or impaired liver or kidney function possibly related to advanced disease.

Pathophysiology

Carcinoma of the breast is not a pathologic entity that develops overnight. It starts with a single cell, which divides or doubles within 30 to 210 days. It takes approximately 16 doubling times for a carcinoma to become 1 cm or greater in size, at which point it becomes clinically apparent. Assuming that it takes 30 days for each doubling time, it would take a minimum of 2½ years for a carcinoma to become palpable. If the doubling time were 210 days, it would take up to 17 years before that carcinoma would be palpable. (The value of mammography is to detect an early carcinoma before it becomes palpable.)

If biopsy and a more definitive procedure are not performed once the carcinoma is discovered, the cancer grows unchecked. If this occurs, the tumor may attach to the chest wall; *peau d'orange* appearance may occur. The tumor can also spread to regional lymph nodes, principally the axillary chain. These can become readily palpable in advanced cases of cancer of the breast. Other sites of lymphatic spread can include subpectoral nodes, subclavicular nodes, Gerota's fascial nodes, internal mammary nodes, and subcuticular nodes on the opposite side. There have been a number of cases in which the patient has breast cancer on the left side with right axillary node metastasis; the disease traveled through the subcutaneous lymphatic channels to the opposite axilla. It is obvious that thorough axillary examinations bilaterally are indicated in patient evaluation (lymphatic drainage of the breast is illustrated in Fig. 46-3). Other common metastatic sites are lungs, liver, bone, and brain. The symptoms of metastases are described in Table 46-2.

Surgical Approaches

The treatment of carcinoma of the breast is removal or destruction of the whole tumor, usually followed by radiation, chemotherapy, or hormonal therapy, or a combination of these. Because of the biologic complexity of this disease, there is no one single approach to management.

Complete removal of the tumor can be accomplished most effectively when the cancer is confined to the breast. This is evidenced by clinical experience, which shows a 5-year survival rate greater than 80% if the tumor is confined to the breast. When cancer cells have spread to the nodes of the axilla, the survival rate falls to as low as 60% or below.

Types of surgical intervention include the following:

1. Lumpectomy (segmental mastectomy) and axillary node dissection followed by a course of cobalt therapy to the remaining breast tissue
2. Quadrantectomy, a resection of the involved breast quadrant, commonly upper outer quadrant, with dissection of axillary lymph nodes and irradiation of the residual breast tissue
3. Simple mastectomy, in which resection extends from the clavicle to the costal margin and from the midline to the latissimus dorsi. The entire axillary tail and the pectoral fascia are removed.
4. Modified radical mastectomy, in which the entire breast tissue

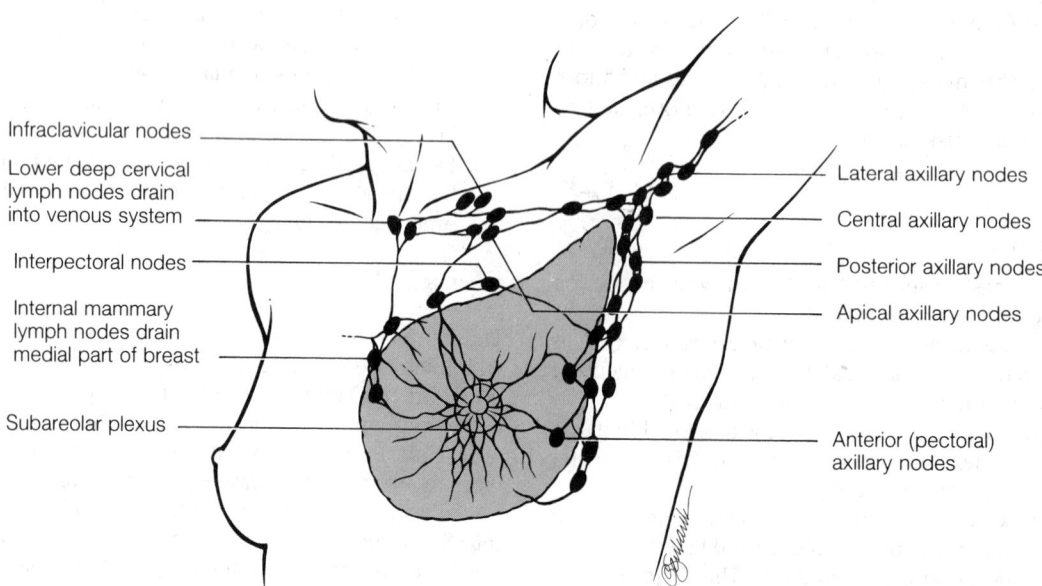

Figure 46-3. Lymphatic drainage of the breast.

TABLE 46-2.   *Common Sites, Signs, and Symptoms of Breast Cancer Metastasis*

Sites	Symptoms	Signs
Bone (particularly spine, proximal long bones)	Initially worse at night Difficult to characterize May be aching, boring	Spinal punch tenderness
Lungs and pleura	Dyspnea Cough Chest pain	Cough Sputum production Diminished breath sounds
Skin	Occasionally pruritus	Firm, discrete flesh-colored papules or nodules May be mildly erythematous Usually painless
Lymph nodes		Nontender enlarged nodes
Liver (unusual as single site of metastasis)	Right upper abdominal discomfort or pain Anorexia	Hepatomegaly Jaundice Ascites
Spinal cord (particularly thoracic and lumbar segments)	Progressive symptoms of cord compression related to level of lesion Localized spinal pain Muscle weakness of lower extremities Sensory loss and paralysis of lower extremities Bowel and bladder dysfunction	Sensory and motor changes corresponding to level of cord lesion Hyperactive reflexes of lower extremities
Central nervous system	Generalized symptoms of increased intracranial pressure Headache Nausea, vomiting Impaired cognitive function Functional changes corresponding to affected cerebral area (*e.g.,* hemiparesis, seizures, visual changes)	Papilledema Corresponding abnormalities in mental status and neurological exam

(Mast M. Primary care of the mastectomy patient. Nurse Pract 1984 Feb; 9[2]:63–78.)

is removed along with axillary lymph nodes. The pectoralis major and pectoralis minor muscles are not removed. This is one of the more common surgical approach to breast cancer treatment.

5. Radical mastectomy, in which the entire breast is removed along with all axillary lymph nodes and both pectoral muscles, including lymph nodes (Table 46-3). This is rarely performed now.

Historical Development of Surgical Treatment.   Surgical management until 25 to 30 years ago consisted of radical mastectomy—removal of both the pectoralis major and pectoralis minor muscles and thorough axillary node dissection. This procedure, developed by Halsted in 1893, had many disadvantages. The morbidity and mortality rates did not improve, and the experience was very distressing for the patient. A modified radical mastectomy was then introduced, which involves mastectomy and axillary node dissection but leaves the pectoralis muscles intact. This procedure was the most common surgical treatment until 5 to 10 years ago. Then, a regimen that included lumpectomy, axillary node dissection, and subsequent irradiation to the remainder of the breast tissue was introduced. Studies showed that 5-year survival statistics were equal to or better than those of the classic Halsted radical mastectomy or the modified radical mastectomy. It has been concluded over the course of multiple studies that lumpectomy, axillary node dissection, and radiation therapy to the remainder of the breast tissue for lesions 4 cm or smaller have, for the most part, proved to be the treatment of choice for cancer of the breast. This has proved to be far more appealing to patients with breast cancer. For lesions that are larger than 4 cm, most surgeons perform a modified radical mastectomy with axillary node dissection.

The approaches to management of breast cancer, with movement away from extensive and often mutilating surgical procedures, have resulted, in large part, from women taking a more active role in their own health care and becoming informed participants in decisions about proposed surgical procedures. Women are encouraged to become informed about the success or failure of the proposed treatment, to ask ques-

TABLE 46-3. *Surgical Treatment of Breast Cancer*

Surgical Procedure	Description

Partial mastectomy
    Lumpectomy
    Wide excision
    Segmental mastectomy
	Relatively synonymous terms to describe removal of varying amounts of breast tissue, including the malignant tissue and some surrounding tissue. Axillary nodes are dissected.

Quadrantectomy	A type of partial mastectomy that may approximate a quadrant. Axillary nodes are dissected.
Axillary node dissection	Removal of some fat-enmeshed axillary nodes for biopsy
Modified radical mastectomy	Removal of all breast tissue and axillary node dissection
Radical mastectomy	Removal of entire breast along with pectoralis major and minor muscles in conjunction with axillary node dissection

tions about treatment options, and to become familiar with the National Cancer Institute's Physician Data Query, a computer access system for current data retrieval.

The approach to treating breast cancer reflects the basic premise that this disease is not local but systemic. Because of this assumption, not only is the local cancer treated, but the micrometastatic cancer, which may be disseminated throughout the body or may be present in surrounding breast tissue, is also treated. More specifically, surgery combined with adjuvant chemotherapy is more effective than surgery alone for some patients. The use of postoperative radiation therapy after simple or modified radical mastectomy reduces local recurrence but does not improve survival. Studies are under way to determine the best strategy, the correct combination of chemotherapeutic agents, and the optimal timing of radiation in the multidisciplinary approach to treatment.

Monoclonal antibodies are becoming helpful adjuncts to treatment and may become more valuable with further research. These synthetic proteins may act like antibodies to cancer cells. They may also act as markers during scans to detect the presence of cancer cells at a very early stage. Flow cytometry, which studies the duplication rate of cells in each phase of growth, is also new and helpful. The number of cells in the S phase (cell division) of the cell cycle is proportional to the aggressiveness of the tumor.

Staging

Clinical staging is a part of the pretreatment evaluation and is performed by histologic examination of the biopsied tissue and axillary specimen to assess the extent of the disease, lymph node involvement, the status of the opposite breast, and the possibility of systemic metastasis (Fig. 46-4).

Stage I consists of a small tumor, less than 2 cm, with negative lymph nodes and no detectable metastases.

Stage II consists of a tumor greater than 2 cm but less than 5 cm with negative or positive unfixed lymph nodes and no detectable metastases.

Stage III is a large tumor, greater than 5 cm, or a tumor of any size with invasion of the skin or chest wall or positive fixed lymph nodes in the clavicular area without evidence of metastases.

Stage IV is a tumor of any size with lymph nodes positive or negative with distant metastases.

This is one type of staging. There are several others in which staging is expressed in TNM symbols; T represents the primary tumor, N describes lymph node involvement, and M describes metastasis, if any (Table 46-4).

Types of Malignancy

The types of malignancy are listed in Table 46-5.

Invasive ductal cancer accounts for about 80% of all breast cancers. Palpably hard, this type may cause dimpling or nipple retraction. It can spread rapidly to lymph nodes, even if the primary lesion is small. The survival rate is good if no lymph nodes are involved and hormonal receptor status is positive (see p. 1303).

Medullary carcinoma makes up 6% of breast cancers and grows in a capsule inside a duct. These can become large but are slow to expand, so the prognosis is often favorable.

Mucinous cancer is a type of ductal carcinoma and accounts for 3% of breast cancers. A mucus producer, it is also slow-growing; thus, it has a more favorable outlook.

Tubular ductal cancer is rare, accounting for only 1.2% of cancers. The outlook is excellent if there is no local extension of the disease.

Lobular cancer of the breast is perhaps the most benign type of cancer of the breast. This type of cancer generally has not invaded adjacent breast tissue and offers a far more favorable prognosis than the other carcinomas previously described. Consensus about treatment has not been reached; however, options that may be given to the patient are careful observation without surgery because this is an *in situ* (local or in place) condition, or bilateral mastectomy as a preventive measure. The incidence of bilateral tumors is about 50%. Often a blind mirror-image biopsy of the opposite breast is done at the time of definitive therapy on the affected breast.

Inflammatory carcinoma is a rare type of breast cancer (1% to 2%) that produces symptoms different from those of other breast cancers. The localized tumor is tender and painful; the breast is abnormally firm and enlarged. The skin over it is red and dusky. Often, edema and nipple retraction occur. These symptoms rapidly increase in severity and usually prompt the

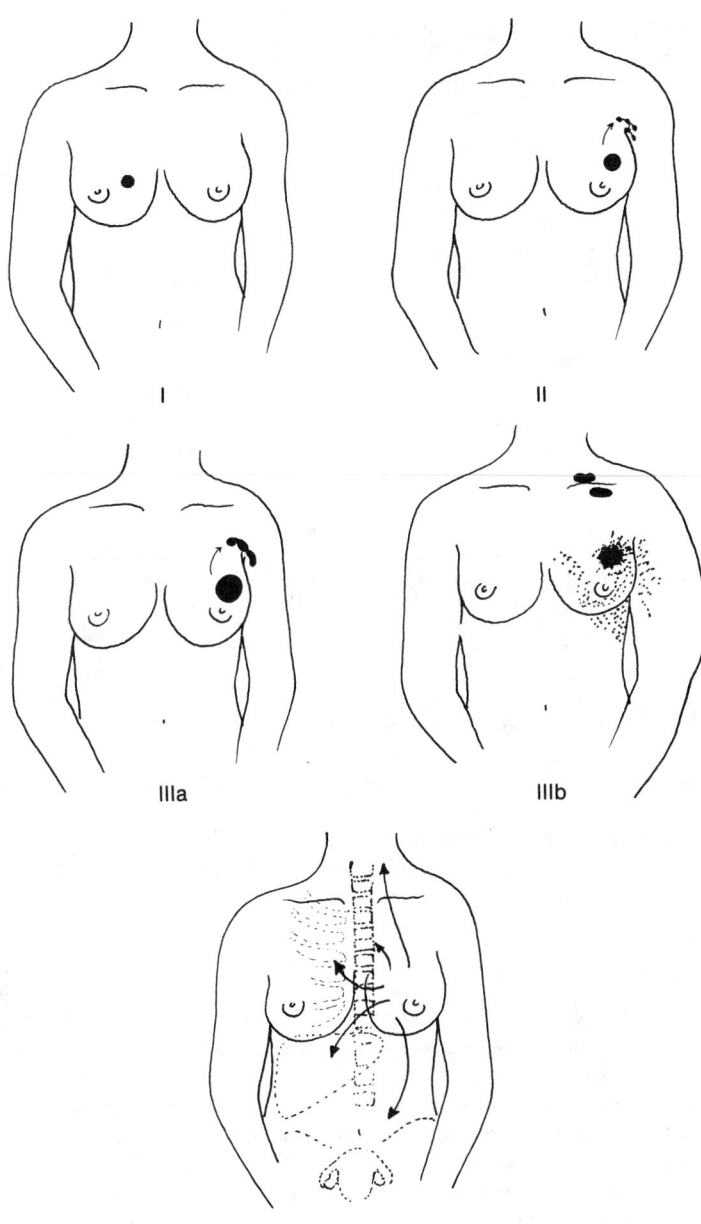

Figure 46-4. Schematic classification of the stages of breast carcinoma has been divided into four clinical stages by The International Union Against Cancer and The American Joint Committee on Cancer. Stage I: Tumors less than 2 cm in diameter that are confined to breast. Stage II: Tumors of less than 5 cm, or smaller tumors with small, mobile axillary lymph nodes. Stage IIIa: Tumors greater than 5 cm, or tumors with enlarged, axillary lymph nodes fixed to one another or adjacent tissues. Stage IIIb: More advanced lesions with satellite nodules, fixation to the skin or chest wall, ulceration, edema, or with clinically apparent supraclavicular or infraclavicular nodal involvement. Stage IV: All tumors with distant metastases. (Dunnihoo D. Fundamentals of Gynecology and Obstetrics. Philadelphia: JB Lippincott, 1990. Adapted from Danforth DN and Scott JR (eds). Obstetrics and Gynecology, 5th ed. Philadelphia, JB Lippincott, 1986.)

woman to seek health care sooner than the woman with a small breast mass. It can spread to other parts of the body rapidly; chemotherapeutic agents play a major role in the attempt to control the progression of this disease. Radiation and surgery are also used to control spread.

Paget's disease of the breast (described on p. 1295) is one of the rarer forms of breast cancer. Burning and itching are frequent symptoms. The tumor itself may be ductal or invasive. Often, a tumor mass cannot be palpated underneath the nipple, where this disease arises. Mammography may be

TABLE 46-4. *Breast Cancer Staging by Tumor, Nodes, and Metastasis (TNM staging)*

Stage I	T (less than 2 cm)	N (no axillary metastasis)	M (no metastasis)
Stage II	T (greater than 2 cm)	N (axillary metastasis nonfixed)	M (no metastasis)
Stage III	T (greater than 5 cm)	N (axillary metastasis fixed)	M (no metastasis)
Stage IV	T (any T)	N (supra- or infraclavicular nodes)	M (distant metastasis)

(Adapted from American Joint Committee on Cancer. Manual for Staging of Cancer, 3rd ed. Philadelphia, JB Lippincott, 1988, pp 145–150.)

TABLE 46–5. *Types of Breast Cancer and Frequency* *

Infiltrating ductal	70.0%
Invasive lobular	10.0
Medullary	6.0
Mucinous or colloid	3.0
Tubular	1.2
Adenocystic	0.4
Papillary	1.0
Carcinosarcoma	0.1
Paget's disease	3.0
Inflammatory	1.0
In situ breast cancer	5.0
Ductal	2.5
Lobular	2.5

* *There can be combinations of any of these types.*
(Henderson C et al. Cancer of the breast. In DeVita VT Jr, Helman S, and Rosenberg SA [eds]. Cancer: Principles and Practice of Oncology, vol 1, 3rd ed. Philadelphia, JB Lippincott, 1989, pp 1204–1206.)

the only diagnostic study that makes the tumor evident. In most instances, a mastectomy is the treatment of choice. In most patients, the primary cancer is an intraductal lesion without local extension. Axillary lymph node dissection is rarely indicated. If the carcinoma extends beyond the ductal area, it becomes an invasive carcinoma, and a modified radical mastectomy is the treatment of choice.

Prognosis

Breast cancer is more unpredictable than most other cancers because of hormone dependence, immune response, host resistance, and other variable and unknown factors. If the lymph nodes are unaffected, the prognosis is better than in those instances when cancer cells are found in the nodes. In clinical assessment, the absence of palpable nodes does not necessarily mean absence of malignancy in the axillary nodes, because the cancer may be microscopic. Tumor spread at the time of treatment is a significant prognostic indicator. The key to improved cure rates is early diagnosis before metastasis has occurred. The nurse who encourages regular BSE, routine breast examinations by a health care professional, and mammograms when appropriate plays a pivotal role in early diagnosis and treatment.

Management of the Patient With Breast Cancer

Because breast cancer is a complex disease with individual variations, there is no single accepted approach to management. Treatment regimens are often complex and vary according to the patient's histologic diagnosis, age, oncologist and surgeon, disease progression, and current protocols.

There has been a gradual but marked departure from radical mastectomy toward more conservative surgery for primary breast tumors. A breast biopsy is rarely followed immediately

by mastectomy. A two-stage approach spares the patient from awakening after a biopsy not knowing whether she has had a mastectomy. Instead, time is taken to confirm the biopsy result and discuss methods of treatment. Modalities differ, depending on stage and type of disease. Therapy may include combinations of surgery, chemotherapy, immunotherapy, hormone therapy, and radiation. Women are often offered choices about type of surgery. The possibility of breast reconstruction is also considered. Nursing actions during decision making include empathetic listening and offering accurate information to facilitate the optimum choice for the patient.

Before surgery, the surgeon plans an incision that will provide maximum opportunity to excise the tumor and the affected nodes. At the same time, efforts are made to avoid a scar that will be visible and restrictive. An objective of treatment is to maintain or restore normal function to the hand, arm, and shoulder girdle on the affected side after surgery. Skin flaps and tissue are handled meticulously to ensure proper viability, hemostasis, and drainage.

After the removal of the tumor mass, bleeding points are ligated and the skin is closed over the chest wall. Skin grafting is performed if the skin flaps are not of sufficient size to close the wound. A nonadherent dressing (Adaptic) permits serum and blood to escape between the strips. A pressure dressing may then be applied. Two drainage tubes may be placed in the axilla and beneath the superior skin flap; portable suction devices may be used. The final dressing may be held in place by wide elastic bandages.

Hormonal Therapy

Decisions about hormonal therapy for breast cancer are based on the index of estrogen and progesterone receptors; an assay is performed on tumor tissue taken at the time of the original biopsy. The tissue requires special handling and a laboratory with expertise in the proper technique for assessment. Normal breast tissue contains receptor sites for estrogen. However, only about one third of breast malignancies are estrogen-dependent or ER-positive (ER+). An ER+ assay indicates that tumor growth depends on estrogen supply and that measures to reduce hormone production would be appropriate for limitation of disease. ER+ tumors may grow more slowly than those that are ER-negative (ER−). Less than 3 fmol/mg is considered negative. Values of 3 to 10 are questionable, and values greater than 10 are considered positive. The greater the value, the more a beneficial effect from hormone suppression can be expected. The best prognosis exists for patients with both estrogen- and progesterone-positive receptors (PR+). Most positive progesterone receptive tumors also have a positive estrogen receptor status, so this factor becomes a prognostic indicator. The loss of progesterone receptors can be a sign of advancing disease. Premenopausal women and perimenopausal women are more likely to have non–hormonal-dependent lesions. Postmenopausal women (more than 5 years) are likely to have hormone-dependent lesions. (Figure 46-5 describes how hormonal status may determine recommendations for treatment.)

Hormonal therapy can be ablative or additive. Ablative therapy includes removal of endocrine glands that produce hormones (*i.e.*, ovary, pituitary, or adrenal glands). Oophorectomy is one treatment option for premenopausal women with estrogen-dependent tumors. Ablative surgery, considered ef-

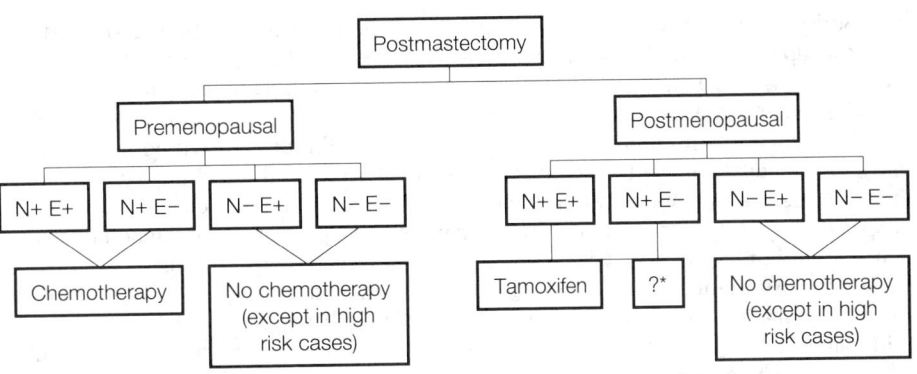

Figure 46–5. Post-mastectomy treatment options. Developed from recommendations of NIH Consensus Development Conference Statement. N+, node-positive; N−, node-negative; E+, estrogen receptor-positive; E−, estrogen receptor-negative. *Chemotherapy should be considered but is not recommended as standard. (Doig B. Adjuvent chemotherapy in breast cancer: A review of the literature. Cancer Nurs 1988 Apr; 11[2]:95.)

fective therapy in the past, is not often performed today because medications can provide the same effect.

Tamoxifen, Megace, DES, Halotestin, and Cytadren are the main hormonal agents used to suppress tumors that are dependent on hormones for growth. Each is described below:

1. *Tamoxifen.* This drug is considered by some to be as effective as oophorectomy and is the most common hormonal method of intervention. It is indicated in postmenopausal patients with positive estrogen receptors and positive axillary nodes. This antiestrogenic agent has few side effects, but some patients may experience nausea, vomiting, hot flashes, fluid retention, and depression. Research may prove this to be a preventive drug for women who are at high risk for development of breast cancer.

2. *DES (diethylstilbestrol).* DES suppresses the release of follicle-stimulating hormone (FSH) and luteinizing hormone (LH); therefore, ovarian production of estrogen and estrogen binding are decreased. This medication is used less frequently than tamoxifen because side effects are more common (*i.e.*, weight gain, fluid retention, nausea).

3. *Megace.* The mechanism of action of Megace is unknown. It may decrease the quantity of estrogen receptors. Increased appetite and weight gain may occur.

4. *Halotestin.* This testosterone derivative suppresses estrogen by suppression of FSH and LH. Side effects include virilization (*i.e.*, increased facial hair, deepened voice, clitoral hypertrophy, and increased libido).

5. *Aminoglutethimide* or *Cytadren.* By blocking conversion of androgens to estrogens, this drug simulates a medical adrenalectomy. It inhibits aromatase, the enzyme responsible for this conversion. Side effects include a rash that may be pruritic. Because suppression of adrenal function may occur, the patient is monitored for signs of adrenal cortical hypofunction; hydrocortisone is administered to prevent its occurrence during this therapy.

All these drugs may cause a "flare" effect, or a worsening of disease after initiation of therapy. Hypercalcemia may occur and may necessitate that therapy be discontinued. Patient education regarding medication and possible reactions is an important issue for nurses working with patients taking hormonal therapy.

Adjuvant Chemotherapy

Chemotherapy is one of the most powerful weapons available to fight cancer. Chemotherapeutic agents interfere with cell reproduction; in the process, however, these agents can also kill normal cells and cause serious side effects. Much of the adverse publicity about this method of treatment is related to the side effects. An overview of chemotherapy is presented in Chapter 19.

The use of chemotherapy to treat carcinoma of the breast after a definitive surgical procedure has been a topic of discussion and debate for many years. Unfortunately, there is no consensus of opinion about which patients should receive chemotherapy and what agents should be used. Many factors, not the least of which is the view of the oncologist administering the chemotherapy, come into play in this decision. Current thinking is that most patients, whether or not they demonstrate evidence of metastatic disease at the time of the discovery of their lesion, should be treated with chemotherapy. This approach is based on research of the Milan group and the National Surgical Adjuvant Breast and Bowel Project (NSABP). Each case is individualized. The diagnosis and treatment of breast cancer require the expertise of a number of specialties. Surgery, radiation, or chemotherapy in isolation is usually not sufficient to ensure the most favorable result for a patient with carcinoma of the breast.

Anticipatory anxiety and dread are common in patients facing chemotherapy treatment. The fear of side effects can be overwhelming but does not often stop patients from participating in treatment. Psychological and educational preparation is important. Written materials along with consultation time with physicians and oncology clinical nurse specialists can help the patient deal with the potential side effects and fears of recurrence of disease when treatment is completed.

Chemotherapy is not combined with radiation concurrently because toxicity and side effects may be exacerbated; however, it may follow or precede radiation. The purpose is to eliminate hidden macro- or micrometastatic spread of the disease. Variables influencing treatment and approach include number of nodes involved, hormonal status of the patient, and size of the tumor.

It is important that chemotherapy be initiated before drug resistance develops. Therefore, the drug must be started shortly after definitive treatment of the neoplasm. Another strategy is to use combined chemotherapy with two or three agents. This treatment seems more effective in premenopausal women. Side effects of chemotherapy include nausea, alopecia, mucositis, dermatitis, hemorrhagic cystitis, constipation, diarrhea, conjunctivitis, malaise, depression, weight gain, and bone marrow depression. Although the cause is unknown, weight gain of more than 10 lb occurs in about half of all patients. This may further threaten a patient's self-image after breast surgery.

Serious complications of chemotherapy include bone marrow suppression leading to systemic infection, toxicity when combined with radiation, hepatotoxicity, coagulation abnormalities, amenorrhea, and ovarian failure.

Physical and emotional feelings related to chemotherapy may have a negative effect on self-esteem, sexuality, and well-being. Nausea and alopecia would be difficult for healthy, unstressed people to tolerate but may be even worse for a patient who is attempting to deal with a potentially life-threatening diagnosis. Assistance from oncology nurses, mental health professionals, and support groups can be helpful with these difficulties.

Aerobic exercise may minimize the amount of weight gained. The sense of well-being that comes from exercise and its anxiety-alleviating effects may also be helpful.

The chemotherapeutic agents used most often to treat breast cancer are Cytoxan (C), methotrexate (M), fluorouracil (F), and Adriamycin (A). A CMF or CAF regimen is often used in a treatment protocol. An oncologist determines which agents should be used in any given patient and uses these drugs in a specific protocol. Again, each treatment plan is strictly individualized.

Some patients may elect to undergo an autologous bone marrow transplant. After 200 to 500 ml of bone marrow is removed, high doses of chemotherapy are given. The patient's bone marrow, spared from the effects of chemotherapy, is then replaced intravenously. This specialized oncologic procedure requires reverse isolation, specialized training, and sensitive patient preparation, education, and support throughout its course.

Side effects may vary with the chemotherapeutic agent used. Adriamycin can be toxic to tissue if it infiltrates out of the vein, so it is usually diluted and used only in a large vein. Nausea and vomiting can occur. Antiemetics and tranquilizers may provide relief, as may visual imagery and relaxation techniques. Adriamycin may cause alopecia. Obtaining a wig prior to hair loss may prevent some of the trauma of this occurrence in women. The use of stylish hats or scarves may also be beneficial. Ice caps, previously thought to prevent hair loss by slowing circulation to the scalp during treatment, have been found ineffective, because they seem to only retard inevitable alopecia. Reassurance that new growth will occur when treatment is completed is helpful, although color and texture of the hair may differ.

Teaching points that should be emphasized to minimize hair loss include:

1. Avoid shampooing daily.
2. Use a mild, protein-based shampoo with conditioner every 4 to 7 days; rinse thoroughly and pat dry.
3. Let hair dry naturally; electric hair dryers, curlers, and curling irons can encourage hair loss. Hair clips, barrettes, bobby pins, hair sprays, and hair dyes should be avoided.
4. Do not brush hair; use a wide-toothed comb.
5. Consider use of eyebrow pencil or false eyelashes if hair loss affects eye areas.

It is important for oncology nurses working with patients receiving chemotherapy to be prepared to assist patients who have difficulty with side effects of treatment. The nurse should have a list of wig suppliers in the patient's geographic region and become familiar with the use of creative scarves and turbans to lessen patient discomfort with hair loss. By encouraging the use of medications to limit nausea, vomiting, and mouth sores, the patient's experience during chemotherapy may be less traumatic than expected. Taking time to explain side effects and possible solutions may alleviate some of the anxiety of women who are uncomfortable asking questions. Because many women are stressed with the additional factors of financial concerns and time away from the family, nursing support and teaching can avert serious emotional distress during treatment.

Because of the diversity of the disease itself, no single option or success/failure rate provides a simple answer to proper treatment. The more knowledge a patient has about her options, the greater her feeling of control and the more educated her choices.

Important aspects of care include communication, support groups, encouragement to ask questions, and, above all, promotion of her trust and faith in care providers. Adequate time for patient discussion must be built into clinical visits. The more informed a patient is about the side effects of chemotherapy and how to manage them, the better she is able to anticipate and deal with them.

Radiation Therapy

Radiation therapy is usually instituted after excision of the tumor mass to decrease the chance of recurrence at the site of surgery and to attempt eradication of any residual cancer. This method of treatment seems to be more effective in eradicating small groups of cells rather than large tumors. One method uses an external source to irradiate the area, including nearby lymph nodes, at specified intervals for several weeks. Tattooing or ink markings are used to delineate the areas to be irradiated. Patients need reassurance and instructions about radiation therapy to lessen anxiety. Patient self-care instructions at this time are based on maintaining skin integrity and include the following: use of mild soap with minimal rubbing, avoidance of perfumed soaps or deodorants, use of hydrophilic lotions (Lubriderm, Aquaphor, Eucerin) for dryness, use of Aveeno soap if pruritus occurs, and avoidance of tight clothes, underwire bras, and excessive temperatures or ultraviolet light. Suggestions for instruction about treatment itself are listed in Table 46-6.

Another method of radiation is to surgically place hollow needles or tubes in the affected area. Radioactive seeds or needles are then inserted for a prescribed time (brachytherapy; Fig. 46-6). On occasion, both methods are used. The purpose of both methods is to destroy migrant or remaining malignant cells. Patients should be advised to use mild soap and no deodorant or powder during treatment, because perfumed products and deodorants may contain a metal residue that could irritate skin treated by radiation.

Boredom, visitor limitation, and minor local discomfort are all problems that patients may encounter during this mode of treatment. Books, television, phone calls, and visitors at different times of the day may be helpful. Teaching patients to minimize sun exposure of the treated area for 1 year and reassuring them that minor twinges and shooting pain in the breast are normal reactions after treatment are important aspects of care.

Benefits of and indications for irradiation have been debated in the literature. Nurses who work in this area, like all nurses, need to stay current regarding research results.

TABLE 46-6. *Suggested Topics for Preparation and Instruction of Patient Before Initiation of Radiation Therapy*

Constant audio and television communication with staff during therapy

Position determined at simulation will be used for all treatments

No pain is associated with actual treatment (like getting an x-ray)

Linear accelerator produces a loud humming noise when on

Length of entire procedure is approximately 15 to 20 minutes

Length of actual treatment is one to two minutes

Verification of treatment area with weekly x-rays

Weekly complete blood counts

Weekly examination by a physician

(Adapted from Harness JK et al [eds]. Breast Cancer: Collaborative Management. Chelsea, MI, Lewis Publishers, 1988.)

Duration of radiation therapy varies, depending on whether the treatment is intended for initial cancer or metastasis, but an average course of treatment is about 6 weeks. Potential complications of radiation therapy include pneumonitis, rib fracture, skin changes, and breast fibrosis. These seem to be rare occurrences. Side effects include a moderate skin reaction, esophagitis, skin telangiectasias, arm edema, fatigue, mild discomfort, and sore throat. The fatigue that occurs with radiation usually begins about 2 weeks after treatment and may last for several weeks after completion of treatment. Fatigue can be depressing, as can be the frequent trips to the oncology clinic. The patient needs to be reassured that the fatigue is normal and not a sign of recurrence. Palliative radiation is used in advanced disease to relieve discomfort related to bone metastases.

Reconstruction

Many women are interested in reconstructive surgery, which has the potential for considerable psychologic benefit to the patient. Support groups provide education and peer support for those patients who are candidates for and interested in breast reconstruction.

Some concerns that women may have about reconstructive surgery are cost, safety, and whether to have immediate or later reconstruction. Cost to the patient may vary depending on insurer, but it is considered rehabilitative surgery and therefore is often covered by insurance reimbursement. The usual surgical risks of infection and potential reaction to anesthesia exist. There is also the potential risk of a cosmetically unsatisfactory reconstructive result. Silicone, the agent used as a coating of some breast expanders and the filler of other prostheses, may result in infection, connective tissue disease, or immune system dysfunction. The FDA has expressed concern about possible adverse effects; no conclusive studies on the long-term effects of silicone implants are available. All women who consider this option should investigate available information and read the package insert on the prosthesis to be used. Obviously, women who have reconstruction with their own tissue do not have to be concerned about reactions to silicone.

If a woman decides to have reconstructive surgery at the time of the mastectomy, she avoids future surgery, although total operative time is lengthened. Some women have found that immediate reconstruction lessens the feelings of loss and disfigurement. Occasionally, reconstruction cannot be done because skin and muscles are too tight. Some women benefit by waiting until later because they are not sure about their choice initially.

Reconstructive surgery is discussed later in this chapter; treatment options are summarized in Table 46-7.

(text continues on page 1308)

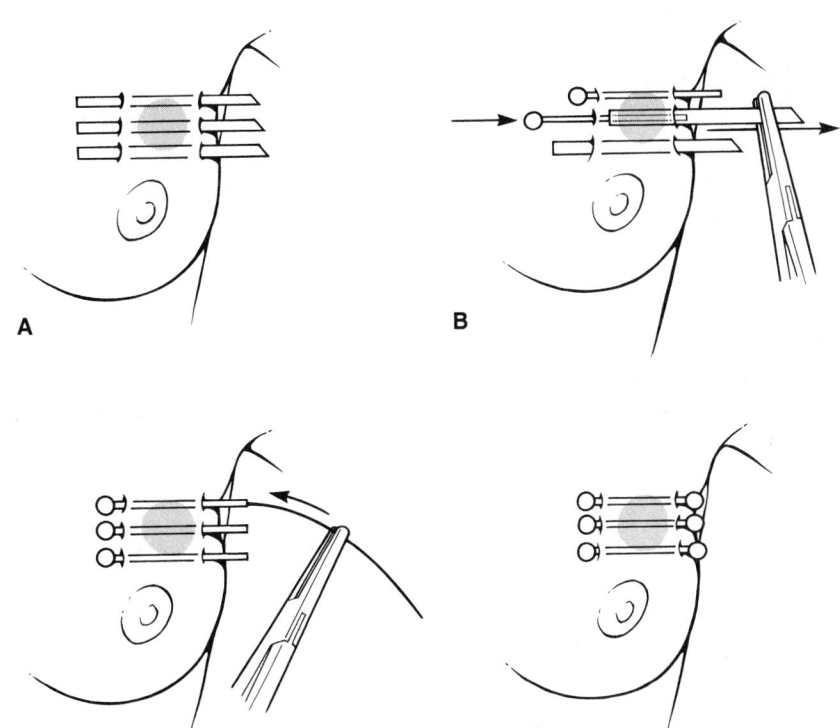

Figure 46-6. Brachytherapy for treatment of breast cancer. (**A**) Hollow metal needles are placed where the tumor was located before surgery. (**B**) Metal needles are replaced by hollow plastic catheters. (**C**) Radioactive material is loaded into the catheters. (**D**) The implant is secured in place with metal buttons. (Redrawn from Mast DE and Mood DW. Preparing patients with breast cancer for brachytherapy. Oncol Nurs Forum 1990; 17:267–270; with permission from the Oncology Nursing Press.)

TABLE 46–7.   Treatment Modalities for Cancer of the Breast*

Type of Treatment	Objectives of Therapy	Possible Concomitant Effects	Nursing Interventions
CHEMOTHERAPY	Decrease or prevent metastasis		Alleviate anxiety and minimize side effects of drugs used
Adriamycin (A)		Mouth sores, nausea, vomiting, diarrhea, decreased appetite, hair loss Can be toxic if infiltration occurs; can be cardiotoxic	Nausea and vomiting—antiemetics, tranquilizers, marijuana, visual imagery relaxation techniques
Cytoxan (C)		Nausea, vomiting, decreased appetite, menstrual irregularities	
Methotrexate (M)		Nausea, vomiting, mouth sores	Mouth sores—avoid commercial mouthwashes. Use baking soda or salt and water rinses
5-Fluorouracil (F)		Mouth sores, nausea, vomiting, diarrhea	Hair loss—obtain wig prior to development of alopecia Encourage use of turbans and scarves Avoid brushing and frequent shampooing
L-Pam		Low blood count, nausea, vomiting	
Velban		Nausea, vomiting, hair loss	
Vincristine (V)		Hair loss, tingling, constipation, headaches, pain at IV site, loss of appetite	Loss of appetite—foods may taste differently, so experimentation with different foods may be helpful Frequent small meals may be tolerated better than three large meals Call the National Cancer Institute for their recipe booklet entitled "Eating Hints"

Combinations
  CMF
  CAF
  CMFVP (prednisone added)
  CA			

HORMONAL THERAPY Androgens, fluoxymesterone (Halotestin) for premenopausal women	Suppress estrogen	Masculinization, fluid retention, cholestatic jaundice, hypercalcemia	Assess for signs of increased libido, deepening voice, facial hirsutism Note serum calcium levels Observe for signs of lethargy, insomnia, thirst, nausea, vomiting, thickened speech, fluid retention, collapse, coma

(continued)

TABLE 46–7. *(Continued)*

Type of Treatment	*Objectives of Therapy*	*Possible Concomitant Effects*	*Nursing Interventions*
Estrogens (diethylstilbestrol) for postmenopausal patients	Suppress FSH and LH		Assess for nausea, vomiting, edema, vaginal bleeding, urinary incontinence, flare, phlebitis, congestive heart failure
Corticosteroids (prednisone)	Suppress estrogen production by the adrenals and decrease urinary estrogenic metabolites	Does not bring about hypercalcemia as does androgen or estrogen therapy It is an effective hormonal treatment for brain metastasis. Induces some degree of Cushing's syndrome: fullness of face, gain in body weight, and edema of lower extremities	
Antiestrogen tamoxifen citrate (Nolvadex)	Effective in palliative treatment in postmenopausal women with positive assays for estrogen receptors May permit delay or avoidance of adrenalectomy or hypophysectomy	Adverse effects usually transient: thrombocytopenia, leukopenia Appears less toxic than other agents	Assess for hot flashes, nausea, vomiting, vaginal bleeding, flare, thrombocytopenia, weight gain, visual loss, edema
Enzyme antagonist (aminoglutethimide)	Inhibition of estrogen synthesis with enzyme antagonists	Adrenal inhibitor	Assess for rash, lethargy, dizziness
Megace	Progestational agent with uncertain action but probably decreases number of estrogen receptors in breast tissue	Weight gain, hot flashes, vaginal bleeding, increased blood pressure, edema, depression, flare	Assess for side effects
RADIATION (see p. 351)	Effective in relieving pain More effective in skeletal metastasis; less effective in visceral metastasis	Depends on area affected: Chest: esophagitis, pneumonitis, shortness of breath, slight cough Abdomen: affects digestion Body: general lethargy	Administer analgesics as required until effects of radiation lessen the need for such drugs Recognize that fatigue and weakness often result from radiation When pain is controlled, instruct patient to take extra precautions in order to avoid pathologic fractures: avoid lifting heavy packages and children and strenuous arm movements, such as those used in sweeping
OOPHORECTOMY	Removes cyclic hormone stimulation of the tumor. Preferred for premenopausal women:		(See Chap. 22 for surgical care)

(continued)

TABLE 46–7.   *(Continued)*

Type of Treatment	Objectives of Therapy	Possible Concomitant Effects	Nursing Interventions
OOPHORECTOMY (continued)	1. Surgical	Immediate estrogen withdrawal	
	2. Radiation	Estrogen withdrawal takes 4–6 weeks	
	If breast cancer is localized to breast, oophorectomy may or may not be advised.		

FSH, follicle-stimulating hormone; LH, luteinizing hormone.
* This listing of drugs, side effects, and nursing interventions is not meant to be exhaustive but is rather a sample of frequently used chemotherapeutic agents for breast cancer.

Pregnancy and Breast Cancer

Two to 5% of breast malignancies occur in pregnant women. Detection of lumps, changes in breast tissue, or masses is more difficult in pregnancy because of the normal physiologic changes that occur during gestation. Because many women discontinue BSE during pregnancy, an important aspect of health teaching is to encourage this practice throughout pregnancy, despite increased difficulty.

If a mass is found during pregnancy, mammography with appropriate shielding, needle aspiration, and biopsy are appropriate. Treatment is basically the same, although radiation is contraindicated in pregnancy. Some oncologists begin chemotherapy as early as the 16th week of pregnancy because fetal organs are formed at this point. If systemic treatment is necessary, a cesarean section is performed as soon as safety allows. If a mass is found while a woman is breast-feeding, weaning is urged to allow the breast to involute (return to its baseline state) before surgery. If aggressive disease is detected early in pregnancy and chemotherapy is advised, termination of the pregnancy is a choice that some patients may consider.

Some surgeons advise a patient to wait 2 years after therapy for breast cancer before considering a pregnancy. In the case of stage II or stage III disease, 4 years may be advised. Pregnancy after treatment for breast cancer does not seem to increase the risk of recurrence of disease.

Active listening is an important nursing function when patients are involved in difficult personal decision making about treatment options, plans for childbearing, or termination of pregnancy.

Anxiety and Breast Cancer

Many women with breast cancer believe that stress was a causative factor in the development of their malignancy. Self-blame can occur and can increase the uncomfortable feelings for these patients. Research on psychologic causation and progression is plentiful, and nurses working with breast cancer patients encounter frequent questions about this factor. Regular perusal of appropriate literature is important because the nurse is a provider of education and reassurance to patients.

Results of animal studies of stress and mammary malignancy are contradictory, but the effects of stress on the immune and endocrine systems are important and may be co-factors in tumor initiation. Personality factors that may increase survival

have been studied. Lack of social support and stress seem to affect survival negatively.

Patients need to be told about the preliminary stage of these findings and discouraged from self-blame. It is important to encourage a positive outlook and participation in care, but patients must also be allowed to grieve their loss.

Female Relatives. Daughters and sisters of patients with breast cancer should not be overlooked by the nurse. These relatives often have concern for their loved one and simultaneously are concerned about their own increased risk of breast cancer because of its increased incidence in female relatives. The nurse is able to provide education, care guidelines, information about BSE, and emotional support.

▶ Nursing Process
The Patient With Breast Cancer

▷ Assessment

The high incidence of this disease, its prognosis, its effects on women's futures, and changing treatment modalities require constant vigilance on the part of the nurse committed to educational preparedness.

The health history includes assessment of the reaction of the patient to the diagnosis and her ability to cope with it. Pertinent questions include the following:

How does the patient feel about having breast cancer?
What coping mechanisms does she use?
What support persons will be assistive?
Is there a partner or significant other available who will be of help in making decisions about treatment choices?
Are there any areas of confusion, misinformation, or irrational guilt that need clarification?
Is the patient in any discomfort?

Family members can be of assistance to the nurse in eliciting data that may be helpful in formulating the nursing care plan. Patients with a history of psychiatric disorders may have more dysfunctional responses to a diagnosis of breast cancer than those with normal coping mechanisms. Patients who have lost close relatives to breast cancer may also have more difficulty coping, because memories of loss and death emerge during their own crisis.

▷ Nursing Diagnoses

Based on the health history and other assessment data, the patient's major nursing diagnoses may include the following:

- Fear and ineffective coping related to the diagnosis of cancer, its treatment, and prognosis
- Body image disturbance related to extensive surgery and side effects of radiation and chemotherapy
- Pain related to surgical trauma
- Self-care deficit related to partial immobility of upper arm on the operative side
- Potential sexual dysfunction related to loss of body part, change in self-image, and fear of partner's reaction to this loss

▷ Planning and Implementation

▷ *Goals:*   The major goals of the patient may include reduction of emotional stress, fear, and anxiety, and improved ability to cope with the diagnosis and treatment; improved self-concept; pain relief; improved self-care; and improved sexual function.

▷ Nursing Interventions

▷ Preoperative

▷ *Reduction of Stress and Improved Coping Ability.*   Emotional preparation of the patient begins at the moment she is informed that hospitalization and treatment will be required. Avoiding delay of treatment is encouraged. Admission to a hospital, even for a same-day stay for a biopsy, is accompanied by a realistic fear of cancer and, for most patients, moderate to severe anxiety. Fear can cause delay and panic and is usually related to concerns about death and disfigurement.

Opportunities are provided to discuss fears and concerns. When a specific treatment plan has been decided upon, all aspects are explained to the patient. She and her partner need to know that a variety of resources and options are available, such as prostheses, reconstructive surgery, groups such as Reach to Recovery, and other services. Anticipatory teaching and counseling are provided prior to each stage of treatment. The details of additional diagnostic methods, treatment, and preoperative preparation are described. Should skin grafting or transplantation of tissue be required, the nature of the incision is explained.

Once the treatment plan has been established, it is initiated promptly with consideration given to promoting the best preoperative physical, psychologic, and nutritional condition possible. The patient is considered an active member of the health care team. Information about the surgery, including the location and extent of the incision and postoperative treatment, are data that the patient needs to cope with the unknown and deal with the present. If blood loss is expected, the patient may need time to donate her own blood or obtain compatible blood from chosen donors. If radiation or chemotherapy is to be initiated, it is important for the patient to meet the radiation oncologist, the medical oncologist, and the oncology nurse clinician to discuss her concerns. Extent and side effects of treatment, nature of the medication, frequency and duration of treatment, and goals are discussed. Methods to compensate for physical changes are discussed and planned (*i.e.,* prostheses and plastic surgery).

▷ Postoperative

Postoperative assessment includes monitoring of pulse and blood pressure, which are valuable indices for the detection of shock and hemorrhage. Blood pressure readings, injections, intravenous infusions, and venipunctures on the operative side are *prohibited* to prevent infection and compromised circulation. Dressings are inspected for bleeding on a regular basis. Drainage is monitored. The patient is encouraged and assisted to turn, cough, and take deep breaths to avoid pulmonary complications. A snug dressing should not inhibit thoracic expansion. Any graft areas are assessed for unusual redness, pain, swelling, or drainage. Monitoring of the operative site alerts the health care team to early signs of infection or other complications.

▷ *Positioning.*   Positioning of the patient depends on the type of dressing used. The semi-Fowler's position is usually desirable. The arm can be elevated to aid gravity in removing fluid via the lymphatic and venous pathways. Lymphedema is usually prevented by each joint being positioned higher than the more proximal joint. The degree of lymphedema is often related to the amount of collateral lymphatic avenues removed during surgery. Whether the arm is flexed or extended depends on the preference of the surgeon.

▷ *Reduction of Stress/Improved Coping Ability.*   If a patient is uncomfortable about the appearance of the operative site, problems may arise. The patient should not be forced to look at the incision if she is not ready or is uncomfortable doing so. Psychologic defenses must be respected. Drawings of the operative site or eliciting assistance from supportive family or friends may promote acceptance of body alteration. Exploration of this sensitive area must be a careful nursing action, and resistance on the part of the patient must be detected and respected.

Ongoing assessment of support systems of the patient and of her spouse is important because they affect postoperative adjustment. The spouse or partner of the patient is often in need of guidance, support, and education from the nurse to cope with the crisis. In addition to available support systems and information, the patient's attitude and religion are important considerations.

▷ *Relief of Pain.*   After the patient has recovered from anesthesia, adequate analgesia is indicated to provide relief for the patient and to encourage deep breathing and movement. Assessment by the nurse for manifestations of discomfort is important because patients experience differing degrees of pain intensity. Moderate elevation of the involved extremity is one measure of pain relief that may prevent lymphedema and fluid accumulation. Patient-controlled analgesia (PCA) may be of considerable assistance in assuring adequate pain relief and comfort (see Chap. 15 for discussion of PCA).

▷ *Improved Self-Care.*   Patients need information about the development of postoperative surgical edema and strategies to prevent it. Cuts, bruises, and infections on the operative side are dangerous precursors to problems. Stress on the suture line must be avoided. Education by the surgeon, reinforced and clarified by the nurse, facilitates assimilation of this information by an anxious patient. Pamphlets, books, and groups may be helpful to patients to supplement information given by professionals. Resources are available at the end of this chapter.

Care of the Incision Site.   Dressing changes present opportunities for the nurse to discuss with the patient (and possibly concerned others) the nature of the incision, how it looks and may feel, and progressive changes in its appearance. The patient needs to know that sensation is decreased in the operative area because of nerve disruption and that gentleness is necessary to avoid injury. Teaching regarding signs of infection or irritation to report to the physician is important. Use of the term *incision* rather than *scar* lessens the feelings of deformity and disfigurement that may accompany physical alteration. When appropriate healing has taken place, gentle massage of the healed incision with cocoa butter or other lotions helps to encourage circulation and increased skin elasticity.

Ambulation is encouraged once the patient is free of postanesthesia nausea and is tolerating fluids. The nurse supports the patient on the nonoperative side. Once drainage tubes are removed, passive range-of-motion exercises are initiated to increase circulation and muscle strength and to prevent joint stiffness. Hand exercises are also important. Self-care, including brushing of teeth, face washing, and hair care, is physically and emotionally therapeutic. Exercises such as climbing the wall with the fingers encourage arm use and prevent the development of contractures. Pain should not accompany therapeutic exercise; mild discomfort, effort, and anxiety, however, may occur initially. If skin grafts or tense, tight surgical incisions exist, exercises must be introduced gradually by the health care members working as a team. Muscle-training exercises are described in Figure 46-7. Bilateral muscle use as well as proper posture is encouraged. If a patient is hunched over, favoring the affected side, any exercise will be ineffective.

Radical mastectomy causes greater difficulty with any arm movement than less extensive procedures. Limitations after simple or modified mastectomies because of lymphedema are unusual, and complete mobility is encouraged postoperatively.

Normal household and work-related arm activities are promoted to maintain muscle tone. Active arm movement when walking, cleanliness of the operative site, avoidance of injury to the hand and arm, and loose, nonconstrictive clothing are all important aspects of patient education.

Follow-up visits or telephone calls can be helpful in the evaluation of incision healing, physical condition, general emotional outlook, and adjustment. Because early discharge from the hospital is common today, follow-up calls can evaluate drainage (if drains remain in place), pain management, and patient and family adjustment. If consultation or assistance is needed from community nurses, the patient's permission to initiate these contacts is obtained.

Lymphedema.   Lymphedema results if functioning lymphatic channels are inadequate to ensure a return flow of lymph to the general circulation. If axillary nodes and the lymph system have been removed, a collateral or auxiliary system must take over their function. This usually occurs within a month's time and is facilitated by movement and exercise with appropriate postoperative education. Most patients do not develop massive lymphedema. Instruction in and encouragement of elevation, massage, and exercise of the affected arm for 3 to 4 months help prevent the development of this disfiguring and possibly disabling swelling. Patient education guidelines are presented in Table 46-8.

If marked lymphedema occurs, the arm is elevated on a pillow so that the elbow is higher than the shoulder. The hand is elevated further to facilitate drainage. Elastic bandages and other constrictions are avoided because these may hinder formation of collateral lymphatic pathways. Some patients wear custom-made elastic sleeves from wrist to shoulder during active hours if necessary in cases of persistent swelling. Marked lymphedema occurred more commonly when a radical mastectomy was performed.

◊   *Improved Sexual Function.*   Change in the patient's body image and self-esteem, the partner's response, and the couple's anxiety level are all factors that may cause changes in sexual practices. Some partners have difficulty looking at the incision, while others seem to be unaffected and comfortable, conveying continuing, unaltered desirability. Either response affects the patient's self-image, sexuality, and acceptance. Discussion about how the patient sees herself and about possible decreased libido related to fatigue, nausea, or anxiety may help clarify issues for her and her partner. Clarification of misconceptions (*i.e.*, that cancer can be transmitted sexually or by fondling) is important. Encouragement of open discussion about fears, needs, and desires may reduce the couple's stress. Suggestions regarding variation in time of day for sexual activity (when the patient is least tired) or positions that are most com-

---

TABLE 46–8.   *Postoperative Care Instructions for Patients Undergoing Axillary Nodal Dissection*

Avoid burns while cooking or smoking

Avoid sunburns

Have all injections, vaccinations, blood samples, and blood pressure tests performed on the other arm

Use an electric razor with a narrow head for underarm shaving to reduce the risk of nicks or scratches

Carry heavy packages or handbags on the other arm

Wash cuts promptly, treat them with antibacterial medication, and cover them with a sterile dressing; check often for redness, soreness, or other signs of infection

Never cut cuticles; use hand cream or lotion

Wear protective gloves when gardening and when using strong detergents, etc.

Use a thimble when sewing

Avoid harsh chemicals and abrasive compounds

Use insect repellent to avoid bites and stings

Avoid elastic cuffs on clothes

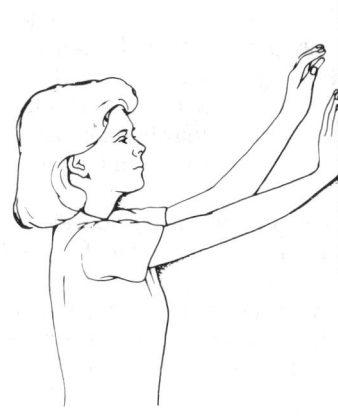

A. *Wall handclimbing.* Stand facing the wall, with the toes as close to the wall as possible—feet apart. With elbows somewhat bent, place the palms on the wall at shoulder level. By flexing the fingers, work hands up the wall until arms are fully extended. Work hands down to starting point.

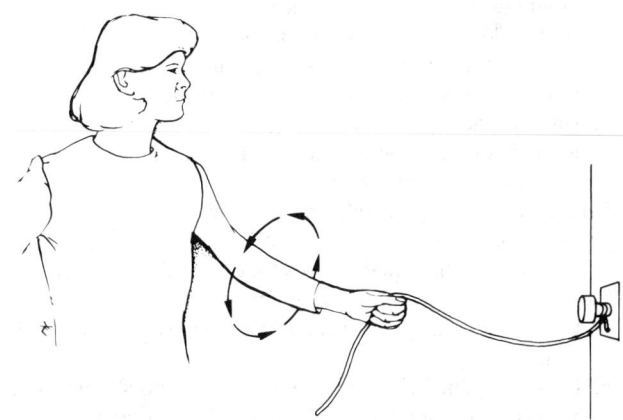

B. *Rope turning.* Stand facing the door. Take free end of light rope in hand of the operated side. Place other hand on hip. With arm extended and held away from the body—nearly parallel with the floor—turn rope, making as wide swings as possible. Slow at first—speed up later.

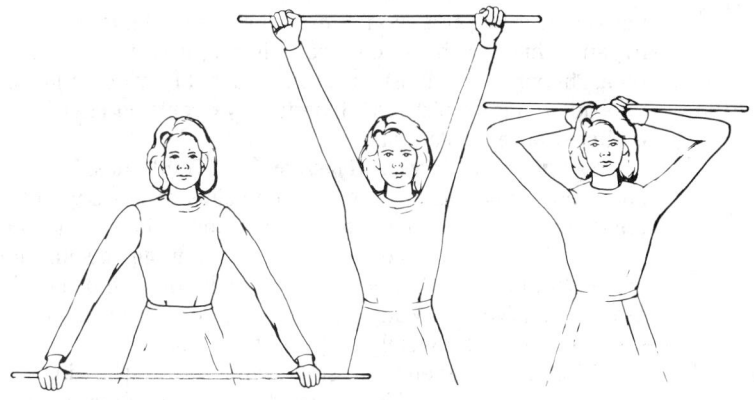

C. *Rod or Broom.* Grasp rod with both hands, held about 2 feet apart. With arms straight, raise rod over the head. Bend elbows lowering rod behind the head. Reverse maneuver, raising rod above the head, then to starting position.

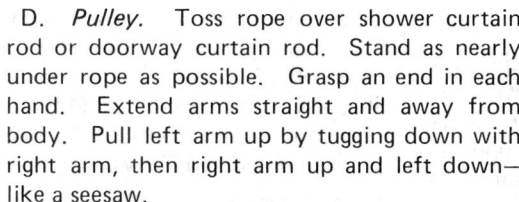

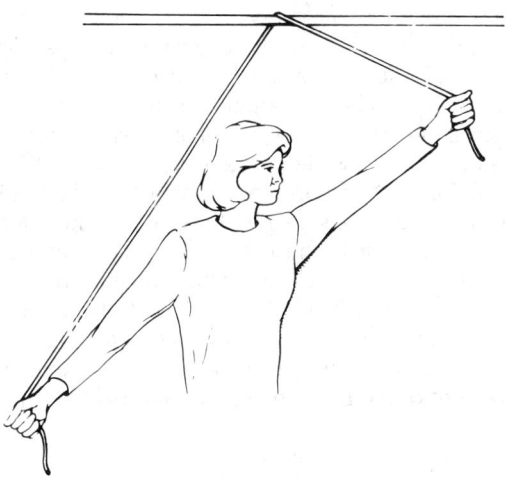

D. *Pulley.* Toss rope over shower curtain rod or doorway curtain rod. Stand as nearly under rope as possible. Grasp an end in each hand. Extend arms straight and away from body. Pull left arm up by tugging down with right arm, then right arm up and left down—like a seesaw.

Figure 46-7. Exercises after mastectomy. The purpose of the exercise program is to secure a complete range of motion of the affected shoulder joint. (Adapted from Radler A. Handbook for Your Recovery. New York, The Society of Memorial Center.)

fortable can be helpful, as are alternative options (*i.e.*, hugging, kissing, manual stimulation).

▷ *Evaluation*

Expected Outcomes

1. Demonstrates willingness to deal with the anxiety of the diagnosis and the impact of surgery on self-image and sexual functioning
   a. Discusses concerns related to future course of disease
   b. States that mastectomy need not have a permanent negative effect on sexuality
2. Experiences little or no discomfort
   a. Is afebrile 48 hours prior to discharge
   b. Reports minimal pain in operative site
   c. Demonstrates a drainage-free incision site
   d. Has satisfactory wound healing
   e. Identifies symptoms of complications (*i.e.*, redness, heat, and pain) to be reported
3. Participates actively in self-care activities
   a. Performs exercises as prescribed
   b. Performs additional exercises that will enhance healing
4. Uses modalities to prevent complications
   a. Lists signs and symptoms that are suggestive of complications
   b. Describes side effects of chemotherapy and strategies or measures to cope with such effects if they occur
   c. Avoids cuts, bruises, infection, and stress on hand and arm on operative side
   d. States rationale for follow-up schedule of physician visits
   e. Explains how to contact appropriate care providers in case of complications

Care of the patient with breast cancer is summarized in Nursing Care Plan 46-1.

Care of the Patient With Advanced Breast Cancer

Follow-up visits after surgery for breast cancer are individualized and often depend on postoperative treatments. Visits every 2 to 3 months for 2 years, followed by every 6 months for 5 years, may proceed to annual examinations, depending on physician preference and patient progress. A disease-free state for as long as possible is the goal. The patient is monitored closely for tumor recurrence or metastasis. Inoperative breast cancer or extensive spread of the disease is monitored by metastatic x-ray series (chest, skull, long bone, and pelvis); liver function tests; mammogram of the remaining breast tissue; and bone, liver, and brain imaging. Half of all patients having recurrence display this as local or regional lymph node recurrence, and one fourth have visceral involvement. Bone involvement of the hips, spine, ribs, and pelvis may occur.

Nursing Interventions

Regression or relief of symptoms is the goal of care. The quality of survival time is an important aspect of nursing intervention.

Assessment of the physical and psychosocial status of the patient is a challenge for the nurse. Information from family members and significant others is valuable. Palliative treatment,

if necessary, is an important aspect of care from care providers. Comfort and pain-free existence, even if a disease-free state is not possible, enhance the quality of remaining life. Bone metastases cause pain and decreased mobility. Hospice and home health care may be indicated for some patients at this time. Specific arrangements for these services may be planned and discussed early, before actually needed, to lessen patient distress.

Severe anxiety and depression may occur. Suicidal ideation is common, but suicide is unusual because the will to survive is strong.

Treatment modes vary and depend on specifics of the patient's condition and modalities available. Refer to Chapter 19, Oncology: Nursing the Patient with Cancer, for further discussion.

Reconstructive and Plastic Surgery of the Breast

Hypertrophy of the Breast

Breasts play an important part in self-image in American culture. Any perceived abnormality may lead to a request for surgical intervention. Variations in the size of the breasts are the most common causes of distress that lead women to seek information regarding alteration. Breasts that are too large are called hypertrophied. If this occurs early in life, it is called virginal breast hypertrophy. It usually is bilateral but may occur just on one side, causing distress. Hypertrophy occurring later in life is almost always bilateral.

Symptoms of Breast Hypertrophy. Tenderness, diffuse pains, and fatigue are common complaints of those with this condition. Premenstrually, tenderness and pain are marked. The weight of an enlarged breast causes a dragging sensation in the shoulder, and support is often futile, despite use of the most expensive bra. Many patients have deep grooves in their shoulders from the weight imposed by bra straps.

Discomfort and embarrassment when wearing bathing suits and participating in athletic events may be limiting; posture can also be affected. Social life can become restricted and insecurity can develop based on poor self-image.

Mammoplasty

After a surgical or plastic surgery consultation, a *reduction mammoplasty* may be performed under general anesthesia. One approach is an incision beneath the breast and a similar curved incision in the skin of the anterior breast. The nipple is transplanted to a new location after excess tissue is removed. Skin edges are approximated with sutures, and the nipple is sutured to its new location. Drains are placed in the incision and remain for 1 to 2 days. Simple gauze dressings are applied, without pressure.

Postoperative Nursing Interventions. After mammoplasty, usual postoperative nursing care is indicated. Patients are up and about fairly quickly and usually describe their surgery as nontraumatic, possibly because of the relief that they have sought. Hypertrophy will not recur, but if weight is gained breast enlargement may result. The new transplanted nipple may turn

(text continues on page 1316)

Nursing Care Plan 46-1

Care of the Patient With Cancer of the Breast

Nursing Interventions	Rationale	Expected Outcomes

Nursing Diagnosis: Fear and ineffective coping related to the diagnosis of breast cancer, its treatment, and prognosis

Goal: Reduction of emotional stress, fear, and anxiety

1. Begin emotional preparation of the patient (and partner) as soon as she is told that hospitalization and treatment are required.	1. The earlier the patient accepts the reality of the situation, the more readily will coping mechanisms be effective.	• Displays a reduction of emotional stress and anxiety and exhibits an ability to cope with the problem.

2. Assess
  a. Personal experience with and knowledge about breast cancer
  b. Coping mechanisms in crisis
  c. Support systems
  d. Affective state re: diagnosis
	2. These factors strongly affect the patient's behavior and ability to deal with the diagnosis, surgery, and follow-up treatment. If a patient has lost close relatives or friends to breast cancer, she will probably react in a manner different from that of the patient who has friends surviving with an excellent quality of life.	• Participates in the treatment plan and asks questions relating to the best choice for her particular needs.
		• States that anger, anxiety, depression, denial, and withdrawal are normal reactions.
		• Responds positively to the information she is accumulating.

3. Inform the patient of recent research and new treatment modalities for breast cancer.	3. Increasing options and improved results both statistically and cosmetically greatly reduce the fear and promote acceptance of the treatment plan.	• Describes her appreciation of social support of family, friends, and women who have had breast surgery as a significant aid in coping with a stressful experience.
4. Describe the experiences the patient will face and encourage her questions.	4. Fear of the unknown is decreased.	• Is aware that husband or significant other has been advised and prepared with regard to supportive role.
5. Acquaint her with the increasing number of available resources to facilitate her recovery.	5. The information about new prosthetics, reconstruction specialists, and other resources confirms that a great deal of attention is being given to newer treatment methods for breast cancer.	• Reads literature provided.

Nursing Diagnosis: Disturbance in self-concept related to nature of surgery and side effects of radiation and/or chemotherapy

Goal: Realistic adaptation to changes that will occur relative to treatment modalities

1. Confirm with the physician the nature of the treatment anticipated.	1. This sets the basis for a cooperative therapeutic plan that will prevent conflicting information from reaching the patient.	• Accepts the treatment plan. • Verbalizes that grief must run its course. • Uses her support system effectively; plans future activities with them.
2. Explain that it is normal to experience grief at the loss of a body part.	2. When this fact is established, the patient can then be free to move to the next level of coping.	• Eventually looks at her incision site and participates in dressing changes.
3. Encourage visits by loved ones and understanding friends.	3. Support systems that are meaningful to the patient are more endurable than those from relative strangers.	• Expresses an understanding of the long-term benefits of chemotherapy/radiation (if prescribed) even though there may be uncomfortable side effects.
4. Tell her that it is normal not to want herself or partner to view the incision (do not refer to this as a "scar"); further reinforce the fact that each day the site will look better.	4. This reduces the feeling that she will never be able to accept her altered body.	
5. Discuss the use of prosthesis, reconstruction possibilities, and clothing adjustment as realistic and attainable expectations.	5. The emphasis on the positive and the availability of adaptations will enhance her self-concept and promote positive acceptance of the treatment plan.	

(continued)

Nursing Care Plan 46-1 *(Continued)*

Care of the Patient With Cancer of the Breast

Nursing Interventions	Expected Outcomes	Expected Outcomes

Nursing Diagnosis: Pain related to tissue trauma from incision(s)

Goal: Absence of pain and discomfort

1. Assess intensity, nature, and location of pain.	1. Provides baseline to assess effectiveness of pain-relief measures.	• Reports when pain is worsening and accepts prescribed pain medication.
2. Administer analgesia by IM, oral, or IV route as prescribed.	2. Promotes pain relief.	• Adjusts her position to relieve discomfort; uses small pillows effectively.
3. Collaborate with physician about use of patient-controlled analgesia.	3. Patient-controlled analgesia results in pain relief and increased comfort and maintains patient's sense of control.	• Exercises frequently; moves affected arm gently and shows progress in moving from passive to active exercises.
4. Explain that nerves are severed or damaged but that analgesics and narcotics are available.	4. Analgesics and narcotics can interrupt nerve pathways to the brain and spinal cord.	• Describes home-related activities that will provide the required range of motion of the affected arm.
5. Proper body positioning will promote comfort, such as semi-Fowler's position and elevation of the arm on the affected side.	5. Stress on the incision site is reduced; gravity reduces fluid accumulation in the arm. (Squeezing ball and wrist flexion begin in first 24 hours.)	• Lists various activities that must be avoided because of potential for injury to the breast site and affected arm.
6. Promote passive and then active exercises of the hand, arm, and shoulder on the affected side.	6. This will stimulate circulation, promote neurovascular competence, and prevent stasis with subsequent stiffening of the shoulder girdle.	• Relates procedures to follow if accidental injury is sustained.
7. Encourage protection and the avoidance of anything that can break through the skin barrier or impose stress on the arm and shoulder (cuts, burns, strong detergents, infections, carrying a heavy bag or purse).	7. Impaired circulation and weakened nerves are vulnerable to sudden or prolonged stress.	• Orders Medic-Alert bracelet when arm lymphedema is diagnosed.
8. Suggest application of an effective cream several times a day.	8. This practice will keep the skin healthy, intact, pliable, and resistant to breakdown.	
9. Instruct patient to contact the physician if the arm or incision site becomes painful, swollen, or red.	9. Early treatment of possible infection or injury will avoid further discomfort and complications.	
10. Suggest the wearing of a Medic Alert tag if there is a potential for edema.	10. A recognized alert tag will serve as a precaution against injections, measurement of blood pressure, and other forms of injury.	

Nursing Diagnosis: Self-care deficit related to partial immobility of upper extremity on side of breast surgery

Goal: Avoidance of impaired mobility and achievement of self-care to the fullest possible level

1. Invite patient's active participation in postoperative care.	1. Patient involvement enhances and facilitates the recovery process.	• Participates in dressing change; expresses interest in working with rehabilitative team including physical therapist.
2. Encourage patient's socialization, particularly with patients who have successfully recovered in similar circumstances.	2. Humans thrive more effectively and happily when they are socially able to relate to others.	• Shows concern about her appearance and accepts suggestions from rehabilitation support groups.

(continued)

Nursing Care Plan 46–1 (Continued)

Care of the Patient With Cancer of the Breast

Nursing Interventions	Expected Outcomes	Expected Outcomes
3. Make progressive modifications in the patient's exercise program as dictated by comfort and tolerance levels. 4. Commend the patient when ingenuity and creativity are in evidence, such as an attractive hair style or make-up application.	3. There is lessened strain on tissues; improvement is steadily consistent. 4. Psychologic well-being complements the effects of optimal physical good health.	• Participates in self-care (*i.e.*, dressing, bathing, grooming). • Verbalizes anticipation and enjoyment of partner's visits and relates her progress.

Nursing Diagnosis: Possible sexual dysfunction related to loss of body part and fear of partner's reaction to this loss

Goal: Identification of alternative satisfying/acceptable sexual experiences

1. Become comfortable in discussing sexuality; display a caring, nonjudgmental supportive attitude. 2. Encourage, at the appropriate time, both partners to discuss their concerns; this can be done before and after major treatment. 3. Arrange for privacy when discussing personal problems with the patient. 4. Describe the incision site and its appearance with the partner before partner actually sees it. 5. Emphasize that behavioral changes take time and should not be interpreted as rejection.	1. The patient will easily sense insincerity, insecurity, lack of knowledge, and inexperience. Nurses new to this area can obtain assistance from the oncology clinical nurse specialist. 2. The patient will not feel that she is alone in facing problems that may concern both partners. 3. Sensitive personal problems are not revealed when people not close to the patient are present. 4. Partner will know what to expect and not likely register shock in front of the patient. 5. The very nature of undergoing any surgery takes time for acceptance, recuperation, and perhaps altered life-style.	• Responds by conveying trust and a desire to obtain assistance; asks appropriate questions. • Includes partner in aspects of the medical problem that concern both. • Expresses appreciation for promoting confidentiality regarding very personal matters. • Accepts the incision site as evidenced by assisting with dressings and using an appropriate prescribed emollient such as cocoa butter. • Expresses awareness that any adjustments take time but that with patience and understanding the desired goals can be approached and possibly reached.

Potential for Complications: Infection, injury, lymphedema, neurovascular deficits

Goal: Avoidance of complications

1. Encourage the elevation of the arm, if not contraindicated, with each joint positioned higher than the more proximal joint. 2. Inform patient to avoid injury, strenuous activity, or infection. 3. Describe and demonstrate exercises in a step-up fashion from simple to more involved. 4. Recommend physical therapy and a weight-reduction program if indicated.	1. Edema is reduced and there is less pressure on the nerves and blood vessels; pain and discomfort are lessened. 2. These can stimulate fluid accumulation and compromise the neurovasculature of the arm. 3. A graduated exercise program will improve muscle tone and hasten full range of activities with avoidance of impairment such as a frozen shoulder. 4. Properly prescribed activities and exercise plus diet modification are general health measures that enhance well-being and thwart complications.	• Demonstrates how to place pillows so that proper elevation of arm is maintained. • Lists activities that are to be avoided, including injections and having blood pressure measured on the affected side. • Gradually moves the arm freely so that hair combing and "climbing the wall" can be achieved with no discomfort. Avoids the discomfort of a frozen shoulder. • Acquires good health habits and avoids complications at the same time.

black and become scab-covered. This is to be expected, and as the nipple regains a new blood supply, the scab falls off and the appearance approximates normal. Lactation may be impossible after this type of surgery; about half of women who have this surgery can breast-feed successfully. Feelings postoperatively may be a mixture of euphoria, relief, sorrow over the loss of a body part, and anxiety over these feelings. Reassurance is important.

Surgery to Enlarge or Uplift the Breasts

Augmentation mammoplasty is requested fairly frequently. This is performed through an incision along the undermargin of the breast, in the axilla, or at the border of the areola and the breast is then elevated and a pocket is formed between the breast and the chest wall. Various types of plastic and synthetic materials are inserted to enlarge and uplift the breast. These procedures may be performed on an outpatient basis with local anesthesia by an experienced plastic surgeon. Complications (*i.e.*, infection) that may occur may require subsequent removal of the implant.

Breast Reconstruction After Mastectomy

Reconstruction after mastectomy in those women with an early cancer and a good prognosis is becoming increasingly common. Looseness and suppleness of the skin and subcutaneous tissue along with sufficient blood supply allow success of this repair. Surgeons and oncologists may differ about the optimal time for reconstruction. Immediate reconstruction was thought to possibly hinder discovery of an early recurrence, but this does not seem to be occurring. Proponents of this technique argue that a delay in diagnosis would be minimal and that the psychologic benefits are important. Criteria for selecting patients for breast reconstruction are being developed to reduce the risk of recurrence of malignancy. Some suggest waiting 5 years after completion of chemotherapy or radiation or 6 months after surgery. Most reconstruction takes place a few months after surgery or after completion of therapy.

Procedures

The choice of surgical procedure for reconstruction is based on the condition of the overlying skin and underlying muscle. Nipple reconstruction may be performed separately. Surgical procedures are described in Figures 46-8 and 46-9.

Silicone implants are used for women with small breasts. However, silicone has been associated with various complications, and its safety is being investigated. Expanders can also be used. An empty bag is inserted during surgery and a small tube remains externally. Small amounts of normal saline are injected over several weeks, and then the expander is replaced by a permanent implant.

Flap surgery is another option. The transrectus abdominal muscle is cut to form a flap, which will accommodate a larger breast reconstruction. The loss of abdominal muscle is a potential problem. If the latissimus dorsi is used, the amount of muscle used is smaller, and so it is less likely to be troublesome. A gluteal flap from the buttocks is another option. All choices involve the risk imposed by any surgery, including bleeding and infection.

Postoperative Nursing Management

Suction tubes to closed drainage are inserted, and measures are used to reduce tension on the incisions. Elevating the head of the bed by 30 degrees and flexing the knees lessen tension on an abdominal incision. Antiemetics are used to control nausea and vomiting; analgesics are used to control discomfort. Assessment of circulation by observation of the color and temperature of the newly reconstructed breast area is an important nursing function. Mottling or an obvious drop in skin temperature is reported to the surgeon immediately. Drainage of more than 50 ml per hour should also be reported.

During ambulation on the first postoperative day, the patient will favor the incision line. Gradually, a more upright position can be accomplished. Bras and breast massage are avoided until the physician indicates that no injury will result. Elevation of the arms above the shoulder and lifting more than 5 lb are avoided for 1 month postoperatively to avoid stress on the incision.

Prophylactic Mastectomy

Some women who are at high risk for the development of breast cancer may be offered the option of prophylactic mastectomy. Possible candidates are those who have a strong family history and very cystic breasts, those who had previous cancer in one breast and progressive nodularity in the other, a woman with lumpy breasts who has a suspicious mammogram, a woman who had a biopsy specimen showing atypical hyperplasia, or a woman with cystic breast changes who has had several biopsies and who is severely affected by fear of breast cancer.

Diseases of the Male Breast

Gynecomastia or overdeveloped breast tissue in the male is the most common male breast condition encountered by health care providers. Adolescent males can be affected by this condition because of hormones secreted by the testes. Gynecomastia usually disappears in 1 or 2 years, but it can occur before or after puberty. It is usually unilateral and presents as a firm, tender mass beneath the areola. In adult males, gynecomastia may be diffuse and can be related to medications (*i.e.*, digitalis, reserpine, ergotamine, and phenytoin). Pain and tenderness are initial symptoms.

Malignancy can occur in the male breast, but this is infrequent. Symptoms can include a painless lump beneath the areola, nipple retraction, and skin ulceration. Average age at the time of diagnosis is about 10 years older than that of women. A mild familial tendency seems to exist if other males in the family have had breast malignancy. Diagnostic and treatment modalities are similar to those used for women. Other risk factors may include mumps orchitis, radiation exposure, and Klinefelter's syndrome (a chromosomal condition with decreased testosterone levels). Most male breast lumps are gynecomastia rather than breast cancer, but gynecomastia may predispose the patient to malignancy, although this theory is unproved.

Treatment usually consists of a radical mastectomy because of pectoral muscle involvement. Radiation therapy may be used postoperatively. Prognosis varies depending on stage at the time of detection. Bone and soft tissue metastases are usually the most common sites of advanced disease. Orchidectomy, adrenalectomy, and hypophysectomy may be used in advanced disease.

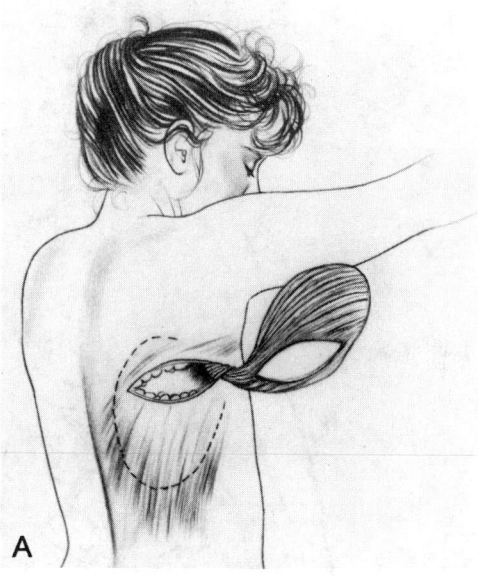

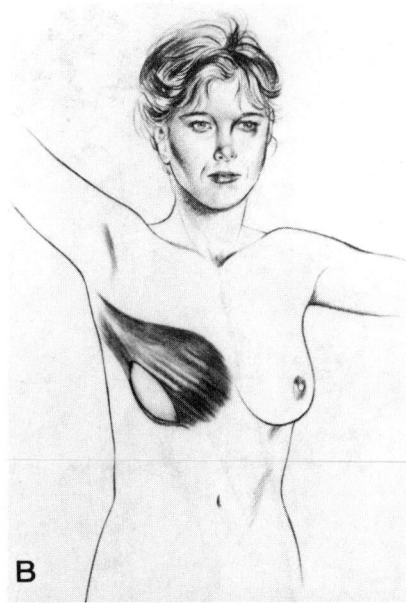

An elliptical incision identifies the skin tissue (island) that will be attached to dissected latissimus dorsi muscle (dissected underneath skin in area of dotted line). When freed but with one end attached, this muscle and skin flap (note arrow) is then threaded through a tunnel under the skin (subaxillary) and brought out at the breast site.

Flap in place after being tunneled from back to front of the chest.

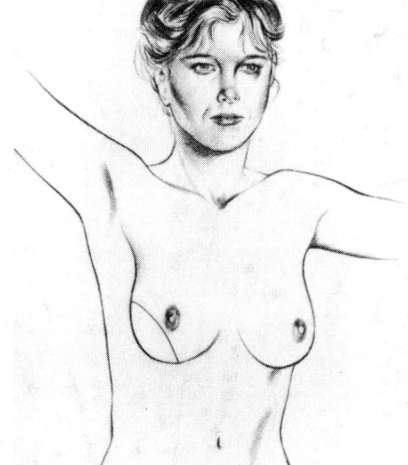

Flap is in place re-creating breast contour with reconstructed nipple and areola.

Figure 46–8. Breast reconstruction: myocutaneous flap procedure using latissimus dorsi muscle. (Adapted from The Breast Cancer Digest, 2nd ed. Bethesda, MD, U.S. Department of Health and Human Services, Public Health Service.)

Chapter Summary

The patient with breast cancer requires nursing care that includes attention to her physiologic needs and emotional reactions to the diagnosis and its treatment. In the early post-operative phase, the patient requires assistance with positioning, self-care activities, and management of pain. Additionally, she needs understanding and assistance in dealing with the diagnosis of breast cancer and its ramifications in terms of treatment options, prognosis, and well-being. The nurse who serves effectively as case manager is able to coordinate the patient's care and identify appropriate support services. Preparation for

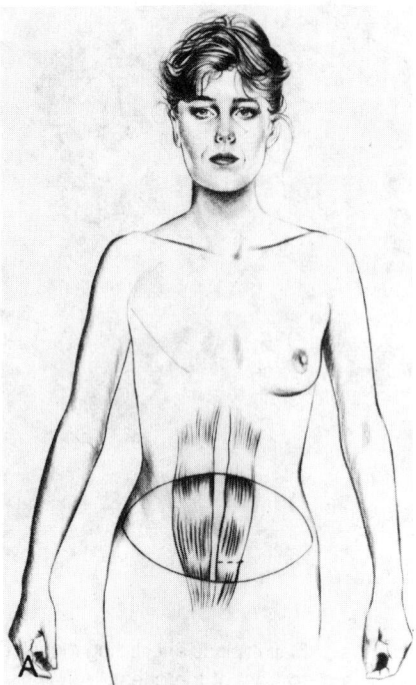

An elliptical lower abdominal incision is made, and one of two vertical abdominal muscles is cut.

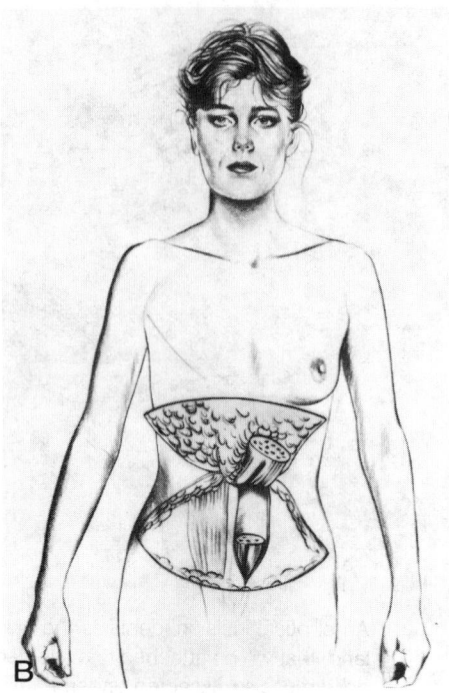

The skin flap including muscle and fat is then tunneled under the skin of upper abdominal and lower chest to the breast site.

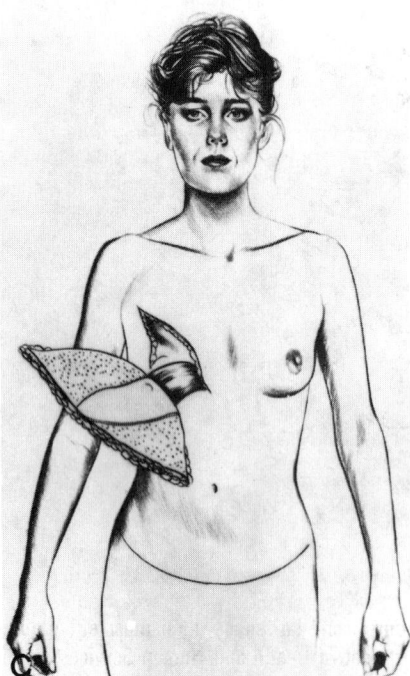

The flap will be positioned and molded to the contour of the breast. Blood supply continues with flap.

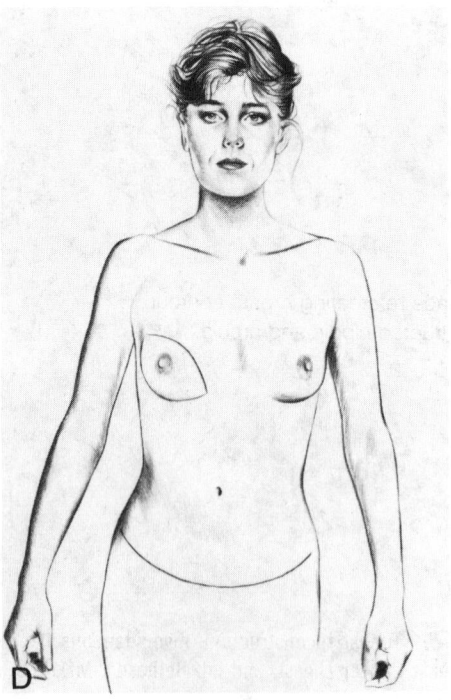

Flap in place re-creating breast contour with reconstructed nipple and areola.

Figure 46–9.   Breast reconstruction: Myocutaneous flap procedure using abdominis rectus muscle. (Adapted from The Breast Cancer Digest, 2nd ed. Bethesda, MD, U.S. Department of Health and Human Services, Public Health Service.)

discharge and for subsequent therapy (*i.e.*, chemotherapy, radiation therapy) assists the patient in coping with these treatments and increases the likelihood of her follow-up with treatment regimens.

The challenge of working with patients who have breast disease has been noted throughout this chapter. Sensitivity to women's feelings and responses to threats to self-esteem, sexuality, and life are considered during care. Rapid changes in treatment modalities and results of research demand constant study. Areas of major change in treatment and prevention include: oncogenes (tumor genes that control cell growth), growth factors (substances released by cancer cells to make the environment more conducive to growth), monoclonal antibodies (synthetic antibodies that fight cancer cells), and lipoprotein research (lipoproteins change in cancer patients, and this may become a method of detection). Biologic response modifiers (*i.e.*, interferon or other substances that help increase the body's immune system response) may be a method of treatment in the near future. Alternative methods of healing and stress-reduction techniques may be used to a greater extent. Optimism and hope for more and better modes of treatment are realistic and should be conveyed to patients. Nurses may play an important part in the reduction of breast malignancy through research, patient care, and commitment to education and prevention. The nurse's role in BSE instruction to all patients may be the key to a decrease in the mortality rate from this disease.

Bibliography

Books
Ariel I and Cleary J. Breast Cancer: Diagnosis and Treatment. New York, McGraw-Hill, 1987.

Ash C and Jenkins J (eds). Enhancing the Role of Cancer Nursing. New York, Raven Press, 1990.

Barger M (ed). Protocols for Gynecologic and Obstetric Health Care. Orlando, Grune & Stratton, 1988.

Bates B. A Guide to Physical Examination, 5th ed. Philadelphia, JB Lippincott, 1991.

Broniatowski-Grundfest S and Esselstyn C. Controversies in Breast Disease. New York, Marcel Dekker, 1988.

Cancer Statistics 1991, American Cancer Society, Atlanta, GA.

Cooper C (ed). Stress and Breast Cancer. New York, John Wiley & Sons, 1988.

Davidson A. Modified Radical and Other Cancer Poems. Palo Alto, CA, Monday Press, 1990.

DeVita V, Hellman S, and Rosenberg SA (eds). Cancer: Principles and Practice of Oncology, 3rd ed. Philadelphia, JB Lippincott, 1989.

Dunnihoo D. Fundamentals of Gynecology and Obstetrics. Philadelphia, JB Lippincott, 1990.

Eating Hints: Recipes and Tips for Better Nutrition During Cancer Treatment. US Dept of Health and Human Services. Public Health Service, National Institutes of Health, National Cancer Institute, Bethesda, MD, 1987. NIH Publication No. 87-2079.

Fogel C and Lauver D. Sexual Health Promotion. Philadelphia, WB Saunders, 1990.

Groenwald S. Cancer Nursing: Principles and Practices. Boston, Jones and Bartlett, 1990.

Haagensen C. Diseases of the Breast, 3rd ed. Philadelphia, WB Saunders, 1986.

Harris J et al. Breast Diseases. Philadelphia, JB Lippincott, 1987.

Henderson C et al. Cancer of the breast. In: DeVita V, Hellman S, and Rosenberg SA. Cancer: Principles and Practice of Oncology, 3rd ed. Philadelphia, JB Lippincott, 1989.

Hindle W. Breast Disease for Gynecologists. Norwalk, CT, Appleton and Lange, 1990.

Holland J and Rowland J. Handbook of Psychooncology. New York, Oxford University Press, 1989.

Kushner R. Alternatives: New Developments in the War on Breast Cancer. New York, Warner, 1986.

Lawrence R. Breastfeeding, 3rd ed. St Louis, CV Mosby, 1989.

Love SM. Dr. Susan Love's Breast Book. Reading, MA, Addison-Wesley, 1990.

Marchant D (ed). Breast Disease. New York, Churchill Livingstone, 1986.

Martin L. Health Care of Women. Philadelphia, JB Lippincott, 1978.

Moosa A, Robson M, and Schimpff S (eds). Complete Textbook of Oncology. Baltimore, Williams & Wilkins, 1986.

Quilligan E and Zuspan F. Current Therapy in Obstetrics and Gynecology 3. Philadelphia, WB Saunders, 1990.

Speroff L, Glass R, and Kase N. Clinical Gynecologic and Endocrinology and Infertility. Baltimore, Williams & Wilkins, 1989.

Stewart F et al. Understanding Your Body. Toronto, Bantam, 1987.

Strax P. Make Sure You Do Not Have Breast Cancer. St. Martin's Press, 1990.

Tenenbaum L. Cancer Chemotherapy: A Reference Guide. Philadelphia, WB Saunders, 1989.

Ziegfeld C (ed). Core Curriculum for Oncology Nursing. Philadelphia, WB Saunders, 1987.

Journals
Asterisks indicate nursing research articles.

General
Moch S. Health within illness: Conceptual evolution and practice. Adv Nurs Sci 1989 July; 11(4):23–31.

Rudolph A and McDermott R. The breast physical examination: Its value in early cancer detection. Cancer Nurs 1987 Feb; 10(2):100–105.

Breast Disorders
Ellerhorst-Ryan J, Turba E, and Stahl D. Evaluating benign breast disease. Nurs Pract 1988 Sep; 13(9):13–28.

Greydanus D, Parks D, and Farrell G. Breast Disorders in Children and Adolescents. Pediatr Clin North Am 1989 Jun; (3):601–637.

Lierman L. Discovery of breast changes: Women's responses and nursing implications. Cancer Nurs 1988 Jun; 11(6):352–361.

Prevention, Breast Self-Examination, and Mammography
Beck S et al. The family high-risk program: Targeted cancer prevention. Oncol Nurs Forum 1988 May/Jun; 15(3):301–306.

Bope E. Screening for breast cancer: Recent increases underscore new urgency. Fem Patient 1989 Mar; 14(3):75–86.

Clarke D and Sandler L. Factors involved in nurses' teaching breast self-examination. Cancer Nurs 1989 Jan; 12(1):41–45.

Cretain G. Motivational factors in breast self-examination: Implications for nurses. Cancer Nurs 1989 Apr; 12(4):250–256.

Crooks C and Jones S. Educating women about the importance of breast screenings: The nurse's role. Cancer Nurs 1989 Jun; 12(3):161–164.

Hamwi D. Screening mammography: Increasing the effort toward breast cancer detection. Nurs Pract 1990 Dec; 15(12):27–32.

Harrison L. Life-saving patient education: Breast self-examination. Matern Child Nurs J 1989 Sep/Oct; 14(5):315.

* Haughey B et al. Breast self-examination: Reported practices, proficiency and stage of disease at diagnosis. Oncol Nurs Forum 1988 Mar; 15(3): 315–319.

Heyman D et al. Is the hospital setting the place for teaching breast self-examination? Cancer Nurs 1991 Feb; 14(1):35–40.

Lauver D. Identifying womens' descriptions of breast tissue for the promotion of breast self examination. Health Care Women Int 1991 Jan/Mar; 12(1):73–83.

* Lauver K and Angerame M. Overadherence with breast self-examination recommendations. Image: J Nurs Scholarship 1990 Fall; 11(3):148–152.

* Lierman L et al. Predicting breast self-examination using the theory of reasoned action. Nurs Res 1990 Mar/Apr; 39(2):97–101.

Nielsen B. The nurse's role in mammography screening. Cancer Nurs 1989 Oct; 12(5):271–275.

* Olson R and Mitchell E. Self-confidence as a critical factor in breast self-examination. J Obstet Gynecol Neonatal Nurs 1989 Nov/Dec; 18(6): 476–481.

Redeker N. Health beliefs, health locus of control, and the frequency of practice of breast self examination in women. J Obstet Gynecol Neonatal Nurs 1989 Jan/Feb; 18(1):45–51.

Rutledge D and Davis G. Breast self-examination compliance and the health belief model. Oncol Nurs Forum 1988 Mar/Apr; 15(2):175–179.

Screening mammography: A missed clinical opportunity? Results of the NCI Breast Cancer Screening Consortium and National Health Interview Survey Studies. JAMA 1990 Jul; 264(1):54–58.

Zapka J et al. Breast cancer screening by mammography: Utilization and associated factors. Am J Public Health 1989 Nov; 79(11):1499–1502.

Cancer

Cady B. New diagnostic, staging and therapeutic aspects of early breast cancer. Cancer 1990 Feb; 65(Suppl):634–647.

Carey R and Jevne R. Development of an information package for post-mastectomy patients on adjuvant therapy. Oncol Nurs Forum 1986 May/Jun; 13(3):78–79.

Clark J and Landis L. Reintegration and maintenance of employees with breast cancer in the workplace. J Am Assoc Occup Health Nurs 1989 May; 37(5):186–196.

Diekman J. Cancer in the elderly: Systems overview. Semin Oncol Nurs 1988 Aug; 4(3):169–177.

* Dodd M. Patterns of self-care in patients with breast cancer. West J Nurs Res 1988 Feb; 10(1):7–24.

Donegan W. Are we positive about node negative cancer. J Surg Oncol 1990 Jan; 43(1):199–202.

Duda R. Pathogenesis, diagnosis and treatment of breast cancer. Compr Ther 1990 Jan; 16(1):43–52.

Fisher B et al. Eight year results of a randomized clinical trial comparing total mastectomy and lumpectomy with or without irradiation in the treatment of breast cancer. N Engl J Med 1989 Mar; 320:822–828.

Fitzsimmons M et al. Hereditary cancer syndromes: Nursing's role in identification and education. Oncol Nurs Forum 1989 Jan; 16(1):87–94.

Fraser M and Tucker M. Late effects of cancer therapy: Chemotherapy related malignancies. Oncol Nurs Forum 1988 Jan/Feb; 15(1):67–77.

Fraser M and Tucker M. Second malignancies following cancer therapy. Semin Oncol Nurs 1989 Feb; 5(1):43–55.

Gambosi J and Ulreich S. Recovering from cancer: A nursing intervention program recognizing survivorship. Oncol Nurs Forum 1990 Feb; 17(2): 215–218.

Breast Cancer

Albrecht S. Season of birth and laterality of breast cancer. Nurs Res 1990 Mar/Apr; 39(2):118–120.

Arathuzik D. Pain experience for metastatic breast cancer patients: Unraveling the mystery. Cancer Nurs 1991 Feb; 14(1):41–48.

Bergvist L et al. The risk of breast cancer after estrogen and estrogen-progestin replacement therapy. N Engl J Med 1989 Aug; 321(5):293–297.

Bonadonna G. Conceptual and practical advances in the management of breast cancer. J Clin Oncol 1989 Oct; 7(10):1380–1397.

Bruera E et al. Asthenia in breast cancer. Am J Nurs 1989 May; 89(5):737–738.

Cawley M et al. Informational and psychosocial needs of women choosing conservative surgery and primary radiation for early stage breast cancer. Cancer Nurs 1990 Apr; 13(2):90–94.

Collins-Hattery A et al. S phase index and ploidy prognostic markers in node negative breast cancer: Information for nurses. Oncol Nurs Forum 1991 Jan/Feb; 18(1):59–62.

Hilton B. The phenomenon of uncertainty in women with breast cancer. Issues Ment Health Nurs 1988 Mar; 9(3):217–238.

Hindle W. Key questions about breast cancer. Contemp Obstet Gynecol 1989 Nov; 34(5):72–78.

Kelsey J and Gammon M. The epidemiology of breast cancer. Ca 1991 May/Jun; 41(3):146–165.

Lindsey A, Dodd M, and Kaempfer S. Endocrine mechanisms and obesity: Influences in breast cancer. Oncol Nurs Forum 1987 Mar/Apr; 14(2): 47–51.

* Loveys B. Breast cancer: Demands of illness. Oncol Nurs Forum 1991 Jan/Feb; 18(1):75–80.

McGee R and White C. Helping employees and families cope with breast cancer treatment. J Am Assoc Occup Health Nurs 1989 May; 37(5): 178–185.

McKenney S. Helping your patient cope with breast cancer. Nursing '88 1988 Dec; 18(12):64.

Moch S. Health within the experience of breast cancer. J Adv Nurs 1990 Dec; 15(12):1426–1435.

Morrow M. Management of nonpalpable breast lesions. Princ Pract Oncol Updates 1990 Jan; 4(1):1–11.

Nettles-Carlson B. Early detection of breast cancer. J Obstet Gynecol Neonatal Nurs 1989 Sep/Oct; 18(5):373–381.

Nielsen B and East D. Advances in breast cancer: Implications for care. Nurs Clin North Am 1990 Jun; 25(2):365–375.

* Northouse L. A longitudinal study of the adjustment of patients and husbands to breast cancer. Oncol Nurs Forum 1989 Jul/Aug; 16(4):511–516.

* Northouse L. The impact of breast cancer on patients and husbands. Cancer Nurs 1989 Oct; 12(5):276–284.

* Northouse L. Social support in patients' and husbands' adjustment to breast cancer. Nurs Res 1988 Mar/Apr; 37(2):91–95.

Rutherford D. Assessing psychosexual needs of women experiencing lumpectomy: A challenge for research. Cancer Nurs 1988 Aug; 11(4): 244–249.

Schover L. The impact of breast cancer on sexuality, body image and intimate relationships. CA 1991 Apr; 41(2):112–120.

Schwartz M. Living with loss: Dreaming of lace. Lears 1990 Oct; 3(8):54–56.

Speroff L. Breast cancer and postmenopausal hormone therapy. Contemp Obstet Gynecol 1990 Jan; 35(1):71–82.

Stein P et al. Breast cancer: Risks, treatment and perioperative patient care. AORN J 1991 Apr; 53(4):938–944.

Stillman M. Evaluation and treatment of pain in breast cancer. Fem Patient 1990 Mar; 15(3):57–72.

Tandon A et al. Cathepsin D and prognosis in breast cancer. N Engl J Med 1990 Feb; 322(5):297–308.

Ward S, Heidrich S, and Wolberg W. Factors women take into account when deciding upon type of surgery for breast cancer. Cancer Nurs 1989 June; 12(6):344–351.

Surgical Treatment of Breast Cancer

Dietrich-Gallagher M and Hyzinski M. Patient education: Teaching patients to care for drains after breast surgery for malignancy. Oncol Nurs Forum 1989 Mar/Apr; 16(2):263–267.

Feather B and Wainstock J. Perceptions of post-mastectomy patients: Social supports and attitudes towards mastectomy. Cancer Nurs 1989 Oct; 12(5):301–309.

Fox K. Ellen's going home: Can she manage without you? Preparing your postmastectomy patient for discharge. Nursing 1989 May; 19(5):80–81.

Kinne D. The surgical management of primary breast cancer. Ca 1991 Mar/Apr; 41(2):71–84.

Love S. Breast removal and reconstruction. Harvard Med School Health Lett 1990 Feb; 15(4):3–6.

Breast Reconstruction

Angelo T and Gorrell C. Breast reconstruction using tissue expanders. Oncol Nurs Forum 1989 Jan/Feb; 16(1):23–27.

Bostwick J. Breast reconstruction following mastectomy. CA 1989; 39(1): 40–49.

Kramer A. Immediate breast reconstruction. Plast Surg Nurs 1988 Winter; 8(4):150–154.

Chemotherapy

Adjuvant chemotherapy of early breast cancer. Med Lett 1990 May 18; 32(818):49–50.

* Brandt B. The relationship between hopelessness and selected variables in women receiving chemotherapy for breast cancer. Oncol Nurs Forum 1987 Mar/Apr; 14(2):35–39.

Cawley M. Recent advances in chemotherapy. Nurs Clin North Am 1990 Jun; 25(2):377–385.

Doig B. Adjuvant chemotherapy in breast cancer: A review of the literature. Cancer Nurs 1988 Feb; 11(2):91–98.

Ehlke G. Symptom distress in breast cancer patients receiving chemotherapy in the outpatient setting. Oncol Nurs Forum 1988 May/Jun; 15(3): 643–646.

Greenspan E. Toward the chemoprevention of breast cancer. Fem Patient 1989 Apr; 14(4):103–110.

Grindel C, Cahill C, and Walker M. Food intake of women with breast cancer during their first six months of chemotherapy. Oncol Nurs Forum 1989 May/Jun; 16(3):401–407.

Hillner B and Smith T. Efficacy and cost-effectiveness of adjuvant chemotherapy in women with node-negative breast cancer. N Engl J Med 1991 Jan; 324(3):160–169.

Love R et al. Side effects and emotional distress during cancer chemotherapy. Cancer 1989 Feb; 63(2):604–612.

* Payne S. Coping with palliative chemotherapy. J Adv Nurs 1990 Jun; 15(6):652–658.

Winningham M and McVicar M. The effect of aerobic exercise on patients' reports of nausea. Oncol Nurs Forum 1988 Jul/Aug; 15(4):447–450.

Winningham M et al. Effect of aerobic exercise on body weight and composition in patients with breast cancer on adjuvant chemotherapy. Oncol Nurs Forum 1989 Sep/Oct; 16(5):683–689.

Hormonal Therapy

Dunne C. Hormonal therapy for breast cancer. Cancer Nurs 1988 May; (11)5:288–294.

Goodman M. Concepts of hormonal manipulation in the treatment of cancer. Oncol Nurs Forum 1988 Sep/Oct; 15(5):639–647.

Radiation Therapy

* Christman N. Uncertainty and adjustment during radiotherapy. Nurs Res 1990 Jan/Feb; 39(1):17–47.

Hassey K. Radiation therapy for breast cancer: A historic review. Semin Oncol Nurs 1985 Aug; 1(3):181–188.

Mast D and Wood D. Preparing patients with breast cancer for brachytherapy. Oncol Nurs Forum 1990 Feb; 17(2):267–270.

Pierce S and Harris J. The role of radiation therapy in the management of primary breast cancer. Ca 1991 Mar/Apr; 41(2):85–96.

Strohl R. Radiation therapy: Recent advances and nursing implications. Nurs Clin North Am 1990 Jun; 25(2):309–328.

Pregnancy and Breast Cancer

Dow K. Breast cancer and fertility. NAACOG's Clinical Issues in Perinatal and Women's Health Nursing 1990; 1(4):444–452.

Greene F. Gestational breast cancer: A ten-year experience. South Med J 1988 Dec; 81:1509–1511.

Hassey K. Pregnancy and parenthood after treatment for breast cancer. Oncol Nurs Forum 1988; 15(4):439–444.

Larkin K. Cancer and pregnancy. NAACOG's Clinical Issues in Perinatal and Women's Health, Vol 1, No. 2. Philadelphia, JB Lippincott, 1990.

Geriatric Considerations

Castiglione M, Gelber R, and Goldhirsch A. Adjuvant systemic therapy for breast cancer in the elderly. J Clin Oncol 1990 Mar; 8(3):519–526.

Ludwick R. Breast examination in the older adult. Cancer Nurs 1988 Feb; 11(2):99–102.

Welch-McCaffrey D and Dodge J. Planning breast self-examination programs for elderly women. Oncol Nurs Forum 1988 Nov/Dec; 15(6): 811–814.

Williams R. Factors affecting the practice of breast self-examination in older women. Oncol Nurs Forum 1988 Sep/Oct; 15(5):611–616.

Information/Resources

Agencies

American Cancer Society
90 Park Avenue
New York, NY 10016
(Extensive professional and patient literature is available, including booklets on reconstruction, radiation, and chemotherapy.)

National Cancer Institute
Public Inquiry Section, Office of Cancer Communications, National Cancer Institute, Building 31, Room 10 A 24, Bethesda, MD 20892
(Patient materials can be ordered on the following topics: biopsies, treatment options, mastectomy, radiation, chemotherapy, reconstruction, diet, and clinical trials.)

National Alliance of Breast Cancer Organizations
1180 Avenue of the Americas, 2nd Floor, New York, NY 10036, (212) 719-0154

Y-ME Breast Cancer Support Program
1757 Ridge Road, Homewood, IL 60430

Reach to Recovery Program—I Can Cope Program
(Information available through local American Cancer Society chapters)

47

Management of Patients With Disorders of the Male Reproductive System

Learning Objectives

On completion of this chapter, the learner will be able to:

1. Describe anatomy and function of the male reproductive system
2. Compare the four types of prostatectomy with regard to advantages and disadvantages
3. Use the nursing process as a framework for care of the patient undergoing prostatectomy
4. Describe the nursing management of patients with cancer of the male reproductive organs
5. Describe the various conditions affecting the testes and penis, their pathophysiology, clinical manifestations, and management
6. Specify the causes and management of erectile dysfunction

In the male, several organs serve as parts of both the urinary tract and the reproductive system. Disease of these organs may produce functional abnormalities of either or both systems. For this reason, diseases of the entire reproductive system in the male usually are treated by the urologist.

Overview

The structures included in the male reproductive system are the testes, the vas deferens (also called ductus deferens) and the seminal vesicles, the penis, and certain accessory glands, such as the prostate gland and Cowper's gland (bulbourethral gland) (Fig. 47-1). The testes are formed in embryonal life within the abdominal cavity near the kidney. During the last month of fetal life, they descend posterior to the peritoneum, to pierce the abdominal wall in the groin. Later they progress along the inguinal canal into the scrotum. In this descent they are accompanied by blood vessels, lymphatics, nerves, and ducts, which, along with supporting tissue, make up the spermatic cord. This cord extends from the internal inguinal ring through the abdominal wall and the inguinal canal to the scrotum. As the testes descend into the scrotum, a tubular extension

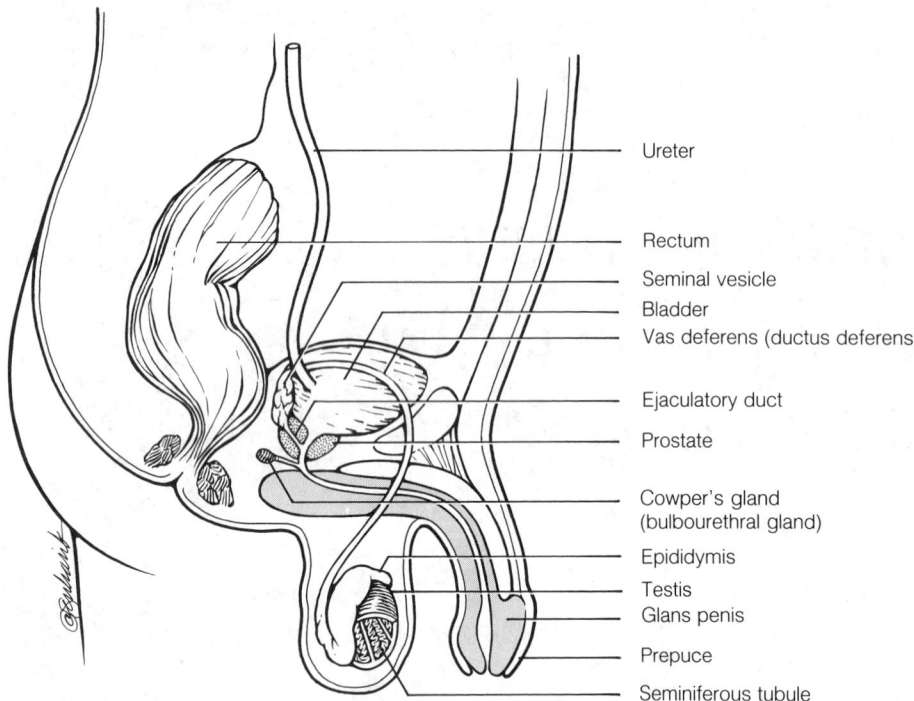

- Ureter
- Rectum
- Seminal vesicle
- Bladder
- Vas deferens (ductus deferens)
- Ejaculatory duct
- Prostate
- Cowper's gland (bulbourethral gland)
- Epididymis
- Testis
- Glans penis
- Prepuce
- Seminiferous tubule

Figure 47–1. Organs of the male reproductive system.

of peritoneum accompanies them. This normally is obliterated, the only remaining portion being that which covers the testes, the *tunica vaginalis.* (When this peritoneal process is not obliterated but remains open into the abdominal cavity, a potential sac remains, into which abdominal contents may enter to form an indirect inguinal hernia.)

The testes are contained in the scrotum, which keeps them at a slightly lower temperature than the rest of the body to allow spermatogenesis. The testes consist of numerous seminiferous tubules in which are formed the male reproductive elements, the spermatozoa. These are transmitted by a system of collecting tubules into the epididymis, which is a hoodlike structure lying on the testes and containing tortuous ducts that lead into the vas deferens. This firm tubular structure passes upward through the inguinal canal to enter the abdominal cavity behind the peritoneum and then extends downward toward the base of the bladder. An outpouching from this structure is the seminal vesicle, which acts as a reservoir for the secretion of the testes. The tract is continued as the ejaculatory duct, which then passes through the prostate gland to enter the urethra. The secretion of the testes is carried by this pathway to the end of the penis in the reproductive act.

The testes have a dual function. The primary function is reproduction—the formation of spermatozoa from the germinal cells of the seminiferous tubules. The testes are also important glands of internal secretion, however. This secretion is produced by the interstitial cells and is called the male sex hormone, or testosterone, which induces and preserves the male sex qualities.

The prostate gland lies just below the neck of the bladder. It surrounds the urethra posteriorly and laterally and is traversed by the ejaculatory duct, the continuation of the vas deferens. This gland produces a secretion that is chemically and physiologically suitable to the needs of the spermatozoa in their passage from the genital glands.

The Cowper's gland lies below the prostate within the posterior aspect of the urethra. This gland empties its secretions into the urethra at the time of ejaculation, providing lubrication.

The penis has a dual function of being the organ of copulation and of urination. Anatomically, it consists of a glans penis, a body, and a root. The glans penis is the soft, rounded portion at the end that retains its soft structure even when erect. The urethra opens at the tip of the glans. The glans normally is covered or protected by an elongation of the skin of the penis—the foreskin—which may be retracted to expose the glans. The body of the penis is composed of erectile tissues that contain numerous blood vessels that may become distended, leading to an erection during sexual excitement. Through it passes the urethra, which extends from the bladder through the prostate to the distal end of the penis.

Congenital Malformations

Of the many disturbances of normal growth that may occur, the most common is a failure of the testes to descend into the scrotum. This condition is called *cryptorchidism.*

Failure of the urethra to form normally in the penis can result in hypospadias or epispadias. *Hypospadias* occurs when the urethral opening is a groove on the underside of the penis; when the urethral opening is on the dorsum of the penis the condition is called *epispadias.* These anatomic abnormalities may be repaired by various types of plastic surgery.

Gerontologic Considerations

As men age, the prostate gland enlarges, prostate secretion decreases, the scrotum hangs lower, the testes become smaller and more firm, and pubic hair becomes sparser and stiffer.

Changes in gonad function include a decline in the concentration of plasma testosterone and a reduction in the amount of progesterone produced.

Male reproductive capability is maintained with advancing age. Although degenerative changes occur in the seminiferous tubules, spermatogenesis (production of sperm) remains. Sexual function, however, involving libido (desire) and potency, lessens. This decline is more evident in men older than 70 years but is also noted in men in their 60s. Sexual function is affected by a number of factors such as psychological problems, illnesses, and medications. In general, the sexual act takes longer. Sexual activity is closely correlated with the man's sexual activity of his earlier years; if he was more active than average as a young man, he will most likely continue to be more active than average in his later years.

Impotence, the difficulty in achieving or maintaining an erection, is usually due to either organic or psychogenic factors. Organic causes include vascular insufficiency, diabetes mellitus, and neuropathy, which cause erectile dysfunction. Drugs also may affect sexual performance. Refer to chapter 17 for a description of sexuality and sexual function.

Conditions of the Prostate

Prostatitis

Prostatitis is an inflammation of the prostate gland caused by infectious agents (bacteria, fungi, mycoplasma) or by a variety of other problems (*e.g.*, urethral stricture, prostatic hyperplasia). Microorganisms usually are carried to the prostate from the urethra. Prostatitis may be classified as bacterial or abacterial, depending on the presence or absence of microorganisms in the prostatic fluid.

The symptoms of prostatitis are many and include perineal discomfort, burning, urgency, frequency, and pain with or after ejaculation. *Prostatodynia* (pain in the prostate) is manifested by pain on voiding or perineal pain symptoms, but there is no evidence of inflammation or bacterial growth in the prostatic fluid.

Acute bacterial prostatitis may produce a sudden onset of fever and chills and perineal, rectal, or low back pain. Urinary symptoms of burning, frequency, urgency, nocturia, and dysuria may be evident. Some patients, however, are asymptomatic.

Diagnosis requires a careful history, culture of prostatic fluid or tissue, and, occasionally, a histologic examination of tissue. To locate the source of the lower genitourinary infection (bladder neck, urethra, prostate), it is necessary to collect a divided urinary specimen for segmental urine culture. After the patient cleanses the glans penis and retracts the foreskin (if present), he voids 10 to 15 ml of urine into the first container. This represents urethral urine. Without interruption of the urinary stream, a second voiding of 50 to 75 ml of urine is then collected in a second container; this represents bladder urine. If the patient does not have acute prostatitis, the physician immediately performs a prostatic massage and any prostatic fluid that is expressed is collected by gravity drainage into a third container. If it is not possible to collect prostatic fluid, the patient voids a small quantity of urine. The specimen may contain the bacteria present in the prostatic fluid. Urinalysis

after prostate examination frequently reveals many white blood cells.

Management. The goal of management is to avoid the complications of abscess formation and septicemia. A broad-spectrum antimicrobial (to which the causative organism is sensitive) is given for a period of 10 to 14 days. Intravenous administration of the drug may be necessary to achieve high serum and tissue levels. The patient it encouraged to remain on bed rest because this alleviates symptoms rapidly. Comfort is promoted with analgesics (relieve pain), antispasmodics, and bladder sedatives (relieve bladder irritability), sitz baths (relieve pain and spasm), and stool softeners (prevent straining at stool, which increases pain).

Swelling of the gland may produce urinary retention. Other complications include epididymitis, bacteremia or septicemia, and pyelonephritis.

Chronic bacterial prostatitis is a major source of relapsing urinary tract infection in men. Symptoms are usually mild, consisting of frequency, urgency, dysuria, and occasional urethral discharge. High fevers and chills are uncommon. The treatment of chronic prostatitis is difficult, because of poor diffusion of most antimicrobials from the plasma into the prostatic fluid. Antimicrobials (trimethoprim-sulfamethoxazole, tetracycline, minocycline, doxycycline) may be given. Continuous suppressive treatment with low-dose antimicrobial drugs may be indicated. The patient is advised of the possibility of relapsing infection. Comfort is promoted with antispasmodics (to relieve bladder irritability), sitz baths, and stool softeners.

The treatment of *nonbacterial prostatitis* is directed toward symptomatic relief: sitz baths, analgesics, etc. The sexual partner should be investigated because of the possibility of cross-infection.

Patient Education. The patient is instructed to take the prescribed antibiotic for the full time. Hot sitz baths (10 to 20 minutes) may be taken several times daily. Fluids are encouraged to satisfy thirst, but fluids are not "forced" because an effective drug level must be maintained in the urine. Foods and drink that have diuretic action or increase prostatic secretions should be avoided: alcohol, coffee, tea, chocolate, cola, and spices. During periods of acute inflammation, sexual arousal and intercourse should be avoided. Ejaculation by sexual intercourse or masturbation may be beneficial in the treatment of chronic prostatitis, however, by reducing the retention of prostatic fluids. The patient should avoid sitting for long periods to minimize discomfort. Medical follow-up is necessary for at least 6 months to 1 year, since recurrence of prostatitis due to the same or different organisms can occur.

Benign Prostatic Hyperplasia

In many patients more than 50 years of age, the prostate gland enlarges, extending upward into the bladder and obstructing the outflow of urine by encroaching on the vesical orifice. This condition is known as benign prostatic hyperplasia (enlargement, or hypertrophy, of the prostate). On examination, the prostate is large, rubbery, and nontender. The cause is uncertain, but evidence suggests a hormonal cause as initiating hyperplasia of the supporting stromal tissue and of glandular elements in the prostate.

Because enlargement of the prostate gland produces an obstruction to flow of urine, a gradual dilatation of the ureters (hydroureter) and kidneys (hydronephrosis) results. The hypertrophied lobes may obstruct the vesical neck or prostatic urethra and thus cause incomplete emptying and urinary retention. Urinary tract infection may result from urinary stasis.

Clinical Manifestations and Diagnostic Evaluation. The obstructive and irritative symptom complex (referred to as *prostatism*) includes increased frequency of urination, nocturia, urgency, hesitancy in starting urination, abdominal straining, a decrease in size and force of urinary stream, interruption of urinary stream, terminal dribbling (in which urine dribbles out after urination), a sensation of incomplete emptying of the bladder, acute urinary retention (postvoiding residual volume of more than 60 ml of urine), and recurrent urinary tract infections. Ultimately, azotemia and renal failure can occur with chronic urinary retention and large residual volumes. Generalized symptoms also may be noted, including fatigue secondary to nocturia, anorexia, nausea, and vomiting due to impaired renal function, and epigastric discomfort may result from a distended bladder.

Other diseases that display similar symptoms include urethral stricture, prostate cancer, neurogenic bladder, and bladder stones.

A physical examination that includes a digital rectal examination and a battery of diagnostic tests may be performed to determine the degree of prostatic enlargement, the presence of any bladder wall changes, and the efficiency of renal function. These tests may include urinalysis and urodynamic studies to determine obstructive flow patterns. Renal function studies including serum creatinine may be obtained to determine if there is renal impairment from prostatic back-pressure and to evaluate renal reserve. A complete hematologic investigation is done. Because hemorrhage is a major postoperative complication, all clotting defects must be corrected. A high percentage of these patients have cardiac or respiratory complications, or both; therefore, cardiac and respiratory function must be assessed.

Management. The plan of treatment depends on the cause, the severity of the obstruction, and the condition of the patient. If a patient is admitted as an emergency because he is unable to void, he is immediately catheterized. The ordinary catheter frequently is too soft and pliable to pass through the urethra into the bladder. A thin wire called a stylet is introduced (by a urologist) into the catheter to prevent the catheter from collapsing when it encounters resistance. In severe cases, metal catheters with a pronounced prostatic curve may be used. Sometimes an incision is made into the bladder (a suprapubic cystostomy) to provide adequate drainage.

Because the hormonal component of benign prostatic hyperplasia has been identified, one method of treatment involves hormonal manipulation with antiandrogen and progestational agents. These medications can help decrease the size of the prostate and improve urinary flow. Side effects of these medications include gynecomastia, erectile dysfunction, and flushing. Surgery to remove the hyperplastic prostatic tissue is frequently necessary to provide permanent relief of the obstruction. The procedure is referred to as a prostatectomy.

The Patient Undergoing Prostatectomy

The preoperative objectives before prostatectomy (removal of the prostate) are to assess the patient's general health status and to establish optimum renal function. The operation should be performed before the development of acute urinary retention and infection and before the upper urinary tract and collecting system are damaged.

Four different approaches are possible in removing the hypertrophied fibroadenomatous portion of the prostate gland (Table 47-1). In all four techniques, all hyperplastic tissue is removed, leaving behind the surgical capsule of the prostate. The transurethral approach is a closed procedure, and the other three are open surgical procedures.

A *transurethral resection* of the prostate (TUR or TURP) is the most common procedure and can be carried out by means of an endoscopic instrument that has ocular and surgical capability. The instrument is introduced directly through the urethra to the prostate, which can be viewed directly. The gland is then removed in small chips with an electrical cutting loop (Fig. 47-2A). The advantage of this method is the absence of an incision. It may be used for glands of varying size (urologists differ on how large the prostate must be before considering an open procedure), and it is ideal for most poor-risk patients with small glands. This approach means a shorter hospital stay; however, strictures are more frequent, and repeat operations may be necessary.

Suprapubic prostatectomy is one method of removing the gland through an abdominal wound. An opening is made into the bladder, and the gland is removed from above (see Fig. 47-2B). Such an approach can be used for a gland of any size, and few complications occur, although blood loss may be greater than with other methods. Another disadvantage is the need for an abdominal incision, with the concomitant hazards of any major abdominal surgical procedure.

Perineal prostatectomy involves the removal of the gland through an incision in the perineum (see Fig. 47-2C). This approach is practical when other approaches are not possible. It is a useful procedure when open biopsy is needed. In the postoperative period, the wound may become contaminated rather easily because of the location of the incision near the rectum. Incontinence, impotence, or rectal injury are more likely sequelae when this approach is used.

Retropubic prostatectomy is another technique and is more common than the suprapubic approach. A low abdominal incision is made, and the prostate gland is approached between the pubic arch and the bladder (without entering the bladder) (see Fig. 47-2D). This procedure is suitable for large glands located high in the pelvis. Blood loss is controlled more easily, and there is better visualization. Infections can readily start in the retropubic space, however.

▶ Nursing Process
The Patient Undergoing Prostatectomy

◊ Assessment

The nurse assesses how benign hyperplasia of the prostate has affected the patient's life style during the past few months. Has he been reasonably active for his age? What is the presenting urinary problem (as described in the patient's words): decreased force of urinary flow, decreased ability to initiate voiding, urgency, frequency, nocturia, dysuria, urinary retention, hematuria? Are there aches or pains associated with the above problems, such as back pain, flank pain, and lower abdominal or suprapubic discomfort? If such discomfort is present, pos-

TABLE 47–1. *Comparison of Surgical Approaches for Prostatectomy*

The surgical approach of choice depends on (1) the size of the gland, (2) the severity of the obstruction, (3) the age of the patient, (4) the condition of patient, and (5) the presence of associated diseases.

Surgical Approach	Advantages	Disadvantages	Nursing Implications
TRANSURETHRAL RESECTION (removal of prostatic tissue by instrument introduced through urethra)	Avoids abdominal incision Safer for surgical-risk patient Shorter period of hospitalization and convalescence Lower morbidity rate Causes less pain	Requires highly skilled operator Recurrent obstruction, urethral trauma, and stricture may develop. Delayed bleeding may occur.	Watch for evidence of hemorrhage (drainage in bag). Observe for symptoms of urethral stricture (dysuria, straining, small urinary stream).
OPEN SURGICAL REMOVAL Suprapubic	Technically simple Offers wide area of exploration Permits exploration for cancerous lymph nodes Allows more complete removal of obstructing gland Permits treatment of associated lesions in bladder	Requires surgical approach through the bladder Control of hemorrhage difficult Urinary leakage around suprapubic tube may occur Convalescence may be prolonged and uncomfortable	Watch for indications of hemorrhage and shock. Give meticulous aseptic attention to area around suprapubic tube.
Perineal	Offers direct anatomic approach Permits gravity drainage Particularly efficacious for radical cancer therapy Allows hemostasis under direct vision Low mortality rate Less incidence of shock Ideal for very old, feeble, and poor surgical risk patient with large prostate	Higher postoperative incidence of impotency and urinary incontinency Problem of damage to rectum and external sphincter Restricted operative field Greater potential for infection	Avoid use of rectal tubes, rectal thermometers, and enemas after perineal surgery. Use drainage pads to absorb excess urinary drainage. Provide foam rubber ring for patient comfort in sitting. Urinary leakage may occur around wound for several days after catheter removal.
Retropubic	Avoids incision into the bladder Permits easier visualization and control of bleeders Shorter period of convalescence Less bladder sphincter damage	Cannot treat associated bladder disease Increased incidence of hemorrhage from prostatic venous plexus; pubic osteitis	Watch for evidences of hemorrhage. Posturinary leakage may occur for several days after catheter is removed.

sible causes might be infection, retention, and possibly renal colic.

The nurse determines the patient's family history of cancer and heart or kidney disease, including hypertension. Has he lost weight? Does he appear pale? Can he raise himself out of bed and return to bed without assistance? This information may help in determining how soon he will be returned to normal activities after prostatectomy.

Nursing Diagnoses

Based on the nursing history and all other assessment data, the patient's major nursing diagnoses may include the following:

Preoperative
- Anxiety related to the inability to void
- Pain related to bladder distention
- Knowledge deficit about factors related to the problem and the treatment protocol

Postoperative
- Pain related to the surgical incision, catheter placement, and bladder spasms
- High risk for infection, related to bacterial invasion of the incision
- Knowledge deficit about postoperative and convalescent management
- Sexual dysfunction

Potential postoperative complications include:
- Hemorrhage and shock
- Infection
- Thrombosis
- Catheter obstruction

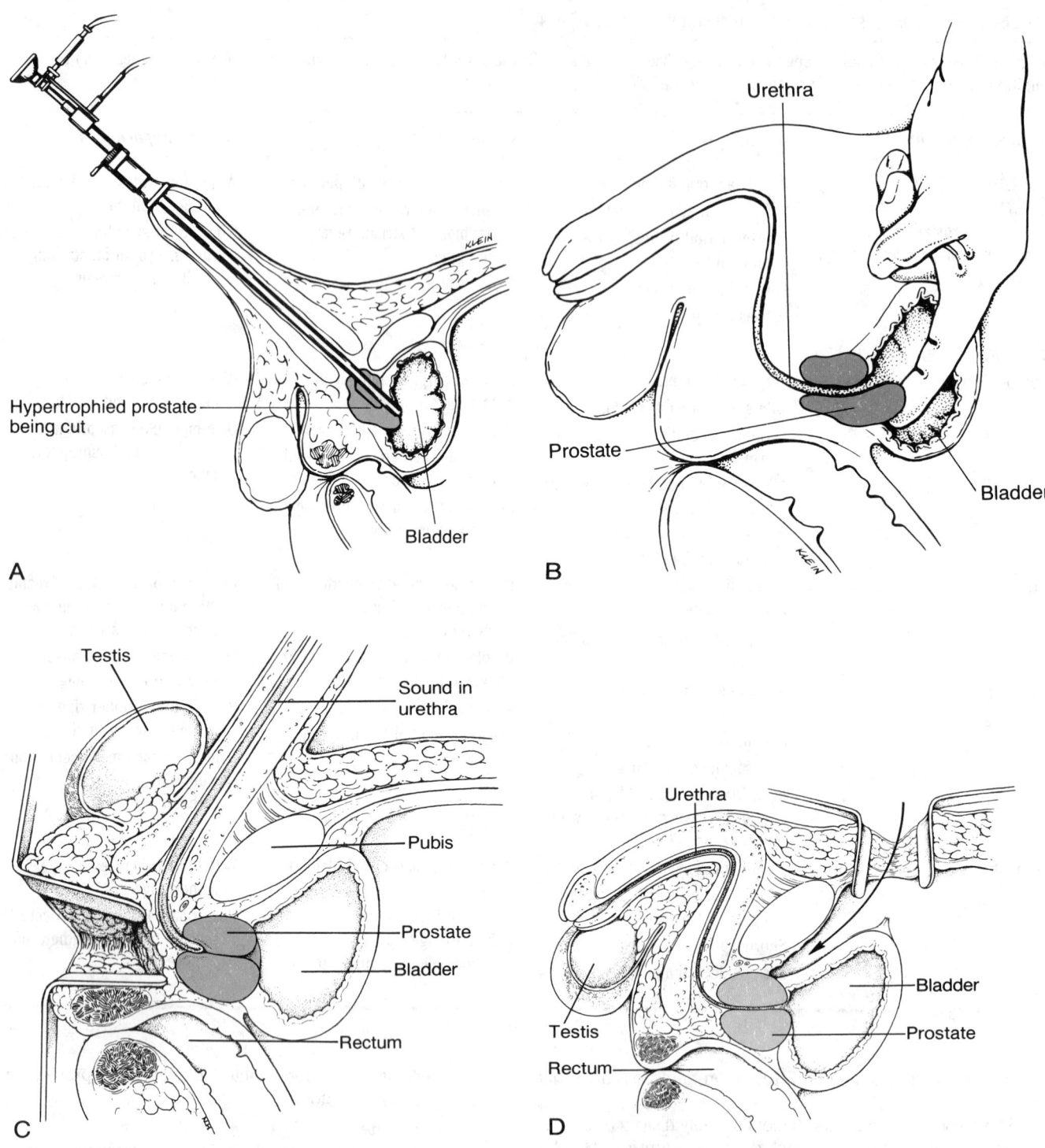

Figure 47–2. Prostatectomy procedures. (**A**) Transurethral resection (TUR). A loop of wire connected with a cutting current is rotated in the cystoscope to remove shavings of prostate at the bladder orifice. (**B**) Suprapubic prostatectomy. Using an abdominal approach, the prostate is shelled out of its bed by the surgeon. (**C**) Perineal prostatectomy. Two retractors on the left spread the perineal incision to provide a view of the prostate. (**D**) Retropubic prostatectomy is done through a low abdominal incision. Note two abdominal retractors and arrow approaching the prostate gland.

▷ Planning and Implementation

▷ **Goals:** The patient's major *preoperative* goals may include reduction of anxiety and learning about his prostate problem and the perioperative experience. His major *postoperative* goals may include correction of fluid volume disturbances, relief of pain and discomfort, prevention of infection, and ability to perform self-care activities.

▷ Nursing Interventions

▷ Preoperative

▷ *Reduction of Anxiety.* The nurse familiarizes the patient with his hospital environment and initiates measures to reduce his anxiety. Communication is established regarding his understanding of his problem and what the physician has already told him. He may be sensitive and embarrassed to discuss problems related to the genitalia and issues of sexuality. Privacy is provided, and a trusting and professional relationship is developed with the patient because he often has related sexual concerns that may need to be discussed. Guilt feelings often surface as he falsely assumes a cause-and-effect relationship between early sexual practices and his current problems. His verbalization of feelings and concerns is encouraged.

▷ *Comfort Measures.* If the patient presents with signs and symptoms of discomfort, he is placed on bed rest, analgesic agents are administered, and measures to relieve his anxiety are initiated. The nurse monitors the patient's voiding patterns, observes for bladder distention, and assists with catheterization. An indwelling catheter is inserted if the patient has continuing urinary retention or if there is evidence of azotemia (accumulation of nitrogenous waste products in the blood). It may be desirable to decompress the bladder gradually over a period of several days, especially if the patient is elderly and hypertensive and has diminished renal function or an excessive amount of urinary retention that has existed for many weeks. The blood pressure may fluctuate, and renal function declines the first few days after bladder drainage is instituted. If the patient cannot tolerate a urethral catheter, he is prepared for a cystostomy (see Chaps. 42 and 43).

▷ *Patient Education.* A convenient time is established for the patient (ensuring his privacy) to review the anatomy of the affected parts and how they function in relation to the urinary and reproductive systems. Diagrams may be effective in the teaching process. The nurse reinforces what will take place as the patient is prepared for diagnostic tests and then for surgery. (The protocol is differentiated as it relates to the specific type of prostatectomy planned for the particular patient.) The nurse describes the nature of the incision because this varies—it could be directly over the bladder, low on the abdomen, in the perineal area, or performed through a resectoscope, in which case there is no external incision. The patient is informed about the type of drainage system that is expected, the type of anesthesia, and the recovery room procedure. The amount of information is individualized based on the patient's needs and questions. Procedures expected during the immediate perioperative period are explained, questions are answered, and support is provided.

▷ *Preoperative Preparation.* When the patient is scheduled for a prostatectomy, the preparation described in Chapter 20 is followed. Antiembolism stockings are applied before the operation and are particularly important if the patient is placed in a lithotomy position during surgery. A preoperative enema may prevent postoperative straining, which can induce postoperative bleeding.

▷ Postoperative

▷ *Pain Relief.* After a prostatectomy, the patient is kept on bed rest for the first 24 hours. If pain occurs, the cause and location must be determined. It may be related to the incision; it may be due to excoriation of the skin at the catheter site; it may be in the flank area, indicating a kidney problem; or it may be due to bladder spasms. Bladder irritability can initiate bleeding and result in clot retention.

When patients are experiencing bladder spasms, they may note urgency to void, pressure or fullness in the bladder, and bleeding from the urethra around the urethral catheter. Smooth muscle relaxant medications can help to ease the spasms, which can be intermittent and severe. Warm compresses applied to the pubis or sitz baths can provide symptomatic relief of the spasms.

Before administering the prescribed medication for pain relief, the patient's vital signs, including blood pressure, are checked; then the drainage tubing is checked and the system is irrigated as prescribed, thus correcting any obstruction that may cause discomfort. Usually, the catheter is irrigated with 50 ml of irrigating fluid at a time, making sure that the same amount is recovered in the drainage receptacle. Securing the catheter to the leg or abdomen can help to decrease tension on the catheter and prevent bladder irritation.

Discomfort may be caused by dressings that are too snug or have become saturated with drainage or are not properly placed.

▷ *Prevention of Infection.* After perineal prostatectomy, the urologist changes the dressing on the first postoperative day; after that dressing changes may become the nurse's responsibility. Careful aseptic technique is used, as the possibility of infection is great. Dressings can be held in place by a double-tailed T-binder bandage or a padded athletic supporter. The tails cross over the incision to give double thickness, and then each tail is drawn up on either side of the scrotum to the waistline and fastened.

Rectal temperatures, rectal tubes, and enemas are avoided because of the risk of causing trauma and bleeding in the prostatic fossa. After the perineal sutures are removed, the perineum is cleansed as indicated. A heat lamp may be directed to the perineal area to promote healing. The scrotum is protected with a towel while the heat lamp is in use. Sitz baths are also used to encourage healing.

▷ *Patient Education and Home Health Care.* When the patient is ambulatory, he is encouraged to walk but not to sit for prolonged periods, as this increases intra-abdominal pressure and increases the possibility of discomfort and bleeding. The bowel movements are kept soft through use of prune juice and stool softeners to prevent excessive straining. If an enema is prescribed, it is administered with caution to avoid possible rectal perforation.

As the patient progresses and drainage tubes are removed, the patient often shows signs of discouragement and depression because he is not able to regain bladder control immediately.

Urinary frequency and burning may occur after the catheter is removed. The following exercises are helpful for regaining urinary control:

- Tense the perineal muscles by pressing the buttocks together; hold this position; relax. This exercise, done 10 to 20 times each hour, can be performed while sitting or standing.
- Try to interrupt the urinary stream after starting to void; wait a few seconds and then continue to void.

Perineal exercises are continued until full urinary control is gained. The patient is instructed to urinate as soon as the *first* desire to do so is felt. It is important for the patient to know that regaining urinary control is a gradual process, and that even though he may continue to "dribble" after being discharged from the hospital, the dribbling should gradually diminish (up to 1 year). The urine may be cloudy for several weeks but should clear as the prostate area heals.

While the prostatic fossa is healing (6 to 8 weeks), the patient should not engage in any Valsalva efforts (straining at stool, heavy lifting), as this increases venous pressure and may produce hematuria. He should avoid long automobile rides and strenuous exercise, which increase the tendency to bleed. He will also benefit from knowing that spicy foods, alcohol, and coffee may cause discomfort. The patient is cautioned to drink enough fluids to avoid dehydration, which increases the tendency for a clot to form and obstruct the flow of urine. Bleeding, passage of blood clots, decrease in the size of urinary stream, urinary retention, or symptoms of urinary tract infections are to be reported to the physician.

◊ *Sexual Dysfunction.* Most surgical approaches for prostatectomy do not result in impotence. (Perineal prostatectomy may cause impotence because of unavoidable damage of the pudendal nerves.) In most instances, sexual activity may be resumed in 6 to 8 weeks, the time required for the prostatic fossa to heal. After ejaculation, the seminal fluid goes into the bladder and is excreted with the urine. (The anatomic changes in the posterior urethra lead to retrograde ejaculation.)

After total prostatectomy (usually for cancer), impotence is almost always expected. For the patient who does not desire to give up sexual activity, a prosthetic penile implant may be used to make the penis rigid for sexual intercourse.

◊ *Assessing for Potential Complications.* After prostatectomy, it is important to observe the patient for major complications such as hemorrhage, infection, thrombosis, and catheter obstruction.

Hemorrhage. Because a hyperplastic prostate gland is very vascular, the immediate dangers after a prostatectomy are

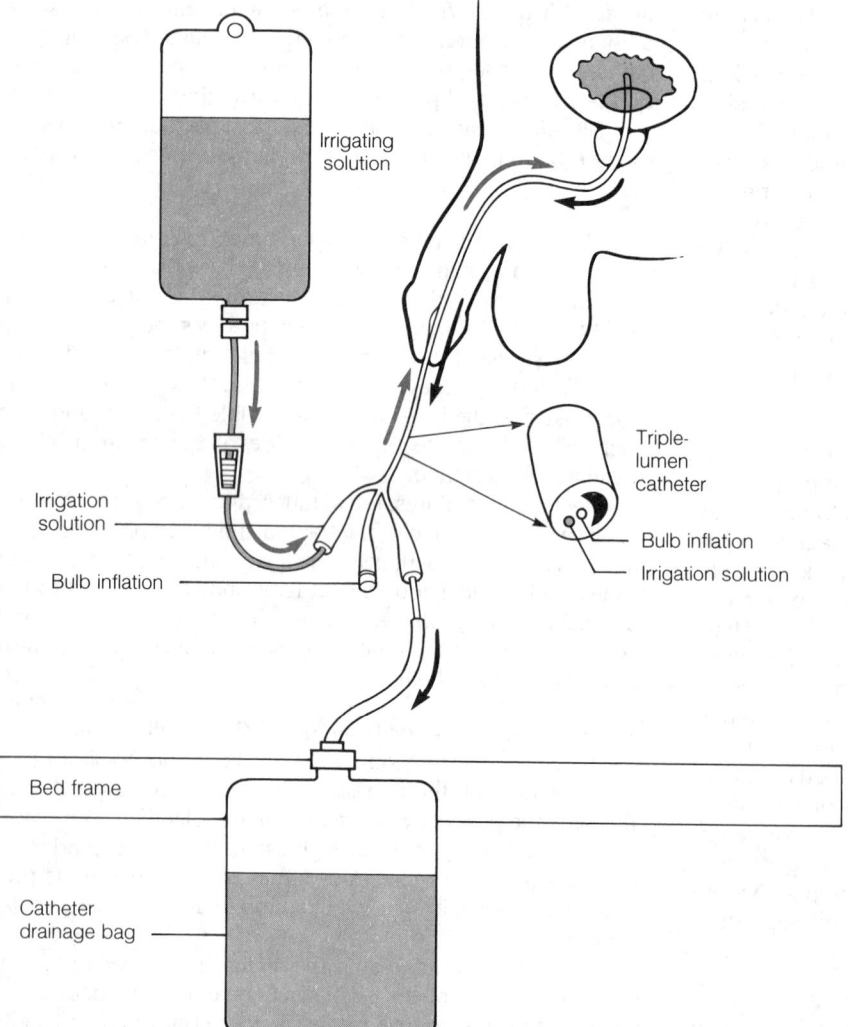

Figure 47–3. A three-way system for bladder irrigation.

bleeding and shock. Bleeding may occur from the bed of the prostate. Bleeding may also result in the formation of clots, which then obstruct the flow of urine. The drainage begins as reddish pink and then clears to a light pink within 24 hours after operation.

- Bright red bleeding with increased viscosity and numerous clots usually indicates arterial bleeding. Venous bleeding appears darker and less viscous.
- Arterial hemorrhage usually requires surgical intervention (*e.g.*, suturing of bleeders or transurethral coagulation of bleeders), whereas venous bleeding may be controlled by applying prescribed traction to the catheter so that the balloon applies pressure to the prostatic fossa.

Infection and Thrombosis. In addition to hemorrhage, urinary tract infections and epididymitis are possible complications after prostatectomy. A vasectomy may be performed during surgery to prevent retrograde spread of infection from the prostatic urethra through the vas and into the epididymis. If epididymitis occurs, it is managed as discussed on p. 1338.

Patients undergoing prostatectomy (with the exception of transurethral resection) have a high incidence of deep-vein thrombosis and pulmonary embolism. Low-dose heparin therapy may be administered prophylactically.

Catheter Obstruction. After a transurethral prostatic resection, *the catheter must drain well*; an obstructed catheter produces distention of the prostatic capsule with resultant hemorrhage. Furosemide may be prescribed to initiate postoperative diuresis, thereby helping to keep the catheter patent.

- The lower abdomen is observed to ensure that no blockage of the catheter occurs. An overdistended bladder presents a distinct rounded swelling above the pubis.
- The drainage bag, dressings, and incision site are checked for evidence of bleeding. The color of the urine is noted and recorded; a change in color from pink to amber indicates lessened bleeding.
- The blood pressure, pulse, and respirations are monitored and compared with the preoperative vital signs to assess for hypotension. The patient is observed for restlessness; cold, sweating skin; pallor; fall in blood pressure; and an increasing pulse rate.

Drainage of the bladder may be accomplished by gravity through a closed sterile system of drainage. A three-way system is useful in cleansing the bladder and preventing clot formation (Fig. 47-3). Some urologists leave an indwelling catheter attached to dependent drainage. Gentle irrigation of the catheter may be prescribed to remove any obstructing clots.

- If the patient complains of pain, the tubing is checked. The drainage system is irrigated if indicated and prescribed to clear any obstruction before administering an analgesic. Usually, the catheter is irrigated with 50 ml of irrigating fluid at a time, making sure that the same amount is recovered in the drainage bag.
- Overdistention of the bladder is avoided, as it can produce secondary hemorrhage by stretching the coagulated vessels in the prostatic capsule.
- An intake and output record is maintained, including the amount of fluid used for irrigation.

The drainage tube (not the catheter) is taped to the shaved inner thigh to prevent traction on the bladder. If a cystostomy catheter is in place, it is taped to the abdomen. The nurse reexplains to the patient the purpose of the catheter and assures him that the urge to void is from the presence of the catheter and bladder spasms. He is cautioned not to pull on the catheter, because this causes bleeding, subsequent plugging of the tubing, and urinary retention.

Catheter Removal. After the catheter is removed (usually when the urine clears), urinary leakage may occur around the wound for several days in patients who have undergone perineal, suprapubic, and retropubic surgery. The cystostomy tube may be removed before or after the urethral catheter is removed. Some urinary incontinence may occur after the catheter is removed. The patient is informed that this will probably disappear in time.

◊ Evaluation

Expected Outcomes

Preoperative

1. Free of anxiety
   a. Verbalizes concerns and accepts solutions offered
   b. Expresses relief that the bladder problem can be treated and that the condition is not a malignant tumor
2. Experiences increased comfort
   a. States pain and discomfort are decreased.
   b. Reports increased ability to rest and sleep
3. Relates understanding of the surgical procedure and preoperative course
   a. Discusses the surgical procedure and expected postoperative course
   b. Practices perineal muscle exercises and other techniques useful in facilitating control of bladder function
   c. Participates in all preoperative preparations for surgery

Postoperative

1. Is free of pain
   a. Relates relief of discomfort
   b. Relates signs and symptoms of problems that are to be reported
2. Is free of infection
   a. Maintains vital signs within normal limits
   b. Exhibits wound healing; no signs of inflammation
   c. Relates what signs are to be reported if an infection is developing
3. Responds positively to self-care measures
   a. Increases activity and ambulation daily
   b. Urinary output within normal ranges and consistent with intake
   c. Uses perineal exercises and interruption of urinary stream to promote bladder control
   d. Drinks adequate amounts of fluids daily
   e. Avoids straining and lifting of heavy objects
4. Verbalizes concerns about sexual functioning
5. Maintains acceptable level of urinary elimination
   a. Maintains optimal drainage of catheter and other drainage tubes
   b. Verbalizes his understanding that urinary incontinence will gradually disappear

In summary, nursing care of the patient undergoing a prostatectomy requires knowledge of the procedure as well as the physiology of the genitourinary system to help the patient through the perioperative period and prepare the patient and family for rehabilitation. The focus of postoperative nursing care is promotion of the patient's comfort, prevention of complications, and return of bladder control. The patient is instructed and encouraged to perform routine perineal exercises to improve bladder control. Erectile dysfunction may occur postoperatively, and issues related to sexuality and self-esteem need to be sensitively addressed.

Cancer of the Prostate

Cancer of the prostate is the most common cause of cancer in men (other than nonmelanoma skin cancer), the second most common cause of cancer deaths in American men older than 55, and the most prevalent cancer overall in black men. With increasing numbers of men in the older age group, greater attention will be focused on this condition.

Clinical Manifestations.   Early cancer of the prostate does not usually produce symptoms. The obstructive symptoms occur late in the disease. This cancer tends to be variable in its course. If the neoplasm is large enough to encroach on the bladder neck and cause obstruction of urine, there are symptoms and signs of obstruction, namely, difficulty and frequency of urination, urinary retention, and decreased size and force of the urinary stream. Prostatic cancer commonly metastasizes to bone, lymph nodes, brain, and lungs. Symptoms due to metastases include backache, hip pain, perineal and rectal discomfort, anemia, weight loss, weakness, nausea, and oliguria. Hematuria may result from urethral or bladder invasion, or both. Unfortunately, these symptoms may be the first overt indications of prostate cancer.

Early Detection.   Every man over age 40 should have a digital rectal examination as part of his regular health checkup. Early detection is the key to a higher cure rate. Routine repeated rectal palpation of the gland (preferably by the same examiner) is important because early cancer may be felt as a nodule within the substance of the gland or as a diffuse induration in the posterior lobe. A digital rectal examination, in addition to being more accurate, readily available, and less costly than other screening tests for prostatic cancer, provides useful clinical information about the rectum, anal sphincter, and quality of stool.

Diagnostic Evaluation.   On rectal examination, an area of increased firmness within the prostate is noted. The more advanced lesion is "stony hard" and fixed. The diagnosis is made on histologic examination of tissue removed surgically by transurethral resection, open prostatectomy, or needle biopsy (perineal or transrectal). Fine needle aspiration is a quick, painless method of obtaining prostate cells for cytologic examination. It is a helpful method for determining staging of the tumor if cancer is present. The serum acid phosphatase level is frequently increased when cancer extends outside the prostatic capsule. (Acid phosphatase is seen in most body tissues but is 1000 times more concentrated in the prostate gland.) Smaller amounts of acid phosphatase can be detected with radioimmunoassay.

The prostate-specific antigen (PSA) is produced by the normal and neoplastic ductal epithelium of the prostate and secreted into the glandular lumen. The concentration of PSA is proportional to the total prostatic mass. Although the PSA indicates the presence of prostate tissue, it does not necessarily indicate malignancy. PSA is routinely used to monitor the patient's response to cancer therapy and to detect local progression and early recurrence of prostate cancer.

Ultrasound studies may help increase the detection of nonpalpable prostate cancers. More commonly, transrectal ultrasound is used as a complement to digital rectal examination to assist with the staging of localized prostate cancer. Biopsies of the prostate are frequently guided by ultrasound.

Other tests include bone scans to detect metastatic bone disease, skeletal radiographs to show osteoblastic metastases, excretory urograms to demonstrate changes from ureteral obstruction, and renal function tests and lymphangiography to seek evidence of metastases to the pelvic nodes.

Management

Treatment selection is based on the stage of the disease and on the patient's age and symptoms. Table 47-2 summarizes the treatment options for the various stages of prostate cancer. A radical prostatectomy (removal of the prostate and seminal vesicles) still remains the standard operative procedure for patients who have potentially curable disease and a life expectancy of 10 years or more. This procedure may be followed by bilateral orchiectomy. Sexual impotency follows radical prostatectomy, and 5% to 10% of the patients have various degrees of urinary incontinence. (See p. 1329 for care of the patient after a prostatectomy.)

If the cancer is found in the early stage, the treatment may be curative radiation therapy, either using teletherapy with a linear accelerator or interstitial irradiation (implantation of radioactive iodine or gold combined with pelvic lymphadenec-

TABLE 47–2.   *Treatment of Prostate Cancer*

Stage A:	Early stage unsuspected on rectal examination but discovered at time of prostatectomy for obstructive symptoms
Treatment:	Stage A$_1$: Observation
	Stage A$_2$: Radical prostatectomy alone or with radiation therapy
Stage B:	Disease limited to prostate and is clinically detectable with palpation: firm nodule in gland or diffuse firmness in lobe
Treatment:	Radical prostatectomy or radiation therapy
Stage C:	More extensive localized disease extending into or beyond the prostatic capsule, bladder neck, or seminal vesicle, without distant metastasis to bone, liver, or lung
Treatment:	Radiation therapy
Stage D:	Metastatic disease
Treatment:	Orchiectomy, diethylstilbestrol, chemotherapy for hormone-refractory disease, and palliative radiation therapy for bone metastases

(Perez CA et al. Carcinoma of the prostate. In DeVita VT, Hellman S, and Rosenberg SA (eds): Principles and Practice of Oncology, 3rd ed. Philadelphia, JB Lippincott, 1989, p 940.)

tomy). Radiation therapy is also used for palliation in patients with late-stage disease. Side effects, which usually are transitory, include proctitis (inflammation of the rectum), enteritis (inflammation of the bowel), and cystitis due to the radiation doses and the proximity of the rectum, bowel, and bladder. There is better preservation of sexual potency with radiation therapy; therefore, younger patients may prefer this treatment modality.

Because approximately half of the patients have locally advanced tumors or evidence of metastatic disease at the time they present for treatment, palliative measures are indicated. Hormonal therapy may be selected to suppress all androgenic stimuli to the prostate. This is accomplished by either orchiectomy (removal of the testes) or administration of estrogens (see below). Hormonal therapy is a method of control rather than cure, as adenocarcinoma of the prostate is hormone dependent. The rationale underlying hormone treatment is that prostatic epithelium becomes atrophied or inactivated when androgen hormones are greatly reduced or inactivated.

Orchiectomy lowers plasma testosterone levels, as 93% of circulating testosterone is of testicular origin. This results in completely removing the testicular stimulus required for continued prostatic growth. Prostatic atrophy occurs after this procedure. Orchiectomy is preferred over hormonal therapy by many urologists because it does not result in the potential side effects of estrogen therapy. Castration carries a significant emotional impact, however. The administration of *estrogen* is thought to inhibit the gonadotropins that are responsible for testicular androgenic activity, thus removing the androgenic hormone, on which the growth of the malignancy depends. Diethylstilbestrol (DES) is the most widely used estrogen at this time.

DES gives symptomatic control, lessens tumor size, lessens pain from metastatic nodules, and imparts an improved sense of well-being. There is evidence that giving higher doses of DES, however, carries a significant risk of thromboembolism, pulmonary embolism, myocardial infarction, and increased risk of stroke. A lower dose apparently is as effective and presents less risk.

Gynecomastia (enlargement of breasts in men) is an annoying complication of estrogen therapy that may be lessened by pretreatment radiation of breast tissue. Impotence almost always occurs after estrogen therapy.

Cryosurgery of the prostate gland has been advocated by some for the poor-risk patient. Chemotherapy may also be tried. Doxorubicin, cisplatin, and cyclophosphamide are under investigation.

For patients failing to respond to conventional therapy, estramustine phosphate (Emcyt), a conjugate of estradiol and nitrogen mustard, has been shown to be promising in giving rapid pain relief. It is based on the premise that a hormone (estrogen) can be used as a carrier to bring a chemotherapeutic agent (nitrogen mustard) to hormone-sensitive tissues (prostate). The drug is available in capsule form. Side effects include nausea, vomiting, and occasionally diarrhea. It is contraindicated in patients who have active thrombophlebitis or thromboembolic disorders and cautiously used in patients with a history of cerebrovascular and coronary artery disease.

To maintain patency of the urethral passage, repeated transurethral resections may have to be performed. When this is impractical, catheter drainage is instituted by way of the suprapubic or transurethral route.

Patients with recurring symptoms are treated symptomatically. Corticosteroids may give relief but do not affect the tumor.

Blood transfusions are given to maintain adequate hemoglobin levels when bone marrow is replaced by tumor. Radiation therapy to skeletal lesions can relieve bone pain. Pain may be controlled by estrogens and narcotics and, if necessary, by severing spinal cord pain fibers through neurosurgery.

In summary, cancer of the prostate is the most common cancer in men. Helping the patient and family to cope with the diagnosis, the alterations in usual activities, and uncertainty of the future is an important component of nursing care. Sensitivity to issues of sexuality as a result of changes due to the disease or therapy assists in the rehabilitation process. See also pp. 264–265, care of the patient with pain; pp. 378–379, care of the patient with advanced cancer; and pp. 1326–1332, care of the patient with a prostatectomy. Care of the patient with cancer of the prostate is summarized in Nursing Care Plan 47-1.

Conditions Affecting the Testes and Adjacent Structures

Undescended Testis (Cryptorchidism)

Cryptorchidism is the absence of one or both testes from the scrotum. The testes may be located in the abdominal cavity or inguinal canal. If the testis does not descend, hormone therapy or surgery (orchiopexy) is used to secure proper positioning.

In orchiopexy, an incision is made over the inguinal canal, and the testis is brought down and placed in the scrotum. To maintain proper position of the testis, traction may be applied to the thigh by means of a suture drawn from the lower end of the scrotum.

Orchitis

Orchitis is an inflammation of the testes (testicular congestion). The cause is usually pyogenic, viral, spirochetal, parasitic, traumatic, chemical, or idiopathic.

When mumps is contracted in the postpubertal man, about one in five develop some form of orchitis 4 to 7 days after swelling of the jaw and neck. The testis may show some atrophy. In past years, sterility and impotence often resulted. Current practice is for the man who has not previously had mumps and is now exposed to the disease to receive gamma globulin immediately. The disease is likely to be less severe, with reduced or no complications.

Management

If the causes of orchitis are bacterial, viral, or fungal, therapy is specific. Rest, elevation of the scrotum, ice packs to reduce scrotal edema, antibiotics, analgesics, and anti-inflammatory medications are recommended.

Epididymitis

Epididymitis is an infection of the epididymis that usually descends from an infected prostate or urinary tract. It also may develop as a complication of gonorrhea. In men under 35 years

Nursing Care Plan 47–1

Care of the Patient With Cancer of the Prostate

Nursing Interventions	Rationale	Expected Outcomes

Nursing Diagnosis: Anxiety related to concern and lack of knowledge about the diagnosis, treatment plan, and prognosis

Goal: Reduced stress and improved ability to cope

Nursing Interventions	Rationale	Expected Outcomes
1. Obtain health history to determine the following: a. Patient's reasons for concerns b. His level of understanding of his health problem c. His past experience with cancer d. Whether he knows his diagnosis of malignancy/prognosis e. His support systems and coping potential	1. Nurse and patient become partners in clarifying information and understanding the patient's ability to cope with his illness.	• Appears more relaxed. • States that anxiety has been reduced or relieved. • Demonstrates understanding of his illness and treatment when questioned. • Engages in open communication with others.
2. Provide education about his diagnosis and treatment plan: a. Explain in simple terms what diagnostic measures he will require; how long they will take, and what he will experience during each test. b. Review treatment plan and allow patient to ask questions.	2. Helping the patient to understand the diagnostic tests and treatment plan will help decrease his anxiety.	
3. Assess his psychological reaction to his diagnosis/prognosis and how he has coped with past stresses.	3. This information provides clues in determining appropriate measures to facilitate his coping ability.	

Nursing Diagnosis: Alteration in urinary elimination patterns related to urethral obstruction secondary to prostatic enlargement/tumor and loss of bladder tone due to prolonged distention/retention

Goal: Improved pattern of urinary elimination

Nursing Interventions	Rationale	Expected Outcomes
1. Determine patient's usual pattern of bladder elimination.	1. Provides a baseline for comparison and goal to work toward.	• Voids at normal intervals. • Reports absence of frequency, urgency, or bladder fullness. • Displays no palpable suprapubic distention after voiding. • Maintains balanced intake and output.
2. Assess for signs and symptoms of urinary retention: amount and frequency of urination, suprapubic distention, complaints of urgency and discomfort.	2. Suspect retention if the patient voids 20 to 30 ml frequently and if output is less than intake.	
3. Catheterize patient to determine amount of residual urine.	3. This is done after voluntary urination is completed to determine amount of urine remaining.	
4. Initiate measures to treat retention: a. Encourage assuming normal position for voiding. b. Recommend using Valsalva maneuver. c. Administer prescribed cholinergic drug. d. Monitor effects of medication.	a. Usual position provides relaxed conditions conducive for voiding. b. By exerting pressure, this has a tendency to force urine out of bladder. c. Stimulates bladder contraction. d. If unsuccessful, another measure may be required.	
5. Consult with physician regarding intermittent or indwelling catheterization; assist with procedure as required.	5. Catheterization will relieve urinary retention until the specific cause is determined; it may be an obstruction that can be corrected only surgically.	

(continued)

Nursing Care Plan 47–1 *(Continued)*

Care of the Patient With Cancer of the Prostate

Nursing Interventions	Rationale	Expected Outcomes
6. Monitor catheter function; maintain sterility of closed system; irrigate as required.	6. Adequate functioning of catheter is to be ensured to achieve purpose and to prevent infection.	
7. Prepare patient for surgery if indicated.	7. Surgical removal of obstruction may be necessary.	

Nursing Diagnosis: Knowledge deficit about a new health problem: cancer, urinary difficulties, and treatment modalities

Goal: Understanding of health problem and ability to care for self

1. Encourage communication with the patient.	1. This is designed to establish rapport and trust	• Discusses his concerns and problems freely.
2. Review the anatomy of the involved area.	2. Orientation to one's anatomy is basic to understanding its function.	• Asks questions and shows interest in his condition.
3. Be specific in selecting information that is relevant to the patient's particular treatment plan.	3. This is based on the treatment plan, as it varies with each patient; individualization is desirable.	• Describes activities that help or harm his recovery.
4. Suggest ways in which pressure on the operative area can be reduced or avoided after the prostatectomy.	4. This is to prevent bleeding; such precautions are in order for 6 to 8 weeks postoperatively.	• Identifies ways of attaining/maintaining bladder control.
a. Avoid prolonged sitting (in a chair, long automobile rides), standing, walking.		• Demonstrates satisfactory technique and understanding of catheter care.
b. Avoid straining, such as during exercises, bowel movement, lifting, and sexual intercourse.		• Lists signs and symptoms that must be reported should they occur.
5. Familiarize patient with ways of attaining/maintaining bladder control	5. These measures will help him to control frequency and dribbling, and aid in preventing retention.	
a. Encourage urination when he feels the need—usually every 2 to 3 hours; discourage his voiding when supine.	a. By sitting or standing, he is more likely to empty his bladder.	
b. Avoid drinking cola and caffeine beverages; urge a cut-off time in the evening for drinking fluids to minimize frequent voiding during the night.	b. Spacing the kind and amount of liquid intake will help to prevent frequency.	
c. Describe perineal exercises to be performed every hour.	c. Exercises will assist him in starting and stopping the urinary stream.	
d. Develop a schedule with patient so that it will fit into his routine.	d. A schedule will assist in developing a workable pattern of normal activities.	
6. Demonstrate catheter care; encourage his questions; stress the importance of position of urinary receptacle.	6. By requiring return-demonstration of care, collection, and emptying of his device, he will become more independent and also can prevent backflow of urine, which can lead to infection.	
7. Alert the patient to those changes that may occur (after he leaves the hospital) that need to be reported:	7. These are signs and symptoms of complications (hemorrhage, infection, obstruction) and are to be reported to health care personnel.	
a. Continued bloody urine; passing of blood clots		
b. Pain; burning around the catheter		

(continued)

Nursing Care Plan 47–1 *(Continued)*

Care of the Patient With Cancer of the Prostate

Nursing Interventions	Rationale	Expected Outcomes

   c. Frequency of urination
   d. Diminishing output
   e. Increasing loss of bladder control

Nursing Diagnosis: Alteration in nutrition related to decreased oral intake because of anorexia, nausea, and vomiting brought on by cancer or its treatment

Goal: Maintain optimal nutritional status

Nursing Interventions	Rationale	Expected Outcomes
1. Assess the amount of food eaten.	1. This assessment will help determine nutrient intake.	• Responds positively to his favorite foods.
2. Routinely weigh patient.	2. Weighing the patient on the same scale under similar conditions can help monitor changes in weight.	• Assumes responsibility for his oral hygiene. • Notes increase in weight after improved appetite.
3. Listen to patient's explanation of why he is unable to eat more.	3. His explanation may present easily corrected practices.	
4. Cater to his individual food requirements (*e.g.,* avoiding foods that are too spicy or too cold).	4. He will be more likely to consume larger servings if food is palatable to him.	
5. Recognize effect of medication or radiation therapy on his appetite.	5. Some chemotherapeutic agents and radiation therapy promote anorexia.	
6. Tell the patient that alterations in taste can occur.	6. Aging and the disease process can reduce taste sensitivity. In addition, smell and taste can be altered as a result of the body's absorption of by-products of cellular destruction (brought on by malignancy and its treatment).	

7. Use measures to control nausea and vomiting.
  a. Administer prescribed antiemetics; around the clock if necessary.
  b. Provide mouth care after vomiting episodes.
  c. Provide rest periods after meals.
	7. Vomiting can decrease appetite.	

8. Provide frequent small meals, and a comfortable and pleasant environment.	8. Smaller portions of food are less overwhelming to the patient.	
9. Assess patient's ability to obtain and prepare foods.	9. Disability or lack of social support can hinder the patient's ability to obtain and prepare foods.	

Nursing Diagnosis: Sexual dysfunction related to effects of therapy: chemotherapy, hormonal therapy, radiation therapy, surgery

Goal: Ability to assume/enjoy modified sexual functioning

Nursing Interventions	Rationale	Expected Outcomes
1. Determine from nursing history what effect patient's medical condition is having on his sexual functioning. (Full assessment follows guidelines in Chap. 17, Human Sexuality).	1. Usually decreased libido and, later, impotence may be experienced.	• Describes the reasons for changes in sexual functioning. • Discusses with appropriate health care personnel what practices have been substituted and appreciated.
2. Inform patient of the effects of prostate surgery, orchiectomy (when applicable), chemotherapy, irradiation, and hormonal therapy, on sexual function.	2. Treatment modalities may alter sexual function, but each is evaluated separately with regard to its effect on a particular patient.	

(continued)

Nursing Care Plan 47–1 *(Continued)*

Care of the Patient With Cancer of the Prostate

Nursing Interventions	Rationale	Expected Outcomes
3. Include his partner in developing understanding and in discovering alternative satisfying close relations with each other.	3. Often the bonds between a couple are strengthened with new appreciation and support that had not been considered before the current illness.	

Nursing Diagnosis: Pain related to progression of disease and treatment modalities

Goal: Relief of pain

1. Evaluate nature of patient's pain and its location.	1. Determining nature and causes of pain helps to select proper relief modality and provide baseline for later comparison.	• Reports control of pain. • Expects exacerbations, reports their quality or intensity, and obtains relief.
2. Avoid activities that aggravate or worsen pain.	2. Bumping the bed is an example of an action that can intensify the patient's pain.	
3. Because pain usually is related to bone metastasis, ensure that patient's bed has a bed board on a firm mattress and protect from falls/injuries.	3. This will provide added support and is more comfortable.	
4. Provide support for affected extremities.	4. The more support coupled with reduced movement of the part helps in pain control.	
5. Prepare patient for radiation therapy if prescribed.	5. Radiation therapy may be effective in controlling pain.	
6. Administer analgesic or narcotic at regularly scheduled intervals as prescribed.	6. Analgesics alter perception of pain and provide comfort. Regularly scheduled analgesics around the clock rather than prn provide more consistent pain relief.	

Nursing Diagnosis: Impaired physical mobility/activity intolerance related to tissue hypoxia, malnutrition, and exhaustion and to spinal cord or nerve compression from metastatic spread

Goal: Improved physical mobility

1. Assess for factors causing limited mobility (*e.g.*, pain, hypercalcemia, limited exercise tolerance).	1. This information offers clues to the cause; if possible, cause is treated.	• Achieves improved physical mobility. • Relates that short-term goals are encouraging him because they are attainable.
2. Provide pain relief by administering prescribed medications.	2. Analgesics/narcotics allow the patient to increase his activity more comfortably.	
3. Encourage use of assistive devices: cane, walker	3. Support may offer the security needed to become mobile.	
4. Involve significant others in helping patient with range of motion exercises, positioning, and walking.	4. Assistance from partner or others encourages patient to repeat activities and achieve goals.	
5. Praise the patient for achieving small gains.	5. Encouragement stimulates improvement of performance.	
6. Assess nutritional status	6. See Nursing Diagnosis: Alteration in nutrition	

of age, the major cause of epididymitis is *Chlamydia trachomatis.* The infection passes upward through the urethra and the ejaculatory duct, and then along the vas deferens to the epididymis.

The patient complains of unilateral pain and soreness in the inguinal canal along the course of the vas deferens, and then develops pain and swelling in the scrotum and the groin.

The epididymis becomes swollen and extremely painful; the temperature is elevated. The urine may contain pus (pyuria) and bacteria (bacteriuria), and the patient may experience resulting chills and fever.

Management.   If the patient is seen within the first 24 hours after onset of pain, the spermatic cord may be infiltrated with a local anesthetic agent to relieve pain. If the epididymitis is chlamydial in origin, the patient and the patient's sexual partners must be treated with antibiotics. The patient is observed for abscess formation. If no improvement occurs within 2 weeks, an underlying testicular tumor should be considered. An epididymectomy (excision of the epididymis from the testis) may be performed for patients with recurrent, incapacitating episodes or for those with chronic, painful conditions. With long-term epididymitis, obstruction of the passage of sperm may occur, and when bilateral, often leads to infertility.

Nursing Considerations.   The patient is placed on bed rest with the scrotum elevated with a scrotal bridge or folded towel to prevent traction on the spermatic cord and to improve venous drainage and relieve pain. Antimicrobials are given as prescribed until all evidence of the acute inflammatory reaction has subsided.

Intermittent cold compresses to the scrotum may help ease the pain. Later, local heat or sitz baths may hasten resolution of the inflammatory process. Analgesics are given for pain relief as prescribed.

Patient Education and Home Health Care.   The patient should avoid straining, lifting, and sexual excitement until the infection is under control. He should be instructed to continue with analgesics and antibiotics as prescribed and to use ice packs if necessary for discomfort. It may take 4 weeks or longer for the epididymis to return to normal.

Tumors of the Testes

Testicular cancer ranks first in cancer deaths among men in the 20- to 35-year age group. Such cancers are classified as *germinal* or *nongerminal.* Germinal tumors arise from the germinal cells of the testes (seminomas, teratocarcinomas, and embryonal carcinomas); nongerminal tumors are from epithelium. Most neoplasms are germinal, with about 40% of these being seminoma. Seminomas tend to remain localized, whereas nonseminomatous tumors are fast growing. The cause of testicular tumors is unknown, but cryptorchidism, infections, and genetic and endocrine factors appear to play a part in their development.

The risk of testicular cancer is 35 times greater for men with any type of undescended testis than for the general population. Testicular tumors are usually malignant and tend to metastasize early, spreading from the testicle to the lymph nodes in the retroperitoneum and to the lungs.

Clinical Manifestations.   The symptoms appear very gradually with a mass or lump on the testicle and generally painless enlargement of the testis. The patient may complain of heaviness in the scrotum, inguinal area, or lower abdomen. Backache (from retroperitoneal node extension), pain in the abdomen, loss of weight, and general weakness may be from metastatic disease.

- The enlargement of the testis without pain is a significant diagnostic finding.

One method of early detection of testicular cancer is self-examination. Part of health promotion practices for men should include testicular self-examination. Teaching men to perform self-examination as depicted in Figure 47-4 is an important intervention for early detection of this disease.

Diagnostic Evaluation. α-Fetoprotein and human chorionic gonadotropin are tumor markers that may be elevated in patients with testicular cancer. (Tumor markers are substances synthesized by the tumor cells and released into the circulation in abnormal amounts.) Newer immunocytochemical techniques have made possible the identification of the cells that apparently produce these markers. These tumor markers are used for diagnosis, staging, and monitoring the response to treatment. Other diagnostic tests include an intravenous urogram to detect ureteral deviation secondary to tumor mass, lymphangiography to assess extent of lymphatic spread of the tumor, and computed tomography of the chest and abdomen to determine the extent of the disease in the lungs and retroperitoneum.

Management.   The goals of management are to eradicate the disease and achieve a cure. Treatment selection is based on the cell type and the anatomic extent of the disease. The testis is removed (orchiectomy) through an inguinal incision with a high ligation of the spermatic cord. Retroperitoneal lymph node dissection (RPLND) to prevent lymphatic spread may be employed after orchiectomy, although controversy exists over this approach. Some believe that the after-effects of the surgical procedure, including ejaculatory dysfunction with resultant infertility and potential ureteral injury, are not justified when more than half of patients have negative lymph nodes. The proponents of RPLND are quick to claim that it may be a curative procedure and as such spares the patient the greater discomforts of chemotherapy should relapse occur. After RPLND, normal libido and orgasm are usually unimpaired, but the patient is not fertile. Postoperative irradiation of the lymph nodes from the iliac region to the diaphragm is the treatment of choice for seminomas. Such radiation is limited to the side of the tumor. The other testis is shielded from radiation to preserve fertility. Radiation is also used to treat patients who do not receive a response to chemotherapy or for whom RPLND is not recommended.

Sperm banking before surgery may be considered for the young man as a hedge against sterility after surgery. A gel-filled prosthesis can be implanted to offset the absence of one testis.

Testicular carcinomas are highly responsive to drug therapy. Multiple chemotherapy using cisplatin with other agents (vinblastine, bleomycin, dactinomycin, cyclophosphamide) gives a high percentage of complete remission. The program of therapy is probably best prescribed by those trained in oncology, as these regimens are toxic and require intensive therapeutic support. Good results may be obtained by combining different types of treatment, including surgery, radiation therapy, and chemotherapy. Disseminated testicular cancer is regarded as a treatable and probably curable disease as a result of advances in diagnosis and treatment.

Patient Education.   The patient may have difficulty in accepting his condition. Issues related to body image and sexuality should be addressed. He needs encouragement to maintain a positive attitude during what may be a long course of therapy. Radiation therapy does not necessarily prevent the patient from fathering children, nor does unilateral excision of a tumor necessarily lessen virility.

A patient with a history of one tumor of the testes has a greater chance of developing subsequent tumors. Follow-up evaluation includes chest films, excretory urography, radioimmunoassay of human chorionic gonadotropins and α-fetoprotein, and examination of lymph nodes to detect recurrence of malignancy.

In summary, although testicular cancer accounts for only 1% of all cancers, it is the major cause of cancer death in men 25 to 35 years of age. Current treatment modalities have sig-

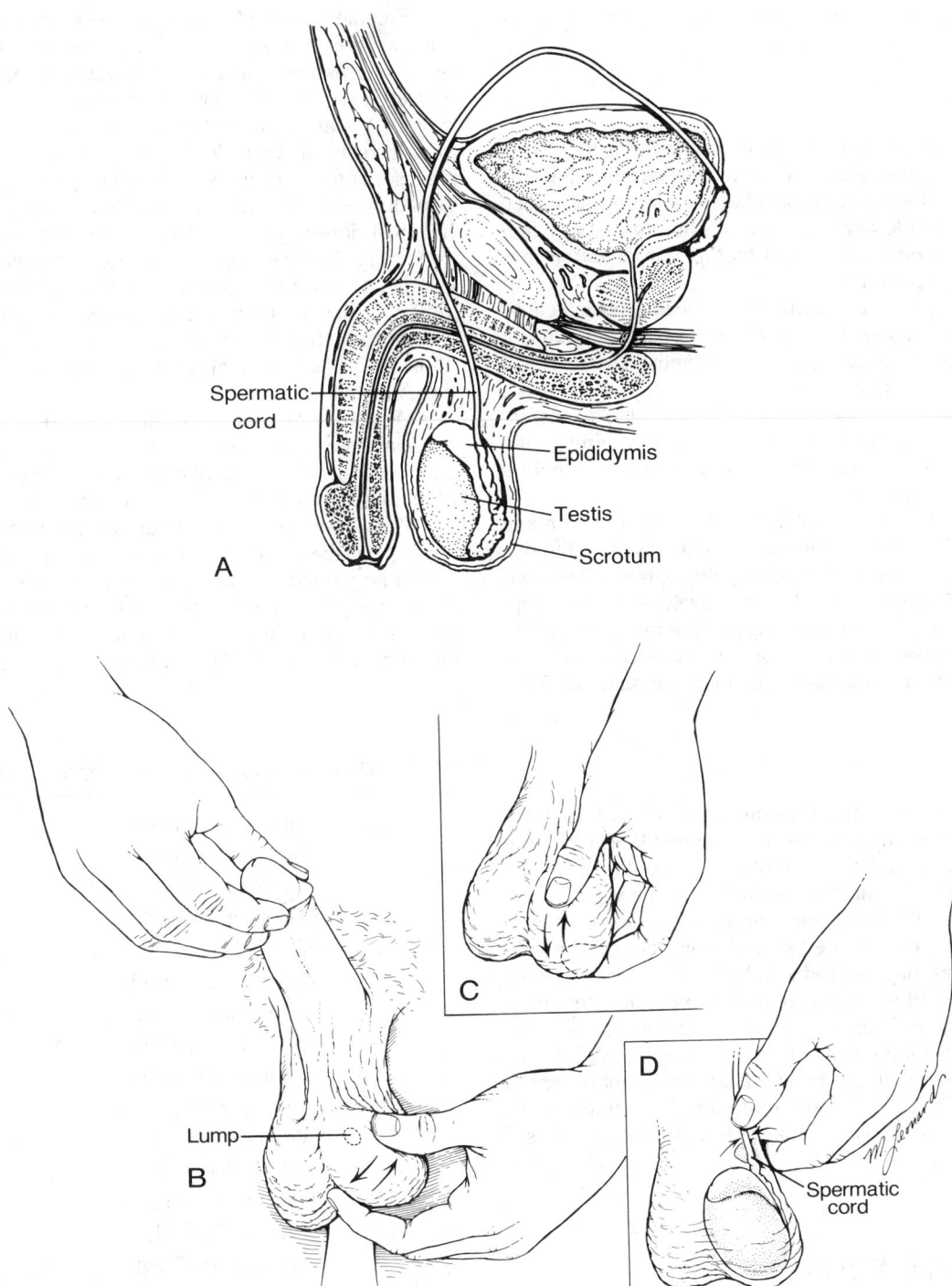

Figure 47–4. Testicular self-examination (TSE) is to be performed once a month; it is neither difficult nor time-consuming. A convenient time is often after a warm bath or shower when the scrotum is more relaxed. Both hands are used to palpate the testis; the normal testicle is smooth and uniform in consistency. (**A**) Normal anatomy. (**B**) With the index and middle finger under the testis and the thumb on top, roll the testis gently in a horizontal plane between the thumb and fingers, feeling for any evidence of a small lump or abnormality. (**C**) Follow the same procedure for palpation in the "vertical" plane. (**D**) Locate the epididymis (cordlike structure on the top and back of the testicle that stores and transports sperm). Repeat the examination for the other testis; it is normal to find one testis larger than the other. Any evidence of a small, pea-sized lump should be checked by a physician. It may be due to an infection or a tumor growth.

nificantly improved survival. Long-term follow-up is necessary for early detection of recurrence.

Hydrocele

A *hydrocele* is a collection of fluid, generally in the tunica vaginalis of the testis, although it also may occur within the spermatic cord. The tunica vaginalis becomes widely distended with fluid. Hydrocele may be acute or chronic and is differentiated from a hernia by the fact that a hydrocele transmits light when transilluminated.

Acute hydrocele occurs in association with acute infectious diseases of the epididymis or as a result of local trauma or systemic infectious diseases, such as mumps. The cause of chronic hydrocele is unknown.

Usually, therapy is not required. Treatment is necessary only if the hydrocele becomes tense and compromises testicular circulation or if the scrotal mass becomes large, uncomfortable, or embarrassing.

In the surgical treatment of hydrocele, an incision is made through the wall of the scrotum down to the distended tunica vaginalis. The sac is resected or, after being opened, is sutured together to collapse the wall. Postoperatively, an athletic supporter is worn for comfort and support. The major complication is the formation of a hematoma in the loose tissues of the scrotum. The nursing management is the same as for a varicocele.

Varicocele

A *varicocele* is an abnormal dilation of the veins of the pampiniform venous plexus in the scrotum (network of veins from the testis and the epididymis, constituting part of the spermatic cord). Varicoceles occur most frequently in the veins on the upper portion of the left testicle in adults. In some men, a varicocele has been associated with infertility. Few, if any, subjective symptoms may be produced by the enlargement of the spermatic vein, and no treatment is required unless fertility is a matter of concern. Symptomatic varicocele (pain, tenderness, and discomfort in the inguinal region) is corrected surgically by ligating the external spermatic vein at the inguinal area. An ice bag may be applied to the scrotum for the first few hours after operation to relieve edema. The patient then wears a scrotal support.

Erectile Dysfunction

Erectile dysfunction, also called impotence, is the alteration of a man's sexual capability to either achieve or maintain an erection sufficient to accomplish intercourse. The man may note a decreased frequency of erections, inability to achieve a firm erection or rapid detumescence (subsiding of erection). Incidence ranges from 25% to 50% in men over 65 years of age. The physiology of erection and ejaculation is complex and involves sympathetic and parasympathetic components. At the time of erection, pelvic nerves carry parasympathetic impulses that dilate the smaller blood vessels of the region and increase blood flow to the penis, expanding the corpora cavernosa.

Erectile dysfunction has both psychogenic and organic causes. Causes of psychogenic impotence include anxiety, fatigue, depression, and cultural pressure to perform sexually. Research suggests, however, that organic impotence may account for a larger percentage of cases of impotence than previously realized. Organic causes include occlusive vascular disease, endocrine disease (diabetes, pituitary tumors, hypogonadism with testosterone deficiency, hyperthyroidism, and hypothyroidism), cirrhosis, chronic renal failure, genitourinary conditions (radical pelvic surgery), hematologic conditions (Hodgkin's disease, leukemia), neurologic disorders (neuropathies, Parkinsonism), trauma to the pelvic or genital area, drugs (alcohol, psychoactive drugs, anticholinergics) and drug abuse. Table 47-3 lists drugs that are commonly associated with erectile dysfunction.

Diagnosis of erectile dysfunction includes sexual and medical history, an analysis of presenting symptoms, physical examination, detailed assessment of all medications taken and drug abuse, as well as various laboratory studies.

The advent of sleep laboratories has made the nocturnal penile tumescence test possible. Changes in penile circumference are monitored (using a mercury strain gauge placed around the penis) and recorded. Research showed that normal men have nocturnal penile erections closely paralleling rapid eye movement (REM) sleep in their occurrence and duration.

TABLE 47–3. *Drugs Associated With Erectile Dysfunction*

Methyldopa (Aldomet)
Guanethidine (Ismelin)
Clonidine (Catapres)
Reserpine (Serpasil)
Spironolactone (Aldactone)
Diuretics (*e.g.,* Diuril)
Chlorthalidone (Hygroton)
Prazosin (Minipress)
Clofibrate (Atromid-S)
Methantheline (Banthine)
Cimetidine (Tagamet)
Propranolol (Inderal)
Methadone (Dolophine)
Baclofen (Lioresal)
Ethionamide (Trecator)
Perhexiline (Pexid)
Hexamethonium (Methium Cl)
Mecamylamine HCl (Inversine)
Trimethaphan camsylate (Arfonad)
Propantheline (Pro-Banthine)
Disulfiram (Antabuse)
Digoxin (Lanoxin)
Cancer chemotherapy agents

(Leiblum SR and Segraves RT. Sex therapy with aging adults. In Leiblum SR and Rosen RC [eds]: Principles and Practice of Sex Therapy: Update for the 1990s, 2nd ed. New York, Guilford Press, 1989, p 365.)

Organically impotent men show inadequate sleep-related erections that correspond to their waking performance. The nocturnal penile tumescence test can help to determine whether erectile impotence has organic or psychological cause.

Arterial blood flow to the penis is measured with the Doppler probe. Nerve conduction tests and psychological evaluation of the patient are part of the diagnostic workup.

Management. Treatment, which depends to some extent on the cause, can be medical, surgical, or a combination of both. A patient's response to nonsurgical therapy, such as treatment of alcoholism and readjustment of hypertensive agents or other medications, is examined. Erectile dysfunction secondary to hypothalamic-pituitary-gonadal dysfunction may be reversible with endocrine therapy. Insufficient penile blood flow may be treated with recently developed vascular surgery procedures. Patients with erectile dysfunction from psychogenic causes are directed to a professional specializing in sex therapy. Patients with erectile dysfunction secondary to organic causes are considered candidates for penile implants.

Two basic types of penile implants are available: the semirigid rod and the inflatable prosthesis. The semirigid rod, such as the Small-Carrion prosthesis, has no moving parts and leaves the man with a permanent semierection. In contrast, the inflatable prosthesis simulates natural erections and natural flaccidity.

Complications after implant procedures include infection, erosion of the prosthesis through the skin (more common with semirigid rod than the inflatable prosthesis), and persistent pain, which may require removal of the implant. Cystoscopic surgery such as TURP is more difficult with a semirigid rod than with the inflatable prosthesis. Choice of prosthesis should include consideration of the patient's activities of daily living, social activities, and expectations of the patient and his partner.

Pharmacologic measures to induce erections can involve injection of vasoactive agents such as papaverine and phentolamine directly into the penis. Untoward effects include priapism (persistent abnormal erection of the penis) and development of fibrotic plaques at the injection sites.

In summary, erectile dysfunction can result from a variety of different factors requiring specific treatment strategies. Regardless of its cause, erectile dysfunction has vast psychological and social implications for most men. Therefore, the nurse must listen and be supportive to both the patient and his partner.

Conditions Affecting the Penis

Phimosis

Phimosis, a condition in which the foreskin is constricted so that it cannot be retracted over the glans, can occur congenitally or as a result of inflammation and edema. There has been a trend away from routine circumcision of newborns. Therefore, the child and adult require early instruction in cleansing of the prepuce. In the adult, when the cleansing of the preputial area is neglected or impossible, the accumulation of normal secretions and subsequent inflammation (*balanitis*) occur. This causes adhesions and fibrosis. The thickened secretions become encrusted with urinary salts and calcify, forming preputial

concretions. In the aged, penile carcinoma may develop. Phimosis is corrected by circumcision (see below). The patient is instructed in proper hygienic care of the foreskin.

Paraphimosis is a condition in which the foreskin is retracted behind the glans and, because of narrowness and subsequent edema, cannot be reduced back to its usual position (covering the glans). It is treated by manual reduction (compressing the glans firmly to reduce its size, and then pushing the glans back as the prepuce is moved forward). Circumcision is usually indicated once the inflammation and edema subside.

Circumcision

Circumcision is the excision of the foreskin (prepuce) of the glans penis. It is usually performed in infancy for hygienic purposes. In adults, it is indicated for phimosis, paraphimosis, recurrent infections of the glans and foreskin, and personal desire of the patient.

Postoperatively, the patient is observed for bleeding. The petrolatum (Vaseline) gauze dressing is changed as indicated. Because adult men may experience a considerable amount of pain after circumcision, analgesics are given when needed.

Cancer of the Penis

Cancer of the penis occurs in men over 60 years of age and represents about 0.5% of malignancies in men in the United States. In some countries, however, the incidence is up to 10%. Cancer of the penis rarely occurs in circumcised individuals. It appears on the skin of the penis as a painless, wartlike growth or ulcer. Cancer of the penis can involve the glans, coronal sulcus under the prepuce, the corporal bodies, urethra, and regional or distant lymph nodes. Bowen's disease is a form of squamous cell carcinoma *in situ* of the penile shaft. Often diagnosis is delayed for more than a year, probably because of guilt, embarrassment, or ignorance. Smaller lesions involving only the skin may be controlled by excisional biopsy. Topical chemotherapy with 5-fluorouracil cream may be one option in selected patients. Radiation therapy or radioactive needle implant produces varying results. Partial penectomy (removal of the penis) is preferred to total penectomy if possible; about 40% of patients are then able to participate in sexual intercourse and to stand for voiding. Total penectomy is indicated when the tumor is not amenable to conservative treatment. Radiation therapy may be used as treatment for small squamous cell carcinomas of the penis or for palliation in advanced tumors or lymph node metastasis.

Patient Education. Circumcision in infancy almost eliminates the possibility of penile cancer, because chronic irritation and inflammation of the glans penis predisposes to penile tumors. Personal hygiene is an important preventive measure in uncircumcised men.

Priapism

Priapism is an uncontrolled, persistent erection of the penis that causes the penis to become large, hard, and often painful. It occurs from either neural or vascular causes, including sickle cell thrombosis, leukemic cell infiltration, spinal cord tumors, and tumor invasion of the penis or its vessels. This condition may result in gangrene and often results in impotence, whether treated or not.

Priapism is considered a urologic emergency. The goal of therapy is to improve venous drainage of the corpora cavernosa to prevent ischemia, fibrosis, and impotence. Initially, treatment is directed at relieving the erection and includes bed rest and sedation. The corpora may be irrigated with an anticoagulant, which allows aspiration of stagnant blood. Shunting procedures to divert the blood from the turgid corpora cavernosa to the venous system (corpora cavernosa–saphenous vein shunt) or into the corpus spongiosum–glans penis compartment may be tried.

Peyronie's Disease

Peyronie's disease involves the buildup of fibrous plaques in the sheath of the corpus cavernosum. These plaques are not visible when the penis is flaccid. When erect, however, curvature of the penis occurs that can be painful and can make sexual intercourse difficult or impossible. Peyronie's disease primarily occurs in middle-aged and older men. Although the plaques may shrink over time, surgical removal of the plaques may be necessary.

Urethral Stricture

Urethral stricture is a condition in which there is a narrowing of a section of the urethra. It can occur congenitally or as a result of a scar along the urethra. Traumatic injury to the urethra such as from instrumentation and infections can result in urethral strictures. Treatment involves dilation of the urethra or in severe cases, surgical removal of the stricture or urethrotomy.

In summary, there are many conditions that can affect the penis. Although usually not life threatening, the patient experiences anxiety as a result of body image changes. It is important to assess for anxiety and provide the necessary support and education to help the patient cope with these changes.

Chapter Summary

Disorders related to the male reproductive system are commonly encountered in nursing practice. The nurse caring for the patient with one of these disorders must understand the complexities of the male urinary and reproductive systems.

Additionally, the nurse must be sensitive to the impact that such disorders and their treatment may have on the patient's self-concept, self-esteem, and sexuality. The nurse must be comfortable in discussing issues related to urinary function and sexuality and cognizant of the importance of teaching patients about health promotion behaviors such as testicular self-examination to permit detection of problems early in their course.

The male patient who is discharged soon after surgery on the reproductive system needs clear verbal and written instructions about what activities are permitted; additionally, providing information about how to contact the nurse or other health care provider if problems arise may be reassuring to the patient and his family.

Bibliography

Books

Corriere JN Jr. Essentials of Urology. New York, Churchill Livingstone, 1986.

Hanno PM and Wein AJ. A Clinical Manual of Urology. Norwalk, CT, Appleton-Century-Crofts, 1986.

Hill GS. Uropathology, Vols 1 and 2. New York, Churchill Livingstone, 1989.

Kaufman JJ. Current Urologic Therapy, 2nd ed. Philadelphia, WB Saunders, 1986.

Kaye JW. Outpatient Urologic Surgery. Philadelphia, Lea & Febiger, 1985.

Leiblum SR and Rosen RC (eds). Principles and Practice of Sex Therapy: Update for the 1990s, 2nd ed. New York, Guilford Press, 1989.

Perez CA et al. Carcinoma of the prostate. In DeVita VT, Hellman S, and Rosenberg SA (eds). Principles and Practice of Oncology, 3rd ed. Philadelphia, JB Lippincott, 1989, pp 1023–1058.

Schover LR. Sexuality and Cancer: For the Man Who Has Cancer, and His Partner. Atlanta, American Cancer Society, Inc, 1988.

Smith DR. General Urology, 11th ed. Los Altos, CA, Lange Medical Publications, 1984.

Swanson JM and Forrest KA. Men's Reproductive Health. New York, Springer-Verlag, 1984.

Walsh PC et al. Campbell's Urology, Vols 1–3, 5th ed. Philadelphia, WB Saunders, 1986.

Journals

Asterisks indicate nursing research articles.

General Articles

Allen DG and Whatley M. Nursing and men's health. Nurs Clin North Am 1986 Mar; 21(1):3–13.

Bansal S. Sexual dysfunction in hypertensive men. A critical review of the literature. Hypertension 1988 Jul; 12(1):1–10.

Baum N. Treatment of impotence. Part 1. Nonsurgical methods. Part 2. Surgical methods. Postgrad Med 1987 May 15; 81(7):133–140.

Cowling WR and Campbell VG. Health concerns of aging men. Nurs Clin North Am 1986 Mar; 21(1):75–83.

Cozad J. Impotence: Psychosocial aspects, evaluation methods, and treatments. Urol Nurs 1988 Oct/Dec; 9(2):10–12.

Forrester DA. Myths of masculinity: Impact upon men's health. Nurs Clin North Am 1986 Mar; 21(1):15–23.

Heller JE and Gleich P. Erectile impotence: Evaluation and management. J Fam Pract 1988 Mar; 26(3):321–324.

Kaiser FE. Impotence in diabetic men. Am J Med 1988 Nov; 85(5A):147–152.

Kaufman DG and Nagler HM. Specific nonsurgical therapy in male infertility. Urol Clin North Am 1987 Aug; 14(3):489–498.

Kniefe-Hardy MJ et al. Managing indwelling catheters in the home. Geriatr Nurs 1985 Sep/Oct; 6(5):280–285.

Mackety CJ. Lasers in urology. Nurs Clin North Am 1990 Sep; 25(3):697–709.

Mastman TJ et al. Erectile dysfunction in men with diabetes mellitus. Urology 1987 Jun; 29(6):589–592.

Meisler AW et al. Success and failure in penile prosthesis surgery: Two cases highlighting the importance of psychosocial factors. J Sex Marital Ther 1988 Summer; 14(2):108–119.

Merrill DC. Clinical experience with the Mentor inflatable penile prosthesis in 301 patients. J Urol 1988 Dec; 140(6):1424–1427.

* Millon-Underwood S and Sanders E. Factors contributing to health promotion behaviors among African-American men. Oncol Nurs Forum 1990 Sep/Oct; 17(5):707–712.

Morrison H. Diabetic impotence. Nurs Times 1988 Aug; 84(22):35–37.

Payton TR. Impotence: A non-prosthetic approach. Urol Nurs 1988 Jul/Sep; 9(1):10–12.

Pedersen B et al. Evaluation of patients and partners 1 to 4 years after penile prosthesis surgery. J Urol 1988 May; 139(5):956–958.

Podell RM. Sexual science: Bridging the disciplines. Urology 1988 Jan; 31(1):90–93.

Rousseau P. Impotence in elderly men. Postgrad Med 1988 May; 83(6):212–219.

Sarosdy MF et al. A prospective double-blind trial of intracorporeal papaverine versus prostaglandin E1 in the treatment of impotence. J Urol 1989 Mar; 141(3):551–553.

Sidi AA. Vasoactive intracavernous pharmacotherapy. Urol Clin North Am 1988 Feb; 15(1):95–101.

Wein AJ and Van Arsdalen KN. Drug-induced male sexual dysfunction. Urol Clin North Am 1988 Feb; 15(1):23–31.

Williams L. Pharmacologic erection programs: A treatment option for erectile dysfunction. Rehabil Nurs 1989 Sep/Oct; 14(5):264–268.

Prostatic Conditions

Barry MJ et al. Watchful waiting vs. immediate transurethral resection for symptomatic prostatism. JAMA 1988 May; 259(20):3010–3017.

Benson MC et al. Prostate cancer in men less than 45 years old: Influence of stage, grade, and therapy. J Urol 1987 May; 137(5):888–890.

Consensus Conference. The management of clinically localized prostate cancer. JAMA 1987 Nov; 258(19):2727–2730.

Early detection and diagnosis of prostate cancer. CA 1989 Nov/Dec; 39(6): 1–69.

Fowler FJ et al. Symptom status and quality of life following prostatectomy. JAMA 1988 May; 259(20):3018–3022.

Geller J. Overview of benign prostatic hypertrophy. Urology 1989 Oct; 34(4 Suppl):57–63.

Gibbons RP et al. Total prostatectomy for clinically localized prostatic cancer: Long term results. J Urol 1989 Mar; 141(3):564–566.

Goodman M. Concepts of hormonal manipulation in the treatment of cancer. Oncol Nurs Forum 1988 Sep/Oct; 15(5):639–647.

Graverson PH et al. Controversies about indications for transurethral resection of the prostate. J Urol 1989 Mar; 141(3):475–481.

Heinrich-Rynning T. Prostatic cancer treatments and their effects on sexual function. Oncol Nurs Forum 1987 May/Jun; 14(3):17–21.

Kirby RS. Alpha-adrenoceptor inhibitors in the treatment of benign prostatic hyperplasia. Am J Med 1989 Aug; 87(2A):26S–30S.

Krieger JN et al. Fast neutron radiotherapy for locally advanced prostate cancer. Urology 1989 Jul; 34(1):1–9.

LaFollette SS. Radical retropubic prostatectomy. AORN J 1987 Jan; 45(1): 57–71.

Libman E and Fichten CS. Prostatectomy and sexual function. Urology 1987 May; 29(5):467–478.

Nielsen KT and Madsen PO. Pathogenesis, diagnosis, and management of benign prostatic hypertrophy. Compr Ther 1988 Nov; 14(11):21–26.

Pilepich MV et al. Definitive radiotherapy in resectable (Stage A_2 and B) carcinoma of the prostate: Results of a nationwide overview. Int J Radiat Oncol Biol Phys 1987 May; 13(5):659–663.

Schellhammer PF et al. Morbidity and mortality of local failure after definitive therapy for prostate cancer. J Urol 1989 Mar; 141(3):567–571.

Schellhammer PF et al. Prostate biopsy after definitive treatment by interstitial ^{125}Iodine implant or external beam radiation therapy. J Urol 1987 May; 137(5):897–901.

Sogani PC. Treatment of advanced prostatic cancer. Urol Clin North Am 1987 May; 14(2):353–371.

Stone NN. Flutamide in treatment of benign prostatic hypertrophy. Urology 1989 Oct; 34(4 Suppl):64–68.

Testicular Conditions

* Blackmore C. The impact of orchidectomy upon the sexuality of the man with testicular cancer. Cancer Nurs 1988 Feb; 11(1):33–40.

Fossa SD et al. Post-chemotherapy lymph node histology in radiologically normal patients with metastatic nonseminomatous testicular cancer. J Urol 1989 Mar; 141(3):557–559.

Geller NL et al. Prognostic factors for relapse after complete response in patients with metastatic germ cell tumors. Cancer 1989 Feb; 63(3): 440–445.

Higgs DJ. The patient with testicular cancer: Nursing management of chemotherapy. Oncol Nurs Forum 1990 Mar/Apr; 17(2):243–249.

Laukkanen E et al. Management of seminoma with bulky abdominal disease. Int J Radiat Oncol Biol Phys 1988 Feb; 14(2):227–233.

* Martin JP. Male cancer awareness: Impact of an employee education program. Oncol Nurs Forum 1990 Jan/Feb; 17(1):59–64.

* Reno DR. Men's knowledge and health beliefs about testicular cancer and testicular self-examination. Cancer Nurs 1988 Apr; 11(2):112–117.

* Rudolf VM et al. The practice of TSE among college men: Effectiveness of an educational program. Oncol Nurs Forum 1988 Jan/Feb; 15(1): 45–48.

Nursing Research Profile for Unit 11

Sexual and Reproductive Problems

Overview

In the area of female reproductive health, nurse researchers have focused on such diverse issues as psychological reactions of couples and spouses to *in vitro* fertilization, premenstrual syndrome, and the diagnosis of breast cancer, women's reactions to invasive and potentially uncomfortable or painful and stressful diagnostic and therapeutic procedures, gastrointestinal symptoms across the menstrual cycle, and readability of written package information provided with prescription and nonprescription contraceptives.

In the area of male reproductive health, nurse researchers have examined knowledge and reported frequency of testicular self-examination and the impact of loss of a testicle by orchidectomy on men's sexuality.

Couples' and Husbands' Reactions Related to in Vitro Fertilization, Premenstrual Syndrome, and Breast Cancer

▷ Milne BJ. *Couples' experiences with in vitro fertilization.* J Obstet Gynecol Neonatal Nurs 1988 Sep/Oct; 17(5): 347–352

One hundred twenty-eight couples who had undergone at least one *in vitro* fertilization (IVF) procedure were interviewed to examine how the procedure is experienced by couples and to identify their needs. A descriptive approach, using a guided interview and participant observation, was used to address these questions. Six closed-ended questions designed to obtain demographic data and 12 open-ended questions about the experience of IVF constituted the interview. Couples initially were asked to describe the IVF experience and to describe the most positive and the most negative aspects of the experience. Data obtained from the interviews were analyzed to identify persistent themes and concepts.

Couples' interactions with IVF team personnel were cited most frequently as the most positive aspect of the IVF experience. Other positive aspects included the friendship, support, and camaraderie that resulted from interaction with other cou-

ples in the same situation. Interestingly, couples' interactions with IVF team personnel were also cited most frequently as the most negative aspect of the IVF experience. Other negative aspects included the depersonalization, impersonal and mechanical aspects of the experience, along with inability to obtain information.

Depersonalization by IVF team members was felt most acutely when couples were in need of support because of treatment failure and subsequent grieving. Men in the study felt helpless, embarrassed, anxious about their wives undergoing laparoscopy, and guilt that their wives were undergoing pain and discomfort.

Implications. Anticipatory counseling for couples going through IVF procedures throughout the process may decrease anxiety and feelings of depersonalization. Information provided to couples should be repeated several times and reinforced with patient literature. This repetition and reinforcement is important for adult learners, as high anxiety levels interfere with information processing. Group interaction and networking also may alleviate anxiety and provide comfort. The nurse may serve as coordinator of support groups or as a resource for those interested in a networking system. The woman and her partner often experience grief with treatment failure and require extra support from the nurse during these times.

▷ Olshansky E. *In vitro fertilization.* Image: Journal of Nursing Scholarship 1988 Fall; 20(3):128–131.

Using open-ended questions to interview 54 patients, Olshansky examined individuals' and couples' experiences, and responses to infertility and treatment. The stated purpose of this study was to increase the understanding of the psychosocial dynamics of infertility.

Ninety- to 120-minute interviews were taped and then transcribed for data analysis. Selective coding was used to detect recurrent themes that then were reviewed by other infertility patients, who validated those themes as making sense to them. Findings include the following themes: intense motivation, described as a "drivenness," difficulty terminating treatment and "getting on with life," aversion to sexual intercourse because of its association with treatment failure, and very unique, individual responses to treatment, along with intense hope followed by intense despair if conception did not occur.

Implications. Nursing care directed toward couples undergoing IVF requires sensitivity to the stresses that develop with "high-tech" infertility treatment. Treatment failure is likely to have a negative impact on couples' self-esteem. The serious emotional stress that results requires anticipatory guidance by the nurse. Further research on nursing models of therapeutic intervention based on the emotional responses found in this study are needed.

▷ *Cortese J and Brown M. Coping responses of men whose partners experience premenstrual symptomatology. J Obstet Gynecol Neonatal Nurs 1989 Sep/Oct; 18(5):405–412.*

Premenstrual syndrome (PMS), a complex clinical entity, can disrupt family life and marital harmony. Cortese and Brown conducted an exploratory study to examine responses of male partners of PMS patients. Their conceptual basis included family systems theory and Lazarus's coping model. Eighty-six couples were recruited from various sources, such as medical practices, newspaper ads, and PMS seminars. Patients were interviewed to categorize coping strategies of partners of those with severe PMS and those with mild or no symptoms, using a premenstrual symptom inventory and a PMS coping inventory.

The types of coping responses used by men whose partners experience moderate to severe premenstrual symptoms were rank-ordered, and data were analyzed to determine if any of the men's coping responses were different in two groups (partners of women with a low level of symptoms and partners of those with a high level of symptoms).

The findings indicate that partners of women with severe PMS symptoms used a wide variety of coping strategies and actively sought out assistance and information about the situation. Men whose partners had a high level of symptoms tended more often than those in the low-level group to try to learn more about the symptoms. Partners of women with severe symptoms tended to use many strategies and more varied responses to their wives' symptoms.

Implications. Nurses in a primary care setting using this information as a sign of possible severe distress in a relationship can offer information, teaching, group support, and counseling. Supportive spouses, involved in constructive assistance and coping, are an important adjunct to any medical treatment. Spouses seeking assistance and information may indicate a high degree of distress and a severe level of symptoms of PMS. Assessment, teaching, and counseling of the woman and her partner are indicated. PMS literature and information on groups can be displayed in the ambulatory gynecologic health care setting. Discussion with male partners about coping strategies may provide alternatives for them while the nurse is screening for any unhealthy coping methods. Referrals are indicated for those who do not respond or whose distress exceeds the nurse's capabilities.

▷ *Norhouse L. A longitudinal study of the adjustment of patients and husbands to breast cancer. Oncol Nurs Forum 1989 Apr; 16(4):511–515.*

The purpose of this study was to assess and compare the ongoing psychosocial adjustment of 41 patients and their husbands to breast cancer at three times: 3 days, 30 days, and 18 months after surgery. Mood, symptom distress, and role function were assessed. Instruments used included the Affects Balance Scale, Brief Symptom Inventory, and Psychosocial Adjustment to Illness Scale. Based on family systems theory, the author states that assessment of the impact of illness over time for the patient and her family is an important nursing function directed toward identifying ways to promote adjustment.

The results of this three-phase descriptive study show similar levels of distress at the three points and indicate that mild to severe distress in patients and their husbands persists more than 18 months after surgery. Most patients had resumed normal life-styles, but those with recurrence of cancer or who were undergoing chemotherapy had more difficulty. Husbands who were younger or married for shorter periods had more negative mood states.

Patients' and husbands' mood scores did not differ significantly from each other over time. Husbands reported as much distress as their wives across the three periods.

Nursing Implications. Assessment of patients with breast cancer and their families must extend over time and not end with treatment. Assessment of family members is important, as their coping affects the family as a system and the patient herself. Problem-solving techniques and assistance in minimizing role disruption may help the family cope with diagnosis and treatment with less anxiety. Further research may indicate specific resources that may be helpful and the length of time that such resources should be available.

Information Needs and Responses to Invasive Procedures

▷ *Barsevick AM and Lauver D. Women's informational needs about colposcopy. Image: Journal of Nursing Scholarship 1990 Spring; 22(1):23–26.*

The purpose of this study was to determine educational needs related to colposcopy examination. This study examined questions asked by 36 women undergoing colposcopy, a visual diagnostic procedure to evaluate cervical or Pap smear abnormalities. The theoretical framework was based on the premise that teaching about threatening procedures and self-care lessens anxiety.

Spontaneous questions were recorded during the visit and were not prompted or elicited by the interviewer. Questions were sorted into those about the procedure and those about results. Fifty-two percent of the questions were related to the examination itself, and 34% were related to the results and their implications for the patient. Fourteen percent of the questions sought to clarify information already given by the physician; 32% of the participants questioned the cause of cervical abnormalities.

The authors noted that although women sought information about the procedure, they did not ask about possible sensations they might experience during the procedure or how to care for themselves after colposcopy.

Nursing Implications. Nurses need to provide concrete, objective information about the colposcopy procedure itself and self-care after it. By anticipating women's needs for information about the procedure and cause of abnormalities along with clarification, if necessary, of previously provided information, anxiety can be lessened. If anxiety is lessened, this may become a mildly uncomfortable and mildly anxiety-producing procedure rather than a crisis.

▷ *Wells N. Management of pain during abortion. J Adv Nurs 1989; 14:56–62.*

Wells examined the effect on pain and distress ratings of 40 patients receiving local anesthesia for discomfort during an abortion when four interventions were added: relaxation, pleasant imagery, analgesic imagery, and a pain discussion group. The last group served as a control group to control for the effects of increased attention on the ratings of pain and distress. The purpose of the study was to determine the effects of cognitive behavioral strategies in pain management. Based on the gate control theory, which proposes that pain is multi-dimensional, the hypotheses proposed that the first three interventions mentioned above would result in less pain and distress and quicker recovery for those instructed in these techniques than for those who do not use these techniques. Outcomes were assessed by subjective measures of pain sensation and distress, length of time for the abortion procedure, length of time in the recovery room, and use of analgesics for the first 24 hours after abortion. Before the procedure, subjects received one of the interventions: instructions and practice with relaxation, pleasant imagery, or analgesic imagery. Subjects in the fourth group participated with the investigator in a discussion of the pain model, previous pain experiences, and previous coping; however, they did not receive instruction in any techniques for pain reduction or relief. During the abortion procedure, the investigator coached the subjects in the technique in which they had received instruction. Pain and distress ratings were obtained at the end of the procedure and in the recovery room. Follow-up phone calls were made the next day to determine the number and type of analgesics taken at home after the procedure.

Results showed that subjectively rated pain, speed of recovery, or use of analgesics did not differ significantly by groups. The small sample size (N = 40), lack of a second data collector who was blind to patients' group assignments, and the emotional reactions associated with abortion may have affected the findings.

Implications. For nurses working in this specific field, a review of this study may generate other options for study. Further investigation and possible use of these techniques with a larger sample is warranted to determine if the techniques may be useful in relieving pain and distress during this procedure and other brief medical procedures.

Gastrointestinal Symptoms Across the Menstrual Cycle

▷ *Heitkemper M, Shaver JF, and Mitchell ES. Gastrointestinal symptoms and bowel patterns across the menstrual cycle in dysmenorrhea. Nurs Res 1988 Mar/Apr; 37(2):108–113*

Because gastrointestinal (GI) alterations such as nausea, vomiting, diarrhea, and other changes may produce symptoms that contribute to distress during the menstrual cycle, Heitkemper and co-workers examined GI symptoms during the menstrual cycle. The purposes of the study were to describe GI function across the menstrual cycle and to compare GI function in women with and without dysmenorrhea. The sample was composed of 34 women. On the basis of self-reports of menstrual cramping, subjects were categorized as dysmenorrheic (N=15) or nondysmenorrheic (N=19). The nondysmenorrheic group was further divided into those taking oral contraceptives (N=9) and those not taking them (N=10). Subjects were studied for two menstrual cycles. A GI diary was used to record daily self-reports of stool frequency and stool consistency, and the occurrence of nausea, vomiting, constipation, and diarrhea. The GI diary contained a daily checklist of six

GI-related symptoms: stomach pain, nausea, diarrhea, constipation, increased food intake, and decreased food intake. Perimenstrual symptoms were retrospectively assessed; these symptoms were categorized into eight factors: pain, impaired concentration, behavior changes, autonomic reactions, fluid retention, negative affect, excitement, and a general complaint of a variety of symptoms.

The dysmenorrheic group tended to have longer menstrual cycles and menses than both nondysmenorrheic groups; however, the difference was significant only for length of the menstrual cycle. All three groups exhibited looser stools during menses, with no differences across groups. Reports of stomach pain were higher at menses than at other phases of the menstrual cycle; nausea and decreased food intake were more frequent in dysmenorrheic women at menses. More dysmenorrheic than nondysmenorrheic women had GI symptoms at menses. Menstrual distress with negative affect, pain, behavior changes, and autonomic reactions were reported more frequently at menses by dysmenorrheic women.

Implications. Alterations in GI function related to hormones or prostaglandins could be explained to patients with dysmenorrhea, possibly alleviating anxiety and further distress. Women taking oral contraceptives who notice a change in stools can be reassured that the change is due to variation in ovarian steroid levels. Knowledge of these changes could be helpful in planning therapeutic interventions.

Readability of Written Contraceptive Information

▷ *Swanson J et al. Readability of commercial and generic contraceptive instructions. Image: Journal of Nursing Scholarship 1990 Summer; 22(2):96–99.*

This study examines the readability of commercially prepared package inserts and those generic instruction inserts prepared by clinic personnel in the use of various contraceptive methods. Because many teenagers and adults function at a lower reading level than expected and because many contraceptive failures result in unintended pregnancies, this review has important implications for nurses who instruct patients in contraceptive use. Previous studies have suggested that functional illiteracy may contribute to noncompliance. Patient package inserts on methods of contraception and generic information written by health care agency staff members and health information publishers were obtained and analyzed using six standard readability formulas.

Results showed that commercially prepared patient package inserts on oral contraceptives were written at a 9th to 11th grade reading level, whereas those using over-the-counter methods had an 11th grade reading level. The clinic material was at a reading ability above 8th grade level. These results suggest that written instructions may be too difficult for young teenagers, especially those who have difficulty reading English.

Implications. Generic information or clinic instruction development must be based on the needs of at-risk populations. Clear information prepared at an appropriate reading level is an important aspect of patient instruction. Patient package inserts alone may be inadequate for clinic populations. Generic inserts also should be provided. Patient package inserts could be rewritten at a lower grade level to accommodate more readers. As an aid to health care personnel, those who write inserts should include the reading level required to comprehend the information provided. Personal instruction by health care providers, reinforced by written materials appropriate to the patient's reading level, may decrease the incidence of unintended pregnancies. Nursing education must prepare students to teach those with low literacy skills and to develop materials for this population. Reading level assessment might be included before patient teaching with a population at risk.

Male Sexual and Reproductive Health

▷ Martin JP. *Male cancer awareness: Impact of an employee education program.* Oncol Nurs Forum 1990 Jan/Feb; 17(1): 59–64.

The effectiveness of a male cancer awareness program was evaluated by Martin. A convenience sample of 663 male employees of an electrical power company in the southwestern United States participated in a cancer education program. This program provided general information about cancer as well as specific information about prostate and testicular cancer; risk factors, signs and symptoms, screening techniques, and testicular self-examination were discussed. Presession and postsession questionnaires were administered to determine previous experience with cancer, early detection practices, and knowledge and attitudes about prostate and testicular cancers.

Eighty-five percent employees who attended the educational program provided information about previous experience with cancer and early detection practices. Of these, only 7.8% reported practicing monthly testicular self-examination and 27.9% reported that they had annual physical examinations. Pre-educational and posteducational session questionnaires were returned from 448 subjects. The knowledge test scores significantly increased, from 70.2% to 86.6% of responses correct, after the educational program. Analysis of the presession questionnaires demonstrated misconceptions related to age risk for testicular cancer and risk factors for prostate cancer. The postsession tests demonstrated that the educational program successfully corrected misconceptions, increased knowledge and awareness about male cancers, and fostered attitudes that positively influenced health-seeking behaviors.

Nursing Implications.   Although knowledge or intention to adopt a health behavior does not assure its adoption, increased knowledge about a potential health problem and methods to detect it is generally considered a first step. Lack of knowledge and misconceptions about cancer in men are common and indicate the need for educational efforts by nurses in school health, occupational health, and settings with elderly adults.

▷ Reno DR. *Men's knowledge and health beliefs about testicular cancer and testicular self-examination.* Cancer Nurs 1988 Apr; 11(2):112–117.

The knowledge of and health beliefs about testicular cancer and testicular self-examination (TSE), the practice of TSE, and demographic characteristics were evaluated by Reno in a convenience sample of 126 male college students (ages 18 to 40 years). Reno proposed that the practice of TSE depended on whether the man believed that he was susceptible to testicular cancer and that his performance of TSE would detect the disease early. A questionnaire that measured knowledge, beliefs about benefits of TSE, and beliefs about susceptibility to testicular cancer was administered.

Of the 126 subjects, 12 reported practicing TSE and 114 subjects did not practice TSE. Of the 12, only 41% practiced TSE once a month and 50% were not sure if they were performing the procedure correctly. The nonpracticers had not heard about TSE, and all subjects reported that no one had shown them how to perform TSE. Of the 114 nonpracticers, 100 responded that if they were given the information, they would practice TSE. There was no significant difference between the perceived susceptibility scores of the two groups. Although the knowledge scores for both groups were low, the practicers' knowledge was significantly higher than that of the nonpracticers. There was a highly significant positive relationship between the belief in susceptibility to testicular cancer (TC) and the belief in benefits of TSE. A significant positive relationship also was found between the belief of susceptibility to TC and the knowledge of TC and TSE. There were no significant differences between the demographic characteristics of practicers and nonpracticers of TSE. The findings support the positive relationship of perceived susceptibility and perceived benefits, and the practice of TSE.

Nursing Implications.   The findings strongly support the need for patient education about testicular cancer, the benefits of testicular self-examination, and the correct technique of performing the examination. The author suggests that men be taught testicular examination techniques during adolescence to promote adoption of this and other health-promoting behaviors.

▷ Blackmore C. *The impact of orchidectomy upon the sexuality of the man with testicular cancer.* Cancer Nurs 1988 Feb; 11(1):33–40.

This study was undertaken to determine if the loss of a testicle by orchidectomy affects the sexuality of the man with testicular cancer. Blackmore compared the sexual function of 16 men with germ cell tumors of the testis treated with unilateral orchidectomy, with five men who had a unilateral orchidectomy for reasons other than testicular cancer. Orchidectomy had been performed within 2 years for both groups. A third group, which served as a control group, consisted of 10 men of the same age group (18 to 45 years); although the sample was obtained through the control subjects' visits to their general practitioner, none had a history of testicular problems.

A self-report questionnaire that focused on affects (anxiety, depression, guilt, hostility, joy, contentment, vigor and affection), body image, symptoms of psychopathology, sexual drive (frequency of intercourse, masturbation, and ideal or preferred frequency of intercourse), and sexual satisfaction was administered. Additionally, subjects in the first and second groups were asked to rate the intensity of their presurgery sexual drive.

No significant differences were found between the three groups; however, sexual problems were reported in all three groups. A significant decrease in *perceived* sexual drive was noted in the men with testicular cancer when postoperative sexual drive was compared with retrospective reports of preoperative sexual drive.

Nursing Implications.   Blackmore recommends that nurses continue to explore methods for assessing sexuality to better assess patients' concerns and to recommend appropriate strategies to deal with alterations in sexuality. Knowledge and understanding of the psychosocial implications of sexuality are important in all areas of nursing practice.

unit 12
Immunologic Function

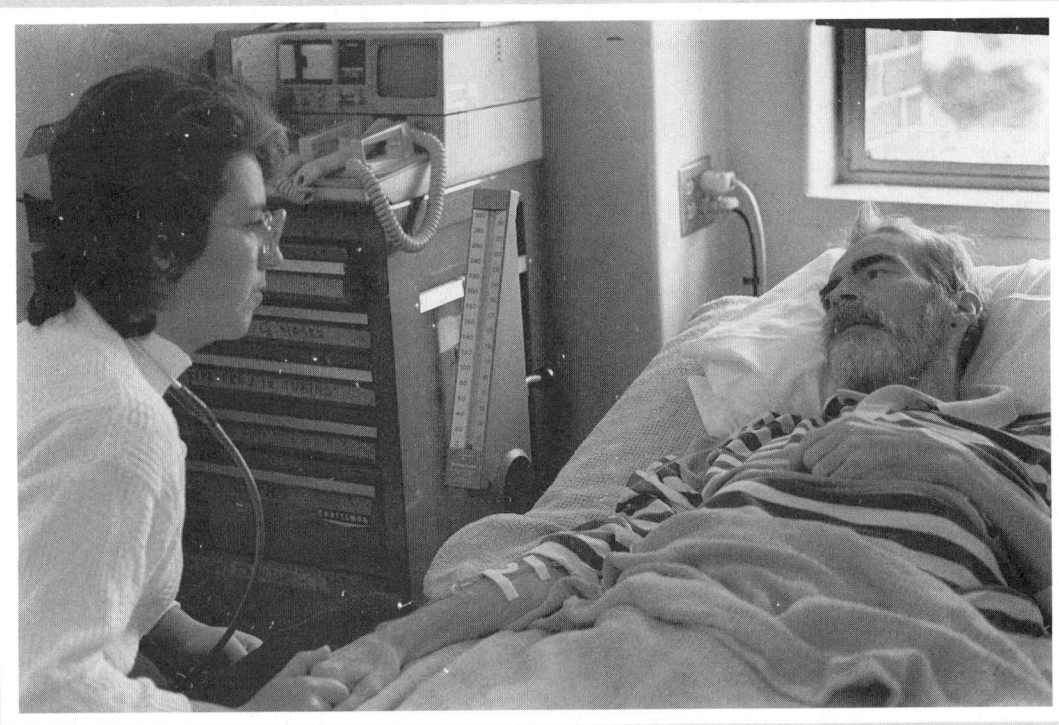

48

The Immune System, Immunopathology, and Immunodeficiency

Learning Objectives

On completion of this chapter, the learner will be able to:

1. Describe the body's general immune responses and the stages of the immune system response
2. Differentiate between cellular and humoral immune responses
3. Describe the stages of hypersensitivity reactions
4. Describe the effects that the following variables have on function of the immune system: age, nutrition, concurrent illness, cancer, medications, and radiation
5. Describe nursing diagnoses common to patients with AIDS
6. Use the nursing process as a framework for care of the patient with AIDS

The term *immunity* refers to the body's specific protective response to an invading foreign agent or organism. However, pathologic developments within the immune system lead to certain disease manifestations. Therefore, the term *immunopathology* is used to describe the study of diseases caused by the *immune reaction*—the protective response that the body initiates but that paradoxically turns against the body and causes tissue damage and disease. *Immunodeficiencies*, on the other hand, are disorders characterized by a defect in the immune system that leads to suppression of the immune response. To understand immunopathology and immunodeficiency, one must first understand how the body's immune system functions normally.

Types of Immunity: Natural and Acquired

There are two general types of immunity: natural immunity and acquired immunity. Natural immunity, which is a nonspecific immunity, is present at birth, while acquired or specific immunity develops after birth. Although each type of immunity plays a distinct role in the defense against harmful invaders, it is important to remember that the various components often act in an interdependent manner.

Natural Immunity

Natural immunity provides a nonspecific response to any foreign invader, regardless of the composition of the invader. The basis of natural defense mechanisms is merely the ability to distinguish between "self" and "nonself." Such natural mechanisms include physical and chemical barriers, the action of white blood cells, and inflammatory responses.

Physical barriers consist of intact skin and mucous membranes, which prevent pathogens from gaining access to the body, and the cilia of the respiratory tract along with coughing and sneezing responses, which act to clear pathogens from the upper respiratory tract before they can invade the body further. *Chemical barriers* such as acid gastric juices, enzymes in tears and saliva, and substances in sebaceous and sweat secretions act in a nonspecific way to destroy invading bacteria and fungi. Viruses are countered by other means, such as interferon (one of the *biologic response modifiers* currently being investigated), which is a nonspecific viricidal substance naturally produced by the body and capable of stimulating the activity of other components of the immune system.

White blood cells, or *leukocytes,* participate in both the natural and the acquired immune responses. Granular leukocytes, or *granulocytes* (so called because of granules in their cytoplasm), include neutrophils, eosinophils, and basophils. *Neutrophils* (also called polymorphonuclear leukocytes or PMNs because their nuclei have multiple lobes) are the first cells to arrive at the site of inflammation. *Eosinophils* and *basophils*, other types of granulocytes, increase in number during allergic reactions and stress responses. Granulocytes assist in fighting invasion by foreign bodies or toxins by releasing cell mediators, such as histamine, bradykinin, and prostaglandins, and engulfing the foreign bodies or toxins. *Nongranular leukocytes* include *monocytes* or *macrophages* (referred to as *histiocytes* when they enter tissue spaces) and lymphocytes. Monocytes also function as phagocytic cells and are able to engulf greater numbers and quantities of foreign bodies or toxins than granulocytes. *Lymphocytes,* consisting of B and T cells, play major roles in humoral and cell-mediated immunity, as will be discussed later.

The *inflammatory response* is a major component of the nonspecific or natural immune system elicited in response to tissue injury or invading organisms. Chemical mediators assist in the inflammatory response to minimize blood loss, wall off the invading organism, activate phagocytes, and promote fibrous scar formation and regeneration of injured tissue. (The inflammatory response is discussed in detail on p. 105.)

Acquired Immunity

Acquired immunity consists of immunologic responses that are not present at birth but are acquired during life. Most acquired immunity develops as a result of contracting a disease or generating a protective immune response through immunization. Weeks or months after exposure to the disease or immunization, an immune response develops sufficiently to prevent contraction of the disease on re-exposure to it. This type of acquired immunity is referred to as *active acquired immunity* because the immunologic defenses are developed by the body of the person being defended. Active acquired immunity generally lasts many years or even the person's lifetime. (Acquired immunity is discussed further in Chap. 49.)

Passive acquired immunity is temporary immunity transmitted from another source that has developed immunity through previous disease or immunization. Gamma globulin and antiserum, obtained from blood plasma of persons with acquired immunity, are used in emergencies to provide passive immunity to diseases when the risk of contracting a specific disease is great and there is not time for a person to develop adequate active immunity.

Both types of acquired immunity involve humoral and cell-mediated (cellular) immunologic responses, described below.

The Immune System

General Immune Responses

When the body is invaded or attacked by bacteria or viruses, it has three means of defending itself—the phagocytic immune response, the humoral or antibody immune response, and the cellular immune response.

The first line of defense, the *phagocytic immune response,* involves the white blood cells (granulocytes and macrophages), which have the ability to ingest foreign particles. These cells can move to the point of attack to engulf and destroy the foreign agents.

The second protective response, the *humoral or antibody response,* begins with the lymphocyte cells, which can transform themselves into plasma cells that manufacture antibodies. It is the antibodies, which are highly specific proteins, that are transported in the bloodstream and have the ability to disable the invaders.

The third mechanism of defense, the *cellular immune response,* also involves the lymphocytes, which, in addition to transforming themselves into plasma cells, can also turn into special cytotoxic T cells that can attack the microbes themselves.

Antigens and Antibodies

The part of the invading or attacking organism that is responsible for stimulating the production of an antibody is called an *antigen* or an *immunogen.** An antigen is a small patch of proteins on the outer surface of the microorganism. A single bacterium, even a single large molecule such as a toxin (diphtheria or tetanus toxin), may have several such antigens or "markers" on its surface and can therefore induce the body to produce a number of different antibodies. Once an antibody is produced, it is released into the bloodstream and carried to the attacking organism, where it combines with the antigen on its surface, binding with it like a complementary piece of a jigsaw puzzle (Fig. 48-1).

Stages of the Immune System Response

There are four well-defined stages in an immune response: recognition, proliferation, response, and the effector stage. An

---

* *The newer term* immunogen *is being used widely as an alternative to* antigen.

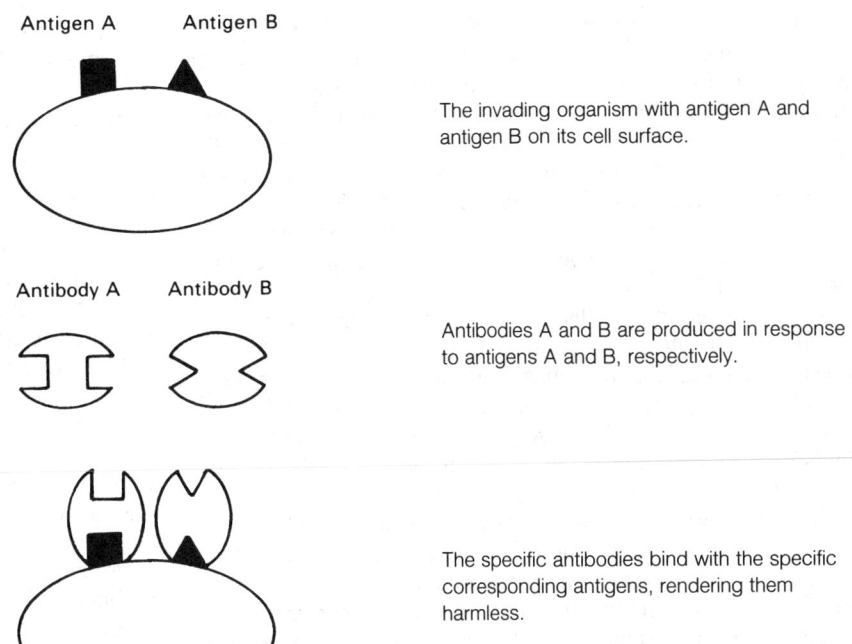

Antigen A   Antigen B

The invading organism with antigen A and antigen B on its cell surface.

Antibody A   Antibody B

Antibodies A and B are produced in response to antigens A and B, respectively.

The specific antibodies bind with the specific corresponding antigens, rendering them harmless.

Figure 48–1. Antibody specificity. Antibodies are produced by B-cell lymphocytes to bind with specific antigens.

overview of these stages is presented here, followed by descriptions of humoral immunity, cell-mediated or cellular immunity, and the complement system.

Recognition

The basis of any immune reaction is, first and foremost, recognition. It is our immune system's ability to recognize antigens on materials as "foreign," or "nonself," that is the initiating event in any immune reaction. The body must first recognize invaders as "foreign" before it can react to them.

Surveillance by Lymph Nodes and Lymphocytes. The body accomplishes its surveillance in two ways. First, the immune system is widely dispersed—distributed close to all of the body's surfaces, internal as well as external, in the form of tiny organs called lymph nodes. Second, small lymphocytes are continuously being discharged from each lymph node into the bloodstream, where they patrol the tissues and vessels that drain the areas served by that node. Basically, it is the lymph nodes and lymphocytes that make up our immune system.

Circulating Lymphocytes. There are lymphocytes in the lymph nodes themselves and lymphocytes that circulate in the blood. Taken in aggregate, the total number of lymphocytes in the body adds up to a mass of cells of impressive size. Radioactive labeling of circulating lymphocytes has shown that these cells recirculate from the blood to lymph nodes and from the lymph nodes back into the bloodstream again, in a never-ending series of patrols. Some circulating lymphocytes can survive for decades. Some of these small, hardy cells maintain their solitary circuits for the lifetime of the person.

The exact way in which circulating lymphocytes recognize antigens on foreign surfaces is not known. At present, the accepted theory is that recognition depends on specific receptor sites on the surface of the lymphocytes. It appears that *macrophages,* a type of nongranular leukocyte found in the tissues of the body, play an important role in helping these circulating lymphocytes to process the antigens. Foreign materials enter the body, and a circulating lymphocyte comes into physical contact with the surfaces of these materials. Upon contact, the lymphocyte, with the help of macrophages, either removes the antigen from the surface or in some way picks up an imprint of its structure. For example, during a streptococcal throat infection, the streptococcal organism gains access to the mucous membranes of the throat, and a circulating lymphocyte moving through the tissues of the neck comes in contact with the organism. The lymphocyte, familiar with the surface markers on the cells of its own body, recognizes the antigens on the microbe as being different (nonself) and the streptococcus as being antigenic (foreign). This triggers the second phase, the immune response—proliferation.

The Proliferation Stage

The circulating lymphocyte containing the antigenic message returns to the nearest lymph node. Once in the node, these "sensitized" lymphocytes stimulate certain of the dormant lymphocytes residing there to enlarge, divide, proliferate, and differentiate into either T lymphocytes or B lymphocytes. Enlargement of the lymph nodes in the neck in conjunction with a sore throat is one example of the immune response.

The Response Stage

In the response stage, the changed lymphocytes will function in either a humoral or a cellular fashion.

Humoral. The production of antibodies to a specific antigen is called a humoral response, *humoral* referring to the fact that the antibodies are released into the bloodstream and so reside in the plasma or fluid fraction of the blood, one of the classical four "humors" of the body. (An explanation of humoral immunity and antibody function can be found on pp. 1354–1356.)

Cellular. The returning sensitized lymphocytes migrate to areas of the lymph node (other than those areas containing lymphocytes programmed to become plasma cells), where they stimulate the residing lymphocytes to become cells that will attack microbes directly rather than through the action of antibodies. These transformed lymphocytes have been given the descriptive name *cytotoxic T cells.* The *T* stands for the fact that during the embryologic development of the immune system, these lymphocytes spent some time in the thymus of the developing fetus, at which time they were genetically programmed to become T cells rather than the antibody-producing B lymphocytes. Viral rather than bacterial antigens induce a cellular response. This response is manifested by the increasing number of lymphocytes seen in the blood smears of people with viral illnesses—for instance, in the lymphocytosis occurring in infectious mononucleosis. (Cellular or cell-mediated immunity is discussed in detail on p. 1357.)

Most immune reactions to antigens involve both humoral and cellular responses, though usually one predominates. During transplantation rejection the cellular reaction predominates, whereas in the bacterial pneumonias and sepsis it is the humoral response that plays the dominant protective role (Chart 48-1).

The Effector Stage

In the effector stage, the antibody of the humoral response or the cytotoxic T cell of the cellular response reaches and couples with the antigen on the surface of the foreign object. The coupling initiates a series of events that in most instances results in the total destruction of the invading microbes or the complete neutralization of the toxin. The events involve an interplay of antibodies (humoral immunity), complement, and action by the cytotoxic T cells (cellular immunity).

Figure 48-2 summarizes the phases of the immune response.

Humoral Immune Response

The humoral response is characterized by production of antibodies by the B-cell lymphocytes in response to a specific antigen. Although the B lymphocyte is ultimately responsible for the production of antibodies, both the macrophages of natural immunity and the special T-cell lymphocytes of cellular immunity are involved in recognition of the foreign substance and in antibody production.

Antigen Recognition

Several theories exist about the mechanisms by which the B cells recognize the invading antigen and produce appropriate antibodies in response. The existence of several theories probably results from the fact that there are several different methods of recognition of antigens by the B lymphocyte or cell. These different means of antigen recognition may also be responsible for different types of antibody response. Some antigens seem to have the ability to trigger antibody formation by the B lymphocytes directly, while others require the assistance of T cells.

T cells, or T lymphocytes, are part of a surveillance system dispersed throughout the body. These lymphocytes recycle through the general circulation, tissues, and lymphatic system. It is suggested that, with the assistance of macrophages, the T lymphocyte recognizes the antigen of a foreign invader. The T lymphocyte picks up the antigenic message or "blueprint" of the antigen and returns to the nearest lymph node with that message.

Antibody Production

B lymphocytes, which are stored in the lymph nodes, are subdivided into thousands of clones, each responsive to a single group of antigens having almost identical characteristics. The T lymphocyte carries the antigenic message back to the lymph node and stimulates specific clones of the B lymphocyte to enlarge, divide, proliferate, and differentiate into plasma cells capable of producing specific antibodies to the antigen. Other B lymphocytes differentiate into B-cell clones with a memory for the antigen. These "memory cells" are responsible for the more exaggerated and rapid immune response in a person who is repeatedly exposed to the same antigen.

Antibody Structure

Antibodies are large proteins that are referred to as *immunoglobulins* because they are found in the globulin fraction of the plasma proteins. Each antibody molecule consists of two subunits, each of which contains a light and a heavy peptide chain (Fig. 48-3). The subunits are held together by a chemical link composed of disulfide bonds. Each subunit has a portion that serves as a binding site for a specific antigen. This site,

Chart 48-1
Comparison of Cellular and Humoral Immunologic Responses

Cell-Mediated Immune Responses	Humoral-Mediated Immune Responses
Transplant rejection	Bacterial phagocytosis and lysis
Delayed hypersensitivity—tuberculin reaction	Anaphylaxis
Contact dermatitis	Allergic hay fever and asthma
Graft-versus-host reactions	Immune complex disease
Tumor surveillance or destruction	Defense against bacterial and some viral infections
Intracellular infections	
Defense against viral, fungal, and parasitic infection	

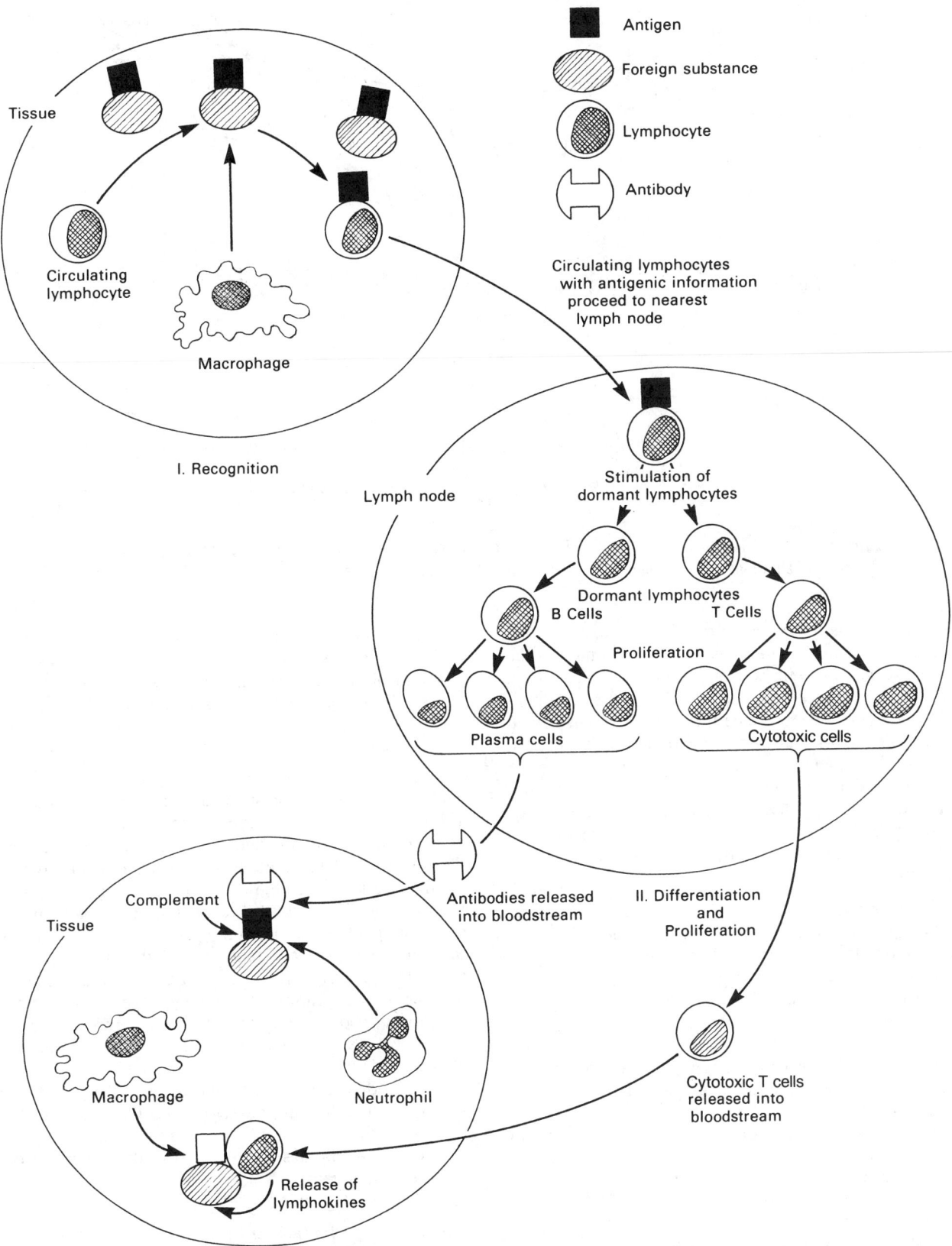

Figure 48–2. The phases of the immune response. I. Recognition of the antigen by circulating lymphocytes and macrophages. II. Stimulation of dormant lymphocytes, and differentiation and proliferation of T cells and B cells with formation and release of antibodies. III. Destruction or neutralization of antigens through the action of antibodies, complement, macrophages, and killer T cells.

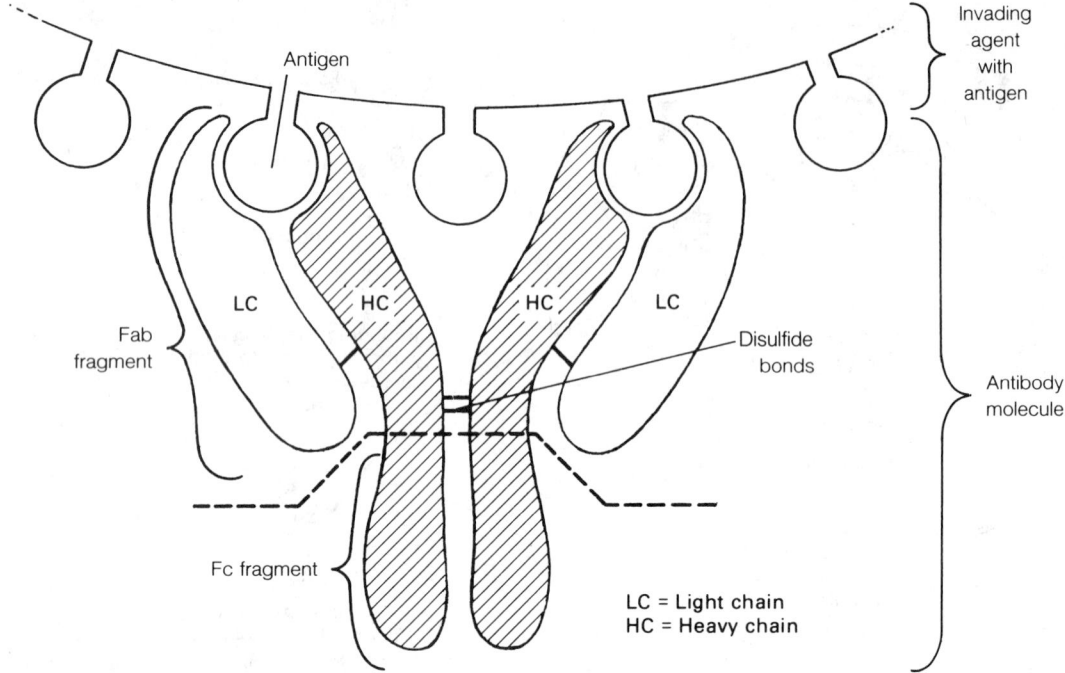

Figure 48–3. An antibody molecule. The Fab fragment serves as the binding site for a specific antigen. The Fc fragment allows the antibody molecule to take part in the complement system.

referred to as the *Fab* fragment, provides the "lock" portion that is highly specific for an antigen. An additional portion, known as the *Fc* fragment, allows the antibody molecule to take part in the complement system (to be discussed later).

The body is able to produce five different types of antibodies or immunoglobulins. Immunoglobulins in general are designated by the symbol *Ig*, and each of the five types, or classes, is identified by a specific letter of the alphabet (IgA, IgD, IgE, IgG, and IgM). Classification is based on the chemical structure and biologic role of the individual immunoglobulin. Some of the outstanding characteristics of the immunoglobulins may be summarized as follows:

1. *IgG* (75% of total)
   - Present in serum and tissues (interstitial fluid)
   - Major role in blood-borne and tissue infections
   - Activates complement system
   - Enhances phagocytosis
   - Crosses placenta
2. *IgA* (15% of total)
   - Present in body fluids (blood; saliva; tears; breast milk; and pulmonary, gastrointestinal, prostatic, and vaginal secretions)
   - Protects against respiratory, gastrointestinal, and genito-urinary infections
   - Prevents absorption of antigens from food
   - Passed in breast milk to protect neonate
3. *IgM* (10% of total)
   - Mostly limited to intravascular serum
   - First immunoglobulin produced in response to bacterial and viral infections
   - Activates complement system
4. *IgD* (0.2% of total)
   - Present in small amounts in serum
   - Role unclear; may influence B-lymphocyte differentiation

5. *IgE* (0.004% of total)
   - Present in serum
   - Involved in allergic and hypersensitivity reactions
   - May help in defense against parasites

Antibody Function

Antibodies defend against foreign invaders in several ways. The type of defense employed depends on the structure and composition of both the antigen and the immunoglobulin. As discussed above, the antibody molecule has at least two combining sites known as the Fab fragments. One antibody can act as a cross-link between two antigens, causing them to bind or clump together. This clumping effect, referred to as *agglutination*, helps in clearing the body of the invading organism by facilitating phagocytosis. Some antibodies have the ability to assist in the removal of offending organisms through the process of *opsonization*. In this process, the antigen–antibody molecule is coated with a sticky substance that also facilitates phagocytosis.

Antibodies also promote the release of vasoactive substances, such as histamine and slow-reacting substance (SRS), two of the chemical mediators of the inflammatory response. In addition, antibodies are involved in the activation of the complement system.

Antigen–Antibody Binding

The portion of the antigen involved in binding with the antibody is referred to as the *antigenic determinant*. The binding of the Fab fragment (antibody binding site) to the antigenic determinant can be likened to a "lock and key" situation (Fig. 48-4). The most efficient immunologic responses occur when the antibody and antigen fit exactly. Poor fit can occur with an

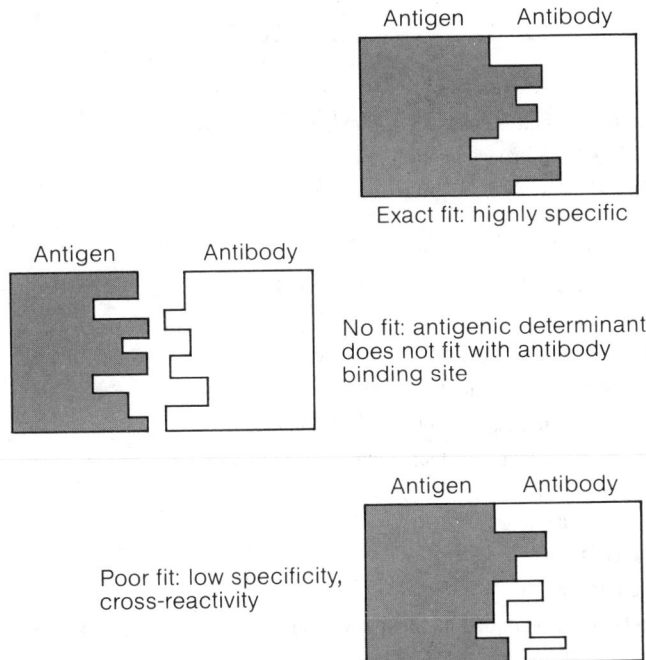

Figure 48–4. Antigen–antibody binding. (**Top**) A highly specific antigen–antibody complex. (**Middle**) No match and therefore no immune response occurs. (**Bottom**) Poor fit or match with low specificity; antibody reacts to antigen with *similar* characteristics, producing cross-reactivity. (Adapted from Kirkwood EM and Lewis CJ. Understanding Medical Immunology. Chichester, England, John Wiley & Sons, Ltd., 1983. Used with permission.)

antibody that was produced in response to a different antigen (Fig. 48-4). This phenomenon is known as *cross-reactivity*. For example, in acute rheumatic fever, the antibody produced against *Streptococcus pyogenes* in the upper respiratory tract may cross-react with the patient's heart tissue, leading to damage to valves of the heart.

Cell-Mediated (Cellular) Immune Response

While the B lymphocytes are the soldiers of humoral immunity, the T lymphocytes, also referred to as T cells, are primarily responsible for cellular immunity. These lymphocytes spend time in the thymus, where they are programmed to become T cells rather than antibody-producing B lymphocytes. There are several types of T cells, each with designated roles in the defense against bacteria, viruses, fungi, parasites, and malignant cells. T cells attack foreign invaders directly rather than through the production of antibodies.

Cell-mediated reactions are initiated by the binding of an antigen with an antigen receptor located on the surface of a T cell. This may occur with or without the assistance of macrophages. The T cells then carry the antigenic message or blueprint to the lymph nodes, where the production of other T cells is stimulated. Some T cells remain in the lymph nodes and retain a memory for the antigen. Other T cells migrate from the lymph nodes into the general circulatory system and ultimately to the tissues, where they remain until they either come in contact with their respective antigens or die.

There are two main classifications of effector T cells that participate in the destruction of foreign organisms. Cytotoxic or killer T cells attack the antigen directly by altering the cell membrane and causing cell lysis. Delayed-type hypersensitivity cells protect the body through the production and release of lymphokines. Lymphokines, which belong to a larger group of glycoproteins known as cytokines, can recruit, activate, and regulate other lymphocytes and white blood cells. These cells then assist in destroying the invading organism (Table 48-1).

Other lymphocytes that assist in combating organisms include the null lymphocyte and the natural killer (NK) cell. Null lymphocytes, a subpopulation of lymphocytes that lack the usual characteristics of B and T cells, destroy antigens already coated with antibody. These cells have special Fc receptor sites on their surfaces that allow them to couple with the Fc end of antibodies (antibody-dependent, cell-mediated cytotoxicity). NK cells, which represent another subpopulation of lymphocytes without the usual characteristics of T and B cells, defend against microorganisms and some types of malignant cells. NK cells are capable of direct cytotoxicity and production of cytokines.

The discovery of T lymphocytes known as helper and suppressor cells has contributed to the understanding that humoral and cellular immune responses are not separate, unrelated processes but branches of the immune response that can and do affect each other. Upon contact with the antigen, helper T cells release cytokines known as interleukins, which stimulate growth and functioning of white blood cells and T- and B-cell lymphocytes.

In addition, helper T cells contribute to the differentiation of null and NK cells. *Suppressor T cells* have the ability to decrease B-cell production, thereby keeping the immune response at a level that is compatible with health (*e.g.,* sufficient to fight infection adequately without attacking the body's healthy tissues).

Complement

The term *complement* refers to circulating plasma proteins made in the liver that can be activated when an antibody couples with its antigen. Once activated, these proteins interact sequentially with one another in a cascade or "falling domino" effect. This causes alterations of the cell membranes on which antigen and antibody complex form, permitting fluid to enter the cell and leading eventually to cell lysis and death. In addition, activated complement molecules attract macrophages and granulocytes to areas of antigen–antibody reactions. These cells continue the body's defense by devouring the antibody-coated microbes and by releasing bacterial agents.

Complement plays a very important role in the immune response. Destruction of an invading or attacking organism or toxin is not achieved merely by the binding of the antibody and antigens; it also requires activation of complement, the arrival of killer T cells, or the attraction of macrophages.

Classical Complement Activation. There are two ways to activate the complement system. One, termed the classical pathway because it was the first method discovered, involves the reaction of the first of the circulating complement proteins (C_1) with the receptor site of the Fc portion of an antibody molecule following formation of an antigen–antibody complex. The activation of the first complement component then acti-

TABLE 48-1. *Cytokines and Their Biologic Effects*

Cytokine*	Effect
Interleukin-1	Promotes differentiation of T and B cells, NK and null cells
Interleukin-2	Stimulates growth of T cells and special activated killer lymphocytes (known as lymphocyte-activated killer cells—LAK cells)
Interleukin-3	Stimulates growth of mast cells and other blood cells
Interleukin-4	Stimulates growth of T and B cells, mast cells, and macrophages
Interleukin-5	Stimulates antibody responses
Interleukin-6	Stimulates growth and function of B cells and antibodies
Permeability factor	Increases vascular permeability, allowing white cells into area
Interferon	Interferes with viral growth, stopping the spread of viral infection
Migration inhibitory factor	Suppresses movement of macrophages, keeping macrophage in area of foreign cells
Skin reactive factor	Induces inflammatory response
Cytotoxic factor (lymphotoxin)	Kills certain antigenic cells
Macrophage chemotactic factor	Attracts macrophages into the area
Lymphocyte blastogenic factor	Stimulates more lymphocytes, recruiting additional lymphocytes into the area
Macrophage aggregation factor	Causes clumping of macrophages and lymphocytes
Macrophage activation factor	Causes macrophages to adhere to surfaces more readily
Proliferation inhibitor factor	Inhibits growth of certain antigenic cells
Cytophilic antibody	A factor that binds to an Fc receptor on macrophages that permits them to bind to antigens

* Cytokines are biologically active substances released by cells to regulate growth and function of other cells within the immune system. Lymphocytes produce lymphokines, and monocytes and macrophages produce monokines. The table above lists some of the cytokines that play a role in immune system functioning.

vates all the other components in the sequence in which the other components were discovered, namely, C_1, C_4, C_2, C_3, C_5, C_6, C_7, C_8, and C_9.

Alternate Pathway of Complement Activation.   The alternative method of complement activation occurs without the formation of antigen–antibody complexes. This alternate pathway can be initiated by the release of bacterial products such as endotoxins. When complement is activated through this pathway, the process bypasses the first three components (C_1, C_4, and C_2) and begins with C_3. Whatever the method of activation, however, once activated, the complement can and does destroy cells by altering or damaging the cell membrane of the antigen, by chemically attracting phagocytes to the antigen (*chemotaxis*), and by rendering the antigen more vulnerable to phagocytosis (*opsonization*). The complement system enhances the inflammatory response by the release of vasoactive substances.

This response is usually therapeutic and can be lifesaving if the cell attacked by the complement system is a true foreign invader, such as a streptococcus or staphylococcus. However, if that cell is in reality part of the person—a cell of the brain or liver, the tissue lining the blood vessels, or the cells of a transplanted organ or skin graft—the result can be devastating

disease and even death. The result of the immune response—the vigorous attack on any material read as foreign, the deadliness of the struggle—is obvious in the purulent material, or pus (the remains of microbes, granulocytes, and macrophages, T-cell lymphocytes, plasma proteins, complement, and antibodies), that accumulates in wound infections and abscesses.

Interferons

Biologic response modifiers are currently under investigation to determine their roles in the immune system and their potential therapeutic effects in disorders characterized by disturbed immune responses. *Interferons*, one example of the compounds known as *biologic response modifiers*, have antiviral and antitumor properties. In addition to responding to viral infection, they are produced by T cells, B cells, and macrophages in response to antigens. They are thought to have a role in modifying the immune response by suppressing antibody production and cellular immunity. They also facilitate the cytolytic role of macrophages and natural killer cells. Interferons are undergoing extensive study to determine their effectiveness in the treatment of tumors and acquired immunodeficiency syndrome (AIDS).

Factors Affecting Immune System Functioning

Age. Persons at the extremes of the life span are more likely to develop problems related to immune system functioning than are those in their middle years. There is an increased frequency and severity of infections in the elderly, which may be a result of a decreased ability to respond adequately to invading organisms. Both the production and the function of T- and B-cell lymphocytes may be impaired. The incidence of autoimmune diseases also increases with aging; this may be related to a decreased ability of antibodies to differentiate between "self" and "nonself." Failure of the surveillance system to recognize mutant, or abnormal, cells may be responsible for the high incidence of cancer associated with increasing age.

Declining function of various organ systems associated with increasing age also contributes to impaired immunity. Decreased gastric secretions and motility allow normal intestinal flora to proliferate and produce infection, causing gastroenteritis and diarrhea. Decreased renal circulation, filtration, absorption, and excretion contribute to urinary tract infections. Prostatic enlargement and neurogenic bladder can hinder the passage of urine and subsequently bacterial clearance through the urinary system. Urinary stasis, common in the elderly, permits the growth of organisms.

Exposure to tobacco and environmental toxins will impair pulmonary function. Prolonged exposure to these agents causes decreased elasticity of lung tissue, decreased effectiveness of cilia, and a decreased ability to cough effectively. These impairments hinder the removal of infectious organisms and toxins, increasing the elderly person's susceptibility to pulmonary infections and malignancies.

Finally, with age the skin becomes thinner and less elastic. Peripheral neuropathy and the accompanying decreased sensation and circulation may facilitate stasis ulcers, pressure ulcers, abrasions, and burns. Impaired skin integrity predisposes the aging person to infection from organisms that are part of normal skin flora.

Nutrition. Adequate nutrition is essential for function of the immune system. Depletion of protein reserves results in atrophy of lymphoid tissues, depression of antibody response, reduction in the number of circulating T cells, and impairment of phagocytic function. As a result, susceptibility to infection is greatly increased. During periods of infection and serious illness, nutritional requirements may be exaggerated further, potentially contributing to protein depletion and an even greater risk of impaired immune response and sepsis.

Existence of Other Organ Diseases. Conditions such as burns or other forms of trauma, infection, and cancer may contribute to altered immune system function. Major burns or other factors cause impaired skin integrity and compromise the body's first line of defense. Loss of large amounts of serum with burn injuries depletes the body of essential proteins, including immunoglobulins. The physiologic and psychologic stressors induced during surgical disruption of tissue integrity stimulate cortisol release from the adrenal cortex; increased serum cortisol also contributes to suppression of normal immune responses.

Chronic illness may contribute to immune system impairments in a variety of ways. Renal failure is associated with a deficiency in circulating lymphocytes. In addition, immune defenses may be altered by acidosis and uremic toxins. An increased incidence of infection in diabetes has been associated with vascular insufficiency, neuropathy, and poor control of serum glucose levels. Recurrent respiratory tract infections are associated with chronic obstructive pulmonary disease (COPD) as a result of altered inspiratory and expiratory effort and ineffective airway clearance.

Cancer. Immunosuppression contributes to the development of malignancies. However, cancer itself is immunosuppressive. Large tumors are able to release antigens into the blood that combine with circulating antibodies and prevent them from attacking the tumor cells. Furthermore, tumor cells may possess special blocking factors that coat tumor cells and prevent destruction by killer T lymphocytes. During the early development of tumors, the body may fail to recognize the tumor antigens as foreign and subsequently fail to initiate destruction of malignant cells.

Hematologic malignancies such as leukemia and lymphoma are associated with altered production and function of white blood cells and lymphocytes.

Medications. Certain drug therapies are capable of causing both desirable and undesirable alterations in immune system functioning. Four major classifications of medications have the potential for causing immunosuppression: antibiotics, corticosteroids, nonsteroidal anti-inflammatory drugs (NSAIDs), and cytotoxic drugs (Table 48-2). Therapeutic use of these agents requires striking a delicate balance between therapeutic benefit and dangerous suppression of host defense mechanisms.

Radiation. Radiation therapy may be used in the treatment of cancer or in the prevention of allograft rejection. Radiation destroys lymphocytes and decreases the population of cells required to replace them. The size or extent of the irradiated area determines the extent of immunosuppression. Whole-body radiation may render the individual totally immunosuppressed.

In summary, the immune system is a complex one that protects the body against foreign substances and the proliferation of malignant cells. The normal immune response is activated by invasion by bacteria or viruses, by ingestion or injection of foreign substances, and by other modes of contact with antigens. Disorders of the immune system occur when the immune response is directed at the body's own tissues (*i.e.*, in autoimmune disorders), when the immune response is excessive (*i.e.*, in anaphylaxis), or when the immune response is depressed (by cancer or radiation; in acquired immunodeficiency syndrome). Immune disorders may be genetically determined, or acquired through infection with bacteria, viruses, and fungal or protozoan infections. Modification of the immune response by medication is necessary if transplantation of organs is to be successful. An altered immune system may occur with

TABLE 48–2.   Drugs That Can Compromise the Inflammatory–Immune Response

Classification and Examples of Drugs	Effects on Inflammatory–Immune Response
ANESTHETICS	
Halothane, ether, nitrous oxide, cyclopropane	Depression of T- and B-cell responses, inhibition of phagocytosis, altered allergic responses
ANTIBIOTICS (IN LARGE DOSES)	
Dactinomycin (Cosmegen)	Decreased antibody production
Chloramphenicol (Chloromycetin)	Hypoplasia of bone marrow
Mitomycin (Mutamycin)	Destruction of normal bacteria flora of gastrointestinal and respiratory tracts, allowing overgrowth of fungi or resistant strains of bacteria
CORTICOSTEROIDS (IN LARGE DOSES)	Decreased antibody production
	Decreased fibroplasia
	Decreased polymorphonuclear (PMN) leukocyte responses
	Decreased prostaglandin synthesis
CYTOTOXIC DRUGS	
Purine Antagonists Mercaptopurine (6-MP) (Purinethol)	Decreased antibody production in presence of antigen
Azathioprine (Imuran)	
Folic Acid Antagonists Methotrexate	Blocked conversion of folic acid to tetrahydrofolic acid, which is necessary for DNA and RNA synthesis, particularly in leukocytes
Alkylating Agents	Decreased antibody production
Mechlorethamine (Mustargen)	Destruction of circulating lymphocytes
Cyclophosphamide (Cytoxan)	Suppression of bone marrow production of leukocytes
Cyclosporine	Inhibition of T-cell function
	Defects in cell-mediated responses, inhibition of T-cell proliferation and activation
ALCOHOL (IN LARGE AMOUNTS)	Depressed bone marrow production of leukocytes
	Decreased Kupffer cell activity
HEROIN ADDICTION	Unknown action
ASPIRIN (IN LARGE DOSES)	Inhibition of prostaglandin synthesis and release
INDOMETHACIN (INDOCIN) (IN LARGE DOSES)	Inhibition of prostaglandin synthesis and release

(Adapted from Jett MF and Lancaster LE. The inflammatory immune response: The body's defense against invasion. Crit Care Nurs 1983 Sept/Oct; 3[5]:64–86.)

medications used to treat other disorders (*i.e.*, antibiotics, corticosteroids, or nonsteroidal anti-inflammatory drugs). Alteration of the immune system also occurs as a result of the aging process.

Disorders of the Immune System

Disorders of the immune system can be divided into two general categories, one related to immunopathology and the other to immunodeficiencies. Disorders related to *immunopathology* are those diseases in which the normally protective immune response paradoxically turns against or attacks the body, leading to tissue damage. Disorders related to *immunodeficiencies* are those diseases in which there is either an unexplained (primary) or explained (secondary) defect in one or more components of the immune response.

Immunopathology

When the body fails to differentiate between self and nonself, *immunopathology* may develop. This is a determining factor that allows the disease-producing potential of the immune response to take precedence over its protective nature. If the antigen is truly foreign, we are protected; if not, autoimmune disease and associated tissue damage result. The underlying problems of immunopathology may involve any component of the immune system in a variety of adverse interactions referred to as *hypersensitivity reactions*.

Allergic/Anaphylactoid Reaction (Hypersensitivity Type I)

An *allergic reaction* is a result of antigen–antibody reactions (specifically IgE) that attract and destroy mast cells and basophils. Basophils are found in the general circulation, and mast cells (fixed basophils) are particularly abundant in connective tissue found in the lungs, intestinal mucosa, skin, and blood vessels. These cells serve as storage sites for potent vasoactive chemicals such as bradykinin, prostaglandins, and serotonin. When the antigen and antibody combine, mast cells and basophils explosively release vasoactive chemicals, causing sneezing, rhinitis, and watery eyes. Anaphylaxis, the most extreme reaction, involves laryngobronchospasm, shock, hypotension, and, potentially, death.

Cytotoxicity Reaction (Hypersensitivity Type II)

A cytotoxicity reaction occurs when the system mistakenly identifies a normal constituent of the body as foreign. Such reactions may be a result of a cross-reacting antibody and eventually lead to cell and tissue damage. An example of this is seen in myasthenia gravis, in which the body mistakenly generates antibodies against normal receptors of nerve endings. Another example is seen in Goodpasture's syndrome, in which antibodies against lung and renal tissue are generated, producing lung damage and renal failure.

In some instances, antigens may bind to the membrane of normal cells within the system and stimulate antibody and complement activation. An example of this is seen in drug-induced hemolytic anemia. The drug can bind to the membrane of a red blood cell and form an antigenic complex with the surface of the red blood cell. Antibody production and complement activation result in red blood cell destruction and severe anemia characterized by fever, weakness, fatigue, and jaundice.

Immune Complex–Mediated Reaction (Hypersensitivity Type III)

Immune complexes (antigen–antibody molecules) normally circulate in the bloodstream during the course of infectious diseases. Usually, these complexes cause no symptoms and eventually disappear from the circulation. However, in some persons these large complexes are deposited in the lining of blood vessels or on tissue surfaces. As a result, the complement system is activated and vasculitis (inflammation of blood vessels) and other tissue damage may occur. The vessels of the joints and kidneys are particularly susceptible to this type of injury. Examples of this process include glomerulonephritis and systemic lupus erythematosus (SLE). Antigen–antibody complexes involving streptococcus are often responsible for glomerulonephritis. In SLE, abnormal suppressor T-cell function may contribute to the development of antibodies generated against the body's own DNA. DNA/anti-DNA complexes may lead to arthritis and a form of glomerulonephritis associated with SLE.

Delayed Hypersensitivity (Hypersensitivity Type IV)

A delayed hypersensitivity reaction may occur as a result of exposure to microbial infections or to skin irritants, such as chemicals found in cosmetics or poison ivy. This type of hypersensitivity is dependent on lymphokines released from T-cell lymphocytes. As a result of the release of the lymphokines, inflammatory reactions can occur, leading to such problems as contact dermatitis, graft rejection, and the formation of granulomas.

In an attempt to isolate, contain, and block an invading microbe, the body may recruit a large mass of cells. This mass of cells surrounds and "walls off" the organism from the rest of the body in order to prevent dissemination and further infection. As a result, a granuloma is formed. An example of this type of response is the body's response to the tubercle bacillus. Unfortunately, as in tuberculosis, large caseating lung abscesses may be formed, compromising organ function.

Management

Treatment of immunopathology falls into two categories: (1) removal of the offending antigens and (2) suppression of the immune response through immunosuppression. Unfortunately, the vast majority of antigens that cause immune disease have not yet been identified or, if known, cannot be removed from the body because they constitute normal cellular elements. Use of immunosuppression has become the most common method for dealing with immune reactions.

Immunosuppressive drugs may be classified according to their chemical structure and/or mechanism of action. Regardless of classification, most immunosuppressive drugs work by interfering with normal cell growth and metabolism. Some of these drugs were first used by cancer specialists in the treatment of malignancies because of their detrimental effects on cancer cells. Immunosuppressive drugs also impede the growth and metabolism of T- and B-cell lymphocytes. For this reason, they are used in the treatment of immunopathology.

Immunosuppressive therapy, however, is not without potential adverse effects. The use of antimetabolites, for example, may increase the risk of infections and malignancies such as leukemia and non-Hodgkin's lymphoma. Steroid therapy may increase the risk of infections or mask the signs and symptoms of infection. In addition, steroids may contribute to the development of hypertension, diabetes, gastrointestinal bleeding, cataracts, changes in appearance, and psychosis.

In view of the potential adverse effects of immunosuppressive therapy, the nurse has a key role in patient education and continuing assessment for potential complications. This role has special importance for nurses involved in the care of the older adult, who is already at risk for immune dysfunction.

Immunodeficiency

The second type of disorder of the immune system is immunodeficiency. Regardless of the underlying cause of immu-

TABLE 48-3.   *Primary Immunodeficiencies*

Immune Component	Underlying Abnormality	Example
Nonspecific immunity	Phagocytic dysfunction: chemotaxis, opsonization, ingestion, and digestion	Chronic granulomatous disease
Humoral immunity	Immunoglobulin production: decrease in or absence of one or all of the immunoglobulins (hypogammaglobulinemia)	Hypogammaglobulinemia
Cellular immunity	Abnormal or absent T-lymphocyte production	DiGeorge syndrome
Combined deficiencies	Abnormalities of more than one component of the immune system	Wiskott–Aldrich syndrome

nodeficiency, the cardinal symptoms include recurrent, severe infections often involving unusual organisms. Immunodeficiencies may be classified as either primary or secondary, and also according to which components of the immune system are affected.

Primary Immunodeficiencies

Immunodeficiencies for which there are no known causes or underlying medical conditions are referred to as primary immunodeficiencies. They may involve one or a combination of components of the immune system (Table 48-3).

Manifestations of immune deficiency disease are related to the role that the deficient component plays. T-cell defects are associated with viral, fungal, or protozoan infections, while B-cell defects are associated with bacterial infections. The prognosis is generally poor because most affected individuals develop overwhelming fatal infections. Treatment options under investigation include bone marrow transplantation, intravenous immunoglobulin replacement, and thymus gland transplantation.

Secondary Immunodeficiencies

Secondary immunodeficiencies, which are more common than primary deficiencies, often occur in the course of underlying disease or health care problems as a result of the treatment or

TABLE 48-4.   *Factors Contributing to Secondary Immunodeficiencies*

Immune Deficit	Examples
Alteration in skin integrity	Venipunctures, burns, trauma
Alteration in nutrition (deficit)	Anorexia, malabsorption, and impaired ingestion, digestion, and assimilation; severe protein losses in urine
Alteration in urinary elimination	Urinary stasis, bladder catheterization
Immunosuppressive therapy	Chemotherapy, antibiotics
Malignancy	Leukemia, lymphoma
Infectious processes	Septicemia, HIV (AIDS)

of the conditions themselves. Persons with secondary immunodeficiencies are immunosuppressed and are often referred to as *immunocompromised hosts*. A variety of factors contribute to the development of secondary immunodeficiency (Table 48-4). The goals of treatment include elimination of the contributing factors and use of sound principles of infection control. AIDS is an example of a devastating secondary immunodeficiency that results in increased susceptibility of the patient to a variety of infections and rare malignancies. This syndrome is discussed in detail in the section that follows.

Acquired Immunodeficiency Syndrome

AIDS is defined as the most severe form of a continuum of illnesses associated with *human immunodeficiency virus* (HIV) infection. HIV has previously been referred to as human T-cell lymphotropic virus type III (HTLV III) and lymphadenopathy-associated virus (LAV). Manifestations of HIV infection range from mild abnormalities in the immune response without overt signs and symptoms to profound immunosuppression associated with a variety of life-threatening infections and rare malignancies.

Pathology

HIV belongs to a group of viruses known as *retroviruses*. The designation of retrovirus indicates that these viruses carry their genetic material in RNA rather than DNA. HIV is known to selectively infect helper T-cell lymphocytes. Through the use of an enzyme known as *reverse transcriptase*, HIV is able to reprogram the genetic materials of the infected T_4 cell. As a result, HIV can use the T_4 cell to produce the virus instead of itself. Consequently, whenever the infected T_4 cell is stimulated to reproduce by invading organisms, HIV is reproduced instead of the T_4 lymphocyte. The newly produced virus can then infect other T_4 lymphocytes.

The rate of HIV production is thought to be associated with the current health status of the infected individual. If the individual is not fighting another infection, such as cytomegalovirus or hepatitis, at the time of HIV infection, HIV reproduction may proceed slowly. If the individual is combating another infection at the time of HIV infection, HIV reproduction appears to be accelerated. This may explain the latent period exhibited by some individuals after transmission and infection with HIV. It has been estimated that 20% to 30% of HIV-infected individuals will develop AIDS within 5 years of infection.

As was discussed earlier in this chapter, the T_4 lymphocyte plays several important roles in the immune response, including recognition of foreign antigens, activation of antibody-producing B-cell lymphocytes, stimulation of cytotoxic T lymphocytes, production of lymphokines, and defense against parasitic infections. When T_4-lymphocyte function is impaired, organisms that do not usually cause disease are given the opportunity to invade and cause serious illness. Infections and malignancies that develop as a result of immune system impairment are referred to as *opportunistic infections or diseases*.

HIV is also able to enter other cells such as monocytes and macrophages. The cell membrane marker on these cells, known as CD4, is very similar to the cell membrane marker found on the T_4 lymphocyte. Monocytes and macrophages serve as reservoirs for HIV, allowing the virus to hide from the immune system and to be transported throughout the system to infect a variety of body tissues. Most of these tissues either contain the CD4 molecule or have the ability to produce it (Fig. 48-5).

Incidence

As of January 1991, there were slightly more than 161,000 cases of AIDS diagnosed in the United States. Current data suggest that as many as 1.5 million people are infected with HIV. The Public Health Services (PHS) has estimated that 390,000 to 480,000 cases of AIDS will have occurred in the United States by the end of 1992, with an associated 285,000 to 340,000 deaths.

In the United States, most (59%) persons with AIDS have engaged in male homosexual behaviors. An increasing percentage (22%) of cases are related to intravenous drug use (IVDU). Other high-risk behaviors or means of exposure include heterosexual contact with sexual partners with HIV infection or at risk for HIV infection (5%) and blood or blood product transfusions with products infected with HIV (especially prior to screening of blood) (2%). Most (84%) of children with AIDS are born to mothers with HIV infection or at risk for HIV infection. As compared to whites, there has been an increasing percentage of AIDS cases in the black and Hispanic populations. It has been suggested that this may be largely related to IVDU and a lack of access to health care and education. Large urban areas continue to report more cases of AIDS than rural areas because of a higher incidence of IV drug use and homosexual practices. HIV is predominantly an infection of young people, with the majority of cases involving persons between 17 and 55 years of age; however, it has also been reported in elderly men and women. The number of women with HIV infection is also growing at an alarming rate. AIDS has reached epidemic proportions in other parts of the world as well.

Transmission

The routes of transmission of HIV are very similar to those of hepatitis type B. In male homosexuals, anal intercourse or manipulation increases chances of trauma to the rectal mucosa and subsequently increases chances of exposure to the virus through body secretions. Increased frequency of this practice and multiple sexual partners have contributed to the spread of this disease. Heterosexual intercourse with individuals who have been directly exposed to HIV is also a mode of transmission that is growing in significance.

Transmission among intravenous drug users occurs through direct blood exposure to contaminated needles and syringes. Although the amount of blood in a syringe is relatively small, the cumulative effect of repeated sharing of contaminated equipment leads to an increased risk of virus transmission.

Blood products, including those used by hemophiliacs, are capable of transmitting HIV to the recipients. The risk associated with transfusions has been greatly reduced as a result of voluntary self-deferral, serologic testing, heat-treating of clotting factor concentrates, and other blood-inactivation methods. The incidence for health care workers who are exposed to HIV through needle-stick injury is estimated to be less than 1%. Transmission of HIV infection to health care workers through mucocutaneous exposure has not been documented. Large-scale studies of exposed health care workers are being conducted by the Centers for Disease Control (CDC) as well as other groups throughout the country. The virus may also be transmitted *in utero* from mother to child and during the postpartum period through breastfeeding.

When an individual is infected with HIV, the immune system responds by producing antibodies against the virus. Antibodies generally develop within 1 to 4 months of exposure but may take as long as 6 to 14 months. Unfortunately, the antibodies for HIV are ineffective and are not able to halt the development of HIV infection. The ability to document the presence of HIV antibodies in the blood has permitted screening of blood products and has facilitated diagnostic evaluations

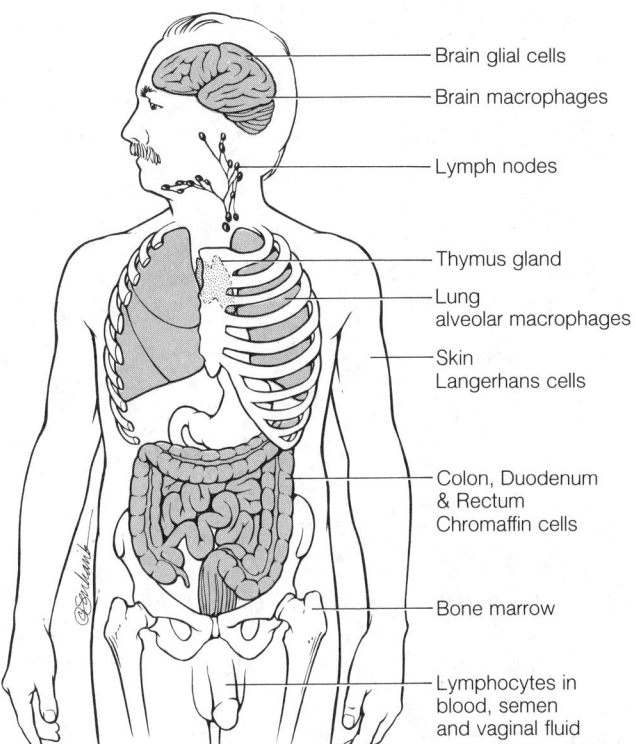

Brain glial cells

Brain macrophages

Lymph nodes

Thymus gland

Lung
alveolar macrophages

Skin
Langerhans cells

Colon, Duodenum
& Rectum
Chromaffin cells

Bone marrow

Lymphocytes in
blood, semen
and vaginal fluid

Figure 48–5.   Potential sites where HIV may be harbored.

of individuals with HIV infection. In 1985, the Food and Drug Administration (FDA) licensed an HIV antibody assay for all blood and plasma donations.

The ELISA (enzyme-linked immunosorbent assay) test determines the presence of antibodies directed specifically against HIV. The ELISA test does not establish a diagnosis of AIDS but rather indicates that the individual has been exposed to or infected with HIV. Persons whose blood contains antibodies for HIV are said to be *seropositive*. The *Western blot assay* is another test that can identify the presence of HIV antibodies and is used to confirm seropositivity as identified by the ELISA procedure. These tests are also used by physicians to assist in diagnosing patients with AIDS.

The results of HIV antibody testing are explained carefully to the patient undergoing testing. The implications of antibody test results are summarized in Chart 48-2. Education concerning transmission is discussed whenever HIV antibody testing is obtained.

Diagnostic Evaluation

The manifestations of HIV infections vary. Diagnosis is based on clinical history, identification of risk factors, physical examination, laboratory evidence of immune dysfunction, identification of HIV antibodies, signs and symptoms, and infections and/or malignancies included in the CDC classification system for HIV infection (Table 48-5). This classification system is intended to help define the spectrum of HIV infection (Table 48-6).

Group I includes those individuals with acute HIV infection. This is characterized by a mononucleosis-type syndrome involving fever, chills, muscle and joint aching, maculopapular rash, abdominal cramps, diarrhea, and enlarged lymph nodes. This phase often is associated with seroconversion. In group II, individuals are generally seropositive but often lack overt signs and symptoms of illness. If examined or tested, these individuals might have enlarged lymph nodes as well as laboratory evidence of immune dysfunction (Chart 48-3). Group III includes those persons with signs and symptoms such as fatigue, fevers, night sweats, laboratory evidence of immune dysfunction, and persistent generalized lymphadenopathy (PGL). PGL refers to the presence of two or more enlarged noninguinal lymph nodes larger than 1 cm in size lasting for 3 months or longer. Group IV encompasses individuals with more serious manifestations of HIV infection, including AIDS. This group is further divided into five categories, including the following: (1) debilitating constitutional symptoms (fever, weight loss greater than 10% of body weight, fatigue, diarrhea, and PGL) previously referred to as AIDS-related complex or ARC, (2) neurologic impairments, (3) opportunistic infections, (4) malignancies, and (5) other conditions such as adrenal insufficiency, HIV nephropathy, and interstitial pneumonitis. Often, individuals with severe HIV infection will have disease manifestations from more than one category. The diagnosis of AIDS is reserved for those persons who develop life-threatening opportunistic infections and malignancies.

Clinical Manifestations

The clinical manifestations of AIDS are widespread and may affect virtually any organ system. Diseases associated with HIV infection and AIDS result from infections, malignancies, and/or the direct effect of HIV on body tissues. The following dis-

---

Chart 48–2
Interpreting Antibody Tests for HIV

HIV antibody is produced by the body in response to HIV infection. Seropositivity does not diagnose AIDS or project future illness. Test results must be interpreted with some caution.

A *Positive Test Result* DOES Mean:
- Antibodies to the AIDS virus are present in your blood.
- You have been infected with the AIDS virus and your body has produced antibodies.
- You probably have active virus in your body and should assume that you are capable of passing the virus to others.

A *Positive Test* DOES NOT Mean:
- You necessarily have AIDS.
- You will necessarily get AIDS in the future.
- You are immune to AIDS.

A *Negative Test* DOES Mean:
- Antibodies to the virus are not present in your blood at this time.
Two possible reasons for this are:
- You have not been infected with the virus OR
- You have been infected with the virus, but have not yet produced antibodies (which takes from 2 weeks to 6 months, or even longer).

A *Negative Test* DOES NOT Mean:
- You have nothing to worry about (you may contact the virus and become infected at a later date).
- You are immune to the virus.
- You have not been infected with the virus (you may have been infected and have not yet produced antibodies).

(Adapted from Carr GS and Gee G. AIDS and AIDS-related conditions: Screening for populations at risk. Nurse Pract 1986 Oct; 11[10]:44.)

TABLE 48-5. *Infections and Malignancies Defining AIDS*

VIRAL
Cytomegalovirus (CMV)
Herpes simplex—chronic mucocutaneous or disseminated
Papovavirus—progressive multifocal leukoencephalopathy

PARASITIC
Cryptosporidiosis
Isosporiasis
Pneumocystis carinii pneumonia
Strongyloidiasis
Toxoplasmosis

FUNGAL
Candidiasis—esophageal or pulmonary
Cryptococcosis
Histoplasmosis

BACTERIAL
Mycobacterium avium-intracellulare (MAI)
Mycobacterium kansasii

NEOPLASMS
Kaposi's sarcoma
Lymphoma, isolated cerebral
Non-Hodgkin's lymphoma

OTHER
Lymphoid interstitial pneumonia (children only)

(Cummings D. Caring for the HIV-infected adult. Nurse Pract 1988 Nov; 13[11]:34.)

cussion is limited to the most common clinical manifestations of severe HIV infection.

Pulmonary. Shortness of breath, dyspnea, cough, chest pain, and fever are associated with a variety of opportunistic infections such as those caused by *Mycobacterium avium-intracellulare* (MAI), cytomegaloviruses, and *Legionella*. However, the most common infection in persons with AIDS is *Pneumocystis carinii* pneumonia (PCP), which has a mortality rate of approximately 60%. *Pneumocystis carinii*, a protozoan, causes disease only in immunocompromised hosts. It invades and proliferates within the pulmonary alveoli, resulting in consolidation of the pulmonary parenchyma.

The clinical presentation of PCP in the AIDS patient is generally less acute than in persons who are immunosuppressed as a result of other conditions. The period of time between the onset of symptoms and the actual documentation of disease may be weeks to months. Patients with AIDS initially develop nonspecific signs and symptoms such as fevers, chills, nonproductive cough, shortness of breath, dyspnea, and occasionally chest pain. PCP may be present despite the absence of crackles or rhonchi. Room air arterial oxygen concentrations may be mildly decreased, indicating minimal hypoxemia. Untreated, PCP will eventually progress to cause significant pulmonary impairment and ultimately respiratory failure. A small number of patients have a dramatic onset and fulminant course, involving severe hypoxemia, cyanosis, tachypnea, and altered

mental status. Respiratory failure can develop within 2 to 3 days of initial onset of symptoms.

PCP can be diagnosed definitively by identifying the organism in lung tissue or bronchial secretions. This is accomplished by sputum induction, bronchial–alveolar lavage, or transbronchial biopsy obtained by using a fiberoptic bronchoscope.

Mycobacterium-avium complex (MAC) disease is emerging as a leading cause of bacterial infections in persons with AIDS. Organisms belonging to MAC include *M. avium, M. intracellulare,* and *M. scrofulaceum.* MAC, a group of acid-fast bacilli, usually cause respiratory infection but are also commonly found in the gastrointestinal tract, lymph nodes, and bone marrow. Most patients with AIDS have widespread disease at the time of diagnosis and are often debilitated. MAC infections are associated with rising mortality rates. Treatment has not been clearly established and involves multidrug regimens which are given over a prolonged period.

Gastrointestinal. The gastrointestinal manifestations of AIDS include loss of appetite, nausea, vomiting, oral and esophageal candidiasis, and chronic diarrhea. *Diarrhea* is a problem for 50% to 90% of all AIDS patients. In some instances, gastrointestinal symptoms may be related to the direct effect of HIV on the cells lining the intestines. Some of the enteric pathogens that occur most frequently, which are identified by stool cultures or intestinal biopsy, include *Cryptosporidium muris, Salmonella,* cytomegalovirus (CMV), *Clostridium difficile,* and *Mycobacterium avium-intracellulare.* For patients with AIDS, the effects of diarrhea can be devastating in terms of profound weight loss (more than 10% of body weight), fluid and electrolyte imbalances, perianal skin excoriation, weakness, and inability to carry out usual activities of daily living. Although many forms of infectious diarrhea respond to treatment, it is not unusual for the infections to recur and become a chronic problem.

Oral candidiasis, a fungal infection, is nearly universal in all patients with AIDS and AIDS-related conditions. The development of oral candidiasis often precedes other life-threatening infections. It is characterized by the presence of creamy white patches in the oral cavity. When untreated, oral candidiasis will progress to involve the esophagus. Associated signs and symptoms include difficult and painful swallowing and retrosternal pain. Some patients also develop ulcerating

TABLE 48-6. *CDC Classification System for HIV Infection*

Group I. Acute infection
Group II. Asymptomatic infection
Group III. Persistent generalized lymphadenopathy
Group IV. Other disease
  Subgroup A. Constitutional disease
  Subgroup B. Neurologic disease
  Subgroup C. Secondary infectious diseases
    Category C-1. Specified secondary infectious diseases listed in the CDC surveillance definition for AIDS
    Category C-2. Other specified secondary infectious diseases.
  Subgroup D. Secondary cancers
  Subgroup E. Other conditions

(Centers for Disease Control, U.S. Department of Health and Human Services. Classification system for human T-lymphotropic virus III/ lymphadenopathy–associated virus infections. Ann Intern Med 1986 Aug; 105[2]:235.)

Chart 48–3
Signs and Symptoms and Laboratory Studies Indicating Immune Dysfunction

Clinical Signs/Symptoms

Chronic condition present for 3 months or longer, *unexplained.*
Lymphadenopathy ≥ 2 noninguinal sites
Fever ≥ 38°C, intermittent or continuous
Unexplained diarrhea
Unexplained fatigue/malaise
Unexplained night sweating

Laboratory Studies

Decreased number of T-helper cells
Decreased ratio of T-helper:T-suppressor lymphocytes
Anemia *or* leukopenia *or* thrombocytopenia *or* lymphopenia
Increased serum globulin levels
Decreased blastogenic response of lymphocytes to mitogens
Cutaneous anergy to multiple skin-test antigens
Increased levels of circulating immune complexes

(Gottlieb MS and Groopman JE [eds]. AIDS. New York, Alan R Liss, 1984. Reprinted with permission.)

---

oral lesions and are particularly susceptible to dissemination of candidiasis to other body systems.

Neurologic. An estimated 50% to 60% of all patients with AIDS experience some form of neurologic involvement during the course of HIV infection. Another 20% to 30% will have neurologic involvement without overt signs or symptoms. Neurologic complications involve central, peripheral, and autonomic functions. Neuropathology results from the direct effects of HIV on nervous system tissue or the immune system response to HIV infection and includes inflammation, atrophy, demyelination, degeneration, and necrosis. Other manifestations are related to infections and malignancies involving the neurologic system.

Cryptococcus neoformans, a fungal infection, is the fourth most common opportunistic infection among patients with AIDS. Cryptococcal meningitis is characterized by symptoms such as fever, headache, malaise, stiff neck, nausea, vomiting, mental status changes, and seizures. Diagnosis is confirmed by examination of cerebrospinal fluid (CSF).

HIV encephalopathy, previously referred to as AIDS dementia complex, occurs in at least 40% to 65% of patients with AIDS. It is a clinical syndrome characterized by a progressive decline in cognitive, behavioral, and motor functions. Signs and symptoms may be subtle and difficult to distinguish from fatigue, depression, or the adverse effects of treatments for infections and malignancies. Early manifestations include memory deficits, headache, difficulty with concentration, progressive confusion, psychomotor slowing, apathy, and ataxia. The later stages of HIV encephalopathy include global cognitive impairments, delay in oral responses, vacant starelike appearance, spastic paraparesis, hyperreflexia, psychosis, hallucinations, tremor, incontinence, seizures, mutism, and death. Confirming the diagnosis of HIV encephalopathy may be difficult. Extensive neurologic evaluation includes a computed tomography (CT) scan that may indicate diffuse cerebral atrophy and

ventricular enlargement. Other tests that may indicate abnormalities include magnetic resonance imaging (MRI), examination of CSF through lumbar puncture, and brain biopsy.

Progressive multifocal leukoencephalopathy (PML) is a central nervous system demyelinating disorder that is associated with AIDS. This disorder, which is caused by a virus, may begin with mental confusion and rapidly progress to include blindness, aphasia, paresis, and ultimately death. Other common infections involving the nervous system include *Toxoplasma gondii* and *Cryptococcus neoformans.*

Other neurologic manifestations include both central and peripheral neuropathies. Vascular myelopathy is a degenerative disorder affecting lateral and posterior columns of the spinal cord, resulting in progressive spastic paraparesis, ataxia, and incontinence. HIV-related peripheral neuropathy is thought to be a demyelinating disorder associated with painful numbness in the extremities, weakness, diminished deep tendon reflexes, orthostatic hypotension, and impotence.

Malignancy. Individuals with AIDS have a higher than normal incidence of cancer. This may be related to HIV stimulation of developing cancer cells or the immune deficiency allowing cancer-causing substances such as viruses to transform susceptible cells into malignant cells. Kaposi's sarcoma and certain types of B-cell lymphomas are included in the CDC classification of AIDS-related malignancies. The following malignancies also occur more frequently than expected in persons with AIDS: carcinomas of the skin, stomach, pancreas, rectum, and bladder.

Kaposi's sarcoma (KS) (pronounced KA-po-sheez), the most common malignancy seen in HIV infection, is a disease involving the endothelial layer of blood and lymphatic vessels. When first noted in 1872, KS characteristically presented as lower-extremity skin lesions in elderly men of Eastern European ancestry. In that population, the disease was slow to progress and easily treated. In the AIDS population, epidemic KS is most

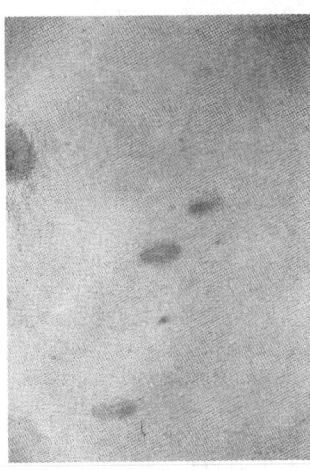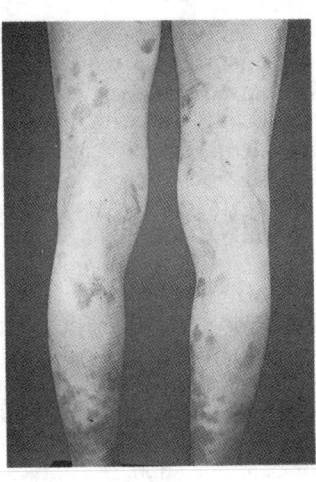

Figure 48-6. Epidemic Kaposi's sarcoma. (**A**) The elongated, pinkish brown macules and early plaque-stage lesions located on the chest are typical of this tumor seen in patients with AIDS. Some of the lesions are slightly hyperpigmented. (**B**) Throughout the course of the disease, increasing numbers of lesions continue to appear, although lesions often remain as flat plaques rather than develop into nodules. In this patient, lesions rapidly increased in number and were widely disseminated, with confluency of neighboring lesions occurring in certain areas. The symmetry of the eruption is typical of the epidemic form of Kaposi's sarcoma. (Redrawn from DeVita VT Jr, Hellman S, and Rosenberg SA [eds]. AIDS: Etiology, Diagnosis, Treatment and Prevention, 2nd ed. Philadelphia, JB Lippincott, 1988.)

often seen in male homosexuals and bisexuals. This form of KS ranges from localized cutaneous lesions to disseminated disease involving multiple organ systems. Cutaneous lesions appearing anywhere on the body are usually brownish pink to deep purple. They may be either flat or raised and surrounded by ecchymosis and edema (Fig. 48-6). Rapid development of lesions involving large areas of skin is associated with extensive disfigurement.

The location and size of some lesions can lead to venous stasis, lymphedema, and pain. Fungating or ulcerative lesions cause disruption in skin integrity and increase patient discomfort and susceptibility to infection. The most common sites of visceral involvement include the lymph nodes, gastrointestinal tract, and lungs. Involvement of internal organs may eventually lead to organ failure, hemorrhage, infection, and death. Diagnosis of KS is confirmed through biopsy of suspected lesions.

B-cell lymphomas are the second most common malignancy occurring in the AIDS population. Lymphomas associated with AIDS often differ from those occurring in the general population. Patients with AIDS are generally much younger than the usual population developing non-Hodgkin's lymphoma. In addition, AIDS-related lymphomas tend to develop outside of the lymph nodes, most commonly in the brain, bone marrow, and gastrointestinal tract. These types of lymphomas are characteristically of a higher grade, indicating aggressive growth and resistance to treatment. The course of AIDS-related lymphomas includes multiple sites of organ involvement and complications related to the development of opportunistic infections.

Integumentary. Cutaneous manifestations are associated with HIV infection and the accompanying opportunistic infec-

tions and malignancies. Kaposi's sarcoma has been previously described. Opportunistic infections such as herpes zoster and herpes simplex are associated with painful vesicles that disrupt skin integrity. Molluscum contagiosum is a viral infection characterized by deforming plaque formation. Seborrheic dermatitis is associated with an indurated, diffuse, scaly rash involving the scalp and face. AIDS patients may also exhibit a generalized folliculitis associated with dry, flaking skin or atopic dermatitis such as eczema or psoriasis. Up to 60% of patients treated with trimethoprim-sulfamethoxazole (TMP/SMZ) for PCP develop a drug-related rash that is pruritic with pinkish red macules and papules. Regardless of the origin of these cutaneous manifestations, patients experience discomfort and are at increased risk for additional infection due to disruptions in skin integrity.

Clinical Manifestations of HIV Infection in Women. Persistent, recurrent vaginal candidiasis may be the first sign of HIV infection in women. Lesions of vaginal candidiasis and genital herpes may be large, deep, painful lesions requiring continuous therapy. Ulcerative sexually transmitted diseases (STDs) are more severe in these women. Human papillomavirus (HPV) and cervical cancer have been reported to have an increased incidence and severity in the woman with HIV infection. Failure of health care providers to consider HIV infection in women may lead to later diagnosis and failure of women to receive appropriate treatment.

Chronic Illness. Almost all AIDS patients develop at least one opportunistic infection during the course of their disease. Although many infections are successfully treated, some persons never fully recover and are at increased risk for developing a second infection or malignancy. Treatment is often complicated by the debilitating signs and symptoms of HIV infection that include unexplained fatigue, headache, profuse night sweats, unexplained weight loss, dry cough, shortness of breath, extreme weakness, diarrhea, and persistent lymphadenopathy. Chronic illness develops when opportunistic diseases and the symptoms of HIV do not resolve.

The effects of chronic illness—repeated and prolonged hospitalizations—can be devastating. Persons who progress to the terminal phases of HIV infection are usually severely immunocompromised. Multiple local and disseminated infections involving several organ systems are common. Many persons become profoundly malnourished as a result of impaired oral intake, gastrointestinal malabsorption, and the effects of opportunistic diseases. Pulmonary, renal, and hepatic failure may develop as a result of infection or malignancy. Skin breakdown related to immobility, profuse diarrhea, and progression of KS is common. Neurologic impairments may progress to coma and eventually death.

Patients in the advanced stages of AIDS are often no longer able to work, maintain current roles or relationships, or care for themselves independently. Although the length of survival varies from months to years, approximately half of all the cases that have occurred since 1981 have resulted in death. Death occurs because either there is no known effective treatment for the opportunistic diseases or the patient no longer responds to standard therapy.

Management

Medical management efforts encompass several approaches, including treatment of HIV-associated infections and malignancies, arresting HIV growth and replication through antiviral agents, and augmentation and restoration of the immune system through the use of immunomodulators. Also essential is supportive care for the debilitating effects of chronic illness, such as malnutrition, skin breakdown, weakness, immobility, and altered mental status. It is hoped that the development of a vaccine in the future will assist in preventing HIV infection.

HIV-*Related Infections.* In the last several years, there have been many advances in the treatment of *Pneumocystis* pneumonia (PCP).

Trimethoprim-sulfamethoxazole (TMP/SMZ) is an antibacterial drug that is used to treat a variety of organisms causing infection. It has long been the treatment of choice for PCP in non-AIDS patients. Unfortunately, AIDS patients with PCP who are treated with TMP/SMZ have experienced an increased incidence of adverse effects, such as rashes, decreased white blood cell counts, and drug-related fevers. These adverse effects have been reported in as many as 65% of all AIDS patients treated with TMP/SMZ. Pentamidine, an antiprotozoal drug, is a second option for combating PCP. Many physicians initiate treatment with TMP/SMZ and change to pentamidine if adverse effects develop or patients do not show evidence of clinical improvement when treated with TMP/SMZ. The adverse effects of pentamidine include the formation of sterile abscesses at the site of intramuscular injection, impaired glucose metabolism, renal damage, and bone marrow suppression.

Recently, aerosolized delivery of pentamidine has proved effective for the prophylaxis and treatment of PCP. The inhaled particles are delivered directly to the alveoli, the site of infection. There are fewer associated side effects because only small amounts of the drug enter the systemic circulation. Patients are instructed on the use of nebulizers for home administration of aerosolized pentamidine. Other drugs being investigated for their role in the treatment of PCP include dapsone, trimethoprim-dapsone, trimetrexate, and clindamycin with primaquine.

The traditional therapy for cryptococcal meningitis has been intravenous amphotericin B administered for at least 4 to 6 weeks. The patient is monitored for serious potential adverse effects of amphotericin B including anaphylaxis, renal and hepatic impairment, electrolyte imbalances, anemia, fevers, and rigors. Frequent relapses and high mortality rates often necessitate prolonged therapy. In some instances, the patient continues to receive intravenous amphotericin in the home setting. The patient's ability to continue therapy at home is evaluated. The patient requires long-term venous access and education concerning intravenous administration of amphotericin and management of adverse reactions. Recently, the FDA approved fluconazole as an antifungal agent to be used as maintenance therapy for cryptococcal meningitis. This medication is available in an oral form and is not associated with serious adverse effects. Investigators continue to examine the role of fluconazole and other antifungal agents in the treatment of cryptococcal infections.

Retinitis caused by cytomegalovirus (CMV) is a leading cause of blindness in individuals with AIDS. Recently, the FDA approved the use of ganciclovir for the treatment of CMV retinitis. Because ganciclovir does not kill the virus, but rather controls its growth, it must be given for the remainder of the patient's life. Discontinuation of the drug is associated with relapse of retinitis within 1 month. Initially, ganciclovir is given intravenously every 8 to 12 hours for 2 weeks. Maintenance therapy is given once a day for 5 to 7 days each week. In some instances, patients will have progression of disease despite

treatment. Adverse effects that necessitate patient teaching and outpatient monitoring include bone marrow suppression producing a decrease in white blood cell and platelet counts, oral candidiasis, and liver and renal impairments. Patients require long-term venous access and education concerning home administration of ganciclovir. Other drugs being investigated for the treatment of CMV retinitis include foscarnet, acyclovir, granulocyte colony-stimulating factor, and beta-interferon.

A variety of antimicrobial drugs are being investigated in the treatment of infections such as *Candida* esophagitis, *Toxoplasmosis gondii*, cryptococcal meningitis, herpes zoster and herpes simplex, and disseminated CMV.

Malignancies. In the past, treatment for Kaposi's sarcoma (KS) has relied on the use of chemotherapeutic agents such as Adriamycin, vinblastine, vincristine, and methotrexate alone or in combination. Use of these drugs has been met with limited success and further compromise of the patient's immune status. Recently, the FDA approved the use of alpha-interferon for the treatment of KS. Interferon (previously discussed in Chap. 19) is known for its antiviral and antitumor effects. It has also been shown to enhance immune system functioning. Response rates have ranged between 30% and 50%, with the best responses seen in patients with limited disease and absence of opportunistic infections. Interferon is administered by either intravenous, intramuscular, or subcutaneous routes. Adverse effects of interferon include fever, chills, chronic fatigue, malaise, muscle pain, headache, and leukopenia. Dose reductions may be necessary because of severe adverse effects. Many patients may either self-administer interferon at home or receive it in an outpatient setting. Education concerning administration and management of adverse effects is provided by the nurse. Radiation therapy is also used for KS lesions that are disfiguring or anatomically inconvenient.

The success of treatment for AIDS-related lymphomas has been limited because of the rapidly progressing nature of these malignancies. Combination chemotherapy regimens and radiation therapy have achieved approximately a 50% response rate with markedly short durations. Because standard regimens for non-AIDS lymphomas have been ineffective, many clinicians have suggested that AIDS-related lymphomas be studied as a separate group in clinical trials.

Antiviral Agents. The discovery of zidovudine (AZT) has been one of the most significant advances in the fight against AIDS. This drug prevents reproduction of HIV by mimicking one of the molecular substances used by HIV to build DNA for new virus particles. By altering the structural components of the DNA chain, new virus production is inhibited. In 1987, the FDA approved AZT for the treatment of severe HIV infection. More recently, the FDA has approved the use of AZT for patients earlier in the course of infection prior to the development of profound immunosuppression. Measurement of the CD4 count is an important parameter used to determine the level of immunosuppression. The CD4 count reflects the number of circulating helper T-cell lymphocytes. Normal CD4 counts range between 700 and 1200. Patients whose CD4 counts are below 500 are given AZT by mouth at a dose of 500 mg/day in equally divided doses. AZT has been shown to slow viral reproduction, improve immune competence, and prolong survival. Patients taking AZT have demonstrated an improved sense of well-being, increased weight, fewer opportunistic infections, and improvement of neurologic functioning within the first few weeks of therapy. Patient education stresses the importance of taking each dose. AZT can be quite toxic to the bone marrow, producing dose-limiting anemia and neutropenia. In some instances the drug must be discontinued. Many clinicians are examining the use of colony-stimulating factors such as erythropoietin and granulocyte colony-stimulating factor (G-CSF) as a means of combating the adverse effects of anemia and neutropenia. Colony-stimulating factors are substances naturally produced by the body to stimulate growth and production of both red and white blood cells.

Other adverse effects of AZT include nausea, abdominal discomfort, fevers, chills, myalgias, headache, and less commonly confusion, somnolence, and seizures. Patient teaching concerning the importance of regular medical examinations and the assessment and management of adverse effects is indicated. Referrals for financial counseling are often needed because the cost of the drug may be as high as $600 per month.

Several other antiviral agents are currently under investigation (Table 48-7). For many patients, dideoxyinosine (ddI) has shown promising results as an alternative to AZT. The mechanisms of action vary with each drug. Some of the drugs act by interfering with HIV's affinity for the T_4 lymphocytes. Others alter the viral membrane and prevent HIV from entering the host's cells. Inhibition of viral reproduction is another mechanism of action. Most of the agents are in various phases

TABLE 48-7. *Antiviral Agents Under Investigation*

Drug	Mechanism of Action	Status*	Adverse Effects
AL721	Alters viral membrane so HIV cannot bind with CD4	Phase I/II	Unclear
Ampligen	Enhances role of interferon	Phase II/III	Minimal
Alpha interferon	Inhibits virus formation	Phase II	Flulike syndrome Decreased white blood cell (WBC) counts
Dideoxycytidine (DDC)	Inhibits reverse transcriptase	Phase II/III	Rash, stomatitis, decreased platelets, neurologic impairments
Dideoxyinosine (ddI)	Inhibits reverse transcriptase	Phase I/III	Unclear
Didehydrodideoxy-thymidine (DT4)	Inhibits reverse transcriptase	Phase I/II	Peripheral neuropathy; hepatic dysfunction
Compound Q (GLQ223)	Impairs cell protein synthesis	Phase I	Red blood cell clumping
Foscarnet (phosphonoformate)	Inhibits reverse transcriptase	Phase I/III	Anemia, increased serum creatinine, elevated liver function tests (LFTs)
Peptide T	Blocks HIV attachment to CD4 receptors	Phase I	Unclear
Recombinant CD4	Provides alternate site for HIV binding	Phase I	Unclear
Dextran sulfate	Inhibits HIV attachment to CD4 receptors	Phase I	Unclear
Ribavirin	May inhibit reverse transcriptase	Phase II/III	Dry mouth, headache, poor concentration, gastrointestinal upset, fatigue, metallic taste, anemia, elevated LFTs
Tumor necrosis factor (TNF)	Causes cell lysis	Phase I/II	Fever; chills; fatigue; headache; pain at injection site; decreased WBC, platelet, and red blood cell counts; increased LFTs, hypotension
Rifabutin	Inhibits reverse transcriptase	Available from CDC on a case-by-case basis	Increased LFTs, renal impairments, decreased WBCs and platelets

* See text for description of clinical trials.
(Adapted from Gee G, Moran T, and Wong R. Current strategies in the treatment of HIV infection. *Semin Oncol Nurs* 1988 May; 4[2]:128.)

of clinical trials where they are being studied for toxicity and maximal tolerated doses (phase I), activity against HIV (phase II), and effectiveness as compared with other drugs (phase III).

Immunomodulators.   Combating AIDS requires not only agents that will inhibit viral growth but also agents that will restore or augment the damaged immune system. Interferon is being studied for its antiviral properties as well as its ability to stimulate macrophages and T-cell lymphocytes. Other substances being evaluated for their role in macrophage and lymphocyte stimulation include interleukin 2, isoprinosine, diethyldithiocarbamate (DTC), lentinan, and granulocyte macrophage colony-stimulating factor. Many of these substances cause a flulike reaction including fevers, chills, arthralgias, myalgias, and headache. In addition, some drugs cause nausea, vomiting, elevated liver enzymes, neutropenia, confusion, and behavioral changes. The nurse plays an important role in this treatment modality by participating in assessment and management of adverse effects, providing patients with appropriate support and education, and participating in collection of data for clinical trials.

Vaccination.   A vaccine is any substance that triggers the body to produce antibodies to destroy the offending organism. Researchers have been working on the development of a vaccine for HIV since the virus was first discovered. Currently there are at least seven vaccines undergoing phase I and II clinical trials. Because of the complex nature and behavior of HIV, most scientists agree that a vaccine for HIV will not be available for use until the late 1990s. Other problems in vaccine development involve the identification of a population suitable for testing. It might be difficult to determine if a decline in infection rate in male homosexuals has resulted from a vaccine or from a change in sexual practices as a result of massive educational efforts. Following intravenous drug users for several years in vaccine trials might be difficult when these individuals often have unstable home situations and are involved in illicit activities. Finally, several legal and ethical concerns may evolve, including liability of manufacturers, potential development of AIDS in the test subjects, development of serious adverse effects, and the development of seropositivity in test subjects.

Supportive Care

Persons who become weak and debilitated as a result of chronic illness associated with HIV infection often require many forms of supportive care. Nutritional support may be as simple as providing assistance for obtaining or preparing meals. For persons with more advanced nutritional impairment that results from decreased intake or gastrointestinal malabsorption associated with diarrhea, parenteral feedings such as total parenteral nutrition may be required. Fluid and electrolyte imbalances that result from nausea, vomiting, and profuse diarrhea often necessitate intravenous replacement. Skin breakdown associated with Kaposi's sarcoma, perianal skin excoriation, and immobility is managed with thorough and meticulous skin care involving turning schedules, cleansing, and application of ointments and dressings as prescribed by the physician. Pulmonary symptoms such as dyspnea and shortness of breath may be related to infection, Kaposi's sarcoma, or fatigue. For these patients, oxygen therapy, relaxation training, and energy conservation techniques may be helpful. Patients with severe respiratory dysfunction may require mechanical ventilation in order to sustain life. Pain associated with skin breakdown, ab-

dominal cramping, or Kaposi's sarcoma is managed by analgesics given at regular intervals around the clock. Relaxation and guided imagery can be helpful in reducing pain and anxiety.

▶ Nursing Process
The Patient With AIDS

The nursing care of persons with AIDS is quite challenging because of the potential for any organ system to be the target of infections or malignancies. In addition, this disease is complicated by several controversial emotional and ethical issues. The plan of care for the patient with AIDS is individualized to meet the needs of the patient.

◊ Assessment

Nursing assessment includes identification of potential risk factors, including sexual history and history of intravenous drug use. The patient's physical status and psychologic status are assessed. All factors reflecting immune system functioning are thoroughly explored.

Nutritional status is assessed by obtaining a dietary history and identifying factors that may interfere with oral intake, such as anorexia, nausea, vomiting, oral pain, or difficulty swallowing. In addition, the patient's ability to purchase and prepare food is investigated. Weight, triceps skin fold measurements, and blood urea nitrogen, serum protein, albumin, and transferrin levels provide objective measurements of nutritional status.

The *skin and mucous membranes* are inspected daily for evidence of breakdown, ulceration, and infection. The oral cavity is monitored for redness, ulcerations, and the presence of white creamy patches indicative of candidiasis. It is especially important to assess the perianal area for excoriation and infection in those patients with profuse diarrhea. Wound cultures are obtained in order to identify infectious organisms.

Respiratory status is assessed by monitoring the patient for cough, sputum production, shortness of breath, orthopnea, tachypnea, and chest pain. The presence and quality of breath sounds are also assessed. Other objective parameters of pulmonary function include chest radiographs, arterial blood gas concentrations, and pulmonary function tests.

Neurologic status is determined by assessing the patient's level of consciousness and orientation to person, place, and time, and the occurrence of memory lapses. The patient is also observed for sensory impairments such as visual changes, headache or numbness, and tingling in the extremities. Motor impairments such as altered gait and paresis may also occur. Finally, the patient is observed for evidence of seizure activity.

Fluid and electrolyte status is assessed by examining the skin and mucous membranes for turgor and dryness. Increased thirst, decreased urine output, low blood pressure or a decline in systolic blood pressure of 15 mm Hg with concurrent rise in pulse when the patient sits up, weak rapid pulse, and specific gravity of 1.025 or more may indicate dehydration. Electrolyte imbalances such as decreased serum sodium, potassium, calcium, magnesium, and chloride often result from profuse diarrhea. The patient is assessed for signs and symptoms of electrolyte depletion. These may include decreased mental status, muscle twitching, muscle cramps, irregular pulse, nausea and vomiting, and shallow respirations.

The patient's *level of knowledge* about the disease and means of transmission is evaluated. In addition, the level of knowledge of family and friends is assessed. The patient's psychologic reaction to the diagnosis of AIDS is important to explore. Reactions vary among individuals and may include denial, anger, fear, shame, withdrawal from any social interactions, and depression. It is often helpful to gain an understanding of how the patient has dealt with illness and major life stressors in the past. The patient's resources for support are also identified.

▷ Nursing Diagnoses

The list of potential nursing diagnoses is quite extensive because of the complex nature of this disease. However, based on assessment data, major nursing diagnoses for the patient may include the following:

- Impaired skin integrity related to cutaneous manifestations of HIV infection
- Impaired perianal skin integrity related to excoriation and diarrhea
- Diarrhea related to enteric pathogens and/or HIV infection
- High risk for infection related to immunodeficiency
- Activity intolerance related to weakness, fatigue, malnutrition, impaired fluid and electrolyte balance, and hypoxia associated with pulmonary infections
- Altered thought processes related to shortened attention span, impaired memory, confusion, and disorientation associated with HIV encephalopathy
- Fluid volume deficit related to losses associated with persistent diarrhea
- Ineffective airway clearance related to *Pneumocystis* pneumonia, increased bronchial secretions, and decreased ability to cough related to weakness and fatigue
- Pain related to diarrhea and impaired perianal skin integrity
- Altered nutrition, less than body requirements, related to decreased oral intake
- Knowledge deficit concerning means of preventing transmission of HIV
- Social isolation related to stigma of the disease, withdrawal of support systems, isolation procedures, and fear of infecting others
- Grieving related to changes in life-style and roles and to unfavorable prognosis

▷ Planning and Implementation

▷ *Goals:* Goals for the patient may include achievement and maintenance of skin integrity, resumption of usual bowel habits, absence of infection, improved activity tolerance, improved thought processes, maintenance of fluid and electrolyte status, improved airway clearance, increased comfort, improvement of nutritional status, increased knowledge concerning means of preventing disease transmission, decreased sense of social isolation, and expression of grief.

▷ Nursing Interventions

▷ *Promotion of Skin Integrity.* Skin and oral mucosa are assessed routinely for changes in appearance, location and size of lesions, and evidence of infection and breakdown. The patient is encouraged to maintain a balance between rest and mobility whenever possible. Patients who are immobile are assisted to change position every 2 hours. Devices such as egg crates, alternating-pressure mattresses, and low- and high-airloss beds are used to assist in preventing skin breakdown. Patients are encouraged to avoid scratching, to use nonabrasive soaps, and to apply nonperfumed skin moisturizers to dry skin surfaces. Routine oral care is also encouraged. Medicated lotions, ointments, and dressings are applied to affected skin surfaces as prescribed by the physician. The use of excessive tape is avoided. Skin surfaces are protected from friction and rubbing by keeping bed linens free from wrinkles and avoiding tight or restrictive clothing. Patients with foot lesions are advised to wear white cotton socks and shoes that do not cause the feet to perspire. Antipruritics, antibiotics, and analgesics are administered as prescribed by the physician.

▷ *Maintenance of Perianal Skin Integrity.* The patient's perianal region is assessed frequently for impairment of skin integrity and infection. The patient is instructed to keep the area as clean as possible. The perianal area is cleaned after each bowel movement with nonabrasive soap and water to prevent further excoriation and breakdown of the skin and infection. If the area is very painful, soft cloths or cotton sponges may prove to be less irritating than washcloths. In addition, sitz baths or gentle irrigation may facilitate cleansing and promote comfort. The area is dried thoroughly after cleansing. The physician is consulted concerning topical lotions or ointments to promote healing. Wounds are cultured if infection is suspected so that the appropriate antimicrobial treatment can be initiated. Debilitated patients may require assistance in maintaining hygienic practices.

▷ *Resumption of Usual Bowel Habits.* The patient's bowel patterns are assessed for signs and symptoms of diarrhea, including frequency and consistency of stools and the presence of abdominal pain or cramping associated with bowel movements. Factors that exacerbate the frequency of diarrhea are also assessed. The quantity and volume of liquid stools are measured in order to document fluid volume losses. Stool cultures are obtained in order to identify pathogenic organisms.

The patient is counseled about ways to decrease diarrhea. Restriction of oral intake may be indicated and recommended by the physician in order to rest the bowel during periods of acute bowel inflammation associated with severe enteric infections. As the patient's dietary intake is advanced, the patient is advised to avoid foods that act as bowel irritants, such as raw fruits and vegetables, popcorn, carbonated beverages, spicy foods, and foods of extreme temperatures. Small, frequent meals will also help to prevent abdominal distention. The physician may prescribe medications such as anticholinergic antispasmodics or opiates, which decrease diarrhea by decreasing intestinal spasms and motility. Antibiotics and antifungal agents may also be prescribed in order to combat offending pathogens that are identified by stool cultures.

▷ *Prevention of Infection.* The patient and caregivers are instructed to monitor for signs and symptoms of infection: fever; chills; night sweats; cough with or without sputum production; shortness of breath; difficulty breathing; oral pain or difficulty swallowing; creamy white patches in the oral cavity; unexplained weight loss; swollen lymph nodes; nausea; vomiting; persistent diarrhea; frequency, urgency, or pain on urination; headache; visual changes or memory lapses; redness, swelling, or drainage from skin wounds; and vesicular lesions on the face, lips, or perianal area. The nurse also monitors laboratory values that indicate the presence of infection, such as the white blood cell count and differential blood cell count. The physician may request culture specimens of wound drainage, skin lesions, urine, stool, sputum, mouth, and blood in order to identify pathogenic organisms and the most appropriate antimicrobial therapy.

The patient will require education about ways of preventing infection. The importance of personal hygiene is emphasized. Kitchen and bathroom surfaces should be cleansed regularly with disinfectants in order to prevent fungal and bacterial growth. Patients with pets are instructed to use gloves when cleaning areas soiled by animals, such as bird cages and litter boxes. Patients are advised to avoid exposure to others who are sick or who have been recently vaccinated. Patients with AIDS and their sexual partners are *strongly* urged to avoid exposure to body fluids during sexual activities and to use condoms for any form of sexual intercourse. Intravenous drug use is *strongly* discouraged because of risk to the patient of other infections and transmission of HIV infection to others. The importance of avoiding smoking and maintaining a balance between diet, rest, and exercise is also addressed. All health professionals must remember to maintain strict aseptic technique when performing invasive procedures such as venipunctures and bladder catheterizations and to use universal precautions in all patient care.

▷ *Improved Activity Tolerance.* Activity tolerance is assessed by monitoring the patient's ability to ambulate and perform activities of daily living. Patients may be unable to maintain usual levels of activity because of weakness, fatigue, shortness of breath, dizziness, and neurologic involvement. Assistance in planning daily routines that maintain a balance between activity and rest may be necessary. In addition, patients benefit from instructions about the use of energy conservation techniques, such as sitting while washing or while preparing meals. Personal items that are frequently used should be kept within the patient's reach so that they can be obtained without walking any distance. Measures such as relaxation and guided imagery may be beneficial in decreasing anxiety that contributes to weakness and fatigue.

▷ *Promoting Improvement of Thought Processes.* The patient is assessed for alterations in mental status that may be related to neurologic involvement, metabolic abnormalities, infection, side effects of treatment, and/or coping mechanisms. Mental status is assessed as early as possible to provide a baseline for monitoring changes in behavior (Table 48-8). Manifestations of neurologic impairment may be difficult to distinguish from psychologic reactions to HIV infection, such as anger and depression.

The patient and family are helped to understand and cope with changes in thought processes. The patient is reoriented to person, place, and time whenever necessary. It is often helpful to have a clock and calendar within the patient's view to facilitate sustained orientation. The patient's family and friends are encouraged to bring favorite objects from home in order to provide a familiar and less threatening environment while the patient is hospitalized. All instructions given to the patient are delivered in a slow, simple, and clear manner. Measures to protect the patient from injury are instituted. These may include placing the call bell within easy reach, keeping side rails up and the bed in a low position, instructing the patient to wear shoes and slippers with nonskid soles, and monitoring the patient who is smoking or shaving.

Strategies for improving or maintaining functional abilities and for providing a safe environment are used for patients with HIV encephalopathy (Table 48-9).

TABLE 48–8. *Mental Status Assessment and Observations*

Category	Definition	Examples of Descriptors
Appearance	Dress, hygiene, physical characteristics	Clean, dirty, neat, disheveled, inappropriate dress for weather, obese, cachectic
Behavior	General behavior during the interview	Agitated, restless, somnolent, cooperative, uncooperative, suspicious, hostile, evasive
Motor activity	Behavior compared with peer group	Loss of precision, slowing, tremors, hyperactive, rigid, falling out of chair, repetitive and/or nonproductive movements
Speech	Cadence, articulation, vocabulary, tone, reality base	Goal-oriented, pressured, slurred, hesitant, rapid, loud, soft, nonstop, absent
Affect	Moment-to-moment emotions expressed	Bland, flat, labile, tearful, blunted, dull, appropriate, inappropriate, fearful
Mood	Predominant and pervasive feeling of the interview	Euphoria, despondent, pensive, hopeless
Perception	How the patient sees the world. Illusions—misinterpretation of actual stimuli. Hallucinations—absence of real stimuli	Auditory, visual, olfactory hallucinations
Thinking	Recent and remote memory, orientation, intellect, judgment, and level of insight	Delusional, confabulating, goal-directed, loose associations, illogical, concrete, thought-blocking, oriented, disoriented, able or unable to do math problems appropriate to level of education, problem-solving ability, knowledge of current events, can identify prominent persons or events

(Hall JM, Koehler SL, and Lewis A. HIV-related mental health nursing issues. Semin Oncol Nurs 1989 Nov; 5[4]:277.)

TABLE 48–9. *Nursing Interventions for HIV Encephalopathy*

Orientation	Use orienting clues such as clocks, calendars, posted schedules, and large-print signs such as "John's Room."
	Keep lights on to help with nighttime confusion.
Environment	Avoid changes by keeping things in the same place.
	Encourage significant others to bring in and display familiar objects such as photos or a favorite bathrobe.
	Keep environment safe and unrestrictive.
Communication	Arrange for continuity of staff or caregivers.
	Keep verbal instructions simple and concrete; give only one instruction at a time.
	If patients comprehend the written word, write orienting information down and refer them to it.
	Recognize that demented patients may have impaired decision-making ability and need to strike a balance between a needless struggle and preservation of autonomy and integrity.
Stimulation	Balance environmental stimuli to maximize awareness without causing confusion.
	If mobility is impaired, consider physical therapy.
	Offer a variety of visual, tactile, and auditory experiences; *e.g.*, alternate stimuli by switching between the radio, television, and periods of exercise.
	Arrange to have pets visit on a regular basis.
Significant others	Encourage the patient to identify those who are significant, then involve those individuals as much as they and the patient choose.
	Refer significant others to support groups; if HIV support groups are unavailable, consider groups for other terminally ill patients and significant others.
	Remember that significant others may also have concerns about HIV.

(Hall JM, Koehler SL, and Lewis A. HIV-related mental health nursing issues. Semin Oncol Nurs 1989 Nov; 5[4]:279.)

▷ *Maintenance of Fluid and Electrolyte Balance.* Fluid and electrolyte status is monitored on an ongoing basis. The skin is assessed for dryness and turgor. Fluid intake and output and specific gravity of urine are measured daily. The patient is also monitored for decreases in systolic blood pressure or increases in pulse associated with sitting or standing. Signs and symptoms of electrolyte disturbances such as muscle cramping, weakness, irregular pulse, decreased mental status, nausea, and vomiting are documented and reported to the physician. Serum electrolyte values are monitored and abnormalities reported to the physician when indicated. The nurse assists the patient in selecting foods that will replenish electrolytes, such as oranges and bananas (potassium) and cheese and soups (sodium). A fluid intake of 2500 ml or more, unless contraindicated, is encouraged in order to regain fluid lost from diarrhea. In addition, measures to control diarrhea are initiated. If fluid and electrolyte imbalances persist, the nurse may administer intravenous fluid and electrolytes as prescribed by the physician. It then becomes important for the nurse to monitor the therapeutic or potentially adverse effects of parenteral therapy.

▷ *Improved Nutritional Status.* Nutritional status is assessed by monitoring weight, dietary intake, anthropometric measurements, and serum albumin, BUN, protein, and transferrin levels. The patient is also assessed for factors that interfere with oral intake, such as anorexia, nausea, pain, weakness, and fatigue. Based on the results of assessment, the nurse can implement specific measures to facilitate oral intake.

When fatigue and weakness interfere with intake, the patient is encouraged to rest prior to meals. In addition, meals should be planned so that they do not occur immediately after painful or unpleasant procedures. The patient with diarrhea and abdominal cramping is encouraged to avoid foods that stimulate intestinal motility and distention, such as foods high in fiber or of extreme temperatures. The dietitian is consulted to determine the patient's nutritional requirements. The patient is instructed about ways in which to supplement nutritional value of meals. The addition of eggs, butter, margarine, and fortified milk to gravies, soups, or milkshakes can provide additional calories and protein. Use of commercial supplements such as puddings, powders, and milkshakes may be advised. Patients who are unable to maintain nutritional status through oral intake often require enteral or parenteral feedings. Instruction is provided to patients and families about how to administer such feedings when patients are able to return home. Community health nurses provide additional teaching and support for these patients after discharge from the hospital. The nurse often consults with social workers in order to identify sources of financial support for patients who are unable to purchase or prepare meals. Referral to the AIDS Task Force or other community resources may be indicated if the patient is unable to shop for or prepare meals. These resources are often able to provide volunteers who can assist patients after discharge from the hospital.

▷ *Patient Education.* Patients, families, and friends are instructed about the routes of transmission of AIDS. All fears and misconceptions are thoroughly discussed. In addition, the nurse discusses precautions necessary to prevent transmission of HIV, including the use of condoms during vaginal or anal intercourse; avoiding oral contact with the penis, vagina, or rectum; avoiding sexual practices that might cause cuts or tears in the lining of the rectum, vagina, or penis; and avoiding sexual contact with multiple partners or individuals known to be HIV-positive, persons who use illicit intravenous (IV) drugs, or sexual partners of persons who use IV drugs (Table 48-10). Patients who are HIV-positive or who use IV drugs are instructed not to donate blood.

▷ *Improved Airway Clearance.*   Respiratory status, including rate, rhythm, use of accessory muscles, and breath sounds; mental status; and skin color must be assessed at least daily. The presence of cough and the quantity and characteristics of sputum are documented. Sputum specimens are tested for the possible presence of infectious organisms. Pulmonary measures (coughing, deep breathing, postural drainage, percussion, and vibration) are provided as often as every 2 hours to prevent stasis of secretions and promote clearance of airways. Because of weakness and fatigue, many patients may require assistance in attaining a position (such as a high or semi-Fowler's) that will facilitate breathing and airway clearance. The provision of adequate rest periods is essential to maximize the patient's energy expenditure and prevent excessive fatigue. The patient's fluid volume status is evaluated so that adequate hydration can be maintained. Unless contraindicated by renal or cardiac disease, intake of 3 to 4 L of fluid daily is encouraged. Humidified oxygen may be prescribed, and nasopharyngeal or tracheal suctioning may be indicated to maintain adequate ventilation. Mechanical ventilation may be necessary for patients who are unable to maintain adequate ventilation as a result of pulmonary infection, fluid and electrolyte imbalance, or respiratory muscle weakness.

▷ *Increased Comfort.*   The patient is assessed for the quality and quantity of pain associated with diarrhea and impaired perianal skin integrity. In addition, the effects of pain on elimination, nutrition, sleep, affect, and communication are explored, along with exacerbating and relieving factors. Cleansing the perianal area as previously described can promote comfort. Topical anesthetics or ointments may be prescribed. Soft cushions or foam pads may be used to increase comfort while sitting. The patient is instructed to avoid foods that act as bowel irritants. Antispasmodics and antidiarrheal preparations may be prescribed to reduce discomfort and frequency of bowel movements. If necessary, systemic analgesics may also be prescribed.

▷ *Decreased Sense of Social Isolation.*   AIDS patients are at risk for "double stigmatization." They have what society often refers to as "a dread disease," and they may have a life-style (homosexuality or drug abuse) that differs from what is considered acceptable to many people. The majority of persons with AIDS are young adults at a developmental stage in which they should be establishing intimate relationships and personal and career goals. Their focus changes as they are faced with a disease that has no cure and a limited life expectancy. In addition, they may be forced to reveal hidden life-styles to family, friends, co-workers, and health care providers. As a result, persons with HIV infection are often flooded with emotions such as anxiety, guilt, shame, and fear. Patients may be faced with multiple losses, such as rejection by family and friends and loss of financial security, normal roles and functions, self-esteem, privacy, ability to control bodily functions, ability to interact meaningfully with the environment, and sexual functioning. Some patients may harbor feelings of guilt because of their chosen life-style or because of the possibility of having infected others in current or previous relationships. Other pa-

---

TABLE 48-10.   *Safer Sex Guidelines*

- Reduce the number of sexual partners, preferably to one.
- Avoid sexual intercourse if possible and especially sexual practices that may injure tissues, *e.g.,* anal intercourse. Avoid oral-genital contact. "Deep" kissing is somewhat controversial because of the presence of virus in saliva; however, no instance of transmission from kissing alone has been reported.
- If sexual intercourse or oral sex is continued, always use a condom to protect partners from contact with body fluids. Intact latex condoms are impermeable to HIV; natural animal-skin condoms are not. The addition of a spermicide containing nonoxynol-9 both inside and outside the condom appears to provide additional protection should the condom break. Avoid the use of oil-based lubricants; they can damage the condom. Vaginal diaphragms are not protective.
- Don't share needles, razors, toothbrushes, sexual toys, or other blood-contaminated articles.
- Inform prospective partners of HIV-positive status.
- Notify present or previous sexual partners (and those who have shared needles) of their possible exposure. If a partner is female and possibly pregnant, she needs an immediate referral for medical evaluation and antibody testing, if she is willing.
- If female, avoid pregnancy.
- Do not donate blood, plasma, body organs, or sperm.
- Inform doctors and dentists of seropositivity for their protection.
- These guidelines are important for the protection of HIV-positive persons as well as HIV-negative, because severity of disease may be related to total viral dose as well as repeated antigenic stimulation.

(Cummings D. Caring for the HIV-infected adult. Nurse Pract 1988 Nov; 13[11]:31.)

tients may feel anger toward sexual partners who may have been responsible for transmission of the virus. Infection control measures used in the hospital or at home may further contribute to the patient's emotional isolation. Any or all of these stressors may cause the AIDS patient to withdraw both physically and emotionally from social contact.

Nurses are in a key position to provide an atmosphere of acceptance and understanding of AIDS patients and their families and partners. A patient's usual level of social interaction is assessed as early as possible, to provide a baseline for monitoring changes in behavior indicative of social isolation (*e.g.*, decreased interaction with staff or family, hostility, noncompliance). Patients are encouraged to express feelings of isolation and aloneness and are assured that these feelings are not unique or abnormal.

Providing information about how to protect themselves and others can help to prevent patients from avoiding social contact. Patients, family, and friends must be assured that AIDS is not spread through casual contact. Educating ancillary personnel, nurses, and physicians will help to reduce factors that might contribute to feelings of isolation. Patient care conferences concerning the psychosocial considerations regarding AIDS patients may help sensitize nurses to patients' needs.

The nurse can help patients explore and identify resources for support and mechanisms for coping. Patients are encouraged to telephone family and friends as well as local or national AIDS support groups and hotlines. If at all possible, barriers to social contact are identified and eliminated. For patients who are able to participate, social interaction with family, friends, or co-workers is encouraged. Patients are also encouraged to engage in their usual diversional activities whenever possible.

▷ *Home Health Care Considerations.* Many persons with AIDS are able to return to the community and resume their usual daily activities. Others who return home are unable to continue employment or maintain their preexisting level of independence. Families or caregivers need assistance in providing supportive care. They must receive instructions about how to prevent disease transmission, including hand washing and methods of safely handling items soiled with body fluids. Caregivers in the home are taught how to administer medications, including intravenous preparations. Guidelines about infection, follow-up care, diet, rest, and activities are also necessary. Both the patient and caregivers will require support and guidance in coping with this debilitating and usually fatal disease.

Community health nurses and hospice nurses are in an excellent position to help provide the support and guidance so often needed in the home setting. As hospital costs continue to rise and insurance coverage continues to undergo major changes, the complexity of home care continues to increase. Community nurses are frequently able to assist in the administration of parenteral antibiotics, chemotherapy, and nutrition. In addition, complicated wound care or respiratory care is often required in the home. Both patients and families are often unable to meet these skilled care needs without the assistance of nurses. Hospice nurses are increasingly called upon to provide emotional support to patients and families as AIDS patients enter the terminal stages of disease. This support takes on special meaning when AIDS patients lose the support of friends and families who have turned away from them because of fear of the disease or anger concerning life-styles adopted by patients.

Nurses may also refer patients to many community programs located in towns and cities throughout the country. These programs offer a range of services for patients, friends, and families, including help with housekeeping, grooming, and meals; transportation and shopping; individual and group therapy; support for caregivers; telephone networks for the homebound; and legal and financial assistance. These services are often provided by both professional and nonprofessional volunteers.

▷ *Prevention of HIV Transmission.* As discussed earlier in this chapter, AIDS is not transmitted by casual contact. Epidemiologic evidence has indicated that HIV is transmitted only through intimate sexual contact, parenteral exposure to infected blood or blood products, and perinatal transmission from mother to neonate. Studies of nonsexual household contacts of AIDS patients as well as nonsexual person-to-person contact that generally occurs in the work place have not demonstrated any increased risk for transmission of AIDS through such contact.

In the interest of public health, the CDC and the Surgeon General of the U.S. have issued recommendations for preventing the transmission of HIV (Chart 48-4). These guidelines apply to health care workers in all settings as well as families and friends providing care in the home. The guidelines, entitled "Universal Blood and Body Fluid Precautions," are intended to prevent parenteral, mucous membrane, and nonintact skin exposures of health care providers to bloodborne pathogens of all patients regardless of HIV status. Although HIV has been isolated from all types of body fluids, the risk of transmission to health care providers is less likely from contact with feces, nasal secretions, sputum, sweat, breast milk, tears, urine, and vomitus unless they contain visible blood. The CDC has suggested that universal precautions be applied to blood; cerebrospinal fluid; synovial, pleural, peritoneal, pericardial, amniotic, and vaginal fluids; and semen. In emergency circumstances when differentiation between fluid types is difficult, all body fluids are considered to be potentially hazardous.

Another isolation system, the Body Substance Isolation System, is used by some institutions as an alternative to Universal Blood and Body Fluid Precautions. This system offers a broader strategy of isolation in order to reduce the risk of disease transmission to patients and health care workers. This system eliminates the need for health care workers to identify particular body fluids. The elements of Body Substance Isolation are listed in Table 48-11.

▷ ## Evaluation

Expected Outcomes
1. Resumes usual bowel habits
2. Experiences no infections
3. Maintains usual level of thought processes
4. Maintains fluid and electrolyte balance
5. Maintains effective airway clearance
6. Experiences increased sense of comfort
7. Maintains skin integrity
8. Maintains adequate nutritional status
9. Understands means of preventing disease transmission
10. Experiences decreased sense of social isolation
11. Maintains adequate level of activity tolerance
12. Progresses through grieving process

Specific outcomes are discussed in Nursing Care Plan 48-1, pp. 1378–1382.

Chart 48–4
Universal Precautions to Prevent Transmission of HIV

- Sharp items (*e.g.,* needles, scalpel blades) should be considered potentially infective and be handled with extraordinary care to prevent accidental injuries.
- Disposable syringes and needles, scalpel blades, and other sharp items should be placed in puncture-resistant containers located as near as is practical to the area in which they were used. Needles should not be recapped, purposely bent, broken, removed from disposable syringes, or otherwise manipulated by hand.
- Protective barriers (gloves, gowns, masks, and protective eyewear) must be used to prevent exposure to blood, body fluids containing visible blood, and other fluids to which universal precautions apply. The type of protective barrier should be appropriate for the procedure being performed and the type of exposure anticipated.
- Immediately and thoroughly wash hands and other skin surfaces that are contaminated with blood, body fluids containing visible blood, or other body fluids to which universal precautions apply.

- To minimize the need for emergency mouth-to-mouth resuscitation, mouth pieces, resuscitation bags, or other ventilation devices must be located strategically and available for use in areas where the need for resuscitation is predictable.
- Health care workers who are pregnant are not known to be at greater risk of contracting HIV infection than those who are not pregnant; however, if a health care worker develops HIV infection during pregnancy, the infant is at increased risk of infection resulting from perinatal transmission. Because of this risk, pregnant health care workers must be especially careful and maintain proper precautions.
- In the home setting, blood and body fluids may be flushed down the toilet.
- Contaminated items that cannot be flushed down the toilet should be wrapped securely in a plastic bag and placed in a second bag before being discarded in a manner consistent with local regulations for solid waste disposal.
- Spills of blood or other body fluids should be cleaned with soap and water or a household detergent. Freshly prepared solutions of sodium hypochlorite (household bleach) in concentrations of 1:10 dilution are effective disinfectants. Persons cleaning spills should wear gloves.

(U.S. Department of Health and Human Services. Update: Universal precautions for prevention of transmission of human immunodeficiency virus, hepatitis B virus and other bloodborne pathogens in health care settings. MMWR 1988 June; 37[24]:377–382.)

Emotional and Ethical Concerns for Nurses

Nurses in all settings may be called upon to provide care for patients with HIV infection. In doing so, nurses encounter not only the physical challenges of this epidemic but also many controversial emotional and ethical concerns. These concerns raised by health care professionals involve issues such as fear of contagion, responsibility for giving care, values clarification, confidentiality, developmental stages of patients and caregivers, and poor prognostic outcomes.

The majority of patients with HIV infection have engaged in "stigmatized" behaviors such as homosexuality and intravenous drug use. Because these practices challenge individual religious and moral values, nurses may be reluctant to provide nursing care for these patients. In addition, health care providers often have fear and anxiety about the possibility of disease transmission despite education concerning infection control and the low incidence of transmission to health care providers. Nurses are encouraged to examine their personal beliefs and utilize a process of values clarification to rationally approach controversial issues. The American Nurses Association's Code for Nurses can also be used to help resolve dilemmas that might affect the quality of care given to HIV-infected patients.

Nurses are responsible for protecting the patient's right to privacy by safeguarding confidential information. Inadvertent disclosure of confidential patient information may result in personal, financial, and emotional hardships for HIV-infected individuals. The controversy surrounding confidentiality concerns the identification of circumstances when information is disclosed to others. Health team members need accurate patient information to conduct assessment, planning, implementation, and evaluation of patient care. Failure to disclose HIV status could compromise the quality of patient care. Sexual partners of HIV-infected patients should know about the potential of infection and the need to engage in safer sex practices as well as the potential need for medical evaluation. Nurses are advised to discuss concerns about confidentiality with nurse administrators and physicians in order to identify the most appropriate courses of action.

AIDS is associated with a very high mortality rate. Most nurses have never been faced with an epidemic where almost everyone will experience serious illness and die within a relatively short period of time. Nurses may struggle with the value and meaning of their professional roles as they witness repeated cases of patient deterioration. Exposure to so many deaths in a population that is at the same developmental stage as many nurses can create feelings of stress. Contributing to stress are the ethical issues previously discussed. Unlike cancer or other diseases, AIDS is associated with controversies challenging our legal and political systems as well as religious and personal beliefs. Nurses feeling stressed and overburdened may experience physical and psychologic manifestations such as fatigue, headache, changes in appetite and sleep patterns, helplessness, irritability, apathy, negativity, and anger.

Many strategies have been used by nurses to cope with stress associated with providing care for AIDS patients. Edu-

TABLE 48-11. *Elements of Body Substance Isolation System*

Categories of Protection	Nursing Action
Handwashing	Wash hands for 10 seconds with soap, running water, and friction before touching patients and any time the hands have been soiled.
Gloves	Put on clean gloves just before contact with mucous membranes and nonintact skin.
	Wear appropriate gloves any time hands are likely to have contact with moist body substances.
	Remove gloves immediately after task is completed.
Gowns or plastic aprons	Wear any time it is likely that clothing or skin will be soiled.
Masks	Wear when working directly over large areas of open skin.
	Wear when it is likely that nasal and oral mucous membranes will be spattered with moist body substances.
Needles and sharps	Discard in rigid, puncture-resistant containers.
	Do not recap used needles by hand.
	Be particularly careful when manipulating small devices such as heparin locks.
Roommate selection	Avoid roommate combinations in which one patient is likely to have contact with the other patient's moist body substances.
	Assign patients with airborne communicable diseases to private rooms or rooms with immunocompetent roommates.
Trash and linen	Bag all soiled trash and linen securely.
	Discard according to facility policy.
	Personnel handling soiled linen and trash should wear gloves and protective garments when necessary.
Housekeeping	Routine cleaning for all rooms should be done on a regular schedule.
	Articles, equipment, and furniture soiled with moist body substances should be cleaned immediately by gloved personnel.
Laboratory specimens	All laboratory specimens should be handled with equal care.
	No special precautionary labels required.
Signs and labels	Signs and labels identifying patients known to have infectious diseases are unnecessary and may encourage a double standard of care.
	The rooms of patients with airborne communicable diseases should be identified so that susceptibility of care providers can be assessed.
Compliance of care providers	A program to ensure that health care workers comply with the infection precautions system is essential.

(Jackson M and Lynch P. Infection prevention and control in the era of the AIDS/HIV epidemic. Semin Oncol Nurs 1989 Nov; 5[4]:240.)

cation and provision of up-to-date information help to alleviate apprehension and prepare nurses to deliver safe, high-quality patient care. Interdisciplinary meetings allow participants to provide support for each other and comprehensive patient care. Staff support groups give nurses an opportunity to problem-solve and explore values and feelings about caring for AIDS patients and their families. They also provide a forum for grieving. Other sources of support include nursing administration, peers, and spiritual leaders.

In summary, acquired immunodeficiency syndrome (AIDS), the clinical syndrome of infection by the human immunodeficiency virus (HIV), is a disorder characterized by severe suppression of the immune system. The virus, a retrovirus, is transmitted by sexual contact, contaminated blood, and perinatal transmission from mother to fetus. The virus enters the helper T lymphocytes, a type of T_4 lymphocyte, where the virus replicates. As these cells are destroyed by the virus, the infected person is unable to mount an immune response against common or ordinarily harmless pathogens or abnormal cells. The result is the appearance of opportunistic infections and neoplasms (cancer).

The severity of physical symptoms, the poor prognosis, and the emotional, psychologic, and social consequences of AIDS exact a toll on the patient, the family, and often the health care provider. The nurse caring for the patient with AIDS

(text continues on page 1382)

Nursing Care Plan 48–1

Care of the Patient With Acquired Immunodeficiency Syndrome (AIDS)

Nursing Interventions	Rationale	Expected Outcomes

Nursing Diagnosis: Diarrhea related to enteric pathogens and/or HIV infection

Goal: Resumption of usual bowel habits

Nursing Interventions	Rationale	Expected Outcomes
1. Assess patient's normal bowel habits.	1. Provides baseline for evaluating effectiveness of measures.	• Bowel habits return to normal.
2. Assess for signs and symptoms of diarrhea: frequent, loose stools; abdominal pain or cramping.	2. Detects changes in status.	• Reports decreasing episodes of diarrhea and abdominal cramping.
a. Measure amount of liquid stools.	a. Quantifies loss of fluids.	• Identifies and avoids foods that irritate the gastrointestinal tract.
b. Identify exacerbating and alleviating factors.	b. Provides basis for nursing measures.	• Appropriate therapy is initiated as prescribed.
3. Obtain stool cultures as prescribed by physician. Administer antimicrobial therapy as prescribed.	3. Identifies pathogenic organism.	• Exhibits normal stool cultures. • Maintains adequate fluid intake.
4. Initiate measures to reduce hyperactivity of bowel:	4. Bowel rest may decrease acute episodes.	• Maintains body weight and reports no additional weight loss.
a. Maintain food and fluid restrictions as prescribed by physician.	a. Reduces stimulation of bowel.	• States rationale for avoiding smoking. • Enrolls in program to stop smoking.
b. Discourage smoking.	b. Nicotine acts as bowel stimulant.	• Uses medication as prescribed.
c. Avoid bowel irritants such as foods high in fat, fried foods, raw vegetables and fruits, nuts, onions, popcorn, carbonated beverages, spicy foods, and foods of extreme temperatures.	c. Prevents stimulation of bowel and abdominal distention.	• Maintains adequate fluid status. • Exhibits normal skin turgor, moist mucous membranes, adequate urine output, and no excessive thirst.
d. Offer small, frequent meals.		
5. Administer anticholinergic antispasmodics as prescribed (propantheline bromide, dicyclomine hydrochloride).	5. Decreases intestinal spasms and motility.	
6. Administer opiates or opiatelike medications as prescribed by physician (tincture of opium, loperamide, or diphenoxylate hydrochloride).	6. Decreases intestinal motility.	
7. Maintain fluid intake of at least 2500 ml unless contraindicated.	7. Prevents hypovolemia.	

Nursing Diagnosis: High risk for infection related to immunodeficiency

Goal: Absence of infection

Nursing Interventions	Rationale	Expected Outcomes
1. Monitor for signs and symptoms of infection: fever, chills, and diaphoresis; cough; shortness of breath; oral pain or painful swallowing; creamy white patches in oral cavity; urinary frequency, urgency, or dysuria; redness, swelling, or drainage from skin wounds; vesicular lesions on face, lips, or perianal area.	1. Early detection of infection is essential for prompt initiation of treatment. Repeated and prolonged infections contribute to patient's debilitation.	• Identifies reportable signs and symptoms of infection. • Reports signs and symptoms of infection if infection does occur. • Exhibits and reports absence of fever, chills, and diaphoresis. • Exhibits normal (clear) breath sounds without adventitious breath sounds.
2. Teach patient or caregiver about need to report above signs and symptoms of infection.	2. Allows early detection of infection.	• Maintains weight. • Reports adequate energy level without excessive fatigue.

(continued)

Nursing Care Plan 48–1 *(Continued)*

Care of the Patient With Acquired Immunodeficiency Syndrome (AIDS)

Nursing Interventions	Rationale	Expected Outcomes

3. Monitor white blood cell count and differential
4. Obtain cultures of wound drainage, skin lesions, urine, stool, sputum, mouth, and blood as prescribed by physician. Administer antimicrobial therapy as prescribed by physician.
5. Instruct patient in ways in which to prevent infection:
  a. Cleanse kitchen and bathroom surfaces with disinfectants.
  b. Cleanse hands thoroughly after exposure to body fluids.
  c. Avoid exposure to others' body fluids or sharing eating utensils.
  d. Turn, cough, and deep breathe, especially when activity is decreased.
  e. Maintain cleanliness of perianal area.
6. Maintain aseptic technique when performing invasive procedures such as venipunctures, bladder catheterizations, and injections.
	3. Elevated WBC is associated with infection.
	4. Offending organism must be identified in order to initiate appropriate treatment.
	
	5. Minimizes exposure of patient to infection and transmission of HIV infection to others.
	
	6. Prevents hospital-acquired infections.
		• Reports absence of shortness of breath and cough.
		• Exhibits pink, moist oral mucous membranes without fissures or lesions.
		• Appropriate therapy is administered.
		• Infection is prevented.
		• States rationale for strategies to avoid infection.
		• Modifies activities to reduce exposure to infection or infectious persons.
		• Practices "safe sex."
		• Avoids sharing eating utensils and toothbrush.
		• Exhibits normal body temperature.
		• Uses recommended techniques to maintain cleanliness of skin, skin lesions, and perianal area.

Nursing Diagnosis: Altered thought processes related to shortened attention span, impaired memory, confusion, restlessness, and disorientation associated with HIV encephalopathy

Goal: Improved thought processes

1. Assess patient for evidence of impaired thought processes such as decreased attention span, impaired memory, confusion, disorientation, agitation, and decreased level of consciousness. 2. Reorient patient to person, place, and time as necessary; keep calender and clock within patient's view; leave low light on at night. 3. Encourage family and friends to bring patient's favorite objects from home to place in hospital room. 4. Repeat instructions slowly as necessary, using simple, clear language. 5. Implement measures to protect patient from injury.	1. HIV is able to invade the CNS, resulting in subacute encephalitis; this is believed to account for approximately 25% of all neurologic symptoms seen in patients with AIDS. 2. Facilitates patient's orientation to environment. 3. Provides familiar and less threatening environment. 4. Prevents overwhelming and frustrating the patient. 5. Prevents injuries from falling, cuts, burns, and other accidents.	• Demonstrates intact orientation to time and place. • Responds appropriately to interactions and conversation of others. • Exhibits interest in events and surroundings. • Experiences no falls or other consequences of trauma. • Explains treatments and other instructions in own words. • Follows recommendations to reduce safety hazards and to protect self and others from injury. • Calls for assistance from others when appropriate.

Nursing Diagnosis: Ineffective airway clearance related to *Pneumocystis* pneumonia, increased bronchial secretions, and decreased ability to cough related to weakness and fatigue

Goal: Improved airway clearance

1. Assess and report signs and symptoms of altered respiratory status: tachypnea,	1. Indicates abnormal respiratory function.	• Maintains normal airway clearance: —Respiratory rate <20/minute

(continued)

Nursing Care Plan 48-1 (Continued)

Care of the Patient With Acquired Immunodeficiency Syndrome (AIDS)

Nursing Interventions	Rationale	Expected Outcomes
use of accessory muscles, cough, color and amount of sputum, abnormal breath sounds, dusky or cyanotic skin color, restlessness, confusion, or somnolence.		—Unlabored breathing without use of accessory muscles and flaring of nares (nostrils)
2. Obtain sputum sample for culture prescribed by physician. Administer antimicrobial therapy as prescribed.	2. Aids in identification of pathogenic organisms.	—Skin color pink (without cyanosis) —Alert and aware of surroundings —Arterial blood gases normal
3. Provide pulmonary care (cough, deep breathing, postural drainage, and vibration) every 2 to 4 hours.	3. Prevents stasis of secretions and promotes airway clearance.	—Normal breath sounds without adventitious breath sounds • Appropriate therapy is initiated.
4. Assist patient in attaining semi- or high Fowler's position.	4. Facilitates breathing and airway clearance.	• Takes medication as prescribed. • Reports improved breathing. • Airway clearance is maintained.
5. Encourage adequate rest periods.	5. Maximizes energy expenditure and prevents excessive fatigue.	• Coughs and takes deep breaths every 2–4 hours as recommended.
6. Initiate measures to decrease viscosity of secretions: a. Maintain fluid intake of at least 2500 ml per day unless contraindicated. b. Humidify inspired air as prescribed by physician. c. Consult with physician concerning use of mucolytic agents delivered through nebulizer or IPPB treatment.	6. Facilitates expectoration of secretions; prevents stasis secretions.	• Demonstrates appropriate positions for postural drainage. • Practices postural drainage every 2–4 hours. • Reports reduced breathing difficulty when in semi- or high Fowler's position. • Practices energy-conserving strategies. • Plans schedule to allow alternating periods of rest and activity.
7. Perform tracheal suctioning as needed.	7. Removes secretions if patient is unable to do so.	• Demonstrates reduction in thickness (viscosity) of pulmonary secretions.
8. Administer oxygen therapy as prescribed.	8. Increases availability of oxygen.	• Reports increased ease in coughing up sputum.
9. Assist with endotracheal intubation; maintain ventilator settings as prescribed.	9. Maintains ventilation.	• Uses humidified air or oxygen as prescribed and indicated. • Indicates need for assistance with removal of pulmonary secretions. • States rationale for endotracheal intubation and use of a mechanical ventilator. • Cooperates with intubation procedure and use of mechanical ventilator. • Verbalizes fears and anxieties about increased respiratory difficulty and need for intubation and mechanical ventilation.

Nursing Diagnosis: Altered nutrition, less than body requirement, related to decreased oral intake

Goal: Improvement of nutritional status

1. Assess patient for evidence of malnutrition through the following: height, weight, age, BUN, serum protein, albumin, transferrin levels, hemoglobin, hematocrit, cutaneous anergy, and anthropometric measurements.	1. Provides objective measurement of nutritional status.	• Deficient values return to normal. • Identifies factors limiting oral intake. • Identifies and uses resources to assist in adequate dietary intake. • Reports increased appetite. • States understanding of nutritional needs.
2. Obtain dietary history, including likes and dislikes and food intolerances.	2. Helps to identify need for nutritional education; assists in planning individualized interventions.	• Identifies ways to minimize factors limiting oral intake. • Rests before meals.

(continued)

> ## Nursing Care Plan 48–1 *(Continued)*

Care of the Patient With Acquired Immunodeficiency Syndrome (AIDS)

Nursing Interventions	Rationale	Expected Outcomes

3. Assess factors that interfere with oral intake.
4. Consult with dietitian to determine patient's nutritional needs.
5. Reduce factors limiting oral intake:
  a. Encourage patient to rest prior to meals.
  b. Plan meals so that they do not occur immediately after painful or unpleasant procedures.
  c. Encourage patient to eat meals with visitors or others in the home when possible.
  d. Encourage patient to prepare simple meals or to obtain assistance with meal preparation if possible.
  e. Serve small, frequent meals: 6 per day.
  f. Limit fluids 1 hour prior to meals and with meals.
  —Provide mouth care prior to eating.
6. Instruct patient in ways to supplement nutritional value of meals: consume foods high in protein (meat, poultry, fish, legumes, dairy products) and carbohydrates (pasta, fruit, breads).
7. Consult with physician about alternate means of providing nutrition, such as enteral feedings or parenteral nutrition.
8. Consult with social worker or AIDS Task Force to identify means of obtaining financial assistance if patient is unable financially to obtain food.
	3. Provides basis and directions for interventions.
	4. Facilitates meal planning.
	
	  a. Minimizes fatigue, which can decrease appetite.
	  b. Decreases noxious stimuli.
	
	  c. Limits social isolation.
	
	  d. Limits energy expenditure.
	
	  e. Prevents overwhelming patient and reduces satiety.
	
	6. Provides additional proteins and calories.
	
	7. Provides nutritional support if patient is unable to take sufficient amounts by mouth.
	8. Increases availability of resources and nutrition.
		• Eats in pleasant, odor-free environment.
		• Arranges meals to coincide with visitors' visits.
		• Reports increased dietary intake.
		• Uses oral hygiene prior to meals.
		• Takes pain medication prior to meals as prescribed.
		• States ways to increase protein and caloric intake.
		• Identifies foods high in protein and calories.
		• Consumes foods high in protein and calories.
		• Reports decreased rate of weight loss.
		• Maintains adequate intake.
		• States rationale for enteral or parenteral nutrition if needed.
		• Demonstrates skill in preparing alternate sources of nutrition.

Nursing Diagnosis: Knowledge deficit related to means of preventing transmission of HIV

Goal: Increased knowledge concerning means of preventing disease transmission

1. Instruct patient, family, and friends about routes of transmission of HIV.
2. Instruct patient, family, and friends about means of preventing transmission of HIV:
  a. Avoid sexual contact with multiple partners.
  b. Use precautions when it is not absolutely certain that the sexual partner has not been exposed to HIV through intravenous drug use, sexual contact, or blood or blood products.
  c. Use condoms during sexual intercourse (vaginal, anal, oral–genital).
  d. Avoid mouth contact with the penis, vagina, or rectum.
	1. Knowledge about disease transmission can help prevent spread of disease; may also alleviate fears.
	
	  a. The risk of infection increases with the number of sexual partners, male or female, and sexual contact with those who engage in high-risk behaviors.
	
	  c. Reduces risk of transmission of HIV.
		• Patient, family, and friends state means of transmission.
		• Reports and demonstrates practices to reduce exposure of others to HIV.
		• Avoids intravenous drug use.
		• Demonstrates safe sexual practices.
		• Identifies means of preventing disease transmission.
		• States that sexual partners are informed about positive HIV antibodies in blood.

(continued)

Nursing Care Plan 48-1 (Continued)

Care of the Patient With Acquired Immunodeficiency Syndrome (AIDS)

Nursing Interventions	Rationale	Expected Outcomes
e. Avoid sexual practices that can cause cuts or tears in the lining of the rectum, vagina, or penis.		
f. Avoid sex with prostitutes and others at high risk.	f. Many prostitutes are infected with HIV through sexual contact with multiple partners or intravenous drug use.	
g. Do not use intravenous drugs; if addicted and unable or unwilling to change behavior, use clean needles and syringes.	g. Clean needles and syringes are the only way to prevent HIV transmission for those who continue to use drugs. Taking precautions is especially important for those who are antibody-positive to prevent transmission of HIV to others.	
h. Women who may have been exposed to AIDS through sexual or drug practices should consult with a physician prior to becoming pregnant.	h. AIDS can be transmitted from mother to child in utero.	

Nursing Diagnosis: Social isolation related to stigma of the disease, withdrawal of support systems, isolation procedures, and fear of infecting others

Goal: Decreased sense of social isolation

1. Assess patient's usual patterns of social interaction.	1. Establishes basis for individualized interventions.	• Shares with others the need for valued social interaction.
2. Observe for behaviors indicative of social isolation, such as decreased interaction with staff or friends and family, hostility, noncompliance, sad affect, and verbalization of feelings of rejection or loneliness.	2. Social isolation may be manifested in several ways.	• Demonstrates interest in events, activities, and communication.
3. Provide instruction concerning means of transmission of HIV.	3. Provision of accurate information corrects misconceptions and alleviates anxiety.	• Verbalizes feelings and reactions to diagnosis, prognosis, and resulting changes in life.
4. Assist patient to identify and explore resources for support and positive mechanisms for coping (*e.g.,* contact with family, friends, AIDS task force).		• Identifies means of transmission of AIDS.
5. Allow time to be with patient other than for medications or procedures.	5. Promotes feelings of self-worth and provides social interaction.	• States ways of preventing transmission of AIDS virus to others while maintaining contact with valued friends and relatives.
6. Encourage participation in diversional activities such as reading, television, or hand crafts.	6. Provides distraction.	• Reveals AIDS diagnosis to others when appropriate.
		• Identifies resources (*i.e.,* supportive family, friends, and support groups).
		• Uses resources when appropriate.
		• Accepts offers of assistance and support from others.
		• Reports decreased sense of social isolation.
		• Maintains contacts with those of importance to self.
		• Develops or continues hobbies that effectively serve as diversion or distraction.

requires expert assessment, communication, and interpersonal skills; the ability to deal with a wide range of physical problems and psychologic reactions; and commitment to and respect for the dignity of patients from all walks of life who have contracted AIDS, often at a young age.

Bibliography

Books

Alyson S (ed). You Can Do Something About AIDS. Boston, The Stop AIDS Project, 1988.

Barrett JT. Textbook of Immunology: An Introduction to Immunochemistry and Immunobiology, 5th ed. St Louis, CV Mosby, 1988.

Bayer R. Private Acts, Social Consequences: AIDS and the Politics of Public Health. New York, The Free Press, Macmillan, 1989.

Coleman RM, Lombard MF, Sicard RE, Rencricca NJ. Fundamental Immunology. Dubuque, WMC Brown, 1989.

Colman W. Understanding and Preventing AIDS. Chicago, Childrens' Press, 1988.

Croenenberger JH and Jennette JC. Immunology: Basic Concepts, Diseases and Laboratory Methods. Norwalk, CT, Appleton and Lange, 1988.

DeVita VT, Hellman S, Rosenberg SA. AIDS: Etiology, Diagnosis, Treatment, and Prevention, 2nd ed. Philadelphia, JB Lippincott, 1988.

Fan H, Conner RF, Villareal LP. The Biology of AIDS. Boston, Jones and Bartlett Publishers, 1989.

Friedman–Kien AE. Color Atlas of AIDS. Philadelphia, WB Saunders, 1989.

Goidl EA (ed). Aging and the Immune Response. New York, Marcel Dekker, 1987.

Gottlieb MS and Groopman JE (eds). AIDS. New York, Alan R Liss, 1984.

Gottlieb MS et al. Current Topics in AIDS, Vol 2. Chichester, England, John Wiley & Sons, 1989.

Griffin JP. Hematology and Immunology: Concepts for Nursing. Norwalk, CT, Appleton–Century–Crofts, 1986.

Hamblin AS. Lymphokines. Oxford, IRL Press, 1988.

Kaslow RA and Francis DP (eds). The Epidemiology of AIDS. New York, Oxford University Press, 1989.

Langman RE. The Immune System. San Diego, Academic Press, 1989.

Leoung G and Mills J (eds). Opportunistic Infections in Patients With AIDS. New York, Marcel Dekker, 1989.

Lewis A. Nursing Care of the Person with AIDS/ARC. Rockville, MD, Aspen Systems, 1988.

Ma P and Armstrong D. AIDS and Infections of Homosexual Men. Boston, Butterworths, 1989.

National Research Council. AIDS: The Second Decade. Washington, DC, National Academy Press, 1990.

Reynolds CW and Wiltgout RH (eds). Functions of the Natural Immune System. New York, Plenum Press, 1989.

Rosen FS, Steines LA, and Unanoe ER. Dictionary of Immunology. London, Macmillan Press Ltd, 1989.

Sell S. Immunology, Immunopathology and Immunity, 4th ed. New York, Elsevier, 1987.

Specter S, Bendinelli M, and Friedman H (eds). Virus-Induced Immunosuppression. New York, Plenum Press, 1989.

Virella G, Goust JM, and Fudenberg HH (eds). Introduction to Medical Immunology, 2nd ed. New York, Marcel Dekker, 1990.

Watstein SB and Laurich RN. Source Book: AIDS and Women. Phoenix, Oryx Press, 1991.

Weismann K et al. Skin Signs in AIDS. Munksgaard, Copenhagen, Year Book Medical Publishers, 1988.

Williams I, Mindel A, and Weller IVD. Pocket Picture Guides: AIDS. Philadelphia, JB Lippincott/Gower Medical Publishing, 1989.

World Health Organization. Guidelines for Nursing Management of People Infected with Human Immunodeficiency Virus (HIV). Geneva, World Health Organization, 1988.

Journals

Asterisks indicate nursing research articles.

Immunology (General)

Buckley RH. Immunodeficiency diseases. JAMA 1987 Nov; 258(20):2841–2850.

Coffman RL. T-Helper heterogeneity and immune response patterns. Hosp Pract 1989 Aug; 24(8):101–133.

DiJulio J. Hematopoiesis: An overview. Oncol Nurs Forum 1991 Mar; 18(2): 3–6.

Heinzel FP. Infections in patients with humoral immunodeficiency. Hosp Pract 1989 Sep; 24(9):99–130.

Murasko DM et al. Immunologic response in an elderly population with a mean age of 85. Am J Med 1986 Oct; 81(4):612–618.

Nossal GJV. Current concepts: Immunology—The basic components of the immune system. N Engl J Med 1987 May 21; 316(21):1320–1325.

Weigle WO. The effects of aging on the immune system. Hosp Pract 1989 Dec; 24(12):112–116, 118, 119.

Young LS. Infections in patients with cellular immunodeficiency. Hosp Pract 1989 Aug; 24(8):191–212.

AIDS

Abernathy E. How the immune system works. Am J Nurs 1987 Apr; 87(4): 456–459.

Alexander MC. Interferon therapy. NITA 1987 Jan/Feb; 10(1):40–42.

Anderson H and MacElveen–Hoehn, P. Gay clients with AIDS: New challenges for hospice programs. The Hospice Journal 1988 Winter; 4(2): 37–54.

Armstrong TBB. The pathophysiology of human immunodeficiency virus infections. J Adv Med Surg Nurs 1988 Dec; 1(1):9–20.

Baird SB and Jassak PF (eds). The biotherapy of cancer. Oncol Nurs Forum 1987 Nov/Dec; 14(6):2–40.

* Barrick B. The willingness of nursing personnel to care for patients with AIDS: A survey study and recommendations. J Prof Nurs 1988 Sep/Oct; 4(5):366–372.

Baver SA, Crocker KS, and Frame P. Home intravenous therapy for cytomegalovirus retinitis: A case report. NITA 1987 Sep/Oct; 6(7):358–365.

* Beaman ML and Strader MK. STD patients' knowledge about AIDS and attitudes toward condom use. J Community Health Nurs 1989; 6(3): 155–164.

Bennett JA. Nurses talk about the challenge of AIDS. Am J Nurs 1987 Sep; 87(9):1148–1155.

Bennett J. Helping people with AIDS live well at home. Nurs Clin North Am 1988 Dec; 23(4):731–747.

Birdsall C and Uretsky S. How do you give pentamidine aerosol for PCP? Am J Nurs 1988 Aug; 88(8):1126, 1128.

Bloom JN and Palestine AG. The diagnosis of cytomegalovirus retinitis. Ann Intern Med 1988 Dec; 109(12):963–969.

Bolle JL. Supporting the deliverers of care: Strategies to support nurses and prevent burnout. Nurs Clin North Am 1988 Dec; 23(4):843–849.

Brown ML. AIDS and ethics: Concerns and considerations. Oncol Nurs Forum 1987 Jan/Feb; 1(14):69–73.

Bryant–Armstrong TB. The pathophysiology of human immunodeficiency virus infections. J Adv Med Surg Nurs 1988 Dec; 1(1):9–20.

Carr GS and Gee G. AIDS and AIDS-related conditions: Screening for populations at risk. Nurse Pract 1986 Oct; 11(10):41–48.

Centers for Disease Control, U.S. Department of Health and Human Services. Classification system for human T-lymphotropic virus type III/lymphadenopathy–associated virus infections. Ann Intern Med 1986 Aug; 105(2):234–237.

Chin J. Epidemiology: Current and future dimensions of the HIV/AIDS pandemic in women and children. Lancet 1990 Jul; 336(8709):221–224.

Clark C et al. Hospice care: A model for caring for the person with AIDS. Nurs Clin North Am 1988 Dec; 23(4):851–862.

Cline RJW. Communication and death and dying: Implications for coping with AIDS. AIDS and Public Policy Journal 1989 Summer; 4(1):40–50.

Corkey KJ, Luce JM, and Montgomery AB. Aerosolized pentamidine for treatment and prophylaxis of Pneumocystis carinii pneumonia: An update. Respir Care 1988 Aug; 33(8):676–685.

Cox PH et al: Outcomes of treatment with AZT of patients with AIDS and symptomatic HIV infection. Nurse Pract 1990 May; 15(5):36–44.

Cummings D. Caring for the HIV-infected adult. Nurse Pract 1988 Nov; 13(11):28–47.

Davis WM. Self care for PWA's: How to teach your patients. AIDS Patient Care 1988 Apr; 2(2):13–16.

Doll DC and Rungenberg QS. Lymphomas associated with infection. Semin Oncol Nurs 1989 Nov; 5(4):255–262.

Donehowes MC. Malignant complications of AIDS. Oncol Nurs Forum 1987 Jan/Feb; 14(1):57–64.

Farrell B. AIDS patients: Values in conflict. Crit Care Nurs Q 1987 Sep; 10(2):74–85.

Fauci A. The human immunodeficiency virus: Infectivity and mechanisms of pathogenesis. Science 1988 Feb; 239(5):617–622.

Figlin RA. Biotherapy with interferon. Semin Oncol 1988 Dec; 15(6-S):3–9.

Friedland GH and Klein RS. Transmission of the human immunodeficiency virus: An updated review. Int Nurs Rev 1988 Mar/Apr; 35(2):44–54.

Gee G. AIDS: Context of care. Semin Oncol Nurs 1989 Nov; 5(4):244–248.

Gee G, Wong R, and Moran T. Current treatment strategies for HIV infection. Semin Oncol Nurs 1989 Nov; 5(4):249–254.

Glatt AE, Chirgwin K, and Landesman SH. Treatment of infections associated with human immunodeficiency virus. N Engl J Med 1988 Jun 2; 318(22):1439–1448.

Govoni LA. Psychosocial issues of AIDS in the nursing care of homosexual men and their significant others. Nurs Clin North Am 1988 Dec; 23(4):749–765.

Grady C. HIV: Epidemiology, immunopathogenesis and clinical consequences. Nurs Clin North Am 1988 Dec; 23(4):683–695.

Haeuber D. Future strategies in the control of myelosuppression: The use of colony-stimulating factors. Oncol Nurse Forum 1991 Mar; 18(2):16–21.

Hall JM, Koehler SL, and Lewis A. HIV-related mental health nursing issues. Semin Oncol Nurs 1989 Nov; 5(4):276–283.

Halloran J, Hughes A, and Mayer DK. AIDS task force: ONS position paper on HIV-related issues. Oncol Nurs Forum 1988 Mar/Apr; 15(2):206–216.

Hannon S. Adaptable nursing care plan for AIDS patients at home. AIDS Patient Care 1990 Apr; 4(2):23–30.

Hardy WD. Comparing options for prophylaxis of Pneumocystis carinii pneumonia. AIDS Medical Report 1988 Jun; 2(6):57–63.

Hendricksen C. The AIDS clinical trials unit experience: Clinical research and antiviral treatment. Nurs Clin North Am 1988 Dec; 23(4):697–705.

Heyward WL and Curran JW. The epidemiology of AIDS. Sci Am 1988 Oct; 259(4):72–81.

Hilton G. AIDS dementia. Neurosci Nurs 1989 Feb; 21(1):24–29.

Hood LE. Interferon. Am J Nurs 1987 Apr; 87(4):459–465.

Hoth DF and Myers MW. Current status of HIV therapy: Antiviral agents. Hosp Pract 1991 Jan; 26(1):174–197.

Jackson MM and Lynch P. Infection prevention and control in the era of the AIDS/HIV epidemic. Semin Oncol Nurs 1989 Nov; 5(4):236–243.

Jacob JL et al. AIDS-related Kaposi's sarcoma: Concepts of care. Semin Oncol Nurs 1989 Nov; 5(4):263–275.

Jassak PF and Spiewak PL. Interleukin-2. Am J Nurs 1987 Apr; 87(4):464–467.

Jordan KS. Assessment of the person with AIDS in the Emergency Department. Int Nurs Rev 1989 Mar/Apr; 36(2):57–59.

Keithly JK and Kohn CL. Managing nutritional problems in people with AIDS. Oncol Nurs Forum 1990; 17(1):23–27.

Kendig NE and Adler WH. The implications of the acquired immunodeficiency syndrome for gerontology research and geriatric medicine. J Gerontol 1990 May; 45(3):77–81.

Kovacs AJ and Masur H. Pneumocystis carinii pneumonia: Therapy and prophylaxis. J Infect Dis 1988 Jul; 158(1):254–259.

Krigel RL and Friedman-Kien AE. Epidemic Kaposi's sarcoma. Semin Oncol 1990 Jun; 17(3):350–360.

Krown SE. Alpha interferon in AIDS-related Kaposi's sarcoma. Biotherapy and Cancer 1988 Dec; 1(4):1, 4, 5.

LaCharite CL and Meinsenbelder JB. Fear of contagion: A stress response to acquired immunodeficiency syndrome. Adv Nurs Sci 1989 Jan; 11(2):29–38.

Larson E. Nursing research and AIDS. Nurs Res 1988 Jan/Feb; 37(1):60–62.

Laskin MEA. Pain management in the patient with AIDS. J Adv Med Surg Nurs 1988 Dec; 1(1):37–43.

Laskin OL et al. Use of ganciclovir to treat serious cytomegalovirus infections in patients with AIDS. J Infect Dis 1987 Feb; 155(2):323–327.

* Lawrence SA and Lawrence RA. Knowledge and attitudes about acquired immunodeficiency syndrome in nursing and non-nursing groups. J Prof Nurs 1989 Mar/Apr; 5(2):92–101.

Levine AM. Non-Hodgkin's lymphoma and other malignancies in the acquired immune deficiency syndrome. Semin Oncol 1987 Jun; 14(2 Suppl):34–39.

Levine AM, Gill PS, and Muggia F. Malignancies in the acquired immunodeficiency syndrome. Curr Probl Cancer 1987 Jul/Aug; 11(4):213–255.

Lunk DL. Antibiotic therapy in the cancer patient: Focus on third generation cephalosporins. Oncol Nurs Forum 1987 Sep/Oct; 14(5):35–41.

Lone P. A place to call home. Am J Nurs 1989 Apr; 89(4):490–492.

Lovejoy NC. The pathophysiology of AIDS. Oncol Nurs Forum 1988 Sep/Oct; 15(2):563–571.

* Lovejoy NC and Moran TA. Selected AIDS beliefs, behaviors and informational needs of homosexual/bisexual men with AIDS or ARC. Int J Nurs Stud 1988 May; 25(3):207–216.

Lynch M, Yanes L, and Todd K. Nursing care of AIDS patients participating in a phase I/II trial of recombinant human granulocyte-macrophage colony stimulating factor. Oncol Nurs Forum 1988 Jul/Aug; 15(4):463–469.

Lyon JC. AIDS: What are the costs? Who will pay? Nurs Econ 1988 Oct; 6(5):241–244.

Marin G. AIDS prevention among Hispanics: Needs, risk behaviors and cultural values. Public Health Rep 1989 Sept/Oct; 104(5):411–415.

Masur H et al. Public Health Service Task Force recommendations for anti-pneumocystis prophylaxis for patients infected with HIV. AIDS Patient Care 1990 Apr; 4(2):5–14.

McArthur JH, Polenicek JG, and Bowersox LL. Human immunodeficiency virus and the nervous system. Nurs Clin North Am 1988 Oct; 23(4):823–841.

McGough KN. Assessing social support of people with AIDS. Oncol Nurs Forum 1990 Jan/Feb; 17(1):31–35.

McMahon KM. The integration of HIV testing and counseling into nursing practice. Nurs Clin North Am 1988 Dec; 23(4):803–821.

McMahon KM and Coyne N. Symptom management in patients with AIDS. Semin Oncol Nurs 1989 Nov; 5(4):289–301.

Melamed AJ. The use of inhaled pentamidine for the prevention and treatment of Pneumocystis carinii pneumonia in AIDS patients. Hosp Pharm 1988 Jan; 23(1):65, 66, 72.

Merz B. Aerosolized pentamidine promising in Pneumocystis therapy, prophylaxis. JAMA 1988 Jun 10; 259(22):3223–3224.

Mills J and Masur H. AIDS-related infections. Sci Am 1990 Aug; 263(2):50–57.

Mitsuyasu RT. The role of alpha interferon in the biotherapy of hematologic malignancies and AIDS-related Kaposi's sarcoma. Oncol Nurs Forum 1988 Nov/Dec; 15(6 Suppl):7–11.

Mitsuyasu RT. The enhanced potential use of recombinant alpha-interferon in the treatment of AIDS-related Kaposi's sarcoma. Oncol Nurs Forum 1989 Nov/Dec; 16(6 Suppl):5–7.

Mitsuyasu RT. Clinical oncology quiz no. 5: Interferon therapy for Kaposi's sarcoma in AIDS patients. Roche Laboratories 1989 Feb; 2(1):1–8.

Mitsuyasu RT. Hematopoietic growth factors may be answer for neutropenia, anemia. AIDS Med Rep 1990 Nov; 3(11):137–141.

* Moran TA et al. Informational needs of homosexual men diagnosed with AIDS or AIDS-related complex. Oncol Nurs Forum 1988 May/June; 15(3):311–314.

The National Institute of Allergy and Infectious Diseases. AZT therapy recommendations for early HIV infection: State-of-the-art conference executive summary. AIDS Patient Care 1990 Jun; 4(3):6–8.

Nily G. AIDS: Opportunistic diseases and their physical assessment. J Adv Med Surg Nurs 1988 Dec; 1(1):27–36.

O'Brien AM, Derlemens-Bunn M, and Blanchfield JC. Nursing the AIDS patient at home. AIDS Patient Care 1987 Jun; 1(1):21–24.

Oerlemans–Bunn M. On being gay, single and bereaved. Am J Nurs 1988 Apr; 88(4):472–476.

Orellana J et al. Combined short and long-term therapy for the treatment of CMV retinitis using ganciclovir (BWB759U). Ophthalmology 1987 Jul; 94(7):831–838.

Otte DM and Allen KS. Ethical principles in the nursing care of the terminally ill adult. Oncol Nurs Forum 1987 Sep/Oct; 14(5):87–91.

Parkinson DR. Interleukin-2 in cancer therapy. Semin Oncol 1988 Dec; 15(6-S):10–26.

Pasacreta JV and Jacobsen PB. Addressing the need for staff support among nurses caring for the AIDS population. Oncol Nurs Forum 1989 Sep/Oct; 16(5):659–663.

Pfeiffer N. Zidovudine resistance. AIDS Patient Care 1991 Feb; 5(1):13–14.

Pfeiffer N. Highlights from the national conference on women and HIV infection. Part I: Early care and policy issues. AIDS Patient Care 1991 Apr; 5(2):67–69.

Pizzi M. Occupational therapy: Creating possibilities for adults with HIV infection, ARC and AIDS. AIDS Patient Care 1989 Feb; 3(1):18–23.

Pizzo PA. Combating infections in neutropenic patients. Hosp Pract 1989 Jul; 24(7):81–96.

Price RW et al. The brain in AIDS: Central nervous system HIV-1 infection and AIDS dementia complex. Science 1988 Feb; 239(5):586–591.

Prichard JG. Human immunodeficiency virus: The best use of serologic tests. Consultant 1988 Nov; 28(11):41–45, 49, 52.

Quinn TC. The Epidemiology of the human immunodeficiency virus. Ann Emerg Med 1990 Mar; 19(3):225–232.

Raphael BG and Knowles DM. AIDS associated non-Hodgkin's lymphoma. Semin Oncol 1990 Jun; 17(3):361–366.

Reisman EC. Ethical issues confronting nurses. Nurs Clin North Am 1988 Dec; 23(4):789–801.

Ripper M. Universal blood and body fluid precautions. J Adv Med Surg Nurs 1988 Dec; 1(1):21–25.

Rogers PL et al. Admissions of AIDS patients to a medical intensive care unit: Causes and outcome. Crit Care Med 1989; 17(2):113–115.

Rosenthal Y and Haneiwich S. Nursing management of adults in the hospital. Nurs Clin North Am 1988 Dec; 23(4):707–717.

Saunders JM. Psychosocial and cultural issues in HIV infection. Semin Oncol Nurs 1989 Nov; 5(4):284–288.

Scherer P. How HIV attacks the peripheral nervous system. Am J Nurs 1990 May; 90(5):66–70.

Scheser YK, Haughey BP, and Wu YWB. AIDS: What are nurses' concerns? Clin Nurse Spec 1989 Spring; 3(1):48–54.

Schofferman J. Hospice care of the patient with AIDS: The Hospice Journal 1988 Winter; 4(2):57–75.

* Scura KW and Whipple B. Older adults as an HIV positive risk group. J Gerontol Nurs 1990 Feb; 15(2):6–10.

Sinclair BP. AIDS in women. NAACOG's Clinical Issues in Perinatal and Women's Health Nursing 1990; 1(1):1–127.

Stern C. AIDS: What office nurses need to know. The Office Nurse 1988 Aug/Sep; 1(3):8–10, 12, 34.

Sticklin LA. Interleukin-2 and killer T cells. Am J Nurs 1987 Apr; 87(11):468–469.

Streckfuss BL and Bergers RM. Infection control for caregivers of AIDS patients (domiciliary). NITA 1987 Jul/Aug; 10(4):282–284.

Task Force on Nutrition Support in AIDS. Guidelines for nutrition support in AIDS. AIDS Patient Care 1989 Aug; 3(4):32–38.

Trimetrexate for PCP. Am J Nurs 1988 Feb; 88(1):158.

U.S. Department of Health and Human Services. AIDS and human immunodeficiency virus infection in the United States. MMWR 1989 May; 38(S-4):1–14.

U.S. Department of Health and Human Services. Coordinated community programs for HIV prevention among intravenous drug users—California, Massachusetts. MMWR 1989 Jun; 38(21):369–374.

U.S. Department of Health and Human Services. HIV epidemic and AIDS: Trends in knowledge—United States, 1987 and 1988. MMWR 1989 May; 38(24):353–358, 363.

U.S. Department of Health and Human Services. Guidelines for prophylaxis against Pneumocystis carinii pneumonia for persons infected with human immunodeficiency virus. MMWR 1989 Jun; 38(S-5):1–9.

U.S. Department of Health and Human Services. Transmission of HIV

through bone transplantation: Case report and public health recommendations. MMWR 1988 Oct; 37(39):597–599.

U.S. Department of Health and Human Services. Revision of the CDC surveillance case definition for AIDS. MMWR 1987 Aug; 36(15):3–15.

U.S. Department of Health and Human Services. Guidelines for prevention of transmission of HIV and hepatitis B virus to health-care and public safety workers. MMWR 1989 Jun; 38(S-6):3–37.

U.S. Department of Health and Human Services. Mortality attributable to HIV infections/AIDS: U.S. 1981–1990. MMWR 1991 Jan; 40(3):41–44.

U.S. Department of Health and Human Services. HIV prevalence estimates and AIDS case projections for the U.S.: Report based upon a workshop. MMWR 1990 Nov; 39(RR-16):1–31.

U.S. Department of Health and Human Services. HIV/AIDS: Surveillance 1991 Jan; 1–22.

Valentine FT. Pathogenesis of the immunological deficiencies caused by infection with the human immunodeficiency virus. Semin Oncol 1990 Jun; 17(3):321–334.

Vlahov D. AIDS: Overview, immunology, virology and informational needs. Semin Oncol Nurs 1989 Nov; 5(4):227–235.

Weber JN and Weiss RA. HIV infection: The cellular picture. Sci Am 1988 Oct; 259(4):101–109.

Whipple B and Scura KW. HIV and the older adult: Taking the necessary precautions. J Gerontol Nurs 1989 Sep; 15(9):15–19.

White K. Highlights from the national conference on women and HIV infection. Part II: Care definition and clinical trend changes. AIDS Patient Care 1991 Apr; 5(2):70–72.

Willoughby A. AIDS in women: Epidemiology. Clin Obstet Gynecol 1989 Sep; 32(3):429–436.

Winich M et al. Guidelines for nutrition support in AIDS. Nutrition 1989 Jan/Feb; 5(1):39–45.

Yarbro CH, Collins JL, and Thaney KM (eds). Biotherapy: A nursing challenge. Semin Oncol Nurs 1988 May; 4(2):81–153.

Young LS and Inderlied CB. *Mycobacterium-avium* complex infections. AIDS Patient Care 1990 Dec; 4(1):13–16.

Patient/Family Resources
Bartel NR and Orlando JE. AIDS: A Guide for Parents. Philadelphia, Jonet Publishers, 1988.

Colman W. Understanding and Preventing AIDS: A Guide for Young People. Chicago, Childrens' Press, 1988.

Dietz SD and Hicks MJP. Take These Broken Wings and Learn to Fly. Tucson, Harbinger House, 1989.

Eidson T (ed). The AIDS Care Givers Handbook. New York, St Martin's Press, 1988.

Langone J. AIDS: The Facts. Boston, Little, Brown, 1988.

Lingle VA and Wood MS. How to Find Information About AIDS. New York, Harrington Park Press, 1988.

Malinowsky RH and Perry GJ (eds). AIDS Information Sourcebook, 2nd ed, 1989–90. Phoenix, Oryx Press, 1989.

Information/Resources

Agencies

AIDS Action Council
    729 Eighth St. SE, Suite 200, Washington, DC 20003, (202) 547-3101
AIDS Clinical Trials Unit (ACTU)
    2300 Eye St., Suite 202, Washington, DC 20037, (202) 994-2417
AIDS Program
    Centers for Infectious Diseases, CDC 1600 Clifton Rd., Atlanta, GA 30333, (800) 342-AIDS
American Red Cross
    AIDS Education Office, 431 18th St NW, Washington, DC 20006, (202) 737-8300 (or local Red Cross)
Gay Men's Health Crisis Network
    P.O. Box 274, 132 West 24th St., New York, NY 10011, (212) 807-6655

Hispanic AIDS Committee for Education and Resources
    1139 W Hildebrant, Suite B, San Antonio, TX 78201, (512) 732-3108
Hispanic AIDS Forum
    c/o APRED, 853 Broadway Suite 2007, New York, NY 10003, (212) 870-1902 or 870-1864
Minority Task Force on AIDS
    c/o New York City Council of Churches, 475 Riverside Dr., Room 456, New York, NY 10115, (212) 749-1214
Mothers of AIDS Patients (MAP)
    c/o Barbara Peabody, 3403 E St., San Diego, CA 92102, (619) 234-3432
National AIDS Information Clearinghouse (NAIC)
    P.O. Box 6003, Rockville, MD 20850, (301) 762-5111
National AIDS Network (NAN)
    2033 M St. NW, Suite 800, Washington DC, 20036, (202) 293-2437
National Association of People with AIDS
    P.O. Box 65472, Washington, DC 20035, (202) 483-7979
National Coalition of Gay Sexually Transmitted Disease Services
    c/o Mark Behar, P.O. Box 239, Milwaukee, WI 53201-0239, (414) 277-7671

National Council of Churches/AIDS Task Force
    475 Riverside Dr., Room 572, New York, NY 10115, (212) 870-2421
National Lawyers Guild AIDS Network
    211 Gough St., 3rd Floor, San Francisco, CA 94102
New York City Department of Health Division of AIDS Program Services
    125 Worth St., Box A/1, New York, NY 10013, (212) 566-7103, Hotline: (718)485-8111
Philadelphia Community Health Alternatives/The Philadelphia AIDS Task Force 1216 Walnut St., Philadelphia, PA 19107, (215) 545-8686
U.S. Public Health Service
    Public Affairs Office, Hubert H. Humphrey Bldg., Room 725-H, 200 Independence Ave. SW, Washington, DC 20201, (202) 245-6867

Telephone Hotlines (Toll Free)

National Gay Task Force AIDS Information Hotline: (800) 221-7044; (212) 807-6016 (NY State)
National Sexually Transmitted Disease Hotline/American Social Health Association: (800) 227-8922
PHS AIDS Hotline: (800) 342-AIDS; (800) 342-2437

49

Assessment and Management of Patients With Allergic Disorders

Learning Objectives

On completion of this chapter, the learner will be able to:

1. Explain the physiology underlying allergic reactions
2. Describe the management and nursing care of patients with allergic disorders
3. Use the nursing process as a framework for care of the patient with allergic rhinitis
4. Describe the prevention and management of anaphylaxis

The human body is menaced by a host of potential invaders—for the most part, microbial organisms—that are constantly threatening its surface defenses. Having penetrated those defenses, these agents compete with the body for its nutrients and, if allowed to flourish unimpeded, disrupt its enzyme systems and destroy its vital tissues. To protect against these agents, the body is equipped with an elaborate blockade system. The first line of defense consists of the epithelial cells that coat the skin and make up the lining of the respiratory, gastrointestinal, and genitourinary tracts. The structure and continuity of these surfaces and the resistance to penetration are initial deterrents to invaders.

One of the most effective of the body's defense mechanisms is its capacity to equip itself rapidly with weapons (*antibodies*) individually designed to meet each new invader, namely, specific protein *antigens*. Antibodies react with antigens in a variety of ways: (1) by coating their surface if they are particular substances, (2) by neutralizing them if they are toxic, or (3) by precipitating them out of solution if they are dissolved. In any event, the antibodies prepare the antigen for action by the phagocytic cells of the blood and the tissues.

Allergic Reaction: Physiologic Overview

Immunity

Some people are born with the ability to resist invasion by certain types of foreign agents. Most persons, however, acquire resistance by actually fighting off the invader. It is also possible to acquire resistance by two other methods: (1) *actively acquired immunization,* whereby an antigenic substance (one that has lost its ability to produce illness but is able to stimulate antibody formation) is injected into the body (*e.g.,* virus vaccine and tetanus toxoid); and (2) *passively acquired immunization,* whereby resistance is brought about by the transfer of antibody-containing serum from a sensitized donor to a normal recipient (*i.e.*, human gamma globulin).

Allergy

Allergy is an inappropriate and often harmful response of the immune system to normally harmless substances. An *allergic reaction* is a manifestation of tissue injury resulting from interaction between an antigen and an antibody. When the body is invaded by the antigen, usually a protein that is recognized as foreign, a series of events takes place with the goal of making the invader harmless, destroying it, and ridding the body of it. When lymphocytes respond to the antigen, antibodies are often produced. Common allergic reactions occur when the immune system of a susceptible person responds aggressively to a substance that is normally harmless (*i.e.*, dust, weed pollen). The production of chemical mediators in such allergic reactions may produce symptoms that range from those that are mild and inconvenient to those that are life-threatening.

The immune system is composed of many cells and organs, and substances that are secreted by these cells and organs; these parts of the immune system must work together to assure adequate defense against invaders (*i.e.*, virus, bacteria, other foreign substances) without destruction of the body's own tissues by an overly aggressive reaction.

B Cells and Immunoglobulins

One type of lymphocyte, the *B cell* or *B lymphocyte,* is programmed to produce one specific antibody. When a B cell encounters a specific antigen, it stimulates production of plasma cells. The plasma cell is the site of antibody production. The response of this mechanism to an antigen is the outpouring of antibody for the purpose of destroying and removing the antigen.

Antibodies that are formed by lymphocytes and plasma cells in response to an immunogenic stimulus constitute a group of serum proteins called *immunoglobulins*. These can be found in the lymph nodes, tonsils, appendix, and Peyer's patches of the intestinal tract, or circulating in the blood and lymph. These antibodies combine with antigens in a very special way, which has been likened to keys fitting into a lock. Antigens (keys) only fit certain antibodies (locks); hence, the term *specificity* has been coined in relation to the specific reaction of an antibody to an antigen. There are many variations and complexities in these patterns.

Antibody molecules are *bivalent*, which means that they have two combining sites. Because of this, the antibody easily becomes a cross-link between two antigen groups, causing them to clump together (*agglutination*). By this action, invaders in the bloodstream are cleared. Agglutination is the means of determining blood group in laboratory tests.

There are five classes of immunoglobulins, designated as follows: IgE, IgD, IgG, IgM, and IgA. Antibodies of the IgM, IgG, and IgA classes have definite and well-established protective functions. These include neutralization of toxins and viruses, and precipitation, agglutination, or lysis of bacteria and other foreign cellular material.

   IgE—IgE levels are elevated in allergic disorders and some parasitic infections. IgE-producing cells are located in the respiratory and intestinal mucosa. Two or more IgE mol-

ecules bind together to an allergen and trigger mast cells or basophils to release histamine, serotonin, kinins, slow-reacting substance of anaphylaxis (SRS-A), and the neutrophil factor. These mediators produce the allergic reaction on the skin, asthma, and hay fever.

   IgD—IgD immunoglobulin functions as a receptor on B lymphocytes. IgD can be found in very small quantities in the serum.

   IgG—IgG is the major immunoglobulin responding after reexposure to an antigen and the second immunoglobulin to respond to an antigen in the immune response. IgG is found in the extravascular fluid spaces of the body, such as lymph, cerebrospinal fluid, synovial fluid, and peritoneal fluid.

   IgM—IgM is the major antibody involved in the immune response and the first to respond to an antigen. One of the major functions of IgM is to bind with viral and bacterial antigens in circulation. IgM and IgG work together as antitoxins in response to tetanus, snake venom, and botulism.

   IgA—IgA exists in two forms: serum IgA and secretory IgA. Serum IgA constitutes 10% to 15% of the entire serum immunoglobulin. Secretory IgA, the major IgA component, is concentrated in exocrine secretions such as saliva, sweat, tears, and colostrum and secretions of the urogenital, gastrointestinal, and respiratory tracts.

T Cells

T cells, or *T lymphocytes*, a second type of lymphocyte with a major role in the immune system, assist the B cells or lymphocytes in the production of antibodies. T cells work by secreting substances known as *lymphokines*, which assist the immune response by encouraging cell growth, promoting cell activation, directing the flow of cell activity, destroying target cells, and stimulating the macrophages. Macrophages digest antigens and present the antigen to the T cells; they initiate the immune response and assist in removal of cells and other debris.

An *antigen* is any substance that stimulates activation of the immune response and reacts with an *antibody* or a sensitized T cell. Antigens that are important in immediate hypersensitivity are divided into two groups: complete protein antigens and low-molecular-weight substances. Complete protein antigens, such as animal dander, pollen, and horse serum, stimulate a complete humoral response. (*Humoral immunity* refers to substances, including antibodies, that circulate primarily in the serum and lymph.)

Low-molecular-weight substances such as drugs function as haptens (incomplete antigens) binding to tissue or serum proteins to produce a carrier complex that initiates an antibody response. The production of antigen-specific IgE antibodies requires active communication between macrophages, T cells, and B cells. Allergen sensitization begins when the allergen is absorbed through the respiratory tract, gastrointestinal tract, or skin. The macrophage processes the antigen and presents it to the appropriate T cell. B cells that are influenced by the T cell mature into an allergen-specific IgE immunoglobulin–secreting plasma cell that synthesizes and secretes antigen-specific IgE antibody (Fig. 49-1).

Allergen stimulation is begun by the cross-linking of two or more cell-bound IgE molecules by an antigen. The mast cell then degranulates, and mediators are released. The important

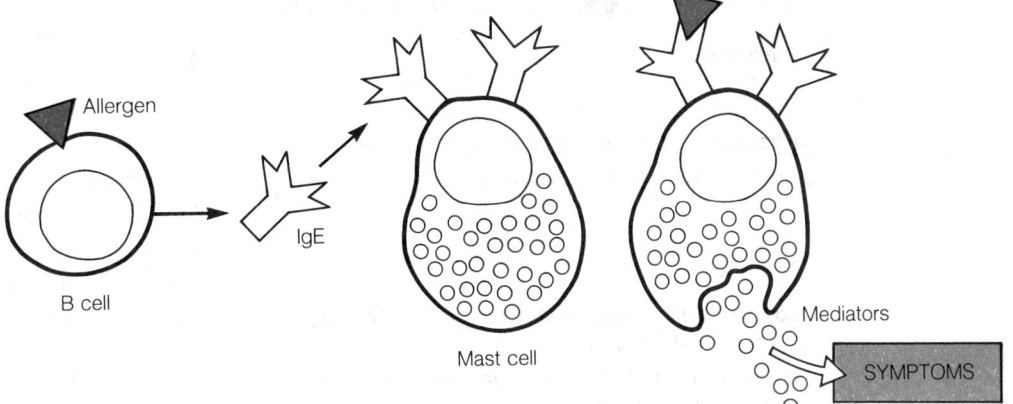

Figure 49-1. Allergen triggers B cell to make IgE antibody, which attaches to mast cell. When that allergen reappears, it binds to the IgE and triggers the mast cell to release its chemicals. (U.S. Dept. of Health and Human Services. Understanding the Immune System. NIH Publication No. 88-529, July 1988, p 19.)

known mediators are histamine, leukotrienes, eosinophil chemotactic factors of anaphylaxis (ECF-A), platelet-activating factor (PAF), bradykinin, serotonin, and prostaglandins that stimulate activation of the complement system. Release of these mediators is responsible for the symptoms associated with allergic reactions. See Table 49-1 for a description of the actions of chemical mediators.

Hypersensitivity

A hypersensitivity reaction usually does not occur after the first exposure to an allergen. The reaction follows a re-exposure after sensitization in a predisposed individual. Sensitization provides the humoral response or buildup of antibodies. Hypersensitivity reactions have been classified by Gell and Coombs (Fig. 49-2) into four specific types of reactions to offer a distinct understanding of the immunopathogenesis of disease. Most allergies are identified as either type I or type IV reactions.

Type I Reaction (Anaphylactic or Immediate Hypersensitivity)

This is an immediate, anaphylactic hypersensitivity; the reaction begins within minutes of exposure to an antigen. When chemical mediators continue to be released, a delayed reaction may continue for up to 24 hours. This reaction is mediated by IgE antibodies (reagins). A type I reaction requires previous exposure to the specific antigen, resulting in the production of IgE antibodies by plasma cells. This takes place in the lymph nodes and is supported by helper T cells. The IgE antibodies bind to membrane receptors on mast cells found in connective tissue and basophils. During re-exposure, the antigen binds to adjacent IgE antibodies, activating a cellular reaction that triggers degranulation and the release of chemical mediators (histamine, leukotrienes, and eosinophil chemotactic factor of anaphylaxis [ECF-A]).

Chemical mediators (see Fig. 49-1) are classified as primary mediators, which are found in mast cells and basophils, or as secondary mediators, which are formed in response to primary mediators. These primary mediators are responsible for the symptoms of type I reactions because of their effects on the skin, lungs, and gastrointestinal tract. Clinical symptoms are determined by the amount of the allergen, the amount of mediator released, the sensitivity of the target organ, and the route

of allergen entry. A type I reaction functions in local and systemic anaphylaxis. Examples of local anaphylaxis are extrinsic bronchial asthma, hay fever, and allergic conjunctivitis. Systemic anaphylaxis, which is more severe, occurs with particular drugs, food allergies, and insect stings. Symptoms include urticaria (hives), angioedema, pruritus, erythema, hypotension, shock, cardiac dysrhythmias, laryngeal edema, nausea, vomiting, diarrhea, and incontinence. (Anaphylactic reactions are described more fully later in this chapter.)

Type II Reaction (Cytotoxic Reactions)

The type II mechanism involves the binding of either IgG or IgM antibody to the cell-bound antigen. The result of antigen–antibody binding is activation of the complement cascade and destruction of the cell to which the antigen is bound. Type II mechanisms are involved in myasthenia gravis, pernicious anemia, Goodpasture's syndrome, immune hemolytic anemia, and Rh hemolytic disease in the newborn.

Type III Reaction (Immune Complex–Mediated Reactions)

Immune complexes are formed when antigens bind to antibodies and are cleared from the circulation by phagocytic action. When these complexes are deposited in tissues or vascular endothelium, two factors contribute to injury: the increased amount of circulating complexes and the presence of vasoactive amines. As a result, there is an increase in vascular permeability and tissue injury. Type III mechanisms are associated with systemic lupus erythematosus, rheumatoid arthritis, serum sickness, certain types of nephritis, and particular elements of bacterial endocarditis.

Type IV Reaction (Delayed Hypersensitivity)

This reaction is also known as delayed or cellular hypersensitivity, and it occurs 24 to 72 hours after exposure to an allergen. It is mediated by sensitized T cells and macrophages. An example of this reaction is the effect of an intradermal injection of tuberculin antigen or purified protein derivative (PPD). Sensitized T cells react with the antigen at or near the injection site. Release of lymphokines attracts, activates, and retains macrophages at the site. Lysozymes are released by macrophages, resulting in tissue damage. Edema and fibrin are responsible for the positive tuberculin reaction. Contact der-

TABLE 49–1.   *Chemical Mediators of Hypersensitivity*

Mediators	Action
PRIMARY MEDIATORS (Preformed and found in mast cells or basophils)	
Histamine (preformed in mast cells)	Vasodilation
	Smooth muscle contraction
	Increased vascular permeability
	Increased mucus secretions
Eosinophil chemotactic factor of anaphylaxis (ECF-A) (preformed in mast cells)	Attracts eosinophils
Platelet-activating factor (PAF) (requires synthesis by mast cells, neutrophils, and macrophages)	Smooth muscle contraction
	Incites platelets to aggregate and release serotonin and histamine
Prostaglandins (chemically derived from arachidonic acid; require synthesis by cells)	D and F series → bronchoconstriction
	E series → bronchodilation
	D, E, and F series → vasodilation
Basophil kallikrein (preformed in mast cells)	Frees bradykinin, which causes: a. Bronchoconstriction b. Vasodilation c. Nerve stimulation
SECONDARY MEDIATORS (Inactive precursors formed or released in response to primary mediators)	
Bradykinin (derived from precursor kininogen)	Smooth muscle contraction
	Increased vascular permeability
	Stimulates pain receptors
	Increased mucus production
Serotonin (preformed in platelets)	Smooth muscle contraction
	Increased vascular permeability
Heparin (preformed in mast cells)	Anticoagulant
Leukotrienes (derived from arachidonic acid and activated by mast cell degranulation) C, D, and E or slow-reacting substance of anaphylaxis (SRS-A)	Smooth muscle contraction
	Increased vascular permeability

matitis results from exposure to allergens such as cosmetics, tape, topical drugs, drug additives, and plant toxins. The primary exposure results in sensitization; re-exposure causes a hypersensitivity reaction composed of low-molecular-weight molecules or haptens that bind with proteins or carriers and are then processed by the Langerhans cells in the skin. The symptoms that occur include itching, erythema, and raised lesions.

Mediators of Immediate Hypersensitivity

When mast cells are stimulated by antigens, powerful chemical mediators are released that cause a sequence of physiologic events resulting in symptoms of immediate hypersensitivity. The most prevalent known mediators are described below.

1. *Histamine.* Histamine plays an important role in regulating the immune response. The physiologic effects of histamine upon major organs include: (1) contraction of bronchial smooth muscle resulting in wheezing and bronchospasm, (2) dilation of small venules and constriction of larger vessels, causing erythema, edema, and urticaria, and (3) an increase in secretion of gastric and mucosal cells, causing diarrhea. Histamine acts on many target organs through two types of receptors: H_1 and H_2 receptors. Histamine receptors appear on different types of lymphocytes, particularly T-lymphocyte suppressor cells as well as basophils. H_1 receptors are found predominantly on bronchiolar and vascular smooth muscle cells and are used for the treatment of allergic diseases. H_2 receptors are found on gastric parietal cells and are used pharmacologically to inhibit gastric secretions in peptic ulcer disease. Antihistamines are categorized by these receptors. Diphenhydramine (Benadryl) is an example of an antihistamine medication displaying an affinity for H_1 receptors, while cimetidine, another pharmacologic agent, targets H_2 receptors.

2. *Leukotrienes.* Leukotrienes are chemical mediators that initiate the inflammatory response. One of these substances,

slow-reacting substance of anaphylaxis (SRS-A), has long been known to produce sustained spasm of the bronchioles. Compared with histamine, leukotrienes are 100 to 1000 times more potent in causing bronchospasm. Many of the manifestations of inflammation can be attributed, in part, to leukotrienes.

3. *Eosinophil chemotactic factor of anaphylaxis (ECF-A).* This chemotactic factor is preformed in mast cells and released upon degranulation to inhibit the action of leukotrienes and histamine.

4. *Platelet-activating factor (PAF).* This factor is responsible for initiating platelet aggregation at sites of immediate hypersensitivity reactions. PAF also causes bronchoconstriction and increased vascular permeability. It also activates factor XII or Hageman factor, which induces the formation of bradykinin.

5. *Bradykinin.* Bradykinin contracts smooth muscles of the bronchi and blood vessels. It causes increased permeability of the capillaries, resulting in edema. Bradykinin stimulates nerve cell fibers and produces pain.

6. *Serotonin.* Serotonin is released during platelet aggregation, causing contraction of bronchial smooth muscle.

7. *Prostaglandins.* Prostaglandins produce smooth muscle contraction as well as vasodilation and increased capillary permeability. The fever and pain that occur with inflammation are due, in part, to the prostaglandins.

(Table 49-1 summarizes the actions of primary and secondary mediators.)

Atopic (Allergic) Disorders

Overview

The atopic diseases are processes mediated by IgE immediate hypersensitivity. In the United States, 10% to 20% of the population is affected by allergic diseases. Genetic factors play a role in susceptibility to these diseases. The disorders characterized as atopic are (1) anaphylaxis, (2) allergic rhinoconjunctivitis, (3) urticaria and angioedema, (4) asthma, (5) gastrointestinal allergy, and (6) atopic dermatitis.

Anaphylaxis. Anaphylaxis is the most serious of the atopic (allergic) diseases. The antigen is usually introduced parenterally (*i.e.*, injection of penicillin or an insect sting) or through ingestion of seafood. It is mediated by IgE antibodies, and the activity occurs in three steps: (1) the antigen attaches to the IgE antibody, which is fixed to the surface membrane of mast cells and basophils, resulting in the cross-linking of these sensitizing antibodies, activating these target cells; (2) activated basophils and mast cells release massive amounts of mediators; and (3) the effects of mediator release cause the clinical picture of bronchospasm, urticaria, and shock.

Allergic rhinoconjunctivitis. Allergic rhinoconjunctivitis is the most common atopic disease, affecting 15% of the population. It is mediated by IgE produced under the mucosal surfaces of the eyes and nose. An airborne antigen contacts mast cells sensitized by IgE and produces degranulation, resulting in local anaphylaxis of the nasal and conjunctival membranes. Symptoms include nasal congestion, a clear watery discharge, paroxysmal sneezing, nasal itching, conjunctival edema, ocular tearing, and itching.

Urticaria and angioedema. Urticaria and angioedema are often self-limited and last approximately 6 weeks. These symptoms are most often related to the ingestion or administration of food or drugs.

Asthma. Asthma is an expression of immediate hypersensitivity reactions of the lung. Bronchospasm develops after natural exposure to antigens and by bronchial challenge studies. (Asthma is discussed in detail in Chap. 26.)

Gastrointestinal allergy. Nausea, cramping, vomiting, and diarrhea are common symptoms following food exposure. Gastrointestinal allergy can be mediated by IgE hypersensitivity.

Atopic dermatitis. Atopic dermatitis exists in up to 10% of the population. These eczematous cutaneous eruptions are often associated with atopic disorders of asthma and allergic rhinitis.

Assessment

A comprehensive allergy history provides data useful for the diagnosis and management of patients with allergic disorders. A standardized assessment sheet (Chart 49-1) is useful for obtaining and organizing this information.

The degree of difficulty and discomfort experienced by the patient because of allergic symptoms and the degree of improvement in those symptoms with and without treatment are assessed and documented. The temporal and spatial relationships of symptoms to exposure to possible allergens are noted.

Diagnostic Evaluation

Assessment of the patient with allergic disorders commonly includes blood tests, smears of body secretions, skin tests, and the RAST (radioallergosorbent test).

Results of laboratory blood studies provide supportive data for various diagnostic possibilities; however, they are not the major criteria for the diagnosis of allergic disease. Initial studies may include the following:

Complete Blood Count With Differential

The white blood cell (WBC) count is usually normal except during infective states. Eosinophils, one type of WBC, normally make up 1% to 3% of the total number of WBC. A level between 5% and 15% is nonspecific but does suggest allergic reaction.

Moderate eosinophilia—15% to 40% of blood leukocytes as eosinophils are found in patients with allergic disorders as well as patients with malignancy, immunodeficiencies, parasitic infections, peritoneal dialysis, and congenital heart disease

Severe eosinophilia—50% to 90% of blood leukocytes as eosinophils are found in the idiopathic hypereosinophilic syndrome.

Total Eosinophil Count

Accurate counts of eosinophils can be obtained by the use of special diluting fluids that hemolyze erythrocytes and stain the eosinophils.

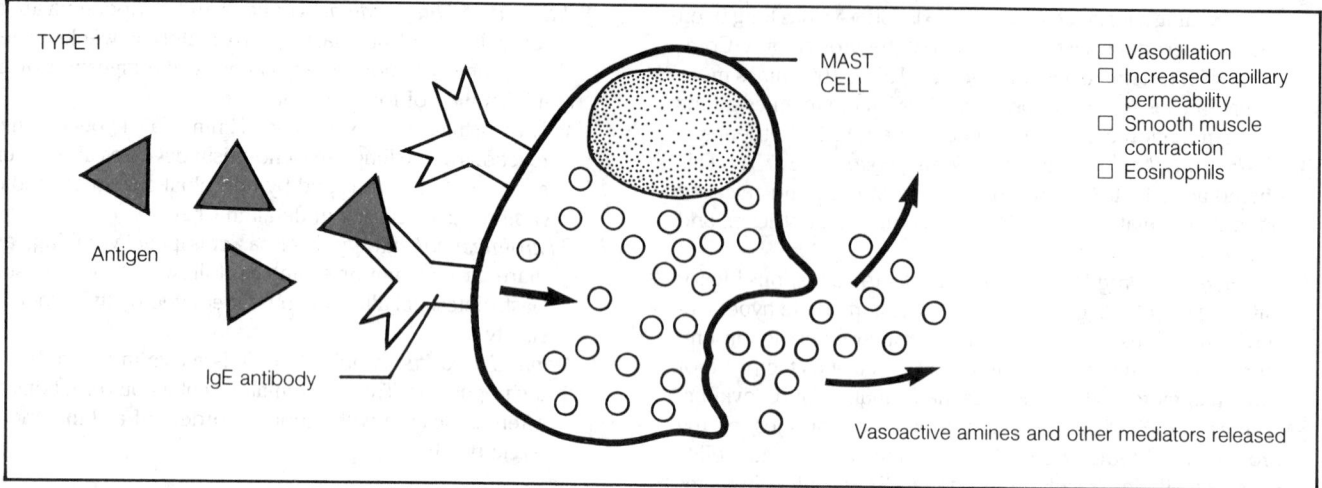

Reactions
Anaphylactic (immediate, atopic, IgE-mediated, reaginic)

Pathophysiology
IgE antibodies bind to certain cells; antigen binding causes release of vasoactive amines and other mediators, resulting in vasodilation, increased capillary permeability, smooth-muscle contraction, and eosinophilia.

Signs and symptoms
Systemic: angioedema; hypotension; bronchial, GI, or uterine spasm; stridor
Local: urticaria

Clinical examples
Extrinsic asthma, seasonal allergic rhinitis, systemic anaphylaxis, reactions to stinging insects, some food and drug reactions, some cases of urticaria, infantile eczema

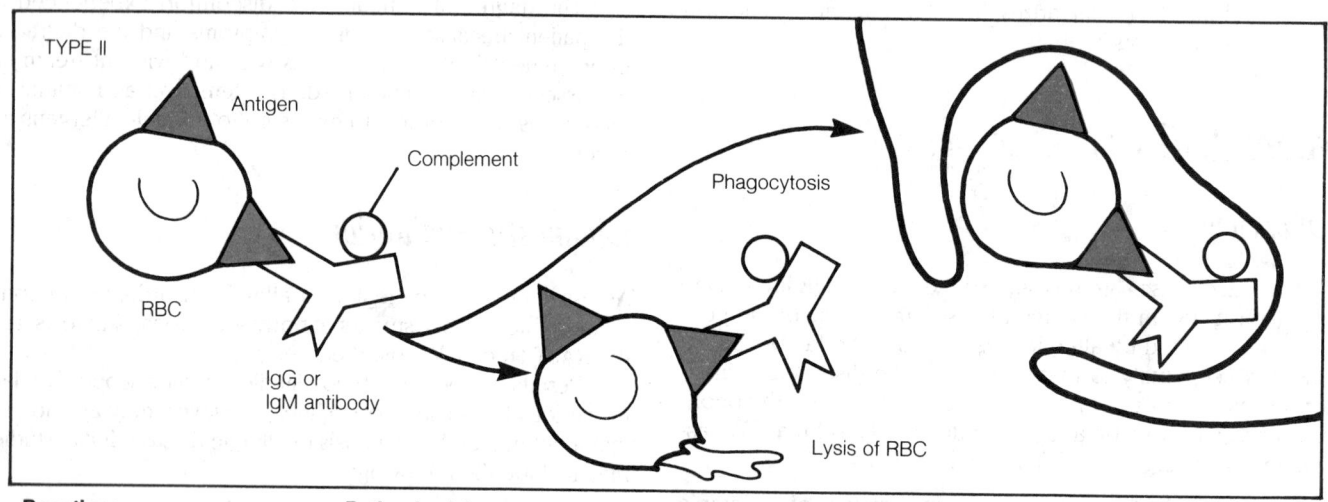

Reactions
Cytotoxic (cytolytic, complement-dependent cytotoxicity, cell-stimulating)

Pathophysiology
IgG or IgM antibodies bind to cellular or exogenous antigens. This can result in activation of complement components through C3 with phagocytosis or opsonization of the cell or activation of the full complement system with cytolysis or tissue damage.

Signs and symptoms
Varies with disease; can include dyspnea, hemoptysis, fever

Clinical examples
Goodpasture's syndrome, autoimmune hemolytic anemia, thrombocytopenia, pemphigus, pemphigoid, pernicious anemia, hyperacute graft rejection of transplanted kidney, transfusion reaction, hemolytic disease of the newborn, some drug reactions

Figure 49–2. Four types of hypersensitivity reactions. (Text of figure from Nurse's Clinical Library. Immune Disorders. Copyright 1985. Springhouse Corp.)

Smears for Eosinophils

During symptomatic episodes, nasal secretions, conjunctival secretions, and sputum of atopic patients usually reveal eosinophils.

Total Serum IgE Levels

High total serum IgE levels support the diagnosis of atopic disease; however, a normal IgE level does not exclude the diagnosis of an allergic disorder. More sensitive tests are the

paper radioimmunosorbent test (PRIST) and the enzyme-linked immunoassay (ELISA). Commercial kits are available for IgE determinations. Indications for determining IgE levels include:

* Evaluation of immunodeficiency
* Evaluation of drug reactions
* Initial laboratory screening for allergic bronchopulmonary aspergillosis
* Prediction of allergy among children with bronchiolitis
* Differentiation of atopic and nonatopic eczema
* Differentiation of atopic and nonatopic asthma and rhinitis

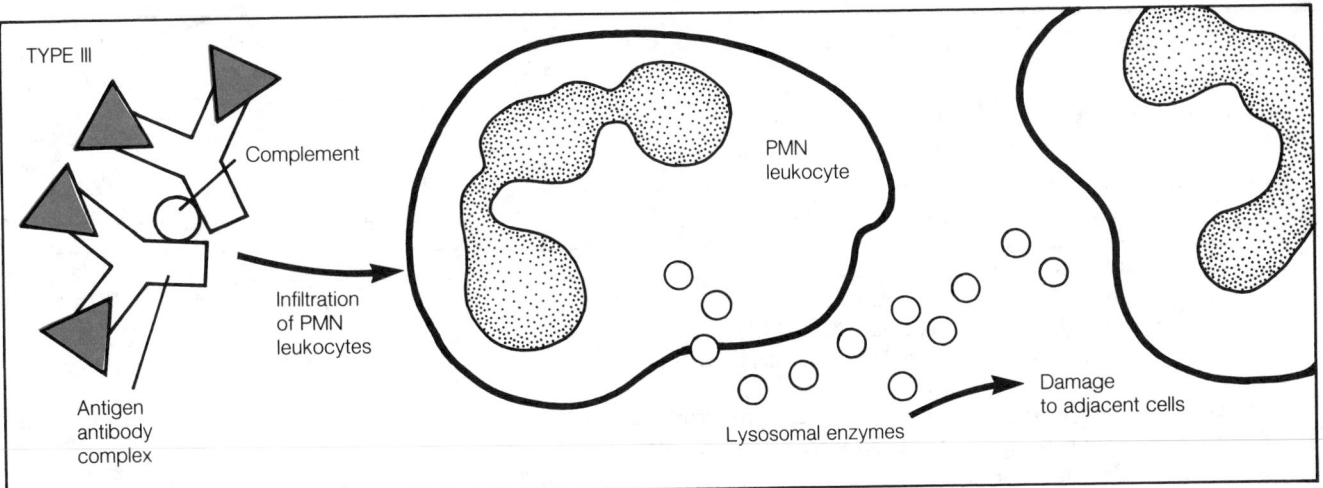

Reactions
Immune complex (soluble complex, toxic complex)

Pathophysiology
IgG or IgM antigen-antibody complexes are deposited in tissue where they activate complement. This reaction is marked by infiltration of polymorphonuclear leukocytes and by release of lysosomal proteolytic enzymes and permeability factors in tissues, which produce an acute, inflammatory reaction.

Signs and symptoms
Urticaria; multiform, scarlatiniform, or morbilliform rash; adenopathy; joint pain; fever; serum sickness-like syndrome

Clinical examples
Systemic: serum sickness due to serum, drugs, or viral hepatitis antigen; acute glomerulonephritis; systemic lupus erythematosus; rheumatoid arthritis; polyarteritis; cryoglobulinemia
Local: Arthus reaction

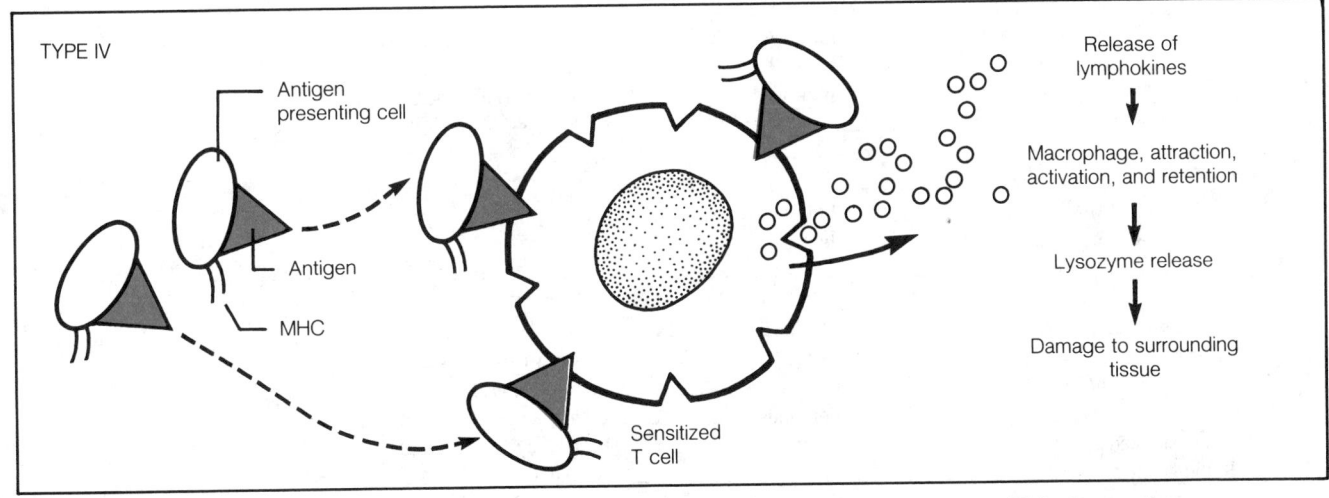

Reactions
Delayed (cellular, cell-mediated, tuberculin-type)

Pathophysiology
An antigen-presenting cell presents antigen to T cells in presence of MHC. The sensitized T cells release lymphokines, which stimulate macrophages; lysozymes are released; and surrounding tissue is damaged.

Signs and symptoms
Varies with disease; can include fever, erythema, and itching.

Clinical examples
Contact dermatitis, graft-versus-host disease, allograft rejection, granuloma due to intracellular organisms, some drug sensitivities, Hashimoto's thyroiditis, tuberculosis, sarcoidosis

Figure 49–2. (Continued)

Skin Tests

Skin testing entails the simultaneous intradermal inoculation (or superficial application), at separate sites, of several solutions. These contain individual antigens representing an assortment of allergens, including pollen, most likely to be implicated in the patient's disease. The clinical significance of positive reactions (wheal and flare) depends on correlation with the history, physical findings, and other laboratory tests.

Skin tests lend important weight to other evidence obtained from the patient's history, indicating which of several antigens are most likely to provoke symptoms and providing some clue to the intensity of the patient's sensitization.

The dosage of the pollen injected is important also. Most patients are hypersensitive not to one but to several pollens, and under testing conditions they may not react to the specific pollens that induce their attacks; however, they usually do so. Ragweed seems to be the most potent of all.

If there is any doubt about the validity of the skin tests, a RAST (see below) or a provocative challenge test may be performed. In the provocative challenge test, the suspected antigen is applied to the sensitive tissue (such as the conjunctiva, nasal

Chart 49–1
Allergy Assessment Sheet

Name _____ Age _____ Sex _____ Date _____

I.   Chief complaint: _____

II. Present illness: _____

III. Collateral allergic symptoms: _____

      Eyes: Pruritus _____ Burning _____ Lacrimation _____

                      Swelling _____ Injection _____ Discharge _____

      Ears: Pruritus _____ Fullness _____ Popping _____

                      Frequent infections _____

      Nose: Sneezing _____ Rhinorrhea _____ Obstruction _____

                      Pruritus _____ Mouth-breathing _____

                      Purulent discharge _____

      Throat: Soreness _____ Postnasal discharge _____

                      Palatal pruritus _____ Mucus in the morning _____

      Chest: Cough _____ Pain _____ Wheezing _____

                      Sputum _____ Dyspnea _____

                      Color _____ Rest _____

                      Amount _____ Exertion _____

      Skin: Dermatitis _____ Eczema _____ Urticaria _____

IV. Family allergies

V.   Previous allergic treatment or testing: _____

      Prior skin testing: _____

      Medications: Antihistamines   Improved _____ Unimproved _____

                  Bronchodilators   Improved _____ Unimproved _____

                  Nose drops   Improved _____ Unimproved _____

                  Hyposensitization   Improved _____ Unimproved _____

                      Duration _____

                      Antigens _____

                      Reactions _____

                  Antibiotics   Improved _____ Unimproved _____

                  Steroids   Improved _____ Unimproved _____

VI. Physical agents and habits: _____

Bothered by:

Tobacco for _____ years   Alcohol _____ Air cond. _____

Cigarettes _____ packs/day   Heat _____ Muggy weath. _____

Cigars _____ per day   Cold _____ Weath. chngs. _____

Pipes _____ per day   Perfumes _____ Chemicals _____

Never smoked _____   Paints _____ Hair spray _____

Bothered by smoke _____   Insecticides _____ Newspapers _____

                                    Cosmetics _____

VII. When symptoms occur: _____

      Time and circumstances of 1st episode: _____

      Prior health: _____

      Course of illness over decades: progressing _____ regressing _____

      Time of year: _____ Exact dates: _____

          Perennial _____

          Seasonal _____

          Seasonally exacerbated _____

      Monthly variations (menses, occupation): _____

      Time of week (weekends vs. weekdays): _____

      Time of day or night: _____

      After insect stings: _____

VIII. Where symptoms occur: _____

      Living where at onset: _____

      Living where since onset: _____

(continued)

Chart 49-1 *(Continued)*

Effect of vacation or major geographic change: _____

Symptoms better indoors or outdoors: _____

Effect of school or work: _____

Effect of staying elsewhere nearby: _____

Effect of hospitalization: _____

Effect of specific environments: _____

Do symptoms occur around: _____

    old leaves _____ hay _____ lakeside _____ barns _____

    summer homes _____ damp basement _____ dry attic _____

    lawnmowing _____ animals _____ other _____

Do symptoms occur after eating:

    cheese _____ mushrooms _____ beer _____ melons _____

    bananas _____ fish _____ nuts _____ citrus fruits _____

    other foods (list) _____

Home: city _____ rural _____

          house _____ age _____

          apartment _____ basement _____ damp _____ dry _____

          heating system _____

          pets (how long) _____ dog _____ cat _____ other _____

Bedroom:	Type	Age	*Living room:*	Type	Age
Pillow	_____	_____	Rug	_____	_____
Mattress	_____	_____	Matting	_____	_____
Blankets	_____	_____	Furniture	_____	_____
Quilts	_____	_____			
Furniture	_____	_____			

    Anywhere in home symptoms are worse: _____

IX. What does patient think makes symptoms worse? _____

X. Under what circumstances is patient free of symptoms? _____

XI. Summary and additional comments: _____

(Patterson R. *Allergic Diseases.* Philadelphia, JB Lippincott.)

---

or bronchial mucosa, or to the gastrointestinal tract by ingestion of allergens) and the response is observed.

The indication for skin testing is a reasonable suspicion that a specific allergen is producing symptoms in an allergic patient. Several precautionary steps, however, must be observed prior to skin testing:

- Testing is not performed during periods of bronchospasm.
- Epicutaneous tests (scratch or prick tests) are performed first to detect the sensitive patient with a minimal risk of systemic reaction.
- Emergency equipment must be available to treat anaphylaxis (see p. 1403).
- The methods of skin testing include prick skin tests, scratch tests, and intradermal skin testing (Fig. 49-3). Following prick skin or scratch tests, intradermal skin testing is performed with allergens that did not elicit positive reactions. A larger antigen challenge is used; therefore, local or systemic reactions could occur if the same antigens that produced positive skin or scratch reactions are used. The patient's back is the most suitable area of the body for skin testing because it permits the performance of many tests.

The Multi-Test applicator (Lincoln Labs) is a commercially available device with multiple test heads that allows simulta-neous administration of antigens by multiple punctures at different sites.

Interpretation of Skin Tests. Consistency and familiarity with a chosen grading system are essential. The grading system used should be identified on a skin test sheet for later interpretation. A positive reaction, evidenced by the appearance of an urticarial wheal (Fig. 49-4) or by localized erythema (redness) in the area of inoculation or contact, is considered indicative of sensitivity to the corresponding antigen.

There may be false-negative results due to improper technique, outdated allergen solutions, and prior use of drugs that suppress skin reactivity. Corticosteroids and antihistamines suppress skin test reactivity and should therefore be withheld 48 to 96 hours before testing, depending on the duration of their activity. False-positive skin tests may result from improper preparation or administration of allergen solutions.

Interpretation of positive or negative skin tests must be based on the patient's history, physical examination, and other laboratory results. The following guidelines are used for the interpretation of skin test results:

1. Skin tests are more reliable for diagnosing atopic sensitivity in patients with allergic rhinoconjunctivitis than in patients with asthma.

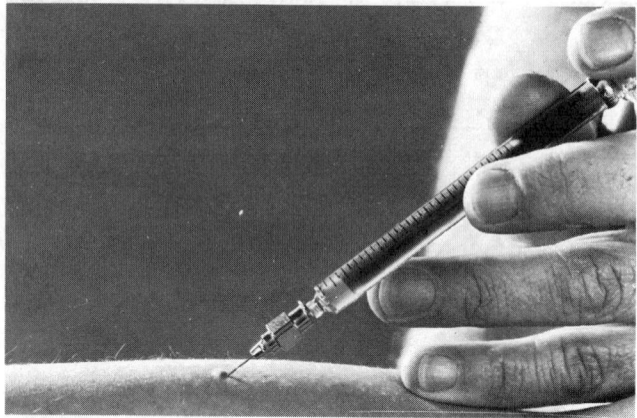

Figure 49–3. Intradermal testing. Cleanse the testing site with alcohol or ether. Tests are made on the volar surface of the lower arm and the outer surface of the upper arm, omitting the antecubital space. Intradermal tests are limited to 10 or 20 at most. (Courtesy of Hollister-Stier Laboratories.)

2. Positive skin tests correlate highly with food allergy.
3. The use of skin tests to diagnose immediate hypersensitivity to drugs is limited because metabolites of drugs, not the drugs themselves, are usually responsible.

Provocative Testing

Provocative testing involves the direct administration of an allergen to the respiratory mucosa with observation of target organ response. This type of testing is helpful in identifying clinically significant allergens in those patients with a large number of positive tests. The major disadvantages of this type of testing are the limitation of one antigen per session and the risk of producing severe symptoms, particularly bronchospasm, in patients with asthma.

Radioallergosorbent Test

The radioallergosorbent test (RAST) is a radioimmunoassay that measures allergen-specific IgE. A sample of the patient's serum is exposed to a variety of suspected allergen particle complexes. If antibodies are present, they will combine with radiolabeled allergens. Following centrifugation, radioimmunoassay detects the allergen-specific IgE antibody. Test results are then compared to control values. As well as detecting an allergen, RAST also indicates the quantity of allergen necessary to evoke an allergic reaction. Values are reported on a scale from 0 to 5; 2+ or greater is considered significant. The major advantages of RAST over other tests include (1) decreased risk of systemic reaction, (2) stability of antigens, and (3) lack of dependence on skin reactivity modified by drugs. The major disadvantages include (1) the limited allergen selection, (2) reduced sensitivity as compared with intradermal skin tests, (3) lack of immediately available results, and (4) cost.

Allergic Rhinitis

Allergic rhinitis (hay fever, chronic allergic rhinitis, pollinosis) is the most common form of respiratory allergy presumed to be mediated by an immunologic reaction. It affects about 8% to 10% of the U.S. population (20% to 30% of adolescents). When untreated, many complications may result, such as allergic asthma, chronic nasal obstruction, chronic otitis media with hearing loss, anosmia (absence of the sense of smell), and, in children, orofacial dental deformities. Consequently, early diagnosis and adequate treatment are strongly recommended.

Because allergic rhinitis is induced by airborne pollens or molds, it is characterized by seasonal occurrences, for example:

Early spring—tree pollen (oak, elm, poplar)
Early summer (rose fever)—grass pollen (Timothy, red-top)
Early fall—weed pollen (ragweed)

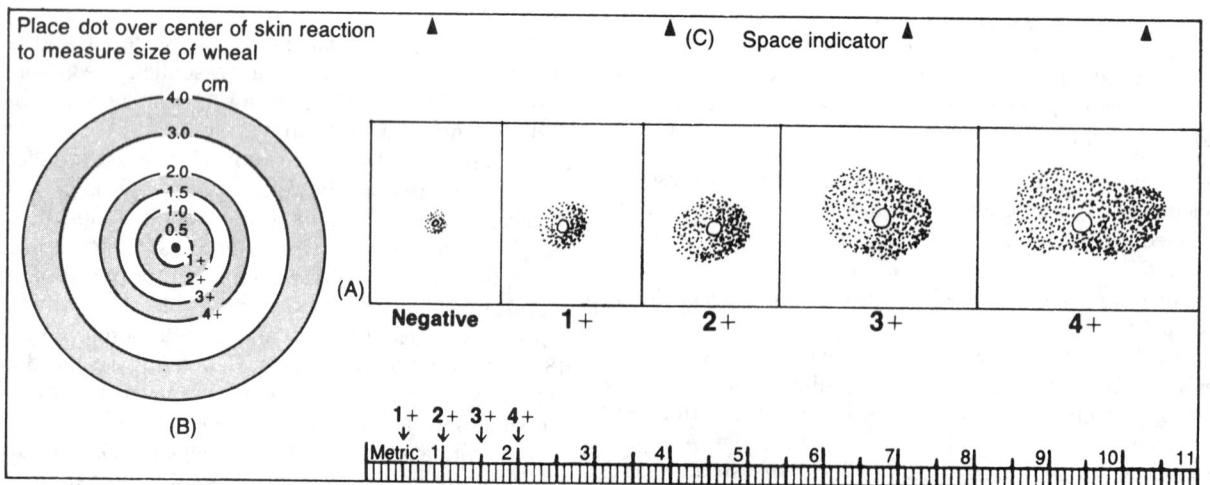

Figure 49–4. Method for evaluating wheals. (**A**) This series of reactions indicates the sizes of wheals as they are referred to by the allergist (1+, 2+, etc). A negative reaction is shown at the left. (**B**) The target wheal guide can be traced on a transparent sheet (acetate or x-ray film) and then placed over the wheal to measure the size in centimeters or according to plus-size. The relationship between the two is indicated on the lower metric scale. (**C**) Showing placement of test sites spaced uniformly. (Patient Care, Sep 15, 1973. Copyright © 1973, Patient Care Corp, Darien, CT. All rights reserved.)

Each year, the attacks begin and end at approximately the same time. Airborne mold spores require warm, damp weather. Although there is no rigid seasonal pattern, these spores appear in early spring, are rampant during the summer, and taper off and disappear by the first frost.

Pathophysiology

Sensitization begins by ingestion or inhalation of an antigen. On re-exposure, the nasal mucosa reacts by the slowing of ciliary action, edema formation, and leukocyte infiltration, primarily of eosinophils. Histamine is the major mediator of allergic reactions in the nasal mucosa. Tissue edema is a result of vasodilation and increased capillary permeability.

Clinical Manifestations

Typical findings of allergic rhinitis include nasal congestion, a clear, watery discharge, intermittent sneezing, and nasal itching. Itching of the throat and soft palate are not uncommon. Drainage of nasal mucus into the pharynx results in multiple attempts to clear the throat, a dry cough, or hoarseness. Headache, pain over the paranasal sinuses, and epistaxis can accompany allergic rhinitis. It is a chronic, recurring condition with symptoms that are dependent upon environmental exposure and intrinsic host responsiveness.

Diagnostic Evaluation

In most cases of seasonal allergic rhinitis, early diagnosis by history and physical exam is necessary. During a diagnostic workup, the following studies may be performed: nasal smears, peripheral blood counts, total serum IgE, epidermal testing, intradermal testing, RAST, food elimination and challenge, and nasal provocation tests.

Management

The goal of therapy is to provide relief from the annoying symptoms just described. Therapy may include one or all of the following interventions: avoidance therapy, pharmacotherapy, or immunotherapy. It is essential that verbal instruction be reinforced by written information to provide the patient with permanent reminders. A knowledge of the general concepts regarding assessment and therapy in allergic diseases is important, because the nurse is likely to have an active role in the management of patients with these disorders and may be in a position to advise patients who are potential candidates for one or another of these procedures.

Avoidance Therapy (Avoidance of Allergens)
In avoidance therapy, every attempt is made to remove those allergens that act as precipitating factors. Simple measures and environmental controls are often effective in decreasing symptoms. Examples of these include use of air conditioners, air cleaners, and humidifiers/dehumidifiers, and smoke-free environments.

Pharmacotherapy
Antihistamines. Antihistamines are classified as H_1- or H_2-receptor antagonists and are associated synonymously with H_1 antagonists. Table 49-2 describes the classification of H_1 antihistamines, side effects, and nursing responsibilities. Antihistamines given orally are readily absorbed. They are most ef-

fective when given at the first occurrence of symptoms because they prevent the development of new symptoms by preventing further histamine release. In actual practice, the effectiveness of these drugs is limited to certain patients with hay fever, vasomotor rhinitis, urticaria (hives), and mild asthma. They are rarely effective in other conditions or in severe conditions of any sort. Antihistamines are the major class of drugs prescribed for the symptomatic relief of allergic rhinitis. The major side effect of this group of drugs is somnolence. Additional side effects include nervousness, dryness of mouth, palpitations, anorexia, nausea, and vomiting. Newer antihistamines do not cross the blood-brain barrier (terfenadine [Seldane]) and therefore cause less sedation.

Adrenergic Agents. Adrenergic drugs are vasoconstrictors of mucosal vessels and are used topically in addition to the oral route. The topical route causes fewer side effects than oral administration; however, topical vasoconstrictors (drops and sprays) are recommended for use for only a few days to avoid rebound congestion. Adrenergic nasal decongestants are used for the relief of nasal congestion when applied topically to the nasal mucosa. They activate the alpha-adrenergic receptor sites on the smooth muscle of the nasal mucosal blood vessels; this reduces local blood flow, fluid exudation, and mucosal edema. Potential side effects include hypertension, dysrhythmias, palpitations, CNS stimulation, irritability, tremor, and tachyphylaxis (acceleration of hemodynamic status).

Examples of adrenergic decongestants and their route of administration include:

- Pseudoephedrine hydrochloride (Sudafed)—oral
- Phenylephrine hydrochloride (Neo-Synephrine)—topical
- Phenylpropanolamine hydrochloride (Propagest)—oral
- Naphazoline hydrochloride (Privine)—topical

Cromolyn Sodium. Cromolyn sodium (Nasalcrom) is a spray that acts by stabilizing the mast cell membrane and inhibiting mediator release. It is used prophylactically before exposure to allergens or therapeutically in chronic allergic rhinitis. The adverse effects are usually mild (*i.e.*, sneezing and local stinging and burning sensations).

Corticosteroids. Topical corticosteroids are indicated for more severe cases of allergic rhinitis. Newer corticosteroids such as Vancenase and Nasalide are very potent and are metabolized rapidly. It is important that patients be informed that full benefit may not be achieved for several days to 2 weeks. Parenteral corticosteroids are used when conventional therapy has failed and symptoms are severe and of short duration.

Patients who receive corticosteroids must be cautioned not to stop taking the medication suddenly and without specific instructions from the physician. The patient is also instructed about side effects of corticosteroids: fluid retention, weight gain, hypertension, gastric irritation, glucose intolerance, and adrenal suppression.

Immunotherapy
Immunotherapy is indicated only when IgE hypersensitivity is demonstrated to specific inhalant allergens that the patient is unable to avoid (house dust, pollens). The goals of immunotherapy include a reduced level of circulating IgE, an increased level of blocking antibody IgG, and reduced mediator cell sensitivity. Immunotherapy has been most effective for ragweed pollen; however, treatment for grass, tree pollen, cat, and house dust mite allergens has also been positive.

TABLE 49–2.   Chemical Classes of H₁ Antihistamines

Classification & Example	Major Side Effects	Nursing Implications
1. Ethanolamines Ex: diphenhydramine (Benadryl)	A. Drowsiness, confusion	A. Teach patient to avoid alcohol, driving, or engaging in any hazardous activities until CNS response to drug treatment is established.
	B. Dry mouth, nausea, vomiting	B. Suggest sucking on hard candy or ice chips for relief of dry mouth.
	C. Photosensitivity	C. Encourage use of sunscreen and hat while outdoors.
	D. Urinary retention	D. Assess for urinary retention; monitor urinary output.
2. Piperazines Ex: hydroxyzine (Atarax)	A. Dulls mental alertness; drowsiness	A. Teach patient to avoid alcohol, driving, or engaging in any hazardous activities until CNS response to drug treatment is established.
	B. Dry mouth	B. Suggest sucking on hard candy or ice chips for relief of dry mouth.
3. Alkylamines Ex: chlorpheniramine (Chlor-trimeton)	A. Causes less CNS depression than other groups. Best class for daytime use.	A. Teach patient to avoid alcohol, driving, or engaging in any hazardous activities until CNS response to drug treatment is established.
4. Ethylenediamines Ex: tripelennamine (PBZ)	A. Produces GI upset	A. Take medication with food or milk to decrease GI distress. Drink plenty of fluids.
	B. Drowsiness	B. Teach patient to avoid alcohol, driving, or engaging in any hazardous activities until CNS response to drug treatment is established.
	C. Palpitations	C. Sit and relax a few minutes before activity.
5. Phenothiazines Ex: promethazine (Phenergan)	A. Produces heavy sedation and drowsiness	A. Teach patient to avoid alcohol, driving, or engaging in any hazardous activities until CNS response to drug treatment is established.
	B. Nasal congestion	B. Use humidification when at home.
	C. Hypotension	C. Rise from a sitting position slowly.

Correlation of a positive skin test with a positive history is an indication for immunotherapy if the allergen cannot be avoided. The value of such injections has been fairly well established in instances of allergic rhinitis and bronchial asthma that are clearly due to sensitivity to one of the common pollens or molds or to house dust. Although immunotherapy is referred to as a "hyposensitization" procedure, the effects are most likely attributable to the opposite process (i.e., immunization), for it appears to stimulate the production of a new antibody with the capacity to neutralize the allergy-provoking properties of the responsible allergen.

Although helpful in most patients, immunotherapy does not cure the condition. Before such a program is launched, the physician discusses with the patient what may be expected from immunotherapy and why it is important to continue the therapy for several years. When skin tests are performed, they are to be correlated with clinical manifestations; the treatment is based on the patient's needs rather than on the skin tests.

The most common method of treatment is the serial injection of one or more antigens that are selected in each particular case on the basis of skin tests. This method provides a simple and efficient technique for determining IgE antibodies to specific antigens. Specific treatment consists of injecting extracts of the pollens or mold spores that cause symptoms in a particular patient. Injections begin with very small amounts and are gradually increased, usually at weekly intervals, until a maximum tolerated dose is attained. Maintenance "booster" injections are then given at 2- to 4-week intervals, frequently for a period of several years, before maximum benefit is achieved.

There are three methods of injection therapy: coseasonal, preseasonal, and perennial. When treatment is given on a co-seasonal basis, it is initiated during the season in which the patient experiences symptoms. This method has been used less widely in recent years because it has been found to be an ineffective form of therapy, and there is increased risk of systemic reactions. Preseasonal therapy injections are given 2 to 3 months before symptoms appear, allowing time for hyposensitization to occur. This treatment is discontinued after the season begins. Perennial therapy is administered all year round, usually on a monthly basis, and is the preferred method because more effective, longer-lasting results are achieved.

Precautions: Because there is a possibility that the injection of an allergen may induce systemic reactions, it is given only in a physician's office where epinephrine is immediately available. Because of the dangers involved, injections should not be given by a lay person or by the patient. The patient remains in the physician's office for a minimum of 30 minutes and is observed for the possible development of systemic symptoms. If a large, local swelling develops at the injection site, the next dose should not be increased, because this may be a warning of a possible systemic reaction. Therapeutic failure is evident when a patient does not (1) experience a decrease of symptoms within 12 to 24 months, (2) develop an increase in tolerance to known allergens, and (3) decrease the use of medications to reduce symptoms. Potential causes of treatment failure include: misdiagnosis of allergies, inadequate doses of allergen, newly developed allergies, and inadequate environmental controls.

▶ Nursing Process
The Patient With Allergic Rhinitis

▷ Assessment

The examination and history of the patient reveal sneezing, often in paroxysms, thin and watery nasal discharge, itching eyes and nose, lacrimation, and occasionally headache. The nursing history includes a personal or family history of allergy. The allergy assessment will identify the nature of antigens, seasonal changes in symptoms, and medication history. The nurse also obtains subjective data about how the patient feels just before symptoms become obvious, such as the occurrence of pruritus, breathing problems, and tingling sensations. In addition to these symptoms, hoarseness, wheezing, hives, rash, erythema, or edema is noted. Any relation between emotional problems or stress and the triggering of allergy symptoms is assessed.

▷ Nursing Diagnoses

Based on the data collected from the patient history and assessment, the patient's major nursing diagnoses may include:

- Potential ineffective breathing pattern related to allergic reaction
- Knowledge deficit about allergy and the modifications in lifestyle and self-care practices
- Impaired adjustment related to chronicity of condition and need for environmental modifications

▷ Planning and Implementation

▷ **Goals:** The patient's goals may include restoration of normal breathing pattern, knowledge about the causes and control of allergic symptoms, and adjustment to alterations and modifications.

▷ Nursing Interventions

▷ *Improved Breathing Pattern.* The patient is instructed and assisted to modify his environment to reduce the severity of allergic symptoms or prevent their occurrence. Additionally, he is instructed to maintain normal breathing patterns by reducing exposure to persons with upper respiratory infections (URIs). If URI occurs, he is encouraged to take deep breaths and cough frequently to assure adequate gas exchange and prevent atelectasis. The patient is instructed to seek medical attention, because allergy symptoms along with URI may compromise adequate lung function. Compliance with medications and other treatment regimens is encouraged and reinforced.

▷ *Increased Knowledge About Allergy and Strategies to Control Symptoms.* Instruction for the patient includes discussion of strategies to minimize exposure to allergens, desensitization procedures, and correct use of medications.

Instruction about other strategies to control allergic symp-

toms is based on the individual needs of the patient as determined by the results of tests, the severity of symptoms, and the motivation of the patient and family to deal with the condition. Some general suggestions for those sensitive to dust and mold in the home include the following:

1. Try to maintain a dust-free environment, particularly in the bedroom:
   a. Reduce contents to barest minimum; remove drapes, curtains, and venetian blinds and replace with pull shades.
   b. Remove carpets; wash woodwork and floor and thereafter dust and vacuum daily. Wood flooring or linoleum is preferable to rugs.
   c. Replace stuffed furniture with wooden pieces that can be dusted easily.
   d. Avoid tufted bedspreads, stuffed toys, feather pillows; replace them with easily washable cotton material.
   e. Cover the mattress with a hypoallergenic cover that can be zippered to fit snugly.
   f. Avoid wearing fabrics that cause itching.
2. Within the house as a whole, reduce dust by the following practices:
   a. Use steam or hot water for heating rather than hot air.
   b. Use filters or air conditioning.
   c. Wear a mask if cleaning is being done.
3. For patients sensitive to pollen or mold, reduce exposure to them:
   a. Determine times of the year when pollen count is highest; reduce exposure at these times.
   b. Avoid barns, weeds, dry leaves, and freshly cut grass.
   c. Wear a mask at times of increased exposure (*e.g.,* windy days, when grass is being cut).
   d. Seek air-conditioned areas at the height of the season.
   e. Take antihistamines as prescribed.
   f. Avoid sprays and perfumes; use hypoallergenic cosmetics.
4. Determine specific foods that may be a problem. Avoid what appears to be troublesome food for a period of time. By trial, one can develop a list of foods that are to be avoided. Examples include fish, nuts, eggs, and chocolate.

If the patient is to undergo desensitization, the nurse reinforces the physician's explanation regarding the purpose and procedure. It is necessary to follow instructions thereafter regarding the subsequent series of inoculations, usually given every 2 weeks or monthly. These include (1) remaining in the physician's office at least 30 minutes after the injection so that emergency treatment may be given if the patient sustains a reaction, (2) avoiding rubbing or scratching the site of the injection, and (3) continuing with the series for the period of time required.

In addition to avoiding situations that bring on the allergic symptoms, the patient needs to understand the rationale, actions, and side effects of all medications prescribed to control the allergy problem and the correct methods of administration.

Because antihistamines often produce drowsiness, the patient is cautioned about this and other side effects of the particular medication. Operating machinery, driving a car, and activities requiring intense concentration should be postponed. The patient is also informed about the dangers of drinking alcohol when taking these drugs, which tend to potentiate the effects of alcohol.

The patient must be aware of the effects caused by *overuse* of the sympathomimetic agents in nose drops or sprays. A condition referred to as *rhinitis medicamentosa* may result (Fig. 49-5). After topical application of the drug, a rebound period may occur in which the nasal mucous membranes become more edematous and congested than they were before the medication was used. Such a reaction encourages the use of more drug. A cyclical pattern of activity results. The topical agent must be discontinued immediately and completely to correct this problem.

◊   *Adjustment to Chronic Disorder.*   Although allergic reactions are infrequently life-threatening, they require constant vigilance for allergens and modifications of the patient's life-style or the environment to prevent recurrence of symptoms. Allergic symptoms are often present year-round and create discomfort and inconvenience for the patient. Although he may not feel ill during allergy seasons, he often does not feel well either. The necessity of being on the alert for possible allergens in the environment and their presence throughout the environment may be tiresome for the patient and place extra burdens on his ability to lead a normal life. Stress related to these difficulties may in turn increase the frequency or severity of symptoms.

To assist the patient in adjusting to these modifications, the nurse must have an appreciation of the difficulties encountered by the patient. The patient is encouraged to verbalize his feelings and concerns in a supportive environment and to identify strategies to deal with them effectively.

◊   Evaluation

Expected Outcomes

1. Exhibits normal breathing patterns
   a. Lungs clear to auscultation
   b. Exhibits absence of adventitious breath sounds (crackles, rhonchi, wheezing)
   c. Demonstrates an effective respiratory rate
   d. Reports no respiratory distress (shortness of breath, difficulty on inspiration or expiration)
2. Demonstrates knowledge about allergy and strategies to control symptoms
   a. Identifies causative allergens, if known
   b. States methods of avoiding allergen and how to control for indoor and outdoor precipitating factors
   c. Describes name, purpose, side effects, and method of administration of prescribed medications
   d. Identifies when to seek immediate medical attention for severe allergic responses
   e. Describes activities that are possible and how involvement in them can be maximized without activating the allergies

3. Experiences relief of discomfort and adapts to the inconveniences of an allergy
   a. Relates the emotional aspects of the allergic response
   b. Removes from the bedroom environment those items that retain dust
   c. Wears a dampened mask if dust or mold may be a problem
   d. Avoids smoke-filled rooms and dust-filled or freshly sprayed areas
   e. Uses air-conditioned areas for a major part of the day
   f. Takes antihistamines as prescribed; participates in hyposensitization program, if applicable

Allergic Dermatoses

Contact Dermatitis

Contact dermatitis (dermatitis venenata) is an inflammatory, often eczematous, condition caused by a skin reaction to a variety of irritating or allergenic materials. There are four basic types: allergic, irritant, phototoxic, and photoallergic (Table 49-3). Almost any substance can produce contact dermatitis. Poison ivy is probably the most common example; cosmetics, soaps, detergents, and industrial chemicals are frequent offenders. The skin sensitivity may develop after brief or prolonged periods of exposure, and the clinical picture may appear hours or weeks after the sensitized skin has been exposed.

The symptoms include itching, burning, erythema, skin lesions (vesicles), and edema, followed by weeping, crusting, and finally drying-up and peeling of the skin. In very severe responses, hemorrhagic bullae may develop. Repeated reactions may be accompanied by thickening of the skin and pigmentary changes. Secondary invasion by bacteria may develop in skin abraded by rubbing or scratching. Usually, there are no systemic symptoms unless the eruption is widespread.

Diagnosis may sometimes be made easily on the basis of the location of the eruption and history of exposure. In cases of obscure irritants or an unobservant patient, however, diagnosis may be extremely difficult, and many trial-and-error procedures may be involved before the cause is correctly determined. Patch tests on the skin with suspected offending agents may clarify the diagnosis. Treatment modalities for each type are outlined in Table 49-3.

Atopic Dermatitis

Atopic dermatitis (Fig. 49-6) is a component of immediate hypersensitivity disorders, which include asthma and rhinoconjunctivitis. A family history is common. The incidence of atopic dermatitis is highest in infants and children. Most patients have significant elevations of serum IgE and peripheral eosinophilia. Pruritus and hyperirritability of the skin are the most consistent features of atopic dermatitis and are related to large amounts of histamine in the skin. Excessive dryness of the skin with resultant itching is related to changes in lipid content, sebaceous gland activity in the skin, and sweating. In response to stroking, immediate redness appears on the skin and is followed in 15 to 30 seconds by pallor, which persists for 1 to 3 minutes. Lesions develop secondary to the trauma of scratching and appear in areas of increased sweating and hypervascularity. Atopic dermatitis is chronic, with remissions and exacerbations; treatment must therefore be individualized to the needs of each patient. Guidelines for treatment include: (1) decreasing itching

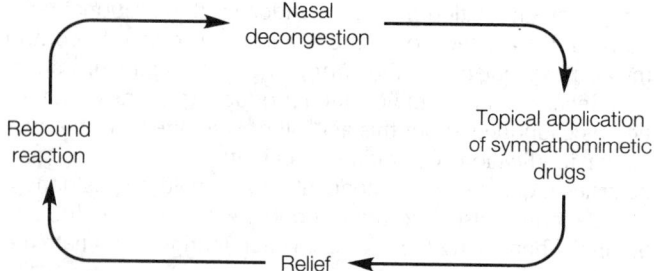

Figure 49-5.   Rhinitis medicamentosa. This cyclic pattern results from overuse of sympathomimetic nose drops or sprays.

TABLE 49-3. *Summary of Characteristics, Diagnostic Testing, and Treatment of Types of Contact Dermatitis*

Type	Etiology	Clinical Presentation	Diagnostic Testing	Treatment
Allergic	A type IV hypersensitivity reaction that results from contact of skin and allergenic substance. It has a sensitization period of 10–14 days.	Vasodilation and perivascular infiltrates on the dermis Intracellular edema Usually seen on dorsal aspects of hand	Patch testing (contraindicated in acute, widespread dermatitis)	Avoid offending material Burow's solution or cool water compress Systemic corticosteroids (prednisone) for 7–10 days Topical corticosteroids for mild cases Oral antihistamines to relieve pruritus
Irritant	Results from contact with a substance that chemically or physically damages the skin on a nonimmunologic basis. Occurs after first exposure to irritant or repeated exposures to milder irritants over an extended time.	Dryness lasting days to months Vesiculation, fissures, cracks Hands and lower arms most common areas	Clinical judgment Appropriate negative patch tests	Identification and removal of source of irritation Application of hydrophilic cream or petrolatum to soothe and protect Topical corticosteroids and compresses for weeping lesions Antibiotics for infection and oral antihistamines for pruritus
Phototoxic	Resembles the irritant type but requires sun and a chemical in combination to damage the epidermis.	Similar to irritant dermatitis	Photopatch test	Same as for allergic and irritant dermatitis
Photoallergic	Resembles allergic dermatitis but requires light exposure in addition to allergen contact to produce immunologic reactivity	Similar to allergic dermatitis	Photopatch test	Same as for allergic and irritant dermatitis

and scratching by wearing cotton fabrics, washing with a mild detergent, humidifying dry heat in winter, maintaining room temperature at 68° to 72°F, using antihistamines such as diphenhydramine (Benadryl) or terfenadine (Seldane), and avoiding animals, dust, sprays, and perfumes; (2) keeping skin moisturized by taking daily baths to hydrate the skin and using topical skin moisturizers; (3) preventing inflammation by using topical corticosteroids on the skin; and (4) treating infection with antibiotics to eliminate *Staphylococcus aureus* whenever necessary.

Drug Reactions (Dermatitis Medicamentosa)

Dermatitis medicamentosa is the term applied to skin rashes induced by the internal administration of certain drugs. While as a rule certain drugs tend to induce eruptions of similar types, individuals react differently to each drug.

In general, drug rashes appear suddenly, have a particularly vivid color, present characteristics that are more spectacular than the somewhat similar eruptions of infectious origin, and, with the exception of bromide and the iodide rashes, disappear rapidly after the drug is withdrawn. Some drug rashes are accompanied by systemic or generalized symptoms. On discovery of a drug allergy, such patients are warned that they have an idiosyncrasy to a particular drug and are advised not to take it again.

The nurse has an important responsibility regarding skin eruptions related to drug therapy, for these lesions suggest more serious idiosyncrasies. Through early assessment of the patient, the nurse is able to report the appearance of the eruption so that early treatment can be initiated.

Urticaria and Angioneurotic Edema

Urticaria (hives) is an allergic reaction of the skin characterized by the sudden appearance of pinkish edematous elevations that vary in size and shape, itch, and cause local discomfort. They may involve any part of the body, including the mucous membranes (especially those of the mouth), the larynx (occasionally with serious respiratory complications), and the gastrointestinal tract. Each hive remains for a period varying from a few minutes to several hours and then disappears. For hours or days, clusters of these lesions may come, go, and return, episodically. If this sequence continues indefinitely, the condition is called *chronic urticaria*.

The swellings of *angioneurotic edema* involve the deeper layers of the skin, resulting in more diffuse swelling rather than the discrete lesions characteristic of hives. Occasionally one may be seen that covers the entire back. The skin over it may appear normal but often has a reddish hue. It does not pit on pressure, as ordinary edema does. The regions most often involved are lips, eyelids, cheeks, hands, feet, genitalia, and

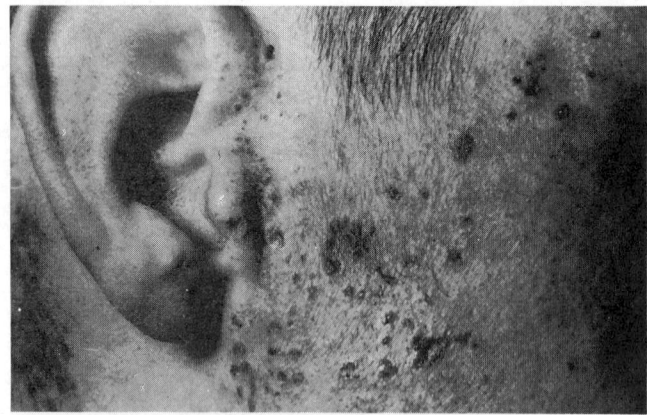
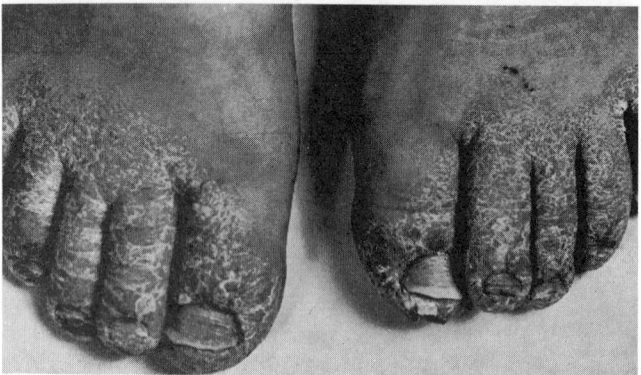

Figure 49–6. Atopic eczema, one form of allergic dermatosis.

this time the patient should be observed carefully for signs of laryngeal obstruction, which may necessitate tracheostomy as a lifesaving measure. Epinephrine, antihistamines, and corticosteroids are usually used in treatment, but the success of these agents is limited.

Food Allergy

Estimates of the incidence of IgE-mediated food allergy range from 0.1% to 7.0% of the population. The clinical symptoms are classic allergic symptoms (urticaria, atopic dermatitis, wheezing, cough, laryngeal edema, angioedema) and gastrointestinal symptoms (itching; swelling of lips, tongue, and palate; abdominal pain; nausea; cramps; vomiting; and diarrhea). Almost any food can cause allergic symptoms. The most common offenders are nuts, peanuts, eggs, milk, soy, wheat, and chocolate. A careful diagnostic workup is needed for any patient with a suspected food hypersensitivity. Included in this workup is a detailed allergy history, a physical examination, and pertinent diagnostic tests. When testing for allergy, skin testing and *in vitro* testing are used for identifying the source of symptoms. Both tests are useful in eliminating specific foods as the causative agents.

Therapy for food hypersensitivity includes elimination or reduction of the sensitive food. Pharmacologic therapy is necessary in patients with uncontrolled exposure to offending foods or patients with multiple food sensitivities not responsive to elimination measures. Drug therapy involves the use of H_1 and H_2 antihistamines, adrenergic agents, corticosteroids, and cromolyn sodium (not approved for oral use).

Many food allergies disappear with time, particularly in children. About a third of proven allergies disappear in 1 to 2 years if the patient carefully avoids the offending food.

tongue; the mucous membranes of the larynx, the bronchi, and the gastrointestinal canal may also be affected, particularly in cases of the hereditary type. An eye may be completely closed; one lip may become so large that eating is impossible; one hand may become so huge that the fingers cannot be flexed. These swellings may appear suddenly, in a few seconds or minutes, or slowly, in 1 or 2 hours. In the latter case, their appearance often is preceded by itching or burning sensations. Seldom does more than a single swelling appear at one time, although one may develop while another is disappearing. Only infrequently do they recur in the same region. The individual lesions usually last from 24 to 36 hours. On rare occasions, they recur with remarkable regularity at intervals of 3 to 4 weeks.

Hereditary Angioedema

Hereditary angioedema, although not an immunologic disorder in the usual sense, is included in this section because of its resemblance to allergic angioedema and because of the seriousness of this condition. Symptoms are due to edema of the skin, the respiratory tract, or the digestive tract. Attacks may be precipitated by trauma or may seem to occur spontaneously.

When the skin is involved, the swelling is usually rather diffuse, does not itch, and is usually not accompanied by urticaria. Gastrointestinal edema may cause abdominal pain severe enough to suggest the need for surgery. Edema of the upper respiratory tract may cause marked swelling of the uvula and of the larynx, resulting in suffocation. Acute laryngeal edema is the most serious manifestation of this disorder and has resulted in death due to asphyxiation in nearly 20% of these patients. Attacks usually subside within 3 to 4 days, but during

Serum Sickness

The illness known as serum sickness, an example of an immune complex–mediated drug reaction or type III reaction, traditionally has resulted from the administration of therapeutic antisera of animal sources for the treatment or prevention of infectious diseases such as tetanus, pneumonia, rabies, diphtheria, and botulism and for bites of venomous snakes and black widow spiders. With the advent of human antitetanus serum and antibiotics, true serum sickness is much less common now than in previous years. However, various drugs, chief of which is penicillin, are now the main cause of a syndrome identical to that caused by foreign sera.

Clinical Manifestations

The symptoms are due to a reaction and immunologic attack upon the serum or the drug. Antibodies appear chiefly to be of the IgE and IgM classes. Early manifestations, beginning 6 to 10 days after the administration of the drug, include an inflammatory reaction at the site of injection of the drug, followed by regional and generalized lymphadenopathy. There is nearly always a skin rash, which may be urticarial or purpuric, and joints are frequently tender and swollen. Vasculitis may occur in any organ but is most commonly observed in the kidney, resulting in proteinuria and, occasionally, casts in the urine. Cardiac involvement, mild to severe in nature, may occur. Peripheral neuritis may cause temporary paralysis of the upper extremities or may be widespread, causing the Guillain-Barré syndrome.

The usual untreated course lasts for several days to a few weeks, but ordinarily the patient responds promptly and completely if treated with antihistamines and corticosteroids. Aggressive therapy including ventilator support may be necessary if peripheral neuritis and Guillain-Barré syndrome occur.

Anaphylaxis

Anaphylaxis is a clinical response to an immediate (type I) immunologic reaction between a specific antigen and an antibody. The reaction results from IgE antibody in the following manner: (1) An antigen attaches to the IgE antibody fixed to the surface membrane of mast cells and basophils, causing these target cells to become activated. (2) Mast cells and basophils then release mediators, causing vascular changes; activation of platelets, eosinophils, and neutrophils; and activation of the coagulation cascade. An anaphylactoid (anaphylaxis-like) reaction is clinically similar to anaphylaxis. It is not mediated by antigen–antibody interactions but rather as a result of substances that act directly on the mast cells or tissues causing the release of mediators. This reaction may occur with medications, food, exercise, and cytotoxic antibody transfusions.

Types of Reactions

Local anaphylactic reactions usually involve urticaria and angioedema at the site of the antigen exposure and can be severe but are rarely fatal. Systemic reactions occur in the following organ systems within about 30 minutes of exposure: cardiovascular, respiratory, gastrointestinal, and integumentary.

The major signs and symptoms of anaphylactic reactions may be categorized as mild, moderate, and severe systemic reactions.

Mild—Mild systemic reactions consist of peripheral tingling and a warm sensation and may be accompanied by a fullness in the mouth and throat. Nasal congestion, periorbital swelling, pruritus, sneezing, and tearing of the eyes can also be expected. The onset of symptoms begins within the first 2 hours of exposure.

Moderate—Moderate systemic reactions may include any of the above symptoms in addition to bronchospasm and edema of the airways or larynx with dyspnea, cough, and wheezing. Flushing is frequently a chief complaint as well as warmth, anxiety, and itching. The onset of symptoms is the same as for a mild reaction.

Severe—Severe systemic reactions have an abrupt onset with the same signs and symptoms described above and progress rapidly to bronchospasm, laryngeal edema, severe dyspnea, and cyanosis. Dysphagia (difficulty swallowing) abdominal cramping, vomiting, diarrhea, and seizures can also occur. Rarely, cardiac arrest and coma result.

Treatment

Specific treatment depends on the severity of the reaction. Initially, respiratory and cardiovascular function are evaluated. If the patient is in cardiac arrest, cardiopulmonary resuscitation is instituted. Oxygen is provided in high concentrations during cardiopulmonary resuscitation or when a patient is cyanotic, dyspneic, or wheezing. Epinephrine, in a solution of 1:1000 dilution, is given subcutaneously in the upper extremity or thigh and may be followed by a continuous infusion. Antihistamines and steroids may also be given to prevent recurrences of the reaction and for urticaria and angioedema. To maintain blood pressure and normal hemodynamic status, volume expanders are used as well as vasopressor agents. Because of the potential for recurrences, patients with mild reactions must be educated concerning this risk, and patients with severe reactions are observed closely for 12 to 14 hours.

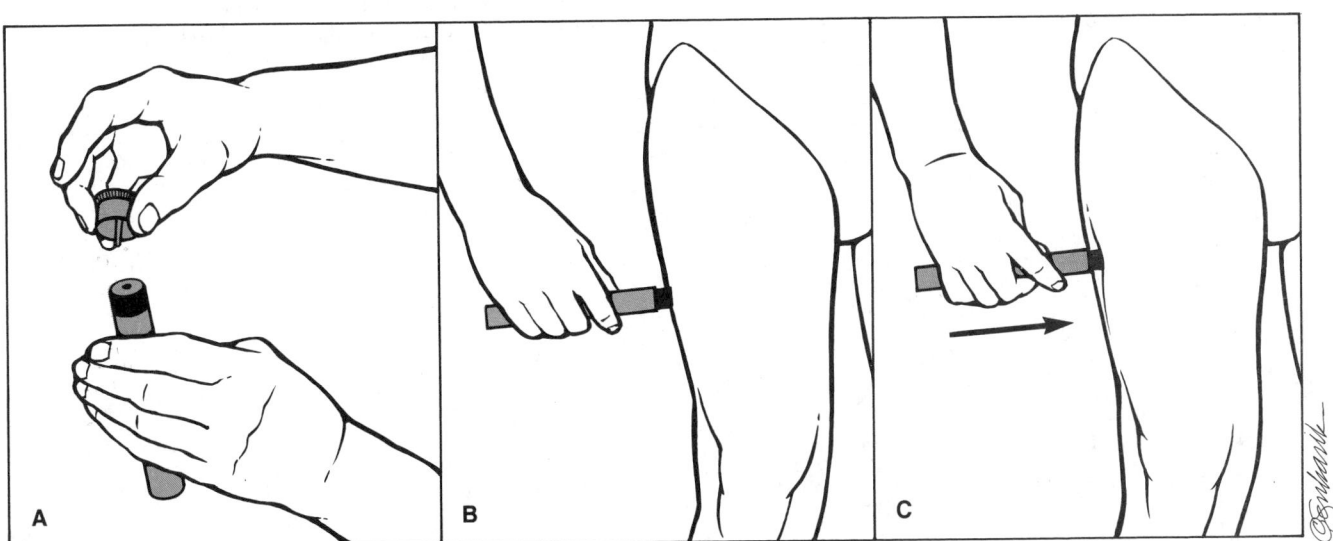

Figure 49-7. Epinephrine autoinjector. (Courtesy of Center Laboratories, Port Washington, NY.)

Prevention

Prevention is the single most important aspect of the management of anaphylaxis. Individuals sensitive to insect bites and stings, and those who have experienced food or drug reactions or idiopathic or exercise-induced anaphylactic reactions, should always carry an emergency kit that contains epinephrine. The Epipen from Center Laboratories is a commercially available first-aid device that delivers premeasured doses of 0.3 mg (Epipen) and 0.15 mg (Epipen Jr.) of epinephrine. The autoinjection system requires no preparation and the self-administration technique is uncomplicated (Fig. 49-7). The nurse provides information and instruction to all patients at risk for potentially fatal anaphylactic reactions. It is important that the patient be given an opportunity to demonstrate the correct technique for use; an Epipen training device is also available to assist in this effort. The patient is provided with verbal and written information about the emergency kit as well as strategies to avoid exposure to threatening allergens.

It is essential that a careful history of any sensitivity to suspected antigens be obtained before administering any medication, particularly a parenteral form, to a patient, because this route is associated with the most severe anaphylaxis.

It is essential to encourage patients predisposed to anaphylaxis to wear some evidence of identification related to drug allergies. One example is the Medic-Alert bracelet.*

Chapter Summary

The nurse's role in the assessment and management of patients with allergic disorders focuses on education. An understanding of allergic reactions and the allergens that trigger these reactions enables the nurse to accurately assess patients for signs and symptoms of hypersensitivity and thus act in preventing or decreasing the reaction process. Allergy is believed to complicate the lives and hamper the life-styles of approximately 40 million children and adults. Patients with allergies often mistake their symptoms for colds and other illnesses, thus ignoring the causes and methods for controlling allergic disorders. Promoting public awareness about allergies is a key nursing goal in facilitating early and accurate diagnosis and treatment.

Bibliography

Books

Bierman CW and Pearlman DS. Allergic Diseases From Infancy to Adulthood. Philadelphia, WB Saunders, 1988.

Lockey RF. Fundamentals of Immunology and Allergy. Philadelphia, WB Saunders, 1987.

Middleton E. Allergy: Principles and Practice. St Louis, CV Mosby, 1988.

U.S. Department of Health and Human Services. Understanding the Immune System. Washington, DC, National Institutes of Health, 1988 (NIH Publication No. 88-529).

Journals

Bahana SL et al. What food allergy is—and isn't. Patient Care 1989 Aug 15; 23(13):94–106.

Cason D. Anaphylactic shock. J Emerg Nurs 1989 Feb; 14(2):42–46, 51–52.

Ebeid MR. An atypical hypersensitivity reaction. Hosp Pract 1989 Nov 15; 24(11):57–60, 62.

Foods as occupational allergens: Part II. National Institute of Allergy and Infectious Diseases Symposium, September 8–9, 1988. Allergy Proc 1990 Mar/Apr; 11(2):59–70.

Roth R. Allergic response. Emergency 1990 June; 22(6):28–32.

Smith TE. Allergy and pseudoallergy. An overview of basic mechanisms. Prim Care 1987 Sep; 14(3):421–434.

Tipton RW. Immunotherapy for allergic diseases. Prim Care 1987 Sep; 14(3):623–629.

VanArsdel PP Jr. et al. Diagnostic tests for patients with suspected allergic disease. Ann Intern Med 1989 Feb 15; 110(4):304–312.

Information/Resources

Agencies

American Academy of Allergy and Immunology
611 E. Wells St., Milwaukee, WI 53202
(For a series of patient-oriented pamphlets, Tips to Remember)
The Asthma and Allergy Foundation of America
1717 Massachusetts Ave. NW, Suite 305, Washington, DC 20036
Center Laboratories
Division of EM Pharmaceuticals, Inc., 35 Channel Dr., Port Washington, NY 11050
National Institute of Allergy and Infectious Diseases
National Institute of Health, Bethesda, MD 20892

---

* *Medic-Alert Foundation, P.O. Box 1009, Turlock, CA 95380*

50

Management of Patients With Rheumatic Disorders

Learning Objectives

On completion of this chapter, the learner will be able to:

1. Describe the assessment and diagnostic evaluation for patients with suspected diagnosis of rheumatic disease

2. Discuss nursing diagnoses that commonly occur with rheumatic disorders and describe appropriate nursing interventions for each diagnosis

3. Compare and contrast the clinical manifestations and diagnostic findings of osteoarthritis and rheumatoid arthritis

4. Use the nursing process as a framework for the care of the patient with rheumatoid arthritis

5. Describe the systemic effects of systemic lupus erythematosus

6. Use the nursing process as a framework for the care of the patient with systemic lupus erythematosus

7. Devise a teaching plan for the patient with osteoarthritis

8. Compare and contrast clinical manifestations, probable nursing diagnoses, and nursing interventions indicated with systemic sclerosis versus gout

Glossary

arthritis—inflammation of a joint

arthrocentesis—needle puncture of a joint with aspiration of fluid

arthrodesis—surgical fusion of a joint

arthrography—x-ray of a joint

arthroplasty—surgical repair of a joint

bursa—a small, fluid-filled sac found near joints between the muscles, bones, ligaments, and tendons; helps absorb shock and reduce friction

bursitis—inflammation of a bursa

cartilage—rubbery material that cushions the ends of the bones and absorbs shock

fibrositis—a condition in which there is generalized pain in the muscles, ligaments, and tendons

flare—a period during which disease symptoms reappear or become worse

(continued)

Glossary *(continued)*

hemarthrosis—*bleeding into a joint*

inflammation—*a reaction of the body to injury or disease, causing pain, swelling, redness, warmth, and sometimes loss of motion in the area affected*

myositis—*inflammation of muscle*

remission—*a period during which disease symptoms are reduced or absent*

rheumatic diseases—*a group of diseases that affect muscles, ligaments, tendons, joints, and sometimes other body parts as well*

rheumatoid disease—*alternative terminology sometimes used for rheumatoid arthritis*

rheumatologist—*a medical doctor specializing in the diagnosis and treatment of people with forms of arthritis or other rheumatic diseases*

synovectomy—*excision of the synovial membrane*

systemic rheumatic disease—*a disease that can affect many organs or body systems, not only the joints*

tophi—*accumulation of urate crystals in tissues near joints due to gout*

Commonly known as arthritis and thought of as one condition, the rheumatic diseases are actually more than 100 different types of disorders. A wide classification of conditions, the rheumatic diseases primarily affect skeletal muscles, bones, and joints. These disorders can affect all ages from infants to the elderly. Some have a more likely onset at a particular time of life or for one sex. The impact of these conditions can be life-threatening or merely an inconvenience. The problems caused by the rheumatic disorders are not only the obvious ones related to muscles, bones, and joints, such as limitations in mobility and activities of daily living; some of the rheumatic diseases also cause systemic effects that result in problems such as pain, fatigue, altered self-image, and sleep disturbances.

Onset of these varied conditions can be acute or insidious, and the course may be marked by remissions and exacerbations. Treatment can be very simple and aimed at localized relief, or it can be very complex when directed toward relieving systemic effects.

The rheumatic diseases are classified in ten categories. Chart 50-1 gives examples of each of the categories. The inclusion of conditions that may also affect the musculoskeletal structure emphasizes the diversity of the rheumatic diseases.

Physiologic Overview

Those rheumatic diseases that are subclassified as diffuse connective tissue diseases share a common pathology, involving disruption of the protein components and collagen portion of the connective tissue. Connective tissue is distributed throughout the body in three forms: loose connective tissue, hematopoietic tissue, and strong supporting connective tissue. *Loose connective tissue* is divided into three major types: *collagen* (the most abundant type), proteins clustered in bundles to increase strength; *elastin,* fibers whose elastic properties allow tissues to stretch; and *reticulin,* delicate networks of fibers that support capillaries, nerve fibers, and the smallest units of organs. *Hematopoietic tissue* includes the bone marrow, blood cells, and lymphatic tissue. *Strong supporting connective tissue* is the main component of cartilage, bone, tendons, ligaments, and serous organ coverings. The function of connective tissue is to provide mechanical support, warmth, structure, and movement.

The systemic nature of the diffuse connective tissue diseases is reflected in the resulting widespread inflammatory process. In the joints, this inflammatory response is manifested as pannus (a proliferation of synovial tissue) extending throughout the joint space and, if persistent, is erosive to the articular cartilage, causing secondary degenerative changes to the joint.

The degenerative processes of other rheumatic diseases in themselves cause secondary inflammation as a response to the remodeling efforts of the cartilage. These conditions are more likely to be localized in nature.

The inflammation that accompanies the crystal-induced conditions or infectious agents is that which is seen with the body's reaction to a foreign or toxic substance, as in the immunologic response.

The degenerative and reactive disease processes do not have a major immunologic basis but are included in this chapter because of their classification as rheumatic diseases.

Gerontologic Considerations

Although arthritis is commonly thought of as synonymous with aging, rheumatic diseases affect people of all ages, from infancy through childhood, adolescence, and maturity. However, the rheumatic diseases do have some special implications for the older adult.

The frequency, pattern of onset, clinical features, severity, and impact on function may be different in the aged. Some of the rheumatic diseases are more prevalent with advancing age (osteoarthritis); one is exclusive to the older person (polymyalgia rheumatica). The severity of some of the rheumatic diseases may be less for the elderly. Rheumatoid arthritis that has its onset in the later years is generally less severe than the disease in a young person who has had it the same length of time. For persons whose rheumatoid arthritis started earlier in life, there are the cumulative effects of the disease over time, as well as the potential severity of the disease. Other conditions (soft tissue problems such as bursitis) are not in themselves impairing but, combined with the natural physiologic processes of aging, may add up to have a significant effect. In most cases, the arthritis is a secondary diagnosis; that is, other medical conditions that the individual has may take precedence. This

Chart 50–1
Classification of the Rheumatic Diseases

I. Diffuse connective tissue diseases
   Rheumatoid arthritis (RA)
   Juvenile rheumatoid arthritis (JRA)
   Systemic lupus erythematosus (SLE)
   Systemic sclerosis (SS)
   Polymyositis/dermatomyositis (PM/DM)
   Necrotizing vasculitis and other vasculopathies
   Sjögren's syndrome
   Overlap syndromes
   Others (polymyalgia rheumatica, erythema nodosum, etc.)
II. Arthritis associated with spondylitis
   Ankylosing spondylitis (AS)
   Reiter's syndrome
   Psoriatic arthritis (PA)
   Arthritis associated with chronic inflammatory bowel disease
III. Degenerative joint disease (DJD) (osteoarthritis [OA], osteoarthrosis)
   Primary (erosive OA)
   Secondary
IV. Arthritis, tenosynovitis, and bursitis associated with infectious agents (bacterial, viral, fungal, parasitic)
   Direct
   Indirect (reactive)
V. Metabolic and endocrine diseases associated with rheumatic states
   Crystal-induced conditions (gout, chondrocalcinosis, etc.)
   Biochemical abnormalities (amyloidosis, scurvy, etc.)
   Endocrine diseases (diabetes mellitus, acromegaly, etc.)
   Immunodeficiency diseases (primary and acquired—AIDS)
   Other hereditary disorders (hypermobility syndromes, etc.)
VI. Neoplasms
   Primary (synovioma, synoviosarcoma)
   Metastatic
   Multiple myeloma
   Leukemia and lymphoma
   Villonodular synovitis
   Osteochromatosis

VII. Neuropathic disorders
   Charcot joints
   Compression neuropathies (carpal tunnel syndrome, radiculopathy, spinal stenosis)
   Reflex sympathetic dystrophy
VIII. Bone, periosteal, and cartilage disorders associated with articular manifestations
   Osteoporosis
   Osteomalacia
   Hypertrophic osteoarthropathy
   Diffuse idiopathic skeletal hyperostosis
   Osteitis
   Osteonecrosis
   Osteochondritis
   Bone and joint dysplasias
   Slipped capital femoral epiphysis
   Costochondritis
   Osteolysis and chondrolyis
   Osteomyelitis
IX. Nonarticular rheumatism
   Myofascial pain syndromes (fibrositis)
   Low back pain and intervertebral disc disorders
   Tendonitis and/or bursitis
   Ganglion cysts
   Fasciitis
   Chronic ligament and muscle strain
   Vasomotor disorders (Raynaud's, erythromelalgia)
X. Miscellaneous disorders
   Associated with arthritis (trauma, internal derangement of joints, sarcoidosis, palindromic rheumatism, erythema nodosum, hemophilia)
   Other conditions (nodular panniculitis, familial Mediterranean fever, Goodpasture's syndrome, chronic active hepatitis, drug-induced rheumatic syndromes, etc.)

(Modified from Schumacher HR [ed]. Primer on the Rheumatic Diseases, 9th ed. Atlanta, Arthritis Foundation, 1988.)

co-morbidity is probably the most difficult issue because the treatment of the arthritis may not be addressed because of the nature of the other medical problem, the lack of awareness of what can be done to treat the arthritis, and the misconception that arthritis and aging are synonymous.

The effects of the condition may lead to considerable changes in the life-style of the individual and may threaten his independence. Decreased vision and altered balance in the elderly make safety factors a concern of the nurse. Special techniques for promoting self-management (memory aids for medications) and concentration may need to be employed. The combination of poor hearing, diminished vision, forgetfulness, and depression contribute to nonadherence to the treatment regimen in the elderly.

The elderly may not seek adequate diagnosis, believing that the manifestations of the rheumatic disease are a consequence of aging. Unfortunately, this belief may also extend to health care providers. Yet, when the disorder is adequately diagnosed, much can be done to improve the quality of life of the older person with arthritis.

Pharmacologic treatment of the rheumatic disease in the older patient is more difficult than for younger patients. If the medications used have an effect on the senses (hearing, cognition), this effect is magnified in the elderly. The cumulative effect of medications is accentuated because of the physiologic changes of aging. For example, decreased renal function in the elderly alters the metabolism of medications. The elderly are more likely to use over-the-counter remedies, to use many different medications (polypharmacy), and to be more susceptible to unproven methods of treatment.

The elderly may unnecessarily accept or endure pain, loss of ambulation, and difficulty with activities of daily living. Their body image and self-esteem, combined with underlying depression, may interfere with the use of assistive devices.

Assessment

Management of rheumatic diseases begins with a complete and accurate assessment of the patient's history of problems and present status of symptoms and a complete physical assessment. The health history is the most valuable diagnostic aid to the physical assessment.

Besides a general medical history, information about the onset of problems, course of disease, family history, and any other contributing factors is gathered. Pain is the symptom that most commonly causes a person to seek medical attention. Other common symptoms include joint swelling, limited movement, stiffness, weakness, and fatigue.

The health history also includes information about the patient's perception of the problem, previous treatment modalities and their effectiveness, the patient's support systems, and the patient's present knowledge base and source of that information.

Inspection of the patient's general appearance occurs during initial contact. Gait, posture, and general musculoskeletal size and structure are observed. Gross deformities and abnormalities in movement are noted. The symmetry, size, and contour of other connective tissues, such as the skin and adipose tissue, are also noted and recorded.

The present status of signs and symptoms is assessed through inspection and interview. Common problems of pain, stiffness, fatigue, sleep/rest habits, and limitations of daily activity are explored. Information about the current medication regimen is elicited.

Because connective tissue is found in nearly all body systems, a complete physical assessment is performed. Special attention is given to the examination of each joint and its adjacent structures.

Chart 50-2 outlines the important areas for consideration during the physical assessment.

Diagnostic Evaluation

In addition to the history and physical assessment, a battery of diagnostic studies is used to confirm or support a tentative diagnosis. The physician determines what tests are necessary based on the presenting symptoms, stage of disease, and the cost factor/benefit ratio.

An *arthrocentesis* is performed to obtain a sample of synovial fluid, usually from the knee or shoulder. The joint is anesthetized locally, and a large-bore needle is inserted into the joint space to obtain a fluid specimen. Because this procedure has the potential for introducing bacteria into the joint, aseptic technique must be followed. After the procedure, no special precautions are necessary, but the patient is observed for signs of infection and hemarthrosis (bleeding into the joint).

The fluid is examined for volume, viscosity, glucose level, white blood cells, and its ability to form a mucin clot. It is examined microscopically for cell count, cell identification, Gram stain, and formed elements. Normally, synovial fluid is clear, viscous, straw-colored, and scanty in volume with few cells. In inflammatory joint disease, the fluid often becomes cloudy, milky, or dark yellow and contains numerous inflammatory cells, such as leukocytes (white blood cells) and complement, a plasma protein associated with immunologic reactions. The viscosity is reduced in inflammatory disease, and copious amounts of fluid may be present. (The removal of joint fluid may also give temporary pain relief.) Blood in the fluid specimen suggests trauma or a tendency to bleed. Diagnostically, this is the most valuable test if joint fluid can be obtained.

X-rays are important in evaluating patients with musculoskeletal conditions. Timing of x-rays should be considered: it is unlikely that a patient with a 2-month history of joint inflammation will have x-ray changes; however, someone with knee crepitus (a grating sound heard on movement) will likely show severe joint degeneration. X-rays can also be used over years to monitor disease activity and progression of disease. Bone films determine gross bone density, texture, erosion, and changes in bone relationships. X-rays of the bone cortex detect widening, narrowing, and signs of irregularity. Joint x-rays reveal the presence of fluid excess, irregularity, bony overgrowth, narrowing, and changes in the joint structure.

A *bone scan* reflects the degree to which the crystal lattice of bone "takes up" a bone-seeking radioactive isotope. An area of increased uptake, such as a joint, is considered abnormal.

A *joint scan* procedure is similar to that of the bone scan and allows determination of joint damage throughout the body. It is the most sensitive study for the detection of early disease.

Electromyography (EMG) may be performed when skeletal muscles or nerves are affected by a connective tissue disease. When an EMG is performed, an electrode is inserted in a muscle by use of a very small needle, and electrical activity is measured.

A *muscle biopsy* is carried out for microscopic examination of skeletal muscle. The procedure may be performed in the operating room under local or general anesthesia. A surgical incision is made, and the desired specimen is obtained. A pressure dressing is applied, and the affected extremity is immobilized for 12 to 24 hours. Muscle biopsy is useful in the diagnosis of myositis.

Magnetic resonance imaging (MRI) is another, more sophisticated approach to diagnose problems involving soft tissue. MRI uses magnetic fields and radio waves to look through bone to examine the underlying soft tissue; a computer then produces the image on a screen. MRI is used to diagnose connective tissue diseases involving the spine, heart, kidneys, brain, etc. A thorough patient history prior to the MRI is necessary to determine if there are any internal metal sources in the body, such as aneurysm clips, pacemaker, shrapnel, or any metal substance. The presence of metal could be hazardous to the patient because the strength of the magnetic fields could cause movement or displacement of these objects.

Arterial biopsy is carried out to examine a specimen of an arterial vessel wall. Most frequently, the temporal artery is selected, but other arteries may undergo biopsy as indicated. The procedure is similar to that for the incisional muscle biopsy but is generally performed under local anesthesia in the operating room. Arterial biopsy most often confirms inflammation of the vessel wall, or *arteritis*, a type of vasculitis.

A *skin biopsy* may be performed to confirm inflammatory connective tissue diseases, such as lupus erythematosus or sys-

Chart 50–2
Physical Assessment

In addition to the head-to-toe assessment or systems review, the following are important areas of consideration to be noted at the time the complete physical assessment is being done.

Manifestation	Nursing Significance
Skin (inspect and inquire)	
1. Rash/lesions	1. Associated with SLE, vasculitides, drug complications
2. Increased bruising	2. Associated with several RDs and drug complications
3. Erythema	3. Sign of inflammation
4. Thinning	4. Drug complication
5. Warmth	5. Sign of inflammation
6. Photosensitivity	6. Associated with SLE, dermatomyositis, drug complications
Hair (inspect and inquire)	
1. Alopecia	1 & 2. Associated with RDs or drug complication
2. Thinning	
Eye (inspect and inquire)	
1. Dryness, grittiness	1. Associated with Sjögren's (commonly occurring with RA and SLE)
2. Decreased acuity or blindness	2. Associated with temporal arteritis, drug complications
3. Cataracts	3 & 4. Drug complications
4. Decreased peripheral vision	
5. Conjunctivitis/uveitis	5. Associated with ankylosing spondylitis and Reiter's syndrome
Ear (inquire)	
1. Tinnitus	1 & 2. Drug complications
2. Decreased acuity	
Mouth (inspect and inquire)	
1. Buccal/sublingual lesions	1. Associated with vasculitis, dermatomyositis, drug complications
2. Altered sense of taste	2. Drug complication
3. Dryness	3. Associated with myositis
4. Dysphagia	4. Associated with myositis
5. Difficulty chewing	5. Associated with decreased ROM in jaw
Chest (inspect and inquire)	
1. Pleuritic pain	1. Associated with RA & SLE
2. Decreased chest expansion	2. Associated with AS
3. Activity intolerance (dyspnea)	3. Associated with pulmonary hypertension in SS
Cardiovascular System (inspect, inquire, palpate)	
1. Blanching of fingers on exposure to cold	1. Associated with Raynaud's phenomenon
2. Peripheral pulses	2. Deficit may indicate vascular involvement or edema associated with drug complications or rheumatic diseases, especially SLE or SS
Abdomen (inquire and palpate)	
1. Altered bowel habits	1. Associated with SS, spondylosis, ulcerative colitis, decreased physical mobility, drug complications
2. Nausea/vomiting/bloating/pain	2. Drug complications
3. Weight change	3. Associated with RA (decreased), drug complications (increased or decreased)
Genitalia (inspect and inquire)	
1. Dryness/itching	1. Associated with Sjögren's syndrome
2. Abnormal menses	2. Drug complication

(continued)

Chart 50–2
Physical Assessment (Continued)

Manifestation	Nursing Significance
3. Altered sexual performance	3. Limited mobility, pain
4. Hygiene	4. Poor hygiene may be related to ADL limitations
5. Urethritis, dysuria	5. Associated with AS
6. Lesions	6. Associated with vasculitis

Neurologic (inspect and inquire)

1. Paresthesias of extremities	1 & 2. Nerve compressions associated with carpal tunnel syndrome, spinal stenosis, etc.
2. Abnormal reflex pattern	
3. Headaches	3. Associated with temporal arteritis, drug complications

Musculoskeletal (inspect and palpate)

1. Joint redness/warmth/swelling/tenderness/deformity—location of first joint involved, pattern of progression, symmetry, acute vs chronic nature	1. Signs of inflammation
2. Joint ROM	2. Decreased ROM may indicate severity or progression of disease

3. Surrounding tissue findings
    Muscle atrophy
    Subcutaneous nodules
    Popliteal cyst
	3. Extra-articular manifestations

4. Muscle strength (grip)	4. Muscle strength decreases with increased disease activity

Lab Values

1. ESR	1. Indicator of inflammation
2. CBC	2. Anemia often associated with systemic disease
3. Platelet count	3. Drug complications (decreased) or associated with SLE
4. Salicylate level	4. Measure of therapeutic level to decrease inflammation

SLE, systemic lupus erythematosus; RD, rheumatoid disease; RA, rheumatoid arthritis; ROM, range of motion; AS, ankylosing spondylitis; SS, systemic sclerosis; ADL, activities of daily living; ESR, erythrocyte sedimentation rate; CBC, complete blood count.

temic sclerosis (scleroderma). A specimen may be lightly scraped from the patient's skin without discomfort. Deeper skin biopsies may need to be carried out when scraping is not sufficient.

Myelography is performed to confirm a diagnosis of nerve root compression or displacement of vertebral structures resulting from degenerative joint disease of the spine or degenerative disc disease. A radiopaque substance, air, or metrizamide (Amipaque), a water-soluble material, is injected into the subarachnoid space of the lumbar or cervical spine. This allows visualization of abnormalities, such as narrowing of the spinal canal.

Arthrography is another diagnostic tool used to detect connective tissue disorders. A radiopaque substance or air is injected into the joint cavity, especially of the knee or shoulder, in order to outline the contour of the joint. The joint is put through passive range of motion while a series of x-rays is taken. After the test, the patient is reassured that the radiopaque substance will be absorbed systemically and joint swelling will consequently subside. No special post-test precautions are necessary, but the patient is instructed to observe for signs of infection and hemarthrosis.

In general, *serum laboratory studies* in rheumatology rely on the theory that most rheumatic diseases are autoimmune.

While many of the tests are highly complex and technical, no one test *sufficiently* supports a diagnosis of a rheumatic disease. In Table 50-1, some of the most common serum studies are listed with corresponding normal value ranges and primary indications. Because many of the tests require special laboratory techniques, they may not be used in every health care facility.

Management

A treatment program involving the multidisciplinary team, including the patient, is the basis for managing any of the rheumatic diseases. The nurse plays a central role because she is often the first of the team members to come in contact with the patient and assists the patient with his most basic needs. The nurse identifies problems that can be affected by the interventions and collaborates with other team members to achieve the expected patient outcomes. Management of the patient with any rheumatic disease begins with patient education regarding self-management principles. Medications, exercise, joint protection techniques, and thermal modalities may be included in the management program. Chart 50-3 outlines

TABLE 50-1. *Common Serum Laboratory Diagnostic Studies for Rheumatic Diseases*

Description	Normal Value	Nursing Significance
SERUM		
Creatinine Metabolic waste excreted through the kidneys	0.6–1.2 mg/dl (SI: 50–110 μmol/L)	Increase may indicate renal damage in SLE, SS, and polyarteritis
Erythrocyte Sedimentation Rate (ESR) Measures the rate at which RBCs settle out of unclotted blood in 1 hour	Westergren = *Men* 0–15 mm/hr, *Women* 0–20 mm/hr Wintrobe = *Men* 0–9 mm/hr, *Women* 0–15 mm/hr	Increase often seen in any inflammatory CTD An increase indicates increased inflammation, resulting in clustering of RBCs, which make them heavier than normal. The higher the sedimentation rate, the greater the inflammatory activity.
Hematocrit Measures the size, capacity, and number of cells present in blood	*Men:* 45–50 vol/dl *Women:* 40–45 vol/dl	Decrease can be seen in chronic inflammation (anemia of chronic disease); also, blood loss through bowel due to medication.
Red Blood Cell Count (RBC) Measures the number of circulating erythrocytes	*Men:* Average 4.8 million/μl *Women:* Average 4.3 million/μl	Decreased in RA, SLE
White Blood Cell Count (WBC) Measures the number of circulating leukocytes	5000–10,000 cells/mm^3	Sometimes decreased in SLE Neutropenia associated with Felty's syndrome
VDRL (Venereal Disease Research Laboratory) Measures antibody to syphilis	Nonreactive	False-positive sometimes found with SLE
Uric Acid Measures level of uric acid in serum	2.5–8 mg/dl (SI: 0.15–0.5 mmol/L)	Increase seen with gout
SERUM IMMUNOLOGY		
Antinuclear Antibody (ANA) Measures the presence of antibodies that react with a variety of nuclear antigens If antibodies are present, further testing determines the type of ANA circulating in the blood (anti-DNA, anti-RNP).	Negative A small number of healthy adults have a positive ANA	Positive test (titer 1:10–1:30) is associated with SLE, RA, SS, Raynaud's disease, Sjögren's syndrome, necrotizing arteritis The higher the titer, the greater the degree of inflammation The pattern of immunofluorescence (speckled, homogeneous, or nucleolar) seen helps determine the diagnosis
Anti-DNA, DNA binding Titer measurement of antibody to double-stranded DNA	Negative	High titer seen in SLE; increases in titer may indicate increase in disease activity
Complement Levels—C_3 C_4 *Complement* is a protein substance that binds with antigen–antibody complexes for the purpose of lysis. When the number of complexes increases markedly, complement is used for lysis, thus depleting the amount available in the blood.	C_3: 55–120 mg/dl (SI: 550–1200 mg/L) C_4: 11–40 mg/dl (SI: 110–400 mg/L)	Decrease may be seen in RA and SLE Decrease indicates autoimmune and inflammatory activity
C-Reactive Protein Test (CRP) Shows presence of abnormal glycoprotein due to inflammatory process	Trace 6 μg/ml	A positive reading indicates active inflammation Often positive for RA, disseminated lupus erythematosus

(continued)

TABLE 50–1. *(Continued)*

Description	Normal Value	Nursing Significance
SERUM IMMUNOLOGY (Continued)		
Immunoglobulin Electrophoresis		
Measures the values of immunoglobulins	IgA 50–300 mg/dl (SI: 0.5–3 g/L)	Increased levels are found in people who have autoimmune disorders
	IgG 635–1400 mg/dl (SI: 6.35–14 g/L)	
	IgM 40–280 mg/dl (SI: 0.4–2.8 g/L)	
Rheumatoid Factor (RF)		
Determines the presence of abnormal antibodies seen in CTD	Negative	Positive titer > 1:80
		Present in 80% of those with rheumatoid arthritis
		Positive RF may also suggest SLE, Sjögren's syndrome, or mixed CTD. The higher the titer (number at right of colon), the greater the degree of inflammation
TISSUE TYPING		
HLA-B27 Antigen		
Measures presence of HLA antigens, which are used for tissue recognition	Negative	Found in 80%–90% of those with ankylosing spondylitis and Reiter's syndrome

SLE, systemic lupus erythematosus; SS, systemic sclerosis; CTD, connective tissue disease; RA, rheumatoid arthritis; RNP, ribonucleoic protein.

the goals and strategies of basic rheumatic disease management. Table 50-2 reviews the various medications used, and Table 50-3 summarizes the exercises appropriate for rheumatic diseases.

▶ Nursing Process
The Patient With a Rheumatic Disease

◊ Nursing Assessment

The health history and physical assessment focus on the patient's current and past symptoms and the effects of these symptoms on his life and life-style. Because the rheumatic disorders affect many body systems, the history and physical assessment include review and examination of all systems, with particular attention given to those areas most commonly affected. Chart 50-2 provides a guide to the physical assessment

of the patient with rheumatic disorders. The patient's psychological and mental status is also assessed, and his ability to participate in activities and manage self-care is addressed during the assessment process.

◊ Nursing Diagnoses

Based on the physical examination and patient history data, the most common nursing diagnoses of the patient with a rheumatic disease may include the following:

- Pain related to inflammation, tissue damage, depression, anxiety, stress, fatigue, immobility, physical activity, increased disease activity
- Fatigue related to increased disease activity, anemia, muscle atrophy, pain, inadequate rest, emotional stress/depression
- Impaired physical mobility related to decreased range of motion, inflammation, pain, contractures, increased stiffness,

(text continues on page 1415)

Chart 50-3
Management of Connective Tissue Diseases

Major Goals
1. Suppression of inflammation and the autoimmune response
2. Pain management
3. Maintenance of/or improved joint mobility
4. Maintenance of/or improved functional status
5. Knowledge regarding the specific disease and self-management techniques
6. Compliance with the therapeutic regimen

Management Strategies
1. Patient education
2. Exercise programs for joint motion and muscle strengthening
3. Joint protection, splints, adaptive devices
4. Anti-inflammatory medications
5. Disease-modifying antirheumatic drugs
6. Thermal modalities
7. Experimental treatments, *e.g.*, plasmaphoresis

TABLE 50–2. *Drugs Used in Rheumatic Diseases*

Drug	Actions, Use, and Indications	Nursing Implications and Assessment for Drug Intolerance
SALICYLATES		
Aspirin (buffered or enteric-coated)	*Actions:* Anti-inflammatory, analgesic, and antipyretic	Should be taken with meals to protect against primary adverse reaction of gastric irritation
Choline magnesium trisalicylate	Acetylated salicylates are platelet aggregation inhibitors	
Choline salicylate	Used in early phase of disease	
Salsalate	Anti-inflammatory dosage will produce blood salicylate levels of 20–30 mg/dl	Assess for complaints of tinnitus, gastric intolerance, or GI bleeding and purpuric tendencies
NONSTEROIDAL ANTI-INFLAMMATORY DRUGS (NSAIDs)		
Propionic Acid Derivatives	*Actions:* Anti-inflammatory, analgesic, antipyretic, platelet aggregation inhibitor	Long-term administration requires monitoring for gastrointestinal, CNS, cardiovascular, renal, hematologic, and skin adverse reactions. Aspirin products should be avoided.
Fenoprofen (Nalfon)		
Ibuprofen (Motrin)	Onset of anti-inflammatory effects—about 4 weeks	
Flurbiprofen (Ansaid)	All NSAIDs are useful for short-term treatment of an acute gouty attack	
Ketoprofen (Orudis)		
Naproxen (Naprosyn)	NSAIDs are used as an alternative to salicylates for a first-line therapy in several rheumatic diseases	Acetaminophen used for headaches, fever
Fenamates		
Meclofenamate (Meclomen)		
Pyrazoles		
Phenylbutazone (Butazolidin)		
Oxyphenbutazone (Tandearil)		
Osicams		
Piroxican (Feldene)		
Acetic Acid Derivatives		
Diclofenac (Voltaren)		
Indene Derivatives:		
Indomethacin (Indocin)		
Sulindac (Clinoril)		
Tolmetin (Tolectin)		
DISEASE-MODIFYING DRUGS		
Gold-Containing Compounds	*Actions:* Anti-inflammatory, mechanism unknown; suppresses synovitis during active stage of rheumatoid disease	Administered concurrently with anti-inflammatory agents until benefits from gold therapy are achieved
Aurothioglucose (Solganal)		
Gold sodium thiomalate (Myochrysine)	IM preparations initially given weekly, then frequency decreases to every 2–4 weeks	Assess for signs/symptoms of drug toxicity: stomatitis, dermatitis, diarrhea, proteinuria, hematuria, bone marrow suppression
Auranofin (Ridaura)	PO gold given daily in capsule form, dosage remains constant	
	Onset of benefit from drug may be 3–6 months	Gold sodium thiomalate may produce nitroid reaction 1–36 hours after injection.
		Blood and urine monitored every other injection
Penicillamine	*Action:* Mechanism unknown, may improve lymphocyte function	Administered concurrently with anti-inflammatory agents
	May take 2–3 months before benefits are seen	Assess for signs/symptoms of toxicity: gastric irritation, decreased taste sensation, skin rash/itching, bone marrow suppression, proteinuria
	Taken on empty stomach	
	Useful in RA and SS	

(continued)

TABLE 50–2. *(Continued)*

Drug	Actions, Use, and Indications	Nursing Implications and Assessment for Drug Intolerance
DISEASE-MODIFYING DRUGS (continued)		
		Blood and urine monitored every 2 weeks until stabilized, then monthly
Hydroxychloroquine (Plaquenil) *Chloroquine (Aralen)*	*Action:* Anti-inflammatory, mechanism unknown Useful in RA and SLE, 200 mg once or twice a day May take 2–4 months before benefits are seen	Administered concurrently with anti-inflammatory agents Assess for signs/symptoms of toxicity: changes in vision, GI disturbance, skin rash, sun sensitivity, bleaching of hair, headaches Ophthalmologic exams required every 6 months
IMMUNOSUPPRESSIVES Methotrexate Azathioprine (Imuran) Cyclophosphamide (Cytoxan)	*Actions:* Used in advanced rheumatoid arthritis or SLE that is unresponsive to conventional therapy These drugs have teratogenic potential Action is believed to result from drug's cytotoxic effects of inhibiting lymphocytes or macrophages and thus interfering with joint inflammation	Highly toxic: Bone marrow depression, GI ulcerations Skin rashes, alopecia Bladder toxicity Reduces patient's resistance to infections Patient must be monitored with weekly blood evaluation and urinalysis Advise patient of contraceptive measures
CORTICOSTEROIDS Prednisone (Deltasone) Prednisolone (Delta-Cortef) Hydrocortisone (Cortef)	Corticosteroids used in treatment of incapacitating active rheumatoid arthritis, SLE, progressive SS, necrotizing arteritis Use of corticosteroids for long periods has wide range of adverse effects Steroids are used with caution and are tapered to minimal maintenance dose if possible Onset of action is rapid, within the first week	Toxic effects with high doses or long-term treatment Osteoporosis, fractures, avascular necrosis Gastric ulcers, psychiatric problems, infection susceptibility Hirsutism, acne, moon facies, abnormal fat deposition, edema, emotional disorders, menstrual disorders Hyperglycemia, hypokalemia Hypertension Cataracts and glaucoma
CORTICOSTEROIDS *Intra-articular Injections*	Given when arthritic reaction has been suppressed and one or two joints are not responding to treatment Given when only one or two joints are affected Given to patient with extremely painful joints so he can undergo physical therapy Relieves pain. Benefit may last from weeks to months No more than three injections in a single joint should be given	An inflamed joint may respond to local injection when it has failed to come under control through other general systemic measures Joints most amenable to corticosteroid injections are ankles, knees, hips, shoulders, and hands Repeated injections can cause joint damage

(continued)

TABLE 50–2. (Continued)

Drug	Actions, Use, and Indications	Nursing Implications and Assessment for Drug Intolerance
AGENTS USED IN GOUT		
Allopurinol (Zyloprim)	Interrupts the breakdown of purines before uric acid is formed. Inhibits xanthinoxidase because it blocks uric acid formation	Side effects include bone marrow depression, vomiting, and abdominal pain
Colchicine	Action is unknown. It does not alter serum or urine levels of uric acid. It lowers the deposition of uric acid and interferes with leukocytes and kinin formation, thus reducing inflammation	Prolonged use may decrease vitamin B$_{12}$ absorption Causes gastrointestinal upset in the majority of patients Must be given when attack first begins. Dosage is increased until pain is relieved or diarrhea develops.
Probenecid (Benemid) (Uricosuric agent)	Inhibits renal reabsorption of urates and increases the urinary excretion of uric acid. Prevents tophi formation	Be alert for nausea, rash, and constipation

RA, rheumatoid arthritis; SS, systemic sclerosis; SLE, systemic lupus erythematosus.

weakness, limited endurance, improper use of ambulatory devices
- Self-care deficit related to contractures, fatigue, impaired mobility, loss of motion, decreased endurance, weakness, stiffness, depression, lack of knowledge, lack of motivation, learned helplessness, secondary gain

Additional nursing diagnoses that are frequently made include:

- Knowledge deficit related to anxiety, previous experience, inadequate pain control
- Sleep pattern disturbance related to pain, fatigue, stiffness, physical activity, depression, anxiety, environmental factors, medication, overstimulation
- Body image, disturbance related to physical changes caused by disease or treatment, loss of significant roles, unrealistic self-expectations, life-style changes
- Ineffective coping, defensive coping, ineffective denial related to actual or perceived life-style change, actual or perceived role change, chronic illness/disability, lack of knowledge, isolation (physical or emotional)
- Altered nutrition less than body requirements or more than

body requirements related to loss of mobility, pain, fatigue, lack of knowledge
- Impaired skin integrity related to contractures, loss of mobility, disease process, treatment

▷ **Planning and Implementation**

▷ *Goals:* The major goals of the patient may include relief of pain and discomfort, relief of fatigue, increased mobility, and maintenance of self-care.

▷ **Nursing Interventions**

An understanding of the underlying disease process (*i.e.,* degeneration, inflammation, as well as degeneration resulting from inflammation or inflammation resulting from degeneration) guides the nurse's thought process. In addition, the nurse's knowledge of whether the condition is localized or more widely systemic influences the scope of the nursing activity.

Some rheumatic diseases (*e.g.,* osteoarthritis) are more localized alterations in connective tissue in which there is the potential to control symptoms such as pain or stiffness. Other

TABLE 50–3.   *Exercise Tolerance Related to Inflammatory Process: Suggested Exercises*

Inflammatory Process/Pain	Recommended Exercise	Patient Performance Level
Acute exacerbation; severe pain	Passive range of motion (ROM)	Unable to perform exercises alone
Subacute; moderate or minimal pain	Active assistive or active ROM within pain tolerance	Can perform with help from another person or an assistive mechanical device
Inactive; remission; minimal pain or absence of pain	Active ROM; isometrics	Can perform alone

rheumatic diseases have a known cause and specific treatment to control the symptoms. An example of this latter type of rheumatic disease is gout. The rheumatic diseases that present the greatest challenge for the nurse are those with systemic manifestations.

Nursing Care Plan 50-1 details the nursing interventions to be considered for each nursing diagnosis. Interventions that are particularly appropriate for a specific rheumatic disease are addressed in the discussion of the specific disorder.

Specific nursing measures that are often used include:

▷ *Relief of Pain*

Warm and Cold Applications. Heat applications are often helpful in relieving pain, stiffness, and muscle spasm. Superficial heat may be supplied in the form of warm tub baths or showers and warm moist compresses. Paraffin baths (dips) offer concentrated heat and are helpful to patients with wrist and small-joint involvement. Therapeutic exercises can be carried out more comfortably and effectively after heat has been applied. In some patients, however, heat may actually increase pain, muscle spasm, and synovial fluid volume. If the inflammatory process is acute, cold applications may be tried in the form of moist packs or an ice bag. Both heat and cold are analgesic to nerve pain receptors and relax muscle spasms.

Pain Relief Strategies. Other strategies of relieving pain and increasing comfort are introduced to the patient. These include muscle relaxation techniques, imagery, self-hypnosis, and distraction. Muscle relaxation techniques reduce muscle tension and anxiety. These techniques involve a sequence of muscle contraction and relaxation exercises in association with controlled breathing exercises. Imagery is used to encourage the patient to concentrate on a pleasant scene or experience so that attention is drawn away from the pain experience. Self-hypnosis is a process whereby the state of consciousness is altered so the patient is able to relax and focus on pleasant images to the exclusion of unpleasant events or painful stimuli. Distraction is often an effective method of pain control in which the patient is encouraged to pay attention to events other than the pain experience.

▷ *Relief of Fatigue.* Rest also helps to reduce fatigue and allay pain. For the systemic rheumatic diseases, the whole patient (and involved systems)—not merely the joints—must be treated. The amount of rest required is indicated by the amount of inflammatory involvement and the comfort of the patient.

Frequent periods of bed rest during the day take the weight off the joints and relieve fatigue. If joint inflammation is severe, the patient may be placed on complete bed rest for a brief period. Range-of-motion exercises should still be carried out.

▷ *Increased Mobility*

Positioning and Posture. Proper body positioning is essential to minimize stress on inflamed joints and prevent deformities. All joints should be supported in a position of optimal function. When in bed, the patient should lie flat on a firm mattress, with feet positioned against a footboard, and only one pillow under the head because of the risk of dorsal kyphosis. A pillow should *not* be placed under the knees, because this promotes flexion contracture of those joints. The patient lies on the abdomen several times daily to prevent hip flexion contracture. Active range-of-motion exercises are encouraged because they prevent joint stiffness. If the patient is unable to actively range the joints, passive range-of-motion should be provided.

Good posture is also important. Proper body posture includes walking erect and the use of chairs that have straight backs so that the feet can rest flat on the floor and the shoulders and hips can rest against the back of the chair.

Assistive and Supportive Devices. Braces and splints can be used to support and immobilize a joint. Cervical collars may be used to support the weight of the head and limit cervical motion. A metatarsal bar or special pads may be put into shoes if foot pain or deformity is present.

Acutely inflamed joints can be rested by applying splints to limit motion. Splints also support the joint to relieve spasm and may help prevent deformity. The knee is splinted at full extension and the wrist at slight dorsiflexion. The joints should not be permitted to "freeze" in positions of flexion, because of the predominant strength of flexor muscles, by regular removal of the splint and putting the joint through a range-of-motion. Splints may need to be modified when changes occur in joint structure.

Canes and crutches can relieve stress from inflamed and painful weight-bearing joints while allowing safe ambulation. The cane should be of a length to allow for only a slight bend of the elbow and should be held in the hand opposite the affected side. Crutches may need to be of the forearm-trough style to protect the upper extremities if there is wrist and hand involvement. This is especially important for the patient rehabilitating from lower extremity joint reconstruction.

▷ *Maintenance of Self-Care* Assistive devices can often be the difference between dependence and independence; however, they may alter the patient's body image and become a barrier to compliance. The nurse must introduce assistive devices by being sensitive to the patient's feelings and attitude and must demonstrate acceptance and positive attitudes about the use of these devices.

▷ Evaluation

Expected Outcomes
1. Experiences relief of pain
   a. Identifies factors that cause or increase pain and discomfort
   b. Uses pain management strategies effectively
   c. Identifies realistic goals for pain relief
   d. Reports decreased pain and increased comfort level
2. Experiences reduction in level of fatigue
   a. Identifies factors that contribute to fatigue
   b. Schedules periodic periods of rest
   c. Reports decreased level of fatigue
3. Increases level of mobility
   a. Identifies factors that impede mobility
   b. Participates in activities and exercises that promote or maintain mobility
   c. Uses assistive devices appropriately
   d. Demonstrates good body alignment and posture
4. Maintains self-care activities
   a. Participates in self-care activities within capabilities
   b. Uses assistive devices to increase participation in self-care activities
   c. Maintains maximum level of mobility and self-care activities

See Nursing Care Plan 50-1 for additional expected outcomes.

(text continues on page 1421)

Nursing Care Plan 50–1

Care of the Patient With a Rheumatic Disease

Nursing Interventions	Rationale	Expected Outcomes

Nursing Diagnosis: Pain related to inflammation, increased disease activity, tissue damage, or immobility

Goal: Improvement in comfort level; incorporation of pain management techniques into daily life

Nursing Interventions	Rationale	Expected Outcomes

1. Provide variety of comfort measures:
   a. Application of heat or cold
   b. Massage
   c. Foam matresss
   d. Supportive pillow
   e. Relaxation techniques
   f. Position changes
   g. Splints
   h. Diversional activities
   i. Resting affected joints
	1. Pain may respond to nondrug interventions such as joint protection, exercise, relaxation, and thermal modalities.	• Identifies factors that exacerbate or influence pain response.
		• Identifies and uses pain management measures.

2. Administer medications as directed:
   a. Anti-inflammatory
   b. Analgesic
   c. Disease-modifying
	2. Pain of rheumatic disease responds to individual or combination drug regimens.	• Verbalizes decrease in pain.
		• Evidences minimal side effects.

3. Instruct in self-administration of medications.		• Demonstrates accurate self-administration of medications.
4. Observe for side effects: GI disturbances, decreased kidney function, bone marrow suppression, etc. (see Table 50–1)		
5. Individualize medication schedule to best meet patient's needs for pain management.		
6. Encourage ventilation of thoughts and feelings on pain and chronicity of disease.	6. The impact of pain on an individual's life often leads to misconceptions about pain and pain management techniques.	• Verbalizes that pain is characteristic of rheumatic disease. • Establishes realistic pain-relief goals.
7. Provide nonthreatening environment		
8. Instruct on pathophysiology of pain and rheumatic disease.		
9. Assist to identify that pain often leads to unproved treatment methods.		• Verbalizes that pain often leads to the use of nontraditional and unproved self-treatment methods.
10. Assess for subjective changes in pain.	10. With rheumatic disease pain, the individual's description of the pain sensation is a more reliable indicator than objective measurements such as change in vital signs, body movement, and facial expression.	• Identifies changes in quality or intensity of pain.

Nursing Diagnosis: Sleep pattern disturbance related to pain, fatigue, physical inactivity, depression, medications, or overstimulation

Goal: Verbalizes an improvement in the quality of sleep

Nursing Interventions	Rationale	Expected Outcomes
1. Instruct in the use of comfort measures to promote sleep. a. Provide heat, massage, proper posi-	1. Increased comfort at bedtime may promote better sleep pattern. Use of bed adaptations (eggcrate mattress, butterfly	• Identifies and uses techniques to induce and/or maintain sleep.

(continued)

Nursing Care Plan 50–1 (Continued)

Care of the Patient With a Rheumatic Disease

Nursing Interventions	Rationale	Expected Outcomes
tioning, relaxation techniques, analgesics, or anti-inflammatory medications prior to sleep. b. Use bed adaptations. c. Adhere to bedtime rituals.	pillow) can increase comfort allowing sleep.	
2. Instruct in the use of antidepressants.	2. Antidepressants in low doses can improve sleep pattern and help manage chronic pain that may be interfering with sleep.	• Verbalizes rationale for use of antidepressants to aid sleep.
3. Discuss factors that can interfere with sleep. a. Decrease food intake and caffeine at bedtime. b. Avoid alcohol at bedtime. c. Increase daytime activity as tolerated. d. Avoid stimulation at bedtime. e. Discourage late afternoon napping.	3. Sleep disturbance often occurs because of factors unrelated to the actual disease process.	• Identifies factors that may interfere with sleep pattern.
4. Administer hypnotic or sedative when other measures fail.	4. Hypnotics alter REM and stage 4 sleep, which may cause a less restful sleep.	• Identifies and uses hypnotics when appropriate.

Nursing Diagnosis: Fatigue related to increased disease activity, pain, inadequate sleep/rest, inadequate nutrition, emotional stress, anemia

Goal: Incorporates as part of daily activities those measures necessary to modify fatigue

1. Instruct in: a. Relationship of disease activity to fatigue b. Relationship of anemia to disease process c. Physical capability will fluctuate with various phases of illness. d. Benefits of increased iron from food or supplements e. Physical and emotional factors can cause fatigue.	1. Generalized fatigue may increase or decrease in relation to disease activity.	• Verbalizes the relationship of fatigue to disease activity. • Differentiates between psychologic and physical factors that may cause fatigue.
2. Supervise adherence to the pharmacologic treatment program.		
3. Provide comfort measures to decrease fatigue. a. Incorporate rest periods into daily schedule. b. Instruct to pace activities. c. Assist with priority setting. d. Instruct in relaxation techniques. e. Instruct in pain management techniques. f. Facilitate development of appropriate activity/rest schedule.	3. Fatigue may be lessened by conserving energy, developing effective coping strategies, controlling the disease process, using appropriate pain management measures.	• Identifies and uses measures to prevent or modify fatigue.

(continued)

Nursing Care Plan 50–1 *(Continued)*

Care of the Patient With a Rheumatic Disease

Nursing Interventions	Rationale	Expected Outcomes

Nursing Diagnosis: Impaired physical mobility related to disease activity, decreased range of motion, limited endurance, improper use of ambulatory devices

Goal: Attains and maintains optimal functional mobility

Nursing Interventions	Rationale	Expected Outcomes
1. Encourage verbalization regarding limitations in mobility.	1. Mobility is not necessarily related to deformity. Pain, stiffness, and fatigue may temporarily limit mobility. The degree of mobility is not synonymous with the degree of independence. Decreased mobility may influence a person's self-concept and lead to social isolation.	• Identifies factors that interfere with mobility.
2. Assess need for OT/PT consult: a. Emphasize ROM of affected joints. b. Reinforce use of ambulatory devices. c. Reinforce use of safe footwear. d. Use individual appropriate positioning/posture.	2. Therapeutic exercises, proper footwear, and/or assistive equipment may improve mobility. Correct posture and positioning are necessary for maintaining optimal mobility.	• Describes and uses measures to prevent loss of motion.
3. Assist to identify environmental barriers.	3. Furniture and architectural adaptations may enhance mobility.	• Identifies environmental (home, school, work, community) barriers to optimal mobility.
4. Encourage independence in mobility and assist as needed. a. Allow ample time for activity b. Provide rest period after activity. c. Reinforce principles of joint protection and work simplification.	4. Changes in mobility may lead to a decrease in personal safety.	• Uses appropriate techniques and/or assistive equipment to aid mobility.
5. Initiate consult to community health agency.	5. The degree of mobility may be slow to improve or may not improve with intervention.	• Identifies community resources available to assist in managing decreased mobility.

Nursing Diagnosis: Self-care deficit related to disease activity, impaired mobility, contractures, depression, lack of knowledge, lack of motivation, learned helplessness

Goal: Achieves self-care independently or with the use of resources

Nursing Interventions	Rationale	Expected Outcomes
1. Assist patient to identify self-care deficits and factors that interfere with ability to perform self-care activities.	1. The ability to perform self-care activities is influenced by the disease activity and the accompanying pain, stiffness, fatigue, muscle weakness, loss of motion, and depression.	• Identifies factors that interfere with the ability to perform self-care activities.
2. Develop plan with patient on how to establish and achieve goals to meet self-care needs, incorporating joint protection, energy conservation, and work simplification concepts. a. Provide appropriate assistive devices. b. Reinforce proper use of assistive devices. c. Allow patient to control timing of self-care activities.	2. Assistive devices may enhance self-care abilities. The degree of deformity does not necessarily reflect the individual's ability to perform self-care activities.	• Identifies alternative methods for meeting self-care needs. • Uses alternative methods for meeting self-care needs.

(continued)

Nursing Care Plan 50-1 *(Continued)*

Care of the Patient With a Rheumatic Disease

Nursing Interventions	Rationale	Expected Outcomes
3. Consult with community health care agencies when individuals have attained a maximum level of self-care yet still have some deficits, especially regarding safety.	3. Individuals differ in ability and willingness to perform self-care activities. Changes in ability to care for self may lead to a decrease in personal safety.	• Identifies and uses other health care resources for meeting self-care needs.

Nursing Diagnosis: Knowledge deficit (regarding self-management decisions) related to lack of previous experience, anxiety, inadequate pain control

Goal: Has necessary information about the disease process and therapy to make self-care management decisions

1. Instruct in basic disease management (cause, treatment, prognosis). a. Assess readiness to learn. b. Assess barriers to individual ability to learn. c. Use variety of methods to teach self-management.	1. The individual's perception of the cause, treatment, and prognosis of the disease may need correction or clarification. Factors such as pain, fatigue, and depression may interfere with the individual's readiness to learn. Physical, psychologic, intellectual, and social barriers may influence the individual's readiness to learn. The way in which information is given, not just the information itself, may influence the individual's behavior.	• Verbalizes general knowledge of disease process and treatment. • Verbalizes sufficient information to meet self-management needs according to personal value system.
2. Instruct in medication regimen and self-administration of medications.	2. An individual may need supervised practice to incorporate self-care management techniques into daily activities. The individual needs accurate information in order to discriminate between proven and unproven methods of treatment.	• Verbalizes general knowledge regarding medications. Demonstrates ability to self-administer medications.
3. Instruct in necessary adaptations in lifestyle. a. Encourage involvement of significant others.	3. Involvement of significant others may influence the individual's ability to make necessary life-style changes.	• Verbalizes concepts of disease management related to life-style.

Nursing Diagnosis: Body image disturbance related to physical changes in body appearance, impaired self-care ability, family's perception of individual

Goal: Achieves a reconciliation between self-concept and the physical and psychologic changes imposed by the rheumatic disease

1. Help patient identify elements of control over disease symptoms and treatment.	1. The individual's self-concept may be altered by the disease or its treatment.	• Verbalizes an awareness that changes taking place in self-concept are normal responses to rheumatic disease.
2. Encourage verbalization of feelings, perceptions, and fears. a. Help to assess present situation and identify problems. b. Assist to identify past coping mechanisms. c. Assist to identify effective coping mechanisms.	2. The individual's coping strategies reflect the strength of his self-concept.	• Identifies strategies to cope with altered self-concept.

Diffuse Connective Tissue Diseases

Rheumatoid Arthritis

Rheumatoid arthritis (RA) is a chronic, systemic, and progressive connective tissue disease. It is an inflammatory disorder that primarily involves the synovial membrane of the joints and is commonly characterized by joint pain, stiffness, decreased mobility, and fatigue. Synovitis presents symmetrically in peripheral joints. The disease manifests itself differently in individual patients, resulting in variable outcomes.

RA can occur at any age and generally increases in incidence with advancing age. With increasing age, the incidence rate for women and men tends to equalize. Research data continue to support the manifestation of symptoms in the second to third decade of life, with peak incidence occurring in the fourth to the sixth decades.

The etiology remains a mystery. Rheumatoid arthritis is believed to be an immune response to unknown antigens of internal or external origin. The stimulus for the immune response may be viral or bacterial, or related to an alteration in the normal production and function of collagen.

There may be a genetic predisposition to the disease. Evidence suggests that individuals who carry the human leukocyte–associated histocompatibility antigen, HLA-DR4, may have a predisposition to RA; however, only a few of those who carry HLA-DR4 actually are affected by the disease. Black Americans with RA do not carry HLA-DR4, which demonstrates that it is possible for individuals without this gene to have RA.

Pathophysiology

To understand the pathophysiology of rheumatoid arthritis, the normal anatomy and physiology of joints must be understood (see Chap. 58). The *diarthrodial* or *synovial* joint is most commonly affected by the inflammation and degeneration seen in rheumatoid arthritis.

The function of the synovial joints is to provide movement. Each synovial joint has a range in which it is capable of being moved. Not everyone has the same range of motion in their movable joints.

Articular cartilage covers the bone end of a joint and provides a smooth, resilient surface for movement. Because the cartilage has no vascular supply, it cannot regenerate. Once the cartilage is damaged, it cannot be repaired.

Synovial membrane lines the inner surface of the fibrous capsule and secretes fluid into the space between the bones. This *synovial fluid* functions as a shock absorber and a lubricant to allow the joint to move freely in the appropriate direction.

The pathologic changes of rheumatoid arthritis are first seen in the synovial tissue, where the immune response tends to localize. Inflammation involves a series of steps that are related. The first step is the triggering event.

The antigen stimulus activates monocytes and T lymphocytes. The immunoglobulin antibodies form immune complexes with antigens. Phagocytosis of the immune complexes is initiated, which generates an inflammatory reaction (joint swelling, pain, and edema) (Fig. 50-1).

During the next step, there is a deviation from the normal immune response. Phagocytosis produces chemicals such as leukotrienes and prostaglandins. Leukotrienes contribute to the inflammatory process by attracting other white cells to the area. Prostaglandins act as modifiers to inflammation; in some cases they increase inflammation and in other cases they slow it down. Leukotrienes and prostaglandins produce enzymes, such as collagenase, that break down collagen, a vital part of a normal joint. The release of these enzymes in the joint causes edema, proliferation of synovial membrane and pannus formation, destruction of cartilage, and erosion of bone (see Fig. 50-1B). The consequence of this is loss of articular surfaces and loss of joint motion. The muscles are affected as the muscle fibers undergo degenerative changes with loss of muscle elasticity and contractile power.

Clinical Manifestations

The clinical picture of rheumatoid arthritis is variable but may generally be determined by the stage and severity of the disease process. Joint pain, swelling, warmth, erythema, and lack of function are classic clinical features of rheumatoid arthritis. Palpation of the joints reveals spongy or boggy tissue. Fluid can usually be aspirated from the inflamed joint.

The characteristic pattern of joint involvement begins with the small joints in the hands, wrists, and feet. As the disease progresses, knees, shoulders, hips, elbows, ankles, cervical spine, and temporomandibular joints are involved. The onset of symptoms is usually acute, bilateral, and symmetric. In ad-

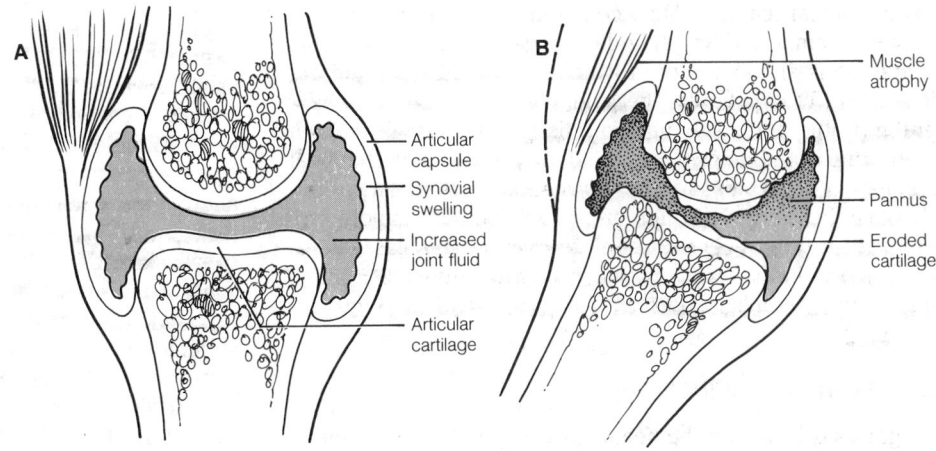

Figure 50–1. Pathophysiology of rheumatoid arthritis. (**A**) Joint structure with synovial swelling and fluid accumulation in joint. (**B**) Pannus, eroded articular cartilage with joint space narrowing, muscle atrophy, and ankylosis.

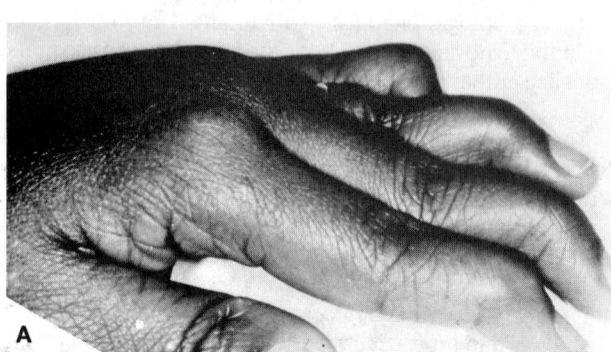
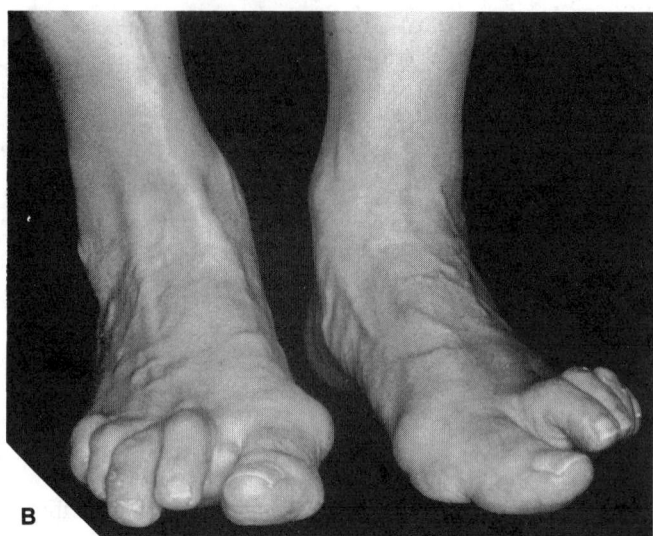

Figure 50–2. Rheumatoid arthritis changes in the hand and foot. (**A**) Example of swan neck deformity, in which the proximal interphalangeal (middle) joint is hyperextended and the distal interphalangeal joint is in flexion. (**B**) Example of hallux valgus and hammer toe deformities. The cockup toe deformities shown are associated with subluxation of the metatarsophalangeal joints. (Teaching Slide Collection, 2nd ed. Copyright 1988. Used by permission of the Arthritis Foundation.)

dition to joint pain and swelling, another classic sign of RA is joint stiffness, especially in the morning, lasting for more than 30 minutes.

Limitation in function can occur even in the early stages of disease before there are bony changes and when there is active inflammation in the joints. Joints that are hot, swollen, and painful are not easily moved, and one tends to guard or protect these joints through immobilization. Immobilization for extended periods can lead to contractures, creating soft-tissue deformity.

Deformities of the hands (Fig. 50-2*A*) and feet (see Fig. 50-2*B*) are common in rheumatoid arthritis. The deformity may be caused by the misalignment resulting from swelling, progressive joint destruction, or subluxation that occurs when slippage of bone over bone eliminates the joint space. *Ulnar drift* occurs when the fingers point to the ulna (inner bone of the forearm, on the side opposite that of the thumb). *Swanneck deformity* occurs when the proximal interphalangeal (PIP) joints hyperextend, and *boutonnière deformity* occurs when the PIP joints develop flexion deformities.

Rheumatoid arthritis is a systemic disease with multiple extra-articular features. Most common are fever, weight loss, fatigue, anemia, and lymph node enlargement. Raynaud's phenomenon is also common. Rheumatoid nodules are present in 20% to 25% of patients. These nodules are usually nontender and movable in the subcutaneous tissue. They usually appear over bony prominences, are varied in size, and can disappear spontaneously. Nodules occur only in individuals with a positive rheumatoid factor and often are associated with rapidly progressive and destructive disease. Other extra-articular features include arteritis, neuropathy, scleritis, pericarditis, splenomegaly, and Sjögren's syndrome (dry eyes and dry mucous membranes).

Diagnostic Evaluation

Diagnosis is based on the health history, physical assessment, and diagnostic studies. Physical examination reveals informa-

tion about the size, symmetry, and movement of involved joints. The presence of rheumatoid nodules can be noted. Joint inflammation is detected on palpation.

Certain serum laboratory studies are significant. Rheumatoid factor (RF) is present in more than 80% of patients with rheumatoid arthritis; however, the test alone is not diagnostic of rheumatoid arthritis. The erythrocyte sedimentation rate (ESR) is significantly elevated with rheumatoid arthritis. The red blood count and C₄ complement component are decreased. The C-reactive protein (CRP) and antinuclear antibody (ANA) tests are positive. An arthrocentesis shows synovial fluid that is cloudy, milky, or dark yellow and contains numerous inflammatory cells, such as leukocytes and complement.

Radiologic studies are performed to diagnose and stage the disease as well as for monitoring the progression of disease. The radiographic examination will show characteristic bony erosions and narrowed joint spaces occurring later in the disease.

Management

Treatment of rheumatoid arthritis requires a multidisciplinary approach to disease management. The goals of treatment include the reduction or suppression of the inflammatory process, establishing a level of comfort, minimizing undesirable side effects, preservation of joint and muscle function, and return to a desirable and productive life.

For early disease, treatment begins with education, a balance of rest and exercise, and referral to community agencies for support. Medication management begins with high doses of salicylates or nonsteroidal anti-inflammatory drugs (NSAIDs). When used in full therapeutic dosages, these drugs provide both anti-inflammatory and analgesic effects. Patients are instructed to maintain a consistent blood level to optimize the effectiveness of the anti-inflammatory drug.

Additional analgesia may be prescribed for periods of extreme pain. Care should be taken to avoid narcotic analgesics, because the patient may become drug-dependent as a result of the chronic need for pain relief. Although salicylates and nonsteroidal anti-inflammatory medications are the foundation of drug therapy, most patients will need additional drugs. When appropriate, the use of antimalarials and gold is begun early in the course of disease, before destruction of the joints occurs. Table 50-2 summarizes the drugs used in the treatment of rheumatoid arthritis. All patients on drug therapy are thoroughly instructed regarding drug type, purpose, dosage, side effects, toxic effects, and procedures for monitoring for side effects. Barriers to compliance are assessed and measures are taken to promote compliance with medications and the comprehensive treatment program.

For *moderate, erosive rheumatoid arthritis*, a formal program with occupational and physical therapy is prescribed to educate the patient in principles of joint protection, pacing of activities, work simplification, range of motion, and muscle-strengthening exercises. Emphasis is placed on active participation by the patient in the management program. Pain management techniques such as thermal modalities, relaxation exercises, and biofeedback are taught. The medication program may have to be reevaluated and appropriate changes made.

Penicillamine (Cuprimine), an oral chelating agent, may be used as an alternative to gold therapy. Like gold, its anti-inflammatory action is not understood, but it has been useful in suppressing the progress of rheumatoid arthritis in some patients. Methotrexate may also be used if gold is unsuccessful. In more active and severe disease, larger doses are used.

For *active, erosive rheumatoid arthritis*, reconstructive surgery and corticosteroids are often prescribed. Reconstructive surgery is indicated when pain cannot be relieved by conservative measures. Surgical procedures include *synovectomy* (excision of the synovial membrane), *tenorrhaphy* (suturing of a tendon), *arthrodesis* (surgical fusion of the joint), and *arthroplasty* (surgical repair of the joint) (see Chap. 59).

Systemic corticosteroids are used when the patient has unremitting inflammation and pain and/or needs a "bridging" medication while waiting for the disease-modifying drug (*i.e.,* gold) to begin working. Low-dose corticosteroid therapy is recommended for the shortest period of time necessary to minimize side effects. Joints that are severely inflamed and fail to respond promptly to the measures outlined above may be treated by the local injection of a corticosteroid.

For *advanced, severe rheumatoid arthritis*, immunosuppressive drugs are prescribed because of their ability to affect the production of antibodies at the cellular level. These include methotrexate, cyclophosphamide, and azathioprine. However, these drugs are highly toxic and can produce bone marrow depression, anemia, gastrointestinal disturbances, and skin rashes. *Plasmapheresis, lymphopheresis,* and total *lymphoid irradiation* are new, controversial procedures that are limited to extreme cases where conventional therapy has failed.

Through all stages of rheumatoid arthritis, depression and sleep deprivation may require the short-term use of low-dose antidepressant medications such as amitriptyline to reestablish an adequate sleep pattern and better manage chronic pain.

Patients with rheumatoid arthritis frequently experience anorexia, weight loss, and anemia. A dietary history will identify usual eating habits and food preferences. The patient is taught how to select foods to include the daily requirements from the basic four food groups, with emphasis on foods high in vitamins, protein, and iron for tissue building and repair. For the extremely anorexic patient, small, frequent feedings with increased protein supplements may be prescribed.

Some medications (oral corticosteroids) used in the treatment of rheumatoid arthritis stimulate the appetite and, when combined with decreased activity, may lead to weight gain.

▶ Nursing Process
The Patient With Rheumatoid Arthritis

▷ Assessment

Data collection begins with an interview and physical examination. During the interview process, the nurse assesses the patient's self-image related to musculoskeletal changes and determines if the patient is experiencing unusual fatigue, generalized weakness, pain, morning stiffness, fever, or anorexia.

Physical examination for a patient with rheumatoid arthritis includes assessment of the cardiovascular, pulmonary, and renal systems as well as the musculoskeletal system. See Chart 50-2 for an outline of the important areas for consideration during the physical assessment.

The nurse focuses the assessment on identifying patient problems and factors that will influence the choice of interventions. When assessing the joints, the nurse inspects, palpates, and inquires about tenderness, swelling, and redness in affected joints. Joint mobility and range of motion are assessed, as well as muscle strength. Any noticeable impairments require further assessment of functional difficulties. The patient is asked to perform specific movements for determination of compensated losses in function.

The nurse also assesses medication compliance and self-management. The information obtained can give insight into the patient's understanding of the medication regimen and may reveal misuse of medications, noncompliance, or use of unproven remedies. Information should also be gathered regarding the patient's understanding, motivation, knowledge, coping abilities, past experiences, preconceptions, and unknown fears. The effects of the disease on the patient's self-concept and coping abilities are also assessed.

▷ Nursing Diagnoses

Based on all the assessment data, major nursing diagnoses for the patient may include the following:

- Pain related to inflammation, tissue damage, and joint immobility
- Fatigue related to increased disease activity
- Impaired physical mobility related to restricted joint movement
- Self-care deficits (feeding, bathing, dressing, toileting) related to fatigue and joint stiffness
- Sleep pattern disturbance related to pain and fatigue
- Knowledge deficit regarding self-management decisions
- Disturbance in self-concept related to the physical and psychologic dependency of chronic illness and loss of independence

▷ Planning and Implementation

▷ *Goals:*   The major goals of the patient may include relief of pain and discomfort, decreased fatigue, increased mobility, achievement of an optimal, individual level of independence in activities of daily living, improved quality of sleep, increased knowledge regarding self-management, and attainment of a positive self-concept.

⊳ Nursing Interventions

Nursing Care Plan 50-1 outlines the basic plan of care for the patient with rheumatoid arthritis.

⊳ *Relief of Pain and Discomfort.*   The pain of rheumatoid arthritis can be unremitting and unpredictable and therefore can have a significant impact on the patient's self-management abilities. The pain can be both acute and chronic in nature. While the frequent assessment of acute pain is appropriate, the assessment of chronic pain should be based on comparison to a baseline measurement of the usual intensity over a period of time. The patient may have difficulty distinguishing pain from stiffness, so careful questioning is necessary. Information about previous pain experiences can be used when planning nursing interventions. The patient's prior experience with pain and effective strategies already used to control pain can be built upon to achieve even more effective pain management.

Pain management techniques are used and taught for immediate or short-term management (*i.e.*, use of heat and cold, joint protection, rest, and analgesics). Education regarding long-term management of pain is also essential. This includes use of anti-inflammatory medications and establishing an exercise regimen for maintaining joint mobility. Relaxation techniques are taught for both immediate and long-term pain management. The nurse provides comfort measures while the patient is receiving care. The patient then incorporates these and other techniques into his self-management program. The family or significant other's involvement may have an effect on the achievement of pain management. The patient learns to communicate his pain needs. Realistic expectations must be set so that the patient and significant others realize that pain can be controlled but that the amount of control may vary depending on disease activity.

⊳ *Reduced Fatigue.*   The fatigue of rheumatoid arthritis can have a major effect on the patient's feeling of lack of control over his disease. The impact of overwhelming fatigue, unrelated to physical activity, is poorly understood and appreciated by caregivers and significant others.

Patient education is focused on the physical and emotional factors related to the disease that cause or contribute to fatigue. The nurse helps the patient learn how to use the amount of fatigue he is experiencing to monitor the disease activity and balance physical activities accordingly.

⊳ *Increased Mobility and Independence in Self-Care Activities.*   Rheumatoid arthritis can result in joint deformity; however, it is essential that the nurse not equate deformity with disability. For example, swollen hands may be more limiting than hands with deformities. Limitations can be determined only by assessing joint motion and functional capabilities.

By relieving persistent pain or morning stiffness, the nurse may significantly increase the patient's mobility and ability to perform self-care activities. For the patient with rheumatoid arthritis, the use of assistive devices such as an elevated toilet seat may be resisted because of accentuation of fears of dependency on others.

⊳ *Improved Sleep.*   Various problems can contribute to sleep disturbance. Fatigue, physical inactivity, and depression may interfere with the patient's ability to fall asleep or remain asleep. Pain and stiffness can interrupt the sleep pattern; medications can disrupt the quality of sleep. Interventions should focus on the cause of the sleep problem. Hypnotics are rarely used; however, adjusting the anti-inflammatory and analgesic administration times may be effective in producing a higher level of comfort prior to sleep and throughout the night. Education regarding relaxation techniques may also be helpful in relieving muscle tension, fatigue, and stress. Adequate sleep is essential in managing pain, fatigue, and the overall disease process.

⊳ *Increased Knowledge Regarding Disease Management.*   Patients are usually unfamiliar with their disease process and treatment regimen and need to verbalize their concerns and ask questions. Pain, fatigue, and depression can interfere with the patient's ability to learn and should be addressed before initiating an educational program. Various educational techniques may be used, depending on the patient's previous knowledge base, interest level, degree of comfort, and social or cultural influences. The nurse instructs the patient on basic disease management, medications, and necessary adaptations in life-style. If hospitalized, the patient is encouraged to practice new self-management skills with support from caregivers and significant others. The nurse reinforces disease management skills during each patient contact.

⊳ *Improved Self-Concept.*   All aspects of the patient's life, including work role, social life, sexual function, and financial status, may be altered because of the unpredictability and uncertainty of the course of the disease. Body-image changes may cause social isolation and depression. The nurse and the family should try to understand the patient's emotional reactions to the disease. Communication should be encouraged so that the patient and family verbalize feelings, perceptions, and fears related to the disease. The nurse helps the patient and family identify elements of control over disease symptoms and treatment. Commitment to the management program is the key to positive outcomes.

⊳ *Home Health Care.*   After the patient's discharge from the hospital, a community nurse can visit the home to make sure the patient is able to function as independently as possible with his mobility problems and to safely manage treatments and pharmacotherapy. The patient/family should be alerted to local support services such as local chapters of the Arthritis Foundation.

⊳ Evaluation

Expected Outcomes

1. Experiences improvement in comfort level
   a. Identifies factors that exacerbate or influence pain response
   b. Identifies and uses pain management measures
2. Incorporates into daily activities those measures necessary to modify fatigue
   a. Verbalizes the relationship of fatigue to disease activity
   b. Identifies and uses measures to prevent or modify fatigue
3. Attains/maintains optimal functional mobility and achieves self-care independently or with the use of resources
   a. Describes and uses measures to prevent loss of motion
   b. Uses appropriate techniques and/or assistive equipment to aid mobility
   c. Identifies and uses alternative methods for meeting self-care needs
4. Experiences an improvement in the quality of sleep
   a. Identifies and uses techniques to induce or maintain sleep

b. Identifies pharmacologic measures to aid sleep and uses them appropriately

5. Attains the necessary information about the disease process and therapy to make self-care management decisions

6. Achieves a reconciliation between self-concept and changes imposed by the disease
   a. Verbalizes acceptance of self-worth
   b. Sets and achieves realistic and meaningful goals
   c. Uses appropriate communication skills and self-management techniques

In summary, rheumatoid arthritis is a progressive, inflammatory disorder that affects connective tissue. Joint pain, swelling, warmth, erythema, and impaired joint function are common symptoms. Deformities of the hands are also common. Rheumatoid arthritis may occur at any age and increases in frequency with advancing age. The goals of nursing and medical management are to relieve pain, reduce inflammation, and maintain or improve mobility and function.

Systemic Lupus Erythematosus

Systemic lupus erythematosus (SLE) is a chronic, inflammatory autoimmune collagen vascular disease that involves multiple body systems. A form of lupus erythematosus affecting only the skin (discoid) may exist alone or be the precursor of the more involved systemic disease. About 500,000 people in the United States are afflicted with this disease. Women tend to be affected 9:1 over men; the average age at onset is 30 years, with predominance in nonwhites.

The etiology of lupus is unknown. Although a genetic link has not been found, there is a familial association that suggests that a genetic predisposition may be related to environmental factors or susceptibility to certain viruses. Certain drugs, such as hydralazine hydrochloride (Apresoline), procainamide hydrochloride (Pronestyl), and some anticonvulsants, have been thought to trigger the onset of symptoms or aggravate an existing disease. A hormonal abnormality is a possible risk factor because an increased incidence has been noted during the childbearing years. Ultraviolet radiation is also considered a possible risk factor.

Pathophysiology

SLE seems to result from a disturbance of immune regulation causing an exaggerated production of autoantibodies. This immunoregulatory disturbance is brought about by some combination of genetic, hormonal (as evidenced by the usual onset during the childbearing years), and environmental factors (sunlight, thermal burns). Certain drugs, such as hydralazine, procainamide, isoniazid, chlorpromazine, and some anticonvulsants, have been implicated, as have foods such as alfalfa sprouts.

The pathophysiology is believed to be related to one or several immune system defects that produce inflammation and local tissue damage subsequent to the clustering of antigens and antibodies (immune complexes). A reduction in the number of T lymphocytes causes the body to synthesize immunoglobulins and autoantibodies, which then form immune complexes that cause tissue damage. Inflammation stimulates antigens, which in turn stimulate additional antibodies, and the cycle continues.

Clinical Manifestations

The onset of SLE may be insidious or acute. For this reason, the patient with SLE may be undiagnosed for many years. The characteristic clinical course is one of exacerbations and remissions.

Clinical features of SLE demonstrate the involvement of multiple body systems. The musculoskeletal system is involved with arthralgias and arthritis (synovitis), which are common presenting features of SLE. Joint swelling, tenderness, and pain on movement are common and are accompanied by morning stiffness.

Several different types of skin manifestations may occur in patients with SLE, such as subacute cutaneous lupus erythematosus (SCLE) and discoid lupus erythematosus (DLE). The most familiar (but occurring in less than 50% of patients) skin manifestation is an acute cutaneous lesion consisting of a butterfly rash across the bridge of the nose and cheeks. There may be only skin involvement in some cases of lupus erythematosus. In some patients, the initial skin involvement may be the precursor to more systemic involvement. The lesions often worsen during exacerbations ("flares") of the systemic disease and may be provoked by sunlight or artificial ultraviolet light.

Oral ulcers may involve the buccal mucosa or the hard palate. They occur in crops, are often associated with exacerbations, and may accompany skin lesions.

Pericarditis is the most common clinical cardiac manifestation and occurs in up to 30% of patients. It may be asymptomatic and is often accompanied by pleural effusions. Myocarditis is also present in up to 25% of patients.

Lung and pleural involvement occurs in 40% to 50% of patients; this is most often manifested by pleuritis or pleural effusions.

The vascular system is involved, with inflammation of the terminal arterioles producing papular, erythematous, and purpuric lesions. These lesions may develop on the fingertips, elbows, toes, and extensor surfaces of the forearms or lateral sides of the hand and may progress to necrosis.

Lymphadenopathy occurs in 50% of all SLE patients at some time during the course of their clinical illness. Renal involvement occurs in about 50% of patients with SLE, and the glomeruli of the kidneys are usually affected. The extent of kidney damage indicates whether or not renal involvement will be reversible.

The varied and frequent neuropsychiatric presentations of SLE are now being more widely recognized. These are generally demonstrated by subtle changes in behavior patterns. The spectrum of central nervous system involvement is wide and encompasses the entire range of neurologic disease. Depression and psychosis are frequent.

Diagnostic Evaluation

Diagnosis is based on a complete history and analysis of blood work. The physician observes for the classic symptoms of fever, fatigue, and weight loss and assesses for arthritis, pleurisy, and pericarditis. There is no single definitive laboratory test in the diagnosis of SLE. Serum testing reveals moderate to severe anemia, thrombocytopenia, and leukocytosis or leukopenia. Other diagnostic immunologic tests support but often do not confirm the diagnosis. (See Table 50-1 for more detailed information.)

Management

Treatment is focused on the principle of management of acute and chronic disease. Acute disease requires interventions directed at the control of increased disease activity or exacerbations that may involve any organ system. Disease activity is a composite of clinical and laboratory features that reflect the presence of active inflammation secondary to SLE. The clinical features include nephritis, cardiopulmonary disease, skin rashes, and more indirect evidence of systemic inflammation (fever, fatigue, and weight loss). The laboratory evidence of a deranged immune system is reflected in the antinuclear antibody, anti-DNA antibodies, and hypocomplementemia. Management of the more chronic condition involves periodic monitoring and recognition of meaningful clinical changes requiring adjustments in therapy. Patient education is extremely important.

The goals of treatment include preventing progressive loss of organ function, reducing the likelihood of acute disease, minimizing disabilities from the disease process, and preventing complications from therapy. Management of systemic lupus erythematosus involves regular monitoring to assess disease activity and effectiveness of therapy.

Drug therapy for SLE is based on the concept that local tissue inflammation is mediated by exaggerated or heightened immune responses, which can vary widely in intensity and require different therapies at different times. The NSAIDs are used for the treatment of minor clinical manifestations of SLE and are often used along with corticosteroids in an effort to minimize corticosteroid requirements.

Corticosteroids are the single most important class of drugs available for SLE treatment. They are used topically for cutaneous manifestations, in low oral doses for minor disease activity, and in high doses for major disease activity. Bolus intravenous administration is regarded as an alternative to traditional high-dose oral use. Antimalarial drugs are effective in the management of cutaneous, musculoskeletal, and mild systemic features of SLE. Immunosuppressive agents (alkylating agents and purine analogs) are used because of their effect on immune function. These drugs are regarded as experimental and are generally reserved for patients with serious forms of SLE for whom conservative therapies have failed.

▶ ## Nursing Process
The Patient With Systemic Lupus Erythematosus

◊ ### Assessment

The nurse performs a thorough, systematic physical assessment of the patient as detailed in Chart 50-2. Careful attention is paid to the integumentary, gastrointestinal, cardiovascular, respiratory, renal, musculoskeletal, and neurologic systems.

The skin is inspected for erythematous rashes. The presence of a classic malar butterfly-shaped rash across the bridge of the nose and cheeks is occasionally noted (Fig. 50-3). Cutaneous erythematous plaques with an adherent scale may be observed on the scalp, face, or neck. Areas of hyperpigmentation or depigmentation may be noted depending on the phase and type of the disease. The patient should be questioned regarding observation of skin changes (because these may be

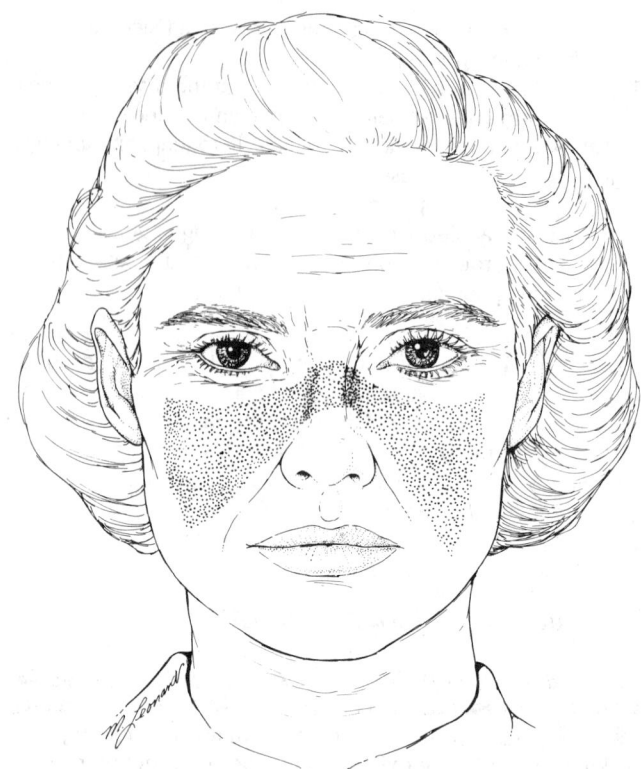

Figure 50-3. Butterfly rash of systemic lupus erythematosus.

transitory) and specifically about sensitivity to sunlight or artificial ultraviolet light. The scalp should be inspected for alopecia. The mouth and throat should be examined for ulcerations reflecting gastrointestinal involvement.

Cardiovascular assessment includes checking for the presence of pericardial friction rub, which may be associated with myocarditis and may accompany pleural effusions. The pleural effusions and infiltrations reflect respiratory insufficiency and are demonstrated by abnormal lung sounds. Papular, erythematous, and purpuric lesions that may become necrotic can indicate vascular involvement. These lesions may develop on the fingertips, elbows, toes, and extensor surfaces of the forearms or lateral sides of the hand.

Joint swelling, tenderness, warmth, pain on movement, and stiffness are signs of musculoskeletal involvement. The joint involvement is often symmetric and similar to that found in rheumatoid arthritis.

Edema and hematuria are indicative of involvement of the renal system. In addition to the physical assessment, confirming evidence of systemic involvement can be found in laboratory findings.

Interactions with the patient and family may provide further evidence of systemic involvement. The neurologic assessment is directed at identifying and describing any central nervous system involvement that might be present. Family members can be questioned regarding behavioral changes, neuroses, or psychosis. Signs of depression should be noted, as well as reports of seizures, chorea, or other CNS manifestations.

Knowledge of the disease process and self-management is assessed. The patient's perception of and coping with fatigue, body image, and other problems caused by the disease are also assessed.

Nursing Diagnoses

Based on the assessment data, nursing diagnoses for the patient with SLE may include the following:

- Impaired skin integrity related to photosensitivity or vasculitis, or as a manifestation of the disease process
- Fatigue related to increased disease activity, pain, inadequate sleep/rest, and emotional stress
- Body image disturbance related to body-image changes
- Lack of knowledge in self-management decisions related to lack of previous experience or anxiety

Other nursing diagnoses may be appropriate, particularly for the patient who is acutely ill with major organ system involvement.

Planning and Implementation

Goals: The major goals of the patient may include maintenance of skin integrity, decreased fatigue, attainment of a positive self-concept, and an adequate information base upon which appropriate self-care management decisions can be based.

Nursing Interventions

Nursing Care Plan 50-1 outlines the basic plan of care for the patient with SLE.

Maintenance of Skin Integrity. The skin rash of SLE is often scaly and itchy. Cool baths may decrease discomfort and scaliness. The skin should be kept clean, and powders and other irritants are avoided.

The nurse reinforces the physician's explanations concerning the need to avoid sunlight and ultraviolet lights (such as fluorescent lighting), which may trigger disease exacerbations or skin eruptions. Long-sleeved clothing, wide-brim hats, and long pants are worn to protect the skin. A sunscreen with the maximum solar protection factor rating should be applied to uncovered skin areas, and sunglasses should be worn to decrease photosensitivity.

The nurse checks for the presence or spread of superficial vasculitic lesions. Appropriate skin hygiene measures, such as keeping the skin clean and dry but moisturized, help to prevent skin breakdown. Because of the high-dose corticosteroids that may be used, there is an increased risk of infection.

Meticulous mouth care is given to prevent and manage oral lesions. Care is taken when brushing the teeth to prevent gum irritation with subsequent bleeding. Antifungal mouth rinses or tablets may be prescribed for secondary oral yeast infections.

Decreased Fatigue. The patient with SLE often experiences severe fatigue. The nurse helps the patient learn to monitor the amount of fatigue as an indicator of disease activity. Nursing Care Plan 50-1 outlines the basic plan of care for the patient with a problem of fatigue.

Promoting a Positive Self-Concept. The presence of the erythematous rash on the face and other parts of the body can cause a major change in body image. Even when the disease is in remission, the rash may not disappear. The patient may be advised to consult a cosmetologist who specializes in skin disorders to help select appropriate cosmetics to cover the rash and make it less noticeable. A wig may be desirable if there is significant hair loss.

The unpredictability of the disease also contributes to a poor self-concept. The nurse and the family should try to understand this reaction and approach the patient in a realistic but optimistic manner. Nursing Care Plan 50-1 provides additional guidance for the nursing care of an SLE patient with self-concept and body-image problems.

Increased Knowledge. The chronic and unpredictable course of SLE requires that the patient have sufficient understanding of his condition to monitor changes and make self-management decisions. This will challenge the nurse because of the importance of the patient having the right information at the appropriate time. The timing of information about SLE is important. The newly diagnosed patient does not usually need detailed information about the management of clinical manifestations from organ involvement. Such information will have little meaning because such involvement may never occur. However, questions that are asked about such systemic features should be answered openly. The extent of systemic involvement cannot be predicted. Nursing Care Plan 50-1 provides a basic nursing care plan that can be individualized to the patient with systemic lupus erythematosus.

The patient with SLE may have little interference with his life-style but has the potential of severe, life-threatening involvement. The expected outcomes will reflect the variability of the disease and will be specific to the nursing diagnoses as described in Nursing Care Plan 50-1.

Evaluation

Expected Outcomes

1. Maintains skin integrity
   a. Applies topical creams or ointments as prescribed
   b. Identifies measures to protect from external factors that contribute to skin alterations
2. Decreases fatigue
   a. Takes measures to control activity of disease
   b. Identifies factors contributing to increased fatigue
   c. Applies principles of energy conservation
3. Attains positive self-concept
   a. Expresses feelings freely to family and members of the health team
   b. Accepts physical appearance
   c. Socializes appropriately with family members, peers, and friends
4. Participates in self-management strategies for control of disease activity appropriately
   a. Complies with prescribed medication program
   b. Practices good health measures, including adequate rest and nutrition
   c. Identifies factors that increase activity of disease

In summary, SLE is a rheumatic disorder characterized by involvement of multiple body systems. Collagen tissue throughout the body is affected, producing a wide spectrum of manifestations ranging from skin and mucous membrane lesions to cardiac involvement and renal failure. The patient is often young and in the childbearing years at the time of onset of the disorder. The treatment may include corticosteroids and immunosuppressive medications. Dialysis may be necessary if renal failure develops. The disease or its treatment may produce dramatic changes in appearance and considerable stress to the patient. These changes and the unpredictable course of SLE necessitate expert assessment skills, expert nursing care, and sensitivity to the psychologic reactions of the patient.

Systemic Sclerosis

Systemic sclerosis is a progressive disease of connective tissue characterized by inflammatory, fibrotic, and degenerative changes associated with immunologic abnormalities.

The skin, blood vessels, synovium, and skeletal muscle are usually affected, as well as internal organs, including the esophagus, intestines, lungs, heart, and kidneys. Systemic sclerosis is divided into three subgroups: *diffuse scleroderma,* which is manifested by widespread skin and visceral involvement; *CREST syndrome,* characterized by limited skin involvement (see further description under Clinical Manifestations); and *overlap syndrome,* the occurrence of systemic sclerosis along with additional connective tissue disorders, such as rheumatoid arthritis or myositis.

It is important to distinguish systemic sclerosis from localized scleroderma because organ involvement is different with each. Localized scleroderma is characterized by hardening of the skin and is an inflammatory condition without the serologic and visceral manifestations. Systemic sclerosis is thought to be an autoimmune disease. The exact cause is unknown and is believed to be related to many factors.

Pathophysiology

Like lupus erythematosus, systemic sclerosis has a variable course with remissions and exacerbations; its prognosis, however, is not as optimistic as that of lupus.

The disease often begins with skin involvement. Mononuclear cells cluster on the skin and stimulate lymphokines to stimulate procollagen. Insoluble collagen is formed and accumulates excessively in the tissues. Initially, the inflammatory response causes edema formation, with a resulting taut, smooth, and shiny skin appearance. The skin then undergoes fibrotic changes leading to loss of elasticity and movement. Eventually the tissue degenerates and becomes nonfunctional. This chain of events, from inflammation to degeneration, also occurs in blood vessels, major organs, and body systems, often resulting in death.

Clinical Manifestations

The disease starts insidiously with Raynaud's phenomenon and swelling in the hands. The skin and the subcutaneous tissues become increasingly hard and rigid and cannot be pinched up from the underlying structures. Wrinkles and lines are obliterated. The skin is dry because sweat secretion over the involved region is suppressed. The extremities become stiff and lose mobility.

The condition spreads slowly. For years, these changes may remain localized in the hands and the feet. The face appears masklike, immobile, and expressionless, and the mouth becomes rigid.

The changes within the body, while not visible directly, are vastly more important than the visible changes. The left ventricle of the heart is involved, manifesting congestive heart failure; the esophagus is hardened, interfering with swallowing; the lungs are scarred, impeding respiration; digestive disturbances occur because of hardening of the intestine; and progressive renal failure may occur.

The patient may manifest a variety of symptoms referred to as the *CREST syndrome.* The letters CREST stand for *c*alcinosis (calcium deposits in the tissues), *R*aynaud's phenomenon, *e*sophageal hardening and dysfunctioning, *s*clerodactyly (scleroderma of the digits), and *t*elangiectasis (capillary dilatation that forms a vascular lesion).

Diagnostic Evaluation

There is no one conclusive test to diagnose progressive systemic sclerosis. A complete history and physical examination are performed to note any fibrotic changes in the skin, lungs, heart, or esophagus. The skin is biopsied to identify cellular changes specific to scleroderma. Lung tests will show ventilation–perfusion abnormalities. An echocardiogram will identify pericardial effusion often present with heart involvement. Studies of the esophagus demonstrate decreased motility in 75% of patients with systemic sclerosis.

The presence of antinuclear antibodies (ANAs) indicates a connective tissue disorder and aids in distinguishing which subgroup of systemic sclerosis is present. A positive ANA with a nuclear pattern is common with diffuse scleroderma. The anticentromere pattern is associated with the CREST syndrome, and the overlap conditions are commonly distinguished with a speckled-pattern ANA.

Management

Treatment is dependent on the clinical manifestations associated with the subgroup classification. All patients require personal counseling in which realistic individual goals are determined. There is currently no pharmacologic drug regimen that has proved effective in controlling systemic sclerosis. Various drugs can be used to treat the symptoms. D-Penicillamine has been the most promising in decreasing skin thickening, reducing the rate of new visceral organ involvement, and prolonging life. Captopril and other potent antihypertensives are effective in controlling hypertensive crises. Anti-inflammatory drugs can be used to control arthralgia, stiffness, and general musculoskeletal discomfort. Vasodilators have not proved to be effective for vascular abnormalities. Supportive measures include decreasing pain and limiting disability. A moderate exercise program is encouraged to prevent joint contractures. Patients are advised to avoid extremes in temperature and to use lotions to minimize excessive skin dryness.

▶ Nursing Process
The Patient With Systemic Sclerosis

▷ Assessment

The nursing assessment begins with observation of the sclerotic changes in the skin. The most predominant changes of the hands and face are easily recognizable. Contractures in the fingers may have already occurred, and color changes or lesions may be present in the fingertips. Assessment of systemic involvement requires a systems review with special attention to gastrointestinal, pulmonary, renal, and cardiac symptoms.

Limitations in mobility and self-care activities should be assessed, as well as the impact the disease has had (or will have) on body image. Refer to Chart 50-2 for a guide to assessment of multisystem problems.

Nursing Diagnoses

Based on all the assessment data, major nursing diagnoses for the patient with systemic sclerosis may include the following:

- Impaired skin integrity related to disruption of the skin surface and tissue layers
- Self-care deficits related to musculoskeletal impairment
- Altered nutrition related to inability to prepare and/or eat food, esophageal dysmotility, intestinal malabsorption, and abnormal excretory function
- Self-concept disturbance related to body-image changes

Planning and Implementation

Goals: The major goals of the patient may include attainment or maintenance of optimum skin integrity, attainment of optimal independence in activities of daily living, attainment or maintenance of optimal nutrition, and attainment of a positive self-concept.

Nursing Interventions

Nursing Care Plan 50-1 outlines the basic plan of care for the patient with systemic sclerosis.

Maintenance of Skin Integrity. Nursing care for a patient with systemic sclerosis includes maintaining skin integrity and suppleness. Although skin elasticity cannot be regained, adequate moisturizing can prevent cracking and scaling of skin. It is essential to maintain body warmth if Raynaud's disease is present, especially in the hands and feet. The increasing tightness of the skin may restrict joint movement, which can be painful. To maintain as much motion as possible and minimize pain, range-of-motion exercises should be done.

Independence in Self-Care. Decreased joint mobility also interferes with self-care activities. Assistive devices can be helpful in maintaining independence.

Improved Nutritional Status. For patients with gastrointestinal involvement, the nurse administers prescribed medications (antacids, antibiotics) and helps patients cope with the discomforts of constipation or diarrhea. The patient with dysphagia needs frequent, small feedings and encouragement to chew food thoroughly. If there is pulmonary involvement, the patient needs encouragement to take periodic deep breaths and to rest at prescribed intervals throughout the day. Vital signs, breath sounds, and fluid intake are evaluated. Oxygen therapy, at a low flow-rate, is administered along with bronchodilators, steroids, and antimicrobials as prescribed. For those who show evidence of renal failure, the nurse assesses daily weight and keeps hourly urinary output records, monitors the urine specific gravity and serum sodium levels, and inspects the skin for signs of excess fluid volume.

Improved Self-Esteem. The patient is also encouraged to verbalize feelings about self-esteem and the impact of living with a chronic illness.

Evaluation

Expected Outcomes

1. Maintains skin integrity and suppleness
   a. Applies moisturizers as indicated
   b. Demonstrates maximal range of motion of joints
   c. Demonstrates range-of-motion exercises
   d. Uses safe measures to maintain warmth of hands and feet
2. Participates in self-care management
   a. Complies with prescribed treatment and exercise program
   b. Demonstrates good health care practices
   c. Uses assistive devices safely
3. Maintains optimal nutritional status
   a. Maintains body weight
   b. Consumes nutritious diet
   c. Drinks adequate fluids
4. Demonstrates positive self-concept
   a. Verbalizes feelings to family and members of the health care team
   b. Participates in activities and events in environment
   c. Acknowledges changes in appearance and functional status

Polymyositis/Dermatomyositis

Polymyositis (PM) and dermatomyositis (DM) are among the least common of the autoimmune connective tissue diseases. These illnesses are noted by proximal limb and neck weakness sometimes associated with muscle pain. Although these conditions are considered primarily diseases of skeletal muscle, the heart, gastrointestinal tract, and lungs are frequently involved. High-dose corticosteroid therapy is usually used initially in treatment; doses are modified in response to muscle enzymes. As the muscle enzymes fall, the dosage is lowered. Reduction of the enzymes may take several months, followed by long-term maintenance treatment. Graded exercise after inflammation has subsided helps restore strength and range of motion.

Nursing interventions are focused on specific patient problems, with particular attention paid to compliance and careful self-management of the corticosteroid therapy. Emotional support as well as high-quality physical care is very important.

Polymyalgia Rheumatica

Polymyalgia rheumatica (PMR), a relatively common clinical syndrome, is characterized by severe aching and stiffness in the neck, shoulder girdle, or pelvic girdle muscle areas. The stiffness is more noticeable in the morning or after periods of inactivity. Because PMR generally occurs in people 50 years of age and older, it may be confused with or disregarded as merely an inevitable occurrence of aging.

Diagnosis is difficult because of the lack of specificity of tests. Diagnosis is more likely to be made by eliminating other potential diagnoses and is highly dependent upon the skills and experience of the diagnostician. The dramatic and immediate response to treatment with corticosteroids is considered by some to be diagnostic. In addition to oral corticosteroids, NSAIDs are used in the treatment of mild disease.

A commonly associated process is giant cell arteritis (GSA). The association between PMR and giant cell arteritis is not completely understood. Headaches, changes in vision, and jaw claudication are warning signs of GSA and should be heeded immediately because of the potential for a sudden and permanent loss of vision. Immediate treatment with adequate doses of corticosteroids can prevent blindness and other vascular complications. Both of these conditions generally run a self-limited course lasting several months to several years.

Nursing care of these patients is aimed at early detection and prevention of complications. Careful patient education of these often elderly patients is essential because of the importance of medication compliance. However, the initial response to corticosteroids produces a masking of the symptoms and may lead to the patient discontinuing treatment prematurely.

Spondyloarthropathies

The spondyloarthropathies are inflammatory disorders of the skeleton that include ankylosing spondylitis, reactive arthritis, and psoriatic arthritis. Spondyloarthritis is also associated with inflammatory bowel diseases such as Crohn's disease and ulcerative colitis.

Ankylosing Spondylitis. Ankylosing spondylitis is a systemic inflammatory disease of unknown etiology that affects the cartilaginous joints of the spine and surrounding tissues. Occasionally the large synovial joints such as hips, knees, or shoulders may be involved. Its most characteristic clinical feature is back pain. Diagnosis is based on a comprehensive history, physical examination, and radiologic studies. Sacroiliac joint changes are considered an early sign. An elevated sedimentation rate and absence of rheumatoid factor are relevant laboratory clues. It is usually diagnosed around the second or third decade of life and is believed to be associated with inherited histocompatibility antigen HLA-B27.

The effects of the disease range from an asymptomatic sacroiliitis to a progressive disease affecting many body systems. As the disease progresses, the entire spine may become ankylosed, causing respiratory compromise and complications. Other manifestations such as iritis (inflammation of the iris) and cardiac conduction disturbances may also occur. The majority of the patient population with significant systemic involvement is usually male. The disease is not usually as severe in women.

Medical management focuses on treating the pain and maintaining mobility by suppressing inflammation. The drugs of choice are salicylates and NSAIDs. Surgical management may include total hip replacement.

In addition to addressing the nursing diagnoses related to pain and self-management, the nurse observes for activities that affect good body positioning and posture. Patient education directed at maintaining range of motion with a regular exercise and muscle-strengthening program is especially important.

Reactive Arthritis. Previously known as Reiter's syndrome, reactive arthritis affects young adult males and is characterized primarily by urethritis, arthritis, and conjunctivitis. Dermatitis and ulcerations of the mouth and penis may also be present. Low back pain is common.

A second type of reactive arthritis is that related to an enteropathic infection following *Shigella-*, *Salmonella-*, *Campylobacter-*, or *Yersinia*-associated diarrhea. The same triad of urethritis, conjunctivitis, and arthritis is usually seen. Symptoms occur after a sexually transmitted or enteric infection. A genetic association with the antigen HLA-B27 has been theorized over the last decade.

The treatment of reactive arthritis is largely symptomatic with salicylates and nonsteroidal anti-inflammatory agents as the basic drugs for the arthritis symptoms. The nurse may need to facilitate discussion with the patient or between the patient and physician about sexual partners and the use of condoms in the sexually acquired form.

Recently, reactive arthritis has been observed in persons with acquired immunodeficiency syndrome (AIDS).

Psoriatic Arthritis. Psoriatic arthritis occurs in less than 5% to 10% of patients who have cutaneous psoriasis and is characterized by synovitis, polyarthritis, and spondylitis. Psoriatic arthritis tends to be slowly progressive. When fingers and toes are involved there is a diffuse swelling, making them look like sausages. Affected joints are often surprisingly functional and only minimally symptomatic.

Salicylates, NSAIDs, and corticosteroids often produce marked improvement in back, skin, and joint symptoms. Methotrexate is also used to control psoriasis as well as joint inflammation.

Degenerative Joint Disease (Osteoarthritis)

Osteoarthritis (OA), also known as degenerative joint disease (DJD), is the most common type of rheumatic disease in the United States.

The prevalence of osteoarthritis increases with age, with the majority of people over the age of 65 being affected. Osteoarthritis is characterized by a progressive loss of the joint cartilage and by reactive changes at the joint margins and on the subchondral bone.

The etiology of osteoarthritis is unknown; however, there are several associated factors. Increasing age directly relates to the degenerative process, which often begins in the third decade of life and peaks between the fifth and sixth decades. By age 70, more than 80% of people have some form of bone degeneration. The disease may be associated with repetitive stress activities, obesity, previous trauma, or strenuous physical labor.

Pathophysiology

Cartilage destruction and new bone formation at the edges of the joints are the most common pathologies seen with osteoarthritis. These pathologies are associated with biomechanical and biochemical changes that occur in response to joint insult. The process initiates the degeneration of the matrix of the cartilage. As a joint undergoes repeated mechanical stress, the elasticity of the joint capsule, articular cartilage, and ligaments is reduced. The articular plate is thinned, and its function as a shock absorber is decreased. There is narrowing of the joint space and loss of stability. When the articular plate disappears, bony spurs form at the edges of the joint surfaces, and the capsule and synovial membranes thicken. The joint cartilage degenerates and atrophies, the bones harden and hypertrophy at their articular surfaces, and the ligaments calcify. As a result, sterile joint effusions and secondary synovitis may be present (Fig. 50-4).

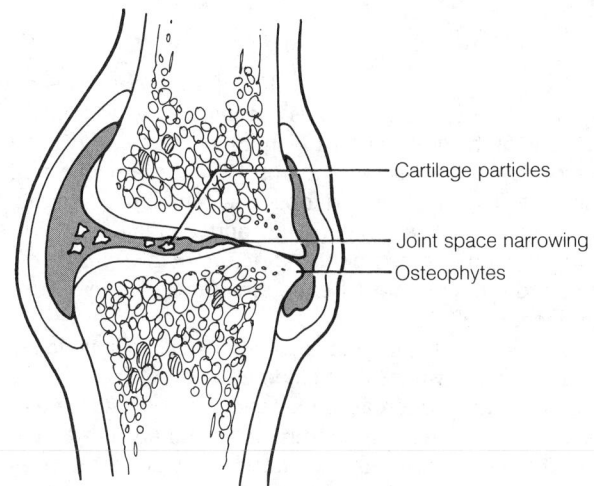

Cartilage particles
Joint space narrowing
Osteophytes

Figure 50–4. Examples of osteoarthritic changes in the joint.

Clinical Manifestations

The primary clinical manifestations are pain, stiffness, and functional impairment. Stiffness, which is most commonly experienced in the morning after awakening, usually lasts less than 30 minutes. Functional impairment is due to pain on movement and limited joint motion, which occurs when structural changes develop in the joints.

Although osteoarthritis occurs most often in weight-bearing joints (hips, knees, cervical and lumbar spine), the distal interphalangeal (DIP) and proximal interphalangeal (PIP) joints are also involved.

Characteristic bony nodes may be present; on inspection and palpation these are usually painless, unless inflammation is present. When present on the distal interphalangeal joints, the nodes are called *Heberden's nodes*. Nodes on the proximal interphalangeal joints are called *Bouchard's nodes* and primarily affect women in their middle years or result from repetitive trauma.

Diagnostic Evaluation

A physical assessment of the musculoskeletal system will show tenderness and enlargement of the joints. Radiographic examination of degenerating joints demonstrates bony hypertrophy, spur formation, cartilage destruction with resulting narrowing of joint spaces, and gross irregularities of the joint structures. Serum laboratory diagnostic studies are not useful in the diagnosis of this disorder.

Management

Medical management focuses on treating the symptoms because there is no treatment available that stops the degenerative joint disease process. Therapeutic modalities consist of pharmacotherapy, supportive measures, and surgical intervention when pain is intractable and function has been lost.

The pharmacologic regimen centers on analgesics and anti-inflammatory agents. Acetaminophen is used for the analgesic effect. When inflammation is present, NSAIDs or aspirin is used. Intra-articular injections of corticosteroids are used cautiously for an immediate, short-term effect when a joint is acutely inflamed.

Conservative measures include the use of heat, weight reduction, joint rest and avoidance of joint overuse, orthotic devices to support inflamed joints (splints, braces), and isometric and postural exercises. Occupational and physical therapy can be helpful in teaching self-management strategies.

▶ Nursing Process
The Patient With Osteoarthritis

▷ Assessment

The health history is structured to obtain information about mobility and the patient's ability to perform activities of daily living. Because osteoarthritis is localized primarily to the weight-bearing joints in the musculoskeletal system, the nurse uses the techniques of inspection, palpation, and joint movement to assess joint function or impairment. The patient's gait and mobility are observed, and muscle spasm and crepitus are noted if present. Joints are palpated for swelling, effusion, enlargement, and the presence of bony nodules. Palpation may elicit a pain response. Pain that tends to worsen with activity and improve with rest is the most common symptom of osteoarthritis and should be assessed thoroughly to determine the effect it has on the patient's attitude and life-style.

Once the joints are inspected and palpated, they are evaluated for range of motion. A decrease in range of motion should prompt further assessment in the area of functional limitations, such as one's ability to perform activities of daily living. Refer to Chart 50-2 for areas of special consideration during the physical assessment.

▷ Nursing Diagnoses

Based on all the assessment data, major nursing diagnoses for the patient with osteoarthritis may include the following:

- Pain related to joint degeneration
- Impaired physical mobility related to limited joint movement
- Self-care deficits related to limited joint movement
- Ineffective coping related to actual or perceived life-style or role changes

▷ Planning and Implementation

▷ *Goals:* The major goals of the patient may include relief of pain and discomfort, increased physical mobility and endurance, and attainment of an optimal level of independence in activities of daily living.

▷ Nursing Interventions

Nursing Care Plan 50-1 outlines the basic plan of care for the patient with osteoarthritis.

▷ *Relief of Pain and Discomfort.* Measures for relief of pain and stiffness include resting the affected joint as well as protecting the area by use of a cane or splint. The application of heat and gentle range of motion movements can reduce the stiffness. A weight-reduction diet may be required to reduce stress on weight-bearing joints.

Patient education includes self-administration of medications and instituting a plan for incorporating principles of pain management.

▷ *Increased Physical Mobility and Endurance.*   Patient education includes the rationale for balancing rest with activity and the importance of exercises to maintain mobility and strength.

▷ *Independence in Self-Care Activities.*   Although gross deformity is not usually present in OA, joint pain decreases joint movement and the ability of patients to care for themselves. Assistive devices such as tonglike reachers and dressing aids such as elastic shoe laces or Velcro fasteners can help the patient with limited joint movement to be more independent.

▷ *Effective Coping.*   The nurse helps the patient identify what impact the disease is having on his life. The patient is taught that degenerative changes are not automatically progressive and that pain and suffering are not expected just because of age. Coping mechanisms are identified, and support of significant others is encouraged.

▷ Evaluation

Expected Outcomes

1. Experiences improvement in comfort level
   a. Identifies factors that exacerbate or influence pain response
   b. Identifies and uses pain management measures
2. Attains/maintains optimal functional mobility and achieves self-care independently or with the use of resources
   a. Describes and uses measures to prevent loss of motion
   b. Uses appropriate techniques and/or assistive equipment to aid mobility
   c. Identifies and uses alternative methods for meeting self-care needs
3. Attains optimal degree of independence in self-care activities
   a. Demonstrates maximum independence in eating, dressing, toileting, and personal care activities
   b. Appropriately uses assistive devices as necessary
4. Attains optimal level of coping
   a. Identifies impact disease is having on life and develops realistic expectations of disease and self
   b. Identifies and uses various coping mechanisms and techniques

In summary, osteoarthritis is a disorder that affects approximately 12% of the U.S. population; its prevalence increases with age. It occurs more frequently in persons who are obese or who have experienced repetitive stress to the joints. Pain, stiffness, and impairment on joint movement are common. Nursing interventions that focus on reducing stress and promoting the patient's self-care often improve function, promote independence, and enhance the patient's self-esteem.

Crystal-Induced Arthropathies

Of the metabolic and endocrine diseases associated with rheumatic states, the most common are the crystal-induced conditions. Such arthritis is caused by the deposition of crystals, such as monosodium urate or calcium pyrophosphate, within joints.

Gout

The best known of the crystal-induced arthropathies is a heterogeneous group of conditions commonly called gout. Manifestations of the gout syndrome include: *acute gouty arthritis* (recurrent attacks of severe articular and periarticular inflammation), *tophi* (crystalline deposits accumulating in articular tissue, osseous tissue, soft tissue, and cartilage), *gouty nephropathy* (renal impairment), and *uric acid urinary calculi*. The disorder occurs most frequently in males in the fourth to sixth decades of life.

The etiology of gout seems to be related to a genetic defect of purine metabolism, with oversecretion of uric acid or a renal defect resulting in decreased excretion of uric acid, or a combination of both. *Hyperuricemia* can be primary, in which case elevated serum urate levels or manifestations of urate deposition appear to be consequences of faulty uric acid metabolism. Primary hyperuricemia may be due to severe dieting or starvation, excessive intake of foods that are high in purines (shellfish, organ meats), or heredity. In secondary hyperuricemia, the gout is a minor clinical feature secondary to any of a number of genetic or acquired processes, including conditions in which there is an increase in cell turnover (leukemia, multiple myeloma, some types of anemias, psoriasis) and an increase in cell breakdown. Altered renal tubular function, either as a major action or as an unintended side effect of certain pharmacologic agents (diuretics such as thiazides and furosemide, low-dose salicylates, and ethanol), can contribute to uric acid underexcretion.

Pathophysiology

Hyperuricemia (serum concentration greater than 7.0 mg/dl) (SI: 0.4 μmol/L) can cause monosodium urate crystal deposition. Attacks of gout seem to be related to sudden increases or decreases of serum uric acid levels. When the urate crystals precipitate within a joint, an inflammatory response occurs and an attack of gout begins.

With repeated attacks, accumulations of sodium urate crystals, called *tophi,* are deposited in peripheral areas of the body, such as the great toe, the hands, and the ear. Renal urate lithiasis (kidney stones) with chronic renal disease secondary to urate deposition may develop.

The finding of urate crystals in the synovial fluid of asymptomatic joints suggests that factors other than the presence of crystals may be related to the inflammatory reaction. Recovered monosodium urate crystals are coated with immunoglobulins that are mainly IgG. IgG enhances crystal phagocytosis, thereby demonstrating immunologic activity.

Clinical Manifestations

Four stages of gout can be identified: asymptomatic hyperuricemia, acute gouty arthritis, intercritical gout, and chronic tophaceous gout.

Hyperuricemia.   Fewer than one in five hyperuricemic individuals will at any point develop clinically apparent urate crystal deposition. The subsequent development of gout is directly related to the duration and magnitude of the hyperuricemia.

Acute Gouty Arthritis.   The acute arthritis of gout is the most common early clinical manifestation. The metatarsophalangeal (MTP) joint of the big toe is the most common (75% of patients) joint affected, but the tarsal area, ankle, or knee may also be targeted.

The acute attack may be triggered by trauma, alcohol ingestion, drugs, surgical stress, or illness. The abrupt onset often occurs at night with the patient awakening with severe pain, redness, swelling, and warmth of the affected joint. Early attacks tend to subside spontaneously over 3 to 10 days even without treatment. The attack is followed by a symptom-free period until the next attack, which may not come for months or years. However, with time, attacks tend to occur more frequently and involve more joints, and also last longer.

Intercritical Gout.   The intercritical stage of gout is that interval between attacks.

Chronic Tophaceous Gout.   Tophi are generally first noted an average of 10 years after the onset of gout. About 50% of inadequately treated patients eventually develop tophaceous deposits. The presence of tophi is generally associated with more frequent and severe inflammatory episodes. Higher serum concentrations of uric acid are also associated with more extensive tophus formation. Tophi most commonly occur in the synovium, olecranon bursa, subchondral bone, infrapatellar and Achilles tendons, subcutaneous tissue on the extensor surface of the forearms, and overlying joints. They have also been found in the aortic walls, heart valves, nasal and ear cartilage, eyelids, cornea, and sclerae. Joint enlargement may cause a loss of motion.

Renal Disease

Parenchymal compromise and renal stones may occur in patients with gout. The risk of urolithiasis is increased in patients with gout. The incidence of renal stones is two times higher for patients with secondary gout than for those with primary gout. Stone formation is related to the increase in serum uric acid, acidity of the urine, and urinary concentration.

Management

Hyperuricemia, tophi, joint destruction, and renal problems are treated after the acute inflammatory process has subsided. Uricosuric agents, probenecid and sulfinpyrazone, correct hyperuricemia and dissolve deposited urate. Allopurinol is also an effective drug, but its use is limited because of the risk of toxicity. When lowering the serum urate level is indicated, the uricosuric agents are the drugs of choice. When the patient has renal insufficiency or stones (or is at increased risk of stones), then allopurinol is the drug of choice.

The nursing care for the patient with gout will reflect the stage of the disease. The nurse is most likely to be directly involved with the patient in an acute gouty attack. Assessment includes a history of the patient's usual alcohol intake, a recent history of dieting, and adherence to any previously prescribed treatment program for the condition. Care must be taken to protect the involved areas from painful trauma, such as bumping the bed or even the added weight of the bed linens. Patient education regarding the condition and self-management of the gout may be required. Lack of compliance with a prophylactic medication program may be a problem at any stage of the disease. During the chronic stage, there may be impairment of skin integrity related to changes in joint structure due to the presence of tophi. Prevention includes meticulous skin hygiene and avoidance of injury to the tophaceous areas.

The expected outcomes of the nursing interventions should include the patient's management of pain in the affected joint, the maintenance of skin integrity, and compliance with the prophylactic medication program.

Calcium Pyrophosphate Dihydrate Crystal Deposition Disease

Calcium pyrophosphate dihydrate (CPPD) *disease,* or pseudogout, is another crystal deposition disease. *Chondrocalcinosis* is the term used to describe the radiologic appearance of calcified joint cartilage. Unlike gout, there is no way to remove CPPD crystals from joints. Acute attacks in large joints can be treated by thorough aspiration and intra-articular corticosteroids. Nonsteroidal anti-inflammatory drugs are often useful.

Nonarticular Rheumatism

Fibromyalgia

Sometimes called fibrositis (a misnomer because inflammation is not present), this is a poorly understood chronic condition characterized by diffuse musculoskeletal aching and pain, fatigue, morning stiffness, and disturbed sleep. Although many patients complain of joint pain and may have some mild joint tenderness, there is no evidence of joint swelling or an inflammatory or degenerative process. Patients do, however, have multiple specific areas of tenderness called "trigger points." Disturbances of non-REM sleep, mechanical stresses on the lumbar and cervical spine, psychologic distress, and disturbance of CNS endorphins and enkephalins are among the hypothesized causes of this disorder. Fibromyalgia is not progressive.

The difficulty in diagnosis and the chronic nature of the pain make the nursing care of these patients especially important. Support includes reassurance that although the pain can be severe at times, fibromyalgia is neither deforming nor crippling, and control of the pain is possible. Tricyclic antidepressants are used at bedtime to increase the amount of non-REM sleep.

The focus is on maintaining activity and helping patients to learn to "work through" (continue activity despite discomfort) the pain. A regular conditioning program, such as walking, keeps muscles toned. Relaxation and stress-management techniques are important treatment modalities.

Soft Tissue Conditions

There are a wide variety of soft tissue conditions, sometimes referred to as rheumatism. These include bursitis and tendonitis, low back pain, psychogenic rheumatism, chronic ligament and muscle strain, and other miscellaneous conditions. Treatment is directed toward local symptoms.

Chapter Summary

In summary, the rheumatic diseases that are systemic in nature are disorders of the autoimmune system. Inflammation is the pathologic process. Those rheumatic diseases that are more localized in nature reflect degeneration of a specific portion of the musculoskeletal system. Other than the crystal arthropathies, such as gout, and infectious arthritis, the etiology is unknown but thought to be some combination of genetic, environmental, and possibly viral factors. The rheumatic diseases include a group of conditions that vary in manifestation and severity. This diversity challenges the nurse in identification of the patient problems, rather than the disease, in the determination of the nursing diagnoses, in the application of appropriate nursing interventions, and in realistic expected outcomes.

Bibliography

Asterisks indicate nursing research articles.

Books

American Nurses Association, Arthritis Health Professions Association. Outcome Standards for Rheumatology Nursing Practice. Kansas City, MO, American Nurses Association, 1983.

Banwell BF and Gall V (eds). Physical Therapy Management of Arthritis. New York, Churchill Livingstone, 1988.

Blau SP (ed). Emergencies in Rheumatoid Arthritis. New York, Futura Publishing Company, 1986.

Ehrlich GE (ed). Rehabilitation Management of Rheumatic Conditions, 2nd ed. Baltimore, Williams & Wilkins, 1986.

* Halfmann T and Pigg JS. Nurses' perceptions of rheumatic disease patient problems as evidenced in nursing diagnoses defining characteristics, etiologies, interventions and expected outcomes. In Kim MJ et al (eds). Classification of Nursing Diagnoses. Proceedings of the Fifth National Conference. St Louis, CV Mosby, 1984.

Kelley WN et al (eds). Textbook of Rheumatology, 3rd ed. Philadelphia, WB Saunders, 1989.

Moskowitz RW and Haug MR. Arthritis and the Elderly. New York, Springer Publishing, 1986.

McCarty D (ed). Arthritis and Allied Conditions, 11th ed. Philadelphia, Lea & Febiger, 1989.

Pigg JS, Driscoll PW, and Caniff R. Rheumatology Nursing: A Problem-Oriented Approach. Albany, Delmar, 1985.

Porth CM. Pathophysiology: Concepts of Altered States, 3rd ed. Philadelphia, J B Lippincott, 1990.

Riggs GK and Gall EP (eds). Rheumatic Diseases: Rehabilitation and Management. Boston, Butterworth, 1984.

Schumacher HR (ed). Primer of Rheumatic Diseases, 9th ed. Atlanta, Arthritis Foundation, 1988.

Utsinger PD, Zvaifler NJ, and Ehrlich GE. Rheumatoid Arthritis: Etiology, Diagnosis, Management. Philadelphia, JB Lippincott, 1985.

Voith AM, Frank AM, and Pigg JS. Validation of fatigue as a nursing diagnosis. In Kim MJ et al (eds). Classification of Nursing Diagnoses. Proceedings of the Seventh National Conference. St Louis, CV Mosby, 1987.

Journals

General

* Bradbury VL and Catanzaro ML. The quality of life in a male population suffering from arthritis. Rehabil Nurs 1989 Jul/Aug; 14(4):187–190.

Bradley LA. Psychological approaches to the management of arthritis pain. Soc Sci Med 1984; 19(12):1353–1360.

Brown GM. The nursing care of rheumatology patients. Nurs RSA 1989 Feb; 4(2):56.

* Burckhardt CS. The impact of arthritis on quality of life. Nurs Res 1985 Jan/Feb; 34(1):11–16.

* Burckhardt CS, Clark SR, and Nelson DL. Assessing physical fitness of women with rheumatic disease. Arthritis Care Res 1988 Mar; 1(1): 38–44.

Carsons S. Newer laboratory parameters for the diagnosis of rheumatic disease. Am J Med 1988 Oct 14; 85(Suppl 4A):34–38.

Cassady JR et al. Rheumatology training enhances students' long-term care skills. Nurs Health Care 1987 Jan; 8(1):39–41.

Chamberlain A. Arthritis: Social problems and practical solutions. Nurs Times 1989 Feb 1–7; 85(5):36–39.

* Collier IC. Assessing functional status of the elderly. Arthritis Care Res 1988 Mar; 1(1):45–52.

* Cornwall CJ and Schmitt MH. Perceived health status, self-esteem and body image in women with rheumatoid arthritis or systemic lupus erythematosus. Res Nurs Health 1990 Apr; 13(2):99–107.

* Goeppinger J et al. A reexamination of the effectiveness of self-care education for people with arthritis. Arthritis Rheum 1989 Jun; 32(6): 706–716.

Goeppinger J et al. A nursing perspective on the assessment of function in persons with arthritis. Res Nurs Health 1988 Oct; 11(5):321–331.

Gran JT. An epidemiological survey of the signs and symptoms of ankylosing spondylitis. Clin Rheumatol 1985 Jun; 4:161–169.

Lawrence RC et al. Estimates of the prevalence of selected arthritis and musculoskeletal diseases in the United States. J Rheumatol 1989 Apr; 16(4):427–441.

* Lorig K et al. Comparison of lay-taught and professional-taught arthritis self-management courses. J Rheumatol 1986 Apr; 13(4):763–767.

* Oermann MG et al. Effectiveness of self-instruction for arthritis patient education. Patient Educ Coun 1986 Sep; 8(3):245–254.

Orr PM. An educational program for total hip and knee replacement patients as part of a total arthritis center program. Ortho Nurs 1990 Sep/Oct; 9(15):61–69, 86.

Pigg JS and Schroeder PM. Frequently occurring problems of patients with rheumatic disease: The ANA outcome standards for rheumatology nursing practice. Nurs Clin North Am 1984 Dec; 19(4):697–708.

Pigg JS. Rheumatology nursing: Evolution of the role and functions of a subspecialty. Arthritis Care Res 1990 Sep; 3(3):109–115.

Soric R, Tepperman PS, and Devlin HTM. Arthritis rehabilitation: A multifaceted process. Postgrad Med 1986 Dec; 80(8):175–182.

Stevens MB. Connective tissue disease in the elderly. Clin Rheum Dis 1986 Apr; 12(1):11–32.

Sudbury F. Rheumatology nursing assessment. Can Orthop Nurs Assoc J 1987 Sep; 9(3):4–8.

Vaidyanathan S, Velayadhan R, and Chandrasekaran TI. Arthritis education. Nurs J India 1988 Aug; 79(8):207–214.

Osteoarthritis

Doyle DV and Lanham JG. Routine drug treatment of osteoarthritis. Clin Rheum Dis 1984 Aug; 10(2):277–291.

* Laborde JM and Powers MH. Life satisfaction, health control orientation, and illness-related factors in persons with osteoarthritis. Res Nurs Health 1985 June; 8(2):183–190.

Mankin JH and Treadwell BV. Osteoarthritis: A 1987 update. Bull Rheum Dis 1986; 36(5):1–10.

Miller B. Osteoarthritis in the primary health care setting. Orthop Nurs 1987 Sep/Oct; 6(5):42–46.

Olivio JL. Developing an exercise program for the elderly with osteoarthritis. Orthop Nurs 1987 May/Jun; 6(3):23–26.

Rheumatoid Arthritis

Arnett FC. Revised criteria for the classification of rheumatoid arthritis. Orthop Nurs 1990 Mar/Apr; 9(2):58–64.

Badley EM and Papageorgiou AC. Visual analogue scales as a measure of pain in arthritis: A study of overall pain and pain in individual joints at rest and on movement. J Rheumatol 1989 Jan; 16(1):102–105.

Bell MJ, Bombardier C, and Tugwell P. Measurement of functional status, quality of life, and utility in rheumatoid arthritis. Arthritis Rheum 1990 Apr; 33(4):591–601.

* Crosby LJ. EEG sleep variables of rheumatoid arthritis patients. Arthritis Care Res 1988 Dec; 1(4):198–204.

Crosby LJ. Stress factors, emotional stress and rheumatoid arthritis disease activity. J Adv Nurs 1988 Jul; 13(4):452–461.

Fuller E. Aggressive drug therapy for RA. Patient Care 1987 Mar 15; 21(5):22–24, 26, 28+.

Fuller E. Diagnosing RA as soon as possible. Patient Care 1987 Apr 15; 21(7):18–21, 24, 26+.

Guccione AA, Felson DT, and Anderson JJ. Defining arthritis and measuring functional status in elders; methodological issues in the study of disease and physical disability. Am J Public Health 1990 Aug; 80(8):945–949.

Harris ED Jr. Rheumatoid arthritis: Pathophysiology and implications for therapy. N Engl J Med 1990 May 3; 322(18):1277–1289.

Lambert VA. Coping with rheumatoid arthritis. Nurs Clin North Am 1987 Sep; 22(3):551–558.

Lindroth Y et al. A controlled evaluation of arthritis education. Br J Rheumatol 1989 Feb; 28(1):7–12.

Mackenzie AH. Differential diagnosis of rheumatoid arthritis. Am J Med 1988 Oct 14; 85(Suppl 4A):2–11.

Minor MA et al. Efficacy of physical conditioning exercise in patients with rheumatoid arthritis and osteoarthritis. Arthritis Rheum 1989 Nov; 32(11):1396–1405.

Papageorgiou AC and Badley EM. The quality of pain in arthritis: The words patients use to describe overall pain and pain in individual joints at rest and on movement. J Rheumatol 1989 Jan; 16(1):106–112.

Parker JC et al. Pain management in rheumatoid arthritis patients. Arthritis Rheum 1988 May; 31(5):593–601.

Pincus T et al. Self-report questionnaire scores in rheumatoid arthritis compared with traditional physical, radiographic, and laboratory measures. Ann Intern Med 1989 Feb 15; 110(4):259–266.

Salmond SW. Stress and stressors in rheumatoid arthritis. J Adv Med Surg Nurs 1989 Sep; 1(4):35–43.

Touger-Decker R. Nutritional considerations in rheumatoid arthritis. J Am Diet Assoc 1988 Mar; 88(3):327–331.

Willkens RF. Rheumatoid arthritis: Clinical considerations in diagnosis and management. Am J Med 1987 Oct 30; 83(Suppl 4B):31–35.

Systemic Lupus Erythematosus and Systemic Sclerosis

Bauman A et al. The unmet needs of patients with systemic lupus erythematosus: Planning for patient education. Patient Educ Couns 1989 Dec; 14(3):235–242.

Blau SP. Systemic lupus erythematosus. In management, less is often more. Consultant 1986 Oct; 26(10):95–108.

Bresnihan B. Outcome and survival in systemic lupus erythematosus. Ann Rheum Dis 1989 Jun; 48(6):443–445.

Callen JP and Klein J. Subacute cutaneous lupus erythematosus. Arthritis Rheum 1988 Aug; 31:1007–1013.

Engle EW et al. Learned helplessness in systemic lupus erythematosus: Analysis using the rheumatology attitudes index. Arthritis Rheum 1990 Feb; 33(2):281–286.

Gatenby PA. Systemic lupus erythematosus and pregnancy. Aust NZ J Med 1989 Jun; 19(3):261–278.

Hess E. Drug-related lupus. N Engl J Med 1988 Jun 2; 318(22):1460–1462.

Hochberg MC and Sutton JD. Physical disability and psychosocial dysfunction in SLE. J Rheumatol 1988 Jun; 15(6):959–964.

Joyce K et al. Health status and disease activity in systemic lupus erythematosus. Arthritis Care Res 1989 Jun; 2(2):65–69.

Klippel JH. Systemic lupus erythematosus: Treatment-related complications superimposed on chronic disease. JAMA 1990 Apr 4; 263(13):1812–1815.

Spondyloarthritides

Arnett FC. Seronegative spondyloarthritides. Bull Rheum Dis 1987; 37(1):1–12.

Felts W. Ankylosing spondylitis: The challenge of early diagnosis. Postgrad Med 1988 Sep; 72(3):184–195.

Winchester RJ, Benstein DH, and Fischer HD. The co-occurrence of Reiter's syndrome and acquired immunodeficiency. Ann Intern Med 1987 Jan; 106(1):19.

Diagnosis and Pharmacotherapy

Benson MD. Arthritis: Effective use of highly regarded and often disregarded tests. Consultant 1985 Sep 15; 25(12):25–39.

Brassell M. Pharmacologic management of rheumatic diseases. Orthop Nurs 1988 Mar/Apr; 7(2):43–51.

Christman C. Protocol for administration and management of chryotherapy. Nurs Pract 1987 Oct; 12(10):30+.

Clegg DO. Slow-acting anti-rheumatic drug therapy for rheumatoid arthritis. Nurse Pract 1987 Mar; 12(3):44–52.

Ignatavicius DD. Meeting the psychosocial needs of patients with rheumatoid arthritis. Orthop Nurs 1987 May/Jun; 6(3):16–21.

Miscellaneous

Cathey MA et al. Functional ability and work status in patients with fibromyalgia. Arthritis Care Res 1988 Jun; 1(2):85–98.

Smeltzer KJ. Fibromyalgia: The frustration of diagnosis and management. Orthop Nurs 1987 May/Jun; 6(3):28–31.

Information/Resources

Agencies

American Lupus Society
  23751 Madison St., Torrance, CA 90505, (213) 542-8891
Ankylosing Spondylitis Association
  511 N. La Cienge, Suite 216, Los Angeles, CA 90048, (800) 777-8189
The Arthritis Foundation
  1314 Spring St., Atlanta, GA 30309, (404) 872-7100
Lupus Foundation of America, Inc.
  1717 Massachusettes Ave. NW, Suite 203, Washington, DC 20036, (703) 660-6523
Lyme Borreliosis Foundation
  P.O. Box 462, Tolland, CT 06084, (203) 871-2900
National Institute of Arthritis and Musculoskeletal and Skin Diseases
  National Institutes of Health, Information Clearinghouse, P.O. Box AMS, 9000 Rockville Pike, Bethesda, MD 20892
Scleroderma International Foundation
  1725 York Ave. #29F, New York, NY 10128, (212) 427-7040
Sjögren's Syndrome Foundation, Inc.
  382 Main St., Port Washington, NY 11050, (516) 767-2866
United Scleroderma Foundation, Inc.
  P.O. Box 399, Watsonville, CA 95077, (408) 728-2202

Nursing Research Profile for Unit 12

HIV Infections and AIDS

Overview

Nursing research studies that focus on human immunodeficiency virus (HIV) infection and the acquired immunodeficiency syndrome (AIDS) are beginning to appear in the literature. Many of these studies have focused on knowledge, attitudes, and beliefs regarding AIDS and high-risk practices among subgroups of the population. The studies reported here have included nurses, other health care personnel, students with non-nursing majors, and individuals at high risk for HIV infection (*i.e.*, homosexual men and persons with sexually transmitted diseases).

▷ Barrick B. *The willingness of nursing personnel to care for patients with* AIDS: A survey study and recommendations. J Prof Nurs 1988 Sep/Oct; 4(5):366–372.

The purpose of this study was to determine the nature of the relationship between attitudes toward gay males and lesbians and willingness to work with patients with AIDS. The hypothesis tested was as follows: nurses with negative attitudes toward gay males and lesbians are less willing to care for patients with AIDS than are nurses with positive attitudes.

Participants in the study were from a general community hospital in northern California. Survey packets were mailed to registered nurses (RNs), licensed vocational nurses (LVNs), licensed psychiatric technicians, and hospital aides and orderlies. In addition to a cover letter, the survey packets included the following: a one-page "unwillingness to care for AIDS patients" instrument (a 9-point Likert scale response set ranging from "strongly disagree" to "strongly agree"), the short form of Herek's Attitudes Toward Lesbians and Gay Men scale, a blank page for opinion statements on AIDS and homosexuals, and a demographic instrument. The instruments were determined to have construct and criterion validity.

Of the 504 packets that were mailed, 208 (44%) were returned and usable. The responses represented 16% males and 86% females ranging in age from 23 to 62 years, with a mean age of 36 years. Eighty-eight percent of the responses were from RNs, 11% were from LVNs and licensed psychiatric tech-

nicians, and 1% were from aides or orderlies. The average length of experience was 12 years.

Analysis of the returned questionnaires revealed a positive correlation between negative attitudes toward gay males and lesbians and unwillingness to work with patients with AIDS. The hypothesis was supported. Analysis of variance revealed no significant difference between attitudes among the various types of health care workers. At least 9% of the sample said they would refuse assignment to a patient with AIDS. The author cautions that factors in addition to antihomosexual attitudes could have influenced this response.

Nursing Implications. A large number of patients with AIDS have been male homosexuals or bisexuals. Nurse managers and educators must recognize caregivers' attitudes about homosexuality and the potential influence of attitudes on willingness or unwillingness to work with AIDS patients. Strategies must be identified to prevent negative attitudes from interfering with quality of patient care.

▷ Beaman ML and Strader MK. STD *patients' knowledge about* AIDS *and attitudes toward condom use.* J Community Health Nurs 1989; 6(3):155–164.

Most educational programs to increase the use of condoms to prevent the transmission of HIV have relied on the provision of information. There has been limited evaluation of the effectiveness of such programs. The authors of this study suggest that attitudes and other factors, rather than information, should be addressed in programs that attempt to facilitate behavior changes. This study investigated knowledge and beliefs about condom use and HIV transmission of patients with sexually transmitted disease (STD), with use of a social–psychologic theoretic framework.

The Theory of Reasoned Action, an attitude behavior model, was used as a conceptual framework for the study. It describes attitudes as a function of either behavioral or normative beliefs. An individual with a favorable attitude toward a behavior believes that performing a certain behavior will lead to positive outcomes. Unfavorable attitudes exist when the individual believes that performing the behavior will lead to negative outcomes. The beliefs that underlie the attitude toward the behavior are termed behavioral beliefs. Normative beliefs are the individual's beliefs that specific persons or groups think he should or should not perform the behavior. Beliefs are seen as the determinants of attitudes.

A convenience sample of 71 racially mixed patients from two STD clinics was used for the study. Open-ended questions were structured to elicit behavioral and normative beliefs underlying attitudes toward condom use during vaginal and anal intercourse and oral–penile contact. In addition, a knowledge questionnaire containing 28 true–false items was used. All questions were read to the participant by one of the investigators because the subjects had difficulty comprehending the instructions. The potentially sensitive nature of the questions may have influenced subjects' responses to verbally presented questions and is a potential limitation of the study. Demographic data including sexual preferences and practices, reasons for the clinic visit, and history of condom use were collected.

Of the 71 participants, 55% were men and 45% were women. Ages ranged from 12 to 40, with a mean age of 19 years. Most of the participants were black (79%), followed by white (21%). Overall, knowledge of AIDS-related facts was high, with a mean score of 22 on the 28-item questionnaire. White subjects had significantly more education and higher scores than did blacks; no differences were found between men and women. Most respondents (89%) knew that condom use lowered the risk of HIV infection. Although 30% reported using condoms for vaginal encounters, they did so for only 25% of their vaginal intercourse experiences. None of the participants used condoms for oral or rectal penile contact. Knowledge did not correlate with condom use behavior.

Beliefs concerning condom use in order of frequency included the following: prevents STDs, prevents pregnancy, decreases feeling, may slip or break, decreases pleasure, makes me feel safe, prevents AIDS, inconvenient to use, and not romantic. Individuals who influenced participants' decisions to use condoms were mothers (34%), fathers (17%), and sexual partners (22%). Of the participants who listed their sexual partners as having a significant influence on their decision to use condoms, 69% stated that the partner held unfavorable beliefs about condom use.

Nursing Implications.   Factual information did not influence behavioral practices. Unfavorable beliefs such as decreased pleasure or inconvenience supported negative attitudes toward condom use. The role of parents and partners was also influential. Nurses should concentrate on educational interventions that focus on the underlying beliefs and attitudes of specific target populations. Careful evaluation of educational interventions is essential.

▷   *Lawrence SA and Lawrence RM. Knowledge and attitudes about AIDS in nursing and nonnursing groups. J Prof Nurs 1989 Mar/Apr; 5(2):92–101.*
The purpose of this study was to determine the difference between knowledge and attitudes about AIDS in nursing and non-nursing groups and to determine the effect that knowledge acquisition would have on attitudes about AIDS. The study was conducted in two phases. The hypotheses for phase 1 of the study were as follows: (1) There are major differences between knowledge and attitudes about AIDS among registered nurses (RNs), baccalaureate nursing students, liberal arts college students, and non-nurse adults; (2) RNs with master's and doctoral degrees will be more knowledgeable and have more positive attitudes about AIDS than will RNs with entry-level preparation; and (3) Persons who have greater knowledge about AIDS will

have more positive attitudes about AIDS. The hypothesis for phase 2 of the study stated that factual information presented by lecture and small group discussion will be effective in improving knowledge and changing attitudes about AIDS.

Of the 182 participants in the study, 60 were RNs, 50 were baccalaureate nursing students, 42 were non-nursing college students, and 30 were non-nurse, employed adults. The authors did not describe the source of the study participants. The mean age was 30.27 years; 94.5% were female and 5.49% were male.

An AIDS knowledge and attitudes assessment instrument, developed by the authors, was administered to the participants. Instrument questions focused on knowledge of incidence, symptoms, infection control procedures, and behavioral practices toward individuals with AIDS. Attitudes concerning issues such as AIDS testing and human rights were also assessed. Content validity and internal consistency were established. Criterion-related validity and construct validity were not determined.

Analysis of data revealed that RNs had more knowledge and more positive attitudes about AIDS than did baccalaureate nursing students. The nursing students had more knowledge about AIDS than did liberal arts students, but their attitudes about AIDS did not differ significantly. Liberal arts college students had more knowledge and more positive attitudes about AIDS than did the non-nurse employed adults. RNs with master's and doctoral degrees had more knowledge and more positive attitudes than did nurses with entry-level preparation. Analysis of data also supported the hypothesis that people who are knowledgeable about AIDS will have more positive attitudes about AIDS. This was established by correlating total knowledge scores and attitude scores. Subjects who understood disease transmission, the purpose of antibody testing, and the nature of health care costs were less likely to believe in social isolation and mandatory testing for all individuals and were more likely to support federal funding to cover financial burdens.

As part of phase 2 of the study, 50 BSN students, 42 liberal arts college students, and 8 RNs were exposed to lecture content on AIDS and given the opportunity to participate in group discussions concerning issues surrounding AIDS. The knowledge and attitude instrument was administered as a pretest and post-test. Analysis of these data supported the hypothesis that factual information does increase knowledge and improve attitudes about AIDS.

Nursing Implications.   This study emphasizes the relationship between knowledge of AIDS and attitudes about AIDS. Other studies have suggested that improving knowledge alone is not a sufficient means of improving attitudes. Further exploration of mechanisms for improving both knowledge and attitudes is needed for nurses as well as non-nurses.

▷   *Moran TA et al. Informational needs of homosexual men diagnosed with AIDS or AIDS-related complex. Oncol Nurs Forum 1988 May/Jun; 15(3):311–314.*
Education about preventing transmission of HIV is currently the single most effective weapon against AIDS. The purpose of this study was to survey patient perceptions of the adequacy of safe sex information provided by primary caregivers during routine outpatient visits in a university-affiliated AIDS clinic in the San Francisco Bay area. A convenience sample included patients with AIDS and AIDS-related symptoms. The sample consisted of 76 patients who were self-identified homosexual or bisexual men. All participants were independent

in their care, were able to read and write English, and had no diagnosed neurologic impairments. The study was conducted in 1985.

The survey consisted of six open-ended questions taken from a survey instrument developed by another author to assess sexual practices of gay men in the San Francisco area. The six questions were designed to obtain the following information: questions the patients would have liked the health care personnel to answer, ways in which the health care provider helped the patient deal with sexual needs, ways in which the health care personnel could have been more helpful, types of educational material that was most helpful, sources of educational materials, and identification of who was most helpful in assisting the patient to change sexual behaviors. The surveys were self-administered in the clinic and at home 2 weeks later to establish test/retest reliability. Data were coded by three oncology nurses with master's or doctoral preparation. The consensus among the nurses for data analysis was 94.7%.

Approximately 52% of the participants felt the need for additional information about safe sex behaviors. Most of the respondents indicated that the health care personnel were not helpful in dealing with sexual needs. Some did state that the health care personnel validated their sexual identity by helping the patients to feel attractive and encouraging them to express their sexuality in a safe manner. Most of the patients could not identify ways in which the health care personnel could be more helpful, although a minority suggested that educational services need to be improved. Pamphlets and brochures published by local community organizations were cited as being the most helpful sources of safe sex information. Those patients who reported that they had changed their sexual practices were most influenced by sources other than the health care personnel, such as friends, lovers, and the media.

Nursing Implications. The results of this survey indicate that patients do want accurate and detailed information. Nurses involved in patient education must be aware that life-threatening illness may make assimilation of information difficult. Repetition of information through written materials and visual aids may be useful. The authors suggest that some patients may need intensive counseling provided by clinical specialists or sexual counselors. Nurses must also work with community organizations to ensure that pamphlets and brochures contain accurate and current information.

▷ *Van Servellen GM, Lewis CE, and Leake B. Nurses' responses to AIDS crisis: Implications of continuing education programs. J Contin Educ Nurs 1988 Jan/Feb; 19(1):4–8.*

The authors note that with the projected increases in the number of AIDS cases, there will be a significant increase in the responsibility of nurses for providing health care for these individuals. The purpose of this study was to identify the fears and attitudes, knowledge, and experiences of nurses regarding AIDS and to obtain a preliminary overview of projected educational needs. A mailed survey was sent to 3000 randomly selected nurses in the state of California, which has the second highest incidence of AIDS. To be eligible for participation, nurses had to be employed in settings where at least a portion of their work included direct care of patients with AIDS. A total of 1019 responses were analyzed.

The survey measured knowledge through questions about symptoms, epidemiology, risk factors, means of transmission, and CDC precautions. Practice-oriented questions asked if nurses conducted sexual histories or counseled patients about ways to decrease transmission. Attitudes and fears were assessed by asking nurses about their discomfort with the care of high-risk patients, their willingness to accept assignments for patients with AIDS, their perceptions of other nurses' discomfort, the right to refuse assignments, and their perceived personal risk for contracting AIDS. Questions were both structured and open-ended. Information concerning the nurses' backgrounds and AIDS education was also assessed. Most of the respondents were white women with an average of 10 to 15 years of nursing experience. Educational preparation was fairly evenly divided among diploma, associate degree, and baccalaureate degree preparation.

The results of the survey indicated that, in general, the nurses lacked accurate information concerning the signs and symptoms of AIDS. Most (68.7%) did know about high-risk behaviors but were unsure about low-risk behaviors. Approximately 81% answered questions concerning appropriate isolation correctly, although at least 10% chose an overcautious approach to isolation precautions. Most of the nurses (91.3%) reported that they did not obtain sexual histories from their patients and did not counsel patients about ways in which to decrease transmission of HIV.

About one fourth of the nurses believed that they were at moderate to high risk for contracting AIDS through occupational exposure. Almost half felt that other nurses were uncomfortable in discussing sexual information with male homosexuals, and 38.4% indicated discomfort in dealing with these patients. About 23% indicated that they would refuse assignments involving patients with AIDS, and 50% thought that nurses should be given this option.

Nursing Implications. The authors concluded that continuing education programs need to focus on the basic facts about AIDS. Without accurate epidemiologic and scientific information, nurses cannot provide appropriate care. The authors also emphasized a need for education concerning counseling practices. Finally, the authors noted that programs were needed to address patients' fears and attitudes concerning sexuality. A lengthy discussion about the role of attitudes and personal values as they relate to education and practice was presented. Future research might address the most beneficial ways in which to achieve these educational objectives.

Rheumatic Disorders

Nursing research related to rheumatic disorders has focused on assessment of the impact of arthritis and other rheumatic disorders on quality of life, physical fitness, functional ability, self-esteem, and sleep. Fewer nursing research studies have focused on assessing the impact of nursing interventions on changes in these variables.

▷ *Bradbury VL and Catanzaro ML. The quality of life in a male population suffering from arthritis. Rehabil Nurs 1989 Jul/Aug; 14(4):187–190.*

The purpose of this study was to describe the relationship of selected physical, psychologic, and social variables on the perception of the quality of life in a group of 38 males suffering from arthritis. The variables of feelings about the illness, perceived support, internal locus of control, severity of functional impairment, life satisfaction, domain satisfaction, and overall quality of life were surveyed with a convenience sample. The subjects had the greatest difficulty with activities that had an impact on joints and required muscular strength. Self-care activities had little impact on the participants' lives.

Nursing Implications. Awareness of the importance of perceptions and feelings of men with arthritis can lead the nurse to careful assessment and exploration with the male patient of topics that might not otherwise be discussed. The finding that a negative attitude toward illness is negatively related to the perception of a good quality of life is important in directing the nursing interventions toward identification of factors that bring about feelings of disappointment, frustration, or discouragement. By explaining the disease process and treatment plan, the nurse may be able to help the patient achieve greater feelings of control over his health.

▷ *Burckhardt CS, Clark SR, and Nelson DL. Assessing physical fitness of women with rheumatic disease. Arthritis Care Res 1988 Mar; 1(1):38–44.*

People with arthritis are increasingly concerned about their physical conditioning, because fitness is seen by society as an important component of health. To knowledgeably direct exercise programs, nurses and other health care professionals need reliable and valid clinically oriented physical fitness assessment tests. Seventy women (ages 20 to 59) with either rheumatoid arthritis (RA), systemic lupus erythematosus (SLE), or fibrositis were tested for flexibility of the lower back, muscle strength of the arms and legs, and cardiovascular endurance. Overall, most of the affected population had low to fair cardiovascular endurance and flexibility when compared to a control group of 40 women and known norms. This study demonstrated that women with rheumatoid arthritis, systemic lupus erythematosus, or fibrositis can safely complete a series of simple, clinically oriented physical fitness tests that are sensitive enough to distinguish several levels of physical fitness.

Nursing Implications. This study demonstrated that the tests used were safe for subjects. This is of interest to the nurse because of the previous concern that increased physical activity might also increase disease activity or be harmful to involved joints for patients with systemic rheumatic diseases such as RA and SLE. The preliminary evidence of the feasibility and safety of several brief, clinically oriented tests of physical fitness for young to middle-aged women with rheumatic diseases can help the nurse in counseling patients who may be concerned about maintaining physical fitness. Physical conditioning for patients with rheumatic diseases may become part of the treatment plan.

▷ *Cathey MA, Wolfe F, and Kleinheksel SM. Functional ability and work status in patients with fibromyalgia. Arthritis Care Res 1988 Jun; 1(2):85–98.*

The functional ability of 176 patients with fibromyalgia was assessed in this study. The performance of patients with fibromyalgia on five standardized work tasks was compared with the performance by patients with RA (N=26) and healthy community controls (N=11). The fibromyalgia patients performed 58.6% and the RA patients 62.1% of the work done by the normal control group. Work status was also examined in 176 fibromyalgia patients. Sixty percent were employed; 9.6% considered themselves disabled (but only 6.2% received dis-

ability payments, none of which was for the specific diagnosis of fibromyalgia). Thirty percent of patients had changed jobs because of their fibromyalgia. Findings indicated that functional ability in fibromyalgia is impaired. Other important correlates of work ability were psychologic status and pain. Pain, psychologic status, and disability status appear to affect work performance in fibromyalgia patients and RA patients, and to approximately the same extent.

Nursing Implications. This study demonstrates that less obvious, less visible conditions, such as fibromyalgia, may affect level of pain, psychologic status, and level of disability as much as do conditions that are visible and demonstrable (*i.e.*, RA). Assessment of the effect of the disorder on the individual patient is more useful and more accurate than general assumptions about the effects of the disorder on the patient's life-style and functional status. Assuming that the degree of disruption of the patient's well-being is correlated with the degree of visible disability may result in an underestimation of the effect of the disorder on the patient.

▷ *Cornwall CJ and Schmitt MH. Perceived health status, self-esteem and body image in women with rheumatoid arthritis or systemic lupus erythematosus. Res Nurs Health 1990 Apr; 13(2):99–107.*

A sample of 26 women with RA, 23 women with SLE, and 28 healthy women was studied to examine the relationship of illness to perceived health status, self-esteem, and body image. Perceived health status differences were found between the women with RA and SLE as compared with the healthy subjects. However, self-esteem differences were not demonstrated. The body image scores of the women who were healthy or who had RA were similar, while the SLE subjects had lower scores. This suggests that persons with some illnesses may maintain a more positive body image. Persons with RA who experience mobility problems and crippling have ambulatory aids and assistive devices to help them maintain independent functioning. These devices and aids may help them to maintain a positive body image. For the person with SLE who may experience more generalized, life-threatening problems, such as kidney dysfunction, there are less amenable compensatory mechanisms. Perceived health status was directly related to self-esteem, but not to body image. As perceived health declined, self-esteem also declined. There was a weak, positive relationship between perceived health status and age and time since diagnosis. In addition, a survey of problems, needs, and fears related to RA and SLE was conducted. The biggest problem cited by the RA subjects was restriction in mobility. SLE subjects identified pain and fatigue followed by avoidance of the sun as their biggest problems. Both groups identified progression of their disease as the most frequent fear. Death was mentioned as a fear by approximately 20% of the SLE subjects but was not mentioned by any of the RA subjects. The investigators noted that the cross-sectional design of this study was a limiting factor in studying the adaptational processes because the course of both RA and SLE produces an uncertain variation in physical status.

Nursing Implications. With knowledge of the findings of this study, the nurse would identify nursing interventions that maintain and augment patients' self-esteem and body image. Other nursing interventions aimed at assisting patients deal with their major problems, fears, and needs associated with their particular chronic rheumatic disease might also be indicated.

▷ *Crosby LJ. EEG sleep variables of rheumatoid arthritis patients. Arthritis Care Res 1988 Dec; 1(4):198–204.*

Poor sleep quality and quantity are frequent complaints of individuals with RA. This research determined electroencephalographic (EEG) sleep variables of RA patients at different stages of RA disease activity. The EEG sleep variables of 15 RA patients were compared to those of an age- and gender-matched control group. The nine female and three male patients were monitored for one night in a sleep laboratory. The RA of five of the patients was in exacerbation, and the RA of 10 of the patients was not in exacerbation. RA patients with exacerbations had statistically significant lower sleep efficiency scores and spent more time awake at night compared with the control group. Both RA patient groups demonstrated fragmented sleep patterns due to frequent awakenings and frequent sleep stage changes. This study concludes that rheumatoid arthritis may further compound a set of existing problems, all of which may manifest as disturbed sleep.

Nursing Implications.   Sleep disturbances have long been overlooked as a significant problem of patients. The findings of this study emphasize the importance and need for assessment of health status and appropriate nursing interventions directed at promotion of sleep for the patient with RA.

▷ *Goeppinger J et al. A nursing perspective on the assessment of function in persons with arthritis. Res Nurs Health 1988 Oct; 11(5):321–331.*

The psychometric properties of two self-administered measures of function were examined: the Disability Score of the Health Assessment Questionnaire (HAQ) and the total Health Score of the Arthritis Impact Measurement Scales (AIMS). Respondents (N = 140) had diagnoses of osteoarthritis, rheumatoid arthritis, or diabetes mellitus; resided in rural and urban areas; and were for the most part elderly, female, and white, with educational levels of high school or below. The findings from the content analyses suggest that the HAQ Disability Score may be preferable because it more thoroughly reflects the nursing diagnoses related to function. An exploratory principal components analysis confirmed that the HAQ is relevant to nursing practice. However, the HAQ was also found to be somewhat less arthritis-specific. The authors maintain that the psychometric findings alone do not indicate the selection of one instrument over another, especially for use in nursing practice and research. The HAQ Disability Score reflects nursing diagnoses as defined in the *Pocket Guide to Nursing Diagnoses* (Kim MJ, McFarland GK, and McLane AM [eds]. Pocket Guide to Nursing Diagnoses. St Louis, CV Mosby, 1984). The authors question whether the nursing diagnoses themselves have content validity, because the inability to take one's medicine, to use public transportation, and to handle money could not be classified yet would seem to reflect self-care deficit, impaired physical mobility, and impaired home maintenance management.

Nursing Implications.   Selection of an assessment tool can provide the basis for nursing care. Several measures are now available for use with the patient with arthritis. Two of the most widely used are the HAQ and AIMS. The nurse who needs assistance in identifying nursing diagnoses may be best served by using the HAQ, recognizing that it is less arthritis-specific.

The AIMS may provide better information relating to mobility and self-care within the limitation of not fitting into current nursing diagnostic criteria.

▷ *Goeppinger J et al. A reexamination of the effectiveness of self-care education for persons with arthritis. Arthritis Rheum 1989 Jun; 32(6):706–716.*

The effectiveness of two models of arthritis self-care intervention (the home study model and the small group model) was examined in this study. A pretest/post-test control group design was used in the initial experimental study. Longitudinal studies used comparison group designs. Three hundred seventy-four subjects completed the interventions and 12 months of research follow-up. The intervention models had a statistically significant positive impact on arthritis knowledge, self-care behavior, perceived helplessness, and pain and were not affected by education level, disease diagnosis and duration, informal social support, or treatment. The small group was more effective in bringing about initial improvements in pain and depression. The home study group was more effective in maintaining improvements in perceived helplessness. Changes in perceived helplessness and self-care behavior appear to explain in part the observed improvement in pain.

Nursing Implications.   The findings of this study suggest that the social support provided by the small group model may be important in initiating changes more quickly and may be more effective in sustaining improvements in depression. The home study model may be more likely to produce and sustain long-term changes in some areas. Because maintenance of positive change over the long term is essential for persons with arthritis, the home study model is of particular interest as an alternative method for teaching patients to deal with their arthritis.

▷ *Joyce K et al. Health status and disease activity in systemic lupus erythematosus. Arthritis Care Res 1989 Jun; 2(2): 65–69.*

This study investigated the relationship between certain physical features of SLE and key components of health status. Physical manifestations of disease activity were measured by the Clinical Activity Index scale (CAI), and the health status of 49 patients was measured by the Arthritis Impact Measurement Scales (AIMS). Scores indicated a relationship between health status and clinical disease activity. The total score of the CAI was significantly correlated with the physical activity, pain, and depression subscales of health status. The total score of the AIMS was significantly correlated with mucocutaneous, musculoskeletal, and general features of the physical status. More specifically, mucocutaneous aspects of SLE were significantly correlated with physical activity and pain. General aspects of the disease, including fatigue, were significantly correlated with physical activity. The results of this study indicated that there is a relationship between certain physical features of SLE and key components of health status. The demonstrated relationship can be interpreted in several ways. First, health status is likely to change as SLE disease activity changes; therefore, there may be improvement in health status after treatment for the disease. Second, other factors (such as disease duration and stress, which were not measured in this study) may influence health status and disease activity. Third, the correlations between health status and disease activity also demonstrated that there were some components of health status (*i.e.*, mobility, dexterity, household activities, activities of daily living) that were affected. This may indicate a functional adaptation by patients with SLE.

Nursing Implications. The demonstrated relationships between certain physical features of SLE and key components of health status are of value to the nurse. This includes the recognition of (and sharing with the patient) the fact that as the disease is controlled, health status will improve. Reduction of stress may influence disease activity and health status. Functional problems may result that can be addressed by the nurse and patient. There are implications of this study for nursing practice. For instance, depression was correlated with the total score for CAI, but only with the mucocutaneous features of SLE disease activity. Nursing interventions can be aimed at patients experiencing skin rashes and alopecia by providing information and support. This study illustrates the complexity of the process of clarifying and measuring the relationship between disease activity and health status in SLE.

unit *13*

Integumentary Function

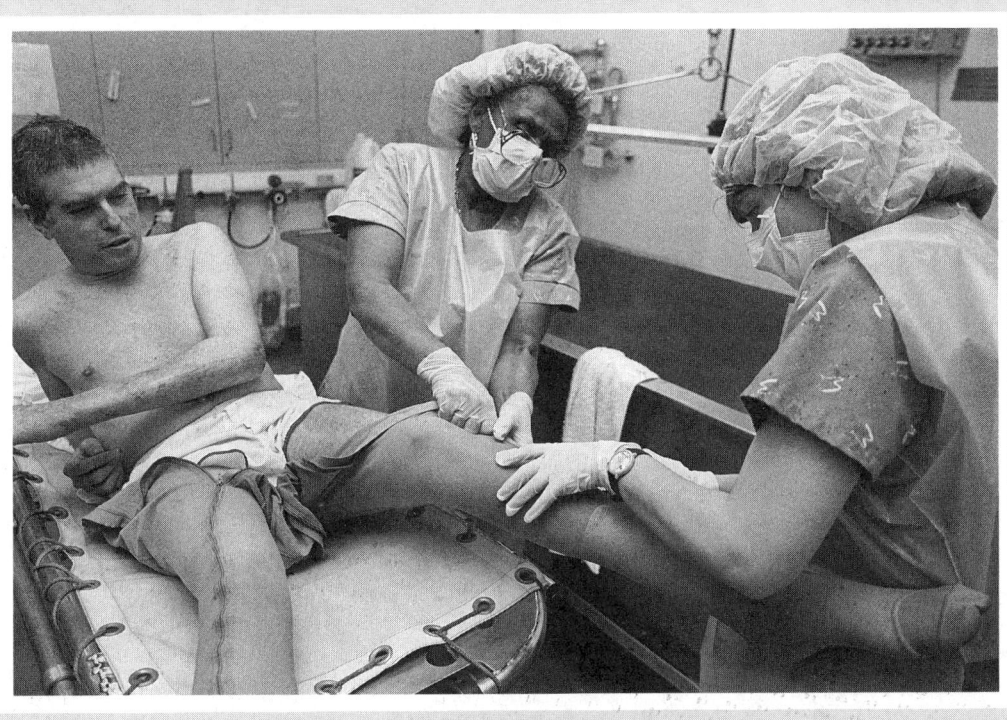

51

Management of Patients With Dermatologic Problems

Chapter Outline

Learning Objectives

On completion of this chapter, the learner will be able to:

1. Describe the functions of the skin
2. Use the nursing process as a framework for care of the patient with an abnormal skin condition
3. Use the nursing process as a framework for care of the patient with acne
4. Describe the health education needs of the patient with infections of the skin and parasitic skin diseases
5. Use the nursing process as a framework for care of patients with noninfectious inflammatory dermatoses
6. Specify the management and nursing care of the patient with cancer of the skin
7. Use the nursing process as a framework for care of the patient with malignant melanoma
8. Use the nursing process as a framework for care of the patient with Kaposi's sarcoma
9. Compare the various types of dermatologic and plastic reconstructive surgeries
10. Compare chemical and surgical planing and the related nursing needs of the patient
11. Use the nursing process as a framework for care of the patient undergoing facial reconstructive surgery

Skin problems are encountered frequently in nursing practice. Skin-related complaints account for 5% to 10% of all ambulatory patient visits in this country. Because the skin mirrors the general condition of the patient, many systemic conditions may be accompanied by dermatologic manifestations.

The psychologic stress of illness or a variety of personal and family problems are frequently exhibited outwardly as dermatologic problems. Any hospitalized patient may suddenly develop itching and a rash secondary to the treatment regimen. In certain systemic conditions, such as hepatitis and cancer, dermatologic manifestations may be the first sign that these disorders are present.

Physiologic Overview

The skin is a structure that is indispensable for human life. It forms a barrier between the internal organs and the external environment and participates in many vital functions of the body. The skin is continuous with the mucous membrane at the external openings of the organs of the digestive, respiratory, and urogenital systems. Because disorders of the skin are readily visible, dermatologic complaints are frequently the primary reason for patient visits.

Anatomy of the Skin

The skin is composed of three layers: the *epidermis*, the *dermis*, and the *subcutaneous tissue* (Fig. 51-1). The *epidermis* is an external layer of squamous epithelial cells that is contiguous with the mucous membranes and the lining of the ear canals. The epidermis consists of live, continuously dividing cells covered on the surface by dead cells that were originally deeper in the dermis but were pushed upward by newly developing cells underneath. This external layer is almost completely replaced every 3 to 4 weeks. The dead cells contain large amounts of *keratin*, an insoluble, fibrous protein that forms the outer barrier of the skin. *Keratin* is the principal ingredient of the hard keratinized structure of the hair and nails.

Melanocytes are special cells of the epidermis primarily involved in producing the pigment *melanin*, which gives color to the skin and hair. The more melanin present, the darker the color. The skin of black persons and the darker areas of the skin on light-skinned persons (*e.g.*, the nipple) contain larger amounts of this pigment. Normal skin color depends on race and varies from light pink to a brown shade. Systemic disease will affect skin color. The skin will appear bluish when there is insufficient oxygenation of the blood, yellow-green in the presence of jaundice, or red or flushed when there is fever. Production of melanin is under the control of a hormone secreted from the hypothalamus of the brain, called melanocyte-stimulating hormone (MSH). It is believed that melanin is capable of absorbing ultraviolet light and thus protecting against the harmful effects of the ultraviolet rays that occur with suntanning.

The epidermis is modified in different areas of the body. Over the palms of the hands and soles of the feet, it is thickened and contains increased amounts of keratin; this is in contrast to the thin epidermis over most of the rest of the body. The thickness of the epidermis can increase with use and can result in callus formation on the hands or feet.

The junction where the epidermis and dermis meet is an area of many undulations and furrows called *rete ridges*. This junction anchors the epidermis with the dermis and permits the free exchange of essential nutrients between the two layers. This interlocking between the dermis and epidermis produces

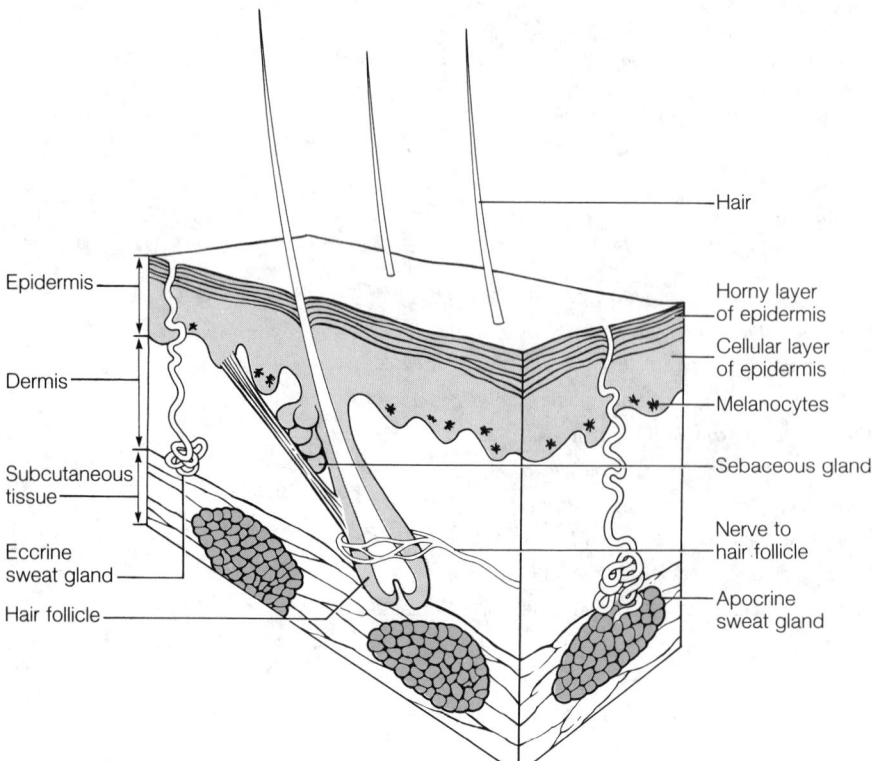

Figure 51–1. Anatomic structures of the skin.

ripples on the surface of the skin. On the fingertips these ripples are called *fingerprints*. They are perhaps a person's most individualistic characteristic and they almost never change.

The *dermis* is a broad layer of connective tissue composed of collagen and elastic fibers, blood and lymph vessels, nerves, sweat and sebaceous glands, and hair roots. The dermis is often referred to as the "true skin."

The *subcutaneous tissue* is primarily adipose tissue. It is here that the skin is anchored to the muscles and bones. Fat is deposited and distributed according to the person's sex and in part accounts for the difference in body shape between men and women. Overeating results in increased deposition of fat beneath the skin. The subcutaneous tissues and amount of fat deposited are important factors in body temperature regulation.

Hair. Hair is present over the entire body except for the palms of the hands and soles of the feet. The hair consists of a root formed in the dermis and a hair shaft that projects beyond the skin. It grows in a cavity called a *hair follicle*. The proliferation of cells in the bulb of the hair causes the hair to form (see Fig. 51-1).

Hair follicles undergo cycles of growth and rest. The rate of growth varies; beard growth is the most rapid, followed by hair on the scalp, axillae, thighs, and eyebrows. The growing phase, *anagen*, may last 3 to 6 years for the scalp before ceasing. During *telogen*, or the resting phase, hair sheds from the body. The hair follicle will recycle into the growing phase spontaneously, or it can be induced by plucking out hairs. New hair growth and resting telogen hair can be found side by side on all parts of the body. About 80% of the hair follicles on a normal scalp are in the growing phase at any one time.

Hairs in different parts of the body serve different functions. The hairs of the eyes (eyebrows and lashes), nose, and ears screen dust, bugs, and airborne debris. Hair of the skin serves as thermal insulation in lower animals. This function is enhanced during cold or fright by the piloerection (hairs "standing on end") caused by contraction of the tiny arrector muscles attached to the hair follicle. The piloerector response that occurs in humans is probably vestigial. The color of hair is due to the presence of varying amounts of melanin within the hair shaft. Gray or white hair is the result of loss of pigment. Growth of hair in certain locations on the body is under the control of sex hormones. The best examples are the hair on the face (beard and mustache) and the hair on the chest and back that are controlled by the presence of the male hormones (androgens).

Hair quantity and distribution can be affected by endocrine conditions. Cushing's syndrome causes *hirsutism* (excessive growth of hair, especially in women); hypothyroidism causes texture changes. Many cancer chemotherapy agents and radiation therapy will cause hair thinning or weakening of the hair shaft, causing partial or complete hair loss (alopecia) from the scalp as well as from other parts of the body.

Nails. On the dorsal surface of the fingers and toes, a hard, transparent plate of keratin, called the *nail*, overlies the skin. The nail grows from its root, which lies under a thin fold of skin called the *cuticle*. The nail helps to protect the fingers and toes, in order to preserve their highly developed sensory function, and aids in the performance of certain fine functions of the fingers, such as picking up small objects.

Nail growth is relatively slow and slows further with aging. Complete renewal of a fingernail takes about 170 days, while a toenail takes about 12 to 18 months.

Glands of the Skin. *Sebaceous glands* are associated with hair follicles. The ducts of the sebaceous glands empty an oily secretion onto the space between the hair follicle and the hair shaft. For each hair there is a sebaceous gland, the secretions of which oil the hair and render the skin soft and pliable (see Fig. 51-1).

Sweat glands are found in the skin over most of the body surface. They are heavily concentrated on the palms of the hands and soles of the feet. Only the glans penis, the margins of the lips, the external ear, and the nail bed are devoid of sweat glands. Sweat glands are subclassified into two categories: *eccrine* and *apocrine*. The eccrine sweat glands are found in all areas of the skin. Their ducts open directly onto the skin surface. The apocrine sweat glands are larger, and, in contrast to that of the eccrine glands, their secretion contains parts of the secretory cells. They are located in the axillae, anal region, scrotum, and labia majora. Their ducts generally open onto hair follicles. The apocrine glands become active at the time of puberty. In the female, they enlarge and recede with each menstrual cycle.

Apocrine glands produce a milky sweat that is broken down by bacteria to produce the characteristic underarm odor. Specialized apocrine glands called *cerumenous glands* are found in the external ear, where they produce wax (*cerumen*).

The thin, watery secretion called *sweat* is produced in the basal coiled portion of the eccrine gland and is released into its narrow duct. Sweat is composed predominantly of water and contains about half of the salt content of the blood plasma. Sweat is released from eccrine glands in response to elevated ambient temperature. The rate of sweat secretion is under the control of the sympathetic nervous system. Excessive sweating of the palms and soles, axillae, forehead, and other areas may occur in response to pain and stress.

Gerontologic Considerations

The major changes in the skin of older people include dryness, wrinkling, uneven pigmentation, and a variety of proliferative lesions. The histologic features of skin associated with aging include a thinning at the junction of the dermis and epidermis, loss of dermal and subcutaneous tissue, reduction of the vascular bed (especially of the capillary loops), marked reduction of the vascular network surrounding hair bulbs and the eccrine, apocrine, and sebaceous glands, and reduced numbers of melanocytes, specialized epidermal cells, and mast cells.

Loss of dermal thickness approaches 20% in elderly persons, accounting for the thin, sometimes nearly transparent quality of their skin. The aging skin, like all other aging organ systems, has a loss of functional capacity. Functions affected include cell replacement, the barrier function, sensory perception, thermoregulation, and sweat and sebum production.

Hair growth diminishes with age, especially over the lower legs and dorsum of the feet. Thinning of hair is common to the scalp, axillae, and pubic areas.

Photoaging or damage from excessive sun exposure adds to the normal aging process of the skin. A lifetime of outdoor work or outdoor activities (construction workers, lifeguards, or sunbathing) without careful use of sunscreens can lead to profound wrinkling, increased loss of elasticity, mottled pigmented areas, cutaneous atrophy, and benign or malignant lesions. Figures 51-2 through 51-4 demonstrate the aging process and effects of excessive and lifetime sun exposure.

In summary, the elderly skin undergoes many physiologic changes associated with the normal aging process. A lifetime of sun exposure, systemic diseases, and medications can also contribute to the range of skin problems and the rapidity with which skin problems appear. The result is an increasing vulnerability to injury and to certain diseases. Skin problems are common among older people.

Functions of the Skin

Protective Function.   The skin protects the body against invasion by bacteria and foreign matter. The thickened skin of the palms and soles protects against the effects of the constant trauma occurring in these areas.

The epidermis is relatively impermeable to most chemical substances. It is this property of skin that allows it to be an effective barrier for protection. Some substances go through the skin more readily than others. A variety of different lipids (fatty substances) may be absorbed through the skin. Fat-soluble vitamins (A and D) and steroid hormones are examples. Substances may enter the skin through the epidermis—the transepidermal route—or via the orifices of the follicles.

Sensory Function.   Stimulation of the receptor endings of nerves in the skin allows us to monitor constantly the conditions of our immediate environment. The primary functions of the receptors in the skin are to sense temperature, pain, light touch, and pressure (or heavy touch). Different nerve endings are responsible for responding to each of the different stimuli. Although the nerve endings are distributed over the entire body, they are more concentrated in some areas than in others. For example, the fingertips are much more densely innervated than the skin of the back.

Water Balance.   Skin forms a barrier that prevents loss of water and electrolytes from the internal environment and also prevents drying out of the subcutaneous tissues. When skin is damaged, as occurs with a severe burn, for example, large quantities of fluids and electrolytes can be lost rapidly, possibly

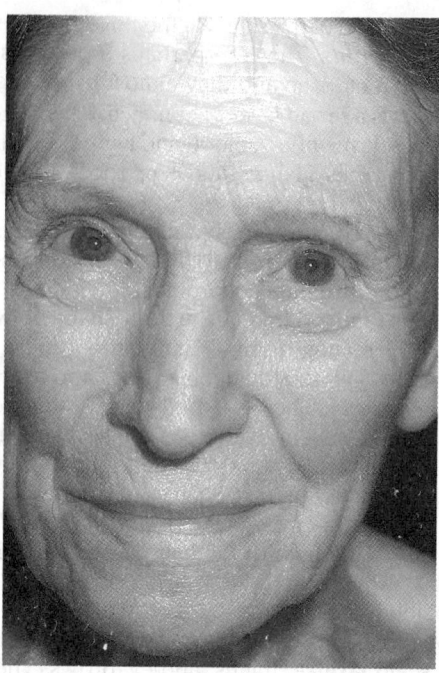

Figure 51–3.   Face of a 90-year-old woman who had avoided sun exposure throughout her life. Note blemish-free skin with marked laxity and deepening of expression lines. (Patterson JA. Aging and Clinical Practice Skin Disorders: Diagnosis and Treatment. New York, Igaku-Shoin Medical Publishers, 1989.)

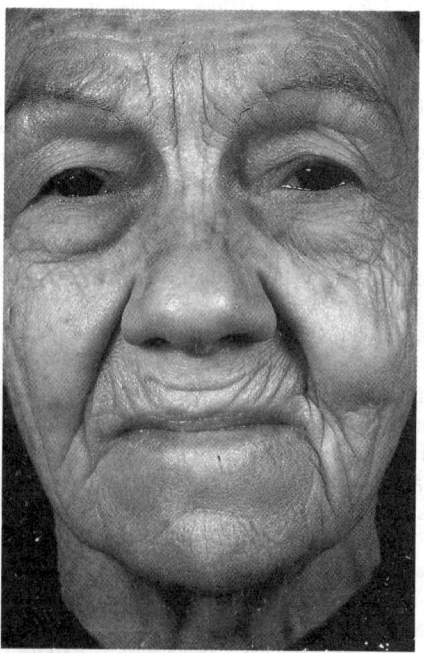

Figure 51–4.   Face of a 70-year-old woman exposed to sun throughout her life. Note mottled hyperpigmentation, fine wrinkles, and deep furrows. (Patterson JA. Aging and Clinical Practice Skin Disorders: Diagnosis and Treatment. New York, Igaku-Shoin Medical Publishers, 1989.)

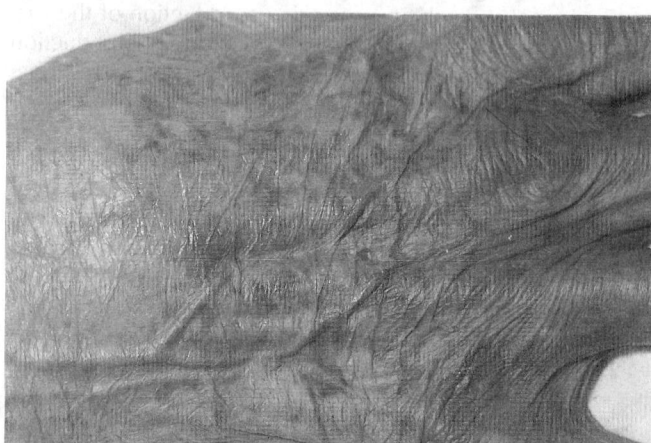

Figure 51–2.   Close-up of dorsum of hand of 90-year-old woman. (Patterson JA. Aging and Clinical Practice Skin Disorders: Diagnosis and Treatment. New York, Igaku–Shoin Medical Publishers, 1989.)

leading to circulatory collapse, shock, and death. On the other hand, the skin is not completely impermeable to water. Small amounts of water continuously evaporate from the skin surface. This evaporation, called *insensible perspiration,* amounts to approximately 500 ml per day for a normal adult. Insensible water loss may vary with the body temperature, and in the presence of fever these losses can increase. During immersion in water, the skin can accumulate water up to approximately three or four times its normal weight. A common example of this is the swelling of the skin after prolonged bathing.

Temperature Regulation.   The body continuously produces heat as a result of the metabolism of foodstuffs to produce energy. This heat is dissipated primarily through the skin. Three major physical processes are involved in loss of heat from the body to the environment. The first process, *radiation,* is the ability of a body to give off its heat to another object of lower temperature situated at a distance. The second process, *conduction,* is the transfer of heat from the body to a cooler object in contact with it. Heat transferred by conduction to the air surrounding the body is removed by the third process, *convection,* which consists of bulk movement of warm air molecules away from the body. Evaporation from the skin aids the process of heat loss by conduction. Heat is conducted through the skin into water molecules on its surface, causing the water to evaporate. The source of the water on the skin surface may be insensible perspiration, sweat, or water from the environment. Normally, all of these mechanisms for heat loss are utilized. When the ambient temperature is very high, however, radiation and convection are not effective, and evaporation from the skin becomes the only means for heat loss.

Under normal conditions, metabolic heat production is exactly balanced by heat loss, and the internal temperature of the body is maintained constant at approximately 37°C (98.6°F). The rate of heat loss depends primarily on the surface temperature of the skin, which is in turn a function of the skin blood flow. Skin is richly supplied with blood vessels that carry heat to the skin from the core of the body. Blood flow through these vessels is controlled primarily by the sympathetic nervous system. Increased blood flow to the skin results in delivery of more heat to the skin and a greater rate of heat loss from the body. On the other hand, decreased skin blood flow decreases the skin temperature and helps conserve heat for the body. When the temperature of the body begins to fall, as occurs on a cold day, the blood vessels of the skin constrict and reduce heat loss from the body.

Sweating is another process by which the body can regulate the rate of heat loss. Sweating is increased when body temperature starts to rise. In extremely hot environments, the rate of sweat production may be as high as 1 L/hr. Under some circumstances, for example with emotional stress, sweating may occur on a reflex basis unrelated to the necessity to lose heat from the body.

Wheal and Flare Reaction.   Stroking the skin with sufficient firmness to cause local injury results in local reddening. This is followed within a few minutes by localized swelling and more diffuse redness around the injury site. The combination of the swelling (called a *wheal*) and the diffuse redness (called a *flare*) constitutes a normal reaction of the skin to injury.

The flare reaction is due to an increased temperature in the area (from the stimulus) and to dilation of the arterioles and venules. It is also dependent upon local nervous mecha-nisms. The wheal is caused by increased capillary permeability induced by trauma. Fluid-containing protein leaks out of the capillaries locally and produces edema at the site of injury.

These responses have also been attributed to the release of some diffusible substance (histamine, bradykinin) by the injured cells.

▶ Nursing Process
The Patient With an Abnormal Skin Condition

When caring for clients with dermatologic disorders, the nurse obtains important information about the client through the health history and direct observations as she cares for the patient. Frequently the client or family is more comfortable talking with the nurse or feels less embarrassed and thus is able to supply pertinent information they may have withheld or forgotten to divulge to the physician or other health care providers. The nurse's skill in physical assessment in conjunction with an understanding of integumentary anatomy and function will ensure that deviations from normal are recognized, reported, and documented.

▷ Assessment

The health history will reveal information regarding the onset, signs and symptoms exhibited, location of pain, and discomfort experienced by the client. Table 51-1 provides a list of questions that will facilitate obtaining appropriate information.

▷ *Physical Assessment*

Assessment of the skin involves the entire skin area, including the mucous membranes, scalp, and nails. The skin is a reflection of a person's overall health, and alterations often correspond to disease in other organ systems.

Inspection and palpation constitute the chief procedures used in examining the skin and require that the room be well lighted and warm. The patient should completely disrobe and should be adequately draped.

The general appearance of the skin is examined by observing color, temperature, moisture, dryness, skin texture (rough or smooth), and the condition of the hair and nails. Skin turgor and elasticity are also determined by palpation.

A thorough examination of the skin includes an assessment of color, lesions, vascularity, temperature, texture, mobility, and the presence of edema. Skin color varies from person to person and ranges from ivory to deep brown. The skin of exposed portions of the body, especially in sunny, warm climates, tends to be more pigmented than that of the rest of the body. The vasodilative effects of fever, sunburn, and inflammation produce a pink or reddish hue to the skin. Pallor is an absence of or decrease in normal skin tones and vascularity and is best observed in the conjunctivae. The bluish hue of cyanosis indicates cellular hypoxia and is easily observed in the nail beds, lips, and mucous membranes. Jaundice, a yellowing of the skin, is directly related to elevations in serum bilirubin and is often noted in the sclerae and mucous membranes.

▷ *Assessing Patients With Dark or Black Skin*
The gradations of color that occur in dark-skinned persons are

TABLE 51-1.   *Patient History: Skin Disorders*

The data base that constitutes the basis of the patient history may be obtained by asking the following questions:

- When did you first notice this skin problem? (onset, duration, intensity)
- Has it occurred previously?
- Are there any other symptoms?
- What site was first affected?
- What did the rash/lesion look like when it first appeared?
- Where and how fast did it spread?
- Are there itching, burning, tingling, or crawling sensations? loss of sensation?
- Is it worse at a particular time? season?
- Do you have any idea how it started?
- Do you have a history of hay fever, asthma, hives, eczema, allergies?
- Does anyone in your family have skin problems or rashes?
- Did the eruptions appear after certain foods were eaten?
- Had there been recent intake of alcohol?
- Was there a relation between a specific event and the outbreak of the rash/lesion?
- What medications are you taking?
- What medication (ointment, cream, salve) have you put on the lesion? (Include over-the-counter medications.)
- What skin products/cosmetics do you use?
- What is your occupation?
- What in your immediate environment (plants, animals, chemicals, infections) might be precipitating this problem? Anything new or any changes in the environment?
- Does anything touching your skin cause a rash?
- Is there anything else you wish to talk about in regard to this problem?

largely determined by genetic transmission; they may be described as light, medium, or dark. In dark-skinned persons, melanin is produced at a faster rate and in larger quantities than in lighter-skinned persons. Healthy, dark skin has a reddish base or undertone. The buccal mucosa, tongue, lips, and nails normally appear pink.

In examining the dark-skinned or black patient, it is important to have good lighting and to look at the skin and the nail beds as well as in the mouth. All suspicious areas are palpated.

The degree of pigmentation of the black patient's skin may affect the appearance of a lesion. Lesions may be black, purple, or gray instead of the tan or red color seen in light-skinned patients.

◊ *Erythema.*   Because there is a tendency for black skin to assume a purplish grayish cast when an inflammatory process is present, it may be difficult to detect *erythema* (redness of skin due to congestion of the capillaries). To determine possible inflammation, the skin is palpated for increased warmth or for signs of smoothness (edema) or hardness. The adjacent lymph nodes are also palpated.

◊ *Rash.*   In instances of itching, the patient should be asked to indicate what areas of the body are involved. The skin is then stretched gently to decrease the reddish tone and make the rash stand out. The differences in skin texture are then palpated by running the tips of the fingers lightly over the skin. Usually, the borders of the rash can be felt. The patient's mouth and ears are included in the examination. (Sometimes rubeola will cause a red cast to appear on the tip of the ears.) Finally, the patient's temperature is checked and the lymph nodes are palpated.

◊ *Cyanosis.*   When a person with black skin goes into shock, the skin usually assumes a grayish cast. To determine signs of cyanosis, the areas around the mouth and lips and over the cheekbones and earlobes should be observed. Other indicative signs to assess for include cold, clammy skin; a rapid, thready pulse; and rapid, shallow respirations. When the conjunctivae of the eyelids are checked for *petechiae* (small red spots due to escape of blood), it is important to realize that deposits of melanin may normally appear in this area and should not be misinterpreted as petechiae.

◊ *Changes in Skin Color.*   Changes in skin color that occur in dark-skinned persons are noticeable and often cause distress to the patient. For example, *hypopigmentation* (loss of or decrease in skin color), which may be due to *vitiligo* (a condition characterized by destruction of melanocytes in limited or extensive skin areas), may cause more concern in the dark-skinned person because it is so readily visible. *Hyperpigmentation* (increase in color) may occur after disease or injury to the skin. A pigmented nasal crease below the eye may be an external sign of allergy. However, pigmented streaks in the nails are considered to be normal.

In general, persons with dark or black skin suffer from the same skin conditions as those with light skin, although they are less apt to have skin cancer and scabies. On the other hand, black and other dark-skinned persons have a greater propensity for keloid or scar formation and for disorders resulting from occlusion or blockage of hair follicles.

◊ *Skin Lesions*

Skin lesions represent the most prominent characteristic of dermatologic conditions. They vary in size, shape, and cause and are classified according to their appearance and origin.

Skin lesions can be described as primary or secondary. *Primary* lesions are the initial lesions and are characteristic of the disease itself. *Secondary* lesions result from external causes, such as scratching, trauma, infections, or changes caused by wound healing (Fig. 51-5). Depending on the stage of development, skin lesions are further divided according to type and appearance (Table 51-2).

A preliminary look at the eruption or lesion should help to identify the type of dermatosis (abnormal skin condition) and indicate whether the lesion is primary or secondary. At the same time, the anatomic distribution of the eruption should be noted because certain diseases tend to affect certain sites of the body and are distributed in characteristic patterns and shapes (Figs. 51-6 and 51-7). To determine the extent of the regional distribution, the left and right sides of the body should be compared while the color and shape of the lesions are noted. Following observation, the lesions are palpated to determine their texture, shape, and border and to see if they are soft or filled with fluid, or hard and fixed to the surrounding tissue.

A metric ruler is used to measure the size of the lesions so that any further extension can be compared with this initial baseline measurement. The dermatosis is then documented on

Primary Lesions

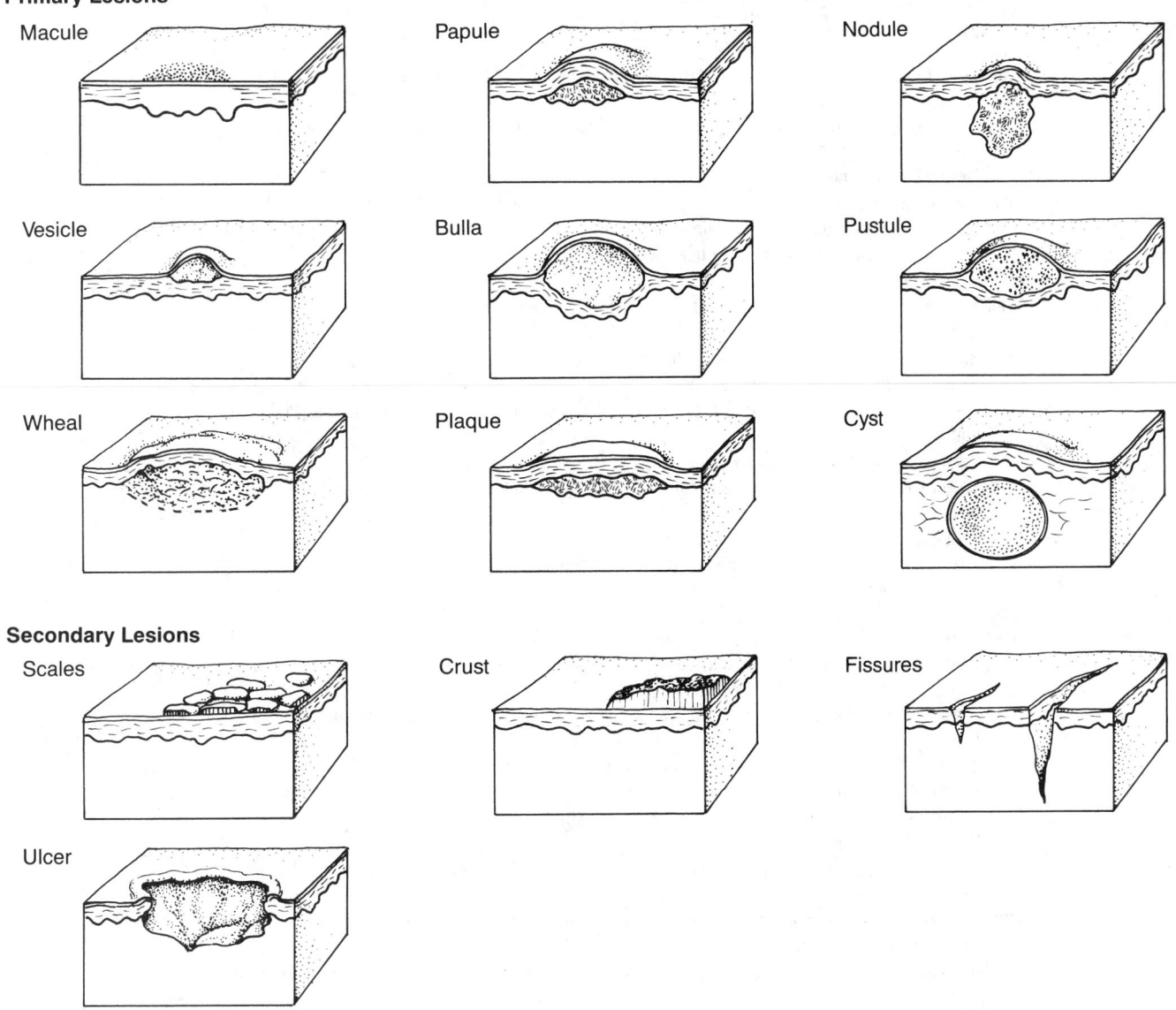

Figure 51–5. Types of skin lesions.

the patient's record; it should be described clearly and in detail, with precise terminology.

After the characteristic distribution of the lesions has been determined, the following information should be obtained and described clearly and in detail:

- What is the color of the lesion?
- Is there redness, heat, pain, or swelling?
- How large an area is involved? Where is it?
- Is the eruption macular, papular, scaling, oozing, discrete, confluent?
- What is the distribution of the lesion—symmetric, linear, circular?

Once the color of the skin has been inspected and lesions have been noted, an assessment of vascular changes in the skin is carried out. A description of vascular changes includes location, distribution, color, size, and the presence of pulsations. Common vascular changes include petechiae, ecchymosis, telangiectasia, angiomas, and venous stars.

Skin moisture, temperature, and texture are assessed primarily by palpation. The elasticity (*turgor*) of the skin, which lessens in normal aging, may be a factor in assessing the hydration status of a patient.

A brief inspection of the nails includes observation of configuration, color, and consistency. Many of the alterations seen in the nail or nailbed reflect local or systemic abnormalities in progress or are the result of past events (Fig. 51-8). Transverse depressions (*Beau's lines*) in the nails may reflect retarded growth of the nail matrix secondary to severe illness or, more commonly, they are the result of local trauma. Ridging, hypertrophy, and other changes may also be visible with local trauma. Inflammation of the skin around the nail (*paronychia*) is usually accompanied by tenderness and erythema. The angle between the normal nail and its base is 160 degrees. When palpated, the base of the nail is usually firm. *Clubbing* is manifested by a straightening of the normal angle (180 degrees or greater) and a softening of the nail base. This softening is perceived as spongelike when palpated.

TABLE 51-2.   *Common Skin Lesions*

PRIMARY LESIONS (INITIAL LESIONS)

Macule—a flat, circumscribed discoloration of the skin on exposed surfaces (hands, forehead)
   Example—freckle or age spot
Papule—a solid, elevated, palpable lesion smaller than 1 cm (0.4 in) in diameter; lesions may vary in color
   Example—wart, nevus
Nodule—a raised, solid lesion larger than 1 cm in diameter and greater than 0.5 cm in height
   Example—tumor (basal cell carcinoma)
Vesicle—a small elevation of the skin filled with clear fluid
   Example—blister
Bulla—a large vesicle or blister larger than 1 cm in diameter
   Example—second-degree burn
Pustule—a lesion that contains pus; may form as a result of purulent changes in a vesicle
   Example—acne, impetigo, or carbuncle
Wheal—transient elevation of the skin caused by edema of the dermis and surrounding capillary dilatation.
   Example—allergic reactions to food, drugs, or insect bites (mosquito bite)
Plaque—a solid, elevated lesion of any color on the skin or mucous membrane larger than 1 cm in its largest diameter
   Example—wart, lesions of psoriasis
Cyst—a tumor that contains semisolid or liquid material
   Example—sebaceous cyst

SECONDARY LESIONS

Secondary lesions are the changes that take place in primary lesions and possibly modify them. Secondary lesions include the following:
Scales—heaped-up, horny layers of dead epidermis; may develop as a result of inflammatory changes
   Example—dandruff or dry skin
Crusts—a covering formed from serum, blood, or pus drying on the skin
   Example—eczema or impetigo
Excoriations—scratch marks or traumatized area of skin
   Example—scratching
Fissures—cracks in the skin, usually from marked drying and long-standing inflammation
   Example—athlete's foot
Ulcers—lesions formed by local destruction of the epidermis and part or all of the underlying dermis
   Example—pressure ulcer.
Lichenification—thickening of the skin accompanied by accentuation of skin markings from chronic scratching
   Example-contact dermatitis, psoriasis
Scar—a fibrotic change in the skin following a destructive process
   Example—healed wound, surgical scar
Atrophy—loss of one or more of the skin components
   Example—loss of hair or sweat glands
Ecchymosis—extravasation of red blood cells into tissue secondary to trauma
   Example—bruise
Petechia—red or purple nonpalpable macule lesions associated with bleeding disorders
   Example—associated with leukemia
Spider angioma—red arteriole lesion with radiating branches from a central core located on the face, neck, trunk, or arms. Associated with liver disease, pregnancy, or vitamin B deficiency

▷ *Psychosocial Assessment*

Because patients with skin conditions (1 in 20 persons) can see and feel their problems, they are more apt to be disturbed by their ailments than are many patients with other conditions. Skin conditions can lead to cosmetic disfigurement, social isolation, and economic hardship. Some conditions are often erroneously associated with immorality and contagion. Some conditions can cost the patient a job, with devastating effects on the person's life. Others may subject the patient to a protracted course of illness, leading to feelings of depression, frustration, self-consciousness, and rejection. Itching and skin irritation may also be a constant annoyance and are common features of most skin diseases. The result of these discomforts may be loss of sleep, anxiety, and depression, all of which reinforce the general distress and fatigue that so frequently

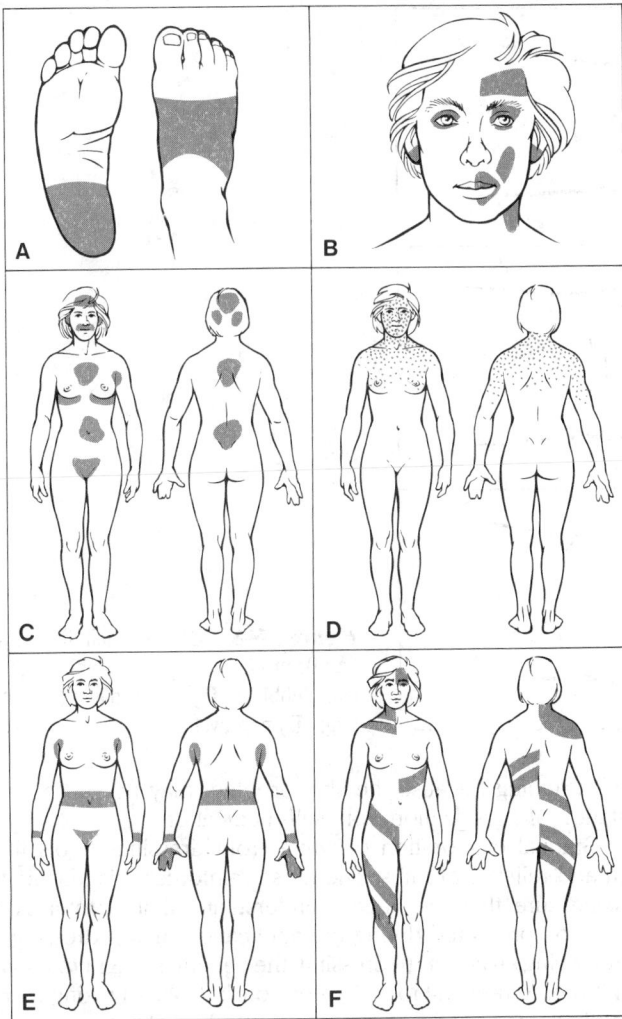

Figure 51–6. Anatomic distribution of common skin disorders: (**A**) contact dermatitis (shoes); (**B**) contact dermatitis (cosmetics, perfumes, earrings); (**C**) seborrheic dermatitis; (**D**) acne; (**E**) scabies; (**F**) herpes zoster.

accompany skin disorders. In addition, skin diseases often present concerns related to self-image and interpersonal relationships.

Patients suffering from such physical and psychologic discomforts require understanding, explanations of the problem and its treatment, nursing support, unending patience, and continual encouragement. It takes time to help patients gain insight into their problems and resolve their difficulties. It becomes imperative, therefore, to overcome any aversion that might be felt when caring for patients with unattractive skin disorders. There must be no sign of hesitancy when approaching these patients. Such behavior would only reinforce the psychologic trauma of the disorder.

▷ Nursing Diagnoses

The nursing diagnoses for patients with dermatoses (abnormal skin conditions) may include the following:

* High risk for impaired skin integrity related to change in barrier function of the skin

* Pain and itching related to skin lesions
* Sleep pattern disturbance related to pruritis
* Body image disturbance related to unsightly appearance of the skin
* Knowledge deficit of the treatment regimen related to length of treatment or the life-style adjustment required

▷ Planning and Implementation

▷ *Goals:* The major goals of the patient may include maintenance of skin integrity, relief of discomfort, achieving restful sleep, development of self-acceptance, and acquiring knowledge of skin care.

▷ Nursing Interventions

▷ *Maintaining Skin Integrity.* Many persons have dry and sensitive skin that is easily irritated. This is especially true of the elderly. Too much or too vigorous washing and scrubbing can increase the problem. Soaps are also irritating. Persons with sensitive skin should be bathed in tepid water with minimal soap, taking care to rinse well and dry by gently patting the skin with a towel. An emollient can be applied to damp skin to trap moisture. Dry air is irritating because it reduces skin moisture, so keeping the environment humidified is also helpful.

Skin problems of the hands are a common complaint. The skin of the back of the hand is thin, accounting for its sensitivity and dryness and its poor resistance to soaps and detergents.

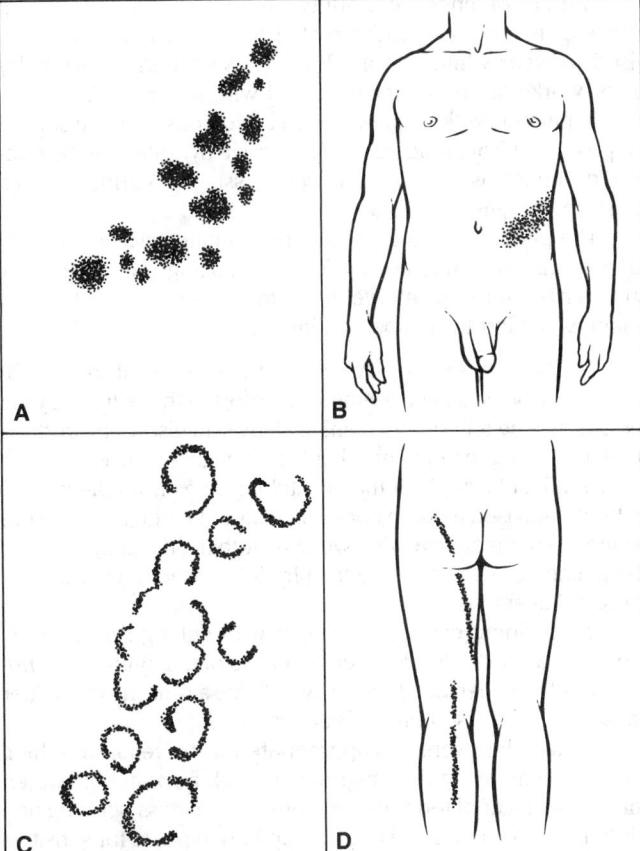

Figure 51–7. Examples of different configurations of skin lesions: (**A**) grouped; (**B**) zosteriform; (**C**) annular (circular) and arciform (arc); (**D**) linear.

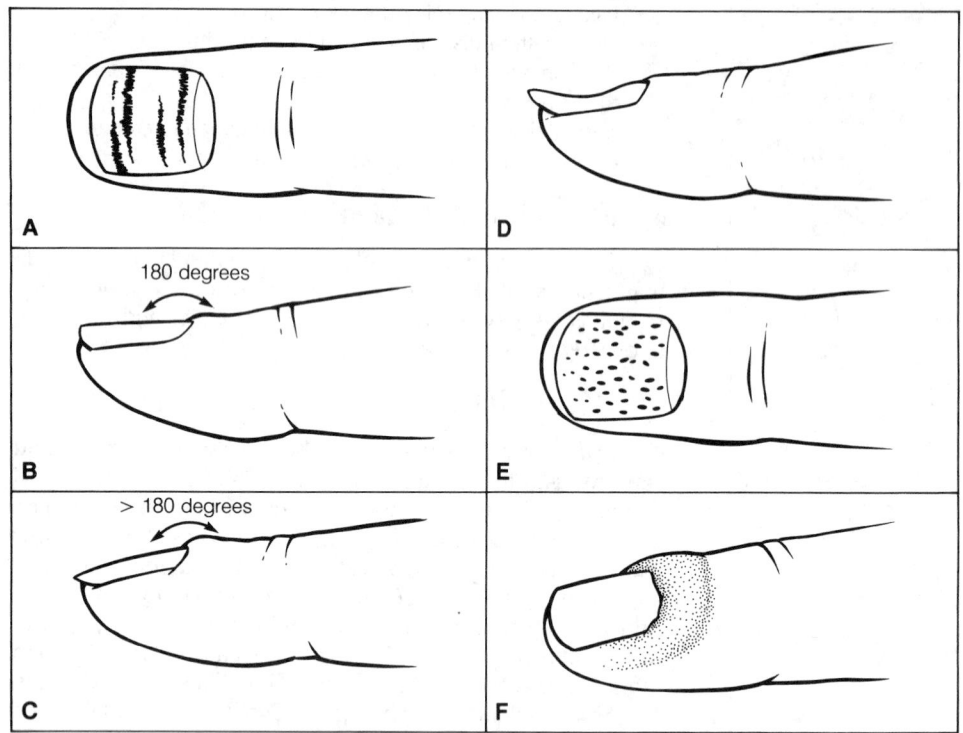

Figure 51–8. Common nail disorders: (**A**) Beau's lines; (**B**) early clubbing; (**C**) late clubbing; (**D**) spoon nails; (**E**) pitting; (**F**) paronychia.

Persons with this problem should protect the hands from contact with soaps, solvents, detergents, and other chemicals by wearing cotton-lined heavy-duty vinyl gloves when handling these agents. Persons with irritations of the hands can be advised to wear white cotton gloves (cosmetic gloves) for dry housework and to minimize contact with water.

In patients with diagnosed skin conditions, the skin should be protected from maceration (excessive hydration of the stratum corneum) when applying wet dressings. Thermal injuries must be prevented.

The patient with a compromised immune system is at increased risk for cutaneous infection. Nursing Care Plan 51-1 summarizes nursing interventions for persons with dry skin changes related to trauma and infection.

▷ *Relieving Discomfort.* A rash that seems trivial to the observer may be causing extreme discomfort to the patient. Cystic lesions may be tender and painful. Many skin disorders produce itching, making the patient irritable and unable to sleep. Itching is a significant symptom that scratching does not relieve. The patient is advised to keep cool, especially at night, and to avoid taking hot baths and wearing woolen clothing. If itching persists, the patient is advised to see the physician, who may prescribe a topical agent.

In providing care for a patient with itching skin lesions, the nurse attempts to discover the cause of discomfort. A *sudden* onset of generalized rash may indicate a drug allergy. Other causes are discussed under Pruritus, p. 1463.

Nursing interventions appropriate for the relief of itching include humidifying the environment with a room humidifier, maintaining a cool temperature, removing excess bedding and clothing, and limiting the use of soap to one made for sensitive skin. The nails are trimmed to decrease skin damage from scratching. Every effort should be made to keep the skin hydrated and moistened to avoid skin breakdown. The patient is advised to refrain from using over-the-counter preparations to relieve itching because the skin problem may be caused by irritation or sensitization from self-medication.

Gradual evaporation of water from dressings cools the skin and relieves pruritus. The nurse reinforces this teaching, making sure that the patient understands that normal skin should be protected during the application of wet dressings. In removing an adherent dressing, the patient is taught to moisten it before removal to relieve discomfort. When taking therapeutic baths (a form of wet dressing), the patient is advised to limit bathing time to no longer than 30 minutes to prevent skin maceration. Generally, therapeutic baths may be taken twice daily.

▷ *Achieving Restful Sleep.* Irritation and itching interfere with normal sleep. The nurse may advise the patient of the following measures to promote sleep:

- Keep a regular schedule for sleeping; go to bed at the same time and get up at the same time.
- Avoid caffeinated drinks late in the evening.
- Use a bedtime routine or ritual to ease the transition from wakefulness to sleep.
- Exercise regularly.

In addition, the bedroom should be well ventilated and humidified. Other measures to promote skin comfort so that the patient may feel more relaxed are found in Nursing Care Plan 51-1.

▷ *Increasing Self-Acceptance.* Physical appearance exerts profound influence in the social world and in the way people are treated. Preferential treatment is often bestowed on someone who is perceived as being attractive. Clean and healthy skin is intimately correlated with one's self-esteem.

Skin diseases can cause emotional suffering and can affect social relationships and business and recreational activities.

(text continues on page 1458)

Nursing Care Plan 51-1

Care of Patients With Dermatoses (Abnormal Skin Conditions)

Nursing Interventions	Rationale	Expected Outcomes

Nursing Diagnosis: Impaired skin integrity related to changes in barrier function of skin

Goal: Maintenance of skin integrity

CHANGES RELATED TO SKIN TRAUMA

Nursing Interventions	Rationale	Expected Outcomes
1. Protect healthy skin from maceration (excessive hydration of stratum corneum) when applying wet dressings.	1. Maceration of healthy skin can cause skin breakdown and extension of the primary condition.	• Maintains skin integrity • Absence of maceration • No signs of thermal injury • Absence of infection • Applies prescribed topical medication • Takes prescribed medication on schedule
2. Remove moisture from skin by blotting gently and avoiding friction.	2. Friction and maceration play a major role in some skin diseases.	
3. Guard carefully against risks of thermal injuries from excessively hot wet dressings and from subtle heat injuries (heating pads, radiators).	3. Patients with dermatoses may have decreased perception of heat.	
4. Advise patient to use sun-screening agents.	4. Many cosmetic problems and virtually all cutaneous malignancies can be attributed to chronic skin damage.	

CHANGES FROM INFECTION (RELATED TO ENTRY OF ORGANISMS THROUGH BREAK IN SKIN)

Nursing Interventions	Rationale
1. Have a high index of suspicion for an infection in patients with compromised immune systems.	1. Any condition that compromises the immune status increases the risk of cutaneous infection.
2. Instruct the patient clearly and in detail about the therapeutic regimen.	2. Effective patient education is dependent on the interpersonal skills of the health professionals and on giving clear instructions reinforced through written instructions.
3. Apply intermittent wet dressings as prescribed to reduce intensity of inflammation.	3. A wet dressing produces evaporative cooling, causing constriction of superficial cutaneous vessels and thereby decreasing erythema and serum production. Wet dressings help in debridement of vesicles and crusts and control inflammatory processes.
4. Provide tub baths and soaks as prescribed.	4. Loosens exudates and scales.
5. Administer prescribed antimicrobial.	5. Used to kill or prevent the growth of the infectious organism.
6. Use topical medications containing corticosteroids as prescribed and as indicated. a. Observe lesion periodically for changes in response to therapy. b. Instruct the patient about possible adverse effects of long-term use of fluorinated topical steroids.	6. Corticosteroids have an anti-inflammatory action, resulting in part from their ability to induce vasoconstriction of the small vessels in the upper dermis. Extensive prolonged use of topical corticosteroids can lead to antiproliferative effects on epidermal cells (loss of hair in area used).
7. Advise patient to stop using any skin agent that makes the problem worse.	7. A contact allergic reaction may develop from any ingredient in the medication.

(continued)

Nursing Care Plan 51-1 *(Continued)*

Care of Patients With Dermatoses (Abnormal Skin Conditions)

Nursing Interventions	*Rationale*	*Expected Outcomes*

Nursing Diagnosis: Body image disturbance related to unsightly skin appearance

Goal: Development of increasing self-acceptance

1. Assess patient for disturbance of self-image (avoidance of eye contact, self-negating verbalizations, expression of disgust about skin condition).	1. Disturbance of body image may accompany any disease or condition that is apparent to the patient. An impression of one's own body has an effect on self-concept.	• Develops increasing acceptance of own body
		• Follows through and participates in self-care measures
2. Identify psychosocial stage of development.	2. There is a relationship between development stage, self-image, and the patient's reaction to and interpretation of skin condition.	• Reports feeling in control of situation
		• Gives self positive reinforcement
		• Verbalizes a more healthy self-regard
3. Provide opportunity for expression. Listen (in an open, nondefensive way) to expressions of grief/anxiety about changes in body image.	3. The patient needs the experience of being heard and understood.	• Appears less self-conscious; is not afraid to socialize and be seen by others
		• Uses concealing and highlighting techniques to enhance appearance
4. Find out what the patient worries about and fears. Assist anxious patient to improve insight and identify and cope with problems.	4. This gives health care personnel opportunity to neutralize undue anxiety and restore reality to the situation. Fear is an element destructive to adaptation.	
5. Support patient's efforts to improve body image (participation in skin treatments; grooming).	5–8. A positive approach and suggestions of cosmetic techniques are often helpful in promoting self-acceptance and socialization.	
6. Help patient toward self-acceptance.		
7. Encourage socialization with others.		
8. Advise patient of available cosmetic measures to conceal disfiguring conditions.		

Nursing Diagnosis: Pain and itching related to skin lesions

Goal: Relief of discomfort

1. Examine area of involvement.		• Achieves relief of discomfort
a. Attempt to discover cause of discomfort.	a. Helps to identify appropriate comfort measures.	• Verbalizes that itching has been relieved
b. Record observations in detail, using descriptive terminology.	b. An accurate description of a cutaneous eruption is necessary for diagnosis and treatment. Many skin conditions appear similar but have different etiologies. Cutaneous inflammatory response may be muted in the elderly.	• Demonstrates absence of skin excoriation and scratch marks
c. Be aware that *sudden* onset of generalized rash may indicate drug allergy.		• Complies with prescribed treatment
		• Keeps skin hydrated and lubricated
		• Demonstrates intact skin; skin regaining healthy appearance
2. Control environmental and physical factors.	2. Itching is aggravated by heat, chemicals, and physical irritants.	
a. Keep humidity about 60%; use a humidifier.	a. At low humidity, the skin loses water.	
b. Maintain a cool environment.	b. Coolness deters itching.	
c. Use mild soap (Dove) or soap made for sensitive skin (Neutrogena, Aveeno)	c. These contain no detergents, dyes, or hardening agents.	

(continued)

Nursing Care Plan 51–1 *(Continued)*

Care of Patients With Dermatoses (Abnormal Skin Conditions)

Nursing Interventions	Rationale	Expected Outcomes
d. Remove excess clothing or bedding. e. Wash bed linens and clothing with mild soap. f. Stop repeated exposures to detergents, cleansers, and solvents.	d. Promotes cool environment. e. Strong soaps can cause skin irritation. f. Any substance that removes water, lipids, or protein from the epidermis alters the barrier function of the skin.	
3. Use skin-care measures to maintain skin integrity. a. Provide tepid cooling baths or cool dressings for itching. b. Treat dryness (xerosis) as prescribed. c. Apply skin lotion/cream immediately after bathing. d. Keep nails trimmed. e. Apply prescribed topical therapy. f. Help the patient accept the prolonged treatment that some conditions require. g. Advise the patient to refrain from using salves/lotions that are commercially available.	3. The skin is an important barrier that must be maintained intact in order to function properly. a. Gradual evaporation of water from dressings cools the skin and relieves pruritus. b. Dry skin can produce areas of dermatitis with redness, itching, scaling, and, in more severe forms, swelling, blistering, cracking, and weeping. c. Effective hydration of the stratum corneum prevents compromise of the barrier layer of the skin. d. Trimming decreases skin damage from scratching. g. The patient's problem may be caused by irritation or sensitization from self-medication.	

Nursing Diagnosis: Sleep pattern disturbance related to pruritus

Goal: Achievement of restful sleep

1. Prevent and treat dry skin. a. Advise patient to keep bedroom well ventilated and humidified. b. Keep skin moisturized. c. Bathe/shower only as absolutely necessary if skin is excessively dry. Use no soap or only mild soap. Apply skin lotion/cream immediately after bathing while skin is damp. 2. Advise patient of the following meaures that may be helpful in promoting sleep: a. Keep a regular schedule for sleeping. Go to bed at the same time; get up at same time.	1. Nocturnal pruritus interferes with normal sleep. a. Dry air will make skin feel scratchy. A comfortable environment promotes relaxation. b. This prevents water loss. Dry, itchy skin can usually be controlled but not cured. c. This will trap some of the water absorbed into the skin surface during bathing. a. Regularity of sleep schedule is important in maintaining sleep hygiene.	• Achieves restful sleep • Reports relief of itching • Maintains appropriate environmental conditions • Avoids caffeine in late afternoon/evening • Identifies measures to promote sleep • Experiences satisfactory rest/sleep pattern

(continued)

Nursing Care Plan 51–1 (Continued)

Care of Patients With Dermatoses (Abnormal Skin Conditions)

Nursing Interventions	Rationale	Expected Outcomes
b. Avoid caffeinated drinks late in the evening.	b. Caffeine has peak effect 2–4 hours after being consumed.	
c. Exercise regularly.	c. Exercise appears to have beneficial sleep effect if done in late afternoon.	
d. Use a bedtime routine or ritual.	d. This eases transition from wakefulness to sleep.	

Nursing Diagnosis: Knowledge deficit about skin care and methods of treating skin ailment

Goal: Understanding of skin care

1. Determine what the patient knows (understands and misunderstands) about the condition.	1. Provides baseline data for developing the teaching plan.	• Acquires understanding of skin care.
2. Keep the patient informed; correct misconceptions/misinformation.	2. Patients need to have a sense that there is something they can do. Most patients benefit from explanations and reassurance.	• Follows treatment as prescribed and can verbalize rationale for measures taken • Carries out prescribed baths, soaks, wet dressings
3. Demonstrate application of prescribed therapy (wet compresses; topical medication).	3. Allows patient the opportunity to visualize the correct way to perform therapies.	• Uses topical medication appropriately • Understands importance of nutrition to skin health
4. Advise the patient to keep skin moist and flexible with hydration and application of skin cream and lotion.	4. The stratum corneum needs water to stay flexible. Application of skin cream or lotion to damp skin prevents dry, rough, cracked, and scaly skin.	
5. Encourage the patient to attain a healthy nutritional status.	5. The appearance of the skin reflects a person's general health. Skin changes may be a feature of abnormal nutrition.	

Persons with eczema often have difficulty convincing others that their disease is not contagious. Those with flaking and scaling conditions may be wary of meeting new people. Comments from strangers may be difficult to deal with. A lowering of self-confidence, excessive fixation on skin defects, and worry about scarring are frequently found in persons with acne. All of these factors can generate negative emotions in the patient.

The nurse understands that body image is a complex psychologic concept that is related to the mental concept of self and self-esteem. Allowing patients to express their feelings freely gives them a sense of support and acceptance. Mutual trust and respect between patient and nurse are necessary to promote communication.

Informed patients are usually less anxious and more cooperative. Thus, teaching them about their condition and its treatment may make them more hopeful, which may reinforce their ability to use their resources effectively.

Self-care, particularly hair and skin care, can make a difference in the perceptions of others. Appropriate cosmetics can bring substantial benefits to a person with a chronic skin condition or disfigurement. A referral to an expert cosmetitian to camouflage birthmarks, mottled skin, scars, and chronic dermatitis can be advantageous. Persons who remain depressed over their condition may benefit from psychologic counseling.

◊ *Patient Education.* A healthy skin reflects one's general health. Principles of good nutrition, exercise, rest, and sleep are emphasized in any teaching program focused on skin care. Each person can learn that sunlight can permanently damage skin, leading to roughening, freckling, wrinkling, and malignant changes. It is not possible to tan without incurring some skin damage.

A patient who is under treatment for a skin condition is usually informed by the physician what the skin condition is, its etiology, and what to expect from treatment. The nurse reinforces this teaching. It may be advisable to have a relative or friend of the patient nearby for emotional support and also to listen to the instructions. Some patients do not listen, do not hear, or hear only part of what is being said.

The patient is taught how to apply topical medication, particularly the amount to be used, the size of the area to be treated, and the frequency of application. The topical medication is massaged gently onto the affected areas, never rubbed vigorously. In general, the medication is not used on normal skin. Potential side effects of the medication are discussed. Printed instruction sheets are provided to reinforce what has been told.

▷ Evaluation

Expected Outcomes

1. Maintains skin integrity
   a. Indicates absence of skin cracking
   b. Protects skin from contact with irritating substances
   c. Applies emollient to skin as prescribed
2. Achieves relief of discomfort
   a. Uses topical medication and treatments as prescribed
   b. Reports relief of itching
3. Achieves more restful sleep
   a. States he is "sleeping better"
   b. Reports an increased feeling of well-being
4. Demonstrates increasing self-acceptance
   a. Voices fewer self-deprecating remarks
   b. Pays attention to appearance
5. Acquires understanding of skin care
   a. Verbalizes rationale of prescribed treatment
   b. Demonstrates ability to perform treatments

Nursing management is discussed further in Nursing Care Plan 51-1.

Diagnostic Evaluation

Dermatology is a visually oriented specialty. In addition to obtaining the patient's history, the examiner inspects the appearance of the primary and secondary lesions and their configuration and distribution. Certain diagnostic procedures may also be used to help in identifying skin conditions.

A *skin biopsy* is performed to obtain tissue for microscopic examination. It may be obtained by scalpel excision or by a skin punch that removes a small core of tissue. Biopsies are performed on skin nodules of uncertain origin to rule out malignancy, on plaques of unusual shapes and colors, and to secure an exact diagnosis in blistering and other disorders.

Immunofluorescence (IF) testing is a technique in which antigen or antibody is combined with a fluorochrome dye and used to localize the site of an immune reaction. (Antibodies can be made fluorescent by attaching them to a dye.) Immunofluorescence tests on skin (*direct IF test*) are techniques to detect autoantibodies directed against portions of the skin. The *indirect IF test* detects specific antibodies in the patient's serum.

Patch testing is performed to identify substances to which the patient has developed an allergy. The suspected allergens are applied to normal skin under occlusive patches. If dermatitis develops, the presence of redness, fine bumps, or itching is considered a *weak* positive reaction; fine blisters, papules, and severe itching indicate a *moderate* positive reaction; and the presence of blisters, pain, and ulceration indicates a *strong* positive reaction.

Explanations to the patient prior to and during the patch test usually include the following:

1. Do not use any cortisone-type medication for 1 week prior to the test date.
2. Small samples of each test material will be applied to a disc. The discs are then taped to the upper back unless contraindicated. The number of test samples applied will vary (20 to 30).
3. The procedure usually takes about 30 minutes.
4. Keep the test area (back) dry while the tape is in place. Showers and swimming are not permitted.
5. Return on date specified (2 to 3 days) to have the discs removed and the test site examined and evaluated.

Skin scrapings are taken of suspected fungal lesions. This is performed with a scalpel blade moistened with oil so that the scraped skin adheres to the blade. The scraped material is transferred to a glass slide, covered with a cover slip, and examined microscopically.

A *Tzanck smear* is used to examine cells from blistering skin conditions, such as herpes zoster, varicella, herpes simplex, and all forms of pemphigus. The secretions from a suspected lesion are applied to a glass slide and examined after staining.

The *Wood's light examination* uses a special lamp for producing long-wave ultraviolet rays (black light) that result in a characteristic dark purple fluorescence. The color of the fluorescent light is best seen in a darkened room, where it is possible to differentiate epidermal from dermal lesions and hypo- and hyperpigmented lesions from normal skin. The patient is reassured that the light is not harmful to skin or eyes.

Clinical photographs are taken to show the nature and extent of the skin condition and to reveal progress or improvement resulting from treatment.

Management of Skin Disorders

Therapeutic modalities used in the treatment of patients with dermatologic problems include topical and systemic medications, wet dressings, other special dressings, and therapeutic baths.

The major objectives of therapy are to (1) prevent damage to the healthy skin, (2) prevent secondary infection, (3) reverse the inflammatory process, and (4) relieve the symptoms.

Preventing Damage to Healthy Skin. Some skin problems are markedly aggravated by soap and water. Therefore, bathing routines are modified according to the condition being treated.

- Denuded skin, whether the area of desquamation is large or small, is excessively prone to damage by chemicals and trauma.

The friction of a towel, if applied with vigor, is sufficient to excite a brisk inflammatory response that causes any existing lesion to flare up and increase in extent. Thus, the essence of skin care and protection in bathing a patient with abnormal skin is to use a mild, superfatted soap or soap substitute and to ensure the complete removal of the soap when rinsing, before blotting the area dry with a soft cloth. Deodorant soaps should be avoided in these patients.

Pledgets saturated with oil will aid in loosening crusts, removing exudates, or freeing an adherent dry dressing. The dressing also may be saturated with sterile saline or another prescribed solution, which softens it and permits it to be pulled away gently.

Preventing Secondary Infection.   Potentially infectious skin lesions should be regarded strictly as such, and proper precautions should be observed until the diagnosis is established. Some lesions with pus contain infectious material. Although some genital lesions are infectious, most are minor irritations.

- The nurse and physician should adhere to universal precautions and wear either clean or sterile gloves when inspecting or changing the dressing. Proper disposal of any contaminated dressing should be carried out according to agency protocol.

Reversing the Inflammatory Process.   The type of skin lesion (oozing, infected, or dry) usually suggests the local medication or treatment that is prescribed. As a rule, if the skin is acutely inflamed (hot, red, and swollen) and is oozing, it is best to apply wet dressings and soothing lotions. In chronic conditions in which the skin surface is dry and scaly, water-soluble emulsions, creams, ointments, and pastes are used. The therapy must be changed as the response indicates. The patient is instructed to contact the physician or clinic if the medication or compresses seem to irritate the dermatosis. Success or failure of skin therapy often depends upon adequate instruction and motivation of the patient and the interest and support of the health personnel.

Wet Dressings

Wet dressings (wet compresses applied to areas of the skin) are usually used for acute, weeping, inflammatory lesions. They may be either sterile or nonsterile, depending on the condition being treated. The purposes of wet dressings are (1) to reduce inflammation by producing constriction of blood vessels (thus decreasing vasodilation and the local blood flow in inflammation); (2) to cleanse the skin of exudates, crusts, and scales; and (3) to maintain drainage of infected areas. Before these dressings are applied, the hands should be washed thoroughly.

Wet dressings are used for vesicular, bullous, pustular, and ulcerative disorders, as well as for acute inflammatory disorders, erosions, and exudative, crusted surfaces.

The solutions generally consist of room-temperature tap water or saline. Other agents used include silver nitrate, aluminum acetate (Burow's solution), potassium permanganate, 5% acetic acid, and sodium hypochlorite (Dakin's solution). Medication may be applied after wet dressings are removed.

Although some dressings must be covered to prevent evaporation, most are allowed to remain open. The *open dressing* requires frequent changes because evaporation is rapid. The *closed dressing* is changed less frequently. However, there is always a danger that it will cause not only softening but actual maceration of the underlying skin. Wet-to-dry dressings are used to remove exudate from erosions or ulcers. The dressing is left in place until dry. It is then removed without soaking so that crusts, exudate, or pus from the cutaneous dermatitis will adhere to the dry dressing and be removed with it.

Areas of normal skin that may be exposed to moisture for any extended period should first be coated with petrolatum jelly, a silicone oil, or zinc oxide paste to avoid skin maceration.

Smooth muslin or cotton materials can be cut and folded to make dressings that are two to four layers thick. The dressing is saturated with the prescribed solution before it is applied. Usually wet dressings are kept cool or at room temperature. Compresses are removed, wrung out of the solution, and reapplied every 5 minutes to ensure their wetness. Wet dressings are usually applied for 15-minute periods three to four times daily during the acute phase unless otherwise prescribed. Medications applied to moist skin immediately after treatment with compresses are absorbed better than when applied to dry skin. If extensive areas are to be treated with wet compresses, the patient must be kept warm, and not more than one-third of the body should be treated at one time.

If warm compresses are prescribed, the area must be observed carefully because the skin may be burned. If a closed dressing is used, it may be covered with sterile towels to hold the dressing in place and further protected with a plastic film. In this way, the temperature can be maintained for a longer period.

Dressing materials such as gauze should be discarded after each use. Usually, the acute stage of dermatitis subsides after 48 to 72 hours of treatment. Wet dressings continued beyond this point can lead to dryness of the skin.

Therapeutic Baths (Balneotherapy)

Baths or soaks are useful when large areas are involved to remove crusts, scales, and old medications and to relieve the inflammation and itching that accompany acute dermatoses. The temperature of the water should be comfortable; and the bath should not exceed 20 to 30 minutes because of the tendency of baths and soaks to produce maceration. For the different types of therapeutic baths and their uses, see Table 51-3.

Pharmacotherapy: Topical Medications

Because skin is the most accessible body organ to treat, the use of topical medications is advantageous over systemic therapy. High concentrations of a medication can be directly applied to the dermatosis site with little systemic absorption and therefore few systemic side effects.

Medications in the form of lotions, creams, ointments, and powders are frequently used to treat skin lesions. In general, wet dressings, with or without medication, are used in the acute stage; lotions and creams are reserved for the subacute stage; and ointments are used when inflammation has become chronic and the skin is dry with scaling and *lichenification* (leathery thickening of the skin).

Lotions are of two types: *suspensions,* consisting of a powder in water that requires shaking before application, and *clear solutions,* in which the active ingredients have been completely dissolved. A lotion, such as *Calamine,* is a suspension that provides a cooling and drying effect on the skin as it evaporates, while leaving a thin medicinal layer of powder on the affected area. Lotions are frequently used to provide replenishment of lost skin oils and relieve pruritus. Lotions must be applied every 2 to 3 hours for sustained therapeutic effect. Because lotions are easy to use, compliance is generally high.

Powders usually have a talc, zinc oxide, bentonite, or cornstarch base and are dusted on the skin with a shaker or with cotton sponges. Although their medical action is brief, powders act as hygroscopic agents, absorbing moisture and

TABLE 51-3. *Types of Therapeutic Baths*

Bath Solution and Medication	Desired Effect	Nursing Interventions for Therapeutic Baths
Water	Same effects as wet dressings	• Fill the tub half full.
Saline	Used for widely disseminated lesions	• Keep the water at a comfortable temperature.
Colloidal—Aveeno (oatmeal)	Antipruritic; soothing	• Do not allow the water to cool excessively.
Sodium bicarbonate	Cooling	• Use a bath mat—*medications may cause tub to be slippery.*
Starch	Soothing	• Apply a lubricating agent to wet skin after bath if emollient action is desired—increases hydration. Because tars are volatile, the bath area should be well ventilated.
Medicated tars—Alma-Tar, Balnetar (follow package directions)	Tar baths are used for psoriasis and chronic eczematous conditions.	
Bath oils—Alpha-Keri, Lubath, Domol	Bath oils are used for antipruritic and emollient actions; used for acute and subacute eczematous eruptions	• Dry by blotting with a towel.
		• Keep room warm to minimize temperature fluctuations.
		• Encourage patient to wear light, loose clothing after the bath.

reducing friction between skin surfaces and between the skin and bedding.

Creams are suspensions of oil and water, are easily applied, and usually are the most cosmetically acceptable to the patient. Creams are generally rubbed into the skin by hand. They are used for their moisturizing and emollient effects.

Gels are semisolid emulsions that become liquid when applied to the skin. They are cosmetically acceptable to the patient because they vanish after application, and they are greaseless and nonstaining. Most topical steroids are prescribed in gel form because the gel appears to penetrate more effectively than other skin preparations.

Pastes are mixtures of powders and ointments and are used in inflammatory conditions. They adhere best to the skin and may need to be removed with mineral oil or olive oil.

Ointments retard water loss, lubricate and protect the skin, and are preferred in the more chronic or localized skin conditions. Both pastes and ointments are applied with a wooden tongue depressor or by hand, with gloves if necessary.

Sprays and *aerosols* may be used on extensive lesions. These evaporate on contact and are used infrequently.

In all types of topical medication, the patient is taught to apply the medication gently but thoroughly and, when necessary, to cover these medications with a dressing to prevent soiling of clothing. Table 51-4 lists commonly used topical preparations.

Corticosteroids are widely used in the treatment of many dermatologic conditions. Topical steroids frequently are used to suppress inflammation, thus relieving pain and itching. The patient is taught to apply this medication sparingly on hydrated skin and to rub it in thoroughly. Topical corticosteroids may be covered with occlusive dressings to enhance skin penetration. However, this can cause obstruction of sweat glands and overgrowth of skin bacteria.

Oral corticosteroids are frequently ordered for the short-term treatment of contact dermatitis or the long-term treatment of chronic dermatosis, such as pemphigus vulgaris.

Wet dressings may be used with topical steroids to enhance steroid absorption by softening and hydrating the skin. Other techniques to enhance skin penetration include the application of hot wet dressings before applying the medication or using a heating pad over a wet dressing on treated skin areas.

When steroids are applied around the eyes, much caution is required, because chronic use around the eyes may cause glaucoma, cataracts, and viral and fungal infections. Also, when strong (fluorinated) steroids are applied to the face, precautions must be taken because they may produce an acnelike dermatitis (*perioral dermatitis*), steroid-induced *rosacea* (characterized by lesions around the nose and cheeks), and *hypertrichosis* (excessive hair growth). Table 51-5 lists topical corticosteroid preparations according to potency.

Intralesional therapy consists of the injection of a sterile suspension of medication (usually a corticosteroid) into or just below a lesion. Although this treatment may have an anti-inflammatory effect, local atrophy may result if the injection is made into subcutaneous fat. Skin lesions treated with intralesional therapy include psoriasis, keloids, and cystic acne. Occasionally, immunotherapeutic and antifungal agents are administered by intralesional therapy.

Systemic medications are also prescribed for skin conditions. These include the corticosteroids, antibiotics, antifungals, antihistamines, sedatives and tranquilizers, analgesics, and cytotoxic drugs.

Dressings for Skin Conditions

Skin dressings are used to keep topical medication in place and to allay itching and pain. One very effective type of dressing is the *occlusive dressing*, which increases the local skin temperature and hydration and enhances the absorption of topically applied medications. Occlusive dressings also promote the retention of moisture, which keeps the medication from evaporating and reduces the expense of topical corticosteroid treatment. An airtight plastic film, such as plastic kitchen wrap, is placed over the medicated skin. Plastic film is advantageous because it is thin and adapts itself readily to anatomic structures of all sizes and shapes. Plastic surgical tape containing corticosteroid in the adhesive layer can be cut to size and applied

TABLE 51–4. *Common Topical Medications*

Bath preparations	Alpha-Keri bath oil
	Neutrogena bath oil
	Aveeno oatmeal bath powder
	Oilated Aveeno bath powder
	Balnetar
	Lubath
Creams	Aquacare
	Acid Mantle Creme
	Curel
	Eucerin
	Moisturel
	Nutraderm
Lotions	Alpha-Keri lotion
	Dermassage
	Lubriderm
Ointments	Aquaphor
	Hydrophilic petrolatum
	Vaseline Petroleum Jelly
	White or yellow petrolatum
Topical anesthetics	Xylocaine (lidocaine) of various strengths in the form of sprays, ointments, lotions
Topical antibiotics	Bacitracin ointment
	Bacitracin and polymyxin B ointment (Polysporin)
	1% Clindamycin phosphate (Cleocin T)
	2% Erythromycin solution (Eryderm, Erymax, T-Stat)
	1% Gentamicin sulfate cream or ointment (Garamycin)
	2% Mupirocin
	1% Silver sulfadiazine cream (Silvadene)

to individual lesions. Plastic wrap should generally be used no more than 10 to 12 hours a day. The patient is given the following instructions: (1) wash the area, then pat dry; (2) rub the medication into the lesion while the skin is moist; (3) cover with plastic wrap (*e.g.*, Saran Wrap, vinyl gloves, plastic bags); and (4) cover with an Ace bandage, dressing, or paper tape to seal the edges.

It is important to remember that prolonged use of occlusive dressings may cause local skin atrophy, *striae* (bandlike streaks), *telangiectasia* (small red lesions caused by dilation of blood vessels), inflammation of hair follicles, nonhealing ulceration or erythema, and systemic absorption of corticosteroids. Dressings should be removed for 12 of every 24 hours to prevent these complications.

There are other forms of dressings that can be used to cover topical medications. The best material is soft cotton cloth. Stretchable cotton dressings (Surgitube, Tubegauze) can be used for fingers, toes, and extremities. The hands can be covered with disposable polyethylene or vinyl gloves, sealed at

the wrists; the feet can be wrapped in plastic bags covered by cotton socks. When large areas of the body must be covered, cotton cloth covered with tubular material can be used. Disposable diapers or cloths folded diaper-fashion are also useful as dressings for the groin and the perineal areas. Axillary dressings can be made of cotton cloth taped in place or held by dress shields. A turban or plastic shower cap is useful for holding dressings on the scalp. A face mask may be made from gauze with holes cut out for the eyes, nose, and mouth and held in place with gauze ties looped through holes cut in the four corners of the mask.

If the patient is troubled with itching at nighttime that interferes with sleep, the nurse can advise that wearing cotton

TABLE 51–5. *Common Topical Corticosteroid Preparations*

Potency	Topical Corticosteroid Preparation
Lowest	0.1% Dexamethasone (Decaderm)
	0.25–2.5% Hydrocortisone (Hytone, Nutraderm, Penecort, Synacort, Cortef)
	0.25 or 1.0% Methylprednisolone acetate (Medrol)
Low	0.01% Betamethasone valerate (Valisone)
	0.1% Clocortolone (Cloderm)
	0.05% Desonide (Tridesilon)
	0.01% Fluocinolone acetonide (Synalar)
	0.025% Flurandrenolide (Cordran)
	0.2% Hydrocortisone valerate (Westcort)
	0.025% Triamcinolone acetonide (Aristocort, Kenalog)
Intermediate	0.025% Betamethasone benzoate (Benisone, Uticort)
	0.1% Betamethasone valerate (Valisone)
	0.05% Desoximetasone (Topicort)
	0.025% Fluocinolone acetonide (Fluonid)
	0.05% Flurandrenolide (Cordran)
	0.025% Halacinonide (Halog)
	0.1% Triamcinolone acetonide (Aristocort, Kenalog)
High	0.1% Amcinonide (Cyclocort)
	0.05% Betamethasone dipropionate (Diprosone)
	0.25% Desoximetasone (Topicort)
	0.2% Fluocinolone (Synalar)
	0.05% Fluocinonide (Lidex)
	0.1% Halcinonide (Halog)
	0.5% Triamcinolone acetonide (Aristocort, Kenalog)
	0.05% Diflorasone diacetate (Florone, Maxiflor)
Highest	0.05% Betamethasone dipropionate (Diprolene)
	0.05% Clobetasol propionate (Temovate)

(Patterson JAK. Aging and Clinical Practice Skin Disorders: Diagnosis and Treatment. New York, Igaku-Shoin Medical Publishers, 1989.)

clothes next to the skin may be helpful. Excessive warmth is avoided, and the room is kept cool and humidified. The fingernails are trimmed to prevent injury from scratching.

Pruritus

Pruritus (itching) is one of the most common complaints in dermatologic disorders, causing alteration in comfort and changes in the integrity of the skin. Although pruritus is most frequently due to primary skin disease, it may also reflect systemic disease. Thus, it may be the first indication of systemic internal disease such as diabetes mellitus, blood disorders, or cancer. Itching may also accompany renal, hepatic, and thyroid diseases. Pruritus may be caused by certain oral medications; by the external application of certain drugs, soaps, and chemicals; by prickly heat (*miliaria*); and by contact with woolen garments. Patients may also experience pruritus as a side effect of radiation therapy, as a reaction to chemotherapy, analgesics, or antibiotic therapy, or as a symptom of infection. Pruritus may occur in the elderly as a result of dry skin. Itching may also be caused by psychologic factors. A rash may or may not be present.

Pruritus usually leads to scratching, which often is more severe at night. Pruritus is reported less frequently during waking hours because the person is involved in daily activities. At nighttime when there are few distractions, the slightest symptom of pruritus cannot be easily overcome. Scratching causes histamine release from the inflamed cells and thus produces more pruritus; a vicious itch–scratch cycle ensues.

The secondary effects include excoriations, redness, raised areas on the skin (*wheals*), infections of the skin, and changes in pigmentation. Severe itching is debilitating.

Management

The cause of pruritus, if known, should be removed. The presence of signs of infection and environmental clues such as warm, dry air or irritating bed linens should be identified. In general, washing with soap and hot water is avoided. The application of a cold compress, ice cube, or cool agents that contain soothing menthol and camphor that constrict blood vessels is helpful.

Bath oils (Lubath, Alpha-Keri bath oil) containing a surfactant that makes the oil mix with water in the bath may be sufficient for cleansing. (However, an elderly patient or a patient with disturbed balance should not add oil to the bath because of the danger of slipping in the bathtub.) Soothing baths containing starch or water-soluble tar derivatives may be prescribed.

Topical steroids may be beneficial as anti-inflammatory agents to decrease itching. Oral antihistamines are even more effective because they can overcome the effects of histamine release from damaged mast cells. Tricyclic antidepressants are prescribed when the pruritus is of a neuropsychogenic origin.

A thorough history and physical examination will provide clues to the cause of the pruritus (hay fever, asthma, recent ingestion of a new medication, change of cosmetics). Unless a definite cause is found, the patient usually will respond to therapy to relieve xerosis (dry skin). If pruritus continues, further investigation into a systemic etiology (malignancy, anemia, metabolic or endocrine cause) is advised.

Nursing Interventions: Patient Education.   The nurse reinforces the reasons for the prescribed therapeutic regimen and guides the patient on specific points of care. If baths have been prescribed, the patient is reminded to use tepid (not hot) water and to shake off the excess water and blot between intertriginous areas with a towel. Rubbing vigorously with the towel is avoided because this overstimulates the skin, causing more itching. It also removes water from the stratum corneum. Immediately after bathing, the skin should be lubricated with an emollient that traps moisture.

Perianal Itching

Pruritus of the anal and genital regions may be caused by small particles of fecal material lodged in the perianal crevices or attached to anal hairs, or by perianal skin damage caused by scratching, moisture, and decreased skin resistance due to steroids or antibiotics. Other possible causes of perianal itching include local irritants such as scabies and lice, local lesions such as hemorrhoids, fungal or yeast infections, and pinworm infestation. Conditions such as diabetes mellitus, the anemias, hyperthyroidism, and pregnancy may also result in perianal pruritus.

Patient Education and Home Health Care.   The patient is instructed to follow proper hygienic measures and to discontinue home and over-the-counter remedies. The perianal area should be rinsed with lukewarm water and the area blotted dry with cotton balls. Premoistened tissues may be used after defecation.

As part of health teaching, the patient is instructed to avoid bathing in water that is too hot and to avoid using bubble baths, sodium bicarbonate, or detergent soaps, all of which aggravate dryness. To keep the perianal skin as dry as possible, patients should avoid wearing underwear made of synthetic fabrics. Local anesthetic agents should not be used because of possible allergenic effects. The patient should avoid vasodilating agents or stimulants that increase emotional tension (alcohol, coffee) and mechanical irritants such as rough or woolen clothing.

Secretory Disorders

The main secretory function of the skin is performed by the sweat glands, which help to regulate body temperature. These glands excrete a fluid, perspiration, which evaporates and thus cools the body. The sweat glands are located in various parts of the body and respond to different stimuli. Those on the trunk generally respond to thermal stimulation; those on the palms and soles respond to nervous stimulation; and those in the axillae and on the forehead respond to both kinds of stimulation.

As a rule, moist skin is warm, and dry skin is likely to be cool. However, this is not a hard and fast rule. It is not unusual to observe cold sweats; warm, dry skin in a dehydrated patient; and very hot, dry skin peculiar to some febrile states.

Seborrheic Dermatoses

Seborrhea is excessive production of sebum (secretion of sebaceous glands) in those areas where glands are normally found in large numbers (face, scalp, eyebrows, eyelids, at the sides of the nose and upper lip, malar or cheek regions, ears, axillae, under the breasts, groin, gluteal crease of the buttocks).

Seborrheic dermatitis is a chronic inflammatory disease of the skin with a predilection for areas that are well supplied with sebaceous glands or lie between folds of the skin, where the bacterial count is high.

The characteristic lesions are remarkably variable, but this is a dermatitis of the seborrheic areas. It may start in childhood with fine scaling of the scalp or other areas and may continue throughout life. The scales may be dry, moist, or greasy. There may be patches of sallow, greasy-appearing skin, with or without scaling, and slight erythema, predominantly on the forehead, nasolabial fold, and scalp, and between adjacent skin surfaces in the regions of the axillae, groin, and breasts.

The dry, flaky desquamation of the scalp with a profuse amount of fine, powdery scales is commonly called *dandruff*. The mild forms of the disease are asymptomatic. When scaling is present, it is often accompanied by pruritus, which may lead to scratching and result in secondary complications, such as infection and excoriation.

Seborrheic dermatitis has a genetic predisposition; hormones, nutritional status, infection, and emotional stress influence its course. There are remissions and exacerbations of this condition, which should be explained to the patient.

Management

Because there is no known cure for seborrhea, the objective of therapy is to control the disorder and allow the skin to repair itself. Seborrheic dermatitis of the body and face may respond to a topically applied corticosteroid cream, which allays the secondary inflammatory response. However, this medication should be used with caution near the eyelids, because it can induce glaucoma in predisposed persons. Patients with seborrheic dermatitis may develop a secondary *Candida* yeast infection in body creases or folds. To avoid this, patients should be advised to ensure maximum aeration of the skin and to carefully cleanse areas where there are creases or folds in the skin. Patients with persistent candidiasis should be evaluated for diabetes.

The mainstay of dandruff treatment is proper shampooing, which should be done frequently (daily or at least three times weekly) with medicated shampoos. Two or three different types of shampoo should be used in rotation to prevent the seborrhea from becoming resistant to a particular shampoo. The shampoo is left on at least 5 to 10 minutes. As the condition gets better, the treatment can be less intense. Antiseborrheic shampoos include those containing selenium sulfide suspension, zinc pyrithione shampoos, salicylic acid sulfur shampoos, and tar shampoos that contain sulfur and salicylic acid.

Nursing Interventions: Patient Education

A person with seborrheic dermatitis is advised to remove external irritants and to avoid excess heat and perspiration; rubbing and scratching prolong the disorder. To avoid secondary infections, the patient should air the skin and keep skin folds clean and dry.

Instructions on the use of medicated shampoo are reinforced for those with dandruff that requires treatment.

The patient is cautioned that seborrheic dermatitis is a chronic problem that tends to wax and wane. The goal is to keep it under control. Patients need to be encouraged to adhere to the treatment program. Those who become discouraged and disheartened by the effect on body image should be treated with sensitivity and an awareness of their need to express their feelings.

Acne Vulgaris

Acne vulgaris is a common follicular disorder affecting susceptible pilosebaceous follicles (hair follicles) most commonly found on the face, neck, and upper trunk. It is characterized by the presence of closed comedones (whiteheads), open comedones (blackheads), papules, pustules, nodules, and cysts.

Acne is the most commonly encountered skin condition, affecting an estimated 85% of the population between 12 and 35 years of age. It becomes more marked at puberty and during adolescence, perhaps because at this age certain endocrine glands of the body that influence the secretions of the sebaceous glands are functioning at peak activity. The etiology of acne appears to be multiple, reflecting an interplay of genetic, hormonal, and bacterial factors.

Pathogenesis

During childhood, the sebaceous glands are small and virtually nonfunctioning. These glands are under endocrine control, especially the androgens. During puberty, the presence of androgen stimulates the sebaceous glands, causing them to enlarge and to secrete a natural oil, *sebum*, which rises to the top of the hair follicle and flows out onto the skin surface. In adolescents who develop acne, androgenic stimulation produces a heightened response in the sebaceous glands. Acne occurs when the pilosebaceous ducts through which the sebum flows become plugged, resulting in an accumulation of the sebaceous material that plugs the duct. This accumulation of material forms comedones.

Clinical Manifestations

The initial lesions of acne are comedones. *Closed comedones* (whiteheads) are obstructive lesions formed from impacted lipids or oils and keratin that plug the dilated follicle. Whiteheads are small, whitish papules with minute follicular openings that generally cannot be seen. These closed comedones may evolve into *open comedones,* in which the contents of the ducts are in open communication with the external environment. Open comedones are termed *blackheads*. The color of the blackhead is *not* due to dirt but to an accumulation of lipid, bacterial, and epithelial debris that obstructs the flow of sebum.

Although the exact cause is not known, some closed comedones may rupture and result in an inflammatory reaction due to the leakage of follicle contents (sebum, keratin, bacteria) into the dermis. This inflammatory response may result from the action of certain skin bacteria, such as *Propionibacterium acnes*, that live in the hair follicles and break down the triglycerides of the sebum into free fatty acids and glycerin. The resulting inflammation is seen clinically as papules, pustules, nodules, cysts, or abscesses.

Management

The goals of management are to reduce colonization by the bacteria, decrease sebaceous gland activity, prevent the follicles from becoming plugged, reduce inflammation, combat secondary infection, minimize scarring, and eliminate factors that may predispose to acne. The therapeutic regimen depends on the type of lesion (comedonal, papular, pustular, cystic).

There is no predictable cure for the disease, but combinations of therapies are available that can control its activity effectively. Topical treatment may be all that is needed to treat mild to moderate lesions as well as superficial inflammatory lesions (papular or pustular).

Topical Therapy

Benzoyl Peroxide. *Benzoyl peroxide* preparations are widely used because they produce a rapid and sustained reduction of inflammatory lesions. They also have an antibacterial effect by suppressing *Propionibacterium acnes*. They depress sebum production and lead to the breakdown of the comedone plugs. Initially, benzoyl peroxide causes redness and scaling, but generally the skin adjusts quickly to its use. Usually the patient applies a gel preparation of benzoyl peroxide once daily. In many instances this will be the only treatment needed. Benzoyl peroxide, benzoyl–erythromycin and benzoyl–sulfur combinations are available over the counter and by prescription.

Vitamin A Acid. Topically applied *vitamin A acid* (tretinoin) is used to clear the keratin plugs from the pilosebaceous ducts. Vitamin A acid speeds up the cellular turnover, forces out the comedones, and prevents occurrence of new comedones. Thus, it is effective in the treatment of comedonal acne. However, the patient should be informed that symptoms may worsen during early weeks of therapy because inflammation may occur during the process. Erythema and peeling are also a frequent result. Improvement may take up to 8 to 12 weeks. Some patients cannot tolerate this therapy. The patient is cautioned against sun exposure while using this topical medication because it may cause an exaggerated sunburn. Package insert directions are to be followed implicitly.

Topical Antibiotics. The use of *topically applied antibiotics* for the treatment of acne has become widespread. Topical antibiotics suppress the growth of *P. acnes*; reduce skin-surface free fatty acid levels; decrease comedones, papules, and pustules; and do not have systemic side effects. Topical preparations containing clindamycin, erythromycin, meclocycline, or tetracycline hydrochloride are frequently used.

Systemic Therapy

Systemic Antibiotics. Oral antibiotics given in small doses over a long period are very effective in the treatment of patients with moderate and severe acne, especially when the acne is inflammatory and results in pustules, abscesses, and scarring. Therapy may be continued for months to years. The patient is advised to take tetracycline at least 1 hour before or 2 hours after meals, because the drug is poorly absorbed with food. Side effects of tetracyclines include photosensitivity, nausea, diarrhea, vaginitis in women, and cutaneous infection in either sex. (In some women, broad-spectrum antibiotics may suppress normal vaginal bacteria and predispose the patient to candidiasis, a fungal infection.)

Oral Retinoids. Synthetic vitamin A compounds (*retinoids*) are being used with dramatic results in patients with nodular cystic acne that is unresponsive to conventional therapy. One compound is *isotretinoin* (Accutane), which is also used for active inflammatory papular pustular acne that has a tendency to scar. Isotretinoin causes a reduction in sebaceous gland size and inhibits sebum production. It also causes the epidermis to shed (*epidermal desquamation*), thereby unseating and expelling existing comedones. The most common side effect, experienced by almost all patients, is *cheilitis* (inflammation of the lips). Drying and chapping of the skin and mucous membranes are also frequently encountered. These changes are reversible with the withdrawal of the medication. Most important, isotretinoin is teratogenic in humans, meaning that it can have an adverse effect on a fetus, causing CNS and cardiovascular defects and structural abnormalities of the face. Therefore, contraceptive measures for females of childbearing age are obligatory during treatment and for about 4 to 8 weeks thereafter. Patients are also cautioned not to take vitamin A supplements while on this medication, to avoid additive toxic effects.

Hormone Therapy. Estrogen therapy (progesterone–estrogen preparations) has been found to suppress sebum production and reduce skin oiliness. It is usually reserved for young women when the acne begins somewhat later than usual and tends to flare at certain times in the menstrual cycle, which is often irregular. Estrogen in the form of estrogen-dominant oral contraceptive compounds may be given on a prescribed cyclic regimen. Estrogen is not given to males because of undesirable side effects. Table 51-6 summarizes the current commonly prescribed treatment modalities for acne vulgaris.

Surgical Treatment

Surgical treatment of acne consists of comedo extraction, injections of steroids into the inflamed lesions, and incision and drainage of large, fluctuant, nodular cystic lesions. *Cryosurgery* (freezing with liquid nitrogen) may be used for nodular and cystic forms of acne. Patients with deep scars may be treated with deep abrasive therapy (*dermabrasion*), in which the epidermis and some superficial dermis are removed down to the level of the scars.

Comedo Extraction. Comedones may be removed with a comedo extractor. The site is first wiped with an alcohol sponge. The comedo is nicked with an 18-gauge needle or scalpel blade to incise the follicular opening, widen the port, and facilitate the removal of the comedo. The opening of the extractor is then placed over the lesion, and direct pressure is applied to cause extrusion of the plug through the expressor.

Removal of comedones will leave areas of erythema, which may take several weeks to subside. Recurrence of comedones after extraction is common because part of the comedone frequently remains in the pilosebaceous canal.

In summary, acne vulgaris is a highly prevalent disease that affects many persons, especially teenagers. Both sexes are affected equally, but males have more severe cases. Most cases of acne subside spontaneously within a few years of symptom onset. The cases that continue into adulthood produce con-

TABLE 51-6. *Commonly Prescribed Treatment Modalities for Acne Vulgaris**

Topical therapy	Benzoyl peroxide
	Benzoyl-erythromycin
	Benzoyl-sulfur
	Topical antibiotics:
	Clindamycin lotion and gel
	Erythromycin lotion, gel, and swabs
	Meclocycline cream
	Tetracycline lotion
	Resorcinol
	Salicylic acid
	Sulfur
	Tretinoin
	Various soaps, cleansers and astringents
Systemic therapy	Oral antibiotics:
	Tetracycline
	Erythromycin
	Minocycline
	Trimethoprim-sulfamethoxazole
	Accutane (isotretinoin)
	Hormones:
	Corticosteroids
	High dose for anti-inflammatory action
	Low dose to suppress androgen action
	Sex hormones (women only)
	Estrogen
	Antiandrogens
Surgical therapy	Extraction of comedonal contents
	Drainage of pustules and cysts
	Excision of sinus tracts and cysts
	Intralesional corticosteroids
	Cryotherapy
	Dermabrasion for scars

* Treatments listed are commonly used but do not include all available forms of therapy.

siderable psychologic and social distress, especially if there are disfiguring scars. At present there is no predictable cure.

▶ Nursing Process
The Patient With Acne

▷ Assessment

Virtually all persons will develop an occasional blemish or lesion during adolescence. The nurse, through observation and listening, finds out how patients perceive their skin condition. One young person will view a small blemish as intolerable, while another teenager will regard more extensive involvement as "normal." Adolescents, who are in their formative years of development, are vulnerable and need to be approached with empathy and compassion as they attempt to deal with acne. The nurse keeps this in mind during her assessment and other contacts with adolescents.

When assessing the patient, the skin is stretched gently and the lesions are inspected. Closed comedones (which are precursors of larger inflammatory lesions) appear as slightly elevated small papules. Open comedones appear flat or slightly raised with a central follicular impaction. The presence of inflammatory lesions (papules, pustules, nodules, or cysts) is documented.

▷ Nursing Diagnoses

Based on the nursing assessment data, major nursing diagnoses for the patient may include the following:

- Impaired skin integrity related to disruptions of epidermal and dermal tissue by lesions and erythema
- Knowledge deficit of cause and treatment of acne
- Body image disturbance related to embarrassment and frustration over appearance

▷ Planning and Implementation

▷ *Goals:* The major goals of the patient include development of knowledge and understanding of the condition, compliance with prescribed therapy, and development of self-acceptance.

▷ Nursing Interventions

▷ *Patient Education and Home Health Care.* Before treatment is initiated, patients are counseled and assured that the problem is not related to uncleanliness, dietary indiscretions, masturbation, sexual activity, or any of the other common misconceptions. It is important to reinforce the concept that acne arises because of a combination of factors, including heredity, large sebaceous glands, and large numbers of *P. acnes* bacteria, all of which are beyond the control of the patient.

When treatment is instituted, it usually takes 4 to 6 weeks or longer for results to be seen. Patients are instructed to wash the face with mild soap and water twice a day to remove the surface oils and prevent obstruction of the oil glands. They are cautioned to avoid scrubbing the face constantly, because acne is not caused by dirt and cannot be washed away. Mild abrasive soaps and drying agents are prescribed to eliminate the oily feeling that troubles many patients. However, excessive abrasion is to be avoided because it only makes acne worse. It is also important to realize that soap itself can be irritating to the skin. The use of a polyester sponge pad (Buf-Puf) provides the mechanical removal of superficial skin cells (*epidermabrasion*) and may be helpful to some patients. Hair should be kept off the face and shampooed daily if necessary.

All forms of friction and trauma are to be avoided: propping the hands against the face, rubbing the face, and wearing tight collars and helmets. Patients are instructed to keep hands away from the face and not to squeeze pimples or blackheads. Squeezing merely worsens the problem, because a portion of the blackhead is pushed down into the skin, which may cause the follicle to rupture. Because cosmetics, shaving creams, and lotions can aggravate acne, these substances are best avoided unless the patient is advised otherwise. There is no evidence that a particular food can cause or worsen acne. In general, a nutritious diet is followed.

Patients are counseled that acne is not something that can be cleared up in a short time and that they must be consistent with treatment *every day*. They are instructed to use the cleansing product prescribed by the physician. It is helpful to reassure them that most acne medications cause some degree of drying and peeling, although the sudden appearance of diffuse redness and vesicles suggests contact allergy. Misconceptions must be corrected because understanding promotes compliance and a better chance of success.

▷ *Development of Self-Acceptance.* The patient is enrolled as a partner in therapy. It is of great importance that the problems be taken seriously and that the patient be given understanding, reassurance, and support. All facets of the emotional factors involved must be taken into account, including the possibility that acne can become a power struggle between teenager and parents. Stressful situations (*e.g.*, final exams) cause exacerbations. Stress reduction techniques may be helpful.

▷ Evaluation

Expected Outcomes

1. Develops increasing understanding of the skin problem
   a. Reviews drawings of obstructive and inflammatory lesions of acne
   b. Reads patient education brochures
   c. Verbalizes that picking and squeezing blemishes/lesions will worsen the condition and may cause scarring
   d. Reads the product information brochure of the prescribed medication
2. Adheres to the prescribed therapy
   a. States he will make a major commitment to required treatment that may take months or years
   b. Verbalizes that he must continue with the treatment when the skin clears
   c. Follows cleansing program
   d. Avoids overcleansing
3. Develops self-acceptance
   a. Identifies someone with whom he can talk over problems
   b. Expresses optimism about outcome of treatment

Infections and Infestations of the Skin

Bacterial Infections (Pyodermas)

Bacterial infections of the skin may be primary or secondary. Primary skin infections originate in previously normal-appearing skin and are usually caused by a single organism. Secondary skin infections arise from a preexisting skin disorder in which several microorganisms may be implicated.

The most common primary bacterial skin infections are impetigo and folliculitis. Folliculitis may lead to furuncles or carbuncles.

Impetigo

Impetigo is a superficial infection of the skin caused by streptococci, staphylococci, or multiple bacteria. The lesions begin as small, red macules, which quickly become discrete, thin-walled vesicles that soon rupture and become covered with a loosely adherent honey-yellow crust (Fig. 51-9). These crusts are easily removed and reveal smooth, red, moist surfaces on which new crusts soon develop. If the scalp is involved, the hair is matted, distinguishing the condition from ringworm.

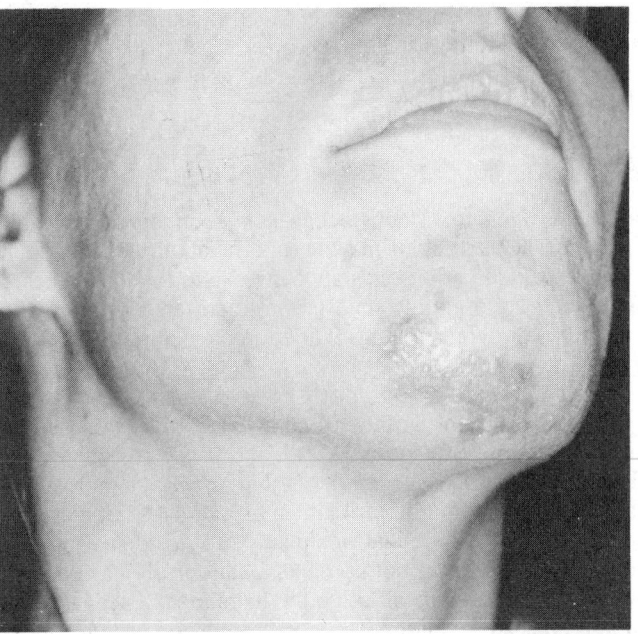

Figure 51-9. Impetigo of the chin. (Courtesy of Mervyn L. Elgart, MD)

The exposed areas of the body, face, hands, neck, and extremities are most frequently involved. Impetigo is contagious and may spread to other parts of the patient's skin or to other members of the family who touch the patient or use towels or combs that are soiled with the exudate of the lesions.

Although impetigo is seen at all ages, it is particularly common among children living in poor hygienic conditions. Often it appears secondary to pediculosis capitis, scabies, herpes simplex, insect bites, poison ivy, or eczema. In adults, ill health, poor hygiene, and malnutrition may predispose to impetigo.

Bullous impetigo, a superficial infection of the skin caused by *Staphylococcus aureus*, is characterized by the formation of bullae from original vesicles. The bullae rupture, leaving a raw, red area.

Management. Systemic antibiotic therapy is the usual treatment. It is used to reduce contagious spread, treat deep infection, and prevent acute glomerulonephritis, which has been known to occur as an aftermath of streptococcal skin diseases. In nonbullous impetigo, benzathine penicillin or oral penicillin may be given. Bullous impetigo is treated with a penicillinase-resistant penicillin (cloxacillin, dicloxacillin).

An antiseptic preparation (povidone-iodine [Betadine]; chlorhexidine [Hibiclens]) may be used to cleanse the skin and reduce bacterial content in the vicinity of the infection to prevent spread.

The lesions are soaked or washed with soap solution to remove the central site of bacterial growth and to give the topical antibiotic an opportunity to reach the infected site. After the crusts are removed, a topical medication (*e.g.*, neomycin, bacitracin) is applied. Topical treatment must be performed several times a day. Gloves should be worn when care is given to these patients.

Patient Education and Home Health Care. The patient and family should be instructed to bathe at least once daily with bactericidal soap. Cleanliness and good hygienic practices help prevent the spread of the lesions from one skin area to another and from one person to another. Each person should have a separate towel and washcloth. Because impetigo is a contagious disorder, an infected child should be kept away from other children.

Folliculitis, Furuncles, and Carbuncles

Folliculitis refers to a staphylococcal infection that arises within the hair follicles. Lesions may be superficial or deep. Single or multiple papules or pustules appear close to the hair follicles. Folliculitis is commonly seen in the beard area of men who shave and on women's legs. Other areas include the axillae, trunk, and buttocks.

Pseudofolliculitis barbae ("shaving bumps") is an inflammatory reaction on the face of curly-haired males caused by ingrowing hairs that pierce the skin and cause an irritative reaction. Curly hair has a curved root that grows at a more acute angle. This is a common problem in black males but may also occur in others. The initial treatment is to avoid shaving and grow a beard. If this is not possible, a handbrush may be used over the facial area to dislodge the hairs mechanically. If the patient must shave, a depilatory cream may be useful.

A furuncle (boil) is an acute inflammation arising *deep* in one or more hair follicles and spreading into the surrounding dermis. It is a deeper form of folliculitis. (*Furunculosis* refers to multiple or recurrent lesions.) Furuncles may occur anywhere on the body but are more prevalent in areas subjected to irritation, pressure, friction, and excessive perspiration, such as the back of the neck, the axillae, or the buttocks.

A furuncle may start as a small, red, raised, painful "pimple." Frequently, the infection progresses and involves the skin and subcutaneous fatty tissue, causing tenderness, pain, and surrounding cellulitis. The area of redness and induration represents an effort of the body to keep the infection localized. The bacteria (usually staphylococcus) produce necrosis of the invaded tissues, followed in a few days by the characteristic pointing of a boil. When this occurs, the center becomes yellow or black, and the boil is said popularly to have "come to a head."

A carbuncle is an abscess of the skin and subcutaneous tissue representing an extension of a furuncle that has invaded several follicles and is larger and more deep-seated. It is usually caused by a staphylococcal infection. Carbuncles appear most commonly in areas in which the skin is thick and inelastic. The back of the neck and the buttocks are common sites. In carbuncles, the extensive inflammation frequently is not associated with a complete walling off of the infection, so absorption occurs, resulting in high fever, pain, leukocytosis, and even extension of the infection to the bloodstream.

Furuncles and carbuncles are more apt to occur in patients with underlying systemic diseases, such as diabetes or hematologic malignancies, and those receiving immunosuppressive therapy for other diseases. Both are more prevalent in hot climates, especially on skin beneath occlusive clothing.

Management.   In the treatment of staphylococcal infections, it is important not to rupture or destroy the protective wall of induration that has localized the infection. Therefore, the boil or pimple should never be squeezed.

The follicular disorders (folliculitis, furuncles, carbuncles) are usually caused by staphylococci. If the immune system is impaired, the causative organisms may be gram-negative bacilli.

Systemic antibiotic therapy, selected by sensitivity study, is generally indicated. Oral cloxacillin, dicloxacillin, and flucloxacillin are first-line drug therapy. Cephalosporins and erythromycin are also effective.

Intravenous fluids, fever sponges, and other supportive modalities are indicated for the very ill and toxic patient. Warm, moist compresses increase vascularization and hasten resolution of the furuncle or carbuncle. The surrounding skin may be cleansed gently with antibacterial soap and followed by the application of an antibacterial ointment.

When the pus has localized and is fluctuant (moving in palpable waves), a small incision with a scalpel will speed resolution by relieving the tension and ensuring a direct evacuation of the pus and slough. The patient is instructed to keep the draining lesion covered with a dressing. Soiled dressings should be handled according to universal precaution guidelines. Nursing personnel should carefully follow isolation precautions in order to avoid becoming staphylococcus carriers. Disposable gloves should be worn when caring for these patients.

- Special precautions must be taken with boils on the face, because the skin area drains directly into the cranial venous sinuses. Sinus thrombosis, with fatal pyemia, has been known to develop after manipulation of a boil in this location.

Bed rest is advised for patients who have boils on the perineum or in the anal region, and a course of systemic antibiotic therapy is indicated to control the spread of the infection.

Patient Education.   To prevent and control staphylococcal skin infections (boils, carbuncles), the staphylococcus must be eliminated from the skin and environment. Efforts must be made to increase the patient's resistance and provide a hygienic environment.

If lesions are actively draining, the mattress and pillow should be covered with plastic material and wiped off with disinfectant daily; the bed linens, towels, and clothing should be laundered after each use; and the patient should shower and shampoo with an antibacterial soap and shampoo for an indefinite period, often for several months. Prevention of recurrent infection has been achieved by prescribed antibiotics such as a daily dose of oral clindamycin to be taken continuously for about 3 months. It is essential that the patient take the full dose for the time prescribed. The purulent exudate (pus) is a source of reinfection or transmission of infection to caregivers.

When the patient has a history of recurrent infections, a carrier state (external nares) may exist, which should be investigated and treated with an antibacterial cream.

Viral Infections

Herpes Zoster (Shingles)

Herpes zoster (shingles) is an inflammatory viral condition in which the virus produces a painful vesicular eruption along the distribution of the nerves from one or more posterior ganglia. It is caused by the varicella virus, commonly known as varicella-zoster virus, which is a member of a group of DNA viruses. (The viruses of chickenpox and zoster are indistinguishable; hence the name varicella-zoster.) It is assumed that herpes zoster represents a reactivation of latent varicella (chickenpox) virus and reflects a lowered immunity. After a case of chickenpox runs its course, it is believed that the varicella-zoster viruses responsible for the outbreak lie dormant inside nerve cells near the brain and spinal cord. Later, when these latent viruses are reactivated, they travel by way of the peripheral nerves to the skin. There, the viruses multiply, creating a red rash of small fluid-filled blisters. About 10% of adults get shingles during their lifetime, usually after the age of 50. There is an increased frequency of herpes zoster in patients with weakened immune systems and malignancies, especially the leukemias and the lymphomas.

Clinical Manifestations. The eruption is generally accompanied or preceded by pain, which may radiate over the entire region supplied by the nerves. The pain may be burning, lancinating (tearing; sharply cutting), stabbing, or aching. In some patients the pain is absent. Some itching and tenderness may occur over the area. At times, malaise and gastrointestinal disturbances precede the eruption.

The patches of grouped vesicles appear on the red and swollen skin. The early vesicles contain serum and later become purulent, rupture, and form crusts. The inflammation is usually unilateral, involving the thoracic, cervical, or cranial nerves in a bandlike configuration. The blisters are usually confined to a narrow region of the face or trunk. The clinical course varies from 1 to 3 weeks. If an ophthalmic nerve is involved, the patient may have a painful eye. Inflammation and a rash on the trunk may cause pain at the slightest touch. The healing time varies between 7 and 26 days.

Herpes zoster in healthy adults is usually localized and benign. However, in immunosuppressed patients, the disease may be severe and the clinical course acutely disabling.

Management. The goals of management are to relieve the pain and to reduce or avoid complications. These include infection, scarring, and postherpetic neuralgia and eye complications.

The pain is controlled with analgesics, because adequate pain control during the acute phase will help prevent persistent pain patterns.

Systemic corticosteroids are prescribed for patients over age 50 to reduce the incidence and duration of postherpetic neuralgia (persistent pain of affected nerve following healing). Healing is usually more rapid in those who have been treated with steroids. Triamcinolone (Aristocort, Kenacort, Kenalog) injected subcutaneously under painful areas is effective as an anti-inflammatory agent.

There is some evidence that infection is arrested if oral acyclovir is administered within 24 hours of the appearance of the eruption. Intravenous acyclovir, if started early, is effective in significantly reducing the pain and halting the progression of the disease. Another antiviral drug, vidarabine, may also be tried.

If the eye is involved, the patient is referred to an ophthalmologist, because keratitis, uveitis, ulceration, and blindness may occur. This is referred to as ophthalmic herpes zoster.

A susceptible person can acquire chicken pox through contact with the infective vesicular fluid of a zoster patient. A person with a previous history of chicken pox is immune and thus not at risk of infection after exposure to zoster patients. In older persons, the pain from herpes zoster may persist as postherpetic neuralgia for months after the skin lesions disappear.

Patient Education and Home Health Care. The nurse assesses the patient's discomfort and response to medication and collaborates with the physician to make necessary adjustments to the treatment regimen. The patient is taught how to apply wet dressings or medication to the lesions and to follow proper hand washing techniques to avoid spreading the herpes zoster virus.

Diversionary activities and relaxation techniques are encouraged to assure restful sleep—all of which help to alleviate discomfort.

Because so many of these patients are elderly, a caregiver may be required to assist with dressings. Relatives, neighbors, or a community health nurse may need to help with dressing changes and food preparation for patients who are unable to care for themselves or prepare nourishing meals.

In summary, herpes zoster is becoming more prevalent in persons who are immunocompromised (post–organ transplant patients, those receiving chemotherapy or radiation therapy for malignancies, or patients with AIDS). These persons are very susceptible to the development of opportunistic infections that may become life-threatening. Prevention of herpes zoster or prompt recognition of those most susceptible is essential for a favorable outcome. Fortunately, herpes zoster is a self-limiting disease even in the immunosuppressed patient.

Mycotic (Fungal) Infections

The fungi, tiny representatives of the plant kingdom that feed on organic matter, are responsible for a variety of common skin infections. In some cases, they affect only the skin and its appendages (*i.e.*, hair and nails), but in others, the internal organs are involved. In the latter instance, fungal disease may be so serious that it constitutes a threat to life. Superficial infections, on the other hand, rarely cause temporary disability and respond readily to treatment. Secondary infection with bacteria or *Candida* or both may occur.

The most common fungal skin disorder is known as tinea or "ringworm." Tinea infections affect the feet (commonly called "athlete's foot") (tinea pedis); the scalp (tinea capitis); the body, including the face, neck, and extremities (tinea corporis); the groin ("jock itch") (tinea cruris); and the nails (tinea unguium). Table 51-7 summarizes the tinea infections.

To obtain material for diagnosis, the lesion is cleaned and a scalpel is used to remove scales from the margin of the lesion. The scales are dropped onto a slide to which potassium hydroxide has been added. The diagnosis is made by examining the infected scales microscopically and by isolating the organism in culture.

Wood's light induces fluorescence of a specimen of infected hair and may be helpful in diagnosing some cases of tinea capitis.

Tinea Pedis (Ringworm of the Feet; Athlete's Foot)

Tinea pedis is the most common fungal infection. It may appear as an acute or chronic infection to the soles of the feet or the space between the toes. The toenail may also be involved with chronic infection. Lymphangitis and cellulitis may be seen occasionally when bacterial superinfection occurs. Sometimes a mixed fungal, bacterial, and yeast infection occurs.

TABLE 51–7.   *Tinea Fungal Infections (Ringworm)*

Type and Location	Clinical Manifestations	Treatment
Tinea capitis (ringworm of scalp)	Contagious infection of the hair shaft. Common in children. Round patches of redness and scaling. Small pustules or papules at edges. Hair brittle; breaks easily at scalp.	Griseofulvin. Shampoo hair 2–3 times a week
Tinea corporis (ringworm of body)	Begins with erythematous macule advancing to rings of papules or vesicles with central clearing. Lesions found in clusters—may extend to scalp, hair, or nails. Pruritic. (Infected pet may be the source.)	Ketoconazole Griseofulvin
Tinea cruris (ringworm of groin— "jock itch")	Pruritus with small, red, scaly patches extending to circular plaques with elevated scaly or vesicular borders.	*Mild conditions:* Topical medications Clotrimazole Miconazole Haloprogin *Severe conditions:* Oral griseofulvin
Tinea pedis (ringworm of feet— "athlete's foot")	Pruritus—soles of feet, spaces between toes affected. Inflamed vesicles (acute) or scaly, dusky, or red rash (chronic).	*Acute infections:* Soak with Burow's solution, saline, or potassium permanganate. Topical antifungals: Miconazole Clotrimazole *Resistant infections:* Griseofulvin
Tinea unguium (ringworm of nails)	More common in toenails. Associated with long-standing fungal infection of feet. Nails thicken, crumble easily, and lack luster. Whole nail may be destroyed.	*Long-term therapy* (6 mo–1 yr): Griseofulvin (for fingernails) Amphotericin B lotion; miconazole; clotrimazole Nystatin (if *Candida albicans* etiology)

Preventive Measures and Patient Education.   Because footwear provides a favorable environment for fungi, the causative fungi may be in the shoes and socks. Because moisture encourages the growth of fungi, the patient is instructed to keep the feet as dry as possible, including the areas between the toes. Small pieces of cotton can be placed between the toes at night to absorb moisture. Socks should be made of absorbent cotton, and hosiery should have cotton feet, because synthetic material does not absorb perspiration as well as cotton. For persons whose feet perspire excessively, perforated shoes permit better aeration of the feet. Plastic- or rubber-soled footwear should be avoided. Talcum powder or antifungal powder applied twice daily helps to keep the feet dry. Several pairs of shoes should be alternated so that they can dry completely before they are worn again.

Management.   During the acute (vesicular) phase, soaks of Burow's solution, saline, or potassium permanganate are used to remove the crusts, scales, and debris and to reduce the inflammation. Topical antifungals (miconazole; clotrimazole) are applied to the infected areas. Topical therapy is continued for several weeks, because there is a high rate of recurrence.

Tinea Corporis (Ringworm of the Body)

Tinea corporis affects the face, neck, trunk, and extremities. Animal varieties (nonhuman variety) are known to cause an intense inflammatory reaction in humans because they are not normally adapted to living on human hosts. The typical "ringed" lesion is produced. Humans make contact with animal varieties through contact with pets or through contact with objects that have been in contact with an animal.

Management.   Topical antifungal medication may be applied to small areas. Griseofulvin is used in extensive cases.

Side effects of griseofulvin include photosensitivity, skin rashes, headache, and nausea. Ketoconazole, an antifungal agent, shows real promise in patients with chronic fungal (dermatophyte) infections, including those resistant to griseofulvin.

Patient Education.   The patient is instructed to use a clean towel and washcloth daily. All areas and skin folds that retain moisture must be dried thoroughly, because fungal infections are fostered by heat and moisture. Clean cotton clothing should be worn next to the skin.

Tinea Capitis (Ringworm of the Scalp)

Ringworm of the scalp is a contagious fungal infection of the hair shafts and a common cause of hair loss in children. Clinically, one or several round patches of redness and scaling are present. Small pustules or papules may be seen at the edges of such patches. As the hairs in the affected areas are invaded by the fungi, they become brittle and often break off at or near the surface of the scalp, resulting in areas of baldness. Most cases of tinea capitis heal without scarring, so the hair loss is only temporary.

Management.   Griseofulvin, an antifungal agent, is prescribed for patients with tinea capitis. Topical agents are not effective as a cure because the infection occurs within the hair shaft and below the surface of the scalp. However, topical agents are often used to inactivate organisms already on the hair. This diminishes contagiousness and eliminates the need to clip the hair. Infected hairs break off anyway, and noninfected ones may be left in place. The hair should be shampooed two to three times weekly, and a topical antifungal preparation should be applied to reduce dissemination of the organisms.

Patient Education and Home Health Care.   Because the disease is contagious, the patient and family should be advised to set up a hygienic regimen for home use. Each person should have a separate comb and brush and should avoid exchanging headgear. All infected members of the family and household pets must be examined because familial infections are relatively common.

Tinea Cruris (Ringworm of the Groin)

Tinea cruris ("jock itch") is ringworm infection of the groin, which may extend to the inner thighs and buttock area. It is commonly associated with tinea pedis. It occurs most frequently in young joggers, obese persons, and those who wear tight underclothing.

Management.   Mild infections may be treated with topical medication such as clotrimazole, miconazole, or haloprogin for at least 3 to 4 weeks to ensure complete eradication of the infection. Oral griseofulvin may be required for more severe infections.

Patient Education and Home Health Care.   Heat, friction, and maceration (from sweating) predispose to the infection. The patient is instructed to avoid as far as possible excessive heat and humidity, nylon underwear, tight-fitting clothing, and the prolonged wearing of a wet bathing suit. The groin area should be cleansed, dried thoroughly, and dusted with a topical antifungal agent (tolnaftate [Tinactin]) as a preventive measure, because the infection is apt to recur.

Tinea Unguium (Onychomycosis)

Tinea unguium (ringworm of the nails) is a chronic fungal infection of the toenails or, less commonly, the fingernails and is usually caused by *Trichophyton* species (*T. rubrum*, *T. mentagrophytes*) or *Candida albicans*. It is usually associated with long-standing fungal infection of the feet. The nails become thickened, friable (easily crumbled), and lusterless. In time, debris accumulates under the free edge of the nail, and ultimately the nail plate becomes separated. Because of the chronic nature of this infection, the entire nail may ultimately be destroyed.

Management.   Griseofulvin is usually prescribed orally for 6 months to a year when the fingernails are involved. Of course, griseofulvin is not of value in treating candidal infections; these must be treated topically with amphotericin-B lotion, miconazole, clotrimazole, nystatin, or other preparations. These products penetrate poorly, and the infections are difficult to treat. Response to griseofulvin in fungal infections of the toenails is poor at best. Frequently, when the treatment is stopped the infection returns.

In summary, fungal infection of the skin is called tinea but is more popularly known as "ringworm." The lesions are usually but not always ring shaped. The fungi grow well in areas of the body that are prone to excessive perspiration (between skin folds, groin, axillae, feet). These fungal infections are contagious and can be spread by direct contact with the infected person or by contact with objects used by the individual (*e.g.*, comb, towel). Scratching is a means of spreading the infection from one body area to another. Treatment includes body cleanliness, thorough drying following bathing, and therapy with antifungal agents.

Parasitic Skin Diseases

Pediculosis (Infestation by Lice)

Lice infestation affects persons of all ages. Three varieties of lice infest humans: *Pediculus humanus capitis* (head louse); *Pediculus humanus corporis* (body louse); and *Phthirus pubis* (pubic, or "crab," louse). Lice are termed *ectoparasites* because they live on the outside of the host's body. They depend on the host for their nourishment, feeding on human blood approximately five times a day. They inject their digestive juices and excrement into the skin, which causes severe itching.

Pediculosis Capitis

Pediculosis capitis is an infestation of the scalp by the head louse, *Pediculus humanus capitis*. The female head louse lays her eggs (nits) close to the scalp. The nits become firmly attached to the hair shafts with a tenacious substance. The young lice hatch in about 10 days and reach maturity in 2 weeks. Head lice are found most commonly along the back of the head and behind the ears. The eggs are visible to the naked eye as silvery, glistening oval bodies that are difficult to remove from the hair. The bite of the insect causes *intense itching*, and the resultant scratching often leads to secondary bacterial infection with pustules, crusts, matted hair, impetigo, and furunculosis. The infestation is more common in children and people with long hair. Head lice may be transmitted by direct physical contact or indirectly by the use of infested combs, brushes, wigs, hats, and bedding.

Management.   Treatment involves washing the hair with a shampoo containing lindane (Kwell) or pyrethrin compounds with piperonyl butoxide (RID or R&C Shampoo). The patient is instructed to shampoo the scalp and hair according to the product directives. After the hair is rinsed thoroughly, it is combed with a fine-toothed comb that is dipped in vinegar to remove any remaining nits or nit shells freed from the hair shafts. These are extremely difficult to remove and may have to be picked off with the fingernails, one by one (hence the expression *nit picking*). All articles, clothing, towels, and bedding that might have lice or nits should be washed in hot water (at least 54°C [130°F]) or dry-cleaned to prevent reinfestation. Upholstered furniture, rugs, and floors should be vacuumed frequently. Combs and brushes are also disinfected with the shampoo. All family members and close contacts are treated.

Complications such as severe pruritus, pyoderma (pus-forming infection of the skin), and dermatitis are treated with antipruritics, systemic antibiotics, and topical corticosteroids.

Patient Education.   The patient is reassured that head lice infestation may happen to anyone and is not a sign of uncleanliness. This condition spreads rapidly, so treatment must be started immediately. Control of school epidemics may be helped by having all of the students shampoo their hair on the same night. Students should be warned not to share combs, brushes, or hats. Each family member should be inspected for head lice daily for at least 2 weeks. The patient should be instructed that lindane may be toxic when not used properly.

Pediculosis Corporis and Pediculosis Pubis

Pediculosis corporis is an infestation of the body by the body louse, *Pediculus humanus corporis*. This is a disease of the unwashed, usually homeless persons or those who live in close quarters such as shelters and do not change their clothing. The body louse lives chiefly in the seams of underwear and clothing, to which it clings as it pierces the skin with its proboscis. Its bites cause characteristic minute hemorrhagic points. Widespread excoriation may appear as a result of intense itching and scratching, especially on the trunk and neck. Among the secondary lesions produced are parallel linear scratches and a slight degree of eczema. In long-standing cases, the skin may become thickened, dry, and scaly, with dark pigmented areas. The areas of the skin chiefly involved are those that come in closest contact with the underclothing (*i.e.*, the neck, trunk, and thighs). The lice may be seen even in the seams of the clothing, so the clothing and bedding must be laundered or dry-cleaned to destroy the parasite and its eggs. A shower should be taken and precautionary methods followed to prevent reinfestation.

Complications such as severe pruritus, pyoderma (pus-forming infection of the skin), and dermatitis are treated with antipruritics, systemic antibiotics, and topical corticosteroids. It is important to remember that body lice are capable of transmitting epidemic disease in humans, namely, rickettsial disease (epidemic typhus, relapsing fever, and trench fever). The causative organism may be in the gastrointestinal tract of the insect and may be excreted on the skin surface of the infested person.

Pediculosis pubis, infestation by *Phthirus pubis* (crab louse), is an extremely common problem that is generally localized in the genital region and transmitted chiefly by sexual contact.

Reddish brown "dust" from the excretions of the insects

may be found in underclothing. Lice may also infest the hairs of the chest, axillary hair, beard, and eyelashes. Gray-blue macules may sometimes be seen on the trunk, thighs, and axillae as a result of either the reaction of the insects' saliva with bilirubin (converting it to biliverdin) or an excretion produced by the salivary glands of the louse. The pubic crease should be examined with a magnifying glass to detect the presence of *Phthirus pubis* crawling down a hair shaft or nits cemented to the hair or at the junction with the skin. Itching is the most common symptom, particularly at night. Infestation by pubic lice may coexist with other sexually transmitted diseases (gonorrhea, candidiasis, syphilis).

Management and Patient Education.   The patient is instructed to bathe with soap and water. Then either lindane (Kwell) or malathion in isopropyl alcohol (Prioderm lotion) is applied to affected areas of the skin and to hairy areas, according to the product information directives. An alternative topical therapy is a pyrethrin-based pediculicide (RID, which is an over-the-counter preparation) or 0.03% copper oleate (Cuprex). If the eyelashes are involved, petrolatum may be thickly applied twice daily for 8 days, followed by mechanical removal of any remaining nits.

All sexual contacts and family members must be treated. The patient and partner must also be scheduled for a diagnostic workup for coexisting sexually transmitted disease. All clothing and bedding should be machine-washed or dry-cleaned.

Scabies

Scabies is an infestation of the skin by the itch mite, *Sarcoptes scabiei*. The disease may be found in poor persons living under substandard hygienic conditions, but it is also common in very clean individuals. It is often found among the sexually active. However, infestations are not dependent on sexual activity, because the mites frequently involve the fingers, and hand contact may produce infection. In children, overnight stays with friends or the exchange of clothes may be a source of infection. Health care personnel who have prolonged "hands on" physical contact with an infected patient may likewise become infected.

The adult female burrows into the superficial layer of the skin and remains there for the rest of her life. With her jaws and the sharp edges of the joints of her forelegs, the mite extends the burrow, laying two to three eggs daily for up to 2 months. She then dies. The larvae (eggs) hatch in 3 to 4 days and progress through larval and nymphal states to form adult mites in about 10 days.

Clinical Manifestations.   It takes approximately 4 weeks from the time of contact for the patient's symptoms to appear. The patient complains of severe itching caused by a delayed type of immunologic reaction to the mite or its fecal pellets. During examination, the patient is asked where the itch is most severe. A magnifying glass and a penlight are held at an oblique angle to the skin while a search is made for the small, raised burrows. The burrows may be multiple, straight or wavy, brown or black, threadlike lesions, most commonly observed between the fingers and on the wrists.

Other sites are the extensor surfaces of the elbows, the knees, the edges of the feet, the points of the elbows, around the nipples, in the axillary folds, under pendulous breasts, and in or near the groin or gluteal fold, penis, or scrotum. Red pruritic eruptions usually appear between adjacent skin areas. The burrow, however, is not always seen. Any patient with a rash may have scabies.

One classic sign of scabies is the increased itching that occurs at night, perhaps because the increased warmth of the skin has a stimulating effect on the parasite. Also, hypersensitivity to the organism and its products of excretion may contribute to the itching. If the infection has spread, other members of the family and close friends will also complain of itching about a month later.

Secondary lesions are quite common and include vesicles, papules, excoriations, and crusts. Bacterial superinfection may result from constant excoriation of the burrows and papules.

The diagnosis is confirmed by recovering *Sarcoptes scabiei* or the mites' by-products from the skin. A sample of superficial epidermis is scraped off the top of the burrows or papules with a small scalpel blade. The scrapings are placed on a microscope slide and examined through a low-powered microscope to demonstrate the presence of any stage of the mite (adult, eggs, egg casings, larva, nymph) and fecal pellets.

Patient Education. The patient is instructed to take a warm, soapy bath or shower to remove the scaling debris from the crusts and then to dry thoroughly and allow the skin to cool.

It is important that the patient understand these directions, because application of a scabicide immediately after bathing and prior to drying and cooling of the skin increases percutaneous absorption of the scabicide and the potential for CNS side effects such as seizures.

A scabicide, such as lindane (Kwell) or crotamiton (Eurax cream and lotion), is applied thinly to the entire skin from the neck down, sparing only the face and scalp (which are not affected in scabies). The medication is left on for 12 to 24 hours, after which the patient is instructed to wash thoroughly. One application may be curative, but it is advisable to repeat the treatment in 1 week.

The patient should wear clean clothing and sleep between freshly laundered bed linens. All bedding and clothing should be washed in very hot water and dried on the hot dryer cycle because the mites are known to survive up to 36 hours in linens away from the host. If bed linen or clothing cannot be washed in hot water it is advised that they be dry-cleaned.

After the treatment is completed, an ointment, such as a topical corticosteroid ointment, is applied to skin lesions because the scabicide may be irritating to the skin. The hypersensitivity state does not cease upon destruction of the mites. Itching may remain a troublesome problem for a few days or weeks, because itching is a manifestation of hypersensitivity, particularly in atopic (allergic) persons. However, this is not a sign that the treatment has failed. The patient is instructed *not* to apply more scabicide (because this will cause more irritation and increased itching) and *not* to take frequent hot showers (because this dries the skin and produces itching).

All family members and close contacts should be treated simultaneously to eliminate the mites. If scabies is sexually transmitted, the patient may require treatment for coexisting sexually transmitted disease. Scabies may also coexist with pediculosis.

Gerontologic Considerations. Although the older patient itches severely, the vivid inflammatory reaction seen in younger people is usually absent. Scabies may not be recognized in the elderly, and the itching may erroneously be attributed to the dry skin of old age or to anxiety.

For patients in extended care facilities, health care personnel should wear gloves when providing hands-on care for a patient suspected of having scabies until the diagnosis is confirmed and treatment accomplished. It is advisable that all residents, staff, and families of patients be treated as described at the same time to prevent reinfection.

In summary, scabies is the result of infestation by the female mite *Sarcoptes scabiei* (*var hominis*). The mite burrows underneath the skin, laying eggs that hatch and reach adult dimensions in 10 days. Clinical symptoms include intense itching between the fingers, on the wrists and trunk, in the axillary folds, under the breasts in women, and on the penile shaft in men. Symptoms are worse at night. The treatment most widely used is 1% gamma benzene hexachloride (lindane) lotion.

Contact Dermatitis

Contact dermatitis (dermatitis venenata) is an inflammatory reaction of the skin to physical, chemical, or biologic agents. The epidermis is damaged by repeated physical and chemical irritations. Contact dermatitis may be of the primary irritant type, in which a nonallergic reaction results from exposure to an irritating substance, or it may be allergic in nature (*allergic contact dermatitis*), resulting from exposure of sensitized persons to contact allergens. (Allergic dermatoses are discussed in Chap. 49.) Common causes of *irritant contact dermatitis* are soaps, detergents, scouring compounds, and industrial chemicals. Predisposing factors include extremes of heat and cold, frequent immersion in soap and water, and a preexisting skin disease.

Clinical Manifestations

The eruptions begin at the point at which the causative agent contacts the skin. The first reactions include itching, burning, and erythema, followed soon by edema, papules, vesicles, and oozing or weeping. In the subacute phase, these vesicular changes are less marked and alternate with crusting, drying, fissuring, and peeling. If repeated reactions occur, or if the patient continually scratches the skin, thickening of the skin (*lichenification*) and pigmentation (*coloration*) occur. Secondary bacterial invasion may follow.

Management

The objectives of management are to rest the involved skin and protect it from further damage. The distribution pattern of the reaction is determined in order to differentiate between allergic contact dermatitis and the irritant type. A detailed history is obtained. Then the offending irritant is identified and removed. Local irritation should be avoided, and soap is not generally used until healing occurs.

There are many preparations advocated for the relief of dermatitis. In general, a bland, unmedicated lotion is used for small patches of erythema. Cool, wet dressings also are applied over small areas of vesicular dermatitis. Finely cracked ice added to the water often enhances its antipruritic effect. Wet dressings usually help clear the oozing eczematous lesions. Then a thin layer of cream or ointment containing one of the steroids may be used. Medicated baths at room temperature are prescribed for larger areas of dermatitis. In more widespread conditions, a short course of systemic steroids may be prescribed.

Patient Education and Home Health Care

The patient is instructed as follows:

- Study the pattern of your dermatitis (location on the skin) and think about things that have touched your skin and may have caused the problem.
- Try to avoid contact with these materials.
- Avoid heat, soap, and rubbing, all of which are external irritants.
- Avoid topical medications except when specifically prescribed.
- Wash the skin thoroughly immediately after exposure to irritants or antigens.
- When gloves are used for washing dishes, use cotton-lined gloves but do not wear them more than 15 to 20 minutes at a time.

The instructions should be followed for at least 4 months after the skin appears to be completely healed, because the resistance of the skin is lowered.

In summary, contact dermatitis is an external inflammatory response by the skin to a chemical or physical irritant where an allergen is not involved. These skin reactions are more common than allergic contact dermatitis. Skin reaction ranges from mild erythema to inflammation, vesicle formation, and pain. Most cases of contact dermatitis are located on the hands, face, and eyelids and remain confined. Removal or avoidance of the irritant usually results in clearing of the skin. Patch testing should be performed cn cases that do not clear within a short time.

Noninfectious Inflammatory Dermatoses

Psoriasis

Psoriasis is a chronic noninfectious inflammatory disease of the skin in which the production of epidermal cells occurs at a rate that is approximately six to nine times faster than normal. The cells in the basal layer of the skin divide too quickly, and the newly formed cells move so rapidly to the skin surface that they become evident as profuse scales or plaques of epidermal tissue. The psoriatic epidermal cell may travel from the basal cell layer of the epidermis to the stratum corneum (skin surface) and be cast off in 3 to 4 days, which is in sharp contrast to the normal 26 to 28 days. As a result of the increased number of basal cells and rapid cell passage, the normal events of cell maturation and growth cannot take place. This abnormal process does not allow formation of the normal protective layers of the skin.

Psoriasis, one of the most common skin diseases, affects approximately 2% of the population. There appears to be a hereditary defect that causes overproduction of keratin. The primary defect is unknown. A combination of specific genetic makeup and environmental stimuli may trigger the onset of the disease. There is some evidence that the cell proliferation is mediated by the immune system. Periods of emotional stress and anxiety aggravate the condition, and trauma, infections, and seasonal and hormonal changes are trigger factors. The onset may occur at any age but is most common between the ages of 10 and 40 years. Psoriasis has a tendency to improve and then recur periodically throughout life.

Clinical Manifestations

The lesions appear as red, raised patches of skin covered with silvery scales. The scaly patches are formed by the buildup of living and dead skin that results from the vast increase in rate of skin-cell growth and turnover (Fig. 51-10). If the scales are scraped away, the dark red base of the lesion is exposed, producing multiple bleeding points. These patches are not moist and may or may not itch. The lesions may remain small, giving rise to the term *guttate psoriasis*. Usually, the lesions enlarge slowly, but after many months they coalesce, forming extensive irregularly shaped patches. Psoriasis may range from a cosmetic source of annoyance to a physically disabling and disfiguring affliction. Particular sites of the body tend to be affected by this ailment; they include the scalp, the area over the elbows and knees, the lower part of the back, and the genitalia. Psoriasis also appears on the extensor surfaces of the arms and legs, on the scalp and ears, and over the sacrum and the intergluteal fold. Bilateral symmetry is a feature of psoriasis. In approximately one quarter to one half of the patients, the nails are involved, with pitting, discoloration, crumbling beneath the free edges, and separation of the nail plate. When psoriasis occurs on the palms and soles, it can cause pustular lesions.

The disease may be associated with asymmetric rheumatoid factor–negative arthritis of multiple joints. The arthritic development can occur either before or after the cutaneous lesions appear.

The relation between arthritis and psoriasis is not understood. Another complication is an exfoliative psoriatic state in which the disease progresses to involve the total body surface.

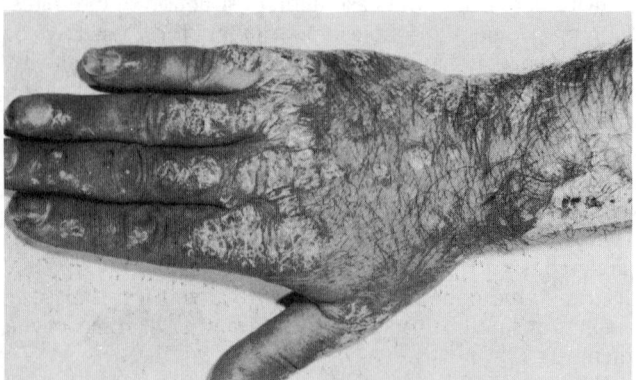

Figure 51-10. Psoriasis of the hand. (Sauer GC. Manual of Skin Diseases, Philadelphia, JB Lippincott.)

Psychologic Considerations

Psoriasis may cause despair and frustration for the patient; observers may stare, comment, ask embarrassing questions, or even avoid the person. The disease can eventually exhaust the patient's resources, interfere with his job, and make life miserable in general. Teenagers are especially vulnerable to the psychologic effects of this ailment. The family, too, is affected, because time-consuming treatments, messy salves, and constant shedding of scales disrupt home life and cause resentment. In many cases, the patient's frustrations are expressed through hostility directed at health care personnel.

Management

The goals of management are to reduce the rapid turnover of epidermis and to promote resolution of the psoriatic lesions. Thus, the goal is limited to control of the problem, because there is no known cure.

The therapeutic approach should be one that the patient understands; it should be cosmetically acceptable and not too disruptive of life-style. It will involve the commitment of time and effort by the patient and possibly the family.

First, any precipitating or aggravating factors are removed. Then an assessment is made of life-style, because psoriasis is significantly affected by stress. The patient must also be advised that treatment of a severe psoriasis can be time-consuming, expensive, and aesthetically unappealing at times.

Therapy can be divided into three types: topical, intralesional, and systemic.

Topical Therapy. Topically applied agents are used to slow down the overactive epidermis without affecting other tissues. Medications include such agents as tar preparations, anthralin, salicylic acid, and corticosteroids. These therapies seem to act by suppressing *epidermopoiesis* (creation of epidermal cells).

Tar is formulated as lotions, ointments, pastes, creams, and shampoos. Tar baths or tar preparations may retard and inhibit the rapid growth of psoriatic tissue. Coal tar preparations are photosensitizing agents, so patients should be warned not to expose treated skin to the sun. This aspect of therapy may be combined with carefully graded doses of ultraviolet-B light, which produces radiation in wavelengths between 280 and 320 nanometers (nm). Ultraviolet-B light seems to potentiate the action of tar. The tar is partially removed prior to ultraviolet light exposure to allow maximum transmission of light. During this phase of treatment, the patient is advised to wear goggles and to protect the eyes. Use of a timer will prevent the danger of severe burns due to overexposure to the light rays. A daily tar shampoo followed by an application of steroid lotion may be used for scalp lesions. The patient is also taught to remove excess scales by scrubbing with a soft brush while bathing.

Anthralin preparations (Anthra-Derm, Dritho-Creme, Lasan) are useful for thick psoriatic plaques that are resistant to other coal tar or steroid preparations. The patient is instructed to apply anthralin medication with a tongue blade or gloved fingers, taking special care not to cover normal skin. The hands must be washed after the medication is handled, because a chemical conjunctivitis can be produced if the patient touches the eyes while medication is still on the hands.

Anthralin stains, leaving a brownish purple skin discoloration that fades once treatment is stopped. Lesions treated with anthralin should be covered in some way (gauze, stockinette, old pajamas) to avoid permanent staining of clothing, furniture, and carpeting. The preparation is left on the skin for 8 to 12 hours.

Topical Corticosteroids. Topical corticosteroids may be applied for their anti-inflammatory activity. Once the medication is applied, the area is covered with an occlusive plastic film dressing to enhance drug penetration and soften the scaly plaques. Tape that is impregnated with corticosteroid medication may be used in patients with relatively few but resistant psoriatic plaques. However, once the steroid treatment is stopped, the psoriasis may quickly reappear (rebound phenomenon) and, in some instances, be more extensive than the original lesions.

When psoriasis involves large areas of the body, topical corticosteroid treatment can become expensive. In this event, other treatment modalities (coal tar, ultraviolet light) may be used in combination. As with anthralin, hand washing is stressed following application. Repeated eye contact with corticosteroid preparations is associated with cataract development. Strict guidelines for applying these drugs should be emphasized, because overuse can result in skin atrophy, striae, and drug resistance.

Occlusive Dressings. Some patients will require hydrocolloid (Duoderm) occlusive dressing over the entire body. For the hospitalized patient, large plastic bags may be used—one for the upper body (with holes cut out for the head and arms) and one for the lower body (with holes for the legs). This leaves only the extremities to wrap. In some dermatologic units, large rolls of tubular plastic are used (such as the kind that dry-cleaners place over clean clothes).

- When these substances are used, it is important to check for flammability.

Some of these thin, plastic films will burn slowly (if touched by a lighted cigarette), whereas others will burst rapidly into flame and may cause severe injury. The patient should be cautioned not to smoke while wrapped in these dressings.

For patients being treated at home, a plastic vinyl jogging suit may be purchased. The medication is applied and the suit simply put over it. The hands can be wrapped in gloves, the feet in plastic bags, and the head in a shower cap.

Intralesional Therapy. Intralesional injections of triamcinolone acetonide (Aristocort, Kenalog-10, Trymex) can be performed directly into highly visible or isolated patches of psoriasis that are resistant to other forms of therapy. Care must be taken to ensure that normal skin is not injected with the medication.

Systemic Therapy. Systemic cytotoxic preparations, such as methotrexate, have been used in treating extensive psoriasis that fails to respond to other forms of therapy. Methotrexate appears to function by inhibiting DNA synthesis in epidermal cells, thereby reducing the turnover time of the psoriatic epidermis. However, the drug can be very toxic, especially to the liver, which can suffer irreversible damage. Thus, laboratory studies must be monitored to ensure that the hepatic, hematopoietic, and renal systems are functioning adequately.

The patient should avoid drinking alcohol while on methotrexate, because this increases the possibility of liver damage. The drug is teratogenic (producing physical defects in the fetus) in pregnant women.

Oral Retinoids.   Oral retinoids (synthetic derivatives of vitamin A and its metabolite, vitamin A acid) modulate the growth and differentiation of epithelial tissue and thus show great promise in treating the patient with severe psoriasis.

Another drug currently being used is hydroxyurea (Hydrea), which inhibits cell replication by affecting DNA synthesis. The patient is monitored for signs and symptoms of bone marrow depression.

Phototherapy.   A treatment for severely debilitating psoriasis is psoralen and ultraviolet A (PUVA) therapy, which involves the patient taking a photosensitizing drug (usually 8-methoxypsoralen) in a standard dose with subsequent exposure to long-wave ultraviolet light when peak drug plasma levels are obtained. Although the mechanism of action is not completely understood, it is assumed that when psoralen-treated skin is exposed to ultraviolet-A light, the psoralen binds with DNA and decreases cellular proliferation. PUVA is not without its hazards; it has been associated with long-term risks of skin cancer, cataracts, and premature aging of the skin.

PUVA therapy requires that psoralen be taken orally, followed in 2 hours by irradiation with high-intensity long-wave ultraviolet light (UVA). (Ultraviolet light is the portion of the electromagnetic spectrum containing wavelengths ranging from 180 to 400 nm.) The PUVA unit consists of a light cabinet containing high-output blacklight lamps and an external reflectance system. The exposure time is calibrated according to the specific unit in use and the anticipated tolerance of the patient's skin. The patient is usually treated two or three times a week until the psoriasis clears. An interim period of 48 hours between treatments is necessary, because it takes this long for any PUVA burns to become evident. The patient is then placed on a maintenance program. Once little or no disease is present, less potent therapies are used to keep minor flare-ups under control.

Ultraviolet B (UVB) light therapy is also used to treat generalized plaque. It is combined with topical coal tar (Goeckerman therapy). Side effects are similar to those of PUVA therapy.

Patient Education During PUVA Therapy.   PUVA treatment produces photosensitization, which means that the patient is sensitive to the sun until methoxsalen has been excreted from the body (about 6 to 8 hours). Therefore, exposure to the sun must be avoided at this time. If exposure is unavoidable, the skin must be protected with sunscreen and clothing. Gray- or green-tinted wraparound sunglasses should be worn to protect the eyes during and after treatment. Ophthalmologic examinations are performed on a regular basis. Nausea, which may be a problem in some patients, is lessened when methoxsalen is taken with food. Lubricants and bath oils may be used to help remove scales and prevent excess dryness. No other creams or oils are to be used except on areas that have been shielded from ultraviolet light. Contraceptives should be used by sexually active women of reproductive age, because the teratogenic risk of PUVA has not been established. The patient must remain under constant and careful supervision and is encouraged to look for unusual changes in the skin. Table 51-8 provides a summary of current treatment modalities.

In summary, psoriasis is a chronic noninfectious dermatosis. It is characterized by unrestricted proliferation of basal cells of the epidermis. This increased production of skin cells results in reddened, thick scales or plaques of epidermal tissue.

The cause is unknown, but heredity may play a role. No cure is possible, but current therapy is capable of controlling lesions. The disease has devastating psychologic effects on the patient's self-esteem and body image, requiring sympathetic concern and support from family and care givers.

▶ Nursing Process
The Patient With Psoriasis

▷ Assessment

The nursing assessment focuses on how the patient is functioning with the skin condition, the appearance of the "normal" skin, and the appearance of the skin lesions. (See Clinical Manifestations, above.) The major manifestations to note are red, scaling papules that coalesce to form oval, well-defined plaques. Silvery white scales are also present. Adjacent skin areas reveal red, smooth plaques with a macerated surface. It is important to examine the areas especially affected by psoriasis: elbows, knees, scalp, gluteal cleft, fingers, and toenails (for small pits).

▷ Nursing Diagnoses

Based on the nursing assessment data, major nursing diagnoses for the patient may include the following:

- Knowledge deficit of the disease process and treatment
- Impairment of skin integrity related to diminished protective function of the stratum corneum
- Disturbance in body image related to embarrassment over appearance and self-perception of uncleanliness

▷ Planning and Implementation

▷ *Goals*:   The major goals of the patient may include acquisition of knowledge about psoriasis and its treatment, achievement of smoother skin with control of lesions, and development of self-acceptance.

▷ Nursing Interventions

▷ *Patient Education and Home Health Care.*   The patient is told with sensitivity that at the present time there is no permanent cure for psoriasis and that lifetime management is necessary, but that the condition can usually be cleared and controlled. The pathophysiology of psoriasis is reviewed as well as the factors that provoke psoriasis: any irritation or injury to the skin (cut, abrasion, sunburn), any current illness (*e.g.*, pharyngeal infection), and emotional stress. It is emphasized that repeated trauma to the skin as well as an unfavorable environment (cold) and any drug (*e.g.*, lithium, beta blockers, indomethacin) may exacerbate psoriasis. The patient should be advised not to pick or scratch the psoriasis areas to avoid injuring the skin. In addition, any topical irritant or allergy-producing substance is to be avoided. The patient should report to the physician any infection that appears to aggravate the psoriasis. The patient is cautioned about taking any medication, because some drugs may worsen a mild psoriasis. It is also important to emphasize the need for a balanced life, including recreation, exercise, and rest.

The patient is encouraged to prevent the skin from drying out, because dry skin causes psoriasis to worsen. Too-frequent

TABLE 51–8. *Summary of Current Treatment Modalities for Psoriasis*

Topical Agents	Use	Agents
Coal tar products	Mild/moderate lesions	Coal tar and salicylic acid ointment
		Aquatar
		Estar gel
		Fototar
		Anthralin (Anthra-Derm, Dritho-Creme)
		Neutrogena T/Derm
		Psori Gel
Topical corticosteroids	Mild/moderate lesions	Aristocort
		Kenalog
		Trymex
		Betamethasone valerate (Betatrex, Beta-Val, Valisone)
	Lesions on face, groin/axillae	DesOwen
		Tridesilon
		Aclovate
Coal tar shampoos	Scalp lesions	Neutrogena T/Gel
		Polytar
		Zetar
		Lasan (pomade)
		Danex
		Head & Shoulders
		Zincon
		Selsun Blue
		Capitrol
		Bakers P&S (emulsifying agent with phenol, saline, and mineral oil)
Occlusive dressings	Body and limb lesions	Hydrocolloid occlusive dressings (Duoderm)
		Restore
		Plastic wrap over corticosteroids
		Cordran (tape impregnated with corticosteroid flurandrenolide)
Intralesional therapy	Thick plaques	Kenalog-10 (only when other therapies fail)
	Nails	Cordran impregnated tape
		Fluoroplex
Systemic therapy	Extensive lesions and nails	Methotrexate
		Methotrexate sodium (Folex, Mexate)
		Hydroxyurea (Hydrea)
		Retinoic acid
		Etretinate (Tegison) (not with pregnant women or during childbearing age)
	Psoriatic arthritis	Oral gold (auranofin)
		Etretinate
		Methotrexate
Phototherapy	Severe disease	UVA or UVB light with topical coal tar preparations (Goeckerman therapy)
		UVB light therapy with topical coal tar (Estar gel) (modified Goeckerman therapy)
		UVB light therapy and anthralin (Ingram therapy)
		Photochemotherapy (PUVA) (combines UVA and oral psoralen tablets or topical tripsoralen or methoxsalen)

washing produces more soreness and scaling. Water should not be too hot, and the skin is dried by patting with a towel rather than vigorous rubbing. Emollients have a moisturizing effect by providing an occlusive body film on the skin surface so that normal water loss through the skin is halted, allowing the trapped water to hydrate the stratum corneum. A bath oil or emollient cleansing agent can give comfort to sore and scaling skin. Softening the skin can prevent fissuring (see also Nursing Care Plan 51-1).

Successful treatment of psoriasis takes persistence and patience, because treatment is constant and expensive. Some patients spend 2 or more hours daily in applying medications and carrying out cosmetic efforts. The patient is taught to use topical therapy appropriately. A therapeutic alliance with health care professionals should be educative and supportive and should help the patient move toward self-acceptance. Mental health professionals can ease emotional strain and give support. Belonging to a support group helps patients acknowledge that they are not alone in experiencing life adjustments in response to a visible, chronic disease. The National Psoriasis Foundation publishes periodic bulletins and reports updating new and relevant developments about this condition (see Bibliography for the address).

◊ *Evaluation*

Expected Outcomes

1. Acquires knowledge and understanding of psoriasis
   a. Describes psoriasis and the prescribed therapy
   b. Verbalizes that trauma, infection, and emotional stress may be trigger factors
   c. Maintains control with appropriate therapy
   d. Demonstrates proper application of topical therapy
2. Achieves smoother skin and control of lesions
   a. No new lesions appear
   b. Keeps skin lubricated and soft
3. Develops self-acceptance
   a. Identifies someone with whom he can discuss his feelings and concerns
   b. Expresses optimism about outcome of treatment

Exfoliative Dermatitis

Exfoliative dermatitis is a serious condition characterized by a progressive inflammation in which erythema and scaling often occur in a more or less generalized distribution. It may be associated with chills, fever, prostration, severe toxicity, and an itchy scaling of the skin. There is a profound loss of stratum corneum (outermost layer of the skin), which causes capillary leakage, hypoproteinemia, and negative nitrogen balance. Because of widespread dilation of cutaneous vessels, large amounts of body heat are lost. Thus, exfoliative dermatitis has a marked effect on the entire body.

Exfoliative dermatitis has a variety of causes. It is considered to be a secondary or reactive process to an underlying skin or systemic disease. It may appear as a part of the lymphoma group of diseases and may actually precede the appearance of lymphoma. Preexisting skin disorders that have been implicated as a cause include psoriasis, atopic dermatitis, and contact dermatitis. It also appears as a severe reaction to a wide number of drugs, including penicillin and phenylbutazone. The etiology is unknown in approximately 25% of cases.

This condition starts acutely as either a patchy or a generalized erythematous eruption accompanied by fever, malaise, and, occasionally, gastrointestinal symptoms. The skin color changes from pink to dark red; then, after a week, the characteristic exfoliation (scaling) begins, usually in the form of thin flakes that leave the underlying skin smooth and red, with new scales forming as the older ones come off. Hair loss may accompany this disorder. Relapses are the rule. The systemic effects include high-output congestive heart failure, intestinal disturbances, breast enlargement (gynecomastia), elevated levels of uric acid in the blood (hyperuricemia), and temperature disturbances.

Management. The objectives of management are to maintain fluid and electrolyte balance and to prevent intercurrent or cutaneous infection. The treatment is individualized and supportive and should be started as soon as the diagnosis is determined.

The patient is hospitalized and placed on bed rest. All medications that may be implicated are discontinued. A comfortable room temperature should be maintained because the patient does not have normal thermoregulatory control as a result of fluctuations in temperature due to vasodilation and evaporative water loss. The fluid and electrolyte balance must be maintained because there is considerable water and protein loss from the skin surface. Plasma expanders may be indicated.

Continual nursing assessment is carried out to detect infection. The erythematous, moist skin is susceptible to infection and becomes colonized with pathogenic organisms, which produce more inflammation. Antibiotics are prescribed if infection is present and are selected on the basis of culture and sensitivity.

- The patient is observed for signs and symptoms of congestive heart failure, because hyperemia and increased cutaneous blood flow can produce a cardiac failure of high-output origin.

Hypothermia may also occur because increased skin blood flow coupled with increased water loss through the skin leads to heat loss by radiation, conduction, and evaporation.

As in any acute dermatitis, topical therapy is used to give symptomatic relief. Soothing baths, compresses, and lubrication with emollients are used to treat the extensive dermatitis. The patient is likely to be extremely irritable because of the severe itching. Oral or parenteral steroids may be prescribed when the disease is not controlled by more conservative therapy. When a specific cause is known, more specific therapy may be used. The patient is advised to avoid all irritants in the future, particularly medications.

Pemphigus Vulgaris

Pemphigus vulgaris is a serious disease of the skin characterized by the appearance of bullae (blisters) of various sizes (1 to 10 cm) on apparently normal skin (Fig. 51-11) and mucous membranes (mouth, vagina).

Available evidence indicates that pemphigus is an autoimmune disease involving IgG, an immunoglobulin. It is thought that the pemphigus antibody is directed against a specific cell-surface antigen in epidermal cells. A blister forms from the

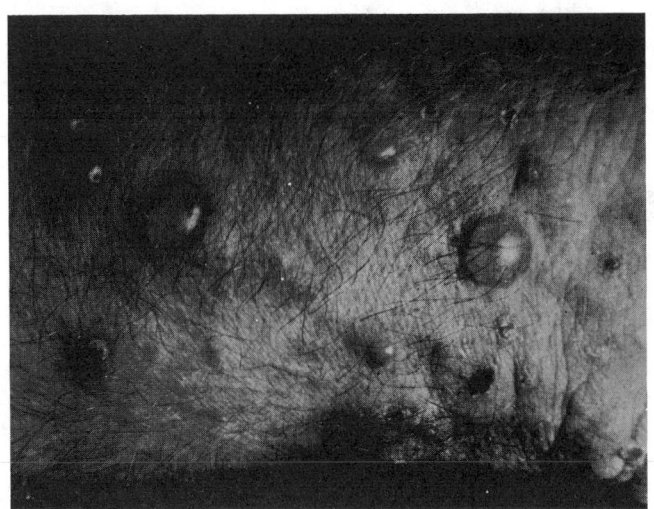

Figure 51–11. Pemphigus vulgaris bullae on the wrist. (Sauer GC. Manual of Skin Diseases, Philadelphia, JB Lippincott.)

antigen–antibody reaction. The level of serum antibody is predictive of disease severity. Genetic factors may also play a role in its development, with the highest incidence in those of Jewish descent. This disorder usually occurs in middle and late adult life.

Clinical Manifestations. The majority of patients initially present with oral lesions appearing as irregularly shaped erosions that are painful, bleed easily, and heal slowly. The skin bullae enlarge, rupture, and leave large, painful eroded areas that are accompanied by crusting and oozing. A characteristic offensive odor emanates from the bullae and the exuding serum. There is blistering or sloughing of uninvolved skin when minimal pressure is applied (Nikolsky's sign). The eroded skin heals slowly, so that eventually huge areas of the body are involved (Fig. 51-12). Bacterial superinfection is common.

Diagnostic Evaluation. A biopsy specimen from the blister and surrounding skin will demonstrate *acantholysis* (separation of epidermal cells from each other because of damage to or an abnormality of the intracellular substance). Circulating antibodies (pemphigus antibodies) may be demonstrated by immunofluorescent studies of the patient's serum.

Management. The goals of therapy are to bring the disease under control as rapidly as possible, to prevent loss of serum and the development of secondary infection, and to promote reepithelialization of the skin.

Corticosteroids are administered in high doses to control the disease and keep the skin free of blisters. The high dosage level is maintained until remission is apparent. Corticosteroids are administered with or immediately after a meal and may be accompanied by an antacid as prophylaxis against gastric complications. Essential to the patient's therapeutic management are daily evaluations of body weight, measurement of blood pressure, testing of blood for glucose, and recording of fluid balance. (High-dosage corticosteroid therapy has its own serious toxic effects.)

Immunosuppressive agents (azathioprine, cyclophosphamide, gold) may be prescribed to help control the disease and reduce the steroid dose. *Plasmapheresis* (reinfusion of specially treated plasma cells) temporarily decreases the serum level of antibodies and has been used with variable success.

In summary, pemphigus vulgaris is an uncommon but serious autoimmune, bullous skin disorder. It is characterized by epidermal bullae that rupture easily, heal poorly, and involve both the mucous membranes and the skin. Incidence is highest in those of Jewish descent. It occurs with equal frequency in men and women in middle to old age. Diagnosis is confirmed by histologic and immunofluorescent examination of skin biopsies. Primary treatment is with systemic oral corticosteroids. Topical steroids are helpful on oral and skin lesions. Adjunct therapy may include cyclosporine, azathioprine (Imuran), and cyclophosphamide (Cytoxan). While a cure is not possible, control of the disease can be achieved. Psychologic and emotional support are vital to help the patient live with the disease and follow the prescribed treatment plan.

▶ **Nursing Process**
The Patient With Pemphigus

▷ **Assessment**

Because patients with pemphigus are invariably hospitalized at one time or another during exacerbations of the disease, the nurse soon discovers that pemphigus is perhaps a cause of significant disability. The constant discomfort and distress of the patient and foul odor of the lesions make effective assessment and nursing management a challenge.

Disease activity is monitored clinically by examining the skin for the appearance of new blisters, which are usually tense and not easily broken. The scalp, chest, and adjacent skin areas are examined for blistering. Particular attention is given to assessing for signs and symptoms of infection.

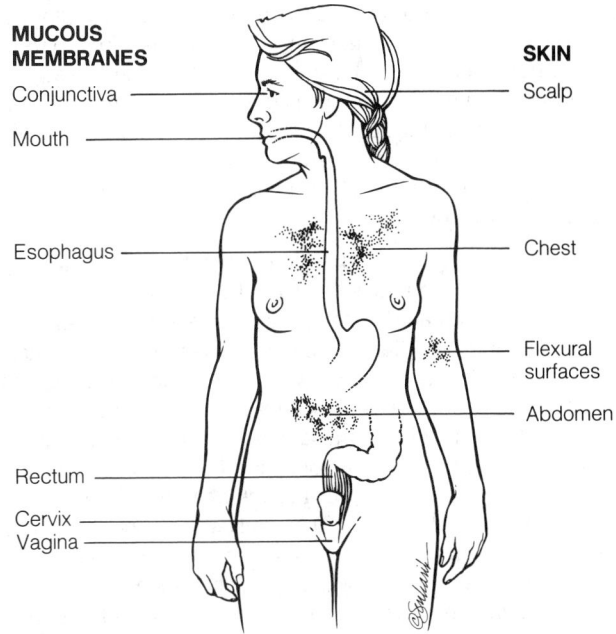

Figure 51–12. Pemphigus vulgaris: distribution of lesions.

Nursing Diagnoses

Based on nursing assessment data, major nursing diagnoses for the patient may include the following:

- Pain of oral cavity and skin related to blistering and erosions
- Impaired skin integrity related to ruptured bullae and denuded areas of the skin
- Infection related to loss of protective barrier of skin and mucous membranes
- Fluid volume deficit and electrolyte imbalance related to loss of tissue fluids
- Anxiety and ineffective coping related to appearance of the skin

Possible problems that might develop include opportunistic infections, psychosis, and hyperglycemia.

Planning and Implementation

Goals: The major goals of the patient may include relief of discomfort from lesions, achievement of skin healing, avoidance of infection, fluid and electrolyte balance, reduction in anxiety, and an improvement in coping capacity.

Nursing Interventions

Relieving Oral Discomfort. The patient's entire oral cavity may be affected with erosions and denuded surfaces. A necrotic slough may develop over these areas, adding greatly to the patient's misery and interfering with food intake. Weight loss and hypoproteinemia may thus result. Meticulous oral hygiene is important to keep the oral mucosa clean and allow for regeneration of epithelium. Prescribed mouth washes are used to rinse the mouth of debris. This is performed frequently to soothe ulcerative areas. Commercial mouth washes are avoided. The lips are kept moist with lanolin, petrolatum, or lip balm. Cool mist therapy is helpful to humidify environmental air.

Cool, nonirritating fluids (*e.g.,* grape or apple juice) are encouraged to maintain hydration. Small, frequent feedings of high-protein, high-calorie foods (Ensure; Sustacal; eggnogs; milkshakes) will help maintain nutritional status. Total parenteral nutrition is considered if the patient is unable to eat.

Secondary infection may be associated with offensive odor from oral lesions. *Candida albicans* of the mouth is frequently seen in patients on high-dose steroid therapy. The oral cavity should be inspected daily and any changes noted and reported. Oral lesions are slow to heal.

Skin Care. Cool, wet dressings or baths are protective and soothing. The patient with painful and extensive lesions should be premedicated with analgesics before skin care is initiated. Patients with large areas of blistering have a characteristic odor that is lessened when secondary infection is controlled. After bathing, the patient's skin is dried carefully and dusted liberally with nonirritating powder, which enables the patient to move freely in bed. Fairly large amounts are necessary to keep the patient from sticking to the sheets. Tape should never be used on the skin because it may produce more blisters. Hypothermia is common, and measures to keep the patient warm and comfortable are priority nursing activities.

The nursing management of patients with bullous skin conditions is similar to that of patients with extensive burns (see Chap. 52).

Control of Infection. The patient is susceptible to infection because the barrier function of the skin is compromised. Bullae are also susceptible to infection, and septicemia may follow. The skin is kept clean to eliminate debris and dead skin and to prevent infection.

Infection is the leading cause of death. Particular attention is given to assessing the patient for signs and symptoms of local and systemic infection. "Trivial" complaints or minimal changes are investigated because corticosteroids mask or alter typical signs and symptoms of infection. The vital signs are taken and temperature fluctuations monitored. The patient is observed for chills, and all secretions and excretions are monitored for changes suggestive of infection. Results of culture and sensitivity tests are followed. Antimicrobials are administered as prescribed, and response to treatment is noted. Health care personnel should employ effective hand-washing techniques. Environmental contamination is avoided as much as possible by having the housecleaning personnel dust with a damp cloth and wash the floor with a wet mop. Protective isolation measures may be employed, and universal precautions are used.

Achieving Fluid and Electrolyte Balance. Extensive denudation of the skin leads also to fluid and electrolyte imbalance. There is significant loss of tissue fluids, and therefore of sodium chloride. This sodium chloride loss is responsible for many of the systemic symptoms associated with the disease and is treated with administration of saline infusions.

A large amount of protein and blood is lost from the denuded skin areas. Blood component therapy may be prescribed to maintain the blood volume as well as the hemoglobin and plasma protein concentrations. The patient is encouraged to maintain adequate oral fluid intake. Serum albumin and protein levels are monitored.

Reducing Anxiety. Critical to the nursing management of the patient with pemphigus is the development of a trusting relationship. This encompasses the way the nurse listens, interacts, and demonstrates a warm and caring concern. The patient has legitimate concerns that may be reduced when the health team shows appropriate concern. The patient is allowed free expression of anxieties, discomfort, and feelings of hopelessness. This is necessary for specific reassurance to be most effective.

Attention to the psychologic needs of this patient require being available, giving expert nursing care, and educating the patient and the family. This provides support from which the patient gains strength. Arranging for a family member or a significant other to spend more prolonged periods of time with the patient can be supportive. When patients receive information about the disease and its treatment, uncertainty is reduced and the patient's capacity to act on his own behalf is enhanced.

A referral for psychologic counseling may be helpful to assist the patient in dealing with fears, anxiety, and depression.

Patient Education. The disease can be characterized by recurrent relapses that require continuing therapy to maintain clinical control. Regular monitoring for the side effects of corticosteroids is necessary. Long-term administration of immunosuppressive drugs is associated with an increased risk of cancer. The patient is encouraged to report for health-care follow-up regularly.

Evaluation

Expected Outcomes

1. Achieves relief from pain of oral lesions
   a. Identifies therapies that reduce pain
   b. Uses mouth washes and anesthetic–antiseptic aerosol mouth spray
   c. Drinks chilled fluids at 2-hour intervals
2. Achieves skin healing
   a. States purpose of therapeutic regimen
   b. Cooperates with soaks/bath regimen
   c. Reminds personnel to use liberal amounts of nonirritating powder on sheets
3. Is free of infection
   a. Cultures from bullae, skin, and orifices are negative for pathogenic organisms
   b. Absence of purulent drainage
   c. Shows signs that skin is clearing
   d. Temperature normal
4. Attains fluid and electrolyte balance
   a. Keeps intake record to assure adequate fluid intake
   b. Verbalizes an understanding of the necessity for intravenous infusion therapy
   c. Urine output is within normal limits
   d. Has serum chemistries within normal limits
5. Experiences decreased anxiety and increased ability to cope
   a. Verbalizes concerns about condition, self, and relationships with others
   b. Participates in self-care

Toxic Epidermal Necrolysis

Toxic epidermal necrolysis (TEN) is a severe, potentially fatal skin disease. Its etiology is unknown, but it is probably linked to the immune system as a reaction to medications or possibly secondary to a viral infection. Antibiotics, barbiturates, hydantoins, butazones, and sulfonamides are the medications most frequently implicated. TEN is characterized by initial signs of conjunctival burning or itching, cutaneous tenderness, fever, headache, extreme malaise, and myalgias. These signs are followed by a rapid onset of erythema, involving much of the skin surface and mucous membranes. Large, flaccid bullae develop in some areas; in other areas, large sheets of epidermis are shed, exposing the underlying dermis. Fingernails, toenails, eyebrows, and eyelashes may all be shed along with the surrounding epidermis. The skin is excruciatingly tender, and the loss of skin leaves a weeping surface similar to that of a total-body second-degree burn; thus, the condition may be referred to as *scalded skin syndrome*.

The patient with TEN is severely ill. High fever, tachycardia, and extreme weakness and fatigue are seen, perhaps as a result of the process of epidermal necrosis, increased metabolic needs, and possible gastrointestinal and respiratory mucosal sloughing.

The major cause of death is infection, and the most common sites of infection are the skin and mucosal surfaces, lungs, and blood. The organisms most frequently involved are *Staphylococcus aureus, Pseudomonas, Klebsiella, Escherichia coli, Serratia,* and *Candida.* The patient is monitored for ophthalmologic complications to avoid keratoconjunctivitis. Hypertrophic scarring of the skin is not unusual.

Frozen histologic studies of peeled skin from a fresh lesion of TEN and cytodiagnosis of collections of cellular material from a freshly denuded area are used for diagnosis.

Management

The goals of treatment are control of fluid and electrolyte balance and prevention of death from infection. Supportive care is the mainstay of treatment.

All nonessential medications are discontinued immediately. It is desirable that the patient be treated in a regional burn center because aggressive treatment similar to that of a severe burn is required. Skin loss may approximate 100% of the total body surface area. Surgical debridement or hydrotherapy in the Hubbard tank may be performed initially to remove involved skin.

Cultures are taken of the nasopharynx, eyes, ears, blood, urine, skin, and unruptured blisters to determine the presence of pathogenic organisms. Intravenous infusions are prescribed to maintain fluid and electrolyte balance. However, because an indwelling intravenous catheter may result in infection, fluid replacement is carried out by nasogastric tube, and orally as soon as possible. Systemic corticosteroids are usually not effective in the treatment of TEN.

Protecting the skin with topical agents is paramount. A variety of topical antibacterial agents are used to prevent wound sepsis, including silver nitrate solution, nitrofurazone, and polymyxin. Temporary biologic dressings (pigskin; amniotic membrane) or plastic semipermeable dressings (Vigilon) may be used to reduce pain, decrease evaporative losses, and prevent secondary infection while awaiting reepithelialization.

In summary, TEN is a severe, potentially fatal skin disease. The total body surface may be involved with widespread sheets of erythema and blisters. The eyes may become very inflamed. Mucous membranes are less commonly involved. Causation is associated with a wide range of drugs, chemicals, and infections. TEN is assumed to be the result of an allergic reaction, possibly of cell-mediated immunity. Mortality rates approach 50% when lesions extend to more than half of the body surface and are accompanied by elevated BUN and creatinine, neutropenia, and old age. Treatment may include systemic corticosteroids early in the disease process only, debridement of necrotic skin, correction of fluid and electrolyte imbalance, and relief of fever and pain.

▶ Nursing Process
The Patient With Toxic Epidermal Necrolysis

◇ Assessment

A careful inspection of the skin is made, with emphasis on its appearance and extent of involvement. The "normal" skin is closely observed to determine if new areas of blistering are developing. Skin seepage is monitored for amount, color, and odor. An inspection of the oral cavity for blistering and erosive lesions is performed daily. The patient's ability to drink fluids is determined.

The patient's vital signs are monitored, with special attention given to the presence and character of fever and the respiratory rate, depth, rhythm, and cough. The character and amount of respiratory secretions are noted. Urine volume, specific gravity, and color are monitored. The intravenous insertion sites are inspected for local signs of infection. The patient's height is noted, and daily weight is recorded.

The patient is questioned about fatigue and pain. An attempt is made to evaluate the patient's level of anxiety. The patient's basic coping mechanisms, which may be altered because of acute illness, are evaluated.

◊ Nursing Diagnoses

Based on all the assessment data, major nursing diagnoses for the patient may include the following:

- Impaired tissue integrity (oral and skin) related to epidermal shedding
- Fluid volume deficit and electrolyte losses related to loss of fluids from denuded skin
- Potential hypothermia related to heat loss secondary to skin loss
- Pain related to raw, denuded skin, oral lesions, and possible infection
- Anxiety related to the appearance of the skin and fear about prognosis

◊ Planning and Implementation

◊ *Goals:* The major goals of the patient may include achievement of skin and oral tissue healing, attainment of fluid balance, prevention of heat loss, relief of pain, and reduction of anxiety.

◊ Nursing Interventions

◊ *Skin Care.* The local care of the skin is a nursing challenge. The skin denudes easily, even when the patient is lifted and turned. It may be necessary to place the patient on a circular turning frame.

Secondary infection can be introduced through the damaged skin surface, which also has a compromised blood supply. Strict protective isolation techniques are employed to reduce the chances of secondary skin infection. Aseptic techniques are used during treatments of denuded skin.

The nurse applies the prescribed topical agents that reduce the bacterial population of the wound surface. Warm compresses, if prescribed, should be applied *gently* to denuded areas. The topical antibacterial agent may be used in conjunction with hydrotherapy in a tank, bathtub, or shower. The hydrotherapy aids in debridement (removal of foreign material and devitalized tissue), reduces pain, and provides a form of physical therapy. The nurse's role is that of monitoring during the treatment and encouraging the patient to exercise the extremities during the hydrotherapy.

The painful oral lesions make oral hygiene difficult. Careful oral hygiene is performed to keep the oral mucosa clean. Prescribed mouth washes are frequently used to rid the mouth of debris and soothe ulcerative areas. The oral cavity is inspected daily, and any changes are noted and reported. Petrolatum (or prescribed ointment) is applied to the lips.

◊ *Attaining Fluid Balance.* The vital signs, urine output, and sensorium are observed for signs of hypovolemia. Mental changes from fluid and electrolyte imbalance or sensory over-

load or deprivation may be manifested. The results of laboratory tests are evaluated, and abnormal results are reported. The patient is weighed daily, with use of a bed scale if necessary.

The nurse regulates intravenous fluids at prescribed infusion rates and assesses for systemic (overinfusion or underinfusion) and local (infection) complications. An indwelling intravenous catheter may result in septicemia, so fluid replacement is provided by a feeding tube, and orally as soon as possible. Oral lesions may result in dysphagia, making tube feeding or even total parenteral nutrition necessary. Daily calorie count and accurate recording of all intake and output are essential.

◊ *Preventing Heat Loss.* A patient with TEN is prone to chilling. Dehydration may be worsened by exposure of denuded skin to a continuous current of warm air. The patient is usually conscious of room temperature changes. As in the care for a burn patient, cotton blankets, ceiling-mounted heat lamps, or heat shields are useful in maintaining the patient's comfort and body temperature. The nurse should work rapidly and efficiently when large wounds are exposed for wound care in order to minimize shivering and heat loss. The patient's temperature is carefully monitored.

◊ *Relieving Pain.* The patient is assessed for the presence and character of pain, behavioral responses, and any factors that influence the pain. The prescribed analgesics are administered, and the nurse observes for pain relief, any side effects, and the activity of the patient. Analgesics are administered before painful treatments. Proper explanations and speaking soothingly to the patient during treatments can alleviate the anxiety that may worsen pain. Emotional support and reassurance and providing measures to promote rest and sleep are essential in achieving pain control. As the pain diminishes and the patient has more physical and emotional energy, self-management techniques for pain relief, such as progressive muscle relaxation and imagery, may be taught.

◊ *Lessening Anxiety.* It is important to remember that the life-style of patients with TEN has been abruptly changed to one of complete dependence. Assessment of their emotional state may reveal anxiety, fear of dying, and depression. Patients can be reassured that these reactions are normal. They need nursing support, honesty, and some hope that their situation can get better. They are encouraged to express their feelings to someone with whom they have developed a trusting relationship. Listening to their concerns and being readily available with skillful and compassionate care are anxiety-relieving interventions.

Emotional support by a psychiatric nurse, chaplain, psychologist, or psychiatrist may be invaluable for promoting coping during the long period of recovery.

◊ Evaluation

Expected Outcomes

1. Achieves increasing skin and oral tissue healing.
   a. Skin reveals areas of healing.
   b. Patient is able to swallow fluids.
2. Attains fluid balance.
   a. Laboratory reports are within normal range.
   b. Urine volume and specific gravity are within acceptable range.
   c. Vital signs are stable.

d. Increases intake of oral fluids without discomfort.
e. Gains weight, if appropriate.
3. Attains thermoregulation.
a. Temperature remains within normal range.
4. Reports lessening of intensity of pain.
a. Uses analgesics as prescribed.
b. Uses self-management techniques for relief of pain.
5. Appears less anxious.
a. Discusses concerns freely.
b. Sleeps at longer intervals.

Ulcers and Tumors of the Skin

Ulcerations

The superficial loss of surface tissue due to death of the cells is called an ulceration. A simple ulcer, such as is found in a small, superficial, second-degree burn, tends to heal by granulation if kept clean and protected from injury. If it is exposed to the air, the serum that escapes will dry and form a scab, under which the epithelial cells will grow and cover the surface completely. Certain diseases cause characteristic ulcers—tuberculous ulcers and syphilitic ulcers are examples.

Ulcers Due to a Deficient Arterial Circulation. Ulcers related to problems with arterial circulation are seen in patients with peripheral vascular disease, arteriosclerosis, Raynaud's disease, and frostbite. In these patients, the treatment of the ulceration must be carried out in conjunction with the treatment of the arterial disease. The danger is from secondary infection. Frequently, amputation of the part is the only effective therapy.

Pressure Ulcers. Pressure ulcers result from continuous pressure on a particular area of the skin (see Chap. 14).

Tumors of the Skin

Cysts

Cysts of the skin are epithelium-lined cavities containing fluid or solid material.

Epidermal cysts (epidermoid) occur frequently and may be described as slow-growing, firm, elevated tumors found most frequently on the face, neck, upper chest, and back. Removal of the cysts provides cure.

Pilar cysts (trichilemmal cysts), originally called sebaceous cysts, are most frequently found on the scalp. They apparently originate from the middle portion of the hair follicle and from the cells of the outer root sheath. The treatment is surgical removal.

Benign Tumors

Seborrheic Keratoses. These tumors are benign, wartlike lesions of varying size and color, ranging from light tan to black. They are usually located on the face, shoulders, chest, and back and are the most common skin tumors seen in middle-aged and elderly persons. They may be cosmetically unacceptable to the patient, and a black keratosis may be erroneously diagnosed as malignant melanoma. The treatment is

removal of the tumor tissue by excision, electrodesiccation, and curettage, or the application of carbon dioxide or liquid nitrogen.

Actinic keratoses are premalignant skin lesions that develop in chronic sun-exposed areas of the body. They appear as rough, scaly patches with underlying erythema. An estimated 10% to 20% of these lesions gradually transform into invasive squamous cell carcinoma.

Verrucae (Warts). Warts are common benign skin tumors caused by infection with the human papilloma virus that belongs to the DNA virus group. All age groups may be affected, but the condition occurs most frequently between the ages of 12 and 16 years. There are many types of warts.

As a rule, warts are asymptomatic, except when they occur on weight-bearing areas, such as the soles of the feet. They may be treated with locally applied laser therapy, liquid nitrogen, salicylic acid plasters, electrodesiccation, or the application of cantharidin.

Venereal Warts. Warts occurring on the genitalia and perianal areas are known as *condyloma acuminata* and have been shown to be sexually transmitted. These are treated with podophyllin in tincture of benzoin, which is applied to the wart and washed off later. Other treatment modalities include liquid nitrogen, cryosurgery, electrosurgery, and curettage.

Angiomas (Birthmarks). Birthmarks are benign vascular tumors involving the skin and the subcutaneous tissues. They may occur as flat, violet red patches (port-wine angiomas) or as raised, bright red nodular lesions (strawberry angiomas). The latter have a tendency to involute spontaneously. Port-wine angiomas, on the other hand, usually persist indefinitely. Most patients use masking cosmetics (Covermark) to camouflage the defect. The argon laser is being used on various angiomas with some success.

Pigmented Nevi (Moles). Moles are common skin tumors of various sizes and shades, ranging from yellowish brown to black. They may be flat, macular lesions or elevated papules or nodules that occasionally contain hair. The great majority of pigmented nevi are harmless lesions. However, in rare cases, malignant changes supervene and a melanoma develops at the site of the nevus. Some authorities feel that all congenital moles should be removed, because these may have a higher incidence of malignant change. Nevi that show a change in color or size or become symptomatic (itch) or develop notch borders should be removed to determine if malignant changes have occurred. Moles that occur in unusual places should be examined carefully for any irregularity and for notching of the border and variation in color. (Early melanomas may frequently show some redness and irritation and areas of bluish pigmentation where the pigment-containing cells have become deeper in the skin.) Nevi larger than 1 cm should be examined carefully. Excised nevi should be examined histologically.

Keloids. Keloids are benign overgrowths of fibrous tissue at the site of a scar or trauma. They appear to be more common among black persons. Keloids are asymptomatic but may cause disfigurement and cosmetic concern. The treatment, which is not always satisfactory, consists of surgical excision, intralesional corticosteroid therapy, and radiation.

Dermatofibroma. A dermatofibroma is a common benign tumor of connective tissue that occurs predominantly on the extremities. It is a firm, dome-shaped papule or nodule that may be skin-colored or have a pinkish brown hue. Excisional biopsy is the recommended method of treatment.

Neurofibromatosis (von Recklinghausen's Disease). Neurofibromatosis is a hereditary condition manifested by pigmented patches (café-au-lait macules), axillary freckling, and cutaneous neurofibromas that vary in size. Developmental changes may occur also in the nervous system, muscles, and bone. Malignant degeneration of the neurofibromas is found in 2% to 5% of the patients.

Cancer of the Skin

Skin cancer is the most common form of cancer in the U.S. If it continues at the present rate, an estimated one of eight fair-skinned Americans may develop skin cancer, especially basal cell carcinoma. Because the skin is accessible to direct visualization, skin cancer is readily detected and is the most successfully treated type of cancer.

Causes and Prevention

Exposure to the sun is the leading cause of skin cancer; incidence is related to the total amount of exposure to the sun. Sun damage is cumulative, and harmful effects may be severe by the age of 20. The increase in skin cancer is probably due to changing life-styles and the emphasis on sunbathing and related activities. Protective measures should be started in childhood and carried on throughout life.

Persons who do not produce sufficient melanin pigment in the skin to give protection to underlying tissue are very susceptible to sun damage. Those at greatest risk are fair, blue-eyed, red-haired persons of Celtic ancestry or persons with ruddy or light complexions, as well as those who suffer prolonged sunburn and do not tan. Others at risk are outdoor workers (such as farmers, sailors, fishermen) and people who are exposed to the sun over a period of time. Elderly persons with sun-damaged skin are also at risk, as are persons who have had a history of x-ray treatment for acne or benign skin lesions. Workers exposed to certain chemical agents (arsenic, nitrates, coal, tar and pitch, oils and paraffins) are also included in the risk group. People who have scars due to severe burns may develop skin cancer 20 to 40 years later. Squamous cell cancer can develop in areas of chronic draining osteomyelitis. Neoplastic changes can develop in chronic fistulae. Chronic ulcers of the lower extremity may be the site of origin of skin cancer. In fact, any condition causing scarring or chronic irritation may lead to cancer. Immunosuppressed patients have an increased incidence of malignant skin tumors. Genetic factors are also involved.

Changes in the ozone layer from the effects of worldwide industrial air pollutants such as chlorofluorocarbons have prompted concern that skin cancers, especially malignant melanoma, will increase in incidence. The ozone is a thin and variable stratospheric layer of bluish explosive gas formed by the sun's ultraviolet radiation on an allotropic form of oxygen. The ozone layer is known to vary in depth with the seasons and is thickest at the North and South Poles and thinnest at the equator. It is believed that it helps protect the earth from the effects of solar ultraviolet radiation. Proponents of this theory predict an increase in skin cancers as a consequence of changes in the ozone layer. Further research should reveal if ozone destruction is a viable concern and a potential health hazard.

Types of Skin Cancer

The most common types of skin cancer are basal cell carcinoma, squamous cell (epidermoid) carcinoma, and malignant melanoma.

Basal cell carcinoma (BCC) arises from the basal cell layer of the epidermis or the hair follicles. This is the most common type of skin cancer. It generally appears on the sun-exposed areas of the body and is more prevalent in regions where the population is subjected to intense and extensive exposure to the sun. The incidence is proportional to the age of the patient (average age of 60) and the total amount of sun exposure and is inversely proportional to the amount of melanin pigment in the skin.

BCC usually presents as a small, waxy nodule with rolled, translucent, pearly borders; telangiectatic vessels may be present. As it grows, it undergoes central ulceration and sometimes crusting (Fig. 51-13). The tumors appear most frequently on the face. Basal cell carcinoma is characterized by invasion and erosion of contiguous (adjoining) tissues, but it rarely metastasizes. However, a neglected BCC can account for the loss of a nose, an ear, or a lip. Other lesions of this disease may appear as shiny, flat, gray, or yellowish plaques.

Squamous cell carcinoma (SCC) is a malignant proliferation arising from the epidermis. Although it usually appears on sun-damaged skin, it may arise from normal skin or from preexisting skin lesions. It is of greater concern than basal cell carcinoma because it is a truly invasive carcinoma. The lesions may be primary, arising on both the skin and mucous membranes, or may develop from a precancerous condition, such as actinic keratosis (lesions occurring in sun-exposed areas), leukoplakia (premalignant lesion of the mucous membrane), or scarred or ulcerated lesions. It appears as a rough, thickened, scaly tumor that may be asymptomatic or may involve bleeding (Fig. 51-14). The border of the lesion may be wider, more infiltrated, and more inflammatory than that of basal cell carcinoma. Secondary infection can occur. Exposed areas, es-

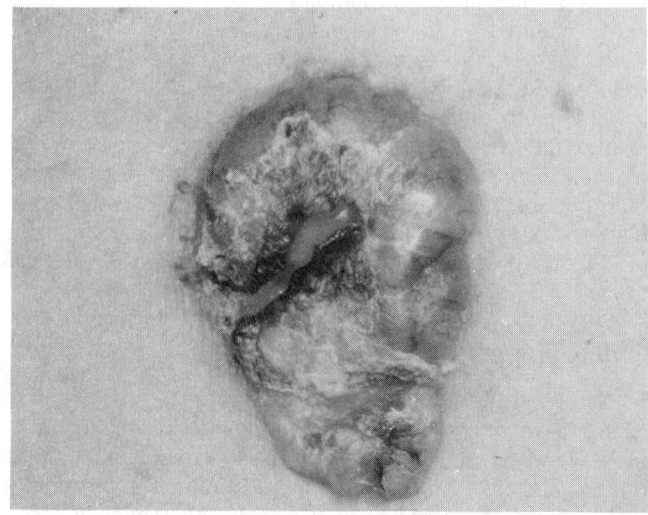

Figure 51–13.   Basal cell carcinoma. (Courtesy of Mervyn L. Elgart, MD)

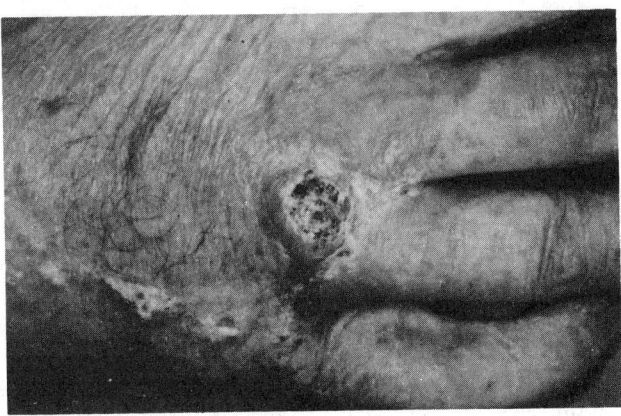

Figure 51–14. Squamous cell carcinoma. (Courtesy of Mervyn L. Elgart, MD)

pecially of the upper extremities and of the face, lower lip, ears, nose, and forehead, are common sites.

Skin cancer is diagnosed by biopsy and histologic evaluation.

The incidence of metastases is related to the histologic type and the level or depth of invasion. Usually, tumors arising in sun-damaged areas are less invasive and rarely cause death, whereas SCC arising without a history of sun or arsenic exposure or scar formation appears to have a greater chance of metastatic spread. The patient should be evaluated subsequently for regional lymph node metastases.

Management of Basal Cell and Squamous Cell Carcinomas

The goal of treatment is to eradicate or completely destroy all the tumor. The method of treatment depends on the tumor location, the cell type (location and depth), the cosmetic desires of the patient, the history of previous treatment, whether or not the tumor is invasive, and the presence or absence of metastatic nodes.

The management of BCC and SCC includes excision, Mohs' micrographic surgery, electrosurgery, cyrosurgery, and radiation therapy.

Surgical Excision. The primary goal is to remove the tumor entirely. The best way to maintain cosmesis is to properly place the incision along natural skin tension lines and natural anatomic body lines. In this way, scars are less noticeable. The size of the incision will depend on tumor size and location but usually involves a length-to-width ratio of 3:1. The adequacy of the surgical excision is verified by microscopic evaluation of sections of the specimen. When the tumor is large, reconstructive surgery with use of a skin flap or skin grafting may be required. The incision is closed in layers to enhance cosmetic effect. A pressure dressing applied over the wound provides support. Infection following a simple excision is uncommon if proper surgical asepsis is maintained during and after the procedure.

Mohs' Micrographic Surgery. Moh's micrographic surgery (MMS) is the most accurate and the most conserving of normal tissue for the removal of malignant cutaneous lesions. When the surgical technique was first introduced, the excision followed an application of zinc chloride paste to the tumor (che-

mosurgery). At the present time, MMS is performed without the initial chemosurgery component. The MMS procedure requires that the tumor be removed layer by layer. The first layer excised includes all evident tumor and a small margin of normal-appearing tissue. The specimen is analyzed by frozen section to determine if all the tumor has been removed. It not, additional layers of tissue are removed and examined until all tissue margins are tumor-free. In this manner, only tumor and a safe normal-tissue margin are removed; thus, MMS is the recommended tissue-sparing procedure. Cure rates for both basal cell carcinoma and squamous cell carcinoma with MMS approach 99%; thus, it is the treatment of choice. This surgical technique is also the most effective for tumors that occur around the eyes, nose, upper lip, and auricular and periauricular areas.

Electrosurgery. Electrosurgery is the destruction or removal of tissue through the use of electrical energy. The current is converted to heat, which is then passed to the tissue from a cold electrode. Electrosurgery may be preceded by curettage. Curettage is carried out by excising the skin tumor by scraping its surface with a curette; electrodesiccation is then applied to achieve hemostasis and to destroy any viable malignant cells at the base of the wound or along its edges. It is useful for small lesions (smaller than 1 to 2 cm [0.4 to 0.8 in] in diameter). This method takes advantage of the fact that the tumor in each instance is softer than surrounding skin and therefore can be outlined by a curette, which "feels" the extent of the tumor. The tumor is removed and the base cauterized. The process is repeated three times. Usually, healing occurs within a month.

Cryosurgery. Cryosurgery employs deep freezing to destroy the tumor tissue selectively. A thermocouple needle apparatus is inserted into the skin, and liquid nitrogen is directed to the center of the tumor until a temperature of $-40°$ to $-60°C$ is reached at the tumor base. Liquid nitrogen has the advantage of having the lowest boiling point of all cryogens tried, is inexpensive, and is easy to obtain.

The tumor tissue is frozen, allowed to thaw, and then refrozen. The site thaws naturally and then becomes gelatinous and heals spontaneously. Swelling and edema follow the freezing. The appearance of the lesion varies. Normal healing may take 4 to 6 weeks, occurring faster in areas with a good blood supply.

Radiation Therapy. Radiation therapy is frequently performed for cancer of the eyelid, the tip of the nose, and areas in or near vital structures (*e.g.,* facial nerve). It is reserved for older patients, because x-ray changes may be seen after 5 to 10 years and malignant changes in scars may be induced by x-rays 15 to 30 years later.

The patient should be informed that the skin may become red and blistered. A bland skin ointment (prescribed by the physician) may be applied to relieve discomfort. The patient should also be cautioned against exposure to the sun.

In summary, skin cancer is the most common human malignancy and is also the most curable if diagnosed early. BCC is increasing because of excessive exposure to ultraviolet radiation and possibly loss of the ozone layer. It is most prevalent in fair-skinned, red-headed, blue-eyed persons who do not tan easily. Most lesions occur on the face and neck. BCC seldom metastasizes but does tend to recur following removal. Treatment for cure is usually excision, electrosurgery and curettage, and cryotherapy.

SCC is the second most common skin malignancy and arises in damaged skin or mucous membrane (lip). SCC has a propensity to metastasize by the blood or lymphatics. Death from SCC approaches 75% when metastasis has occurred. Treatment is similar to that described for basal cell carcinoma.

Nursing Management

Because many skin cancers are removed by excision, patients are treated in outpatient surgical units. The role of the nurse is that of teaching the patient postoperative self-care activities.

The wound is usually (but not always) covered with a dressing to protect the site from physical trauma, external irritants, and contaminants. The patient is advised when to report for a dressing change or is given written and verbal information on how to change dressings—including what type of dressing to purchase, how to remove dressings and apply fresh ones, and the importance of hand washing before and after the procedure.

The patient is advised to watch for excessive bleeding and dressings so tight that circulation is compromised. If the lesion is in the perioral area, the patient is instructed to drink liquids through a straw and limit excess talking and facial movement.

After the sutures are removed, an emollient cream may be used to help reduce dryness. Use of sunscreens over the wound is advised to prevent postoperative hyperpigmentation if the patient spends time outdoors.

Patient Education. The follow-up treatment should be regular, including palpation of the adjacent nodes. The following points of emphasis should be made part of patient education:

1. Do not try to tan if your skin burns easily, never tans, or tans poorly.
2. Avoid unnecessary exposure to the sun, especially during times when ultraviolet radiation light is most intense (10 AM to 3 PM).
3. *Do not become sunburned.*
4. Apply a protective sunscreen if you must be in the sun; sunscreens block out harmful sun rays.
   a. Sunscreens are rated in strengths from 4 (weakest) to above 15 (ultra sun protection). This number is called SPF (solar protection factor) and is printed on the bottle. Use a sunscreen with an SPF of 15 or greater.
   b. Water-resistant sunscreens should be reapplied after swimming or during prolonged sun exposure.
   c. Oils applied before or during sunning do *not* protect against sunburn or sun damage.
5. Use a lip balm that contains a sunscreen with the highest SPF number.
6. Wear appropriate protective clothing (*e.g.,* broad-brimmed hat, long-sleeved clothing). However, clothing does not provide complete protection, because up to 50% of the sun's damaging rays can go through clothes. Ultraviolet rays also penetrate clouds.
7. Do not use sun lamps for indoor tanning; avoid commercial tanning booths.
8. Have moles treated that are subject to repeated friction and irritation.
9. Watch for indications of potential malignancy in moles (*e.g.,* increase in size, ulceration, bleeding, or serious exudation).
10. Have follow-up evaluation throughout lifetime. Watch for development of new lesions. (There is also an incidence of internal malignancy associated with SCC.)
11. Caution your children and grandchildren, especially those with fair skin, to avoid excessive exposure to the sun and to use sunscreen to prevent later skin cancers.

Malignant Melanoma

A malignant melanoma is a malignant neoplasm in which atypical *melanocytes* (pigment cells) are present in both the epidermis and the dermis (and sometimes the subcutaneous cells). It is the most lethal of all the skin cancers.

It can occur in one of several forms: superficial spreading melanoma, lentigo-maligna melanoma, nodular melanoma, and acral-lentiginous melanoma. These types have certain clinical and histologic features as well as different biologic behaviors. Most melanomas derive from cutaneous epidermal melanocytes, but some appear in preexisting nevi (moles) in the skin or develop in the uveal tract of the eye. Melanomas frequently appear simultaneously with cancer of other organs.

The incidence of melanoma has doubled during the past few decades, a rise that is probably related to increased recreational sun exposure. The incidence of melanoma is increasing faster than that of almost any other cancer, and the mortality rate is increasing faster than that of any other cancer except lung cancer.

Clinical Manifestations

The *superficial spreading melanoma* occurs anywhere on the body and is the most common form of melanoma. It usually affects persons of middle age and occurs most frequently on the trunk and lower extremities. The lesion tends to be circular with irregular outer portions. The margins of the lesion may be flat or elevated and palpable (Fig. 51-15). This type of melanoma may appear in a combination of colors, with hues of tan, brown, and black mixed with gray, bluish black, or white. Sometimes there is a dull pink rose color in a small area within the lesion.

The *lentigo-maligna melanomas* are slowly evolving pigmented lesions that occur on exposed skin areas, especially the head and neck in elderly people. Often the lesions are present for many years before they are examined by the physician. They first appear as tan, flat lesions and in time undergo changes in size and color.

The *nodular melanoma*, the second most common type, is a spherical, blueberry-like nodule with a relatively smooth surface and relatively uniform blue-black color (Fig. 51-15). It may be dome-shaped with a smooth surface. It may have other shadings of red, gray, or purple. Sometimes nodular melanomas appear as irregularly shaped plaques. The patient may describe this as a blood blister that fails to resolve. A nodular melanoma invades directly into adjacent dermis (vertical growth) and hence has a poorer prognosis.

Acral-lentiginous melanoma is a form of melanoma that occurs in areas not excessively exposed to sunlight and where hair follicles are absent. It is found on the palms of the hands, on the soles, in the nail beds, and in the mucous membranes in black and other dark-skinned persons. These melanomas appear as irregular pigmented macules that develop nodules. They may become invasive early.

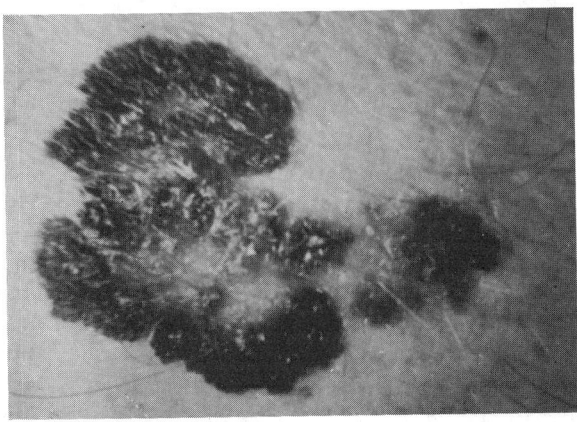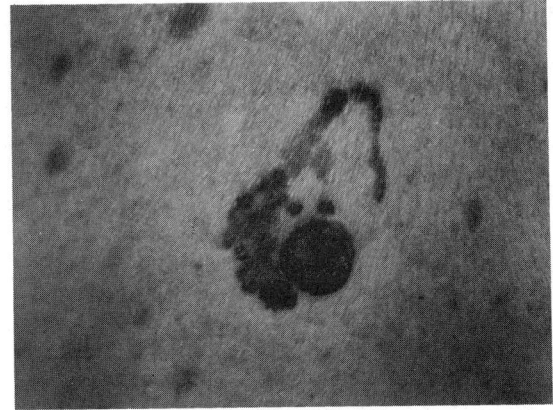

Figure 51–15. Malignant melanoma. (**Left**) Superficial melanoma. (**Right**) Nodular melanoma. (Courtesy of Mervyn L. Elgart, MD.)

An excision biopsy specimen is taken to gain histologic information on the type, level of invasion, and thickness. In addition, the patient is thoroughly examined to determine the extent of the disease.

Prognosis

The prognosis is related to the depth of dermal invasion and the thickness of the lesion. The deeper and thicker the melanoma, the greater the likelihood of metastases. If the melanoma is growing radially (horizontally) and is characterized by peripheral growth with minimal or absent dermal invasion, the prognosis is favorable. When the melanoma progresses to the vertical growth phase (decimal invasion), the prognosis is poor. The presence of ulceration correlates with a poor prognosis. Malignant melanoma can spread through both the bloodstream and the lymphatic routes and can metastasize to every organ of the body. Melanomas of the trunk appear to have a poorer prognosis than those of other sites, perhaps because the network of lymphatics in the trunk permits metastasis to regional nodes.

Causes and Persons at Risk

The etiology is unknown, but ultraviolet rays are strongly suspected. In general, at greatest risk are patients with fair complexions, blue eyes, red or blonde hair, and freckles. These persons synthesize melanin more slowly. Persons of Celtic or Scandinavian origin are at greater risk. Persons who burn and do not tan are also at risk. In areas where sunlight is intense, there is a disproportionate increase in incidence. Older Americans retiring to the Southwestern sunbelt appear to have a higher incidence. Others at risk have had a melanoma in the past, have a family history of melanoma, have giant congenital nevi, or have a significant history of severe sunburn.

Up to 10% of melanoma patients are members of melanoma-prone families who have multiple changing moles (dysplastic nevi) that are susceptible to malignant transformation. Persons with *dysplastic nevus syndrome* have been found to have unusual moles, larger and more numerous moles, lesions with irregular outlines, and pigmentation located all over the skin. Microscopic examination of dysplastic moles shows disordered, faulty growth.

Management

The therapeutic approach to the treatment of malignant melanoma depends on the level of invasion and the measurement of thickness.

Surgery. Small superficial lesions are treated by local excision. Deeper lesions require wide local excision and coverage with a skin graft. This is the primary mode of treatment at this time. A regional node dissection may be performed.

Regional Perfusion for Melanoma of the Extremities. The regional perfusion method consists of isolating an anatomic region (*e.g.*, the leg) by mechanically controlling its arterial inflow and venous outflow. A chemotherapeutic agent is perfused directly into the area that contains the melanoma. The limb is perfused for 1 hour with high concentrations of the chemotherapy agent at temperatures of 39° to 40°C with a perfusion pump. The use of hyperthermia enhances the effect of the chemotherapy drug so that a smaller total dose can be used.

This approach allows delivery of a high concentration of cytotoxic drugs while avoiding the systemic toxic effects of these higher doses. Regional perfusion can achieve excellent control of metastases and the primary tumor itself, especially when used in combination with surgical excision of the primary lesion and with regional lymph node dissection.

Immunotherapy. The term *immunotherapy* encompasses treatment methods that modify not only immune but other biologic responses to cancer.

There have been some encouraging results from several forms of immunotherapy (bacillus Calmette-Guérin vaccine [BCG], *Corynebacterium parvum*, levamisole). Research is currently under way to investigate the effects of biologic response modifiers (alpha interferon, interleukin-2), adaptive immunotherapy (lymphokine-activated killer cells), and monoclonal antibodies directed at melanoma antigens.

In summary, malignant melanoma is the most dangerous of all skin cancers, causing about 2% of all cancer deaths. The incidence is doubling every 10 years. Melanoma occurs as a result of transformation of precursor lesions (lentigo maligna, congenital melanocyte nevus, and dysplastic nevus). The lighter and fairer the skin, the greater the risk. Risk factors include fair skin, red hair, blue eyes, skin that freckles easily, family or personal history of melanoma or dysplastic nevi, and sun exposure.

The peak incidence for melanoma is between 20 and 45 years of age. Males have a tendency to develop melanoma on the back, while females develop it on the lower legs. Treatment includes primary resection of the melanoma with or without lymph node dissection, isolation limb perfusion technique with chemotherapy infusion in the involved limb, chemotherapy, and immunotherapy. At present there is no cure.

▶ Nursing Process
The Patient With Malignant Melanoma

◇ Assessment

An assessment of the patient with malignant melanoma is based on the history and symptomatology. The patient is asked specifically about pruritus, tenderness, and pain, which are *not* features of a benign nevus. He is also questioned about changes in preexisting moles or the development of new pigmented lesions. Persons at risk are assessed carefully.

A magnifying lens in good lighting is used to examine the skin for *irregularity* and *changes* in the mole. Signs that suggest malignant changes include the following:

1. *Variegated color*
   - Colors that may indicate malignancy in a brown or black lesion are shades of red, white, and blue; shades of blue are considered ominous.
   - White areas within a pigmented lesion are suspicious.
   - Some malignant melanomas are not variegated but instead are uniformly colored (bluish black, bluish gray, bluish red).
2. *Irregular border*
   - Angular indentation or notch in the border of the mole is noted.
3. *Irregular surface*
   - Uneven elevations of the surface (irregular topography) may be palpable or visible. The change in the surface may be from smooth to scaly.
   - Some nodular melanomas have a smooth surface.

The common sites of melanomas are the skin of the back, the legs (especially in women), between toes and on the feet, face, scalp, fingernails, and backs of hands. In black persons, melanomas are most apt to occur in the less pigmented sites: palms, soles, subungual areas, and mucous membranes.

The diameter of the mole is measured, because melanomas are often larger than 6 mm. Satellite lesions (those situated near the mole) are noted.

◇ Nursing Diagnoses

Based on the nursing assessment data, major nursing diagnoses for the patient may include the following:

- Pain related to surgical excision and grafting
- Anxiety and depression related to possible life-threatening consequences of melanoma and disfigurement
- Knowledge deficit about early signs of melanoma

◇ Planning and Implementation

◇ *Goals:* The major goals of the patient may include relief of pain and discomfort, reduction of anxiety, and absence of recurrence.

◇ Nursing Interventions

◇ *Relief of Pain and Discomfort.* Surgical removal of melanoma in different locations (head and neck, eye, trunk, abdomen, extremities, central nervous system) presents different challenges, taking into consideration the removal of the primary melanoma, the intervening lymphatics, and the lymph nodes to which metastases may spread. Nursing management of the patient having surgery in these regions is discussed in the appropriate chapters.

Nursing intervention following surgery for a malignant melanoma centers on promoting comfort, because wide excision surgery may be necessary. A split-thickness or full-thickness skin graft may be necessary when large defects are created by surgical removal of a melanoma. Anticipating the need for and administering appropriate analgesic medication are important.

◇ *Reduction of Anxiety.* Psychologic support is essential when disfiguring surgery is performed. Support includes allowing patients to express feelings about the seriousness of this cutaneous neoplasm, understanding their anger and depression, and conveying understanding of these feelings. During the diagnostic workup and staging of the depth, type, and extent of the tumor, the nurse answers questions, clarifies information, and helps clear up misconceptions. Learning that they have a melanoma can cause patients considerable fear and anguish. Pointing out patients' resources, past effective coping mechanisms, and social support systems helps them to cope with the problems associated with diagnosis, treatment, and continuing follow-up.

◇ *Patient Education.* The best hope of controlling the disease lies in the education of patients regarding the *early* signs of melanoma. Patients at risk are taught to examine their skin monthly in an orderly manner, including scalp examination (Fig. 51-16). The following are points to stress in patient education:

1. Use a full-length mirror and a small hand mirror to aid in examination.
2. Learn where moles and birthmarks are located.
3. Inspect all moles and other pigmented lesions; report to the physician/clinic immediately moles that *change* colors, enlarge, become raised or thicker, itch, or bleed.
4. Have a physician examine your skin at least twice yearly. A person who has had a malignant melanoma should have lifelong follow-up. A person developing a malignant melanoma has a higher risk of developing a second one.

A key factor in the development of malignant melanoma is exposure to sunlight. See p. 1484 for preventive measures.

◇ Evaluation

Expected Outcomes
1. Experiences relief of pain and discomfort
   a. States pain has lessened and is diminishing

b. Exhibits healing of surgical scar with no evidence of heat, redness, or swelling
2. Achieves reduction of anxiety
   a. Expresses fears and fantasies
   b. Asks questions about medical condition
   c. Requests repetition of facts about melanoma
   d. Identifies family member or significant other for positive reinforcement
3. Demonstrates an understanding of the means for detecting melanoma
   a. Demonstrates how to conduct self-examination of skin on a monthly basis
   b. Verbalizes the following danger signals of melanoma: change in size of mole, color of mole, mole surface, shape or outline of mole, or skin around mole
   c. Recalls measures to protect self from sun

Metastatic Skin Tumors

The skin is an important, although not a common, site of metastatic cancer. All types of cancer may metastasize to the skin, but carcinoma of the breast is the primary source of cutaneous metastases in women. Other sources include cancer of the large intestine, ovaries, and lungs. In men, the primary site is most commonly the lungs, large intestine, oral cavity, kidneys, or stomach. Skin metastases from melanomas are found in both sexes. The clinical appearance of metastatic skin lesions is not distinctive, except perhaps in some cases of breast cancer in which diffuse, brawny hardening of the skin of the involved breast is seen ("cancer en cuirasse"). In most instances, metastatic lesions occur as multiple cutaneous or subcutaneous nodules of varying size that may be skin-colored or show different shades of red.

Other Malignancies of the Skin

Kaposi's Sarcoma

First described by Moritz Kaposi in 1872, Kaposi's sarcoma (KS) has received renewed attention since its recent association with acquired immunodeficiency syndrome (AIDS). Its occurrence with AIDS has demonstrated a more varied and aggressive form of KS, and this is generally referred to as epidemic Kaposi's sarcoma (EKS). This discussion will emphasize EKS, with only a general background review of classic KS. See Chapter 48 for a full discussion of AIDS.

Clinical Manifestations

Classic Kaposi's Sarcoma.   KS was once a rare type of malignancy found predominantly in three population groups: (1) elderly Jewish males from Eastern Europe and the Mediterranean areas of Europe, (2) adults and children in various areas of Africa affected by endemic KS, and (3) persons with immunodeficiency from an immunologic disorder or from treatment with immunosuppressive therapy.

The clinical manifestations and disease course for each of these three groups have distinct characteristics. In the first group, KS generally presents in the form of slow-growing cutaneous lesions of the extremities (ankle, foot, hand, forearm) and rarely results in the death of the individual. In endemic African KS, the clinical presentation varies with the age group: children generally have lymph node involvement, which can progress rapidly to involve internal organs, and adults have symptoms and lesions that are often the same as those described for the first group. In persons with immune suppression (post–kidney transplant) or an immunodeficiency disorder (lupus erythematosus), KS is very aggressive and involves widely disseminated areas. In this type of KS, if immunosuppressive therapy is discontinued, the lesions usually disappear and the disease spread is halted.

Epidemic Kaposi's Sarcoma.   Today EKS is the malignancy most often associated with acquired immunodeficiency syndrome. EKS is much more aggressive than the classic form and its response to therapy is quite different from that of the classic form, being less predictable and less responsive to treatment. EKS often progresses to a fatal outcome for the patient. The patient presents with nonpruritic, painless, single or multiple cutaneous lesions anywhere on the body that range in color from blue-violet to red-brown. These lesions may begin as nodules, then progress to plaques, and eventually cause extensive erosion and ulceration of the involved area. In addition, EKS patients may initially present with lesions involving the lymph nodes and visceral organs (GI tract, liver, spleen, lungs) and bones. This systemic involvement may or may not be accompanied by fever, weight loss, and night sweats.

Diagnosis and Prognosis

Histologic examination of the lesions of KS and EKS shows that they are indistinguishable, and the etiology of both is still under investigation. Multiple theories for the causation of EKS have been suggested: viral, genetic, and environmental. One factor that does appear common to both KS and EKS is a probable defect in the immune system resulting in immune depression. In EKS, the cytomegalovirus (CMV) and possibly the human immunodeficiency virus (HIV) may also be etiologic agents or co-factors.

No universally accepted staging system now exists; however, survival for patients with EKS generally is based on the degree of skin and systemic involvement that exists at the time of diagnosis. The best survival is achieved when lesions are limited in number and confined to the skin in one area of the body. When there are cutaneous lesions as well as visceral organ invasion, the outlook is considered poor. If fever, weight loss, and night sweats are present or if there is a history of prior opportunistic infectious processes, the patient's prognosis is very unfavorable.

Persons at Risk

EKS was initially believed to be a disease of male homosexuals who were infected with HIV. It is now known that other persons or groups who are at risk of acquiring AIDS can also develop EKS. These include intravenous drug users, bisexual males, and women and children. Women are at increased risk if they have sexual contact with bisexual men or if they are themselves intravenous drug users. The number of blacks with EKS is now steadily rising.

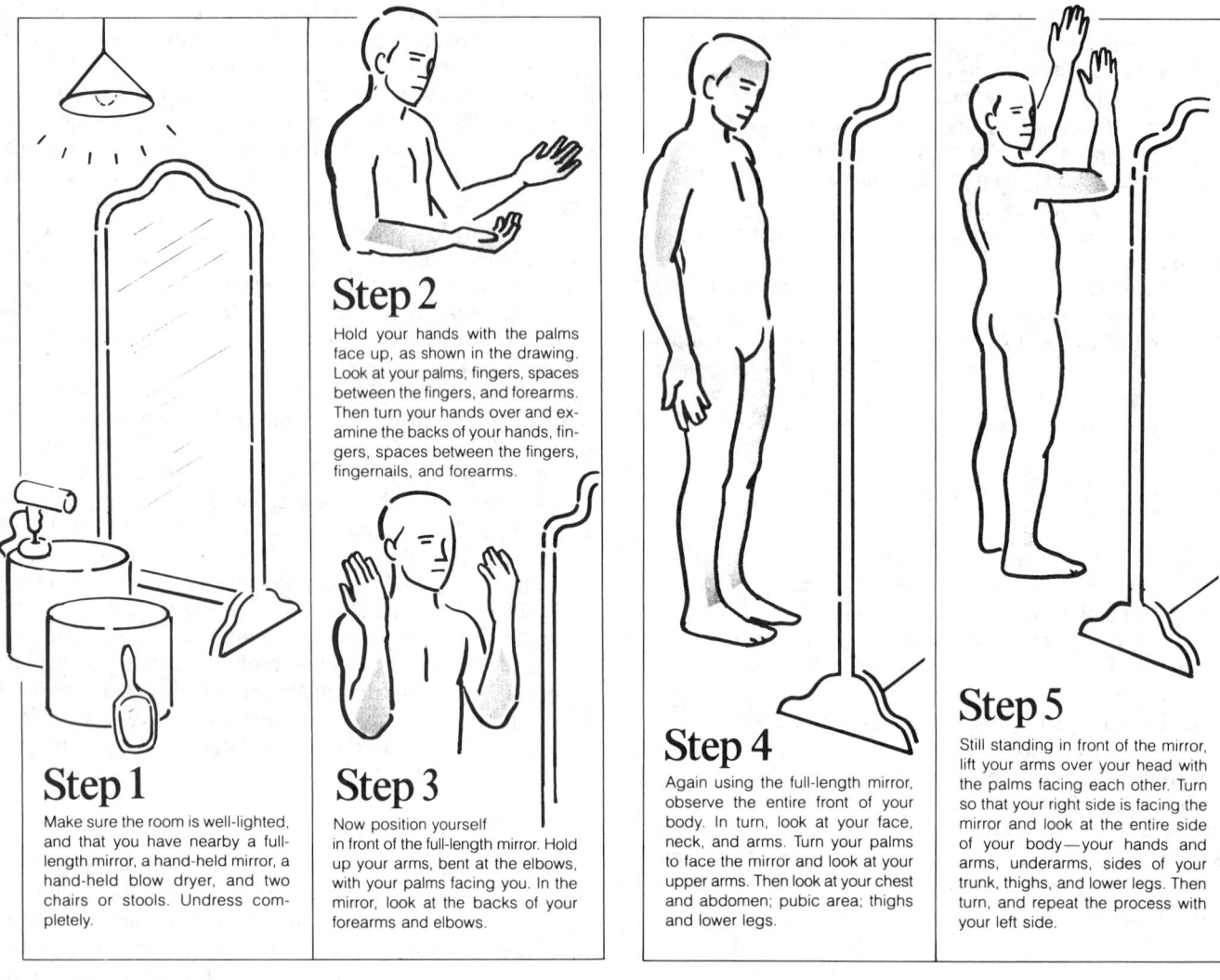

Step 1

Make sure the room is well-lighted, and that you have nearby a full-length mirror, a hand-held mirror, a hand-held blow dryer, and two chairs or stools. Undress completely.

Step 2

Hold your hands with the palms face up, as shown in the drawing. Look at your palms, fingers, spaces between the fingers, and forearms. Then turn your hands over and examine the backs of your hands, fingers, spaces between the fingers, fingernails, and forearms.

Step 3

Now position yourself in front of the full-length mirror. Hold up your arms, bent at the elbows, with your palms facing you. In the mirror, look at the backs of your forearms and elbows.

Step 4

Again using the full-length mirror, observe the entire front of your body. In turn, look at your face, neck, and arms. Turn your palms to face the mirror and look at your upper arms. Then look at your chest and abdomen; pubic area; thighs and lower legs.

Step 5

Still standing in front of the mirror, lift your arms over your head with the palms facing each other. Turn so that your right side is facing the mirror and look at the entire side of your body—your hands and arms, underarms, sides of your trunk, thighs, and lower legs. Then turn, and repeat the process with your left side.

Figure 51–16. Technique for self-examination of the skin. (Courtesy of the American Cancer Society.)

Management

The therapeutic modalities used to treat EKS depend on the location and extent of the disease process.

Radiation Therapy. Lesions treated with radiation therapy are usually confined to those causing a cosmetically undesirable appearance or those that obstruct lymphatics, nerves, or vessels, resulting in edema and pain (especially in the soles of the feet and the oral cavity). Radiation therapy is not curative but does provide temporary relief of distressing appearance and discomfort.

Chemotherapy. The use of single-agent medications has resulted in decreased symptoms. Single-agent regimens include the *Vinca* alkaloids (vincristine, vinblastine), bleomycin, etoposide (VP-16), and doxorubicin. Various combinations of these agents have been used with varying success rates, and their effects are palliative at best. Because these agents depress the bone marrow, infections are a major problem. Clinical trials using various chemotherapeutic agents and antiviral agents (zidovudine [AZT]) are under way at the present time.

Other Treatment Modalities. The use of recombinant alpha interferon in recent clinical trials has provided tumor regression in some patients, but the response remains only as long as therapy is sustained. Relapses can occur after therapy is discontinued.

Future treatments that show promise but are still in the research stage include: recombinant interleukin-2; granulocyte macrophage colony-stimulating factor (GM-CSF) to assist in more rapid recovery of the bone marrow following chemotherapy; and erythropoietin to stimulate red blood cell production.

In summary, KS is a neoplastic disease first described in 1872. Once thought to be a rare disease, it is now the most frequent malignancy associated with AIDS. AIDS-related EKS is a more aggressive form of the disease compared with the classic form. Classic KS has most often been identified in individuals of Jewish descent from eastern Europe and the area around the Mediterranean. An endemic form has also been found in specific regions of Africa.

Histologically, AIDS-related EKS and classic KS are identical. The clinical course, however, is different: EKS manifests with a more aggressive and potentially fatal clinical course and has variable success with treatment (radiation and chemotherapy). Signs and symptoms exhibited in KS most commonly include cutaneous skin lesions found primarily on the extrem-

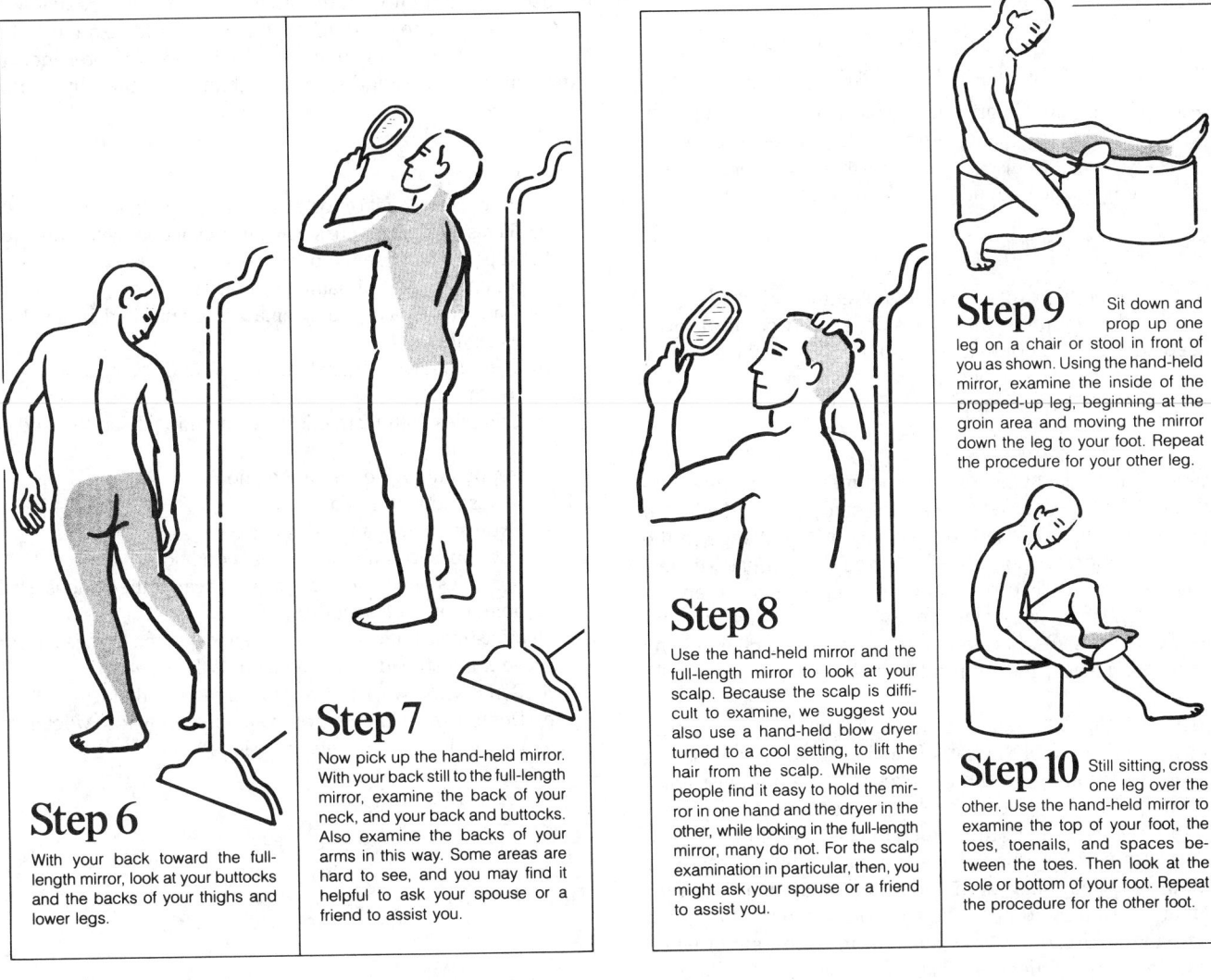

Step 6

With your back toward the full-length mirror, look at your buttocks and the backs of your thighs and lower legs.

Step 7

Now pick up the hand-held mirror. With your back still to the full-length mirror, examine the back of your neck, and your back and buttocks. Also examine the backs of your arms in this way. Some areas are hard to see, and you may find it helpful to ask your spouse or a friend to assist you.

Step 8

Use the hand-held mirror and the full-length mirror to look at your scalp. Because the scalp is difficult to examine, we suggest you also use a hand-held blow dryer turned to a cool setting, to lift the hair from the scalp. While some people find it easy to hold the mirror in one hand and the dryer in the other, while looking in the full-length mirror, many do not. For the scalp examination in particular, then, you might ask your spouse or a friend to assist you.

Step 9   Sit down and prop up one leg on a chair or stool in front of you as shown. Using the hand-held mirror, examine the inside of the propped-up leg, beginning at the groin area and moving the mirror down the leg to your foot. Repeat the procedure for your other leg.

Step 10   Still sitting, cross one leg over the other. Use the hand-held mirror to examine the top of your foot, the toes, toenails, and spaces between the toes. Then look at the sole or bottom of your foot. Repeat the procedure for the other foot.

Figure 51–16.   (Continued)

ities. A more systemic variation can invade internal organs. EKS also presents with cutaneous lesions but more commonly demonstrates systemic involvement of the GI tract, spleen, liver, lungs, and bone.

The cause remains unclear for both EKS and KS; however, both involve impairment of the immune system. Several theories of causation for EKS include genetic, environmental, and viral factors. In AIDS-related EKS, HIV and the CMV may be factors in the etiology. There is a need for continued research into the areas of causation and identification of the best treatment modalities.

▶ Nursing Process
The Patient With Epidemic Kaposi's Sarcoma

◇ Assessment

The assessment of the patient with EKS should begin with a thorough history. Of importance is the determination of the presence and location of cutaneous lesions and evidence of

any systemic involvement. A close look at genetic, environmental, and life-style factors that might contribute to the etiology is imperative. Suspicion of EKS should be aroused if the information reveals a history of organ transplant surgery, previous transfusion of blood or blood products, the use of intravenous drugs, a previous or present infectious process (fever, weight loss, night sweats), or sexual practices that place the patient at risk for HIV infection.

The nurse uses universal precautions, including gloves, when examining cutaneous lesions for size, color, and location. The entire skin surface should be observed with a good lighting source. Typical lesions of EKS generally present as nonpruritic and painless. Lesions that change in size or color and spread to other parts of the body need to be well documented. A thorough examination of the oral cavity may reveal the initial invasion of lesions to the GI tract. An abdominal examination is performed to elicit signs and symptoms of involvement of other abdominal cavity organs in addition to the GI tract. Symptoms that might indicate spread within the abdomen include nausea, vomiting, weight loss, fever, and pain or tenderness on palpation or percussion. The patient with lung involvement may complain of breathing difficulties or a history of recurrent respiratory infections.

▷ Nursing Diagnoses

Based on the nursing assessment data, major nursing diagnoses for the patient may include the following:

- Alteration in skin integrity related to cutaneous lesions
- Pain related to lymphatic, nerve, or blood vessel obstruction
- Anxiety related to disease state, treatment, and prognosis
- Knowledge deficit about treatment and self-care

▷ Planning and Implementation

▷ *Goals*: The major goals of the patient may include resolution or reduced spread of lesions, increased comfort level, reduced anxiety, and compliance with the therapeutic regimen.

▷ Nursing Interventions

▷ *Resolution or Reduced Spread of Lesions and Promotion of Comfort.* The nurse observes and documents the patient's response to therapy. Cutaneous lesions treated with radiation or chemotherapy are assessed for any observable change in the size and number of lesions or evidence that spread of new lesions has ceased. The resolution of lymphedema in an extremity is a positive sign. Daily measurement of the diameter of the extremity should be recorded to verify any changes. As swelling diminishes, the comfort level of the patient should improve.

The nursing interventions during radiation and chemotherapy include care of the skin of the irradiated area, ensuring adequate nutritional and fluid intake, and the administration of prescribed medications for relief of discomfort. Close observation of any change in temperature is vital. Fever in the already immunocompromised patient receiving radiation or chemotherapy may suggest the presence of an infectious process that, if not treated immediately, could result in the death of the patient. Use of reverse isolation may be helpful when there is threat of an infection. The nurse monitors the patient's blood values, especially the CBC, which will reveal the status of bone marrow function and the ability of the patient to withstand an infectious process.

▷ *Reduction in Anxiety.* AIDS-related Kaposi's sarcoma is a life-threatening disease. It is associated with great anxiety and fear about the prognosis. In addition, there is a social stigma that occurs with the diagnosis of AIDS. The patient may suffer guilt from past or present life-style practices and feelings of isolation when denied the support of family and friends.

Changes in body image and self-esteem are common. Disfiguring lesions are readily visible, and excessive weight loss cannot be easily hidden. There is fear of job discrimination or loss of employment, which often leads to financial problems. The nurse must consider the psychologic, spiritual, social, and physical needs of the patient. Referrals to the chaplain, social worker, or a local support group are interventions the nurse can easily provide.

▷ *Patient Education.* Prevention and education are the two most important means of dealing with AIDS-related EKS. Those who are at high risk of acquiring AIDS and EKS should be informed of their risk factors. Preventive measures should be well defined and attainable so that the patient will understand and be able to comply. Those already diagnosed with EKS need education on ways to prevent further extension of the disease and instructions they can follow to protect sexual partners or family. They should be taught how to examine their body skin surface and mucous membranes for presence or extension of lesions and to report changes to the physician.

▷ Evaluation

Expected Outcomes

1. Experiences reduction or elimination of cutaneous lesions
   a. States that lesions are smaller in size or completely resolved
   b. Reports the absence of new lesions
2. Experiences relief of painful symptoms
   a. States that pain and edema are diminished in involved extremity
   b. Demonstrates understanding of and compliance with treatment
   c. Complies with instructions for nutritional support and/or skin care
   d. Reports no evidence of infection
3. Achieves reduction of anxiety
   a. Expresses fears and anxieties
   b. Asks questions about medical condition
   c. Identifies family member or significant other who is available to provide support
4. Demonstrates understanding and acceptance of measures to prevent the spread and extension of the disease
   a. Can discuss ways to prevent spread to others
   b. Demonstrates method of examining body for evidence of new lesions or changes in lesions

Dermatologic and Plastic Reconstructive Surgery

The word *plastic* comes from a Greek word meaning "to form." Plastic or reconstructive surgery is performed to reconstruct or alter congenital or acquired defects in order to restore or improve the body's form and function. (Often the terms *plastic* and *reconstructive* are used interchangeably.) This type of surgery includes closure of wounds, removal of skin tumors, repair of soft-tissue injuries or burns, correction of deformities of the breast, and repair of cosmetic defects. Frequently, plastic surgery is performed primarily for aesthetic and cosmetic improvement, but it can be used to repair many parts of the body and numerous structures, such as bone, cartilage, fat, fascia, mucous membrane, muscle, nerve, and cutaneous structures. Bone inlays and transplants for deformities and nonunion can be performed; muscle can be transferred; nerves can be reconstructed and spliced; and cartilage can be replaced. Last, but as important as any of these measures, is the reconstruction of the cutaneous tissues around the neck and the face; this is usually referred to as *aesthetic* or *cosmetic surgery*.

Wound Coverage: Grafts and Flaps

Skin Grafts

Skin grafting is a technique in which a section of skin is detached from its own blood supply and transferred as free tissue to a distant (recipient) site. Skin grafting can be used to repair almost any type of wound and is the most common form of reconstructive surgery. In dermatology, skin grafts are commonly used to repair defects that result from excision of skin tumors, to cover areas denuded of skin, and to cover wounds in which insufficient skin is available to permit wound closure. They are also used when primary closure of the wound increases the risk of complications or when primary wound closure will interfere with function.

Skin grafts may be classified as autografts, allografts, or xenografts. *Autografts* are grafts performed with tissue transplanted from the patient's own skin. *Allografts* involve the transplant of tissue from one individual to another individual of the same species. These grafts are also called *allogeneic* or *homograft*. A *xenograft* or *heterograft* involves the transfer of tissue from another species.

Grafts are also referred to by their thickness. A skin graft may be split-thickness (thin, intermediate, or thick) or full-thickness, depending on the amount of dermis included in the specimen. A split-thickness graft can be cut at varying thicknesses and is commonly used to cover large wounds or defects for which a full-thickness graft or flap is impractical (Fig. 51-17). A full-thickness graft consists of epidermis and the entire dermis without the underlying fat. It is used to cover wounds that are too large to be closed directly.

Application of the Graft.   A graft is obtained by a variety of instruments: razor blades, skin-grafting knives, electric- or air-powered dermatomes, or drum dermatomes. The skin graft is taken from the "donor" or "host" site and applied to the wound/ulcer site, called the "recipient" site or "graft bed."

For a graft to survive and be effective, certain conditions must be met: (1) the recipient bed must have an adequate blood supply so that normal physiologic function can resume; (2) the graft must be in close contact with its bed (to avoid accumulation of blood or fluid); (3) the graft must be fixed firmly (immobilized) so that it remains in place on the recipient site; and (4) the area must be free of infection.

The graft, when applied to the recipient site, may or may not be sutured in place. It may be slit and spread apart to cover a greater area. The process of revascularization and reattachment of a skin graft to a recipient bed is referred to as a "take."

After a skin graft is put in place, the graft may be left exposed (in areas that are impossible to immobilize) or covered with a light dressing or a pressure dressing, depending on the area.

Patient Education and Home Health Care.   The patient is instructed to keep the affected part immobilized as much as possible. For a facial graft, strenuous activity must be avoided. A graft on the hand or arm may be immobilized with a splint. When a graft is placed on a lower extremity, the part is kept elevated because the new capillary connections are fragile and excess venous pressure may cause rupture. When ambulation is permitted, the patient wears an elastic stocking to counteract venous pressure.

The patient or family member is instructed to inspect the dressing daily. Unusual drainage or an inflammatory reaction

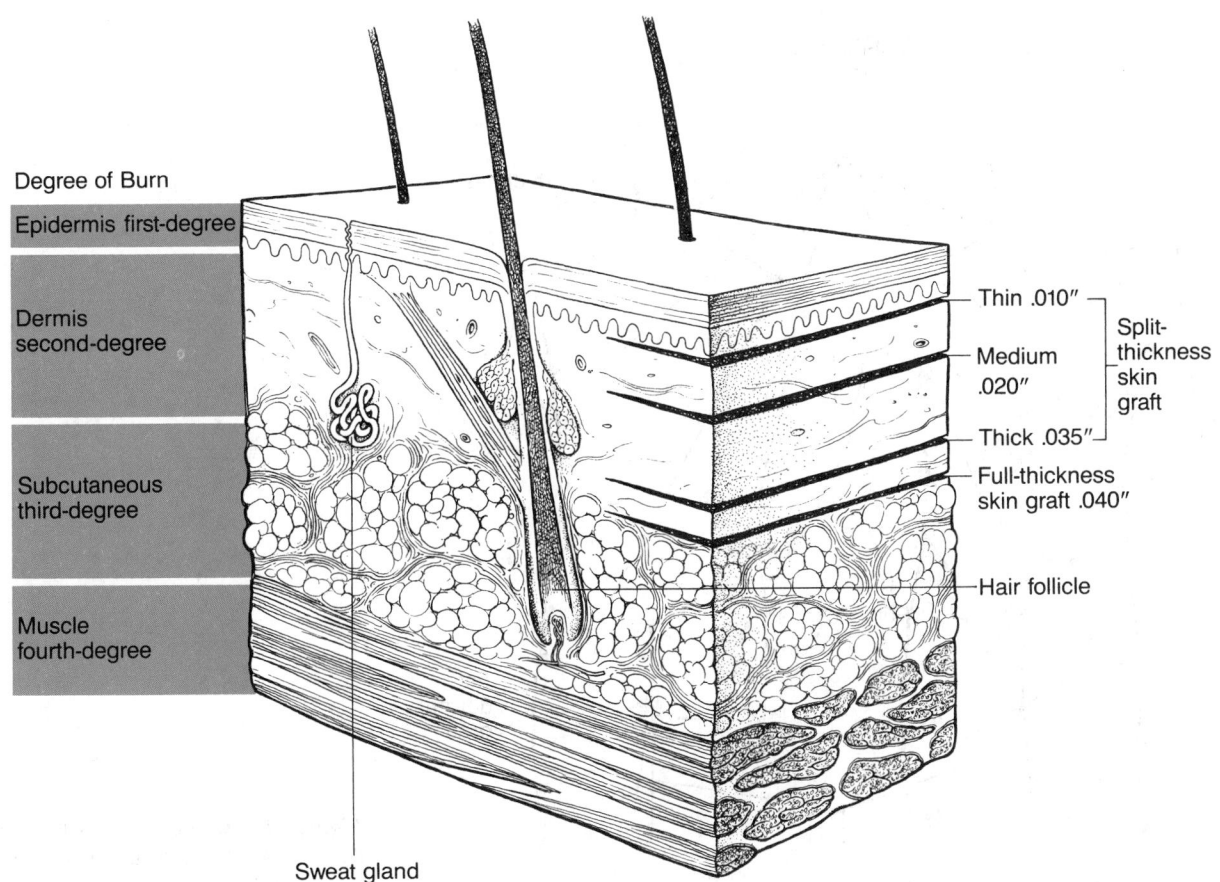

Figure 51–17.   Layers of skin showing split-thickness graft.

around the wound margin suggests infection and should be reported to the physician. Any fluid, purulent drainage, blood, or serum that has collected will be gently evacuated by the surgeon, because accumulation of this material would cause the graft to separate from its bed.

When the graft appears pink, it apparently is vascularized. After 2 to 3 weeks, mineral oil or a lanolin cream is massaged into the wound to moisten the graft and stimulate circulation. Because there may be loss of feeling or sensation in the grafted area for a prolonged period, the application of heating pads and exposure to sun are avoided to prevent burns and further skin trauma.

Donor Site for Skin Grafting

Selection Criteria. The donor site is selected with several criteria in mind: (1) to obtain the closest possible color match in keeping with the amount of skin graft required; (2) to match the texture and hair-bearing qualities; (3) to obtain the thickest possible skin graft without jeopardizing the healing process of the donor site (Fig. 51-18); and (4) to consider the cosmetic effects of the donor site after healing, so that it is in an inconspicuous location.

Donor Site Care. Detailed attention to the donor site is just as important as the care of the recipient area. The donor site heals by reepithelialization of the raw, exposed dermis. Usually a single layer of nonadherent fine-mesh gauze is placed directly over the donor site. Absorbent gauze dressings are then placed on top to absorb blood or serum from the wound. A membrane dressing may be used (Op-Site) and provides

certain advantages: it is transparent and allows the wound to be checked without disturbing the dressing, it permits the patient to shower without fear of saturating the dressing with water, and it is virtually painless.

After healing, the patient is instructed to keep the donor site soft and pliable with cream (lanolin, olive oil). Extremes in temperature, external trauma, and sunlight are to be avoided for both donor sites and grafted areas because these areas are sensitive, especially to thermal injuries.

Flaps

Another form of wound coverage may be provided by flaps. A *flap* is a segment of tissue that has been left attached at one end (called a *base* or *pedicle*) while the other end has been moved to a recipient area. It is dependent for its survival on functioning arterial and venous blood supplies and lymphatic drainage in its pedicle or base. A flap differs from a graft in that a portion of the tissue is attached to its original site and retains its blood supply. (An exception is the free flap, described below.) Flaps may consist of skin, mucosa, muscle, adipose tissue, omentum, and bone. They are used for wound coverage and provide bulk, especially when bone, tendon, blood vessels, or nerve tissue is exposed. Flaps are used to repair defects caused by congenital deformity, trauma, or tumor ablation in an adjacent part of the body.

Flaps have the advantage of offering the best aesthetic solution, because a flap retains the color and texture of the donor area, is more apt to survive than a graft, and can be

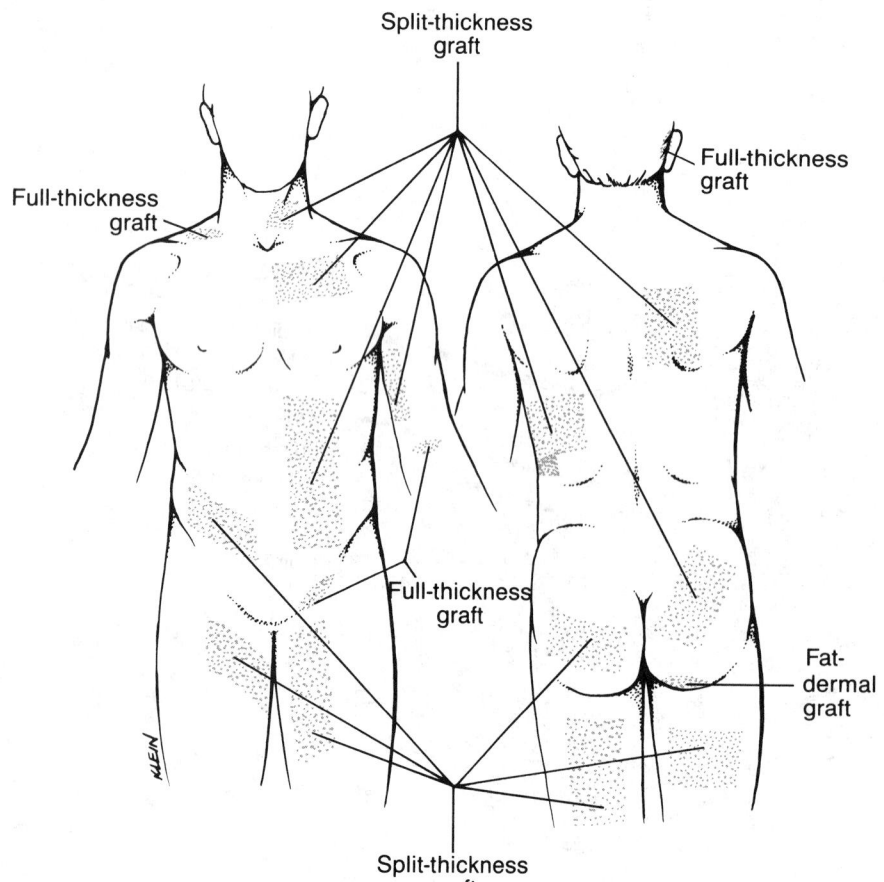

Figure 51-18. Commonly employed sites for donor areas of skin grafts. (Converse JM and Brauer RA. Reconstructive Plastic Surgery. Philadelphia, WB Saunders.)

used to cover nerves, tendons, and blood vessels. However, several operations are usually required to move a flap. The major complication is necrosis of the pedicle or base due to failure of the blood supply.

Free Flaps.   A striking advance in reconstructive surgery is the use of *free flaps* or *free-tissue transfer*, achieved by means of microvascular techniques. A free flap is completely severed from the body and transferred to another site, and it receives early vascular supply from microvascular anastomosis with vessels at the recipient site. Thus, the procedure is generally completed in one step, eliminating the need for a series of operations to move the flap. Microvascular surgery has provided for an era that allows surgeons to use a variety of donor sites for tissue reconstruction.

Chemical Face Peeling

Chemical face peeling involves the application of a chemical mixture to the face for the purpose of causing superficial destruction of the epidermis and the upper layers of the dermis. It is used to treat fine wrinkles and superficial blemishes. It is not a substitute for face-lifting because skin folds remain intact.

Pretreatment medication (analgesic and tranquilizer) is designed to control pain and apprehension. Prior to surgery, the skin is cleansed thoroughly, and any soap and oily residue are removed with ether or acetone wipes.

The type of chemicals used depends on the planned depth of the peel. A phenol-based chemical in an oil–water emulsion is frequently used in the procedure because it causes a controlled, predictable chemical burn. The chemical is carefully applied in a systematic manner to the face with cotton-tipped applicators. The patient will experience a burning sensation at this time. A mask of waterproof adhesive may then be applied directly to the skin and molded closely to the contours of the face, thereby acting as an occlusive dressing that increases the chemical penetration and action. (Some surgeons feel that equally good results can be obtained without occlusive tape.) After the tape mask is applied, the burning sensation returns. Frequent small doses of analgesics and tranquilizers are prescribed to keep the patient as comfortable as possible.

Complications may arise when control of the chemically induced burn cannot be sustained. Complications include pigment changes, infection, milia (small inclusion cysts that disappear after several months), scarring, atrophy, sensitivity changes, and long-term erythema (4 to 5 months) and pruritus.

Nursing Interventions

After 6 or 8 hours, the face becomes edematous and the eyelids often swell shut. The patient should be reassured that this reaction is normal. The patient is cautioned to move the mouth as little as possible so that the tape stays adherent to the skin. The head of the bed is elevated, and liquids are administered through a straw.

By the second day, the patient may feel moisture under the dressings as serous exudate seeps from the chemically treated skin.

Most of the burning sensation and discomfort subside after the first 12 to 24 hours. The dressings are removed after 48 hours, exposing skin similar to that of a second-degree burn. The patient may become alarmed by the appearance of the

skin and should be reassured again. After the tape mask is removed, some surgeons dust the treated skin surface with thymol-iodide powder because of its drying and bacteriostatic effects. The powdered surface is left open and dry for a period of time, during which a thin, yellow-brown crust forms. An ointment is prescribed to cover the face in order to soften and loosen the crust. After several days, the patient is advised to wash the face with lukewarm water and to lubricate the face with an ointment between washings.

Patient Education and Home Health Care.   The nurse reinforces the physician's explanation that the redness of the skin gradually decreases over the next 4 to 12 weeks. Although a line between treated and untreated skin may be noted, makeup is usually permitted after the first few weeks. The patient is cautioned to avoid direct or reflected sunlight, because the treatment has reduced the natural protection of the skin from sun. The skin will probably never tan evenly again. Blotchy pigmentation can occur if sunlight is not avoided.

Dermabrasion

Dermabrasion (skin planing) is a form of skin abrasion used to correct acne scarring, aging, and sun-damaged skin. A special instrument (motor-driven wire brush, diamond-impregnated disk, serrated wheel) is used in the procedure. The epidermis and some superficial dermis is removed, while enough of the dermis is preserved to allow reepithelialization of the dermabraded areas. Results are best in the face because it is rich in intradermal epithelial elements.

Patient Instruction and Preparation.   The primary reason for undergoing dermabrasion is to improve appearance. The surgeon explains to the patient what can be expected from dermabrasion. The patient should also be informed about the nature of the postoperative dressing, what discomfort may be experienced, and how long it will be before the tissues look normal. Dermabrasion may be performed in the office, the operating room, or an outpatient setting. It is performed under local or general anesthesia. During the procedure, some dermatologic surgeons use refrigerant anesthetics to turn the skin into a numb, solid mass of rigid tissue and to provide a momentarily bloodless surgical field. During and after planing, the area is irrigated with copious amounts of saline solution to remove debris and allow the surgeon to see the area. A dressing impregnated with ointment is usually applied to the abraded surface.

Patient Education and Home Health Care.   The nurse instructs the patient about the after-effects of the surgery. Edema occurs during the first 48 hours and may cause the eyelids to close. The head of the bed is elevated to hasten fluid drainage. Erythema occurs and can last for weeks or months. After 24 hours, the dressing may be removed (upon physician directives). When the serum oozing from the skin begins to gel, the patient applies the prescribed ointment to the face several times a day to prevent hard crusting and to keep the abraded areas soft and flexible. Clear water cleansing/soaking of the face is started with physician approval to remove crusts from the healing skin.

The patient is advised to avoid extreme cold and heat and excessive straining or lifting, which may bruise delicate new capillaries. Direct or reflected sunlight is avoided for 3 to 6 months, and a sunscreen should be used.

Management of the Patient With Facial Reconstructive Surgery

Reconstructive procedures on the face are designed to suit the individual patient and to repair deformities or restore normal function as much as possible. They may vary from closure of small defects to complicated procedures involving implantation of prosthetic devices to conceal a large defect or replace a lost part of the face (e.g., nose reconstruction, ear reconstruction; resection of the mandible). Each surgical solution is custom-tailored and involves a variety of incisions, flaps, and grafts.

In correcting a primary defect, the surgeon may have to create a secondary defect. Although the operation may restore some function, such as eating or talking, the cosmetic or aesthetic results are sometimes limited. The original appearance of a patient with severe damage to soft tissue and bone structure can seldom be restored. Multiple surgical procedures may be required. The process of facial reconstruction is often slow and tedious.

▶ Nursing Process
The Patient With Facial Reconstructive Surgery

◊ Assessment

The face is a part of the body that every person desires to keep at its best or improve because most human interactions center on the face. When the face loses its appearance and function (e.g., by accident or cancer), an emotional reaction occurs. Changes in appearance frequently cause anxiety and depression. Patients with facial changes frequently mourn for the lost part, suffer a loss of self-esteem due to reactions or rejection by others, and withdraw and isolate themselves. Health care personnel can legitimize these emotions by acknowledging that anxiety and depression are appropriate for what the patient is experiencing.

In addition to assessing emotional responses, the nurse identifies strengths as well as usual coping mechanisms to determine how the patient will handle the surgical procedure. Any area in which the patient and family will need extra support is also highlighted.

Preoperative Nursing Management

The patient is prepared as thoroughly as possible for the extent of disfigurement and improvement that can be anticipated. The nurse is in a better position to reinforce factual information and clarify misconceptions when the surgeon has fully informed the patient about the procedure, the functional defects that may result, the possible need for a tracheostomy and/or other prosthesis, and the necessity for additional surgery.

Preoperative teaching also includes an explanation of intravenous feedings, the use of a nasogastric tube to allow gastric decompression and prevent vomiting, and the frequent and lengthy dressing periods that may be necessary to care for wounds, flaps, and skin grafts. Extra time is needed when presenting this information to anxious patients because they may not listen, may not comprehend, or may distort what is being said.

◊ Nursing Diagnoses

Based on the nursing assessment data, major nursing diagnoses for the patient may include the following:

- Ineffective airway clearance related to tracheobronchial secretions
- Pain related to facial edema and effects of the procedure
- Potential altered nutrition (less than body requirements) related to changed physiology of oral cavity, dribbling, impairment of chewing and swallowing, or excision surgery affecting the tongue
- Impaired verbal communication related to trauma/surgery producing anatomic and physiologic abnormalities of speech
- Body image disturbance related to disfigurement
- Altered family processes related to grief reaction and disruption of family life

◊ Planning and Implementation

◊ *Goals:* The major goals of the patient may include maintenance of a patent airway and pulmonary function, achievement of increased comfort, attainment and maintenance of adequate nutritional status, development of a form of effective communication, reinforcement of positive self-concept, and achievement of effective family coping.

◊ Nursing Interventions

◊ *Maintaining Airway and Pulmonary Function.* The immediate postoperative concern following facial reconstruction is maintenance of an adequate airway. If the patient has regained consciousness, mental confusion with combative anxious behavior is a sign of anoxia. Sedatives or narcotics are not given in this situation because they may impair oxygenation. If the patient shows signs of restlessness, the airway is carefully inspected to see if there is laryngeal edema or accumulation of tracheobronchial mucus. Secretions are suctioned as necessary until the patient can manage the secretions without help. If a tracheostomy is used, suctioning is performed with sterile technique to prevent infection and cross-contamination. (See Chap. 25 for care of the patient with a tracheostomy.)

◊ *Achieving Comfort.* Edema of the face is uncomfortable and is a consequence of this type of surgery. The patient's head and upper torso are kept slightly elevated (if the blood pressure is stable) to help reduce facial edema. Suction catheters attached to closed drainage may be in place to keep the tissue in close apposition and to remove serous discharge. If extensive reconstruction has been performed, the patient's head should be properly aligned and supported so that minimal stress is placed on the suture line.

Mild doses of analgesics as prescribed will usually control pain. If bone grafts have been used for reconstruction, there can be considerable pain in the donor area. Pain may be more severe if secondary infection occurs, a complication that may be minimized if frequent oral hygiene is practiced. The mouth is inspected to note the location of sutures so that they are not accidentally disturbed during the cleansing process. The mouth is cleansed according to the type of surgery. Loose clots may be removed by gentle swabbing. The patient is advised not to loosen clots with the tongue, because this may provoke fresh bleeding.

If the patient has head and neck cancer with increasing levels of pain, more sophisticated modalities of nursing management will be required. (See Chap. 15, The Person Experiencing Pain.)

▷ *Maintaining Adequate Nutrition.*   After oral and pharyngeal edema have diminished, the incisional areas and flaps are healed, and the patient is able to swallow saliva, fluids may be offered, followed gradually by soft foods. If the patient cannot eat enough to satisfy nutritional needs, enteral alimentation (infusion of nutrients, water, and vitamins into the stomach or proximal small intestine via tube) is employed. The formula strength and the feeding rate are gradually increased until the desired daily caloric level is attained. (See Chap. 35 for nursing management of the patient requiring enteral feedings.) Patients who have had radical operations for large, encroaching neoplasms will have to learn to eat again. Positive nutrition is reflected in weight gain, and nutritional status is monitored by daily checks of weight and periodic checks of serum protein and electrolyte levels.

▷ *Enhancing Communication.*   Communication problems can present a major difficulty and may range from little or no problem to loss of oral speech. Some tumors and trauma require aggressive surgical treatment that involves the larynx, tongue, and mandible. Paper, pen or pencil, and a firm writing surface should be provided. If the patient cannot write, a pictograph board may be used.

The family may become frustrated by the patient's inability to communicate. The patient soon senses this, and both parties may withdraw. Allowing the family to vent their feelings and fears (away from the patient) is supportive.

▷ *Improving Self-Concept.*   Success in rehabilitation of the patient undergoing reconstructive surgery is dependent upon the relationship between the patient and the nurse, the physician, and other health care personnel. Mutual trust, respect, and clear lines of communication are essential for an effective relationship. Unhurried care provides emotional reassurance and support.

Often the kinds of dressings that must be worn, the unusual positions that have to be maintained, and the temporary incapacities that must be experienced can be upsetting to the most stable person. Honest reinforcement of the patient's coping and fortitude improves self-esteem. If prosthetic devices are to be used, the patient is taught how to use and care for them in order to gain a sense of greater independence. Once involved in self-care activities, the patient may feel some control over what was previously an overwhelming situation.

Patients with severe disfigurement are encouraged to socialize in the hospital to experience the reactions of others in a more protected environment. Gradually they can widen this sphere of contact. Every effort is made to cover or mask defects. Patients may require support by members of the mental health team to accept their changed appearance.

▷ *Helping Family Coping.*   The family is informed about the patient's appearance following surgery, the presence of supportive equipment, and ways that the equipment aids in recovery. It is helpful to join the family for a few minutes during their first postoperative visit to help them cope with the changes they will see.

A major nursing task is to support the family in their decision to participate (or not to participate) in the patient's treatment. Nursing interventions also include helping the family members communicate by suggesting techniques for reducing anxiety and stress and promoting problem solving and decision making. These activities encourage nurturance and growth of family members.

▷ ## Evaluation

Expected Outcomes
1. Maintains patent airway
   a. Demonstrates respiratory rate within normal limits
   b. Has normal breath sounds
   c. Has no signs of choking or aspiration
2. Is free of complications
   a. Demonstrates vital signs within normal limits
   b. Undergoes normal wound healing
   c. Is free of signs of infection
3. Attains adequate nutrition
   a. Consumes adequate amounts of foods and fluids
   b. Progressively gains weight, with gradual approach toward normal weight range
   c. Serum protein and electrolyte levels within normal range
4. Achieves increasing comfort
   a. Reports decreasing pain
   b. Demonstrates lessening facial edema
   c. Adheres to oral hygiene regimen to prevent infection/subsequent pain
5. Communicates effectively
   a. Uses appropriate aids to enhance communication
   b. Interacts with health team members and family/support persons
6. Develops positive self-image
   a. Express positive feelings about surgical changes
   b. Demonstrates increasing independence in self-care activities
   c. Uses prosthetic devices independently (when appropriate)
   d. Verbalizes plans for resumption of pre-illness activities (*e.g.*, work, recreation)
7. Family copes with situation
   a. Demonstrate lessening anxiety and conflict among family members
   b. Verbalize what to expect

Cosmetic Dermatology Surgery

Rhytidectomy (face lift) is an operation on the face to remove soft tissue folds and minimize cutaneous wrinkles. It is performed to improve and create a more youthful appearance.

Psychologic preparation requires that the person recognize the limitations of surgery and the fact that miraculous rejuvenation will not occur. The patient is informed that the face may appear bruised and swollen after the dressings are removed and that several weeks may pass before the edema subsides.

The procedure is performed under local or general anesthesia; the outpatient setting has become an increasingly popular site for the surgery. The incisions are placed in areas of concealment (natural skin folds and creases and areas hidden by hair). The loose skin, separated from underlying muscle, is pulled upward and backward. Excess skin that overlaps the incision line is removed. More recently, liposuction-assisted rhytidectomy is being performed, in which fat is suctioned via a cannula through a small incision.

Patient Education. The patient is encouraged to rest quietly for the first 2 postoperative days until the dressings are removed. The head of the bed is elevated and neck flexion is discouraged to avoid compromising the circulation and the suture line. There is some degree of tightness of the face and neck due to pressure created by the newly tightened muscles, fascia, and skin. Analgesics may be prescribed for discomfort. A liquid diet may be given by means of straws, and a soft diet is permitted if chewing is not too uncomfortable.

When the dressings are removed, the skin is gently cleansed of crusting and oozing and coated with the prescribed topical ointment. Any hair matted with drainage may be combed with warm water and a wide-toothed comb.

The patient is advised not to lift or bend for 7 to 10 days because this activity may increase edema and provoke bleeding. Activities are gradually resumed. When all sutures are removed, the hair may be shampooed and blown dry with *warm*, not hot, air to avoid burning the ears, which may be numb for a period of time. Sudden pain indicates that blood is accumulating underneath the skin flaps, and it should be reported to the surgeon immediately. Complications include sloughing of the skin, deformities of the face and neck, and partial facial paralysis. Cigarette smoking has been implicated as a cause of skin slough in some patients.

The effects of a face lift will not stop the aging process. With time, the tissues drift downward. Some patients have two or more face lifts.

Laser Treatment of Cutaneous Lesions

Lasers are devices that amplify or generate highly specialized rays of potent light. They are capable of mobilizing immense heat and power when focused at close range and are a valuable tool in surgical procedures. Several types of lasers (the argon laser, carbon-dioxide laser, and tunable pulse-dye laser) have application in dermatologic surgery.

Argon Laser

The argon laser produces a blue-green light that is absorbed by vascular tissue and hence is useful in treating vascular lesions: port-wine stains, telangiectasias, vascular tumors, and pigmented lesions. The argon beam is capable of penetrating approximately 1 mm of skin and reaches the pigmented layer, causing protein coagulation in this area. An immediate effect is that tiny blood vessels under the skin are coagulated, causing the area to turn a much lighter color. A crust forms within a few days.

During the procedure, the patient may require local anesthesia (lidocaine) only if the lesion, such as a port-wine stain, is greater than 0.5 cm in diameter. (It is necessary that all personnel and the patient wear orange-colored, argon light-absorbing, polycarbonate safety glasses to prevent possible damage to the retina of the eye during the procedure.)

Patient Education and Home Health Care. Cold compresses are usually applied over the treatment area for approximately 6 hours to minimize edema, exudate, and loss of capillary permeability. The patient is advised that swelling will subside in 1 to 2 days to be followed by a crust that will last 7 to 10 days. The patient should avoid picking at the crust. An antibacterial ointment is applied sparingly until the crust separates. Makeup is not applied until after the wound has healed. Sun exposure of the treated area is avoided to prevent development of hypopigmentation, and sunscreen is to be used when exposure is unavoidable.

Carbon Dioxide Laser

The carbon dioxide (CO_2) laser emits light in the infrared spectrum that is absorbed at the skin surface because of the high water content of the skin and the long wavelength of the CO_2 light. As the laser beam strikes human tissue, it is absorbed by the intra- and extracellular water, which vaporizes, destroying the tissue. The CO_2 laser is a precise surgical instrument for use in vaporizing and excising tissue with minimal tissue damage. Because of the ability of the beam to seal blood and lymphatic vessels, it creates a dry surgical field that makes many procedures easier and quicker. It is therefore safe to use on patients with bleeding disorders or those receiving anticoagulant therapy. It is useful for the removal of epidermal nevi, tattoos, certain warts, skin cancer, ingrown toenails, and keloids. Incisions made with the laser heal in much the same way as those made by a scalpel.

During treatment with the CO_2 laser, the patient and all personnel must wear clear plastic safety glasses to prevent possible damage to the cornea of the eye. In addition, it is advisable that the patient and personnel wear laser-grade surgical masks.

Patient Education and Home Health Care. The wound is covered with antibacterial ointment and a nonstick dressing. The patient is instructed to keep the wound dry and apply the prescribed ointment and dressing.

Because nerve endings and lymphatics are sealed by the laser, there is less edema and pain following the procedure than there would be with conventional surgery. Some patients, however, do develop discomfort about 3 days after treatment, which can be relieved by analgesics. It is important that the patient be informed about this possible delayed reaction.

After reepithelialization is complete, the dressing is removed. A steroid ointment may be prescribed at this stage to reduce chances of hypertrophic scarring.

Pulse-Dye Laser

The tunable pulse-dye laser (varying wavelengths) is the newest laser available for dermatologic surgery. It is especially useful in treating cutaneous vascular lesions (port-wine stains, telangiectasia). Eye protection used for the argon and carbon-dioxide lasers is not sufficient when the pulse-dye laser is in use. Special eyeglasses, such as those made of Didymium glass, are required for the patient and all personnel. The procedure itself is generally painless. For those requiring anesthesia, lidocaine without epinephrine is sufficient because local vasoconstriction is not necessary.

Patient Education and Home Health Care. After treatment, there may be a sensation of "stinging" in the treated area for several hours. Ice to the area and a light application of an antibacterial ointment followed by a nonstick dressing (Telfa) are usually sufficient to ease any discomfort. If crusting occurs, the patient is advised to wash the area gently with soap and water and reapply the antibacterial cream twice daily until the crust disappears. Makeup should not be applied until all crust is removed. Sun exposure should be avoided. Sunscreens with an SPF of 15 or higher should be used for 3 to 4 months after the treatment. Complete removal of the lesion, especially a port-wine stain, is not anticipated. The patient should be informed that several treatments may be necessary.

Hair Disorders

Alopecia

Alopecia is baldness or loss of hair. It may occur as a result of illness, drug therapy, hormonal imbalance, or nutritional problems. In many of these events, it usually can be reversed when the underlying disorder is corrected. Other causes include the aging process, excessive traction on the hair (from braiding too tightly), excessive use of dyes, straighteners, and oils, fungus infection of the scalp, and moles or cancer on the scalp.

The most common cause of alopecia is male pattern baldness, affecting more than half of the male population. This is believed to be caused by a combination of factors, including heredity, increasing age, and androgen (male hormone) levels. (The presence of androgen is necessary for male pattern baldness to develop.) The pattern of hair loss begins with receding of the hairline in the frontal–temporal area and progresses to gradual thinning and complete loss of hair over the top of the scalp and crown. See p. 1447 for an overview of the anatomy and physiology of the hair.

Management

There are literally hundreds of over-the-counter products claiming to promote hair growth or prevent hair loss. Most, if not all, of these products are ineffective. Research continues for a suitable antiandrogen to prevent hair loss.

Topical minoxidil is currently receiving a great deal of publicity as a method for treating baldness. The medication is applied to the scalp twice daily. It stimulates hair growth in some men with male pattern baldness, presumably by increasing the blood supply to the scalp.

Minoxidil's effectiveness is still in question. It appears to provide the most benefits when used on young men who have a small area of balding of the vertex and whose hair loss is less than 5 years in duration. It takes almost a year of constant treatment before any evidence of hair growth can be observed. Hair growth is maintained only while treatment continues; therefore, long-term use of minoxidil can become very expensive.

Natural-appearing hairpieces have been developed that allow the wearer to feel more attractive.

Hair Transplantation Surgery. Hair transplantation surgery (hair replacement surgery) involves transplanting hair-bearing skin from the sides and posterior portions of the scalp to recipient spaces in the bald areas. This redistributes the patient's remaining hair as naturally and evenly as possible over the bald scalp area and is accomplished by punch grafting, scalp reduction, or the use of flaps of various kinds.

Punch grafting is the transplantation of small plugs of hair-bearing scalp from the uninvolved areas at the back and side of the head to the bald areas. It is performed in four or more sessions, 1 to 2 months apart, and is an office outpatient procedure.

Scalp reduction is a surgical procedure in which the bald portion of the scalp is reduced by staged surgical excisions. It is usually the procedure of choice for baldness of the vertex (top of head) and anterior vertex regions.

Hair-bearing *flaps* can be transposed from adjacent areas into bald areas. This procedure may be performed in several stages over a period of several months. With the use of flaps, 200 to 250 hairs per square centimeter, about normal density, can be transferred. Thus, hair is obtained instantly as soon as the flap is rotated over the bald area. Infection and bone necrosis can occur in scalp operations.

Bibliography

Books

Baden H. Diseases of the Hair and Nails. Chicago, Year Book Medical Publishers, 1987.

Cunliffe WJ. Acne. Chicago, Year Book Medical Publishers, 1989.

Dahl MV. Clinical Immunodermatology, 2nd ed. Chicago, Year Book Medical Publishers, 1988.

Dover JS, Arndt KA, and Geronemus RG et al. Illustrated Cutaneous Laser Surgery: A Practitioner's Guide. Norwalk, CT, Appelton and Lange, 1990.

Draelas ZK. Cosmetics in Dermatology. New York, Churchill Livingstone, 1990.

Gonzalez–Ulloa M et al (eds). Aesthetic Plastic Surgery. Vol 1. St Louis, CV Mosby, 1988.

Greer KE. Common Problems in Dermatology. Chicago, Year Book Medical Publishers, 1988.

Krusinski P and Flowers F. Life Threatening Dermatoses. Chicago, Year Book Medical Publishers, 1987.

Lebwohl M (ed). Difficult Diagnoses in Dermatology. New York, Churchill Livingstone, 1988.

Monk BE, Graham–Brown RAC, and Sarkany I. Skin Disorders in the Elderly. Oxford, Blackwell Scientific Publications, 1988.

Parish CL and Lask GP. Aesthetic Dermatology. New York, McGraw–Hill, 1991.

Patterson J. Aging and Clinical Practice Skin Disorders. New York, Igaku–Shoin Medical Publishers, 1989.

Sams WM and Lynch PJ (eds). Principles and Practices of Dermatology. New York, Churchill Livingstone, 1990.

Scher R and Daniel CR. Nails: Therapy, Diagnosis, Surgery. Philadelphia, WB Saunders, 1990.

Shelley W and Shelley ED. Advanced Dermatologic Therapy. Philadelphia, WB Saunders, 1987.

Tromovitch TA, Stegman SJ, and Glogau RG. Flaps and Grafts in Dermatologic Surgery. Chicago, Year Book Medical Publishers, 1989.

Ziegler JL and Darfman RE (eds). Kaposi's Sarcoma: Pathophysiology and Clinical Management. New York, Marcel Dekker, 1988.

Journals

Assessment and Treatment

Bloch B and Hunter ML. Teaching physiological assessment of black persons. Nurse Educator 1981 Jan/Feb; 24–27.

Cuzzell JZ. Clues: Pain, burning, and itching. Am J Nurs 1990 Jul; 90 (7): 15–16.

Gupta MA and Voorhees JJ. Psychosomatic dermatology. Is it relevant? Arch Dermatol 1990 Jan; 126(1):90–93.

Roach L. Assessment: Color changes in dark skin. Nursing 1977 Jan; 7(1): 48–51.

Taylor CR et al. Photo aging/photo damage/and photo protection. J Am Acad Dermatol 1990 Jan; 22(1):1–15.

Acne

Cunliffe WJ. Evolution of a strategy for the treatment of acne. J Am Acad Dermatol 1987 Mar; 16(3pt1):591–599.

Drake LA et al (Committee on Guidelines of Care). Guidelines of care for acne vulgaris. J Am Acad Dermatol 1990 Apr; 4:676–680.

Alopecia

Burke KE. Hair loss. What causes it and what can be done about it. Postgrad Med 1989 May 1; 85(6):52–58, 67–73, 77.

Dover JS and Arndt KA. Dermatology. JAMA 1989 May 19; 261(19):2838–2839.

Gilhar A, Pillar T, and Etzioni A. Topical cyclosporine in male pattern alopecia. J Am Acad Dermatol 1990 Feb; 22(2pt1):251–253.

Keller JF and Blausey LA. Nursing issues and management in chemotherapy-induced alopecia. Oncol Nurs Forum 1988 Sep/Oct; 15(5):603–607.

Nordstrom R. Tissue expansion for surgical correction of male pattern baldness. Br J Plast Surg 1988 Mar; 41(2):154–159.

Weiner MS, Amara IA, and Long ER. Five-year follow-up of men with androgenetic alopecia treated with topical minoxidil. J Am Acad Dermatol 1990 Apr; 22(4):643–646.

Blistering Diseases

Bystryn JC. Plasmapheresis therapy of pemphigus. Arch Dermatol 1988 Nov; 124(11):1702–1704.

Korman N. Pemphigus. J Am Acad Dermatol 1988 Jun; 18(6):1219–1238.

Rasmussen JE. Conspectus: Causes, diagnosis, and management of toxic epidermal necrolysis. Compr Ther 1989 May; 3–6.

Tan–Lim R and Bystryn JC. Effect of plasmapheresis therapy on circulating levels of pemphigus antibodies. J Am Acad Dermatol 1990 Jan; 22(1):35–40.

Rice MJ and Hall RP. Pemphigus: New insights on an old disease. Hosp Med 1989 Nov; 125–136.

Weber DJ and Salazar JE. Bullous eruption in a psoriatic patient. Bullous pemphigoid and psoriasis. Arch Dermatol 1989 May; 125(5):690, 693–694.

Cancer of the Skin, Melanoma, and Kaposi's Sarcoma

Brozena SJ, Waterman G, and Fenske NA. Malignant melanoma: Management guidelines. Geriatrics 1990 Jun; 45(6):55–58.

Goodman J, Chapman R, and Meiri E. Clinical review of epidemic Kaposi's sarcoma with focus on treatment modalities. Henry Ford Hosp Med J 1987; 35(1):26–28.

Ho VC and Sober AJ. Therapy for cutaneous melanoma: An update. J Am Acad Dermatol 1990 Feb; 22:159–176.

Kaminester LH. Skin cancer: Diagnosis and treatment. Hosp Med 1990 Mar; 99, 100, 102, 105–109, 113–116.

Loggie B and Eddy J. Solar considerations in the development of cutaneous melanoma. Semin Oncol 1988 Dec; 15(6):494–499.

Mitsuyasu RT. Clinical variants and staging of Kaposi's sarcoma. Semin Oncol 1987 Jun; 14(3)(Suppl 3):13–18.

Mitsuyasu RT. Kaposi's sarcoma in the acquired immunodeficiency syndrome. Infect Dis Clin North Am 1988 Jun; 2(2):511–523.

Safai B. Pathophysiology and epidemiology of epidemic Kaposi's sarcoma. Semin Oncol 1987 Jun; 14(2, Suppl 3):7–12.

Contact Dermatitis

deGroat AC, Bruynzeel DP, Bos JD, et al. The allergens in cosmetics. Arch Dermatol 1988 Oct; 124(10):1525–1529.

Oxholm A and Maibach HI. Causes, diagnosis, and management of contact dermatitis. Comprehens Ther 1990; 16(5):18–24.

Uehara M and Swai T. A longitudinal study of contact sensitivity in patients with atopic dermatitis. Arch Dermatol 1989 Mar; 125(3):366–368.

Psoriasis

Abel EA, Pincus SH, and Stern R. Insights into psoriasis management. Patient Care 1989 Nov; 30:102–131.

Dunn ML, Cockerline EB, and Rice MR. Treatment options for psoriasis. Am J Nurs 1988 Aug; 88(8):1082–1087.

Lombardo B et al. Group support for derm patients. Am J Nurs 1988 Aug; 88(8):1088–1091.

Surgery

Brody HJ. Complications of chemical peeling. J Dermatol Surg Oncol 1989 Sep; 15:1010–1019.

Goldberg DJ. Laser surgery of the skin. Am Fam Phys 1989 Nov; 40(5):109–116.

Hartwig PA. Lasers in dermatology. Nurs Clin North Am 1990 Sep; 25(3):657–666.

Roenigk RK and Roenigk HH. Current surgical management of skin cancer in dermatology. J Dermatol Surg Oncol 1990 Feb; 16:136–151.

Information/Resources

Agencies

American Cancer Society, Inc
1599 Clifton Rd NE, Atlanta, GA 30329

National Institute of Arthritis and Musculoskeletal and Skin Diseases
National Institutes of Health, Bethesda, MD 20892

National Psoriasis Foundation
6415 SW Canyon Court, Suite 200, Portland, OR 97221

Skin Cancer Foundation
575 Park Ave S, New York, NY 10016

52

Management of Patients With Burn Injury

Chapter Outline

Learning Objectives

On completion of this chapter, the learner will be able to:

1. Describe the local and systemic effects of a major burn injury
2. Describe first-aid measures for the person who experiences a burn injury
3. Describe the three phases of burn care and the priorities of care for each phase
4. Compare and contrast the potential fluid and electrolyte derangements of the three phases of burn management
5. Describe the nurse's role in the following areas of management:
   Pain management
   Restrictions of activity and joint motion
   Psychologic support of the patient and his family
   Nutritional support
   Pulmonary care
6. Describe the goals of the following aspects of burn wound care and the nurse's role in each of the following:
   Wound cleansing
   Dressing changes
   Grafting of burn wound
   Topical antibacterial therapy
   Débridement
7. Use the nursing process as a framework for care of the patient during the emergent/immediate phase, the acute/intermediate phase, and the rehabilitation/long-term phase of burn care
8. Identify community services and resources that may be used by the patient discharged from the hospital with a major burn injury

Approximately 2,000,000 people experience burn injury in the United States annually. Of this group, 200,000 require outpatient treatment and 75,000 are hospitalized. About 12,000 people die from burns and related inhalation injuries. More than half of burn injuries leading to hospital admissions could have been prevented. Nurses can play an active role in preventing fires and burns by teaching prevention concepts and promoting legislation related to the use of smoke detectors, space heaters, and fire-retardant fabrics.

Young children and the elderly are at particularly high risk for burn injury. Adolescent males and men of working age also are burned more frequently than would be expected by their representation in the total population. Most burn injuries occur in the home. Cooking, heating, or the use of electrical appliances is usually involved. Industrial settings also account for a large number of burn injuries.

The National Institute for Burn Medicine, which collects statistical data from burn centers throughout the United States, notes that most patients (75%) are victims of their own actions. Scalds in toddlers, match play in school-age children, electrical injury in adolescent males, and cigarette smoking and alcohol use in adults all contribute to this fact.

There are four major goals relating to human burns:

1. Prevention
2. Institution of lifesaving measures for the severely burned person
3. Prevention of disability and disfigurement through early, specialized, individualized treatment
4. Rehabilitation of the individual through reconstructive surgery and rehabilitative programs

Pathophysiology of Burns

Burns are caused by a transfer of energy from a heat source to the body. Heat may be transferred through conduction or electromagnetic radiation. Burns can be categorized as thermal, radiation, electrical, or chemical. Tissue destruction results from coagulation, protein denaturation, or ionization of cellular contents. The skin and the mucosa of the upper airways are the sites of tissue destruction. Deep tissues, including the viscera, can be damaged by electrical burns or through prolonged contact with the burning agent.

The depth of the injury depends on the temperature of the burning agent and the duration of contact with the agent. For example, in the case of scald burns, hot tap water at a temperature of 68.9°C (156°F) may in the course of 1 second result in a burn that destroys both epidermis and dermis (full-thickness injury). Fifteen seconds of exposure to hot water at 56.1°C (133°F) results in a similar full-thickness injury (Fig. 52-1).

Systemic Response

The initial systemic event following a major burn injury is hemodynamic instability (burn shock), resulting from loss of capillary integrity and a subsequent shift of fluid from the intravascular space into the interstitial spaces (Fig. 52-2). Cardiac output decreases before any significant change in blood volume

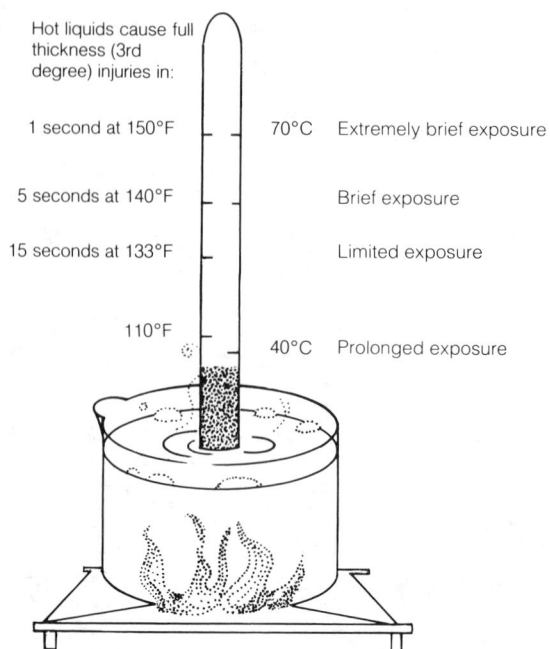

Hot liquids cause full thickness (3rd degree) injuries in:

1 second at 150°F	70°C Extremely brief exposure
5 seconds at 140°F	Brief exposure
15 seconds at 133°F	Limited exposure
110°F	40°C Prolonged exposure

Figure 52–1. Extent of tissue damage from hot liquids.

is evident. As fluid loss continues and fluid volume in the vascular system decreases, cardiac output continues to fall and a drop in blood pressure becomes evident. The response of the sympathetic nervous system to this burn shock is an increase in peripheral resistance, reflected in decreased pulse pressure and an increase in pulse rate. Prompt fluid resuscitation allows blood pressure to stay in the low normal range.

Generally, the fluid leak occurs in greatest magnitude over the first 24 to 36 hours postburn, peaking by 12 hours postinjury. As the capillaries begin to regain their integrity, fluid returns to the vascular compartment and the patient moves into the acute stage of burn care. As fluid is reabsorbed from the interstitial tissue into the vascular compartment, blood volume increases. An extra strain is placed on the heart and, if renal function is adequate, urinary output is greatly increased. Diuresis continues for several days to 2 weeks.

During this period, the elderly patient or the patient with previous cardiovascular pathology is at risk for fluid overload and may require cardiotonic drugs and diuretics to support circulatory function and prevent congestive heart failure. Fluid restriction may be needed to prevent pulmonary edema.

It should be noted that in burns involving less than 30% of the total body surface area (BSA), the loss of capillary integrity and shift of fluid are localized to the burn itself, resulting in blister formation and edema only in the area of the injury.

Fluid, Electrolyte, and Blood

Evaporative fluid loss through the burn wound may reach 3 to 5 liters or more per 24-hour period. The need for water replacement can be measured by monitoring serum sodium and potassium; a sodium reading higher than the normal level of 140 to 144 mEq/L (140 to 144 mmol/L) suggests the need for water. More frequently, *serum hyponatremia* (sodium below 132 mEq/L [132 mmol/L]) occurs between the third and the tenth day with rapid movement of fluid from the burned area.

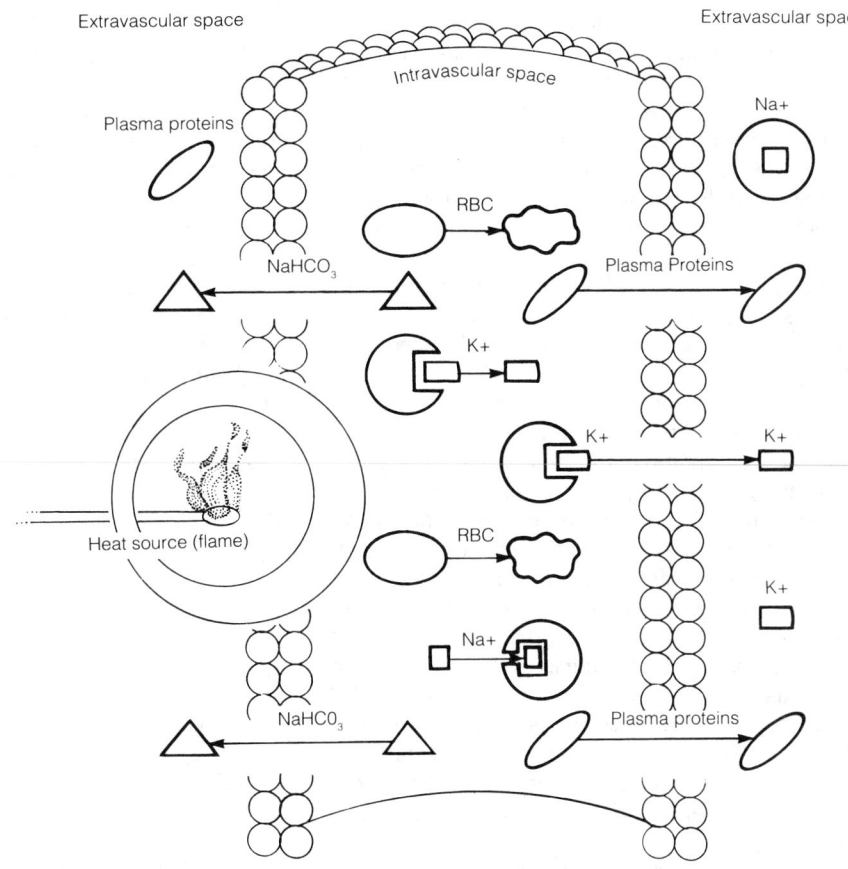

The capillary wall separates (loss of integrity), leading to increased capillary permeability resulting in massive fluid losses.

- Potassium excess
  Massive cellular trauma causes K+ to be released into the extracellular fluid. K+ is usually intracellular.

- Sodium deficit
  Na+ in large amounts is lost in edema fluid and by shifts into the cell. Na+ is usually extracellular.

- Metabolic Acidosis
  Loss of bicarbonate ions as they accompany Na+ ions

- Hemoconcentration
  Blood components lost into extravascular space. Damage to RBCs from the intense heat at the time of injury resulting in crenation of RBC.

Figure 52-2. Fluid and electrolyte changes in the initial postburn period.

Hyperkalemia occurs with massive cell destruction. *Hypokalemia* may occur later with fluid shifts and inadequate potassium intake.

Other indications helpful in determining water replacement needs are urinary output and weight loss, which should not exceed 1 kg per day. If the patient is not able to stand on a scale at the bedside, a bed scale is used.

At the time of burn injury, some red blood cells may be destroyed and others damaged, resulting in anemia. Blood loss during operative procedures, wound care, diagnostic studies, and hemolysis as a result of infection further contribute to anemia. (Abnormalities in coagulation, including a decrease in platelets [thrombocytopenia] and prolonged clotting and prothrombin times, occur with burn injury.) Blood transfusions are required periodically to maintain hemoglobin above 10 gm/dl (1.55 mmol/L) and hematocrit above 30 vol % (volume fraction: 0.3).

Pulmonary

One third of all burn patients will present with a pulmonary component to their burn injury. Inhalation injury is the leading cause of death in fire victims. It is estimated that half of these deaths could have been prevented by the use of smoke detectors.

Pulmonary injuries fall into several categories: upper airway injury, smoke inhalation injury, and restrictive defects. Upper airway injury is the result of direct heat or edema formation. It is manifested by mechanical obstruction of the upper airway. Direct heat injury does not occur below the level of the bronchus unless live steam is inhaled. This is a physiologic impossibility because of the cooling effect of rapid vaporization in the pulmonary tract. The treatment of upper airway injury is early nasotracheal or endotracheal intubation.

Smoke inhalation injury results from the inhalation of the products of incomplete combustion. The injury is a direct result of chemical irritation of the pulmonary tissues at the alveolar level. These products include carbon monoxide, sulfides, aldehydes, cyanide, benzene, and halogens. Smoke inhalation causes loss of ciliary action and severe mucosal edema. Surfactant activity is reduced, resulting in atelectasis. Expectoration of carbon particles in the sputum is the cardinal sign of this injury.

Carbon monoxide is a prominent cause of inhalation injury. The pathophysiologic effects are due to tissue hypoxia. Carbon monoxide combines with hemoglobin to form carboxyhemoglobin, which competes with oxygen for available hemoglobin-binding sites. The affinity of hemoglobin for carbon monoxide is 200 times greater than that for oxygen. Treatment usually consists of early intubation and ventilation. However, some patients may require only oxygen therapy, depending on the extent of the injury and the edema.

Restrictive defects arise from full-thickness burns encircling the neck and thorax, resulting in edema of great magnitude. Chest excursion may be greatly restricted, resulting in decreased tidal volume. Release of the constricting eschar is a necessity. Release is accomplished by surgical escharotomy (the making of a longitudinal incision through the eschar under sterile conditions).

Pulmonary abnormalities are not always immediately apparent. More than half of burn victims with pulmonary involvement do not initially demonstrate pulmonary signs and symptoms. Airway obstruction may occur very rapidly or may take hours to develop. Decreased lung compliance, decreased PaO_2, and respiratory acidosis may occur gradually.

Indicators of possible pulmonary damage include the following:

- A history indicating that the burn occurred in an enclosed area
- Burns of the face or neck
- Singed nasal hair
- Hoarseness, voice change, dry cough, sooty sputum
- Bloody sputum, labored respiration, erythema, and blisters of the oral or pharyngeal mucosa

Diagnosis of inhalation injury is an important priority for many burn victims. Blood carbon monoxide levels, arterial blood gases, and bronchoscopy are frequently used to aid diagnosis in the early postburn period. Lung scans and pulmonary function studies may also be useful in diagnosing decreased lung compliance or obstruction of air flow.

Other Systemic Effects of Burns

Renal function may be altered as a result of decreased blood volume. Destruction of red blood cells at the injury site results in free hemoglobin in the urine. If there is inadequate blood flow through the kidney, the result is tubular necrosis. Adequate fluid volume replacement restores renal blood flow, increasing glomerular filtration rate and urine volume.

The immunologic defenses of the body are greatly altered by burn injury. The obvious loss of skin integrity is compounded by abnormal inflammatory factors, altered levels of immunoglobulins and serum complement, and a reduction in lymphocytes (*lymphocytopenia*).

Loss of skin also results in an inability to regulate body temperature. Burn patients may therefore manifest low body temperatures in the early hours postburn. As hypermetabolism resets core temperatures, burn patients become hyperthermic for much of the postburn period, even in the absence of infection.

Decreased peristalsis and bowel sounds are manifestations of paralytic ileus resulting from burn trauma. Gastric distention and nausea may lead to vomiting unless gastric decompression is initiated. Gastric bleeding may be manifested through occult blood in the stool, regurgitation of coffee-ground material from the stomach, or definite signs of bloody vomitus. These signs provide evidence of gastric or duodenal erosion.

Extent of Burns and Local Response

Burn Depth

Burns are classified according to the depth of tissue destruction and are identified as superficial partial-thickness injuries, deep partial-thickness injuries, or full-thickness injuries. Corresponding descriptive terms are first-, second-, and third-degree burns.

The local response to burn injury is dependent on the depth of tissue destruction.

- In a *superficial partial-thickness (first-degree) injury*, the epidermis is destroyed or injured and a portion of the dermis may be injured. The wound may be painful and may appear red and dry, as in the case of sunburn, or it may be blistered.
- A *deep partial-thickness (second-degree) injury* involves destruction of the epidermis and upper layers of the dermis and injury to deeper portions of the dermis. The wound is painful, appears red, and exudes fluid. Blanching of the burned tissue is followed by capillary refill; hair follicles remain intact.
- A *full-thickness (third-degree) injury* involves total destruction of epidermis and dermis and, in some cases, underlying tissues as well. The color of the wound varies widely from white to red, brown, or black. The burn is painless because of destruction of nerve fibers and has a leathery appearance. Hair follicles and sweat glands are destroyed.

Table 52-1 describes these wounds in detail. Generally, the burn wound is not of uniform depth. When assessed, it is noted that there are areas of superficial injury at the periphery with increasing depth proximally. This description is more characteristic of flame and electrical injuries than of injuries caused by hot liquids.

In determining the depth of a burn, it is important to consider the following factors:

- A history of how the accident occurred
- The causative agent, such as flame or a scalding liquid
- The temperature of the burning agent
- The duration of contact with the agent
- The thickness of the skin

The presence of hemoglobin and myoglobin in the urine suggests deep burns. The depth and extent of the burn are considered in determining the appropriate health care site for treatment (Table 52-2).

TABLE 52–1. *Evaluation of Depth of a Burn*

Cause of Burn	Skin Involvement	Symptoms	Appearance	Course
SUPERFICIAL (FIRST-DEGREE)				
Sunburn Low-intensity flash	Epidermis	Tingling Hyperesthesia Painful Soothed by cooling	Reddened; blanches with pressure Minimal or no edema	Complete recovery within a week Peeling
PARTIAL-THICKNESS (SECOND-DEGREE)				
Scalds Flash flame	Epidermis and part of dermis	Painful Hyperesthesia Sensitive to cold air	Blistered, mottled red base; broken epidermis; weeping surface Edema	Recovery in 2 to 3 weeks Some scarring and depigmentation Infection may convert to third-degree
FULL-THICKNESS (THIRD-DEGREE)				
Flame Prolonged exposure to hot liquids Electric current	Epidermis, entire dermis, and sometimes subcutaneous tissue	Painless Symptoms of shock Hematuria and hemolysis of blood likely Entrance and exit wounds	Dry; pale white, leathery, or charred Broken skin with fat exposed Edema	Eschar sloughs Grafting necessary Scarring and loss of contour and function Loss of digits or extremity possible

TABLE 52–2. *Types of Burn Injuries and Recommended Treatment Site*

Type of Injury	Definition/Description	Recommended Treatment Site
MINOR BURN INJURY	*2nd-degree* (partial-thickness) —less than 15% in adults *3rd-degree* (full-thickness) —less than 2%	Hospital emergency department B (basic level)
MODERATE UNCOMPLICATED BURN INJURY	*2nd-degree* (partial-thickness) —15–25% in adults —10–20% in children or elderly *3rd-degree* (full-thickness) —less than 10%	Burn program or burn unit/center I (intermediate level)
MAJOR BURN INJURY	*2nd-degree* (partial-thickness) —more than 25% *3rd-degree* (full-thickness) —more than 10% Smaller burns at extremes of age (<2 or >60 years) Burns involving face, hands, feet, perineum Burns with inhalation injury Electrical burns Burns with other trauma or illness	Burn unit/center A (advanced level)

Percent (%) refers to percentage of body surface area (BSA) burned.
(Data from *Specific Optimal Criteria for Hospital Resources for Care of Patients With Burn Injury.*
American Burn Association.)

Intravenous fluorescein may be used to determine the functional circulation in the skin, and it makes it possible to differentiate between full-thickness, deep dermal, and superficial burns. Burn wound biopsy and histologic examination also indicate the depth of tissue destruction.

A transcutaneous flow Doppler offers a noninvasive method to assess red blood cell flow within the capillary with laser fiberoptics and may prove effective in helping to determine burn depth.

Extent of Surface Area Burned

Rule of Nines.   An estimation of the total BSA involved as a result of a burn is simplified by using the Rule of Nines (Fig. 52-3). The Rule of Nines measures the percentage of the body burned by dividing the body into multiples of nine. The initial evaluation is made upon arrival at the hospital and is revised on the second and third postburn days, because the demarcation usually is not clear until then.

Berkow Method.   A more reliable method of estimating the extent of burned surface area is the Berkow method, which is based on Lund and Brower's recognition that the percentage of body surface area of various anatomic parts, especially the head and legs, changes with growth. By dividing the body into very small areas and providing an estimate of the proportion of body surface area accounted for by such body parts, one is able to obtain a very reliable estimate of total surface area involved. This is helpful in estimating fluid requirements and determining prognosis and surgical intervention.

Survival Prediction.   The very young and the older person are at risk of mortality following burn injuries. The chances of survival are greater in children (over 5 years of age) and young adults (40 years of age or younger). Table 52-3 shows the effects that age and percent of body surface burned have on survival rate. Prognosis depends on the depth and extent of the burn as well as on the preinjury health status and age of the patient.

Phases of Burn Care

The pathophysiology and management of a burn can be divided into three phases. Although priorities exist for each of the phases, it is imperative to remember that these phases overlap and that assessment and management of specific problems and complications are *not* limited to these phases but take place throughout the course of burn care. The three phases and the priorities for care are summarized in Table 52-4.

Emergent/Immediate Phase

Emergency Management

On-the-Scene Care

- *When clothes catch on fire*, the flames can be extinguished if the victim falls to the floor or ground and rolls ("drop and roll"); anything available to smother the flames, such as a blanket, rug, or coat, may be used. Standing still would force the victim to breathe flames and smoke, and running would fan the flames.
- After the flames are extinguished, the burned area and adherent clothing are soaked with cold water, briefly, to cool the wound. Although adherent clothing may be left in place, other clothing and all jewelry should be removed to allow for assessment and to prevent constriction secondary to rapidly developing edema.

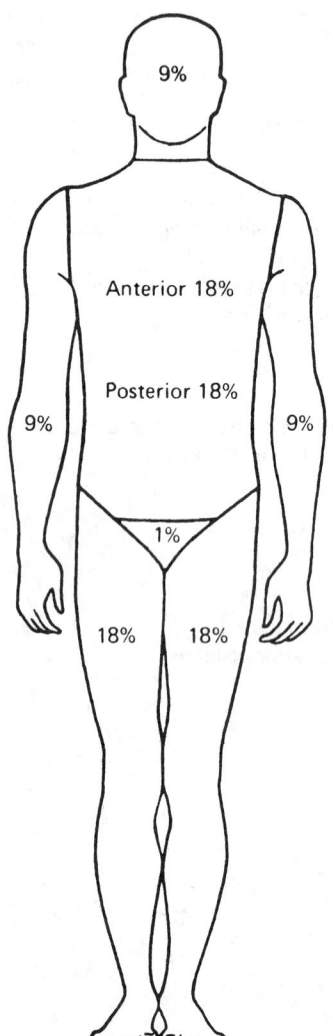

Figure 52-3. The Rule of Nines used for estimating the percentage of body burns in the adult.

TABLE 52-3. *Survival Rate in Relation to Age and Percentage of Burn*

Age	Portion of Body Burned	Survival Rate
5 and under	50%	66%
5–40	50%	80%
40–60	50%	51%
Over 60	50%	9%

TABLE 52-4. *Phases of Burn Care*

Phase	Duration	Priorities
Emergent/Immediate Resuscitative Phase	From onset of injury to completion of fluid resuscitation	• First aid • Prevention of shock • Prevention of respiratory distress • Detection and treatment of concomitant injuries • Wound assessment and initial care
Acute/Intermediate Phase	From beginning of diuresis to near completion of wound closure	• Wound care and closure • Prevention and treatment of complications, including infection • Nutritional support
Rehabilitation/Long-Term Phase	From major wound closure to return to individual's optimal level of physical and psychosocial adjustment	• Prevention of scars and contractures • Physical, occupational, and vocational rehabilitation • Functional and cosmetic reconstruction • Psychosocial counseling

• Once a burn has been sustained, the application of cold is the best first-aid measure. Soaking the burn area intermittently in cool water or applying cold towels gives immediate and striking relief from pain and restricts local tissue edema and damage. However, one should not apply ice directly to the burn or use cold soaks or dressings for longer than several minutes; such a procedure may worsen the tissue damage and lead to hypothermia in patients with large burns.

• The burn should also be covered as quickly as possible to minimize bacterial contamination and decrease pain by preventing air from coming into contact with the injured surface. Sterile dressings are best, but any clean, dry cloth can be used as an emergency dressing.

• Ointments and salves are not used. In fact, other than the dressing, no medication or material should be applied to the burn wound.

• *Chemical burns*, which result from contact with a corrosive material, are irrigated immediately. Most chemical laboratories have a high-pressure shower for such emergencies; if such an injury occurs at home, all areas of the body that have come in contact with the chemical should be rinsed in a shower or other source of continuously running water.

• If a chemical gets in or near the eyes, the eyes should be flushed with cool, clean water immediately.

Airway, Breathing, Circulation. Although the local effects of a burn are the most evident, the systemic effects pose a greater threat to life. Therefore, it is important to remember the ABCs of all trauma care during the early postburn period:

• *A*irway
• *B*reathing
• *C*irculation

Breathing must be assessed and a patent airway established immediately during the initial minutes of emergency care. Many burn victims sustain some degree of concomitant pulmonary dysfunction, as previously described.

• Immediate therapy is directed toward establishing an airway, possibly through oropharyngeal suctioning followed by the administration of 100% oxygen. If such a high concentration of oxygen is not available under emergency conditions, oxygen by mask or nasal prongs is given initially.

In mild cases, inspired air is humidified and the patient is encouraged to cough so that secretions can be suctioned. For more severe situations, it is necessary to remove secretions by bronchial suctioning and to administer bronchodilators and mucolytic agents.

• When edema of the airway is present, it may be necessary to intubate the patient. Hyperinflation hourly with an Ambu-bag helps to prevent atelectasis. Continuous positive airway pressure and mechanical ventilation may also be required.

Authorities differ on the administration of antibiotics. Gram stains of the sputum will help in determining antibiotic use; if gram-positive organisms and large numbers of neutrophils are present, penicillin or penicillinase-resistant antibiotics are given. Usually, steroids are not given because their disadvantages outweigh their advantages. Meticulous aseptic technique in all aspects of tracheal care is required in this infection-prone patient.

The circulatory system must also be assessed quickly. Apical pulse and blood pressure are monitored frequently. Tachycardia and slight hypotension are expected in the untreated patient early postburn.

Prevention of Shock. Prevention of shock in a person with a major burn is imperative. Therefore, intravenous fluid therapy is initiated promptly.

• *Nothing* is given by mouth, and the patient is placed in a position that will prevent aspiration of vomitus, because nausea and vomiting often occur as a result of paralytic ileus resulting from the stress of injury.

• In *very rare* instances in which definitive care is markedly delayed, an effective first-aid measure is to give fluids orally to the conscious patient who can tolerate them. To a quart of water (1 liter), add 1 teaspoon (3 g) of salt and a half teaspoon (1.5 g) of soda bicarbonate. (Salt provides sodium, and soda bicarbonate helps to combat acidosis.)

Usually, an emergency medical technician (EMT) or ambulance or fire personnel will take steps to cool the wound, establish an airway, supply oxygen, and start an IV line.

Emergency Department Management

The patient is transported to the nearest emergency department. The hospital and physician are alerted that the patient is enroute to the emergency department. Thus, lifesaving measures can be initiated immediately by a trained team, with no time lost.

After adequate respiratory and circulatory status has been established, attention is directed to the burn wound itself. All smoldering clothing and jewelry are removed. Flushing of chemical burns with water is continued. The patient is checked for the presence of contact lenses; these are removed immediately if chemicals have contacted the eyes or if facial burns have occurred. It is important to validate the history of the burn scenario provided by the patient, witnesses at the scene, and paramedics and to assess the patient for cervical spinal injuries or head injury if an explosion, a fall, a jump, or an electrical injury has occurred.

Assessment of the extent of body surface area burned and the depth of the burn is carried out by the physician and nurse. Full- and partial-thickness burns are noted and documented on burn assessment diagrams (Fig. 52-4). These assessments are performed after soot and debris have been gently cleansed from the burn wound. Assessment is repeated frequently during the course of burn wound care. Figure 52-5 presents guidelines for the assessment and initial care of patients with severe burns.

Overview of Immediate Patient Care

When the patient is admitted to the hospital, clothes are carefully removed, weight and height are recorded, and the patient is placed on or between sterile or pathogen-free (freshly laundered) sheets. Because this patient is usually frightened and may be in emotional shock, those in attendance should demonstrate concern. Reassurance and support are provided and explanations are given. If the patient wants to see a spiritual advisor, one is notified.

Careful attention must be given to aseptic technique. Attending personnel wear masks, caps, and gowns; sterile gloves are worn when the burn area is handled. The physician evaluates the patient's general condition, assesses the burn, determines the priorities, and directs the individualized plan of treatment, which is divided into systemic management and local care of the burned area.

Photographs may be taken of the burn areas at this time and periodically throughout the treatment. In this way, the progress of healing may be determined quickly. Such evidence is invaluable in insurance claims and courts of law.

Environment Preparation.   When a bed is prepared for a burn patient, the mattress is completely covered with a plastic sheet, which is covered in turn with a sterile bottom sheet. Sterile Microdon sheeting (3M Company) on top of this bedding prevents the patient from sticking to the sheets as a result of the oozing of exudate from the burn. Caps, masks, and sterile gowns and gloves are worn by those attending the patient. The equipment most likely to be required should be in the room, including intravenous therapy equipment, with polyethylene central venous catheters and fluids (*e.g.*, plasmanate and lactated Ringer's solution); blood withdrawal syringes, needles, and tubes; catheterization tray and drainage equipment; urine testing devices; tracheostomy set; intubation equipment; venesection set; suction and oxygen therapy equipment; fresh, pathogen-free linens; over-bed cradle; and side rails. The particular procedure to be followed in wound care determines additional needs.

Transfer to a Burn Center

If the patient is to be transported to a burn center, the following measures are instituted prior to transfer: a secure IV line is in

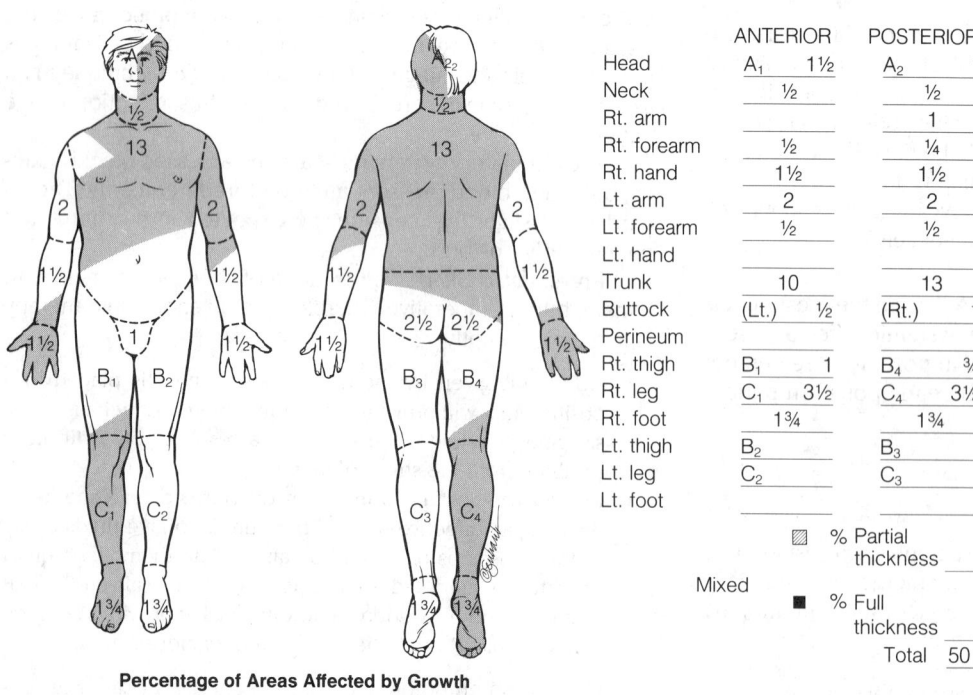

	ANTERIOR	POSTERIOR
Head	A₁ 1½	A₂ 1
Neck	½	½
Rt. arm		1
Rt. forearm	½	¼
Rt. hand	1½	1½
Lt. arm	2	2
Lt. forearm	½	½
Lt. hand		
Trunk	10	13
Buttock	(Lt.) ½	(Rt.) 1
Perineum		
Rt. thigh	B₁ 1	B₄ ¾
Rt. leg	C₁ 3½	C₄ 3½
Rt. foot	1¾	1¾
Lt. thigh	B₂	B₃
Lt. leg	C₂	C₃
Lt. foot		

▨ % Partial thickness ___

Mixed

■ % Full thickness ___

Total 50

Percentage of Areas Affected by Growth

	0	1 yr	5 yr	10 yr	15 yr	Adult
A = ½ head	9½	8½	6½	5½	4½	3½
B = 1 thigh	2¾	3¼	4	4¼	4½	4¾
C = ½ leg	2½	2½	2¾	3	3¼	3½

Figure 52–4. Example of burn evaluation chart for estimating percentage of body surface burned (indicated by shading). (Courtesy of Crozer–Chester Medical Center, Philadelphia, PA.)

ASSESSMENT AND INITIAL CARE OF SEVERE BURN PATIENTS
Guidelines for Hospital Emergency Departments

1. **STOP BURNING PROCESS**
   Remove or cool hot clothing
   Extensive lavage of chemical burns

2. **ADMINISTER CPR AS NEEDED**

3. **MAINTAIN VENTILATION**
   Look for signs of inhalation injury
   (cough, singed nasal hair, soot, or
   edema in upper airway)
   Establish open airway
   FOR RESPIRATORY INSUFFICIENCY:
   Administer high concentration of humidified
   oxygen until carbon monoxide is
   proven to be below toxic level
   Monitor ABG's
   Use endotracheal tube and respirator if
   necessary

4. **ESTABLISH CIRCULATION**
   Install I.V. line (#16 or #18 plastic cannula)
   Use Ringer's lactate, without glucose
   (2-4cc/kg body weight / % BSA burned)
   Objective: At least 50cc urine/hr in adults,
   1 ml urine/kg/hr in children
   For electrical injury, at least
   100cc urine/hr in adults
   FOR BURNED EXTREMITY:
   Elevate, remove rings, bracelets, etc.
   Monitor pulses in circumferentially
   burned limb

5. **REVIEW FOR MAJOR TRAUMA**
   Assess for head or spinal trauma, blunt
   and penetrating injuries and stabilize

6. **MAINTAIN BODY TEMPERATURE**
   Avoid systemic hypothermia or chill,
   using dry blankets.

7. **HISTORY AND PHYSICAL**
   Type, area and depth of burn
   Other injuries (fractures, lacerations, etc.)
   Details of accident
   Pre-existing illness (e.g. diabetes)
   Use of alcohol, tobacco, drugs
   Allergies, medications

8. **PREVENT ILEUS COMPLICATIONS**
   Keep patient N.P.O.
   Nasogastric tube to drainage
   –for nausea, vomiting or distention
   –for burns over 25% BSA

9. **RELIEVE PAIN**
   Give narcotics, 2-4 mg. morphine or
   equivalent, I.V. only, to achieve
   desired effect
   (Restlessness may be from hypoxia)

10. **TREAT BURN WOUND**
    Maintain irrigation of eye wounds
    Stabilize other injuries (fractures, etc.)
    For patients being transferred to burn
    center, remove wet dressing and cover
    with clean dry sheet
    For all other burn patients, cleanse
    gently with soap and water or saline

11. **TETANUS PROPHYLAXIS**

12. **COMFORT PATIENT AND FAMILY**

BURN REFERRAL CHECKLIST
(Use sheet from pocket to collect
information needed when preparing to
refer a burn patient)

**FOR ADDITIONAL COPIES OF
BURN REFERRAL CHECKLIST
WRITE OR CALL BURN FOUNDATION**

FOR TRANSFER TO BURN CENTER CALL:
Crozer-Chester Medical Center
215 / 447-2800
Saint Agnes Medical Center
215 / 339-4339
The Allentown Hospital–
Lehigh Valley Hospital Center
215 / 776-8111
St. Christopher's Hospital for Children
215 / 427-5323

BURN CENTER TRIAGE CRITERIA
Burned Area 2° and 3° (age <10 or >50): 10%
Burned Area 2° and 3° (age >10 or <50): 20%
Burned Area 3°: >5% at any age
Chemical Burn
Electrical Injury
Burn of Face, Hands, Feet or Perineum
Burn Accompanied By:
– Significant Associated Injury or Pre-Existing Disease
– Airway or Inhalation Injury
– Suspected Child Abuse

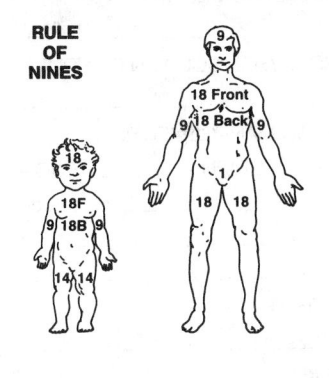

RULE
OF
NINES

BurnFoundation
1311 Chancellor Street, Philadelphia, PA 19107   (215) 735-4050
5000 Tilghman Street, Allentown, PA 18104   (215) 481-9810

Rev. 3/89

Figure 52–5. Guidelines for hospital emergency departments: Assessment and initial care of severe burn patients. (Used with permission of the Burn Foundation, Philadelphia, PA.)

place, with fluid infusing at the rate required to attain urine output of at least 30 ml per hour; a patent airway is ensured; adequate pain relief is attained; and adequate peripheral circulation in the burned extremities is established. Wounds are covered with sterile, dry dressings and the patient is kept comfortably warm. Assessments and treatments are documented (Fig. 52-6), and this information is provided to the burn center.

Management of Fluid Loss and Shock

Next to handling respiratory difficulties, the most urgent need is to replace lost fluid and to prevent irreversible shock (Table 52-5). Therefore, immediate management of the burn patient includes the following:

- An intravenous route is established, preferably through an unburned area.
- Blood specimens are drawn for hematocrit, electrolyte, and blood gas determinations, and for typing, cross-matching, and screening. These parameters must be followed closely in the immediate postburn (resuscitation) period.

- An indwelling urinary catheter is inserted so that urine volume and specific gravity can be monitored hourly. The amount of urine first obtained is recorded, because it may assist in determining the extent of renal function. Urine is also tested for the presence hemoglobin. Urine volumes of less than 30 ml/hr (10 ml in children) are reported.
- The patient's vital signs are monitored at frequent intervals: temperatures above 38.3°C (101°F) or below 36.1°C (97°F) are reported.

Fluid Replacement

There is no known way to stop movement of fluid into the interstitial spaces, but replacement of fluids is possible. The projected fluid requirements for the first 24 hours are calculated by the physician by evaluating the patient's burn injury. Some combination of fluid categories may be appropriate: (1) *colloids*—whole blood, plasma, and plasma expanders and (2) *electrolytes*—physiologic sodium chloride, Ringer's solution, Hartmann's solution.

Formulas have been developed for estimating fluid loss

BURN FOUNDATION
BURN REFERRAL CHECKLIST

(Use this form to collect essential information when preparing to refer a burn patient)

....

NAME _____ AGE _____ WT. _____

DATE/TIME OF BURN _____ %BSA _____

TYPE OF BURN: (circle) FLAME   SCALD   ELEC.   CHEM.   CONTACT

SPECIAL AREAS AFFECTED: RESP.   FACE   HANDS   FEET   PERIN.

CIRCUMFERENTIAL AREAS: THORAX   ARMS: L R   LEGS: L R

CAUSE OF INJURY _____

_____

ACCOMPANYIING TRAUMA _____

PMH _____ ALLERGIES _____

INITIAL MANAGEMENT *(complete as applicable)*

A) INHALATION INJURY:

ETT # _____ NASAL _____ O$_2$ THERAPY _____

CARBOXYHEMOGLOBIN (PURPLE TOP ON ICE) _____

ABG _____ CXR _____

B) FLUID MANAGEMENT:

IV LINES: PERIPH # _____ CVC # _____ (CONFIRMED BY CXR _____)

IV FLUIDS _____ cc/hr. UO _____ cc/hr.

FOLEY # _____ NPO _____

LAB STUDIES _____

C) OTHER

VS:T _____ P _____ RR _____ BP _____

NGT # _____ NGT TO SUCTION _____

TETANUS TOXOID _____ HYPERTET _____

IV ANALGESIA _____

ACCEPTING BURN CENTER _____

CONTACT PERSON/PHONE _____

MODE OF TRANSPORT _____ BURN TEAM ETA _____

Figure 52–6. Burn Referral Checklist. (Used with permission of the Burn Foundation, Philadelphia, PA.)

based on the estimated percentage of body surface area burned and the weight of the patient. These are individualized to meet the requirements of each patient. The various formulas are discussed in the following paragraphs and summarized in Chart 52-1.

The Consensus Formula. At the NIH Consensus Development Conference on Supportive Therapy in Burn Care in November 1978, it was agreed that salt and water are essential requirements of burn patients but that colloid may or may not be useful during the first 24 to 48 hours postburn.

The consensus formula provides for the volume of balanced salt solution to be administered in the first 24 hours in a range of 2 to 4 ml per kilogram per percent (ml/kg/%) burn. The volume should be started at the lower level of this range, because the overall goal of fluid therapy is to maintain vital organ function at the least immediate or delayed physiologic cost.

Generally, 2 ml/kg/% burn of lactated Ringer's solution may be used for adults, while children may require 3 ml/kg/% burn. As with the other formulas, half of the calculated total

should be given over the first 8 hours postburn, and the other half should be given over the next 16 hours. The rate and volume of the infusion must be regulated according to the patient's response.

Studies have demonstrated that with large burns there is a failure of the sodium–potassium pump at the cellular level. Thus, persons with very large burns may need proportionately more milliliters of fluid per percent burn than those with smaller burns.

Fluid Replacement Example: 70-kg patient with 50% body surface area (BSA) burn

1. Consensus formula: 2 to 4 ml/kg/% BSA
2. Calculate $2 \times 70 \times 50 = 7000$ ml/24 hours
3. Plan to administer: First 8 hours = 3500 ml = 437 ml/hr; next 16 hours = 3500 ml = 219 ml/hr

The Evans Formula. According to the Evans formula, second- to third-degree burns totaling more than 50% BSA are calculated on the basis of 50% BSA.

TABLE 52–5. *Water and Electrolyte Changes in the Emergent Phase of Burn Care* (First 48 Hours After Major Burns)

Fluid Accumulation Phase (Shock Phase)
Plasma → Interstitial Fluid (Edema at Burn Site)

Observation	Explanation
Generalized dehydration	Plasma leaks through damaged capillaries.
Reduction of blood volume	Secondary to plasma loss, fall of blood pressure, and diminished cardiac output
Decreased urinary output	Secondary to: Fluid loss Decreased renal blood flow Sodium and water retention caused by increased adrenocortical activity (Hemolysis of red blood cells, causing hemoglobinuria and myonecrosis or myoglobinuria)
Potassium excess	Massive cellular trauma causes release of K^+ into extracellular fluid (ordinarily, most K^+ is intracellular).
Sodium deficit	Large amount of Na^+ is lost in trapped edema fluid and exudate and by shift into cells as K^+ is released from cell (ordinarily most Na^+ is extracellular).
Metabolic acidosis (base bicarbonate deficit)	Loss of bicarbonate ions accompanies sodium loss.
Hemoconcentration (elevated hematocrit)	Liquid blood component is lost into extravascular space.

(Adapted from Metheny NM and Snively WD. Nurses' Handbook of Fluid Balance. Philadelphia, JB Lippincott.)

1. *Colloids* (blood, plasma, dextran): 1 ml × kg body weight × % BSA burned
2. *Electrolytes* (saline): 1 ml × kg body weight × % BSA burned
3. *Glucose* (5% in water): 2000 ml (for insensible losses)

A maximum of 10,000 ml of total fluids is given in a 24-hour period. Half of the calculated fluid is given in the first 8 hours postburn; the remainder is spread evenly over the next 16 hours.

On the second postburn day, the patient receives half of the colloid, half of the electrolyte, and all of the insensible replacement.

The Brooke Army Hospital Formula. This formula differs from the Evans formula only in that the colloid fraction is reduced from 1 to 0.5 ml and the electrolyte fraction is increased from 1 to 1.5 ml. Instead of saline, the electrolyte preferred is lactated Ringer's solution because of its lower chloride content.

On the second postburn day, the patient receives one-half of the colloid, one-half of the electrolyte, and all insensible replacement.

The Parkland or Baxter Formula. The patient is given 4 ml/kg/% burn of lactated Ringer's solution. Half is given in the first 8 hours, and the rest over the next 16 hours.

Hypertonic Saline. This method utilizes concentrated solutions of sodium chloride and lactate so that the resulting solution has a concentration of 300 mEq of sodium. It is administered at a rate sufficient to maintain a desired urinary output. The rate is *not* usually increased during the first 8 hours

postburn. The major therapeutic effects are a result of the sustained hypernatremia and the increase in serum osmolality that occur. Edema is reduced and lung complications from fluid loading are decreased.

- *Remember:* Formulas are a guide. Patient response evidenced by heart rate, blood pressure, and urine output is the primary determinant of actual fluid therapy and must be assessed at least hourly.

Fluid Therapy

The amount and speed of fluid given through an indwelling plastic vein cannula are gauged by the urinary output and the blood pressure and pulse rate. Urine flow from an indwelling catheter should be maintained at 30 to 50 ml/hr. This means that the flow from the indwelling catheter must be collected, measured, and recorded every hour. Pulse rate should be lower than 110 per minute.

These parameters are far more important in resuscitation than any formula. Indeed, the patient's individual response *is* the "formula."

The following observations must be reported:

- The presence of hematuria
- Urine output below 30 ml/hr—this suggests an inadequate rate of fluid resuscitation
- Urine output above 100 ml/hr, which may precede pulmonary edema or imminent water intoxication (suggested by the fol-

Chart 52-1
Guidelines and Formulas for Fluid Replacement in Burn Patients

Consensus Formula

Lactated Ringer's solution (or other balanced salt solution): 2-4 ml × kg body weight × % body surface area (BSA) burned. Half to be given in first 8 hours; second half to be given over next 16 hours

Evans Formula

1. *Colloids:* 1 ml × kg body weight × % BSA burned
2. *Electrolytes (saline):* 1 ml × kg body weight × % BSA burned
3. *Glucose* (5% in water): 2000 ml for insensible loss
    Day 1: Half to be given in first 8 hours; second half over next 16 hours.
    Day 2: Half of previous day's colloids and electrolytes; 2000 ml for insensible fluid replacement

Brooke Army Formula

1. *Colloids:* 0.5 ml × kg body weight × % BSA burned
2. *Electrolytes (lactated Ringer's solution):* 1.5 ml × kg body weight × % BSA burned
3. *Fluids:* Same as Evans formula
    Day 1: Same as Evans formula
    Day 2: Half of colloids; half of electrolytes; all of insensible fluid replacement

Parkland/Baxter Formula

Lactated Ringers' solution: 4 ml × kg body weight/% BSA burned. Half to be given in first 8 hours; half to be given over next 16 hours

Hypertonic Saline

Concentration solutions of NaCl and lactate with concentration of 300 mEq of sodium, administered at a rate sufficient to maintain a desired urinary output volume. *Goal:* Increase serum sodium level and osmolality to reduce edema and pulmonary complications.

---

lowing signs: tremor, twitching, nausea, diarrhea, salivation, and disorientation)
• Blood pressure below 90/60

If all extremities are burned, blood pressure determination may become difficult. A sterile dressing applied under the blood pressure cuff will protect the wound from contamination. A Doppler (ultrasound) device, an electronic blood pressure device, or other noninvasive means of monitoring may be helpful. An arterial catheter is used in severe burns for blood pressure measurement and accessibility for collection of specimens for measuring blood gases.

The Doppler is a useful tool in monitoring peripheral pulses. A more sophisticated method of determining tissue pressure levels to permit early intervention in the event of compartment syndrome is the use of the Wick catheter, connected to a transducer.

Additional gauges of the fluid requirements include hematocrit and hemoglobin determinations. Blood samples for these examinations and for the determination of electrolyte balance are obtained at frequent intervals. If the hematocrit and hemoglobin levels decrease, or if the urinary output is greater than 50 ml of urine per hour, the rate of intravenous fluid administration may be decreased.

Although the nurse is not responsible for calculating the patient's fluid requirements, she needs to know the maximal amount of fluid the patient should receive. Infusion pumps and rate controllers are a useful adjunct to the correct delivery of a complex regimen of prescribed intravenous fluids. With the addition of piggy-back IVs for medication infusion and total parenteral nutrition, monitoring intravenous therapy is a major nursing responsibility.

▶ Nursing Process
Burn Care During the Emergent/Immediate Phase

◇ Assessment

Assessment data obtained by prehospital providers are shared with the physician and nurse in the emergency department. Nursing assessment in the emergent phase of burn injury focuses on the major priorities for assessment of any trauma patient, with the wound as a secondary consideration.

If a patent airway and spontaneous respirations are noted, the nurse assesses further for signs of inhalation injury. Apical, carotid, and femoral pulses are checked. Cardiac monitoring is useful if there is a history of cardiac disease, electrical injury, or respiratory problems, or if the pulse is dysrhythmic and the rate is abnormally slow or rapid.

Vital signs are checked frequently with a Doppler or Dynamapp device, because increasing edema makes cuff pressures difficult to detect. Signs of hypovolemia are reported to the physician. Peripheral pulses on burned extremities are checked hourly. As edema increases in circumferential burns, pressure on small blood vessels and nerves in distal extremities causes obstruction to blood flow and ischemia. The physician may need to perform an *escharotomy* (surgical incision into the eschar) to relieve the constricting effect of the burned tissue.

Large-bore intravenous lines and an indwelling urinary catheter are inserted, and the nurse's assessment includes monitoring of fluid intake and output. Urine output is an excellent indicator of circulatory status; it is monitored carefully and measured hourly. Urine specific gravity, *p*H, glucose, acetone, protein, and hemoglobin levels are assessed frequently.

A burgundy color of the urine may indicate the presence of hemochromogen and myoglobin in the urine as a result of muscle damage from deep burns associated with electrical injury or prolonged contact with flames. Glucosuria is a common finding in the early hours postburn and is due to the release of stored glucose from the liver in response to stress.

Nursing assessment includes reviewing results of laboratory and radiologic tests. Although chest x-ray and arterial blood gases may be normal initially, changes will often occur with time and progression of inhalation injury. It is essential to note the presence of increased hoarseness, stridor, abnormal respiratory rate and depth, or mental changes caused by hypoxia. These may signal the need for intubation, mechanical ventilation, or escharotomy to relieve constriction from circumferential chest burns.

Body temperature, body weight, history of preburn weight, allergies, tetanus immunization, past medical and surgical problems, current illnesses, and use of medication are assessed. A head-to-toe assessment is performed, looking for signs and symptoms of concomitant illness or injury.

Assessment of the burn wound continues, with use of the anatomic diagrams described previously. In addition, the nurse works with the physician to assess the depth of the wound, noting areas of full- and partial-thickness injury.

The neurologic assessment focuses on the patient's level of consciousness, psychologic status, and behavior. The patient's and family's understanding of the injury and treatment are assessed.

Nursing Diagnoses

Based on assessment data, clinical manifestations, and laboratory data, nursing diagnoses in the emergent (immediate) postburn phase may include the following:

- Impaired gas exchange related to carbon monoxide poisoning, smoke inhalation, and upper airway obstruction
- Ineffective airway clearance related to edema and effects of smoke inhalation
- Fluid volume deficit related to increased capillary permeability and evaporative fluid loss from burn wound
- Altered tissue perfusion related to peripheral burn wound edema and circumferential full-thickness burns
- High risk for altered body temperature: hypothermia related to loss of skin microcirculation and open wounds
- Altered nutrition: less than body requirements related to increased nutritional requirements secondary to thermal injury and altered gastrointestinal function

Planning and Implementation

Goals: The major goals of the patient may include maintenance of a patent airway, ventilation, and tissue oxygenation; establishment of optimal fluid and electrolyte balance and perfusion of vital organs; maintenance of normal body temperature; and attainment of optimal nutrition.

Nursing Interventions

Maintaining Oxygenation and a Patent Airway. Assessment for signs of upper airway obstruction or a compromised lower airway is an essential nursing activity. Aggressive pulmonary care measures—including turning, coughing, deep breathing, periodic forceful expiration using spirometry, and tracheal suction as needed—are particularly important in the burn patient with inhalation injury. Proper positioning to decrease the work of breathing and promote optimal chest expansion and the provision of humidified oxygen or mechanical ventilation may further decrease metabolic stress and ensure adequate tissue oxygenation. The nurse reports promptly to the physician any signs of respiratory compromise resulting from edema and prepares to assist with naso- or endotracheal intubation, tracheotomy, or escharotomy as required. Asepsis is maintained to prevent contamination of the respiratory tract and to prevent infection that increases metabolic requirements.

Establishing Fluid and Electrolyte Balance. Rapid fluid shifts and losses during the early postburn period require that nurses frequently assess vital signs and urinary output, as well as central venous pressure, pulmonary artery pressure, and cardiac output if required. Intravenous fluids are provided as prescribed and may need to be titrated with urinary output. Meticulous documentation of intake and output and daily weight is required. The patient must be monitored for early signs of hypovolemic shock or fluid overload, including altered mental status, change in respirations, and hemodynamic parameters.

The extremities are assessed carefully, particularly if burns are circumferential, to detect compromised circulation resulting from increased edema or a constricting effect of eschar formation in full-thickness burns. Elevating affected extremities may be indicated to help reduce edema.

Maintaining Normal Body Temperature. Burn patients are prone to chilling and hypothermia because a loss of the skin microcirculation in the burned areas decreases the patient's ability to retain body heat. The room temperature is adjusted according to the patient's needs. An environment that is too warm may cause fluid loss through perspiration and in addition may promote bacterial growth. Overcooling of a room, which can easily occur when staff members turn on air conditioners to keep themselves comfortable, will chill the patient and increase metabolic demands. A patient who is allowed to control environmental room temperature will select a temperature of approximately 32.2° to 32.8°C (90° to 91°F). Cotton blankets, ceiling-mounted heat lamps, and aluminum-coated "space" blankets are helpful in maintaining the patient's comfort. Heat shields with sensors and blanket-draped bed cradles to deflect drafts are also useful. An efficient approach for removing the dressing and caring for the wound shortens the time during which patients are exposed to the ambient temperature and reduces shivering and metabolic stress.

As a result of episodes of bacteremia and septicemia, fever is also common in burn patients. A resetting of core body temperature in severely burned persons causes them to have a body temperature a few degrees higher than normal for several weeks postburn. Bacteremia and septicemia also cause fever in many patients. Acetaminophen and hypothermia blankets may be required to keep body temperature in a range of 37.2° to 39.4°C (99° to 103°F) and to reduce metabolic stress.

▷ *Improving Nutritional Status.* Following a thermal injury, the patient's nutritional requirements are dramatically increased. However, in the early postburn period, the patient is usually unable to take nutrients orally because of gastrointestinal responses to the injury. Gastric dilatation and paralytic ileus frequently occur in the early postburn period and are indicated by nausea and distention. A nasogastric tube is inserted early in the treatment to prevent vomiting and aspiration of gastric contents into the lungs. The tube is connected to low intermittent suction until bowel sounds return.

If oral alimentation is initiated after the immediate or emergent burn phase, oral fluids should be administered slowly. The patient's tolerance is noted. If vomiting and distention do not occur, fluids may be increased gradually and the patient advanced to a normal diet or tube feedings.

Severely burned patients are prone to gastric and duodenal ulcers because of hypersecretion of gastric acid and erosion of the gastric mucosa in response to the stress of the burn injury. Gastric pH should be assessed regularly in the patient with a nasogastric tube and maintained at a level less acidic than usual through antacid therapy. Histamine blockers such as cimetidine (Tagamet) or ranitidine (Zantac) are administered as prescribed to prevent gastric erosion and the formation of bleeding ulcers.

▷ Evaluation

Expected Outcomes

1. Maintains patent airway, adequate ventilation, and oxygenation
   a. Breathes spontaneously with adequate tidal volume
   b. Is free of dyspnea or shortness of breath
   c. Exhibits respiratory rate between 12 and 20
   d. Has pulmonary function parameters within normal limits
   e. Lungs sound clear on auscultation
   f. Chest x-ray is normal
   g. Is free of cerebral signs of hypoxia
   h. Arterial blood gases are within normal limits
   i. Respiratory secretions are minimal, colorless, and thin
   j. Uses humidified oxygen as prescribed
   k. Coughs and breathes deeply hourly
2. Regains optimal fluid and electrolyte balance and perfusion of vital organs
   a. Intake, output, and body weight correlate with pattern of physiologic pathology and expected results of therapy
   b. Serum electrolytes are within normal limits
   c. Urine output is between 0.5 ml/kg/hr and 1.0 ml/kg/hr
   d. Blood pressure is within patient's normal range (usually higher than 90/60)
   e. Heart rate is within patient's normal range (usually below 110/min)

   f. Heart is in sinus rhythm
   g. Sensorium is clear
   h. Is free of thirst
   i. Shows normal reflexes and muscle tone indicative of electrolyte balance
   j. BUN and creatinine are normal
   k. Urine is clear yellow; protein, sugar, acetone, pH, and specific gravity are within normal limits
   l. Hemoglobin and hematocrit are normal
   m. Is free of paresthesias or symptoms of ischemia of nerves and muscles (compartment syndrome)
3. Demonstrates acceptable body temperature
   a. Body temperature is in range of 37.2° to 38.3°C (98.6° to 101°F)
   b. Reports comfort without chills or shivering
4. Achieves adequate nutritional status
   a. Bowel sounds are normal
   b. Gastric aspirate is normal, with no indication of blood present
   c. Tolerates oral or nasogastric feedings
   d. Stools negative for occult blood
   e. Reports absence of abdominal pain or feeling of abdominal fullness or bloating
   f. Exhibits no abdominal distention on palpation

Care of the patient during this emergent/immediate phase of burn care is delineated in Nursing Care Plan 52-1.

In summary, the emergent phase of burn care focuses on fluid replacement (fluid resuscitation) and correction of acute life-threatening problems, such as compromised pulmonary, cardiovascular, and renal status. Collaboration among multiple disciplines is essential to care for the patient with major burns as well as elderly persons with moderate burns and other patients with pre-existing health problems that compromise physiologic status.

Although the most critical aspects of management at this stage focus on life-saving strategies and restoring or maintaining pulmonary, cardiovascular, and renal function, interventions to prevent later complications (*i.e.*, sepsis, contractures, disabilities) must be initiated in the early phases of burn management. Expertise in assessment is critical in identifying concomitant problems and in the early detection of changes in the patient's physiologic status. Dealing with the psychologic reaction of the patient and his family to a burn injury requires effective communication skills to assist them in dealing with the psychologic trauma of a major burn while life-saving measures are undertaken.

Acute/Intermediate Phase

General Care Considerations

The acute or intermediate phase of burn care follows the emergent or immediate phase of burn care and begins 48 to 72 hours after the burn injury. During this phase, attention is directed toward continued assessment and maintenance of respiratory and circulatory status, fluid and electrolyte balance, and gastrointestinal function. Burn wound care is a major focus of this stage.

Nursing Care Plan 52-1

Care of the Patient During the Emergent/Immediate Phase of Burn Care

Nursing Interventions	Rationale	Expected Outcomes

Nursing Diagnosis: Alteration in gas exchange and airway clearance

Goal: Assure patent airway and adequate respiratory function

Nursing Interventions	Rationale	Expected Outcomes
1. Maintain patent airway through proper positioning, removal of secretions, and artificial airway if indicated.	1. Ensures patent airway	• Breathes spontaneously • Is free of dyspnea or shortness of breath • Exhibits respiratory rate between 12 and 20 breaths/min • Has pulmonary function parameters within normal limits • Shows lungs clear on auscultation • Is free of cerebral effects of hypoxia • Has arterial blood gases within normal limits • Exhibits respiratory secretions that are minimal, colorless, and thin
2. Provide humidified oxygen through appropriate mode.	2. Provides humidity to injured tissues and adequate oxygen supply	
3. Assess breath sounds and respiratory rate, rhythm, and depth, chest excursion, and signs of hypoxia.	3. Provides baseline for further assessment and evidence of increasing respiratory compromise	

4. Observe for the following:
  a. Erythema or blistering of lips or buccal mucosa
  b. Singed nares
  c. Burns of face, neck, or chest
  d. Increasing hoarseness
  e. Soot in sputum or tracheal tissue in respiratory secretions
	4. Indicate injury to respiratory tree and/or risk of respiratory dysfunction	

5. Monitor arterial blood gases.	5. Increasing Pco_2 and decreasing Po_2 may indicate need for mechanical ventilation	
6. Monitor patient on mechanical ventilation; check settings and patient responses as determined by arterial blood gases.	6. Respiratory dysfunction/pulmonary obstruction changes may occur quickly or gradually	
7. Encourage patient to turn, take deep breaths, cough, and use incentive spirometry; suction as needed.	7. Reduces risk of atelectasis and promotes removal of increased secretions	

Nursing Diagnosis: Alteration in fluid and electrolyte balance

Goal: Restore optimal fluid and electrolyte balance; maintain perfusion of vital organs and adequate circulation to extremities

Nursing Interventions	Rationale	Expected Outcomes
1. Observe vital signs (including central venous pressure or pulmonary artery pressure, if indicated), urine output, and signs of hypovolemia or fluid overload.	1. Hypovolemia is a major risk immediately after the burn injury; as mobilization of fluid occurs, there is increased risk of fluid overload and congestive heart failure	• Exhibits intake, output, and body weight that correlate with pattern of physiologic pathology and expected results of therapy • Has serum electrolytes within normal limits • Exhibits urine output between 0.5 and 1.0 ml/kg/hr • Has blood pressure higher than 90/60 • Shows heart rate less than 110/min • Exhibits clear sensorium • Is free of excessive thirst • Shows normal reflexes and muscle tone indicative of electrolyte balance
2. Monitor urine output at least hourly and weigh patient daily.	2. Provides information about renal perfusion, adequacy of fluid replacement, and fluid requirement and fluid status	
3. Monitor mental status and sensorium.	3. Provides information about adequacy of cerebral perfusion and oxygenation	
4. Maintain IV lines and regulate fluids at appropriate rates, as prescribed.	4. Adequate fluids are necessary to maintain fluid and electrolyte status and adequate perfusion of vital organs	
5. Observe for symptoms of deficiency or excess serum sodium, potassium, calcium, phosphorus, and bicarbonate. Note results of laboratory tests, and report abnormal values to physician.	5. Rapid shifts in fluid and electrolyte status are possible in the postburn period	
6. Elevate head of patient's bed and elevate burned extremities.	6. Promotes venous return	

(continued)

Nursing Care Plan 52–1 (Continued)

Care of the Patient During the Emergent/Immediate Phase of Burn Care

Nursing Interventions	Rationale	Expected Outcomes

Nursing Diagnosis: High risk for infection

Goal: Absence of infection and sepsis

1. Use asepsis in all aspects of patient care:
  a. Wash hands carefully with antibacterial cleansing agent before and after patient care.
  b. Wear isolation gown or plastic apron for patient contact.
  c. Cover hair and use mask when patient's wounds are exposed or during sterile procedures.
  d. Use clean or sterile gloves in patient care.
  e. Use aseptic technique for wound care and invasive procedures.
  f. Change IV lines and tubing and other equipment as recommended.
	1. Minimizes risk of cross-contamination and spread of bacterial contamination	• Is free of signs of local or systemic infection
		• Has negative blood cultures
		• Has negative wound, sputum, and urine cultures

2. Administer antibiotics and topical antibacterial agents as prescribed.	2. An adequate concentration of the agent is necessary to treat or prevent infection effectively	
3. Assess wounds daily for local signs of infection: swelling and redness, purulent drainage, discoloration.	3. Indicative of bacterial contamination and infection	
4. Observe mental status, respiratory rate, bowel sounds.	4. Decreased mentation and peristalsis and increased respiratory rate are early signs of septicemia	
5. Assess for increased pulse, decreased BP, changes in urine output, facial flushing, fever.	5. These are later signs of septicemia	
6. Provide adequate nutrition.	6. Adequate nutrition is essential for immunologic response (functioning of white blood cells and lymphocytes) and healing	
7. Assist with or promote optimal personal hygiene (e.g., daily cleaning of unburned areas, meticulous care of teeth and mouth, shampooing hair).	7. Reduces bacterial contamination from areas adjacent to burn	

Nursing Diagnosis: Altered body temperature: hypothermia/hyperthermia

Goal: Maintenance of adequate body temperature

1. Provide a warm environment through use of heat shield, space blanket, heat lights or blankets.	1. Minimizes evaporative heat loss	• Body temperature in range of 36.1° to 38.3°C (97° to 101°F) • Exhibits no shivering • States room temperature is not too warm or too cold
2. When wounds must be exposed for wound care, work quickly.	2. Minimizes heat loss through the burn wound	
3. Monitor rectal temperature.	3. Allows frequent assessment of body temperature	
4. Administer antipyretics for elevated body temperature as prescribed.	4. Reduces metabolic stress	

(continued)

> ## Nursing Care Plan 52–1 *(Continued)*

Care of the Patient During the Emergent/Immediate Phase of Burn Care

Nursing Interventions	Rationale	Expected Outcomes

Nursing Diagnosis: Altered nutritional status: less than body requirements related to increased nutritional requirements and altered gastrointestinal function

Goal: Improved nutritional status

1. Maintain nasogastric tube on low intermittent suction until bowel sounds return.	1. Burn injury often produces paralytic ileus, which results in gastric and abdominal distention; nasogastric suction removes gastric secretions and prevents vomiting	• Exhibits bowel sounds • Shows normal gastric aspirate; no bleeding • Tolerates oral or nasogastric feedings • Has negative stools for occult blood
2. Auscultate for bowel sounds every 4 hours.	2. Absent bowel sounds and decreased peristalsis may indicate paralytic ileus, obstruction, or sepsis	
3. Prior to tube feedings, aspirate stomach contents to check for residual amount and pH of gastric contents.	3. Large residual volume of gastric contents indicates inadequate absorption; low pH indicates need for histamine blockers or antacids	
4. Administer histamine blockers and antacids as prescribed.	4. Reduces risk of gastric ulceration common in burn patients	
5. Test stools and gastric aspirate contents for occult bleeding.	5. May indicate presence of gastric or duodenal ulcer	

Nursing Diagnosis: Pain and anxiety

Goal: Reduction in pain and anxiety

1. Assess patient for pain, and differentiate from hypoxia.	1. Assessment of pain provides baseline for evaluating pain relief measures	• Shows that comfort level permits adequate rest and active participation in required activities • Requires analgesics primarily prior to dressing changes and potentially painful treatments
2. Administer narcotic analgesics intravenously as prescribed; monitor respiratory response to narcotics.	2. Intravenous administration is necessary because of altered absorption and circulation resulting from the burn	
3. Introduce relaxation techniques, imagery, or other adjuncts to analgesics.	3. Relaxation and imagery complement analgesia and reduce anxiety	
4. Provide emotional support and reassurance.	4. Emotional support and reassurance are essential to reduce extreme fear and anxiety resulting from burn injury, treatments, and outcomes	
5. Give honest information regarding status and medical care required for optimal response.	5. Promotes trust needed for patient's emotional well-being and acceptance of painful treatments	

Airway obstruction as a result of upper airway edema can take as long as 48 hours to develop. Changes in x-rays and blood gases may occur as the effects of resuscitative fluid and the chemical reaction of smoke ingredients with lung tissues become apparent. The patient's arterial blood gases and other parameters serve as a guide to determine the need for intubation, tracheostomy, or mechanical ventilation.

As capillaries regain their integrity, in 48 hours or more postburn, and fluid moves from the interstitial to the vascular compartment, diuresis begins (Table 52-6). If cardiac or renal function is not adequate, fluid overload occurs and symptoms of congestive heart failure may result. Detection of early signs allows for early intervention and careful titration of fluid intake.

Cardiotonic drugs and diuretics may be necessary at this time to prevent congestive heart failure.

Cautious administration of fluids and electrolytes continues during this phase of burn care because of the shifts in fluid from interstitial to vascular compartments, losses of fluid from large burn wounds, and the patient's physiologic responses to the burn injury. If blood transfusions are necessary to treat blood loss and anemia, the patient is monitored closely for a possible transfusion reaction.

Central venous, peripheral arterial, Swan-Ganz, or thermal-dilution catheters may be required for monitoring venous and arterial pressures, pulmonary wedge pressures, or cardiac output. Generally, however, invasive lines are avoided unless ab-

TABLE 52-6.   *Water and Electrolyte Changes in the Acute/Intermediate Phase of Burn Care (Beginning 48 Hours After Major Injuries)*

Fluid Remobilization Phase (State of Diuresis)
Interstitial Fluid → Plasma

Observation	*Explanation*
Hemodilution (decreased hematocrit)	Blood cell concentration is diluted as fluid enters the vascular compartment; loss of red blood cells destroyed at burn site.
Increased urinary output	Fluid shift into intravascular compartment increases renal blood flow and causes increased urine formation.
Sodium deficit	With diuresis, sodium is lost with water; existing serum sodium is diluted by water influx.
Potassium deficit (occurs occasionally in this phase)	Beginning on the fourth or fifth postburn day, K^+ shifts from extracellular fluid into cells.
Metabolic acidosis	Loss of sodium depletes fixed base; relative carbon dioxide content increases.

(Adapted from Metheny NM and Snively WD. Nurses' Handbook of Fluid Balance. Philadelphia, JB Lippincott.)

solutely necessary because they provide an additional portal for infection in this already greatly compromised patient.

Infection is the major cause of death in patients who have survived the first few days following extensive burns. The infection begins within the burn site and then is carried into the bloodstream. Because of the danger of infection, cultures are taken of the burn wound to monitor colonization of the wound by microbial organisms. These may be swab cultures or tissue biopsy cultures (Fig. 52-7). A major part of the nurse's role during this and other phases of burn care is detection and prevention of infection. Several parenteral antimicrobial agents may be used to treat or prevent infection and sepsis. It is important that these medications be given as scheduled to maintain proper blood concentrations.

The Burn Wound

The burn wound is unique among surgical wounds because it involves a large amount of dead tissue (eschar) that remains in place for a prolonged period of time. It is rapidly colonized by pathogenic bacteria; exudes large quantities of water, protein, and electrolytes; and frequently requires that tissue be mobilized through skin grafting from another part of the body to achieve permanent closure.

Threat of Infection

Despite aseptic precautions and the use of topical antimicrobial agents, the burn wound represents an excellent medium for

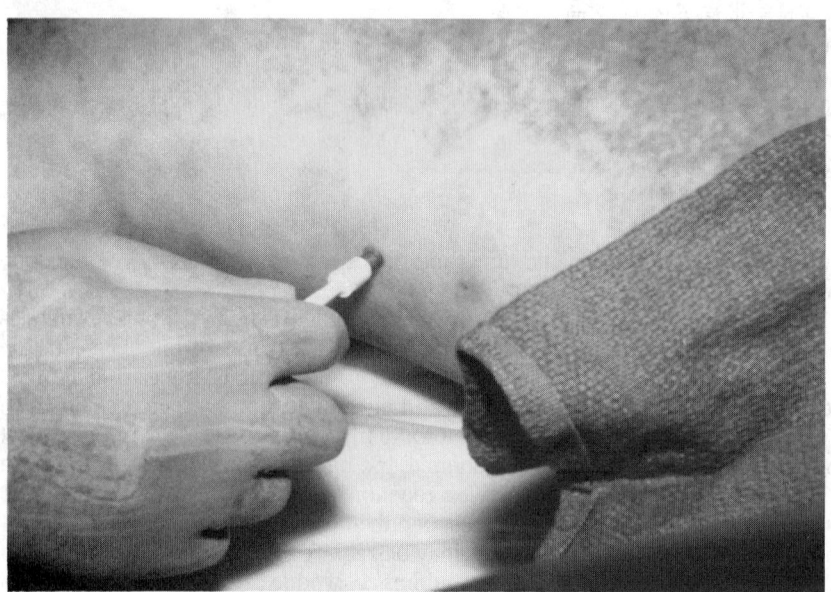

Figure 52-7.   Punch biopsy. This biopsy technique permits assessment for burn wound sepsis.

bacterial growth and proliferation. Bacteria such as *Staphylococcus, Proteus, Pseudomonas, Escherichia coli,* and *Klebsiella* enterobacteria find optimal conditions for growth within the burn. The burn eschar is a nonviable crust with no blood supply, so polymorphonuclear leukocytes and antibodies, as well as systemic antibiotics, cannot reach the area. Phenomenal numbers of bacteria—over one billion per gram of tissue—may appear and subsequently spread to the bloodstream or release their toxins, which reach distant sites.

During the time in which the burn wound is healing through spontaneous reepithelialization or being prepared for skin grafting, it must be protected from burn wound sepsis. Burn wound sepsis has these characteristics:

1. 10^5 bacteria per gram of tissue
2. Inflammation
3. Sludging and thrombosis of dermal blood vessels

If not appropriately treated, burn wound sepsis can progress to systemic sepsis.

The primary source of bacterial infection appears to be the patient's own intestinal tract. A major secondary source is the environment. Antibiotics are seldom given prophylactically today because of the tendency to promote resistant strains. There is documentation that streptococcal infection can be prevented by prophylactic administration of penicillin; this should be continued only through the edema phase (48 to 72 hours). Systemic antibiotics are administered thereafter when there is documentation of burn wound sepsis or other positive cultures such as urine, sputum, or blood. Sensitivity to antibiotics should be determined prior to administration. Serum antibiotic levels are monitored for evidence of maximal effectiveness; the patient is monitored for toxic side effects. Combination drug regimens may be used.

Localized infection must be identified and eliminated. A prime objective is to guard against burn wound infection by maintaining strict isolation precautions.

- A mask and sterile gloves are worn while caring for the patient with extensive burns in order to prevent infection. Aseptic technique, with cap and gown, is used when caring directly for burn wounds.

Because burns are contaminated wounds, tetanus prophylaxis is given. If the patient has been immunized or has had no booster dose in the preceding 4 years, a booster dose of tetanus toxoid is administered. If the patient has never had immunizing toxoid, then tetanus immune globulin (TIG) should be given. The extent of the burn and the environment in which the injury occurred are taken into consideration. If the patient was rolled on the ground or has been lying on the ground, the danger of tetanus is increased.

Wound Care

Wound care includes cleansing and débridement, application of topical antimicrobial agents, and dressings. Gauze, biologic, biosynthetic, and synthetic materials may be used. Split-thickness skin grafts are required to close full-thickness and deep partial-thickness wounds.

Wound Cleansing

A variety of measures can be taken to cleanse the burn wound. Total immersion hydrotherapy is performed in some settings; bedside baths are performed in others; and some use a procedure in which the patient is suspended on a vinyl stretcher over a tub and showered. A walk-in bath, a tub, or a whirlpool may be used. The agitation in the whirlpool aids in cleansing and gently massaging the tissues. Because of the high risk of infection and sepsis, plastic liners are used in hydrotherapy equipment to prevent cross-contamination. Tap water alone, saline, or antiseptic solutions such as dilute iodine preparations may be used.

The temperature of the bath is maintained at 37.8°C (100°F), and the temperature of the room should be between 26.6° and 29.4°C (80° to 85°F).

During the bath, the patient is encouraged to carry out as much activity as possible. Hydrotherapy provides an excellent medium for exercising the extremities and cleaning the entire body. When the patient is removed from the tub following the bath, any residue adhering to the body is washed away with a spray or shower of clear water.

Hydrotherapy should be limited to a 20- to 30-minute period to prevent chilling and additional metabolic stress.

Unburned areas including the hair must be washed regularly as well. At the time of wound cleansing, all skin is examined for any hints of redness, breakdown, or local infection. Hair in and around the burn area should be clipped short. Intact blisters may be left, but the fluid should be aspirated with a needle and syringe and discarded.

Conscientious management of the burn wound is of vital importance. When nonviable loose skin is removed, aseptic conditions must be established. Borderline normal skin near the burn wound is shaved to prevent possible contamination from hair follicles.

Wound cleansing is usually done at least daily in wound areas that are not undergoing surgical intervention. When the eschar begins to separate from the viable tissue beneath, approximately 1½ to 2 weeks postburn, more frequent cleansing and débridement may be in order.

After a tub bath, wounds are gently patted dry with sterile towels and the prescribed method of wound care is employed. Physician preferences, the skill level of the nursing staff, and resources in terms of number of personnel, supplies, and time must be considered in choosing the best method for a given patient. Whatever the method, the goal is to protect the wound from overwhelming proliferation of pathogenic organisms and invasion of deeper tissues until either spontaneous healing or skin grafting can be achieved. Patient comfort and ability to participate in the prescribed method of treatment are also important considerations.

Topical Antibacterial Therapy

There is general agreement that some form of antimicrobial therapy applied to the burn wound is the best method of local care in extensive burn injury. Topical antibacterial therapy does not sterilize the burn wound but simply reduces the number of bacteria so that the overall microbial population can be controlled by the body's host defense mechanisms. Topical therapy buys time during which vigorous efforts must be made to convert the open, dirty wound to a closed, clean one.

No single agent is universally effective. Use of different agents at different times in the postburn period may be necessary. Effectiveness is based on cultures of the burn wound. Before the topical agent is reapplied, the previously applied topical agent is thoroughly removed. The nurse should be aware of the length of time the topical agents are effective and the prescribed concentration of each agent. The number of times the dressings are changed and soaked is planned to promote optimal therapeutic use of the topical agent.

Bacteriologic cultures are required to monitor the effect of topical medications. Swab cultures or surface cultures may be used. These procedures are noninvasive, simple, and painless, but resulting data apply only to the area sampled. Wound biopsy cultures (invasive) may be required for quantitative sampling. Systemic antibiotics are used sparingly but are essential for pulmonary or other concomitant infections.

Criteria for topical agents include the following: (1) it is effective against gram-negative organisms, *Pseudomonas aeruginosa, Staphylococcus aureus,* and even fungi; (2) it is clinically effective; (3) it penetrates the eschar but is not systemically toxic; (4) it does not lose its effectiveness, thereby permitting another infection to develop; (5) it is cost-effective, available, and acceptable to the patient; and (6) it is easy to apply, minimizing nursing care time.

Silver Sulfadiazine (Silvadene)

Silver sulfadiazine, a common topical medication used in burn treatment, is synthesized by reacting silver nitrate with sodium sulfadiazine. It is available as a water-soluble cream in concentrations of 1% and is bactericidal for gram-negative and gram-positive bacteria as well as yeast.

Evidence indicates that the *Pseudomonas* cells may split the agent so that silver is bound but sulfadiazine is released. This binding action may account for the potent inhibition of bacterial growth.

Compared with mafenide acetate and other antibacterial agents, silver sulfadiazine is more effective in controlling infection; causes no pain on application; does not disturb acid–base balance, electrolytes, or renal function; and does not stain.

Leukopenia (WBC count less than 5000) has been associated with Silvadene within 2 to 4 days of initiating treatment. However, leukocyte levels rebound without discontinuation of treatment within 2 to 3 days.

It is applied with a sterile gloved hand, one sixteenth of an inch thick, once or twice daily. The medicated burn area can be left open or covered with a dressing. When silver sulfadiazine is applied to dermal burns, a proteinaceous gel (several millimeters thick) forms on the wound surface; after 72 hours this pseudoeschar can be easily removed. It is believed by some burn care specialists that this gel slows reepithelialization and dressings should be removed and wounds cleansed every 8 hours to prevent this pseudoeschar from forming.

It has been reported that a significant number of gram-negative bacilli can become highly resistant to sulfadiazine as a result of protracted use of this agent.

Silver Sulfadiazine–Cerium Nitrate.   Cerium (a lanthanide element) has been incorporated into silver sulfadiazine to enhance clinical effectiveness. A combination of just under 1% of silver sulfadiazine and 2.2% of cerium nitrate provides a thin cream that can be applied topically. It appears to be most effective against gram-negative bacteria and has been credited with lowering mortality rates. Occasionally, methemoglobinemia has been noted; however, on the whole the drug seems effective and safe.

Cerium Nitrate Solution.   Cerium nitrate solution (1.74%) can be used alone or in conjunction with the combination silver sulfadiazine–cerium nitrate cream as a wet soak to enhance the effectiveness of the antibacterial action of these agents. It must be rewet every 4 hours and applied with a bulky dressing for maximal effectiveness and to assist in maintaining the patient's body temperature at optimal levels. A dry top covering, such as a layer of stockinette or cotton bath blanket, helps to reduce evaporative heat loss.

Silver Nitrate Solution (0.5% Aqueous Solution)

Silver nitrate is an effective agent in preventing eschar contamination; in concentrations of 0.5% it does not injure tissue and is effectively bacteriostatic. However, because the drug is unable to penetrate the eschar, infection can occur in the subeschar region. Therefore, it is necessary to inspect the wound frequently and débride as necessary.

The treatment begins soon after the patient reaches the hospital. The wounds are cleansed and then covered with gauze dressings thoroughly soaked with 0.5% silver nitrate solution. These dressings are kept wet with the silver nitrate solution, which is applied by means of a bulb syringe or catheters incorporated into the layers of the dressing. The wet dressings are covered with layers of dry gauze, held in place with nonelastic outer dressings. They are remoistened every 2 to 4 hours and changed daily.

The patient is covered with dry sheets and a dry blanket. These dry layers reduce the heat loss produced by vaporization from the wet dressings and from the burned surface.

The use of 0.5% silver nitrate solution dressings is not without danger; because the solution is hypotonic, electrolytes, especially sodium and potassium, are withdrawn from the body fluids and pass into the dressings impregnated with silver nitrate solution. The withdrawal of sodium may occur very rapidly, especially in patients with extensive burns and in children, producing an acute electrolyte imbalance.

- In the early phases of the burn treatment, blood must be drawn at frequent intervals to determine sodium, chloride, potassium, and calcium levels. These electrolytes must be replaced, usually by the intravenous administration of Ringer's lactate solution.

Once the patient can take a normal diet, salt is added to the diet. Hypocalcemia is treated by the addition of calcium lactate or gluconate to the diet (usually within a few days postburn), and potassium depletion is treated by the administration of potassium chloride elixir. Deficits in these constituents of the blood electrolytes naturally are more marked in more extensive burns (constituting 50% to 80% of the body surface).

The silver nitrate solution has the disadvantage of turning black in the sunlight. This means that everything touched by the solution is stained black, including clothes, hands, floors, and other objects. The nurse attending a patient being treated with silver nitrate solution must wear rubber gloves as a protection against the silver nitrate stains. (Such stains may be prevented by applying an organic iodine preparation, such as Wescodyne or Betadine solutions, to objects that have come in contact with the silver solution and then rinsing them in water.) Stain-resistant floor and wall coverings are available, but such materials increase the cost of care.

Mafenide Acetate (Sulfamylon Acetate)

Mafenide acetate (10%) in cream form with a hydrophilic base diffuses rapidly through the devitalized tissue. It is the topical agent of choice in electrical burns because of its ability to penetrate the thick eschar associated with this type of injury. It is effective against a broad range of gram-positive and gram-negative organisms in the subeschar area. It is limited in use to the treatment of localized invasive burn wound sepsis caused by organisms sensitive to this agent.

The cream is applied in a thin layer once or twice daily; the wound is frequently left open, but dressings may be applied and changed every 6 hours. Although it is relatively nontoxic, mafenide acetate is a strong carbonic anhydrase inhibitor and may adversely affect the blood pH level, causing a reduction of the renal tubular buffering mechanism. With continued use, severe metabolic acidosis may occur, making it necessary to monitor the respiratory rate, blood gases, and pH. Chest x-rays also may be justified because of possible pulmonary failure. The occurrence of these problems may require that mafenide be discontinued.

Another disadvantage of this form of treatment is the burning pain experienced by the patient for a few minutes following application of the cream. Thus, analgesics may be required before the ointment is applied. Mafenide may delay eschar separation, thereby delaying skin grafting unless the eschar is aggressively débrided. Mafenide 5% solution is effective for use after skin grafting or to dress newly excised areas before grafts are applied.

Other Topical Agents

Povidone-iodine ointment (10%) and *Betadine solution* are effective against a wide variety of gram-negative and gram-positive organisms as well as yeasts, fungi, and viruses. These dressings are usually changed every 6 hours. Iodine preparations may be painful to patients when first applied. Some patients are allergic to iodine. Iodine also has the property of staining bed linens.

Gentamicin sulfate is a bactericidal aminoglycoside available in a 0.1% cream for topical use. It is useful for short periods of time in small areas of invasive infection. Superinfection with resistant bacterial strains has been reported, indicating the need for very careful monitoring when this agent is used.

Nitrofurazone (Furacin) is a synthetic nitrofuran available in ointment or cream and is bactericidal against most bacteria commonly causing surface burn wound infections. The polyethylene glycol–based ointment may be absorbed through the wound and not normally excreted by the compromised kidney, leading to symptoms of renal impairment such as elevated BUN and metabolic acidosis. Use of nitrofurazone may result in bacterial or fungal superinfections or nonsusceptible organisms.

All topical agents must be used with consideration given to the microbial population found in the burn wound. Prudent use of antimicrobial agents results in less-resistant strains of bacteria, greater effectiveness of the agents, and a decreased risk of sepsis for the patient.

Dressing Changes

Dressings are changed in the patient's unit, hydrotherapy room, or treatment area approximately 20 minutes after the administration of an analgesic. They may also be changed in the operating room after the patient is anesthetized. A mask, hair cover, disposable plastic apron or cover gown, and gloves are worn by health care personnel when removing the dressings. The outer dressings are slit with blunt scissors, and the soiled dressings are removed and disposed of following established procedures for contaminated materials.

Dressings that adhere to the wound can be removed more comfortably if they are moistened with saline or if the patient is allowed to soak for a few moments in the tub. The remaining dressings are *carefully* and *gently* removed with forceps or gloved hands. The patient may participate in the removal of dressings, providing him with some degree of control over this painful procedure. The wounds are then cleansed and débrided to remove debris, any remaining topical agent, exudate, and devitalized skin. Sterile scissors and forceps may be employed to trim loose eschar and encourage separation of devitalized skin. During this procedure, the wound and surrounding skin are carefully inspected. The color, odor, size, exudate, signs of reepithelialization, and character of the eschar and any changes from the previous dressing change are noted. Because wound care procedures, particularly tub baths, are metabolically stressful, the patient is assessed for signs of chilling, fatigue, changes in hemodynamic status, and pain unrelieved by predressing analgesics or relaxation techniques.

Following wound cleansing, the burned areas are patted dry and the prescribed topical agent is applied. The wound is then covered with several layers of dressings (Fig. 52-8). A light dressing is used over joint areas to allow for motion (unless the patient has undergone grafting of the area and motion is contraindicated) and over areas for which a splint has been designed to conform to the body contour for proper positioning.

Close communication and cooperation among the patient, surgeon, nurse, and other health team members are essential for optimal burn wound care. Different wound areas on a given patient may require a variety of wound care techniques. Use of a diagram, updated daily by the nurse responsible for the patient's care, helps to inform all those concerned about the latest wound care procedures in use for the patient. Diagrams posted at the bedside are also useful to inform staff of the current prescription for splints to be applied over dressings and the exercise regimen to be followed before dressings are reapplied.

Exposure Versus Occlusive Dressing

Exposure Method

Occasionally a wound is treated with the exposure method. Wound care proceeds in the described manner, a topical agent is applied (mafenide most frequently), but no dressings are applied. The success of the exposure method depends on keeping the immediate environment free of organisms. Some practitioners maintain that everything coming in contact with the patient must be sterile. Linens are sterile; those who come

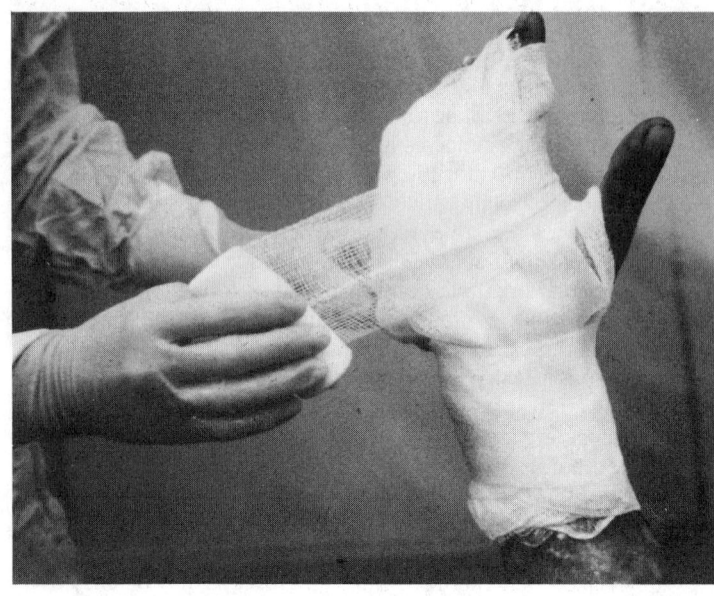

Figure 52-8. Application of dressing to a hand burn.

in direct contact with the patient wear masks, sterile gowns, and gloves; and visitors are instructed to wear gowns and masks and not to touch the bed or hand the patient anything. Other practitioners maintain a clean environment and rely on the efficiency of the topical antibacterial agents to limit burn wound infection.

The patient's room must be maintained at a comfortably warm temperature with 40% to 50% humidity to prevent excessive evaporative fluid losses as well as to maintain the patient's body temperature. A cradle may be placed over the patient to prevent sheets from coming in contact with the burn area, to minimize the effects of air currents to which a burn patient is unusually sensitive, and to provide some covering.

Generally small areas such as the face, neck, or perineum may also be effectively treated with the exposure method, while other areas of the wound may be dressed.

Occlusive Dressings

There is a role for occlusive dressings in the treatment of specific wounds. Occlusive dressings are most often seen over areas that have been newly skin grafted. These dressings are applied under sterile conditions in the operating room. Their purpose is to protect the graft, promoting an optimal condition for adherence of the graft to the recipient site. Ideally, these dressings remain in place for 5 days, at which time they are removed by the physician for examination of the graft.

When these dressings are applied, precautions are taken to prevent two body surfaces from touching, such as fingers or toes, ear and scalp, the areas under the breasts, any point of flexion, or between the genital folds. Functional body alignment positions are maintained with the use of splints or positioning.

Débridement

Débridement is another facet of burn wound care. This technique has two goals:

- To remove tissue contaminated by bacteria and foreign bodies, thus protecting the patient from invasive infection
- To remove devitalized tissue or burn eschar in preparation for grafting and wound healing

After partial- and full-thickness burns, bacteria that are present at the interface of the burned tissue and the viable tissue underneath gradually liquefy the collagen fibrils that hold the eschar in place for the first week or two postburn. This occurs because of the action of proteolytic and other natural enzymes.

With *natural débridement*, the dead tissue separates from the underlying viable tissue spontaneously. The use of antibacterial topical agents, however, tends to slow down this natural process of eschar separation. It is advantageous to the patient to speed this process through other means, such as mechanical or surgical débridement, and thus reduce the time during which bacterial invasion and other iatrogenic problems may arise.

Mechanical débridement involves the use of surgical scissors and forceps to separate and remove the eschar. This technique can be performed by physicians or experienced nurses and physical therapists and is usually done with daily dressing changes and wound cleansing procedures. Débridement by this means is carried out to the point of pain and bleeding. Hemostatic agents or pressure can be used to stop small-vessel bleeding.

Dressings are also helpful as débriding agents. Course-mesh dressings applied dry or wet-to-dry (applied wet and allowed to dry) will slowly débride the wound of exudate and eschar when they are removed. Topical enzymatic agents such as sutilains (Travase), a proteolytic enzyme derived from *Bacillus subtilis* and supplied in a petrolatum base, can also be helpful in débriding burn wounds. Because such agents are not antibacterial in themselves, they should be used in conjunction with topical antibacterial therapy to protect the patient from bacterial invasion.

Surgical débridement is an operative procedure that employs either primary excision of the full thickness of the skin down to the fascia (tangential excision) or the shaving of burned skin layers gradually down to freely bleeding, viable tissue. This may be initiated a few days postburn, or as soon as the patient is hemodynamically stable and edema has decreased. The wound is then covered immediately by a skin graft or dressing. A temporary biologic dressing or biosynthetic dressing may be used until a skin graft can be applied during a subsequent operation.

The use of excision is selective, particularly with large burns, for the following reasons: The procedure carries with it high risk due to extensive blood loss (as much as half a unit [or 100 to 125 ml] of blood per percent of body surface area excised) and lengthy operative and anesthesia time. However, when used, excision results in shorter hospital stays and may decrease potential complications from invasive burn wound sepsis. It has recently become an increasingly effective and successful approach to burn wound management.

Grafting the Burn Wound

If wounds are deep (full-thickness) or large, spontaneous re-epithelialization is not possible. Therefore, a skin transplant or graft with use of the patient's own skin (autograft) is required. Priority areas for skin grafting include the face, for cosmetic and psychologic reasons; the hands and other functional areas such as the feet; and areas that involve joints. Grafting permits earlier functional ability and reduces the development of contractures. When burns are very extensive, the chest and abdomen may be grafted first to reduce the extent of the burn surface.

During wound healing, granulation tissue develops. It fills the space created by the wound, creates a barrier to bacteria, and serves as a bed for epithelial cell growth.

Richly vascular granulation tissue is pink, firm, shiny, and free of exudate and debris. It should have a bacterial count of less than 100,000 per gram of tissue in order to optimize graft take. A preoperative culture is mandatory before autografting, because enzymes of bacteria can dissolve a graft and lead to failure of the graft. Beta-hemolytic *Streptococcus* is of particular significance in terms of graft failure.

Types of Autograft

Autografts can be split-thickness, full-thickness, or pedicle flaps. The last two types are more commonly used for reconstructive surgery, months or years after the initial injury. Split-thickness autografts can be applied in sheets or in postage-stamp pieces, or they can be expanded by meshing so that, for a given amount of donor site area, an area 1½ to 9 times greater can be covered.

Skin meshers, which enable the surgeon to cut tiny slits into a sheet of donor skin, make it possible to cover large areas of total body surface area with smaller amounts of donor skin. Expanded grafts cling to the recipient site more easily than sheet grafts and prevent the accumulation of blood, serum, air, or purulent material under the graft. It must be recognized that any graft other than a sheet graft will contribute to scar formation as it heals. The use of expanded grafts is often necessary in large wounds but should always be viewed as a compromise in terms of cosmetic effects.

If blood, serum, air, fat, or necrotic tissue lies between the recipient site and the graft, there may be either partial or total loss of the graft. Infection and mishandling of the graft, as well as trauma occurring during dressing changes, account for most other instances of graft loss.

The use of split-thickness grafts allows the remaining donor site to retain sweat glands and hair follicles and allows for rapid healing (within 10 to 14 days).

Care of Patients With Autografts

Occlusive dressings are often used after grafting to immobilize the grafts. Homografts, heterografts, or synthetic dressings may also be used to protect the grafts (see below). The graft may be left open, using skin staples to immobilize it while affording close observation of the graft's progress.

The first dressing change is usually performed by the surgeon 3 to 5 days postoperatively, or earlier if purulent drainage or a foul odor is noted. If the graft is dislodged, sterile saline compresses will help prevent drying of the graft until the physician reapplies it. The patient begins exercise 7 to 10 days after grafting.

Care of Donor Site

A moist gauze dressing is applied during the operative period to maintain pressure and stop any oozing. A thrombostatic agent such as thrombin or epinephrine may be applied directly to the site as well. The donor site may be treated in a number of ways, from single-layer gauze impregnated with petrolatum, scarlet red, or bismuth to new biosynthetic dressings. Ultimately, because it is a partial-thickness wound, given proper care it will heal spontaneously within 7 to 14 days.

Biologic Dressings

Biologic dressings consist of homografts (or allografts) and heterografts (or xenografts). *Homografts* are skin obtained from living or recently deceased humans. The amniotic membrane (*amnion*) from the human placenta may also be used as a biologic dressing. *Heterografts* consist of skin taken from animals (usually pigs).

Homografts tend to be the most expensive biologic dressings. They are available from several skin banks in various regions of the country. Homograft is available in both fresh and cryo-preserved forms and is considered by most surgeons to provide the best infection control of all the biologic or biosynthetic dressings available.

Amnion is low in cost and is available in hospitals with burn centers and specialized tissue-banking facilities, which obtain and process it in cooperation with obstetric services.

Pigskin is available from a number of commercial suppliers. It is available fresh, frozen, or lyophilized for longer shelf-life. Pigskin impregnated with a topical antibacterial such as silver nitrate is also available.

Biologic dressings can be used for several purposes. In a large burn, biologic dressings can be lifesaving by providing temporary wound closure until autografting is complete. They provide immediate coverage for clean, superficial burns and decrease the wound's evaporative water loss and protein loss. They decrease pain by protecting nerve endings and are an effective barrier to water and bacteria. When applied to superficial partial-thickness wounds, they appear to speed the healing process.

Biologic dressings protect the granulation tissue during completion of wound débridement or while waiting for donor sites to heal and be reused. This is common in patients with large areas of burn and little remaining normal skin suitable for donor sites.

Biologic dressings are used to débride untidy wounds after eschar separation. With each biologic dressing change, débridement takes place. Once the biologic dressing appears to be "taking," or adheres to the granulating surface with a minimum of underlying exudation, the patient is ready for permanent placement of the patient's own skin, an autograft. Another major use of these dressings is temporary coverage of wounds following excision while awaiting autografting.

Biologic materials can be left open or covered. They are usually changed every 2 to 5 days to avoid systemic and local signs of tissue rejection.

Biosynthetic and Synthetic Wound Coverings

Problems with availability, sterility, and cost have prompted the search for synthetic skin substitutes, which may eventually replace biologic dressings as temporary wound coverings. The most widely used currently is Biobrane, which is composed of a nylon, Silastic membrane combined with a collagen derivative. The material is semitransparent and sterile. It has an indefinite shelf-life and is less costly than homograft or pigskin.

Biobrane adheres to wound fibrin, which binds to the nylon–collagen material. Within 5 days, cells migrate into the nylon mesh. Generally, adherence to the wound surface has been shown to correlate directly with low bacterial counts. When the Biobrane dressing adheres to the wound, as in the "take" of an allograft without vascularization, the wound remains stable and the Biobrane is left in place for periods of 3 to 4 weeks. Biobrane II dressings (Fig. 52-9) readily adhere to donor sites and meticulously clean débrided partial-thickness wounds; they will remain until spontaneous epithelialization and wound healing occur. Biobrane can be laid on top of wide-meshed autograft to protect the wound until the autograft epithelium grows out to close the interstices. The Biobrane gradually separates and is trimmed, leaving a healed wound.

Biobrane is also useful for intermediate or long-term closure of a surgically excised wound until autograft becomes available. Just as with biologic dressings, Biobrane should not be used over grossly contaminated or necrotic wounds. Removal of Biobrane after several weeks is similar to but easier than removal of vascularized allograft and leaves a bleeding granulation bed that readily accepts autograft.

There are a number of other synthetic dressings available for burn wound care. Op-Site, a thin, transparent, polyurethane elastic film, can be used to cover clean partial-thickness wounds and donor sites. This dressing is occlusive and waterproof yet permeable to water vapor and air. This permeability still provides for protection from microbial contamination and also allows for the exchange of gases that occurs much more quickly in a moist environment. Other synthetic dressings used for burn wounds include Tegaderm, N-TERFACE, and Duo-Derm.

Artificial skin was developed in Boston in 1979. Clinical evaluations continue, and mass production is being undertaken. Artificial skin may soon be commercially available under the trade name "Integra." Artificial skin is composed of two main layers. The epidermal layer, consisting of Silastic, acts as a bacterial barrier and prevents water loss from the dermis. The dermal layer is composed of animal collagan. It interfaces with the open wound surface and allows migration of fibroblasts and capillaries into the material. This "neodermis" becomes a permanent structure. The artificial dermis is biodegraded and resorbed. The epidermal layer is removed 2 to 3 weeks after application and is replaced with the patient's own skin. It is

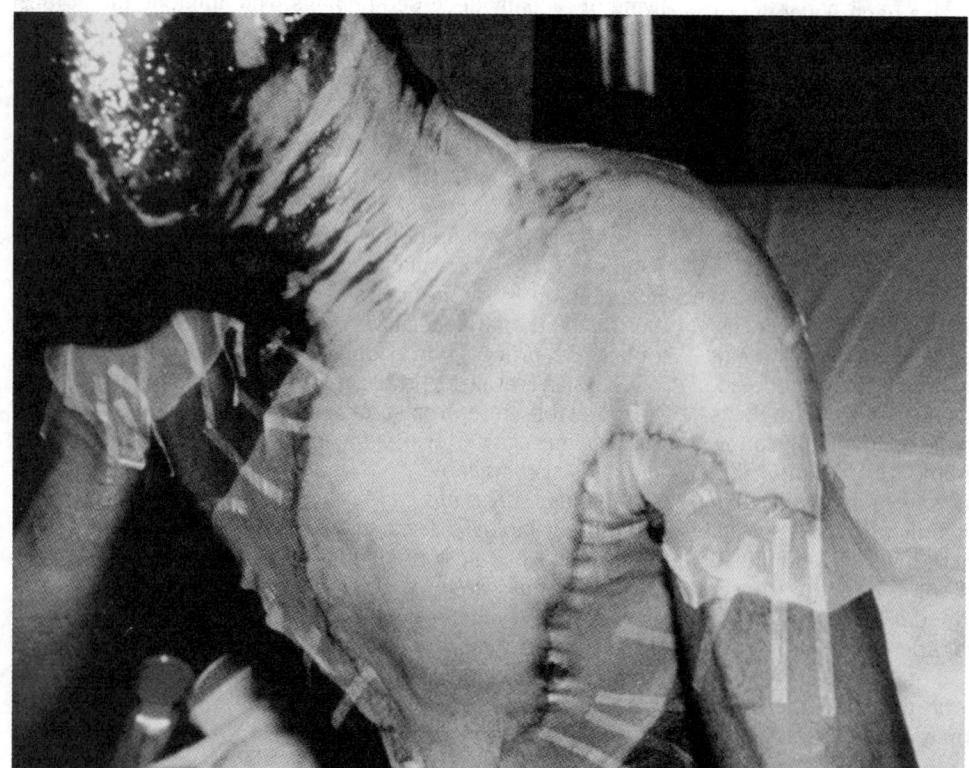

Figure 52–9. BIOBRANE II immediately after application to a superficial to partial thickness burn injury of the claviopectoral and supraclavicular area. (Used with permission of Winthrop Pharmaceuticals Wound Care Division, New York.)

reported that contracture has been minimal with no hypertrophic scar. The appearance resembles normal skin.

Pain Management

The outstanding features of burn pain are its intensity and long duration. Necessary wound care carries with it the anticipation of pain and anxiety; the pain experienced is often severe.

In a typical burn pain trajectory, there are many peaks and valleys. The primary pain from the burn itself is very intense in the initial acute postburn phase. This primary pain gradually subsides, but for weeks thereafter, until the skin heals or skin grafts are applied and "take," the pain level remains high because of treatment-induced pain. Wound cleansing, dressing change, débridement, and physical therapy are often performed simultaneously or serially, inflicting intense pain. Even when grafts are applied, making the burn site more comfortable, donor sites are created and may be exquisitely painful for several days. Discomfort related to tissue healing, such as itching, tingling, and tightness of contracting skin and joints, further adds to the duration if not the intensity of pain over many weeks or months.

Because pain cannot be eliminated short of complete anesthesia, the goal is to minimize the pain through analgesia before the patient faces wound care procedures. With adequate staff working gently, swiftly, and skillfully, the duration of pain from wound care can be shortened. Bolus doses of morphine or meperidine (Demerol) are often used. Ketamine anesthesia administered intravenously is also used for some wound care procedures in burn units.

Patient-controlled analgesia (PCA), continuous morphine drips at 2 to 3 mg/hr, and sustained-release oral morphine, given every 12 hours with an additional dose prior to wound care, have been found to be helpful for burn patients. Self-administered nitrous oxide also helps to make dressing changes more tolerable for those patients who have sufficient hand function to hold a mask to their faces intermittently during dressing changes.

Early surgical excision with grafting under anesthesia is perhaps the best way to reduce the overall pain experience for burn patients.

Disorders of Wound Healing

Disorders of wound healing in the burn patient result from excessive abnormal healing or inadequate new tissue formation. Hypertrophic scarring and keloid formation are the result of excessive, abnormal healing.

Scars. Hypertrophic scars and wound contractures are more likely to occur if the initial burn injury extends below the level of the deep dermis. Healing of these deep wounds results in the replacement of normal integument with highly metabolically active tissues lacking the normal architecture of the skin. In the collagen layer beneath the epithelium, many fibroblasts gradually proliferate. Myofibroblasts, cells that have the ability to contract, are also present in immature wounds. As these elements contract, the collagen fibers, which normally are laid down in flat bundles, tend to form a wavy pattern. Eventually the collagen bundles take on a supercoiled appearance and collagen nodules develop. The scar becomes very red (because of its hypervascular nature), raised, and hardened.

The wound is in a dynamic state for 1½ to 2 years after the burn occurs. If appropriate measures are instituted during this active period, the scar tissue loses its redness and softens. The application of elastic pressure garments (Fig. 52-10) induces loosening of collagen bundles and encourages parallel orientation of the collagen to the skin surface with the disap-

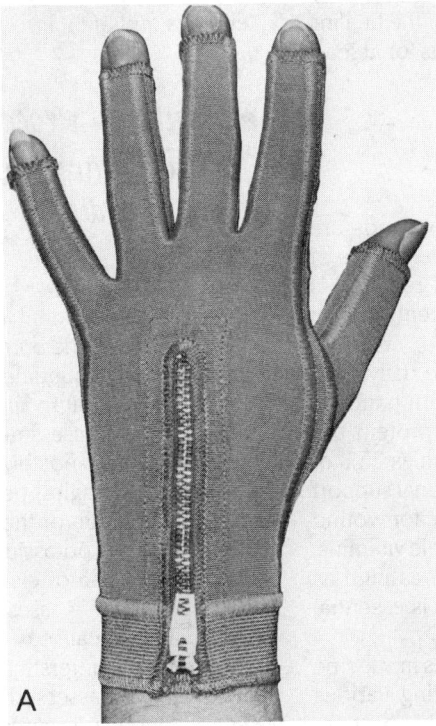
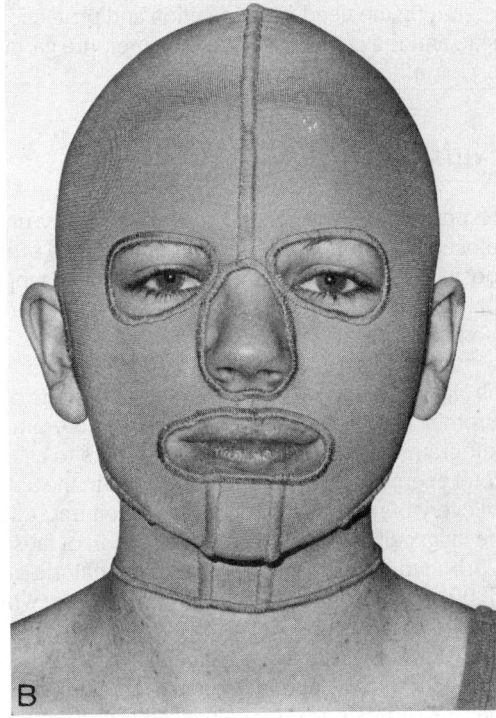

Figure 52-10. Elastic pressure garments. Application of pressure garments prevents hypertrophic burn scarring. (**A**) Elastic pressure glove. (**B**) Elastic pressure face mask. (Illustrations courtesy of Jobst Institute, Inc, Toledo, OH.)

pearance of the dermal nodules. With the application of pressure, there is a restructuring of the collagen and a decrease in vascularity and cellularity.

Hypertrophic scarring may cause severe contracture across involved joints. However, these scars are limited to the area of injury and will gradually regress over time.

Keloids.   In other patients, a large heaped-up mass of scar tissue develops and may extend beyond the wound surface. This is called a *keloid*. Keloids tend to be found in darkly pigmented persons, grow outside of wound margins, and are more likely to recur after surgical excision.

Failure to Heal.   Failure of the wound to heal may be related to many factors, including infection and inadequate nutrition. Serum albumin below 2 g/dl (20 g/L) is frequently a factor in impaired healing in the burn patient.

Contractures.   Contractures are another concern as wounds heal. The burn wound will shorten because of the force exerted by the fibroblasts and the flexion of muscles as a natural part of wound healing. An opposing force in the form of splints, traction, and purposeful movement and positioning must be used to counteract deformity caused by this process in burns that occur across joints.

Much of the long-term care of healed burns will be carried out by the patient and significant others at home. Patients commonly leave the hospital with small areas of clean, open wounds that are slowly healing. These areas should be washed daily with mild soap and water, and the prescribed topical agent or dressing should be applied. Healed areas that are prone to hypertrophic scarring require the use of pressure garments. Examples of such areas are partial-thickness wounds that require more than 2 weeks to heal and the edges of grafted skin. The physical therapist or a representative of the manufacturer of elastic pressure garments measures the patient for correct fit. While awaiting the arrival of the garment, soft, tubular, knit elastic pressure bandages can be used to help desensitize the patient's skin, protect healing areas, provide pressure, and promote venous return. Patients must be educated regarding the need for lubrication and protection of the healing skin and the necessity of wearing pressure garments for at least a year after the injury.

Nutritional Support

Hypermetabolism persists after burn injury until wounds are closed. The goal of nutritional support is to promote a state of positive nitrogen balance. The nutritional support required is based on the patient's preburn status and the extent of total body surface area burned.

A number of formulas exist for estimating the daily metabolic expenditure and caloric requirements of burn patients. Protein requirements may range from 3.0 gm of protein per kilogram of body weight every 24 hours to as much as 25% of total energy needs. Lipids are included in the nutritional support of every burned patient because of their importance for wound healing, cellular integrity, and absorption of fat-soluble vitamins. Carbohydrates are included to meet caloric goals as high as 5000 calories per day and to spare protein, which is essential for wound healing.

Current research is bringing about rapid changes in specific guidelines for estimating energy expenditure during various phases of postburn recovery. The proportions of fat, protein,

and carbohydrate are carefully planned for maximal utilization. Overfeeding can also be detrimental. Therefore, a dietitian familiar with current concepts in nutrition for burn patients should be consulted for all patients with major burns.

As soon as gastrointestinal function returns after the patient's condition stabilizes, nutritional support begins. The enteral route is preferred, and many burn patients will tolerate oral fluids and food. In patients with large burns, tube feeding may be employed to ensure a certain number of calories per day. In this case, high-protein, high-calorie snacks and fluids may be offered as supplements to the essential tube feedings. A diet containing semisolid or solid food is usually begun toward the end of the first week when the patient's tolerance for food improves.

Patients lose a great deal of weight in the process of recovering from severe burns. Reserve fat deposits are mobilized during the recovery, fluids have been lost, and calorie intake may have been limited. Because burns cause low resistance to infection and disease, the nutritional state must be improved even though the patient has a poor appetite and is still weak.

Indications for total parenteral nutrition include weight loss greater than 10% of normal body weight, inadequate intake of enteral nutrition due to clinical status, prolonged wound exposure, and malnutrition or debilitated condition prior to injury. The risk of infection of the central catheter required by this method must be considered. While solutions commonly used may provide 1000 or more calories per liter, they are deficient in fatty acids. Therefore, intravenous fat solutions will also have to be given periodically.

Ulcers of the gastric or duodenal mucosa are a common complication of burn injury (Curling's ulcer). This condition is manifested by hemorrhage, detected in the bloody contents from nasogastric suction or in the stool. A sudden drop in hemoglobin concentration may be diagnostic even before the hemorrhage is evident. Gastric surgery may be indicated. Use of histamine blockers (ranitidine [Zantac]) continues during this phase to prevent this serious problem. Small, frequent feedings and antacids are also included in the patient's care.

▶ Nursing Process
Burn Care During the Acute/ Intermediate Phase

▷ Assessment

Continued assessment of the burn patient during the early weeks following the burn focuses on hemodynamic alterations, the process of wound healing, and detection of complications. Vital signs, including apical pulse, are assessed frequently.

Continued assessment of peripheral pulses is essential for the first few days postburn while edema continues to increase, potentially damaging peripheral nerves and restricting blood flow. Observation of the ECG may give clues to dysrhythmias that result from potassium imbalance, preexisting cardiac disease, or sequelae of electrical injury or burn shock.

The patient is assessed for fluid overload and congestive heart failure because of the mobilization of fluid and shifts of fluid from the interstitial to the vascular compartment. The neck veins are assessed for fullness, and arterial, wedge, and central venous pressures are monitored closely.

The patient's respiratory status is monitored closely for increased difficulty in breathing, change in respiratory pattern, and appearance of adventitious sounds. Assessment of the patient's respiratory status is also important because it is frequently at this stage that signs and symptoms of injury to the respiratory tract become apparent. As described previously, decreased breath sounds, wheezing, tachypnea, stridor, and sputum tinged with soot (or in some cases containing sloughed tracheal tissue) are among the many possible findings that can be auscultated or observed. Patients on mechanical ventilation must be assessed for a decrease in tidal volume and lung compliance.

Assessment of residual volumes and *p*H of gastric fluid of the patient with a nasogastric tube is also important and gives clues to early sepsis or the need for antacid therapy. Evidence of blood in gastric fluid or stool should also be noted and reported.

Assessment of the burn wound is a daily activity that requires an experienced eye, hand, and nose. Some of the characteristics of the wound that are assessed include size, color, odor, presence of eschar or exudate, presence of abscess formation under the eschar, presence of *epithelial buds* (small pearl-like clusters of cells on the wound surface), bleeding, nature of granulation tissue, progress of grafts and donor sites, and quality of the surrounding skin. Any significant changes in the wound are reported to the physician, because they often indicate burn wound or systemic sepsis and require immediate intervention.

The signs of systemic sepsis are listed in Table 52-7. Some are rather subtle and require a high index of suspicion and very close monitoring of changes in the patient's mental status, a gradual increase in gastric residual volumes, and an increased respiratory rate. As with many observations of the burn patient, one needs to look for patterns or trends in the data.

Other ongoing assessments significant in burn care include daily patient weights, records of caloric intake, assessment of general hydration, and serum electrolyte, hemoglobin, and hematocrit levels. Weekly audiometry may be indicated for patients on long-term ototoxic antibiotics. Careful attention must also be paid to signs or reports of pain related to deep muscle ischemia in patients with electrical burns. The nurse is alert to signs of necrosis of visceral organs injured by electricity and of hemorrhage from blood vessels adjacent to areas of surgical exploration and débridement in patients with serious electrical burns.

◊ Nursing Diagnoses

Based on the assessment data, nursing diagnoses in the acute/intermediate phase of burn care may include the following:

- High risk for fluid volume excess related to resumption of capillary integrity and fluid shift from interstitial to vascular compartment
- High risk for infection related to loss of skin barrier and dysfunctional host defense mechanisms
- Altered nutrition: less than body requirements related to hypermetabolism
- Impaired skin integrity related to thermal injury
- Pain, itching, and skin and joint tightness related to exposed nerves and wound healing
- Impaired physical mobility related to burn wound edema, pain, and joint contractures

◊ Planning and Implementation

◊ *Goals:* The major goals of the patient may include restoration of normal fluid balance, absence of infection, attainment of anabolic state and normal weight, improved skin integrity, reduction of pain and discomfort, and achievement of optimal physical mobility.

◊ Nursing Interventions

◊ *Restoring Normal Fluid Balance.* To reduce the risk of fluid overload and congestive heart failure, the nurse closely monitors the patient's intravenous and oral fluid intake, using intravenous infusion pumps to minimize the risk of inadvertent rapid infusion of fluids. To monitor changes in fluid status, careful intake and output records are kept and the patient is weighed daily. Changes in arterial, wedge, and central venous pressures, as well as in blood pressure and pulse rate, are

TABLE 52-7. *Clinical Features of Septic Shock**

Early Stage	Middle Stage	Late Stage
VITAL SIGNS	*VITAL SIGNS*	*VITAL SIGNS*
Full, bounding pulse	Rapid pulse	Markedly increased pulse; weak, thready pulse
Normal or increased blood pressure	Decreased blood pressure	Falling blood pressure
Increased pulse pressure		Decreased pulse pressure
HYPERDYNAMIC STATE	*NORMODYNAMIC STATE*	*HYPODYNAMIC STATE*
Increased cardiac output	Decreased cardiac output	Marked fall in cardiac output
Increased urinary output	Falling urinary output or renal failure	Renal failure
Hyperthermia		Pale, moist, cool skin
Warm, dry, flushed skin		
Restlessness		

* Signs and symptoms may be variable and nonspecific.

reported to the physician. Cardiotonics and diuretics may be prescribed to promote increased urine output. The nurse's role is to administer these medications as prescribed and to observe the patient's response to them.

Increased difficulty with respiration is reported promptly to the physician. In the meantime, the patient is positioned comfortably, with the head of the bed raised (if not prohibited by other treatments or burn injuries) to promote lung expansion and gas exchange.

◊   *Preventing Infection.*   Aside from monitoring fluid requirements and providing constant care, the nurse is responsible for providing a clean and safe environment and for closely scrutinizing the wound in order to detect early manifestations of infection.

Aseptic technique is used for wound care procedures and for any invasive procedures such as insertion of intravenous lines, urinary catheters, or tracheal suctioning. The nurse protects the patient from sources of cross-contamination, including other patients, staff members, visitors, and equipment. Antibiotics must be administered on schedule to maintain appropriate blood levels. Wound and blood cultures are obtained as prescribed, and results of significance are reported to the physician immediately. The nurse also observes for early signs of septicemia and promptly intervenes, administering prescribed intravenous fluids and antibiotics to prevent septic shock, a complication with a high mortality rate.

Tube feeding reservoirs and drainage containers are changed regularly. Visitors are screened to prevent the introduction of pathogens to the severely immunocompromised burn patient. Barrier gowns or disposable aprons are worn when working at the bedside and changed when leaving the room. Hair covers, masks, and sterile gloves are required when wounds are exposed or central venous catheters are inserted. Meticulous hand washing prior to and following each patient contact is also an essential component of nursing care.

◊   *Maintaining Adequate Nutrition.*   The nurse collaborates with the dietitian to plan a diet that is high in protein and calories and acceptable to the patient. Family members may be encouraged to bring nutritious favorite foods to the hospital. Milkshakes and sandwiches made with peanut butter, meat, and cheese may be offered as snacks between meals and late in the evening. Caloric intake must be documented.

If caloric goals cannot be met by oral feeding, a nasogastric tube is inserted and used for continuous or bolus feedings of specific formulas. The volume of residual gastric secretions should be checked to ensure absorption. Total parenteral nutrition may also be required and provides the nurse with a new challenge in making frequent assessments related to the expected and untoward effects of this therapy.

Patients should be weighed each day and a graph of their weight maintained. This can be used to help patients set goals for their own nutritional intake and to monitor weight loss and gain. Ideally, the patient will lose no more than 5% of preburn weight if aggressive nutritional management is employed. Vitamins A and D, trace elements such as copper and zinc, and fatty-acid supplements may also be required, particularly for patients receiving parenteral nutritional support.

The patient who is experiencing anorexia requires encouragement and considerable support from the nurse to increase food intake. The patient's surroundings should be as pleasant as possible during meals. Catering to food preferences and offering snacks high in protein and vitamins are ways of tempting a person to gradually increase intake.

◊   *Improving Skin Integrity Through Wound Care.*   Wound care is often the single most time-consuming element of burn care after the emergent period has passed. The surgeon will prescribe the desired topical antibacterial agents and specific biologic, biosynthetic, or synthetic wound coverings and will plan for surgical excision and grafting. The nurse has an opportunity to make astute assessments of wound status, to use creative approaches to wound dressing, and to support the patient during the emotionally distressing and very painful experience of wound care.

The nurse serves as the coordinator of the complex aspects of wound care and dressing changes for the patient. Nursing functions include assessing and recording any changes or progress in wound healing and keeping all members of the health care team informed of changes in the patient's burn wounds and in the treatment regimen. The nurse also assists the patient and family through instruction, support, and encouragement to take an active part in dressing changes and wound care when appropriate. Home care needs are anticipated early in the course of burn management, and the strengths of the patient and family are assessed and used in preparing for eventual discharge and home care.

◊   *Relieving Pain and Discomfort.*   Pain is more severe in second-degree burns than in third-degree burns because the nerve endings are not destroyed. Exposed nerve endings are sensitive to cool, moving air; therefore, a sterile covering can help to reduce pain.

- Symptoms of restlessness and anxiety, often attributed to pain, may actually be due to hypoxia. Therefore, careful respiratory assessment is essential before giving analgesics in the early postburn period. Intravenous morphine or other narcotics are prescribed as needed, but large doses are avoided because of the danger of respiratory depression and the possibility of masking other symptoms. Subcutaneous or intramuscular routes are not recommended because the impaired circulation in the injured tissue makes absorption erratic and unpredictable.

Nursing interventions such as teaching the patient relaxation techniques, giving the patient some control over wound care and analgesia, and providing frequent reassurance are helpful. Imagery has been used effectively to moderate patients' perceptions of and responses to pain. Hypnosis, biofeedback, and behavioral modification have also been used successfully by staff experienced in these modalities. Minor tranquilizers are administered in conjunction with analgesics as prescribed. Frequent assessment of pain and discomfort is essential.

The nurse works quickly to complete treatments and dressing changes in order to reduce pain and discomfort. She encourages the patient to use analgesic medications before painful procedures and assesses their effectiveness in making the pain and discomfort more tolerable.

Healing burn wounds are often described by patients as "itchy" and "tight." Oral antipruritic agents, a cool environment, frequent lubrication of the skin with water or silica-based lotion, exercise and splinting to prevent skin contracture, and diversional activities are helpful in promoting comfort in this phase.

◊ *Promoting Physical Mobility.* An early priority is to prevent complications resulting from immobility. Deep breathing, turning, and proper repositioning are essential nursing practices to prevent atelectasis and pneumonia, to control edema, and to prevent pressure ulcers and contractures. These interventions are modified to meet the individual patient's needs. Air-fluidized beds and rotation beds may be useful. Early ambulation is encouraged.

Whenever the lower extremities are involved, elastic pressure bandages should be applied before the patient is placed in an upright position.

The burn wound is in a dynamic state for a year or more after wound closure. During this time, aggressive efforts must be made to prevent contracture and hypertrophic scarring of the wound area. Both passive and active range-of-motion exercises are initiated from the day of admission and are continued after grafting within prescribed limitations.

Splints or functional devices may be applied to extremities for contracture control. The nurse monitors for signs of vascular insufficiency and nerve compression. Pressure garments are worn to prevent hypertrophic scarring (see Fig. 52-10).

◊ *Evaluation*

Expected Outcomes

1. Achieves optimal fluid balance
   a. Intake, output, and body weight correlate with expected pattern.
   b. Vital signs and arterial, wedge, and central venous pressures remain within designated limits.
   c. Exhibits no respiratory distress; is able to recline flat without increased respiratory distress
   d. Lungs are clear to auscultation.
   e. Demonstrates increased urine output in response to diuretics and cardiotonics
   f. Receives intravenous and oral fluids as prescribed
   g. Exhibits no increase in neck vein distention
   h. Heart rate is lower than 110/min and in normal sinus rhythm.
2. Is free of pathogenic organisms
   a. Has no signs of local systemic infection
   b. Blood cultures are negative.
   c. Exhibits negative wound, sputum, and urine cultures
3. Demonstrates anabolic nutritional status; normal weight
   a. Gains weight daily after initial loss due to fluid diuresis and NPO status
   b. Has no signs of protein, vitamin, or mineral deficiencies
   c. Meets required nutritional needs entirely by oral intake
   d. Consumes diet high in carbohydrate and protein
   e. Participates in selection of diet with prescribed nutrients
   f. Exhibits normal serum protein levels
4. Majority of wounds are closed; small, open wounds are clean and healing; scars are minimal.
   a. Skin is generally intact and free of infection, signs of pressure, and trauma.
   b. Open wound areas are pink, reepithelializing, and free of infection.
   c. Donor sites are clean and reepithelializing.
   d. Healed wounds feel soft and smooth.
   e. Skin is lubricated and elastic, with no scales or other signs of dryness.
   f. Skin pigmentation is near normal preburn color.

5. Experiences minimal pain, itching, or skin tightness
   a. Requests analgesics only for specific wound care procedures or physical therapy activities
   b. States pain is minimal when assessed
   c. Gives no physiologic or nonverbal cues that pain is moderate or severe
   d. Uses pain control measures such as nitrous oxide, relaxation techniques, and imagery to assist with coping with pain
   e. Is able to sleep without being disturbed by pain or itching
   f. Does not scratch skin
   g. Reports skin is comfortable, with no itching or tightness
6. Demonstrates optimal physical mobility
   a. Improves range of motion of joints daily
   b. Demonstrates preinjury range of motion of all joints
   c. Has no signs of periarticular calcification
   d. Participates in activities of daily living as desired

Nursing care of the patient in the acute/intermediate phase of burn management is further discussed in Nursing Care Plan 52-2.

In summary, the acute or intermediate phase of burn care begins 48 to 72 hours after the burn injury has occurred and extends to the point at which the burn wounds are satisfactorily closed. Because infection is the major cause of death in patients who have survived the emergent phase of a major burn injury, prevention of infection and sepsis is a major priority of management. Advanced assessment skills and burn wound care skills are among the critical care nursing skills needed to prevent and detect infection and sepsis. The patient in the acute/intermediate phase of burn care is critically injured and requires care by nurses and other health care providers with highly specialized critical care skills in the management of pulmonary, cardiovascular, and renal complications. Pain management, nutritional support, and early mobilization require attention from all personnel with a view toward immediate and long-term outcomes. Psychologic assistance and support become of paramount importance as the patient and his family begin to realize that a long course of recovery and rehabilitation will be necessary.

Rehabilitation/Long-Term Phase

Although longer-term aspects of burn care are discussed last, it is important to remember that rehabilitation begins *immediately* after the burn has occurred—as early as the immediate postburn phase.

In the aftermath of the acute stages of illness, the burn patient increasingly focuses on the alterations in self-image and life-style that may be required. Reconstructive surgery to improve cosmetic and functional results may be needed. Counseling, both psychologic and vocational, may be valuable. Significant others will also need support and guidance in assisting the patient in returning to optimal health.

Follow-up care planned by the burn team will be necessary. In the case of children, such follow-up care is needed for many years. Preparations for this reality should begin during the earlier stages of care. It is a great challenge to the health care team

(text continues on page 1532)

Nursing Care Plan 52–2

Care of the Patient During the Acute/Intermediate Phase of Burn Care

Nursing Interventions	Rationale	Expected Outcomes

Nursing Diagnosis: High risk for infection of burn wound and burn wound sepsis

Goal: Reduced risk of burn wound sepsis

1. Wash hands prior to all patient contacts.	1. Minimizes risk of cross-contamination	• Exhibits clean, small, open wounds
2. Assess for early signs of shock and sepsis.	2. Enables detection of signs of shock, so that treatment can be initiated	• Exhibits open wound areas that are pink, reepithelializing, and free of infection
3. Prevent pressure on wounds.	3. Minimizes trauma and ensures adequate perfusion to burn wounds	• Shows clean reepithelializing donor sites
4. Apply topical antibacterials as prescribed.	4. Promotes adequate antibacterial effects of topical agents	• Exhibits negative burn wound cultures
5. Prevent cross-contamination.	5. Reduces risk of bacterial colonization	
6. Remove possible reservoirs of infection.	6. Reduces or eliminates source of bacteria and contamination	
7. Use barrier gowns, gloves, masks, and hair covers when wounds are exposed or when in direct contact with patient or bed.	7. Minimizes contamination of wound by normal or pathogenic bacteria from health care providers	

Nursing Diagnosis: Impaired skin integrity related to open burn wounds

Goal: Improved skin integrity and wound healing

1. Cleanse wound and rest of body, including hair, daily.	1. Reduces potential bacterial contamination, a common cause of impaired wound healing	• Demonstrates that most wounds are closed
2. Apply topical antibacterial agents and dressing as prescribed.	2. Reduces bacterial colonization and promotes healing	• Has completed or nearly completed skin grafting
3. Prevent pressure, infection, and mobilization of autografts.	3. Avoids trauma of grafts necessary for wound closure	• Over 80% of body covered with intact skin
4. Provide donor site care.	4. Promotes healing of donor site	
5. Observe and report any signs of poor graft take or loss of skin integrity after healing.	5. Grafted or healed burn wounds are susceptible to trauma	
6. Provide adequate nutritional support.	6. Adequate nutrition is essential for normal granulation and healing.	

Nursing Diagnosis: Pain and discomfort related to painful burn wound, treatments, debridement, and surgical interventions

Goal: Relief of pain and discomfort

1. Assess patient's pain carefully.	1. Provides baseline for assessment of pain relief measures	• Obtains relief of pain
2. Offer analgesics and relaxation breathing, transcutaneous nerve stimulator, or other appropriate measures.	2. Provides multiple interventions that offer relief of pain and anxiety related to fear of pain	• Requests analgesics only occasionally, and specifically for muscle and joint pain
3. Assess and document patient's response to interventions.	3. Promotes use of effective pain relief measures	• Verbally reports minimal pain
4. Assist patient with appropriate means of expressing pain.	4. Allows/encourages patient to express extended pain and discomfort that accompany repeated painful treatments	• Is free of physiologic and nonverbal indicators of moderate or severe pain
5. Educate patient about the usual pain trajectory in burn recovery.	5. Reduces fear of the unknown, and may provide some measure of control to the patient	

(continued)

Nursing Care Plan 52-2 *(Continued)*

Care of the Patient During the Acute/Intermediate Phase of Burn Care

Nursing Interventions	Rationale	Expected Outcomes

Nursing Diagnosis: Altered nutrition: less than body requirements

Goal: Improved nutritional status

1. Provide high-calorie, high-protein diet by appropriate route.	1. Provides nutrients for healing and to meet increased metabolic requirements for calories	• Demonstrates optimal nutritional status • Demonstrates daily weight gain (by weight curve)
2. Administer total parenteral nutrition according to protocol.	2. May be necessary to provide adequate nutrition to anorexic patient	• Is free of signs of protein, vitamin, or mineral deficiencies
3. Give supplemental vitamins and minerals as prescribed.	3. Necessary for normal healing and function	• Has increasing energy level • Meets required nutritional needs by oral intake entirely
4. Weigh patient daily; record in graphic form.	4. Provides record of trends in weight	• Exhibits normal serum protein levels
5. Report intolerance manifested by abdominal distention, diarrhea, osmotic diuresis, dehydration.	5. May indicate abnormal gastrointestinal function or need for alteration in dietary prescription	

Nursing Diagnosis: Body image disturbances related to burn wound and changes in role and life-style

Goal: Improved body image and acceptance of alterations required as a result of burn injury

1. Assess patient's readiness to express feelings regarding alteration in body image or life-style.	1. Helps to determine patient's awareness of effects of burn injury and ability to begin to deal with these changes	• Has realistic concept of changes in body image and alterations required in daily activities as a result of burn injury
2. Provide opportunity for expression of thoughts and feelings.	2. Allows patient to express and verbalize feelings regarding burn injury, its effects, and outcomes	• Verbalizes an accurate description of alterations in body image postburn
3. Maintain positive but honest approach in responding to questions.	3. Encourages patient to voice concerns and ask questions in a trusting atmosphere	• Discusses changes in life-style and daily activities that may be required postdischarge
4. Use significant others, counselors, and appropriate resource persons to help patient cope.	4. Provides multiple sources of support	• Demonstrates interest in resources that may be able to positively affect cosmetic and functional results of injury
5. Support effective premorbid coping mechanisms.	5. Encourages patient to use familiar coping mechanisms that have been successful in the past	• Is free of withdrawal and depression

Nursing Diagnosis: Immobility related to possible development of flexion contractures and muscle atrophy

Goal: Increased mobility and participation in activities of daily living

1. Position patient carefully to prevent flexed position in burned areas.	1. Reduces risk of flexion contractures	• Demonstrates range of joint motion that approaches preburn range
2. Implement range-of-motion exercises several times daily.	2. Minimizes muscle atrophy	• Shows joint motion that permits activities of daily living
3. Assist with ambulation.	3. Encourages increased mobility and use of muscles	• Improves range of motion of contracted joints daily
4. Use splints and exercise devices recommended by occupational and physical therapists.	4. Encourages activity while maintaining proper position of joints	• Is free of periarticular calcification
5. Encourage self-feeding and turning and moving in bed.	5. Encourages independence and self-care while encouraging activity and exercise	

(continued)

Nursing Care Plan 52-2 (Continued)

Care of the Patient During the Acute/Intermediate Phase of Burn Care

Nursing Interventions	Rationale	Expected Outcomes

Nursing Diagnosis: Knowledge deficit about surgical procedures and postoperative course

Goal: Increased knowledge about procedures and own role in them

1. Review surgical procedures and post-operative course with patient and family.	1. Prepares patient for procedures and own role in them	• Verbalizes understanding of treatments and surgical procedures and participates appropriately in care
2. Explore patient's previous experience with hospitalization and surgery.	2. Provides basis for explanations and indication of patient's expectations	• Expresses concerns about surgery and treatments with health team members and family
3. Tailor information given to patient's questions and nonverbal cues to anxiety level.	3. Promotes adequacy of explanations to patient without excessively increasing anxiety level	• Describes surgical procedures and treatments accurately
4. Define expectations of required patient participation for optimal results.	4. Provides specific directions and goals for patient	

to prepare a person for independent functioning after such a major traumatic event.

A program including elastic pressure garments, splints, and exercise under the supervision of an experienced physiatrist and physical and occupational therapy team is recommended for optimal functional and cosmetic results. As the inpatient phase of burn recovery gets shorter and shorter, much of the rehabilitation of the burn patient takes place on an outpatient basis or in a rehabilitation center.

The focus on maintaining fluid and electrolyte balance and improving nutritional status continues. The electrolyte changes that occur in the rehabilitative or long-term phase of care are described in Table 52-8.

▶ Nursing Process
Burn Care During the Rehabilitation/ Long-Term Phase

◊ Assessment

Information about the patient's educational level, cultural background, religion, previous dietary habits and preferences, and self-concept is obtained early in the care of the burn patient. Other important information areas for assessment include the patient's occupational history and preference for leisure activities, family interactions, and communication with significant others by both the patient and family members.

The patient's mental status, emotional response to the injury and hospitalization, level of intellectual functioning, previous hospitalizations, response to pain and pain relief measures, and sleep pattern are also essential components of a comprehensive assessment. Information about general self-concept and how the patient has coped with stressful situations in the past will be valuable in addressing emotional needs.

Ongoing assessments related to rehabilitation goals include range of motion of affected joints, functional abilities in activities of daily living, early signs of skin breakdown from splints

or positioning devices, evidence of neuropathies, activity tolerance, and quality of healing skin. The patient's participation in care and ability to demonstrate self-care in such areas as ambulation, feeding, wound cleansing, and application of pressure wraps are also documented on a regular basis.

In addition to the assessment parameters identified above, many of which apply to all patients with major burns, specific complications and treatments require specific assessments. For example, the patient undergoing primary excision requires postoperative assessment; the patient receiving nutritional support requires continuous monitoring of metabolic response to total parenteral nutrition.

Recovery from burn injury involves every system of the

TABLE 52–8. *Electrolyte Changes in the Rehabilitation/Long-Term Phase of Burn Care*

Observation	Explanation
Calcium deficit	Calcium may be immobilized at the burn site in the slough and early granulation phase of burns; symptoms of calcium deficit occur rarely.
Potassium deficit	Extracellular K^+ moves into the cells, leaving a deficit of K^+ in the extracellular fluid.
Negative nitrogen balance (present for several weeks following burns)	Secondary to: Stress reaction Immobilization Inadequate protein intake Protein losses in exudate Direct destruction of protein at burn site

(Adapted from Metheny NM and Snively WD. Nurses' Handbook of Fluid Balance. Philadelphia, JB Lippincott.)

body, so assessment of the burn patient must be comprehensive and continuous. Specific parameters may take priority during one phase and be less important in another. Understanding the physiologic and pathologic processes that underlie the injury and the body's response to it provides a basis for early detection of significant signs and symptoms. Early detection leads to early intervention and enhances the potential for optimal patient outcomes.

◊ *Nursing Diagnoses*

Based on the assessment data, nursing diagnoses in the rehabilitation/long-term phase of burn care may include the following:

- Activity intolerance related to metabolic demands, pain, muscle wasting
- Knowledge deficit related to need for continuing care of burn wounds and healing skin
- Ineffective individual coping related to fear and anxiety, grieving, and forced dependence on health care providers
- Body image disturbance related to altered body image, self-esteem, role performance, and personal identity

◊ *Planning and Implementation*

◊ *Goals:* The major goals of the patient may include increased participation in activities of daily living; increased understanding of the injury, treatment, and planned follow-up care; use of appropriate coping strategies; and adaptation and adjustment to alterations in self-concept and life-style.

◊ *Nursing Interventions*

◊ *Promoting Rest.* Nursing interventions that must be carried out according to a set regimen and the pain that accompanies movement each take their toll on burn patients. They may become confused and disoriented and lack the energy to participate optimally in their own care. The nurse must plan the care for each patient in a manner that permits some unbroken periods for sleep. A good time for planned patient rest is after the stress of dressing changes and exercise, while pain interventions and sedation may still be effective. This plan must be communicated to family members and other care providers. Hypnotics given in the evening, as prescribed, may promote sleep at night. Because burn patients frequently have nightmares related to the burn injury, the nurse listens to and reassures the patient when such nightmares, or other fears and anxieties about the outcome of the injury, cause insomnia.

◊ *Planning Activity.* Reduction of metabolic stress by relieving pain, preventing chilling, and promoting physical integrity of all body systems will help the patient to conserve energy for therapeutic activities and wound healing. The nurse incorporates physical therapy exercises in the patient's care to prevent muscular atrophy and maintain the mobility required for daily activities. A gradual increase in the patient's activity tolerance, strength, and endurance will occur if activity is planned for time periods of increasing duration. Fatigue, fever, and pain tolerance are monitored and used to determine the amount of activity to be encouraged on a daily basis. Scheduling activities such as family visits, recreational or play therapy, listening to the radio, or walking to the patient lounge can provide diver-

sion, improve the patient's psychologic outlook, and increase tolerance for physical activity as well.

◊ *Patient Education.* Patients will be better able to participate in their care if they are aware of the consequences of the injury, the goals of planned treatment, and their role in ongoing care. This education begins in the emergency department and continues throughout rehabilitation. Families are included in planning and carrying out care to the extent allowed by their interest and ability and the patient's needs.

◊ *Strengthening Coping Strategies.* Depression, regression, and manipulative behavior are common coping mechanisms used by burn patients. Withdrawal from participation in required treatments and regression must be viewed with an understanding that such behavior helps the patient cope with an enormously stressful event. Much energy goes into maintaining vital physical functions and wound healing in the early weeks postburn, leaving little emotional energy for coping in a mature and effective manner. Nurses can assist patients to develop effective coping strategies through setting specific expectations for behavior, promoting truthful communication to build trust, helping patients practice appropriate strategies, and giving positive reinforcement when appropriate. Family members must also be informed about these behavioral patterns so they will not be hurt by unexpected patient behavior and so they will be able to participate in the health team's approaches to the patient.

Patients are very dependent on health team members during the long period of acute illness. However, even when physically unable to contribute much to self-care, they can be included in decisions regarding care and encouraged to assert their individuality in terms of preferences and recognition of their unique identities. As patients improve in mobility and strength, the nurse works with them to set realistic expectations for self-care, including self-feeding, assistance with wound care procedures, exercise, and planning for the future. Many patients respond positively to the use of contractual agreements and other strategies that recognize their independence and their specific role as part of the health care team moving toward the goal of self-care.

Burn patients frequently suffer profound losses. These include not only loss of their own previous body image due to disfigurement but also losses of personal property, their homes, their loved ones, and their ability to perform in their occupations. They lack the benefit of anticipatory grief often seen in a patient approaching elective surgery or a person dealing with the terminal illness of a loved one. In addition to being available as a listener and counselor, the nurse can refer patients to a support group, such as those usually available at regional burn centers or through organizations such as the Phoenix Society. Through participation in such groups, patients will meet others with similar experiences and learn to develop coping strategies to help them deal with their losses.

◊ *Assisting With Psychologic Adjustments.* As care progresses, the burn victim becomes aware of daily improvement and begins to exhibit basic concerns: Will I be disfigured? How long will I have to be in the hospital? What about my job and family? Will I ever be independent again? How can I pay for my care? Was this the result of my carelessness? As the patient expresses such concerns, the nurse should take time to listen and be encouraging.

In addition to showing signs of fear, the patient frequently ventilates feelings of anger. At times the anger may be directed inward because of a sense of guilt—perhaps for causing the fire, or even for surviving when loved ones perished; or the anger may reach outward toward those who escaped unharmed or even to those who are now providing care. One way to help the patient handle these emotions is to find someone to whom the patient can vent feelings without fear of retaliation. A nurse, social worker, or clergy member who is not involved in direct care activities may fill this role successfully.

A major responsibility of the nurse is to constantly assess the patient's psychosocial reactions. Why is the patient fearful? Is it fear of losing control of bodily care, or sanity itself? Is it fear of rejection by family and loved ones? Is it fear of being unable to cope with pain, or physical appearance? Is it concern about sexual function? Being aware of these anxieties and understanding the basis of the patient's fears will enable the nurse to provide support and to cooperate with other members of the health care team in developing a plan to assist the patient to handle these feelings.

▷ *Improving Self-Concept.*   When caring for burn patients, the nurse needs to be aware that there are prejudices and misunderstandings in our society about those who differ from "the norm." Opportunities available to others are often denied to those who are disfigured, including social participation, means of employment, prestige, various roles, and status. It is the disfigured persons who must show others who they are, how they function, and how they want to be treated.

The nurse can help patients practice their responses to people who may stare or inquire about their injury once they are discharged from the hospital. The nurse can build self-esteem in patients by recognizing their uniqueness through small gestures such as providing a birthday cake, combing the patient's hair before visiting hours, sharing information on the availability of a cosmetician to enhance appearance, and teaching the patient to direct attention away from a disfigured body toward the self within. Consultants such as psychologists, social workers, vocational counselors, and teachers are valuable participants in the care of burn patients during rehabilitation.

▷ Evaluation

Expected Outcomes

1. Demonstrates activity tolerance required for desired daily activities
   a. Obtains sufficient sleep each 24 hours
   b. Reports no nightmares or sleep disturbances
   c. Shows gradually increasing tolerance and endurance in physical activities
   d. Is able to concentrate during conversations
   e. Has energy available to sustain desired daily activities
2. Demonstrates knowledge of self-care and follow-up care required
   a. Describes surgical procedures and treatments accurately
   b. Verbalizes detailed plan for follow-up care
   c. Demonstrates ability to do wound care and exercise
   d. Returns to clinic and physical/occupational therapy appointments as scheduled
   e. Lists resource people and agencies to contact for specific problems
3. Uses appropriate coping strategies to deal with postburn problems
   a. Verbalizes reactions to burns, therapeutic procedures, losses
   b. Identifies coping strategies used previously in stressful situations
   c. Accepts dependency on health care providers during acute illness
   d. Demonstrates denial, anger, regression, and depression in pattern common to postburn illness
   e. Verbalizes realistic view of problems resulting from burn injury and plans for future
   f. Cooperates with health care providers in required therapy
   g. Asks relevant questions regarding burn injuries and outcomes
   h. Participates in decision making regarding care
   i. Demonstrates interest in resources that may be able to positively affect cosmetic and functional results of injury
4. Adapts and adjusts to alterations in self-concept and life-style
   a. Verbalizes an accurate description of alterations in body image postburn
   b. Discusses changes in life-style and daily activities that may be required after discharge
   c. Adapts to and accepts appearance
   d. Uses cosmetics, wigs, and prostheses as desired to achieve acceptable appearance
   e. Socializes with significant others, peers, and usual social group
   f. Seeks and gains employment or return to role in family, school, or community as contributing member
   g. Is free of withdrawal and depression
   h. Resolves grief over losses resulting from burn injury and circumstances surrounding injury (*e.g.,* death of others; damage to house or other property)
   i. States realistic objectives for plastic surgery, further medical intervention, and results
   j. States abilities and goals that can be achieved
   k. Has hopeful attitude toward future

Nursing care of the patient during the rehabilitation/long-term phase is discussed in Nursing Care Plan 52-3.

Home Care and Follow-Up

As hospital stays become shorter, outpatient and home care of burn patients take on increasing importance. Patients and families must gradually be educated during the course of the hospital stay to care for the burn wound by active participation in this process as early as possible. Looking at the wound and touching the wound may be difficult and even frightening to some family members and patients. However, with encouragement and support, the majority of patients and family members can handle follow-up wound care with little need for professional care on a daily basis.

Follow-up care for the burn patient is carefully planned by all disciplines involved in the patient's care prior to hospital discharge. The nurse is often responsible for coordinating all aspects of care and ensuring that all the needs of the patient are met in a holistic manner. Many patients require outpatient physical and/or occupational therapy, often several times per week. Information related to specific exercises and use of elastic pressure garments and splints is fully reviewed with both the patient and responsible significant others. Written instructions are also provided.

Nursing Care Plan 52-3

Care of the Patient During the Rehabilitation/Long-Term Phase of Burn Care

Nursing Interventions	Rationale	Expected Outcomes

Nursing Diagnosis: Ineffective individual coping related to increased emotional and physical dependence on others

Goal: Improved coping and increased independence

Nursing Interventions	Rationale	Expected Outcomes
1. Be alert for verbal and nonverbal cues of patient regarding rehabilitation and adaptation to altered self-image.	1. Provides information about patient's understanding, awareness, and acceptance of changes in body image and life	• Achieves emotional and physical independence
2. Assist patient to set achievable short-term goals for increased independence in activities of daily living.	2. These are often easier to identify and to meet than long-term goals that seem unrealistic and unachievable to the patient.	• Participates fully in activities of daily living • Is equipped with and knowledgeable about use of prostheses or assistive devices
3. Provide positive feedback and support.	3. Encourages continued progress toward independence	• Verbalizes realistic view of self and plans for future
4. Consult with appropriate health team members for assistance with regressive behavior.	4. Uses knowledge and expertise of others	• Reports ability to participate in family, social, and vocational spheres
5. Assist with physical and occupational therapy as outlined by physical medicine staff.	5. Provides assistance to the patient while encouraging independence	

Nursing Diagnosis: Pain and discomfort related to skin tightness, dryness, and itching

Goal: Relief of discomfort and achievement of soft, lubricated, comfortable skin

Nursing Interventions	Rationale	Expected Outcomes
1. Assist patient with application of cocoa butter, Nivea, or other cream to healed wounds several times daily.	1. Lubricates and softens the skin	• Exhibits soft, comfortable, lubricated skin • Demonstrates no evidence of scratching of skin
2. Use mild soap for daily bathing.	2. Avoids use of harsh, drying soaps	• Sleeps without being disturbed by itching
3. Maintain cool, comfortable environment.	3. Minimizes discomfort and itching	• Reports minimal or no itching
4. Administer antipruritic medication.	4. Prevents or minimizes itching	• Skin feels soft and smooth
5. Recommend white cotton underwear under street clothing.	5. Avoids direct contact of skin with irritating dyes in clothes	• Demonstrates no scales or dryness

Nursing Diagnosis: Activity intolerance related to pain on exercise, limited joint mobility, fatigue, and low endurance

Goal: Increased activity and independence

Nursing Interventions	Rationale	Expected Outcomes

1. Relieve pain:
  a. Assess and document pain.
  b. Use analgesics, transcutaneous nerve stimulator, relaxation therapy, or other appropriate nursing interventions prior to exercise periods.
	1. Permits evaluation of baseline of pain and pain's contribution to inactivity	• Exhibits no pain
		• Requests no analgesics
		• Reports no pain on exercise
		• Sleeps without being disturbed by pain
		• Achieves activity tolerance and endurance consistent with desired levels

2. Increase activity tolerance and endurance	2. Promotes pain relief while encouraging exercise and activity	• Participates in activities of daily living as desired
3. Collaborate with physical and occupational therapists to plan for exercise requiring gradually increasing energy levels.	3. Helps to identify graded increases in exercise and activity within patient's current limitations	• Has stamina required for usual activities • Obtains optimal joint mobility • Has normal range of motion in all joints
4. Plan daily activities to maximize energy required for specific treatments in which patient must actively participate.	4. Promotes conservation of energy for its expenditure on required tasks and activities	
5. Plan care to provide rest period during day and 8 hours of sleep during night.	5. Encourages rest to decrease fatigue and increase exercise tolerance level	

(continued)

Nursing Care Plan 52–3 *(Continued)*

Care of the Patient During the Rehabilitation/Long-Term Phase of Burn Care

Nursing Interventions	Rationale	Expected Outcomes
6. Promote full range of joint motion.	6. Exercises affected joints and minimizes the risk of flexion contractures	
7. Encourage patient to follow exercise schedule planned by physical therapists.	7. Permits exercise while maintaining position of joints needed to prevent flexion contractures	
8. Apply splints as prescribed to reduce contractures. Administer analgesics if required prior to major physical therapy treatments.	8. Minimizes pain and discomfort during physical therapy treatments, and encourages full participation in exercises and treatments	
9. Use creative approaches to encourage patient to move joints in activities of daily living and self-care activities.	9. Promotes exercise while maintaining patient's independence	

Nursing Diagnosis: Dysfunctional grieving and depression related to inability to cope with alterations in appearance, life-style, body image, and self-image

Goal: Reduction of grieving and depression to an appropriate level

1. Employ concepts of psychiatric nursing to explore and improve depressed affect.	1. Interaction and communication skills are necessary to assist the grieving, depressed patient.	• Returns to preburn or better level of social and vocational functioning
2. Help patient employ short-term goals and a "one day at a time" philosophy.	2. Short-term goals are easier to identify and achieve than long-term goals that seen unachievable to the grieving, depressed person	• Socializes with significant others, peers, usual social group
		• Is able to seek and gain employment or return to role in school or community as contributing member of the group
3. Recognize need for grieving over losses.	3. Provides for a normal grief response to injury	• Has adapted to and resolved grief over losses resulting from burn injury and circumstances surrounding the injury (*e.g.*, death of others involved; damage to house, other property)
4. Have patient talk with other patients who are making good progress after similar injury.	4. Provides encouragement and a model for patient	
5. Obtain psychiatric consultation and administer prescribed mood elevators if depression lasts abnormally long.	5. Additional intervention may be necessary to help the patient cope with losses while continuing activity without jeopardizing progress and recovery	• Has hopeful attitude toward the future
6. Explain that depression is a normal sequela of major trauma but is relieved with general improvement in health.	6. Communicates that the patient's response is normal and is likely to abate as physical condition improves	

Nursing Diagnosis: Impaired skin integrity related to hypertrophic scarring

Goal: Prevention of hypertrophic scarring and achievement of optimal cosmetic result

1. Apply elastic bandages or pressure garments over healed areas prone to scarring.	1. These measures restructure the collagen and decrease vascularity and cellularity of the burned area, thus reducing hypertrophic scarring	• Achieves optimal cosmetic results
		• Adapts to and accepts appearance
		• Utilizes cosmetics, wigs, prostheses as desired to achieve acceptable appearance
2. Instruct patient in proper use and care of elastic garments for optimal results.	2. Provides information for patient to use correctly to promote the optimal result	• Has met plastic surgery goals
		• Exhibits minimal hypertrophic scarring
3. Provide information and referral for use of cosmetics and other aids to minimize impact of burn wounds.	3. Provides other resources and aid for the patient and improves body image	• States interest in acquiring information about cosmetics and other aids

Patients who receive care in a burn center usually return to a burn clinic periodically for evaluation of their status by the burn team, modification of home care instructions, and planning for reconstructive surgery. Others will be followed by the general or plastic surgeon who cared for them during hospitalization. Other patients require the services of a rehabilitation center and may be transferred to such a facility for aggressive rehabilitation prior to going home. A referral to the patient's regular physician is required for continuing care of any preexisting or new medical problems.

Some persons, particularly those without competent family members or friends available to help, will need referral to a community health nurse who can provide assistance with wound care and exercises at home. Patients with severe or long-lasting depression or difficulty adjusting to their social and/or occupational roles may require referral to a psychologist, psychiatrist, or vocational counselor.

There are a number of burn patient support groups and other organizations located throughout the United States that offer services for burn victims. They provide caring persons (often recovered burn victims) who can visit a burn patient in the hospital or home or telephone a patient and family periodically to provide support and counseling about skin care, use of cosmetics, and problems related to psychosocial adjustment. Such organizations, and many regional burn centers, sponsor group meetings and social functions at which outpatients are welcome. Some also provide school reentry programs and are active in burn-prevention activities.

In summary, although the earlier phases of burn care did not specifically focus on rehabilitation, rehabilitation begins as the patient enters the health care system and may extend for years following major burn injury. Attention to fluid and electrolyte status, nutrition, activity, and psychologic status continues through the rehabilitation/long-term phase. Additionally, a major role of the nurse at this phase of burn management is coordination of services and preparation of the patient and family for discharge from the acute care hospital and continuation of care at home. Knowledge about community services, supports, and other resources is necessary for the nurse to make appropriate referrals for the patient and family. Social services, occupational and physical therapy, home care nursing, and psychologic counseling are only a few of the services that may be required for reintegration of the patient into the community and continuity of care for the patient.

Gerontologic Considerations

The morbidity and mortality associated with burns are often much greater in the elderly than they are in younger patients. Reduced mobility, changes in vision, and decreased sensation in the feet and hands associated with the older age group are significant factors related to the inability of a person to avoid a preventable burn injury. Furthermore, thinning and loss of elasticity of the skin in the elderly predispose them to a deep injury from a thermal insult that might cause a less severe burn in a younger person.

Chronic illnesses decrease the aged person's ability to withstand the multisystem stresses of burn injury. Decreased

function of the cardiovascular and renal systems and lung disease increase the need for very close observation of elderly patients with even relatively small burns during the emergent and acute phases. Acute oliguric renal failure is much more common than in those under 40 years of age. The margin of difference between hypovolemia and fluid overload is very small. Suppressed immunologic response, a high incidence of malnutrition, and the inability to withstand metabolic stressors such as a cold environment further compromise the elderly person's ability to respond to burn injury.

Eschar separation in full-thickness burns is often delayed in the elderly. Because older persons are frequently poor risks for operative excision, prolonged hospitalization and immobilization and associated nosocomial problems may ensue.

Nursing assessment of the elderly should include particular attention to pulmonary function, response to fluid resuscitation, and signs of mental confusion or disorientation. A careful history of preburn medications and preexisting illnesses is essential. Nursing care promotes early mobilization, aggressive pulmonary care, and attention to reducing the potential for breakdown of normal skin. Because of lowered host resistance, the danger of burn wound sepsis and systemic septicemia is not only increased but also most likely to be lethal in the elderly. Fever may not be present in the elderly to signal such events. Therefore, surveillance for other signs of infection becomes even more important.

For stable patients, early operative intervention may be preferred to remove eschar and to facilitate wound covering with biologic dressings or autograft before infection and other problems cause deterioration of the patient. Rehabilitation takes into account preexisting functional abilities and problems such as arthritis and low activity tolerance. Lack of significant others available and able to provide home care is common. It is imperative that social services and community nursing services be contacted to provide for optimal care upon hospital discharge.

Chapter Summary

The severity and extent of a burn injury can vary from a superficial burn resulting from touching a finger to a hot stove, to a full-thickness burn covering most of the body surface and accompanied by massive tissue damage and destruction. Although the survival of patients experiencing severe burns has increased, the course of postburn injury care is often long and complex. The patient with extensive burns has a multisystem injury and often requires multiple surgeries to close the burn wound and complete skin grafting and improve joint mobility. Nursing care of the patient with severe burns requires critical care nursing skills combined with an equal focus on the rehabilitation needs of the patient. Astute assessment skills are essential to detect subtle changes in the patient's physical status and to evaluate the effects of treatment methods.

The nurse who works with burn patients requires expertise in dealing with the emotional responses of the patient and his family to life-threatening burns and complications and the resulting disruptions in family life, altered participation in work or school, and significant changes in life-style. Collaboration and cooperation among all members of the health care team are essential to provide quality care and continuity throughout the postburn course. Referral to mental health professionals and use of community resources often assist the patient in the transition from the hospital to home and aid in reintegration of the patient to his family and to the home, community, and work setting.

Bibliography

Books

Achauer B. Management of the Burned Patient. Norwalk, CT, Appleton and Lange, 1987.

Bayley EW and Martin MT (eds). A Curriculum for Basic Burn Nursing Practice, 4th ed. Galveston, TX, University of Texas Medical Branch and Shriners Burns Institute for the American Burn Association, 1985.

Bernstein NR and Robson MC. Comprehensive Approaches to the Burned Person. New Hyde Park, Medical Examination Publishing Co, 1983.

Demling RH. Management of the Burned Patient. In Textbook of Critical Care, 2nd ed. Philadelphia, WB Saunders, 1989.

Dolecek R et al. Endocrinology of Thermal Trauma: Pathophysiological Mechanisms and Clinical Interpretation. Philadelphia, PA, Lea & Febiger, 1990.

Dressler, Hozid JL, and Nathan D. Thermal Injury, St Louis, CV Mosby, 1988.

Haponick EF and Munster AM. Respiratory Injury: Smoke Inhalation and Burns. New York, McGraw-Hill, 1990.

Martin JAJ. Acute Management of the Burned Patient. Philadelphia, WB Saunders, 1990.

Journals

Asterisks indicate nursing research articles.

Bartle EJ et al. Cancers arising from burn scars: A literature review and report of twenty-one cases. J Burn Care Rehabil 1990 Jan/Feb; 11(1): 46–49.

Baxter CR and Weeckerle JF. Emergency treatment of burn injury. Ann Emerg Med 1988 Dec; 17(12):1305–1315.

Bayley EW et al. Standards for burn nursing practice. J Burn Care Rehabil 1989 Jul/Aug; 10(4):362–372.

Bayley EW and Smith GA. The three degrees of burn care. Nursing 1987 Mar; 17(3):34–42.

Bayley EW. Wound healing in the patient with burns. Nurs Clin North Am 1990 Mar; 25(1):205–222.

Boswick JA (ed). Burns. Surg Clin North Am 1987 Feb; 67(1):1–89.

Bowden ML. Factors influencing return to employment after burn injury. Arch Phys Med Rehabil 1989 Oct; 70(10):772–774.

*Brown B et al. Gender differences in variables associated with psychosocial adjustment to a burn injury. Res Nurs Health 1988 Feb; 11:23–30.

Bush A. What to look for when the patient suffers an electrical injury. RN 1987 Sep; 50(9):39–43.

Cella DF et al. Stress and coping in relatives of burn patient: A longitudinal study. Hosp Community Psychiatry 1988 Feb; 39(2):159–166.

Choinière M et al. The pain of burns: Characteristics and correlates. J Trauma 1989 Nov; 29(11):1531–1539.

Cobb N, Maxwell G, and Silverstein P. Patient perception of quality of life after burn injury. J Burn Care Rehabil 1990 Jul/Aug; 11(4):330–333.

Concilus R et al. Continuous intravenous infusion of methadone for control of burn pain. J Burn Care Rehabil 1989 Sep/Oct; 10(5):406–409.

Cooper DM. Optimizing wound healing: A practice within nursing's domain. Nurs Clin North Am 1990 Mar; 25(1):163–180.

Daniels SM et al. Self-inflicted burns: A ten year retrospective study. J Burn Care Rehabil 1991 Mar/Apr; 12(2):144–147.

Deitch EA (ed). Burns. Trauma Q 1989 Aug; 5(4):1–18.

Delaney AR, Damato RA, and Ikeda CJ. Delayed autograft loss in HIV patients: Two cases. J Burn Care Rehabil 1990 Jan/Feb; 11(1):67–70.

Dobner D and Mitani M. Community re-entry program. JBurn Care Rehabil 1988 Jul/Aug; 9(4):420–421.

Doherty D and Austin E. Effective management of cultured epithelial cells: Two case reports. J Burn Care Rehabil 1986 Jan/Feb; 7(1):33–34.

Dyer C. Burn wound management: An update. Plast Surg Nurs 1988 Spring; 8(1):6–12.

Dyer C and Roberts D. Thermal trauma. Nurs Clin North Am 1990 Mar; 25(1):85–117.

Hammond J and Ward CG. Decision not to treat/do not resuscitate order for the burn patient in the acute setting. Crit Care Med 1989 Feb; 117(2):136–138.

Heggers J et al. The efficacy of nystatin combined with microbial agents in treatment of burn wound sepsis. J Burn Care Rehabil 1989 Nov/Dec; 10(6):508–511.

Herbert K and Lawrence JC. Chemicals burns. Burns 1989 Dec; 15(6):381–384.

Ireton-Jones C. Use of indirect calorimetry in burn care. J Burn Care Rehabil 1988 Sep/Oct; 9(5):526–529.

Jarlsberg CR. Burns of the neck and chest. Nursing 1990 Jan; 20(1):33.

Johnson CL. Wound healing and scar formation. Top Acute Care Trauma Rehabil 1987 Apr; 1(4):1–14.

Jones JD et al. Alcohol use and burn injury. J Burn Care Rehabil 1991 Mar/Apr; 12(2):148–152.

Klein DG and O'Malley P. Topical injury from chemical agents: Initial treatment. Heart Lung 1987 Jan; 16(1):48–54.

Krings J. Hyperbaric oxygen therapy and critical burned patients. Nurs Manage 1987 Sep; 18(9):80A, 80D, 80H.

Madden MR et al. Grafting of cultured allogenic epidermis on 2nd and 3rd degree burns on 26 patients. J Trauma 1986 Nov; 26(11):955–962.

Mark MW et al. Burn management: Role of tissue expansion. Clin Plast Surg 1987 Jul; 14(3):543–548.

Martin LM. Nursing implications of today's burn care techniques. RN 1989 May; 52(5):26–33.

Marvin JA. Pain management in the burn patient. Top Acute Care Trauma Rehabil 1987 Apr; 1(4):15–24.

McCabe CJ, et al. Electrical and chemical burns. Emerg Care Q 1985 Nov; 1(3):31–40.

Merrel SW et al. The declining incidence of fatal sepsis following thermal injury. J Trauma 1989 Oct; 29(10):1326–1366.

Miller L et al. Sildimal: A new delivery system for silver sulfadiazine in the treatment of full thickness burn injuries. J Burn Care Rehabil 1990 Jan/Feb; 11(1):35–41.

Mosley S. Inhalation injury: A review of the literature. Heart Lung 1988 Jan; 17(1):3–9.

Neff J. Standard of care for the adult patient with thermal injury. J Emerg Nurs 1987 Jan/Feb; 13(1):59–63.

Nevelle C et al. Discharge planning for burn patients. J Burn Care Rehabil 1988 Jul/Aug; 9(4):414–420.

Norwicki CR and Sprenger CK. Temporary skin substitute for burn patients: A nursing perspective. J Burn Care Rehabil 1988 Mar/Apr; 9(2):209–215.

O'Neil CE, Hutsler D, and Hiddreth MD. Basic nutritional guidelines for pediatric burn patients. J Burn Care Rehabil 1989 May/Jun; 10(3):278–284.

Ostrow LB et al. Burns in the elderly. Am Fam Physician 1987 Jan; 35(1):149–154.

Patterson DR. Psychologic management of the burn patient. Top Acute Care Trauma Rehabil 1987 Apr; 1(4):25–39.

Patterson DR et al. Post-traumatic stress disorder in hospitalized patients with burn injuries. J Burn Care Rehabil 1990 May/Jun; 11(3):181–184.

Peck MD. Does early excision of burn wounds change the pattern of mortality? J Burn Care Rehabil 1989 Jan/Feb; 10(1):7–10.

Perry SW et al. Pain perception vs pain response in burn patients. Am J Nurs 1987 May; 87(5):698.

Phillips LG, Robson MC, and Heggers JP. Treating minor burns. Ice, grease or what? Postgrad Med 1989 Jan; 85(1):219–231.

Phillips LG et al. Uses and abuses of biosynthetic dressing for partial skin thickness burns. Burns 1989 Aug; 15(4):254–256.

Phillips LG et al. Meshed biobrane: A dressing for difficult topography. J Burn Care Rehabil 1990 Jul/Aug; 11(4):347–351.

Punch JD, Smith DJ, and Robson MC. Hospital care of major burns. Postgrad Med 1989 Jan; 85(1):205–215.

Purdue GF and Hunt JL. Multiple trauma and the burn patient. Am J Surg 1989 Dec; 158(6):536–539.

Rivers EA. Vocational considerations with major burn patients. Top Acute Care Trauma Rehabil 1987 Apr; 1(4):74–80.

Roberts D and Appleton V. Psychosocial care of burn injured patients. Plast Surg Nurs 1989 Summer; 9(2):62–65.

*Roberts JG. Analyses of coping responses and adjustment: Stability of conclusions. Nurs Res 1987 Mar/Apr; 36(2):94–97.

Sawhney CP. Amniotic membrane as a biological dressing in the management of burns. Burns 1989 Oct; 15(5):339–342.

Schmidt MA, French L, and Kalil ET. How soon is safe? Ambulation of the patient with burns after lower extremity skin grafting. J Burn Care Rehabil 1991 Jan/Feb; 12(1):33–37.

Shane J, Golde M, and Siverstein P. Comparison of energy expenditure measurement techniques in severely burned patients. J Burn Care Rehabil 1987 Sep/Oct; 8(5):366–370.

Shenkman B and Stechmiller J. Patient and family perception of projected function after discharge from burn unit. Heart Lung 1987 Sep; 16(5):490–496.

Slater AL, Slater H, and Goldfarb IW. Effect of aggressive surgical treatment of older patients with burns. J Burn Care Rehabil 1989 Nov/Dec; 10(6):527–530.

Smith GA and Bozinko GS. Giving emergency care for burns. Nursing 1989 Sep; 19(9):55–62.

Stearns G and Kahn A. The rehabilitation nurse: An able but often overlooked member of the burn team. J Burn Care Rehabil 1988 Jul/Aug; 9(4):422.

Talley MA and Luterman A. Myths and facts about burns. Nursing 1989 Jan; 19(1):21.

Tempereau CE. Volitional collapse (loss of the will to live) in patients with burn injuries: Treatment strategies. J Burn Care Rehabil 1989 Sep/Oct; 10(5):464–468.

Thompson PD et al. Hydrotherapy: A survey of burn hydrotherapy in the US. J Burn Care Rehabil 1990 Mar/Apr; 11(2):151–155.

van der Does AJW. Patients' and nurses' ratings of pain and anxiety during burn wound care. Pain 1989 Oct; 39(1):95–101.

Ward RS et al. Sensory loss over grafted areas in patients with burns. J Burn Care Rehabil 1989 Nov/Dec; 10(6):536–538.

Wasserman D et al. Use of topically applied silver sulfadiazine and cerium nitrate in major burns. J Burn Care Rehabil 1989 Aug; 15(4):257–260.

Wilding P. Care of a burn injured patient. Nurs Times 1988 Aug 24; 84(34):70–75.

Woodly DT. Covering wounds with cultured keratinocytes. JAMA 1989 Oct 20; 262(15):2140–2141.

Zawacki B. Tongue-tied in the burn intensive care unit. Crit Care Med 1989 Feb; 17(12):198, 199.

Note: Also see issues of The Journal of Burn Care and Rehabilitation and BURNS—The Journal of the International Society for Burn Injuries.

Information/Resources

Agencies

Alisa Ann Ruch Burn Foundation
20944 Sherman Way, Suite 115, Canoga Park, CA 91303, (818) 883-7700

American Burn Association
c/o The Shriners Burns Institute, 202 Goodman St., Cincinnati, OH 45219, Attn: Glenn D. Warden, MD, (513) 751-3900

Burn Foundation
1311 Chancellor St., Philadelphia, PA 19107

National Institute for Burn Medicine
909 E. Ann St., Ann Arbor, MI 48104

Northern California Burn Council
c/o Andrew McGuire, Director, Trauma Foundation, Trauma Center, Building 1, San Francisco General Hospital, San Francisco, CA 94110

Phoenix Society
11 Rust Hill Rd., Levittown, PA 19056

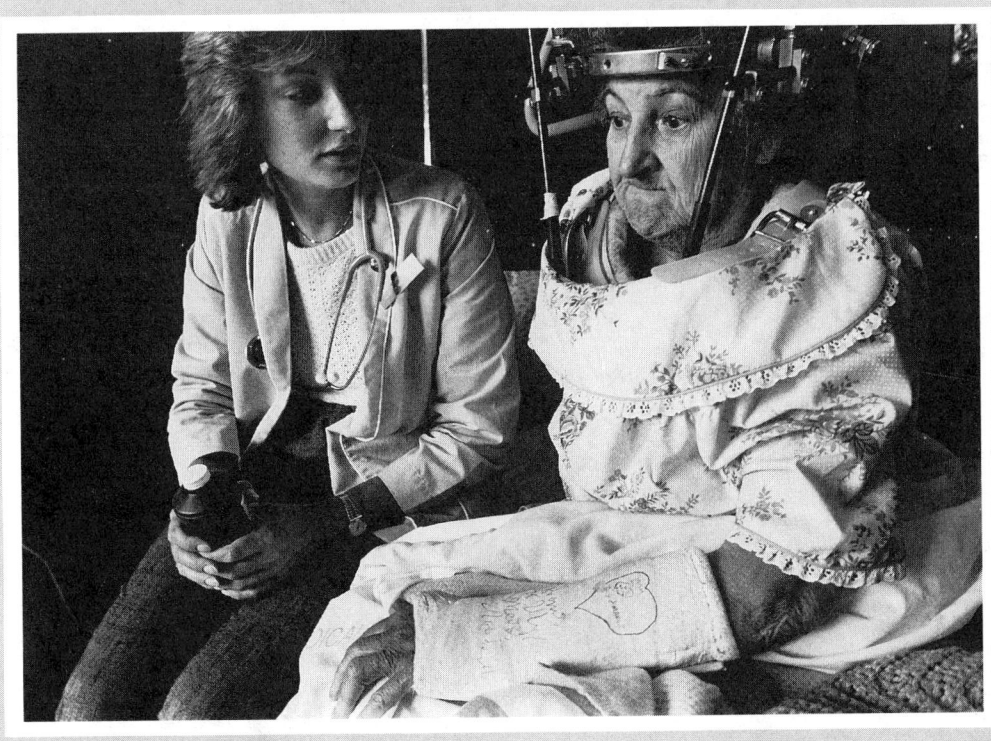

53

Assessment and Management of Patients With Vision Problems and Eye Disorders

Chapter Outline

Learning Objectives

On completion of this chapter, the learner will be able to:

1. Specify diagnostic tests used for assessment of the eyes and of vision
2. Describe the care and precautions necessitated by contact lenses
3. Specify the procedures used for daily care of patients with eye disorders
4. Use the nursing process as a framework for care of patients with eye disorders
5. Describe the nursing care of patients having surgery for corneal disorders and for detached retina
6. Use the nursing process as a framework for care of patients with glaucoma
7. Use the nursing process as a framework for care of patients undergoing surgery for cataract removal
8. Describe the emergency care of patients who have sustained trauma to the eye
9. Describe the health care needs of blind persons
10. Describe the nursing responsibilities related to sensory deprivation that results from loss of sight
11. Identify the components of health education directed toward preventive eye care

Glossary

Ocular Anatomy

anterior chamber—space in the eye filled with aqueous humor, bounded in front by the cornea and in back by the iris and lens

aqueous humor—clear, watery fluid circulating in the anterior and posterior chambers of the eye

blind spot—gap in the visual field that corresponds to the point where the optic nerve enters the eye

canal of Schlemm—aqueous drainage channel encircling the periphery of the anterior chamber

canaliculus—small tear drainage tube in the inner aspect of the upper

(continued)

Glossary *(continued)*

and lower lids leading from the puncta to the common canaliculus and then to the tear sac.

canthus—the angle at either end of the space between the eyelids

choroid—vascular pigmented middle layer of the eye between the retina and sclera

ciliary body—portion of uveal tract between base of iris and anterior part of choroid; consists of ciliary processes and ciliary muscle

cones and rods—two types of retinal receptor cells. Cones are concerned with visual acuity and color discrimination; rods are concerned with peripheral vision in decreased illumination.

conjunctiva—mucous membrane that lines the eyelids (palpebral) and is reflected onto the eyeball (bulbar)

cornea—clear, transparent anterior part of the fibrous coat of the eyeball

crystalline lens—transparent biconvex structure separating the aqueous from the vitreous humor spaces. Its function is to refract rays of light and bring them to focus on the retina.

epicanthus—vertical fold of skin covering the inner canthus

fovea centralis retinae—a pit in the middle of the macula lutea adapted for most acute vision

fundus oculi—posterior inner portion of the eye seen through an ophthalmoscope

iris—colored, circular, contractile membrane located between the cornea and crystalline lens and perforated in the center by the pupil

lacrimal sac—dilated proximal end of each of the two nasolacrimal ducts

lens—see crystalline lens

limbus—the edge of the cornea where it joins the sclera

macula lutea retinae—depression at the center of the retina surrounding the fovea, lateral to and slightly below the optic disc; responsible for acute central vision

optic disc (disk)—area in the retina where the optic nerve enters; blind spot; the intraocular position of the optic nerve formed by fibers converging from the retina.

optic nerve—second cranial nerve that carries visual impulses from the retina to the brain

palpebral—relating to the eyelid

posterior chamber—space filled with aqueous humor anterior to the lens and posterior to the iris

puncta—tear drainage opening in the medial aspect of the margin of each eyelid allowing flow into the lacrimal duct

pupil—circular, contractile opening in the center of the iris that regulates the amount of light that enters the eye

retina—innermost layer of the eye wall composed of nervous tissue; contains light-sensitive rods and cones that receive images of external objects and transmit visual impulses through the optic nerve to the brain

rods—see cones and rods

sclera—white part of the eye; tough, fibrous, opaque layer continuous with the cornea, which together form the external protective coat of the eye.

uvea—the middle, pigmented, vascular coat of the eye; includes the iris, ciliary body, and the choroid

vitreous—transparent, colorless, gelatinous mass filling the rear two thirds of the eye between the crystalline lens and the retina

zonule—numerous fine tissue strands that stretch from the ciliary processes to the crystalline lens and hold the lens in position

Eye Disorders

aphakia—absence of the crystalline lens of the eye

astigmatism—refractive error in which the light rays are prevented from coming to a single point of focus on the retina because of an unequal curvature of the cornea and lens

blepharitis—inflammation of the edges of the eyelids

cataract—loss of transparency of the crystalline lens

chalazion—a meibomian cyst

dacryocystitis—inflammation of the lacrimal sac

diplopia—seeing one object as two (double vision)

ectropion—turning out (eversion) of the eyelid

emmetropia—normal vision; refractive condition in which parallel rays focus exactly on the retina without the aid of accommodation

endophthalmitis—intraocular infection

entropion—turning in (inversion) of the eyelid

epiphoria—excessive production of tears

esotropia—inward deviation of one eye (crossed eyes)

exophthalmos—abnormal protrusion of the eyeballs

exotropia—outward deviaiton of one eye (wall eyes)

glaucoma—group of diseases of the eye characterized by increased intraocular pressure, which cause pathologic changes in the optic disc and progressive defects in the field of vision

hemianopia—blindness in half the field of vision

hordeolum, external (sty)—infection of the glands of Moll or Zeis

hordeolum, internal—infection of meibomian gland

hyperopia, hypermetropia—farsightedness

hypertropia—upward deviation of one eye

hyphema—blood in the anterior chamber of the eye

hypopyon—pus in the anterior chamber of the eye

hypotony—abnormally low intraocular pressure

keratitis—inflammation of the cornea

keratoconus—cone-shaped deformity of the cornea with central non-inflammatory thinning

myopia—nearsightedness

nystagmus—repetitive involuntary rapid movement of the eyeball

optic atrophy—degeneration of the optic nerve

papilledema—swelling of the optic disc

photophobia—abnormal sensitivity to light

presbyopia—lessening of the power of accomodation due to the aging process

pterygium—thick, triangular growth of tissue of the conjunctiva, which may extend onto the cornea

ptosis—drooping of the upper eyelid

retinal detachment—separation of the sensory retina from the underlying pigmented epithelial layer

(continued)

Glossary (continued)

retinitis pigmentosis—*hereditary progressive bilateral degeneration of the retina*

strabismus—*misalignment of the eyes caused by extraocular muscle imbalance; both eyes do not fixate on the object being observed*

sty—*see hordeolum, external*

sympathetic ophthalmia—*uveitis of the uninjured eye due to sensitization to uveal pigment after a penetrating injury of the other eye*

trabeculum—*meshwork in the anterior chamber angle through which the aqueous humor flows to leave the eye*

trachoma—*severe, chronic bacterial (Chlamydia trachomatis) infection of the conjunctiva and cornea*

uveitis—*inflammation of the iris, ciliary body, or choroid*

xerosis—*abnormal dryness of the conjunctiva and cornea caused by deficiency of tears*

Ophthalmic Agents

cycloplegic—*an agent that paralyzes the ciliary muscle*

miotic—*an agent that causes pupillary contraction*

mydriatic—*an agent that causes pupillary dilation*

Anatomy and Physiology

The eye is the organ of vision. It is an intricate structure with a complex function that allows for interpretation of objects and events both near and far. Vision, or sight, is made possible by the conversion of light rays into nerve impulses. Light rays enter the eye through the cornea and pass through the pupil, crystalline lens, and vitreous body to the retina. The light rays stimulate the sensory receptors in the retina to send impulses to the brain through the optic nerve to the occipital cortex, where the impulses are registered as visual sensations.

In front of the eye are the eyelids, two movable muscu-lofibrous folds that can open and close to protect the eye. The space between the open lids is called the palpebral fissure, which terminates at the medial canthus at the nasal side and at the lateral canthus at the temporal side. The lids are lined with the conjunctiva, a thin transparent mucous membrane that lies over the anterior sclera to the margins of the cornea (Fig. 53-1).

Tears, produced by the lacrimal glands, are distributed by the blinking of the lids; this keeps the cornea and the conjunctiva moist. Tears leave the eye through the puncta, two small openings in the upper and lower aspects of each lid on the nasal side. From there they pass through the canaliculi to the lacrimal sac and finally into the nose.

Two kinds of tears are normally produced: lubricating tears,

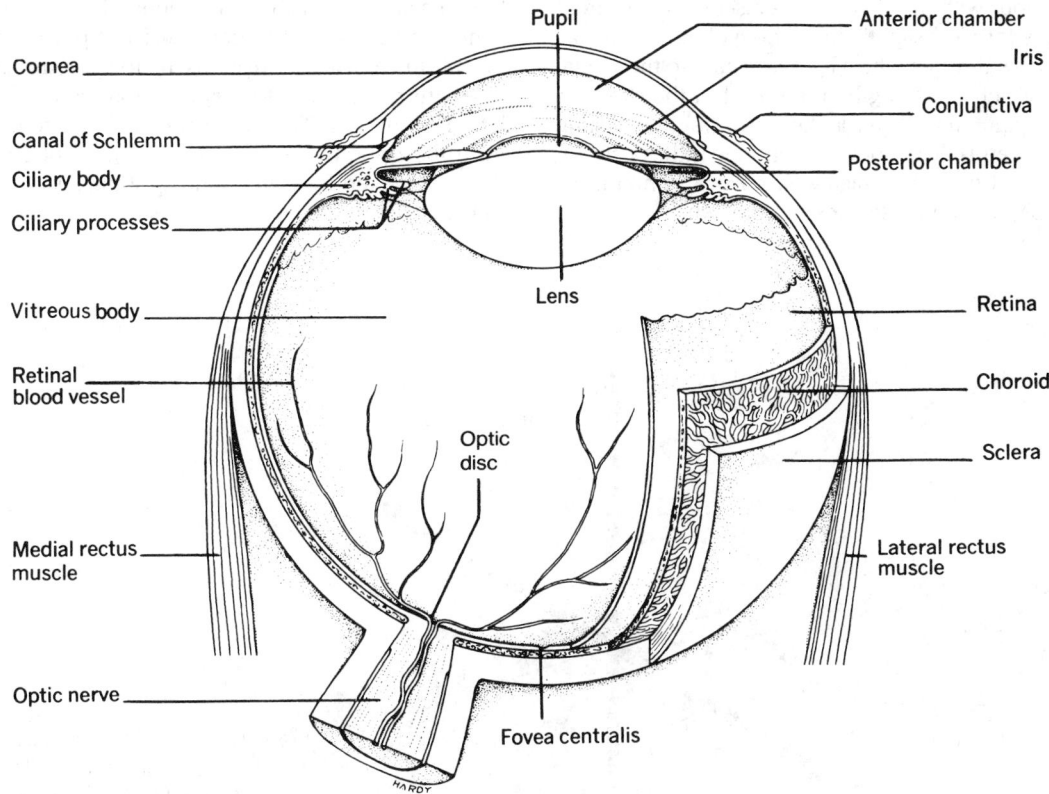

Figure 53–1.   Transverse section of eye. (Chaffee EE and Greisheimer EM. *Basic Physiology and Anatomy.* Philadelphia, JB Lippincott.)

which consist of oil, water, and mucus, and tears produced in response to emotion or irritation, which contain only water. Excessively watery tears do not adhere to the eyes and thus overflow onto the check. Production of lubricating tears decreases with age and may diminish to the point where there is not enough moisture to keep the eyes protected and comfortable. Symptoms of dry eyes are burning, redness, pain, scratchiness, difficulty in moving the lids, and stringy mucus. The eyes respond by increasing the amount of watery tears, which, ironically, results in tearing but does not help the lubrication problem. When dry eyes are accompanied by a dry mouth and arthritis, the condition is known as Sjögren's syndrome.

Inadequate tear formation or faulty lid closure results in drying and eventual scarring of the cornea. Artificial tears are instilled to replace the natural ones. Patients are advised to avoid irritants, such as a smoky room, and to add humidity to their environment. Ointment at bedtime is often helpful.

Movement of the eye is controlled by six extraocular muscles (Fig. 53-2), which insert into the sclera. The lateral rectus muscle abducts and the medial rectus muscle adducts the eye. The superior rectus muscle elevates and adducts and the inferior rectus muscle depresses and adducts. The superior oblique muscle directs the eye laterally and inferiorly, and the inferior oblique muscle directs it superiorly and laterally.

The eyeball is a spherical organ situated in a protective bony cavity called the orbit; it is surrounded by a cushion of orbital fat. It is composed of three layers: the sclera, uvea, and the retina.

The sclera is the dense, white fibrous protective coating of the eye. Posteriorly it has an opening through which the optic nerve and the central retinal vessels pass. Anteriorly it becomes continuous with the cornea, an avascular, transparent tissue that bulges forward slightly from the globe. It serves as a refracting window through which light rays pass to the retina, and it provides structural strength to the front of the eye.

The middle pigmented layer is the uveal tract consisting of the choroid, iris, and ciliary body. The choroid is the posterior portion of the uveal tract. It is highly vascular and nourishes the retina. The pigmented muscular structure, which gives the

characteristic color to the eyes, is the iris. The iris is the anterior aspect of the tract and divides the space between the cornea and the lens into an anterior and posterior chamber. It is a thin, circular, muscular diaphragm that has at its center a circulation aperture, the pupil. The pupil changes size as the iris spontaneously adapts, by dilation or constriction. These changes control the amount of light entering the eye to give the best visual function under varying degrees of light intensity. The peripheral border of the iris is attached to the ciliary body, which is composed of muscle fibers that contract and relax the lens zonules. The ciliary body plays a role in maintaining intraocular pressure (IOP) by secreting *aqueous humor*, a watery, transparent liquid, which fills the anterior and posterior chambers and exits through the trabecular meshwork through the canal of Schlemm. The constant flow of this liquid is responsible for maintaining the IOP, normally in the range of 12 to 21 mm Hg.

The crystalline lens is a biconvex, avascular, colorless, and transparent structure suspended behind the iris by the zonules. Contraction and relaxation of the zonules changes the shape of the lens and allows it to focus light on the retina. This process is known as *accommodation.*

The vitreous body is the clear, transparent avascular, gelatinous fluid that fills the space in the posterior portion of the eye bounded by the lens, retina, and optic disc. It plays an important part in maintaining the transparency and form of the eye.

The retina is the thin, semitransparent layer of nerve tissue that lines the eye wall. The rods and cones within the retina are receptors that respond to light energy and initiate the neural response that eventually is interpreted in the brain. The cones are responsible for visual acuity and color discrimination, and the rods are responsible for peripheral vision under decreased light conditions. In the center of the posterior retina is the macula lutea, which surrounds the fovea centralis. These structures are responsible for acute vision, color vision, and resolution of images. The nerve fibers of the retina converge to form the optic nerve. The head of the optic nerve, or optic disc, is referred to as the blind spot because it is not sensitive to light.

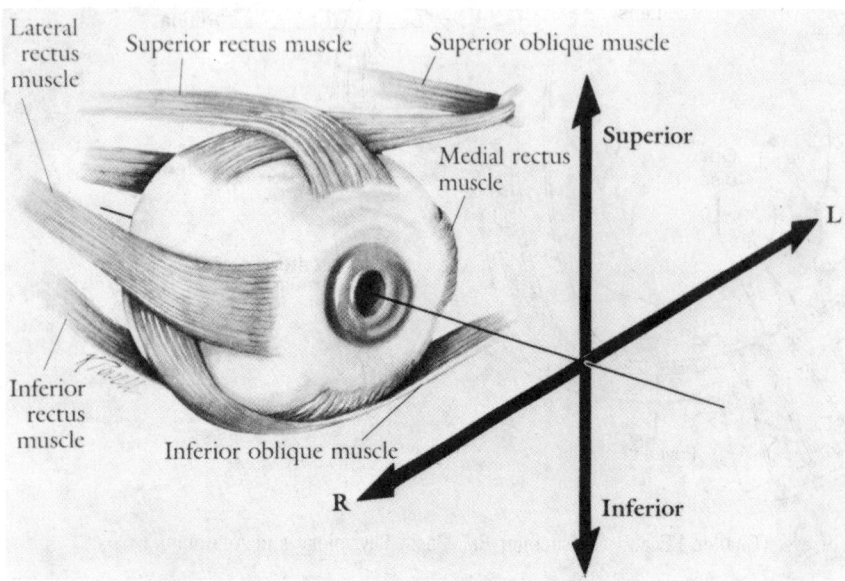

Figure 53–2. The extraocular muscles and their insertions onto the right eye. The arrows and the line to the pupil indicate the six cardinal positions of gaze. (Gittinger JW Jr. Ophthalmology. Boston, Little, Brown.)

Disease or trauma may interrupt the passage of light rays or their conversion and transmission as nerve impulses; this results in impaired vision or blindness. Fortunately, many pharmacologic, medical, and surgical treatments are available that can preserve or restore sight.

Gerontologic Considerations

As a person ages, vision becomes less efficient. The pupil becomes less responsive to light because of sclerosis of the pupillary sphincter, which results in a decrease in pupil size. The lens becomes more opaque, and the visual field decreases, making peripheral vision more difficult. Eyes adapt to darkness less rapidly; therefore, vision at night or in dimly lit areas is less clear in older people. With advancing years, there is a slowing in the process of accommodation as the lens gradually loses its elastic nature and becomes a relatively solid mass. *Presbyopia* refers to the loss of the ability to accommodate due to aging. Ciliary muscles with time also become less flexible and functional. Because near vision requires the greatest work by the ciliary muscles, near vision is compromised earliest, a condition that requires the wearing of reading glasses, bifocal lenses, and even trifocal lenses.

With advancing age, clumping of collagen materials of the vitreous body occurs; such clumping produces "floaters," which may be apparent in the field of vision. The retina shows fewest changes with aging, except for the macula. The macula is a small yellow spot in the center of the retina that contains the fovea, which functions as the area of most acute vision (central vision). Very small sclerotic changes in the macula result in impaired vision.

Eye Care Specialists

An *ophthalmologist* is a medical physician who specializes in the diagnosis and treatment, both medical and surgical, of diseases of the eye, visual disorders, and injuries of the eye. In addition to the general ophthalmologist, there are those who specialize in specific eye problems such as pediatric conditions, corneal disease, retinal and vitreal disease, glaucoma, oculoplastic surgery, and low vision.

An *optometrist* is a doctor of optometry and is licensed to examine, diagnose, manage and treat vision problems, diseases, and other abnormalities of the eyes and related structures.

An *optician* is licensed to fit, adjust, and dispense eyeglasses and other optical devices on the written prescription of an ophthalmologist or optometrist.

An *ocularist* is a technician who makes artificial eyes and other ophthalmic prostheses.

The following abbreviations are frequently used in the ophthalmology specialties:

OD (oculus dexter) or RE—right eye
OS (oculus sinister) or LE—left eye
OU (oculi unitas)—both eyes together
D—diopter, the unit of measurement of strength or refractive power of lenses (a 1-D lens brings parallel light rays to a focus 1 m from the lens)
HT—hypertropia

ST—esotropia
IOP—intraocular pressure
IOL—intraocular lens
EOM—extraocular lens
ICCE—intracapsular cataract extraction
ECCE—extracapsular cataract extraction

Examination of the Eye and Assessment of Vision

Examination of the eye is an essential component of the physical examination, not only because of the importance of the function of the eye to the well-being of the patient but also because the eye is reflective of the general state of health. The retina, which may be viewed with the ophthalmoscope, is the only site in the human body where the vascular bed may be examined directly. Diseases such as hypertension and diabetes produce changes that are readily observable. The pupil may be said to be a window to the human microcirculation.

History

A thorough history is obtained from the patient. This history includes any visual impairment, headaches, including location and frequency, vertigo, ocular or brow pain, and any eye discharge. Pain is assessed with regard to location, onset, duration, visual changes associated with pain, circumstances when pain occurs, relief measures, and severity. Use of corrective lenses and response to these lenses should be noted.

The health history should include questions about glaucoma, diabetes, hypertensive disease, eye trauma, eye surgery, and other disorders and diseases that can effect vision. It is important to identify the dates of onset of these conditions.

Life-style—type of work, leisure and sports activities, risk factors, and environmental exposure to airborne irritants—should also be evaluated.

Family history is also assessed. Family history should include questions about glaucoma, blindness, hypertensive disease, cataracts, and diabetes, as well as response to treatment for these diseases.

Visual Acuity. Formal testing of visual acuity is a part of the database of every patient. Visual acuity is tested with an eye chart placed 6 meters (20 feet) from the patient. The patient is instructed to cover one eye with a card, to keep both eyes open, and to read each line of the chart until he is no longer able to distinguish the details for a given size of print. If the patient wears glasses, his acuity should be assessed with and without corrective lenses.

Illiteracy may be circumvented by the use of charts that display the letter *E* in four different positions. This also enables one to assess the vision of children as young as 5 years of age.

Visual acuity is expressed in a ratio that relates what a person with normal vision sees at 20 feet to what the patient can see at 20 feet. Acuity of 20/50 means that the patient can see at 20 feet what he should see at 50 feet; 20/200, the boundary of legal blindness, indicates that the patient can see at 20 feet what he should be able to see at 200 feet. Such patients can only discern with accuracy the large letter at the top of the chart.

The patient whose visual acuity is less than 20/20 when corrected by his own glasses should be referred to an ophthalmologist or an optician.

Near vision is not routinely assessed unless the patient is complaining of difficulty in reading at close range or if he is over 40 years of age. After age 40, the lens may become rigid and incapable of accommodating its shape to close-range vision (presbyopia). Having a patient read newsprint at a distance of 30.5 cm (12 in) provides a general screening for this disorder. Patients who experience difficulty with this examination are referred to a specialist for further evaluation.

External Evaluation of the Eye.   The external structures of the eye are assessed primarily by inspection. These structures include the eyebrow, eyelid, eyelashes, lacrimal apparatus, conjunctiva, cornea, anterior chamber, iris, and pupil. The examination begins with an assessment of the position and alignment of the eyes. The eyebrows are observed for the quantity and distribution of the hair. The position of the lids in relation to the eyeballs is noted. With the eyes open, no sclera should be visible above the corneas. *Ptosis* (drooping of the lid) may be due to lid edema, muscle weakness, congenital defect, or involvement of the third cranial nerve. The eyelids are also inspected for color, swelling, lesions, and the presence and direction of eyelash growth. Common abnormalities of the lids are discussed later in this chapter.

The region of the lacrimal gland in the upper lateral orbit is inspected. If enlargement is suspected, the upper lid is everted to expose the lacrimal gland for further inspection. Next, the lacrimal apparatus is inspected for swelling. Obstruction or inflammation of the nasolacrimal duct can often be identified by pressing on the medial aspect of the lower lid just inside the orbital rim. The area is palpated for tenderness, and regurgitation of fluid from the puncta is noted.

The sclera and bulbar conjunctiva are inspected concurrently. The lids are separated by placing the index finger on the patient's upper orbital rim and the thumb on the lower rim. As the lids are separated, the patient is instructed to look up, down, and to each side. Small capillaries are normally visible in the conjunctiva, and the white, fibrous sclera is normally clearly visible. In dark-skinned persons, however, the sclera is often yellowish; this is a normal finding, not to be confused with jaundice. The palpebral conjunctiva of the lower lid is readily inspected by having the patient look upward while the lower lid is gently everted.

To inspect the cornea and anterior chamber for opacities, the examiner shines a light from a penlight held at an oblique angle. Normally, the cornea is smooth and transparent. Irregularities are often detected by defects in the light reflection through the cornea. Shadows cast on the iris may be indicative of a corneal lesion or forward displacement of the anterior chamber. The iris is inspected for continuity and unusual markings.

The pupils are normally round, regular, and equal in diameter and in their reaction to light. Although a small percentage of the population may have unequal pupils that may be considered normal, this phenomenon is sufficiently unusual that it should lead to thorough examination to ascertain that the inequality is not due to central nervous system (CNS) disease. When subjected to light, the normal pupil promptly constricts in a regular concentric fashion. The unstimulated opposite pupil constricts as well. This pupillary reaction is assessed by instructing the patient to focus on a distant object while the examiner shines a bright light on each pupil, in turn.

Constriction of the stimulated pupil is called the *direct light reflex*, whereas constriction of the opposite pupil is termed *consensual light reflex*. Exploration of this phenomenon allows one to distinguish between blindness due to damage to the optic nerve and blindness due to more central disease. Direct light stimulation of the nerve-damaged eye results in neither a direct nor a consensual light reflex. Stimulation of the uninvolved eye, however, results in consensual constriction of the pupil of the damaged eye, because the consensual reflex is not dependent on transmission through the optic nerve.

Pupillary reaction to accommodation (adjustments that occur when vision is shifted from near to far objects or vice versa) is best observed by asking the patient to focus on an object in the distance and then at the examiner's finger, which is positioned 7.5 to 12.5 cm (3 to 5 in) from the patient's nose. A normal response is for the pupil to constrict as the eyes converge to focus on the examiner's finger.

Autonomic disease due to syphilis or to diabetes may result in a pupil that is incapable of responding to light but that retains its capacity to respond to accommodation. Such a pupil is known as an *Argyll Robertson pupil*.

Ocular Tension.   An increase in intraocular tension is the cardinal manifestation of glaucoma, a disease responsible for more than one fifth of the blindness in the United States. A general determination of IOP can be made by applying gentle finger pressure over the sclera of the closed eye. The tips of both forefingers are placed on the closed upper lid. One finger gently presses inward while the adjacent finger senses the amount of pressure exerted against it. Some examiners then compare the tension felt or perceived in the patient's eye to their own. At best, this maneuver is a general estimation. When a more accurate measurement is required, tonometry is indicated.

Assessment of Extraocular Muscles.   The extraocular muscles (see Fig. 53-2) are six small muscles attached to each eye. They are innervated by three of the cranial nerves. Synergistic (correlated) action of the extraocular muscles of both eyes results in parallel gaze. The mechanism by which this takes place is highly complex, and analysis of abnormality requires physician consultation.

Parallel alignment of the eyes may be easily detected by shining a light directly into the face while the patient is staring at the light source. The light should be reflected from the pupils of both eyes identically. Light reflexes that vary from one pupil to the other indicate disturbance in parallax vision. Despite normal alignment of both eyes when they function together, the tendency of either eye to drift to the nasal or temporal side (and the necessity to involuntarily compensate for this with effort) may be assessed by the *cover test*. One eye is covered by a card or by the hand of the examiner, and the patient is asked to focus the free eye on a stationary object while keeping the covered eye open. The card or hand is abruptly removed from the covered eye, which is then observed for any abnormal movement. If the eye, when covered, has drifted to the temporal side, it will snap back into alignment when the cover is removed. Conversely, if it has drifted to the nasal side, the reverse phenomenon will occur. The tendency of an eye to drift, when covered, to the temporal side is called an *exophoria;* a tendency of an eye to drift to the nasal side is called an *esophoria.*

Integrity of the nervous control of the muscles of the eye may be assessed by directing the patient to move his eyes in the six cardinal positions of gaze (see Fig. 53-2) while following an object. The object is moved laterally to either side along the horizontal axis and then along two oblique axes, each of which makes a 60-degree angle with the horizontal axis. Each of the cardinal positions of gaze represents the function of one of the six extraocular muscles attached to each eye. If *diplopia*, or double vision, develops during the transition to any one of the cardinal positions of gaze, the examiner has an indication that one or more of the extraocular muscles are failing to function properly.

When extraocular movements are checked, the eye is observed for *nystagmus*, an irregular jerking movement of the eyes as gaze is shifted to a lateral position. Nystagmus has two components: a quick component in one or the other direction, and a slower subsequent component that brings the eye back to the intended position. Nystagmus on extreme lateral gaze is a normal finding, however, and can be avoided by not placing the object too far laterally beyond binocular gaze. A number of conditions cause nystagmus. Although many of these conditions are benign, others may reflect severe pathologic processes.

Assessment of Field of Vision.   Although the visual field (Fig. 53-3) can be assessed with a high degree of precision by an ophthalmologist, a rough estimate may be made in the office or at the patient's bedside when the examiner is concerned with any general disturbance of the visual field. Such a circumstance may arise, for example, in assessing the patient with a stroke. Such patients commonly lose one fourth or one half of the visual fields of both eyes.

A simple and reliable method of testing the fullness of the visual field is direct confrontation. The examiner and patient sit directly facing each other at a distance of 60 cm (2 feet). The patient is instructed to cover one eye with a card while looking directly at the examiner's nose. The examiner in turn covers one eye as a method of comparison. If the patient has covered his left eye, for instance, the examiner covers his or her right eye. The examiner then takes an object (pen, finger) in his right hand and moves it along a plane halfway between the examiner and the patient. The nasal, temporal upward, and downward fields are assessed by bringing the object into view from various peripheral points. During each maneuver, the patient informs the examiner the moment he is able to see the object. To test the nasal fields of gaze for the same eye, the examiner switches the object from the right hand to the left hand. The entire procedure is reversed for an assessment of the fields of the left eye. When confrontation testing shows

decreases in visual fields, or blind spots, the patient is referred immediately to an ophthalmologist for further evaluation.

Ophthalmoscopy.   The internal eye is referred to as the *fundus* and is composed of the retina, optic disc, macula, and retinal vessels. It is visualized with the aid of an instrument called an *ophthalmoscope*. With practice and repetition, the nurse can become proficient in the use of the ophthalmoscope. The ophthalmoscope is an instrument that projects light through a prism and bends the light at 90 degrees, allowing the observer to view the retina through a lens in such a way that the line of vision is parallel to the bent ray of light. A number of lenses are available and are arranged on a wheel so that they may be chosen by rotating the wheel with the index finger without interrupting the inspection. The small, unfiltered aperture is appropriate and most useful for standard ophthalmoscopy.

To avoid a confrontation of noses, the right eye of the patient is examined with the right eye of the examiner, the left eye of the patient with the left eye of the examiner (Fig. 53-4A). The room is darkened so that the pupil dilates. The patient is instructed to hold the eyes still and focus on a real or imaginary distant object. The ophthalmoscope is gripped firmly in the hand, with the index finger resting on the lens wheel. The head of the ophthalmoscope is braced within the angle made by the brow and the nose. The lens chosen for initial inspection should be the one labeled zero unless the examiner is knowingly correcting his or her own defect in visual acuity. If the examiner wears glasses, it may be better to remove the glasses and become familiar with which lens is analogous to zero for the examiner with 20/20 vision; or the examiner may prefer to keep the glasses on and use the zero lens setting. Provided that the patient has 20/20 vision, the zero lens should enable the examiner to obtain a precise focus on the retina. If the retina is out of focus, the lens wheel is rotated until it is brought into focus. The use of a lens labeled with a red numeral implies that one is focusing farther away than normal; the use of a lens labeled with a black numeral implies that one is focusing nearer to the examiner. The examiner chooses lenses among the red series for patients who are *hyperopic* (farsighted) and lenses in the black series for patients who are *myopic* (nearsighted).

With the room in darkness, with the patient appropriately gazing into the distance, and with the ophthalmoscope properly positioned within the cradle of the brow and nose, the examiner now approaches the patient. The examiner stands about 37.5 cm (15 in) from the patient and about 15 degrees lateral to

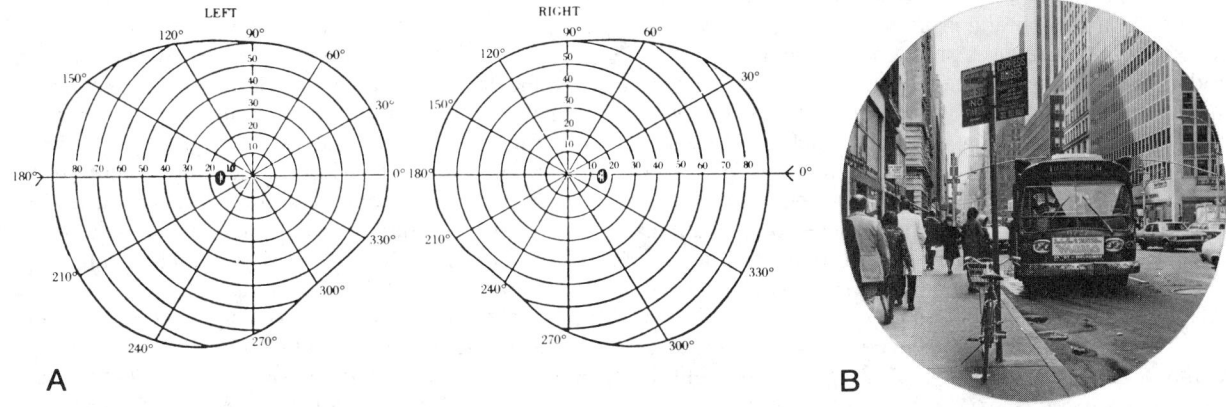

Figure 53–3.   (**A**) Visual field charts showing peripheral vision of 180 degrees with both eyes. (**B**) Photograph representing a street scene as viewed by a person with normal (20/20) vision. (Photo courtesy of The Lighthouse, The New York Association for the Blind.)

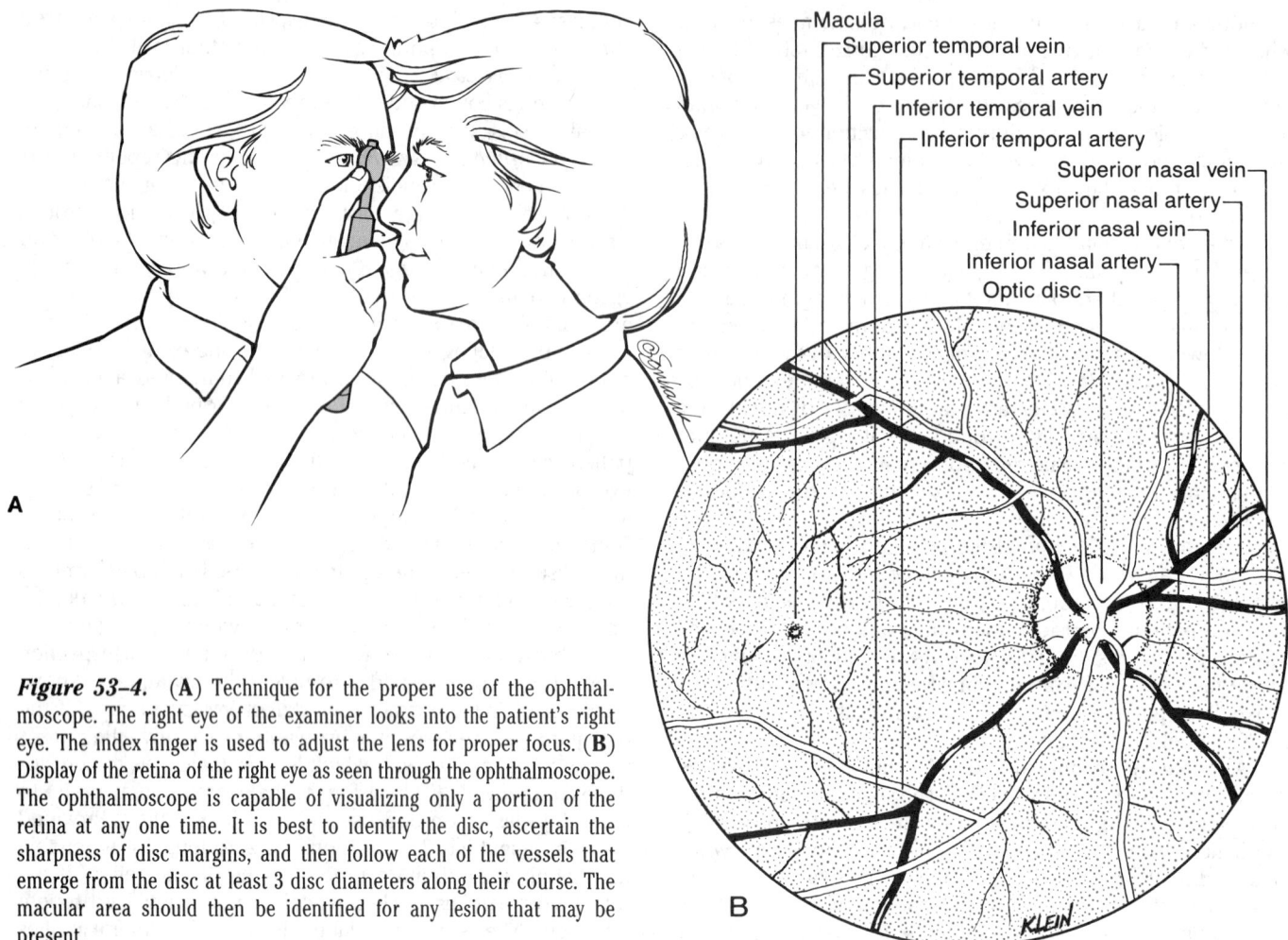

A

B

- Macula
- Superior temporal vein
- Superior temporal artery
- Inferior temporal vein
- Inferior temporal artery
- Superior nasal vein
- Superior nasal artery
- Inferior nasal vein
- Inferior nasal artery
- Optic disc

KLEIN

Figure 53–4. (**A**) Technique for the proper use of the ophthalmoscope. The right eye of the examiner looks into the patient's right eye. The index finger is used to adjust the lens for proper focus. (**B**) Display of the retina of the right eye as seen through the ophthalmoscope. The ophthalmoscope is capable of visualizing only a portion of the retina at any one time. It is best to identify the disc, ascertain the sharpness of disc margins, and then follow each of the vessels that emerge from the disc at least 3 disc diameters along their course. The macular area should then be identified for any lesion that may be present.

the patient's gaze. When the light is focused on the pupil, the retina glows red through the dilated pupil opening. This is known as the *red reflex.* The examiner then approaches the patient until the examiner's forehead touches his or her left hand, which has been placed on the patient's forehead (see Fig. 53-4*A*). At this point, provided that the proper lens has been selected, the retina should be in focus, and the venules and arterioles that course through the retina are readily apparent (see Fig. 53-4*B*). In scanning the surface of the retina, it is important that the examiner hold the scope firmly and move his or her head rather than the instrument.

The examiner first focuses on the optic disc. In the event that the disc is not in view when the retina is first visualized, the veins that are within the field of vision should be followed down their tributaries toward the disc from which the arterioles emerge and the venules enter. This is analogous to following the limbs of a tree until one sees the trunk. The optic disc is examined for size, shape, color, and sharpness of its margin. Normally the disc is circular and yellowish pink. The margin is sharp and occasionally surrounded by a rim of dark pigment (choroidal crescent). One must become familiar with what is regarded as a normal-sized disc. In the center of the disc there is frequently a small physiologic cup into which the central vein of the retina recedes. To focus on the base of this cup accurately, one may have to choose another lens in the direction of the red sequence. A deep cup is seen in glaucoma.

Edema of the optic disc (papilledema) with concomitant blurring of the disc margin is seen with increased intracranial pressure. The disc becomes pink, and accurate focus may require shifting to a lens in the direction of the black sequence. *Optic atrophy* is characterized by extreme pallor of the disc and reduction of its size.

The remainder of the retina is now examined. Abnormalities are precisely located for other observers by using a standard nomenclature that makes reference to an imaginary clock face and by referring to the diameter of the disc to delineate distance. Thus, a hemorrhage may be documented as half of the disc diameter in size, located two disc diameters away from the disc margin at the 2 o'clock position. Another observer is then able to replicate this finding.

The examiner now follows each of the major vessels from the margin of the disc. The arterioles are lighter in color and narrower than the venules. Under normal circumstances, arterioles are two thirds to four fifths the diameter of veins. The walls of the vessels are essentially transparent, and what is being observed is the blood column itself. The size and character of the arteriovenous crossings is noted, as well as any lesions in the retina. The retinal changes associated with diabetes are distinctive and are discussed in Chapter 39.

Lastly, the macular area of the retina is visualized by having the patient look directly at the light source. This causes the patient slight discomfort and tearing and provides the examiner with only a brief second or two during which to inspect the small, circular, red area of the macula. The glistening reflection of its center is called the *fovea centralis retinae.* Any edema, hemorrhages, or lesions are noted and brought to the attention of an ophthalmologist.

All of the techniques that have been discussed for the examination of the eye are not performed on every patient. Routinely, one inspects the conjunctiva, the cornea, and the pupil and assesses extraocular motion. Ophthalmoscopic examination is a part of every complete physical examination. Although visual acuity is a part of the data base, it need not be assessed more often than once every year or two, except in the elderly and in persons with symptoms or conditions known to affect vision, such as diabetes mellitus.

Assessment of Visual Acuity. The most widely accepted method of screening for visual problems is the letter chart (Snellen). Its accuracy is limited, however. Other devices are available, including a BVAT microprocessor and echography. A BVAT (Mentor) microprocessor produces an E of 30 different sizes on a television monitor. A computer monitors the responses the patient makes with a hand-held response box. A computer printout provides the mean visual acuity and standard deviation computed from 20 trials. The time required is about 8 minutes.

Letter Chart/Microprocessor. In echography (ultrasound, ultrasonography), high-frequency pulses of ultrasound are emitted from a small probe placed on the eye. After striking the ocular tissues, the sound energy is reflected to the probe, which in turn is displayed on an oscilloscope. Two primary types of ultrasound are used in ophthalmology:

A-scan—Oscilloscopic reflection is a vertical deflection from the baseline (one-dimensional).
B-scan—Oscilloscopic reflections are lines or dots (two-dimensional).

When used jointly, over 100 lesions or groups of lesions may be detected and differentiated in the orbital and periorbital region. Measurements for intraocular lenses (IOLs) can be performed by ultrasound and analyzed by computer; this enables the surgeon to determine lens power for an implant and postoperative refractive power.

This procedure is painless but requires the instillation of topical anesthetic eyedrops. After the examination, the patient is cautioned not to rub his eyes, because corneal lesions may occur.

Endothelial Cell Counter. An endothelial cell counter is a photographic instrument that can be attached to a slit lamp and used to produce high resolution, revealing subtle details of endothelial cell morphology: cell size, cell shape, cell population density, nature of cell boundary, and presence of intercellular bodies and pathologic processes. This is a valuable test preoperatively because if a compromised endothelium is observed, it may suggest an increased risk of postoperative complications.

Optics and Refraction

Minor defects and alignments of the eyes can be seen in almost everyone. Refractive correction is unnecessary for most of these defects. When refractive correction is necessary, however, it is for the purpose of relieving symptoms such as blurred vision, headache, or eye fatigue, and not for improving the health of the eye. Several types of corneal refractive surgery are available to correct myopia, hyperopia, and astigmatism. The procedures may eliminate the need for eye glasses or reduce the strength of the prescription required to correct vision.

Refractive errors include myopia (nearsightedness), hyperopia (farsightedness) (Fig. 53-5), anisometropia (unequal focus of the two eyes), astigmatism (asymmetric focus), and presbyopia (inability to change focus).

Refractive errors and their treatment are best understood when related to the process of accommodation. Accommodation is produced when the ciliary muscles contract, increasing the curvature of the lens. This causes the refractive power of the eye to increase (accommodation) and results in the eye being able to focus on near objects. When the ciliary muscles relax, the refractive power of the eye is at its lowest possible strength.

As a person ages, the ability of the eye to accommodate gradually decreases. After age 40 the decreased ability to accommodate becomes more noticeable, especially with regard to close work. Presbyopia is the loss of accommodation because of age.

When the normal eye is focused for distance, without accommodation, it is known as emmetropia. The eye clearly sees objects in the distance without effort and, using accommodation, it can focus on close objects.

With myopia, the eye has excessive reactive power and focuses light from distant objects in front of the retina. The myopic eye is unable to clearly see objects in the distance because the eye has no way to reduce this excessive refractive power. Decreased distant vision is the only symptom apparent with myopia.

With hyperopia, the eye has insufficient reactive power to focus light on the retina. It is a condition that causes the rays of light entering the eye to be focused behind the retina. Impairment of near vision results.

Astigmatism results from unequal curvature of the cornea. The focus of light rays is distorted and the patient is not able to focus horizontal and vertical rays on the retina at the same time. Vision is generally blurred, and the patient often complains of eye discomfort. Either hyperopia or myopia may coexist with astigmatism. Astigmatism cannot be eliminated by accommodation but can generally be corrected by glasses ground to neutralize the unequal curvature.

Refractive Errors

Assessment

The strength and type of lens that will overcome refractive errors are determined by means of a *retinoscope,* which measures the refractive error. On the basis of this examination, an appropriate corrective lens is selected and then further refined by having the patient read letters on the Snellen chart through several different lenses.

Automated refractors, which rely on photoelectric devices sensitive to light, may also be used. The patient sits in front of the instrument and is instructed to look steadily at a target. A printout on a card or graph indicates the refractive error to be

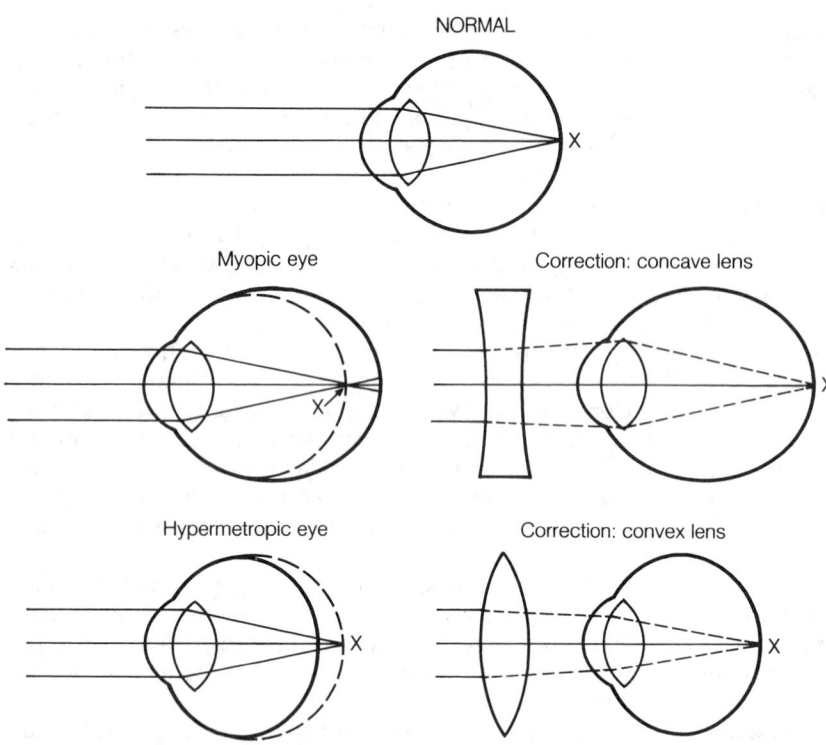

NORMAL

Myopic eye

Correction: concave lens

Hypermetropic eye

Correction: convex lens

Figure 53–5. Normal vision, myopia, and hypermetropia. (Suddarth DS. The Lippincott Manual of Nursing Practice. Philadelphia, JB Lippincott, 1991.)

corrected. Other types of automated refractors require the patient to make focusing adjustments by turning a knob.

Correction

Refractive errors may be corrected with eyeglasses, contact lenses (Table 53-1), or IOLs. If the refractive error is relatively slight, the patient may elect not to use glasses. A more significant refractive error can result in the patient's wearing prescription glasses. Others may elect to wear contact lenses.

An advance in prescription eye glasses is the progressive power lenses. Progressive power lenses provide distance, intermediate, and near corrections without the visual dividing line usually seen in bifocals and trifocals. The advantages of progressive power lenses are that clear vision is obtained at all distances without abrupt power changes and the absence of visible line segments. The disadvantages are prescription limitations, optical aberrations, and fitting difficulties.

Contact lenses are lightweight, paper-thin plastic discs. When properly fitted, contact lenses float on the fluid layer of the eyeball and are held loosely in place by the capillary attraction of the tears and the upper lid. The lens moves with the eye and is centered over the cornea.

Contact lenses have many advantages over framed lenses; they do not steam up when the wearer goes from a cold environment to a warm room; they are automatically cleaned with each blink of the eyelid; they can be worn safely during sports; they provide increased peripheral vision; and they do not break easily.

There are basically two types of contact lenses—hard and soft. Hard contact lenses can either be non–gas permeable or gas permeable. With the non–gas-permeable lens, oxygen that is dissolved in the tears surrounding the lens flows under the lens during blinking, thus supplying the cornea with the oxygen needed to properly function.

Gas-permeable lenses are more popular because of comfort. The oxygen dissolved from the tears is mixed with atmospheric oxygen, which is passed directly through the lens to the cornea.

Soft contact lenses are gas permeable and are available as either extended-wear, flexible (daily) wear, or disposable lenses. Because of the thickness and design of the lens, differing amounts of gas pass through the lens. The soft contact lenses are soft and flexible because of absorption of water.

Extended-wear lenses are those lenses made with newer plastic and silicone materials that allow more oxygen to pass through to the cornea. Extended-wear lenses are so named because they can be worn for several weeks at a time without removal. This is particularly helpful for the elderly, those patients who have a difficult time inserting lenses, and those patients who are nearsighted.

Irritation of the surface of the cornea, conjunctivitis, chemical sensitivity, and corneal infection are possible complications associated with all contact lenses but especially with extended-wear lenses. Often these lenses need to be replaced more frequently than the lenses designed for daily wear because of the accumulation of deposits and film from the eye. To reduce the chance of complications it is recommended that the extended-wear lenses be worn for no longer a period than that prescribed by the ophthalmologist.

Removal of Contact Lenses

Contact lenses are designed to be worn only while the person is awake and fully conscious (the exception is extended-wear lenses). They should be removed as a safety measure if the wearer is incapacitated due to accident, sickness, or other cause. If the patient is conscious or semiconscious, he is questioned regarding whether or not he is wearing contact lenses. Depending on his condition, he may be able to remove the

TABLE 53-1.   Types of Corrective Lenses

Durability	Advantages	Disadvantages
EYEGLASSES (SPECTACLES)		
Excellent	Excellent vision correction	Fogging in cool weather
	Easily cared for	Some cosmetic objections
		Unsuitable for certain activities and sports; some occupational drawbacks
		May need to be replaced more frequently than soft contact lenses
HARD CONTACT LENSES		
With care, may last 15–20 years	Excellent vision correction	Uncomfortable for some
	Usually less costly than other types	Require period of adaptation
	Effective for persons with astigmatism	Possibility of eventual intolerance
		May pop out of position
SOFT CONTACT LENSES		
May require more frequent replacement (usually replaced every 1–3 years)	More comfortable than hard lenses	Require time daily for sanitation
	Can be worn longer than hard lenses	Greater risk of eye irritation and infection
		Not as effective for astigmatism
		Possibility of eventual intolerance
EXTENDED-WEAR LENSES		
Most fragile of all lenses	Provide corrected vision around the clock	Expensive
May have to be replaced every 6 months or more often	May be worn for an extended period.	More frequent visits to eye physician
		Risk of corneal injury
		May not correct vision as well as other lenses
		Possibility of eventual intolerance

lenses himself or with some assistance. Unconscious patients need to be assessed as to whether they are wearing contact lenses. This assessment can be made by gently separating the eyelids and shining a light on the eye from the side. A nurse who wears contact lenses may be of help in removing the lenses of these patients.

The nurse removes the patient's contact lenses if he cannot do so himself. The following procedure is used:

- With clean hands, one thumb is positioned on the upper eyelid and one thumb on the lower eyelid, with thumbs near the margin of each eyelid.
- The eyelids are separated.
- A visible lens should slide easily with a gentle movement of the eyelids.
- If the lens does not drop out easily, the position of the lens is identified.
- Force should not be used.
- If the lens is seen but cannot be removed, it is gently slid onto the sclera, where it can remain with relative safety until experienced help is available.

If the patient is wearing soft contact lenses, it is best to wait until someone experienced in removing these types of lenses is available to lend assistance. If soft lenses are left in place for many hours, they do little harm.

Nursing Care of Patients With Eye Disorders

The eye is such an important organ that its care and protection are major considerations from the day of birth. The nurse, as an important member of the health team and as a teacher and a practitioner of sound health habits, can provide excellent health education in eye care and in the prevention of eye diseases.

Sound principles of safe care need to be stressed at an early age. Such problems as headache, dizziness, tiredness after close eye work ("the letters run together"), and scratchy or itchy eyes should be checked by a health care provider. Also significant are inflamed or watery eyes; red-rimmed, encrusted, or puffy lids; recurring sties; crossed eyes; and unequal pupils. Unusual behavior should be noted, such as holding a book too closely, frowning, blinking, squinting, rubbing the eyes, and failing in school or study work.

The importance of eye care has been recognized by industries that require workers to wear protective devices during activities that pose a danger of injury from foreign objects. Safety glasses should be worn when the task warrants it. Eyes should be protected from bright sun, sunlamps, ultraviolet rays, and aerosols such as hair spray. In the home, ammonia and alkali products, such as lye, present a particularly dangerous hazard for both children and adults and should be stored in safe places out of reach and used with care.

Eyes need to rest after being used for close work for a time. Occasionally glancing out the window or around the room provides relaxation.

The importance of adequate and well-placed light in preventing eyestrain is essentially no longer a medical problem but one of general, industrial, and social concern.

Medical management of patients with eye conditions has changed drastically in recent years and has resulted in less frequent need for hospitalization. For example, a patient with a cataract no longer needs to stay in the hospital for several days on extended bed rest, which can result in sensory deprivation as well as complications such as thrombophlebitis, pulmonary embolism, and pneumonia. Cataract surgery and many other ophthalmic operations, are performed in same-day surgery units, on an outpatient basis, thus allowing the patient to return home on the same day as the surgery. Such brief contact with the patient or family allows the nurse only a short time for observation, assessment, nursing interventions, and patient evaluation. Therefore, any teaching sessions or demonstrations of self-care procedures must be performed in such a way as to ensure that the patient and family understand their responsibilities for self-care and can recognize those signs and symptoms that may require professional consultation and intervention. Although outpatient surgery is common for some eye disorders, many eye problems do require more prolonged hospital care.

General Management Modalities

Ophthalmic Medication

A wide variety of ophthalmic medications are available for both diagnostic and therapeutic use (Table 53-2). Nurses, patients, and their family members must understand the correct techniques for using these medications. The label should be read before each instillation and the appropriate eye identified to verify the correctness of both the medication and the site. The hands are washed immediately before treatment. To avoid injury to the eye, the tip of the bottle or tube should never touch the eye. Contaminated medications are discarded.

The puncta should be occluded to avoid systemic absorption. If more than one medication is to be used, there should be at least 30 seconds between each because the eye is not capable of holding more than one drop at a time. Containers should be tightly capped when not in use. Old medications, as evidenced by the expiration date, color change, or sediment, are discarded.

Eyedrops

Various drug solutions are instilled into the eyes in the treatment of nearly every kind of eye disorder.

Before drops are instilled, it is important to make sure that the correct drug is being given. Some drugs (*e.g.*, miotics and mydriatics) act in exactly opposite ways (Fig. 53-6). Therefore, if one of these drugs is indicated in the treatment of a certain eye disease, the other is contraindicated. For this reason, it is imperative that eye drop containers are clearly labeled

and that the labels are carefully checked prior to use of the medications.

In addition, the solution should be checked for color changes and sedimentation, which indicate that the solution is decomposing. If this is present, the solution is discarded and a fresh one obtained. Patients are especially warned to avoid using medication of any kind that has been in the medicine cabinet at home for months or years. Patients should be instructed to check the medication expiration date and discard those medications that are outdated.

Instillation

Handwashing before instillation of medication is imperative. If a dressing is present, the procedure to follow is as follows: (1) The hands are washed before the dressing is removed. (2) The dressing is removed. (3) The hands are washed again before instilling the eye drops. Before the medication is instilled into the eyes (Fig. 53-7A), the lids and the lashes are cleansed. The patient's head then is tilted backward and inclined slightly to the side, so that the solution runs away from the tear duct and the other eye, preventing contamination. This latter precaution is especially necessary when toxic solutions such as atropine are used, because systemic absorption of the excess fluid by way of the nose and the pharynx may lead to adverse effects. In most patients, it is appropriate to press the inner angle of the eye after instilling the drops to prevent the excess solution from entering the nose.

- The lower lid is depressed with the finger of one hand; the patient is told to look upward, and, using the other hand, the solution is dropped on the everted lower lid, not on the cornea. In the unanesthetized eye, if the cornea is touched the patient is startled; this increases the probability that the patient will jump and contaminate the dispensing tip of the eye dropper and possibly cause injury to the eye.
- Care must be taken that the tip of the dropper bottle does not touch any part of the eye or the lids to guard against contamination of the dropper and injury to the eye.
- After the drops (one or two at most) are placed in the eye, the lid is released, and any excess fluid is sponged gently from the lids and the cheeks with a tissue.
- After the medication is instilled, the patient is instructed to close his eyes gently; patients often have a tendency to squeeze their eyes closed, thereby expelling the medication. When the lids are kept closed as directed, the pumping action of the eyelids (to remove fluids from the eye) is stopped. This keeps the medication in the eye longer.
- Patients who have difficulty using eye medication without touching the dropper bottle to the eye should have the eye medication instilled by another person to avoid contamination or injury. The nurse includes the other person when teaching the patient eye care.

Ointments

Ointments of various kinds are used frequently in the treatment of inflammatory diseases of the lids, the conjunctiva, and the cornea. Those prescribed most commonly are antibiotics, anti-inflammatory agents, and various combinations of the two.

Ointments are applied by gently pulling down the lower lid and expressing a small amount of the ointment from the

(text continues on page 1558)

TABLE 53–2. *Frequently Used Ophthalmic Medications*

Medication	Action/Advantage
LOCAL ANESTHETICS	
Tetracaine hydrochloride (Pontocaine), 0.5%	Commonly used topical anesthetic
	Anesthesia occurs in 5–9 minutes
Proparacaine hydrochloride (Ophthaine, Alcaine, 0.5%)	Least irritating of the local anesthetics
	Anesthesia occurs in 20 seconds
MYDRIATICS	
(Dilates pupil. Because mydriatics and cycloplegics dilate the pupil, they should not be given to patients who are known to have narrow angles, since they can precipitate an acute glaucoma episode)	
Phenylephrine hydrochloride (Neo-Synephrine), 2.5%–10%	Most commonly used
	Action lasts 3 hours
Hydroxyamphetamine hydrobromide ophthalmic solution (Paredrine), 1%	Action lasts 3 hours; useful in those with allergy to phenylephrine
Epinephrine hydrochloride (Adrenalin), 1:1,000 (Glaucon) 0.5%, 1%, and 2%	Lowers intraocular pressure in open-angle glaucoma (increases aqueous humor outflow)
CYCLOPLEGICS	
(Parasympatholytics)	
(Dilates pupil and paralyzes power of accommodation; contraindicated for patients with glaucoma)	
Homatropine hydrobromide, 2% and 5%	A popular drug for cycloplegic refraction
	Action lasts 24–36 hours
	Allergic reactions rare
Scopolamine hydrobromide (Isopto Hyoscine), 0.2% to 0.5%	Used in children's refraction
	Used in treating uveitis
	Because of low allergic reaction, it is preferred to atropine
	May cause dizziness and disorientation in older persons
Atropine sulfate, 0.25%, 0.5%, 1%, and 2%	Most powerful of this group
	Action lasts 10–14 days, during which eyes must be protected from bright light
	Used in treating uveitis
	Used in refraction of children
	5% of persons are sensitive to it (symptoms: difficulty in swallowing; dizziness; flushed skin with circumoral pallor; rapid, full pulse; delirium)
Cyclopentolate hydrochloride (Cyclogyl), 0.5% and 1%	Action is less than 24 hours
	Popular drug for cycloplegic refraction
Tropicamide (Mydriacyl), 0.5% and 1%	Newer, shorter acting—action lasts 6 hours
MIOTICS	
(Parasympathomimetics) (Constricts pupil)	
Pilocarpine hydrochloride, 0.5%, 1%, 2%, 3%, 4%, and 6%	Frequently used in glaucoma
	Action lasts 6–8 hours
Carbachol (Carbacel) 1.5% to 3%	Used if pilocarpine is ineffective

(continued)

TABLE 53–2. *(Continued)*

Medication	Action/Advantage
Physostigmine salicylate (Eserine), 0.25% and 0.5%	Action lasts 6–8 hours Because it is allergenic, unstable, and short in its action, it is gradually being replaced by echothiophate
Echothiophate iodide (Phospholine iodide), 0.06%, 0.125%, and 0.25%	Water-soluble Causes less local irritation than physostigmine
Isoflurophate (diisopropyl fluorophosphate) (DFP) (Floropryl), 0.025% ophthalmic ointment; 0.1%-ophthalmic solution	Oil-soluble miotic May produce side effects; observe for vomiting, diarrhea, tenesmus

ADRENERGIC

(Sympathomimetic) (Decreases intraocular pressure)

Medication	Action/Advantage
Epinephrine (Epitrate), 1%–2%	Action lasts 12 hours
Epinephrine hydrochloride (Adrenalin), 1:1,000; (Glaucon) 0.5%, 1%, and 2%	Lowers intraocular pressure in open-angle glaucoma (increases aqueous humor outflow)

BETA-ADRENERGIC ANTAGONISTS

(Lowers IOP)

Medication	Action/Advantage
Timolol maleate (Timoptic), 0.25%–5%	Most widely used medication to reduce intraocular pressure Reduces aqueous humor formation within 30 minutes
Levobunolol hydrochloride (Betagan) 0.5%	Similar action as timolol maleate

CARBONIC ANHYDRASE INHIBITOR

(Carbonic anhydrase is an enzyme present in body tissues. In the ciliary body, it is directly involved in the production of aqueous humor)

Medication	Action/Advantage
Acetazolamide (Diamox)	Effective in decreasing production of aqueous humor by ciliary body in glaucoma

HYPEROSMOTIC AGENTS

(Lowers IOP by making plasma hypertonic, thereby drawing aqueous humor from the eye)

Medication	Action/Advantage
Mannitol (20% solution in water)	Lowers intraocular pressure; used before glaucoma surgery (trabeculectomy)
Glycerin (Glyrol, Osmoglyn)	Lowers intraocular pressure

OPHTHALMIC DRUGS USED INTRAOPERATIVELY

Medication	Action/Advantage
Lacri-lube ointment	Widely used for comatose patients or patients undergoing general anesthesia to keep cornea moist Prevents corneal irritation and drying *Not* used on operative eye
Alpha-Chymotrypsin (Alpha Chymar)	An enzyme used to dissolve the zonules in intracapsular cataract surgery
Miochol (Acetylcholine 1:100) (acethylcholine 20 mg and mannitol 100 mg)	Used to constrict the pupil rapidly after removal of the lens in cataract surgery
Sodium hyaluronate (Healon)	Viscous jelly used in anterior segment surgery to prevent damage and adhesion formation Deepens anterior chamber to prevent corneal endothelial damage By maintaining anterior chamber pressure during cataract extraction, decreases risk of vitreous moving forward.

(continued)

TABLE 53–2. *(Continued)*

Medication	Action/Advantage
ANTIMICROBIALS AND ANTIBIOTICS	
Neomycin sulfate with polymyxin and bacitracin (Neosporin)	Broad-spectrum, ointment or solution Only disadvantage is its allergenic nature (allergy is to neomycin)
Bacitracin, 500 units/g ointment	Effective as a penicillin substitute for local eye uses against gram-positive organisms
Erythromycin, 1% ointment	Effective as a penicillin substitute against resistant staphylococcal organisms

Sulfonamides:
  Sulfisoxazole (Gantrisin), 4% solution or ointment
  Sulfacetamide sodium (Sulamyd sodium)
	Used in treatment of conjunctivitis; sometimes effective against larger viruses

Gentamicin sulfate (Garamycin)	Used when gram-negative organisms are suspected
Tobramycin	Used for gram-negative and gram-positive organisms
Tetracycline	Used for gram-negative and gram-positive bacteria
Polymyxin B	Used for gram-positive bacteria
Cefazolin	Used for gram-negative and gram-positive bacteria
ANTIFUNGAL AGENTS	
Natamycin (Natacyn)	Effective against filamentary and yeast forms of fungus Initial drug of choice for most mycotic corneal ulcers
Amphotericin B (Fungizone)	Used when Natacyn is ineffective
ANTIVIRAL AGENTS	
Idoxuridine (Dendrite Herptex, IDU), 0.1%	Used in treatment of keratitis caused by the herpes simplex virus (HSV)
Adenine arabinoside (Ara-A, Vira-A), 3% ointment	Used in treatment of acute keratoconjunctivitis and recurrent epithelial keratitis due to HSV types I and II.
Acyclovir (Zovirax)	Available in Europe; presently not available in the U.S. for ophthalmic use. Shows promise in the treatment of herpes simplex and herpes zoster infections.
CORTICOSTEROIDS	
(Effective in treating inflammatory conditions of the eye: uveitis, episcleritis, chemical burns. Decreases vascularization and scarring after burns, trauma, and severe inflammation)	
Cortisone acetate, 0.5%–2.5%-suspension; 1.5%-ointment	Least expensive
Hydrocortisone, 0.5%–2.5%-suspension; 1.5%-ointment	Greater potency than cortisone, so it can be used in lower concentrations
Prednisone, prednisolone, dexamethasone	These are thought to be more potent than hydrocortisone.

NOTE: Corticosteroids are dangerous when used in the presence of herpes simplex keratitis. All patients receiving these medications must be under the care of an ophthalmologist. All steroids are now known to produce glaucoma in certain predisposed patients. Use of steroids locally or systemically must be carefully supervised.

(continued)

TABLE 53–2. *(Continued)*

Medication	Action/Advantage
DYES	
(Will stain corneal epithelia defects a bright green) (Used for corneal staining to detect superficial abrasions)	Used to determine extent of corneal injury, fit of a contact lens, or in applanation tonometry
Fluorescein sodium, 0.5%–2%	Used in retial photography to determine pathology
	NOTE: Because *Pseudomonas aeruginosa*, highly pathogenic for corneal tissue, grows well in fluorescein solutions, the sterile single-dose containers or sterile *Kimura fluorescein* papers are recommended.
Rose bengal, 1% and 2%	Selective dye to stain conjunctiva; mucus shreds stain more brilliantly than with fluorescein
TEAR REPLACEMENT AND LUBRICATING AGENTS	
Hydroxypropyl methylcellulose Polyvinyl alcohol	Used as artificial tears, ophthalmic lubricants, and in contact lens solutions, and gonioscopic lens solutions
DECONGESTANTS/VASOCONSTRICTORS	
(Constricts the superficial vessels of the conjunctiva and relieves redness; sooths minor surface irritation and itching of the conjunctiva)	
The active ingredients in these agents are either ephedrine 0.123%, naphazoline 0.012%, or tetrahydrozoline 0.5%–0.15%	

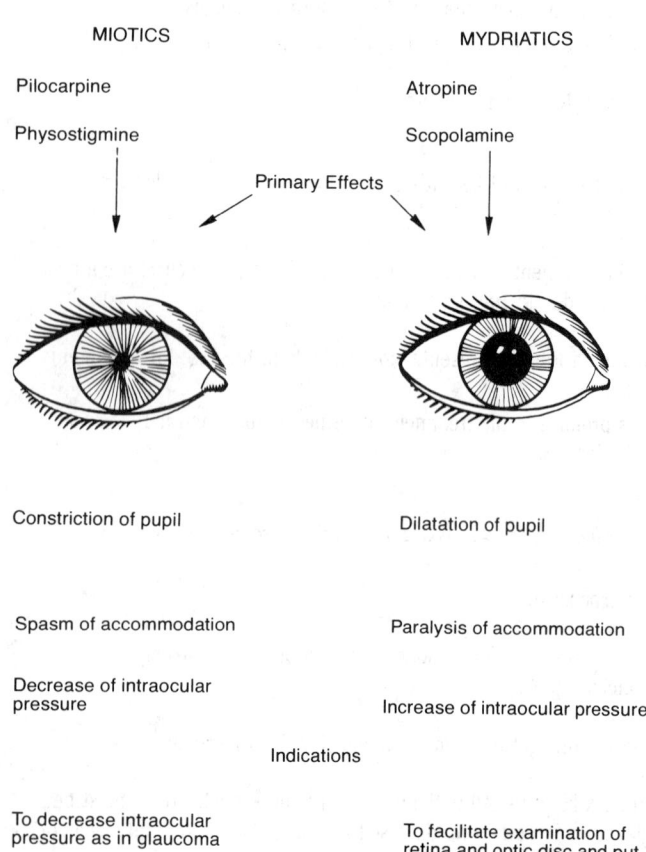

Figure 53–6. Effects and indications for miotics and mydriatics.

tube onto the conjunctiva of the lower lid (see Fig. 53-7*B*). Ointment is applied from inner to outer canthus. Care is taken not to touch the eye or the eyelid with the tube. The lid then may be massaged gently in such a way as to distribute the ointment over the surface of the eye.

Ocular Irrigations

Ocular irrigations are indicated in treating various inflammations of the conjunctiva, in preparing the patient for eye surgery, and in removing inflammatory secretions. They are also used for their antiseptic effect. The fluid to be used depends on the condition present. The irrigating apparatus is simple, consisting of a commercially prepared irrigating bottle containing sterile ophthalmic solution (Blinx, Dacriose) and a small, curved basin, gloves, and cotton for catching the fluid and the secretions. Each patient should have his own solutions in a plastic dispenser with a cap and label.

- The patient lies flat on his back or sits with the head tilted backward and inclined slightly toward the side. The basin may be held by the patient if he is sitting or placed so that when he is lying down it will catch the fluid as it runs from the eye. The nurse stands in front of the patient.
- After the lids are carefully cleansed to remove dust, secretions, and crusts, the lids are held open with the thumb and the fingers of one hand, and the eye is flushed gently, directing the stream away from the nose. The fluid is never directed toward the nose, because of the danger that it may spill over into the other eye. The procedure is continued until the eye is entirely free of secretions.
- It must be remembered that little force is to be used, because of the danger of injury. For the same reason, and to prevent

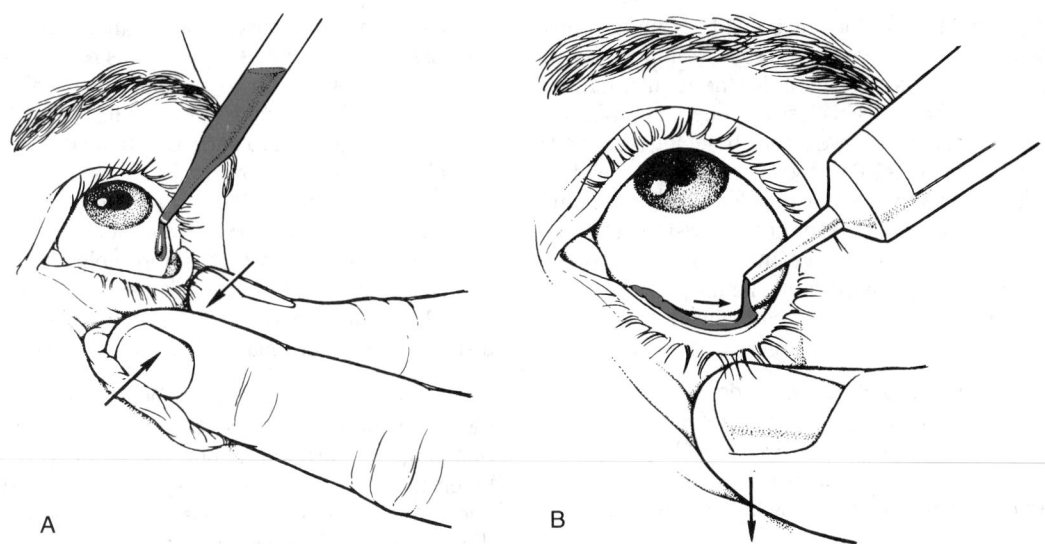

Figure 53–7.   Instillation of eye drops. (**A**) When instilling eye drops, the patient is instructed to look upward; then the lower lid is lightly pinched to form a receptacle for the dropped medication. (**B**) In applying ointment, the patient is instructed to look upward; then the lower lid is depressed and the ointment is gently squeezed along the everted lid, beginning at the inner canthus (close to the nose) and then moving outward.

contamination, no part of the irrigator should touch the eye, the lid, or the lashes.

- When the irrigation has been completed, the eye and the cheek are dried gently with cotton.

Continuous Irrigation of the Eye

Continuous irrigation is indicated in chemical burns, resistant corneal ulcers, uveitis, socket infections after enucleation, or conditions in which constant medication or debridement is indicated. Before irrigation, a local anesthetic is instilled.

Warm Wet Compresses

Heat relieves pain and increases the circulation, thereby promoting absorption and reducing tension in the eye. It is especially valuable for conjunctivitis accompanied by excessive secretions. Heat is best applied in the form of compresses composed of seven or eight layers of gauze or cotton just large enough to cover the eye.

- The patient is moved to the side of the bed, and a towel is used to cover the chest. A protective layer of cold cream or petrolatum jelly may be applied to the skin of the lid and the adjacent cheek.
- The compresses then are moistened in a basin of water or other prescribed solution that has been heated.
- The fluid, which should be kept at a temperature between 46° and 49°C (115° to 120°F), is expressed or squeezed from the pad, and the compress, after being tested for temperature, is placed gently over the closed lid.
- The pads are changed every 30 to 60 seconds for 10 to 15 minutes, and the application is repeated every 2 or 3 hours.
- At the completion of the period of application, the lid is dried gently with cotton.
- New pads are used for each application, and if the eye has a purulent secretion, the compresses are applied to one eye at a time, the solution and the basin being changed between

applications so as not to transfer infection from one eye to the other.

Cold Compresses

Cold causes a capillary constriction that tends to reduce the amount of secretion and relieve pain during the early stages of acute inflammatory conditions of the conjunctiva. Cold compresses are useful in relieving itching due to allergic conjunctivitis.

The patient is prepared in the same manner as for the application of hot compresses. The pads are moistened in the prescribed solution and placed over the closed eye. Latex gloves or small plastic bags filled with ice can be used to maintain the cold temperature. These are placed on top of the moistened pads. They are applied to the closed lids and are changed every 15 to 30 seconds for a period of 5 to 15 minutes each hour.

- Cold compresses are never used in the treatment of inflammations of the eye (iritis, keratitis), because cold, by constricting the capillaries, interferes with the nutrition of the cornea.

▶ Nursing Process
The Patient With Eye Disorders

◊ Assessment

An initial health history is taken to determine the patient's primary problem, such as difficulty in reading, blurred vision, a burning sensation in the eyes, watering of the eyes, double vision, spots before the eyes, and isolated areas of lost vision (scotomas, itching, myopia, or hyperopia). The nurse should determine whether the problem is in one or both eyes and how long the patient has had this difficulty.

It is also important to ascertain the patient's general ocular condition or status: Does he wear glasses or contact lenses? When were they checked last? Is he under the regular care of an ophthalmologist? When was his last eye checkup? Was his eye pressure checked? Does he have difficulty seeing (focusing) at close range or at a distance? Does he have problems reading or watching television? What about problems differentiating colors, or problems with lateral or peripheral vision? Has the patient had any past eye trauma or eye infections? If so, when? What eye problems exist in the patient's family?

A pertinent past ocular history is essential. What past illnesses has the patient had?

Childhood—strabismus, amblyopia, injuries?

Adult—glaucoma, cataract, eye trauma, refractive errors— how corrected? Any previous eye surgery? Hypertension, diabetes, thyroid disorders, sexually transmitted diseases, allergies, cardiovascular and collagen diseases, neurologic condition?

Family illnesses—Is there a history of eye disorders in parents or grandparents?

The patient's understanding of eye care and treatment is elicited to identify misconceptions or misinformation that can be corrected early.

▷ Nursing Diagnoses

Based on the nursing assessment data, the patient's major nursing diagnoses may include the following:

- Pain related to injury of or pressure in the eye
- Fear and anxiety related to impaired vision and potential for further loss of sight
- Alteration in visual sensory perception related to ocular trauma, inflammation, infection, tumor, or degeneration
- Self-care deficit related to impaired vision and limited knowledge regarding eye care
- Social isolation related to limited ability to participate in diversional and social activities secondary to impaired vision

▷ Planning and Implementation

▷ *Goals:* The major goals of the patient may include relief of pain, control of anxiety, prevention of further visual deterioration and acceptance of treatment, accomplishment of self-care activities including medication administration, and avoidance of social isolation with participation in diversional activities.

▷ Nursing Interventions

Regardless of the cause of a visual problem, measures can be initiated in an attempt to control as well as to prevent further progression of deterioration. This can be accomplished by putting the eye at rest, restricting activities, wearing dark glasses, or instilling a prescribed local anesthetic. If the problem is related to an infection, an antibiotic or antimicrobial medication may be prescribed.

▷ *Relieving Pain, Fear, and Anxiety.* Pain may be due to trauma, such as a scratched cornea or increasing pressure within the eye. An eye patch helps to limit eye movement. It must be remembered, however, that the uncovered eye should also rest because eyes move in synchrony.

Because light causes pain in many eye conditions, and because the eyes should be rested as much as possible before and after an operation to facilitate the healing process, it is best to maintain subdued lighting in the room. If those assisting the patient need light to carry out their activities, then dimmed artificial lights may be used.

Prescribed analgesics and antibiotics help to control discomfort. Avoiding emotional disturbances and physical stresses promotes relaxation, which in turn helps to relieve pain.

After a physical examination and diagnostic studies, a diagnosis is determined; anxieties are frequently lessened when a specific treatment plan to correct the problem is in place.

▷ *Decreasing Sensory Deprivation.* When the eyes are bandaged, distortions in perception can occur, such as "eye-patch delirium," inappropriate behavior, and loss of position sense. Often these problems are magnified and become frightening and upsetting. One way to assist the patient in overcoming these unsettling feelings is to reorient him periodically to reality and offer reassurance, explanations, and understanding. Anyone entering the patient's room should speak and identify himself so as not to startle the patient.

▷ *Preoperative Nursing Management.* The preparation of the patient for an ophthalmic operation must be carried out with scrupulous care so that complications are minimized, comfort is achieved, and delay is minimized. The type of anesthesia often determines how the patient is prepared. For example, if general anesthesia is used, the lower intestinal tract is evacuated the morning of the operation and only a liquid diet is given after that. Before the eyes are prepared for surgery, the patient's hair is covered with a cap and the face is cleansed. If the eyelashes are to be cut, this is done in the operating room; the scissors are coated lightly with petrolatum so that the lashes adhere to the scissors and do not fall into the eye. An antibiotic is usually prescribed before surgery, while the patient is awake. The patient is encouraged to discuss his concerns so that they may be addressed before surgery.

▷ *Postoperative Nursing Management.* After surgery in which both eyes are bandaged, the patient is placed in bed in a supine position with a small pillow under his head. Pillows may be placed on each side of the head to keep it still, and siderails are set in place to promote safety and a sense of security. The patient is provided with a call bell or light and instructed to ask for help rather than move or strain in an attempt to be self-sufficient.

If a local anesthesia is used during the operation, the patient is usually ambulatory in a few hours after surgery.

The ophthalmologist is notified immediately if the patient has excessive pain or if the dressings are disturbed.

- Morphine is never given to ophthalmic patients unless it is certain that vomiting will not injure the eye.

▷ *Enhancing Self-Care Activities.* The patient is encouraged to carry out as much self-care as possible to promote a feeling of self-sufficiency. Nursing assistance is provided as needed. A patient who cannot see is assisted with eating, but if he is accustomed to feeding himself, he is encouraged to do so. Elimination is promoted by proper diet, stool softeners, or enemas, as prescribed. Patients are not to read, smoke, or shave unless given permission by the physician. They must be cautioned against rubbing their eyes or wiping them with a soiled handkerchief. All patients receiving dilating medications should wear dark glasses.

Medication bottles and instructions should be labeled in large letters and used where there is plenty of light. Before the patient uses any medication, he must wash his hands. When instilling eye drops, the patient is supervised so that he develops a technique specific to his needs. He may find it convenient to rest the base of the hand that is holding the medicine dropper against his forehead. With his other hand, he can lightly pinch the lower lid to form a V-trough to catch the eye drop.

The patient's home environment is assessed for safety. The patient or a family member is encouraged to remedy any safety hazards. In addition, lighting is adapted to the patient's needs. Light is regulated so that it is not bright and does not produce a glare.

▷ *Promoting Coping Mechanisms and Socialization.* The anxiety frequently experienced by the ophthalmic patient requires as much consideration as his physical condition. A person's dependence on sight is emphasized when one faces a temporary or possibly permanent loss of this vital sense. Worry, fear, and depression are common reactions; tension, resentment, anger, and rejection also may occur. By encouraging the patient to express his feelings, the nurse can then take steps to help the patient to cope and adjust to his situation.

The patient should be encouraged to have visitors and to socialize. Depending on his interests and preferences, suggestions can be made for diversional activities. When permissible, the radio and occupational therapy may be used to keep the patient's mind occupied. Although it is important not to be oversolicitous, showing interest, empathy, and understanding enhances the patient's sense of well-being. Because of differences of personality, the approaches in overcoming the anxiety of individual patients vary. When permanent blindness is apparent, re-education may be done by specially trained personnel or similarly afflicted persons.

▷ Evaluation

Expected Outcomes

1. Experiences less pain
   a. Takes prescribed medication to counteract irritation, to rest the eyes, and to treat or prevent any infection; also takes medication (sedation) for body relaxation
   b. Applies prescribed cold or warm compresses.
   c. Reduces eye activity by applying appropriate eye dressing and resting
   d. Protects eye from additional injury by using a protective shield
2. Shows evidence of calmness and absence of anxiety
3. Copes with limitations in sensory perception
   a. Oriented to time, place, and surroundings
   b. Responds appropriately to others
4. Accepts treatment regimen and carries out recommendations
   a. Washes his hands before using eye drops and taking medications
   b. Reports any untoward signs such as accumulation of granulations, watering of eyes, and pain
   c. Reduces eye activity by using an eye patch if prescribed
   d. Keeps a diary about his progress and jots down questions to ask when he next visits his physician

5. Practices self-care activities effectively
   a. Demonstrates how he manages treatments; forms a V-trough in lower lid to receive eye drops
   b. Cleans lenses effectively as taught
   c. Lists safety measures to prevent falls, such as being aware of loose carpeting and cluttered steps
   d. Describes proper lighting for reading and hand crafts
6. Participates in diversional and social activities

Laser Surgery

Ophthalmic laser surgery is one of the most important developments during the past decade in the treatment of many conditions of the eye. This procedure offers a noninvasive alternative to incisional surgery, decreased risk of infection, shorter postoperative course, and less expense. Therapy is usually performed on an outpatient basis with topical anesthetics. This avoids the risks and complications of general or retrobulbar anesthesia required for conventional surgery.

The term *laser* is an acronym for *l*ight *a*mplification by *s*timulated *e*mission of *r*adiation. The laser machine produces energy and emits a narrow, uniform beam of light that can be precisely focused on selected tissue. Depending on the type of laser used, heat coagulation, cutting, or microexplosion can be produced. The laser may be used to treat retinal breaks, diabetic retinopathy, retinal vein occlusion, macular degeneration, glaucoma, some tumors, and opacities of the posterior capsule after cataract surgery with IOL implantation.

The most recent addition to the laser field is the eximer laser, which is currently in the investigational phase. It offers the possibility of altering the focusing strength of the eye by computer-controlled recontouring of the cornea, thereby correcting refracting errors.

Possible complications of laser surgery include iritis, cataract formation, hyphema, corneal damage, and retinal burns. There may also be increased IOP, which is usually transient. Patients who are at risk for increased IOP after therapy require monitoring for 1 to 2 hours after the procedure. Contraindications for laser procedures are target tissue that cannot be visualized, corneal edema, or an uncooperative patient or one who is unable to sit still.

The patient and family members should be prepared for the procedure by informing them about what will be experienced. Many people are fearful of lasers, and this anxiety may cause agitation, movement, or syncope during the procedure. Patients should be informed that anesthetic drops will be administered before treatment, that they will be seated comfortably with the head positioned in a headrest, and that the surgeon will stabilize the eye. They need to know to expect a tingling sensation, a flash of light, and a clicking sound with each application. Patients are informed to tell the surgeon immediately if they feel faint.

Postoperatively the patient can expect some blurring of vision for about an hour and light flashes. Therefore, arrangements must be made for transportation home. Post-treatment headache may be relieved by acetaminophen. There are usually no restrictions on activity or diet.

Several treatment sessions may be necessary when the patient's condition requires an extensive number of laser burns.

Excessive treatment at one time can cause uveitis, macular edema, exudative retinal detachment or shallowing of the anterior chamber with angle-closure.

In summary, the eye is an organ of vision. It provides one of the five senses, sight. The various parts of the eye work in harmony to allow light rays to enter, converge, and register as nerve impulses, thus producing an image. Disease, trauma, and the aging process all account for changes in vision.

Visual function as well as changes in vision can be assessed in different ways. Ocular, health, and family history should be reviewed as well as the patient's life-style. Various instruments and tests are used to assess vision and eye movement. Visual acuity or the clearness with which the patient sees is probably the most important test that can be performed. Other tests include those for assessment of ocular tension, the extraocular muscles, field of vision, and the internal eye.

Refractive errors, problems in focusing light rays (*e.g.,* presbyopia, myopia, hyperopia, and astigmatism), are corrected by lenses. Correction of these errors can be made with eyeglasses, contact lenses, or IOLs.

The nurse, as a primary caregiver, can provide reassurance, physical comfort, and ophthalmic nursing care. Above all, the nurse must use good handwashing technique to avoid cross-contamination. The nurse ensures that the environment is safe and that the patient and family members are taught self-care. Instructions about eye drops, ointments, irrigations, and compresses are provided with specific detail.

One of the most recent developments in the treatment of many eye conditions is ophthalmic laser surgery. This procedure is noninvasive and less costly than conventional procedures in terms of length of postoperative course and decreased chance of infection.

Conditions of the Eyelids

Blepharitis
Blepharitis is an inflammation of the lid margins. It may be due to seborrhea (nonulcerative), the most common form, or staphylococcal infection (ulcerative), or both. The chief symptoms are irritation, burning, and itching of the lid margins with red-rimmed eyes. Many scales or granulations cling to the lashes. Treatment includes cleaning the lid margins using a cotton-tipped applicator and mild baby shampoo, warm compresses, and topical antibiotic ointments.

Chalazion
Chalazion is a sterile granulomatous inflammation of the meibomian gland in which there is painless localized swelling that develops over a period of weeks. Treatment may include warm compresses, massage and expression of the glandular secretions, or antibiotic or corticosteroid drops or injections. Excision is indicated if it becomes large enough to distort vision or be a cosmetic blemish.

Sty (External Hordeolum)
A sty is an infection of the superficial lid glands of Zeis or Moll, usually caused by *Staphylococcus aureus*. The principle symptoms are subacute pain, redness, and swelling of a localized area of the lid. Treatment consists of warm, moist compresses

for 10 to 15 minutes, three or four times a day. If the condition does not begin to resolve within 48 hours, incision and drainage may be indicated. Topical and systemic antibiotics may be prescribed.

In summary, the eyelids protect and cover the eyeball. They are movable folds of skin over the eye. Blepharitis, chalazion, and hordeolum are the most common conditions of the eyelids for which treatment is sought.

Conditions of the Conjunctiva/ Lacrimal Sac and Uveal Tract

Conjunctivitis
Conjunctivitis, or inflammation of the conjunctiva, has many origins. It may be infectious (bacterial, chlamydial, viral, fungal, parasitic), immunologic (allergic), irritative (chemical, thermal, electrical, radiational [*i.e.,* ultraviolet light]) or associated with systemic disease. Signs and symptoms may include hyperemia (redness), discharge, edema, tearing, itching, burning, scratching, or foreign body sensation.

Depending on the causative factor, treatment may include systemic or topical antibiotics, anti-inflammatory agents, eye irrigation, lid cleansing, or warm compresses. When the conjunctivitis is caused by microorganisms, the patient should be instructed in ways to prevent cross-contamination to the unaffected eye and to other people: avoidance of rubbing the affected eye and then touching the unaffected eye, handwashing after touching the affected eye, and use of separate washcloths, towels, and handkerchiefs.

Trachoma
Trachoma, a chlamydial conjunctivitis, is an infectious disease that affects more than 400 million of the world's population. It is the world's leading cause of preventable blindness and primarily affects people in Africa, the Middle East, and Asia. It is rare in the United States except among American Indians, where it is now becoming less prevalent. It is usually bilateral. Without prompt treatment trachoma will involve the cornea, resulting in scarring and, often, blindness. It is spread by direct contact, fomites, and, possibly, insect vectors. Trachoma can be prevented by proper sanitation and education.

Assessment and Clinical Manifestations. The principal symptoms are mild itching and irritation. After an acute inflammatory process, follicles appear on the conjunctiva. Blurring of vision and increasing discomfort occur. The upper palpebral conjunctiva are affected.

The progress of the disease has been classified into four stages: in stage I (incipient trachoma), immature follicles are present, especially in the upper tarsal conjunctiva. At the top of the cornea there is incipient pannus (abnormal vascularization). Stage II (established trachoma) consists of two types—type A and type B. In type A, follicular hypertrophy is predominant, while in type B, papillary hypertrophy is predominant (acute trachoma). In stage III, early conjunctival scarring is observed as fine, white lines; corneal pannus also increases. In stage IV, smooth scarring of the tarsal conjunctiva occurs and vascular pannus becomes inactive. Secondary bacterial conjunctivitis increases the hazard of corneal ulceration, and this in turn leads to blindness.

Management. Trachoma is spread by direct contact; therefore, personal cleanliness is a key factor in prevention. Isolating known cases and initiating antibiotic therapy early may help control the disease. If untreated, it lasts for months or years. Medical treatment consists of a 3- to 4-week course of tetracycline or sulfonamides. The World Health Organization is making great strides in eliminating this curable disease.

Pterygium

Pterygium is a triangular connective tissue overgrowth of the intrapalpebral bulbar conjunctiva with extension to the cornea. It is thought to be an irritative and degenerative phenomenon caused by ultraviolet light because it is common among people who spend a lot of time out of doors, especially in tropical areas. Surgical removal is indicated if the pterygium encroaches on the visual axis or causes significant discomfort.

Dacryocystitis

Dacryocystitis is an infection of the lacrimal sac secondary to nasolacrimal duct obstruction. It is a common acute or chronic disease usually seen in infants or in adults over the age of 40. The condition usually responds well to antibiotic therapy. Chronic conditions, however, require probing of the lacrimal system or dacryocystorhinostomy (surgical procedure to create an outflow channel into the nose) to relieve the obstruction.

Uveitis

Uveitis is the inflammation of one or all three of the structures of the uveal tract. Because the uvea contains many of the blood vessels that nourish the eye and because it borders many other parts of the eye, inflammation of this layer may threaten vision. Causative factors include allergens, bacteria, fungi, viruses, chemicals, trauma, and systemic illness such as sarcoidosis or ulcerative colitis. Acute anterior uveitis (iritis) is the most common type, and is characterized by a history of pain, photophobia, blurring of vision, and red eye. Dilating drops are instituted immediately to prevent scar formation, which could cause glaucoma by impending aqueous outflow. Local corticosteroids are used to decrease the inflammation, and sunglasses and pain management provide symptomatic relief.

Intermediate uveitis (pars planitis, chronic cyclitis) presents with "floating spots" in the field of vision. Topical or injected corticosteroids are used in severe cases.

Posterior uveitis (inflammation affecting the choroid or retina) is usually associated with some form of systemic disease, such as acquired immunodeficiency syndrome (AIDS), herpes simplex or zoster, toxoplasmosis, tuberculosis, or sacroidosis. The patient complains of decreased or distorted vision. Redness and pain may present. Systemic corticosteroids are indicated to reduce the inflammation, along with treatment of the underlying systemic condition.

Sympathetic Ophthalmia

Sympathetic ophthalmia is a rare but devastating bilateral uveitis that occurs after a latent period of days to years after a penetrating injury to the uveal tract. The cause is unknown, but it is probably related to a hypersensitivity to uveal pigment. Initially, the injured eye becomes inflamed, followed by inflammation of the unaffected (sympathetic) eye. If untreated, the disease will progress to bilateral blindness. Enucleation of the sightless eye within 10 days of an injury is usually recommended to reduce the risk of sympathetic disease in the other eye. Such a drastic step is usually not undertaken the day of injury. Instead, the wounds are closed and the patient is allowed time to give informed consent. In patients whose eyes are not severely injured and for whom there is hope of some useful vision, enucleation is not a consideration. If sympathetic ophthalmia does develop, it is treated with local and systemic corticosteroids and dilating drops. Cytotoxic drugs may be required.

In summary, conditions of the conjunctiva, the lacrimal sac, and the uveal tract include the following conditions that prompt the patient to seek medical treatment. Conjunctivitis is the inflammation of the conjunctiva. Trachoma, a chlamydial conjunctivitis, is seen most often in third-world countries. Pterygium is an outgrowth of tissue extending to the cornea, thought to be caused by ultraviolet light. Dacryocystitis is an infection of the lacrimal sac secondary to nasolacrimal duct obstruction. Uveitis is the inflammation of one or all three structures of the uveal tract. Sympathetic ophthalmia is an inflammation of the uveal tract of the fellow eye occurring after injury to the uveal tract of one eye.

Conditions of the Cornea

The cornea functions as a mechanically tough, chemically impermeable, protective membrane and is an important part of the refractive system. Its functions require integrity of the surface layers, adequate smoothness, transparency, and spherical shape. To prevent damage to the epithelium surface, the cornea must be kept moist. To function as an optical lens, it must be kept smooth. The film of tears, evenly spread by the blinking eyelids, provides both moisture and smoothing. Transparency is due to the cornea's uniform structure, avascularity, and relative dehydration.

The cornea consists of five layers: the epithelium, Bowman's layer, stroma, Descemet's membrane, and the endothelium. The epithelium, the outermost layer, has four to six layers of cells endowed with sensitive nerve endings. It is the only layer capable of regeneration and is completely replaced approximately every 7 days. The endothelium, a single-cell layer, is responsible for pumping fluid from the inner structures of the cornea.

Because there are many nerve fibers in the cornea, most corneal lesions cause pain, photophobia, and tearing. Pain may be severe and may seem disproportionate to the amount of damage. Movement of the lids over the cornea increases pain, which usually persists until healing is complete. Although topical anesthetics relieve this discomfort, they also interfere with healing and are therefore contraindicated for long-term use. Because corneal lesions interfere with the cornea's ability to transmit and refract light, there is usually blurring of vision.

The cornea is examined with the aid of a *slit lamp*, which provides magnification and illumination. Alternatively, the cornea may be viewed using a flashlight. Local anesthetic drops are used to facilitate the procedure. Fluorescein staining is helpful in outlining superficial epithelial defects.

Trauma, infection, congenital anomalies, tumors, and inherited or acquired disorders of the cornea may impair its function. Scarring, opacifications, and alteration in corneal architecture may result in mild to severe visual loss.

Corneal Abrasions

Corneal abrasions are defects in the epithelial layer that may be caused by trauma, foreign bodies, contact lenses that are worn for a prolonged time, defects in the tear film, difficulty with lid closure, or malposition of the lids or lashes. Corneal abrasions and foreign bodies are more fully discussed in the section on ocular trauma (p. 1582). Recurrent corneal abrasions, which may be a result of rubbing the eye, are treated with artificial lubricant ointment at bedtime or a bandage soft contact lens (a nonprescription contact lens that is used to protect the cornea from irritation due to lid movement).

Microbial Keratitis

Microbial keratitis (infection of the cornea) can be caused by a variety of bacterial, viral, fungal or parasitic organisms. Whenever the epithelium is damaged, the cornea becomes quite susceptible to infection. Even small abrasions provide a point of entry for bacteria. Most infections of the cornea occur as a result of trauma or compromised systemic or local defense mechanisms. Corticosteroids modify the immune reaction, and their long-term use allows opportunistic organisms to invade the cornea.

Marked inflammation of the globe, sensation of a foreign body in the eye, mucopurulent discharge with the lids stuck together in the morning, epithelial ulceration, and hypopyon (pus in the anterior chamber of the eye) may indicate corneal infection. In advanced disease, there may be perforation of the cornea, extrusion of the iris, and endophthalmitis. Culture and sensitivity tests are necessary to confirm the diagnosis and to identify the causative pathogen.

Patients with severe corneal infections are usually hospitalized to allow frequent administration (as often as every 30 minutes) of antimicrobial drops and regular examination by the ophthalmologist. Meticulous handwashing is imperative. Gloves are worn whenever nursing interventions involve the eye. The lids are kept clean, and cool compresses may be ordered. The patient is monitored for signs of increased IOP. Acetaminophen may be required for pain management. Cycloplegics and mydriatics may be prescribed to alleviate pain and inflammation. Patching and bandage soft contact lenses are avoided until after the infectious process has been controlled, because they encourage microbial growth. They then may be required to facilitate healing of epithelial defects.

Exposure Keratitis

Exposure keratitis may develop whenever the cornea is not adequately moistened and protected by the eyelids. Corneal drying occurs and may be followed by ulceration and secondary infection. Exposure of the cornea may occur as a result of conditions such as exophthalmos, paresis of the seventh cranial nerve (facial nerve), or Bell's palsy, but it also may be of concern in the patient who is comatose or anesthetized. Taping shut the lids of those in the latter group protects the cornea. For others, a bandage soft contact lens may be indicated.

A bandage soft contact lens is fitted to preserve the corneal surface, encourage healing of epithelial defects, and provide comfort. Its use may be indicated in corneal dystrophies, persistent epithelial erosions, complications after corneal surgery, infectious keratitis (after the infectious process is controlled), dry eyes, and chemical burns. Contraindications are active infection, immunologically suppressed patients, and those who are bedridden or practice poor hygiene. The patient must be reliable and able to meet a follow-up examination schedule.

Possible complications of bandage soft contact lenses include infection, corneal infiltrates, hypopyon, corneal edema, corneal neovascularization, and contact lens deposits.

A collagen shield may be used when short-term corneal protection is required. The shield resembles a contact lens in shape but is made from a porcine scleral collagen that has been dehydrated and sterilized. The eye is anesthetized before application. Once the shield is applied, it conforms to the shape of the cornea and absorbs fluid from the tears. It dissolves over a 24- to 72-hour period, depending on the type, providing lubrication and protection to the cornea without the complications of a contact lens.

The collagen shield also may be initially hydrated with antibiotic solution to provide high, sustained antibiotic levels over a long period. Subsequent topical medications also may be administered. Collagen shields are used to protect the cornea after injury, and to deliver medications after cataract extraction and penetrating keratoplasty and to facilitate treatment of severe infection.

Corneal Dystrophies

Corneal dystrophies are inherited, bilateral alterations of the cornea with abnormal deposition of substances. They are of unknown origin. The effects on vision depend on the type of dystrophy, age of the patient, and occurrence of complications such as recurrent erosions.

Fuchs's Dystrophy

Fuchs's dystrophy affects the corneal endothelium and compromises its pump mechanism. Endothelial decomposition results in corneal edema, opacification, scarring, and visual impairment. The disorder manifests during the third or fourth decade and is slowly progressive. Females are more often affected than males.

Keratoconus

Keratoconus is a noninflammatory, progressive thinning of the cornea, which assumes a conical configuration. It usually becomes evident during puberty and affects females more frequently than males. Blurring and distortion of vision are the earliest symptoms. As the disease progresses, irregular astigmatism and high myopia cannot be corrected with eye glasses. The patient must use contact lenses or undergo surgical intervention. Patients are advised to avoid rubbing their eyes, because vigorous rubbing can contribute to the disease process.

Corneal Transplantation

Penetrating keratoplasty, or corneal transplantation, is the microsurgical, full-thickness replacement of the cornea with tissue from a deceased donor (Fig. 53-8). Trephines (circular blades) are used to incise both the damaged recipient and the donor cornea. The new cornea button is secured in the recipient eye with very fine suture (10-0). This procedure may be combined with cataract extraction or IOL insertion. Patients who require corneal transplantation are placed on a computerized Eye Bank waiting list. When a suitable cornea becomes available, surgery is scheduled on an urgent basis. For best results, the graft should be removed within 8 to 10 hours after the death of the donor (to prevent softening of the cornea).

Penetrating keratoplasty is used to restore vision in patients with corneal dystrophies, corneal degenerations, keratoconus, resolved microbial keratitis, traumatic scarring, corneal pigmentation, and chemical burns. Possible complications of sur-

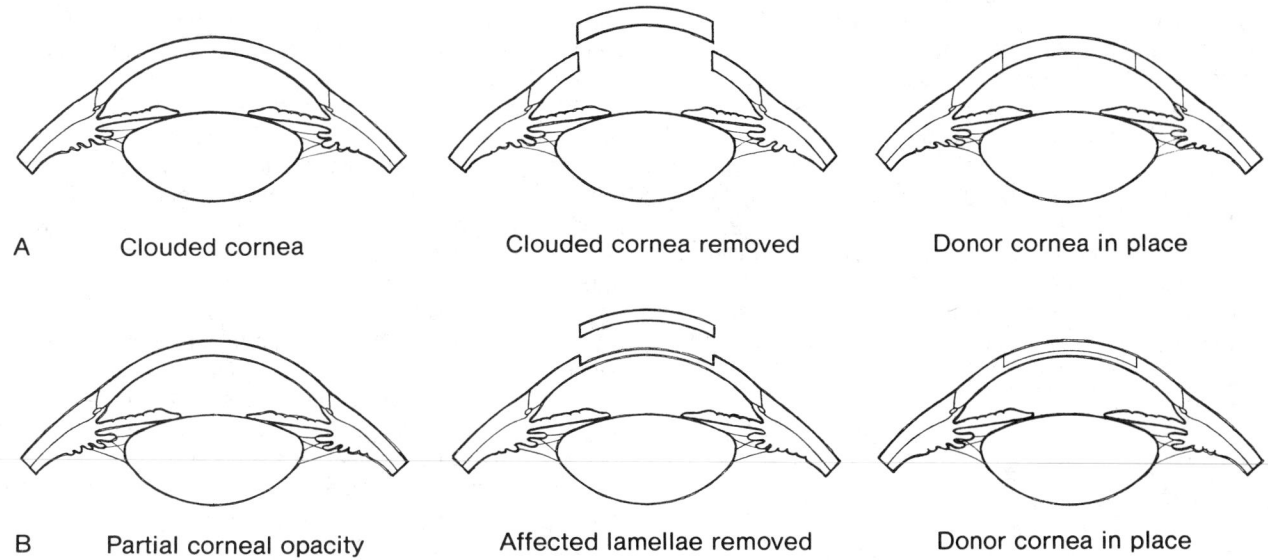

A   Clouded cornea   Clouded cornea removed   Donor cornea in place

B   Partial corneal opacity   Affected lamellae removed   Donor cornea in place

Figure 53–8. Corneal transplantation (keratoplasty). (**A**) Penetrating keratoplasty: a full-thickness (7- to 8-mm) disc is removed from the host and replaced with a matching full-thickness button from the donor. (**B**) Lamellar keratoplasty: a thin layer of corneal tissue is excised from the host eye. Stroma and entire endothelium are spared.

gery include hemorrhage, epithelial defects, wound leaks, glaucoma, and graft rejection.

Preoperative Nursing Interventions. Because keratoplasty is elective surgery, the patient is probably aware of the nature of the operation and is usually optimistic about the likelihood of improved vision. The nurse, nevertheless, must allow time for the expression of concerns or questions that the patient may still have. Physically, the patient should be free from respiratory or eye infections to promote postoperative healing.

Postoperative Nursing Interventions. Goals for postoperative patient care are (1) to monitor for and avoid activities that will cause an elevation of IOP as well as pressure on the operated eye, (2) to rest the eye so that healing progresses smoothly, and (3) to institute measures that will prevent infection of the eye.

Elevated IOP constricts the vascular supply and can cause optic nerve atrophy and damage to the graft. To prevent pressure from increasing within the eye, the nurse must be cognizant of those activities that can elevate pressure (sneezing, coughing, straining during defecation, or lifting heavy objects). Loss of aqueous humor through the suture line could cause prolapse of the iris, adhesions of the iris to the cornea, or malformation of the anterior chamber. IOP can be measured by sensitive electronic applanation tonometers. If the pressure is elevated, pharmacologic control can be achieved with such medications as acetazolamide, which inhibits the production of aqueous humor.

Healing is slow because the cornea is avascular, which also increases the possibility of infection. Thus, meticulous sterile technique is followed in dressing changes to protect the susceptible corneal epithelium from infection. Another means of reducing the chance of infection is to provide the patient with antibiotic ointments or drops or a collagen shield hydrated with antibiotic solution.

Eye Donation

Corneal transplantation surgery has restored sight for many people with corneal damage or disease. But there are many others who would benefit from this highly successful procedure if donor tissue were available. Nurses can play a vital role, both in their professional and private lives, in educating the public about the need for eye donation. It is important for people to know that they can make a critical difference by providing the gift of sight and that anyone may become an eye donor by completing a donor card or filling out the back of the driver's license. The decision to become a future donor should be shared with significant others so that they can take the appropriate action when needed. If this decision was not made and documented before death, the next of kin may consent to the donation of the eyes of their deceased family member. They may be reassured by knowing the following:

- There will be no visible sign of disfigurement after procurement.
- The body will be treated with respect.
- The donation will not interfere with funeral arrangements.
- There is no cost to the family.
- The donation will remain confidential.

The following criteria are used for selecting donors for corneal transplantation:

- Known time of death (eyes should be obtained within 6 hours of death)
- Probable cause of death (no sepsis or transmissible infectious disease)
- Over 26 weeks of gestation. No upper age limit

Eye care for donor eyes includes instillation of physiologic solution every 4 hours, keeping the lids closed by taping the eyelids shut, and securing a moist gauze to the lids. The use of ointments is contraindicated.

Any eyes not suitable for transplantation can be used in one of many valuable eye research projects.

In summary, the cornea, which refracts light rays, is examined with the aid of a slit lamp. Corneal abrasions are defects in the epithelial layer. Microbial keratitis is infection of the cornea; exposure keratitis may develop whenever the cornea is not adequately moistened and protected by the eyelids. Corneal dystrophies are inherited, bilateral alterations of the cornea with abnormal deposition of substances. Fuchs's dystrophy affects the corneal endothelium and compromises its pump mechanism. Keratoconus is a noninflammatory, progressive thinning of the cornea.

Corneal transplantation or penetrating keratoplasty is used to restore vision in many patients suffering from the above-mentioned corneal conditions. Corneal transplantation surgery has restored sight for many people. Many others could also be helped if more donor tissue were available.

Glaucoma

Glaucoma is one of the leading causes of blindness in Western society. It is estimated that in the United States 2 million people have been diagnosed as having glaucoma. Of these, almost half are visually impaired, with 70,000 legally blind; 5500 additional people become legally blind each year.

When glaucoma is diagnosed early and managed properly, blindness is almost always preventable. Most cases of glaucoma, however, are asymptomatic until extensive and irreversible damage has already occurred. Therefore, routine eye examinations and screening clinics play a vital role in the detection of this disease. It is recommended that all who are at risk for developing glaucoma and those over 35 years of age have periodic examinations by an ophthalmologist to assess IOP and evaluate the optic nerve head.

Glaucoma affects people of all ages but is more prevalent with age, affecting about 2% of those over 35 years of age. Others at risk are diabetics, blacks, those with a family history of glaucoma, and people who have had previous eye trauma or surgery or who have received long-term steroid treatment.

Although there is no cure for glaucoma, it can most often be controlled with medication. Laser or conventional (incisional) surgery may also be required. The goal of treatment is to arrest the progression of the condition or to slow it enough to maintain good lifetime vision. This is usually accomplished by reducing the IOP.

The term *glaucoma* refers to a group of diseases that differ in their pathophysiology, clinical presentation, and treatment. They are generally characterized by visual field loss due to damage to the optic nerve. This damage is related to the level of IOP, which is too high for proper functioning of the optic nerve. The higher the pressure, the more rapidly optic nerve damage progresses. The increased IOP results from pathologic changes that prevent normal circulation of aqueous humor (Fig. 53-9).

Aqueous Humor Dynamics
The ciliary body is the portion of the uveal tract that lies between the iris and the choroid. The iris inserts into the anterior side of the ciliary body and divides the aqueous space into the anterior and posterior chambers. The lens is attached to the ciliary body by the zonules, which separate the aqueous compartment anteriorly from the vitreous compartment posteriorly.

Smooth muscles in the ciliary body are responsible for movement in the zonules, trabecular meshwork, and Schlemm's canal.

The ciliary processes produce aqueous humor, which serves a circulatory function for the avascular tissues of the eye (cornea, lens, trabecular meshwork). The aqueous humor brings essential nutrients to, removes metabolites from, and provides the proper chemical environment for the eye. It is also responsible for maintaining IOP, which is important for optical and structural integrity.

There is a constant flow of aqueous humor from the ciliary processes into the posterior chamber, through the pupil between the lens and the iris, into the anterior chamber and out the trabecular meshwork, Schlemm's canal, and the venous plexus. The trabecular meshwork and Schlemm's canal are located in the anterior chamber angle at the junction of the iris, cornea, and sclera and are visible by means of gonioscopy (see p. 1568).

IOP results from the balance between aqueous humor formation and the resistance of aqueous humor outflow. IOP is not constant. It fluctuates over the course of the day and can be affected by the seasons of the year, exercise, postural changes, eyelid movement, foods, and medications. Conditions that increase IOP may result in progressive structural and functional damage to the eye.

Classification

The classifications of glaucoma relate to the configuration of the anterior chamber angle and the age at onset. These are:
I. Open-angle glaucoma
  A. Primary
  B. Normal-tension
  C. Secondary
II. Angle-closure glaucoma
  A. Primary
    1. With pupillary block
      a. Acute
      b. Subacute
      c. Chronic
    2. Without pupillary block
  B. Secondary
    1. With pupillary block
    2. Without pupillary block
III. Combined-mechanism glaucoma
IV. Developmental/congenital glaucoma

Primary Glaucomas
The term *primary glaucoma* denotes a type of glaucoma not associated with any known ocular or systemic condition that contributes to the abnormal level of IOP. It is usually bilateral and is thought to have an hereditary component.

Secondary Glaucomas
Secondary glaucomas are associated with ocular or systemic disorders that are responsible for the elevation in IOP. They are often unilateral.

In secondary open-angle glaucoma, elevated IOP is due to an increased resistance to aqueous humor outflow through the trabecular meshwork, Schlemm's canal, and the episcleral venous system. This increased resistance may be a result of a

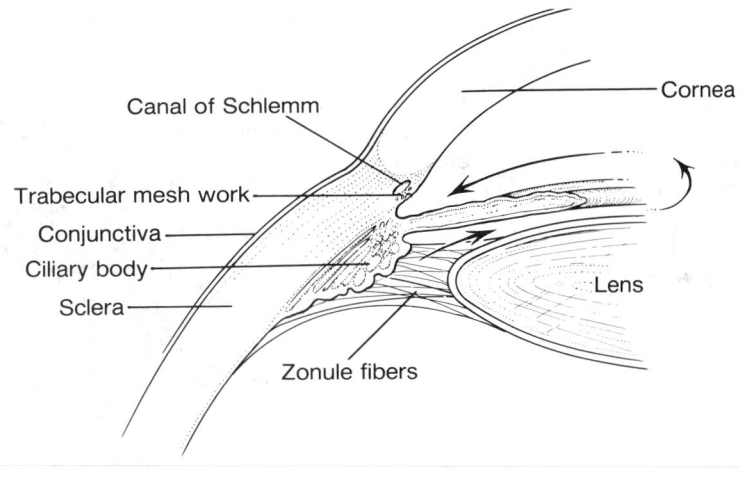

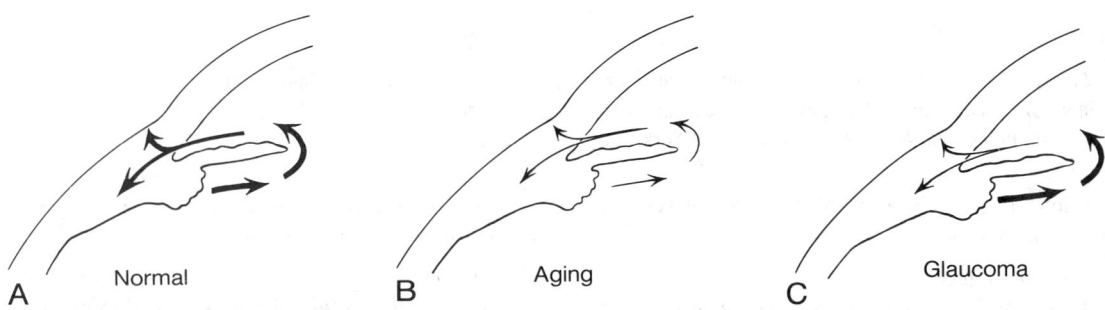

Figure 53–9. Effects of aging and of glaucoma on secretion of aqueous humor. Normal anatomy is identified in the upper illustration. (**A**) Arrows indicate the secretion of aqueous humor from the ciliary body to the posterior chamber, through the pupil into the anterior chamber, and out through the trabecular meshwork to the canal of Schlemm and then into the venous system. (**B**) The same pathway is followed in the aging person, except that the amount of fluid is reduced. (**C**) In glaucoma, more fluid enters the anterior chamber than leaves it. This accounts for hardness of the eyeball due to the increase of pressure.

number of conditions: long-term corticosteroid use, intraocular tumors, uveitis from diseases such as herpes simplex or herpes zoster, or trabecular meshwork blockage by lens material, viscoelastic substance (used in cataract surgery), blood, or pigment. Elevation in episcleral venous pressure from conditions such as chemical burns, retrobulbar tumors, thyroid disease, arteriovenous fistulas, or jugular superior vena cava, or pulmonary venous obstruction can also result in increased IOP. In addition, open-angle glaucoma may be seen after cataract extraction, IOL implantation (especially anterior chamber lenses), scleral buckling, vitrectomy, posterior capsulotomy, or trauma.

In secondary angle-closure glaucoma, increased resistance to aqueous humor outflow is due to blockage of the trabecular meshwork by the peripheral iris. The central iris normally overlies the anterior lens surface, which causes slight resistance to aqueous humor flow from the posterior chamber through the pupil to the anterior chamber. When flow through the pupil is blocked (pupillary block) by close apposition of the iris to the middle part of the lens, however, the resulting increase in pressure in the posterior chamber balloons the peripheral iris forward into contact with the trabecular meshwork. This can narrow or completely close the anterior chamber angle and causes elevated IOP (Fig. 53-10). Pupillary block also may be a result of posterior synechia (iris adherent to the lens), which may

result from scleral buckling surgery or from a swollen, dislocated, or abnormally shaped lens.

Persons with an anatomic predisposition to angle-closure glaucoma with pupillary block may have an episode precipitated by moderate pupillary dilation or marked pupillary miosis. Dilation may result from emotional episodes such as fear or pain, dim illumination, or a variety of topical or systemic medications, including pupillary dilators, vasoconstrictors, bronchodilators, tranquilizers, and anti-Parkinson's agents. Activities, such as reading, that cause forward movement of the lens, and miotic therapy may also be precipitating factors. A glaucomatous episode often occurs in anatomically predisposed people who previously had completely normal eye examinations or who were, up to that point, totally asymptomatic. Those with a family history of this type of glaucoma should have a slit-lamp examination and gonioscopy to evaluate the anterior chamber angle.

Normal-Tension Glaucoma and Ocular Hypertension
Normal intraocular levels are defined by population statistics. For some people, pressures in the normal range may be too high for continued health of the optic nerve. At the other end of the scale are instances of elevated IOP without evidence of optic nerve damage, where the optic nerve head seems resistant to higher than normal pressures that are withstood for a re-

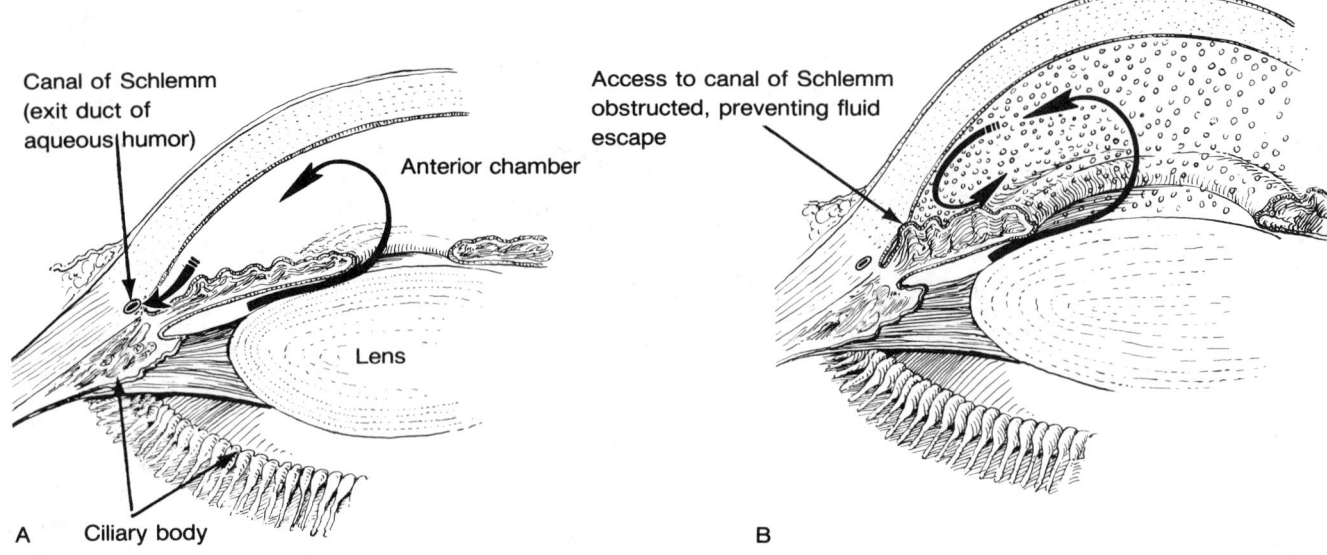

Figure 53–10. Obstruction of flow of aqueous fluid in glaucoma. (**A**) Normal flow of aqueous fluid through canal of Schlemm. (**B**) Obstruction to the flow of fluid, causing narrow-angle glaucoma. (Lechliger M and Moya F. Introduction to the Practice of Anesthesia, 2nd ed. New York, Harper & Row.)

markably long time. Eventually some of these people will develop glaucomatous damage.

Combined-Mechanism Glaucoma

Some people may have a combination of two or more forms of disease. Open-angle glaucoma complicated by angle-closure glaucoma (or narrowing of the angles that impede outflow of aqueous) is the most common form of combined-mechanism glaucoma.

Clinical Evaluation

A glaucoma diagnostic workup involves examination of the eye, a number of diagnostic tests, and ocular and medical histories.

Tonometry

Tonometry is a simple and painless test to measure IOP. There are two types of tonometric devices used for assessment: applanation and indentation. An applanation, or Goldmann, tonometer is the most accurate device and measures the force required to flatten a small, standard area of the cornea. The pneumotonometer, or air puff tonometer, is similar to the Goldmann tonometer. It is not as accurate but has the advantage of not requiring the instrument to actually touch the eye. An indentation tonometer measures the deformation of the globe in response to a standard weight placed on the cornea. Normal IOP is 11 to 21 mm Hg.

In glaucoma, IOP is usually, but not always, elevated above 21 mm Hg. Because the IOP is not constant in any one eye, a single normal reading does not rule out the possibility of glaucoma. Conversely, a single high reading does not indicate the presence of glaucoma but does require further evaluation.

Perimetry

Perimetry is used to measure the scope of the field of vision. Loss of visual field is the major clinical manifestation of optic nerve damage from glaucoma and is, therefore, used both in the diagnosis of glaucoma and in the evaluation of the response to treatment. A perimeter is used to plot the topography of the

island of vision and is used to recognize any variations from normal in either localized areas or the overall visual field.

Gonioscopy

Gonioscopy is the technique used to directly visualize the anterior chamber angle of the eye using binocular magnification (slit lamp) and a goniolens (specialized mirror contact lens). Gonioscopy is important in determining if the angle is open or closed.

Ophthalmoscopy

An ophthalmoscope is used to examine the optic nerve head for color and shape. Glaucoma causes damage to the optic nerve, either by ischemia or mechanical compression, which can be recognized by atrophy and cupping of the optic nerve head.

History

Ocular and health histories are valuable in providing clues to the diagnosis, classification, and management of glaucoma. Important aspects of the ocular history include symptoms of elevated IOP, uveitis, trauma, surgery, prolonged use of systemic or topical corticosteroids, or a family history of glaucoma.

In a review of systems, special attention is given to the following conditions that can cause, aggravate, or mimic glaucoma: diabetes mellitus, cardiovascular disease, systemic hypertension, an episode of shock, cerebrovascular disease, thyroid disease, respiratory disease, or demyelinating disease.

Current medications are recorded, noting those that are associated with glaucoma: tricyclic antidepressants, antihistamines, phenothiazides, monoamine oxidase inhibitors, anticholinergic and antispasmodic agents, and anti-Parkinsonian drugs.

Clinical Manifestations

Primary open-angle glaucoma is the most common type of glaucoma, yet it is the most difficult to recognize early because it is asymptomatic until late in its course. It is insidious in onset, slowly progressive, and small areas of peripheral vision loss may go unnoticed. By the time visual field loss becomes apparent to the patient, extensive irreversible damage to the optic nerve has usually already occurred. Routine ocular examinations are necessary to diagnose the disease early enough to provide appropriate treatment to prevent significant visual loss and blindness. Primary open-angle glaucoma is a bilateral disease, but damage is often asymmetric. One eye frequently is involved earlier and more severely than the other.

Symptoms of acute closed-angle glaucoma include pain, halo vision, blurred vision, redness, and a change in the eye's appearance. Ocular pain may be caused by a rapid rise in IOP, by inflammation, or by drug-induced side effects (*e.g.*, ciliary muscle spasm). Severe ocular pain may be accompanied by nausea, vomiting, sweating, or bradycardia. Redness may be associated with acute iritis, drug reaction, neovascular glaucoma, hyphema, subconjunctival hemorrhage, or elevated episcleral venous pressure. Corneal edema, as a result of a rapid rise in IOP or corneal epithelial decompensation, may produce halo vision, which is a sensation of colored halos around incandescent lights. Episodic blurring of vision may also be noted. Some patients notice a change in the appearance of the eye, including haziness of the cornea, ocular displacement, and alteration in pupil position, size, or shape.

Management

The objective of treatment for glaucoma is to lower the IOP to a level consistent with retention of visual function. The treatment varies depending on the classification of the disease and response to therapy. Medication therapy, laser surgery, and conventional surgery may be used in the attempt to control progression of damage resulting from glaucoma.

Medication therapy is the initial and principle mode of treatment for primary open-angle glaucoma. If this therapy fails to adequately decrease the IOP, the next therapeutic option for most patients is laser trabeculoplasty with continued medication administration. For some patients, a trabeculectomy is required. Laser or incisional surgery, however, is usually an adjunct to, rather than replacement for, medication therapy.

Acute angle-closure glaucoma with pupillary block is a surgical emergency. Medications are used to reduce the IOP as much as possible before laser or incisional iridectomy. In some instances, medications alone may terminate the attack, but there is a high incidence of recurrence. In addition, there is a high incidence of later involvement of the other eye. Bilateral laser iridectomy is therefore recommended.

Treatment of secondary glaucomas is directed at the underlying condition as well as the elevated IOP. For example, glaucomas caused by steroid therapy are managed by discontinuing the medication. Lens-induced glaucomas require lens extraction or removal of residual lens material. Uveitis with glaucoma is treated with anti-inflammatory agents. Antiviral agents, cycloplegics, and topical corticosteroids are prescribed for glaucoma associated with herpes simplex and herpes zoster.

Pharmacotherapy

Patients with open-angle glaucoma usually require a lifetime of medication therapy, which often changes depending on the response to treatment and the occurrence of side effects. These medications must be administered routinely to be effective in preventing optic nerve damage. In general, the safest topical drugs are prescribed first in the lowest possible dosage that will control IOP at the desired level. If the reduction of IOP by the initial medication in the maximally tolerated dosage is inadequate, different or additional topical and, possibly, systemic medications may be prescribed.

- Use of pupillary dilating (mydriatic) medication is contraindicated for patients with glaucoma.

Most medications have some side effects, which often subside after 1 to 2 weeks. In some instances, however, a drug may need to be discontinued because of intolerance. Common side effects of topical medications include blurring of vision, dimming of vision, especially at night, and difficulty focusing. Occasionally, heart rate and breathing are affected. Systemic agents may cause tingling of fingers or toes, drowsiness, loss of appetite, bowel irregularities, and, occasionally, kidney stones. Patients should be informed about possible side effects. Those who are warned in advance are more likely to cope successfully with the situation.

Beta-Adrenergic Antagonists. Topical beta-adrenergic antagonists are now the most widely used hypotensive agents because they are effective in many types of glaucoma and do not produce some of the side effects frequently seen with other drugs. Beta-adrenergic antagonists, such as timolol, reduce IOP by decreasing aqueous humor formation.

Cholinergic Agents. Topical cholinergic medications (*e.g.*, pilocarpine hydrochloride) are used in the short-term management of glaucoma with pupillary block because of their effect on the parasympathetic receptors in the iris and ciliary body. The result is constriction of the pupillary sphincter, tightening of the iris, decrease of the iris tissue volume in the angle, and pulling of the peripheral iris away from the trabecular meshwork. These changes allow aqueous humor to reach the outflow channels and, therefore, reduce IOP.

Adrenergic Agonists. Topical adrenergic agonists reduce IOP by increasing aqueous humor outflow. Epinephrine eye drops are widely used in the treatment of open-angle glaucoma.

Carbonic Anhydrase Inhibitors. Carbonic anhydrase inhibitors (*e.g.*, acetazolamide [Diamox]) are administered systemically to lower IOP by decreasing aqueous humor formation. They are used in the long-term management of open-angle glaucoma, short-term treatment of acute angle-closure glaucoma, and self-limiting glaucomas such as those that develop after trauma. They also may be required after iridectomy to control residual glaucoma.

Osmotic Diuretics. Oral (*e.g.*, glycerol) or intravenous (*e.g.*, mannitol) hyperosmotic agents reduce IOP by increasing the osmolality of the plasma and drawing water from the eye into the vascular circulation. Hyperosmotic medications are helpful in the short-term treatment of acute glaucoma. They are used to lower IOP preoperatively so that surgery can be performed on a more normotensive eye. They also may prevent the need for surgery in transient glaucoma.

Laser Surgery

Laser surgery may be indicated as the primary treatment for glaucoma or it may be required when medication therapy is poorly tolerated or ineffective in lowering IOP. Lasers can be used to perform many procedures related to the treatment of glaucoma.

Peripheral iridectomy—creates a full-thickness hole in the iris to allow aqueous humor to flow from the posterior chamber to the anterior chamber. Indications for this procedure include:

Acute primary angle-closure glaucoma with pupillary block

Fellow eye of a patient who has had an attack of acute primary angle-closure glaucoma

Chronic, subacute, or intermittent primary angle-closure glaucoma

Prophylactic treatment of anatomically narrow anterior chamber angle glaucoma

Combined-mechanism glaucoma

Secondary angle-closure glaucoma, including ciliary block and aphakic (absence of a crystalline lens) pupillary block glaucoma

Trabeculoplasty—modifies the trabecular meshwork to increase aqueous humor outflow. It is employed when medication therapy alone is insufficient to control IOP in open-angle glaucoma.

Gonioplasty—contracts the peripheral iris to eliminate contact with the trabecular meshwork. It is performed when iridectomy does not resolve the problem of iris blockage at the angle.

Pupilloplasty—enlarges miotic pupillary area by contracting the iris fibers and stretching the pupil opening.

Synechiolysis—pulls lightly adherent adhesions away from the angle wall of the cornea.

Sphincterotomy—creates radial cuts in the iris sphincter muscle to allow pupillary enlargement.

Cyclophotocoagulation—destroys some of the ciliary processes to reduce aqueous humor production.

Goniophotocoagulation—eradicates new vessels in anterior chamber neovascularization. It is used with panretinal photocoagulation to treat neovascular glaucoma.

Laser surgery can also be performed to treat ciliary block (malignant) glaucoma, reopen failed filtering sites, sever sutures after trabeculectomy, and rupture cysts of the iris or ciliary body.

Conventional Surgery

Conventional surgical procedures are performed when laser techniques are unsuccessful, laser equipment is unavailable, or when the patient is not a good candidate for laser surgery (*e.g.*, a patient who is unable to sit still or follow instructions).

A *peripheral* or a *sector iridectomy* is performed to remove a portion of the iris to allow aqueous humor flow from the posterior chamber to the anterior chamber. It is indicated in the treatment of glaucoma with pupillary block if laser treatment is unsuccessful or unavailable.

A *trabeculectomy* (filtering procedure) is performed to create a new drainage pathway through the sclera. This is accomplished by dissecting a half-thickness flap of sclera hinged at the limbus. A segment of trabecular tissue is removed, the scleral flap is reapproximated, and the conjunctiva is securely sutured to prevent leakage of aqueous fluid. Trabeculectomy increases aqueous humor outflow by bypassing the usual drainage structures. As fluid flows through this new channel, a bleb (blister or bubble) is formed that can be observed on examination of the conjunctiva. Complications after filtering procedures have been reported to include hypotony (abnormally low IOP), hyphema (blood in the anterior chamber of the eye), infection, and failure of the filtration.

Seton procedures involve the use of various types of synthetic devices to maintain a patent drainage fistula. An open tube is implanted in the anterior chamber and connects to an episcleral drainage field. These devices are most often used in eyes with high pressures, extremely poor surgical risk, or failure of a previous filtration. Possible complications of drainage implants include cataract formation, hypotony, corneal decompensation, and erosion of the apparatus.

The patient may require a short hospital stay after surgery. Progressive ambulation is allowed, depending on the patient's age and physical condition. Vigorous activity and movements that cause a Valsalva effect (with resulting increased IOP) such as straining, lifting, and bending, are to be avoided for 1 week. The patient is not permitted to drive for 1 week. The eye is patched for 24 hours or longer if needed. Water should be kept out of the eye. Broad-spectrum antibiotic drops may be instilled for 4 to 5 days, and a topical steroid may be used for many weeks to reduce inflammation and scarring. Occasionally, more potent antifibrinolytic or anti-inflammatory agents, such as 5-fluorouracil (5-FU) and oral steroids, may be indicated. Because aspirin may induce bleeding, it is contraindicated, and pain is usually managed with acetaminophen. Reading causes rapid, jerky eye movements; thus it is discouraged until permitted by the physician.

Patient Education and Home Health Care

Patients diagnosed with glaucoma are faced with learning how to live with a chronic health condition. Members of the health care team can help them with this difficult adjustment by providing the information needed to understand the disorder, its treatment, and their responsibilities in its management. An informed patient is more likely to take an active role in his own care; this involvement is imperative because optimum reduction of IOP and control of glaucomatous damage depend on the patient's adherence to his medication regimen and attendance at follow-up examinations.

Patients are given written instructions to explain the name of each medication, a description of the containers (*e.g.*, green top, yellow label), and the frequency and times of administration. They should understand the expected action and the possible side effects. The importance of making medication administration a part of the daily routine is stressed so that doses are not missed. Patients need to understand that medications are to be continued even when IOP is under control.

Patients should be aware that their responsibilities include good eye care, maintenance of good physical health, and a life-style consistent with low levels of stress. Eye care involves keeping the eyes clean and free of irritants, avoiding rubbing, using nonallergenic cosmetics, and wearing goggles while swimming and protective glasses while playing sports or working in the yard or other potentially hazardous areas. Noting how the eyes look and feel is important. Unusual changes that should be reported to the physician include excessive irritation, watering, blurring, cloudy vision, discharge, rainbows around lights at night, flashes of light, and floating objects in the field of vision.

Because the treatment of glaucoma is a matter of control rather than cure, it usually involves lifelong management. Follow-up examinations are necessary to determine the efficacy of therapy and include monitoring of the IOP and assessment of visual field and optic disc. The frequency of follow-up visits depends on the level and stability of IOP and the extent of damage. Patients who are newly diagnosed, or who have a highly elevated IOP and wide fluctuations from visit to visit, extensive optic nerve head cupping or visual field loss, or only one eye with visual function, require more frequent examination.

An explanation is given regarding the importance of timely follow-up examinations. It may be helpful for patients to know what each diagnostic study is designed to demonstrate.

Maintaining good health and limiting stress may have a positive effect on eye pressure. Proper nutrition, salt restriction, avoiding excessive fluid intake, maintaining an appropriate weight level, exercising, and taking time for fun and relaxation may be helpful. Sharing feelings and concerns with family and friends or talking with other patients with glaucoma may be useful in learning how to live with glaucoma.

Gerontologic Considerations

Most patients with glaucoma are in the older age group. Often dimming vision is accepted as part of the aging process, and medical assistance is not sought. Therefore, as part of the physical examination of anyone over age 35, tonometry should be recommended and eye pressure periodically checked thereafter.

A major concern of health care providers caring for patients with glaucoma is the tendency of these patients to stop taking their eye drops, claiming that it does not help. They must be helped to understand that the eye drops keep glaucoma from worsening. Discontinuing the medication will allow the glaucoma to continue insidiously until blindness occurs. Other problems often experienced by elderly patients such as arthritis, loneliness and depression, constipation (straining on defecation), and potential for falling and accidents must be considered when caring for the patient with glaucoma.

In summary, glaucoma is the leading cause of blindness in the United States. Although there is no cure for glaucoma, it can often be controlled with medication. Laser or incisional surgery may be required; the goal of these procedures is to arrest the progression of the condition.

The term *glaucoma* refers to a group of diseases that differ in their pathophysiology, clinical presentation, and treatment. The classifications of glaucoma relate to the configuration of the anterior chamber angle and the age at onset. Diagnostic tests often include tonometry, perimetry, and use of gonioscopy and the ophthalmoscope. Acute closed-angle glaucoma occurs when there is blockage of the angle of the anterior chamber by iris tissue, causing a rise in IOP. Primary open-angle glaucoma develops slowly, is asymptomatic initially, and is more commonly seen than closed-angle glaucoma.

The clinical manifestations of acute glaucoma are extreme ocular pain, blurred vision, red eyes, and a dilated pupil. Nausea and vomiting may occur. Permanent blindness occurs within 2 to 5 days if the condition goes untreated.

Gradual loss of peripheral vision is usually the only symptom of open-angle glaucoma. Later, central blindness may occur.

Acute closed-angle glaucoma is a surgical emergency. Medications are used preoperatively to decrease IOP. Chronic open-angle glaucoma is most frequently treated with miotic eye drops such as pilocarpine. The objective of treatment is to lower IOP to a level consistent with retention of visual function.

It is imperative that the nurse stress to the patient and his family the importance of regular eye examinations and the consistent and proper use of medications prescribed for glaucoma. See Nursing Care Plan 53-1 for care of the patient with glaucoma.

Cataracts

A cataract is an opacification of the normally clear, transparent crystalline lens (Fig. 53-11). It is usually a result of aging but occasionally occurs at birth (congenital cataract). It may also be associated with blunt or penetrating trauma, medications such as corticosteroids used over a long period, systemic disease such as diabetes mellitus or hypoparathyroidism, radiation exposure, or other eye disorders such as anterior uveitis. Studies have shown that long hours of bright sunlight (ultraviolet light) have an effect on cataract formation.

Pathophysiology

The normal lens is a clear, transparent, buttonlike structure lying in back of the iris; it possesses strong refractive powers. The lens consists of three anatomic components. In the central zone is the *nucleus*, peripherally is the *cortex*, and surrounding both is a *capsule*. With aging, the nucleus takes on a yellowish brown hue. Surrounding opacities are spokelike white densities occurring anteriorly and posteriorly to the nucleus. Opacity of the posterior capsule is the most significant form of cataract— it looks like frost on a window.

Physical and chemical changes may produce a loss of transparency of the lens. Changes in the multiple fine fibers (zonules) that extend from the ciliary body to the outer circumference of the lens, for example, may cause a distortion of the image. A chemical change in lens protein may cause coagulation, thereby producing cloudy vision by blocking the passage of light to the retina. One theory postulates that a breakdown in normal lens protein occurs with an influx of water into the lens. This process disrupts the tight lens fibers and interferes with the transmission of light. Another theory is that an enzyme plays a part in protecting the lens from degeneration. It decreases with aging and is absent in many patients with cataracts.

Clinical Manifestations

As the lens becomes opaque, it scatters light instead of transmitting a sharply focused image on the retina. The result is a disabling glare, dimmed or blurred vision with distortion of images, and poor night vision (see Fig. 53-11). The pupil, which is normally black, may appear yellowish, gray, or white. Cataracts usually develop gradually over a period of years, and as the cataract worsens, stronger glasses no longer improve sight.

People with cataracts often develop strategies to avoid the disabling glare that is caused by extraneous light. Some find it helpful to rearrange the seating arrangement in their homes so that lights do not shine directly in their eyes. Wearing a wide-

Nursing Care Plan 53–1

Care of Patient With Glaucoma/Increased Intraocular Pressure

Nursing Interventions	Rationale	Expected Outcomes

Nursing Diagnosis: Alteration in visual sensory perception related to progressive nature of glaucoma

Goal: Adjustment to altered visual status

Nursing Interventions	Rationale	Expected Outcomes
1. Encourage patient to maintain independence. 2. Instruct patient regarding effects of pupillary constriction. 3. Refer patient to appropriate agencies if home assistance is needed. 4. Instruct patients about signs and symptoms to report to ophthalmologist. 5. Provide information about medications both verbally and in writing to the patient and significant other. 6. Explain and demonstrate techniques of general eye care.	1. Independence and self-reliance promote feelings of self-worth. 2. Visual acuity is decreased in early morning and at dusk. 3. Resources available for home health services, shopping, and transportation are invaluable for persons with significantly impaired vision. 4. Headache, brow pain, nausea and vomiting, blurred vision, halos around lights indicate increased IOP. 5. Understanding use of medications increases compliance. Consistent, on time use is important even when asymptomatic, with IOP under control. 6. Understanding proper eye care increases compliance.	• Adjustments made in home environment to allow for visual limitation. • Plans outdoor activities in mid part of day. • Calls community resources and arranges for appropriate services. • Signs and symptoms of increased IOP are reported immediately to ophthalmologist. • Uses proper technique for instillation of medications. • Keeps medication in special, visible place at home. • Reports to ophthalmologist abnormal effects, inconvenient, uncomfortable, or expensive medication. • Keeps reserve bottle of medication at home. • Carries eye drops on person when away from home. • Carries card identifying condition of glaucoma and current eye medications, or wears medic alert bracelet. • Uses antihistamines or sympathomimetics only with medical supervision. • Schedules medication around daily routines such as waking, mealtime, bedtime. • If oral medication is not taken on schedule, checks with ophthalmologist to see if it should be taken when it is remembered or wait until next scheduled time. • Avoids stress. • Avoids excessive fluid intake. • Complies with follow-up visits at recommended intervals. • Avoids rubbing eyes. • After eye surgery, wears goggles for swimming and protective glasses for yard work and sports. • Reports having glaucoma to all health care providers.

Nursing Diagnosis: Pain related to rapid increase in pressure within the eye

Goal: Relief of pain and discomfort

Nursing Interventions	Rationale	Expected Outcomes
1. Assess pain; notify physician of any changes in eye pain; administer medications as prescribed.	1. Medications prescribed to decrease intraocular pressure will promote comfort.	• Experiences relief of pain. • Uses prescribed medications to relieve pain.

(continued)

Nursing Care Plan 53–1 *(Continued)*

Care of Patient With Glaucoma/Increased Intraocular Pressure

Nursing Interventions	Rationale	Expected Outcomes
Nursing Diagnosis: Anxiety or fear related to possible or actual loss of vision		
Goal: Reduction of anxiety and fear and coping with decrease in vision		
1. Identify fears and concerns of patient. Help patient to understand that progressive damage of glaucoma can usually be controlled with medication and/or surgery. Recognize that learning to live with glaucoma as a chronic health condition involves a commitment to its treatment, but drastic changes in life style are not indicated.	1. As patient has understanding of disease, anxiety and fear are lessened.	• Asks questions about condition and prognosis • Talks about fears and concerns. • Shares feelings with family or significant others. • Uses relaxation techniques. • Uses diversional activities that promote relaxation.
2. Instruct patient in relaxation techniques	2. Relaxation techniques help to reduce stress and anxiety	
Nursing Diagnosis: Self-care deficit related to impaired vision		
Goal: increases or maintains self-care skills		
1. Encourage patient's personal grooming.	1. Visual blurring may decrease one's interest in personal appearance.	• Maintains personal grooming. • Receives positive reinforcement from family or significant other. • Light fixtures placed to provide maximum illumination. • Furniture arranged to maximize safety. • Makes use of support systems. • Seeks assistance from family or significant others in adapting home environment to meet individual needs.
2. Instruct patient in ways to modify environment for safety and efficiency.	2. Safe and efficient environment promotes self-care.	
3. Instruct family or significant others regarding special needs of patient.	3. Support systems are important for compliance.	
Nursing Diagnosis: Potential social isolation related to fear of injury that might further complicate visual problem		
Goal: Participates in social activities within limitations		
1. Encourage patient to maintain social contacts with family and friends.	1. Socialization promotes positive attitude and self-worth.	• Maintains social contacts with family and friends. • Participates in diversional activities.
2. Encourage patient to identify activities/hobbies that can be accomplished and enjoyed.	2. Persons with visual limitations often can learn to enjoy new activities that do not require full sight.	

brimmed hat or sunglasses and lowering the visor while driving during the day are strategies commonly used by patients with cataracts.

Diagnostic Evaluation

In addition to the usual eye tests, keratometry, and slit-lamp and ophthalmoscopic examination, A-scan ultrasound (echography) and the endothelial cell counter are particularly useful diagnostic tools. With an endothelial cell count of 2000 cells/ mm^3, the patient is a good candidate for phacoemulsification and insertion of an IOL.

Management

There is no medical treatment for cataracts, and they cannot be removed with laser surgery. Two surgical techniques are available for cataract removal: intracapsular and extracapsular extraction (Fig. 53-12). The indications for surgical intervention are loss of vision that interferes with the patient's normal activities or a cataract that is causing glaucoma or interfering with the diagnosis and treatment of other ocular disorders such as diabetic retinopathy.

Cataract surgery is the most frequently performed operation in people over the age of 65. Today cataracts are most often removed under local anesthesia on an outpatient basis,

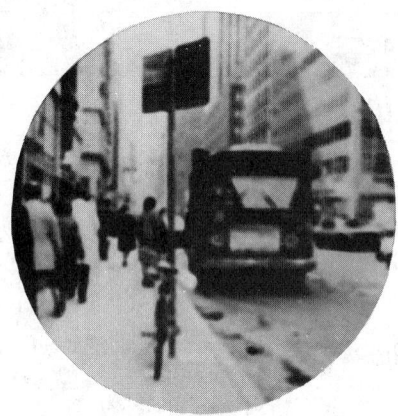

Cataract Diminished acuity from an opacity of the lens. The field of vision is unaffected. There is no scotoma, but the person has an overall haziness of the view, particularly in glaring light conditions.

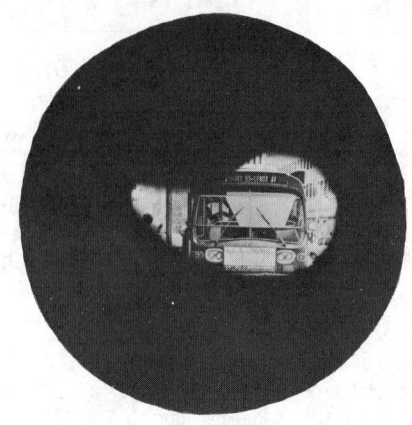

Glaucoma Advanced glaucoma involves loss of peripheral vision but the individual still retains most of his central vision.

Figure 53–11. Effects of cataract and glaucoma on vision. Photographs representing the eye diseases are taken as if the camera were the right eye. (Photos courtesy of The Lighthouse, The New York Association for the Blind.)

although patients may be hospitalized when it is medically indicated. Successful return to useful vision is accomplished in more than 95% of patients.

Intracapsular Extraction

Intracapsular cataract extraction (ICCE) is the removal of the entire intact lens as a unit. It is removed by a cryoprobe, which is placed directly on the lens capsule.

Cryosurgery is a surgical technique in which freezing temperatures are used. The cryosurgical instrument operates on the principle that a cold metal adheres to a moist object. A thin, pencil-like instrument with a metal-probe tip (straight or curved) is activated so that the temperature of the tip ranges from −30° to −40°C. The cryosurgical instrument is placed directly on the lens capsule. An ice ball forms in seconds, causing the capsule to adhere to the probe. A gentle upward

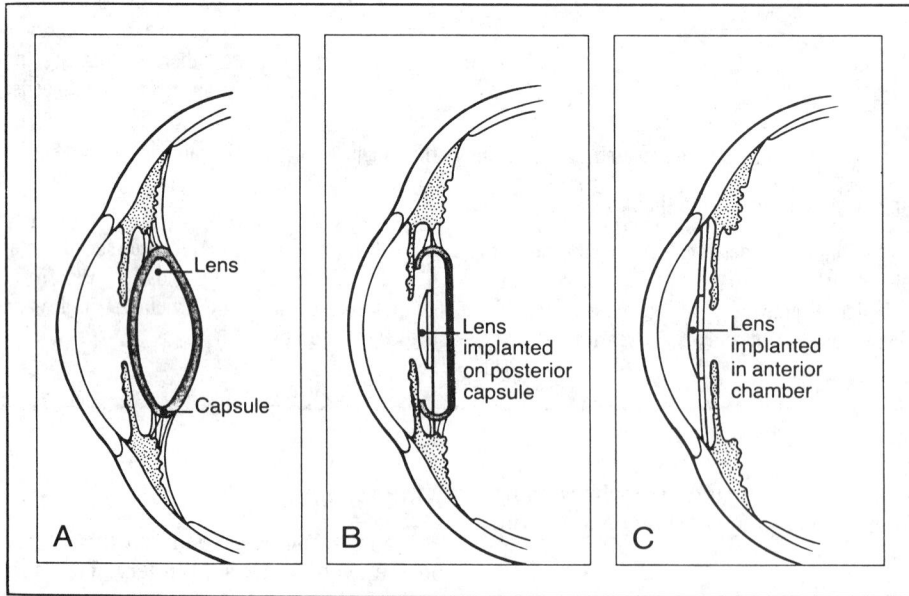

Figure 53–12. (**A**) Normal eye anatomy. Basic surgical techniques for cataract removal are the extracapsular method (**B**) and the intracapsular method (**C**). During extracapsular extraction, the contents of the lens are removed but the posterior capsule is left intact, leaving a suitable site for attachment of an intraocular lens. During intracapsular extraction, both the lens contents and the capsular bag are removed entirely and an intraocular lens must be placed in the anterior chamber. The extracapsular method, perceived as safer and less prone to complications, is now the more popular method. (Reproduced with permission from Patient Care, August 15, 1986. Copyright © 1986, Patient Care Communications, Inc, Darien, CT. Artist, Paul J. Singh-Roy. All rights reserved.)

and then sideward force frees and delivers the lens. The corneal flap is sutured back in place.

Extracapsular Extraction

Extracapsular cataract extraction (ECCE) is currently the more preferred technique and accounts for about 98% of cataract surgeries. A microscope is used for visualization during the surgery. The procedure involves removing the anterior capsule, expressing the lens nucleus, and aspirating the remaining soft cortical fragments with the use of a special irrigation-aspiration machine. By leaving the posterior capsule and lens zonules intact, the architecture of the posterior portion of the eye is preserved, thus reducing the incidence of serious complications.

Phacoemulsification is the most recent innovation in extracapsular extraction. It permits the removal of the lens through a smaller incision by using a high-frequency ultrasound device to fragment the lens nucleus and cortex into small particles that are then aspirated through the same handpiece, which also provides continuous irrigation. This technique requires less convalescent time and has a decreased incidence of postoperative astigmatism. Both the irrigation-aspiration and phacoemulsification techniques preserve the posterior capsule, which is used to support a posterior chamber IOL.

Cataract extraction and IOL implantation also can be performed in conjunction with corneal transplantation or surgery for glaucoma.

Because the crystalline lens is responsible for one third of the focusing power of the eye, whenever the lens is removed, the patient requires optical correction. This correction can be provided by one of three methods: aphakic spectacles, contact lenses, or an IOL implant.

Aphakic spectacles provide good central vision. The 25% to 30% magnification, however, results in a corresponding reduction in and distortion of peripheral vision, which causes difficulty in evaluating spatial relations. Objects seem much closer than they really are. These eye glasses also cause spherical aberrations, turning straight lines into curves. Binocular vision is not possible unless the lens has been removed from both eyes. There is often a lengthy period of adjustment until the patient is able to coordinate movements, judge distances, and function safely with a limited visual field.

Contact lenses are far less visually disabling. There is no significant magnification (5% to 10%), no spherical aberration, no decrease in visual field, and no false spatial orientation. These lenses provide almost complete visual rehabilitation for those who can master insertion, removal, and maintenance and who can wear them comfortably. Many elderly people, however, do not possess the manual dexterity or the hygiene practices to use daily-wear contact lenses. For some of these people, extended wear lenses may provide a reasonable alternative; however, extended wear lenses require frequent office visits for removal and cleaning. They are also expensive and often need replacement because of loss or breakage. Another disadvantage is the risk of infectious keratitis.

IOL implants have become the optical correction of choice largely because of the refinements in microsurgical techniques and the improvements in lens design. An IOL is a plastic permanent lens that is surgically implanted in the eye. It produces images that are normal in size and shape. Because IOLs eliminate the disabling optical effects of aphakic spectacles and the inconvenience of contact lenses, about 97% of cataract surgeries are performed in conjunction with their insertion— more than a million per year.

About 95% of IOLs are positioned in the posterior chamber, and the remaining 5% in the anterior chamber. Anterior chamber lenses are used for patients who have had an intracapsular extraction or who have had the posterior capsule inadvertently ruptured during an extracapsular procedure. The combination of extracapsular extraction and posterior lens insertion is preferred because it carries a lower incidence of sight-threatening complications.

A recent development in IOL design is a lens that can be folded for insertion, allowing it to be passed through the smaller incision made for phacoemulsification while preserving a full-size lens body after implantation.

There are a number of contraindications for IOL implantation, including recurrent uveitis, proliferative diabetic retinopathy, and neovascular glaucoma.

Although there is an excellent chance for full visual recovery after cataract extraction or IOL implantation, there is some risk of complications. Corneal endothelial damage, pupillary block, glaucoma, hemorrhage, wound fistula, cystoid macular edema, choroidal detachment, uveitis, and endophthalmitis have been observed. The IOL may become malpositioned. It may be repositioned with the sequential use of dilating drops, head positioning and the use of constricting drops, or the patient may require additional surgery to reposition or remove the IOL.

A common complication of surgery is the formation of secondary membranes, which usually occur within 3 to 36 months after surgery. They are often erroneously referred to as an opacification of the posterior capsule or as second cataracts. These membranes are formed as a result of proliferation of residual lens epithelium and interfere with vision by impeding the passage of light and increasing glare disability. An opening through the membranes can be made with a needle or laser surgery to reestablish good vision.

After a brief postoperative recovery period after cataract extraction or IOL implantation, the patient is discharged with instructions for eye medications, cleansing and protection, activity level and restrictions, diet, pain control, positioning, office appointments, information regarding the expected postoperative course, and a list of symptoms that are to be reported immediately to the surgeon (Chart 53-1).

Patients usually progress rather quickly to a return to normal daily activities. Bending and lifting heavy objects are restricted. An eye shield worn at night and eye glasses (sunglasses when outdoors in bright light) during the day are necessary for about 2 weeks to protect the eye from injury. This need for protection must be stressed because many patients who have had cataracts removed are elderly and at risk for falling; blunt trauma to the eye could cause rupture of the globe and loss of vision. Patients are usually given a new prescription for eye glasses in 6 to 8 weeks after surgery.

In summary, a cataract is a progressive condition of the lens of the eye generally resulting from aging. The lens is normally clear and transparent. Any opacity of the lens is called a cataract. As the lens opacifies, vision is blurred or dimmed with distortions of images and poor night vision.

Severe visual loss and eventual blindness will occur unless surgery is performed. The timing of cataract surgery is determined by the patient's needs. When the loss of sight interferes

Chart 53–1
Patient Education for Self-Care After Cataract Surgery

Note: To be reviewed with patient or significant other or caregiver. Print directions in large letters using felt-tipped pen for strong contrast.

Activity Limitations

Permissible

- Watch television; read if necessary but use moderation
- Do everything in moderation
- At first, "sponge bath"; later, use tub or shower (with assistance)
- Do not bend over sink or tub; tilt head slightly backward when washing hair
- Sleep with protective perforated metal eye shield at night; wear glasses during the day
- When sleeping, lie on back or side, not abdomen
- Sedentary activities
- Wear sunglasses for comfort
- Kneel or squat when picking up something from the floor

Avoid

- Sleeping on operative side
- Rubbing eyes; squeezing eyelids shut
- Straining at bowel movements
- Getting soap near eyes
- Lifting anything heavier than 15–20 pounds
- Sexual relations until (date)
- Driving, if possible
- Coughing, sneezing, and vomiting
- Bending head down below waist; bend knees only and keep back straight to pick up something from the floor

Medications and Eye Care

- Use medications as directed.
- Wash hands before and after instilling eye medications.
- Clean around eye with sterile cotton balls or gauze sponges moistened with sterile water (eye stream); wipe lid gently from inner corner to outer corner.
- To instill eye drops, be seated and tilt head back; gently pull down lower lid margin.
- Wear protective, perforated metal eye shield at night; wear glasses during the day.
- At follow-up visit, take all eye medication so that dosages can be checked and adjusted.

Report Unusual Signs and Symptoms

- Pain in and around eyes
- Any pain not relieved by pain medication prescribed
- Pain accompanied by ocular redness, swelling, or drainage
- Sudden onset of brow pain
- Changes in vision
- Changes in visual acuity, blurring, diplopia (double vision), a film over visual field, light flashes, showers or spots before eyes
- Halos around lights
- Persistent headaches
- Inflammation, discharge from eyes

with the patient's life-style, surgery is indicated. Two surgical techniques used to remove cataracts are intracapsular and extracapsular extraction. Intracapsular cataract extraction involves the removal of the entire intact lens with a cryoprobe. Extracapsular cataract extraction is used for about 98% of cataract surgeries. The phacoemulsification and irrigation-aspiration techniques preserve the posterior capsule, which is used to support a posterior chamber IOL. See Nursing Care Plan 53-2 for care of the perioperative patient.

Because the focusing power of the eye is altered after removal of the cataract, correction is made by aphakic spectacles, contact lenses, or an IOL implant.

Postoperative teaching includes instructions for eye medications, cleansing, protection, activity level, restrictions, pain control, follow-up appointments, and a list of symptoms that should be reported immediately to the physician. An eye shield or eye glasses must be worn as protection. Protection must be stressed because of the patient's risk for falling.

Retinal and Vitreous Body Disorders

Retinal Detachment

Retinal detachment occurs when there is a separation of the neurosensory retina from the underlying pigment epithelium layer of the retina. Because the neurosensory retina, the part

Nursing Care Plan 53–2

Care of the Perioperative Patient (Cataract, Retinal, Glaucoma, Corneal Procedures)

Nursing Interventions	Rationale	Expected Outcomes

Nursing Diagnosis: Fear or anxiety related to sensory impairment and lack of understanding

Goal: Reduction of emotional stress, fear, and depression; acceptance of surgery

1. Assess degree and duration of visual impairment. Encourage conversation to determine patient's concerns, feelings, and level of understanding. Answer questions, offer support, assist patient to devise methods for coping. 2. Orient patient to new surroundings. 3. Explain perioperative routine. *Preoperative:* Level of activity, dietary restriction, medications. *Intraoperative:* Importance of lying still during surgery or giving surgeon warning if needs to cough or change position. Face covered with drapes, and air/O_2 provided. Unfamiliar noises from equipment. Monitoring, including frequent BP measurements. *Postoperative:* Positioning, patching, level of activity, importance of assistance with ambulation until stable and vision adequate. 4. Explain interventions in detail; announce yourself with each interaction; interpret unfamiliar sounds; use touch to assist with verbal communication. 5. Encourage to carry out ADL as ability allows. Order finger foods for those who can not see well enough or do not have the coping skills to use implements. 6. Encourage participation of family or significant others in patient care. 7. Encourage participation in social and diversional activities as allowed (visitor, radio, audio tapes, book tapes, TV, crafts, games).	1. Information can replace fear of the unknown. Coping mechanisms can help patients to deal with worry, fear, depression, tension, resentment, anger, and rejection. 2. Familiarity with environment helps to decrease anxiety and increase safety. 3. An informed patient is more likely to accept treatment and comply with instructions. 4. Patients who are visually impaired depend on other sensory input for information. 5. Self-care and independence will promote feelings of well-being. 6. Patient may not be able to perform all tasks related to treatment and self-care. 7. Social isolation and prolonged unoccupied time may result in negative feelings.	• Verbalizes understanding of received information. • Uses methods for coping and is able to relax. • Is able to locate call bell, foods on dinner tray, furnishings, bathroom. • Verbalizes understanding of perioperative events and complies with directions and therapeutic regimen. • Is not startled or frightened by interactions or environment. • Participates in ADL as ability allows. • Recognizes limitations. • Family or significant others assist patient with care as needed. • Participates in social and diversional activities of interest as allowed or able.

Nursing Diagnosis: High risk for injury related to visual impairment or knowledge deficit

Goal: Prevention of injury

1. Assist patient when able to ambulate postoperatively until stable and has adequate vision or coping skills (remember that bilaterally patched patients are unable to see). 2. Assist patient in arranging environment. Do not rearrange furnishings without reorienting patient.	1. Reduces risk of falling or injury when gait unsteady or without coping skills for visual impairment. 2. Facilitates independence and reduces risk of injury.	• Requests assistance with ambulation when indicated. • Able to maneuver safely in environment. • Wears appropriate eye protective device during prescribed timeframe. • Manipulation of the lids is accomplished by resting fingers only on the bony orbits (see section on eye trauma).

(continued)

Nursing Care Plan 53–2 (Continued)

Care of the Perioperative Patient (Cataract, Retinal, Glaucoma, Corneal Procedures)

Nursing Interventions	Rationale	Expected Outcomes
3. Discuss need for wearing metal shield or glasses when ordered.	3. Metal shield or glasses protect the eye from injury.	• No injury occurs to eye.
4. Apply *no* pressure to the traumatized eye.	4. Pressure on the eye could result in serious further damage.	
5. Use proper procedure to administer eye medications.	5. Injury may result if the medication container is allowed to touch the eye.	

Nursing Diagnosis: Potential for complications related to surgical intervention.

Goal: Complications will be avoided or reported promptly to the physician.

Nursing Interventions	Rationale	Expected Outcomes
1. Maintain rigorous aseptic technique; perform frequent handwashing.	1. Will minimize risk of infection.	• No signs of infection.
2. Observe for and report immediately to the physician signs and symptoms of complications, ie, hemorrhage; increased IOP—sudden brow pain; infection—redness, edema, purulent drainage; pain not relieved by prescribed medication; light flashes; changes or decrease in visual function; changes in eye structure—iris prolapse, pear-shaped pupil, wound dehiscence; adverse reactions to medications.	2. Early recognition of complications may reduce the risk of permanent visual loss.	• Signs and symptoms of complications are recognized early and reported immediately. • Required position is maintained. • Activity limitations are observed. • Avoids restricted actions. • Demonstrates proper technique for administration of eye medications
3. Explain prescribed position.	3. Head elevation and avoiding lying on the operative side will decrease amount of edema. Maintaining the prescribed position when a gas bubble has been placed in the vitreous body will promote retinal reattachment and reduce the risk of cataract formation or corneal endothelial damage.	
4. Instruct the patient regarding activity limitations—bed rest, with bathroom privileges; increase in activities gradually as tolerated.	4. Activity limitations may be prescribed to facilitate healing and avoid further damage to the eye or injury.	
5. Explain actions to be avoided, as prescribed—coughing, sneezing, vomiting (request medication for), bending, excessive straining at defecation, lifting heavy objects (more than 20 pounds), squeezing eyes shut, rubbing eyes, fast jerky head motions.	5. May produce complications such as vitreal prolapse or wound dehiscence due to increased wound tension on very fine sutures.	
6. Administer medications as prescribed, following prescribed technique.	6. Medications administered other than as prescribed may compromise healing or cause complications. If the container is allowed to touch the eye, there is an increased risk for infection from the contaminated medication.	

(continued)

Nursing Care Plan 53-2 *(Continued)*

Care of the Perioperative Patient (Cataract, Retinal, Glaucoma, Corneal Procedures)

Nursing Interventions	Rationale	Expected Outcomes

Nursing Diagnosis: Pain related to trauma, increased IOP, surgical intervention, or instillation of dilating drops.

Goal: Reduction of pain and IOP.

1. Administer medications for pain and IOP control as prescribed.	1. Use of prescribed medication relieves pain and IOP and increases comfort.	• Verbalizes that pain and IOP are reduced.
2. Apply cold compresses as ordered for blunt trauma.	2. Decrease in edema reduces pain.	• Edema relieved.
3. Reduce light levels; light dimmed, shades/drapes drawn.	3. Lower light levels may be more comfortable after surgery.	• Verbalizes increase in comfort.
4. Encourage use of dark glasses in strong light.	4. Strong light causes discomfort after the use of dilating drops.	• Wears dark glasses after instilling dilating drops.

Nursing Diagnosis: Potential for self-care deficit related to altered visual status.

Goal: Adjustment to altered visual status.

1. Instruct patient and significant other regarding signs and symptoms of complications to be reported immediately to the physician.	1. Early recognition and treatment of complications may reduce the risk for further damage.	• Verbalizes signs and symptoms to be reported.
2. Provide verbal and written instructions for patient and significant other on proper technique to administer medications. Discuss indications for use of medication as well as normal and abnormal responses. Suggest methods for identifying containers (red top, green label).	2. Use of proper technique will reduce the risk of infection and injury to the eye. Knowledge of normal drug responses may increase compliance. Knowledge of abnormal responses will help in decision regarding reportable changes. Written instructions are used for enforcement after discharge.	• Patient and significant other verbalize or demonstrate understanding of correct technique for administering medications and the normal and abnormal drug responses. • Identifies needs for assistance. • Appropriate referrals made.
3. Evaluate need for assistance after discharge. Ascertain availability of help by significant others or arrange for appropriate referrals.	3. Resources are available for home health, escort, and companion services.	

---

of the retina containing the rods and cones, is detached from the nourishing retinal pigment epithelial layer, these photosensitive cells cannot perform their visual function, and loss of sight results. Retinal detachment may be caused by congenital malformations, metabolic disorders, vascular disease, intraocular inflammation, neoplasms, trauma, or degenerative changes in the vitreous or retina. Most commonly, they are caused by the mechanical forces associated with posterior vitreous detachment and retinal tear formation. Retinal holes, which affect 5% to 13% of the population, and lattice degeneration, which is present in about 8% of the population, are asymptomatic retinal degenerative defects that require periodic examinations because they predispose to retinal detachment.

Inflammatory detachments are usually treated medically. Some exudative or serous retinal detachments (which are due to an associated process such as a tumor or inflammation that produces subretinal fluid without a retinal break) respond to laser photocoagulation. Diabetic traction or post-traumatic traction retinal detachments may require vitreous surgery to relieve the tractional forces. Radiation therapy may be of benefit in treating retinal detachments associated with intraocular tumors.

Rhegmatogenous (tear-induced) detachments are the most common detachments, with an incidence of 1:10,000 of the population each year, primarily in the 40- to 70-year-old age group. There is a male preponderance thought to be related to trauma. Predisposing conditions include high myopia (nearsightedness), lattice degeneration, aphakia (surgical removal of part or all of the crystalline lens), and trauma. Degenerative changes (liquefaction) in the vitreous, causing traction on the retina, are often responsible for these retinal tears.

The vitreous body is a meshwork of collagen fibers filled with hyaluronic acid and water, and it is attached to the inner retinal surface. Although the vitreous is originally gelatinous in consistency, the hyaluronic acid concentration decreases with age, and the vitreous becomes more liquefied. As this occurs, the individual often notices a few clear floaters, a normal finding. This liquefaction process deprives the collagen fibers of their support and causes them to collapse and move forward. When the vitreous collapses, it usually separates easily from the posterior retina, but in some cases the vitreous is adherent to a portion of the posterior retina and pulls on the retina as it collapses, causing a tear.

If left untreated, rhegmatogenous detachments usually become total and may progress to retinal atrophy, secondary cataract formation, chronic uveitis, hypotony, and phthisis bulbi (atrophy of the eyeball with blindness).

Assessment and Clinical Manifestations.   The patient usually presents with a history of floaters or flashing lights or both. The floaters may be perceived as tiny dark spots or cobwebs. These floating particles consist of retinal cells and blood that are released at the time of the tear and cast shadows on the retina as they drift by (Fig. 53-13). Later the patient may notice a spreading shadow or curtain moving across the field of vision, resulting in blurred vision and loss of visual field. Decreased central acuity or loss of central vision indicates that the macula is involved.

A patient with suspected retinal detachment is urgently referred to a retinal specialist. The pupil is dilated and the fundus is examined with an indirect ophthalmoscope and a hand-held condensing lens. This method of examination provides a wide field of view so that the entire retina may be examined and all tears identified.

Surgical Management.   Patients with a confirmed diagnosis of retinal detachment are usually admitted to the hospital the same day. Depending on the extent or location of the retinal detachment, the patient may require emergency surgery or ocular rest in preparation for surgery. Ocular rest includes bilateral eye patching and bed rest and is instituted to facilitate settling of the retina and to prevent the detachment from spreading. The affected eye is maximally dilated before surgery to permit adequate visualization of the fundus.

Scleral buckling is the primary surgical procedure performed to reattach the retina. Transscleral cryotherapy is applied around each retinal tear, producing a chorioretinal adhesion that seals the break so that liquid vitreous can no longer pass through into the subretinal space. A piece, or pieces, of silicone (the buckle) are sutured and infolded into the sclera, physically indenting, or buckling, the sclera, choroid, and retinal pigment epithelium toward the retina, supporting the breaks.

When the retina is thus brought into contact with the underlying tissue, normal physiologic function is restored. Often, external drainage of subretinal fluid is necessary to bring the detached retina closer to the buckled area so that the retina can be reattached.

During surgery it may be necessary to inject inert gas (*e.g.*, sulfahexafluoride SF6, octofluroptopane C3F8, or air bubble) into the vitreous body to maintain IOP or to assist in the flattening of the retina. Depending on which gas is used, the bubble will be reabsorbed and replaced by aqueous fluid in 3 days to 2 months.

Some 90% to 95% of retinal detachments can be reattached and achieve good visual acuity with scleral buckling, although more than one procedure may be needed. Full visual recovery may not be achieved, even with successful reattachment, in patients with chronic retinal detachments or those in which the macula is involved. Detachments that cannot be reattached by scleral buckling may require vitreous surgery.

Postoperative Management.   Postoperative activity may be restricted to bed rest with bathroom privileges. If the patient's eyes are bilaterally patched, or if vision in the unaffected eye is low, he requires assistance when out of bed to prevent falls and jarring. If there is a gas bubble in the eye, it is important that the prescribed position be maintained so that the gas effectively tamponades the retinal break. It is also important that the patient not assume a flat supine position for any length of time because the gas bubble would rise and push the iris forward, causing acute glaucoma in aphakic patients (those who have had the crystalline lens removed). In other patients, the bubble would rest against the crystalline lens, causing cataract formation. Pupillary dilation is maintained to facilitate postoperative examination. Often the eyelashes are trimmed in the operating room; the nurse can assure the patient that they will grow back in about 6 to 8 weeks.

Early possible complications after retinal surgery include increased IOP, glaucoma, infection, choroidal detachment, failure of the retina to reattach, or redetachment of the retina. The nurse monitors the patient for the following signs and symptoms, which are reported to the physician: pain that does not respond to medication, purulent or excessive mucoid drainage, severe nausea and vomiting, redness, swelling, cloudy vision, halos around lights, or any symptoms of retinal detachment.

Late complications include infection, extrusion of the

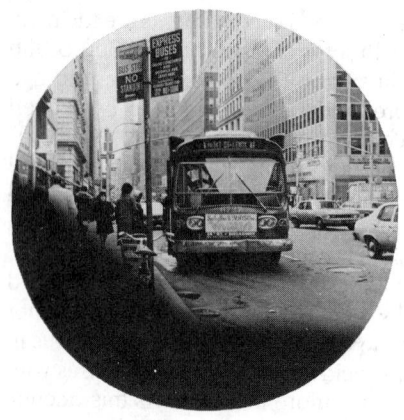

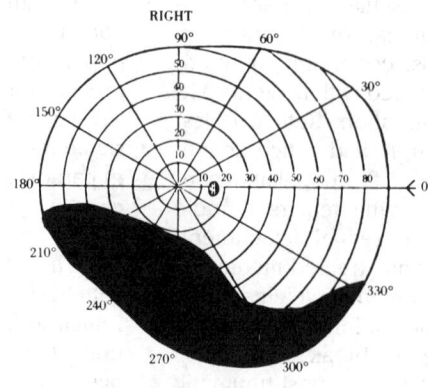

Figure 53-13. Retinal detachment causes a field of vision defect. Detachments are most often superior so the shadow or defect is perceived as inferior. (Photo courtesy of The Lighthouse, The New York Association for the Blind.)

buckling material through the conjunctiva or erosion though the globe, proliferative vitreoretinopathy (scar tissue formation involving the retina), diplopia, refractive errors, or astigmatism.

Infectious Endophthalmitis

Infectious endophthalmitis is an abscess of the vitreous body. It may occur as a result of endogenous infection, such as emboli from endocarditis, or exogenous seeding from penetrating injuries or surgery. The patient may present with complaints of eye pain and loss of vision. Clouding of the normally transparent structures of the eye may be seen. Treatment may include intraocular injection of antibiotics and vitrectomy.

Surgical Management.   *Vitrectomy* is the surgical procedure performed to remove part or all of the vitreous gel. Indications for this surgical intervention, in addition to infectious endophthalmitis, include unresolved hemorrhage, traction and giant retinal detachment, failure of the retina to reattach after scleral buckling, epiretinal membranes, diabetic retinopathy, penetrating injury, and intraocular foreign body.

After removal of the vitreous gel, fluid, air, inert gas, or silicone oil is used to replace the vitreous. The postoperative considerations and management are similar to those for scleral buckling.

Diabetic Retinopathy

Diabetic retinopathy is a frequent complication of diabetes mellitus and is caused by damage to or occlusion of the blood vessels that nourish the retina as a result of inadequate blood glucose control. Weakened vessels become hyperpermeable and leak, causing microhemorrhages, retinal swelling, or exudative deposits. Progressive retinal ischemia stimulates the formation of new vessels (neovascularization), which may proliferate on the vitreal surface. These new vessels are fragile and may rupture, causing hemorrhage into the vitreous body. Also, they may form fibrovascular bands that contract, resulting in traction retinal detachment.

If fluid collects in the macula, central vision blurring is noted. Vitreous hemorrhage results in cloudy or hazy vision of sudden onset. Most people with diabetic retinopathy eventually develop visual problems. Diabetic retinopathy is the leading cause of new blindness among adults in the United States.

In some self-limiting cases, treatment is not indicated; in most cases, however, laser surgery is useful. The intense beam of laser light is used to seal off leaking blood vessels and destroy abnormal new ones. If there is vitreous hemorrhage or traction detachment of the retina, vitrectomy may be required to remove the bloody vitreous, release the traction, or remove membranes.

The risk of developing diabetic retinopathy is greater for patients who have had diabetes for a long time. Diabetics should be made aware of this risk and encouraged to comply with their diets, medications, and exercise regimens in an effort to control blood glucose levels and hypertension. They also should be directed to seek regular eye examinations because the ophthalmologist may detect signs of diabetic retinopathy long before symptoms are evident to the patient. Early diagnosis and treatment by a retinal specialist can greatly reduce the risk of severe visual loss. For additional discussion of diabetic retinopathy see pages 1057–1060.

Age-Related Macular Degeneration

Age-related macular degeneration is a condition that results in the progressive loss of central vision, often leading to legal blindness. It is caused by damage to or deterioration of the photoreceptor cells in the area of the macula. It is probably hereditary.

Age-related macular degeneration is the leading cause of severe visual loss for people over 65 years of age. There are approximately 165,000 new cases in the United States each year. About one third of the people over the age of 50 have some degree of macular degeneration. If the fovea is damaged, the symptoms include distortion or blurring of central vision, loss of contrast sensitivity, increased glare, dimming of color vision, and even total loss of central vision.

There is no treatment available for most types of macular degeneration, but in a few cases early diagnosis and laser treatment may stabilize or improve the condition. Magnifying devices, high-contrast print, and strong illumination may be helpful.

Retinitis Pigmentosa

Retinitis pigmentosa refers to a group of familial disorders characterized by progressive visual field loss and night blindness due to degeneration of the retina. Onset usually occurs in youth or young adulthood, although it can be seen at any age. The disease course typically is 30 to 40 years or more from onset and results in total or near-total loss of vision at age 60 or 70.

Patients should be followed closely by the ophthalmologist because other treatable diseases, such as glaucoma, may develop. Genetic counseling should be obtained to determine the risk factors to other family members or future offspring. Low vision aids are usually indicated. These are discussed in the section on low vision and blindness (see pp. 1583–1585).

Defective Color Vision

Defective color vision (color blindness) is usually a hereditary disorder. Normally there are three types of cones in the retina: red, green, and blue. They all work together to help us perceive a wide range of colors. In 8% of men and 0.4% of women, however, there is an abnormal gene that may slightly alter or completely eliminate one, two, or all three types of cones. Red-green defects are the most common. Persons with these defects are insensitive to deep red light and confuse shades of red, green, and yellow. Because the choice of occupation may depend on the ability to correctly perceive color, testing should be done at an early age.

Defective color vision may also be acquired. It can be caused by retinal disease, poisoning, some medications, or aging. Persons with acquired defective color vision should be referred to an ophthalmologist for diagnosis and management of the causative disorder.

In summary, conditions of the adult retina and vitreous body include retinal detachment, infections endophthalmitis, diabetic retinopathy, age-related macular degeneration, retinitis pigmentosa, and defective color vision.

Retinal detachment is the separation of the neurosensory retina from its underlying pigmented epithelial layer. Rhegmatogenous detachments (tear-induced) are the most common type of detachment. The retinal tear allows liquid vitreous to enter the subretinal space causing separation of the retinal layers. Surgery is required to repair the defect.

Scleral buckling is the primary surgical procedure performed to reattach the retina. Activity may be limited postoperatively to insure settling of the retina. After instillation of inert gas, it is important that the prescribed position be maintained to facilitate effective tamponade of the retinal break by the gas bubble. The nurse should be alert to pain, drainage, nausea and vomiting, cloudy vision, or halos, which are symptoms of retinal detachment.

Diabetic retinopathy, a frequent complication of diabetes mellitus, is a disorder of the retinal blood vessels. Progressive retinal ischemia stimulates the formation of new vessels, which are fragile and may rupture, causing hemorrhage into the vitreous body. Most people with diabetic retinopathy develop visual problems; therefore, persons with diabetes should be encouraged to have regular eye examinations.

Age-related macular degeneration is a condition that is caused by damage to or deterioration of the photoreceptor cells in the area of the macula. It is the leading cause of severe visual loss of people older than 65 years. No treatment is available for most types of macular degeneration.

Retinitis pigmentosa is a group of rare conditions that are familial and caused by degeneration of the retina. It is characterized by progressive visual field loss as the cones become involved and night blindness results. There is no treatment available at this time.

Defective color vision is usually a hereditary disorder. It is an abnormal condition characterized by an inability to clearly distinguish colors of the spectrum. Red-green defects are the most common. The patient should be referred to an ophthalmologist for diagnosis and management.

Ocular Trauma

Trauma is a common cause of unilateral visual loss in young people. It is often a result of accidents in and around the home, battery explosions, auto accidents, or sports injuries. Examination of the injured eye should proceed with great caution to avoid further injury.

Assessment and Clinical Manifestations

When evaluating a patient with ocular trauma, the first priority is to obtain a history of the mechanism of injury and associated visual changes. This is followed by evaluation and documentation of visual acuity and mobility of both eyes and a visual inspection of the outer structures.

Inspection of the outer structures of the eyes that discloses relatively minor damage does not preclude the possibility of severe injury. The eyelids are thin, and a laceration of the lid could also involve the cornea or sclera. A small painless wound in the lid may be the only external evidence of a penetrating injury with an intraocular foreign body. The force sufficient to cause the lid hemorrhage of a "black eye" may also cause intraocular bleeding, retinal detachment, or rupture of the globe.

Whenever there is reason to suspect laceration, penetrating injury, or rupture of the globe, either by the mechanism of injury or the evidence of external trauma, *no pressure* should ever be directed on the eye. Such pressure could cause extrusion of intraocular contents and irreparable damage. Separation of the lids can be safely accomplished by resting the thumb and forefinger against the upper and lower orbital margins. In addition, the patient should be warned not to squeeze the lids shut.

Signs of possible severe injury to the globe include:

Pain (although small penetrating wounds may be painless)
Subconjunctival hemorrhage
Conjunctival laceration
Enophthalmia (abnormal displacement of the eye backward due to loss of contents or orbital fracture)
Iris defect
Pupil displacement; may be caused by anterior chamber collapse
Hyphema (blood in the anterior chamber)
Lowered IOP (soft eye)—*do not palpate the eye*
Extrusion of ocular contents (iris, lens, vitreous, retina)
Hypopyon (purulent material in the anterior chamber)—a late sign of trauma

If severe injury of the globe is suspected, further manipulation of the eye is avoided until the time of surgery. A light dressing is applied (*no pressure*), and a metal shield that rests on the orbital bones is taped from the forehead to the cheek. If there is a protruding foreign body, only the shield is applied. Bilateral patching may be helpful because movement of the eyes should be kept to a minimum. Parenteral antibiotics are initiated and analgesics, antiemetics, and tetanus antitoxin are administered as prescribed.

When rupture of the globe is ruled out, examination of the other structures of the eye can be accomplished. Laceration of the lids may require simple suturing, antibiotic ointment, and a dressing. Depending on the extent and involvement of other structures, surgery may be required.

Patients with foreign bodies of the conjunctiva may present with a foreign body sensation, especially with lid movement, profuse tearing, and conjunctival injection (redness). The inner surface of the lower lid should be inspected and the upper lid should be everted and examined. Nonpenetrating foreign bodies under the upper lid may be removed by lifting the upper lid over the lower lid, which allows the lashes of the lower lid to brush the object off the inside of the upper lid.

Alternatively, the object may be removed by irrigation; care is used to avoid touching the cornea. If the foreign body cannot be removed in this fashion, the eye should be closed and patched and the patient referred to an ophthalmologist. One of the dangers of a conjunctival foreign body is the threat of damage to the cornea.

Corneal Abrasions

Corneal abrasions are common ocular injuries in which epithelial cells are lost. Abrasions can be caused by scratches from objects such as a mascara brush, twig, or fingernail. They also may be a result of a foreign body, or overworn contact lenses. The patient presents with sudden onset of pain, which is often intense, photophobia, foreign body sensation, and tearing. Visual acuity may be normal or decreased, depending on the site of the lesion.

Topical anesthetics are used only during the initial treatment because their prolonged use causes delay in healing and can mask further damage that could lead to permanent corneal scarring. The use of steroids is also avoided. Topical antibiotics are prescribed prophylactically, and a short-acting cycloplegic is administered topically to alleviate pain. A pressure eye patch is used to immobilize the lids and promote comfort and healing. Patching of the other eye and bed rest for 24 hours may be indicated for extensive abrasions. If the underlying layers of the cornea are not involved, healing occurs without scarring, usually within 24 to 48 hours.

Superficial foreign bodies of the cornea may only require irrigation to remove them. Embedded foreign bodies require the attention of an ophthalmologist. Fluorescein staining is often used to outline superficial epithelial defects. A topical anesthetic is given before the removal of the foreign body, which is accomplished with an instrument. A cotton-tipped applicator is not used because it rubs off too large an area of epithelium. Deeply embedded materials may require surgery.

When the corneal epithelium, which is a natural barrier to microorganisms, is compromised, the eye is vulnerable to infection. A corneal wound, therefore, should be inspected daily for evidence of infection until it has healed completely.

Chemical Burns

Chemical burns to the conjunctiva or cornea should be irrigated with copious amounts of physiologic solution or water immediately. The easiest and quickest way to flush the eye is to have the patient hold his head under a faucet and allow the water to run over the eye and wash it out. It is often more satisfactory, however, to flush the eye with a syringe, if available, taking care not to contaminate the other eye if it has not already been contaminated. Continuous flushing for at least 15 minutes is desirable. Plain tap water is adequate under such circumstances. The use of topical anesthetic drops before irrigation relieves pain. A lid speculum and standard IV tubing and solution are used for irrigation. Neutralizing agents are avoided because the heat from their reaction with the chemical could cause further injury. If the irritant is alkaline, irrigation should continue for at least 1 hour; these substances remain in the tissues longer than acids and continue to cause additional damage for hours after exposure.

After irrigation, the eye is dilated and antibiotics are instilled as prescribed. Collagenase inhibitors such as acetylcysteine (Mucomyst) or sodium edetate (EDTA) are prescribed to treat severe alkali burns. A soft contact lens may be used as a bandage lens to facilitate healing and decrease the abrasive effect of blinking. This is not removed for the instillation of medications. Persistent pain may be an indication to discontinue the use of the contact lens. Bilateral eye patching may provide the patient with more comfort than patching of the affected eye alone because both eyes move together; however, this advantage needs to be weighed against the disadvantage of the loss of vision. Patients with chemical burns are followed by an ophthalmologist because of the possibility of complications such as infection and corneal perforation.

Ocular Emergencies

The following is a list of ocular emergencies. Patients with these conditions should be seen immediately by an ophthalmologist. A few hours' delay in treatment may lead to permanent damage.

Trauma
 Corneal abrasions and foreign bodies
 Lacerations of the eyewall
 Intraocular foreign bodies
 Rupture of the globe
Corneal ulcer/infection
Severe conjunctivitis
Orbital cellulitis
Chemical burns
Acute iritis
Acute glaucoma
Occlusion of the central retinal artery
Retinal detachment
Endophthalmitis

Those conditions that should receive treatment as soon as possible but in which a delay of a few days may not be an immediate threat to sight, include:

Chronic glaucoma
Vitreous hemorrhage
Unilateral exophthalmos of recent origin
Acute dacryocystitis
Ocular tumors
Optic nerve disorders

Enucleation

Enucleation is the complete surgical removal of the eyeball. Indications for this procedure are blindness after penetrating injury, blindness with recalcitrant (stubbornly resistant) infection, painful blind eyes that are unresponsive to medical treatment, and selected tumors of the eye. The procedure is accomplished by incising the conjunctiva, disinserting the extraocular muscles, severing the optic nerve, and removing the eye. The muscles are then reapproximated over a ball implant that maintains the volume of the orbit. The conjunctiva is closed and a plastic conformer is positioned to maintain the fornices of the conjunctival sac during healing. Later the patient will be referred to an ocularist for removal of the conformer, prosthesis fitting, and training in its use.

Postoperatively, antibiotic and steroid ointments may be prescribed. A pressure dressing is often used to control swelling; ice compresses may be used. Mucous that collects over the surface of the conformer may require gentle irrigation. The eyelids are to be kept clean. Complications of surgery include hemorrhage, infection, and extrusion of the implant.

Patients requiring an enucleation require considerable emotional and psychological support. Because they no longer have binocular vision, they also need assistance in relearning how to judge distances with the remaining eye (monocular vision) and how to move forward with a panning motion (move from right to left scanning the panorama) so that they can see around them.

Low Vision and Blindness

The term *legally blind* is used to refer to those persons whose best visual acuity (with glasses, if needed) is 20/200 or worse in the better eye or whose visual field is restricted to 20 degrees. Many of these people have some useful vision, so the term *blind* can be misleading. Each individual requires assessment to determine if he has any functional vision and, if so, how much.

Low vision and *partially sighted* are terms used to describe visual impairment that cannot be corrected with ordinary eyeglasses, contact lenses, or intraocular implants. It may be a result of birth defects, inherited diseases, glaucoma, cataract, macular degeneration, retinal detachment, or aging. It is estimated that 11.4 million people in the United States have some type of visual impairment. Of these, approximately 1.4 million have a vision loss that interferes with normal living. More than one million of these 1.4 million are visually impaired rather than totally blind.

Low vision treatment should be started at whatever stage the patient experiences difficulty with customary visual tasks. The responsibility of health care providers, however, does not end with the diagnosis, prevention, and treatment of the ocular disorder that results in visual impairment, irreversible progressive visual loss, or blindness. Despite this sensory loss, patients can live meaningful and rewarding lives, but it is important that they receive early referral for rehabilitation, counseling, or financial assistance. It is therefore important for health care providers to know what referral sources are available and how to use them. Individuals and agencies with expertise in the area of low vision treatment include:

Low vision specialist in ophthalmology
Local State Commission for the Blind and Visually Impaired
Low vision clinics
American Foundation for the Blind
National Association for Visually Handicapped
National Center for Vision and Aging, *The Lighthouse*
National Federation of the Blind

Low vision services are designed to enable the person to lead as normal a life as possible. They can include:

Assessment of visual condition
Clinical examination
Orientation and mobility training
Employment and financial consultation
Educational, vocational, and psychological counseling
Vocational rehabilitation
Adaptive training skills for independent living
Special education
Support groups
Training in the use of low vision aids

The low vision aids that follow are designed to make the most of the available vision (those in italics can also be used by persons who are blind):

Magnifying eye glasses
Hand and stand magnifiers
Telescopes
Large-print books, newspapers, and magazines
Talking books
Braille
Closed-circuit TV—produces highly magnified image
Tactually marked watches and clocks
Tactually modified table top games
Enlarged telephone dials

Kitchen implements, tools, medication devices
Talking clocks, timers, scales, calculators, and computers
Text scanner—converts text to audio mode or braille
Speech synthesizer
Flashlight eye sonar devices
Canes, including laser canes
Seeing eye dogs

Many of the devices for the visually handicapped are expensive.

In addition to low vision devices, adequate lighting is imperative. For greatest visibility, the light source should be close to the work. High-intensity lights with adjustable arms work well for this purpose.

Blindness, which is the absence of any functional vision, may be caused by trachoma, diabetic retinopathy, cataract, glaucoma, injury, leprosy, or xerophthalmia. Many of the low vision aids can be used by those who are blind.

When a patient has marked visual impairment or is newly blind, he needs a great deal of help in making a healthy adjustment. For the most part, this help is entrusted to those skilled in such rehabilitation. The nurse, however, can follow certain practices when caring for such a patient.

The nurse recognizes that there are stages through which this person moves:

1. Denial—Do not discredit this phase of the sightless person's experience, because it is a normal response to loss.
2. Value changes—adapting to aids that he thought he would never use
3. Independence–dependence conflict—attempting to accept his condition without becoming completely dependent
4. Coping with stigma—This person must cope with the unfortunate stigma that is so prevalent among the sighted toward the sightless, such as the belief that they are helpless, unemployable, completely dependent, or depressed.
5. Learning to communicate in social settings without visual cues

The major goals for the patient are to adjust to the sightless or nearly sightless condition:

1. Adaptation to the use of auxiliary aids
2. Acceptance of his new condition without becoming completely dependent
3. Continuing with physical self-care
4. Coping with the social climate and stigmata that are prevalent
5. Learning to communicate without visual cues
6. Adherence to the prescribed therapeutic regimen

Nursing Interventions

The nurse is able to assist the patient in several ways: (1) patient teaching, (2) patient support, (3) patient care, and (4) collaboration with the physician.

By monitoring what the physician has told the patient about the diagnosis, anticipated treatment, and prognosis, the nurse is able to reinforce this information, answer questions, provide support, and relay to the ophthalmologist the reaction of the patient and his family. If information is withheld, such as little hope for recovery of vision, this interferes with the patient's adjustment and rehabilitation. The nurse is often helpful in determining when the time is right for conveying such information. Fears are to be described because they can unearth misinformation. Frequently, self-imposed limitations are more restricting than physical disabilities. Attitudes and beliefs of the nurse can have a direct or indirect effect on the patient. A positive attitude by those who care for patients affects the patient's self-esteem and body image in a beneficial way.

A blind person should always be treated with the dignity accorded any other person. Expressions of pity are to be avoided. Ensuring that the patient has someone with whom he can talk and that he has diversional activities can be helpful. He can be helped to gain self-confidence as he performs simple activities.

If he is allowed out of bed, the blind person should survey his room by walking around and touching the furniture. Thereafter, the nurse should be sure that the furniture remains in the same position. A door should not be left half open; it should be either open or shut. When walking with a blind person, the patient follows the nurse by lightly touching the nurse's elbow. When the patient walks alone, he should learn to use a lightweight walking stick to warn him of obstacles.

Personal appearance is a significant part of the patient's care. He should be encouraged to dress by himself; a woman can learn to fix her hair and use cosmetics. Activities such as table etiquette and writing can be acquired with practice.

Familiarity with resources that are available to help the patient is a nursing responsibility. When a patient is declared legally blind, he should be referred to the state blindness agency. A directory of agencies serving the visually handicapped in the United States is available from the American Foundation for the Blind. In most states, the only way to obtain rehabilitation training is through a state agency for the blind.

Interesting and effective aids are devices that "talk," such as clocks, calculators, thermometers, and scales. There also is an optical scanner that when passed over lines of text in a book sends signals to a computer (programmed to recognize letters) that turns them into words and pronounces them. Another similar device scans words and records the shape of letters, which are then converted into vibrations felt by the fingertips of the user.

Technology continues to provide devices that are becoming available and useful in expanding the world of those with limited vision.

Preventive Eye Care

The nurse, as an important member of the health care team, and as a teacher and a practitioner of sound health habits, can provide education in eye care, eye safety, and the prevention of eye disease. The nurse can help people to learn how to prevent cross-contamination or spread of infectious diseases to others through the practice of good hygiene. The nurse can encourage people to have periodic eye examinations and can recommend ways to prevent eye injury.

When and how often a person's eyes should be examined depends on the person's age, risk factors for pathology, and the presence of ocular symptoms. Individuals with ocular symptoms should have immediate eye examination. Those without symptoms, but who are at high risk of having ocular disease, should have periodic eye examinations. Patients taking medications that can affect the eyes, such as corticosteroids, hydroxychloroquine sulfate, thioridazine HCl, or amiodarone

should also be examined regularly. All others should have a routine glaucoma evaluation at age 35 and periodic re-evaluations every 2 to 5 years.

Ocular signs and symptoms requiring examination at any age include:

Loss, dimness, or distortion of vision
Double vision
Pain in or around the eyes
Swelling of the eyelids or protrusion of the eye
Excessive tearing or discharge from the eyes
Floaters or flashes of light
Halos around lights
Sudden crossing or deviation of the eye
Change in the color of the iris

Risk factors for ocular disease and frequency of examination include:

Diabetes—at diagnosis and annually thereafter
Family history of glaucoma, cataracts, retinal detachments, or other hereditary or familial eye conditions—annually
Hypertension: at diagnosis and annually thereafter
Age 65 years or more—every 2 years

It is estimated that 90% of all eye injuries are preventable. Recommendations of the American Academy of Ophthalmology for prevention of eye injuries are presented in Table 53-3. These are important for people of all ages.

In summary, safety precautions are the best prevention for ocular trauma, since trauma is often the result of accidents. Once injury is suspected, it is imperative *not* to apply pressure to the eye globe. Inspection of the outer structures of the eye may indicate a minor injury; however, this should be treated as a serious injury until severe ocular injury can be excluded.

Corneal abrasions in which epithelial cells are lost are common ocular injuries. After initial treatment of the corneal abrasion, the eye should continually be assessed for infection.

Chemical burns are a true ocular emergency and the eyes should be immediately flushed with copious amount of water or irrigating solution such as normal saline. Visual acuity should be checked after no less than 20 minutes of continuous irrigation. Complaints of pain should be monitored by the nurse and reported to the physician. The use of topical anesthetics are contraindicated because they interfere with healing.

Enucleation is the complete surgical removal of the eyeball. A pressure dressing is applied postoperatively for 24 to 48 hours to help reduce the swelling. Ice compresses also may be used to decrease the swelling. A long-term complication of enucleation may be a sunken orbit, which can be managed by the ocularist or reconstructive surgery. Patients undergoing enucleation require considerable emotional and psychological support.

Legally blind refers to visual acuity (with glasses) that is 20/200 or worse in the better eye, or when the visual field is restricted to a 20-degree diameter. Low vision or partially sighted refers to visual impairment that cannot be corrected by framed or contact lenses. Low vision treatment should be initiated when the patient experiences problems in his daily life. It is vital that the patient be referred to appropriate health care providers and agencies that will help with the adjustment needed for the patient to live as normal a life as possible.

Prevention continues to remain the primary measure in

TABLE 53–3. *Guidelines for Preventing Eye Injuries*

IN AND AROUND THE HOUSE

Make sure that all spray nozzles are directed away from you before you press down on the handle.

Read instructions carefully before using cleaning fluids, detergents, ammonia, or harsh chemicals. Wash hands thoroughly after use.

Use grease shields on fry pans to decrease spattering.

Wear special goggles to shield your eyes from fumes and splashes when using powerful chemicals.

When opening carbonated beverage containers (*e.g.*, soda bottle, champagne bottle) direct them away from yourself and others.

IN THE WORKSHOP

Protect yourself from flying fragments, fumes, dust particles, sparks, and splashed chemicals by wearing safety glasses.

Read instructions thoroughly for tools and chemicals you are using and observe precautions for their use.

AROUND CHILDREN

Pay attention to age and responsibility level of a child when selecting toys and games. Avoid projectile toys such as darts and pellet guns.

Teach children the correct way to handle potentially dangerous items such as scissors and pencils, and supervise their play.

IN THE GARDEN

Do not let anyone stand on the side or in front of a moving lawn mower.

Pick up rocks and stones before going over them with the lawn mower. These stones can hurl out of the rotary blades and rebound off curbs or walls, causing severe injury to the eye.

Make sure that pesticide spray can nozzles are directed away from your face.

Avoid low-hanging branches.

AROUND THE CAR

Before opening the hood of the car, put out all smoking materials and matches. Use a flashlight, not a match or lighter, to illuminate the battery at night.

Wear goggles when grinding metal, or striking metal against metal while performing auto body repair.

When using jumper cables to start the car, wear goggles; make sure the cars are not touching one another; make sure the jumper cable clamps never touch each other; never lean over the battery when attaching cables. *Never* attach a cable to the negative terminal of the dead battery.

IN SPORTS

Wear protective safety glasses, especially for sports such as racquetball, squash, tennis, baseball, and basketball.

Wear protective caps, helmets, or face protectors when appropriate, especially for sports such as ice hockey.

AROUND FIREWORKS

Wear eye glasses or safety goggles.

Do not use explosive fireworks.

Never allow children to ignite fireworks.

Do not stand near others when lighting fireworks.

Do not try to relight duds. Douse them in water.

IN BRIGHT SUNLIGHT

Wear 100% ultraviolet light-absorbing sunglasses, preferably with wraparound sides, and a wide-brimmed hat.

Use opaque goggles to avoid burns from sunlamps.

During eclipse of the sun, avoid looking directly at the sun.

(Reprinted with permission of the American Academy of Ophthalmology.)

---

reducing damage to the eye. As a teacher and practitioner of sound health habits, the nurse plays a major role in promoting eye care and safety.

Bibliography

Books

Benson WE. Retinal Detachment Diagnosis and Management, 2nd ed. Philadelphia, JB Lippincott, 1988.

Boyd-Monk H. Nursing Care of the Eye. East Norwalk, CT, Appleton & Lange, 1987.

Clayman HM (ed). Atlas of Contemporary Surgery. St Louis, CV Mosby, 1990.

Doxanas MT and Anderson RL. Clinical Orbital Anatomy. Baltimore, Williams & Wilkins, 1984.

Gittinger JW Jr. Manual of Clinical Problems in Ophthalmology. Boston, Little, Brown, 1988.

Gittinger JW Jr. Ophthalmology. Boston, Little, Brown, 1984.

Gruendemann BJ and Meeker MH. Alexander's Care of the Patient in Surgery, 6th ed. St Louis, CV Mosby, 1989.

Havener WH. Synopsis of Ophthalmology, 6th ed. St Louis, CV Mosby, 1984.

Heckenlively JR. Retinitis Pigmentosa. Philadelphia, JB Lippincott, 1988.

Hersh PS. Ophthalmic Surgical Procedures. Boston, Little, Brown, 1988.

Hilton GF et al. Retinal Detachment, 5th ed. San Francisco, American Academy of Ophthalmology, 1989.

Hoskins HD and Kass MA. Becker-Shaffer's Diagnosis and Therapy of the Glaucomas, 6th ed. St Louis, CV Mosby, 1989.

Jaffe NS (ed). Atlas of Ophthalmic Surgery. Philadelphia, JB Lippincott, 1990.

Jaffee NS et al. Cataract Surgery and Its Complications, 5th ed. St Louis, CV Mosby, 1990.

Kaufman HE (ed). The Cornea. New York, Churchill Livingstone, 1988.

Krupin T. Manual of Glaucoma. New York, Churchill Livingstone, 1988.

Mackety CJ. Perioperative Laser Nursing: A Practical Guide. Thorofare, NJ, Charles B Slack, 1984.

Roy FH. Ocular Syndromes and Systemic Diseases, 2nd ed. Philadelphia, WB Saunders, 1989.

Smith JF and Machazel DP. Ophthalmologic Nursing. Boston, Little, Brown, 1980.

Spoor TC (ed). Management of Ocular, Orbital, and Adnexal Trauma. New York, Raven Press, 1988.

Spoor TC (ed). Medical Management of Ocular Diseases. Thorofare, NJ, Charles B Slack, 1986.

Tuttle DW. Self-Esteem and Adjusting With Blindness. Springfield, IL, Charles C Thomas, 1984.

Vaughan D et al. General Ophthalmology. Norwalk, Appleton & Lange, 1989.

Walsh JB et al (eds). Physicians Desk Reference for Ophthalmology. Oradell, Med Economics Company Inc, 1990.

Yanoff M. Ocular Pathology: A Color Atlas. Philadelphia, JB Lippincott, 1988.

Yanoff M. Ocular Pathology, 3rd ed. Philadelphia, JB Lippincott, 1989.

Journals

Assessment

Bostater SS. Assessment tool for low vision patients. J Ophthalmic Nurs Technol 1986 Nov/Dec; 5(6):216–218.

Boyd-Monk H. The structure and function of the eye and its adnexa. J Ophthalmic Nurs Technol 1987 Sep/Oct; 6(5):176–183.

Garber N et al. Model eye for teaching application tonometry. J Ophthalmic Nurs Technol 1986 Nov/Dec; 5(6):214–215.

Gould D. The biology of aging: The special senses. Geriatr Nurs Home Care 1987 Feb; 7(2):15–19.

Hall PS and Wick BC. Simple procedures for comprehensive vision screening. J School Health 1988 Feb; 58(2):58–61.

Kallman H and Vernon MS. The aging eye. Postgrad Med 1987 Feb; 81(2):108–130.

Kosnik W et al. Visual changes in daily life throughout adulthood. J Gerontol 1988 Mar; 43(3):63–70.

Makes DJ. Photographic artifacts: Make the diagnosis and correct the problem. J Ophthalmic Nurs Technol 1987 Jan/Feb; 6(1):29–32.

Millette JM and Drascic EA. Vision in aging. J Ophthalmic Nurs Technol 1987 Nov/Dec; 6(6):234–237.

Pinholt EM et al. Functional assessment of the elderly. Arch Intern Med 1987 Mar; 147(3):484–488.

Sanderson D. Ocular screening. Canadian Nurs 1986 Feb; 82(2):19–20.

Walker ML. Growing old. AORN J 1986 Apr; 43(4):887–890.

Contact Lens

Arentsen JJ. A review of complications associated with soft contact lenses. J Ophthalmic Nurs Technol 1987 Nov/Dec; 6(6):230–233.

Childress CM et al. A review of contact lens induced giant papillary conjunctivitis. J Ophthalmic Nurs Technol 1988 Jan/Feb; 7(1):12–17.

Cotgreave JT et al. Part of your daily routine: Teaching good contact lens care. Prof Nurse 1989 Jun; 4(9):446–449.

Donzis P et al. Microbial contamination of contact lens care systems. Am J Ophthalmol 1987 Oct; 104(4):325–333.

Ficker L et al. Acanthamoeba keratitis occurring with disposable contact lens wear. Am J Ophthalmol 1989 Oct; 108(4):4532.

Goldstein J. Contact lens care products: Uses and actions of ingredients. J Ophthalmic Nurs Technol 1987 Mar/Apr; 6(2):70–72.

Grutzmacher RD. Ocular disease from wearing contact lens. Postgrad Med 1989 Sep; 86(4):90–100.

Insler M et al. Visual field constriction caused by colored contact lens. Arch Ophthalmol 1988 Dec; 106(12):1680–1682.

Kershner RM. Infectious corneal ulcer with overextended wearing of disposable contact lens. JAMA 1989 Jun; 261(24):3549–3550.

Kirn TF. As number of contact lens users increases, research seeks to determine risk factors: How best to prevent potential eye infections. JAMA 1987 Jul; 258(1):17–18.

Kirn TF. Contact lenses need tender, loving care, ophthalmologist warn, as infection may result. JAMA 1987 Jul; 258(1):18.

Koenig S et al. Acanthamolba keratitis associated with gas-permeable contact lens wear. Am J Ophthalmol 1987 Jun; 103(6):832.

Koidau-Tsiligianni A et al. Ulcerative keratitis associated with contact lens wear. Am J Ophthalmol 1989 Jul; 108(1):64–67.

MacRae S et al. Guidelines for safe contact lens wear. Am J Ophthalmol 1987 Jun; 103(6):832–833.

Mobley CL. New extended wear materials: A safer modality for patients. J Ophthalmic Nurs Technol 1988 Sep/Oct; 7(5):170–173.

Rakow PL. Bausch & Lomb Research Symposium Focuses on RGP Lenses. J Ophthalmic Nurs Technol 1987 Nov/Dec; 6(6):249–250.

Rakow PL. Bifocal contact lenses: Are they coming of age? J Opthalmic Nurs Technol 1986 Nov/Dec; 5(6):232–233.

Rakow PL. Breakthroughs in lens design and care. J Ophthalmic Nurs Technol 1988 Jan/Feb; 7(1):36–37.

Rakow PL. Disposable lenses: A Pandora's box? J Ophthalmic Nurs Technol 1988 Mar/Apr; 7(2):72–24.

Rakow PL. Giving credit where credit is due. J Ophthalmic Nurs Technol 1987 Jul/Aug; 6(4):159.

Rakow PL. Perspective on Contact Lenses. J Ophthalmic Nurs Technol 1987 Mar/Apr; 6(2):83–84.

Rakow PL. RGP Lenses: Proceed with caution: Rigid gas permeable. J Ophthalmic Nurs Technol 1988 May/Jun; 7(3):108–110.

Olson CM. Increasing use of contact lenses prompts issuing of infection-prevention guidelines. JAMA 1989 Jan; 261(3):343–344.

Poggio E et al. The incidence of ulcerative keratitis among users of daily-wear and extended-ware soft contact lenses. N Engl J Med 1989 Sep; 321(12):779–783.

Randolph SA. Contact lens survey implications for the occupational health nurse. AAOHN J 1987 Jan; 35(1):6–12.

Schein O et al. The relative risk of ulcerative keratitis among users of daily-wear and extended-wear contact lenses. N Engl J Med 1989 Sep; 321(12):773–778.

Smith RE and MacRae SM. Contact lenses convenience and complications. N Engl J Med 1989 Sep; 321(12):824–826.

To K. Artificial tears or lens cleaner. Am J Ophthalmol 1989 Nov; 108(5):610.

Tolbert M et al. Are your contact lenses as safe as you think? FDA Consum 1987 Apr; 21(3):16–19.

Udell IJ et al. Treatment of contact lens-associated corneal erosions. Am J Ophthalmol 1987 Sep; 104(3):306–307.

Cataracts

Andrews CL. Nursing care of the cataract patient in an ambulatory surgery center. Ophthalmic Nurs Forum 1987 Mar; 3(3):1–8.

Applegate WB et al. Impact of cataract surgery with lens implantation on vision and physical function in elderly patients. JAMA 1987 Feb; 257(8):1064–1066.

Balyeat HD. Cataracts surgical removal and lens implantation. Consultant 1986 Nov; 26(1):151–154.

Brady SE et al. Diagnosis and treatment of chronic postoperative bacterial endophthalmitis. J Ophthalmic Nurs Technol 1990 Jan/Feb; 9(1):22–26.

Brown B. Preoperative evaluation of cataract patients. J Ophthalmic Nurs Technol 1988 Nov/Dec; 7(6):204–208.

Capino D et al. The elderly patient with cataract. Hosp Pract 1987 Mar; 22(3):19–26.

Carner JA. Cataract care made plain. Am J Nurs 1987 May; 87(5):626–630.

Donnelly D. Instilling eyedrops: Difficulties experienced by patients following cataract surgery. J Adv Nurs 1987 Feb; 12(2):235–243.

Elam JT et al. Functional outcome one year following cataract surgery in elderly persons. J Gerontol Med Sci 1988 May; 43(5):122–126.

Frank A et al. ECCE with phacoemulsification and flexible IOL implantation: Extracapsular cataract extraction. J Ophthalmic Nurs Technol 1988 Mar/Apr; 7(2):62–67.

Gottsch D et al. Cataracts: Diagnosis and treatment. Hosp Med 1987 Apr; 23(4):21–29.

Hale E. Lifting the clouds of cataracts. FDA Consum 1990 Jan; 23(6):6–8.

Hutchinson BT. Cataracts. Harvard Medical School Health Lett 1988 Apr; 13(6):6–8.

Jampel HD et al. A computerized analysis of astigmatism after contract surgery. J Ophthalmic Nurs Technol 1987 May/Jun; 6(3):100–105.

Maltzman BA et al. Penlight Test for Glare Disability of Cataracts. J Ophthalmic Technol 1988 Jul/Aug; 7(4):137–139.

Rigler S. Personalizing "routine" cataract and IOL surgery: Intraocular lens. Todays OR Nurse 1987 Nov; 9(11):20–21, 44–46.

Sagaties MJ. Preparing patients for cataract surgery. Nursing 1987 Jun; 17(6):324.

Smith S. Day-care cataract surgery: The patient's perspective. J Ophthalmic Nurs Technol 1987 Mar/Apr; 6(2):50–56.

Sutherland A and Karlinsky H. Abrupt recognition of age-related physical changes in appearance following cataract surgery. J Am Geriatr Soc 1989 May; 37(5):117–119.

West K. ABCs of cataract surgery preparation: Assessment, briefing and counseling. J Ophthalmic Nurs Technol 1987 Jul/Aug; 6(4):156–158.

Zavon B et al. A surgical counseling plan for patients undergoing cataract surgery. J Ophthalmic Nurs Technol 1988 Mar/Apr; 7(2):68–71.

Cornea

Binder PS. Radical keratotomy in the United States. Arch Ophthalmol 1987 Jan; 105(1):37–39.

Boyd-Monk H. Need for donor organs and tissues. J Ophthalmic Nurs Technol 1987 Jul/Aug; 6(4):133.

Coburn MA. Hypopyon keratitis with subsequent evisceration: A nursing care study. J Ophthalmic Nurs Technol 1988 Nov/Dec; 7(6):209–219.

Garber N. Model eye for teaching keratometry. J Ophthalmic Nurs Technol 1987 Mar/Apr; 6(2):73–74.

Kaye B. Corneal transplantation: Guidelines for the refraction of patients with corneal transplantation. J Ophthalmic Nurs Technol 1987 Mar/Apr; 6(2):61–65.

Lambrix KK. Epikeratophaxia: Correcting visual deficits with corneal tissue. AORN J 1987 Aug; 46(2):218–225.

Lee PP et al. Cornea donation laws in the United States. Arch Ophthalmol 1989 Nov; 107(11):1585–1589.

Lundergan MK et al. What patients should know about radical keratotomy. AFP 1986 May; 33(5):169–172.

Parker P. Moraxella corneal ulcer. J Ophthalmic Nurs Technol 1988 May/Jun; 7(3):87–89.

Pflugfelder SC et al. Peripheral corneal ulceration in a patient with AIDS-related complex. Am J Ophthalmol 1987 Nov; 104(5):542–543.

Sawelson H and Marks RG. Three-year results of radial keratotomy. Arch Ophthalmol 1987 Jan; 105(1):81–85.

Torento C et al. Pseudophakic bullous keratopathy and the nursing implication. Ophthalmic Nurs Forum 1988 Mar; 4(3):1–12.

Diabetes

Bernbaum M et al. Promoting diabetes self-management and independence in the visually impaired: A model clinical program. Diabetes Educ 1988 Jan/Feb; 14(1):51–54.

Bernbaum M et al. Psychosocial profiles in patients with visual impairment due to diabetic retinopathy. Diabetes Care 1988 Jul/Aug; 11(7):551–557.

Collins JW. Proposed criteria for referring diabetic retinopathy. Nurse Pract 1988 Apr; 13(4):21–28.

Davis MD. Eye care focus on prevention: Diabetic retinopathy. Diabetes Forecast 1987 Jan; 40(1):28–31.

Davis MD. Eye care focus on treatment. Part 2. Diabetes Forecast 1987 Mar; 40(3):56–61.

Forrest RD et al. Screening for diabetic retinopathy: Comparison of a nurse and a doctor with retinal photography. Diabetes Res 1987 May; 5(1):39–42.

Goldberg RE et al. The equation: A photo essay acquainting the diabetic patient with the goals of pars plana vitrectomy for proliferative diabetic retinopathy. J Ophthalmic Nurs Technol 1987 May/Jun; 6(3):95.

Hampton LA et al. Choosing and using helpful aids. Nursing 1989 Jun; 19(6):70–71.

Hector M et al. Diabetic retinopathy: Recommendations for primary care management. Geriatrics 1987 Dec; 42(12):51–60.

Herget MJ et al. New aids for low-vision diabetics. Am J Nurs 1989 Oct; 89(10):1319–1322.

Minaker KL. Aging and diabetes mellitus as risk factors for vascular disease. Am J Med 1987 Jan; 82(Suppl 1B):47–53.

Packer AJ. Diabetic retinopathy. Postgrad Med 1987 May; 81(6):191–198.

Roach VG. What you should know about diabetic retinopathy. J Ophthalmic Nurs Technol 1989 Sep/Oct; 7(5):166–169.

Robertson C. Coping with chronic complications: Diabetes. RN 1989 Sep; 52(9):34–43.

Rogell GD. Vitrectomy for diabetic retinopathy. Diabetes Forecast 1987 Nov; 40(11):18–20.

Rosenthal JL. Timely recognition of diabetic retinopathy. Emerg Med 1989 Jun; 21(11):87–90.

Wulsin LR et al. Psychosocial aspects of diabetic retinopathy. Diabetes Care 1987 May/Jun; 10(3):367–373.

Glaucoma

Anderson DR. Glaucoma: The damage caused by pressure. XLVI Edward Jackson Memorial Lecture. Am J Ophthalmol 1989 Nov; 108(5):485–495

Capino DO et al. Glaucoma: Screening, diagnosis, and therapy. Hosp Pract 1990 May; 25(5A):73–86.

Everitt DE and Avorn J. Systemic effects of medications used to treat glaucoma. Ann Intern Med 1990 Jan; 112(2):120–125.

Hamrick S et al. Therapeutic ultrasound: A precise noninvasive therapy for glaucoma. AORN J 1988 Apr; 47(4):950–955+.

Hanson CM and Hodnicki DR. Glaucoma screening: An important role for NPs. Nurse Pract 1987 Dec; 12(12):14–21.

Langseth FG. Transscleral cyclophotocoagulation: A laser treatment for glaucoma. AORN J 1988 Dec; 48(6):1122–1127.

Skolink NS. Screening for open-angle glaucoma in a primary care setting. Hosp Pract 1987 Sep; 22(9):57–63.

Vader L. End-stage glaucoma and enucleation: An ophthalmic nursing challenge. Ophthalmic Nurs Forum 1987 Apr; 3(4):1–8.

Laser

Bessette FM and Nguyen LC. Laser light: Its nature and its action in the eye. Can Med Assoc J 1989 Dec; 141(11):1141–1148.

Mackety C. Nursing laser safety recommendation: Ophthalmology. Laser Nurs 1986–1987; 1(1):2–5.

Spadoni D and Cain CL. Laser blepharoplast. AORN J 1988 May; 47(5):1184–1194.

Ticho U and Nesher R. Laser trabeculoplasty in glaucoma. Arch Ophthalmol 1989 Jun; 107(6):844–846.

Yannuzzi LA et al. Lasers in ophthalmology. J Ophthalmic Nurs Technol 1988 Nov/Dec; 7(6):199–203.

Medication

Aspirin: Risk of blindness in the elderly? Nurses Drug Alert 1988 Jul; 12(7):49.

Goldstein J. Pharmacology of ophthalmic drugs. J Ophthalmic Nurs Technol 1987 Jul/Aug; 6(4):146–150.

Goldstein J. Pharmacology of ophthalmic drugs: Part II. J Ophthalmic Nurs Technol 1987 Sep/Oct; 6(5):193–197.

Hahn K. Administering eye medication. RN 89 Sep; 19(9):80.

Misuse of steroid eye medications. Nurses Drug Alert 1987 Jan; 11(1):7.

OTC eye drops and blindness. Nurses Drug Alert 1988 Jul; 12(7):56.

Timolol eye drop overdosing. Nurses Drug Alert 1989 Aug; 13(8):57

Retina

Bloom JN and Palestine AG. The diagnosis of cytomegalovirus retinitis. Ann Intern Med 1988 Dec; 106:963–969.

Michels RG. Scleral buckling methods for rhegmatogenous retinal detachment. Retina 1986 Jan; 6(1):1–49.

Taylor HR. Protect eyes from ultraviolet light to prevent cataract rather than retinal damage. JAMA 1989 Jun; 261(24):3550.

Miscellaneous

Alvern MT. Ophthalmic prosthetics: A guide for nurses. J Ophthalmic Nurs Technol 1987 Nov/Dec; 6(6):218–223.

Arentsen JJ. The dry eye. J Ophthalmic Nurs Technol 1987 Jul/Aug; 6(4):134–137.

Barker-Stotts K. Action STAT: Hyphema. Nursing 1988 Dec; 18(12):33.

Boyd-Monk H. Eye trauma; A close-up on emergency care. RN 1989 Dec; 19(12):22–29.

Boyd-Monk H. Spectacles: Goggles or face shields. J Ophthalmic Nurs Technol 1988 May/Jun; 7(3):84–86.

Burns FR et al. Prompt irrigation of chemical eye injuries may avert severe damage. Occup Health Saf 1989 Apr; 58(4):33–36.

Clanton C et al. Retinal reattachment quality and appropriateness of care. J Ophthalmic Nurs Technol 1988 Jul/Aug; 7(4):130–133.

Clark RB et al. Eye emergencies and urgencies. Patient Care 1989 Jan; 23(1):24–38.

Curtain JW et al. Cosmetic surgery update: The face. Patient Care 1987 Sep; 21(9):30–44.

Donshik PC et al. Eye to eye with systemic disease. Patient Care 1989 Jun; 23(1):34–46.

Ernest DT. 20/20 is not enough: Psychosocial aspects of patient care. Arch Ophthalmol 1987 Aug; 105(8):1028.

Finn SM et al. Ocular complications of AIDS. Ophthalmic Nurs Forum 1987 Jan; 3(1):2–4.

Goldman R. For your eyes only: Eye injuries. Emergency 1987 Dec; 15(12): 27–29.

Goldsmith MF. Computers star in new communication concepts for physically disabled people. JAMA 1989 Mar; 261(9):1256–1259.

Kahrman BD and Warfield CA. Eye pain: Ocular and nonocular causes. Hosp Pract 1987 Dec; 22(12):33–50.

Lawlor MC. Common ocular injuries and disorders: Red eye. Part 2. J Emerg Nurs 1989 Jan/Feb; 15(1):36–43.

Mansir JH et al. Intraocular inflammatory disease (uveitis). Ophthalmic Nurs Forum 1988 Jan; 4(1):1–8.

Melamed M. The injured eye at first sight. Emerg Med 1988 Oct; 20(17): 86–98.

Neger RE. The evaluation of dyplopia in head trauma. J Head Trauma Rehabil 1989 Jun; 4(2):27–34.

Newsome DA. Noninfectious ocular complications of AIDS. Int Ophthalmol Clin 1989 Summer; 29(2):95–97.

Pederson KM et al. Herpes zoster ophthalmicus. J Ophthalmic Nurs Technol 1987 Jul/Aug; 6(4):151–155.

Pigassou-Albouy R. A discussion of prism therapy for strabismus. J Ophthalmic Nurs Technol 1988 Jan/Feb; 7(1):18–25.

Shingleton BJ. A clearer look at ocular emergencies. Emerg Med 1989 May; 21(9):52–64.

Springer M. Sight-saving month calls attention to eye care. Arch Ophthalmol 1988 May; 106(5):593.

Sridama V and DeGroat LJ. Treatment of Graves' disease and the course of ophthalmopathy. Am J Med 1989 Jul; 87(7):70–73.

Tarail J. Sjogrens syndrome: A dry-eyed diary. Am J Nurs 1987 Mar; 87(3): 324–326.

Taylor PB and Nozik RA. Conjunctivitis: Causes and management. Hosp Med 1987 Dec; 23(12):58–78.

Toglia JP. Visual perception of objects: An approach to assessment and intervention. Am J Occup Ther 1989 Sep; 43(9):587–595.

Teutsch E and Hill M. Adding moisture to your life. Am J Nurs 1987 Mar; 87(3):326–329.

Walker KF. Clinically relevant features of the visual system. J Head Trauma Rehabil 1989 Jun; 4(2):1–8.

Wolfe CP. Tonography. J Ophthalmic Nurs Technol 1987 Sep/Oct; 6(5): 203–206.

Zegeer LJ. Oculacephalic and vestibuloocular responses: Significance for nursing care. J Neurosci Nurs 1989 Feb; 21(1):46–55.

Zito M. Effects of two gravity inversion methods on heart rate, septalic brachial pressure, and ophthalmic artery pressure, . . . ankle or thigh suspension. Phys Ther 1988 Jan; 68(1):20–25.

Vision Loss

Allen MN. Adjusting to visual impairment. J Ophthalmic Nurs Technol 1990 Mar/Apr; 9(2):47–51.

Allen MN. The meaning of visual impairment to visually impaired adults. J Adm Nurs 1989 Aug; 14(8):640–646.

Capino DG and Leibowitz HM. Age-related macular degeneration. Hosp Pract 1988 Mar; 23(3):23–42.

Edmonds SE. Resources for the visually impaired. J Ophthalmic Nurs Technol 1990 Jan/Feb; 5(1):14–15.

Ehrenberg M. Blindness prevention. AAOHN J 1987 May; 35(5):243–245.

Holt JE and Selhorst JB. Differential diagnosis of vision loss. Patient Care 1987 Jan; 21(1):61–72.

Jones DA et al. Visual disability and associated factors in the elderly. Health Visit 1987 Aug; 60(8):256–257.

Kupfer C. A decade of progress in the prevention of blindness. Am J Ophthalmol 1987 Jul; 104(1):80–83.

Lawlor MC. Common ocular injuries and disorders. Part 1: acute loss of vision. J Emerg Nurs 1989 Feb; 15(1):32–36.

Maloney CC. Identifying and treating the client with sensory loss. Phys Occup Ther Geriatr 1987 Spring; 5(4):31–46.

Norris RM. Commonsense tips for working with blind patients. Am J Nurs 1989 Mar; 89(3):360–361.

Pesci BR. When the patient's problem is really poor vision. RN 1986 Oct; 49(10):22–25.

Smith-Brewer S and Singerman LJ. Vision loss in age-related maculopathy: primary care referral guide. Geriatrics 1987 Sep; 42(9):99–106.

Spencer RE. Transitions: Reflections on going blind in a sighted world. J Ophthalmic Nurs Technol 1988 Nov/Dec; 7(6):220–222.

Stones MJ et al. Balance and age in the sighted and blind. Arch Phys Med Rehabil 1987 Feb; 68(2):85–89.

Information/Resources

Agencies

American Academy of Ophthalmology
   655 Beach St, San Francisco, CA 94109

American Council of the Blind (ABC)
   1010 Vermont Ave, Suite 1100 NW, Washington, DC 20005

American Foundation for the Blind
   15 West 16th St, New York, NY 10011

American Optometric Association (AOA)
   243 Lindbergh Blvd, St Louis, MO 63141

American Society of Ophthalmic Registered Nurses, Inc (ASORN)
   P.O. Box 3030, San Francisco, CA 94119

Better Vision Institute Inc (BVI)
   1800 N Kent St Suite 1220, Rosslyn, VA 22209

Braille Institute
   741 N Vermont Ave, Los Angeles, CA 90029

Contact Lens Society of America (CLSA)
   523 Decatur St, Suite 1, New Orleans, LA 70130

Eye-Bank Association of America (EBAA)
   1725 I St NW, Washington, DC 20006–2403

Leader Dogs for the Blind
   1039 Rochester Rd, Rochester, MI 48063

National Association for Visually Handicapped (NAVH)
   305 E 24th St, New York, NY 10010

National Braille Association (NBA)
   1290 University Ave, Rochester, NY 14607

National Federation of the Blind (NFB)
   1800 Johnson St, Baltimore, MD 21230

National Society to Prevent Blindness (NSPB)
   500 E Remington Rd, Schaumburg, IL 60173

Recording for the Blind (RFB)
   20 Roszel Rd, Princeton, NJ 08540

Seeing Eye (SE)
   P.O. Box 375M, Washington Valley Rd, Morristown, NJ 07960

Taping for the Blind (TFTB)
   3935 Essex Lane, Houston, TX 77027

54

Assessment and Management of Patients With Hearing Problems and Ear Disorders

Learning Objectives

On completion of this chapter, the learner will be able to:

1. Describe methods used to assess hearing ability
2. Identify ways to communicate effectively with a person who has a hearing impairment
3. Describe the management of problems of the external ear
4. Compare the problems of infection of the external ear with infection of the middle ear
5. Compare the various types of tympanoplasty and the nursing care of patients undergoing these procedures
6. Use the nursing process as a framework for care of patients undergoing ear surgery
7. Describe the clinical manifestations, diagnosis, and management of the patient with Ménière's disease

Glossary

Ear Anatomy

acoustic—pertaining to sound or to the sense of hearing

acoustic nerve—the eigth cranial nerve, which consists of two separate divisions, the vestibular nerve and the cochlear nerve; auditory nerve; vestibulocochlear nerve

auditory tube—eustachian tube

auricle—the outer part of the external ear; the pinna

cerumen—brown waxlike secretion found in the external ear canal; earwax

cochlea—the winding, cone-shaped tube that forms a portion of the inner ear and contains the organ of Corti, the receptor for hearing

endolymph—the pale transparent fluid within the labyrinth of the ear

eustachian tube—the 3- to 4-cm auditory tube that extends from the middle ear to the nasopharynx

external ear—the portion of the ear that consists of the pinna (auricle) and external auditory canal; it is separated from the middle ear by the tympanic membrane

(continued)

Glossary (continued)

incus—the middle portion of the three ossicles of the middle ear; the anvil

internal (inner) ear—the portion of the ear that consists of the cochlea, which contains the sensory receptors for hearing, and the vestibule and semicircular canals, which contain the receptors for equilibrium and the sense of position; the labyrinth

labyrinth—the inner ear

malleus—the largest of the three ossicles in the middle ear; it is attached to the eardrum and articulates with the incus; the hammer

mastoid—a process of the temporal bone

middle ear—the tiny air-filled cavity located in the temporal bone and containing three small bones (ossicles)—the malleus, incus, and stapes; the typanum

organ of Corti—the terminal acoustic apparatus in the cochlea

ossicle—one of the three small bones (the malleus, incus, and stapes) of the middle ear

oval window—the oval aperature in the middle ear

pinna—the outer part of the external ear, which collects and directs sound waves into the external auditory canal for passage to the tympanic membrane; the auricle

presbycusis—progressive hearing loss associated with aging

semicircular canals—the superior, posterior, and interior passages that form part of the inner ear

stapes—one of the three ossicles in the middle ear; it articulates with the incus, and its footplate fits into the oval window; the stirrup

tympanic membrane—the membrane that serves as the lateral wall of the tympanic cavity and that separates it from the external ear; eardrum

tympanum—the middle ear

vestibular apparatus—the middle part of the inner ear that is composed of the membranous saccule, urticle, and semicircular canals; it detects changes in the body's equilibrium

Ear Disorders and Treatments

endolymphatic hydrops—Ménière's disease

labyrinthitis—inflammation of the labyrinth; Ménière's disease

Ménière's disease—a condition of the inner ear characterized by recurrent and usually progressive symptoms including vertigo, tinnitus, a sensation of pressure in the ears, and neurosensory hearing loss

myringotomy—an incision made into the tympanic membrane for the purpose of draining pus from a middle ear infection and relieving pressure

otalgia—pain in the ear; earache

otitis media—infection of the middle ear

otosclerosis—a condition characterized by chronic progressive deafness caused by the formation of abnormal spongy bone in the labyrinth that results in ankylosis of the stapes and prevention of sound transmission

tinnitus—ringing sound in the ear

tympanoplasty—any of several sugical procedures designed to restore function to middle ear structures that have become diseased or that are congenitally deformed

---

The ear is a sensory organ with dual, complex functions—hearing and the maintenance of equilibrium. The early detection and the accurate diagnosis of ear and hearing disorders are important. Among those who help diagnose auditory disorders are pediatricians, otolaryngologists, psychiatrists, neurologists, nurses, psychologists, speech pathologists, educators, and audiologists. Disorders due to birth injury, childhood infections, toxic drug effects, and physiologic aging are only a few of the problems that require assessment, treatment, and rehabilitation.

Physiologic Principles Underlying Sound Conduction

The conductive function of the eardrum and the ossicles transforms sound waves from airborne vibrations to mechanical stimulation of the endolymphatic fluids. The vibrations of the large tympanic membrane are transmitted through the lever action of the ossicles to the smaller oval window and then on to the endolymphatic fluid (Fig. 54-1). During this transmission, the sound waves encounter progressively smaller mass, which results in increasing amplitude (or loudness) of the sound. Defects in the tympanic membrane or interruption of the ossicular chain disturb that mass relationship to the oval window and cause a loss of the sound–pressure ratio, resulting in hearing loss.

The functional physiology of the round and oval windows plays an important role as well. The oval window is bordered by the annular ligament, and the unimpeded motility of the stapedial footplate receives impulses transmitted by the incus and the malleus from the eardrum membrane. The round window, opening on the opposite side of the cochlear duct, permits motion of the endolymphatic fluids by sound wave stimulation. With the normally intact tympanic membrane, sound waves stimulate the oval window first, and a lag occurs before the terminal effect of the stimulus reaches the round window. This lag phase, normally present with an intact eardrum, is changed when a perforation of the eardrum is large enough to allow sound waves to impinge on both the round and oval windows simultaneously. This effect cancels the lag and prevents the maximal effect of labyrinth fluid motility and its subsequent effect in stimulating the hair cells in the organ of Corti. The result is a reduction in hearing ability.

Pathophysiology. Pathologic sequelae of ear disorders vary and result in minimal or large defects remaining in the tympanic membrane. In protracted or virulent infections, necrotic involvement of the ossicles may occur. Impairment of freedom of motion of one or all parts of the ossicular chain may occur as a result of fibrosis or necrosis. The malleus commonly is involved, the handle being destroyed by osteonecrosis as the perforation in the eardrum enlarges. The lenticular process of the incus often is involved because of its limited blood supply. Osteonecrosis may involve the entire ossicular chain, so that the stapedial footplate is the only portion remaining. The oval and round windows may be impeded functionally by granuloma, polyps, and fibrous or bony plaques. Otosclerosis

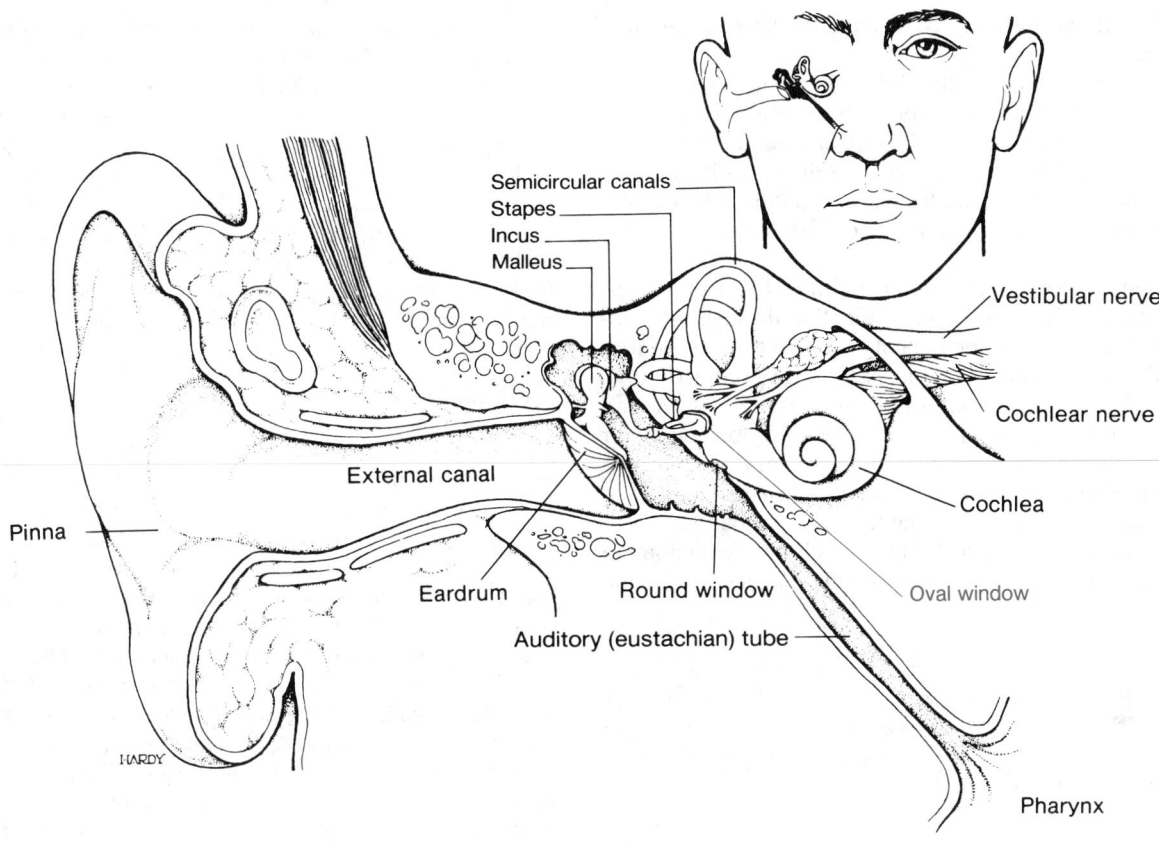

Figure 54–1. Anatomy of the ear.

may exist along with the pathologic sequelae of otitis media. Obstruction of the orifice of the auditory tube by tissue deposits or fibrotic stenosis may result in dysfunction of this structure.

Assessment of Hearing Ability

Examination of the Ear

The ear is examined by inspection and palpation of the external and middle ear. Assessment of auditory acuity, a vital part of an examination, is also included in every physical examination.

Auditory Acuity.   A general estimation of the patient's hearing is effectively screened by assessing the patient's ability to hear a whispered phrase or a ticking watch. A soft whisper can be produced if the examiner begins to whisper after a full exhalation. One ear is tested at a time, followed by testing of the other ear. To exclude one ear from the testing, the examiner covers the untested ear with the palm of the hand. From a distance of 30.5 to 61 cm (1 to 2 feet) from the unoccluded ear and out of visual range, the patient with normal acuity can correctly repeat what was whispered. If a ticking watch is used, the examiner holds the watch at a distance of 7.5 cm (3 in) from the auricle. Because a watch produces a higher-pitched sound than the whispered voice, it is less reliable and is not used as the sole means of assessing auditory acuity.

Hearing normally occurs over two pathways. The sounds that are transmitted by way of the air-filled external and middle ear travel by way of *air conduction*. The sounds transmitted through bone directly to the inner ear travel by means of *bone conduction*. Normally air conduction is the more efficient pathway.

Hearing loss is generally one of two types. The first type is a *conductive* loss and usually results from an external ear disorder, such as impacted cerumen, or middle ear disorders, such as otitis media or a perforated tympanic membrane. In such instances, the transmission of sound by air to the inner ear, where it is converted to a neural impulse, is blocked. The second type of loss is a *sensorineural*, or *perceptive*, loss and involves damage to the eighth cranial nerve. These losses may be distinguished through the use of a tuning fork selected for frequencies within the conversational voice range (512 or 1024 cycles per second [cps] or Hertz [Hz]).

In addition to conductive loss and sensorineural (perceptive) loss, there is also combined hearing loss as well as psychogenic hearing loss. A combined hearing loss indicates that the patient has both a conductive and sensorineural loss.

Psychogenic hearing loss is a nonorganic or functional loss. This type is unrelated to detectable structural changes in the hearing mechanisms and is usually a manifestation of an emotional disturbance, but the loss is frequently total.

The *Weber test* uses bone conduction to test lateralization of sound. The tuning fork is set in motion by grasping it firmly by its stem and tapping it lightly. It is then placed on the forehead or on the center of the top of the patient's head. The patient is asked if he can hear a sound. Where does he perceive the sound? In one ear? In both ears? If there is a conductive loss (cerumen plug, otitis media) in one ear, the sound is heard better in the affected ear. This is because the obstruction obliterates the room noise, thus enhancing bone conduction. If a sensorineural loss exists, however, the sound is not perceived in the affected ear. Instead, the sound lateralizes to the unaffected ear.

In the *Rinne test*, the stem of a vibrating tuning fork is placed on the mastoid process of the temporal bone until the patient can no longer hear it. The fork is then quickly moved to within 2.5 cm (1 in) from the opening of the auditory canal. Under normal circumstances, the patient continues to hear the sound, demonstrating that air conduction lasts longer than bone conduction.

In conductive hearing loss, bone conduction exceeds air conduction. That is, once bone conduction through the temporal bone has died out, the patient is unable to hear the fork through the usual conductive mechanism. In contrast, nerve deafness or sensorineural loss permits sounds to be conducted by air better than by bone, although neither is a good conductor and all sounds may be perceived to be distant and faint. Use of the Weber and Rinne tests enables one to distinguish conductive loss from nerve loss when hearing is impaired. These tests are not a part of the usual screening physical examination but are useful if a more discrete assessment is needed for the patient.

In summary, conductive hearing loss results from an impairment of the outer ear, middle ear, or both. (The inner ear is not involved in this type of loss; it can analyze clearly the sounds that come to it.) A sensorineural (perceptive) hearing loss is produced from a disorder of the inner ear or nerve pathways that impairs sensitivity to and discrimination of sounds. Sounds may be conducted properly through the external and middle ear but are not analyzed correctly in the inner ear. Various tests are available using the tuning fork that help assess the origin of the hearing loss.

External Ear.   Inspection of the external ear is a simple procedure and is often overlooked. The auricle and surrounding tissues are inspected for deformities, lesions, or discharges. Movement of the auricle does not normally elicit pain. If this maneuver is painful, acute external otitis is suspected. Tenderness in the area of the mastoid may indicate mastoiditis or inflammation of the posterior auricular node. Occasionally, sebaceous cysts and tophi (subcutaneous mineral deposits) may be present on the pinna. A flaky scaliness on or behind the auricle usually indicates seborrheic dermatitis and may be present on the scalp and facial structures as well.

Otoscopic Examination.   Proper inspection of the ear canal and tympanic membrane (eardrum) requires that the canal be free of cerumen. If the membrane cannot be visualized because of cerumen, the ear canal may be gently irrigated with warm tap water. In the event that adherent cerumen is present, a small amount of mineral oil or similar commercial preparation may be instilled within the ear canal and the patient instructed to return for subsequent removal of the wax and inspection of the ear. (The use of the cerumen spoon for wax removal is reserved for physicians and nurses with specialized training because of the danger of perforation of the tympanic membrane.) Cerumen buildup demands attention because it is a common cause of hearing deficit and of local irritation.

To examine the ear canal and tympanic membrane, the patient's head is tipped away from the examiner. The auricle is grasped firmly and pulled upward, backward, and slightly outward (Fig. 54-2). This straightens the canal in the adult, allowing better visualization. The largest speculum that the canal can accommodate is used and is guided gently down into the canal and slightly forward. Because the distal portion of the canal is bony and covered by a sensitive layer of epithelium, only light pressure may be used without causing pain.

Any discharge, inflammation, or foreign body in the ear canal is noted. The healthy tympanic membrane is pearly gray and is positioned obliquely at the base of the ear canal. The landmarks are identified if visible (Fig. 54-3): the pars tensa and cone of light, the umbo, the manubrium of the malleus, and its short process. A slow movement of the speculum allows further visualization of the malleolar folds and periphery. The position and color of the membrane, as well as any unusual markings or deviation in the cone of light, are noted.

Audiogram

In the detection of deafness, the audiometer is the single most important diagnostic instrument. The unit of measure of loudness of intensity of sound is the decibel (dB). Audiometric testing is of two kinds: (1) *pure-tone audiometry*, in which the sound stimulus consists of a pure or musical tone (the louder the tone before the patient perceives it, the greater the hearing loss); and (2) *speech audiometry*, in which the spoken word is used to determine the ability to hear and discriminate sounds.

The patient wears earphones and is instructed to signal when he hears the tone and again when he no longer hears it. When the tone is applied directly over the external auditory opening, air conduction is measured. When the stimulus is applied to the mastoid bone, bypassing the conductive mechanism, nerve conduction is tested. For accuracy, audiometric tests are performed in a soundproof room.

The normal human ear perceives sounds ranging from 20 to 20,000 Hz; however, only the frequencies from 500 to 2000 Hz are important in understanding everyday speech. Clinically, this range is referred to as *speech range*. The critical level of loudness is approximately 30 dB. In treating patients surgically to improve hearing loss, the aim is to improve the hearing level to 30 dB or better within the speech frequencies (Figs. 54-4 and 54-5).

Gerontologic Considerations

With aging, changes occur in the ear that may eventually lead to hearing deficits. Little change occurs in the external ear, except that cerumen tends to become harder and there is a greater chance of impaction. In the middle ear, the tympanic membrane may atrophy or sclerose. The inner ear changes with a degeneration of cells at the base of the cochlea. This is manifested by a loss in the ability to hear high-frequency sounds followed in time by the loss of middle and lower frequencies. The term *presbycusis* is used to describe this progressive hearing loss.

Early signs of hearing loss may include tinnitus, increasing inability to hear at group meetings, and a need to turn up the volume of the television. Presbycusis may progress rapidly over a few years or slowly over a decade.

Other factors affect hearing in the elderly, such as lifelong exposure to loud noises (*e.g.*, jets, guns, heavy machinery in the workplace). Certain drugs, such as streptomycin, neomycin, and even aspirin, may have ototoxic effects because renal changes in the older person result in delayed drug excretion. Psychogenic factors and other disease processes (*e.g.*, diabetes) also may be partially responsible for sensory changes.

Hearing impairment should not be assumed to be a normal

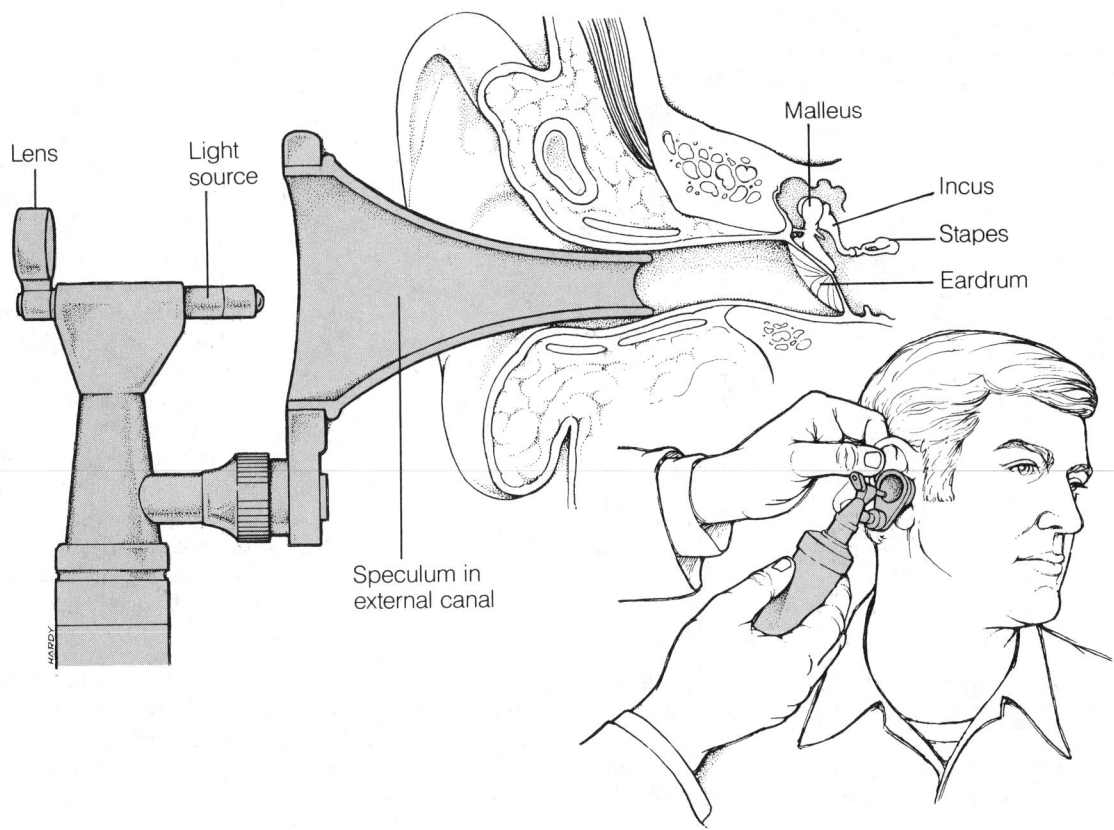

Figure 54–2. Technique for using the otoscope.

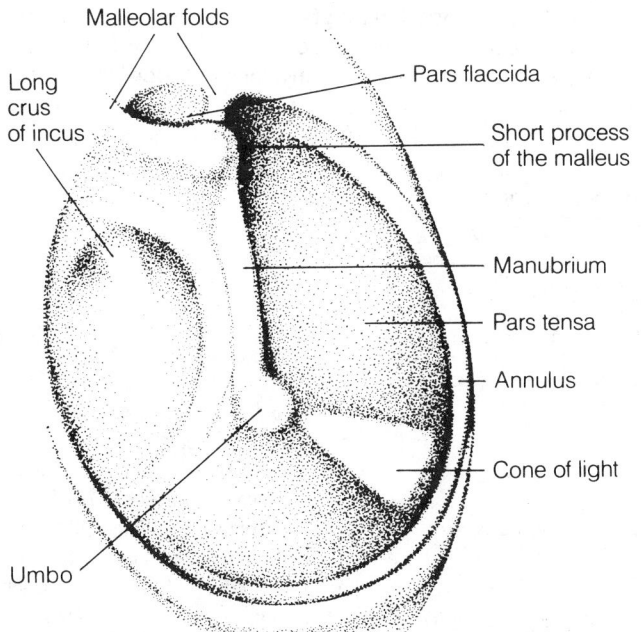

Figure 54–3. Illustration of the right eardrum as it would be seen through the otoscope.

consequence of aging and thus ignored. When a problem occurs, an audiometric evaluation should be performed. Hearing aids should not be purchased without a medical referral.

Even with the best of medical care, the older person has to learn to adjust to varying degrees of hearing loss. Care of elderly patients includes recognizing emotional reactions related to hearing loss such as (1) being suspicious of others because of an inability to hear adequately, (2) frustration and anger with repeated statements such as "I didn't hear what you said," and (3) feeling insecure because of the inability to hear the telephone or alarms. Hearing aids help to a certain point, but hearing problems in the elderly are often compounded by difficulty in discriminating speech. As a result, hearing aids frequently are not used.

By understanding what type of hearing loss a patient has, the nurse will more successfully be able to communicate with him. Trying to speak in a loud voice to a person who cannot adequately hear high-frequency sounds only makes matters worse. Talking into the least impaired ear, using sign language, gestures, and facial expressions may help.

Noise and Its Effect on Hearing

Noise (unwanted and unavoidable sound) has been identified as one of the environmental hazards of the 20th century. The sheer volume of noise that surrounds us daily has increased from a simple annoyance into a potentially dangerous source of physical and psychological damage.

In terms of physical impact, loud, persistent noise has been found to cause constriction of peripheral blood vessels, increases in blood pressure and heart rate (because of increased secretion of adrenalin), disturbances in equilibrium, and increased gastrointestinal activity. Additional research is required to answer many questions regarding the overall effects of noise on the human body. One thing seems certain, however—a

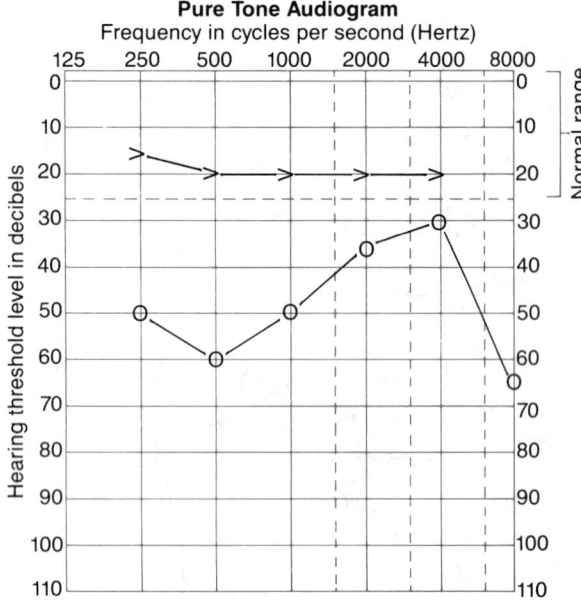

Pure Tone Audiogram
Frequency in cycles per second (Hertz)

Audiogram Code

Ear	Air		Bone	
	Un-masked	Masked	Un-masked	Masked
R	O---O	Δ---Δ	]---]	>-->
L	×---×	□---□	[---[	<---<

Figure 54–4. An audiogram presents a graphic outline of the person's hearing as measured by tones of different pitches ranging from 125 through 8000 cycles per second (cps) or Hertz (Hz). This audiogram of the right ear shows a conductive loss. Thresholds for these different tones as heard by air and bone conduction are plotted. The information is important for determining the type of hearing loss. Also, by testing through the critical speech range (approximately 300 to 3000 Hz), one can predict how much difficulty there may be in hearing and understanding speech. The code box to the right indicates the signs used on the chart. (Dayal VS. Clinical Otolaryngology. Philadelphia, JB Lippincott, 1981.)

quiet environment is more conducive to peace of mind. A person who is ill feels more at ease when noise is kept to a minimum.

Sound Intensity and Frequency. Scientists measure sound *intensity* (pressure exerted by sound) in decibels (dB). For example, the shuffling of papers in quiet surroundings represents about 15 dB; a low conversation, 40 dB; and a jet plane 100 feet away, about 140 dB. Sound above 80 dB begins to grate harshly on the human ear. Sound that is uncomfortable to the ear can be damaging to the ear.

Over the past several decades, the loudest sounds to which humans are exposed have increased from 120 dB (the roar of a small, two-engine prop plane) to more than 150 dB (the blast of a giant, four-engine jet). Some music concerts exceed 180 dB. Experiments have shown that 160 dB is lethal for small fur-bearing animals. Research at many universities shows that exposure to noise of 90 dB or more can cause the skin to flush, the abdominal muscles to constrict, and tempers to be short.

Frequency refers to the number of sound waves emanating from a source per second—cycles per second or Hertz. *Pitch* is the term used to describe frequency; a tone with 100 Hz is considered of low pitch; a tone of 10,000 Hz is considered of high pitch.

Hearing Loss

Psychosocial Considerations

Impairment of hearing may cause changes in personality and attitude, in the ability to communicate, in the awareness of surroundings, and even in the ability to protect oneself. In a classroom, a student with impaired hearing may show disinterest, inattention, and failing grades. A person at home may feel isolated because he no longer can hear the clock chime, the refrigerator hum, the birds sing, or the traffic pass. A pe-

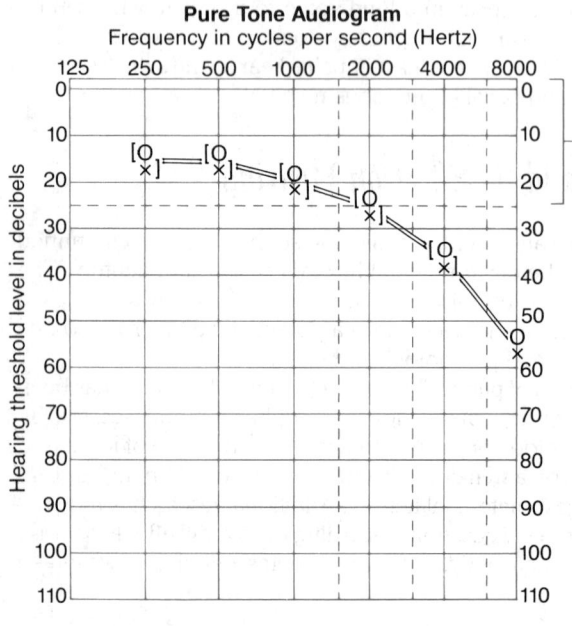

Pure Tone Audiogram
Frequency in cycles per second (Hertz)

Audiogram Code

Ear	Air		Bone	
	Un-masked	Masked	Un-masked	Masked
R	O---O	Δ---Δ	]---]	>-->
L	×---×	□---□	[---[	<---<

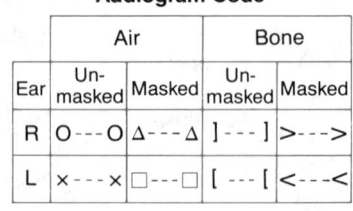

Speech Audiometry

	Right	Left
SRT	20 dB	20 dB
Discrim.	96% at 50 dB	96% at 50 dB

Figure 54–5. Audiogram of right ear shows a sensorineural hearing loss. In this audiogram, speech tests used are speech reception threshold (SRT) and speech discrimination. If the ability of this patient to understand speech is poor, a hearing aid will be of little or no benefit to him, nor will he benefit from reconstructive surgery to correct the conductive hearing loss. (Dayal VS. Clinical Otolaryngology. Philadelphia, JB Lippincott, 1981.)

destrian may attempt to cross the street at the wrong time because of failure to hear an approaching car. The person with a hearing loss may miss parts of a conversation and may believe that people are talking about him. Many people are not even aware that their hearing is gradually becoming impaired.

More than 20 million people in the United States suffer from some form of hearing loss. Most of these people can be helped with medical or surgical therapies or with a hearing aid. The nurse and the family physician play a major role in diagnosing hearing loss and guiding patients toward assistance. Although some hearing difficulty may be due to impacted cerumen (wax), which is readily treated, proper assessment is best performed by an otologist.

The *otologist* is a physician who specializes in the diagnosis and treatment of problems of the ear. An *otolaryngologist* is a physician who specializes in problems relating to the ear, nose, and throat. An *audiologist* is a person who specializes in nonmedical evaluation and rehabilitation of hearing disorders.

The symptoms of hearing loss are varied, complex, and often subtle, as is indicated in the danger signals listed in Chart 54-1. The signs of significant ear disease that require referral to an otolaryngologist have been identified by the National Hearing Aid Society (NHAS):

1. Visible congenital or traumatic deformity of the ear
2. Active drainage from the ear within the previous 90 days
3. Sudden or rapidly progressive hearing loss
4. Acute or chronic dizziness or tinnitus
5. Unilateral hearing loss of sudden or recent onset
6. Significant air–bone hearing gap (which can be recognized only from hearing tests)
7. Visible evidence of cerumen accumulation or a foreign body in the ear canal
8. Pain or discomfort in the ear

Not infrequently, a person with a hearing loss refuses to seek medical attention; because of fear that hearing loss is a sign of advancing age, many people refuse to wear a hearing aid. Others feel self-conscious when they do wear an aid. These attitudes and behaviors should be taken into account when counseling patients who need hearing assistance.

Rehabilitation

It is important to identify the type of hearing impairment a person has so that rehabilitative efforts can be directed at meeting a particular need. With a conductive loss, correction of the problem may be all that is necessary to treat and improve this type of impairment (Fig. 54-6). If the problem cannot be corrected, the patient benefits greatly from a hearing aid, because in most instances he requires only amplification of sounds. In sensorineural (perceptive) loss, because of poor sensitivity to sound, hearing aids are not as helpful as they are to those with conductive loss. A hearing aid should not be ruled out, however, until the patient's hearing is evaluated and until a variety of aids are tested against hearing loss.

The Conference of Executives of American Schools for the Deaf proposed the following classification of hearing impairment based on (1) time of onset of hearing loss and (2) functional status of hearing:

1. The deaf—those in whom the sense of hearing is nonfunctional for ordinary purposes of life. This general group is made up of two distinct classes:
   a. The congenitally deaf—those who lose hearing before speech is developed.
   b. The adventitiously deaf—those who are born with normal

Chart 54-1
Symptoms of Hearing Loss

Speech deterioration—If a person slurs his words or drops word endings, or if speech is flat sounding, he may not be hearing correctly. The ears guide the voice, both in loudness and pronunciation.

Fatigue—If a person tires easily when listening to conversation or to a speech, fatigue may be the result of straining to hear. Under these circumstances, he may become irritable very easily.

Indifference—It is easy for a person to become depressed and disinterested in life in general when he cannot hear what others are saying.

Social withdrawal—Not being able to hear what is going on around him causes the hearing impaired person to withdraw from situations that might prove embarrassing.

Insecurity—Lack of self-confidence and fear of mistakes create a feeling of insecurity in many hearing impaired persons. No one likes to say the wrong thing or do something that might tend to make him look foolish.

Indecision-Procrastination—Loss of self-confidence makes it increasingly difficult for a hearing impaired person to make decisions.

Suspiciousness—Because he often hears only part of what is being said, the hearing impaired person may suspect that others are talking about him or that portions of the conversation relating to him are deliberately spoken softly so that he will not hear them!

False pride—The hearing impaired person wants to conceal his hearing loss. Consequently, he often pretends he is hearing when he actually is not.

Loneliness and unhappiness—Although everyone wishes for quiet now and then, *enforced* silence can be boring and even somewhat frightening. People with a hearing loss often feel isolated.

Tendency to dominate the conversation—Many hearing impaired people tend to dominate the conversation, knowing that as long as it is centered on them and they can control it they are not so likely to be embarrassed by some mistake.

(Courtesy of Maico Hearing Instruments.)

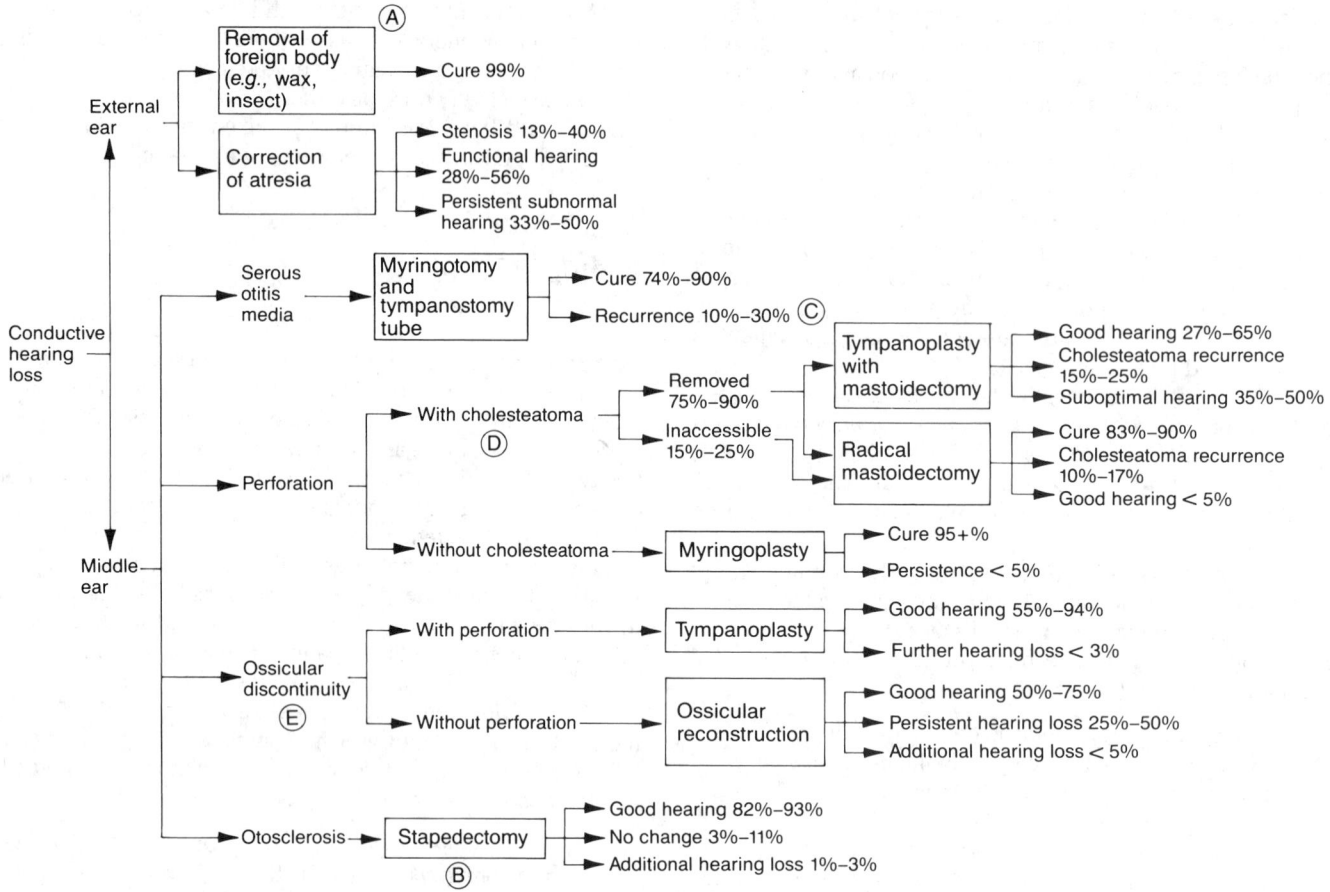

Figure 54–6. Conductive hearing loss. When a patient presents with this problem, the above flow chart indicates how the diagnosis determines the management of the patient and further predicts the outcome. (Jafek BW and Balkany TJ. Conductive hearing loss. In Eiseman B. Prognosis of Surgical Disease. Philadelphia, WB Saunders.)

hearing but then suffer some illness or accident that causes their hearing to become nonfunctional.

2. The hard of hearing—those in whom hearing, although defective, is serviceable with or without a hearing aid.

Hearing Aids

A hearing aid is an instrument through which sounds, both speech and environmental, are received by a microphone, converted into electrical signals, amplified, and reconverted to acoustical signals. Many aids available for nerve deafness depress the low tones and give better hearing for the high tones. When the hearing loss is more than 30 dB in the range of 500 to 2000 Hz in the better ear, the patient may benefit from a hearing aid. A variety of aids are available; the best aid must be selected for the individual patient (Table 54-1). Even a good match does not ensure optimal benefit from a hearing aid because psychological factors, such as vanity, may be involved.

A hearing aid makes speech louder, but it does not always make it clear enough for the deaf person to understand what is said. A problem with most hearing aids is that background noise is also amplified, which may be disturbing to the wearer. Binaural aids (*i.e.*, one for each ear) may be indicated. The wearer must experiment and adjust the controls for optimal

results. It may be necessary for the patient to receive auditory training and lessons in speech reading (lipreading) to make the new hearing aid effective. In auditory training, speech discrimination and listening skills are emphasized. Speech reading can help fill in the gaps of those words that might be missed. With such assistance, the person can learn to interpret sounds and use to his advantage whatever hearing remains.

The patient needs to know that the aid will not restore hearing to the level of normal hearing but that it will improve hearing in the range of 300 to 3500 Hz (range of primary speech).

FDA Regulations. The Food and Drug Administration (FDA) has established the following regulations on hearing aids to protect the health and safety of people with hearing impairments:

1. A medical evaluation of the impairment by a licensed physician (preferably one specializing in diseases of the ear) must be obtained within 6 months before the purchase of a hearing aid.
   a. Such a written statement from a physician, however, may be waived by the client (a fully informed adult 18 years of age or older) on signing a document to this effect.
   b. Children must be evaluated by a physician.
2. Health professionals who dispense hearing aids are required to refer prospective users to a physician if any of eight spec-

TABLE 54-1. *Types of Hearing Aids*

Site/Range of Hearing Loss	Advantages	Disadvantages
Body (40–110 dB)	Separation of receiver and microphone prevents acoustic feedback, allowing high amplification	Bulky; requires long wire, which may be cosmetically displeasing; some loss of high-frequency response
Behind the ear (25–80 dB)	Cosmetically good because easily hidden by hair; comfortable; no long wires	Proximity of microphone and receiver limits the amount of amplification because of feedback
In the ear (25–55 dB)	Smallest; most easily concealed	Very close proximity of amplifier and microphone and size limitations on power make aid suitable only for mild to moderate losses
Eyeglasses (25–70 dB; greater range with special modifications)	Conceals most of the aid with frame of glasses; allows wires separating microphone and receiver to be hidden within glasses	Requires wearing glasses, usually with bulky, stylistically limited frame

(Sataloff RT. Choosing the right hearing aid. Hosp Pract; 16[5]:32E)

ified otologic conditions are evident: visible congenital or traumatic ear deformity, drainage from the ear within the preceding 90 days, history of sudden or rapidly progressive hearing loss within the preceding 90 days, complaints of dizziness, unilateral hearing loss that occurred suddenly or within the preceding 90 days, audiometric air–bone gap equal to or greater than 15 dB at 500, 1000, and 2000 Hz, significant accumulation of cerumen or a foreign body in the ear canal, pain or discomfort in the ear.

3. A *user instructional brochure* is to accompany every hearing aid device. In this brochure, the following information is presented:
   a. Specification that good health practice requires a medical evaluation before purchasing a hearing aid
   b. Notification that any of the eight designated otologic conditions should be investigated by a physician before purchase of a hearing aid
   c. Instructions for proper use, maintenance, and care of the hearing aid as well as instructions for replacing or recharging the batteries
   d. Repair service information
   e. Description of avoidable conditions that could adversely effect or damage the hearing aid
   f. Specification of any known side effects that may warrant physician consultation (*e.g.*, skin irritation, accelerated cerumen accumulation)

Care of a Hearing Aid.   A hearing aid must be cared for carefully. The ear mold, the only part of the instrument that may be washed, is washed daily in soap and water, and the cannula is cleansed with a small applicator or pipe cleaner. (The mold must be dry before it is snapped into the receiver.) The transmitter usually is worn behind the ear or in the frame of eyeglasses. Spare parts should be available to the wearer.

When a hearing aid is not functioning properly, inadequate amplification, whistling noise, or pain from the mold may occur (Chart 54-2). If the hearing aid still does not work after checking for malfunctions (*e.g.*, switch is on, batteries are positioned correctly, cord is intact and plugged in correctly), the patient should notify the local service agency. If the unit requires extended time for repair, the agency from whom it was purchased may lend the patient a hearing aid until the repair can be accomplished.

Hearing Guide Dogs

Specially trained dogs are available to assist the person with hearing loss. Persons who live alone are eligible to apply for a dog trained by International Hearing Dog Inc. At home, the dog reacts to the sound of a telephone, a doorbell, an alarm clock, a baby's cry, a knock at the door, a smoke alarm, or an intruder. The dog does not bark but alerts his master by physical contact; the dog then runs to the source of the noise. In public, the dog positions itself between the hearing impaired person and any potential hazard that the person cannot hear, such as an oncoming vehicle or a hostile person.

The dog wears an orange collar, and the person carries a certification card that reads: "The dog has been professionally trained by Hearing Dog Inc. in auditory awareness to serve its hearing-impaired master. Therefore, as with guide dogs for the blind, this dog shall accompany its master at all times." In many states, a hard of hearing person with a certified hearing guide dog is legally permitted access to public transportation, public eating places, and stores, including grocery markets.

Communication With a Person Who Has a Hearing Impairment

Use of the following suggestions promotes better communication with deaf persons whose speech is difficult to understand*:

1. Devote full attention to what the person is saying. Look and listen—do not try to give attention to another task while listening.
2. Engage him in conversation when it is possible for you to anticipate his replies. This enables you to become accustomed to any peculiarities in speech patterns.
3. Try to determine the essential context of what is being said; you can often fill in the details from context.
4. Do not try to appear as if you understand when you do not.
5. If you cannot understand at all or have serious doubt about your ability to understand what is being said, have the person write his message rather than risk misunderstanding. Having

---

* *Terry FJ et al. Rehabilitation Nursing. St Louis, CV Mosby.*

Chart 54-2
Hearing Aid Problems

Whistling Noise

Loose Ear Mold
  Improperly made
  Improperly worn
  Worn out

Improper Aid Selection
  Too much power required in aid with inadequate separation
    between microphone and receiver
  Open mold used inappropriately

Inadequate Amplification

Dead batteries
Wax in ear
Wax or other material in mold
Wires or tubing disconnected from aid
Aid turned off or volume too low
Improper mold
Improper aid for degree of loss

Pain From Mold

Improperly fitted mold
Ear skin or cartilage infection
Middle ear infection
Ear tumor
Unrelated causes:
  Temporomandibular joint
  Throat or larynx
  Other

(Sataloff RT. Choosing the right hearing aid. Hosp Pract 16[5]:32A.)

---

him repeat his message in speech, after you know its content, also aids you in becoming accustomed to his pattern of speech.

Suggestions for better communication with a deaf person who lip-reads are as follows:

1. When speaking, always face the person as directly as possible.
2. Make sure your face is as clearly visible as possible; locate yourself so that your face is well-lighted; avoid being silhouetted against strong light; do not obscure that person's view of your mouth in any way; avoid talking with any object held in your mouth.
3. Be sure the patient knows the topic or subject of your verbal expression before going ahead with what you plan to say—this enables him to use contextual clues in his lipreading.
4. Speak slowly and distinctly, pausing more frequently than you would normally.
5. If you question whether the patient has understood some important direction or instruction, check to be certain that he has the full meaning of your message.
6. If for any reason your mouth must be covered (as with a mask) and you must direct or instruct the patient, there is no alternative but to write the message for him.

Problems of the External Ear

The auricle or external ear aids in the collection of sound waves and their passage into the external auditory canal. The *external auditory canal* is an elastic cartilaginous and dense fibrous framework to which thin skin is attached, ending at a disclike structure, the tympanic membrane (eardrum). The skin of the canal contains highly specialized glands that secrete a brown, waxlike substance called *cerumen* (ear wax). The ear's self-cleaning mechanism moves old skin cells and cerumen to the outer part of the ear. The cerumen seems to have antibacterial properties and serves as a protection for the skin.

Otalgia is pain in the ear (earache). Because the ear is innervated by a rich nerve supply (cranial nerves V, VII, IX, and X as well as the second and third cervical nerve roots), the skin is extremely sensitive. Otalgia is a symptom that can arise from irritation from a number of conditions, including referred pain from disorders of the larynx or pharynx.

Infections (External Otitis)

Bacterial or fungal infections may result from an abrasion of the ear canal or from swimming in contaminated water; they appear more commonly during the summer. Such infections are painful.

The goals of management are directed toward relieving the discomfort, reducing the swelling in the ear canal, and eradicating the infection. Even touching or moving the auricle increases pain. (In a middle ear infection, movement of the auricle does not increase pain.) Aspirin, codeine, and applications of heat provide comfort. If the tissues are edematous, it may be necessary to insert a wick of cotton gently through the canal to the eardrum so that liquid medications (such as Burow's solution [5% aluminum acetate] or antibiotics) may be introduced. These medications may also be administered by dropper at room temperature. Such medications usually are combinations of antibiotics and agents to soothe the inflamed membranes. Systemic antibiotic therapy also may be required. Patients are also reminded to avoid self-cleaning of the ear (cotton-tipped applicators are not to be used).

Another precaution is for the patient to avoid swimming or allowing water to enter the ear when shampooing or showering. Those prone to "swimmer's ear" should wear specially fitted ear plugs made from plastic material molded to exact measure.

The chronic form of external otitis is often due to a dermatosis such as psoriasis, eczema, or seborrheic dermatitis. Even allergic reactions to hair spray, hair dye, and permanent wave lotions can cause dermatitis, which clears when the offending agent is removed.

Furuncle of the External Canal

Infections of the skin and the subcutaneous tissue of the external canal usually result in a great deal of pain in the affected ear. There may be fever, severe headache, and enlargement of the local lymph nodes. This disorder may be mistaken for mastoid infection. The early administration of antibiotics and application of hot packs usually result in resolution of the furuncle. Incision and drainage are rarely performed because such measures may result in perichondritis or chondritis. It is better for the furuncle to localize (point) and open spontaneously or resolve by itself.

Cerumen in the Ear Canal

Ear wax normally accumulates in the ear in varying amounts and color. Although it does not ordinarily need to be removed, on occasion it may become impacted, causing *otalgia* (earache), dizziness, a sensation of fullness in the ear, and decreased hearing. Research has shown that accumulation of cerumen is especially significant in geriatric patients as a cause of hearing deficits. Attempts to clear the external auditory canal with matches, hair pins, and other implements are dangerous because trauma to the skin may result in infection or damage to the eardrum.

Management. Wax deposits may be removed by irrigation, suction, or instrumentation. Unless there is a history of perforated tympanic membrane or there is inflammation of the external ear (otitis externa), irrigation is the procedure of choice when the cerumen is impacted. If irrigation is not completely successful or if there is an incomplete impaction of the wax, direct visual, mechanical removal may be performed on the patient who is cooperative.

Wax deposits may be softened by instilling a few drops of warmed glycerin, mineral oil, half-strength hydrogen peroxide, or sodium bicarbonate drops for 30 minutes before removal. Cerumenolytic agents, such as peroxide in glyceryl (Debrox) or Cerumex, are also available; however, these compounds may cause an allergic reaction in the form of a dermatitis and should be avoided if the wax is so hard that it cannot be removed in a limited time. In such patients, mineral oil may be instilled and left in place for 2 or 3 days before the wax is removed. If the wax deposit cannot be dislodged by these methods, the cerumen may be removed by a physician with specific instruments such as a cerumen spoon used under magnification.

Foreign Bodies in the External Canal

Objects are, at times, inserted into the ear accidentally by adults, who may have been trying to clean the external canal or relieve itching, and intentionally by children, who introduce the object themselves. The effects may range from no symptoms at all to symptoms of profound pain and decreased hearing. An insect entering the ear may be disturbing but usually can be dislodged by instilling oil drops that smother the insect and allow it to be floated or flushed out.

There are three standard methods of removing foreign bodies from the external canal: irrigation, suction, and instrumentation. Irrigation is the first choice for most patients presenting in the emergency department. However, vegetable foreign bodies (*e.g.*, beans, peas) have a tendency to swell, so irrigation is contraindicated. Many foreign bodies in which irrigation is not an appropriate treatment may be removed with suction. If instrumentation is used, direct visualization of the canal is necessary to prevent damage. Attempts at removal of any foreign body from the external canal may be dangerous in unskilled hands. The object may be pushed completely into the bony portion of the canal, lacerating the skin and perforating the eardrum. Serious infections of the middle ear and the mastoid, with ensuing deafness, may result.

Irrigation of the External Auditory Canal

Irrigation of the ear canal is used less frequently today than in the past. When it is used, the purposes are (1) to carry out the caloric test for labyrinthine function, (2) to facilitate surgery on the external ear, and (3) to remove impacted cerumen (done by the physician).

The solutions for irrigating the ear should be at a temperature of about 40.6° to 43.3°C (105° to 110°F). Solutions that are too hot or too cold or that are used with too much force may cause pain or dizziness. The patient may sit or lie with his head tilted toward the side of the affected ear. A curved basin can be supported under the ear to catch the solution. To be effective, the fluids must reach the eardrum. To achieve this end, the auricle is pulled upward and backward to straighten the external auditory canal. (In children, this canal may be straightened by pulling the auricle down and back.) Extreme gentleness is used, and care must be taken that the fluid has free exit so that it is not driven into the middle ear. After the irrigation, the external opening is plugged lightly with sterile cotton, which is changed when necessary. After the procedure, the patient is instructed to lie on the affected ear so that gravity facilitates drainage.

- If injury to the tympanic membrane is suspected, irrigation should not be performed.

Problems of the Middle Ear

The middle ear, with its ossicles and ligaments and their connection to the eardrum, is vital to the function of hearing. The middle ear connects with the posterior portion of the nose by means of the auditory (eustachian) tube. Normally the tube is closed, but it opens by action of the muscles of the palate on yawning or swallowing. The tube serves as a drainage channel for normal and abnormal secretions of the middle ear and equalizes pressure in the middle ear to that of the atmosphere. When the membrane of this tube is inflamed, it offers an easy passage for infection into the middle ear.

Sound waves transmitted by the eardrum to the ossicles of the middle ear are transferred to the *cochlea*, the organ of hearing, lodged in the labyrinth or inner ear. An important ossicle is the stapes, which rocks and sets up vibrations (waves) in fluids contained in the labyrinth. These fluid waves, in turn, cause movement of the basilar membrane to occur that then stimulates the hair cells of the organ of Corti to move in a wavelike manner. The movements of the membrane set up electrical currents that stimulate the various areas of the cochlea. The hair cell sets up a neural impulse that is encoded and then transferred through the auditory cortex in the brain, where it is decoded into a sound message.

Trauma to the Tympanic Membrane (Perforation)

Permanent perforation of the tympanic membrane may occur as a result of vehicular accidents with skull fracture or from ear infections. Other causes of traumatic damage may be from intense compression, such as the blast effects of explosives or a severe blow on the ear. Perforations of the eardrum that fail to heal are often the end result of acute or chronic suppurative otitis media. The eardrum also may be burned by a spark from a welder's equipment.

Less frequently, perforation is caused by foreign objects, burns of the face that include the external ear and the eardrum, postmyringotomy defects, or scuba diving. Perforations also may occur when people, using cotton-tipped applicators to clean their ears, insert one into the external ear, pushing the applicator deep into the ear. If the tip is bumped or is pushed into the canal, severe destruction of the eardrum, ossicles, and even the inner ear may occur. Thus, all attempts to clean the ear with applicator sticks must be discouraged.

Management.   Most accidental perforations of the eardrum membrane heal spontaneously. Some persist because of the growth of scar tissue over the edges of the perforation, thus preventing extension of the epithelial areas across the margins and final healing.

- In suspected traumatic perforation, the patient is warned against irrigating the ear. He is instructed to cleanse the outer ear carefully with sterile cotton but to leave the ear canal alone until an otologist can aspirate blood and inspect the eardrum for evidence of perforation.

If the patient has sustained a head injury, he is kept under observation to detect any evidence of cerebrospinal fluid otorrhea, such as clear, watery drainage. Such fluid can be examined in the laboratory to determine whether its source is the cerebrospinal canal.

Middle Ear Effusion (Serous Otitis Media)

Secretory Otitis Media.   Because this condition is found primarily in children, the reader is directed to pediatric nursing texts.

Aerotitis Media.   *Aerotitis media* is a form of serous otitis media in which noninfective fluid or air is trapped in the middle ear because of sudden pressure changes such as descending in an airplane (barotrauma). The condition usually lasts a short time, but it may continue for days. For this reason, people may avoid flying when they have an upper respiratory tract infection because the normal functions of the eustachian tube are decreased when the tube is swollen. Preventive measures that allow equalization of middle ear pressure and relief of the annoying symptoms include chewing gum, sucking on hard candy, yawning, swallowing, or performing the Valsalva maneuver during the descent of the plane.

Acute Otitis Media (Purulent or Suppurative Otitis Media)

Acute otitis media is an acute infection of the middle ear (Table 54-2). The primary cause of acute otitis media is the entrance of pathogenic bacteria into the normally sterile middle ear when the host's resistance is lowered, or when the virulence of the organism is great enough to produce inflammation, or when there is eustachian tube obstruction that prevents drainage. Eustachian tube obstruction may be caused by upper respiratory infections, inflammations of surrounding structures (*e.g.*, sinusitis or enlarged adenoids), or by allergic reactions (*e.g.*, allergic rhinitis). Bacteria commonly found as the causative organisms are *Streptococcus pneumoniae, Hemophilus influenzae, Branhamella catarrhalis,* and *Staphylococcus.* Certain viruses also may be causative agents but are difficult to culture. The mode of entry of the bacteria in most patients is the auditory canal or the eustachian tube, from contaminated secretions in the nasopharynx.

Clinical Manifestations.   The symptoms of otitis media may vary with the severity of the infection and may be either very mild and transient or very severe. The condition is usually unilateral, affecting one ear in adults. Pain in and about the ear (otalgia) is one of the first symptoms and may be intense. It is relieved after spontaneous perforation of the eardrum or after myringotomy (see below). Fever, another symptom, varies and in severe cases may range between 40.0° and 40.6°C (104° to 105°F). The tympanic membrane often is bulging, opaque, and has decreased mobility; however, retracted or concave tympanic membranes have been visualized on pneumatic otoscopy. Deafness, ear noises, headache, loss of appetite, nausea, and vomiting are other symptoms that accompany the condition.

Management.   The outcome of otitis media is dependent on the efficiency of the therapy (*i.e.*, the prescribed dose of antibiotic and the duration of therapy), the virulence of the bacteria, and the resistance of the patient. With early and appropriate wide-spectrum antibiotic therapy, otitis media may clear with no serious sequelae.

It is important to note that symptoms may be masked by antibiotic therapy and that during the course of treatment of an acute middle ear infection, symptoms such as headache, slow pulse, vomiting, and vertigo should be evaluated by an otologist. The appropriate antibiotic is important for eventual cure and should be taken for the complete course of treatment. Research has shown that certain antibiotics have a problem penetrating the affected area because capillary permeability

TABLE 54–2. *Clinical Features of Acute Diffuse External Otitis and Acute Otitis Media*

Feature	External Otitis	Otitis Media
Pain	Persistent	Subsides in 6–9 hours
	Aggravated by moving jaw	Relieved immediately if tympanic membrane ruptures
		Aggravated by swallowing, belching
Tenderness	Prominent	Absent
Systemic symptoms	Usually absent	Fever, rhinitis, sore throat
Hearing loss	Conductive type	Conductive type
Swelling of ear canal	Prominent	Absent
Discharge	Foul odor	No odor
	Pus, never profuse	
Tympanic membrane	Inflamed but intact	May be perforated
	No middle ear fluid	Fluid in middle ear

(Farmer HS. A guide for the treatment of external otitis. Am Fam Physician 21[6]:98. Published by the American Academy of Family Physicians.)

decreases as inflammation subsides. Therefore, it is imperative that prescribed doses of antibiotics be adequate and that all of the prescribed medicine is taken.

The condition may become subacute (*i.e.*, lasting 3 weeks to 3 months), with persistent purulent discharge (otorrhea) from the ear. Healing may take place with permanent deafness.

Perforation of the eardrum may persist and develop into a chronic otitis media. Secondary complications, with involvement of the mastoid, and other serious intracranial complications, such as meningitis or brain abscess, may result.

Myringotomy (Tympanotomy).   An incision of the tympanic membrane is known as myringotomy or tympanotomy. An incision is made into the tympanic membrane to relieve pressure and to drain serous or purulent fluid from the middle ear behind the eardrum (see Fig. 54-6). In mild cases of otitis media, treated effectively, a myringotomy may not be necessary; however, if pain persists, this procedure is important for promoting surgical drainage. It also allows the organism to be identified, and its sensitivity to antibiotic agents can be determined.

The incision heals rapidly and hearing usually is not impaired. Although performed less frequently than it was before the advent of antibiotic therapy, if a myringotomy is done, a plastic tube is temporarily inserted through the eardrum to prevent accumulation of fluid or chronic otitis media.

In summary, acute otitis media is caused by pathogenic bacteria that cause infection and inflammation in the normally sterile middle ear. Although symptoms vary, pain is common, accompanied by earache, and sometimes hearing loss. Appropriate early antibiotic therapy is important for cure and is the treatment of choice. Tympanic membrane perforation (spontaneous or by surgical procedure) relieves the pain and also allows for drainage. If acute otitis media is not treated, it can progress to a subacute or chronic stage in which surrounding structures can be affected and intracranial complications may occur.

Chronic Otitis Media

Chronic otitis media results from repeated attacks of otitis media, causing persistent perforation of the eardrum. It is due to particular virulence of the infecting organisms or to bacterial resistance to antibiotic therapy. The chronically infected ear is characterized by persistent or recurrent purulent discharge, with or without pain, and varying degrees of deafness, usually conductive or mixed type. Most chronic otitis media begins in childhood and may persist into adult life.

Classification.   Chronic suppurative middle ear infection has been classified into five groupings, as indicated in Table 54-3.

Clinical Manifestations.   The symptoms of chronic otitis media may be minimal, with varying degrees of deafness and the presence of a persistent or intermittent foul-smelling discharge of variable quantity. Pain may or may not be present. Symptoms such as sudden facial paralysis, unusually profound deafness or dizziness, onset of headache with dizziness, and stiff neck may herald a beginning meningitis or brain abscess or erosion into the semicircular canals. The diagnosis is supported by the physical findings; in addition, x-ray films of the mastoid usually show pathologic changes.

Management.   Local treatment consists of careful cleansing of the ear and instillation of antibiotic drops or application of antibiotic powder. Tympanoplastic procedures may be required early to prevent further damage to hearing and more serious complications.

In summary, otitis media can become a chronic problem, resulting from repeated infections causing persistent perforation of the eardrum and recurrent purulent discharge. Pain may or may not be present, along with varying degrees and types of deafness. Extending intracranial symptoms, such as headache with dizziness and stiff neck, may suggest meningitis. Management consists of careful cleaning, antibiotic therapy, and

TABLE 54-3.   *Classification of Chronic Otitis Media*

Type	Specific Condition	Involvement	Manifestation
I	Chronic otitis media simplex	Central perforation of the tympanic membrane	Mucoid serous discharge
II	Chronic otitis media with cholesteatoma*	Usually, attic perforation (posterior superior part of eardrum)	Usually, odorous discharge
		With or without perforation	
III	Chronic adhesive otitis media	Marked retraction of tympanic membrane	No discharge
			Marked hearing loss
IV	Chronic otitis media with tympanosclerosis	Tympanosclerosis, a degenerative process in eardrum and middle ear	Severe hearing loss
		Plaque of amorphous connective tissue	No discharge
V	Chronic serous otitis media	If untreated or neglected, may result in severe deafness, chronic adhesive otitis media, cholesteatoma,* or tympanosclerosis	Repeated bout of serous or fluid ear

* Cholesteatoma *is due to the ingrowth of the skin of the external ear canal (squamous epithelium) into the middle ear. The skin from the external canal forms the outer sac, which fills with degenerated skin and sebaceous material. The sac is attached to the structures of the middle ear and mastoid and produces changes by pressure necrosis.*
(Woodrow D. Schlesser, MD, personal communication.)

x-rays to assess for further structural involvement. Tympanoplasty may prevent serious complications.

Mastoiditis and Mastoidectomy

Mastoiditis is an inflammation of the mastoid resulting from an infection of the middle ear; if it is untreated, osteomyelitis may occur. Symptoms are pain and tenderness behind the ear, discharge from the middle ear, and swelling of the mastoid. Usually, this is successfully treated with antibiotics; occasionally myringotomy is required.

When there is recurrent or persistent tenderness, fever, headache, and discharge from the ear, it may be necessary to remove the mastoid process (mastoidectomy). However, this procedure is seldom required because the infection usually responds to appropriate antibiotics.

Preoperative Management.   Preparation of the patient is important. Depending on the procedure to be performed—for example, closed (or simple) mastoidectomy performed through the ear with a tympanoplasty, or an open (modified or radical) mastoidectomy—the patient must be instructed on specific preoperative and postoperative expectations. Hospital admission may be expected if the patient is in poor general health and if previous outpatient surgeries or other treatments have been ineffective in clearing the infection.

During the operation, the infection is removed completely from the mastoid process by removing the mastoid cells, and the middle ear is drained (myringotomy), thus preventing spread of the infection to surrounding tissues.

Postoperative Management.   Analgesics usually are indicated after the operation and during the first 1 or 2 postoperative days to control pain and restlessness. Fluids are given freely when the patient is alert. A bulky mastoid dressing is changed when sutures are removed; a smaller dressing is applied if drainage is still present and is changed by the patient as required. Antibiotics are continued for several days.

A possible complication after mastoidectomy is facial pa-

ralysis. The nurse may be the first to note this serious indication of facial nerve inflammation or injury. Symptoms may include the patient's inability to close the eye and drooping of the mouth on the affected side, as well as the inability to whistle, or drink without fluid dripping out of the mouth. Any evidence of facial paralysis is reported immediately to the physician. The patient may be taken back to surgery, the wound opened, and repair of the facial nerve performed. Other possible complications are meningitis or brain abscess.

In summary, the inflammation of the mastoid (mastoiditis) is usually treated in a clinic or outpatient setting. Infection is controlled primarily by antibiotic therapy; however, various surgical procedures may be used after other treatments are found ineffective. Patients should be prepared for the specific surgery and carefully instructed about postoperative expectations. Analgesics and oral antibiotics are continued after surgery to control pain, restlessness, and to prevent new infection. Dressings to the surgical site are changed as necessary after sutures are removed. Possible complications include facial paralysis, meningitis, or brain abscess.

Tympanoplasty

Tympanoplasty refers to the reconstruction of the middle ear bones. The goal is to provide better continuity from the eardrum to the oval window through which sound waves pass. Several reconstructive procedures that can be performed on middle ear structures that have been destroyed by chronic infections or disease, or which are congenitally deformed, are noted in Table 54-4. Using an illuminated microscope and specialized instruments, the otologist is able to visualize and reconstruct defective conductive mechanisms to maintain or improve hearing.

Procedure.   Tympanoplasty is performed to reestablish functions of the middle ear. The outcome depends on the extent of middle ear physiologic changes and structural damage

TABLE 54-4. *Tympanoplastic Procedures*

Type	Damage of Middle Ear	Methods of Repair
I	Perforated tympanic membrane with normal ossicular chain	Closure of perforation; same as myringoplasty
II	Perforation of tympanic membrane with erosion of malleus	Closure with graft against incus or remains of malleus
III	Destruction of tympanic membrane and ossicular chain *but with* intact and mobile stapes	Graft contacts normal stapes; also gives sound protection to round window
IV	Similar to type III, but head, neck, and crura of stapes missing; footplate mobile	Mobile footplate left exposed; air pocket between round window and graft provides sound protection for round window
V	Similar to type IV plus *fixed* footplate	Fenestra in horizontal semicircular canal; graft seals off middle ear to give sound protection for round window

(DeWeese DD and Saunders WH. Textbook of Otolaryngology, 6th ed. St Louis, CV Mosby.)

and how well three aspects of middle ear physiology are supported. The three aspects are (1) the transformer action, (2) sound protection for the round window, and (3) normal size of the space within the middle ear. An ear that remains dry and free from infection postoperatively is necessary for the procedure to be successful. Five types of tympanoplastic procedures have been described (see Table 54-4).

Indications. The simplest surgical procedure, tympanoplasty type I (myringoplasty) is designed to close perforations in the tympanic membrane and is a one-stage operation. The other types of procedures, types II through V, involve more extensive repair of middle ear structures and may involve two stages—the first is to clear any infection or to remove pathology, and the second is for the reconstructive process. The structures and the degree of involvement may differ, but part of all tympanoplasty procedures includes restoring the continuity of the sound transmission mechanism. Ossicular interruption is most frequent in otitis media, but problems of reconstruction occur with malformations of the middle ear and ossicular dislocations due to head injuries.

Dramatic improvement in hearing may result from closure of a perforation if there is no involvement of the ossicles. When the patching of a perforation of the eardrum is not followed by audiometric improvement, one must consider involvement of the ossicular chain. During the surgical repair of the perforation, a careful inspection of the middle ear contents, with particular attention to the continuity of the ossicles, is important.

Surgery is performed almost exclusively in an outpatient environment. If the patient has had previous, unsuccessful operations for the existing problem or if the patient has a chronic health problem (*e.g.*, diabetes mellitus), the surgery may be performed in an inpatient environment.

Contraindications. It is generally accepted that closure of perforations of the eardrum in the presence of an active infection is contraindicated. Also, if there is chronic inadequate drainage from the middle ear due to malfunction of the auditory canal (eustachian tube), surgery is contraindicated. Involvement of the nasopharynx because of chronic infectious discharge from sinusitis of an allergy, plus a history of acute exacerbations of otitis media, also may be a contraindication for surgery.

Management. The goals of treatment are to create a closed middle ear cavity by placing a graft over the perforation and to improve hearing. Antibiotic therapy is usually continued for a specified time after the surgery. Dressings are left undisturbed except for external dressings, which may be changed if soiled from drainage.

Safety is a primary concern for the patient and must be provided because dizziness and nystagmus may occur. The patient is assisted the first time out of bed. Medications to combat vertigo and nausea may be prescribed. Teaching is extremely important for the patient. The patient is cautioned to avoid blowing his nose or wetting the dressings during bathing. Once discharged from the surgical facility, the patient must avoid getting moisture in the ear. Eventually, showering and other activities are permitted.

Clinical Results. Better results are generally achieved with younger patients than with older patients. The simpler the surgery, the better the chance for improvement of hearing; this, of course, relates directly to the functional integrity of the ossicular chain and the efficiency of the newly created tympanic covering.

Clinical failures due to infections and tissue rejection of graft or prosthesis have been reported. Continued research is being conducted to improve tympanoplasty procedures.

Otosclerosis

Otosclerosis, or otospongiosis, is a term applied to a form of progressive deafness caused by the formation of new, abnormal spongy bone in the labyrinth that eventually immobilizes the stapes. The transmission of sound is then prevented because the stapes is unable to vibrate and carry the stimulus of the vibrating malleus and incus to the inner ear fluids.

Etiology.   The cause of the condition is unknown, but it may have a hereditary basis. Other possible causes include vitamin deficiency or otitis media. It occurs most commonly in women, beginning in early teens, and seems to worsen with pregnancy.

The condition, which involves both ears, but unequally, begins with insidious loss of hearing and a ringing or buzzing in the ears. The patient gives a history of progressive hearing loss without middle ear infection. Sound transmission by air is markedly reduced. The bone conduction is better than air conduction when tested by the Rinne's test. Diagnosis is made from the findings of audiometry.

Stapedectomy.   There is no known medical treatment for the deafness that accompanies otosclerosis other than the help offered by amplification with an electric hearing aid or by a stapedectomy. A stapedectomy involves removing the otosclerotic lesion at the footplate of the stapes and creating a suitable implant with a prosthesis to replace this portion of the conductive mechanism (Fig. 54-7). The otologic binocular microscope coupled to a laser is of distinct value in this operation. A variety of lasers have been used for stapedectomy and stapedectomy revisions in correcting conductive hearing loss secondary to otosclerosis. Prosthetic materials have included the use of steel wires with fat implants, Gelfoam, or a segment of vein. These materials help bridge the gap between the incus and the inner ear, thus providing better sound conduction.

▶ Nursing Process
The Patient Undergoing Ear Surgery

Many surgical procedures on the ear are performed under local anesthesia in an outpatient setting.

◊ Assessment

The health history includes a description of the ear problem, for example, earache, discharge, or hearing loss. Data are collected about causation, intensity of the problem, and duration, as well as previous treatment. Information is obtained about other health problems and all medications that the patient is taking. When discomfort is apparent, gentleness is necessary when touching or manipulating the ear. Swelling, redness, lesions, drainage, and odor of any discharge are noted. One ear is compared with the other.

◊ Nursing Diagnoses

Based on the assessment data, the patient's major nursing diagnoses may include:

- Anxiety about the surgical procedure and the postoperative course
- Pain related to the surgical procedure
- High risk for injury related to vertigo
- High risk for infection related to contamination of the operative area
- Altered auditory sensory perception related to preoperative hearing loss and postoperative interference with sound transmission (dressings, blood, drainage, packing)
- Knowledge deficit about the nature of the operation, and postoperative care and expectations

◊ Planning and Implementation

◊ *Goals:*   The major goals of the patient may include reduction of anxiety and acquisition of knowledge, freedom from discomfort (pain, nausea, and vomiting), prevention of infection and absence of injury, improved hearing/minimal hearing loss, and knowledge regarding the surgical procedure and follow-up care.

◊ Nursing Interventions

◊ *Reducing Anxiety.*   The nurse reinforces information the surgeon has discussed with the patient regarding the nature of the anesthesia, the location of the incision, and the expected surgical results. Information about the operating room environment is important for the patient to know before surgery. Discussing postoperative expectations helps to decrease anxiety about the unknown. Before surgery, the patient is informed that he will be expected to rest quietly for the first 24 hours (off the operative side) to prevent dislodgement of the prosthesis.

◊ *Relieving Pain and Preventing Injury.*   Pain may last for a few hours postoperatively; therefore, it is desirable for the patient to take the prescribed analgesic.

Vertigo occurs because the semicircular canals and vagus nerve are manipulated and stimulated during surgery. Dizziness after a stapedectomy is common but usually resolves within the first 3 days. The head of the bed is usually elevated to help drainage. Sudden movement of the head is undesirable; therefore, rising slowing is advisable and sneezing or coughing are to be avoided. (If sneezing and coughing are unavoidable, the patient is instructed to open his mouth and sneeze and cough as gently as possible.) Blowing the nose, straining during defecation, and bending at the waist also must be avoided. All motions are to be performed slowly. Antiemetic or anti–motion sickness medication can be prescribed in case the patient becomes nauseated or dizzy. The nurse monitors the patient for effects of the medication to see if the desired results have been obtained. The patient should be instructed on the expected effects also. Safety measures such as assisted ambulation are carried out to prevent the patient from falling should he experience vertigo or disturbances in equilibrium.

◊ *Preventing Infection.*   Measures are initiated to prevent infection in the operative ear. Packing may be impregnated with an antibiotic solution before instillation, and prophylactic antibiotics are given as prescribed. Visitors with upper respiratory tract infections are discouraged. Aseptic technique is required when changing dressings. The patient is instructed to avoid touching his dressings to prevent contamination and to avoid getting his ear or dressings wet when washing his face because moisture helps to transmit contaminants. No shampoos are permitted until the physician determines that their use is safe, usually about 2 weeks. The patient is reminded not to blow his nose or sneeze because such actions may force organisms through the auditory canal to the middle ear. Any signs of infection such as temperature elevation and the presence of purulent, foul-smelling drainage are observed for and reported. The patient should be instructed to report increasing ear pressure or pain and any evidence of facial paralysis: drooping of the mouth on the operative side, altered taste, drooling when drinking, and excessive mouth dryness. Loss of taste or facial

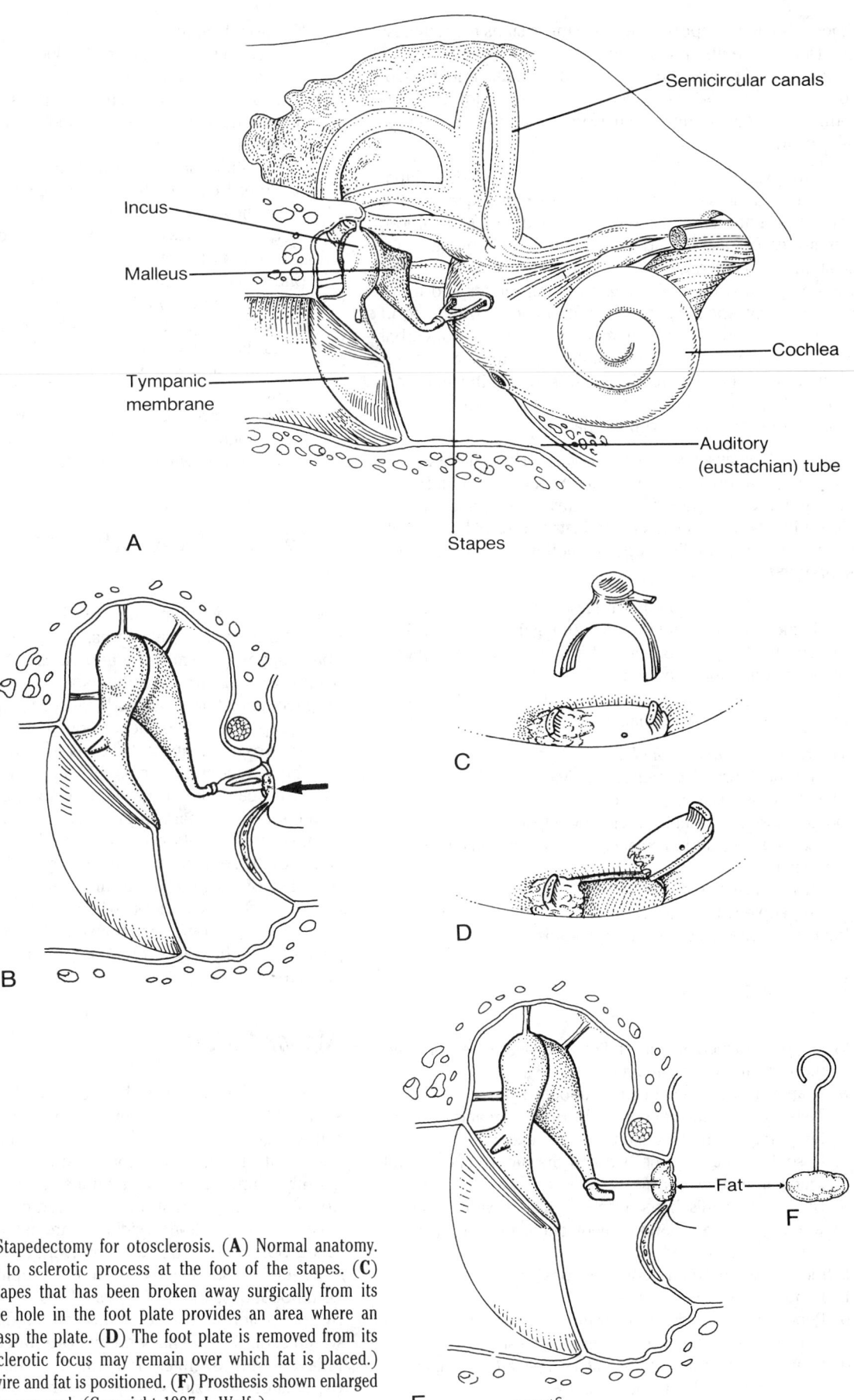

Figure 54-7. Stapedectomy for otosclerosis. (**A**) Normal anatomy.
(**B**) Arrow points to sclerotic process at the foot of the stapes. (**C**)
Enlargement of stapes that has been broken away surgically from its
diseased base. The hole in the foot plate provides an area where an
instrument can grasp the plate. (**D**) The foot plate is removed from its
base. (Some otosclerotic focus may remain over which fat is placed.)
(**E**) Prosthesis of wire and fat is positioned. (**F**) Prosthesis shown enlarged
with fat attached to one end. (Copyright 1987 J. Wolfe)

weakness should be reported because these signs may suggest trauma to the seventh cranial nerve.

Should facial nerve damage occur, fluid intake is increased. If drooling occurs, a straw is used and frequent mouth care is performed. The patient must be reassured that these symptoms usually resolve.

▷ *Improving Communication.*   The patient must be advised that hearing in the ear undergoing surgery will be reduced for several weeks because of edema, accumulation of drainage or blood, and dressings or packing. Thus, measures to improve communication are initiated, such as reducing environmental noise, facing the patient when speaking, speaking louder and more slowly than usual, speaking into the better ear, providing good lighting if the patient relies on lipreading, and using nonverbal clues such as facial expression, pointing, gestures, and other forms of communication. Family members or significant others must be instructed regarding effective practices so they may communicate successfully with the patient.

▷ *Patient Education for Self-Care at Home.*   The patient is usually discharged a few hours after surgery and may require assistance at home. The person accompanying the patient home should be involved in the discharge instructions also. The following are examples of discharge instructions for patients after ear surgery:

To Prevent Dislodgement of Prosthesis
- Avoid blowing nose and sneezing during the first week. This protects the tympanic membrane from air pressure changes.
- Avoid sudden rapid movements.
- Do not bend at the waist or strain on defecation. Do not lift objects that weigh more than 5 pounds.

To Prevent Infection in the Ear
- Do not touch dressings unnecessarily.
- Change dressings as instructed.
- Do not wash hair until instructed by physician.
- Do not shower, fly in a plane, or swim until instructed by physician.
- Cover the ear when outside.
- Avoid people with colds.
- Report any unusual signs and symptoms.

▷ Evaluation

Expected Outcomes
1. Verbalizes lessened anxiety and can explain the reasons and methods of his care or treatment
   a. Shares knowledge with family about treatment protocol
   b. Tells nurse he can accept results of surgery and adjust to temporary hearing impairment, if necessary
   c. Describes treatment he had and the time frame he will follow in recovery phase
   d. Discusses the discharge plan formulated with the nurse with regard to rest periods, medication, and activities permitted and restricted
2. Is free of discomfort and complications
   a. Reports absence of dizzy spells
   b. Reports no taste distortion or mouth dryness
   c. Lists ways to prevent dislodging prosthesis
   d. Identifies symptoms of possible complications that are to be reported to health care person
   e. Specifies methods for preventing ear infections

3. Has no infection or injury
   a. Practices acceptable technique when changing dressings
   b. Is afebrile on discharge
   c. Postpones showers and shampoos as advised
   d. Modifies environment to avoid falls (*e.g.*, lights on at night; no clutter on steps)
4. Demonstrates improved hearing
   a. Verbalizes that sounds unable to be heard before treatment are heard postoperatively
   b. Expresses pleasure about progressive hearing gain noticed from day to day
5. Understands (as confirmed by conversation) what is expected of him in self-care/follow-up care
   a. Reiterates limitations in activities and for how long regarding showering, swimming, lifting, and air flights
   b. Demonstrates how to move when getting in and out of bed
   c. Lists symptoms that should be reported to health care personnel
   d. Keeps follow-up appointments

Problems of the Inner Ear

Body balance is maintained by the cooperation of muscles, joints, tendons, visceral senses, eyes, and the inner ear or vestibular apparatus. The inner apparatus of the ear provides feedback regarding the movements and the position of the head in space, coordinates all body muscles, and positions the eyes during rapid motion or head movement.

The vestibular apparatus consists of the utricle, the saccule, and the semicircular canals, of which there are three in each ear. Each canal lies in a plane at right angles to the others, with the entire apparatus grouped in working pairs for the accomplishment of its complex functions. The mechanism of action of the semicircular canals may be likened to the cochlea or organ of hearing. Here, also, fluids are set in motion by head or body movement, which in turn stimulate extremely delicate nerve fibers that transmit messages as electrical impulses along the nerve to centers in the brain, where they are interpreted.

Motion Sickness

Motion sickness is a disturbance of equilibrium caused by constant motion, such as occurs aboard a ship or boat, riding on a merry-go-round or swing, or even riding a distance in the back seat of a car. Symptoms are dizziness, nausea, and frequently vomiting. These manifestations may persist several hours after the stimulation stops. Medications that prevent and treat vertigo and motion sickness are helpful in providing some relief. Some side effects of antivertigo medications may be experienced, such as dry mouth, cycloplegia (paralysis of accommodation), and drowsiness. These side effects are reduced by administering the medication with a disc (Transderm V) in which scopolamine has been incorporated. Dry mouth can be relieved with lozenges. Patients must be warned that if they experience drowsiness they must avoid potentially hazardous activities such as driving a car.

TYPE	SYMPTOMS AND SIGNS

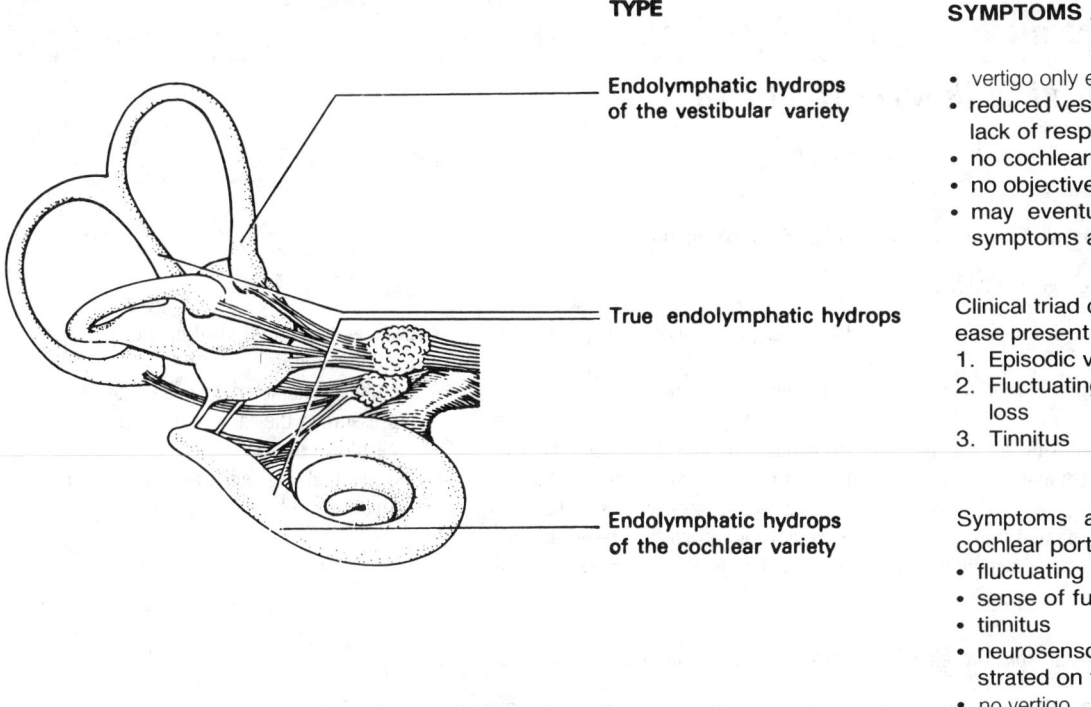

Endolymphatic hydrops of the vestibular variety

- vertigo only episodic
- reduced vestibular response or total lack of response in affected ear
- no cochlear symptoms
- no objective hearing loss
- may eventually develop cochlear symptoms and signs

True endolymphatic hydrops

Clinical triad of typical Ménière's disease present
1. Episodic vertigo
2. Fluctuating neurosensory hearing loss
3. Tinnitus

Endolymphatic hydrops of the cochlear variety

Symptoms and signs confined to cochlear portion of labyrinth
- fluctuating hearing loss
- sense of fullness in ear
- tinnitus
- neurosensory hearing loss demonstrated on testing
- no vertigo
- normal vestibular labyrinthine tests
- may eventually develop vestibular symptoms and signs

Figure 54–8.   A practical classification of Ménière's disease.

Endolymphatic Hydrops (Ménière's Disease)

Ménière's disease is an inner ear problem stemming from a labyrinthine dysfunction, the cause of which has not been definitely established. Many theories have been advanced, such as abnormal hormonal and neurochemical influences on the blood flow to the labyrinth, electrolyte disturbance within labyrinthine fluids, an allergic reaction, or autoimmune disorders. Some attribute the impairment of the microvasculature of the inner ear to abnormal metabolites (glucose, insulin, triglycerides, and cholesterol) in the bloodstream.

Clinical Manifestations.   Ménière's disease is most frequently characterized by the presence of a triad of symptoms: paroxysmal whirling vertigo with nausea and vomiting, tinnitus, and neurosensory hearing loss. Some add a fourth manifestation, a sense of pressure in the ear. At the onset of the condition, perhaps only one or two of these symptoms are manifested; however, the disease is not diagnosed as Ménière's syndrome until all three signs are present (Fig. 54-8).

Vertigo, the outstanding symptom of Ménière's disease, occurs as a sudden attack, appearing at irregular intervals and possibly persisting for several hours. Early in this condition, weeks or months pass between attacks, but the time is gradually reduced so that they may be experienced every 2 or 3 days. The attacks can last several hours, with residual symptoms remaining for days. Usually, only one ear is involved, although bilateral involvement has been reported. Nystagmus and ataxia also may be apparent. Tinnitus is characteristically a low, fluctuating, buzzing sound in the ears. It is often louder preceding

and during an attack. Sensorineural loss applies to low tones and usually occurs unilaterally. It becomes progressively worse and may cause severe cochlear damage if untreated.

Diagnostic Evaluation.   Because Ménière's disease simulates signs and symptoms of acoustic neuroma and other cerebellopontine angle tumors, careful diagnostic evaluation is required, including an audiogram, head scan (magnetic resonance imaging), and allergy evaluation. Early in the course of the condition, patients are evaluated for glucose intolerance and for abnormal insulin levels. If results are abnormal, these patients are regarded as prediabetic and are managed by a controlled-carbohydrate weight-reduction diet.

Electronystagmography is the preferred test; it measures the electropotential of eye movements when nystagmus is produced and provides a graphic record of labyrinthine function.

Auditory Dehydration Test.   Endolymphatic hydrops is verified when a hearing gain occurs after the intake of a hyperosmolar substance (glycerol or urea). A baseline audiogram is performed, and a serum osmolality value is obtained. The patient eats a light breakfast about 2 hours before drinking the prescribed amount of the hyperosmolar substance, which is usually mixed with unsweetened fruit juice. Serum osmolalities are taken hourly and measured on an osmometer. A positive audiometric fluctuation at any hour constitutes a positive test.

Management.   The goals of treatment are to eliminate vertigo and improve or stabilize the patient's hearing. This is accomplished by a combination of methods to avoid severe hearing loss. Treatment approaches may include medical, surgical, rehabilitative, and dietary strategies and are prescribed according to the underlying cause. Medications are used that (1) suppress the vestibular system (*i.e.*, benzodiazepines [an-

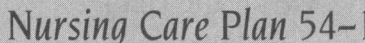

Nursing Care Plan 54–1

Care of the Patient With Ménière's Disease

Nursing Interventions	Rationale	Expected Outcomes

Nursing Diagnosis: High risk for injury related to labyrinth dysfunction

Goal: Freedom from vertigo and falling

1. Encourage patient to lie down; side rails up on bed.	1. Decreases possibility of falling and injury.	• Assumes horizontal position when dizzy.
2. Place pillow on each side of head to restrict movement.	2. Movement aggravates vertigo.	• Keeps head still.
3. Assist patient in identifying aura that suggests an attack is coming.	3. Recognition of aura may trigger the need to react before an attack occurs, thereby minimizing the severity or effects.	• Identifies a characteristic fullness or sense of pressure in the ear as occurring before a full-blown attack.
4. Recommend that the patient close his eyes when lying down and experiencing vertigo.	4. Sensation of vertigo decreases and motion decelerates if eyes are kept closed.	• Reports that closing eyes helps reduce vertigo.

Nursing Diagnosis: Social isolation related to attacks of vertigo and hearing loss

Goal: Renewal of social contacts; control, and preferably elimination of vertigo, tinnitus; return to usual life-style.

1. Administer prescribed vestibular suppressants for motion sickness and vertigo.	1. Decreasing attacks of vertigo will allow for more movement and socialization.	• Takes prescribed medications. Reports less vertigo.
2. Review salt-restricted dietary regimen.	2. Salt restriction helps some patients by decreasing symptoms.	• Follows recommended low-salt dietary plan. Reports fewer symptoms of vertigo.
3. Instruct patient about taking prescribed diuretics, vasodilators, and other drugs.	3. Medications help relieve fullness in the ear and abate symptoms. Patient knowledge of drug actions promotes compliance.	• Resumes usual activities. Verbalizes medication actions and schedule.

Nursing Diagnosis: Self-care deficit: feeding, bathing/hygiene, dressing/grooming, toileting, related to labyrinth dysfunction and episodes of vertigo.

Goal: Ability to care for self.

1. Administer antiemetic and other prescribed medications to relieve nausea and vomiting.	1. Antiemetics and sedative-type drugs depress stimuli in vomiting center.	• Carries out necessary functions during symptom-free periods. Takes medications to relieve nausea or vomiting.
2. Encourage patient to care for bodily needs when free of vertigo.	2. Spacing activities is important because episodes of vertigo vary in occurrence.	• Carries out daily activities without vertigo.
3. Review diet with patient and other care givers. Offer fluids as necessary.	3. Sodium restriction helps decrease vertigo in some patients. Fluids help prevent dehydration.	• Accepts dietary plan and reports its effectiveness. Drinks fluids in sufficient amounts.

Nursing Diagnosis: Anxiety related to disabling effects of condition and concern about progressive hearing loss.

Goal: Freedom from worry and acceptance of outcome of treatment.

1. Provide comfort measures and avoid stress-producing activities.	1. Stressful situations may exacerbate symptoms of the disease.	• Avoids upsetting encounters.
2. Instruct patient in all aspects of treatment regimen.	2. Patient knowledge helps to decrease anxiety.	• Repeats instructions given and verbalizes understanding of treatments.

(continued)

▶ **Nursing Care Plan 54-1** *(Continued)*

Care of the Patient With Ménière's Disease

Nursing Interventions	Rationale	Expected Outcomes

Nursing Diagnosis: Altered sensory perception (auditory) related to labyrinth dysfunction

Goal: Improved hearing with freedom from complications

1. Assist patient in preparing for diagnostic tests.	1. Data promote diagnosis of problem.	• Accepts the preparation for tests and verbalizes understanding of audiometric tests and blood work.
2. Prepare patient for surgery if this is indicated.	2. Endolymphatic sac surgery may be performed to relieve symptoms.	
3. Observe for potential complications.	3. Infection, increased loss of hearing, spinal fluid leakage, speech paralysis may occur.	• Expresses hope that surgery may help but recognizes that some hearing may be lost.
		• Has no postoperative complications; absence of infection, exhibits normal speech.
4. Assist the unsteady patient as required; expect vertigo and nausea after labrinthectomy.	4. Structures of equilibrium may be damaged during surgery. Edema may cause vertigo postoperatively. Safety is important after surgery.	• Develops an understanding of what to expect postoperatively. Uses safety precautions to avoid falls.
5. Arrange for psychosocial and family support as necessary.	5. Support is needed after prolonged or major disorders.	• Responds positively to support systems and modifies life-style. Learns to read lips.
6. Provide patient and family with the appropriate hearing aid service information.	6. Some improvement in hearing may be realized with a hearing aid.	• Indicates that the recovery process is slow and that patience is required.

tianxiety agents], anticholinergics, and antihistamines); (2) cause diuresis; and (3) control nausea. Steroids such as prednisone may be used to maintain hearing and to decrease dizziness. Use of streptomycin sulfate in autoimmune disorders causing bilateral aural symptoms has been documented. Vasodilating drugs, such as nicotinic acid, tolazoline hydrochloride (Priscoline), and methantheline bromide (Banthine), improve tinnitus. The patient's vital signs and general condition are monitored, along with any evidence of untoward effects of the medications (*e.g.*, ataxia and kidney dysfunction).

Dietary management is controversial, but many patients respond when treated with a salt-free diet and a diuretic. Alcohol, excessive smoking, and caffeine are avoided. Food allergy is investigated and may require that certain foods be eliminated from the diet.

Surgical Management. A variety of treatments exist for Ménière's disease. Research continues in an effort to find the cause of this syndrome, which will more clearly suggest definitive therapy. Some of the surgical therapies used in the treatment are listed below.

An endolymphatic subarachnoid shunt is a procedure favored by many otolaryngologists. The procedure is successful in providing relief to patients without destroying function. It involves decompressing the endolymphatic sac and sectioning the vestibular nerve.

An endolymphatic system–mastoid shunt with valve implant is a procedure performed instead of a destructive labyrinthectomy. This type of surgery, first performed in Sweden and then in the United States in the late 1970s, appears to be more promising for those having surgery before the endolymphatic sac is obliterated by the disease process.

Ultrasonic surgery is another technique that has been tried. A mastoidectomy incision is made to gain access to the horizontal semicircular canal. Ultrasonic vibrations then are applied directly to the bone in the canal by means of a probe. The destructive effects of these vibrations last for only a few days, and proponents claim that hearing is preserved while vertigo is eliminated.

Total labyrinthectomy (destruction of the inner ear) is another procedure sometimes used when medical management fails and the patient has had progressive hearing loss and experiences severe vertigo attacks. This is performed through the ear canal: the stapes is removed and the endolabyrinth is aspirated with suction.

Postoperatively, the patient who has had surgical destruction of the labyrinth may experience vertigo for a few days, after which it gradually subsides and permits him to get out of bed. Some unsteadiness and vertigo may persist as long as 1 or 2 months, but this may be controlled if the patient moves carefully. Nursing care for the patient with Ménière's disease is presented in Nursing Care Plan 54-1.

Cochlear Implant

A cochlear implant is an auditory prosthesis used for people who are profoundly deaf and designated as untreatable by other methods. A cochlear implant system marketed by 3M was granted FDA approval in 1984 (Fig. 54-9). Another system, developed in Australia and approved in 1986, is sold by the Cochlear Corporation. An implant is an inner ear device that helps a person detect medium to loud environmental sounds

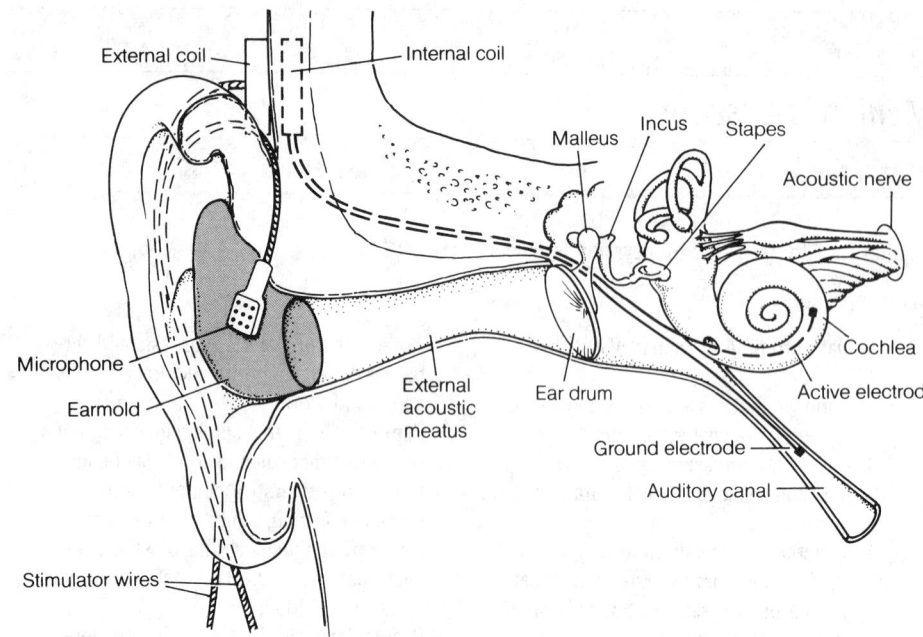

Figure 54–9. The cochlear implant. The internal coil has a stranded electrode lead. The electrode is inserted through the round window into the scala tympani of the cochlea. The external coil (the transmitter) is held in alignment with the internal coil (the receiver) by a magnet. The microphone receives the sound. The stimulator wire receives the signal after it has been filtered, adjusted, and modified so that the sound is at a comfortable level for the patient. Sound is passed by the external transmitter to the inner coil receiver by magnetic conduction and is then carried by the electrode to the cochlea.

and, perhaps, some conversation. It does not restore normal hearing.

Candidates are selected after careful screening by otologic history, physical examination, and audiologic assessment. Some patients do best when a combination of a hearing aid in one ear and an implant in the other ear is used. There are several issues that are being addressed presently in research that may affect uses of cochlear implants. Such issues include the need for preimplant versus postimplant speech training, as well as the decision of which ear should be implanted (*i.e.*, the "better hearing ear" or the "poorer hearing ear"). Evaluation of the effectiveness of cochlear implants needs to be standardized.

A patient who has a cochlear implant undergoes a surgical procedure in which a small receiver is implanted in the bone behind the ear and electrodes are surgically inserted into the inner ear. The microphone and transmitter, which are the external portion of the system, are fitted several weeks later. By way of a signal processor, sounds are transmitted to the inner ear, where sensory cells are helped to stimulate the auditory nerve. These signals are then relayed to the brain, where they are interpreted. A patient may need several weeks or months to learn to properly interpret these sounds.

During rehabilitation, the patient learns about the use and care of the implant, determines the appropriate settings for the signal processor, and attends auditory training sessions. These sessions, which are conducted by a multidisciplinary team, are an important part of the whole process to ensure that the implant is used and that the person has made progress in differentiating sounds. The patient is able to differentiate between one kind of sound and another (*e.g.*, a doorbell and a telephone); however, there are wide variations of success.

There has been continued development of these devices as well as others as aids to help the hearing impaired. Extracochlear implants are being researched, and improvements are being made in their performance. The simplified procedure, usually performed in an outpatient setting, may become an alternate procedure that will help patients with sensory hearing loss. The dedication of researchers will undoubtedly lead to greater advancements in this facet of care.

Bibliography

Books

Alberti PW and Ruben RJ (eds). Otologic Medicine and Surgery. Vols 1 and 2. New York, Churchill Livingstone, 1988.

Ballenger JJ. Diseases of the Nose, Throat, Ear, Head and Neck. Philadelphia, Lea & Febiger, 1985.

Bates B. A Guide to Physical Examination and History Taking, 5th ed. Philadelphia, JB Lippincott, 1991.

Bernstein JM and Ogra P (eds). Immunology of the Ear. New York, Raven Press, 1987.

Bluestone CD and Klein JO. Otitis Media in Infants and Children. Philadelphia, WB Saunders, 1988.

Brooks DN (ed). Adult Aural Rahabilitation. London, Chapman & Hall, 1989.

Halper AS and Burns MS. Treatment materials for auditory comprehension and reading comprehension. Rockville, MD, Aspen Publishers, 1989.

Lubin MF et al. Medical Management of the Surgical Patient, 2nd ed. Stoneham, MA, Butterworths, 1988.

Noble J (ed). Textbook of General Medicine and Primary Care. Boston, Little, Brown, 1987.

Olin BR (ed). Drug Facts and Comparisons. Philadelphia, JB Lippincott, 1988.

Swartz JD (ed). Imaging of the Temporal Bone. New York, Thieme Medical Publishers, 1986.

Journals

Asterisks indicate nursing research articles.

General

Abbas PJ. Electrophysiology of the auditory system. Clin Phys Physiol Meas 1988, 9(1):1–31.

Adamson PA et al. Otoplasty: An update. J Otolaryngol 1987 Aug; 16(4): 258–262.

Bailie GR and Neal D. Vancomycin ototoxicity and nephrotoxicity: A review. Med Toxicol Adverse Drug Exp 1988 Sep/Oct; 3(5):376–386.

Bailey BJ. Otolaryngology—Head and neck surgery. JAMA 1989 May 19; 261(19):2870–2872.

Baker MD. Foreign bodies of the ears and nose in childhood. Pediatr Emerg Care 1987 Jun; 3(2):67–70.

Barrlere SL. Aminoglycosides: A reassessment of their therapeutic role. Clin Pharm 1988; 7(5):385–390.

Crabtree JA and Maceri DR. Tympanoplasty and ossicular reconstruction: An update. Am J Otolaryngol 1988 Jul; 9(4):334–339.

Dobbin M. Loud noise from little headphones. US News World Rep 1987 Oct 12; 103(15):77–78.

Dreschler WA et al. Role of high-frequency audiometry in the early detection of ototoxicity. II. Clinical aspects. Audiology 1989; 28(4):211–220.

Hagerty JW. The amino-glycosides. Focus Crit Care 1989 Apr; 16(2):104–108.

Harrison RK. Hearing conservation: Implementing and evaluating a program. AAOHN J 1989 Apr; 37(4):107–111.

Hazel JW. Tinnitus: II. Surgical management of conditions associated with tinnitus and somatosounds. J Otolaryngol 1990 Feb; 19(1):6–10.

Hollinger LM. Communicating with the elderly: Nurse's touch and the verbal responses of the hospitalized elderly. J Gerontol Nurs 1986 Dec; 44(3):8–13.

Jackson CG. Antimicrobial prophylaxis in ear surgery. Laryngoscope 1988 Oct; 98(10):1116–1123.

Jahnke K. Advances in middle ear surgery. Adv Otorhinolaryngol 1988 Jan; 39:65–82.

Jones IH. Military medicine and surgery: The ear and aviation. 1917 [reprint]. Aviat Space Environ Med 1989 Apr; 60(4):378–382.

Kerr AG. Blast injury to the ear: A review. Rev Environ Health 1987 Jan/Jun; 7(1-2):65–79.

Luxford WM et al. Otoscope update. Patient Care 1987 Sep 15; 21(14):85–107.

Mahoney DF. One simple solution to hearing impairment. Geriatr Nurs 1987 Sep/Oct; 8(5):242–245.

Mancino DJ. Overview of occupational safety and health hazards and right to know legislation. J NY State Nurs Assoc 1987 Aug; 18(3):4–10.

Moloy PJ and Brackmann DE. Control of venous bleeding in otologic surgery. Laryngoscope 1986 May; 96(5):580–582.

Murphy JE. Aminoglycosides: Another look at current and future roles in antimicrobial therapy. Pharmacotherapy 1990; 10(3):217–221.

Sheehy JL. Acquired cholesteatoma in adults. Otolaryngol Clin North Am 1989 Oct; 22(5):967–979.

Simon C et al. Bacteriological findings after premature rupture of the membranes. Arch Gynecol Obstet 1989; 244(2):69–74.

Song YG and Zhuang HX. One-stage total reconstruction of the ear with simultaneous tympanoplasty. Clin Plast Surg 1990 Apr; 17(2):251–261.

Stefanatos GA et al. Neurophysiological evidence of auditory channel anomalies in developmental dysphasia. Arch Neurol 1989 Aug; 46(8):871–875.

Timms MS et al. Experience with a new topical anaesthetic in otology. Clin Otolaryngol 1988 Dec; 13(6):485–490.

Votey S and Dudley JP. Emergency ear, nose, and throat procedures. Emerg Med Clin North Am 1989 Feb; 7(1):117–154.

Assessment

Bellucci RJ. Selection of cases and classification of tympanoplasty. Otolaryngol Clin North Am 1989 Oct; 22(5):911–926.

Blair KA. Aging: Physiological aspects and clinical implications. Nurs Pract 1990 Feb; 15(2):14–23.

Cook N and Hopson B. Pearls for practice: Quick and easy ear cleaning. J Am Acad Nurse Pract 1989 Jul/Sept; 1(3):98.

Karmy SJ. Audiometry: Why and how. Occup Health 1990 Feb; 42(2):39–43.

Nelson GB. Assessment and intervention for communication problems in home health care. J Home Health Care Pract 1988 Nov; 1(1):61–76.

Nomura Y et al. Walking through a human ear. Acta Otolaryngol (Stockh) 1989 May/Jun; 107(5-6):366–370.

Rambur BA. Sudden hearing loss. Nurs Pract 1989 Jan; 14(1):8–14.

Reich ND. Ear infections. Emerg Med Clin North Am 1987; 5(2):227.

Regan D and Regan MP. The transducer characteristic of hair cells in the human ear; A possible objective measure. Brain Res 1988 Jan 12; 438(1-2):363–365.

Turkiak TW. Ear trauma. Emerg Med Clin North Am 1987 May; 5(2):243–251.

Warwick-Brown NP. Wax impaction in the ear. Practitioner 1986 Apr; 230(1414):301.

Hearing Conditions/Problems

Belal A Jr and Glorig A. The aging ear. A clinico-pathological classification. J Laryngol Otol 1987 Nov; 101(11):1131–1135.

Bernstein LE et al. Speech training aids for hearing-impaired individuals: I. Overview and aims. J Rehabil Res Dev 1988 Fall; 25(4):53–62.

Bluestone CD. Modern management of otitis media. Pediatr Clin North Am 1989 Dec; 36(6):371–387.

Chovaz C. Nursing the hearing impaired patient. Can Nurse 1989 Mar; 85(3):34–36.

Cunha BA. Case studies in infectious diseases: Otitis media. Emerg Med 1988 May 15; 20(9):164–172.

Curtis HD. Congenital malformations of the ear. Otolaryngol Clin North Am 1988 May; 21(2):317–336.

Dudley JP. Ear, nose, throat, and sinus infections. Top Emerg Med 1989 Jan; 10(4):43–51.

Farrior JB. Surgical approaches to cholesteatoma. Otolaryngol Clin North Am 1989 Oct; 22(5):1015–1028.

Fireman P. Newer concepts in otitis media. Hosp Pract 1987 Nov 30; 22(11):85–91.

Flood J. Glue-ear: Accumulation of fluid in the middle ear. Nurs Times 1989 Sep; 85(36):38–41.

Goldsmith MM. The punch myringotomy system. Otolaryngol Head Neck Surg 1989 Jun; 100(6):642–643.

Harrison CJ. Tympanostomy tubes: To use or not to use. Consultant 1987 Mar; 27(3):143–144.

LaMarte FP and Tyler RS. Noise-induced tinnitus. AAOHN J 1987 Sep; 35(9):403–406.

Lambert PR. Major congenital ear malformations: Surgical management and results. Ann Otorhinolaryngol 1988 Nov/Dec; 97(6):641–649.

*Lewis-Cullinan C and Jankin JK. Effect of cerumen removal on the hearing ability of geriatric patients. J Adv Nurs 1990 May; 15(5):594–600.

Mandel EM et al. Myringotomy with and without tympanostomy tubes for chronic otitis media with effusion. Arch Otolaryngol Head Neck Surg 1989 Oct; 115(10):1217–1224.

Muchnik C et al. Validity of tympanometry in cases of confirmed otosclerosis. J Laryngol Otol 1989 Jan; 103(1):36–38.

Paparella MM et al. Dizziness. Primary Care 1990 Jun; 17(2):299–308.

Paparella MM et al. Survey of interactions between middle ear and inner ear. Acta Otolaryngol Suppl (Stockh) 1989; 457:9–24.

Rubin W. Noise-induced deafness: Major environmental problem. Hosp Med 1987 Jul; 23(7):19–32.

Schwartz RH. A practical approach to chronic otitis. Patient Care 1987 Jul 15; 21(12):91–103.

Silverstein H et al. Routine intraoperative facial nerve monitoring during otologic surgery. Am J Otol 1988 Jul; 9(4):269–275.

Tonkin JP. Deafness: Diagnosis and management. Med J Aust 1990 Jun; 152(12):659–663.

Tortora ML. Noise-induced hearing loss: Prevention and environment. AAOHN J 1987 Jun; 35(6):271–273.

Verney A. The patient with hearing impairment. J Clin Practice Educ Management 1989 Mar; 3(35):17–19.

Whittet HB et al. An evaluation of topical anaesthesia for myringotomy. Clin Otolaryngol 1988 Dec; 13(6):481–484.

Stapedectomy

Dickins JRE and Graham SS. Otologic surgery in the outpatient versus the hospital setting. Am J Otol 1989 May; 19(3):252–255.

Lesinsik SG and Stein JA. Stapedectomy revision with the CO_2 laser. Laryngoscope 1989; 99(Suppl 46):13–20.

Ross JK et al. A silastic foam dressing for the protection of the post-operative ear. Br J Plast Surg 1987 Mar; 40(2):213–214.

Smalley PJ. Lasers in otolaryngology. Nurs Clin North Am 1990 Sep; 25(3): 645–656.

Williams L and Peters CR. Otoplasty. Plast Surg Nurs 1989 Fall; 9(3):132–135.

Ménière's Disease

Barna BP and Hughes GB. Autoimmunity and otologic disease: Clinical and experimental aspects. Clin Lab Med 1988 Jun; 8(2):385–398.

Cleveland PJ and Morris J. Ménière's disease: The inner ear out of balance. RN 1990 Aug; 53(8):28–32.

Darmstadt GL and Harris JP. Luetic hearing loss: Clinical presentation, diagnosis, and treatment. Am J Otolaryngol 1989 Nov/Dec; 10(6):410–421.

Dickins JR and Graham SS. Ménière's disease—1983–1989. Am J Otol 1990 Jan; 11(1):51–65.

Estrem SA and Davis WE. Ménière's disease: Recent advances. Mod Med 1988 Mar; 85(3):151–154.

Farber SD. Living with Ménière's disease: An occupational therapist's perspective. Am J Occup Ther 1989 May; 43(5):341–343.

Horowitz M et al. Cryosurgical treatment of endolymphatic hydrops. J Laryngol Otol 1989 May; 103(5):481–484.

Jackler RK and Dillon WP. Computed tomography and magnetic resonance imaging of the inner ear. Otolaryngol Head Neck Surg 1988 Nov; 99(5):494–504.

McKennis AT. Vestibular neurectomy: Midfossa approach for Ménière's disease. AORN J 1989 Oct; 50(4):784–795.

Pesznecker S et al. Vestibular disorders: A common cause of dizziness. J Soc Otorhinolaryngol Head Neck Nurs 1989 Spring; 7(2):6–11.

Slater R. Vertigo. How serious are recurrent and single attacks? Postgrad Med 1988 Oct; 84(5):58–67.

Smith WC and Pillsbury HC. Surgical treatment of Ménière's disease since Thomsen. Am J Otol 1988 Jan; 9(1):39–43.

Wackym PA et al. Re-evaluation of the role of the human endolymphatic sac in Ménière's disease. Otolaryngol Head Neck Surg 1990 Jun; 102(6):732–744.

Ylikoski J. Delayed endolymphatic hydrops syndrome after heavy exposure to impulse noise. Am J Otol 1988 Jul; 9(4):282–285.

Hearing Devices and Cochlear Implants

Bennington S. Cochlear implants. Can Oper Room Nurs J 1987 Oct; 5(5):6–11.

Henrichsen J et al. In-the-ear hearing aids. The use and benefit in the elderly hearing-impaired. Scand Audiol 1988; 17(4):209–212.

Mahshie JJ et al. Speech training aids for hearing-impaired individuals: III. J Rehabil Res Dev 1988 Fall; 25(4):69–82.

Mitchell VL. Cochlear implantation: A nursing perspective. J Soc Otorhinolaryngol 1987 Summer; 5(2):11–15.

National Institutes of Health. Cochlear Implants. Consensus Development Conference Statement. 1988 May 4; 7(4):1–9.

Page JC. Selecting a hearing protective device. AAOHN J 1988 Jan; 36(1):40–41.

Pulec JL et al. Multichannel extracochlear implant. Am J Otol 1989 Mar; 10(2):84–90.

Weinstock CP. Hearing aids: A link to the world. A reprint from FDA consumer magazine, 1990 Feb DHHS Publ No. (FDA) 90–4242.

Youngblood J and Robinson S. Ineraid (Utah) multichannel cochlear implants. Laryngoscope 1988 Jan; 98(1):5–10.

Information/Resources

Agencies

Alexander Graham Bell Association for the Deaf, Inc
   3417 Volta Place NW, Washington, DC 20007
American Academy of Facial Plastic and Reconstructive Surgery
   1101 Vermont Ave NW, Suite 304, Washington, DC 20005
American Academy of Otolaryngology—Head and Neck Surgery
   One Prince St, Alexandria, VA 22314
American Speech-Language-Hearing Association
   10801 Rockville Pike, Rockville, MD 20852
American Tinnitus Association
   PO Box 5, Portland, OR 97207
International Hearing Dog Inc.
   5901 East 89th Avenue, Henderson, CO 80640
National Association for Hearing and Speech Action
   10801 Rockville Pike, Rockville, MD 20852
National Association for the Deaf
   814 Thayer Ave, Silver Spring, MD 20910
National Bureau of Standards and FDA
   1390 Piccard Dr, Rockville, MD 20850
National Hearing Aid Society (NHAS)
   20361 Middlebelt, Livonia, MI 48152
National Hearing Association (DEAF) (NHA)
   Butterfield Ridge Office Center, 1430 Branding Lane, Suite 122, Downers Grove, IL 60515
Self-Help for Hard of Hearing People (DEAF) (SHHH)
   7800 Wisconsin Ave, Bethesda, MD 20814
The National Hearing Conservation Association
   900 Des Moines St, Suite 200, Des Moines, IA 50309
The Deafness Research Foundation
   55 East 34th St, New York, NY 10016
US Department of Health and Human Services
   Public Health Service, National Institute of Health, Bethesda, MD 20892

55

Assessment of Neurologic Function

Learning Objectives

On completion of this chapter, the learner will be able to:

1. Differentiate between pathologic changes that affect motor control and those that affect sensory pathways
2. Compare the functioning of the sympathetic and parasympathetic nervous systems
3. Describe the significance of physical assessment to the diagnosis of neurologic dysfunction
4. Describe changes in neurologic function with aging and their impact on neurologic assessment findings.
5. Specify diagnostic tests used for assessment of neurologic function and the related nursing implications

Glossary

Nervous System Anatomy

autonomic nervous system—the branch of the nervous system that functions without conscious control. It governs the innervation of smooth and cardiac muscle, and the body's glands.

Broca's area—the area for speech in the frontal lobe.

central nervous system (CNS)—part of the nervous system that consists of the spinal cord and brain

cerebellum—second largest part of the brain, it is primarily concerned with coordinating body movements

chiasm—the X-like crossing of the two optic nerves in the forebrain

circle of Willis—the anastomotic loop of arteries at the base of the brain

corpus callosum—large mass of white matter located at the bottom of the longitudinal fissure that connects the two hemispheres of the brain

dominant hemisphere—the cerebral hemisphere that controls speech

foramen magnum—opening in the base of the skull (occipital bone) where the brain is connected to the spinal cord

frontal lobe—the area of the brain located at the front on both sides. This area plays a role in controlling emotions, motivation, social skills, expressive language, and the inhibition of impulses. The motor strip, which controls movement and motor integration, runs along the posteior of this lobe.

ganglia—a group of nerve cells outside the central nervous system

limbic system—a set of structures, usually considered part of the temporal lobe, that play an important role in memory, attention, emotions, and behavior

lower motor neuron—cells and fibers of the nervous system that pass from the anterior horn to the muscle

medulla—the lowest portion of the brain stem

neuron—the nerve cell, its fibers, and all its branches

nervous system—all nerve tissue and associated supporting tissue; divided into the CNS and the peripheral nervous system

occipital lobe—the posterior (back) part of each side of the brain, involved in perceiving and understanding visual information

parietal lobe—the upper middle lobe of each side of the brain, involved in perceiving and understanding visual information

pons—part of the brain stem lying between the medulla and the midbrain

spinal cord—part of the CNS that lies in the spinal canal. It is composed of gray matter on the inside, white matter on the outside.

synapse—site of contact between neurons, at which site one neuron is excited or inhibited by another neuron

(continued)

Glossary *(continued)*

temporal lobe—*the lower middle part of each side of the brain. It is involved in receiving information from the auditory system and in memory.*

tract—*collection of nerve fibers in the CNS having similar functions*

Nervous System Characteristics, Reflexes, Conditions, and Disorders

agnosia—*loss of ability to recognize objects through a particular sensory system. Visual agnosia refers to the inability to name an object even though it may be familiar. There are also auditory and tactile agnosias*

agraphia—*inability to express thoughts in writing due to a lesion of the CNS*

aneurysm—*a weakening or bulge in an arterial wall*

anopsia—*nonuse or suppression of vision in one eye*

aphasia—*loss of the ability to express oneself or to understand language. Receptive aphasia is the inability to understand what someone else is saying. This is often associated with damage to the temporal lobe area. Expressive aphasia is the inability to express oneself. Many patients know what it is they wish to say, but are unable to form the words. This type of aphasia is often associated with the left frontal lobe area.*

apraxia—*inability to perform purposeful movement when paralysis is not present*

ataxia—*inability to coordinate muscle movements, resulting in difficulty in walking, talking, and performing self-care tasks.*

Babinski reflex (sign)—*a reflex action of the toes, indicative of abnormalities in the motor control pathways leading from the cerebral cortex*

cerebral hemorrhage—*a hemorrhage into an area of the brain that results in loss of function for that part of the brain; commonly referred to as a cerebrovascular accident (CVA) or stroke*

corneal reflex—*normal blinking on touching of the cornea*

dementia—*organic loss of intellectual function*

diplopia (double vision)—*seeing two images of a single object*

dysarthria—*difficulty in forming or articulating words. This may be caused by damage to the motor areas of the cerebrum or damage to the brain stem. This term encompasses speech that is slurred, too fast or slow, or of abnormal pitch*

electroencephalography (EEG)—*a method of recording, in graphic form, the electrical activity of the brain*

electromyography (EMG)—*a method of recording, in graphic form, the electrical activity of the muscle*

upper motor neurons—*the motor cells and fibers running from the cerebral cortex to cranial nerve nuclei and anterior horn cells*

ventricles—*four cavities interconnected in the brain, which contain CSF*

flaccid—*limp, floppy, lacking tone*

focal—*arising from, or limited to, one part*

hemiplegia or paresis—*weakness of one side of the body, or part of it, due to an injury to the motor areas of the brain*

infarction—*a zone of tissue deprived of blood supply*

monoplegic (paresis)—*paralysis (weakness) of one limb*

multiple sclerosis—*demyelination of the white matter of the brain and the spinal cord*

myelography (myelogram)—*a radiologic study of the spinal cord after injection of a contrast medium into the subarachnoid space*

myopathy—*any degenerative disease of a muscle*

nuchal rigidity (neck stiffness)—*a sign of irritation or infection of the meninges*

neuralgia—*pain in a nerve or along the course of one or more nerves*

oculomotor—*concerned with eye movement*

otorrhea—*fluid (usually CSF) draining from the ear*

paraplegia (paraparesis)—*paralysis (weakness) of both legs and the lower part of the trunk*

photophobia—*the inability to tolerate light*

position (postural) sense—*knowledge of where each part of the body is without looking at it*

ptosis—*drooping of an eyelid*

quadriparesis—*a weakness that involves all four extremities*

quadriplegia—*paralysis of all four extremities*

reflex—*an automatic response to stimuli*

rhinorrhea—*fluid (usually CSF) draining from the nose*

spasticity—*an abnormal increase in muscle tone, causing the muscles to resist being stretched. A patient with spasticity may look "curled up," with his arms held close to his chest, or he may appear to be stiff.*

stroke, cerebral—*see cerebral hemorrhage*

tinnitus—*ringing in the ears*

tone—*the tension present in a muscle at rest*

xanthochromic—*yellow in color; used in reference to CSF*

Physiologic Overview

The nervous system consists of the brain, the spinal cord, and the peripheral nerves. Its function is to control and to coordinate cellular activities throughout the body. It controls these activities through the transmission of electrical impulses. These impulses are routed by way of nerve fibers and nerve pathways that are direct and continuous. The responses elicited are practically instantaneous, because changes in electrical potential transmit the signals.

The Brain

The brain has been described in many ways. It can be divided anatomically or by functions. If the brain is discussed anatomically, it is divided into the three large categories of fossas. A fossa is an anatomic landmark that allows for easy referencing. The three fossas are:

Anterior—contains the frontal and cerebral hemispheres
Middle—contains the parietal, temporal, and occipital lobes
Posterior—contains the brain stem and the medulla

The anterior and middle fossas sit above the tentorium, a

membranous structure that separates the cerebral hemispheres from the brain stem and cerebellum.

The brain is enclosed in a rigid bony compartment called the skull or cranium (Fig. 55-1). To assess neurologic function, one must understand the functions of the brain. Starting from the area closest to the skull, the different areas and their functions are described.

Beneath the skull, the brain is covered by three membranes or *meninges*. The meninges are fibrous connective tissue whose job it is to protect, support, and provide small amounts of nourishment to the brain. The three meninges are as follows:

Dura mater—the outermost layer; covers the brain and the spinal cord. It is a Latin word that translated means "tough mother." It is tough, thick, nonelastic, fibrous, and gray. There are two extensions of the dura: the falx cerebri, which separates the two hemispheres in a longitudinal plane, and the *tentorium*, which is an infolding of the dura that forms a tough membranous shelf. This shelf supports the hemispheres and keeps them separate from the lower part of the brain (the posterior fossa). When herniation occurs, it is because the tentorium has weakened and the hemispheres have collapsed onto the brain stem.

Arachnoid—the middle membrane; a flimsy, delicate membrane that closely resembles a spiderweb, hence the name *arachnoid*. It is white in color because it has no blood supply. The arachnoid layer contains the choroid plexus, which is responsible for the production of cerebrospinal fluid (CSF). This membrane also has unique fingerlike projections, called arachnoid villi, which absorb CSF. In the normal adult, some 500 ml of CSF is produced each day; all but 150 ml is absorbed by the villi. Villi absorb CSF; thus when blood enters the system (from trauma, a ruptured aneurysm, stroke, and so forth), they become ob-

structed. When the arachnoid villi become obstructed, hydrocephalus (increased size of ventricles) can result.

Pia mater—the innermost membrane, which translated from Latin means "tender sweet mother." It is a thin, transparent layer that hugs the brain closely and extends into every fold of the brain's surface.

The *cerebrum* consists of two hemispheres and four lobes. The gray matter is in the external or outer layer of the cerebrum, and the white matter makes up the internal layer of the cerebrum. *Gray matter* is composed principally of nerve cell bodies that are concentrated in the cerebral cortex, the nuclei, and basal ganglia. *White matter* is composed of nerve cell processes, which form tracts or commissures connecting various parts of the brain with each other. The cerebral hemispheres contain the largest amount of central nervous system (CNS) tissue. This area is responsible for an individual's function and intelligence. It is the area where high motor function occurs. The four lobes are as follows:

Frontal—the largest lobe; located in the anterior fossa. This area controls an individual's affect, judgment, personality, and inhibitions.

Parietal—a pure sensory lobe. This area allows one to interpret sensation. The only sense that does not interact here is smell. The parietal lobe allows an individual to know the position and space of his body. Patients with damage to this area may experience hemineglect syndrome.

Temporal—contains the sensations of taste, smell, and hearing. Short-term memory is found in the temporal lobe area.

Occipital—the posterior lobe of the cerebral hemisphere, responsible for visual interpretation.

The middle fossa or diencephalon contains the thalamus, hypothalamus, and the pituitary gland. The *thalamus* lies on

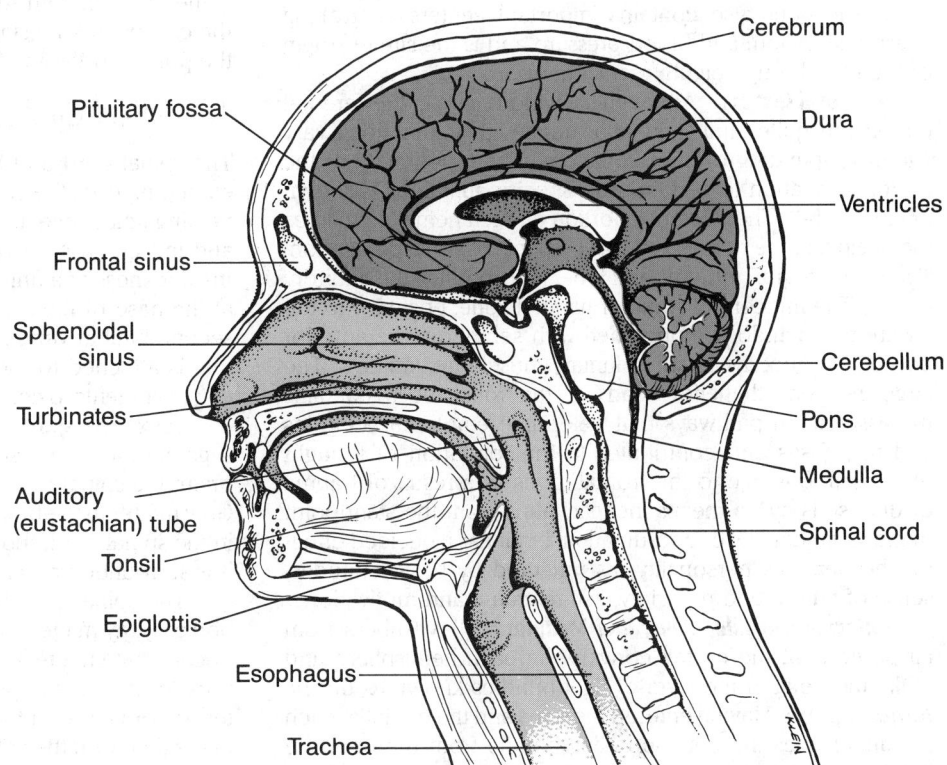

Figure 55-1. Cross-sectional view showing the anatomic position and the relation of structures of the head and neck.

either side of the third ventricle and acts primarily as a relay station for all sensation except for smell. All memory, sensation, and pain impulses pass through this section.

The *hypothalamus* is involved in a wide variety of functions. It controls and regulates the autonomic nervous system. It works with the pituitary to maintain water regulation, and it maintains temperature regulation by promoting vasoconstriction or vasodilation. The hypothalamus is the site of the hunger center and is involved in weight control. It houses the sleep regulator, the blood pressure regulator, and the center for emotional responses (*i.e.*, blushing, rage, depression, panic, and fear).

The *pituitary* gland is considered the master gland because of the number of hormones and functions it controls. The pituitary with its hormones is able to control the function of the kidneys, pancreas, reproductive organs, and others. The pituitary is the third most common site for brain tumors in adults; frequently they are detected by physical signs and symptoms that can be traced to the pituitary. The anterior lobe of the pituitary produces growth hormone and adrenocorticotropic hormone (ACTH). The posterior lobe stores antidiuretic hormone (ADH), which allows the kidneys to either release or retain water. The two most common syndromes associated with ADH abnormalities are diabetes insipidus (DI) and syndrome of inappropriate ADH (SIADH).

The *posterior fossa* contains the brain stem and the medulla oblongata. The *brain stem* consists of the midbrain and the pons. The *midbrain* connects the pons and the cerebellum with the cerebral hemispheres. The *pons* is situated in front of the cerebellum between the midbrain and the medulla and is a bridge between the two halves of the cerebellum as well as between the medulla and the cerebrum.

The *medulla oblongata* transmits motor fibers from the brain to the spinal cord and sensory fibers from the spinal cord to the brain. Most of these fibers cross, or decussate, at this level. The pons also contains important centers controlling heart, respiration, and blood pressure and is the site of origin of the fifth through eighth cranial nerves.

Cerebral Cortex.   Although the various cells in the cerebral cortex are quite similar in appearance, their functions vary widely, depending on their locations. The topography of the cortex in relation to certain of its specific functions is shown in Figure 55-2. The posterior portion of each hemisphere (*i.e.*, the occipital lobe) is devoted to all aspects of visual perception. The lateral region, or temporal lobe, incorporates the auditory center. The midcentral zone, or parietal zone, posterior to the fissure of Rolando, is concerned with sensation; the anterior portion is concerned with voluntary muscle movements. The large area beneath the forehead (*i.e.*, the frontal lobes) contains the association pathways that determine emotional attitudes and responses and contributes to the formation of thought processes. Damage to the frontal lobes as a result of trauma or disease is by no means incapacitating from the standpoint of muscular control or coordination, but it has a decided effect on the person's personality, as reflected by basic attitudes, sense of humor and propriety, self-restraint, and motivations.

Internal Capsule, Pons, and Medulla.   Nerve fibers from all portions of the cortex converge in each hemisphere and make their exit in the form of tight bundles known as the *internal capsule*. Having entered the pons and the medulla, each bundle crosses the corresponding bundle from the opposite side. Some of these axons make connections with axons from

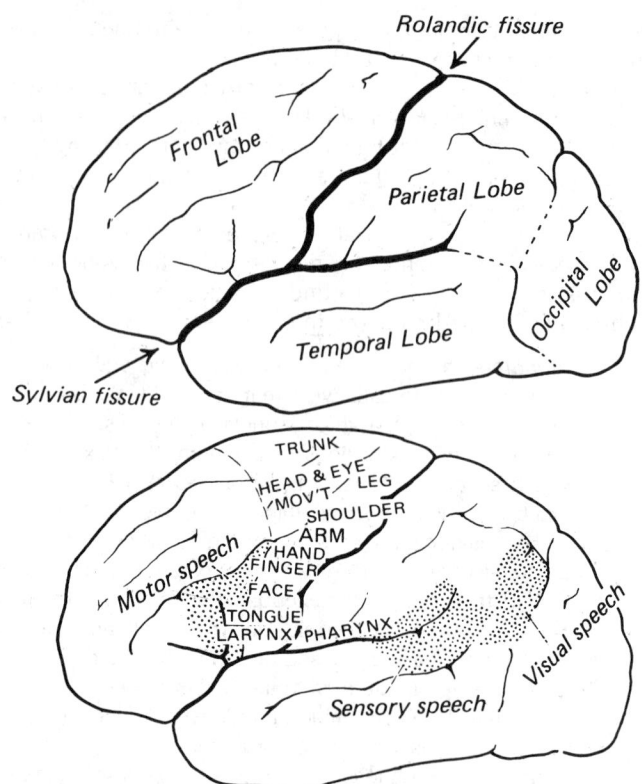

Figure 55–2. (**Top**) Diagrammatic representation of the cerebrum, showing relative locations of various lobes of the brain and the principal fissures. (**Bottom**) Diagrammatic representation of cerebral localization for motor movements of various portions of the body.

the cerebellum, basal ganglia, thalamus, and hypothalamus; some connect with the cranial nerve cells. Other fibers from the cortex and the subcortical centers are channeled through the pons and the medulla into the spinal cord.

The Spinal Cord and Its Connections

The spinal cord and brain stem form a continuous structure extending from the cerebral hemispheres and serving as a connecting link between the brain and the periphery (such as skin and muscles). Approximately 45 cm (18 in) long and about the thickness of a finger, it extends from the foramen magnum at the base of the skull to the upper level of the body of the second lumbar vertebra, where it terminates in a fibrous band that is attached to the coccyx. The spinal cord is composed of 31 segments: 8 cervical, 12 thoracic, 5 lumbar, 5 sacral, and 1 coccyx. The spinal cord has 31 pairs of spinal nerves; each segment has 1 for each side of the body (Fig. 55-3). Like the brain, the spinal cord consists of both gray and white matter. Gray matter in the brain is external and white matter is internal; in the spinal cord, though, the gray matter is in the center and it is surrounded on all sides by white fibers.

The spinal cord is an H-shaped structure with nerve cell bodies (gray matter) surrounded by ascending and descending tracts (white matter) (Fig. 55-4). The lower portion of the H is broader than the upper portion and it corresponds to the anterior horns. It is in these horns that the cells lie that have the fibers that form the anterior (motor) root end and are essential for the voluntary and reflex activity of the muscles supplied by

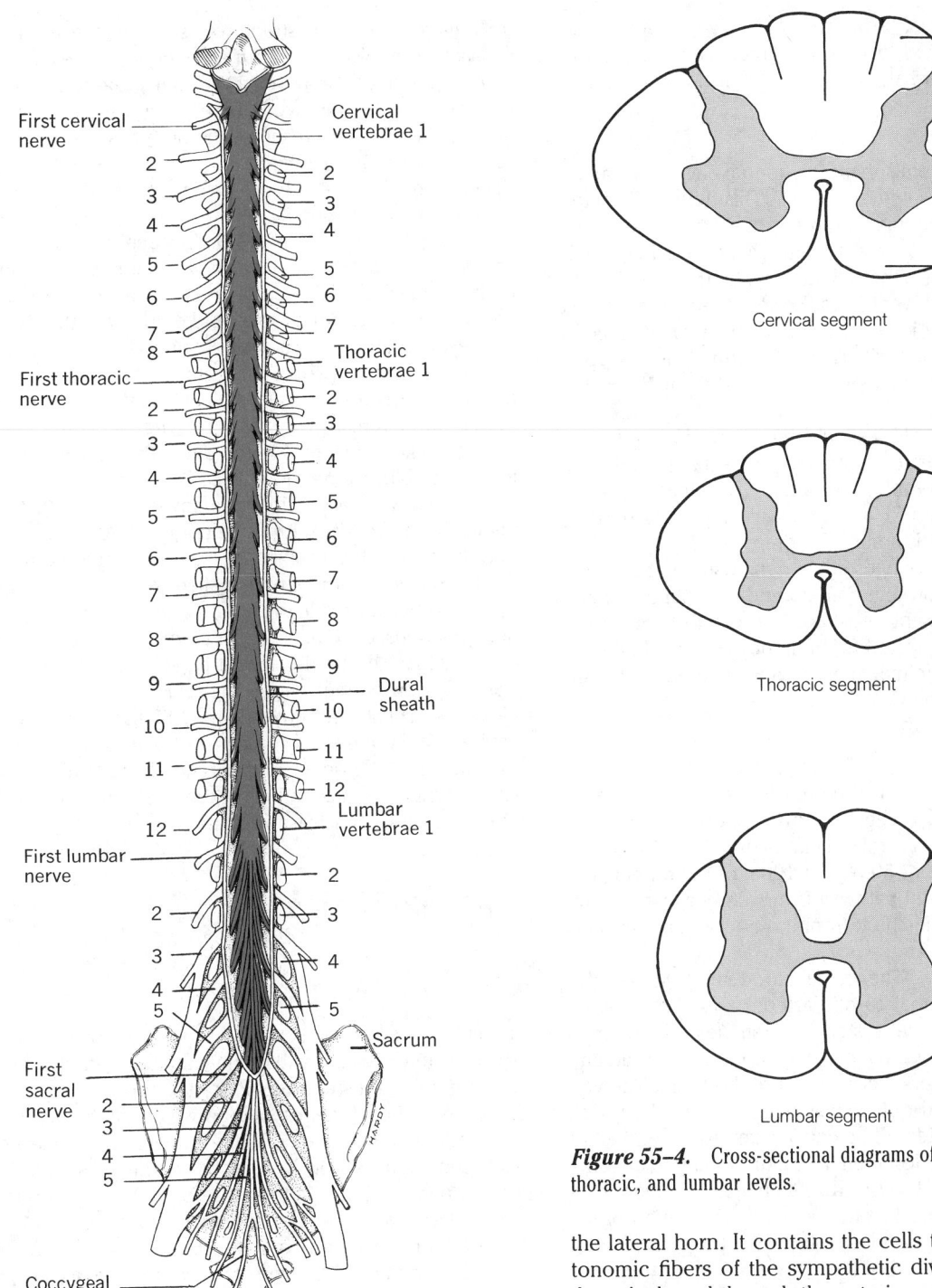

Figure 55–3. Spinal cord lying within the vertebral canal; spinous processes and laminae have been removed; dura and arachnoid have been opened. Spinal nerves are numbered on the left side; vertebrae are numbered on the right side. (Chaffee EE and Greisheimer EM. Basic Physiology and Anatomy, 4th ed. Philadelphia, JB Lippincott.)

Figure 55–4. Cross-sectional diagrams of the spinal cord at cervical, thoracic, and lumbar levels.

them. The thinner posterior (upper horns) portions contain cells with fibers that enter over the posterior (sensory) root end and thus form a relay station in the sensory/reflex pathway.

In the thoracic region of the spinal cord is a projection from each side at the crossbar of the H of gray matter called the lateral horn. It contains the cells that give rise to the autonomic fibers of the sympathetic division. The fibers leave the spinal cord through the anterior roots in the thoracic and upper lumbar segments.

The white matter forms the greater part of the spinal cord and can be subdivided simply into three groups of fibers called tracts or pathways. The *posterior tract* conducts sensation, principally the perception of touch, pressure, vibration, position, and passive motion from the same side of the body. Before reaching the cerebral cortex, these fibers cross to the opposite side in the medulla oblongata. The *spinothalamic tract* (the fibers of which cross to the opposite side immediately after entering the spinal cord and then ascend) transmits pain and temperature impulses to the thalamus and cortex. The *lateral (pyramidal, corticospinal) tract* conducts motor impulses to the anterior horn cells from the opposite side of the brain.

These descending fibers, the nerve cells of which are found in the precentral cortex, cross in the medulla oblongata in what is called the decussation of the pyramids.

Cerebrospinal Fluid

Within each cerebral hemisphere is a central cavity, the lateral ventricle, which is filled with clear CSF. This fluid is extracted from the blood as it circulates through the capillaries of the choroid plexus. If then passes through well-defined channels from the lateral ventricles through narrow, tubular openings to the third and the fourth ventricles. From this narrow cavity it flows to the subarachnoid space to bathe the entire surface of the brain and the spinal cord. The CSF normally is absorbed by the large venous channels of the skull and along the spinal and the cranial nerves.

CSF is clear and colorless and has a specific gravity of 1.007. The average patient's ventricular and subarachnoid systems contain about 150 ml of this fluid. The organic and inorganic contents of the CSF are similar to that of the plasma, but their concentration is somewhat different.

Disease produces changes in the composition of the CSF. Determinations of the protein content and the quantity of glucose and chloride present constitute the chief chemical examinations. CSF is also tested for immunoglobulins. In a state of health, there are a minimal number of white blood cells and no red blood cells in the CSF.

Cerebral Circulation

A constant flow of blood must be maintained for the proper functioning of cerebral tissue. Blood transports oxygen and nutrients to the brain. Cerebral circulation requires 15% of cardiac output at all times, or 50 ml per 100 g of brain tissue per minute. The brain's blood pathway is unique because it flows against gravity; its arteries fill it from the bottom and its veins drain it from the top.

Cerebral Blood Flow.   The arterial blood supply to the brain is provided by two internal carotid arteries and two vertebral arteries and their extensive system of branches. The internal carotids arise from the bifurcation of the common carotid and supply much of the anterior circulation of the brain. The vertebral arteries branch from the subclavian arteries, flow back and upward on either side of the cervical vertebrae, and enter the cranium through the foramen magnum. Joining to become the basilar artery at the level of the brain stem, the vertebrobasilar arteries supply most of the posterior circulation of the brain. The basilar artery divides to form the two branches of the posterior cerebral arteries.

At the base of the brain surrounding the pituitary gland, a ring of arteries is formed between the vertebral and internal carotid arterial chains. This ring is called the *circle of Willis* and is formed from the branches of the internal carotid arteries, anterior and middle cerebral arteries, and anterior and posterior communicating arteries. Blood flow from the circle of Willis directly affects the anterior and the posterior cerebral circulation. The arteries of the circle of Willis provide alternative routes of blood flow if one of the major arteries leading to it becomes occluded.

The arterial anastomosis along the circle of Willis is a frequent site of aneurysms. An aneurysm can be congenital. It can be formed when blood pressure at a weakened arterial wall causes the artery to balloon out. An aneurysm can press on adjacent cerebral structures, such as the optic chiasm, causing visual disturbances. If an artery becomes occluded by vasospasm, an embolus, or a thrombus, the neurons distal to the occlusion are deprived of their blood supply and the cells quickly die. The end result of the above is a stroke (cerebral vascular accident or infarction). The effects of the occlusion depend on which vessels are involved and which areas of the brain these vessels supply.

Venous drainage for the brain does not accompany the arterial circulation as in other body structures. The veins of the brain reach the brain's surface and join larger veins. These cross the subarachnoid space and empty into the larger dural sinuses, which are the vascular channels lying within the tough dura mater. The network of the sinuses carries venous outflow for the brain and empties into the internal jugular vein back to the central circulatory system. Cerebral veins are unique because, unlike other veins in the body, they do not have valves to prevent blood from flowing backwards.

The CNS is inaccessible to many substances that circulate in the blood (*i.e.*, dyes, drugs, antibiotics). After being injected into the blood these substances do not reach the neurons of the CNS; this phenomenon is called the *blood–brain barrier.* The endothelial cells of the brain's capillaries form continuous tight junctions, creating a barrier to macromolecules and many compounds. The barrier to the large molecules entering the CSF is the low permeability of the secretory cells of the choroid plexus. All substances entering the CSF must filter through the capillary membranes of the choroid plexus. Often altered by trauma, cerebral edema, and cerebral hypoxemia, the blood–brain barrier has implications in the treatment and medication selection for CNS disease processes.

Pathophysiology

Vision and Cortical Blindness

It has been said that the eyes are the windows of the brain. Through the eyes an astute clinician can detect subtle clues about the patient's neurologic status. There is a definite area in the rear of each hemisphere in which the fibers of the corresponding optic nerve end. It is through these receiving cells that vision is possible. The eyes may be normal and the optic nerves perfect; if the cells of the optic nerves in one of the hemispheres are diseased, however, the person is half-blind and has cortical blindness. The individual has no vision on one side of the midline. This type of vision is known as hemianopsia (half-blindness).

The patient's visual acuity is tested using Snellen charts and ordinary newsprint. If the patient wears corrective lenses, he should be tested both with and without them.

To conduct the test for visual fields, the patient should cover one eye and look at the examiner's nose. Starting at the periphery of each quadrant of vision, the examiner moves his finger or a cotton-tipped applicator in front of the patient toward the center of vision. The patient is asked to indicate as soon as he sees the finger or applicator. The test is performed for each eye. This procedure reveals gross defects. If more information is desired, the patient is referred for more specific testing. Visual extinction may be tested by moving the fingers simultaneously in opposite sides of the visual fields.

The tests for visual fields may demonstrate disturbances in function along the optic pathways, including sense organs and neurons in the retina, fibers of the optic nerve and tract, and the occipital lobe.

Cortical blindness of one optic area (*e.g.*, of the posterior tip of one cerebral hemisphere) always affects both eyes equally. Total blindness in one eye may be due to a disease of the eye itself or to its optic nerve. Just behind the two eyes, however, the optic nerves become confluent (the optic chiasm); then they separate and continue to the brain as two optic tracts.

In each of these tracts is just half of each optic nerve, so that if one tract is injured, there is blindness of exactly one half of each eye. For example, if the right tract is injured, the patient is blind on the right half of each retina, so that with that eye he can see nothing to his left but can see perfectly to his right. An optic nerve lesion produces partial or complete blindness in the eye that the nerve serves. A complete lesion of one optic tract results in blindness in the opposite half of both visual fields. An abnormality in the temporal lobe may produce blindness in the upper quadrants of both visual fields on the side opposite the lesion. A lesion in the parietal lobe may produce contralateral blindness in the corresponding lower quadrants of both eyes. In a lesion of the occipital lobe,

contralateral blindness may occur in the corresponding half of each visual field, but central vision is intact (Fig. 55-5).

The pituitary gland is located just beneath the chiasm; a pituitary tumor often disturbs the optic chiasm and produces blindness of both inner halves of the retinas, because it is only the fibers in the nasal halves of the optic nerves that cross. In many cases, visual problems may lead a patient to seek medical attention and, through a complete ophthalmic examination, neurologic diseases are detected.

Motor Controls: Paralysis and Dyskinesia

A vertical band of cortex on each cerebral hemisphere governs the voluntary movements of the body. This region, known as the *motor cortex*, can be located accurately.

The exact location within the brain in which the voluntary movements of the muscles of the face, the thumb, the hand, the arm, the trunk, or the leg originate are known. Before a person can move a muscle, these particular cells must send the stimulus down along their fibers. If these cells are stimulated with an electric current, the muscles they control contract.

En route to the pons, as described previously, the motor fibers converge into a tight bundle known as the *capsule*. A comparatively small injury to the capsule causes paralysis in

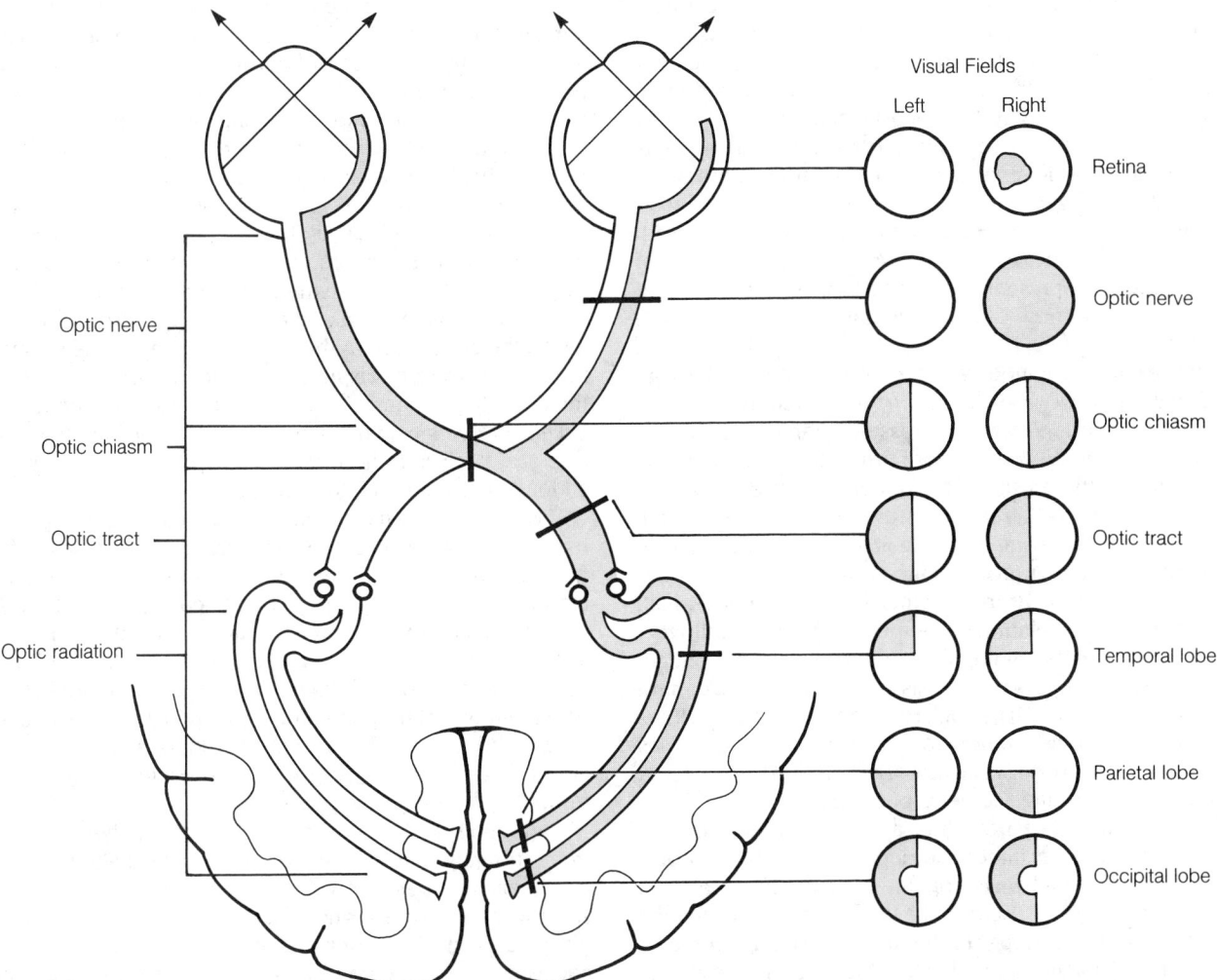

Figure 55-5.   Visual field defects and sites of lesions. Shaded areas indicate areas without vision.

more muscles than does a much larger injury to the cortex itself.

The brain is like a telephone station, in which one blow of an ax can sever all the wires at the point where they leave the building, but a similar blow on the switchboard would sever only a few.

A common cause of a stroke, followed by paralysis of half of the body (hemiplegia), is usually a small hemorrhage from a blood vessel in the capsule. A much larger hemorrhage nearer to or in the cortex might paralyze one extremity. Hemiplegia may be due to the rupture of a microaneurysm of a tiny artery running to the internal capsule or to the occlusion of this artery by a thrombus or an embolus, and the subsequent death of the fibers that it supplies with blood.

Immediately after a stroke, half of the body is often paralyzed. Then, gradually, the person recovers the use of certain muscles, usually those of the leg, often those of the upper arm, least often those of the hand. Although the hemorrhage actually destroys the fibers of only a few nerves, it temporarily injures all those in its surrounding area, perhaps by the pressure of the escaped blood or by the edema. As the swelling from the hemorrhage diminishes, these latter fibers resume their function, but those actually destroyed never do.

Within the medulla, the motor axons from the cortex form two well-defined bands known as the *corticospinal* or *pyramidal tracts*. Here, most of these fibers cross (or decussate) to the opposite side, continuing thereafter as the *crossed* pyramidal tract. The remaining fibers then enter the spinal cord on the original side as the *direct* pyramidal tract, each fiber in this tract finally crossing to the opposite side of the cord near the point of termination and coming to an end within the gray matter constituting the anterior horn on that side, in proximity to a motor nerve cell. Fibers of the crossed pyramidal tract terminate within the anterior horn and make connections with anterior horn cells on the same side. All of the motor fibers of the spinal nerves represent extensions of these anterior horn cells, with each of these fibers communicating with only one particular muscle fiber.

Thus, each muscle fiber is under voluntary control through a combination of two nerve cells. One is located in the motor cortex, its fiber in the direct or crossed pyramidal tract, and the other is located in the anterior horn of the spinal cord, its fiber running to the muscle. The former is referred to as the *upper motor neuron*; the latter, as the *lower motor neuron*. Every motor nerve serving a muscle is a bundle composed of several thousand lower motor neurons.

Several motor nerve tracts, other than the corticospinal, are contained in the spinal cord. Some represent the pathways of the so-called extrapyramidal system, establishing connections between the anterior horn cells and the automatic control centers located in the basal ganglia and the cerebellum. Others are components of reflex arcs, forming synaptic connections between anterior horn cells and sensory fibers that have entered adjacent or neighboring segments of the cord.

Motor Paralysis.   Paralysis of a muscle may be due to pathologic changes in either the upper or the lower motor neuron. The motor pathways from the brain to the spinal cord as well as from the cerebrum to the brain stem are formed by neurons referred to as upper motor neurons. The upper motor neurons are contained entirely within the CNS, in contrast to the lower motor neurons, which begin in the CNS but terminate

in the muscle. An individual is considered to have *lower motor neuron* damage if a motor nerve is cut somewhere between the muscle and the spinal cord, thus destroying the final common pathway to a muscle. The end result of lower motor neuron damage is that the muscle becomes paralyzed and the person is unable to move that muscle. The nerve takes no part in reflex movements, and the muscle becomes limp, wastes away, or atrophies due to disuse. If the patient has injured the spinal trunk and it is able to heal, the patient may regain the use of the muscles connected to that section of the spinal cord. If the anterior horn motor cells are destroyed, however, the nerves cannot regenerate, and the muscles are never useful again. This sequence of events occurs in anterior poliomyelitis. Flaccid paralysis and atrophy of the affected muscles are the principle signs of lower motor neuron disease.

If the *upper motor neuron* is destroyed, a different condition exists in the muscle. It is paralyzed as far as voluntary movement is concerned but not necessarily for reflex (involuntary) movements, because these originate in the nerve cells in the cord or the medulla. The muscle does not atrophy, and it will not become limp; on the contrary, it remains permanently more tense than normal. This paralysis seldom affects a part of one muscle, one single muscle, or only a few muscles; it usually affects a whole extremity, both extremities, or an entire half of the body.

An example of upper motor neuron disease is the spastic paralysis of infants who during birth receive some mechanical injury that may have caused an intracerebral bleed or a hematoma. The long-continued pressure of the escaped blood may injure large areas of the brain, causing these children to have neurologic deficits and learning disabilities. When these children begin to walk, their legs and arms are stiff. During their lifetime, body movements are awkward, stiff, and weak. Because those muscles that draw the feet and the knees toward each other (the adductor muscles) are naturally stronger than those that spread those extremities apart (the abductor muscles), these patients walk by a cross-legged progression, also called the *scissors gait*; that is, in each step the leg is moved not only forward but is also swung round across the front of the other leg. When both legs are paralyzed, the condition is called *paraplegia;* and when the arm and the leg on the same side are paralyzed, the term *hemiplegia* is used. Paralysis of all four extremities is *quadriplegia.*

Hemiplegia is an example of upper motor neuron paralysis. If a hemorrhage, an embolus, or a thrombus destroys the fibers from the motor area in the internal capsule, the arm and the leg of the opposite side promptly become stiff and more or less paralyzed, and the reflexes are exaggerated. Another illustration of upper neuron disease is seen in adults with spastic paraplegia, a chronic stiffness of both legs due to a gradual degeneration of the fibers in the pyramidal tract. The person so afflicted walks stiffly, as though wading through water, the knees always touching each other and the feet scarcely raised from the ground (the spastic gait).

An upper and a lower motor neuron paralysis may result from an injury that crushes, transects, or somehow destroys the spinal cord. An individual, for example, who dives into shallow water, strikes his head, fractures his neck, and transects his spinal cord with a bony fragment would have both an upper and a lower motor neuron paralysis. The vertebrae are no longer properly aligned and the spinal cord has been manipulated in such a way that its motor and sensory tracts cannot receive, transmit, or act on stimuli. The hunchback deformity caused by the bone destruction of tubercle bacilli accomplishes the same thing, only more slowly. This can still be seen in some people, particularly those who have come from countries where standards for pasteurization of milk and tuberculin testing of cattle are not rigid, or elderly who contracted it before the advent of antituberculosis drugs. The result of such deformities of the spinal cord leads to a rigid paralysis on both sides of all muscles whose nerves leave the cord below the damaged area.

Flaccid paralysis also occurs in those muscles whose motor nerve fibers come from cells in the deformed area. There is also a loss of sensation to the skin below the damaged area, because the sensory fibers from below the injury are no longer able to reach the brain. The sometimes violent leg spasms of complete spinal cord injury result from the preserved capabilities of the reflex arc along the spinal cord below the level of injury, again a hallmark of upper motor neuron disease. Lower motor neuron disease, however, occurs at the level of injury and is exhibited in the flaccid, atrophied muscles of the hand as in a cervical cord injury at the fifth cervical vertebrae. Tumors of the spinal cord ultimately cause this same clinical picture. In the initial stages of tumor growth, only the part of the spinal cord directly involved is disturbed, but as the tumor grows, it may completely destroy the spinal cord.

Extrapyramidal Motor Controls. The smoothness, the accuracy, and the strength that characterize the muscular movements of a normal person are attributable to the influence of the cerebellum and the basal ganglia.

The cerebellum (see Fig. 55-1), nestled beneath the posterior lobe of the cerebrum, is responsible for coordinating, balancing, timing, and synergizing with precision all muscular movements that originate in the motor centers of the cerebral cortex. Through the action of the cerebellum, the contractions of opposing muscle groups are adjusted in relation to each other to maximal mechanical advantage; muscular contractions can be sustained evenly at the desired tension and without significant fluctuation, and reciprocal movements can be reproduced at high and constant speed, in stereotyped fashion, and with relatively little effort.

The basal ganglia are masses of gray matter in the midbrain beneath the cerebral hemispheres. These border or project into the lateral ventricles and lie in proximity to the internal capsule. It is their function to control habitual or automatic acts and to maintain a postural background against which voluntary movements are performed. These ganglia, aided by their connections with the organs of special sense, keep the contractile tone of every muscle in the trunk and the extremities in a constant state of adjustment, so that a person is able to keep his balance regardless of the posture of his body, in darkness as well as in light. Moreover, because of the basal ganglia, the person is equipped to react swiftly, appropriately, and automatically to any smell, sight, or sound that demands an immediate response.

Dyskinesias. Loss of cerebellar function, which may occur as a result of an intracranial injury or some type of an expanding mass (*i.e.*, a hemorrhage, abscess, or tumor), results in a loss of muscle tone, weakness, and fatigue. The patient exhibits a coarse involuntary tremor that increases in intensity in association with voluntary movements. He is unable to control his movements accurately or to coordinate his muscles

efficiently or smoothly; every act is performed in disjointed fashion. The patient is incapable of performing fine, rapidly repeated coordinated movements with speed or uniformity. The above characteristics are called *adiadochokinesis* and signal that there is a problem with the cerebellar section of the brain. When the patient walks, he staggers from side to side because his gait is unsteady. His gait is similar to that of an individual who is intoxicated and attempting to walk (*i.e.*, feet wide apart and the steps short).

Destruction or dysfunction of the basal ganglia does not lead to paralysis but to muscular rigidity, with consequent disturbances of posture and movement. Such patients are afflicted by a tendency to display involuntary movements. These may take the form of coarse tremors, characterized by approximately 6 oscillations per second; *athetosis*, namely, movement of a slow, squirming, writhing, twisting type; or *chorea*, marked by spasmodic, purposeless, and grotesque motions of the trunk and the extremities, and facial grimacing. Clinical syndromes based on lesions involving the basal ganglia include parkinsonism (see Chap. 57); Huntington's disease (see Chap. 57); Wilson's disease, or hepatolenticular degeneration; and spasmodic torticollis.

Sensory Pathways and Disturbances

The Thalamus. The thalamus, a major receiving and transmitting center for the afferent sensory nerves, is a large structure located in the middle fossa (midbrain). It lies next to the third ventricle, forming its lateral wall, and it forms the floor of the lateral ventricle. It is also in proximity to the basal ganglia and adjacent to the internal capsule. The thalamus serves to integrate sensory impulses, as in the recognition of pain or variation in temperature or touch. The thalamus is responsible for allowing the sense of movement and position and the ability to recognize size, shape, and quality of objects. It is also responsible for the routing of all sensory stimuli to their destinations, including the cerebral cortex, which receives them and translates them automatically into appropriate responses.

Sensory Pathways. The transmission of sensory impulses from their points of origin to their cerebral destinations involves three neuron relays; moreover, there are three major pathways by which they may be routed, depending on the type of sensation that is registered. Specific knowledge of these paths is of great importance from the standpoint of neurologic diagnoses, being indispensable for the accurate localization of brain and cord lesions in many patients.

The axon of the nerve in which the sensory impulse originates enters the spinal cord by way of the posterior root. Axons conveying sensations of heat, cold, and pain immediately enter the posterior gray column of the cord, where they make connections with the cells of secondary neurons. Pain and temperature fibers cross immediately to the opposite side of the cord and course upward to the thalamus. Fibers carrying sensations of touch, light pressure, and localization do not connect immediately with the second neuron but rather ascend the cord for a variable distance before entering the gray matter and completing this connection. The axon of the secondary neuron crosses the cord and proceeds upward to the thalamus.

The third category of sensation, produced by stimuli arising from muscles, joints, and bones, includes position sense and vibratory sense. These stimuli are conveyed, uncrossed, all the way to the brain stem by the axon of the primary neuron. In the medulla, synaptic connections are made with cells of the secondary neurons, whose axons then cross to the opposite side and proceed to the thalamus.

Sensory Losses.   Severance of a sensory nerve results in total loss of sensation in its area of distribution. Transection of the spinal cord yields complete anesthesia below the level of injury. Selective destruction or degeneration of the posterior columns of the spinal cord, a characteristic of combined system disease, is responsible for a loss of position sense in segments distal to the lesion, unaccompanied by loss of touch, pain, or temperature perception. Those persons with such disorders of the posterior columns, unless they look, cannot tell where their feet are or in what direction they are pointing. Moreover, they cannot perceive vibrations in the affected area. A lesion, such as a cyst, in the center of the cord causes dissociation of sensation, that is, loss of pain at the level of the lesion. This is explainable on the basis that the fibers carrying pain and temperature cross the cord immediately on entering; thus, any lesion that divides the cord longitudinally divides these fibers likewise. Other sensory fibers ascend the cord for variable distances, some even to the medulla itself, before crossing, thereby bypassing the lesion and avoiding destruction.

Dysesthesias.   Irritative lesions affecting the posterior spinal nerve roots may cause intermittent severe pains that are referred to their areas of distribution. This phenomenon explains the pains of tabes dorsalis. The sensation of tingling of the fingers and the toes constitutes a prominent symptom of combined systems disease, presumably due to degenerative changes in the sensory fibers that extend to the thalamus (*i.e.*, belonging to the spinothalamic tract).

Autonomic Nervous System

The contractions of muscles that are not under voluntary control, including the heart muscle, the secretions of all digestive and sweat glands, and the activity of certain endocrine organs as well, are controlled by a major component of the nervous system known as the autonomic nervous system. The term *autonomic* refers to the fact that the operations of this system are independent of the desires and the intentions of the person. The autonomic nervous system is not subject to his will—that is, it is in a sense autonomous.

To the extent that the autonomic nervous system is not subject to regulation by the cerebral cortex, it resembles the extrapyramidal systems that are centered in the cerebellum and the basal ganglia. However, in other respects it is unique. First, its regulatory effects are exerted not on individual cells but on large expanses of tissue and on entire organs. Second, the responses that it elicits do not appear instantaneously, but only after a lag period. These responses are sustained far longer than other neurogenic responses, a type of response that is calculated to ensure maximal functional efficiency on the part of receptor organs, such as the blood vessels and the hollow viscera. The autonomic nervous system regulates visceral effectors to maintain or quickly restore homeostasis.

The quality of these responses is explained by the fact that the autonomic nervous system transmits its impulses only partly by way of nerve pathways, the remainder of the route being serviced by chemical mediators, resembling in this respect the

endocrine system. Electrical impulses, conducted through nerve fibers, stimulate the formation of specific chemical agents at strategic locations within the muscle mass, the diffusion of these chemicals being responsible for the contraction.

The Hypothalamus.   Overall supervision of the autonomic nervous system is considered a function of the hypothalamus. The hypothalamus is a portion of the diencephalon (interbrain) located immediately beneath and lateral to the lower portion of the wall of the third ventricle. It includes among its components the optic chiasm; the tuber cinereum; the pituitary stalk, which originates from the latter; and the pituitary gland itself. Large cell groups in adjacent portions of the hypothalamus have the role of autonomic regulation. These centers are richly endowed with connections linking the autonomic system with the thalamus, the cortex, the olfactory apparatus, and the pituitary gland. Here reside the mechanisms for the control of visceral and somatic reactions that were originally important for defense or attack, but in humans these are associated with emotional states (*i.e.*, fears, anger, anxiety); for the control of metabolic processes, including fat, carbohydrate, and water metabolism; for the regulation of body temperature, arterial pressure, and all muscular and glandular activities of the gastrointestinal tract; for control of the genital functions; and for the sleep rhythm. The proximity, histologic similarity, and multiple connections between the pituitary gland, master gland of the endocrines, and this portion of the brain suggest that the hypothalamus controls the endocrine and autonomic nervous systems, commanding all vital processes.

Sympathetic and Parasympathetic Nervous Systems

The autonomic nervous system contains two divisions that are anatomically and functionally distinct—the sympathetic and the parasympathetic nervous systems. Most of the tissues and the organs under autonomic control are innervated by both systems. Sympathetic stimuli are mediated by norepinephrine, and parasympathetic impulses are mediated by acetylcholine. These chemicals produce opposing and mutually antagonistic effects, as indicated in Table 55-1.

Sympathetic Nervous System.   A unique function of the sympathetic division of the autonomic nervous system is to serve as an emergency preparedness system. Under stress conditions from either physical or emotional causes, sympathetic impulses increase greatly. The body prepares for the "fight or flight" reflex when threatened. As a result of this reflex, bronchioles dilate for easier gas exchange; the heart's contractions are stronger and faster; the arteries to the heart and voluntary muscles dilate, carrying more blood to them; peripheral blood vessels constrict, making the skin feel cool but shunting blood to essential active organs; the pupils dilate; the liver releases glucose for quick energy; peristalsis slows down; hair stands on end; and perspiration increases. This sudden increase in sympathetic discharge is the same as if the body has been given an injection of adrenalin; hence the term *adrenergic nervous system* is sometimes used when referring to this condition.

Sympathetic neurons are located in the thoracic and the lumbar segments of the spinal cord; their axons, called *preganglionic fibers*, emerge by way of all anterior nerve roots from the eighth cervical or first thoracic segment to the second or third lumbar segment, inclusive. A short distance from the

TABLE 55-1. Comparison of Parasympathetic and Sympathetic Effects
on Specific Organs and Tissues

Organ or Tissue	Parasympathetic Effects (Cholinergic)	Sympathetic Effects (Adrenergic)
VESSELS		
Cutaneous		Constriction
Muscular		Variable
Coronary	Constriction	Dilatation
Salivary gland	Dilatation	Constriction
Buccal mucosa		Dilatation
Pulmonary	Variable	Variable
Cerebral	Dilatation	Constriction
Of abdominal and pelvic viscera		Constriction
Of external genitalia	Dilatation	Constriction
HEART	Inhibition	Acceleration
EYE		
Iris	Constriction	Dilatation
Ciliary muscle	Contraction	Relaxation
Smooth muscle of orbit and upper lid		Contraction
BRONCHI	Constriction	Dilatation
GLANDS		
Sweat		Secretion
Salivary	Secretion	Secretion
Gastric	Secretion	Inhibition?
		Secretion of mucus
PANCREATIC		
Acini	Secretion	
Islets	Secretion	
LIVER		Glycogenolysis
ADRENAL MEDULLA		Secretion
SMOOTH MUSCLE		
Skin		Contraction
Stomach wall	Contraction (predominantly)	Inhibition (predominantly)
Small intestine	Increased tone and motility	
Large intestine	Increased tone and motility	Inhibition
Bladder wall (detrusor muscle)	Contraction	Inhibition
Trigone and sphincter	Inhibition	Contraction
Uterus, pregnant	None	Contraction
Uterus, nonpregnant	None	Inhibition

(Best CH and Taylor NB. Physiological Basis of Medical Practice, 6th ed. Baltimore, Williams & Wilkins.)

cord, these fibers diverge to join a chain composed of 22 linked ganglia that extends the entire length of the spinal column, flanking the vertebral bodies on both sides. Some form multiple synapses with nerve cells within the chain. Others traverse the chain without making connections or losing continuity to join large ''prevertebral'' ganglia in the thorax, the abdomen, or the pelvis or one of the ''terminal'' ganglia in the vicinity of an organ, such as the bladder or the rectum. Postganglionic nerve fibers originating in the sympathetic chain rejoin the spinal nerves that supply the extremities and are distributed to blood vessels, sweat glands, and smooth muscle tissue in the skin. Postganglionic fibers from the prevertebral plexuses (*i.e.*, the cardiac, pulmonary, splanchnic, and pelvic plexuses) supply structures in the head and the neck, the thorax, the abdomen, and the pelvis, respectively, having been joined in these plexuses by fibers from the parasympathetic division.

The adrenals, the kidneys, the liver, the spleen, the stomach, and the duodenum are under the control of the giant celiac plexus, familiarly known as the *solar plexus*. This receives its sympathetic nerve components by way of the three splanchnic nerves, composed of preganglionic fibers from nine segments of the spinal cord (*i.e.*, T4 to L1), and is joined by the vagus nerve, representing the parasympathetic division. From the celiac plexus, fibers of both divisions travel along the course of blood vessels to their target organs.

Parasympathetic Nervous System.   The parasympathetic system functions as the dominant controller for most visceral effectors much of the time. During quiet, nonstressful conditions, impulses from parasympathetic fibers (cholinergic) predominate. The fibers of the parasympathetic system, are located in two sections, one in the brain stem and the other from spinal segments below L2. Because of the location of these fibers, the parasympathetic system is referred to as the *craniosacral* division, as distinct from the *thoracolumbar* division of the autonomic nervous system.

The cranial parasympathetics arise from the midbrain and the medulla oblongata. Fibers from cells in the midbrain travel with the third oculomotor nerve to the ciliary ganglia, where postganglionic fibers of this division are joined by those of the sympathetic system. Forming the ciliary nerve, these innervate the ciliary muscles of the eye to control the size of the pupil. Parasympathetic fibers from the medulla travel with the seventh (facial), ninth (glossopharyngeal), and tenth (vagus) cranial nerves. Those from the facial nerve end in the sphenopalatine ganglion, from which emanate the fibers that innervate the lacrimal glands, the ciliary muscle, and the sphincter of the pupil. Those from the glossopharyngeal nerve innervate the parotid gland. The vagus nerve carries preganglionic parasympathetic fibers without interruption to the organs that it innervates, joining ganglion cells within the myocardium and within the walls of the esophagus, the stomach, and the intestine.

Preganglionic parasympathetic fibers from the anterior roots of the sacral nerves coalesce to become the pelvic nerves, consolidate and regroup in the pelvic plexus, and terminate around ganglion cells in the musculature of the pelvic organs. These innervate the colon, the rectum, and the bladder, inhibiting the muscular tone of the anal and the bladder sphincters and dilating the blood vessels of the bladder, the rectum, and the genitalia.

The vagus, splanchnic, pelvic, and other autonomic nerves carry impulses generated in the viscera to the dorsal nucleus of the vagus, where connections are made with efferent parasympathetic neurons, forming a series of reflex arcs. These provide the basis for self-regulation, a cardinal feature of the autonomic nervous system, and one reason for autonomy.

Autonomic Functions and Dysfunctions.   A detailed listing of the effects produced by the two divisions of the autonomic nervous system is supplied in Table 55-1. This listing identifies the scope and the importance of autonomic activity in relation to all bodily functions and from the standpoint of survival itself. Both sympathetic and parasympathetic divisions are in a constant state of activity, the activity of each relative to the other being one of controlled opposition, with a delicate balance maintained between the two at all times.

Sympathetic Syndromes.   Certain syndromes are distinctive of diseases of the sympathetic nerve trunks. Among these are dilatation of the pupil of the eye on the same side as a penetrating wound of the neck (evidence of disturbance of the cervical sympathetic cord); temporary paralysis of the bowel (indicated by the absence of peristaltic waves and the distention of the intestine by gas) after fracture of any one of the lower dorsal or upper lumbar vertebrae with hemorrhage into the base of the mesentery; and the marked variations in pulse rate and rhythm that often follow compression fractures of the upper six thoracic vertebrae.

The Neurologic Examination

The neurologic examination is a sophisticated and subtle process, comprising a large number of tests of highly specialized function. Although the neurologic examination is often limited to a simple screening, it is necessary for the examiner to be able to conduct a thorough neurologic assessment when the history or other physical findings warrant it.

The brain and spinal cord cannot be inspected, percussed, palpated, and auscultated as directly as other systems of the body. A neurologic assessment is divided into five components: *cerebral function, cranial nerves, motor system, sensory system,* and *reflex status*. As in other facets of the physical assessment, the neurologic examination follows a logical sequence and is pursued from higher levels of cortical function through to a determination of the integrity of peripheral nerves.

Much of the patient's neurologic function is assessed during the history and during the routine of the earlier parts of the physical examination. One can learn much about speech patterns, mental status, gait, stance, motor power, and coordination. The simple act of shaking a patient's hand as he enters the room conveys an enormous amount of information to the alert observer.

Cerebral Function

Cerebral abnormalities may cause disturbances in communication, intellectual functioning, and in patterns of emotional behavior. Adequate cerebral functioning is determined by assessing the patient's *mental status*. The examiner observes the patient's appearance and behavior, noting the patient's dress, grooming, and personal hygiene. Observation of posture, gestures, movements, facial expressions, and motor activity often provides important information about the patient. The manner of speech and the patient's level of consciousness are also observed: Is his speech clear and coherent? Is he alert and responsive, or drowsy and stuporous?

Intellectual function is tested when doubts exist about the patient's intellectual competence. Often, patients in a toxic state or those who have destruction of the frontal cortex appear superficially normal until or unless one or more tests of integrative capacity are performed. First, the examiner determines whether the patient is oriented to time, place, and person. Does the patient know what day it is, what year it is, or who is the president of the United States? Is the patient aware of where he is? Is the patient aware of who you are and of his purpose for being in the room? Is the capacity for immediate memory intact? A person with an average IQ is able to repeat seven digits without faltering and is able to recite five digits backward. The examiner might ask the patient to count backward from 100, or to subtract 7 from 100, then 7 from that, then 7 from that, and so forth. The capacity to interpret well-known proverbs tests abstract reasoning, which is a higher intellectual function. For example, does the patient know what is meant by "the early bird catches the worm?"

It is important to determine the patient's thought content during the course of the interview. Are his thoughts spontaneous, natural, and clear? Are his ideas relevant and coherent? Does he have any fixed ideas, illusions, or preoccupations? What are his insights into these thoughts? Preoccupation with death or morbid events, evidence of hallucinations, and paranoid ideation are all important and require further evaluation.

An assessment of cerebral functioning also includes the patient's emotional status. Is the patient's affect natural and even, or is he irritable and angry, anxious, apathetic, or euphoric? Does his mood fluctuate normally, or does he unpredictably swing from joy to sadness during the interview? Is his affect appropriate to his words and thought content? Are his verbal communications consistent with his nonverbal communications?

The examiner may now consider more specific areas of higher cortical function. *Agnosia* is the inability to interpret or recognize objects seen through the special senses. The patient may see a pen but not know what it is called or what to do with it. He may even be able to describe it but not to interpret its function. The patient may experience auditory or tactile agnosia, as well as visual agnosia. Each of the dysfunctions implicates a different part of the cortex. (Chart 55-1).

To screen for agnosia, the examiner tests the patient's cortical sensory interpretation. The patient is shown a familiar object and asked to identify it by name. Next, he is confronted with a familiar sound (bell) and asked to identify its source. Tactile interpretation is easily assessed by placing a familiar object (*e.g.*, key, coin) in the patient's hand and having him identify it while his eyes are closed.

An assessment of cortical motor integration is carried out by asking the patient to perform a skilled act (throw a ball, move a chair). Successful performance hinges on the person's ability to understand the activity desired. He also must have normal motor strength. Failures signal cerebral dysfunction.

Lastly, language function is assessed. The person with normal neurologic function is able to understand and communicate in spoken and written language. Does the patient answer questions relevantly? Can he read a sentence from a newspaper

Chart 55–1
Types of Agnosia and Corresponding Sites of Lesions

Type of Agnosia	Affected Cerebral Area
Visual	Occipital lobe
Auditory	Temporal lobe (lateral and superior portions)
Tactile	Parietal lobe
Body parts and relationships	Parietal lobe (postero-inferior regions)

and explain its meaning? Can he write his name or copy a simple figure that the examiner has drawn? A deficiency in language function is called *aphasia*. Different types of aphasia result from injury to different parts of the brain (Chart 55-2).

Interpretation of neurologic abnormalities is a highly sophisticated and technical process. It is the obligation of the examiner to record and report what is found. Analysis and the conclusions that may be drawn from these findings usually depend on the physician's extensive knowledge of neuroanatomy, neurophysiology, and neuropathology.

The nurse includes in her assessment of neurologic function the impact the neurologic impairment will have on the individual's current life style. This nursing perspective examines two issues: the limitations imposed by the neurologic deficit within the context of the patient's role in society and a plan of care that will support adaptation to the neurologic insult within the individual's support system.

Examination of the Cranial Nerves

Twelve pairs of cranial nerves emerge from the undersurface of the brain. They are designated by Roman numerals I to XII, according to the order of their location. The cranial nerves are

Chart 55–2
Types of Aphasia and Region of Brain Involved

Type of Aphasia	Brain Area Involved
Auditory-receptive	Temporal lobe
Expressive speaking	Inferior posterior frontal areas
Visual-receptive	Parietal-occipital area
Expressive writing	Posterior frontal area

often assessed during a complete head and neck examination. These nerves, their functions, and the tests for their measurement are outlined in Table 55-2.

Examination of the Motor System

The motor system is complex, and the end result of motor function is a synthesis of the integrity of the corticospinal tracts, the extrapyramidal system, and cerebellar function. A motor impulse traverses two neurons. The *upper motor neuron* begins in the cortex of the opposite side of the brain, descends through the internal capsule, crosses to the opposite side in the brain stem, descends through the corticospinal tract, and synapses with the *lower motor neuron* in the cord. The lower motor neuron receives the impulse in the posterior part of the cord and runs to the myoneural junction. The other two systems, the extrapyramidal system and the cerebellar system, act as modifiers.

A thorough examination of the motor system includes an assessment of muscle size, muscle tone, muscle strength, coordination, and balance. The patient is instructed to walk across the room while the examiner notes his posture and gait. The muscles are inspected, and palpated if necessary, for their size and symmetry. Any evidence of atrophy or involuntary movements (tremors, tics) is noted. Muscle tone is evaluated by palpating various muscle groups at rest and during passive movement. Resistance to these movements is assessed and documented. Abnormalities in tone include spasticity, rigidity, or flaccidity.

Muscle strength is tested by assessing the patient's ability to flex or extend his extremity against resistance. The function of an individual muscle or group of muscles is evaluated by placing the muscle at a disadvantage. The quadriceps, for example, is a powerful muscle responsible for straightening the leg. Once the leg is straightened, it is exceedingly difficult for the examiner to flex the knee. Conversely, if the knee is flexed, and the patient is asked to straighten the leg against resistance, a more subtle disability can be elicited. It is critically important to compare the two sides to detect subtle changes in muscle strength.

Most authorities advocate the use of a five-point scale for strength of motor power. A 5 would indicate full power of contraction; a 4 would indicate fair, but not full, strength; a 3 would imply just sufficient strength to overcome the force of gravity; a 2 indicates the ability to move but not to overcome the force of gravity; a 1 indicates minimal contractile power; a 0 implies no contraction whatsoever.

Assessment of motor power can be as detailed as necessary. One may quickly test the strength of the proximal muscles of the upper and lower extremities, comparing the two. The motor capacity of the finer muscles that control the function of the hand and of the foot can then be assessed.

Cerebellar influence on the motor system is reflected in balance control and coordination. Coordination in the hands and upper extremities is tested by having the patient perform *rapid, alternating movements* and *point-to-point testing*. First, the patient is instructed to pat his thigh as fast as he can with his hand. Each hand is tested separately. Then he is instructed to turn his hands from a supine to a prone position as rapidly as possible. Lastly, he is asked to touch each of his fingers with his thumb in a consecutive motion. Speed, symmetry, and degree of difficulty are noted.

Point-to-point testing is accomplished by having the patient touch the examiner's extended finger and then his own nose. This is repeated several times. This assessment is then carried out with the patient's eyes closed.

Coordination in the lower extremities is tested by having the patient run his heel down the anterior surface of his tibia. Each leg is tested in turn. Inability to perform these maneuvers is referred to as *ataxia*. The presence of ataxia or tremors (rhythmic, involuntary movements) during these movements suggests cerebellar disease.

It is not necessary to carry out each of these assessments for coordination. During a routine examination, it is advisable to perform a simple screening of the upper and lower extremities by having the patient perform either rapid, alternating movements or point-to-point testing. When abnormalities are observed, a more thorough examination is indicated.

The *Romberg test* is a screening measurement for balance. The patient stands with his feet together, arms extended in front of him, and eyes closed. The examiner stands close to the patient and reassures him that he will be supported if he begins to lose his balance. Slight swaying is normal. Additional cerebellar tests for balance in the ambulatory patient include hopping in place, alternating knee bends, and heel-to-toe walking.

Examination of the Reflexes

The motor reflexes are involuntary contractions of muscles or muscle groups in response to abrupt stretching near the site of the muscle's insertion. The tendon is struck directly with a reflex hammer, or indirectly by striking the examiner's thumb, which is placed firmly against the tendon. Testing these reflexes enables the examiner to assess involuntary reflex arcs that depend on the presence of afferent stretch receptors, spinal synapses, efferent motor fibers, and a variety of modifying influences from higher levels. Common reflexes that may be tested include the biceps, the brachioradialis, the triceps, the patellar, and the ankle (or Achilles) reflexes (Fig. 55-6).

A reflex hammer is used to elicit a deep tendon reflex. The stem of the hammer is held loosely between thumb and index finger, allowing a full swinging motion. The wrist motion is similar to that used during percussion. The extremity is positioned so that the tendon is slightly stretched. This requires a sound knowledge of the location of muscles and their tendon attachments. The tendon is then struck briskly and the response compared with the corresponding reflex on the opposite side of the body. Wide variation in reflex response may be considered normal. It is more important, however, that the reflexes be symmetrically equivalent. When the comparison is made, both sides should be equivalently relaxed and each tendon struck with equal force.

Valid findings depend on several factors: proper use of the reflex hammer, proper positioning of the extremity, and a relaxed patient. If the reflexes are symmetrically diminished or absent, the examiner may use a technique called *reinforcement* to increase reflex activity. This involves the isometric contraction of other muscle groups. If lower extremity reflexes are diminished or absent, the patient is instructed to lock his fingers together and pull in opposite directions. Having the patient clench his jaw or press his heel against the floor or examining table may likewise elicit more reliable biceps, triceps, or brachioradialis reflexes.

The absence of reflexes is significant, although ankle jerks (Achilles reflex) may be absent in older people.

TABLE 55–2. *Cranial Nerves*

Cranial Nerve	Function	Clinical Examination
I (olfactory)	Sense of smell	With his eyes closed, the patient identifies familiar odors (coffee, tobacco). Each nostril is tested separately.
II (optic)	Visual acuity	Snellen eye chart; visual fields; ophthalmoscopic examination
III (oculomotor) IV (trochlear) VI (abducens)	Cranial nerves III, IV, and VI function in the regulation of eye movements; CN III also innervates the levator muscle of the eyelid, the constrictor muscle of the pupil, and the ciliary muscle, which controls accommodation.	Test for ocular rotations, conjugate movements, nystagmus. Test for pupillary reflexes, and inspect eyelids for ptosis.
V (trigeminal)	Facial sensation	Have patient close his eyes. Touch cotton to forehead, cheeks, and jaw. Opposite sides of face are compared. Sensitivity to superficial pain is tested by using the sharp and dull ends of a broken tongue blade. Alternate between the sharp point and the dull end. Patient reports "sharp" or "dull" with each movement. If responses are incorrect, test for temperature sensation. Test tubes of cold and hot water are used alternately.
	Corneal reflex	While the patient looks up, *lightly* touch a wisp of cotton against the temporal surface of each cornea. A blink and tearing is a normal response.
	Mastication	Have the patient clench his jaw and move it from side to side. Palpate the masseter and temporal muscles, noting strength and equality.
VII (facial)	Facial muscle movement Facial expression Tear and saliva secretion	Observe for symmetry while the patient performs facial movements: smiles, whistles, elevates eyebrows, frowns, tightly closes eyelids against resistance (examiner attempts to open them). Observe face for flaccid paralysis (shallow nasolabial folds).
	Taste: anterior two thirds of tongue	Patient extends his tongue. His ability to discriminate between sugar and salt is tested.
VIII (vestibulocochlear)	Hearing and equilibrium	Whisper or watch-tick test
		Test for lateralization (Weber)
		Test for air and bone conduction (Rinne)
IX (glossopharyngeal)	Taste: posterior third of tongue	Assess patient's ability to discriminate between sugar and salt on posterior third of the tongue.
X (vagus)	Pharyngeal contraction	Depress a tongue blade on posterior tongue, or stimulate posterior pharynx to elicit gag reflex.
	Symmetric movement of vocal cords.	Note any hoarseness in voice.
	Symmetric movement of soft palate	Have patient say "ah." Observe for symmetric rise of uvula and soft palate.
	Movement and secretion of thoracic and abdominal viscera	
XI (spinal accessory)	Movement of sternocleidomastoid and trapezius muscles	Palpate and note the strength of the trapezius muscles while the patient shrugs his shoulders against resistance.
		Palpate and note the strength of each sternocleidomastoid muscle as the patient turns his head against opposing pressure of the examiner's hand.
XII (hypoglossal)	Movement of the tongue	While the patient protrudes his tongue, any deviation or tremors are noted. The strength of the tongue is tested by having the patient move his protruded tongue from side to side against a tongue depressor.

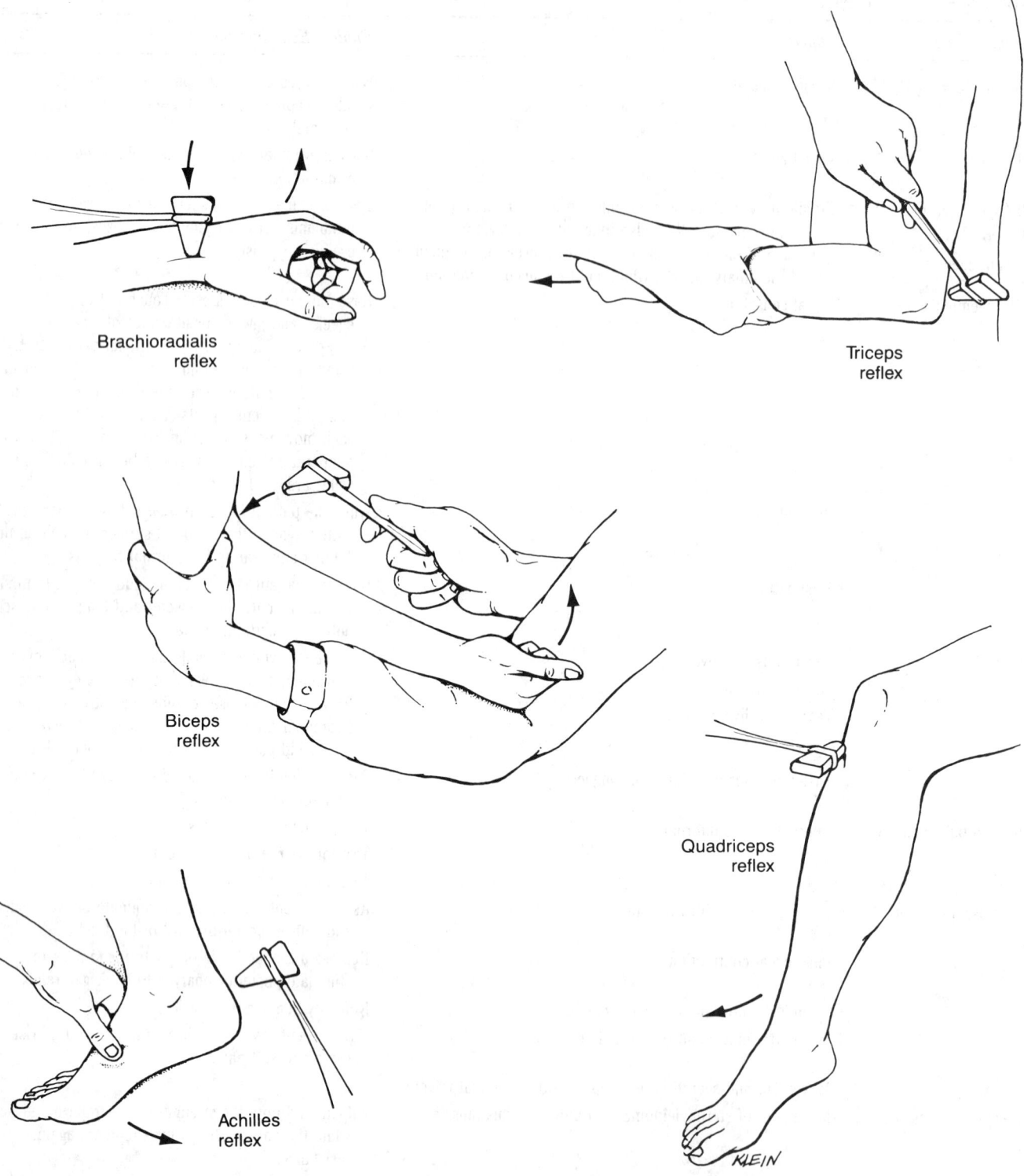

Brachioradialis
reflex

Triceps
reflex

Biceps
reflex

Quadriceps
reflex

Achilles
reflex

KLEIN

Figure 55–6. The proper technique for eliciting the major tendon reflexes. The tendon can be struck *directly* with the reflex hammer or *indirectly* by striking the examiner's thumb, which is placed on the tendon. Arrows indicate the normal extremity motion expected.

Reflex responses are often graded on a 0 to 4 scale:

4—hyperactive with sustained clonus
3—hyperactive
2—normal
1—hypoactive
0—absent

Recording plus or minus to the grade, unless well defined, only confuses the accuracy of the examination.

As was previously mentioned, scale ratings are highly subjective. When used, the findings are recorded as a fraction, indicating the scale range (*e.g.,* 2/4). Some examiners prefer to use the terms *present, absent,* and *diminished* when describing reflexes.

The *biceps reflex* is elicited by striking the biceps tendon of the flexed elbow. The examiner supports the forearm with one arm while placing the thumb against the tendon and striking the thumb with the reflex hammer. The normal response is flexion at the elbow and contraction of the biceps.

To elicit a *triceps reflex*, the patient's arm is flexed at the elbow and positioned in front of the chest. The examiner supports the patient's arm and identifies the triceps tendon by palpating 2.5 to 5 cm (1 to 2 in) above the elbow. A direct blow on the tendon normally produces contraction of the triceps muscle and extension of the elbow.

With the patient's forearm resting on the lap or across the abdomen, the *brachioradialis reflex* is assessed. A gentle strike of the hammer 2.5 to 5 cm (1 to 2 in) above the wrist results in flexion and supination of the forearm.

The *patellar reflex* is elicited by striking the patellar tendon just below the patella. The patient may be in a sitting or a lying position. If the patient is supine, the examiner supports the legs to facilitate relaxation of the muscles. Contraction of the quadriceps and knee extension are normal responses.

To facilitate an *ankle reflex*, the foot is dorsiflexed at the ankle and the hammer strikes the stretched Achilles tendon. This reflex normally produces plantar flexion. If the examiner is unable to elicit the ankle reflex and suspects that the patient is unable to relax, the patient is instructed to kneel on a chair or similar elevated, flat surface. This position places the ankles in dorsiflexion and reduces any muscular tension in the gastrocnemius. The Achilles tendons are struck in turn, and plantar flexion is usually demonstrated.

When reflexes are exceedingly hyperactive, a phenomenon called *clonus* may be elicited. If the foot is abruptly dorsiflexed, it may continue to "beat" two or three times before it settles into a position of rest. Occasionally, in CNS disease, this activity persists, and the foot does not come to rest while the tendon is being stretched but persists in repetitive activity. The unsustained clonus associated with normal but hyperactive reflexes is not considered pathologic. Sustained clonus always indicates the presence of CNS disease and requires evaluation by a physician.

Certain superficial reflexes may be elicited by scratching the skin of the abdominal wall, or the inside of the thigh in men. The former results in involuntary contraction of the abdominal muscles, and the latter results in retraction of the scrotum. Although interesting phenomena, they have little clinical significance.

A well-known reflex, indicative of CNS disease affecting the corticospinal tracts, is the *Babinski response*. If the lateral aspect of the sole of the foot of a person with an intact CNS is stroked, the toes contract and are drawn together. In patients who have CNS diseases of the motor system, the toes fan out and are drawn back. This is normal in newborns but represents serious abnormality in adults. A variety of other reflexes convey similar information. Many of them are interesting but not particularly informative.

Sensory Examination

The sensory system is even more complex than the motor system because sensory modalities are carried in different tracts, located in different portions of the spinal cord. The sensory examination is largely subjective and requires the cooperation of the patient. It is recommended that the examiner become familiar with dermatomes that represent the distribution of the peripheral nerves that arise from the spinal cord. Most sensory deficits result from peripheral neuropathy and follow anatomic dermatomes. Exceptions to this include major destructive lesions of the brain; loss of sensation, which may affect an entire side of the body; and the neuropathies associated with alcoholism, which occur in a glove and stocking distribution.

Assessment of the sensory system involves tests for tactile sensation, superficial pain, vibration, and proprioception. Throughout the sensory assessment, the patient's eyes are closed. The cooperation of the patient is encouraged by simple directions and reassurance that the examiner will not hurt or startle the patient.

Tactile sensation is assessed by lightly touching a cotton wisp to corresponding areas on each side of the body. The sensitivity of proximal parts of the extremities is compared with that of distal parts.

Pain and temperature sensations are transmitted together in the lateral part of the cord. Thus, it is not necessary to test for temperature sense in most circumstances. Superficial pain can be assessed by determining the patient's sensitivity to a sharp object. The patient is asked to differentiate between the sharp and dull ends of a broken wooden cotton swab or tongue blade; using a safety pin should be avoided because it breaks the integrity of the skin. Both the sharp and dull sides of the object are applied with equal intensity at all times, and the two sides are tested symmetrically.

Vibration and proprioception (the subjective sense of joint position) are transmitted together in the posterior part of the cord. Vibration may be evaluated through the use of a low-frequency (128- or 256-Hertz) tuning fork. The handle of the vibrating fork is placed against a bony prominence and the patient is asked whether he feels a sensation. He is instructed to signal the examiner when the sensation ceases. If the patient does not perceive the vibrations at the distal bony prominences, the examiner progresses upward with the tuning fork until the vibrations are perceived by the patient. As with all measurement of sensation, side-to-side comparison is made.

Position sense may be determined by asking the patient to close his eyes and indicate, as the toes are moved, in which direction movement has taken place. Vibration and position sense are often lost together, frequently in circumstances where all others remain intact.

Having tested peripheral sensation, one now asks whether *integration of sensation* in the brain is being carried out properly. This may be performed by testing two-point discrimination. That is, if the patient is touched with two sharp objects simultaneously, are they perceived as two or as one? If a patient is touched simultaneously on opposite sides of the body, he should normally recognize that he has been touched in two places. If he recognizes only one, the one not recognized is said to demonstrate *extinction*. A good test of higher cortical sensory ability is that of *stereognosis*. The patient is instructed to close his eyes and identify a variety of objects (*e.g.*, keys, coins) that are placed in his hand by the examiner.

Gerontologic Considerations

The nervous system of older adults undergoes many changes from the normal aging process and is extremely vulnerable to general systemic illness. Changes throughout the nervous system vary in degree as the person ages. Nerve fibers that connect directly to muscles show little decline in function with age, as do simple neurologic functions that involve a number of connections in the spinal cord. Disease processes that complicate the normal aging processes often make it difficult to distinguish normal from abnormal changes.

The elderly often assume a flexed posture and display muscle rigidity, tremor, and a slowness in movements. Among the known structural alterations that occur with increasing age are a decrease in brain weight and a decrease in the number of synapses. The loss of neurons occurs in select layers and regions of the brain but is not consistent throughout the CNS. Memory loss, particularly for recent events, and slower reaction times may be annoyances to the elderly person, and he may have trouble choosing among several responses to a situation unless given enough time to reach a decision. Sensory isolation due to visual and hearing loss causes confusion, anxiety, disorientation, misinterpretation, and a feeling of inadequacy. Sensory alterations may require modification of the home environment and extra orientation to new surroundings. Simple explanations of routines, the location of the bathroom, and how to operate the call bell in the hospital are just a few examples of information the elderly patient needs.

In addition, a number of other neurologic alterations occur with the aging process. For example, the pupillary response becomes more sluggish or may not appear at all if the individual has cataracts. Other changes include diminished or absent Achilles reflexes, loss of strength, and muscle wasting. Other manifestations of neurologic changes are related to temperature regulation and the ability to feel pain. The geriatric patient usually feels cold more easily than heat and may require extra covering when in bed; a room temperature somewhat higher than usual may be desirable. Perception of a reaction to painful stimuli may be decreased with age. Because pain is an important warning signal, for safety the nurse must use caution when applying hot or cold packs or any therapeutic interventions. The geriatric patient may be burned or suffer frostbite before being aware of any discomfort.

More accurate assessment of physical signs and symptoms may be necessary to alleviate conditions underlying complaints of pain, such as abdominal discomfort or chest pain, which may be more serious than the patient's perception might indicate.

The acuity of the taste buds decreases with age, which along with an altered olfactory sense causes a decreased appetite. Extra seasoning often increases food intake, as long as it does not cause gastric irritation. The reduced olfactory sense arises from the atrophy of the olfactory organs and increased hair in the nostrils.

A decreased sense of smell may present a safety hazard, because elderly persons living alone may be unable to detect household gas leaks or fires if they occur.

Another neurologic alteration in the elderly patient is the dulling of tactile sensation as a result of a decrease in the number of areas of the body responding to all stimuli and in the number and sensitivity of sensory receptors. There may be difficulty in identifying objects by touch, and because fewer tactile cues are received from the bottom of the feet, the person may get confused as to his position and location. These factors combined with sensitivity to glare, decreased peripheral vision, and a constricted visual field may result in disorientation, especially at night when there is little or no light in the room.

Because the elderly person takes longer to recover visual sensitivity when moving from a light to dark area, night lights and a safe and familiar arrangement of furniture are essential.

Mental status is evaluated while the history is obtained, and areas of judgment, intelligence, memory, affect, mood, orientation, speech, and grooming are assessed. Changes in mental status may be discerned by family members who bring the patient to the health care setting. Drug toxicity should always be suspected as a causative factor when the patient has a change in mental status. Delirium (mental confusion, usually with delusions and hallucinations) is seen in elderly patients who have underlying CNS damage or are experiencing an acute condition such as infection or dehydration. Dementia (deterioration of intellectual function) may be reversible and treatable (as in drug toxicity or thyroid disease) or chronic and irreversible. Depression may produce impairment of attention and memory.

Nursing care for the patient with an aging nervous system should include the modifications previously described. In addition, patient teaching is also affected because the nurse must understand the altered responses and the changing needs of the elderly patient before beginning health education.

When caring for the elderly patient, the nurse adapts activities such as preoperative teaching, diet therapy, instruction about new medications, their timing and doses, to the changes in the aging nervous system. The nurse considers the aged person's difficulty with fine motor movement and failing vision. When using visual aids, adequate lighting without glare, contrasting colors, and large print are used to offset visual difficulties caused by rigidity and opacity of the lens in the eye and slower pupillary reaction. Procedures and preparation needed for diagnostic tests are explained, taking into account the possibility of impaired hearing and slowed responses in the elderly. Even with hearing loss, the elderly patient often hears adequately if the health care provider uses a low-pitched, clear speaking voice; shouting only makes it harder for the patient to understand the spoken voice. Providing auditory and visual cues aids understanding. Teaching at an unrushed pace and using reinforcement enhances learning and retention. Material should be short in length, concise, and concrete. Vocabulary is matched to the patient's ability, and terms are clearly defined. The elderly patient requires adequate time to receive and to respond to stimuli, to learn, and to react. These measures allow comprehension, memory, and formation of association and concepts.

As more research is carried out on the healthy geriatric population, the effects of normal aging on the nervous system will be distinguished from the effects of disease processes. Identification of the normal aging process may then open avenues for research into the prevention of degenerative nervous system changes that impair motor functions in the elderly.

Diagnostic Tests and Procedures

Imaging Procedures

Computed Tomography Scanning. Computed tomography (CT) makes use of a narrow beam of x-ray to scan the head in successive layers. The images that are produced provide cross-sectional views of the brain, with distinguishing differences in tissue densities of the skull, cortex, subcortical structures, and ventricles. The brightness of each portion, or "slice," of brain in the final image is proportional to the degree to which it absorbs x-ray. The image is displayed on an oscilloscope or TV monitor and is photographed.

Lesions in the brain are seen as variations in tissue density differing from the surrounding normal brain tissue. Abnormalities of tissue indicate possible tumor masses, brain infarction, displacement of the ventricles, and cortical atrophy. Whole-body CT scanners allow visualization of sections of the spinal cord. The injection of water-soluble iodinated contrast material into the subarachnoid space through lumbar puncture permits improved visualization of the spinal and intracranial contents on these films. The CT scanner has replaced the myelogram as a diagnostic procedure for the diagnosis of herniated lumbar discs.

CT scanning is usually performed first without contrast material and then with intravenous contrast enhancement. The patient lies on an adjustable table, with his head held in a fixed position, while the scanning system rotates around the head. (The patient serves as the axis, and the machine is rotated around this axis, resulting in a cross-sectional image). The patient must lie with the head held perfectly still and with a careful effort not to talk or move the face, because head motion may cause considerable distortion of the image.

CT is noninvasive, painless, and has a high degree of sensitivity for detecting lesions. As newer versions are developed and physicians become more and more sophisticated at interpreting them, the number of diseases and injuries that are able to be diagnosed is increasing, and the need for invasive diagnostic procedures is decreasing.

Positron Emission Tomography. Positron emission tomography (PET) is a computer-based nuclear imaging technique that can produce pictures of actual organ functioning. The patient either inhales a radioactive gas or is injected with a radioactive substance that emits positively charged particles. When these positrons combine with negatively charged electrons (normally found in the body's cells), the resultant gamma rays can be detected by a scanning device. In the scanning equipment, detectors are arranged in a ring and produce a series of two-dimensional views at various levels of the brain. This information is integrated by computer and gives a composite picture of the brain at work.

PET permits the measurement of blood flow, tissue composition, and brain metabolism. The brain is one of the most metabolically active organs, consuming 80% of the glucose the body uses. PET measures this activity in specific areas of the brain and is able to detect changes in glucose use. This test is useful in showing metabolic changes in the brain (Alzheimer's disease), in locating lesions (brain tumor, epileptogenic lesions), in identifying blood flow and oxygen metabolism in stroke patients, in evaluating new therapies for brain tumors, as well as in revealing biochemical abnormalities associated with mental illness.

Patient preparation involves teaching the patient about inhalation techniques and the possible sensations (*i.e.*, dizziness, lightheadedness, headache) that may occur. The intravenous injection of the radioactive substance produces similar side effects.

Single Photon Emission Computed Tomography. Single photon emission computed tomography (SPECT) is a three-dimensional imaging technique using nuclear medicine procedures that employ radionuclides and instruments that emit and detect, respectively, single photons. Gamma photons are emitted from a radiopharmaceutical agent administered to the patient and are detected by a rotating gamma camera or cameras; the image is sent to a minicomputer. This approach allows viewing behind overlying structures or background, which greatly increases the contrast between normal and abnormal tissue. It is relatively inexpensive, and patient participation time is similar to that of CT scanning.

SPECT is useful in detecting the extent and location of abnormally perfused areas of the brain, thus allowing detection, localization, and sizing of stroke (before it is visible by CT), localization of seizure foci in epilepsy, and evaluation of perfusion before and after neurosurgical procedures.

Magnetic Resonance Imaging. Magnetic resonance imaging (MRI) uses a powerful magnetic field to obtain images of different areas of the body (Fig. 55-7). Magnetized photons (hydrogen nuclei) within the body align like small magnets in this magnetic field. After bombardment with radiofrequency pulses, the protons emit signals; these are converted to images. MRI has the potential for identifying cerebral abnormality earlier and more clearly than other diagnostic tests. It can provide information about the chemical changes within cells, thus allowing the physician to monitor a tumor's response to treatment. It does not require ionizing radiation.

Before the patient is taken to the room where the MRI is to be performed, he must remove all metallic objects (jewelry, including wedding rings, watches, hair pins) from his person, as well as credit cards (the magnetic field can erase them). A complete history should also be taken so that there is no metal inside the patient that could cause harm (*e.g.*, aneurysm clips, orthopedic hardware, artificial heart valves, intrauterine devices) The patient lies on a flat platform that is moved into a tube containing the magnet. The scanning process is painless, but the patient hears the thumping of the magnetic coils as the magnetic field is being pulsed. Because the MRI scanner is a narrow tube, patients may experience claustrophobia. Patient preparation should include teaching the patient relaxation techniques and informing him that he will be able to talk to the staff by means of a microphone located inside the scanner.

Cerebral Angiography

Cerebral angiography is a radiologic study of the cerebral circulation after the injection of contrast material into a selected artery. Cerebral angiography is a valuable tool for investigating vascular disease, aneurysms, and arteriovenous malformations. It is frequently performed before a patient undergoes a craniotomy so that the cerebral arteries and veins are visualized and to determine the site, size, and nature of the pathologic processes. It also demonstrates the patency and adequacy of the cerebral circulation.

Most cerebral angiograms are performed by threading a catheter through the femoral artery in the groin and up to the desired vessel. The procedure may also be accomplished by direct puncture of the carotid or vertebral artery or by retrograde injection of contrast medium into the brachial artery.

Patient Preparation. The patient should be well hydrated, and clear liquids are usually permitted up to the time of the study. Before going to the radiology department, the patient is instructed to void. The locations of the appropriate peripheral

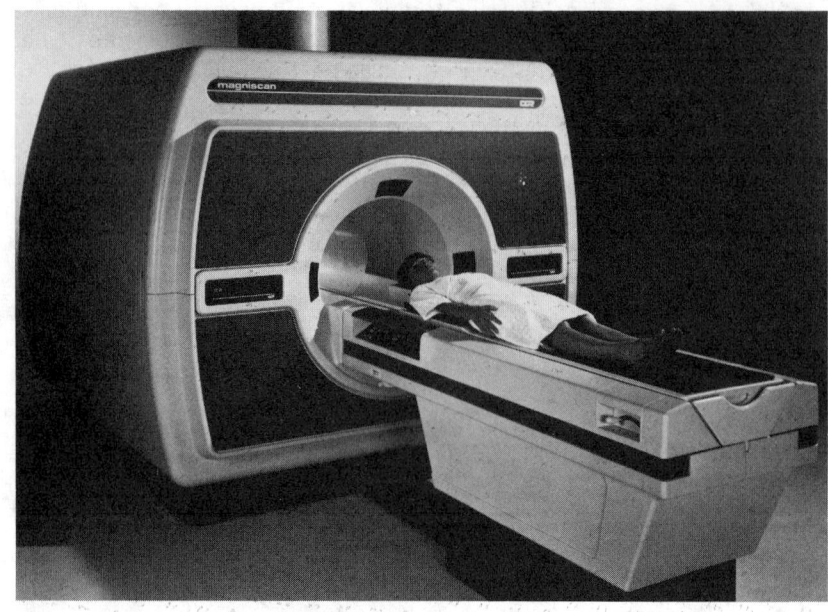

Figure 55–7. Magnetic resonance imaging (MRI). In central nervous system conditions, MRI has the potential for identifying cerebral pathology earlier and more clearly. (Courtesy of Thomson-CGR Corporation.)

pulses are marked with a felt-tip pen. The patient is asked to try to remain immobile during the film sequence. He is told to expect a brief feeling of warmth in the face, behind the eyes, or in the jaw, teeth, tongue, and lips, and a metallic taste when the contrast material is injected.

After the groin is shaved and prepared, a local anesthetic is administered for patient comfort and for reduction of arterial spasm. A catheter is introduced into the femoral artery, flushed with heparinized saline, and filled with contrast material. Under fluoroscopic guidance, the catheter is advanced to the appropriate vessels. During injection of the contrast medium, radiographs are made of the arterial and venous phases of circulation through the brain.

Postprocedure Nursing Management. In some instances, patients may experience major or minor arterial block due to embolism, thrombosis, or hemorrhage, producing a neurologic deficit. Signs of such an occurrence include alterations in the level of responsiveness and consciousness, weakness on one side of the body, motor or sensory deficits, or speech disturbances. Therefore, it is necessary to observe the patient frequently for these signs and to report them immediately if they occur.

The injection site is observed for hematoma formation (a localized collection of blood), and an ice cap may be applied intermittently to the puncture site to relieve swelling and discomfort. Because a hematoma at the puncture site or embolization to a distant artery affects the peripheral pulses, these pulses are monitored frequently. The color and temperature of the involved extremity are also assessed to detect possible embolism.

Digital Subtraction Angiography

In digital subtraction angiography, x-ray images of the area in question are obtained before and after the injection of contrast material. The computer "subtracts" the second set of films and produces an enhanced image of the carotid and vertebral arterial systems. This procedure is less invasive than arteriography, because the injection can be given through a peripheral venous access.

Myelography

A myelogram is a radiograph of the spinal subarachnoid space taken after a contrast medium or air is injected into the spinal subarachnoid space through a spinal puncture. It outlines the spinal subarachnoid space and shows any distortion of the spinal cord or spinal dural sac caused by tumors, cysts, herniated vertebral discs, or other lesions.

After the contrast medium is injected, the head of the table is tilted down and the course of the contrast medium is observed radioscopically. The contrast medium may be water soluble or oil based. Metrizamide is a water-soluble contrast agent that is absorbed by the body and excreted by the kidneys. It does not have to be removed by the needle route from the spinal canal because it is highly soluble and clears relatively quickly from the CSF. Side effects include headache, which is most probably due to CNS irritation by the metrizamide.

If iophendylate (Pantopaque), an oil-based iodine compound, is used for myelography, the radiologist may remove it by syringe and needle aspiration. The patient may complain of sharp pain down the leg during aspiration if a nerve root is affected. This is remedied by rotating the needle point or adjusting the depth of the needle.

Nursing Management. Because most patients have some misconceptions about this procedure, the nurse can answer questions and clarify the explanation offered by the physician. The patient should be aware that the x-ray table may be tilted in varying positions during the study. The meal that would normally be eaten before the procedure is omitted. The patient may be given a light sedative to help him cope with a rather lengthy test.

After myelography, when a water-soluble medium has been used, the patient lies in bed with the head of the bed elevated 15 to 30 degrees to reduce the rate of upward dispersion of the medium. The patient may be ambulatory or remain in bed as prescribed by the physician.

After a procedure in which an oil-based medium has been used, the patient should lie in a recumbent position for the amount of time specified by the physician (usually 12 to 24 hours) to reduce CSF leakage and decrease the frequency of headache. Usually, he is permitted to turn from side to side.

The patient is encouraged to drink liberal amounts of fluid for rehydration and replacement of CSF and to decrease the incidence of postlumbar puncture headache. The blood pressure, pulse, respiratory rate, and temperature are monitored, as well as the patient's ability to void. Other untoward signs include fever, stiff neck, photophobia (sensitivity to light), or signs of chemical or bacterial meningitis.

Myelography is performed less frequently today because of the sensitivity of CT scanning and MRIs.

Lumbar Epidural Venography

In lumbar epidural venography, a catheter is inserted percutaneously into the femoral vein and guided into the ascending lumbar vein or internal iliac vein. The contrast medium is injected to fill the epidural veins overlying the disc spaces and to opacify the epidural venous plexus. The procedure may be useful in the diagnosis of herniated lumbar discs that are not demonstrated by myelography. It shows deviation or compression of the epidural veins due to a herniated disc or tumor. The procedure is relatively easy to perform, well tolerated, fairly painless, and not associated with arachnoiditis. Lumbar epidural venography and myelography may be performed as complementary diagnostic studies. After the test, the site is observed for evidence of hematoma formation.

Radionuclide Imaging Studies (Brain Scan)

Radionuclide imaging is based on the principle that a radiopharmaceutical agent may diffuse through the blood–brain barrier at a point where the barrier has been disrupted and collect in abnormal cerebral tissue. (Normal brain tissue is relatively impermeable.) There is increased uptake of radioactive material at the site of pathology.

In this procedure, the patient is given an intravenous injection of a radiopharmaceutical agent. The radioactivity subsequently transmitted through the skull is traced by a scanner that prints out a picture, or a gamma camera is used to monitor the passage of the radiopharmaceutical agent through the cerebral circulation to gain information about cerebral blood flow.

Brain scanning is particularly useful in evaluating vascular lesions of the brain and meninges and in locating vascular neoplasms and brain tumors. It is useful in the early detection and evaluation of stroke, abscess, and follow-up of surgical or radiation therapy of the brain. Newer techniques permit the evaluation of cerebral circulation during the brain scan. However, CT scanning is replacing traditional radioisotope scanning.

Echoencephalography

Echoencephalography is the recording of sound waves reflected by the structures of the brain in response to ultrasound signals created by a transducer positioned over specific areas of the head. Echoencephalography is a rapid and useful technique to determine the position of midline structures of the brain and the distance from the midline to the lateral ventricular wall or the third ventricular wall. Therefore, it is performed to detect a shift of the cerebral midline structures caused by subdural hematoma, intracerebral hemorrhage, massive cerebral

infarction, and neoplasms. It is useful in the evaluation of hydrocephalus, because it can detect dilation of the ventricles.

The nurse explains that this is a noninvasive test, and that some type of water-soluble jelly is used to eliminate the air gap between the hand-held transducer and the patient's head.

Noninvasive carotid flow studies use ultrasound imagery and Doppler measurements of arterial blood flow to evaluate carotid and deep orbital circulation. These tests are often obtained before arteriography, which carries combined risks of strokes and death (0.5% to 2%). Carotid Doppler studies, carotid ultrasonography, oculoplethysmography, and ophthalmodynamometry are four common noninvasive vascular studies that analyze the arterial blood flow and detect arterial stenosis, occlusion, and plaques. There are no special preparations for these studies except for patient education. To reduce the patient's anxiety, he should be informed that a hand-held transducer will be placed over the neck and orbits of the eyes and that some type of water-soluble jelly is used on the transducer.

Air Studies

The CSF spaces in and around the brain may be seen on x-ray examination when the fluid is replaced with a gas. This is based on the principle that gas inserted in the ventricular and subarachnoid systems serves as a contrast medium, because air is less dense than fluid to x-rays. The CSF may be partially replaced with air through *pneumoencephalography* and *ventriculography*.

Pneumoencephalography is a diagnostic procedure in which air or gas is instilled through a lumbar puncture as a means of demonstrating the ventricular system and subarachnoid space overlying the hemispheres and basal cisterns. A small amount of CSF is removed and an equal amount of air injected. A special chair allows the patient to be rotated in all directions so that air may be placed selectively in the desired cavities. Films are then taken and studied.

A ventriculogram is a radiograph taken of the lateral ventricles after withdrawal of CSF and injection of air or gas into the lateral ventricles through openings in the skull.

These studies are rarely performed since the advent of CT and MRI scanning.

Electrophysiologic Tests

Electroencephalography

An electroencephalogram (EEG) represents a record of the electrical activity generated in the brain and obtained through electrodes applied on the scalp surface or through microelectrodes placed within the brain tissue. It provides physiologic assessment of cerebral activity. EEG is a useful test for diagnosing seizure disorders such as the epilepsies and is a screening procedure for coma or organic brain syndrome. It also serves as an indicator of brain death. Tumors, abscesses, brain scars, blood clots, and infection may cause electric activity to differ from normal patterns of rhythm and rate.

Electrodes are arranged on the scalp to record the electrical activity in various regions of the head. The amplified activity of the neurons between any two of these electrodes is recorded on a continuously moving paper sheet; this record is the encephalogram. For a baseline recording, the patient lies quietly with his eyes closed. Then he may be asked to

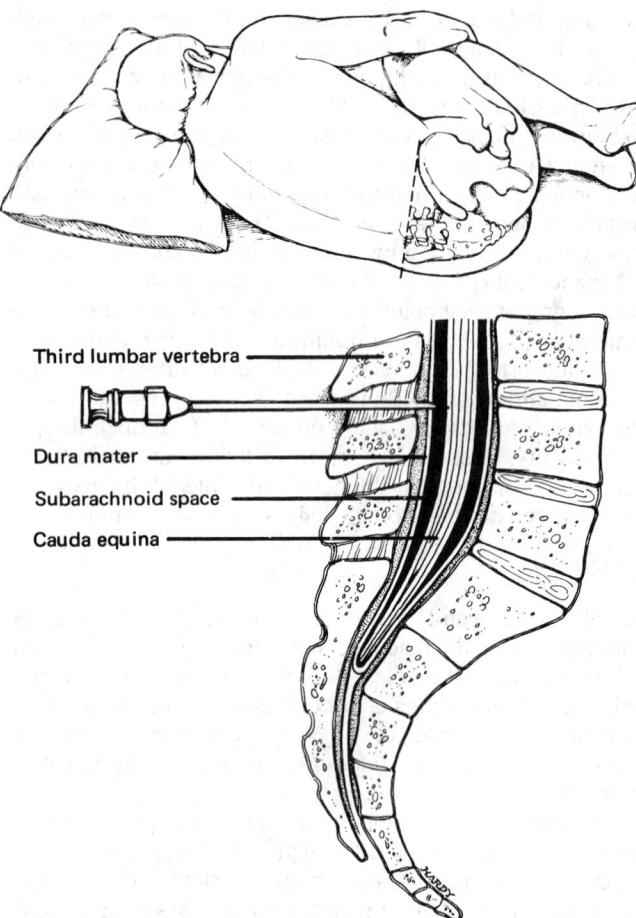

Third lumbar vertebra

Dura mater

Subarachnoid space

Cauda equina

Figure 55–8. Technique of lumbar puncture. The interspaces between L3 and L5 are just below the line connecting the anterosuperior iliac spines.

hyperventilate for 3 to 4 minutes and then to look at a bright, flashing light for photic stimulation. These are activation procedures performed to evoke abnormal electrical discharges, especially seizure potentials. A sleep EEG may be recorded after sedation because some abnormal brain waves are seen only when the patient is asleep. If the epileptogenic area is inaccessible to the conventional scalp electrodes, nasopharyngeal electrodes may be used.

Depth recording of EEG is performed by introducing electrodes stereotactically into a target area of the brain, as dictated by the patient's seizure pattern and scalp EEG. It is used to select patients who may benefit from surgical excision of epileptogenic foci.

Patient Preparation. To increase the chances of recording seizure activity, it is sometimes recommended that the patient be sleep deprived on the night before the EEG. Tranquilizers and stimulants should be withheld 24 to 48 hours before an EEG, because these medications can alter the EEG wave patterns or mask the abnormal wave patterns of seizure disorder. Coffee, tea, chocolate, and cola drinks are omitted in the meal before the test because of their stimulating effect. The meal is not omitted, however, because an altered blood glucose level can also cause changes in the brain wave patterns.

The patient is informed that the standard EEG takes 45 to 60 minutes or longer if a sleep EEG is performed. At the same

time, the patient is assured that the procedure does not cause an electric shock and that the EEG is a diagnostic test and not a form of treatment. Special transsphenoidal, mandibular, and nasopharyngeal electrodes can be placed; and videorecording combined with EEG monitoring and telemetry is used in hospital settings to capture epileptiform abnormalities and their sequelae. Some epilepsy centers provide long-term ambulatory EEG monitoring with portable cassette recorders.

Evoked Potential Studies

Evoked potential studies evaluate the changes and responses in brain waves recorded from scalp electrodes that are evoked (elicited) by the introduction of an external stimulus of peripheral sensory receptors. Evoked changes are detected with the aid of computerized devices that extract the signal, display it on an oscilloscope, and store the data on magnetic tape or disc. These studies are based on the concept that any insult or dysfunction that can alter neuronal metabolism or disturb membrane function may change evoked responses in brain waves. In neurologic diagnosis they reflect conduction times in the peripheral nervous system. In clinical practice, the visual, auditory, and somatosensory systems are most often tested.

In *visual evoked responses*, the patient looks at a visual stimulus (flashing lights, a checkerboard pattern on a screen). The average of several hundred stimuli is recorded by EEG leads placed over the occiput. The transit time from the retina to the occipital area is measured using computer-averaging methods.

To measure *auditory evoked responses* or brain stem evoked responses, an auditory stimulus (a repetitive auditory click) is given and the transit time up the brain stem into the cortex is measured. Specific lesions in the auditory pathway modify or delay the response.

In *somatosensory evoked responses*, the peripheral nerves are stimulated (electrical stimulation through skin electrodes), and the transit time up the spinal cord to the cortex is measured and recorded from scalp electrodes. This test is used to detect a deficit in spinal cord conduction and to monitor cord function during operative procedures. Because myelinated fibers conduct impulses at a higher rate of speed, nerves with intact myelin sheath record the highest velocity. Demyelination of nerve fibers leads to a decrease in conduction velocity as found in Guillain-Barré syndrome, multiple sclerosis, and polyneuropathies.

There is no specific patient preparation other than reassurance and encouragement of relaxation. The patient is advised to remain perfectly still throughout the recording to prevent artifacts (potentials not generated by the brain) that interfere with the recording and interpretation of the test.

Electromyography

An electromyogram (EMG) is obtained by introducing needle electrodes into the skeletal muscles to measure changes in the electrical potential of the muscles and the nerves leading to them. The electrical potentials are shown on an oscilloscope and amplified by a loudspeaker so that both the sound and appearance of the waves can be analyzed and compared simultaneously. EMGs are useful in determining the presence of a neuromuscular disorder and myopathies. They help to distinguish weakness due to neuropathy (functional or pathologic changes in the peripheral nervous system) from weakness due to other causes.

No special patient preparation is required. The patient is informed that he will experience a sensation similar to that of an intramuscular injection as the needle is inserted into the muscle. The muscles examined may ache for a short time after the procedure.

Nerve Conduction Studies

Nerve conduction studies are performed by stimulating a peripheral nerve at several points along its course and recording the muscle action potential or the sensory action potential that results. Surface or needle electrodes are placed on the skin over the nerve to stimulate the nerve fibers. This test is useful in the study of peripheral nerve neuropathies.

Special Procedures

Lumbar Puncture and Examination of Cerebrospinal Fluid

A lumbar puncture (spinal tap) is carried out by insertion of a needle into the lumbar subarachnoid space to withdraw CSF for diagnostic and therapeutic purposes. The purposes are to obtain spinal fluid for examination, to measure and relieve spinal fluid pressure, to determine the presence or absence of blood in the spinal fluid, to detect spinal subarachnoid block, and to administer antibiotics intrathecally in certain cases of infection.

The needle is usually inserted into the subarachnoid space through the third and fourth lumbar interspace. Because the spinal cord divides into a sheaf of nerves at the first lumbar vertebra, the needle is inserted below the level of the third lumbar vertebra to prevent the spinal cord from being punctured (Fig. 55-8).

A successful lumbar puncture requires that the patient be relaxed; an anxious patient is a tense patient and the increased anxiety may cause an increase in the pressure reading. The normal range of spinal fluid pressure with the patient in a lateral recumbent position is 70 to 200 mm H_2O. Pressures over 200 mm H_2O are considered abnormal.

A lumbar puncture may be quite dangerous in the presence of an intracranial mass lesion. The danger is because intracranial pressure is decreased by the removal of CSF and the brain may herniate downward through the tentorium and the foramen magnum.

A lumbar manometric test (Queckenstedt's test) may be performed by compressing the jugular veins on each side of the neck during the lumbar puncture. The increase in the pressure caused by the compression is noted. Then the pressure is released and pressure readings are made at 10-second intervals. Normally, the CSF pressure rises rapidly in response to compression of the jugular veins and returns quickly to normal when the compression is released. A slow rise and fall in pressure indicates a partial block due to a lesion compressing the spinal subarachnoid pathways. If there is no pressure change, a complete block is indicated. This test is not performed if an intracranial lesion is suspected.

Nursing Intervention. During the initial explanations, the patient must be assured that inserting a needle into the spine will not result in paralysis. Before the lumbar puncture, the bladder and bowel should be emptied. The patient is placed on his side with his back toward the physician. The thighs and head are flexed as much as possible to increase the space between the spinous processes of the vertebrae and afford easier entry into the subarachnoid space. A pillow fixed between the legs prevents the upper leg from rolling forward. A small pillow is placed under the patient's head so that the spine is maintained in a horizontal position. The nurse may assist the patient to maintain the position to avoid sudden movement, which can produce a traumatic (bloody) tap. During the procedure, the patient is instructed to breathe normally because hyperventilation may lower an elevated pressure. After the procedure, the patient is encouraged to lie prone for the first 3 hours to separate the alignment of the dural and arachnoid needle punctures in the meninges, to reduce the leakage of CSF. It is also suggested that fluids be encouraged to reduce the potential of postpuncture headache; however, the value of this in preventing headache is not proved.

Examination of the Cerebrospinal Fluid. CSF should be clear and colorless. Pink, blood-tinged, or grossly bloody CSF may indicate a cerebral contusion, laceration, or subarachnoid hemorrhage. Sometimes if it has been a difficult lumbar puncture, the CSF initially is bloody because of local trauma but then becomes clearer. Usually, specimens are sent to the laboratory for cell count, culture, glucose, and protein. The specimens should be sent immediately, because changes will take place and alter the result if the specimens are allowed to stand. (See Appendix for the normal values of CSF.)

Post–Lumbar-Puncture Headache. A post–lumbar-puncture headache, ranging from mild to severe, may appear in a few hours to several days after the procedure. This is the most frequently encountered complication, occurring in 11% to 25% of patients. It is a throbbing bifrontal or occipital headache, dull and deep in character, that is particularly severe when the patient sits or stands upright but that lessens or disappears when he lies down in a horizontal position.

Headache is caused by the leakage of CSF at the puncture site. The fluid continues to escape into the tissues by way of the needle tract from the spinal canal. It is then absorbed promptly by the lymphatics, never having accumulated in sufficient volume to be detected. As a result of this leak, the supply of CSF in the cranium is depleted to a point at which it is insufficient to maintain proper mechanical stabilization of the brain. This leakage of CSF allows settling of the brain when the patient assumes an upright position. This produces tension and stretching of venous sinuses and pain-sensitive structures. Both traction and pain are lessened and the leakage reduced when the patient lies down.

The postpuncture headache is usually managed by bed rest, analgesics, and hydration. Occasionally, if the postpuncture headache persists, the epidural blood patch technique may be used. Blood is withdrawn from the patient's antecubital vein and injected into the epidural space, usually at the site of the previous spinal puncture. The rationale is that the blood acts as a gelatinous plug to seal the hole in the dura, thus preventing continuing loss of CSF.

The lumbar puncture headache may be avoided if a needle with a small gauge is used and if the patient is encouraged to remain prone after the procedure. When large volumes of fluid (> 20 ml) are collected, the patient is positioned prone for 2 hours, then flat in a side-lying position for 2 hours, and then supine or prone for 6 more hours. Keeping the patient flat overnight may reduce the incidence of headaches.

Other complications of a spinal puncture include herniation of the intracranial contents, traumatic complications, spinal epidural abscess, spinal epidural hematoma, and meningitis.

Chapter Summary

The nervous system is one of the most complex and fascinating systems in the human body. The neurologic evaluation of a patient is an integral component of the nursing assessment. Patients who suffer from a neurologic disease process offer one of the most challenging experiences for nurses. For the nurse to gather accurate information, background knowledge of basic neurologic anatomy and physiology is necessary, as well as awareness of what a normal neurologic examination entails. The patient frequently offers only subtle clues that there is any type of disease process occurring. It is often the nurse who first notices the subtle changes, because more then any other health care professional, the nurse interacts with the patient and uses a holistic approach to render care rather then a disease- or system-specific one. Basic neuroanatomy and physiology are reviewed in this chapter, and assessment of the more common neurologic deficits and disease processes is discussed. Diagnostic testing of neurologic disorders is reviewed because the nurse plays a key role in the success of these procedures through patient preparation and education. The nervous system changes throughout the life span; thus, the nurse must be aware not only of developmental changes but also of the aging process when evaluating the patient.

Bibliography

Books

Bernat JL and Vincent FM. Neurology Problems in Primary Care. Oradell, NJ, Medical Economics Books, 1987.

Burggraf V and Stanley M. Nursing the Elderly: A Care Plan Approach. Philadelphia, JB Lippincott, 1989.

Curtis BA. Neurosciences: The Basics. Philadelphia, Lea & Febiger, 1990.

Davis RL and Robertson DM. Textbook of Neuropathology. Baltimore, Williams & Wilkins, 1990.

DeGroot J. Correlative Neuroanatomy, 20th ed. East Norwalk, CT, Appleton & Lange, 1988.

Godwin-Austen RB. The Neurology of the Elderly. London, Springer-Verlag, 1990.

Joseph R. Neuropsychology, Neuropsychiatry and Behavioral Neurology. New York, Plenum Press, 1990.

Lechtenberg R. Synopsis of Neurology. Philadelphia, Lea & Febiger, 1991.

Marshall S et al. Neuroscience Critical Care: Pathophysiology and Patient Management. Philadelphia, WB Saunders, 1990.

Mettler F. Imaging 1990. Boston, Little, Brown, 1990.

Mettler F et al. Clinical Magnetic Resonance: Imaging and Spectroscopy. Chichester, NY, Wiley, 1990.

Mitchell P et al. AANN's Neuroscience Nursing-Phenomena and Practice. Norwalk, CT, Appleton & Lange, 1988.

Olson WH et al. Handbook of Symptom-Oriented Neurology. Chicago, Yearbook Medical Publishers, 1989.

Pansky B and Allen D. Review of Neuroscience. New York, Macmillan, 1980.

Swearingen PL et al. Manual of Critical Care Nursing, 2nd ed. St Louis, CV Mosby, 1990.

Wasserman P and Grefsheim S. Encyclopedia of Health Information Sources. Detroit, Gale Research Company, 1987.

Williams A and Haughton V. Cranial Computer Tomography: A Comprehensive Test. St Louis, CV Mosby, 1985.

Wood JH. Cerebral Blood Flow. Physiologic and Clinical Aspects. New York, McGraw-Hill, 1987.

Yurick A et al. The Aged Person and the Nursing Process, 3rd ed. Norwalk, CT, Appleton & Lange, 1989.

Journals

Asterisks indicate nursing research articles.

Bass B and Vandervoost MK. Post-lumbar puncture headache: Review of the literature and nursing implications. Axon 1988 Mar; 9(3):30–34.

Chaudhuri G et al. Computerized axonal tomography head scans as predictors of functional outcome of stroke patients. Arch Phys Med Rehabil 1988 Jul; 69(7):496–498.

Cook T et al. Bed rest and post-lumber puncture headache: The effectiveness of 24 hours recumbency in reducing the post-lumber puncture headache. Anesthesia 1989 May; 44(5):389–391

*Dilorio C. An analysis of trends in neuroscience research. J Neurosci Nurs 1990 Jun; 22(3):139–146.

Evans RL et al. Family intervention after stroke: Does counseling or education help? Stroke 1988 Oct; 19(10):1243–1249.

Flaaten H et al. Postdural puncture headache: A comparison between 26- and 29-gauge needles in young patients. Anesthesia 1989 Dec; 35(12): 1052–1054.

Ford CD et al. A simple treatment of post lumbar-puncture headache. J Emerg Med 1989 Jan/Feb; 7(1):29–31.

*Foreman MD. Reliability and validity of mental status questionnaires in elderly hospitalized patients. Nurs Res 1987 Jul/Aug; 36(4):216–220.

Frawley P. Neurological observations. Nurs Times 1990 Aug/Sep; 86(35): 29–32.

Frost EAM. Controversies in neuroanesthesia. Curr Rev Nurse Anesth 1989 Dec 14; 12(14):111–120.

Kalbach LR. Spinal headache: Cause and care. Orthop Nurse 1989 Mar/ Apr; 8(2):51–55.

Kaufman J. Nurse's guide to assessing the 12 cranial nerves. Nursing 1990 Jun; 20(6):56–58.

Kernich CA and Robb G. Development of a stroke family support and education program. J Neurosci Nurs 1988 Jun; 20(3):193–197.

Lundgren JP. Computerized EEG: Applications and interventions. J Neurosci Nurs 1990 Apr; 22(2):100–112.

March K. Transcranial Doppler sonography: Noninvasive monitoring of intracranial vasculature. J Neurosci Nurs 1990 Apr; 22(2):113–116.

National Institutes of Health. Magnetic resonance imaging. Consensus Development Conference Statement. 1987 Oct; 6(14):1–10.

Osberg JS et al. Predicting long-term outcome among post rehabilitation stroke patients. Am J Phys Med Rehabil 1988 Jun; 67(3):94–103.

Richmond TS. Spinal cord injury. Nurs Clin North Am 1990 Mar; 25(1): 57–69.

Sand T. Which factors affect reported headache incidences after lumbar myelography? A statistical analysis of publications in the literature. Neuroradiology 1989; 31(1):55–59.

*Smith CA. The effect of ambulation on post-myelography headache in patients injected with metrizamide. J Neurosci Nurs 1990 Feb; 22(1): 32–35.

Sullivan J. Neurologic assessment. Nurs Clin North Am 1990 Dec; 25(4): 795–809.

Vilming ST et al. The significance of age, sex and cerebrospinal fluid pressure in post-lumbar-puncture headache. Cephalagia 1989 Jun; 9(2):99–106.

Wahlquist GL. Evaluation and primary management of spasticity. Nurse Pract 1987 Mar; 12(3):27–32.

56

Management of Patients With Neurologic Dysfunction

Chapter Outline

Learning Objectives

On completion of this chapter, the learner will be able to:

1. Specify the special nursing needs of patients with neurologic dysfunction
2. Use the nursing process as a framework for care of the patient with neurologic dysfunction
3. Identify the early and late clinical manifestations of increased intracranial pressure
4. Use the nursing process as a framework for care of the patient with increased intracranial pressure
5. Describe the multiple needs of the unconscious patient
6. Use the nursing process as a framework for care of the unconscious patient
7. Describe the various types of aphasia and the nursing management of the aphasic patient
8. Identify the risk factors of stroke and related measures for stroke prevention
9. Compare the various types of stroke: their causes, clinical manifestations, and nursing and medical management
10. Use the nursing process as a framework for care of the patient with stroke
11. Use the nursing process as a framework for care of the patient undergoing intracranial surgery
12. Compare the various types of neurosurgical procedures used to treat intractable pain

Scope of Neurologic Nursing

Neurologic illness is the principal cause of chronic disease in our society. The final common pathway of many neurologic disorders is musculoskeletal dysfunction. Patients with these disorders are prone to deconditioning that increases functional losses from weakness, immobility, impaired postural reflexes, painful joints, and depression of the patient and his family.

A damaged brain cannot be completely restored. Neurologic tissue that has been injured by trauma or bleeding cannot tolerate much compression by blood clot or edema. The resultant pressure on neighboring tissue may displace vital centers or disrupt the function of adjacent tissue. Paralysis, coma, and chronic pain are frequently seen after central nervous system (CNS) injury. Many brain diseases are manifested by disorders in behavior and a high incidence of psychiatric disorders. Recovery is slow and unpredictable. Neurologic problems change over time and affect every aspect of living.

Neuroscience nursing has become a specialty and requires an understanding of neuroanatomy, neurophysiology, neurodiagnostic testing, critical care nursing, and rehabilitation nursing. In addition to ongoing assessment of the patient's neurologic function and health needs, the nurse's role is to help the patient identify problems, set mutual goals, direct a course of action, use appropriate nursing interventions (including teaching, counseling, and coordinating activities), and evaluate the outcomes of care.

Although sometimes the patient's body may be damaged, his brain impaired, his vision and speech changed, and his self-esteem diminished, the nurse and health care team can take a fresh look, redefine problems, suggest other options, and help the patient gain control, while tapping all available educational and support resources. The goals of helping the patient achieve as high a level of function as possible and the enhancement of the quality of life for the patient and family may be realized in this area of nursing practice.

▶ Nursing Process
The Patient With Neurologic Dysfunction

▷ Assessment

The patient with a neurologic dysfunction undergoes a thorough neurologic examination that is described in Chapter 55, Assessment of Neurologic Function. The neurologic examination involves tests of several major areas of functioning, including cerebral, cranial nerve, motor system and sensory system function, and reflex responses. The patient's movements are observed, and he is questioned about changes in sensation. When assessing the patient's neurologic dysfunction, the nurse observes his level of alertness and determines whether there is a disturbance of consciousness. Alterations in the patient's mental and emotional status are elicited. Cognitive function is tested by determining if the patient is oriented to person, place, and time. Intellectual functions are evaluated by asking questions of general knowledge, ascertaining reasoning ability, and assessing recent and remote memory. An assessment is also made of the person's language abilities. Loss of function and certain alterations in function indicate deterioration and are reported to the physician. These indices are described further in the discussions of specific types of neurologic dysfunctions that follow.

▷ Nursing Diagnoses

There is no known cure for a large number of neurologic illnesses. The nursing goal is to help the patient to adapt to his dysfunction and continue with his life in as meaningful a way as possible. Nursing interventions include knowing and accepting the patient's self-protective responses, providing information, helping the patient set achievable goals, reinforcing positive coping skills, and offering ongoing support.

Many patients with neurologic conditions face a wide range of possible nursing diagnoses, including the following:

- Ineffective breathing pattern
- Impaired swallowing
- Impaired skin integrity
- Impaired physical mobility
- Self-care deficits
- Pain
- Altered oral mucous membranes
- Impaired tissue integrity: cornea
- Altered nutrition: less than body requirements
- Altered urinary and bowel elimination
- Altered thought processes
- Sexual dysfunction
- Ineffective individual coping
- Altered family processes

▷ Nursing Interventions

▷ *Impaired Breathing.*   Patients with neuromuscular disorders such as Guillain-Barré syndrome and myasthenia gravis and neurologic disorders such as cervical spinal cord injury may have weakness of the diaphragm, intercostal muscles, and accessory muscles of respiration that compromises ventilation. When the diaphragm is paralyzed the patient is in danger while supine, when hypoventilation may be particularly severe. Additionally, the patient's inability to breathe deeply and cough results in retained secretions and atelectasis. The end result may be respiratory insufficiency and failure.

Nursing interventions include monitoring the adequacy of alveolar ventilation by frequent measurements of the respiratory rate, vital capacity, and inspiratory force. Measures to promote chest expansion include elevating the head of the bed 30 degrees and working with the respiratory therapist in assessing the effectiveness of incentive spirometry and positive-pressure breathing. If the disorder appears to be progressing (increasing respiratory rate; vital capacity less than 15 ml/kg of body weight; or inspiratory force less than −25 cm H_2O), the patient may require intubation and mechanical ventilation. In many instances the neuromuscular weakness is reversible, but the patient often requires prolonged ventilatory support.

In patients with depressed states of consciousness, a common cause of airway obstruction is the posterior displacement of oropharyngeal soft tissue structures; the tongue becomes flaccid and falls back against the posterior pharyngeal wall. An immediate nursing intervention is to extend the patient's head or elevate the mandible. It may be necessary to insert an oropharyngeal tube or airway. Placing the patient on his side allows the tongue to fall to the side and away from the back of the pharynx.

▷ *Swallowing Problems.*   Neurologic disorders that impair breathing often cause swallowing dysfunctions. These patients are at risk of aspiration of secretions or regurgitated gastric contents. The awake patient is observed for paroxysms of coughing or nasal regurgitation when swallowing liquids. The patient with impaired swallowing, laryngeal function, and cough reflexes is placed in a lateral position. Respiratory function may be improved by clearing the obstructed airway by means of suctioning and by correcting the hypoxia by immediate ventilation. Patients with swallowing dysfunctions may require nasogastric tube feedings to prevent aspiration and ensure adequate nutrition. The nurse's responsibilities in feeding are to place the patient in an upright position, to check the position of the tube before feeding, or to ensure that the cuff of the endotracheal tube is inflated and to give the tube feeding slowly.

▷ *Maintenance of Skin Integrity.* Special nursing challenges arise when the patient is paralyzed and has sensory disturbances or altered mental status (confusion, depression, stupor, or coma). Patients with chronic neurologic conditions usually have some physical defect and are at high risk for pressure ulcers. Prevention is the hallmark of management. For the patient with impaired neurologic function, prevention includes inspecting the skin for signs of pressure, having properly fitted wheelchair cushions, and wearing a wrist watch with a buzzer alarm (for auditory cueing) as a reminder to the patient to shift position to relieve pressure. An additional discussion of the prevention of pressure ulcers is presented in Chapter 14.

▷ *Physical Mobility.* Any paralyzed extremity deserves careful attention. Care must be taken to see that the patient does not lie on the extremity too long and that the circulation to the part is not impeded. To prevent contractures, the nurse ensures that the patient is positioned correctly and that the joints are moved either actively or passively through their range of motion several times daily.

Muscle weakness (lack of strength) is seen in clinical conditions that have resulted from lesions of the cortex, brain stem, spinal cord, anterior horn cells, peripheral nerve, neuromuscular junction, or muscle. In general, therapeutic exercises are carried out to increase strength. The patient should not work to the point of fatigue because weakness may occur from overuse. Patients with neurologic conditions have increased energy demands resulting from motor involvement, the secondary effects of deconditioning, and the emotional stress of living with a disability.

▷ *Promoting Self-care.* An impairment of neuromuscular function can interfere with activities that are necessary for caring for personal needs. The nurse, working collaboratively with other rehabilitation team members, evaluates the patient's joint range of motion, sensation, muscle strength, endurance, and coordination, as well as his ability to learn. The patient is taught self-care skills and compensatory techniques to enhance his abilities (see Chap. 14).

▷ *Relief of Pain.* As in any other condition, the nursing assessment of the patient who is complaining of pain due to neurologic dysfunction focuses on how the patient is functioning. The nurse works with the patient to determine the location of the pain, its distribution, the degree of limitation, its intensity, and its adverse effects on the patient's life. The nurse listens to the patient's description of pain and identifies factors that increase and decrease the pain. Patients with chronic pain from neurologic conditions become depressed and anxious and are subject to insomnia. In addition, they may limit their activities because of the pain, which causes a generalized fatigue.

Nursing interventions include establishing a trusting relationship with the patient, teaching the patient about pain and its relief, decreasing noxious stimuli, providing distraction from pain, being with the patient, and using assistance from other professionals. The nurse administers the prescribed pharmacologic agent and monitors the patient's response. Nursing interventions also include appropriate reassurance to relieve the anxiety that often occurs with pain. Maximum function within the framework of the patient's disability is encouraged. Explanations of the deleterious effects of prolonged inactivity are provided.

A patient with neurologic dysfunction is at risk for painful contractures because as he lies in bed his feet drop into plantar flexion and his knees and hips flex (if the head of the bed is raised). Fibrous tissue stiffening within muscles occurs, and painful spasticity accentuates the problem. Prevention is the key to this type of pain by positioning and the use of appropriate range-of-motion exercise of each joint several times a day. Encouraging the patient to participate in self-care is important.

Specific nursing interventions for the relief of pain and discomfort are found in the sections of the book on headache, intracranial and spinal surgery, head injuries, and the neurosurgical relief of pain.

▷ *Oral Hygiene.* The unconscious patient is at risk of developing parotitis (inflammation of the parotid gland) if the mouth is not kept clean. The condition of the patient's oral mucous membranes is assessed frequently, because buccal structures tend to become exceedingly dry after a short period of mouth breathing. The lips, tongue, and gums are cleansed and lubricated at frequent intervals, and the patient's fluid intake is maintained at an adequate level. A patient who is intubated requires frequent oral care, suctioning, and repositioning of the endotracheal tube to prevent oral ulceration.

▷ *Eye Care.* When facial paralysis, from any cause, makes it impossible for the patient to shut his eyes, or the patient has an impaired corneal reflex, the cornea is left exposed, which can lead to keratitis and corneal ulceration. Gentle cleansing of the eyelids with sterile warm water or normal saline every few hours removes discharge and debris. Artificial tears or a lubricant may be instilled when prescribed. An eye shield or patch is worn when necessary.

Care should be taken to ensure that the eyelid is closed when the patch is worn, to prevent the cornea from ulcerating further from friction caused by the eye patch. The nurse inspects the eyes regularly for signs of inflammation. Patients who are conscious and able can administer their own eye care with proper instruction and supervision.

▷ *Adequate Nutrition.* Patients with neurologic dysfunction are at risk for nutritional disorders. Depression, so commonly encountered in patients with neurologic conditions, may suppress the appetite. Nutritional problems also arise if there is impairment of chewing and swallowing.

Some patients require gastrostomy feedings, usually ingesting foods that have been prepared in a food blender. The blenderized meal is tolerated well, because the patient's gastrointestinal tract is accustomed to this type of diet. In addition to initiating a referral to the dietitian for nutritional counseling, the nurse works with the occupational therapist to obtain eating utensils that assist the patient to compensate for a physical disability.

▷ *Urinary and Bowel Elimination.* Many patients with CNS disease initially or eventually, temporarily or permanently, exhibit urinary and fecal incontinence. The hygienic care of patients with incontinence is an important nursing priority.

The management of bladder disturbances due to a lesion of the nervous system is discussed in Chapter 14. The management of urinary incontinence from other causes is discussed in Chapter 42. Promotion of a bowel training program is described in Chapter 14.

▷ *Cognitive Function.*   Some patients with brain tumors, head injuries, and strokes, for example, experience cognitive impairment characterized by deficits in memory or abstract thinking, judgment, and intellectual performance. This profoundly affects not only the patient but also the caregiver and the family.

In general, the nurse counsels the family to provide a stable, dependable environment, to minimize confusion, to provide sensory cues, to give information simply and in a positive manner, and to readjust tasks to fit the patient's level of functioning. When the patient becomes agitated and displays undesirable behavior, the use of motor distraction (giving him something to hold) and reducing environmental stimulation (turning off the television) can be effective. Management of patients with brain damage involves a combination of psychiatric nursing skills and neuroscience nursing skills.

▷ *Managing Sexual Dysfunction.*   Sexual dysfunction may be due to a lesion in the neural pathways in which there is loss of erection, lubrication, ejaculation, or emission. The nurse encourages expression of beliefs and feelings; sexual counseling by one skilled in sexual counseling of the disabled can be initiated (see Chap. 17).

▷ *Promoting Effective Coping.*   Patients with neurologic dysfunctions are faced with multiple stresses: serious and often unpredictable outcomes; assault of self-image; and, in many instances, a long-term illness. The patient and his family experience reactive responses to the crisis of diagnosis and prolonged treatment. The patient may react to these stresses with a variety of psychological responses, including regression, depression, anger, denial, and anxiety.

▷ *Supporting Family Functioning.*   The family faces the disruption caused by illness, which means an alteration in life style, role changes, and possible intrafamilial conflicts. Denial or nonacceptance by the family can produce enormous strains on its individual members. The family requires time to deal with their feelings of powerlessness, ambivalence, anger, and guilt. They should be included and educated about the patient's therapy, understand the nature of the neurologic dysfunction and the meaning of remissions and exacerbations, and have some awareness of present and future changes.

Commonly encountered nursing diagnoses, nursing interventions and rationales, and expected outcomes of patients with impaired neurologic function are summarized in Nursing Care Plan 56-1.

Special Problems of Patients With Neurologic Dysfunction

The Patient With Increased Intracranial Pressure

Pathophysiology

Intracranial pressure (ICP) is the result of the amount of brain tissue, intracranial blood volume, and cerebrospinal fluid (CSF) within the skull at any one time. The normal ICP varies de-

pending on the position of the patient and is considered to be less than or equal to 15 mm Hg.

The rigid cranial vault contains brain tissue (1400 g), blood (75 ml), and CSF (75 ml). The volume and pressure of these three components are usually in a state of equilibrium. Because there is limited space for expansion within the skull, an increase of any one of these components causes a change in the volume of the other, by either displacing or shifting CSF, increasing the absorption of CSF, or decreasing cerebral blood volume. Under normal circumstances, minor changes in blood volume and CSF volume occur constantly when there are changes in intrathoracic pressure (coughing, sneezing, straining), posture, and blood pressure, and fluctuations in arterial blood gas levels.

Pathologic conditions such as head injury, stroke, inflammatory lesions, brain tumor, or intracranial surgery alter the relationship between intracranial volume and pressure. Increased ICP may significantly reduce cerebral blood flow. The resultant ischemia stimulates the vasomotor centers, and the systemic pressure rises to maintain cerebral blood flow. Usually this is accompanied by a slow bounding pulse and respiratory irregularities. These changes in blood pressure, pulse, and respiration are of importance clinically because they are clues to the existence of increased ICP. The ultimate effect of raised ICP is cerebral ischemia. The brain is vulnerable to ischemia and generally does not recover function if it is subjected to more than 3 to 5 minutes of complete ischemia.

The concentration of carbon dioxide in the blood and in brain tissues also has a role in the regulation of cerebral blood flow. A rise in carbon dioxide partial pressure (Pco_2) causes the cerebral blood vessels to dilate, leading to increased cerebral blood flow and increased ICP, whereas a fall in Pco_2 has a vasoconstrictor effect. Decreased venous outflow may also increase cerebral blood volume, thus raising ICP.

Cerebral swelling or edema occurs when there is an increase in the water content of the CNS. Certain brain tumors are associated with the development of large quantities of water. Even a small tumor may create a great increase in ICP. Table 56-1 identifies the factors that cause an increase in ICP and the associated physiology and nursing interventions.

Although an elevated ICP is most commonly associated with head injury, an elevated pressure may be seen as a secondary effect in a variety of other conditions: brain tumors, subarachnoid hemorrhage, and toxic and viral encephalopathies. Thus, increased ICP is the summation of a number of physiologic processes. Increased ICP from any cause affects cerebral perfusion and produces distortion and shifts of brain tissue.

There are two stages of cerebral adjustment to the increase in ICP—compensation and decompensation. During the compensation phase, the brain and its components are able to alter their volume to allow for the expanding volume of brain tissue. The ICP, during this phase, is less than the arterial pressure, thus maintaining cerebral perfusion pressure. The patient at this point does not exhibit changes in mental status.

At a certain volume, the ability of the brain to compensate for an increase in pressure becomes ineffective and the decompensation phase begins. In this phase, the patient exhibits a change in his mental status and changes in vital signs: bradycardia, widening pulse pressure, and respiratory changes. At this point, herniation of the brain stem occurs and occlusion of the cerebral blood flow ensues if therapeutic intervention is not initiated.

(text continues on page 1647)

Nursing Care Plan 56-1

Care of the Patient With Impaired Neurologic Function

Nursing Interventions	Rationale	Expected Outcomes

Nursing Diagnosis: Ineffective breathing pattern related to neurogenic pulmonary dysfunction (head trauma, intracranial pressure variations)

Goal: Attains/maintains effective respirations

1. Evaluate the abnormal breathing pattern.
  a. Auscultate lungs.
  b. Assess ventilatory status and ability to clear airway.
	1. Respiratory function is impaired in the presence of abnormal breathing patterns if there are prolonged periods of apnea (Cheyne-Stokes respiration; ataxic breathing) or if the work of breathing is associated with elevated oxygen consumption (hyperthermia, central neurogenic hyperventilation)	• Exhibits improved respiratory status.
		• Shows adequate ventilatory function.
		• Has blood gas values within acceptable range.
		• Absence of crackles.
		• Reports signs and symptoms of early respiratory impairment.

2. Prepare for ventilatory support for management of respiratory dysfunction.	2. Ventilatory support maintains the patency of the airway, helps ensure adequate oxygen uptake in the lungs, prevents carbon dioxide retention, and decreases the work of breathing.	
a. Controlled mechanical ventilation—usually employed with severe head trauma.	a. Mechanical ventilation permits control and maintenance of patient's ventilation.	
b. Intermittent mandatory ventilation—allows progressive transition from mandatory ventilation by the ventilator to spontaneous breathing.	b. Adequate gas exchange is essential to maintain intracranial homeostasis as near normal as possible.	
c. Continuous positive airway pressure (CPAP)—used when patient has inadequate alveolar ventilation and when intubation is necessary for airway control and positive airway.	c. Positive airway pressure is used to prevent alveolar collapse and atelectasis.	

Nursing Diagnosis: Impaired swallowing related to cranial nerve involvement and muscle weakness

Goal: Regains/develops ability to swallow within limits imposed by neurologic dysfunction

1. Assess patient's ability to handle his secretions; position upright with neck slightly flexed.	1. Patients with drooling and swallowing deficits are at risk for aspiration.	• Secretions are managed; aspiration is avoided.
2. Suction as necessary, using great care.	2. Care is needed because suctioning can raise intracranial pressure.	
3. Before suctioning, hyperventilate and hyperoxygenate the patient.	3. These procedures produce respiratory alkalosis, increase O_2 levels, and reduce the negative effects of suctioning on ICP.	
4. Ensure adequate hydration.	4. Adequate hydration loosens pulmonary secretions and helps replenish fluid losses.	

Nursing Diagnosis: High risk for impaired skin integrity related to neurologic impairment (inability to shift position, immobility, motor paralysis, decreased sensory awareness, abnormal posture secondary to spasticity)

Goal: Attains and maintains healthy, intact skin

1. Monitor for signs of pressure, especially on weight-bearing areas.	1. Excessive pressure is the initiating factor for pressure ulcers. Pressure causes tis-	• Has healthy appearing, intact skin. • Monitors self for pressure areas.

(continued)

Nursing Care Plan 56–1 *(Continued)*

Care of the Patient With Impaired Neurologic Function

Nursing Interventions	Rationale	Expected Outcomes
	sue damage by closure of blood vessels, resulting in ischemic necrosis.	• Adheres to turning and positioning schedule.
2. Assess for signs and symptoms of pressure (redness, warmth, tenderness, edema) after change in position.	2. Pressure ulcers are encountered on weight-bearing areas in different positions.	
3. Use interventions to relieve pressure (reposition every 2 hours; use cushions, special beds or mattresses; establish turning schedule).	3. Skin and subcutaneous compression, blood flow obstruction, and tissue ischemia are relieved. Cushions and mattress provide greater pressure distribution.	
4. Teach patient to inspect for potential pressure areas.		

Nursing Diagnosis: Impaired physical mobility related to central nervous system deficit/injury, weakness, and fatigue

Goal: Gains mobility within limits imposed by neurologic dysfunction

1. Determine activity level.		
2. Initiate passive/active range of motion; teach family these techniques. Maintain a functional range of motion for all joints.	2. Passive range of motion helps prevent painful contractures. Range-of-motion exercises maintain muscle length and joint flexibility, help stimulate circulation, and give the patient sensory feedback.	• Demonstrates improving joint mobility. • Absence of contractures. • Caregiver demonstrates ability to perform range-of-motion exercises. • Uses adaptive equipment.
3. Instruct patient in self range-of-motion and transfer techniques.		
4. Use safety precautions when teaching patient transfer techniques.	4. Patients with lower extremity paralysis should be trained as wheelchair travelers.	
5. Work collaboratively with physical and occupational therapists to activate the patient (see Chap. 14, Principles and Practices of Rehabilitation).	5. Many neurologic lesions cause mental dulling and loss of initiative. Loss of muscle strength occurs quickly. Deliberate stimulation and cooperative action by the health care team are required to prevent deterioration.	

Nursing Diagnosis: Self-care deficits related to neurologic impairment, unilateral neglect, inattention, confusion, cognitive and perceptual dysfunction

Goal: Achieves self-care within limits of neurologic dysfunction

1. Assess patient's ability to perform activities of daily living (ADL).	1. The long range goal is maximal independence in as many self-care activities as possible. ADL should be within the patient's functional limitations.	• Functions as independently as possible within limitations imposed by neurologic dysfunction. • Identifies goals for self-care. • Shows beginning ability to perform self-care.
2. Assist patient to identify small achievable goals.		
3. Explain and demonstrate specific ADL skills.		
4. Discuss and demonstrate adaptive equipment.		
5. Encourage patient and show him extent of his progress on ADL record.	5. Encouragement helps patient gain confidence and feelings of self-worth.	

(continued)

Nursing Care Plan 56–1 *(Continued)*

Care of the Patient With Impaired Neurologic Function

Nursing Interventions	Rationale	Expected Outcomes

Nursing Diagnosis: Social isolation related to limits imposed by neurologic dysfunction

Goal: Participates in social relationships and social system

Nursing Interventions	Rationale	Expected Outcomes
1. Determine pre-illness activities and coping skills.	1. Neurologic impairment increases vulnerability to loneliness and social isolation. A restricted environment causes sensory and social deprivation.	• Seeks diversional activities. • Works with occupational therapist. • Continues with social contacts via the telephone. • Has information and phone numbers of support persons and groups.
2. Listen for expressions that may indicate underlying loneliness, fear, sadness, boredom, dread; observe behavior indicating the presence of these feelings.	2. Social isolation can be used (inappropriately) to protect from loss of self-esteem, rejection, and feelings of worthlessness. Human companionship is essential for physical and emotional well-being.	
3. Encourage patient to discuss his problems with a confidant.	3. Good relationship with a confidant may help reduce psychological stress.	
4. Encourage patient to develop social network.	4. Through interactions the patient attains/maintains internal and external harmony and balance.	
5. Encourage individual and group counseling, joining mutual self-help group, and participation in church, civic, and social groups.	5. These can be growth-producing interactions.	

Nursing Diagnosis: Pain related to damage of neuronal structures, stimulation of pain receptors, compression or infiltration by tumor, stretching or compression of nerve roots, consequences of therapy (surgery, radiation, chemotherapy)

Goal: Achieves relief of pain

Nursing Interventions	Rationale	Expected Outcomes
1. Assess for pain, including history of pain experience and evaluation of physical and psychosocial factors.	1. Provides baseline and background for selecting interventions.	• Achieves relief of pain. • Identifies factors and situations that induce and relieve pain. • Uses measures to prevent pain. • Sleeps during most of night. • Appears more relaxed.
2. Encourage verbalization of fears and concerns.	2. Anxiety, depression, and sleeplessness commonly accompany pain.	
3. Administer prescribed analgesics for acute pain.	3. The management of *acute* neurologic pain usually requires drug therapy.	
4. Instruct patient in noninvasive pain-relieving techniques (relaxation training, biofeedback, cognitive training).	4. The management of pain from neurologic causes requires a multidisciplinary approach that includes analgesic drug therapy; behavioral techniques; neurosurgical procedures (placement of epidural, intrathecal, and intraventricular catheters for narcotic drug delivery); and supportive care. Behavioral methods are aimed at promoting an increased sense of control by reducing the helplessness and hopelessness.	

(continued)

Nursing Care Plan 56-1 *(Continued)*

Care of the Patient With Impaired Neurologic Function

Nursing Interventions	Rationale	Expected Outcomes

Nursing Diagnosis: Alteration in family processes related to uncertainty, changes in family member's (patient's) ability to function, preexisting interpersonal problems, and inadequate financial resources

Goal: Family members gain control over their lives

Nursing Interventions	Rationale	Expected Outcomes
1. Assess family strengths as a family unit, signs of stress, interactions with patient, and interactions with one another.	1. Family needs can be met using a collaborative approach, building on each member's strengths. An enabling family provides support, maintains patient's valued role, involves patient in decision making, and encourages adherence to the therapeutic program.	• Demonstrates increasing ability to cope with situation. • Demonstrates a more optimistic outlook. • Maintains ongoing positive contact with patient. • Able to accurately describe patient's condition. • Demonstrates increasing ability to assist in patient's care when appropriate. • Seeks support through counseling when necessary. • Uses appropriate referrals and community resources.
2. Provide opportunity for verbalization of concerns and fears.		
3. Acknowledge their fears; convey hope. Give accurate information. Model appropriate behavior when interacting with patient/family.	3. Information is essential for problem solving.	
4. Reassure family that health care professionals are accessible.	4. Reduces family's sense of isolation.	
5. Encourage family to obtain adequate rest and sleep.	5. Sleep deprivation causes mood disturbances, irritability, and cognitive impairment.	
6. Make appropriate referrals for financial service and psychological counseling.	6. Some families may be alienated, overprotective, neglectful, punitive, and withdrawn. Family may need assistance in deciding when and where to ask for help.	
7. Arrange for contact with other patients/families/support groups.	7. Contact with others offers opportunity for exchange of information, attention, and support.	

Nursing Diagnosis: Sexual dysfunction related to stroke, transient ischemic attack, intracranial surgery, hematomas, or head injury

Goal: Resumes sexual activity commensurate with ability and interest

Nursing Interventions	Rationale	Expected Outcomes
1. Assess the patient's sexual history.	1. The patient's past sexual history will allow the nurse to assist the patient and significant other in meeting the sexual needs or discovering new methods of meeting those needs.	• Verbalizes the ability to participate in sexual intercourse. • Discusses positions and identifies alternatives for meeting sexual needs. • Verbalizes feelings concerning body. • Seeks support and guidance in discussing his fears and concerns. • Discusses if the alternative methods are meeting his needs.
2. Encourage the patient to verbalize feelings about body changes.	2. Provides the patient with the opportunity to explore his feelings concerning the changes of his body. The patient may feel that he may no longer be able to perform sexually.	
3. Acknowledge fears and frustration relating to sexual abilities.	3. The patient will be able to share his concerns, which may be able to be resolved.	
4. Discuss methods of meeting sexual needs.	4. By identifying alternative methods of meeting the patients sexual needs, the patient will hopefully adjust and be sexually satisfied.	

TABLE 56-1. *Increased ICP and Nursing Interventions*

Factor	Physiology	Nursing Intervention	Rationale
Cerebral edema	Can be caused by water intoxication (hypo-osmolality); alteration in the blood–brain barrier (protein leaks into the tissue causing water to follow); contusion, tumor, or abscess	Administer osmotic diuretics as prescribed (monitor serum osmolality) Maintain head of bed elevated 30 degrees Maintain alignment of the head	Promotes venous return Prevents impairment of venous return through the jugular veins
Hypoxia	A decrease in the PaO_2 causes cerebral vasodilation at less than 60 mm Hg	Maintain PaO_2 greater than 60 mm Hg Maintain oxygen therapy Monitor ABGs Suction the patient when needed Maintain a patent airway	Prevents hypoxia and vasodilation
Hypercapnea (elevated CO_2)	Causes vasodilation	Maintain $PaCO_2$ within the ordered range (normally 25–30), through hyperventilation	Avoid decreases in the $PaCO_2$, which causes vasoconstriction and reduces the cerebral blood volume
Impaired venous return	Increases the cerebral blood volume	Maintain head alignment Elevate head of bed 30 degrees	Hyperextension, rotation, or hyperflexion cause a decrease in venous return
Increase in intrathoracic or abdominal pressure	Increase in these pressures due to coughing, PEEP, Valsalva maneuver causes a decrease in venous return	Monitor ABGs and keep PEEP as low as possible Provide humidified oxygen Administer laxatives as ordered	To keep secretions loose and easy to suction or expectorate Soft bowel movements will prevent straining or Valsalva maneuver

Clinical Manifestations

When ICP increases to the point where the brain's ability to adjust has reached its limits, neural function is impaired and may be manifested by changes in the level of consciousness and by abnormal respiratory and vasomotor responses.

The level of responsiveness/consciousness is the most important indicator of the patient's condition.

- The earliest sign of increasing ICP is *lethargy*. Slowing of speech and delay in response to verbal suggestions are early indicators.

Any sudden change in condition, such as shifting from quietness to restlessness (without apparent cause), shifting from orientation to confusion, or increasing drowsiness, has neurologic significance. These signs may result from compression of the brain due to either swelling from hemorrhage or edema, an expanding intracranial lesion (hematoma or tumor), or a combination of both.

As pressure increases, the patient may react only to loud auditory or painful stimuli. At this stage, serious impairment of brain circulation is probably taking place, and immediate surgical intervention may be required. If the stupor deepens, the patient responds to painful stimuli by moaning but may not attempt to withdraw. As the condition worsens, the extremities become flaccid and reflexes are absent. The jaw sags and the tongue becomes flaccid, airway obstruction and inadequate respiratory exchange may occur. When the coma is profound, with the pupils dilated and fixed and the respirations impaired, a fatal outcome is usually inevitable.

Management

Increased ICP constitutes a true emergency and must be treated promptly. As pressure rises, the brain substance is compressed. Secondary phenomena caused by circulatory impairment and edema may lead to death.

The immediate management for relief of increased ICP is based on reducing the size of the brain by decreasing cerebral edema, lowering the volume of CSF, or decreasing blood volume. These goals are accomplished by administering osmotic diuretics and corticosteroids, restricting fluids, draining CSF, hyperventilating the patient, controlling fever, and reducing cellular metabolic demands.

Osmotic diuretics (mannitol, glycerol) may be given to dehydrate the brain and reduce cerebral edema. They act by drawing water across intact membranes, thereby reducing the volume of brain and extracellular fluid. An indwelling catheter is usually inserted into the bladder for monitoring urinary output and for management of the ensuing diuresis. A patient who is receiving osmotic diuretics should have a serum osmolality drawn to assess hydration status.

Corticosteroids (such as dexamethasone) help reduce edema surrounding brain tumors when a brain tumor is the cause of increased ICP.

CSF drainage is frequently employed because the removal of even a small amount of CSF may dramatically reduce ICP and restore cerebral perfusion pressure.

Hyperventilation (with a volume ventilator) produces respiratory alkalosis, which in turn causes cerebral vasoconstriction. The result of this action is a reduction in cerebral blood volume and lowering of ICP. It is considered a short-term means of control.

Temperature control is aimed at preventing an elevation of temperature, because fever increases cerebral metabolism and the rate at which cerebral edema forms. Cardiac output is monitored if measures are taken to reduce the patient's temperature.

Reduction of cellular metabolic demands may also be accomplished through the administration of high doses of barbiturates when the patient is not responsive to conventional treatment. The mechanism by which barbiturates decrease ICP and protect the brain is uncertain, but the resultant comatose state is thought to reduce metabolic requirements of the brain, thus providing some protection.

- The patient receiving high doses of barbiturates experiences loss of all neurologic clinical parameters. Barbiturates are significant cardiorespiratory depressants. Thus, prolonged barbiturate anesthesia requires a high level of nursing surveillance and support, because the patient is totally dependent and vulnerable to many complications. The patient is transferred to the intensive care unit, and the following parameters are monitored: ICP, electroencephalogram (EEG), electrocardiogram (ECG), arterial pressures, and blood and serum barbiturate levels. An endotracheal tube is inserted and the patient receives mechanical ventilation.

▶ Nursing Process
The Patient With Increased Intracranial Pressure

◊ Assessment

The Glasgow Coma Scale encompasses three types of behaviors that are used to assess the patient's level of responsiveness: verbal response, motor response, and eye opening. The criteria that best reflect the patient's responses are selected, and a numerical value is assigned to those criteria.

The ratings of the three responses are used to assess the patient's level of responsiveness and for comparison. The Glasgow Coma Scale score ranges from 3 to 15. Three indicates a severe impairment of neurologic function; a score of 15 indicates that the patient is responsive to the three criteria (see p. 1733 and Fig. 57-10.)

Eye opening can assist in the determination of the cause of a neurologic deficit. If the patient is in a coma but has spontaneous eye opening, the problem may be metabolic, whereas if the patient had no eye opening there could be a neurologic problem.

When assessing the patient's verbal response, the nurse must be careful not to assume that because the patient responds, he is oriented. The examiner needs to further assess the patient's orientation to time, place, and person.

The motor response includes spontaneous movement, movement caused by noxious stimuli, such as an injection or pinch, and posturing. The two types of posturing are decelerate and decorticate. These are both discussed later in the chapter. Occasionally, these responses cannot be assessed because of the patient being intubated, eyes swollen shut, or a language barrier. In this case, the total assessment is not completed and the reason is documented.

Patients with increased ICP have other changes that may herald the further increase in ICP. They are subtle changes, changes in vital signs, headache, pupillary changes, and vomiting.

◊ *Subtle Changes.*   Restlessness, headache, forced breathing, purposeless movements, and mental cloudiness may be early clinical indications of rising ICP.

◊ *Changes in Vital Signs.*   Alterations in vital signs may be a late sign of increased ICP. As the ICP increases, the pulse rate and respiratory rate decrease and the blood pressure and temperature rise. Special signs to observe for include arterial hypertension, bradycardia, and respiratory irregularity; the development of any of these signs warrants further investigation. Cheyne-Stokes breathing (rhythmic waxing and waning of rate and depth of respirations alternating with brief periods of apnea) and ataxic breathing (irregular breathing with a random sequence of deep and shallow breaths) are frequently observed respiratory irregularities.

The vital signs of the patient compensate as long as the major circulation of the brain is preserved. If, as a result of brain compression, the major circulation begins to fail, the pulse and respirations become rapid and the temperature usually rises but does not follow a consistent pattern. The pulse pressure (the difference between the systolic and the diastolic pressure) widens; this is considered a serious development. Immediately preceding this reversal of clinical responses there is usually a period of rapid fluctuations in the pulse, varying from a slow rate to a rapid one. Immediate surgical intervention is indicated or death ensues.

The vital signs may not always be altered, even in the event of increased ICP. The patient is assessed for changes in the level of responsiveness and for the presence of shock; these manifestations aid in evaluation.

◊ *Headache.*   The headache is constant, increasing in intensity, and aggravated by movement or straining.

◊ *Pupillary Changes.*   Increasing pressure or an expanding clot can displace the brain against the oculomotor or optic nerves, producing pupillary changes.

- The pupils are periodically inspected with a penlight to evaluate size, configuration, and reaction to light. Both eyes are compared for similarities or differences.
- Gaze is evaluated as to whether it is conjugate (paired; working together) or dysconjugate.
- The ability of the eyes to abduct and adduct is assessed to evaluate cranial nerve function.

- The retina and optic nerve are inspected for hemorrhage and papilledema.

▷ *Vomiting.*   Recurrent or projectile vomiting may occur with increased pressure on the reflex center for vomiting located in the medulla.

Clinical assessment is not always a reliable guide in recognizing increased ICP, especially in comatose patients. In certain situations, ICP monitoring is an essential part of management (see p. 1650).

▷ Nursing Diagnoses

Based on the assessment data, the patient's major nursing diagnoses may include the following:

- Altered cerebral tissue perfusion related to the effects of increased ICP
- Ineffective breathing patterns related to neurologic dysfunction (brain stem compression, structural displacement)
- Ineffective airway clearance related to accumulation of secretions secondary to depression of level of responsiveness.
- High risk for fluid volume deficit related to dehydration procedures.
- Altered urine and bowel elimination related to effects of medication, indwelling urethral catheter, and diminished fluid/food intake.
- High risk for infection related to ICP monitoring system (intraventricular catheter)

Other relevant nursing diagnoses could include altered oral mucous membranes related to mouth-breathing, absence of pharyngeal reflex, and inability to ingest fluids; potential for impairment of skin integrity related to immobility and constraints imposed by ICP monitoring system; impaired tissue integrity (cornea) related to diminished or absent corneal reflex; and altered family process related to crisis situation. (These diagnoses are discussed in the sections on the patient undergoing intracranial surgery, p. 1679, and the patient with a head injury, Chap. 57.)

▷ Planning and Implementation

▷ *Goals:*   The goals for the patient may include achievement of cerebral tissue perfusion through reduction in ICP, normalization of respiration, achievement of airway clearance, restoration of fluid balance, normal urine and bowel elimination, and absence of infection.

▷ Nursing Interventions

▷ *Achieving Cerebral Tissue Perfusion.*   In addition to ongoing nursing surveillance, the following nursing strategies may be employed to reduce factors contributing to the elevation of ICP:

- The patient is monitored for bradycardia and a rising blood pressure, which are signs of increasing ICP.
- Any activity interfering with venous drainage of blood from the head raises jugular venous pressure and with it, ICP.
  The patient's head is kept in a neutral (midline) position, which is maintained with the use of a cervical collar if necessary.
  Slight elevation of the head is maintained to aid in venous drainage unless otherwise prescribed.
  Extreme rotation of the neck and flexion of the neck are avoided because compression or distortion of the jugular veins increases ICP.
- Extreme hip flexion is avoided because this position causes an increase in intra-abdominal and intrathoracic pressures, which can produce a rise in ICP.
- The Valsalva maneuver, which can be produced by straining at defecation or even moving in bed, is to be avoided. Stool softeners may be prescribed. If the patient is alert and able to eat, a diet high in fiber may be indicated.
  The patient can be instructed to exhale (which opens the glottis) while being moved or turned passively.
- Isometric muscle contractions are also contraindicated, because they raise the systemic blood pressure and hence the ICP.
- Relatively minor changes in the patient's position may significantly affect ICP. If monitoring parameters demonstrate that turning the patient raises his ICP, rotating beds and turning sheets may be used and the patient's head may be held by the nurse's hands during turning to minimize the stimuli that increase ICP.
- Before suctioning is instituted, the patient should be hyperventilated with a resuscitator bag or by using the sigh mode on the ventilator with 100% oxygen. Suction should not last longer than 15 seconds.
- Nursing activities that raise ICP should be avoided if possible. Spacing the occurrence of nursing interventions may prevent transient increases in ICP.
- During nursing interventions the ICP should not rise above 25 mm Hg and should return to baseline levels within 5 minutes.
- Emotional stress and frequent arousal from sleep are to be avoided. A calm atmosphere is maintained. Environmental stimuli (noise, conversation) should be minimal.
- Abdominal distention, which increases intra-abdominal and intrathoracic pressure and ICP, should be noted. Enemas and cathartics are avoided if possible.

▷ *Attaining Normal Respiratory Pattern.*   The nurse monitors the patient constantly for respiratory irregularities. Increased pressure on the frontal lobes or deep midline structures may result in Cheyne-Stokes respirations, whereas pressure in the midbrain may cause hyperventilation. When there is involvement of the lower portion of the brain stem (the pons and medulla), respirations become irregular and eventually cease.

When hyperventilation therapy is used to reduce ICP (by causing cerebral vasoconstriction and a decrease in cerebral blood volume), the nurse collaborates with the respiratory therapist in monitoring the arterial carbon dioxide pressure ($PaCO_2$), which is usually maintained between 25 and 30 mm Hg.

- A neurologic observation record (see Fig. 57-10) is maintained and all observations are made in relation to the patient's baseline condition. Repeated assessments of the patient are made (sometimes minute by minute) so that improvement or deterioration may be noted immediately. If the patient's condition deteriorates, preparations are made for surgical intervention.

▷ *Achieving Airway Clearance.*   The patency of the airway is assessed. If secretions are obstructing the airway, they must be suctioned with care, because transient elevations of ICP occur with suctioning. It may be necessary to oxygenate the patient before and after suctioning to maintain adequate oxygenation. Hypoxia caused by poor oxygenation leads to poor cerebral perfusion. Coughing is discouraged because coughing and straining also increase ICP. The lung fields are auscultated at least once every 8 hours to determine the presence of adventitious sounds or any areas of congestion. Elevating the head of the bed may aid in clearing secretions as well as improving venous drainage of the brain.

◊ *Attaining Fluid Balance.* The administration of various dehydrating agents is part of the treatment protocol. Corticosteroids are used to reduce cerebral edema; also, fluids may be restricted. All of these treatment modalities promote the development of dehydration.

The patient's skin turgor, mucous membranes, serum, and urine osmolality are monitored for signs of dehydration. If fluids are given intravenously, the nurse makes sure that they are administered at a slow to moderate rate with a drip-monitoring device to prevent too rapid administration. For the patient receiving mannitol, the nurse observes for the possible development of congestive heart failure and pulmonary edema due to the ability of mannitol to shift fluid from the intracellular compartment to the intravascular system.

Patients undergoing dehydrating procedures require monitoring of their vital signs, including blood pressure, to assess fluid volume status. These patients also need careful oral hygiene because dehydration is associated with mouth dryness. Frequent rinsing of the mouth, lubrication of the lips, and removal of encrustations relieve dryness and promote comfort.

◊ *Attaining Normal Urine and Bowel Elimination.* The urine is tested for specific gravity and monitored for glucose. A complication of steroid therapy is hyperglycemia. An indwelling urethral catheter is usually inserted to permit assessment of renal function and fluid status. The nurse observes for purulent drainage and encrustation at the urinary meatus, maintains the patency of the catheter and an unobstructed flow of urine by proper positioning of the tubing and drainage bag, uses measures to prevent cross-contamination (*e.g.*, handwashing, keeping infected patients separate from other patients), and monitors urine for the presence of infection (cloudy, bloody, or foul-smelling urine).

The patient's lower abdomen is assessed for signs of bowel distention and the area is auscultated for bowel sounds. Usually the stools are tested for blood if the patient is on high doses of steroids because gastrointestinal bleeding is a complication of this therapy. The patient is cautioned to avoid straining while having a bowel movement because the Valsalva maneuver can increase ICP.

◊ *Preventing Infection.* The nurse is aware that infection is the greatest risk of ICP monitoring with an intraventricular catheter. Most health care facilities have written protocols for managing these systems, and strict adherence to these guidelines must be observed.

The dressing over the ventricular catheter must be kept dry because a wet dressing is conducive to bacterial growth. Aseptic technique is used when managing the system and changing the ventricular drainage bag. The drainage system is also checked for loose connections because they cause leaking and contamination of the system and CSF as well as inaccurate readings of ICP. The patient is monitored for signs and symptoms of meningitis: fever, chills, nuchal (neck) rigidity, and increasing or persisting headache.

◊ **Evaluation**

Expected Outcomes

1. Achieves improved cerebral tissue perfusion
   a. Becomes increasingly oriented to time, place, and person
   b. Follows verbal commands; answers questions correctly
2. Attains normal respirations
   a. Breathes in a normal pattern
   b. Attains or maintains arterial blood gas values within acceptable range
3. Is free of excessive airway secretions
4. Attains improved fluid balance
   a. Takes fluids orally
   b. Serum and urine osmolality are within acceptable range
5. Attains normal urine and bowel elimination
6. Has no sign of infection
   a. Has no fever
   b. Has no purulent drainage from ventricular drainage system

Monitoring Intracranial Pressure

ICP monitoring is the recording of the pressure exerted within the skull by the brain, cerebral blood, and CSF. The volume of any of these elements can expand as a result of tumor, trauma, edema, bleeding, and cerebral vessel dilatation. ICP monitoring provides a continuous reflection of the intracranial state.

The purposes of ICP monitoring are to (1) identify increased pressure early in its course (before cerebral damage occurs), (2) quantitate the degree of abnormality, (3) initiate appropriate treatment, (4) have access to CSF for sampling and drainage, and (5) evaluate the effectiveness of treatment.

ICP is not in a steady state but fluctuates, as indicated by waves of high pressure and troughs of relatively normal pressure. These waves have been classified as A waves (plateau waves), B waves, and C waves (Fig. 56-1). The *plateau waves (A waves)* are transient, paroxysmal, recurring elevations of ICP that may last from 5 to 20 minutes and range in amplitude between 50 and 100 mm Hg. Plateau waves have clinical significance and indicate vascular volume changes within the intracranial compartment that are beginning to compromise cerebral perfusion. They may increase in amplitude and frequency, reflecting cerebral ischemia and brain damage that can occur before overt signs and symptoms of raised ICP are seen clinically. This is especially true in the unconscious patient. Rapid variations of pressure waves may also indicate a potentially serious intracranial situation. Therefore, ICP monitoring provides a more objective evaluation of early or changing trends of ICP than other forms of observation.

B waves are of shorter duration (30 seconds to 2 minutes) with smaller amplitude (up to 50 mm Hg). They have less clinical significance but, if seen in runs in a patient with depression of consciousness, may precede the appearance of A waves. B waves may be seen in patients with intracranial hypertension and decreased intracranial compliance.

C waves are small, rhythmic oscillations with frequencies of approximately six per minute. They appear to be related to rhythmic variations of the systemic arterial blood pressure and respirations.

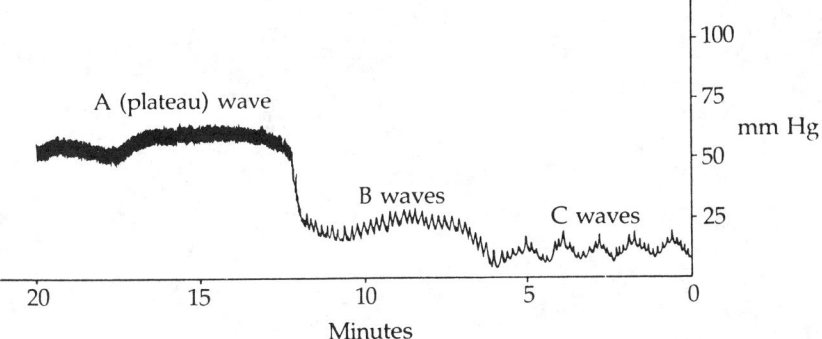

Figure 56–1. Intracranial pressure waves. Composite diagram of A (plateau) waves, B waves, and C waves. (Holloway NM. Nursing the Critically Ill Adult, 2nd ed. Menlo Park, California, Addison-Wesley, 1984.)

Monitoring Devices. ICP is monitored by measuring CSF pressure within the lateral ventricle, the subarachnoid space, and the epidural space. A large number of devices are available that monitor ICP by means of sensors or transducers that are either connected to an intraventricular catheter or implanted in the skull (Fig. 56-2). The three main types are the intraventricular catheter, subarachnoid screw or bolt, and epidural pressure-recording devices.

Ventricular Catheter Monitoring. Ventricular catheter monitoring (see Fig. 56-2) involves the insertion of a fine catheter into a lateral ventricle, using either a twist drill or burr hole opening. It is connected by way of a fluid-filled system to a transducer. In addition to obtaining continuous ICP recordings, the ventricular catheter allows for drainage of CSF, particularly during acute rises in pressure. The ventriculostomy can be used also to drain the ventricle of blood.

This method of monitoring is useful in patients with infratentorial brain tumors and aneurysms. Also, continuous drainage of ventricular fluid under pressure control is an effective method of treating intracranial hypertension. Another advantage of an indwelling ventricular catheter is the route it provides for the intraventricular administration of drugs and the instillation of air or contrast medium for ventriculography. Complications include ventricular infection, meningitis, ventricular collapse, occlusion of the catheter by brain tissue or blood, and problems with the monitoring system.

Subarachnoid Screw. The subarachnoid screw (or bolt) is a hollow screw that is inserted through the skull and dura mater to the cranial subarachnoid space (see Fig. 56-2). It has the advantage of not requiring a ventricular puncture. The subarachnoid screw is inserted through a small hole in the skull under local anesthesia; it is attached to a pressure transducer, and the output is recorded on an oscilloscope for continuous monitoring. The hollow screw technique is useful in patients with head trauma and those with supratentorial brain tumors. It has the additional advantage of avoiding complications from brain shift and small ventricle size. Complications include blockage of the screw by clot or brain tissue, which leads to loss of pressure tracing and a decrease in accuracy at high ICP readings.

A disposable stopcock network is used for both the ventricular catheter and hollow screw monitoring systems to connect the patient to a pressure transducer and display system. The network contains a three-way stopcock attached to the screw or ventricular catheter, a nondistensible saline-filled tubing leading from one outlet of the three-way stopcock to a manifold containing the pressure transducer. The pressure transducer transmits a waveform through the electrical circuitry to a display system for continuous monitoring. The system is flushed with sterile saline at varying intervals to keep the device patent.

Epidural Monitoring. Another method of ICP monitoring requires implantation of a miniature transducer in the epidural space, usually through a burr hole in the skull. One type of epidural ICP-monitoring mode is the pneumatic flow sensor that functions on a nonelectrical basis. This pneumatic epidural monitoring system has a low incidence of infection and complications and appears to read pressures accurately. Calibration of the system is maintained automatically, and abnormal pressure waves trigger an alarm system. One disadvantage to the epidural catheter is the inability to withdraw CSF for analysis.

Clinical Implications. ICP is expressed by ventricular fluid pressures that normally fluctuate in the range of 0 to 10 mm Hg (110 to 140 mm H_2O). Sustained elevations above 15 mm Hg (200 mm H_2O) are generally considered abnormal.

Nursing Implications of ICP Monitoring. The trend of ICP measurements over time is an important indication of the underlying state of the patient. The measurement of ICP is only one parameter of patient assessment, however. Repeated neurologic checks and clinical examinations are important.

Strict aseptic techniques are used when handling any part of the monitoring system. The insertion site is inspected for signs of infection. The patient's temperature, pulse, and respirations are closely monitored for systemic signs of infection. All connections and stopcocks are checked for leaks because small leaks can distort pressure readings.

When recording the ICP, the transducer is zeroed at a particular reference point, usually 2.5 cm (1 in) above the ear in the supine patient; this point corresponds to the level of the foramen of Monro (Fig. 56-3). (CSF pressure readings depend on the patient's position.) For subsequent pressure readings, the patient's head should be in the same position relative to the transducer.

Whenever technology is associated with patient management, the nurse must be certain that the technology remains functioning. The most important concern is that there is a patient attached to the technology. Talking in a soothing tone and stroking the patient's hand or cheek may be helpful in reducing emotional stress.

The patient with an increase in ICP can initially be alert and oriented without apparent neurologic deficit, or may be unresponsive with a neurologic deficit. The ICP may increase with risk of a life-threatening event. Astute observation, comparison of previous examinations, and interventions can assist

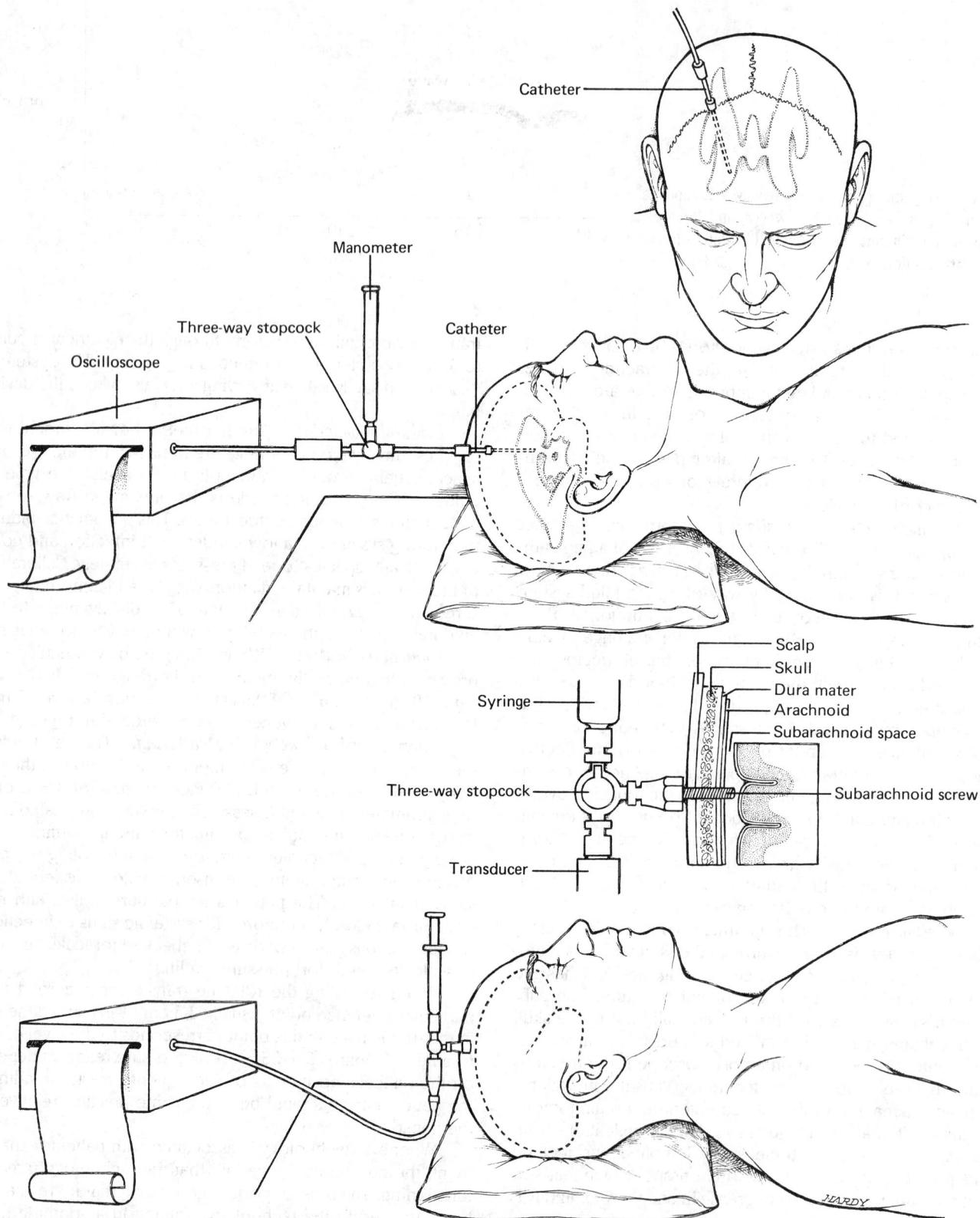

Figure 56–2.   Intracranial pressure monitoring. (**Top**) Ventricular catheter. (**Center**) Subarachnoid or hollow screw. (**Bottom**) Monitoring system connected to pressure transducer and display system.

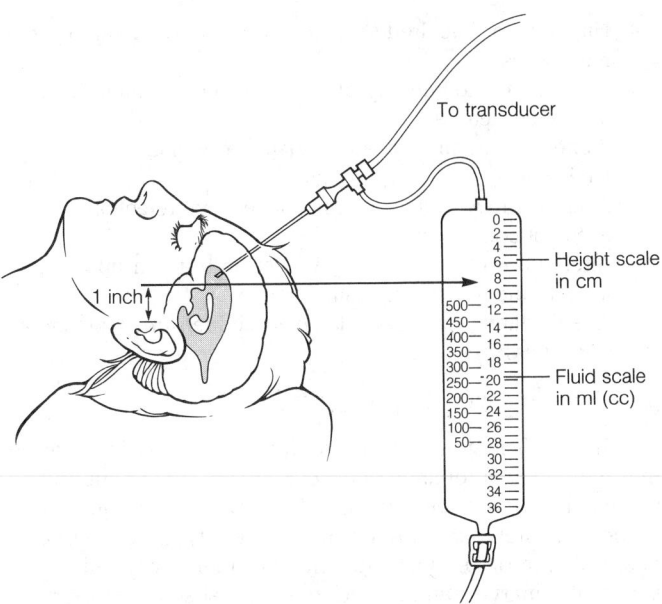

Figure 56–3. Location of foramen of Monroe for calibration of ICP monitoring system.

in preventing such an event. Assessment of the patient includes the Glasgow Coma Scale, pupil changes, posturing, and ICP measurement.

Gerontologic Considerations. Geriatric patients with an increase in ICP may present with an alteration in their mental status. The altered mental status may be the result, not of the change in ICP, but of the aging process. The nurse needs to involve the patient's family in obtaining a baseline assessment of mental status. On radiologic examination, the geriatric patient may have a chronic or old hematoma. This may be frustrating for the family who is unaware of falls when the patient is alone. The family should be included in the treatment plan as much as possible, because of the possible need for assistance at home or the need for a long-term care facility.

Other Monitoring Modalities (Electrophysiologic Monitoring). Evoked potential monitoring is accomplished by measurement of electrical potentials produced by nerve tissue in response to external stimulation. The external stimulation can be either auditory, visual, or sensory. This diagnostic test is useful for following the course of a patient in drug-induced coma, one receiving muscle relaxants, or in any condition in which clinical examination is unreliable. Special EEG recording devices are useful in evaluating some forms of abnormal EEG activity. The major nursing responsibility is ensuring that the electrodes are not displaced during patient care interventions.

Hyperthermia

Because of damage to the heat-regulating center in the brain or severe intracranial infection, neurologic and neurosurgical patients often develop very high temperatures. Such temperature elevations must be controlled, because the increased metabolic demands by the brain will overburden brain circulation and oxygenation, resulting in cerebral deterioration. Persistent hyperthermia is indicative of brain stem damage and indicates a poor prognosis.

Hyperthermia is also seen in the neurologically impaired patient with CNS, respiratory, urinary, and wound infections. Drug reactions may also be the cause. It has been shown that body temperatures well below normal decrease cerebral edema, reduce the quantity of oxygen and metabolites required by the brain, and protect the brain from continued ischemia. Also, the collateral circulation in the brain may be able to provide an adequate blood supply to the brain if the body metabolism can be lowered.

Nursing Considerations. The induction and maintenance of hypothermia is a major clinical procedure and requires knowledge and skilled nursing observation and management. It is desirable to begin treatment before the patient's temperature gets too high.

- All bedding over the patient should be removed (with the possible exception of a light sheet or small drape).
- Repeated doses of aspirin or acetaminophen are given as prescribed.
- Alcohol or cool water sponging and an electric fan blowing over the patient to increase surface cooling may be helpful.
- The use of the hypothermia blanket and equipment is usually effective in controlling neurogenic hyperthermia.

Frequent temperature monitoring is indicated to assess the patient's response to the therapy and to prevent an excessive decrease in temperature and shivering.

The Unconscious Patient

Unconsciousness is a condition in which there is a depression of cerebral function, ranging from stupor to coma. In *stupor*, the patient shows symptoms of annoyance when stimulated by something unpleasant, such as a pinprick or loud clapping of hands. He may draw back or make facial grimaces or unintelligible sounds. *Coma* is a clinical state of unconsciousness in which the patient is unaware of himself and his environment. *Akinetic mutism* is a state of unresponsiveness to the environment in which the patient makes no movement or sound but sometimes has his eyes open. A *persistent vegetative state* is one in which the patient is described as wakeful but devoid of conscious content, without cognitive or effective mental function.

The causes of unconsciousness may be neurologic (head injury, stroke), toxicologic (drug overdose, alcohol intoxication), or metabolic (hepatic or renal failure, diabetic ketoacidosis).

Diagnostic Evaluation

Laboratory tests that may be helpful in diagnosing the cause of unconsciousness include tests for blood glucose, electrolytes, serum ammonia, blood urea nitrogen, osmolality, calcium, prothrombin time, serum ketones, and arterial blood gases.

Management

The first priority is assessment and stabilization of the airway to ensure respiration and ventilation. The circulatory status (carotid pulse, heat rate and impulse, blood pressure) is assessed because perfusion of the brain depends on the ability of the heart to maintain adequate cardiac output. An intravenous line is established and dextrose in water is administered to prevent and treat hypoglycemia, which causes an altered mental status and CNS damage.

Oxygen may be administered until the cause of unconsciousness or the arterial blood gas measurements are known. An indwelling catheter is usually inserted.

The neurologic examination is repeated frequently to determine whether the cause of coma is increased ICP or metabolic encephalopathy (reaction of brain in response to generalized change in the metabolism of the brain or in its extracellular environment) due to acidosis, drug overdose, or toxic exposure. Specific therapies are administered for increased ICP and metabolic abnormalities.

▶ Nursing Process
The Unconscious Patient

▷ Assessment

The level of responsiveness (consciousness) is assessed by evaluating eye-opening responses, verbal responses, and motor responses to a command or painful stimulus. These measurements are assessed and graded using the Glasgow Coma Scale rating (see p. 1733). The pupils are evaluated as to size, equality, and reaction to light. In addition, the movement of the eyes is noted. Facial symmetry, swallowing reflexes, and deep tendon reflexes are elicited. If the patient is not responding to commands, motor response is tested by applying a painful stimulus (firm but *gentle* pressure) on the supraorbital notch or to the nailbed or by squeezing a muscle. If the patient attempts to push away or withdraw, the response is recorded as purposeful or appropriate. An inappropriate or nonpurposeful response is random and aimless. The unconscious patient with severely impaired cerebral function may respond to a stimulus with *decorticate posturing* (arms flexed, adducted, and internally rotated and legs in extension) or *decerebrate posturing* (extremities extended and reflexes exaggerated) (Chart 56-1). Decerebrate posturing indicates a more severe alteration in responsiveness. The patient with flaccid motor response has the most neurologic involvement. This patient is unable to move any extremity and has no muscle tone in all four extremities. Paralysis or stroke must be ruled out as a cause of flaccidity.

Body functions (circulation, respiration, elimination, fluid and electrolyte balance) are examined in a systematic manner.

If the patient is comatose and localized signs are severe, it is assumed that neurologic disease is present until proved otherwise. If the patient is comatose and a pupillary light reflex is preserved, a toxic or metabolic disorder is suspected.

Important signs to evaluate in assessing the unconscious patient are noted in Chart 56-1 and in Chapter 57 in the section on the assessment of the patient with a head injury.

▷ Nursing Diagnoses

Based on the assessment data, the patient's major nursing diagnoses may include the following:

- Ineffective airway clearance related to inability to clear respiratory secretions
- High risk for fluid volume deficit related to inability to ingest fluids
- Altered oral mucous membranes related to mouth-breathing, absence of pharyngeal reflex, and inability to ingest fluids

- High risk for impaired skin integrity related to immobility or restlessness
- Impaired tissue integrity of cornea related to diminished or absent corneal reflex
- Ineffective thermoregulation related to damage to hypothalamic center
- Altered urinary elimination (incontinence or retention) related to the unconscious state
- Altered bowel elimination (diarrhea and/or constipation) related to the unconscious state
- Altered family process related to sudden crisis of unconsciousness

▷ Planning and Implementation

▷ *Goals:* The goals of care during the unconscious period may include maintenance of a clear airway, attainment of fluid volume balance, achievement of intact oral mucous membranes, maintenance of normal skin integrity, absence of corneal irritation or keratitis, attainment of thermoregulation, absence of urinary retention and infection, absence of diarrhea or fecal impaction, and maintenance of intact family or support system.

The quality of nursing care given an unconscious patient may literally mean the difference between life and death, because the patient's protective reflexes are impaired. The nurse must assume responsibility for the patient until the basic reflexes return (coughing, blinking, and swallowing) and the patient becomes conscious and oriented. Thus, the major nursing goal is to assume these protective reflexes for the patient until he is aware of himself and can function consciously.

▷ Nursing Interventions

▷ *Maintaining the Airway.* The most important consideration in the management of the unconscious patient is establishment of an adequate airway and ventilation. Circulation to the brain must be ensured. Obstruction of the airway is a risk facing the unconscious patient, because the epiglottis and tongue may relax, occluding the oropharynx, or the patient may aspirate vomitus or nasopharyngeal secretions.

- The patient is positioned in a lateral or semiprone position, which permits the jaw and tongue to fall forward and thus facilitates drainage of secretions.
- An unconscious patient must not be allowed to remain on his back.
- The accumulation of secretions in the pharynx presents a serious problem. Because the patient is unable to swallow and lacks pharyngeal reflexes, these secretions must be removed to eliminate the danger of aspiration.
- Elevating the head of the bed to a 30-degree angle helps prevent aspiration of secretions.
- The patient requires frequent suctioning and oral hygiene.
- Suction is employed to remove secretions from the posterior pharynx and upper trachea. With the suction turned off, a whistle-tip catheter is lubricated with a water-soluble lubricant and inserted to the desired level. Then the suction is turned on (negative pressure) while the aspirating catheter is withdrawn with a twisting motion of the thumb and forefinger. This twisting maneuver prevents the suctioning end of the catheter from irritating the tracheal or pharyngeal mucosa, because irritation increases secretions and produces mucosal trauma and bleeding.

Chart 56–1
Nursing Assessment of the Unconscious Patient

Examination	Clinical Assessment	Clinical Significance
Level of responsiveness or consciousness	Eye opening; verbal and motor responses; pupils (size, equality, reaction to light)	Obeying commands is a favorable response and demonstrates a return to consciousness
Pattern of respiration		Disturbances of respiratory center of brain may result in various respiratory patterns
	Cheyne-Stokes respiration	Suggests lesions deep in both hemispheres; area of basal ganglia and upper brain stem
	Hyperventilation	Suggests onset of metabolic problem or brainstem damage
	Ataxic respiration with irregularity in depth/rate	Ominous sign of damage to medullary center
Eyes		
Pupils (size, equality, reaction to light)	Equal normally reactive pupils	Suggests that coma is toxic or metabolic in origin
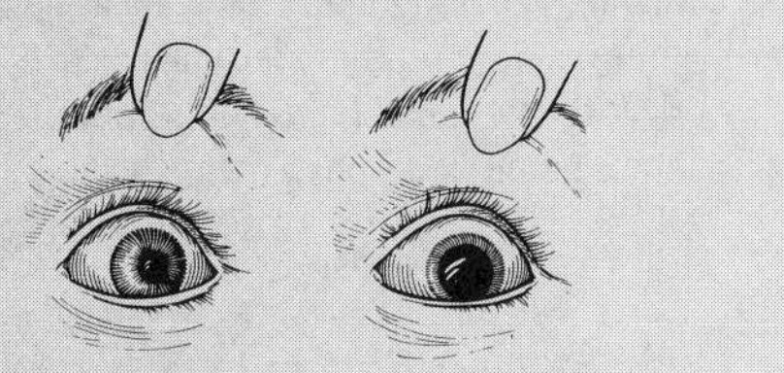	Equal or unequal diameter	Localizing sign
	Progressive dilatation	Indicates increasing intracranial pressure
	Fixed dilated pupils	Indicates injury at level of midbrain
Eye movements	Normally eyes should move from side to side	Functional and structural integrity of brain stem is assessed by inspection of extraocular movements; usually absent in deep coma
Corneal reflex 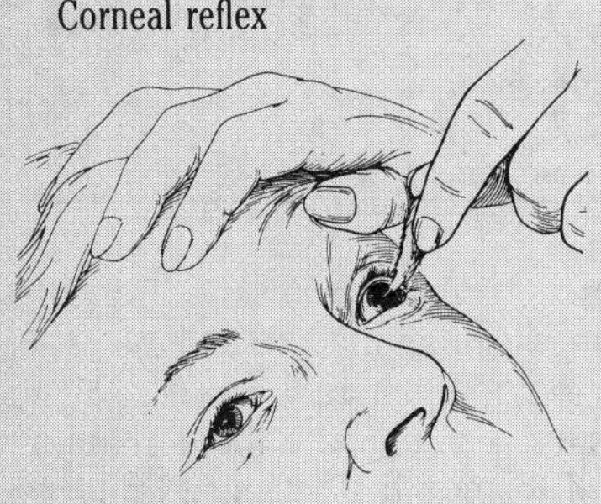	When cornea is touched with a wisp of clean cotton, blink response is normal	Tests cranial nerves V and VII; localizing sign if unilateral; absent in deep coma
Facial symmetry	Asymmetry (sagging, decrease in wrinkles)	Sign of paralysis
Swallowing reflex	Drooling versus spontaneous swallowing	Absent in coma
		Paralysis of cranial nerves X and XII
Neck	Stiff neck	Subarachnoid hemorrhage, meningitis
	Absence of spontaneous neck movement	Fracture or dislocation of cervical spine
Response of extremity to noxious stimuli	Firm pressure on a joint of the upper and lower extremity	Asymmetrical response in paralysis
		Absent in deep coma
	Observe spontaneous movements	
Deep tendon reflexes 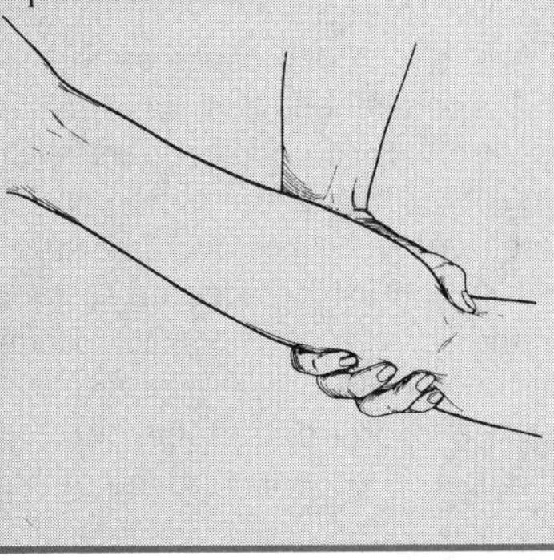	Tap patellar and biceps tendons	Brisk response may have localizing value
		Asymmetric response in paralysis
		Absent in deep coma

(continued)

Chart 56-1 (Continued)

Examination	Clinical Assessment	Clinical Significance
Pathologic reflexes	Firm pressure with blunt object on sole of foot moving along lateral margin and crossing to the ball of foot	Flexion of the toes, especially the great toe, is normal except in newborn Dorsiflexion of toes (especially great toe) indicates contralateral pathology of corticospinal tract (Babinski reflex) Localizing signs
Abnormal posture	Observation for posturing (spontaneous or in response to noxious stimuli) Flaccidity with absence of motor response Decorticate posture (flexion and internal rotation of forearms and hands; see *A* below) Decerebrate posture (extension and external rotation; see *B* below)	Deep extensive brain lesion Seen with cerebral hemisphere pathology and in metabolic depression of brain function Decerebrate posturing indicates deeper and more severe dysfunction than does decorticate posturing; implies brain stem pathology; poor prognostic sign

A   B

| **Muscle tone** | Flexor or extensor rigidity or extremity flaccidity | Indicates paralysis |

- The chest is auscultated at least every 8 hours for crackles, rhonchi, or absence of breath sounds.
- The patient may require intubation and mechanical ventilation. The nurse must maintain the patency of the endotracheal tube or tracheostomy, provide frequent oral care, monitor arterial blood gases, and maintain ventilator settings.

▷ *Attaining Fluid and Nutritional Balance.* The patient is assessed for hydration status; the mucous membranes are examined, and the skin is assessed for tissue turgor. The fluid needs of this patient are initially met by giving the required fluids intravenously and then by nasogastric or gastrostomy feedings.

- Intravenous solutions and blood transfusions for patients with intracranial conditions must be administered slowly. If given too rapidly, they may increase the ICP. The quantity of fluids administered may be restricted to minimize the possibility of producing cerebral edema.
- Fluids are never given by mouth to the patient who cannot swallow. One way of testing to see whether the patient is able to swallow without choking is to give him a wet swab to suck.
- A nasogastric tube may be inserted so that the patient can be given liquid and blenderized feedings.

▷ *Maintaining Healthy Oral Mucous Membranes.*   The patient's mouth is inspected for dryness, inflammation, and the presence of crusting. The unconscious patient requires conscientious oral care because there is a risk of parotitis if the mouth is not kept scrupulously clean. The mouth is cleansed and rinsed carefully to remove secretions and crusts and to keep the membranes moist. A thin coating of petrolatum on the lips prevents drying, cracking, and the formation of encrustations. If the patient has an endotracheal tube, the sides of the mouth and lips should be assessed for ulcerations.

▷ *Maintaining Skin Integrity.*   Preventing skin breakdown requires continuing nursing assessment and intervention. Special attention is given to unconscious patients because they are insensitive to external stimuli. This includes a regular schedule of turning to avoid pressure, which can cause necrosis of the skin. Turning also provides kinesthetic (sensation of movement), proprioceptive (awareness of position), and vestibular (equilibrium) stimulation. After turning, the patient is carefully repositioned to prevent ischemic necrosis over pressure areas. Dragging the patient up in bed must be avoided because this creates a shearing force and friction on the skin surface.

  Maintaining correct body position is important; equally important is passive exercise of the extremities so that contractures are prevented. The use of a footboard or high-top sneakers aids in the prevention of footdrop and eliminates the pressure of bedding on the toes. Trochanter rolls supporting the hip joints keep the legs in good position. The arms should be in abduction, the fingers lightly flexed, and the hands in a position of slight supination. The patient's heels and feet should be assessed for pressure areas.

◊ *Maintaining Corneal Integrity.*   Some unconscious patients lie with their eyes open and have inadequate or absent corneal reflexes. The cornea is likely to become irritated or scratched, leading to keratitis and corneal ulcers.

The eyes may be cleansed with cotton balls moistened with sterile normal saline to remove debris and discharge. It may be necessary to instill artificial tears every 2 hours. (This is an interdependent action requiring consultation with the physician.) Often, periocular edema (swelling around the eyes) occurs after cranial surgery. Cold compresses may be prescribed, and care must be exerted to avoid contact with the cornea. Eye patches should be used cautiously because of the potential to cause further corneal abrasions from the cornea coming in contact with the eye patch.

◊ *Attaining Thermoregulation.*   High fever in the unconscious patient may be caused by infection of the respiratory tract or urinary tract, drug reactions, or damage to the hypothalamic temperature-regulating center. A slight elevation of temperature may be caused by dehydration. The temperature of the environment is determined by the patient's condition. An elevated body temperature would call for a minimum amount of bedding—a sheet or perhaps only a small drape.

The room may be cooled to 18.3°C (65°F). If the patient is elderly and does not have an elevation of temperature, however, a warmer atmosphere is needed. Regardless of the temperature, the air should be fresh and free from odors.

- The body temperature of an unconscious patient is *never* taken by mouth. Rectal temperature is preferred to the less accurate axillary temperature.

Hyperthermia is treated by measures described on p. 1653. Shivering is avoided.

◊ *Preventing Urinary Retention.*   The unconscious patient is either incontinent or has urinary retention. The patient's bladder is palpated at intervals to determine whether urinary retention is present, because a full bladder may be an overlooked cause of incontinence. If there are signs of urinary retention, initially an indwelling catheter attached to a closed drainage system is inserted. Because the catheter is a major cause of urinary infection, the patient is observed for fever and cloudy urine. The area around the urethral orifice is inspected for suppurative drainage. The urinary catheter is usually removed when the patient has a stable cardiovascular system and if no problems with diuresis, sepsis, or voiding dysfunction existed before the onset of coma. Although many comatose patients urinate spontaneously after catheter removal, the patient's bladder periodically should be palpated for urinary retention. An external penile catheter (condom catheter) for the male patient and absorbent pads for the female patient can be used for the unconscious patient who can urinate spontaneously, although involuntarily. As soon as consciousness is regained, a bladder training program is initiated.

The incontinent patient is monitored frequently for irrita-tion and skin breakdown. Appropriate skin care is implemented to prevent these complications.

◊ *Promoting Bowel Function.*   Abdominal distention is evaluated by listening for bowel sounds and measuring the girth of the abdomen with a tape measure. There is a risk of diarrhea from infection, antibiotics, and hyperosmolar fluids. Frequent loose stools are also an indication of fecal impaction. Commercial fecal collection bags are available for patients with fecal incontinence.

Immobility and lack of dietary fiber may cause constipation. The nurse monitors the number and consistency of bowel movements and performs a rectal examination for signs of fecal impaction. The patient may require an enema every other day to empty the lower colon. Enemas may be contraindicated, however, if the Valsalva maneuver increases a compromised ICP. A glycerin suppository stimulates bowel emptying. Stool softeners may be prescribed and can be administered with the tube feedings.

◊ *Supporting the Family.*   The family of the unconscious patient may be thrown into a sudden state of crisis and go through the process of high anxiety, denial, anger, remorse, grief, and reconciliation. To assist family members to mobilize their own adaptive capacities, the nursing personnel can reinforce and clarify information about the patient's condition, permit the family to be involved in the care of their loved one, and listen and encourage ventilation of feelings and concerns while supporting them in their decision-making process concerning posthospitalization management and placement.

◊ *Other Nursing Interventions*

◊ *Safety.*   For the protection of the patient, padded siderails are provided. Every measure that is available and appropriate for calming and quieting a disturbed patient should be carried out. Any form of restraint is likely to be countered by resistance, which may lead to self-injury or to a dangerous increase in ICP.

◊ *Promoting Sensory Stimulation.*   Continuing sensory stimulation is provided to help overcome the profound sensory deprivation of the unconscious patient. Efforts are made to maintain the sense of daily rhythm by keeping the usual day and night patterns for activity and sleep. The nurse touches and talks to the patient and encourages family members and friends to do the same. Communicating with the patient is extremely important and includes touching him and spending enough time with him to become sensitive to his needs. It is also important to avoid making any negative comments about the patient's status or prognosis in his presence. The patient is oriented to time and place at least once every 8 hours. Sounds from the patient's home and workplace may be introduced by means of a tape recorder. In addition, family members can read to the patient from a favorite book and may suggest radio and television programs that he previously enjoyed as a means of enriching the environment and providing meaningful input. When the patient has regained consciousness, videotaped family or social events may assist the patient in recognizing family and friends and allow him to be a part of missed events.

◊ *Attaining Self-care.*   The unconscious patient is dependent on the nursing staff for all his activities of daily living (ADL). As soon as consciousness returns, the nurse begins to teach, support, encourage, and supervise these activities until the patient gains independence. (See Activities of Daily Living in Chap. 14.) A summary of the nursing management of the unconscious patient is found in Nursing Care Plan 56-2.

◊ Evaluation

Expected Outcomes

1. Maintains clear airway
   a. Has no adventitious breath sounds
2. Attains/maintains adequate fluid status
   a. Has no clinical signs of dehydration
   b. Demonstrates normal range of serum electrolytes
3. Attains/maintains healthy oral mucous membranes
   a. Has moist and intact oral mucosa
4. Maintains normal skin integrity
5. Has no corneal irritation
6. Attains or maintains thermoregulation
   a. Temperature within acceptable range
   b. Skin of normal temperature and texture
7. Has no urinary retention
8. Has no diarrhea or fecal impaction
9. Family members coping with crisis
   a. Verbalize fears and concerns
   b. Participate in patient's care
   c. Provide sensory stimulation through talking and touching

Aphasia

Aphasia is a disturbance of language function resulting from injury or disease of the brain centers. It may involve impairment of the ability to read and write as well as to speak, listen, calculate, comprehend, and understand gestures (Chart 56-2). Some 1 to 1.5 million adults in this country have a chronic disabling aphasia. The major causes are stroke, head injury, and brain tumor. An estimated 20% of stroke patients develop aphasia. The number of aphasic patients is growing because more patients are surviving stroke.

The cortical area that is responsible for integrating the myriad association pathways required for the comprehension and formulation of language measures little more than 1 square inch in size. The principal speech center, called *Broca's area*, is located in a convolution adjoining the middle cerebral artery. Here are stored the combinations of muscular movements necessary to speak each word. They are not the cells that govern the muscles of speech; these cells are in the motor area itself. Each word requires for its utterance a combination or sequence of combinations of muscular contractions. Not only must the muscles of the vocal cords contract, but also those of the throat, the tongue, the soft palate, the lips, and the chest wall. These combinations are stored in the cells of Broca's convolution. They direct the cells of the motor area, which make the muscles contract at the proper time and with the proper force.

Broca's area is so near the left motor area that a disturbance in the motor area often affects the speech area. This is the reason that so many patients paralyzed on the right side (due to damage or injury to the left side of the brain) are unable to speak, whereas in those paralyzed on the left side, speech disturbances are less common. Some patients are not affected, but these usually are left-handed persons whose speech area is located in the right hemisphere.

▶ Nursing Process
The Patient With Aphasia

◊ Assessment

The speech-language pathologist in cooperation with the neurologist assesses the communication abilities of the patient. Information is obtained regarding the patient's pre-illness speech-language skills and interests. Formalized, standardized tests and observational methods are used to evaluate comprehension, mathematical, reading, and residual language skills.

(text continues on page 1664)

Chart 56-2
Glossary of Selected Terms Relating to Aphasia*

acalculia; dyscalculia—difficulty in dealing with mathematical processes or numerical symbols in general

agnosia—failure to recognize familiar objects perceived by the senses
   Auditory agnosia—inability to recognize significance of sounds
   Color agnosia—inability to recognize differences in color
   Tactile agnosia—inability to recognize familiar objects by touch or feel
   Visual object agnosia—inability to recognize objects; visual acuity may or may not be intact

agraphia; dysgraphia—disturbances in writing intelligible words

alexia; dyslexia—difficulty in reading

anomia; dysnomia—difficulty in selecting appropriate words, particularly nouns

apraxia—inability to perform previously learned purposeful motor acts on a voluntary basis
   Verbal apraxia—difficulty in forming and organizing intelligible words although the musculature is intact

dysarthria—defects of articulation due to neurologic causes

hemianopia—blindness of one half of the field of vision in one or both eyes

paraphasia—a frequently observed characteristic in many aphasic patients; uses wrong words, word substitutions, grammatical errors, faults in word usage; may be observed in both oral and written language

perseveration—continued and automatic repetition of an activity or word or phrase that is no longer appropriate

* The prefix *a* means "without" or "absence." The prefix *dys* refers to "difficulty" or "disordered." These prefixes are frequently used interchangeably in these conditions.

Nursing Care Plan 56–2

Care of the Unconscious Patient

Nursing Interventions	Rationale	Expected Outcomes

Note: The basic nursing principles underlying the care of an unconscious patient are applicable to any unconscious patient, regardless of the clinical cause. There are two major threats to the patient; (1) the disease or trauma that produced unconsciousness and (2) the threat of the unconscious state. The primary problem is that the patient's normal protective reflexes are impaired. The nursing goal is to assume these protective mechanisms for the patient until he is aware of himself and can function in his environment

Nursing Diagnosis: Ineffective breathing pattern related to unconscious state

Goal: Attainment of normal breathing

Nursing Interventions	Rationale	Expected Outcomes

1. Establish and maintain an adequate airway, respiratory exchange, and circulation.
  a. Place the patient in a three-fourths prone position or in a lateral position with his head turned to one side. (In the event of increased intracranial pressure, the head of the bed may be elevated as prescribed.)
  b. Note the respiratory rate and pattern.
 	
  c. Insert oral airway if tongue is paralyzed or is obstructing the airway.
 	
  d. Provide oxygen and other therapies as prescribed.
 	
  e. Keep the airway free of secretions by efficient suctioning.
 	
  f. Prepare for insertion of cuffed endotracheal tube if patient's condition requires (inefficient cough reflex, respiratory failure).
 	
  g. Use humidified oxygen, positive-pressure assisted breathing techniques, or mechanical ventilation when there is indication of impending respiratory failure.
  h. Evaluate pulses (radial, carotid, apical, pedal): measure blood pressure.
	1. a. Inadequate respiratory exchange promotes carbon dioxide retention, which can produce diffuse cerebral edema. Airway obstruction will aggravate cerebral swelling and may be a cause of continuing or deepening unconsciousness.
	
	  b. The respiratory pattern reflects activity throughout the brain and spinal cord. Disordered respiration is an indication of brain dysfunction; prompt initiation of respiratory support is indicated.
	  c. A noisy airway is an obstructed airway. (An obstructed airway increases intracranial pressure.) The use of an oropharyngeal airway is considered a short-term measure.
	  d. Oxygen therapy increases the amount of oxygen available to the brain and systemic circulation.
	  e. With the absence of the cough and swallowing reflexes, secretions rapidly accumulate in the posterior pharynx and upper trachea and can pave the way to fatal respiratory complications.
	  f. Endotracheal intubation is more effective in permitting positive-pressure ventilation. The cuffed tube seals off the digestive tract, thus preventing aspiration, and allows efficient removal of tracheobronchial secretions.
	  g. When arterial blood gas measurements reveal that patient has insufficient ventilation and gas exchange, respiratory failure may quickly ensue.
	  h. These are measures of circulatory adequacy/inadequacy and give clues to the cause of the unconscious state.
		• Attains normal breathing.
		• Respirations quiet and appear effortless.
		• Absence of excessive respiratory secretions.
		• Respirations within normal range.
		• Peripheral pulses are of normal amplitude.
		• Has blood pressure within acceptable range for condition.
		• Has less than 50 ml of gastric aspirate before NG feeding.

(continued)

Nursing Care Plan 56-2 *(Continued)*

Care of the Unconscious Patient

Nursing Interventions	Rationale	Expected Outcomes
i. Assist with passage of a nasogastric (NG) tube. (The cuffed endotracheal tube should be in place before passage of NG tube.)	i. Aspiration of gastric contents is common in unconscious patients secondary to the loss of protective pharyngeal reflexes, decreased gastric motility, and regurgitation. An NG tube permits suctioning of stomach contents and provides a route for oral feeding.	

Nursing Diagnosis: Alteration in cerebral tissue perfusion related to unconscious state

Goal: Achievement of cerebral tissue perfusion to maintain cerebral homeostasis

Nursing Interventions	Rationale	Expected Outcomes
1. Maintain a constant assessment of patient's level of consciousness and changes in responsiveness.	1. The level of consciousness is the most sensitive indicator of improvement or deterioration. Unconscious patients can deteriorate rapidly from numerous clinical causes.	• Begins to open eyes, responds to commands. • Pupils of normal size, equality, and reaction. • Appears more alert, less restless. • Moves extremities appropriately in response to commands or noxious stimuli. • Vital signs within acceptable limits.
2. Record the patient's exact reactions: eye opening, verbal response, movements, and quality of speech. Describe the stimuli required to elicit the patient's responses.	2. The Glasgow Coma Scale depicts these modes of behavior. An unconscious patient is unable to obey commands or utter recognizable words.	
3. Examine pupils of eyes for size, shape, and reaction to light.	3. Pupillary abnormalities are important in localizing the cause of unconsciousness.	
4. Assess movements of extremities in response to verbal commands or painful stimulus.	4. No response or a delayed or unequal response is an unfavorable clinical sign. Obeying commands is a favorable response and indicates a return to consciousness.	
5. Evaluate the progression of vital signs: a. Know the patient's baseline (initial) vital signs, and alert the physician if there are significant fluctuations of blood pressure and instability of the pulse and respiratory cycles.	5a. Fluctuations of vital signs indicate a change in intracranial homeostasis. Monitoring of vital signs is also essential to detect hidden bleeding.	
b. Obtain blood pressure readings, pulse, respiratory rate and patterns, and temperature at frequently specified intervals until there is clinical evidence of stabilization.	b. Obtaining and recording of temperature is mandatory because temperature-regulating mechanisms may be impaired. Hyperthermia is an unfavorable prognostic sign. The systolic blood pressure must be adequate to maintain cerebral perfusion pressure. Brain injury can both elevate and depress blood pressure. A slow pulse, rising blood pressure, and slowing respirations are associated with cerebral compromise.	

(continued)

Nursing Care Plan 56–2 *(Continued)*

Care of the Unconscious Patient

Nursing Interventions	Rationale	Expected Outcomes

Nursing Diagnosis: Fluid volume deficit related to inability to ingest oral fluids secondary to unconscious state

Goal: Maintain fluid balance

1. Observe for signs of overhydration or dehydration. Administer intravenous fluids as indicated.	1. Serial laboratory electrolyte evaluations are made when the patient is maintained on intravenous fluids to ensure proper balance.	• Laboratory evaluations within acceptable range. • Skin turgor is normal.

Nursing Diagnosis: Altered nutritional status (less than required) related to unconscious state

Goal: Meet nutritional requirements

1. Prepare for nasogastric feedings.	1. Feeding through a gastric tube ensures better nutrition than does intravenous feeding. Paralytic ileus is fairly frequent in unconscious patients, and a nasogastric tube to suction may be necessary for gastric decompression.	• Tolerates NG feedings well. • No evidence of aspiration.
a. Insert gastric tube through nose into stomach.		
b. Aspirate the stomach before each feeding.	b. If aspirated residual exceeeds 50 ml, the patient may be developing an ileus. Gastric distention and vomiting may result.	
c. Elevate the patient's head and thorax and give 100 to 150 ml blenderized feeding slowly. Give small amount at first and gradually increase until 400 to 500 ml is given at each feeding.	c. Elevation of the patient's head before, during, and after feeding reduces likelihood of esophageal reflux, regurgitation, and aspiration.	
d. Give 2000 to 2500 ml of water through the tube daily.	d. An unconscious patient requires adequate fluids daily. High-protein feedings can produce a solute diuresis that will produce dehydration and hyperosmolar coma unless enough fluid intake is ensured. Fever, excessive sweating, or fluid loss elsewhere in the body increases fluid requirements.	
e. Follow the tube feeding with water after each feeding. Keep tube feeding refrigerated.	e. Administering water keeps the tube patent and provides fluid to prevent dehydration.	
2. Prepare for gastrostomy or total parenteral nutrition if patient is expected to remain comatose for an indefinite period.	2. Prolonged nasogastric intubation can cause esophagitis (from gastric reflux) and erosion of the nasal septum.	

Nursing Diagnosis: Incontinence related to unconscious state

Goal: Attain/maintain bladder continence as soon as possible

1. Observe the patient for indications of an overdistended bladder.	1. Most unconscious patients are incontinent but empty their bladders regularly.	• Absence of bladder distention. • Absence of skin breakdown.
a. Use external sheath catheter (condom catheter) for male patient. An in-	a. Containment of urine protects the skin from maceration and breakdown.	

(continued)

Nursing Care Plan 56–2 (Continued)

Care of the Unconscious Patient

Nursing Interventions	Rationale	Expected Outcomes
dwelling catheter is avoided because of the risk of urinary tract infection.		
b. Send urine culture to laboratory at specified intervals.	b. Culture can detect urinary infection.	

Nursing Diagnosis: Constipation and/or diarrhea related to unconscious state

Goal: Attainment of bowel continence

1. Assess for constipation or diarrhea.	1. Constipation results from immobilization and lack of dietary fiber. Diarrhea occurs from infection, antibiotics, hyperosmolar feedings, and fecal impaction.	• Has soft, formed stool.
2. Place patient on bowel program (see Chap. 14) as soon as possible.		

Nursing Diagnosis: High risk for impaired skin integrity related to immobility or restlessness

Goal: Maintenance of normal skin integrity

1. Keep the skin clean, dry, and free of pressure.	1. Comatose patients are susceptible to the formation of pressure ulcers. All of these activities are to prevent formation of pressure ulcers on pressure-sensitive areas.	• Absence of skin breakdown. • Skin appears healthy with normal turgor.
2. Turn patient frequently.	2. To relieve pressure.	
3. Lubricate skin with emollient lotions.	3. Prevents irritation from sheet, dryness, chafing, and cracking.	
4. Inspect pressure areas for evidence of skin redness and breakdown.	4. See Chapter 14 for other preventive measures for pressure ulcers.	
5. Clip patient's fingernails to prevent skin excoriation by accidental or reflex scratching.		

Nursing Diagnosis: Potential impaired tissue integrity (cornea) related to unconscious state

Goal: Preservation of sight

1. Protect the eye from corneal irritation.	1. The cornea functions as a shield. If the eyes remain open for long periods, corneal drying, abrasion, and secondary infection and ulceration are likely to result.	• Eyes appear normal; absence of redness, purulent drainage, or signs of irritation or infection.
a. Make sure patient's eye is not rubbing against the bedding.		
b. Routinely inspect the size of pupils and condition of eyes using a penlight.		
c. Irrigate eyes with prescribed solution and instill sterile ophthalmic drops or ointment in each eye.	c. Removes discharge and helps prevent glazing and corneal ulceration.	
d. Seal eyelids shut with plastic tape or prepare for temporary suturing of eyelids in closed position if unconscious state is prolonged.		

(continued)

Nursing Care Plan 56–2 *(Continued)*

Care of the Unconscious Patient

Nursing Interventions	Rationale	Expected Outcomes

Nursing Diagnosis: High risk for injury related to occurrence of seizures and restlessness

Goal: Protection from injury

Nursing Interventions	Rationale	Expected Outcomes
1. Protect the patient from self-injury.	1. A patient with head trauma is a potential candidate for seizures.	• No evidence of injury or trauma. • No undue restlessness noted.
a. See Chapter 57 for nursing interventions.		
b. Observe the patient during the seizure and record observations.		
c. Administer prescribed anticonvulsant medications via nasogastric tube.		
2. Administer nursing support as the patient's changing condition indicates. Be aware of the varying phases of restlessness.	2. A certain degree of restlessness may be favorable, since it may indicate that the patient is regaining consciousness. However, restlessness is quite common in cerebral hypoxia or when there is a partially obstructed airway, distended bladder, overlooked bleeding, or fracture; it may be a manifestation of brain injury.	
a. Have adequate lighting in the room to prevent hallucinations in the patient who is regaining consciousness.		
b. Pad side rails, apply mitts or boxing gloves.	b. To prevent injury.	
c. Avoid oversedating the patient.	c. Sedatives and narcotics depress the level of responsiveness, which is a guide to clinical assessment. Certain drugs affect pupillary size and reaction, which are important signs.	

Nursing Diagnosis: Sensory-perceptual alteration related to unconsciousness

Goal: Promotion of sensory stimulation

Nursing Interventions	Rationale	Expected Outcomes
1. Provide for environmental stimulation and social contacts.	1. Introducing meaningful sounds stimulates the cortical levels.	• Family visiting and interacting with patient.
a. Direct conversation to the patient; encourage family to talk to the patient.	a. Attempting to stimulate the patient's senses helps overcome sensory deprivation.	• Family initiate reading-aloud session; have planned television/radio sessions taking into consideration patient's previous interests.
b. Arouse patient; touch him; stimulate his senses.		• Asks questions and listening to responses.
c. Introduce sounds from the patient's home and work environment via a tape recorder to "normalize" the environment.	c. Determine the patient's preferences in music, radio, TV, and patterns of daily living.	
2. Give the patient an explanation of what has happened during the period of unconsciousness. Permit him to question and talk about the experience of unconsciousness.	2. This will help the patient to cope with anxieties, mobilize psychological defenses, and promote psychological recovery.	

The nursing assessment of the aphasic patient includes *listening* to him, asking him to follow simple directions (*e.g.*, "Pick up the book"), and observing him cope with his dysfunction.

▷ Nursing Diagnoses

Based on the assessment data, the patient's major nursing diagnoses may include the following:

- Self-esteem disturbance related to loss of ability to communicate
- Impaired communication related to brain damage
- Ineffective family coping related to sudden disruption in life style and lack of understanding of brain damage and how to help the patient

▷ Planning and Implementation

▷ *Goals:*   The major goals of the patient may include development of a more positive self-esteem, improved communication abilities, and improved family coping.

▷ Nursing Interventions

▷ *Developing a Positive Self-Esteem.*   A patient with aphasia should be given as much psychological security as possible. The same manner is used with this patient as with a young child learning to speak. At the same time, the patient is treated as an adult. A kind, unhurried manner combined with encouragement, patience, and a willingness to invest time are required. Relearning speech and language skills may take several years.

An aphasic person may become depressed because of the inability to talk to others. Not being able to talk on the telephone or answer a question or being excluded from conversation causes anger, frustration, fear of the future, and a sense of hopelessness.

The nurse must accept the patient's behavior and feelings, relieve his embarrassment, and give support by assuring him that there is nothing wrong with his intelligence and that the nurse realizes he knows what he wants to say. The environment should be relaxed and permissive, and the patient should be encouraged to socialize with family and friends. Often the aphasic person has almost an obsession with orderliness. Thus, nurses and family members should return items in the room to their proper place.

▷ *Improving Communication Abilities.*   It is essential that aphasic patients be guided in their efforts to improve their communication skills. Listening skills as well as speaking skills are emphasized in the rehabilitation program. The patient may also benefit from a communication board, which has pictures of commonly requested needs and phrases. The board may be translated into several languages. The patient should be encouraged to verbalize his needs and to use the board when he is unable to express his needs.

Increasing Auditory Stimulation: First the patient is encouraged to *listen*. Speaking is thinking out loud, and the emphasis is on *thinking*. The patient must think and sort out incoming messages and formulate a response. Listening requires mental effort; yet the patient must struggle against mental inertia and needs time to organize an answer.

In working with the aphasic patient, the nurse must re-

member to *talk to* the patient while caring for him. This provides social contact for the patient.

- It is best to face the patient and establish eye contact, at the same time speaking in a normal manner but in short phrases, pausing between phrases. The emphasis here is on ensuring that the patient understands what is being said.
- Conversation should be confined to practical and concrete matters and supplemented with gestures, pictures, and objects.
- As the patient handles and uses the object, the word should be stated; it helps when words are matched with actions.
- Consistency is important and the same wording and gestures are used each time instructions are given and questions are asked.
- Because the patient is easily fatigued and distracted, extraneous noises and sounds must be kept to a minimum; the patient cannot sort out messages when there is too much noise and confusion in the environment.

Restoring Speech: When the patient attempts to communicate, the nurse must make a real effort to understand him and must treat him as an intelligent adult. It is important to behave in a way that shows acceptance of the patient as a worthwhile person. The patient should never be forced to correct his mistakes because this merely adds to his frustration, nor should the nurse rush to finish sentences for him. During periods of emotional lability, the patient should be approached in a calm, accepting, and deliberate manner, because frustration and depression are frequent reactions to the inability to communicate. Because speech that is motivated by emotions usually comes first (*i.e.*, swearing), the content of this speech should be ignored by the nursing personnel.

Patients with aphasia must be stimulated both internally and externally to action. Therapy is based on a recognition of the patient's needs, previous interests, drives, and motivation. If the patient's speech is unintelligible or filled with jargon, his gestures may offer a clue to his intent.

- The nurse continues to listen to him.
- The nurse nods and makes neutral statements occasionally.

If necessary, the topic is shifted to gain another point of interest and frame of reference.

The environment should provide sensory input, with auditory stimulation supplemented with visual stimulation. Reading is encouraged for a few minutes at a time, and the patient can look at pictures while another person talks about them. Games stimulate the mind and help organize the thoughts. The nurse can try to elicit responses from the patient, asking him to nod his head if he understands. Every correct response should be reinforced. For more relaxed forms of communication, the television, radio, electronic games, and tape recorder can be used. Too much sensory, auditory, or visual stimulation may overload and further frustrate the patient.

▷ *Helping the Family Cope.*   Helping the family cope with irrevocable changes in their life style is accomplished by talking about the stroke or head injury, acknowledging the changes that have occurred, focusing on the patient's abilities, and informing them of support systems. The attitude of the family is an important factor in helping the patient adjust to this deficit. Family members are encouraged to act naturally and treat the patient in the same manner as before his illness. They should be aware that the patient's ability to speak may vary from day to day and that fatigue has an adverse effect on speech. They also should be aware that the patient may strike out verbally when his emotional controls are lowered. The patient is likely to become frustrated. Tears and laughter may flow without apparent cause, and frequent mood shifts are common.

Support groups such as Stroke Clubs and group therapy for aphasic patients can help in the socialization and motivation of the patient as well as aid in the relief of anxiety and tension. The strain of the constant adjustment to the patient's illness, demands, and needs, as well as the financial drain and the change in life style, can produce explosive pressures on the family. Members of the family actually go through a period of mourning. In addition to the family learning as much as possible about the support of the patient with aphasia, they should also be counseled to continue a life of their own and to seek the aid of a social worker, clergyman, or psychologist if they need additional help in dealing with their frustrations and pressures. (See bibliography at the end of the chapter for resources for patients with aphasia.)

◊ Evaluation

Expected Outcomes

1. Demonstrates improvement in self-esteem
   a. Participates in decision making
   b. Returns to a few former activities
   c. Attends and participates in support group
2. Communicates with others according to his ability/disability
   a. Practices relaxation techniques
   b. Attempts to read aloud; repeats words
3. Family members improve coping abilities
   a. Include patient in activities and social affairs
   b. Demonstrate an encouraging attitude toward patient
   c. Modify their expectations of patient
   d. Continue to pursue their own interests

Neurologic Deficits Due to Cerebrovascular Disease

Cerebrovascular disease refers to any functional abnormality of the CNS caused by interference with the normal blood supply to the brain. The pathology may involve an artery, a vein, or both, when the cerebral circulation becomes impaired as a result of partial or complete occlusion of a blood vessel or hemorrhage resulting from a tear in the vessel wall. The blood vessel most frequently associated with cerebrovascular disease is the internal carotid artery.

Vascular disease of the CNS may be caused by arteriosclerosis (most common), hypertensive changes, arteriovenous malformations, vasospasm, inflammation, arteritis, or embolism. As a result of vascular disease, blood vessels lose their elasticity, become hardened, and develop atheromatous deposits, or plaques, which may be the source of an embolus. The lumen of the vessel may gradually close, causing impairment of cerebral circulation and ischemia of the brain. If cerebral ischemia is transient, as in transient ischemic attacks (TIA), there is usually no lasting neurologic deficit. Occlusion of a large vessel, however, produces cerebral infarction (Fig. 56-4). The vessel may rupture and produce hemorrhage.

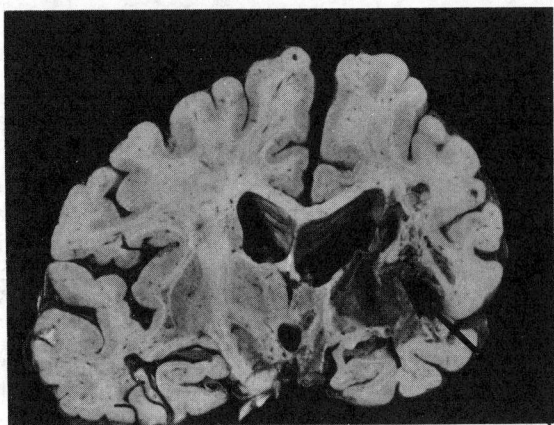

Figure 56-4. Impairment of cerebral circulation leading to a stroke. The arrow points to the area of cerebral infarction. (Armed Forces Institute of Pathology. Neg. No. 55-13956.)

Transient Ischemic Attacks

A TIA is a transient or temporary episode of neurologic dysfunction commonly manifested by a sudden loss of motor, sensory, or visual function, lasting a few seconds or minutes but no longer than 24 hours. Complete recovery usually occurs between attacks. A transient ischemic attack may serve as a warning of impending stroke, which has its greatest incidence in the first month after the first attack. The cause of this clinical entity is a temporary impairment of blood flow to a specific region of the brain due to a variety of reasons, including atherosclerosis of the vessels supplying the brain, obstruction of cerebral microcirculation by a small embolus, a fall in cerebral perfusion pressure, cardiac dysrhythmias, and so on.

The most common sites of atherosclerosis in the extracranial arteries are located at the bifurcation of the common carotid and at the origin of the vertebral arteries. Among the intracranial arteries, the middle cerebral artery is the most common location of atherosclerosis.

Clinical Manifestations

The classic symptom of carotid artery disease is *amaurosis fugax* (fleeting blindness) occurring without warning in which there is sudden, painless loss of vision of one eye or dimming or graying out of the field of vision of one eye. This is suggestive of retinal ischemia due to insufficiency of the homolateral ophthalmic or carotid artery. If the ischemia occurs in the vertebral basilar system, vertigo, diplopia, disturbances of consciousness, and various signs of motor and sensory impairment may occur.

Diagnostic Evaluation

A *bruit* (abnormal sound heard on auscultation resulting from interference with normal blood flow) may be heard over the carotid artery. There are diminished or absent carotid pulsations in the neck.

Carotid phonoangiography may be performed, which provides auscultation, direct visualization, and photographic recording of carotid bruits. *Oculoplethysmography* (OPG) measures pulsation in blood flow through the ophthalmic artery. *Carotid angiography* visualizes intracranial and cervical vessels.

Digital subtraction angiography is used to define carotid artery obstruction and provide information on patterns of cerebral blood flow.

Management

Patients who are not candidates for surgical intervention may be placed on anticoagulant therapy to prevent future attacks and a possible massive cerebral infarction. Platelet-inhibiting drugs (particularly aspirin) are useful in decreasing the occurrence of cerebral infarction in patients who have experienced multiple TIAs.

Surgical intervention procedures in common use are endarterectomy (see below) and angioplasty, in which a balloon on a catheter is inserted in the artery to break up the plaque and dilate the artery.

Carotid Endarterectomy. A carotid endarterectomy is the removal of an atherosclerotic plaque or thrombus from the carotid artery to prevent stroke in patients with occlusive disease of the extracranial cerebral arteries. (Most ischemic strokes are associated with lesions of the extracranial arteries.)

- After endarterectomy, a neurologic flow sheet is kept to maintain close assessment of the patient's neurologic status. The neurosurgeon is notified immediately if the patient develops a neurologic deficit. Formation of a thrombus at the side of endarterectomy can be suspected if there is a sudden increase in neurologic deficits, such as weakness on one side of the body. The patient should be prepared for reoperation.
- The primary complications of carotid endarterectomy are stroke, cranial nerve injuries, infection or hematoma of the wound, and carotid artery disruption.
- It is important to maintain adequate blood pressure levels in the immediate postoperative period. Hypotension is avoided, to prevent cerebral ischemia and thrombosis.
- Excessive hypertension may precipitate cerebral hemorrhage. Edema, hemorrhage in the operative wound, or disruption of the arterial reconstruction also may result from excessive hypertension. Sodium nitroprusside is commonly used to bring the blood pressure to previous levels.
- Difficulty in swallowing, hoarseness, or other signs of cranial nerve dysfunction must be assessed. Some swelling in the neck after surgery is expected. Swelling and hematoma formation, however, if large enough, can obstruct the patient's airway. A tracheostomy set must be available.
- Close cardiac monitoring is necessary because these patients have a high incidence of coronary artery disease.
- Long-term complications include recurrent stroke and myocardial infarction.

Stroke (Cerebrovascular Accident)

A stroke is a sudden loss of brain function resulting from a disruption of the blood supply to a part of the brain. Frequently it is the culmination of cerebrovascular disease of many years' standing.

Stroke is the primary neurologic problem in the United States and in the world. Although preventive efforts have brought about a steady decline in the incidence in the past decade, stroke is the third ranking cause of death, striking over 510,000 people annually in this country, with an overall mortality rate of 18% to 37% for the first stroke and as high as 62%

for subsequent strokes. There are approximately 2 million people surviving strokes who have some disability; of these, 40% need assistance with ADL.

Causes of Stroke

A stroke usually results from one of four events: (1) thrombosis (a blood clot within a blood vessel of the brain or neck), (2) cerebral embolism (a blood clot or other material carried to the brain from another part of the body), (3) ischemia (decrease of blood flow to an area of the brain), and (4) cerebral hemorrhage (rupture of a cerebral blood vessel with bleeding into the brain tissue or spaces surrounding the brain). The result is an interruption in the blood supply to the brain, causing temporary or permanent loss of movement, thought, memory, speech, or sensation.

Cerebral Thrombosis. Cerebral arteriosclerosis and slowing of the cerebral circulation are major causes of cerebral thrombosis, which is the most common cause of stroke.

Headache is rather uncommon at the onset of cerebral thrombosis. Some patients may experience dizziness, mental disturbances, or convulsions, and some may have an onset indistinguishable from that of intracerebral hemorrhage or cerebral embolism. In general, cerebral thrombosis does not develop abruptly, and a transient loss of speech, hemiplegia, or paresthesias in one half of the body may precede the onset of a severe paralysis by a few hours or days.

Cerebral Embolism. Pathologic abnormalities of the left side of the heart, such as infective endocarditis, rheumatic heart disease, and myocardial infarction, as well as pulmonary infections, are the sites where emboli originate. It is possible that the insertion of a prosthetic heart valve may precipitate a stroke, because there seems to be an increased incidence of embolism after this procedure. The incidence of stroke after this procedure can probably be reduced with postoperative anticoagulant therapy. Pacemaker failure, atrial fibrillation, and cardioversion for atrial fibrillation are other possible causes of cerebral emboli and stroke.

The embolus usually lodges in the middle cerebral artery or its branches, where it disrupts the cerebral circulation.

- Sudden onset of hemiparesis or hemiplegia with or without aphasia or loss of consciousness in a patient with cardiac or pulmonary disease is characteristic of cerebral embolism.

Cerebral Ischemia. Cerebral ischemia (insufficiency of the blood supply to the brain) is due mainly to atheromatous constriction of the arteries supplying the brain. The most common manifestation is transient ischemic attacks.

Cerebral Hemorrhage. In the 24-year Framingham Study on Heart Disease and Stroke, hemorrhage was found to be the mechanism of stroke in 15% of the patients. Hemorrhage may occur outside the dura mater (extradural or epidural hemorrhage), beneath the dura mater (subdural hemorrhage), in the subarachnoid space (subarachnoid hemorrhage), or within the brain substance (intracerebral hemorrhage). Figure 56-5 illustrates the locations of epidural, subdural, and intracerebral hematomas.

Extradural Hemorrhage. Extradural hemorrhage (epidural hemorrhage) is a neurosurgical emergency that requires urgent care. It usually follows skull fracture with a tear of the middle artery or other meningeal artery. If the patient is not treated within hours of the accident, he has little chance of survival. (This is discussed in the section on head injury in Chap. 57.)

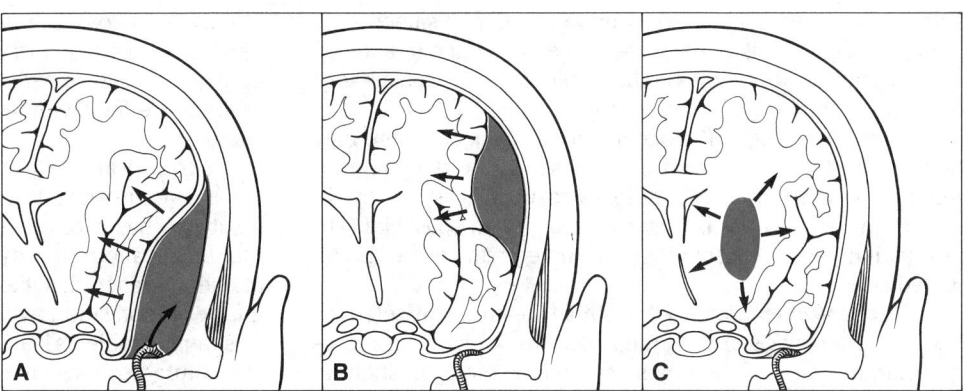

Figure 56–5. (**A**) Epidural or extra-dural hematoma—bleeding between the inner skull and the dura, compressing the brain underneath. (**B**) Subdural hematoma—bleeding between the dura mater and arachnoid membrane. (**C**) Intracerebral hemorrhage—bleeding in the brain or the cerebral tissue with displacement of surrounding structures.

Subdural Hemorrhage. Subdural hemorrhage (excluding *acute* subdural hemorrhage) is basically the same as an epidural hemorrhage, except that in subdural hematoma usually a bridging vein is torn. Thus, a longer period (longer lucid interval) is required for the hematoma to form and cause pressure on the brain. (This is discussed in the section on head injury in Chap. 57.)

Subarachnoid Hemorrhage. Subarachnoid hemorrhage (hemorrhage occurring in the subarachnoid space) may occur as a result of trauma or hypertension, but the most common cause is a leaking aneurysm in the area of the circle of Willis and congenital arteriovenous malformations of the brain. Any artery within the brain can be the site of an aneurysm. (The treatment of intracranial aneurysms is discussed in Chap. 57.)

Intracerebral Hemorrhage. Hemorrhage or bleeding into the brain substance is most common in patients with hypertension and cerebral atherosclerosis, because degenerative changes due to these diseases usually cause rupture of the vessel. Strokes frequently occur in the 40- to 70-year-old age group. In persons younger than 40, intracerebral hemorrhages are usually caused by arteriovenous malformations and hemangioblastomas.

The bleeding is usually arterial and occurs particularly around the basal ganglia. Intracerebral hemorrhage also may be due to certain types of arterial pathology, presence of brain tumor, and the use of medications (oral anticoagulants, amphetamines, and a variety of addictive drugs). The clinical picture and the prognosis depend mainly on the degree of hemorrhage and brain damage. Occasionally, the bleeding ruptures the wall of the lateral ventricle and causes intraventricular hemorrhage, which is frequently fatal.

Usually, the onset is abrupt, with severe headache. As the hematoma enlarges, a more pronounced neurologic deficit occurs in the form of decreased alertness and abnormalities in the vital signs. If the bleeding is limited or develops gradually, there may be no significant pressure effects. Conversely, the full deficit may evolve in a matter of hours. A marked reduction in consciousness (stupor/coma) in the early phase of the bleeding episode usually has an ominous prognosis.

The treatment of intracerebral hemorrhage is controversial. If the hemorrhage is small, the patient is treated conservatively and symptomatically.

- The blood pressure is carefully lowered with antihypertensive drugs. The patient's neurologic deficit may worsen if the blood pressure is dropped too low or lowered too rapidly. The most

effective form of treatment is the prevention of hypertensive vascular disease.

Risk Factors and Prevention of Stroke

Prevention of stroke is the best possible approach. Steps are taken to alter those factors and human conditions that predispose certain people to stroke or increase their risk of having a stroke.

- Control of hypertension, the major risk factor, is the key to prevention of stroke.
- Patients with cardiovascular disease (rheumatic heart disease, rhythm abnormalities [particularly atrial fibrillation], congestive heart failure, left ventricular hypertrophy) are at increased risk because cerebral embolism may originate in the heart.
- A high normal hematocrit level is related to an increased incidence of cerebral infarction.
- Diabetes is associated with accelerated atherogenesis.
- There appears to be an increased risk of stroke among women taking oral contraceptives, which is enhanced by coexisting hypertension, age over 35 years, cigarette smoking, and high estrogen levels.
- An excessive or prolonged fall of blood pressure after shock, hemorrhage, surgery, diagnostic procedures, and ingestion of certain drugs may cause general cerebral ischemia. In these instances, the patient requires careful monitoring.
- Drug abuse is a cause of stroke, particularly in adolescents and young adults.
- In younger persons, attention should be directed at controlling blood lipids (particularly cholesterol), blood pressure, cigarette smoking, and obesity.
- There appears to be a link between alcohol consumption and stroke.

Clinical Manifestations

A stroke causes a wide variety of neurologic deficits, depending on the location of the lesion (which vessels are obstructed), the size of the area of inadequate perfusion, and the amount of collateral (secondary or accessory) blood flow. The damaged brain cannot be fully restored.

Motor Loss. Stroke is a disease of the upper motor neurons and results in loss of voluntary control over motor movements. Because the upper motor neurons decussate (cross), a disturbance of voluntary motor control on one side of the body may reflect damage to the upper motor neurons on the opposite side of the brain. The most common motor dysfunction is hemiplegia (paralysis of one side of the body) due to a lesion of the opposite side of the brain. Hemiparesis, or weakness of one side of the body, is another sign.

In the early stage of stroke, the initial clinical feature may be flaccid paralysis and loss or decrease in the deep tendon reflexes. When these deep reflexes reappear (usually by 48 hours), increased tone is observed along with spasticity (abnormal increase in muscle tone) of the extremities on the affected side.

Communication Loss.   Other brain functions affected by stroke are language and communication. Stroke or cerebrovascular accident is the most common cause of aphasia. Dysfunction of language and communication may be manifested by:

- *Dysarthria* (difficulty in speaking), as demonstrated by poorly intelligible speech caused by paralysis of the muscles responsible for producing speech
- *Dysphasia* or *aphasia* (defective speech or loss of speech), which is mainly expressive or receptive
- *Apraxia* (inability to perform a previously learned action), as may be seen when a patient picks up a fork and attempts to comb his hair with it

Aphasia and its nursing management are discussed in detail on p. 1658.

Perceptual Disturbances.   Perception is the ability to interpret sensation. Visual perceptual dysfunctions are due to disturbances of the primary sensory pathways between the eye and visual cortex. *Homonymous hemianopia* (loss of half of the visual field) may occur from stroke and may be temporary or permanent. The affected side of vision corresponds to the paralyzed side of the body. The patient's head turns away from the affected side of his body, and he tends to neglect that side and the space on that side. In such instances, the patient is unable to see food on half of the tray, and only half of the room is visible.

To assess for hemianopia, the nurse requests the patient to look at her face. The nurse's examining finger is placed about 30 cm (12 in) from the patient's ear on the unaffected side and is moved inward toward his field of vision. Inability to detect movement on one or both sides suggests visual neglect and hemianopia. This decreased field of vision must be kept in mind during all rehabilitation procedures. Personnel should approach the patient on the side where visual perception is intact. All visual stimuli (clock, calendar, television) should be placed on this side. The patient can be taught to turn his head in the direction of the defective visual field to compensate for this loss. The nurse should make eye contact with the patient and draw his attention to his affected side by encouraging him to move his head. Increasing the natural or artificial lighting in the room and providing his eyeglasses are important in increasing vision.

Disturbances in visual-spatial relationships (perceiving relationship of two or more objects in spatial areas) are frequently seen in patients with left hemiplegia. The patient may not be able to dress himself because of his inability to match his clothing to his body parts. To assist this patient, the nurse can take steps to keep his environment organized and uncluttered because the patient with a perceptual problem is easily distracted. He is told to slow down and gently reminded where an object is located.

Sensory losses from stroke may take the form of slight impairment of touch or be more severe with loss of proprioception (inability to perceive position and motion of body parts) as well as difficulty in interpreting visual, tactile, and auditory stimuli.

Impairment of Mental Activity and Psychological Effects. If damage has occurred to the frontal lobe, then learning capacity, memory, or other higher cortical intellectual functions may be impaired. Such dysfunction may be reflected in a limited attention span, difficulties in comprehension, forgetfulness, and a lack of motivation, which cause these patients to encounter frustrating problems in their rehabilitation programs. Depression is a natural response to such a catastrophic illness. Other psychological problems are myriad and are manifested by emotional lability, hostility, frustration, resentment, and lack of cooperation.

Bladder Dysfunction.   After a stroke the patient may have transient urinary incontinence due to confusion, inability to communicate his needs, and inability to use the urinal/bedpan because of impaired motor and postural controls. Occasionally after a stroke the bladder becomes atonic with impaired sensation in response to bladder filling. Sometimes control of the external urinary sphincter is lost or diminished. During this period, intermittent catheterization with sterile technique is carried out. When muscle tone increases and deep tendon reflexes return, bladder tone increases and spasticity of the bladder may develop. Because the patient's sense of awareness is clouded, persistent urinary incontinence or urinary retention may be symptomatic of bilateral brain damage. Continuing bladder and bowel incontinence may reflect extensive neurologic damage.

Management of the Acute Phase of a Patient With Stroke

A patient who is in deep coma on admission to the hospital is considered to have a poor prognosis. Conversely, a fully conscious patient faces a more favorable outcome. The acute phase usually lasts 48 to 72 hours. The principles underlying the management of the unconscious patient are summarized on p. 1653. Maintaining the airway and adequate ventilation are priorities in the acute phase. Table 56-2 reviews the neurologic deficits frequently seen in patients with strokes. Table 56-3 compares the symptoms seen in right hemispheric stroke with those seen in left hemispheric stroke. Approximately 90% of the population have left hemisphere dominance, which would control the right side of the body. There are a small number of left-handed people who have left hemisphere dominance, rather than right hemispheric dominance.

Medical treatment for the patient with acute stroke may include diuretics to reduce cerebral edema, which reaches maximum levels 3 to 5 days after cerebral infarction. Anticoagulants may be given to prevent further development or propagation of the thrombosis or embolization from elsewhere in the cardiovascular system. Antiplatelet drugs may be given because platelets play a major role in thrombus formation and embolization.

Treatment is also aimed at improving cerebral blood flow and metabolism.

- A patent airway and circulation to the brain are maintained.
- Adequate oxygenation of blood to the brain is necessary to

TABLE 56-2. *Neurologic Deficits of Stroke: Manifestations and Nursing Implications*

Neurologic Deficit	Manifestation	Nursing Implications/Patient Teaching Applications
VISUAL FIELD DEFICITS:		
Homonymous hemianopsia (Loss of half of the visual field)	• Unaware of persons or objects on side of visual loss • Neglect of one side of the body • Difficulty judging distances	Place objects within the patient's intact field of vision. Approach the patient from side of his intact field of vision. Teach and remind the patient to turn his head in the direction of visual loss to compensate for loss of visual field. Encourage the use of eye glasses if available. When teaching the patient, do so within patient's intact visual field.
Loss of peripheral vision	• Difficulty seeing at night • Unaware of objects or the borders of objects	Place objects in the patient's center of vision Encourage the use of a cane or other object to identify objects in the periphery of the visual field. Avoid night driving or any other risky activity in the darkness.
Diplopia	• Double vision	Explain to the patient the location of an object when placing it near the patient. Consistently place patient care items in the same location.
MOTOR DEFICITS:		
Hemiparesis	• Weakness of the face, arm, and leg on the same side (due to a lesion in the opposite hemisphere)	Place objects within the patient's reach on the nonaffected side. Instruct the patient to exercise and increase the strength on the unaffected side.
Hemiplegia	• Paralysis of the face, arm and leg on the same side (due to a lesion in the opposite hemisphere)	Encourage the patient to provide range-of-motion exercises to the affected side. Provide immobilization as needed to the affected side. Encourage neutral body alignment. Exercise unaffected limb to increase mobility, strength, and use.
Ataxia	• Staggering, unsteady gait • Unable to keep feet together, needs a broad base to stand	Support patient during the initial ambulation phase. Provide supportive device for ambulation, (*i.e.*, walker, crutches, cane). Instruct the patient not to walk without assistance or supportive device.
Dysarthria	• Inability to form words	Provide the patient with alternative methods of communicating. Allow the patient sufficient time to respond to verbal communication. Support patient and family to alleviate frustration related to difficulty in communicating.
Dysphagia	• Difficulty in swallowing	Test the patient's pharyngeal reflexes before offering food or fluids. Assist the patient with meals. Place food on the unaffected side of the mouth. Allow ample time to eat.
SENSORY DEFICITS:		
Paresthesia (occurs on the side opposite the lesion)	• Numbness and tingling of body parts • Difficulty with proprioception	Instruct the patient to avoid using this body part as the dominant limb. Provide range of motion to affected areas and apply corrective devices as needed. Place patient care items toward the nonaffected side.

(continued)

TABLE 56-2.   *(Continued)*

Neurologic Deficit	Manifestation	Nursing Implications/Patient Teaching Applications
VERBAL DEFICITS:		
Expressive aphasia	• Unable to form words that are understandable; may be able to speak in single-word responses	Encourage patient to repeat sounds of the alphabet.
Receptive aphasia	• Unable to comprehend the spoken word; is able to speak but may not make sense	Speak slowly and clearly to assist the patient in forming the sounds.
Global aphasia	• Combination of both receptive and expressive aphasia	Speak clearly and in simple sentences; use gestures or pictures when able.
COGNITIVE DEFICITS:	• Short- and long-term memory loss • Decreased attention span • Impaired ability to concentrate • Poor abstract reasoning • Altered judgment	Reorient patient to time, place, and situation frequently. Use verbal and auditory cues to orient patient. Provide familiar objects (family photographs, favorite objects). Use noncomplicated language with the patient. Match visual tasks with a verbal cue: holding a toothbrush, simulate brushing of teeth while saying, "I would like you to brush your teeth now." Minimize distracting noises and views when teaching the patient. Repeat and reinforce instructions frequently. Ask questions concerning abstract reasoning and judgment that are appropriate to the patient's educational and cultural background, such as, "How are an apple and an orange alike?"; "What should you do if there is a fire?"
EMOTIONAL DEFICITS:	• Loss of self-control • Emotional lability • Decreased tolerance to stressful situations • Depression • Withdrawal • Fear, hostility, and anger • Feelings of isolation	Support patient during uncontrollable outbursts. Discuss with the patient and family that the outbursts are due to the disease process. Encourage patient to participate in group activity. Provide stimulation for the patient. Control stressful situations, if possible. Provide a safe environment. Encourage patient to express feelings and frustrations related to disease process.

minimize cerebral damage. Brain function is absolutely dependent on available oxygen being delivered to the neuronal tissues. The blood pressure and cardiac output must be maintained to sustain cerebral blood flow, and hydration (intravenous fluids) must be ensured to reduce blood viscosity and improve cerebral blood flow. Oxygen therapy, if necessary, should be given at an adequate perfusion pressure.

• The patient is placed in a lateral or semiprone position with the head of the bed slightly elevated to lower cerebral venous pressure.
• Endotracheal intubation and mechanical ventilation are necessary for patients with massive stroke, because respiratory arrest is usually the life-threatening factor in this situation.
• The patient is monitored for pulmonary complications (aspiration, atelectasis, pneumonia), which may be due to loss of airway reflexes, immobility, or hypoventilation.
• The heart is examined for abnormalities in size, rhythm, and signs of congestive failure.

A dysrhythmia may have caused a cerebral embolus and must be corrected. Cerebral embolism may occur after myocardial infarction or atrial fibrillation or may originate from a prosthetic heart valve.

The blood pressure is not allowed to drop precipitously because brain ischemia or myocardial ischemia may result. Hypertension is prevented and treated.

▶ Nursing Process
The Patient With a Stroke
◊ Assessment

A neurologic flow sheet is maintained to reflect the following nursing assessment parameters:

1. A change in the level of responsiveness as evidenced by movement, resistance to changes of position, and response to stimulation; orientation to time, place, and person

TABLE 56-3. *Comparison of Left-Sided Versus Right-Sided Hemispheric Stroke**

Left Hemispheric Stroke	Right Hemispheric Stroke
Expressive, receptive, or global aphasia	Difficulty in perceptual or spatial interpretation
Alteration in intellectual ability	Easily distractable
Deficit in right visual field	Impulsive behavior
	Deficit in the left visual field

* *Associated clinical manifestations and nursing interventions can be found in Table 56-2.*

2. Presence or absence of voluntary or involuntary movements of the extremities; the tone of the muscles; the body posture; and the position of the head
3. Stiffness or flaccidity of the neck
4. Eye opening, the comparative size of the pupils and pupillary reactions to light, and ocular position
5. The color of the face and the extremities; the temperature and the moisture of the skin
6. The quality and the rates of pulse and respiration; arterial blood gases as indicated, body temperature, and arterial pressure
7. Ability to speak
8. Volume of fluids ingested or administered and the volume of urine excreted each 24 hours

When the patient begins to regain consciousness, signs of extreme fatigue and confusion are apparent as a result of the cerebral edema that follows a stroke. To offset any anxiety, efforts should be made at frequent intervals to orient the patient to time and place and to reassure him.

If the lesion occurs in the dominant hemisphere, the patient is likely also to have aphasia. A nondominant hemispheric lesion may result in apraxia (inability to perform previously learned movements).

After the acute phase, the nurse assesses the following functions: mental status (memory, attention span, perception, orientation; affect, speech/language), sensation/perception (usually patient has decreased awareness of pain and temperature); motor control (upper and lower extremity movement); bladder function.

Nursing assessment continues to focus on the impairment of function in the patient's daily activities because the quality of life after stroke is closely related to the patient's functional status.

Nursing Diagnoses

Based on the assessment data, the patient's major nursing diagnoses may include the following:

- Impaired physical mobility related to hemiparesis, loss of balance and coordination, spasticity, and brain injury
- Pain (painful shoulder) related to hemiplegia and disuse
- Self-care deficits (hygiene, toileting, transfers, feeding) related to stroke sequelae
- Altered urinary elimination (incontinence) related to flaccid bladder, detrusor instability, confusion, difficulty in communicating

- Altered thought processes related to brain damage, confusion, inability to follow instruction
- Impaired verbal communication related to brain damage
- High risk for impaired skin integrity related to hemiparesis/hemiplegia, decreased mobility
- Altered family processes related to catastrophic illness and caregiving burdens

▷ Planning and Implementation (Rehabilitation Phase)

Although rehabilitation begins on the day the patient has the stroke, the process is intensified during the convalescent phase and requires a coordinated team effort. The team has to know what the patient was like before this catastrophic illness: what he was able to do, his mental and emotional state, behavioral characteristics, and ADL.

▷ *Goals:* The major goals of the patient (and family) may include improvement of mobility, avoidance of shoulder pain, achievement of self-care, attainment of bladder control, improvement of thought processes, achievement of some form of communication, maintenance of skin integrity, and restoration of family functioning.

▷ Nursing Interventions

▷ *Improving Mobility: Preventing Deformities.* A hemiplegic patient has unilateral paralysis. When control of the voluntary muscles is lost, the strong flexor muscles exert control over the extensors. The arm tends to adduct (adductor muscles are stronger than abductors) and to rotate internally. The elbow and the wrist tend to flex, the affected leg tends to rotate externally at the hip joint and flex at the knee, and the foot at the ankle joint supinates and tends toward plantar flexion (Fig. 56-6).

Positioning: Correct positioning in bed is of prime importance (Fig. 56-7) to prevent contractures; measures are used to relieve pressure, assist in maintaining good body alignment, and prevent compressive neuropathies, especially of the ulnar and peroneal nerves. A bed board under the mattress provides firm support for the body. The patient should remain flat in bed except when engaged in ADL. Maintaining the upright position in bed for extended periods is one of the greatest contributors to hip flexion deformity. A footboard may be used at intervals during the flaccid period after a stroke to keep the feet at right angles to the legs when the patient is in a supine (dorsal) position. This prevents footdrop and the heel cords from shortening as a result of contracture of the gastrocnemius muscles.

The patient may also wear high-top sneakers. Care should be employed to prevent pressure areas on the heels and ankles. As soon as spasticity develops, a footboard is generally not used because it may worsen spasticity and a plantar flexion deformity. If the affected extremity is spastic, a bed cradle is used to keep the bedding off the extremity.

Because flexor muscles are stronger than extensor muscles, it may be necessary to apply a posterior splint at night to prevent flexion of the affected extremity. The posterior splint is used only at night to maintain correct positioning during sleep.

To prevent external rotation at the hip joint, a trochanter roll is used, extending from the crest of the ilium to the mid-thigh, because the hip joint lies between these two points (see

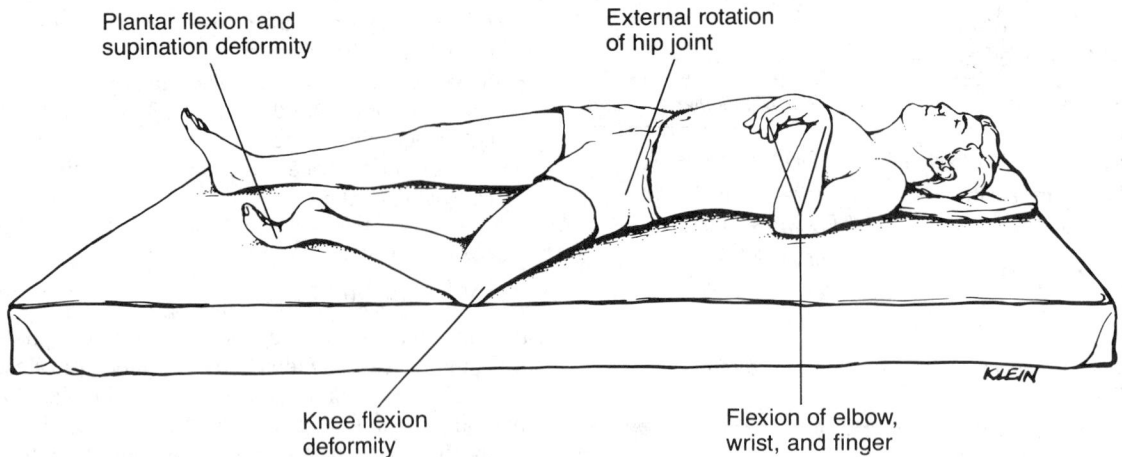

Plantar flexion and supination deformity

External rotation of hip joint

Knee flexion deformity

Flexion of elbow, wrist, and finger

KLEIN

Figure 56–6. Hemiplegic deformities. The involved leg immediately falls into external rotation. The knee almost invariably flexes. As soon as knee flexion occurs, abduction of the upper leg follows. The foot falls into plantar flexion, so that there is always a footdrop and a shortening of the Achilles tendon. This position of the leg is assumed whether the leg is flaccid or spastic. The arm of the affected side is held against the body. Often, a flail arm is placed across the body for convenience in handling the patient, but if spastic, the elbow flexes to about 90 degrees. With the arm across the body, the wrist is dropped. If the arm is spastic, the fingers curl into a fist, with the thumb adducted and flexed under the fingers. (After Covalt NK. Preventive technics of rehabilitation for hemiplegic patients. GP 17:131.)

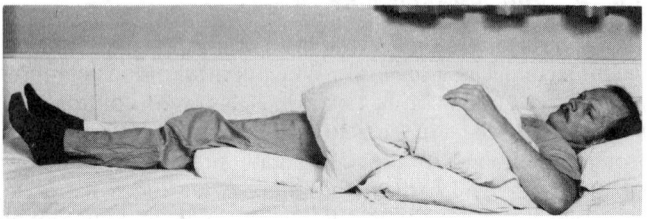

1. A pillow is placed in the axilla to prevent adduction of the affected shoulder. Pillows are placed under the arm, which is in a slightly flexed position with each joint positioned higher than the preceding one.

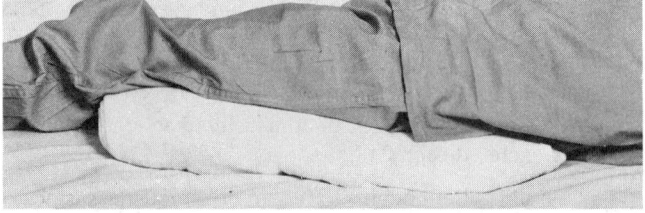

2. The trochanter roll should extend from the crest of the ilium to the midthigh, since the hip joint lies between these two points. The trochanter roll acts as a mechanical wedge under the projection of the greater trochanter and prevents the femur from rolling.

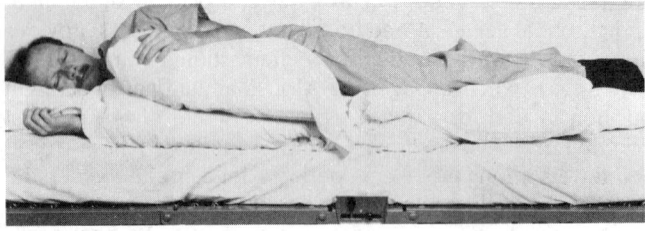

3. Lateral or side-lying position. The patient should be turned on his unaffected side. The upper thigh should not be acutely flexed.

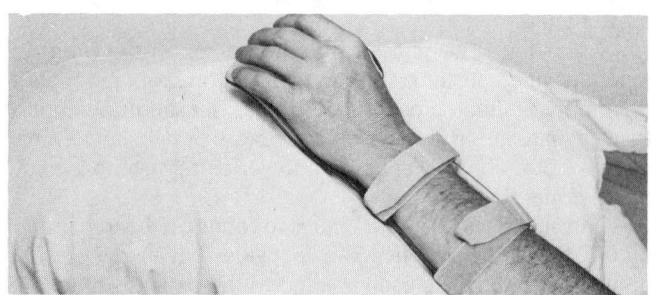

4. A volar resting splint may be used to support the wrist and hand if the upper extremity is flaccid.

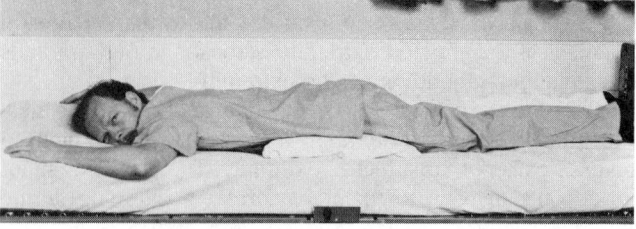

5. Prone position. A pillow is placed under the pelvis to help promote hyperextension of the hip joints, which is essential for normal gait. Note position of arms.

Figure 56–7. Positioning for a patient after a stroke. (*Dark side of clothes represents affected or hemiplegic side.*)

Fig. 56-7*B*). A sandbag applied at the side of the leg will not prevent external rotation, inasmuch as this motion originates in the ball and socket joint of the hip. The knee has no such rotating function. The trochanter roll acts as a mechanical wedge under the projection of the greater trochanter and prevents the femur from rolling.

To prevent adduction of the affected shoulder, a pillow is placed in the axilla when there is limited external rotation (see Fig. 56-7*A*). This keeps the arm away from the chest. A pillow is placed under the arm, and the arm is placed in a neutral (slightly flexed) position, with each joint positioned higher than the preceding one. Thus, the elbow is higher than the shoulder and the wrist is higher than the elbow. The elevation of the arm helps to prevent edema and the resultant fibrosis that will prevent normal range of motion if the patient regains control of the arm.

The fingers are positioned so that they are barely flexed. The hand is placed in slight supination (palm faces upward), which is its most functional (*i.e.*, useful) position. If the upper extremity is flaccid, a volar resting splint can be used to support the wrist and hand in a functional position. If the upper extremity is spastic, a hand roll is *not* desirable because it stimulates the grasp reflex. In this instance a dorsal wrist splint is useful in allowing the palm to be free of pressure. Every effort is made to prevent hand edema.

Changing Positions: The patient's position should be changed every 2 hours. To place a patient in a lateral (side-lying) position, a pillow is placed between the legs before the patient is turned. The upper thigh should not be acutely flexed. The patient may be turned from side to side, but the amount of time spent on the affected side should be limited because of impaired sensation. Lying on the affected side, however, is thought to increase the patient's awareness of the side and allows use of the unaffected hand.

If possible, it is desirable to place the patient in a prone position for 15 to 30 minutes several times a day. A small pillow or a support is placed under the pelvis, extending from the level of the umbilicus to the upper third of the thigh (see Fig. 56-7*E*). This helps to promote hyperextension of the hip joints, which is essential for normal gait and helps prevent knee and hip flexion contractures. The prone position also helps to drain bronchial secretions and prevents contractural deformities of the shoulders and knees.

◊ Retraining the Affected Extremities

Exercise. The affected extremities are exercised passively and put through a full range of motion four or five times a day to maintain joint mobility, to regain motor control, to prevent development of a contracture in the paralyzed extremity, to prevent further deterioration of the neuromuscular system, and to enhance circulation. Exercise is helpful in the prevention of venous stasis, which may predispose to thrombosis and pulmonary embolus.

Repetition of an activity forms new pathways in the CNS and therefore encourages new patterns of motion. At first, the extremities are usually flaccid. If tightness occurs in any area, the range-of-motion exercises should be performed more frequently. (See Chap. 14 for techniques of range-of-motion exercises.) Signs to observe for include shortness of breath, chest pain, cyanosis, and increasing pulse rate during the exercise period.

Frequent short periods of exercise always are preferable to longer periods at infrequent intervals. *Regularity* in exercise is most important. Improvement in muscle strength and maintenance of range of motion can be achieved only through daily exercise.

The patient is encouraged and reminded to exercise the unaffected side at intervals throughout the day. It is helpful to work out a written time schedule that can be used to remind the patient of the exercise activities. The nurse has the responsibility of supervising and supporting the patient during these activities. The patient can be taught to put the unaffected leg under the affected one to move it when turning and exercising. Flexibility, strengthening, coordination, endurance, and balancing exercises prepare the patient for ambulation and give the patient a goal. Quadriceps muscle setting and gluteal setting exercises are started early to improve the muscle strength needed for walking. These are performed at least five times daily for 10 minutes at a time.

Quadriceps setting—The patient is instructed to contract the quadriceps muscle (on the anterior portion of the thigh) while raising the heel and pushing the popliteal space against the mattress. The muscle contraction is held until the count of 5, then relaxed until the count of 5 and repeated. This exercise is performed with each extremity.

Gluteal setting—Gluteal setting is performed in the following manner: contract or pinch the buttocks together until the count of 5; relax until the count of 5; repeat.

Biofeedback. Electromyographic (EMG) biofeedback is being used in neuromuscular re-education for improving muscle strength and reducing spasticity.

◊ Preparing for Ambulation.

As soon as possible, the patient is assisted out of bed. Usually, when hemiplegia has resulted from a thrombosis, an active rehabilitation program is started as soon as the patient regains consciousness; a patient who has had a cerebral hemorrhage cannot participate actively until all evidence of bleeding is gone.

Sitting Balance. A hemiplegic patient tends to lose his sense of balance and needs to learn to maintain balance in a sitting position before learning to balance himself in the standing position.

- Before the patient attempts to rise from a recumbent position, blood pressure should be checked because orthostatic hypotension may occur. A fall in blood pressure may further damage the ischemic area.
- To develop sitting balance, the head of the bed is raised to an upright position and the patient is instructed to hold the bedrail with his unaffected hand.

The patient is then helped to come to a sitting position on the edge of the bed. This may be achieved in the following manner:

1. The bed is adjusted to the low position.
2. The patient is instructed to place the unaffected leg beneath the weak leg and lift it toward the side of the bed.
3. The patient is instructed to press the strong elbow that is flexed to a 90-degree angle into the mattress and come to a sitting position by transferring weight to the forearm and then to the hand, while lifting the unaffected leg with the strong leg over the edge of the bed. The force of gravity, set in motion by pushing against the hand and moving the legs, is sufficient to pivot the patient's torso on the buttocks.

4. The patient extends his strong arm with his hand flat on the bed behind him to assist in balancing.

5. The nurse stands in front of the patient to observe and, if necessary, to help him to maintain this posture.

- A change in color, shortness of breath, increasing pulse rate, or profuse perspiration is an indication that the patient should be placed in bed again. The sitting time is increased as rapidly as the patient's condition permits.

Standing Balance.   As soon as the patient is able to balance while sitting, he is taught standing balance. He should wear walking shoes with a strong shank for all ambulation activities. Tape on the shoe or colored shoelaces help identify the affected foot and leg if the patient is having perceptual problems.

- The patient is seated on the edge of the bed, and straightback chairs are positioned on each side of him (Fig. 56-8).
- The patient is assessed for dizziness before assisting him to a standing position.
- The patient is assisted to a standing position by the nurse supporting his lower back with her hands and positioning her knees on the outside of the patient's knees. This gives the patient maximum support in the standing position and prevents his knees from buckling. The patient should be reminded to lean forward when he comes from a sitting to a standing position. The patient's arms must be left free for balance and support.
- The nurse stands behind the patient and stabilizes him at his waist. A waistband or a belt, (an abdominal binder can serve as a waistband) is placed around the patient's waist and grasped for patient support.

- Dizziness, pallor, and an increasing pulse rate indicate that the patient should be permitted to rest in a sitting position. If the symptoms continue, the patient should be put back in bed. With repeated effort, the patient can tolerate this activity for longer periods.
- The patient is assisted to practice standing and shifting weight from one leg to another.
- After the patient learns to sit and stand, a portable commode is used instead of the bedpan.

If the patient has difficulty in achieving standing balance, a tilt table can help him assume an upright position. This helps the patient in weight bearing, provides a sense of being upright, and increases endurance in the upright position. There should be frequent periods of standing before walking is started.

Walking.   The patient is usually ready to walk as soon as standing balance is achieved. Parallel bars are useful when the patient first starts to walk. A chair or wheelchair should be readily available in the event of sudden fatigue or vertigo. The following method is one way to ambulate the patient:

1. The patient is instructed to stand between the parallel bars or beside one rail with his weight evenly distributed on both feet and his strong arm on the rail about 10 cm (4 in) in front of his body.

2. The patient shifts the weight to the strong leg and advances the involved leg while pushing *down* on the rail.

3. The patient then shifts the weight to the weak leg. (If the

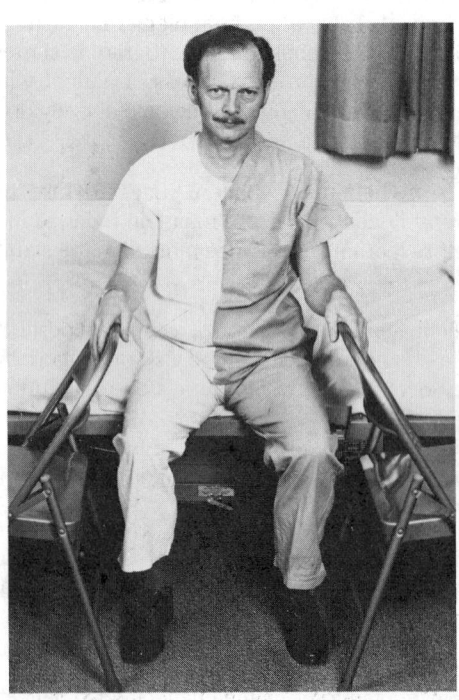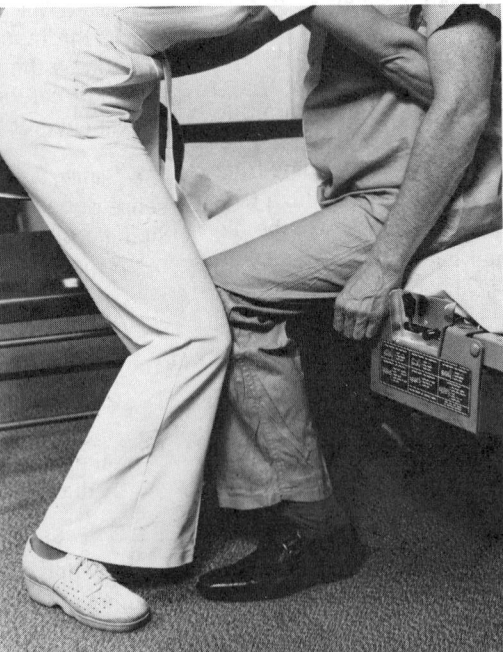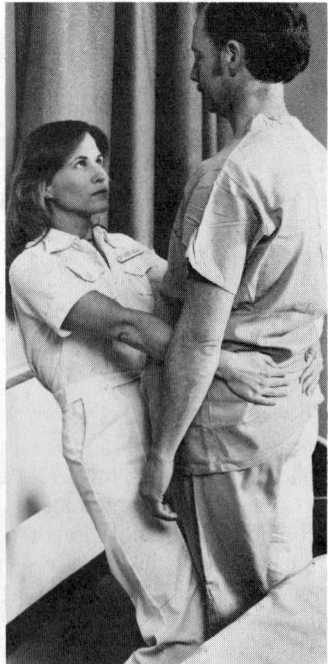

Figure 56–8.   Procedure for getting the patient out of bed following a stroke. (*Dark side of clothes represents affected or hemiplegic side.*) (**Left**) Place the bed in the low position so that the patient's feet are resting on the floor. Observe the patient's reaction and increase the sitting time as rapidly as the patient's condition permits. (**Center**) Getting ready to rise to a standing position. Positioning the nurse's knees on the outside of the patient's knees will prevent the patient's knees from buckling. (**Right**) Stabilizing the patient as he assumes a standing position. Note that the nurse is (1) stabilizing the patient's lower back and knees and (2) assessing his reaction to standing. (Courtesy of Washington Adventist Hospital; Glenn Dalby, photographer.)

patient has poor muscle tone and cannot advance his involved leg, functional electrical stimulation may be used. Stimulating muscles electrically may increase strength, reverse atrophy, and enhance voluntary control.)

4. The patient is encouraged to look at his feet occasionally because proprioceptive loss may accompany hemiplegia.

The training periods for ambulation should be short and frequent. As the patient gains in strength and confidence, he can begin to walk with an adjustable aluminum cane. Generally a three- or four-prong cane provides a stable support in the early phases of this training program.

Orthotic devices (braces) may be necessary to give adequate joint support and stability. An ankle–foot orthosis of lightweight thermoplastic material provides ankle and knee stability. If the patient's knee tends to buckle, a small rubber cushion placed in the heel of the shoes decreases the impact of the heel striking the floor as the patient walks. A small lift on the opposite shoe is helpful if the patient drags the affected leg. After time has elapsed, the patient is evaluated to determine if he needs to be fitted with a short or a long leg brace.

Wheelchair. If the patient needs a wheelchair, the folding type with hand brakes is the most practical because it allows the patient to manipulate the chair. The chair should be low enough so that the patient can propel it with the uninvolved foot and narrow enough to permit it to be used in the home. To propel the wheelchair, the patient places the strong hand on the hand rim and the stronger foot on the floor to guide and direct the chair.

When the patient is transferred from the wheelchair, the brakes are applied on both sides of the chair. The technique a patient uses for transferring from a wheelchair placed on his unaffected side is as follows:

- Lift the foot pedals out of the way and move forward in the chair, placing weight on the strong leg.
- Push up with the strong arm and foot.
- Place most of the weight on the strong leg while keeping the weak knee locked.
- Pivot in the direction of the stronger leg; bring weak leg over to stronger leg. Maintain standing position for a few minutes.
- Lower body onto bed or chair gradually, using strong arm and leg.

Wheelchair mobility provides greater independence in self-care activities. When a permanent wheelchair is needed, it is ordered with specific modifications and instructions for the individual patient.

▷ *Preventing Shoulder Pain.* Up to 70% of stroke patients suffer from severe pain in the shoulder that prevents them from learning new skills, because shoulder function is essential in achieving balance and performing transfers and self-care activities. Three problems can occur: painful shoulder, subluxation of the shoulder, and shoulder–hand syndrome.

A flaccid shoulder joint may be overstretched by the use of excessive force in turning the patient or from overstrenuous arm and shoulder movement. To prevent *shoulder pain*, the nurse should never lift the patient by the flaccid shoulder or pull on the affected arm or shoulder. If the arm is paralyzed, *subluxation* (incomplete dislocation) at the shoulder can occur from overstretching of the joint capsule and musculature by the force of gravity when the patient sits or stands in the early

stages after a stroke. This results in severe pain. *Shoulder–hand syndrome* (painful shoulder and generalized swelling of the hand) can cause a frozen shoulder and ultimate atrophy of subcutaneous tissues. When a shoulder becomes stiff, it is usually more painful.

These problems can be prevented by proper patient movement and positioning. The flaccid arm is positioned on a table or pillows while the patient is seated. Some authorities advocate a properly worn sling when the patient first becomes ambulatory to prevent the paralyzed upper extremity from dangling without support. Range-of-motion exercises are important in preventing painful shoulder. Overstrenuous arm movements are avoided. The patient is instructed to interlace his fingers, place his palms together, and push his clasped hands slowly forward to bring the scapulae forward. He then raises his hands above his head. This is repeated throughout the day. The patient is instructed to flex the affected wrist at intervals and move all the joints of the affected fingers. He is encouraged to touch, stroke, rub, and look at his hands. Pushing the heel of the hand firmly down on a surface is useful. Elevation of the arm and hand is also important in preventing dependent edema of the hand.

▷ *Achieving Self-Care.* As soon as the patient is able to sit up, he is encouraged to assist in his personal hygiene. He is helped to set realistic goals and, if feasible, a new task is added daily. The first step is to have the patient carry out all self-care activities on the unaffected side. Such activities as combing the hair, brushing the teeth, shaving with an electric razor, bathing, and eating can be carried out with one hand and are suitable for self-care. Although the patient may feel awkward at first, the various motor skills can be learned by repetition and the unaffected side will become stronger with use. The nurse must be sure that he does not neglect his affected side. Assistive devices will help make up for some of the patient's deficits. A small towel is easier to control while drying after bathing, and boxed paper tissues are easier to use than a roll of toilet tissue.

Dressing Activities: The patient's morale will improve if ambulatory activities are carried out while he is fully dressed. The family is instructed to bring in clothing that is preferably a size larger than that normally worn. Clothing fitted with front or side fasteners or Velcro closures is the most suitable. The patient has better balance if most of the dressing activities are done in a seated position.

The clothing is placed on his affected side in the order in which the garments are to be put on. Using a large mirror while dressing helps make the patient aware of what he is putting on his affected side. Each garment is put on the affected side first. The patient has to make many compensatory movements when dressing that can produce fatigue and painful twisting of the intercostal muscles. He requires support and encouragement to prevent overfatigue and discouragement. Even with intensive training, not all patients are able to achieve independence in dressing skills.

▷ *Attaining Bladder Control.* Most stroke patients have bladder problems in the early stage, but bladder control is usually quickly regained. The patient's voiding pattern is analyzed and the urinal/bedpan offered on this pattern or schedule. The upright posture and standing position is helpful for male patients during this aspect of rehabilitation. (See also p. 42 for a bladder retraining program.)

▷ *Improvement of Thought Processes.* After a stroke, the patient may have problems with cognitive, behavioral, and emotional deficits related to brain damage. In many instances, however, there can be considerable recovery of functioning because not all areas are equally damaged; some remain more intact and functional than others.

After assessment procedures that delineate and describe the patient's problems, the neuropsychologist, interacting when possible with the psychologist, psychiatrist, nurse, and other professionals, structures a training program using cognitive-perceptual retraining, visual imagery, reality orientation, and cueing procedures to compensate for losses.

The role of the nurse is supportive. The nurse reviews the results of neuropsychologic testing, observes the patient's performance and progress, gives positive feedback, and, most important, conveys an attitude of confidence and hopefulness. Interventions capitalize on the patient's strengths and what he can still do, while attempting to improve performance of affected functions. Other interventions are similar to those for improvement of cognitive functioning after a head injury (see p. 1737).

▷ *Achieving Communication.* Aphasia impairs the patient's ability to communicate both in understanding what is being said and in the ability to express himself. The speech-language pathologist assesses the communication needs of the stroke patient, describes the precise deficit, and suggests the best overall method of communication for the patient. There are many language intervention strategies for the adult aphasic person, and the program is individually tailored. Goals are established with the patient, and he is expected to take an active part.

Nursing interventions include doing everything possible to make the atmosphere conducive to communication. This includes being sensitive to the patient's reactions and needs and reacting to them in an appropriate manner, always keeping in mind that the patient is treated as an adult. The nurse lends strong moral support and understanding to allay anxiety. A consistent schedule, routines, and repetitions help the patient to function in spite of significant deficits. He may be given a written copy of his schedule, a folder of personal information (birth date, address, names of relatives), checklists, and an audiotaped list to help his memory and concentration. Reviewing an album of snapshots with him can be stimulating. Surrounding the patient with familiar objects and caring people is reassuring.

When talking with the patient, the nurse must make sure she has the patient's attention, must speak slowly, and must keep the language of instruction consistent. One instruction is given at a time, and time is allowed for the patient to process what has been said. The use of gestures may enhance comprehension. Other nursing strategies for helping the aphasic patient are found on p. 1658.

▷ *Maintenance of Skin Integrity.* The patient who suffers a stroke may be at risk for skin and tissue breakdown because of altered sensation and inability to respond to pressure and discomfort by turning and moving. Therefore, preventing skin and tissue breakdown requires frequent assessment of the skin, with particular emphasis on bony areas and dependent parts of the body. A regular turning and positioning schedule must be followed to minimize pressure and prevent skin breakdown. Pressure-relieving devices may be used but must not be used in place of regular turning and positioning. The turning schedule (at least every 2 hours) must be adhered to even if pressure-relieving devices are used to prevent tissue and skin breakdown. When the patient is positioned or turned, care must be used to minimize shear and friction forces, which cause damage to tissues and predispose the patient to breakdown. The patient's skin must be kept clean and dry; gentle massage of healthy skin and maintenance of adequate nutrition are other factors that help to maintain normal skin and tissue integrity.

▷ *Improving Family Coping Through Health Teaching.* Members of the patient's family play an important role in the patient's recovery. Some type of counseling and support system should be available to them to prevent the care of the patient from taking a significant toll on their health and interfering too radically with their life style. Respite care, which is planned short-term care to ease the burden of the family in providing continuous 24-hour care, may be available from an adult day care center. Some hospitals also offer weekend respite care.

Family coping is also facilitated by involving others in the patient's care, stress management techniques, and maintenance of personal health.

The family may have difficulty in accepting the patient's disability and may be unrealistic in their expectations. They are given advice concerning the expected outcomes of the patient's stroke and are counseled to avoid doing for the patient those things that he can do for himself. They are assured that their loving and warm interest is part of the patient's therapy. The family needs to be informed that the rehabilitation of the hemiplegic patient requires many months and that progress may be slow. The gains made by the patient during hospitalization must be maintained. All should approach the patient with a supportive and optimistic attitude, focusing on the abilities that remain. The rehabilitation team, the medical and nursing team, the patient, and his family all must be involved in developing attainable goals for the patient when he is home. Most relatives of stroke patients have problems with the emotional aspects of care. The family should be prepared to expect occasional episodes of emotional lability. The patient may laugh or cry easily. He may be irritable and demanding or depressed and confused. The nurse can explain to the family that the patient's laughing does not necessarily mean he is glad, nor does crying mean that he is sad, and that emotional lability usually improves with time.

▷ *Home Health Care.* Some of the patient's emotional problems are related to speech dysfunction. A *speech therapist* coming to the home allows the family to be involved and gives them practical instructions to help the patient between speech therapy sessions.

The family is advised that the patient will tire easily, will become irritable and upset by small events, and is likely to show less interest in things. Because a stroke frequently occurs in the later stages of life, there is the possibility of intellectual decline related to dementia.

Asking the patient what he would like to do gives insight into establishing new goals. Depression is a common and serious problem in the post-stroke patient. The nurse can discuss this event with the physician because antidepressant therapy may help if depression dominates the patient's life. As progress is made in the rehabilitation program, some problems will diminish. The family can help by continuing to support the patient and giving honest praise for progress that is made.

The *occupational therapist* makes a home assessment and recommends modifications to help the patient to become more independent. A shower is more convenient than a tub for the hemiplegic patient, because most patients do not gain sufficient strength to get up and down from a tub. Sitting on a stool of medium height with rubber suction tips permits him to wash with greater ease. A long-handled bath brush with a soap container is helpful to the patient who has only one functional hand. If a shower is not available, a stool may be placed in the tub and a portable shower hose attached to the faucet. Handrails may be attached beside the bathtub and the toilet. There are numerous self-help devices available that can assist the patient in the ADL. Community-based stroke clubs give the patient a feeling of belonging and fellowship with others who have similar problems. He is encouraged to continue with hobbies, recreational and leisure interests, and contact with friends to prevent social isolation.

▷ *Sexual Function.* Sexual functioning can be profoundly altered by disability. A stroke is such a catastrophic illness that the patient often experiences loss of self-esteem and value as a sexual being. Although research in this area of stroke management is limited, it appears that post-stroke patients believe that sexual function is important, but most experience sexual dysfunction after stroke (see Sexuality and the Disabled in Chap. 14).

All nurses coming in contact with the patient, whether as members of the hospital health care team, community health nurses, or office or occupational health nurses, should encourage the patient to *keep active*, faithfully adhere to the exercise program, and confidently continue to remain as self-sufficient as possible.

Gerontologic Considerations. The person who sustains a stroke is often elderly and may have several residual effects of a stroke: impaired mobility, altered communication, memory loss, visual defects, altered bowel, bladder and sexual function, and altered thought processes. The extent of these changes may vary from slight impairment to major alterations that necessitate complete care, including feeding, bathing, turning, and bowel and bladder care. The effects of stroke in the elderly can be moderated by early and prompt attention to rehabilitation. Nursing care that is directed toward maximal recovery, along with speech therapy and physical and occupational therapy, may be employed to assist the patient regain skills that enable him to participate in self-care activities. The patient's age is not and should not be a reason for failure to initiate a full rehabilitation program.

In many instances, it is the patient's spouse who assumes a major role in post-stroke care of the patient. The spouse may require assistance and instruction in techniques that promote optimal care to the affected person. The nurse's coordination of services for the stroke patient and his spouse as well as attention to the physical and emotional health of the caregiving spouse, who is often also elderly, may enable continued care of the patient in the home.

▷ **Evaluation**

Expected Outcomes
1. Achieves improved mobility
   a. Avoids deformities; absence of contractures and footdrop
   b. Participates in prescribed exercise program
   c. Achieves sitting balance

   d. Increases walking time
   e. Uses unaffected side to compensate for loss of function of hemiplegic side
2. Has no complaints of shoulder pain
   a. Demonstrates shoulder mobility
   b. Elevates arm and hand at intervals
   c. Exercises shoulder; no evidence of hand edema
3. Achieves self-care
   a. Is able to perform hygienic care
   b. Uses adaptive equipment
4. Attains bladder continence
5. Participates in cognitive improvement program (see Head Injury, Chap. 57)
6. Demonstrates improved communication (see Aphasia Evaluation, p. 1665)
7. Exhibits normal skin integrity
   a. Maintains intact skin without breakdown
   b. Demonstrates normal skin turgor
   c. Participates in turning and position activities
8. Family members demonstrate a positive attitude and coping mechanisms
   a. Encourage patient in exercise program
   b. Take an active part in rehabilitation process
   c. Help patient set new goals

In summary, the patient immediately after the stroke and during the rehabilitation phase requires much support and guidance. This is a difficult period for the family as well. The plans for their future have been altered and the realization of reaching old age may impede the patient's progress. The nurse needs to support and assist the patient and family in addressing the issues related to the stroke and begin to plan for the rehabilitation phase. The deficits from a stroke vary, depending on the area of involvement, which influences the patient's recovery.

The Patient Undergoing Intracranial Surgery

In recent years, certain technological advances have helped to refine existing neurologic procedures and develop newer ones. Superior neuroradiologic techniques have made it possible to localize intracranial lesions. Improved illumination and magnification have made it possible to obtain a three-dimensional view of the field of operation. Lasers enable neurosurgeons to remove tumors precisely with minimal trauma to surrounding tissue; this is of utmost importance in neurosurgery. It is possible to coagulate vessels adjacent to structures without causing injury to the structures themselves. Microsurgical instruments allow delicate tissue to be separated without trauma. Ultrasonic dissecting systems permit rapid and gentle removal of certain brain and spinal cord tumors with precision. Probes placed deep into brain tissue can be used for application of interstitial radiation, hyperthermia, or chemotherapy; before the development of these probes, many lesions were inaccessible to treatment. Suture material smaller than a strand of human hair permits very small nerves and vessels to be sutured and anastomosed.

Surgical Approaches

A *craniotomy* is the surgical opening of the skull to gain access to intracranial structures. This procedure is performed to remove a tumor, relieve ICP, evacuate a blood clot, and control hemorrhage. The skull is opened by making a bony flap that is replaced after surgery and fixed in position by periosteal or wire sutures. In general, two approaches through the skull are used: (1) above the tentorium (supratentorial craniotomy) into the supratentorial compartment and (2) below the tentorium into the infratentorial (posterior fossa) compartment (Fig. 56-9). A transsphenoidal approach is used to gain access to the pituitary gland.

Table 56-4 compares the three different surgical approaches: supratentorial, infratentorial, and transsphenoidal. The intracranial structures may be approached through *burr holes* (Fig. 56-10), which are circular openings made in the skull by either a hand drill or an automatic craniotome (which has a self-controlled system to stop the drill when the bone is penetrated). Burr holes are made for exploration or diagnosis. They may be used to determine the presence of cerebral swelling and injury and the size and position of the ventricles. They are also a means of evacuating an intracranial hematoma or abscess, making a bone flap in the skull, and allowing access to the ventricles for decompression purposes, ventriculography, or shunting procedures.

Other cranial procedures include *craniectomy* (an excision of a portion of the skull) and *cranioplasty* (repair of a cranial defect by means of a plastic or metal plate).

Diagnostic Evaluation

Preoperative diagnostic procedures may include computed tomography (CT scanning) to demonstrate the lesion and show the degree of surrounding brain edema, the ventricular size, and the displacement. Magnetic resonance imaging (MRI) provides information similar to that of the CT scan, with the additional advantage of examining the lesion in other planes. Cerebral angiography may be used to study the tumor blood supply or give information about vascular lesions.

Preoperative Management

Usually patients are placed on anticonvulsant medication (phenytoin) before surgery to reduce the risk of postoperative seizures. Preoperative steroids (dexamethasone) are introduced before surgery to reduce cerebral edema. Fluids may be restricted. A hyperosmotic agent (mannitol) and a diuretic (furosemide) may be given intravenously immediately before and sometimes during surgery if the patient tends to retain water, as many do who have intracranial dysfunction. An indwelling urethral catheter is inserted before the patient is taken to the operating room to drain the bladder during the administration of diuretics and measure urinary output and for periodic measurements of urine specific gravity and glucose. The patient may be given antibiotics if there is a chance of cerebral contamination.

The scalp is shaved immediately before surgery (usually in the operating room) so that any resultant superficial abrasions do not have time to become infected. Most patients find this alteration in their appearance distressing. Reassuring the patient that his head will be covered with a head dressing after surgery will help him cope. He may be given diazepam preoperatively to allay anxiety.

Postoperative Management

An arterial line and a central venous pressure (CVP) line may be in place for blood pressure monitoring and CVP measurements. Oxygen is usually administered. Drug therapy for cerebral edema includes the administration of mannitol, which increases serum osmolality and draws free water from areas of the brain (with an intact blood–brain carrier). The fluid is

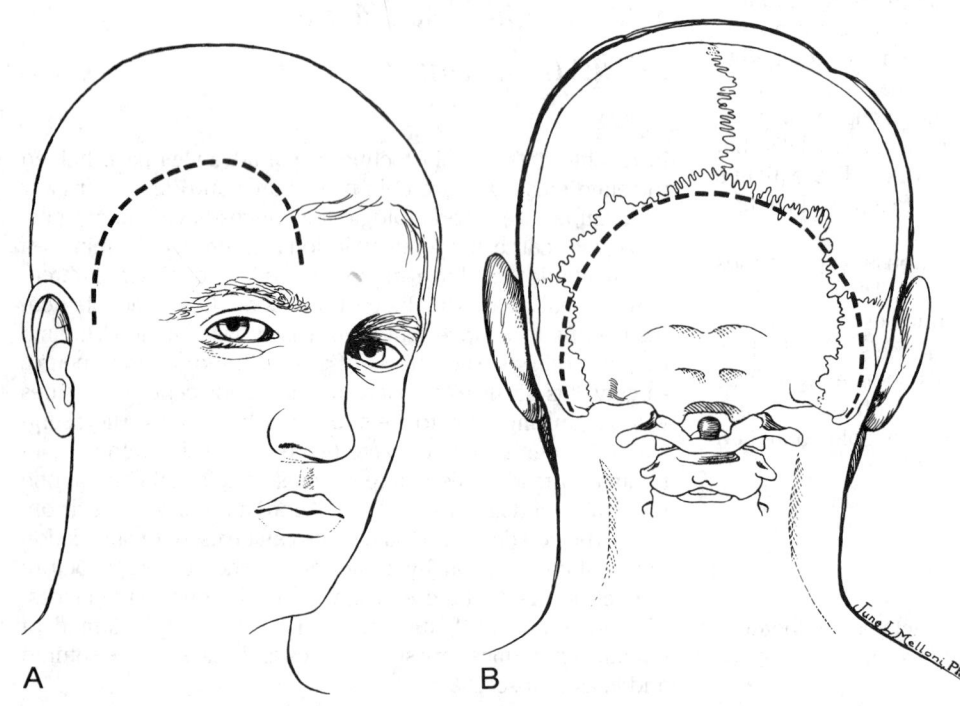

Figure 56–9. Surgical approaches for craniotomy (surgical opening of the cranial cavity). The dashed lines indicate scalp incisions. (**A**) Supratentorial approach. (**B**) Infratentorial approach.

TABLE 56-4. *Comparison of Cranial Surgical Approaches*

	Supratentorial	**Infratentorial**	**Transsphenoidal**
Site of surgery	Above the tentorium	Below the tentorium, brain stem	Sella turcica and small pituitary tumors
Incision location	Incision is made above the area to be operated on; is usually located behind the hairline	Incision is made at the nape of the neck, around the occipital lobe	Incision is made beneth the upper lip to gain access into the nasal cavity
Selected nursing interventions	Maintain head of bed elevated 30–45 degrees. Position the patient on either side or back. (Avoid placing patient on operative side if a large tumor has been removed.)	Maintain neck in straight alignment. Avoid flexion of the neck to prevent possible tearing of the suture line. Position the patient on either side. (Avoid positioning the patient on his back; this may be a surgeon's preference.)	Maintain nasal packing in place and reinforce as needed. Instruct patient to avoid blowing his nose. Provide frequent oral care. Keep head of bed elevated to promote venous drainage and drainage from the surgical site.

then excreted by osmotic diuresis. Dexamethasone may be administered intravenously every 6 hours for 24 to 72 hours; subsequently the dosage is tapered.

Acetaminophen is usually given for temperature over 99.6°F (37.5°C) and for pain. Frequently the patient may have a headache after a craniotomy; it is usually attributed to stretching or irritation of the nerves of the scalp that occurs during operation. Codeine, given parenterally, is usually sufficient to relieve headache. Anticonvulsant medication (phenytoin, diazepam) is given to patients who have undergone supratentorial craniotomy, because of the high risk of epilepsy after supratentorial neurosurgical procedures. Serum levels are monitored to keep the drug within therapeutic range.

A ventricular catheter, or some type of drainage, is frequently inserted in patients undergoing surgery for tumors of the posterior fossa. The catheter is connected to an external drainage bottle. The patency of the catheter is noted by the pulsations of the fluid in the tubing. In addition, the degree of ICP can be determined by the height of the fluid level in the tube above the level of the ventricle. The catheter is removed when the ventricular pressure is normal. The neurosurgeon should be notified if at any time the catheter appears to be obstructed.

Ventricular shunting is sometimes performed before certain operations to control intracranial hypertension, particularly in patients with posterior fossa tumors.

▶ Nursing Process
The Patient Undergoing Intracranial Surgery

◊ Preoperative Assessment/Preparation

Proper assessment of the postoperative status of the patient requires an awareness of the patient's signs and symptoms so that a comparison may be made between the preoperative and postoperative conditions. Included in this assessment are evaluation of the level of responsiveness or consciousness and the presence of any neurologic deficits. Observations of paralysis, visual dysfunction, alterations in personality or speech, and bladder and bowel disturbances are made. Motor function of the hands can be tested by the strength of the hand grip. Observations of leg movement should be especially noted if the patient is not ambulatory.

If there is paralysis of the extremities, trochanter rolls are applied to both extremities, and the feet are positioned against a footboard. Patients who have speech difficulties, failing vision, and hearing loss are a challenge to the nurse's ingenuity. If the patient is aphasic, writing materials or picture and word cards showing the bedpan, glass of water, blanket, and other frequently used items may be supplied to help improve communication. If the patient is able to ambulate, he is encouraged to do so in an unhurried way.

The emotional preparation of the patient is also important,

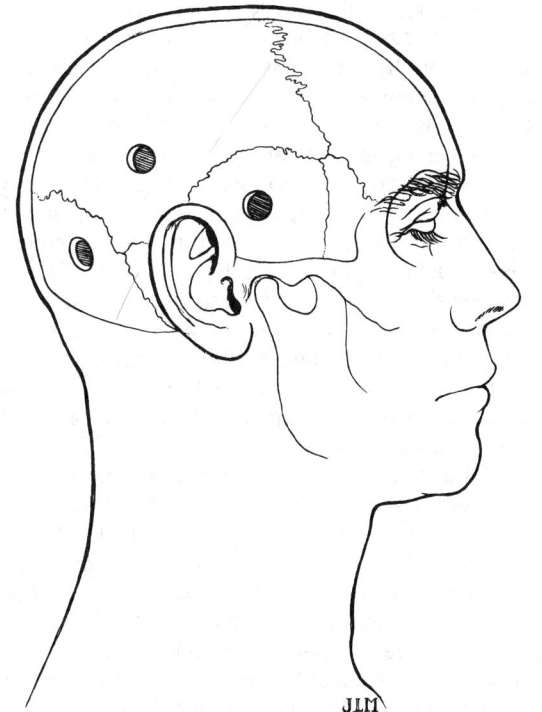

Figure 56-10. Burr holes may be used in neurosurgical procedures to make a bone flap in the skull, to aspirate a brain abscess, or to evacuate a hematoma.

including informing him of postoperative expectations. The large head dressing applied after surgery may impair his hearing ability temporarily. He will have difficulty seeing if his eyes are swollen shut. If he has a tracheostomy or endotracheal tube, he will be unable to talk. Thus, an alternate method of communication should be developed before surgery.

The patient's altered cognitive state may make him unaware that he is about to undergo surgery. Even so, encouragement and attention to his needs usually reinforce his confidence. Whatever the state of awareness of the patient, the family needs reassurance and consideration, because they recognize the seriousness of a brain operation.

▷ Postoperative Assessment

The frequency of postoperative nursing monitoring of the patient undergoing intracranial surgery is determined minute by minute or hour by hour, depending on his clinical status. Assessment of respiratory status is essential because small degrees of hypoxia can aggravate cerebral ischemia. The respiratory rate and patterns of respiration are monitored, and arterial blood gas values are reviewed. Fluctuations of the patient's vital signs are carefully monitored and documented because they indicate increased ICP. The patient's rectal temperature is measured at intervals to evaluate for hyperthermia that may result from damage to the hypothalamus.

Neurologic checks are made frequently to detect increased ICP resulting from edema or bleeding after intracranial surgery. A change in the level of responsiveness or consciousness may be the first sign of increasing ICP. Assessment of neurologic status includes determining the level of responsiveness or consciousness, eye signs, motor response, and vital signs. The nurse carefully observes for the insidious development of any neurologic deficit, such as diminished response to stimuli, speech problems, difficulty in swallowing, weakness or paralysis of an extremity, visual changes (diplopia, blurred vision), and paresthesias. The patient is observed for restlessness, which may reflect a return to consciousness or may be due to pain, confusion, an obstructed urinary drainage system, or other stimuli. Any evidence of seizure activity is reported immediately.

The patient's head dressing is inspected to determine the presence of bleeding and CSF drainage. In patients undergoing transsphenoidal surgery, the nasal packing is checked for signs of bloody or CSF drainage.

The intravenous infusion drip rate monitoring device is checked to see that it is working properly to prevent too rapid infusion of fluids. The infusion site is observed for redness, pain, swelling, or purulent drainage.

Patient positioning depends on the surgical approach used. The patient's neck should be in a straight line, however, because neck flexion may interfere with cerebral drainage.

The nurse is always alert to the development of complications (p. 1684), and all assessment is carried out with these problems in mind.

▷ Nursing Diagnoses

Based on the assessment data, the patient's major nursing diagnoses after intracranial surgery may include the following:

- Altered cerebral tissue perfusion related to cerebral edema.
- Potential for ineffective thermoregulation related to damage to the hypothalamus, dehydration, and infection

- Altered fluid and electrolyte balance related to possible metabolic or hormonal dysfunction
- Sensory-perceptual alterations (visual, auditory, possibly speech) related to periorbital edema, head dressing, endotracheal tube, and effects of ICP
- High risk for infection (intracranial and other) related to neurosurgical procedure (brain exposure; bone exposure, removal and replacement; wound hematomas)
- Potential for impaired gas exchange related to hypoventilation, aspiration, and immobility
- Body image disturbance related to change in appearance or physical disabilities

Other nursing diagnoses may include impaired communication (aphasia) related to insult to brain tissue and high risk for impaired skin integrity related to immobility, pressure, and incontinence. There may be impaired physical mobility related to a neurologic deficit secondary to the neurosurgical procedure.

▷ Planning and Implementation

▷ *Goals:* The major goals of the patient may include achievement of neurologic homeostasis to improve cerebral tissue perfusion, achievement of thermoregulation, achievement or maintenance of fluid and electrolyte balance, ability to cope with sensory deprivation, avoidance of intracranial infection, avoidance of pulmonary infection, and restoration of confidence concerning body image. A summary of the nursing management of the patient having intracranial surgery is given in Chart 56-3.

Nursing Interventions

▷ *Achieving Neurologic Homeostasis.* Attention to the respiratory status is essential because even slight deficiencies in oxygen supply (hypoxia) can aggravate cerebral ischemia. Nursing assessment and monitoring affect the clinical course. The endotracheal tube is left in place until the patient shows signs of awakening and is breathing spontaneously, as evaluated clinically and by arterial blood gas analysis. Secondary brain damage can result from impaired cerebral oxygenation.

Cerebral edema is an increase in the water content of brain tissue leading to an increase in brain volume. Some degree of cerebral edema occurs after brain surgery, and it tends to be maximal 24 to 36 hours postoperatively. This is why there may be a slump in the patient's level of responsiveness on the second postoperative day. The control of cerebral edema is discussed on p. 1647. The nursing strategies employed to eliminate factors contributing to the elevation of ICP are found on p. 1649. Intraventricular drainage is carefully monitored, using strict asepsis if any part of the system is handled.

The vital signs and neurologic checks (level of responsiveness, pupillary and motor responses) are made every 15 minutes to 1 hour and recorded. Extreme head rotation is avoided, as this raises ICP. After a supratentorial operation, the patient is placed on his back or side (unoperated side if a large lesion was removed) with one pillow under his head. The head of the bed may be elevated 20 to 30 degrees according to the level of the ICP and the neurosurgeon's directives. (Usually, the patient is kept in relatively the same position as during the operation.) After a posterior fossa operation (in-

Chart 56–3
Summary: Nursing Management of the Patient Having Intracranial Surgery

Postoperative Interventions

Nursing Diagnosis: Potential for ineffective breathing pattern related to postoperative cerebral edema

Goal: Achievement of adequate respiratory function
1. Establish proper respiratory exchange to eliminate systemic hypercarbia and hypoxia, which increase cerebral edema.
   a. Unless contraindicated, place the patient in a lateral or a semiprone position to facilitate respiratory exchange until consciousness returns.
   b. Employ tracheopharyngeal aspiration cautiously to remove secretions; suctioning can raise intracranial pressure.
   c. Maintain patient on controlled ventilation if prescribed to maintain normal ventilatory status; monitor arterial blood gas results to determine respiratory adequacy.
   d. Elevate the head of the bed 30.5 cm (12 in) after patient is conscious to aid venous drainage of the brain.
   e. Administer nothing by mouth until active coughing and swallowing reflexes are demonstrated; this prevents regurgitation.
   f. Ensure cardiovascular stability.

Potential Complication: Cerebral edema secondary to intracranial surgery

Goal: Prevention of cerebral edema
1. Assess patient's level of responsiveness/consciousness; the diminution of the level of consciousness may be the first sign of increased intracranial pressure.
   a. Eye opening (spontaneous, to sound, to pain); pupillary reactions to light
   b. Response to commands
   c. Assessment of spinal motor reflexes (pinch Achilles tendon, arm, or other body site)
   d. Observation of patient's spontaneous activity
2. Keep a neurologic flow sheet for sequentially assessing and documenting neurologic status, fluid administration, therapeutic agents, and laboratory data.
3. Evaluate for signs and symptoms of increasing intracranial pressure, which can lead to ischemia and further impairment of brain function.
   a. Assess patient minute by minute, hour by hour, for:
      1) Diminished response to stimuli
      2) Fluctuations of vital signs
      3) Restlessness
      4) Weakness and paralysis of extremities
      5) Increasing headache
      6) Changes or disturbances of vision; pupillary changes
   b. Modify nursing management to prevent further increases in intracranial pressure (see p. 1649).
4. Control postoperative cerebral edema as prescribed.
   a. Administer steroids and osmotic dehydrating agents when prescribed in postoperative period to reduce brain swelling.
   b. Monitor fluid intake; basic fluid requirements are usually precisely calculated; care is taken not to overload the patient.

c. Maintain a normal temperature during the postoperative period. Temperature control may be lost in certain neurologic states, and fever increases the metabolic demands of the brain.
   1) Monitor rectal temperature at specified intervals. Assess temperature of extremities, which may be cold and dry due to paralysis of heat-losing mechanisms (vasodilation and sweating).
   2) Employ measures as prescribed to reduce excessive fever when present: ice bags to axillae and groin; tepid or cool water sponges; hypothermia blanket. Use ECG monitoring to detect dysrhythmias during hypothermia procedures.
d. Employ hyperventilation when prescribed (results in respiratory alkalosis, which causes cerebral vasoconstriction and reduces circulation, which therefore reduces intracranial pressure).
e. Elevate head of bed to reduce intracranial pressure and facilitate respirations.
f. Avoid excessive stimuli.
g. Use intracranial pressure monitoring if patient is at risk for intracranial hypertension.

Nursing Diagnosis: Potential alteration in fluid volume related to intracranial pressure or diuretics

Goal: Attainment of fluid and electrolyte balance
1. Monitor for polyuria especially during first postoperative week; diabetes insipidus may develop in patients with lesions around the pituitary or hypothalamus
   a. Measure urinary specific gravity at intervals.
   b. Monitor serum and urinary electrolyte levels.
2. Evaluate patient's electrolyte status, because after certain major procedures patients have a tendency to retain water and sodium.
   a. Early postoperative weight gain indicates fluid retention; a greater than estimated weight loss indicates negative water balance.
   b. Loss of sodium and chloride will produce weakness, lethargy, and coma.
   c. Low potassium will cause confusion and decreased level of responsiveness.
3. Weigh patient daily; keep intake and output record.
4. Administer prescribed intravenous fluids with care—rate and composition depend on fluid deficit, urine output and composition, and blood loss. Fluid intake and fluid losses should remain relatively equal.

Nursing Diagnosis: Alteration in sensory perceptions (visual/auditory) related to periorbital edema and head dressings

Goal: Compensate for sensory deprivation
1. Perform supportive measures until the patient is able to care for himself.
   a. Change position as indicated; be aware that position changes can increase intracranial pressure.

(continued)

Chart 56-3 *(continued)*

Postoperative Interventions

    b. Administer prescribed analgesics (codeine) that do not mask the level of responsiveness.

2. Employ prescribed measures to relieve signs of periocular edema.
    a. Lubricate eyelids and around eyes with petrolatum.
    b. Apply light, cold compresses over eyes at specified intervals.
    c. Observe for signs of keratitis if cornea has no sensation.

3. Put extremities through range of motion exercises.

4. Evaluate and support patient during episodes of restlessness.
    a. Evaluate for airway obstruction, distended bladder, meningeal irritation from bloody cerebrospinal fluid.
    b. Pad patient's hands and bed rails to protect him from injury.

5. Reinforce blood-stained dressings with sterile dressing; blood-soaked dressings act as a culture medium for bacteria.

6. Orient patient frequently to time, place, and person.

Monitoring the Patient for Complications

1. *Intracranial hemorrhage*
    a. Postoperative bleeding may be intraventricular, intracerebellar, subdural, or extradural.
    b. Observe for progressive impairment of state of responsiveness and other signs of increasing intracranial pressure.
    c. Prepare deteriorating patient for reoperation and evacuation of hematoma.

2. *Increased intracranial pressure; cerebral edema* (see p. 1648)

3. *Seizures* (There is a greater risk with supratentorial operations.)
    a. Administer prescribed anticonvulsants; monitor anticonvulsant blood levels.
    b. Observe for status epilepticus, which may occur after any intracranial operation.

4. *Infections*
    a. Urinary tract infections
    b. Pulmonary infections related to aspiration secondary to depressed level of responsiveness; may result in atelectasis and bronchopneumonia
    c. CNS infections (postoperative meningitis, cerebrospinal fluid shunt infection)
    d. Wound infections/septicemia

5. *Venous thrombosis*

6. *Leakage of cerebrospinal fluid*
    a. Differentiate between cerebrospinal fluid and mucus.
      1) Collect fluid on Dextrostix; if cerebrospinal fluid is present, the indicator will have a positive reaction, as cerebrospinal fluid contains glucose.
      2) Assess for moderate elevation of temperature and mild neck rigidity.
    b. Caution patient against nose blowing or sniffing.
    c. Elevate head of bed as prescribed.
    d. Assist with insertion of lumbar subarachnoid drainage catheter that is inserted to lower spinal fluid pressure.
      1) Ventricular catheters may be inserted in the patient undergoing surgery of the posterior fossa (ventriculostomy); the catheter(s) is connected to a closed reservoir system.
      2) Administer antibiotics as prescribed.

7. *Gastrointestinal ulceration;* monitor for signs and symptoms of hemorrhage, perforation, or both (probably caused by stress response).

Evaluation

Expected Outcomes

1. Demonstrates normal breathing pattern
    a. Absence of crackles
    b. Demonstrates active swallowing and coughing reflexes

2. Demonstrates improved neurologic function
    a. Opens eyes on request
    b. Obeys commands
    c. Has appropriate motor responses
    d. Shows increasing alertness

3. Attains/maintains fluid balance
    a. Takes fluids orally
    b. Maintains weight within expected range

4. Compensates for sensory deprivation
    a. Makes needs known
    b. Demonstrates improvement of vision

5. Reveals absence of complications
    a. No evidence of increased intracranial pressure
    b. No evidence of rhinorrhea, otorrhea, or spinal fluid seepage
    c. Absence of fever
    d. No evidence of inflammation or infection around wound
    e. Absence of seizures

fratentorial), the patient is kept flat on his side (off his back) with his head on a small, firm pillow. He may be turned on either side, but his head should not be flexed on his chest. When the patient is being turned, his body should be turned as a unit to prevent strain on the wound and possible tearing of the sutures.

The patient's position is changed every 2 hours and skin care is given frequently. If the position is changed too frequently, the intracranial monitoring equipment is disrupted. A turning sheet from the head to the mid-thigh level makes it easier to move the patient.

▷ **Temperature Regulation.** Moderate levels of fever can be expected after intracranial operations because of reaction to blood at the operative site or in the subarachnoid. Injury to the hypothalamic centers that control heat-conserving mechanisms can occur during surgery. High fever is treated vigorously to combat the effect of increasing temperature on brain metabolism and function. Nursing interventions include taking the temperature at specified intervals and employing measures to reduce excessive fever: removing blankets, applying ice caps to axilla and groin areas, administering tepid to cold sponges, allowing a fan to blow on the patient to increase surface cooling, and using a hypothermia blanket as directed.

Conversely, hypothermia may be seen after lengthy neurosurgical procedures. Therefore, frequent measurements of rectal temperature are necessary.

▷ *Maintaining Fluid and Electrolyte Balance.* The postoperative fluid regimen depends on the type of neurosurgical procedure and is calculated on an individual basis. The volume and composition of fluids are adjusted according to daily electrolyte determinations and intake and output.

Electrolyte imbalance, particularly sodium imbalance, may contribute to the development of cerebral edema. Sodium retention is observed in the immediate postoperative period in certain intracranial operations. Serum and urine electrolytes, blood urea nitrogen, blood glucose, weight, and clinical status are monitored. The intake and output are measured in view of losses incurred from fever, respiration, and ventricular or spinal drainage. Fluids may have to be restricted in patients with cerebral edema.

Oral fluids are usually resumed in a short period, and the body's own homeostatic mechanisms regulate electrolyte balance. Some patients with posterior fossa tumors may have impaired swallowing, however, and fluids may have to be administered by way of alternate routes.

Patients having surgery for brain tumors may be on large doses of corticosteroids and thus may have a tendency to develop hyperglycemia. Serum glucose levels are then measured every 4 hours. Because these patients are prone to gastric ulcers, antacids or H_2-receptor blockers may be prescribed to reduce the secretion of gastric acid.

After surgery in and around the pituitary gland and hypothalamus, the patient may develop symptoms of diabetes insipidus, which is characterized by excessive urinary output. The urine specific gravity is measured hourly, and fluid intake and output charts are monitored.

The syndrome of inappropriate secretion of antidiuretic hormone (SIADH), resulting in water retention with hyponatremia and serum hypo-osmolality, occurs in a wide variety of CNS dysfunctions (brain tumor, head trauma) causing fluid disturbances. Fluid intake must compensate for the increased urine output to prevent dehydration. Electrolytes need to be monitored frequently, especially serum potassium levels. Nursing management of this syndrome requires careful intake and output measurements, specific gravity determinations of urine, and monitoring of serum and urine electrolyte studies, while following directives for fluid restriction. This syndrome is usually self-limiting.

▷ *Coping With Sensory Deprivation.* Periorbital edema is a common consequence of intracranial surgery because fluid drains into the dependent periorbital areas when the patient has been positioned in a prone position during surgery.

When drainage catheters are not used, a hematoma frequently forms under the scalp and spreads down to the orbit, producing an area of ecchymosis (black eye). Sometimes the eyes cannot be opened for a few days because of edema of the eyelids.

Preoperatively, the patient is warned that one or both eyes may close temporarily after operation. The head-up position and cold compresses over the eyes help reduce the edema. If it worsens significantly, however, it may indicate that a postoperative clot is developing or that there is increasing ICP and poor venous drainage. The surgeon is then notified. Health care personnel should announce their presence when entering the room to avoid startling the patient.

▷ *Preventing and Managing Intracranial and Other Infections.* There is an increased risk for infection in patients who undergo lengthy intracranial operations, those with external ventricular drains left in place longer than 48 to 72 hours, and those with neurosurgical procedures in the region of the third ventricle of the hypothalamus. A CSF leak carries the threat of infection and meningitis.

An early rise in temperature after surgery may be due to the reaction to blood at the operative site. This usually resolves in a few days.

The incision site is monitored for evidence of redness, tenderness, bulging, separation, or foul odor. The dressing is often stained with blood in the immediate postoperative period. It is important to reinforce the dressing with sterile pads so that contamination and infection may be avoided. (Blood is an excellent culture medium for bacteria.) If the dressing is heavily stained or displaced, it should be reported immediately. (A drain is sometimes placed in the craniotomy wound to facilitate drainage.)

After suboccipital operations, CSF may leak through the wound. This complication is dangerous because of the possibility of meningitis. Any sudden discharge of fluid from a cranial or spinal wound is reported at once because a massive leak requires direct surgical repair. Attention should be paid to the patient complaining of a salty taste in his mouth because this can be due to CSF trickling down his throat. He is warned against coughing, sneezing, or nose blowing, which may cause CSF leakage by creating pressure on the operative site.

Other causes of infection in the patient having intracranial surgery are similar to those of other postoperative patients: phlebitis, deep vein thrombosis, and urinary tract infections.

▷ *Improving Gas Exchange.* Neurosurgical patients are at risk for impaired gas exchange and pulmonary infections because of immobility, immunosuppression, decreased levels of awareness, and fluid restriction. Immobility compromises the respiratory system by causing pooling and stasis of secretions in dependent areas and the development of atelectasis. Underhydrated patients may be more vulnerable to atelectasis as a result of inability to expectorate thickened secretions. Pneumonia is frequently seen in neurosurgical patients, possibly related to aspiration.

The patient is observed for signs of respiratory infection: rise in temperature, increase in pulse rate, and changes in respirations. The lungs are auscultated for decreasing breath sounds and the presence of adventitious sounds.

Nursing interventions include repositioning the patient every 2 hours to mobilize secretions and prevent stasis; encouragement of yawning, sighing, deep breathing, and coughing to open up collapsed alveoli; and suctioning secretions that cannot be raised by cough. It is important to remember that coughing and suctioning raise ICP. Humidification of the air may be helpful. The nurse works interdependently with the respiratory therapist to monitor the effects of pulmonary physical therapy.

▷ *Assessing for Postoperative Complications.*   Complications that may develop within hours after surgery include intracranial bleeding or hematoma, cerebral edema, and water intoxication. These problems require close collaboration between the nurse and the surgeon.

- A drop in blood pressure, a rapid pulse and respiration, and a pale and cold body are usually manifestations of hypovolemic shock after long operations. This type of shock is best treated by blood component therapy.
- Conversely, an increase in blood pressure and decrease in pulse with respiratory failure may indicate increased ICP.
- An accumulation of blood under the bone flap (extradural, subdural, intracerebral) may pose a threat to life. A clot must be suspected in any patient who does not waken as expected or whose condition deteriorates. An intracranial hematoma is suspected if the patient has any new postoperative neurologic deficits (especially a dilated pupil on the side of surgery). In these events, the patient is returned to the operating room immediately for evacuation of the clot if indicated.
- Cerebral edema, infarction, metabolic disturbances, and hydrocephalus are conditions that may simulate the clinical manifestations of a clot.

Interdependent nursing functions include monitoring the patient for these complications, reporting early signs and trends in clinical status to the surgeon, initiating treatments promptly, and assisting in evaluating the patient's response to treatment. Additionally, the nurse provides support to the patient and family.

In addition to the immediate postoperative complications, other complications may occur during the first 2 weeks or later and may endanger the patient's recovery. The most important of these are thromboembolic complications (deep vein thrombosis, pulmonary embolism), pulmonary infection, urinary infection, and pressure ulcers. Most of these complications may be avoided by frequent change of position, adequate suctioning of secretions, observation and auscultation for pulmonary complications, observation for urinary complications, and skin care.

Postoperative Seizures.   Seizures and epilepsy may be complications after any intracranial neurosurgical procedure. Preventing seizures is essential to avoid further cerebral edema. Administering the prescribed anticonvulsant medication before and immediately after the operation may prevent the appearance of seizures in subsequent months and years. Status epilepticus (occurrence of prolonged seizures without recovery of consciousness in the intervals between seizures) may occur after craniotomy and also may be related to the development of complications (hematoma, ischemia). The management of status epilepticus is described in Chapter 57.

General Postoperative Interventions.   Patients without complications are ambulated with assistance as soon as possible, whereas those with depressed levels of responsiveness require nursing management similar to that for the unconscious patient (p. 1659). Postneurosurgical patients with motor deficits require nursing management similar to that after a stroke (p. 1670). Those with postoperative intellectual and speech impairment require psychological evaluation, speech therapy, and rehabilitation. The nurse works collaboratively with these health care professionals to achieve as complete a rehabilitation of the patient as is possible.

Achieving Self-acceptance.   The patient is encouraged to verbalize his feelings and frustrations about his changed appearance. Nursing support is based on the patient's feelings and their expression. Factual information may need to be provided if the patient has misconceptions about puffiness about the face, periorbital bruising, and hair loss. Attention to grooming, the use of his own clothing, and covering the head with a turban (and ultimately a wig until hair growth occurs) are encouraged. Social interaction with close friends, family, and hospital personnel may increase his sense of self-worth.

It takes time for the acquisition of a good body image. As the patient begins to take more responsibility for self-care and participates in more experiences, he gains a sense of control and personal competence. The patient's family and social support system can help sustain him until adaptation is fully made.

Patient Education and Home Health Care.   The convalescence at home of a neurosurgical patient depends on the extent of the procedure and its success. The family is made aware of the patient's strengths as well as limitations and their part in promoting his recovery. Because remembering to take the anticonvulsant medication is a priority, the patient and family are advised to have a check-off system to make sure the medication is taken. The patient may need to be accompanied while walking if he has sudden attacks of dizziness or seizures.

Usually the patient does not have any dietary restrictions unless there is another health problem requiring a special diet. He may take a shower or tub bath but should avoid getting his scalp wet until all the sutures have been removed. A clean scarf or cap may be worn until a wig or hairpiece is purchased. If skull bone has been removed, the neurosurgeon may suggest a protective helmet.

After a craniotomy, the patient is usually more sensitive to loud noises. Television noise can be irritating to the convalescing person. If the patient is aphasic, speech therapy may be necessary. This is likely to become a long-term and time-consuming project. It demands great patience and continuing encouragement on the part of all who are working with the patient.

When tumor, injury, or disease is of such a nature that the prognosis is poor, care is directed toward making the patient as comfortable as possible. With return of the tumor or cerebral compression, the patient becomes less alert and aware. Other possible sequelae include paralysis, blindness, and seizures. If the family is not able to give this type of care, the community health nurse and social worker plan together with the family in making arrangements for additional home health care or in placing the patient in an extended-care or hospice facility. (See also section on cerebral metastases in Chap. 57.)

▷ *Evaluation*

Expected Outcomes

1. Achieves neurologic homeostasis/improved cerebral tissue perfusion
   a. Opens eyes on request; utters recognizable words progressing to normal speech
   b. Obeys commands with appropriate motor responses
2. Attains thermoregulation and normal body temperature
3. Attains fluid and electrolyte balance
   a. Demonstrates serum chemistries within acceptable limits for a patient undergoing intracranial surgery

b. Complies with fluid restriction
4. Copes with sensory deprivation
5. Has no intracranial infection
6. Has normal gas exchange
7. Demonstrates an improving self-concept
   a. Pays attention to grooming
   b. Visits and interacts with others

Transsphenoidal Surgery

Pituitary tumors (which represent 10% to 20% of all intracranial tumors) may be treated by surgery or irradiation. Surgical removal may be carried out through an open craniotomy (usually transfrontal) or by the transsphenoidal approach. The choice is determined by anatomic considerations and the extent and nature of the pathologic process.

Tumors located within the sella turcica and small adenomas of the pituitary can be removed by way of the transsphenoidal approach (Fig. 56-11). The incision is made beneath the upper lip, and entry is then gained successively into the nasal cavity, sphenoidal sinus, and sella turcica. Although the initial opening may be made by an otorhinolaryngologist, the neurosurgeon completes the opening into the sphenoidal sinus and exposes the floor of the sella. Microsurgical techniques provide improved illumination, magnification, and visualization so that nearby vital structures can be avoided.

This approach, which is being used with increased frequency, offers direct access to the sella with minimal risk of trauma and hemorrhage. It avoids many of the risks of craniotomy, and the postoperative discomfort is similar to that of other transnasal operations. It is also used for pituitary ablation (removal) in patients with disseminated breast or prostatic cancer.

Preoperative Evaluation. The preoperative workup includes a series of endocrine tests, rhinologic evaluation (to assess status of the sinuses and nasal cavity), and neuroradiologic studies. Funduscopic examination and visual field determinations are performed, because the most serious effect of pituitary tumor is localized pressure on the optic nerve or chiasm. In addition, the nasopharyngeal secretions are cultured because a sinus infection is a contraindication to an intracranial procedure through this approach. Cortisone may be given preoperatively and postoperatively (because the source of adrenocorticotropic hormone is removed). Antibiotics may or may not be administered prophylactically. Deep breathing is taught preoperatively. The patient is instructed to avoid vigorous coughing and sneezing because they may cause a CSF leak after surgery. He is instructed to apply pressure on the inner aspect of both sides of the nose to control sneezing.

Postoperative Management

Because there has been disruption of the oral and nasal mucous membranes, management focuses on preventing infection and promoting healing. Medications given to the patient include antimicrobials (which are continued until the nasal packing is removed), corticosteroids, analgesics for discomfort, and agents for the control of diabetes insipidus, when necessary.

The nasal packing is removed in 24 hours to several days. The area around the nares is cleaned with the prescribed solution to remove crusted blood and moisten the mucous membranes.

Postoperative Nursing Interventions

The vital signs are measured to monitor hemodynamic, cardiac, and ventilatory status. Because of the anatomic proximity of the pituitary gland to the optic chiasm, visual acuity is assessed at regular intervals. One method is to ask the patient to count the number of fingers held up by the nurse. Evidence of decreasing visual acuity suggests an expanding hematoma.

The major discomfort of the patient is related to the nasal

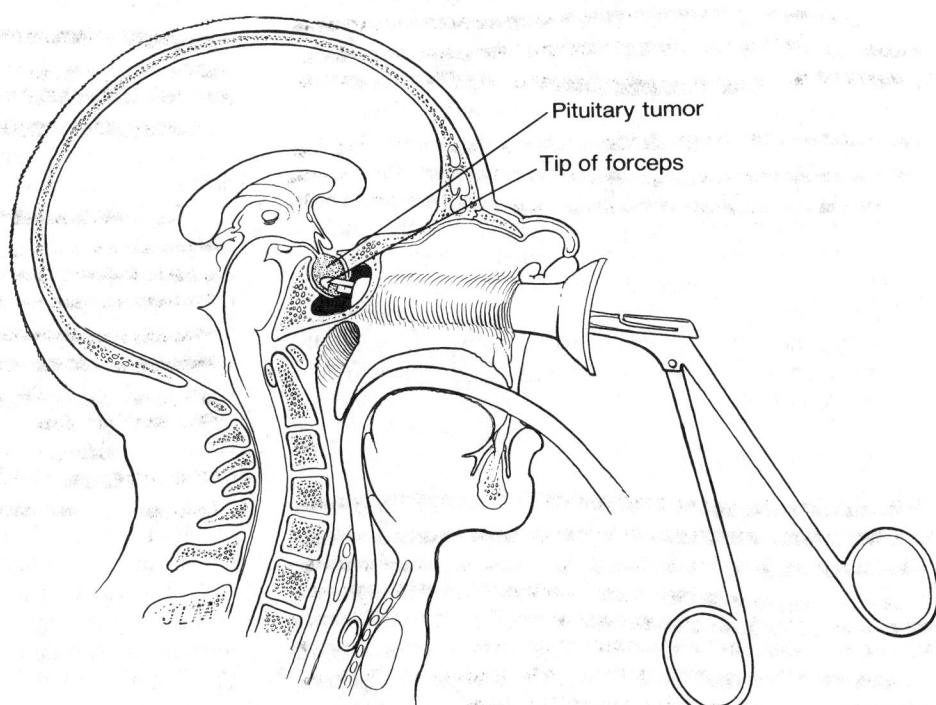

Figure 56-11. Transsphenoidal approach to the pituitary. A special nasal speculum is used to view the sinus cavity. After the dura is opened, the tumor is removed using microcurettes or other specially designed instruments.

packing and to mouth dryness and thirst from mouth-breathing. Oral care is provided every 4 hours or more frequently. Usually, the patient's teeth are not brushed until the incision above the teeth has healed. The use of warm saline mouth rinses, dental floss, and occasionally a cool mist vaporizer is helpful. Petrolatum is soothing when applied to the lips. A room humidifier assists in keeping the patient's mucous membranes moist.

The head of the bed is raised to decrease pressure on the sella turcica and to promote normal drainage. The patient is cautioned against blowing his nose or engaging in any activity that raises ICP, such as bending over or straining during urination or defecation.

The intake and output are measured as a guide to fluid and electrolyte replacement. The urinary specific gravity is measured after each voiding. The patient's daily weight is monitored. Fluids are generally given when nausea ceases, and the patient then progresses to a regular diet.

Complications

Manipulation of the posterior pituitary gland during operation may produce transient diabetes insipidus of several days' duration that is treated with vasopressin. Occasionally, there is more persistent diabetes insipidus. Other complications include CSF leakage, postoperative meningitis, and SIADH.

The patient is advised to have a room humidifier when he returns home. This keeps the membranes moist and soothes irritation. Keeping the head of the bed elevated for at least 2 weeks after surgery is helpful.

Neurosurgical Treatment of Pain

The management of long-term pain requires a multidisciplinary approach. (See Chap. 15 for a discussion of the basic theories of the psychophysiology of pain and its management.)

Intractable pain refers to pain that cannot be relieved satisfactorily by drugs without causing addiction or incapacitating sedation. Such pain usually is the result of malignancy (especially of the cervix, bladder, prostate, and lower bowel), but it does occur in many other conditions, such as postherpetic neuralgia, trigeminal neuralgia, spinal cord arachnoiditis, and uncontrollable ischemia and other forms of tissue destruction.

Neurosurgical methods available for pain relief include (1) stimulation procedures: intermittent electric stimulation of a tract or center to inhibit the transfer of pain information, (2) administration of intraspinal opiates, and (3) interruption of the tracts conducting the pain between the periphery and the cerebral integration centers. The latter are destructive or ablative procedures.

Stimulation Procedures

Electrical stimulation, or neuromodulation, is a method of suppressing pain by applying controlled low-voltage electrical pulses to the different parts of the nervous system. Electrical stimulation is thought to relieve pain by preventing messages from reaching the brain by blocking small afferent-fiber input at the dorsal horn or by stimulating the release of endogenous opiates (natural pain-relieving peptides). This pain-modulating technique is administered by many modes. Transcutaneous electrical nerve stimulation and dorsal column stimulation are the procedures most frequently performed. In addition, there are also brain stimulators in which stimulating electrodes are implanted in the periventricular area of the posterior third ventricle, allowing self-stimulation of the periventricular gray area to produce analgesia.

Transcutaneous Electric Nerve Stimulation

Transcutaneous electric nerve stimulation (TENS) is the passage of small electrical currents through the skin for the purpose of controlling localized pain. The stimulating electrodes are placed over the site of pain or along the course of the major peripheral nerves innervating the area, or over the peripheral plexus. The patient operates the amplitude control until stimulation, detected by a vibration, buzzing, or tapping sensation, is felt within the deeper tissue. The amplitude is increased slowly until the sensation is perceived at the site or origin of pain or along radiating pathways. The patient controls the amplitude, frequency, and duration of stimulation. It appears useful to the well-instructed patient in the early management of acute pain as well as for the patient with chronic pain. It is best used as an adjunct to a comprehensive rehabilitation program for relief and elimination of pain.

Patient Education for TENS. The patient is given the instruction booklet provided by the manufacturing company that explains care of the skin, electrodes, and generator. The skin is cleansed and electrode gel is applied to the electrodes, which are then placed over the nerves that innervate the painful area. The electrodes are secured with hypoallergenic tape. The major problem of TENS is skin irritation from the tape (from mechanical stresses created by shearing forces between tape and skin), gels, or electrodes. The patient is advised to keep a record evaluating the effectiveness of TENS. If there is a progression of pathology (as in advanced cancer), changes in amplitude may be necessary.

Dorsal Column Stimulation

Dorsal column stimulation (DCS) is a technique used for the relief of chronic intractable pain in which a surgically implanted device allows the patient to apply pulsed electrical stimulation to the dorsal aspect of the spinal cord to block pain impulses. (The largest accumulation of afferent fibers is found in the dorsal column of the spinal cord.)

The dorsal column stimulation unit consists of a radio frequency stimulation transmitter, a transmitter antenna, a radio frequency receiver, and a stimulation electrode. The battery-powered transmitter and antenna are worn externally while the receiver and electrode are implanted. A laminectomy is performed above the highest level of pain input, and the electrode is placed in the epidural space over the posterior column of the spinal cord. (The placement of the stimulating systems is varied.) The subcutaneous pocket is constructed over the clavicular area or some other site for placement of the receiver. The two are connected by a subcutaneous tunnel.

Postoperative Nursing Management. The postoperative nursing management is similar to that after a laminectomy. The patient is assessed for evidences of paraplegia, quadriplegia, and urinary incontinence. The extremities are evaluated for movement. The laminectomy site is assessed for leakage of CSF because the dura is opened during surgery. The implant site is also assessed for signs of infection. As soon as the patient is fully alert, the dorsal column stimulation system may be tested, although initial testing may not be accurate because a bandage may cover the receiver site. Complications include infection, cord trauma, CSF leakage, and pain around the implantation site.

Patient Education and Home Health Care.   The patient is given the manufacturer's booklet to become acquainted with the system. Proper skin care is taught as well as the method for attaching the antenna to the skin, connecting the transmitter, and adjusting the settings. Different stimulation frequencies should be tried to determine which one gives the best pain relief. A record is to be kept of the stimulation used. The patient is also instructed to keep several batteries in reserve. (Battery life depends on the extent of use.) The transmitter and antenna are cleaned according to the manufacturer's directions.

Percutaneous Epidural Neurostimulation

Percutaneous epidural neurostimulation is a method of neurostimulation in which electrodes are inserted percutaneously into the spinal epidural space. It appears effective in treating arachnoiditis and postamputation neuroma.

Deep Brain Stimulation

Deep brain stimulation is performed for special pain problems when the patient does not respond to the usual techniques of pain control. With the patient under local anesthesia, electrodes are introduced through a burr hole and inserted into a selected site in the brain, depending on the location or type of the patient's pain. After the effectiveness of stimulation is confirmed, the implanted electrode is connected to a radio frequency device or pulse generator system operated by external telemetry.

Immediate postoperative complications include infection and transient neurologic deficits after insertion of the electrodes. Failure of the stimulating system and development of tolerance may occur later. Nursing interventions include teaching the patient and family about the system, encouraging the patient to keep a record of amplitude and frequency settings and the relief obtained, and monitoring for complications.

Intraspinal Opiates

Opiate receptors have been demonstrated not only in the brain but also in the substantia gelatinosa of the spinal cord. These receptors can combine with locally administered opiates (morphine) injected epidurally or intrathecally to produce long-lasting pain relief with little or no blunting of the patient's level of responsiveness and no losses of sensory, motor, or sphincter function.

There are numerous techniques employed, but most include placing a catheter in the epidural or subarachnoid space with a spinal needle and inserting the catheter as near as possible to the spinal segment where the pain is projected. Small doses of preservative-free morphine diluted in saline are injected into the system at 6- to 24-hour intervals. If the patient requires long-term management, an implantable programmable pump is used.

After the procedure the patient is evaluated for the degree of pain relief, which ranges from good to excellent. The puncture site is examined for evidence of infection.

With this method, the patient may be at home. The necessary dose of drug is small, the patient's mind is clear, and he is usually able to function at a relatively high level. He may complain of generalized itching and urinary retention (self-limited) for several days. With long-term use there can be tolerance buildup and mechanical failure (catheter obstructed, dislodged, broken) of the administration system. If the patient has rapid tumor growth, the dosage of morphine is increased, but the doses needed are low in comparison to those required for systemic administration for intractable pain.

Destructive or Ablative Procedures

Pain-conducting fibers can be interrupted at any point from their origin to the cerebral cortex. There is destruction of some part of the nervous system that can result in varying amounts of neurologic deficit and incapacity. In time, pain usually returns as a result of either regeneration of axonal fibers or the development of alternative pain pathways.

Cordotomy.   Cordotomy is the division of certain tracts of the spinal cord. It may be performed percutaneously, by the open method after laminectomy, or by other techniques.

Percutaneous cordotomy uses radio frequency currents to produce lesions in the anterolateral surface of the spinal cord. With the patient under local anesthesia, a needle is inserted into the neck below and behind the mastoid process. It is guided into the spinal cord under x-ray control, and then an electrode is inserted through it. By means of radio frequency currents, a lesion is made at the desired spinal cord level.

Verification of electrode placement is determined by the patient's response to stimulation. The procedure is tolerated by emaciated and debilitated patients.

An *open cordotomy* is the surgical division of the anterolateral columns of the spinal pain fibers high in the thoracic or cervical region. This procedure interrupts or destroys conduction of pain and temperature sensation, while touch and position sense are preserved. The spinal cord is exposed by laminectomy. Cordotomy is used most frequently in controlling the severe pain of terminal cancer, especially of the thorax, abdomen, or lower extremities. Because a significant percentage of cordotomies lose their effectiveness in 1 to 5 years, the procedure is used for pain associated with conditions in which survival time is limited.

Postoperative Nursing Management.   The principles of nursing management after a laminectomy are applicable in the postoperative and rehabilitation requirements of this patient (see Chap. 57). After a cordotomy, the patient may be kept flat for the prescribed time, because there is less tension on the incision when this position is assumed. A patient with a thoracic cordotomy may be turned to the prone position. In instances of a cervical incision, pillows should not be used when the patient is in a supine position. Trauma to the surgical site is eliminated when the neck is kept in a neutral position. The patient is turned as a unit (log fashion) by two persons using a turning sheet to avoid twisting the body and putting pressure on the incision.

Assessment for Complications.   The patient is monitored for respiratory complications, as well as for signs of fatigue and weakening of the voice. The patient may ventilate adequately while awake but may experience progressive hypercarbia and hypoxia while asleep. Therefore, arterial blood gases are monitored, and assisted mechanical ventilation is initiated if required.

Because hemorrhage may result in motor and sensory loss, the motion, strength, and sensation of each extremity must be tested every few hours, or more frequently if necessary, during the first 48 hours postoperatively. If hemorrhage is suggested or detected, immediate surgical intervention is imperative. Because the patient has no sense of temperature, the skin should be palpated at intervals to ascertain any changes in temperature. Because pressure ulcers may develop without the patient realizing it, the patient is taught to inspect his skin using a hand mirror to view the hard-to-see areas and to change position frequently. Urinary retention may occur. There is usually a slow return to normal voiding, but this cannot be guaranteed. If there is permanent loss of urinary control from a high cervical procedure, a bladder training program is started.

Rhizotomy. Rhizotomy is the surgical division of the spinal roots and is used in controlling severe chest pain of lung cancer and for pain relief in head and neck malignancies.

Because many patients with metastatic malignancies may not be able to tolerate an open rhizotomy, a *percutaneous rhizotomy* may be performed, whereby a radio frequency current is used to selectively coagulate the pain fibers, while the fibers concerned with touch and proprioception are preserved.

A *chemical rhizotomy* is one in which alcohol, phenol, or a mixture of drugs is injected into the subarachnoid space. The medication is maneuvered over the affected nerve roots by tilting the patient to the desired level. This renders the sensory nerve roots functionless. The patient's perception of pain is absent, but the motor nerve roots are usually not affected.

Psychosurgical Approaches

The purpose of psychosurgical procedures is to alter the patient's response to pain. A *thalamotomy* is the destruction (either unilateral or bilateral) of the specific cell groups within the thalamus. Burr holes are made in the skull, electrodes are placed in the target area by stereotaxic techniques, and a radiofrequency current is then directed through the electrodes to create the lesion. This procedure represents the highest level in the CNS in which pain pathways can be interrupted and is usually performed for malignancy of the head and neck.

Cingulotomy is a unilateral or bilateral interruption of the anterior cingulate bundle in the frontal lobe of the brain. It is accomplished either by an open or stereotaxic approach. It tends to modify the patient's affective reaction to pain.

Chapter Summary

Neurologic disorders may be acute and life threatening; they also may be chronic disorders that alter the function and well-being of the patient. Rarely do neurologic disorders affect only the patient; they often have a direct influence on the functioning and well-being of the patient's family as well. Although many neurologic disorders are treatable through surgery or medical regimens, the potential consequences of many neurologic disorders are frequently within the domain of independent nursing practice. It is often the nurse, in collaboration with other members of the health care team, who works most closely with the patient and family to identify and coordinate the resources and services (*i.e.*, physical therapy, occupational therapy, home health care nurse, social worker, speech therapist) that will promote the patient's rehabilitation.

The patient with neurologic dysfunction may initially exhibit a poor clinical prognosis, which may improve over time. The patient's neurologic status is continuously assessed for any changes, which may alter the outcome. The nurse needs to act swiftly and expediently to implement a plan of care, based on the patient's needs. The patient with neurologic deficits usually requires a plan of care that involves almost every other body system. The patient and family need to be supported and encouraged during the critical and rehabilitative periods. The patient who is neurologically dysfunctional needs rehabilitation and supportive care to promote his recovery and ability to complete ADL.

Bibliography

Books

Archer-Copp L (ed). Perspectives on Pain. New York, Churchill Livingstone, 1985.

Bannister R. Brain's Clinical Neurology, 6th ed. New York, Oxford University Press, 1985.

Barnett H et al. Stroke: Pathophysiology, Diagnosis and Management. New York, Churchill Livingstone, 1986.

Barr M and Kiernan J. The Human Nervous System: An Anatomical Viewpoint, 5th ed. Philadelphia, JB Lippincott, 1988.

Bates B. A Guide to the Physical Examination, 5th ed. Philadelphia, JB Lippincott, 1991.

Bonica J. The Management of Pain, 2nd ed. Philadelphia, Lea & Febiger, 1990.

Brandstater M and Basmajian J (ed). Stroke Rehabilitation. Baltimore, Williams & Wilkins, 1987.

Britt B. Malignant Hyperthermia. Boston, Kluwer Academic Publishers, 1987.

Burns M. Speech/Language Treatment of the Aphasias: An Integrated Clinical Approach. Rockville, MD, Aspen Publishers, 1988.

Chusid J. Correlative Neuroanatomy and Functional Neurology. Los Altos, CA, Lange Medical Publications, 1985.

Crockard A et al (eds). Neurosurgery: The Scientific Basis of Clinical Practice. Boston, Blackwell Scientific, 1985.

Davies P. Steps to Follow: A Guide to the Treatment of Adult Hemiplegia. New York, Springer-Verlag, 1985.

Decker BC. Current Therapy in Neurological Surgery. St Louis, CV Mosby, 1985.

Donnell F (ed). Clinical Management of Neurogenic Communicative Disorders, 2nd ed. Boston, Little, Brown, 1985.

Echternach J (ed). Pain. New York, Churchill Livingstone, 1987.

Fein J and Flamm E. Cerebrovascular Surgery. New York, Springer-Verlag, 1985.

Freidberg S. The neurosurgeon's approach to pain, evaluation and treatment of chronic pain. In Aronoff G (ed). Baltimore, Urban & Schwarzenberg, 1985, pp 319–331.

Gilroy J. Basic Neurology. New York, Pergamon Press, 1990.

Gunderson C. Essentials of Clinical Neurology. New York, Raven Press, 1990.

Heldick-Smith M. Neurologic Problems in the Elderly. Philadelphia, Bailliere Tindall, 1985.

Henning R and Jackson D. Handbook of Critical Care Neurology and Neurosurgery. New York, Praeger Scientific, 1985.

Henry G and Little N. Neurologic Emergencies: A Symptom-Oriented Approach. New York, McGraw-Hill, 1985.

Hickey J. The Clinical Practice of Neurological and Neurosurgical Nursing, 2nd ed. Philadelphia, JB Lippincott, 1986.

Johnstone M. The Stroke Patient: A Team Approach. New York, Churchill Livingstone, 1987.

Kaplan P and Cerullo L. Stroke Rehabilitation. Boston, Butterworths, 1986.

Lundgren J. Acute Neuroscience Nursing: Concepts and Care. Boston, Jones & Bartlett, 1986.

Marshall SB et al. Neuroscience Critical Care: Pathophysiology and Patient Management. Philadelphia, WB Saunders, 1990.

McCaffery M and Bebe A. Pain: Clinical Manual for Nursing Practice. St Louis, CV Mosby, 1989.

McLeod J. Introductory Neurology, 2nd ed. Chicago, Year Book Medical Publishers, 1989.

Millikan C. Stroke. Philadelphia, Lea & Febiger, 1987.

Pallett P and O'Brien M. Textbook of Neurological Nursing. Boston, Little, Brown, 1985.

Prithvi-Raj P (ed). Practical Management of Pain: Special Emphasis on Physiology of Pain Syndromes and Techniques of Management. Chicago, Year Book Medical Publishers, 1986.

Roper A and Kennedy S. Neurological and Neurosurgical Intensive Care, 2nd ed. Rockville, MD, Aspen Publishers, 1988.

Rosenbeck J et al. Aphasia: A Clinical Approach. Boston, Little, Brown, 1989.

Rowland LP (ed). Merritt's Textbook of Neurology, 8th ed. Philadelphia, Lea & Febiger, 1989.

Rudy E. Advanced Neurological and Neurosurgical Nursing. St Louis, CV Mosby, 1984.

Ryalls J (ed). Phonetic Approaches to Speech Production in Aphasia and Related Disorders. Boston, Little, Brown, 1987.

Salcman M (ed). Neurologic Emergencies: Recognition and Management, 2nd ed. New York, Raven Press, 1990.

Samuels M. Manual of Neurologic Therapeutics. Boston, Little, Brown, 1986.

Skinner P and Shelton R. Speech, Language and Hearing: Normal Processes and Disorders, 2nd ed. New York, John Wiley & Sons, 1985.

Smith G and Covino B. Acute Pain. Boston, Butterworths, 1985.

Spetzler R et al. Cerebral Revascularization for Stroke. New York, Thieme-Stratton, 1985.

Tindall G et al. Disorders of the Pituitary. St Louis, CV Mosby, 1986.

Umphred D. Neurological Rehabilitation. St Louis, CV Mosby, 1985.

Vogt G et al. Mosby's Manual of Neurological Care. St Louis, CV Mosby, 1985.

Wade D et al. Stroke: A Critical Approach to Diagnosis, Treatment, and Management. London, Chapman & Hall, 1985.

Weiner W and Goetz CG (ed). Neurology for the Non-Neurologist, 2nd ed. Philadelphia, JB Lippincott, 1989.

Weinstein P and Faden A. Protection of the Brain from Ischemia. Baltimore, Williams & Wilkins, 1989.

Wilkins R and Rengachary S. Neurosurgery. New York, McGraw-Hill, 1985.

Youmans J (ed). Neurological Surgery: A Comprehensive Reference Guide to the Diagnosis and Management of Neurosurgical Problems, 3rd ed. Philadelphia, WB Saunders, 1990.

Journals
Asterisks indicate nursing research articles.

Care of the Neurosurgical Patient

* Boortz-Marx R. Factors affecting intracranial pressure: A descriptive study. Journal of Neurosurgical Nursing 1985 Apr; 17(2):89–94.

Bouma G and Muizelaar J. Relationship between cardiac output and cerebral blood flow in patients with intact and with impaired autoregulation. J Neurosurg 1990 Sep; 73(3):368–374.

Cammermeyer M and Evans J. A brief neurobehavioral exam useful for early detection of postoperative complications in the neurosurgical patients. J Neurosurg Nurs 1988 Oct; 20(5):314–323.

Carpenter R. Infections and head injury: A potentially lethal combination. Crit Care Nurs Q 1987; 10: 1–11.

Chase M and Whelan-Decker E. Nursing management of a patient with subarachnoid hemorrhage. Neurosurg Nurs 1984; 16(1):23–29.

* Cunha B and Tu R. Fever in the neurosurgical patient. Heart Lung 1988 Nov; 17(6):608–611.

Dauch W and Bauer S. Circadian rhythms in the body temperatures of intensive care patients with brain lesions. J Neurol Neurosurg Psychiatry 1990 Apr; 53(4):345–347.

Diamond S. Headaches that herald intracranial emergencies. Emerg Med 1988; 20(2):20–24.

Dilorio C. An analysis of trends in neuroscience nursing research: 1960–1988. J Neurosci Nurs 1990 Jun; 22(3):139–146.

Flannery J. Guilt: A crisis within a crisis, a catostophic neurologic event. J Neurosci Nurs 1990 Apr; 22(2):83–88.

Gronert G et al. Aetiology of malignant hyperthermia. Br J Anaesth 1988 Feb; 60(13):253–267.

Grotta J. Current medical and surgical therapy for cerebrovascular disease. N Engl J Med 1987 Dec; 317(24):1505–1516.

Hannegan L. Transient cognitive changes after craniotomy. J Neurosurg Nurs 1989 Jun; 21(3):165–170.

Harper J. The use of steroids in cerebral edema: Therapeutic implications. Heart Lung 1988 Jan; 17(1):70–73.

Hendrickson S. Psychological care of the patient with neurological dysfunction. J Neurosurg Nurs 1984 Aug; 16(4):202–207.

Hinshaw A. Exciting challenges ahead: Neuroscience nursing research. J Neurosci Nurs 1990 Jun; 22(3):137–138.

Kruger L. Complications of transsphenoidal surgery. J Neurosurg Nurs 1985 Jun; 17(3):179–183.

McCash A. Meeting the Challenge of Craniotomy Care. RN 1985 Jul; 48(6): 26–33.

Miller J. Assessing patients with head injury. Br J Surg 1990 Mar; 77(3): 241–224.

* Morgan S. A comparison of three methods of managing fever in the neurologic patient. J Neurosci Nurs 1990 Feb; 22(1):19–24.

Nikas D (ed). Head trauma. Part 2. Nursing issues and controversies. Crit Care Nurse Q 1987 Jun; 10(1):3.

Norris M. Malignant hyperthermia. Nursing 1990 Jun; 20(6):33.

Reimer M. Head-injured patients: How to detect early signs of trouble. Nursing 1989 Mar; 19(3):34–42.

Resio M. Nursing diagnosis: Alteration in oral/nasal mucous membranes related to trauma of transsphenoidal surgery. J Neurosci Nurs 1986 Jun; 18(3):112–115.

Sloan T. Neurological monitoring. Crit Care Clin 1988(Jul); 4(3):543–557.

Smejkal C and Hill F. Life sustaining treatment: A legal-ethical dilemma. J Nurs Admin 1990 Jul/Aug; 20(7/8):49–52.

Wilberger J et al. Acute subdural hematoma: Morbidity and mortality related to timing of operative intervention. J Trauma 1990 Aug; 30(8):933—940.

Wolcott K and McDonnell A. Malignant hyperthermia: Nursing implications. Crit Care Nurse 1990 Mar; 10(3):78–85.

Stroke

Albert M et al. Diagnosis and treatment of aphasia. Part I. JAMA 1988 Feb; 259(7):1043–1047.

Albert, M. et al. Diagnosis and treatment of aphasia. Part II. JAMA 1988 Feb; 259(8):1205–1210.

Burgener S et al. Sexuality concerns of the post-stroke patient. Rehab Nurs 1989 Jul/Aug; 14(4):178–181.

Bonita R et al. Predicting survival after stroke: A three year follow-up. Stroke 1988 Jun; 19(6):669–673.

Byers V et al. Predictive risk factors associated with stroke patient falls in acute care settings. J Neurosci Nurs 1990 Jun; 22(3):147–154.

Carr E and Hawthorn P. Lip function and eating after a stroke: A nursing perspective. J Adv Nurs 1988; 13: 447–451.

Carr J et al. A motor learning model for stroke rehabilitation. Physiotherapy 1989 Jul; 75(7):72–80.

Doolittle N. Stroke recovery: Review of the literature and suggestions for future research. J Neurosurg Nurs 1988 Jun; 20(3):169–173.

Gorelick P. Cerebrovascular disease: Pathophysiology and diagnosis. Nurs Clin North Am 1986; 21(2):275–288.

Grosswasser Z et al. Rehabilitation outcome after anoxic brain damage. Arch Phys Med Rehabil 1989 Mar; 70(3):186–188.

Hagen C. Treatment of aphasia: A process approach. J Head Trauma Rehab 1988 Jun; 3(2):95–96.

Kasuya A and Holm K. Pharmacologic approach to ischemic stroke management. Nurs Clin North Am 1986; 21(2):289–296.

Keller C et al. Psychological respiration in aphasia: Theoretical considerations and nursing implications. J Neurosci Nurs 1989 Oct; 21(5): 290–294.

Kinkel W. Classification of stroke by neuroimaging technique. Stroke 1990 Sep; 21(9):117–118.

Pasquarello M. Measuring the impact of an acute stroke program on patient outcomes. J Neurosci Nurs 1990 Apr; 22(2):76–82.

Pinel C. Cerebrovascular accidents. Nursing (London) 1989 Jan; 3(33): 24–27.

Printz-Feddersen V. Group process effect on caregiver burden. J Neurosci Nurs 1990 Jun; 23(3):164–168.

Rao N. The art of medicine: Subjective measures as predictors of outcome in stroke and traumatic brain injury. Arch Phys Med Rehabil 1988 Mar; 69(3):179–182.

Rothrock J. Clinical evaluation and management of transient ischemic attacks. West J Med 1987 Apr; 146(4):452–460.

Smith A et al. Relationships between perceptions and language deficits in stroke patients. Br J Occup Ther 1989 Jan; 52(1):8–10.

Stroke, but which kind? Emerg Med 1989 Aug; 21(14):112–116.

Swaffield L. Striking back at strokes. Community Outlook 1989 Jun; 25–33.

Trueblood P et al. Pelvic exercise and gait in hemiplegia. Phys Ther 1989 Jan; 69(1):18–26.

Weingarten S et al. The principle of parsimony: Glasgow Coma Scale Score predicts mortality as well as the APACHE II score for stroke patients. Stroke 1990 Sep; 21(9):1280–1282.

Yanagihara T et al. Brief loss of consciousness in bilateral carotid occlusive disease. Arch Neurol 1989 Aug; 46(8):858–861.

Increased Intracranial Pressure

* Allen D. Intracranial pressure monitoring: A study of nursing practice. J Adv Nurs 1989 Feb; 14(2):127–131.

Barker E. Avoiding increased intracranial pressure. Nursing 1990 May; 20(5): 64Q–64RR.

Barker E. Myths and facts about increased intracranial pressure. Nursing 1988 Dec; 18(12):20.

* Bruya M. Planned periods of rest in the ICU: Nursing activities and ICP. J Neurosurg Nurs 1981 Aug; 13:184–194.

Constantini S et al. Intracranial pressure monitoring after elective intracranial surgery. J Neurosurg 1988 Oct; 69(4):540–544.

Davenport-Fortune P and Dunnam L. Professional nursing care of the patient with an increased intracranial pressure: Planned or "hit and miss." J Neurosci Nurs 1985 Dec; 17(6):367–379.

Drummond B. Preventing increased intracranial pressure: Nursing care can make the difference. Focus 1990 Apr; 17(2):116–122.

* Hendrickson SL. Intracranial pressure changes and family presence. J Neurosci Nurs 1987 Feb; 19(1):206–209.

Hickman M et al. Intracranial pressure monitoring: A review of risk factors associated with infection. Heart Lung 1990 Jan; 19(1):84–90.

Hinkle J. Treating traumatic coma. Am J Nurs 1986 May; 86(5):551–556.

Horner A and Mechsner W. Bedside insertion of ICP monitoring devices. Crit Care Nurse 1985 Jul/Aug; 5(4):21–27.

* Lee S. Intracranial pressure changes during positioning of patients with severe head injury. Heart Lung 1989 Jul; 18(4):411–414.

Lehman L. Intracranial pressure monitoring and treatment: A contemporary view. Ann Emerg Med 1990 Mar; 19(3):295–303.

Pollack-Latham C. Intracranial pressure monitoring. Part I. Physiologic principles. Crit Care Nurse 1987 Oct; 7(5):40–52.

Reimer M. Head injured patients: How to detect early signs of trouble. Nursing 1989 Mar; 19(3):34–42.

Shepard R and Hotter A. Evaluating an ICP epidural catheter. Crit Care Nurse 1989 Feb; 9(2):74–80.

Pain

Barker E. Pain. J Neurosurg Nurs 1987 Oct; 19(5):233–234.

Copp L. Multidisciplinary pain policy model: the Wisconsin initiative. J Prof Nurs 1987 Mar/Apr; 3(2):83, 125.

Coyle N. Analgesics and pain: Current concepts. Nurs Clin North Am 1987 Sep; 22(3):699.

Dubuisson D. Neurosurgery for pain of malignancy. Hosp Pract 1988 June 15; 23(6):41–54.

Edwards R. Pain and the ethics of pain management. Soc Sci Med 1984: 18(6):515–523.

Escobar P. Management of chronic pain. Nurse Pract 1985 Jan; 10(1):24–32.

Fordyce W et al. The behavioral management of chronic pain: A response to the critics. Pain 1985 Jun; 22(2):113–125.

Greipp M and Thomas A. Reflex sympathetic dystrophy syndrome: Pain that doesn't stop. J Neurosci Nurs 1986 Feb; 18(1):23–25.

Harrison M and Cotanch P. Pain: Advances and issues in critical care. Nurs Clin North Am 1987 Sep; 22(3):691–697.

Lamb S and Barbaro N. Neurosurgical approaches to the management of chronic pain syndromes. Orthop Nurs 1987 Jan/Feb; 6(1):33–40.

Levy R et al. Treatment of chronic pain by deep brain stimulation: Long term follow-up and review of the literature. Neurosurgery 1987 Dec; 21(6):885–893.

Magni G. On the relationship between chronic pain and depression when there is no organic lesion. Pain 1987 Oct; 31(1):1–21.

Puntillo. Phenomenon of pain and critical care nursing. Heart Lung 1988 May; 17(3):262–273.

Radwin L. Autonomous nursing interventions for treating the patient in acute pain. Nurs Clin North Am 1987 Sep; 22(3):705.

Raja S et al. Peripheral mechanisms of somatic pain. Anesthesiology 1988 Apr; 68(4):571–590.

Wilton L. Thalmic pain syndrome. J Neurosurg Nurs 1989 Dec; 21(6):362–365.

Unconsciousness and Coma

Done A. Encephalopathic presentation. Emerg Med 1988 Oct; 20(17): 154–163.

Gadow S. Clinical subjectivity. Advocacy with silent patients. Nurs Clin North Am 1989 Jun; 24(2):384–386.

Gavin J. Neurologic emergencies. Emerg Med Serv 1988 Aug; 17(7):40–42.

Glanutsus R. Rehabilitation optometric services for persons emerging from coma. J Head Trauma Rehab 1989 Jun; 4(2):17–25.

Hinkle J. Treating traumatic coma. Am J Nurs 1986 May; 86(5):551–556.

Hunter C. Cardiopulmonary cerebral resuscitation: Nursing interventions. Crit Care Nurse 1987 May/Jun; 7(3):46–56.

Ingersoll G et al. Glasgow coma scale for patients with head injuries. Crit Care Nurse 1987 Sep/Oct; 7(5):26, 28–32.

Johnson S. Coma stimulation: A challenge to occupational therapy. Br J Occup Ther 1988 Mar; 51(3):88–90.

* Johnson S et al. Effects of conversation of the ICP in comatose patients. Heart Lung 1989 Jan: 18(1):56–63.

Klingbeit G. Airway problems in patients with traumatic brain injury. Arch Phys Med Rehabil 1988 Jul; 69(7):493–495.

Levin H et al. Duration of impaired consciousness in relation to side of lesion after severe head injury. NIH Traumatic Coma Data Bank Research Group. Lancet 1989 May; 1(8645):1001–1003.

Ogata J et al. Primary brainstem death: A clinico-pathological study. J Neurol Neurosurg Psychiatry 1988 May; 51(5):646–650.

Ross D et al. Brain shift, level of consciousness, and restoration of consciousness in patients with acute intracranial hematoma. J Neurosurg 1989 Oct; 71(4):498–502.

* Sisson R. Effects of auditory stimuli on comatose patients with head injury. Heart Lung 1990 Jul; 19(4):373–378.

Tosch P. Patient's recollection of their post-traumatic coma. J Neurosci Nurs 1988 Aug; 20(4):223–228.

Vilkki J et al. Memory disorder related to coma duration after head injury. J Neurol Neurosurg Psychiatry 1988 Nov; 51(11):1452–1454.

57

Management of Patients With Neurologic Disorders

Chapter Outline

Learning Objectives

On completion of this chapter, the learner will be able to:

1. Compare the various types and causes of headache

2. Use the nursing process as a framework for care of patients with migraine headaches

3. Describe brain tumors: their classification, clinical manifestations, diagnosis, and management

4. Use the nursing process as a framework for care of patients with cerebral metastases or inoperable brain tumors

5. Describe subarachnoid precautions and their application to the patient with a cerebral aneurysm

6. Use the nursing process as a framework for care of patients with multiple sclerosis

7. Use the nursing process as a framework for care of patients with Parkinson's disease

8. Compare myasthenia gravis, amyotrophic lateral sclerosis, and muscular dystrophy: their pathophysiology, clinical manifestations, and nursing and medical management

9. Describe disorders of the cranial nerves, their manifestations, and indicated nursing interventions

Headache

Possibly the most common of all human afflictions is headache or *cephalgia* ("condition of head pain"). Headache is actually considered a symptom rather than a disease entity. The symptom of headache may indicate organic disease (neurologic or other disease), a stress response, vasodilation (migraine), skeletal muscle tension (tension headache), or a combination of the above.

Classification

Categorizing and defining diseases have historically been difficult tasks; this is particularly true with headache. There is little pathophysiologic evidence or diagnostic testing that can support the diagnosis of headache. Headaches may change within individuals over the course of a lifetime, and manifestations of the same type of headache vary significantly among different individuals.

The Headache Classification Committee of the International Headache Society has revised the classification of headaches; this revised classification may aid in both diagnosis and communication.

1. Migraine (with and without aura)
2. Tension-type headache
3. Cluster headache and paroxysmal hemicrania
4. Miscellaneous headaches associated with structural lesion
5. Headache associated with head trauma
6. Headache associated with vascular disorders (*e.g.*, subarachnoid hemorrhage)
7. Headache associated with nonvascular intracranial disorders, *e.g.,* brain turmor
8. Headache associated with use of chemical substances or their withdrawal
9. Headache associated with noncephalic infection
10. Headache associated with metabolic disorder (*e.g.*, hypoglycemia)
11. Headache or facial pain associated with disorder of the head, neck, or their structures (*e.g.*, acute glaucoma)
12. Cranial neuralgias (persistent pain of cranial nerve origin)

Frequently headache is not associated with either a structural or inflammatory process but falls either into the category of tension headache or migraine headache. The following discussion focuses on migraine headache as a prototype for assessment and management of the patient with headache.

Assessment

When data are obtained for the health history, patients should be given a chance to describe their headache *in their own words* as related to the following questions:

- How old were you when these headaches started? Under what circumstances did they start?
- What is the location? Is it unilateral or bilateral? Does it radiate?
- What is the quality—dull, aching, steady, boring, burning, intermittent, continuous, paroxysmal?
- How many headaches occur during a given time?
- Are there any precipitating factors (environmental, such as sunlight and weather change; foods; exertion; other)?
- What makes the headache worse (coughing, straining)?
- What time (day/night) does it occur?
- Are there any associated symptoms (facial pain, lacrimation, scotomas (blind spots in field of vision)?
- What usually relieves the headache (aspirin, ergot preparation, food, heat, rest, neck massage)?
- Is there nausea, vomiting, weakness, numbness in the extremities?
- Does the headache interfere with your daily activities?
- Do you have any allergies?
- Do you have insomnia, poor appetite, loss of energy?
- Is there a family history of headache? "Sick" headache?
- What is the relationship of the headache to the life style: physical/emotional stress?
- What is your medication history?

Vascular Headache

Vascular headaches result from dilation, compression, edema, or inflammation of the intracranial or extracranial arteries.

Migraine

Migraine is a symptom-complex characterized by periodic and recurrent attacks of severe headache. The cause of migraine has not been clearly demonstrated, but it is primarily a vascular disturbance that occurs more commonly in women and has a strong familial tendency.

Pathophysiology

The cerebral signs and symptoms of migraine are the result of cortical ischemia of varying degree. The typical attack begins with vasoconstriction affecting the arteries of the scalp and certain cerebral or retinal vessels. Extracranial and intracranial blood vessels dilate, causing pain and discomfort. Studies suggest that the dilated artery becomes hyperpermeable and that sterile local inflammatory reactions occur in the vicinity of the painful, dilated arteries. It is proposed that vasoactive substances (histamine, serotonin, plasmokinins) participate in this sterile inflammatory reaction.

Clinical Manifestations.   Often the headache begins on awakening, but it can occur at any time. The classic migraine attack can be divided into three phases: the aura, the headache, and the recovery phases. The aura lasts for up to 30 minutes and when it occurs it may provide enough time for the patient to take the prescribed medication to avert a full-blown attack (described in later section). This period is characterized by sensory manifestations, predominantly visual disturbances (light flashes). Other symptoms that may follow include numbness and tingling of the face or hands, mild confusion, slight weakness of an extremity, and dizziness. This period of aura corresponds to the painless vasoconstriction that is the initial physiologic change characteristic of classic migraine. Cerebral blood flow studies performed during migraine headaches demonstrate that during all phases of the attack cerebral blood flow is reduced throughout the brain, with subsequent loss of autoregulation and impaired CO_2 responsiveness.

As these symptoms begin to recede, they are followed by a unilateral (in two thirds of patients) and throbbing headache. This headache is severe and incapacitating and is often associated with photophobia, nausea, and vomiting. Its duration varies, ranging from several hours to a day or longer.

The recovery phase is a period of muscle contraction in the neck and scalp with associated muscle ache and point (localized) tenderness. Exhaustion is common, and any physical exertion exacerbates the headache pain. During this postheadache phase, patients may sleep for extended periods.

Diagnostic Evaluation. For patients with abnormalities on the neurologic examination, computed tomography (CT) or magnetic resonance imaging (MRI) may be used to detect underlying causes such as tumor or aneurysm. Other diagnostic tests may be indicated for patients with persistent or disabling pain.

Management. Therapy for migraine headache is divided into abortive (symptomatic) and preventive approaches. The symptomatic approach is best employed in patients who suffer frequent attacks and is aimed at relieving or limiting a headache at the onset or while it is in progress. The preventive approach is used in patients who experience frequent attacks at regular or predictable intervals and may have medical conditions that preclude the use of abortive therapies.

Management of Acute Attack. Ergotamine preparations (taken orally, sublingually, subcutaneously, intramuscularly, by rectum, or by inhalation) may be effective in aborting the headache if taken *early* in the migraine process. Ergotamine tartrate acts on smooth muscle, causing prolonged constriction of the cranial blood vessels. Each patient's dosage is titrated according to individual needs. Side effects include aching muscles, paresthesias, nausea, and vomiting. During the acute attack, the patient may find relief by lying quietly in a darkened room with the head slightly elevated. Drinking black coffee also may be helpful in counteracting the attack. Symptomatic therapy for migraine includes analgesics, sedatives, antianxiety agents, and antiemetics.

Management Between Attacks. The most widely used and important drug for the prevention of migraine is propranolol (Inderal). Beta-blocking drugs such as propranolol stop the activities of beta-receptors—cells in the heart and brain that control the dilation of blood vessels. The ability of beta-blockers to halt the dilation of blood vessels in the brain is believed to be a major reason for their antimigraine action.

Methysergide is an effective prophylactic agent in preventing frequent and severe migraine attacks; before the widespread use of propranolol in migraine prevention, it was the drug of choice. It is thought to inhibit or block the effects of serotonin, a substance possibly involved in the mechanism of vascular headaches. Troublesome side effects include abdominal discomfort, muscle cramps, edema, numbness, tingling of extremities, and depression. There should be a medication-free interval of at least 1 to 2 months after every 6-month course of treatment because of the potential complication of retroperitoneal fibrosis and pleuropulmonary and cardiac fibrosis.

Preventive medical management of migraine employs the daily use of one or more agents that are thought to block the physiologic events leading to an attack. Drug therapy is carried out at intervals of 3 to 6 months and is gradually tapered, because natural remissions of migraine do occur. Treatment regimens vary greatly, as do patient responses; thus close monitoring is indicated.

Additional drug therapy includes the use of antidepressants, barbiturates, and tranquilizers. These medications should be used cautiously and only on a short-term basis because of the dependency considerations.

▶ Nursing Process
The Patient With a Migraine Headache

▷ Assessment

The physical examination includes a detailed history, a physical assessment of the head and neck, a neurologic examination including cranial nerve testing, evaluation of the size and reaction of the pupils, a funduscopic examination of the eyes, and testing of motor and sensory functions.

The health history is focused on assessment of the headache itself, with particular emphasis on precipitating or provoking factors. Patients are encouraged to describe their headaches in their own words. History can be obtained according to the following outline.

▷ *General History.* Because headache can often be the presenting symptom of a wide variety of both physiologic and psychological disturbances, a general health history is an essential component of the patient database. General review questions include major medical and surgical illness as well as a body systems review. Headache may be a symptom of endocrine, hematologic, gastrointestinal, infectious, renal, cardiovascular, psychiatric, or hemologic disease.

A complete medication review is important. Medication history can provide insight into the patient's overall health status. Antihypertensives, such as hydralazine, diuretics, anti-inflammatory drugs, and monoamine oxidase inhibitors are a few of the categories of drugs that can provoke headaches. Although sometimes exaggerated in importance, emotional factors can play a role in the precipitation or development of many headaches. Stress is thought to be a major initiating factor in migraine headaches; therefore, sleep patterns, level of stress, recreational interests, appetite, emotional problems, and family stressors are relevant.

▷ *Family History.* There is a strong familial tendency for headache disorders. A positive family history is strongly suggestive of the diagnosis of migraine headache.

▷ *Occupational History.* A direct relationship may exist between exposure to toxic substances and headache. Careful questioning may be required to identify a comprehensive list of the chemicals to which workers are exposed. Under the Right to Know law, employees should have access to the Material Safety Data Sheets for all the substances to which they come in contact in the workplace. In addition, the occupational history includes the workplace as a source of stress.

▷ *Headache History.* A complete description of the headache itself is crucial. The patient's age at onset of headache, its frequency, location, duration, type of pain, factors that relieve and precipitate the event, and associated symptoms are reviewed.

◊ Nursing Diagnosis

Based on the assessment data, the potential nursing diagnoses for the patient with a migraine headache may include:

- Pain related to vascular changes
- Knowledge deficit about the headache:
  Preventive strategies
  Precipitating and relieving factors

◊ Planning and Implementation

◊ *Goals:* The patient's goals may include relief of pain and discomfort during an acute attack and increased knowledge about headache and those factors that precipitate and relieve it.

◊ Nursing Interventions

When migraine headache has been diagnosed, the goals of nursing management are to treat the acute event of the headache and to prevent recurrent episodes. Prevention involves patient education regarding precipitating factors, possible lifestyle or habit changes that may be helpful and pharmacologic measures.

◊ *Relief of Pain.* Nursing care is directed toward treatment of the acute episode. A migraine headache in the early phase requires abortive drug therapy instituted as soon as possible. Some headaches actually may be prevented if the appropriate medications are taken before the onset of pain. Early administration of Cafergot, a combination preparation of ergotamine and caffeine can arrest or reduce the headache severity in 90% of migraine sufferers. Nursing care during a fully developed attack includes comfort measures such as a quiet, dark environment and elevation of the head of the bed 30 degrees. In addition, symptomatic treatment such as antiemetics may be indicated.

◊ *Knowledge About Precipitating and Alleviating Factors.* Although there is a wide variation in the personality types of those who are subject to migraine, there is some evidence that the hard-driving, somewhat compulsive perfectionist is most vulnerable to this condition. Migraine headaches are likely to occur when a person is ill, overtired, or feeling stressed. Stress is believed to be a factor in the precipitation of migraine. Instruction about the importance of proper diet, adequate rest, and coping strategies may help the patient deal with his stress. Identifying circumstances that precipitate headaches may assist the patient in the development of alternate means of coping.

Patients can be helped to develop insight into their feelings, behavior, and conflicts and to make the necessary modifications in life style on the basis of these analyses. Regular periods of exercise and relaxation are suggested, and any offending or provoking factors (allergens, fatigue, foods, environmental stresses) are removed or reduced to obtain relief.

A discussion of the patient's problems, instead of the headache, can be helpful. To obtain long-term relief, he needs to understand the source of any emotional conflicts and attempt to change or adapt to stressful and anxiety-producing situations. This requires supportive counseling and education, including biofeedback and relaxation techniques. (Cognitive restructuring teaches people to change their attitudes to stress.)

The nurse's role is one of supportive care during physical or emotional distress, listening, instructions, and positive reinforcement so that a beneficial outcome will be achieved. The patient is encouraged to use moderation in all activities.

Certain foods containing tyramine, monosodium glutamate, milk products, or nitrite may trigger headaches. Therefore, aged cheese, chocolate, and many processed foods should be avoided. Potential headache-causing substances should be avoided. Long intervals between meals should also be avoided. The patient is advised to awaken at the same time each day, as disruption in the normal sleeping pattern provokes a migraine in many patients. Birth control pills increase the frequency and severity of the attacks in some women.

A record may be kept of the circumstances surrounding the attack (*e.g.*, activities, food, feelings) to determine if there is a pattern to the migraine episodes. If so, a change in the pattern may help avoid the attacks.

The National Headache Foundation (see bibliography) provides a list of clinics in the United States and the names of physicians in specific areas who specialize in headache and who are members of the American Association for the Study of Headache.

◊ Evaluation

Expected Outcomes
1. Experiences reduced pain and discomfort
   a. Reports reduction in level of headache pain
   b. Uses medication appropriately as prescribed
   c. Initiates comfort techniques as instructed
   d. Maintains close follow-up with the health care provider
2. Is knowledgeable regarding possible precipitating and relieving factors related to headache
   a. Establishes a program of rest and exercise
   b. Initiates stress-relieving techniques
   c. Reports reduced level of stress
   d. Identifies factors that precipitate headache and reports efforts to alter these factors
   e. Reports decreased frequency and severity of headache

Cluster Headache

Cluster headaches are another severe form of vascular headache. They are seen most frequently in men. The attacks come in clusters or groups, with excruciating pain localized in the eye and orbit and radiating to the facial and temporal regions. The pain is accompanied by watering of the eye and nasal congestion. Each attack lasts from 15 minutes to 2 hours and may have a crescendo–decrescendo pattern.

One theory is that this type of headache is due to dilatation of orbital and nearby extracranial arteries. Cluster headaches may be precipitated by alcohol, nitrites, vasodilators, and histamines. Eliminating these factors helps in preventing the headaches. Cluster headache responds to vasoconstricting agents (ergotamine tartrate). The serotonin antagonist methysergide and the beta-blocker propranolol also may provide relief. Chlorpromazine may also be effective. Inhalation of 100% oxygen eases the pain of cluster headache by reducing blood flow to the brain.

Cranial Arteritis

Inflammation of the cranial arteries is characterized by a severe headache localized in the region of the temporal arteries. The inflammation may be generalized, in which cranial arteritis is part of a vascular disease, or of a focal type, in which only the cranial arteries are involved. Cranial arteritis is a cause of headache in the older population, reaching its greatest incidence in those over the age of 70.

Often the disease begins with general manifestations, such as fatigue, malaise, weight loss, and fever. Clinical manifestations associated with inflammation (heat, redness, swelling, tenderness, or pain over the involved artery) are usually present. Sometimes a tender, swollen, or nodular temporal artery is visible. Visual problems are caused by ischemia of the involved structures.

Cranial arteritis is thought to represent an immune vasculitis in which immune complexes are deposited within the walls of affected blood vessels, producing vascular injury and inflammation. A biopsy may be performed on the involved artery to confirm or refute the diagnosis.

Treatment consists of early administration of a corticosteroid drug to prevent the possibility of loss of vision due to vascular occlusion or rupture of the involved artery. The patient is instructed not to stop the medication abruptly because this can lead to relapse. Analgesic agents are given for comfort.

Tension Headache (Muscle Contraction Headache)

Emotional or physical stress may cause contraction of the muscles in the neck and scalp, resulting in tension headache. The headache may be characterized by a steady, constant feeling of pressure that usually begins in the forehead, the temple, or the back of the neck. It is often bandlike or may be described as "a weight on top of my head." Tension headaches tend to be more chronic than severe and are probably the most common type of headache. The patient needs reassurance that the headache is not due to a brain tumor. This is a common unspoken fear. Symptomatic relief may be obtained by local heat, massage, analgesics, antidepressants, and muscle relaxants.

In summary, headache is a symptom that can be a consequence of increased stress and tension in one's life, or it may be an indication of serious underlying pathology. Regardless of its cause, headache is often disruptive and at times incapacitating. Supportive counseling and education, including biofeedback and relaxation techniques, may be helpful if the patient's headache is primarily stress related. Extensive diagnostic evaluation and treatment may be warranted for headache due to vascular changes and structural abnormalities. The patient undergoing diagnostic testing is often anxious about possible diagnostic findings and requires support and an opportunity to verbalize his concerns.

Brain Tumors

A brain tumor is a localized intracranial lesion that occupies space within the skull and tends to cause a rise in intracranial pressure (ICP). In adults, most brain tumors originate from *glial cells.* (Glial cells generally make up the structure and support system of the brain and spinal cord.) The highest incidence of brain tumors in adults occurs in the fifth, sixth, and seventh decades, and most of these are *supratentorial* (above the covering of the cerebellum) in location. Brain tumors rarely metastasize outside the central nervous system but cause death by impairing vital functions, either by direct involvement or by increasing ICP.

Classification

Brain tumors may be classified into several groups: (1) those arising from the coverings of the brain, such as dural meningioma; (2) those developing in or on the cranial nerves, best exemplified by acoustic neuroma and optic nerve spongioblastoma polare; (3) those originating in the brain tissue, such as the various gliomas; and (4) metastatic lesions originating elsewhere in the body (Chart 57-1). The major concerns are the location and the histologic character of the tumor. Tumors may be benign or malignant. Because a benign tumor may occur in a vital area, however, it may have effects as serious as those of a malignant tumor.

Specific Tumors

Gliomas. Malignant glioma is the most frequent brain neoplasm. Usually, these tumors cannot be totally removed because they spread by infiltrating into the surrounding neural tissue.

Pituitary Adenomas. The *pituitary gland*, also called the *hypophysis*, is a relatively small gland located in the sella turcica. It is attached to the hypothalamus by a short stalk (hypophyseal stalk) and is divided into two lobes: the anterior (adenohypophysis) and the posterior (neurohypophysis). The anterior lobe secretes growth hormone, adrenocorticotrophic hormone (ACTH), thyroid-stimulating hormone (TSH), prolactin and the gonadotropic hormones, follicle-stimulating hormone (FSH), and luteinizing hormone (LH). The posterior pituitary stores and releases antidiuretic hormone (vasopressin) and oxytocin.

Pituitary tumors may cause symptoms due to mass (pressure) effects on adjacent structures or to hormonal changes (hyperfunction or hypofunction of the pituitary). The mass effects of adenomas of the pituitary gland are caused by pressure on the optic nerves, optic chiasm, or optic tracts, or on the hypothalamus or the third ventricle when the tumors invade the cavernous sinuses or expand into the sphenoid bone. These pressure effects produce headache, visual dysfunction, hypothalamic disorders (*e.g.,* disorders of sleep, appetite, temperature, emotions), increased ICP, and enlargement and erosion of the sella turcica.

Functioning pituitary tumors can produce one or more hormones normally produced by the anterior pituitary. These hormones may cause prolactin-secreting pituitary adenomas (prolactinomas), growth hormone-secreting pituitary adenomas that produce acromegaly in adults, and ACTH-producing pituitary adenomas that give rise to Cushing's disease. Adenomas secreting TSH or FSH-LH occur infrequently, whereas adenomas that produce both growth hormone and prolactin are relatively common.

The female patient whose pituitary gland is secreting excessive quantities of prolactin presents with amenorrhea or galactorrhea (excessive or spontaneous flow of milk). Male patients with prolactinomas may present with impotence and hypogonadism.

Chart 57-1
Classification of Brain Tumors

Tumors Originating in the Brain Tissue

Gliomas—infiltrating tumors that may invade any portion of the brain; most common type of brain tumor

Astrocytomas (grades 1 and 2)
Glioblastomas (grades 3 and 4 astrocytomas)
Ependymomas
Medulloblastomas   } Subclassified according to cell type
Oligodendrogliomas
Colloid cysts

Tumors Arising From Covering of Brain

Meningioma—encapsulated, well-defined, growing outside the brain tissue; compresses rather than invades brain

Tumors Developing in or on the Cranial Nerves

Acoustic neuroma—derived from sheath of acoustic nerve
Optic nerve spongioblastoma polare

Metastatic Lesions

Most commonly from lung and breast

Tumors of the Ductless Glands

Pituitary
Pineal

Blood Vessel Tumors

Hemangioblastoma
Angioma

Congenital Tumors

Acromegaly, caused by excess growth hormone, produces enlargement of the hands and feet, distortion of the facial features, and pressure on peripheral nerves (entrapment syndromes).

The clinical features of Cushing's disease, a condition associated with prolonged overproduction of cortisol occurs with excessive production of ACTH. Manifestations include a form of obesity with redistribution of fat to the facial, supraclavicular, and abdominal areas, hypertension, purple striae and ecchymoses, osteoporosis, glucose intolerance, and emotional disorders.

Most pituitary adenomas are treated by transsphenoidal microsurgical removal (see Chap. 56), whereas the remainder of tumors that cannot be removed completely are treated by radiation.

Angiomas. Brain angiomas (masses composed largely of abnormal blood vessels) are found either in or on the surface of the brain. Some persist throughout life without causing symptoms; others give rise to symptoms of brain tumor. Occasionally, the diagnosis is suggested by the presence of another angioma somewhere in the head or by a *bruit* (an abnormal sound) audible over the skull. Because the walls of the blood vessels in angiomas are thin, these patients are at risk for a cerebral vascular accident (stroke). In fact, cerebral hemorrhage in persons under 40 years of age should suggest the possibility of an angioma.

Acoustic Neuroma. An acoustic neuroma is a tumor of the eighth cranial nerve, the nerve for hearing and balance. It usually arises just within the internal auditory meatus, where it frequently expands before filling the cerebellopontine recess.

An acoustic neuroma may grow slowly and attain considerable size before it is correctly diagnosed. The patient usually experiences loss of hearing, tinnitus, and episodes of vertigo and staggering. As the tumor becomes larger, painful sensations of the face may occur on the same side as a result of the tumor's compression of the fifth cranial nerve.

With improved radiologic techniques and the use of the operating microscope and microsurgical instrumentation, even large tumors can be removed through a relatively small craniotomy.

Clinical Manifestations

Brain tumors produce clinical manifestations when they cause increased ICP or produce localizing signs and symptoms as a result of the tumor interfering with specific regions of the brain.

Increasing Intracranial Pressure Symptoms. Symptoms of increased ICP are caused by a gradual compression of the brain due to the growth of the tumor. The effect is to disrupt the equilibrium that exists between the brain, the cerebrospinal fluid, and the cerebral blood—all located within the skull. As the tumor grows, adjustment may occur through compression of intracranial veins, through reduction of cerebrospinal fluid volume (by increased absorption or decreased production), through a modest decrease of cerebral blood flow, and through reduction of intracellular and extracellular brain tissue mass. When these compensatory mechanisms fail, the patient develops signs and symptoms of increased ICP.

The most common symptoms produced by this pressure are headache, vomiting, *papilledema* (choked disc or edema of the optic nerve), personality changes, and a variety of focal deficits including motor, sensory, and cranial nerve dysfunction. Headache, although not always present, is most common in the early morning and is made worse by coughing, straining, or sudden movement. It is thought to be caused by the tumor's invading, compressing, or distorting the pain-sensitive structures or by the edema that accompanies the tumor.

Headaches are usually described as deep or expanding or as dull but unrelenting. Frontal tumors usually produce a bilateral frontal headache; pituitary gland tumors produce pain radiating between the two temples (bitemporal); in cerebellar tumors the headache may be located in the suboccipital region at the back of the head.

Vomiting, seldom related to food intake, is usually due to irritation of the vagal centers in the medulla. If the vomiting is of the forceful type, it is described as projectile vomiting.

Papilledema (edema of the optic nerve) is present in 70% to 75% of patients and is associated with visual disturbances such as decreased visual acuity, diplopia, and visual field deficits.

Localizing Symptoms. Localizing symptoms occur when specific regions of the brain are disrupted, resulting in locally referable signs, such as sensory and motor abnormalities, visual alterations, and convulsive seizures.

Because the functions of the different parts of the brain are known, the location of the tumor can be determined, in part, by identifying functions that are affected by the presence of the tumor. For example, a tumor of the motor cortex manifests itself by causing convulsive movements localized on one side of the body, called *Jacksonian seizures*. Symptoms of occipital lobe tumors tend to be visual, contralateral homonymous hemianopsia (visual loss in one half of the visual field on the opposite side of the tumor) and visual hallucinations. Tumors of the cerebellum cause dizziness, an ataxic or staggering gait with a tendency to fall toward the side of the lesion, marked muscle incoordination, and *nystagmus* (involuntary rhythmical eye movements) usually in the horizontal direction. Tumors of the frontal lobe frequently produce personality disorders, changes in emotional state and behavior, and a disinterested mental attitude. The patient often becomes extremely untidy and careless and may use obscene language.

Personality changes, confusion, speech dysfunction, and disturbances of gait occur more frequently in elderly patients with intracranial tumors. The most frequent tumor types in the elderly are meningiomas, glioblastomas, and cerebral metastases from other sites.

Tumors of the cerebellopontine angle usually originate in the sheath of the acoustic nerve and give rise to a sequence of symptoms that is the most characteristic of all brain tumor symptomatology. First, tinnitus and vertigo appear, soon followed by progressive nerve deafness (eighth nerve dysfunction); next there is numbness and tingling of the face and the tongue (due to involvement of the fifth nerve); still later, weakness or paralysis of the face develops (seventh nerve involve-

ment); and finally, because the enlarging tumor presses on the cerebellum, abnormalities in motor function may be present.

Many tumors are not so easily localized, because they lie in the so-called *silent areas* of the brain (*i.e.*, areas in which functions are not definitely determined).

The *progression* of the signs and symptoms is important, because it indicates tumor growth and expansion.

Diagnostic Evaluation

The history of the illness and the manner in which the symptoms evolved are important. A neurologic examination indicates the areas of the central nervous system involved. To assist in the precise localization of the lesion, a battery of tests is performed. CT imaging gives specific information concerning the number, size, and density of the lesions and the extent of secondary cerebral edema. It also provides information about the ventricular system. MRI, when available, is helpful in the diagnosis of brain tumors. Its use has resulted in the detection of smaller lesions, and it is particularly helpful in detecting tumors in the brain stem and pituitary regions, where bone interferes with CT imaging (Fig. 57-1). Computer-assisted stereotactic (three-dimensional) biopsy is being used to diagnose deep-seated brain tumors and to provide a basis for treatment and prognostic information. Cerebral angiography provides visualization of cerebral blood vessels and can localize most cerebral tumors.

An electroencephalogram can detect abnormal brain waves in regions occupied by a tumor and can enable evaluation of temporal lobe seizures.

Cytologic studies of the cerebrospinal fluid may be performed to detect malignant cells, because tumors of the central

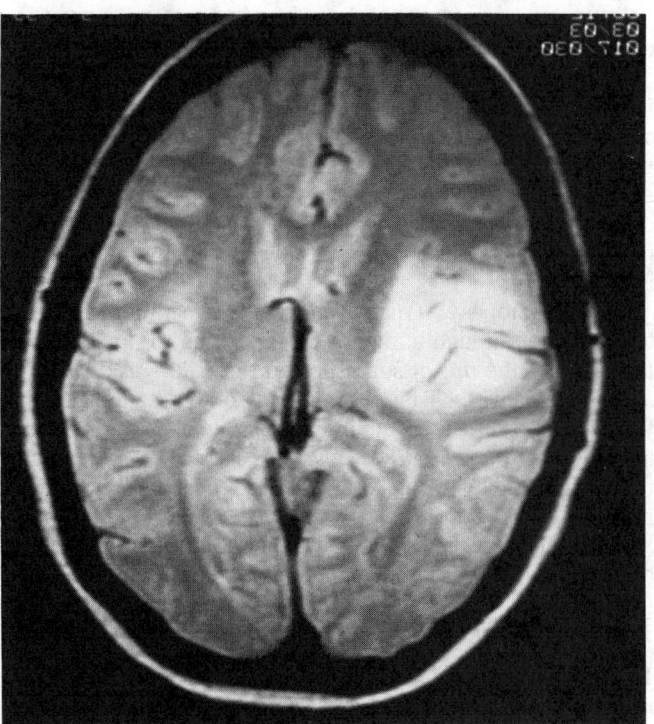

Figure 57-1. Low-grade glioma. MRI image of the brain shows a mass of abnormal density in the right temporal lobe. This lesion corresponds exactly to the lesion seen on the CT scan (not shown). (Courtesy of the Hospital of the University of Pennsylvania, Nuclear Medicine Section.)

nervous system are capable of shedding cells into the cerebrospinal fluid.

Management

An untreated brain tumor ultimately leads to death, either from increasing ICP or from the brain damage it causes. Patients with possible brain tumor should be evaluated and treated as soon as possible before irreversible neurologic damage occurs.

The objective of management is to remove all of the tumor or as much as possible without increasing the neurologic deficit (paralysis, blindness) or to achieve relief of symptoms by partial tumor removal (decompression), radiation therapy, chemotherapy, or a combination of these. Most patients with brain tumors undergo a neurosurgical procedure, when possible, followed by radiation therapy and possibly chemotherapy. Corticosteroids are highly effective in combating cerebral edema, thus allowing for a thorough diagnostic workup and a carefully planned surgical approach. (Also, appropriate dosages of corticosteroids are used to prevent postoperative swelling and facilitate a smoother, more rapid recovery.) In general, patients with meningiomas, acoustic neuromas, cystic astrocytomas of the cerebellum, colloid cyst of the third ventricle, congenital tumors such as dermoid cyst, and some of the granulomas can be cured by surgical removal of the tumor. A complete extirpation (removal) of the infiltrating gliomas is not possible. In these patients, the treatment consists of biopsy to establish the diagnosis, partial removal, and radiation therapy. Certain chemotherapeutic agents combined with radiation therapy are also being used. More recently, deep-seated brain tumors have been removed using the carbon dioxide laser with CT scanning and stereotactic techniques.

Intravenous autologous bone marrow transplantation is used in some patients who will receive chemotherapy or radiation because it has the potential to "rescue" the patient from the marrow toxicity associated with high dosages of drugs and radiation. A fraction of the patient's bone marrow is aspirated, usually from the iliac crest, and stored. The patient is exposed to large doses of chemoradiotherapy for the purpose of destroying large numbers of malignant cells. The patient's marrow is then reinfused intravenously after chemoradiotherapy is completed.

Radioisotopes (^{125}I) can be implanted directly into the brain tumor to permit high total doses of radiation to the localized tumor. With the use of sophisticated three-dimensional guidance systems with CT monitoring and computer graphics, the tumor can be visualized and interstitial radioisotopes precisely implanted (*brachytherapy*). This helps avoid radiation toxicity to the surrounding normal brain, but prognosis using this technique is unchanged from conventional radiation therapy.

Newer drugs are continually being evaluated, and there is hope that these will eventually be more successful.

Nursing Interventions

The patient with a brain tumor may have problems with aspiration related to cranial nerve dysfunction. Preoperatively, the gag reflex and ability to swallow are evaluated. If there is a diminished gag response, the plan of care includes teaching the patient to direct food and fluids toward the unaffected side, placing the patient upright to eat, offering a semisoft diet, and having suction readily available. Function should be reassessed postoperatively, as changes can occur.

The problems of increased ICP caused by the tumor mass are reviewed on Chapter 56. The nurse performs neurologic checks, monitors vital signs, maintains a neurologic flow record, spaces nursing interventions to prevent rapid increase in ICP, and reorients the patient when necessary to person, time, and place. Patients with changes in cognition caused by the lesion require frequent reorientation and the use of orienting devices (personal possessions, photographs, lists, clock), supervision of and assistance with self-care, and ongoing monitoring and intervention for prevention of injury. Patients with seizures are carefully monitored.

Motor function is checked at intervals because specific motor deficits may be involved, depending on the tumor's location. Sensory disturbances are assessed. The patient's speech function is evaluated. Eye movement and pupillary size and reaction may be affected by cranial nerve involvement.

The major treatment of brain tumor is surgery. The nursing process applied to the patient undergoing neurosurgery is found in Chapter 56.

Cerebral Metastases

A significant number of patients suffer central nervous system complications as a result of systemic cancer and neurologic deficits caused by cerebral metastases. Cancer of the lung commonly metastasizes to the brain, as do tumors of the breast, kidney, prostate gland, uterus, thyroid, skin (melanoma), and gastrointestinal tract.

Neurologic symptoms and signs include headache, disturbances of gait, deterioration of vision, personality changes, altered mentation (memory loss and confusion), focal weakness, paralysis, aphasia, and seizures. These problems can be devastating to both patient and family.

Management

The treatment is palliative and involves eliminating or reducing serious symptomatology. Even when palliation is the goal, distressing signs and symptoms can be resolved, thereby improving the quality of life for both patient and family. Patients with intracerebral metastases who are not treated have a steady downhill course with a very limited survival time, whereas those who are treated may survive for slightly longer periods.

The therapeutic approach includes radiation therapy, which is the foundation of treatment, surgery (usually for a single intracranial metastasis), chemotherapy, or a combination of these methods. Adrenocorticosteroid hormones may be helpful in relieving headache and alterations of consciousness. It is thought that corticosteroids (dexamethasone, prednisone) reduce inflammatory reaction around the metastatic deposits and decrease the edema surrounding them. Other drugs include osmotic agents (mannitol, glycerol) to decrease the water content of the brain, which leads to a decrease in ICP. Anticonvulsant drugs (phenytoin) are used to prevent and treat seizures. There have been encouraging results in the treatment of metastatic lesions with chemotherapeutic agents such as carmustine (BCNU).

If the patient has severe pain, morphine can be infused into the epidural or subarachnoid space with a spinal needle and insertion of a catheter as near as possible to the spinal segment where the pain is projected. Small doses of morphine are injected into the system at prescribed intervals (see Chap. 15).

▶ Nursing Process
The Patient With Cerebral Metastases or Incurable Brain Tumor

◊ Assessment

The nursing assessment focuses on how the patient is functioning, moving and walking, adapting to weakness or paralysis, visual loss, and speech loss, and dealing with seizures.

A dietary history is taken to assess dietary intake and food intolerances and preferences. Anthropometric measurements confirm the loss of subcutaneous fat and lean body mass. Biochemical measurements (albumin, transferrin, total lymphocyte count, creatinine index, and urinary tests) are reviewed to assess the degree of malnutrition, impaired cellular immunity, and electrolyte balance.

Cachexia (weak and emaciated condition) is seen in patients with metastases and is characterized by anorexia, pain, weight loss, altered metabolism, muscle weakness, malabsorption, and diarrhea. The patient may have altered taste sensation secondary to dysphagia, weakness, and depression. Smell distortions and diminution of smell (*anosmia*) frequently occur among these patients.

Assessment is made for symptoms that cause distress to the patient, including pain, respiratory problems, problems with elimination and urination, disturbances in sleep, and impairment of skin integrity, fluid balance, and temperature regulation. These problems may be caused by tumor invasion, compression, or obstruction.

The nurse may discuss with the social worker the impact of the patient's illness on the family in terms of home care, altered relationships, financial problems, time pressures, and intrafamily problems. This information is important in helping family members strengthen their coping skills.

◊ Nursing Diagnoses

Based on the assessment data, the patient's major problems may include the following:

- Self-care deficits related to loss or impairment of motor and sensory function and decreased cognitive abilities
- Altered nutrition, less than body requirements, related to cachexia due to treatment and tumor effects, decreased nutritional intake, and malabsorption
- Anxiety related to anticipation of death, uncertainty, change in appearance, discontinuity in life style
- Potential for altered family processes related to anticipatory grief and the burdens imposed by the care of the person with a terminal illness.

Other nursing diagnoses of the patient with cerebral metastases may include pain related to tumor compression; impaired gas exchange related to dyspnea; constipation related to decreased fluid and dietary intake and medications; alteration in urinary elimination related to reduced fluid intake, vomiting, and reactions to medications; sleep pattern disturbances related to discomfort and fear of dying; impairment of skin integrity related to cachexia, poor tissue perfusion, and decreased mobility; potential or actual fluid volume deficit related to fever, vomiting, and low fluid intake; impaired thermal regulation related to hypothalamic involvement, fever, and chills. The reader is referred to Chapter 19 for appropriate assessment and nursing interventions for the patient with cancer.

◊ Planning and Implementation

◊ *Goals:* The goals of the patient may include compensating for self-care deficits, attaining improved nutrition, relief of anxiety, and enhancing of family coping skills.

◊ Nursing Interventions

◊ *Compensating for Self-Care Deficits.* The patient may have difficulty in participating in goal-setting, as the tumor metastasizes and affects mental capabilities. It is important to encourage the family to keep the patient mobile and at the highest level of functioning possible. Increasing assistance with self-care activities will be required. The patient with cerebral metastasis (and the family) lives with uncertainty. They are encouraged to plan for each day and make that day count. The tasks and challenges are to assist the patient to find useful coping mechanisms, adaptations, and compensations in solving problems that arise. This helps patients maintain some sense of control. An individualized exercise program helps maintain strength, endurance, and range of motion. Eventually referral may have to be made for home health care assistance.

◊ *Improved Nutrition.* Patients with nausea, vomiting, breathlessness, and pain are disinterested in eating. These symptoms must be managed or controlled by assessment, planning, and appropriate nursing and medical interventions.

The nurse teaches the family optimum positioning of the patient for comfort during meals. The timing of meals is important. Food is offered when the patient is more rested and in less distress from pain or effects of treatment. The patient needs to be clean, comfortable, and free of pain, with an environment that is as attractive as possible. This requires planning to minimize offensive sights, sounds, and odors. Oral hygiene helps to improve oral intake. The family is taught to keep a daily weight chart. It may be necessary to record the quantity of food eaten to determine the daily calorie count. Nursing ingenuity is called for to make food more palatable, provide enough fluids, and increase opportunities for socialization. This involves communication and interaction with the dietician, physician, patient, and family.

Dietary supplements, as preferred by the patient, can be encouraged to take care of increased caloric needs. If the patient refuses to eat the foods needed, it may be wise to offer whatever diet is accepted.

When the patient shows marked deterioration as a result of tumor growth and effects, some other form of nutritional support (tube feeding, total parenteral nutrition) may be used. Nursing interventions include assessment to ensure patency of the central and intravenous line or feeding tube, monitoring the insertion site for infection, checking the infusion rate, monitoring intake and output, and changing the IV tubing and dressing. These techniques can be taught to the caregivers at home. Additionally, programs are available for total parenteral nutrition.

The quality of life for the patient may serve to guide in the selection, institution, and maintenance of nutritional support.

The patient may become weary with all the urging to eat and the discussions about food, and may not desire aggressive nutritional intervention. The subsequent course of action should be ethical and humane, taking into consideration the wishes of the patient and family.

▷ *Relief of Anxiety.*   Persons with cerebral metastases may be restless, with changing moods that may include intense depression, euphoria, paranoia, severe anxiety, and a sense of impending doom. The response of patients to terminal illness reflects their pattern of reaction to other crisis situations. Serious illness imposes additional strains that often bring other unresolved problems to light. Learning to use patients' own coping strategies to help them deal with their feelings can be very beneficial. This requires experience and sensitivity to the patients' stated concerns.

Patients need the opportunity to exercise some control over their situation. A sense of intellectual mastery can be gained as they learn to understand the disease and its treatment, and how to deal with their feelings. The presence of family, friends, clergy, and health professionals may be supportive. Support groups such as Make Today Count may provide a feeling of support and strength.

Time spent with patients is helpful. It is important to allow time to talk and to communicate their worries. Communication has been called the "final comfort." Sponsoring open communication and acknowledging fears are therapeutic. Touch is also a form of communication. These patients need assurance of the continuation of the relationship with the nurse and that they will not be abandoned. Life becomes more endurable when others share in the experience of dying.

If a patient's emotional reactions are very intense or prolonged, additional help from a member of the clergy, social worker, mental health professional, occupational therapist, or recreational therapist may be indicated.

▷ *Enhanced Family Coping.*   The family needs to be reassured that their loved one is receiving optimal care and that attention will be paid to the patient's changing symptoms and to their problems. When the patient can no longer engage in self-care, the family is helped with the essentials of the patient's physical care and assisted in finding support systems (social worker, home health aid, community nurse, hospice care). The nursing goal is to keep their anxiety at manageable levels.

▷ Evaluation

Expected Outcomes

1. Engages in self-care activities as long as possible
   a. Uses assistive devices
   b. Accepts assistance
   c. Demonstrates optimal hygiene
   d. Schedules periodic rest periods to permit maximal participation in self-care
2. Demonstrates improvement in nutritional status
   a. Shows no additional weight loss
   b. Has increased calorie intake
   c. Accepts assistance with meals if indicated
3. Appears less anxious
   a. Seems less restless and is sleeping better
   b. Verbalizes concerns
   c. Participates in activities that are important to him
   d. Demonstrates an interest in events and activities in the environment

4. Family members seek help as needed
   a. Demonstrate ability to bathe, feed, and care for patient
   b. Express feelings and concerns to appropriate health professionals

Meningitis

Meningitis is an inflammation of the meninges (membranes surrounding the brain and spinal cord) and is caused by a viral, bacterial, or fungal organism. Further classification of meningitis frequently seen in the clinical setting includes aseptic, septic, and tuberculous. Aseptic refers to either viral meningitis or cases of meningial irritation from other causes such as brain abscess, encephalitis, lymphoma, leukemia, or blood in the subarachnoid space. Septic meningitis refers to meningitis caused by bacterial organisms such as meningococcus, staphylococcus, or influenza bacillus. Tuberculous meningitis is caused by the tubercle bacillus.

Meningeal infections generally originate in one of two ways: either through the bloodstream as a consequence of other infections such as cellulitis or by direct extension such as might occur after a traumatic injury to the facial bones. In a small number of cases the cause is iatrogenic or secondary to invasive procedures (*e.g.*, lumbar puncture) or invasive devices (*e.g.*, ICP monitoring devices).

Bacterial Meningitis

By far the most significant form of meningitis is the bacterial type. The bacteria most frequently encountered in acute bacterial meningitis are *Neisseria meningitidis* (meningococcal meningitis), *Streptococcus pneumoniae* (in adults), and *Haemophilus influenzae* (in children and young adults). These three organisms account for about 75% of the cases of bacterial meningitis. The mode of transmission is by direct contact, including droplets and discharges from the nose and throat of carriers (most often) or infected persons. Of those exposed to it, most do not develop the infection but become carriers. There has been an increased incidence of meningitis caused by enteric gram-negative bacteria in the elderly, as well as in those who have had neurosurgery or who have a compromised immune response.

Bacterial meningitis is endemic in the United States and throughout the world, and occurs most frequently in the winter and spring months. Epidemics are most apt to occur in people who live in crowded quarters, notably in cities, crowded institutions, military installations, or prisons, but the disease also occurs in rural regions.

Bacterial meningitis starts as an infection of the oropharynx and is followed by septicemia, which extends to the meninges of the brain and upper region of the spinal cord.

Pathophysiology

Predisposing factors include upper respiratory tract infections, otitis media, mastoiditis, sickle cell anemia and other hemoglobinopathies, recent neurosurgical procedures, head trauma, and immunologic defects. The venous channels serving the posterior nasopharynx, middle ear, and mastoid drain toward the brain and are near the veins draining the meninges; these channels favor bacterial proliferation.

The organism enters the bloodstream and causes an inflammatory reaction in the meninges and underlying cortex, which may result in vasculitis with thromboses and reduced cerebral blood flow. The cerebral tissue is metabolically impaired from the presence of meningeal exudate, vasculitis, and underperfusion. A purulent exudate may spread over the base of the brain and spinal cord. The inflammation spreads also to the membrane lining the cerebral ventricles. Bacterial meningitis is associated with profound alterations in intracranial physiology, including increased permeability of the blood–brain barrier, cerebral edema, and raised ICP.

In acute infections, however, the patient dies from the toxin of the bacteria before meningitis develops. In these patients the infection is overwhelming, with adrenal damage, circulatory collapse, and associated widespread hemorrhages (Waterhouse-Friderichsen syndrome) occurring as a result of endothelial damage and vascular necrosis caused by the meningococci.

Clinical Manifestations

The symptoms of meningitis result from infection and increased ICP. Headache and fever are frequently the initial symptoms. The headache associated with meningitis is considered severe and is the result of irritation. Fever is generally present and remains high throughout the course.

Changes in level of consciousness are associated with bacterial meningitis. Disorientation and memory impairment are common early in the course of the illness. The changes that occur are dependent on the severity of illness as well as the individual response to the physiologic changes. Behavioral manifestations are also common. As the illness progresses, lethargy, unresponsiveness, and coma may develop.

Meningeal irritation results in a number of well-recognized signs commonly seen in all types of meningitis. Nuchal rigidity (stiff neck) is an early sign. Any attempts at flexion of the head are difficult because of the presence of spasm in the muscles of the neck. Forceful flexion causes severe pain. Other signs of meningeal irritation include the following:

Positive Kernig's sign: When the patient is lying with his thigh flexed on the abdomen, he cannot completely extend his leg.

Positive Brudzinski's sign: When the patient's neck is flexed, flexion of the knees and hips is produced; when passive flexion of the lower extremity of one side is made, a similar movement is seen for the opposite extremity.

Also, for reasons that are unknown, these patients complain of photophobia (aversion to light).

Seizures and increased ICP are also associated with meningitis. Convulsions occur secondary to focal areas of cortical irritability. Signs of increasing ICP secondary to purulent exudate or cerebral edema include the characteristic vital sign changes (widened pulse pressure and bradycardia), respiratory irregularity, headache, vomiting, and depressed levels of consciousness. A striking feature of meningococcal meningitis (neisseria meningitidis) is the development of a rash. About half of all patients with this type of meningitis develop skin lesions ranging from a petechial rash with purpuric lesions to large areas of ecchymosis.

In about 10% of patients with meningococcal meningitis,

a fulminating infection occurs, with signs of overwhelming septicemia: an abrupt onset of high fever, extensive purpuric lesions (over face and extremities), shock, and signs of disseminated intravascular coagulopathy. Death may occur within a few hours of onset of the infection.

The infecting organisms can usually be identified through a culture of the cerebrospinal fluid and blood. Counter immunoelectrophoresis is widely used to detect bacterial antigens in body fluids, particularly cerebrospinal fluid and urine.

Management

Successful management depends on the administration of an antibiotic that crosses the blood–brain barrier into the subarachnoid space in sufficient concentration to halt the multiplication of bacteria. When the cerebrospinal fluid (CSF) and blood cultures are obtained, antimicrobial therapy is immediately started. Penicillin, ampicillin, or chloramphenicol, or one of the cephalosporins, may be used. Other antibiotics may be used if resistant strains of bacteria are identified. The patient is maintained on large intravenous doses of the appropriate antibiotic.

Dehydration or shock is treated with fluid volume expanders. Seizures, which may occur in the early course of the disease, are controlled with diazepam or phenytoin. An osmotic diuretic (*e.g.*, mannitol) may be used to treat cerebral edema.

Nursing Interventions

The patient's prognosis may depend on the supportive care given. The patient is very ill, and the combination of fever, dehydration, alkalosis, and cerebral edema may predispose to seizures. Airway obstruction, respiratory arrest, or cardiac dysrhythmias may follow. Thus, some of the nursing interventions are collaborative with those of the physician.

- In meningitis of all causes, the patient's clinical status and vital signs are constantly assessed, as altered consciousness may lead to airway obstruction. Arterial blood gas determinations, insertion of a cuffed endotracheal tube (or tracheostomy), and mechanical ventilation may be prescribed. Oxygen may be given to maintain the arterial partial pressure of oxygen (Po_2) at desired levels.
- The central venous pressure is monitored to assess for incipient shock, which precedes cardiac or respiratory failure. Generalized vasoconstriction, circumoral cyanosis, and cold extremities may be noted. The high fever must be reduced to decrease the load on the heart and the brain's oxygen demand. See Nursing Care Plan 62–1, p. 1905, for nursing interventions for the patient with an infectious disease.
- Rapid intravenous fluid replacement may be prescribed, but care is taken not to overhydrate the patient because of risk of cerebral edema.
- The body weight, serum electrolytes, urine volume and specific gravity, and osmolality of urine are closely monitored, especially if inappropriate antidiuretic hormone (ADH) secretion is suspected.
- Continuing nursing management requires ongoing assessment of the patient's clinical status, attention to skin and oral hygiene, promotion of comfort, and protection during seizures (p. 1723) and while comatose.
- Discharge from the nose and mouth is considered infectious. Respiratory isolation is advised for 24 hours after the start of antibiotic therapy.

Prevention and Patient Education. Persons having close contact with the patient should be considered candidates for antimicrobial prophylaxis (rifampin). Close contacts are observed and immediately examined if fever or other signs and symptoms of meningitis develop.

A meningococcal vaccine currently licensed in this country includes the polysaccharides of groups A, C, W135, and Y, and is used primarily in military recruits. Vaccine may be of benefit for some travelers visiting countries that are experiencing epidemic meningococcal disease. Vaccination should also be considered as an adjunct to antibiotic chemoprophylaxis for anyone living with a patient who has meningococcal disease.

A polysaccharide vaccine (Haemophilus b Polysaccharide Vaccine) against invasive *Haemophilus influenzae* type b has been licensed in the United States and is now used routinely in pediatrics for the prevention of meningitis.

Meningitis in AIDS. Aseptic, cryptococcal, and tuberculous meningitis have been reported in patients with acquired immunodeficiency virus (AIDS). Acute and chronic forms of aseptic meningitis may occur with AIDS; both are accompanied by headache, but signs of meningeal irritation generally occur with the acute form. Aseptic meningitis with AIDS may be accompanied by cranial nerve palsies. The meningitis is thought to be related to direct human immunodeficiency virus (HIV) infection of the central nervous system, as the virus can be isolated from the CSF.

Cryptococcal meningitis is the most common fungal infection of the central nervous system in patients with AIDS. Patients may experience headache, nausea, vomiting, seizures, confusion, and lethargy. Some patients develop few if any symptoms because of blunted inflammatory response occurring in the immunocompromised patient; others develop atypical features. The treatment of crytococcal meningitis is intravenous administration of amphotericin B, which may be used with or without 5-flucytosine. Maintenance therapy with amphotericin may be necessary to prevent relapse.

Intracranial Infection: Brain Abscess

A brain abscess is a collection of infectious material within the substance of the brain itself. It may occur by *direct invasion of the brain* from intracranial trauma or surgery; by *spread of infection from nearby sites* such as the sinuses, ears, and teeth (paranasal sinus infections, otitis media, dental sepsis); or by *spread of infection from other organs* (lung abscess, infective endocarditis); and can be a complication associated with some forms of meningitis. Brain abscess is a complication encountered increasingly in patients whose immune systems have been suppressed through either therapy or disease. To prevent brain abscesses, otitis media, mastoiditis, sinusitis, dental infections, and systemic infections should be treated promptly.

Assessment

Clinical Manifestations. The clinical manifestations of a brain abscess result from alterations in intracranial dynamics (edema, brain shift), infection, or the location of the abscess. Headache, usually worse in the morning, is the patient's most continuing symptom. Vomiting is also common. Focal neu-

rologic signs (weakness of an extremity, decreasing vision, seizures) may occur, depending on the site of the abscess. There may be a change in the patient's mental status, as reflected in lethargic, confused, irritable, or disoriented behavior. Fever may or may not be present.

Diagnostic Evaluation. Repeated neurologic examinations and continuing assessment of the patient are necessary to determine accurately the location of the abscess. CT is invaluable in showing the site of the abscess, after the evolution and resolution of suppurative lesions, and determining the optimum time for surgical intervention.

Management

The goal of management is to eliminate the abscess. Brain abscess is treated with antimicrobial therapy and surgical incision or aspiration. Antimicrobial treatment is given to eliminate the causative organism or reduce its virulence. Large intravenous doses are usually prescribed preoperatively to penetrate brain tissue and brain abscess. The therapy is continued postoperatively. Corticosteroids may be given to help reduce the inflammatory cerebral edema if the patient shows evidence of an increasing neurologic deficit.

Anticonvulsant medications (phenytoin, phenobarbital) may be given as a prophylaxis against seizures.

Multiple abscesses may be treated with appropriate antimicrobial therapy alone, with close monitoring by CT scans.

Neurologic deficits after treatment of brain abscess may include hemiparesis, seizures, visual defects, and cranial nerve palsies because of possible interference with brain tissue. Relapse is common, with a high mortality rate.

Intracranial Aneurysm

An intracranial (cerebral) aneurysm is a dilation of the walls of a cerebral artery that develops as a result of weakness in the arterial wall. The cause of aneurysms is unknown, although research is ongoing in an attempt to understand this problem (Fig. 57-2). An aneurysm may be due to atherosclerosis, resulting in a defect in the vessel wall with subsequent weakness of the wall; a congenital defect of the vessel wall; hypertensive vascular disease; head trauma; or advancing age. The cerebral arteries most commonly affected by an aneurysm are the internal carotid, anterior cerebral, anterior communicating, and middle cerebral arteries. A small percentage develop in the vertebrobasilar area. Multiple cerebral aneurysms are not uncommon.

Pathophysiology

Symptoms are produced when the aneurysm enlarges and presses on nearby cranial nerves or brain substance, or more dramatically, when the aneurysm ruptures, causing *subarachnoid hemorrhage* (hemorrhage into the cranial subarachnoid space). Normal brain metabolism is disrupted by the brain being exposed to blood; by an increase in ICP resulting from the sudden entry of blood into the subarachnoid space, which compresses and injures brain tissue; or by ischemia of the brain resulting from the reduced perfusion, pressure, and vasospasm that frequently accompany subarachnoid hemorrhage.

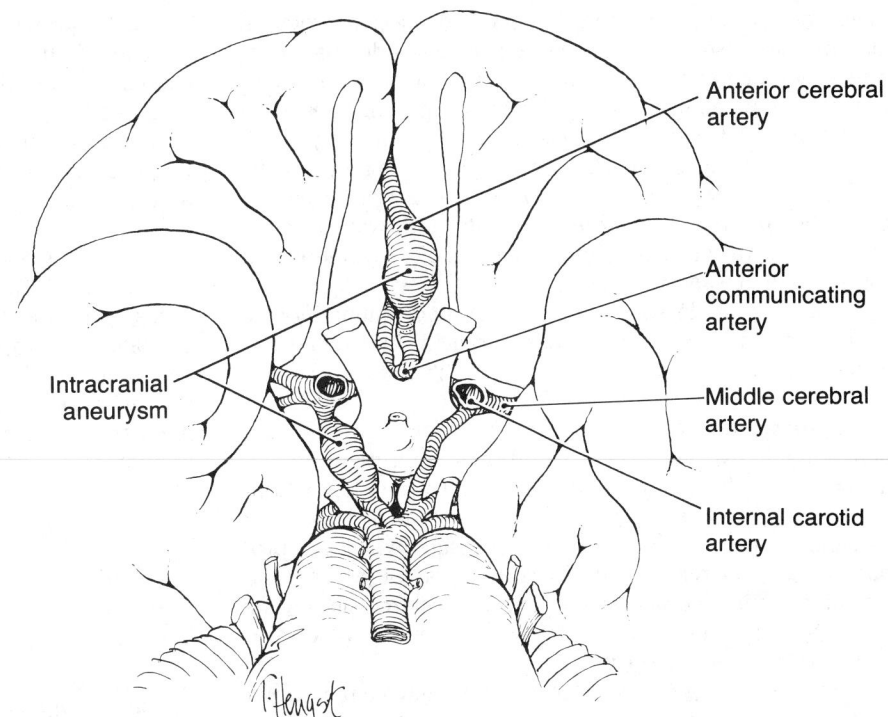

Figure 57-2. Intracranial aneurysm.

In addition to aneurysms, other causes of subarachnoid hemorrhage include arteriovenous malformations, tumors, trauma, blood dyscrasias, and unknown causes.

Clinical Manifestations

Rupture of the aneurysm usually produces a sudden, unusually severe headache and often loss of consciousness for a variable period. There may be pain and rigidity of the back of the neck and spine due to meningeal irritation. Visual disturbances (visual loss, diplopia, ptosis) occur when the aneurysm is adjacent to the oculomotor nerve. Tinnitus, dizziness, and hemiparesis also may occur.

At times, an aneurysm "leaks" blood, leading to the formation of a clot that seals the site of rupture. In this instance, the patient may show little neurologic deficit, or there may be severe bleeding, resulting in cerebral damage followed rapidly by coma and death. The mortality corresponds to the level of consciousness and neurologic deficit, but there is a high *immediate* mortality. Prognosis depends on the neurologic condition of the patient, age, associated diseases, and the extent and location of the aneurysm. Subarachnoid hemorrhage from an aneurysm is truly a catastrophic event.

Diagnostic Evaluation

The diagnosis is confirmed by CT scan; lumbar puncture, which discloses blood in the cerebrospinal fluid; and cerebral angiography, which shows the location and size of the aneurysm and gives information about the affected artery, adjoining vessels, and vascular branches.

Management

The goals of treatment are to allow the brain to recover from the initial insult (bleeding), to prevent or minimize the risk of rebleeding, and to prevent or treat other complications. These include rebleeding; cerebral vasospasm resulting in cerebral ischemia; acute hydrocephalus, which results when free blood obstructs the reabsorption of cerebrospinal fluid by the arachnoid villi; epilepsy; and anxiety.

Management consists of bed rest with sedation to prevent agitation and stress, management of the vasospasm, and surgical or medical treatment to prevent rebleeding.

Vasospasm. The development of cerebral vasospasm (narrowing of the lumen of the involved cranial blood vessel) is a serious complication of subarachnoid hemorrhage and often is correlated with a poor clinical condition and prognosis. The mechanism responsible for the spasm is not clear, but the occurrence of vasospasms correlates with increasing amounts of blood in the subarachnoid cisterns and cerebral fissures, as visualized by CT scan. Vasospasm leads to increased vascular resistance, which impedes cerebral blood flow and causes brain ischemia and infarction. The signs and symptoms exhibited by the patient reflect the areas of the brain involved. Vasospasm is often heralded by a worsening headache, a decrease in level of responsiveness (confusion, lethargy, disorientation), or the appearance of a new focal neurologic deficit (aphasia, hemiparesis [partial paralysis affecting one side of the body]). Vasospasm frequently occurs within the 4th to 12th day after the initial hemorrhage. It is during this time that the clot undergoes the lytic process (dissolution), and this increases the chances of rebleeding.

It is believed by many neurosurgeons that early operation to clip the aneurysm will prevent rebleeding, and that the removal of blood from the basal cisterns around the major cerebral arteries may prevent the development of vasospasm. In addition, the intravenous administration of the calcium-blocker nimodipine during the critical time in which vasospasm may develop may offer protection against delayed ischemic deterioration.

Increased Intracranial Pressure. An increase in ICP almost always follows a subarachnoid hemorrhage, probably because of disturbed circulation of CSF caused by blood in the basal cisterns. If the patient shows evidence of deterioration from increased ICP (due to cerebral edema, herniation, hydroceph-alus, or vasospasm), CSF drainage is instituted by lumbar punc-ture or ventricular catheter drainage, and mannitol is given to reduce ICP. When mannitol is used as a long-term measure to control ICP, dehydration and disturbances in electrolyte bal-ance (hyponatremia/hypernatremia; hypokalemia/hyperkale-mia) may occur. Mannitol acts by osmotically pulling water out of the brain as well as by reducing total body water through diuresis. The patient is monitored for signs of dehydration and for rebound elevation of ICP.

If surgery is delayed or contraindicated, antifibrinolytic agents (aminocaproic acid; tranexamic acid) may be admin-istered to delay or prevent dissolution of the clot at the site of the aneurysmal rupture.

Systemic Hypertension.   Efforts are made to prevent sud-den systemic hypertension. If blood pressure is elevated, an-tihypertensive therapy (nitroprusside) may be prescribed. Con-stant blood pressure monitoring by arterial line is carried out to avoid a precipitous drop in blood pressure, which can pro-duce brain ischemia. Because seizures cause blood pressure elevation, anticonvulsant agents are administered prophylac-tically. Stool softeners are used to prevent straining, which also can elevate the blood pressure.

Analgesics (codeine, acetaminophen) may be prescribed for head and neck pain. The patient is fitted with graded pres-sure elastic stockings to prevent deep vein thrombosis, a threat to any patient who is on bed rest.

Surgical Management

The patient is prepared for surgical intervention as soon as his condition is deemed suitable. The nursing management of the patient after a craniotomy is discussed in Chapter 56.

The goal of surgery is to prevent further bleeding. This is accomplished by isolating the aneurysm from its circulation or by strengthening the arterial wall. An aneurysm may be treated by excluding it from the cerebral circulation by means of a ligature or a clip across its neck (Fig. 57-3). If this is not ana-tomically possible, the aneurysm can be reinforced by wrap-ping it with plastic, muscle, or some other substance. An extracranial–intracranial arterial bypass may be performed to establish collateral blood supply to allow surgery on the aneu-rysm. Alternatively, an extracranial method may be used, whereby the carotid artery is gradually occluded in the neck

to reduce pressure within the blood vessel. After ligation of the carotid artery, there is some risk of cerebral ischemia and sudden hemiplegia because during the operative procedure there is a temporary occlusion of the blood supply to the brain (unless a temporary inlying bypass shunt is used). In anticipa-tion of these complications, measurements of cerebral blood flow and internal carotid pressure may be taken to identify those patients who are at risk for postoperative ischemic episodes.

Other postoperative complications include the appearance of psychological symptoms (disorientation, amnesia, Korsa-koff's syndrome, personality impairment), intraoperative em-bolization, postoperative internal artery occlusion, fluid and electrolyte disturbances (from dysfunction of the neurohypo-physeal system), and gastrointestinal bleeding. (The manage-ment of the patient after intracranial surgery is discussed in Chapter 56.)

▶ Nursing Process
The Patient With a Cerebral Aneurysm

▷ Assessment

A complete neurologic assessment is performed initially and should include an evaluation of the following:

    Level of consciousness
    Pupillary reaction
    Motor and sensory function
    Cranial nerve deficits (extraocular eye movements, facial
        droop, presence of ptosis)
    Speech difficulties, visual disturbance or other neurologic def-
        icits, headache

Neurologic assessment findings are documented and re-ported as indicated. Frequency of these assessments varies and is determined by the patient's condition. Any changes in the patient's condition require reassessment and thorough documentation; changes should be reported immediately.

Alteration in level of consciousness is often the earliest sign of deterioration in a patient with a cerebral aneurysm. Because nurses have the most frequent contact with patients, it is often the nurse who is the first to detect what may be subtle changes. Mild drowsiness and slight slurring of speech may be early signs that the patient's level of consciousness is

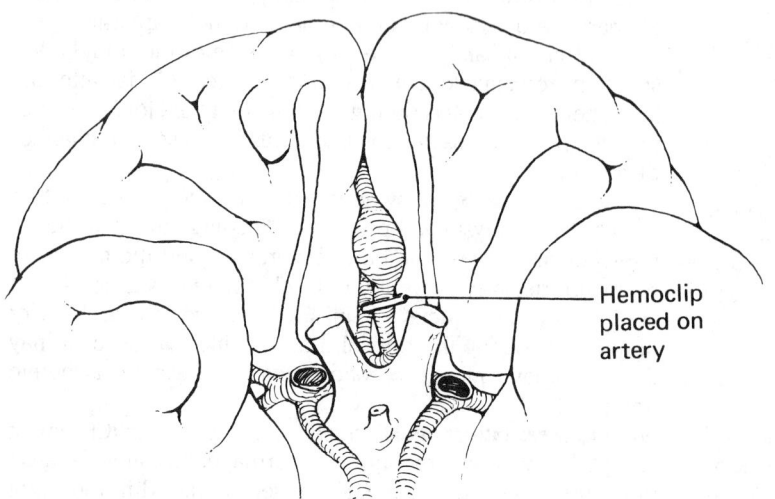

Figure 57–3. Cerebral aneurysm isolated by means of a hemoclip.

Hemoclip placed on artery

deteriorating. Frequent nursing assessment is critical in the patient with known or suspected cerebral aneurysm.

▷ Nursing Diagnoses

Based on the assessment data, the patient's nursing diagnoses may include the following:

- Altered cerebral perfusion due to bleeding from the aneurysm
- Sensory/perceptual alteration due to the restrictions of subarachnoid precautions
- Anxiety due to illness or restrictions of subarachnoid precautions

▷ *Potential Problems.* Based on the assessment data, potential problems that are addressed jointly by members of the health care team include the following:

- Seizures
- Vasospasm

▷ Planning and Implementation

▷ *Goals:* The goals for the patient may include improved cerebral tissue perfusion, relief of sensory/perceptual deprivation, relief of anxiety, and the absence of seizure activity and vasospasm.

▷ Nursing Interventions

▷ *Improved Cerebral Tissue Perfusion.* The patient is monitored continually for neurologic deterioration occurring from recurrent bleeding, increasing ICP, or vasospasm. A neurologic flow record is kept. The blood pressure, pulse, level of responsiveness (an indicator of cerebral perfusion), pupillary responses, and motor function are checked hourly. The respiratory status is monitored, since reduction in PO_2 in brain areas with impaired autoregulation increases the chances of a cerebral infarction. Any changes are reported immediately.

Subarachnoid precautions are implemented to provide a nonstimulating environment and prevent increases in intracranical pressure and further bleeding. The patient is placed on immediate and absolute bed rest in a quiet, nonstressful setting because activity, pain, and anxiety elevate the blood pressure, which increases the risk of bleeding. Visitors, except for family, are restricted.

The head of the bed is elevated moderately to provide venous drainage and decrease ICP. Some neurologists, however, prefer that the patient remain flat to increase cerebral perfusion.

Any activity that suddenly increases the blood pressure or obstructs venous return is avoided. This includes the Valsalva maneuver, straining, forceful sneezing, pulling up in bed, acute flexion or rotation of the head and neck (which compromises the jugular veins), and cigarette smoking. Any activity requiring exertion is contraindicated. The patient is instructed to exhale through the mouth during voiding or defecation to decrease strain. No enemas are permitted but stool softeners and mild laxatives are prescribed. Both prevent constipation, which would cause an increase in ICP, as would enemas. Dim lighting is helpful, because photophobia (visual intolerance of light) is common. Coffee and tea, unless decaffeinated, are usually eliminated.

All personal care is administered by the nurse. The patient is fed and bathed to prevent any exertion that might raise the blood pressure. External stimuli are kept to a minimum, including no television, no radio, no reading, and maintenance of visitor restriction. Visitors are restricted in an effort to keep the patient as quiet as possible. This precaution must be individualized based on patient condition and response to visitors. A sign indicating this restriction should be placed on the door of the room, and the restrictions should be discussed with both patient and family.

▷ *Relief of Sensory Deprivation.* Sensory stimulation is kept to a minimum. In patients who are awake, alert, and oriented, an explanation of the restrictions helps reduce the patient's sense of isolation. Reality orientation is provided to help in maintaining orientation.

▷ *Relief of Anxiety.* The purpose of subarachnoid precautions should be thoroughly explained to both patient (if possible) and family. Keeping the patient well informed of the plan of care provides reassurance and helps minimize anxiety. Appropriate reassurance helps relieve the patient's fears and anxiety. The family also requires information and support.

▷ *Reduced Seizure Activity.* Seizure precautions are maintained for every patient who may be at risk for seizure activity. These include fully functioning suction equipment at the bedside, including suction catheter, a padded tongue blade, and an oral airway. Padded siderails are provided to protect the patient from possible injury. Should a seizure occur, maintaining the patient's airway and preventing injury are the primary initial goals. Drug treatment is initiated at this time if it has not already been initiated. The drug of choice is phenytoin (Dilantin), as this drug usually provides adequate anticonvulsant action while causing no drowsiness at therapeutic levels.

▷ *Reduced Vasospasm.* The management of vasospasm remains difficult and controversial. Currently a popular explanation for vasospasm is that it is caused by an increased influx of calcium into the cell; thus drug therapy is designed to block or antagonize this action and may prevent or reverse the action of vasospasm already present. Two calcium blockers are approved and available, including verapamil (Isoptin) and nifedipine (Procardia). Other therapy for vasospasm aimed at minimizing the deleterious effects of the associated cerebral ischemia include fluid volume expanders and induced arterial hypertension, normotension, or hemodilution. These treatments remain somewhat experimental but have shown promise. The practice of fluid restriction in these patients is currently being questioned and has been discontinued in many institutions.

▷ Evaluation

Expected Outcomes

1. Demonstrates intact neurologic status
   a. Is alert and oriented to time, place, and person
   b. Demonstrates normal speech patterns and intact cognitive processes
   c. Demonstrates normal and equal strength, movement, and sensation of all four extremities
   d. Exhibits normal deep tendon reflexes and pupillary responses
   e. Exhibits normal vital signs and respiratory pattern
   f. Participates in procedures to reduce intracranial bleeding (on bed rest in quiet, nonstimulating environment; avoids

straining, excess rotation or flexion of head and neck, and smoking)

2. Demonstrates normal sensory perceptions
   a. States rationale for subarachnoid precautions
   b. Verbalizes psychological effects of restrictions on self and family
   c. Exhibits clear thought processes
3. Exhibits reduced anxiety level
   a. States that he is less anxious
   b. Reports moderate level of anxiety
   c. Verbalizes concern for family
   d. Is less restless
   e. Exhibits absence of physiologic indicators of anxiety (*i.e.*, normal vital signs; normal respiratory rate; absence of excessive, fast speech)
   f. Reports that he is sleeping and resting at intervals
4. Exhibits absence of seizure activity
   a. Exhibits normal neuromuscular activity without seizures
   b. Verbalizes understanding of seizure precautions
   c. Participates in seizure precautions, including adhering to medication regimen
5. Exhibits absence of vasospasm
   a. Exhibits normal mental status
   b. Exhibits normal motor and sensory status
   c. Has normal vital signs
   d. Reports no visual changes

In summary, a cerebral aneurysm is a dilation of the walls of a cerebral artery. Signs and symptoms may occur as the aneurysm enlarges and impinges on nearby intracranial structures or when the aneurysm ruptures, causing hemorrhage. With massive hemorrhage, severe neurologic deficit results, and the mortality rate is high. Other patients may experience less severe bleeding rather than massive hemorrhage. In these patients, efforts are initiated to prevent sudden increases in bleeding by minimizing the risk of vasospasm, hypertension, and increased ICP. Subarachnoid precautions are implemented and require minimization of sensory stimulation. The nurse provides all physical care and uses communication skills to reduce the anxiety level of the patient and his family. Expert assessment skills are essential to detect subtle changes in the patient's neurologic status.

Multiple Sclerosis

Multiple sclerosis (MS) is a chronic, degenerative progressive disease of the central nervous system characterized by the occurrence of small patches of demyelination in the brain and spinal cord. (*Demyelination* refers to the destruction of myelin, the fatty and protein material that surrounds certain nerve fibers in the brain and spinal cord.) Demyelination results in a disorder in the transmission of nerve impulses.

The cause of MS is not known. Research evidence suggests that myelin damage is the primary event, and that it results from a viral infection early in life that becomes apparent as an immune process later in life. Although some form of viral infection may be the initiating mechanism, a defective immune response probably plays a major role in the pathogenesis of MS.

Epidemiologic findings indicate that MS is more common in people living in the northern temperate climate zones. It is one of the most disabling neurologic diseases of young adults (20 to 40 years of age) in this country, affecting twice as many women as men. Its occurrence in patients who are young increases the medical, psychological, social, and economic problems encountered by both patient and family.

Pathophysiology

In MS, the demyelination is scattered irregularly throughout the central nervous system (Fig. 57-4). Myelin is lost from the axis cylinders, and the axons themselves degenerate. The plaques or patches in the involved areas become sclerosed, interrupting the flow of nerve impulses and resulting in a variety of manifestations, depending on which nerves are affected. The areas most frequently affected are the optic nerves, chiasm, tracts, the cerebrum, the brain stem and cerebellum, and the spinal cord.

Clinical Manifestations

The course of MS may take on many different patterns. Most patients who are young at the onset of symptoms begin with a relapsing–remitting course with complete recovery between relapses. Other patients have a chronic progressive course from the outset with a progressive decline in function. A rapidly progressive course is much less frequent. Other patients' disease follows a benign course with a normal life span and symptoms so mild that patients do not seek health care and treatment.

The signs and symptoms of MS are varied and multiple, reflecting the location of the lesion (plaque) or combination of lesions. The symptoms most commonly reported are fatigue, weakness, numbness, difficulty in coordination, and loss of balance. About 75% of patients in one survey had visual disturbances due to lesions in the optic nerves or their connections: blurring of vision, patchy blindness (*scotoma*), or total blindness. Spastic weakness of the extremities and loss of the abdominal reflexes are due to involvement of the main motor pathways (*pyramidal tracts*) of the spinal cord. Disruption of the sensory axons may produce sensory dysfunction. Cognitive and psychosocial problems may reflect frontal or parietal lobe involvement. Involvement of the cerebellum or basal ganglia can produce *ataxia* (impaired coordination of movements) and tremor. Emotional lability and euphoria result from loss of the control connections between the cortex and the basal ganglia and may occur in patients with MS. Bladder, bowel, and sexual problems also occur if the process involves the cord pathways connected with the pontine micturition center and the sacral plexus.

Secondary manifestations are related to complications: urinary tract infections, constipation, pressure ulcers, contracture deformities, dependent pedal edema, pneumonia, and reactive depressions. Emotional, social, marital, economic, and vocational problems may result as a consequence of the disease.

MS is characterized by exacerbations (the appearance of new symptoms and worsening of existing ones) and remissions (periods in which symptoms decrease or disappear). Relapses may be associated with periods of emotional and physical stress. As evidenced by MRI, however, many plaques do not produce serious symptoms, and many patients are not seriously incapacitated but have long periods of remission between ep-

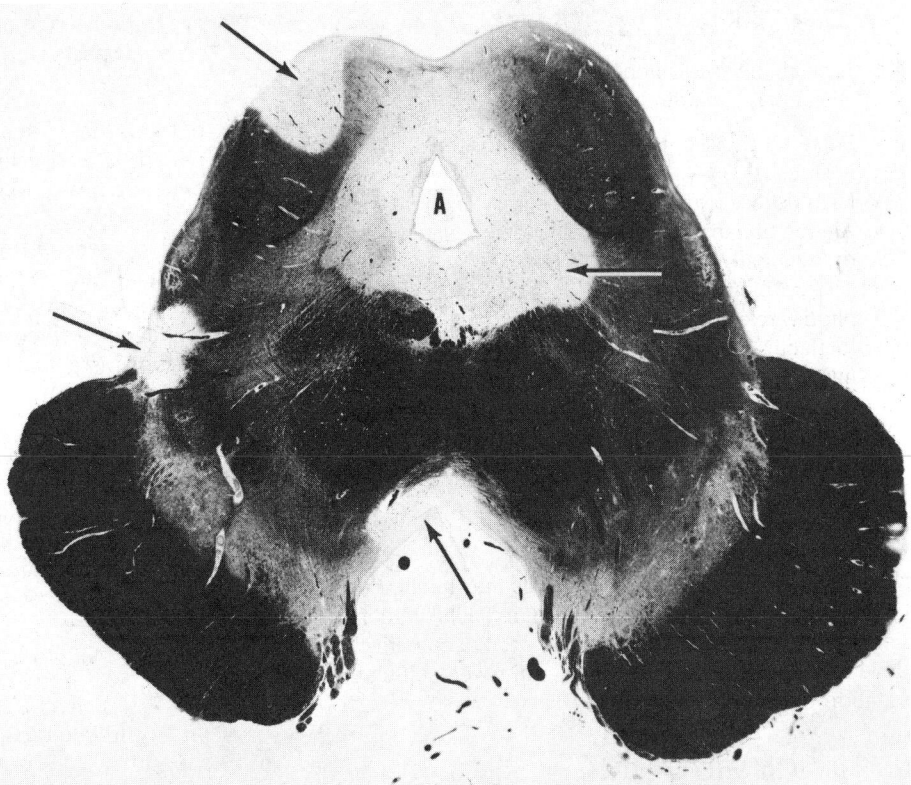

Figure 57–4. Cross section from the midbrain (enlarged approximately three times) of a patient with chronic MS. Specimen stained to show myelin (*black*). The four white areas indicated by the arrows are typical plaques in which the myelin has been destroyed. The plaque to the right of the aqueduct (A) impinges upon periaqueductal gray matter. The nerve fibers in these plaques have lost their myelin sheaths, and as a consequence, conduction of stimuli in these areas would be impeded or lost. (Courtesy of Cedric S. Raine, MD, Professor of Pathology [Neuropathology] and Neuroscience, Albert Einstein College of Medicine of Yeshiva University.)

isodes. There is evidence that remyelination occurs in some patients.

Diagnostic Evaluation

Electrophoresis study of the CSF usually discloses the presence of *oligoclonal banding* (several bands of gamma G immunoglobulin [IgG]), reflecting immunoglobulin abnormalities. In fact, abnormal IgG antibody appears in the CSF of up to 95% of patients with MS. Evoked potential studies are carried out to help define the extent of the disease process and monitor changes. CT scans may show cerebral atrophic changes. MRI has become a primary diagnostic tool for visualizing small plaques and for evaluating the course of the disease and effect of the treatment. Underlying bladder dysfunction is diagnosed by urodynamic studies. Neuropsychological testing may be indicated to assess cognitive impairment. A sexual history helps to identify specific areas of concern.

Management

At this time there is no cure for MS. An individualized, organized, and rational treatment program is indicated to relieve the patient's symptoms and provide continuing support. Many patients with MS are in stable condition and only require intermittent treatment aimed at controlling symptoms; others experience steady progression of their disease.

Corticosteroids or ACTH is used as an anti-inflammatory agent that may improve the nerve conduction. Because immune mechanisms may be a factor in the pathogenesis of MS, a number of pharmacologic agents are being tried to modulate the immune response and reduce the rate at which the disease progresses and the frequency and severity of the exacerbations. These drugs include azathioprine, cyclophosphamide, and interferon. Other immunosuppressive modalities (*e.g.*, radiation)

are currently under investigation as possible treatments for progressive forms of MS.

Baclofen is the current treatment of choice for spasticity. Patients with severe spasticity and contractures may require nerve blocks and surgical intervention to prevent further disability.

Management of bladder and bowel control are among the patient's most difficult problems. Generally, bladder symptoms fall into the following categories: (1) inability to store urine (hyperreflexic; uninhibited); (2) inability to empty the bladder (hyporeflexic; hypotonic); and (3) a mixture of both types. Although a variety of drugs are used to treat these problems, intermittent self-catheterization is an effective treatment of bladder dysfunction. Often urinary tract infection is superimposed on the underlying neurologic dysfunction. Ascorbic acid may be given to acidify the urine, making bacterial growth less likely. Antibiotics are prescribed when appropriate.

▶ Nursing Process
The Patient With Multiple Sclerosis

◊ Assessment

Nursing assessment is carried out with an awareness of actual and potential problems associated with the disease, including neurologic problems, secondary complications, and the impact of the disease on the patient and family. The patient's movements and walking are observed to determine if he is in danger of falling. The patient's function is assessed when he is well rested and when fatigued. The patient is assessed for weakness, spasticity, visual impairment, and incontinence. How has this condition affected his life style? How well is the patient coping? What would the patient like to do better?

Nursing Diagnoses

Based on all the assessment data, the patient's potential nursing diagnoses may include the following:

- Impaired physical mobility related to weakness, muscle paresis, spasticity
- High risk for injury related to sensory and visual impairment
- Altered urinary and bowel elimination related to spinal cord dysfunction
- Altered thought processes (loss of memory, dementia, euphoria) related to cerebral dysfunction
- Ineffective coping
- Impaired home maintenance management related to physical, psychological, and social limits imposed by MS
- Potential for sexual dysfunction related to spinal cord involvement or psychological reactions to condition

Planning and Implementation

Goals:
The patient's major goals may include promotion of physical mobility, avoidance of injury, achievement of bladder and bowel continence, improvement of cognitive function, development of coping strengths, improved self-care and adaptation to sexual dysfunction.

Nursing Interventions

An individualized program of physical therapy, rehabilitation, and education is combined with emotional support. The nursing interventions also focus on the social and psychological problems of the person with chronic disease.

Physical Mobility.
Relaxation and coordination exercises promote muscle efficiency for the person with MS. Progressive resistive exercises are used to strengthen weak muscles, because diminishing muscle power is a significant problem for these patients. The patient is encouraged to work up to the point just short of fatigue. Vigorous physical exercise is *not* advisable, because it raises the body temperature and may aggravate symptoms. Prolonged exercise that tires an extremity may cause paresis, numbness, or incoordination. The patient is advised to take frequent short rest periods, preferably lying down. Extreme fatigue may be a contributing factor in exacerbation of symptoms.

Walking exercises improve the gait, particularly when there is loss of position sense of the legs. If certain muscle groups are irreversibly affected, other muscles can be trained to take over their actions.

Muscle spasticity is common and, in its later stages, is characterized by severe adductor spasm of the hips with flexor spasm of the hips and knees. If this is not relieved, fibrous contractures of these joints with resultant pressure ulcers over the sacrum and hips (due to inability to properly position the patient) occur. Warm packs may be beneficial, but hot baths should be avoided because of risk of burn injury secondary to loss of sensation. Daily exercises for muscle stretching are prescribed to minimize joint contractures. Special attention is given to hamstrings, gastrocnemius muscles, hip adductors, biceps, and wrist and finger flexors. Muscle spasticity is common and interferes with normal function. A stretch-hold-relax routine is helpful for relaxing and treating muscle spasticity. Swimming and stationary bicycling are useful, and progressive weight-bearing can relieve spasticity in the legs. The patient should not be hurried in any of these activities, because hurrying increases spasticity.

Prevention of Injury.
If motor dysfunction causes problems of incoordination and clumsiness, or if ataxia is apparent, the patient is at risk for falling. To overcome this disability, the patient is taught to walk with feet wide apart to widen the base of support and increase walking stability. If there is loss of position sense, the patient is taught to watch the feet while walking. Gait training may require aids (walker, cane braces, crutches, parallel bars) and physical therapy. If the gait remains inefficient, a wheelchair may be the solution. The occupational therapist is a valuable resource person in suggesting and securing aids to promote independence. If incoordination is a problem, and tremor of the upper extremities occurs when voluntary movement is attempted (*intention tremor*), weighted bracelets or wrist cuffs are helpful. The patient is trained in transfer and activities of daily living.

Because sensory loss may occur in addition to motor loss, pressure ulcers are a continuing threat to skin integrity. Confinement to a wheelchair compounds the threat. (See pp. 236–240 for a discussion of the prevention and treatment of pressure ulcers.)

Promotion of Bladder and Bowel Control.
The patient with urinary frequency, urgency, or incontinence requires special support. The sensation of the need to void must be heeded immediately, so the bedpan or urinal should be readily available. A voiding time schedule is set up (every 1½ to 2 hours initially, with gradual lengthening of the time intervals). The patient is instructed to drink a measured amount of fluid every 2 hours and then attempt to void 30 minutes after drinking. An alarm clock may be set for the patient who does not have enough sensation to warn of the need to empty the bladder. The nurse encourages the patient to take the prescribed medications to treat bladder spasticity, as this allows greater independence. Intermittent self-catheterization has been successful in maintaining bladder control.

If the female patient has permanent urinary incontinence, urinary diversion procedures are considered. The male patient may wear a condom appliance for urine collection.

Bowel problems include constipation, fecal impaction, and incontinence. Adequate fluids, dietary fiber, and a bowel-training program are frequently effective in solving these problems. (see pp. 240–242).

Improved Sensory and Cognitive Function.
Measures may be taken if visual and speech defects occur (the cranial nerves relating to sight and speech may be affected by MS). An eye patch or an eyeglass occluder may be used to block visual impulses of one eye when the patient has *diplopia* (double vision). Prism glasses may be helpful for the bedridden patient who is having difficulty reading in the supine position. Persons with any physical limitations preventing them from reading regular print materials are eligible for the free talking book services of the Library of Congress (see Bibliography for address).

When the cranial nerves controlling the mechanisms of speech are involved, *dysarthrias* (defects of articulation) marked by slurring, low volume of speech, and difficulties in phonation are seen. There are also problems with shallow breathing. A speech-language pathologist teaches the patient, family, and health team members about communication problems and the use of compensatory techniques.

MS imposes numerous stresses on the patient and family. Although not common, cognitive impairment may occur early in the disease. Embarrassing and humiliating symptoms may result in "inappropriate" responses by the patient. As there may be organic changes in the brain, MS patients may be forgetful and easily distracted and may exhibit emotional lability. Patients adapt to illness in a variety of ways, which may include denial (with euphoria), depression, withdrawal, and hostility. MS patients frequently conceal their emotions behind a smiling or flat, unsmiling mask. Compassion and significant emotional support are required to help patients adapt to a new self-image and cope with the disruption in their lives. The patient is assisted to set meaningful and realistic goals to achieve a sense of purpose, to remain as active as possible, and to keep up social interests and activities. Hobbies may help the patient's morale and provide satisfying interests if the disease progresses to the stage in which normal activities cannot be pursued.

The family should be made aware of the nature and degree of cognitive impairment. The environment is kept structured, and lists and other memory aids are used to help the patient move ahead in the daily routine.

▷ *Strengthened Coping Mechanisms.*   The family faces almost overwhelming frustrations and problems. MS strikes individuals who are in the developmental stage of life concerned about career and family responsibilities. Family conflict, disintegration, separation, and divorce are not uncommon. Often very young family members assume the responsibility of caring for a disabled parent. Nursing interventions in this area include alleviating stress and making appropriate referrals for counseling and support to minimize the adverse effects of dealing with chronic illness.

The nurse, mindful of these complex problems, initiates home care through several channels and coordinates a network of services: social services, speech therapy, physical therapy, homemaker services, and the like. To strengthen the patient's coping skills, as much information as possible is provided. People who live with chronic illness need an updated list of aids and resources that are available.

Coping through problem-solving involves helping the patient define the problem and develop alternatives for its management. Careful planning, staying flexible, and maintaining a hopeful attitude are useful for psychological and physical adaptation.

▷ *Improved Self-Care.*   MS can affect every facet of daily living. Once certain abilities are lost, they are almost impossible to regain. Physical abilities may vary from day to day. Modifications that allow continuance of self-care activities should be sought (raised toilet seat, bathing helps, telephone modifications, long-handled comb, tongs, modified clothing). Physical and emotional stresses should be avoided as much as possible, because these worsen symptoms and impair performance. Exposure to heat appears to increase fatigue, and fatigue lessens motor power. Air-conditioning in at least one room is recommended. Exposure to extreme cold may increase spasticity. The patient must remain under continuing medical supervision.

The patient with MS is encouraged to contact the local chapter of the National Multiple Sclerosis Society for services, publications, and contact with others with MS. Local chapters give direct services to patients. Through group participation, the patient has an opportunity to identify with others having similar problems, gain relief and release, and learn self-help methods in a social environment.

▷ *Adaptation to Sexual Dysfunction.*   Patients with MS and their partners face problems that interfere with sexual activity, arising not only as a direct consequence of nerve damage but also from psychological reactions to the disease. Easy fatigability, conflicts arising from dependency and depression, emotional lability, and loss of self-esteem and feelings of self-worth compound the problem. Erectile and ejaculatory disorders in males and orgasmic dysfunction and adductor spasms of the thigh muscles in females can make intercourse difficult or impossible. Bladder and bowel incontinence and urinary tract infections add to the difficulties.

An experienced sexual counselor helps bring into focus the patient's or partner's sexual resources and suggests relevant information and supportive therapy. Sharing and communicating feelings, planning for sexual activity (to counteract fatigue), exercising different sexual options, and demonstrating a willingness to experiment may open up a wide range of sexual enjoyment and experiences.

▷ Evaluation

Expected Outcomes

1. Adapts to impaired mobility and spasticity
   a. Participates in gait-training and rehabilitation program
   b. Establishes a balanced program of rest and exercise
   c. Uses assistive devices
   d. Identifies measures to conserve energy; arranges schedule to accommodate periods of higher energy levels
2. Avoids injury
   a. Uses visual cues to compensate for decreased sense of touch or position
   b. Asks for assistance when necessary
3. Attains/maintains improved bladder and bowel control
   a. Monitors self for urine retention
   b. Demonstrates intermittent self-catheterization technique, if indicated
   c. Identifies the signs and symptoms of urinary tract infection
   d. Maintains adequate fluid and fiber intake
   e. Shows no fecal soiling
4. Compensates for cognitive dysfunction
   a. Uses lists to compensate for memory losses
   b. Discusses problems with trusted advisor–friend
   c. Substitutes new activities for those that have been given up
5. Demonstrates improvement of coping strengths
   a. Maintains sense of control
   b. Makes plans to redesign life style
   c. Verbalizes desire to pursue goals and developmental tasks of adulthood
6. Adapts to sexual dysfunction
   a. Is able to discuss problem with partner and appropriate health professional
   b. Identifies alternate means of sexual expression

Parkinson's Disease

Parkinson's disease is a progressive neurologic disorder affecting the brain centers that are responsible for control and regulation of movement. It is characterized by *bradykinesia* (slowness of movement), tremor, and muscle stiffness or rigidity.

Pathophysiology

The major lesion appears to result in a loss of pigmented neurons, particularly those in the substantia nigra of the brain (Fig. 57-5). (The *substantia nigra* is a collection of midbrain nuclei that project fibers to the corpus striatrum.) One of the major neurotransmitters in this area of the brain, and in other parts of the central nervous system, is dopamine, which has an important inhibiting function in the central control of movement. Although dopamine normally exists in high concentration in certain parts of the brain, in Parkinson's disease it is depleted in the substantia nigra and the corpus striatum. Depletion of dopamine levels in the basal ganglia is associated with bradykinesia, rigidity, and tremors.

Regional cerebral blood flow is reduced in patients with Parkinson's disease, and there is a high prevalence of dementia. Biochemical and pathologic data suggest that demented patients with Parkinson's disease may have coexistent Alzheimer's disease.

In most patients, the cause of the disease is unknown. Arteriosclerotic parkinsonism is seen more frequently in older age groups. It may follow encephalitis, poisoning or toxicity (manganese, carbon monoxide), or hypoxia, or may be drug induced.

The disease is most prevalent among persons in their 60s and is the second most common neurologic disorder of the elderly.

Clinical Manifestations

The chief manifestations of Parkinson's disease are impaired movement, muscular rigidity, resting tremor, muscle weakness, and loss of postural reflexes. Early signs include a stiffening of the extremities and a waxlike rigidity in the performance of all movements. The patient has difficulty in initiating, maintaining, and performing motor activities, and experiences some delay in carrying out normal activity.

As the disease progresses, the tremor begins, frequently in one hand and arm, then the other, and later in the head, although the tremor may remain unilateral (Fig. 57-6). The tremor is characteristic: it is a slow, turning motion (pronation–supination) of the forearm and the hand, and a motion of the thumb against the fingers as if rolling a pill between the fingers. It increases when the patient is concentrating or feeling anxious, and is present while the patient is at rest.

Other characteristics of the disease affect the face, stature, and gait. There is loss of normal arm swing. Eventually, the rigid extremities become definitely weaker. Because there is limited movement in the muscles, the face has so little expression that it is said to be masklike (with infrequency of blinking), a feature that can be recognized at a glance.

There is a loss of postural reflexes, and the patient stands with head bent forward and walks with a propulsive gait. Difficulty in pivoting and loss of balance (either forward or backward) may lead to frequent falls.

Frequently these patients show signs of depression, and it has not been established whether the depression is a reaction to the disorder or related to a biochemical abnormality. Mental manifestations may appear in the form of cognitive, perceptual, and memory deficits. A number of psychiatric manifestations (personality changes, psychosis, dementia, acute confusion) are particularly common among the elderly. Complications from immobility (pneumonia, urinary tract infection) and the consequences of falls and accidents are major causes of death.

Diagnostic Evaluation

Early diagnosis of Parkinson's disease can be difficult, as the patient can rarely pinpoint when symptoms started. Often someone close to the patient notices a change such as stooped posture, a stiff arm, a slight limp, or tremor. Handwriting changes may be an early diagnostic clue. A diagnosis of Parkinson's disease can usually be made with certainty when there is evidence of tremor, rigidity, and bradykinesia (abnormally slow movements). The results of the patient's history and neurologic examination are carefully evaluated.

Management

The goal of treatment is to enhance dopamine transmission. Drug therapy includes antihistamines, anticholinergics, amantadine, levodopa, monoamine oxidase (MAO) inhibitors, and antidepressants. Many of these drugs can cause psychiatric side effects in the elderly.

Antihistamine Drugs.   Antihistamines have mild central anticholinergic and sedative effects, and may be helpful in allaying tremors.

Anticholinergic Therapy.   Anticholinergic drugs (trihexyphenidyl, procyclidine, and benztropine mesylate) are effective for controlling the tremor and rigidity of parkinsonism. These drugs may be used in combination with levodopa. They counteract the action of acetylcholine in the central nervous system. Side effects of these drugs include blurred vision, flushing, rash, constipation, urinary retention, and acute confusional states. Intraocular pressure is closely monitored because these

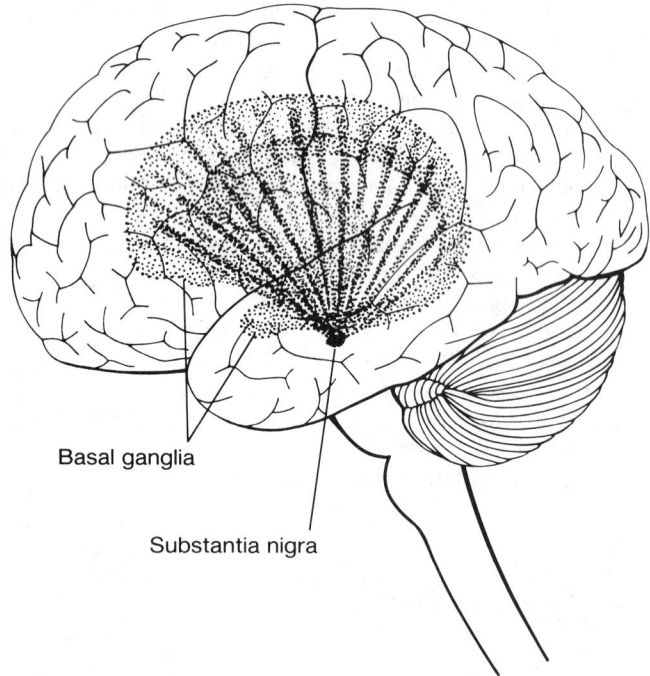

Figure 57–5.   The loss of dopamine nerve cells from the brain's substantia nigra is thought to be responsible for the symptoms of parkinsonism. (Courtesy of the National Institutes of Health.)

Basal ganglia

Substantia nigra

CLINICAL FEATURES

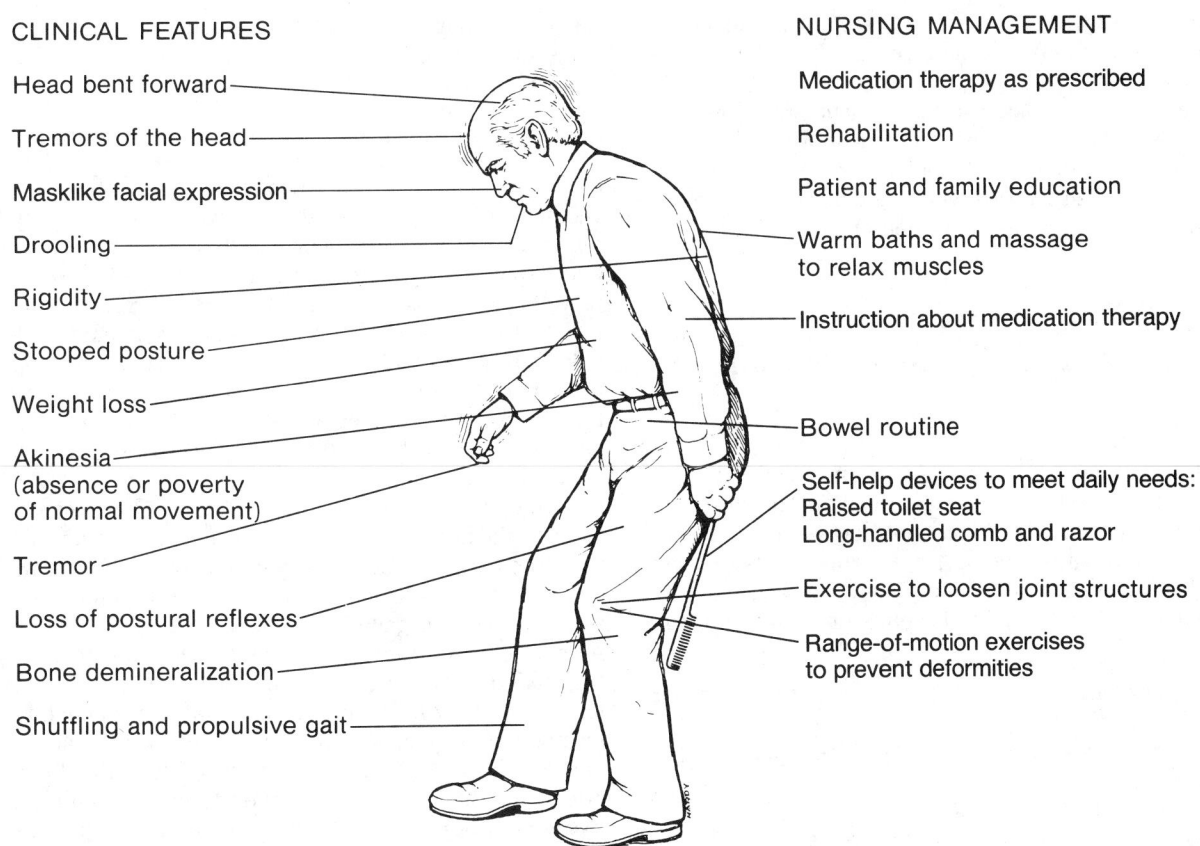

Head bent forward

Tremors of the head

Masklike facial expression

Drooling

Rigidity

Stooped posture

Weight loss

Akinesia
(absence or poverty
of normal movement)

Tremor

Loss of postural reflexes

Bone demineralization

Shuffling and propulsive gait

NURSING MANAGEMENT

Medication therapy as prescribed

Rehabilitation

Patient and family education

Warm baths and massage
to relax muscles

Instruction about medication therapy

Bowel routine

Self-help devices to meet daily needs:
Raised toilet seat
Long-handled comb and razor

Exercise to loosen joint structures

Range-of-motion exercises
to prevent deformities

Figure 57–6. Clinical manifestations and nursing management of the patient with parkinsonism.

drugs are contraindicated in patients with narrow-angle glaucoma. Patients with prostatic hyperplasia are monitored for signs of urinary retention.

Amantadine Hydrochloride. Amantadine hydrochloride (Symmetrel), an antiviral agent, is used early in the treatment of Parkinson's disease to reduce rigidity, tremor, and bradykinesia. It is thought to act by releasing dopamine from neuronal storage sites. Adverse reactions include psychiatric disturbances (mood changes, confusion, hallucinations), nausea, epigastric distress, headache, and visual impairment.

Levodopa Therapy. Levodopa, although not a cure, is currently the most effective agent for the treatment of Parkinson's disease. It is presumably converted from L-dopa to dopamine in the basal ganglia to relieve the patient's symptoms.

The beneficial effects of levodopa are most pronounced in the first few years of treatment. Benefits to the patient begin to wane, and adverse side effects become more severe with the passage of time. Confusion, hallucinations, depression, and sleep alterations are associated with prolonged use. The patient may experience an on/off reaction in which sudden periods of near immobility ("off effect"), lasting minutes to hours, are followed by a sudden return of effectiveness ("on effect"). *Dyskinesias* (abnormal involuntary movements) are fairly common side effects, and include facial grimacing, rhythmic jerking movements of the hands, head bobbing, chewing and smacking movements, and involuntary movements of the trunk and extremities. This is probably due to the body's failure to readjust properly to the disappearance of dopamine. One method of dealing with on/off fluctuations is to give a "drug holiday" by taking the patient off the drug. This requires hospitalization and expert medical and nursing care.

Levodopa is usually given in combination with a decarboxylase inhibitor, carbidopa (Sinemet), which allows a greater concentration of levodopa to reach the brain and decrease the peripheral side effects.

Dopamine-Agonist–Ergot Derivatives. These agents (bromocriptine and pergolide) are thought to be dopamine receptor agonists, and are useful when added to levodopa and in patients experiencing on/off reactions to smooth out clinical fluctuations.

Pergolide (Permax) is the newest of this classification. It is 10 times more potent than bromocriptine, although therapeutically this is of no particular advantage. Patient response to these drugs is quite individual, and for reasons not well understood response to one drug may be better than to the other.

MAO Inhibitors. Eldepryl (called Deprenyl in Europe, marketed in the United States as Selegilene) is one of the most exciting developments in the pharmacotherapy of Parkinson's disease. This medication inhibits dopamine breakdown; thus increased amounts of dopamine are available. It has been found to smooth out the fluctuations in function that occur in this disease; unlike the other forms of therapy it may actually slow the progression of the disease.

Antidepressant Drugs. Tricyclic antidepressants may be given to alleviate the depression that is so common in Parkinson's disease.

Surgical Intervention. In some patients with disabling tremor or with severe levodopa-induced dyskinesia, surgery may be considered. Although surgery provides a certain amount of relief in selected patients, it does not alter the course of Parkinson's disease or assure permanent improvement. The purpose of the surgery is to destroy a part of the thalamus (*stereotaxic thalamotomy*) to relieve certain types of excessive muscle contraction.

The stereotaxic technique allows the neurosurgeon to position precisely and localize a small target deep within the brain. Special guiding instruments and rapid x-rays are used to place an electrode or freezing probe with pinpoint precision in the target area of the brain. A lesion is then created at that point.

▶ Nursing Process
The Patient With Parkinson's Disease

▷ Assessment

The health history and assessment focus on how the disease has affected the patient's activities and functional abilities. The patient is observed for what he can do and what changes in function occur throughout the day, and his responses after the administration of medications. The patient is asked what he would like to do better. The following questions may be helpful:

- Do you have leg or arm stiffness?
- Have you experienced any irregular jerking of your arms or legs?
- Have you ever been "frozen" or rooted to the spot and unable to move?
- Does your mouth water excessively?
- Have you (or others) noticed yourself grimacing or making faces or chewing movements?
- What specific activities do you have difficulty doing?

During this assessment, the patient is observed as he rolls over in bed, gets out of bed and a chair, walks, drinks, and eats.

▷ Nursing Diagnoses

Nearly every patient with a movement disorder has some functional alteration and may have some type of behavioral dysfunction. Based on the assessment data, the patient's major nursing diagnoses may include the following:

- Impaired physical mobility related to muscle rigidity and weakness
- Self-care deficits (eating, drinking, dressing, hygiene) related to tremor and motor disturbance
- Constipation related to medication and reduced activity
- Altered nutrition, less than body requirements, related to tremor, slowness in eating, difficulty in chewing and swallowing
- Impaired verbal communication related to decreased speech volume, slowness of speech, inability to move facial muscles
- Ineffective coping related to depression and dysfunction due to disease progression

Other nursing diagnoses may include sleep pattern disturbances, knowledge deficit, alteration in thought processes, and ineffective family coping.

▷ Planning and Implementation

▷ *Goals:* The patient's goals may include improvement of mobility, attainment of independence in activities of daily living, achievement of adequate bowel elimination, attainment and maintenance of satisfactory nutritional status, achievement of communication, and development of positive coping mechanisms.

▷ Nursing Interventions

▷ *Improved Mobility* A progressive program of daily exercise will increase muscle strength, improve coordination and dexterity, reduce muscular rigidity, and prevent contractures that occur when muscles are not used. Walking, riding a stationary bicycle, swimming, and gardening are all exercises that help maintain joint mobility. Stretching exercises (stretch-hold-relax) help loosen the joint structures. Postural exercises are important to counter the tendency of the head and neck to be drawn forward and down. Special walking techniques must also be learned to offset the shuffling gait and the tendency to lean forward.

The patient also may walk off balance because of the rigidity of the arms. (Arm swinging is necessary in normal walking.) The patient is taught early in the course of the disease to concentrate on walking erect, to watch the horizon, and to use a wide-based gait (*i.e.*, walking with the feet separated). A conscious effort must be made to swing the arms and raise the feet while walking and to use a heel-toe, heel-toe gait in fairly long strides. The patient is advised to practice walking to marching music or to the sound of a ticking metronome, because this provides sensory reinforcement. Breathing exercises while walking help to move the rib cage and transport oxygen to poorly aerated parts of the lungs. Frequent rest periods aid in preventing frustration and fatigue.

Warm baths and massage in addition to passive and active exercises help relax muscles and relieve painful muscle spasms that accompany rigidity.

▷ *Enhanced Self-Care Activities.*   Teaching and support of the patient during activities of daily living promote self-care. (See Chap. 14 for rehabilitation techniques.)

Environmental modifications are necessary to compensate for functional disabilities. These patients have difficulty turning in bed and getting in and out of bed. Bedside rails, an overbed frame with a trapeze if the patient has a hospital bed at home, or a rope tied to the foot of the bed provide assistance in pulling up without help.

▷ *Improved Bowel Elimination.*   A patient with parkinsonism may have severe problems with constipation. Among the factors causing this condition are weakness of the muscles used in defecation, lack of exercise, an inadequate fluid intake, and decreased autonomic nervous system activity. The drugs used for the treatment of the disease also inhibit normal intestinal secretions. A regular bowel routine may be established by encouraging the patient to follow a regular time pattern, consciously increase fluid intake, and eat foods with a moderate fiber content. A raised toilet seat is a useful device to facilitate toilet activities, because the patient has difficulty in moving from a standing to a sitting position.

▷ *Adequate Nutrition.*   Patients with parkinsonism have a problem in maintaining their weight. They become embarrassed by their slowness and untidiness in eating. Their mouths are dry from the medications, and they experience difficulty in chewing and swallowing. They are at risk for aspiration due to decreased cough reflexes. They may not be aware that they are aspirating, and may develop bronchopneumonia. Some patients have saliva buildup because of a slow rate of swallowing. Because of problems in eating, they may eventually show a considerable weight loss.

Swallowing disorders are also due to tongue tremor, hesitancy in initiating swallowing, difficulty in shaping food into a bolus, and disturbances in pharyngeal motility. To offset these problems, the patient should sit in an upright position during mealtime. A semisolid diet with thick liquids is easier to swallow than solids and thin liquids. Thin liquids should be avoided. It is helpful for patients to think through the swallowing sequence. The patient is taught to place the food on the tongue, close lips and teeth, lift the tongue up and then back, and swallow. He is encouraged to chew first on one side of the mouth and then on the other. To control the buildup of saliva, the patient is reminded to hold the head upright and make a conscious effort to swallow. Massaging the facial and neck muscles before meals may be beneficial.

An electrical warming tray keeps food hot and permits the patient to rest during the prolonged time that it takes to eat. Special utensils also assist at mealtime. A plate that is stabilized, a nonspill cup, and eating utensils with built-up handles are useful self-help devices. Supplementary feedings augment caloric intake. Monitoring weight on a weekly basis indicates whether caloric intake is sufficient.

▷ *Improved Communication.*   Speech disorders are present in most patients with Parkinson's disease. Their low-pitched, monotonous, soft speech requires that they make a conscious effort to speak slowly, with deliberate attention to what they are saying. Patients are reminded to face the listener, exaggerate the pronunciation of words, speak in short sentences, and take a few deep breaths before speaking.

A speech-language pathologist may be helpful in designing speech improvement exercises and assisting health care personnel to develop a method of communication to meet the patient's needs. Having the patient speak into a tape recorder periodically is useful in monitoring the patient's progress. A small electronic amplifier is helpful if the patient has difficulty in being heard.

▷ *Positive Coping Abilities.*   Faithful adherence to an exercise and walking program helps to delay the progress of the disease. Encouragement and reassurance can be given by praising the patient for perseverance and pointing out that activities are being maintained through active participation. A combination of physiotherapy, psychotherapy, drug therapy, and sociotherapy may be necessary to help combat the depression that so often accompanies this condition.

Patients with Parkinson's disease often feel embarrassed, apathetic, inadequate, bored, and lonely. These feelings may be due, in part, to physical slowness and the great effort that even small tasks require. Patients are assisted and encouraged to set achievable goals (*e.g.,* improvement of mobility). Because parkinsonism tends to lead to withdrawal and depression, patients must be *active* participants in their therapeutic program, including social and recreational events. There should be a planned program of activity throughout the day to prevent too much daytime sleeping as well as disinterest and apathy.

Every effort should be made to encourage patients to carry out the tasks involved in coping with their own daily needs and to retain independence. "Doing things" for the patient merely to save time runs contrary to this basic goal of improvement of coping abilities.

▷ *Patient Education and Home Health Care.*   The need for information about Parkinson's disease is ongoing as adaptations and concessions are made to the illness. Every effort is made to explain the nature of the disease and its management to offset anxieties and fears that may be as disabling as the disease itself. The American Parkinson's Disease Foundation publishes booklets and a newsletter for patient education.

The family is under considerable stress from living with a disabled member. Giving them information about treatment and care prevents many unnecessary problems. The caregiver is included in the plan; the caregiver is counseled to learn stress reduction techniques, to include others in the care-giving process, to obtain periodic relief from responsibilities, and to have a yearly health assessment. Giving family members "permission" to express feelings of frustration, anger, and guilt is often helpful to them.

▷ Evaluation

Expected Outcomes
1. Strives toward improved mobility
   a. Participates in exercise program daily
   b. Avoids hurrying
   c. Walks with wide base of support; exaggerates arm swinging when walking
   d. Takes prescribed medications faithfully
2. Progresses toward self-care
   a. Plans for and allows time for self-care
   b. Uses self-help devices
3. Maintains bowel function
   a. Consumes adequate fluid intake
   b. Increases dietary intake of fiber
   c. Reports regular pattern of bowel function
4. Attains improved nutritional status
   a. Swallows without chocking
   b. Takes time while eating
5. Achieves a method of communication
   a. Communicates needs
   b. Practices speech exercises
6. Copes with effects of Parkinson's disease
   a. Sets realistic goals
   b. Demonstrates persistence in meaningful activities
   c. Verbalizes feelings to appropriate person

Huntington's Disease

Huntington's disease (HD) is a chronic, progressive, hereditary disease of the nervous system that results in progressive involuntary choreiform (dancelike) movement and dementia. It affects men and women of all races. Because it is transmitted as an autosomal dominant genetic disorder, each child of a parent with Huntington's disease has a 50% risk of inheriting the illness.

Pathophysiology

The basic pathology involves premature death of cells in the basal ganglia, the region deep within the brain involved in the control of movement. There is also loss of cells in the cortex, which is associated with thinking, memory, perception, and judgment. Research suggests that the disease may be related to a lack of important brain chemicals (gamma-aminobutyric acid [GABA] and acetylcholine [ACh]) that inhibit nerve action. Onset usually occurs between the ages of 35 and 45; the patient slowly progresses toward death in 10 to 15 years. About 10% of victims are children.

A genetic marker for HD has been located through the use of recombinant deoxyribonucleic acid (DNA) technology. As a result, researchers can now identify presymptomatic individuals who will develop this disease. Although this presymptomatic test for HD can remove the uncertainty, it offers no hope of cure or even specific determination of its onset.

Clinical Manifestations

The most prominent clinical features of the disease are abnormal involuntary movements (*chorea*), intellectual decline, and, often, emotional disturbance. As the disease progresses, a constant writhing, twisting, uncontrollable movement may involve the entire body. These motions are devoid of purpose or rhythm, although patients may try to turn them into purposeful movement. All of the body musculature is involved. Facial movements produce tics and grimaces. Speech is affected, becoming slurred, hesitant, often explosive, and eventually unintelligible. Chewing and swallowing are difficult and there is a constant danger of choking and aspiration. Like speech, the gait becomes disorganized to the point that ambulation eventually is impossible. Although independent ambulation should be encouraged for as long as possible, a wheelchair is usually necessary at some point. (Eventually, the patient is confined to bed, as the chorea interferes with walking, sitting, and all activities.) Control of bladder and bowel is lost. Likewise, the sensorium is usually involved. There is progressive intellectual impairment, although the patient is generally aware that the disease is responsible for the myriad dysfunctions that are occurring.

The mental and emotional changes may be more devastating to the patient and family than the abnormal movements. Patients may be nervous, clumsy, irritable, or impatient. Particularly in the early stages of the illness, patients are subject to uncontrollable fits of anger, profound, often suicidal depression; apathy; or euphoria. Judgment and memory are impaired and dementia eventually ensues. Hallucinations, delusions, and paranoid thinking may even precede the appearance of disjointed movements. Emotional symptoms often become less acute as the disease progresses. Despite a ravenous appetite, often for sweets, patients usually become emaciated and exhausted. Eventually, patients succumb from heart failure, pneumonia, or infection, or die as a result of a fall or choking.

Management

Although no treatment halts or reverses the underlying process, several methods of management have fairly good palliative action. The phenothiazines, butyrophenones, and thioxanthenes, which predominantly block dopamine receptors, improve the chorea in many patients. Chorea is also lessened by reserpine (acts by depleting presynaptic dopamine) and tetrabenazine (reduces dopaminergic transmission).

The patient's motor signs must be assessed and evaluated on a continuing basis so that optimal therapeutic drug levels may be reached. *Akathisia* (motor restlessness) in the overmedicated patient is a danger because it may be mistaken for the restless fidgetiness of the illness and consequently be overlooked.

In certain types of the disease in which hypokinetic motor impairment resembles parkinsonism, some benefit may be obtained from antiparkinsonism therapy (see p. 1710). Patients who have emotional disturbances, particularly depression, may be helped by antidepressant medications. The threat of suicide is always present. Psychotic symptoms usually respond to antipsychotic drugs. Psychotherapy aimed at allaying anxiety and reducing stress may be beneficial. It is imperative that nurses look beyond the disease to focus on the patient's needs and capabilities (Chart 57-2).

▷ *Patient and Family Teaching.*   A program combining medical, psychological, social, occupational, speech, and physical rehabilitation services is needed to help the patient and family cope with this severely disabling illness. More than most disorders, Huntington's disease exacts enormous emotional, physical, social, and financial tolls on every member of the patient's family. Entire families often live under a heavy burden of uncertainty, anxiety, and guilt.

Individuals of childbearing age may wish information about their risk for Huntington's disease when considering a family, or couples who would consider abortion may consider the testing at the time of an amniocentesis. For most people the benefits of testing remain questionable and controversial.

Not only is genetic counseling crucial, but patients and their families also require access to long-term psychological counseling, marriage counseling, and emotional, financial, and legal support. Regular follow-up helps to allay fear of abandonment. Some form of home care assistance, work and recreation day centers, respite care, and eventually skilled long-term care is necessary to help the patient and family cope with the constant strain of the illness. Although nothing can stop the relentless progression of the disease, families who have had supportive care have benefited tremendously.

Voluntary health organizations are major aids to families and have been largely responsible for bringing the illness to national attention. The Huntington's Disease Foundation of America (see Bibliography for address) is oriented toward helping patients and their families by providing information, referrals, family and public education, and support for research.

Alzheimer's Disease

Alzheimer's disease, or senile dementia of the Alzheimer's type, is a chronic, progressive, and deteriorative brain disorder accompanied by profound effects on memory, cognition, and ability for self-care. Approximately 4% of the population over the age of 65 is affected, and the prevalence reaches 20% by age 80. It is one of the most feared disorders of modern times because it has catastrophic consequences for the victim and family, who experience what has been termed an "endless funeral."

The cause of Alzheimer's disease remains unknown. A variety of factors that may contribute to the development of the disease have been suggested, including age; familial, genetic, and chromosomal factors; metabolic abnormalities; and perhaps a virus.

Chart 57–2
The Challenges of a Patient With Huntington's Disease

Problem/Challenge	Nursing Interventions
Constant movement Skin excoriation Abrasions or pressure ulcers Falls	Pad the sides and head of the bed; ensure that the patient can see over the sides of bed. Use lamb's wool padding for heel and elbow protection. Keep the skin meticulously clean. Apply emollient cleansing agent and skin lotion frequently. Use *soft* sheets and bedding. Have patient wear football or other padding. Encourage ambulation with assistance to maintain muscle tone. Restrain the patient (only if absolutely necessary) in bed or chair with padded protective devices, making sure that they are loosened frequently. Remove objects that the patient can trip over.

Feeding
Constant movement
Difficulty in chewing or swallowing
Choking/Aspiration
Malnutrition/Emaciation
Dehydration
	Administer phenothiazines as prescribed before meals (appears to calm some patients)
	Use a warming tray.
	Talk to the patient before mealtime to promote relaxation; use mealtime for social interaction. Provide undivided attention. Help the patient enjoy the mealtime experience.
	Learn the position that is best for *this* patient. Keep patient as close to upright as possible while feeding. Stabilize patient's head gently with one hand while feeding.
	Show the food and tell the patient what the foods are (*e.g.*, whether hot or cold).
	Encircle the patient with one arm and get as close as possible to provide stability and support. Use pillows and wedges for additional support.
	Do not interpret stiffness, turning away, or sudden turning of the head as rejection; these are uncontrollable choreiform movements.
	For feeding, use a long-handled spoon (iced-tea spoon). Place spoon on middle of tongue and exert slight pressure.
	Place bite-sized food between teeth. Serve stews, casseroles, thick liquids; avoid too many milk drinks (produces mucus).
	Disregard messiness. Treat the person with dignity.
	Wait for the patient to chew and swallow before introducing another spoonful. Make sure that bite-sized food is small.
	Give between-meal feedings. Constant movement uses more calories. Patients are often voracious, particularly for sweets.
	Use *blenderized meals* if patient cannot chew; do not repeatedly give the same strained baby foods; gradually introduce increased textures and consistencies to the diet.
	For swallowing difficulties:
	  Apply gentle deep pressure around the patient's mouth.
	  Rub fingers in circles on the patient's cheeks.
	  Rub fingers simultaneously down each side of the patient's throat.
	Develop skill in Heimlich maneuver (to be used in the event of choking).

Psychological support and communication Grimacing Unintelligible speech	Approach from the front and avoid startling the patient. Respect the patient as an individual with rights and needs. Use eye contact. Touch the patient. *Talk,* even though the patient may not be able to answer.

(continued)

Chart 57–2 *(Continued)*

Problem/Challenge	Nursing Interventions
	Read to the patient.
	Employ biofeedback and relaxation therapy to reduce stress.
	Use speech and language therapy to help maintain and prolong communication abilities.
	Try to devise a communication system, perhaps using cards with words or pictures of familiar objects, before verbal communication becomes too difficult. Patients can indicate correct card by hitting it with hand, grunting, or blinking the eyes.
	Learn how this particular patient expresses needs and wants—particularly nonverbal messages (widening of eyes, responses).
	Patients can understand even if unable to speak. Do not isolate patients by ceasing to communicate with them.
Progressive intellectual impairment and emotional disturbance	Have a clock, calendar, and wall posters in view.
	Interact with the patient in a *creative* manner.
	Use every opportunity for one-to-one contact.
	Use music for relaxation.
	Reorient the patient after awakening.
	Have the patient wear an identification bracelet with name, telephone number, and "memory impaired" on it.
	Keep the patient in the social mainstream.
	Recruit and train volunteers for social interaction. Set a good example.
	Do not abandon a patient because the disease is eventually terminal. Patients are *living* until the end.

Possible risk factors include the occurrence of either dementia or Down's syndrome in other family members, birth to a mother older than 40, and head trauma with loss of consciousness.

Pathophysiology

Evidence indicates that a number of neuronal systems are involved in this disease. The distinguishing microscopic feature is an accumulation of *neurofibrillary tangles* (abnormal tangled fibers) and the occurrence of *senile plaques* (round or ovoid structures composed of destroyed dendrites and synapses that are imbedded in a central amyloid core) in the brains of patients with Alzheimer's disease. There is a marked loss of nerve cells from the cerebral cortex with a corresponding atrophy of the brain. The cell death is accompanied by a corresponding reduction in blood flow in the brain. Research scientists report that there is evidence of a significant and progressive decrease in the activity of the enzyme choline acetyltransferase in the brain tissue. Choline acetyltransferase is a crucial ingredient in the chemical process that produces *acetylcholine*, a neurotransmitter involved in learning and memory.

Clinical Manifestations

Although the onset may be insidious, family members usually notice that the patient has significant forgetfulness and memory impairment. Gradually there is deterioration of higher cognitive function, with loss of ability to read, to write, to calculate, and even to communicate intelligently. Personality changes may be marked. In time, disorders of motor function, including disorders of gait, occur.

The family, who are the "other victims" of this dementing illness, report that the patient's restlessness, neglect of self-care, confusion, urinary incontinence, falls, and episodes of rage are particularly troublesome burdens.

Diagnostic Evaluation

At this time Alzheimer's disease can only be confirmed with certainty by microscopic examination of neural tissue, usually at autopsy. CT scans in patients demonstrate progressive reduction in brain volume (atrophy) in excess of that occurring in normal aging. Positron emission tomography (PET) shows decreased regional metabolism of glucose and oxygen and decreased blood flow in cortical areas. Serial evaluations of neuropsychological testing provide information on the rate of deterioration.

Probable Alzheimer's disease diagnosis is based on clinically determined progressive dementia (confirmed by neuropsychological tests), two or more cognitive deficits, progressive worsening of memory or other cognitive functions, no disturbances of consciousness, and absence of systemic disorders or other brain disorders that could cause progressive deficits in memory and cognition.

The nursing process applied to the management of the patient with Alzheimer's disease is found in Chapter 12.

In summary, MS and Parkinson's, Huntington's, and Alzheimer's diseases are described as chronic, progressive degenerative disorders. Although the classic picture of each of these disorders is that of progressive loss of physical or cognitive function, not all patients follow the usual or predictable course. Therefore, each patient should be approached as an individual and provided all opportunities to receive available treatment, nursing care, and rehabilitative services.

The patient and his family require assistance, including counseling and education, about the disorder and the possible variations in its course to be able to cope with changes and make plans. The nurse is often in the ideal position to assist the patient and family in identifying needs for supportive services and in coordinating and evaluating those services. Regardless of the degree of physical or cognitive deterioration, the patient must be afforded a continuing key role in the decision-making process.

Neuromuscular Diseases

Myasthenia Gravis

Myasthenia gravis is a disorder affecting the neuromuscular transmission of the voluntary muscles of the body; it is characterized by excessive weakness and fatigability particularly of voluntary muscles and those innervated by cranial nerve function. It affects younger women; men who develop the disease do so later in life.

Pathophysiology

The basic abnormality in myasthenia gravis is a defect in the transmission of impulses from nerve to muscle cells due to loss of available or normal receptors on the postsynaptic membrane of the neuromuscular junction. Myasthenia gravis is considered an autoimmune disease in which antibodies directed against acetylcholine receptor (AChR) impair neuromuscular transmission.

Clinical Manifestations. The disease is characterized by *extreme muscular weakness* and easy fatigability, which generally is worse after effort and is relieved by rest. Patients with this disease tire on such slight exertion as combing the hair, chewing, and talking, and must stop for rest. Symptoms vary according to the muscles affected. Symmetric muscles are involved, first and foremost those innervated by cranial nerves. Because of the involvement of the ocular muscles. *diplopia* (double vision) and *ptosis* (drooping of the eyelids) are early symptoms. The patient has a sleepy, masklike expression because the facial muscles are affected. Laryngeal involvement produces a *dysphonia* (voice impairment) in the form of a nasal sound of the voice or difficulty in articulation. Weakness of the bulbar muscles causes problems with chewing and swallowing and presents a danger of choking and aspiration. Some 15% to 20% of patients complain of weakness of arm and hand muscles and, less commonly, of leg muscle weakness, which makes these patients subject to falls.

- Progressive weakness of the diaphragm and intercostal muscles may produce respiratory distress or myasthenic crisis, which is an acute emergency.

Diagnostic Evaluation. The signs and symptoms of myasthenia gravis are sometimes so striking that a presumptive diagnosis can be made on the basis of the patient's history and physical examination. An injection of edrophonium (Tensilon), a drug that facilitates the transmission of impulses at the myo-

neural junction, is used to confirm the diagnosis. Within 30 seconds of an intravenous injection of edrophonium, most patients improve substantially but only temporarily. Improvement in muscle strength after administration of this agent represents a positive test and usually confirms the diagnosis of myasthenia. Demonstration of the anti-AChR antibodies in the serum is found in nearly 90% of patients with generalized myasthenia and in about 70% of those with symptoms restricted to the eye muscles (ocular form).

Electromyography (EMG) is used to measure the electrical potential of muscle cells but is not considered specifically diagnostic for myasthenia gravis.

Management

Management of myasthenia gravis is directed at improving remaining function through the administration of anticholinesterase medications and reducing and removing circulating antibodies. Therapy includes anticholinesterase drugs and immunosuppressive therapy, including plasmapheresis, and thymectomy.

Anticholinesterase drugs act by increasing the relative concentration of available acetylcholine at the neuromuscular junction. They are given to increase the response of the muscles to nerve impulses and to improve strength. They provide only symptomatic relief, however.

Drugs in current use include pyridostigmine bromide (Mestinon), ambenonium chloride (Mytelase), and neostigmine bromide (Prostigmin).

Most patients prefer pyridostigmine because it produces less marked side effects. The dosage is increased gradually until maximal benefits are obtained (additional strength, less fatigue), although normal muscle strength may not be achieved and the patient will likely have to adapt to some disability. Anticholinesterase medications are given with milk, crackers, or other buffering substances. Their side effects include abdominal cramps, nausea, vomiting, and diarrhea. Small doses of atropine, given once or twice daily, may ameliorate or prevent these side effects. Other side effects of anticholinesterase therapy include adverse effects on skeletal muscles, such as fasciculations (fine twitching), spasm, and weakness. The effects on the central nervous system include irritability, anxiety, insomnia, headache, dysarthria, syncope, convulsions, and coma. Increased salivation and lacrimation, increased bronchial secretions, and moist skin may also be noted.

- The nursing (and patient) priority is to give the drug prescribed according to an exact time schedule to control the patient's symptoms. *Any delay in drug administration may result in the patient's inability to swallow.* An increase in muscle strength within 1 hour after the administration of the anticholinesterase drug is expected.

After the initial medication doses have been adjusted, the patient learns to take the medication according to his needs and time plan. Further adjustments may be necessary in the presence of physical or emotional stress and intercurrent infection.

Immunosuppressive Therapy. Immunosuppressive therapy is directed toward reducing the production of antireceptor antibody or its direct removal by plasma exchange (explained below). Included in immunosuppressive therapy are corticosteroids, plasmapheresis, and thymectomy. Corticosteroid therapy may benefit the patient with severe generalized myasthenia. Steroids exert their effect by suppressing the patient's immune response. thus decreasing the amount of blocking antibody. The anticholinesterase dosage is lowered while the patient's ability to maintain effective respirations and to swallow is monitored. The steroid dosage is gradually increased and the anticholinesterase medication is slowly reduced. Prednisone, taken on alternate days to lower the incidence of side effects, appears to be successful in suppressing the disease. Sometimes the patient shows a marked decrease in muscle strength right after steroid therapy is started, but this is usually only temporary. The patient can be given a call bell to use in emergency situations and should be closely monitored for signs of respiratory distress.

Plasma Exchange. Plasma exchange is a technique that permits selective removal of the patient's plasma and plasma components. The remaining cells are reinfused. Plasma exchange produces a temporary reduction in the titer of circulating antibodies. This process has caused remarkable improvement in some patients but does not treat the underlying abnormality (production of antireceptor antibody) over the long term.

Surgical Management

In myasthenia gravis patients the thymus seems to be involved in the process of AChR antibody production. *Thymectomy* (surgical removal of the thymus) causes substantial remission of the disease, especially in patients with tumor or hyperplasia of the thymus gland. Thymectomy is carried out through the sternum because the entire thymus must be removed.

It is thought that thymectomy *early* in the course of the disease is specific therapy, as it prevents formation of antireceptor antibodies. After surgery, the patient is monitored in an intensive care unit; special attention is given to ventilatory function.

Myasthenic Crisis Versus Cholinergic Crisis

Myasthenic crisis is the sudden onset of muscular weakness in patients with myasthenia and is usually the result of undermedication or no cholinergic medication at all. In addition, myasthenic crisis may result from progression of the disease itself, emotional upset, systemic infections, certain drugs, surgery, or trauma. It is manifest by the sudden onset of acute respiratory distress and an inability to swallow or speak. Weakness of respiratory, laryngeal, and bulbar musculature can cause respiratory depression and airway obstruction if not treated promptly.

Cholinergic crisis is caused by overmedication with cholinergic or anticholinesterase drugs. In addition to the muscle weakness and respiratory depression of myasthenic crisis, these patients experience a variety of gastrointestinal symptoms, including nausea, vomiting, and diarrhea, as well as sweating, increased salivation, and bradycardia.

▶ Nursing Process
The Patient With Myasthenia Gravis

▷ Assessment

The patient with myasthenia gravis is usually managed as an outpatient unless hospitalization is required for diagnostic test-

ing or to manage symptoms or complications. The health history and assessment focus on the patient and family's knowledge about the disease and the drug treatment program that has been established. The more knowledgeable they are, the less likely the patient is to develop complications. It is important to determine what the patient's drug therapy schedule was while at home, as this same schedule is likely to be the one of choice at the time of discharge. In addition, an assessment of the patient's functional capability and support system assists in determining discharge needs for services.

▷ Nursing Diagnosis

Based on the assessment data, the patient's potential nursing diagnosis may include the following:

- Ineffective breathing pattern related to respiratory muscle weakness
- Impaired physical mobility due to voluntary muscle weakness
- High risk for aspiration related to weakness of bulbar muscles

Other nursing diagnoses of the patient with myasthenia gravis may include high risk for injury related to voluntary muscle weakness; activity intolerance; ineffective airway clearance; anxiety; altered nutrition, less than body requirements; and body image disturbance.

▷ *Potential Problems.* Based on the assessment data and knowledge of the disease process, potential problems may include:

- Myasthenic crisis
- Cholinergic crisis

▷ Planning and Implementation

▷ *Goals:* The patient's major goals may include improved respiratory function, increased physical mobility, avoidance of aspiration, and avoidance or management of myasthenic and cholinergic crises.

▷ Nursing Interventions

▷ *Improved Respiratory Function.* For a patient with diminishing ventilatory capacity, the nurse assesses respiratory rate, depth, and breath sounds, and studies the results of pulmonary function tests (tidal volume, vital capacity, inspiratory force) at very frequent intervals to detect pulmonary problems before changes in arterial blood gas levels become clinically apparent. When there is severe weakness of abdominal, intercostal, and pharyngeal muscles, the patient is unable to cough and breathe deeply or clear secretions. Chest physical therapy, including postural drainage to mobilize secretions and suctioning to remove secretions, may have to be performed frequently.

The patient with insufficient air exchange experiences anxiety sometimes bordering on panic. This is compounded by an inability to communicate verbally and by a tendency to choke. Acknowledging the patient's fears can give assurance that the nurse understands his concerns. The patient gains some sense of control through skilled care and the calm support of the nurse.

A number of drugs aggravate myasthenia gravis, and the patient is advised to consult with the physician before taking any new medications, including certain antibiotics, cardiovascular drugs, anticonvulsant and psychotrophic drugs, morphine, quinine and related agents, beta-blockers, and nonprescription drugs. Novocain should be avoided, and the patient's dentist so advised.

▷ *Increased Physical Mobility.* The patient's goal is improvement of strength and endurance. To be a participant in treatment, the patient must learn the basic facts about anticholinergic drugs—their action, timing, dosage adjustment, symptoms of overdose, and toxic effects. The importance of taking the medication on time is emphasized. The patient is encouraged to keep a diary to determine fluctuation of symptoms and to know when the medication is wearing off.

In addition, it may be helpful to include the following:

- Taking medication 30 minutes before meals for maximal muscle strength
- Planning adequate rest periods throughout the day
- Setting a realistic schedule daily and spacing activities
- Wearing appropriate shoes to minimize weakness and prevent injury

Certain factors may increase weakness and precipitate a myasthenic crisis: emotional upset, infections (particularly respiratory infections), vigorous physical activity, and exposure to heat (hot baths, sun bathing) and cold. These situations should be avoided. To avoid the risk of fatigue, it is best to rest *before* becoming too tired. A cervical collar is useful for patients with weak neck muscles. Adaptive or self-help devices are available and are useful in helping the patient handle the disease more effectively and live as full a life as possible. The patient is also advised to wear an identification bracelet such as Medic Alert.

The weakened speech muscles in patients in myasthenic crisis interfere with communication. Techniques for improving communication include listening to patients; repeating what they have tried to communicate, to clarify and verify information; and asking patients to blink their eyes or wiggle their fingers or toes for yes and no answers. After the period of myasthenic crisis has resolved, patients are usually able to make their needs known.

Impaired vision results from ptosis of one or both eyelids, decreased eye movement, or double vision. Nursing interventions to help the patient cope include taping the eyes open for short intervals, instilling artificial tears to prevent corneal damage when eyelids do not close completely, placing a patch over one eye when double vision is a problem, and keeping the patient informed while giving care.

Applying a thin adhesive tape over the upper eyelid helps relieve ptosis. Sunglasses diminish the effects of bright light that frequently increase eye problems.

Indicating that the crisis should pass and that the patient will not be left alone may help to make the situation bearable.

▷ *Avoidance of Aspiration.* Decreased ability to chew and swallow may result in choking and aspiration. The patient is assessed for drooling, regurgitation through the nose, and choking while attempting to swallow. Standby suction should be available. Rest before meals is encouraged to lessen muscle fatigue. The patient is placed in an upright position with neck slightly flexed to facilitate swallowing. Soft foods in gravy or sauces appear to be swallowed more easily than liquids. If the patient is taking an anticholinesterase agent, the nurse makes sure it is given 1 hour before mealtime to ensure maximum muscle strength. Because muscles of mastication may be

stronger in the morning, the calorie intake can be increased at breakfast. The patient is encouraged to rest after eating.

Mealtimes should coincide with the peak effects of anticholinesterase if the patient has difficulty in swallowing. If choking occurs frequently, blenderized food may be easier to swallow. Standby suction should be available at home as well as during hospitalization and the patient and family instructed in its use. Gastrostomy feedings may be necessary.

▷ *Prevention of Complications*

▷ *Management of Myasthenic and Cholinergic Crises.* Respiratory distress combined with varying signs of dysphagia (difficulty in swallowing), dysarthria (difficulty in speaking), eyelid ptosis, diplopia, and prominent muscle weakness are symptoms of crisis of either type.

- Providing adequate ventilatory assistance takes precedence in the immediate management of the patient with myasthenic crisis.
- The patient is suctioned, because aspiration is a common problem. Arterial blood is drawn for arterial blood gas analysis. Endotracheal intubation and mechanical ventilation may be needed (see Chap. 25). The patient is placed in an intensive care unit for constant monitoring, as this condition is marked by intense and sudden fluctuations.

Intravenous edrophonium (Tensilon) is used to differentiate the type of crisis. It improves the condition of the patient in myasthenic crisis, temporarily worsens that of the patient in cholinergic crisis, and is unpredictable in brittle crisis. If the patient is in true myasthenic crisis, neostigmine methylsulfate (Prostigmin) is administered intramuscularly or intravenously.

If the edrophonium (Tensilon) test is inconclusive or there is increasing respiratory weakness, all anticholinesterase drugs are withdrawn and atropine sulfate is given to reduce excessive secretions.

Other supportive measures include the following:

- Arterial blood gases, serum electrolytes, input and output, and daily weight are monitored.
- If the patient is unable to swallow, nasogastric tube feedings may be prescribed (200 ml at a time). (Postural drainage should not be performed for half an hour after feeding.)
- Sedatives and tranquilizing drugs are avoided because these agents aggravate hypoxia and hypercapnia and can cause respiratory and cardiac depression.

▷ **Evaluation**

Expected Outcomes
1. Achieves adequate respiratory function
   a. Exhibits normal respiratory rate and depth and normal muscle strength
   b. Adheres to established medication schedule
   c. States that manual resuscitation bag and portable suction are available for home use
   d. Avoids situations that may predispose to colds and infections, which might exacerbate symptoms.
2. Adapts to impaired mobility
   a. Establishes a balanced program of rest and exercise
   b. Identifies measures to conserve energy; paces self
   c. Uses assistive devices

d. Establishes and adheres to a medication schedule that maximizes muscle strength
3. Experiences no aspiration
   a. Exhibits normal breath sounds
   b. Eats slowly and selects appropriate (soft) diet
   c. Establishes a medication schedule that coincides with mealtime
4. Exhibits absence of myasthenic and cholinergic crises
   a. Lists signs and symptoms of crisis
   b. Adheres to medication regimen
   c. Wears Medic-Alert bracelet

The Myasthenia Gravis Foundation has materials written for both lay and professional readers, available on request (see Bibliography for address).

Amyotrophic Lateral Sclerosis

Amyotrophic lateral sclerosis (ALS) is a disease of unknown cause in which there is a loss of motor neurons (nerve cells controlling muscles) in the anterior horns of the spinal cord and the motor nuclei of the lower brain stem. As these cells die, the muscle fibers that they supply undergo atrophic changes. The degeneration of the neurons may occur in both the upper and lower motor neuron systems.

ALS affects more men than women, with onset occurring usually in the fifth or sixth decade. In this country, it is often referred to as Lou Gehrig's disease after the famous ballplayer who suffered from it.

Clinical Manifestations.   The clinical manifestations of ALS depend on the location of the affected motor neurons, because specific neurons activate specific muscle fibers. The chief symptoms are progressive muscle weakness, atrophy, and fasciculations (twitching). Loss of motor neurons in the anterior horns of the spinal cord results in progressive weakness and atrophy of the muscles of the arms, trunk, or legs. Spasticity is usually present, and the stretch reflexes become brisk and overactive. Usually the anal and bladder sphincters are not affected because the spinal nerves that control muscles of the rectum and urinary bladder are preserved. In about 25% of patients, weakness starts in the musculature supplied by the cranial nerves and there is difficulty talking, swallowing, and ultimately breathing. When the patient ingests liquids, the soft palate and upper esophageal weakness cause the liquid to be regurgitated through the nose. Weakness of the posterior tongue and palate impairs the ability to laugh, cough, or even blow the nose. When bulbar muscles are impaired, there is progressive difficulty in speaking and swallowing, and aspiration becomes a problem. The voice assumes a nasal sound and speech articulation becomes so disrupted that the patient's speech is unintelligible. Some emotional lability may be present, but intellectual function is not impaired. Eventually respiratory function is compromised.

The prognosis generally is based on the area involved and the speed with which the disease progresses. Death usually occurs as a result of infection, respiratory failure, or aspiration. The average time from onset of the disease to death is approximately 3 years. A small number may survive for longer periods.

Diagnostic Evaluation.   ALS is diagnosed on the basis of the signs and symptoms, because no clinical or laboratory tests are specific for this disease. Electromyographic studies of the affected muscle indicate reduction in the number of motor units.

Management

No specific treatment for ALS is available. Symptomatic treatment and rehabilitative measures are employed to support the patient and improve the quality of life. Baclofen or diazepam may be useful for patients troubled by spasticity, because spasticity causes pain and interferes with self-care. Quinine therapy may be prescribed for painful muscle cramps. High doses of thyrotropin-releasing hormone, a naturally occurring hormone produced by the brain and found in the motor neurons of the spinal cord, are being used investigationally to improve function. Interferon, a compound that appears to stimulate the body's defense system, is another investigational drug. A patient experiencing problems with aspiration and swallowing may require nasogastric feedings. A cervical *esophagostomy* (opening into the esophagus) or a gastrostomy may be performed to bypass the larynx, to prevent aspiration, and for long-term nutritional support.

Mechanical ventilation is considered when alveolar hypoventilation develops. The decision for the use of life support measures is made by the patient and family and should be based on a thorough understanding of the disease, the prognosis, and the implications of initiating such therapy. Patients who decide against ventilation therapy may consider making a "living will" to preserve their autonomy.

▶ Nursing Process
The Patient With Amyotrophic Lateral Sclerosis

◊ Assessment

The focus of the nursing assessment is to determine how ALS is affecting the patient's functioning. Ongoing assessment is directed at detecting incipient respiratory difficulties. A history of present eating habits is obtained. The foods the patient can manage are identified. The facial muscles are inspected for bilateral weakness. The patient's ability to safely drink fluids is assessed by having him drink a small amount of water; as he drinks, he is observed for incomplete lip closure, poor head position, pooling of secretions, difficulty in swallowing, choking, and regurgitation of fluids through the nose. Loss of tongue coordination, which causes difficulty in moving solids back toward the pharynx, is documented. Speech abnormalities also indicate oral or palatal dysfunction.

The patient is asked to cough, clench the jaw, and hold his breath. He is observed for muscle wasting and the ability to perform self-care and activities such as turning a page of a book.

◊ Nursing Diagnoses

Based on all the assessment data, the patient's major nursing diagnoses may include the following:

- Impaired physical mobility related to muscle weakness and wasting

- Altered nutrition, less than body requirements, related to inability to chew and swallow
- Impaired communication related to disturbance in muscular control of speech mechanisms
- Ineffective breathing pattern related to impaired intercostal, thoracic, and diaphragmatic muscle function/bulbar paralysis with aspiration/asphyxiation
- Ineffective family coping related to overwhelming physical and emotional demands imposed by the disease

▷ *Planning and Implementation*

▷ *Goals:* The patient's goals may include compensation for muscle weakness and wasting, improvement of nutritional intake, development of an alternative communication system, and recognition of and dealing with respiratory dysfunction. The family's goals are adaptation to and coping with prolonged illness.

▷ *Nursing Interventions*

▷ *Compensation for Muscle Weakness and Atrophy.* An important nursing goal is to assist the patient in maximizing independence. The patient should remain active as long as possible without tiring the involved muscles. Active exercises and range-of-motion exercises help to strengthen uninvolved muscles and maintain muscle power at optimum levels. Stretching exercises (stretch-hold-relax) are beneficial. Exercise is stopped short of fatigue. Such devices as ankle–foot orthoses for the patient with weak dorsiflexors (which impair dorsiflexion of the ankle) help keep the patient mobile. Hand splints can provide a stronger grip and more effective use of the hand, and other devices to support weakened extremities or neck muscles can maintain optimum joint position.

As the muscles grow weaker, the patient may use a wheelchair for activities outside the house. Assistive devices are used to help the patient function independently for as long as possible. The patient is taught energy conservation and work-simplification methods. When the illness has progressed to the point where the patient is confined to a wheelchair, an electrically powered model can be used. At this stage, the prevention of contractures is important. When the patient becomes dependent, a mechanical lift for bed, toilet, and tub transfers is needed, and special instructions will need to be given to the family concerning the best way to position the patient for the greatest comfort. (See pp. 236–240 for prevention of pressure ulcers.)

▷ *Improved Nutritional Intake.* Nutrition is very important, especially in the patient with progressive bulbar involvement that affects the swallowing mechanism and causes choking and difficulty in swallowing and speaking. Aspiration is a constant danger. Standby suction should be available. The patient is encouraged to rest before meals to alleviate muscle fatigue, which increases swallowing difficulty. The patient is placed in an upright position with his neck slightly flexed to facilitate swallowing, and should remain in the upright posture for 15 to 30 minutes after eating. Foods with consistency (soft foods in gravy) seem to be more easily swallowed than liquids. Weakened swallowing muscles allow fluid and food to become entrapped in the throat. Washing down solid foods with liquids is avoided, as this may cause choking and aspiration. The family is taught procedures for dislodging food in the event of choking.

A soft cervical collar is useful if the patient has difficulty holding the head erect.

▷ *Improved Communication.* The patient will require an alternate communication system as the disease relentlessly progresses and speech is lost. Practical methods can be selected by a speech-language pathologist to maximize the patient's remaining potential for speech. For patients who can use their hands, small computers are available with artificial speech articulation. A pointer held in the teeth may be used with a picture or word chart. There are ingenious high-tech instruments that can assist ALS patients to speak through a computer's synthesizer by moving the muscles of the eyebrows. A predetermined code using eye blinks for yes and no may eventually be the patient's only means of communication.

▷ *Improved Respiratory Function.* Central respiratory drive may be reduced during sleep, causing restless sleep, multiple awakenings, and daytime drowsiness. The most serious complication in the later stages of the disease is respiratory dysfunction, because all muscles involved in breathing may be affected. The patient with ALS should be evaluated periodically with pulmonary function testing. Techniques to enhance pulmonary function include upright positioning, breathing exercises, suctioning of excessive secretions, chest physical therapy, and the use of incentive spirometry. Decisions about whether or not to use assisted ventilation are based on respiratory assessment and patient desire. Improved technology and lightweight portable units have made the home use of ventilators more practical. (See Chap. 25 for discussion of ventilators.)

▷ *Family Coping and Home Health Care.* The patient and family facing this progressive disease need compassionate caring and support. It is often agonizing to discuss this disease with them, but information about the disease and the teaching of nursing procedures and comfort measures are essential for the management of the patient in the home care setting. The family will require ongoing assistance and supervision. Professionals can help in making practical suggestions and in giving information about home health care products and equipment, services, and support groups. Arranging for respite care for the family and providing emotional support and reliable backup in the event of emergencies are part of caring for the caregivers. It is desirable that a social worker or counselor support the patient and family throughout the course of the illness. This helps keep stress within manageable limits.

The ALS Association has broad programs of research funding, patient and clinical services, patient information and support, and medical and public information (see Bibliography for address.) The ALS Association Quarterly Newsletter is filled with practical information.

▷ *Evaluation*

Expected Outcomes
1. Copes with impaired mobility
   a. Maintains activities within physical limitations
   b. Family uses mechanical lift, wheelchair, and other aids
   c. Patient maintains interest in reading and in listening to "talking books" and tapes as a means of diversion
2. Attempts to maintain nutritional status
   a. Avoids empty calories
   b. Chooses food that he is able to swallow
   c. Eats and drinks foods and liquids slowly and deliberately

d. Maintains body weight
e. Patient and family make informed decisions regarding alternative methods of taking foods and liquids (*i.e.*, gastrostomy tube)

3. Uses alternative communication system
   a. Seeks consultation from speech-language pathologist
   b. Reviews information about computer programs

4. Is aware of danger of respiratory failure
   a. Verbalizes risk of further deterioration of respiratory function
   b. Exhibits clear breath sounds
   c. Family members can verbalize signs and symptoms of respiratory dysfunction.
   d. Patient and family make informed decisions about treatment options. (*i.e.*, tracheostomy, negative pressure ventilator, positive-pressure ventilator)

5. Patient and family members use coping mechanisms
   a. Have adequate backup system of trained family, friends, health professionals
   b. Use community and other resources appropriately

The Muscular Dystrophies

The muscular dystrophies are a group of chronic muscle disorders characterized by progressive weakening and wasting of the skeletal or voluntary muscles. Most of these diseases are inherited.

The pathologic features include degeneration and loss of muscle fibers, variation in muscle fiber size, phagocytosis and regeneration, and replacement of muscle tissue by connective tissue.

The common characteristics of these diseases include varying degrees of muscle wasting and weakness; abnormal elevation in serum creatine phosphokinase, indicating a leakage of muscle enzymes; a myopathic EMG pattern; and myopathic findings on muscle biopsy. The differences center around the pattern of inheritance, the muscles involved, the age of onset, and the rate of progression.

Management

There is no specific treatment at this time for the muscular dystrophies. The objectives of supportive management are to keep the patient as active and functioning as normally as possible and to minimize functional deterioration. A therapeutic exercise program is prescribed for the individual patient to prevent muscle tightness, contractures, and disuse atrophy. Night splints and stretching exercises are used to delay contractures of the joints, especially the ankles, knees, and hips. Braces may compensate for muscle weakness.

Spinal deformity is a severe problem. Weakness of trunk muscles and spinal collapse occur almost routinely in patients with severe neuromuscular disease. In the battle against spinal deformity, the patient is fitted with an orthotic jacket to improve sitting stability and reduce trunk deformity. This measure also supports cardiovascular status. In time, spinal fusion is performed to maintain spinal stability. Other surgical procedures may be carried out to correct deformities.

Compromised pulmonary function may be due either to progression of the disease or to deformity of the thorax secondary to severe scoliosis. Intercurrent illnesses, upper respiratory infections, and fractures from falls must be vigorously treated in a way that minimizes immobilization, because joint contractures will become worse if the patient's activities are restricted more than usual. Aside from muscle weakness and contractures, a variety of other difficulties may be manifested in relation to the underlying disease. Dental and speech problems may result from weakness of the facial muscles, which makes it difficult to attend to dental hygiene and to speak coherently. Additional problems may affect the gastrointestinal tract, resulting in gastric dilatation, rectal prolapse, and fecal impaction. Finally, cardiomyopathy appears to be a common complication in all forms of muscular dystrophy.

Because of the genetic nature of this disease, parents and siblings of the patient are advised to seek genetic counseling. The Muscular Dystrophy Association works to combat neuromuscular disease through scientific research, programs of patient services and clinical care, and professional and public education (see Bibliography for address).

Nursing Interventions and Home Health Care

The goals of the patient and the nurse are to maintain function at optimal levels and to enhance the quality of life. This is accomplished in part by attending to the patient's physical requirements, which are considerable, without losing sight of emotional needs. The patient and family are actively involved in decision making.

Both the neuromuscular disease and the associated deformities may progress in adolescence and adulthood. Self-help devices can assist in achieving a greater degree of independence. Additional self-help devices become necessary as more muscle groups become affected. The patient is encouraged to continue with range-of-motion exercises to prevent contractures, which are particularly disabling. The family is taught to monitor the patient for respiratory problems. As respiratory difficulties develop, patients and their families need information regarding appropriate respiratory support. Options currently exist that can provide ventilatory support (negative pressure devices, positive-pressure ventilators) while allowing mobility. Patients can remain relatively independent in a wheelchair, for example, while being maintained on a ventilator at home.

Practical adaptations must be made to cope with the effects of chronic neuromuscular disability. To maximize functional independence, the patient at various stages of the disease may require a manual or an electric wheelchair, gait aids, upper and lower extremity and spinal orthoses, seating systems, bathroom equipment, lifts, ramps, and additional ADL aids. This requires a team approach. The home health nurse assesses how the patient and family are managing, makes referrals, and coordinates the activities of the physical therapist, occupational therapist, and social services.

Of great concern to the patient are the issues surrounding the threat of increasing disability. The patient is faced with a drawn-out, progressive loss of powers, leading eventually to death. Helplessness and powerlessness are central in the course of prolonged illness. Each functional loss involves a period of grieving and mourning. The patient is assessed for signs of depression, prolonged anger, bargaining, or denial. A psychiatric nurse clinician or other mental health professional is invaluable in helping the patient cope and adapt to chronic disease. By understanding and providing for the physical and psychological needs of the patient and family, the nurse can communicate strength to the patient and help provide a hopeful, supportive, and nurturing environment.

In summary, the neuromuscular disease (myasthenia gravis, ALS, and the muscular dystrophies) are characterized by muscle weakness. Respiratory dysfunction secondary to this muscle weakness is a major concern that requires astute assessment; collaboration among the patient, family, and health care team; and advanced planning. Discussion of treatment options to manage respiratory dysfunction and failure should take place before the patient with ALS or muscular dystrophy faces a respiratory crisis. The patient and family require assistance and support in the difficult decision-making process involved in acceptance or rejection of use of a respirator. The patient's role in decision making is maintained and promoted throughout the process.

Convulsive Disorders

Seizures

Seizures are episodes of abnormal motor, sensory, autonomic, or psychic activity (or a combination of these) as a consequence of sudden excessive discharge from cerebral neurons. A part or all of the brain may be involved. The seizures are usually sudden and transient.

The causes are varied and are classified as idiopathic (genetic, developmental defects) and acquired. Among the causes of acquired seizures are hypoxemia of any cause, including vascular insufficiency, fever (childhood), head injury, hypertension, central nervous system infections, metabolic and toxic conditions (*e.g.*, renal failure, hyponatremia, hypocalcemia, hypoglycemia, pesticides), brain tumor, drug withdrawal, and allergies. Stroke and cerebral metastasis are the leading causes of seizures in the elderly.

Often there is memory loss for the convulsive episode and for a short time thereafter. Brain damage may occur when seizures are severe or prolonged. The patient is at risk for hypoxia, vomiting, and pulmonary aspiration or persistent metabolic abnormalities.

The immediate therapeutic goal is to control the seizure, and the long-term goal is to determine and control the cause.

Nursing Assessment During a Seizure

A major responsibility of the nurse is to observe and to record the sequence of symptoms. The nature of the seizure usually indicates the type of treatment that is used. Before and during an attack, the following should be noted:

1. Description of the circumstances before the attack (visual stimuli, auditory stimuli, olfactory stimuli, tactile stimuli, emotional or psychological disturbances, sleep, hyperventilation)
2. The first thing the patient does in an attack—where the movements or the stiffness starts, position of the eyeballs and the head at the beginning of the attack. This information gives clues as to the location of the epileptogenic focus in the brain. (In recording, always state whether or not the beginning of the attack was observed.)

3. The type of movements in the part of the body involved
4. The areas of the body involved. (Turn back bedding and expose patient.)
5. The size of both pupils. Are the eyes open? Did the eyes/head turn to one side?
6. Whether or not automatisms (involuntary motor activity such as lip smacking or repeated swallowing) were observed
7. Incontinence of urine or feces
8. Duration of each phase of the attack
9. Unconsciousness, if present, and its duration
10. Any obvious paralysis or weakness of arms or legs after the attack
11. Inability to speak after the attack
12. Movements at the end of the seizure
13. Whether or not the patient sleeps afterward
14. Whether or not the patient was confused after the attack

Nursing Management During a Seizure

During a convulsive seizure, the nursing goal is to prevent injury to the patient. This includes not only physical support but psychological support as well.

- Provide privacy and protect the patient from curious onlookers. (The patient who has an *aura* [warning of an impending seizure] may have time to seek a safe place.)
- Ease the patient to the floor, if possible.
- Protect the head with a pad to prevent injury (from striking a hard surface).
- Loosen constrictive clothing.
- Push aside any furniture that may injure the patient during the attack.
- If the patient is in bed, remove pillows and elevate siderails.
- If an aura precedes the seizure, insert a padded tongue blade between the teeth to reduce the possibility of the tongue or cheek being bitten.
- *Do not attempt to pry open jaws that are clenched in a spasm to insert* anything. Broken teeth and injury to the lips and tongue may result from such an action.
- No attempt should be made to restrain the patient during the seizure, because muscular contractions are strong, and restraint can produce injury.
- If possible, place the patient on one side with head flexed forward, which permits the tongue to fall forward and facilitates drainage of saliva and mucus. If suction is available, use it if necessary to clear secretions.
- After the seizure, keep the patient turned on one side to prevent aspiration. Make sure the airway is patent.
- There is usually a period of confusion after epileptic seizures.
- A short apneic period may occur during or immediately after a generalized seizure.
- The patient, on awakening, should be reoriented to the environment.
- If the patient experiences severe excitement after a seizure (postictal), try to handle the situation with calm persuasion and gentle restraint.

The Epilepsies

The epilepsies are a symptom-complex of several disorders of brain function characterized by recurring seizures. There may be associated loss of consciousness, excess or loss of muscle tone or movement, and disturbances of behavior, mood, sensation, and perception. Thus, epilepsy is not a disease but a symptom.

The basic problem is thought to be an electrical disturbance (dysrhythmia) in the nerve cells in one section of the brain, causing them to emit abnormal, recurring, uncontrolled electrical discharges. The characteristic epileptic seizure is a manifestation of this excessive neuronal discharge.

Incidence.   An estimated 1% of the population (more than 2 million people) in the United States have epilepsy, with some 100,000 new patients diagnosed each year. There has been an increasing incidence of this condition, probably due to a number of factors. Improved obstetric and pediatric care salvages babies who experience respiratory, circulatory, and other distress during delivery; these infants may be predisposed to intermittent seizures. The improved medical, surgical, and nursing management of patients with head injuries, brain tumors, meningitis, and encephalitis saves those whose conditions may produce cerebral changes with resultant seizures. Also, advances in electroencephalography have aided in the identification of patients with epilepsy. Education has served to enlighten the general public and has lessened the stigma associated with the condition, so that more persons are more willing to admit that they have epilepsy.

Altered Physiology.   Messages from the body are carried by the neurons (nerve cells) of the brain by means of discharges of electrochemical energy that sweep along them. These impulses occur in bursts whenever a nerve cell has a task to perform. Sometimes these cells or groups of cells continue firing after a task is finished. During the period of unwanted discharges, parts of the body controlled by the errant cells may perform erratically. Resultant discomfort and dysfunction range from mild to incapacitating, and usually cause unconsciousness. When these uncontrolled, abnormal discharges occur repeatedly, a person is said to have epilepsy. The erratic physical movements are called *seizures*.

Causes.   No one knows what makes brain cells in some people cause epilepsy. Scientists have produced seizures in experimental animals through surgical injury or chemical or electrical stimulation. Epilepsies often follow birth trauma, asphyxia neonatorum, head injuries, some infectious diseases (bacterial, viral, parasitic), toxicity (carbon monoxide and lead poisoning), circulatory problems, fever, metabolic and nutritional disorders, and drug or alcohol intoxication. They are also associated with brain tumors, abscesses, and congenital malformations. In most cases of epilepsy, the cause is unknown (idiopathic). There is evidence that susceptibility to some types may be inherited. Epilepsy strikes before the age of 20 in over 75% of patients.

The epilepsies have little to do with intelligence in most cases. Persons with epilepsy who do not have other brain or nervous system disabilities fall within the same intelligence ranges as does the overall population. Epilepsy is not synonymous with mental retardation or illness. However, many who are retarded because they have serious neurologic damage often have epilepsy too, thus pulling the mean IQ for all epilepsy victims below that of the so-called normal range.

Prevention.   A full-scale attack incorporating a wide range of measures must be mounted for the prevention of epilepsy. Because the infants of epileptic mothers who take certain antiepileptic medications are at risk, these women need careful monitoring, including blood studies to detect the level of an-

tiepileptic drugs taken throughout pregnancy. High-risk mothers (teenagers, women with histories of difficult deliveries, drug addicts, those with diabetes and hypertension) should be identified and supervised closely during pregnancy because brain lesions or injury that ultimately causes epilepsy may occur to the fetus during pregnancy and delivery.

Childhood infections (measles, mumps, bacterial meningitis) should be controlled with appropriate vaccination. Lead poisoning is another preventable cause of epilepsy. Parents with a child who has had a febrile convulsion should be instructed about methods to control fever (cool sponging, antipyretic medications).

Head injury is one of the main causes that can be prevented. Through highway safety programs and occupational safety precautions, not only can lives be saved, but the possible development of epilepsy from head injury can be prevented.

Screening programs to detect children with seizure disorders at an early age, and seizure prevention programs with the judicious use of antiepileptic medications and modification of life style are part of this prevention plan.

Clinical Manifestations.   Depending on the location of the discharging neurons, seizures may range from a simple staring spell to prolonged convulsive movements with loss of consciousness. The variations in seizures have been classified internationally according to the area of the brain involved, and have been identified as partial, generalized, and unclassified. *Partial* seizures are focal in origin and affect only part of the brain. *Generalized* seizures are nonspecific in origin and affect the entire brain simultaneously. *Unclassified* seizures are so termed because of incomplete data. (See Chart 57-3 for the international classification of seizures.)

The initial pattern of the seizures indicates the region of the brain in which the seizure originates. Also it is important to determine if the patient has had an *aura*, a premonitory or warning sensation before an epileptic seizure, which may indicate the origin of the seizure (*e.g.*, seeing a flashing light may indicate the seizure originated in the occipital lobe).

In *simple partial seizures*, only a finger or hand may shake, or the mouth may jerk uncontrollably. The person may talk unintelligibly, may be dizzy, and may experience unusual or unpleasant sights, sounds, odors, or tastes, but without loss of consciousness.

In *complex partial seizures*, the person either remains motionless or moves automatically but inappropriately for time and place, or may experience excessive emotions of fear, anger, elation, or irritability. Whatever the manifestations, the person does not remember the episode when it is over.

Generalized seizures, more commonly referred to as *grand mal seizures*, involve both hemispheres of the brain, causing both sides of the body to react. There may be intense rigidity of the entire body followed by jerky alternations of muscle relaxation and contraction (generalized tonic–clonic contraction). The simultaneous contractions of the diaphragm and chest muscles may produce a characteristic epileptic cry. Often the tongue is chewed and the patient is incontinent of urine and stool. After 1 or 2 minutes, the convulsive movements begin to subside; the patient relaxes and lies in deep coma, breathing noisily. The respirations at this point are chiefly abdominal. In the postictal state (after the seizure), the patient is often confused and hard to arouse, and may sleep for hours. Many patients complain of headache or sore muscles.

Diagnostic Evaluation.   The diagnostic assessment is

aimed at determining the *type* of seizures, their frequency and severity, and the factors that precipitate them. A development history is taken, including events of pregnancy and childbirth, to seek evidence of preexisting injury. A search is made for illnesses or head injuries that may have affected the brain. In addition to a physical and neurologic examination, diagnostic examinations include biochemical, hematologic, and serologic studies. CT imaging is used to detect lesions in the brain, focal abnormalities, cerebrovascular abnormalities, and cerebral degenerative changes.

The electroencephalogram (EEG) furnishes diagnostic evidence in a substantial proportion of patients with epilepsy and aids in classifying the type of seizure. Abnormalities in the EEG usually continue to be apparent between seizures, or, if concealed, may be brought out by hyperventilation or during sleep. In addition, microelectrodes can be inserted deep in the brain to probe the action of single brain cells. It should be noted, however, that some persons with seizures may have normal EEGs, whereas persons who have never had seizures may have abnormal EEGs. Telemetry and computer equipment developed by space technology are used to take and store EEG readings on computer tapes while patients pursue their normal activities. Videorecording of seizures taken simultaneously with EEG telemetry is useful in determining the type of seizure as well as its duration and magnitude. This type of intensive monitoring

is revolutionizing the treatment of severe epilepsy in this country.

Management

The management of epilepsy is planned according to a long-range program, one that is tailored to meet the special needs of each patient and not just to manage and prevent seizures. There is no simple solution, because some forms of epilepsy arise from brain damage and others depend on alterations of brain chemistry.

Drug Therapy. Many antiepileptic drugs are available to control seizures, although the mechanisms of their actions are still unknown. The objective of drug therapy is to achieve seizure control with minimal side effects. Drug therapy is a form of control, not cure. The drug is selected according to the type of seizure being treated and the effectiveness and safety of the drug. If properly prescribed and taken, these drugs cause seizure control in 50% to 60% of patients with recurring seizures, and partial control in another 15% to 35%. The condition of some 15% to 35% of patients is not improved by any available drug.

Usually treatment is started with a single drug. The starting dose and the rate at which the dosage is increased depend on whether or not side effects develop. The drug levels are monitored in the blood, because the rate of drug absorption varies among people. Changing to another drug may be necessary if seizure control is not achieved or when toxicity makes it impossible to increase the dosage. The drug may need to be adjusted because of concurrent illness, weight gain, or increases in stress. Sudden withdrawal of antiepileptic medication can cause seizures to occur with greater frequency or can precipitate the development of status epilepticus (see p. 1528).

The side effects of these medications may be divided into three groups: (1) idiosyncratic or allergic disorders, which present primarily as skin reactions; (2) acute toxicity, which may be manifested when the drug is initially prescribed; or (3) chronic toxicity, which occurs late in the course of drug therapy. The manifestations of drug toxicity are variable, and any organ system may be involved. Periodic physical examinations and laboratory tests are performed for patients receiving drugs known to have toxic effects on the hematopoietic, genitourinary, or hepatic systems. Thorough oral hygiene after each meal, regular dental care, and regular gum massage are important for the patient taking phenytoin (Dilantin) to prevent or control gingival hyperplasia. Table 57-1 summarizes the antiepileptic/anticonvulsant medications in current use.

Surgery for Epilepsy. Surgery is indicated for patients whose epilepsy results from intracranial tumors, abscess, cysts, or vascular anomalies.

Some patients have intractable seizure disorders that do not respond to drug therapy. There may be a focal atrophic process secondary to trauma, inflammation, stroke, or anoxemia. If the seizures originate in a reasonably well-circumscribed area of the brain that can be excised without producing significant neurologic deficits, the removal of the epileptogenic focus generating the seizures seems to give long-term control and improvement. This type of neurosurgery has been aided by several modern advances, including microsurgical techniques, depth electroencephalography, improved illumination and hemostasis, and the introduction of neuroleptanalgesic agents (droperidol and fentanyl). These techniques, combined with local infiltration

TABLE 57–1. *Major Antiepileptic/Anticonvulsant Drugs*

Generic Name	Dose-Related Side Effects	Toxic Effects
CARBAMAZEPINE	Dizziness; drowsiness	Severe skin rash
	Unsteadiness; nausea and vomiting	Blood dyscrasias
	Diplopia; mild leukopenia	Hepatitis
PRIMIDONE	Lethargy; irritability	Skin rash
	Diplopia; ataxia	
	Sexual impotence	
PHENYTOIN	Visual problems	Severe skin reaction
	Hirsutism	Peripheral neuropathy
	Gingival hyperplasia	Ataxia; drowsiness
	Dysrhythmias	Blood dyscrasias
PHENOBARBITAL	Sedation; irritability	Skin rash
	Diplopia	
	Ataxia	
ETHOSUXIMIDE	Nausea and vomiting	Skin rash
	Headache	Blood dyscrasias
	Gastric distress	Hepatitis
		Lupus erythematosus
VALPROATE	Nausea and vomiting	Hepatotoxicity
	Weight gain	Skin rash
	Loss of hair	Blood dyscrasias
		Nephritis

PATIENT COUNSELING

1. Take medication daily to keep the blood level constant to prevent seizures.
2. Report to the laboratory for blood sampling before taking morning medication when testing is prescribed.
3. Do not stop taking the drug abruptly; sudden withdrawal of medication may cause seizures.
4. Avoid alcohol; check with physician before taking additional prescription or over-the-counter medications.
5. Avoid activities that require alertness and coordination (*e.g.*, driving, operating machinery) until after the effects of the drug have been evaluated.
6. Maintain oral hygiene and have regular dental care.
7. Carry a personal identification card stating the name of the drug you are taking.

of scalp incisions, enable the neurosurgeon to perform surgery on an alert and cooperative patient. With special testing devices, electrocortical mapping, and the patient's response to stimulation, the boundaries of the epileptogenic focus are determined. Any abnormal epileptogenic cortex (*i.e.*, abnormal area of the brain) is then removed.

▶ Nursing Process
The Patient With Epilepsy

▷ Assessment

The nurse serves as an historian and observer to elicit information about the patient's seizure history. The patient is asked about the factors or events that may precipitate the seizures.

His alcohol intake is documented. The effects of epilepsy on his life style are assessed: Does the patient have a recreational program? Social contacts? Is work a positive experience? What coping mechanisms are used? What are the limitations imposed by the seizure disorder?

Observation and neurologic nursing assessment during and after a seizure are important for determining the type of seizure and its management.

▷ Nursing Diagnoses

Based on the assessment data, the patient's major nursing diagnoses may include the following:

- Fear related to the ever-present possibility of having seizures
- Ineffective coping related to stresses imposed by epilepsy

- Knowledge deficit about epilepsy and its control
- High risk for injury during seizures

The major potential problem of patients with epilepsy is status epilepticus.

▷ Planning and Implementation

▷ *Goals:* The major goals of the patient may include maintenance of control of seizures, achievement of a satisfactory psychosocial adjustment, and acquisition of knowledge and understanding about the condition. The long-term goal is to achieve a satisfactory life adjustment and to prevent or manage episodes of status epilepticus.

▷ Nursing Interventions

▷ *Seizure Control.* Fear that a seizure may occur unexpectedly can be reduced by the patient's compliance with the prescribed treatment. The complete cooperation of the patient and family is of the utmost importance. They must have confidence in the value of the regimen that is prescribed. It must be emphasized that the prescribed antiepileptic drug must be taken on a continuing basis and that it's not a habit-forming drug. It may be taken without fear, for many years if necessary, if the patient is under health supervision and following instructions faithfully.

The control of seizures depends in part on the patient's understanding and cooperation. Life style and environment are examined to determine whether certain factors precipitate the seizures: emotional disturbances, new environmental stresses, onset of menstruation in female patients, or fever. The patient is encouraged to follow a regular and moderate routine in life style, diet (avoiding excessive stimulants), exercise, and rest. (Sleep deprivation may lower the patient's threshold to seizures.) Moderate activity is good therapy, but excessive expenditure of energy is to be avoided. Some patients need to avoid photic stimulation (bright flickering lights, television viewing). Wearing dark glasses or covering one eye may help control this problem. Tension states (anxiety, frustration) induce seizures in some patients. Classes in stress management may be of value. Because seizures are known to follow alcohol intake, alcoholic beverages are restricted. All in all, the best therapy is to follow the therapeutic program.

▷ *Improved Coping Mechanisms.* It has been noted that the social, psychological, and behavioral problems frequently accompanying epilepsy can be more of a handicap than the actual seizures. Epilepsy imposes feelings of fear, alienation, depression, and uncertainty. The patient must cope with the constant fear of a seizure and its embarrassing consequences. Children with epilepsy may be ostracized and excluded from school and peer activities. These problems are compounded in the teen years and add to the challenges of dating, not being able to drive, and feeling different. Adults face all of these problems plus the burden of finding employment, decisions concerning marriage and childbearing, noninsurability, stigma, and legal barriers. Alcohol abuse may complicate matters. The burden on the family is great, and family problems run the gamut of outright rejection to overprotection. As a result of all these factors, many persons with epilepsy have psychological and behavioral problems.

Counseling is a must for helping the individual and the family to understand the condition and the limitations imposed by it. Social and recreational opportunities are necessary for good mental health. Some persons are not able to cope with epilepsy; others have psychological problems resulting from brain damage. Those with seizures originating in the temporal lobes of the brain (areas controlling thought and emotions) have particular emotional problems. Symptoms of schizophrenia and impulsive or irritable behavior may be due to brain damage associated with temporal lobe seizures. These patients require comprehensive mental health services.

▷ *Patient Education.* Of all the services that are contributed by the nurse in the care of the person with epilepsy, perhaps the most valuable are efforts to modify the attitudes of the patient and family toward the disease itself.

For the observer, an epileptic seizure is a terrifying or repulsive spectacle; thus, for the person who has them, every seizure is inevitably a source of humiliation and shame. This in turn breeds anxiety, depression, hostility, secrecy, and deceit, to which the public reacts with abhorrence, and the vicious cycle is complete. The reaction of shame and denial is not confined merely to persons with epilepsy but extends to their families as well.

To escape from this vicious cycle, patients who have epilepsy, their families, and the public at large need factual information. Epilepsy is not a mysterious disease; it does not reflect the supernatural. Epilepsy is no more disgraceful than diabetes, pernicious anemia, or hyperthyroidism. It is not a form of insanity. It does not tend to get worse with time. It can be controlled effectively. It should not keep the adult from work. *Activity tends to inhibit, not stimulate, epileptic seizures.* Some 50% to 60% of patients with epilepsy now may have their symptoms controlled.

Enlightenment of the public will give new hope to those facing centuries-old prejudices. Continuing encouragement should be given patients to mobilize their inner resources to overcome feelings of inferiority and self-consciousness resulting from seizures. The licensing of persons with epilepsy to drive automobiles varies from state to state. The patient with epilepsy should carry an emergency medical identification card in wallet or purse or wear an identification bracelet around the wrist.

Hereditary transmission of epilepsy has not been proved. The matter of marriage and children must be decided on an individual basis, but this right should not be denied to persons with epilepsy merely because they have the disease. Genetic counseling is advised, however.

▷ *Patient Resources.* Because epilepsy is a long-term disorder, the continuous use of expensive medications may present a sizable burden to the patient and family. The Epilepsy Foundation of America offers a mail-order program to provide medications at minimum cost and access to life insurance. This organization serves as a referral source through which a person with epilepsy obtain special services (see Bibliography for address).

For many, employment problems still remain the greatest handicap of epilepsy. Studies have demonstrated that the person with epilepsy who is properly placed in work has a satisfactory job performance. The director of each State Vocational Rehabilitation agency can provide information about vocational rehabilitation. The Epilepsy Foundation of America has developed a training and placement service. If the individual's seizures are not well controlled, information about sheltered workshops or home employment programs may be obtained.

Counseling and job training are provided for qualified persons through the Veterans' Administration. The US Civil Service Commission now grants government jobs to individuals if seizures are controlled and the person is otherwise qualified. The Rehabilitation Act helped to end job discrimination of the handicapped. Private firms are becoming knowledgeable, and the number of employers who knowingly hire persons with epilepsy is increasing.

The Commission for the Control of Epilepsy and Its Consequences makes recommendations covering all aspects of the problem of epilepsy in the United States—social, legal, scientific, economic, and humanitarian. Epilepsy International sponsors international congresses, publishes *Epilepsia* (the international journal on epilepsy), and has ongoing projects of international significance.

Persons who have uncontrollable seizures and psychological and social maladaptation with other overwhelming problems can be referred to comprehensive epilepsy centers where continuous television and EEG monitoring, specialized treatment, and rehabilitation services are available.

▷ Prevention of Complications: Status Epilepticus

▷ Prevention and Management of Status Epilepticus

Status epilepticus (acute prolonged seizure activity) is a series of generalized convulsions that occur without full recovery of consciousness between attacks. The term has been broadened to include continuous clinical or electrical seizures lasting at least 30 minutes, even without impairment of consciousness. It is considered a major medical emergency. Status epilepticus produces cumulative effects. Vigorous muscular contractions impose a heavy metabolic demand and can interfere with respirations. There is some respiratory arrest at the height of each seizure that produces venous congestion and hypoxia of the brain. Repeated episodes of cerebral anoxia and swelling may lead to irreversible and fatal brain damage.

Common factors that precipitate status epilepticus include withdrawal of antiepileptic medication, fever, and intercurrent infection.

Management

The goals of treatment are to stop the seizures as quickly as possible, to ensure adequate cerebral oxygenation, and to maintain the patient in a seizure-free state. An airway and adequate oxygenation are established. If the patient remains deeply unconscious, a cuffed endotracheal tube is inserted. Intravenous diazepam is given slowly in an attempt to halt seizures immediately. Other antiepileptic drugs (phenytoin, phenobarbital) are given as prescribed after diazepam is administered to maintain a seizure-free state, because the anticonvulsant effect of diazepam is short lived.

An intravenous line is established and blood samples are obtained to monitor electrolytes, blood urea, and glucose. EEG monitoring may be useful in determining the nature of epileptogenic activity. Vital signs and neurologic signs are monitored on a continuing basis. An intravenous infusion of dextrose is given if hypoglycemia has caused the seizure. If initial treatment is unsuccessful, general anesthesia with a short-acting barbiturate may be used.

Serum concentration of the antiepileptic drug is measured, because a low level suggests that the patient was not taking the medication or that the dosage was too low. Patients recovering from status epilepticus may die within a few days from cardiac involvement or respiratory depression. There is also the potential for postictal (after a seizure) cerebral swelling.

Nursing Interventions

The nurse provides ongoing assessment and monitoring of respiratory and cardiac function. There may be delayed depression of respiration and blood pressure induced by the medications given to halt the seizures. Nursing assessment also includes monitoring the seizure type and the general condition of the patient.

The patient is moved to the semiprone position, if possible, to assist in draining pharyngeal secretions. Standby suction equipment must be available because there is danger of aspiration. The intravenous line is closely monitored because it may become dislodged during seizures.

A person with epilepsy who is receiving long-term anticonvulsant therapy has a significant incidence of fractures resulting from bone disease. Chronic treatment with anticonvulsant drugs leads to a combination of osteoporosis, osteomalacia, and hyperparathyroidism. Thus, during seizures the patient is protected from injury with padded side rails and is kept under constant observation. No effort should be made to restrain movements. The patient having seizures can inadvertently injure attending persons, so nurses should take care to protect themselves. Other nursing interventions for the person having seizures are discussed on p. 1723.

▷ Evaluation

Expected Outcomes

1. Maintains control of seizures
   a. Complies with drug regimen
   b. Verbalizes the need to take prescribed antiepileptic drug; can relate the hazards of drug stoppage
   c. Recalls the side effects of drugs
   d. Keeps laboratory appointment after hospital discharge for serum level determination of antiepileptic drug
   e. Avoids factors/situations that may precipitate seizures (flickering light, hyperventilation)
   f. Follows a healthful life style by
      (1) Getting enough sleep
      (2) Eating meals at regular times to avoid hypoglycemia
   g. Wears an identification bracelet
2. Strives to improve psychosocial adjustment
   a. Identifies significant other with whom to talk
   b. Is able to discuss feelings
   c. Identifies rights under Federal law
   d. States knowledge that job counseling/job placement services are available
3. Gains knowledge and understanding of epilepsy
   a. Reads pamphlets/books about epilepsy
   b. Answers most questions about epilepsy correctly
4. Exhibits absence of status epilepticus
   a. Is seizure free
   b. Complies with drug regimen

In summary, seizures can result from a variety of causes. Although the sudden onset of seizure activity may be an indication of underlying structural abnormalities (*i.e.*, brain tumors), many seizure disorders are of unknown origin. Although those due to brain tumors likely require surgical intervention, many other seizures can be adequately controlled with medication and avoidance of seizure-inducing activities.

Nursing management during a seizure focuses on maintenance of the airway, protection of the patient from injury, minimization of the patient's embarrassment about the seizure, and observation and description of the seizure.

Seizures and seizure disorders are often frightening and anxiety provoking to the patient and his family. In some families, seizures also may be considered a stigma. In these circumstances, it is particularly important for the nurse to assess patient and family attitudes about seizure disorders, as family fears and pressures may lead the patient to stop taking anticonvulsant medication because it is a constant reminder that he has a seizure disorder.

Head Injuries

Injuries to the head involve trauma to the scalp, skull, and brain. Head injuries are among the most frequent and serious neurologic disorders, and have reached epidemic proportions as a result of traffic accidents. An estimated 100,000 persons die annually from head injuries, and more than 700,000 have injuries severe enough to require hospitalization. Of this group, between 50,000 and 90,000 people a year are left with intellectual or behavioral deficits that preclude their return to normal life. Two thirds of these are below the age of 30, with males outnumbering females. Detectable blood alcohol levels have been found in more than 50% of head-injured patients treated in emergency departments. At least half of all severely head-injured patients have significant injuries to other parts of the body. Hypovolemic shock in a head-injured patient is usually due to injuries to other parts of the body.

Scalp and Skull Injuries

Scalp Injury

Because of its many blood vessels, the scalp can bleed profusely when injured. Scalp wounds are also a portal of entry for intracranial infections. Trauma may result in an abrasion (brush wound), contusion, laceration, or avulsion. A subcutaneous injection of procaine makes it easier for the wound to be cleaned and treated. The area is irrigated to remove foreign material and minimize the chance of infection before lacerations are closed.

Fractures of the Skull

A skull fracture is a break in the continuity of the skull caused by trauma (Fig. 57-7). It may occur with or without damage to the brain. The presence of a skull fracture usually means that there was considerable force on impact. Skull fractures are classified as open or closed. In an *open* fracture, the dura is torn, and in a *closed* fracture, the dura is not torn.

Clinical Manifestations. The symptoms, aside from those of the local injury, depend on the amount and the distribution of brain injury. Pain, persistent or localized, usually suggests

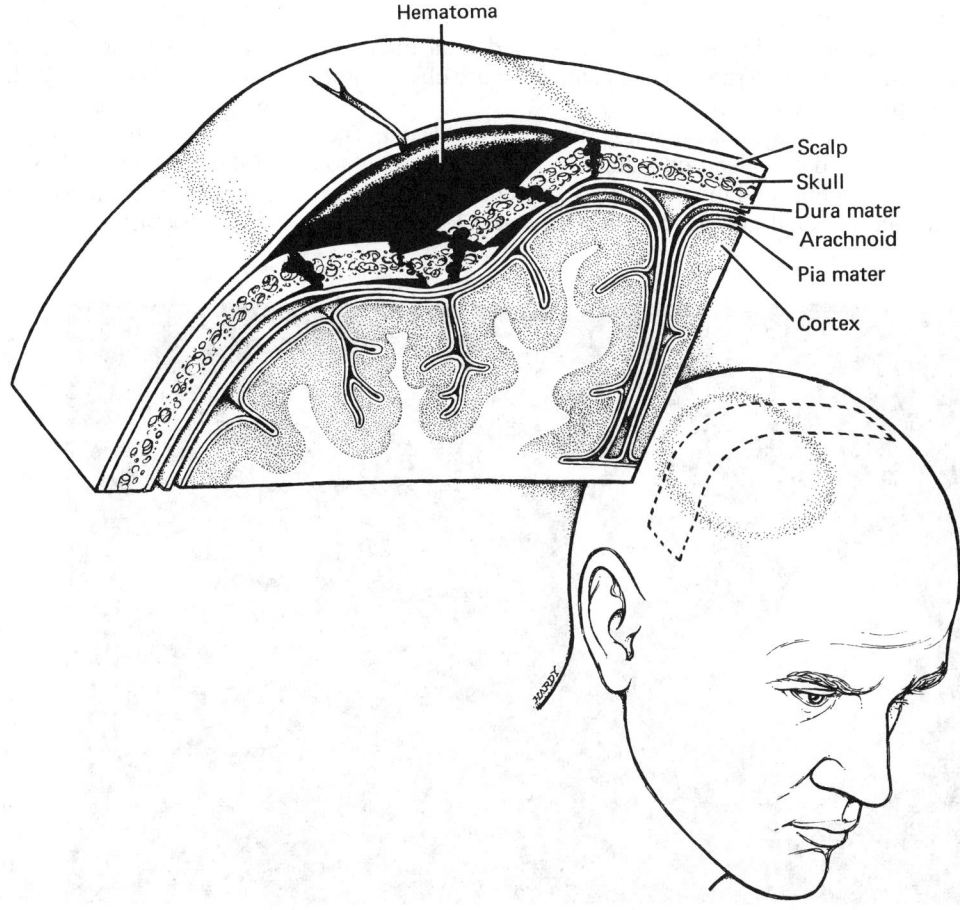

Figure 57–7. Depressed fracture of the skull.

that a fracture is present. Fractures of the cranial vault produce swelling in the region of the fracture, and for this reason an accurate diagnosis cannot be made without an x-ray. Fractures of the base of the skull tend to traverse the paranasal sinus of the frontal bone or the middle ear located in the temporal bone; thus, they frequently produce hemorrhage from the nose, the pharynx, or the ears, and blood may appear under the conjunctivae. An area of *ecchymosis*, or bruising, may be seen over the mastoid (Battle's sign). The escape of CSF from the ears (*cerebrospinal fluid otorrhea*) and the nose (*cerebrospinal rhinorrhea*) suggests basal skull fracture. Drainage of cerebrospinal fluid is a serious problem because infection such as meningitis can occur if organisms gain access to the cranial contents through the nose, ear, or sinus through a tear in the dura. Bloody spinal fluid, if present, suggests brain laceration or contusion.

Diagnostic Evaluation. Although a rapid physical examination and evaluation of neurologic status demonstrate the more obvious brain injuries, the less apparent abnormalities found in head injuries may be detected by cranial CT, which can differentiate subtle changes in the degree to which the soft tissue absorbs x-rays. It is accurate and safe in showing the presence, nature, location, and extent of the lesion as well as in disclosing cerebral edema, contusion, intracerebral or extracerebral hematoma, subarachnoid and intraventricular hemorrhage, and late traumatic changes (infarction, hydrocephalus). Where available, MRI is also being used to evaluate patients with head injury (Fig. 57-8).

If CT is not available, cerebral angiography demonstrates the presence of supratentorial, extracerebral, and intracerebral hematomas and cerebral contusion. Lateral and anteroposterior views of the skull are obtained.

Management. In general, nondepressed skull fractures usually do not require surgical treatment, but close observation of the patient is essential.

For depressed skull fractures, surgery is indicated. The scalp is shaved and cleansed with large amounts of saline to remove all debris, and the fracture is exposed. The skull fragments are elevated and the area is debrided. Closure of the

dura is carried out if possible, and the wound is closed. Large defects in the skull can be repaired later with metallic or plastic plates if necessary. In instances of a clean wound and an intact dura, the elevated fragments can be replaced, at the time of the initial surgery, making a later cranioplasty unnecessary. Penetrating wounds require surgical debridement to remove foreign bodies and devitalized brain tissue and to control hemorrhage. Antibiotic treatment is instituted immediately, and blood component therapy is administered if indicated.

Fractures of the base of the skull are serious because they are usually open (involving the paranasal sinuses or middle or external ear) and there is the possibility of leakage of cerebrospinal fluid. A combination of blood surrounded by a yellowish stain is referred to as the halo sign. Seen on bed linens or dressing material, it is highly suggestive of a cerebrospinal fluid leak. The nasopharynx and the external ear should be kept clean, and usually a plug of sterile cotton is placed in the ear or a sterile cotton pad may be taped loosely under the nose or against the ear to collect the draining fluid. The patient who is conscious is cautioned against sneezing or blowing the nose. The head is usually elevated 30 degrees to reduce ICP and promote spontaneous closure of the leak. (Some neurosurgeons prefer that the bed be kept flat.) Persistence of spinal fluid rhinorrhea or otorrhea usually requires surgical intervention.

Brain Injury

The most important consideration in any head injury is whether or not the brain has been injured. Even ''minor'' injury can cause permanent brain damage. The brain is unable to store oxygen and glucose to any significant degree. The cerebral cells need an uninterrupted blood supply for these nutrients. The brain dies when its blood supply is interrupted for only a few minutes; there is no regeneration of damaged neurons.

Serious brain injury may occur, with or without fracture of the skull, after blows or injuries to the head that produce contusions, laceration, and hemorrhage of the brain.

Concussion. A cerebral concussion after a head trauma

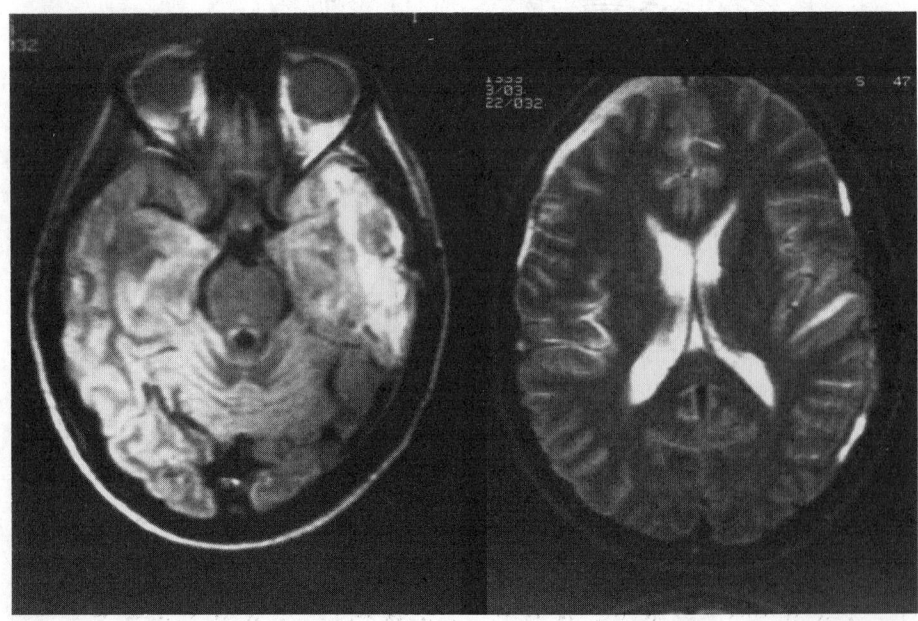

Figure 57–8. Head injury. MRI demonstrates subdural hematomas in the right frontal and left temoral areas. Also, significant contusion is seen in the left temporal lobe and to some degree in the right temporal lobe. (Courtesy of the Hospital of the University of Pennsylvania, Nuclear Medicine Section.)

is a temporary loss of neurologic function from which there is complete recovery. There is no apparent structural damage, and recovery occurs quickly. A concussion generally involves a period of unconsciousness lasting from a few seconds to a few minutes. The jarring of the brain may be so slight as to cause only dizziness and spots before the eyes (spoken of as "seeing stars"), or there may be complete loss of consciousness for a time. If the brain tissue in the frontal lobe is affected, the patient may exhibit bizarre irrational behavior, whereas disruption of brain tissue in the temporal lobe can produce temporary amnesia or disorientation.

The treatment of concussion is to observe the patient for headache, dizziness, irritability, and anxiety (*postconcussion syndrome*), which may follow this type of injury. Giving the patient information, explanations, and encouragement may reduce some of the problems of postconcussion syndrome.

The patient is discharged from the hospital in a relatively short time after a head injury. The family is instructed to look for the following signs and to notify the physician or clinic or bring the patient back to the Emergency Department if they occur: difficulty in awakening, difficulty in speaking, confusion, severe headache, vomiting, or weakness of one side of the body. The patient is advised to resume normal activities slowly.

Contusion.   A cerebral contusion is a more severe cerebral injury in which the brain is bruised, with possible surface hemorrhage. The patient is unconscious for a considerable period. The symptoms, as would be expected, are more marked. The patient may lie motionless; the pulse is feeble, the respirations shallow, and the skin cold and pale. Often there is involuntary evacuation of the bowels and the bladder. The patient may be aroused with effort but soon slips back into unconsciousness. The blood pressure and the temperature are subnormal, and the picture is somewhat similar to that of shock.

In general, persons with widespread injury who have abnormal motor function, abnormal eye movements, and elevated ICP have a poor outcome. Conversely, the patient may recover consciousness completely and perhaps pass into a stage of cerebral irritability.

In the stage of cerebral irritability, the patient is no longer unconscious but, on the contrary, is easily disturbed by any form of stimulation, noises, light, and voices, and may become hyperactive at times. Gradually, the pulse, respirations, temperature, and other body functions return to normal. However, recovery is not complete at once. Residual headache and vertigo are common, and often impaired mentality or epilepsy occurs as a result of irreparable cerebral damage.

Intracranial Hemorrhage

The most common serious results of brain injuries are *hematomas* (collections of blood) that develop within the cranial vault (Fig. 57-9). The hematoma is referred to as epidural, subdural, or intracerebral, depending on its location. The main effects are frequently delayed until the hematoma is large enough to cause distortion and herniation of the brain and increased ICP.

- The signs and symptoms of brain ischemia resulting from

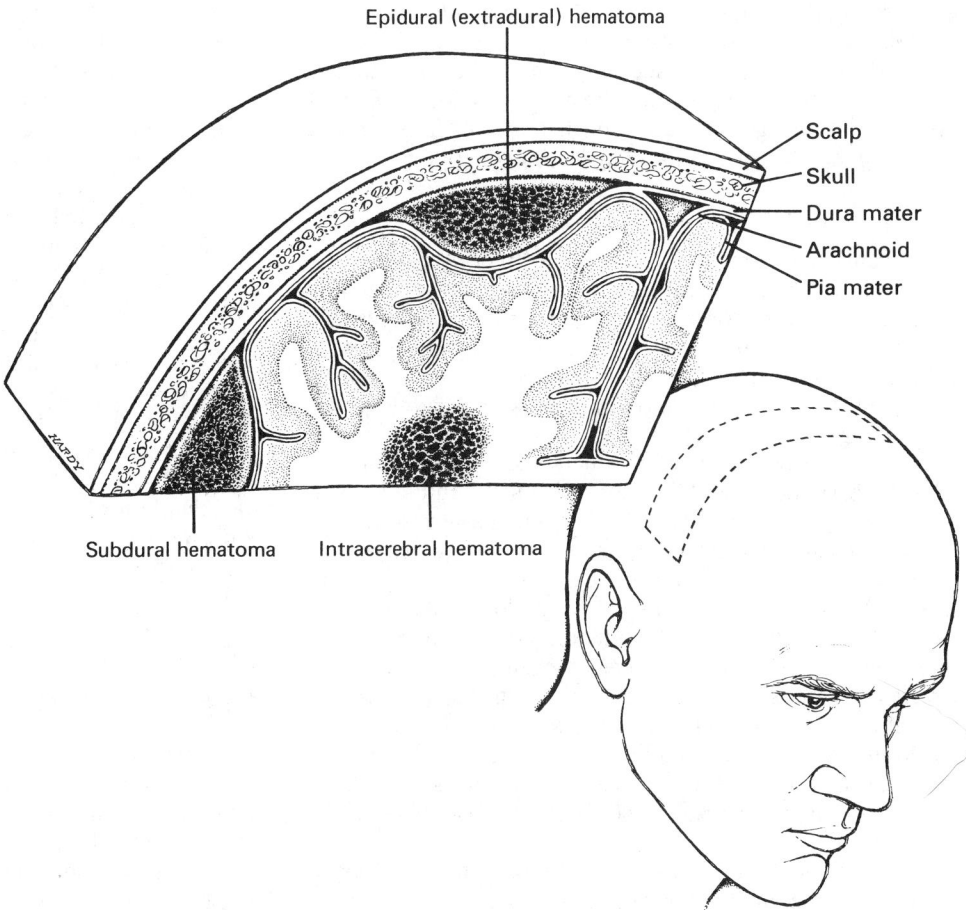

Figure 57-9. Diagrammatic views showing epidural, subdural, and intracerebral hematomas.

compression caused by a hematoma are variable and depend on the speed with which vital areas are encroached on or the changes that involve the underlying brain.

In general, a small hematoma that develops rapidly may be fatal, whereas a more massive hematoma that develops slowly may allow the patient to adapt.

Epidural Hematoma (Extradural Hematoma or Hemorrhage)

After a head injury, blood may collect in the epidural (extradural) space between the skull and the dura. This often results from fractures of the skull that cause rupture or laceration of the middle meningeal artery, which runs between the dura and the skull located just inferior to a thin portion of temporal bone; hemorrhage from this artery causes pressure on the brain.

The symptoms are caused by the expanding hematoma. There is usually a momentary loss of consciousness at the time of injury, followed by an interval of apparent recovery (lucid interval). It should be noted that although the lucid interval is characteristic of an extradural hematoma, it does not occur in approximately 15% of patients with this lesion. During the lucid interval, compensation for the expanding hematoma takes place by rapid absorption of CSF and decreased intravascular volume, which maintains a normal ICP. When these mechanisms can no longer compensate, even a small increase in the volume of the blood clot produces a marked elevation of ICP. Then, often suddenly, signs of compression appear (usually deterioration of consciousness and signs of focal neurologic deficits such as dilation and fixation of a pupil or paralysis of an extremity), and the patient deteriorates rapidly.

Management.   An epidural hematoma is considered an extreme emergency, as marked neurologic deficit or even cessation of breathing may occur within minutes. The treatment consists of making openings through the skull (*burr holes*), removing the clot, and controlling the bleeding point.

Subdural Hematoma

A subdural hematoma is a collection of blood between the dura and the underlying brain, a space normally occupied by a film of fluid. The most common cause is trauma, but it may also occur in various bleeding diatheses and aneurysms. A subdural hemorrhage is more frequently venous in origin and is attributed to the rupture of small vessels that bridge the subdural space.

A subdural hematoma may be acute, subacute, or chronic, depending on the size of the involved vessel and the amount of bleeding present. Acute subdural hematomas are associated with major head injury involving contusion or laceration. Usually the patient is comatose, and the clinical signs are similar to those of epidural hematoma. A rising blood pressure with slowing of pulse and respirations indicates a rapidly increasing hematoma. Subacute subdural hematoma is the sequela of less severe contusions and is suspected in patients failing to regain consciousness after head trauma. Signs and symptoms are similar to those of an acute subdural hematoma.

The mortality rate for patients with acute subdural hematomas is high, because frequently there is associated brain damage.

If the patient can be transported rapidly to the hospital, an immediate craniotomy is performed to open the dura, allowing for the solid subdural clot to be evacuated. Successful outcome also depends on the control of ICP and careful monitoring of respiratory function (see The Patient Undergoing Intracranial Surgery in Chap. 56).

Chronic subdural hematomas can develop from seemingly minor head injuries and are seen most frequently in the elderly. The time between injury and onset of symptoms may be lengthy (*e.g.*, months), so the actual insult may be forgotten. Symptoms may appear weeks after what may have seemed to be a minor injury.

A chronic subdural hematoma imitates other conditions and may be mistaken for a stroke. The bleeding is less profuse and there is compression of the intracranial contents. The blood within the brain changes in character in 2 to 4 days, becoming thicker and darker. In a few weeks, the clot breaks down and has the color and consistency of motor oil. Eventually, calcification or ossification of the clot takes place. The brain adapts to this foreign body invasion, and the patient's clinical signs and symptoms fluctuate. There may be severe headache, which tends to come and go; alternating focal neurologic signs; personality changes; mental deterioration; and focal seizures. Unfortunately, the patient may be labeled neurotic or psychotic if the cause of the symptoms is overlooked.

The treatment of a chronic subdural hematoma consists of surgically evacuating the clot by suctioning or irrigating the area. The procedure may be carried out through multiple burr holes, or a craniotomy may be performed for a sizable subdural mass lesion that cannot be drained through burr holes.

Intracerebral Hemorrhage/Hematoma

Intracerebral hemorrhage is bleeding into the substance of the brain. It is commonly seen in head injuries in which force is exerted to the head over a small area (missile injuries or bullet wounds; stab injury). These hemorrhages within the brain may also result from systemic hypertension, which causes degeneration and rupture of a vessel; from rupture of a saccular aneurysm; from vascular anomalies; from intracranial tumors; from systemic causes, including bleeding disorders such as leukemia, hemophilia, aplastic anemia, and thrombocytopenia; and from complications of anticoagulant therapy.

There may be an insidious development with the onset of neurologic deficits followed by headache. Medical therapy involves careful administration of fluids and electrolytes, antihypertensive medications, control of ICP, and supportive care. Surgical intervention by craniotomy or craniectomy permits removal of the blood clot and provides opportunity for control of the sites of hemorrhage but may not be possible either because of the inaccessible location of the bleeding or the lack of a clearly circumscribed area of blood that can be removed. Physical therapy is usually required for the rehabilitation of these and all head injury patients.

General Approach to Head Injuries

Clinical Manifestations

Brain trauma affects every system of the body. The clinical manifestations of brain injury include disturbances of consciousness, confusion, pupillary abnormalities, sudden onset of neurologic deficits, and changes in vital signs. There may be visual impairment, hearing impairment, sensory dysfunction, spasticity, headache, vertigo, movement disorders, seizures, and many other effects. The presence of hypovolemic shock suggests the possibility of multisystem injury, because CNS injury alone is not likely to produce shock.

Diagnostic Evaluation

The initial physical and neurologic examinations are the baseline on which all future examination comparisons are made. CT is the primary neuroimaging diagnostic tool, and is useful in the evaluation of soft-tissue injuries.

Management

A person with a head injury is presumed to have a cervical spine injury until proven otherwise. The patient is transported from the scene of the accident on a board, with head and neck maintained in alignment with the axis of the body. Slight traction should be maintained on the head, and a cervical collar in place until negative cervical spine films have been obtained.

The initial brain injury is not amenable to treatment, and all therapy is directed toward the preservation of brain homeostasis and prevention of secondary brain damage. This includes stabilization of cardiovascular and respiratory function to maintain adequate cerebral perfusion. Hemorrhage is stopped, hypovolemia is corrected, and blood gas values are maintained at their physiologic values.

As the damaged brain swells with edema or a collection of blood forms, a rise in ICP can be expected and requires aggressive treatment. Increased ICP is monitored closely and is managed by maintaining adequate oxygenation, administering mannitol, which reduces brain water by osmotic dehydration; hyperventilation; the use of steroids; a head-up position in bed; and possibly neurosurgical intervention. Surgery is required for evacuation of blood clots, debridement and elevation of depressed fractures of the skull, and suture of severe scalp lacerations. Insertion of devices to monitor ICP can be performed during surgery or at the bedside using aseptic technique in patients not requiring surgical intervention.

Treatment also includes ventilatory support, prevention of seizures, and maintenance of fluid, electrolyte, and nutritional balance. Patients with severe head injury who are in coma are intubated and placed on mechanical ventilation to control and protect the airway. Controlled hyperventilation also induces hypocapnia, which causes vasoconstriction, lowers cerebral blood flow, decreases cerebral blood volume, and thus reduces ICP.

Because seizures are common after head injury and can cause secondary brain damage from hypoxia, anticonvulsant therapy may be started.

If the patient is very agitated, chlorpromazine may be prescribed to quiet the patient without deepening the consciousness level. A nasogastric tube may be inserted, as reduced gastric motility and reverse peristalsis are associated with head injury, making regurgitation common in the first few hours.

▶ Nursing Process
The Patient With a Head Injury

▷ Assessment

The health history may include the following questions:

> At what time did the injury occur?
> What caused the injury? A high velocity missile? An object striking the head? A fall?

What was the direction and force of the blow?
Was there a loss of consciousness? What was the duration of the unconscious period? Could the patient be aroused? (A history of unconsciousness or amnesia after a head injury indicates a significant degree of brain damage, whereas subsequent changes can reflect recovery or indicate the development of secondary brain damage.)

▷ *Assessment of Level of Consciousness/Responsiveness.* The level of consciousness/responsiveness is regularly assessed because an alteration in the level of consciousness precedes all other changes in vital and neurologic signs. A practical means of monitoring changes in the level of consciousness is the Glasgow Coma Scale, which is based on three aspects of the patient's behavior: eye opening, verbal responses, and motor responses to a verbal command or painful stimulus. These elements are further subdivided into different levels of response, and the best responses the patient makes to predetermined stimuli are recorded as follows:

Eyes Open:

Spontaneously	4
To speech	3
To pain	2
No response	1

Best Motor Response:

Obeys	6
Localizes pain	5
Withdraws	4
Abnormal flexion	3
Extends	2
Nil	1

Verbal Response

Oriented	5
Confused conversation	4
Inappropriate words	3
Incomprehensible sounds	2
Nil	1

Total: 3–15

Each response is given a number (high for normal and low for impaired), and the summation of these figures gives an indication of the severity of coma and a prediction of possible outcome. The lowest score is 3 (least responsive), and the highest is 15 (most responsive). A score of 7 or less is generally accepted as coma and requires appropriate nursing intervention for the comatose patient.

Figure 57-10 is a neurologic observation chart that incorporates the Glasgow Coma Scale, vital signs, pupillary size and reactivity, and extremity movement and strength, which provides a comprehensive record of the patient's neurologic status at any given time. This or any other standardized format for obtaining and recording neurologic status is recommended to standardize and facilitate care and communication between caregivers.

▷ *Monitoring Vital Signs.* Although deterioration of the patient's level of consciousness is the most sensitive neurologic indication of impending danger, vital signs are monitored at frequent intervals to assess the intracranial status.

• Signs of increasing ICP include slowing of the pulse, increasing systolic pressure, and widening pulse pressure.

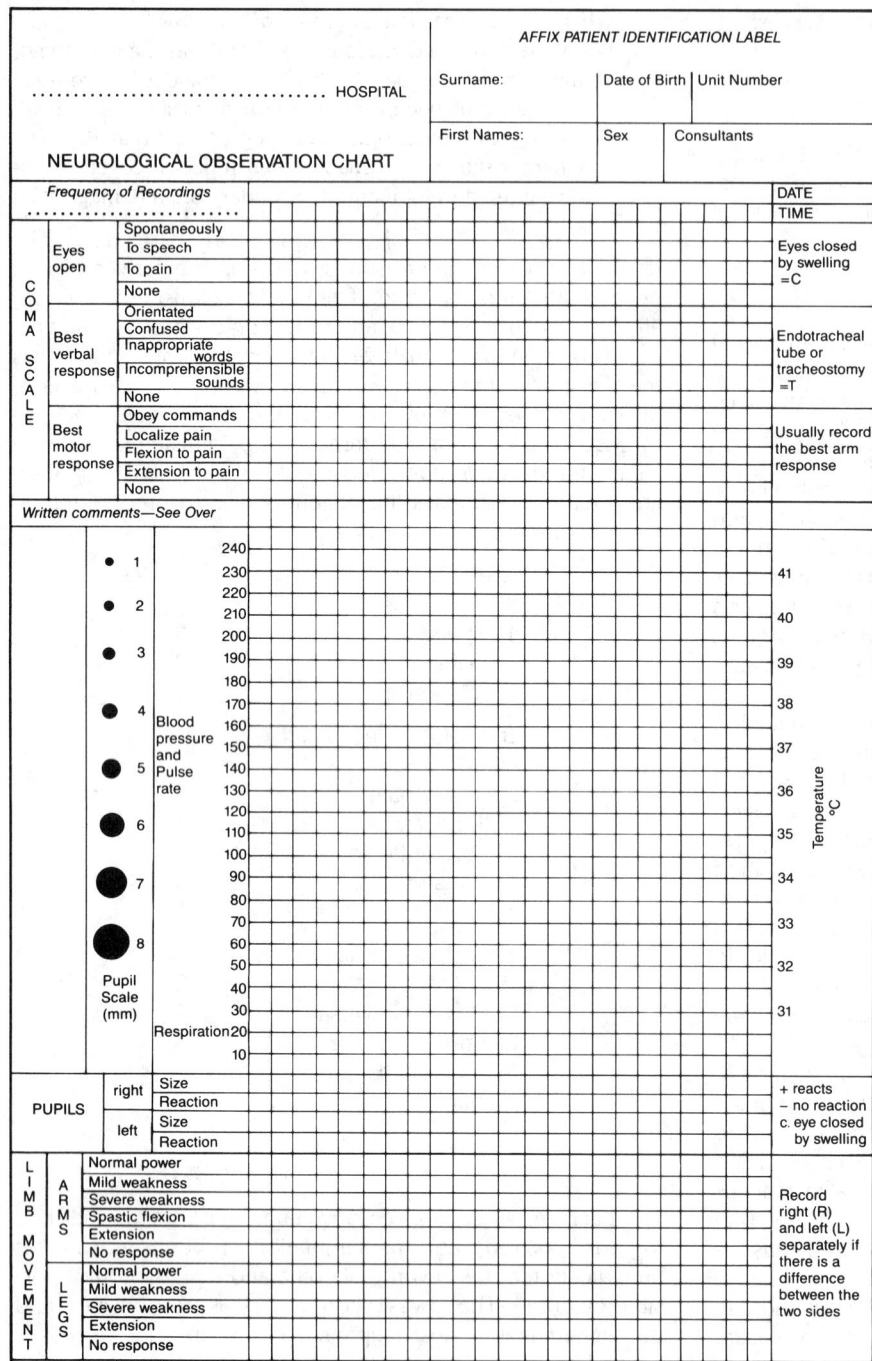

Figure 57–10. Example of neurologic observation chart that includes the Glasgow Coma Scale. (Reproduced by courtesy of Butterworth and Company, London, from Campkin and Turner, *Neurosurgical Anaesthesia and Intensive Care.*)

• As brain compression increases, the vital signs tend to be reversed—the pulse and respiration become rapid, and the blood pressure may decrease. This is an ominous development, as is a rapid fluctuation of vital signs.
• A rapid rise in body temperature is regarded as unfavorable, because hyperthermia increases the metabolic demands of the brain. The temperature is kept below 38°C (100.4°F).
• Tachycardia and arterial hypotension may indicate that bleeding is occurring somewhere in the body.

▷ *Motor Function.* Motor function is assessed frequently by observing spontaneous movements, asking the patient to raise and lower the extremities, and comparing the power of the

hand grasp at periodic intervals. The presence or absence of spontaneous movement of each extremity is noted.

• If the patient does not demonstrate spontaneous movement, determine responses to painful stimuli. Abnormal responses (lack of motor response; extension responses) carry a poorer prognosis.
• Also determine the patient's ability to speak, and note the quality of speech. The capacity to speak indicates a high level of brain function.

▷ *Eye Signs*
• Determine whether the patient is opening his eyes spontaneously.

- Evaluate the size of the pupils and their reaction to light. A unilaterally dilated and poorly responding pupil may indicate a developing hematoma with subsequent pressure on the third cranial nerve due to shifting of the brain. If both pupils become fixed and dilated, overwhelming injury and intrinsic damage to the upper brain stem usually are indicated, a poor prognostic sign.

▷ *Assessment of Complications.*   Deterioration in the patient's condition may be due to an expanding intracranial hematoma and progressive brain edema. Other complications after traumatic head injuries include systemic infections (pneumonia, urinary tract infection, septicemia) and neurosurgical infections (wound infection, osteomyelitis, meningitis, ventriculitis, brain abscess).

After injury, these patients may develop focal nerve palsies such as *anosmia* (lack of sense of smell) or eye movement abnormalities and focal neurologic deficits such as aphasia, memory defects, and post-traumatic seizures/epilepsy. Patients may be left with organic psychosocial deficits (impulsiveness, emotional lability, or uninhibited, aggressive behaviors) and, as a consequence of the impairment, lack insight into their emotional responses.

▷ Nursing Diagnoses

Based on all the assessment data, the patient's major nursing diagnoses may include the following:

- Ineffective airway clearance and ventilation related to hypoxia
- Fluid volume deficit related to disturbances of consciousness and hormonal dysfunction
- Altered nutrition, less than body requirements, related to metabolic changes, fluid restriction, and inadequate intake
- High risk for violence (self-directed and directed to others) related to disorientation, restlessness, and brain damage
- Altered thought processes (deficits in intellectual function, communication, memory, information processing) related to results of head injury
- Potential for ineffective family coping related to unresponsiveness of patient, unpredictability of outcome, prolonged recovery period, and patient's residual physical and emotional deficit

The nursing diagnoses for the unconscious patient and the patient with increased ICP also apply (both are discussed in Chapter 56).

▷ Planning and Implementation

▷ *Goals:*   The patient's goals may include attainment of a patent airway, achievement of fluid and electrolyte balance, achievement of adequate nutritional status, prevention of injury, improvement of cognitive function, and accomplishment of effective family coping behaviors.

▷ Nursing Interventions

As soon as the initial assessment and diagnostic tests are made, a neurologic flow record is started and maintained (see Fig. 57-10). Figure 57-11 is a flow chart including ongoing nursing assessments, priorities for nursing interventions, and anticipatory and rehabilitation nursing of the patient with a head injury.

▷ *Airway Maintenance.*   One of the most important nursing goals in the management of the patient with a head injury is to establish and maintain an adequate airway. The brain is extremely sensitive to hypoxia, and a neurologic deficit can worsen if the patient is hypoxic. Therapy is directed toward maintenance of adequately oxygenated circulation so that there is a supply of oxygenated blood to the brain to preserve cerebral function. An obstructed airway causes CO_2 retention and hypoventilation, which produces cerebral vessel dilatation and increases ICP.

Therapeutic and nursing activities to ensure an adequate exchange of air are summarized in Chapter 56 and include the following:

- Keep the unconscious patient in a position that facilitates drainage of oral secretions, with the head of the bed elevated about 30 degrees to decrease intracranial venous pressure.
- Establish effective suctioning procedures. (Pulmonary secretions produce coughing and straining, which increase ICP.)
- Guard against aspiration and respiratory insufficiency.
- Monitor arterial blood gases to assess adequacy of ventilation. (The goal is to keep blood gases within normal range to ensure adequate cerebral blood flow.)
- Monitor the patient on mechanical ventilation.

▷ *Fluid and Electrolyte Balance.*   Brain damage can produce metabolic and hormonal dysfunctions. The monitoring of serum electrolyte concentrations is important, especially in patients receiving osmotic diuretics, those with inappropriate antidiuretic hormone secretion, and those with post-traumatic diabetes insipidus.

- Serial studies of blood and urine electrolytes and osmolality are carried out because head injuries may be accompanied by disorders of sodium regulation. Sodium retention may last several days, followed by sodium diuresis. Increasing lethargy, confusion, and convulsions may be due to electrolyte imbalance.
- Endocrine dysfunctions are evaluated by monitoring serum electrolytes, glucose values, and intake and output.
- Urine is tested regularly for acetone.
- A record of daily weight is kept, especially if the patient has hypothalamic involvement and must be observed for the development of diabetes insipidus.

▷ *Adequate Nutrition.*   Head injury results in metabolic changes that increase calorie consumption and nitrogen excretion. Steroid therapy also increases the catabolic state. As soon as the patient's condition has stabilized, nasogastric feedings are started unless there is discharge of CSF from the nose (*cerebrospinal rhinorrhea*).

Small, frequent feedings lessen the possibility of vomiting and diarrhea. Elevating the head of the bed and aspirating the tube before feeding (for evidence of residual feeding in the stomach) are measures used to prevent distention, regurgitation, and aspiration. A continuous-drip infusion or controlling pump may be used to regulate the feeding. The principles and technique of nasogastric feedings are discussed in Chapter 35. The feeding tube is usually kept in place until the swallowing reflex returns.

▷ *Prevention of Injury.*   As the patient emerges from coma, there is a period of lethargy and stupor followed by a period of agitation. Each stage is variable, depending on the individual,

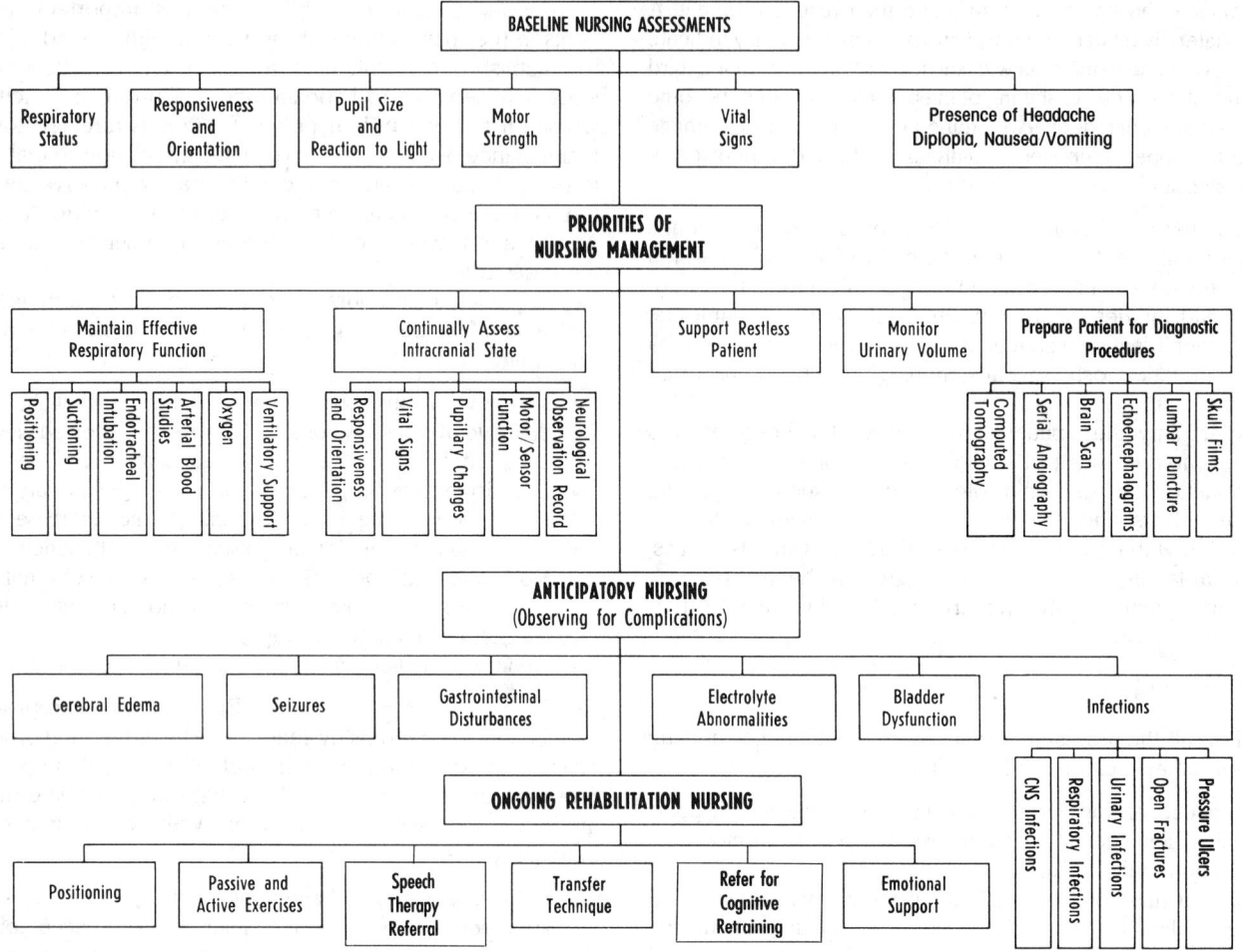

Figure 57–11. Nursing intervention for the patient with a head injury.

the depth and duration of coma, and the patient's age. The patient emerging from a coma may become increasingly agitated toward the end of the day. Restlessness may be due to hypoxia, fever, pain, or a full bladder. It may indicate injury of the brain but is also a sign that the unconscious patient is regaining consciousness. (Some restlessness may be beneficial because the lungs and extremities are exercised.) Agitation may also be due to annoyance from an indwelling urinary catheter, intravenous lines, restraints, and repeated neurologic checks.

- The patient is assessed to ensure that the airway is adequate and the bladder is not distended. Likewise, bandages and casts should be checked for constriction.
- To protect the patient from self-injury and dislodging of body tubes, siderails are padded and the patient's hands may be wrapped in mitts. Restraints are avoided when possible because straining against them can increase ICP or cause other injury.
- Restlessness should not be controlled with narcotics, because these substances depress respiration, constrict the pupils, and alter the level of the patient's responsiveness.
- The use of a floor bed (floor mattresses surrounded by a wall of mattresses) allows freedom of movement and promotes patient safety.
- Environmental stimuli should be kept to a minimum by keeping the room quiet, limiting visitors, speaking calmly, and providing frequent orientation information (*e.g.*, explaining where the patient is and what is being done).
- Adequate lighting may prevent visual hallucinations.
- The patient's sleep–wake cycles should not be interrupted.
- The skin is lubricated with oil or emollient lotion to prevent irritation due to rubbing against the sheet.
- If incontinence is a problem, an external sheath catheter may be used on the male patient. Because prolonged use of an indwelling catheter inevitably produces infection, the patient may be placed on an intermittent catheterization schedule.

▷ *Improved Cognitive Functioning.* Although many brain-damaged victims survive because of resuscitative and supportive technology, they frequently sustain significant mental sequelae that may not be noticed during the acute phase of injury. Cognitive impairment includes memory deficits, decrease in ability to focus and sustain attention to a task (easily distracted), reduced ability to process information, and slowness in thinking, perceiving, communicating, reading, and writing. An estimated 25% to 38% of these persons develop psychiatric problems. Such psychosocial, behavioral, and emotional impairments are devastating to the family as well as to the patient.

These problems require collaboration among many disciplines. A *neuropsychologist* (specialist in evaluating and treating cognitive problems) plans a program and initiates therapy or counseling that is designed to help the patient reach maximum potential. Cognitive rehabilitation activities are directed at redeveloping the patient's ability to devise new problem-solving strategies. The retraining is carried out over an extended period, and includes the use of computer-training programs, video games, sensory stimulation and reinforcement, behavior modification, and reality orientation. Assistance from many disciplines is necessary during this phase of recovery. Intellectual ability may not improve after time, but social and behavioral aspects may improve.

The nurse needs to be aware that there are fluctuations in the orientation and memory of such patients. They are easily distracted. If they are pushed to a level greater than their impaired cortical functioning allows, symptoms of fatigue and stress (headache, dizziness) may occur.

▷ *Patient and Family Education.* Serious head injury can produce a great deal of prolonged stress in the family because of the patient's physical and emotional deficits, the unpredictable outcome, and altered family relationships. Families report difficulties in dealing with changes in temperament, behavior, and personality. These are associated with disruption in family cohesion, loss of leisure pursuits, and loss of work capacity, as well as the social isolation and entrapment of the caretaker. The family may experience such feelings as anger, grief, guilt, and denial in recurring cycles.

The family is asked how the patient is different at this time. What has been lost? What is most difficult about coping with this situation? Helpful interventions include providing family members with accurate and honest information, and encouraging them to continue to set well-defined, mutual, short-term goals. Family counseling helps deal with overwhelming feelings of loss and helplessness and gives guidance to the management of inappropriate behaviors. Support groups are available to provide a forum for sharing problems, developing insight, referring information, networking, and gaining assistance in maintaining realistic expectations and hope.

The National Head Injury Foundation serves as a clearinghouse for information and resources for patients with head injuries and their families, including specific information on coma, rehabilitation, behavioral consequences of head injury, and family issues. This organization can provide names of facilities and professionals who work with persons with head injuries and can assist families in organizing local support groups.

The patient is encouraged to continue the rehabilitation program after discharge, because improvement in status may continue up to 3 or more years after injury. Headache may be the most reliable guide to recovery. A second pillow or backrest at night may be helpful to alleviate some head discomfort.

Because posttraumatic seizures occur frequently, anticonvulsants may be prescribed for 1 to 2 years after injury. The patient is encouraged to return to normal activities gradually.

▷ Evaluation

Expected Outcomes
1. Attains/maintains effective airway clearance, ventilation, and brain oxygenation
   a. Achieves normal blood gas values
   b. Has normal breath sounds on auscultation
   c. Mobilizes and clears secretions

2. Achieves satisfactory fluid and electrolyte balance
   a. Demonstrates serum electrolytes within normal range
   b. Has no clinical signs of dehydration or overhydration
3. Attains adequate nutritional status
   a. Has less than 50 ml of aspirate in stomach before each tube feeding
   b. Is free of gastric distention and vomiting
   c. Shows minimal weight loss
4. Avoids injury
   a. Shows lessening agitation and restlessness
   b. Is oriented to time, place, and person
5. Shows cognitive progression
   a. Demonstrates lessening of inappropriate behaviors
   b. Shows improved memory
   c. Verbalizes realistic plans
6. Family members demonstrate adaptive coping mechanisms.
   a. Have joined support group
   b. Are willing to identify problem areas
   c. Share their feelings with appropriate health-care personnel

In summary, head injury may be severe and life threatening or mild with few lasting signs or symptoms. The consequences of severe injury may be complete loss of voluntary and involuntary functions, loss of cognitive function, or instantaneous death at the scene of the injury. Less severe head injury may result in persistent headache, memory loss, and sleep disturbances. Patients with severe head injuries are usually managed in intensive care units; they may be discharged to special units with services designed to rehabilitate patients with brain injuries. Those with less severe injuries may not be hospitalized for an extended time or may be treated and discharged from the emergency department.

The nurse caring for the patient with severe head injury requires specialized assessment skills and expert skills in meeting the needs of the critically injured patient. Additionally, the nurse considers the long-term and rehabilitative needs of the patient and initiates nursing care directed toward long-term recovery of the patient. The occurrence of severe head injury usually creates a crisis for the family; the nurse must also assist the family in dealing with this crisis.

The nurse who cares for the patient with mild or moderate head injury must keep in mind the more subtle symptoms that are possible and prepare the patient and family for their occurrence.

Spinal Cord Injury

Spinal cord injury is a major health problem affecting 150,000 to 500,000 persons in this country, with an estimated 10,000 new injuries occurring each year. Half of these injuries result from motor vehicle accidents; most of the others occur from falls, sporting and industrial accidents, and gunshot wounds. Two thirds of the victims are 30 years of age or younger. The estimated total annual cost of these injuries exceeds $2 billion a year. There is a high frequency of associated injuries and medical complications. The vertebrae most frequently involved in spinal cord injuries are the 5th, 6th, and 7th cervical (neck), the 12th thoracic, and the 1st lumbar vertebrae. These vertebrae are the most susceptible because there is a greater range of mobility in the vertebral column in these areas.

Prevention.   To prevent this devastating and catastrophic injury, the following steps should be taken: (1) reduction in driving speed, (2) use of a seat belt/shoulder harness, (3) wearing of helmets by motorcyclists, (4) educational programs directed against driving while intoxicated, (5) water safety instruction, (6) prevention of falls, and (7) use in sports of protective devices and proper coaching techniques. Paramedical personnel are taught the importance of properly removing a car-crash victim from a motor vehicle and of following proper methods in transporting the victim to a hospital emergency department to avoid further and possibly permanent damage to the spinal cord.

Pathogenesis.   Damage to the spinal cord ranges from transient concussion (from which the patient fully recovers) to contusion, laceration, and compression of the cord substance (either alone or in combination), to complete transection of the cord (which renders the patient paralyzed below the level of the injury). When hemorrhage occurs in the area of the spinal cord, the blood may seep into the extradural, subdural, or subarachnoid spaces of the spinal canal. Immediately after a contusion or tear injury, the nerve fibers begin to swell and disintegrate. Blood circulation to the gray matter of the spinal cord is curtailed. Not only is there injury to the spinal cord vasculature, but there also appears to be a pathogenic process responsible for the progressive damage of the acute spinal cord injury. A secondary chain of events produces ischemia, hypoxia, edema, and hemorrhagic lesions, which in turn result in destruction of myelin and axons.

These secondary reactions, believed to be the principal causes of spinal cord degeneration at the level of injury, are now thought to be reversible 4 to 6 hours after injury. Therefore, if the cord has not suffered irreparable damage, some method of *early* treatment is needed to prevent partial damage from developing into total and permanent damage. Dexamethasone, given as an anti-inflammatory agent; mannitol, given to decrease edema; and dextran, given to prevent the blood pressure from dropping and to improve capillary blood flow, are being investigated. Naloxone, a drug that has shown promise in treating animal models of spinal cord injury, has minimal side effects and may promote neurologic improvement in humans. The effectiveness of using cooling techniques or hypothermia perfusion on the injured area of the spinal cord to counteract the autodestructive forces that follow this type of injury is also being investigated. The administration of high-dosage steroids promptly after injury has been found to improve prognosis and reduce disability.

Emergency Management

The immediate management of the patient at the scene of the accident is critical, because improper handling can cause further damage and loss of neurologic function. Any victim of a motor vehicle or driving accident, a contact sport injury, falls, or any direct trauma to the head and neck must be considered to have a spinal cord injury until such an injury is ruled out.

- At the scene of the accident, the victim must be immobilized on a spinal (back) board, with head and neck in a neutral position, to prevent an incomplete injury from becoming complete.
- One member of the team must assume control of the patient's head to prevent flexion, rotation, or extension.

- The hands are placed on both sides of the head about at the ear to maintain traction and alignment while a spinal board or cervical immobilizing device is applied.
- At least four persons should slide the victim carefully onto a board for transfer to the hospital. Any twisting movement may irreversibly damage the spinal cord by causing a bony fragment of the vertebra to cut into, crush, or sever the cord completely.

It is desirable that the patient be referred to a regional spinal injury or trauma center because of the multidisciplinary personnel and support services required to counteract destructive changes that occur in the first few hours after injury.

Transferring the Patient.   During treatment in the emergency and radiology departments, the patient is kept on the transfer board. The transfer of the patient to a bed presents a definite nursing problem.

- The patient must always be maintained in an extended position. No part of the body should be twisted or turned, nor should the patient be allowed to assume a sitting position.

The patient should be placed on a Stryker or other turning frame when transfer to a bed is planned. Later, if it has been proved that there is no cord injury, the patient can always be moved to a conventional bed without harm; the reverse, however, is not true. If a Stryker or other turning frame is not available, the patient should be placed on a firm mattress with a bedboard under it. The patient may be transferred from the board to the Stryker or turning frame in the following manner.

- The board on which the patient is strapped is placed directly on the posterior frame.
- The patient is unstrapped from the board, but the head strappings are not removed.
- A blanket roll is placed between the legs.
- The anterior frame is positioned and secured.
- The frame is turned so that the patient is in the prone position.
- The frame straps and the posterior frame are removed. The head strapping is removed with care. The transfer board is removed.

Clinical Manifestations

If conscious, the patient usually complains of acute pain in the back or neck, which may radiate along the involved nerve. Often the patient speaks of fear that the neck or back is broken. *The consequences of spinal cord injury depend on the level of injury of the cord* (Fig. 57-12). *Neurologic level* refers to that lowest level at which sensory and motor functions are normal. There is total sensory and motor paralysis below the neurologic level, loss of bladder and bowel control (usually with urinary retention and bladder distention), loss of sweating and vasomotor tone below the neurologic level, and marked reduction of blood pressure from loss of peripheral vascular resistance.

Respiratory problems are related to compromised respiratory function, the severity of which depends on the level of injury. The muscles contributing to respiration are the abdominals, intercostals (T1–T11), and the diaphragm. In high cervical cord injury, acute respiratory failure is the leading cause of death.

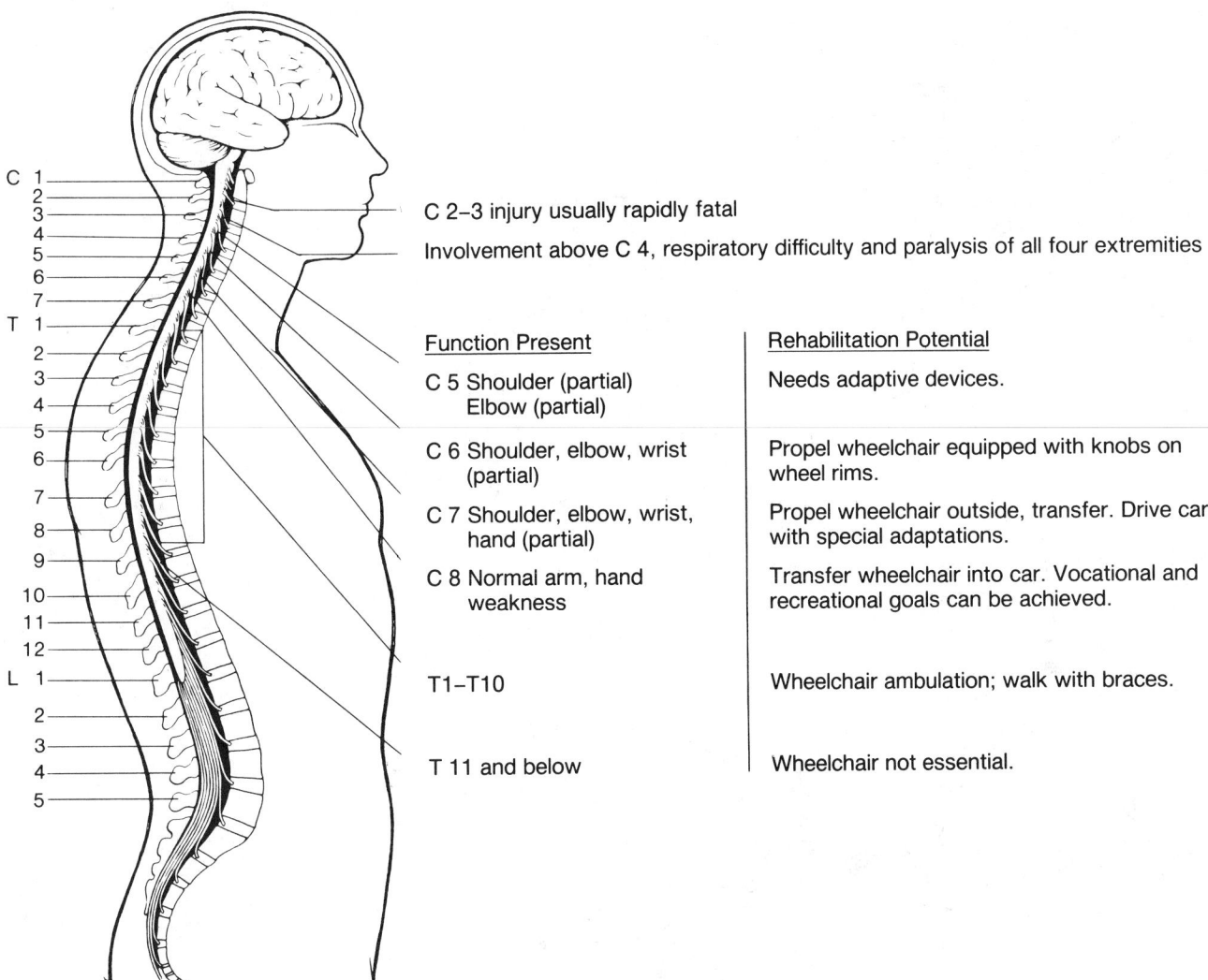

C 2–3 injury usually rapidly fatal

Involvement above C 4, respiratory difficulty and paralysis of all four extremities

Function Present	Rehabilitation Potential
C 5 Shoulder (partial) Elbow (partial)	Needs adaptive devices.
C 6 Shoulder, elbow, wrist (partial)	Propel wheelchair equipped with knobs on wheel rims.
C 7 Shoulder, elbow, wrist, hand (partial)	Propel wheelchair outside, transfer. Drive car with special adaptations.
C 8 Normal arm, hand weakness	Transfer wheelchair into car. Vocational and recreational goals can be achieved.
T1–T10	Wheelchair ambulation; walk with braces.
T 11 and below	Wheelchair not essential.

Figure 57–12. Sequelae of spinal cord injury and rehabilitation challenges. (The vertebrae are numbered on the left side of the drawing and the spinal nerves are numbered on the right.)

Diagnostic Evaluation

A detailed neurologic examination is performed. Radiographic examination (lateral cervical spine x-rays and CT scanning) is carried out. A search is made for other injuries because spinal trauma is associated with multiple injuries, commonly affecting the head and chest. Continuous ECG monitoring may be indicated, because *bradycardia* (slow heart rate) and *asystole* (cardiac standstill) are common in acute cervical injuries.

Management of Cervical Spine Injuries (Acute Phase)

The goals of management are to prevent further spinal cord injury and to observe for symptoms of progressive neurologic deficits.

The patient is resuscitated as necessary, and oxygenation and cardiovascular stability are maintained. High-dose steroids may be administered to counteract cord edema. It has recently been reported that the administration of high doses of steroid (methylprednisolone) within 8 hours of the injury and continuous infusion for 24 hours can reduce the extent of damage and disability. Oxygen is administered to maintain a high arterial Po_2, because anoxemia can create or worsen a neurologic deficit of the spinal cord. If endotracheal intubation is necessary, extreme care is taken to avoid flexing or extending the neck, which can result in an extension of the injury. *Diaphragm pacing* (electrical stimulation of the phrenic nerve) may be considered for the patient with a high cervical lesion but is usually carried out after the acute phase.

Management of cervical spinal injury requires *immobilization*, and *reduction* of dislocations (restoration of normal position), and *stabilization* of the vertebral column. To reduce the fracture dislocation and maintain alignment of the cervical spine, some form of skeletal traction such as skeletal tongs/calipers or the halo-vest technique is used (Fig. 57-13). A variety of skeletal tongs are available, all of which involve fixation in the skull in some manner. The Gardner-Wells tongs require no

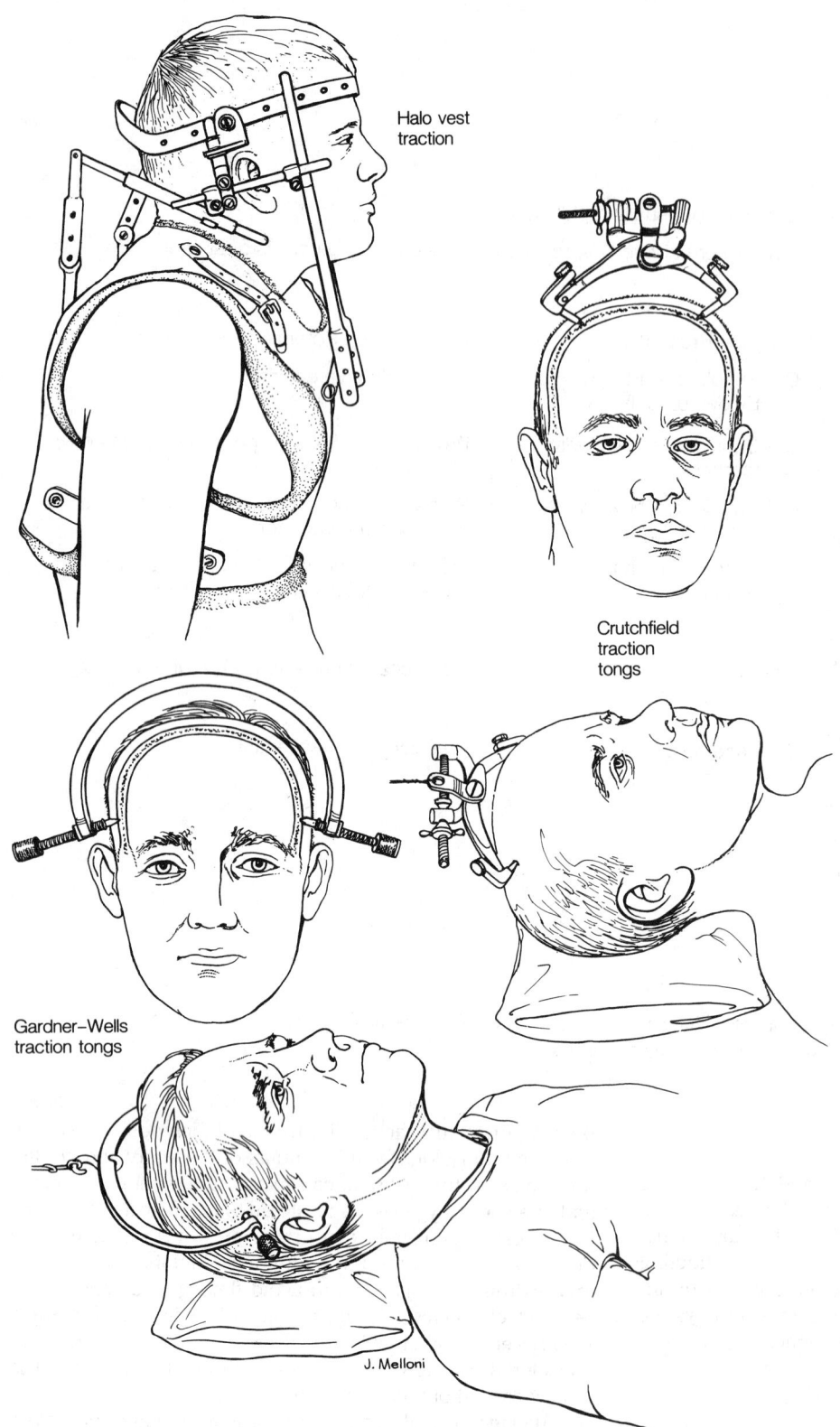

Halo vest
traction

Crutchfield
traction
tongs

Gardner–Wells
traction tongs

J. Melloni

Figure 57–13. Methods of cervical traction. (Suddarth DS. The Lippincott Manual of Nursing Practice, 5th ed. Philadelphia, JB Lippincott, 1991.)

predrilled holes in the skull. Crutchfield and Vinke tongs are inserted through holes made with a special drill under local anesthesia.

Traction is applied to the tongs by weights, the amount depending on the patient's size and the degree of fracture

displacement. The traction force is exerted along the longitudinal axis of the vertebral bodies, with the neck in a neutral position. Then the traction is gradually increased by the addition of more weights. As the amount of traction is increased, the spaces between the intervertebral discs widen, and the vertebrae slip back into position. Reduction usually takes place after correct alignment has been restored. Once reduction is achieved, as verified by cervical spine films and neurologic examination, the weights are gradually removed until the amount of weight needed to maintain the alignment is obtained. The weights should hang freely so as not to interfere with the traction. The patient is placed on a Stryker or other turning frame if one is available. (See p. 1738 for a method of transfer to the turning frame.)

A halo device may be used initially with traction or may be applied after removal of the tongs. It consists of a stainless steel halo ring that is fixed to the skull by four pins. The ring is attached to a removable halo vest, which suspends the weight of the unit circumferentially around the chest. A metal frame connects the ring to the chest. Halo devices provide immobilization of the cervical spine while allowing early ambulation.

Surgical Intervention.   If the patient's deformities cannot be reduced by traction, if there is significant instability of the cervical spine, or if the patient's neurologic status is deteriorating, surgery is performed to reduce the spinal fracture or dislocation or decompress the cord.

A *laminectomy* (excision of the posterior arches and spinous processes of a vertebra) may be indicated in the presence of progressive neurologic deficit, suspicion of epidural hematoma, or penetrating injuries that require surgical debridement, or to permit direct visualization and exploration of the cord. (The care of the patient following a laminectomy is discussed on p. 1747.)

Management of Spinal Shock

Spinal shock represents a sudden depression of reflex activity in the spinal cord (*areflexia*) below the level of injury. In this condition, the muscles innervated by the part of the cord segment situated below the level of the lesion become completely paralyzed and flaccid, and the reflexes are absent. The blood pressure falls, and the parts of the body below the level of the cord lesion are paralyzed and without sensation. With injuries to the cervical and upper thoracic spinal cord, the innervation to the major accessory muscles of respiration is lost and respiratory problems develop: decreased vital capacity, retention of secretions, increased partial pressure of carbon dioxide (PCO_2), decreased PO_2, respiratory failure, and pulmonary edema. The reflexes that initiate bladder and bowel function are also affected. (The management of the patient with a neurogenic bladder—*i.e.*, a bladder disturbance due to a lesion of the central nervous system—is discussed in Chap. 42.) Bowel distention and paralytic ileus caused by depression of the reflexes may be treated with intestinal decompression. The patient does not perspire on the paralyzed portions of his body, because sympathetic activity is blocked, so close observation is required for early detection of an abrupt onset of fever. (Hyperthermia is treated as outlined in Chap. 56.)

- The patient's body defenses are supported and maintained until spinal shock abates and the system has recovered from the traumatic insult (3 to 6 weeks). Special attention must be directed also to the respiratory system. There may not be enough intrathoracic pressure for the patient to cough effectively. Chest physical therapy is used to help clear pulmonary secretions.

▶ Nursing Process
The Patient With Spinal Cord Injury

◊ Assessment

The breathing pattern is observed, the strength with which the patient coughs is assessed, and the lungs are auscultated because paralysis of abdominal and respiratory muscles diminishes coughing and makes it difficult to clear bronchial and pharyngeal secretions. Ventilation is also affected when these muscles decrease the ventilatory excursion of the chest.

The patient is monitored constantly for any changes in motor or sensory function and symptoms of progressive neurologic damage. It may be impossible in the early stages of cord injury to determine whether the cord has been transected, because signs and symptoms of cord edema are indistinguishable from those of cord transection. Edema of the spinal cord may occur with any severe cord injury, and may further compromise spinal function.

Motor and sensory function is determined by careful neurologic examination. These findings are recorded so that changes in or progression from the baseline neurologic status can be evaluated accurately.

- Motor ability is tested by asking the patient to spread the fingers, squeeze the examiner's hand, and move the toes or turn the feet.
- Sensation is evaluated by pinching the skin or pricking it with the broken end of a cotton swab, starting at the shoulder level and working down both sides of the extremities. The patient is asked where the sensation is felt.
- Any decrease in neurologic function is reported immediately.

The patient is also assessed for the presence of spinal shock, in which there is complete loss of all reflex, motor, sensory, and autonomic activity below the level of the lesion. This causes bladder distention from paralysis of the bladder. The area over the bladder is palpated for signs of urinary retention and overdistention of the bladder. Further assessment is made for gastric dilatation and ileus due to an atonic bowel, a result of autonomic disruption.

Temperature is monitored because the patient may have periods of hyperthermia as a result of alteration in temperature control due to autonomic disruption.

◊ *Assessment for Complications.*   In addition to monitoring for respiratory complications (respiratory failure; pneumonia) and *autonomic hyperreflexia* (which is characterized by pounding headache, profuse sweating, nasal congestion, piloerection [gooseflesh], bradycardia, and hypertension [see p. 1747]), constant surveillance is maintained for signs and symptoms of pressure ulcers and infection (urinary; respiratory; local infection at the pin sites).

Deep vein thrombosis with pulmonary embolism is a common complication of immobility; its clinical manifestations include pleuritic chest pain, anxiety, shortness of breath, and changes in blood gas values. Thigh and calf measurements are made daily. The patient is prepared for venography if there is a significant increase in the circumference of one extremity.

◊ Nursing Diagnoses

Based on all the assessment data, the patient's major nursing diagnoses may include the following:

- Ineffective breathing patterns related to weakness/paralysis of abdominal and intercostal muscles and inability to clear secretions
- Impaired physical mobility related to motor and sensory impairment
- High risk for impaired skin integrity related to immobility, sensory loss
- Urinary retention related to inability to void spontaneously
- Constipation related to presence of atonic bowel as a result of autonomic disruption
- Pain and discomfort related to treatment and prolonged immobility

◊ Planning and Implementation

◊ *Goals:*   The patient's goals may include improvement of breathing pattern, improvement of mobility, maintenance of skin integrity, relief of urinary retention, improvement of bowel function, and promotion of comfort.

◊ Nursing Interventions

◊ *Adequate Breathing.*   Possible impending respiratory failure is detected by observing the patient, measuring vital capacity, and monitoring arterial blood gas values. Early and vigorous attention to clearing bronchial and pharyngeal secretions can prevent retention of secretions and resultant atelectasis. Suctioning may be indicated, but caution must be employed during suctioning because this procedure can stimulate the vagus nerve, producing bradycardia, which can result in cardiac arrest. If the patient cannot cough effectively because of decreased inspiratory volume and inability to develop sufficient expiratory pressure, chest physical therapy may be indicated. Specific breathing exercises are supervised by the nurse to increase strength and endurance of inspiratory muscles, particularly the diaphragm. The nurse also ensures proper humidification and hydration to prevent secretions from becoming thick and difficult to cough up. The patient is assessed for signs of respiratory infection: cough, fever, and dyspnea. Smoking is discouraged because it increases bronchial and pulmonary secretions and damages cilia.

◊ *Improved Mobility.*   Proper body alignment is maintained at all times. The patient is placed in the dorsal or supine position as follows:

- The feet are positioned against a padded footboard to prevent footdrop. There should be a space between the end of the mattress and the footboard to allow free suspension of the heels. A wooden block on either end of the mattress prevents the mattress from pushing against the footboard.
- Trochanter rolls are applied from the crest of the ilium to the midthigh of both extremities to prevent external rotation of the hip joints.

Patients with lesions above the midthoracic level have loss of sympathetic control of peripheral vasoconstrictor activity, leading to hypotension. These patients may tolerate changes in position poorly and require monitoring of blood pressure when positions are changed. Usually the patient is turned every 2 hours. If not on a turning frame, the patient should not be turned unless the physician has indicated that it is safe to do so. Directives for turning a patient not on a turning frame are found in Chart 57-4. Adequate preparation and time must be made for turning the patient, maintaining a gentle, firm, and steady touch.

Contractures develop rapidly in association with immobility and muscle paralysis. Atrophy of the extremities results from disuse. To avoid these complications, passive range-of-motion exercises may be prescribed within 48 to 72 hours after injury. These exercises preserve joint motion and stimulate circulation. A joint that is immobilized too long becomes fixed as a result of contractures of the tendon and joint capsule. Toes, meta-

---

Chart 57-4
Turning the Patient With Crutchfield Tongs

If Crutchfield tongs are used and the patient is not on a turning frame, a directive from the physician must be obtained before the patient is turned. The patient's head *should never be flexed,* either forward or laterally, and at all times must be kept in a direct line with the axis of the cervical spine.

To Turn the Patient

- Three persons should turn the patient in a logrolling fashion, making sure that the shoulder turns with the head and the neck. One nurse should support the head; the second nurse or assistant, the shoulders; and the third person, the hips and the legs.
- The nurse supporting the head gives the commands for turning.
- A pillow is placed between the legs of the patient to prevent the upper leg from slipping forward and jarring the patient's head.
- A pillow is placed longitudinally on the chest, with the patient's upper arm resting on it. The pillow prevents the shoulder from sagging and pulling on the neck as the patient is turned.
- As the patient is turned in a logrolling fashion, the traction should be moved carefully to keep it in a direct line with the cervical spine. The patient's position should be adjusted so that the traction, the patient's head, and the cervical spine are in correct alignment.
- While the nurse still supports the head in the lateral position, a small pillow is placed under the head to maintain cervical alignment.

tarsals, ankles, knees, and hips should be put through a full range of motion at least 4, and ideally 5, times daily. Range-of-motion exercises can prevent many complications.

▷ *Skin Integrity.*   Because the patient with a spinal cord injury is immobilized and has loss of feeling, there is an ever-present, life-endangering threat of pressure ulcers. In areas of local tissue ischemia where there is continuous pressure and where the peripheral circulation is inadequate as a result of the spinal shock and recumbency, pressure ulcers have been known to develop within 6 hours. The most common sites are over the ischial tuberosity, the greater trochanter, and the sacrum.

- The patient's position is changed at least every 2 hours. Turning not only aids in the prevention of pressure ulcers but also prevents the pooling of blood and tissue fluid in the dependent areas.
- Careful inspection of the skin is made each time the patient is turned. The skin over the pressure points is assessed for redness or breaks in the skin; the perineum is checked for soilage, and the catheter is observed for adequate drainage. The patient's general body alignment and comfort are assessed.
- Every few hours the patient's skin should be washed with a mild soap, rinsed well, and *blotted* dry. Pressure-sensitive areas should be kept well lubricated and soft with bland cream or lotion. Massage should be performed gently with a circular motion.
- The patient must know the danger of pressure ulcers and accept responsibility for prevention. (See Chap. 14 for other aspects of the prevention of pressure ulcers.)

▷ *Urinary Elimination.*   Immediately after a spinal cord injury, the urinary bladder becomes atonic and cannot contract by reflex activity. Urinary retention is the immediate result of spinal cord injury. Because the patient has no sensation of bladder distention, overstretching of the bladder and detrusor muscle may occur and delay the return of bladder function.

Intermittent catheterization is carried out to avoid overstretching and infection. If this is not feasible, an indwelling catheter is inserted. At an early stage, family members are shown how to carry out the procedure and encouraged to participate in this facet of care, because they will be involved in long-term follow-up and must be able to recognize complications so that treatment can be instituted.

The patient is taught to note and write down fluid intake, voiding pattern, amounts of residual urine after catheterization, quality of urine, and any unusual feelings that may be occurring. The management of a neurogenic bladder is discussed in detail in Chap. 42.

▷ *Improved Bowel Function.*   Immediately after spinal cord injury, the patient usually develops a paralytic ileus due to neurogenic paralysis of the bowel. The nurse monitors the patient's reactions to gastric intubation, which is prescribed to relieve gastric distention and prevent aspiration.

Bowel activity usually returns within the first week. As soon as bowel sounds are heard by auscultation, the patient is given a high-calorie, high-protein, and high-fiber diet, with the amount of food gradually increased. The nurse administers the prescribed stool softener to counteract the effects of immobility and pain medications. A bowel program is instituted as early as possible (see Chap. 14).

▷ *Comfort.*   When tongs or calipers are in place, the patient's skull is assessed for signs of infection, including drainage around the tongs. The back of the head is checked periodically for signs of pressure and is massaged at intervals, with care being taken not to move the neck. The hair around the tongs is shaved to facilitate inspection. Probing under encrusted areas is avoided.

Halo Traction.   The patient may experience a slight headache or discomfort around the skull pins for several days after the pins are inserted. The patient may not initially appreciate the rather startling appearance of this apparatus but can readily adapt to it because the device provides comfort for the unstable neck. The patient may complain of being caged in and of noise created by any object coming in contact with the steel frame but can be reassured that adaptation to such annoyances will occur.

The areas around the pin sites are cleansed daily and observed for redness, drainage, and pain. The pins are observed for loosening, which is apt to contribute to infection. If one of the pins becomes detached, the patient's head is stabilized in a neutral position while another person notifies the neurosurgeon. A torque screwdriver should be readily available in case the screws on the frame need tightening.

The skin under the halo vest is inspected for excessive perspiration, redness, and skin blistering, especially on the bony prominences. The vest is opened at the sides to allow the patient's torso to be washed. The liner of the vest is not allowed to become wet, because dampness causes skin problems. Powder is not used inside the vest, because it may contribute to the development of pressure ulcers.

▷ *Ambulation.*   For patients with a cervical fracture without neurologic deficit, reduction in traction followed by rigid immobilization for about 16 weeks restores skeletal function in most patients. These patients are allowed to move gradually to an erect position. A four-poster neck brace or molded collar is applied when the patient is mobilized after traction is removed.

The rehabilitation of the patient with a permanent spinal cord injury (*i.e.*, the paraplegic patient) is discussed in the next section.

▷ Evaluation

Expected Outcomes
1. Demonstrates improvement in gas exchange and clearance of secretions
   a. Demonstrates normal breath sounds on auscultation without adventitious sounds
   b. Reports absence of shortness of breath
   c. Performs hourly deep breathing exercises
   d. Demonstrates effective cough
   e. Reports ability to clear pulmonary secretions
   f. Exhibits absence of respiratory infection (*i.e.*, has normal temperature, respiratory rate and pulse, normal breath sounds, absence of purulent sputum)
2. Moves within limits of the dysfunction
   a. Describes turning schedule; reminds health care personnel of it
   b. Describes importance of exercise program

c. Demonstrates completion of exercises within functional limitations
3. Demonstrates optimal skin integrity
   a. Demonstrates skin free of reddened areas or breaks of skin
   b. Exhibits normal skin turgor and clear dry skin
   c. States importance of skin care; reminds caregiver of it
   d. Participates in skin care and monitoring procedures within functional limitations
4. Regains urinary bladder function
   a. Exhibits no signs of urinary tract infection (*i.e.*, has normal temperature, voids clear, dilute urine)
   b. Consumes an adequate fluid intake
   c. Monitors own fluid intake and output
   d. Participates in bladder training program within functional limitations
5. Regains bowel function
   a. Reports regular pattern of bowel movement
   b. Consumes adequate dietary fiber and oral fluids
   c. Participates in bowel training program within functional limitations
6. Reports absence of pain and discomfort
   a. Reports absence of localized pain or discomfort at pin sites
   b. States rationale for immobilization

In summary, the patient with a spinal cord injury is at risk for complications that affect almost every body system. Most patients with spinal cord injury have difficulty dealing with the sudden loss of body functions, including mobility, bowel and bladder function, sexual and reproductive functions, and the ability to care for themselves. Because they are usually young, persons who experience spinal cord injury often have not yet developed effective coping skills. Therefore, in addition to dealing with the physical changes that occur, the nurse caring for them must also assist the patient in coming to terms with the consequences of the injury.

Care for the patient with spinal cord injury must involve members from all the health care disciplines (nursing, medicine, rehabilitation, respiratory therapy, physical therapy, and so forth). The nurse is often in a key position to serve as coordinator of the management team and serve as liaison with rehabilitation centers and home care agencies. The patient and family often require assistance in dealing with the psychological impact of the spinal cord injury and its consequences; referral to a psychiatric clinical nurse specialist or other mental health care professional is often helpful.

The Paraplegic Patient

Paraplegia refers to loss of motion and sensation in the lower extremities and all or part of the trunk as a result of damage to the thoracic or lumbar spinal cord or to the sacral root. It most frequently follows trauma due to accidents and gunshot wounds but may be the result of spinal cord lesions (intervertebral disc, tumor, vascular lesions), MS, infections and abscesses of the spinal cord, and congenital defects.

Diagnostic Evaluation

Evaluation includes the observations and studies performed for the patient with a spinal cord injury: full neurologic examination, x-ray studies, and ECG monitoring.

Management

The patient faces a lifetime of great disability, requiring ongoing follow-up and care and the expertise of a number of health professionals, including the physician, psychiatrist, rehabilitation nurse, occupational therapist, physical therapist, psychologist, social worker, rehabilitation engineer, and vocational counselor at different times as the need arises. As the years go by, these patients also have the same medical problems as others in the aging population. Additionally, they face the threat of complications associated with paraplegia. Usually the patient is encouraged to attend a spinal clinic when problems arise. Lifetime care includes assessment of the urinary tract at prescribed intervals, because there is likelihood of continuing alteration in detrusor and sphincter function and the patient is prone to urinary tract infections.

Management includes observing and caring for any alteration in physiologic status and psychological outlook, and the prevention and management of complications.

Prevention of Complications

Complications of Paraplegia.   Long-term complications of paraplegia include autonomic dysreflexia (see below), bladder and kidney infections (which are discussed under Neurogenic Bladder in Chap. 42), pressure ulcers with complications of sepsis, osteomyelitis, fistulas, and depression. Flexor muscle spasms may be particularly disabling. *Heterotopic ossification* (overgrowth of bone) occurs in 20% to 40% of spinal cord injury patients in the hips, knees, shoulders, and elbows. This complication can produce a loss of range of motion. The nursing role is that of emphasizing the need for vigilance in self-assessment and care.

▶ Nursing Process
The Patient With Paraplegia

▷ Assessment

Patients with paraplegia have experienced varying degrees of loss of motor power, deep and superficial sensation, vasomotor control, bladder and bowel control, and sexual function. They are faced with threats of dysfunction related to paraplegia, including immobility, skin breakdown and pressure ulcers, recurring urinary infection, contractures, and psychosocial problems. Nurses in any health care setting must be cognizant of these potential problems in the lifetime management of these persons. Assessment focuses on the patient's general condition, observation for complications, and determining how the patient is managing at this particular time.

▷ *Psychosocial Assessment.*   It is usually some time before these patients comprehend the magnitude of their disability. They may go through stages of adjustment, including shock and disbelief, denial, depression, grief, and acceptance. During the acute phase of the injury, denial can be a protective mechanism to shield patients from the overwhelming reality of what has happened. As they realize the finality of paraplegia (or quadriplegia), the grieving process may be prolonged and all-encompassing because of the awareness of "what will never be." A period of depression follows as the patient experiences a loss of self-esteem in areas of self-identity, sexual functioning, and social and emotional roles. Self-esteem is related to being strong, loved, and lovable—all of which are threatened.

◊ *Nursing Diagnoses*

Based on all the assessment data, the major nursing diagnoses of the patient with paraplegia may include the following:

- Immobility related to inability to walk
- Impairment of skin integrity related to permanent sensory loss and immobility
- Urinary retention related to level of spinal cord injury
- Constipation related to effects of spinal cord disruption
- Sexual dysfunction related to neurologic dysfunction
- Ineffective individual coping related to impact of dysfunction on daily living

◊ *Potential Problems* Based on all the assessment data, possible complications or paraplegia include:

- Autonomic dysreflexia

◊ *Planning and Implementation*

◊ *Goals*: The goals for the patient may include attainment of some form of mobility, maintenance of healthy, intact skin, achievement of bladder management without infection, achievement of bowel control, achievement of sexual expression, strengthening of coping mechanisms, and management of autonomic dysreflexia.

◊ *Nursing Interventions*

The patient requires extensive rehabilitation, which is less difficult if appropriate nursing management has been carried out during the acute phase of the injury or illness. (See Management of Cervical Spine Injuries [Acute Phase], p. 1739.) The nursing care is one of the determining factors in the success of the rehabilitation program. The main objective is for the patient to live as independently as possible in the home community.

◊ *Mobility*

Weight-Bearing Activities. A patient with complete severance of the cord can begin weight-bearing early, because no further damage can be incurred. The sooner muscles are strengthened, the less is the chance of disuse atrophy. The earlier the patient is brought to a standing position, the less opportunity there is for osteoporotic changes to take place in the long bones. Weight-bearing also reduces the possibility of formation of renal calculi and enhances many other metabolic processes.

Exercise Program. The unaffected parts of the body are built up to optimal strength to enable the patient to ambulate with braces and crutches. The muscles of the hands, arms, shoulders, chest, spine, abdomen, and neck must be strengthened, because the patient must bear full weight on these muscles. The triceps and the latissimus dorsi are important muscles used in crutch walking. The muscles of the abdomen and the

back also are necessary for balance and the maintenance of the upright position.

To strengthen these muscles, the patient can do push-ups when in a prone position and sit-ups when in a sitting position. Extending the arms while holding weights (traction weights can be used) also develops muscle strength. Squeezing rubber balls or crumbling newspaper promotes hand strength.

Through the encouragement of all of the members of the rehabilitation team, the patient develops the increased exercise tolerance needed for gait training and ambulation activities.

Managing Postural Hypotension. Because vasomotor tone is lacking in the lower extremities, the patient may become hypotensive when placed in an upright position. Profound postural hypotension is seen in all patients with lesions above the mid-thoracic level. Postural hypotension results because the reflex arcs that normally produce vasoconstriction in the upright position have been interrupted. There is pooling of blood in the peripheral veins and splanchnic bed from lack of muscle tone and poor skin turgor. Reduced venous return to the heart, orthostatic hypotension, and decreased cerebral blood flow also occur.

To counteract this problem, a tilt table may be used to help the patient overcome vasomotor instability and tolerate the upright posture. Other possible measures include using elastic stockings to facilitate venous return in the legs and applying an abdominal binder to alleviate the pooling of blood in the abdominal area.

When a tilt table is used, the patient is gradually elevated to an upright position. At first the patient may be able to tolerate only an elevation of 45 degrees (or less), but gradually the angle of elevation is increased. The patient is observed closely for signs of intolerance, including nausea, perspiration, pallor, dizziness, and syncope. Blood pressure is taken before the patient is allowed up and when positioned on the tilt table, as periods of recumbency also favor the development of orthostatic hypotension.

If no tilt table is available, a high-back reclining wheelchair with extension leg rests may be used. To overcome the effects of hypotension, the backrest is raised slowly and the leg rests are lowered gradually over a period of 7 to 10 days. While in the wheelchair, the patient may experience dizziness, tachycardia, hypotension, and blackouts. If dizziness develops, the brakes should be placed in the on position and the wheelchair tilted back for several minutes. If hypotension is prolonged, cerebral anoxia with the possibility of a cerebrovascular accident is a distinct threat and must be avoided.

Mobilization. When the spine is stable enough to allow the patient to assume an upright posture, mobilization activities are initiated. A brace or vest may be used, depending on the level of the lesion. Braces and crutches enable some patients to ambulate for short distances and even to drive manually operated automobiles. Crutch ambulation in paraplegics requires high energy expenditure. Modern technological developments, such as motorized wheelchairs and specially equipped vans, are contributing to the greater independence and mobility of patients with high-level spinal cord injuries.

A major goal of nursing management is to help these patients overcome their sense of futility and to encourage them in the emotional adjustment that must be made before they are willing to venture into the outside world. To achieve this goal, it is important to realize that an excessively sympathetic attitude may cause patients to develop an overdependence that defeats the purpose of the entire rehabilitation program.

The patient is taught and assisted when necessary, but effort is made not to take over activities that patients can do for themselves with a little effort. This type of nursing care more than repays itself in the satisfaction of seeing a completely demoralized and helpless patient begin to find meaning in a newly emerging life style.

▷ *Skin Integrity.*   Because paraplegic patients spend a great portion of their lives in a wheelchair, pressure ulcers are an ever-present threat. Contributing factors are permanent sensory paralysis and loss of sensation over pressure areas, immobility that makes relief of pressure difficult, trauma from bumps (against the wheelchair, toilet) that cause unperceived abrasions and wounds, loss of protective function of the skin from excoriation and maceration due to excessive perspiration and possible urine and fecal incontinence, and poor general health (anemia, edema, malnutrition) leading to poor tissue perfusion.

The prevention and management of pressure ulcers are discussed in detail in Chapter 14 and under the care of the patient with a spinal cord injury (p. 1743).

The person with paraplegia must take responsibility for monitoring his skin condition. This involves relieving pressure and avoiding holding any position for longer than 2 hours, in addition to seeing that the skin receives meticulous attention and cleanliness. The patient is taught that ulcers develop over bony prominences exposed to unrelieved pressure in the lying and sitting positions. The most vulnerable areas are pointed out, and the patient is instructed to use mirrors to inspect these areas morning and night, observing for redness, slight edema, or any abrasions. While in bed the patient should turn at 2-hour intervals and then inspect the skin again for redness that does not fade on pressure. The foundation sheet should be checked for wetness and for creases.

The patient is taught to relieve pressure in the wheelchair by doing pushups, leaning from side to side to relieve ischial pressure, and tilting forward while leaning on a table. Each person requires a wheelchair cushion prescribed to meet individual needs, which may change in time with changes in posture, weight, and skin tolerance. A referral can be made to a rehabilitation engineer, who can measure pressure levels while the patient is sitting and then tailor the cushion and other necessary aids and appliances to the individual patient's needs.

The diet for the patient with paraplegia should be high in protein, vitamins, and calories to ensure minimal wasting of muscle, well-functioning kidneys, and the maintenance of healthy skin.

▷ *Bladder Management.*   The effect of the spinal lesion on the bladder depends on the level of the cord injury, degree of cord damage, and length of time after injury. A patient with paraplegia usually has either a reflex or a nonreflex bladder, which are discussed under Neurogenic Bladder in Chapter 42. Both problems increase the risk of urinary tract infection.

The nurse emphasizes the importance of maintaining an adequate flow of urine by encouraging the drinking of about 2.5 liters of liquids daily, emptying the bladder frequently so there is minimal residual urine, and giving attention to personal hygiene because infection of the bladder and kidneys almost always occurs by the ascending route. The perineum is to be kept clean and dry and attention given to perianal skin after defecation. Underwear should be cotton (more absorbent) and changed at least daily.

If an external catheter (condom catheter) is used, the sheath is removed nightly; the penis is cleansed to remove urine and dried carefully because warm urine on the periurethral skin promotes growth of bacteria. Attention is also given to the collection bag. The nurse emphasizes the importance of monitoring for indications of urinary tract infection: cloudy, foul-smelling urine or *hematuria* (blood in the urine), fever, or chills.

The female patient who cannot achieve reflex bladder control or self-catheterization may need to wear pads or waterproof undergarments. Surgical intervention may be necessary in the form of a urinary diversion procedure.

▷ *Bowel Control.*   The objective of a bowel training program is to establish bowel evacuation through reflex conditioning. This technique is described in Chapter 14. If a cord injury occurs above the sacral segments or nerve roots and there is reflex activity, the anal sphincter may be massaged to stimulate defecation. (If the cord lesion involves the sacral segment or nerve roots, anal massage is not performed because the anus may be relaxed and lack tone. Massage is also contraindicated if there is spasticity of the anal sphincter.) The anal sphincter is massaged by inserting a gloved finger (which has been adequately lubricated) 2.5 to 3.7 cm (1 to 1.5 in) into the rectum and moving it in a circular motion or from side to side. It soon becomes apparent which area triggers the defecation response. This procedure should be performed at the same time (usually every 48 hours), after a meal, and at a time that is convenient for the patient on returning home. The patient is also taught the symptoms of impaction (frequent loose stools; constipation) and cautioned to watch for the development of hemorrhoids. A diet with sufficient fluids and fiber is essential to a bowel training program.

▷ *Sexual Expression.*   Most patients with cord injury can have some form of meaningful sexual relationship, although some modifications will have to be made. The patient and partner benefit from counseling on the range of sexual expression possible, special techniques, positions, exploration of body sensations offering sensual feelings, and urinary and bowel hygiene as related to sexual activity. Penile prostheses are available for men with erectile failure. Sexual education and counseling services are being included in the rehabilitation services at spinal centers. Small group meetings in which the patients can share their feelings, receive information, and discuss sexual concerns and practical aspects are helpful in producing effective attitudes and adjustments.

▷ *Coping Mechanisms.*   The impact of the full realization of their disability and loss becomes marked when patients return home. Each time something new enters their life (*e.g.*, a new relationship, going to work), they are reminded anew of their limitations. Grief reactions and depression are frequently encountered.

To be able to work through this depression, patients must be able to see some hope for relief in the future. Thus, they are guided toward a sense of confidence in their ability to achieve self-care and relative independence. The role of the nurse ranges from caretaker during the acute phase to teacher, counselor, and facilitator, as patients gain mobility and independence.

Adjustment to the disability leads to the development of realistic goals for the future, making the best of those abilities that are left intact, and reinvesting in other activities and relationships. Rejection of the disability causes self-destructive neglect and noncompliance with the therapeutic program. This leads to more frustration and depression. Crises for which interventions may be sought include social, psychological, marital, sexual, and psychiatric problems. The family usually requires counseling, social services, and other support systems to help them cope with the changes in their life style and socioeconomic status. (The psychological implications of a disability are discussed also in Chap. 14.)

▷ *Management of Autonomic Dysreflexia.* Autonomic dysreflexia (autonomic hyperreflexia) is an acute emergency that occurs as a result of exaggerated autonomic responses to stimuli that are innocuous in normal individuals. This syndrome is characterized by severe, pounding headache with paroxysmal hypertension, profuse sweating (most often of the forehead), nasal congestion, and bradycardia. It occurs among patients with cord lesions above the T6 level (the sympathetic visceral outflow level), generally after spinal shock has subsided. The sudden rise in blood pressure may cause a rupture of one or more cerebral blood vessels or lead to an increase in ICP. A number of stimuli may trigger this reflex: distended bladder (the most common cause), distended bowel, stimulation of the skin (tactile, pain, thermal stimuli), or distention or contraction of the visceral organs, especially the bowel (from constipation, impaction). Because this is an emergency situation, the objective is to remove the triggering stimulus and to avoid the possibly serious complications.

The following measures are carried out:

- Place the patient in a sitting position to lower the blood pressure.
- Drain the bladder with the catheter. If the catheter is not patent, irrigate it with a small amount of irrigating solution or insert another catheter.
- After the symptoms subside, the rectum is examined for a fecal mass. If one is present, dibucaine ointment is inserted 10 to 15 minutes before the mass is removed, because visceral distention or contraction can cause autonomic dysreflexia.
- Any other stimulus that can be the triggering event, such as an object on the skin or a draft of cold air, must be removed.
- If these measures do not relieve the patient's hypertension and excruciating headache, a ganglionic blocking agent (hydralazine hydrochloride [Apresoline]) is prescribed and given slowly intravenously.
- The patient's chart should be tagged with an allergic marker.
- Instruct the patient in prevention and management measures.

Any patient with a lesion above the T6 segment should be informed that such an episode is possible and may even occur many years after the initial injury.

▷ *Patient Education and Home Health Care.* Patients with a spinal injury are at special risk during the first few weeks after their return home. Urinary infections and deconditioning resulting in contractures may appear and require rehospitalization. For the rest of their lives, patients are at risk of developing pressure ulcers that pose a serious threat to life. To avoid these complications, the patient and a family member are taught skin care, catheter care, range-of-motion exercises, and other care techniques while the patient is still in the hospital. The teaching is reinforced during home visits by the home care nurse. Environmental modifications are made and specialized equipment is purchased before the patient goes home. Other complications during the extended care period may include lower extremity edema, ankle and feet contractures, pain, and alcohol abuse.

The community health nurse provides continuing follow-up evaluation to reinforce previous teaching and to determine if further physical help is needed. The patient's self-esteem and body-image perceptions may be very low at this time.

It has been shown that persons with high levels of social support who are satisfied with their social contacts and believe that they have high levels of control generally report feelings of well-being despite the presence of a major disability. Thus it is beneficial for the nurse to assess and promote further development of the support system of each patient.

The local counselor for the Division of Vocational Rehabilitation works with the patient with respect to job placement or additional educational or vocational training.

The patient requires continuing, lifelong follow-up by the physician, physical therapist, and other rehabilitation team members, because the neurologic deficit is permanent and new problems can erupt that require prompt attention before they take their toll in additional physical impairment, time, morale, and money.

▷ *Evaluation*

Expected Outcomes. See pp. 1743–1744 for other expected outcomes.

1. Attains some form of mobility
2. Maintains healthy, intact skin
3. Achieves bladder control, absence of urinary tract infection
4. Achieves bowel control
5. Reports sexual satisfaction
6. Shows improved adaptation to environment and others
7. Exhibits absence of autonomic dysreflexia
8. Reports understanding of the precipitating factors

Intraspinal Tumors

Tumors within the spine are classified according to their anatomic relation to the spinal cord. They include *intramedullary* lesions (within the spinal cord), *extramedullary-intradural* lesions (within the subarachnoid space), and *extradural* lesions (outside the dural membrane). Tumors that occur within the spinal cord or exert pressure on it cause symptoms ranging from weakness and loss of reflexes above the tumor level and localized or shooting pains, to progressive loss of motor function and paralysis. Usually sharp pain occurs in the area that is innervated by the spinal roots that arise from the cord in the region of the tumor. In addition, increasing paralysis develops below the level of the lesion.

The diagnosis is made by neurologic examination and myelography in combination with CT scanning and MRI.

Preoperative Management

The patient is assessed for weakness, muscle wasting, spasticity, and sensory or sphincter disorders. A search is made for potential pulmonary problems, especially if a cervical tumor is present. The patient is also evaluated for coagulation deficiencies. A history of aspirin intake is obtained because its use may create problems with hemostasis postoperatively. Breathing exercises are taught and demonstrated preoperatively.

Surgical Management

The removal of the tumor is usually desired but not always feasible. The goal is to remove as much tumor as possible while sparing intact portions of the spinal cord. Microsurgical techniques have improved the prognosis for surgical treatment of intramedullary tumors. The prognosis is related to the degree of neurologic impairment at the time of surgery, the speed of occurrence of symptoms, and the tumor's origin. Patients with large neurologic deficits before surgery usually do not make significant functional recovery after successful tumor removal.

Other treatment modalities include subtotal removal of the tumor, decompression of the spinal cord, chemotherapy, and radiation therapy.

If the patient has epidural spinal cord compression resulting from metastatic cancer (from breast, prostate, or lung), high-dose dexamethasone combined with radiation therapy is effective in relieving pain.

Postoperative Nursing Interventions

The nursing management is similar to that after disc surgery (see p. 1752). The patient is monitored for deterioration in neurologic status. A sudden onset of neurologic deficit is a sinister sign. It may be due to vertebral collapse associated with spinal cord infarction. Neurologic checks are made, with emphasis on evaluating arm and leg movement, strength, and sensation. Sensory function is checked by pinching the skin of the arms, legs, and trunk to determine if there is loss of feeling and, if so, at what level. Vital signs are monitored at intervals. If the tumor was in the cervical area, there is always the possibility of postoperative respiratory compromise. Chest movement is observed for symmetry and abdominal breathing, and the chest is auscultated for abnormal breath sounds. In the instance of a high cervical lesion, the endotracheal tube is left in place until respiratory function is assured. Deep breathing and coughing are encouraged.

The area over the patient's bladder is palpated for urinary retention. Incontinence may be present. Urinary dysfunction usually implies significant decompensation of spinal cord function. An intake and output record is maintained. Additionally, the abdomen is auscultated for bowel sounds.

The prescribed pain medication should be given in adequate amounts and at appropriate intervals to relieve pain and prevent its recurrence. Pain is the hallmark of spinal metastasis. Patients with sensory root involvement or vertebral collapse may suffer excruciating pain.

The bed is usually kept flat. The patient is turned as a unit, keeping shoulders and hips aligned. The back is kept straight. The side-lying position is usually the most comfortable because

it avoids pressure on the wound. A pillow is placed between the knees of the patient in a side-lying position, and extreme knee flexion is avoided.

Staining of the dressing may indicate leakage of CSF. Any CSF leakage from the area of operation may lead to disastrous infection or to an inflammatory reaction in the surrounding tissues that can cause severe pain in the postoperative period.

Patient Education

Patients with residual sensory involvement are cautioned about the dangers of extremes in temperature. They should be alert to the dangers of heating devices (*e.g.*, space heaters, fireplaces). The patient is taught to check skin integrity daily.

A patient who has impaired motor function related to motor weakness or paralysis may require training in activities of daily living and an ambulatory aid such as a cane or walker.

Herniation or Rupture of an Intervertebral Disc

The intervertebral disc is a cartilaginous plate that forms a cushion between the vertebral bodies. This tough, fibrous material is incorporated in a capsule. A ball-like condensation in the disc is called the *nucleus pulposus*. In herniation of the intervertebral disc (ruptured disc), the nucleus of the disc protrudes into the annulus (the fibrous ring around the disc), with subsequent nerve compression. Protrusion or rupture of the nucleus pulposus is usually preceded by degenerative changes that occur with aging. Loss of protein polysaccharides in the disc decreases the water content of the nucleus pulposus. The development of radiating cracks in the annulus weakens resistance to nucleus herniation. After trauma (falls, accidents, and repeated minor stresses, such as lifting), the cartilage may be injured.

In most patients, the immediate symptoms of trauma are short lived, and those resulting from injury to the disc do not appear for months or years. Then, with degeneration in the disc, the capsule pushes back into the spinal canal, or it may rupture and allow the nucleus pulposus to be pushed back against the dural sac or against a spinal nerve as it emerges from the spinal column (Fig. 57-14). This sequence produces pain due to pressure in the area of distribution of the involved nerve endings. Continued pressure may produce degenerative changes in the involved nerve, such as changes in sensation and reflex action.

Clinical Manifestations.   A herniated disc with accompanying pain may occur in any portion of the spine: cervical, thoracic (rare), or lumbar. The clinical manifestations depend on the location, the rate of development (acute or chronic), and the effect on the surrounding structures.

Diagnostic Evaluation.   A myelogram usually demonstrates the area of pressure and localizes the herniation of the disc. CT scans may identify small disc protrusions. MRI is complementary to CT scans. A neurologic examination is carried out to determine if there is reflex, sensory, or motor impairment

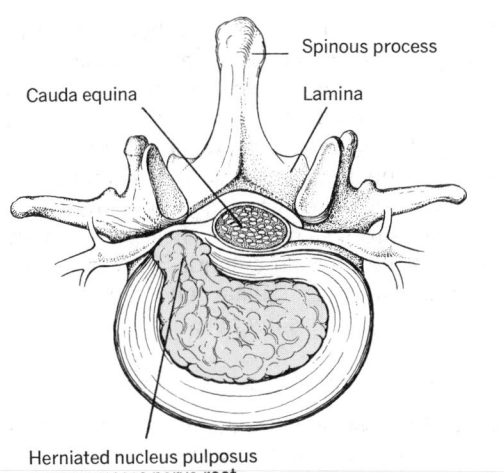

Spinous process

Cauda equina   Lamina

Herniated nucleus pulposus
compresses nerve root

Figure 57–14.   Ruptured vertebral disc. (Chaffee EE and Greisheimer
EM. Basic Physiology and Anatomy, 3rd ed. Philadelphia, JB Lippincott.)

from root compression. Electromyography may be used to localize the specific spinal nerve roots involved.

Management

Herniations of the cervical and the lumbar discs occur most
commonly, and these are usually managed conservatively. The
specific conservative management and surgical interventions
for each form of herniation are discussed in detail.

Disc Surgery.   In general, surgical excision of a herniated
disc is performed when there is evidence of a progressing neurologic deficit (muscle weakness and atrophy, loss of sensory
and motor function, loss of sphincter control) and continuing
pain and sciatica that are unresponsive to conservative management. The goal of surgical treatment is to relieve pressure
on the nerve root to relieve pain and reverse neurologic deficits.
Microsurgical techniques are making possible the precise removal through a small incision of only that amount of tissue
that is absolutely necessary. This approach better preserves
the integrity of normal tissue and imposes less trauma on the
body. During these procedures, spinal cord function can be
monitored electrophysiologically.

To achieve the goal of pain relief, several operative techniques are used, depending on the type of disc herniation,
operative morbidity, and overall results of surgery:

Discectomy—removal of herniated or extruded fragments of
   intervertebral disc
Laminectomy—removal of the lamina to expose the neural
   elements in the spinal canal; allows the surgeon to inspect
   the spinal canal, identify and remove pathology, and relieve
   compression of the cord and roots
Laminotomy—division of the lamina of a vertebra
Discectomy with fusion—a bone graft (from iliac crest/bone
   bank) is used to fuse the vertebral spinous process; the
   object of spinal fusion is to bridge over the defective disc
   to stabilize the spine and reduce the rate of recurrence.

Surgeries for herniated cervical disc and lumbar disc are
discussed in detail in the sections that follow.

Herniation or Rupture of a Cervical Intervertebral Disc

The cervical spine is subjected to stresses that result from disc
degeneration (from aging, occupational stresses) and *spon-
dylosis* (degenerative changes occurring in disc and adjacent
vertebral bodies). Cervical disc degeneration may lead to lesions that can cause damage to the spinal cord and its roots.

A cervical disc herniation usually occurs at the C5–C6 and
C6–C7 interspaces. Pain and stiffness may occur in the neck,
the top of the shoulders, and the region of the scapulae. Sometimes patients interpret these signs as symptoms of heart trouble
or bursitis. Pain may also occur in the upper extremities and
head, accompanied by paresthesia and numbness of the upper
extremities. The diagnosis is usually confirmed by cervical
myelography.

Management

The goals of treatment are (1) to rest and immobilize the cervical spine to give the soft tissues time to heal, and (2) to
reduce inflammation in the supporting tissues and the affected
nerve roots in the cervical spine. Bed rest (usually 2 weeks) is
important, because it eliminates the stress of gravity and frees
the cervical spine from having to support the weight of the
head. It also reduces inflammation and edema in soft tissues
around the disc, relieving pressure on the nerve roots. Proper
positioning on a firm mattress may bring dramatic relief from
pain.

The cervical spine may be rested and immobilized by a
cervical collar, cervical traction, or a brace. A collar allows
maximal opening of the intervertebral foramina and holds the
head in a neutral or slightly flexed position. The patient may
have to wear the collar 24 hours a day during the acute phase.
The skin site under the collar is inspected for irritation. When
the patient is free of pain, cervical isometric exercises are
started to strengthen the muscles in the neck.

Cervical traction is accomplished by means of a head halter
attached to a pulley and weight. It increases vertebral separation
and thus relieves pressure on the nerve roots. The head of the
bed is elevated to provide countertraction. If the skin becomes
irritated, the halter can be padded. Experience has shown that
a male patient may suffer more skin irritation if he shaves; the
beard offers a natural form of padding.

Hot, moist compresses (for 10 to 20 minutes) applied to
the back of the neck several times daily increase blood flow
to the muscles and help to relax the spastic muscles as well
as the patient. Analgesics are given during the acute phase to
relieve pain, and sedatives may be administered to control the
anxiety often associated with cervical disc disease. Muscle relaxants are administered to interrupt the cycle of muscle spasm
and to allow for patient comfort. Anti-inflammatory drugs (aspirin, phenylbutazone [Butazolidin]) or corticosteroids are
given to treat the inflammatory response that usually occurs in
the supporting tissues and affected nerve roots. Occasionally
an injection of a corticosteroid drug into the epidural space
may be tried as a means of relieving radicular pain. Food and
antacids are given with anti-inflammatory agents to prevent
gastrointestinal irritation. Periodic blood evaluations should be

carried out to detect the development of blood dyscrasias because hematologic toxicity to phenylbutazone can occur.

Surgical Management

Surgical excision of the herniated disc may be necessary when there is a significant neurologic deficit, progression of a neurologic deficit, evidence of cord compression, or pain that either fails to improve or worsens. A cervical discectomy, with or without fusion, may be performed to alleviate symptoms. In the cervical area, an anterior approach may be used through a transverse incision in the neck to remove disc material that has herniated into the spinal canal and foramina, or a posterior approach may be used at the desired level of the cervical spine.

Potential Postoperative Complications

Potential complications for the anterior approach include carotid or vertebral artery injury, recurrent laryngeal nerve dysfunction, esophageal perforation, and airway obstruction. Complications of the posterior approach include damage to the nerve root or to the spinal cord due to retraction or contusion of either of these structures, resulting in weakness of muscles supplied by the nerve root or cord.

▶ Nursing Process
The Patient Undergoing a Cervical Discectomy

▷ Assessment

The patient is asked about past injuries to the neck (whiplash), because unresolved trauma may cause persistent discomfort, pain, and tenderness and the development of arthritis in the injured joint of the cervical spine. Assessment of the patient's problems includes determining the onset, location, and radiation of pain, paresthesias, limited movement, and diminished function of the neck, shoulders, and upper extremities. It is important to determine whether or not the symptoms are bilateral because, with large herniations, bilateral symptoms may be due to cord compression. Examination of the area around the cervical spine includes palpation to assess muscle tone and tenderness.

Range of motion in the neck and shoulders is evaluated. The patient is also queried about any health problems that may influence the postoperative course. The nurse determines the patient's need for information about the operative procedure and reinforces what has been explained by the physician. Strategies that have been used in the past for pain management are elicited.

▷ *Postoperative Assessment.*   Assessment includes monitoring the blood pressure and pulse for evaluation of the cardiovascular status. The patient is evaluated for bleeding that is manifested by the complaint of excessive pressure in the neck or severe pain in the incisional area. The dressing is inspected for serosanguineous drainage, which suggests a dural leak. In this event, meningitis is a threat. A complaint of headache requires careful evaluation. Neurologic checks are made for

upper and lower extremity weakness because cord compression may produce rapid or delayed onset of paralysis. Throughout the postoperative course, the vital signs are monitored frequently to detect any signs of respiratory difficulty. Occasionally, during surgery, the recurrent laryngeal nerve may be injured by retractors, resulting in hoarseness and inability to cough effectively. The elimination of pulmonary secretions then becomes a problem requiring chest physical therapy. One sign to observe for after an anterior cervical discectomy is a sudden return of radicular (spinal nerve root) pain, which may indicate that the spine has become unstable.

▷ Nursing Diagnoses

Based on all the assessment data, the patient's major nursing diagnoses may include the following:

* Pain related to the surgical procedure
* Impaired physical mobility related to postoperative surgical regimen
* Knowledge deficit relative to the postoperative course and home care management

Other nursing diagnoses (which may be encountered in any surgical patient) may include preoperative anxiety and a number of postoperative concerns, as follows: constipation related to the procedure; urinary retention related to dehydration and the operative procedure; self-care deficits related to neck orthosis; and sleep pattern disturbance related to disruption in life style.

▷ Planning and Implementation

▷ *Goals:*   The goals of the patient may include relief of pain, attainment of improved mobility, and increased knowledge and self-care ability.

▷ Nursing Interventions

▷ *Pain Relief.*   The patient may be kept flat in bed for 12 to 24 hours. If the patient has had a bone fusion in which bone has been removed from the iliac crest, considerable pain may be experienced. Nursing interventions consist of monitoring the donor site for hematoma formation, giving the prescribed postoperative analgesic according to the patient's needs, positioning for comfort, and reassuring the patient that the pain can be controlled. If the patient experiences a sudden reappearance of radicular pain, extrusion of the graft may have occurred, a situation requiring reoperation and surgical repositioning of the graft.

Usually the major complaint of the patient is a sore throat, hoarseness, or dysphagia that may be related to temporary edema. These complaints may be relieved by throat lozenges, voice rest, and room humidification. A blenderized soft diet may be given if the patient is experiencing some dysphagia.

▷ *Improved Mobility.*   A cervical collar (neck orthosis) is usually worn after the procedure, which contributes to limited neck motion and altered mobility. Patients are taught to turn the body instead of the neck when looking from side to side. The neck should be kept in a neutral (midline) position. Patients are assisted during positional changes, making sure that head, shoulders, and thorax are aligned during turning. When assisting a patient to a sitting position, the nurse provides support behind the neck and shoulders. Patients should wear shoes when ambulating to increase stability.

▷ *Patient Education and Home Health Care.* The cervical collar is usually worn for about 6 weeks. Patients are cautioned against flexing, extending, or rotating the neck in any extreme manner while stretching, exercising, or working. While sleeping, the prone position should be avoided. The head is to be kept in a neutral position. Patients should be cautioned not to prop themselves up in bed with several pillows, because this produces unwanted neck flexion.

Patients are advised to monitor themselves for signs and symptoms of infection: fever, wound drainage, or increased pain. If any of these appear, medical attention should be sought.

Sitting or standing for more than 30 minutes can induce considerable neck strain. Patients are advised to alternate tasks in which the body does not move (*e.g.*, reading) with tasks that require greater body movement. Long automobile rides should generally be avoided, because vibration associated with such trips has an adverse effect on the spine. Patients are instructed to report for reevaluation at prescribed intervals to document the disappearance of old symptoms and for examination of range of motion of the neck.

▷ Evaluation

Expected Outcomes

1. Achieves increasing comfort
   a. Is able to get out of bed
   b. States that pain is lessening
2. Attains improved mobility
   a. Walks in hallway
   b. Turns body when looking in a lateral direction
3. Acquires knowledge for self-care
   a. Asks questions; gives positive feedback
   b. Knows the signs and symptoms to be reported

Herniation of a Lumbar Disc

Most lumbar disc herniations occur at the L4–L5 or the L5–S1 interspaces. A lumbar disc produces low back pain accompanied by varying degrees of sensory and motor impairment. The patient complains of low back pain with muscle spasms, which is followed by radiation of the pain into one hip and down into the leg (*sciatica*). Pain is aggravated by actions that increase intraspinal fluid pressure (bending, lifting, straining, as in sneezing and coughing) and is usually relieved by bed rest. There is usually some type of postural deformity, because pain causes an alteration of the normal spinal mechanics. If the patient lies on the back and attempts to raise a leg in a straight position, pain radiates into the leg because this maneuver (*straight leg raising test*) stretches the sciatic nerve. Additional signs include muscle weakness, alterations in tendon reflexes, and sensory loss.

Diagnostic Evaluation

The diagnosis of lumbar disc disease is based on the history and physical findings and the use of imaging techniques, myelography, or CT scanning and MRI. Dynamic studies, such as lateral bending and flexion of the spine, are used to enhance the value of the myelogram.

Management

The objectives of treatment are to relieve the pain and slow the progression of the disease and to increase the functional ability of the patient. Bed rest on a firm mattress (to limit spinal flexion) is encouraged to reduce the weight load and gravitational forces, thereby freeing the disc from stress. The patient is allowed to assume a comfortable position; usually, a semi-Fowler's position with moderate hip and knee flexion to relax the back muscles is most satisfactory. While in the side-lying position, a pillow is placed between the legs. To get out of bed, the patient lies on his side while pushing up to a sitting position.

Because muscle spasm is prominent during the acute phase, muscle relaxants are used. Anti-inflammatory drugs and systemic steroids may be administered to counter the inflammation that usually occurs in the supporting tissues and the affected nerve roots. Moist heat and massage help to relax spastic muscles and produce a sedating effect on the patient. See also Nursing Process: The Patient With Low Back Pain in Chapter 61 for nursing interventions.

Surgical Management

In the lumbar region, surgical treatment includes lumbar disc excision through a posterolateral laminotomy and the newer techniques of microdiscectomy and percutaneous discectomy.

Microdiscectomy incorporates the use of the operating microscope to visualize the offending disc and compressed nerve roots; it permits a smaller incision (2.5 cm [1 in]) and minimal blood loss, and takes about 30 minutes of operating time. Generally it involves a shorter hospital stay, and the patient makes a more rapid recovery.

Percutaneous discectomy is an alternative treatment for herniated intervertebral discs of the lumbar spine at the L4–L5 level. One approach in current use is through a 2.5-cm (1-in) incision just above the iliac crest. A tube, trocar, or cannula is inserted under x-ray guidance through the retroperitoneal space to the involved disc space. Specially lengthened instruments are used to remove the disc. The operating time is about 15 minutes. Blood loss and postoperative pain are minimal, and the patient is generally discharged within 2 days after surgery.

The disadvantage of this procedure involves the possibility of damage to structures located in the surgical pathway.

Preoperative Nursing Management

Most patients fear surgery on any part of the spine, and therefore need assurance (that surgery will not weaken the back) and explanations all along the way. When data are being collected for the health history, any complaints of pain, paresthesia, and muscle spasm are recorded to provide a baseline for comparison after surgery. Preoperative assessment should also include an evaluation of movement in the extremities as well as bladder and bowel function. To facilitate the postoperative turning procedure, the patient is taught to turn as a unit (logrolling), as part of the preoperative preparation. Other facets of the postoperative regimen that should be practiced before the operation are deep-breathing, coughing, and muscle-setting exercises, which will help maintain muscle tone.

Postoperative Nursing Management

After lumbar disc excision, the vital signs are checked frequently and the wound is inspected for evidence of hemorrhage, because vascular injury is a complication of disc surgery. Because postoperative neurologic deficits may occur from nerve root injury, the sensation and motor power of the lower extremities are evaluated at specified intervals, along with the color and temperature of the legs and sensation of the toes. Another important sign to check for is possible urinary retention.

Most patients walk to the bathroom the same day (the day of surgery), and all but a few are home by the second postoperative day. They are instructed in how to turn in bed (see below) and taught an exercise routine. Sitting is discouraged except for defecation.

To position the patient, a pillow is placed under the head, and the knee rest is elevated slightly, because slight knee flexion relaxes the muscles of the back. When the patient is lying on one side, however, extreme knee flexion must be avoided. The patient is encouraged to move from side to side to relieve pressure, but he is first reassured that no injury will result from moving. When the patient is ready to turn, the bed is placed in a flat position and a pillow is placed between the legs. Turning is performed with the body as a unit (logrolling), without twisting the back.

To get out of bed, the patient lies on one side while pushing up to a sitting position. At the same time, a second person eases the patient's legs over the side of the bed. Coming to a sitting or standing posture is accomplished by one long, smooth motion.

In cases requiring discectomy with fusion, the patient has an additional wound if bone fragments are taken from the iliac crest or fibula to serve as wedges in the spine. The recovery period is somewhat slower than for those patients who have undergone removal of the ruptured portion of the disc without a spinal fusion, because bony union must take place.

Complications of Disc Surgery

A person having a disc procedure at one level may have degenerative process at other levels of the vertebral column. A herniation relapse may occur at the same level or elsewhere, so that the patient is apt to become a candidate for another disc procedure. *Arachnoiditis,* (inflammation of the arachnoid membrane) may occur after operation (and after myelography); it involves an insidious onset of diffuse, frequently burning pain in the lower back, radiating into the buttocks. Disc excision can leave adhesions and scarring around the spinal nerves and dura, which then produce inflammatory changes that can create chronic neuritis and neurofibrosis. Disc surgery may relieve pressure on the spinal nerves, but it does not reverse the effects of neural injury and scarring and the pain that ensues.

Failed disc syndrome (recurrence of sciatica after lumbar discectomy) remains a common cause of disability.

Patient Education and Home Health Care

The patient is advised that, because it takes up to 6 weeks for the ligaments of the muscles to heal, activity is to be gradually increased up to the point of tolerance. Excessive activity may result in spasm of the paraspinal muscles.

Activities that produce flexion strain on the spine (*e.g.,* driving a car) should be avoided until healing has taken place. Heat may be applied to the back to soothe and relax muscle spasms and help absorb exudates in the tissues. Scheduled rest periods are important. Usually the patient is advised to avoid heavy work for 2 to 3 months after surgery. Exercises are prescribed to strengthen the abdominal and erector spinal muscles. A back brace or corset may be necessary if back pain persists (see also Patient Education for Low Back Pain in Chap. 61).

Cranial Nerve Disorders

There are 12 pairs of cranial nerves that emerge from the lower surface of the brain and pass through the *foramina* (openings) in the skull. They are classified as motor, sensory, and mixed nerves. The cranial nerves are numbered in the order in which they arise from the brain. The names of the cranial nerves suggest their primary function or some anatomic characteristic. Most cranial nerves originate in the brain stem and innervate the head, neck, and special organs.

The cranial nerves are examined separately and in sequence (see Chap. 55). Some cranial nerve deficits can be detected by observing the patient's face, eye movements, speech, and swallowing. Electromyography is used to investigate motor and sensory dysfunction. MRI produces excellent images of the cranial nerves and brain stem.

Because the brain stem and cranial nerves control vital motor, sensory, or autonomic functions of the body, they may be involved in conditions arising primarily within these structures or in secondary extension from adjacent disease processes. The following discussions center on trigeminal neuralgia, a condition affecting the fifth cranial nerve, and on Bell's palsy, caused by involvement of the seventh cranial nerve.

An overview of disorders that may affect each of the cranial nerves, including clinical manifestations and nursing interventions, is presented in Table 57-2, and the cranial nerves are illustrated in Figure 57-15.

Trigeminal Neuralgia (Tic Douloureux)

Trigeminal neuralgia is a condition of the fifth cranial nerve characterized by paroxysms of pain similar to an electric shock or a lancinating burning sensation in the area innervated by one or more branches of the trigeminal nerve. The pain ends as abruptly as it starts. Each pain episode can be described as stabbing, lasting from a few seconds to minutes and produces contraction of some of the facial muscles, such as a sudden closing of the eye or a twitch of the mouth; hence the name *tic douloureux* (painful twitch). The cause is not certain, but chronic compression or irritation of the trigeminal nerve or degenerative changes in the gasserian ganglion are suggested causes. Some investigators believe that the condition may be due to vascular pressure from structural abnormalities (loop

TABLE 57-2.   *Disorders of Cranial Nerves*

Disorder	Clinical Manifestations	Nursing Interventions
OLFACTORY NERVE—I Head trauma Intracranial tumor Intracranial surgery	Unilateral or bilateral anosmia (temporary or persistent) Diminished taste for food	Assess for CSF rhinorrhea if patient has sustained head trauma.
OPTIC NERVE—II Optic neuritis Increased intracranial pressure Pituitary tumor	Lesions of optic tract produce homonymous hemianopia.	Assess level of visual acuity. Restructure environment to prevent accidents. Teach patient to accommodate for visual loss.

OCULOMOTOR NERVE—III
TROCHLEAR NERVE—IV
ABDUCENS NERVE—VI
Vascular
  Brain stem ischemia
  Hemorrhage/infarction
Neoplasm
Trauma
Infection
	Dilation of pupil with loss of light reflex on one side
	Impairment of ocular movement
	Diplopia
	Gaze palsies
	Ptosis of eyelid
		Assess extraocular movement and for nonreactive pupil.

TRIGEMINAL NERVE—V Trigeminal neuraliga Head trauma Cerebellopontine lesion Sinus tract tumor/metastatic disease Compression of trigeminal root by tumor	Pain in face Facial membrane Diminished/loss of corneal reflex Chewing dysfunction	Assess for pain and triggering mechanisms for pain. Assess for difficulty in chewing. Discuss trigger zones and pain precipitants with patient. Protect cornea from abrasion. Ensure good oral hygiene. Educate patient about medication regimen.
FACIAL NERVE—VII Bell's palsy Facial nerve tumor Intracranial lesion Herpes zoster	Facial dysfunction; weakness and paralysis Hemifacial spasm Diminished/absent taste	Recognize facial paralysis as emergency; refer for treatment as soon as possible. Teach protective care for eyes. Select easily chewed foods; patient should eat and drink from unaffected side of mouth. Emphasize importance of oral hygiene. Provide emotional support for changed appearance of face.
VESTIBULOCOCHLEAR NERVE—VIII Tumors/acoustic neuroma Vascular compression of nerve Meniere's syndrome	Tinnitus Vertigo Hearing difficulties	Assess pattern of vertigo Provide for safety measures to prevent falls. Patient should obtain balance before ambulating. Caution patient to change positions slowly. Assist with ambulation. Encourage use of ADL aids.

(continued)

TABLE 57–2.   *(Continued)*

Disorder	Clinical Manifestations	Nursing Interventions
GLOSSOPHARYNGEAL NERVE—IX		
Glossopharyngeal neuralgia from neurovascular compression of IXth and Xth nerves	Pain at base of tongue	Assess for paroxysmal pain in throat, decreased or absent swallowing, gag and cough reflexes.
Trauma	Difficulty in swallowing	
	Loss of gag reflex	Monitor for dysphagia, aspiration, nasal dysarthric speech.
Inflammatory conditions	Palatal, pharyngeal, and laryngeal paralysis	
Tumor		Position patient upright for eating or tube feeding.
Vertebral artery aneurysms		
VAGUS NERVE—X		
Spastic palsy of larynx; bulbar paralysis; high vagal paralysis	Voice changes (temporary or permanent hoarseness)	Assess for airway obstruction/provide airway management.
Guillain-Barré syndrome	Vocal paralysis	Prevent aspiration.
Carotid endarterectomy	Dysphagia	Support patient having voice reconstruction procedures.
Vagal body tumors		
Nerve paralysis from malignancy, surgical trauma		
SPINAL ACCESSORY NERVE—XI		
Spinal cord disorder	Drooping of affected shoulder with limited shoulder movement	Support patient undergoing diagnostic tests.
Amyotrophic lateral sclerosis		
Trauma	Weakness/paralysis of head rotation, flexion, extension; shoulder elevation	
Guillain-Barré syndrome		
HYPOGLOSSAL NERVE—XII		
Medullary lesions	Abnormal movements of tongue	Observe swallowing ability.
Amyotrophic lateral sclerosis	Weakness/paralysis of tongue muscles	Observe speech pattern.
Polio and motor system disease may destroy hypoglossal nuclei.	Difficulty in talking, chewing, and swallowing	Be aware of attendant swallowing/vocal difficulties.
Multiple sclerosis		Prepare for alternate feeding methods (tube feeding) to maintain nutrition.
Trauma		

of an artery) encroaching on the trigeminal nerve, gasserian ganglion, or root entry zone.

Early attacks, appearing most often in the fifth decade of life, are usually mild and brief. Pain-free intervals may be measured in terms of minutes, hours, days, or longer. With advancing years, the painful episodes tend to become more and more frequent and agonizing. The patient lives in constant fear of attacks.

The pain of this neuralgia is felt in the skin, not in the deeper structures, but it is more severe at the peripheral areas of distribution of the affected nerve, notably over the lip, the chin, the nostrils, and in the teeth. Paroxysms are aroused by any stimulation of the terminals of the affected nerve branches, such as washing the face, shaving, brushing the teeth, eating, and drinking. A draft of cold air and direct pressure against the nerve trunk may also cause pain. Certain areas are called *trigger points*, because the slightest touch immediately starts a paroxysm. To avoid stimulating these areas, patients with trigeminal neuralgia try not to touch or wash their faces, shave,

chew, or do anything else that might cause an attack. Behavior of this type is a clue to diagnosis.

Management

The antiepileptic agents carbamazepine (Tegretol) and phenytoin (Dilantin), by reducing the transmission of impulses at certain nerve terminals, relieve pain in most patients. Carbamazepine is taken with meals, in dosages gradually increased until relief is obtained. Side effects include nausea, dizziness, drowsiness, and hepatic dysfunction. The patient is monitored for bone marrow depression during long-term drug therapy. Phenytoin also produces such side effects as nausea, dizziness, somnolence, ataxia, and skin allergies.

When medication fails to provide pain relief, a number of surgical options are available, as described in the following paragraphs. Patients should participate in choosing the procedure that best suits their health status.

Alcohol injection of the gasserian ganglion and peripheral

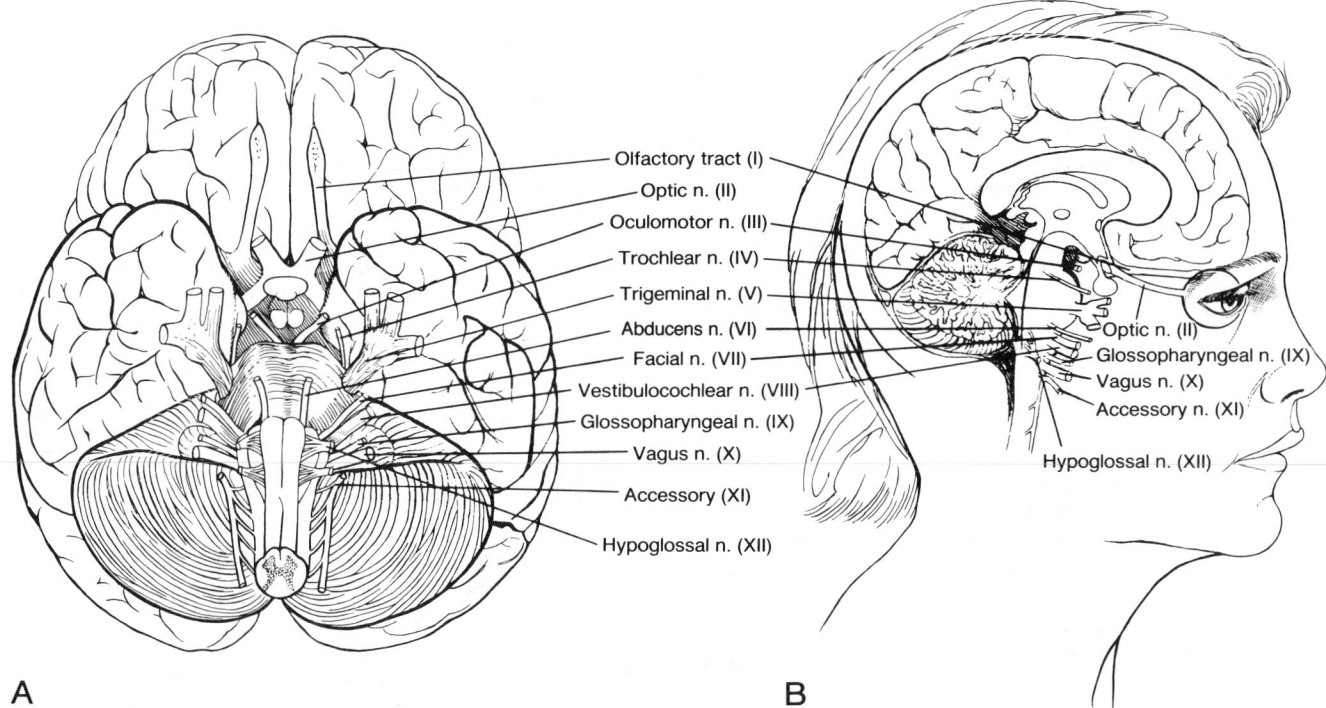

A   **B**

Figure 57–15.   The cranial nerves. (**A**) Inferior view of the brain showing the cranial nerves. (**B**) Lateral view of the brain showing a schematized version of the cranial nerves.

branches of the trigeminal nerve relieves pain for several months. However, the pain returns after the nerve regenerates.

Percutaneous Radiofrequency Trigeminal Gangliolysis. Percutaneous radiofrequency interruption of the gasserian ganglion, whereby the small unmyelinated and thinly myelinated fibers that conduct the pain are thermally destroyed, is becoming the surgical procedure of choice for trigeminal neuralgia.

Under local anesthesia, the needle is introduced through the cheek on the affected side. Under fluoroscopic control, the needle electrode is guided through the foramen magnum into the Gasserian ganglion. The divisions of the Gasserian ganglion (mandibular, maxillary, and ophthalmic) are encountered sequentially. The nerve is stimulated with a small current, while the patient is awake. The patient then reports when a tingling sensation is felt. When the electrode needle is in the desired position, the patient is anesthetized briefly and a radiofrequency current (heating current to destroy the nerve) is passed in a controlled manner to thermally injure the trigeminal ganglion and rootlets. The patient is then awakened from the anesthetic and examined for sensory deficits. Repeat lesions may be produced until the desired effect is achieved. The operative procedure takes less than 1 hour and gives permanent pain relief in most patients. Touch and proprioceptive functions are left intact.

Microvascular Decompression of the Trigeminal Nerve. An intracranial approach can be used to decompress the trigeminal nerve, because the pain may be caused by vascular compression of the entry zone of the trigeminal root by an arterial loop and occasionally by a vein. With the aid of an operating microscope, the artery loop is lifted from the nerve to relieve the pressure, and a small prosthetic device is inserted to prevent recurrence of impingement on the nerve. This procedure relieves facial pain while preserving normal sensation. It is a major procedure, involving a craniotomy. The postoperative management is the same as for any intracranial operation (see Chap. 56).

Nursing Interventions

Preoperative management of a patient with trigeminal neuralgia includes recognizing that certain factors may aggravate excruciating facial pain, such as food that is too hot or too cold or jarring the bed. Even washing the face, combing the hair, or brushing the teeth may produce acute bouts of pain. The nurse can lessen these discomforts in a variety of ways—by using cotton pads and room-temperature water to wash the patient's face, instructing the patient to rinse the mouth after eating when tooth brushing causes pain, and performing personal hygiene during pain-free intervals. The patient is advised to take food and fluids at room temperature, to chew on the unaffected side, and to ingest soft foods when maintenance of nutrition is a problem. The nurse is aware that anxiety, depression, and insomnia often accompany chronic painful conditions and uses appropriate interventions and referrals.

Bell's Palsy

Bell's palsy (facial paralysis) is due to peripheral involvement of the seventh cranial nerve on one side, which results in weakness or paralysis of the facial muscles. The cause is unknown, although possible causes may include vascular ischemia, viral disease (herpes simplex, herpes zoster), autoimmune disease, or a combination of all of these factors.

Pathophysiology

Bell's palsy is considered by some to represent a type of pressure paralysis. The inflamed, edematous nerve becomes compressed to the point of damage, or its nutrient vessel is occluded to the point of producing ischemic necrosis of the nerve within its long canal—a channel in which the fit at best is very snug. There is distortion of the face from paralysis of the facial muscles; increased lacrimation (tearing); and painful sensations in the face, behind the ear, and in the eye. The patient may experience speech difficulties and may be unable to eat on the affected side because of relaxation of the facial muscles.

Management

The objectives of treatment are to maintain the muscle tone of the face and to prevent or minimize denervation. The patient should be reassured that no stroke has occurred and that spontaneous recovery occurs within 3 to 5 weeks in most patients.

Steroid therapy (prednisone) may be given to reduce inflammation and edema, which in turn reduces vascular compression and permits restoration of blood circulation to the nerve. Early administration of the drug appears to diminish the severity of the disease, relieve the pain, and help prevent or minimize denervation.

Facial pain is controlled with analgesics. Heat may be applied to the involved side of the face to promote comfort and the flow of blood through the muscles.

Electrical stimulation may be applied to the face to prevent muscle atrophy. Although most patients recover with conservative treatment, surgical exploration of the facial nerve may be undertaken in patients who are suspected of having a tumor or for surgical decompression of the facial nerve and for surgical rehabilitation of a paralyzed face.

Patient Education and Home Health Care

While the paralysis lasts, the involved eye must be protected. Frequently, the patient's eye does not close completely, and the blink reflex is diminished so that the eye is vulnerable to dust and foreign particles. Corneal irritation and ulceration are potential complications in these patients. Sometimes there is an overflow of tears down the cheek (*epiphora*) from keratitis caused by drying of the cornea and absence of the blink reflex. The laxity of the lower lid alters the proper drainage of tears. To manage these problems, the eye should be covered with a protective shield at night. The eye patch may abrade the cornea, however, because there is some difficulty in keeping the partially paralyzed eyelids closed. The application of eye ointment at bedtime causes the eyelids to adhere to one another and remain closed during sleep. The patient can be taught to close the paralyzed eyelid manually before going to sleep. Wraparound sunglasses or goggles are worn to decrease normal evaporation from the eye.

If the nerve is not too sensitive, the face may be massaged several times daily to maintain muscle tone. The technique is to massage the face with a gentle upward motion. Facial exercises, such as wrinkling the forehead, blowing out the cheeks, and whistling, may be performed with the aid of a mirror and are intended to prevent muscle atrophy. The face should be kept warm.

Disorders of the Peripheral Nervous System

Peripheral Neuropathies

A peripheral neuropathy is a disorder affecting the peripheral motor, sensory, or autonomic nerves. Peripheral nerves, by connecting the spinal cord and brain to all other organs, transmit motor impulses outward and relay sensory impulses to encode sensation in the brain. A *mononeuropathy* affects a single peripheral nerve, whereas the involvement of multiple single peripheral nerves or their branches is termed *multiple mononeuropathy or mononeuritis multiplex*. *Polyneuropathies* are characterized by bilaterally symmetric disturbance of function, usually beginning in the feet and hands. (Most nutritional, metabolic, and toxic neuropathies take this form.)

The most common causes of peripheral neuropathy are diabetes, alcoholism, and occlusive vascular disease. Many bacterial and metabolic toxins and exogenous poisons also affect the structure and function of the peripheral nerves. Because of the growing use of chemicals in industry, agriculture, and medicine, the number of substances known to cause peripheral neuropathies is increasing. In the developing countries, leprosy is a major cause of severe nerve disease because *Mycobacterium leprae* invade the peripheral nervous system.

The major symptoms of peripheral nerve disorders are loss of sensation, muscle atrophy, weakness, diminished reflexes, pain, and paresthesia (tingling, prickling) of the extremities. The patient frequently describes some part of the extremity as numb. Autonomic features include decreased or reduced sweating, orthostatic hypotension, nocturnal diarrhea, tachycardia, impotence, and atrophic skin and nail changes.

Peripheral nerve disorders are diagnosed by electromyography and the recording of the nerve and muscle responses evoked when electrical stimulation is applied to a nerve.

Mononeuropathy

Mononeuropathy is limited to a single peripheral nerve and its branches. It arises when the trunk of the nerve is compressed or entrapped (as by carpal tunnel syndrome, Chap. 61); traumatized, as when bruised by a blow, or overstretched, as in cases of dislocation of a joint; punctured by a needle used to inject a drug, or damaged by the drugs thus injected; or inflamed because an adjacent infectious process extends to the nerve's trunk. Mononeuropathy is frequently seen in the patient with diabetes.

Pain is seldom a conspicuous symptom of mononeuropathy when the condition is due to trauma, but in patients with complicating inflammatory conditions, such as arthritis, this feature is prominent. Such pain is increased by all body movements that tend to stretch, strain, or cause pressure on the injured nerve, and by all sudden jarrings of the body, such as those associated with coughing and sneezing. The skin in the areas supplied by nerves that are injured or diseased may become reddened and glossy; its subcutaneous tissue may become edematous, and the nutrition of the nails and the hair in this area defective. Chemical injuries to a nerve trunk, such as those caused by drugs injected into or near it, often are permanent.

Management.   The objective of treatment of mononeuropathy is to remove the cause, if possible, such as by freeing the compressed nerve. Local steroid injections may lessen inflammation, resulting in less pressure on the nerve. Pain may be relieved by aspirin or codeine.

Causalgia

Causalgia (Greek word for heat and pain) refers to the group of signs and symptoms that follow peripheral nerve injuries. The nerves most often affected, in order of frequency, are the median, the ulnar, the radial, and the internal and external popliteals.

The chief symptom of causalgia is severe burning pain along the course of the injured nerve. The pain may be described as hot, burning, stabbing, or crushing. This is more or less persistent but becomes severe after such physical stimuli as the contact of clothes. The skin over the affected extremity becomes hot, shiny, and, at times, swollen; it shows abnormalities in sweating, and eventually undergoes atrophic changes involving the nails also. The patient holds the extremity quiet, because each movement tends to increase the pain.

Sympathetic nerve blocks, repair of local nerve lesions, and aggressive physical therapy are part of the treatment program. Experience with war-related injuries showed that active and passive exercises with very early mobilization appeared to reduce the incidence of causalgia after wounds of the extremities.

Guillain-Barré Syndrome (Polyradiculoneuritis)

Guillain-Barré syndrome is a clinical syndrome of unknown cause involving the peripheral and cranial nerves. In most patients, the syndrome is preceded by an infection (respiratory or gastrointestinal) 1 to 4 weeks before the onset of neurologic deficits. In some instances, it has occurred after vaccination or surgery. It may be due to a primary viral infection, an immune reaction, some other process, or a combination of processes. One hypothesis is that a viral infection induces an autoimmune reaction that attacks the myelin of the peripheral nerves. (*Myelin* is a substance that surrounds or ensheaths the axons of certain nerves and plays an important role in the transmission of nerve impulses.)

Proximal portions of the nerves tend to be affected most often, and the nerve roots within the subarachnoid space are commonly involved. Autopsy findings have shown inflammatory edema and demyelination with some lymphocytic infiltration that is especially prominent in the spinal nerve roots.

Clinical Manifestations

There is variation in the mode of onset. The initial neurologic symptoms are *paresthesia* (tingling and numbness) and muscle weakness of the legs, which may progress to the upper extremities, trunk, and facial muscles. Muscle weakness may be followed quickly by complete paralysis. The cranial nerves are frequently affected, leading to paralysis of the ocular, facial, and oropharyngeal muscles and thus causing marked difficulty in talking, chewing, and swallowing. Autonomic dysfunction frequently occurs and takes the form of over-reactivity or under-reactivity of the sympathetic or parasympathetic nervous systems, as manifested by disturbances of heart rate and rhythm, blood pressure changes (transient hypertension, orthostatic hypotension), and a variety of other vasomotor disturbances. There may be severe and persistent pain in the back and calves of the legs. Frequently the patient exhibits loss of position sense as well as diminished or absent tendon reflexes. Sensory changes are manifested by paresthesias.

Most patients make a full recovery over several months to a year, but about 10% are left with a residual disability.

Diagnostic Evaluation

The spinal fluid shows an increased protein concentration with a normal cell count. Electrophysiologic testing demonstrates marked slowing of nerve conduction velocity.

Management

Guillain-Barré syndrome is considered a medical emergency, and the patient is managed in an intensive care unit. A patient with respiratory problems requires mechanical ventilation, sometimes for prolonged periods. *Plasmapheresis* (plasma exchange), which produces a temporary reduction in circulating antibodies, may be used in the severely affected and deteriorating patient to limit the deterioration and demyelination. Continuous ECG monitoring may be required because of possible alteration in heartbeat. Cardiac dysrhythmias associated with autonomic abnormalities are treated with propranolol to prevent tachycardia and hypertension. Atropine may be administered to avoid episodes of bradycardia during endotracheal suctioning and physical therapy.

▶ Nursing Process
The Patient With Guillain-Barré Syndrome

◇ Assessment

Careful and continuing assessment of respiratory function is essential because respiratory insufficiency and failure due to weakness or paralysis of the intercostal and diaphragm muscles may develop *quickly*. In fact, this is the main threat to life. The patient's vital capacity is monitored around the clock to anticipate respiratory insufficiency. A decreasing vital capacity along with weakness of the muscles used in swallowing, which causes difficulty in coughing and swallowing, indicates deterioration of respiratory function. Signs to watch for are breathlessness while talking, shallow and irregular breathing, increasing pulse rate, use of accessory muscles while breathing, and any *change* in the respiratory pattern.

Because the diaphragm is the prime muscle of inspiration, the patient is observed for paradoxical inward movement of the upper abdominal wall while in a supine position. This is a sign of weakness and impending paralysis of the diaphragm.

▷ *Assessment for Complications.* Assessment for complications of Guillain-Barré syndrome involves constant monitoring for the life-threatening problem of acute respiratory failure. Other complications include cardiac dysrhythmias, which necessitate ECG monitoring and observing the patient for signs of deep vein thrombosis and pulmonary embolism, ever-present threats to any immobilized and paralyzed patient.

▷ Nursing Diagnoses

Based on the assessment data, the patient's major diagnoses may include the following:

- Ineffective breathing pattern and gas exchange related to rapidly progressive weakness and impending respiratory failure
- Impaired physical mobility related to paralysis
- Altered nutrition, less than body requirements, related to inability to swallow, which is secondary to cranial nerve dysfunction
- Impaired verbal communication related to cranial nerve dysfunction
- Fear related to loss of control and paralysis

▷ Planning and Implementation

▷ *Goals:* The major goals of the patient may include attainment of respiratory function and spontaneous breathing, achievement of mobility, accomplishment of normal nutrition, achievement of communication, and resolution of fear.

▷ Nursing Interventions

▷ *Respiratory Function.* The patient with Guillain-Barré syndrome is absolutely dependent on nursing surveillance and care for recovery. Mechanical ventilation probably is required if serial measurements of the patient's vital capacity show progressive deterioration, indicating worsening of respiratory muscle power. A particularly dangerous situation occurs when the patient has difficulty in coughing and swallowing, which may cause aspiration of saliva and precipitate acute respiratory failure. The management of the patient requiring mechanical ventilation is a team effort and is discussed in Chapter 25. Chest physical therapy is usually indicated if crackles are heard on auscultation.

▷ *Promotion of Mobility.* The paralyzed extremities are supported in functional positions and given passive range-of-motion exercises at least twice daily. The nurse collaborates with the physical therapist to prevent contracture deformities by using careful positioning and range-of-motion exercises. Deep vein thrombosis and pulmonary embolism are threats to the paralyzed patient, who is unable to move his extremities. Nursing interventions include ensuring adequate hydration, assisting with physical therapy, and administering the prescribed anticoagulant regimen.

A paralyzed person has the potential to develop compression neuropathies, most often of the ulnar and peroneal nerves. Padding may be placed over the elbows and head of the fibula to prevent this problem. The prevention of pressure ulcers is a major nursing challenge. For severely paralyzed patients, the principles of nursing management of the unconscious patient (Chap. 56) may be applied, although these patients are in full possession of their mental faculties.

When recovery begins to take place, these patients may experience orthostatic hypotension (from autonomic dysfunction) and probably require the use of a tilt table to help them assume an upright posture.

▷ *Adequate Nutrition.* Attention is paid to adequate nutrition and prevention of muscle wasting. Paralytic ileus may result from insufficient parasympathetic activity. In this event, intravenous feedings are prescribed by the physician and monitored by the nurse until bowel sounds are heard. If the patient is unable to swallow, nasogastric tube feedings may be prescribed. When the patient can swallow normally, oral feeding is gradually resumed.

▷ *Improved Communication.* Because of paralysis, tracheostomy, and intubation, the patient is unable to talk, laugh, or cry, and thus has no outlet for emotional expression. These problems are compounded by boredom, dependency, isolation, and frustration. To establish some form of communication, lipreading and the use of picture cards, combined with a system of blinking the eyes to indicate yes or no, may be tried. If the patient remains on the ventilator for a prolonged period, a referral to a speech-language pathologist may be made. Diversional therapy (television, cassette tapes, visits from the family) can alleviate some of the frustrations that are encountered.

▷ *Relief of Anxiety and Fear.* Involving the family and friends with selected patient care activities, reading aloud, and the like will reduce the sense of isolation of the patient. Nursing interventions that are helpful in increasing the patient's sense of control (and hence reduction of fear) include giving him information about his condition, emphasizing a positive appraisal of coping resources, involving him in relaxation exercises and distraction techniques, and giving positive feedback. The attitude and atmosphere created by the nurse, physical therapist, and occupational therapist are important. Giving expert nursing care, explanations, and reassurance helps the patient gain some control over his situation.

▷ *Patient Education.* After discharge from the hospital, patients are encouraged to continue with the exercise program. A walker may be required for ambulation. Patients are cautioned about becoming fatigued and overworking muscles. "Take one day at a time" is good advice when the patient feels overwhelmed with problems of fatigue. The Guillain-Barré support group offers emotional support and information booklets.

▷ Evaluation

Expected Outcomes
1. Attains spontaneous breathing and normal respiratory function
   a. Has vital capacity within normal range
   b. Has been weaned from mechanical ventilation
2. Shows increasing mobility
   a. Is able to move all extremities
   b. Participates in rehabilitation program
3. Demonstrates ability to swallow
   a. Expresses desire for food
   b. Consumes oral fluids and food
4. Demonstrates recovery of speech
   a. Talks without undue breathlessness
   b. Can make needs known

5. Shows lessening fear
   a. Sleeps at longer intervals
   b. Appears more relaxed; does not appear anxious

Chapter Summary

The complexity of the central nervous system and its important role in mediating cognitive, motor, and sensory function make neurologic disorders particularly devastating to patients and their families. Neurologic disorders range from occasional headache that may cause no disruption in activities to acute and chronic disorders that may be debilitating and life threatening. The nurse caring for the patient with a neurologic disorder must have an appreciation of the complex functions of the nervous system, highly developed assessment skills, and an understanding of and sensitivity to the anxiety and fear experienced by the patient and his family. Although many patients with neurologic disorders are initially treated in acute care facilities, including neurologic/neurosurgical intensive care units, they also require consideration of their rehabilitation needs from the moment of entry into the health system.

Management of the patient with neurologic disorders requires the collaboration and cooperation of all members of the health care team; the health care team is frequently involved in the care of an individual for many years and that care often extends into the home and community. An important role for the nurse is coordination of the services required by the patient and his family, as it is often easy to lose sight of the complex regimens that are often required of patients and their families as they cope with neurologic disorders.

Bibliography

Books

Adams R and Victor M. Principles of Neurology, 4th ed. New York, McGraw-Hill, 1989.

Adler CS. Psychiatric Aspects of Headache. Baltimore, Williams & Wilkins, 1987.

Albert M (ed). Clinical Neurology of Aging. New York, Oxford University Press, 1984.

Becker DP et al. Head Injury. Philadelphia, WB Saunders, 1989.

Block R and Basbaum M. Management of Spinal Cord Injuries. Baltimore, Williams & Wilkins, 1986.

Brandstater ME. Stroke Rehabilitation. Baltimore, Williams & Wilkins, 1987.

Cook SD (ed). Handbook of Multiple Sclerosis. New York, Marcel Dekker, 1990.

Cooper P (ed). Head Injury, 2nd ed. Baltimore, Williams & Wilkins, 1987.

Crompton R. Closed Head Injury: Its Pathology and Legal Medicine. London, Williams & Wilkins, 1988.

Dalessio D. Wolf's Headache and Other Pain, 5th ed. New York, Oxford University Press, 1987.

Dipple R and Hutton JT (eds). Caring for the Parkinson's Patient: A Care Giver Guide. New York, Golden Age Books, 1989.

Drachman DB (ed). Myasthenia Gravis: Biology and Treatment. New York, Academy of Science, 1987.

Ferrari MD and Fataste X (eds). Migraine and Other Headaches. Park Ridge, NJ, Parthenon, 1989.

Frieschmann RB. Spinal Cord Injuries: Psychological, Social and Vocational Rehabilitation. New York, Demos Publishing Inc, 1988.

Frowein RA et al (eds). Head Injuries. New York, Springer-Verlag, 1989.

Grant J and Kennedy-Caldwell C. Nutrition Support in Nursing. Philadelphia, Grune & Stratton, 1988.

Griffin M. Going the Distance: Living a Full Life with Multiple Sclerosis and other Debilitating Diseases. New York, Dutton, 1989.

Hickey JV. The Clinical Practice of Neurological and Neurosurgical Nursing, 2nd ed. Philadelphia, JB Lippincott, 1986.

Jennett HB and Teasdale G. Management of Head Injuries. Philadelphia, FA Davis, 1981.

Lechtenberg R. Seizure Diagnosis and Management. Philadelphia, FA Davis, 1990.

McDonald WI and Silberberg DH (eds). Multiple Sclerosis. Stoneham, MA, Butterworths, 1986.

Plum F and Posner J. The Diagnosis of Stupor and Coma, 3rd ed. Philadelphia, FA Davis, 1982.

Richardson T and McKinlay W. Clinical and Neuropsychological Aspects of Closed Head Injury. New York, Taylor & Francis, 1990.

Rose FC (ed). The Management of Headache. New York, Raven Press, 1988.

Rosenthal M et al (eds). Rehabilitation of the Adult and Child with Traumatic Brain Injury, 2nd ed. Philadelphia, FA Davis, 1990.

Scheinberg LC and Holland NJ (eds). Multiple Sclerosis: A Guide for Patients and Their Families, 2nd ed. New York, Raven Press, 1987.

Stern M and Hurtig H (eds). The Comprehensive Management of Parkinson's Disease. Great Neck, PMA Publishing Corp, 1988.

Wirth F and Ratcheson R. Neurosurgical Critical Care. Baltimore, Williams & Wilkins, 1987.

Whiteman S and Herman BP (eds). Psychopathology in Epilepsy: Social Factors. New York, Oxford University Press, 1987.

Yahr M and Bergmann K (eds). Parkinson's Disease. New York, Raven Press, 1987.

Journals
Asterisks indicate nursing research articles.

Amyotrophic Lateral Sclerosis

Ashford W. ALS. Cleaning up the confusion about this paralytic disease can lead to better care of the patient. RNABC News 1987 Jan/Feb; 19(1):14–15.

Bay EJ. George wasn't ready to die. Nursing 1988 Aug; 18(8):52–53.

Beisecker AE et al. Patient's perspectives of the role of care providers in amyotrophic lateral sclerosis. Arch Neurol 1988 May; 45(5):553–556.

Carpenter J. Once a coach . . . always a coach: ALS patient "coaches" students through home health clinicals . . . amyotrophic lateral sclerosis. J Pract Nurs 1988 Dec; 38(4):32–33.

Evans R et al. Motor neurone disease. Nursing (Lond) 1989 Jan; 3(33):9–11.

Knapp MT. Jim's new world. Nursing 1987 Jul; 17(7):96.

Peters B. MND: A personal profile: Motor neurone disease. Aust Nurses J 1989 Mar; 18(8):8–10.

Preikschas J. ALS. A case study: Caring for ALS patients. RNABC News 1987 Jan/Feb; 19(1):17–18.

Roche J. Spirituality and the ALS patient. Rehabil Nurs 1989 May/Jun; 14(3):139–141.

Sebring DL et al. Amyotrophic lateral sclerosis: Psychosocial interventions for patients and their families. Health Soc Work 1987 Spring; 12(2):113–201.

Stone N. Amyotrophic lateral sclerosis: A challenge for constant adaptation. 1987 Jun; 19(3):166–173.

Taylor SG. Nursing theory and nursing process: Orem's theory in practice. Nurs Sci Q 1988 Aug; 1(3):111–119.

Woy D. In Lynne's eyes. Nursing 1987 Nov; 17 (11):152.

Aneurysm and Subarachnoid Hemorrhage

Asby D. Ruptured cerebral aneurysm: Case studies. J Post Anesth Nurs 1986 Feb; 1(1):57–59.

Bisnaire D. Cerebral aneurysms and subarachnoid hemorrhage: An overview. Axon 1987 Mar; 8(3):73–78.

Fode NC. Subarachnoid hemorrhage from a ruptured intracranial aneurysm. Am J Nurs 1988 May; 88(5):673–679.

Stewart-Amidei C. Hypervolemic hemodilution: A new approach to subarachnoid hemorrhage. Heart Lung 1989 Nov; 18(6):590–595.

Willis D et al. A fatal attraction: Cocaine related subarachnoid hemorrhage. J Neurosci Nurs 1989 Jun; 21(3):171–174.

Brain Tumor

Bonner K and Siegel KR. Pathology, treatment and management of posterior fossa brain tumors in childhood. J Neurosci Nurs 1988 Apr; 20(2): 84–93.

Hodges K. Meningioma, astrocytoma and germinoma: Case presentations of three intracranial tumors. J Neurosci Nurs 1989 Apr; 21(2):113–121.

Kinash RG. Malignant brain tumors: Therapies and nursing interventions. Axone 1987 Sep; 9(1):7–11.

Koch F et al. Targeting cerebral tumors: Combining image-guided stereotactic endoscopy with laser therapy. AORN J 1989 Mar; 49(3):740–741, 743, 745–747.

Leclerc DB. Infusion of intra-arterial chemotherapy through superselective cerebral catheterization. Axone 1987 Sep; 9(1):18–21.

Randal TM et al. Neuro-oncology update: Radiation safety and nursing care during interstitial brachytherapy. J Neurosci Nurs 1987 Dec; 19(6): 315–320.

Resio MH and DeVroom HL. Spiromustine and intracarotid artery cisplatin in the treatment of glioblastoma multiforme. J Neurosci Nurs 1986 Feb; 18(1):13–22.

Shpritz DW. Neurologic aspects of critical care: Brain tumor basics. Crit Care Nurs 1986 Sep/Oct; 6(5):94–96.

Welsh DM and Zumwalt CB. Volumetric interstitial hyperthermia: Nursing implications for brain tumor treatment. J Neurosci Nurs 1988 Aug; 20(4):229–235.

Werner M and Schold S. Primary intracranial neoplasms in the elderly. Clin Geriatr Med 1987 Nov; 3(4):765–780.

Wicker P. Discussion group summary: When caring doesn't mean curing. NLN 1988 Oct; (15-2237):53–55.

Willis A. The final journey. Nurs Times 1988 Dec; 84(50):26–28.

Guillain-Barré Syndrome

A man alone—and afraid: Caring for a patient with Guillain-Barré Syndrome. Nursing grand rounds. Nursing 1989 Dec; 17(12):44–48.

Fawcett M. Lessons from a patient. AD Nurse 1987 Nov/Dec; 2(6):11–13.

George MR. Neuromuscular respiratory failure: What a nurse knows may make the difference. J Neurosci Nurs 1988 Apr; 20(2):110–117.

Sic S et al. Immobility syndrome: Use it or lose it. AD Nurse 1987 Nov/Dec; 2(6):6–10.

Uprichard E et al. Guillian-Barré syndrome: Patients' and nurses' perspectives. Intens Care Nurs 1987 Mar 2; (3):123–134.

Yarnin M et al. Guillian-Barré syndrome: A nursing challenge. Aust Nurses J 1988 May; 17(10):8–10.

Headache

Daroff R. New headache classification. Neurology 1988 Jul; 8(7):1138–1139.

Derman H. Migraine headache: Old, newer and new treatments. Consultant 1988 Sep; 28(A):31–38.

Headache Classification Committee of the International Headache Society. Classification and diagnostic criteria for headache disorders, cranial neuralgias and facial pain. Cephalgia 1988 Aug; 8(7):9–96.

*Kunzar MB. Marital adjustment of headache sufferers and their spouses. J Psychosoc Nurs Ment Health Serv 1987 May; 25(5):12–17.

Smith LS. Evaluation and management of muscle contraction headache. Nurse Pract 1988 Jan; 13(1):20–23, 26–27.

Whitney C and Daroff R. An approach to migraine. J Neurosci Nurs 1988 Oct; 20(5):284–289.

Head Injury

Anderson BJ. The metabolic needs of head trauma victims. J Neurosci Nurs 1987 Aug; 19(4):211–215.

Baggerly J. Rehabilitation of the adult with head trauma. Nurs Clin North Am 1986 Dec; 21(4):577–587.

Batchelor J et al. Cognitive rehabilitation of severely closed-head injured patients using computer-assisted and noncomputerized treatment techniques. J Head Trauma Rehabil 1988 Sep; 3(3):78–85.

Bell TN. Nurses' attitudes in caring for the comatose head-injured patient. J Neurosci Nurs 1986 Oct; 18(5):279–289.

Blackerby WF. Practical token economics . . . Neurologically impaired. J Head Trauma Rehabil 1988 Sep; 3(3):33–45.

Brotherton FA et al. Social skills training in the rehabilitation of patients with traumatic closed head injury. Arch Phys Med Rehabil 1988 Oct; 69(10):827–832.

Burns PG. Reentry of the head injured survivor into the educational system: First steps. J Community Health Nurs 1987 Mar; 4(3):145–152.

Bush GW. The National Head Injury Foundation: Eight years of challenge and growth. J Head Trauma Rehabil 1988 Dec; 3(4):73–77.

Byrnes MB et al. FIM: Its use in identifying rehabilitation needs in the head-injured patient. J Neurosci Nurs 1989 Feb; 21(1):61–63.

Campbell CH. Needs of relatives and helpfulness of support groups in severe head injury. Rehabil Nurs 1988 Nov/Dec; 13(6):520–525.

Carpenter R. Infections and head injury: A potentially lethal combination. Crit Care Nurs Q 1987 Dec; 10(3):1–11.

Cline DM et al. Observation of head trauma patients at home: A prospective study of compliance in the rural south. Ann Emerg Med 1988 Feb; 17(2):127–131.

*Crosby L et al. Clinical neurologic assessment tool: Development and testing of an instrument to index neurologic status. Heart Lung 1989 Mar; 18(2):121–129.

Date E et al. Relatives familiar faces. Nurs Times 1987 Sep 16–22; 83(37): 26–27.

Davidoff G et al. Closed head injury in acute traumatic spinal cord injury: Incidence and risk factors. Arch Phys Med Rehabil 1988 Oct; 69(10): 869–872.

Davidson L. The forgotten injury. Nurs Times 1989 Jan; 85(4):31–32.

DeChancie H et al. An enclosure for the disoriented head-injured patient. J Neurosci Nurs 1987 Dec; 19(6):34.

Diktaban T et al. Face the challenge. Emergency 1988 Nov; 20(11):42–45.

Do HK et al. Head trauma rehabilitation: Program evaluation. Rehabil Nurs 1988 Mar/Apr; 13(2):71–75.

Eames P. Behavior disorders after severe head injury: Their nature and causes and strategies for management. J Head Trauma Rehabil 1988 Sep; 3(3):1–6.

Frye B. Head injury and the family: Related literature. Rehabil Nurs 1987 May/Jun; 12(3):135–136.

Gerold KB. Special problems in post trauma respiratory management: Maxillofacial, head and chest injuries. Crit Care Nurs Q 1988 Sep; 11(2):59–62.

Gibbs J et al. Rehabilitation in head injury: A case study. Rehabil Nurs 1987 May/Jun; 12(3):137–138.

Guentz SJ. Cognitive rehabilitation of the head injured patient. Crit Care Nurs Q 1987 Dec; 10(3):51–60.

Hannegan L. Transient cognitive changes after craniotomy. J Neurosci Nurs 1989 Jun; 21(3):165–170.

Hinkle JL et al. Restoring social competence in minor head injury patients. J Neurosci Nurs 1986 Oct; 18(5):268–271.

Hogan RT. Behavior management for community reintegration. J Head Trauma Rehabil 1988 Sep; 3(3):62–71.

Holosko MJ et al. Perceived social adjustment and social support among a sample of head injured adults. Can J Rehabil 1989 Spring; 2(3): 145–154.

Howard ME. Behavior management in the acute care rehabilitation setting. J Head Trauma Rehabil 1988 Sep; 3(3):14–22.

Hugo M. Alleviating the effects of care on the intracranial pressure (ICP) of head injured patients by manipulating nursing care activities. Intens Care Nurs 1987 Feb; 3(2):78–82.

Ingersoll GL et al. The Glasgow Coma Scale for patients with head injuries. Crit Care Nurse 1987 Sep/Oct; 7(5):26–32.

Jacobs HE. The Los Angeles Head Injury Survey: Procedures and initial findings. Crit Care Nurse 1987 Sep/Oct; 7(5):26–32.

Johnson D et al. Head injury: Early rehabilitation of head-injured patients. Nurs Times 1989 Jan; 85(4):25–28.

*Kater KM. Response of head-injured patients to sensory stimulation. West J Nurs Res 1989 Feb; 11(1):20–33.

Katz N et al. Loewenstein Occupational Therapy Cognitive Assessment (LOTCA) battery for brain injured patients: Reliability and validity. Am J Occup Ther 1989 Mar; 43(3):184–192.

Kolpan KL. Medical malpractice. 1989 Jun; 4(2):79–80.

*Kozak GS et al. A comparison of teaching methods for ED discharge instruction after head injury. J Emerg Nurs 1989 Jan/Feb; 15(1):18–22.

Krefting L. Reintegration into the community after head injury: The results of an ethnographic study. Occup Ther J Res 1989 Mar/Apr; 9(2):67–83.

*Lee S. Intracranial pressure changes during positioning of patients with severe head injury. Heart Lung 1989 Jul; 18(4):411–414.

London PS. A long look at head injuries. Br J Occup Ther 1989 Mar; 52(3):43–50.

Lynch W. Memory assessment: The next step. J Head Trauma Rehabil 1988 Dec; 3(4):100–102.

MacKay-Lyons M. Low-load, prolonged stretch in treatment of elbow flexion contractures secondary to head trauma. Phys Ther 1989 Apr; 69(4):292–296.

McGinley WJ. SNF-based care for the head injured. Provider 1988 Aug; 14(8):28, 30.

McKinlay WW et al. How can families help in the rehabilitation of the head injured? J Head Trauma Rehabil 1988 Dec; 3(4):64–72.

McPhee AT. Let the family in. J Emerg Nurs 1987 Mar/Apr; 13(2):120–121.

Milton SB. Management of subtle cognitive communication. J Head Trauma Rehabil 1988 Jun; 3(2):1–11.

Moore HS et al. Emergency care of the patient with neurogenic pulmonary edema. J Emerg Nurs 1987 Jul/Aug; 13(4):244–248.

Moore TH et al. The use of tone-reducing casts to prevent joint contractures following severe closed head injury. J Head Trauma Rehabil 1989 Jun; 4(2):63–65.

Neger RE. Evaluation of diplopia in head trauma. J Head Trauma Rehabil 1989 Jun; 4(2):27–34.

Nikas DL. Prognostic indicators in patients with severe head injury. Crit Care Nurs Q 1987 Dec; 10(3):25–34.

Patterson TS and Sargent M. Behavioral management of the agitated head trauma client. Rehabil Nurs 1990 Sep/Oct; 15(5):248–253.

Rees R. How some families cope and why some families do not. J Head Trauma Rehabil 1988 Sep; 3(3):72–77.

Reimer M. Head injured patients: How to detect early signs of trouble. Nursing 1989 Mar; 19(3):34–42.

Rudy EB et al. The relationship between endotracheal suctioning and changes in intracranial pressure: a review of the literature. Heart Lung 1986 Sep; 15(5):488–494.

Shordone RJ. Assessment and treatment of cognitive–communicative impairments in the closed head injured patient: A neurobehavioral systems approach. J Head Trauma Rehabil 1988 Jun; 3(2):55–62.

*Smith KA. Head trauma: Comparison of infection rates for different methods of intracranial pressure monitoring. J Neurosci Nurs 1987 Dec; 19(6):310–314.

Sparadeo FR et al. Effects of prior alcohol use on head injury recovery. J Head Trauma Rehabil 1989 Mar; 4(1):75–81.

Stavros MK. Family issues in moderate to severe head injury. Crit Care Nurs Q 1987 Dec; 10(3):73–82.

Stevens SA et al. A simple step-by-step approach to neurologic assessment Part I. Nursing 1988 Sep; 18(9):53–61.

Stewart-Amidei C. What to do until the neurosurgeon arrives. J Emerg Nurs 1988 Sep/Oct; 14(5):296–301.

Talbot RJ. Headway: The first nine years, 1979 to 1988. J Head Trauma Rehabil 1988 Dec; 3(4):78–81.

Temple AP et al. Management of acute head injury. Implications for perioperative nurses. AORN J 1987 Dec; 46(6):1066–1076.

Turnbull J. Perils (hidden and not so hidden) for the token economy . . . Behavior modification. J Head Trauma Rehabil 1988 Sep; 3(3):46–52.

Well T et al. Action Stat! Closed head injury. Nursing 1988 Nov; 18(11):33.

Winslade WJ et al. Prognosis in head injury: Legal and ethical issues. Crit Care Nurs Q 1987 Dec; 10(3):35–42.

Woody S. Episodic dyscontrol syndrome and head injury: A case presentation. J Neurosci Nurs 1988 Jun; 20(3):180–184.

Zarski JJ et al. Traumatic head injury: Dimensions of family responsibility. J Head Trauma Rehabil 1988 Dec; 3(4):31–41.

Zucker L. Transport of the neurologically injured patient. Emerg Care Q 1989 Feb; 4(4):40–47.

Huntington's Disease

Clark M and Zabarsky M. Decoding a killer disease Huntington's disease. Newsweek 1983 Nov 21; 102(21):107.

Hunt VP. Dysphagia in Huntington's disease. J Neurosci Nurs 1989 Apr; 21(2):92–95.

Jackson L. A predictive test for Huntington's disease: Recombinant DNA technology and implications for nursing. J Neurosci Nurs 1987 Oct; 19(5):244–250.

Levine J et al. Do they really want to know? A new test confounds potential Huntington's disease victims. Time 1986 Oct 20; 128(16):80.

Peacock IW. A physical therapy program for Huntington's disease patients. Clin Manage Phys Ther 1987 Jan/Feb; 7(1):22–23.

Small O. Huntington's chorea. Nurs Times 1986 Apr; 82(15):32–33.

Meningitis and Brain Abscess

Coderre C. Meningitis: Dangers when the diagnosis is viral. RN 1989 Aug; 52(8):50–54.

Gilliland K. Epidural abscesses of the spine: Case comparisons. J Neurosci Nurs 1989 Jun; 21(3):185–189.

Grabbe LL et al. Identifying neurologic complications of AIDS. Nursing 1989 May; 19(5):66–68.

Gryfinski J. Intramedullary spinal cord abscesses. J Neurosci Nurs 1988 Feb; 20(1):34–38.

McArthur JH et al. Human immunodeficiency virus and the nervous system. Nurs Clin North Am 1988 Dec; 23(4):823–841.

Prendergast V. Bacterial meningitis update. J Neurosci Nurs 1987 Apr; 19(2):95–99.

*Smith KA. Head trauma: Comparison of infection rates for different methods of intracranial pressure monitoring. J Neurosci Nurs 1987 Dec; 19(6):310–314.

Strampfer MJ et al. Laboratory aids in the diagnosis of bacterial meningitis. Winthrop University Hospital Infectious Disease Symposium. Heart Lung 1988 Nov; 17(6):605–607.

Travers GR et al. Neurological complications in acquired immune deficiency syndrome. Axone 1987 Jun; 8(4):107–111.

Wilson J. Paediatric bacterial meningitis. Aust Nurses J 1987 Jun; 16(11):46–48.

Multiple Sclerosis

Asburn A et al. An approach to the management of multiple sclerosis. Physiother Pract 1988 Sep; 4(3):139–145.

Allan S. ARMS extended. Nurs Times 1987 Oct/Nov; 83(43):44–45.

Birk K et al. Pregnancy and multiple sclerosis. Semin Neurol 1988 Sep; 8(3):205–213.

Coffey K. Multiple sclerosis: The inner world. Home Health Nurse Sep/Oct 1987; 5(5):33–36.

Csesko PA. Sexuality and multiple sclerosis. J Neurosci Nurs 1988 Dec; 20(6):353–355.

Dewis ME et al. Sexual dysfunction in multiple sclerosis. J Neurosci Nurs 1989 Jun; 21(3):175–179.

Feeney S. A family affair: Considering the wide-ranging effects of chronic illness in the family. NZ Nurs J 1988 Aug; 81(8):28–30.

Ferguson JM. Helping an MS patient live a better life. 1987 Dec; 40(12): 22–27.

Francabandera FL et al. Multiple sclerosis rehabilitation: Inpatient vs outpatient. Rehabil Nurs 1988 Sep/Oct; 13(5):251–253.

Friedemann M et al. Multiple sclerosis and the family. Arch Psychiatr Nurs 1987 Feb; 1(1):47–54.

Gingrich V. Another gift given: Living with multiple sclerosis, learning about myself. Can Nurse 1988 Nov; 84(10):32–33.

*Goodkin DE et al. Upper extremity function in multiple sclerosis: Improving assessment sensitivity with box and block and nine-hole peg tests. Arch Phys Med Rehabil 1988 Oct; 69(10):850–854.

*Gulick EE. Model confirmation of the MS-related symptom checklist. Nurs Res 1989 May/Jun; 38(3):147–153.

Halper, J. The functional model in multiple sclerosis. Rehabil Nurs 1990 Mar/Apr; 15(2):77–79, 85.

Henderson JS. A subcoccygeal exercise program for simple urinary stress incontinence: Applicability to the female client with multiple sclerosis. J Neurosci Nurs 1988 Jun; 20(3):185–188.

Henderson JS. Intermittent clean self-catheterization in clients with neurogenic bladder resulting from multiple sclerosis. J Neurosci Nurs 1989 Jun; 21(3):160–164.

Henderson JS et al. The cobblestones of Scotland: Enjoying Edinburgh in a wheelchair. Kans Nurs 1988 Mar; 53(3):3.

Jones IH. Helping hands. Labor of love. Nurs Times Dec/Jan 1988; 83(51): 32–34.

Kassires MR et al. Pain in multiple sclerosis. Am J Nurs 1987 Jul; 87(7): 968–969.

Kassires MR et al. Pain in chronic multiple sclerosis. J Pain Symptom Manage 1987 Spring; 2(2):95–97.

Kelly B and Mahon SM. Nursing care of the patient with multiple sclerosis. Rehabil Nurs 1988 Sep/Oct; 13(5):238–243.

Kurtzke JF. The disability status scale for multiple sclerosis: Part I. Neurology 1989 Feb; 39(2):291–302.

Larsen, PD. Psychosocial adjustment in multiple sclerosis. Rehabil Nurs 1990 Sep/Oct; 15(5):242–246.

MacLellan M. Community care of the patient with multiple sclerosis. Nursing 1989 Jan; 3(33):28–32.

McBride EV et al. Explaining diagnostic tests for MS. Nursing 1988 Feb; 18(2):68–72.

Melia K. Everyday ethics for nurses: Whose morals are they, anyway? Nurs Times 1987 Jan/May; 83(21):44–46.

Molitor RE et al. Home intravenous administration of adrenocorticotropic hormone in patients with multiple sclerosis. J Intraven Nurs 1988 Jul/Aug; 11(4):249–251.

Oligiati R et al. Increased energy cost of walking in multiple sclerosis: Effect of spasticity, ataxia and weakness. Arch Phys Med Rehabil 1988 Oct; 69(10):846–849.

Oliver H. Continence. The treatment of choice. Nurs Times 1988 Aug; 84(31):70.

*Pollock SE et al. Responses to chronic illness: Analysis of psychological and physiological adaptation. Nurs Res 1990 Sep/Oct; 39(5):300–304.

*Sammonds RH et al. Perceptions of body image in subjects with multiple sclerosis: A pilot study. J Neurosci Nurs 1989 Jun; 21(3):190–194.

Schmitt DM. Helping Gwen to keep going. Nursing 1989 Mar; 19(3):54–56.

Shaw CA. Spasticity: Its functional implication in multiple sclerosis. Axon 1988 May; 9(4):63–65.

*Smeltzer SC et al. Pulmonary function and dysfunction in multiple sclerosis. Arch Neurol 1988 Nov; 45(11):1245–1249.

*Smeltzer SC et al. Testing of an index of pulmonary dysfunction in multiple sclerosis. Nurs Res 1989 Nov/Dec; 38(6):370–374.

Smithers K. Practical problems of mothers who have multiple sclerosis. Midwife Health Visit Community Nurse 1988 May; 24(5):165, 167–168.

*Storm DS et al. Achieving self-care in the ventilator-dependent patient: A critical analysis of a case study. Int J Nurs Stud 1987 Feb; 24(2):95–106.

Sutcliffe P. Thumbnail sketches of disabling diseases encountered by community staff, Part 2. Br J Occup Ther 1988 Jul; 51(7):235.

Thornton NG et al. Multiple sclerosis and female sexuality. Can Nurse 1989 Apr; 85(4):16–18.

Weinstein MS et al. Carbon dioxide cystometry and postural changes in patients with multiple sclerosis. Arch Phys Med Rehabil 1988 Nov; 69(11):923–927.

Wenola M. Cyclophosphamide in chronic progressive multiple sclerosis. NITA 1987 May/Jun; 10(3):219–223.

*Wineman NM. Adaptation to multiple sclerosis. The role of social support, functional disability, and perceived uncertainty. Nurs Res 1990 Sep/Oct; 39(5):294–299.

Winter S et al. A nurse-managed multiple sclerosis clinic: Improved quality of life for persons with MS. Rehabil Nurs 1989 Jan/Feb; 14(1):13–16.

Woodall L. Multiple sclerosis and patients' feelings. AARN News Lett 1988 Apr; 44(4):27.

Myasthenia Gravis

Bell J. Understanding and managing myasthenia gravis. Focus Crit Care 1989 Feb; 16(1):57–65.

Gamburg C et al. Neuromuscular diseases, myopathies and anesthesia. Curr Rev Nurse Anesth 1989 Jul 28; (11)4:26–32.

George MR. Neuromuscular respiratory failure: What the nurse knows may make the difference. J Neurosci Nurs 1988 Apr; 20(2):110–117.

Rhynsburger J. How to fight MG fatigue: Myasthenia gravis. Am J Nurs 1989 Mar; 89(3):337–340.

Parkinson's Disease

Adrenal medullary transplantation in Parkinson's disease. Nurses Drug Alert 1989 Apr; 13(4):28.

Alerman C. Parkinson's disease. Nurs Stand 1988 May; 2(32):26.

*Athlin E et al. Aberrant eating behavior in elderly Parkinsonian patients with and without dementia: Analysis of video-recorded meals. Res Nurs Health 1989 Feb; 12(1):41–51.

Baker M. The Parkinson's Disease Society. Geriatr Nurs Home Care 1988 Jan; 8(1):17–18.

Barker E. Parkinsonism: Surgical treatment requires new nursing management (editorial). J Neurosci Nurs 1987 Aug; 19(4):181.

Burford K. The physiotherapist's role in Parkinson's disease. Geriatr Nurs Home Care 1988 Jan; 8(1):14–16.

Calne S. Parkinson's disease problems in nursing management related to medications. Axon 1988 May; 9(4):55–58.

Delgado JM et al. Care of the patient with Parkinson's disease: Surgical and nursing interventions. J Neurosci Nurs 1988 Jun; 20(3):142–150.

Diet modifications may improve response to levodopa. Nurses Drug Alert 1988 Dec; 12(12):95–96.

Goetz CG et al. Update on Parkinson's disease. Patient Care 1989 Apr; 23(7):124–138.

Goto L and Braun K. Nursing home without walls. J Gerontol Nurs 1987 Jan; 3(1):18–21.

*Hurwitz A. The benefit of a home exercise regimen for ambulatory Parkinson's disease patients. J Neurosci Nurs 1989 Jun; 21(3):180–184.

Kierans CA. Parkinson's disease: A nursing challenge. Perspectives 1988 Summer; 12(2):10–14.

Looney KM. The respite care alternative. J Gerontol Nurs 1987 May; 13(5): 18–21.

Lyall J. Brave new world. Nurs Times 1988 May 25–31; 84(21):19.

Mitchell PH et al. Group exercise: A nursing therapy in Parkinson's disease. Rehabil Nurs 1987 Sep/Oct; 12(5):242–245.

Norberg A et al. The interaction between the parkinsonian patient and his care giver during feeding: A theoretical model. J Adv Nurs 1987 Sep; 12(5):545–550.

Norberg A et al. A model for the assessment of eating problems in patients with Parkinson's disease. J Adv Nurs 1987 Jul; 12(4):473–481.

Pednault E. Home care of patients with Parkinson's disease. Prim Care 1987 Sep; 4(3):485–498.

Pentland B. The management of Parkinson's disease. Geriatr Nurs Home Care 1988 Jan; 8(1):12–14.

Sargent SM et al. Autologous adrenal medulla transplant. Investigational treatment for Parkinson's disease. AORN J 1988 Mar; 47(3):682–694.

Swindin J. Never alone. Nurs Stand 1988 May; 2(32):27.

Topp B. Toward a better understanding of Parkinson's disease. Geriatr Nurs (New York) 1987 Jul/Aug; 8(4):180–182.

Van Dillen LR et al. Interrater reliability of a clinical scale of rigidity. Phys Ther 1988 Nov; 68(11):1679–1681.

Van Oteghen SL. An exercise program for those with Parkinson's disease. Geriatr Nurs (New York) 1987 Jul/Aug; 8(4):183–184.

Williams V. Parkinson's disease: Autotransplantation of adrenal medulla to caudate nucleus of the brain. J Neurosci Nurs 1987 Jun; 19(3): 174.

Peripheral Neuropathy

Bild DE et al. Lower extremity amputation in people with diabetes: Epidemiology and prevention. Diabetes Care 1989 Jan; 12(1):24–31.

Cosgrove JL et al. A prospective study of peripheral nerve lesions occurring in traumatic brain-injured patients. Am J Phys Med Rehabil 1989 Feb; 68(1):15–17.

Identifying heavy metal poisoning. Emerg Med 1989 Apr; 21(8):81.

Pease WS et al. Monopolar needle stimulation: Safety consideration. Arch Phys Med Rehabil 1989 May; 70(5):412–414

Seizure Disorders

Bare MA. Hemispherectomy for seizures. J Neurosci Nurs 1989 Feb; 21(1): 18–23.

Bernat JL. Getting a handle on an adult's first seizure. Emerg Med 1989 Jan 15; 21(1):20–28.

Callanan M. Epilepsy: Putting the patient back in control. RN 1988 Feb; 51(2):48–56.

Conley NJ et al. Current controversies in pregnancy and epilepsy: A unique challenge to nursing. J Obstet Gynecol Neonatal Nurs 1987 Sep/Oct; 16(5):321–328.

Counselman FL. When fevers lead to seizures. Emerg Med 1989 Jun 15; 21(11):186–192.

De Vroom HL et al. Advances in the localization of epileptic loci for surgical resection. J Neurosci Nurs 1987 Apr; 19(2):77–82.

Dieter DC. Corpus callostomy: The role of the nurse in family decision making. J Neurosci Nurs 1989 Aug; 21(4):234–240.

Foxton W. Managing epilepsy. Nurs Stand 1988 Jan 18; 2(37):35.

Friedman D. Taking the scare out of caring for seizure patients. Nursing 1988 Feb; 18(2):52–60.

Friedman D. Controlling epilepsy with surgery. RN 1988 Feb; 51(2):52–53.

Graham O et al. A model for ambulatory care of patients with epilepsy and other neurological disorders. J Neurosci Nurs 1989 Apr; 21(2): 108–112.

Jastremski MS et al. What to look for in seizure workups. Patient Care 1988 Oct 15; 22(16):68–76.

Koplan KL. Can a physician be held liable for certifying a person with a seizure history fit to drive? J Head Trauma Rehabil 1988 Jun; 3(2): 97.

McCormick KB. Pregnancy and epilepsy nursing implications. J Neurosci Nurs 1987 Apr; 19(2):66–76.

Mitchell A et al. Temporal lobectomy: An increasingly viable option for seizure patients. Axon 1989 Mar; 10(3):69–71.

Morrison JL. Obtaining a seizure history: Discovering a pattern. RN 1988 Feb; 51(2):54–55.

Phenobarbital for status epilepticus. Emerg Med 1988 Oct 30; 20(18):45–49.

Richardson E. Surgery for epilepsy. Nursing (Lond) 1989 Jan; 3(33):20–23.

Ross D. Dealing with epilepsy. Occup Health (Lond) 1988 Dec; 40(12): 741–743.

Santilli N et al. Advances in the treatment of epilepsy. J Neurosci Nurs 1987 Jun; 19(3):141–157.

Sneed RC et al. Interference of oral phenytoin absorption by enteral tube feedings. Arch Phys Med Rehabil 1988 Sep; 69(6):682–684.

Wiseman E et al. AANA Journal Course: Advanced scientific concepts update for nurse anesthetists: Anesthesia for patients on anticholinesterase and antiepileptic drugs. AANA J 1989 Feb; 57(1):78–87.

Spinal Disease

Allison RE et al. Spinal fixation: Using the Steffee pedicle screw and plate system. AORN J 1989 Apr; 49(4):1016–1024.

Cramer C. Lumbar laminectomy: PACU standard or malpractice? J Post Anesth Nurs 1987 Aug; 2(3):149–158.

Grashion LA. Physiotherapy management of internal fixations of the spine with the Hartshill system. Physiotherapy 1989 Jun; 75(6):364–366.

Jones AG et al. Side effects following metrizamide myelography and lumbar laminectomy. J Neurosci Nurs 1987 Apr; 19(2):90–94.

Kruszewski MA et al. Harrington rod instrument and spinal fusion: Postoperative care plan. Crit Care Nurse 1985 Nov/Dec; 5(6):77–78.

Nazaroff KS et al. Halo-body jacket immobilization in rheumatoid arthritis patients with cervical myelopathy. Nurs Clin North Am 1989 Mar; 24(1):209–223.

Neatherlin JS et al. Factors determining length of hospitalization for patients having laminectomy surgery. J Neurosci Nurs 1988 Feb; 20(1):39–41.

Quast LM. Thoracic disc disease: Diagnosis and surgical treatment. J Neurosci Nurs 1987 Aug; 19(4):198–204.

Quattro LS. Spinal stabilization. An introduction to Cotrel-DuBousset instrumentation. AORN J 1987 Jul; 46(1):54–63.

Reid DC et al. Contraindications and precautions to spinal joint manipulations: A review. Specific spinal conditions. Part 1. Can J Rehabil 1988 Fall; 2(1):19–30.

Reid DC et al. Contraindications and precautions to spinal joint manipulations: A review. Selected patient groups and special conditions. Part 2. Can J Rehabil 1988 Winter; 2(2):71–78.

Stearns HC. Radiology review. Orthop Nurs 1986; Sep/Oct; 5(5):43–44.

Stuckey PA et al. Oncology alert for the home care nurse: Spinal cord compression. Home Health Nurse 1987 Mar/Apr; 5(2):29–31.

Wilkowski J. Spinal cord compression: An oncologic emergency. J Emerg Nurs 1986 Jan/Feb; 12(1):9–12.

Spinal Injury

Adamson T et al. Spinal injuries: Rehabilitation. NZ Nurs J 1989 Apr; 82(3): 28–30.

Adelstein WM. Cost containment in spinal cord injuries. Rehabil Nurs 1988 Jan/Feb; 13(1):32–37.

Adelstein W. C1–C2 fractures and dislocations. J Neurosci Nurs 1989 Jun; 21(3):149–159.

Annear D. Assessing the spinal cord injured patient. Axon 1988 Dec; 10(2): 42–44.

*Balmaseda MT et al. The value of the ice water test in the management of the neurogenic bladder. Am J Phys Med Rehabil 1988 Oct; 67(4): 225–227.

Balmaseda MT et al. Posttraumatic syringomyelia associated with heavy weightlifting exercises: Case report. Arch Phys Med Rehabil 1988 Nov; 69(11):970–972.

Balmaseda MT et al. An unusual presentation of gluteal hematoma during anticoagulation therapy for deep venous thrombosis in spinal cord injury. Am J Phys Med Rehabil 1988 Dec; 67(6):261–263.

Barker E et al. Managing a suspected spinal cord injury. Nursing 1989 Apr; 19(4):52–59.

Barker E et al. Rescuing an SCI victim from a pool: Spinal cord injuries. Nursing 1989 May; 19(5):58–64.

Black J. Autonomic dysreflexia/hyperreflexia in spinal cord injury. Urol Nurs 1988 Apr/Jun; 8(4):12.

Blake S et al. Spinal injuries: First aid and acute nursing part 2. NZ Nurs J 1989 Mar; 82(2):26–27.

Bloom KK et al. Tibial nerve somatosensory evoked potentials in spinal cord hemisection. Am J Phys Med Rehabil 1989 Apr; 68(2):59–65.

*Borkowski C. A comparison of pulmonary complications in spinal cord-injured patients treated with two modes of spinal immobilization. J Neurosci Nurs 1989 Apr; 21(2):79–85.

*Boschen KA. Housing options and preferences among urban-dwelling spinal cord injured young adults. Can J Rehabil 1988 Fall; 2(1):31–40.

Bourdon SE. Psychological impact of neurotrauma in the acute care setting. Nurs Clin North Am 1986 Dec; 21(4):629–640.

Bowers JE et al. Analysis of a support group for young spinal cord-injured males. Rehabil Nurs 1987 Nov/Dec; 12(6):313–315, 322.

Brady S. Implications of aging in spinal cord injury. Sci Nurs 1986 Fall; 3(4):43–44.

Cooley W. Facilitating change. Sci Nurs 1986 Summer; 3(3):34–36.

Coyle M. Incontinence: Now you're paralyzed. Nurs RSA 1987 Sep; 2(9):21–23.

Davidoff G et al. Closed head injury in acute traumatic spinal cord injury: Incidence and risk factors. Arch Phys Med Rehabil 1988 Oct; 69(10):869–872.

Dewis ME. Spinal cord injury: Responses of adolescents and young adults to body changes. Axon 1987 Dec; 9(2):9–12.

*Dewis ME. Spinal cord injured adolescents and young adults: The meaning of body changes. J Adv Nurs 1989 May; 14(5):389–396.

Dillingham TR. Prevention of complications during acute management of the spinal cord-injured patient: First step in the rehabilitation process. Crit Care Nurs Q 1988 Sep; 11(2) 71–77.

Doloresco LG. Recruitment and retention of nurses for spinal cord injury. Sci Nurs 1988 Spring; 5(2):18–20.

Drayton-Hargrove S et al. Rehabilitation and long-term management of the spinal cord injured adult. Nurs Clin North Am 1986 Dec; 21(4):599–610.

Duci B et al. SCI home care: Transitional rehabilitation as a composite of follow-up care. Sci Nurs 1986 Winter; 3(1):6–9.

Egerton J et al. ABC of spinal cord injury. Br Med J 1986 Feb; 3(1):6–9.

*Ferington FE. Personal control and coping effectiveness in spinal cord injured persons. Res Nurs Health 1986 Sep; 9(3):257–265.

Formal C et al. Burns after spinal cord injury. Arch Phys Med Rehabil 1989 May; 70(5):380–381.

Frost F et al. Intrathecal Baclofen infusion: Effect on bladder management programs in patients with myelopathy. Am J Phys Med Rehabil 1989 Jun; 68(3):112–115.

Gardenshire M. Quality assurance monitoring: A rewarding step in the development of the nurse researcher. Sci Nurs 1988 Spring; 5(2):22–24.

Gribble MJ et al. Pyuria: Its relationship to bacteriuria in spinal cord injured patients on intermittent catheterization. Arch Phys Med Rehabil 1989 May; 70(5):376–379.

Hegde S et al. Thoracic disc herniation and spinal cord injury. Am J Phys Med Rehabil 1988 Oct; 67(5):228–229.

Hooker EZ et al. A method for quantifying the area of closed pressure sores by sinography and digitometry. J Neurosci Nurs 1988 Apr; 20(2):118–127.

Hooker EX. Problems of veterans spinal cord injured after age 55: Nursing implications. J Neurosci Nurs 1986 Aug; 18(4):188–195.

Jaeger RJ et al. Rehabilitation technology for standing and walking after spinal cord injury. Am J Phys Med Rehabil 1989 Jun; 68(3):128–133.

Jones IH. Walking tall. Nurs Times 1987 Apr/May; 83(17):44–46.

*Koehler ML. Relationship between self-concept and successful rehabilitation. Rehabil Nurs 1989 Jan/Feb; 14(1):9–12.

Lae S et al. Risk factors for heterotopic ossification in spinal cord injury. Arch Phys Med Rehabil 1989 May; 70(5):387–390.

Laven GT et al. Nutritional status during the acute stage of spinal cord injury. Arch Phys Med Rehabil 1989 Apr; 70(4):277–282.

Little JW et al. Lower extremity manifestations of spasticity in chronic spinal cord injury. Am J Phys Med Rehabil 1989 Feb; 68(1):32–36.

Little NE. In case of a broken neck. Emerg Med 1989 May; 21(9):22–32.

Lloyd EE et al. An examination of variables in spinal cord injury patients with pressure sores. Sci Nurs 1986 Spring; 3(2):19–22.

*Lyons M. Immune function in spinal cord injured males. J Neurosci Nurs 1987 Feb; 19(1):18–23.

Mackelprang RW et al. Ecological factors in rehabilitation of patients with severe spinal cord injuries. Soc Work Health Care 1987 Jan; 13(1):23–38.

Mahon-Darby J et al. Powerlessness in cervical spinal cord injury patients. DCCN 1988 Nov/Dec; 7(6):346–355.

Markman LJ. Bladder and bowel management of the spinal cord injured patient. Plast Surg Nurs 1988 Winter; 8(4):141–145.

Mawson AR et al. Sensation-seeking and traumatic spinal cord injury: Case-control study. Arch Phys Med Rehabil 1988 Dec; 69(12):1039–1043.

McGibbon J. Paramedical aspects of spinal cord injured patients. Paraplegic 1987 Jun; 25(3):270–274.

McGuire A. Issues in the prevention of neurotrauma. Nurs Clin North Am 1986 Dec; 21(4):549–554.

McKenna ME et al. Acute care of the patient with spinal cord injury. CONA J 1989 Spring; 11(1):5–10.

McKenna ME et al. Nursing management of the patient with a spinal fracture. CONA J 1988 Sep; 10(3):4–9.

Merli GJ et al. Deep vein thrombosis: Prophylaxis in acute spinal cord injured patients. Arch Phys Med Rehabil 1988 Sep; 69(9):661–664.

Meyers AR et al. Predictors of medical care utilization by independently living adults with spinal cord injuries. Arch Phys Med Rehabil 1989 Jun; 70(6):471–476.

Minchington S et al. Specialized care at the Christchurch spinal unit. Part 1. NZ Nurs J 1989 Feb; 82(1):26–27.

Moak E. Perioperative care of the spinal cord injured patient. Today's OR Nurse 1989 Jan; 11(1):12–15, 36–38.

Molitor L. An adult male with spinal cord injury and hypotension and bradycardia. J Emerg Nurs 1988 Sep/Oct; 14(5):324–325.

Murphy SS. First impressions on a spinal cord injury unit. Sci Nurs 1988 Spring; 5(2):21.

Nemeth L et al. Intensive care of the spinal cord-injured patient; Focus on early rehabilitation. Crit Care Nurs Q 1988 Sep; 11(2):79–84.

Novak PP et al. Professional involvement in sexuality counseling for patients with spinal cord injuries. Am J Occup Ther 1988 Feb; 42(2):105–112.

O'Brien J. Vasogenic shock: Lost connections and overwhelming infection. JEMS 1989 Mar; 14(3):32–42.

Page JO. Anatomy of a lawsuit: The real-world aftermath of a spinal injury. JEMS 1989 Apr; 14(4):36–40.

Pervin-Dixon L. Sexuality and the spinal cord injured. J Psychosoc Nurs Ment Health Serv 1988 Apr; 26(4):31–34.

Pontier M. Investigating bladder complaints: Complications following spinal cord injury. Nurs RSA 1988 Apr; 3(4):31–32.

Reid DC et al. Contraindications and precautions to spinal joint manipulations: A review of specific spinal conditions. Part 1. Can J Rehabil 1988 Fall; 2(1):19–30.

Richards JS et al. Spinal cord injury and concomitant traumatic brain injury: Results of a longitudinal investigation. Am J Phys Med Rehabil 1988 Oct; 67(5):211–216.

Richmond T et al. Psychosocial responses to spinal cord injury. J Neurosci Nurs 1986 Aug; 18(4):183–187.

Rodriguez GP et al. Collagen metabolite excretion as a predictor of bone and skin related complications in spinal cord injury. Arch Phys Med Rehabil 1989 Jan; 70(6):442–444.

Romeo JH. The critical minutes after spinal cord injury. RN 1988 Apr; 51(4):61–67.

Romeo JH. Spinal cord injury: Nursing the patient toward a new life. RN 1988 May; 51(5):31–35.

Roye WP et al. Cervical spinal cord injury: A public catastrophe. J Trauma 1988 Aug; 28(8):1260–1264.

Rucker B et al. Legal, ethical and religious issues related to fertility enhancement of men with spinal cord injuries. Can J Rehabil 1988 Summer; 1(4):225–231.

Segatore M et al. Spinal cord testing development of a screening tool. J Neurosci Nurs 1988 Feb; 20(1):30–33.

Simor AE et al. Molecular and epidemiologic study of multiresistant serratia marcescens infections in a spinal cord injury rehabilitation unit. Infect Control 1988 Jan; 9(1):20–27.

Smith M et al. Ties that bind: Immobilizing the injured spine. JEMS 1989 Apr; 14(4):28–35.

Smith R. Mouth stick design for the client with spinal cord injury. Am J Occup Ther 1989 Apr; 43(4):251–255.

Spica MM. Sexual counseling standards for the spinal cord-injured. J Neurosci Nurs 1989 Feb; 21(1):56–60.

Stover SL et al. Urinary tract infection in spinal cord injury. Phys Med Rehabil 1989 Jan; 70(1):47–54.

Taylor J. Care of the ventilator dependent spinal cord injured patient and their families in the acute rehabilitation stage. Axon 1988 Dec; 10(2): 45–47.

Urey JR et al. Prediction of marital adjustment among spinal cord injured persons. Rehabil Nurs 1987 Jan/Feb; 12(1):26–30.

Verghese M. Autonomic dysreflexia: A life threatening emergency. Nurs J India 1989 May; 80(5):134–135.

Villeneuve MJ. Sexual function and fertility: The impact of spinal cord injury. CONA J 1989 Spring; 11(1):12–17.

Warms CA. Health promotion services in post-rehabilitation spinal cord injury health care. Rehabil Nurs 1987 Nov/Dec; 12(6):304–308.

Waters JD. Learning needs of spinal cord–injured patients. Rehabil Nurs 1987 Nov/Dec; 12(6):309–312.

Weber W. Spinal cord cooling: A nursing perspective. Axon 1987 Dec; 9(2):13–16.

Zucker L. Transport of the neurologically injured patient. Emerg Care Q 1989 Feb; 4(4):40–47.

Information/Resources

Agencies

Governmental

Division for the Blind and Physically Handicapped
    Library of Congress, Washington, DC 20542
National Institute of Neurological and Communicative Disorders and Stroke
    National Institutes of Health, Bethesda, MD 20892

Voluntary

American Cancer Society
    90 Park Ave, New York, NY 10016

American Parkinson's Disease Association
    116 John St, Suite 417, New York, NY 10038
American Speech-Language-Hearing Association
    10801 Rockville Pike, Rockville, MD 20852
Amyotrophic Lateral Sclerosis Association
    15300 Ventura Blvd, Suite 315, PO Box 5951, Sherman Oaks, CA 91403
Epilepsy Foundation of America
    4351 Garden City Dr, Landover, MD 20785
Guillain-Barré Syndrome Support Group
    PO Box 262, Wynnewood, PA 19096
Hereditary Disease Foundation
    9701 Wilshire Blvd, Suite 1204, Beverly Hills, CA 90212
Huntington's Disease Foundation of America
    140 West 22nd St, 6th Floor, New York, NY 10011
Muscular Dystrophy Association
    810 Seventh Ave, New York, NY 10019
Myasthenia Gravis Foundation
    53 West Jackson Blvd, Chicago, IL 60604
National Easter Seal Society
    2023 West Ogden Ave, Chicago, IL 60612
National Head Injury Foundation
    333 Turnpike Rd, Southborough, MA 01772
National Headache Foundation
    5252 North Western Ave, Chicago, IL 60625
National Multiple Sclerosis Society
    205 E 42nd St, New York, NY 10017
National Parkinson Foundation
    1501 NW Ninth Ave, Miami, FL 31316
National Spinal Cord Injury Association
    600 West Cummings Park, Suite 2000, Woburn, MA 01801
Paralyzed Veterans of America
    801 18th St NW, Washington, DC 20006
Parkinson's Disease Foundation
    Columbia Presbyterian Medical Center, 640 W 168th Street, New York, NY 10032

Nursing Research Profile
for Unit 14

Neuroscience Nursing

Overview

Research in neuroscience nursing continues to focus mainly on the nursing considerations, management, and implications for patients with head and spinal cord injuries, stroke, and multiple sclerosis. These catastrophic events for both patient and family require intensive nursing management and deserve the attention of nurse researchers. The effects of nursing interventions on intracranial pressure continue to be studied, but few other aspects of the care of these patients have been investigated. A number of studies have focused on family and caregiver issues. Investigation of neurologic problems should continue to yield important implications for future nursing practice.

Assessment

▷ Cammermeyer M and Evans J. A *brief neurobehavioral exam useful for early detection of postoperative complications in neurosurgical patients.* J Neurosci Nurs 1988 Oct; 20(5): 314–323.

This article describes data collected from 11 patients before and after neurosurgical intervention for treatment of brain tumor, subdural hematoma, and hydrocephalus. Results of serial examinations and case studies are presented to illustrate the clinical relevance to patient management of a brief, standardized cognitive status evaluation. The Neurobehavioral Cognitive Status Examination (NCSE) was administered preoperatively and postoperatively. The NCSE assesses eight areas of cognitive function, including level of consciousness, orientation, attention, and language. Improvement was documented by this instrument in 6 of 11 patients postoperatively. In the other five patients there was evidence of deterioration of cognitive function. Clinical and diagnostic reevaluation of these patients determined the need for repeat surgery, which was performed. According to the authors, follow-up evaluation with the NCSE after a second surgical procedure was helpful in determining treatable versus nontreatable causes of cognitive decline in three patients (presented as case studies).

Nursing Implications. The authors believe that the use of the NCSE may have expedited effective diagnostic evaluation and thus improved patient care. Subtle changes in cognitive functioning may be early indicators of increased intracranial pressure or surgical complications (according to the researchers) and can be detected with a standardized neurologic assessment tool such as the NCSE. It is not mentioned whether these patients with cognitive changes also had other clinical changes such as lethargy, confusion, or memory decline detectable on standard neurologic (clinical) examinations. Standardized tools such as this one and the Mini Mental State Examination (MMSE), which are easily administered, pragmatic, and objective, are valuable clinical aides. An earlier finding by Williams and co-workers (Res Nurs Health 1985 Mar; 8[1]:31–40) that revealed that the most important predictor of cognitive impairment is the mental status questionnaire score. As the authors suggest, the NCSE may be a valuable instrument for nurse researchers interested in patient care and rehabilitation issues.

▷ Foreman M. Reliability and validity of mental status questionnaires in elderly hospitalized patients. Nurs Res 1987 Jul/Aug; 36(4):216–220.

This study tested the reliability and validity of three mental status questionnaires—the Short Portable Mental Status Questionnaire (SPMSQ), the MMSE, and the Cognitive Capacity Screening Examination (CCSE). The study population consisted of 66 elderly (at least 65 years old), hospitalized medical–surgical patients. In general, mental status questionnaires have not undergone vigorous psychometric testing. Most psychometric and clinical studies have been conducted with psychiatric patients, and the performance of these three questionnaires in assessing patients has not been compared, making selection of a tool difficult. Both the SPMSQ and the MMSE were developed and tested with psychiatric patients, while only the CCSE was developed with the use of nonpsychiatric subjects.

The SPMSQ is a 10-item, easily administered instrument that takes 5 to 10 minutes. The MMSE is an 11-item cognitive screening examination that takes 5 to 10 minutes to administer. The CCSE is a 30-item questionnaire that is easy to administer and takes 5 to 15 minutes (though Cammermeyer and Evans state that it takes 15 to 30 minutes to administer).

All three tools were found to be internally consistent. With use of a variety of parameters, the reliability and validity of the three mental status questionnaires were found to be relatively consistent, but the CCSE provides the most comprehensive measure of mental status, followed by the MMSE and SPMSQ.

Nursing Implications. This study is valuable to clinicians for a number of reasons. Clinicians need to use caution when utilizing instruments developed in dissimilar populations. This author has validated the use of three popular tools commonly used in medical–surgical settings. Though the results indicate that the CCSE may be the most comprehensive measure available, all three tools are reliable measures of mental status.

In a clinical setting, the MMSE and the SPMSQ may be more practical to use because they are short and can be administered quickly.

Discharge Teaching

▷ *Sanguinetti M and Catanzaro M. A comparison of discharge teaching on the consequences of brain injury. J Neurosci Nurs 1987 Oct; 19(5):271–275.*

The authors of this study developed a discharge teaching video tape that reviewed the most common cognitive dysfunctions experienced by post–brain injury patients that are likely to affect activities of daily living. This study involved 29 head-injured patients. One family member per patient was selected for study participation. Subjects were randomly assigned to either a control group (video-taped standard discharge instructions) or an experimental group (standard discharge instructions plus the experimental video tape). Both groups received a post-test designed to determine the caregiver's ability to extrapolate appropriate patient care techniques after receiving discharge teaching. Results demonstrated a statistically significant difference between the experimental group's ability to repeat information learned from the video tape presentation and their understanding of the information as it applied to everyday functioning.

Nursing Implications. The authors suggest that follow-up research is needed to determine whether the caregiver's behavior also changes as a result of the discharge instructions.

▷ *Morgan S. Comparison of three methods of managing fever in the neurologic patient. J Neurosci Nurs 1990 Feb; 22(1):19–24.*

An increase in body temperature can be detrimental to the neurologically impaired patient. It is estimated that a patient's metabolic rate can increase 7% for each degree above the normal temperature; this in turn increases cellular metabolism, oxygen requirements, and carbon dioxide levels. One consequence of this sequence is vasodilation of the cerebral vasculature. The purpose of this study was to compare three methods of temperature control in adults: (1) acetaminophen, (2) acetaminophen and tepid water sponging, and (3) acetaminophen and hypothermia blanket. In each case, 650 mg of acetaminophen was administered orally or rectally. The three cooling methods were examined for their effectiveness in reducing patients' temperature and for the effect of each on patient shivering.

With use of a quasi-experimental study design, 21 neurologic patients with a fever of 101°F or greater were randomly assigned to one of the three methods of temperature control on admission to the hospital. Patients who developed fever (defined as a rectal temperature of ≥101°F) received the previously assigned method of temperature control. The assigned protocol was initiated when patients first became febrile. In groups 2 and 3, the tepid water sponging and hypothermia blanket were initiated when the patient's temperature was 102°F or greater. Patients' rectal temperatures were monitored every 15 minutes until the temperature was 100°F. The amount of time required for the temperature to reach 100°F was recorded. Patients were also observed for shivering.

Temperature reduction from 101° to 100°F with acetaminophen took only an average of 110 minutes. Temperature reduction from 102° to 100°F with tepid sponging and the hypothermia blanket (along with acetaminophen) took 144 and 100 minutes, respectively. Analysis indicates that these differences are not statistically significant. The only group to experience shivering was the hypothermia group, which had four patients with shivering.

Nursing Implications. For the neurologically impaired patient, rapid reduction of temperature is a nursing priority. Use of the hypothermia blanket would be the method of choice in terms of speed of reducing patients' temperature. However, the risk of shivering is greatest with this method.

Stroke

▷ *Printz-Feddersen V. Group process effect on caregiver burden. J Neurosci Nurs 1990 Jun; 22(3):164–168.*

The patient who has sustained a stroke frequently requires assistance with many of the activities of daily living; it is often the patient's spouse or another family member who assumes the role of primary care provider for the patient. Attendance at support groups, such as stroke club meetings, has been suggested as one strategy that may assist the caregiver in coping with the changes that occur as one assumes the role of caregiver. The purpose of this study was to determine if caregivers (of patients who survived a stroke) who participated in a stroke club had the same experiences as those who had not participated in a stroke club. An ex post facto design was used for the comparison.

A sample of 40 caregivers of stroke patients, randomly selected from a private neurology practice, constituted the first group—those who did not participate in a stroke club. A convenience sample of 40 caregivers identified as participants in a stroke club constituted the second group. The patient with the stroke had to be at least 55 years of age and had to be 6 months poststroke. Four areas previously shown to increase the caregiver's burden were evaluated: degree of difficulty in performing the caregiver's tasks, depression, financial concerns, and social restriction. Four tools were used: Demographic Inventory, PCRI (Physical Caregiving Responsibility Inventory), the Geriatric Depression Scale, and CADET (Communication, Ambulation, Daily Activities, Excretion, and Transfer). The CADET measured the caregiver's perception of the stroke patient's dysfunction. The PCRI measured the amount of perceived physical responsibility of the caregiver and the level of difficulty. The Geriatric Depression Scale evaluated the emotional health of the caregiver.

A questionnaire comprised of the four tools was mailed to each caregiver; those caregivers who did not respond within 15 days were removed from the study. Forty-three (53%) of the questionnaires were returned; nine did not meet the criteria, one patient had died, and two patients had no residual deficits and required no assistance from a caregiver. The final sample size of the control group was 21; there were 17 caregivers in the group of stroke club participants. There was no significant difference between the two groups on the variables of age, financial status, caregivers' perceptions of stroke patients' level of dysfunction, caregivers' perceptions of responsibility, or level of depression. However, approximately 22% of the caregivers in both groups did have scores indicative of depression, although the overall score indicated that depression was not perceived as a burden.

The results of this study demonstrated no difference in the perception of the burden of caregiving between those caregivers who attended a support group and those who did not. There are several factors that may have contributed to these results, including: (1) the stroke club group was not a random sample but rather was comprised of those caregivers who elected to participate, and (2) a minimal level of care and assistance was required by the stroke patients. The caregivers felt that their own health problems were not a hindrance but were rather a part of the aging process, and they rated themselves as being in good health. There was an average income of greater than $10,000 per year, and the caregivers did not see finances as a burden. Forty-seven percent of the caregivers did report a decrease in their social activities.

Nursing Implications.   Although the findings of this study do not reveal differences in the perception of caregiving burden between those who attended a stroke club and those who did not, these findings should not lead nurses to the conclusion that support groups make no difference in patients' or caregivers' ability to cope with an acute or chronic disorder. Further study with prospective research designs and greater control over the selection and assignment of subjects to groups would enable nurses to evaluate the impact of participation on caregivers.

▷ *Pasquarello M. Measuring the impact of an acute stroke program on patient outcomes. J Neurosci Nurs 1990 Apr; 22(2):76–82.*

Little research has been conducted on outcomes of stroke patients in the acute care setting. This research was conducted to examine the outcomes of patients admitted to a nurse-managed stroke program in an acute care setting. The nurse-managed stroke program consisted of inpatient care, patient education, family care including a support group, coordinated discharge care, postdischarge telephone contact, and education of other nurses in the setting.

An ex post facto retrospective chart review was conducted, with a random sample of 25 pre–stroke-program patients in the control group and 25 post–stroke-program patients in the experimental group. A chart review tool was developed by a clinical nurse specialist to assess the following: length of stay, return to either the emergency department or ambulatory care center within 3 months, disposition on discharge, complications, timeliness in initiating rehabilitation, compliance with the medical regimen, and compliance with follow-up appointments 3 months after discharge. The newly developed tool was reviewed by another clinical nurse specialist and nursing administrator for content validity. Charts of patients admitted before implementation of the stroke program were compared to those of patients admitted after implementation of the program.

The two groups were similar in gender, race, and baseline health status. The patients in the nurse-managed stroke program

tended to be younger than those in the comparison group. Fewer complications (N=5) were identified in patients in the nurse-managed program than in those in the comparison group (N=16). Length of stay for subjects in the program was 8 days and for those in the comparison group was 17 days. There was a 62% increase in the number of patients discharged to home and a 300% increase in the number of patients discharged to a rehabilitation facility when patients in the nurse-managed program were compared to those not in the program. There were 20% fewer hospital readmissions and 100% fewer returns to the emergency department or ambulatory care center in patients in the program than in those not in the program. Those patients who were part of the stroke program had greater compliance with medication regimens and clinic appointment visits.

The author concludes that the nurse-managed stroke program is likely to have produced many of the positive changes demonstrated in this study. However, as the author points out, those patients who were part of the nurse-managed program may have had a better prognosis than did those in the second group because of their younger age. Lack of statistical analysis in the study precludes conclusions that the differences reported by the author are statistically significant.

Nursing Implications.   Many of the strategies identified as part of the nurse-managed stroke program are part of standard nursing practice. The preliminary findings of this study support their importance in practice and the need for nurses to initiate nursing measures and other rehabilitative strategies early in patients' hospitalizations and to encourage family members to become involved in patients' care.

▷ *Byers V, Arrington M, and Finstuen K. Predictive risk factors associated with stroke patient falls in acute care settings. J Neurosci Nurs 1990 Jun; 2(3):147–154.*

This retrospective study evaluated the risk factors associated with falls in stroke patients in the acute care setting in an effort to increase accuracy in prediction of those at risk. A retrospective chart review was conducted on 313 patients from two medical centers with use of the Fall Risk Assessment Inventory (FRAI), developed for this study. The FRAI was used to assess (1) demographic characteristics, (2) neurologic function, (3) objective measures of clinical status (*i.e.,* vital signs, medications, laboratory results), and (4) activity level and fall precautions in effect. The FRAI was pilot tested before use in this study.

Of the 313 patients whose charts were reviewed, 212 had sustained a stroke and fell; 111 patients had a stroke but did not fall. The stroke fall group was identified from incident reports, while subjects in the comparison group (those who did not fall) were randomly selected by computer from diagnostic codes of stroke. With use of the FRAI, charts of patients who fell and met the criteria for inclusion in the study were reviewed at three points in time: at the time of the patient's admission, 24 hours prior to the fall, and at the time of the fall.

Analysis of demographic data indicated that the two groups were relatively similar in age, gender, race, and the period of time that had elapsed between the stroke and the study period. The two groups were similar in incidence of previous stroke, site of the stroke, and secondary medical diagnoses. Of the patients in the fall group, 11% were described as physically restrained and almost 20% sustained an injury. Falls occurred more on the night shift than on the evening or day shift. Mental status factors that were significant predictors of falls included impaired decision-making ability and restlessness.

Motor and sensory status factors associated with falls included greater generalized weakness, fatigue, and constructional apraxia. Paralysis and balance were not significant predictors of falls. General status and vital signs showed that 22% of those in the fall group had experienced a previous fall, while only 12% of the nonfall group had a previous fall. Medications showed that 36% of the fall group were taking cardiac medications, compared with 24% of the nonfall group. For the laboratory data, 60% of the patients who had falls had a low hematocrit, while only 45% of the nonfall patients did.

The profile of the stroke patient at risk for falls in acute care facilities includes: history of falls, impaired decision-making ability, restlessness, generalized weakness, abnormal hematocrits, and those who are easily fatigued.

Nursing Implications.   To reduce the incidence of falls in stroke patients hospitalized in acute care facilities and prevent the complications that may occur as a result of those falls, the nurse can identify patients who have a greater risk of falls. Increased surveillance of the stroke patient who fits the at-risk profile is indicated to reduce the occurrence. Improved lighting, more frequent observation of the patient, especially during the night, moving the at-risk patient closer to the nurses' station, and assisting with ambulation may reduce the occurrence of falls in this vulnerable population.

Intracranial Pressure

▷   **Franges EZ and Beideman ME. Infections related to intracranial pressure monitoring. J Neurosci Nurs 1988 Apr; 20(2):94–103.**

In this study, the researchers retrospectively reviewed 52 patients who underwent intracranial pressure (ICP) monitoring at a community hospital. Twelve variables possibly related to infection were studied: diagnosis, type of monitor, date and place of insertion, duration of monitoring, drainage, frequency of system change or irrigation and personnel involved, dressing changes, range of patient temperatures, culture results, concurrent infections, and antibiotic therapy. Seventy-one percent of the study group had intraventricular catheters in place for an average of 5.5 days, while 29% had subarachnoid bolts inserted and in place for 3.4 days.

A total of three infections (8.1%) occurred in those with intraventricular catheters, and one site infection (6.9%) was documented in the subarachnoid bolt group. The overall infection rate at this institution was 7.1%. Data analysis suggested that the length of time the monitoring device was in place and patient age did not play a role in the risk of infection. The authors noted that the patients with ventricular catheters who became infected all had the diagnosis of hemorrhage, a finding previously reported in the literature. Pooled blood increases the inflammatory reaction and sets up an ideal medium for bacterial growth; thus, this patient group may be at higher risk for developing infections. Data regarding other variables were not presented.

Nursing Implications.   In this study, those patients with intracranial pressure monitoring–related infections were those with a diagnosis of hemorrhage. Although lack of statistical analysis is a weakness of this study, the results do suggest that careful monitoring of the patient for infection and scrupulous care in manipulation of the ICP monitoring system are critical, especially with patients with a diagnosis of intracranial hemorrhage.

▷   **Prins MM. The effect of family visits on intracranial pressure. West J Nurs Res 1989 Jun; 11(3):281–297.**

Nursing care, including turning and positioning, suctioning, blood pressure monitoring, and daily hygiene, has been documented to cause an increase in ICP. Verbal and auditory stimuli have also been reported to increase ICP. Anecdotal reports have suggested that family members' voices may have a calming effect on the patient, thereby reducing the patient's ICP. A descriptive study was conducted to address the following research questions: (1) Do visits by family members affect a patient's ICP? (2) Does the quality of a family visit alter the ICP?

A Patient/Family Interaction Scale (PFIS) was developed by the researcher to evaluate the effect of family members' visits at the bedside of patients undergoing ICP monitoring. The scale identified the body part touched, mode of touching, verbal behavior, verbal volume, positioning behavior, and conversation content. With use of a Likert scale, each criterion was broken down into specific actions and given a numerical value. A low score indicated that there was much patient/family interaction or contact and that it was a supportive visit. A high score indicated little contact during the family's visit at the bedside and that the visit was nonsupportive.

Continuous ICP monitoring was performed for 5 minutes before the family visit (previsit). During the patient/family interaction, the ICP was monitored every 2 minutes for a total of 10 minutes. Continuous ICP monitoring was then obtained for 5 minutes following the family's visit. Data were also obtained on those variables that are known to affect patients' ICP readings: $PaCO_2$, and administration of mannitol and Decadron.

A convenience sample included 15 patients with a total of 47 patient/family "interactions" observed. All the families were observed in the same nine-bed neurologic intensive care unit by the same nurse researcher using the PFIS. Of the 15 patients, 8 had ICP monitoring by an intraventricular catheter, while the remaining 7 had ICP monitoring by a subarachnoid bolt. Patients' diagnoses included arteriovenous malformation, tumors, intraventricular hemorrhage with cerebral edema, and subarachnoid hematoma. The age range was 16 to 81 years, with an average age of 55 years. The Glasgow Coma Scale scores ranged from 3 to 15. No nasotracheal or endotracheal suctioning was performed within 1 hour before the family visit. No other nursing intervention was provided during the observation period; if nursing interventions were necessary during an observation period, that observation was not included in the study.

The mean previsit ICP was 9.52, the visit ICP was 8.75, and the postvisit ICP was 9.48. No significant differences were found in previsit, visit, or postvisit ICP readings. There were significant correlations between ICP during visit and postvisit and $PaCO_2$ and mannitol and Decadron use, suggesting that these variables may have acted as intervening variables; that is, they may have had an effect on patients' responses to family visits.

The author points out that this study should be considered a pilot study; this is supported by the author's statement that the scoring of patients' responses on the Glasgow Coma Scale was recorded inconsistently. Further work on the scale developed to assess patient/family interaction during family visits also appears warranted.

Nursing Implications.   Although the findings of this pilot study did not support previous findings that indicated that family visits do decrease ICP, they do demonstrate that family visits at the bedside do not increase ICP. Therefore, visits from patients' family members should not be restricted because of concern that they will distress the patient and compromise his neurologic status. Permitting family members to visit the patient may alleviate some of his anxiety.

Demyelinating Disorders

▷ **Smeltzer SC et al. *Pulmonary function and dysfunction in multiple sclerosis*. Arch Neurol 1988 Nov; 45(11):1245–1249.**

This study evaluated pulmonary function in 25 patients with clinically definite multiple sclerosis. The subjects had disability ranging from ataxia to quadriplegia, with three patients ambulatory without assistance. Seven required assistance for ambulation (*e.g.*, cane, walker, or crutches), seven were wheelchair-bound, and eight were bedridden. Pulmonary function was assessed in two ways. First, a variety of clinical assessments were made. An interview was conducted to obtain information regarding symptoms of respiratory dysfunction or illness. Patients were asked to cough, and the examiner's rating of normal, decreased, or absent cough was compared to the patient's own report of cough ability. A disability scale was used to assess the level of neurologic disability. Second, pulmonary function tests were performed, including flow rates, lung volumes, and maximal respiratory pressure measures (assess inspiratory and expiratory muscle strength).

The results of this study indicate that patients with multiple sclerosis who are ambulatory are unlikely to have significant respiratory muscle dysfunction; patients who are bedridden or wheelchair-bound with or without upper extremity weakness often have severely compromised respiratory muscle function. Surprisingly, few patients reported shortness of breath or other respiratory problems despite the evidence of significant respiratory muscle weakness on assessment.

Nursing Implications. The findings of this study demonstrate that there is pulmonary compromise earlier in the course of multiple sclerosis than was previously thought. The impact of this dysfunction on life-style is offset in many cases by the fact that these patients are so "slowed" by the disease process that exertional symptoms (*e.g.*, dyspnea) are not problematic.

Nevertheless, caregivers need to be aware that the patient's self-report of some significant symptoms (*e.g.*, cough) is not reliable and that thorough history and assessment of respiratory muscle function are necessary to identify patients who may be at risk for pulmonary complications.

▷ **Smeltzer SC et al. *Testing of an index of pulmonary dysfunction in multiple sclerosis*. Nurs Res 1989 Nov/Dec; 38(6):370–374.**

This study evaluated the reliability and validity of an Index of Pulmonary Dysfunction in Multiple Sclerosis. The items included in the Index were derived from previously obtained clinical data; thus, this study is an extension of the first study by Smeltzer and co-workers. The Index is comprised of four items. The first two items of the Index are obtained through direct questioning of the patient and include self-reported difficulty clearing or handling mucus and cough strength. The third item is the patient's ability to generate a strong cough on demand. The fourth item assesses the patient's ability to count aloud on a single exhalation following inhalation to total lung capacity.

Forty patients with multiple sclerosis performed pulmonary function tests and underwent clinical evaluation to determine whether or not the Index correctly identified those patients with pulmonary dysfunction. The Index correctly predicted the presence or absence of significant respiratory muscle weakness in 80% of the subjects. In all subjects who had normal expiratory muscle strength, the Index correctly classified them; however, not all patients with isolated expiratory muscle weakness were correctly identified. Test–retest reliability, interrater reliability, and internal consistency of the Index were all acceptable.

Nursing Implications. The authors state that the Index has acceptable validity and reliability for use in clinical practice to identify those neurologic patients with expiratory muscle weakness. The levels of sensitivity, specificity, and accuracy of the Index in discriminating patients who have normal respiratory muscle strength from those with abnormal strength suggest that it may be useful in screening patients with multiple sclerosis. It provides a method of identifying patients with this disease who may be at risk for pulmonary complications because of respiratory muscle weakness but who do not report pulmonary symptoms.

unit 15
Musculoskeletal Function

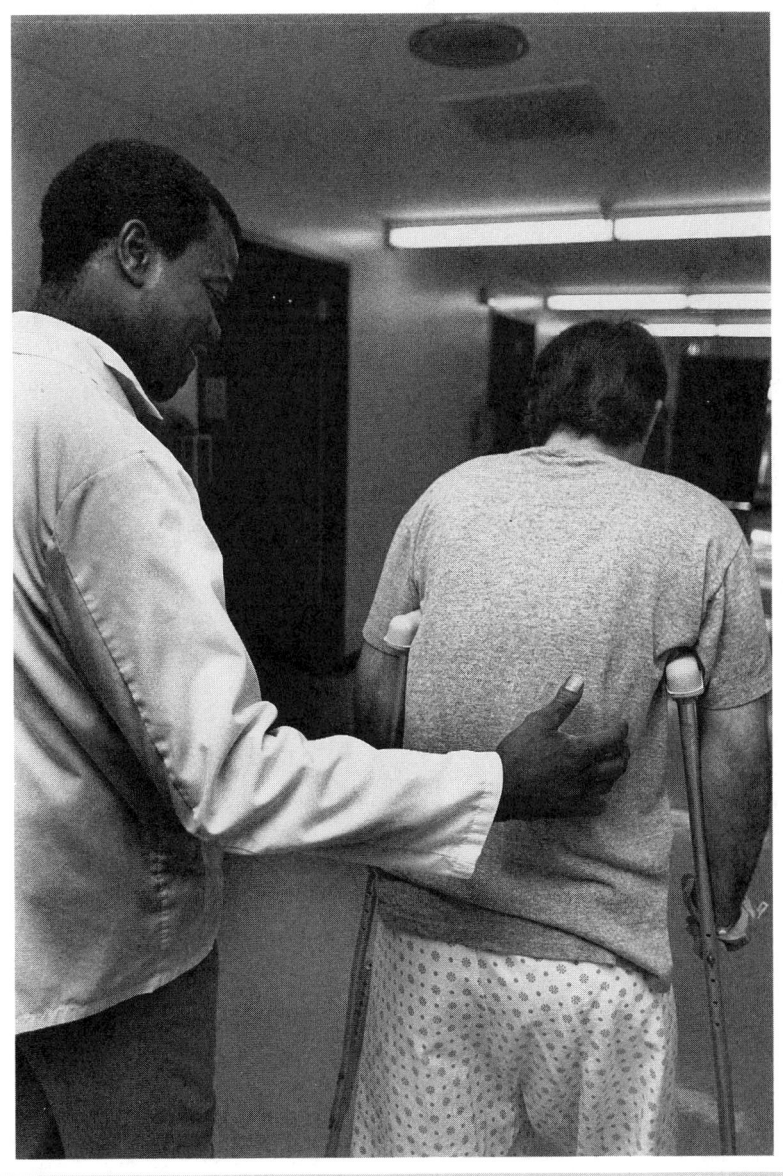

58

Assessment of Musculoskeletal Function

Learning Objectives

On completion of this chapter, the learner will be able to:

1. Describe the physiology of the skeletal, articular, and skeletal muscle systems
2. Describe the physiology of bone healing
3. Describe the significance of physical assessment to the diagnosis of musculoskeletal dysfunction
4. Specify the diagnostic tests used for assessment of musculoskeletal function
5. Identify nursing diagnoses common to patients with musculoskeletal disorders

The musculoskeletal system includes the bones, joints, muscles, tendons, ligaments, and bursae of the body. The occurrence of problems associated with these structures is very common and affects all age groups. Problems with the musculoskeletal system are generally not life-threatening, but they have a significant impact on one's normal activities and productivity. Problems associated with the musculoskeletal system will be encountered by the nurse practicing in any field of nursing and during daily living experiences.

Physiologic Overview

The musculoskeletal system is collectively the largest organ system in the body. Bony structures and connective tissue ac-

count for approximately 25% of the body weight, and muscle accounts for approximately 50% of the body weight. The health and functions of the musculoskeletal system are interdependent with the rest of the body systems.

The functions of the musculoskeletal system include protection, support, locomotion, mineral storage, hematopoiesis, and heat production. The bony structure provides protection for vital organs, including the brain, heart, and lungs. The bony skeleton supports body structures by providing a strong and sturdy framework. The muscles attached to the skeleton allow the body to move. Calcium, phosphorus, magnesium, and fluoride are among the minerals deposited and stored in the bone matrix. More than 99% of the total body calcium is present in bone. The red bone marrow located within the bone cavity is responsible for the production of red and white blood cells. Muscle contraction results in mechanical action for movement as well as heat production to maintain body temperature.

The Skeletal System

Anatomy of the Skeletal System. There are 206 bones in the human body, divided into four categories: *long bones* (*e.g.,* the femur), *short bones* (*e.g.,* the tarsals), *flat bones* (*e.g.,* the sternum), and *irregular bones* (*e.g.,* the vertebrae). The shape and construction of a specific bone are determined by its function and the forces exerted on the bone.

Bones are constructed of *cancellous* (trabecular or spongy) or *cortical* (compact) bone tissue. *Long bones* are shaped like rods or shafts with rounded ends. The shaft, or *diaphysis,* is primarily cortical bone. The ends of the long bones are called *epiphyses* and are primarily cancellous bone. The *epiphyseal plate* separates the epiphyses from the diaphysis and is the center for longitudinal growth in children. In the adult, it is calcified. The ends of long bones are covered by articular cartilage at the joints. Long bones are constructed for weight-bearing and movement. *Short bones* consist of cancellous bone covered by a layer of compact bone. *Flat bones* are important sites for *hematopoiesis* (formation of blood) and frequently provide vital organ protection. They are made of cancellous bone layered between compact bone. *Irregular bones* have unique shapes related to their function. Generally, irregular bone makeup is similar to that of flat bones.

Bone is composed of cells, protein matrix, and mineral deposits. The cells are of three basic types—osteoblasts, osteocytes, and osteoclasts. *Osteoblasts* are involved in bone formation by secreting *bone matrix*. The matrix is 98% collagen and 2% ground substances (glucosamine glycans [acid polysaccharides] and proteoglycans). The matrix is a framework in which inorganic mineral salts are deposited. *Osteocytes* are mature bone cells involved in bone maintenance functions and are located in *osteons* (bone matrix units). *Osteoclasts* are multinuclear cells involved in bone destruction, resorption, and remodeling.

The osteon is the microscopic functioning unit of mature bone. The center of the osteon contains a capillary. Around the capillary are circles of bone matrix called *lamellae*. Within the lamellae are *osteocytes* (mature, living bone cells). The osteocytes are nourished through processes that extend into tiny *canaliculi* (canals that communicate with blood vessels less than 0.1 mm away).

Covering the bone is a dense, fibrous membrane known as the *periosteum*. The periosteum functions in the nutrition and growth of bone and provides for the attachment of tendons and ligaments. The periosteum contains nerves, blood vessels, and lymphatics. The layer closest to the bone contains osteoblasts, which are bone-forming cells.

Endosteum is a thin, vascular membrane covering the marrow cavity of long bones and the spaces in cancellous bone. *Osteoclasts*, which dissolve bone to maintain the marrow cavity, are located near the endosteum and in *Howship's lacunae* (indentations on bone surfaces).

Bone marrow is a vascular tissue located in the medullary (shaft) cavity of long bones and in flat bones. Red bone marrow is responsible for the production of red and white blood cells. In the adult, the red bone marrow in the long bone cavity is replaced mostly by fatty, yellow marrow. Red bone marrow in the adult is located mainly in the sternum, ilium, vertebrae, and ribs.

Bone tissue is well vascularized. Cancellous bone receives a rich blood supply through metaphyseal and epiphyseal vessels. Periosteal vessels carry blood to compact bone through minute *Volkmann canals*. In addition, *nutrient arteries* penetrate the periosteum and enter the medullary cavity through *foramina* (small openings). Nutrient arteries supply blood to the marrow and bone. The venous system may accompany arteries or may exit independently.

Bone Formation. Bone begins to form long before birth. *Ossification* is the process by which the bone matrix (*e.g.,* collagen fibers and ground substance) is formed and hardening minerals (*e.g.,* calcium salts) are deposited on the collagen fibers in an electronegative environment. The collagen fibers give tensile strength to the bone, and the calcium provides compressional strength.

There are two basic models of ossification: intramembranous and endochondral. *Intramembranous ossification,* in which bone develops within membrane, occurs in the bones of the face and skull. Therefore, when the skull heals, it is by fibrous union. The other kind of bone formation is known as *endochondral ossification,* in which a cartilage model exists. Cartilage-like (osteoid) tissue is formed, resorbed, and replaced by bone. Most bones in the body are formed and heal by endochondral ossification.

Bone Maintenance. Bone is a dynamic tissue in a constant state of turnover (resorption and reforming). Calcium in bone in an adult is replaced at the rate of about 18% a year. The important regulating factors that determine the balance between bone formation and bone resorption include local stress, vitamin D, parathyroid hormone, calcitonin, and circulation.

Vitamin D functions to increase the amount of calcium in the blood by promoting absorption of calcium from the gastrointestinal tract and accelerating mobilization of calcium from the bone.

Parathyroid hormone and calcitonin are the major hormonal regulators of calcium homeostasis. Parathyroid hormone regulates the concentration of calcium in the blood, in part by promoting movement of calcium from the bone. Excessive mobilization of calcium due to excess parathyroid hormone results in demineralization of the bone and formation of bone cysts. Calcitonin, from the thyroid gland, increases the deposit of calcium in bone.

Blood supply to the bone also affects bone formation. With diminished blood supply or *hyperemia* (congestion), osteogenesis is reduced and the bone becomes osteoporotic. Bone necrosis occurs when the bone is deprived of blood.

Bone Healing

Most fractures heal through endochondral ossification. When the bone is injured, the bone fragments are not merely patched together with scar tissue. The bone regenerates itself. There are several stages in fracture healing: (1) inflammation, (2) cellular proliferation, (3) callus formation, (4) callus ossification, and (5) remodeling into mature bone.

Inflammation. With a fracture, the body's response is similar to that of injury elsewhere in the body. There is bleeding, extravasation of blood, and the formation of a fracture hematoma. The area exhibits edema, inflammation, and pain. The fracture fragment ends become devitalized because of the interrupted blood supply. The injured area is invaded by macrophages (large white blood cells), which débride the area. The inflammatory stage lasts several days, and resolution of the inflammatory response is characterized by a decrease in pain and swelling.

Cellular Proliferation. Within about 5 days, the fracture hematoma undergoes organization. Fibrin strands form within the clot, creating a network for revascularization and invasion by fibroblasts and osteoblasts.

Fibroblasts and osteoblasts (developed from osteocytes, endosteal cells, and periosteal cells) produce collagen and proteoglycans for a collagen matrix at the fracture. Cartilage and fibrous connective tissue develop. From the periosteum, a collar of growth is in evidence. This is the beginning of an external cartilaginous callus, also known as osteoid tissue. Callus formation is stimulated by minimal micromotion at the fracture site. Excessive motion disrupts the callus structure. Actively growing bone exhibits electronegative potentials.

Callus Formation. Tissue growth continues and the cartilage collar from each bone fragment grows toward the others until the fracture gap is bridged. The fracture fragments are joined by fibrous tissue, cartilage, and immature fiber bone. An internal callus also develops and invades the remaining blood clot. The shape of the callus and the volume of tissue required to bridge the defect are directly proportional to the amount of bone damage and displacement. It takes 3 to 4 weeks for fracture fragments to be united by cartilage or fibrous tissue. Clinically, the fragments are no longer easily moved.

Ossification. Ossification of the developed callus begins within 2 to 3 weeks of fracture through the process of endochondral ossification. The mineral deposition continues and produces a firmly reunited bone. The callus surface continues to be electronegative. With major adult long bone fractures, ossification takes 3 to 4 months.

Remodeling. The final stage of fracture repair consists of removal of any remaining devitalized tissue and reorganization of the new bone into its former structural arrangement. Bone architecture is related to its function. Compact bone and cancellous bone develop according to functional stresses. Depending on the extent of bone modification needed, remodeling may take months to years. Cancellous bone heals and remodels more rapidly than compact cortical bone, especially at points of direct contact. When remodeling is complete, the fracture surface charge is no longer negative.

The progress of bone healing is monitored by serial x-rays. Adequate immobilization is essential until there is radiologic evidence of callus. Progression of the therapeutic regimen (*e.g.*, application of a cast brace to a patient who has had a femur fracture reduced and immobilized by skeletal traction) is determined by evidence of healing of the fracture.

Bone Healing With Fragments Firmly Approximated. When fractures are treated with open rigid fixation techniques, the bony fragments can be placed in direct contact. Motion at the fracture is eliminated. In this situation, the stages of bone healing are modified. Hematoma formation is not essential and is not observed. Little or no external cartilaginous callus develops. Primary bone healing occurs.

Immature bone develops from the endosteum. There is an intensive regeneration of new osteons. The new osteons develop in the fracture line by a process similar to normal bone maintenance. Fracture strength is obtained when the new osteons have become established. With rigid internal fixation, the bone heals through cortical bone remodeling. This process is slower than bone healing by callus formation.

Local stress (weight-bearing) acts to stimulate local bone formation and remodeling. Weight-bearing bones are thick and strong. When weight-bearing or stress is prevented, as in prolonged bed rest, calcium is lost from the bone (resorption) and the bone becomes osteoporotic (less dense) and weak. Local stress may stimulate extensive remodeling of bone, resulting in straightening of deformed bones. However, if the stress on the bone is excessive, fracture or bone necrosis will occur.

The Articular System

The bones of the body are joined together at *joints* or *articulations* that allow for a variety of movements. Regardless of the amount of movement possible, the junction of two or more bones is called a joint. There are three basic kinds of joints: synarthrosis, amphiarthrosis, and diarthrosis joints. *Synarthrosis joints* are immovable, as exemplified by the skull sutures. *Amphiarthroses*, such as the vertebral joints and symphysis, allow some limited motion. The bones are separated by fibrous cartilage. *Diarthroses* are freely movable joints.

Types of Diarthrosis Joints
- *Ball and socket joints*, best exemplified by the hip or the shoulder, permit full freedom of movement.
- *Hinge joints* permit bending in one direction only and are best exemplified by the elbows and knees.
- A *saddle joint* allows movement in two planes at right angles to each other. The joint at the base of the thumb is a saddle, biaxial joint.
- The *pivot joint* is characterized by the articulation between the radius and the ulna. It permits rotation for such activities as turning a doorknob.
- *Gliding joints* allow for limited movement in all directions and are located at the joints of carpal bones in the wrist.

At a typical movable joint, the ends of the articulating bones are covered with a smooth hyaline cartilage. The articulating bones are surrounded by a tough, fibrous sheath, the *joint capsule*. The capsule is lined with a membrane, the *synovium*, which secretes the lubricating and shock-absorbing *synovial fluid* into the joint capsule. Therefore, the bone surfaces do not come in direct contact. In some synovial joints, fibrocartilage discs are located between the articular cartilage surfaces. They provide shock absorption.

Ligaments (fibrous connective tissue bands) bind the articulating bones together. Ligaments and muscle tendons, which pass over the joint, provide joint stability. In some joints, interosseous ligaments (*e.g.*, the cruciate ligaments of the knee) are found within the capsule and add stability to the joint.

Bursae are additional structures associated with some joints. A bursa is a sac filled with synovial fluid that is located at a point of friction. Bursae are generally found cushioning the movement of tendons, ligaments, and bones at the elbow, shoulder, knee, and other joints.

The Skeletal Muscle System

Anatomy of Skeletal Muscles. Skeletal (striated) muscles are involved in body movement, posture, and heat-production functions (see Chart 58-1). Muscles are attached by *tendons* (cords of fibrous connective tissue) or *aponeuroses* (broad,

---

Chart 58–1
Skeletal Muscle Terminology

Sarcomere—contractile unit of muscle cell
Myofibril—muscle cell; contains sarcomeres
Fasciculi—parallel groups of muscle cells (myofibrils)
Fascia (epimysium)—tough fibrous tissue encasing striated muscle(s)
Tendon—cord of fibrous tissue connecting muscle to bone
Aponeurosis—broad band of fibrous tissue connecting muscle to bone, connective tissue, other muscles, soft tissue, or skin

---

flat sheets of connective tissue) to bones, connective tissue, other muscles, soft tissue, or skin. Muscles contract to bring the two points of attachment closer together. Muscles vary in shape and size according to the activity for which they are responsible. Muscles develop and are maintained when actively used. Age and disuse cause loss of muscular function as fibrotic tissue replaces the contractile muscle tissue.

The muscles of the body are composed of parallel groups of muscle cells (*fasciculi*) encased in fibrous tissue called *epimysium* or *fascia*. The more fasciculi contained in a muscle, the more precise the movements.

The speed of the muscle contraction is variable. *Myoglobulin*, a hemoglobin-like protein pigment, is present in striated muscle cells and transports oxygen from the blood capillaries to the muscle cell mitochondria for cellular metabolic needs. Muscles containing large quantities of myoglobulin (*red muscle*) have been observed to contract slowly and powerfully (*e.g.*, respiratory and postural muscles). Muscles containing little myoglobulin (*white muscles*) contract quickly and for extended periods of time (*e.g.*, extraocular eye muscles). Most body muscles contain both red and white muscle fibers.

Each muscle cell (also referred to as a *muscle fiber*) contains *myofibrils*, which in turn are composed of a series of *sarcomeres*, the actual contractile units of skeletal muscle. The components of the sarcomeres are known as thick and thin filaments. The thin filaments are composed mainly of a protein known as actin. The thick filaments are composed mainly of myosin, another protein material.

Skeletal Muscle Contraction.   Contraction of a muscle is due to the contraction of each of its component sarcomeres. The contraction of a sarcomere is due to interactions between the myosin in the thick filaments and the actin in the thin filaments, brought about by a local increase in the calcium ion concentration. The thick and thin filaments slide across one another. When calcium concentration in the sarcomere subsequently falls, the myosin and actin filaments cease to interact and the sarcomere returns to its original resting length (relaxation). Interaction between actin and myosin does not occur in the absence of calcium.

Muscle fibers contract in response to electrical stimulation. When stimulated, muscle cells generate an action potential in a manner similar to that described for nerve cells. These action potentials propagate along the muscle cell membrane and lead to the release in the muscle cell of calcium ions that are stored in specialized organelles called the *sarcoplasmic reticulum*. The calcium allows the interaction of actin and myosin in the sarcomere. Very shortly after the muscle cell membrane is depolarized, it recovers its resting membrane voltage. Calcium is rapidly removed from the sarcomeres by active reaccumulation in the sarcoplasmic reticulum, and the muscle relaxes.

Depolarization of the muscle cells normally occurs in response to a stimulus delivered by a nerve cell. The communication between the nerve cell and the muscle cell takes place at the *motor end plate*. The neurons that control the activity of skeletal muscle cells are called *lower motor neurons*, which originate in the anterior horn of the spinal cord.

Energy is consumed during muscle contraction and relaxation. The rate of energy used by skeletal muscle varies; it increases markedly during exercise. The source of energy for the muscle cells is adenosine triphosphate (ATP) that is generated through cellular oxidative metabolism. Creatine phosphate, also present in muscle cells, functions as a second reservoir of metabolic energy; it can be converted to ATP when necessary. At low levels of activity, the skeletal muscle synthesizes ATP from the oxidation of glucose to water and carbon dioxide. During periods of high activity, when sufficient oxygen may not be available, glucose is metabolized primarily to lactic acid. Although ATP is generated during the production of lactic acid, the process is inefficient compared with that of oxidative pathways. Therefore, increased amounts of glucose are required and are supplied by muscle glycogen. *Glycogen* is a starch that is produced from glucose, stored in the cells during periods of rest, and utilized during periods of activity. Muscle fatigue is thought to be caused by depletion of glycogen and energy stores and accumulation of lactic acid. As a result, the cycle of muscle contraction and relaxation cannot continue.

During muscle contraction, the energy released from ATP is not completely utilized by the contractile apparatus. This excess energy is dissipated in the form of heat. During isometric contraction, almost all the energy is released in the form of heat; during isotonic contraction, some of the energy is expended in mechanical work. In some situations, such as shivering, the need for generation of heat is the primary stimulus for muscle contraction.

Types of Muscle Contractions.   The contraction of muscle fibers can result in either isotonic or isometric contraction of the muscle. In *isometric contraction*, the length of the muscles remains constant but the force generated by the muscles is increased. An example of this is when one pushes against an immovable wall. *Isotonic contraction*, on the other hand, is characterized by shortening of the muscle with no increase in tension within the muscle. An example of this is flexion of the forearm. In normal activities, many muscle movements are a combination of isometric and isotonic contraction. For example, during walking, isotonic contraction results in shortening of the leg, and, during isometric contraction, the stiff leg pushes against the floor.

Muscle Tone.   Relaxed muscles demonstrate a state of readiness to respond to contraction stimuli. This state of readiness is known as *muscle tone* (tonus) and is due to the maintenance of some of the muscle fibers in a contracted state. Sense organs in the muscles (*muscle spindles*) monitor muscle tone. Muscle tone is found to be minimal during sleep and increased when the person is anxious. A muscle that has less than normal tonus is known as *flaccid*. *Spastic* describes the muscle with greater than normal tonus. In lower motor neuron destruction (*e.g.*, polio), denervated muscle becomes *atonic* (soft and flabby) and atrophies.

Muscle Actions.   Muscles accomplish movement only by contraction. They cannot push. Through the coordination of muscle groups, the body is able to perform a wide variety of movement. The *prime mover* is the muscle that causes a particular motion. The muscles assisting the prime mover are known as *synergists*. The muscle causing movement opposite to that of the primary mover is known as the *antagonist*. The antagonist must relax to allow the prime mover to contract, producing motion. For example, when contraction of the biceps causes flexion of the elbow joint, the biceps is the prime mover and the triceps is the antagonist. With muscle paralysis, a person may be able to retrain functioning muscles within a synergistic group to coordinate in such a way as to effect the needed movement. Secondary movers then become the primary mover.

The body movements that muscle contractions can produce are many. *Flexion* is characterized by bending at a joint (*e.g.*, elbow). The opposite movement is *extension* or straightening at a joint. *Abduction* is the action of moving away from the midline of the body. To move toward the midline is *adduction*. *Rotation* describes turning around a specific axis (*e.g.*, shoulder joint). *Circumduction* is the conelike movement of the thumb. Special body movements include *supination* (turning the palm up), *pronation* (turning the palm down), *inversion* (turning the sole of the foot inward), *eversion* (the opposite of inversion), *protraction* (the jaw is pulled forward), and *retraction* (the jaw is pulled backward). (See Chart 14-2, pp. 221–223, and Chart 14-4, p. 226.)

Exercise, Disuse, and Repair.   Muscles need to be exercised to maintain function and strength. When a muscle repeatedly develops maximum or close to maximum tension over a long period of time, as in regular exercise with weights, the cross-sectional area of the muscle increases (*hypertrophies*). This is due to an increase in the size of individual muscle fibers without an increase in the number of muscle fibers. Hypertrophy will persist only if the exercise is continued.

The opposite phenomenon occurs with disuse of muscle over a long period of time. The decrease in the size of a muscle is called *atrophy*. Bed rest and immobility will cause loss of muscle mass and strength. When immobility is due to a treatment mode (*e.g.*, casting or traction), the patient can decrease the effects of immobility by isometric exercise of the muscles of the immobilized part. Quadriceps setting exercises (tightening the muscles of the thigh) and gluteal setting exercises (tightening of the muscles of the buttocks) help maintain the larger muscle groups that are important in ambulation. Active and weight-resistant exercises of uninjured parts of the body prevent muscle atrophy.

When muscles are injured, they need rest and immobilization until tissue repair occurs. The healed muscle then needs progressive exercise to resume its preinjury functional and strength status.

Gerontologic Considerations

Multiple changes in the musculoskeletal system, including osteoporotic bones, enlarged joints, sclerosed tendons, limited range of motion, thinned intervertebral discs, and weakened muscles, occur with aging. Bone mass peaks at about age 35, after which there is a universal gradual loss of bone. Numerous metabolic changes, including menopausal withdrawal of estrogen and decreased activity, contribute to the loss of bone mass (*osteoporosis*). Women lose more bone mass than men. By the age of 75, the average women has lost 25% of her cortical (compact) bone and 40% of her trabecular (cancellous) bone. Additionally, bones change in shape and have reduced strength. If a fracture occurs, fibrous tissue develops more slowly in the aged.

In the elderly, the ability of the collagen structures to absorb energy is reduced. The articular cartilage degenerates in weight-bearing areas and has a reduced ability to heal. This contributes to the development of osteoarthritis.

Likewise, muscle mass and strength are diminished. There is an actual loss in the number of muscle fibers due to myofibril atrophy with fibrous tissue replacement, which begins in the fourth decade.

In addition, remote musculoskeletal problems for which the patient has compensated may become new problems with age-related changes. For example, patients who have recovered from polio and who have been able to function normally by using synergistic muscle groups may discover increasing incapacity. They have a reduced compensatory ability.

Many of the effects of aging can be overcome if the body is kept healthy and active.

Physical Assessment

An examination of the musculoskeletal system ranges from a basic assessment of functional capabilities to sophisticated physical examination maneuvers that facilitate diagnosis of specific muscle and joint disorders. The nurse examiner's assessment is primarily a functional evaluation. Techniques of inspection and palpation are employed to evaluate the patient's bone integrity, posture, joint function, muscle strength, gait, and ability to perform activities of daily living.

The musculoskeletal assessment is commonly integrated into the routine progression of the physical examination. This system relates closely to the neurologic and cardiovascular systems, and thus assessments of all three systems are often carried out together. The basis of the assessment is a comparison of symmetric regions of the body. The extent of the assessment depends on the patient's physical complaints and health history and any physical clues detected by the examiner that warrant further exploration.

When specific symptoms or physical findings of musculoskeletal dysfunction are apparent, the examination findings are carefully documented and the information is shared with the physician, who may decide that a more extensive examination and diagnostic workup are necessary.

Assessment of the Bony Skeleton.   The bony skeleton is assessed for deformities and alignment. Abnormal bony growths due to bone tumors may be observed. Shortened extremities, amputations, and body parts out of anatomic alignment are noted. Abnormal angulation of long bones or motion at points other than joints is frequently indicative of fracture. *Crepitus* (grating sensation) at the point of abnormal motion may be detected. Movement of bony fragments must be minimized to avoid additional injury.

Assessment of the Spine.   Inspection of the spine is carried out with the patient's gown open to expose the entire back, buttocks, and legs. The examiner stands behind the patient, noting any differences in the height of the shoulders or iliac crests. The gluteal folds are normally symmetric. Shoulder and hip symmetry, as well as the straight line of the vertebral column, are inspected with the patient erect and bending forward (*flexion*). Loss of height occurs with loss of vertebral cartilage in the aged.

The normal curvature of the spine is convex through the thoracic portion and concave through the cervical and lumbar portions. Common deformities of the spine that may be noted include *scoliosis* (a lateral curving deviation of the spine), *kyphosis* (an increased roundness of the thoracic spine curve), and *lordosis* (swayback; exaggeration of the lumbar spine curve). Kyphosis is frequently seen in the elderly patient with osteoporosis and in some patients with neuromuscular diseases. Scoliosis may be congenital, idiopathic, or a result of damage to the paraspinal muscles, as in poliomyelitis. Lordosis is frequently seen during pregnancy as the woman adjusts for changes in her center of gravity.

Assessment of the Articular System. The articular system is evaluated by noting range of motion, deformity, stability, and nodular formation. Range of motion is evaluated both actively (joint is moved by the muscles surrounding the joint) and passively (joint is moved by the examiner). The examiner is familiar with the normal range of motion of major joints as defined by the American Academy of Orthopedic Surgeons. Precise measurement of range of motion can be made by a *goniometer* (a protractor designed for evaluating joint motion). If maximum extension of a joint reveals residual flexion, the range of motion is said to be limited. Limited range of motion may be due to skeletal deformity, joint pathology, or contracture of surrounding muscles and tendons. In elderly persons, limitations of range of motion associated with degenerative joint pathology may reduce their ability to perform activities of daily living.

In the event that joint motion is compromised or the joint is painful, the joint is examined for the presence of excessive fluid within its capsule (*effusion*), swelling, and increased temperature that might reflect active inflammation. An effusion is suspected when the joint is swollen in size and the normal bony landmarks are obscured. The most common site for joint effusion is the knee. If a small amount of fluid is present in the joint spaces beneath the patella, it may be identified by the following maneuver: The physician firmly milks the medial and lateral aspects of the extended knee in a downward motion. This displaces any fluid downward. As pressure is exerted against the medial or lateral side, the physician observes the opposite side for a bulge below the patella. When larger amounts of fluid are present, the patella becomes elevated from the femur during knee extension. When inflammation or fluid is suspected in a joint, physician consultation is indicated.

Joint deformity may be due to *contracture* (shortening of surrounding joint structures), *dislocation* (complete separation of joint surfaces), *subluxation* (partial separation of articular surfaces), or *disruption of structures* surrounding the joint. Weakness or disruption of joint-supporting structures may result in a joint that is too weak to function as designed, and it may therefore require external supporting appliances.

Palpation of the joint while it is passively moved provides information concerning the integrity of the joint. Normally, the joint moves smoothly. A snap or a crack may indicate that a ligament is slipping over a bony prominence. Slightly roughened surfaces, as in arthritic conditions, will result in *crepitus* (an audible or palpable crunching sound) as the irregular surfaces of the joint are moved across one another.

Joints and the tissues surrounding them are examined for nodule formation. Rheumatoid arthritis, gout, and osteoarthritis produce characteristic nodules. The subcutaneous nodules of rheumatoid arthritis are soft and occur within and along tendons that provide extensor function to the joints. Usually, involvement of the joints assumes a symmetric pattern. The nodules of gout are hard and lie within and immediately adjacent to the joint capsule itself. Frequently, they rupture, exuding white uric acid crystals onto the skin surface. The nodules of osteoarthritis are hard and painless and represent bony overgrowth that has resulted from destruction of the cartilaginous surface of bone within the joint capsule. These are frequently seen in older adults.

Often the size of the joint is exaggerated by the atrophy of muscles proximal and distal to that joint. When the joint is kept immobile to avoid the pain that may arise from moving it, the muscles that provide function for the joint atrophy from disuse. This is seen in rheumatoid arthritis of the knees, in which the quadriceps muscle may atrophy dramatically. (See Chap. 50, Management of Patients With Rheumatic Disorders.)

Assessment of the Muscular System. The muscular system is assessed by noting the patient's ability to change position, his muscular strength and coordination, and the size of individual muscles. Muscular weakness of a group of muscles might indicate a variety of conditions, such as polyneuropathy, electrolyte disturbances (particularly potassium and calcium), myasthenia gravis, poliomyelitis, and muscular dystrophy. By palpating the muscle while passively moving the relaxed extremity, the nurse can determine the muscle tone. Muscle strength can be estimated by having the patient perform certain tasks with and without added resistance. For example, the biceps can be tested by requesting the patient to fully extend the arm and then flex it while the nurse applies resistance to prevent the arm from flexing. A simple handshake provides an indication of grasp strength.

Muscle clonus (rhythmic contractions of a muscle) may be elicited in the ankle or wrist by sudden, forceful, sustained dorsiflexion of the foot or extension of the wrist. *Fasciculations* (involuntary twitching of muscle fiber groups) may be observed.

The girth of an extremity must be measured at times to monitor increased size due to edema or bleeding into the muscle or to detect a decrease in size due to atrophy. The unaffected extremity is measured and used as the reference standard. Measurements are to be taken at the maximum circumference of the extremity. It is important that the measurements be at the same location on the extremity and with the extremity in the same position with the muscle at rest. Distance from a specific anatomic landmark (*e.g.*, 10 cm below the medial aspect of the knee for measurement of the calf muscle) should be indicated in the patient's chart so that subsequent measurements are made at the same point. For ease of serial assessment, the point of measurement can be indicated by marking the skin. Variations in size must be greater than 1 cm to be considered significant.

Gait Assessment. An assessment of gait is performed by having the patient walk normally for a short distance away from the examiner. The examiner observes the gait for smoothness and rhythm. Any unsteadiness or irregular movements (frequently noted in elderly patients) are considered abnormal. When a limping motion is noted, it is most likely due to painful weight-bearing. In such instances, the patient can usually pinpoint the area of discomfort, thus guiding a further examination. When one extremity is shorter than another, a limp may also be observed as the patient's pelvis drops downward on the affected side with each step. Limited joint motion may affect gait. A variety of neurologic conditions are associated with abnormal gaits (*e.g.*, spastic hemiparesis gait—stroke; steppage gait—lower motor neuron disease; shuffling gait—Parkinson's disease).

Assessment of Skin and Peripheral Circulation. In addition to assessing the musculoskeletal system, the nurse must inspect the skin and assess peripheral circulation. Cuts, bruises, skin color, and evidence of decreased circulation or infection can influence nursing management. Palpation of the skin can reveal if any areas are warmer or cooler than others and if edema is present. Peripheral circulation is evaluated by assessing peripheral pulses, color, temperature, and capillary refill time.

Diagnostic Evaluation

Nursing Implications

Preparation for diagnostic studies includes assessment of the patient for indicators (*e.g.*, pregnancy, claustrophobia, metal implants, ability to tolerate required positioning due to age, debility, deformity) that may affect the patient undergoing the study. The nurse must communicate with the physician and the appropriate department concerning identified problems related to completion of the prescribed diagnostic test.

Specific Studies

Radiologic and Imaging Procedures

X-rays are important in evaluating patients with musculoskeletal disorders. Bone films determine bone density, texture, erosion, and changes in bone relationships. Multiple x-ray views are needed for full assessment of the structure being examined. X-ray of the cortex of the bone reveals the presence of any widening, narrowing, and signs of irregularity. Joint x-rays will reveal the presence of fluid, irregularity, spur formation, narrowing, and changes in the joint structure.

Tomography shows in detail a specific plane of involved bone. *Computed tomography* (CT) scan can be useful in orthopedic diagnosis by revealing tumors of the soft tissue or injuries to the ligaments or tendons. It is helpful in identifying the location and extent of fractures in areas difficult to define (*e.g.*, the acetabulum). Studies may be performed with or without contrast and last about an hour.

Magnetic resonance imaging (MRI) is a noninvasive, special imaging technique that uses magnetic fields, radio waves, and computers to demonstrate abnormalities (*i.e.*, tumors or narrowing of tissue pathways through bone) of soft tissue such as muscle, tendon, and cartilage. Because an electromagnet is used, patients with any metal implants, braces, or pacemakers are not candidates for this procedure. Jewelry must be re-

moved. Patients who experience claustrophobia are unable to tolerate the confinement of MRI.

Angiography is the study of the vascular structures. *Arteriography* is the study of the arterial system. A radiopaque contrast medium is injected into the selected artery, and serial films are taken of the supplied arterial system. The procedure is useful for determining arterial perfusion and aids in determining the amount of an extremity that must be amputated.

Digital subtraction angiography (DSA) uses computer technology to demonstrate the arterial system from a venous catheter access. *Venogram* is a study of the venous system frequently used to detect venous thrombosis.

Myelography, the injection of contrast medium into the subarachnoid space of the lumbar spine, is carried out to determine disc herniation, *spinal stenosis* (narrowing of the spinal canal), or the site of a tumor. This technique is discussed under Myelography in Chapter 55.

Discography is a study of the intervertebral discs in which a contrast medium is injected into the disc and its distribution is noted.

Arthrography is the injection of a radiopaque substance or air into the joint cavity in order to outline soft-tissue structures and the contour of the joint. The joint is put through its range of motion while a series of radiographs are taken. Arthrography is useful in identifying acute or chronic tears of the joint capsule or supporting ligaments of the knee, shoulder, ankle, hip, or wrist. (If a tear is present, the contrast medium will leak out of the joint and will be evident on radiographs.)

Following the arthrogram, the joint is usually immobilized for 12 to 24 hours and a compression elastic bandage is applied for 2 to 5 days as prescribed. Comfort measures are provided as prescribed.

Other Studies

An *arthrocentesis* is carried out to obtain synovial fluid for purposes of examination. Using aseptic technique, the physician inserts a needle into the joint and aspirates fluid. Following aspiration, no special precautions are necessary.

Normally, synovial fluid is clear, pale, straw-colored, and scanty in volume. The fluid is examined grossly for volume, color, clarity, viscosity, and formation of mucin clot. It is examined microscopically for cell count, cell identification, Gram's stain, and formed elements. Examination of synovial fluid is helpful in the diagnosis of rheumatoid arthritis and other inflammatory arthropathies and will reveal the presence of *hemarthrosis* (bleeding into the joint cavity), which suggests trauma or a tendency to bleed.

Arthroscopy is an endoscopic procedure that allows direct visualization of a joint. The procedure is carried out in the operating room under sterile conditions and following the injection of a local anesthetic into the joint or a general anesthesia. A large-bore needle is inserted and the joint is distended with saline. The arthroscope is introduced and the joint is visualized, including the synovium, articular surfaces, and joint structures. The puncture wound is covered with a sterile dressing and the joint is wrapped with a compression dressing that is worn for 24 to 48 hours for support.

Generally the joint is kept in extension and elevated to reduce swelling, and neurovascular function is monitored. The patient is advised to limit activity following the procedure. Complications are rare but may include infection, hemarthrosis (blood in the joint cavity), thrombophlebitis, stiffness, and delayed wound healing.

A *bone scan* reflects the degree to which the matrix of bone "takes up" a bone-seeking radioactive isotope that is injected into the system. The scan is done 4 to 6 hours after the isotope is injected. The degree of nuclide uptake is related to the metabolism of the bone. An increased uptake of isotope is seen in primary skeletal disease (osteosarcoma), metastatic bone disease, inflammatory skeletal disease (osteomyelitis), and certain types of fractures.

No activity restrictions related to the study are needed. To increase excretion of the isotope, the patient is encouraged to drink plenty of fluids. Other radionuclide tests are not scheduled for 1 to 2 days.

Thermography measures the degree of heat radiating from the skin surface. Inflammatory conditions such as arthritis and infections, as well as neoplasms, may be evaluated. Serial studies may be used to document inflammatory episodes and the patient's response to anti-inflammatory drug therapy.

Electromyography provides information about the electric potential of the muscles and the nerves leading to them. The purpose of the procedure is to determine any abnormal physiology involving the motor unit. Needle electrodes are inserted into selected muscles, and responses to electrical stimuli are recorded on an oscilloscope.

Single and dual *photon absorptiometry* are noninvasive tests to determine bone mineral content at the wrist or vertebrae. Osteoporosis may be monitored with this type of densitometry.

Bone biopsy may be performed to determine the structure and composition of bone tissue, which may be helpful in diagnosing specific diseases. The biopsy site must be monitored for bleeding.

Laboratory Studies

Examination of the patient's blood and urine can provide information concerning a primary musculoskeletal problem (*e.g.*, Paget's disease), information about a developing complication (*e.g.*, infection), baseline information for instituting therapy (*e.g.*, anticoagulant therapy), or information regarding response to therapy. The complete blood count will provide information concerning the hemoglobin level (frequently lower after bleeding associated with trauma) and the white blood cell count. Prior to surgery, coagulation studies are performed to determine bleeding tendencies, because bone is a very vascular tissue.

Blood chemistry studies provide data about a wide variety of musculoskeletal conditions. Serum calcium levels are altered in osteomalacia, parathyroid function, Paget's disease, metastatic bone tumors, and with prolonged immobilization. Serum phosphorus levels are inversely related to calcium levels and are diminished in rickets associated with malabsorption syndrome. Serum enzyme levels of creatine kinase (CK) and serum glutamic-oxaloacetic transaminase (SGOT) become elevated with muscle damage. Alkaline phosphatase is elevated during fracture healing and in diseases with increased osteoblastic activity (*e.g.*, metastatic bone tumors). Bone metabolism may be evaluated through thyroid studies and determination of calcitonin, parathyroid hormone (PTH), and vitamin D levels.

Urine calcium levels increase with bone destruction (*e.g.*, parathyroid dysfunction, metastatic bone tumors, multiple myeloma).

Nursing Assessment and Diagnosis Considerations

Assessment of the patient's functional status and health care needs is an integral part of the nursing assessment. Nursing diagnoses and the care plan are developed and modified according to the identified patient needs.

Initially, the patient with a musculoskeletal problem will require support and nursing care during the period of examinations and testing. There will be a need for physical and psychologic preparation. Patient education prior to the tests (including what is to be done; why it is being done; what the patient can expect to experience, including tactile, visual, and auditory sensations; and what patient participation is expected) will reduce anxiety and enable the patient to be an active participant in care.

The resulting medical diagnosis and prescribed treatment regimen will affect the nursing management of the patient. The nursing plan of care will reflect nursing measures that will facilitate the resolution of the patient's health problems.

The nursing assessment will enable the nurse to identify the health problems that can be improved by nursing interventions. Actual and potential nursing diagnoses common to patients with musculoskeletal disorders include the following:

- Impaired physical mobility
- Pain—acute or chronic
- Actual or high risk for impaired skin integrity
- Constipation
- Altered peripheral tissue perfusion
- High risk for infection
- Knowledge deficit about the disease process and treatment regimen
- Self-care deficits
- Disturbance in body image, self-esteem, role performance
- Ineffective individual coping
- Altered family processes
- Potential for sexual dysfunction
- Powerlessness
- Sleep pattern disturbance
- Diversional activity deficit
- Potential for altered nutrition—less than body requirements

In collaboration with the patient, health goals and nursing strategies are formulated to resolve the identified nursing diagnoses.

Chapter Summary

The nurse assesses the functional integrity of the musculoskeletal system. The bony skeleton protects vital organs, supports body structures, and stores minerals. Blood cells are produced in the bone marrow. The muscles contract to move the body, maintain posture, and maintain body temperature. Tendons attach muscles to bones. Joints allow for and control the extent of movement. Ligaments provide stability to the musculoskeletal system. Movement and muscle tone are coordinated through the nervous system.

Bone is highly vascular, living tissue that is maintained and repaired by bone cells (*i.e.*, osteocytes, osteoblasts, osteoclasts). Healing of fractured bone generally occurs in stages: inflammation, cellular proliferation, callus formation, callus ossification, and remodeling. Exercise maintains muscle strength and function. Atrophy and contracture occur with immobility and disuse. Aging is reflected in the musculoskeletal system by the development of osteoporosis, decreased range of motion, thinned intervertebral discs, and weakened muscles.

In addition to physical assessment, multiple diagnostic studies are used to evaluate the musculoskeletal system. The nurse prepares and supports the individual undergoing various diagnostic procedures and reviews the diagnostic findings for nursing care implications.

Loss of functional integrity of the musculoskeletal system affects the person's ability to carry out activities of daily living. The nurse and the patient with a musculoskeletal problem develop strategies to meet the patient's basic human needs that have been compromised by alterations in the musculoskeletal system.

Bibliography

Books

Adams JC. Outline of Orthopaedics, 10th ed. Edinburgh, Churchill–Livingstone, 1986.

Albright J and Brand R (eds). The Scientific Basis of Orthopaedics, 2nd ed. Norwalk, CT, Appleton and Lange, 1987.

American Nurses Association and National Association of Orthopaedic Nurses. Orthopaedic Nursing Practice. Kansas City, MO, American Nurses Association, 1986.

Birnbaum JB. The Musculoskeletal Manual, 2nd ed. Orlando, Grune & Stratton, 1986.

Cittadine TJ. Orthopedic Terminology: Including Sports Medicine. Thorofare, NJ, Slack, 1988.

Dee R, Mango E, and Hurst LC (eds). Principles of Orthopaedic Practice. New York, McGraw–Hill, 1988.

Eliopoulos C. Gerontological Nursing, 2nd ed. Philadelphia, JB Lippincott, 1987.

Farrell J. Illustrated Guide to Orthopedic Nursing, 3rd ed. Philadelphia, JB Lippincott, 1986.

Footner A. Orthopaedic Nursing. London, Bailliere Tindall, 1987.

Gartland JJ. Fundamentals of Orthopaedics, 4th ed. Philadelphia, WB Saunders, 1987.

Hadler NM. Clinical Concepts in Regional Musculoskeletal Illness. Orlando, Grune & Stratton, 1987.

Horowitz M. Stress Response Syndromes. Northvale, NJ, Aronson, 1986.

Lewis MM and Weiner LS. Orthopaedics. Philadelphia, JB Lippincott, 1989.

Lewis RC. Primary Care Orthopedics. New York, Churchill–Livingstone, 1988.

Magee DJ. Orthopedic Physical Assessment. Philadelphia, WB Saunders, 1987.

Mercies LR. Practical Orthopedics, 2nd ed. Chicago, Year Book Medical Pub, 1987.

Miller TR. Evaluating Orthopedic Disability: A Commonsense Approach, 2nd ed. Oradell, NJ, Medical Economics Books, 1987.

Mourad LA and Droste MM. The Nursing Process in the Care of Adults with Orthopaedic Conditions, 2nd ed. New York, John Wiley & Sons, 1988.

Salmond S et al (eds). Core Curriculum for Orthopaedic Nursing, 2nd ed. Pitman, NJ, National Association of Orthopaedic Nurses, 1991.

Schoen D. The Nursing Process in Orthopaedics. Norwalk, CT, Appleton–Century–Crofts, 1986.

Smith C. Orthopaedic Nursing. London, Heinemann Nursing, 1987.

Stearns CM and Brunner NA. Opcare: Orthopaedic Patient Care. A Nursing Guide, Vols. 1, 2, 3. Rutherford, NJ, Howmedica, 1987.

Journals

Asterisks indicate nursing research articles.

Assessment/Diagnostic Procedures

Amadio PC. Pain dysfunction syndromes. J Bone Joint Surg [Am] 1988 Jul; 70(6):944–949.

Bigos DM et al. Idiopathic radial tunnel syndrome: Surgical treatment and nursing care. AORN J 1987 Aug; 46(2):255, 258, 260+.

Bonafeds RP and Bennett RM. Shoulder pain. Postgrad Med 1989 Jul; 82(1):185–193.

Edeiken J and Karasick D. Imaging in bone cancer. CA 1987 Jul/Aug; 37(4):239–245.

Gavant ML. Digital subtraction angiography of the foot in atherosclerotic occlusive disease. South Med J 1989 Mar; 82(3):328–334.

Hodges DL, McGuire TJ, and Kumar VN. Diagnosis of hip pain: An anatomical approach. Orthop Rev 1987 Feb; 16(2):109–113.

* Holmes R et al. Nutrition know how: Combating pressure sores—nutritionally. Am J Nurs 1987 Oct; 87(10):1301–1303.

Infante MC et al. Interactive aspects of pain assessment. Orthop Nurs 1987 Jan/Feb; 6(1):31–34.

Kyba FN et al. Magnetic resonance imaging: The latest in diagnostic technology. Nursing 1987 Jan; 17(1):44–47.

Maher AB. Early assessment and management of musculoskeletal injuries. Nurs Clin North Am 1986 Dec; 21(4):717–727.

Mann RA. Pain in the foot. Postgrad Med 1987 Jul; 82(6):154–162.

Mulvey T. Anatomy and physiology of the shoulder complex. Orthop Nurs 1988 May/Jun; 7(3):23–28.

Schon L and Zuckerman JD. Hip pain in the elderly: Evaluation and diagnosis. Geriatrics 1988 Jan; 43(1):48–62.

Wapner KL. Diagnosis of foot pain. Hosp Med 1987 Nov; 23(11):69, 70, 79–86, 92+.

Zubay R. Understanding magnetic resonance imaging from a nursing perspective. Orthop Nurs 1988 Nov/Dec; 7(6):17–23.

Responses to Injury

American Pain Society. Relieving pain: An analgesic guide. Am J Nurs 1988 Jun; 88(6):815–825.

Dunwoody CJ. Patient controlled analgesia: Rationale, attributes, and essential factors. Orthop Nurs 1987 Sep/Oct; 6(5):31–36.

Horowitz M. Stress response syndromes: A review of posttraumatic and adjustment disorders. Hosp Community Psychiatry 1986 Mar; 37(3): 241–249.

Moore K and Thompson D. Posttraumatic stress disorder in the orthopaedic patient. Orthop Nurs 1989 Jan/Feb; 8(1):11–19.

Payne MB. Utilizing role theory to assist the family with sudden disability. Rehabil Nurs 1988 Jul/Aug; 13(4):191–194.

Rubin M. The physiology of bedrest. AJN 1988 Jan; 88(1):50–56.

Sculco T. Approaches to senior care. Orthop Rev 1988 Mar; 17(3):239–240.

Bone Metabolism

Chambers JK. Metabolic bone disorders. Imbalances in calcium and phosphorus. Nurs Clin North Am 1987 Dec; 22(4):861–872.

Hansel MJ. Fractures and the healing process. Orthop Nurs 1988 Jan/Feb; 7(1):43–50.

Loder RT. The influence of diabetes mellitus on the healing of closed fractures. Clin Orthop 1988 Jul; (232):210–216.

Agencies

National Institute of Arthiritis and Musculoskeletal and Skin Diseases National Institutes of Health, Bethesda, MD 20892

59

Management Modalities for Patients With Musculoskeletal Dysfunction

Learning Objectives

On completion of this chapter, the learner will be able to:

1. Use the nursing process as a framework for care of the patient with musculoskeletal dysfunction
2. Use the nursing process as a framework for care of the patient with a cast
3. Describe the preventive and health teaching needs of the patient with a cast
4. Describe the various types of traction and the principles of effective traction
5. Specify the preventive nursing care needs of the patient in traction
6. Use the nursing process as a framework for care of the patient in traction
7. Use the nursing process as a framework for care of the patient undergoing orthopedic surgery
8. Compare the nursing needs of the patient undergoing total hip replacement with those of the patient undergoing total knee replacement

▶ Nursing Process Overview
◇ Assessment

The nursing assessment of the patient with musculoskeletal dysfunction includes an evaluation of the impact of the musculoskeletal problem on the patient. The nurse is concerned with assisting persons with musculoskeletal problems to maintain their general health, accomplish their activities of daily living, and manage their treatment modalities. Systemic homeostasis is assured; optimal nutrition is encouraged; and problems related to immobility are prevented. The nurse helps the patient to achieve a balance between periods of exercise and rest through an individualized plan of care.

◇ *Initial Interview.* In the initial interview, the nurse obtains a general impression of the patient's health status. The nurse obtains subjective data from the patient concerning the onset of the problem and how it has been managed to this point. The patient's perceptions and expectations related to the health problems may affect restoration of health. The existence of concurrent health problems (*e.g.,* diabetes, heart disease, upper respiratory infection) needs to be noted for consideration when developing the plan of care. A history of medication use and response to pain medication will aid in designing drug management regimens.

Allergies are noted, and their description should include the type of reaction the patient has experienced. The use of tobacco, alcohol, and other drugs is assessed to evaluate the effects of these agents on patient care. Notations of the patient's ability to learn, economic status, and current occupation are needed for discharge planning and for rehabilitation. Additions to the initial interview data will be made as the nurse interacts with the patient. Such data allow for adjustment of the individualized plan of care.

◊ *Physical Assessment.* The nurse is interested in identifying the functional abilities of the patient, the effects that any disabilities and medical treatment have on the patient's ability to meet his needs effectively, and the ability of the patient to perform activities of daily living. A general inspection of the body will disclose any gross deformity, asymmetry of contours or size, swelling, edema, bruising, or breaks in the skin. Observing the patient's posture, movement, and gait will provide information concerning alterations in ability to move, the existence of discomfort, or the presence of involuntary movements (fasciculations or twitches). (See Chap. 58.)

Any deviations from normal are noted. A baseline for noting and evaluating changes in the person's abilities is established.

◊ *Subjective Assessment Data.* During the interview and physical assessment, the patient may report the presence of pain, tenderness, tightness, and abnormal sensations. This information is assessed and documented.

Pain

Most patients with diseases and traumatic conditions of muscles, bones, and joints experience pain. *Bone pain* is characteristically described as a dull, deep ache that is boring in nature, whereas *muscular pain* is considered sore and aching and is frequently referred to as "muscle cramps." *Fracture pain* is sharp and piercing and is relieved by immobilization. Sharp pain may also result from *bone infection* with muscle spasm or pressure on a sensory nerve.

Most musculoskeletal pain is relieved by rest. Pain that increases with activity may indicate joint sprain or muscle strain, whereas steadily increasing pain points to a progression of an infectious process (osteomyelitis), a malignant tumor, or vascular complications. Radiating pain is seen in conditions in which pressure is exerted on a nerve root. Pain is variable, and its assessment and nursing management must be individualized.

Assessment of Pain and Related Factors
- What was the patient doing before the complaint of pain?
- Is the body in proper alignment?
- Is there pressure from traction, bed linen, a cast, or other appliances?
- Is the position of a muscle mass causing tension on the skin at a pin site?
- Is the patient overly tired from lack of sleep, exciting stimuli, or too much activity?
- Can the pain be localized?
- How does the patient describe it?
- What was the manner of onset?
- Is there radiation of pain? If so, in what direction does it occur?
- Is there pain in any other part of the body?
- What is the character of the pain (sharp, dull, boring, shooting, throbbing, cramping)?
- Is it constant?
- What relieves it?
- What makes it worse?

Pain and discomfort are important to the patient and must be managed successfully. Not only is pain exhausting, but if prolonged it can force the patient to become increasingly preoccupied and dependent.

Altered Sensations

Sensory disturbances are frequently associated with musculoskeletal problems. The patient may describe the presence of *paresthesias* (burning or tingling sensations) and numbness. These sensations may be due to pressure on nerves or circulatory impairment. Soft tissue swelling or direct trauma to these structures can impair their function. Loss of function can result from impaired nerves and circulatory structures located throughout the musculoskeletal system. Assessment of the neurovascular status of the involved musculoskeletal area provides information for planning interventions.

Assessment of Neurovascular Integrity
- Is the patient experiencing any abnormal sensations or numbness?
- When did this begin? Is it getting worse?
- Is the patient also experiencing pain?
- What is the color of the part distal to the problem? Pale? Dusky? Cyanotic?
- Is there a pulse present distal to the problem?
- Is there rapid capillary refill? (Compress the patient's nail and release. When pressure is released, the color of the nailbed should quickly assume a pink hue.)
- Is the motor component of the nerve intact? Is the patient able to move the innervated part?
- Is edema present?
- Is any constrictive device or clothing causing nerve or vascular compression?
- Are symptoms decreased by elevation of the affected part or modification of position?

◊ Nursing Diagnoses

Based on the nursing assessment data, the major nursing diagnoses for a patient with musculoskeletal dysfunction may include the following:

- Anxiety related to changes in body integrity
- Knowledge deficit about the therapeutic regimen
- Pain related to musculoskeletal disorder
- Altered peripheral tissue perfusion related to physiologic responses to injury, swelling, or increased pressure within a closed space (*i.e.*, muscle compartment; constrictive dressing, or cast)
- Impaired physical mobility related to musculoskeletal impairment

◊ Planning and Implementation

◊ *Goals:* The major goals of the patient with musculoskeletal dysfunction may include reduced anxiety, understanding of the therapeutic regimen, relief of pain, maintenance of adequate tissue perfusion, and improved physical mobility.

◊ Nursing Interventions

◊ *Reduced Anxiety.* Musculoskeletal problems may be due to an acute traumatic injury or may be of a persistent, recurrent, long-term nature. The psychological and social/economic impact of the problem causes a variety of reactions in these patients. The nurse assists the patient in coping with the problems associated with musculoskeletal dysfunction and the associated therapies.

Most patients with acute musculoskeletal problems are anxious and have pain. They experience a mixture of fear and anticipation before definitive therapy begins. People who have long-term disabilities frequently undergo repeated reconstructive operations. They are familiar with the routines of the hospital and are concerned with the ultimate outcome of the procedure. Their patience and hope may be limited. Such patients with musculoskeletal problems need an understanding, supportive nurse. (See Nursing Care Plan 10–1, Care of the Patient With Anxiety.)

▷ *Patient Education.* Preparatory education increases the patient's understanding. The patient needs to be informed so that he can actively participate in the development and implementation of the therapeutic regimens. Information about what to expect, including sensations during and after the therapy, will encourage active participation in the therapeutic regimen. When possible, specific information concerning anticipated equipment (*e.g.*, casts, traction), mobilization aids (*e.g.*, trapeze, walker, crutches), exercises (*e.g.*, quadriceps setting, deep breathing), and medications (*e.g.*, analgesics, antibiotics) should be shared with the patient. Cognitive preparations facilitate active participation in the plan of care. At times patients can practice recuperative activities, such as using a urinal in a recumbent position, before they are immobilized and must tend to basic bodily functions in unusual positions.

Before the time of discharge, patients should have explicit instructions that they understand, indicating those activities they may and may not perform. It is not enough to say "take it easy." Patients must know any untoward signs and symptoms that should be reported to the physician. They must be aware of the importance of follow-up visits. If they have any difficulties, they should know where and how to get help. The nurse has a major part of the responsibility for educating these patients before they leave the hospital (see Chap. 14, Principles and Practices of Rehabilitation).

▷ *Relief of Pain.* Patients who have bone and joint problems frequently experience severe pain. Often the person who has undergone surgery to correct a foot condition is much more uncomfortable than one who has had extensive abdominal surgery. Narcotics and other pain-relieving measures are given as prescribed, taking into consideration the patient's age and body size as well as the type and the site of the musculoskeletal problem. Generally, elderly patients require less pain medication. In the patient with persistent pain over an extended period, drug dependence may occur and may pose a considerable problem.

Pain may result from either the primary musculoskeletal problem or associated problems (*e.g.*, pressure over bony prominences, muscle spasm, swelling). Prolonged pressure over bony prominences (*e.g.*, heel, head of fibula, tibial tuberosity) may cause a burning type of pain. Relieving the pressure is necessary to relieve the pain and prevent further tissue damage.

Muscle spasm is another associated cause of pain. When a muscle is injured, the natural response of the muscle is to contract, thereby splinting and protecting the injured area. Prolonged muscle contraction is painful. Relaxation techniques, traction, or medications may be used to reduce pain from muscle spasm.

Usually swelling can be controlled and compartment syndrome (see p. 1792) avoided by elevating the injured part and intermittently applying an ice pack to the injury for 20 to 30 minutes.

Additional information and guidelines to nursing management of the patient with pain are presented in Chapter 15.

▷ *Improved Tissue Perfusion.* Swelling usually accompanies musculoskeletal injury. If the swelling occurs in a confined space (*e.g.*, cast, constrictive dressing, muscle fascia sheath), a *compartment syndrome* may develop. Excruciating pain and loss of motion and sensory function may result from tissue anoxia. The blood supply can be assessed by determining nail bed capillary refill (*i.e.*, the nail is gently squeezed until it blanches; pressure is released and the amount of time for color to return to normal is noted. Color normally returns quickly, within 3 seconds.) In addition, if the tissue perfusion is diminished, the skin will feel cool to the touch and will appear dusky, pale, or blue. Tissue pressure may be elevated and can be measured directly with a tissue pressure-monitoring device (Fig. 59–1). Sensory and motor function may be altered or diminished.

▷ *Improved Mobility.* The immobility necessitated by some treatment modalities must not result in undue deterioration. Throughout the treatment period, the nurse is concerned with health maintenance and ultimate restoration of function. Exercise of nonimmobilized muscles and joints helps maintain their strength and function, minimizes cardiovascular deterioration, and prevents disuse osteoporosis. Isometric exercises of immobilized extremities help to maintain muscle strength.

Involvement in activities of daily living (*e.g.*, hygiene, dressing, eating) provides a sense of independence and accomplishment. Coordinating nursing interventions with special therapy approaches (*e.g.*, physical therapy, occupational therapy) makes it easier for the patient to learn and practice the therapeutic regimens. Emphasis is placed on what the patient is able to do within the limits of the treatment modalities.

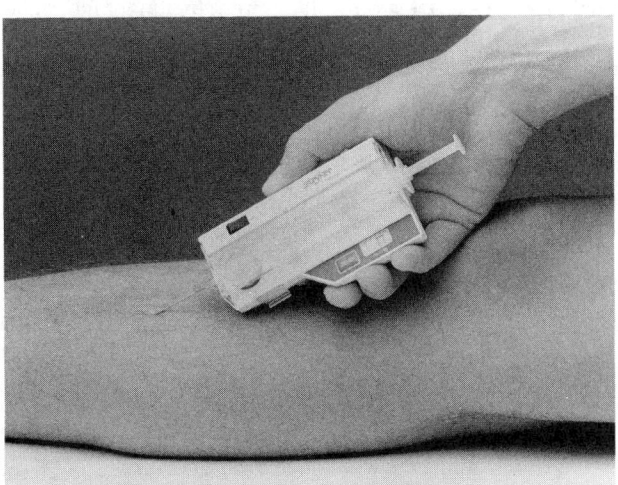

Figure 59–1. Tissue pressure monitoring device. (Courtesy of Stryker Surgical.)

▷ Evaluation

Expected Outcomes
1. Exhibits minimal anxiety
   a. Appears relaxed and confident in abilities
   b. Uses effective coping strategies
   c. Participates in care
2. Relates plan for continued health management
   a. Describes planned treatment regimen
   b. States signs and symptoms to report to physician
   c. Makes appointment for follow-up care
3. Achieves pain relief
   a. Controls discomfort with occasional oral medications
   b. Moves with minimal discomfort
   c. Uses positioning to increase comfort
4. Maintains adequate tissue perfusion
   a. Controls swelling
   b. Demonstrates normal capillary refill
   c. Reports normal sensations
   d. Demonstrates motor function
5. Demonstrates improved physical mobility
   a. Transfers self independently or with minimal assistance
   b. Participates in activities of daily living
   c. Uses mobility aids safely

In summary, individuals with musculoskeletal dysfunction must be assessed by the nurse to determine the impact of the musculoskeletal problem on their ability to maintain health, accomplish activities of daily living, and manage the treatment modality. Using knowledge of various treatment modalities, the nurse applies the nursing process to assist the patient in meeting identified health needs. Nursing diagnoses frequently applicable for patients who have musculoskeletal problems include anxiety related to changes in body integrity; knowledge deficit about the therapeutic regimen; pain related to musculoskeletal disorder; altered peripheral tissue perfusion related to physiologic response to injury or increased pressure within a closed space (*i.e.*, muscle compartment; constrictive dressing or cast); and impaired physical mobility related to musculoskeletal dysfunction.

Treatment modalities frequently used with musculoskeletal dysfunction include casts, external fixation devices, traction, and surgery.

Through an awareness of usual patient problems and potential problems associated with different treatment modalities, the nurse can assist the patient with a musculoskeletal dysfunction to meet the identified health needs and avoid potential health problems.

Management of the Patient in a Cast

A cast is a rigid external immobilizing device that is molded to the contours of the body to which it is applied. The purpose of a cast is to immobilize a body part in a specific position and to apply uniform pressure on encased soft tissue. It may be used to immobilize a reduced fracture, correct a deformity, apply uniform pressure to underlying soft tissue, or provide support and stability for weakened joints. Generally, casts permit mobilization of the patient while restricting movement of some body part.

Types of Casts

The condition being treated influences the type and thickness of the cast applied. Generally speaking, the joints proximal and distal to the area to be immobilized are included in the cast. With some fractures, however, cast construction and molding may allow movement of a joint while immobilizing a fracture (*e.g.*, three-point fixation in a patellar tendon weight-bearing cast).

Figure 59–2 illustrates some of the common types of cylindrical casts and areas in which pressure problems commonly occur.

Short arm cast—extends from below the elbow to the palmar crease, secured around the base of the thumb. If the thumb is included, it is known as a *thumb spica* or *gauntlet cast*.
Long arm cast—extends from the upper level of the axillary fold to the proximal palmar crease; the elbow usually is immobilized at a right angle
Short leg cast—extends from below the knee to the base of the toes. The foot is at a right angle in a neutral position.
Long leg cast—extends from the junction of the upper and middle third of the thigh to the base of the toes. The knee may be slightly flexed.
Walking cast—a short- or long-leg cast reinforced for strength. It might incorporate a walking heel.
Body cast—encircles the trunk
Spica cast—incorporates a portion of the trunk and one or two extremities (single or double spica cast)
   Shoulder spica cast—a body jacket that encloses the trunk and the shoulder and elbow
   Hip spica cast—encloses the trunk and a lower extremity; may be a single or double hip spica cast

Casting Materials

Plaster. The traditional cast is made of plaster. Plaster bandages mold very smoothly to the body contours. Rolls of crinoline are impregnated with powdered, anhydrous calcium sulfate (gypsum crystals). When wet, a crystallizing reaction occurs and heat is given off (an exothermic reaction).

• The heat given off during this reaction can be uncomfortable. Therefore, the water used should be cool. The cast needs to be exposed to allow maximum dissipation of the heat. Most casts are cool after about 15 minutes.

The crystallization produces a rigid dressing. The speed at which the reaction occurs varies from a few minutes to 15 to 20 minutes. The orthopedist will determine what setting speed is appropriate for the cast being applied.

After the plaster has set, the cast is still wet and somewhat soft. It does not have its full strength until dry. While damp, it can be dented if handled with the fingertips instead of the palms of the hand or if allowed to rest on hard surfaces or sharp edges. These dents produce pressure areas on the skin under the cast. The cast requires 24 to 72 hours to dry, depending on the thickness of the cast and the environmental drying conditions. A freshly applied cast should be exposed to circulating air to dry. Clothing or bed linens restrict the escape of moisture. A dry cast is white and shiny, resonant, and odorless as well as firm; a wet cast is gray and dull in

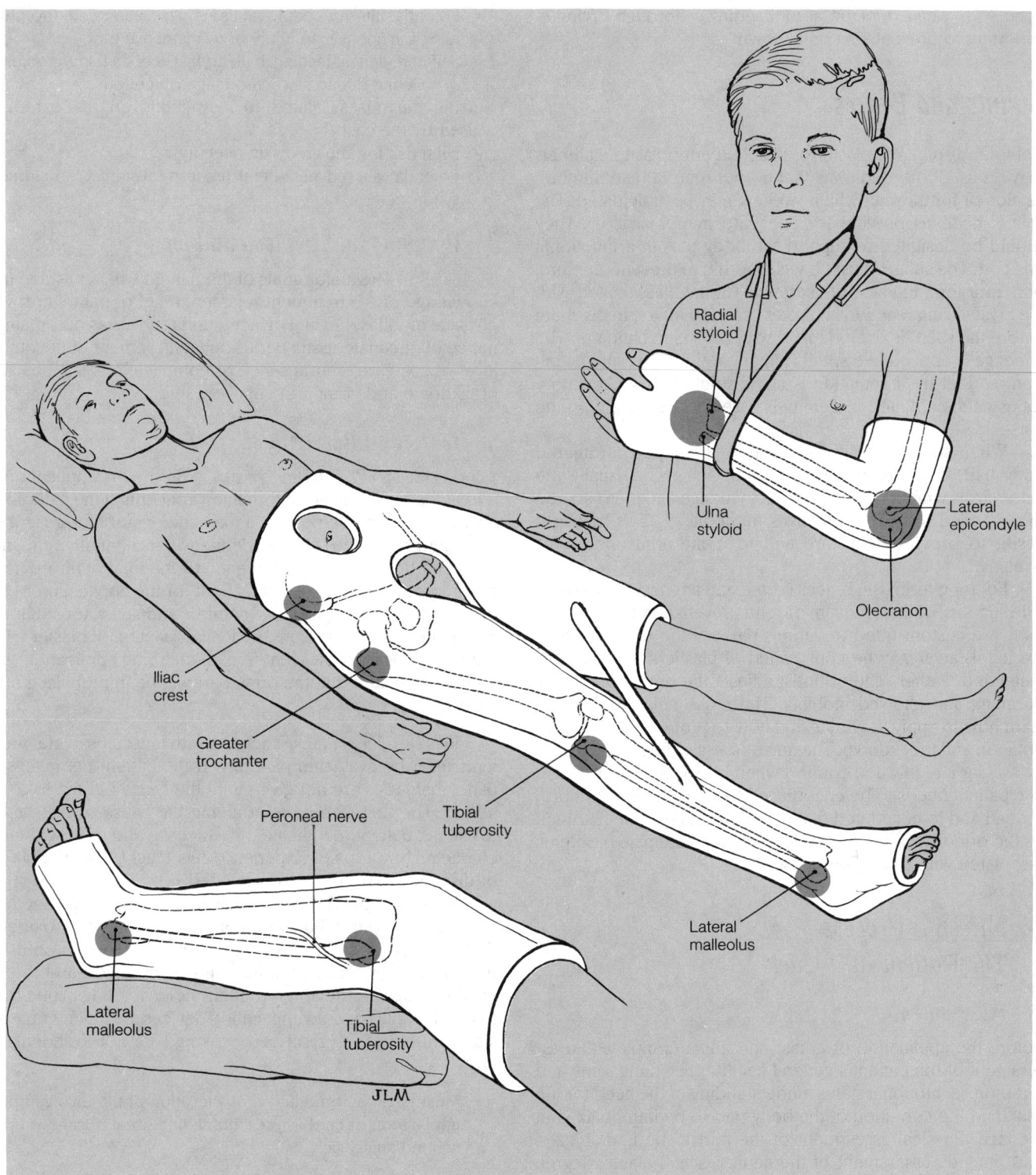

Figure 59–2. Pressure areas in different types of casts. (Suddarth DS. The Lippincott Manual of Nursing Practice, 5th ed. Philadelphia, JB Lippincott, 1991.)

appearance, is dull to percussion, feels damp, and has a musty odor.

Nonplaster. Generally referred to as *fiberglass casts*, these water-activated polyurethane materials have the versatility of plaster and the additional advantages of being of lighter weight and increased strength, water resistant, and durable.

They are made of an open-weave, nonabsorbent fabric impregnated with hardeners that reach full rigid strength in minutes.

Nonplaster casts are porous and therefore diminish skin problems. They do not soften when wet, which allows for *hydrotherapy* (use of water for treatment). When wet, they are dried with a hair drier on a cool setting. Thorough drying is important to prevent skin breakdown.

Splints and Braces

Contoured splints of plaster or pliable thermoplastic materials may be used for conditions that do not require rigid immobilization or for those in which swelling may be anticipated. The splints need to provide for adequate immobilization. They should be designed to support the body part in a functional position. The splints must be well padded to prevent pressure, skin abrasion, and skin breakdown. The heat associated with the crystallizing reaction in plaster casts is allowed to dissipate before the splint is overwrapped with an elastic bandage. The bandage is applied in a spiral fashion, and the pressure is uniform so that the circulation is not restricted. The circulatory status of the splinted extremity is assessed frequently by the nurse.

When soft immobilizers are used to support an injured body part, rigid immobilization is not achieved. Usually the extremity is wrapped with an elastic bandage and then secured to a padded, contoured, canvas immobilizer. This makes it easier to provide skin care and to make adjustments for swelling.

For long-term use, braces (*orthoses*) are designed to provide support, control movement, and prevent additional injury. They are custom fitted to various parts of the body, such as the leg. Braces may be constructed of plastic materials or of metal and leather. The orthotist adjusts the brace for fit, positioning, and allowed mobility. The nurse helps the patient learn how to apply the brace and how to protect the skin from irritation and breakdown. The nurse assesses the patient's neurovascular integrity and comfort when he is wearing the brace. The patient needs to be encouraged to wear the brace as prescribed and to be assured that minor adjustments of the brace by the orthotist will increase comfort and minimize problems associated with its long-term use.

▶ Nursing Process
The Patient in a Cast

▷ Assessment

Before the application of a cast, the nurse completes an assessment of the patient's general health, presenting signs and symptoms, emotional status, understanding of the need for the cast, and the condition of the body part to be immobilized in the cast. Physical assessment of the part to be immobilized must include assessment of the neurovascular status, degree and location of swelling, bruising, and presence of skin abrasions or lacerations.

▷ Nursing Diagnoses

Based on the assessment data, major nursing diagnoses for the patient may include:

- Knowledge deficit about the management regimen
- Pain related to the disease process
- Impaired physical mobility related to disease process and cast
- Impaired skin integrity related to lacerations and abrasions

- Potential altered peripheral tissue perfusion related to physiologic responses to injury or to restrictive cast
- Self-care deficit: feeding, bathing/hygiene, dressing/grooming, or toileting due to restricted range of motion

Nursing diagnoses related to restrictions on the extremity caused by the cast:

- High risk for impaired skin integrity
- Potential altered peripheral tissue perfusion: Compartment syndrome

▷ Planning and Implementation

▷ *Goals:*   The major goals of the patient with a cast include knowledge of the treatment regimen, relief of pain, improved physical mobility, healing of lacerations and abrasions, maintenance of adequate tissue perfusion, achievement of maximum level of self-care, and absence of complications such as skin breakdown and compartment syndrome.

▷ Nursing Interventions

▷ *Knowledge of Treatment Regimen.*   Before the application of a cast, the patient needs information concerning the pathologic problem and the purpose and expectations of the prescribed treatment regimen. This knowledge will facilitate the patient's active participation and adherence to the treatment program. It is important to prepare the patient for the application of the cast by describing the sights, sounds, and sensations that are anticipated (*e.g.*, heat from hardening reaction of plaster). The patient needs to know what to expect during application (see Table 59–1), and that the body part will be immobilized after casting.

▷ *Relief of Pain.*   Pain associated with musculoskeletal problems must be evaluated carefully. If the patient complains of pain, analgesics are not given until the cause of pain is determined. The first step in determining the cause of the pain is to ask the patient to indicate the exact site and to describe the character of the pain. Experience has taught that complaints of discomfort must not go unheeded.

Pain associated with the disease process (*e.g.*, fracture) is frequently controlled by immobilization. Pain due to edema that is associated with trauma, surgery, or bleeding into the tissues can frequently be controlled by elevation and, if prescribed, application of intermittent cold. Ice bags (one-third to one-half full) or cold application devices are placed on each side of the cast, if prescribed, making sure not to indent the cast.

- Most pain can be relieved by elevation of the involved part, application of cold as prescribed, and usual dosages of prescribed analgesics.

Pain may be indicative of development of complications: *skin breakdown* due to pressure on the tissues or bony prominences or *compartment syndrome* due to impairment of circulation. Severe pain over a bony prominence warns of an impending pressure ulcer. *Pain decreases when ulceration occurs.* Discomfort due to pressure on the skin may be relieved by elevation that controls edema and positioning that alters pressure, or it may require modification of the cast or recasting by the physician. Pain associated with compartment syndrome is relentless and not controlled by modalities such as elevation, application of cold, and usual dosages of analgesics.

TABLE 59–1. *Application of a Cast*

Procedure	Rationale
1. Support part to be casted.	1. Minimizes movement; maintains reduction and alignment; increases comfort
2. Position and maintain part to be casted in desired position during casting procedure.	2. Facilitates casting; reduces incidence of complications (*e.g.*, malunion, nonunion, contracture)
3. Drape patient.	3. Avoids undue exposure; protects other body parts from contact with casting materials.
4. Wash and dry part to be casted.	4. Reduces incidence of skin breakdown.
5. Place knitted material* (*e.g.*, stockinette) over part to be casted. Apply in smooth and nonconstrictive manner. Allow additional material.	5. Protects skin from casting materials. Protects skin from pressure. Folds over edges of cast when finishing application; creates smooth, padded edge; protects skin from abrasion.
6. Wrap soft, nonwoven roll padding* smoothly and evenly around part.	6. Protects skin from pressure of cast.
Use additional padding around bony prominences (see Fig. 59–2) and at nerve grooves (*e.g.*, head of fibula, olecranon process).	Protects skin at bony prominences. Protects superficial nerves.
7. Apply plaster or nonplaster casting material evenly on body part. Choose appropriate width bandage. Overlap preceding turn by half the width of the bandage. Use continuous motion, maintaining constant contact with body part. Use additional casting material (splints) at joints and at points of anticipated cast stress.	7. Creates smooth, solid, well-contoured cast. Facilitates smooth application. Creates smooth, solid, immobilizing cast. Shapes cast properly for adequate support. Strengthens cast.
8. "Finish" cast: • Edges smooth; • Trim and reshape with cast knife or cutter.	8. Protects skin from abrasion. Assures full range of motion of adjacent joints.
9. Remove particles of casting materials from skin.	9. Prevents particles from loosening and sliding underneath cast.
10. Support cast during hardening and drying.	10. Casting materials harden in minutes. Maximum hardness of nonplaster cast occurs in minutes. Maximum hardness of plaster cast occurs with drying (24 to 72 hours, depending on thickness of cast and environment).
Handle hardening casts with palms of hands; do not rest on hard surfaces or on sharp edges; avoid pressure on cast.	Avoids denting of cast and pressure areas.

* *Nonabsorbent materials are used with nonplaster casts.*

- The complaints of pain from the patient in a cast must never be ignored; a pressure ulcer or tissue perfusion problems must be suspected.
- Unrelieved pain must be reported immediately to the physician to avoid possible necrosis and paralysis.

▷ *Improved Mobility.* Every joint that is not immobilized should be exercised and moved through its range of motion to maintain function. If the patient has a leg cast, toe exercise is encouraged. If the patient has an arm cast, finger exercise is encouraged. The patient is encouraged to actively participate in his care.

While in a cast, the patient is taught to tense or contract muscles (*e.g.*, isometric muscle contraction) without moving the part to reduce muscle atrophy and maintain muscle strength. If the patient has a leg cast, the nurse places her hand under the knee and instructs the patient to "push down." If the patient has an arm cast, he is encouraged to "make a fist." Muscle setting exercises (*e.g.*, quadriceps setting and gluteal setting exercises) are important in maintaining muscles essential for walking (Chart 59–1). Isometric exercises should be done at least hourly while the patient is awake.

At times, portable electrical muscle stimulators may be attached to the skin over large muscles before cast application. Muscle contractions are electrically stimulated for about 8 hours a day to prevent the development of disuse atrophy.

▷ *Healing of Skin Abrasions.* Before the application of a cast, skin lacerations and abrasions must be treated to enhance healing. The skin is cleansed thoroughly and treated as prescribed. Sterile dressings are used to cover the injured skin. If the skin wounds are extensive, an alternative method (*e.g.*, external fixator) may be chosen to immobilize the body part.

During the time that the cast is on, the patient is observed for development of systemic signs of infection, odors from the cast, and purulent drainage staining the cast. If problems develop the physician must be notified.

▷ *Maintenance of Adequate Tissue Perfusion.* Swelling and edema are natural responses of the tissue to trauma and surgery. The patient may complain that the cast is too tight. Vascular insufficiency and nerve compression due to unrelieved swelling can reduce blood supply to an extremity and result in peripheral nerve damage. Generally the extent of swelling can be controlled by elevating the injured area. If not controlled, the

Chart 59–1
Muscle Setting Exercises

Isometric contraction of the muscle maintains muscle mass and strength and prevents atrophy.

Quadriceps-Setting Exercises

- Position patient supine with leg extended.
- Instruct patient to push knee back onto the mattress by contracting the anterior thigh muscles.
- Encourage patient to hold the position for 5 to 10 seconds.
- Let patient relax.
- Repeat exercise 10 times each hour when patient is awake.

Gluteal-Setting Exercises

- Position patient supine with legs extended, if possible.
- Instruct patient to contract muscles of buttocks and abdomen.
- Encourage patient to hold the contraction for 5 to 10 seconds.
- Let patient relax.
- Repeat exercise 10 times each hour when patient is awake.

swelling can result in increased tissue pressure, ultimate occlusion of the blood supply, and subsequent anoxia resulting in loss of both nerve and muscle tissue. If this complication occurs it is known as *compartment syndrome*.

In promoting tissue perfusion, the nurse monitors the affected extremity for pain, swelling, discoloration (paleness or blueness), paresthesia (tingling or numbness), diminished or absent pulses, paralysis, and coldness of the extremity. Fingers or toes of the casted limb are assessed and compared with the opposite limb. Normal findings include minimal discomfort, pink in color, warm to touch, rapid capillary refill response, ability to move fingers or toes, and normal sensations. The patient is encouraged to move fingers and toes hourly to stimulate circulation.

Swelling indicates edema and reduced venous return. Blue-tinged nail beds suggest venous congestion. White and cold phalanges suggest arterial obstruction. Reduced pulse indicates arterial insufficiency. Reduced motor abilities and occurrence of paresthesia (*e.g.,* abnormal sensations such as tingling) indicate nerve ischemia due to tissue pressure or nerve injury. Sensations in the fingers and toes and ability to move toes provide indications of specific sensory and motor function. Normal sensation in thumb and index finger indicates function of the sensory branch of the musculocutaneous nerve—cervical nerve root 6. Asking the patient to dorsiflex his great toe facilitates assessment of the function of the motor component of the peroneal nerve.

Tissue pressure can be measured directly by tissue pressure-monitoring devices when the muscle is accessible (see Fig. 59–1). Generally indirect measures reflecting tissue perfusion must be used.

Early recognition of diminished circulation and nerve function is essential. Frequent, regular assessments of neurovascular status must be done. When data indicate a potential compartment syndrome (*e.g.,* progressive unrelieved pain, pain on passive stretch, paresthesia, motor loss, sensory loss, coolness, paleness, slow capillary refill, sensation of tightness), the nurse adjusts the extremity so that it is no higher than heart level to enhance arterial perfusion, *notifies the physician at once*, and anticipates release of restrictive dressings (*e.g.,* bivalving cast).

▷ *Achievement of Maximum Level of Self-Care.* Self-care deficits occur when a portion of the body is immobilized, resulting in reduced self-care abilities. The nurse must assist the patient in identifying areas of self-care deficit and devise mechanisms for optimizing independence in activities of daily living. The patient's participation in planning and accomplishing activities of daily living is important in promotion of self-care, independence, maintenance of control, and avoidance of untoward psychological reaction such as depression.

▷ *Management of Skin Breakdown.* Pressure of the cast on soft tissues causes tissue anoxia and pressure ulcers. Sites most susceptible to pressure on the lower extremity are the heel, malleoli, dorsum of the foot, head of the fibula, and anterior surface of the patella. On the upper extremity, the main pressure sites are located at the medial epicondyle of the humerus and the ulnar styloid (see Fig. 59–2).

Generally the patient complains of pain and tightness in the area. If the pressure is not relieved, the necrotic area may drain, stain the cast, and emit a odor. Discomfort may not be present when a pressure ulcer develops. Extensive loss of tissue may occur if signs and symptoms of pressure ulcer development are not monitored and reported.

To visually inspect the area in question, the physician may bivalve (cut in half while maintaining alignment) or "window" (cut an opening) the cast.

The procedure for bivalving a cast is as follows:

1. A longitudinal cut is made in the cast, dividing it into two halves.
2. The underlying padding is also cut, as blood-soaked padding may shrink and cause constriction of circulation.
3. The cast is spread apart sufficiently to relieve constriction.
4. The anterior and posterior parts of the cast may be held together with an elastic compression bandage.
5. After the cast is bivalved, the extremity is elevated (no higher than heart level) until the circulation is restored, swelling diminishes, and pain is relieved.

After the affected areas are inspected and possibly treated, the portions of the cast are replaced and held in place by an elastic compression dressing or tape. This is important to prevent the underlying tissue from swelling through the window and forming of pressure areas around its margins.

▷ *Management of Compartment Syndrome.* Compartment syndrome occurs when there is an increase of tissue pressure within a limited space (*e.g.*, cast, muscle compartment) that compromises the circulation and the function of the tissue within the confined area.

- Unrelieved pain, excessive swelling, poor capillary refill response, inability to move toes or fingers, and elevated tissue pressure indicate compartment syndrome and must be reported to the physician at once.

To relieve the pressure, the cast must be bivalved and the extremity elevated (no higher than heart level). If pressure is not relieved and circulation restored, a fasciotomy may be necessary to relieve the pressure within the muscle compartment.

Patient Education and Home Health Care.   When the cast is dry, the patient is instructed as follows:

1. Move about as normally as possible. Avoid excessive use of the injured extremity.
2. Perform the prescribed exercises regularly, as scheduled.
3. Elevate the casted extremity to heart level frequently to prevent swelling.
4. Keep the cast dry.
   a. Wetness destroys the hardness of plaster casts.
      (1) Do not cover the cast with plastic or rubber, as this causes condensation and wetting of the cast.
      (2) Avoid walking on wet floors or sidewalks.
   b. Fiberglass casts, after being wet, must be dried thoroughly with a hair dryer on a cool setting to avoid skin problems.
5. Cushion rough edges of the cast with tape.
6. Report to the physician if the cast breaks; do not attempt to fix it yourself.
7. To clean a cast:
   a. Remove surface soil with a damp cloth.
   b. Stained areas may be touched up with a thin layer of white shoe polish.
8. Do not attempt to scratch the skin under the cast. This may cause a break in the skin and result in the formation of a cast sore. Cool air from a hair dryer may alleviate an itch.

9. Note odors about the cast, stained areas, warm spots, and pressure spots. Report them to the physician.
10. Report to the physician: persistent pain, swelling that does not respond to elevation, changes in sensation, decreased ability to move exposed fingers or toes, and changes in skin color and temperature.

When the cast is to be removed or changed (Table 59–2), the patient needs to be prepared for the experience through explanation of what to expect. The cast is cut using a *cast cutter*, which oscillates to cut the cast. The patient will feel the vibration and pressure applied during its use. The cutter will not hurt the patient's skin. The cast padding is then cut with scissors.

The body part that has been casted will be weak from disuse, stiff, and may appear atrophied. Therefore, it requires support when the cast is removed. The skin is usually dry and scaling because of the accumulated dead skin and is vulnerable to injury from scratching. The skin needs to be washed gently and lubricated with an emollient lotion.

The patient is taught to gradually resume activities within the prescribed therapeutic regimen. Because the muscles are weak from disuse, the body part that has been casted is not able to withstand normal stresses immediately. In addition, the patient may notice swelling of the affected extremity after the cast is removed and he is taught to continue to elevate it to control swelling until normal muscle tone and use are reestablished.

◊ Evaluation

Expected Outcomes
1. Patient actively participates in therapeutic regimen
   a. Elevates affected extremity
   b. Exercises according to instructions
   c. Keeps cast dry
   d. Reports any problems that develop
   e. Keeps follow-up clinic or physician appointments

TABLE 59–2.   *Cast Removal*

Procedure	Rationale
1. Inform the patient about the procedure.	1. Facilitates cooperation and reduces fear about the procedure.
2. Assure patient that the electric saw or cast cutter will not cut him.	2. Reduces anxiety. (Blade oscillates to cut cast.)
3. The cast is bivalved using a series of alternating pressures and linear movements of blade along the line to be cut.	3. Cuts cast in halves. Avoids burning sensation from prolonged contact of oscillating blade with padding.
4. Wear eye protection (patient and cast cutter operator).	4. Protects eyes from flying cast particles.
5. Cut padding with scissors.	5. Releases all of the casting materials.
6. Support body part as it is removed from the cast.	6. Reduces stresses on body part that has been immobilized.
7. Gently wash and dry area that has been immobilized.* Apply emollient lotion.	7. Removes dead skin that has accumulated during immobilization. Keeps skin supple.
8. Teach patient to avoid rubbing and scratching skin.	8. Prevents skin breakdown.
9. Teach patient to gradually resume active use of body part within the guidelines of prescribed therapeutic regimen.	9. Protects weakened part from excessive stress. Progressive exercises reduce stiffness, restore muscle strength and function.
10. Teach patient to control swelling by elevation of extremity or use of elastic bandage if prescribed.	10. Facilitates circulation (*i.e.,* venous return) and controls fluid pooling.

* *If a new cast is to be applied, follow guidelines for application of a cast and associated nursing care.*

2. Reports less pain
   a. Elevates extremity that is in the cast
   b. Repositions self
   c. Uses occasional oral analgesic
   d. Appears comfortable
3. Demonstrates increased mobility
   a. Uses mobility aids safely
   b. Exercises to increase strength
   c. Changes position frequently
   d. Performs range of motion exercises of joints not in the cast
4. Exhibits healing of abrasions and lacerations
   a. Demonstrates no systemic signs or symptoms of infection
   b. Demonstrates no local signs of infection (*i.e.*, local discomfort, purulent drainage, staining, odor)
   c. Demonstrates intact skin when cast is removed
5. Maintains adequate circulation to affected extremity
   a. Exhibits normal skin color and temperature
   b. Experiences minimal swelling
   c. Achieves satisfactory capillary refill on testing
   d. Demonstrates active movement of fingers or toes
   e. Reports normal sensations in casted body part
   f. Reports pain is controllable
6. Exhibits absence of complications
   a. Develops no pressure ulcers
   b. Demonstrates normal neurovascular status of casted extremity
   c. Reports pain is controlled

Arm Casts

The patient whose arm is immobilized in a cast must readjust to many routine tasks. The unaffected arm must assume all the upper extremity activities. The patient may experience muscle fatigue due to the additional activities and the weight of the cast. Frequent rest periods are necessary.

To diminish and control swelling when the patient is lying down, the arm is elevated, with each joint positioned higher than the preceding proximal joint (*e.g.*, elbow higher than the shoulder, hand higher than the elbow). To minimize venous congestion and edema, the extremity should be slightly higher than the level of the heart.

When the patient begins to ambulate, a sling may be used. Slings should distribute the supported weight over a large area and not on the back of the neck. Triangular cloth slings, when used, need to be pinned at the sides and not tied with a knot behind the neck, to prevent pressure on the cervical spinal nerves. The patient should be encouraged to remove the arm from the sling frequently and elevate it.

Circulatory disturbances in the hand may become apparent with signs of cyanosis, swelling, and an inability to move the fingers. One serious effect of circulatory constriction in an arm cast is *Volkmann's contracture*, a compartment syndrome (Fig. 59-3). Contracture of the fingers and wrist occurs as the result of ischemia due to the obstruction of arterial flow to the forearm and hand. The patient is unable to extend the fingers, describes abnormal sensation (*e.g.*, unrelenting pain, pain on passive stretch), and presents signs of diminished circulation to the hand.

This serious complication can be prevented with nursing surveillance and proper care. Neurovascular checks need to

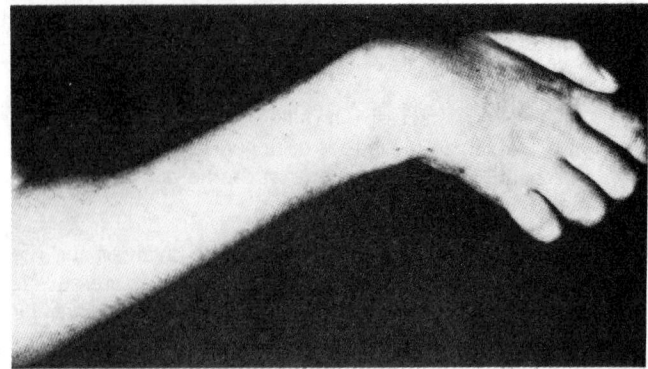

Figure 59-3. The forearm and hand of a patient with late Volkmann's ischemic contracture. (Rockwood CA and Green DP [eds]. Fractures, Vol 1. Philadelphia, JB Lippincott.)

be made frequently. Tissue pressure within muscle compartments may be measured directly, using pressure-monitoring devices (see Fig. 59-1). Management of compartment syndrome includes bivalving the cast to remove constricting cast and dressings. A fasciotomy may be necessary to improve vascular status. Permanent damage develops within a few hours if not action is taken.

Leg Casts

The application of a leg cast imposes a degree of immobility on the patient. The leg cast may be a short leg cast, extending to the knee, or a long leg cast, extending to the groin. The fresh cast must be handled in a manner that will not cause denting or disruption. The leg is supported on soft pillows to heart level to control swelling. Ice packs as prescribed may be applied over the fracture site for the first day or two.

As with other cast applications, the leg must be assessed for adequate circulation and normal nerve function. The circulation is assessed by observing the color, temperature, and capillary refill of the exposed toes. Nerve function is assessed by observing the patient's ability to move the toes and by asking about the sensations in the foot. Numbness, tingling, and burning may be due to peroneal nerve injury from pressure at the head of the fibula.

- Injury to the peroneal nerve as a result of pressure is a common cause of footdrop.

When the cast is dry, the patient is taught how to transfer and ambulate safely with walking aids (*e.g.*, crutches, walker). The gait to be used depends on whether or not the patient's problem allows weight-bearing. If weight-bearing is allowed, the cast will be reinforced to withstand the body weight. A walking heel (a rubber pad) may be incorporated into the bottom of the cast, or the patient may be given a cast boot to wear over the casted foot (Fig. 59-4). Cast boots are preferred to walking heels because they provide a broader support surface and do not disturb the patient's balance or posture by elevating the injured leg.

After ambulation begins, elevation of the cast is encouraged when the patient is seated. Several times during the day, the patient should lie down, because a sitting position does not promote complete drainage. If the skin has become irritated

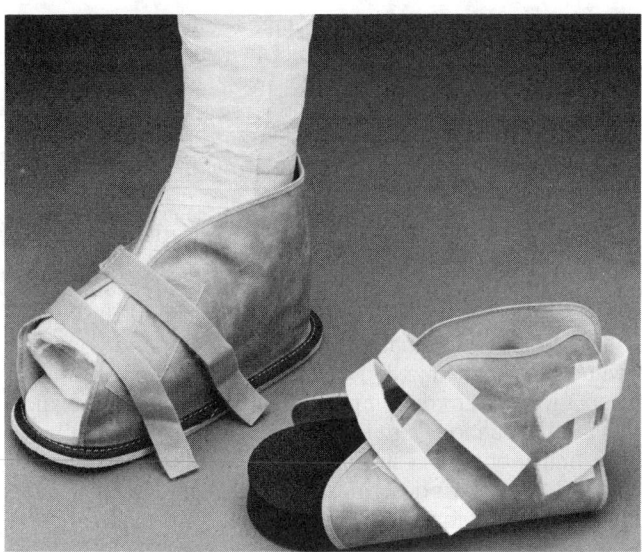

Figure 59–4. Cast boots. (Courtesy of Srouse Manufacturing, Inc., Ligonier, IN.)

at the cast edges, moleskin padding may be added around the edges of the cast.

Cast Brace

A cast brace is a special type of cast in which hinges are incorporated to allow for joint motion while providing adequate alignment and immobilization (Fig. 59–5). Some cast braces

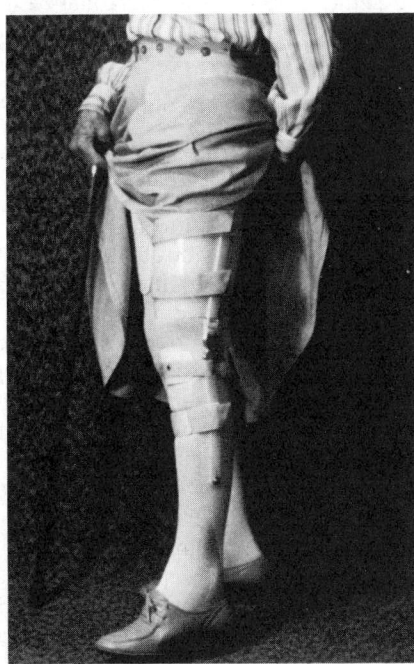

Figure 59–5. A type of cast brace. This molded plastic knee–ankle-foot orthosis with total contact femoral section orthosis is useful when long-term (greater than 6 months) immobilization is required. It is removable by the patient. (Courtesy of the University of Texas Health Science Center at Dallas.)

are constructed with hinges at the hip, knee, ankle, elbow, or wrist. Most frequently, cast braces are used for femoral shaft fractures. Usually the patient has been in skeletal traction for a few weeks. Initial bone healing is evident and thigh swelling is minimal.

Fracture healing is enhanced with cast braces. Weight-bearing (stress) and hydraulic pressure on the soft tissues stimulate bone healing. Cast brace use promotes physiologic homeostasis, maintains muscle strength and joint mobility, and promotes rehabilitation.

A cast brace requires the application of a circumferential thigh cast and a short leg walking cast. Hinges (metal or polypropylene) that allow flexion are placed on each side of the knee and incorporated into the cast. After the cast is dry (about 48 hours for plaster cast braces), the patient can ambulate with crutches, using a three-point gait (see p. 233), progressing from partial to full weight-bearing on the fractured extremity.

Problems that the patient may have after cast brace application include angulation deformity of the fracture site (malalignment of bone resulting in a bend in the bone), edema about the knee, skin breakdown on the thigh as a result of pressure from the edge of the cast, and soiling of the thigh cast. The patient is monitored for excessive swelling, neurovascular problems, and skin breakdown.

To promote venous return and to control edema, the patient is encouraged to elevate his leg when not walking. Because the cast may extend to the groin, measures should be taken to protect this area of the cast from becoming soiled with urine and feces.

Body or Spica Casts

Casts that encase the trunk *(body cast)* and portions of the trunk and one or two extremities *(spica cast)* require special nursing techniques. Body casts may be used in situations requiring spinal immobility. *Hip spicas* are used for patients after femoral fractures and some hip joint surgeries. *Shoulder spica* casts are used for some humeral neck fractures. Patient preparation, turning, and skin and hygienic care and monitoring for cast syndrome are nursing responsibilities.

Explaining the procedure will help reduce the patient's apprehension about being encased in a large cast. Often the patient has been immobilized in traction for weeks, and anticipates recurrence of pain while being moved for casting. Also, the fracture table used for large cast application looks like a torture device. Saying that the patient will be cared for by several people during the application and that support for the injured body will be adequate and as gentle as possible may help to allay fear. Medications for pain and relaxation administered before the procedure will help the patient to relax and cooperate during the procedure.

After cast application, the patient needs to be supported by flexible, waterproof pillows until the cast is dry to prevent it from being dented. Inadequate cast support will cause a soft cast to crack or become dented, resulting in subsequent pressure points. The bed must have firm mattress support. Three pillows placed crosswise on the bed will suffice for the body cast; for a hip spica, one pillow placed crosswise at the waist and two pillows placed lengthwise for the affected leg are necessary. If both legs are involved, two additional pillows are necessary. It is important that the pillows be next to each other, because any spaces in between the pillows will allow the damp cast to sag, become weak, and possibly break. It is also important to make sure that a pillow is not placed under the head and shoulders (of a patient in a body cast) while the cast is drying, as this causes pressure on the chest.

Patients are turned every 2 hours to relieve pressure and to allow the cast to dry (Table 59–3). The patient is turned as a unit toward the uninjured side. Twisting the patient's body within the cast is avoided. Sufficient personnel (at least three people) are needed when the patient is turned so that the fresh cast can be adequately supported with the palms of the hands. Vulnerable points in the cast are located at body joints and need to be supported to prevent the cast from cracking. The patient is encouraged to assist in the repositioning by using the trapeze or bedrail. An abduction bar might be incorporated in spica casts to stabilize cast positioning. This bar is *not* to be used as a turning device. Pillows are readjusted so that support is provided and no pressure areas are present.

The patient is turned to a prone position, twice daily if tolerated, to provide postural drainage of the bronchial tree and relieve pressure on the back. A small pillow under the abdomen will be an added comfort measure. Placing a pillow lengthwise under the dorsum of the feet will prevent the toes from being forced into the mattress. The toes are allowed to hang over the edge of the mattress.

The skin around the edges of the cast must be inspected frequently for signs of irritation. Some of the area under the cast can be inspected by pulling the skin taut and using a flashlight. Reaching under the cast edges with the fingers allows for removal of cast crumbs and massage of the skin. Accessible skin should be bathed carefully and massaged with an emollient.

The perineal opening must be large enough for hygienic care. If it is not, the cast must be adjusted. To protect the cast from excreta soiling, clean dry plastic sheeting can be inserted under the cast and brought over the cast edge before each elimination. Generally, fracture bed pans are easier than regular bed pans for hip spica patients to use. When the cast has dried, the perineum is protected with a towel and the cast around the perineum is sprayed with a plastic protective spray to make the cast resistant to soiling.

Cast Syndrome

Patients immobilized in large casts may develop psychological and physiologic responses to the confinement. The psycho-

logical component of cast syndrome is similar to a claustrophobic reaction. The patient exhibits an acute anxiety reaction characterized by behavioral changes and autonomic responses (eg, increased respiratory rate, diaphoresis, dilated pupils, increased heart rate, elevated blood pressure). The nurse needs to recognize the anxiety reaction and provide an environment in which the patient feels secure.

The physiologic responses to large casts are associated with the imposed immobility. With decreased physical activity, gastrointestinal motility decreases. With accumulation of intestinal gases, pressure increases and ileus occurs. The patient has distention, abdominal discomfort, nausea, and vomiting. As with other adynamic ileus situations, the patient is treated conservatively with decompression (nasogastric intubation connected to suction) and intravenous fluid therapy until gastrointestinal motility is restored. If the cast restricts the abdominal distention, a window must be cut in the cast over the abdominal area. Otherwise, the distention may place traction on the superior mesenteric artery, reducing the blood supply to the bowel. The bowel may become gangrenous, requiring surgical intervention.

The nurse needs to be aware of the possible development of cast syndrome in patients with large body casts and plan interventions for its prevention or resolution.

In summary, casts are rigid, external immobilizing devices that encase a body part to maintain a specific position. They are most frequently used to treat fractures and to support weakened joints and muscles. They may be used for immobilization after orthopedic surgery (*i.e.*, bone grafting, bone fusion, internal fixation). Nursing diagnoses applicable to the patient in a cast might include high risk for impaired skin integrity due to pressure on the skin. Because casting contributes to the development of disuse atrophy, the nurse teaches the patient muscle setting exercises and gradual resumption of activities when the cast is removed.

External Fixators

External fixation devices are used to manage open fractures with soft-tissue damage and provide stable support for severe comminuted fractures while permitting active treatment of damaged soft tissue (Fig. 59–6). Complicated fractures of the humerus, forearm, femur, tibia, and pelvis are managed with external skeletal fixators. The fracture is reduced, aligned, and immobilized by a series of pins inserted in the bone fragments. The pins are maintained in position through attachment to a portable frame. The fixators facilitate patient comfort, early mobility, active exercise of adjacent uninvolved joints, and shortened hospitalization. In addition, complications related to disuse and immobility are minimized.

Psychological preparation for application of the external fixator is important. The apparatus looks clumsy and foreign to the patient. Reassurance that the discomfort associated with the device is mild and that early mobility is anticipated aids in the acceptance of the device. Involvement of the patient in the care associated with the fixator after it is applied will also promote the patient's acceptance.

After application of the external fixator, the extremity is elevated to reduce swelling. The neurovascular status of the

---

TABLE 59–3.   *Turning the Patient in a Hip Spica Cast*

1. The patient is moved with a steady, even, pulling motion to the side of the bed.
2. Pillows are placed along the other side of the bed for cast support.
3. Instruct the patient to assist by using the arm on the involved side to pull the shoulder over when turning.
4. Two nurses are on the side to which the patient is being turned to provide support for the cast while rolling the patient toward them.
5. The third nurse assists in rolling the patient from behind, adjusts the patient's shoulder, and adjusts the pillows.
6. The patient's body should be turned as a unit and positioned comfortably in good alignment.

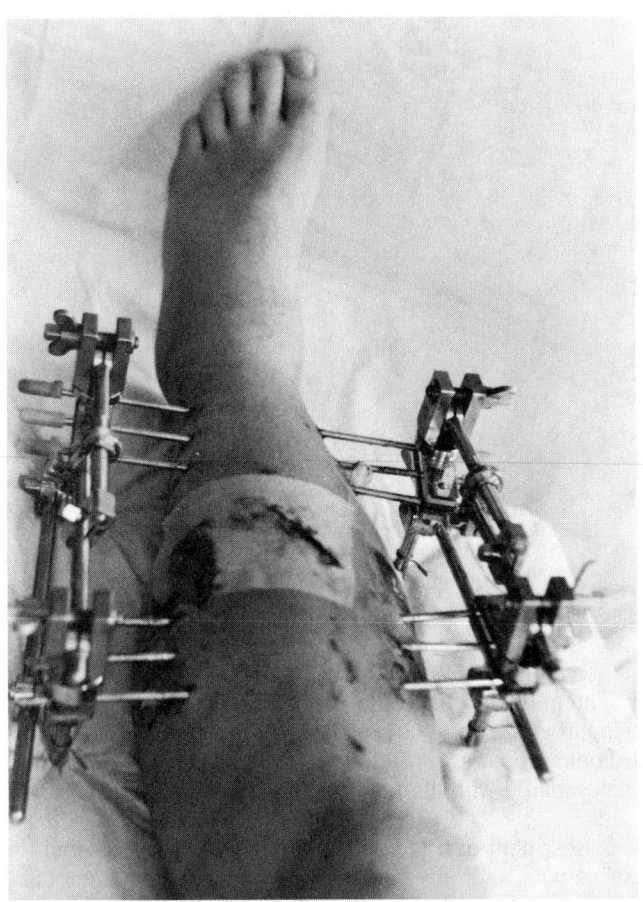

Figure 59–6. External fixation device. Pins are inserted into bone fragments. The fracture is reduced and aligned. The reduction is stabilized by attaching the pins to a rigid portable frame. The device facilitates treatment of soft tissue damaged in complex fracture situations.

extremity is monitored frequently. The injured area and pin sites are checked for signs of infection. Some serous drainage from the pin sites is to be expected.

Each pin site is assessed for redness, drainage, tenderness, pain, and loosening of the pin.

- The clamps on the external fixator frame are *never* adjusted.

Pin care to prevent pin tract infection is carried out according to the prescribed routine. Crusts should not form at the pin site, and the fixator must be kept clean.

Isometric and active exercises are encouraged within the limits of tissue damage. The nurse must be alert for potential problems due to pressure by the device on the skin, nerves, or blood vessels, and prevent device-induced injury by covering any sharp points on the fixator or pins. When the swelling has subsided, the patient is mobilized within the limits of any other injuries. Weight-bearing limits are prescribed to minimize the chance of the pins loosening when stress is applied at the bone–pin interface.

The fixator is removed when the soft tissue has healed; the fracture may be stabilized by cast or molded orthosis until the bone has healed by callus formation.

The *Ilizarov* external fixator is a special device using tension wires to attach the fixator rings, which are joined by telescoping rods. The Ilizarov device is used for correction of an-

gulation and rotational defects, treatment of nonunion, and limb lengthening. Callus and bone formation is stimulated by prescribed daily adjustment of the telescoping rods. The patient is taught how to adjust the telescoping rods and perform skin care. Weight-bearing is generally encouraged. When the desired correction has been achieved, no additional adjustments are made and the fixator is left in place until bone healing occurs.

In summary, external fixators are special frames attached to the bone by pins or wires. They are used primarily for treatment of open fractures. Special fixators (*e.g.,* Ilizarov device) may be used for correction of deformity and nonunion and may be used for limb lengthening. Pin care to prevent infection is important when these devices are used.

Management of the Patient in Traction

Traction is the application of a pulling force to a part of the body. Traction is used to minimize muscle spasms; to reduce, align, and immobilize fractures; to lessen deformity; and to increase space between opposing surfaces within a joint. Traction must be applied in the desired direction and magnitude to obtain its therapeutic effects. Factors that reduce the effective pull of the traction must be eliminated.

At times, the traction needs to be applied in more than one direction to achieve the desired line of pull. When this is done, part of one of the lines of pull counteracts the other line of pull. These lines of pull are known as the *vectors of force*. The actual resultant pulling force is somewhere between the two lines of pull (Fig. 59–7). The effects of applied traction are evaluated with x-ray, and adjustments may be necessary. As the muscle and soft tissue relax, the amount of weight used may be changed to obtain the desired pulling force.

Types of Traction

Straight or running traction applies the pulling force in a straight line with the body part resting on the bed. Buck's extension traction (Fig. 59–8) and pelvic traction (see Fig. 61–2) are examples of straight traction.

Balanced suspension traction (Fig. 59–9) supports the affected extremity off the bed and allows for some patient mobility without disruption of the line of pull.

Traction may be applied to the skin *(skin traction)* or directly to the bony skeleton *(skeletal traction)*. The mode of application is determined by the purpose of the traction.

Traction can be applied with the hands *(manual traction)*. This is a very temporary traction that may be used when applying a cast, giving skin care under a Buck's extension foam boot, or adjusting traction apparatus.

Principles of Effective Traction

Whenever traction is applied, the *countertraction* must be considered. Countertraction is the force acting in the opposite direction. (Newton's third law of motion states that for every action there is an equal and opposite reaction.) Generally, the

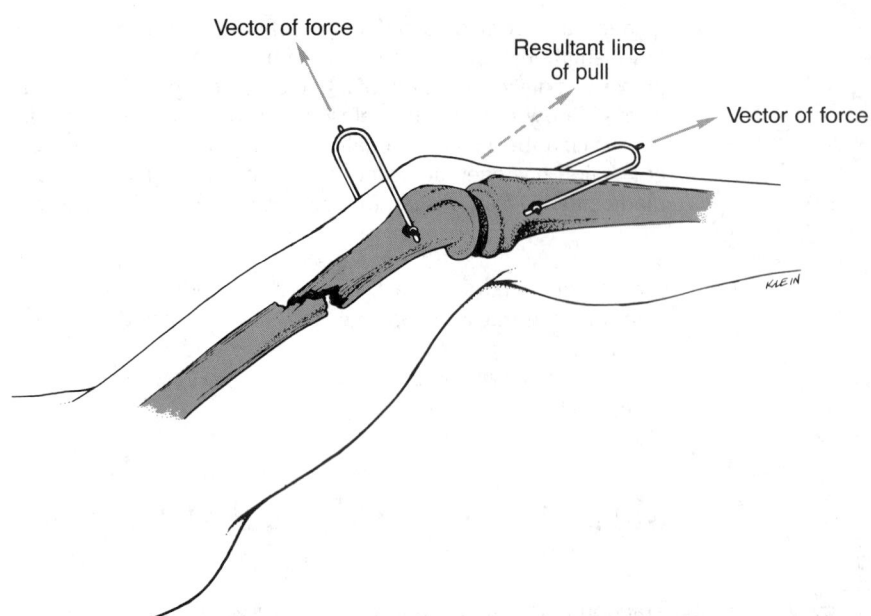

Vector of force

Resultant line of pull

Vector of force

KLEIN

Figure 59–7. Traction may be applied in different directions to achieve the desired therapeutic line of pull. Adjustments in applied forces may be prescribed over the treatment period.

patient's body weight and bed position adjustments supply the needed countertraction.

- Countertraction must be maintained for effective traction.

For traction to be effective in reducing fractures and in providing immobilization, it must be *continuous*. Pelvic and cervical skin tractions are frequently used to reduce muscle spasm and are usually prescribed as an intermittent traction.

- Skeletal traction is *never* interrupted.
- Weights are not removed unless the traction is prescribed intermittently.

Maintain the line of pull. Any factor that might reduce the pull or alter its resultant line of pull must be eliminated.

- The patient is centered in bed and in good body alignment when traction is applied.
- Weights must hang free and not rest on the bed or floor.
- Ropes must be unobstructed
- Knots in the rope or the footplate must not touch the pulley or the foot of the bed.

▶ Nursing Process
The Patient in Traction

◊ Assessment

The psychological and physiologic impact of the musculoskeletal problem, traction device, and immobility must be considered.

Traction restricts one's mobility and independence. The equipment often looks threatening, and its application can be a frightening experience. Confusion, disorientation, and behavioral problems may develop in patients who are confined in a limited space for an extended time. Therefore, the patient's anxiety level and psychological responses to traction must be assessed and monitored.

The body part to be placed in traction must be assessed. The neurovascular status (*i.e.*, color, temperature, capillary refill, edema, pulses, sensations, ability to move) is evaluated and compared with the unaffected extremity. Skin integrity is noted.

Assessment of body system functioning is completed for baseline data, and ongoing assessment is indicated. Immobility may contribute to the development of integumentary, respiratory, gastrointestinal, urinary, and cardiovascular system problems. Pressure ulcers may develop. Lung congestion and stasis pneumonia may occur. Constipation and loss of appetite accompany immobility. Urinary stasis and urinary tract infections may occur. Reports of calf tenderness or a positive Homan's sign (discomfort in the calf when the foot is forcibly dorsiflexed) suggest the development of deep vein thrombosis. Early identification of preexisting or developing problems facilitates prompt interventions to resolve the problems.

◊ Nursing Diagnoses

Based on the nursing assessment, the patient's major nursing diagnoses related to traction may include the following:

- Knowledge deficit about the treatment regimen
- Anxiety related to health status and traction device
- Pain and discomfort related to traction and immobility
- Impaired physical mobility related to disease process and traction devices restricting mobility
- Self-care deficit related to traction devices.

Nursing diagnoses related to the immobility imposed by the traction include:

- High risk for impaired skin integrity
- Potential ineffective airway clearance
- Potential constipation and decreased appetite
- Potential altered urinary elimination
- Potential altered peripheral tissue perfusion

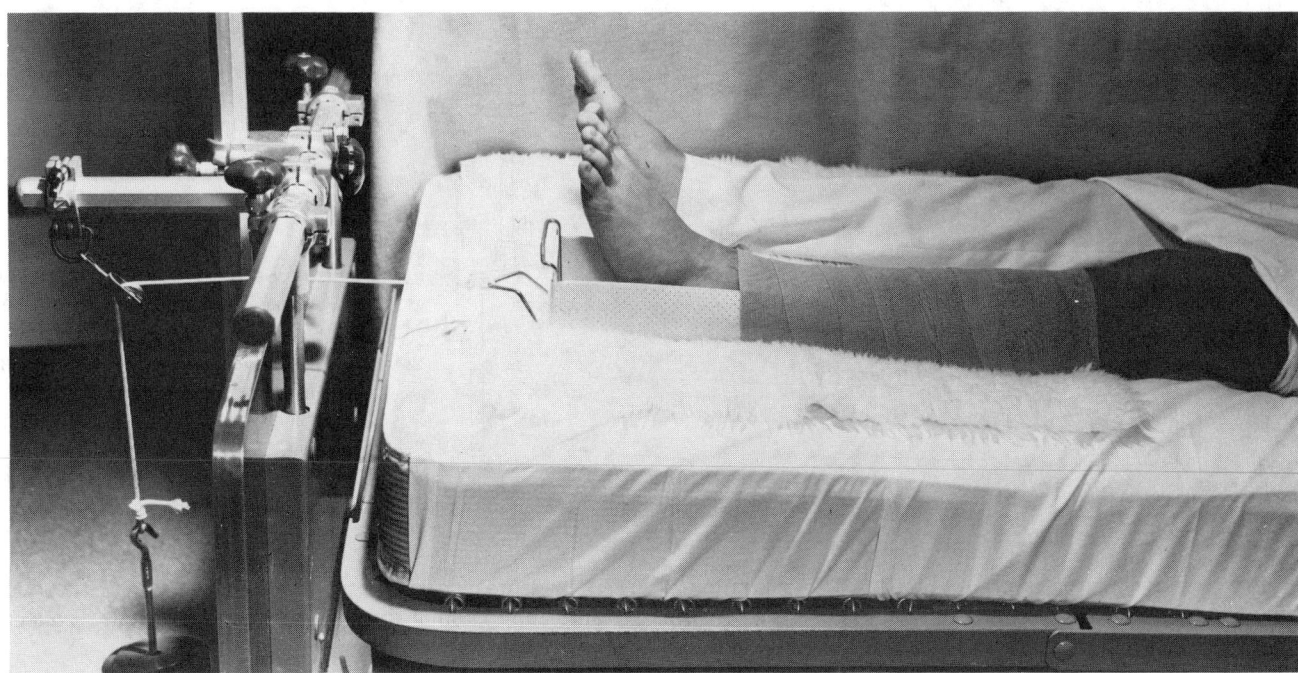

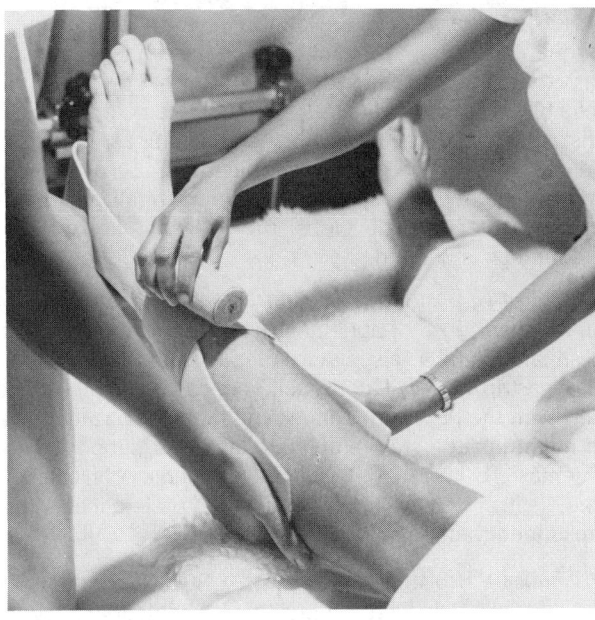

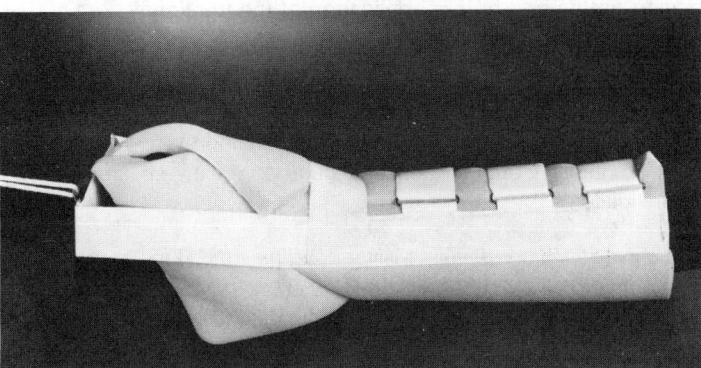

Figure 59–8. Buck's extension. (**A**) Lower extremity in Buck's extension traction. (**B**) Applying elastic bandage for Buck's extension traction. (**C**) Prepadded boot that may be used in Buck's extension. (Photo of boot courtesy of All Orthopedic Appliances.)

▷ Planning and Implementation

▷ *Goals:* The major goals of the patient in traction may include understanding of the treatment regimen, reduced anxiety, maximum comfort, achieving maximum mobility within therapeutic limits of traction, maximum level of self-care, and avoidance of the development of potential problems (*e.g.,* pressure ulcers, lung congestion, constipation, decrease of appetite, urinary stasis, urinary tract infection, deep vein thrombosis).

▷ Nursing Interventions

▷ *Understanding of Treatment Regimen.* The patient must understand the pathologic problem being treated and must ac-

curately perceive the rationale for the traction therapy. The information may need to be repeated and reinforced frequently. With increased understanding of the therapy, the patient will become an active participant in his health care.

▷ *Reduced Anxiety.* Before the application of any traction, the patient needs to be informed about the procedure, its purpose, and its implications. Talking to the patient about what is being done, and why, helps to allay apprehension. After being in traction for a period, the patient may react to being confined to a limited space. Frequent visits by the nurse will reduce feelings of isolation and confinement. Family and friends should be encouraged to visit frequently for the same reason. Diversional activities that can be done within the limits of the traction are encouraged.

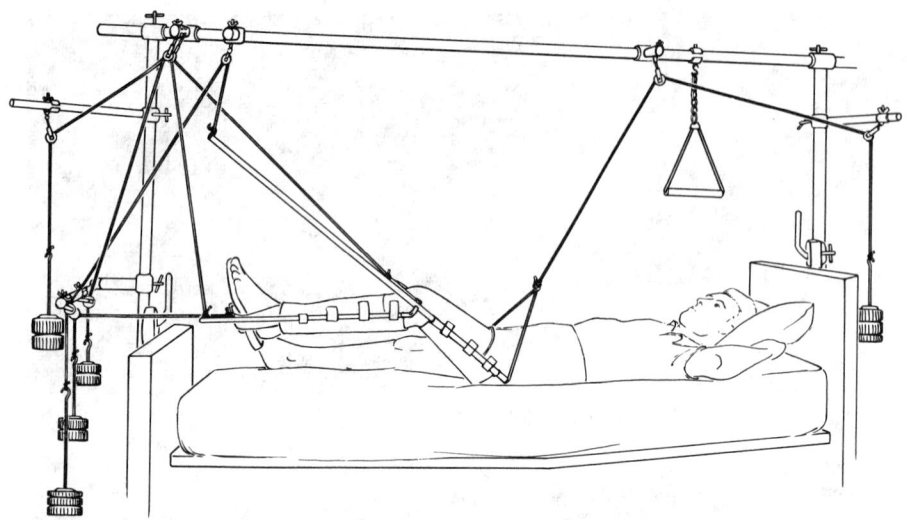

Figure 59–9. Balanced suspension traction with Thomas leg splint. Vertical movement of the patient is permitted as long as resultant line of pull is maintained. In the nursing management of the patient in traction, one has to understand the direction in which the force is operating. Study the line drawing carefully. Notice that the force produced by the weights is changed in direction by the pulleys.

▷ *Achievement of Maximum Level of Comfort.* Because the patient will be immobilized in bed, the mattress needs to be firm and supported with a bed board. Special mattress pads designed to minimize the development of pressure ulcers should be placed on the bed before application of the traction.

- Pressure on dependent body parts can be relieved by turning and by positioning the patient for comfort within the limits of the traction.
- The bed linens need to be kept wrinkle-free and dry.
- Every complaint of the patient in traction is to be investigated immediately.

▷ *Attainment of Maximum Mobility Within the Limits of Traction.* During traction therapy, the patient needs to exercise nonimmobilized muscles and joints to diminish their deterioration due to immobilization. Active motion of all unaffected joints is encouraged. The physical therapist can be consulted to design bed exercises that minimize loss of muscle strength. The nurse needs to encourage the patient to exercise. During exercising, the nurse must ensure that traction forces are maintained and that the patient is properly positioned to prevent complications resulting from poor alignment.

▷ *Attainment of Maximum Level of Self-Care.* Initially the patient may require assistance with self-care activities. The nurse helps the patient learn how to provide for such needs as eating, bathing, dressing, and toileting while immobilized in the traction device. Patient aids such as reachers and an overbed trapeze may facilitate self-care. The patient will feel less dependent and less frustrated and will experience improved self-esteem with resumption of self-care activities.

Some assistance will be required throughout the period of immobility; however, the nurse and the patient can creatively develop routines that will maximize the patient's independence.

▷ *Prevention of Pressure Ulcers.* The patient's skin is examined frequently for evidence of pressure or friction, especially over bony prominences. Early intervention is necessary to relieve pressure by frequent patient repositioning and use of skin protective devices (*e.g.*, elbow protectors). If the risk of skin breakdown is high, such as with a multi-trauma patient, the nurse may consult with the physician concerning the use of a specialized bed to prevent the development of skin breakdown.

If a pressure ulcer occurs, the nurse consults with the physician (and enterostomal therapist if one is available) concerning treatment.

▷ *Prevention of Respiratory Problems.* The patient's lungs are auscultated to determine his respiratory status. The patient is taught deep breathing and coughing exercises that aid in full expansion of the lungs and move respiratory secretions. If the patient's history and baseline assessment indicate that he is at high risk for developing respiratory complications, the nurse should consult with the physician concerning use of specific therapies (*e.g.*, incentive spirometer). If a respiratory complication (*e.g.*, infection) develops, prompt institution of prescribed therapy is needed.

▷ *Prevention of Gastrointestinal Problems.* The problems of constipation and loss of appetite are related to reduced gastrointestinal motility. Diets high in fiber and fluids may help to stimulate gastric motility. If constipation does develop, the nurse consults with the physician concerning therapeutic measures, which might include stool softeners, laxatives, suppositories, and enemas. To improve the patient's appetite, consultation with the dietitian often helps to identify food preferences within the prescribed therapeutic diet.

▷ *Prevention of Urinary Tract Problems.* Because of the position of the patient in bed, emptying of the bladder may be incomplete, predisposing the patient to the development of urinary tract infection. In addition the patient may find use of the bedpan uncomfortable and restrict fluids to minimize frequency of urination. The nurse must monitor the fluid intake and the character of the urine. The nurse teaches the patient to consume adequate amounts of fluid and to empty his bladder every 2 to 3 hours. If the patient exhibits signs or symptoms of urinary tract infection, the nurse consults with the physician concerning treatment of the problem.

▷ *Prevention of Circulatory System Problems.* Venous stasis occurs with immobility. The nurse teaches the patient to do ankle and foot exercises within the limits of the traction therapy on a regular basis throughout the day to prevent the development of deep vein thrombosis. The patient is encouraged to drink fluids to prevent dehydration and associated hemoconcentration, which contribute to stasis. The nurse monitors the patient for development of signs of deep vein thrombosis and reports findings promptly to the physician for definitive evaluation and therapy.

▷ Evaluation

Expected Outcomes

1. Demonstrates understanding of traction regimen
   a. Describes purpose of traction
   b. Participates in plan of care
2. Exhibits reduced anxiety
   a. Appears relaxed
   b. Uses effective coping mechanisms
   c. Expresses concerns and feelings
3. States increased level of comfort
   a. Requests occasional oral analgesia
   b. Repositions self frequently
4. Demonstrates increased mobility
   a. Performs prescribed exercises
   b. Uses assistive devices
5. Performs self-care activities
   a. Requires minimal assistance with feeding, bathing, dressing, and toileting
6. Exhibits absence of complications
   a. Intact skin
   b. Clear lungs
   c. No reports of shortness of breath
   d. No productive cough
   e. Regular bowel evacuation pattern
   f. Appetite normal
   g. Clear, yellow, nonconcentrated urine of adequate amount
   h. No signs or symptoms of deep vein thrombosis

Specific Traction Applications

Skin Traction

Skin traction is accomplished by a weight pulling on tape, sponge rubber, or canvas materials that have been attached to the skin. Traction on the skin transmits traction to the musculoskeletal structures. Only limited traction can be applied with skin traction, however. The amount of weight applied must not exceed the tolerance of the skin. No more than 2 to 3 kg (4.5 to 7 lb) of traction can be used on an extremity. Pelvic traction is generally 4.5 to 9 kg (10 to 20 lb), depending on the weight of the patient. Therefore, when prolonged or heavy traction weight is necessary, skeletal traction is used rather than skin traction.

Two forms of skin traction used for adults are *Buck's extension traction* and *Russell's traction.*

Buck's Traction.   Buck's extension (unilateral or bilateral) is a form of skin traction in which the pull is exerted in one plane when partial or temporary immobilization is desired (see Fig. 59-8A). It is used for injuries to the hip while the patient is awaiting surgical fixation.

Before the traction is applied, the skin is inspected for abrasions and circulatory disturbances, as the skin and circulation must be in healthy condition to tolerate the traction. The extremity should be clean and dry before the traction tape or a foam boot is applied (see Fig. 59-8B, C).

To apply Buck's traction with tape, foam-rubber–padded straps are applied with the foam surface against the skin on each side of the affected leg. A loop of tape about 10 to 15 cm (4 to 6 inches) long is extended beyond the sole of the foot. A spreader is applied to the distal end of the tape to prevent pressure along the side of the foot. The malleolus and proximal fibula are protected with cast padding to prevent pressure ulcers and skin necrosis. While one person elevates and supports the extremity under the patient's heel and knee, another person wraps the elastic bandage circumferentially over the traction tape, beginning at the ankle and wrapping up to the tibial tubercle. The elastic bandage helps the tape to adhere to the skin and prevents slipping. A rope is attached to the spreader and passed over a pulley fastened to the end of the bed. Then a weight is attached to the rope. A sheepskin pad is placed under the leg to reduce the friction of the heel against the bed.

Russell's Traction.   Russell's traction, which may be used for fractures of the tibial plateau, supports the flexed knee in a sling and applies the horizontal pulling force to the lower leg. If prescribed, the leg may be supported by a pillow to assure proper knee flexion and to prevent pressure on the heel.

Ensuring Effective Traction

To ensure effective traction, wrinkling and slipping of the traction bandage are avoided and countertraction is maintained. Proper positioning must be maintained to keep the leg or arm in a neutral position. To prevent bony fragments from moving against one another, the patient should not turn from side to side.

Potential Problems

Skin Breakdown.   Skin traction can irritate the skin. Sensitive skin must be identified during the initial assessment. Reaction of the skin to contact with tape and foam must be monitored closely. The skin traction must be applied firmly enough to ensure contact of the tapes or foam device with the skin. Shearing forces on the skin must be avoided. The area over the traction tapes should be palpated daily to detect pressure points. With the lower extremity, the area over the Achilles tendon should be inspected several times a day.

- The foam boots and wrappings are removed to inspect the skin three times a day. A second nurse is needed to support the extremity during the inspection.
- Special back care is given to the patient at regular intervals to avoid pressure ulcer development. The patient must remain in a supine position, which increases the chance of pressure ulcer development.
- Special care mattresses may be indicated to minimize development of skin ulcers.

Nerve Pressure.   Skin traction can place pressure on peripheral nerves.

Care must be taken to avoid pressure on the peroneal nerve at the point at which it passes around the neck of the fibula just below the knee. Pressure at this point can cause footdrop (see Fig. 59-2). The patient is questioned about sensation and requested to move the toes and foot.

Dorsiflexion of the foot demonstrates function of the peroneal nerve. Weakness of dorsiflexion or foot movement and inversion of the foot might indicate pressure on the common peroneal nerve. Planter flexion demonstrates function of the tibial nerve.

When skin traction is applied to the arm, the area around the elbow where the ulnar nerve is located should not be wrapped tightly. Ulnar nerve function can be assessed by active abduction of the little finger and sensation on the ulnar side of the little finger.

- Sensation and motion must be assessed regularly.
- Any complaint of burning sensation under the traction bandage or boot must be investigated immediately.
- Altered sensation and motor function must be reported to the physician promptly.

Circulatory Impairment.   After application of skin traction, the foot or hand is inspected for circulatory difficulties within a few minutes and then every 2 hours.

- Peripheral pulses and the color, capillary refill, and temperature of the fingers or toes are assessed.
- The patient is assessed for calf tenderness and for a positive Homan's sign for indications of deep vein thrombosis.
- Active foot exercise is encouraged hourly.

Skeletal Traction

Skeletal traction is applied directly to the bone. This method of traction is used most frequently in the treatment of fractures of the femur, the humerus, the tibia, and the cervical spine. The traction is applied directly to the bone by use of a metal pin or wire (*e.g.*, Steinmann's pin; Kirschner wire) that is inserted through the bone distal to the fracture, avoiding nerves, blood vessels, muscles, tendons, and joints. Head tongs (*e.g.*, Gardner–Wells tongs) are fixed in the skull to apply traction that immobilizes cervical fractures.

Patient preparation is important and contributes to the patient's comfort and cooperation. Skeletal traction may be applied under local or general anesthesia.

Skeletal traction is applied under surgical asepsis. The insertion site is prepared with a surgical scrub such as povidone-iodine. A local anesthetic is administered at the insertion site and periosteum. A small skin incision is made and the sterile pin or wire is drilled through the bone. The patient feels pressure during this procedure and possibly some discomfort when the periosteum is penetrated.

After insertion, the pin or wire is attached to the traction bow or caliper. The ends of the wire are covered with corks or tape to prevent injury to the patient or personnel. The weights are attached to the pin or wire bow by a rope–pulley system that exerts the appropriate amount and direction of pull for effective traction. Skeletal traction frequently uses 7 to 12 kg (15 to 25 lb) to achieve the therapeutic effect. The weights applied initially must overcome the shortening spasms of the affected muscles. As the muscles relax, the traction weight is reduced to prevent fracture dislocation and to promote fracture healing.

Often skeletal traction is balanced traction, which supports the affected extremity and facilitates patient independence and nursing care while maintaining effective traction.

The *Thomas splint with the Pearson attachment* is frequently used with skeletal traction in fractures of the femur (see Fig. 59–9). It may be used with skin traction and other balanced suspension apparatus. Because upward traction is required, an overbed frame is used. Figure 59–10 shows suspension traction using slings.

Maintaining Effective Traction.   When traction is being used, the apparatus is checked to see that the ropes are in the wheel grove of the pulleys; that the ropes are not frayed; that the weights hang freely; and that the patient has not slipped down in bed, causing ineffective traction. The knots in the rope must be tied securely.

- Weights should never be removed from a patient with skeletal traction unless a life-threatening situation occurs. If the weights are removed, the whole purpose of their use has been defeated and injury may result.

Positioning.   The alignment of the patient's body in traction must be maintained as prescribed to promote an effective

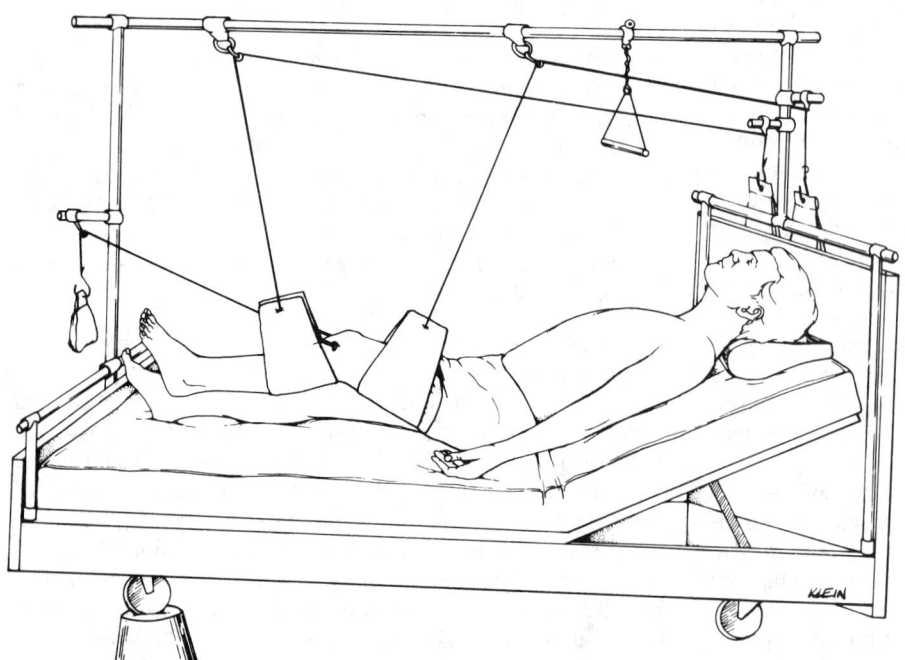

Figure 59–10.   Balanced suspension traction using slings. Skeletal traction is applied to the patient's injured leg, which is supported in slings.

line of pull. The foot should be positioned to avoid *footdrop* (plantar flexion), inward rotation (*inversion*), or outward rotation (*eversion*). The patient's foot may be supported in a neutral position by orthopedic devices (*e.g.,* foot supports).

Skin Care. When traction frames are used, a trapeze may be suspended overhead within easy reach of the patient. This apparatus is of great help in assisting the patient to move about in bed and on and off bedpans. It is also a help to the nurse in caring for these patients.

The patient's elbows frequently become sore, and nerve injury may occur if most repositioning is done by pushing on the elbows. Often patients use the heel of the good leg to act as a brace when they raise themselves. This digging of the heel into the mattress may cause injury to the tissues; hence the heel must be protected and inspected for pressure areas.

Specific pressure points need to be checked for redness and skin breakdown. Pressure areas caused by the traction apparatus may include the ischial tuberosity, popliteal space, Achilles tendon, and heel.

When a patient is not permitted to turn on one side or the other, the nurse must make a special effort to provide back care and to keep the bed dry and free of crumbs and wrinkles. The patient can assist by holding onto the overhead trapeze and raising his hips off the bed. If the patient is unable to raise himself off the mattress, the nurse can push down on the mattress with one hand, leaving space for the other hand to massage the back and bony prominences.

Neurovascular Status. Neurovascular assessment of the immobilized extremity is conducted at least every 2 hours initially and then several times a day. Prompt recognition of a developing neurovascular problem is essential so that corrective measures can be instituted promptly.

Pin Site. The wound at the insertion site requires attention. Initially the site is covered with a sterile dressing. Subsequent care of the pin site is individually prescribed. The area must be kept clean. The drainage and pin site are assessed for signs of infection such as purulent drainage, inflammation, and pain. The goal is to avoid infection and development of osteomyelitis. Slight serous oozing at the pin site is to be expected and decreases bacteria in the pin tract. Crusting should be prevented and the pin site should be kept clean. Discomfort at the pin site may be due to traction on the skin caused by an unsupported muscle.

- The pin site is inspected daily for signs of inflammation and evidence of infection.

Exercise. Patient exercises are valuable in maintaining muscle strength and tone and in promoting circulation. Exercises need to be planned within the therapeutic limits of the traction. Active exercises frequently encouraged include pulling up on the trapeze, flexing and extending the feet, and range-of-motion and weight-resistance exercises for noninvolved joints. The immobilized extremity benefits from isometric exercises. Quadriceps- and gluteal-setting exercises (see Chart 59–1) are important to maintain strength in major ambulatory muscles. Without bed exercises, the patient will lose much muscle mass and strength, and rehabilitation time will be greatly extended.

Development of deep vein thrombosis is a significant risk for anyone immobilized for a time. Active flexion–extension ankle exercises and isometric contracting of the calf muscles (calf pumping exercises) 10 times an hour while awake are encouraged to decrease venous stasis. In addition, antiembolic stockings, sequential compression devices, and anticoagulant therapies may be prescribed to help prevent thrombus formation.

Pin Removal. When x-ray studies demonstrate the presence of callus, skeletal traction is discontinued. The extremity is gently supported while the weights are removed. The pin is cut close to the skin and removed by the physician. Casts or splints are used to support the healing bone.

Summary of Nursing Interventions

When the patient is in traction, the nurse's responsibilities include the following:

1. Assess the neurovascular status of the extremity frequently.
2. Ensure that effective traction is maintained (*e.g.,* ropes and pulleys are freely movable; patient positioning is correct).
3. Maintain continuous traction unless prescribed otherwise.
4. Observe for skin irritation and breakdown.
5. Observe for pressure under the sling and equipment and at common pressure points (*e.g.,* ischial tuberosity, popliteal space, heel)
6. Encourage active foot exercises; use foot supporters as needed.
7. Encourage exercises to minimize deconditioning of the immobilized patient.
8. Involve the patient in care to help avoid depression and boredom that frequently accompany weeks of traction therapy.
9. Assess the patient for signs or symptoms of complications (*e.g.,* pin tract infection; deep vein thrombosis)

In summary, traction is the application of a pulling force to the skin or bony skeleton to minimize muscle spasm; to reduce, align, and immobilize fractures; to lessen deformity; and to increase space between opposing joint surfaces. Traction must be applied in the desired direction and appropriate magnitude to achieve the therapeutic effect. Skin traction such as pelvic and cervical traction used to reduce muscle spasm is usually prescribed as intermittent traction. Conversely, *skeletal traction is not to be interrupted and must be continuous.* Nursing diagnoses applicable to the patient in traction include impaired physical mobility related to the disease process and the traction devices; related potential problems include high risk for skin breakdown, infection of the pin site, respiratory problems, constipation and loss of appetite, urinary stasis and urinary tract infection, and deep vein thrombosis. Preventive nursing interventions and monitoring for the development of these problems are included in the nursing plan of care.

Management of the Patient Undergoing Orthopedic Surgery

Many patients who have musculoskeletal dysfunction need to undergo surgery to correct the problem. Problems that may be corrected by surgery include impaired function due to unstabilized fracture, deformity, or joint disease; necrotic or infected tissue; impaired circulation (*e.g.,* compartment syndrome); and tumors or growths. Frequent surgical procedures include *open reduction with internal fixation* for fractures; *arthroplasty, meniscectomy,* and *joint replacement* for joint problems; *amputation* for severe extremity problems (*e.g.,* gangrene, massive trauma); *bone graft* for joint stabilization, defect-filling, or stimulation of healing; and *tendon transplants* for improvement of motion. The goals of most orthopedic surgery include improving function by restoring motion and stability and relieving pain and disability.

Types of Surgery

Orthopedic surgery generally falls into the following categories:

Open reduction—the reduction and alignment of the fracture after surgical dissection and exposure of the fracture

Internal fixation—the stabilization of the reduced fracture by the use of metal screws, plates, nails, and pins

Bone graft—the placement of bone tissue (autologous or homologous grafts) to promote healing, stabilization, or replacement of diseased bone

Amputation—the removal of a body part

Arthroplasty—the repair of joint problems through the operating arthroscope (an instrument that allows the surgeon to operate within a joint without a large incision) or through open joint surgery

Meniscectomy—the excision of damaged joint fibrocartilage

Joint replacement—the substitution of joint surfaces with metal or plastic materials

Total joint replacement—the replacement of both articular surfaces within a joint with metal or synthetic materials

Tendon transfer—the movement of tendon insertion to improve function

Fasciotomy—the cutting of the muscle fascia to relieve muscle constriction or to reduce fascia contracture

▶ Nursing Process
Preoperative Care of the Patient Undergoing Orthopedic Surgery

◊ Assessment

The nurse assesses the patient for adequate hydration, current medication history, and possible infection.

Adequate hydration is an important goal for orthopedic patients. Immobilization and bed rest contribute to urinary stasis and associated bladder infections and to stone formation. Adequate hydration assures adequate urine flow and helps to prevent the occurrence of urinary tract problems. To avoid preoperative dehydration, the nurse assesses the skin, vital signs, urinary output, and laboratory values for evidence of dehydration.

It should be determined whether the patient has undergone previous therapy with corticosteroids. The person with rheumatoid arthritis or chronic pulmonary disease frequently has had steroid medications to control the disease. Steroid therapy, whether current or past, may adversely affect the body's ability to withstand the stress of surgery. The steroid should be given preoperatively as prescribed to assure adequate corticosteroid levels and prevent occurrence of Addisonian crisis in patients with suppressed adrenal function.

The patient may be on other long-term medications, such as anticoagulants, cardiovascular drugs, or insulin. All of these need to be documented and discussed with the surgeon and anesthesiologist.

The patient is questioned specifically about the existence of colds, dental problems, urinary tract infections, and other possible sites of infection occurring in the 2 weeks before surgery. Osteomyelitis could develop from spread of infection through the bloodstream. Permanent disability can result if infection occurs within a bone or joint. Preexisting infections must be resolved prior to elective orthopedic surgery.

Other areas of preoperative assessment are similar to those for any patient undergoing surgery. The "on-call" preoperative medications are injected into an uninvolved area because tissue absorption is better in a nontraumatized area.

◊ Nursing Diagnoses

Based on the nursing assessment data, the patient's major preoperative nursing diagnoses related to his orthopedic status may include the following:

- Pain related to fracture, swelling, or inflammation
- Potential altered peripheral tissue perfusion related to swelling, constricting devices, or impaired venous return
- Altered health maintenance related to loss of independence
- Impaired physical mobility related to pain, swelling, and possibly an immobilizing device
- Altered body image, self-esteem, or role performance related to impact of musculoskeletal problem

◊ Planning and Implementation

◊ *Goals:* The major goals of the patient before orthopedic surgery may include relief of pain, adequate tissue perfusion, health maintenance, improved mobility, and improved self-concept.

◊ Nursing Interventions

◊ *Relief of Pain.* Physical, pharmacologic, and psychological management techniques to control pain are useful in the preoperative period. Specific methods selected are tailored to the individual patient. Immobilization of a fractured bone or injured, inflamed joint will decrease discomfort. Elevation of a swollen extremity will promote venous return and reduce associated discomfort. Ice, if prescribed, will relieve swelling and directly reduce discomfort by diminishing nerve stimulation. Analgesics are frequently prescribed to control the acute pain of musculoskeletal injury and associated muscle spasm. During the immediate preoperative period, the nurse needs to discuss and coordinate administration of analgesic medications with the anesthesiologist and surgeon. Alternative methods of pain control (*e.g.,* distraction, focusing, guided imagery, quiet environment, back rubs) may be used to decrease pain perception.

◊ *Maintenance of Adequate Tissue Perfusion.* Trauma, swelling, or immobilization devices may interrupt tissue perfusion. Venous return is promoted by avoiding pressure on the popliteal area and by using antiembolic stockings as prescribed. The neurovascular status (*i.e.,* color, temperature, capillary refill, pulse, pain, edema, paresthesia, motion) of the extremity must be assessed frequently. If compromised circulation is noted, measures to restore adequate circulation are instituted. The physician is notified promptly, the extremity is elevated, and constricting wraps and casts are released as prescribed.

◊ *Health Maintenance.* The nurse needs to assist the patient in activities that will promote health during the perioperative and rehabilitative periods. Nutritional needs and hydration are assessed. Generally, nutrition for orthopedic patients is a reflection of their normal eating patterns. It may be appropriate to discuss ways of modifying the diet or to refer the patient to the dietitian. The preoperative fasting regimen is usually tolerated well. If the patient is diabetic, elderly and frail, or the victim of multiple trauma, special provisions may be necessary. Abnormal urinalysis findings and complaint of burning on urination require further investigation before surgery. At times patients will decide to limit their fluid intake to minimize the use of a bedpan. A small fracture pan may be more comfortable for the patient to use. The nurse monitors fluid intake and urinary output. The use of an indwelling catheter should be avoided to reduce the risk of urinary tract infection.

Smoking should be stopped during the preoperative period to facilitate optimum respiratory function. Coughing, deep breathing, and use of the incentive spirometer are practiced preoperatively for improved respiratory function during the postoperative period. Preoperative teaching facilitates postoperative compliance.

Exercises are taught during the preoperative period. Gluteal-setting and quadriceps-setting isometric exercises are taught for maintenance of the muscles needed for ambulation. Unless contraindicted, isometric contraction of the calf muscles and ankle exercises are practiced to minimize venous stasis and prevent deep vein thrombosis. Active range-of-motion exercises of uninvolved joints are encouraged. The patient who will be using ambulatory aids may exercise to strengthen the upper extremities and shoulders. If possible, assistive devices (*e.g.*, trapeze) are used and transfer techniques are practiced before surgery.

Skin care is provided, with special attention to pressure points. The use of pressure-reducing surfaces (*e.g.*, convoluted foam or air mattress, alternating air mattress) needs to be instituted before surgery for those at risk for skin breakdown.

To minimize the risk of infection, meticulous nontraumatizing cleaning of the skin with soap and water is done the day before surgery. If the operation is elective, the orthopedic surgeon may advise the patient to begin the skin cleansing with a germicidal soap before hospitalization.

◊ *Improved Mobility.* Preoperatively, the patient's mobility is impaired by pain, swelling, and immobilizing devices (*e.g.*, splints, casts, traction). The nurse must gently assist the patient in moving the injured part while providing adequate support. Swollen extremities are elevated and adequately supported with hands and pillows. Pain is controlled before an injured part is moved by splinting it and by administering medication in time to take effect before the injured part is moved. Movement within the limits of therapeutic immobility is encouraged. If mobility aids (*e.g.*, crutches, walker, wheelchair) are to be used postoperatively, practice with the devices preoperatively facilitates the patient's safe use of the aids postoperatively and promotes earlier independent mobility.

◊ *Improved Self-Concept.* Preoperative orthopedic patients may need assistance in accepting changes in body image, di-

minished self-esteem, or inability to perform the responsibilities of their life roles. The degree of assistance required in this area varies greatly, depending on the events preceding hospitalization, the surgery and rehabilitation planned, the temporary or permanent nature of the altered body image, and the extent of changes required in role performance. The nurse promotes a trusting relationship for patients to express concerns and anxieties, and helps them examine their feelings about changes in self-concept. The nurse can clarify any misconceptions patients may have, and help them work through modifications that may be necessary because of alterations in physical capacity and self-concept.

◊ **Evaluation**

Expected Outcomes

1. Reports controlled pain
   a. Uses multiple approaches to reduce pain
   b. States medication is effective in controlling pain
   c. Moves with greater comfort
2. Exhibits adequate tissue perfusion
   a. Skin color normal
   b. Skin warm
   c. Capillary refill response normal
   d. Sensation and motion normal
   e. Demonstrates reduced swelling
   f. Uses antiembolism stockings if prescribed
3. Promotes health
   a. Eats balanced diet appropriate to meet nutritional needs
   b. Maintains adequate hydration
   c. Abstains from smoking
   d. Practices respiratory exercises
   e. Repositions self to relieve skin pressure
   f. Engages in strengthening and preventive exercises
4. Maximizes mobility within the therapeutic limits
   a. Requests assistance when moving
   b. Elevates swollen extremity after transfer
   c. Uses immobilizing devices and assistive devices as prescribed
5. Expresses positive self-concept
   a. Acknowledges temporary or permanent changes in body image
   b. Discusses role performance changes
   c. Views self as valuable and capable of assuming responsibilities

▶ **Nursing Process**
Postoperative Care of the Patient Undergoing Orthopedic Surgery

◊ **Assessment**

After orthopedic surgery, the nurse continues the preoperative care plan, modifying it to the current postoperative status. The nurse reassesses the patient's needs in relation to pain, tissue perfusion, health promotion, mobility, and self-concept.

Skeletal trauma and surgery performed on bones, muscles, and joints can produce significant pain, especially during the first several postoperative days.

Tissue perfusion must be monitored closely because edema and bleeding into the tissues may compromise circulation and result in a compartment syndrome. Assessment of respiratory, gastrointestinal, and urinary function provides data for promoting function of these systems. General anesthesia and immobility can result in altered functioning of these systems.

Prescribed limits on mobility are noted. The nurse assesses the patient's understanding of these limits. Reassessment of the patient's self-concept facilitates modification of the preoperative plan of care.

In addition, the nurse is concerned with assessing and monitoring the patient for potential problems related to the surgery. Frequent assessment of vital signs, level of consciousness, wound drainage, breath sounds, bowel sounds, fluid balance, and pain will provide the nurse with data that suggest the possible development of a potential problem. Abnormal findings are reported to the physician promptly.

With major orthopedic surgery, shock may be a problem. Persistent bleeding may occur with orthopedic surgery. Muscle dissection frequently produces wounds in which hemostasis is poor. Wounds that are closed under tourniquet control may bleed during the postoperative period. The nurse must be alert for signs of shock (*e.g.*, rising pulse rate, falling blood pressure, restlessness).

Changes in the pulse rate, respiratory rate, or in the patient's color may indicate pulmonary or cardiac complications. The pulmonary complications of atelectasis and pneumonia are frequently seen and may be related to preexisting pulmonary disease, deep anesthesia, minimal activity, analgesics, and reduced respiratory reserve due to advanced age or an underlying musculoskeletal disorder (*e.g.*, restrictive lung expansion secondary to kyphosis related to osteoporosis).

Voiding in unnatural positions may contribute to urinary retention. In addition, elderly men usually have some degree of prostatism and may already have difficulty in voiding. Therefore it is important to monitor urinary output.

Elevated temperature may be related to a pulmonary problem, a urinary problem, dehydration, or an infection. Temperature elevations within the first 48 hours are frequently related to atelectasis or other respiratory problems. Temperature elevations during the next few days are frequently associated with urinary tract infections. Superficial wound infections take about 5 to 9 days to develop. Phlebitis-associated temperatures generally occur during the second week.

Thromboembolic disease (see Deep Vein Thrombosis, p. 462, and Pulmonary Embolism, p. 587) is one of the most common and most dangerous of all complications occurring in the postoperative orthopedic patient. Advancing age, hemostasis, lower extremity orthopedic surgery, and immobilization are significant risk factors. The nurse assesses the patient's legs daily for calf tenderness, calf edema, and a positive Homan's sign. Abnormal findings are reported to the physician promptly.

In addition, *fat embolus* (p. 1826) may occur with orthopedic surgery. The nurse must be alert to changes in respirations, behavior, and level of consciousness that might indicate the development of fat embolus.

▷ Nursing Diagnoses

Based on all assessment data, the patient's major nursing diagnoses after orthopedic surgery may include the following:

- Pain related to the surgical procedure, swelling, and immobilization

- Potential for altered peripheral tissue perfusion related to swelling, constricting devices, impaired circulation
- Altered health maintenance related to loss of independence
- Impaired physical mobility related to pain, swelling, surgical procedure, presence of immobilizing device (splint, traction, cast, external fixator, dressing)
- Altered body image, self-esteem, or role performance related to impact of musculoskeletal problems.

Nursing diagnoses related to potential complications of orthopedic surgery include:

- High risk for fluid volume deficit
- Potential ineffective airway clearance
- Potential urinary retention
- High risk for infection
- Potential altered peripheral tissue perfusion

▷ Planning and Implementation

▷ *Goals:*   The major goals of the patient after orthopedic surgery may include relief of pain, adequate tissue perfusion, health maintenance, improved mobility, improved self-concept, and absence of complications such as shock, pulmonary problems, urinary retention, infection, and thromboembolic disease.

▷ Nursing Interventions

▷ *Relief of Pain.*   After orthopedic surgery, pain can be intense. Edema, hematomas, and muscle spasms contribute to the pain experienced. At times the patient will indicate that the pain is less than that experienced preoperatively, and only moderate amounts of analgesics are needed. The patient's pain level and response to therapeutic measures are monitored closely. Every effort is made to relieve the pain and provide comfort to the patient.

Multiple pharmacologic approaches to pain management exist. Patient-controlled analgesia (PCA) and epidural analgesia may be prescribed to control the pain. If intramuscular and oral analgesics are prescribed, the patient needs to understand that he should request the pain medication before the pain reaches a severe intensity. It should be administered promptly within the prescribed intervals. Intramuscular injection sites should be rotated, avoiding the operative hip and thigh. The medications may be administered on a preventive basis within the prescribed intervals if the onset of pain can be predicted (*e.g.*, a half hour before planned activity such as transfer or exercise).

In addition to pharmacologic approaches to controlling pain, elevation of the operative extremity and application of cold, if prescribed, help to control edema. Portable suction of the wound decreases fluid accumulation and hematoma formation. The nurse may find that repositioning, relaxation, distraction, and guided imagery techniques are helpful in reducing and controlling the patient's pain.

Increasing and uncontrollable pain suggests that a problem exists. This needs to be reported to the orthopedic surgeon for evaluation. Pain should diminish rapidly after the initial postoperative period. After 3 to 4 days, most patients require only occasional oral analgesia for residual muscle soreness and spasm.

▷ *Maintenance of Adequate Tissue Perfusion.*   The preoperative plan of care is continued. The nurse monitors the neurovascular status of the involved body part and notifies the physician promptly of findings indicative of diminished tissue perfusion. In addition the nurse reminds the patient to perform muscle-setting, ankle, and calf-pumping exercises hourly while awake to enhance circulation.

▷ *Health Maintenance.* The preoperative plan of care is continued. The preoperative teaching and exercise programs promote health and encourage the patient to participate in the postoperative treatment regimen.

Well-balanced diets with adequate protein and vitamins are needed for healthy tissue and wound healing. The patient is placed on a normal diet as soon as possible. Large amounts of milk should not be given to orthopedic patients who are on bed rest, however, because this only adds to the calcium pool in the body and requires that more calcium be excreted by the kidneys, which can lead to formation of urinary calculi.

The nurse monitors the patient for evidence of pressure ulcers, which are a constant threat to any patient who must spend an extended period in bed or who is elderly, malnourished, or unable to move without assistance. Turning, washing, drying, and massaging the skin are necessary to avoid skin breakdown.

▷ *Improved Physical Mobility.* Patients are frequently afraid to move after orthopedic surgery. Establishing a therapeutic relationship with the patient helps to secure full participation of the patient in frightening, uncomfortable therapeutic activities designed to improve the level of physical mobility. With reassurance that movement within therapeutic limits will benefit them, that assistance will be provided by the nurse, that discomfort can be controlled, and that activity goals are attainable, patients are usually receptive to increasing their mobility.

Soft tissue heals more rapidly than bone. Even though the incision appears healed, the underlying bone needs additional time to repair and regain normal strength. Some orthopedic procedures require prolonged protection from excessive stress (*e.g.*, weight-bearing restrictions: immobilizing splints, cast, braces). This is especially important to remember in surgeries of the lower extremities.

Metal pins, screws, rods, and plates used for internal fixation are designed to maintain the position of the bone until ossification occurs. They are not designed to support the body's weight and can bend, loosen, or break if stressed. The estimated strength of the bone, the stability of the fracture, reduction and fixation, and the amount of bone healing are important considerations in determining the stress the bone can withstand after surgery. The orthopedic surgeon will prescribe the weight-bearing limits and use of protective devices (orthosis), if necessary, after surgery.

- Weight-bearing limits and use of protective devices are discussed with the orthopedic surgeon before transfer and ambulation.

The exercise program is tailored to the individual's clinical problem. The goal is to return the patient to the highest level of function in the shortest time consistent with the surgical procedure. Rehabilitation involves progressively increasing the patient's activities and instituting progressive exercises as prescribed. Frequently some form of walking aid (crutches, walker) is used for postoperative mobility. Preoperative practice with mobility aids helps the patient use them postoperatively. Within the prescribed weight-bearing limits (determined by the type of surgery), the nurse monitors the patient's gait, making sure

that it is safe. (Crutch walking and using a walker are discussed in Chapter 14.)

▷ *Improved Self-Concept.* The preoperative plan of care is continued. The nurse and the patient set realistic goals. Increasing self-care activities within the limits of the therapeutic regimen and resumption of roles facilitate recognition of abilities and promote self-esteem, personal identity, and role performance. Altered body image is gradually accepted with the support of the nurse, family, and others.

▷ *Management of Shock.* The nurse monitors the patient after surgery for the development of shock. Excessive loss of blood during surgery or excessive postoperative drainage can result in shock. The nurse identifies early signs and symptoms of shock and reports the findings to the orthopedic surgeon for appropriate management. (See pp. 457–462 for management of shock.)

▷ *Prevention of Pulmonary Problems.* The nurse monitors the patient's lung sounds and encourages deep breathing and coughing exercises. Full expansion of the lungs prevents accumulation of respiratory secretions. If incentive spirometry is prescribed, the nurse encourages its use. If signs of respiratory problems develop, the nurse reports the findings to the surgeon for appropriate management.

▷ *Prevention of Urinary Retention.* Monitoring the urinary output after surgery provides information concerning possible retention. Suggesting that the patient attempt to void every 3 to 4 hours may prevent the bladder from becoming overly distended. Privacy must be provided during toileting. Because the patient may need to void in an unusual position, the nurse assists the patient with positioning. Fracture bedpans may be more comfortable. Voiding in the side-lying position may be helpful to the male patient. At times the male patient can only void if standing, and clarification of the activity prescription may be needed before assisting the patient to a standing position. If the patient is unable to void, intermittent catheterizations may be prescribed until the patient is able to void independently.

▷ *Management of Infection.* Infection is a potential problem after any surgery. It is of particular concern for the postoperative orthopedic patient because of the high risk for osteomyelitis. Osteomyelitis is difficult to treat, requiring prolonged courses of intravenous antibiotics. At times the infected bone, prosthesis, and internal fixation devices must be surgically removed. Therefore, prophylactic systemic antibiotics are frequently prescribed during the perioperative and immediate postoperative period. The nurse assesses the patient's response to these antibiotics. When changing dressings and emptying wound drainage devices, aseptic technique is essential. The nurse monitors the patient's vital signs, assesses the appearance of the wound, and notes the character of the drainage. Also, because urinary retention is common after orthopedic surgery, the character of the urine is monitored for signs of urinary tract infection. Prompt recognition and reporting to the physician of an apparent infective process is necessary. Patient education concerning reporting of the signs and symptoms of infection, handwashing, and wound care reduces the development of infections.

▷ *Prevention of Thromboembolic Disease.* Preventive measures (*e.g.*, ankle and calf pumping exercises; use of antiembolic elastic stockings or sequential compression devices; adequate hydration; early mobilization) are included in the nursing care plan. Prophylactic warfarin or adjusted-dose heparin may be prescribed. Aspirin has no apparent venous thromboembolism prophylactic effect in the orthopedic patient. The nurse monitors the patient for the development of signs of deep vein thrombosis and promptly reports findings to the physician for management.

Evaluation

Expected Outcomes

1. Reports controlled pain
   a. Uses multiple approaches to reduce pain
   b. Uses occasional oral medication to control discomfort
   c. Elevates extremity to control swelling and discomfort
   d. Moves with greater comfort
2. Exhibits adequate tissue perfusion
   a. Skin color normal
   b. Skin warm
   c. Capillary refill response normal
   d. Sensation and motion normal
   e. Demonstrates reduced swelling
3. Promotes health
   a. Eats balanced diet appropriate to meet nutritional needs
   b. Maintains adequate hydration
   c. Abstains from smoking
   d. Practices respiratory exercises
   e. Repositions self to relieve skin pressure
   f. Engages in strengthening and preventive exercises
   g. Uses antiembolism stockings or sequential compression devices if prescribed.
4. Maximizes mobility within the therapeutic limits
   a. Requests assistance when moving
   b. Elevates swollen extremity after transfer
   c. Uses immobilizing devices as prescribed
   d. Complies with prescribed weight-bearing limitation
5. Expresses positive self-concept
   a. Acknowledges temporary or permanent changes in body image
   b. Discusses role performance changes
   c. Views self as valuable and capable of assuming responsibilities
   d. Actively participates in planning care and in the therapeutic regimen
6. Exhibits absence of complications
   a. Does not experience shock
   b. Maintains normal vital signs and blood pressure
   c. Lung sounds clear
   d. Wound heals without signs of infection
   e. Wound drainage is not purulent
   f. Does not experience urinary retention
   g. Urine clear
   h. Exhibits no signs of thromboembolism disease

In summary, surgical approaches (i.e., open reduction, internal fixation, bone grafting, amputation, arthroplasty, meniscectomy, joint replacement, tendon transfer, fasciotomy) are used to treat a variety of musculoskeletal disorders. Care of the patient having orthopedic surgery includes measures to prevent potential problems—shock, pulmonary problems, urinary retention, infection, thromboembolic disease. In the early postoperative period, the nurse focuses on management of pain, promotion of tissue perfusion, and promotion of homeostasis. High risk for infection is a major concern with any orthopedic surgery. In addition, orthopedic patients are at a high risk for thromboembolic disease, and preventive measures (i.e., ankle and calf pumping exercises, hydration, early mobilization, elastic stockings or sequential compression devices) are important components of the nursing plan of care.

Orthopedic treatment plans contain specific mobility and weight-bearing prescriptions that are based on the patient's condition and therapeutic procedure. Care must be taken not to disrupt therapeutic treatment by improper positioning (e.g., resulting in dislocation of a joint prosthesis) or excessive stress (e.g., resulting in disruption of internal immobilization).

Reconstructive Joint Surgery

At times, the impact of joint disease or deformity will necessitate surgical intervention to relieve pain, improve stability, and improve function. Surgical therapies used for joint disease include excision of damaged and diseased tissue, repair of damaged structures (e.g., ruptured tendon), removal of loose bodies (debridement), immobilizing fusion of a joint (arthrodesis), and replacement of all or part of the joint surfaces (e.g., arthroplasty, prosthesis, total joint).

Total joint replacement is the replacement of both articular surfaces within a joint capsule (e.g., total hip replacement refers to implantation of both femoral and acetabular prostheses). Hemiarthroplasty refers to the replacement of one of the articular surfaces (e.g., in a hip hemiarthroplasty the femoral head and neck are replaced with a femoral prosthesis—the acetabulum is not replaced).

The procedure is selected according to the patient's underlying problems, general physical health, impact of joint disability on life, and age. Timing of these procedures is important for gaining maximum function. Surgery should be performed before surrounding muscles become contracted and atrophied and serious structural abnormalities occur. The patient must be carefully evaluated so that the procedure with the best chance of success and best long-range benefits is selected.

Joint Replacement

Patients with severe pain and disability associated with the joint may be selected for joint replacement. Conditions contributing to joint degeneration include rheumatoid arthritis, osteoarthritis (degenerative joint disease), trauma, and congenital deformity. At times, joint replacement is a salvage procedure because of disruption of the blood supply and subsequent avascular necrosis. Joints frequently replaced include the knee, the hip (Fig. 59–11), shoulder, and finger joints. Less frequently, more complex joints (elbow, wrist, ankle) are replaced. The procedure is usually an elective one.

Most joint replacements consist of metal and high-density polyethylene components. Finger prostheses are generally silastic. The joint implants may be cemented in the prepared bone with methyl methacrylate (a bone-bonding agent), which has properties similar to bone. Loosening of the prosthesis due to cement failure in 5 to 15 years is the most common reason

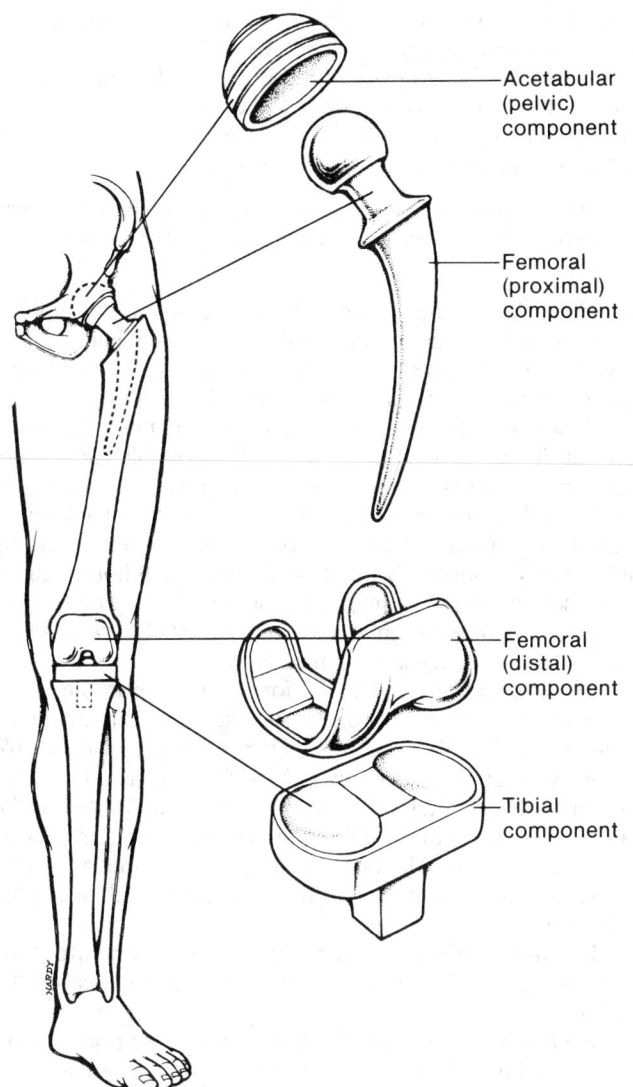

Acetabular (pelvic) component

Femoral (proximal) component

Femoral (distal) component

Tibial component

Figure 59-11. Hip and knee replacement.

for prosthesis failure. Newer techniques and materials seem to reduce the failure rate. Ingrowth prostheses (porous-coated, cementless, artificial joint components) that allow the patient's bone to grow into and securely fix the prosthesis are being used more frequently. They are expected to last longer than cemented components. Accurate fitting and the presence of healthy bone stock with adequate blood supply are important in the use of cementless components.

With joint replacement, excellent pain relief is obtained in 85% to 90% of patients. Return of motion and function depends on preoperative soft tissue condition, soft tissue reactions, and general muscle strength. Early failure of joint replacement is associated with high levels of activity and prereplacement joint pathology.

Preoperative Assessment

Assessment of the patient and preoperative management are aimed at having the patient in optimal health at the time of surgery. A complete preoperative evaluation is carried out, with emphasis on cardiovascular, respiratory, renal, and hepatic function. Age, obesity, preoperative leg edema, history of deep vein thrombosis, and varicose veins increase the risk of

postoperative deep vein thrombosis and pulmonary embolism. Every effort is made to prevent deep vein thrombosis and pulmonary embolism, the most common cause of postoperative mortality in patients over 60 years of age undergoing total hip replacement.

Preoperatively, the nurse assesses the neurovascular status of the extremity undergoing joint replacement. Postoperative assessment data are compared with preoperative assessment data to identify changes and deficits. Nerve palsy can occur during surgery. An absent pulse postoperatively is of concern unless the pulse was also absent preoperatively.

Preventing Infection

Infection is a major concern with joint replacements. Careful preoperative assessment of the patient for sites of infection is necessary. Any infection 2 to 4 weeks before planned surgery may result in postponement of surgery. Preoperative urine cultures may be taken, because urinary tract infection is a frequent portal of entry for bacteria. It has been observed that infection occurs nearly twice as often in patients with rheumatoid arthritis as in those the osteoarthritis. (This may be associated with a deficit in polymorphonuclear leukocyte function observed in many patients with rheumatoid arthritis.)

Preoperative skin preparation frequently begins a day or two before the surgery. Research suggests that the majority of deep infections are caused by bacteria that are implanted into the wound at the time of surgery, mostly from airborne sources. During the operation, there is strict adherence to aseptic principles and the operating area is controlled and made as nearly bacteria-free as possible.

Prophylactic antibiotics may be administered just before surgery or started intraoperatively. Culture of the joint during surgery, before intraoperative antibiotic therapy is begun, may be important in identifying and treating subsequent infections.

Osteomyelitis is difficult to treat. Infection of the prosthesis generally requires removal of the implant and joint revision, a complex procedure. Also, it is not always possible to achieve a functional joint when the reconstruction procedure has to be repeated.

Ambulation After Surgery

Ambulation is started within a day or two after surgery, depending on the patient's condition. The goal is independent ambulation. At first the patient may be only able to stand for a brief period because of orthostatic hypotension. As the patient is able to tolerate more activity, transferring to a chair several times a day for short periods is encouraged.

Specific weight-bearing limits on the prosthesis are determined by the physician based on the patient's condition, the procedure, and the fixation method. Generally, cemented prostheses can have weight-bearing as tolerated by patient comfort. If the patient has an ingrowth prosthesis, weight-bearing may be limited immediately after surgery; this minimizes micromotion of the prosthesis in the bone, in an attempt to prevent disruption of bone ingrowth.

Total Hip Replacement

Total hip replacement is the replacement of a severely damaged hip with an artificial joint. The following conditions are amenable to this type of surgery: arthritis (degenerative joint disease, rheumatoid arthritis), femoral neck fractures, failure of previous reconstructive surgeries (failed prosthesis, osteotomy, femoral head replacement), and problems resulting from congenital hip disease. A variety of total hip prostheses are available. Most consist of a metal femoral component topped by a spherical ball fitted into a plastic acetabular socket (see Fig. 59–11). The surgeon selects the prosthesis most suited to the individual, considering various factors including skeletal structure and activity level.

The operation is usually reserved for patients over age 60 with unremitting pain or irreversibly damaged hip joints. With the advent of improved prosthetic materials and operative techniques, life of the prosthesis is extended and younger patients with severely damaged painful hip joints are undergoing total hip replacement.

Specific Nursing Care Considerations

The nurse must be aware of specific potential problems associated with total hip replacement and include them in the nursing care plan. The primary potential problems include dislocation of the hip prosthesis, excessive wound drainage, thromboembolism, and infection.

Dislocation of the Hip Prosthesis. Positioning activities that will ensure positioning of the femoral head component in the acetabular cup are essential. The patient is taught about positioning the leg in *abduction*, which helps to prevent dislocation of the prosthesis. The use of abduction splints, wedge pillows (Fig. 59–12), or two or three pillows between the legs keep the hip in abduction. When turning a patient in bed, the operative hip must be kept in abduction and the entire length of the leg is supported by pillows.

The hip is not to be flexed more than 45 to 60 degrees. Therefore the head of the bed should not be elevated more than 45 degrees to prevent acute flexion of the hip. When using the fracture bedpan, the patient is instructed to flex the unoperated hip and use the trapeze to lift the pelvis onto the pan; he is also reminded not to flex the operated hip.

Limited flexion is maintained during transfers and when sitting. When the patient is initially assisted out of bed, an abduction splint or pillows are kept between the legs. The patient is encouraged to keep the operative hip in extension. The patient is instructed to pivot on the unoperated leg while the nurse assists him in moving and protects the operative leg from adduction, flexion, and excessive weight-bearing. Semireclining wheelchairs and toilet seat extenders may be used to minimize hip joint flexion.

The patient is taught protective positioning. Until otherwise instructed, to maintain abduction, the patient should use a pillow between the legs when lying in a supine or side-lying position and when turning. The patient is not to sleep on the operated side until this position is cleared with the surgeon.

At no time should the patient cross his legs. Stooping and acute flexion of the hip are to be avoided.

Dislocation may occur with positioning that exceeds the limits of the prosthesis. If dislocation of the prosthesis occurs it needs to be recognized and reduced early so that circulatory and nerve damage to the leg do not occur.

- The indicators of dislocation are shortening of the leg, inability to move it, malalignment, abnormal rotation, and increased discomfort.

If a prosthesis becomes dislocated, the surgeon must be notified to reduce and stabilize the hip. As the muscles and joint capsule heal, the chance of dislocation diminishes. Stresses to the new hip joint should be minimal for the first 3 to 6 months.

Wound Drainage. Fluid and blood accumulating at the surgical site are generally drained with a portable suction device. This prevents accumulation of fluid, which could contribute to discomfort and could provide a site for infection. Drainage of 200 to 500 ml in the first 24 hours is expected; by 48 hours postoperatively, the total drainage in 8 hours usually decreases to 30 ml or less, and the suction device is then removed. Drainage volumes greater than anticipated must be reported to the physician promptly.

Thromboembolism. The risk for thromboembolism is particularly great after hip reconstructive surgery. The incidence of deep vein thrombosis is 45% to 70%. Of these patients, 20% develop pulmonary emboli, with 1% to 3% being fatal. Therefore the nurse must institute preventive measures and monitor the patient closely for the development of deep vein thrombosis and pulmonary emboli. Measures to promote circulation and decrease venous stasis are priorities for the patient having hip reconstruction.

Infection. Infection is a serious complication after total hip replacement. Deep infection may require removal of the implant.

Patients who are diabetic, elderly, obese, or poorly nourished, who have rheumatoid arthritis, or who have concurrent infections (*e.g.*, urinary tract infections, dental abscesses) or develop large hematomas are at high risk for infection.

Because total joint infections are so disastrous, all efforts are undertaken to minimize their occurrence. Potential sources of infection are scrupulously avoided. Prophylactic antibiotics are used. If used, indwelling urinary catheters and portable wound suction devices are removed as soon as possible to avoid infection. Prophylactic antibiotics may be prescribed if the patient needs any future surgical instrumentation, such as tooth extraction or cystoscopic examination.

Classic signs of infection may be present, or the patient may at some time months to years after the surgery experience return of discomfort in the hip, which could mean a late infection. Acute infections may occur within 3 months of surgery, and are associated with progressive superficial infections or draining hematomas. Delayed surgical infections may appear 4 to 26 months after surgery. Infections occurring more than 2 years after surgery are attributed to the spread of infection through the bloodstream from another place in the body.

If an infection occurs, antibiotics are used to treat the infection. Severe infections may require surgical debridement or removal of the prosthesis.

Other Complications. Other complications of total hip replacement include those associated with immobility, loosening of the prosthesis, *heterotrophic ossification* (formation of bone

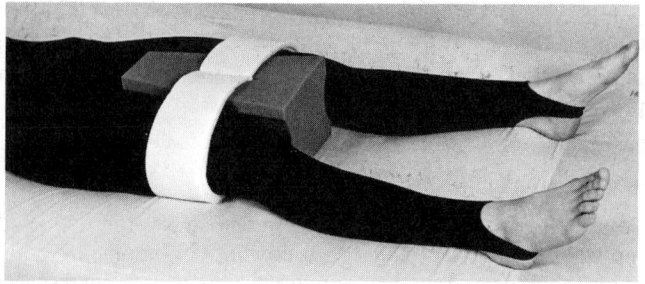

Figure 59–12. An abduction pillow may be used after a total hip replacement to prevent dislocation of the prosthesis.

in the periprosthetic space) and *avascular necrosis* (bone death caused by loss of blood supply). Methods for improved cement fixation, ingrowth prosthesis, and bone grafts are aimed at reducing the change of prosthesis loosening.

Patient Education for Continuing Care

Before the patient prepares to leave the acute care setting, the nurse provides a thorough teaching program to promote continuity of the therapeutic regimen and progress toward full rehabilitation. The patient must accept the responsibility for being the primary rehabilitation resource.

The patient is advised to be faithful in the daily exercise program to maintain the functional motion of the hip joint and strengthen the abductor muscles of the hip. It will take time to strengthen and reeducate the muscles.

Ambulatory aids (crutches, walker, or cane) are used for a time. When sufficient muscle tone has developed to permit a normal gait without discomfort, the cane may be abandoned. Walking efficiency after total hip replacement is improved because of the acquired painless normal gait. In general, by 3 months the patient is able to resume all routine daily living activities. Generally, stair climbing is avoided during the first 3 months after surgery and kept to a minimum for the next 3 months. Frequent walks, swimming, and use of a high rocking chair are excellent for hip exercises. Sexual activities should be carried out in the dependent position for 3 to 6 months to avoid adduction and flexion of the new hip.

At no time should the patient cross his legs or assume positions of acute flexion, more than 90 degrees. Assistance in putting on shoes and socks may be needed. Low chairs are avoided, as well as sitting for more than 30 minutes at a time, to minimize hip flexion and the risk of prosthetic dislocation and to prevent hip stiffness and flexion contracture. Traveling long distances is to be avoided unless frequent changes in position are possible. Other activities to avoid include overexertion, lifting heavy loads, and excessive bending and twisting (lifting, shoveling snow, forceful turning).

After successful surgery and rehabilitation, the patient can expect a hip joint that is free or nearly free of pain, has good motion, is stable, and that usually permits normal or near normal ambulation.

Nursing Care Planning

Based on the nursing assessment of the patient's needs and knowledge of care of the patient undergoing orthopedic surgery, specifically total hip replacement, the nurse develops with the patient a plan of care to meet his needs and to monitor for potential problems. A model nursing care plan for the patient having a total hip replacement is presented in Nursing Care Plan 59–1.

Total Knee Replacement

Total knee replacement surgery is considered for patients who have severe pain and functional disabilities related to joint surfaces destroyed by arthritis (rheumatoid arthritis, osteoarthritis, posttraumatic arthritis) and hemophilia. There are a large variety of metal and acrylic prostheses that are designed to provide the patient with a functional, painless, stable joint. If the patient's ligaments have weakened, a fully constrained (hinged) or semiconstrained prosthesis may be used to provide joint stability. A nonconstrained prosthesis depends on the patient's ligaments for joint stability.

Postoperative Management.   Postoperatively, the knee is dressed with a compression bandage. Ice may be applied to control edema and bleeding. The neurovascular status of the leg is assessed. Active flexion of the foot is encouraged. Efforts are directed at preventing complications (thromboembolism, peroneal nerve palsy, infection).

A wound suction drain removes fluid accumulating in the joint. Drainage during the first 8 hours after surgery is about 200 ml; it diminishes to less than 25 ml by 48 hours postoperatively. The drains are then removed by the surgeon.

Frequently the patient's leg is placed on a continuous passive motion (CPM) device (Fig. 59–13) in the postanesthesia area. This device promotes healing by increasing circulation and movement of the knee joint. The rate and amount of extension and flexion are prescribed. Usually 10 degrees of extension and 50 degrees of flexion are initiated, and increased to 90 degrees of flexion by discharge. The patient is encouraged to use the device most of the time. The physical therapist supervises exercises for strength and range of motion. If satisfactory flexion is not achieved, gentle manipulation of the knee joint under general anesthesia may be done about 2 weeks after surgery.

The patient is assisted with transfers out of bed the day after surgery. The knee is usually protected with a knee immobilizer and is elevated when the patient sits in a chair. Weight-bearing limits are prescribed by the physician. Progressive ambulation, using ambulatory aids and within the prescribed weight-bearing limits, is begun a day or two after the surgery.

After discharge from the hospital, the patient may continue to use the CPM at home as well as to do physical therapy on an outpatient basis. Late complications that may occur include infection and loosening and wear of prosthetic components. Generally, the patient is able to achieve a pain-free, functional joint and participate more fully in life activities.

In summary, joint replacement is frequently an elective surgical procedure to reduce pain and disability. A variety of

(text continues on page 1815)

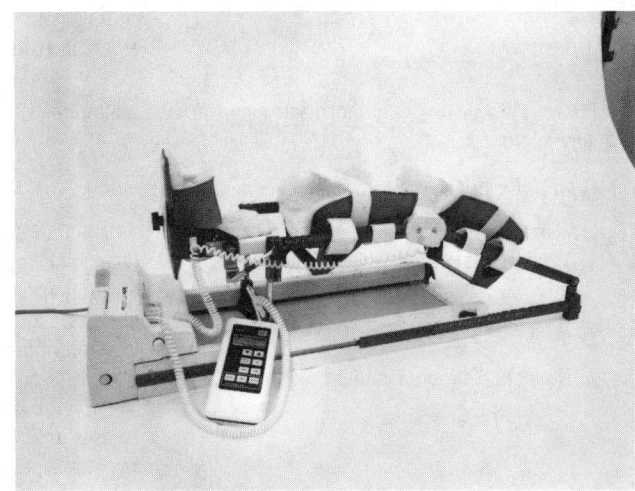

Figure 59–13.   Continuous passive motion device used for postoperative total knee arthroplasty patients to facilitate joint range of motion. (Courtesy of Sutter Biomedical Inc.)

Nursing Care Plan 59–1

Care of the Patient With a Total Hip Replacement

Nursing Interventions	Rationale	Expected Outcomes
Nursing Diagnosis: Pain related to total hip replacement		
Goal: Relief of pain		
1. Assess patient for pain.	1. Pain is expected after a surgical procedure because of the surgical trauma and tissue-response. Muscle spasms occur after total hip replacements. Immobility causes discomfort at pressure points.	• Patient describes discomfort. • Expresses confidence in efforts to control pain • States pain is reduced • Appears comfortable and relaxed • Uses physical, psychological, and pharmacologic measures to reduce discomfort
2. Ask patient to describe discomfort.	2. Pain characteristics may help to determine cause of discomfort. Pain may be due to complication (hematoma, infection, flatus). Pain is an individual experience—it means different things to different people.	
3. Acknowledge existence of pain; inform patient of available analgesics or muscle relaxants.	3. Reduces the stress experienced by patient by communicating concern and availability of assistance to help patient deal with the pain	
4. Use pain-modifying techniques. a. Use analgesics.	a. Patient will require parenteral narcotics during the first 24–48 hours, and then will progress to oral analgesics.	
b. Change position within prescribed limits.	b. Use pillows to provide adequate support; relieve pressure on bony prominences.	
c. Modify environment.	c. Interactions with others, distractions, and sensory overload or deprivation may affect pain experience.	
d. Notify surgeon if necessary.	d. Surgical intervention may be necessary if pain is due to hematoma or excessive edema.	
5. Evaluate and record discomfort and effectiveness of pain-modifying techniques.	5. Effectiveness of action is based on experience; notations provide data concerning pain experiences, management, and pain relief	

Potential Problems: Hemorrhage; neurovascular compromise; dislocation of prosthesis; deep vein thrombosis; infection related to surgery

Goal: Experiences an absence of complications

Hemorrhage

1. Monitor vital signs, observing for shock.	1. Changes in pulse, blood pressure, and respirations may indicate development of shock. Blood loss and stress of surgery may contribute to development of shock.	• Vital signs stabilize within normal limits. • Amount of drainage decreases • No bright red bloody drainage • Hematology values are within normal limits.
2. Note character and amount of drainage.	2. Within 48 hours, bloody drainage collected in portable suction device decreases to 25–30 ml per 8 hours. Excessive drainage (more than 250 ml in first 8 hours after surgery) and bright red drainage may indicate active bleeding.	

(continued)

Nursing Care Plan 59–1 *(Continued)*

Care of the Patient With a Total Hip Replacement

Nursing Interventions	Rationale	Expected Outcomes
3. Notify surgeon if patient develops shock or excessive bleeding.	3. Corrective measures need to be instituted.	
4. Note hemoglobin and hematocrit values.	4. Anemia due to blood loss may develop. Blood replacement therapy may be needed.	

Neurovascular Compromise

Nursing Interventions	Rationale	Expected Outcomes
1. Assess affected extremity for color and temperature.	1. The skin becomes pale and feels cool with decreased tissue perfusion. Venous congestion may produce cyanosis.	• Color normal • Extremity warm • Normal capillary refill
2. Assess toes for capillary refill response.	2. After compression of the nail, rapid return of pink color indicates good capillary perfusion.	• Moderate edema and swelling; tissue not palpably tense • Pain is controllable
3. Assess extremity for edema and swelling. Listen to patient complaints of leg tightness.	3. The trauma of surgery will cause edema. Excessive swelling and hematoma formation can compromise circulation and function.	• No pain with passive dorsiflexion • Normal sensations • No paresthesia
4. Elevate extremity (keep lower than hip when in chair).	4. Minimizes dependent edema.	• Normal motor abilities • No paresis or paralysis
5. Assess for deep, throbbing, unrelenting pain.	5. Surgical pain can be controlled; pain due to neurovascular compromise is refractory to treatment.	• Pulses strong and equal
6. Assess for pain on passive flexion of foot.	6. With nerve ischemia, there will be pain on passive stretch. Additionally, pain may indicate deep vein thrombosis—positive Homan's sign.	
7. Assess for sensations and numbness.	7. Diminished pain and paresthesia may indicate nerve damage. Sensation in web between great and second toe—peroneal nerve; sensation on sole of foot—tibial nerve	
8. Assess ability to move foot and toes.	8. Dorsiflexion of ankle and extension of toes indicate function of peroneal nerve. Plantar flexion of ankle and flexion of toes indicate function of tibial nerve.	
9. Assess pedal pulses in both feet. Notify surgeon if diminished neurovascular status is noted.	9. Indicator of extremity circulation. Function of extremity needs to be preserved.	

Dislocation of Prosthesis

Nursing Interventions	Rationale	Expected Outcomes
1. Position patient as prescribed.	1. Hip component positioning (femoral component in acetabular component) needs to be maintained.	• Prosthesis not dislocated
2. Use abductor splint or pillows to maintain position and to support extremity.	2. Keep hip in abduction and in a neutral rotation to prevent dislocation.	
3. Support leg and place pillows between legs when patient is turning and sidelying; turn to the unaffected side.		
4. Avoid acute flexion of hip (head of bed at 45°).		
5. Avoid crossing legs.		

(continued)

Nursing Care Plan 59–1 *(Continued)*

Care of the Patient With a Total Hip Replacement

Nursing Interventions	Rationale	Expected Outcomes
6. Assess for dislocation of prosthesis (extremity shortens, internally or externally rotated, severe hip pain, patient unable to move extremity)	6. Findings may indicate dislocation of prosthesis.	
7. Notify surgeon of possible dislocation.	7. Joint dislocations compromise neurovascular status and future function of extremity.	
Deep Vein Thrombosis		
1. Use antiembolic stocking or sequential compression device as prescribed.	1. Aid in venous blood return and prevent stasis.	• Wears antiembolism stockings/uses compression device
2. Remove stockings for 20 minutes twice a day and provide skin care.	2. Skin care is necessary to avoid breakdown. Extended removal of stockings defeats purpose of stockings.	• No skin breakdown • Pulses equal and strong • Skin temperature normal
3. Assess popliteal, dorsalis pedis, and posterior tibial pulses.	3. Pulses indicate arterial perfusion of extremity.	• Negative Homan's sign • Changes position with assistance and supervision.
4. Assess skin temperature of legs.	4. Local inflammation will increase local skin temperature.	• Participates in exercise regimen
5. Assess for Homan's sign every 8 hours.	5. Pain on dorsiflexion of ankle may indicate deep vein thrombosis.	• No chest pain; lungs clear to auscultation; no evidence of pulmonary emboli
6. Avoid pressure on popliteal blood vessels from appliances or pillows.	6. Compression of blood vessels diminishes blood flow.	
7. Change position and increase activity as prescribed.	7. Activity promotes circulation and diminishes venous stasis.	
8. Supervise ankle exercises hourly.	8. Muscle exercise promotes circulation.	
9. Monitor body temperature.	9. Body temperature elevates with inflammation.	
10. Assess lung status; encourage coughing, deep breathing, and use of incentive spirometer.	10. Provides for optimal ventilation	
Wound Infection		
1. Monitor vital signs.	1. Temperature, pulse, and respirations elevate in response to infection. (Magnitude of response may be minimal in an elderly patient.)	• Vital signs normal • Well-approximated incision without drainage or excessive inflammatory response • Minimal discomfort; no hematoma • Patient tolerates antibiotics.
2. Use aseptic technique for dressing changes and emptying of portable drainage.	2. Avoid introducing organisms.	
3. Assess wound appearance and character of drainage.	3. Red, swollen, draining incision is indicative of infection.	
4. Assess complaints of pain.	4. Pain may be due to wound hematoma—a possible locus of infection—that needs to be surgically evacuated.	
5. Administer prophylactic antibiotics if prescribed, and observe for side effects.	5. Infected prosthesis is to be avoided.	

Nursing Diagnosis: Impaired physical mobility related to enforced bed rest after hip replacement

Goal: Achieves pain-free, functional, stable hip joint.

1. Maintain proper positioning of hip joint (abduction, neutral rotation, limited flexion).	1. Prevents dislocation of hip prosthesis.	• Prescribed position maintained • Patient assists in position changes.

(continued)

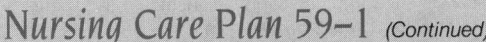

Nursing Care Plan 59-1 *(Continued)*

Care of the Patient With a Total Hip Replacement

Nursing Interventions	Rationale	Expected Outcomes
2. Instruct and assist in position changes and transfers.	2. Encourage patient's active participation while preventing dislocation.	• Shows increased independence in transfers
3. Instruct and supervise isometric quadriceps and gluteal setting exercises.	3. Strengthens muscles needed for walking	• Exercises hourly
4. In consultation with physical therapist, instruct and supervise progressive safe ambulation within limitations of weight-bearing prescription.	4. Amount of weight-bearing depends on patient's condition and prosthesis; ambulatory aids are used to assist the patient with nonweight-bearing and partial weight-bearing ambulation.	• Participates in progressive ambulation program • Actively participates in exercise regimen • Uses ambulatory aids correctly and safely
5. Offer encouragement and support exercise regimen.	5. Reconditioning exercises can be uncomfortable and fatiguing; encouragement helps patient comply with exercise program.	
6. Instruct and supervise safe use of ambulatory aids.	6. Prevents injury from unsafe use.	

Nursing Diagnosis: Potential impaired home maintenance management related to total hip replacement

Goal: Cares for self at home.

1. Assess home environment for discharge planning.	1. Physical barriers (especially stairs, bathrooms) may limit patient's ability to ambulate and care for self at home.	• Home is accessible for patient at time of discharge.
2. Encourage patient to express concerns about care at home; explore together possible solutions to the problem.	2. Patient may have special problems that need to be identified and resolved.	• Patient appears relaxed and develops strategies to deal with identified problems. • Personal assistance is available.
3. Assess availability of physical assistance for health care activities.	3. Because of limitation of mobility and limited hip range of motion, patient may require some assistance in routine health care.	• Patient demonstrates ability to provide necessary assistance within therapeutic prescription.
4. Teach caregiver home health care regimen.	4. Understanding of rehabilitative regimen is necessary for compliance.	• Complies with home care program • Keeps follow-up health care appointments

5. Instruct patient on posthospital care:
  a. Activity limitations (avoid stressing prosthesis)
  b. Reinforce exercise instructions.
  c. Safe use of ambulatory aids
  d. Wound care
  e. Measures to promote healing
  f. Medications, if any
  g. Potential problems
  h. Continuing health care supervision and management
	5. Lack of knowledge and poor preparation for care at home contribute to patient anxiety, insecurity, and nonadherence to therapeutic regimen.	

prostheses are available and may be surgically implanted using cement or cementless approaches.

A comprehensive health assessment of the individual undergoing joint replacement is performed to identify potential risk factors for postoperative complications. Age, obesity, preoperative leg edema, history of deep vein thrombosis, and varicose veins increase the risk of thrombosis and pulmonary emboli.

The orthopedic surgeon prescribes weight-bearing and motion limits to prevent prosthesis dislocation. Indicators of hip prosthesis dislocation include shortening of the leg, inability to move it, malalignment, abnormal rotation, and increased discomfort.

Other major postoperative problems include infection and excessive wound drainage, as well as problems related to major surgery (*e.g.*, pain, pulmonary problems, urinary retention). In the plan of care the nurse includes measures to reduce the incidence of postoperative complications and monitors the patient for indicators of these complications.

Patient education is important for continuing care. The patient is encouraged to participate actively in the progressive rehabilitation program.

Bibliography

Books

American Nurses Association and National Association of Orthopaedic Nurses. Orthopaedic Nursing Practice. Kansas City, MO, American Nurses Association, 1986.

Booth RE et al. Total Hip Arthroplasty. Philadelphia, WB Saunders, 1988.

Brashear HR Jr and Raney RB Sr. Handbook of Orthopaedic Surgery, 10th ed. St Louis, CV Mosby, 1986.

Chapman MW (ed). Operative Orthopaedics. Philadelphia, JB Lippincott, 1988.

Crenshaw AH (ed). Campbell's Operative Orthopaedics, 7th ed. St Louis, CV Mosby, 1987.

Epps CH Jr. Complications in Orthopaedic Surgery, 2nd ed. Philadelphia, JB Lippincott, 1986.

Farrell J. Illustrated Guide to Orthopedic Nursing, 3rd ed. Philadelphia, JB Lippincott, 1986.

Footner A. Orthopaedic nursing. London, Bailliere Tindall, 1987.

Gerhardt JJ et al (ed). Interdisciplinary Rehabilitation in Orthopedic Medicine. Toronto, Han Huber, 1987.

Hughes SPF et al (eds). Orthopaedics: The Principles and Practice of Musculoskeletal Surgery and Fractures. Edinburgh, Churchill Livingstone, 1987.

Laurin CA et al (eds). Atlas of Orthopaedic Surgery. Chicago, Year Book Medical Publishers, 1989.

Mourad LA and Droste MM. The Nursing Process in the Care of Adults with Orthopaedic Conditions, 2nd ed. New York, John Wiley & Sons, 1988.

Powell M (ed). Orthopaedic Nursing and Rehabilitation, 9th ed. Edinburgh, Churchill Livingstone, 1986.

Reynolds D and Freeman M (eds). Osteoarthritis in the Young Adult Hip: Options for Surgical Management. Edinburgh, Churchill Livingstone, 1989.

Rodrigo J. Orthopaedic Surgery: Basic Science and Clinical Science. Boston; Little, Brown, 1986.

Salmond S et al (eds). Core Curriculum for Orthopaedic Nurses, 2nd ed. Pitman, NJ, National Association of Orthopaedic Nurses, 1991.

Schlossberg D. Orthopedic Infection. New York, Springer-Verlag, 1988.

Scott WN. Total Knee Revision Arthroplasty. Orlando, Grune & Stratton, 1987.

Smith C. Orthopaedic Nursing. London, Heinemann Nursing, 1987.

Stearns CM and Brunner NA. Opcare: Orthopaedic Patient Care. A Nursing Guide, Vols 1-3. Rutherford, NJ, Howmedica, 1987.

Yaremchuck MJ et al. Lower Extremity Salvage and Reconstruction. New York, Elsevier, 1989.

The Zimmer Traction Handbook, Warsaw, IN, Zimmer, 1989.

Journals
Asterisks indicate nursing research articles.

Treatment Modalities

Bach BR et al. Surgical arthroscopy for anterior cruciate ligament reconstruction. Todays OR Nurs 1990 Feb; 12(2): 4-9, 28-30.

Berg EE. Progress in orthopaedic surgery: The 1980's in review. Orthop Nurs 1990 May/Jun; 9(3): 29-31.

Calhoun JH and Burke EE. Orthopaedic rehabilitation at home. Phys Med Rehabil 1988 Aug; 2(3): 415-459.

Christie J et al. Intramedullary locking nails in the management of femoral shaft fractures, J Bone Joint Surg [Br] 1988 Mar; 70(2): 206-210.

Collins R et al. Reduction in fatal pulmonary embolism and venous thrombosis by perioperative administration of subcutaneous heparin. N Engl J Med 1988 May 5; 318(18): 1162-1170.

Dobberstein K. Orthopaedic surgery: What patients need to know. Am J Nurs 1987 Jul; 87(7): 961.

Friedlaender GE. Bone Grafts. J Bone Joint Surg [Am] 1987 Jun; 69(5): 786-790.

Friedlaeder GE (ed). Bone grafting. Orthop Clin North Am 1987 Apr; 18(2).

Funk JR et al. Tibial osteotomy. Orthop Nurs 1990 Mar/Apr; 9(2): 29-34.

Gamron RB. Taking the pressure out of compartment syndrome. Am J Nurs 1988 Aug; 88(8): 1076-1080.

Genge ML. Epidural analgesia in the orthopaedic patient. Orthop Nurs 1988 Jul/Aug; 7(4): 11-19.

Goldhaber BZ. Venous thromboembolism: How to prevent a tragedy. Hosp Pract 1988 Oct 15; 23(10): 164-174.

Griffin PP. Orthopedic surgery 1947-1987. Postgrad Med 1987 Jul; 82(1): 147-152.

* Groth F. Effects of wheat bran in the diet of post surgical orthopaedic patients to prevent constipation. Orthop Nurs 1988 Jul/Aug; 7(4): 41-46.

Hampel G. Closed interlocking nailing in the lower extremity: Indications and positioning. AORN J 1988 May; 47(5): 1203-1209.

Hines NA and Bates MS. Discharging the patient in skeletal traction. Orthop Nurs 1987 Jul/Aug; 6(4): 21-24.

* Hoshiko B. Valsalva maneuver as a possible risk factor for pulmonary embolism. Orthop Nurs 1990 Jan/Feb; 9(1): 56-62.

Jackson MF. High risk surgical patients. J Gerontol Nurs 1988 Jan; 14(1): 8-15, 36-37.

* Jones-Walton P. Clinical standards in skeletal traction pin site care. Orthop Nurs 1991 Mar/Apr; 10(2): 12-16.

Lavine LS and Grodzinsky AJ. Electrical stimulation in repair of bone. J Bone Joint Surg [Am] 1987 Apr; 69(4): 626-630.

Lhowe DW and Hansen ST. Immediate nailing of open fractures of the femoral shaft. J Bone Joint Surg [Am] 1988 Jul; 70(6): 812-820.

Mather MLS. The secret to life in a spica cast. Am J Nurs 1987 Jan; 87(1): 56-58.

Miller B and Eden-Kilgour S. Preventing peroneal nerve damage. Orthop Nurs 1987 Jul/Aug; 6(4): 41-46.

Moore TJ et al. Complications of surgically treated supracondylar fractures of the femur. J Trauma 1987 Apr; 27(4): 402-406.

Morris L et al. Special care for skeletal traction. RN 1988 Feb; 51(2): 24-29.

Morris L et al. Nursing the patient in traction. RN 1988 Jan; 51(1): 26-31.

Newschwander GE and Dunst RM. Limb lengthening with Ilizarov internal fixator. Orthop Nurs 1989 May/Jun; 8(3): 15-21.

Osborne LJ and DiGiacomo I. Traction: A review with nursing diagnoses and interventions. Orthop Nurs 1987 Jul/Aug; 6(4): 13-19.

Paley D et al. Ilizarov treatment of tibial nonunions with bone loss. Clin Orthop 1989 Apr; (241): 146-165.

Peimer C. Compression neuropathies of the upper extremity. Orthop Rev 1987 Jun; 16(6): 379-385.

Ritter MA et al. The exogenous sources and controls of microorganisms in the operating room. Orthop Nurs 1988 Jul/Aug; 7(4): 23-28.

Roberts SL. Pulmonary tissue perfusion altered: Emboli. Heart Lung 1987 Mar; 16(2): 128-138.

Ross D. Acute compartment syndrome. Orthop Nurs 1991 Mar/Apr; 10(2): 33-38.

Rubin M. The physiology of bedrest. Am J Nurs 1988 Jan; 88(1): 50-56.

* Schmeltzer M. Effectiveness of wheat bran in preventing constipation of hospitalized orthopaedic surgery patients. Orthop Nurs 1990 Nov/Dec; 9(6): 55-59.

Schonholtz GJ. Arthroscopic debridement of the knee joint. Orthop Clin North Am 1989 Apr; 20(2): 257-263.

* Teter K et al. Patient controlled analgesia and GI dysfunction. Orthop Nurs 1990 Jul/Aug; 9(4): 51-56.

Thal ER. Embolism—Clot, fat, or air. Emerg Med 1987 Oct 15; 19(17): 31-32, 35.

Wienki VK. Pressure sores: Prevention is the challenge. Orthop Nurs 1987 Jul/Aug; 6(4): 26-30.

Zagorski JB et al. Diaphyseal fractures of the humerus. Treatment with prefabricated braces. J Bone Joint Surg [Am] 1988 Apr; 70(4): 607–610.

Joint Replacement

Ajemian E et al. Hospital acquired infections after arthroscopic knee surgery: A probable environmental source. Am J Infect Control 1987 Aug; 15(4): 159–162.

Apley AG. The prevention of deep sepsis in joint replacement. J Bone Joint Surg [Br] 1987 Aug; 69(4): 517–518.

Basso MD et al. Comparison of two continuous passive motion protocols for patients with TM implants. Phys Ther 1987 Mar; 67(3): 360–363.

Beisaw NE et al. Dihydroergotamine/heparin in the prevention of deep-vein thromposis after total hip replacement. J Bone Joint Surg [Am] 1988 Jan; 70(1): 2–10.

Bray TJ et al. The displaced femoral neck fracture. Internal fixation versus bipolar endoprosthesis. Clin Orthop 1988 May; (230): 127–140.

A conversation with William L Bargar, MD. Custon cementless total hip replacement. Orthop Rev 1987 Jan; 16(1): 27–35.

Cooke PH and Newman JH. Fractures of the femur in relation to cemented hip prothesis. J Bone Joint Surg [Br] 1988 May; 70(3): 386–389.

Cushner FD and Friedman PJ. Osteonecrosis of the femoral head. Orthop Rev 1988 Jan; 17(1): 29–32.

Doheny M and Ceccio CM. Total shoulder replacement: Preparing patients for discharge. Orthop Nurs 1988 May/Jun; 7(3): 13–21.

Dunajcik LM. The hip: When the joint must be replaced. RN 1989 Apr; 52(4): 62–71.

Ecker ML and Lotke PA. Postoperative care of the total knee patient. Orthop Clin North Am 1989 Jan; 20(1): 55–62.

Enis JE. Total hip arthroplasty in the geriatric patient. Hosp Med (Suppl) 1987 Apr; 23(4): 41.

Figgie HE and Goldberg VM. Some success rates of revision total knee arthroplasty. Orthop Rev 1988 May; 17(5): 464–466.

Finlay J. Uncemented total hip arthroplasty. Can Oper Room Nurs J 1987 Dec; 5(6): 22–24, 26.

Follman D. Nursing care concerns in total shoulder replacement. Orthop Nurs 1988 May/Jun; 7(3): 29–31.

Gill KP. Cementless total hip arthroplasty. Can Nurse 1987 Nov; 83(10): 18–20.

Goldberg VM et al. Total elbow arthroplasty. J Bone Joint Surg [Am] 1988 Jun; 70(5): 778–783.

Green A. Hip replacement: What's happening to hips. Nurs Times 1989 Nov 15–21; 85(46): 32–33.

Haddad RJ et al. Biological fixation of porous-coated implants. J Bone Joint Surg [Am] 1987 Dec; 69(9): 1459–1466.

Haug J et al. Efficacy of neuromuscular stimulation of the quadriceps femoris during continuous passive motion following total knee arthroplasty. Arch Phys Med Rehabil 1988 Jan; 69(6): 423–424.

Hughes SPF. The use of antibiotics in orthopaedic surgery: Total joint single vs multiple dose prophylaxis. Orthop Rev 1987 Apr; 16(4): 209–214.

Kozinn SC et al. Adult hip disease and total hip replacement. Clin Symp 1987; 39(5): 2–32.

Lotkr PA (ed). Reconstructive knee surgery. Orthop Clin North Am 1989 Jan; 20(1).

Lynch AF et al. Deep-vein thrombosis and continuous passive motion after total knee arthroplasty. J Bone Joint Surg [Am] 1988 Jan; 70(1): 11–14.

Nelson CL. Infected joint implants: Principles of treatment. Orthop Rev 1987 Apr; 16(4): 215–223.

Orthopaedic nursing surgical guide: Total hip replacement. Orthop Nurs 1987 Jul/Aug; 6(4): 57–59.

Podesta L et al. Knee bracing. Orthop Clin North Am 1988 Oct; 19(4): 737–745.

Radin EL. Loosening of total hip replacement prosthesis. Orthop Rev 1989 Mar; 16(3): 134–136.

* Selman S. Impact of total hip replacement on quality of life. Orthop Nurs 1989 Sep/Oct; 8(5): 43–49.

Salvati EA (ed). Long term results of cemented joint replacement: Is cement obsolete? Orthop Clin North Am 1988 Jul; 19(3).

Smith C. Total hip replacement. Nurs Times 1989 Nov 15–21; 85(46): 28–31.

Smith JE. Applying the continuous passive motion device. Orthop Nurs 1990 May/Jun; 9(3): 54–56.

Spaulding JM et al. Total ankle arthroplasty: A procedural review. AORN J 1988 Aug; 48(2): 201–203; 206–207.

Total knee replacement. Orthop Nurs 1987 May/Jun; 6(3): 37–39.

Viadero A et al. Post operative care of the TSR patient . . . Total shoulder replacement. Clin Manage Phys Ther 1987 Jul/Aug; 7(4): 14–15.

External Fixation

Alanso J et al. External fixation of femoral fractures: Indications and limitations. Clin Orthop 1989 Apr; 241: 83–88.

Browner CM et al. Halo immobilization brace care: An innovative approach. J Neurosci Nurs 1987 Feb; 19(10): 24–29.

Edwards CC et al. Severe open tibial fractures. Results treating 202 injuries with external fixation. Clin Orthop 1988 May; 230: 98–115.

Garfin SR et al. Subdural abscess associated with halo-pin traction. J Bone Joint Surg [Am] 1988 Oct; 70(9): 1338–1340.

Goldberger DK et al. A survey of external fixator pin care techniques. Clin Nurse Spec 1987 Winter; 1(4): 166–169.

Javernig Sr P. Organizing and implementing an Ilizarov program. Orthop Nurs 1990 Sep/Oct; 9(5): 47–55.

* Jones–Walton P. Effects of pin care on pin reactions in adults with extemity fracture treated with skeletal traction and external fixation. Orthop Nurs 1988 Jul/Aug; 7(4): 29–33.

Liang GY and Wu JW. Fracture of the patella treated by open reduction and external compression skeletal fixation. J Bone Joint Surg [Am] 1987 Jan; 69(1): 83–89.

Paley D et al. Ilizarov treatment of tibial nonunions with bone loss. Clin Orthop 1989 Apr; 241: 146–165.

Schuind F et al. External fixation of clavicle fracture for non-union in adults. J Bone Joint Surg [Am] 1988 Jun; 70(5): 692–695.

Agencies

Arthritis Foundation
    1314 Spring Street NW, Atlanta, GA 30309
National Institute of Arthritis and Musculoskeletal and Skin Diseases
    National Institutes of Health, Bethesda, MD 20892

60

Management of the Patient With Musculoskeletal Trauma

Learning Objective

On completion of this chapter, the learner will be able to:

1. Differentiate between contusions, strains, sprains, and dislocations
2. Specify the clinical manifestations of a fracture and the emergency management of the patient with a fracture
3. Describe the principles and methods of fracture reduction, fracture immobilization, and management of open fractures
4. Use the nursing process as a framework for care of the patient with a simple fracture
5. Describe the prevention and management of immediate and delayed complications of fractures
6. Describe the rehabilitative needs of patients with fractures of the clavicle, upper and lower extremities, pelvis, hips, ribs, and thoracolumbar spine
7. Use the nursing process as a framework for care of the elderly patient with fracture of the hip
8. Describe the rehabilitative and health education needs of the patient who has had an amputation
9. Use the nursing process as a framework for care of the patient with an amputation

Injury to one part of the musculoskeletal system usually produces injury or dysfunction of adjacent structures and of structures enclosed or supported by them. If the bones are broken, the muscles cannot function; if the nerves do not send impulses to the muscles, as in paralysis, the bones cannot move; if the joint surfaces do not articulate normally, neither the bones nor the muscles can function properly. Thus, although a fracture primarily affects the bone, it may also produce injury to the muscles, the blood vessels, and the nerves in the vicinity of the fracture.

In the treatment of injury of the musculoskeletal system, support is provided for the injured part until healing is complete. Support may be accomplished by bandages, adhesive strapping, splints, or casts, applied externally. Support may be applied directly to the bone in the form of pins or plates. At times, traction must be applied to correct deformity or shortening.

After the immediate and the painful effects of the injury have passed, consideration must be given to the prevention of fibrosis and the resulting stiffness in the injured muscles and the joint structures. *Activity by the patient is the best form of treatment to guard against this disability.* In some cases, the support applied may permit activity almost from the start. The healing process and recovery of function may be hastened by various forms of physical therapy.

Contusions, Strains, and Sprains

A *contusion* is an injury of the soft tissues, produced by blunt force (*e.g.,* a blow, kick, fall). There is always some bleeding into the injured part *(ecchymosis)*, due to the rupture of many small vessels. This produces the well-known discoloration of the skin (bruising), which gradually turns to brown and then to yellow, and finally disappears as absorption becomes complete. When the bleeding is sufficient to cause an appreciable collection of blood, it is called *hematoma.* The local symptoms (pain, swelling, and discoloration) are easily explained.

A *strain* is a "muscle pull" due to overuse, overstretching, or excessive stress. Strains are microscopic, incomplete muscle tears with some bleeding into the tissue. The patient experiences gradual soreness or sudden pain and then local tenderness. Pain is experienced with muscle use and isometric contraction.

A *sprain* is an injury to the ligamentous structures surrounding a joint, caused by a wrench or a twist. The function of a ligament is to maintain stability while permitting mobility. A torn ligament loses its stabilizing ability. As is the case with contusions, blood vessels are ruptured, and ecchymosis and edema occur. The joint is tender and movement of the joint becomes painful. The degree of disability and pain increases during the first 2 to 3 hours after the injury because of the associated swelling and bleeding. To be certain that there is no bone injury, the patient should have an x-ray examination. *Avulsion fracture* (a bone fragment is pulled away by a ligament or tendon) may be associated with sprains.

Management.   Treatment of contusions, strains, and sprains consists of elevating the affected part, application of cold, and use of an elastic compression bandage. Elevation controls the swelling. Moist or dry cold applied intermittently for 20 to 30 minutes during the first 24 hours after injury produces vasoconstriction, which decreases bleeding, edema, and discomfort. An elastic compression bandage also controls bleeding, reduces edema, and provides support for the injured tissues. The neurovascular status of the injured extremity is monitored frequently. If the sprain is severe (torn muscle fibers and disrupted ligaments), surgical repair or cast immobilization is necessary so that the joint will not lose its stability.

During the recovery phase, the injured muscles, ligaments, or tendons must be allowed to rest and repair themselves. Moist heat applied intermittently (15 to 30 minutes, 4 times a day) promotes vasodilation, absorption, and repair. Patient education must emphasize minimal exercise until healing has taken place, and then gradual progression of activity. Excessive exercise early in the course of treatment will delay recovery. Severe strains and sprains take about a month to heal, at which time active exercise can be gradually resumed.

Joint Dislocations

A dislocation of a joint is a condition in which the articular surfaces of the bones forming the joint are no longer in ana-tomic contact. The bones are literally "out of joint." A *sub-luxation* is a partial dislocation of the articulating surfaces. Traumatic dislocations are orthopedic emergencies, because the associated joint structures, blood supply, and nerves are distorted and severely stressed. *Avascular necrosis* (tissue death due to anoxia and diminished blood supply) and nerve palsy may occur.

Dislocations may be (1) *congenital* (present at birth, due to some maldevelopment, most often noted at the hip); (2) spontaneous or *pathologic,* due to disease of the articular or the periarticular structures; and (3) *traumatic* due to injury, such as the application of force in such a manner as to produce disruption of the joint.

The signs and symptoms of a traumatic dislocation are (1) pain, (2) change in contour of the joint, (3) change in the length of the extremity, (4) loss of normal mobility, and (5) change in the axis of the dislocated bones.

X-ray films confirm the diagnosis and should be made in every case, because frequently there is an associated fracture.

Management.   The affected part needs to be immobilized while the patient is transported. The dislocation is reduced (*i.e.,* displaced parts brought into normal position), usually under anesthesia. The head of the dislocated bone is manipulated back into the joint cavity. The joint is immobilized by bandages, splints, casts, or traction and is maintained in a stable position. With a stable reduced dislocation, gentle active motion three or four times a day is begun several days to weeks after reduction. This is to preserve range of motion. The joint is supported between exercise sessions.

Nursing concerns are directed at providing comfort, evaluating the neurovascular status, and protecting the joint during healing. The patient needs to learn how to manage the immobilizing devices and how to protect the joint from reinjury.

Sports Injuries

More and more people are participating in recreational sports. These recreational athletes may push themselves beyond the level of their physical conditioning and incur sports injuries. Injuries to the musculoskeletal system may be of an acute nature (sprains, strains, dislocations, fractures) or may result from gradual overuse (chondromalacia patella, tendinitis, stress fractures). Professional athletes are also susceptible to injury, even though their training is supervised closely to minimize the occurrence of injury and to enhance the development of athletic performance.

Musculoskeletal contusions result from direct falls or blows from sporting equipment. The initial dull pain becomes greater, with edema and stiffness occurring by the next day. Sprains commonly occur in fingers, ankles, and knees. If the ligamentous damage is major, the joint becomes unstable and surgical repair may be required. An avulsion fracture may exist. Strains present with a sharp, stabbing pain from bleeding and immediate protective muscle contraction. Tennis players often suffer calf muscle strains; soccer players often experience quadriceps strains; and swimmers, weight lifters, and tennis players often suffer shoulder strains. *Tendinitis* (inflammation of a tendon) is due to overuse and is seen in tennis players (epicondylar tendinitis), runners and gymnasts (Achilles tendinitis), and runners and basketball players (infrapatellar tendinitis). Meniscal injuries of the knee occur with excessive rotational stress.

Dislocations are seen with throwing and lifting sports. Fractures occur with falls. Skaters and bikers frequently suffer Colles's fractures of the wrist when they fall on outstretched arms; ballet dancers and field and track athletes may experience metatarsal fractures. Stress fractures occur with repeated bone trauma from activities such as jogging, gymnastics, basketball, and aerobics. The tibias, fibulas, and metatarsals are most vulnerable.

Management.   Generally, musculoskeletal injuries need to be recognized and managed early to facilitate healing and to minimize residual disabilities. Basic to the management of most soft-tissue injuries is ICE (*ice*, *compression*, *elevation*). The ice is applied for 20 to 30 minutes intermittently during the first 24 hours to control swelling and relieve pain. The area is wrapped with an elastic compression bandage to minimize effusion, support the area, and provide comfort. The wrap must not be constricting. Monitoring the neurovascular status of the extremity becomes an important nursing function. The injured extremity is elevated to the heart to control swelling and to promote rest. Depending on the site and the severity of the injury, the extremity may be immobilized or surgical intervention may be required. Arthroscopic surgery may be required for meniscus tears and other joint injuries that limit joint function and contribute to articular cartilage wear.

Patients who have experienced a sports-related injury are highly motivated to return to their previous level of activity. Compliance with restriction of activities and resumption of them on a *gradual, progressive* timetable may be a real problem for these patients. They need to be taught how to avoid further injury or new injury. With recurrence of symptoms, they need to learn to diminish the level and intensity of activity to a comfort level and to treat (ICE) the symptoms. Recovery from sports-related injury can take a few days to 6 or more weeks.

Prevention of sports-related injuries can be achieved by use of appropriate equipment (*e.g.*, running shoes) and by training and conditioning the body. Changes in activities and stresses should occur gradually. The athlete needs to be taught to "tune in" to body symptoms indicating stress and to modify activities to minimize injury and to promote healing.

Internal Derangement of the Knee

Injury to most joints consists of a tear of the supporting ligaments. In the knee joint, however, there may also be a displacement or tear of the *semilunar cartilages*, which are two crescent-shaped cartilages attached to the edge of the shallow articulating surface of the head of the tibia. They normally move slightly backward and forward to accommodate the condyles of the femur when the leg is flexed or extended.

Normally, little torsion movement is permitted in the knee joint. In sports or accidents, twisting of the knee with the foot fixed may result in either tearing the cartilage or tearing the cartilage from its attachment to the head of the tibia.

These injuries leave loose cartilage in the knee joint that may slip between the femur and the tibia, preventing full extension of the leg. If this happens during walking or running, patients often describe the disability as their "leg giving way" under them. Patients may hear or feel a click in the knee when they walk, especially when they extend the leg that is bearing weight, as in going upstairs. When the cartilage is attached front and back, but torn loose laterally (bucket-handle tear), it may slide between the bones to lie between the condyles

and prevent full flexion or extension. As a result, the knee "locks."

These injuries, *internal derangements* of the knee joint, produce disturbing disabilities because the patients never know when their knee will malfunction. The treatment usually consists of surgical removal of the damaged cartilage through an incision into the knee joint or through an arthroscope.

After surgery, a pressure dressing is applied; a knee-immobilizing splint may be required. The leg is elevated on pillows to minimize edema. The most common complication is an effusion into the knee joint, which produces marked pain. If this occurs, the physician should be notified. Relief can be obtained by loosening the pressure dressing. The physician may need to aspirate the joint to remove fluid and relieve the pressure.

To prevent atrophy of the thigh muscles, these patients are taught quadriceps setting exercises. Additional exercises help to restore full function, stability, and strength.

Arthroscopic surgery is frequently an outpatient procedure. The patient resumes activities in 1 to 2 days and sports can be resumed in several weeks, as prescribed by the physician.

Rupture of the Achilles Tendon

Traumatic rupture of the Achilles tendon, generally within the tendon sheath, occurs during activities when there is a sudden contraction of the calf muscle with the foot fixed firmly to the floor. The patient experiences pain and is unable to plantar flex the foot. Immediate surgical repair usually obtains satisfactory results. In some situations, conservative management with a plantar-flexed cast for 6 to 8 weeks may be used instead of surgery.

In summary, injury to the musculoskeletal system includes not only trauma to the bones and muscles, but also to associated soft tissues (*i.e.*, cartilage, tendons, ligaments, blood vessels, nerves). Treatment includes immobilization of the injured part and measures to control edema.

Contusions from blunt blows result in bleeding into the soft tissues. Strains are "muscle pulls." Sprains are injuries to the ligament structures surrounding a joint. All of these soft tissue injuries require immobilization and elevation to control edema. Gradual resumption of activities is essential for rehabilitation.

Joint dislocations are medical emergencies because of possible injury to associated blood vessels and nerves. Prompt reduction and gradual resumption of activities are necessary for restoration of joint function.

Sports injuries are most common in individuals participating in recreational sports without adequate training. Proper equipment (*e.g.*, running shoes) and conditioning can help prevent sports injuries. Patients who experience sports-related injuries are highly motivated to return to preinjury level of activity. Compliance with gradual resumption of prescribed activities is essential for healing.

Fractures

A fracture is a break in the continuity of bone and is defined according to type and extent (Fig. 60–1). Fractures occur when the bone is subjected to stress greater than it can absorb. Frac-

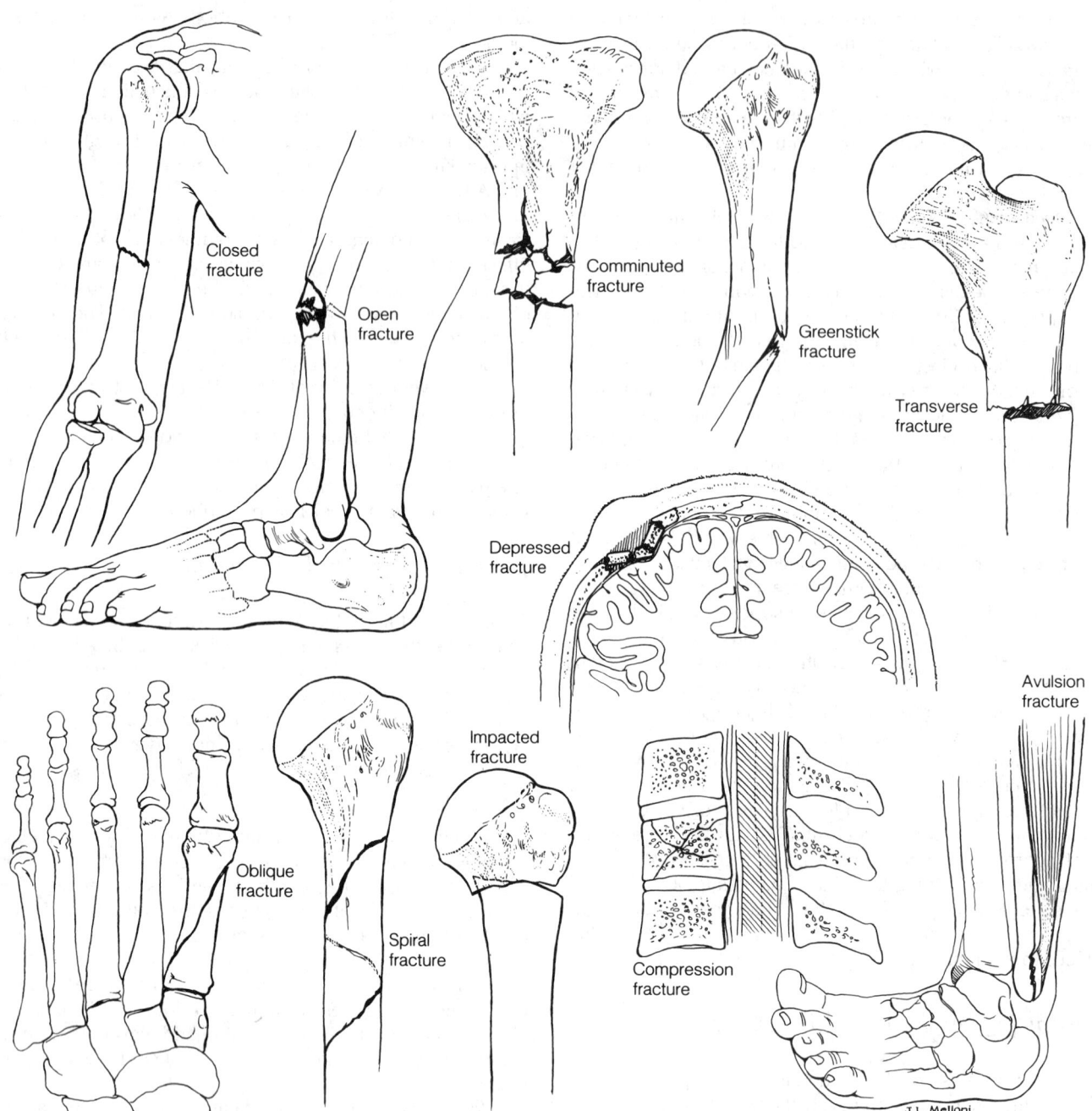

Figure 60-1. Types of fractures. (Suddarth DS. The Lippincott Manual of Nursing Practice, 4th ed. Philadelphia, JB Lippincott, 1991.)

tures can be caused by direct blow, crushing force, sudden twisting motion, and even extreme muscle contraction.

Although the bone is the part most directly affected, other structures also may be involved, resulting in soft-tissue edema, hemorrhage into the muscles and joints, joint dislocations, ruptured tendons, severed nerves, and damaged blood vessels. Body organs may be injured by the force that caused the fracture or by the fracture fragments.

Types of Fractures

A *complete fracture* involves a break across the entire cross section of the bone and is frequently displaced (removed from normal position). In an *incomplete fracture*, the break occurs through only part of the cross section of the bone.

A *closed fracture* (simple fracture) does not produce a break in the skin. An *open fracture* is one in which the skin or mucous membrane wound extends to the fractured bone. Open fractures are graded: Grade I is a clean wound less than 1 cm long; grade II is a larger wound without extensive soft-tissue damage; and grade III is the most severe, with extensive soft-tissue damage.

Fractures may also be described according to anatomic placement of fragments — *displaced/nondisplaced fracture*.

The following are specific types of fractures (see Fig. 60-1):

Greenstick—a fracture in which one side of a bone is broken and the other side is bent

Transverse—a fracture that is straight across the bone

Oblique—a fracture occurring at an angle across the bone (less stable than transverse)

Spiral—a fracture twisting around the shaft of the bone

Comminuted—a fracture in which bone has splintered into several fragments

Depressed—a fracture in which fragments are driven inward (seen frequently in fractures of skull and facial bones)

Compression—a fracture in which bone has been compressed (seen in vertebral fractures)

Pathologic—a fracture that occurs through an area of diseased bone (bone cyst, Paget's disease, bony metastasis, tumor)

Avulsion—a pulling away of a fragment of bone by a ligament or tendon and its attachment

Epiphyseal—a fracture through the epiphysis

Clinical Manifestations

The clinical manifestations of a fracture are pain, loss of function, false motion, deformity, shortening, crepitation, local swelling, and discoloration.

1. The *pain* is of a continuous type and increases in severity until the bone fragments are immobilized. The muscle spasm that accompanies fracture is natural splinting to minimize further movement of the fracture fragments

2. After the break, the part cannot be used and tends to move unnaturally (false motion) instead of remaining rigid as it normally would. The displacement of the fragments in a fracture of the arm or leg causes a deformity (either visible or palpable) of the extremity, detectable when it is compared with the normal extremity. The extremity cannot function properly because normal function of the muscles depends on the integrity of the bones to which they are attached.

3. In fractures of long bones, there is actually shortening of the extremity because of the contraction of the muscles that are attached above and below the site of the fracture. The fragments may often overlap as much as 2.5 to 5 cm (1 to 2 in).

4. When the extremity is examined with the hands, a grating sensation, called *crepitus*, can be felt because of the rubbing of the fragments one on the other. (Testing for crepitation can produce further tissue damage.)

5. Localized swelling and discoloration of the skin occur as a result of trauma and hemorrhage that follow a fracture. These signs may not develop for several hours or days after the injury.

All of these signs and symptoms are not necessarily present in every fracture. Many are not present with *linear* or *fissure fractures* and with *impacted fractures* (fractured surfaces are driven together).

The diagnosis of a fracture depends on the symptoms of the patient, the physical signs, and x-ray examination. Usually, the patient reports that he sustained an injury to the area.

Emergency Management

Immediately after injury, a person may be in a state of confusion, be unaware of a fracture, and attempt to walk on a fractured leg. Therefore, when a fracture is suggested, it is important to immobilize that body part immediately before the patient is moved. If an injured patient must be removed from a vehicle before splints can be applied, the extremity is supported above and below the fracture site, and traction is applied in accordance with the line of the long axis of the bone to prevent rotation as well as angular motion. Movement of fracture fragments will cause additional pain, soft-tissue damage, and additional hemorrhage.

The pain associated with a fracture is severe and can be reduced by preventing movement of the bone fragments and joints adjacent to the fracture. Adequate splinting is essential to prevent damage to the soft tissue by the bony fragments.

Immobilization is established by applying temporary, well-padded splints, which are then firmly bandaged over the clothing. Immobilization of the long bones of the lower extremities also may be accomplished by bandaging the extremities together, with the unaffected extremity serving as a splint for the injured one. In an upper extremity injury, the arm may be bandaged to the chest, or an injured forearm may be placed in a sling.

The peripheral pulses distal to the injury should be palpated to ensure that circulation has not been compromised and that tissue perfusion is sufficient.

In an *open fracture*, the wound is covered with a clean (sterile) dressing to prevent contamination of deeper tissues. No attempt is made to reduce the fracture, even if one of the bone fragments is protruding through the wound. Splints should be applied as described above.

In the emergency department, the patient is evaluated completely. With care and gentleness the clothes are removed, first from the uninjured side of the body and then from the injured side. Sometimes the patient's clothing must be cut away on the injured side. The fractured extremity is moved as little as possible to avoid causing more damage.

Principles of Fracture Management

The principles of fracture treatment include reduction, immobilization, and regaining of normal function and strength through rehabilitation (Chart 60–1).

Fracture Reduction and Immobilization. Reduction of a fracture ("setting" the bone) refers to restoration of the fracture fragments into anatomic rotation and alignment.

Before fracture reduction and immobilization, the patient is prepared for the procedure; permission for the procedure is obtained, and an analgesic is administered as prescribed. At times the patient may need anesthesia when a fracture is reduced and immobilized. The extremity that is to be manipulated must be handled gently to avoid additional damage.

After the fracture has been reduced, bone fragments must be immobilized or held in correct position and alignment until union has had time to take place. Immobilization may be accomplished by external or internal fixation. Methods of *external fixation* include bandages, casts, splints, continuous traction, pin and plaster technique, or external fixators. *Internal fixation* devices (metal implants) include nails, plates, screws, wires, and rods. These serve as internal splints to hold the fractured bone in alignment while healing takes place.

Several methods are used to obtain reduction of a fracture; the method selected depends on the nature of the fracture. Variations of these methods are carried out, but the underlying principles are the same. Usually, fractures are reduced as soon

Chart 60-1
The Treatment of Fractures

Goals of Fracture Treatment

1. Restore fracture fragments to their normal anatomic position (reduction).
2. Maintain reduction in place until healing occurs (immobilization).
3. Promote regaining of normal function and strength of the affected part (rehabilitation).

Methods for Obtaining Fracture Reduction

1. Closed reduction
2. Traction
3. Open reduction

Methods for Maintaining Immobilization

1. External devices
   a. Splint
   b. Brace
   c. Cast
   d. Pins in plaster
   e. External fixator
   f. Traction
   g. Bandage
2. Internal devices
   a. Nails
   b. Plates
   c. Screws
   d. Wires
   e. Rods

Maintaining and Restoring Function

1. Maintain reduction and immobilization
2. Elevate to minimize swelling
3. Monitor neurovascular status
4. Control anxiety and pain
5. Isometric and muscle-setting exercises
6. Participation in activities of daily living
7. Gradual resumption of activities

---

fragments. As the fracture heals, evidence of callus formation is noted radiologically. When the callus is well established, a cast is frequently used for the immobilization technique. Traction therapy and the nursing management of a patient in traction are discussed more fully on pp. 1797–1803.

Open Reduction. Some fractures require open reduction. Through a surgical approach, the fracture fragments are reduced (put into alignment). Internal fixation devices in the form of metallic pins, wires, screws, plates, nails, or rods may be used to hold the bone fragments in position until solid bone healing occurs. Internal fixation devices may be attached to the sides of bone or inserted through the bony fragments or directly into the medullary cavity of the bone (Fig. 60–2). These devices assure firm approximation and fixation of the bony fragments.

Maintaining and Restoring Function. (See Chap. 59 for Nursing Process: The Patient in a Cast; The Patient in Traction; The Patient Undergoing Orthopedic Surgery)

Efforts are directed toward facilitating bone and soft tissue healing. Reduction and immobilization are maintained as prescribed. Swelling is controlled by elevating the injured extremity

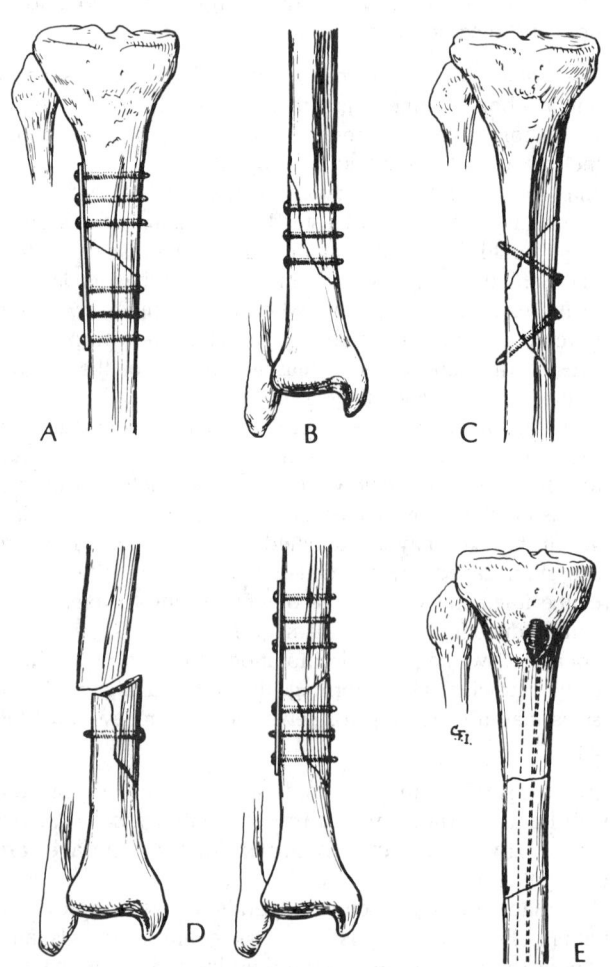

Figure 60–2. Techniques of internal fixation. (**A**) Plate and six screws for a transverse or short oblique fracture. (**B**) Screws for a long oblique or spiral fracture. (**C**) Screws for a long butterfly fragment. (**D**) Plate and six screws for a short butterfly fragment. (**E**) Medullary nail for a segmental fracture. (Smith H. Fractures. In Crenshaw AH [ed]. Campbell's Operative Orthopaedics, Vol 1. St Louis, CV Mosby.)

---

as possible because tissues may lose their elasticity if infiltrated by edema or hemorrhage. In most cases, fracture reduction becomes more difficult as the injury begins healing.

Closed Reduction. In most instances, closed reduction is accomplished by bringing the bone fragments into apposition (ends in contact) by *manipulation* and *manual traction*.

The extremity is held in the desired position while it is being immobilized by cast, splint, or other device by the physician. The immobilizing device maintains the reduction and stabilizes the extremity for bone healing. X-rays are obtained to determine that the bone fragments are in correct alignment.

Traction. Traction may be used to effect fracture reduction and immobilization. Adjustments of the magnitude of traction are made as muscle spasm is overcome. X-rays are used to monitor the fracture reduction and approximation of the bony and applying ice as prescribed. Frequent neurovascular monitoring (*i.e.*, assessment of circulation, pain, sensation, movement) is done, and the orthopedist is notified immediately if neurovascular compromise is identified. Restlessness, anxiety, and discomfort are controlled with a variety of approaches (*i.e.*, reassurance, position changes, pain-modifying techniques, including pain medications). Isometric and muscle setting exercises are encouraged to minimize disuse atrophy and to promote circulation. Patients are encouraged to participate in activities of daily living, which promote independent functioning and self-esteem. Gradual resumption of activities is promoted within the therapeutic prescription. Usually internal fixation allows for early mobilization. The surgeon estimates the stability of the fracture fixation, determines the amount of movement and stress the extremity can withstand, and prescribes the level of activity and weight-bearing.

Factors Affecting Healing of Fracture. Weeks to months are required for most fractures to heal. Many factors influence the speed with which fractures heal (Chart 60-2). The reduction of the displaced fracture fragments must be accurate and successfully maintained to ensure healing. The affected bone must have an adequate blood supply. The age of the patient and the type of fracture also affect healing time. In general, fractures of flat bones (pelvis, scapula) heal quite rapidly. Fractures at the ends of long bones where the bone is more vascular and cancellous heal more quickly than do fractures in areas where

the bone is dense and less vascular (midshaft). Weight-bearing will stimulate healing of stabilized fractures of the long bones in the lower extremities. In addition, activity minimizes the development of immobility-related *osteoporosis* (a reduction of total bone mass, producing porous and fragile bones because of imbalance in homeostatic bone turnover). Table 60-1 shows the approximate immobilization times necessary for union of the most common types of fractures.

If fracture healing is disrupted, the bone union time may be delayed or stopped completely. Factors that may interrupt fracture healing include loss of fracture hematoma by debridement, devitalization of adjacent tissue by inadequate blood supply, extensive space between bone fragments, interposition of soft tissue between bone ends, inadequate fracture immobilization, infection, complications from the treatment, and metabolic problems.

Care of the Patient With a Simple Fracture

Patients with simple fractures are encouraged to return to their usual activities as rapidly as possible. Fracture healing and restoration of full strength and mobility may take months. Patients

---

Chart 60-2
Factors Affecting Fracture Healing

Factors Enhancing Fracture Healing

- Immobilization of fracture fragments
- Maximum bone fragment contact
- Sufficient blood supply
- Proper nutrition
- Exercise—weight-bearing for long bones
- Hormones—growth hormone, thyroid, calcitonin, insulin, vitamins A and D, anabolic steroids
- Electric potential across fracture

Factors Inhibiting Fracture Healing

- Extensive local trauma
- Bone loss
- Inadequate immobilization
- Space/tissue between bone fragments
- Infection
- Local malignancy
- Metabolic bone diseases (*e.g.*, Paget's)
- Irradiated bone (radiation necrosis)
- Avascular necrosis
- Intra-articular fracture (synovial fluid contains fibrolysins, which lyse the initial clot and retard clot formation)
- Age (elderly persons heal more slowly)
- Corticosteroids (inhibit the repair rate)
- Denervation

TABLE 60-1. *Approximate Immobilization Time Necessary for Union*

Fracture Site	Number of Weeks
Phalanx (finger)	3-5
Metacarpal	6
Carpal	6
Scaphoid	10 (or until x-ray shows union)
Radius and ulna	10-12
Humerus:	
Supracondylar	8
Midshaft	8-12
Proximal (impacted)	3
Proximal (displaced)	6-8
Clavicle	6-10
Vertebra	16
Pelvis	6
Femur:	
Intracapsular	24
Intratrochanteric	10-12
Shaft	18
Supracondylar	12-15
Tibia:	
Proximal	8-10
Shaft	14-20
Malleolus	6
Calcaneus	12-16
Metatarsal	6
Phalanx (toe)	3

(Compere EL et al. Pictorial Handbook of Fracture Treatment, 5th ed. Chicago, Year Book Medical Publishers.)

are taught how to control swelling and pain associated with the fracture and soft-tissue trauma. They are encouraged to be active within the limits of the fracture immobilization. Bed rest is kept at a minimum. Exercises are begun to maintain health of unaffected muscles and to increase strength of muscles needed for transferring and for using ambulatory aids. Patients are taught how to use these devices safely. Planning is done to help patients modify their home environment as needed and secure personal assistance if necessary. Patient teaching includes self-care, medication information, monitoring for potential problems, and the need for continuing health care supervision.

Nursing Care Plan 60–1 outlines the basic nursing care for the patient who has sustained a simple fracture.

Care of the Patient With an Open Fracture

In an open fracture (one associated with an open wound extending through the skin surface and down to the area of bone injury), there is risk of *infection* — osteomyelitis, gas gangrene, and tetanus. The objectives of management are to minimize the chance of infection of the wound, soft tissue, and bone and to promote healing of soft tissue and bone.

The patient is taken to the operating room, where the wound is cleansed, debrided (foreign matter and devitalized tissue removed), and irrigated. The wound is swabbed for culture and sensitivity studies. Devitalized bone fragments are usually removed. Bone grafting may be done to bridge the defect, provided that the recipient tissue is healthy and able to facilitate union. The fracture is carefully reduced and stabilized by external fixation (see External Fixators in Chap. 59). Repair of damage to blood vessels, soft tissue, muscles, nerves, and tendons is completed.

The extremity is elevated to minimize the development of edema. Neurovascular status is assessed frequently. The temperature is taken at regular intervals and the patient is observed for signs of infection.

Primary closure may not be accomplished because of edema and potential ischemia, restricted wound drainage, and anaerobic infection. A heavily contaminated wound may be left open, dressed with sterile gauze, and not closed until it is clear that the area is not infected. Tetanus prophylaxis is given. Usually, intravenous antibiotics are prescribed to prevent or treat serious infection. The wounds are closed by suture or by autogenous skin or flap grafts in 5 to 7 days.

Complications of Fractures

Early Complications
The early complications after fracture are *shock*, which may be fatal within a few hours after injury; *fat embolism*, which may occur within 48 hours or later; and *compartment syndrome*, which may result in permanent loss of extremity function if not treated promptly. Other early complications associated with fracture are *infection; thromboembolism* (pulmonary embolism), which may cause death several weeks after injury; and *disseminated intravascular coagulopathy*.

Shock.   Hypovolemic or traumatic shock, resulting from hemorrhage (both external and nonvisible blood loss) and loss of extracellular fluid into damaged tissues, may occur in frac-

tures of the extremities, thorax, pelvis, and spine. Because the bone is very vascular, large quantities of blood may be lost as a result of trauma, especially in femoral and pelvic fractures.

Treatment consists of replacing the depleted blood volume, relieving the patient's pain, providing adequate splinting, and protecting the patient from further injury.

Fat Embolism Syndrome.   After fracture of long bones or pelvis, multiple fractures, or crush injuries, fat emboli may develop, especially in the young adult (20 to 30 years old) male. At the time of fracture, innumerable fat globules may move into the blood because the marrow pressure is greater than the capillary pressure or because catecholamines elevated by the patient's stress reaction cause mobilization of fatty acids and the development of fat globules in the bloodstream. The fat globules combine with platelets to form emboli, which then occlude the small blood vessels that supply the brain, lungs, kidneys, and other organs. The onset of symptoms may occur a few hours after injury to a week after injury, but usually occurs within 48 hours after injury. The onset of symptoms is rapid.

The presenting feature is usually cerebral disturbance manifested by mental status changes varying from mild agitation and confusion to delirium and coma that occur in response to hypoxia, due to the lodging of fat emboli in the brain. In addition, tachycardia is noted.

The respiratory response includes tachypnea, dyspnea, crackles, wheezes, and large amounts of thick, white sputum. Blood gases show PO_2 below 60 mm Hg, with an early respiratory alkalosis and later respiratory acidosis. The chest x-ray exhibits a typical "snow storm" infiltrate.

With systemic embolization the patient appears pale. Petechiae are noted in the buccal membranes and conjunctival sacs, on the hard palate, on the fundus of the eye, and over the chest and anterior axillary folds. Free fat may be found in the urine when emboli reach the kidneys.

- Personality changes, restlessness, irritability, or confusion in a patient who has sustained a fracture is an indication that immediate blood gas studies should be done. Occlusion of a large number of small vessels causes the pulmonary pressure to rise, possibly resulting in acute right heart failure. Edema and hemorrhages in the alveoli impair oxygen transport, leading to hypoxia. There is an increase in respiratory rate, precordial chest pain, cough, dyspnea, and acute pulmonary edema.

Management.   Immediate immobilization of fractures, minimal fracture manipulation, and adequate support for fractured bones during turning and positioning are measures that may reduce the incidence of fat emboli. Frequently, fat emboli syndrome becomes apparent through subtle changes in the patient's mental status. Monitoring high-risk patients will aid in the early identification of this problem. Prompt initiation of respiratory support is essential.

The objectives of management are to support the respiratory system and to correct homeostatic disturbances. Arterial blood gas analysis is done to determine the degree of respiratory impairment, as respiratory failure is the most common cause of death. Respiratory support is provided with oxygen given in high concentrations. Controlled volume ventilation with positive end-expiratory pressure (PEEP) may be employed to decrease and inhibit the formation of pulmonary edema. Steroids may be given to treat the inflammatory lung reaction and to control cerebral edema. Low-molecular-weight dextran may improve pulmonary and capillary flow because of its de-

> ## Nursing Care Plan 60-1
>
> ## Care of the Patient With a Simple Fracture

Nursing Interventions	Rationale	Expected Outcomes

Nursing Diagnosis: Pain related to fracture

Goal: Relief of pain

1. Encourage patient to describe type and location of discomfort.	1. Pain and tenderness are expected with fracture and tissue damage; muscle spasms occur in response to injury and immobilization.	• Patient describes discomfort • Keeps injured extremity elevated • Uses ice during first 24 hours • Controls edema; neurovascular status intact
2. Assess patient's discomfort.	2. Pain assessment provides basis for planning nursing interventions.	• Uses relaxation techniques. • Demonstrates methods to control pain and swelling
3. Use measures to control pain: a. Splint and support injured area.	a. Prevents additional injury; minimizes movement of fracture fragments.	• Performs active and passive range-of-motion exercises on nonimmobilized joints; changes position frequently

b. Perform position changes gently.
  c. Elevate injured extremity to heart level.
  d. Apply ice, if prescribed.
	b. Decreases muscle spasms.
	c. Controls edema by promoting drainage.
	d. Ice decreases pain and controls bleeding and edema.
		• Obtains pain relief

e. Monitor swelling and neurovascular status.	e. Edema and bleeding into the traumatized tissues cause discomfort; unrelenting pain may indicate compartment syndrome.	
f. Administer pain medications as prescribed early in pain experience.	f. Oral analgesics provide pain relief after fracture; control techniques are more effective early in pain cycle.	
g. Suggest relaxation techniques.	g. Modifies pain experience.	
4. Offer explanation of nursing measures to control pain, swelling, and additional tissue damage.	4. Damaged tissues cause pain; immobilization decreases discomfort from movement of fracture fragments; understanding of cause of pain reduces patient's perception of pain.	
5. Encourage active and passive range-of-motion exercises for nonimmobilized joints; encourage position changes as permitted within limits of immobilizing device.	5. Pressure on bony prominences and disuse contribute to discomfort.	
6. Minimize the time the injured extremity is in dependent position.	6. Swelling will occur in injured tissues when dependent; swelling contributes to discomfort.	

Nursing Diagnosis: High risk for injury related to neurovascular compromise, pressure, and disuse

Goal: Achievement of uncomplicated healing

1. Assess for the development of neurovascular compromise:
  a. Increasing pain
  b. Cool skin temperature
  c. Increasing swelling
  d. Decreased motor abilities
  e. Abnormal sensations
  f. Diminished capillary refill
	1. Early recognition of circulation and nerve problems due to compartment syndrome is needed to prevent loss of function.	• Neurovascular status distal to fracture is intact
		• Describes signs and symptoms of neurovascular compromise
		• Shows no evidence of skin breakdown
		• Describes signs and symptoms of skin breakdown

(continued)

Nursing Care Plan 60–1 *(Continued)*

Care of the Patient With a Simple Fracture

Nursing Interventions	Rationale	Expected Outcomes
		• Participates in activities that will minimize diminished muscle function and loss of joint motion
2. Teach the signs and symptoms of neurovascular compromise.	2. Any indication of neurovascular compromise must be reported to the physician promptly.	
3. Assess for the development of skin breakdown: a. Skin abrasion b. Cast "hot spots" c. Drainage d. Irritation sensations	3. Pressure of casts and appliances can cause skin breakdown.	
4. Teach the signs and symptoms of skin breakdown.	4. Patient education is needed for self-care.	
5. Encourage active exercise and range-of-motion exercise of body parts not immobilized.	5. Disuse results in atrophy of muscles and loss of joint motion.	
6. Encourage isometric exercises of immobilized muscles.	6. Maintains muscle function and promotes self care.	

Nursing Diagnosis: Self-care deficit related to disruption of ability to perform activities of daily living

Goal: Patient demonstrates satisfactory adjustment to altered performance of activities of daily living.

1. Encourage patient to express concerns and to discuss injury and problems associated with injury. Listen actively.	1. Fractures result from accidents and affect one's ability to perform activities of daily living. Life style is interrupted. Time loss from employment occurs.	• Patient discusses injury and its impact on life • Uses available resources and coping mechanisms to modify emotional stress • Participates in development of health care plan • Participates in activities of daily living • Demonstrates safe use of treatment modalities and mobilization aids • Achieves appropriate level of self-care at home
2. Support use of coping mechanisms.	2. Sudden disruption of routines and plans requires use of coping mechanisms.	
3. Involve significant others and support services as needed and appropriate.	3. Others can assist patient with activities of daily living.	
4. Modify home environment as necessary.	4. Accommodations for home management of fracture may be necessary to promote self care and safety.	
5. Engage patient in development of treatment regimen.	5. Patient regains independence by active participation in treatment plan decisions.	
6. Explain various facets of treatment regimen.	6. Patient education and understanding of rationale increase compliance.	
7. Encourage active participation in activities of daily living within therapeutic limits.	7. Self-esteem is enhanced through self-care activities.	
8. Teach safe use of treatment modalities and mobilization aids. Supervise use to assure safety.	8. Injury from unsafe use of modalities or mobilization aids can be prevented through education.	
9. Evaluate patient's ability to care for self at home: a. Planned treatment regimen b. Recognition of potential problems c. Recognition of unsafe situations d. Continued health supervision	9. Ensures patient's ability to manage fracture at home. Lack of knowledge and poor preparation for self-care at home contribute to anxiety and nonadherence to therapeutic regimen.	

sludging effect. Heparin may be used for its lipolytic action (breakdown of fat globules), but its anticoagulant effect may cause hemorrhage at the fracture site. To allay apprehension and decrease pain, morphine may be prescribed for the patient on a ventilator.

Fat emboli are a major cause of death in patients with fractures. Respiratory support must be instituted early. Response to therapy frequently occurs within 48 hours.

Compartment Syndrome.   Compartment syndrome is a problem that develops when tissue perfusion in the muscles is less than that required for tissue viability. This can be due to (1) reduction of the muscle compartment size because the enclosing muscle fascia is too tight or a cast or dressing is constrictive, or (2) an increase in muscle compartment contents because of edema or hemorrhage associated with a variety of problems (*e.g.*, ischemia, crush injuries, injection of tissue-destroying [toxic] substances, fractures). The forearm and the leg muscle compartments are involved most frequently. Permanent function can be lost if the situation continues for more than 6 to 8 hours and *myoneural* (muscle and nerve) ischemia and necrosis occur. Volkmann's contracture (see Fig. 59–3) is an example of this complication.

The patient complains of deep, throbbing, unrelenting pain, which is not controlled by narcotics. Palpation of the muscle, if that is possible, will show it to be swollen and hard. The actual tissue pressure can be monitored by inserting a fluid-filled needle or wick catheter into the suspected compartment and determining the pressure with a pressure transducer monitoring setup (see Fig. 59–1). (Normal pressure is up to 8 mm Hg.) Nerve and muscle tissues deteriorate as compartment pressure increases. Passive stretching movement of the muscle will cause acute pain. If it does not, the patient's pain may be due to nerve ischemia. Diminished capillary refill, cyanotic nailbeds, paralysis, and paresthesia may be present. The pulse may be obscured by swelling. Usually, major arteries are not occluded by compartment syndrome.

Prevention and Management.   Compartment syndrome can be prevented by elevating the injured extremity and by applying ice after injury as prescribed. If compartment syndrome occurs, restrictive dressings must be released. A fasciotomy may be needed if conservative measures have not restored tissue perfusion and relieved pain within an hour. After fasciotomy, the wound is not sutured. The wound is covered with moist sterile saline dressings. The limb is splinted in a functional position and passive range-of-motion exercises are usually prescribed every 4 to 6 hours. In 3 to 5 days when the edema has resolved and tissue perfusion has been restored, the wound is debrided and closed.

Other Early Complications.   Thromboembolism, infection (all open fractures are considered to be contaminated), and disseminated intravascular coagulopathy *(DIC)* are other possible complications of fractures. Disseminated intravascular coagulopathy includes a group of bleeding disorders with diverse causes, including massive tissue trauma. Manifestations include ecchymoses, unexpected bleeding after surgery, and bleeding from the mucous membranes, venipuncture sites, and gastrointestinal and urinary tracts. The treatment of DIC is discussed on p. 811.

Delayed Complications

Delayed Union and Nonunion.   Delayed union occurs when healing does not advance at a normal rate for the location and type of fracture. *Nonunion* results from failure of the ends of a fractured bone to unite. The patient complains of persistent discomfort and movement at the fracture site. Factors contributing to union problems include infection at the fracture site; interposition of tissue between the bone ends; inadequate immobilization or manipulation, which disrupts callus formation; excessive space between bone fragments (bone gap); limited bone contact; and restricted blood supply that results in avascular necrosis.

In nonunion, fibrocartilage or fibrous tissue exists between the bone fragments; no bone salts have been deposited. A false joint *(pseudarthrosis)* often develops at the site of the fracture. Fractures of the middle third of the humerus, of the neck of the femur in elderly people, and of the lower third of the tibia most frequently result in nonunion.

Nonunion may be managed by *bone grafting*. Surgically, the fractured bone fragments are freshened, infection if present is removed, and a bone graft, frequently from the iliac crest, is placed in the bony defect. The bone graft provides a lattice work for invasion by bone cells. After grafting, rigid immobilization is required.

Electrical Stimulation of Osteogenesis.   Osteogenesis in nonunion may be stimulated by electrical impulses, and is approximately as effective as bone grafting. It is not effective with large bone gaps or synovial pseudarthrosis. The electrical stimulation modifies the tissue environment, enhancing mineral deposition and bone formation.

In some situations, pins that act as cathodes are inserted percutaneously directly into the fracture site, and direct current is passed over the fracture continuously. Direct current methods cannot be used when infection is present.

Another method is noninvasive inductive coupling. Pulsing electromagnetic fields (PEMFs) are delivered to the fracture for 10 to 12 hours a day by an electromagnetic coil implanted in the dressing over the nonunion site (Fig. 60–3). During the electrical stimulation treatment period, rigid fracture fixation with adequate support is needed.

Avascular Necrosis of Bone.   Avascular necrosis occurs when the bone loses its blood supply and dies. It may follow a fracture (especially of the femoral neck), dislocations, prolonged high-dosage steroid therapy, chronic renal disease, sickle cell anemia, and other diseases. The devitalized bone may collapse or reabsorb and be replaced by new bone. The patient develops pain and limitation of movement. X-ray demonstrates calcium loss and structural collapse. Treatment generally consists of attempts to revitalize the bone with bone grafts, prosthetic replacement, or *arthrodesis* (joint fusion).

Reaction to Internal Fixation Devices.   Internal fixation devices may be removed after bony union has taken place, but for the majority of patients a device is not removed unless it produces symptoms. Pain and decreased function are the prime indicators that a problem has developed. Such problems may include mechanical failure (inadequate insertion and stabilization); material failure (faulty or damaged internal fixation devices); corrosion of the device, causing local inflammation; allergic response to the metallic alloy used; and osteoporotic remodeling adjacent to the fixation device (stress needed for bone strength is carried by the device, causing a disuse osteoporosis). If the device is removed, the bone needs to be protected from refracture related to osteoporosis, altered bone structure, and accident. Bone remodeling reestablishes the bone's structural strength.

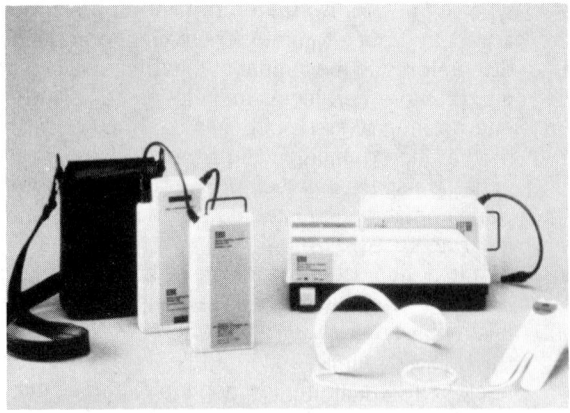

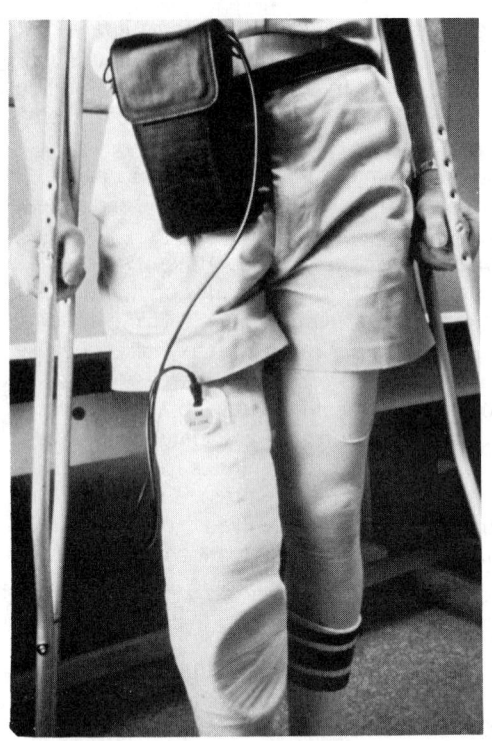

Figure 60-3. Electromagnetic bone-healing stimulator. Pulsed electromagnetic fields generated through coils included in the cast produce bone growth (osteogenesis) at the fracture site. The system is portable and battery powered. The therapy is used for 10 to 12 hours a day (Courtesy of EBI Medical Systems, Inc, Fairfield, NJ.)

Fractures of Specific Sites

An injury to the skeletal structure may vary from a simple linear fracture to a severe crushing injury. The therapeutic program is determined by the type and location of the fracture and the degree of involvement of surrounding structures. Maximum functional recovery is the goal of fracture management.

Appendicular Skeletal Fractures

Clavicle Fractures

Fracture of the clavicle (collar bone) is a common fracture that results from a fall or a direct blow to the shoulder. Associated head or cervical spine injuries are often seen with these fractures.

The clavicle helps to hold the shoulder upward, outward, and backward from the thorax. Therefore, when the clavicle is fractured, the patient assumes a protective position—slumping the shoulders and immobilizing the arm to prevent shoulder movements. The objective of management is to hold the shoulder in its normal position by means of closed reduction and immobilization.

More than 80% of these fractures occur in the middle or inner two thirds of the clavicle. A modified shoulder spica (clavicular cast) or a figure-of-eight bandage or a commercially available clavicular strap (Fig. 60-4) may be used to reduce the fracture, pull the shoulders back, and hold them in that position. When a clavicular strap is used, the axillae are well padded to prevent a compression injury to the brachial plexus and axillary artery. Circulation and nerve function of both arms are monitored.

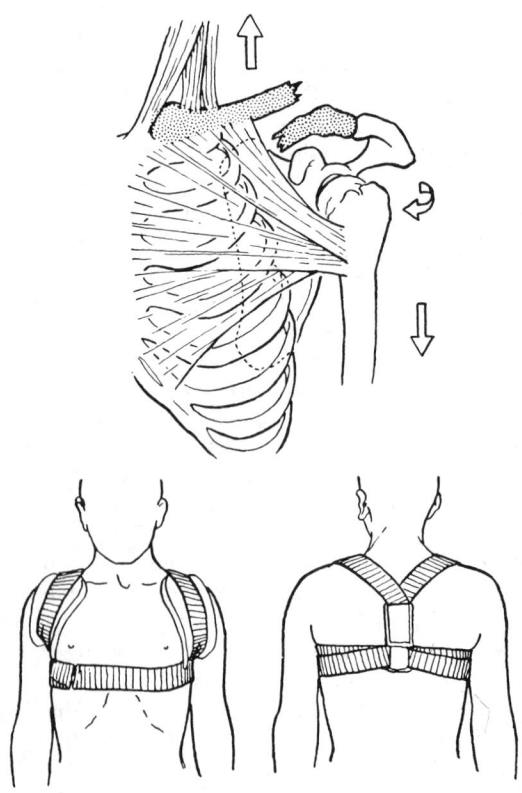

Figure 60-4. Fracture of the clavicle. (**Top**) Anteroposterior view, showing typical displacement of midclavicle fracture. (**Bottom**) Method of immobilization with a clavicular strap. (Hardy JD. Rhoads' Textbook of Surgery. Philadelphia, JB Lippincott.)

Fracture of the distal third of the clavicle without displacement and ligament disruption is treated with a sling and restricted use of the arm. When a fracture in the distal third is accompanied by a disrupted coracoclavicular ligament, there is displacement, which may be treated by open reduction and internal fixation to achieve healing.

Complications of clavicular fractures include trauma to the nerves of the brachial plexus, injury to the subclavian vein or artery from a bony fragment, and malunion. Malunion may be a cosmetic problem when low-neckline clothing is worn.

Patient Education and Home Health Care. The patient is cautioned not to elevate the arm above shoulder level until the fracture has united (about 6 weeks) but is encouraged to exercise the elbow, wrist, and fingers as soon as possible. When the patient is able, shoulder exercises (Fig. 60–5) are prescribed to obtain full shoulder motion. Vigorous activity is limited for 3 months.

Upper Extremity Fractures

Fractures of the Humeral Neck. Fractures of the proximal humerus may occur through either the anatomic or the surgical neck of the humerus. The anatomic neck is located just below the humeral head. The surgical neck is the region below the tubercles. Impacted fractures of the surgical neck of the humerus are seen most frequently in older women after a fall on an outstretched arm. These are essentially nondisplaced fractures. Active middle-aged patients may suffer severely displaced humeral neck fractures with associated rotator cuff damage.

The patient presents with the affected arm hanging limp at the side and supported by the uninjured hand. Neurovascular assessment of the involved extremity is essential to fully evaluate the extent of injury and possible involvement of the neurovascular bundle (nerves and blood vessels) of the arm.

Many impacted fractures of the surgical neck of the humerus are not displaced and do not require reduction. The arm is supported and immobilized by a sling and swathe that secure the supported arm to the trunk (Fig. 60–6). A soft pad is placed in the axilla to absorb moisture and avoid skin breakdown. Limitation of motion and stiffness of the shoulder occur from disuse. Therefore, *pendulum exercises* are begun as soon as tolerated by the patient. (In pendulum or circumduction exercises, the patient is instructed to lean forward and to allow the affected arm to abduct and rotate [see Fig. 60–5].) Early motion of the joint does not displace the fragments if motion is carried out within the limits imposed by pain.

These fractures require 6 to 8 weeks to heal, and the patient should avoid vigorous activity, such as tennis, for an additional 4 weeks. Residual stiffness, aching, and some limitation of range of motion may persist for 6 or more months.

When a humeral neck fracture is displaced, treatment consists of closed reduction under x-ray control, open reduction, or replacement of the humeral head with a prosthesis. In this type of fracture, there must be a specified period of immobilization before exercises are started.

Fractures of the Shaft of the Humerus. Fractures of the shaft of the humerus are most frequently caused by (1) direct trauma that results in a transverse, oblique, or comminuted fracture, or (2) an indirect twisting force that results in a spiral fracture. The nerves and brachial blood vessels may be injured with these fractures. Wrist drop is indicative of radial nerve injury. Initial neurovascular assessment is essential to differentiate between trauma from the injury and complications from treatment.

Frequently, the weight of the arm helps to correct any displacement so that surgery is not required. With oblique, spiral, or displaced fracture that has resulted in shortening of the humeral shaft, a hanging cast may be used. This cast is designed so that its weight provides traction to the arm when

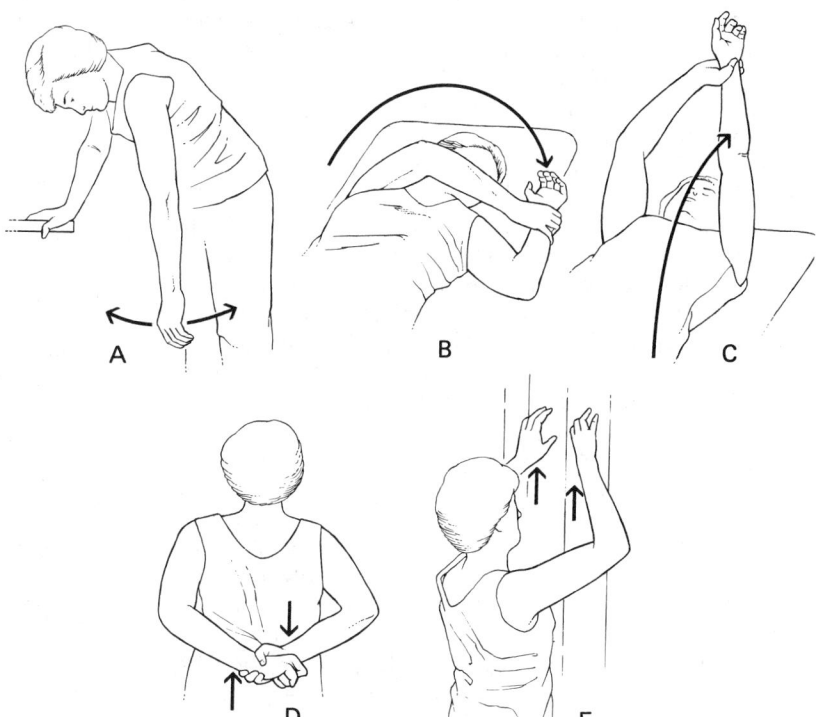

Figure 60–5. Exercises to develop range of motion of shoulder. (**A**) Pendulum exercise. (**B**) External rotation. (**C**) Elevation. (**D**) Internal rotation. In all of these, the unaffected arm is used for power. (**E**) Wall climbing.

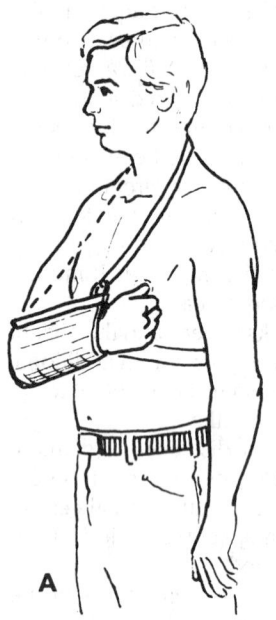
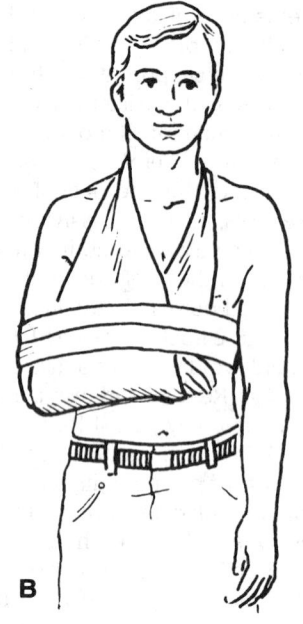
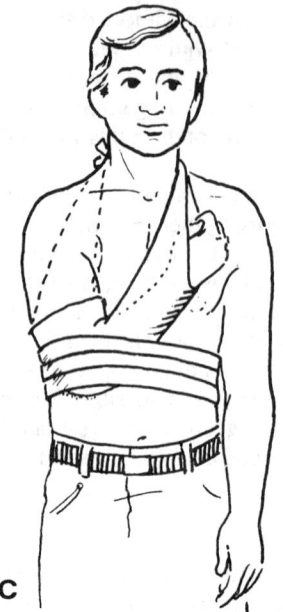

Figure 60-6. The types of immobilizing dressings used for proximal humeral fractures. (**A**) A commercial sling and swathe that permits easy removal of the arm for hygiene and is comfortable on the neck. (**B**) A conventional sling and swathe. (**C**) A stockinette Velpeau and swathe are used when there is an unstable surgical neck component, because this position relaxes the pectoralis major. (Redrawn from Rockwood CA and Green DP. Fractures. Philadelphia, JB Lippincott.)

the patient is upright, thereby reducing and immobilizing the fracture. The hanging cast must be dependent (allowed to hang free without support), because the weight of the cast is the means by which continuous traction is applied to the long axis of the arm. The patient is advised to sleep in an upright position so that traction from the weight of the cast is maintained constantly. Problems encountered with this mode of therapy are fracture distraction (pulling fracture fragments too far apart) due to the weight of the cast, and fracture angulation due to excessive fracture motion.

Finger exercises are started as soon as the cast is applied, and pendulum-shoulder exercises are done as directed to provide active movement of the shoulder, thereby preventing adhesions of the shoulder joint capsule. Isometric exercises may be prescribed to prevent muscle atrophy.

After the cast is removed, a sling is applied and exercises of the shoulder, elbow, and wrist are begun. Humeral fractures require about 10 weeks to heal when treated with hanging casts.

Elderly patients may not tolerate a cast. A sling and swathe (see Fig. 60-6) may provide adequate comfort and immobilization. Shoulder exercises are begun in about 3 weeks.

Functional bracing is another form of treatment being used for these fractures. A hanging cast is applied for about 1 week, and then a contoured thermoplastic sleeve is secured in place with Velcro closures around the upper arm. As swelling decreases, the Velcro is tightened, applying uniform pressure and stability to the fracture. Functional bracing allows active use of muscles, shoulder and elbow motion, and good approximation of fracture fragments. The callus that develops is substantial, and the sleeve can be discontinued in about 9 weeks.

Shoulder spica casts may be used during early treatment of unstable humerus fractures. Generally, the patient is uncomfortable and feels quite awkward.

Skeletal traction may be appropriate for patients who must remain in bed because of other injuries (Figs. 60-7 and 60-8). Active exercises of the hand and wrist are encouraged.

Open fractures of the humeral shaft are frequently treated by external fixators (see Chap. 59). Open reduction of a humerus fracture is necessary with evidence of nerve palsy, pathologic fractures, or when other systemic or neurologic disease (*e.g.*, Parkinson's disease) would make management with a hanging cast inappropriate.

Fractures at the Elbow. Fractures of the distal humerus result from automobile accidents, from falls on the elbow or the flexed elbow, or by direct blow. These fractures may result in nerve damage from injury to the median, radial, or ulnar nerves. The patient is evaluated for paresthesias and also for signs of compromised circulation in the forearm and hand. The most serious complication of a supracondylar fracture of the humerus is *Volkmann's ischemic contracture*, which results from antecubital swelling or damage to the brachial artery (see Fig. 59-3).

The nurse must:

- Observe the hand for swelling, skin color, nailbed capillary refill, and temperature. Compare it with the unaffected hand.
- Assess for paresthesias (prickling and burning sensations) in the hand, because they may indicate nerve injury or impending ischemia.
- Assess for ability to move fingers.
- Evaluate the radial pulse. If it weakens or disappears, the orthopedic surgeon must be informed *immediately* because irreversible ischemia may result.
- Directly measure tissue pressure as prescribed.
- Report indications of diminished nerve function or diminished circulatory perfusion promptly before irreparable damage occurs. Fasciotomy may become necessary.

Other problems that may occur are damage to the joint articular surfaces and *hemarthrosis* (blood in the joint). With hemarthrosis, the physician may aspirate the joint to remove the blood, relieving the pressure and pain.

The goal of fracture therapy is prompt reduction and stabilization of the fracture, followed by controlled active motion when swelling has subsided and healing has begun. If the fracture is not displaced, the arm is immobilized in a cast or pos-

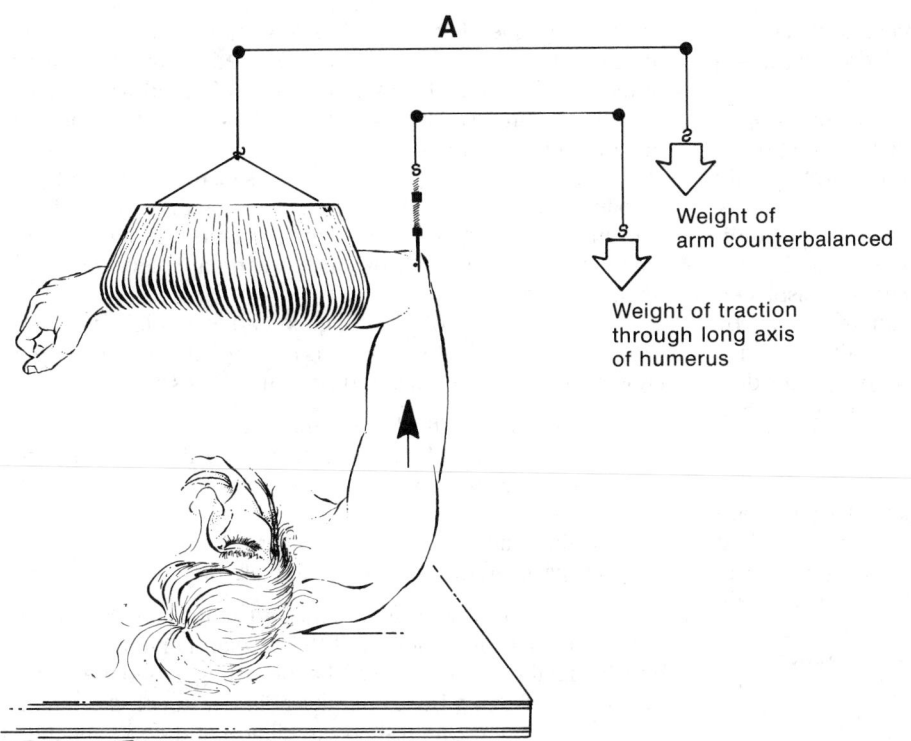

Figure 60-7. Over-the-face traction for supracondylar fracture reduces swelling by creating a very effective elevation of the extremity. (Lewis RC. Handbook of Traction, Casting and Splinting Techniques. Philadelphia, JB Lippincott.)

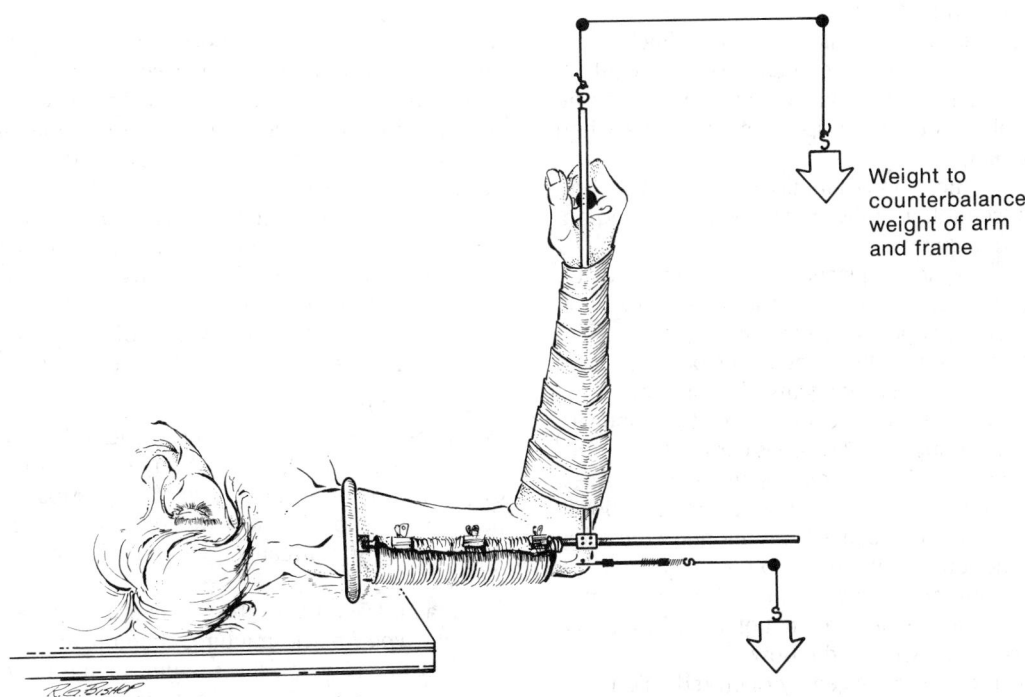

Figure 60-8. Balanced side-arm traction. The arm is passed through the ring, which is then passed up so that it encompasses the shoulder. The upright attachment for the forearm may be moved in either direction to accommodate the length of the humerus. A cloth sling is placed on the horizontal segment to provide a surface on which the arm may rest. The olecranon extends just past the vertical extremity, so that the pin drilled through the olecranon will be clear and allow unimpeded traction. The forearm is placed between the two upright supports, and is usually held there with a circumferentially applied elastic bandage. A rope is attached to the vertical section and is passed through pulleys. A weight is attached to exactly counterbalance the weight of the arm and the frame. Skeletal traction is then applied in the desired amount through the pin in the olecranon. The entire extremity is counterbalanced so that a balanced traction system is created. (Lewis RC. Handbook of Traction, Casting and Splinting Techniques. Philadelphia, JB Lippincott.)

terior splint with the elbow at 45 to 90 degrees of flexion, or the elbow may be supported with a pressure dressing and a sling.

A displaced fracture is usually treated by traction or open reduction and internal fixation. Sometimes the bone fragments are excised. Additional external support with a plaster splint is then applied.

Active finger exercises are encouraged. Gentle range-of-motion exercise of the injured joint is begun about 1 week after internal fixation and after 2 weeks with nondisplaced closed reduction. Motion aids healing of injured joints by movement of synovial fluid into the articular cartilage. Active exercise of the elbow is carried out when prescribed, as residual limitation of motion is common without an intensive rehabilitation program.

Radial and Ulnar Fractures

Fractures of the Radial Head.   Radial head fractures are common, and are usually produced by a fall on the outstretched hand with the elbow in extension. If blood has collected in the elbow joint *(hemarthrosis)*, it is aspirated to relieve pain and allow early range of motion. Immobilization for these undisplaced fractures is accomplished by a sling. Active joint motion may be prescribed as early as 1 to 2 days after injury.

If the fracture is displaced, surgery is required, with excision of the radial head when necessary. Postoperatively, the arm is immobilized in a posterior plaster splint and sling. The patient is encouraged to carry out a program of active motion of the elbow and forearm when prescribed.

Fractures of the Shafts of the Radius and Ulna.   Fractures of the shaft of the bones of the forearm occur most frequently in children. Either the radius, the ulna, or both bones may be broken at any level. Frequently, displacement occurs when both bones are broken.

The forearm has the unique functions of pronation and supination, and those motions must be preserved by good anatomic position and alignment.

If the fragments are not displaced, the fracture is treated by closed reduction with a long arm cast applied from the upper arm to the proximal palmar crease. A loop may be incorporated in the cast near the elbow and a sling pulled through it to prevent the cast from sagging against the forearm.

The circulation, sensation, and motion of the hand are assessed after the cast is applied. The arm is elevated to control edema. Frequent finger flexion and extension are encouraged to reduce edema. Active motion of the involved shoulder is essential. The reduction and alignment are monitored closely by x-ray to ensure adequate immobilization.

The fracture is immobilized for about 12 weeks; during the last 6 weeks the arm may be in a functional forearm brace that allows exercise of the wrist and elbow.

Displaced fractures are managed by open reduction with internal fixation, using a compression plate with screws, intramedullary nails, or rods. The arm is usually immobilized in a plaster splint, cast, or pressure dressing. Open fractures may be managed with external fixation devices. The arm is elevated to control swelling. Neurovascular status is monitored. Elbow, wrist, and hand exercises are begun as permitted by the immobilization device.

Fractures of the Wrist

A fracture of the distal radius (Colles's fracture) is a common fracture and is usually the result of a fall on an open dorsiflexed hand. It is frequently seen in elderly women with osteoporotic bones and weak soft tissues that do not dissipate the energy of the fall. The patient presents with a deformed wrist, radial deviation, pain, swelling, weakness, limited finger range of motion, and numbness.

Treatment usually consists of closed reduction and immobilization with a cast. For more severe fractures, a Kirschner wire may be inserted or an external fixation device used to maintain reduction. The wrist and forearm are elevated for 48 hours after reduction.

Active motion of the fingers and shoulder is begun promptly. The patient is taught to do the following finger exercises to reduce swelling and prevent stiffness:

1. Hold the hand at the level of the heart.
2. Move the fingers from full extension to flexion. Hold and release. (Repeat above at least 10 times every half hour when awake).
3. Use the hand in functional activities.
4. Actively exercise the shoulder and elbow.

Fingers may swell from diminished venous and lymphatic return. The sensory function of the median nerve is assessed by pricking the distal aspect of the index finger, and the motor function is assessed by testing the ability to touch the thumb to the little finger. Diminished circulation and nerve function must be treated promptly by release of constricting casts and bandages.

Fracture of the Hand

Because trauma to the hand can be a complex problem, requiring extensive reconstructive surgery, the reader is referred to specialized books on the hand. The objective of treatment is always to regain maximum function of the hand.

For an undisplaced fracture of the distal phalanx (finger bone), the finger is splinted for 3 to 4 weeks to relieve pain and to protect the fingertip from further trauma. Displaced fractures and open fractures may require open reduction with internal fixation, using wires or pins.

Neurovascular status of the injured hand is evaluated. Swelling is controlled by elevation of the hand. Functional use of the uninvolved portions of the hand is encouraged.

Pelvic Fractures

The sacrum, coccyx, ilium, pubis, and ischium bones form the pelvic bone, a fused, stable, bony ring in adults. The severity of pelvic fractures varies (Fig. 60–9). Most fractures of the pelvis heal rapidly because the innominate bone (hip bone) is made up mostly of cancellous bone, which has a rich blood supply.

Stable fractures of the pelvis are classified as type I and type II. *Type I* pelvic fractures, fractures of a single ramus of the pubis or ischium, the sacrum, or the coccyx, exhibit no break in the pelvic ring. The most common *type II* fracture (single break in the pelvic ring) is the fracture of two ipsilateral rami. Stable fractures are treated with bed rest using a bedboard under the mattress for additional firmness until the discomfort resolves. Log rolling increases patient comfort. The patient with a fractured sacrum should be monitored for bowel sounds. The patient with fractures of the coccyx experience pain on sitting and with defecation. Sitz baths and stool softeners may be prescribed. Full activity is resumed in 10 to 16 weeks.

Unstable fractures of the pelvis, *type III*, exhibit a double break in the pelvic ring. They are rotationally unstable—the

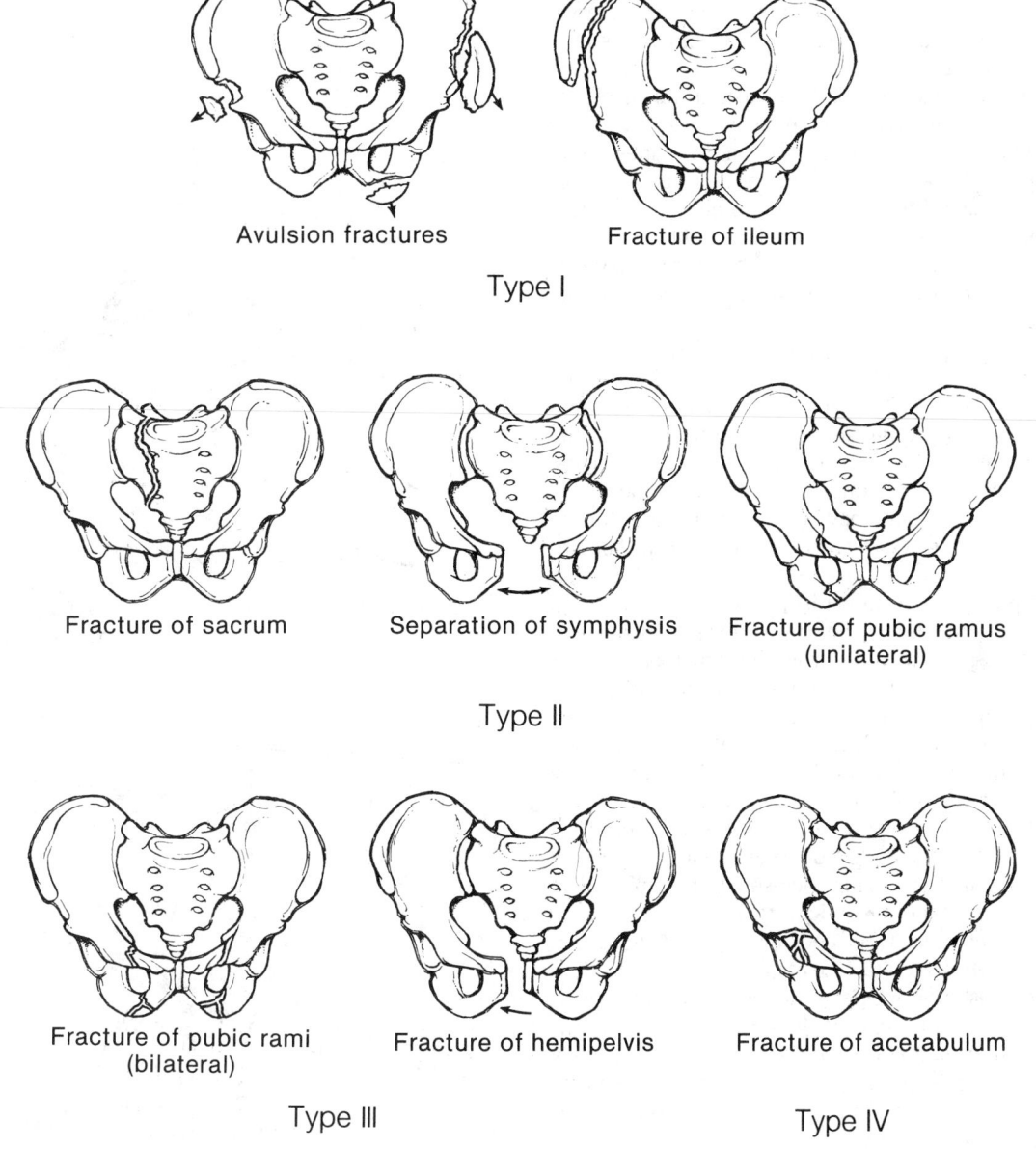

Figure 60–9. Fractures of the pelvis.

open book type (separation occurs at the symphysis pubis), or vertically unstable—the *vertical shear* type (superior-inferior displacement of the sides of the pelvis).

Unstable fractures of the pelvic ring occur as a result of automobile accidents, crush injuries, and falls from buildings and scaffolds. General symptoms include deformity, local swelling, ecchymosis, tenderness over the symphysis pubis, anterior iliac spines, iliac crest, sacrum, or coccyx, and inability to bear weight without discomfort. In addition, shock and hemorrhage may occur.

Pelvic fractures are serious because at least two thirds of these patients have significant and multiple injuries. (The care of the patient with multiple injuries is discussed in Chap. 63.) Therefore, a high mortality rate accompanies these fractures. Death may ensue from local hemorrhage in view of the rich blood supply to the pelvis and the possibility of massive and hidden bleeding in the retroperitoneal region.

Bleeding arises from the cancellous surfaces of the fracture fragments, laceration of veins and arteries by bone spicules, and possibly from a torn iliac artery. The peripheral pulses of both lower extremities are palpated; absence of pulses may indicate a torn iliac artery or one of its branches. The patient is handled gently to minimize further bleeding and shock. A peritoneal lavage may be performed to detect intra-abdominal hemorrhage.

In addition to hemorrhage, the bladder, the urethra, or the intestines may be lacerated, resulting in conditions that can prove to be more serious than the fracture itself. There is a high mortality rate associated with pelvic fractures from hemorrhage, pulmonary complications, fat emboli, intravascular coagulation, thromboembolic complications, and infection.

To assess for possible damage to the urinary tract, the patient's urine is examined for blood. A voiding cystourethrogram and an intravenous urogram may be performed. Laceration of the urethra is suspected in males with anterior fracture of the pelvis and blood at the urethral meatus. (Females rarely experience lacerated urethra.) A catheter should not be inserted until the status of the urethra is known.

Hemorrhage, thoracic, intra-abdominal, and cranial injuries have priority over treatment of fractures. The nurse continues to assess for injuries to the bladder, rectum, intestines, intra-abdominal organs, and pelvic vessels and nerves. Paralytic ileus may accompany pelvic fractures and immobility. In addition, thrombophlebitis is a threat with immobility and bed rest.

Unstable fractures may be treated with bed rest, external fixation, open reduction and internal fixation, skeletal traction, or pelvic sling. A pelvic sling immobilizes the pelvis into a single unit so that the patient can move in bed with less pain. The pelvic sling lifts the weight of the pelvis very slightly from the mattress (Fig. 60–10*A*). The sling may be folded back over the buttocks to permit the patient to use the bedpan. (Some orthopedists permit the sling to be loosened for certain nursing care activities if the patient's condition permits.) Because skin care is a problem, sheep skin may be used to line the sling to prevent excoriation. It is necessary to reach under the sling to give skin care.

If separation of the symphysis pubis has occurred, a compression force may be applied by an external fixator or pelvic sling, by crossing the ropes from the sling (see Fig. 60–10*B*), which exerts a compression effect from the sides over the trochanteric region and corrects the separation of bones. Pelvic slings are not used with fractures that have collapsed inward or when the acetabulum is fractured. The patient may become quite uncomfortable in the pelvic sling.

The use of an external fixator stabilizes the pelvis, controls hemorrhage, and allows for early mobilization out of bed. Open reduction and internal fixation may be used for multiple pelvic fractures where stabilization is difficult to achieve.

Undisplaced fractures of the acetabulum (*type IV* fractures) are seen after motor vehicle accidents in which the femur is jammed into the dashboard. Open reduction and fixation with multiple screws or direct lateral skeletal traction by insertion of a large trochanter screw into the femoral head is usually necessary. Traction is maintained for 6 weeks, followed by non–weight-bearing for another 6 weeks. Internal fixation permits earlier motion and function.

During the period of immobility, exercises (leg, respiratory, range-of-motion, and strengthening), elastic stockings, and elevation of the foot of the bed to aid venous return are appropriate measures to help diminish the effects of prolonged bed rest. When bony healing has taken place in a pelvic fracture, the patient is mobilized with a method of progressive weight-bearing, usually with crutches. Long-term complications of pelvic fractures include malunion, nonunion, residual gait disturbances, and back pain from ligament injury.

Lower Extremity Fractures

The objectives of management of a fracture of the lower extremity are (1) to obtain adequate bony union with full length and normal alignment and without rotational or angular deformity, (2) to restore muscle power and joint motion, and (3) to restore the preinjury ambulatory status of the patient.

Because practically all fractures of the lower extremity require the use of crutches, walker, or cane during convalescence, adjustable equipment should be acquired for the patient. The safe use of these ambulatory aids is discussed in Chapter 14.

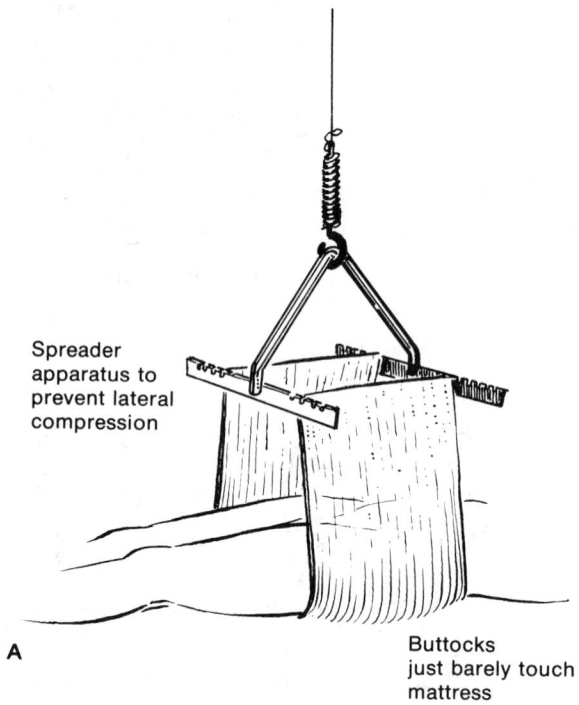

Spreader apparatus to prevent lateral compression

A

Buttocks just barely touch mattress

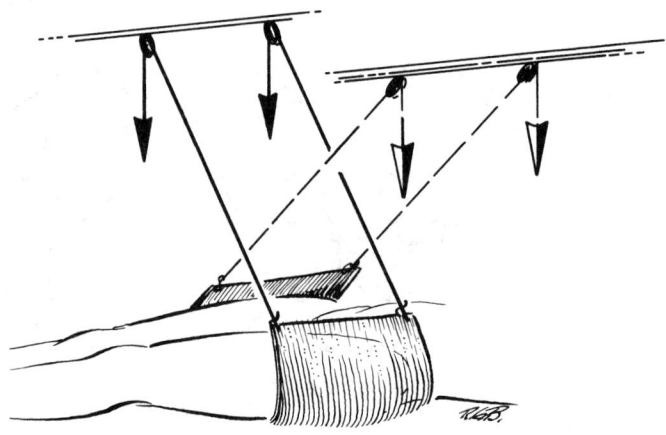

B

Figure 60–10. Pelvic sling suspension for fractures of the pelvis. (**A**) A suspension of the pelvis without an attempt at compression. The sling is suspended by means of a large metal frame, and weight is applied so that the pelvis is largely counterbalanced and becomes, to a certain extent, "weightless." Movement can then occur without moving the pelvic fragments. (**B**) The method for applying compression when there has been separation of the anterior pelvic ring, particularly at the symphysis pubis. This suspension compresses the pelvis from side to side to correct any diastasis that may have occurred. Pain developing at pressure points over the trochanters is unavoidable; it will often limit the duration of time that compression traction is useful. (Lewis RC. Handbook of Traction, Casting and Splinting Techniques. Philadelphia, JB Lippincott.)

Edema is a common problem. Therefore, a fractured lower extremity is not placed in a dependent position for prolonged periods. The patient is encouraged to exercise regularly all joints that do not cause movement of the bone fragments. When the patient becomes ambulatory, the extremity is elevated for intervals to minimize recurrence of edema. It is best

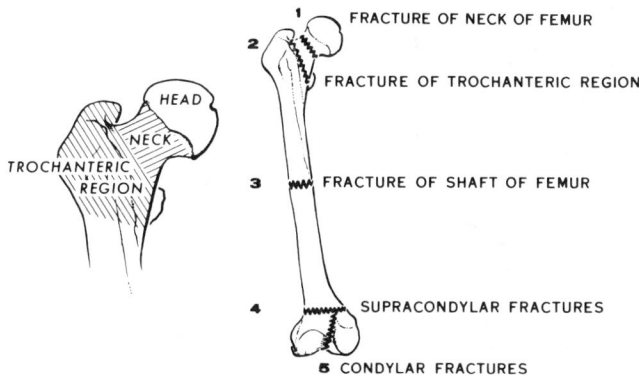

Figure 60–11. Sites of fracture of the femur.

for the patient to lie down when elevating the healing leg. After the immobilizing device is removed, elastic stockings can be worn to support venous circulation, thus reducing the problem of edema.

Femur Fractures. Fractures of the femur can occur at several sites (Fig. 60–11). When the head, neck, or trochanteric region of the femur is involved, a hip fracture results. Fractures also occur in the femoral shaft and in the region of the knee (supracondylar and condylar fractures).

Hip Fractures

There is a high incidence of hip fractures among elderly people. Their bones are brittle from osteoporosis (particularly women). They fall frequently. Weak quadriceps muscles, general frailty due to age, and conditions that produce decreased cerebral arterial perfusion (transient ischemic attacks, anemia, emboli, cardiovascular disease, drug effects) contribute to the incidence of falls. The patient who has sustained a hip fracture frequently has associated medical (*i.e.*, cardiovascular, pulmonary, renal, endocrine) disorders. A hip fracture is viewed by the patient and the family as a catastrophic event that will have a negative impact on the patient's life style.

Classification. There are two major types of hip fractures. *Intracapsular fractures* are fractures of the neck of the femur. *Extracapsular fractures* are fractures of the trochanteric region (between the base of the neck and the lesser trochanter of the femur) and the subtrochanteric region.

Fractures of the neck of the femur are more difficult to heal than those of the trochanteric region, because the vascular system supplying blood to the head and the neck of the femur may be damaged with the fracture. The nutrient vessels within the bone may be interrupted, and the bone cells may die. For this reason, nonunion or aseptic necrosis is common in patients with these types of fractures.

Extracapsular intertrochanteric fractures have an excellent blood supply and heal readily. There is, however, a fairly high mortality rate after intertrochanteric hip fractures, mainly because the patients are elderly (ages 70 to 85) and are poor operative risks. In addition, extensive soft tissue damage may occur at the time of injury, and it is not uncommon for the fracture to be comminuted and unstable.

Clinical Manifestations. Because of the fracture, the leg is shortened, adducted, and externally rotated. The patient may complain of slight pain in the groin or in the medial side of the knee. With most fractures of the femoral neck, the patient is in pain, is unable to move the leg without significant increase in pain, and is able to achieve some comfort with the leg slightly flexed in external rotation. Impacted femoral neck fractures cause moderate discomfort even with movement, may allow the patient to bear weight, and may not demonstrate obvious shortening or rotational changes. With extracapsular femoral fractures, the extremity is significantly shortened, presents external rotation to a greater degree than intracapsular fractures, exhibits muscle spasm that resists positioning of the extremity in a neutral position, and has an associated large hematoma or area of ecchymosis.

The diagnosis of fractured hip is confirmed with x-ray films.

Gerontologic Considerations. Hip fractures are the most frequent cause of traumatic death after the age of 75.

Many elderly persons are confused, not only as a result of the stress of the trauma and unfamiliar surroundings, but also because of underlying systemic illness. Confusion that develops in some elderly patients may be due to mild cerebral ischemia.

Examination of the legs may reveal edema due to congestive heart failure and absent peripheral pulses due to arteriosclerotic vascular disease. Similarly, chronic respiratory problems may be present and contribute to the possible development of inadequate pulmonary ventilation. Coughing and deep-breathing exercises are encouraged. Frequently the elderly are taking cardiac, blood pressure, or respiratory medications that need to be continued and the patient's responses monitored.

Dehydration and poor nutrition may be present. At times elderly persons who live alone are unable to summon help at the time of injury. A day or two may pass before assistance is provided, and as a result dehydration occurs. Dehydration contributes to hemoconcentration and predisposes to thromboembolism problems. Therefore the patient needs to be encouraged to consume adequate fluids and a balanced diet.

Muscle weakness and wasting may have contributed to the fall and fracture. Bed rest and immobility will cause an additional loss of muscle strength. The nurse needs to encourage movement of all joints except the involved hip and knee. Patients are encouraged to use their arms and the overhead trapeze to reposition themselves, thereby improving arm and shoulder strength, which are required for walking with ambulatory aids.

Management. Temporary skin traction in the form of Buck's extension may be applied to reduce muscle spasm, to immobilize the extremity, and to relieve pain. Sand bags or a trochanter roll may be used to control the external rotation.

The goal of surgical treatment of hip fractures is to obtain a satisfactory fixation so that the patient can be mobilized quickly and thereby avoid secondary medical complications. Operative treatment consists of (1) reduction of the fracture and internal fixation, or (2) replacement of the femoral head with a prosthesis (*hemiarthroplasty*). Surgical intervention is carried out as soon as possible after injury. The preoperative objective is to ensure that the patient is in as favorable a condition as possible for the surgery. Displaced femoral neck fractures may be treated as elective emergencies, and reduction and internal fixation are done within 12 to 24 hours after fracture. This minimizes the effects of diminished blood supply and the development of avascular necrosis.

After general or spinal anesthesia, the femoral neck fracture is reduced under radiographic control, using an image intensifier. A stable fracture is usually fixed with nails, a nail-and-plate combination, multiple pins, or compression screw devices (Figs. 60–12 and 60–13). The choice of fixation device is de-

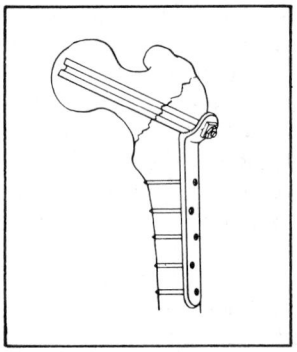

Smith-Petersen nail
with McLaughlin plate

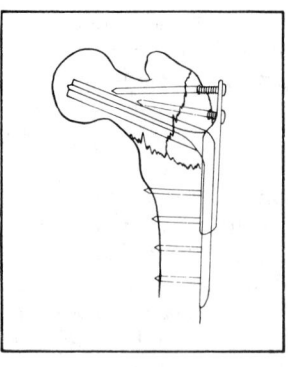

Jewett nail
with overlay plate

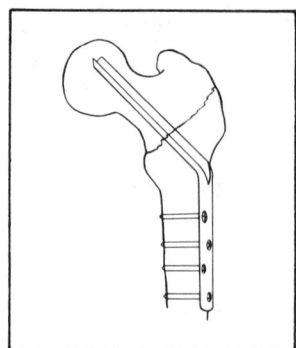

Neufeld nail

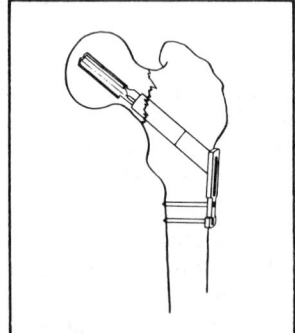

Massie nail assembly

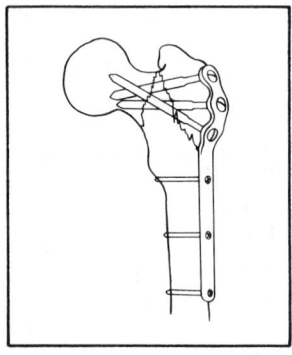

Moe intertrochanteric plate

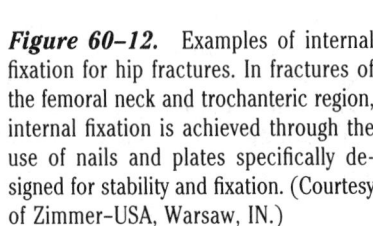

Figure 60–12. Examples of internal fixation for hip fractures. In fractures of the femoral neck and trochanteric region, internal fixation is achieved through the use of nails and plates specifically designed for stability and fixation. (Courtesy of Zimmer–USA, Warsaw, IN.)

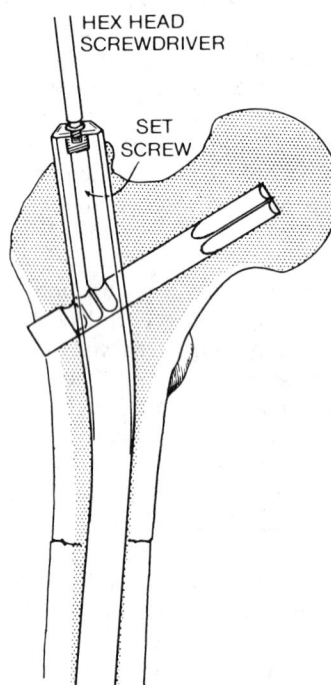

HEX HEAD
SCREWDRIVER

SET
SCREW

Figure 60–13. Zickel nail for subtrochanteric fractures. The triflanged nail is locked in the Zickel rod by a set screw. The Zickel nail fixation controls rotation and maintains alignment, permitting early active hip movement and early progressive weight-bearing ambulation. (Courtesy of Howmedica, Inc.)

termined by the fracture site and the preference of the orthopedic surgeon. A Zickel nail is particularly useful with subtrochanteric fractures, permitting earlier weight-bearing (see Fig. 60–13). Adequate reduction is important for fracture healing. (The better the reduction, the better the healing.)

Replacement of the head of the femur with a prosthesis is usually reserved for a fracture that cannot be satisfactorily reduced or securely nailed. Some orthopedists prefer this method because nonunion and avascular necrosis of the head of the femur are common complications of internal fixation techniques. Salvage of the hip is usually preferred to prosthetic replacement. Total hip replacement (see p. 1809) may be used in selected patients with acetabular defects.

Postoperative Interventions. The immediate postoperative care of a patient with a hip fracture is similar to that for other major surgery patients. (See Care of the Patient Undergoing Orthopedic Surgery in Chap. 59.) Additional attention is given to preventing secondary medical problems, however, and to early mobilization of the patient so that independent functioning can be restored.

During the first 24 to 48 hours, attention is given to the relief of pain and the prevention of complications. Deep breathing, coughing, and foot flexion exercises are encouraged each hour. Prescribed intravenous prophylactic antibiotics are administered. Hydration, general nutrition, and output are monitored. Activity in bed is encouraged. A pillow is used between the legs to maintain alignment and to provide needed support when turning the patient.

Turning. The patient may be turned on the unaffected extremity by the following method:

- A pillow is placed between the legs to keep the affected leg in an abducted position. The patient is then turned onto the unaffected side. After initial soreness has decreased and the incision has healed, the patient usually may be turned in the same manner on the affected hip.

Exercise. It is important that the patient exercise as much as possible by means of the overbed trapeze. This helps strengthen the triceps and shoulders in preparation for ambulatory activities.

On the first or second postoperative day, the patient is generally fairly comfortable and can transfer to a chair with assistance. The following day, assisted ambulation can begin. The amount of weight-bearing that can be permitted depends on the stability of the fracture reduction and the location of the fracture. The physician will prescribe the amount of weight-bearing permitted and the rate at which the patient can progress to full weight-bearing. Physical therapists will work with the patient on transfers, ambulation, and the safe use of walker and crutches.

The patient who has experienced a fractured hip can anticipate discharge with the use of an ambulatory aid. Some modifications in the home to permit safe use of walkers and crutches and for the patient's continuing care may be needed.

Potential Problems. Elderly persons who suffer hip fractures are particularly prone to developing complications that may require more vigorous treatment than the fracture itself. In some instances, the shock of the injury may prove fatal. Hemorrhagic shock after surgery is possible. Achievement of homeostasis after injury and surgery is accomplished through careful monitoring of patient responses and collaborative discussion of data and adjustment of therapeutic interventions as prescribed.

Neurovascular complications may occur because of direct injury of nerves and blood vessels or from increased tissue pressure. With hip fracture, bleeding into the tissues is expected. Excessive edema may be observed. Therefore, monitoring of the neurovascular status of the affected leg is important.

Thromboembolism is the most common complication. To prevent thromboembolism, ankle and foot exercises are encouraged. Elastic stockings, sequential compression devices, and prophylactic anticoagulant therapy may be prescribed. The patient's legs are assessed at least every 2 hours for evidence of thrombophlebitis.

Pulmonary complications are a threat to elderly patients undergoing hip surgery. Deep-breathing exercises, a change of position at least every 8 hours, and the use of an incentive spirometer help to prevent the development of respiratory complications. Breath sounds should be assessed for the development of adventitious or diminished sounds.

Because patients with hip fractures generally have poor circulation and tend to remain in one position, pressure ulcers frequently develop. Giving proper skin care, especially to the back and heels and under the hips and shoulders, helps relieve the constant pressure. A convoluted foam or other special mattress may provide protection by relieving pressure.

Loss of bladder control (incontinence) may occur. In general, the routine use of an indwelling catheter is to be avoided because of the associated high incidence of urinary tract infection. Urinary retention frequently occurs after surgery, and the patient's voiding patterns must be assessed. To assure

proper urinary tract function, liberal fluid intake, within the cardiovascular tolerance of the patient, is important.

Delayed complications of hip fractures include infection, nonunion, avascular necrosis of the femoral head (particularly with intracapsular fractures), metal fatigue failure of the fixation device, and protrusion of the fixation device through the acetabulum. Infection is suspected if the patient complains of moderate discomfort in the hip and has a mildly elevated sedimentation rate.

The nursing management of the elderly patient with a hip fracture is summarized in Nursing Care Plan 60–2.

Fractures of the Shaft of the Femur. Considerable force is required to break the shaft of the femur in adults. Most of these fractures are seen in young men who have been involved in a vehicular accident or have fallen from a height. Frequently, these patients have associated multiple trauma problems.

The patient presents with an enlarged, deformed, painful thigh. The patient cannot move the hip or the knee. The fracture may be transverse, oblique, spiral, or comminuted. Frequently, the patient is in impending shock, as the loss of 2 to 3 units of blood into the tissues with this fracture is common. Expanding diameter of the thigh may indicate continued bleeding.

Assessment includes checking neurovascular status of the extremity, especially circulatory perfusion of the foot. (Popliteal and pedal pulses and toe capillary refill are assessed.) A Doppler ultrasound monitoring device may be needed to assess blood flow.

Dislocation of the hip and knee may accompany these fractures. Knee effusion suggests ligament damage and possible instability of the knee joint.

Management. Continued neurovascular monitoring is needed. Treatment is begun with skin traction for comfort and to immobilize the fracture so that additional soft-tissue damage does not occur. Generally, skeletal traction (Fig. 60–14) (suspension traction with Thomas splint and Pearson attachment or with slings, Bohler-Baum frame, or Neufield roller traction) is used for a while to achieve separation of the fracture fragments (which facilitates the operative procedure) for internal fixation or to achieve reduction and immobilization of the fracture site for subsequent cast bracing.

An external fixator may be used if the patient has experienced a Grade III fracture, has extensive soft-tissue trauma, has lost bone, has an infection, or also has hip and tibial fractures.

Internal fixation is generally carried out 7 to 10 days after injury. Intramedullary nailing using a Küntschner rod, Schneider rod, or Sampson rod obtains adequate internal fixation, which allows for early mobilization. The active muscle movement is important for increasing blood supply and electrical potentials at the fracture site, which enhances healing. A thigh cuff may be used for external support. Dual compression plates may be used, but need external support from a cast brace for stability. Intramedullary implant and compression plates should be removed after 18 months. When plates are being removed, the resultant osteoporosis needs to be considered. A thigh cuff orthosis is used for several months after the removal of plates to provide support while the bone remodels.

A cast brace is commonly used for fractures of the mid- and distal shaft (*supracondylar*). Two to four weeks after the injury, when pain and swelling have subsided, the patient is removed from skeletal traction and placed in a *cast brace.*

(text continues on page 1846)

Nursing Care Plan 60–2

Care of the Elderly Patient With a Fractured Hip

Nursing Interventions	Rationale	Expected Outcomes

Nursing Diagnosis: Pain related to fracture, soft-tissue damage, muscle spasm, and surgery

Goal: Relief of pain

Nursing Interventions	Rationale	Expected Outcomes
1. Encourage patient to describe type and location of pain.	1. Pain is expected after fracture; soft-tissue damage and muscle spasm contribute to discomfort; pain is subjective and is evaluated through description of characteristics and location, which are important for determining cause of discomfort and for proposing interventions. Continuing pain may indicate development of neurovascular problems.	• Patient describes discomfort • Expresses confidence in efforts to control pain • Expresses little discomfort with position changes • Expresses comfort when fracture is positioned and immobilized • Minimizes movement of extremity before reduction and fixation • Uses physical, psychological, and pharmacologic measures to reduce discomfort • Relates a decrease in pain in 24–48 hours after surgery • Requests pain medications and uses pain relief measures early in pain cycle • States that positioning provides comfort • Appears comfortable and relaxed • Moves with increasing comfort as healing progresses
2. Acknowledge existence of pain; inform patient of available analgesics; record discomfort.	2. Reduces stress experienced by the patient by communicating concern and availability of help in dealing with pain. Notation provides data on pain experience.	
3. Handle the affected extremity gently, supporting it with hands or pillow.	3. Movement of bone fragments is painful; muscle spasms occur with movement; adequate support diminishes soft-tissue tension.	
4. Apply Buck's traction as prescribed. Use trochanter roll.	4. Immobilizes fracture to decrease pain and additional tissue trauma; decreases muscle spasm and external rotation of hip.	
5. Use pain-modifying strategies.	5. Pain perception can be diminished by distraction and refocusing of attention.	
a. Modify the environment.	a. Interaction with others, distraction, and sensory overload or deprivation may modify pain experiences.	
b. Administer prescribed pain medications as needed.	b. Analgesics reduce the pain; muscle relaxants may be prescribed to decrease discomfort associated with muscle spasm.	
c. Encourage patient to use pain relief measures before pain is "unbearable."	c. Mild pain is easier to control.	
d. Evaluate and record patient's response to medications and pain-reduction techniques.	d. Notation of effectiveness of measures provides basis for future management interventions; early identification of adverse reactions is necessary for corrective measures and care plan modifications.	
e. Consult with physician if relief of pain is not obtained.	e. Change in treatment plan may be necessary.	
6. Position for comfort and function.	6. Alignment of body facilitates comfort; positioning for function diminishes stress on musculoskeletal system.	
7. Assist with frequent changes in position.	7. Change of position relieves pressure and associated discomfort.	

(continued)

Nursing Care Plan 60–2 *(Continued)*

Care of the Elderly Patient With a Fractured Hip

Nursing Interventions	Rationale	Expected Outcomes
Nursing Diagnosis: Potential alteration in thought process related to age, stress of trauma, unfamiliar surroundings, and drug therapy.		
Goal: Remains oriented and participates in decision making.		
1. Assess orientation status.	1. Evaluate presenting orientation of patient; confusion may result from stress of fracture, unfamiliar surroundings, coexisting systemic disease, cerebral ischemia, or other factors. Baseline data are important for determining change.	• Patient establishes effective communication • Demonstrates orientation to time, place, and person • Participates in self-care activities • Remains mentally alert • Avoids episodes of confusion
2. Interview family regarding patient's orientation and cognitive abilities before injury.	2. Provides data for evaluation of current findings.	
3. Assess patient for auditory and visual deficits.	3. Diminished vision and auditory acuity frequently occur with aging; glasses and hearing aid may increase patient's ability to interact with environment.	
4. Assist patient with use of sensory aids and interacting with environment.	4. Aids must be in good working order and available for use; nonverbal clues, simple direct statements, and control of environmental distractors facilitate communication.	
5. Orient to and stabilize environment a. Use orientation activities and aids (*e.g.*, clock, calendar, pictures, introduction of self).	5. Short-term memory may be faulty in the elderly; frequent reorientation helps.	
b. Minimize number of staff working with patient.	b. Consistency of caregivers promotes trust.	
6. Give simple explanations of procedures and plan of care.	6. Short-term memory may be faulty.	
7. Encourage participation in hygiene and nutritional activities.	7. Participation in routine activities promotes orientation; increases awareness of self.	
8. Provide for safety a. Keep side rails up when patient in bed b. Keep light on at night. c. Have call bell available d. Provide prompt response to requests for assistance.	8. Side rails decrease chance for additional injury from falls; mechanism for securing assistance is available to patient; independent activities based on faulty judgment may result in injury.	
9. Assess mental responses to medications, especially sedatives and analgesics.	9. Elderly persons tend to be more sensitive to medications; abnormal responses (*e.g.*, hallucinations, depression) may occur.	
Nursing Diagnosis: Potential ineffective individual coping related to injury, anticipated surgery, and dependence		
Goal: Uses effective coping mechanisms to modify stress		
1. Encourage patient to express concerns and to discuss meaning of fractured hip.	1. Verbalization helps patient deal with problems and feelings. Clarification of thoughts and feelings promotes problem-solving.	• Patient describes feelings concerning fractured hip and implications for lifestyle

(continued)

Nursing Care Plan 60-2 (Continued)

Care of the Elderly Patient With a Fractured Hip

Nursing Interventions	Rationale	Expected Outcomes
2. Support use of coping mechanisms. Involve significant others and support services as needed.	2. Coping mechanisms modify disabling effects of stress; sharing concerns lessens the burden and facilitates necessary modification.	• Uses available resources and coping mechanisms; develops health promotion strategies • Uses community resources as needed • Participates in development of health care plan
3. Contact social services, if needed.	3. Anxiety may be related to financial or social problems; facilitates management of problems associated with continuing care.	
4. Explain anticipated treatment regimen and routines to facilitate positive attitude in relation to rehabilitation.	4. Understanding of plan of care helps to diminish fears of the unknown.	
5. Encourage patient to participate in planning.	5. Participating in care provides for some control of self.	

Potential Problems: Hemorrhage; neurovascular compromise; deep vein thrombosis; pulmonary complications; pressure ulcers related to surgery and immobility.

Goal: Patient experiences an absence of potential problems.

Hemorrhage

1. Monitor vital signs, observing for shock.	1. Changes in pulse, blood pressure, and respirations may indicate development of shock; blood loss and stress may contribute to development of shock.	• Vital signs stabilized within normal limits • Experiences no excessive or bright red drainage • Exhibits hematology values within normal limits
2. Consider preinjury blood pressure values and management of coexisting hypertension, if present.	2. Necessary for interpretation of current blood pressure determinations.	
3. Note character and amount of drainage.	3. Excessive drainage and bright red drainage may indicate active bleeding.	
4. Notify surgeon if patient develops shock or excessive bleeding.	4. Corrective measures need to be instituted.	
5. Note hemoglobin and hematocrit values and report decreases in values.	5. Anemia due to blood loss may develop; bleeding into tissues after hip fracture may be extensive; blood component therapy may be needed.	

Neurovascular Compromise

1. Assess affected extremity for color and temperature.	1. The skin becomes pale and feels cool with decreased tissue perfusion. Venous congestion may cause cyanosis.	• Patient has normal color and the extremity is warm • Demonstrates normal capillary refill response • Exhibits moderate swelling; tissue not palpably tense • States pain is controllable • Reports no pain with passive dorsiflexion • Reports normal sensations and no paresthesia • Demonstrates normal motor abilities and no paresis or paralysis • Has strong and equal pulses
2. Assess toes for capillary refill response.	2. After compression of the nail, rapid return of pink color indicates good capillary perfusion.	
3. Assess extremity for edema and swelling.	3. The trauma of surgery will cause swelling; excessive swelling and hematoma formation can compromise circulation and function; edema may be due to coexisting cardiovascular disease.	
4. Elevate extremity.	4. Minimizes dependent edema.	
5. Assess for deep, throbbing, unrelenting pain.	5. Surgical pain can be controlled; pain due to neurovascular compromise is refractory to treatment with analgesics.	

(continued)

Nursing Care Plan 60-2 *(Continued)*

Care of the Elderly Patient With a Fractured Hip

Nursing Interventions	Rationale	Expected Outcomes
6. Assess for pain on passive flexion of foot.	6. With nerve ischemia, there will be pain on passive stretch. Additionally, pain may indicate deep vein thrombosis (positive Homan's sign).	
7. Assess for sensations and numbness.	7. Diminished pain and paresthesia may indicate nerve damage. Sensation in web between great and second toe—peroneal nerve; sensation on sole of foot—tibial nerve.	
8. Assess ability to move foot and toes.	8. Dorsiflexion of ankle and extension of toes indicate function of peroneal nerve. Plantar flexion of ankle and flexion of toes indicate functioning of tibial nerve.	
9. Assess pedal pulses in both feet.	9. Indicator of circulatory status of extremities.	
10. Notify surgeon if diminished neurovascular status occurs.	10. Function of extremity needs to be preserved.	

Deep Vein Thrombosis

Nursing Interventions	Rationale	Expected Outcomes
1. Apply thigh-high elastic stockings or sequential compression device as prescribed.	1. Compression aids venous blood return and prevents stasis.	• Wears thigh-high elastic stockings. Uses sequential compression device
2. Remove stockings for 20 minutes twice a day and provide skin care.	2. Skin care is necessary to avoid skin breakdown. Extended removal of stocking or device defeats purpose.	• Experiences no skin breakdown • Experiences no more warmth than usual in skin areas
3. Assess popliteal, dorsalis pedis, and posterior tibial pulses.	3. Pulses indicate arterial perfusion of extremity. With coexisting arteriosclerotic vascular disease, pulses may be diminished or absent.	• Demonstrates a negative Homan's sign • Changes position with assistance and supervision
4. Assess skin temperature of legs.	4. Local inflammation will increase local skin temperature.	• Participates in exercise regimen • Experiences no chest pain; has lungs clear to auscultation; presents no evidence of pulmonary emboli
5. Assess for Homan's sign every 8 hours.	5. Pain in calf on dorsiflexion of ankle may indicate deep vein thrombosis.	• Exhibits no signs of dehydration; has normal hematocrit
6. Avoid pressure on popliteal blood vessels from appliances or pillows.	6. Compression of blood vessels diminishes blood flow.	• Maintains normal body temperature
7. Change position and increase activity as prescribed.	7. Activity promotes circulation and diminishes venous stasis.	
8. Supervise ankle exercises hourly.	8. Muscle exercise promotes circulation.	
9. Assess lung status; encourage coughing and deep breathing and use of incentive spirometer.	9. Adventitious breath sounds, respiratory pain, shortness of breath, blood-tinged sputum, cough, etc., indicate possible pulmonary emboli.	
10. Ensure adequate hydration.	10. Elderly persons may become dehydrated because of low fluid intake, resulting in hemoconcentration.	
11. Monitor body temperature.	11. Body temperature increases with inflammation (magnitude of response minimal in elderly).	

Pulmonary Complications

Nursing Interventions	Rationale	Expected Outcomes
1. Assess lung status. Respiratory rate, depth, and duration. Breath sounds. Monitor temperature.	1. Anesthesia and bed rest diminish respiratory effort and cause pooling of respiratory secretions.	• Patient has clear breath sounds • Breath sounds present in all fields

(continued)

Nursing Care Plan 60–2 (Continued)

Care of the Elderly Patient With a Fractured Hip

Nursing Interventions	Rationale	Expected Outcomes
2. Report adventitious and diminished breath sounds and elevated temperature.	2. Elevated temperature in the early post-operative period may be due to a respiratory problem.	• Exhibits no shortness of breath, chest pain, or elevated temperature • PO_2 on room air within normal limits • Performs respiratory exercises; uses incentive spiromenter as instructed • Changes position frequently • Consumes adequate fluids
3. Supervise deep breathing and coughing exercises. Encourage use of incentive spirometer if prescribed.	3. Promote optimal ventilation. Coexisting respiratory conditions diminish lung expansion.	
4. Administer oxygen as prescribed.	4. Reduced ventilatory efforts may diminish PO_2 when patient is on room air.	
5. Turn and reposition patient at least every 2 hours. Mobilize patient (assist patient out of bed) as soon as possible.	5. Promotes optimal ventilation. Diminishes pooling of respiratory secretions.	
6. Ensure adequate hydration.	6. Liquefies respiratory secretions. Facilitates expectoration.	

Pressure Ulcers

Nursing Interventions	Rationale	Expected Outcomes
1. Monitor condition of skin at pressure points (e.g., heels, sacrum, shoulders).	1. Elderly patients are subject to skin breakdown at points of pressure because of diminished subcutaneous tissue.	• Patient exhibits no signs of skin breakdown • Skin remains intact • Repositions self frequently • Uses protective devices
2. Reposition patient at least every 2 hours. Avoid skin shearing.	2. Avoids prolonged pressure and trauma to the skin.	
3. Administer skin care, especially to pressure points.	3. Immobility causes pressure at bony prominences; massage and position changes relieve pressure.	
4. Use special care mattress and other protective devices (e.g., heel protectors).	4. Devices minimize pressure on skin at bony prominences.	
5. Institute care according to protocol at first indication of potential skin breakdown.	5. Early interventions prevent tissue destruction and prolonged rehabilitation.	

Nursing Diagnosis: Actual impairment of skin integrity related to surgical incision

Goal: Achieves wound healing.

Nursing Interventions	Rationale	Expected Outcomes
1. Monitor vital signs.	1. Temperature, pulse, and respirations increase in response to infection. (Magnitude of response may be minimal in elderly patients.)	• Patient maintains vital signs within normal range • Exhibits well-approximated incision without drainage or excessive inflammatory response • Relates minimal discomfort; demonstrates no hematoma • Tolerates antibiotics; exhibits no evidence of osteomyelitis
2. Use aseptic dressing changes.	2. Avoid introducing infectious organisms.	
3. Assess wound appearance and character of drainage.	3. Red, swollen, draining incision is indicative of infection.	
4. Assess complaint of pain.	4. Pain may be due to wound hematoma, a possible locus of infection, which needs to be surgically evacuated.	
5. Administer prophylactic antibiotic if prescribed, and observe for side effects.	5. Osteomyelitis is to be avoided.	

Nursing Diagnosis: Potential alteration in patterns of urinary elimination related to immobility

Goal: Maintains normal urinary elimination patterns.

Nursing Interventions	Rationale	Expected Outcomes
1. Monitor intake and output.	1. Adequate fluid intake ensures hydration; adequate urinary output minimizes urinary stasis.	• Intake and output are adequate; patient exhibits normal voiding patterns

(continued)

Nursing Care Plan 60–2 (Continued)

Care of the Elderly Patient With a Fractured Hip

Nursing Interventions	Rationale	Expected Outcomes
		• Demonstrates no evidence of urinary tract infection
2. Avoid use of indwelling catheter.	2. Source of bladder infection.	

Nursing Diagnosis: Impaired physical mobility related to fractured hip

Goal: Achieves pain-free, functional, stable hip

1. Maintain neutral positioning of hip.	1. Prevents stress on fixation.	• Patient engages in therapeutic positioning
2. Use trochanter roll.	2. Minimizes external rotation.	• Uses pillow between legs when turning
3. Place pillow between legs when turning.	3. Supports leg; prevents adduction.	• Assists in position changes; shows increased independence in transfers
4. Instruct and assist in position changes and transfers.	4. Encourages patient's active participation while preventing stress on hip fixation.	• Exercises hourly
5. Instruct in and supervise isometric, quadriceps- and gluteal-setting exercises.	5. Strengthens muscles needed for walking.	• Uses trapeze
6. Encourage use of trapeze.	6. Strengthens shoulder and arm muscles necessary for use of ambulatory aids.	• Participates in progressive ambulation program
7. In consultation with physical therapist, instruct in and supervise progressive safe ambulation within limitations of weight-bearing prescription.	7. Amount of weight-bearing depends on the patient's condition, fracture stability, and fixation device; ambulatory aids are used to assist the patient with non–weight-bearing and partial–weight-bearing ambulation.	• Actively participates in exercise regimen
8. Offer encouragement and support exercise regimen.	8. Reconditioning exercises can be uncomfortable and fatiguing; encouragement helps patient comply with the program.	• Uses ambulatory aids correctly and safely
9. Instruct in and supervise safe use of ambulatory aids.	9. Prevents injury from unsafe use.	

Nursing Diagnosis: Potential impaired home maintenance related to fractured hip and impaired mobility

Goal: Cares for self at home

1. Assess home environment for discharge planning.	1. Physical barriers (especially stairs, bathrooms) may limit patient's ability to ambulate and care for self at home.	• Home is accessible for patient at time of discharge
2. Encourage patient to express concerns about care at home; explore with patient possible solutions to problems.	2. Patient may have special problems that need to be identified and dealt with.	• Patient appears relaxed and develops strategies to deal with identified problems
3. Assess availability of physical assistance for health care activities.	3. Because of limitation of mobility, patient may require some assistance in routine health care.	• Has personal assistance available
4. Teach caregiver the home health care regimen.	4. Understanding of rehabilitative regimen is necessary for compliance.	• Demonstrates ability to use necessary assistance within therapeutic prescription
5. Instruct patient in posthospital care.	5. Lack of knowledge and poor preparation for care at home contribute to patient anxiety, insecurity, and nonadherence to therapeutic regimen.	• Complies with home care program; keeps follow-up health care appointments
a. Activity limitations		
b. Reinforce exercise instructions.		
c. Safe use of ambulatory aids		
d. Wound care		
e. Measures to promote healing (nutrition, wound care)		
f. Medications, if any		
g. Potential problems		
h. Continuing health care supervision and management		

The cast (fracture) brace is a total contact device that holds the reduced fracture. The muscle, through hydrodynamic compression, stabilizes the bone and stimulates healing. Minimal partial weight-bearing is begun and is progressed to full weight-bearing as tolerated. Functional ambulation stimulates fracture healing. The cast brace is worn for 12 to 14 weeks. In management of femoral shaft fractures, a major goal is rapid functional healing with sufficient strength to support the multiple stresses placed on the femur.

To preserve muscle strength, the patient should exercise the lower leg, foot, and toes on a regular basis. A common complication after fracture of the femoral shaft is restriction of knee motion. Thus, quadriceps-setting exercises should be started early. Active and passive knee exercises are done as soon as possible, depending on the stability of the fracture and knee ligaments. Progressive strengthening exercises for the upper extremities are needed to prepare for ambulation.

Fractures of the Tibia and Fibula. The most common fracture below the knee is a fracture of the tibia (and fibula) that results from a direct blow, falls with the foot in a flexed position, or a violent twisting motion. Fractures of the tibia and fibula often occur in association with each other. The patient presents with pain, deformity, obvious hematoma, and considerable edema. Frequently, these fractures involve severe soft-tissue damage because there is little subcutaneous tissue in the area.

Peroneal nerve functioning needs to be assessed for baseline data. If nerve function is impaired, the patient is unable to dorsiflex the great toe and has diminished sensation in the first web space. Tibial artery damage is assessed by testing the capillary refill response. Development of an anterior compartment syndrome could occur. (Symptoms include intense pain, paresthesia, pain on passive movement, and diminished cap-

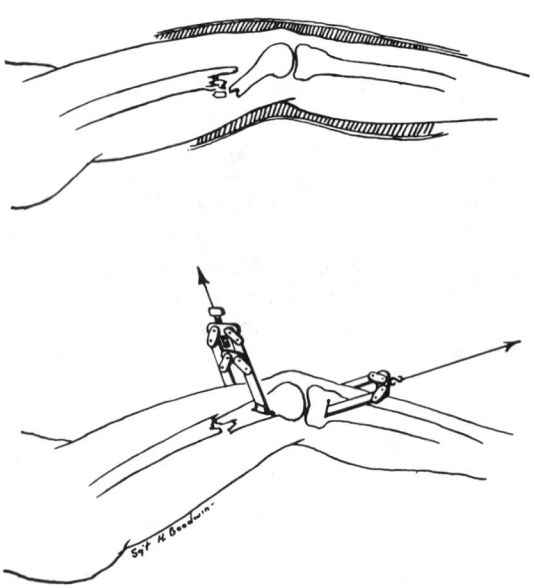

Figure 60–14. Two-wire skeletal traction for fracture of the femur in distal third. (**Top**) Deformity on admission to hospital. (**Bottom**) Adequate reduction when additional wire is inserted in lower femoral fragment and vertical lift is secured. (Hampton OP Jr. Wounds of the Extremities in Military Surgery. St Louis, CV Mosby.)

illary refill.) Articular fracture may be complicated by hemarthroses or ligament damage.

Most closed tibial fractures are treated with closed reduction and initial immobilization in a long leg-walking or patellar-tendon–bearing cast. Reduction must be relatively accurate in relation to angulation and rotation. At times it is difficult to maintain reduction, and percutaneous pins may be placed in the bone and held in position by a plaster cast (*i.e.*, pins-in-plaster technique). Partial weight-bearing is usually prescribed in 7 to 10 days. Activity decreases edema and increases circulation. The cast is changed to a short leg cast or brace in 3 to 4 weeks, which allows for knee motion. Fracture healing takes 16 to 24 weeks.

Open or comminuted fractures may be treated with skeletal traction, internal fixation with rods, plates, or nails, or external fixation. External plaster support may be used with internal fixation. Foot and knee exercises are encouraged within the limits of the immobilizing device. Weight-bearing is begun when prescribed, usually in about 6 weeks.

As with other lower extremity fractures, the leg should be elevated to control edema. Continued neurovascular evaluation is needed. The development of compartment syndrome requires prompt recognition and resolution or there will be a permanent functional deficit.

Axial Skeletal Fractures

Fractures of the skull and cervical spine have been described in Chapter 56. Fracture of the mandible is discussed in Chapter 34.

Rib Fractures

Uncomplicated fractures of the ribs occur frequently in adults, and usually result in no impairment of function. Because fractures of the ribs produce painful respirations, the patient tends to decrease respiratory excursions and refrains from coughing. As a result, tracheobronchial secretions are not coughed up, aeration of the lung is diminished, and a predisposition to pneumonia and atelectasis is created. To help the patient cough and take deep breaths, the nurse may splint the chest with her hands. Intercostal nerve blocks may be done by the physician to relieve respiratory pain and permit productive coughing.

Chest strapping to immobilize the rib fracture is not usually used, because decreased chest expansion may result in respiratory complications of pneumonia and atelectasis. The pain associated with rib fracture diminishes significantly in 3 or 4 days, and the fracture is healed in 6 weeks.

Other serious problems may result from rib fractures. Multiple rib fractures may lead to a flail chest. Rib fractures may result in puncture of the lung with the escape of air into the pleural space (*pneumothorax*) or of blood into the pleural space (*hemothorax*). The management of these patients is discussed in Chapter 26.

Fractures of the Thoracolumbar Spine

Fractures of the thoracolumbar spine may involve (1) the vertebral body, (2) the lamina and articulating processes, and (3) the spinous processes or transverse processes. The T12 to L2 area of the spine is most vulnerable to fracture. Fractures are generally due to indirect trauma caused by excessive loading, sudden muscle contraction, or excessive motion beyond physiologic limits. Osteoporosis contributes to vertebral body collapse.

The patient with a spinal fracture presents with acute tenderness, swelling, paravertebral muscle spasm, and possibly change in normal curves or gap between spinous processes. Pain is greater when moving, coughing, or weight-bearing.

Immobilization is essential until initial assessments have determined if there is any spinal cord injury and if the fracture is stable or unstable. Few spinal fractures are associated with neurologic deficits. However, if spinal cord injury with neurologic deficit occurs, it usually requires immediate surgery (laminectomy with spinal fusion) to decompress the spinal cord.

Stable spinal fractures are due to flexion, extension, lateral bending, or vertical loading. The anterior structural column (vertebral bodies and discs) or the posterior structural column (neural arch, articular processes, ligaments) has been disrupted. Stable spinal fractures are treated conservatively with bed rest until the acute pain subsides (several days to 2 or 3 weeks). Analgesics are prescribed to control pain. The patient is monitored for the development of a transient ileus due to associated retroperitoneal hemorrhage. Sitting is avoided until the pain subsides. A spinal brace or plastic thoracolumbar orthosis may be used for support during progressive ambulation and resumption of activities.

Unstable fractures occur with fracture–dislocations and exhibit disruption of both anterior and posterior structural columns. The potential for neural damage exists. The patient with an unstable fracture is placed on a side-to-side turning frame (*e.g.*, Stryker). Neurologic status is monitored closely during the preoperative and postoperative periods. Within 24 hours of fracture, open reduction and fixation with spinal fusion and Harrington or Luque rod stabilization are usually accomplished. Postoperatively the patient continues to be cared for on the turning frame. Progressive ambulation is begun about 2 weeks after surgery, with the patient using a body jacket cast or brace.

Patient education emphasizes good posture, good body mechanics, and, when healing is sufficient, back-strengthening exercises.

In summary, fractures are breaks in the continuity of the bone and occur when the stress on the bone is greater than the bone can absorb. Adjacent soft tissues as well as the bone are injured with fractures. Clinical manifestations of fracture include pain, loss of function, false motion, deformity, shortening, crepitation, local swelling, and discoloration. Treatment of fracture includes reduction (reestablishment of length and alignment) and immobilization (*e.g.*, cast, traction, splint, brace, bandage, external fixator, internal fixation). Open fractures and comminuted fractures present special management problems. The nurse monitors for the development of fracture complications (*e.g.*, shock, neurovascular compromise, compartment syndrome, thromboembolism, fat embolism, nonunion, malunion, infection, disuse syndrome, avascular necrosis, reaction to internal fixation device). Resumption of activities depends on the location of the fracture and specific rehabilitation prescription.

Specific considerations related to fractures of the appendicular and axial skeleton, with specific nursing care considerations for a patient with a simple fracture, pelvic fracture, or hip fracture, are reviewed.

Amputation

Amputation of an extremity is often necessary as a result of progressive peripheral vascular disease, trauma (crushing injuries, burns, frostbite, electrical burns), congenital deformities, or malignant tumor. Of all these causes, peripheral vascular disease accounts for the majority of amputations of lower extremities.

The loss of an upper extremity presents different problems to the patient than does the loss of a lower extremity, because the upper extremity has such highly specialized functions. The major reasons for upper extremity amputation are severe trauma (acute injury, electrical burns, frostbite), malignant tumors, infection (fulminating gas gangrene, chronic osteomyelitis), and congenital malformations.

Amputation can be considered reconstructive surgery designed to improve the patient's quality of life. It is used to relieve symptoms and to facilitate improved function. If the health care team is able to communicate a positive attitude, the patient will adjust to the amputation and actively participate in the rehabilitative plan.

The loss of an extremity requires major adjustments. The patient's perception of the amputation must be understood by the health care team. The patient must adjust to a permanent change in body image, which must be incorporated in such a way that self-esteem is not lost. Physical mobility or ability to perform activities of daily living are altered, and the patient needs to learn how to modify activities and the environment to accommodate the use of mobility aids and assistive devices. The rehabilitation team is multidisciplinary (patient, nurse, physician, social worker, psychologist, prosthetist, vocational rehabilitation worker) and helps the patient achieve the highest possible level of function and participation in life activities.

Factors Affecting Amputation

Patients who require amputation are usually either young with severe extremity trauma or tumor, or elderly with peripheral vascular disease. *The young* are generally healthy, heal rapidly, and participate in a vigorous rehabilitation program. Because the amputation is usually the result of an injury, much psychological support is needed in accepting the sudden change in body image and in dealing with the stresses of hospitalization, long-term rehabilitation, and modification of life style. These patients need time to work through their feelings about their permanent loss. Their reactions are unpredictable and can include open, bitter hostility.

Conversely, *the elderly* with peripheral vascular disease frequently have concurrent health problems. These cardiovascular, respiratory, or neurologic problems may limit their rehabilitation progress. Therapeutic amputations for long-standing problems may relieve a patient of pain, disability, and dependency. These patients have had time to work through some feelings and come to terms with the amputation. Adjusting to the change in body image may be easier. Planning for psychological and physiologic rehabilitation is started before the amputation.

Levels of Amputation

Amputation is performed at the most distal point that will heal successfully. The site of amputation is determined by two factors: circulation in the part and the requirements of the prosthesis.

The circulatory status of the extremity is evaluated through physical examination and specific studies. Muscle and skin perfusion are important for healing. Doppler flowmetry, segmental blood pressure determinations, and transcutaneous partial pressure of oxygen (PaO_2) are valuable studies. Angiography may be done, especially if revascularization is considered to be an option.

The objective of surgery is to conserve as much extremity length as possible consistent with eradicating the disease process. Preservation of knee and elbow joints is desired. (Figure 60–15 shows the different levels at which an extremity may be amputated.) Almost any level of amputation can be fitted with a prosthesis.

Energy requirements and resultant cardiovascular demands for mobility increase as the patient progresses from using a wheelchair to a prosthesis or to crutch-walking without a prosthesis. Therefore, careful cardiovascular and nutritional monitoring is essential so that physiologic limits and demands can be met.

The amputation of toes and portions of the foot causes minor changes in gait and balance. A *Syme's* amputation (modified ankle disarticulation amputation) is done most frequently for extensive foot trauma, and produces a painless, durable extremity end that can withstand full weight-bearing. Below-knee amputations are preferred to above-knee amputations because of the importance of the knee joint and the energy requirements for walking. Preserving the knee joint of an elderly patient can mean the difference between walking with aids or being confined to a wheelchair. Knee disarticulations are most successful with young, active patients who are able to develop precise control of the prosthesis. When above-knee amputations are done, all possible length is preserved, muscles are stabilized and shaped, and hip contractures are prevented for maximum ambulatory potential. If a hip disarticulation amputation is done, most people must rely on a wheelchair for mobility.

Upper-extremity amputations are performed to preserve the maximum functional length. The prosthesis is fitted early for maximum function.

Amputation Approaches

The major surgical objective is to achieve uncomplicated healing of the amputation wound, resulting in a nontender residual limb (stump) with healthy skin for prosthesis use. The elderly may have slower healing because of preexisting poor nutrition and other health problems. Healing is enhanced by gentle han-

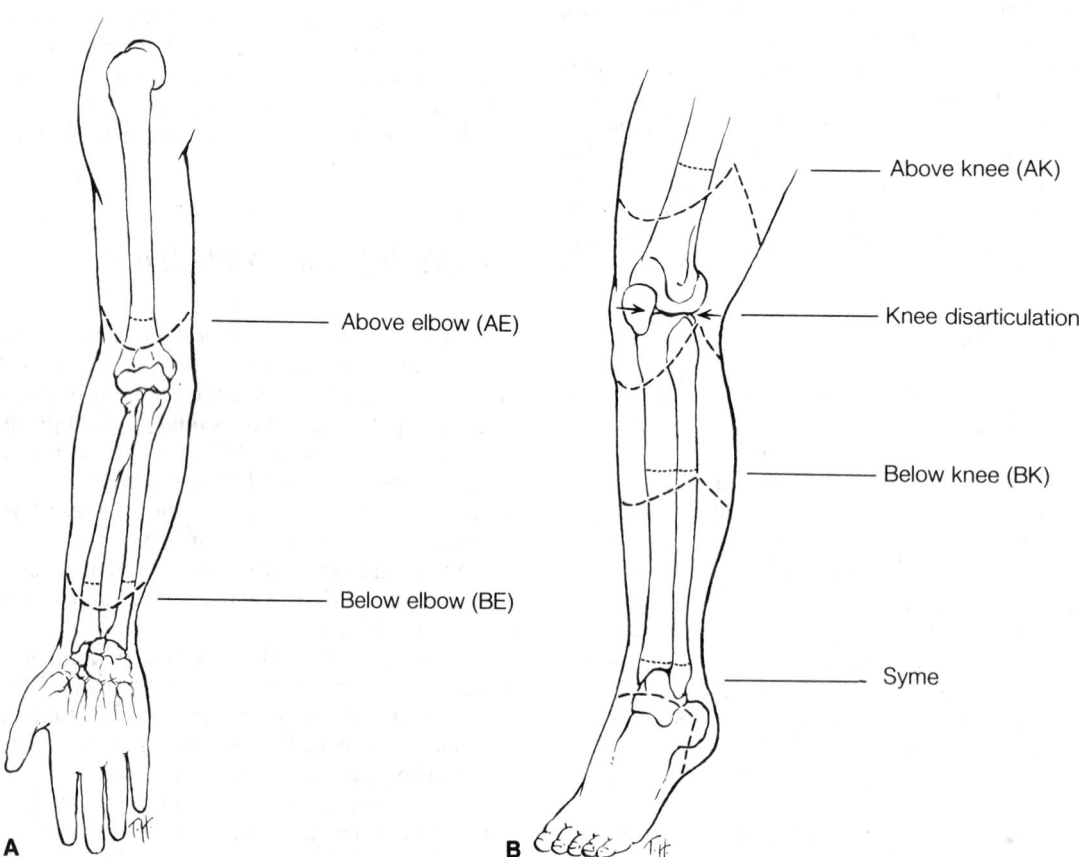

Figure 60–15. Levels of amputation are determined by circulatory adequacy, type of prosthesis, function of the part, and muscle balance. (**A**) Levels of amputation of upper extremity. (**B**) Levels of amputation of lower extremity.

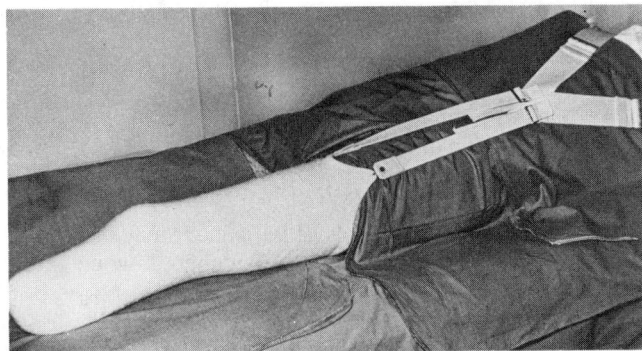

A

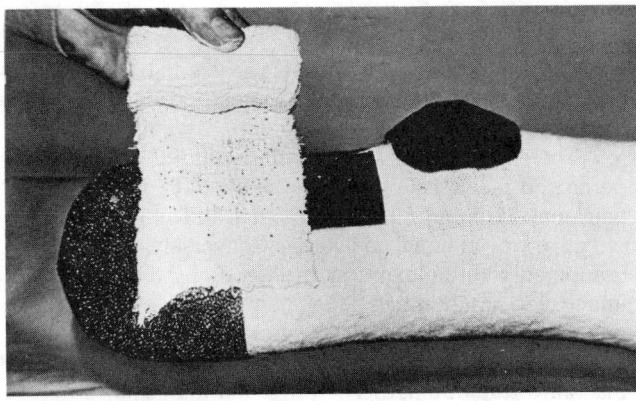

B

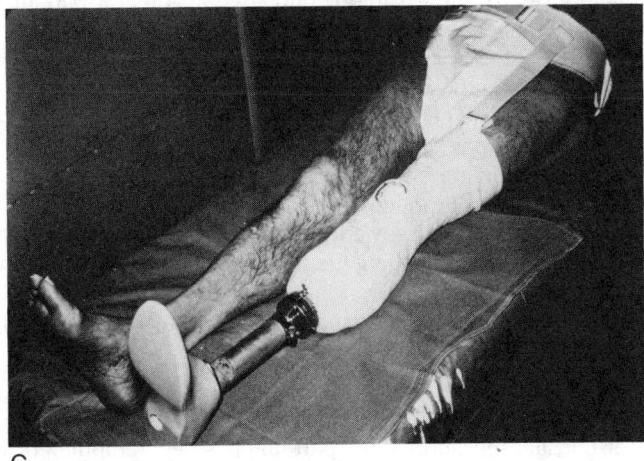

C

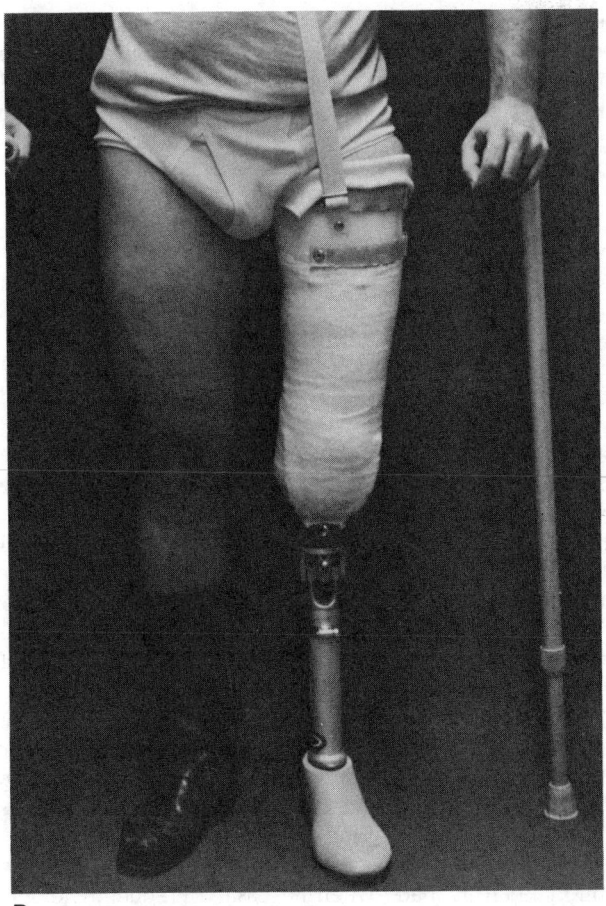

D

Figure 60–16. Immediate prosthetic fitting after amputation. (**A**) Sterile stocking held under firm tension as the rigid dressing is applied. (**B**) Pressure relief pads and distal polyurethane pad in place prior to application of the plaster of paris rigid dressing. (**C**) Complete assembly of components for the immediate postsurgical prosthetic fitting of the above-knee amputee. (**D**) Ambulation with temporary prosthetic extension (pylon) and an artificial foot. (Courtesy of the Prosthetics Research Study, Veterans Administration Contract V663P-784.)

dling of the residual limb, controlling residual limb edema through rigid or soft compression dressings, and using aseptic technique in wound care to avoid infection.

Rigid Cast Dressings. A closed *rigid cast dressing* is frequently used to provide uniform compression, to support soft tissues and thereby control pain, and to prevent contractures. Immediately after surgery, a rigid plaster dressing is applied and is equipped to attach a temporary prosthetic extension (pylon) and an artificial foot (Fig. 60–16). A sterilized residual limb sock is applied to the residual limb. Felt pads are placed over pressure-sensitive areas. Starting from the distal end, the residual limb is wrapped with elastic plaster of paris bandages while firm, even pressure is maintained. Care is taken not to constrict circulation. This rigid dressing technique is used as a

means for creating a socket for immediate postoperative prosthetic fitting. The length of the prosthesis is tailored to the individual patient.

The original cast may be left on for 10 to 14 days unless contraindicated by factors such as elevated body temperature, severe pain, or loose-fitting cast. A second cast is then applied, and changed, usually 10 to 14 days after the initial cast is changed.

Soft Dressings. When frequent inspection of the residual limb (stump) is desired, a *soft dressing*, with or without compression, may be used. An immobilizing splint may be incorporated in the dressing. Stump (wound) hematomas are controlled with wound drainage devices to minimize infection.

Staged Amputation. A staged amputation may be used

when gangrene and infection exist. Initially, a guillotine amputation is done to remove the dead and septic tissue. The wound is debrided and allowed to drain. The sepsis is treated with systemic antibiotics. In a few days, when the infection has been controlled and the patient has stabilized, a definitive amputation with skin closure is done.

▶ Nursing Process
The Patient Undergoing an Amputation

▷ Assessment

Before surgery, the neurovascular and functional status of the extremity must be evaluated through history and physical assessment (*e.g.*, color, temperature, palpable pulses, hair distribution, condition of skin, responses to positioning, sensations, pain, function). A Doppler (a hand-held ultrasonic instrument) may be used to evaluate arterial blood flow. Limitation of range of motion and presence of hip and knee flexion contractures may affect the function and fit of the prosthesis. The circulatory status and function of the unaffected extremity also are assessed.

If infection or gangrene exists, the patient may have associated enlarged lymph nodes, fever, and purulent drainage. A culture is taken to determine appropriate antibiotic therapy. If the patient has experienced a traumatic amputation, the function and condition of the residual limb are assessed.

The patient's nutritional status is evaluated and a plan for nutritional care is made when necessary. Frequently, elderly persons are poorly nourished, obese, or on special diets because of concurrent health problems. For wound healing, a balanced diet with adequate vitamins and protein is essential.

Any concurrent health problems (*e.g.*, dehydration, anemia, cardiac insufficiency, chronic respiratory problems, diabetes mellitus) need to be identified and treated so that the patient is in the best possible condition to withstand the trauma of surgery. The use of steroids, anticoagulants, vasoconstrictors, or vasodilators may influence management and wound healing.

An assessment of the patient's psychological status is very important. Determination of the patient's emotional reaction to amputation is essential for nursing care. Grief response to a permanent alteration in body image is appropriate. Even if the amputation decreases pain and increases functioning, major adjustments are needed. Coping will be facilitated by the presence of an adequate support system and professional help.

▷ Nursing Diagnoses

Based on the assessment data, the patient's major nursing diagnoses may include the following:

- Pain related to surgery
- Sensory/perceptual alteration: phantom limb sensations related to amputation
- Impaired skin integrity related to surgical amputation
- Body image disturbance related to amputation of body part
- Dysfunctional grieving related to loss of body part
- Self-care deficit: feeding, bathing, dressing, grooming, and toileting, related to loss of body part
- Impaired physical mobility related to loss of extremity

Nursing diagnoses related to potential complications of the surgery include:

- Altered tissue perfusion due to postoperative hemorrhage
- High risk for infection
- Impaired skin integrity

▷ Planning and Implementation

▷ *Goals:*   The major goals of the patient may include relief of pain, absence of altered sensory perceptions, wound healing, improved body image, resolution of grieving process, independence in self care, restoration of physical mobility, absence of complications such as hemorrhage, infection, and skin breakdown.

▷ Nursing Interventions

▷ *Relief of Pain.*   Surgical pain is located at the incision and can be readily controlled with analgesics or evacuation of the hematoma or accumulated fluid.

The expression of pain is individual. If the patient has experienced much discomfort before surgery, the postoperative pain may be interpreted as minimal and may be controlled effectively by minimal analgesics. Conversely, the pain may be combined with the expression of grief and alteration of body image, and not modified adequately by analgesics. Severe pain may be due to excessive pressure on a bony prominence or hematoma. The surgeon must be notified and the cause of the discomfort determined. The physician may split the cast and examine the residual limb. Evaluation of the patient's pain and responses to chosen interventions is an integral part of the nurse's management of pain.

Patients who are managed with a cast dressing experience less pain than those with soft dressings. Within a few days, the surgical pain is generally controlled effectively with oral analgesics and pain-modifying techniques.

Early minimal weight-bearing on the residual limb with the pylon attached produces little discomfort.

Muscle spasms may add to the patient's discomfort during convalescence. Changing the patient's position, application of heat, or placing a light sandbag on the residual limb to counteract the muscle spasm may improve the patient's level of comfort.

▷ *Absence of Altered Sensory Perceptions.*   Amputees often experience *phantom pain*, in which the patient describes pain or unusual sensation in the part that has been amputated. The sensation creates a feeling that the extremity is present and possibly crushed, cramped, or twisted in an abnormal position. These sensations are real and need to be accepted by the patient and the caregivers.

Phantom sensation will eventually disappear, but while it lasts it can have a disquieting effect on the patient. The pathogenesis of phantom limb phenomena is unknown. Keeping the patient active helps decrease the occurrence of phantom limb pain. Phantom limb pain may occur 2 to 3 months after amputation, and occurs more frequently in above-knee amputations.

When patients describe phantom pains or sensations, the nurse needs to acknowledge these disquieting feelings and help patients modify their perception of them. Distraction techniques and activity are helpful. Transcutaneous electrical nerve stimulation (TENS) may provide relief for some patients.

▷ *Promotion of Wound Healing.*   Skin integrity has been altered by the surgical amputation. Potential healing problems may exist in relation to associated peripheral vascular, nutritional, or other concurrent health problems such as diabetes mellitus.

To promote healing of the incision, edema is controlled by means of the cast dressing or compression dressing. This helps to reestablish the circulation and lymph drainage.

- *A most important consideration is that the residual limb remain in the plaster cast socket during the patient's entire hospitalization.* If the cast inadvertently comes off, the residual limb must immediately be wrapped with an elastic compression bandage and the surgeon notified so that another cast can be applied. Excessive edema will develop in a very short time and will result in a delay in rehabilitation.

The residual limb must be handled gently. Whenever the dressing is changed, aseptic technique is required to prevent wound infections and possible osteomyelitis.

When amputations of the leg are performed on elderly, debilitated patients, especially those with diabetes and arteriosclerosis, these patients may become incontinent of urine and feces. The dressing and the wound of the residual limb may become soiled. Plastic material secured by a wide adhesive strip around the leg above the dressing has proven to be a good method of protecting the residual limb from becoming soiled.

Residual limb shaping is important for prosthesis fitting. The patient needs to be taught how to wrap the residual limb with elastic dressings (Figs. 60–17 and 60–18). When the incision is healed, the patient is taught to care for the residual limb.

▷ *Enhanced Body Image.*   Although amputation is a reconstructive procedure, it alters the patient's body image. The patient will need to accept the irreversible changes. The nurse establishes a trusting relationship with the patient and communicates acceptance of the patient who has experienced an amputation. The patient is encouraged to look at, feel, and then care for the residual limb. Strengths of and resources available to the patient are identified to facilitate rehabilitation. Care is provided to assist the patient to regain the previous level of independent functioning. When patients perceive that others accept them as whole persons and they are able to resume responsibility for self-care, their self-concept improves and changes in body image are accepted. This process may take months.

▷ *Resolution of Grieving.*   The realization that an extremity has been removed may come as a shock even though the patient had been prepared preoperatively. The patient's behavior (*e.g.*, crying, withdrawal, apathy, anger) and expressed feelings (*e.g.*, depression, fear, helplessness) will demonstrate how the patient is beginning to cope with the loss and work through the grieving process. The nurse acknowledges the reality of the loss by listening and providing support.

Acceptance and support of the patient and family through a trusting relationship during all phases of the process will assist them in dealing with the loss. The patient and family are encouraged to express and share their feelings concerning the loss of an extremity and to work through the grief process.

Support available from family and friends promotes acceptance of the loss. The nurse helps the patient deal with immediate needs and become oriented to realistic rehabilitation goals and future independent functioning.

▷ *Independent Self-Care.*   Amputation of an extremity affects the patient's ability to care for himself. The patient is encouraged to be an active participant in self-care. The patient needs time to accomplish these tasks, and must not be hurried. Practicing an activity with consistent supportive supervision in a relaxed environment will enable the person to learn self-care skills. The patient and nurse need to maintain positive attitudes and minimize fatigue and frustration during the learning process.

Independence in dressing, toileting, and bathing (shower or tub) depends on balance, transfer abilities, and physiologic tolerance of the activities. The nurse works with the physical therapist and occupational therapist in teaching and supervising the patient in these self-care activities.

The upper-extremity amputee will have self-care deficits in feeding, bathing, and dressing. Assistance is provided only as needed; the patient is encouraged to learn to do the task without help and to learn how to use feeding and dressing aids for eventual independent activities of daily living. The nurse, therapists, and prosthetist work with the patient to achieve maximum independence.

▷ *Restored Physical Mobility.*   If the amputation is not an emergency procedure, efforts should be made preoperatively to strengthen the upper extremities as well as the trunk and the abdominal muscles. The extensor muscles in the arm and the depressor muscles in the shoulder especially need to be strengthened, as these muscle groups play an important part in crutch walking. The patient may flex and extend the arms while holding weights. Doing push-ups while in a prone position and sit-ups while seated will strengthen the triceps muscles. In addition, the patient should be taught to crutch walk before the surgical procedure to prepare for postoperative mobility.

Postoperative positioning to prevent development of hip or knee contracture is important. According to the surgeon's preference, the residual limb may be placed in an extended position or elevated for a brief period after surgery. If the residual limb is to be elevated, the foot of the bed should be raised.

- The residual limb should not be placed on a pillow because a flexion contraction of the hip may result. A contracture of the next joint above the amputation is a frequent complication.

In a lower extremity amputation, the patient should be encouraged to turn from side to side after the first 24 to 48 hours and to assume a prone position to stretch the flexor muscles and to prevent flexion contracture of the hip. A pillow may be placed under the abdomen and the residual limb, with the foot resting over the edge of the mattress. The legs should remain close together while the patient is in the prone position to prevent an abduction deformity.

Postoperative Exercises.   Postoperatively, range-of-motion exercises are started early because contracture deformities develop rapidly. Range of motion exercises are carried out to the hip and knee for below-the-knee amputations and to the hip for above-the-knee amputations. It is important that the patient

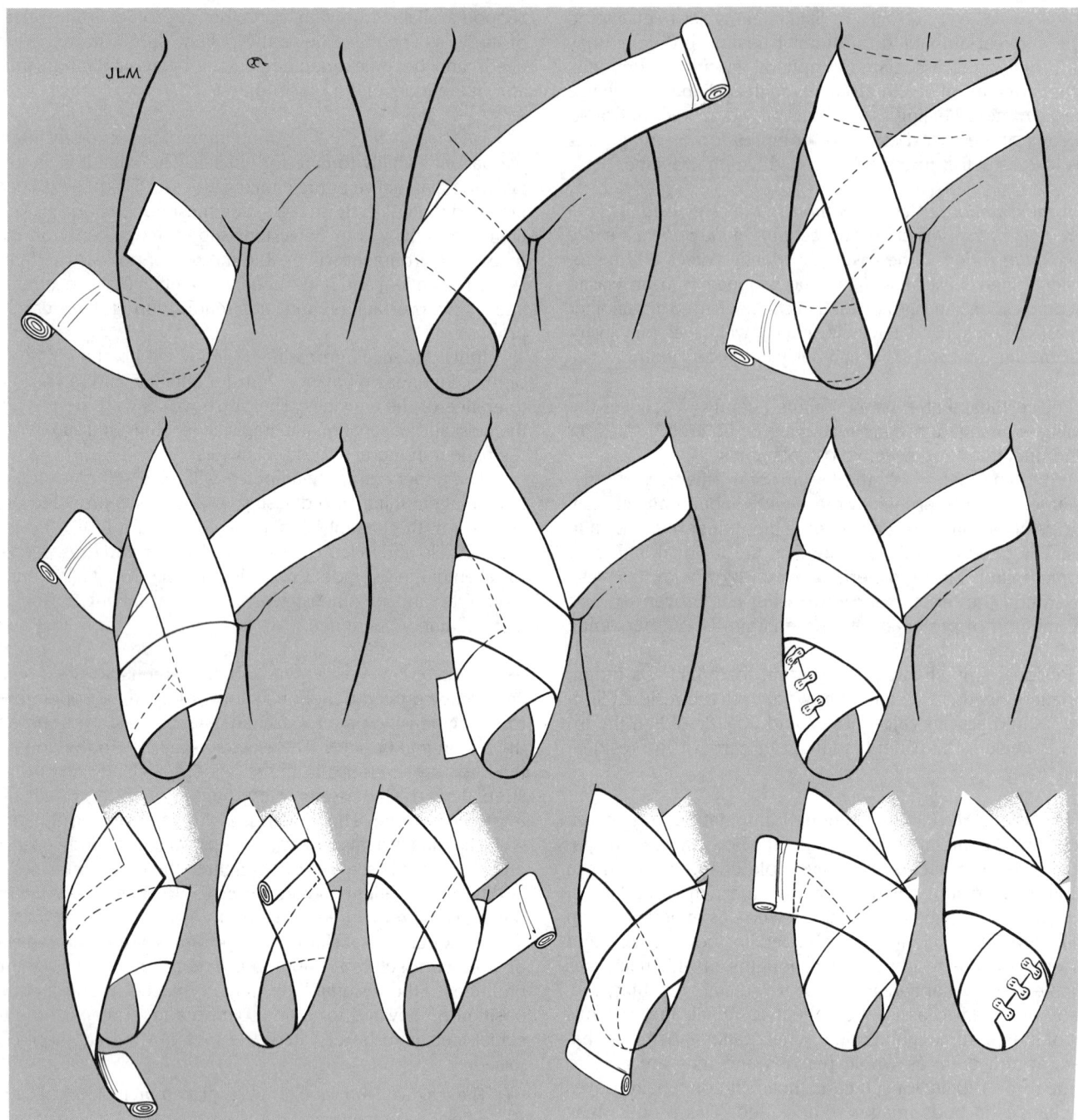

Figure 60–17. Wrapping above-knee residual limb. Elastic bandaging reduces edema and shapes the residual limb in a firm conical form for the prosthesis. (Suddarth DS. The Lippincott Manual of Nursing Practice, 5th ed. Philadelphia, JB Lippincott, 1991.)

recognize the value of moving the residual limb. Sitting for prolonged periods must be discouraged.

An overhead trapeze can be used by the patient to change position and strengthen the biceps. The triceps, necessary in crutch walking, can be strengthened by pressing the palms against the bed while pushing the body upward (push-up exercises). Exercises such as hyperextension of the residual limb, conducted under the supervision of the physical therapist, also aid in strengthening muscles as well as increasing circulation, reducing edema, and preventing atrophy.

Strength and endurance are assessed, and activities are increased gradually to prevent fatigue. As the patient progresses to independent use of the wheelchair, ambulation with aids, or ambulation with prosthesis, safety considerations are emphasized. Environmental barriers (*e.g.,* steps, inclines, doors, wet surfaces) are identified, and methods of managing them are practiced. Problems associated with the use of the mobility aids (*e.g.,* pressure on the axilla from crutches, skin irritation of the hands from wheelchair use, residual limb irritation from prosthesis) are identified and managed.

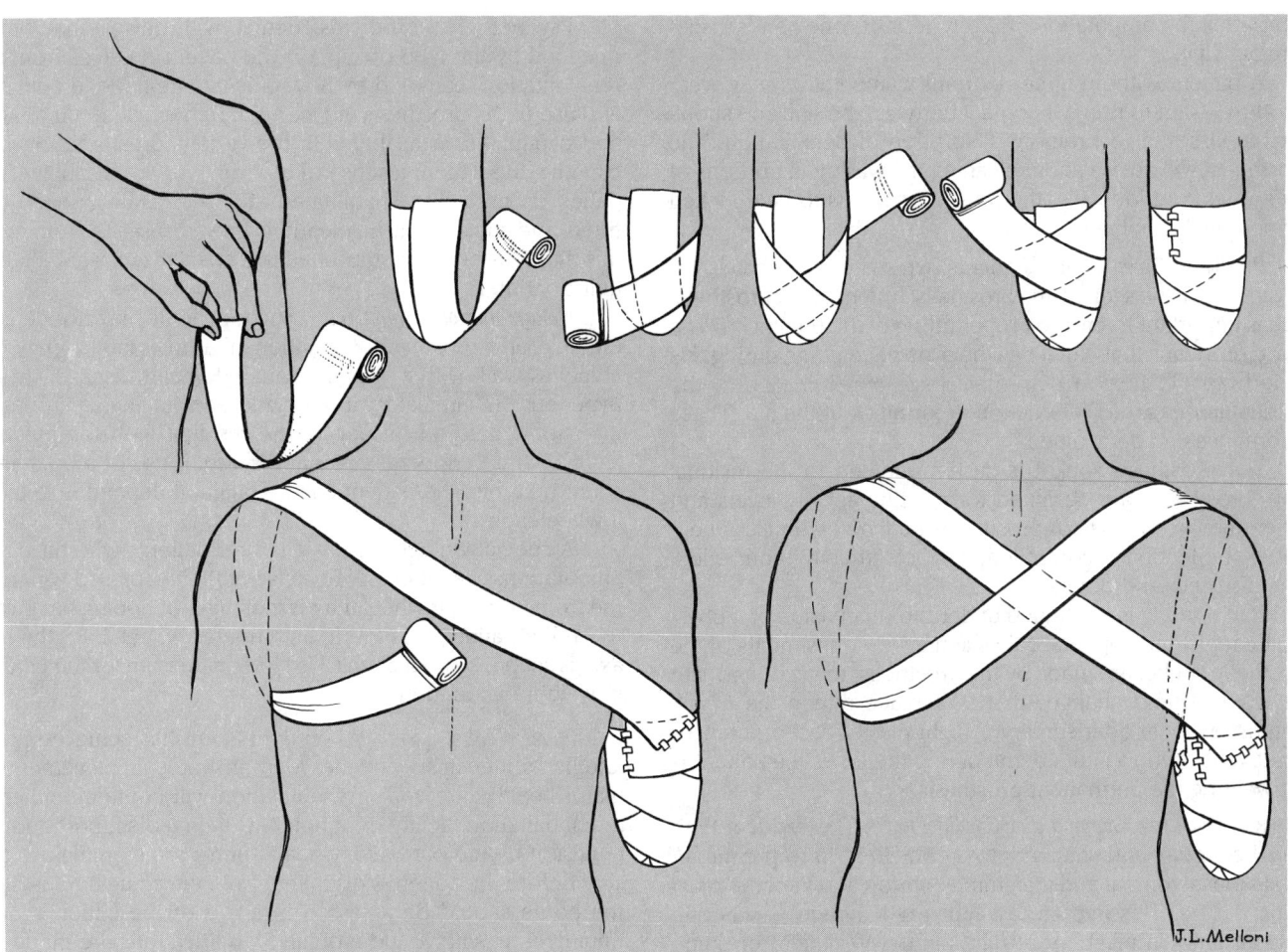

Figure 60–18.   Wrapping above-elbow residual limb. An elastic bandage wrapping for an above-elbow residual limb minimizes edema and shapes it for a prosthesis. The bandage may need to be secured by wrapping across the back and shoulders. (Suddarth DS. The Lippincott Manual of Nursing Practice, 5th ed. Philadelphia, JB Lippincott, 1991.)

Because an upper extremity amputee uses both shoulders to operate the prosthesis, the muscles of both shoulders are exercised. A patient with an above-the-elbow amputation or shoulder disarticulation is likely to develop a postural abnormality caused by loss of weight of the amputated extremity. Thus, postural exercises are helpful.

Ambulation.   Amputation changes the center of gravity, so the patient may need to practice position changes (*e.g.*, standing from sitting and standing on one foot). A well-fitting shoe with a nonslip sole should be worn. During position changes, the patient should be guarded and possibly stabilized with a transfer belt at the waist to prevent falling.

The patient is taught transfer techniques early. When the patient gets out of bed, good posture must be maintained. As soon as possible, the patient may stand between parallel bars or be raised to an upright position on a tilt table to allow extension of the temporary prosthesis to the floor with *minimal* weight-bearing.

- Excessive pressure on the residual limb is to be avoided because it may compromise wound healing.

How soon after surgery the patient is allowed to "touch down" the artificial foot depends on such factors as age and physical status and the condition of the other foot. Patients who are debilitated or have severe diabetes or peripheral vascular disease may not be able to tolerate the degree of pressure required to "touch down" the foot, and thus must wait for a longer period before starting this activity.

The patient usually stands between parallel bars twice daily. As endurance increases, ambulation is started within the parallel bars, but full weight-bearing is not permitted on the amputated side. Crutch walking is started when stable balance is achieved.

While crutch walking, the patient should learn to use a normal gait. The residual limb should move back and forth while the patient is walking with the crutches. To prevent a permanent flexion deformity from occurring, the residual limb should not be held up in a flexed position.

The patient with an upper extremity amputation is instructed in how to carry out the activities of daily living with one arm. The patient is started on one-handed self-care activities as soon as possible. The use of the temporary prosthesis is encouraged. The patient who learns to use the prosthesis soon after the amputation will rely less on one-handed self-care activities.

A patient with an upper extremity amputation may wear a cotton T-shirt to prevent contact between the skin and shoulder harness and to promote absorption of perspiration. The prosthetist will advise about cleaning the washable portions of the harness. Periodically, the prosthesis needs to be checked for potential problems.

Prosthesis Preparation. Patients who are candidates for prosthesis will be seen by the prosthetist. Effective preprosthetic care is important to ensure proper fitting of the prosthesis. The major problems that can delay the prosthetic fitting during this period are (1) flexion deformities, (2) nonshrinkage of the residual limb, and (3) abduction deformities of the hip. These deformities can be avoided.

The prosthesis socket is custom-molded to the residual limb. Prostheses are designed for specific activity levels and patient abilities. Types of prostheses include hydraulic, pneumatic, biofeedback-controlled, myoelectrically controlled, synchronized, and others.

Gait training is continued under the supervision of a physical therapist until optimal gait is achieved. Adjustments of the prosthetic socket are made by the prosthetist to accommodate the residual limb changes that take place during the first 6 months to a year after surgery. A light plaster cast or a tensor bandage is used to limit edema during the times the patient is not wearing the permanent prosthesis.

Residual Limb Shaping and Conditioning. The residual limb must be shrunk and shaped into a conical form to permit accurate measurement and maximum comfort and fit of the prosthetic device. This is done by applying bandages, an elastic residual limb shrinker, or an air splint. The patient or some member of the family can be taught the correct method of bandaging.

Bandaging supports the soft tissue and minimizes the formation of edematous fluid while the residual limb is in a dependent position. The bandage is applied in such a manner that the remaining muscles required to operate the prosthesis are as firm as possible, while those muscles that are no longer useful will atrophy (see Figs. 60–17 and 60–18). An improperly applied elastic bandage contributes to circulatory problems and a poorly shaped residual limb.

To "toughen" the residual limb in preparation for a prosthesis, activities to condition the residual limb are usually prescribed. The patient begins by pushing the residual limb into a soft pillow, then into a firmer pillow, and finally against a hard surface. The patient is taught to massage the residual limb to mobilize the scar, decrease tenderness, and improve vascularity. Massage is usually started when healing takes place, and is first done by the physical therapist. Skin inspection and preventive care are taught.

▷ *Rehabilitation.* The complete rehabilitation of a patient who has had an amputation requires the concerted efforts of the entire rehabilitation team. The orthopedic surgeon, the nurse, the physiatrist, the prosthetist (limb maker), the physical therapist, and the occupational therapist all unite their efforts to condition and train the patient to make a satisfactory adjustment to the prosthesis. The establishment of prosthetic clinics has improved the outlook of patients. With vocational counseling and job retraining where necessary, many of these patients can return to work.

Psychological problems (denial, withdrawal) may be influenced by the type of support the patient receives from the rehabilitation team and by how quickly one-handed activities and use of the prosthesis are learned. Knowing the full options and capabilities available with the various prosthetic devices can give the patient a sense of control over the disability. The patient is not fully rehabilitated until a prosthesis has been fitted and the patient has learned how to use it. Training of this nature is best accomplished in a specialized rehabilitation unit or center.

Nonambulatory Amputees. Some patients may not be candidates for a prosthesis. Conditions that may limit a patient's ability to walk with a prosthesis include heart disease, stroke, hypertension, circulatory insufficiency, advancing age, obesity, infections, delayed healing of the residual limb (amputation stump), and peripheral vascular disease. If use of a prosthesis is not possible, the patient can be taught independence using a wheelchair.

A special wheelchair designed for patients who have had amputations is advocated. Because of the decreased weight in the front, a regular wheelchair is in danger of tipping backward when the patient sits in it. In an amputee wheelchair, the rear axle is set back about 5 cm (2 in) to compensate for the change in weight distribution.

▷ *Home Health Care.* When the patient has achieved physiologic homeostasis and has demonstrated achievement of major health care goals, rehabilitation will continue either in a rehabilitation facility or at home. Continued support and supervision by the community health nurse are essential.

Before the patient's discharge from the acute care facility, the home should be assessed in terms of the patient's continuing care, safety, and mobility. Modifications are made according to the individual patient's needs. An overnight or weekend experience at home may be tried to identify problems that were not identified on the assessment visit. Physical therapy and occupational therapy may continue in the home or on an outpatient basis. Transportation to continuing health care appointments must be arranged. The social service department of the hospital or community agency managing continued health care may be of great assistance in securing personal assistance and transportation services.

During follow-up health visits, the nurse evaluates the patient's physical and psychosocial adjustment. Periodic preventive health assessments are necessary. Frequently, an elderly spouse is unable to provide the assistance required, and additional help at home is needed. Modifications in the care plan are made on the basis of such findings. Often, the patient and family find involvement in an amputee support group to be of value. Here they are able to share problems, solutions, and resources. Talking with those who have successfully dealt with a similar problem may help the patient develop a satisfactory solution.

▷ *Absence of Complications.* After any surgery, efforts are made to reestablish homeostasis and prevent problems related to surgery, anesthesia, and immobility.

Assessment of body systems (*e.g.*, respiratory, gastrointestinal, genitourinary) for problems associated with immobility (*e.g.*, pneumonia, anorexia, constipation, urinary stasis) is needed, and corrective management is instituted. Avoiding problems associated with immobility and restoring physical activity are necessary for maintenance of health.

Absence of Hemorrhage. The most threatening problem is massive hemorrhage due to a loosened ligature. The patient is monitored carefully for any signs or symptoms of bleeding. The patient's vital signs are monitored, and suction drainage is observed frequently.

- Immediate postoperative bleeding may develop slowly or take the form of a massive hemorrhage resulting from a loosened ligature.
- A large tourniquet should be in plain sight at the patient's bedside so that, if severe bleeding occurs, the tourniquet can be applied to the residual limb to control the hemorrhage.
- The surgeon is notified immediately in the event of excessive bleeding.

Absence of Infection. The nurse needs to observe for drainage, odor, and increasing discomfort, which may indicate infection or necrosis. These problems should be reported to the surgeon promptly. Systemic indicators of infection need to be monitored. Patients who have undergone amputation frequently have poor circulation, contaminated wound, or concurrent health problems that may contribute to wound infections.

Absence of Skin Breakdown. Immobilization and pressure from various aids may contribute to skin breakdown. The prosthesis may cause pressure areas to develop. The nurse assesses the skin for breaks.

Careful skin hygiene is essential to prevent skin irritation, infection, and breakdown. The residual limb is washed and dried (gently) at least twice daily. The skin is inspected for pressure areas, dermatitis, and blisters. If present, they must be treated before a major problem develops. Usually, a residual limb sock is worn to absorb perspiration and avoid direct contact between the skin and the prosthetic socket. The residual limb sock is changed daily and must fit smoothly to prevent the irritation caused by wrinkles. The socket of the prosthesis is washed with a mild detergent, rinsed, and dried thoroughly with a clean cloth. The patient is advised that the socket must be thoroughly dry before the prosthesis is applied.

▷ Evaluation

Expected Outcomes

1. Experiences absence of pain
   a. Appears relaxed
   b. Verbalizes comfort
   c. Uses measures to increase comfort
   d. Participates in self-care and rehabilitative activities
2. Experiences absence of phantom limb pain
   a. Reports not perceiving sensations from amputated part
   b. Verbalizes absence of abnormal sensation in residual limb
3. Achieves wound healing
   a. Controls residual limb edema
   b. Achieves healed, nontender, nonadherent scar
   c. Demonstrates residual limb care
4. Demonstrates improved body image
   a. Acknowledges change in body image
   b. Participates in self-care activities
   c. Demonstrates increasing independence
   d. Projects self as a whole person
   e. Resumes role-related responsibilities
   f. Reestablishes social contacts
   g. Demonstrates confidence in abilities
5. Exhibits resolution of grieving
   a. Expresses grief
   b. Uses family and friends to work through feelings
   c. Focuses on future functioning
6. Achieves independent self-care
   a. Asks for assistance when needed
   b. Uses aids and assistive devices to facilitate self-care
   c. Verbalizes satisfaction with abilities to perform activities of daily living
7. Achieves maximum independent mobility
   a. Avoids positions contributing to contracture development
   b. Demonstrates full active range of motion
   c. Maintains balance when sitting and transferring
   d. Increases strength and endurance
   e. Demonstrates safe transferring technique
   f. Achieves functional use of prosthesis
   g. Overcomes environmental barriers to mobility
   h. Uses community services and resources as needed
8. Exhibits absence of complications of hemorrhage, infection, skin breakdown
   a. Does not experience excessive bleeding
   b. Maintains normal blood values
   c. Is free of local and systemic signs of infection
   d. Repositions self frequently
   e. Is free of pressure-related problems
   f. Reports any skin discomfort and irritations promptly

In summary, amputations may be necessary because of progressive peripheral vascular disease, trauma, congenital deformity, or malignant tumor. Amputation is considered to be reconstructive surgery designed to improve the patient's quality of life. Problems that the patient may encounter associated with amputation include pain, phantom limb sensations, altered skin integrity, disturbed body image, grieving, self-care deficit, and impaired mobility as well as hemorrhage, infection, and skin breakdown. Rehabilitation after amputation is a multidisciplinary effort. The nurse focuses on the patient's physical and psychological responses and adjustment to the amputation and promotion of health.

Bibliography

Books

Adams JC. Outline of Fractures, 9th ed. Edinburgh, Churchill Livingstone, 1987.

American Nurses Association and National Association of Orthopaedic Nurses. Orthopaedic Nursing Practice. Kansas City, MO, American Nurses Association, 1986

Apley AG and Solomon L. Concise System of Orthopaedics and Fractures. London, Butterworths, 1988.

Bohne WHD. Atlas of Amputation Surgery. New York, Thieme Medical Publishers, 1987.

Dandy DJ. Essential Orthopaedics and Trauma. Edinburgh, Churchill Livingstone, 1989.

Dee R et al. Principles of Orthopaedic Practice, Vols 1 & 2. New York, McGraw–Hill, 1988.

Farrell J. Illustrated Guide to Orthopedic Nursing, 3rd ed. Philadelphia, JB Lippincott, 1986.

Gates SJ and Mooar PA. Orthopaedics and Sports Medicine for Nurses. Baltimore, Williams & Wilkins, 1989.

Garhardt JJ et al. Interdisciplinary Rehabilitation in Orthopedic Medicine. Toronto, Han Huber, 1987.

Hughes SPF et al (eds). Orthopaedics; The Principles and Practice of Musculoskeletal Surgery and Fractures. Edinburgh, Churchill Livingstone, 1987.

Iversen LD and Clawson DK. Manual of Acute Orthopaedic Therapeutics, 3rd ed. Boston, Little Brown, 1987.

Mears DC and Rubash HE. Pelvic and Acetabular Fractures. Thorofare, NJ, Slack, 1986.

Mourad LA and Droste MM. The Nursing Process in the Care of Adults with Orthopaedic Conditions, 2nd ed. New York, John Wiley & Sons, 1988.

Paton DF. Fractures and Orthopaedics. Edinburgh, Churchill Livingstone, 1988.

Powell M (ed). Orthopaedic Nursing and Rehabilitation, 9th ed. Edinburgh, Churchill Livingstone, 1986.

Salmond S et al (eds). Core Curriculum for Orthopaedic Nurses, 2nd ed. Pitman, NJ, National Association of Orthopaedic Nurses, 1991.

Smith C. Orthopaedic Nursing. London, Heinemann Nursing, 1987.

Stearns CM and Brunner NA. Opcare: Orthopedic Patient Care: A Nursing Guide, Vols 1–3. Rutherford, NJ, Howmedica, 1987.

Journals

Asterisks indicate nursing research articles.

Musculoskeletal Injuries

Cabot A. Tennis elbow: A curable affliction. Orthop Rev 1987 May; 16(5): 322–326.

Clark S et al. Rotator cuffs: Tears, repairs, and care. CONA J 1987 Sep; 9(3): 9–13.

Diamond JE. Rehabilitation of ankle sprains. Clin Sports Med 1989 Oct; 8(4): 13–18.

Folcik MA. Winter sports injuries: An overview. Orthop Nurs 1988 Nov/Dec; 7(6): 25–28.

Hoshowsky VM. Chronic lateral ligament instability of the ankle. Orthop Nurs 1988 May/Jun; 7(3): 33–40.

McInerney VR et al. Rehabilitation of the sports-injured patient. Orthop Clin North Am 1988 Oct; 19(4): 725–735.

Montgomery JB. Dislocation of the knee. Orthop Clin North Am 1987 Jan; 18(1): 149–156.

Nemeth VA. Ankle sprains: Recognition and management. Hosp Med 1987 Jun; 23(6): 146, 148–149.

Norris TR. Recurrent posterior shoulder subluxations. Hosp Med 1990 Apr; 26(4): 45+.

Spalj N et al. The school nurse's role in managing athletic injuries. J Sch Health 1989 Aug; 59(6): 271–273.

* Wild E et al. Analysis of wrist injuries in workers engaged in repetative tasks. AAOHN J 1987 Aug; 35(8): 356–366.

Fractures

American Pain Society. Relieving pain: An analgesic guide. Am J Nurs 1988 Jun; 88(6): 815–825.

Antrum R and Solomkin J. A review of antibiotic prophylaxis of open fractures. Orthop Rev 1987 Apr; 16(4): 246–254.

Bach AW and Hansen ST Jr. Plates versus external fixation in severe open tibial shaft fractures. Clin Orthop 1989 Apr; 261: 89–94.

Bone L and Bucholz R. The management of fractures in the patient with multiple trauma. J Bone Joint Surg (Am) 1986 Jun; 68A(6): 945–949.

Burgess AR et al. Pedestrian tibial injuries. J Trauma 1987 Jun; 27(6): 596–601.

Burgess AR et al. Management of open grade III tibial fractures. Orthop Clin North Am 1987 Jan; 18(1): 85–93.

Carlson DC. Common fractures of the extremities: How to recognize and treat them. Postgrad Med 1988 Mar; 83(4): 311–317.

Cochran S. Action STAT! Open fracture. Nursing 1987 May; 17(5): 33.

Dellinger EP et al. Risk of infection after open fracture on the arm or leg. Arch Surg 1988 Nov; 123(11): 1320–1327.

Dellinger EP et al. Duration of preventive antibiotic administration for open extremity fractures. Arch Surg 1988 Mar; 123(3): 333–339.

Fractured fewer with internal fixation. Orthop Nurs 1987 Mar/Apr; 6(2): 38–41.

Gabel GT et al. Intraarticular fractures of the distal numerous in the adult. Clin Orthop 1987 Mar; (216): 99–108.

Gershuni DH et al. Fracture of the tibia complicated by acute compartment syndrome. Clin Orthop 1987 Apr; (217): 221–227.

Harper MC and Hardin G. Posterior malleolar fractures of the ankle associated with external rotation-abduction injuries. Results with the without internal fixation. J Bone Joint Surg [Am] 1988 Oct; 70(9): 1348–1356.

Herron DG and Nance J. Emergency department nursing management of patients with orthopedic fractures resulting from motor vehicle accidents. Nurs Clin North Am 1990 Mar; 25(1): 73–83.

Johnson KD (ed.). Complicated fractures. Orthop Clin North Am 1987 Jan; 18(1).

Matta JM and Merritt PO. Displaced acetabular fractures. Clin Orthop 1988 May; (230): 83–97.

Mayo KA. Fractures of the acetabulum. Orthop Clin North Am 1987 Jan; 18(1): 43–51.

Merritt K. Factors increasing the risk of infection in patients with open fractures. J Trauma 1988 Jun; 28(6): 823–827.

Mims BC. Fat embolism syndrome: A variant of ARDS. Orthop Nurs 1989 May/Jun; 8(3): 22–28.

Mooney V and Stills M. Continuous passive motion with joint fractures and infections. Orthop Clin North Am 1987 Jan; 18(1): 1–9.

Ross D. Acute compartment syndrome. Orthop Nurs 1991 Mar/Apr; 10(2): 33–38.

Seyfer AE and Lower R. Later results of free muscle flaps and delayed bone grafting in the secondary treatment of open distal tibial fractures. Plast Reconstr Surg 1989 Jan; 83(1): 77–84.

Srabo RM and Weber SC. Comminuted intraarticular fractures of the distal radius. Clin Orthop 1988 Mar; 230: 39–48.

tenDuis HJ et al. Fat embolism in patients with an isolated fracture of the femoral shaft. J Trauma 1988 Mar; 28(3): 383–390.

Waldrop J et al. Fractures of the posterolateral tibial plateau. Am J Sports Med 1988 Sep/Oct; 16(5): 492–498.

Hip Fractures

Barangen J. Factors that influence recovery from hip fracture during hospitalization. Orthop Nurs 1990 Sept/Oct; 9(5): 19–29.

Barnes B et al. Functional outcomes after hip fracture. Phys Ther 1987 Nov; 67(11): 1675–1679.

Billing N et al. Hip fracture, depression, cognitive impairment: A follow-up study. Orthop Rev 1988 Mar; 17(3): 315–320.

Cummings SR et al. Recovery of function after hip fracture: The role of social supports. J Am Geriatr Soc 1988 Sep; 36(9): 801–806.

Dubrouskis V et al. Hip fracture in the elderly: Program planning puts these patients on their feet again. Can Nurse 1988 May; 84(5): 20–22.

Felson DT. Prevention of hip fractures. Hosp Pract 1988 Sep; 23(9A): 23–32, 37–38.

* Gleit C and Graham B. Secondary data analysis: A valuable resource. Nurs Res 1989 Nov/Dec; 38(5): 380–381.

Furstenberg A. Attributions of control by hip fracture patients. Health Soc Work 1988 Winter; 13(1): 43–48.

Gustafson V et al. Acute confusional states in elderly patients treated for femoral neck fracture. J Am Geriatr Soc 1988 Jun; 36(6): 525–530.

Jette AM et al. Functional recovery after hip fracture. Arch Phys Med Rehabil 1987 Oct; 68(10): 735–740.

Kauffman TL et al. Rehabilitation outcomes after hip fracture in persons 90 years old or older. Arch Phys Med Rehabil 1987 Jun; 68(6): 369–371.

Krug BM. The hip: Nursing fracture patients to full recovery. RN 1989 Apr; 52(4): 56–61.

Nelson L et al. Improving pain management for hip fractured elderly. Orthop Nurs 1990 May/Jun; 9(3): 79–83.

Palmer RM et al. The impact of the prospective payment system on the treatment of hip fractures in the elderly. Arch Intern Med 1989 Oct; 149(10): 2237–2241.

Reinhard S. Case managing community services for hip fractured elders. Orthop Nurs 1988 Sep/Oct; 7(5): 42–49, 71.

Pryor GA. Rehabilitation after hip fractures. J Bone Joint Surg [Br] 1989 May; 71B(3): 471–474.

Pryor GA et al. Team management of the elderly patient with hip fracture. Lancet 1988 Feb 20; 1(8582): 401–403.

Schoen DC. Assessing a fractured hip. Nursing 1987 Mar; 17(3): 97–98.

* Wells DL et al. Voiding dysfunction in geriatric patients with hip fracture: Prevalence rate and tentative nursing intervention. Orthop Nurs 1986 Nov/Dec; 5(6): 25–28.

Pelvic Fractures

Coyer HM et al. Pelvic fracture classification: Correlation with hemorrhage. J Trauma 1988 Jul; 28(7): 973–980.

Denis F et al. Sacral fractures: An important problem. Clin Orthop 1988 Feb; (227): 67–81.

Johnson L. Operative management of unstable pelvic fractures. Orthop Nurs 1989 Jul/Aug; 8(4): 21–25.

Kellan JF et al. The unstable pelvic fracture: Operative treatment. Orthop Clin North Am 1987 Jan; 18(1): 25–41.

Lin PS et al. Acute bowel entrapment and perforation following operative reduction of pelvic fracture. J Trauma 1987 Jun; 27(6): 684–686.

Lowe MA et al. Risk factors for urethral injuries in men with traumatic pelvic fractures. J Urol 1988 Sep; 140(3): 506–507.

Meyer PS. Urologic complications associated with pelvic fractures. Orthop Nurs 1989 Jul/Aug; 8(4): 41–44.

Mucha P Jr and Welch TJ. Hemorrhage in major pelvic fractures. Surg Clin North Am 1988 Aug; 68(4): 757–773.

Polando G et al. PASG use in pelvic fracture immobilization . . . Pneumatic antishock garments. JEMS 1990 Mar; 15(3): 48–49, 51–52, 55+.

Peter NK. Care of patients with traumatic pelvic fractures. Crit Care Nurs 1988 May; 8(3): 62–70.

Seibel RW and Flint L. Management of complicated pelvic fractures. Curr Surg 1986 Sep/Oct; 43(5): 391–394.

Spirnak JP. Pelvic fracture and injury to the lower urinary tract. Surg Clin North Am 1988 Oct; 88(5): 1057–1069.

Tile M. Pelvic ring fractures: Should they be fixed? J Bone Joint Surg [Br] 1988 Jan; 70(1): 1–12.

Unkle D and Delong W. Abdominal trauma associated with pelvic fractures. Orthop Nurs 1989 Jul/Aug; 8(4): 27–30.

Ward EF et al. Open reduction and internal fixation of vertical shear pelvic fractures. J Trauma 1987 Mar; 27(3): 291–295.

Amputation

Adler JC et al. Treadmill training program for a bilateral below-knee amputee patient with cardiopulmonary disease. Arch Phys Med Rehabil 1987 Dec; 68(12): 858–861.

Barker-Stotts KA. Action STAT! Traumatic amputation. Nursing 1988 May; 18(5): 51.

Beekman C and Antell L. Prosthetic use in elderly patients with dysvascular above-knee and through knee amputations. Phys Ther 1987 Oct; 67(10): 1510–1516.

Bild DE et al. Lower-extremity amputation in people with diabetes: Epidemiology and prevention. Diabetes Care 1989 Jan; 12(1): 24–31.

Broadhurst C. Adjusting to amputation. Nurs Times 1989 Oct 25–31; 85(43): 55–57.

Ceccio CM et al. Teaching the elderly amputee to meet the world. RN 1988 Sep; 51(9): 70–77.

Colen LB. Limb salvage in the patient with severe peripheral vascular disease. Plast Reconstr Surg 1987 Mar; 79(3): 389–395.

Cotter DHB. Artificial limbs. Br Med J 1988 Apr 23; 296(6630): 1185–1187.

Finsen V et al. Transcutaneous electrical nerve stimulation after major amputation. J Bone Joint Surg [Br] 1988 Jan; 70B(1): 109–112.

Gavant ML. Digital subtraction angiography of the foot in atherosclerotic occlusive disease. South Med J 1989 Mar; 82(3): 328–334.

Huber PM et al. Prosthetic problem inventory scale. Rehabil Nurs 1988 Nov/Dec; 13(6): 326–329.

* Medhat A et al. Factors that influence level of activities in persons with lower extremity amputation. Rehabil Nurs 1990 Jan/Feb: 15(1): 13–18.

Miller RA et al. Immediate postop prosthesis. Am J Nurs 1987 Mar; 87(3): 310–311.

Moore TJ et al. Prosthetic usage following major lower extremity amputation. Clin Orthop 1989 Jan; (238): 219–242.

Mouratoglou VM. Amputees and phantom limb pain: A literature review. Physiother Pract 1986 Dec; 2(4): 177–185.

Pinzur MS et al. Psychological testing in amputation rehabilitation. Clin Orthop 1988 Apr; (229): 236–240.

Osterman HM et al. Amputation: Last resort or new beginning? Geriatr Nurs 1987 Sep/Oct; 8(5): 246–248.

Stern PH. Occlusive vascular disease of lower limbs: Diagnosis, amputation surgery and rehabilitation. Am J Phys Med Rehabil 1988 Aug; 67(4): 145–154.

Wyss CR et al. Transcutaneous oxygen tension as a predictor of success after an amputation. J Bone Joint Surg [Am] 1988 Feb; 70A(2): 203–207.

Agencies

Amputees in Motion
  P.O. Box 2703, Escondido, CA 92025
Amputee Shoe and Glove Exchange
  P.O. Box 27067, Houston, TX 77227
Association for the Handicapped (Sports Program)
  350 Fifth Ave., Suite 1829, New York, NY 10017
National Amputation Foundation
  1245 150th Street, Whitestone, NY 11357
National Easter Seal Society
  70 E. Lake Street, Chicago, IL 60601
National Handicapped Sports and Recreation Association
  1145 19th Street NW, Suite 717, Washington, DC 20036
National Institute of Arthritis and Musculoskeletal and Skin Diseases
  National Institutes of Health, Bethesda, MD 20892
National Odd Shoe Exchange
  P.O. Box 56845, Phoenix, AZ 85079

61

Management of Patients With Musculoskeletal Disorders

Learning Objectives

On completion of this chapter, the learner will be able to:

1. Use the nursing process as a framework for care of the patient with low back pain
2. Describe the rehabilitation and health education needs of the patient with low back pain
3. Use the nursing process as a framework for care of the patient undergoing surgery of the hand or wrist
4. Use the nursing process as a framework for care of the patient undergoing foot surgery
5. Use the nursing process as a framework for care of the patient with spontaneous vertebral fracture related to osteoporosis
6. Use the nursing process as a framework for care of the patient with osteomalacia
7. Specify the drug therapy program for the patient with Paget's disease
8. Use the nursing process as a framework for care of the patient with osteomyelitis
9. Use the nursing process as a framework for care of the patient with a bone tumor

Common Musculoskeletal Problems

Low Back Pain

Back pain is a major health problem. An estimated 80% of the population will experience low back pain sometime during their lifetime. Impairment of the back and spine is the third leading cause of disability of people in their employment years. The limitations imposed by low back pain on the individual are severe. The economic cost, in terms of loss of productivity, is in the billions of dollars. The number of medical visits resulting from low back pain is second only to those for upper respiratory illnesses.

Low back pain may be caused by a large variety of conditions. Most low back pain is caused by musculoskeletal problems (*e.g.*, acute lumbosacral strain, unstable lumbosacral ligaments and weak muscles, osteoarthritis of the spine, spinal stenosis, intervertebral disc problems, inequality of leg length). Older patients may have back pain associated with osteoporotic vertebral fractures or bone metastasis. Other causes include kidney disorders, pelvic problems, retroperitoneal tumors, abdominal aneurysms, and psychosomatic problems. Most back pain due to musculoskeletal disturbances is aggravated by activity, whereas pain due to other considerations is not influenced by activity.

Obesity, stress, and occasionally depression may contribute to low back pain. Patients with chronic low back pain may develop a dependence on alcohol or analgesics.

Pathophysiology

The spinal column can be considered as an elastic rod constructed of rigid units (vertebrae) and flexible units (intervertebral discs) that are held together by complex facet joints, multiple ligaments, and paravertebral muscles. The unique construction of the back allows for flexibility while providing maximum protection for the spinal cord. The spinal curves absorb vertical shocks from running and jumping. The trunk helps to stabilize the spine. The abdominal and thoracic muscles are important in lifting activities. Disuse weakens these supporting structures. Obesity, postural problems, structural problems, or overstretching of the spinal supports may result in back pain.

The intervertebral discs change in character as the person ages. In the young, the disc is mainly fibrocartilage with a gelatinous matrix. It becomes dense, irregular fibrocartilage in the elderly. Disc degeneration is a common cause of back pain. Lower lumbar discs, L4–L5 and L5–S1, are subject to the greatest mechanical stress and the greatest degenerative changes. Disc protrusion (herniated nucleus pulposa) or facet joint changes can cause pressure on nerve roots as they leave the spinal canal, which results in pain that radiates along the nerve. About 12% of the people with low back pain have herniated nucleus pulposa. (Management of intervertebral disc disease is discussed on p. 1749.)

Clinical Manifestations

The patient complains of either acute back pain (present less than 3 days) or chronic back pain (lasting more than 2 months without improvement) and fatigue. During the initial interview, the location of the pain, its character, and whether it radiates along a nerve root (*sciatica*) are assessed. If the pain is of musculoskeletal origin, movement usually accentuates the pain.

The patient's gait, spinal mobility, reflexes, leg length, motor strength, and sensory perception are evaluated, along with the degree of discomfort experienced. Straight leg raising that causes pain indicates spinal root irritation.

Physical examination may disclose *paravertebral muscle spasm* (greatly increased muscle tone of the back postural muscles) with a loss of the normal lumbar lordotic curve and possible spinal deformity. When the patient is examined in a prone position, paraspinal muscles relax and any deformity caused by spasm disappears.

If the patient has *radiculopathy* (nerve root problem) or chronic back pain, multiple diagnostic studies may be necessary.

At times, an organic basis for the back pain cannot be identified. Anxiety and stress may evoke muscle spasms and pain. Chronic low back pain may be a manifestation of depression or mental conflict or a reaction to environmental and life stressors.

When working with individuals with chronic low back pain, the nurse needs insight into family relationships, environmental variables, and work situations. In addition, the impact of chronic pain on the emotional well-being of the patient is assessed. The nursing care plan for the patient with chronic back pain may include psychiatric interventions to help the patient deal effectively with depression and psychosocial stressors that contribute to the chronic pain.

Diagnostic Evaluation

Multiple diagnostic tests may be performed to accurately diagnose the cause of back pain and nerve root compression and pain. The nurse must prepare the patient for these studies, provide the necessary support during the testing period, and monitor him for any adverse responses to the procedures.

The following diagnostic procedures may be prescribed for the patient with low back pain. An x-ray of the spine may demonstrate the presence of fracture, dislocation, infection, osteoarthritis, or scoliosis. Computed tomography (CT) is useful in identifying underlying problems such as obscure soft-tissue lesions adjacent to the vertebral column and problems of vertebral discs. Ultrasound helps to diagnose narrow spinal canals. Magnetic resonance imaging (MRI) aids in visualizing the nature and location of spinal pathology. Myelogram and *discogram* (in which a small amount of contrast medium is injected into the intervertebral disc) may be performed to demonstrate degenerative disc or disc protrusions. Epidural venograms assess lumbar disc disease by demonstrating displacement of epidural veins. Electromyogram (EMG) and nerve conduction studies are used to evaluate radiculopathies.

▶ Nursing Process
The Patient With Low Back Pain

▷ Assessment

The patient with low back pain is encouraged to describe the discomfort. Descriptions of how the problem occurred, with a specific action (*e.g.*, opening a garage door) or with an activity in which weak muscles were overused (*e.g.*, weekend gardening) and how the patient has dealt with it will suggest areas for intervention and patient teaching. If this is a recurrent problem, information about previous successful pain control helps in planning current management. Additionally the patient may indicate how this back problem is affecting his life style. Information about job and recreational activities helps to identify areas for back health education.

During the interview, the nurse observes the patient's posture, position changes, and gait. Generally, the patient guards his movements, keeping the back as still as possible, and selects a chair for support with arms and a standard seat height. The patient may sit and stand in an unusual position, leaning away from the most painful side, and may ask for assistance when undressing because back movements are uncomfortable.

On physical examination the spinal curves, pelvic crest, and shoulder symmetry are assessed. The paraspinal muscles are palpated, and spasm and tenderness are noted. The patient is asked to bend forward and laterally; discomfort and limitations in movement are noted. The effect of these limitations in movement on activities of daily living is determined. The patient is evaluated for nerve irritation by asking about abnormal sensations (*e.g.*, paresthesia, paresis), by testing for muscle weakness or paralysis, and by assessing for back and leg pain with straight leg raises (*e.g.*, with the patient supine, the patient's leg is lifted upward with the knee in extension).

The patient is assessed for obesity. Excess weight can contribute to low back pain. A nutritional assessment is completed.

◊ Nursing Diagnoses

Based on the assessment data, the patient's major nursing diagnoses may include the following:

- Pain related to musculoskeletal problems
- Impaired physical mobility related to pain, muscle spasms, and decreased flexibility
- Altered role performance related to immobility and chronic pain
- Knowledge deficit about back-conserving body mechanics techniques
- Altered nutrition: More than body requirements, related to obesity

◊ Planning and Implementation

◊ *Goals:* The major goals of the patient may include relief of pain, improved physical mobility, improved role performance, use of back-conserving body mechanics techniques, and modified nutrition for weight reduction.

◊ Nursing Interventions

◊ *Relief of Pain.* Most back pain improves with stress reduction, relaxation, bed rest, and inactivity. The patient is confined to bed on a firm, nonsagging mattress. (A bedboard may be used.) Bathroom privileges may be permitted, but all other out-of-bed activities (*e.g.*, answering the phone, checking on the children, general activity due to restlessness) are to be avoided. Acute muscle spasms subside in 3 to 7 days. The patient is positioned to increase lumbar flexion, which reduces compression of the lumbar nerve roots. The head of the bed is elevated 30 degrees and the knees are slightly flexed (Fig. 61–1) or a lateral position with knees and hips flexed (curled position) with a pillow between the knees and legs and a pillow under the head. A prone position is avoided because it accentuates lordosis.

Frequently, the patient is unable to comply with a bed rest regimen at home and is hospitalized for "active conservative" treatment. Intermittent pelvic traction, 15 to 30 pounds of traction, is usually prescribed. Traction promotes additional lumber flexion (Fig. 61–2). The patient becomes an active participant in care by scheduling use of traction around basic self-care activities.

Patients can be taught to control and modify the perceived pain through behavior therapies that reduce muscular and psychological tension. Diaphragmatic breathing and relaxation help reduce muscle tension contributing to low back pain. Diversion of attention from the pain to other activity (*e.g.*, reading, conversation, watching TV) is another method of reducing pain perception. Guided imagery, in which the relaxed patient learns to focus on a very pleasant event and thus block the perception of pain, may be effective.

Gentle soft-tissue massage is useful to decrease muscle spasm, increase circulation, relieve congestion, and reduce pain. Physical therapy may be prescribed to decrease pain and muscle spasm. Forms of therapy used are therapeutic cold, infrared radiant heat, hot moist packs, ultrasound, diathermy, whirlpool, and traction. Each treatment mode is matched to the patient. Impaired circulation, diminished sensation, and trauma are contraindications for hotpacks.

Whirlpool therapy may be contraindicated for patients with cardiovascular problems because these patients are not able to tolerate the associated massive peripheral vasodilation. Ultrasound produces deep heat, which may increase discomfort because of swelling in the acute stages. Additionally, it is contraindicated if the patient has cancer or bleeding disorders

The degree of pain relief obtained supports continuation of the modality. If the patient has had previous episodes of back pain, information concerning the modality that was successful previously is valuable for selection of current treatment modality.

Acute pain may be treated with prescribed drug therapy. Narcotic analgesics interrupt the pain cycle. Muscle relaxants and tranquilizers relax the patient and muscles in spasm, thereby providing pain relief. Anti-inflammatory agents, including aspirin and nonsteroidal anti-inflammatory drugs, are helpful in reducing the pain. Short-term corticosteroids decrease the inflammatory response of the nerves and prevent the development of neurofibrosis, which results from ischemic changes. The nurse assesses the patient's response to each drug. As the acute pain subsides, medications are reduced as prescribed to decrease dependence on habituating drugs.

The physician may use epidural steroid injections, infiltrate paraspinal muscles with local anesthetics, or inject facet joints with steroids to achieve pain relief.

Transcutaneous electrical nerve stimulation (TENS) is a portable, noninvasive pain-reduction device that allows the patient to participate in activities comfortably without medication. The TENS unit is thought to afford pain relief by overriding pain input (gate theory of pain control) and stimulating endorphins.

Nurses need to understand the device and its pain relief potential. Electrodes are attached to areas of the body where

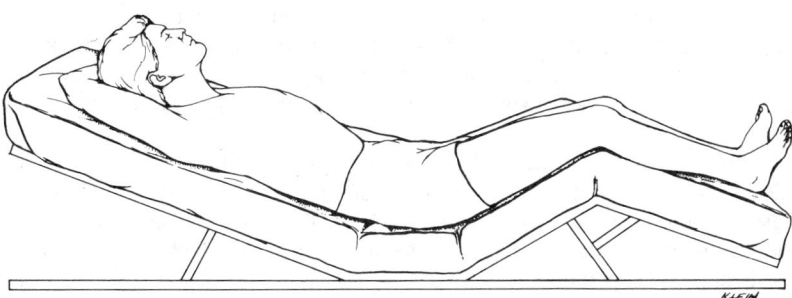

Figure 61–1. Positioning to provide lumbar flexion.

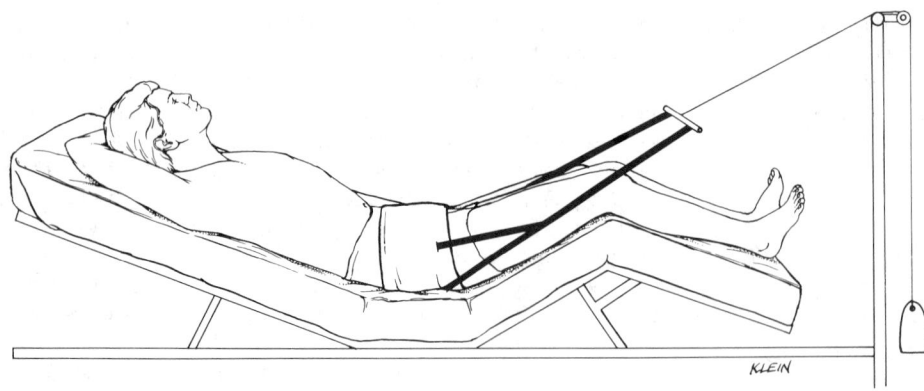

Figure 61–2. Pelvic traction with lumbar flexion to alleviate low back pain.

the patient is able to achieve maximum pain relief. The patient adjusts the stimulator's wave length and intensity to achieve comfort (see p. 259). Patients who use cardiac pacemakers should not use TENS because of the risk of causing dysrhythmias. Those who operate machinery need to be aware of the potential for accidental shocks. Generally, the patient uses the device for 1 to 2 months and gradually decreases its use as pain subsides and the back muscles are strengthened through graduated exercises.

▷ *Improved Physical Mobility.*   The nurse assesses how the patient moves and stands. As the back pain subsides, self-care activities are resumed with minimal strain on the injured structures. Position changes should be made slowly and carried out with assistance as required. The patient should learn to get out of bed with the least possible amount of discomfort. Twisting and jarring motions are avoided. The patient is encouraged to alternate lying, sitting, and walking activities and is advised to avoid sitting, standing, and walking for long periods. Planning for recumbent rest periods several times throughout the day is important in minimizing stress on the back.

As the patient achieves comfort at rest, activities can be gradually resumed and an exercise program initiated as prescribed. The goal is to increase mobility, muscle strength, and flexibility. Hyperextension exercises strengthen the paravertebral muscles; flexion exercises increase back movement and strength; and isometric flexion exercises strengthen trunk muscles.

The exercise program is carried out under the direction of the physical therapist and is adapted to the individual patient. The exercise period begins with relaxation.

The nurse needs to encourage patient adherence to the exercise program. Erratic exercising is ineffective. For most exercise programs, it is suggested that the person exercise twice a day, increasing the number of exercises gradually. Prescribed exercises are designed to strengthen abdominal and trunk muscles, to reduce lordosis, and to reduce strain on the back. Long-term adherence to an exercise program is difficult. Improvement of posture and regular use of good body mechanics, along with regular enjoyable exercise activities such as walking, bike riding, or swimming, help to maintain a healthy back.

Recreational activities that the patient enjoys can be substituted for specific exercises. Activities should not cause excessive lumbar strain, twisting, or discomfort. They may be increased gradually as tolerated. Horseback riding and weight-lifting should be avoided.

▷ *Improved Role Performance.*   As recovery from acute low back pain and immobility progresses, the patient may resume former role-related responsibilities. If these activities contributed to the development of low back pain, however, it may be difficult to resume such responsibilities without risking chronic low back pain syndrome with associated disability and depression. The patient may need help in coping with specific stressors and in learning how to control stressful situations. Once people successfully deal with stress, they learn to give themselves positive reinforcement for their success and develop confidence in their abilities to manage other stressful situations.

Dependency is another problem associated with low back pain. Because of the immobility associated with low back pain, the patient will need to depend on others to do various tasks. Dependency may continue beyond physiologic needs and become a way to fulfill psychosocial needs. Assisting both the patient and support persons in recognizing extended dependency needs helps the patient to identify and cope with the real reason for continued dependency.

Referral to a back clinic or a pain clinic may be needed. These clinics use multidisciplinary approaches to help the patient with the pain and with resumption of role-related responsibilities. Working with these patients is a challenge because major adjustments are coupled with the cure. If the patient has developed secondary gains associated with the low back disability (*e.g.,* workman's compensation, easier life-style or work load, increased emotional support), a "low back neurosis" may develop. Psychotherapy or counseling will be needed to assist the person in resuming a full, productive life.

▷ *Proper Body Mechanics.*   Prevention of recurrence of acute low back pain is a major component of nursing care. The patient must be taught how to stand, sit, lie, and lift properly. Good body mechanics and posture are essential to avoid recurrence of back pain. Providing the patient with a list of suggestions will help in making these long-term changes. If the patient wears high heels, low heels are suggested.

When sitting, the knees and hips should be flexed, and the knees should be level with the hips or higher to minimize lordosis. The feet should be on the floor. The back needs to be supported. Bending forward for long periods is to be avoided.

If long periods of standing are required, the patient should shift his weight frequently and should rest one foot on a low stool, which decreases lumbar lordosis. The patient can check his posture by looking in a mirror to see if the chest is up and the stomach is tucked in. Locking the knees when standing is to be avoided. The patient is instructed in the correct way to lift objects—using the strong quadriceps muscles of the thighs and minimal use of weak back muscles. The object should be held as close to the body as possible.

The patient should sleep on one side with knees and hips flexed, or supine with knees supported in a flexed position. Sleeping prone is to be avoided.

It takes about 6 months for a person to readjust postural habits. Practicing these protective and defensive postures, positions, and body mechanics results in natural strengthening of the back and diminishes the chance of a recurrence of back pain.

Low back supports and braces may be prescribed to limit spinal motion, to correct posture, and to diminish stress on the lower lumbar spine. Long-term use of these devices is discouraged, as they may have the negative effects of promoting disuse muscle atrophy and weakness and decreased muscle elasticity. People with jobs that require heavy lifting may wear wide leather belts (trochanter belts) to decrease the strain on their backs. An individual exercise program is essential so that eventually the needed back support can be supplied by the muscles.

Patient Education and Home Health Care

Standing
- Avoid prolonged standing and walking.
- When standing for any length of time, rest one foot on a small stool or box to relieve lumbar lordosis.
- Avoid forward-flexion work positions.

Sitting
Stress on the back may be greater in the sitting position than in the standing position.

- Avoid sitting for prolonged periods.
- Sit in a straight-back chair with back well supported. Use a foot stool to position knees higher than hips if necessary.
- Eradicate the hollow of the back by sitting with the buttocks "tucked under."
- Avoid knee and hip extension. When driving a car, have the seat pushed forward as far as possible for comfort.
- Maintain back support.
- Guard against extension strains—reaching, pushing, sitting with legs straight out.
- Alternate periods of sitting with walking.

Lying
- Rest at intervals, because fatigue contributes to spasm of the back muscle.
- Place a firm bedboard under the mattress.
- Avoid sleeping in a prone position.
- When lying on the side, place a pillow under the head and one between the legs, which should be flexed at the hips and knees.
- When supine, use a pillow under the knees to decrease lordosis.

Lifting
- When lifting, keep the back straight and hold the load as close to the body as possible. Lift with the large leg muscles, not the back muscles.
- Squat down while keeping the back straight when it is necessary to pick something off the floor.

- Avoid twisting the trunk of the body, lifting above waist level, and reaching up for any length of time.

Exercise
- Daily exercise is important in the prevention of back problems.
- Walking outdoors with progression in distance and pace is recommended.
- Do prescribed back exercises twice daily, increasing exercises gradually.
- Avoid jumping.

▷ **Modification of Nutrition for Weight Reduction.** Obesity contributes to back strain by stressing the relatively weak back muscles. Exercises are less effective and more difficult to perform when overweight. With low back pain there may be a need to undertake a weight-reduction program to decrease the body weight and stresses on the low back. Weight reduction is based on a sound nutritional plan that includes a change in eating habits to maintain desirable weight. Incorporation of weight reduction into the overall supervised plan is important. Monitoring weight reduction, noting achievement, and continuing encouragement facilitate adherence. Frequently the back problems resolve as normal weight is achieved.

▷ **Evaluation**

Expected Outcomes
1. Experiences relief of pain
   a. Rests comfortably
   b. Changes positions comfortably
   c. Obtains relief through use of physical modalities, psychological techniques, and medications
   d. Avoids drug dependency
2. Demonstrates resumption of physical mobility
   a. Resumes activities gradually
   b. Avoids positions that cause discomfort and muscle spasm
   c. Plans recumbent rest periods throughout day
3. Assumes role-related responsibilities
   a. Uses coping techniques to deal with stressful situations
   b. Demonstrates decreased dependence on others for self-care
   c. Resumes occupation as low back pain resolves
   d. Resumes full, productive life style
4. Demonstrates back-conserving body mechanics
   a. Improves posture
   b. Positions self to minimize stress on the back
   c. Demonstrates use of good body mechanics
   d. Participates in exercise program
5. Achieves desired weight
   a. Identifies need to lose weight
   b. Sets realistic goals
   c. Participates in development of weight reduction plan
   d. Complies with weight reduction regimen

In summary, low back pain is experienced by many individuals during their lives. Low back pain affects the individual's well-being and economic productivity. The most frequent of the multiple causes of low back pain is musculoskeletal. The cause of the pain is assessed and therapeutic regimens are aimed at correcting the underlying problem. Frequently the pain is due to strain of weak back muscles as a result of using improper body mechanics. The conservative initial therapy is bed rest to promote healing of weakened structures and progressive strengthening exercises with body mechanics and weight reduction education as appropriate. Anti-inflammatory, antispasmodic, and analgesic medications are useful in reducing the discomfort. At times a multidisciplinary approach is needed to modify pain perception and to modify behaviors related to alterations in role performance contributing to prolonged disability from low back pain. Nursing goals for the patient with low back pain may include relief of pain, improved physical mobility, improved role performance, use of back-conserving body mechanics techniques, and modification of nutrition for weight reduction.

Common Problems of the Upper Extremity

Painful Shoulder Syndrome.   The structures in and near the shoulder are frequently the sites of painful syndromes. With aging, degenerative alterations occur in all joints, including the articulations that make up the shoulder joint (glenohumeral, sternoclavicular, and acromioclavicular). Pain may arise from supraspinatus tendonitis or bicipital tendonitis, with the inflammation spreading to the tendon sheaths, other tendons and their sheaths (*tenosynovitis*), and the bursa, capsule, synovium, cartilage, bone, and surrounding muscles. Syndromes frequently encountered are listed in Table 61–1.

Patient Education.   The nurse provides guidelines for general care and instructs the patient in how to carry out measures that will promote healing. Patient education includes the following:

1. Rest the joint in a position that minimizes stress on the joint structures during the acute phase to prevent further damage and the development of adhesions.
2. Support the affected arm on pillows while sleeping, to keep from rolling over on the shoulder.
3. At first, apply cold intermittently, and then apply heat intermittently, to reduce discomfort and facilitate mobilization. Cold applications help reduce swelling, and heat promotes circulation.
4. Gradually resume motion and use of the joint. Assistance with dressing and other activities of daily living may be needed.
5. Avoid working and lifting above shoulder level or pushing an object against a "locked" shoulder.
6. Perform the prescribed daily range-of-motion exercises to strengthen the shoulder girdle and muscles.

Epicondylitis ("Tennis Elbow").   Tennis elbow is a chronic painful condition that is due to excessive pronation and supination activities of the forearm that result in damage to the tendons of the medial or lateral radial and ulnar epicondyles (*e.g.,* tennis, sculling, using a screwdriver). The pain characteristically radiates down the extensor (dorsal) surface of the forearm. The patient has a weakened grasp. Most often, relief is obtained by resting the arm in a molded splint, applying moist heat, and taking analgesics. In some instances, local injection of a corticosteroid or procaine is prescribed. Gentle daily exercises help to prevent elbow stiffness.

Ganglion.   A ganglion is a round, firm, cystic swelling, usually near the wrist. It is a collection of gelatinous material near the tendon sheaths and joints. Ganglions develop through defects in the tendon sheath or capsule. Ganglions occur most frequently in women under the age of 50. The ganglion is tender and may cause an aching pain. When a tendon sheath is involved, weakness of the finger occurs.

Carpal Tunnel Syndrome.   Carpal tunnel syndrome is an entrapment neuropathy that occurs when the median nerve at the wrist is compressed by a thickened flexor tendon sheath, skeletal encroachment, or soft-tissue mass on the median nerve at the wrist. The patient experiences pain, numbness, paresthesia, and possibly weakness along the median nerve (thumb, first and second fingers). Night pain is common. Rest splints, avoidance of work that requires flexion of the wrist, and cortisone injections may relieve the symptoms. Surgical release of the transverse carpal ligament may be necessary.

Dupuytren's Contracture.   Dupuytren's deformity is a slowly progressive contracture of the palmar fascia that causes flexion of the little finger, the ring finger, and frequently the middle finger, which renders them more or less useless (Fig. 61–3). It is a fairly common abnormality, occurring most frequently in men over the age of 50 who are of Scandinavian or Celtic origin. It may be caused by an inherited autosomal dominant trait. It starts as a tender nodule of the palmar fascia. The tenderness resolves, and the nodule may not change, or it may progress where the fibrous thickening extends to involve the skin in the distal palm and produces a contracture of the fingers. This condition always starts in one hand, but eventually both become deformed symmetrically. Surgery consists of limited palmar and digital fasciectomies that improve function. The recurrence and extension rate is 45% to 80%.

▶ ## Nursing Process
The Patient Undergoing Surgery of the Hand or Wrist

▷ ### Assessment

Surgery of the hand or wrist is generally an ambulatory surgery procedure. Before surgery, the nurse assesses the patient's level and type of discomfort and limitations in function caused by the ganglion, carpal tunnel syndrome, Dupuytren's contracture, or other condition of the hand. After surgery, the nurse assesses the patient for swelling, neurovascular status (circulation, sensation, motion), pain, and function. Pain may be related to edema, restrictive bandages, hematoma formation, or surgery.

▷ ### Nursing Diagnoses

Based on the assessment data, the nursing diagnoses for the patient with surgery of the hand or wrist may include the following:

- Pain related to inflammation and swelling
- Self-care deficit related to bandaged hands
- High risk for infection related to surgical procedure/break in skin

▷ ### Planning and Implementation

▷ *Goals:*   The goals of the patient may include relief of pain, improved self-care, and absence of infection.

▷ ### Nursing Interventions

▷ *Relief of Pain.*   To control swelling, the hand is elevated to heart level with pillows. When higher elevation is prescribed, an elevating sling may be attached to an IV pole or overhead frame. If the patient is ambulatory, the arm is elevated in a conventional sling.

TABLE 61-1. *Painful Shoulder Syndromes*

Syndromes	Clinical Features	Clinical Manifestations	Management
Supraspinatus tendonitis and tenosynovitis	Reaction to mechanical stress and strain plus a degenerative process with traumatic inflammation	Pain in shoulder; "catching" sensation Patient grabs affected shoulder with opposite hand Night pain; inability to lie on affected side Painful arc beyond 60-degree abduction (as tendons and cuff impinge under coracoacromial arch)	Intermittent heat/cold applications Pendulum exercises Anti-inflammatory medications—salicylates (aspirin) to tolerance Local injection of steroid or anesthetic agent into shoulder joint
Calcific tendonitis	Calcium deposits develop in tendons; cause reaction in overlying bursa. Calcium tendonitis and bursitis often coexist.	Occurs in younger and more active persons Abrupt onset of severe aching pain, 1 to 4 days All shoulder and arm movement is painful. Acute phase followed by pain relief	Infiltration of subacromial area and aspiration of deposit Analgesics for pain Anti-inflammatory agents (aspirin, phenylbutazone, indomethacin) Applications of heat/cold Injection with local anesthetic agent and steroid Operative treatment may be necessary for excision of calcified deposits.
Tears and rupture of rotator cuff	Tears occur at the insertion of rotator cuff into the bone, probably from degenerative changes.	Occur most commonly after age 50 Abrupt shoulder pain in deltoid area Weakness/inability to abduct shoulder "Clicking" sensation felt in shoulder on abduction/rotation	Partial rupture usually responds to conservative management Infiltration with local anesthetic to relieve pain Confirmation of defect by arthrogram Surgical repair for complete rupture
Bicipital syndromes (lesions on the long head of biceps muscle): tendonitis and tenosynovitis	Long head of biceps is affected by arm and shoulder movement.	Chronic pain in anterolateral area of shoulder associated with muscle spasm and pain in trapezius, scalenus, deltoid	Rest of the extremity Gentle exercises within tolerance Salicylates Heat applications to reduce inflammation Avoid movements that put biceps tendon on stretch.
Bursitis	Almost all cases of subacromial bursitis have preceding tendonitis and tenosynovitis in the rotator cuff, biceps tendon, and sheath or an inflammatory process in bone or joint; the spread of inflammation to bursa is a secondary event.	Deep-seated ache in shoulder Pain on rotation of arm	Treatment consists of locating and treating the primary process causing the bursitis.

(Adapted from Bateman JE. The Shoulder and Neck. Philadelphia, WB Saunders.)

Intermittent ice packs to the surgical area during the first 24 to 48 hours may be prescribed to control swelling. Active extension and flexion of the fingers promote circulation and are encouraged, even though movement is limited by the bulky dressing.

Neurovascular assessment of the exposed fingers every hour for the first 24 hours is essential for monitoring function of the nerves and perfusion of the hand. The patient is asked to describe the sensations in the hands and to demonstrate finger mobility. The patient's nerve function is observed care-

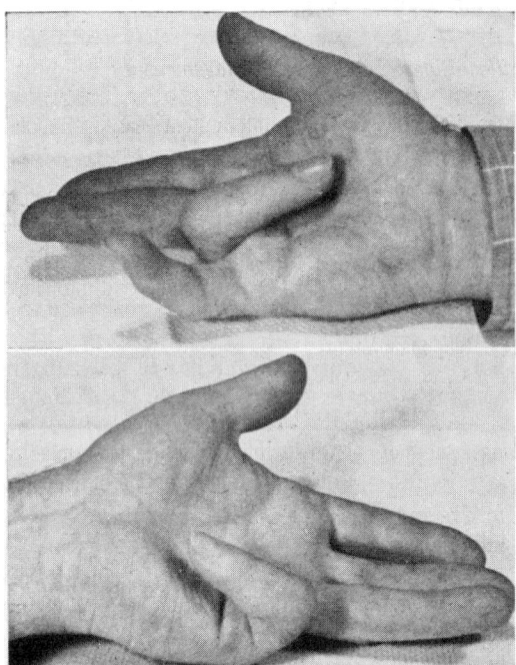

Figure 61–3. Dupuytren's contracture. (Boyes JH. Bunnell's *Surgery of the Hand*, 5th ed. Philadelphia, JB Lippincott.)

fully preoperatively because this information is needed for interpreting function after surgery. Compromised neurovascular functioning can contribute to pain.

Generally, the discomfort can be controlled by oral analgesics. The nurse evaluates the patient's response to the pain medications and to other pain-control measures. Patient education concerning the analgesics is done by the nurse.

▷ *Improved Self-Care.*   During the first few days after surgery, the patient will need assistance with activities of daily living because one hand is bandaged and function is impaired. The patient may need to arrange for assistance with feeding, bathing/hygiene, dressing, grooming and toileting. Within a few days, the patient develops skills in one-handed activities of daily living and is able to function with minimal assistance. As rehabilitation progresses, the patient will resume use of the injured hand. Adherence to the therapeutic regimen is emphasized.

▷ *Absence of Infection.*   As with all surgery, there is a potential for infection. The patient is taught to monitor temperature and pulse for elevations that may indicate a possible infection. He is instructed to keep the dressing clean and dry. Any drainage, foul odor associated with the dressing, or increased pain and swelling are reported. Patient education concerning aseptic wound care may be appropriate as well as education related to prescribed prophylactic antibiotics.

▷ *Evaluation*

Expected Outcomes
1. Achieves relief of pain
   a. Reports increased comfort
   b. Controls edema through elevation of the hand
   c. Experiences no discomfort with movement

2. Demonstrates independent self-care
   a. Secures assistance with activities of daily living during first few days postoperatively
   b. Adapts to one-handed activities of daily living
   c. Uses injured hand functionally
3. Develops no infection
   a. Maintains temperature and pulse within normal limits
   b. Experiences no purulent wound drainage
   c. Experiences no wound inflammation

In summary, several problems commonly affect the upper extremity. Painful shoulder syndrome and "tennis elbow" respond to rest, thermal therapies, and gradual resumption of activities after healing has occurred. Other common problems are of a structural nature (*i.e.*, tear and rupture of rotator cuff, ganglion, carpal tunnel syndrome, Dupuytren's contracture) and may require surgery to relieve the symptoms. After surgery on the hand or wrist, the nurse assists the patient in controlling the pain, performing self-care activities of daily living, and preventing complications such as infection.

Common Foot Problems

Disabilities of the human foot not only develop from poorly fitting shoes but may be the result of hereditary influence. Probably the foot would cause little pain or disability on its own account if it were not for modern civilization, which disregards the physiology of the foot. Fashion, vanity, and eye appeal, rather than function, are for the most part the determining factors in the design of footwear. The restriction of ill-fitting shoes distorts normal anatomy while inducing deformity and pain.

The discomfort of foot strain can be treated by rest, elevation, physiotherapy, supportive strappings, and orthotic devices. Foot exercises in which active motion occurs will benefit the circulation and help strengthen the feet. Walking in properly fitting shoes is considered the best form of exercise.

Common Foot Ailments

A *corn* is an area of *hyperkeratosis* (overgrowth of a horny layer of epidermis) produced by pressure from within (the underlying bone is prominent because of congenital or acquired abnormality, commonly arthritis) or by external pressure (shoes). The usual sites are the lesser toes, mainly the fifth toe, but all toes may be involved.

Corns are treated by soaking and scraping off the horny layer with an instrument by a podiatrist, by applying a protective shield or pad, or by surgical removal of the underlying offending osseous structure.

Soft corns are located between the toes and are kept soft by moisture and maceration. Treatment consists of drying the affected web spaces and separating the affected toes. Usually, a podiatrist will be needed to treat the underlying cause.

A *callus* is a discretely thickened area of the skin that has been exposed to persistent pressure or friction. Faulty foot mechanics usually precede the formation of a callus. Treatment consists of eliminating the underlying causes and having the callus pared by a podiatrist if it is painful. A keratolytic ointment may be applied and a thin plastic cup worn over the heel if the callus is on this area. Felt padding with adhesive backing is also used to prevent and relieve pressure. Orthotic devices can be made to remove the pressure from the bony protuberance. The protuberance may be excised.

An *ingrown toenail* (onychocryptosis) is a condition in which the free edge of a nail plate has penetrated the surrounding skin, either laterally or anteriorly. It may be accompanied by secondary infection or granulation tissue. This painful condition is caused by improper self-treatment, external pressure (tight shoes or stockings), internal pressure (deformed toes; growth under the nail), trauma, and infection. Trimming the nails properly can prevent this problem. Active treatment consists of relieving the pain by decreasing the pressure on the surrounding soft tissue by the nail plate. Warm, wet soaks help to drain an infection. A toenail may have to be surgically excised if there is severe infection.

Common Deformities of the Foot

Flatfoot.   Flatfoot (pes planus) is a common disorder in which the longitudinal arch of the foot is diminished. It may be due to congenital abnormalities or associated with bone or ligament injury, muscle and posture imbalances, excessive weight, muscle fatigue, poorly-fitting shoes, or arthritis. Symptoms include burning sensation, fatigue, clumsy gait, edema, and pain.

Exercises to strengthen the muscles and to improve posture and walking habits are helpful. A number of foot devices are available to give the foot additional support. Severe flatfoot problems are usually treated by an orthopedic surgeon or a podiatrist.

Hammer Toe.   Hammer toe is a flexion deformity of the interphalangeal joint and may involve several toes (Fig. 61–4). The condition is usually an acquired deformity. Tight socks or shoes may push an overlying toe back into the line of the other toes. The toes usually are pulled upward, forcing the metatarsal joints (ball of foot) downward. Corns develop on top of the toes, and tender calluses develop under the metatarsal area. The treatment consists of conservative measures: carrying out manipulative exercises, wearing open-toed sandals or shoes that conform to the shape of the foot, and protecting the protruding joints with pads. Surgical correction is necessary for an established deformity.

Hallux Valgus.   Hallux valgus (bunion) is a progressive deformity in which the great toe deviates laterally (Fig. 61–4).

Associated with this is a marked prominence of the medial aspect of the first metatarsal–phalangeal joint, with osseous

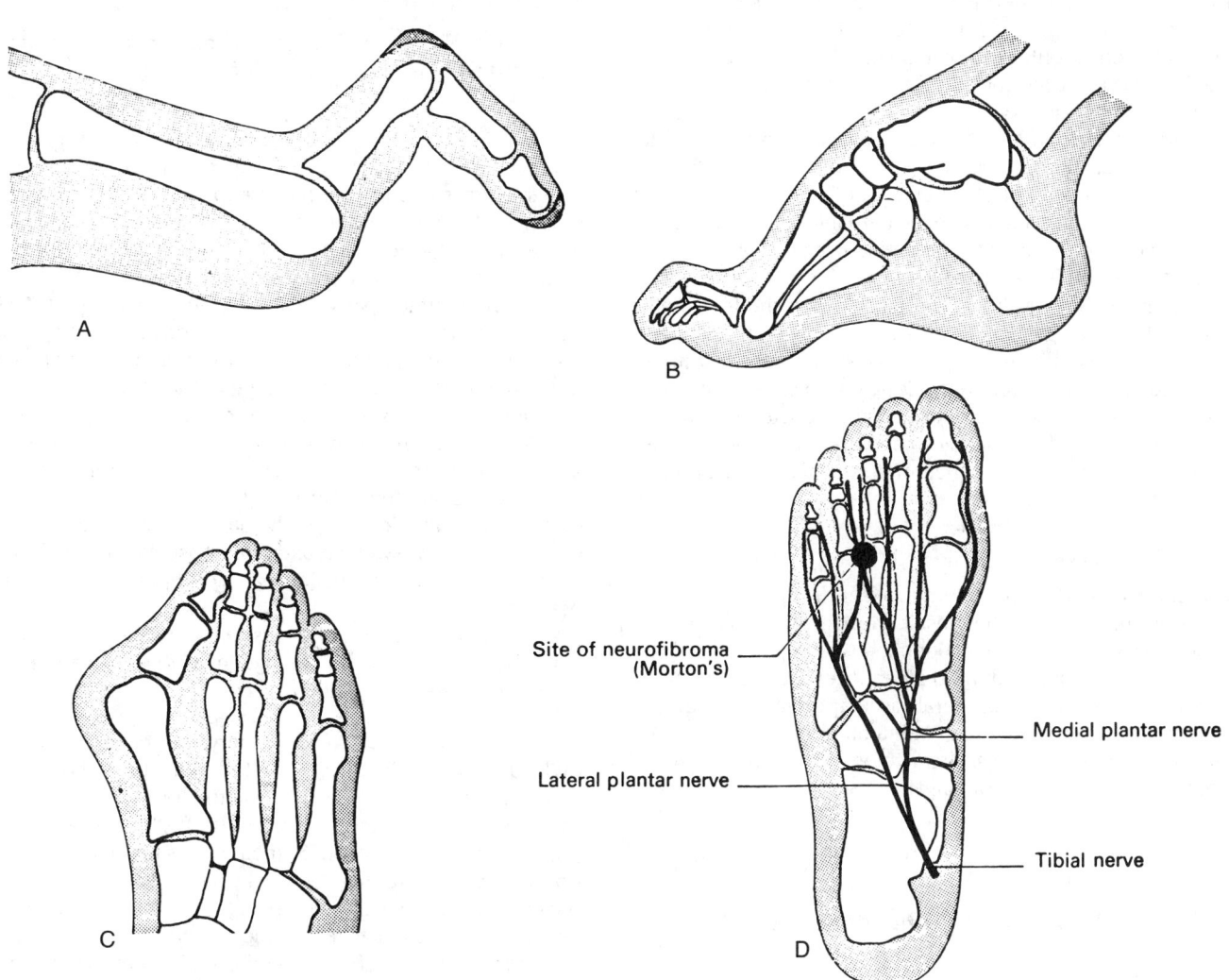

Figure 61–4.   Common foot deformities. (**A**) Hammer toe. (**B**) Clawfoot (pes cavus). (**C**) Hallux valgus. (**D**) Site for Morton's neuroma.

enlargement of the medial side of the first metatarsal head, over which a bursa may form (secondary to pressure and inflammation). Acute bursitis symptoms include a reddened area, edema, and tenderness. Causative factors include heredity, narrow shoes, arthritis, and flatfoot.

Treatment depends on the patient's age, the degree of deformity, and the severity of symptoms. If a bunion deformity is uncomplicated, wearing a shoe that conforms to the shape of the foot or one that is molded to the foot to prevent pressure on the protruding portions may be all the treatment that is needed. If not, surgical removal of the bunion and realignment of the toe may be required.

Postoperatively, the patient may have intense throbbing pain at the operative site, requiring rather liberal doses of analgesic medication. The operated foot is elevated to the level of the heart to decrease edema and pain. The neurovascular status of the toes is assessed. The duration of immobility and initiation of ambulation depend on the procedure used. After surgery, exercises are initiated to flex and extend the toes, because toe flexion is essential in walking. Shoes that do not stress the foot are recommended.

Clawfoot. Clawfoot (pes cavus) refers to a foot with an abnormally high arch (see Fig. 61-4). This causes shortening of the foot and increased pressure that produces calluses on the metatarsal area and on the dorsum (bottom) of the foot. Exercises are prescribed to manipulate the forefoot into dorsiflexion and relax the toes. In severe cases, osteotomies are done to reshape the feet.

Morton's Neuroma. Morton's neuroma (plantar digital neuroma; neurofibroma) is a swelling of the third (lateral) branch of the median plantar nerve (see Fig. 61-4). The third digital nerve, which is located in the third intermetatarsal space, is most commonly involved. Microscopically, digital artery changes cause an ischemia of the nerve.

The result is a throbbing, burning pain in the foot that is usually relieved when the patient rests. Pain sometimes radiates up the leg. Conservative treatment consists of inserting innersoles, metatarsal bars, and pads designed to spread the metatarsal heads and balance the foot posture. Local injections of hydrocortisone and a local anesthetic may give relief. If these fail, surgical excision of the neuroma is necessary. Pain relief is immediate and permanent.

Other Foot Problems

Several systemic diseases affect the feet. In the case of rheumatoid arthritis, deformities result. Persons with diabetes are prone to develop corns and peripheral neuropathies with diminishing sensation, leading to ulcers over pressure points of the foot. Persons with peripheral vascular disease and arteriosclerosis complain of burning and itching feet with attendant scratching and excoriations. Dermatologic problems commonly affect the feet in the form of fungal infections and plantar warts.

▶ Nursing Process
The Patient Undergoing Foot Surgery

▷ Assessment

Surgery on the foot may be necessary because of a variety of conditions, including neuromas and foot deformities (bunion,

hammer toe, clawfoot). Generally, foot surgery is performed on an outpatient basis. The nurse assesses the patient's ambulatory ability and balance and the neurovascular status of the foot before surgery. Additionally, assessment of the availability of assistance at home after surgery and the structural characteristics of the home may help in planning for care during the first few days after surgery. These data, in addition to knowledge of the usual management of the problem, are used by the nurse in formulating appropriate nursing diagnoses. After surgery, the nurse assesses the patient for swelling, neurovascular function, (circulation, motion, sensation), pain, wound status, and mobility.

▷ Nursing Diagnoses

Based on the assessment data, the nursing diagnoses for the patient undergoing foot surgery may include the following:

- Pain related to inflammation, and swelling
- Impaired physical mobility related to the foot immobilizing device
- High risk for infection related to surgical procedure/break in skin

▷ Planning and Implementation

▷ *Goals:*   The goals of the patient may include relief of pain, improved mobility, and absence of infection.

▷ Nursing Interventions

▷ *Relief of Pain.*   Pain experienced by patients who have had foot surgery is related to inflammation and edema. Formation of a hematoma may contribute to the discomfort. To control the swelling, the foot should be elevated on several pillows when the patient is sitting or lying.

Intermittent ice packs to the surgical area during the first 24 to 48 hours may be prescribed to control swelling and to provide some pain relief. As activity increases, the patient will find that the dependent positioning of the foot will be uncomfortable. Simply elevating the foot relieves the discomfort.

Neurovascular assessment of the exposed toes every 1 to 2 hours for the first 24 hours is essential to monitor the function of the nerves and the perfusion of the tissues. If the surgery is done on an outpatient basis, the patient and family are taught how to assess for swelling and neurovascular status. Compromised neurovascular function can contribute to the pain experienced.

Additionally, oral analgesics may be used to control the pain. The nurse provides the patient with information about the use of these medications.

▷ *Improved Mobility.*   After surgery, the patient will have a bulky dressing on the foot, protected by a light cast or a special protective boot. Weight-bearing on the foot will be prescribed by the surgeon; it varies according to the procedure and the preference of the surgeon. Some patients are allowed to walk on the heel and progress to weight-bearing as tolerated; other patients are restricted to non–weight-bearing. An ambulatory aid may be needed to assist the patient. Choice of the aid depends on the patient's general condition and balance and on the weight-bearing prescription. Safe use of the ambulatory aid must be ensured through adequate patient education and practice with the ambulatory aid before discharge. Problems of moving around the house safely while using the ambulatory aid are discussed with the patient. As healing progresses, the patient gradually resumes ambulation within prescribed limits. Adherence to the therapeutic regimen is emphasized.

▷ *Absence of Infection.* As with all surgery, there is a potential for infection. Because the foot is on or near the floor, care must be taken to protect it from soiling, dirt, and moisture. When bathing, the patient can prevent the dressing from getting wet by securing a plastic bag over the dressing and by keeping the foot out of the shower or tub. Patient instruction concerning aseptic wound care may be appropriate.

The patient is taught to monitor temperature and pulse for elevations that could indicate a possible infection. Additionally, drainage on the dressing, foul odor, or increased pain and swelling could be indicators of infection and should be reported promptly to the physician.

If prophylactic antibiotics are prescribed, education related to these will be needed.

▷ Evaluation

Expected Outcome
1. Achieves relief of pain
   a. Elevates foot to control edema
   b. Applies ice to foot as prescribed
   c. Uses oral pain medications as needed and prescribed
   d. Reports increased comfort
2. Demonstrates increased mobility
   a. Uses ambulatory aids safely
   b. Resumes weight-bearing gradually as prescribed
   c. Exhibits diminished disability associated with preoperative condition
3. Develops no infection
   a. Maintains temperature and pulse within normal limits
   b. Experiences no purulent drainage or wound inflammation
   c. Keeps dressing clean and dry
   d. Takes prophylactic antibiotics as prescribed

In summary, common foot ailments (*i.e.*, corns, callus, ingrown toenails) and common deformities of the foot (*i.e.*, flatfoot, hammer toes, bunion, clawfoot, Morton's neuroma) affect the individual's comfort and mobility. Therapies are designed to correct the underlying problem. Frequently, appropriate supportive footwear is needed to relieve the discomfort and to promote mobility. If surgery is the therapy of choice, the nurse assists the patient in controlling pain, improving mobility through the safe use of ambulatory aids, and preventing complications such as infection.

Metabolic Bone Disorders

Osteoporosis

Osteoporosis is a disorder in which there is a reduction of total bone mass. There is a change in the normal homeostatic bone turnover; the rate of bone resorption is greater than the rate of bone formation, resulting in a reduced total bone mass. The bones become progressively porous, brittle, and fragile. They fracture easily under stresses that would not break normal bone.

Osteoporosis frequently results in compression fractures (Fig. 61–5) of the thoracic and lumbar spine, fractures of the neck and intertrochanteric region of the femur, and Colles's fractures of the wrist. Multiple compression fractures of the vertebrae result in skeletal deformity (*kyphosis*).

A gradual collapse of a vertebra may be asymptomatic; it is observed as progressive kyphosis. With the development of kyphosis ("dowager's hump"), there is an associated loss of height (Fig. 61–6). Some postmenopausal women may lose 2.5 to 15 cm (1 to 6 inches) in height from vertebral collapse. The postural changes result in relaxation of the abdominal muscles and hence a protruding abdomen. The deformity may also produce pulmonary abdomen. Many patients complain of fatigue.

Loss of bone mass is a universal phenomenon associated with aging. Women develop osteoporosis more frequently, earlier, and more extensively than do men. Black women, who have a greater bone mass than white women, experience less osteoporosis. Small-framed, nonobese white women are at greatest risk for osteoporosis. More than half of all women over the age of 45 show evidence of osteoporosis on x-ray.

Early identification and education of persons at risk for developing osteoporosis is needed to prevent fractures and associated disability.

Gerontologic Considerations

The prevalence of osteoporosis in women over age 75 is 90%. The average 75-year-old woman has lost 25% of her cortical bone and 40% of her trabecular bone. With the aging of the population, the incidence of fractures (1.3 million per year), pain, and disability associated with osteoporosis is rising.

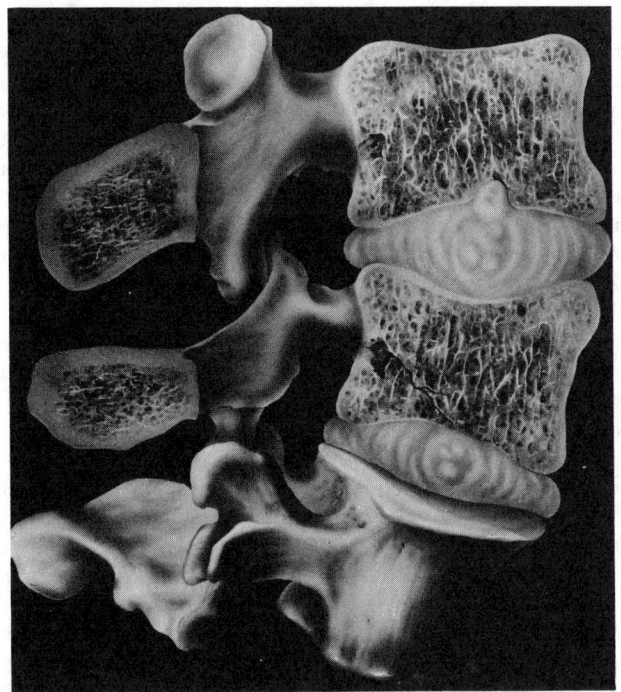

Figure 61–5. Artist's conception of progressive osteoporotic bone loss and compression fractures. (Courtesy of Ayerst Laboratories, New York, New York.)

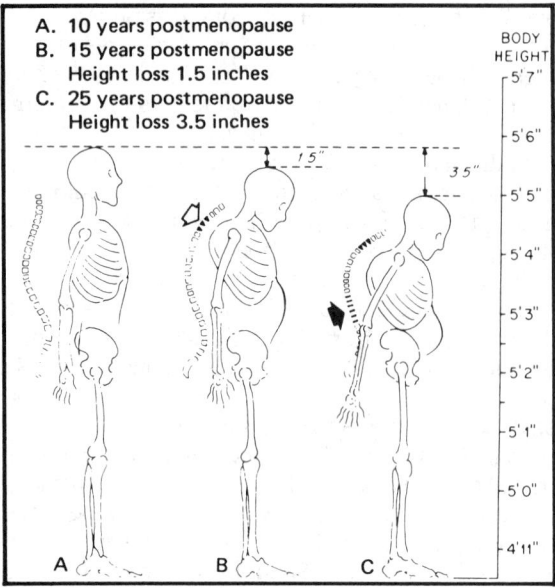

A. 10 years postmenopause
B. 15 years postmenopause
    Height loss 1.5 inches
C. 25 years postmenopause
    Height loss 3.5 inches

BODY HEIGHT
5' 7"
5' 6"
5' 5"
5' 4"
5' 3"
5' 2"
5' 1"
5' 0"
4' 11"

Figure 61–6. Typical loss of height associated with osteoporosis and aging. (Courtesy of Wilson Research Foundation.)

Pathogenesis

Normal bone remodeling in the adult results in increased bone mass until about age 35. Genetics (*e.g.*, small-framed, fair-skinned, caucasian women of European ancestry), nutrition, life-style choices (*e.g.*, smoking, caffeine and alcohol consumption), and physical activity influence the peak bone mass. Age-related loss begins soon after the peak bone mass is achieved. The withdrawal of estrogens at menopause and with oophorectomy causes an accelerated bone resorption that continues during the postmenopause years. Men have a greater peak bone mass and do not experience sudden hormonal changes. As a result, the incidence of osteoporosis is lower in men.

Nutritional factors contribute to the development of osteoporosis. Vitamin D is necessary for calcium absorption and for normal bone mineralization. Dietary calcium and vitamin D must be adequate to maintain bone remodeling and body functions. Inadequate intake of calcium or vitamin D over a period of years results in decreased bone mass and the development of osteoporosis. The recommended daily allowance (RDA) of calcium has been increased for adolescents and young adults (age 11 to 24) to 1200 mg to maximize peak bone mass. The RDA for an adult remains at 800 mg. The actual estimated average daily intake is 300 to 500 mg. To compound the situation, elderly persons absorb dietary calcium less efficiently and excrete it more readily through their kidneys. Postmenopausal women and the elderly actually need to consume liberal amounts of calcium. The best source of calcium and vitamin D is fortified milk.

Endogenous (produced by the body) and *exogenous* (from an external source) catabolic agents can cause osteoporosis. Excessive corticosteroids, Cushing's syndrome, hyperthyroidism, and hyperparathyroidism contribute to bone loss. The degree of osteoporosis is related to the length of glucocorticoid therapy. When the therapy is discontinued or the metabolic problem is corrected, the progression of osteoporosis is stopped, but restoration of lost bone mass usually does not occur.

Coexisting medical conditions (*e.g.*, malabsorption syndromes, lactose intolerance, alcohol abuse, renal failure, liver failure, endocrine disorders) contribute to the development of osteoporosis. Medications (*e.g.*, isoniazid, heparin, tetracycline, aluminum-containing antacids, furosemide, anticonvulsants, corticosteroids, and thyroid supplements) affect calcium use and metabolism.

Immobility contributes to the development of osteoporosis. Bone formation is enhanced by the stress of weight and muscle activity. When immobilized by casts, paralysis, or general inactivity, the bone is resorbed faster than it is formed, and osteoporosis occurs.

Diagnostic Evaluation

Osteoporosis is identified on routine x-ray when there has been 25% to 40% demineralization. There is a radiolucency to the bone. Vertebrae collapse—thoracic vertebrae become wedge shaped and lumbar vertebrae become biconcave.

Laboratory studies (*e.g.*, serum calcium, serum phosphate, alkaline phosphatase, urine calcium excretion, urinary hydroxyproline excretion, hematocrit, erythrocyte sedimentation rate) and x-rays are used to exclude other possible medical diagnoses (*e.g.*, multiple myeloma, osteomalacia, hyperparathyroidism, malignancy) that contribute to bone loss.

Single-photon absorptiometry is used to monitor bone mass of the cortical bone in the wrist. Dual-photon absorptiometry and computed tomography (CT scan) provide information on bone mass at the spine and hip. These are useful in identifying osteoporotic bone and assessing response to therapy.

▶ Nursing Process
The Patient With a Spontaneous Vertebral Fracture Related to Osteoporosis

◌ Assessment

Health promotion, identification of people at risk for developing osteoporosis, and recognition of problems associated with osteoporosis form the basis for nursing assessment. The interview includes questions concerning the occurrence of osteoporosis in the family, previous fractures, dietary consumption of calcium, exercise patterns, onset of menopause, and use of steroids. Any symptoms the patient is experiencing such as back pain, constipation, or altered body image are explored.

Physical examination may disclose a fracture, kyphosis of the thoracic spine, or shortened stature. Occasionally problems in mobility and breathing may exist as a result of changes in posture and weakened muscles. Constipation may be present because of inactivity.

◌ Nursing Diagnoses

Based on the assessment data, the major nursing diagnoses for the patient who experiences spontaneous vertebral fracture related to osteoporosis may include the following:

- Knowledge deficit about the osteoporotic process and treatment regimen
- Pain related to fracture and muscle spasm

- Constipation related to immobility or development of ileus
- High risk for injury: fracture, related to osteoporotic bone

▷ **Planning and Implementation**

▷ *Goals:* The major goals of the patient may include knowledge about osteoporosis and the treatment regimen, relief of pain, improved bowel elimination, absence of additional fracture.

▷ **Nursing Interventions**

▷ *Knowledge of Osteoporosis and Treatment Regimen.* Patient teaching focuses on factors influencing the development of osteoporosis, interventions to arrest or slow the process, and measures to relieve symptoms. Adequate dietary or supplemental calcium, regular weight-bearing exercise, and modification of life-style, if necessary (*e.g.*, reduced use of caffeine, cigarettes, and alcohol), help to maintain bone mass. Exercise and physical activity are the primary keys to developing high-density bones that are resistant to becoming osteoporotic. An adequate, balanced dietary intake rich in calcium and vitamin D throughout life, with an increased calcium intake beginning in the middle years, protects against skeletal demineralization.

This would include three glasses of skim or whole vitamin D milk or other foods high in calcium (*e.g.*, Swiss cheese, steamed bokchoy, canned salmon with bones) daily. A calcium preparation (calcium carbonate) may be taken to add sufficient calcium to the diet, as many older persons frequently suffer from a deficiency in dietary calcium.

At menopause, estrogen/progesterone replacement therapy may be prescribed to retard bone loss and prevent occurrence of additional fractures. A woman who has had her ovaries removed or has undergone a premature menopause may develop osteoporosis at a fairly young age. Estrogen replacement is considered for this patient. Estrogens decrease bone resorption but do not increase bone mass. Estrogens do not diminish the rate of bone loss indefinitely, however, and are of little value in long-term care. Estrogen therapy has been associated with a slightly increased incidence of breast and endometrial cancer. Therefore, during estrogen therapy, the patient must examine her breasts monthly and have a pelvic examination, including a Papanicolaou smear and endometrial biopsy, one or two times a year.

Elderly persons continue to need sufficient calcium, vitamin D, sunshine, and exercise to minimize the osteoporosis process.

▷ *Relief of Pain.* Relief of back pain may be accomplished by resting in bed in a supine or side-lying position for several days to a week. The mattress should be firm and nonsagging. Knee flexion increases comfort by relaxing muscles. Intermittent local heat and back rubs promote muscle relaxation. The patient is instructed to move the trunk as a unit, avoiding twisting. Good posture is encouraged, and body mechanics are taught. When the patient is helped out of bed, a lumbosacral corset may be worn for temporary support and immobilization, although such a device is frequently uncomfortable and poorly tolerated by elderly persons. As the patient spends more time out of bed, daily intermittent recumbent rest periods are encouraged to relieve discomfort and reduce the stress of abnormal posture on weakened muscles.

Oral narcotic analgesics may be needed for the first few days after the onset of back pain. After a few days, nonnarcotic analgesics afford relief.

▷ *Improved Bowel Elimination.* Constipation is a problem related to immobility, medications, and age. Early institution of a high-fiber diet, increased fluids, and the use of prescribed stool softeners help to prevent or minimize constipation. If the vertebral collapse involves a T10–L2 vertebra, the patient may develop an ileus. The nurse therefore monitors the patient's intake, bowel sounds, and bowel activity.

▷ *Prevention of Injury.* Physical activity is essential to strengthen muscles, prevent disuse atrophy, and retard progressive bone demineralization. Isometric exercises can be used to strengthen trunk muscles. Walking, good body mechanics, and good posture are encouraged. Sudden bending, jarring, and strenuous lifting are to be avoided. Daily weight-bearing activity, preferably outdoors in the sunshine to enhance the body's ability to produce vitamin D, is necessary.

▷ *Gerontologic Considerations.* Elderly people fall frequently as a result of environmental hazards, neuromuscular disorders, diminished senses and cardiovascular responses, and responses to drugs. Hazards must be identified and eliminated. Supervision and assistance should be readily available.

The patient and family need to be included in planning for continued care and preventive management regimens. The home environment is assessed for potential hazards (*e.g.*, scatter rugs, cluttered rooms, pets underfoot) and a safe environment is created (*e.g.*, well-lighted staircases with secure hand rails, grab-bars in the bathroom, properly fitting footwear).

▷ **Evaluation**

Expected Outcomes

1. Acquires knowledge about osteoporosis and the treatment regimen
   a. States relationship of calcium intake and exercise to bone mass
   b. Consumes adequate amounts of dietary calcium
   c. Increases level of exercise
   d. Takes prescribed hormonal therapy
   e. Undergoes prescribed screening procedures
2. Achieves relief of pain
   a. Experiences pain relief at rest
   b. Experiences minimal discomfort during activities of daily living
   c. Demonstrates diminished tenderness at fracture site
3. Demonstrates normal bowel elimination
   a. Bowel sounds active
   b. Bowel movements regular
4. Experiences no new fractures
   a. Maintains good posture
   b. Uses good body mechanics
   c. Consumes balanced diet high in calcium and vitamin D
   d. Engages in weight-bearing exercises (walks daily)
   e. Rests by lying down several times a day
   f. Participates in outdoor activities
   g. Creates a safe home environment
   h. Accepts assistance and supervision as needed

Osteomalacia

Osteomalacia is a metabolic bone disease characterized by inadequate mineralization of bone. (A similar condition in children is called *rickets*.) In these patients, a large amount of osteoid or remolded bone does not calcify. It is thought that the primary defect is a deficient supply of calcium and phosphate from the extracellular fluid to the calcification sites in the bones. As a result of this faulty mineralization, there is softening and weakening of the skeleton, causing pain, tenderness to the touch, bowing of the bones, and pathologic fractures. In adults, the condition is chronic, and skeletal deformities are not as severe as in children because skeletal growth has been completed.

Pathophysiology

There are a variety of causes of osteomalacia resulting from a generalized disturbance in mineral metabolism. Risk factors for the development of osteomalacia include dietary deficiencies, malabsorption problems, gastrectomy, chronic renal failure, prolonged anticonvulsant therapy (phenytoin, phenobarbital), and insufficient vitamin D (dietary, sunlight).

Osteomalacia may occur as a result of inadequate dietary intake of calcium or phosphate ions, failure of these ions to be absorbed, or excessive loss of these materials from the body.

The malnutrition type (deficiency in vitamin D often associated with poor intake of calcium) is mainly due to poverty, but food faddism and lack of knowledge of nutrition may be factors. It occurs most frequently in parts of the world where vitamin D is not added to food and where dietary deficiencies exist and sunlight is scarce.

Gastrointestinal disorders in which fats are inadequately absorbed are likely to produce osteomalacia through loss of vitamin D (along with other fat-soluble vitamins) and calcium, the latter being excreted in the feces in combination with fatty acids. Such disorders include celiac disease, chronic biliary tract obstruction, chronic pancreatitis, and small bowel resections or operative shunts that involve the small intestine.

Severe renal insufficiency results in acidosis. The available calcium is used to combat the acidosis, and the parathyroid hormone continues to cause a release of skeletal calcium in an attempt to reestablish a physiologic pH. During this continual drain of skeletal calcium, bony fibrosis occurs and bony cysts form. Chronic glomerulonephritis, obstructive uropathies, and heavy metal poisoning result in a reduced serum phosphate level and demineralization of bone.

In addition, liver and kidney diseases can produce a lack of vitamin D, as these are the organs that convert vitamin D to its active form. Finally, hyperparathyroidism leads to skeletal decalcification, and thus to osteomalacia, through the promotion of phosphate excretion in the urine.

Gerontologic Considerations.   In elderly persons who are economically and socially deprived, special attention to a nutritious diet is important. Adequate intake of calcium and vitamin D is promoted. Because sunlight is necessary, older people should be encouraged to spend some time in the sun.

Prevention, identification, and management of osteomalacia in the elderly are essential to reduce the incidence of fractures. When osteomalacia is combined with osteoporosis, the incidence of fracture in the elderly increases.

Clinical Manifestations

The most common and distressing symptoms of osteomalacia are bone pain and tenderness. As a result of calcium deficiency, there is usually muscle weakness. The patient develops a waddling or limping gait. In the more advanced disease, the legs become bowed (because of body weight and muscle pull). The softened vertebrae become compressed, thus shortening the patient's trunk and deforming the thorax (kyphosis). The sacrum is forced down and forward, and the pelvis is compressed laterally. These two deformities explain the characteristic shape of the pelvis that often necessitates cesarean section in pregnant women affected with this disease. Weakness and unsteadiness present a danger of falls and fractures.

Diagnostic Evaluation

On radiography, generalized demineralization of bone is evident. Studies of the vertebrae may show compression fracture with indistinct vertebral end-plates. Laboratory studies show low serum calcium and phosphorus levels and a moderately elevated alkaline phosphatase level. Urine calcium and creatinine excretion is low.

▶ Nursing Process
The Patient With Osteomalacia

▷ Assessment

Patients with osteomalacia usually complain of generalized bone pain in the low back and extremities, with an associated tenderness. The description of the discomfort may be vague. The patient may present with a fracture. During the interview, information concerning coexisting diseases (e.g., malabsorption syndrome) and dietary habits is obtained.

On physical examination, skeletal deformities are noted. Spinal deformities and bending deformities of the long bones may give patients an unusual appearance and a waddling gait. Muscular weakness may be present. These patients may be uncomfortable with their appearance.

▷ Nursing Diagnoses

Based on the assessment data, the patient's major nursing diagnoses may include the following:

- Knowledge deficit about the disease process and the treatment regimen
- Pain related to bone tenderness and possible fracture
- Body image disturbance related to bowing legs, waddling gait, spinal deformities

▷ Planning and Implementation

▷   *Goals:*   The major goals of the patient with osteomalacia may include knowledge of disease process and treatment regimen, relief of pain, and improved body image.

▷ Nursing Interventions

▷   *Knowledge about the Disease Process and Treatment Regimen.* Patient education focuses on the cause of osteomalacia and approaches to controlling it. The underlying cause is corrected as far as possible.

If osteomalacia is dietary in origin, a normal diet with adequate protein and increased calcium and vitamin D is provided. The patient is instructed about dietary sources of calcium and vitamin D. Safe use of supplements is reviewed. High doses of vitamin D are toxic and enhance the risk of hypercalcemia. The importance of monitoring the serum calcium levels is stressed.

Therapeutic use of vitamin D may be prescribed. Vitamin D raises the concentration of calcium and phosphorus in the extracellular fluid and thus makes these ions available for mineralization of bone.

If osteomalacia is due to a malabsorption problem, larger doses of vitamin D as well as supplemental calcium are usually prescribed. Exposure to sunlight for ultraviolet radiation to transform a cholesterol substance (7-dehydrocholesterol) present in the skin into vitamin D may be recommended.

Frequently skeletal problems associated with osteomalacia resolve themselves when the underlying nutritional deficiency or pathologic process is adequately treated. Long-term monitoring of the patient is appropriate to ensure stabilization or reversal of the osteomalacia process. Some persistent orthopedic deformities may need to be treated with braces or surgery (osteotomy for long bone deformity).

▷ *Relief of Pain.* Physical, psychological, and pharmaceutical measures are used to help the patient reduce discomfort. Because the patient has both skeletal pain and tenderness, gentle assistance needs to be provided when changing positions. Frequent position changes will decrease the discomforts from immobility. A convoluted foam mattress and soft pillows will support the body and conform to existing deformities. Diversional activities and focusing attention on conversation, television, and other such distractions will decrease the patient's perception of pain. At times, analgesics will be needed as prescribed to decrease the discomfort. The patient's response to the medications is monitored. As the condition responds to the therapy, the skeletal discomforts will diminish.

▷ *Improved Body Image.* In an established, trusting relationship, the patient is encouraged to discuss any changes in body image and methods for coping with the changes. The patient is encouraged to recognize and use existing strengths, and he is included in planning of care. Being an active participant promotes self-control and improves feelings of self-worth. Interactions with family and friends are encouraged. Social interactions help provide a feeling of being accepted regardless of physical changes.

▷ **Evaluation**

Expected Outcomes
1. Describes disease process and treatment regimen
   a. Describes specific factors contributing to disease process
   b. Consumes therapeutic amount of calcium and vitamin D
   c. Exposes self to sunlight
   d. Has serum calcium level monitored throughout therapy
   e. Keeps follow-up health care appointments
2. Achieves relief of pain
   a. Reports feeling comfortable
   b. Reports less bone tenderness
3. Demonstrates improved body image
   a. Demonstrates confidence in abilities
   b. Increases level of activity
   c. Increases social interactions

Paget's Disease

Paget's disease (osteitis deformans) is a disorder of localized increased bone remodeling, affecting most commonly the skull, femur, tibia, pelvic bones, and vertebrae. There is a primary proliferation of osteoclasts, which produces bone resorption. This is followed by a compensatory increase in osteoblastic activity that repairs the bone. As bone turnover continues, a classic mosaic pattern of bone matrix develops. The bone formed is high in mineral content but poorly constructed. The bones are structurally weak. Frequently the legs bow. This causes malalignment of the hip, knee, and ankle joints, which contributes to the development of arthritis and pain.

Paget's disease occurs in approximately 3% of the population over age 50. The incidence is slightly greater in men than women and the incidence increases with aging. A family history has been noted, with siblings developing the disease. The cause of Paget's disease is not known. A viral cause is being actively researched.

Clinical Manifestations

The disease is insidious. Most patients with the disease never know they have it. Some patients are asymptomatic but have skeletal deformity. A few patients have symptomatic problems. The condition is most frequently identified when x-rays have been done at a routine physical examination or in the course of workup for another problem. There are sclerotic changes, skeletal deformities (*e.g.*, bowing of femur and tibia, enlargement of the skull) and cortical thickening of the long bones. Bone scans may detect the disease quite early.

In the majority of patients, skeletal deformity involves the skull or long bones. The skull may be thickened and the patient may complain that a hat no longer fits. In some cases of Paget's disease, the cranium is much enlarged, but not the face, which therefore appears small and triangular in shape. Most patients with skull involvement have impaired hearing. Cranial nerve dysfunction may occur because of compression of the nerves. Occasionally, obstructive hydrocephalus may occur.

The femurs and tibiae tend to bow, producing a waddling gait. The spine is bent forward and is rigid; the chin rests on the chest. The thorax is compressed and immobile on respiration. The trunk is flexed on the legs to maintain equilibrium; the arms, which are bent outward and forward and appear long in relation to the shortened trunk, give the patient an apelike appearance. As a result of the kyphosis and the bowing of the legs, the patient's height may be reduced as much as 30 cm (12 in).

Pain and tenderness may be noted in the bones. The pain is mild to moderate, deep, aching pain that increases with weight-bearing if the lower extremities are involved. Such discomfort may precede the skeletal changes of Paget's disease by years; the discomfort is often wrongly attributed by the patient to old age or arthritis.

There is an increase in skin temperature overlying the bone because of increased vascularity of the bone. Patients with very large, highly vascular lesions may develop a high-output cardiac failure because of the increased vascular bed and metabolic demands.

Diagnostic Evaluation

The serum alkaline phosphatase and the level of urinary hydroxyproline excretion are usually increased, reflecting increased osteoblastic activity. The higher these values, the more active the disease. The patients have normal blood calcium levels. Malignant degeneration and osteosarcomas are seen in some patients with Paget's disease.

Management

Usually, no particular treatment is recommended in the patient without symptoms. Pain usually responds to nonsteroidal anti-inflammatory drugs.

Patients with a moderate to severe form of the disease may benefit from suppressive therapy. These patients have severe pain, neurologic deficits, or extensive skeletal involvement. At present, there are several agents that are potent inhibitors of bone resorption and under certain conditions may permit replacement of diseased bone with normal lamellar bone.

Calcitonin, a polypeptide hormone, retards bone resorption by decreasing the number and availability of osteoclasts. Calcitonin therapy facilitates remodeling of abnormal pagetoid bone into normal lamellar bone, relieves bone pain, and helps alleviate neurologic and biochemical complications. Calcitonin is given subcutaneously. Side effects of flushing of the face and nausea can be managed by taking the drug before bedtime or concurrently with an antihistamine, and tend to decrease with time. Calcitonin therapy is continued for about 3 months.

Disodium etidronate (EHDP), a diphosphonate compound, produces rapid reduction in bone turnover and relief of pain. It also reduces elevated serum alkaline phosphatase and urinary hydroxyproline levels. Food inhibits absorption. Side effects of nausea, cramping, and diarrhea may occur and can be alleviated by spacing the doses. Large doses may inhibit fracture healing and may contribute to osteomalacia. Calcitonin and EHDP may be combined and given to patients with very active disease.

Plicamycin (Mithracin), a cytotoxic antibiotic, may be used to control the disease. It is a toxic drug and is reserved for severely affected patients with neurologic compromise or for patients who are resistant to other measures. This drug has dramatic effects on pain reduction and on the serum calcium, alkaline phosphatase, and urinary hydroxyproline levels. It is given by intravenous infusion and requires that hepatic, renal, and bone marrow function be monitored during therapy. Clinical remissions may continue for months after the drug is discontinued.

Fractures are managed according to location. Healing does occur if reduction, immobilization, and stability are adequate. Nonunion of a femoral neck fracture requires treatment with an endoprosthesis.

Loss of hearing is managed with hearing aids and communication techniques used with the hearing-impaired person (*e.g.*, lip reading, body language).

Gerontologic Considerations

Careful assessment of the patient's complaints of discomfort is necessary. Frequently, elderly persons have discomfort associated with arthritis that may be accentuated by the bone deformities. Pain may indicate fracture. Patient education is important to help the patient compensate for altered neurologic functioning. The home environment needs to be assessed for safety to prevent falls and to reduce the incidence of fracture.

In summary, metabolic bone disorders (osteoporosis, osteomalacia, and Paget's disease) affect the quantity and quality of bone. Osteoporosis is a common disorder in which there is a reduction in total bone mass that results in vertebral compression fractures, fractures of the hip, and fractures of the wrist, particularly in small-framed, nonobese, postmenopausal white women. Preventive education includes intake of adequate dietary calcium during the bone-forming years, avoidance of smoking, caffeine, and alcohol, which contribute to bone mass loss, weight-bearing exercise such as walking, and prevention of falls. At menopause, estrogen/progesterone replacement therapy may be prescribed to retard bone loss and prevent occurrence of fractures in women at risk. When a fracture occurs, efforts are directed at pain relief, stabilization and healing of the fracture, and prevention of future fractures.

Osteomalacia is due to inadequate mineralization of bone in which the bone softens and the skeleton weakens, causing pain, bowing of the bones, and pathologic fractures. Malnutrition, gastrointestinal disorders, and liver and kidney conditions contribute to the development of osteomalacia. Therapy is directed at the cause of the problem. The nurse assists the patient to modify his pain experience and accept changes in body image. Positive self-concept is promoted.

Paget's disease is another metabolic bone disorder characterized by increased bone abnormal remodeling. The bones are deformed, structurally weak, and subject to pathologic fracture. Thickening of the skull may result in loss of hearing. Symptoms are varied and treatment approaches are designed for the individual patient. Pain can frequently be controlled by nonsteroidal anti-inflammatory drugs; severe cases may require suppressive therapy. Fractures are treated according to location.

Musculoskeletal Infections

Osteomyelitis

Osteomyelitis is an infection of the bone. Bone infections are more difficult to cure than soft-tissue infections because of the limited blood supply. Osteomyelitis may become a chronic problem that affects quality of life or loss of an extremity.

The infection may be due to *hematogenous* (blood-borne) spread from other foci of infection (*e.g.*, infected tonsils, boils, infected teeth, upper respiratory infections). Osteomyelitis due to hematogenous spread occurs in a bone area where there has been trauma or where there is lowered resistance, possibly due to subclinical (nonapparent) trauma.

Osteomyelitis may be associated with extension of soft-tissue infection (*e.g.*, infected pressure or vascular ulcer; middle ear infection) or direct bone contamination (*e.g.*, open fracture; gunshot wound; bone surgery).

Patients who are at risk for developing osteomyelitis include poorly nourished, elderly, obese, or diabetic patients. In addition, patients who have rheumatoid arthritis, have been hospitalized for a long time, have required long-term corticosteroid therapy, have had surgery on a joint previously operated on, or have a concurrent sepsis are susceptible.

Other patients at risk are those who have undergone lengthy orthopedic surgery, have prolonged wound drainage, have marginal incisional necrosis or wound dehiscence, or require evacuation of postoperative hematomas.

Prevention

Prevention of osteomyelitis is the goal. Treatment of focal infections diminishes hematogenous spread. Management of soft-tissue infections controls erosion to the bone. Careful patient selection and attention to the surgical environment and technique can reduce the incidence of postoperative osteomyelitis.

Prophylactic antibiotics, administered to achieve adequate tissue levels at the time of surgery and for 24 to 48 hours after surgery, are helpful. Aseptic postoperative wound care techniques reduce the incidence of superficial infections and the potential development of an associated osteomyelitis.

Pathophysiology

Staphylococcus aureus causes 70% to 80% of bone infections. Other pathogenic organisms frequently found in osteomyelitis include *Proteus, Pseudomonas,* and *Escherichia coli.* There has been an increasing incidence of penicillin-resistant, nosocomial, gram-negative, and anaerobic infections.

The onset of osteomyelitis after orthopedic surgery may occur during the first 3 months (*acute fulminating—stage 1*) and is frequently associated with hematoma drainage or superficial infection. *Delayed onset* (*stage 2*) infections occur between 4 and 24 months after surgery. *Late onset* (*stage 3*) osteomyelitis is generally due to hematogenous spread and occurs 2 or more years after surgery.

The initial response to infection is one of inflammation, increased vascularity, and edema. After 2 or 3 days, thrombosis of the blood vessels occurs in the area, resulting in ischemia with bone necrosis due to increasing tissue and medullary pressure. The infection extends into the medullary cavity and under the periosteum. Infective pus may spread the infection into adjacent soft tissues and joints. Unless the infective process is controlled early, a bone abscess forms.

In the natural course of events, the abscess may spontaneously drain, but, more often, incision and drainage are performed by the surgeon. The resulting abscess cavity has in its walls areas of dead tissue, as in any abscess cavity; however, dead bone tissue (the *sequestrum*) does not easily liquefy and drain. The cavity cannot collapse and heal, as occurs in soft-tissue abscesses. A bone sheath (the *involucrum*) forms and surrounds the sequestrum. Thus, although healing appears to take place, a chronically infected sequestrum remains that is prone to producing recurring abscesses throughout the life of the individual. This is the so-called *chronic* type of osteomyelitis.

Clinical Manifestations

When the infection is carried by the blood, the onset is usually sudden, occurring often with the clinical manifestations of septicemia (*e.g.,* chills, high fever, rapid pulse, and general malaise). The systemic symptoms at first may overshadow the local signs completely. As the infection extends from the marrow cavity through the cortex of the bone, it involves the periosteum and the soft tissues, with the extremity becoming painful, swollen, and extremely tender. The patient may describe a constant, pulsating pain that intensifies with movement and is due to the pressure of the collecting pus.

When osteomyelitis occurs from spread of adjacent infection or direct contamination, there are no symptoms of septicemia. The area is swollen, warm, painful, and tender to touch.

The patient with a chronic osteomyelitis presents with a continuously draining sinus or experiences recurrent periods of pain, inflammation, swelling, and drainage. The low-grade infection thrives in the scar tissue with its reduced blood supply.

Diagnostic Evaluation

With acute osteomyelitis, early x-rays will show only soft-tissue swelling. In about 2 weeks, areas of irregular decalcification, periosteal elevation, and new bone formation will be evident. Blood studies will reveal elevated leukocytes and an elevated sedimentation rate. Blood cultures and cultures of the abscess are needed for proper antibiotic therapy.

With chronic osteomyelitis, large, irregular cavities, raised periosteum, sequestra, or dense bone formations are seen on x-ray. Bone scans may be performed to identify areas of infection. The sedimentation rate is elevated. The abscess is cultured to determine the infective organism and appropriate antibiotic therapy.

▶ Nursing Process
The Patient With Osteomyelitis

◊ Assessment

The patient presents with an acute onset of symptoms (*e.g.,* localized pain, swelling, erythema, fever) or recurrent draining of an infected sinus with associated pain, swelling, and low-grade fever. The patient is assessed for risk factors (*e.g.,* older age, diabetes, or long-term steroid therapy) and for previous injury, infection, or orthopedic surgery. The patient avoids pressure on the area and guards movement. In acute osteomyelitis, the patient will have generalized weakness due to the systemic reaction to the infection.

Physical examination reveals an inflamed, markedly swollen, warm area that is tender. Purulent drainage may be noted. The patient will have an elevated temperature. With chronic osteomyelitis, the temperature elevation may be only minimal, occurring in the afternoon or evening.

Laboratory studies will show an elevated white blood cell count and usually an elevated erythrocyte sedimentation rate. Blood and drainage cultures may be positive. Wound cultures will indicate the causative organisms and sensitivity to various antibiotics. X-rays may be negative until destruction, bone necrosis, and elevation of the periosteum occur.

◊ Nursing Diagnoses

Based on the nursing assessment data, the nursing diagnoses for the patient with osteomyelitis may include the following:

- Pain related to inflammation and swelling
- Impaired physical mobility associated with pain, immobilization devices, and weight-bearing limitations
- High risk for extension of infection: bone abscess formation
- Knowledge deficit about the treatment regimen

◊ Planning and Implementation

◊ *Goals:* The goals of the patient may include relief of pain, improved physical mobility within therapeutic limitations, control and eradication of infection, and knowledge of treatment regimen.

◊ *Relief of Pain.* The affected part may be immobilized with a splint to decrease pain and muscle spasm. The joints above and below the affected part should be gently placed through the range of motion. The wounds themselves are frequently very painful and must be handled with great care and gentleness.

Elevation reduces swelling and associated discomfort. The neurovascular status of the affected extremity is monitored. Warm saline soaks for 20 minutes several times a day may be prescribed to increase circulation. Techniques for reducing pain perception and prescribed analgesics may be useful.

▷ *Improved Physical Mobility.* Treatment regimens restrict activity. The bone is weakened by the infective process and must be protected by immobilization devices and avoidance of stress on the bone. The patient should be taught the rationale for the activity restrictions. Full participation in activities of daily living within the physical limitations is encourage to promote general well-being.

▷ *Control of the Infectious Process.* The initial goal of therapy is to control and arrest the infective process. Blood cultures and abscess fluid smears and cultures are done to identify the organism and select the best antibiotic. Frequently, the infection is caused by more than one pathogen.

As soon as the culture specimens have been obtained, intravenous antibiotic therapy is begun, assuming a *Staphylococcus* infection that is sensitive to a semisynthetic penicillin or cephalosporin. The aim is to control the infection before the blood supply to the infection diminishes as a result of thrombosis. Around-the-clock dosage administration is necessary to achieve a sustained high therapeutic blood level of the antibiotic. The nurse monitors the patient's response to antibiotic therapy and observes the intravenous site for evidence of phlebitis or infiltration. An antibiotic to which the causative organism is more sensitive is prescribed when the culture reports are known. When the infection appears to be controlled, the antibiotic may be administered orally and continued for up to 3 months. To enhance absorption of oral antibiotics, they should not be administered with food.

If the patient does not respond to antibiotic therapy, the involved bone is surgically exposed, the purulent and necrotic material removed, and the area irrigated directly with sterile physiologic saline solution. Antibiotic therapy is continued.

In chronic osteomyelitis, antibiotics are adjunctive therapy to surgical debridement. A *sequestrectomy* (removal of enough involucrum to enable the surgeon to remove the sequestrum) is performed. Often, sufficient bone is removed to convert a deep cavity into a shallow saucer (*saucerization*). All dead, infected bone and cartilage must be removed before permanent healing takes place.

The wound is either closed tightly to obliterate the dead space or packed to be closed later by granulation or possibly by grafting. A closed suction irrigation system may be used to control the hematoma and remove debris. Physiologic saline solution is usually used for irrigation for 7 to 8 days. The development of superimposed infection may occur with prolonged irrigation.

The debrided cavity may be packed with cancellous bone graft to stimulate healing. With a very large defect, the cavity may be filled with a vascularized bone transfer or *muscle flap* (in which a muscle is moved from an adjacent area with blood supply intact). These microsurgery techniques enhance the blood supply; improved blood supply facilitates bone healing and eradication of the infection. These surgical procedures may be staged over time to ensure healing. Saucerization weakens the bone, which then may need stabilization or support from internal fixation or external supportive devices. During the postoperative period, measures are taken to ensure adequate circulation (wound suction to prevent fluid accumulation, elevation of the area to promote venous drainage, avoidance of pressure on grafted area), to maintain needed immobility, and to comply with weight-bearing restrictions.

The general health and nutrition of the patient are monitored and enhanced. Fluids and a balanced diet high in protein, vitamin C, and vitamin D are desired to ensure a positive nitrogen balance and to promote healing.

▷ *Knowledge of the Therapeutic Regimen.* Management of osteomyelitis may require wound care and intravenous antibiotic therapy at home. The patient must be medically stable and motivated, and the family must be supportive. The home environment needs to be conducive to promotion of health and compliance with the therapeutic regimen.

It is important that the patient and family understand the antibiotic protocol. In addition, aseptic dressing changing and warm compress techniques are taught. Patient education before discharge from the hospital and adequate supervision and support systems are important for successful home management of osteomyelitis.

These patients need to be monitored carefully for development of additional painful areas or sudden increases in temperature. The patient is instructed to observe and report elevated temperature, drainage, odor, and increased inflammation.

▷ **Evaluation**

Expected Outcomes

1. Experiences relief of pain
   a. Reports decreased pain
   b. Experiences no tenderness in area of previous infection
   c. Experiences no discomfort with movement
2. Increases physical mobility
   a. Participates in self-care activities
   b. Maintains full function of unimpaired extremities
   c. Demonstrates safe use of immobilizing device and ambulatory aid
3. Absence of infection
   a. Takes antibiotic as prescribed
   b. Temperature normal
   c. Absence of swelling
   d. Absence of drainage
   e. WBC and sedimentation rate return to normal
   f. Wound cultures negative
4. Conveys an understanding of the health care program
   a. Takes medications as prescribed
   b. Protects weakened bones
   c. Demonstrates proper wound care
   d. Reports problems promptly
   e. Eats a balanced diet that is high in protein and vitamins C and D
   f. Keeps follow-up health appointments
   g. Reports increased strength
   h. Reports no elevation of temperature or recurrence of pain, swelling, or other symptoms at the site

Septic (Infectious) Arthritis

Joints can become infected by spread of infection from other parts of the body (*hematogenous spread)* or directly by trauma or surgical instrumentation. Previous trauma to joints, coexisting arthritis, and diminished host resistance contribute to the development of an infected joint. *Gonococci* and *staphylococci* cause most adult joint infections. Prompt recognition and treatment of an infected joint are important because accumulating pus results in *chondrolysis* (destruction of hyaline cartilage), which heals poorly.

Clinical Manifestations.   The patient with an acute septic arthritis usually presents with a warm, painful, swollen joint with decreased range of motion. Systemic chills and fever may be present. Assessment for a primary locus of infection (*e.g.*, a carbuncle) is performed. Elderly patients and persons taking corticosteroids or immunosuppressive drugs may not exhibit typical clinical manifestations of infection.

Diagnostic Evaluation.   Diagnostic studies include aspiration, examination, and culture of the synovial fluid. Arthrograms may disclose damage to the joint lining. Radioisotope scanning is useful in localizing the process and distinguishing between a joint infection and an overlying cellulitis.

Management.   Prompt treatment is essential. Antibiotics, such as nafcillin, cephalosporin, and gentamicin, should be started promptly by intravenous infusion. Penicillin G is used for gonococcal septic arthritis. The parenteral antibiotics are continued until symptoms disappear. The synovial fluid is monitored for sterility and decrease in white blood cells.

In addition to prescribing antibiotics, the physician may aspirate the joint to remove the excessive joint fluid, exudate, and debris. Occasionally, arthrotomy or arthroscopy is used to drain the joint and remove dead tissue.

The inflamed joint is supported and immobilized by a splint in a functional position that increases the patient's comfort. Codeine may be prescribed to control pain. After the infection has responded to antibiotic therapy, nonsteroidal anti-inflammatory drugs may be prescribed.

The patient's nutrition and fluids are monitored to promote healing. Progressive range of motion exercises are prescribed when the infection subsides.

If septic joints are treated early, recovery of normal function should occur. The patient is assessed periodically for recurrence. If the articular cartilage was damaged during the inflammatory reaction, joint fibrosis and diminished function may result.

In summary, musculoskeletal infections include osteomyelitis and septic arthritis. Prevention of infection is the goal because osteomyelitis may affect the quality of life or result in the loss of an extremity. Osteomyelitis may be associated with direct bone contamination (*e.g.*, open fracture, bone surgery), extension of soft-tissue infection, or hematogenous spread. Prophylactic antibiotics and conscientious aseptic techniques reduce the incidence of osteomyelitis, which may be evident soon after orthopedic injury or surgery or may not become evident for months or years after the surgery. The nurse assists the patient to understand and comply with the therapeutic regimen, which may include long courses of antibiotic therapy and surgical debridement, pain management, and mobility limitations to prevent pathologic fractures. Septic arthritis requires prompt treatment to preserve joint function.

Bone Tumors

Neoplasms of the musculoskeletal system are of a variety of types. They include osteogenic, chondrogenic, fibrogenic, muscle (rhabdomyogenic), and marrow (reticulum) cell tumors as well as nerve, vascular, and fatty cell tumors. They may be primary tumors or metastatic tumors from primary cancers elsewhere in the body (*e.g.*, breast, lung, prostate, kidney). Metastatic bone tumors occur more frequently in older patients.

Benign Bone Tumors

Benign bone tumors generally are slow growing and well circumscribed, present few symptoms, and are not a cause of death. Benign primary neoplasms of the musculoskeletal system include osteochondroma, enchondroma, osteoid osteoma, bone cyst (*e.g.*, aneurysmal bone cyst), rhabdomyoma, and fibroma. Benign tumors of the bone and soft tissue are more common than malignant tumors. Some benign tumors such as giant cell tumors have the potential of undergoing malignant transformation.

Bone cysts are expanding lesions within the bone. *Aneurysmal bone cysts* are seen in young adults, and present with a painful, palpable mass of the long bones, vertebrae, or flat bones. *Unicameral bone cysts* occur in children and cause mild discomfort and possible pathologic fractures of the upper humerus and femur. These may heal spontaneously.

Osteochondroma is the most common benign bone tumor, and usually occurs as a large projection of bone at the end of long bones (at the knee or shoulder). It develops during growth and then becomes a static bony mass. The cartilage cap of the osteochondroma may undergo malignant transformation after trauma, and a chondrosarcoma may develop.

Enchondroma is a common tumor of the hyaline cartilage that develops in the hand, ribs, femur, tibia, humerus, or pelvis. Generally, the only symptom is a mild ache. Pathologic fractures may occur.

A painful tumor that occurs in children and young adults is the *osteoid osteoma*. The neoplastic tissue is surrounded by reactive bone formation that assists in its radiologic identification.

Giant cell tumors (osteoclastoma) are benign for long periods, but may invade local tissue and cause destruction. They occur in young adults and are soft and hemorrhagic. Eventually giant cell tumors may undergo malignant transformation and metastasize.

Malignant Bone Tumors

Primary malignant musculoskeletal tumors are relatively rare and arise from connective and supportive tissue cells (*sarcomas*) or bone marrow elements (*myelomas*). Malignant primary musculoskeletal tumors include osteosarcoma, chondrosarcoma, Ewing's sarcoma, and fibrosarcoma. Soft-tissue sarcomas include liposarcoma, fibrosarcoma of soft tissue, and rhabdomyosarcoma. Bone tumor metastasis to the lungs is common.

Osteogenic sarcoma (osteosarcoma) is the most common and most often fatal primary malignant bone tumor. It is characterized by early hematogenous metastasis to the lungs. The tumor carries a high mortality rate because the sarcoma often has spread to the lungs by the time the patient seeks help. Osteogenic sarcoma appears most frequently in males in the age group between 10 and 25 (in bones that grow rapidly) and in older persons with Paget's disease or as a sequela of ionizing radiation. It is manifested by pain, swelling, limitation of motion, and weight loss (which is considered an ominous finding). The bony mass may be palpable, tender, and fixed, with an increase in skin temperature over the mass and venous distention. The primary lesion may involve any bone; the most common sites are the distal femur, the proximal tibia, and the proximal humerus.

Malignant tumors of the hyaline cartilage are called *chondrosarcomas* and are the second most common primary malignant bone tumor. They are large, bulky, slow-growing tumors that affect adults (men more frequently than women). The usual tumor sites include the pelvis, ribs, femur, humerus, spine, scapula, and tibia. Metastasis to the lungs occurs in fewer than half the patients. If these tumors are well differentiated, large block excision or amputation of the affected extremity results in increased survival rate. These tumors may recur.

Metastatic Bone Cancer

Metastatic bone carcinoma (secondary bone tumor) is more common than any primary malignant bone tumor. Tumors arising from tissues other than the bone may invade the bone and produce localized bone destruction, with results that are clinically quite analogous to those occurring in primary bone tumors. Tumors that metastasize to bone most frequently include carcinomas of the kidney, the prostate, the lung, the breast, the ovary, and the thyroid. Metastatic tumors most frequently attack the skull, spine, pelvis, femur, and humerus.

Pathophysiology

The presence of a tumor in the bone causes the normal bone tissue to react by *osteolytic* response (bone destruction) or by *osteoblastic* response (bone formation). Some of the bone tumors are common and some are exceedingly rare. Some present no problem, whereas others rapidly become life threatening.

Clinical Manifestations.   Patients with a bone tumor present with a wide range of associated problems. They may be asymptomatic or may have pain (mild and occasional to constant and severe); varying degrees of disability; and, at times, obvious bone growth. Weight loss, malaise, and fever may be present. The tumor may be diagnosed incidentally after pathologic fracture.

Diagnostic Evaluation.   Differential diagnosis is based on the history, physical examination, x-rays (including tomograms, bone scans, and arteriography) (Fig. 61-7), biochemical assays of the blood and urine (alkaline phosphatase is frequently elevated with osteogenic sarcoma; with metastatic carcinoma of the prostate, serum acid phosphatase is elevated), and, finally, surgical biopsy for histologic identification. Extreme care is taken during biopsy to prevent seeding and recurrence after excision of the tumor. Radiologic studies of the chest are done to determine the presence of lung metastasis. Staging is based on tumor size, grade, and location as well as on metastasis.

During the diagnostic period, the nurse provides explanations of the diagnostic tests and psychological and emotional support to the patient and his family. Coping behaviors are assessed and use of support systems are encouraged.

▶ # Nursing Process
The Patient With a Bone Tumor
▷ ### Assessment

The patient is encouraged to discuss the problem, and the onset and course of symptoms. During the interview, the nurse notes the patient's understanding of the disease process, how the patient and the family have been coping with the problem, and how the patient has managed the pain.

On physical examination, the mass is palpated gently; its size and associated soft-tissue swelling, pain, and tenderness are noted. Assessment of the neurovascular status and range of motion of the extremity provides baseline data for future comparisons. The patient's mobility and ability to perform activities of daily living are evaluated.

▷ ### Nursing Diagnoses

Based on the nursing assessment data, the major nursing diagnoses for the patient with a bone tumor may include the following:

- Knowledge deficit about the disease process and the therapeutic regimen
- Pain related to pathologic process and surgery
- High risk for injury: pathologic fracture related to tumor
- Ineffective coping related to fear of the unknown, perception of disease process, and inadequate support system
- Disturbance in self-esteem related to loss of body part or alteration in role performance

Nursing diagnoses related to potential complications include the following:

- Impaired tissue integrity with delayed wound healing related to surgery, radiation, or chemotherapy, and to immobility
- Altered nutrition related to chemotherapy or radiation
- High risk for infection related to immunosuppression caused by chemotherapy or radiation

▷ ### Planning and Implementation

▷ *Goals:*   The major goals of the patient include knowledge of disease process and treatment regimen, control of pain, absence of pathologic fractures, effective patterns of coping, improved self-esteem, and absence of complications such as impaired tissue integrity with delayed wound healing, altered nutrition, and infection.

▷ ### Nursing Interventions

The nursing care of a patient who has undergone excision of a bone tumor is similar in many respects to that for other patients who have had skeletal surgery. Vital signs are monitored; blood loss is assessed; observations are made to assess for the development of complications such as deep vein thrombosis, pulmonary emboli, infection, contracture, and disuse atrophy. The operative part should be elevated to control swelling; the neurovascular status of the extremity should be assessed. Generally, the area is immobilized by splints, casts, or elastic bandages until the bone heals.

▷ *Knowledge of Disease Process and Treatment Regimen.*   Patient and family education about the disease process and diagnostic and management regimens is essential. Explanation of diag-

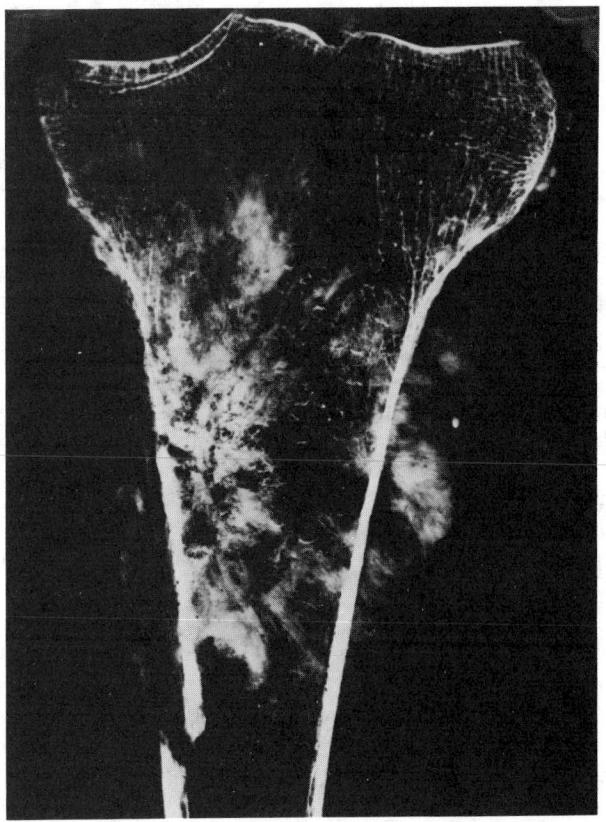
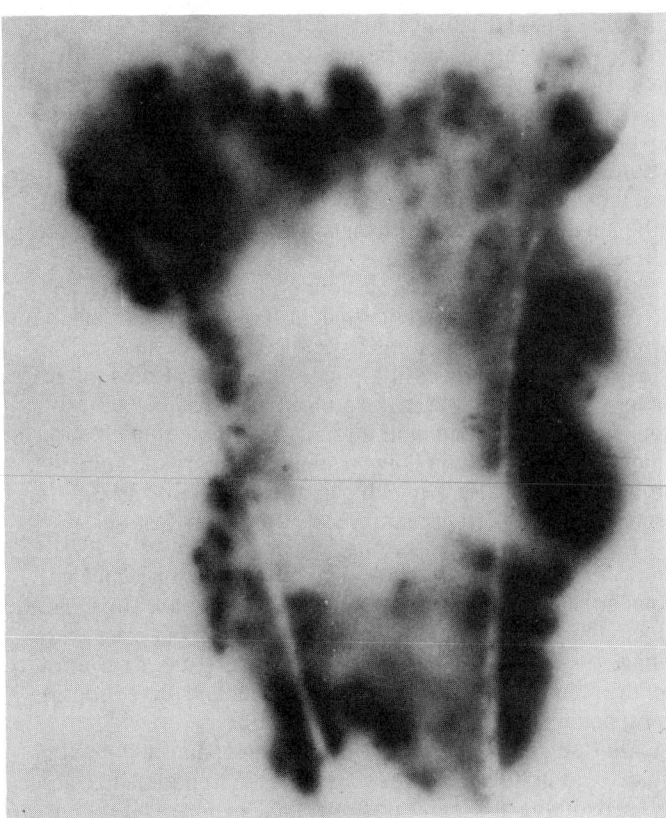

Figure 61–7. Bone scan of a patient with osteosarcoma. (**Left**) X-ray showing osteosarcoma at the proximal end of the tibia. Note the destruction of the normal anatomy of the bone. (**Right**) Contact autoradiograph of the same patient. The patient has received ^{85}Sr (strontium) intravenously for bone scanning. Note the high uptake (*black areas*) in the peripheral growing margin and the relative lack of uptake centrally. (Armed Forces Institute of Pathology. Negative 67-4-8, 67-4-9.)

nostic tests, treatments (*e.g.*, wound care), and expected results (*e.g.*, decreased range of motion, numbness, change of body contours) helps the patient deal with the procedures and changes. Cooperation and adherence to the therapeutic regimen are enhanced through understanding. The nurse can most effectively reinforce and clarify information provided by the physician by being present during these physician–patient discussions.

The goal of treatment is to destroy or remove the tumor tissue by the most effective method. Management of bone tumors includes surgical excision (ranging from local excision to amputation and disarticulation), radiation when the tumor is radiosensitive, and chemotherapy (preoperative, postoperative, and adjunctive for possible micrometastasis). Major gains are being made in using wide block excision with restorative grafting technique. Survival and quality of life are important considerations in procedures that attempt to save the involved extremity.

Surgical removal of the tumor frequently requires amputation of the affected extremity, with the amputation extending well above the bone tumor to achieve local control of the primary lesion. (See Nursing Process: The Patient Undergoing an Amputation, p. 1850.)

Limb-sparing (salvage) procedures remove the tumor and adjacent tissue. The resected portion is replaced by a custom-ized prosthesis, total joint arthroplasty, or bone tissue from the patient or cadaver donor. Soft tissue and blood vessels may need grafting because of the extent of the excision. Complications that may develop include infection, loosening or dislocation of the prosthesis, allograft nonunion, fracture, devitalization of the skin and soft tissues, joint fibrosis, and recurrence of the tumor. Function and rehabilitation after limb salvage depend on reducing the risk of complications and positive encouragement.

Because of the real danger of metastasis with malignant tumors, combined chemotherapy is started before and continued after surgery in an effort to eradicate micrometastatic lesions. The hope is that combined chemotherapy will have a greater effect at a lower toxicity rate, while reducing resistance to the drugs. There is an improved (60%) long-term survival rate when a localized osteosarcoma is removed and chemotherapy (doxorubicin hydrochloride and cisplatin or methotrexate) is initiated.

Soft-tissue sarcomas are treated with radiation, limb-sparing excision, and adjuvant chemotherapy. Additional therapies are consistent with methods used to treat the original cancer.

The treatment of metastatic bone cancer is palliative, and the therapeutic goal is to relieve the patient's discomfort as much as possible. Internal fixation of pathologic fractures minimizes associated disability and pain. At times, large bone metastatic lesions are strengthened by prophylactic internal fixation.

The patient is encouraged to be as independent as possible and function as long as possible. Surgery may be indicated for fractures of long bones.

Preparation for and coordination of continuing health care are begun early as a multidisciplinary effort. Patient education is directed at medication, dressing, and treatment regimens, as well as physical and occupational therapy programs. The safe use of special equipment is taught. The patient and family learn the signs and symptoms of possible complications. The patient is advised to have the phone numbers of persons to contact readily available in case problems arise. Frequently, arrangements are made with a home health care agency for home care supervision. Follow-up appointments are scheduled. The need for long-term health supervision is emphasized to ensure cure or to detect tumor recurrence or metastasis.

▷ *Controlling Pain.*   Psychological, pharmacologic, and environmental pain management techniques are useful. The nurse works with the patient in designing the most effective pain management regimen, thereby increasing the patient's control over the pain. The nurse prepares the patient and gives support during painful procedures.

After surgery, the patient experiences pain at both the surgical and graft donor sites. Prescribed narcotic analgesics are used during the early postoperative period. Later, oral, nonnarcotic analgesics are usually adequate to control discomfort.

▷ *Absence of Pathologic Fracture.*   Bone tumors weaken the bone to a point where normal activities or position changes can result in fracture. During nursing care, the affected bones must be supported and handled gently. External supports (*e.g.,* splints) may be used for additional protection. Prescribed weight-bearing restrictions must be followed. The patient is taught how to use ambulatory aids safely and how to strengthen unaffected extremities.

▷ *Achieving Effective Patterns of Coping.*   The patient and family must be encouraged to express their feelings honestly. They need to be supported and to feel accepted as they come to grips with the impact of the malignant bone tumor. Feelings of shock, despair, and grief are expected. Referral to health care professionals for specific psychological help may be appropriate.

▷ *Improving Self-Esteem.*   Independence versus dependence is an issue with the patient who has a malignancy. Life style is dramatically changed, at least temporarily. The family is supported in working through the adjustments that must be made. Changes in body image due to surgery and possibly amputation need to be recognized. Realistic reassurance about the future and about resumption of role-related activities is provided. Self-care and socialization are encouraged. The patient should help plan daily activities. Involvement of the patient and family throughout the treatment process promotes confidence, restoration of self-concept, and a sense of being in control of one's life.

▷ *Promotion of Tissue Integrity.*   Wound healing may be delayed because of tissue trauma from surgery or previous radiation. Pressure on the wound site is minimized to promote cir-

culation to the tissues. An aseptic, nontraumatic wound dressing promotes healing. Monitoring and reporting of laboratory findings facilitate prescription of interventions (*i.e.,* blood transfusion; electrolyte balance) to promote homeostasis. Balanced nutritional intake is encouraged to promote wound healing.

Repositioning the patient at frequent intervals reduces the incidence of skin breakdown due to pressure. Tissue that has been exposed to radiotherapy is very susceptible to breakdown. At times the nutritional status, pain, and avoidance of movement contribute to potential for skin breakdown. Special therapeutic beds may be needed to prevent skin breakdown.

▷ *Achieving Adequate Nutritional Status.*   Monitoring of balanced nutrition is necessary for health promotion. Frequently a side effect of therapeutic interventions (*i.e.,* chemotherapy; radiation therapy) is loss of appetite, nausea, and vomiting. Antiemetics and relaxation techniques reduce the gastrointestinal reaction. Stomatitis is controlled with anesthetic or antifungal mouthwash. Adequate hydration is essential. Nutritional supplements or total parenteral nutrition may be prescribed to achieve adequate nutrition.

▷ *Absence of Infection.*   Osteomyelitis is a concern. Prophylactic antibiotics and strict aseptic dressing techniques are used to diminish the occurrence of this dreaded complication. During healing, other infections (*e.g.,* upper respiratory infections) need to be avoided so that hematogenous spread does not result in an osteomyelitis.

If the patient is receiving chemotherapy, the patient's white blood cell count is monitored and the patient is taught to avoid persons with colds and infections.

▷ ## Evaluation

Expected Outcomes
1. Describes disease process and treatment regimen
   a. Describes pathologic problem
   b. States goals of the therapeutic regimen
   c. Complies with prescribed regimen (*i.e.,* takes prescribed medications, continues physical and occupational therapy programs)
   d. Seeks clarification of information
   e. Acknowledges need for long-term health supervision
   f. Keeps follow-up health care appointments
   g. Reports occurrence of symptoms of complications
2. Achieves control of pain
   a. Uses multiple pain control techniques, including prescribed medications
   b. Experiences no pain or decreased pain at rest, during activities of daily living, or at surgical sites
3. Experiences no pathologic fracture
   a. Avoids stress to weakened bones
   b. Uses ambulatory aid safely
   c. Strengthens uninvolved extremities
4. Demonstrates effective coping patterns
   a. Verbalizes feelings
   b. Identifies strengths and abilities
   c. Makes decisions
   d. Requests assistance as needed
5. Demonstrates positive self-concept
   a. Assumes responsibilities
   b. Exhibits confidence in own abilities
   c. Demonstrates acceptance of altered body image
   d. Demonstrates independence in activities of daily living

6. Exhibits absence of complications
   a. Demonstrates wound healing
   b. Experiences no skin breakdown
   c. Maintains or increases body weight
   d. Experiences no infections
   e. Manages side effects of therapies
   f. Reports symptoms of drug toxicity or complications of surgery

In summary, bone tumors may be benign (slow growing and well circumscribed), malignant (sarcomas arising from connective and supportive tissue cells), or metastatic carcinomas. Symptoms as well as therapy depend on the nature of the bone tumor. The goal of therapy for primary bone tumors is the destruction or removal of the tumor tissue by the most effective method (surgery, radiation, or chemotherapy). Wide-block excision with restorative grafting and limb-sparing procedures frequently can be used, avoiding amputation. Care of a patient who has had orthopedic surgery for bone tumor is similar in many respects to that for patients who have had skeletal surgery. The goal of therapy for metastatic bone tumors is palliative to control the patient's pain and prevent pathologic fracture. The nurse assists the patient to understand the disease process, comply with the therapeutic regimen, control the pain, use effective coping techniques, improve self-esteem, and avoid pathologic fracture and other potential complications. Because of the multiple needs of the patient with a bone tumor, an interdisciplinary approach to care of the patient can be beneficial to the rehabilitation of the patient.

Bibliography

Books

American Nurses Association and National Association of Orthopaedic Nurses. Orthopaedic Nursing Practice. Kansas City, MO, American Nurses Association, 1986.

Avioli LV. The Osteoporotic Syndrome, 2nd ed. Orlando, Grune & Stratton, 1987.

Borenstein DB and Wiesel SW. Low Back Pain. Philadelphia, WB Saunders, 1989.

Buckle P. Musculoskeletal Disorders at Work. London, Taylor & Francis, 1987.

Cailliet R. Low Back Pain Syndrome, 4th ed. Philadelphia, FA Davis, 1988.

Coombs R and Fitzgerald RH Jr (ed). Infection in the Orthopaedic Patient. London, Butterworths, 1989.

D'Ambrosia RD and Marier RL (ed). Orthopaedic Infections. Thorofare, NJ, Slack, 1989.

Dahlin DC and Unni KK. Bone Tumors, 4th ed. Springfield, IL, Charles C Thomas, 1986.

Farrell J. Illustrated Guide to Orthopedic Nursing, 3rd ed. Philadelphia, JB Lippincott, 1986.

Footner A. Orthopaedic Nursing. London, Ballière Tindall, 1987.

Giles LGF. Anatomical Basis of Low Back Pain. Baltimore, Williams & Wilkins, 1989.

Gustilo RB et al (ed). Orthopaedic Infection: Diagnosis and Treatment. Philadelphia, WB Saunders, 1989.

Hughes SPF and Fitzgerald RH. Musculoskeletal Infections. Chicago, Year Book Medical Publishers, 1986.

Kirkaldy-Willis WH (ed). Managing Low Back Pain, 2nd ed. New York, Churchill Livingstone, 1988.

Lewis MM. Bone Tumor Surgery: Limb Sparing Techniques. Philadelphia, JB Lippincott, 1988.

Mourad LA and Droste MM. The Nursing Process in the Care of Adults With Orthopaedic Conditions, 2nd ed. New York, John Wiley & Sons, 1988.

Salmond S et al (eds). Core Curriculum for Orthopaedic Nurses, 2nd ed. Pitman, NJ, National Association for Orthopaedic Nurses, 1991.

Schlossberg D. Orthopedic Infection. New York, Springer-Verlag, 1988.

Siom FH. Diagnosis and Management of Metastatic Bone Disease: A Multidisciplinary Approach. New York, Raven Press, 1988.

Smith C. Orthopaedic Nursing. London, Heinemann Nursing, 1987.

Tam CS et al. Metabolic Bone Disease: Cellular and Tissue Mechanisms. Boca Raton, FL, CRC Press, 1989.

Tollison CD and Kriegel ML (ed). Interdisciplinary Rehabilitation of Low Back Pain. Baltimore, Williams & Wilkins, 1989.

Yaremchuk MJ et al. Lower Extremity Salvage and Reconstruction. New York, Elsevier, 1989.

Journals
Asterisks indicate nursing research articles.

Low Back Pain

Anderson L. Educational approaches to management of low back pain. Orthop Nurs 1989 Jan/Feb; 8(1): 43–46.

Boachie-Adjei D. Conservative management of low back pain: An evaluation of current methods. Postgrad Med 1988 Sep; 84(3): 127–133.

Dwyer AP. Backache and its prevention. Clin Orthop 1987 Sep; 222: 35–43.

Evans C et al. A randomized controlled trial of flexion exercises, education, and bedrest for patients with acute low back pain. Physiother Can 1987 Mar/Apr; 39(2): 96–101.

Fast A. Low back disorders: Conservative management. Arch Phys Med Rehabil 1988 Oct; 69(10): 880–891.

Gottlieb H et al. Self management for medication reduction in chronic low back pain. Arch Phys Med Rehabil 1988 Jun; 69(6): 442–448.

Harvey BL. Self care practices to prevent low back pain. AAOHN J 1988 May; 36(5): 211–217, 246–248.

Jameson RN et al. Treatment outcome in low back pain patients: Do compensation benefits make a difference. Orthop Rev 1988 Dec; 17(12): 1210–1215.

Klein HA et al. Low back pain. Clin Symp 1987; 39(6): 2–32.

Lanier DC and Stockton P. Clinical predictors of outcome of acute episodes of low back pain. J Fam Pract 1988 Nov; 27(5): 483–489.

Lee CK. Office management of low back pain. Orthop Clin North Am 1988 Oct; 19(4): 797–804.

*Lisanti P. Perceived body space and self-esteem in adult males with and without chronic low back pain. Orthop Nurs 1989 May/Jun; 8(3): 49–56.

McQuadek et al. Physical fitness and chronic low back pain: An analysis of the relationships among fitness, functional limitations, and depression. Clin Orthop 1988 Aug; 233: 198–204.

Posner JB. Back pain and epidural spinal cord compression. Med Clin North Am 1987 Mar; 71(2): 185–205.

Rosen CD et al. A retrospective analysis of the efficacy of epidural steroid injections. Clin Orthop 1988 Mar; 228: 270–272.

Smith IW et al. Nontechnologic strategies for coping with chronic low back pain. Orthop Nurs 1990 Jul/Aug; 9(4): 26–32.

Stauffer JD. Antidepressants and chronic pain. J Fam Pract 1987 Aug; 25(2): 167–170.

Swezey RL. Low back pain in the elderly: Practical management concerns. Geriatrics 1988 Feb; 43(2): 39–44.

Tollison CD and Kriegel ML. Physical exercise in treatment of low back pain, Part I. Orthop Rev 1988 Jul; 17(7): 724–729; Part II. Orthop Rev 1988 Sep; 17(9): 913–923; Part III. Orthop Rev 1988 Oct; 17(10): 1002–1006.

Uhl JE et al. Aching backs? A glimpse into the hazards of nursing. AAOHN J 1987 Jan; 35(1): 13–17.

Warfield CA. Facet syndrome and the relief of low back pain. Hosp Pract 1988 Oct 30; 23(10A): 41–42; 47–48.

Common Foot Problems

Flemming LL (ed). Management of foot problems. Orthop Clin North Am 1989 Oct; 20(4).

Osterman H and Stuck R. The aging foot. Orthop Nurs 1990 Nov/Dec; 9(6): 43–47.

Osteoporosis

Ausenhus MK. Osteoporosis: Prevention during the adolescent and young adult years. Nurs Pract 1988 Sep; 13(9): 42, 45, 48.

Barth RW and Lane JM. Osteoporosis. Orthop Clin North An 1988 Oct; 19(4): 845–858.

Barzel US. Estrogens in prevention and treatment of postmenopausal osteoporosis: A review. Am J Med 1988 Dec; 85(6): 847–850.

Bellantioni MF and Blackman MR. Osteoporosis: Diagnostic screening and its place in current care. Geriatrics 1988 Feb; 43(2): 63–70.

Carter LW. Calcium intake in young adult women: Implications for osteoporosis risk assessment. J Obstet Gynecol Neonatal Nurs 1987 Sep/Oct; 16(5): 8301–8308.

Cauley J et al. Endogenous estrogen levels and calcium intakes in postmenopausal women. JAMA 1988 Dec 2; 260(21): 3150–3155.

Cerrato PL. Piecing together the osteoporosis puzzle. RN 1990 Apr; 53(4): 77–82.

Chambers JK. Metabolic bone disorders. Imbalances of calcium and phosphorus. Nurs Clin North Am 1987 Dec; 22(4): 861–872.

Finn S. Osteoporosis: A nutritionist's approach. Health Values 1987 Jul/Aug; 11(4): 20–23.

Holm K and Dudas S. Osteoporosis: Implications for critical care. DCCN 1987 May/Jun; 6(3): 158–164.

Kaplan FS. Osteoporosis: Pathophysiology and prevention. Clin Symp 1987; 39(1): 2–32.

Ladage E et al. Osteoporosis and calcium. J Urol Nurs 1988 Jan/Mar; 7(1): 364–368.

Lamb K et al. Falls in the elderly: Causes and prevention. Orthop Nurs 1987 Mar/Apr; 6(2): 45–49.

Lane JM et al. Osteopenic syndromes. Orthop Rev 1988 Dec; 17(12): 1231–1235.

Lindsay R. Osteoporosis: An updated approach to prevention and management. Geriatrics 1989 Jan; 44(1): 45–54.

Lindsay R. Prevention of osteoporosis. Clin Orthop 1987 Sep; 222: 44–59.

Madson S. How to reduce the risk of postmenopausal osteoporosis. J Gerontol Nurs 1989 Sep; 15(9): 20–24.

Marcus R. Understanding and preventing osteoporosis. Hosp Pract 1989 Apr; 15; 24(4):189–215.

Martin AD and Houstin CS. Osteoporosis, calcium, and physical activity. Can Med Assoc J 1987 Mar 15; 136(6): 587–593.

McKenna MJ and Frame B. Hormonal influences on osteoporosis. Am J Med 1987 Jun 26; 82(1B): 61–67.

Pak CVC et al. Safe and effective treatment of osteoporosis with intermittent slow-release sodium fluoride: Augmentation of vertebral bone mass and inhibition of fractures. J Clin Endocrinol Metab 1989 Jan; 68(1): 150–159.

Perry BR. Living with osteoporosis: Early awareness and attention to lifestyle can delay or prevent osteoporosis. Geriatr Nurs 1988 May/Jun; 9(3): 174–176.

Raisz LB. Local and systemic factors in the pathogenesis of osteoporosis. N Engl J Med 1988 Mar 31; 318(13): 818–828.

Resnick NM and Greenspan SL. "Senile" osteoporosis reconsidered. JAMA 1989 Feb 17; 261(7): 1025–1029.

Rodysill KJ. Postmenopausal osteoporosis: Intervention and prophylaxis. J Chronic Dis 1987; 40(8): 743–760.

Santora AC II. Role of nutrition and exercise in osteoporosis. Am J Med 1987 Jan 26; 82(1B): 73–79.

Silverberg SJ and Lindsay R. Postmenopausal osteoporosis. Med Clin North Am 1987 Jan; 71(1): 41–57.

Simak M. Exercise and osteoporosis. Arch Phys Med Rehabil 1989 Mar; 70(3): 220–229.

Skolnick A. It's important, but don't bank on exercise alone to prevent osteoporosis, experts say. JAMA 1990 Apr 4; 263(13): 1751–1752.

Skolnick A. New doubts about benefit of sodium fluoride. JAMA 1990 Apr 4; 263(13): 1752–1753.

Skolnick A. New osteoporosis therapies appear close. JAMA 1990 Apr 4; 263(13): 1753.

Solomon DH et al. New issues in geriatric care. Ann Intern Med 1988 May; 108(5): 718–732.

Thorneycroft IH. The role of estrogen replacement therapy in the prevention of osteoporosis. Am J Obstet Gynecol 1989 May; 160(Suppl 2): 1306–1310.

Walden O. The relationship of dietary and supplemental calcium intake to bone loss and osteoporosis. J Am Diet Assoc 1989 Mar; 89(3): 397–400.

Watts NB. Osteoporosis. Am Fam Physician 1988 Nov; 38(5): 193–207.

Metabolic Bone Disorders

Cagel RF et al. Treatment of Paget's disease of bone with salmon calcitonin nasal spray. J Am Geriatr Soc 1988 Nov; 36(11): 1010–1014.

Chambers JK. Metabolic bone disorders. Imbalances in calcium and phosphorus. Nurs Clin North Am 1987 Dec; 22(4): 239–245.

Freeman DA. Paget's disease of bone. Am J Med Sci 1988 Feb; 295(2): 144–158.

Krozy RE. Paget's disease: Implications for home nursing. Home Health Nurs 1987 Mar/Apr; 5(2): 324.

Lando M et al. Stabilization of hearing loss in Paget's disease with calcitonin and etidronate. Arch Otolaryngol Head Neck Surg 1988 Aug; 114(8): 891–894.

Rosenthal MJ et al. Paget's disease of bone in older patients. J Am Geriatr Soc 1989 Jul; 37(7): 639–650.

Osteomyelitis

Bamberger DM et al. Osteomyelitis in the feet of diabetic patients. Am J Med 1987 Oct; 83(4): 653–660.

Dimant J and Tanael L. Decubitus ulcers: When to suspect osteomyelitis. Geriatrics 1987 Jun; 42(6): 74, 79, 83.

Esterhai JL et al. Treatment of chronic refractory osteomyelitis with adjunctive hyperbaric oxygen. Orthop Rev 1988 Aug; 17(8): 809–815.

Esterhai JL et al. Adjunctive hyperbaric oxygen therapy in the treatment of chronic refractory osteomyelitis. J Trauma 1987 Jul; 27(7): 763–768.

Gabb G et al. Hyperbaric oxygen therapy in search of diseases. Chest 1987 Dec; 92(6): 1074–1082.

Gentry LO. Home management of osteomyelitis. Bull NY Acad Med 1988 Jul/Aug; 64(6): 565–569.

Martin ME. Oral antibiotics for treatment of patients with chronic osteomyelitis. Orthop Nurs 1989 May/Jun; 8(3): 35–38.

Perry CR et al. Local antibiotic administration in a inplantable pump for treatment of chronic osteomyelitis. Hosp Formul 1988 Apr; 23(4): 342–351.

Musculoskeletal Tumors

Barker C. Is it drug toxicity—Or something else? Nursing 1989 Apr; 19(4): 84–86.

Bone tumors: Evaluation and treatment. Orthop Clin North Am 1989 Jul; 80(3).

Common soft tissue tumors. Clin Symp 1990; 42(1): 2–32.

Edeiken J and Karasick D. Imaging in bone cancer. CA 1987 Jul/Aug; 37(4): 239–245.

Lang JM (ed). Pathological fractures in metabolic bone disease. Orthop Clin North Am 1990 Jan; 21(1).

Lewis MM (ed). Bone tumors: Evaluation and treatment. Orthop Clin North Am 1989 Jul; 20(3).

Lord CF et al. Infection in bone allografts: Incidence, nature, and treatment. J Bone Joint Surg (Am) 1988 Mar; 70A(3): 369–376.

Nicholson S. Femoral-tibial replacement for osteosarcoma. Nurs Times 1988 Feb 17–23; 84(7): 34–37.

Osteogenic sarcoma: Incidence and distribution. Hosp Med 1987 Jun; 23(6): 19, 22.

Raconlin, AA and Present D. Osteochondral allografts for limb salvage. Orthop Nurs 1989 Mar/Apr; 8(2): 35–39.

Sartoris D et al. New concepts in bone grafting. Orthop Rev 1987 Mar; 16(3): 154–164.

Siegal RD et al. Osteosarcoma in adults. Clin Orthop 1989 Mar; 240: 261–269.

Simon MA. Limb salvage for osteosarcoma. J Bone Joint Surg [Am] 1988 Feb; 70(2): 307–310.

Springfield DS et al. Surgical treatment for osteosarcoma. J Bone Joint Surg [Am] 1988 Sep; 70(8): 1124–1130.

Stine KC et al. Systemic doxorubicin and intraarterial cisplatin preoperative chemotherapy plus postoperative chemotherapy in patients with osteosarcoma. Cancer 1989 Mar 1; 63(5): 848–853.

Taylor WF et al. Prognostic variables in osteosarcoma: A multi institutional study. J Natl Cancer Inst 1989 Jan 4; 81(1): 21–30.

Welch–McCaffrey. Metastatic bone cancer. Cancer Nurs 1988 Apr; 11(2): 103–111.

Agencies

American Chronic Pain Association
257 Old Haymaker Road, Monroeville, PA 15146

National Committee on the Treatment of Intractable Pain
c/o Wayne Coy, Jr., Cohn & Marks, 1333 New Hampshire Ave. NW, Washington, DC 20036

National Easter Seals Society
2023 West Ogden Ave., Chicago, IL 60612

National Institute of Arthritis and Musculoskeletal and Skin Diseases
National Institutes of Health, Bethesda, MD 20892

National Osteoporosis Foundation
2100 M Street NW, Suite 602, Washington, DC 20037

Osteogenesis Imperfecta Foundation, Inc.
P.O. Box 14807, Clearwater, FL 34629-4807

Paget's Disease Foundation
165 Cadman Plaza East, Brooklyn, NY 11202

Texas Back Institute
3801 West 15th Street, Plano, TX 75075

Nursing Research Profile for Unit 15

Orthopedic Research Profile

Nursing research related to problems that patients with musculoskeletal conditions may encounter is found primarily in specialty nursing journals. The research conducted by nurses in this specialty is gradually growing. The following studies focus on issues related to nursing management of individuals with orthopedic conditions and some of the physical and psychosocial factors related to musculoskeletal disorders.

▷ Hoshiko B. *Valsalva maneuver as a possible risk factor for pulmonary embolism.* Orthop Nurs 1990 Jan/Feb; 9(1): 56–62.

Orthopedic patients are at high risk for pulmonary emboli. The hemodynamics of the Valsalva maneuver were reviewed. Activities that reflect Valsalva maneuvers and that would be recorded in patient records were identified. These indicators included ones that were gastrointestinal/urinary-related (*e.g.*, straining at stool), lifting-related (*e.g.*, use of trapeze, self-move), respiratory-related (*e.g.*, coughing), and others (*e.g.*, pain).

The study used a case-control retrospective design to describe the frequency of Valsalva maneuvers in individuals prior to experiencing pulmonary emboli and the frequency of Valsalva maneuvers in individuals who did not experience pulmonary emboli in a comparable time span. The sample was selected from computer listings of patients. Each subject who experienced pulmonary embolism as a complication of hospitalization was matched according to age, gender, and year of hospitalization (1979–1986) with two randomly selected subjects who did not experience pulmonary embolism. A total of 30 subjects were in the pulmonary embolism group and 60 subjects were in the control group.

A Valsalva maneuver indicator tool was developed for the purposes of the study. The overall frequency of Valsalva maneuver and the frequencies of gastrointestinal/urinary-related and lifting-related Valsalva maneuvers were found to be significantly higher for the pulmonary emboli subject group than for the control group. In addition, the level of activity of the groups differed significantly. Subjects experiencing pulmonary emboli were primarily on bed rest, and the subjects of the control group were out of bed more than 4 hours a day. This

was an uncontrolled confounding variable. Other limitations in the study included use of a newly developed Valsalva maneuver indicator tool without established validity and reliability, difficulty in measuring some of the specific indicators (*e.g.*, coughing, constipation, straining) through retrospective chart audits, and lack of intrarater consistency and reliability (research bias).

Nursing Implications. The investigator suggested that Valsalva maneuvers may be related to the incidence of pulmonary emboli. The combination of Valsalva maneuvers and bed rest may increase the risk of pulmonary emboli. Further studies, with matching of activity levels of subjects in the two study groups, are needed to substantiate these conclusions.

Orthopedic patients are especially at risk for the development of pulmonary emboli. Nursing interventions that reduce the incidence of Valsalva maneuvers in combination with other strategies designed to reduce the incidence of deep vein thrombosis (*e.g.*, mobilization, elastic stockings, anticoagulants) may be safe, effective pulmonary emboli prophylaxis.

▷ Jones-Walton P. *Effects of pin care on pin reactions in adults with extremity fracture treated with skeletal traction and external fixation.* Orthop Nurs 1988 Jul/Aug; 7(4):29–33.

A major concern with skeletal traction and subcutaneous pins is the development of uncomfortable reactions and osteomyelitis. Multiple approaches to prevent the occurrence of pin reactions are used. These are based on institutional protocol or surgeon preference. This retrospective study was designed to identify the characteristics of pin reaction and to describe the pin care protocols. Pin reactions were defined as adverse tissue response to the pin and were classified as either minor or major depending upon whether the pin had to be removed for improvement of the condition. Host factors, including age, sex, medication therapy, and health history, were considered.

Twelve records of adults who had sustained a single upper or lower extremity fracture, who were treated with skeletal traction or external fixation within 48 hours of admission, and who were maintained in the device for at least 3 weeks were included in this study. Nine of the subjects received some type of hydrogen peroxide treatment for the pin site; the remaining three subjects received no pin site care.

Seven of the 12 subjects were identified as having no significant pin reaction activity. Six of the seven nonreactive cases had closed fractures. The length of time the pin was in place was significantly longer in the reactive group. Minor and major reactions occurred in five of the nine individuals who had received pin care, and no reaction occurred in those who received no pin care. The researcher concluded that routine pin care with a hydrogen peroxide protocol did not deter development of pin reactions. Host factors identified did not present significant patterns.

Nursing Implications.   No conclusions concerning the efficacy of pin care rituals can be made based on this small study. Studies are needed to address the factors that affect the incidence of pin site reactions and to identify nursing care protocols that reduce pin reactions. Current practices of pin care are not based on scientific evidence. Host factors may be more important variables in the incidence of pin reactions than the pin care that is administered.

▷   *Selman S. Impact of total hip replacement on quality of life.*
    Orthop Nurs 1989 Sep/Oct; 8(5):43–49.

Chronic illness affects multiple aspects of life, including physiologic functioning, self-concept, role function, and interdependence. This retrospective, descriptive study examined the impact of total hip replacement in individuals with osteoarthritis on these aspects of their lives and the dimensions of quality of life.

The accessible population included patients between the ages of 30 and 90 who had osteoarthritis, who had undergone total hip replacement within the past 12 to 24 months, and who were patients of eight orthopedic surgeons. The convenience sample of 46 patients completed a 57-item, modified Arthritis Impact Measurement Scales questionnaire. Qualitative information on general satisfaction with having a total hip replacement was secured through a Likert scale. Reliability and validity of the tools were not fully established.

The study findings revealed that the subjects experienced positive changes in physiologic functioning, self-concept, and role function following total hip replacement. In the area of interdependence, approximately half of the subjects reported a positive change, while the others reported no change or a negative change. Significant positive correlations were found among all variables; physiologic variable correlations with all other variables were strongest. The study also examined the impact of age, sex, and marital status on the four dimensions. Comments regarding general satisfaction with total hip replacement were overwhelmingly positive.

Generalization of the findings of this study is limited by the design and sampling process. Replication of the study with the use of probability sampling is needed.

Nursing Implications.   The nurse can refer to this study when supporting the decision of the individual with osteoarthritis to have total joint replacement. An optimistic attitude focused on an improved quality of life is to be fostered. During the rehabilitative stages, the nurse encourages the patient to achieve the maximum potential and physiologic functioning.

▷   *Wild E et al. Analyses of wrist injuries in workers engaged in*
    repetitive tasks. AAOHN J 1987 Aug; 35(8):356–366.

An increased incidence of wrist injuries, including carpal tunnel syndrome, ganglion cysts, sprains, tendonitis, and tenosynovitis, was identified among female workers classified as "flyers" at a paper products manufacturing company. Their work activities included handling, inspecting, and packing cartons in shipping boxes. These tasks required repeated wrist

motions, including forceful hyperextension, flexion, twisting, and ulnar deviation, as well as lifting.

This retrospective epidemiologic study examined wrist injuries in 45 employees. Past time period (*i.e.*, the time prior to 12 months before the study) and present time period (*i.e.*, the 12 months preceding and including the study time) were studied. Demographic data, employment history, attitudes toward the job, medical and surgical history, and symptoms and conditions experienced in the two time frames were collected through self-administered questionnaires. The work site was evaluated also.

Twenty percent of the subjects reported work-related injuries documented by physicians. More than half of the subjects reported problems with their forearms, wrists, or hands during the study time periods. Symptoms reported most frequently included numbness, tingling, pain, aching weakness, loss of feeling, and prickling sensation. The left hand was affected more frequently than the right. No association was found between health status and incidence of reported symptoms and problems. Through analysis of age, height, length of employment, and length of time in the job category, the younger, shorter employee who had been in this job category less than 4 years was most susceptible to wrist and forearm injury.

Nursing Implications.   This study has multiple implications for nurses, particularly the occupational health nurse. The study findings suggest that the workplace needs to be ergonomically designed to optimize human efficiency and well-being. By designing the workplace ergonomically and modifying the speed and stress impact of the task, the incidence of work-related injury may be reduced.

▷   *Gleit C and Graham B. Secondary data analysis: A valuable*
    resource. Nurs Res 1989 Nov/Dec; 38(6):380–381.

This descriptive study compared 456 individuals who had sustained a hip fracture with a control group matched according to age and sex who had not sustained a hip fracture. The purpose of the study was to compare the two groups with regard to activities of daily living, family support, level of satisfaction with health status, physical mobility, and use of community resources. An attempt was made to correlate these variables with incidence of falls and resulting hip fractures. The sample was obtained from the National Center for Health Statistics, National Health Interview Survey, Supplement on Aging, a national random stratified sample of 16,148 individuals over 55 years old.

The study findings confirmed results of previous studies and generated new information. Both groups reported several falls within the past year; however, the hip fracture group experienced more falls than the control group. The hip fracture group reported more visual and hearing problems, which may have contributed to the incidence of falls. The hip fracture group had reduced physical mobility, more osteoporosis, and arthritis. The hip fracture group was less active; however, exercise patterns were similar to those of the control group. Episodes of confusion and forgetfulness were similar for the two groups. The hip fracture group worried more about their health; however, perceived control over health was similar in the two groups.

The use of community services (*e.g.*, special transportation, home meal delivery, homemaker services, telephone checks, adult day care) was similar for both groups. The hip fracture group used visiting nurses and home health aides and attended senior centers more frequently than did the control group.

Nursing Implications. A combination of factors, including diminished vision and hearing, osteoporosis, and reduced physical mobility due to conditions such as arthritis, may contribute to falls and the incidence of fractured hips in the elderly. Health education by the nurse to compensate for diminished visual and auditory acuity and promotion of physical mobility in a hazard-free environment may reduce the incidence of hip fracture.

▷ Medhat A et al. *Factors that influence level of activities in persons with lower extremity amputation*. Rehabil Nurs 1990 Jan/Feb; 15(1):113–118.

The premise of this study was that diminished abilities in one aspect of one's life affect all other dimensions. The researchers described and compared the impact of above-the-knee and below-the-knee amputation on aspects of "normal life-style."

The specified dimensions studied were activities of daily living, social participation, sexual functioning, and athletic participation. Need fulfillment and adaptation interactions are manifested in these dimensions. Success in the performance of activities of daily living promotes fulfillment of expected functional roles and independence. Social interaction enhances one's sense of self-worth. The need for intimacy is fulfilled through expressions of sexuality. Participation in physical activities promotes self-expression and achievement.

The study sample was selected from a veterans hospital and a large university medical center. The 131 subjects were 24 to 90 years old (mean, 58 years) and had lower limb amputations as a result of peripheral vascular disease, trauma, gangrene, diabetes, malignancy, and infection. Ninety-three percent of the subjects were male. Only 6% of the sample reported never using a prosthesis.

The subjects completed the Prosthetic Problems Inventory Scale questionnaire designed for this study to assess the dimensions of activities of daily living, social participation, sexual functioning, and athletic participation. Reliability and validity of the instrument were not reported.

The study demonstrated a significantly greater level of functioning by the individuals with below-the-knee amputation on the social participation dimension. Activities of daily living that posed major problems for both groups were showering, yard care, and gardening. The individuals with above-the-knee amputations reported additional difficulty with shopping, floor maintenance, and dressing. Low-level sexual performance difficulty was described by both groups. Difficulty with athletic activities requiring use of the lower limbs was reported by both groups.

Generalization of the findings of this study is limited by the sampling process and descriptive design. Replication of the study is needed.

Nursing Implications. The study supports the use of holistic nursing assessment to design a rehabilitation program that helps the client achieve the rehabilitative goal of highest level of independent physical, psychological, and social functioning. The findings suggest that development of balance, facilitation of visual and proprioceptive adaptation, and coordination of movement may promote a high level of independence in activities of daily living. Amputee self-help groups may be helpful to facilitate reintegration of individuals by promoting coping skills and problem-solving strategies in safe social situations. Sexuality issues may not be expressed freely but need to be evaluated, with guidance provided as appropriate. Opportunities for physical activity need to be shared with the individual who has experienced an amputation. Specific, individualized conditioning programs may be helpful in promoting endurance and confidence for participation in athletic activities.

▷ Lisanti P. *Perceived body space and self-esteem in adult males with and without chronic low back pain*. Orthop Nurs 1989 May/Jun; 8(3):49–56.

Individuals with chronic low back pain were compared with individuals with the chronic health problem of hypertension. This comparative study examined differences between the groups in perceived body space as measured by a topographic instrument, and self-esteem as measured by a self-report instrument. A depression inventory was administered also. Male clients between the ages of 35 and 45 years participating in ambulatory care programs were recruited for the purposive sample. The low back pain group consisted of 42 subjects and the comparative group consisted of 43 subjects with hypertension.

The researcher hypothesized that the subjects with chronic pain would perceive larger body space and lower self-esteem than those who did not experience chronic pain. This hypothesis was not supported. Depression scores for both groups were within the nondepressed range. In both groups, Pearson correlation coefficients were significant for depression and self-esteem and depression and social status. The chronic pain group demonstrated a significant correlation between social status and self-esteem.

Previous studies were cited that described low self-esteem associated with chronic pain. The researcher suggests that the inconsistencies between this study and previous studies may be related to the subjects' intact social support systems, active employment, and involvement with life. The chronic low back pain group did not demonstrate the characteristics of invalidism and disability frequently described. Additional research related to the impact of chronic health problems on overall well-being is needed.

Nursing Implications. Promotion of self-esteem in individuals with chronic health problems is a nursing responsibility. The nurse assists the patient to recognize responses to chronic health problems, strengths, limitations, and available social support. The effects of chronic pain on self-esteem may be reduced with adequate social support and involvement in life activities.

unit 16
Other Acute Problems

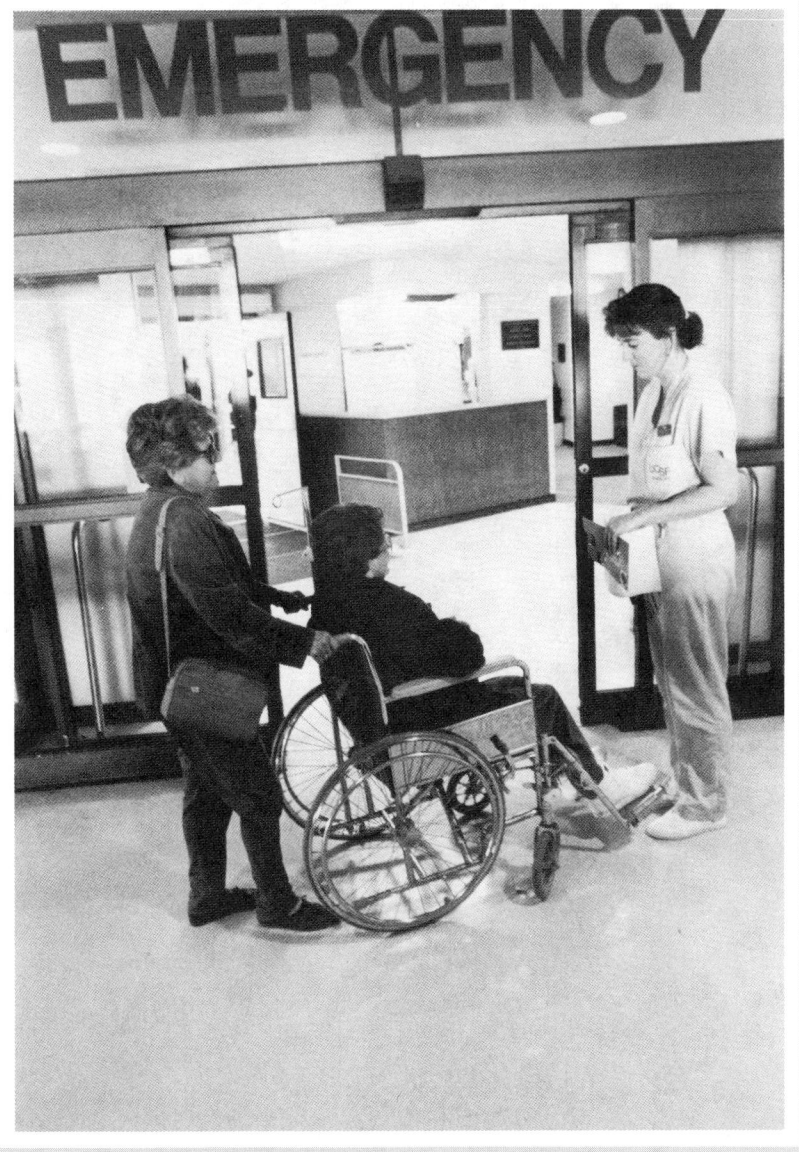

62

Management of Patients With Infectious Diseases

Chapter Outline

Learning Objectives

On completion of this chapter, the learner will be able to:

1. Identify the chain of events responsible for the spread of infectious diseases
2. Specify the parameters used in the assessment of patients for presence of infectious disease
3. Compare active and passive immunity
4. Describe the significance of universal precautions in preventing the spread of infection
5. Use the nursing process as a framework for care of patients with infectious disease
6. Specify the etiology and incidence of sexually transmitted diseases
7. Compare gonorrhea, syphilis, and acquired immunodeficiency syndrome—their pathophysiology, clinical manifestations, complications, management, and prevention
8. Use the nursing process as a framework for care of patients with sexually transmitted disease
9. Use the nursing process as a framework for care of patients with septic shock

(continued)

Learning Objectives (Continued)

10. Use the nursing process as a framework for care of patients with tuberculosis
11. Compare the various viral infections: their etiology, clinical manifestations, management, and prevention
12. Compare the various protozoan infections: their etiology, clinical manifestations, management, and prevention
13. Identify the significance of prevention and health education for the control of fungal and helminthic infections

Glossary

antigen—agent that is capable of producing antibodies when introduced into the body of a susceptible person

antiserum—a serum containing antibodies given to provide immunity against a specific disease; usually regarded as temporary protection

antitoxin—an antibody that neutralizes a bacterial toxin

attenuation—weakening of the toxicity or virulence of an infectious agent

bacteremia—presence of bacteria in the circulating blood

bactericidal—lethal to bacteria

carrier—one who harbors an infectious agent causing a specific disease, although he gives no evidence of having the disease

case—a particular instance of disease

communicable (contagious)—transmissible from person to person, directly or indirectly

contact—a person known or believed to have been exposed to an infectious disease

contaminated—having come in contact with infectious agents or materials

disinfection—destruction (or rendering inert) of pathogenic organisms by chemical or physical means

endemic—occurring habitually within a given geographic area

endogenous—caused by microbes derived from the host's own flora

epidemic—a disease attacking many people in a community simultaneously

exanthem—an eruption on the skin

exogenous infection—infection caused by microbes derived from outside the host

fomites—inanimate vehicles other than food, milk, water, and air that may harbor or be the means of transmission of organisms

immune—protected against disease

incidence—number of new cases of a disease (or event) occurring in a specified time, usually a year

incubation period—the development of an infection from the time it gains entry into the body until the appearance of the first signs and symptoms

infectious—capable of causing infection or disease

infestation—invasion of body by arthropods, including insects, mites, mosquitos, and ticks, and by helminths

in vitro—within a test tube

in vivo—within a living body

morbidity rate—the number of cases of illnesses compared with the total population; may be measured in incidence or prevalence

mortality rate—the number of deaths compared with the total population

nosocomial infection—infection acquired during hospitalization; not present or incubating at the time of admission to hospital

pandemic—affecting a large portion of the population; extensive epidemic

pathogenic—disease producing

prevalence—ratio of the total number of all individuals who have a disease at a particular time to the population at risk of having the disease

prodromal—occurring at the beginning stage of the disease (e.g., prodromal symptoms)

prophylaxis—measures taken to prevent disease

surveillance—dynamic system of collecting, tabulating, analyzing, and reporting data on the occurrence and distribution of disease

toxin—a poisonous substance produced by bacterial action

toxoid—a modified toxin capable of stimulating the production of antibodies

vaccine—a suspension of attenuated or killed microorganisms or their components given to build up an active immunity against an infectious disease

The Challenge of Infectious Diseases

An infectious disease is any disease caused by growth of pathogenic organisms in the body. It may or may not be communicable (contagious).

Infectious diseases are still the major health problem of most people worldwide. In developing countries, the principal causes of death are infectious and parasitic diseases. These diseases impair the ability of people to work and to learn. The major tropical diseases endemic in many areas are actually increasing in number. The increased number of US citizens traveling abroad has contributed to the resurgence of interest in infectious diseases. The conquering of these diseases is necessary for economic self-sufficiency, national development, and the well-being of the world's populations.

In the industrialized countries, the mortality from infectious diseases has declined dramatically, but these diseases still account for a large portion of the cost of health care. Even in highly developed countries where many diseases have been eliminated, new diseases are being introduced by invasive diagnostic techniques, immunosuppressive therapies, changing cultural, behavioral, and sexual patterns, and the creation of high-risk environments such as intensive care units and day care centers. The new sexually transmitted diseases (STDs) (infections caused by *Chlamydia trachomatis,* genital papillomaviruses, and so forth) have caused epidemics throughout the world; the most awesome problem is the global spread of acquired immunodeficiency syndrome (AIDS). Also, people whose normal host defenses have been compromised are susceptible to organisms that are considered minimally pathogenic. Included in this group are the elderly, patients treated with corticosteroids or chemotherapy, and individuals who are positive for the HIV virus.

There is an increase in the number of organisms that are resistant to a variety of antimicrobials. Subsequently, the advances in modern science have led to the development of more antimicrobial drugs, antiviral chemotherapy, and the ability to grow viruses in tissue cultures, as well as an increased knowledge about immunity.

The Infectious Process

Epidemiology is the science concerned with the study of the history and occurrence of a disease, and those factors that may directly or indirectly promote the development of a disease. Table 62-1 provides an overview of infectious diseases, their sources, and their treatment.

An unbroken chain of events is necessary for the spread of an infectious disease (Fig. 62-1):

- A causative agent
- A reservoir
- A portal or mode of escape or exit
- A mode of transmission
- A mode of entry
- A susceptible host

The chain begins with a *causative agent* or invading organism, which may be bacterial, viral, rickettsial, protozoal, fungal, or helminthic. Infection by each type of organism gives rise to specific reactions in the infected organism.

The second link in the chain is a *reservoir,* a place where the invading organisms live and multiply. The reservoir is the environment in which the agent is found, whether it be human, arthropod, plant, soil, or inanimate matter; for example, humans are the reservoir for syphilis, soil is the reservoir for tetanus, and animals are the reservoir for brucellosis. In humans, infectious diseases most often develop from contact with infected persons.

The next link is the *mode of escape* (or portal of exit) from the reservoir. Organisms may exit through various body systems, such as the respiratory tract (most common when the reservoir is human), intestinal tract, and genitourinary tract, or through skin lesions. In addition, the agent may escape from the bloodstream or tissues of the host by means of insect bites, hypodermic needles, or surgical instruments.

After the infectious organism has escaped from its reservoir, it is dangerous only if it reaches a host. This *mode of transmission* may be direct, as in person-to-person contact,

exposure to an animal bite, and exposure to droplet spray, or indirect through an intermediate vehicle, such as water, serum, or contaminated fomites such as contaminated hands or needles. An example of an organism spread by indirect transmission is the typhoid bacillus, which is able to survive for a long period of time outside the body. Diseases may also be transmitted by the vehicle route (contaminated food, water, drugs, blood), by air (droplets), or by vector (arthropod).

The fifth link in the chain is the *mode of entry* of organisms into the human body. This corresponds somewhat to the mode of escape and includes the respiratory tract, gastrointestinal tract, genitourinary tract, direct infection of mucous membranes, or entry through a break in the skin.

The sixth link in the chain is a *susceptible host.* The presence of an infectious agent does not inevitably produce disease. Whether or not the person becomes ill following the entry of infectious organisms into the body depends on numerous factors, including the number of organisms to which the host is exposed; the duration of the exposure; the person's age and general physical, mental, and emotional health and nutritional state; the status of the hematopoietic system; the absence of immunoglobulins (or the presence of abnormal immunoglobulins); and the number of T-lymphocytes and their ability to function.

In summary, infectious diseases are spread through a series of six links in a chain of events. Removal of any one of the links halts the spread of infection; therefore, it is the purpose of public health plans for infection control to eliminate one of these links. Controlling the spread of infection decreases the mortality rates of susceptible patients, minimizes health care costs and lengths of hospital stay, and increases the capabilities of individuals to lead healthy, productive lives.

Principles of Management

Immunity and Immunization

Immunity is the resistance that a person has against disease. *Specific immunity* to a particular organism implies that an individual either has generated the appropriate antibody in his own body or has received ready-made antibodies from another source. Immunity may be natural (resistance not acquired through previous contact with the infectious agent) or acquired (resistance acquired by the host as a result of previous exposure to the infectious agent). Humoral and cellular immunity are discussed in Chapter 48.

Active Immunization

Active immunization is produced by natural or acquired stimulation, so that the body produces its own antibodies. It may result from clinical or subclinical (inapparent) infection (*e.g.,* the person "gets the disease"), or it may be produced by administering live or killed microorganisms or their antigens, or inactivated vaccines and toxoids.

Active immunization is the most important and effective tool in preventive medicine. It has been most effective with

(text continues on page 1899)

TABLE 62-1. *Epidemiology, Therapy, and Control of Communicable Infections*

	Infective Organism	Infectious Sources	Entry Site	Method of Spread	Incubation Period	Chemotherapy*	Prophylaxis
Acquired immunodeficiency syndrome (AIDS)	Human immunodeficiency virus	Blood and body fluids of HIV-infected persons	Vaginal, rectal, and urethral mucosa; bloodstream	Direct sexual or blood contact; use of contaminated hypodermic needles	Variable (weeks to 15 years)	Zidovudine (AZT). (No cure is available)	Detection of HIV-infected persons with case finding; barrier precautions with sexual or blood contact with infected persons
Amebiasis	Entamoeba histolytica	Contaminated water and food	Gastrointestinal tract	Patients and carriers; fecal–oral route; oral and sexual contact	Variable	Metronidazole; diloxanide furoate; iodoquinol; chlortetracycline	Detection of carriers and their removal from food handling; plumbing safeguards
Bacillary dysentery (Shigellosis)	Shigella group	Contaminated water and food	Gastrointestinal tract	Patients and carriers; fecal–oral route	24–48 hours	Ampicillin; chloramphenicol; tetracycline, trimethoprim–sulfamethoxazole	Detection and control of carriers; inspection of food handlers, decontamination of water supplies
Brucellosis	Brucella melitensis and related organisms	Milk, meat, tissues, and blood from infected cattle, goats, horses, and pigs	Gastrointestinal tract	Ingestion of or contact with infective material	5–30 days (variable)	Tetracycline and streptomycin	Milk pasteurization; control of infection in animals
Chancroid	Haemophilus ducreyi	Human cases and carriers	Genitalia	Direct sexual contact	3–5 days	Erythromycin or trimethoprim–sulfamethoxazole	Effective case-finding and treatment of infection
Chickenpox (varicella)	Varicella-zoster (V-Z) virus	Human cases	Probably nasopharynx	Probably respiratory droplets	13–17 days	Acyclovir (?)	Varicella-zoster immune globulin (VZIG) primarily for immunocompromised children and certain neonates exposed in utero
Diphtheria	Corynebacterium diphtheriae	Human cases and carriers; fomites; raw milk	Nasopharynx	Nasal and oral secretions; respiratory droplets	2–5 days	Diphtheria antitoxin; penicillin; erythromycin	Active immunization with diphtheria toxoid
Encephalitis, Epidemic (eastern and western equine)	Viruses	Chicken and wild-bird mites; horses	Skin	Mosquitoes	Variable	None	Destroy larvae; eliminate breeding of mosquitoes Eastern equine encephalitis vaccine for those under

Disease	Agent	Reservoir	Portal of entry	Mode of transmission	Incubation period	Treatment	Prevention/Control
Gonorrhea	*Neisseria gonorrhoeae*	Urethral and vaginal secretions	Urethral or vaginal mucosa; pharynx; rectum	Sexual activity	2–7 days	Aqueous procaine penicillin G, with probenecid or alternative regimen outlined by Public Health Service	...continued and intensive exposure Examination of culture; treatment of sexual partners
Granuloma inguinale	*Calymmatobacterium granulomatis*	Infectious exudate	External genitalia; inguinal and anal region	Direct contact with lesions during sexual activity	Unknown, presumably 8–80 days	Tetracyclines; trimethoprim-sulfamethoxazole	Chemotherapy of carriers and contacts; case-finding and treatment of patients
Infectious mononucleosis	Epstein–Barr virus	Human cases and carriers	Mouth	Probably oral-pharyngeal route; via blood transfusion in susceptible recipients	2–6 weeks	None	None
Influenza	Virus	Human cases	Respiratory tract	Respiratory	24–72 hours	Amantadine; rimantadine	Influenza virus vaccine
Lyme disease	*Borrelia burgdorferi*	Cattle, deer, sheep, and mice	Skin	Ixodid ticks	4–20 days	Tetracycline; penicillin	Wearing protective clothing when in wooded areas; examination and removal of ticks from self and household pets
Lymphogranuloma venereum	*Chlamydia trachomatis*	Human cases	External genitalia; urethral or vaginal mucosa	Sexual intercourse; indirect contact with contaminated articles/clothing	5–21 days	Tetracyclines	Case-finding and treatment of infection
Malaria	*Plasmodium vivax*, *P. falciparum*, *P. malariae*, and *P. ovale*	Human cases	Skin	Mosquitoes (*Anopheles*)	Variable, depending on strain	Chloroquine; primaquine; amodiaquine; quinine	Coordinated measures for wide-scale mosquito control; prompt detection and effective treatment of cases; suppressive drugs in malarious areas
Measles	Virus	Human cases	Respiratory mucosa	Nasopharyngeal secretions	8–13 days	None	Measles vaccine

(continued)

TABLE 62–1. (Continued)

	Infective Organism	Infectious Sources	Entry Site	Method of Spread	Incubation Period	Chemotherapy*	Prophylaxis
Meningococcal meningitis	Neisseria meningitidis	Human cases and carriers	Nasopharynx; tonsils	Respiratory droplets	2–10 days	Penicillin; ampicillin; chloramphenicol	Meningococcal polysaccharide vaccine for persons at risk; rifampin/sulfadiazine for carriers or contacts
Mumps	Virus	Human cases (early)	Upper respiratory tract	Respiratory droplets	2–4 weeks (avg. 18 days)	None	Live mumps vaccine
Paratyphoid fever	Salmonella paratyphi A, B, and C, and related organisms	Contaminated food, milk, water	Gastrointestinal tract	Infected feces or rarely urine	7–21 days	Chloramphenicol; ampicillin; trimethoprim–sulfamethoxazole	Control of public water sources, food vendors, food handlers; treatment of carriers
Pneumococcal pneumonia	Streptococcus pneumoniae	Human carriers; patient's own pharynx	Respiratory mucosa	Respiratory droplets	Variable	Penicillin G; erythromycin	Polyvalent pneumococcal vaccine; control of upper respiratory infections; avoidance of alcoholic intoxication
Poliomyelitis	Polioviruses (types I, II, III)	Human cases and carriers	Gastrointestinal tract	Pharyngeal secretions; fecal-oral	7–14 days	None	Oral polio vaccine (OPV), the live attenuated vaccine containing all three strains of poliovirus—produces long-lasting immunity in most recipients
Rocky Mountain spotted fever	Rickettsia ricksetsii	Infected wild rodents, dogs, wood ticks, dog ticks	Skin	Tick bites	3–14 days	Tetracyclines; chloramphenicol	Avoidance of tick-infested areas, or wearing of protective clothing in such areas; frequent search for, and prompt removal of, ticks from body; specific vaccination of exposed persons
Rubella (German measles)	Virus	Human cases	Respiratory mucosa	Nasopharyngeal secretions	14–23 days	None	Rubella virus vaccine; immune globulin

Disease	Organism	Reservoir	Portal of Entry	Mode of Transmission	Incubation Period	Treatment	Prevention and Control
							(human) given to contacts of persons with rubella
Syphilis	*Treponema pallidum*	Infected exudates, body fluids, and secretions (saliva, semen, blood, vaginal secretions)	External genitalia; cervix; mucosal surfaces; placenta	Sexual activity; contact with open lesions; blood transfusion; transplacental inoculation	10–70 days	Penicillin; tetracycline	Case-finding by means of routine serologic testing and other methods; adequate treatment of infected individuals
Tetanus	*Clostridium tetani*	Contaminated soil	Penetrating and crush wounds	Feces of barnyard animals	4–21 days (avg. 10 days)	Tetanus immune globulin (human—TIG) and tetanus toxoid; penicillin	Wound débridement; toxoid booster injections for patients previously immunized; tetanus toxoid and tetanus immune globulin (separate sites and separate syringes) for nonimmune persons
Trichinosis	*Trichinella spiralis*	Infected pigs	Gastrointestinal tract	Ingestion of infected pork, undercooked	2–28 days	Steroids; thiabendazole	Regulation of hog breeders; adequate meat inspection; thorough cooking of pork
Tuberculosis	*Mycobacterium tuberculosis*	Sputum from human cases; milk from infected cows (rare in United States)	Respiratory mucosa	Sputum; respiratory droplets	Variable	Isoniazid; ethambutol; rifampin; streptomycin; pyrazinamide	Early discovery and adequate treatment of active cases; milk pasteurization
Tularemia	*Francisella tularensis*	Wild rodents and rabbits	Eyes; skin; gastrointestinal tract	Handling infected animals; ingestion of undercooked, infected meat; drinking contaminated water; bites from infected flies, ticks	1–10 days	Streptomycin; tetracyclines; chloramphenicol	Use of rubber gloves when skinning/handling potentially infectious wild animals; avoidance of contact with potentially infected rodents; adequate cooking of wild rabbit dishes; vaccination of hunters, butchers, and laboratory workers risking heavy exposure

(continued)

TABLE 62–1. (Continued)

	Infective Organism	Infectious Sources	Entry Site	Method of Spread	Incubation Period	Chemotherapy*	Prophylaxis
Typhoid fever	Salmonella typhi	Contaminated food and water	Gastrointestinal tract	Infected urine and feces	1–3 weeks	Chloramphenicol; ampicillin; sulfatrimethoprim	Decontamination of water sources; milk pasteurization; individual vaccination of high-risk persons; control of carriers
Typhus, endemic	Rickettsia typhi (mooseri)	Infected rodents	Skin	Flea bites	1–2 weeks	Tetracyclines; chloramphenicol	Delousing procedures; case quarantine
Whooping cough (pertussis)	Bordetella pertussis	Human cases	Respiratory tract	Infected bronchial secretions	Commonly 7 days	Erythromycin; ampicillin	Active immunization with vaccine; case isolation

* Research developments produce changes in drug therapy. The reader is referred to drug brochures and digests to keep abreast of changing dosages and uses.

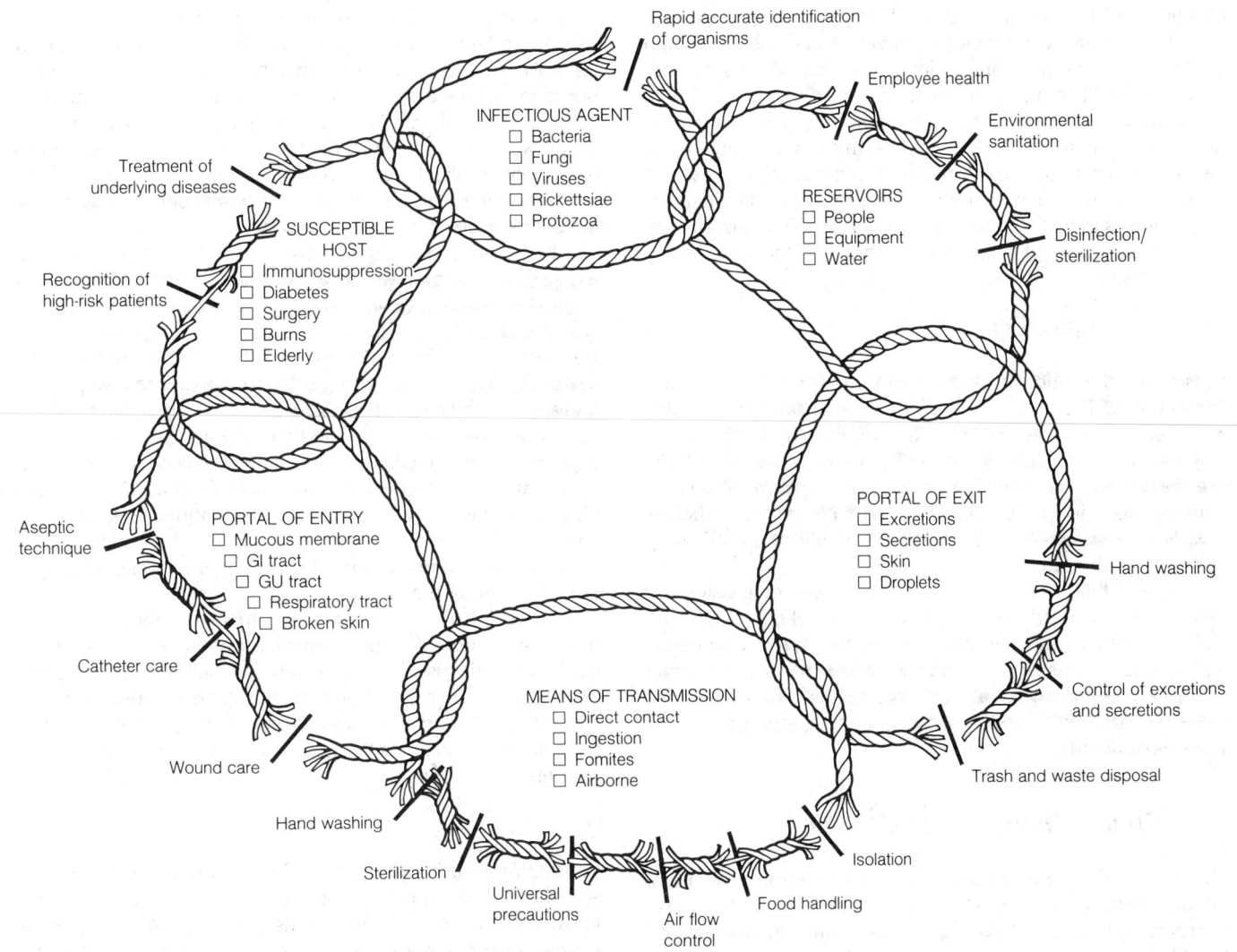

Figure 62-1. Health care workers' interventions used to break the chain of infection transmission.

bacterial exotoxins (diphtherial and tetanus toxoids) and with viruses. Most live-virus vaccines produce antibody responses that consist of prompt but transient production of specific immunoglobulins (IgM followed by a sustained production of specific IgG). Live-virus vaccines may produce mild clinical illness, with fever and rash appearing in some patients.

Inactivated vaccines and toxoids give a less complete response after a single injection and may require repeated administrations according to a prescribed schedule for long-lasting immunoglobulin response and sustained protection against infection. After injection with inactivated vaccines and toxoids, there may be a mild local reaction at the site of injection and occasional systemic symptoms of fever, malaise, and headache.

Depending on age and health status, susceptible persons between the ages of 18 and 24 years should be given tetanus and diphtheria toxoids and vaccines against measles, mumps, and rubella. Persons between 25 and 64 years of age should receive a booster dose of tetanus and diphtheria toxoids every 10 years, and susceptible individuals in this group should be given measles, mumps, and rubella vaccines. It is recommended that persons who are 65 years or older be given a tetanus and diphtheria toxoid booster every 10 years, influenza vaccine annually, and pneumococcal polysaccharide vaccine one time (if they have not previously received this vaccine). Travelers to developing countries may require additional appropriate vaccines.

Current recommendations for the administration of vaccines and other biologicals used in the prevention of disease are available from the Advisory Committee on Immunization Practices of the U.S. Public Health Service, Centers for Disease Control (CDC), Atlanta, Georgia 30333.

Nursing Considerations. Before a vaccine is administered, the person is questioned about possible allergies, because some vaccines may contain trace amounts of substances to which some people are allergic. For example, persons with a known allergy to eggs should not receive influenza vaccine because this vaccine is propagated in embryonated chicken eggs.

All vaccines have some side effects. Usually, immunosuppressed individuals or pregnant women are not given live-virus vaccines, and those persons with febrile illnesses are not vaccinated.

The nurse should be aware that young adults may fall into the immunization gap for measles and rubella. Adults born after 1959 and before 1967 grew up when such vaccines were first licensed but not mandatory. This group may be unprotected and at risk for developing measles and rubella, which may cause different manifestations and more serious complications in adults than in children.

Members of low-income groups often do not receive the protection of immunization programs; this is a challenge to all health care professionals. A person's acceptance of this type of preventive care may help him to accept other medical services. Nurses must listen to the fears and possible misconceptions of these people and inform them of the benefits of immunization.

Passive Immunization

Passive immunization provides temporary protection from a disease. It is produced by the injection of serum that contains antibodies that have been formed in another host. The serum is given for immediate but temporary protection against a disease when active immunizing agents are not available (*e.g.,* immune globulin for hepatitis A) or when there is insufficient time for the person to acquire active immunization following exposure to disease.

Several types of preparations are in use for passive immunization: standard immune globulin, special immune serum globulins with a known antibody content for specific illnesses, and animal serums or antitoxins. Products made with animal serum may cause an anaphylaxis-like reaction or serum sickness; therefore, products made with human serum are given whenever possible.

Reporting Communicable Diseases

Incidences of communicable diseases are reported to local public health authorities. This is important for tracking these diseases and initiating investigative or control measures. The local health department forwards the information to the state health department, which transmits weekly reports to the CDC in Atlanta, where data about communicable and chronic diseases are compiled and published in the *Morbidity and Mortality Weekly Report.* This publication provides an up-to-date picture of epidemiologic notes, trends, and reports, and it disseminates this information to local health departments, people in the field, and others with a need for the information. Thus, the occurrence of any local communicable disease becomes part of a huge network of health surveillance. The CDC operations include epidemiology and disease surveillance, laboratory methods, health education, and organized disease prevention and control programs and training.

The World Health Organization (WHO) receives data about communicable diseases from all countries. Regional epidemiologists track regional disease trends and disseminate this information to the appropriate people and services within the various countries.

Controlling Infectious Diseases in the Health Care Setting

Universal Precautions

In 1987, the CDC expanded previous recommendations to prevent the spread of human immunodeficiency virus (HIV), hep-

atitis B virus (HBV), and other blood-borne pathogens. Previously, certain isolation precautions were recommended only for those patients who were known or suspected to have blood-borne infectious diseases. Because of the growing number of persons infected with HIV and the high mortality rates associated with AIDS, Universal Blood and Body Fluids Precautions (or simply universal precautions) were developed. Under these new recommendations, *all* patients are considered potentially infectious for blood-borne infections.

Universal precautions recommend that all health care workers who come into contact with a patient's blood or body fluids that contain visible blood should wear an appropriate type of barrier (*e.g.,* gloves, masks, and gowns) to prevent the spread of blood-borne pathogens. Other body fluids for which barrier protection is recommended include semen, vaginal secretions, cerebrospinal fluid (CSF), synovial fluid, pleural fluid, pericardial fluid, and amniotic fluid. The type of exposure determines the specific barrier that should be used. For example, a nurse who must inspect an intravenous (IV) site that is clearly bleeding would wear gloves. A nurse suctioning a patient who has blood-tinged sputum would wear, in addition to gloves, protective eye wear and a mask if the patient frequently coughs during the procedure.

Universal precautions are designed to augment, not replace, standard infection control procedures such as hand washing and the use of gloves when touching obviously infected materials. These precautions are designed to prevent the inadvertent transmission of blood-borne pathogens from infected patients to the skin and mucous membranes of health care workers.

Isolation

In addition to using the universal precautions for all patients, specific isolation precautions are used for patients who are known to have specific infectious diseases. Isolation precautions are used to prevent the transmission of infectious agents among patients, health care personnel, and visitors. Isolation precautions are used to isolate the infection rather than the patient. Systems for isolation precautions designed by the CDC include category-specific isolation precautions, in which diseases are grouped by categories, and disease-specific isolation Precautions, in which only the particular precautions for interrupting transmission of the specific disease are recommended.

Isolation precautions may also be established by an individual health care agency. The infection control committee of the agency determines which of the alternative systems of isolation precautions is used. Each hospital prepares a manual that includes the specific sections of the CDC guidelines that pertain to the approach that has been adopted, and incorporates the information into the procedure manual used by each patient care area. Standards of practice are evaluated in light of new information and changing situations. Isolation recommendations are reviewed regularly and revised as appropriate.

Techniques for Isolation Precautions
Hand Washing.   Hand washing is the single most important means of preventing the spread of infection. It can markedly reduce or eliminate the spread of pathogenic organisms by the hands. Lathering the hands and vigorously rubbing together all lathered surfaces, followed by thorough rinsing under a stream of water, suspends and rinses away microorganisms. Plain soaps or detergents should be used for routine hand washing. Anti-

septics are recommended for hand washing when the patient being cared for has been infected with virulent or epidemiologically important microorganisms, especially in intensive care units. Hand washing must be performed before and after direct contact with patients, performance of invasive procedures, and contact with body fluids.

Private Room.   A private room is indicated for patients with conditions that are highly contagious or those caused by microorganisms that are likely to be virulent when transmitted. A private room is also indicated if the patient has poor hygiene habits that contaminate the environment (*e.g.*, carelessness with excretions). A private room may also be required for patients colonized with microorganisms of special clinical or epidemiologic significance (*e.g.*, multiple resistant bacteria), or for patients whose blood is infective, and if profuse bleeding is likely to expose people in the area to contamination. Private rooms may be used as a protective strategy for patients who are especially susceptible to infections: severely immunosuppressed patients such as those receiving chemotherapy, patients diagnosed with AIDS, or recent transplant recipients.

Masks, Gowns, and Gloves.   Except for patients routinely requiring strict isolation, in which cases masks, gowns, and gloves are uniformly indicated, the health care worker who assigns isolation precautions to the patient has the responsibility to decide when such precautionary attire is necessary. This decision is based on the likelihood of exposure to infectious material. For example, a nurse who comes in close contact with a patient who is coughing decides if it is necessary to wear a mask when giving care to the patient. If clothing may become soiled with infectious secretions or excretions, the nurse may decide to wear a gown. If infected materials (excretions, secretions, blood, body fluids) will be touched, gloves must be worn. This approach allows health care workers more responsibility in ensuring their own safety.

General Management

The key to management of the patient who has an infection is identifying the specific organism and instituting specific therapy appropriate for that organism. The drug of choice is usually the drug that is most active against the pathogenic organism or the least toxic alternative. Supportive therapy includes monitoring the patient's response to therapy; ensuring hydration, fluid balance, and oxygenation; continually observing for complications; and providing comfort and information to both the patient and family.

▶ Nursing Process
The Patient With an Infectious Disease

▷ *Assessment*

Many early symptoms of infectious diseases are nonspecific. The illness may begin with malaise and all its attendant sequelae—listlessness, lightheadedness, headache, anorexia, arthralgia. As the disease progresses there is usually fever, although elderly people in general do not have as vigorous a febrile response as younger people, nor do patients who have previously received antibiotics or who are taking immunosuppressive agents.

Other clinical features that are suggestive of infection include chills, myalgia, photophobia, pharyngitis, acute lymphadenopathy, nausea, and vomiting. Because the signs and symptoms associated with infection are a result of the host's inflammatory response as well as the direct response to the pathogen, they can be nonspecific. (The reader is referred to chapters on specific organs or systems for signs and symptoms that suggest infection of a particular organ site.)

In obtaining the health history, it is important to ask the following questions specifically correlated with infectious diseases:

- History of fever? Chills? (Abrupt onset of fever is associated with chills.)
- Night sweats? (Associated with intermittent fever)
- Back pain? General myalgias? Arthralgias? Headache? (All are commonly associated with fever.)
- Sore throat?
- Diarrhea? Vomiting? Abdominal pain?
- Dysuria? Purulent discharge?
- Evidence of local infection: Redness? Heat? Swelling? Pain?
- Contact with an ill person or with his secretions or excretions?
- Insect bite? Animal bite? Cat scratch? Exposure to rodents or birds?
- Medications, especially antibiotics or corticosteroids, being taken? Alcohol intake? Drug use?
- History of sexual practices?
- Travel to or from a developing country or abroad?
- Place of work?
- Vaccination history?

While performing the physical examination, the nurse observes for the manifestations common to many infectious diseases: breaks in the skin, skin rashes, skin and mucous membrane lesions, productive cough, breathing difficulties, purulent drainage from any site, and lymph node enlargement.

To analyze the assessment data, the nurse needs to have knowledge about specific organisms, where and when they occur, how they can be controlled or eliminated, who is at risk, and some information about the patient's environment. In reviewing the findings, one of the nursing decisions is to determine if the patient is at risk for infecting himself or others.

▷ *Gerontologic Considerations.*   Many elderly people with infections develop the typical signs and symptoms. However, infection in those who do not develop these signs and symptoms may come to the attention of the health care provider as a result of other health problems that appear in any illness of the elderly, such as incontinence, confusion, immobility, or falling. Diagnostic evaluation for infection and use of appropriate therapy are essential so that the underlying infectious condition can be managed concurrently with the presenting problem.

▷ *Nursing Diagnoses*

▷ *Ineffective Breathing Patterns.*   An altered breathing pattern in the patient with an infectious disease may result from the disease itself or occur when the normal respiratory defense mechanisms have become impaired or overwhelmed by microbial assault. Also, patients with impaired cell-mediated immunity are susceptible to bacterial, viral, and fungal pneumonias.

▷ *Alteration in Body Temperature.*   Fever is a common symptom of infection. It may occur as a result of an infection acquired outside the hospital, a nosocomial infection related to invasive devices used to monitor and support the patient, or it may be of unknown origin. Fever can be a protective response of the body to fight infectious organisms or it can be a result of a large inflammatory response by the body to injury.

▷ *High Risk for Fluid Volume Deficit.*   Fluid volume deficits in patients with infectious illnesses can result from excessive fever, sweating, and watery diarrhea. Inability to ingest fluids is another cause and can lead to serious dehydration.

▷ *Altered Oral Mucous Membranes.*   The oral tissues are bathed by the patient's own microbial flora and by other organisms that enter the mouth by way of food, water, and other substances. The normal flow of saliva and the motion of the lips, cheeks, and tongue help maintain the integrity of the oral mucosa. The combination of fever, dyspnea, and inability to ingest fluids and food can cause dryness and cracking of the mucous membranes. Viral infections affect the oral mucosa, beginning as vesicles and rapidly developing into ulcers. The patient receiving chemotherapy may have painful mouth ulcers from the toxic effects of the drug or may be increasingly susceptible to infection. Fungal infection involving the oral mucosa is also found in patients receiving chemotherapy and those with compromised immune function. The treatment of the cause of the oral lesions is individualized, and the problems encountered by the patient, such as oral discomfort, can be relieved by appropriate nursing interventions.

▷ *Diarrhea.*   Normal bowel flora plays an important protective role. Anytime the bowel flora is altered (*e.g.*, by taking broad-spectrum antibiotics), diarrhea may ensue. The normal flora of the bowel can be overcome by large numbers of virulent organisms such as occurs in salmonellosis. Acute-onset diarrhea is caused by a variety of bacterial, parasitic, and viral agents and is discussed with the appropriate conditions.

▷ *Altered Nutrition: Less Than Body Requirements.*   A severe and prolonged infection greatly increases a patient's nutritional needs well beyond what is normal for his height and weight. Patients whose protein intake and caloric intake do not meet these needs experience muscle wasting and weight loss, because protein is being catabolized for energy. Those patients who have been acutely ill and who have been without protein and calorie intake for several days, or who were malnourished at the onset of their illness, require extra nutritional support.

▷ *Knowledge Deficit.*   One major goal in the health education of all people is for them to acquire a sense of responsibility for their own health and for avoiding injury to others. Additionally, the person with an infectious disease is taught about his specific disease and the therapeutic regimen, and in some instances he is instructed about personal hygiene and the maintenance of the home environment to prevent the spread of infection. Patients who have immigrated from developing countries may have diseases that reflect crowding and poor sanitation. This situation requires specific teaching.

▷ *High Risk for Infection Spread to Others.*   When caring for those with infectious diseases, all health care personnel must prevent the spread of infection to others. The types of infection control precautions used are based on the mode of transmission of the disease. Universal Precautions must be instituted for all patients, whether or not infectious diseases are suspected.

▷ *Social Isolation.*   The patient with an acute illness may exhibit anxiety and ineffective coping strategies that are related to physiologic and organic disturbances brought about by the illness, his underlying emotional state, the effects of hospitalization (isolation), and inadequate explanation or understanding of the health problem or disease condition. These factors can cause a combination of problems, including social isolation.

The nursing diagnoses described above are applicable to patients with infectious diseases; however, they are not meant to be an exhaustive list. Patients with multiple medical problems or other complications may have additional nursing diagnoses. Likewise, the severity of the infection and the patient's individual response to the infectious disease require constant assessment and revisions of the nursing diagnoses and the plans of care.

▷ Planning and Implementation

▷ *Goals:*   The major goals of the patient may include attainment of normal breathing pattern, attainment of normal body temperature, achievement of fluid balance, achievement of intact and healthy oral mucous membranes, attainment of normal bowel elimination, improvement of nutritional status, acquisition of knowledge about the condition, prevention of the spread of infection, and achievement of social participation.

▷ Nursing Interventions

▷ *Attaining a Normal Breathing Pattern.*   Health care personnel must assess patients at high risk for pulmonary infection and subsequent ineffective breathing patterns. Patients with pre-existing illness (*e.g.*, immunosuppression, alcoholism, drug overdose) tend to have impaired lung clearance. Viral infections and hematologic malignancies depress the cellular defenses of the lungs. Pulmonary compliance is decreased in aging patients. Pulmonary infection also occurs as a result of mechanical disruption of pulmonary defenses, as is seen in the patient with endotracheal intubation. General anesthesia interrupts the normal respiratory process and thus interferes with spontaneous lung expansion.

The nurse monitors these high-risk patients for cough, shortness of breath, change in skin color, and use of accessory muscles for breathing. Respiratory rate, depth, and pattern and chest expansion are assessed. The patient's chest is auscultated for breath sounds. Crackles are indicative of fluid in the lungs; wheezes are indicative of thicker secretions.

Turning the patient and changing his position help to drain secretions and thus reduce the potential for retention of secretions and infection. Yawning, taking deep breaths, and coughing help expand alveolar sacs. If the patient is not able to raise secretions effectively, suctioning is indicated. A high fluid intake (within limits of the patient's cardiac reserve) is encouraged because adequate hydration thins mucus and serves as an effective expectorant. The air may be humidified to loosen secretions and improve ventilation. As soon as his condition permits, the patient is encouraged to ambulate, because this activity helps mobilize secretions and expand the lungs.

If the patient shows signs of respiratory insufficiency, arterial blood gas values are obtained and recorded on a flow sheet so that comparisons can be made over time. Blood gases should not be obtained within 30 minutes to 1 hour of patient suctioning procedures. Suctioning procedures, designed to clear airway secretions and improve ventilation, initially result in a temporary hypoxic episode for the patient. A blood gas report obtained immediately after suctioning would reveal this temporary hypoxia, not the overall oxygenation state of the patient over time.

▷ *Attaining Normal Body Temperature.* The patient's temperature is monitored at regular intervals to determine the type of fever (continuous, remittent, or intermittent). These checks also help assess the severity and duration of the infectious process and the patient's response to therapy. Because some infected patients do not develop a febrile response, the patient is assessed for signs and symptoms of infection: headache, joint pain, muscle aches, backache, cough, diarrhea, and enlarged lymph nodes.

Oral fluids are encouraged because an adequate fluid intake is important to replace fluid losses due to fever, diaphoresis, dehydration, and dyspnea. Nursing interventions to combat the generalized discomfort that accompanies fever include helping the patient change positions, giving back massages, changing bed linens, providing intermittent cool compresses for headache, and encouraging rest to reduce metabolic activity. Oral hygiene promotes comfort and may help prevent oral complications, because many bacterial, mycotic, and viral infections affect the oral cavity.

Although fever occurring during infection may be beneficial and may enhance host defenses, there are times when fever may be deleterious; high fever can permanently damage body tissues. Tepid water sponging of the entire body cools the body through evaporation of water.

The elderly patient with fever requires special nursing surveillance. Fever increases the heart rate, decreases diastolic filling time, and reduces stroke volume. The resulting decreased cardiac output in the elderly may cause reductions in perfusion and in the delivery of oxygen to the brain and kidneys. However, the nurse must remember that many older patients may have serious infections with minimal or no elevation in temperature.

▷ *Attaining Fluid Balance.* The patient is assessed for signs of dehydration: thirst, dryness of mucous membranes, loss of skin turgor, muscle cramping, reduced peripheral pulses, and decreasing urine output. Skin turgor is evaluated by pinching the skin over the sternum, the inner aspects of the thighs, the forehead, or the dorsum of the hand. If the patient has a fluid volume deficit, the skin flattens more slowly after the pinch is released. The patient's oral cavity is inspected for dryness, and the tongue is examined for longitudinal furrows. The patient's weight is monitored because changes in weight indicate fluid volume changes. A rapid loss of weight occurs when the total fluid intake is less than the total fluid output. A sudden gain or loss of 1 kg (2.2 lb) is indicative of a gain or loss of about 1000 ml of fluid, respectively. Serum electrolyte values are monitored because dehydration may produce a deficit or elevation of some electrolytes. The nurse also keeps an intake and output record and monitors urine specific gravity. Concentrated scanty urine indicates a lack of fluids. When oliguria (low urine output in relation to fluid intake) is present, urinary specific gravity increases.

Oral administration of fluids is preferable to IV administration. Varying the type and temperature of oral fluids is helpful if the patient is reluctant to take fluids. If the patient is vomiting or critically ill, IV fluids are prescribed. Nursing interventions include informing the patient about the procedure, selecting a suitable vein, regulating and maintaining the proper rate of infusion flow, ensuring patient comfort, and monitoring the patient for untoward effects of IV therapy. IV sites are assessed at regular intervals for signs of local infection: pain, heat, redness, edema, or drainage.

▷ *Integrity of Oral Mucous Membranes.* Infectious diseases may be accompanied by changes in and lesions of the oral cavity. The patient's oral cavity is inspected for color, edema, the presence of lesions, cracks, coatings, bleeding or purulent drainage.

The patient is taught the importance of oral hygiene and assisted with it when necessary. Warm normal saline or warm water rinsing of the mouth removes debris and helps keep the oral mucosa clean and moist. Strong mouthwashes and antiseptic gargles are avoided. Petrolatum, water-soluble jelly, or mineral oil may be applied to cracked, dry lips to keep them soft and moist. Frequent toothbrushing and flossing remove plaque and help prevent gingivitis. Patients already manifesting pain or lesions of the oral cavity should avoid the use of toothbrushes and use sponge toothettes to prevent further trauma to the mouth.

A high-calorie liquid diet is given when ingestion of solid food is difficult because of painful oral lesions. If oral discomfort persists, a topical anesthetic agent may be prescribed. Chewing is important for oral health, and the patient is encouraged to resume a normal diet as soon as he is able.

▷ *Attaining Normal Bowel Elimination.* Most of the diarrheal illnesses that occur are mild and self-limiting. Diarrhea may be antibiotic-induced colitis, traveler's diarrhea, food- or waterborne diarrhea, or the type of diarrhea seen in immunosuppressed persons. In taking the health history, the nurse determines whether the patient has taken an antibiotic recently, has traveled to a developing country, or is immunosuppressed.

The patient is asked about the number, color, and consistency of his stools and whether blood and mucus are present. The existence of other clinical manifestations, such as nausea, vomiting, fever, and abdominal pain, is elicited. The number of stools in 24 hours gives a clue as to how disabling the patient's diarrhea is. In addition, the patient is assessed for signs of dehydration. The patient's intake, output, and weight are monitored and recorded.

An important nursing function is the collection of stool specimens. Universal Precautions are required, because there is a wide range of viral, bacterial, and parasitic causes of diarrhea. (Negative cultures do not rule out infectious etiology.)

Fluids and electrolytes are essential for patients with diarrhea. Oral fluids (oral glucose and electrolyte-containing rehydration solutions) are given when the patient is able to tolerate them. Parenteral fluid replacement is prescribed if severe dehydration is present.

The patient is instructed to cleanse the perianal area with mild soap and water and to blot the area dry after each bowel movement. This promotes comfort and prevents skin excoriation. The perianal area is inspected for signs of skin breakdown.

Universal precautions are used for the patient with infectious diarrhea. Proper hand washing and the practice of good personal hygiene are emphasized. Other nursing interventions include promoting patient comfort and advising rest for the patient who is having frequent bouts of watery diarrhea.

▷ *Improving Nutritional Status.* An assessment is made of what the patient is actually eating (both amounts and types of foods), because the generalized malaise, discomfort, and anorexia that accompany infections may cause a lack of interest in food. Additionally, the patient with fever has increased catabolism and loss of nutrients. The patient's weight is monitored.

For patients with fever, a high-calorie, high-protein diet is necessary to meet the energy needs created by increased metabolism and restlessness. Increased protein is needed to counteract the loss of nitrogen. Increased fluids are necessary to replenish losses due to perspiration and increased respiratory rate.

A referral may be made to the dietitian so that a diet plan can be tailored to the patient's condition and food preferences. The patient is helped to understand that he will require optimal nutrition during and beyond convalescence to replenish nutrient losses associated with an acute infectious disease, even one of short duration. The patient is also encouraged to monitor his weight.

▷ *Patient Education.* Interaction with the patient gives the nurse an opportunity to learn what he knows about his illness and treatment and to detect and correct misunderstandings and misinformation.

Brief and focused explanations can be made about the infectious organism and how it is spread, how the illness is treated, the importance of personal hygiene and environmental cleanliness, and the importance of seeking health care promptly in the event of an infectious disease. Knowledge of his specific illness and treatment imparts a sense of control to the patient and helps him become an active participant in his care. The nurse encourages the patient to ask questions because they serve as a guide to topics that need further clarification.

Health care personnel serve as educators in the prevention of infectious diseases. The program of instruction includes teaching about the spread of infectious diseases, methods of avoiding spread, the importance and availability of immunizations, the role of nutrition in health maintenance, and the control of environmental contaminants, insects, rodents, and other animal vectors and reservoirs of human infections.

▷ *Preventing the Spread of Infection.* Efforts are directed toward controlling the infectious agent at its source. These include proper hand washing, using a gown when clothing is likely to become soiled with infectious secretions or excretions, and using gloves when coming into contact with body fluids. Needles and syringes are handled with extreme caution because it is frequently not known if a patient's blood is contaminated with hepatitis or HIV viruses. Because accidental needle puncture can occur, needles must never be recapped or broken by hand after use. They must be disposed of in receptacles specifically designed for this purpose. Wastes must also be handled with all due precautions.

Dissemination of infectious droplets can be controlled by teaching the patient to cover his nose and mouth when coughing or sneezing, by bagging and labeling used paper tissues according to agency policy, and by handling soiled linen as little as possible.

Environmental cleanliness is maintained by damp dusting of furniture and wet vacuuming of floors, and by reducing to a minimum the activity of personnel in the area. The door to the room should be kept closed in the case of an infectious disease that can be spread by aerosolized droplets.

▷ *Promoting Social Participation.* Patients with infectious diseases may experience heightened states of anxiety, fear, and depression. These dysfunctional emotions reduce the patient's ability to cope with his illness.

An assessment is made of how the patient is reacting to his illness. The patient's family may have a valuable stress-reducing effect on the patient and are encouraged to visit. Ongoing and regular visits by health care personnel demonstrate to the patient that he is cared for. Being available, answering questions, exploring anxieties that prompt questions, and employing empathetic listening can be therapeutic and can relieve the patient's sense of isolation. Skilled nursing care promotes the patient's well-being. Stress reduction techniques may be useful.

The patient with an STD requires an understanding and sensitive approach. Fear of AIDS is widespread and particularly devastating to the patient. Coping with the illness is extremely stressful. The nurse's compassionate care, which includes providing information about financial and other entitlements and community resources, can fortify the patient. Crisis intervention and mental health services are available and may be appropriate to help the patient and his family begin the process of adaptation and acceptance.

▷ ## Evaluation

Expected Outcomes

1. Exhibits normal breathing pattern
2. Absence of elevated body temperature
3. Attains fluid balance
4. Attains/maintains healthy and intact oral mucous membranes
5. Attains normal defecation pattern
6. Achieves improved nutritional status
7. Acquires knowledge about the infectious process
8. Uses appropriate methods to prevent the spread of infection
9. Achieves reduction of stress imposed by social isolation

Nursing Care Plan 62-1 summarizes the care of the patient with an infectious disease and provides detailed expected outcomes.

In summary, the management of patients diagnosed with infectious diseases is a challenge to all health care professionals. Vigorous hand washing and the use of universal precautions and disease-specific isolation procedures aid in the prevention of the spread of infections. These techniques are essential to decrease the occurrences of infectious diseases, considering the high mortality rates and health care costs associated with them. In an attempt to contain communicable diseases, many are reported to appropriate health agencies for tracking and treatment.

Initial nursing assessments are designed to identify the sources, associated signs and symptoms, and communicable nature of infections. Nursing interventions support effective breathing, nutrition, and elimination patterns of infected patients. Patient comfort is maintained through control of body temperature and effective oral hygiene. Patient teaching is designed to contain the spread of infectious diseases and relieve

(text continues on page 1912)

Nursing Care Plan 62-1

Care of the Patient With an Infectious Disease

Nursing Interventions	Rationale	Expected Outcomes

Nursing Diagnosis: Ineffective breathing pattern related to an inflammatory or infectious process

Goal: Attainment of normal breathing pattern

Nursing Interventions	Rationale	Expected Outcomes
1. Assess patients at risk for pulmonary infection:	1. Patients with predisposing illness (immunosuppression, alcoholism, drug overdose) tend to have impaired mechanical lung clearance.	• Performs deep-breathing exercises. • Coughs at prescribed intervals. • Chest clear on auscultation. • Respirations regular. • Free of shortness of breath with activities of daily living. • Arterial blood gas results within normal limits.
a. Immunosuppressed; pre-existing pulmonary problems.	a. These patients are at high risk for pulmonary infection	
b. Elderly.	b. Lung compliance is decreased in the elderly.	
c. Immobilized.	c. Immobility promotes retention of respiratory secretions, resulting in atelectasis and generalized hypoxia.	
d. Decreased level of awareness with CNS depression.	d. Depression of respiratory centers in medulla and pons results in decreased responses to breathing reflexes.	
e. Viral infections, hematologic malignancies.	e. These depress cellular defenses of lung.	
f. Anesthetized; endotracheal intubation.	f. Pulmonary infection occurs from mechanical disruption of pulmonary defenses.	
g. Malnutrition.	g. Malnutrition increases susceptibility to infection by interfering with the immune system.	
2. Conduct ongoing pulmonary assessment: cough, shortness of breath, change in skin color, use of accessory muscles. a. Auscultate for breath sounds. b. Assess respiratory rate, depth, pattern, and chest expansion. c. Evaluate ABG results.	2. Promotes early detection of signs and symptoms of respiratory infection.	
3. Turn patient at least every 2 hours, more frequently for high-risk patients.	3. Turning and changing position help drain secretions; drainage of airway secretions reduces potential for retention of secretions and infection.	
4. Encourage patient to cough every 2–4 hours; suction his secretions if necessary.	4. Helps expand alveoli and prevents atelectasis.	
5. Instruct and demonstrate how to yawn, take deep breaths, and cough every 2–4 hours.	5. Helps expand alveoli and prevents atelectasis.	
6. Ambulate patient as soon as condition permits; evaluate patient's tolerance.	6. Ambulation helps mobilize secretions and expand the lungs.	

Nursing Diagnosis: Altered body temperature (fever) related to the presence of infection

Goal: Attainment of normal body temperature

Nursing Interventions	Rationale	Expected Outcomes
1. Monitor temperature, pulse, and respiration at regular intervals.	1. This helps determine the type (continuous, remittent, intermittent) of fever. It also helps monitor the severity and duration of the infectious process.	• Body temperature within normal limits. • Maintains adequate intake and output. • Absence of signs of fever: tachypnea, tachycardia, elevated blood pressure, and

(continued)

Nursing Care Plan 62–1 (Continued)

Care of the Patient With an Infectious Disease

Nursing Interventions	Rationale	Expected Outcomes
2. Monitor for localizing symptoms and physical findings (headache, pain, tenderness; cough, diarrhea, adenopathy).	2. Not all infected patients have a febrile response.	flushed/diaphoretic skin. • Absence of chills and sweats.
3. Pay special attention to the elderly patient with fever.	3. Elderly patients may have serious types of infection with minimal or no rise in temperature, or they may be hypothermic. Fever increases the heart rate, decreases diastolic filling time, and decreases stroke volume; thus, reduced cardiac output in the elderly may cause unacceptable perfusion and delivery of oxygen to the brain and kidneys.	
4. Encourage increased oral intake of fluids of 2000–3000 ml/day (unless contraindicated).	4. An adequate fluid intake is important to replace insensible losses via sweat and lungs and also to prevent the complications of infection (shock, renal failure).	
5. Use tepid water sponging of the entire body to lower the body temperature, when fever itself may be deleterious.	5. Fever occurring during infection may benefit the host defense. Tepid water sponging cools the body by evaporation of water.	

6. Combat generalized discomfort.
  a. Help patient change position and suggest positions of comfort.
  b. Provide oral hygiene 3 times/day.
 	
  c. Apply cold compresses for headache intermittently.
  d. Use massage as necessary.
  e. Plan rest periods 3 times a day and limit physical activity.
  f. Change linen when patient is diaphoretic.
	a. Promotes rest and relaxation; helps to prevent circulatory stasis.
	b. A large number of bacterial, mycotic, and viral infections may produce oral manifestations. Oral hygiene helps prevent oral complications and promotes comfort.
	c. Promotes vasoconstriction of superficial vessels
	d. Promotes muscle relaxation
	e. Resting lowers the metabolic activity.
	
	f. Dry linen improves patient comfort.	

Nursing Diagnosis: High risk for fluid volume deficit related to body's response to infectious process (excessive sweating, fever, watery diarrhea)

Goal: Attainment of fluid balance

1. Assess for dehydration (thirst, dryness of mucous membranes, loss of skin turgor, muscle cramping, reduced peripheral pulses, and urine output more than 30 ml/hr).	1. These are signs and symptoms of serious dehydration, which can lead to mental obtundation and circulatory collapse.	• Attains fluid balance (output approximates intake). • Mucous membranes appear moist; normal skin turgor. • Ingests 2000–3000 ml of fluids orally (unless contraindicated). • Serum electrolytes and urine specific gravity within normal limits.
2. Monitor temperature and daily weight.	2. Fever increases loss of fluids (from perspiration, increased respirations). Changes in weight indicate fluid volume changes.	
3. Monitor serum electrolytes, urine specific gravity, and intake and output every shift.	3. Dehydration produces a deficit of some electrolytes. Concentrated scanty urine	

(continued)

Nursing Care Plan 62–1 *(Continued)*

Care of the Patient With an Infectious Disease

Nursing Interventions	Rationale	Expected Outcomes
Include all drainage and diarrhea in calculation of fluid output. 4. Offer oral fluids every 2–4 hours in the event of excessive fluid loss through diarrhea or excessive sweating. 5. If patient is critically ill or vomiting, prepare for administration of intravenous fluids (usually dextrose and normal saline) as required.	indicates lack of fluids; urinary specific gravity increases when oliguria is present. 4. Oral hydration is preferable, because this can be done at home. Fruit juices contain sugar and potassium; bouillon provides salt. 5. Glucose facilitates intestinal reabsorption of electrolytes.	

Nursing Diagnosis: Altered oral mucous membranes related to loss of fluids (fever, sweating) and anorexia

Goal: Achievement of intact and healthy oral mucous membranes

1. Inspect oral cavity for color, edema, presence of lesions, cracks, coatings, bleeding, or purulent drainage.
2. Emphasize the importance of oral hygiene; assist patient when necessary.
  a. Use oral mouthwashes (*e.g.,* warm normal saline, sodium bicarbonate rinses).
  b. Apply petrolatum, water-soluble jelly, or mineral oil to dry, cracked lips.
  c. Encourage frequent toothbrushing and flossing.
3. Offer oral fluids every 2–4 hours.
 	
4. Offer small portions of food 4–6 times/day.
	1. Infectious organisms can present with intraoral manifestations.
	
	  a. Rinsing removes debris and helps keep oral mucosa clean, moist, and intact.
	  b. Lubrication of lips keeps them soft, moist, and intact.
	  c. Brushing and flossing remove plaque and help prevent gingivitis.
	3. Hydration is necessary for healthy moist mucous membranes.
	4. Chewing is important for oral health.
		• Attains/maintains moist, pink, and intact oral mucous membranes.
		• Absence of oral lesions and pain.
		• Performs oral hygiene.
		• Eats foods without difficulty.

Nursing Diagnosis: Diarrhea related to infectious agent

Goal: Achievement of normal bowel elimination

1. Conduct a health history to determine if patient
  a. Has taken an antibiotic recently.
  b. Has traveled abroad.
  c. Is immunosuppressed.
 	
2. Assess patient's signs and symptoms, and assess stools for character and consistency.
  a. Related clinical manifestations: nausea? vomiting? fever? (how long?) abdominal pain?
  b. Stools: soft? formed? bloody? watery?
3. Assess for severity and intensity of acute diarrhea. Determine how disabling the patient's diarrhea is; number of unformed stools/24 hr.
	1. Most of the diarrheal illnesses that occur are mild and self-limiting. Diarrhea may be antibiotic-induced colitis, traveler's diarrhea, or food- or water-borne diarrhea, or it may be related to immunosuppression.
	2. Observation of color, form, and presence of blood and mucus in stool may help determine the cause of diarrhea. Other clinical manifestations can also give clues to the cause of diarrhea.
	
	3. Diarrhea of more than 3 or 4 stools/24 h is usually of infectious origin.
		• Achieves normal defecation pattern.
		• Has stools of normal color and consistency.
		• Absence of cramping and abdominal pain.
		• Absence of signs and symptoms of dehydration.
		• Intact perianal skin.

(continued)

Nursing Care Plan 62–1 (Continued)

Care of the Patient With an Infectious Disease

Nursing Interventions	Rationale	Expected Outcomes
4. Assess for thirst, dryness of mucous membranes, loss of skin turgor and elasticity, muscle cramps, reduced peripheral pulses, and decreased urine output.	4. These are manifestations of dehydration; severe dehydration leads to mental obtundation and circulatory collapse.	
5. Using universal precautions, collect and send stool specimens to the laboratory for examination.	5. There is a wide range of viral, bacterial, and parasitic causes of diarrhea in different settings. When the history or fecal leukocyte findings indicate an infectious process, a culture for invasive pathogens is usually performed.	
6. Offer oral fluids (oral glucose and electrolyte-containing rehydration solution) every 2–4 hours.	6. Fluids and electrolytes represent the essential therapy. Some enteropathogens cause a derangement of fluid and electrolyte balance.	
7. Maintain careful surveillance if patient is immunocompromised.	7. In the immunocompromised patient, infection may not be contained and systemic spread occurs.	
8. Cleanse perianal area with mild soap and water after each bowel movement; blot area dry. Inspect for skin breakdown.	8. This promotes comfort and prevents skin excoriation and breakdown.	
9. Instruct patient and family in hand-washing techniques.	9. Hand washing is the foundation of infection control to prevent the spread of infection.	
10. Teach patient and family to a. Monitor consistency and number of stools.	a. Acute diarrhea is often self-limited, but if the patient does not improve and watery stools continue, re-examination is required. An antimicrobial agent for specific pathogens may be necessary.	
b. Monitor weight and intake and output.	b. Weight changes indicate fluid volume changes (loss or gain); 1 kg (2.2 lb) equals approximately 1000 ml of fluid.	
c. Report to physician/clinic if fever recurs or if patient has persistent or bloody diarrhea.		
11. Include diarrhea stools in output measurements.	11. Significant amounts of fluid can be lost with diarrhea.	

Nursing Diagnosis: Altered nutrition (less than body requirements) related to increased metabolic needs from infection and to lack of interest in food

Goal: Improvement in nutritional status

1. Perform a nutritional assessment. a. Assess for decrease in food intake; institute a calorie count.	a. Generalized malaise, discomfort, and anorexia accompany infections, causing disinterest in food.	• Verbalizes beginning understanding of nutritional needs accompanying an infectious illness. • Maintains weight. • Ingests number of calories appropriate for size and health status.
b. Monitor progress of fever.	b. With fever there are increases in catabolism and loss of nutrients; the	

(continued)

Nursing Care Plan 62-1 *(Continued)*

Care of the Patient With an Infectious Disease

Nursing Interventions	Rationale	Expected Outcomes
	catabolic response and magnitude of loss are proportional to severity and duration of fever.	
c. Monitor weight	c. Any infectious illness causes metabolic and biochemical changes and triggers the stress response, with accompanying hypermetabolism and negative balances of nitrogen, potassium, phosphorus, and magnesium, and consequent weight loss.	
2. Offer high-calorie, high-protein diet; offer small liquid feedings at first, gradually adding foods that are readily digested as tolerated.	2. Sufficient calories are necessary for patients with fever to replenish energy used by increased metabolism and restlessness. Increased protein is required to counteract the loss of nitrogen.	
3. Offer a variety of oral fluids (2000–3000 ml/day).	3. Increased fluids are necessary to replenish losses through perspiration, increased respiratory rate, and losses from the GI tract.	
4. Provide patient education		
a. Encourage patient to continue with optimum plan of nutrition during (and beyond) convalescence.	4a. It may take several weeks to replenish nutrient losses associated with an acute infection of short duration.	
b. Continue to monitor weight.	b. If infection is severe and prolonged, there will be muscle wasting and weight loss because protein is catabolized for energy.	
c. Take vitamin supplements as prescribed.	c. Fever increases vitamin requirements (B complex vitamins, ascorbic acid, vitamin A). Antibiotics may interfere with intestinal synthesis of B complex vitamins.	

Nursing Diagnosis: Knowledge deficit about cause of infection, treatment, and preventive measures

Goal: Acquisition of knowledge of infectious process

1. Listen carefully to what the patient says about his illness and treatment.	1. Listening allows for detection and correction of misunderstanding and misinformation.	• Relates cause of problem and therapy at a level consistent with intellectual and emotional states.

2. Keep explanations brief and focused about:
  a. Organism and method of spread.
  b. Where and when occurs.
  c. How treated.
  d. Importance of environmental cleanliness and personal hygiene.
  e. Importance of seeking health care in the event of a febrile illness or skin eruption.
	2. Knowledge of his specific illness and treatment promotes a sense of control and makes the future more predictable and manageable as well as makes the patient an active participant in his care. The act of explanation is in itself reassuring.	• Actively participates in treatment.
		• Complies with procedures of infection control.

3. Allow for opportunities for questions and discussions.	3. The patient's questions can serve as a guide to topics that need clarification.	

(continued)

Nursing Care Plan 62–1 *(Continued)*

Care of the Patient With an Infectious Disease

Nursing Interventions	Rationale	Expected Outcomes

4. Teach the patient and family about
   a. Availability and importance of prophylactic immunization.
   b. Manner in which infectious illnesses are spread and methods of avoiding spread.
   c. Means of preventing the contamination of food and water supplies.
   d. Importance of adequate nutrition and housing.
   e. Knowledge of insect, rodent, and other animal vectors and reservoirs of human infections and the importance of eliminating them.

4. Education can change human behavior and is an effective way of reducing the risk of infection.

Nursing Diagnosis: High risk for infection (spread of infection to others)

Goal: Prevention of spread of infection

1. Prevent spread of infection.

   a. Wash hands immediately after contact with each patient and after every contact with material that may be contaminated and potentially infectious.
   b. Use gown when indicated; use gown once and discard in appropriate receptacle.

   c. Use masks as indicated.

   d. Use gloves when indicated by the patient's condition:
     (1) Disposable single-use gloves are preferable.
     (2) Use once and discard in appropriate receptable.
     (3) Wash hands after gloves are removed.
   e. Handle needles and syringes with extreme caution. Never recap needles or bend or break by hand after use.

1. Control efforts are directed toward controlling the agent at its source.
   a. Hand washing is the most important procedure for preventing infection.

   b. Gowns are indicated when clothes are likely to be soiled with body secretions or when patients have infections that, if transmitted in hospitals, frequently cause serious illness.

   c. In general, masks are used to prevent transmission of infectious agents through the air. If infection is transmitted by large-particle aerosols, masks may be worn by those close to the patient. If infection (small-particle aerosols) is transmitted over longer distances, masks are worn by all persons entering the room.
   d. Wearing gloves is indicated for touching excretions, secretions, blood, or body fluids.

   e. It is usually not known if the patient's blood is contaminated with hepatitis virus or HIV. Accidental needle puncture may occur. Caution must be exercised when handling any used needle.

- No evidence of signs of infection.
- Temperature within normal limits.
- Negative culture reports.
- Takes proper precautions to prevent spread of infection to others.

(continued)

Nursing Care Plan 62–1 *(Continued)*

Care of the Patient With an Infectious Disease

Nursing Interventions	Rationale	Expected Outcomes
f. Handle wastes with all due precautions; double-bag waste per isolation procedures.	f. Proper handling of wastes prevents spread of infection.	
g. Control dissemination of infectious droplets. (1) Teach patient to cover his nose and mouth when coughing or sneezing. (2) Bag and label soiled paper tissues and dispose according to agency policy.	g. Containment of infectious secretions prevents spread of infection.	
h. Handle soiled linen as little as possible; avoid shaking bed linens.	h. This prevents gross microbial contamination of the air and of persons handling the linen.	
i. Maintain environmental cleanliness by requiring damp dusting of furniture, wet vacuuming of floors, washing visible soil from walls as soon as it appears, and reducing to a minimum the activity of personnel in the patient's room.	i. Appropriate cleaning procedures and methods are designed to remove organic material and soil. Individual agency policies can identify whether cleaning, disinfecting, or sterilizing an item is necessary. Items that ordinarily do not touch the patient (or touch only intact skin) rarely, if ever, transmit disease; washing with a detergent may be sufficient.	
j. Keep the door to the room closed.		

Nursing Diagnosis: Social isolation related to nature of disease

Goal: Achievement of social participation

Nursing Interventions	Rationale	Expected Outcomes
1. Assess verbal and nonverbal communication between patient and significant others. 2. Provide psychosocial support. a. Be available. b. Answer questions. c. Explore anxieties that prompt questions. d. Employ empathetic listening. e. Educate family about acceptable tactile contact with patient.	1. The patient's family/support system can have a valuable stress-reducing effect for the patient. 2. Ongoing and regular visits by health care personnel can have a valuable stress-reducing effect. Willingness to listen and ability to understand can relieve sense of loneliness.	• Shares feelings and anxieties of alienation. • Recalls previous reactions to stressful events. • Establishes/reinvests in relationships. • Involves self in care and activities.
3. Integrate a caring relationship in all nursing strategies; suggest ways to relieve boredom; teach stress-reduction techniques.	3. Interpersonal relationships and personal support are basic for reduction of stress and social isolation. Self-regulation emerges when isolation and loneliness are relieved.	
4. Employ a nonjudgmental approach to the patient with a sexually transmitted disease.	4. If the patient perceives negative verbal or nonverbal communication, he may feel anxious and guilty, which would interfere with the nurse–patient relationship.	

anxiety. Nursing interventions and patient outcomes are evaluated for effectiveness.

Sexually Transmitted Diseases

STDs are diseases acquired through sexual contact with an infected person. These diseases include the traditional venereal diseases (gonorrhea, syphilis, chancroid, lymphogranuloma inguinale, and lymphogranuloma venereum) and a complex array of infections and clinical syndromes that make up a new generation of STDs, of which the newest and most serious is AIDS.

The term *sexually transmitted disease* has replaced *venereal disease* as the term of choice. STDs are the most common infections in the United States and are epidemic in most parts of the world. Portals of entry of STD microorganisms and sites of infection include the skin and mucosal linings of the urethra, cervix, vagina, rectum, and oropharynx. Diseases classified as sexually transmitted diseases are listed in Table 62-2. These diseases are of great concern because of the changing nature of sexual practices and attitudes, personal mobility, the decreasing age at which sexual activity begins, the practice of nonbarrier methods of contraception (*e.g.,* oral contraceptives), and the problem of locating and providing treatment for the carriers of these infections. Those at high risk for acquiring STDs are sexual partners of infected persons (including homosexual and bisexual men), and those with multiple sex partners. In the developing countries, prostitution is the major reservoir for syphilis, chancroid, and gonorrhea.

Problems and Risk Factors

The problems and complications of STDs are challenging. They frequently exist without causing symptoms. A high incidence of co-infection places individuals with one STD at risk for concurrent infection (*e.g.,* gonorrhea together with chlamydial infection). Although some of the organisms that cause STDs are sensitive to antimicrobial therapy, other pathogens demonstrate resistance to treatment. Another problem is that certain drugs used in treatment predispose the patient to superinfection. Diseases that occur in genital mucosal areas may also occur in nongenital mucosal areas that are used for sexual activity (*e.g.,* the pharynx).

Sexual practices associated with risk of infection are seen among women and among heterosexual, homosexual, and bisexual men. The incidence of many STDs is particularly high among those who practice oral and anal sex and among those who have unprotected sexual contact with multiple partners.

STDs are a major health problem of women. Many women with these diseases are asymptomatic, and they have no way of knowing whether they or their sexual partners are infected. Many of the severe complications of STDs are experienced by women. Genital herpes may be a precursor of cervical dysplasia and cancer. Pelvic inflammatory diseases (diseases caused by acute ascending genital tract infections) are significant complications of STDs and may involve more than one infectious organism. Women make up the fastest growing risk group for HIV infection in the United States and around the world. The incidence of AIDS, the clinical syndrome of HIV infection, has increased more rapidly in women than in other major segments of the U.S. population. Women are at risk for HIV infection through heterosexual transmission and transmission through IV drug use.

Preventing the Spread of STDs

Emergency departments, outpatient clinics, college health services, and women's health facilities should be equipped to diagnose and treat STDs to reduce their spread. Most patients require counseling about the transmission and manifestations of these diseases as well as advice about treatment, follow-up, and the importance of referring sexual contacts for treatment. Women need to be informed that untreated male partners and multiple sex partners increase their risk of developing these infections. The risk of infertility is greater with each subsequent recurrence of pelvic inflammatory disease. The use of barrier methods of contraception, specifically condoms, reduces the risk of acquiring certain infections.

Adolescents are not always aware of the cause-and-effect relationship between sexual intercourse and STDs. In addition, denial and risk-taking behaviors are often characteristic of adolescents. Therefore, health care personnel should intensify efforts to reinforce and expand the knowledge of adolescents. Programs designed to help teenagers deal with social and peer pressures may be an alternative approach to prevention of STDs.

Acquired Immunodeficiency Syndrome

AIDS is a severe disorder of the immune system function and results in an impairment of the body's ability to fight disease. Severe damage imposed on the immune system predisposes the patient to life-threatening infections by opportunistic organisms and to Kaposi's sarcoma and other unusual neoplasms.

A retrovirus, designated HIV, has been implicated as the causative agent in AIDS. This virus has its greatest effect on a subpopulation of lymphocytes, the T-4 or T-helper cells, which control the body's response to infections caused by bacteria, viruses, protozoans, fungi, and parasites. The virus is transmitted through intimate sexual contact, sharing of contaminated needles, and transfusion of blood or blood components. The virus can also be transmitted by an infected mother to her child before, at, or shortly after the time of birth.

Persons at risk include those who engage in receptive anal sex such as sexually active homosexual men, persons with multiple sexual partners, IV drug users, persons with hemophilia, and sexual partners of individuals infected with the virus. As the number of persons infected with HIV increases, the number of individuals at risk also increases. To date, there are no cures or vaccines for AIDS, and the culmination of the syndrome is usually death by opportunistic infections.

Increasing evidence suggests that STDs, especially those characterized by ulceration, increase the risk of transmission of HIV if one engages in sexual activity with an infected person. HIV infection and AIDS, in turn, increase the risk of STDs because of the altered and failing immune system associated with HIV infection and AIDS. Studies have suggested that STDs that are characterized by genital ulcers increase the risk of acquiring HIV by allowing penetration of HIV through the ulcerative lesions. Those STDs in which there are excessive inflammatory vaginal secretions may promote HIV transmission because of

TABLE 62-2. *Most Important Sexually Transmitted Pathogens and the Disorders They Cause*

Pathogens	*Disease/Disorder/Syndrome*
BACTERIAL AGENTS	
Neisseria gonorrhoeae	Urethritis, epididymitis, cervicitis, proctitis, pharyngitis, conjunctivitis, endometritis, perihepatitis, bartholinitis, amniotic infection syndrome, disseminated gonococcal infection, premature delivery and premature rupture of membranes, salpingitis and related sequelae (infertility, ectopic pregnancy, recurrent salpingitis)
Chlamydia trachomatis	Urethritis, epididymitis, cervicitis, proctitis, salpingitis, inclusion conjunctivitis, infant pneumonia, otitis media, trachoma, lymphogranuloma venereum, perihepatitis, bartholinitis, Reiter's disease, fetal and neonatal mortality
Mycoplasma hominis	Postpartum fever, salpingitis
Ureaplasma urealyticum	Urethritis, chorioamniotitis, low birth-weight
Treponema pallidum	Syphilis
Gardnerella hemophilus vaginalis	Vaginitis
Haemophilus ducreyi	Chancroid
Calymmatobacterium granulomatis	Donovanosis (granuloma inguinale)
Shigella, Campylobacter sp.	Enterocolitis (among those who practice oral–anal sexual activity)
Group B β-hemolytic streptococcus	Neonatal sepsis, neonatal meningitis
VIRAL AGENTS	
Human T-lymphotropic viruses	Acquired immunodeficiency syndrome (AIDS)
Herpes simplex virus	Primary and recurrent genital herpes, aseptic meningitis, neonatal herpes with associated mortality or neurologic sequelae, carcinoma of the uterine cervix, spontaneous abortion and premature delivery
Hepatitis B virus	Acute, chronic, and fulminant hepatitis, with associated immune complex phenomena
Cytomegalovirus	Congenital infection: gross birth defects and infant mortality, cognitive impairment (*e.g.,* mental retardation, sensorineural deafness), heterophile-negative infectious mononucleosis, cervicitis, protean manifestations in the immunosuppressed host
Human papilloma virus (HPV)	Condyloma acuminata, laryngeal papilloma in infants, cervical dysplasia
Molluscum contagiosum viruses	Genital molluscum contagiosum
PROTOZOAN AGENTS	
Trichomonas vaginalis	Vaginitis, urethritis, balanitis
Entamoeba histolytica	Amebiasis (sexually transmitted especially among those with oral–anal sexual practices)
Giardia lamblia	Giardiasis (sexually transmitted especially among those with oral–anal sexual practices)
Fungal Agents	
Candida albicans	Vulvovaginitis, balanitis
Ectoparasites	
Phthirus pubis	Pubic louse infestation ("crabs")
Sarcoptes scabiei	Scabies

(Reproduced with permission from the Annual Review of Public Health, Vol 6, 1985. Copyright by Annual Reviews, Inc.)

the presence of large numbers of virus-infected cells (lymphocytes) in the genital tract. Patients who have persistent and recurrent STDs that require continuous therapy should be evaluated for evidence of deterioration of the immune system.

AIDS has become a major public health problem in the United States and abroad. Knowledge about the spread, distribution, and natural course of the disease is still evolving. Because AIDS affects the immune system, it is discussed in greater detail in Chapter 48.

Chlamydial Infections

Genital chlamydial infections caused by *Chlamydia trachomatis* are now recognized as the most prevalent and among the most damaging of all STDs seen in the United States. These infections cause inflammation of the urethra and epididymis in men, and inflammation of the cervix with a mucopurulent discharge and an alarming increase in pelvic infections in women. These complications contribute significantly to the increase in the number of women who experience ectopic pregnancies. Chlamydial infections have been linked to infertility in both sexes and have been associated with many other health problems (see Chap. 45).

Genital Herpes Infections

Genital herpes is among the most common and most psychologically distressing of the STDs. Because there is no cure for this disease, infected individuals often experience social isolation. Although symptoms can be treated, there is a high risk of spreading the infection to sexual partners. Some 5 to 10 million Americans are affected, and the number is growing by almost a million cases annually. Genital herpes is epidemiologically significant because it can be transmitted to the newborn and because of its possible link to genital cancer (see Chap. 45).

Management of STDs

Primary prevention is the most important aspect of managing STDs because some of these diseases are not readily cured by antibiotics. Infected persons must be promptly identified and given effective available treatment. Recommendations for the treatment of STDs are periodically updated by the CDC. Antibiotic regimens are now fairly well standardized for some infections, although treatment changes as the various pathogens develop resistance to specific drugs.

Because no antimicrobial regimen is 100% effective, all patients require reexamination and retesting after treatment. Follow-up times vary with the disease.

HBV is the only STD for which an effective vaccine is available.

Gonorrhea

Gonorrhea is an infection involving the mucosal surface of the genitourinary tract, rectum, and pharynx. It is caused by the gonococcus *Neisseria gonorrhoeae* and is an infectious disease that is transmitted sexually (the exception being gonococcal ophthalmia of the newborn). It may be acquired through sexual intercourse and by orogenital or anogenital contacts between members of the opposite sex as well as members of the same sex.

The worldwide incidence of gonorrhea continues to rise. Factors contributing to the rapid spread of gonorrhea are its short incubation period and the large number of persons, both male and female, harboring the gonococcus who are asymptomatic (silent) carriers. Another factor is the use of nonbarrier methods of contraception, such as the contraceptive pill. Barrier methods (condoms with vaginal spermicides) may prevent the spread of some STDs. Gonococcal infection among homosexual males is becoming a major health problem. In addition, gonorrhea frequently coexists with other STDs. Another complicating factor is the development of resistance by infected individuals to penicillin, tetracycline, and other antibiotics.

The highest rate of gonorrhea occurs among persons between the ages of 15 and 24, although there is a rapid rise of the disease in teenagers younger than 15 years of age.

Pathophysiology

The gonococcus causes a surface infection, ascending, in almost all cases, by way of the lower genital tract. The primary infection takes place in or near the urethra in males, and in the cervix, urethra, or rectum in females. If drainage is good, the infection subsides spontaneously and clears in the course of a few days or weeks. However, infection of the prostatic urethra in the male and of the female urethral and vaginal glands predisposes to chronic infection, with occasionally serious sequelae. Females are apt to contract secondarily a mixed infection of the endometrium and fallopian tubes, constituting pelvic infection, with resultant pelvic peritonitis. The upward spread of the infection into the reproductive tract is precipitated by such factors as menstruation, douches, and the trauma associated with sexual intercourse or instrumentation.

Clinical Manifestations and Complications

After an incubation period of 2 to 7 days, most men develop dysuria or a urethral discharge, which may be a scanty clear fluid or a purulent copious drainage. The infection may extend to the prostate, seminal vesicles, and epididymis, causing prostatitis, inguinal lymphadenitis, pelvic pain, and fever. Postgonococcal urethritis develops in one fourth to one third of men treated for gonorrhea. Many cases of nongonococcal urethritis are secondary to chlamydial infections. A particularly serious problem is men with asymptomatic infection who are carriers of gonorrhea. These men are often not discovered by the usual gonorrhea control measures. They remain infected, untreated, and asymptomatic but can infect their sexual partners.

In females, the infection is frequently silent, so a large percentage of women are asymptomatic and unaware that they are infected. A small number have vaginal discharge, urinary frequency, and dysuria. The sites most frequently involved are the urethra and cervix. As the endocervical gonococcal infection spreads upward into the reproductive tract, it causes pelvic infection (pelvic inflammatory disease), with endometritis, salpingitis, or pelvic peritonitis. An estimated 10% to 15% of women infected with the gonococcus develop pelvic infection, as evidenced by abdominal pain, fever, and vaginal discharge. There is marked pelvic tenderness on movement of the cervix and uterus during bimanual pelvic examination. Pelvic infection causes adhesions in the area of the pelvic organs and rectum. This is a major direct cause of infertility. It also leads to ectopic pregnancy and chronic pelvic inflammation, the sequelae of which require surgical intervention.

Other Manifestations of Gonorrhea. *Anal manifestations* consist of anal itching and irritation (from erythema and edema of the anal crypts), a sensation of rectal fullness, rectal bleeding or diarrhea, mucus in the stools, and painful defecation. Anorectal gonorrhea is reported in 28% to 55% of homosexual males attending STD clinics.

Oral manifestations may be the result of the direct contact of the infecting organisms with the pharynx, or of their transmission to the oral cavity from infection elsewhere in the body. Although most pharyngeal infections are asymptomatic, the following oral manifestations are seen: sore throat; painful, ulcerative inflammation of the lips; reddened, spongy, and tender gingivae; reddened, dry tongue; and redness and edema of the soft palate and uvula. The oropharynx may be covered with vesicles.

Systemic manifestations may become apparent, because secondary foci of infection may develop in any organ system, causing disseminated gonococcal infection (gonococcal bacteremia). Disseminated gonococcal infection occurs when the gonococci invade the bloodstream from one of the primary sites of infection. The patient presents with tenosynovitis of the small joints and hemorrhagic skin rash. Two to 3 weeks later, untreated patients develop septic arthritis, exhibiting hot, red, and swollen joints.

Other systemic complications include gonococcal endocarditis, meningitis, and fulminant gonococcemia.

Assessment

Physical Assessment. The patient is inspected for lesions, rashes, adenopathy, and urethral, vaginal, and rectal discharges.

Diagnostic Evaluation. There are a variety of ways of identifying gonorrhea through laboratory diagnosis. The gram-negative intracellular diplococci may be found in smears or through direct fluorescent antibody tests, or may be cultured with selective media. The pharyngeal and anal sites should be cultured in persons who engage in oral or anal sex. In the male, specimens may be obtained from the urethra, anal canal, and pharynx, depending on the patient's sexual history. In the female, cultures are collected from the endocervix, pharynx, and anal canal. Sterile, disposable gloves are worn by the nurse when obtaining these cultures. As a rule, lubricating jellies are not used for the vaginal examination because they may contain

---

Chart 62–1
Obtaining Cultures for Diagnosis of Gonorrhea

For Female Patient

Oropharynx Culture
Swab the posterior pharynx and tonsillar crypts with a cotton-tipped applicator.

Cervical Culture
1. Moisten vaginal speculum with warm water. Do not use any other lubricant.
2. Separate labia. Depress the perineum and posterior vaginal wall with the finger of one hand.
3. Gently insert a bivalve vaginal speculum.
4. Remove excessive cervical mucus with a cotton ball held in ring forceps.
5. Insert sterile cotton-tipped swab into endocervical canal (see Fig. 62-2*A*).
    a. Move from side to side in cervix.
    b. Allow 30 seconds for absorption of organisms by the swab.

Anal Canal Culture (Rectal Culture)
1. Obtain anal specimen *after* obtaining cervical specimen.
2. Insert sterile cotton-tipped swab approximately 2.5 cm (1 in) into the anal canal (Fig. 62-2*B*).
3. Move swab from side to side in anal canal.
4. Allow 10 to 30 seconds for absorption of organism by the swab.

For Male Patient

Oropharynx Culture
Same as in women.

Urethral Culture
Use a sterile bacteriologic wire loop or a sterile calcium alginate urethral swab to obtain a specimen from the anterior urethra by gently scraping the mucosa (see Fig. 62-2*C*). Do not insert loop or swab more than 2 cm.

Anal Canal Culture
Same as in women.

substances that inhibit growth or kill some pathogens. Water is used as the lubricant instead.

See Chart 62-1 and Figure 62-2 for the methods of obtaining cultures and inoculating the culture plate. The *Neisseria* gonococci are susceptible to environmental changes; therefore, specimens must be delivered to the laboratory immediately after they are obtained.

Management

The goals of treatment are to eradicate the organism and educate the patient about his condition. These goals are achieved through screening procedures, drug therapy, and patient education.

For uncomplicated gonorrhea, the CDC recommends treatment regimens that include one of the following: amoxi-

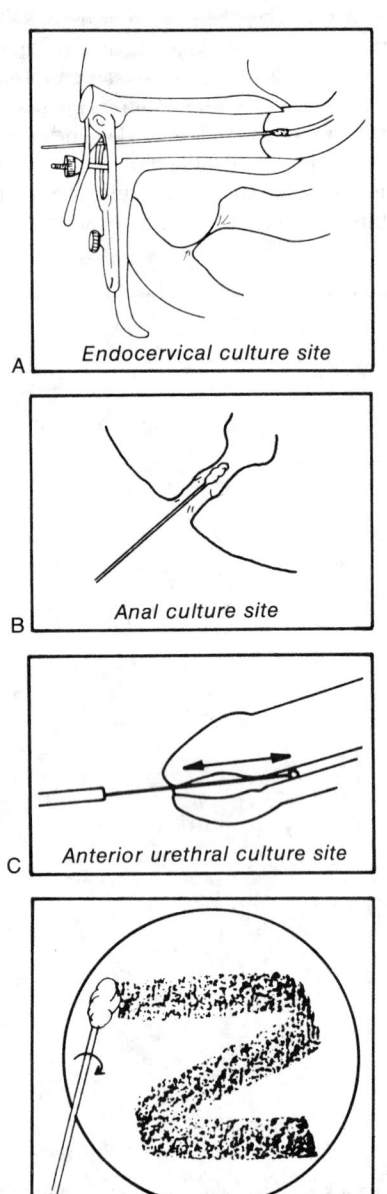

Figure 62-2. Obtaining specimens for culture in the diagnosis of gonorrhea. (Criteria and Techniques for the Diagnosis of Gonorrhea. U.S. Public Health Service, Centers for Disease Control.)

cillin, ampicillin, aqueous procaine penicillin G, ceftriaxone plus tetracycline, or doxycycline. Amoxicillin, ampicillin, and penicillin (but not ceftriaxone) are prescribed with oral probenecid to increase the serum concentration of the penicillins. New antimicrobials are becoming available that may also prove to be effective.

An important concern in the treatment of gonorrhea is coexisting chlamydial infection, documented in up to 45% of gonorrhea cases when chlamydial cultures are performed. Because chlamydiae are resistant to penicillin, a tetracycline or doxycycline regimen is recommended. Other treatment regimens are available for patients who are allergic to penicillin and for those with penicillin-resistant *N. gonorrhoeae*. The treatment of complications (endocarditis, disseminated gonococcal infection) is individualized.

All patients with gonorrhea should undergo serologic testing for syphilis and be screened for other STDs, including HIV infection, at the time of diagnosis. Patients with both gonorrhea and syphilis are given additional treatment, depending on the stages of the diseases.

It is imperative that follow-up cultures be obtained from infected sites 3 to 7 days after the treatment is completed, because no therapy is 100% effective. In addition, cultures are obtained from the rectum of women who have been treated for gonorrhea.

Each patient is interviewed for names of sexual contacts. Public health programs are geared to trace contacts and prevent further spread, which they accomplish through reporting, diagnosis, treatment, and follow-up. Contacts should be investigated and treated within 10 days. The patient is instructed to avoid reinfection by untreated sexual contacts until those contacts have been treated.

Nursing Interventions

Infected discharge from a patient with gonorrhea can be spread to the eyes from contaminated fingers. When examining a patient or coming in contact with vaginal or urethral discharge, the nurse must wear gloves, avoid touching her face, and practice careful hand washing. Universal Precautions must be utilized with specimens.

If penicillin is administered, the patient is instructed to remain in the clinic or office for 30 minutes following injection for monitoring of any untoward reaction.

Points to emphasize for patient education are summarized on p. 1919.

Syphilis

Syphilis is an acute and chronic infectious multisystem disease caused by *Treponema pallidum* (a spirochete). It is acquired through sexual contact or may be congenital in origin.

T. pallidum produces effects locally and is killed quickly by exposure to drying, heat, or air. A *chancre* (primary sore) in syphilis appears at the site (or sites) where the treponemes entered the body. Because these open, untreated lesions contain spirochetes, the disease can be transmitted through contact with the lesions. In the pregnant woman, the fetus is infected from the mother by way of the placenta. Most cases are contracted through sexual activity; the danger of transmission is greatest in the early stage of syphilis.

Epidemiology

People known to have syphilis are interviewed and asked to identify their sexual contacts so that these contacts can be examined and treated within a minimal time period. Statistics indicate that syphilis is most prominent among homosexuals, teenagers, young adults, and members of lower socioeconomic groups.

Each person with syphilis is a potential source for a small outbreak. Studies indicate that each infected individual has an average of three different sexual contacts who are at risk for contracting syphilis. Case reporting of early infectious syphilis is required.

Clinical Manifestations

Syphilis is capable of destroying tissues in almost any organ in the body, resulting in a wide variety of clinical manifestations. Some of the manifestations of syphilis are designated as early and others as late. The time interval between early and late syphilis is about 4 years, during which period the patient develops a partial immunity and an altered tissue response to the spirochete. (If syphilis occurs in a person who is HIV-infected, the course of the syphilis may be altered; the tertiary stage may follow the primary stage.)

Stages of Syphilis

Primary Stage. The incubation period is 10 to 90 days, with an average of 21 days. During the primary (early) stage, also the most infectious stage, the chancre (primary sore) appears at the site or sites where the treponemes entered the body: genitalia, anus, rectum, lips, oral cavity, breasts, or fingers (Fig. 62-3). The sites are generally related to the pattern of sexual activity. The typical chancre is an indurated painless nodule that breaks down, forming a shallow ulcer. The lymph nodes draining the ulcer become enlarged, firm, and nontender. Untreated, the primary lesion heals in a few weeks.

Secondary Stage (Stage of Systemic Involvement). Within a few weeks or months, the treponemes have begun to spread throughout the body, and a variable systemic illness develops, characterized by low-grade fever, malaise, sore throat, headache, lymphadenopathy, arthralgia, and skin or mucosal rash.

The skin manifestations, which prompt many patients to seek health care, may simulate practically every known skin disease. The rash typically is macular (nonelevated discoloration) or maculopapular (elevated lesions) but can become pustular. It can be anywhere on the body, but often the palms and soles are involved. If untreated, the rash gradually fades. At the same time the hair may drop out, sometimes in patches, giving the scalp a moth-eaten appearance.

The lesions that appear on the mucous membranes of the mouth and tongue are glistening, slightly elevated, flat, circumscribed patches that are usually covered with a yellowish exudate. These so-called mucous patches contain large numbers of spirochetes. The lesions that develop in areas where skin is adjacent to skin (in the area of the vagina and anus) take the form of flat wartlike plaques (condylomata); these plaques contain large numbers of spirochetes and are therefore capable of transmitting infection.

Tertiary Stage (Late Syphilis). After the secondary stage, there is a period of latency in which the patient shows no signs or symptoms of syphilis. This stage may last for months or years, and many patients have no further trouble, with or with-

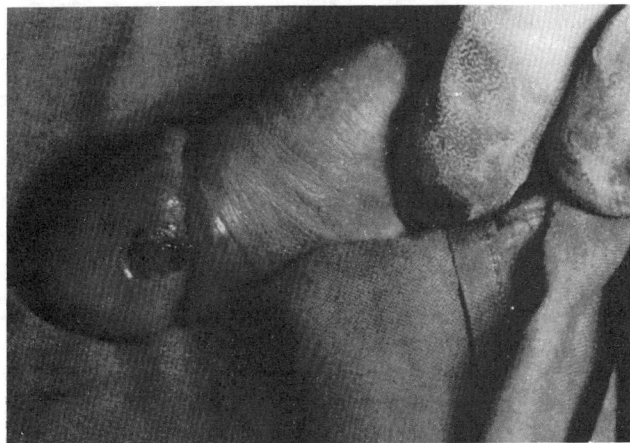
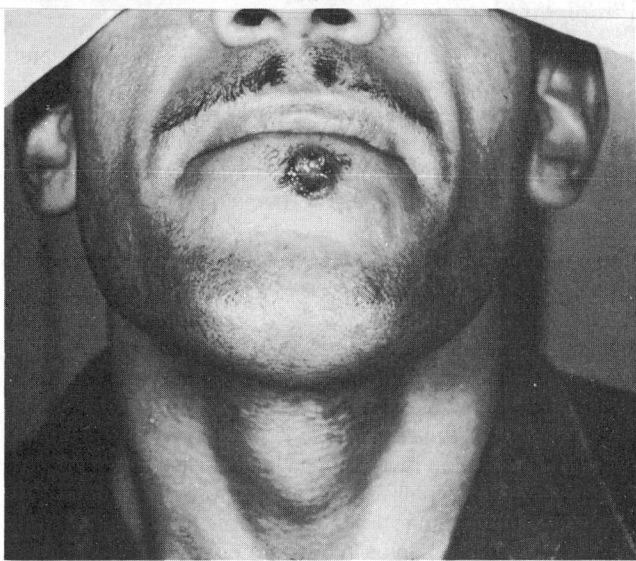

Figure 62–3. (**Top**) Syphilitic chancre on the external surface of the prepuce. (Elliott H and Rhyz K. Venereal Diseases: Treatment and Nursing. London, Balliere Tindall.) (**Bottom**) Primary syphilis: Typical Hunterian chancre on lower lip. (Syphilis: A Synopsis. U.S. Department of Health, Education and Welfare, Public Health Service.)

out treatment. Late syphilis is a slowly progressive inflammatory disease that may involve almost any organ. In cardiovascular syphilis, the inflammatory reaction may involve the heart and great vessels, with lesions occurring in the aorta, pulmonary artery, or great vessels arising from the aorta, resulting in aortitis and aneurysms. In neurosyphilis, disabling lesions occur in the central nervous system, giving rise to a variety of neurologic symptoms. Destructive noninfectious granulomatous lesions of the skin, viscera, bone, and mucosal surfaces can occur, which may impair health and shorten life.

Diagnostic Evaluation

Because syphilis is the great imitator of many diseases, the clinical history and laboratory evaluation are important. A number of serologic tests are used in the diagnosis and management of syphilis; three are nontreponemal and two are treponemal.

- *Nontreponemal or reagin tests* measure antibodies formed in response to products of tissue destruction (called reagin) in the serum of infected patients. The most widely used are the Venereal Disease Research Laboratory (VDRL) slide flocculation test, the rapid plasma reagin circle card test (RPR-CT), and the automated reagin test (ART). These tests are reliable, simple to perform, and inexpensive.
- *Treponemal tests* are tests to measure specific antibodies to *T. pallidum*. These tests are recommended for patients who have reactive reagin tests and atypical signs of primary or secondary syphilis and for diagnosis of late syphilis. The treponemal tests are the fluorescent treponemal antibody absorption test (FTA-ABS) and the microhemagglutination test (MHA-TP).

Management

The treatment guidelines established by the CDC are updated on a regular basis. The current treatment of all stages of syphilis is administration of antibiotics. Penicillin G benzathine is the drug of choice for early syphilis or latent syphilis of less than 1 year's duration. It is given by intramuscular injection at a single session. Patients who are allergic to penicillin are treated with tetracycline.

The optimal treatment regimens for syphilis of greater than 1 year's duration have been less well established than those for early syphilis. In general, syphilis of longer duration requires more prolonged therapy.

Although therapy is recommended for established cardiovascular syphilis, antibiotics may not reverse the pathology (loss of elastic tissues in the aortic wall) associated with this disease.

CSF examination is performed in patients with suspected symptomatic neurosyphilis and is also desirable in other patients with syphilis greater than 1 year's duration, to exclude asymptomatic neurosyphilis. In late syphilis, no treatment can repair structural damage that has already occurred.

The *Jarisch-Herxheimer reaction* is a reaction appearing within hours of the initiation of therapy for syphilis, particularly in the secondary stage. It consists of transient fever and flulike symptoms of malaise, chills, headache, and myalgia that subside within 24 hours. The reaction is thought to be due to the sudden release of large amounts of treponema antigen with subsequent antigen–antibody reaction in the patient. It is managed with bed rest, aspirin, and reassurance.

Nursing Interventions

Chancres contain large numbers of spirochetes and are contagious through direct contact. Universal precautions and strict hand washing must be employed. The patient treated with penicillin is monitored for 30 minutes after the injection to watch for a possible allergic reaction. The following are important preventive and patient education factors:

- Patients exposed to syphilis within the preceding 3 months should be treated for early syphilis.
- All patients with early syphilis should return for repeat follow-up testing. Follow-up should include evaluation and treatment of sexual partners. Patients with syphilis of more than 1 year's duration should, in addition, have a serologic test 24 months after treatment.
- The patient with primary syphilis is assured that, with proper treatment and follow-up, the chancre will disappear (within

a week or two) and the blood test will, in most cases, become nonreactive within a year. Those with secondary syphilis see the rapid disappearance of their rash, and the blood test becomes nonreactive within 2 years.

- The patient is instructed to refrain from sexual contact with previous partners not under treatment.

▶ Nursing Process

The Patient With a Sexually Transmitted Disease

◊ Assessment

A sexual history is taken, including dates of exposure, symptoms, location of lesions, discharges, past history of STD, and self-treatment. Although there are a variety of clinical manifestations, depending on the disease, the most common are dysuria and urethral or vaginal discharge. At the time the patient enters the health care system, every effort is made to learn the names of the patient's sexual partners so they can be treated.

To be most helpful to the patient, the nurse must confront her own anxiety about sexual matters and approach the patient with honesty and sensitivity. Because the patient may be fearful of the health professional, it is important to listen patiently and carefully without passing judgment or moralizing so that the person is not placed on the defensive about life-style and does not find it necessary to hide information that is important in the diagnostic process.

Confidentiality is important when sexual issues are involved. Privacy is assured during information-gathering sessions, and interruptions are avoided. To avoid confusion and negative implications, the nurse uses terms that the patient understands, asks open-ended questions, and uses sensitivity when asking questions about persons with whom the patient has had sexual contact.

During the physical examination, the skin is examined for signs of irritation and itching and for burrows from scabies. The body and pubic hair are inspected for lice. In addition, the skin is assessed for rashes, lesions, drainage, and trauma. The mouth and throat are examined for signs of infection, and the inguinal nodes are palpated for size and consistency.

Gloves are always worn while the genitalia are examined. Any discharge, secretion, or pus is considered to be potentially infectious. The body fluids and tissues of patients with systemic STDs (AIDS, HBV, cytomegalovirus infection, syphilis, disseminated gonorrhea) are regarded as potentially infectious.

The genitalia are examined for redness, swelling, lesions, rashes, warts, and drainage. The urethra (in both men and women) and the vagina are inspected for mucopurulent discharge. (Is there an odor? Any itching?) The patient can be requested to point to the exact area of perineal discomfort. The presence of vaginal discharge and uterine tenderness suggest pelvic infection. The rectal area is examined for tenderness, discharge, and signs of trauma.

When digital vaginal and rectal examinations are performed in a woman with a suspected STD, gloves should be changed after the vaginal examination, to prevent the transmission of gonococci, chlamydiae, or herpes simplex virus from the cervix or vagina to the rectum.

Nursing Diagnoses

Based on the assessment data, the patient's major nursing diagnoses may include the following:

- Anxiety related to embarrassment and fear
- Noncompliance with treatment related to the stigmatizing nature of the disease and lack of understanding
- Knowledge deficit about the nature of the disease and the high risk for spread of infection and for other STDs, including HIV infection
- Potential for reinfection

Other nursing diagnoses could include social isolation and disturbance of self-esteem related to the nature of the disease.

Planning and Implementation

Goals: The major goals of the patient may include reduction of anxiety, compliance with the treatment program, acquisition of knowledge of the nature and treatment of the disease, prevention of recurrence and prevention of the spread of infection.

Nursing Interventions

Reducing Anxiety. The patient may fail to seek treatment because of anxiety, embarrassment, or the hope that the infection will go away. Anxiety may also cause the patient to withhold information, thereby interfering with understanding and hence compliance with treatment. A vaginal or urethral discharge can cause increased anxiety and a poor self-image.

Comfort and privacy without interruption as well as verbal and nonverbal assurances of confidentiality are essential in establishing and maintaining rapport. The patient is encouraged to express frustrations and feelings; talking helps to relieve anxiety and gain insight into problems.

Patient Education. The treatment regimen for most STDs is made as simple as possible to ensure compliance. The patient is informed of the consequences, especially to personal health and the health of the partner, if the condition is not properly treated.

The patient is taught how the disease is transmitted, how to recognize the major signs and symptoms, how long the infectious period lasts, how the disease is treated, and how to prevent its spread. The importance of taking the prescribed medication is emphasized. The patient is advised to continue taking the medication, even after the symptoms disappear. The possible adverse effects of the medication are discussed. The patient is encouraged to abstain from unprotected sexual activity until posttreatment examinations verify an effective treatment.

The control of the spread of an STD requires considerable patient involvement, education, and compliance. The following are important points to stress:

- An STD is acquired by sexual contact (vaginal sexual intercourse, anal intercourse, oral sex) and by close and direct contact with an infected person.
- A person who thinks that he or she may have an STD or who has been exposed to someone who might be infected should have a checkup. Immediate treatment should be sought if symptoms develop.

- Anyone who is sexually active with a number of sexual partners should have regular checkups.
- Washing the sex organs (before and after sexual contact) and using a condom may give limited protection.
- Birth control pills and IUDs provide *no* protection against STDs.
- Gonorrhea and syphilis are different diseases, caused by different organisms; they attack the body in different ways but are spread in the same manner. A person may have both gonorrhea and syphilis as well as other STDs at the same time.
- There appears to be no natural or acquired immunity to gonorrhea and syphilis. A person can get gonorrhea and syphilis again and again.
- A pregnant woman with syphilis may pass the infection to her unborn child. A pregnant woman with gonorrhea may pass it to her baby during childbirth.
- Bacteria from gonorrhea may enter the bloodstream and affect joints, joint linings, heart valves, and other tissues.
- The STD National Hotline (1-800-227-8922 [nationwide]; 1-800-982-5883 [California]) provides toll-free information and referral services for STDs. Confidentiality is maintained.

Preventing Recurrence. The patient is encouraged to persuade his partner or partners to be examined and tested promptly (usually within 24–48 hours). Reinfection can often be traced to the person who was the source of the original infection. Preventing recurrences includes modification of sexual activity. This may mean practicing monogamy (having sexual relations with only one person) or reducing the number of sex partners, avoiding partners known to have multiple partners, and questioning and inspecting partners before sexual activity. Avoiding certain types of sexual practices (anorectal intercourse; oral–anal and digital–anal activity) reduces the likelihood of infection. The use of the barrier methods of contraception (condoms) protects the partner from contact with semen, urethral discharge, or penile lesions, and vaginal spermicides may chemically inactivate some infectious agents.

Evaluation

Expected Outcomes

1. Demonstrates a less anxious demeanor
2. Complies with treatment
   a. Achieves effective treatment.
   b. Reports for follow-up examination
3. Acquires knowledge and understanding of STDs
   a. Recalls signs and symptoms of the most common STDs
   b. Inspects self for lesions, rashes, and discharge
4. Participates in a program to prevent recurrence of disease
   a. Identifies sexual partners for examination and treatment
   b. Recalls risk factors for recurrence

In summary, STDs vary greatly, both in ease of detection and effectiveness of available treatment. As a group, they are the most common infections occurring in the United States today. Preventing the spread of STDs is the most effective method of controlling them. Patient teaching is essential to decrease anxiety and to reinforce an understanding of the nature, treatment, and prevention of the disease.

Specific Bacterial Infections

Nosocomial (Hospital-Aquired) Infections

A nosocomial infection is an infection acquired during hospitalization. Nosocomial infections occur in about 5% to 6% of all hospital patients in the United States, accounting for an incidence of 2 million hospital-acquired infections per year. These infections prolong the hospital stay (an average of 13 days for each infection) and represent a direct economic liability of 5 to 10 billion dollars annually. Nosocomial infections are a significant cause of death among hospitalized patients.

The major cause of these infections is gram-negative bacteria. (For the particular species, see the following section on septic shock.) Such infections arise from the patient's own flora or from opportunistic organisms that gain access to the patient during hospitalization or that are acquired from other sources. The syndrome of septic shock is a complication of gram-negative bacteremia (bacteria in the bloodstream).

Host Susceptibility

Most gram-negative bacilli are not invasive in normal hosts but become invasive in hospitalized patients who have underlying disease and altered host defenses.

The risk of developing nosocomial infection parallels the severity of the underlying disease. Gram-negative infections occur in the very young; the elderly; patients with impaired immune systems, blood dyscrasias, burns, trauma, or poorly controlled diabetes; those undergoing prolonged procedures that result in extensive tissue damage; or those in whom a foreign body has been implanted. Any procedure involving the insertion of a tube into a normally sterile site (catheter into bladder; IV cannula into vein) may cause infection by allowing organisms to enter the sterile site through either the lumen or the outer surface of the tube or catheter. Potent immunosuppressive and cytotoxic drugs, corticosteroids, and radiation further diminish the patient's defense mechanisms. Antibiotics add to the problem by altering the patient's normal flora and encouraging overgrowth of hospital pathogens that are resistant to antibiotics. New pathogens continue to emerge as nosocomial opportunists. In fact, almost any organism can become a nosocomial pathogen, especially in an immunocompromised person.

Thus, the susceptible patient who is exposed to invasive diagnostic and monitoring equipment is predisposed to develop a gram-negative infection. In some patients, however, the original source of bacteremia cannot be identified.

Prevention

Awareness of the possible risk of infection among hospitalized patients is the first step in preventing such infections.

Fundamental to the control of infection are correct hand washing procedures, use of Universal Precautions for all patients, and strict aseptic technique applied to all diagnostic and therapeutic procedures involving the use of catheters, cardiac pacing, IV therapy, endotracheal and tracheostomy tubes, drainage tubes, and wound care.

Catheter-associated urinary tract infections are the leading cause of hospital-associated infections and are the most common predisposing factors in fatal gram-negative sepsis in hospitals. As indicated many times throughout this text, an indwelling catheter should be used *only when absolutely necessary*. A patient can be infected with his own bowel flora, by cross-contamination with other patients or hospital flora, or by exposure to contaminated solutions or nonsterile equipment. If possible, the use of indwelling catheters is avoided; alternative forms of drainage, such as condom drainage, use of a suprapubic catheter, or intermittent catheterization, are associated with less risk of urinary tract infection. In many cases, the need for an indwelling catheter can be avoided by careful attention to the toileting needs of patients, especially incontinent patients. If an indwelling catheter must be used, it should be removed promptly when no longer needed. Nurses can be especially instrumental in assisting with early removal of catheters by assessing urine output and signs of urinary tract infections and making recommendations to the physician.

Pulmonary infections account for about 15% of all hospital-acquired infections. Endotracheal and tracheostomy tubes bypass normal defense mechanisms, allowing organisms to enter the lungs. A grave problem with ventilator-related respiratory infections is aspiration around the tube. Great care must be exercised in using and sterilizing respiratory therapy equipment. Every precaution should be taken to reduce the possibility of aspiration. Patients restricted to bed rest or those experiencing thoracic or abdominal pain must be encouraged to turn, cough, and deep breathe every 1 to 2 hours while awake to prevent atelectasis and pulmonary secretion stasis.

Prolonged IV therapy should be avoided; when used, the IV catheter should be securely anchored to prevent it from moving in the vein. Scrupulous attention should be paid to inserting the needle properly, protecting the needle site, and observing and caring for the IV setup. Evidence indicates that most septicemias from intravascular devices originate from the patient's own flora or from the hands of the person inserting the device. IV sites must be assessed every shift for signs of infection: redness, edema, pain, heat, and drainage. Site locations should be rotated according to the policy of the health care institution.

Wound infections are more likely to occur in operations lasting longer than 2 hours, in abdominal operations, in contaminated or "dirty" operations (those involving gross spillage from the gastrointestinal tract or perforated viscera), or in patients with multiple diagnoses. Most wound infections are caused by endogenous organisms, for example, the bacteria being spread to the wound from the flora of the patient's own skin, nose, perineum, or gastrointestinal tract. Thus, host factors play a predominant role. The nurse must be aware of those patients who may be at risk.

Every hospital should have infection control personnel, including an infection control nurse, to monitor infection control procedures. Every health care provider should use all surveillance and preventive methods known to provide the safest possible environment for patients, personnel, and visitors.

Gram-Negative Bacteremia and Septic Shock

Gram-negative bacteremia (invasion of the bloodstream by a variety of bacterial species) causes a life-threatening state of inadequate tissue perfusion called septic shock. (The terms *septic shock*, *gram-negative shock*, and *endotoxin shock* are used interchangeably.) Most cases occur when the body's normal protective mechanical barriers are disrupted or when the person's defenses against infection are impaired. The organisms most frequently associated with gram-negative bacteremia and septic shock are *Escherichia coli, Klebsiella-Enterobacter-Serratia* species, *Pseudomonas aeruginosa, Proteus* species, *Neisseria meningitidis,* and *Bacteroides fragilis.* Gram-positive bacteria (*Staphylococcus aureus, Streptococcus pneumoniae*) have also been incriminated in septic shock.

Pathophysiology

The pathophysiology of septic shock is complex and poorly understood. It is thought that when gram-negative organisms invade the bloodstream, shock results in reaction to an endotoxin that initiates a number of events: cell injury, extracellular release of lysosomal enzymes from leukocytes, changes and interactions among the coagulation and fibrinolytic systems, and metabolic injury due to tissue anoxia.

Septic shock produces arteriolar and venous spasm, leading to pooling of blood in the pulmonary, splanchnic, renal, and peripheral tissues. This localized alteration in circulating blood results in anoxia and acidosis of the cells. Systemically, there is a decrease in venous return (resulting in a decreased preload) and a decreased cardiac output. Decreased cardiac output begins a cycle of decreased blood flow to the tissues, resulting in further anoxia and acidosis.

Initially, blood pressure, pulse rate, respiratory rate and cardiac output increase as a result of the body's compensatory mechanisms:

- Decreased blood pressure stimulates the sympathetic nervous system, resulting in increased rate and force of myocardial contraction and peripheral vasoconstriction, with resulting increase in blood pressure.
- Decreased *p*H (acidosis) and increased levels of carbon dioxide in the blood stimulate the respiratory center to increase the rate and depth of respirations.
- Vasoconstriction of the renal vessels stimulates the renin–angiotensin system to promote retention of sodium and water.
- Fluid shifts from the tissues into the capillary beds because of the changes of hydrostatic pressures at the cellular level.

If the infection progresses untreated, the body's compensatory mechanisms eventually begin to fail to maintain hemodynamic stability. Cardiac output and blood pressure decrease, and tissues and vital organs are inadequately perfused with oxygenated blood. Capillary damage causes leakage of fluid into the tissues, further decreasing circulating blood volume and resulting in peripheral edema.

Gram-negative bacilli or their endotoxins can activate Hageman factor (factor XII) of the intrinsic coagulation system, which in turn can result in intravascular coagulation, fibrinolysis, and shock.

Clinical Manifestations

The onset of septic shock may be abrupt with a shaking chill and rapid rise in temperature. (Temperature elevation may be blunted in the elderly or those receiving corticosteroids.) The patient has warm, dry skin. Respirations are increased (resulting in respiratory alkalosis) secondary to anoxia and increased lactic acid production.

As shock develops, the patient experiences tachypnea, tachycardia, profound hypotension, cool extremities, mental

obtundation (depression of cerebral function), and oliguria. Various abnormalities of intravascular coagulation (disseminated intravascular coagulopathy [DIC], thrombocytopenia) are frequently observed. A variety of skin lesions may be encountered. Nausea, vomiting, and diarrhea are often present. Patients with pre-existing cardiac disease may experience angina and dysrhythmias.

Gerontologic Considerations. In the elderly patient, septic shock may be manifested in atypical or confusing clinical signs. Septic shock should be suspected in any elderly person who develops an unexplained acute confused state, tachypnea, or hypotension.

Diagnostic Evaluation

The patient is examined to identify the source of sepsis. The etiologic agent is isolated and identified through blood cultures. Other smears and cultures are taken from any possible site of infection. Urinalysis is performed to detect the presence of pyuria, hematuria, casts, and bacteria.

White blood cell counts are elevated, with a shift to the left (a rise in the number of neutrophils) indicating an acute infection. Decreased circulating fluid volumes are indicated by elevated blood urea nitrogen, serum creatinine, and urine specific gravity values. Thrombocytopenia and other abnormal clotting values may be present.

Management

The patient usually is too ill to await the results of culture and sensitivity tests. Therapy is started immediately with agents effective against a broad spectrum of bacteria and with consideration given to the prevalence of resistant strains of bacteria in the hospital. IV antibiotics are prescribed to provide high levels of the drug in the blood, tissues, and body cavity fluids. Serum levels of antibiotics are monitored to ensure adequate doses and to prevent toxicity. When available, culture and sensitivity reports are compared to antibiotic therapy.

Any possible sources of infection, such as IV or urinary catheters, are removed and cultured. Surgical drainage of localized infection (abscess) and débridement of necrotic tissues are undertaken.

Aggressive fluid volume replacement with IV fluids and plasma expanders is a priority to ensure perfusion of vital organs and to correct fluid and electrolyte disturbances. Shock is treated with fluid replacement, vasoactive drugs (to alter the capacity of the vessels to overcome abnormalities of blood flow), and inotropic drugs such as Dopamine, dobutamine, and isoproterenol. Hemodynamic monitoring is essential with late septic shock. Oxygen is administered to keep arterial Po_2 at the desired level, although additional respiratory support with intubation and assisted ventilation may be necessary when arterial hypoxemia complicates shock. Sodium bicarbonate may be administered for severe acidosis.

▶ Nursing Process
The Patient With Septic Shock

◊ Assessment

The patient's health history may indicate the origin of the septic shock (*e.g.,* previous use of urinary catheter, cytotoxic therapy or immunotherapy). In addition to continuous blood pressure, pulse, and electrocardiographic monitoring, the nurse observes the patient for hyperventilation, apprehension, prostration, vomiting, and diarrhea. Reduced blood flow to cerebral vessels impairs mental status and may cause restlessness or confusion. The skin may be dry and warm or moist and pale, depending on the type of circulatory derangement. Hourly urinary output is monitored; oliguria may be evidence of circulatory insufficiency. Hemodynamic monitoring (pulmonary capillary wedge pressure or central venous pressure, cardiac output) is part of assessment because respiratory failure and cardiac failure are important causes of death in patients with septic shock. Rectal temperatures are obtained every 2 to 4 hours. Lab values are reviewed as indicated.

◊ *Nursing Diagnoses*

Based on all assessment data, the patient's major nursing diagnoses may include the following:

- Altered body temperature (fever) related to infectious process
- Altered tissue perfusion (cerebral, renal, peripheral) related to vasoconstriction from septic shock
- Ineffective breathing pattern (tachypnea, hyperpnea) related to pulmonary complications
- Altered urinary elimination (oliguria) related to decrease in circulating blood volume

Potential complications include DIC, respiratory failure, cardiac failure, renal failure, and metabolic acidosis.

◊ *Planning and Implementation*

◊ *Goals:* The major goals of the patient may include reduction of fever, improvement of tissue perfusion, normalization of breathing, attainment of adequate urinary output, and avoidance/management of complications.

◊ *Nursing Interventions*

◊ *Reduction of Fever.* The patient's temperature is carefully monitored, and measures are used to decrease temperature elevations that exceed 38.8°C (101°F) rectally. This control is important because elevated temperature increases the body's metabolic activity and oxygen demands. Such increases further compromise the hemodynamic instability of the patient with septic shock.

When the patient's temperature is elevated, bedding over the patient is removed, with the exception of a light sheet. Cool water bathing of the patient increases surface cooling and may be helpful. Acetaminophen is administered as prescribed for temperature elevation.

Antibiotics must be administered as scheduled to treat the cause of sepsis. Blood cultures are obtained as prescribed, and cultures are made of any catheter insertion sites (*e.g.*, IV catheter sites) and incisions with suspicious drainage, redness, or swelling. Culture and sensitivity reports are communicated to the physician so that antibiotic therapy can be altered as necessary.

◊ *Enhancing Tissue Perfusion.* The nurse monitors those parameters that relate to tissue perfusion: state of responsiveness; skin temperature, moisture, color, and turgor; appearance of mucous membranes and nails; respiratory rate; temperature; pulse; blood pressure; heart and lung sounds; peripheral pulses; intake; and urinary output. The assessment focuses on *trends* and *patterns of change.*

The IV catheter sites are assessed for signs of infection and adequacy of flow. IV infusions of vasoactive and inotropic drugs are closely monitored to prevent infiltration and assess patient response. Central venous pressure measurements provide a gauge for the rate and amount of volume replacement. The Swan–Ganz catheter measures pulmonary capillary wedge pressure, which is an estimate of left ventricular function and provides valuable information about the patient's fluid status. The nurse keeps in mind that fluid deficits may occur from fever, vomiting, diaphoresis, and diarrhea and uses appropriate interventions (see Nursing Care Plan 62-1).

The lung fields are auscultated when fluid is being administered to detect inspiratory and expiratory wheezes, and moist fine crackles, which may indicate impending pulmonary edema.

◊ *Promoting Adequate Breathing Patterns.* Arterial blood gas and *p*H measurements are monitored to determine if the patient requires assisted ventilation, because inadequate respiratory exchange is a frequent cause of death. (Severe shock and metabolic acidosis require correction with bicarbonate.) These measures represent a collaborative function with the physician. Nursing interventions for the patient requiring assisted ventilation are found in Chapter 25.

The patient is instructed to cough frequently and may need to be suctioned when a productive cough is present. Turning and changing position reduce the potential for retention of secretions and infection.

◊ *Ensuring Adequate Urinary Output.* Urinary output is monitored because kidney function deteriorates when circulating blood volume is shunted to other, more vital organs. The specific gravity of urine is measured at prescribed intervals. Urinary specific gravity increases when oliguria is present, signifying the kidneys' efforts to conserve fluid. An increase in urine output (more than 30 ml/hr) usually indicates that tissue perfusion and hence renal perfusion are improving.

◊ *Managing Complications.* When shock occurs in the course of bacteremia, there is an immediate threat to life, with a 60% to 80% mortality rate. Nursing support requires continuing patient assessment and strict adherence to hand washing and aseptic techniques. The nursing management for DIC, respiratory failure, cardiac failure, renal failure and metabolic acidosis is found in the appropriate sections of this book.

◊ *Evaluation*

Expected Outcomes
1. Attains normal body temperature
   a. Temperature within normal limits
   b. Negative blood cultures
   c. Negative cultures of catheter insertion sites and incisions
2. Demonstrates adequate tissue perfusion
   a. Cardiac output, blood pressure, and pulse rate within normal limits
   b. No evidence of angina or dysrhythmias
   c. Warm, dry, normal-color skin
   d. Oriented to person, place, and time
   e. Peripheral pulses strong
   f. Urine output greater than 30 ml/h
3. Demonstrates normal breathing pattern
   a. Respiratory rate and rhythm within normal limits
   b. No evidence of shortness of breath or use of accessory muscles for respiration

c. Arterial blood gas results within normal limits
4. Maintains adequate urine output
   a. Urine specific gravity within normal limits
   b. Urine output greater than 30 ml/hr
5. Demonstrates absence of complications
   a. Coagulation studies within normal limits
   b. Vital signs within normal limits
   c. Performance of activities of daily living

In summary, nosocomial infections are most commonly caused by gram-negative bacteria. Nurses have a great responsibility to help prevent the development of these infections. Strict hand washing, aseptic technique, and universal precautions are essential.

A large percentage of patients who develop bacterial septicemia progress to septic shock states. Patients diagnosed with septic shock often have multiple system involvement requiring constant assessment, intervention, and evaluation by both nursing and medical personnel. Intensive nursing assessments note subtle and acute changes in the patient's status. Enhancing tissue perfusion and maintaining adequate breathing patterns and urinary output guide the nursing interventions for the patient with septic shock.

Staphylococcal Infections

Staphylococci are widely distributed in nature, with humans serving as the predominant reservoir. These bacteria constitute a significant part of the common body flora and are found on the skin surface and in the mouth, nose, and throat. Transmission is by contact with a person who is an asymptomatic carrier or who has a draining lesion. Food may become contaminated by a carrier who is a food handler. Staphylococci are also transmitted through the air (thereby contaminating a wound during dressing changes), by way of contaminated needles, and through animal sources.

When the continuity of the skin has been disrupted or bypassed (abrasions, wounds, surgical incisions, burns, cutaneous viral infections), the patient is susceptible to infection by staphylococci. The patient's own skin may be the source of infection when the organism enters a disrupted portion of the skin.

Staphylococci are responsible for most human skin infections. The furuncle, or common boil, is almost always a staphylococcal abscess, and carbuncles found on the back of the neck or buttocks represent a coalition of staphylococcal abscesses. Most staphylococcal abscesses are located in superficial subcutaneous tissues and do not extend beyond the original site. Eventually, their purulent contents, under mounting pressure, perforate the overlying skin and are evacuated externally, leaving the empty cavities to fill in with granulation tissue, close over, and heal.

Systemic Staphylococcal Infections

If the peripheral defenses are unable to contain the staphylococcus, the infection may spread or invade the bloodstream, attended by profound toxemia. Invasion of the lymphatics may result in axillary, cervical, mediastinal, retroperitoneal, or subdiaphragmatic abscesses. Bloodstream invasion may produce acute bacterial endocarditis, staphylococcal pneumonia, empyema, perinephric abscess, hepatic abscess, staphylococcal enteritis, pyogenic arthritis, meningitis, osteomyelitis, or septic shock.

Irrespective of location, staphylococcal lesions possess many characteristics in common, including varying degrees of necrosis, a tendency to localize, and a tendency to persist, despite intensive chemotherapy, until the exudate finds an escape route or is evacuated.

Its resistance to therapy is explained in part by the extraordinary ability of the staphylococcus to adapt itself to an unfavorable environment. Resistance to the commonly used antibiotics is frequently observed in strains of staphylococci. Thus, initial responsiveness to antibiotic therapy may diminish to the point of true refractoriness.

Methicillin-resistant *S. aureus* (MRSA) denotes a group of strains of *S. aureus* that have developed resistance to treatment with semisynthetic penicillins such as methicillin. The strains of MRSA are extremely virulent, often colonizing in patients and health care personnel. Those at high risk for developing MRSA include: elderly patients who are hospitalized or cared for in nursing homes, burn patients, patients with multisystem diseases, patients in intensive care units with prolonged lengths of stay, patients previously treated with multiple antibiotics, and patients with surgical wounds and invasive lines.

Management

Control Measures and Prevention. The major means by which staphylococci are transmitted within the hospital is person-to-person transmission. The prevention of hospital staphylococcus requires infection control procedures such as Universal Precautions, excellent hand washing and aseptic techniques, and immediate isolation of patients with staphylococcal infections.

Control measures for patients infected with MRSA are more intense. All cases are reported to the infection control team of the institution for daily surveillance and tracking of the infection. Patients at high risk for acquiring MRSA are often cultured prophylactically before symptoms develop. Patients with MRSA are placed in private rooms (or with other patients infected with MRSA). Full isolation procedures are utilized, including gowns, gloves, and strict hand washing when coming into contact with infected patients. Some institutions recommend terminal cleaning of patient rooms after patients with MRSA have vacated them.

Treatment. Treatment for severe staphylococcal infection is an antistaphylococcal antibiotic (penicillinase-resistant penicillin). An alternative antimicrobial agent (*e.g.*, cephalosporin) is considered if the patient has a penicillin allergy. IV administration is the route usually selected when large doses are required. Serious staphylococcal infections may require prolonged treatment to prevent infection of the heart valves.

MRSA strains do not respond to treatment with penicillins, cephalosporin, aminoglycoside, tetracycline, or erythromycin. The drug of choice for the treatment of MRSA is vancomycin. Some patients do not respond to this therapy, and vancomycin can produce severe side effects, including ototoxicity and nephrotoxicity.

Nursing Interventions. The nurse monitors the patient's response to the prescribed therapy. If the patient experiences continuing or recurring fever, the cause may be a drug resistance, drug allergy, or superinfection (infection with a second organism resistant to the antibiotic in use).

Careful observations are made of the patient because fatal complications may develop during the early period of anti-microbial therapy. The promotion of comfort in the patient with fever is discussed in Nursing Care Plan 62-1.

When caring for patients with MRSA, nurses must adhere to the isolation procedures outlined above. In addition, the nurse must monitor visitors and other health care personnel to ensure compliance with these procedures. Patients in isolation often experience a sense of social as well as physical isolation. Patients and families require emotional support and education regarding the purpose and procedures of isolation.

Streptococcal Infections

There are many strains of hemolytic streptococci, but group A streptococci account for most pathogenic infections in humans. Included in this group are the beta-hemolytic streptococci, which gain entrance to the body primarily through the upper respiratory tract from persons with streptococcal infections or those who are asymptomatic carriers. Included in these infections are streptococcal pharyngitis, scarlet fever, sinusitis, otitis media, peritonsillar abscess, pericarditis, pneumonia and empyema, and various wound and skin infections—impetigo, puerperal infections, and erysipelas. Rheumatic fever and acute glomerulonephritis may occur as a sequela to group A streptococcal infection.

Streptococcal Pharyngitis

The most common type of streptococcal infection is streptococcal pharyngitis (strep throat) caused by group A streptococcus.

Clinical Manifestations.   The organism establishes itself in the lymphoid tissues and produces an abrupt onset of illness, with sore throat, fever (38.2°C [101°F]), chills, and headache. The patient may complain of throat pain that is aggravated by swallowing or even turning the head.

On inspection, the pharynx shows varying degrees of redness and edema and may be covered with an exudate. The presence of tender anterior cervical lymph nodes is a significant finding. Although these are the usual symptoms associated with streptococcal pharyngitis, most patients have some, but not all, of these symptoms.

In some cases a rash appears, starting over the neck and chest and spreading over the skin of the abdomen and extremities. If the rash becomes pronounced, the patient has scarlet fever. This presentation of group A streptococcus is uncommon today.

Diagnostic Evaluation.   The presence of an exudate suggests streptococcal pharyngitis. A throat culture is taken to confirm the presence of streptococcus.

Management

Penicillin, in a variety of forms, is the drug of choice for treating streptococcal infections (except for enterococcal group D infections). If the patient is sensitive to penicillin, a course of erythromycin may be used. Therapy is continued for at least 10 days to eliminate the organisms, prevent relapses, reduce the frequency of suppurative complications, and prevent most cases of rheumatic fever. Unfortunately, the risk of developing acute glomerulonephritis, which is also a complication of streptococcal pharyngitis, has not been shown to be altered by treatment of the initial infection.

Patient Education

The patient must understand the importance of *completing the entire course of antibiotic treatment* as prescribed to prevent the development of complications, namely, rheumatic fever and suppurative complications: otitis media, sinusitis, peritonsillar abscess, and cervical adenitis.

During the course of febrile illness, the patient is encouraged to rest. He should be noncontagious to others 24 to 48 hours after treatment is started. A liberal fluid intake is important, especially if the patient is febrile. Oral hygiene adds greatly to patient comfort and aids in preventing the development of fissures of the lips. Warm saline gargles may relieve some of the throat soreness. The patient is advised to monitor his temperature and is informed of the symptoms of possible complications.

Prevention.   Ongoing health education programs are needed to emphasize the relationship of streptococcal infections to heart disease and glomerulonephritis. Persons with these conditions, especially rheumatic heart disease, are at risk and may require long-term prophylaxis with penicillin. Hospitalized patients who are at risk—and this includes the obstetrical patient—must be protected from personnel or visitors with respiratory or skin infections. For the health of the public at large, food handlers should be instructed about hygienic procedures and closely monitored to ensure compliance.

Pulmonary Tuberculosis

Tuberculosis is an infectious disease caused by *Mycobacterium tuberculosis*, and rarely by *Mycobacterium bovis* or *Mycobacterium avium*. It usually involves the lungs, but it may spread to almost any part of the body, including the meninges, kidneys, bones, and lymph nodes. The organisms multiply slowly and are characterized as acid-fast aerobic organisms that can be killed by heat, sunshine, drying, and ultraviolet light.

In contrast with most infectious agents, the bacillus of tuberculosis, once it has gained a foothold in the body, is likely to remain there, quiescent, for years after the forces of immunity have controlled the original infection. If, during this quiescent period, the immunity of the host is diminished as a result of malnutrition, immunosuppression, and so forth, the organisms at once begin to multiply, causing any one of several tuberculous diseases. If the patient's body proves able to recover from this illness, the tubercle bacilli again become dormant.

Transmission and Risk Factors

Tuberculosis is transmitted from a person with active pulmonary disease who expels the organisms while talking, coughing, sneezing, or singing. A susceptible person inhales the droplets and becomes infected.

Persons at high risk for acquiring the infection are as follows:

- Those who have been previously infected
- Those who harbor live, though dormant, tuberculous bacilli
- Those in close contact with someone who has infectious tuberculosis

- Those whose tuberculin skin tests have recently converted to show a significant reaction
- Those with lowered resistance because of factors such as alcoholism
- Elderly persons who live in nursing homes and have healed dormant infections, diabetes, malignancy, or who are treated with corticosteroid therapy
- Persons receiving corticosteroid or immunosuppressive therapy
- Persons with chronic renal failure undergoing maintenance hemodialysis
- Persons who have had intestinal bypass surgery for obesity
- Persons who are homeless or who live in shelters, especially those who are poorly nourished
- Persons with HIV infection and AIDS

Most cases arise from those persons who are already infected. Crowded living conditions, low income, substandard housing, and inadequate health care contribute to the spread of tuberculosis. Tuberculosis is a common infectious disease throughout the world, because so many people throughout the world live in poverty. In the United States, newly arrived immigrants, refugees, and migrant workers constitute a large number of persons with tuberculosis. The homeless are another infection-prone group. There is an increased incidence of patients infected with both HIV and tuberculosis.

Pathophysiology

Once inhaled by a susceptible host, the tuberculosis bacilli, in the form of droplet nuclei, pass through the airways and are deposited on the alveolar surface where they begin to multiply.

Tuberculosis is a granulomatous disease; that is, when the organism invades normal tissues, the response is the formation of new tissue masses, which are called *infectious granulomas*.

Another more diffuse and equally characteristic tissue reaction occurs in response to the tuberculosis bacillus. The bacilli, transported by the lymph and bloodstream, lodge in susceptible tissues in small clumps, or *tubercles*. The neighboring tissue cells quickly accumulate around each of these clumps, forming a protective wall that checks their further spread. If immunity is successful, the germs die, and the tubercle becomes transformed into a tiny mass of fibrous tissue. However, the tissue of the tubercle may become necrotic and transformed into a cheesy mass. If this occurs, the germs are liberated and lymph transports them into the surrounding tissues, which respond by enclosing these freed germs in new tubercles. In this way, tubercles grow into larger and larger irregular masses. The prognosis of the patient depends on which of these two processes prevails.

Host Defense Mechanisms. Individuals who have experienced a primary tuberculosis infection are sensitized to the chemical constituents of the organism. Henceforth, contact with the bacillus, whether it is alive or killed, produces an acute local tissue inflammation. This is the basis of the tuberculin test, in which a suspension of ground-up killed tuberculosis bacilli obtained from a culture is injected beneath the skin. If the patient is sensitive (*i.e.*, has at one time had tuberculous infection) a local skin reaction results; if there is no sensitivity, no reaction is obtained.

A similar inflammatory reaction develops in the lungs of a person who has been previously sensitized to the tubercle bacillus if the lungs are invaded later by more organisms than the immune processes can control at the time. In contrast with the relatively bland, silent, primary type of pulmonary tuberculosis, the course of the reinfection type is complicated by necrosis, with resulting ulceration of the infected lung tissue. Clusters of tubercles, as in the primary type of tuberculosis, form at once around the nest of organisms, but now, because of the tissue sensitivity, these become surrounded by zones of inflammatory reaction. The alveoli in the area become filled with exudate; in other words, a tuberculous bronchopneumonia develops. The tuberculous tissue in this area gradually becomes caseous and ulcerates into a bronchus. As the ulcerations heal, considerable scar tissue forms locally. The pleura over the infected lobe, more often an upper lobe, becomes inflamed, then thickened and retracted by scar tissue.

This cycle of inflammatory bronchopneumonia proceeds to ulceration, followed by scarring. Unless the process can be arrested, it spreads slowly downward toward the hilum and later extends into adjacent lobes. The activity of the process may be prolonged and characterized by long remissions, when the disease may appear to be arrested, only to be followed by periods of renewed activity.

Clinical Manifestations

Chronic pulmonary tuberculosis is insidious in its onset and course. Most patients present with fever, loss of strength, productive cough with mucopurulent sputum, and weight loss. If the patient does not seek treatment until late in the disease, systemic symptoms are marked—daily recurring fever with chills, weight loss, anemia, hemoptysis, and large numbers of bacilli in the sputum.

Gerontologic Considerations. Tuberculosis may have atypical manifestations in the elderly, such as changes in behavior or mentation, organ dysfunction or fever, anorexia, and weight loss. It is being increasingly encountered in the nursing home population.

Diagnostic Evaluation

The initial diagnostic evaluation includes a tuberculin skin test, examination of a sputum sample (smear and culture), and chest radiograph. Most new cases of active tuberculosis arise from previously quiescent lesions that have become activated.

Tuberculin Skin Test. The intracutaneous test (Mantoux test) is the standard test used to identify the infected person. Tubercle bacillus extract (tuberculin) is injected into the intradermal layer of the inner aspect of the forearm. Intermediate strength of purified protein derivative (PPD) is usually used. The tuberculin syringe should be held close to the skin, so that the hub of the needle (26 or 27 gauge) touches it as the needle is introduced, bevel up. This reduces the needle angle at the skin surface and facilitates the injection of tuberculin just beneath the surface of the skin, to form a wheal (Fig. 62-4). The injection site is usually marked by circling the site with a pen to ensure accurate readings. The test is read 48 to 72 hours after injection; because tuberculin skin tests are tests of delayed hypersensitivity, this is when the induration (hardening or thickening of tissues) is the most evident.

Test reactions should be read in a good light, with the forearm slightly flexed at the elbow. After the area is inspected for the presence of induration, it is lightly palpated across the injection site, from the area of normal skin to the margins of induration. Then the diameter of the induration (*not erythema*)

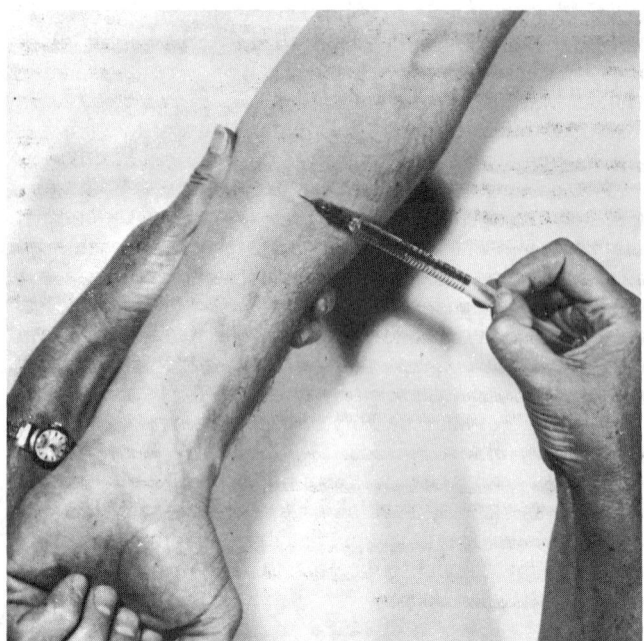

Figure 62-4. The Mantoux intracutaneous test. A tuberculin syringe and a subcutaneous needle, with the bevel up, are used to inject tubercle bacillus extract into the skin of the forearm to form a wheal. (American Lung Association.)

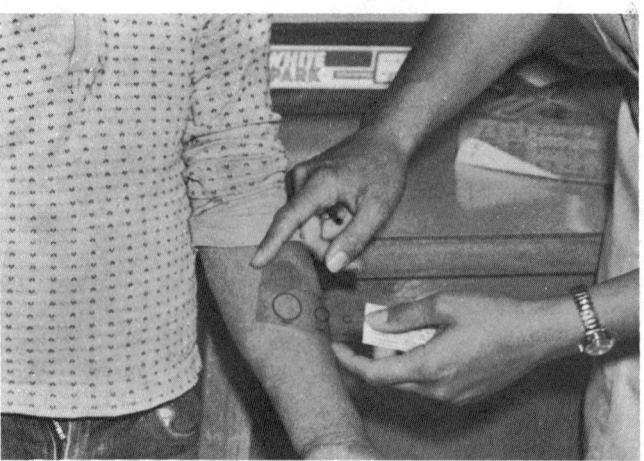

Figure 62-5. Interpretation of Mantoux test. The area of induration is measured most accurately with the aid of a plastic ruler containing concentric circles of specific diameters. (American Lung Association.)

is measured in millimeters, at its widest part (Fig. 62-5). Erythema or redness without induration is generally considered to be of no significance. The size of the induration is documented, as well as the antigen strength, the date the testing was conducted, the date when the reading was taken, and the lot number used, if available.

Interpretation of Skin Test. An area of induration measuring 10 mm or more in diameter is interpreted as significant.

Inconclusive reactions measure 5 to 9 mm and require that the test be repeated at a different site. (Individuals who are close contacts of persons with active tuberculosis and who have reactions in the 5- to 9-mm range should be considered significant reactors and should receive preventive treatment.) Usually, an induration of 0 to 4 mm is not considered significant. This indicates either a lack of tuberculin sensitivity or low-grade sensitivity that probably is not caused by *M. tuberculosis.*

- *A significant reaction indicates that a patient has been exposed to* Mycobacterium tuberculosis *recently or in the past. It does not necessarily mean that active disease is present in the body.* Most (more than 90%) people who are tuberculin-significant reactors do *not* develop clinical tuberculosis. (However, all significant reactors are candidates for active tuberculosis.)

In general, the more intense the reaction, the greater the likelihood of an active infection. A nonsignificant (negative) skin test does not exclude tuberculous infection or disease.

Other Skin Tests. Multiple-puncture skin tests are used for surveying and screening large groups and are not intended to establish positive diagnosis, because there is no way to standardize the amount of tuberculin introduced. The test introduces tuberculin into the skin either by puncturing with a device with points coated with dried tuberculin or by puncturing

through a film of liquid tuberculin. The test is read 48 to 72 hours after administration. If the reaction is in the form of papules, the diameter of the largest single papule or the largest diameter of coalescent induration is measured. If vesiculation is present, the person is sensitive to the tuberculin and is termed a *reactor.* However, not all reactors are infected with tuberculosis. All reactors should be retested with the Mantoux test and should have chest radiographs made.

Sputum Testing. Diagnosis is also confirmed by finding the acid-fast bacilli in smears of sputum. Sputum can be coughed up directly or induced by inhaling aerosols, which irritate the trachea and produce coughing. Bronchoscopic aspiration and transtracheal aspiration are other possible means of obtaining a sputum specimen. An early-morning specimen has pooled overnight secretions and is more likely to be productive and less contaminated. Tubercle bacilli may also be obtained and cultured from ascitic fluid, pleural fluid, CSF, urine, and pus that has been aspirated or drained from abscesses. Tissue such as liver, bone marrow, and lymph nodes may also be cultured.

Chest Radiograph. Tuberculosis is a possibility in anyone with an abnormal chest radiograph. Certain patterns, such as patchy infiltrates, are suggestive of tuberculosis.

Management

The goals of management are (1) to relieve pulmonary and systemic symptoms by eliminating all viable tubercle bacilli; (2) to return the patient to health, work, and family life as quickly as possible; and (3) to prevent transmission of the infection.

- Every active case of tuberculosis must be reported to the local health department so that close contacts may be examined and followed. Contacts are usually placed on preventive therapy (usually isoniazid) to prevent the development of active disease.

Chemotherapy. Active tuberculosis is usually treated with simultaneous administration of a combination of drugs to which the organisms are susceptible. Such therapy is continued until the disease is brought under control. Multiple drug regimens are used to destroy as many viable microbial organisms as possible as quickly as possible and to minimize the emergence of organisms resistant to the various antituberculosis drugs. Although the tubercle bacillus is susceptible to several drugs, there are no drugs to which it cannot develop resistance. Such resistance results from genetic mutations of the organism. The use of a variety of drugs enables one agent to destroy those mutants that are resistant to the initial drug.

In the United States, a 9-month regimen consisting of isoniazid and rifampin is frequently used. Pyrazinamide is frequently added for the initial 2 months of therapy. Other accepted regimens include isoniazid combined with streptomycin or ethambutol. (See Table 62-3 for further information about these drugs.)

The patient is instructed to have a sputum examination every 2 to 4 weeks until two successive cultures are free of bacilli, verifying the patient's noninfectious state.

Surgical Treatment. Since the advent of chemotherapy, surgical intervention is rarely necessary for tuberculosis. Pulmonary resection may be performed when the possibility of cancer coexists. It may also be carried out to eliminate lesions that have ceased to decrease in size after several months of therapy. Surgical procedures may be performed for thoracic drainage of empyema, decompression of constrictive pericarditis, or drainage of a paravertebral abscess.

Preventive Treatment. Eradicating tuberculosis depends on prevention, detection, health education, and improved living conditions. Most cases of tuberculosis occur in persons known to be significant tuberculin reactors. These patients are the reservoir from which more than 90% of active disease develops. Infected persons must be identified, and preventive therapy (isoniazid prophylaxis) must be given to those at risk for developing disease and becoming carriers of the disease. The following groups may benefit from preventive therapy with isoniazid:

- Contacts of newly discovered cases of tuberculosis
- Newly infected persons

TABLE 62-3. *Treatment of Mycobacterial Disease in Adults and Children*

Commonly Used Agents	Most Common Side Effects*	Tests for Side Effects*	Drug Interactions†	Remarks*
Isoniazid (INH)	Peripheral neuritis, hepatitis, hypersensitivity	SGOT/SGPT	Phenytoin–synergistic Antabuse	Bactericidal to both extracellular and intracellular organisms. Pyridoxine as prophylaxis for neuritis.
Rifampin (RMP)	Hepatitis, febrile reaction, purpura (rare)	SGOT/SGPT	Rifampin increases metabolism of oral contraceptives, quinidine, corticosteroids, Coumarin drugs and methadone, digoxin, oral hypoglycemics; PAS may interfere with absorption of rifampin.	Bactericidal to all populations of organisms. Orange urine and other body secretions. Discoloring of contact lenses.
Streptomycin (STM)	8th cranial nerve damage (may lead to deafness), nephrotoxicity	Vestibular function, audiograms,‡ BUN and creatinine	Neuromuscular blocking agents— may be potentiated to cause prolonged paralysis	Bactericidal to extracellular organisms. Use with caution in older patients or those with renal disease.
Pyrazinamide (PZA)	Hyperuricemia, hepatotoxicity	Uric acid, SGOT/SGPT		Bactericidal to intracellular organisms. Combination with an aminoglycoside is bactericidal.
Ethambutol (EMB)	Optic neuritis (may lead to blindness; very rare at 15 mg/kg), skin rash	Red-green color discrimination and visual acuity.‡ Difficult to test in a child under 3 years.		Bacteriostatic to both intracellular and extracellular organisms, primarily used to inhibit development of resistant mutants. Use with caution with renal disease or when eye testing is not feasible.

* *Check product labeling for detailed information on dose, contraindications, drug interaction, adverse reactions, and monitoring.*
† *Reference should be made to current literature, particularly on rifampin, because it induces hepatic microenzymes and therefore interacts with many drugs.*
‡ *Initial examination should be performed at start of treatment.*
(Modified from American Thoracic Society. Treatment of tuberculosis and other mycobacterial diseases. Am Rev Respir Dis 127[6]:791.)

- Tuberculin reactors with radiographic abnormalities
- Tuberculin reactors with certain clinical problems (*e.g.*, certain neoplasms, silicosis, chronic renal insufficiency)
- Tuberculin-positive persons age 35 years and younger with no other factors that increase risk

Isoniazid, for preventive therapy, is given in a single daily dose for 1 year. The most significant adverse reaction is hepatitis; this risk is increased if the person drinks alcohol on a daily basis. All persons taking isoniazid for preventive therapy should be seen in a health care facility on a regular basis to allow for detection of reactions to the medication and to provide personnel with an opportunity to encourage compliance with medication.

▶ Nursing Process
The Patient With Tuberculosis

▷ Assessment

The health history and assessment focus on the patient's fatigue, cough, sputum expectoration, weight loss, chills, and fever. It is important to determine if the patient has experienced hemoptysis. The patient's emotional readiness to learn, his perceptions and understanding of tuberculosis, and his educational level are evaluated. Because therapy may be prolonged, his social support system is assessed.

The results of the physical and laboratory evaluations are reviewed.

▷ Nursing Diagnoses

Based on the assessment data, the patient's major nursing diagnoses may include the following:

- Knowledge deficit about the disease, medications, and self-care techniques
- High risk for infection (spread of infection to others)
- Noncompliance with treatment regimen related to life-style, financial limitations, or other factors (*e.g.*, alcoholism) that limit ability to comply

▷ Planning and Implementation

▷ *Goals:* The major goals of the patient may include acquisition of knowledge and understanding of the disease and its treatment, prevention of spread of infection to others, and compliance with the treatment regimen.

▷ Nursing Interventions

▷ *Patient Education and Prevention of Spread of Infection.* Evidence suggests that patients probably forget at least half of what they are told, especially when anxiety levels are high. The role of the nurse is pivotal in building a trusting relationship so that patient education is an ongoing process and behavioral changes are made.

Although tuberculosis is a communicable disease, effective chemotherapy is the most effective means of preventing transmission. This fact bears frequent repetition.

- A major reason for treatment failure is that patients do not take their medications regularly and for the time prescribed. One of the teaching functions of the community health nurse

is to stress the importance of taking the medicine faithfully and exactly as prescribed.

All details of drug therapy are carefully explained. The nurse observes the patient's reactions and determines if he understands and agrees with the instructions. The American Lung Association has an array of patient teaching aids that can be used to reinforce teaching and learning. Written instructions may provide a valuable reference for patients.

The patient is usually treated at home, except in rare instances where social circumstances or drug-resistant organisms pose a threat to the community. In the patient treated on an outpatient basis, isolation is usually not necessary because the hazard to the family already occurred before the disease was diagnosed. The patient is instructed to cover his mouth and nose with double-ply tissue when he coughs or sneezes; these are to be placed in a paper bag and discarded. (Covering the mouth with the bare hand does not stop small droplets.) Hand washing is demonstrated and stressed.

The patient and family are instructed carefully about possible complications, including hemorrhage, pleurisy, and other untoward symptoms that are indicative of a possible recurrence of tuberculous activity.

Usually, the patient can return to his former employment. However, he should avoid exposure to excessive amounts of silicone dioxide (dusty jobs in foundry, rock quarry, sandblasting), because silicone dioxide dust may be harmful to the lungs.

In the hospitalized patient, universal precautions are used for body fluids, including sputum. Further restrictions are defined by each institution's disease-specific isolation precautions.

- Hands must be washed after touching the patient or potentially contaminated articles and before taking care of other patients.

▷ *Minimizing Noncompliance.* Tuberculosis is often seen in patients who are economically and socially disadvantaged. A significant percentage of these patients fail to take their medication as prescribed or abandon treatment altogether. Their lives may be marked by social upheaval, alcoholism, and drug use. Many are poorly motivated to participate in their treatment. Those patients who are noncompliant should receive their medications under direct supervision.

Most patients with tuberculosis report to the health care facility as outpatients. They require time, support, and, as previously mentioned, education. It is important to try to fit the medication regimen into the patient's routine or life-style, because new habits are difficult to establish. Linking the time of medication to some daily habit (*e.g.*, morning cup of coffee) is often helpful. Uncomfortable side effects of a drug may be a reason the patient discontinues the treatment. If the prescribed medication is causing problems, these should be discussed with the physician to see if a change or adjustment of medication is in order.

An ongoing supportive relationship is built not on dependency but on valuing the patient's beliefs and strengthening his self-confidence to change his health behaviors in a positive manner.

▷ Evaluation

Expected Outcomes

1. Acquires knowledge and understanding of tuberculosis
   a. Answers questions about tuberculosis correctly

b. Knows names of medications he is receiving and schedule for taking them
c. Names expected side effects of medications
2. Prevents spread of infection to others
   a. Continues medication therapy
   b. Uses tissues correctly when coughing and sneezing; disposes of them as instructed.
   c. Reports for sputum monitoring
   d. Encourages persons who are close contacts to report for examination
3. Complies with treatment regimen
   a. Attends appointments
   b. Takes medications exactly as prescribed

Miliary Tuberculosis

Miliary tuberculosis is the result of bloodstream invasion by the tubercle bacillus. It is usually a consequence of late reactivation of dormant infection in the lung or elsewhere, with blood-borne dissemination to multiple organs. It is the most serious form of tuberculosis. The origin of the bacilli that enter the bloodstream is either some chronic focus that has ulcerated into a blood vessel, or multitudes of miliary tubercles lining the inner surface of the thoracic duct. The organisms migrate from these foci into the bloodstream, are carried throughout the body, and disseminate throughout all tissues, with myriad tiny miliary tubercles developing in the lungs, spleen, liver, kidneys, meninges, and other organs.

The clinical course of miliary tuberculosis may vary from an acute, rapidly progressive infection with high fever to an indolent process with low-grade fever, anemia, and debility. At first there may be no localizing signs except for an enlarged spleen and a reduced number of leukocytes. Within a few weeks, however, the chest radiograph reveals small densities scattered diffusely throughout both lung fields; these are the miliary tubercles, which gradually increase in size. Few physical signs may be elicited on physical examination of the chest, but at this stage the patient suffers from a severe cough, dyspnea, and cyanosis. Treatment is the same as that described for pulmonary tuberculosis.

Legionnaires' Disease

Legionnaires' disease is an acute respiratory infection caused by a gram-negative bacterium, *Legionella pneumophila*. It was named after an outbreak of the disease that occurred in Philadelphia in 1976 among people attending the state convention of the American Legion.

Epidemiologic evidence indicates that Legionnaires' disease is transmitted by inhalation of organisms in an aerosol form of infected water from environmental sources. Legionellae are ubiquitous (everywhere) in water, and the organisms have been found in plumbing fixtures, drinking water, and air conditioning systems in hotels and hospitals.

It is proposed that one way in which the aerobic gram-negative bacillus finds its way into humans is through the cooling towers and evaporative condensers of large air conditioners, where the bacteria multiply and are discharged as an infectious aerosol through fans and exhaust vents. The disease is not considered highly communicable. Persons at risk are middle-aged and older men, especially those who smoke, consume alcohol, work in or near construction sites, or are immunosuppressed from disease or medications that affect cellular immunity.

Pathophysiology. Autopsy specimens from tissues of patients with Legionnaires' disease have shown different amounts of lung consolidation in varying distributions. The histologic pattern has been that of an acute fibrinopurulent pneumonia, which resembles a stage of lobar pneumonia. An exudate containing neutrophils, macrophages, and fibrin is found in the alveolar spaces.

Clinical Manifestations. The target organ appears to be the lungs. The earliest symptoms are profound malaise, myalgias, mild headache, and a dry cough. Within a day, the patient experiences a rapidly rising fever and chills. The fever remains high and unremitting, 39° to 41°C (102° to 105°F), until specific therapy is started. Occasionally, diarrhea precedes other symptoms. Associated manifestations include pleuritic pain, confusion, and impaired renal function. A chest radiograph documents evidence of pneumonia. Tachypnea and dyspnea may reflect the extent of the pneumonic process. There may be clinical and laboratory evidence of abnormalities of the gastrointestinal, musculoskeletal, hepatic, renal, and central nervous systems. The diagnosis is made on the basis of an increase in specific serum antibodies and by culture of the organisms on appropriate culture media.

Management. Erythromycin (administered early) is the drug of choice in treatment. These patients may be seriously ill. Death may occur from intractable shock and hemodynamic collapse.

Nursing Interventions. The nursing management is that described for the patient with pneumonia (see Chap. 26). Universal precautions are recommended for sputum and other body fluids.

Salmonella Infections (Salmonellosis)

Salmonellosis is infection caused by bacteria of the genus *Salmonella*. Clinically, salmonellosis is seen in four forms: gastroenteritis (the most common form), enteric fever (such as typhoid and paratyphoid disease), bacteremia with and without focal extraintestinal infection, and asymptomatic carrier state. Infection caused by *Salmonella typhi* (typhoid fever) is discussed on p. 1930. *Salmonella typhimurium* is the most commonly reported type in the United States. In this country, salmonellae are implicated in 3% of cases of gastroenteritis; they cause 3% to 5% of infectious diarrheas in developing countries.

Salmonella organisms may penetrate the epithelial cells of the small intestine and colon, producing an intestinal inflammatory response. The patient is infected by ingesting the organism in food contaminated by infected human or animal feces, in whole eggs and egg products, in meat and meat products, in poultry (especially turkey), and in pharmaceutical agents of animal origin. It has been proposed that large numbers of eggs and chickens on the market are contaminated by *Salmonella* microorganisms. Common foods causing *Salmonella* infections include commercially processed meat pies, poultry, sausages, foods containing eggs or egg products, and unpasteurized milk and other dairy products.

Clinical Manifestations. Symptoms usually develop within 8 to 48 hours of ingestion of contaminated food. The patient experiences headache, abdominal discomfort, low-grade fever, and watery diarrhea that may contain blood and mucus. Some patients have only a headache and occasional loose stools. The infectious agent may localize and cause necrosis in any body tissue, producing abscesses, cholecystitis, arthritis, endocarditis, meningitis, pericarditis, pneumonia, and pyelonephritis. Petechiae, splenomegaly, and leukopenia may also occur. *Salmonella* infection complicated by bacteremia is seen in the elderly, who often have other pre-existing diseases.

Diagnosis of *Salmonella* infection is made by finding the organism in feces and blood.

Management. Rehydration of the patient with fluids and essential electrolytes is the foundation of treatment. Oral intake of fluids is sufficient in most patients. Fruit juices and soft drinks are effective even in severe diarrhea. (Glucose is absorbed in the small intestine.) The patient should avoid beverages with caffeine, which causes increased intestinal motility.

Antimotility drugs (anticholinergics, paregoric) may be counterproductive, because a slowed peristaltic activity may extend the period of infection by interfering with an effective cleansing mechanism.

Patients with moderate to severe illness (those requiring hospitalization) may be treated with trimethoprim-sulfamethoxazole or chloramphenicol. Universal Precautions are indicated.

Prevention and Patient Education. There is no active or passive immunization. Raw eggs and egg drinks should not be eaten, nor should dirty or cracked eggs be used, because salmonellae can penetrate cracked eggs. All foods from animal sources, especially poultry, egg products, and meat, should be *thoroughly cooked*. Food service workers should be instructed about food-borne illnesses and given guidelines on avoiding food contamination, storing and preparing food, cleaning food preparation and service areas (contaminated countertops can serve as a means of transmission), and practicing good personal hygiene. Foods should be refrigerated during storage and protected against insects and rodents. Chickens, ducks, and turtles (as well as other domestic pets) are sources of infection.

The patient must wash his hands after going to the bathroom, particularly during illness and carrier state (several months), to prevent transmission of infection to others.

Typhoid Fever

Typhoid fever is an acute systemic bacterial disease resulting from infection with *Salmonella typhi*. The organism gains access to the body through ingestion of food or water that has been contaminated by infected feces or urine. In the United States, it is spread chiefly by carriers, patients who have recovered from the disease but whose stools or urine may spread the bacilli for years. Because it is eliminated in the stools and urine of patients, the organism can be transmitted into food and water through sewage, flies, and the hands of carriers handling raw fruits, vegetables, and other food. Another source of infection is the ingestion of oysters and shellfish harvested from polluted waters. Typhoid fever, although rare in the United States, is a serious public health problem in regions of the world where there is neither a safe water supply nor adequate sewage disposal.

Pathophysiology. The organism enters the body by way of the mouth and invades the walls of the gastrointestinal tract. There, multiplying rapidly, it gives rise to a massive bacteremia that continues for about 10 days. The chief localization of the organism is in the mesenteric lymph nodes and the masses of lymphatic tissue in the mucous membrane of the intestinal wall. The blood vessels become thrombosed, and the swollen mass of lymphatic tissue dies and sloughs away, leaving clean ulcers in the mucous membrane, the floor of which may be the muscularis, or even the peritoneum. If the latter, they may perforate, causing peritonitis.

Clinical Manifestations. The onset of typhoid fever is gradual, with headache, fever, malaise, somnolence, and abdominal pain. The patient may not seek health care at this time because these are nonspecific symptoms. At the end of the first week, rose spots (a cluster of pink lesions that initially blanch with pressure) may be found on the chest and abdomen. Without therapy, the temperature rises steadily, reaching its highest level—usually 40° to 41°C (104° to 105°F)—in 3 to 7 days. During this period of rising temperature, most patients suffer with a severe headache and a nonproductive cough. During the second week, if the patient is not treated, the temperature remains consistently high. During the third week, however, it becomes more and more remittent, a little lower each morning and not so elevated each afternoon. The pulse rate may be relatively slow despite high fever. Other clinical manifestations are an enlarged liver and spleen, delirium, and intestinal bleeding.

Diagnostic Evaluation. The diagnosis is made by recovery of the causative agent from blood samples, bone marrow aspirate, or stool.

Management

Chloramphenicol, ampicillin, amoxicillin, or trimethoprim-sulfamethoxazole is used in the treatment of typhoid fever. The fever usually subsides in 3 to 5 days following initiation of antibiotic therapy. However, bacteriologic cure is not achieved in all patients. Relapses have occurred and positive stool cultures have been obtained after one course, and even repeated courses, of antibiotic therapy. Thus, while chloramphenicol has reduced the fatality rate of typhoid fever significantly and has curtailed the excretion of typhoid bacilli during convalescence, it has not reduced the frequency of complications or the incidence of the chronic carrier state following typhoid fever.

Nursing Interventions

The goals of nursing management are to give supportive care and to monitor for complications.

Delirium is common in the severe form of the disease, and the patient requires special support during this period. He may be drowsy, indifferent to his surroundings, and incontinent of urine and feces. Universal precautions are used. Patient safety must be maintained with the use of side rails, the bed in the low position, sedation, and soft restraints if necessary.

Tepid water sponges are administered for temperatures over 40°C (104°F). A high fluid intake is encouraged to prevent dehydration from fluid losses due to fever, perspiration, and poor oral intake.

It is important to observe for bladder distention, because the patient may lose the urge to void during the toxic state. Retention of feces may also pose a problem. Enemas, if indicated, are administered *under low pressure* to diminish the chance of intestinal perforation.

Monitoring for Complications. Many structures may become infected in the course of typhoid fever, including the lungs, the pleura, the pericardium, the heart, the kidneys, and the bones. However, the most common of the dangerous complications are intestinal hemorrhage and perforation of the bowel, with resultant peritonitis.

Intestinal hemorrhages, secondary to bacterial invasion of the mucous membranes, which leads to necrosis, ulceration, and erosion of blood vessels, occur in 4% to 7% of patients, usually during the third week. Signs of hemorrhage include apprehension; sweating; pallor; weak, rapid pulse; hypotension; and bloody or tarry stools. Hemorrhage is generally managed by supportive measures, including blood component therapy. Operative intervention (bowel resection) is sometimes necessary.

Intestinal perforation, the most serious complication, may occur at any time but most often occurs during the third week. The perforation usually takes place in the lower ileum. It occurs when the ulcer causing the slough involves the entire thickness of the bowel wall. The intestinal contents pour into the abdominal cavity, causing peritonitis. The patient usually experiences acute abdominal pain. There is associated abdominal tenderness and rigidity and a silent abdomen (*i.e.*, absence of bowel sounds). However, the pain may last only a few seconds and then stop. If such signs occur, a nasogastric tube is passed and IV fluids are administered to correct fluid and electrolyte imbalance. Surgical closure of the perforation is usually necessary.

Other complications of typhoid fever may occur when the typhoid bacilli localize in specific tissues, causing hepatitis, meningitis, cholecystitis, pneumonitis, or pericarditis. During the course of the disease, the gallbladder and bile ducts are routinely infected.

Patient Education. The process of recovery from typhoid fever may be slow. Once a patient has recovered, stools must be checked to determine if he has become a carrier. Carriers harbor the organism and excrete it in their urine and stools. The presence of Vi-agglutinins in the blood of suspected carriers has strong predictive value for the carrier state. A positive stool or urine culture for a year or more indicates a carrier state. Carriers may be given ampicillin or amoxicillin with probenecid in an attempt to abolish the carrier state.

Public health agencies maintain surveillance of carriers, because the occurrence of typhoid fever in the United States is almost always traceable to a known or undetected carrier.

Prevention. There is no substitute for good sanitation. The eradication of typhoid fever depends on the availability of safe water and sewer systems. The detection of carriers and restriction of their occupations are also essential. It is imperative that patients with typhoid fever, convalescents, and carriers always wash their hands after defecation. All persons handling food should use proper hand washing techniques. Flies must be controlled by screening and spraying, and their breeding must be controlled by adequate collection and disposal of garbage. Shellfish should be obtained from an approved source. Scrupulous cleanliness in the preparation and storage of food is vital.

Typhoid vaccination is no longer recommended for people in the United States. It is, however, recommended for those living with chronic typhoid carriers and is considered for persons traveling to countries where typhoid is common. On the basis of the above recommendation, adults may be given typhoid vaccine subcutaneously on two occasions separated by 4 or more weeks.

Shigellosis (Bacillary Dysentery)

Shigellosis is an acute bacterial disease of the intestinal tract. There are some 40 serotypes of shigellae, divided into four groups or species: *Shigella sonnei* (most common serotype isolated in industrialized countries), *Shigella dysenteriae, Shigella flexneri,* and *Shigella boydii.* The source of infection is feces from an infected person, with the route of spread being the fecal–oral route. *Shigella* species are gaining prevalence as agents of STDs. Shigellosis may be passed through toilet paper onto the fingers The bacilli have also been recovered from milk, eggs, cheese, and shrimp.

While encountered in all countries, bacillary dysentery is endemic to the tropics, where serious epidemics are frequent. It continues to pose a substantial problem for people in the United States, especially those with a substandard environment and those living in a closed-group population—day care centers, military installations, nursing homes, and other resident care centers.

Pathogenesis. The pathology of shigellosis, in severe cases, consists of organisms reaching the small intestine, where they multiply and release a toxin that initiates secretion of water and electrolytes from the jejunal area. The invading pathogens are capable of initiating an intense inflammatory response in the mucosa, followed by small patches of ulceration, which may coalesce to form large ulcers.

Clinical Manifestations. Initially there is fever, cramping, and abdominal pain. Watery diarrhea soon appears, often followed by frank dysentery, with the passage of variable amounts of blood, mucus, and pus. There may be high fever. At the peak of the active infection, the symptoms are severe and the prostration is profound. The patient has a constant desire to defecate, and the straining is severe during the attempts. The disease is usually self-limited in healthy adults, and improvement is noted in about 1 week. Some cases last 2 or 3 weeks, and chronic cases last several months, or even years, unless adequately treated. In severe cases, shock, volume depletion, and electrolyte imbalance may supervene.

Management. The objectives of treatment are to maintain fluid and electrolyte balance and to prevent the spread of shigellosis to the patient's contacts (*e.g.*, eliminate the carrier state). To eliminate the spread of shigellosis, infected patients are questioned about travel to underdeveloped countries, exposure to crowded institutions, swimming in contaminated water, and oral–anal sexual activity. Inquiries are made concerning water supplies and food eaten at home and in restaurants. Local and state authorities are notified of all cases.

The organism may be cultured from the stool; sensitivity tests are performed to determine the appropriate antibiotic, because the organism may be resistant to certain antibiotics. Treatment of shigellosis with antibiotics is important in shortening the period of fecal excretion and in arresting the course of illness. Antibiotics that are absorbed from the intestinal tract and to which the shigellae are sensitive (ampicillin, trimethoprim-sulfamethoxazole) may shorten the clinical course and decrease the period of intestinal shedding of the organisms, thus decreasing the period of communicability. The use of antimotility drugs (*e.g.,* Lomotil) to control diarrhea prolongs the symptoms and the presence of the organism in the intestines and is therefore not recommended.

IV fluids are administered to maintain the electrolyte balance and prevent profound dehydration due to an excessively large loss of water and electrolytes (sodium, potassium, chloride, bicarbonate) in the diarrheic stools. The patient may require supplemental potassium.

Nursing Interventions.   The patient is assessed for weight loss, skin turgor, and dryness of mucous membranes, and his vital signs and urinary output are monitored. Clear fluids are offered by mouth during the acute stage.

Prevention and Patient Education.   Dysentery bacilli are spread by drinking water polluted by infected human excreta, by sexual transmission, and by food handled carelessly by shigella carriers, some of whom have the active disease, others being entirely asymptomatic. Thus, the same precautions must be observed, and the same control of water sources and food handling enforced, in the prevention of shigellosis as in that of typhoid fever. This includes proper hand washing, effective sanitation, adequate sewage disposal, a program for fly control, and the detection of carriers. Untreated sexual partners, particularly those of homosexual men, may reinfect the patient.

Meningococcal Meningitis (Bacterial Meningitis)

Meningitis is inflammation of the membranes surrounding the brain and spinal cord and is caused by a variety of bacteria, viruses, protozoa, or fungi. The most common form is bacterial.

The bacteria most frequently encountered in acute bacterial meningitis are *N. meningitidis, S. pneumoniae* (in adults), and *H. influenzae* (in children and young adults). The mode of transmission is by direct contact, including droplets and discharges from the nose and throat of carriers (most often) or infected persons. Of those exposed to it, most do not develop the infection but become carriers. There has been an increased incidence of meningitis caused by enteric gram-negative bacteria in persons older than 60 as well as in those who have had neurosurgery or who have a compromised immune status.

Meningococcal disease is endemic in the United States and throughout the world and occurs most frequently in the winter and spring months. Epidemics are most likely to occur in people who live in crowded quarters, notably in cities, crowded institutions, military installations, or prisons, but the disease also occurs in rural regions.

Bacterial meningitis starts as an infection of the oropharynx and is followed by meningococcal septicemia, which extends to the meninges of the brain and upper region of the spinal cord. It can be one of the most fulminating (coming on suddenly with severity) of all diseases.

Pathophysiology

Predisposing factors include upper respiratory tract infections, otitis media, mastoiditis, sickle cell anemia and other hemoglobinopathies, recent neurosurgical procedures, head trauma, and immunologic defects. The venous channels serving the posterior nasopharynx, middle ear, and mastoid drain toward the brain and are near the veins draining the meninges; these channels favor bacterial proliferation.

The meningococci enter the bloodstream and cause an inflammatory reaction in the meninges and underlying cortex, which may result in vasculitis with thromboses and reduced cerebral blood flow. The cerebral tissue is metabolically impaired due to the presence of meningeal exudate, vasculitis, underperfusion, and cerebral edema. A purulent exudate may spread over the base of the brain and spinal cord. The inflammation spreads also to the membrane lining the cerebral ventricles. Bacterial meningitis is associated with profound alterations in intracranial physiology, including increased permeability of the blood–brain barrier, cerebral edema, and increased intracranial pressure.

In acute infections, however, the patient dies from the toxin of the bacteria before meningitis develops. In these patients, meningococcemia is overwhelming, with adrenal damage, circulatory collapse, and associated widespread hemorrhages (Waterhouse–Friderichsen syndrome) occurring as a result of endothelial damage and vascular necrosis caused by the meningococci.

Clinical Manifestations

The symptoms of meningitis result from infection and increased intracranial pressure. Usually the patient experiences a sudden onset of severe headache, myalgia, back pain, photophobia, fever, and neck pain and stiffness (from spasm of the extensor muscles due to meningeal irritation). Frequently, aggressive behavior is displayed. Another striking feature is a rash ranging from petechiae (small red spots) to a combination of petechiae and ecchymoses (large bruiselike areas) occurring in about two-thirds of patients with meningococcal disease.

On physical examination, there is resistance to neck flexion. Other signs of meningeal irritation include the following:

> *Positive Kernig's sign*—When the patient is lying with his thigh flexed on the abdomen, he cannot completely extend his leg.
> *Positive Brudzinski's sign*—When the patient's neck is flexed, flexion of the knees and hips is produced; when passive flexion of the lower extremity of one side is made, a similar movement is seen for the opposite extremity.

In about 10% of patients, a fulminating infection occurs, with signs of overwhelming septicemia: an abrupt onset of high fever, extensive purpuric lesions (over face and extremities), shock, and signs of intravascular coagulation. Death may occur within a few hours of onset. The infecting organisms can usually be identified through a smear and culture of the CSF and blood.

Management

Successful management depends on the administration of an antibiotic that crosses the blood–brain barrier into the subarachnoid space in sufficient concentration to halt the multiplication of bacteria. Immediately after the CSF and blood cultures are obtained, antimicrobial therapy is started. Penicillin, ampicillin, or chloramphenicol, or one of the cephalosporins, may be used. Other antibiotics may be used if resistant strains of bacteria are identified.

Dehydration and shock are treated with fluid volume expanders. Seizures, which may occur in the early course of the disease, are controlled with diazepam or phenytoin. An osmotic diuretic (*e.g.*, mannitol) may be used to treat cerebral edema.

Nursing Interventions

The patient's outcome depends on the supportive care given. The patient is very ill, and the combination of fever, dehydration, alkalosis, and cerebral edema may predispose him to seizures. Airway obstruction, respiratory arrest, or cardiac dysrhythmias may follow. Thus, some of the nursing interventions are collaborative with those of the physician.

- In meningitis of all causes, the patient's clinical status and vital signs are constantly assessed, because altered consciousness may lead to airway obstruction. Arterial blood gas determinations, insertion of a cuffed endotracheal tube (or tracheostomy), and mechanical ventilation may be indicated. Oxygen may be administered to maintain the arterial Po$_2$ at desired levels.
- Hemodynamic stability is monitored with central venous pressure or Swan–Ganz catheters to assess for incipient shock, which precedes cardiac or respiratory failure. Generalized vasoconstriction, circumoral cyanosis, and cold extremities may be noted. The high fever must be reduced to decrease the load on the heart and the brain's oxygen demand. See Nursing Care Plan 62-1 for appropriate nursing interventions.
- Rapid IV fluid replacement may be prescribed, but care is taken not to overhydrate the patient because of risk of cerebral edema.
- The body weight, serum electrolytes, urine output and specific gravity, and osmolality of urine are closely monitored, especially if syndrome of inappropriate antidiuretic hormone secretion (SIADH) is suspected.
- Continuing nursing management requires ongoing assessment of the patient's clinical status, attention to skin and oral hygiene, promotion of comfort, and protection during seizures (p. 1723) and while comatose.
- Discharges from the nose and mouth are considered infectious. Universal Precautions are used. Disease-specific isolation is advised for 24 hours after the start of antibiotic therapy.

Prevention and Patient Education. Persons who have close contact with the patient should be considered candidates for antimicrobial prophylaxis (rifampin). Close contacts are observed and immediately examined if fever or other signs and symptoms of meningitis develop.

The meningococcal vaccine licensed in this country is used primarily in military recruits. Vaccines may be of benefit for some travelers visiting countries that are experiencing epidemic meningococcal disease. Vaccination should also be considered as an adjunct to antibiotic chemoprophylaxis for anyone in close contact with a patient who has meningococcal disease.

Tetanus (Lockjaw)

Tetanus is an acute disease caused by the tetanus bacillus, *Clostridium tetani,* whose spores are introduced into the body when an injury is contaminated with soil, street dust, or animal or human feces. The bacillus is an anaerobe (it cannot live in the presence of oxygen). It is found most commonly in patients with wounds with small external openings and in IV drug users. Wounds may be minor injuries, scratches, bee stings, lacera-

tions, frostbite, animal injuries, abortions, circumcision, surgery, or dental and orofacial trauma. The incidence is greatest among low-income groups (who often have not been immunized), among women, and among the elderly who never were immunized as children or have lost their immunity.

Pathophysiology

Tissues with low oxygen tension (due to infection or foreign material, or damaged blood supply) provide conditions in which the spores become vegetative forms, multiply, and produce toxins. These toxins are absorbed by the peripheral nerves and carried to the spinal cord, where they produce a reaction that amounts to a stimulation of the nervous tissue. The sensory nerves become sensitive to the slightest stimuli, and the hypersensitive motor nerves carry impulses that produce spasms of the muscles that they supply.

Clinical Manifestations

Early symptoms include irritability, restlessness, headache, low-grade fever, and muscle rigidity. The jaw muscles are the first group affected, making it difficult to open the mouth because of spasms of the masticatory muscles (trismus). This characteristic symptom has given the disease the common name *lockjaw.* The spasms of the facial muscles produce a distorted grin (*risus sardonicus*), which is characteristic of the disease and persists even during convalescence.

The spasm rapidly involves other groups of muscles until the whole body is affected, with tightness of the chest and rigidity of the abdominal wall, back, and extremities. The spasm is continuous, but the least stimulus—a door banging, a loud voice, or a bright light—may cause a generalized convulsion, with every muscle in violent contraction. In fact, fractures of the vertebral bodies can occur during severe spasms. Because the extensor muscles are stronger than the flexors, the head is retracted, the feet are extended fully, and the back is arched, so that during a convulsion the whole body may be supported on the back of the head and the feet. This condition is called *opisthotonos.* The patient is alert and in pain from muscle spasms. Death may occur from asphyxia, due to spasm of the respiratory muscles, and from pneumonia.

Management

The goals of management are to provide a patent airway to prevent respiratory and cardiovascular complications and to neutralize the residual circulating toxins.

The patient with established tetanus is immediately given tetanus immune globulin (TIG) 1 to 2 hours before wound débridement so that the neurotoxin released into the circulation during débridement cannot attach to nerve endings. Active immunization with tetanus toxoid is also started at the beginning of the treatment because even severe tetanus produces no immunity. When tetanus toxoid and TIG are given concurrently, separate syringes and separate sites should be used.

The wound is débrided because necrotic tissue favors the growth of tetanus bacillus. The wound is irrigated copiously to wash out tissue fragments and foreign bodies; it may be left open to promote drainage.

Immune globulin may also be infiltrated into the wound site. Usually, penicillin G (or an alternative antibiotic) is administered IV or intramuscularly in high doses to eradicate persisting *C. tetani* and other pathogens from the wound.

Diazepam is used to reduce restlessness and apprehension (which can induce spasm), for its amnesic effect, and to provide muscle relaxation to treat spasm. Neuromuscular blocking agents (metocurine iodide [Metubine]) are prescribed for treatment of severe tetanus.

The overactivity of the sympathetic nervous system may lead to sympathetic crisis and death. Isolated tachycardia, temporary hypertension, premature ventricular contractions, and diaphoresis require aggressive physiologic monitoring and pharmacologic treatment. Propranolol may be prescribed to control tachycardia, while phentolamine is administered to control hypertensive episodes.

Nursing Interventions

In severe tetanus infection, one of the most important nursing objectives and priorities is constant supportive care of the patient to ensure effective respiratory function. Convulsive paroxysms, especially those involving the respiratory muscles, impair pulmonary gas exchange by preventing normal swallowing and by obstructing the airway. Tetanic spasms of the larynx, pharynx, and respiratory muscles usually occur during convulsions and can lead to asphyxiation and death. Rigidity and spasm of the trunk muscles also contribute to ventilatory failure. In fact, ventilation ceases during a tetanus convulsion.

The patient requires expert respiratory management in an intensive care unit, with early endotracheal intubation and mechanical ventilation. Oral secretions are usually constant and profuse, requiring frequent suctioning. The nursing management of the patient with seizures is discussed in Chapter 57. See Chapter 25 for the management of the patient requiring respiratory intensive care.

Overactivity of the sympathetic nervous system, as manifested by tachycardia, dysrhythmias, labile blood pressure, hyperpyrexia, and excessive diaphoresis and salivation, may eventually lead to circulatory failure and death. A significant increase in the heart rate and mean arterial blood pressure may indicate a need for an adrenergic blocking agent (propranolol) to lessen the possibility of catecholamine-induced myocardial damage. Therefore, cardiac monitoring is essential.

Because the slightest stimulation may trigger paroxysmal spasm, sudden stimuli and light must be avoided. The patient is placed in a quiet, semidark environment to avoid stimulating reflex spasms. Nursing activities are carried out during the periods when sedation has its maximum effect so that the patient is disturbed as little as possible, because tactile stimulation often provokes spasms. Usually, a vein is kept open for emergency situations, such as cardiac or respiratory arrest, and for infusions to maintain careful fluid and electrolyte balance. Insensible fluid losses in the form of sweat and saliva are large and result in dehydration, which, in the presence of impaired cardiovascular control and overactivity of the sympathetic nervous system, can predispose to deep vein thrombosis and pulmonary embolism. Parenteral nutrition may be required, because aspiration pneumonia during oral food intake is a hazard.

Constant attention is given to the eyes, mouth, skin, and bladder and bowels. The patient is monitored for signs of infection (skin, urinary tract, lungs).

The patient is assessed for urinary retention, which occurs when perineal muscles are affected. Pressure ulcers and contractures can be the outcome of prolonged immobility; therefore, preventive nursing interventions are necessary (see Chap.

14). Even with expert care, the mortality rate of tetanus may be 50% or greater.

Prevention and Patient Education. Tetanus can be prevented through proper immunization programs; immunization establishes basal immunity before exposure to the risk of tetanus. For primary immunization of adults, three doses of adult-type tetanus and diphtheria toxoids are prescribed, followed by a booster dose every 10 years to maintain adequate immunity. About two thirds of the tetanus cases in the United States occur in persons over age 50; these persons are least likely to have been immunized as children.

- The most important step in the prevention of tetanus is the thorough washing and cleaning of the wound, with removal of all foreign material and devitalized tissue. This helps eliminate tetanus bacilli from wounds and removes the medium in which tetanus spores can develop.
- Every break in the skin must be considered a potential portal of entry for *C. tetani.*

After injury, the immunization status of the patient determines whether to provide active immunization with tetanus toxoid and passive immunization with tetanus immune globulin. The nature and age of the wound, the conditions under which it was incurred, and the treatment are considered on an individual basis. All individuals are encouraged to keep an up-to-date record of their immunization status.

Clostridial Myonecrosis (Gas Gangrene)

Gas gangrene is a severe infection of skeletal muscle caused by several species of gram-positive clostridia that may complicate trauma, compound fractures, contusions, or lacerated wounds by producing exotoxins that destroy tissue. These organisms (*Clostridium perfringens, Clostridium novyi, Clostridium septicum,* and others) may produce gas gangrene. They are anaerobes that are found normally in the intestinal tract of humans and in soil. Their growth occurs primarily in deep wounds where the oxygen supply is reduced, a situation enhanced by the presence of foreign bodies or necrotic tissue, which leads to further reduction of oxygen tension in wounds.

In contaminated wounds in which the vascular supply may be impaired, the environment is suited for the growth of spores and the production of exotoxins that adversely affect the blood and cause vessel thrombosis and damage to the myocardium, liver, and kidneys.

Spores formed by anaerobic bacilli are highly resistant to heat, cold, sunlight, drying, and many chemical agents. Because the gas bacillus is an inhabitant of the human intestinal tract, it is likely to be the infecting organism in thigh wounds after amputations, especially if the patient is incontinent. Patients with chronic arterial disease and diabetes mellitus are at risk for developing gas gangrene following amputation of the leg because these conditions favor the development of local tissue anoxia necessary for the development of gas gangrene.

Clinical Manifestations

The onset of gas gangrene is usually manifested by sudden, severe pain at the site of injury, which is caused by gas and edema in the tissues, usually occurring 1 to 4 days following the injury. The wound is tender. The surrounding skin initially appears normal, or white and tense, but later becomes bronzed, brown, or even black in color. Vesicles filled with red, watery fluid appear, and crepitus (crackling) produced by gas in the tissue may be felt. Frothy fluid with a foul, sweetish odor may escape from the wound. The gas and edema fluid increase local pressure and impair the blood supply and drainage. The involved muscles become black or reddish purple (necrotic). Amputation of an affected extremity is sometimes necessary. The infection may spread quickly, resulting in systemic toxicity.

The patient is pale, prostrated, and apprehensive but usually alert. Pulse and respirations are rapid, but the temperature usually does not exceed 38.3°C (101°F). Anorexia, diarrhea, vomiting, and vascular collapse may occur. Death from toxemia is frequent.

Management

Prevention. Gas gangrene may be prevented if all devitalized and infected tissue is excised and débrided, with wide incisions made to render the wound unsuitable for the growth of clostridium.

Treatment. Treatment usually involves surgery, antibiotics, and sometimes hyperbaric oxygen. Once infection has developed, extensive incisions in the affected part allow air to inhibit the growth of anaerobic organisms. Antibiotic therapy is combined with prompt surgical débridement of the wound.

Hyperbaric oxygen (oxygen administered under pressure greater than atmospheric) has proved extremely effective in treating gas gangrene. This increases the dissolved oxygen in the arterial system by increasing the partial pressure of oxygen breathed by the patient. With hyperbaric oxygen therapy, it may not be necessary to amputate the extremity.

Nursing Interventions

The nursing functions are collaborative with those of the surgeon. The patient is acutely ill, because the infection produces an intense toxemia. The pulmonary capillary wedge pressures, central venous pressures, and urinary output are closely monitored. IV fluids are administered as prescribed to support the cardiovascular system and to maintain fluid and electrolyte balance. Blood component therapy may be necessary and is prescribed to maintain adequate hematocrit levels. Hemolysis and tissue destruction can lead to hyperkalemia; thus, potassium levels are closely monitored. Enteral nutrition is critical in establishing nutritional balance.

Botulism

Botulism is a type of food poisoning that affects the central nervous system. It is caused by eating food in which the bacterium *Clostridium botulinum* has grown and produced toxins. These toxins are extremely potent and are rapidly absorbed by the gastrointestinal tract, becoming bound to neural tissue and producing a neuroparalytic syndrome. Toxic effects usually follow ingestion of contaminated foods: home-canned, dried, or smoked foods or poorly processed foods. Local, state, and federal public health officials are notified when a case of botulism is diagnosed.

Clinical Manifestations. The symptoms appear 12 to 36 hours after ingestion of the contaminated food. If the symptoms appear less than 24 hours after ingestion, a more severe illness and a higher fatality rate are usually encountered. Nausea and vomiting may occur within hours of ingestion of contaminated food. The toxin causes paralysis of skeletal muscles, interfering with release of acetylcholine.

Cranial nerve symptoms include diplopia, ptosis and blurred vision (extraocular muscle involvement), dysphagia and pharyngeal pain, and dysphonia (involvement of larynx). Paralysis then occurs, slowly descending through the body and affecting all muscle groups, usually in a symmetric fashion. Throughout the ordeal, the patient's mind remains clear. Almost three fourths of the patients have respiratory problems.

Diagnostic Evaluation. The diagnosis is confirmed by finding the toxin in the serum, gastric contents, stools, and incriminated food. There are also characteristic electrophysiologic abnormalities in clinically involved muscle groups.

Management. Ventilatory equipment and emergency drugs must be readily available in the event of a life-threatening reaction to the toxins. Organisms and unabsorbed toxin are eliminated from the gastrointestinal tract by means of gastric lavage, cathartics, and enemas. In instances of respiratory paralysis or an ileus, these procedures may not be prescribed. A botulism antitoxin to neutralize any toxin that may be in the circulation is available from the CDC.

Nursing Interventions. Because the neurotoxins produced by *C. botulinum* may result in neuroparalytic syndromes, the patient is given respiratory care and support as the basic management to prevent the pulmonary complications that are responsible for most fatalities due to botulism. The patient is prepared for endotracheal intubation and mechanical ventilation. (The respiratory care of the paralyzed patient is discussed in detail in Chap. 25.)

The patient's heart is monitored to detect dysrhythmias. Skin care and positioning are also important facets of management to prevent pressure ulcers and musculoskeletal complications. The patient is monitored for urinary retention; if this occurs, an indwelling catheter may be necessary. The appearance of fever usually indicates a nosocomial infection.

After the acute phase of illness, there is a high prevalence of persistent symptoms (fatigue, weakness, dyspnea) that may last a year or more. The patient and family are informed of the need for rest periods throughout the day, energy-saving techniques, and the importance of follow-up care.

Prevention and Patient Education. Home-processed foods pose a serious danger of *C. botulinum,* because this microorganism is a spore-bearer and is not killed rapidly at boiling temperature. Reliable commercial packing houses sterilize their products at 120°C (248°F), which kills all the spores. Preserved foods in which this microorganism has been growing often look soft, contain gas bubbles, and give off an odor of decay; however, contaminated food items may have a normal appearance and taste. Canned foods should be heated at temperatures over 80°C (176°F) for 30 minutes or boiled for 10 minutes, because the toxins are heat-labile and are destroyed by proper cooking of food. The use of the pressure cooker method of canning at high altitudes is advised.

Persons are also cautioned not to use punctured and swollen cans or jars with defective seals. Canned commercial products that are damaged or swollen should not be used.

Leprosy (Hansen's Disease)

Leprosy is a chronic infectious disease caused by *Mycobacterium leprae,* a bacillus that produces lesions in the skin tissues and peripheral nerves. It is not known exactly how leprosy bacilli enter the body, but it is known that a high percentage of people living with leprosy patients have the disease. Large numbers of organisms are disseminated when a person with leprosy sneezes. It is possible that the organism gains entrance through the upper respiratory tract or through broken skin.

As the bacilli multiply, they invade adjoining skin areas and find their way into the axis cylinders of nerves by way of the axon-plasma filaments (the ultimate terminals of the nerves supplying the skin). As the infection spreads, organisms break out of the nerves at various points in the skin to produce macules and papules. These are painless, because the bacilli that caused them to form have already destroyed the nerve supply.

Incidence.   An estimated 12 million people throughout the world suffer from this ancient, feared, and disfiguring disease. It is most prevalent in developing countries, which have inadequate human and financial resources to cope with leprosy. In the United States, the influx of immigrants and increasing world travel by US citizens are factors in its occurrence. It is endemic in California, Hawaii, Texas, Florida, Louisiana, Puerto Rico, and New York City.

Clinical Manifestations.   The earliest manifestation of leprosy is a skin lesion, located anywhere on the body. Some lesions are colorless or reddish brown. The earliest symptom is usually a loss of feeling in a small area of the skin, as a result of damage to the dermal nerves. Nerve involvement can lead to damage of muscles and bones. Other forms of skin lesions include macules, papules, nodules, or plaques appearing over most of the body. These lesions resemble skin tumors or sores. When the face is involved, the lesions, together with the loss of the eyebrows and eyelashes, give the face a typical leonine appearance. Because the lesions are easily infected, giving rise to deep ulcers that heal slowly, scars deform the face. This process often dissects the nose, fingers, and toes and destroys sight.

Diagnostic Evaluation.   Diagnosis is made on the basis of the appearance of the lesions and the discovery of the leprosy bacilli, obtained from slit-scrape smears of the skin lesions and smears from nasal mucosa.

Management.   The goals of management are to give specific chemotherapy until cure is attained and to prevent and treat deformities. Leprosy is best treated with dapsone plus one or more additional drugs (rifampin, clofazimine) to prevent the emergence of resistant mutant strains.

Mucosal lesions respond most readily, disappearing within a few months, resulting in relief of nasal obstruction and clearing of laryngeal lesions. The smaller nodular lesions in the skin shrink and are absorbed, leaving only pigment spots. Larger lesions disperse, with eventual scar formation. However, bacilli can persist after treatment, resulting in relapse at a later date.

Reconstructive surgery and rehabilitation to restore damaged hands, feet, face, and other affected areas require the services of plastic surgeons, physical therapists, orthopedists, and others. Because the disfigurement of leprosy is such a stigma, surgery may be necessary if the patient is to return to society.

To counter the crippling effects of the disease, the patient must realize the importance of maintaining mobility of the affected extremities and preventing fixed deformities. The principles are similar to those stressed in patient education for rheumatoid arthritis. The patient is encouraged to inspect sites of potential injury (eyes, hands, feet) daily, because these areas are not sensitive and injuries can be neglected. The skin is kept hydrated and an emollient is applied to maintain suppleness and pliancy.

The Public Health Service maintains a hospital in Carville, Louisiana (National Hansen's Disease Center), that serves as a treatment, research, and training facility. Research is still being conducted in the hope of finding a specific skin test for leprosy. No isolation precautions are required, because the infection declines rapidly under chemotherapy. Segregation is no longer required in any state of the United States.

Ornithosis (Psittacosis)

Ornithosis is an infectious and atypical form of pneumonia or systemic febrile illness transmitted to humans by infected birds. The causative organisms, *Chlamydia psittaci,* are transmitted to humans inhaling the etiologic agent from dried droppings of infected birds, or directly from infected birds (*i.e.*, workers in food processing plants), or rarely from person to person. Birds of the parrot family (parakeets, parrots, cockatoos, budgerigars), as well as many other species of birds (canaries, sparrows, pigeons, turkeys), may be infected.

Clinical Manifestations.   The illness may appear as a transient, influenza-like illness or a severe pneumonia, or it may be asymptomatic. After an incubation period lasting 4 to 15 days (it may be as long as 6 weeks in humans), the disease begins abruptly, with malaise, headache, photophobia, and chills. Its course is characterized by high fever, extreme weakness, marked depression, and delirium, with surprisingly slow pulse and respiratory rates. Cough is a prominent symptom. The lungs become involved, with edema, mononuclear cells, and lymphocytes appearing in the alveoli and interstitial areas. Chest radiography may reveal an interstitial pneumonitis. Convalescence is likely to be prolonged.

Management.   Ornithosis responds to the tetracyclines. Supportive therapy includes bed rest, oxygen (when necessary), and measures to reduce the fever. Relapses are common.

Prevention.   Persons at risk are those who work in pet shops or around poultry and pigeons, bird fanciers, workers who may handle infected birds in the food processing and marketing business, and veterinarians. Care should be taken to avoid dust from feathers and bird-cage contents. Infected birds should be treated or destroyed. No protective vaccination is available.

Spirochetal Infections

Syphilis

See p. 1916.

Lyme Disease

Lyme disease is a multisystem inflammatory disorder caused by the recently recognized spirochete *Borrelia burgdorferi*. It is transmitted by the bite of ticks, which have a wide range of hosts, including sheep, cattle, deer, and mice. In the United States it is endemic along the East Coast from Massachusetts to Virginia, and in Wisconsin, Minnesota, California, and Oregon.

Clinical Manifestations. The early manifestations occur from spring through late fall. The most characteristic finding is an expanding skin lesion, erythema chronicum migrans, that may be accompanied by flulike symptoms. The skin manifestations generally appear 4 to 20 days after a tick bite and may be located anywhere on the body. The skin lesion at the site of the tick bite starts as a red macule or papule and expands to become an annular erythema. The skin manifestations may be followed weeks to months later by central nervous system abnormalities (aseptic meningitis, encephalitis), cardiac abnormalities (atrioventricular block), and joint abnormalities (arthritis). Serologic tests show a rise in antibodies directed against the spirochete.

Management. Tetracycline or penicillin given as early as possible shortens the duration and prevents recurrence of the skin manifestations. High-dose penicillin administered IV is the treatment for other organ involvement.

Prevention and Patient Education. See section on Rocky Mountain spotted fever, p. 1939.

Viral Infections

Influenza

Influenza is an acute infectious disease caused by an RNA-containing myxovirus. It is characterized by respiratory and constitutional symptoms. It sweeps through the entire world approximately every 20 years, attacking as many as 40% of the people in the affected areas. The striking features of these epidemics have been the speed with which the disease has spread and the extremely high attack rate.

Typical epidemics of influenza have been characterized by three successive waves, separated by brief intermissions. The first wave lasts from 3 to 6 weeks and is explosive in outbreak, widespread, and mild in form in most cases, with few complications. The second wave also is widespread but lasts longer; the cases are more severe, and the complications are serious. The third wave lasts still longer (8 to 10 weeks) and involves fewer persons, but the complications are severe. During the years following a major epidemic, scattered local waves of decreasing severity follow, with sporadic cases of influenza during the intervals.

Etiology. The primary factor in the etiology of influenza is a filtrable virus, of which there are numerous variant types. It is difficult to control influenza because the surface antigens of the virus have the capacity to change. Major changes in these viruses and new influenza strains arise from time to time. Therefore, previously acquired antibodies against earlier influenza strains may not be effective against the newly emerging strain, depending on the extent of the surface change. It has been observed that when a new influenza virus strain becomes prevalent throughout the country, the old virus strain disappears.

Transmission is by close contact or by droplets from the respiratory tract of an infected person. The virus is airborne and multiplies in the upper respiratory tract, invading the nasal, tracheal, and bronchial mucosal cells.

Clinical Manifestations. In most patients, influenza begins after a short incubation period (24 to 72 hours) with an abrupt onset of chills, fever, headache, backache, and malaise. Respiratory features include a dry cough, sore throat, and nasal obstruction and discharge. Other patients' symptoms begin with acute sinusitis, bronchitis, pleurisy, or bronchopneumonia. These symptoms are always abrupt in onset and prostrating. In still another group, there are gastrointestinal symptoms of nausea, vomiting, abdominal pain, and diarrhea; and finally, in each epidemic, cases develop without local symptoms but with chills or a continuous fever. The patient usually recovers within a week if there are no complications.

Complications. Persons at risk of developing the complications of influenza are those over 65, persons with chronic pulmonary or cardiac disease (especially rheumatic valve disease), and those with diabetes, chronic metabolic disorders, or chronic renal disease. The influenza virus damages the ciliated epithelium of the tracheobronchial tree, rendering the patient vulnerable to the development of secondary invaders such as pneumococci or staphylococci, *H. influenzae,* various streptococci, and other organisms.

Dyspnea early in the course of the disease points to bronchopneumonia, which is potentially life-threatening. This pneumonia may be viral, mixed viral, or bacterial in origin. Significant mortality occurs not only as a result of pneumonia but also from cardiopulmonary or other chronic diseases that are exacerbated during influenza infection. Other complications include myocarditis, myositis, and meningoencephalitis.

Management

The goals of management are to relieve symptoms and to prevent and treat complications.

The troublesome symptom of cough is treated with an expectorant–antitussive combination. The patient may be advised to take acetaminophen for headache and myalgias. Children and teenagers are not given aspirin because of its association with Reye's syndrome. Antiviral therapy (amantadine hydrochloride), if given early, can shorten the course of illness and reduce the titer of virus excreted.

The patient is encouraged to rest at home, not only to relieve malaise and headache but also to reduce spread of the infection. Transmission of infection to others is most likely to occur early in the illness.

A liberal fluid intake (water, juices, carbonated beverages) is encouraged to thin secretions and help reduce fever. A vaporizer increases air humidity and reduces irritation of the respiratory mucosa. The patient is advised to avoid respiratory irritants, particularly smoking, because smoking interferes with clearance of secretions by impairing ciliary function. Alcoholic beverages are discouraged because they can increase viscosity of secretions.

If acetaminophen is prescribed, the patient is advised to take it regularly to avoid marked swings of temperature with sweating and chills, which can lead to dehydration and exhaustion.

Prevention and Patient Education

The Immunization Practices Advisory Committee of the Public Health Service recommends annual influenza vaccinations (flu shots) for adults with chronic cardiovascular and pulmonary disorders that are severe enough to require regular medical follow-up or that have required hospitalization during the previous year. In addition, residents of nursing homes and other long-term care facilities, as well as health care personnel who have extensive contact with high-risk patients (*e.g.,* staff of intensive care units), are encouraged to have annual flu shots. The composition of the vaccine is changed annually to match any new antigenic variation of the virus. It is recommended that influenza vaccine be administered in the months of October or November.

The risk of developing influenza is related to crowding and close contact of groups of individuals. Therefore, visiting privileges within health care facilities and nursing homes should be restricted during epidemics to minimize any chance of introducing influenza. Elective admissions and surgery are avoided as much as possible during an influenza outbreak.

Amantadine, an antiviral drug, can prevent clinical infection with influenza A virus. It blocks an early step in the replication of this virus. It is given only to certain high-risk patients, because most persons exposed to influenza require no prophylaxis. Amantadine does not protect against endemic influenza or influenza B. Amantadine is also given for the treatment of symptomatic influenza A infection and may shorten the duration and diminish the severity of illness. Adverse effects, occurring mainly in the elderly, include central nervous system toxicity, confusion, dizziness, slurred speech, headache, sleep disturbances, and visual hallucinations. To be effective, amantadine should be given prior to, and for the duration of, exposure to type A influenza virus.

Infectious Mononucleosis

Infectious mononucleosis (mono) is an acute infectious disease of the lymphatic system caused by the Epstein-Barr virus (EBV), a DNA virus of the herpesvirus group. Another virus, cytomegalovirus, can cause virtually identical symptoms. A third infecting organism, *Toxoplasma* (a protozoan), can also produce a similar clinical picture.

The basic pathology is an intense proliferative response of the lymphoid tissue and organs (lymph nodes, spleen, tonsils), but all organs can be affected. Infectious mononucleosis is usually self-limited, but in rare instances complications and even death do occur.

Epidemiology.   Infectious mononucleosis is encountered most frequently in the 15- to 25-year age group. It has been shown that when natural primary infection with EBV develops in childhood, a mild and nonspecific or inapparent illness occurs, and the child has immunity for many years. Infectious mononucleosis occurs only in individuals without antibody to EBV. If natural primary infection does not take place in childhood and a susceptible person (adolescent or young adult) acquires the infection, clinical manifestations of infectious mononucleosis develop in about half of patients. Infectious mononucleosis is more frequently encountered in countries with a high standard of living; in developing countries or among deprived socioeconomic groups, primary infection almost always occurs in early childhood, so that the disease is virtually unknown in adults. In this country, in persons of college age, the rate of clinical attack is three to five times that of the population at large.

Transmission of infectious mononucleosis is by oral contact, thus the name "the kissing disease." The virus may persist in the pharynx for weeks or months. This suggests that a large number of young adults are probably convalescent carriers of this disease. The virus can also be spread by blood transfusion. The incubation period ranges from 30 to 50 days.

Clinical Manifestations.   The early clinical manifestations are usually vague and masquerade as those of streptococcal sore throat, leukemia, and hepatitis. The triad of fever, sore throat, and cervical lymph node enlargement suggests infectious mononucleosis. A typical attack begins with fever and chills, anorexia, sore throat, and myalgia. Headache and diarrhea are often seen. On the second or third day, the lymph nodes begin to swell and become tender, usually the posterior cervical group first, then the anterior groups. This causes pain in the neck area. Generalized lymphadenopathy may occur. Early in the course of the disease, supraorbital edema occurs and the spleen enlarges in most patients. Although hepatomegaly occurs in less than 25% of patients, most patients have abnormal liver function tests. A faint erythematous or maculopapular eruption may appear on the trunk and proximal extremities in the early stage of the disease.

Evidence suggests that the clinical syndrome of chronic EBV infection does occur. These patients complain of chronic fatigue, recurrent sore throat, and nonspecific symptoms (swollen glands, musculoskeletal pains, headaches, difficulty with concentration).

Diagnostic Evaluation.   The diagnosis is made on the basis of the typical picture of clinical illness, as well as such laboratory findings as lymphocytosis with many atypical lymphocytes, detection of heterophile antibodies, and positive EBV-specific antibody test results.

Management.   The treatment is symptomatic and supportive. The patient is encouraged to remain on bed rest while fever lasts and to rest at intervals during recovery. Aspirin or acetaminophen is given for headache and muscle pains. Constipation (which leads to straining and a sudden increase in portal venous pressure) is avoided. Corticosteroids may be used when severe or life-threatening complications develop, such as marked hepatic dysfunction, neurologic manifestations, thrombocytopenia, hemolytic anemia, and airway obstruction. Most patients recover in 1 to 3 weeks, although illness may be prolonged in some, with complaints of fatigue, poor exercise tolerance, and depression predominating for as long as 1 year.

Patient Education.   The patient is advised of the need for additional rest and sleep for a period of time. Strenuous physical activity and competitive sports are discouraged until recovery is complete because the enlarged spleen of the patient with infectious mononucleosis is vulnerable to injury and may rupture if subjected to relatively mild trauma. For the athlete, this may mean up to 6 months. However, the exact length of time is uncertain, because the spleen may rupture even after clinical, hematologic, and serologic evidence reveals recovery.

Rabies

Rabies is a severe viral infection of the central nervous system communicated to humans from the saliva of infected animals and commonly transmitted by a bite or by contact of the animal's saliva with mucous membranes or open wounds such as cuts, scratches, or abrasions. In the United States, the disease occurs mainly among wildlife: skunks, raccoons, foxes, and bats. The number of rabid dogs has decreased markedly as a result of organized canine rabies vaccination and leash laws. In some parts of the country, however, there has recently been an increased incidence of rabies in some wild animals (*e.g.,* raccoons).

The etiologic agent is the rhabdovirus that is present in the saliva and the central nervous system of rabid animals. In humans, the virus is spread from the wound to the local muscle cells and then invades the peripheral nerves, spreading to the central nervous system, and resulting in rabies viral encephalitis.

Management of the Biting Animal.   The animal inflicting the bite is captured (if possible) and kept under surveillance by veterinarians or animal control personnel. This may enable the bitten person to avoid undergoing unnecessary rabies vaccination. If the animal remains healthy for about 10 days, it is assumed that it was not infective.

Early signs of rabies in animals include altered behavior, fever, loss of appetite, and a change in the tone of bark (in dogs). If the animal becomes sick, the health department is notified.

Prophylactic Management of the Patient

Local Treatment of the Wound.   Animal bites on the face, neck, and hands present the highest risk because of the rich nerve supply in these regions. The bite wounds should be cleansed immediately with thorough and prolonged washing with soap and water to remove the saliva, to dilute viral exposure, and for the virucidal benefits of soap. The patient is then taken immediately for emergency treatment, at which time the wound is again flushed and cleansed. Tetanus prophylaxis and antimicrobial therapy are administered as indicated to counter any other possible infection transmitted by the animal.

Postexposure Prophylaxis.   Postexposure prophylaxis is designed to prevent the development of rabies illness in an exposed person. The decision to give postexposure treatment is made on an individual basis and depends on the circumstances surrounding the exposure incident, whether the animal was captured, the vaccination status of the animal, and the presence of rabies in the region.

A combination of passive and active immunization is recommended when postexposure treatment is deemed necessary. Two types of immunizing products are used concurrently: (1) globulin, providing rapid protection; and (2) vaccine, which induces an active immune response that develops more slowly. As soon as possible, rabies immune globulin (RIG), which is made from the serum of immunized donors and is free of the danger of animal antiserum, is administered. (Part of the RIG dose is infiltrated around the wound, and the rest is administered intramuscularly). At the same time the single dose of RIG is given, human diploid cell rabies vaccine (HDCV) is given intramuscularly in a separate site with use of a separate syringe, followed by four more vaccine doses given on days 3, 7, 14, and 28 after the first dose.

HDCV appears to produce immunity more quickly than previous rabies vaccines and causes substantially fewer side effects. After the completion of the series of inoculations, a serum specimen for rabies antibody testing is drawn to ensure that active immunity has been achieved. Serum antibody testing is arranged through the state health department.

Development of Rabies in Humans

Diagnostic Evaluation.   The diagnosis of rabies is made on the basis of the history of exposure (the patient was bitten or exposed to animal saliva), the development of characteristic symptoms, and the demonstration of rabies antibodies in the patient's blood.

Clinical Course in Humans.   The incubation period in humans is extremely variable, depending on the location and severity of the wound and the length of the nerve over which the virus must travel before it reaches the brain. The incubation period may be only 10 days to several weeks for bites around the face, or from 60 to 90 days and up to a year for a bite in another part of the body.

There are several clinical phases of rabies in humans. During the prodromal phase of the illness, there are abnormal sensations around the site of infection, and the individual experiences general anxiety accompanied by depression and irritability. Headache, nausea, sore throat, and loss of appetite may occur, or unusual sensitivity to sound, light, and changes in temperature may be noted.

The next phase is the stage of excitement. There are episodes of irrational excitement alternating with periods of alert calm. During this stage, seizures occur. Attempting to swallow or even looking at liquids induces such severe and painful spasms of the muscles of swallowing and respiration that the patient writhes, and the ensuing choking may produce apnea. Death usually occurs in this stage from cardiac or respiratory failure.

If the patient survives this stage, the muscle spasms and agitation cease. The paralytic phase is one of usually progressive ascending paralysis terminating in coma and death.

Management

The care of the patient is supportive because there is no specific treatment for rabies. The patient is placed in the intensive care unit and receives continuing cardiac and pulmonary monitoring. The room should be quiet and darkened. The outcome is usually fatal.

- It must be remembered that the rabies virus is contained in the saliva of patients with this disease, constituting a distinct hazard to personnel caring for him. All personnel must be on guard against being bitten by such a patient and must use universal precautions to prevent saliva from contaminating a skin abrasion. If this occurs, personnel must receive postexposure prophylactic treatment.

Rickettsial Infection: Rocky Mountain Spotted Fever

Rocky Mountain spotted fever (tick-borne typhus fever) is characterized by a continuous fever. It is caused by the bite of an infected tick, by an infected tick being crushed on the skin, or by the conjunctiva becoming contaminated with infected tick secretions. The organism responsible is *Rickettsia rickettsii*. The most common vectors for transmitting the disease to humans are the wood tick and the dog tick. The incidence of infections increases in April and reaches its highest level in May and June.

Pathophysiology and Clinical Manifestations

During infection in humans, *R. rickettsii* organisms invade both the endothelial and smooth muscle cells of blood vessels, causing a generalized vasculitis. Cell damage may lead to alterations in capillary permeability, thrombosis, and hemorrhage.

This generalized vasculitis accounts for the manifestations of the disease, both the cutaneous lesions and visceral disturbances. It may involve virtually every organ.

Early symptoms, appearing several days after an infected tick bite, include severe headache, malaise, anorexia, photophobia, slight fever, and muscle and joint pain. Within a few days, the fever, rash, and edema are pronounced. The rash is the most specific manifestation of the infection and consists of rose-colored macules (nonelevated discolorations) of variable size that appear on the wrists, ankles, soles, and palms, gradually spreading over the entire body. The rash becomes papular (consisting of solid elevated lesions), darker red, and slightly dusky; after a few days it develops a petechial or purpuric character (Fig. 62-6). In some cases, however, the rash appears in the terminal stages of illness or not at all. Large subcutaneous hemorrhages may appear. In severe forms of the disease, areas of skin necrosis appear as a result of endarteritis (inflammatory blockage of arterioles). This necrosis may involve the ear lobes, fingers, toes, and scrotum—those areas at the extreme periphery of the vascular system. There may be marked thrombocytopenia due to inflammation of the vessels communicating with the bone marrow. As a result of generalized vascular involvement and resulting escape of serum, generalized edema occurs.

Restlessness, insomnia, and hyperesthesias are distressing symptoms of this disease. Neurologic manifestations, generally attributed to the effects of vasculitis on brain tissue, include altered mental status (confusion, delirium), headache, and stiff neck. The spleen is large and tender. Gastrointestinal symptoms include abdominal tenderness, pain, and muscular rigidity. Pneumonia may occur. Mental confusion, deafness, and visual disturbances are common and may last for weeks.

Diagnostic Evaluation

Early diagnosis is important and is almost always made on a high suspicion for the disease during tick season and on clinical grounds. Laboratory confirmation of Rocky Mountain spotted fever is made by serologic or other methods.

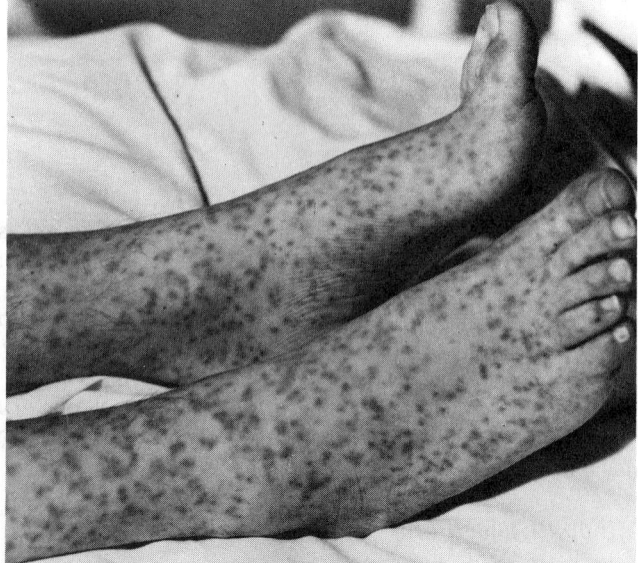

Figure 62–6. The rash of Rocky Mountain spotted fever. (Armed Forces Institute of Pathology photograph, negative N-67987-3.)

Management

The tetracyclines and chloramphenicol are specific rickettsiostatic drugs if administered in the *early stages* of the disease. Rocky Mountain spotted fever can run a rapid and fulminating course, but most patients recover if treated early.

Because Rocky Mountain spotted fever is an infectious vasculitis, the patient may display marked physiologic disturbances, including circulatory collapse, hypotension, oliguria, hypoproteinemia, and edema. Central venous pressure measurements are used to guide fluid and electrolyte replacement. The patient may be given transfusions of packed red blood cells and platelets. Severe coagulation disturbances may be treated with heparin.

Nursing Interventions

Supportive nursing measures are used to combat fever, restlessness, and pain, and to promote comfort (see Nursing Care Plan 62-1). The patient is positioned carefully because he may have severe edema and necrosis from vasculitis. The circumferences of the abdomen, arms, and leg are measured at prescribed intervals to determine the extent of the edema. Intake and output records are kept and evaluated to assess for oliguria, because the patient may develop renal failure as a result of poor tissue perfusion from vascular degeneration.

Prevention and Patient Education.   Rocky Mountain spotted fever is the most commonly reported rickettsial infection in the United States, with most cases occurring in the southern Atlantic and western south-central states. The disease has almost vanished from its original home in the Rockies.

As increasing numbers of Americans participate in backpacking and other camping activities, more people will be exposed to this disease. Important aspects of prevention are wearing protective clothing and conscientiously searching for and removing ticks. Persons living in tick-infested areas or visiting such places should examine their scalp, skin, and clothing for ticks two to three times each day. This is important, because an infected tick must usually be attached and feeding several hours before it can transmit the disease. Tick repellent should be applied to the exposed parts of the body and clothing, especially socks and trouser cuffs and any openings in the clothing (neck, top of pants, button areas).

Ticks may be removed from the body by grasping the tick with tweezers as close to the point of attachment as possible and pulling slowly and steadily. Fingers, protected with facial tissue, may be used when tweezers are not available. Other means of removing a tick are to touch it with gasoline or cover it with a thick ointment to lessen the tick's hold on the skin. Care should be taken not to crush the tick to avoid contaminating the broken skin with infectious tick secretions. The tick bite is disinfected immediately, and the hands are washed immediately after tick removal.

Household pets should be examined for ticks on a regular basis.

Protozoan Infections

Malaria

Malaria is an acute infectious disease caused by protozoa that are transmitted by way of an intermediate host, the bite of an infective female *Anopheles* mosquito. Malaria has also been transmitted through blood transfusions and from the needles and syringes shared by IV drug users.

Incidence.   Malaria affects an estimated 300 million people in the world annually. It causes more disability and a heavier economic burden than any other parasitic disease. International travel and the recent influx of Asian and Middle Eastern immigrants have been responsible for a resurgence of malaria in many nontropical countries. In addition, more than 20 species of anopheline mosquitoes have become resistant to commonly used insecticides.

Types of Malaria.   There are four species of malarial parasites, grouped under the generic name *Plasmodium*, each causing a different type of malaria: *Plasmodium falciparum* (which poses the greatest danger), *Plasmodium vivax, Plasmodium malariae,* and *Plasmodium ovale.* Each malarial parasite lives within a red blood cell, using the hemoglobin as food. When full grown, it divides (segments) into 10 to 20 small, young parasites, called *hyalines* (segments), which burst the cell; this bursting of cells causes chills in the patient. Most of these hyalines die, but a few find their way into new red blood cells, and the process is repeated.

Clinical Manifestations.   Most patients present with paroxysms of chills, fever, and sweating. Nausea, fatigue, and dizziness are present, along with intense headache and muscle pains. Paroxysms of chills and fever may last about 12 hours, after which the cycle may be repeated daily, every other day, or every third day.

Complications occur most frequently with *P. falciparum*. Patients with severe malaria of any form may become comatose and die (pernicious malaria); they may develop renal failure (due to the precipitation of free hemoglobin in the kidney tubule), a serious gastrointestinal disturbance, or cerebral symptoms (due to an accumulation of the parasites in the blood vessels of the affected organ).

Diagnostic Evaluation.   The patient should be asked about travel outside the United States, because most cases in this country are brought in by travelers. Travel or residence in an area where malaria is endemic is an important diagnostic clue. The diagnosis is confirmed by the finding of the parasites in stained peripheral blood smears. More than one blood examination may be required, because the diagnosis can be missed on a routine smear.

Management

The goal of treatment is to destroy the blood trophozoites and schizonts of *Plasmodium* that cause the clinical manifestations and the pathologic effects that characterize the disease.

The use of antimalarial drugs depends on the stage of the life cycle of the parasite. The species of parasite infecting the patient is determined by means of a blood smear.

Chloroquine is prescribed for infections caused by *P. vivax, P. ovale,* and *P. malariae,* followed by a course of primaquine to eliminate the hepatic form of these species. Quinine is given with pyrimethamine-sulfadoxine (Fansidar) to patients with malaria in areas known to be resistant to chloroquine or for malaria due to *P. falciparum* strains.

Cerebral malaria, which occurs in about 2% of patients with acute falciparum malaria, is the most feared complication. It produces changes in consciousness, behavioral changes, seizures, and cerebral edema. Patients with acute *P. falciparum*

are critically ill and must be hospitalized because the infection can be so overwhelming. In fact, acute malaria of this type is considered a medical emergency. Quinine is administered via the intravenous route intermittently. Because neurologic toxicity can occur from the quinine infusion, the patient is monitored for twitching, delirium, confusion, convulsions, and coma. Oxygen is administered to counter tissue anoxia. The patient may have jaundice as a result of the density of malarial parasites in the blood and abnormalities in hepatic function. The degree of anemia present is related to the severity of the infection. Abnormal bleeding (nosebleeds, oozing of blood from venipuncture sites, passage of blood in the stool) may occur as a result of either decreased production of clotting factors by a damaged liver or DIC.

Universal precautions are instituted. Further restrictions are defined by each institution's disease-specific isolation procedures.

Prevention and Patient Education.   The essence of malaria control is the eradication of malaria as an endemic disease. In several areas of the world, this goal has been achieved. To escape malaria, one must avoid *Anopheles* mosquitoes. This includes remaining in well-screened areas, using mosquito nets, and wearing clothes that cover most of the body. The application of mosquito repellent to exposed skin decreases the chance of being bitten. Travelers should be advised to try to reduce contact with mosquitoes between dusk and dawn because malarial transmission occurs primarily in these hours as a result of nocturnal feeding habits.

The CDC publishes *Health Information for International Travel,* which lists the areas of the world where there is risk of infection with malaria, and also the areas with strains of *P. falciparum* that are resistant to chloroquine. Persons planning a visit to areas where malaria is endemic are advised to obtain the most recently recommended prophylactic medication, usually chloroquine, which is taken before entry into the area and continued for a specified time after returning to the United States. In areas where there is chloroquine resistance, advice from the CDC should be obtained.

The traveler is also advised that regardless of the prophylactic regimen used, it is still possible to contract malaria. The onset of fever, chills, and headache should not be attributed to flu, and medical advice should be sought *promptly*. Travelers to areas where malaria is prevalent should not donate blood for up to 3 years.

Giardiasis

Giardiasis is a protozoan infection of the small intestine caused by the flagellate *Giardia lamblia.* This water-borne parasite is found in two forms: cysts and trophozoites. Transmission depends on the ingestion of cysts that are excreted in the feces of a human or animal host. It is transmitted to humans by inadequately treated water, by animal excretion into water, and by person-to-person contact.

Giardiasis is the cause of traveler's diarrhea in many countries, both underdeveloped and modern, and is usually associated with inadequately treated drinking water. In this country, outbreaks have occurred in mountainous regions (Rockies, Appalachians, Pacific Northwest) where the pathogen affects campers, hikers, and mountainous communities where drinking water comes from streams or rivers without a water filtration system. Person-to-person transmission occurs by hand-to-mouth transfer of cysts from the feces of an infected person and is responsible for outbreaks in day care centers, nursing homes, and other institutions. The incidence is high among those who practice oral–anal sexual activity.

Clinical Manifestations.   Patients with a mild infection report only a constant bloated feeling or abdominal pain without diarrhea. Other patients have persistent diarrhea with loose, watery, foul-smelling stools, abdominal cramping, and weight loss. Malabsorption of fats and fat-soluble vitamins may occur. The disease is usually self-limiting, lasting 2 to 6 weeks, but it may recur intermittently and persist for months or even years.

Giardiasis is diagnosed by finding *Giardia lamblia* in feces. The trophozoites may be found in duodenal fluid obtained by having the patient swallow a weighted nylon string that passes to the bowel and is later withdrawn (enterotest). Alternatively, a sample of mucosa may be obtained by small intestine biopsy.

Management.   The treatment of giardiasis for adults is either quinacrine or metronidazole.

Prevention and Patient Education.   Travelers and hikers should boil water or treat it with commercially available iodine compound. Raw, unpeeled fruits and vegetables should not be eaten in areas where giardiasis is endemic. Control of person-to-person transmission requires personal cleanliness, careful hand washing, and sanitary disposal of feces.

Amebiasis (Amebic Dysentery)

Amebae are protozoa, larger than leukocytes, that move by ameboid action. Only a few amebae infect humans. One of the most important of these is *Entamoeba histolytica,* the cause of amebic dysentery. These amebae survive outside the body in resistant encysted forms.

Amebiasis is a worldwide parasitic disease of the large intestine. It is acquired through ingestion of the cyst stage of *E. histolytica* in food or water contaminated by infected human feces, flies, or the hands of infected food handlers who may be carriers. The infection may also be transmitted through oral–anal or oral–genital sexual contact (both heterosexual and homosexual).

It is estimated that 10% of the world's population is infected, and in some tropical countries the infection rate may exceed 30%. In the United States it is becoming more common as a result of increased numbers of carriers. Persons at risk in this country are immigrants and visitors from developing countries, travelers returning from these areas, those who practice oral–anal sexual activity, and contacts with infected persons living in poor sanitary conditions.

Pathophysiology.   The amebae burrow their way into the intestinal mucosa, where they feed mainly on bacteria. Pus pockets may form, with only a small orifice opening into the bowel from which numerous burrows extend for considerable distances in all directions under the mucous membrane. Abscesses form in the mucous membrane and eventually slough off, exposing an underlying ulcer that may enlarge to 1 to 2 cm in diameter. The large bowel may be so covered by such ulcers that little normal mucous membrane is left. Usually, the floor of these ulcers is the muscle wall of the bowel, but they may perforate its entire wall and cause fatal peritonitis.

In the small intestine, the organism may erode intestinal mucosa, invade the bloodstream, and gain access to the liver through the portal vein.

Clinical Manifestations and Course.   Most infected individuals are asymptomatic. The clinical manifestations depend on the site of involvement. Amebiasis may present as an intestinal or extraintestinal disease. When the amebae become invasive in the intestines, the chief symptom is diarrhea, with abdominal cramping and pain. Diarrhea may be mild, with loose stools, or there may be severe dysentery with stools containing considerable amounts of blood, exudate, and mucus. Persons with chronic disease usually have associated weight loss and anemia. Amebiasis may mimic irritable bowel syndrome. The illness may present as appendicitis, abdominal mass, or partial intestinal obstruction.

The two important features of this disease are its chronicity (one attack of acute dysentery following another, separated by periods of constipation that last for months) and the tendency of the infection to cause liver abscess, as a result of dissemination to the liver by way of the portal vein. Complications include peritonitis, abscess formation, hemorrhage, and extraintestinal disease.

Diagnostic Evaluation

The diagnosis is made by finding trophozoites or cysts in a freshly purged stool specimen, in a nonpurged, warm stool specimen, or in proctosigmoidoscopic material or abscess contents. Rectal biopsy may reveal the organism. There are serologic tests (indirect hemagglutination test and indirect fluorescent antibody test) to diagnosis amebiasis.

Management

The objectives of treatment are to eradicate the organism, to give symptomatic relief, to prevent spread of amebae to other tissues, and to replace fluids and electrolytes.

There is uncertainty about what constitutes the best treatment, and a significant number of patients require multiple courses of therapy. Usually two drugs are used—one to rid the intestines of the trophozoites and the other to dispose of the cysts. Metronidazole (Flagyl) followed by iodoquinol (active against the cyst form) is a standard form of treatment. Universal Precautions are utilized.

To support the patient's general condition, IV fluids are prescribed as required to correct fluid and electrolyte imbalance resulting from severe diarrhea. If diarrhea is acute, the patient remains on bed rest and is offered low-residue, bland foods. Follow-up study of the stools is necessary, because relapses are common.

Control and Patient Education

Transmission of *E. histolytica* is principally by ingestion of contaminated food or water. Methods of control include sanitary disposal of human feces, protection of the public water supply, raising and preparing food free of contamination, and an ongoing program of health education, including emphasis on meticulous hand washing after defecation and before preparing and eating food. In areas of high prevalence, fresh fruits and vegetables that cannot be peeled may be a source of contamination. Contacts of recently diagnosed patients should be examined. Patients should abstain from oral–anal and oral–

genital sexual practices while they are under treatment. Sexual partners of infected patients should have a stool examination.

Amebic Liver Abscess

Amebic liver abscess represents the most common extraintestinal complication of amebiasis. It occurs when the amebae invade the liver tissue and form abscesses that increase in size, progressively damaging the liver.

In most patients, the right lobe of the liver is involved, and the abscess may be single or multiple. The major complaints are pain in the right upper abdomen (caused by the liver's rapid enlargement and stretching of its capsule), right upper chest pain (due to the liver's enlarging in an upward direction), fever, anorexia, and loss of weight. Physical examination reveals an enlarged, tender liver (due to hepatic abscess) and auscultatory abnormalities of the right lung field (from direct extension or rupture of a contiguous liver abscess). If the abscess is in the left lobe of the liver, a tender epigastric mass is noted. There is also diaphoresis, weight loss, and pallor. A CT scan of the liver suggests the diagnosis and is useful in identifying the site, size, and number of lesions as well as in following the resolution of the abscess. Ultrasound is used. Immunologic techniques, mainly serologic methods, are also used in diagnosis. One point to be emphasized is that not infrequently the abscesses are found unexpectedly in patients who have had few or no symptoms suggesting amebiasis.

Usually, the patient responds promptly to amebicidal therapy. Metronidazole (Flagyl) has generally been successful, and it may be combined with other drugs. Needle drainage of the abscess may be necessary if there is concern that the abscess may rupture and cause peritonitis, or after rupture to reduce further spread of infection, or when clinical illness persists after adequate drug therapy. The supportive treatment is that outlined for amebiasis.

Systemic Mycotic Infections (Fungal Infections)

Fungi are primitive organisms that take their nourishment from living plants and animals and decaying organic material. Fungi have the ability to exist as yeasts or as molds and may alternate between the yeast and mold form. The fungi present difficult problems in control because they are so widespread in nature— in soil, decaying vegetation, and bird excreta. Although there are thousands of known species of fungi, 100 or more species are generally recognized as pathogens to humans. The three main types of mycoses (fungal infections), as determined by the tissue level at which the fungus settles, are as follows:

1. Systemic or deep mycoses involving primarily the internal organs, with a primary focus in the lungs.
2. Subcutaneous mycoses that involve the skin, subcutaneous tissue, and sometimes the bone.
3. Superficial or cutaneous mycoses that grow in the outer layer of skin (epidermis), hair, and nails.

Systemic infections are usually acquired by accidental inhalation (spores carried on wind currents), occasionally by traumatic implantation (from contaminated soil or plant materials), or by the pathologic takeover of a normal inhabitant when the resistance of the host is lowered. The responsible fungi commonly spread to other organs by either the hematogenous or, less frequently, the lymphatic route. These infections are not transmitted from person to person.

Persons at Risk. The systemic mycoses are occurring more frequently because they are more common in patients with impaired immunologic resistance (*e.g.*, patients with AIDS) and in patients receiving immunosuppressive agents (corticosteroids, antilymphocyte serum, chemotherapy for cancer). Many patients who are receiving such treatment, or who are debilitated or severely ill and have reduced defenses, become prey to invasion by fungi that they could ordinarily withstand.

In addition to those receiving immunosuppressive agents, patients at risk for invasive fungal infections are those with certain immunologic deficiencies, those with advanced malignancies, kidney or other organ-transplant patients, open heart surgery patients, severely burned patients, patients receiving prolonged IV feedings, and those with renal failure and diabetes.

Histoplasmosis

Histoplasmosis is a chronic systemic fungal infection caused by a spore-bearing mold, *Histoplasma capsulatum*. This highly infectious mycosis is transmitted by airborne dust that contains *H. capsulatum* spores. Partially decayed droppings of pigeons, chickens, bats, and birds offer an excellent medium for growth of this fungus.

Clinical Manifestations. The patient may have no detectable illness or he may have signs and symptoms of a mild respiratory disease: fever, malaise, headache, myalgias, and anorexia. If the infection is more severe, signs and symptoms resemble those of pulmonary tuberculosis: fever, cough, dyspnea, anorexia, and loss of weight and strength. Fungal infections mimic symptoms of other diseases, and the patient may present with symptoms of malignant lymphoma, including anemia, thrombocytopenia, splenomegaly, and hepatomegaly.

Management. Most patients do not require treatment, because a mild self-limited course is the rule. Patients are followed clinically and radiologically to determine the course of the disease. Amphotericin B has traditionally been the mainstay of treatment for disseminated or acute pulmonary disease, because it has a wide spectrum of activity against fungal infections. It is given IV and is reserved for serious infections, because this agent has significant toxicity. Severe toxic reactions include nausea, vomiting, chills, fever, diarrhea, hypokalemia, and phlebitis.

Ketoconazole is an antifungal agent that is orally absorbable and effective against the etiologic agents of systemic mycoses. It has been associated with hepatic toxicity, thus requiring close patient monitoring.

Health Education. Stirring up dust by raking and sweeping around bird roosting sites is to be avoided. Exposure to dust in a contained, enclosed environment (chicken coop) should be minimized. Spraying the area with water reduces dust.

Helminthic Infestations

Major helminthic (worm) infections are among the most prevalent of the human infectious diseases. They are global in distribution and have profound effects on the nutritional status of humans and animals and on the physical and mental development of children. Three major groups of helminths are intestinal parasites in humans: the nematodes (roundworms), the cestides (tapeworms), and the trematodes (flukes).

Trichinosis (Trichinellosis)

Trichinosis is infestation by the parasite *Trichinella spiralis,* one of the roundworms. It is acquired by consuming infected meat, usually pork.

Clinical Manifestations and Course.   Trichinosis is a disease of pigs in the continental United States and of bears in Alaska. Tiny embryos of *T. spiralis* become encysted in the muscle fibers of an infected pig. These calcified cysts, barely visible to the naked eye, appear in the meat like tiny grains of sand. If such pork is insufficiently cooked and then eaten, the embryos are set free by the gastric juice and develop in the intestine during the following week into adult worms about 3 to 4 mm in length. These worms make their way into the mucous membrane and there produce myriad embryos. The intestinal phase starts about 24 hours after larval ingestion, causing symptoms of gatrointestinal disturbance: nausea, vomiting, diarrhea, and abdominal pain.

The embryos, carried by the bloodstream and by their own activity, migrate to all parts of the body. The patient's symptoms, arising from muscle invasion (due to an inflammatory process in the muscles), include edema of the eyelids, scleral hemorrhages, pain on eye motion, and generalized pain and soreness of muscles. High fever occurs. Peripheral eosinophilia is a constant finding. Occasional cardiac dysrhythmias (due to trichinae in the heart muscle) may be seen and may be fatal. Difficulties in breathing, chewing, swallowing, or speaking may also occur.

Diagnostic Evaluation.   A biopsy specimen taken from a painful muscle (deltoid, biceps, gastrocnemius) reveals the larvae. Serologic tests may be positive, with demonstrable titers 3 to 4 weeks after the infection. Usually, the eosinophil count begins to rise in the second week. A skin test based on an extract of trichinae as the test antigen becomes positive after 16 to 20 days and may be positive for years afterward.

Management.   The treatment of trichinosis is symptomatic. Mebendazole (Vermox) is used in both the intestinal and muscular stages of infection. The patient is advised to rest, and analgesics are administered to relieve muscle pain. Corticosteroids may be prescribed for critically ill patients during the acute phase.

Electrocardiograms are used to monitor the patient for evidence of myocarditis.

Prevention and Patient Education.   The public should be educated about the importance of thoroughly cooking all pork and pork products, especially sausage. There should be no trace of pink in cooked pork. Cooking pork in a microwave oven may fail to kill larvae. Smoking, pickling, seasoning, or spicing does not make pork safe unless it is cooked. Beef hamburger may be contaminated by a meat grinder that has been used for pork.

Hookworm Disease (Ancylostomiasis)

Hookworm disease is the result of infestation of the small intestine by one or two similar roundworms about 1.2 cm (0.5 in) long. Two species are parasitic in the human intestinal tract: *Necator americanus* (predominant US species) and *Ancylostoma duodenale.* The infection is usually acquired by walking barefoot, whereby infected larvae of the worms penetrate the skin.

Incidence.   Some 700 to 900 million persons are infected with hookworm. It is found mainly in tropical and subtropical regions, notably Asia, the Mediterranean area, South America, Africa, and in most of the western hemisphere. In the United States, hookworm infections are more prevalent in the southeastern states.

Pathology and Clinical Course.   The embryos of this worm, hatched from eggs passed in human feces onto the ground, live in dirt, sand, and clay and easily infest humans. They enter by mouth when food is eaten with dirty hands, or they bore through the skin of bare feet, causing itching and burning followed by vesicular eruption (ground itch). Having gained access to the blood or lymph vessels, they are carried by the bloodstream to the lungs and migrate from the pulmonary capillaries into the alveolar sacs. The larvae migrate up the bronchi and trachea and then pass over the epiglottis, down the esophagus, and into the bowel. The worms attach themselves to the intestinal mucosa and suck the blood of the host. The effect of the blood-sucking and hemorrhages at the attachment sites is iron-deficiency anemia. A patient with severe infection and with inadequate dietary iron may develop profound anemia. He presents with lassitude, dyspnea, anorexia, and pedal edema. Severe anemia may cause cardiac symptoms. Maturation of the worms in the intestine may cause diarrhea and other gastrointestinal symptoms. A dry cough and dyspnea develop when the larvae rupture through the capillary bed and are spread throughout the bronchial tree.

Management.   Both mebendazole and pyrantel pamoate (Antiminth) are effective for hookworm disease. The patient should be placed on a nutritious diet, because hookworm disease occurs in persons suffering from malnutrition. Protein and iron supplementation is administered to aid in the correction of the anemia.

Prevention.   The prevention of hookworm disease depends on sanitary disposal of human excreta, proper hand washing, and the wearing of shoes. Human excrement (night soil) and sewage effluents should not be used for fertilizer.

Ascariasis (Roundworm Infestation)

Ascariasis is an infection by the nematode *Ascaris lumbricoides* (intestinal roundworm). This is the most common worm parasitizing the human intestine, with an estimated 1 billion infections worldwide. In the United States, ascariasis is more common in the southeastern states.

This disease is usually found in overcrowded areas with poor sanitation. Contamination of the soil by human feces is a factor in its spread. Humans are infected by ingestion of the eggs in contaminated raw vegetables and drinking water. Infection may be contracted from eating raw vegetables when night soil is used for fertilizer. Water pollution may cause water transmission.

Life Cycle and Clinical Features. The eggs are swallowed and pass into the intestine, where they hatch as larvae. The larvae enter the bloodstream and pass through the pulmonary circulation, migrate through the lungs, and return to the gastrointestinal tract, where they grow, mature, and mate. Large numbers of worms may migrate into various organs of the body and cause obstruction to the trachea, bronchi, bile duct, appendix, and pancreatic duct. Masses of worms in the intestine cause gastointestinal discomfort, severe abdominal pain, and vomiting. Fever, chills, dyspnea, cough, and pneumonia may develop from invasion of the lungs by large numbers of larvae. Adult worms may migrate into the ampulla of Vater and then to the pancreatic or biliary ducts, causing acute and agonizing pain. Ascariasis is diagnosed by detecting ova or worms in the feces.

Management. Mebendazole (Vermox) given twice daily for 3 days is the drug of choice. Piperazine (Antepar) and pyrantel pamoate (Antiminth) are also effective drugs. Universal Precautions are instituted.

Prevention. Preventive measures include providing adequate toilet facilities and teaching the importance of personal hygiene. All patients with the infestation should be treated.

Chapter Summary

In summary, many infectious diseases are virulent, life-threatening illnesses that may be primary conditions or conditions secondary to other disease entities. Prevention of the spread of infections by breaking the chain of transfer is the key to successful treatment.

Universal precautions have been developed over the past few years, representing a change in the philosophy of treatment. Rather than waiting for infectious diseases to be diagnosed with cultures, all body fluids are handled as if they were infectious. These changes have come about mainly because of the development of life-threatening infectious diseases that do not have cures associated with them.

Pharmacologic advances continue to be studied through research. New medications are continually developed, often only to be followed by resistant strains of infectious diseases. Hospital populations continue to grow older, with many patients diagnosed with multisystem diseases. These populations are more susceptible to infections because of their debilitation and their exposure to infectious organisms.

The challenge to the nursing profession in the area of infectious diseases will continue to grow. Expert skills of assessment, planning, intervention, and evaluation are required to care for these patients.

Bibliography

Books

Cundy KR. Infection Control: Dilemmas and Practical Solutions. New York, Plenum Press, 1990.

DeVita VT, Hellman S, and Rosenberg SA (eds). AIDS: Etiology, Diagnosis, Treatment, and Prevention, 2nd ed. Philadelphia, JB Lippincott, 1988.

Dick G. Practical Immunization. Boston, MTP Press Limited, 1986.

Felman YM. Sexually Transmitted Diseases. New York, Churchill Livingstone, 1986.

Heaton WH. Infection Control Policy and Procedure Manual. Baltimore, National Health Publications, 1990.

Hoeprich PD and Jordan MC. Infectious Diseases, 4th ed. Philadelphia, JB Lippincott, 1989.

Mandell GL et al (eds). Principles and Practice of Infectious Diseases, 3rd ed. New York, Churchill Livingstone, 1990.

Pickering LK and DuPont HL. Infectious Diseases of Children and Adults. Menlo Park, CA, Addison-Wesley, 1986.

Valanis B. Epidemiology in Nursing and Health Care. Norwalk, CT, Appleton-Century-Crofts, 1986.

Journals
Infection Control

Allen U and Ford-Jones EL. Nosocomial infections in the pediatric patient: An update. Am J Infect Control 1990 Jun; 18(3):176–193.

Bence L. Disease-specific isolation: The alternative method. Nurs Manage 1989 Apr; 20(4):16–18.

Cadwallader H. Setting the seal on standards: Infection control. Nurs Times 1989 Sep; 85(37):71–72.

Centers for Disease Control. Update: Universal precautions for prevention of transmission of human immunodeficiency virus, hepatitis B virus, and other bloodborne pathogens in health-care settings. MMWR 1987; 37(24):377–383.

Centers for Disease Control. Recommendations for prevention of HIV transmission in health-care settings. MMWR 1987; 36(Suppl 25):25–185.

Coleman D. The when and how of isolation. RN 1987 Oct; 50(10):50–59.

Crow RA et al. Nursing procedures and their function as policies for effective practice. Int J Nurs Stud 1988; 25(3):217–224.

Ferwerda HE. Getting on top of infection control problems. Am J Nurs 1989 Sep; 89(9):1191.

Ford-Jones EL et al. Satellite infection control committees within the hospital: Decentralizing for action. Infect Control Hosp Epidemiol 1989 Aug; 10(8):368–370.

Jackson MM et al. Why not treat all body substances as infectious. Am J Nurs 1987 Sep; 87(9):1137–1139.

Jenner E. Preaching safe practice . . . to protect staff from blood-borne infections. Nurs Times 1990 Mar 28; 86(13):66–69.

Lynch P et al. Implementing and evaluating a system of generic infection precautions: Body substance isolation. Am J Infect Control 1990 Feb; 18(1):1–12.

MacKellaig JM. A study of the psychological effects of intensive care with particular emphasis on patients in isolation. Intens Care Nurs 1987 Apr; 2(4):176–185.

Martin MT. Wound management and infection control after trauma: Implications for the intensive care setting. Crit Care Nurs Q 1988 Sep; 11(2):43–49.

McFarland A. Infection control: Reducing the risk to medical patients. Prof Nurse 1989 Apr; 4(7):344–348.

Patterson CH. Perceptions and misconceptions regarding the Joint Commission's view of quality monitoring. Am J Infect Control 1989 Oct; 17(5):231–240.

Robertson MM et al. Infection control rounds: A method for evaluating safety. J Nurs Qual Assur 1988 Nov; 3(1):46–56.

Santangelo J et al. Universal precautions still necessary. Calif Nurse 1988 Sep; 84(7):20.

Bacterial Infections

Aly R et al. Restriction of bacterial growth under commercial catheter dressings. Am J Infect Control 1988 Jun; 16(3):95–100.

Barthel JS. Gastritis and peptic ulcer disease: Bacterial agents as a treatable cause. Consultant 1990 Aug; 30(8):61–69.

Brumfitt W and Hamilton-Miller J. Methicillin-resistant *Staphylococcus aureus*. N Engl J Med 1989 May; 320(18):1188–1196.

Currier RW et al. Salmonella enteritidis in eggs (letter). Infect Control Hosp Epidemiol 1989 Aug; 10(8):343–344.

Dupont HL et al. Infectious diarrhea from A to Z. Patient Care 1987 Nov 15; 21(18):98–101.

Hancock BG and Eberhard NK. The pharmacologic management of shock. Crit Care Nurs Q 1988 Jun; 11(1):19–29.

Jong EC. Travel-related infections: Prevention and treatment. Hosp Pract 1989 Nov 15; 24(11):145–148.

Lee BC. Be ready for Lyme disease in your own backyard. RN 1989 Apr; 52(4):26–29.

Littleton MT. Pathophysiology and assessment of sepsis and septic shock. Crit Care Nurs Q 1988 Jun; 11(1):30–47.

Ma M. Brush up on antibacterial agents. Nursing 1989 Jan; 19(1):76–83.

McKenna DF. Lyme disease: A review for primary health care providers. Nurse Pract 1989 Mar; 14(3):18–22.

Neu HC. Antibacterial therapy: Problems and promises. Part 1. Hosp Pract 1990 May; 25(5):63–74.

Neu HC. Antibacterial therapy: Problems and promises. Part 2. Hosp Pract 1990 Jun; 25(6):181–194.

Prendergast V. Bacterial meningitis update. J Neurosci Nurs 1987 Apr; 19(2):95–99.

Raad I et al. Annual tuberculin skin testing of employees at a university hospital: A cost-benefit analysis. Infect Control Hosp Epidemiol 1989 Oct; 10(10):455–459.

Ribner BS et al. Outbreak of multiply resistant *Staphylococcus aureus* in a pediatric intensive care unit after consolidation with a surgical intensive care unit. Am J Infect Control 1989 Oct; 17(5):244–249.

Steinberg DG et al. Dangerous pyrogenic skin infections. Hosp Pract 1989 Oct; 24(10):101–106.

Suppaiah L. Pseudomembranous colitis induced by *Clostridium difficile*. Crit Care Nurse 1988 Jul/Aug; 8(5):65–72.

Thomas JC et al. Transmission and control of methicillin-resistant *Staphylococcus aureus* in a skilled nursing facility. Infect Control Hosp Epidemiol 1989 Mar; 10(3):106–110.

Wahl SC. Septic shock: How to detect it early. Nursing 1989 Jan; 19(1):52–60.

Young LS. Infections in patients with cellular immunodeficiency. Hosp Pract 1989 Aug; 24(8):191–194.

Protozoan Infections

Brillman JC. Preparing for the diseases of travel. Emerg Med 1990 May; 22(10):56–72.

Grossman RJ. PCP and other protozoal infections. Patient Care 1989 Oct 30; 23(17):89–97.

Newman MD. Infectious diarrhea: Major pathogens. Part 2. Physician Assist 1988 Feb; 12(2):119–128.

Sheahan SL et al. Management of common parasitic infections encountered in primary care. Nurse Pract 1987 Aug; 12(8):19–25.

Sexually Transmitted Diseases

Barrick B. Caring for AIDS patients is a challenge you can meet. Nursing 1988; 18(11):50–60.

Benoit JA. Sexually transmitted diseases in pregnancy. Nurs Clin North Am 1988 Nov; 23(4):937–945.

Bromelow L. Special contacts . . . venereal disease . . . VD clinic nurse. Nurs Times 1990 May 16; 86(20):48–49.

Cates W et al. Sexually transmitted disease: An overview of the situation. Prim Care 1990 Mar; 17(1):1–27.

Featherston WE. Sexual identity and practices relating to the spread of sexually transmitted diseases. Prim Care 1990 Mar; 17(1):29–45.

Fishman JA. An approach to pulmonary infection in AIDS. Hosp Pract 1988 Apr; 23(4):196–203.

Grady C. HIV: Epidemiology, immunopathogenesis, and clinical consequences. Nurs Clin North Am 1988 Dec; 23(4):683–696.

Hammerschiag MR et al. When to suspect chlamydia. Patient Care 1987 Nov 15; 21(18):64–78.

Holmes KK et al. The increasing frequency of heterosexually acquired AIDS in the United States. Am J Public Health 1990 Jul; 80(7):858–863.

Nettina SL and Kauffman FH. Diagnosis and management of sexually transmitted genital lesions. Nurse Pract 1990 Jan; 15(1):20–24.

Noble RC. Sequelae of sexually transmitted diseases. Prim Care 1990 Mar; 17(1):173–181.

Rolfs RT. Risk factors for syphilis: Cocaine use and prostitution. Am J Public Health 1990 Jul; 80(7):853–857.

Soloman MZ et al. Preventing AIDS and other STDs through condom promotion: A patient education intervention. Am J Public Health 1989 Apr; 79(4):453–458.

Swanson JM and Chenitz WC. Psychosocial aspects of genital herpes: A review of the literature. Public Health Nurs 1990 Jun; 7(2):96–104.

Talashek ML et al. Sexually transmitted diseases in the elderly: Issues and recommendations. J Gerontol Nurs 1990 Apr; 16(4):33–42.

Viral Infections

Berlinberg CD et al. Occupational exposure to influenza: An introduction of an index case to a hospital. Infect Control Hosp Epidemiol 1989 Feb; 10(2):70–73.

Ford R et al. Bone marrow transplant: Recent advances and nursing implications. Nurs Clin North Am 1990 Jun; 25(2):405–422.

LaBrecque DR. Medical ostriches: Hepatitis B transmission. Infect Control Hosp Epidemiol 1990 Mar; 11(3):126–128.

Spence MR et al. Hepatitis B: Perceptions, knowledge, and vaccine acceptance among registered nurses in high-risk occupations in a university hospital. Infect Control Hosp Epidemiol 1990 Mar; 11(3):129–133.

Stehlin D. Available vaccine safe but underused. FDA Consum 1990 May; 24(4):14–17.

Vargo RL et al. Complications after cardiac transplantation: The role of immunosuppression. Crit Care Nurs Clin North Am 1989 Dec; 1(4):741–752.

Wallace M et al. Nursing management of patients with high risk blood borne virus disease in a psychiatric institution. Infect Control Can 1988 May/Jun; 3(2):18–22.

Other Infections

Overturf GD. Bacterial and rickettsial zoonosis associated with tick and flea bites. Emerg Med 1989 Jan; 10(4):67–79.

Sheahan SL and Seabolt JP. Management of common parasitic infections encountered in primary care. Nurse Pract 1987 Aug; 12(8):19–20.

Agencies

International

World Health Organization
   Avenue Appia, CH 1211 Geneva 27, Switzerland
World Health Organization Collaborating Center on AIDS
   c/o Centers for Disease Control, 1600 Clifton Road, NE, Atlanta, GA 30333.

Governmental

Centers for Disease Control (Center for Prevention Services
   Center for Environmental Health, Center for Health Promotion and Education, Center for Infectious Diseases), 1600 Clifton Road NE, Atlanta, GA 30333
National Institute of Allergy and Infectious Diseases
   National Institutes of Health, Bethesda, MD 20892
US Department of Health and Human Services, Public Health Service, 200 Independence Ave., SW, Washington, DC 20201

Voluntary

American Lung Association
   1740 Broadway, New York, New York 10019
American Public Health Association
   1015 Fifteenth Street NW, Washington DC 20005
American Social Health Association
   VD National Hotline, 260 Sheridan Ave., Suite 307, Palo Alto, CA 94306
American Venereal Disease Association
   Box 22349, San Diego, CA 92122
National Foundation for Infectious Diseases
   P.O. Box 42022, Washington, DC 20015

63

Emergency Nursing

Chapter Outline

Learning Objectives

On completion of this chapter, the learner will be able to:

1. Describe emergency care as a holistic concept that includes the patient and his family and significant others

2. Specify emergency resuscitation measures

3. Describe the emergency management of patients with hemorrhage due to trauma and hypovolemic shock

4. Describe the emergency management of patients with intra-abdominal injuries

5. Compare the immediate management of patients with fractures to long-term management

6. Describe the emergency management of patients with heat stroke, cold injuries, and anaphylactic reaction

7. Specify the emergency management of patients with swallowed, inhaled, and injected poisons, snakebites, and food poisoning

8. Describe the emergency management of patients with drug abuse and those with alcohol abuse

9. Differentiate between the emergency care of patients who are overactive, violent or depressed, and suicidal

10. Specify the significance of crisis intervention in the care of the rape victim

Nursing in Emergency Conditions

The term *emergency management* has traditionally referred to the care given to patients with urgent and critical needs. However, hospital emergency departments and emergency clinics are increasingly being used for nonurgent problems; the phi-losophy of emergency care has broadened to include the concept that an emergency is whatever the patient or his family considers it to be. The staff have an obligation to treat the patient with understanding and to respect the anxiety that he undoubtedly feels. If they do not, the therapeutic process may be threatened.

A large number of people seek emergency help for serious

life-threatening cardiac conditions, such as myocardial infarction, acute congestive heart failure and pulmonary edema, and cardiac dysrhythmias. The priorities of management of such cardiac conditions, as well as the electrocardiographic (ECG) patterns evoked by the dysrhythmias, are discussed in Chapters 28 and 29. This chapter deals mainly with the emergency management of trauma and other conditions not found elsewhere in this book. *It is assumed that treatment is provided under the direction of a physician.*

The Nursing Process in the Emergency Department

The nursing process provides a logical framework for problem solving in the time-limited and pressured environment of the emergency department. The nurse in the emergency department, through specialized education, training, and experience, has expertise in assessing and identifying patients' health care problems in crisis situations, establishing priorities, monitoring acutely ill and injured patients, supporting and attending to families, supervising allied health personnel, and teaching patients and families. Nursing interventions are accomplished interdependently with consultation or direction from the physician. The strengths of nursing and medicine are especially complementary in an emergency situation. The nurse anticipates appropriate nursing and medical interventions based on the assessment data and works as a team member in performing the high-tech, high-touch skills necessary in the care of emergency patients.

Patients in the emergency department have a wide variety of actual or potential problems. The patient's condition may change from minute to minute, and nursing assessment must be continuous. Thus, the nursing diagnoses change just as rapidly. Although a patient may have several diagnoses at a given time, the following discussions focus on the most immediate and assume both independent and interdependent nursing interventions.

Gerontologic Considerations

The elderly are major consumers of health care in the emergency department, accounting for 20% to 35% of visits to urban emergency facilities. Many of these are nonurgent visits, with skin, cardiovascular, and abdominal problems predominating. Elderly clients have multifaceted problems and often arrive in the emergency department with one or more presenting conditions that, although not considered urgent in the younger person, can readily become life-threatening in the aged if untreated. Acute illness may be manifested in the aging person by nonspecific symptoms such as weakness and fatigue, falling episodes, incontinence, and change in mental status.

Social service support may need to be initiated during the visit to the emergency department. The aged client may perceive the emergency as a crisis, since it may signal the end of an independent life-style or even result in death.

Infection Control Considerations

The increasing presence of human immunodeficiency virus (HIV) infection increases the risk that health care providers will be exposed to blood or other body fluids from HIV-infected patients. This is particularly true in emergency settings where life-threatening injuries and conditions necessitate immediate intervention and treatment. It is essential that all care givers in the emergency department consider all patients as potentially infected with blood-borne pathogens and strictly adhere to universal infection control precautions for minimizing exposure.

Psychological Management of Patients and Families in Emergencies and Crisis Situations

Approach to the Patient

Sudden illness or trauma is an insult to both physiologic and psychological homeostasis and requires both physiologic and psychological healing.

An assessment of the patient's psychological functioning includes evaluation of his emotional expression, degree of anxiety, and cognitive functioning (oriented to time, place, and person). In addition, a rapid physical examination, focusing on the clinical problem that caused the patient to seek help, is performed. The nursing diagnoses may include anxiety related to the uncertain potential outcomes of the illness or trauma and ineffective individual coping related to acute situational crisis. The first major goal is reduction of anxiety, which is prerequisite to recovering the ability to cope.

Interventions

Patients experiencing sudden injury or illness are often overwhelmed by anxiety, because they have not had time to mobilize their resources to adapt to the crisis. They experience real and terrifying fear—of death, mutilation, immobilization, and other assaults on their personal identity and body integrity. Those caring for the patient should act confidently and competently to help relieve anxiety. Speaking, reacting, and responding to the patient in a warm manner promote a sense of security. In addition, explanations should be given on a level that the patient can grasp; an informed patient is able to cope more positively with psychological and physical stress. Ongoing human contact helps reduce the panic of the severely injured person, and reassuring words aid in dispelling fear of the unknown. The emotionally distressed patient and family can more effectively mobilize their own psychological resources when the emergency department staff conveys optimism and concern for the welfare of the patient in a calm and reassuring manner.

If the patient is unconscious, he should be treated as if he were conscious: by touching him, calling him by name, and explaining every procedure that is being done. As soon as the patient regains consciousness, a primary concern is to orient him by stating his name, the date, and the place. If necessary, this basic information should be repeated over and over in a calm, reassuring way.

Approach to the Family

In the admitting area, the family is told where the patient is and is informed that he is receiving expert care. When crises of trauma, severe disfigurement, and sudden death are confronted, the family goes through several stages, beginning with anxiety and progressing through denial, remorse, grief, anger, and reconciliation. In addition to anxiety, the nursing diagnoses may include grieving and alterations in family processes related to acute situational crises.

The family members are encouraged to recognize and talk about their feelings of anxiety. The approach is to tune into the family's thinking and to deal with reality as gently and as quickly as possible. Although denial is an ego-defense mechanism that protects one from recognizing painful and disturbing aspects of reality, prolonged denial is not encouraged or supported, because the family must be prepared for the reality of what has happened and for what may come.

Expressions of remorse and guilt are frequently heard, with family members accusing themselves (or each other) of negligence or minor omissions. The nursing approach is to allow expressions of remorse, over and over if need be, until the family members realize that there was probably little that they could have done to prevent the accident or illness.

Expressions of anger are common in crisis situations; they are a way of handling the anxiety. The anger is frequently directed at the patient, but it is also often expressed toward the physician, the nurse, or admitting personnel. Without condemnation or rejection, the therapeutic approach is to allow the anger to be ventilated to help the family identify their feelings of frustration.

Grief is a complex emotional response to anticipated or actual loss. In this stage, the nursing intervention is to help family members work through their grief and to support their usual coping mechanisms, letting them know that it is normal and acceptable for them to cry and feel this way.

The following are guidelines for crisis intervention when helping a family deal with sudden death in the emergency department:

- Take the family to a private place.
- Talk to the family together, so that they can mourn together.
- Assure the family that everything possible was done; inform them of the treatment rendered.
- Avoid using euphemisms such as "passed on." Show the family that you care by touching, offering coffee, and so forth.
- Allow the family members to talk about the deceased and what he meant to them; this permits ventilation of feelings of loss. Encourage the family to talk about events preceding admission to the emergency department.
- Encourage family members to support each other and to express emotions freely (grief, loss, anger, helplessness, tears, disbelief).
- Avoid volunteering unnecessary information (*e.g.*, patient was drinking).
- Avoid giving sedation to family members; this may mask or delay the grieving process, which is necessary to achieve emotional equilibrium and to prevent prolonged depression.
- Encourage the family to view the body if they wish to do so; this action helps to integrate the loss. Cover mutilated areas before the family sees the body. Go with the family to see the body. Show acceptance of the body by touching, to give the family "permission" to touch.
- Spend a few minutes with the family, listening to them and identifying any needs that they may have for which the nursing staff can be helpful.

Posttraumatic Stress Disorder

Posttraumatic stress disorder is the development of characteristic symptoms after a psychologically stressful event that is generally outside the range of human experience (rape, combat, car accident, natural catastrophe). The symptoms of this disorder include intrusive thoughts and dreams, phobic avoidance reaction (avoidance of activities that arouse recollection of the traumatic event), heightened vigilance and exaggerated startle reaction, generalized anxiety, and social withdrawal. Posttraumatic stress disorder may be acute, chronic, or delayed.

Assessment includes an evaluation of the patient's pretrauma history, the trauma itself, and posttrauma functioning.

Interventions

The patient's goal is to organize and begin to integrate his experience to return to his pretrauma level of functioning as soon as possible. The nurse carries out a wide range of interventions including crisis intervention strategies, establishing a trusting and sharing relationship, and educating the patient and family about stress management and support services available in the community.

Priorities and Principles of Emergency Management

Priorities of Emergency Management

When care is being given to a patient in an emergency situation, many crucial decisions must be made. Such decisions require sound judgment based on an understanding of the condition that produced the emergency and its effect on the person.

The major goals of emergency medical treatment are (1) to preserve life, (2) to prevent deterioration before more definitive treatment can be given, and (3) to restore the patient to useful living.

When the patient is first received into the emergency department, the goal is to determine the extent of injury or illness and to establish priorities for the initiation of treatment. These priorities are determined by the comparative threat to the person's life. Injuries or conditions interfering with vital physiologic function (obstructed airway, massive bleeding) take precedence. Usually, injuries of the face, neck, and chest that impair respiration are the highest priorities. The members of the emergency team work together to provide comprehensive, individualized patient care.

Principles of Emergency Management

The following principles are applicable to the emergency management of any patient:

1. Maintain a patent airway and provide adequate ventilation, employing resuscitation measures when necessary. Assess for chest injuries with subsequent airway obstruction.
2. Control hemorrhage and its consequences.
3. Evaluate and restore cardiac output.
4. Prevent and treat shock; maintain or restore effective circulation.

5. Carry out a rapid initial and ongoing physical examination; the clinical course of the injured or seriously ill patient is not static.
6. Assess whether or not the patient can follow commands; evaluate the size and reactivity of the pupils and motor responses.
7. Start ECG monitoring if appropriate.
8. Splint suspected fractures, including fractures of the cervical spine in patients with head injuries.
9. Protect wounds with sterile dressings.
10. Check to see if the patient has a Medic-Alert tag or similar identification designating allergies and other health problems.
11. Start a flow sheet of the patient's vital signs, blood pressure, and neurologic status, to guide decision making.

Obtaining Data From the Patient

If possible, a brief history of the accident or illness is obtained from the patient or the person accompanying him to the emergency department. As part of the history, the following questions should be asked and the answers documented:

1. What were the circumstances, precipitating events, location, and time of the injury or illness?
2. When did the symptoms appear?
3. Was the patient unconscious after the accident?
4. How did the patient reach the hospital?
5. What was the health status of the patient before the accident or illness?
6. Is there a history of illness? of admissions to the hospital?
7. Is the patient currently taking any medications, especially hormones, insulin, digitalis, anticoagulants?
8. Does the patient have any allergies?
9. Does the patient have any bleeding tendencies?
10. When was the last meal eaten? (Important if an anesthetic is to be given.)
11. Is the patient under a physician's care? Name of physician?
12. What was the date of the patient's most recent tetanus immunization?

Recording of Data

Consent to examine and treat the patient is part of the emergency department record. Invasive procedures (*e.g.*, angiography, lumbar puncture) should be specifically consented to by the patient. If the patient is unconscious and brought to the emergency department without family or friends, this fact should be documented. Ongoing monitoring of the patient's condition and all treatment modalities instituted must be documented. After treatment, a notation is made on the record about the patient's condition on discharge or transfer and about the patient education instructions that are given for follow-up care.

Emergency Resuscitation Measures

The first priority in the treatment of any emergency condition is the establishment of the airway. If the airway is obstructed, the ensuing hypoxia produces permanent brain damage or death within 3 to 5 minutes, depending on the age of the patient.

- *Complete airway obstruction* is readily recognized: the patient suddenly stops breathing, becomes cyanotic, and becomes unconscious for no apparent reason.
- *Partial airway obstruction* that interferes with air flow produces an apprehensive appearance, inspiratory and expiratory stridor, labored use of accessory muscles (suprasternal and intercostal retraction), flaring nostrils, and progressive anxiety, restlessness, and confusion. Cyanosis of the earlobes and nail beds may be a late sign. Partial obstruction of the airway can produce progressive hypoxia and hypercarbia and can lead to respiratory and cardiac arrest.

Emergency Management of Airway Obstruction

1. Gently shake the victim and shout, "Are you okay?" to prevent injury from attempted resuscitation of a person who is not truly unconscious.
2. Place the patient supine on a firm, flat surface; if he is lying face down, turn his body as a unit so that the head, shoulders, and torso move simultaneously with no twisting.
3. Methods for opening the airway
   a. Head-tilt/chin-lift maneuver
      (1) Place one hand on the victim's forehead and apply firm backward pressure with the palm to tilt the head back.
      (2) Place the fingers of the other hand under the bony part of the lower jaw near the chin and lift, bringing the chin forward and the teeth almost to occlusion, thus supporting the jaw and helping to tilt the head back.
   b. Jaw-thrust maneuver: Grasp the angles of the victim's lower jaw and lift with both hands (one on each side), displacing the mandible forward while tilting the head backward. (This is a safe approach to opening the airway of a victim with suspected neck injury, because it can usually be accomplished without extending the neck.)
4. Remove any foreign body obstructing the airway.
5. Start cardiopulmonary resuscitation (CPR) immediately (see Chap. 29) to provide oxygen to the brain, heart, and other vital organs until definitive medical treatment can restore normal heart and ventilatory action. (CPR consists of establishing an effective airway and providing artificial ventilation and external cardiac compression.)

Airway management is discussed in detail in Chapter 25.

Management of Foreign Body Upper Airway Obstruction

Obstruction of the upper airway by food ("café coronary") is a cause of unconsciousness and cardiopulmonary arrest. Foreign bodies may cause either partial or complete airway obstruction. In adults, a piece of meat is the most common cause of obstruction. Factors associated with choking on food include large, poorly chewed pieces of food, alcohol consumption, and the presence of upper or lower dentures.

Assessment reveals that the victim is unable to speak, breathe, or cough. He may clutch his neck between the thumb and fingers (universal distress signal). The first response to this person should be to ask if he is choking.

Emergency Management

For partial obstruction (if patient is breathing and able to cough spontaneously):

1. Encourage the victim to cough forcefully; there may be some wheezing between coughs.
2. Continue to encourage the victim to persist with spontaneous coughing and breathing efforts as long as good air exchange persists.
3. If patient demonstrates a weak, ineffective cough, high-pitched noise while inhaling, increased respiratory difficulty, and possibly cyanosis, he is managed as if it were complete airway obstruction.

For complete obstruction, see Chart 63-1 for management of foreign body airway obstruction.

Gerontologic Considerations

In extended care facilities, sedatives and hypnotic drugs as well as diseases affecting motor coordination (Parkinson's disease) and mental functioning (senility, mental retardation) are risk factors for asphyxiation by food. Nursing staff involved in the care of elderly patients must be acutely aware of the symptoms of upper airway obstruction; skill in performing the Heimlich maneuver is essential.

Methods for Providing a Patent Airway

Insertion of an Oropharyngeal Airway

An oropharyngeal airway is a semicircular-shaped tube or tubelike device of plastic or rubber that is inserted over the back of the tongue into the lower posterior pharynx in a spontaneously breathing, unconscious patient; it prevents the tongue from falling back against the posterior pharynx and obstructing the airway, and it allows for suctioning of secretions.

Guidelines for Insertion of an Oropharyngeal Airway

1. Extend the patient's head by placing one hand beneath the neck close to the occiput and gently lifting the neck; simultaneously, with the other hand, tilt the head backward by applying pressure on the forehead.
2. Open the patient's mouth.
3. Insert the oropharyngeal airway with the tip facing up toward the roof of the mouth until it passes the uvula; then rotate the tip 180 degrees so that the tip is pointed down toward the pharynx (Fig. 63-1).
4. The distal end of the oropharyngeal airway is in the hypopharynx, and the flange is approximately at the patient's lips; make sure that the tongue has not been pushed into the airway.

Insertion of an Esophageal Obturator Airway

The esophageal obturator airway (EOA) is a ventilatory device used in respiratory emergencies for resuscitation. Its primary use is in prehospital care. It consists of (1) a face mask to seal off the nose and mouth and anchor the airway, (2) a flexible tube with openings at the level of the pharynx to permit ventilation of the lungs, and (3) a balloon on the distal end of the

tube to block the esophagus, thus reducing the possibility of aspirating gastric contents. The purpose of the EOA is to ventilate the apneic, unconscious patient when endotracheal intubation is not possible.

The tube is inserted through the mouth and advanced into the esophagus just below the bifurcation of the trachea. The proximal part of the tube has air holes at the level of the pharynx through which air or oxygen is blown into the lungs.

The esophageal gastric tube airway (EGTA) (Fig. 63-2) is a modification of the EOA. It has a central lumen that permits passage of a nasogastric tube so that suctioning of the stomach can be accomplished without interfering with ventilation.

Guidelines for Insertion of an EOA. This procedure is contraindicated in conscious or semiconscious patients and in those with corrosive poisoning, esophageal disease, or a foreign body in the trachea.

The required equipment is an EOA, a 50-ml syringe, water-soluble gel, and a manual resuscitation bag with mask. The procedure is as follows:

1. Inflate the cuff to make sure it assumes a symmetric shape and holds air volume without leakage; then maximally deflate the cuff.
2. Lubricate the tube and attach the face mask to the tube by the snap lock.
3. Place the patient's head in a neutral position.
4. Using the left hand, insert the thumb as deeply as possible over the back of the patient's tongue, pulling on it while using the fingers to lift the jaw upward and away from the posterior pharyngeal wall.
5. Insert the EOA tip into the mouth, carefully guiding the tube over the tongue and past the pharynx; rotate the tube 180 degrees into the esophagus.
6. Stop advancing the tube when the mask reaches the face; press the mask firmly against the face.
7. Ventilate the patient by using manual resuscitator. *If the tube is correctly positioned in the esophagus, the chest will rise.*
8. If the chest does not rise or no breath sounds are heard, the airway is possibly blocking the trachea; remove airway. Continue ventilating the patient (by bag-mask ventilation) and prepare for and proceed with second attempt at insertion.
9. Auscultate over both lung fields to check that *both* lungs are receiving adequate ventilation and that the EOA is in the esophagus and *not* in the trachea.
10. Inflate the cuff (balloon) with about 20 ml of air. Inflating the cuff results in occlusion of the esophagus, minimizes the incidence of regurgitation, and prevents air leakage.
11. Connect the end of the EOA to a bag-mask or mechanical ventilator, and continue ventilating the patient.
12. Do not remove the EOA until the patient regains consciousness or has a gag reflex, or until endotracheal intubation has been accomplished. The EOA tube must be deflated before it is removed. If the tube is taken out prematurely, regurgitation and aspiration are almost inevitable.
13. To remove the tube: Have suction available. Turn the patient's head to the side; deflate the cuff and remove the tube.

Emergency Endotracheal Procedures

Endotracheal Intubation. The purpose of endotracheal intubation is to establish and maintain the airway in patients with respiratory insufficiency or hypoxia. Endotracheal intubation is indicated for the following reasons: (1) to establish

Chart 63–1
Guidelines: Management of Foreign Body Airway Obstruction

Action	Rationale/Amplification
Assess for Airway Obstruction	Air movement is absent in the presence of *complete airway obstruction*. Oxygen saturation in the blood decreases rapidly because the obstructed airway prevents entry of air into the lungs. Thus, oxygen deficit occurs in the brain, resulting in unconsciousness, with death following rapidly.
Victim may clutch his neck between his thumb and fingers. Weak, ineffective cough; high-pitched noises on inspiration. Increased respiratory distress. Inability to speak, breathe, or cough. Collapse.	
Heimlich Maneuver (subdiaphragmatic abdominal thrusts)	The term *Heimlich maneuver* is used for the sake of uniformity. The terms *subdiaphragmatic abdominal thrusts* and *abdominal thrusts* are used interchangeably, depending on the circumstances.
For Standing or Sitting Conscious Patient	
1. Stand behind the patient; wrap your arms around his waist and proceed as follows:	
2. Make a fist with one hand, placing the thumb side of the fist against the patient's abdomen, in the midline slightly above the naval and well below the xiphoid process. Grasp the fist with the other hand.	
3. Press your fist into the patient's abdomen with a quick upward thrust. Each new thrust should be a separate and distinct maneuver.	A subdiaphragmatic abdominal thrust, by elevating the diaphragm, can force air from the lungs to create an artificial cough intended to move and expel an obstructing foreign body in the airway.
With Patient Lying (Unconscious)	
1. Position patient on his back.	
2. Kneel astride the patient's thigh, facing his head.	
3. Place the heel of one hand against the patient's abdomen, in the midline slightly above the navel and well below the tip of the xiphoid; place the second hand directly on top of the first.	
4. Press into the abdomen with a quick upward thrust.	
Finger Sweep	
1. Open patient's mouth by grasping both the tongue and lower jaw between the thumb and fingers and lifting the mandible (tongue–jaw lift).	This maneuver is to be used *only in the unconscious patient*. This action draws the tongue away from the back of the throat and away from the foreign body that may be lodged there.
2. Insert the index finger of the other hand down along the inside of the cheek and deeply into the throat to the base of the tongue.	
3. Use a hooking action to dislodge the foreign body and maneuver it into the mouth for removal.	Use care not to force the object deeper into the throat.
Chest Thrusts With Conscious Patient Standing or Sitting	
1. Stand behind patient with arms under patient's axillae to encircle patient's chest.	This technique is to be used *only in the advanced stages of pregnancy or in the markedly obese person.*
2. Place thumb side of your fist on middle of patient's sternum, taking care to avoid xiphoid process and margins of rib cage.	
3. Grasp your fist with the other hand and perform backward thrusts until the foreign body is expelled or patient becomes unconscious.	Each thrust should be administered with the intent of relieving the obstruction.
Chest Thrust With Patient Lying (Unconscious)	
1. Place the patient on his back and kneel close to the side of his body.	This maneuver is used *only in the advanced stages of pregnancy or when the rescuer cannot apply the Heimlich maneuver effectively to the unconscious, markedly obese person.*
2. Place the heel of your hand on the lower half of the sternum.	
3. Deliver each chest thrust slowly and distinctly with the intent of relieving the obstruction.	

(Adapted from Healthcare Provider's Manual for Basic Life Support. Dallas, American Heart Association, 1988.)

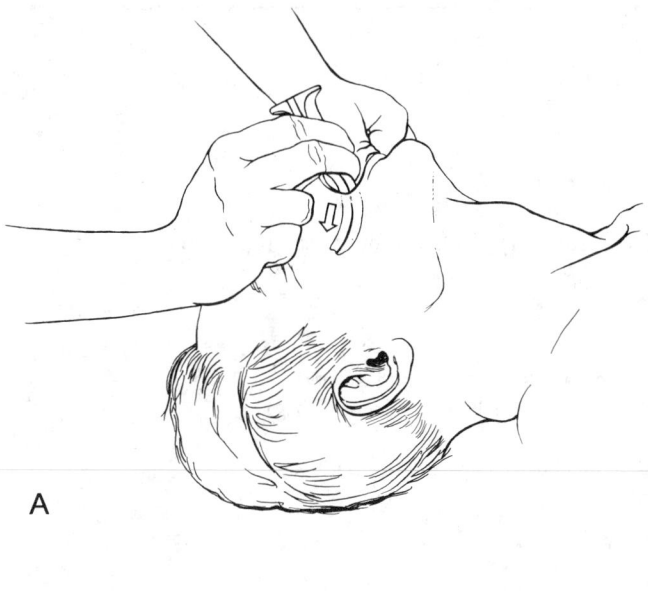

A

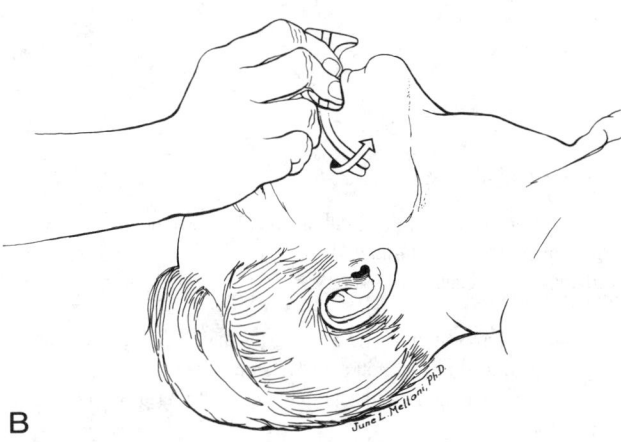

B

Figure 63-1. Insertion of an oropharyngeal airway. (**A**) Place the airway in the mouth of the unconscious patient with the tip pointing up. (**B**) Rotate the airway 180 degrees, pointing the tip down toward the pharynx. This displaces the tongue anteriorly, and the patient then breathes through and around the airway.

an airway for patients who cannot be adequately ventilated with an oropharyngeal airway, (2) to bypass an upper airway obstruction, (3) to prevent aspiration, (4) to permit connection of the patient to a resuscitation bag or mechanical ventilator, and (5) to facilitate the removal of tracheobronchial secretions.

Because the procedure requires skill, endotracheal intubation may be performed only by those who have had intensive training in which they have practiced the technique on a mannequin. It should be performed under expert clinical supervision.

Details for emergency endotracheal intubation are outlined in Chart 63-2 and Figure 63-3.

Cricothyroidotomy (Cricothyroid Membrane Puncture)

Cricothyroidotomy is the puncture or incision of the cricothyroid membrane to establish an airway. This procedure is used in certain emergency situations in which endotracheal intubation and tracheostomy are either not possible or contraindicated, as in airway obstruction from extensive maxillofacial trauma, cervical spine injuries, laryngospasm, laryngeal edema (after an allergic reaction), hemorrhage into neck tissue, or obstruction of the larynx.

Emergency Medical Management

1. With the patient in a supine position, extend the neck so that the cricothyroid membrane can be palpated readily. Place a towel roll beneath the shoulders.
2. Identify the prominent thyroid cartilage (Adam's apple) as shown in Figure 63-4, and allow your finger to descend in the midline to the depression between the lower border of the thyroid cartilage and the upper border of the cricoid cartilage. This depression represents the cricothyroid membrane.
3. Insert a needle or any sharp instrument at a 10- to 20-degree caudal direction in the midline just above the upper part of the cricoid cartilage.
   a. Listen for air passing back and forth through the needle synchronously with the patient's respiration.
   b. Direct the needle downward and posteriorly.
   c. Tape the needle with adhesive for stability.
4. After the patient is stabilized, a more permanent means of ventilatory support is implemented; prepare for endotracheal intubation or tracheostomy.
5. Monitor for potential complications: vocal cord injury, subcutaneous emphysema, bleeding, aspiration.

Special Resuscitation Situation: Near-Drowning

Near-drowning is survival for at least some period of time after suffocation from submersion in water.

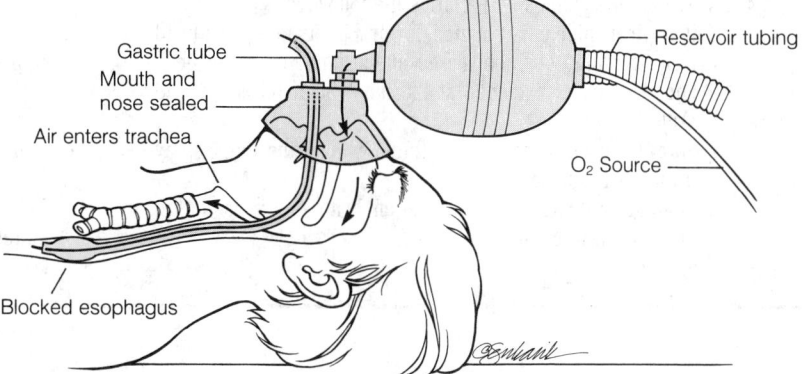

Figure 63-2. The esophageal gastric tube airway (EGTA), a modification of the esophageal obturator airway.

Chart 63–2
Assisting With Emergency Endotracheal Intubation

Clinical Indications for Intubation

1. Respiratory arrest
2. Respiratory insufficiency—marked respiratory effort, substernal retraction, nostril flaring, increasing or decreasing pulse rate, increasing or decreasing respiratory rate, changing color (*cyanosis is a late sign*)
3. Airway obstruction (asphyxia)

Equipment

1. Laryngoscope with curved and straight blades and working light source (check batteries and bulb regularly)
2. Endotracheal tubes with low-pressure cuffs (to seal airway) and adapter (to connect tube to ventilator or bag)
3. Stylet to guide endotracheal tube
4. Oral airway (assorted sizes) or bite block (to keep patient from biting into and occluding endotracheal tube)
5. Adhesive tape or tube fixation system
6. Sterile anesthetic lubricant jelly (water-soluble)
7. Syringe
8. Suction source
9. Resuscitation bag and mask connected to oxygen source
10. Anesthetic spray
11. Sterile towel
12. Gloves
13. Goggles or other eye protection

Action	Rationale/Amplification
1. Remove the patient's dental bridgework and plates.	1. May interfere with insertion; will not be able to remove dentures easily once patient is intubated.
2. Remove headboard of bed (optional).	2. Provides easy access to the head.
3. Prepare equipment.	
a. Ensure function of resuscitation bag and mask, and suction.	3. a. Patient may require ventilatory assistance prior to and/or during procedure. Suction apparatus must be readily available, because gagging and emesis may occur during procedure.
b. Assemble the laryngoscope; make sure the lightbulb is tightly attached and functional.	
c. Select an endotracheal tube of the appropriate size (6–9 mm for average adult).	
d. Place the endotracheal tube on a sterile towel.	d. Although the tube will pass through the contaminated mouth or nose, the airway below the vocal cords is sterile, and efforts must be made to prevent iatrogenic contamination of the distal end of the tube and cuff. The proximal end of the tube may be handled, because it will reside in the upper airway.
e. Inflate the cuff to make sure it assumes a symmetric shape and holds volume without leakage. Then deflate maximally.	e. Malfunction of the cuff must be ascertained *before* tube placement occurs.
f. Lubricate the distal end of tube liberally with the sterile anesthetic water-soluble jelly.	f. Aids in insertion.
g. Insert the stylet into the tube (if oral intubation is planned; nasal intubation does not employ use of the stylet).	g. Stiffens the soft tube, allowing it to be more easily directed into the trachea.
4. Assist the physician as he performs the following:	
a. If cervical spine is not injured, for oral intubation place head in a "sniffing" position: flexed at the junction of the neck and thorax and extended at the junction of the spine and skull.	4. a. Upper airway is open maximally in this position and mouth of the unconscious patient will often open.
b. Spray the back of the patient's throat with an anesthetic spray if time is available.	b. This will decrease gagging.
c. Ventilate and oxygenate the patient with the resuscitation bag and mask before intubation.	c. This decreases the likelihood of cardiac dysrhythmias or respiratory distress secondary to hypoxemia.

(continued)

Chart 63–2 *(Continued)*

Action	*Rationale/Amplification*
d. Hold the handle of the laryngoscope in the left hand and hold the patient's mouth open with the right hand by placing crossed fingers on the teeth.	d. Leverage is improved by crossing the thumb and index fingers when opening the patient's mouth (scissor-twist technique).
e. Insert the curved blade of the laryngoscope along the right side of the tongue, push the tongue to the left, and use right thumb and index finger to pull patient's lower lip away from lower teeth.	e. Rolling the lip away from teeth prevents injury from the lips being caught between teeth and blade.
f. Lift laryngoscope forward (toward ceiling) to expose the epiglottis.	f. Do not use teeth as a fulcrum; this could lead to dental damage.
g. Lift laryngoscope upward and forward at a 45-degree angle to expose glottis and visualize vocal cords.	g. This stretches the hypoepiglottis ligament, folding the epiglottis upward and exposing the glottis.
h. As the epiglottis is lifted forward (toward ceiling), the vertical opening of the larynx between the vocal cords will come into view.	h. Do not use wrist; use shoulder and arm to lift epiglottis.
i. Once vocal cords are visualized, insert tube into the right corner of the mouth and pass the tube—guided by blade, but keeping vocal cords in constant view.	i. Make sure you do not insert tube into esophagus; the esophageal mucosa is pink and the opening is horizontal rather than vertical.
j. Gently push the tube through the triangular space formed by the vocal cords and back wall of trachea.	j. If the vocal cords are in spasm (closed), wait a few seconds before passing tube.
k. Stop insertion just after the tube cuff has disappeared from view beyond the cords.	k. Advancing tube further may lead to its entry into a main-stem bronchus (usually the right bronchus), causing collapse of the unventilated lung.
l. Withdraw laryngoscope while holding endotracheal tube in place. Disassemble mask from resuscitation bag and ventilate the patient.	l. Provides for resumption of oxygenation of the patient.
m. Inflate cuff with the minimal amount of air required to occlude the trachea.	m. The amount of air used for cuff inflation depends on the size of the cuff and the diameter of the patient's trachea. Occlusion occurs when no air is felt or heard passing through the patient's nose or mouth.
n. Insert oral airway or bite block if necessary.	n. This keeps patient from biting down on the tube and obstructing the airway.
o. Ascertain expansion of both sides of the chest by observation and auscultation of breath sounds.	o. Observation and auscultation help in determining that tube remains in position and has not slipped into the right mainstem bronchus.
p. Mark proximal end of tube with marking pen or tape at the point where the tube reaches the corner of the patient's mouth.	p. This allows for detection of any later change in tube position.
q. Secure tube to the patient's face with adhesive tape or apply a commercially available endotracheal tube stabilization device.	q. The tube must be fixed securely to ensure that it will not be dislodged. Dislodgement of a tube with an inflated cuff may result in damage to the vocal cords.
r. Obtain chest radiograph.	r. Verifies correct position of tube.
s. Measure cuff pressure with manometer; adjust pressure. Make adjustment in tube placement on the basis of chest x-ray results.	s. The tube may be advanced or removed several centimeters for proper placement on the basis of the chest x-ray result.
t. Record tube type and size, cuff pressure, and patient tolerance of the procedure. Auscultate breath sounds every 1 to 2 hours or if signs and symptoms of respiratory distress occur. Assess arterial blood gases after intubation if requested by physician.	t. Arterial blood gases may be prescribed to ensure adequacy of ventilation and respiration. Tube displacement outward may result in extubation (cuff above vocal cords). Tube displacement forward may result in tube touching carina (causing paroxysmal coughing) or intubation of a main-stem bronchus (resulting in collapse of the unventilated lung).

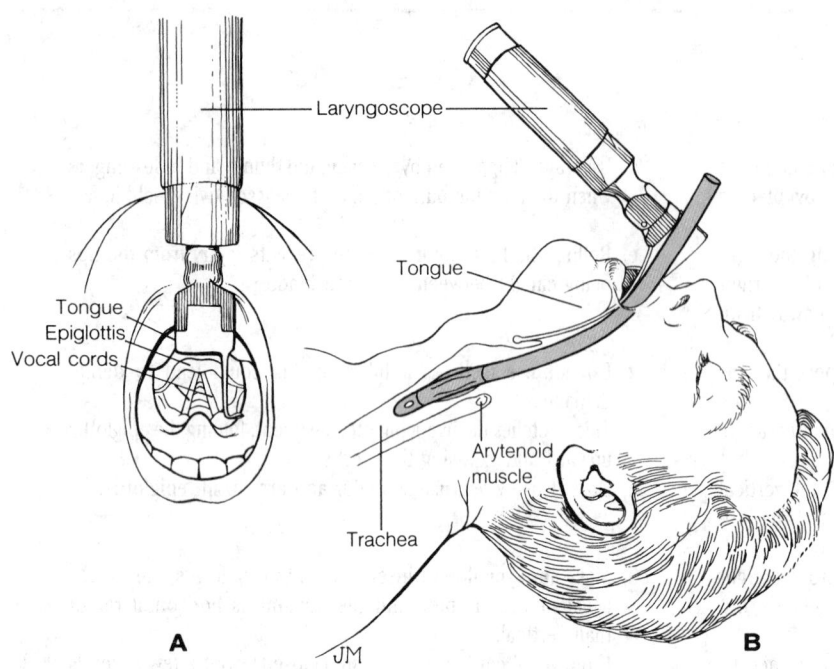

A

B

Figure 63–3. Endotracheal intubation. (**A**) The primary glottic landmarks for tracheal intubation as visualized with proper placement of the laryngoscope. (**B**) Positioning the endotracheal tube. (Suddarth DS. The Lippincott Manual of Nursing Practice, 5th ed. Philadelphia, JB Lippincott, 1991.)

Drowning is one of the three leading causes of accidental death; an estimated 9,000 fatalities from drowning and 80,000 near-drownings occur yearly in the United States. Factors associated with drowning and near-drowning include alcohol ingestion, inability to swim, diving injuries, hypothermia, and exhaustion. Efforts to save the victim should not be abandoned too soon, because successful resuscitation with full neurologic recovery has occurred in near-drowning victims with prolonged submersion in cold water.

After resuscitation, the primary problems of a victim who has nearly drowned are hypoxia and acidosis, which require immediate intervention in the emergency department. The resultant pathophysiologic changes and pulmonary injury depend on the type of fluid (fresh water or salt water) and the volume

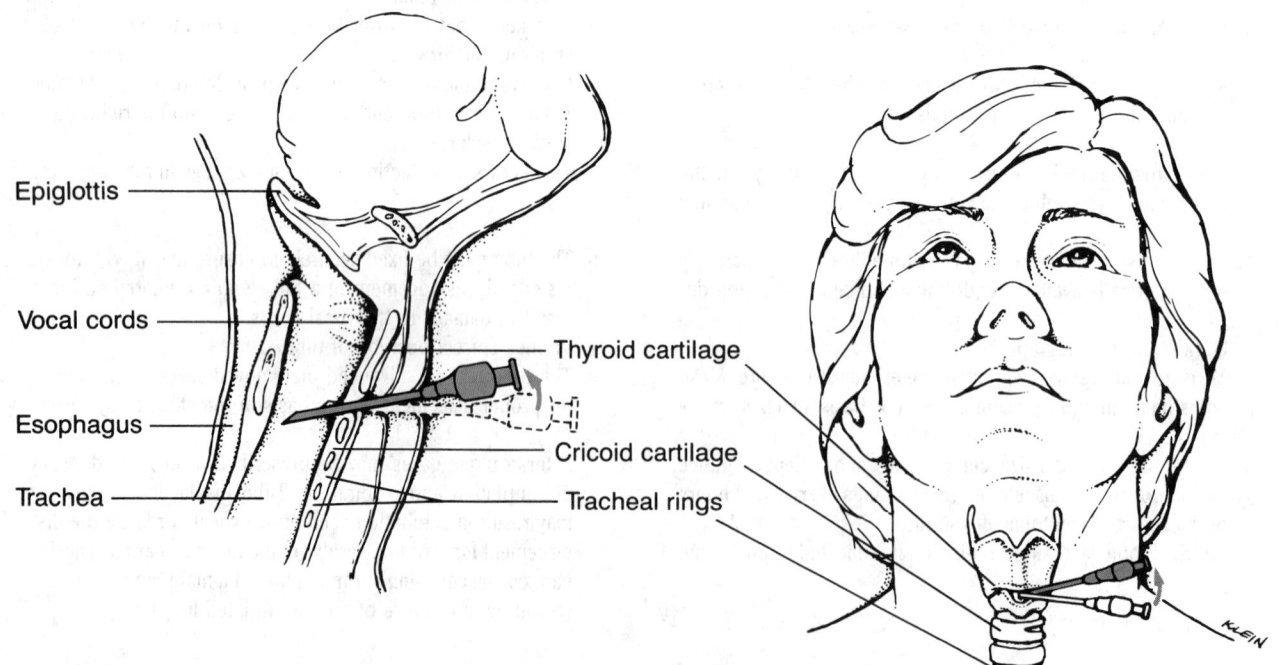

Figure 63–4. Cricothyroidotomy (cricothyroid membrane puncture) is the puncture or incision of the cricothyroid membrane to establish an emergency airway. The needle is inserted at a 10- to 30-degree angle, caudal direction, in the midline just above the upper part of the cricoid cartilage. The cricothyroid membrane is an accessible route for the establishment of an emergency airway in a minimal amount of time. This procedure is generally reserved for patients in whom intubation cannot be safely accomplished.

of aspiration. When water has been aspirated, alterations of pulmonary function may be anticipated. After a person has survived immersion, acute adult respiratory distress syndrome with hypoxia, hypercarbia, and respiratory or metabolic acidosis can occur.

Emergency Management in the Emergency Department. Therapy is aimed at maintaining cerebral perfusion and adequate oxygenation to prevent further damage to vital organs.

1. Ensure adequacy of the airway, respiration, and peripheral perfusion.
    a. Use a rectal probe to determine the degree of hypothermia if the patient has been submerged in cold water.
    b. Start rewarming procedures during resuscitation as prescribed (extracorporeal warming, warmed peritoneal dialysis, inhalation of warm aerosolized oxygen, surface warming); the choice is determined by the severity and duration of hypothermia and available resources.
2. Draw arterial blood to evaluate oxygen and carbon dioxide tensions, *p*H, and bicarbonate levels; these parameters determine the type of ventilatory support required and the subsequent dosage of sodium bicarbonate to be given.
    • Hypotension and impaired tissue perfusion are managed by intravascular volume expansion and inotropic agents.
3. Improve ventilation and oxygenation. Assist with endotracheal intubation with positive pressure ventilation (with positive end expiratory pressure [PEEP]) to improve oxygenation, to prevent aspiration and to correct intrapulmonary shunting and ventilation–perfusion abnormalities (caused by aspiration of water). Continue with supplemental oxygen by way of a mask (if patient is breathing spontaneously) or with an endotracheal tube (if patient is not breathing spontaneously).
    • Respiratory acidosis is managed by improving ventilation.
4. Initiate ECG monitoring, because dysrhythmias occur frequently.
5. Assist with nasogastric intubation to empty the stomach, to prevent the patient from regurgitating gastric contents.
6. Continue to monitor the patient closely: vital signs, serial arterial blood gas values, *p*H, ECG, intracranial pressure, serum electrolytes, serial chest radiographs.
7. Insert an indwelling catheter to determine urinary output; metabolic acidosis may compromise renal function.
8. The patient is admitted to an ICU; the appearance of the patient may be deceptive. Complications of near-drowning that can lead to death include the following:
    a. Hypoxic or ischemic cerebral injury.
    b. Acute respiratory distress syndrome and pulmonary damage secondary to aspiration.
    c. Cardiac arrest.

Control of Hemorrhage Due to Trauma

One of the primary causes of shock is the reduction in circulating blood volume. Only a few conditions, such as obstructed airway or a sucking wound of the chest, take precedence over the immediate control of hemorrhage. Stopping the bleeding is essential to the care and the survival of patients in an emergency or a disaster situation. However, minor bleeding, which is usually venous, generally stops spontaneously unless the patient has a bleeding disorder.

The patient is assessed for cool, moist skin (resulting from poor peripheral perfusion), falling blood pressure, increasing heart rate, and decreasing urine volume. The nursing diagnoses may include fluid volume deficit, decreased cardiac output, and altered tissue perfusion. The goals of emergency management are to control the bleeding, maintain an adequately circulating blood volume for tissue oxygenation, and prevent shock. The nursing interventions are carried out collaboratively with other members of the health care team.

Emergency Management
1. Cut the patient's clothing away quickly to identify the area of hemorrhage, and carry out a rapid physical assessment.
2. Apply direct, firm pressure over the bleeding area or the artery involved (Fig. 63-5). Almost all bleeding can be stopped by direct pressure (except when a major artery has been severed). Unchecked arterial bleeding produces death.
3. Apply a firm pressure dressing. Elevate the injured part to stop venous and capillary bleeding. Immobilize an injured extremity to control blood loss.
4. Insert a large-bore needle or intravenous (IV) cannula to provide a means for fluid and blood replacement.
    a. Withdraw blood samples for analysis, typing, and cross-matching.
    b. Administer replacement fluids as prescribed, including isotonic electrolyte solutions, plasma or plasma protein fractions, or blood component therapy (depending on clinical estimates of the type and volume of fluid lost).
        (1) Fresh blood is infused when there is massive blood loss.
        (2) Additional platelets and clotting factors are given when large amounts of blood are needed, since replacement blood is deficient in clotting factors.
        (3) The blood may be warmed, using a commercial warmer or basin of warm water (massive blood replacement has a cooling effect that can cause cardiac arrest).
        (4) The rate of infusion depends on the severity of blood loss and clinical evidence of hypovolemia.
5. Take the following steps for internal bleeding:
    a. Suspect internal bleeding in patients with hypovolemic shock with no external signs of bleeding: tachycardia rising pulse rate; falling blood pressure; thirst; apprehension; cool, moist skin.
    b. Administer whole blood or plasma expanders as prescribed at the rate of blood loss.
    c. Apply an antishock garment (pneumatic counterpressure device), if available, to control internal bleeding and to facilitate the blood flow to vital areas (Fig. 63-6). (Its primary use is for hypovolemic shock secondary to bleeding in the lower part of the body.) Deflate the device in the emergency department after sufficient volume expansion in a controlled environment.
    d. Prepare the patient immediately for surgical intervention.
    e. Monitor the patient's hemodynamic responses.
    f. Obtain arterial blood for blood gas determination; establish hemodynamic pressure monitoring as an index of the amount of fluid the patient can tolerate.
    g. Maintain patient in supine position until hemodynamic or circulatory parameters improve.
6. Apply a tourniquet on an extremity only as a *last resort*, when the hemorrhage cannot be controlled by any other method.

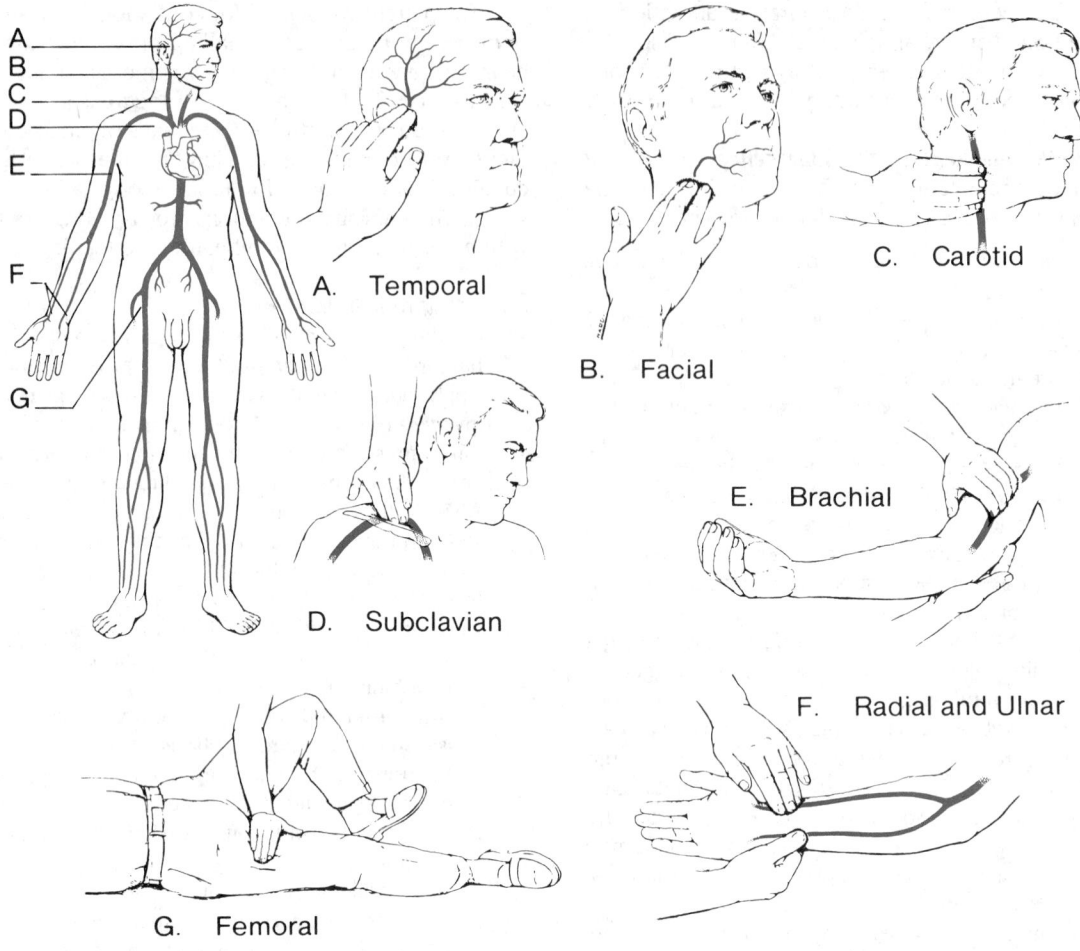

Figure 63–5. Pressure points for control of hemorrhage.

Anticipate loss of an extremity if a tourniquet is applied.

a. Apply the tourniquet just proximal to the wound; tie it tightly enough to control the arterial blood flow.

b. Tag the patient with a skin-marking pencil or on adhesive tape on his forehead with a T, stating the location of the tourniquet and the time applied.

c. Loosen the tourniquet as directed to prevent irreparable vascular or neurologic damage if the patient is in an emergency facility. If there is no arterial bleeding, remove the tourniquet and again try a pressure dressing.

d. In the event of a traumatic amputation, leave the tourniquet applied until the patient is in the operating room.

7. Observe for cardiac arrest; patients who hemorrhage are candidates for cardiac arrest caused by hypovolemia with secondary anoxia.

8. See p. 462 for further discussion of hemorrhage.

Control of Hypovolemic Shock

Shock is a condition in which there is loss of effective circulating blood volume. Inadequate organ and tissue perfusion results,

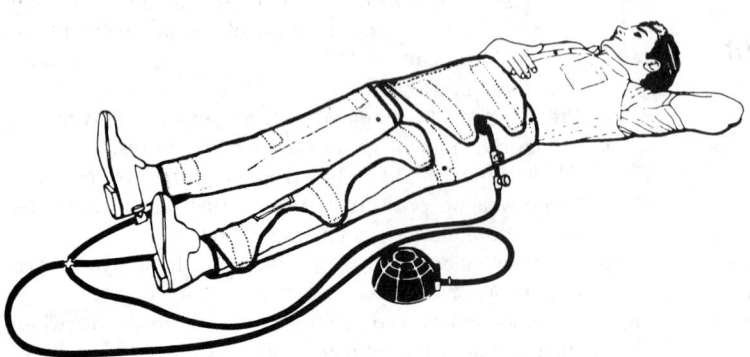

Figure 63–6. The medical antishock trouser (MAST) is a garment designed to correct internal bleeding and hypovolemia by the application of counterpressure around the legs and abdomen. This creates an artificial peripheral resistance and helps sustain coronary perfusion. It should be applied as soon as possible after injury, preferably before the patient is transferred to the emergency department. (Courtesy of David Clark Co, Inc, Worcester, MA.)

ultimately causing cellular metabolic derangements. In any emergency situation, it is wise to anticipate shock before it develops. Any injured person should be assessed immediately to determine the presence of shock. Its underlying cause must be discovered (hypovolemic, cardiogenic, neurogenic, or septic shock). Hypovolemia is the most common cause of shock (see pp. 457–462).

Assess for the following signs and symptoms, which in varying combinations indicate that the patient is in some degree of hypovolemic shock: decreasing arterial pressure; increasing pulse rate; cold, moist skin; pallor; thirst; diaphoresis; altered sensorium; oliguria; metabolic acidosis; and hyperpnea. Of these, the most dependable criterion is the level of arterial blood pressure.

The nursing diagnoses may include altered tissue perfusion related to failing circulation; impaired gas exchange related to ventilation–perfusion imbalance; altered urinary elimination (oliguria or anuria) related to decreased renal perfusion; and decreased cardiac output related to decreased circulating blood volume.

The goals of treatment are to restore and maintain tissue perfusion and to correct physiologic abnormalities.

Emergency Management

1. Ensure a patent airway and maintain breathing and circulation. Give additional ventilatory assistance as required.
2. Restore the circulating blood volume with rapid fluid and blood replacement as prescribed to optimize cardiac preload, correct hypotension, and maintain tissue perfusion.
   a. A central venous pressure catheter is inserted in or near the right atrium to serve as a guide for fluid replacement. Continuous central venous pressure (CVP) readings give the direction and degree of change from baseline readings; the catheter also is a vehicle for emergency fluid volume replacement.
   b. Large-gauge IV needles or catheters are inserted into peripheral veins. Two or more catheters may be necessary for rapid fluid replacement and reversal of hemodynamic instability; the emphasis is on volume replacement.
      (1) Establish IV lines in both upper and lower extremities if there is suspicion that a major vessel in the chest or abdomen has been disrupted.
      (2) Withdraw blood for specimens: arterial blood gases, chemistry studies, typing and cross-matching, and hematocrit.
3. Start IV infusion at a rapid rate until CVP rises to a satisfactory level above the baseline measurement or until there is improvement in the patient's clinical condition.
   a. Infusion of lactated Ringer's solution is useful initially, since it approximates plasma electrolyte composition and osmolality, allows time for blood typing and cross-matching, restores circulation, and serves as an adjunct to blood component therapy.
   b. Start transfusion of blood component therapy as prescribed, especially when blood loss has been severe or when the patient continues to hemorrhage.
   c. Control hemorrhage; hemorrhage compounds the shock state. Carry out serial hematocrit examinations if continued bleeding is suspected.
   d. Maintain the systolic blood pressure at a satisfactory level by administering fluids and blood as prescribed.
4. Insert an indwelling urinary catheter; record urinary output every 15 to 30 minutes. Urinary volume reveals adequacy of kidney perfusion.
5. Carry out a rapid physical assessment to determine the cause of shock.
6. Maintain ongoing nursing surveillance of the *total patient*—blood pressure, heart and respiratory rates, skin temperature, color, CVP, arterial blood gases, ECG, hematocrit, hemoglobin, coagulation profile, electrolytes, and urinary output—to assess patient response to treatment. Keep a flow sheet of these parameters; trend analysis reveals improvement or deterioration of patient.
7. Elevate the feet slightly to improve cerebral circulation and promote return of venous blood to the heart. (*This position is contraindicated in patients with head injuries.*) Avoid unnecessary movement.
8. Give specific pharmacologic agents as prescribed (*e.g.*, inotropic drugs such as dopamine) to improve cardiovascular performance.
9. Support the defense mechanisms of the body.
   a. Reassure and comfort the patient; sedation may be necessary to relieve apprehension.
   b. Relieve pain by *cautious* use of analgesics or narcotics.
   c. Maintain the body temperature.
      (1) Too much heat produces vasodilation, which counteracts the body's compensatory mechanisms of vasoconstriction and also increases fluid loss by perspiration.
      (2) A patient who is in septic shock should be kept cool, because high fever increases the cellular metabolic effects of shock.

Wounds

Wounds (injury to tissues) vary from minor lacerations to severe crushing injuries. Life-threatening problems, such as airway obstruction, hemorrhage, and shock, must be dealt with before the wound is treated.

Assessment

1. Determine *when* as well as *how* the wound occurred; a delay in treatment of more than 3 hours increases the risk of infection.
2. Inspect the wound, using aseptic technique, to determine the extent of damage to underlying structures.
3. Assess for sensory, motor, or vascular complications.

The nursing diagnoses may include impaired skin integrity (puncture wound, laceration) related to injury and high risk for infection.

The patient's goal is restoration of the physical integrity and function of the injured tissue without the development of infection and with minimal scarring.

Emergency Management

1. Clip hairs or shave around the wound (with the exception of eyebrows) only if directed (this is done when it is anticipated that hairs will interfere with wound closure).
2. Cleanse around the wound with prescribed agent. Do not allow the cleansing solution to get into the wound, since it may be injurious to exposed tissues.

3. The area is infiltrated with a local anesthetic intradermally through the wound margins or by regional block. (Patients with soft tissue injuries usually have pain localized at the site of injury.)
4. Assist the physician to cleanse and débride the wound.
   a. Irrigate gently and copiously with isotonic sterile saline to remove surface dirt.
   b. Remove devitalized tissue and foreign matter, which impair the wound's ability to resist infection.
   c. Clamp and tie small bleeding vessels, or achieve hemostasis with a cautery.
5. Suture the wound (usually done by the physician) if primary closure is indicated. (This depends on the nature of the wound, the time since the injury was sustained, the degree of contamination, and the vascularity of tissues.)
   a. Subcutaneous fat is approximated loosely with a few sutures to close off the dead space.
   b. The subcuticular layer is then closed.
   c. The epidermis is closed; sutures are placed close to the wound edge with the skin edges leveled carefully to promote optimal healing.
   d. Sterile strips of reinforced microporous tape may be used to close clean, superficial wounds.
6. Apply nonadherent dressing to protect the wound. (The dressing may serve as a splint and as a reminder to the patient that he has sustained an injury.)
7. For delayed primary closure:
   a. A thin layer of gauze (to ensure drainage and prevent pooling of exudate) covered by an occlusive dressing may be used, or split-thickness cadaver or porcine xenografts may be used since they simulate the function of epithelium.
   b. Splint the wound in a position of rest to prevent motion.
   c. The wound is closed (using local anesthesia) when there are no signs of suppuration.
8. Administer antimicrobial treatment as prescribed. (Use of antibiotics depends on how the injury occurred, the age of the wound, the presence of soil-infection potential, and so forth.)
9. Immobilize the site if the wound is contaminated; elevate the site to limit accumulation of fluid in wound interstitial spaces.
10. Give tetanus prophylaxis as prescribed, based on the condition of the wound and the patient's immunization status.
11. Inform the patient to contact the physician or clinic if there is sudden or persistent pain, fever or chills, bleeding, rapid swelling, foul odor, drainage, or redness surrounding the wound.

In summary, the patient experiencing a life-threatening condition is a priority in emergency nursing. Because patients can present with a variety of signs and symptoms, emergency department nurses must have sharply refined skills of observation and assessment. The nursing process provides a logical framework for problem-solving within the time-limited and pressured environment of the emergency department.

The major goals of emergency treatment are (1) to preserve life, (2) to prevent deterioration before more definitive treatment can be given, and (3) to restore the patient to useful living. To this end, specific principles of emergency management are adhered to by health care providers. Establishing a patent airway is a first priority; there are a variety of methods that can be used depending on the patient's condition.

While an airway is being established, assessment for signs of hemodynamic alterations can be made. The most important threat to hemodynamic stability is blood loss, whether internal or external. Specific guidelines for blood loss management are followed.

Wounds account for a significant number of emergency department visits. Wounds may vary from minor lacerations to severe crush injuries. Protocols developed by emergency nurses and physicians define the steps in wound management.

Trauma

Trauma is now the third leading cause of death in the United States, after atherosclerosis and cancer. Trauma is the leading cause of death in children and adults under the age of 44. Alcohol and drug abuse have been implicated as factors in blunt and penetrating trauma as well as accidental and violent crime-related behavior.

Intra-Abdominal Injuries

Penetrating Abdominal Injuries

Penetrating abdominal injuries (gunshot wounds, stab wounds) are serious and usually require surgery. In penetrating injuries, the most important factor is the velocity with which the missile entered the body. High-velocity missiles (bullets) create extensive tissue damage. Almost all gunshot wounds require surgical exploration. Stab wounds may be managed more conservatively.

Assessment for Abdominal Injuries

- Obtain a history of the mechanism of the injury: Penetrating force (gunshot, stab)? Blunt force (blow)?
- Inspect the abdomen for obvious signs of injury: Penetrating injuries, bruises, and exit sites.
- Auscultate for the presence or absence of bowel sounds and record baseline data so changes can be noted. (Absence of bowel sounds is an early sign of intraperitoneal involvement; if signs of peritoneal irritation are present, an immediate exploratory laparotomy [surgical incision into the abdominal cavity] is usually performed.)
- Assess the patient for progression of abdominal distention, involuntary guarding, tenderness, pain, muscular rigidity or rebound tenderness, diminished bowel sounds, hypotension, and shock.
- Observe for chest injuries, which frequently accompany intra-abdominal injuries; observe for associated injuries.
- Record all physical signs as the patient is examined.

The nursing diagnoses may include impaired skin integrity related to penetrating injuries and high risk for infection related to disruption of skin integrity. The goals of the patient may include control of bleeding, maintenance of blood volume, and prevention of infection of wounds.

Emergency Management

1. Start resuscitation procedures (restoration of airway, breathing, circulation) as indicated.
2. Keep the patient on the stretcher or backboard, since movement may cause fragmentation of a clot in a large vessel and produce massive hemorrhage.

a. Ensure patency of the airway and stability of the respiratory, circulatory, and nervous systems.

b. If the patient is comatose, splint the neck until after cervical neck radiographs are made.

c. Cut the clothing away from the wound.

d. Count the number of wounds.

e. Locate entrance and exit wounds.

3. Assess for signs and symptoms of hemorrhage. *Hemorrhage frequently accompanies abdominal injury*, especially if the liver and spleen have been traumatized.

4. Control the bleeding and maintain the blood volume until surgery can be performed.

a. Apply compression to external bleeding wounds and occlusion of chest wounds.

b. Insert indwelling large-bore IV catheter for rapid fluid replacement to restore circulatory dynamics.

c. Watch for the occurrence of shock after an initial response to transfusion therapy; this is often the first sign of internal hemorrhage.

d. The physician may perform a paracentesis to identify the site of bleeding.

5. Aspirate the stomach contents with a nasogastric tube. This procedure also helps detect gastric wounds, lessens contamination of the peritoneal cavity, and prevents lung complications due to aspiration.

6. Cover protruding abdominal viscera with sterile, moist saline dressings to prevent the viscera from drying.

a. Flex the patient's knees, because this position prevents further protrusion.

b. Withhold oral fluids to prevent increased peristalsis and vomiting.

7. Insert an indwelling urethral catheter to ascertain the presence of hematuria and to monitor the urinary output.

8. Maintain an ongoing flow sheet of the patient's vital signs, urinary output, central venous pressure readings (when indicated), hematocrit values, and neurologic status.

9. Prepare for paracentesis or peritoneal lavage (Chart 63-3) when there is uncertainty about intraperitoneal bleeding.

10. For stab wounds, prepare for sinography to determine whether there is peritoneal penetration.

a. A purse-string suture is placed around the wound.

b. A small catheter is introduced through the wound.

c. A contrast medium is introduced through the catheter; radiographs are made and reveal whether peritoneal penetration has taken place.

11. Administer tetanus prophylaxis as directed.

12. Administer a broad-spectrum antibiotic as prescribed to prevent infection, since trauma predisposes to infection (by disruption of mechanical barriers; by exogenous bacteria from the environment at the time of accident; by diagnostic and therapeutic maneuvers [nosocomial infection]).

13. Prepare the patient for surgery if he exhibits continuing evidence of shock, blood loss, free air under the diaphragm, evisceration, or hematuria.

Blunt Abdominal Trauma

Blunt trauma to the abdomen may result from automobile accidents, falls, and blows to the abdomen. Patients with blunt trauma are a challenge because of potential hidden injuries that may be difficult to detect. The incidence of delayed trauma-related complications is greater than that associated with penetrating injuries. This is especially true of blunt injuries involving the liver, kidneys, spleen, or blood vessels, which can lead to substantial blood loss into the peritoneal cavity. Blunt abdominal trauma is frequently associated with extra-abdominal injuries to the chest, head, or extremities, and the evaluation and treatment of these injuries may take precedence over the abdominal injury.

Assessment

1. Obtain a detailed history (although this is frequently unobtainable, inaccurate, or misleading). Obtain all possible data about the following:

a. Method of injury

b. Time of onset of symptoms

c. Passenger location if in an automobile accident (driver frequently sustains rupture of the spleen or liver.) Seat belts on or off, type of restraint

d. Time of last food or fluid intake

e. Bleeding tendencies

f. Concurrent diseases and medications

g. Immunization history, with attention to tetanus

h. Allergies

2. Perform a rapid examination of the entire patient to detect life-threatening problems.

The clinical manifestations of blunt abdominal trauma include pain (especially on movement), rebound and maximal point tenderness (may indicate peritoneal irritation from blood or gastrointestinal fluid), muscle guarding, and diminishing or absent bowel sounds.

Emergency Management

1. Begin resuscitation procedures as indicated and evaluation of the patient simultaneously.

2. Carry out ongoing physical assessment: inspection, palpation, auscultation, and percussion of the abdomen. The changes noted in subsequent examinations may reveal an undetected abdominal injury.

a. Avoid moving the patient until the initial assessment has been completed. Movement may fragment a clot in a large vessel and produce massive hemorrhage.

b. Expect a wide variety of signs and symptoms resulting from blood loss, bruising and tearing of solid organs, and leaking of secretions from hollow abdominal viscera.

c. Observe for chest injuries, especially for fractures of the lower ribs.

d. Inspect the front of the body, flanks, and back for bluish discoloration, asymmetry, abrasion, and contusion.

e. Evaluate for signs and symptoms of hemorrhage, which frequently accompany abdominal injury, especially if the liver and spleen have been traumatized. Massive intraperitoneal bleeding is associated with shock.

f. Note tenderness, rebound tenderness, guarding, rigidity, and spasm. Rebound tenderness is assessed as follows:

(1) Press the area of maximal tenderness (let the patient point to the area).

(2) Remove the fingers quickly; pain at the suspected point indicates peritoneal irritation.

g. Observe for increasing abdominal distention. Measure the abdominal girth at the umbilical level on admission; this serves as a baseline from which changes can be determined.

Chart 63-3
Assisting With Peritoneal Lavage

Peritoneal lavage is a technique of irrigation of the peritoneum and examination of the irrigating fluid to evaluate the effects of trauma to the abdomen.

Purposes
1. To test for intra-abdominal bleeding after trauma
2. To test patients with equivocal abdominal findings
3. To avoid unnecessary operation, especially in patients with altered states of consciousness (from head injuries, drugs, alcohol) and when physical findings are unreliable (spinal cord injuries)

Equipment
Peritoneal dialysis tray
Sterile solution (lactated Ringer's solution, normal saline)
IV tubing, IV pole
Peritoneal dialysis catheter (multiple perforations)
Local skin anesthetic, sterile gloves

Procedure

Nursing Action	Rationale/Amplification
Preparatory Phase	
1. Explain the procedure to the patient; make certain that the consent form has been signed.	1. Explanation of the procedure helps to decrease fear and anxiety and provides information necessary for informed consent.
2. Empty the bladder (by catheter if necessary).	2. To prevent puncture of the urinary bladder.
3. Insert a nasogastric tube as directed.	3. To decompress the stomach.
4. Prepare the abdomen as for surgery.	4. To minimize or eliminate surface bacteria and decrease the possibility of wound contamination and infection.
5. Fill the IV tubing with solution, using aseptic technique.	
Performance Phase (by the Physician)	
1. The skin is infiltrated 2 to 3 cm (0.7 to 1.2 in) below the umbilicus in the midline with local anesthetic.	1. The midline area is relatively avascular. Epinephrine may be injected with the local anesthetic to produce capillary constriction and prevent a false-positive tap.
2. A vertical incision is made down to the linea alba.	
3. Local pressure is applied to suppress capillary leakage. Bleeding vessels are carefully ligated.	3. Ligation of vessels helps avoid a false-positive lavage.
4. The peritoneum is opened under direct vision, and a peritoneal dialysis catheter is inserted into the peritoneal cavity.	
5. A syringe is attached to the catheter, and the peritoneal cavity is aspirated.	5. If gross blood, bile, or intestinal contents are obtained, the tap shows positive findings; the patient is then prepared for immediate laparotomy (incision into the abdominal cavity).
6. If no blood is present, the catheter is attached to the IV tubing; 500 to 1000 ml of solution is infused into the peritoneal cavity through the intravenous tubing attached to the dialysis catheter.	6. If not contraindicated by the patient's condition, he may be turned from side to side to mix the peritoneal contents with the solution.
7. After the solution is infused, remove the empty IV bag from the pole and lower it below the abdominal level (near the floor).	7. Lowering the bottle creates a siphon effect to drain the excess fluid. As much of the fluid as possible is siphoned from the peritoneal cavity by gravity.
8. The peritoneal dialysis catheter is removed and the wound is closed (unless laparotomy is necessary).	
9. The fluid recovered from the peritoneal cavity is examined visually and is usually sent to the laboratory for cell counts and microscopic inspection of spun-down sediment.	
Interpretation of Lavage Fluid	
1. *Gross examination (visual):* Visually apparent blood is sufficient evidence to indicate a laparotomy.	1. If the test results are positive, a laparotomy is usually performed. If the test results are negative, the catheter is removed and the wound closed.

(continued)

Chart 63-3 *(Continued)*

Nursing Action	Rationale/Amplification

2. *Laboratory evaluation (positive tests):* Free aspiration of blood/grossly bloody fluid.
   RBC greater than 100,000/mm³
   WBC greater than 500/mm³
   Bacteria—pathologic when present
   Bile—pathologic when present
	2. If the test results are questionable, the catheter may be left in place and the lavage repeated. If the test results are weakly positive, the patient may have echography and arteriography if his condition is stable.

Follow-Up Phase 1. Assess the patient for complications.	1. Complications include wound hematoma, perforated bowel or bladder, laceration of major vessel, infection.
2. Observe the patient closely for any change in condition.	2. Repeated physical examinations of the abdomen should be carried out when intra-abdominal injury is suspected.

h. Ask about referred pain. (This is helpful in detecting intraperitoneal injury. Pain in the left shoulder may be encountered in a patient bleeding from a ruptured spleen; pain in the right shoulder can result from laceration of the liver.)

i. Auscultate for bowel sounds. (Silent abdomen accompanies peritoneal irritation.)

j. Note loss of dullness over the solid organs (liver or spleen)—indicates presence of free air. (Dullness over regions normally containing gas indicates presence of blood.)

3. Assist with rectal or vaginal examination for diagnosis of injury to the pelvis, bladder, and intestinal wall.
4. Avoid giving narcotics during the observation period, because they may mask the clinical picture.
5. Monitor vital signs frequently and carefully. This may be the only clue to intra-abdominal bleeding.
6. Prepare the patient for diagnostic procedures.
   a. Laboratory studies
      (1) Urinalysis: as a guide to possible urinary tract injury (hematuria).
      (2) Serial hematocrit levels: trend reflects presence or absence of bleeding.
      (3) Complete blood count (CBC): white blood cell count is elevated with trauma in general.
      (4) Serum amylase determinations: rising level may indicate pancreatic injury or perforations of gastrointestinal tract.
   b. Radiographic studies
      (1) Computed tomography scans: permit detailed evaluation of abdominal contents and retroperitoneal examination.
      (2) Abdominal and chest radiographs: may reveal free air beneath diaphragm, indicating a ruptured hollow viscus (a large interior organ).
7. Prepare for peritoneal lavage to test for intraperitoneal bleeding (see Chart 63-3); organ laceration or bleeding may be diagnosed by gross and microscopic examination of fluid returned after peritoneal lavage.

8. Assist with insertion of a nasogastric tube to prevent vomiting and subsequent aspiration. It is also helpful in decompressing (removing fluid and air from) the gastrointestinal tract.
9. Complications
   a. Immediate: hemorrhage, shock, and associated injuries
   b. Delayed: infectious complications

Crush Injuries

Crush injuries occur when a person is crushed beneath debris, run over by a moving vehicle, or compressed by machinery.

Assessment. Observe for the following:

- Oligemic shock due to extravasation of blood and plasma into injured tissues after compression has been released
- Paralysis of a part
- Erythema and blistering of skin
- Damaged part (usually an extremity) becomes swollen, tense, and hard
- Renal dysfunction (prolonged hypotension causes kidney damage and acute renal insufficiency; myoglobinuria secondary to muscle damage can cause acute renal failure)

Emergency Management
1. Control shock.
2. Observe carefully for acute renal insufficiency. Injury to the back may cause severe kidney damage.
3. Splint major soft tissue injuries early to control bleeding and pain.
4. Elevate the extremity. To relieve the pressure of extravasated fluid, it may be necessary for the physician to incise the fascia.
5. Administer medication for pain and anxiety as prescribed.

Multiple Injuries

The patient with multiple injuries requires a team approach, with one person responsible for coordinating the treatment. Multiple trauma potentially affects every body system.

Assessment.   Evidence of gross trauma may be slight or absent. The injury regarded as the least significant may be the most lethal. After trauma, there may be general depression of body functions leading to such complications as reduced blood pressure, oxygen deficiency in the blood and primary organ systems, dysrhythmias, and respiratory and cardiac failure. It is thought that the defense mechanisms of the body become depressed, contributing to total organ failure. Mortality in patients with multiple injuries is related to the severity of the injuries and the number of systems and organs involved.

Emergency Management.   The goals of treatment are to determine the extent of injuries and to establish priorities of treatment. Any injury interfering with a vital physiologic function

(*e.g.*, airway, breathing, circulation) is an immediate threat to life and has the highest priority for immediate treatment. *Imperative lifesaving procedures are performed simultaneously by the emergency team.* As soon as the patient is resuscitated, the clothes are usually cut off and a rapid physical assessment is performed. Critically traumatized patients should not be moved from the stretcher or backboard until they are stable. Treatment in a level I trauma center is appropriate for major trauma patients.

Treatment priorities are as follows (Fig. 63-7):

1. Carry out a *rapid* physical examination to determine if the patient is breathing, bleeding, or in shock; determine the status

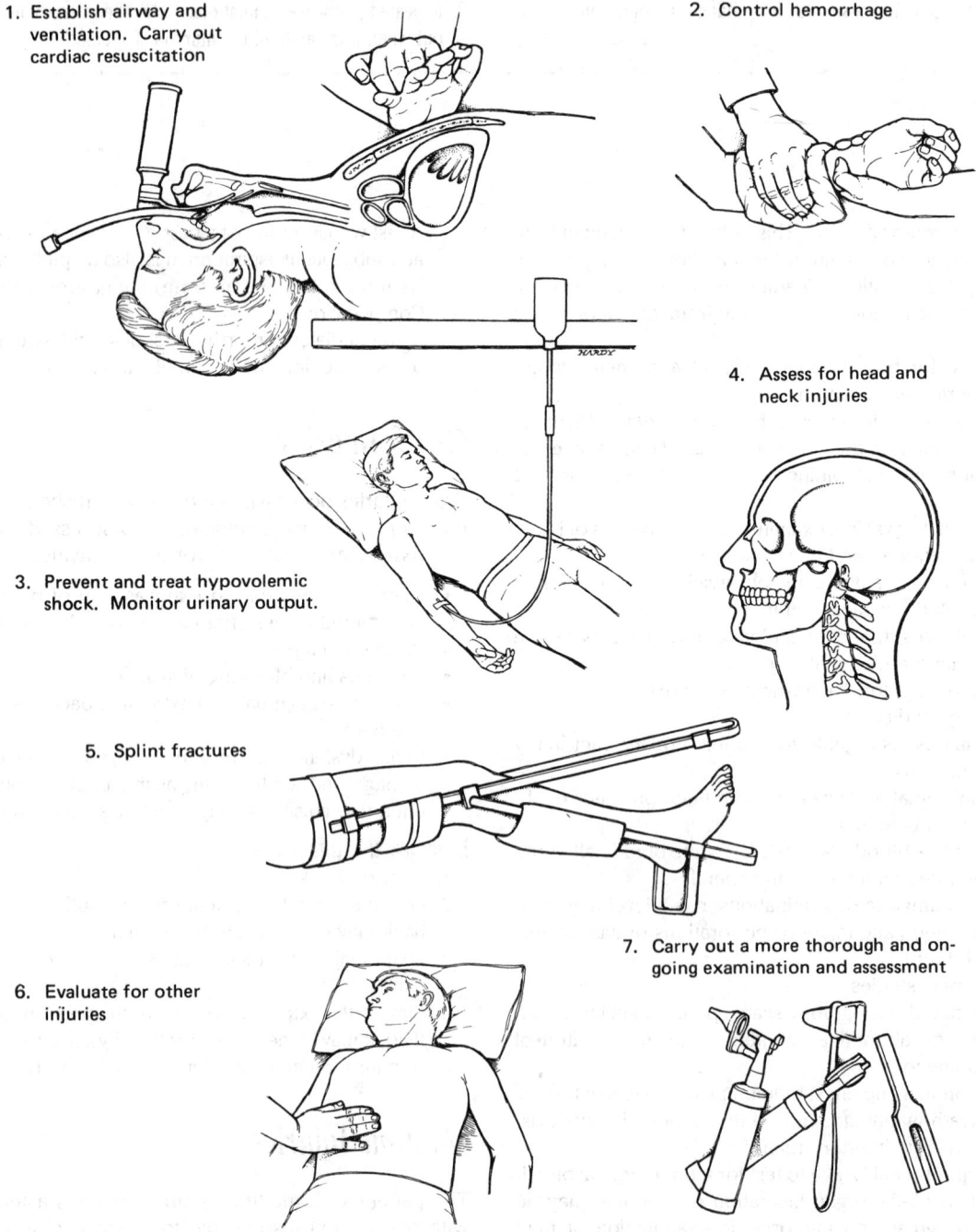

1. Establish airway and ventilation. Carry out cardiac resuscitation

2. Control hemorrhage

3. Prevent and treat hypovolemic shock. Monitor urinary output.

4. Assess for head and neck injuries

5. Splint fractures

6. Evaluate for other injuries

7. Carry out a more thorough and ongoing examination and assessment

Figure 63-7.   Management of the patient with multiple injuries.

of his responsiveness and if he has severe wounds or fracture deformities.*

2. Start resuscitation procedures (*i.e.*, airway, breathing, circulation) simultaneously while another team member is conducting a physical assessment.*
   a. Note the character and symmetry of chest wall motion and the pattern of breathing. Auscultate the chest.
   b. Ask the conscious patient if he is having difficulty breathing. Ask if he has chest pain.
   c. Apply suction to clear the trachea and bronchial tree.
   d. Insert an oropharyngeal airway to prevent occlusion by the tongue.
   e. Ventilate the patient (bag-mask system) to alleviate hypoxia.
   f. Prepare for endotracheal intubation if an adequate airway cannot be maintained.
   g. Suspect serious intrathoracic injuries if respiratory distress continues after an adequate airway has been established. (See Chap. 26 for management of chest injuries.)
3. Assess cardiac function and treat cardiac arrest; hypoxia, metabolic acidosis, and chest trauma may precipitate cardiac arrest.*
   a. For cardiac arrest, start closed chest compression and ventilation (see Chap. 29).
   b. If the chest wall is unstable (flail chest), emergency thoracotomy and manual compression may be necessary.
   c. Give sodium bicarbonate (IV) as prescribed to compensate for acidosis; severely traumatized patients with respiratory and circulatory embarrassment have some degree of metabolic acidosis.
4. Control hemorrhage.*
   a. Apply pressure over bleeding points if hemorrhage is overt.
   b. Expect significant blood loss in the patient with a fracture of the shaft of the femur, with multiple fractures, or with major pelvic trauma.
   c. Use tourniquets on extremities for massive arterial bleeding that cannot be halted with pressure.
   d. Prepare for immediate surgical intervention if the patient is bleeding internally.
5. Prevent and treat hypovolemic shock.
   a. Insert at least two (sometimes four) large-bore IV lines as prescribed. Venous cutdown may be necessary.
   b. Draw blood for laboratory studies as directed (typing and cross-matching, baseline CBC, electrolytes, blood urea nitrogen, glucose, prothrombin time).
   c. The physician may introduce a central venous catheter (multilumen catheter preferred) to monitor the patient's response to fluid infusion, to prevent fluid overload, and as a route for fluid infusion.
   d. Start IV infusions.
      (1) Lactated Ringer's solution is usually indicated for volume replacement until blood is available.
      (2) Give IV infusions rapidly enough to keep central venous pressure readings at 5 to 15 cm H_2O; monitor the rate and direction of change (important parameters).
   e. Administer blood component therapy as prescribed. Massive transfusions have a cooling effect that can cause cardiac irritability and arrest; blood may be warmed.

   f. Insert an indwelling urethral catheter and monitor urinary output to aid in diagnosis of shock and to monitor effectiveness of therapy and renal function. Do not force the catheter, because the patient may have a ruptured urethra.
   g. Monitor the ECG to detect changes.
   h. Carry out ongoing clinical evaluation to observe for improvement or deterioration; improvement in the level of responsiveness, skin warmth, speed of capillary filling, and so forth, shows a reversal of the shock state.
   i. Prepare for immediate surgical intervention if the patient does not respond to fluids or blood. Inability to restore blood pressure and circulatory volume in the patient usually indicates major internal bleeding.
6. Assess for head and neck injuries.
   a. Determine the baseline neurologic status of the patient: level of responsiveness, size and reactivity of pupils, motor power, reflexes.
   b. Neck (and chest) films may be taken; apply rigid cervical collar until radiographs rule out the possibility of cervical spine injury.
   c. Intracranial pressure monitoring may be instituted.
7. Administer dexamethasone as directed; corticosteroids appear to protect pulmonary function in patients with multiple injuries and to help prevent posttraumatic pulmonary insufficiency. (However, this therapy is considered controversial.)
8. Splint fractures to prevent further trauma to soft tissues and blood vessels and to relieve pain; note the presence or absence of pulses in fractured extremities.
9. Assess the patient for gastrointestinal injuries.
   a. Examine the patient repeatedly for abdominal pain, muscular rigidity, tenderness, rebound tenderness, diminished bowel sounds, hypotension, and shock.
   b. Prepare for peritoneal lavage to assess for intraperitoneal bleeding.
   c. Assist with insertion of a nasogastric tube if upper gastrointestinal bleeding is suspected or if gaseous distention of the stomach develops; this decreases the incidence of vomiting and aspiration.
   d. Prepare for laparotomy if the patient shows continuing signs of hemorrhage and deterioration.
10. Continue to monitor urinary output hourly; urinary output reflects cardiac output and state of perfusion of visceral organs.
    a. Assess for hematuria and oliguria.
    b. Record measurements on a flow sheet.
11. Evaluate patient for other injuries and institute appropriate treatment, including tetanus immunization.
12. Carry out a more thorough physical examination after resuscitation and management of the above priorities.

In summary, traumatic injuries are on the increase; injuries classified as traumatic include penetration and blunt intra-abdominal wounds, multiple injuries, and crush injuries. An example of a penetrating intra-abdominal wound is a gunshot wound to the abdomen. The velocity of the missile penetrating the tissue is an important factor, because high-velocity missiles cause extensive tissue damage. In contrast, a blunt intra-abdominal injury may provide no external clues until significant complications from the primary injury evolve, such as a ruptured spleen bleeding into the peritoneal cavity, causing shock.

A crush injury results when an individual is compressed by debris or machinery. Controlling systemic shock is a priority of management.

---

* Imperative lifesaving procedures are performed simultaneously by the emergency team.

Multiple injuries usually require a team approach since several major problems may need to be managed simultaneously. A physician is usually the team coordinator who prescribes the care based on clearly defined protocols.

An ability to make rapid assessments and to provide technically proficient nursing care is essential for nurses working with patients experiencing traumatic injuries.

Fractures

The immediate management of a fracture may determine the patient's outcome and make the difference between recovery and disability. When examining the patient for fracture, the part is handled gently and as little as possible. Clothing is cut off to minimize trauma to the part. Assessment for pain over or near a bone, swelling (from blood, lymph, and exudate infiltrating the tissue), and circulatory disturbance is conducted. The patient is assessed for ecchymosis, tenderness, and crepitation. *It must be remembered that the patient may have multiple fractures accompanied by head, chest, and other serious injuries.*

Emergency Management

1. Give immediate attention to the patient's general condition. If there is any question of multiple injury, the patient needs to be completely undressed, draped, and continuously monitored.
   a. Evaluate for respiratory difficulties from edema due to facial and neck injuries, accumulation of secretions in the respiratory tract, and so forth.
      (1) Examine the chest for evidence of sucking chest wounds, pneumothorax, flail chest, and other such signs.
      (2) Prepare for tracheal intubation or emergency tracheostomy as indicated.
   b. Control hemorrhage.
      (1) Control venous bleeding by applying direct pressure on the site along with digital pressure over the artery nearest to the bleeding area.
      (2) Suspect internal hemorrhage (pleural, pericardial, or abdominal) in the event of continuing shock and in the presence of injuries to the chest and abdomen.
   c. Treat for shock, which, in patients with fractures, is usually the result of blood loss.
      (1) Assess for falling blood pressure; cold, clammy skin; and rapid, thready pulse.
      (2) Keep in mind that a large amount of blood loss may accompany fractures of the femur and pelvis.
      (3) Maintain the blood pressure with IV infusions, plasma, or plasma expanders as prescribed.
      (4) Administer blood transfusion or blood component therapy as prescribed as soon as blood is available.
      (5) Administer oxygen, because cardiopulmonary embarrassment causes a decreased oxygen supply to the tissues and circulatory collapse.
      (6) Administer an analgesic as prescribed to control pain. (Splinting the extremity and controlling pain are essential in treating shock accompanying fractures.)
      (7) Observe for evidence of head, chest, and other injuries.
2. Inspect the fractured part.
   a. Observe the entire body using a systematic head-to-toe physical examination; inspect for lacerations, swelling, and deformities.
   b. Observe for *angulation* (bending), *shortening*, and *rotation.*
   c. Palpate the pulse distal to the extremity fracture and all peripheral pulses.
   d. Assess for coolness, blanching, decreased sensation and motor function, and diminished or absent pulses; these indicate injury to nerves or to blood supply.
   e. Handle the part gently and as little as possible.
3. Apply the splint before the patient is moved; splinting relieves pain, improves circulation, prevents further tissue injury, and prevents a closed fracture from becoming an open one.
   a. Immobilize the joint above and below the fracture. Place one hand distal to the fracture and apply some traction while placing the other hand beneath the fracture for support.
   b. Extend the splints well beyond the joints adjacent to the fracture.
   c. Check the vascular status of the extremity after splinting; check color, temperature, pulse, blanching of nail bed.
   d. Assess for neurologic deficits caused by the fracture.
   e. Apply a sterile dressing if the fracture is an open one.
4. Investigate any complaint of pain or pressure.
5. Transport the patient carefully and gently.
6. See Chapter 60 for a complete discussion of the treatment of fractures at specific sites.

Temperature Emergencies

Heat Stroke

Heat stroke is an acute medical emergency caused by failure of the heat-regulating mechanisms of the body during extended heat waves, especially with high humidity. Persons at risk are those not acclimatized to heat exposure, those with advanced age, those who are unable to care for themselves, those with chronic and debilitating diseases, and those who are taking certain medications (major tranquilizers, anticholinergics, diuretics, beta-adrenergic blocking agents). Another form of heat stroke, *exertional heat stroke*, or exercise in extreme heat and humidity can cause death. It occurs in healthy individuals during sports or work when heat loss is inadequate to prevent hyperthermia.

Gerontologic Considerations. Most heat-related deaths occur in the aged, because their circulatory systems are unable to compensate for the stress imposed by heat.

Assessment. Heat stroke causes thermal injury at the cellular level and resulting widespread damage to the heart, liver, kidney, and blood coagulation systems. Patient history reveals exposure to elevated ambient temperature or excessive exercise. When assessing the patient, the following are noted: profound central nervous system dysfunction (manifested by confusion, delirium, bizarre behavior, coma); elevated body temperature (40.6°C [105°F] or more); hot, dry skin; usually anhidrosis (absence of sweating); and tachypnea.

The nursing diagnoses may include ineffective thermoregulation related to inability of the body's homeostatic mechanisms to maintain normal body temperature. The patient's goal is reduction of the high temperature as quickly as possible, because mortality is directly related to the duration of hyperthermia.

Emergency Management

1. Remove the patient's clothing.
2. Reduce the core (internal) temperature to 39°C (102°F) as rapidly as possible. Use one or more of the following as directed:
   a. Use cool sheets and towels or continuous sponging with cool water.
   b. Apply ice to the skin while spraying with tepid water.
   c. Use cooling blankets.
   d. Iced saline lavage of stomach or colon may be prescribed if the temperature does not decrease.
3. Massage the patient to promote circulation and maintain cutaneous vasodilation during the cooling procedure.
4. Place an electric fan so that it blows on the patient to augment heat dissipation by convection and evaporation.
5. Monitor the patient's temperature constantly by a thermistor probe in the rectum or esophagus (monitors core temperature); avoid hypothermia; hyperthermia may recur spontaneously within 3 to 4 hours.
6. Monitor the patient carefully; vital signs, ECG, CVP, and level of responsiveness change with rapid alterations in body temperature; a seizure may be followed by recurrence of hyperthermia
7. Administer oxygen to supply tissue needs exaggerated by the hypermetabolic condition. Assist in intubating the patient with a cuffed endotracheal tube and attach to a ventilator if necessary to support failing cardiorespiratory systems.
8. Start IV infusion as directed to replace fluid losses and maintain adequate circulation; give slowly because of the dangers of myocardial injury from high body temperature and poor renal function.
9. Measure urinary output; acute tubular necrosis is a complication of heat stroke.
10. Give supportive care as prescribed:
    a. Diuretics (mannitol) to promote diuresis. (Monitor the blood pressure carefully, because hypotension may be precipitated.)
    b. Dialysis for renal failure.
    c. Anticonvulsant agents to control seizures.
    d. Potassium for hypokalemia and sodium bicarbonate to correct metabolic acidosis, depending on laboratory results.
11. Continue to monitor ECG for possible myocardial ischemia, myocardial infarction, dysrhythmias.
12. Carry out serial testing for bleeding diatheses (disseminated intravascular coagulopathy) and serum enzymes to estimate thermal hypoxic injury to the liver and muscle tissue.
13. Admit the patient to the intensive care unit; permanent liver, cardiac, and central nervous system damage may occur.

Patient Education

1. Advise the patient to avoid immediate re-exposure to high temperatures; he may remain hypersensitive to high temperatures for a considerable length of time.
2. Emphasize the importance of maintaining an adequate fluid intake, wearing loose clothing, and reducing activity in hot weather.
3. Advise athletes to monitor fluid losses, replace fluids, and use a gradual approach to physical conditioning, allowing sufficient time for acclimatization.
4. Direct the frail elderly living in urban settings with high environmental temperatures to centers where air conditioning is available (shopping mall, library, church).

Cold Injuries

Frostbite

Frostbite is trauma from exposure to freezing temperatures and actual freezing of the tissue fluids in the cell and intracellular spaces, resulting in vascular damage. The body parts most frequently affected by frostbite are the feet, hands, nose, and ears. A frozen extremity may be hard, cold, and insensitive to touch and appear white or mottled blue-white. The extent of injury from exposure to cold is not always known when the patient is seen initially.

Nursing diagnoses may include hypothermia, high risk for infection, altered tissue perfusion, and sensory alteration: tactile.

Emergency Management. The goal of management is to restore normal body temperature.

1. Do not allow the patient to walk if the lower extremities are involved.
2. Remove all constricting clothing that can impair circulation; rings and watches are removed.
3. Rewarm the extremity by controlled and rapid rewarming, 37° to 40°C (98.6° to 104°F), usually in a whirlpool, until the tips of the injured part flush (about 30 to 45 minutes); flush indicates that circulatory flow is reestablished. Early rewarming appears to decrease the amount of tissue loss.
   a. Administer an analgesic for pain as prescribed; the rewarming process may be very painful.
   b. Handle the part gently to avoid further mechanical injury. *Do not massage.*
   c. Protect the rewarmed part; do not rupture blebs, which develop 1 hour to a few days after rewarming.
   d. Place sterile gauze or cotton between affected fingers or toes to prevent maceration.
   e. Elevate the part to help control swelling.
   f. Use a foot cradle to prevent contact with bedclothes if the feet are involved.
4. Conduct physical assessment to observe for concomitant injury (soft tissue injury, dehydration, alcohol coma, fat embolism).
5. Restore electrolyte balance; dehydration and hypovolemia occur frequently in frostbite victims.
6. Use strict aseptic technique during dressing changes; frostbite injuries make the patient susceptible to infection.
7. Give tetanus prophylaxis as prescribed if there is associated trauma.
8. The following may be carried out when appropriate:
   a. Whirlpool bath for the affected extremity to aid circulation, débride dead tissue, and help prevent infection.
   b. Escharotomy (incision through the eschar) to prevent further tissue damage, to allow for normal circulation, and to permit joint motion.
   c. Fasciotomy (incision in fascia to release pressure on the muscles, nerves, blood vessels) to treat compartment syndrome.

9. Encourage hourly active motion of the affected digits to promote maximum restoration of function and to prevent contractures.
10. Advise patient not to use tobacco because of the vasoconstrictive effects of nicotine, which further reduce the already deficient blood supply to injured tissues.

Accidental Hypothermia

Accidental hypothermia is a condition in which the core (internal) temperature is 35°C (95°F) or below as a result of exposure to cold. *Urban hypothermia* (extreme exposure to cold in an urban setting) is associated with a high mortality rate; elderly people, infants, persons with concurrent illnesses, and the homeless are particularly susceptible. Susceptibility is increased after alcohol ingestion.

In assessing the patient, the following factors are kept in mind. Hypothermia leads to physiologic changes in all organ systems. There is progressive deterioration with apathy, poor judgment, ataxia, dysarthria, drowsiness, and eventually coma. Shivering may be suppressed below a temperature of 32.2°C (90°F). Below this temperature, the body's self-warming mechanisms become ineffective. The heartbeat and the blood pressure may be so weak that the peripheral pulsation becomes undetectable. Cardiac irregularities also may occur. Other physiologic abnormalities include hypoxemia and acidosis.

Emergency Management.   Management consists of continual monitoring, rewarming, and supportive care.

1. Monitor the patient: vital signs, CVP, urinary output, arterial blood gases, blood chemistry determinations (BUN, creatinine, glucose, electrolytes), chest radiograph.
   a. Monitor body temperature with an esophageal or rectal thermistor probe.
   b. Employ continuous ECG monitoring; cold-induced myocardial irritability leads to conduction disturbances, especially ventricular fibrillation.
   c. Maintain an arterial line for recording blood pressure and to facilitate blood sampling.
2. Rewarm the patient. Rewarming methods include active core (internal) rewarming, active external rewarming, and passive or spontaneous rewarming. The optimal method has not been determined.
3. Supportive care during rewarming includes the following as directed:
   a. External cardiac compression if indicated.
   b. Electrical cardioversion of ventricular fibrillation.
   c. Mechanical ventilation with PEEP and heated humidified oxygen, to maintain tissue oxygenation.
   d. IV fluids (warmed) to correct hypotension and maintain urinary output.
   e. Sodium bicarbonate to correct metabolic acidosis.
   f. Antidysrhythmic drugs as necessary.
   g. Indwelling urethral catheter to monitor fluid status.
   h. Prophylactic antibiotics. (A large percentage of hypothermic patients have serious infections.)

Anaphylactic Reaction

An anaphylactic reaction is an acute systemic hypersensitivity reaction that occurs within seconds to minutes after exposure to a variety of foreign substances, for example, drugs (penicillin, iodinated contrast material) and stinging insects (*Hymenoptera* [bee, wasp, yellow jacket, hornet]). Repeated administration of parenteral or oral therapeutic agents also may precipitate an anaphylactic reaction.

An anaphylactic reaction is the result of an antigen–antibody interaction in a sensitized individual who, as a consequence of previous exposure, has developed a special type of antibody (immunoglobulin) that is specific for this particular allergen. The antibody immunoglobulin IgE is responsible for most of the immediate type of human allergic responses: the individual becomes sensitive to a particular antigen after production of IgE to this antigen.

Assessment.   Anaphylactic reaction produces a wide range of clinical manifestations.

- *Respiratory signs* include (1) nasal congestion, itching, sneezing and coughing; (2) possible respiratory distress that progresses rapidly and is caused by bronchospasm or edema of the larynx; (3) tightness of the chest; and (4) other respiratory difficulties, such as wheezing, dyspnea, and cyanosis.
- *Skin manifestations* appear in the form of flushing with a sense of warmth and diffuse erythema. *Generalized itching over the entire body indicates that a general systemic reaction is developing.* Urticaria (hives) may also appear. When massive facial angioedema develops, upper respiratory edema may occur.
- *Cardiovascular manifestations* include tachycardia or bradycardia and peripheral vascular collapse as indicated by pallor, imperceptible pulse, decreasing blood pressure, and circulatory failure, leading to coma and death.
- *Gastrointestinal problems* may occur, such as nausea, vomiting, and colicky abdominal pains or diarrhea.

Nursing diagnoses may include decreased cardiac output, impaired gas exchange, high risk for fluid volume deficit, and anxiety.

Emergency Management

1. Establish an airway. (This is performed while another person administers epinephrine.)
   a. Turn the face to one side; support the angles of the mandible.
   b. An oropharyngeal or endotracheal tube is inserted; apply oropharyngeal suction for excessive secretions.
   c. Employ resuscitative measures (especially for patients with stridor and progressive pulmonary edema).
   d. If glottic edema is present, an incision through the cricothyroid membrane provides an airway.
   e. Administer positive pressure oxygen therapy by mask and resuscitation bag.
   f. Closed chest cardiac massage is administered if necessary.
2. Administer aqueous epinephrine as prescribed to provide rapid relief of hypersensitivity reaction. (This should be done simultaneously while another person is establishing the airway.) Epinephrine may be repeated if necessary as prescribed. Judgment is used in choosing the route for administration of epinephrine:
   a. Subcutaneous injection for mild, generalized symptoms.
   b. Intramuscular injection when the reaction is more severe and progressive, and when there is concern that vascular collapse will inhibit absorption.
   c. IV route (aqueous epinephrine diluted in saline and given *slowly*), used in rare instances in which there is complete

loss of consciousness and severe cardiovascular collapse. This method may precipitate cardiac dysrhythmias; *monitor ECG and have defibrillator available.*

3. Apply a tourniquet above the injection site if an anaphylactic reaction followed an injection (medication to which the patient is allergic) or insect sting, to retard antigen absorption.
   a. Infiltrate the injection site with epinephrine as directed.
   b. Loosen the tourniquet at regular intervals to allow adequate circulation to the extremity.
4. Start an IV infusion of saline for emergency access to a vein and for hypotension.

Additional Treatments as Indicated

1. Give antihistamine drugs as prescribed, for example, diphenhydramine hydrochloride (Benadryl, IM) to block further histamine binding at target cells.
2. Give aminophylline IV *slowly* as prescribed over a period of time for patients with severe bronchospasm and wheezing that is refractory to other treatment. Monitor vital signs.
3. Treat prolonged hypotension as prescribed with crystalloids or colloids and possibly vasopressors; monitor blood pressure. A patient with reduced cardiac output may respond to an infusion of isoproterenol or dopamine.
4. Administer oxygen if significant respiratory or cardiovascular deficits are present.
5. Observe for dysrhythmias and cardiorespiratory arrest.
6. If the patient is having a seizure, administer short-acting barbiturate or diazepam IV as prescribed over a period of several minutes.
7. Administer corticosteroids as prescribed if the patient is having a prolonged reaction and persistent hypotension or bronchospasm.
8. The patient is usually admitted to the hospital after the symptoms abate.

Preventive Measures and Patient Education

1. Be aware of the danger of anaphylactic reactions and the early signs of anaphylaxis.
2. Ask about the patient's previous allergies to medications.
3. Question the patient before giving a foreign serum or other types of antigenic agents to determine whether he has had it at some earlier time.
4. Question the patient about previous allergic reactions to food or pollen.
5. Avoid giving drugs to patients with hay fever, asthma, and other allergic disorders unless absolutely necessary.
6. Avoid giving parenteral medications unless absolutely necessary. Anaphylactic reactions are more likely to occur when the agent is given parenterally.
7. Do skin testing before administration of certain materials known to produce anaphylactic reactions, such as horse serum. It must be remembered that skin testing can precipitate anaphylaxis in highly sensitive individuals.
   a. A negative skin test does not always indicate safety.
   b. Have epinephrine, IV infusions, and intubation and tracheostomy equipment available as precautionary measures.
8. If the patient is being treated as an outpatient, keep him in the office, hospital, or clinic at least 30 minutes after injection of any agent. Caution the patient to return if symptoms develop.
9. Caution patients who are sensitive to insect bites to carry kits equipped to treat insect stings (tourniquet, epinephrine); instruct the patient and his family and significant others in the use of the emergency supplies.

10. Encourage allergic persons to wear identification tags or bracelets.

Poisoning

A poison is any substance that, when ingested, inhaled, absorbed, applied to the skin, or produced within the body in relatively small amounts, causes injury to the body by its chemical action. Poisoning from inhalation and ingestion of toxic materials, both accidental and by design, constitutes a major health hazard. The problem is one of real magnitude; about 7% of all emergency department visits are the direct result of toxic problems.

Ingested (Swallowed) Poisons

The goals of emergency treatment are (1) to remove or inactivate the poison before it is absorbed, (2) to give supportive care to maintain vital organ systems, (3) to use the specific antidote to neutralize the poison, and (4) to give treatment to hasten the elimination of the absorbed poison.

General Management.*

1. Attain control of the airway, ventilation, and oxygenation; in the absence of cerebral or renal damage, the patient's prognosis depends largely on successful management of respiratory and circulatory systems.
   a. Assess adequacy of ventilation by observing ventilatory effort, through blood gas analysis, or by the use of spirometry.
   b. Assess cardiovascular function by measurement of pulse, blood pressure, central venous pressure, and temperature (core and peripheral).
   c. Prepare for mechanical ventilation if respirations are depressed. Positive expiratory pressure applied to the airway (bag-mask) may help keep the alveoli inflated.
   d. Administer oxygen for respiratory depression, unconsciousness, cyanosis, and shock.
   e. Prevent aspiration of gastric contents by positioning (on side with head down), use of oropharyngeal airway, and suctioning.
   f. Stabilize cardiovascular function and monitor ECG.
   g. Insert an indwelling urinary catheter to monitor renal function.
   h. Obtain blood specimen to test for concentration of drug or poison.
   i. Monitor neurologic status (including cognitive function); monitor the course of vital signs and neurologic status over time.
   j. Conduct a rapid physical examination.
2. Try to determine the product taken, amount, time since ingestion, symptoms, age and weight of the patient, and pertinent health history. Call the poison control center in the area if an unknown toxic agent has been taken, or if it is necessary to identify an antidote for a known toxic agent.
3. Treat shock appropriately; it may be due to cardiodepressant

---

* *Many of these measures are performed simultaneously by the emergency department team.*

action of the drug ingested, venous pooling in lower extremities, or a reduction in circulating blood volume due to increased capillary permeability.

4. Remove the toxin or decrease its absorption. Use gastric emptying procedures as prescribed; the following may be used:
   a. Induction of emesis with syrup of ipecac for the alert patient.

   • Do not induce emesis after ingestions of caustic substance or petroleum distillates.

   b. Gastric lavage (Fig. 63-8 and Chart 63-4 for the obtunded patient). Save gastric aspirate for toxicology screens.
   c. Activated charcoal administration if poison is one that is absorbed by charcoal.
   d. Cathartic, when appropriate.
5. Give specific therapy. Administer the specific chemical antagonist or physiologic antagonist as early as possible to reverse or diminish effects of the toxin.
6. Support the patient having seizures; many poisons excite the central nervous system, or the patient may have seizures from oxygen deprivation.
7. Assist in carrying out procedures to promote the removal of the ingested substance if the above are not effective:
   a. Diuresis for agents excreted by the renal route.
   b. Dialysis.
   c. Hemoperfusion (process of passing blood through an extracorporeal circuit and a cartridge containing an adsorbent [such as charcoal or resins], after which the detoxified blood is returned to the patient).
   d. Multiple doses of charcoal.
8. Monitor central venous pressure as indicated.
9. Monitor for fluid and electrolyte imbalance.
10. Reduce elevated temperature.
11. Cautiously give analgesics as prescribed for pain; severe pain causes vasomotor collapse and reflex inhibition of normal physiologic functions.
12. Assist in obtaining specimens of blood, urine, stomach contents, and vomitus.
13. Provide constant nursing surveillance and attention to the patient in a coma; coma from poisoning results from interference with brain cell function or metabolism.
14. Monitor and treat for complications such as hypotension, cardiac dysrhythmias, and seizures.
15. If the patient is discharged, give written instructions of signs and symptoms of potential problems and procedures for callback or return.
    a. Obtain psychiatric consultation if poisoning was a suicide attempt.
    b. In cases of accidental ingestion of poison provide poison prevention and home poison-proofing instructions to the patient or family.

Corrosive Poisons

Corrosive poisons include alkaline and acid agents that can cause tissue destruction after coming in contact with mucous membranes.

- *Alkaline products*: Lye, drain cleaners, toilet bowl cleaners, bleach, nonphosphate detergents, oven cleaners, button batteries (batteries used to power watches, calculators, cameras), Clinitest tablets
- *Acid products*: Toilet bowl cleaners, swimming pool cleaners, metal cleaners, rust removers, battery acid

Assessment
1. Obtain history of type and quantity of agent ingested.
2. Assess for severe pain and burning sensations in mouth and throat, pain on swallowing, inability to swallow, vomiting, drooling, hematuria.

The nursing diagnoses may include altered oral mucous membranes related to swallowing corrosive poison, and high risk for self-directed violence.

Emergency Management
1. Give water (or milk) to drink for dilution.
   a. Dilution is *not* attempted if patient has acute airway swelling or obstruction or if there is clinical evidence of esophageal, gastric, or intestinal perforation.
   b. *Do not induce vomiting if the patient has consumed a strong acid, alkali, or other corrosive substance.*
2. The patient is usually admitted to the hospital for observation and elective endoscopy to evaluate for the presence of burns and deep ulceration.

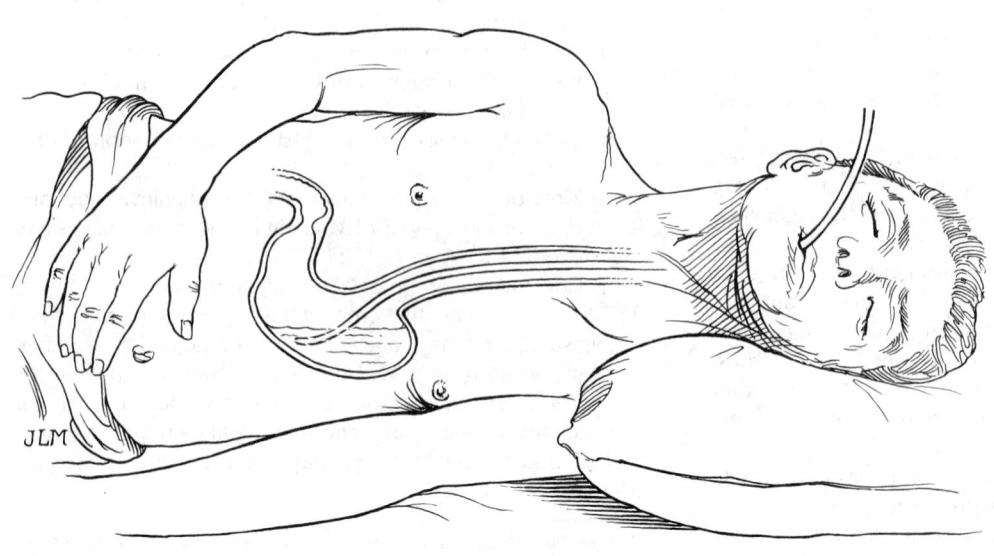

Figure 63–8. Gastric lavage. During gastric lavage the patient is positioned on his left side to allow pooling of the gastric contents and decrease the passage of fluid into the duodenum during lavage.

Chart 63–4
Assisting With Gastric Lavage

Gastric lavage is the aspiration of the stomach contents and washing out of the stomach by means of a gastric tube. Gastric lavage is contraindicated after acid or alkali ingestion, in the presence of seizures, or after ingestion of hydrocarbons or petroleum distillates. It is particularly dangerous after ingestion of strong corrosive agents.

Purposes
1. For urgent removal of ingested substance in order to decrease systemic absorption
2. To empty the stomach before endoscopic procedures
3. To diagnose gastric hemorrhage and to arrest hemorrhage

Equipment
Large-bore/nasogastric tubes or large-bore Ewald tube
Large irrigating syringe with adapter
Large plastic funnel with adapter to fit tube
Water-soluble lubricant
Tap water or appropriate antidote (milk, saline solution, sodium bicarbonate solution, fruit juice, activated charcoal)
Container for aspirate
Mouth gag, nasotracheal or endotracheal tubes with inflatable cuffs
Containers for specimens

Procedure

Action	Rationale/Amplification
1. Remove dentures and inspect the oral cavity for loose teeth.	1. This will prevent accidental aspiration of teeth.
2. Measure the distance between the bridge of the nose and the xiphoid process. Mark the tube with indelible pencil or tape.	2. This distance is a rule-of-thumb measurement of the distance the tube is passed to reach the stomach. This avoids curling and kinking of excess tubing in the stomach.
3. Lubricate the tube with water-soluble lubricant.	3. Lubrication eases insertion of the tube.
4. If comatose, the patient is intubated with a cuffed nasotracheal or endotracheal tube.	4. A cuffed nasotracheal or endotracheal tube prevents aspiration of gastric contents.
5. Place the patient in a left lateral position with the head lowered about 15 degrees downward.	5. This position decreases passage of gastric contents into the duodenum during lavage and minimizes the possibility of aspiration into the lungs.
6. Pass the tube by the oral route while keeping the head in a neutral position. Pass the tube to the adhesive marking or about 50 cm (20 in). After the lavage tube is passed, the head of the table is lowered. Have standby suction available.	6. The depth of insertion of the tube will vary with the size of the patient. If the tube enters the trachea instead of the esophagus, the patient will experience coughing, dyspnea, stridor, and cyanosis.
7. Auscultate the stomach during injection of air with a syringe to confirm gastric location.	7. One method for detection of tube inadvertently placed in trachea; positive confirmation of tube placement can be accomplished with a radiograph.
8. Aspirate the stomach contents with the syringe attached to the tube before instilling water or an antidote. Save the specimen for analysis.	8. Aspiration is carried out to remove the stomach contents.
9. Remove the syringe. Attach the funnel to the end of the tube, or use a 50-ml syringe to inject lavage solution in the gastric tube. The volume of fluid placed in the stomach should be small.	9. Overfilling the stomach may cause regurgitation and aspiration or force the stomach contents through the pylorus.
10. Elevate the funnel above the patient's head and pour approximately 150 to 200 ml of solution into the funnel.	
11. Lower the funnel and siphon the gastric contents into the bucket.	11. The fluid should flow in freely and drain by gravity.
12. Save samples of the first two washings.	12. Keep the first washing sample isolated from other washings for toxicologic analysis.
13. Repeat the lavage procedure until the returns are relatively clear and no particulate matter is seen.	13. This usually requires a total volume of at least 2 liters; some clinicians advocate the use of 5 to 20 liters.
14. At the completion of lavage: a. The stomach may be left empty.	

(continued)

Chart 63-4 (Continued)

Procedure

Action	Rationale/Amplification
b. An adsorbent (powder form of activated charcoal mixed with water to form slurry, the consistency of thick soup) may be instilled in the tube and allowed to remain in the stomach.	14. b. Activated charcoal reduces absorption by adsorbing (attaching to its surface) a wide range of substances; it renders the poison inaccessible to the circulation, thereby reducing its toxicity.
c. A saline cathartic may be instilled in the tube.	c. A cathartic may be given to hasten the elimination of remaining ingested material.
15. Pinch off the tube during removal or maintain suction while the tube is being withdrawn.	15. Pinching off the tube prevents aspiration and the initiation of the gag reflex. Keeping the patient's head lower than the body also helps to prevent initiation of the gag reflex.
16. Warn the patient that his stools will turn black from the charcoal.	

3. Refer the patient for psychiatric evaluation if poisoning was a suicide attempt.

Inhaled Poisons

General Management

1. Carry the patient to fresh air immediately; open all doors and windows.
2. Loosen all tight clothing.
3. Initiate CPR if required.
4. Prevent chilling; wrap the patient in blankets.
5. Keep the patient as quiet as possible.
6. Do not give alcohol in any form.

Carbon Monoxide Poisoning

Carbon monoxide poisoning may occur as an industrial or household accident or as an attempted suicide. It is implicated in more deaths than any other toxic agent except alcohol. Carbon monoxide exerts its toxic effect by binding to circulating hemoglobin to reduce the oxygen-carrying capacity of the blood. Hemoglobin absorbs carbon monoxide more than 200 times more readily than it absorbs oxygen. Carbon monoxide–bound hemoglobin, called *carboxyhemoglobin* is unavailable to transport oxygen.

Clinical Manifestations and Assessment.   The central nervous system has a critical need for oxygen and shows signs of carbon monoxide toxicity. A person suffering from carbon monoxide poisoning appears intoxicated (from cerebral hypoxia). Other signs and symptoms include headache, muscular weakness, palpitation, dizziness, and mental confusion, which can progress rapidly to coma. The skin color is not a reliable sign; the skin may be pink, cherry red, or cyanotic and pale. History of exposure to carbon monoxide justifies immediate treatment.

Nursing diagnoses may include impaired gas exchange and high risk for self-directed violence.

Emergency Management.   The goals of management are to reverse cerebral and myocardial hypoxia and to hasten carbon monoxide elimination.

1. Administer 100% oxygen at atmospheric or hyperbaric pressures to reverse hypoxia and accelerate the elimination of carbon monoxide.

2. Draw blood for carboxyhemoglobin levels; oxygen is administered until the carboxyhemoglobin level is less than 5%.
3. Observe the patient constantly. Psychoses, spastic paralysis, ataxia, visual disturbances, and deterioration of personality may persist after resuscitation and may be symptoms of permanent central nervous system damage.
4. When unintentional carbon monoxide poisoning occurs, the health department should be contacted and the dwelling or building in question should be inspected.
5. Obtain psychiatric consultation if poisoning was a suicide attempt.

Skin Contamination Poisoning (Chemical Burns)

Injuries from exposure to chemicals are challenging because there are a large number of offending agents with diverse actions and metabolic effects. The severity of a chemical burn is determined by the mechanism of action, penetrating strength and concentration, and amount and duration of exposure of the chemical to the skin.

Emergency Management

1. Drench the skin with running water from a shower, hose, or faucet.
2. Continue to apply a stream of water to the skin while removing the clothing; the skin of health care personnel should be appropriately protected if the burn is extensive or the agent significantly toxic.
3. Apply *prolonged* lavage with tepid water in copious amounts.
4. For appropriate future treatment, try to determine the identity and characteristics of the chemical agent.
5. Provide the standard burn treatment appropriate for the size and location of the wound (antimicrobial treatment, tetanus prophylaxis as prescribed).
6. Instruct the patient to have the affected area reexamined at 24 and 72 hours and 7 days; there is a significant risk of underestimating these types of injuries.

Injected Poisons: Stinging Insects

A person may have an extreme sensitivity to the venoms of the *Hymenoptera* (the stings of bees, hornets, yellow jackets, and wasps). It is thought that venom allergy is an IgE-mediated reaction; this constitutes an acute emergency. Stings of the head and neck are especially serious, although stings in any area of the body can result in anaphylaxis.

The clinical response may range from generalized urticaria, itching, malaise, and anxiety to laryngeal edema, severe bronchospasm, shock, and death. In general, the shorter the time between the sting and the onset of severe symptoms, the worse the prognosis.

Emergency Management

1. Administer epinephrine (aqueous) as directed. Massage the site to hasten absorption. If the sting is on an extremity, apply a tourniquet with sufficient compression to occlude venous and lymphatic flow.
2. See p. 1968 for treatment of anaphylactic shock.
3. Counsel all persons known to be sensitive to *Hymenoptera* venom to carry a commercially available self-treatment kit containing a tourniquet, injectable and inhalant forms of epinephrine, an oral antihistamine, and written instructions; the kit is available on prescription. Instruct the patient to do the following if he is stung:
   a. Inject himself with epinephrine immediately.
   b. Remove the stinger with one quick scrape of the fingernail. Do not squeeze the venom sac; this may cause additional venom to be injected.
   c. Cleanse the area with soapy water and apply ice.
   d. Apply a tourniquet proximal to the sting.
   e. Report to the nearest health care facility for further examination.
4. All allergic individuals should wear medical warning bracelets indicating hypersensitivity.
5. Hyposensitization therapy should be given to persons who have had systemic or large local reactions.

Patient Education.   Instruct the patient and his family and significant others to limit exposure to stinging insects by the following measures:

- Avoiding locales with stinging insects (camp and picnic sites).
- Avoiding insect feeding areas (flower beds, ripe fruit orchards, garbage, fields of clover).
- Not going barefoot outdoors (yellow jackets may nest on the ground).
- Avoiding perfumes, scented soaps, and bright colors, which attract bees.
- Keeping car windows closed.
- Spraying garbage cans with rapid-acting insecticide.
- Securing a professional exterminator to dispose of wasp and hornet nests or beehives in the home area.
- Remaining motionless if an insect buzzes around him. (Motion, especially running, increases the likelihood of being stung.)
- Learning self-injection of epinephrine.

Snakebites

Venomous (poisonous) snakes cause some 8,000 of the 45,000 snakebites that occur each year in the United States. Nine to 15 deaths per year are attributed to these snakebites. Children between the ages of 1 and 9 years are the most likely victims. The greatest number of bites occur during daylight hours in summer months. Venomous snakebites are medical emergencies.

Venomous snakes are found in every part of the country. Different parts of the country and the world have different types of snakes. Because snakebites are medical emergencies, the nurse should be familiar with the types of snakes that are common to her geographic region.

Snake venom consists primarily of proteins that have a broad range of physiologic effects. Multiple organ systems, especially the neurologic, cardiovascular, and respiratory systems, may be affected.

Initial first aid at the site of the snakebite includes putting the victim at rest, removing constrictive items such as rings, providing warmth, cleansing the wound, covering the wound with a light sterile dressing, and immobilizing the injured part below the level of the heart. Ice or a tourniquet *is not* to be applied.

The initial evaluation in the emergency department is performed quickly and includes:

- Determination of whether the snake was venomous or nonvenomous
- Determination of where and when the bite occurred and the circumstances of the bite
- Establishment of the sequence of events, signs and symptoms
- Determination of the severity of envenomation (poisonous effects)
- Monitoring of vital signs
- Measurement and recording of the circumference of the bitten extremity or area at several points
- Obtaining appropriate laboratory data (*i.e.*, CBC, urinalysis, and clotting studies)

The course and prognosis of snakebites depend on the kind and amount of venom injected, where on the body the bite occurred, and the general health, age, and size of the victim. There is no one specific protocol for treatment of snakebites. General guidelines include the following:

1. Obtain baseline laboratory data.
2. *Do not* use ice, tourniquets, heparin, or steroids during the acute stage. Corticosteroids are contraindicated in the first 6 to 8 hours after the bite because they may depress the patient's antibody production and hinder the action of antivenin (antitoxin for the snake venom).
3. Parenteral fluids may be used for treatment of hypotension. If vasopressors must be used to treat hypotension, their use should be short-term.
4. Surgical exploration of the bite is rarely indicated.
5. Observe the patient closely for at least 6 hours; the patient is *never* left unattended.

Administration of Antivenin (Antitoxin).   Antivenin is most effective if administered within the first 12 hours of the snakebite. The dosage depends on the type of snake and the estimated severity of the bite. Children may require more antivenin than adults because their smaller bodies make them more susceptible to the toxic effects of the venom. A skin test should be performed prior to the initial dose.

Before administration of the antivenin and every 15 minutes thereafter, the circumference of the affected part is measured proximally. Antivenin should be administered as an IV drip whenever possible, although intramuscular administration can be used. Depending on the severity of the bite, the antivenin should be diluted in 500 to 1000 ml of normal saline; the fluid volume may be reduced for children. The infusion should be started slowly and the rate increased after 10 minutes if there is no reaction. The total dose should be infused during the first 4 to 6 hours after envenomation. The initial dose is repeated until symptoms decrease. After the symptoms decrease, the circumference of the affected part should be measured every 30 to 60 minutes for the next 48 hours.

The most common cause of serum reaction is a too rapid infusion of antivenin, although 3% of patients with negative skin tests develop reactions not related to infusion rate. Reactions may consist of a feeling of fullness in the face, urticaria, pruritus, malaise, and apprehension. These symptoms may be followed by tachycardia, shortness of breath, hypotension, and shock. In this situation, the infusion should be stopped immediately and IV diphenhydramine administered. Vasopressors should be used in the presence of shock. Emergency resuscitation equipment must be on standby while the antivenin is infusing.

Food Poisoning

Food poisoning is a sudden, explosive illness that may occur after ingestion of contaminated food or drink. Botulism, a serious form of food poisoning, is discussed on p. 1935, because the treatment differs and the patient requires continual surveillance.

Emergency Management
1. Determine the source and type of food poisoning.
   a. Have the family bring the suspected food to the medical facility.
   b. Obtain the history:
      (1) How soon after eating did the symptoms occur? (Immediate onset suggests chemical, plant, or animal poisoning.)
      (2) What was eaten in the previous meal? Did the food have any unusual odor or taste? (Most foods causing bacterial poisoning *do not* have unusual odor or taste.)
      (3) Did anyone else become ill from eating the same food?
      (4) Did vomiting occur? What was the appearance of the vomitus?
      (5) Did diarrhea occur? (Diarrhea is usually absent with botulism and with shellfish or other fish poisoning.)
      (6) Are any neurologic symptoms present? (These occur in botulism and in chemical, plant, and animal poisoning.)
      (7) Does the patient have a fever? (Fever is seen in salmonella, favism [ingestion of fava beans], and some fish poisoning.)
      (8) What is the patient's appearance?
2. Collect food, gastric contents, vomitus, serum, and feces for examination.
3. Monitor vital signs on a continuing basis.
   a. Assess respiration, blood pressure, sensorium, CVP (if indicated), and muscular activity.
   b. Weigh the patient for future comparisons.
4. Support the respiratory system. Death from respiratory paralysis can occur with botulism, fish poisoning, and so forth.
5. Maintain fluid and electrolyte balance. Severe vomiting produces alkalosis, and severe diarrhea produces acidosis; large amounts of electrolytes and water are lost by vomiting and diarrhea.
   a. Observe for hypovolemic shock from severe fluid and electrolyte losses.
   b. Evaluate for lethargy, rapid pulse, fever, oliguria, anuria, hypotension, and delirium.
   c. Carry out blood electrolyte studies.
6. Correct and control hypoglycemia.
7. Control the nausea.
   a. Give an antiemetic drug parenterally as prescribed if the patient cannot tolerate fluids or medications by mouth.
   b. Give sips of weak tea, carbonated drinks, or tap water for mild nausea.
   c. Give clear liquids 12 to 24 hours after nausea and vomiting subside.
   d. Progress to a low-residue, bland diet gradually.

In summary, the emergency nurse clinician needs to know the immediate treatment for many different health problems. Fractures, thermal and cold injuries, and anaphylaxis are only a few of the conditions that the emergency nurse encounters regularly. Priorities of care are well defined by protocols that are adhered to to promote quality of care.

Substance Abuse

Substance abuse is the misuse of specific substances to alter mood or behavior and includes drug abuse and alcohol abuse.

Drug Abuse

Drug abuse is the use of drugs for other than legitimate medical purposes. The clinical manifestations may vary with the drug used, but the underlying principles of management are essentially the same. Table 63-1 notes the most commonly abused drugs, listing their clinical manifestations and therapeutic management.

Drug users tend to take a variety of drugs simultaneously (*e.g.*, alcohol, barbiturates, narcotics, and tranquilizers) that may have additive effects. IV drug users are at increased risk for HIV infection, acquired immunodeficiency syndrome (AIDS), and hepatitis B, and are the most frequent victims of tetanus in the United States.

The treatment goals for a patient suffering from drug overdose are to support the respiratory and cardiovascular functions and to enhance the clearance of the agent.

Emergency Management of Acute Drug Reaction
1. Assess the presence and adequacy of respirations. Attain control of the airway, ventilation, and oxygenation.
   a. Use a cuffed endotracheal tube and provide assisted ventilation in a severely depressed patient with absent gag or cough reflexes.
   b. Measure arterial blood gases for hypoxia due to hypoventilation and acid–base abnormalities.
   c. Administer oxygen.
2. Stabilize the cardiovascular system. (This is done simultaneously with airway management.)
   a. Begin external cardiac compression and ventilation in the absence of heartbeat.

(text continues on page 1978)

TABLE 63-1.   *Emergency Management of Drug Abuse Patients and Patients with Drug Overdose*

Drug	Clinical Manifestations	Therapeutic Management
NARCOTICS		

Cocaine
  Intranasally ("snorting"): inhaled into nostrils through straws
  By smoking ("freebasing"): cocaine hydrochloride dissolved in ether to yield a pure cocaine alkaloid base (called "crack"); smoking in a small pipe delivers large quantities of cocaine to lungs
  Intravenously
	Cocaine is a CNS stimulant that can increase heart rate and blood pressure and cause hyperpyrexia, seizures, and ventricular dysrhythmias. It produces intense euphoria, then anxiety, sadness, insomnia, and sexual indifference; cocaine hallucinosis with delusions; psychosis with extreme paranoia with ideas of persecution; and hypervigilance. Chronic psychotic symptoms may persist.	1. Ensure airway and ventilation.
		2. Control seizures.
		3. Monitor cardiovascular effects; have lidocaine and defibrillator available.
		4. Treat for hyperthermia.
		5. Refer for psychiatric evaluation and treatment in an inpatient unit that eliminates access to the drug.

Heroin Opium or paregoric Morphine, codeine, synthetic derivatives (methadone, meperidine) Fentanyl (Sublimaze)	Acute intoxication (overdose) Pinpoint pupils (may be dilated with severe hypoxia); decreased blood pressure Marked respiratory depression Stupor → coma Fresh needle marks along course of any superficial vein; skin abscesses	1. Support respiratory and cardiovascular functions. 2. Establish an IV line; withdraw blood for chemical and toxicologic analysis. Patient may be given bolus of glucose to eliminate possibility of hypoglycemia 3. Give narcotic antagonist (naloxone hydrochloride [Narcan]) as prescribed to reverse severe respiratory depression and coma. 4. Continue to monitor level of responsivenes and respirations, pulse, and BP. Duration of action of naloxone hydrochloride is shorter than that of heroin; repeated dosages may be necessary. 5. Send urine for analysis; opiates can be detected in urine. 6. Obtain an ECG. 7. Do not leave patient unattended; he may lapse back into coma rapidly. Clinical status may change from minute to minute. Hemodialysis may be indicated for severe drug intoxication. 8. Monitor for pulmonary edema, which is frequently seen in patients who abuse/overdose on narcotics. 9. Refer patient for psychiatric evaluation prior to discharge.

BARBITURATES
Pentobarbital (Nembutal)
Secobarbital (Seconal)
Amobarbital (Amytal)
	Acute intoxication (may mimic alcohol intoxication):
	  Respiratory depression
	  Flushed face
	  Decreased pulse rate; decreased blood pressure
	  Increasing nystagmus
	  Depressed tendon reflexes
	  Decreasing mental alertness
	  Difficulty in speaking
	  Poor motor coordination
	  Coma, death
		1. Maintain airway and give respiratory support.
		2. Endotracheal intubation or tracheostomy is considered if there is any doubt about the adequacy of airway exchange.
		  a. Check airway frequently.
		  b. Perform suctioning as necessary.
		3. Support cardiovascular and respiratory functions; most deaths result from respiratory depression or shock.
		4. Start intravenous infusion through large-gauge needle or intravenous catheter to support blood pressure; coma and dehydration result in hypotension and respond to infusion of intra-

(continued)

TABLE 63–1.   *(Continued)*

Drug	Clinical Manifestations	Therapeutic Management
		venous fluids with elevation of blood pressure. Sodium bicarbonate may be prescribed to alkalinize urine; it promotes excretion of barbiturates.
5. Evacuate stomach contents or lavage as soon as possible to prevent absorption; repeated doses of activated charcoal may be administered.
6. Assist with hemodialysis for severely overdosed patient.
7. Maintain neurologic and vital sign flow sheet.
8. Patient awakening from overdose may demonstrate hostility; this can stimulate automatic angry response by health care personnel.
9. Refer for psychiatric consultation to evaluate suicide potential and drug abuse.

AMPHETAMINE-TYPE DRUGS (PEP PILLS, "UPPERS," "SPEED", "CRYSTAL," "METH")

Drug	Clinical Manifestations	Therapeutic Management
Amphetamine (Benzedrine)
Dextroamphetamine (Dexedrine)
Methamphetamine (Desoxyn)
MDMA ("Ecstasy," "Adam")
MDEA ("Eve")
MDA	Nausea, vomiting, anorexia, palpitations, tachycardia, increased blood pressure, tachypnea, anxiety, nervousness, diaphoresis, mydriasis
Repetitive or stereotyped behavior
Irritability, insomnia, agitation
Visual misperceptions, auditory hallucinations
Fearful anxiety/depression, cold, distant hostility, paranoia
Hyperactivity, rapid speech, euphoria
Seizures, coma, hyperthermia, cardiovascular collapse	1. Provide airway support, ventilation, cardiac monitoring; insert IV line.
2. Employ gastrointestinal decontamination in cases of oral overdose; activated charcoal, gastric lavage.
3. Keep in calm, quiet environment; elevated temperature potentiates amphetamine toxicity.
4. Use small doses of diazepam (IV) as prescribed for CNS and muscular hyperactivity.
5. Administer appropriate pharmacologic therapy as prescribed for severe hypertension and ventricular dysrhythmias.
6. Try to communicate with patient if delusions, hallucinations, are present
7. Place in a protective environment (preferably psychiatric security room with video monitoring) to observe for suicide attempt.
8. Refer for psychiatric evaluation.

HALLUCINOGENS OR PSYCHEDELIC-TYPE DRUGS

Drug	Clinical Manifestations	Therapeutic Management
Lysergic acid diethylamide (LSD)
Phencyclidine HCl (PCP, "angel dust")
Mescaline, psilocybin	Nystagmus, mild hypertension
Marked confusion bordering on panic
Incoherence, hyperactivity
Hazardous behavior: delirium, mania, self-injury
Hallucinations, body image distortion
Hypertension, hyperthermia, renal failure
Flashback: recurrence of LSD-like state without having taken the drug; may occur weeks or months after drug was taken
Convulsions, coma, circulatory collapse, death	*Emergency Management*
1. Evaluate and maintain patient's airway, breathing, and circulation.
2. Determine whether the patient has ingested hallucinogenic drug or has a toxic psychosis.
3. Try to communicate with the patient; reassure him.
a. "Talking down" involves understanding the process through which the patient is proceeding and helping him overcome his fears while establishing contact with reality.
b. Remind the patient that fear is common with this problem.
c. Reassure the patient that he is not losing his mind—that he is experiencing effect of drugs and that this will wear off.
d. Instruct the patient to keep his eyes open; this reduces intensity of reaction.

(continued)

TABLE 63–1.   *(Continued)*

Drug	Clinical Manifestations	Therapeutic Management

		e. Reduce sensory stimuli: minimize noise, lights, movement, tactile stimulation.
		f. Do not leave the patient alone.
		4. Sedate the patient as prescribed if his hyperactivity cannot be controlled; diazepam (Valium) or a barbiturate may be prescribed.
		5. Search for evidences of trauma; hallucinogen users have a tendency to "act out" their hallucinations.
		6. Manage seizures.
		7. Observe patient closely; his behavior may become hazardous.
		8. Monitor for hypertensive crisis if patient has prolonged psychosis due to drug ingestion.
		9. Place patient in a protected environment under proper medical supervision to prevent self-inflicted bodily harm.
		
		Management for Phencyclidine Abusers
		1. Place patient in a calm, supportive environment to minimize stimuli; protect from self-injury.
		2. Avoid talking down.
		3. Do not leave patient unobserved. Treat symptoms as they occur.
		  a. Drug effects are unpredictable and prolonged.
		  b. Symptoms are likely to exacerbate; patient becomes out of control.
		4. Refer patient for psychiatric evaluation.

DRUGS PRODUCING SEDATION, INTOXICATION, OR PSYCHOLOGIC AND PHYSICAL DEPENDENCE (NONBARBITURATE SEDATIVES)

Drug	Clinical Manifestations	Therapeutic Management

Diazepam (Valium)
Chlordiazepoxide (Librium)
Oxazepam (Serax)
Lorazepam (Ativan)
	Acute intoxication:
	  Respiratory depression
	  Decreasing mental alertness
	  Confusion
	  Slurred speech, decreased blood pressure
	  Ataxia
	  Pulmonary edema
	  Coma, death
		Management
		1. Endotracheal tube is inserted as a precaution; use assisted ventilation to stabilize and correct respiratory depression. Observe for sudden apnea and laryngeal spasm (especially in patients dependent on glutethimide [Doriden]).
		2. Assess for hypotension.
		  a. Insert indwelling catheter for comatose patient; decreased urinary volume is an index of reduced renal flow associated with reduced intravascular volume or vascular collapse.
		  b. Start volume expansion with saline or dextrose as prescribed.
		3. Evacuate stomach contents; emesis; lavage; activated charcoal; cathartic.
		4. Start ECG monitoring. Observe for dysrhythmias.

SALICYLATE POISONING

Drug	Clinical Manifestations	Therapeutic Management
Aspirin (present in compound analgesic tablets)	Restlessness, tinnitus, deafness, blurring of vision Hyperpnea, hyperpyrexia, sweating Epigastric pain, vomiting, dehydration	1. Treat respiratory depression. 2. Induce gastric emptying: emesis or lavage. 3. Give activated charcoal to adsorb aspirin; a cathartic may be administered with charcoal to help assure intestinal cleansing.

(continued)

TABLE 63-1.   (Continued)

Drug	Clinical Manifestations	Therapeutic Management
	Respiratory and metabolic acidosis Disorientation, coma, cardiovascular collapse	4. Support patient with intravenous infusions as prescribed to establish hydration and correct electrolyte imbalances. 5. Enhance elimination of salicylates as directed by forced diuresis, alkalinization of urine or peritoneal dialysis, or hemodialysis, according to severity of intoxication. 6. Monitor serum salicylate level for efficacy of treatment. 7. Administer specific prescribed pharmacologic agent for bleeding and other problems.

b. Start ECG monitoring.

c. Draw blood samples for testing glucose, electrolytes, BUN, creatinine, and appropriate toxicologic screen.

d. Start IV fluids.

3. Give a specific drug antagonist as prescribed if the drug is known. Naloxone hydrochloride (Narcan) is frequently used; 50% dextrose in water is also used (for hypoglycemia).

4. Remove the drug from the stomach as soon as possible.

a. Induce vomiting if the patient is seen early after ingestion; save the vomitus for toxicologic study.

b. Use gastric lavage if the patient is unconscious or if there is no way to determine when the drug was ingested.

   • In patients with absent gag or cough reflexes, carry out this procedure *only* after intubation with a cuffed endotracheal tube to prevent aspiration of the stomach contents.

c. Activated charcoal may be a useful adjunct to therapy and is used after emesis or lavage.

d. Save gastric aspirate for toxicologic analysis.

5. Provide supportive care.

a. Take rectal temperature; extremes of thermoregulation (hyperthermia and hypothermia) must be recognized and treated.

b. Treat seizures as directed; initiate seizure precautions.

c. Assist with hemodialysis and peritoneal dialysis for potentially lethal poisoning.

d. Insert an indwelling catheter to maintain a free urine flow, because the drug or metabolites are excreted by the urine.

6. Perform a thorough physical examination to rule out insulin shock, meningitis, subdural hematoma, stroke, and other possible causes.

a. Assess for needle marks and external evidence of trauma.

b. Carry out a rapid neurologic assessment (level of responsiveness, pupil size and reaction, reflexes, focal neurologic findings).

c. Keep in mind that many drug users take multiple drugs simultaneously.

d. Be aware that there is a high incidence of HIV infection and hepatitis B among IV drug users, which is the result of communal use of unsterile needles and syringes.

e. Examine the patient's breath for the characteristic odor of alcohol, acetone, and so forth.

7. Try to obtain a history of the drug experience (from the person accompanying the patient or the patient himself).

a. Adopt a supportive and realistic relationship with the patient.

b. Do not leave the patient alone; there is the potential for the patient to harm himself or emergency department staff.

8. Admit the patient to ICU if unconscious; if the patient has deliberately overdosed, psychiatric consultation is necessary.

9. Make every effort to enroll the patient in a drug treatment program (detoxification and rehabilitation) to intervene in a life-style that fosters addiction.

Alcohol Abuse

Acute Alcohol Intoxication

Alcohol is a psychotropic drug affecting mood, judgment, behavior, concentration, and consciousness. A significant number of heavy drinkers are young adults as well as people over 60 years of age. There is a high prevalence of alcoholism in emergency patients. Because alcoholic patients return frequently to the emergency department, they are often exasperating, taxing the endurance of the health professionals caring for them. Thus, their management requires patience as well as thoughtful and correct treatment.

Assessment.   *Ethanol* (alcohol) is a direct multisystem toxin and central nervous system depressant that causes drowsiness, incoordination, slurring of speech, sudden mood changes, aggression, belligerency, grandiosity, and uninhibited behavior. It can cause stupor and coma and even death if taken in excessive amounts.

The patient must be assessed for head injury, hypoglycemia (which mimics intoxication), and other health problems. The nursing diagnoses may include ineffective breathing pattern related to central nervous system depression, and high risk for violence (self-directed or directed at others) related to severe intoxication from alcohol.

Emergency Management of the Acutely Intoxicated Patient.   The treatment involves (1) detoxification of the acute poisoning; (2) recovery, or "drying out"; and (3) rehabilitation.

1. Approach the patient in a nonjudgmental manner, without condemnation or reproach.

a. Expect the patient to use mechanisms of denial and defensiveness.

b. Adopt a firm, consistent, accepting, and reasonable attitude.

c. Speak calmly and slowly; alcohol interferes with thought processes.

d. If the patient appears intoxicated, he is probably drunk even though he denies alcohol intake.

2. Obtain a sample for a blood alcohol test as directed.

3. Allow the drowsy patient to sleep off the state of alcoholic intoxication.

a. Observe for symptoms of central nervous system depression; maintain observation of the patient.

b. Maintain a patent airway.

c. Undress the patient and cover him with a blanket.

4. Sedate the noisy, belligerent patient as directed.

a. *Monitor the patient carefully*; observe for hypotension and decreased level of consciousness.

b. Monitor cardiac and respiratory rates and blood pressure.

5. Examine the patient for injuries and organic disease, which can easily be masked by alcoholic intoxication. (Persons with alcoholism suffer more injuries than does the general population. Also, acute alcohol intoxication is the cause of trauma for many people who are not alcoholics.)

a. Assess neurologic status; observe for symptoms of head injury.

b. *Assess for alcoholic coma, which is a medical emergency.*

c. Monitor carefully for seizures.

d. Evaluate for pulmonary infection.

(1) Pulmonary infections are more common in patients with alcoholism, resulting from respiratory depression, an impaired defense system, and a tendency toward gastric aspiration.

(2) The patient may show little increase in temperature or white blood cell count.

e. Observe for hypoglycemia.

6. Hospitalize the patient if necessary or admit him to a detoxification center; an effort should be made to examine the problems underlying the substance abuse.

Alcohol Withdrawal Delirium (*Delirium Tremens*)

Alcohol withdrawal delirium is an acute toxic state that follows a prolonged bout of steady drinking or sudden withdrawal from prolonged intake of alcohol. It may be precipitated by acute injury or infection (pneumonia, pancreatitis, hepatitis).

Clinical Manifestations and Assessment. Patients suspected of alcohol withdrawal delirium show signs of anxiety, uncontrollable fear, tremor, irritability, agitation, insomnia, and incontinence. They are talkative and preoccupied, and experience visual, tactile, olfactory, and auditory hallucinations that are frequently terrifying. Autonomic overactivity occurs and is evidenced by tachycardia, dilated pupils, and profuse perspiration. Usually, all vital signs are elevated in the alcoholic toxic state. Alcohol withdrawal delirium is life-threatening and carries a high mortality rate.

Emergency Management. The goals of management are to give proper sedation and support to enable the patient to rest and recover without danger of injury or peripheral vascular collapse.

1. Monitor the blood pressure, because the patient's subsequent medication may depend on blood pressure readings.

2. Perform a physical examination to identify pre-existing or contributing illnesses or injuries (*e.g.*, head injury, pneumonia).

3. Obtain a drug history to elicit information that may facilitate adjustment of sedative requirement.

4. Sedate the patient as directed with a sufficient dosage of medication to establish and maintain sedation to reduce agitation, prevent exhaustion, and promote sleep.

a. A variety of drugs and combinations of drugs are used, for example, chlordiazepoxide, diazepam, paraldehyde. Haloperidol may be given for severe acute alcohol withdrawal delirium.

b. The dosage is adjusted according to the patient's symptoms (agitation, anxiety) and blood pressure response.

5. Place the patient in a private room and observe closely.

a. Keep the room lighted to minimize potential for illusions and hallucinations.

b. Close closet and bathroom doors to eliminate shadows.

c. Keep the environment calm and nonstressful.

d. Observe the patient closely; homicidal or suicidal responses may result from hallucinations.

e. Have someone stay with the patient as much as possible; the presence of another person has a reassuring and quieting effect and helps the patient maintain contact with reality.

f. Explain visual misrepresentations (illusions) to strengthen the link with reality.

g. Explain in detail every procedure being performed.

h. Eliminate loud noises.

i. Call the patient by name.

j. Use protective devices/restraints as prescribed if necessary, if the patient is not under direct and constant observation.

• Precaution: The least restrictive device that will prevent the patient from injuring himself and others is used. Caution is taken to ensure that restraints are applied properly and that they are not applied in such a way that they impair circulation to any part of the body or interfere with respirations. Physical observation (*e.g.*, skin integrity, circulatory status, respiratory status) is ongoing, and the patient's response is documented.

6. Maintain electrolyte balance and hydration by way of the oral or IV route as prescribed. Fluid losses may be present from gastrointestinal losses (diarrhea) and profuse perspiration, and from the respiratory tract (hyperventilation). Or the patient may be overhydrated as a result of the effect of alcohol on antidiuretic hormone.

7. Record temperature, pulse, respiration, and blood pressure frequently (every 30 minutes in severe forms of delirium) in anticipation of peripheral circulatory collapse or hyperthermia (the two most lethal complications).

8. Administer phenytoin (Dilantin) or other anticonvulsant drugs as prescribed to prevent or control repeated withdrawal seizures.

9. Assess the respiratory, hepatic, and cardiovascular status; infections (pneumonia), trauma, hepatic failure, hypoglycemia, and cardiovascular problems are complications.

a. Hypoglycemia may accompany alcoholic withdrawal, because alcohol depletes liver glycogen stores and impairs gluconeogenesis; also, many patients with alcoholism suffer from malnutrition.

b. Administer parenteral dextrose as prescribed if liver glycogen is depleted. Give orange juice, Gatorade, or other carbohydrates to stabilize the blood sugar and to counteract tremulousness.

10. Provide supplemental vitamin therapy and a high-protein diet as prescribed; these patients are usually vitamin deficient.

11. Refer the patient to an alcoholic treatment center for subsequent follow-up and rehabilitation.

Psychiatric Emergencies

A psychiatric emergency is an urgent, serious disturbance of behavior, affect, or thought that makes the patient unable to cope with life situations and interpersonal relationships. A patient presenting with a psychiatric emergency may be (1) overactive or violent, (2) underactive or depressed, or (3) suicidal.

The most important concern of the emergency department personnel is whether the patient is likely to cause personal harm or injury to others. In general, the aim is to try to maintain the patient's self-esteem (and life, if necessary) while carrying out assessment and management. The patient is asked if he is currently under psychiatric treatment.

Overactive Patients

Patients in the overactive category display disturbed, uncooperative, and paranoid behavior, as well as anxiety and panic-like feelings. They may be prone to assaultive and destructive impulses and abnormal social behavior. Intense nervousness, depression, and crying are also evident in some patients. Their disturbed and noisy behavior may be compounded by alcohol or drug intoxication.

Emergency Management

1. Determine from the family or another reliable source the events that led to the crisis; whether the patient has had past mental illness, hospitalizations, injuries, or serious illnesses; whether he uses alcohol or drugs; and whether he has experienced crises in interpersonal relationships or intrapsychic conflicts.
   a. Be aware that abnormal thoughts and behavior may be manifestations of an underlying physical disorder, such as hypoglycemia, stroke, epilepsy, and drug or alcohol toxicity.
   b. Perform a physical assessment when feasible.
2. Attempt to gain control of the situation.
   a. Approach the patient with a calm, confident, and firm manner; this attitude is therapeutic and has a calming effect.
   b. Introduce yourself by name.
   c. Tell him, "I am here to help you."
   d. Repeat the patient's name from time to time.
   e. Speak in one-thought sentences. Be consistent.
   f. Give the patient space. Let him slow down by himself and allow him to become compliant.
   g. Be interested in and listen to the patient; encourage him to talk about his thoughts and feelings.
   h. Offer appropriate explanations. Tell the truth.
3. Administer a psychotropic agent for emergency management of functional psychosis as prescribed. Chlorpromazine (Thorazine) or haloperidol (Haldol) acts specifically against psy-

chotic symptoms of thought fragmentation and perceptual and behavioral aberrations.
   a. The initial dosage depends on the patient's body weight and the severity of the symptoms.
   b. Observe the patient for 1 hour after the initial dose to determine the degree of change in psychotic behavior.
   c. Subsequent dosages depend on the patient's reaction.
   d. If the behavior is caused by hallucinogens (*e.g.*, LSD), psychotropic drugs (exerting an effect on the mind) are not used.
4. Use restraints only as a last resort and as prescribed.
5. The patient is admitted to a psychiatric unit, or psychiatric outpatient treatment is arranged.

Violent Patients

Violent and aggressive behavior is usually episodic and is a means of expressing feelings of anger, fear, or hopelessness about a situation. Usually, the patient has a history of outbursts of rage, temper tantrums, or generally impulsive behavior. Persons with a tendency to violence frequently lose control when intoxicated with alcohol or drugs. Family members are the most frequent victims of their aggression. Patients with a propensity for violence include those intoxicated by drugs or alcohol; those going through drug or alcohol withdrawal; and those with acute paranoid schizophrenic state, acute organic brain syndrome, acute psychosis, a paranoid character, a borderline personality, or an antisocial personality.

A specially designated room with at least two exits should be used for the interview. No objects that could be used as weapons should be in sight. If the interviewer feels anxious or uneasy about the patient's response, security staff, a family member, or another health care worker should be asked to remain in the hall nearby in the event that additional help is needed.

The nursing diagnoses could include high risk for violence (self-directed or directed at others) related to acute paranoid schizophrenic state. The goal is to bring this violence under control.

Emergency Management

1. Keep the door of the room open and be in clear view of the staff. Remain between the patient and the door. Do not block the patient's exit to the door; the patient may feel closed in and threatened.
2. Help the patient bring his violence under control.
   a. Give the patient space. Do not make any sudden movement.
   b. If the patient is carrying a weapon, ask him to surrender it.
   c. If the patient is unwilling to surrender his weapon, call the security staff; they may seek assistance from the local police department.
3. Do not leave the patient alone; this can be interpreted as rejection, or the patient may try to harm himself.
4. Adopt a calm, noncritical approach and remain in control of the situation. External calm and structure may help the patient to gain control.
5. Talk and listen to the patient.
   a. Crisis intervention is best done with an attitude of interest in the patient's well-being and with an attempt to tune in to the patient while at the same time remaining firm.

b. Acknowledge the patient's state of agitation, for example, "I want to work with you to relieve your distress."

c. Give the patient the opportunity to ventilate his anger verbally; avoid challenging the delusional patient.

d. Try to hear what the patient is saying.

e. Convey an expectation of appropriate behavior and make him aware that help is available to help him to gain control.

    (1) Let the patient know that his behavior may be frightening to those around him and that violence is not acceptable.

    (2) Describe the help available in crisis situations: clinic, emergency department, mental health facility.

6. Allow the security personnel or police to intervene if the patient does not become calm.

a. Offer protection of hospitalization; this is usually welcomed by the patient who fears losing control or harming himself or others.

b. If the above fails to attenuate the patient's tension, administer medication as prescribed (rapid tranquilization with haloperidol, diazepam, or chlorpromazine) to reduce tension, anxiety, and hyperactivity.

c. Use restraints when necessary but with a minimum of force. Obtain a physician's order for the restraints.

    (1) Use restraints with verbal intervention to calm the patient and make him more compliant.

    (2) Have appropriate personnel available when applying restraints.

      • Precaution: The least restrictive device that will prevent the patient from injuring himself and others is used. Caution is taken to ensure that restraints are applied properly and that they are not applied in such a way that they impair circulation to any part of the body or interfere with respirations. Physical observation (*e.g.*, skin integrity, circulatory status, respiratory status) is ongoing, and the patient's response is documented.

7. Refer the patient for further mental health treatment after combativeness, agitation, and fear have decreased.

Depressed Patients

In the emergency department, depression may be seen as the primary condition bringing the patient to the health care facility, or depression may be masked by anxiety and somatic complaints.

The depressed person has some sort of mood disturbance. Assessment includes observing for sadness, apathy, feelings of worthlessness, self-blame, suicidal thoughts, desire to escape, avoidance of simple problems, anorexia and weight loss, lessened interest in sex, sleeplessness, and ceaseless activity or reduction in activity.

The agitated depressed individual may exhibit motor restlessness and severe anxiety.

Emergency Management

1. Listen to the patient in a calm, unhurried manner.

a. The patient benefits from ventilating his feelings.

b. Give the patient an opportunity to talk about his problems.

c. Anticipate that the patient may be suicidal.

d. Attempt to find out if the patient has thought about or attempted suicide: "Have you ever thought about taking your own life?" The patient is generally relieved because of the opportunity to discuss his feelings.

e. Find out if there is an illness, perceived or real.

f. Assess whether there has been sudden worsening of depression.

g. Notify relatives about a seriously depressed patient. Do not leave the patient alone, since suicide is usually committed in solitude.

2. Give antidepressant and antianxiety agents as prescribed.

3. Emphasize to the patient that depression is treatable.

4. Be aware of crisis and supportive services in the community: mental health center, telephone counseling and referral, suicide prevention centers, group therapy, marital and family counseling, befriending programs.

5. Refer the patient for psychiatric consultation or to a psychiatric unit.

Suicidal Patients

Attempted suicide is an act that stems from depression (the loss of a loved one, the loss of body integrity or status, poor self-image) and can be viewed as a cry for help and intervention. Those at risk include elderly people; males; young adults; people who are enduring unusual loss or stress; those who are unemployed, divorced, widowed, or living alone; those who are showing significant depression (weight loss, sleep disturbances, somatic complaints, suicidal preoccupation); and those who have a history of previous suicidal attempt or completed suicide in the family, or who have a psychiatric illness.

Prevention

1. Be aware of persons at risk.

2. Determine whether a person has communicated *suicidal intent*, such as preoccupation with death or talking of someone else's suicide:

    "I'm tired of living."

    "I've put my affairs in order."

    "I'm better off dead."

    "I'm a burden to my family."

3. Determine whether he has ever attempted suicide; the risk is much greater in these cases.

4. Is there a family history of suicide?

5. Was there loss of a parent at an early age?

6. Does he have a specific plan for suicide? A means to carry out the plan?

Emergency Management

1. Treat the consequences of the suicide attempt (*e.g.*, gunshot wound, drug overdose).

2. Prevent further self-injury; a patient who has made a suicidal gesture may do so again.

3. Employ crisis intervention (a form of brief psychotherapy) to determine suicidal potential; discover areas of depression and conflict; find out about the patient's support system; and determine whether hospitalization, or psychiatric referral, is warranted.

4. Arrange for admission to ICU if condition warrants, arrange follow-up care, or arrange for admission to the psychiatric unit, depending on the assessment of suicide potential.

Sexual Assault

Legally, *rape* is defined as carnal knowledge of a female by force or the threat of force against one's will. It is one of the fastest growing crimes of violence. The feminist movement has focused on the rights and care of rape victims, and law enforcement agencies are becoming increasingly sensitive and aggressive in the management of these crimes. Rape can also happen to males, especially young males. Rape crisis centers offer extensive support and education of victims and help them through the subsequent courtroom experience.

The manner in which the patient is received and treated in the emergency department is important to his or her future psychological well-being. Crisis intervention should begin when the patient enters the health facility. The patient should be seen immediately on entrance into the emergency department. Most hospitals have a written protocol that reflects consideration for the victim's physical and emotional needs as well as concern for meeting requirements for subsequent legal proceedings.

The patient's reaction to rape has been termed the *rape trauma syndrome* and is seen as an acute stress reaction to a life-threatening situation. The nurse performing the assessment is aware that the patient may go through several phases of psychological reactions:

1. An acute disorganization phase that may be manifested in two ways:

- Expressed state, in which shock, disbelief, fear, guilt, humiliation, anger, and other such emotions are encountered.
- Controlled state, in which feelings are masked or hidden and the victim appears composed.

2. A phase of denial and unwillingness to talk about the incident, followed by a phase of heightened anxiety, fear, flashbacks, sleep disturbances, hyperalertness, and psychosomatic reactions.

3. A phase of reorganization, in which the incident is put into perspective. Some victims never fully recover, and they develop chronic stress disorders and phobias.

The nursing diagnoses may include rape trauma syndrome related to a life-threatening situation. The patient's goal is to regain control over his or her life.

Emergency Management. The goals of management are to give sympathetic support, to reduce the emotional trauma of the patient, and to gather available evidence for possible legal proceedings.

1. Respect the privacy and sensitivity of the patient; be kind and supportive.
   a. Reassure the patient that anxiety is natural and that appropriate support is available from professional and community resources. Contact Rape Victim Companion Program, if available in the community, and request services of a volunteer.
   b. Accept the emotional reactions of the patient (*e.g.*, hysteria, stoicism, overwhelmed feeling).
   c. Do not leave the patient alone.
2. Assist with the physical examination.
   a. Secure written, witnessed informed consent from the patient (or parent or guardian if the patient is a minor) for examination and for taking of photographs if necessary, and for release of findings to police.
   b. Take history only if the patient has not already talked to a police officer, social worker, or crisis intervention worker. Do not ask the patient to repeat the history. Record the history of the event in the patient's own words.

c. Ask if the patient has bathed, douched, brushed teeth, changed clothes, urinated, or defecated since the attack; this may alter interpretation of subsequent findings.
d. Record the time of admission, time of examination, date and time of alleged rape, and general appearance of the patient.
   (1) Document any evidence of trauma: discoloration, bruises, lacerations, secretions, torn and bloody clothing.
   (2) Document emotional state.
e. Assist the patient to undress; drape properly.
   (1) Ask the patient to place each item of clothing in a separate paper bag. (Plastic bags promote moisture retention, which may lead to the formation of mold and mildew, which can destroy evidence.)
   (2) Label bags appropriately; give to appropriate law enforcement authorities.
f. Examine the patient (from head to toe) for injuries, especially to the head, neck, breasts, thighs, back, and buttocks.
   (1) Assess for external evidence of trauma (bruises, contusions, lacerations, stab wounds).
   (2) Assess for dried semen stains (appearing as crusted, flaking areas) on the patient's body or clothes.
   (3) Inspect fingers for broken nails and tissue and foreign materials under nails.
   (4) Assist in conducting oral examination. Secure a specimen of saliva; take prescribed cultures of gum and tooth areas.
   (5) Document evidence of trauma with body diagrams and photographs.
3. Assist with pelvic and rectal examinations.
   a. Advise the patient of the nature and necessity of each procedure; give the rationale for each question asked.
      (1) Examine perineum (and other areas) with a Woods lamp or other filtered ultraviolet light; areas that are found to fluoresce may indicate semen stains.
      (2) Note color and consistency of any discharge present.
      (3) Use a water-moistened vaginal speculum for examination; do not use lubricant, which contains chemicals that may interfere with later forensic testing of specimens and acid phosphatase determinations.
   b. Assist with securing laboratory specimens.
      (1) Collect vaginal aspirate, which is examined for presence or absence of motile and nonmotile sperm.
      (2) Use a sterile swab to draw secretions from the vaginal pool for acid phosphatase, blood group antigen of semen, and precipitin test against human sperm and blood.
      (3) Obtain separate smears from the oral, vaginal, and anal areas.
      (4) Obtain culture of body orifices for gonorrhea.
      (5) Obtain blood serum for syphilis; a sample of serum may be frozen and saved for future testing.
      (6) Conduct a test for pregnancy if there is a possibility that the patient may be pregnant.
      (7) Collect foreign material (leaves, grass, dirt) and place in a clean envelope.
      (8) Comb the pubic hairs with a prepackaged clean comb. Trim areas of pubic hair suspected of containing semen. Obtain several pubic hairs with follicles; place in separate containers and identify these as patient's pubic hairs.

(9) Examine rectum for signs of trauma, blood, semen stains.

(10) Label each specimen with name of patient, date, time of collection, body area from which specimen was obtained, and names of personnel collecting specimens to preserve chain of evidence; give to designated person (*e.g.*, crime laboratory) and obtain an itemized receipt.

(11) Photographs are taken by designated person.

4. Treat associated injuries as indicated. Give the patient the option of prophylaxis against sexually transmitted disease.

a. Intramuscular ceftriaxone (Rocephin) administered with 1% xylocaine may be prescribed as prophylaxis for gonorrhea.

b. Doxycycline (Vibramycin) taken for 10 days may be prescribed as prophylaxis for syphilis and chlamydia.

5. Antipregnancy measures may be considered if the patient is of childbearing age, is using no contraceptives, and is at high risk in her menstrual cycle.

a. A postcoital contraceptive drug may be prescribed after a pregnancy test: Ovral contains estrogen ethinyl estradiol and progestin norgestrel.

b. To promote effectiveness, it is preferable that Ovral be administered within 12 to 24 hours and no later than 72 hours after intercourse; the 21-day package rather than the 28-day package is prescribed so that the patient does not take the inert tablets by mistake.

c. An antiemetic may be given as prescribed to decrease discomfort from side effects.

6. Offer cleansing douche, mouthwash, and fresh clothing.

7. Provide for follow-up services:

a. Make an appointment for follow-up surveillance for pregnancy and sexually transmitted disease and HIV testing.

b. Inform the patient of counseling services to prevent long-term psychological effects; counseling services should be made available to both the patient and the family; referral is made to the Rape Victim Companion Program if available.

c. Encourage the patient to return to the previous level of functioning as soon as possible.

d. The patient should be accompanied by a family member or friend when leaving the health care facility.

Management of patients who present to emergency departments with acute drug abuse, psychiatric emergencies, or after sexual assault is complex and requires a multidisciplinary team approach. The patient's physiologic and psychological and emotional status are continuously assessed and managed. Precautions are taken to assure the safety of both the patient and the hospital personnel involved in his care. In addition, specific protocols are followed for victims of sexual assault; these provide for crisis intervention and for measures that ensure that the requirements for subsequent legal proceedings are met. Once the patient's acute needs have been met, provisions are made for ongoing treatment as appropriate.

Bibliography

Books

American Academy of Orthopedic Surgeons. Emergency Care and Transportation of the Sick and Injured, 4th ed. Park Ridge, IL, American Academy of Orthopedic Surgeons, 1987.

American Association of Critical Care Nurses. Outcome Standards for Nursing Care of the Critically Ill. Laguna Niguel, CA, American Association of Critical Care Nurses, 1990.

American Heart Association. Textbook of Cardiac Life Support, 2nd ed. Dallas, American Heart Association, 1987.

Biros MH and Sterner S (eds). Handbook of Urgent Care Medicine. Rockville, MD, Aspen Publishers, 1990.

Cardiopulmonary Emergencies. Springhouse, PA, Springhouse Corporation, 1990.

Cardona VD et al (eds). Trauma Nursing: From Resuscitation Through Rehabilitation. Philadelphia, WB Saunders, 1988.

Galli RL, Spaite DW, and Simon RR. Emergency Orthopedics: The Spine. Norwalk, CT, Appleton & Lange, 1989.

Harwood-Nuss A et al. The Clinical Practice of Emergency Medicine. Philadelphia, JB Lippincott, 1990.

Ho MT and Saunders CE (eds). Current Emergency Diagnosis and Treatment, 3rd ed. Norwalk, CT, Appleton & Lange, 1990.

Holloway NM. Nursing the Critically Ill Adult. Menlo Park, CA, Addison-Wesley, 1988.

Kitt S and Kaiser J (eds). Emergency Nursing: A Physiologic and Clinical Perspective. Philadelphia, WB Saunders, 1990.

Lanros NE. Assessment and Intervention in Emergency Nursing, 3rd ed. Norwalk, CT, Appleton & Lange, 1988.

Mallon B et al. Orthopaedics for the House Officer. Baltimore, Williams & Wilkins, 1990.

Mlynczak-Callahan B (ed). Case Studies in Emergency Nursing. Baltimore, Williams & Wilkins, 1990.

Moore S. Ready Reference for Emergency Nursing. Baltimore, Williams & Wilkins, 1990.

Moore S and Charlson DA. Clinical Guidelines for Emergency Nursing: Standardized Care Plans. Rockville, MD, Aspen Publishers, 1987.

Mowad L and Ruhle DC (eds). Handbook of Emergency Nursing: The Nursing Process Approach. Norwalk, CT, Appleton & Lange, 1988.

Richardson JD and Polk HC. Trauma: Clinical Care and Pathophysiology. Chicago, Year Book Medical Publishers, 1987.

Rogers JH et al. Emergency Nursing: A Practice Guide. Baltimore, Williams & Wilkins, 1989.

Rosen P et al (eds). Emergency Medicine: Concepts and Clinical Practice, 2nd ed. St Louis, CV Mosby, 1988.

Schwartz GR et al. Principles and Practice of Emergency Medicine: The Essential Update. Philadelphia, WB Saunders, 1989.

Sheehy SB et al. Manual of Clinical Trauma Care: The First Hour. St Louis, CV Mosby, 1989.

Skeet M (ed). Emergency Procedures and First Aid for Nurses. Chicago, Year Book Medical Publishers, 1988.

Stine RJ and Marcus RH (eds). A Practical Approach to Emergency Medicine. Boston, Little, Brown, 1987.

Strange JM (ed). Shock Trauma Care Plans. Springhouse, PA, Springhouse Corporation, 1987.

Vincent J (ed). Update in Intensive Care and Emergency Medicine. New York, Springer-Verlag, 1989.

Welton RH and Shane KA (eds). Case Studies in Trauma Nursing. Baltimore, Williams & Wilkins, 1989.

Wilkins E et al (eds). MGH Textbook of Emergency Medicine: Scientific Foundations and Current Practice: Emergency Care as Practiced at the Massachusetts General Hospital. Baltimore, Williams & Wilkins, 1989.

Yvorra JG (ed). Mosby's Emergency Dictionary: Quick Reference for Emergency Responders. St Louis, CV Mosby, 1989.

Journals

Infection Control

Dickerson M. Protecting yourself from AIDS: Infection control measures. Crit Care Nurse 1989 Nov/Dec; 9(10):26–28.

Halpern J. Precautions to prevent transmission of human immunodeficiency virus infections in emergency settings. J Emerg Nurs 1987 Sep/Oct; 13(5):298–300.

Jordan KS. Assessment of the person with acquired immunodeficiency syndrome in the emergency department. J Emerg Nurs 1987 Nov/Dec; 13(6):342–345.

Recommendations for prevention of HIV transmission in health care settings. JAMA 1987 Sep; 258(10):1293–1305.

Geriatrics

Anderson G. Would you know what caused these geriatric emergencies? RN 1988 Aug; 52(8):26–32.

Brenner ZR. Nursing elderly cardiac clients. Crit Care Nurse 1987 Mar/Apr; 7(2):78–87.

Greenstien RA and Hess DE. Psychiatric emergencies in the elderly. Emerg Med Clin North Am 1990 May; 8(2):429–441.

Martin RE and Tiberian G. Multiple trauma and the elderly patient. Emerg Med Clin North Am 1990 May; 8(2):411–420.

Miller MD. Orthopedic trauma in the elderly. Emerg Med Clin North Am 1990 May; 8(2):325–339.

Resuscitation

Bartz C. Pharmacologic augmentation of cardiac output following cardiac arrest. Crit Care Nurs Q 1988 Mar; 10(4):43–49.

Cheney R. Defibrillation. Crit Care Nurs Q 1988 Mar; 10(4):9–15.

Cuzzel JZ and Rodriquez LA. How to use a bag-valve-mask device for artificial ventilation. Am J Nurs 1989 Jul; 89(7):932–933.

DeAngelis R and Lessig NL. Physical augmentation of cardiac output. Crit Care Nurs Q 1988 Mar; 10(4):33–42.

Jost P. The role of antidysrhythmics in cardiac arrest. Crit Care Nurs Q 1988 Mar; 10(4):63–67.

Middaugh RE, Middaugh DJ, and Menk EJ. Current considerations in respiratory and acid-base management during cardiopulmonary resuscitation. Crit Care Nurs Q 1988 Mar; 10(4):25–33.

Sarsany S. Are you ready for this bedside emergency? Sudden loss of consciousness. RN 1988 Nov; 51(11):47–48.

Sheehy SB. A quick overview of the new standards and guidelines for cardiopulmonary resuscitation and emergency cardiac care. J Emerg Nurs 1987 Jan/Feb; 13(1):47–49.

Skootsky SA and Abraham E. Continuous oxygen consumption during initial emergency department resuscitation of critically ill patients. Crit Care Med 1988 Jul; 16(7):706–709.

Control of Hemorrhage Due to Trauma

Halfman-Franey M. Current trends in hemodynamic monitoring of patients in shock. Crit Care Nurs Q 1988 Jun; 11(1):9–18.

Perry A. Shock complications. Crit Care Nurs Q 1988 Jun; 11(1):1–8.

Sarsany S. Are you ready for this bedside emergency? Massive bleeding. RN 1988 Feb; 51(2):36–38.

Shock

Burnett DA and Rikkers LF. Nonoperative emergency treatment of variceal hemorrhage. Surg Clin North Am 1990 Apr; 70(2):291–306.

Hancock BG and Eberhard NK. The pharmacologic management of shock. Crit Care Nurs Q 1988 Jun; 11(1):19–29.

Meyers KA and Hickey MK. Nursing management of hypovolemic shock. Crit Care Q 1988 Jun; 11(1):57–67.

Rice V. Shock, a clinical syndrome: An update. Part 1. Crit Care Nurse 1991 Apr; 11(4):20–27.

Rice V. Shock, a clinical syndrome: An update. Part 2. Crit Care Nurse 1991 May; 11(5):74–82.

Rice V. Shock, a clinical syndrome: An update. Part 3. Crit Care Nurse 1991 Jun; 11(6):34–39.

Rice V. Shock, a clinical syndrome: An update. Part 4. Crit Care Nurse 1991 July; 11(7):28–40.

Trauma

Alexander MH. Mechanism and pattern of injury associated with use of seat belts. J Emerg Nurs 1988 Jul/Aug; 14(4):214–216.

Amidei CS. What to do until the neurosurgeon arrives . . . J Emerg Nurs 1988 Sep/Oct; 14(5):296–301.

Ammons AA. Cerebral injuries and intracranial hemorrhages as a result of trauma. Nurs Clin North Am 1990 Mar; 25(1):23–33.

Andrews J. Difficult diagnoses in blunt thoraco-abdominal trauma. J Emerg Nurs 1989 Sep/Oct; 15(5):399–404.

Ansio JA et al. Trauma: A systematic approach to management. Am Fam Physician 1988 Sep; 38(3):97–112.

Atkins J, Piazza D, and Pierce J. Overlooked gunshot wound in a motor vehicle accident victim: Clinical and legal risks. J Emerg Nurs 1988 May/Jun; 14(3):142–144.

Beaver BM. Care of the multiple trauma victim: The first hour. Nurs Clin North Am 1990 Mar; 25(1):11–21.

Bryson BL et al. Trauma to the aging cervical spine. J Emerg Nurs 1987 Nov/Dec; 13(6):334–341.

Cunningham JL. Assessment and care of the patient with myocardial contusion. Crit Care Nurse 1987 Mar/Apr; 7(2):68–75.

Fontaine DK. Physical, personal, and cognitive responses to trauma. Crit Care Nurs Clin North Am 1989 Mar; 1(1):11–22.

Gough JE, Allison EJ, and Raju VP. Flail chest: Management implications for emergency nurses. J Emerg Nurs 1987 Nov/Dec; 13(6):330–333.

Halpern JS. Mechanisms and patterns of trauma. J Emerg Nurs 1989 Sep/Oct; 15(5):380–388.

Hammond SG. Chest injuries in the trauma patient. Nurs Clin North Am 1990 Mar; 25(1):35–43.

Herron DG and Nance J. Emergency department nursing management of patients with orthopedic fractures resulting from motor vehicle accidents. Nurs Clin North Am 1990 Mar; 25(1):71–83.

Huggins B. Trauma physiology. Nurs Clin North Am 1990 Mar; 25(1):1–10.

Kite JH. Cardiac and great vessel trauma: Assessment, pathophysiology, and intervention. J Emerg Nurs 1987 Nov/Dec; 13(6):346–351.

Kleeman KM. Families in crisis due to multiple trauma. Crit Care Nurs Clin North Am 1989 Mar; 1(1):23–31.

Lindenbaum GA et al. Patterns of alcohol and drug abuse in an urban trauma center: The increasing role of cocaine use. J Trauma 1989 Dec; 29(12):1654–1658.

Loomis J. Traumatic amputation and successful replantation of the left hand after an industrial accident. J Emerg Nurs 1987 Sep/Oct; 13(6):269–271.

McGonigal MD, Lucas CE, and Legerwood AM. The effects of treatment of renal trauma on renal function. J Trauma 1987 May; 27(5):471–475.

Merlotti GJ et al. Peritoneal lavage in penetrating thoraco-abdominal trauma. J Trauma 1988 Jan; 28(1):17–23.

Michal DM. Nursing management of hypothermia in the multiple trauma patient. J Emerg Nurs 1989 Sep/Oct; 15(5):116–121.

Neff JA. Blunt abdominal trauma. J Emerg Nurs 1987 Mar/Apr; 13(2):114–117.

Oakely L and Johnson J. Traumatic injury during pregnancy. Crit Care Nurse 1991 Jun; 11(6):64–71.

O'Hara MM. Emergency care of the patient with a traumatic amputation. J Emerg Nurs 1987 Sep/Oct; 13(6):272–277.

Ordog GJ, Wasserberger J, and Balasubramaniam S. Shotgun wound ballistics. J Trauma 1988 May; 28(5):624–631.

Pearce WH and Whitehill TA. Carotid and vertebral arterial injuries. Surg Clin North Am 1988 Aug; 68(4):705–723.

Proehl JA. Compartment syndrome. J Emerg Nurs 1988 Sep/Oct; 14(5):283–291.

Richmond TS. Spinal cord injury. Nurs Clin North Am 1990 Mar; 25(1):57–69.

Romeo JH. The critical minutes after spinal cord injury. RN 1988 Apr; 51(4):61–67.

Sedlack SK and Mace D. Hidden problems with bleeding in trauma patients. J Emerg Nurs 1989 Sep/Oct; 15(5):422–426.

Smeltzer SC. Research in trauma nursing: State of the art and future directions. J Emerg Nurs 1988 May/Jun; 14(3):145–153.

Smith LG and Glowac BS. New frontiers in the management of the multiple injured patient. Crit Care Nurs Clin North Am 1989 Mar; 1(1):1–9.

Soderstrom CA and Cowley RA. A national alcohol and trauma center survey. Missed opportunities, failures of responsibility. Arch Surg 1987 Sep; 122(12):1067–1071.

Sommers MS. Blunt renal trauma. Crit Care Nurse 1990 Mar; 10(3):38–48.

Stewart PB. Maxillofacial trauma: Implications for critical care. Crit Care Nurse 1989 Jun; 9(6):44–57.

Turner JT. Cardiovascular trauma. Nurs Clin North Am 1990 Mar; 25(1):119–130.

Wagner MM. The patient with abdominal injuries. Nurs Clin North Am 1990 Mar; 25(1):45–55.

Weiskittel P and Sommers MS. The patient with lower urinary tract trauma. Crit Care Nurse 1989 Jan; 9(1):53–64.

White KM. Injuring mechanisms of gunshot wounds. Nurs Clin North Am 1989 Mar; 1(1):97–103.

Temperature Emergencies

Iced peritoneal lavage for heat stroke. Emerg Med 1990 May 30; 22(10):83–84.

Michal DM. Nursing management of hypothermia in the multiple-trauma patient. J Emerg Nurs 1989 Sep/Oct; 15(5):416–421.

Neff J. Standard of care for the adult patient with thermal injury. J Emerg Nurs 1987 Jan/Feb; 13(1):60–63.

Sahdev P et al. Hypothermia in the prehospital environment. Emerg Care Q 1990 Feb; 5(4):61–71.

Poisonings

Dailey MA. Carbon monoxide poisoning. J Emerg Nurs 1989 Mar/Apr; 15(2):120–123.

Joubert DW. Use of emetic, adsorbent, and cathartic agents in acute drug overdose. J Emerg Nurs 1987 Jan/Feb; 13(1):49–51.

Martindale LG. Carbon monoxide poisoning: The rest of the story. J Emerg Nurs 1989 Mar/Apr; 15(2):101–104.

Meyer D. Ethylene glycol poisoning. Focus Crit Care 1988 Dec; 15(6):54–57.

Newton M et al. Descriptive outline of major poisoning treatment modes. J Emerg Nurs 1987 Mar/Apr; 13(2):102–106.

Newton M et al. General treatments of household poisonings. J Emerg Nurs 1987 Jan/Feb; 13(1):12–15.

Newton M et al. Specific treatments of poisoning by household products and medications. J Emerg Nurs 1987 Jan/Feb; 13(1):16–26.

O'Neal L. Acute methyl bromide toxicity. J Emerg Nurs 1987 Mar/Apr; 13(2):96–98.

Robinson D. Ethylene glycol toxicity. Crit Care Nurse 1989 Jun; 9(6):70–74.

Scherb BJ. Carbon monoxide poisoning: Hyperbaric oxygenation preparations. Dimens Crit Care Nurs 1990 May/Jun; 9(3):143–149.

Turnbull TL et al. Emergency department screening for unsuspected carbon monoxide exposure. Ann Emerg Med 1988 May; 17(5):478–483.

Substance Abuse

Kellerman AL et al. Utilization and yield of drug screening in the emergency department. Am J Emerg Med 1988 Jan; 6(1):14–20.

Lowery DW and Galli RL. Street drugs: Recognition and management of the acutely intoxicated patient. Emerg Care Q 1990 Oct; 6(3):45–53.

Merigian KS et al. Use of abbreviated mental status examination in the initial assessment of overdose patients. Arch Emerg Med 1988 Sep; 5(3):139–145.

Povenmire KI and House MA. Acute crack cocaine intoxication: A case study. Focus Crit Care 1989 Apr; 16(2):112–119.

Rich J. Action stat! Acute alcohol intoxication. Nursing 1989 Sep; 19(9):33.

Stewart W. Can we keep Jane alive until an antidote arrives? RN 1988 Jan; 51(1):32–34.

Weaver DA. Cocaine-induced chest pain and myocardial ischemia. J Emerg Nurs 1988 Jul/Aug; 14(4):203–205.

Psychiatric Emergencies

Dreyfus JK. Nursing assessment of the ED patient with psychiatric symptoms: A quick reference. J Emerg Nurs 1987 Sep/Oct; 13(5):278–282.

Kurlowicz LH. Violence in the emergency department. Am J Nurs 1990 Sep; 90(9):34–40.

Sarsany S. Are you ready for this bedside emergency? Violent behavior. RN 1988 Sep; 51(9):64–68.

Miscellaneous

Adams G. The forgotten victims of a medical crisis. RN 1988 Apr; 51(4):30–33.

Adamski DB. Assessment and treatment of allergic response to stinging insects. J Emerg Nurs 1990 Mar/Apr; 16(2):77–80.

Bell NK. Ethical dilemmas in trauma nursing. Nurs Clin North Am 1990 Mar; 25(1):143–154.

Dickerson M. Anaphylaxis and anaphylactic shock. Crit Care Nurs Q 1988 Jun; 11(1):68–74.

Dyer C and Roberts D. Thermal trauma. Nurs Clin North Am 1990 Mar; 25(1):85–117.

Golden H. Near-drowning. Nursing 1988 Jul; 18(7):33.

Hicks DJ. The patient who's been raped. Emerg Med 1988 Nov; 20(20):106–122.

McKinley MG. Near drowning: A nursing challenge. Crit Care Nurse 1989 Nov/Dec; 9(10):52–60.

Minton SA. Present tests for detection of snake venom: Clinical applications. Ann Emerg Med 1987 Sep; 16(9):932–937.

Pennell TC, Babu SS, and Meredith JW. The management of snake and spider bites in the southeastern United States. Am Surg 1987 Apr; 53(4):198–204.

Solursh DS. The family of the trauma victim. Nurs Clin North Am 1990 Mar; 25(1):155–162.

Wasserman GS. Wound care of spider and snake envenomations. Ann Emerg Med 1988 Dec; 17(12):1331–1335.

When a snake strikes. Emerg Med 1990 Jun; 22(12):21–43.

Appendix:
Diagnostic Studies
and Their Meaning

Abbreviations

Conventional Units

kg = kilogram
g = gram
mg = milligram
μg = microgram
$\mu\mu$g = micromicrogram
ng = nanogram
pg = picogram
dl = 100 milliliters
ml = milliliter

mm^3 = cubic millimeter
fl = femtoliter
mM = millimole
nM = nanomole
mOsm = milliosmole
mm = millimeter
μm = micron or micrometer
mm Hg = millimeters of mercury
U = unit
mU = milliunit
μU = microunit
mEq = milliequivalent
IU = International Unit
mIU = milliInternational Unit

SI Units

g = gram
L = liter
d = day
hr = hour
mol = mole
mmol = millimole
μmol = micromole
nmol = nanomole
pmol = picomole

From Goodman D. Appendix I: Diagnostic Studies and Their Meaning. In The Lippincott Manual of Nursing Practice, 5th ed. Philadelphia, JB Lippincott, 1991.

Reference Ranges—Hematology*

Determination	Reference Range		Clinical Significance
	Conventional Units	SI Units	
A₂ hemoglobin	1.5%–3.5% of total hemoglobin	Mass fraction: 0.015–0.035 of total hemoglobin	Increased in certain types of thalassemia
Bleeding time	2–8 min	2–8 min	Prolonged in thrombocytopenia, defective platelet function, and aspirin therapy
Factor V assay (proaccelerin factor)	60%–140%		
Factor VII assay (anti-hemophiliac factor)	50%–200%		Deficient in classical hemophilia
Factor IX assay (plasma thromboplastin component)	75%–125%		Deficient in Christmas disease (pseudohemophilia)
Factor X (Stuart factor)	60%–140%		Deficient in Stuart clotting defect
Fibrinogen	200–400 mg/dl	2–4 g/dl	Increased in pregnancy, infections accompanied by leukocytosis, nephrosis. Decreased in severe liver disease, abruptio placentae
Fibrin split products	<10 mg/L	<10 mg/L	Increased in disseminated intravascular coagulopathy
Fibrinolysins (whole blood clot lysis time)	No lysis in 24 hr		Increased activity associated with massive hemorrhage, extensive surgery, transfusion reactions
Partial thromboplastin time (activated)	20–45 sec		Prolonged in deficiency of fibrinogen, factors II, V, VIII, IX, X, XI, and XII, and in heparin therapy
Prothrombin consumption	>20 sec		Impaired in deficiency of factors VIII, IX, and X
Prothrombin time	9.5–12 sec		Prolonged by deficiency of factors, I, II, V, VII, and X, fat malabsorption, severe liver disease, coumarin-anticoagulant therapy
Erythrocyte count	Males: 4,600,000–6,200,000/mm³	$4.6–6.2 \times 10^{12}$/L	Increased in severe diarrhea and dehydration, polycythemia, acute poisoning, pulmonary fibrosis
	Females: 4,200,000–5,400,000/mm³	$4.2–5.4 \times 10^{12}$/L	Decreased in all anemias, in leukemia, and after hemorrhage, when blood volume has been restored
Erythrocyte indices			
Mean corpuscular volume (MCV)	80–94 (μm^3)	80–94 fl	Increased in macrocytic anemias; decreased in microcytic anemia
Mean corpuscular hemoglobin (MCH)	27–32 $\mu\mu$g/cell	27–32 pg	Increased in macrocytic anemias; decreased in microcytic anemia
Mean corpuscular hemoglobin concentration (MCHC)	33%–38%	Concentration fraction: 0.33–0.38	Decreased in severe hypochromic anemia
Reticulocytes	0.5%–1.5% of red cells	Number fraction: 0.005–0.015	Increased with any condition stimulating increase in bone marrow activity (i.e., infection, blood loss [acute and chronic]); after iron therapy in iron deficiency anemia, polycythemia rubra vera

* Laboratory values vary according to the techniques used in different laboratories.

(continued)

Reference Ranges—Hematology* (Continued)

Determination	Reference Range		Clinical Significance
	Conventional Units	SI Units	
			Decreased with any condition depressing bone marrow activity, acute leukemia, late stage of severe anemias
Erythrocyte sedimentation rate (ESR)—Westergren method	Males under 50 yr: <15 mm/hr	<15 mm/hr	Increased in tissue destruction, whether inflammatory or degenerative; during menstruation and pregnancy; and in acute febrile diseases
	Males over 50 yr: <20 mm/hr	<20 mm/hr	
	Females under 50 yr: <20 mm/hr	<20 mm/hr	
	Females over 50 yr: <30 mm/hr	<30 mm/hr	
Erythrocyte sedimentation ratio—Zeta centrifuge	41%–54% in both sexes	Fraction: 0.41–0.54	Significance similar to ESR
Hematocrit	Males: 42%–50%	Volume fraction: 0.42–0.5	Decreased in severe anemias, anemia of pregnancy, acute massive blood loss
	Females: 40%–48%	Volume fraction: 0.4–0.48	Increased in erythrocytosis of any cause, and in dehydration or hemoconcentration associated with shock
Hemoglobin	Males: 13–18 g/dl	2.02–2.79 mmol/L	Decreased in various anemias, pregnancy, severe or prolonged hemorrhage, and with excessive fluid intake
	Females: 12–16 g/dl	1.86–2.48 mmol/L	Increased in polycythemia, chronic obstructive pulmonary diseases, failure of oxygenation because of congestive heart failure, and normally in people living at high altitudes
Hemoglobin F	<2% of total hemoglobin	Mass fraction: <0.02	Increased in infants and children, and in thalassemia and many anemias
Leukocyte alkaline phosphatase	Score of 40–100		Increased in polycythemia vera, myelofibrosis, and infections. Decreased in chronic granulocytic leukemia, paroxysmal nocturnal hemoglobinuria; hypoplastic marrow, and viral infections, particularly infectious mononucleosis
Leukocyte count Neutrophils Eosinophils Basophils Lymphocytes Monocytes	Total: 5,000–10,000/mm^3 60%–70% 1%–4% 0%–0.5% 20%–30% 2%–6%	$5-10 \times 10^9$/L Number fraction: 0.6–0.7 Number fraction: 0.01–0.04 Number fraction: 0.00–0.05 Number fraction: 0.2–0.3 Number fraction: 0.02–0.06	Elevated in acute infectious diseases, predominantly in the neutrophilic fraction with bacterial diseases, and in the lymphocytic and monocytic fractions in viral diseases. Elevated in acute leukemia, following menstruation, and following surgery or trauma. Depressed in aplastic anemia, agranulocytosis, and by toxic agents such as chemotherapeutic agents used in treating malignancy. Eosinophils elevated in collagen disease, allergy, intestinal parasitosis

(continued)

Reference Ranges—Hematology* (Continued)

Determination	Reference Range		Clinical Significance
	Conventional Units	SI Units	
Osmotic fragility of red cells	Increased if hemolysis occurs in over 0.5% NaCl Decreased if hemolysis is incomplete in 0.3% NaCl		Increased in congenital spherocytosis, idiopathic acquired hemolytic anemia, isoimmune hemolytic disease, ABO hemolytic disease of newborn Decreased in sickle cell anemia, thalassemia
Platelet count	100,000–400,000/mm^3	0.1–0.4 × 10^{12}/L	Increased in malignancy, myeloproliferative disease, rheumatoid arthritis, and postoperatively; about 50% of patients with unexpected increase of platelet count will be found to have a malignancy Decreased in thrombocytopenic purpura, acute leukemia, aplastic anemia, and during cancer chemotherapy, infections, and drug reactions

Reference Ranges—Serum, Plasma, and Whole Blood Chemistries

Determination	Normal Adult Reference Range		Clinical Significance	
	Conventional Units	SI Units	Increased	Decreased
Acetoacetate	0.2–1.0 mg/dl	19.6–98 μmol/L	Diabetic acidosis Fasting	
Acetone	0.3–2.0 mg/dl	51.6–344.0 μmol/L	Toxemia of pregnancy Carbohydrate-free diet High-fat diet	
Adrenocorticotropic hormone (ACTH) (plasma)—RIA*	Less than 50 pg/ml	Less than 50 mg/L	Pituitary-dependent Cushing's syndrome Ectopic ACTH syndrome Primary adrenal atrophy	Adrenocortical tumor Adrenal insufficiency secondary to hypopituitarism
Aldolase	3–8 Sibley-Lehninger U/dl at 37°C	22–59 mU/L at 37°C	Hepatic necrosis Granulocytic leukemia Myocardial infarction Skeletal muscle disease	
Aldosterone (plasma)—RIA	Supine: 3–10 ng/dl Upright: 5–30 ng/dl Adrenal vein: 200–800 ng/dl	0.08–0.30 nmol/L 0.14–0.90 nmol/L 5.54–22.16 nmol/L	Primary aldosteronism (Conn's syndrome) Secondary aldosteronism	Addison's disease
Alpha-1-antitrypsin	200–400 mg/dl	2–4 g/L		Certain forms of chronic lung and liver disease in young adults
Alpha-1-fetoprotein	None detected		Hepatocarcinoma Metastatic carcinoma of liver Germinal cell carcinoma of the testis or ovary	

* By radioimmunoassay.

(continued)

Reference Ranges—Serum, Plasma, and Whole Blood Chemistries *(Continued)*

Determination	Normal Adult Reference Range		Clinical Significance	
	Conventional Units	*SI Units*	*Increased*	*Decreased*
			Fetal neural tube defects— elevation in maternal serum	
Alpha-hydroxybutyric dehydrogenase	Up to 140 U/ml	Up to 140 U/L	Myocardial infarction Granulocytic leukemia Hemolytic anemias Muscular dystrophy	
Ammonia (plasma)	40–80 μg/dl (enzymatic method); varies considerably with method	22.2–44.3 μmol/L	Severe liver disease Hepatic decompensation	
Amylase	60–160 Somogyi U/dl	111–296 U/L	Acute pancreatitis Mumps Duodenal ulcer Carcinoma of head of pancreas Prolonged elevation with pseudocyst of pancreas Increased by drugs that constrict pancreatic duct sphincters: morphine, codeine, cholinergics	Chronic pancreatitis Pancreatic fibrosis and atrophy Cirrhosis of liver Pregnancy (2nd and 3rd trimesters)
Arsenic	6–20 μg/dl; if 50 μg/dl, suspect toxicity	0.78–2.6 μmol/L	Accidental or intentional poisoning Excessive occupational exposure	
Ascorbic acid (vitamin C)	0.4–1.5 mg/dl	23–85 μmol/L	Large doses of ascorbic acid as a prophylactic against the common cold	
Bilirubin	Total: 0.1–1.2 mg/dl	1.7–20.5 μmol/L	Hemolytic anemia (indirect)	
	Direct: 0.1–0.2 mg/dl	1.7–3.4 μmol/L	Biliary obstruction and disease	
	Indirect: 0.1–1 mg/dl	1.7–17.1 μmol/L	Hepatocellular damage (hepatitis) Pernicious anemia Hemolytic disease of newborn	
Blood gases Oxygen, arterial (whole blood)				
Partial pressure (PaO₂) Saturation (SaO₂)	95–100 mm Hg 94%–100%	12.64–13.30 kPa Volume fraction: 0.94–1	Polycythemia Anhydremia	Anemia Cardiac decompensation Chronic obstructive pulmonary disease
Carbon dioxide, arterial (whole blood): partial pressure (PaCo₂)	35–45 mm Hg	4.66–5.99 kPa	Respiratory acidosis Metabolic alkalosis	Respiratory alkalosis Metabolic acidosis
pH (whole blood arterial)	7.35–7.45	7.35–7.45	Vomiting Hyperpnea Fever Intestinal obstruction	Uremia Diabetic acidosis Hemorrhage Nephritis

(continued)

Reference Ranges—Serum, Plasma, and Whole Blood Chemistries (Continued)

Determination	Normal Adult Reference Range		Clinical Significance	
	Conventional Units	SI Units	Increased	Decreased
Calcitonin	Basal: nondetectable 400 pg/ml	400 ng/L	Medullary carcinoma of the thyroid Some nonthyroid tumors Zollinger-Ellison syndrome	
Calcium	8.5–10.5 mg/dl	2.125–2.625 mmol/L	Tumor or hyperplasia of parathyroid Hypervitaminosis D Multiple myeloma Nephritis with uremia Malignant tumors Sarcoidosis Hyperthyroidism Skeletal immobilization Excess calcium intake: milk-alkali syndrome	Hypoparathyroidism Diarrhea Celiac disease Vitamin D deficiency Acute pancreatitis Nephrosis After parathyroidectomy
CO_2 venous	Adults: 24–32 mEq/L Infants: 18–24 mEq/L	24–32 mmol/L 18–24 mmol/L	Tetany Respiratory disease Intestinal obstruction Vomiting	Acidosis Nephritis Eclampsia Diarrhea Anesthesia
Carcinoembryonic antigen (CEA)—RIA	0–2.5 ng/ml	0–2.5 µg/L	The repeatedly high incidence of this antigen in cancers of the colon, rectum, pancreas, and stomach suggests that CEA levels may be useful in the therapeutic monitoring of these conditions.	
Catecholamines (plasma)—RIA	Epinephrine, random: up to 90 pg/ml Norepinephrine, random: 100–550 pg/ml Dopamine, random: up to 130 pg/ml	Up to 490 pmol/L 590–3240 pmol/L Up to 850 pmol/L	Pheochromocytoma	
Ceruloplasmin	30–80 mg/dl	300–800 mg/L		Wilson's disease (hepatolenticular degeneration)
Chloride	95–105 mEq/L	95–105 mmol/L	Nephrosis Nephritis Urinary obstruction Cardiac decompensation Anemia	Diabetes Diarrhea Vomiting Pneumonia Heavy metal poisoning Cushing's syndrome Burns Intestinal obstruction Febrile conditions
Cholesterol	150–200 mg/dl	3.9–5.2 mmol/L	Lipemia Obstructive jaundice Diabetes Hypothyroidism	Pernicious anemia Hemolytic anemia Hyperthyroidism Severe infection Terminal states of debilitating disease

(continued)

Reference Ranges—Serum, Plasma, and Whole Blood Chemistries (Continued)

Determination	Normal Adult Reference Range		Clinical Significance	
	Conventional Units	*SI Units*	*Increased*	*Decreased*
Cholesterol esters	60%–70% of total	Fraction of total cholesterol 0.6–0.7		The esterified fraction decreases in liver diseases
Cholinesterase	Serum: 0.6–1.6 delta pH Red cells: 0.6–1 delta pH	0.6–1.6 U 0.6–1 U	Nephrosis Exercise	Nerve gas intoxication (greater effect on red cell activity) Insecticides, organic phosphates (greater effect on plasma activity)
Chorionic gonadotropin, beta subunit—RIA	0–5 IU/L	0–5 IU/L	Pregnancy Hydatidiform mole Choriocarcinoma	
Complement, human C_3	Males: 88–252 mg/dl Females: 88–206 mg/dl	880–2520 mg/L	Some inflammatory diseases	Acute glomerulonephritis Disseminated lupus erythematosus with renal involvement
Complement C_4	14–51 mg/dl	140–510 mg/L	Some inflammatory diseases	Often decreased in immunologic disease, especially with active systemic lupus erythematosus Hereditary angioneurotic edema
Complement, total (hemolytic)	90%–94% complement		Some inflammatory diseases	Acute glomerulonephritis Epidemic meningitis Subacute bacterial endocarditis
Copper	70–165 μg/dl	11–25.9 μmol/L	Cirrhosis of liver Pregnancy	Wilson's disease
Cortisol—RIA	8 AM: 7–25 μg/dl 4 PM: 2–9 μg/dl	193–690 nmol/L 55–248 nmol/L	Stress: infectious disease, surgery, burns, etc. Pregnancy Cushing's syndrome Pancreatitis Eclampsia	Addison's disease Anterior pituitary hypofunction
C peptide reactivity	1.5–10 ng/ml	1.5–10 μg/L	Insulinoma	Diabetes
Creatine	0.2–0.8 mg/ml	15.3–61 μmol/L	Pregnancy Skeletal muscle necrosis or atrophy Starvation Hyperthyroidism	
Creatine phosphokinase (CPK)	Males: 50–325 mU/ml Females: 50–250 mU/ml	50–325 U/L 50–250 U/L	Myocardial infarction Skeletal muscle diseases Intramuscular injections Crush syndrome Hypothyroidism Alcohol withdrawal delirium Alcoholic myopathy Cerebrovascular disease	
Creatine phosphokinase isoenzymes	MM band present (skeletal muscle); MB band absent (heart muscle)		MB band increased in myocardial infarction, ischemia	

(continued)

Reference Ranges—Serum, Plasma, and Whole Blood Chemistries (Continued)

Determination	Normal Adult Reference Range		Clinical Significance	
	Conventional Units	SI Units	Increased	Decreased
Creatinine	0.7–1.4 mg/dl	62–124 μmol/L	Nephritis Chronic renal disease	Kidney diseases
Creatinine clearance	100–150 ml of blood cleared of creatinine per min	1.67–2.5 ml/sec		
Cryoglobulins, qualitative	Negative		Multiple myeloma Chronic lymphocytic leukemia Lymphosarcoma Systemic lupus erythematosus Rheumatoid arthritis Infective subacute endocarditis Some malignancies Scleroderma	
11-Deoxycortisol	1 μg/dl	<0.029 μmol/L	Hypertensive form of virilizing adrenal hyperplasia due to an 11-β-hydroxylase defect	
Dibucaine number	Normal: 70%–85% inhibition Heterozygote: 50%–65% inhibition Homozygote: 16%–25% inhibition			Important in detecting carriers of abnormal cholinesterase activity who are susceptible to succinyldicholine anesthetic shock
Dihydrotestosterone	Males: 50–210 ng/dl Females: none detectable	1.72–7.22 nmol/L		Testicular feminization syndrome

Estradiol—RIA	Females:
	  Follicular:
	    10–90 pg/ml
	  Midcycle:
	    100–500 pg/ml
	  Luteal:
	    50–240 pg/ml
	  Follicular phase:
	    2–20 ng/dl
	  Midcycle:
	    12–40 ng/dl
	  Luteal phase:
	    10–30 ng/dl
	  Postmenopausal:
	    1–5 ng/dl
	Males:
	  0.5–5 ng/dl
		37–370 pmol/L
		
		367–1835 pmol/L
		
		184–881 pmol/L
			Pregnancy	Depressed or failure to peak—ovarian failure

Estriol—RIA	Nonpregnant females: <0.5 ng/ml Pregnant females: 1st trimester: up to 1 ng/ml 2nd trimester: 0.8–7 ng/ml	<1.75 nmol/L Up to 3.5 nmol/L 2.8–24.3 nmol/L	Pregnancy	Depressed or failure to peak—ovarian failure

(continued)

Reference Ranges—Serum, Plasma, and Whole Blood Chemistries (Continued)

Determination	Normal Adult Reference Range		Clinical Significance	
	Conventional Units	SI Units	Increased	Decreased
Estrogens, total—RIA	3rd trimester: 5–25 ng/ml	17.4–86.8 nmol/L	Pregnancy	Fetal distress
	Females: cycle days:		Measured on a daily basis, can be used to evaluate response of hypogonadotrophic, hypoestrogenic women to human menopausal or pituitary gonadotropin	Ovarian failure
	Days 1–10: 61–394 pg/ml	61–394 ng/L		
	Days 11–20: 122–437 pg/ml	122–437 ng/L		
	Days 21–30: 156–350 pg/ml	156–350 ng/L		
	Males: 40–115 pg/ml	40–115 ng/L		
Estrone—RIA	Females:		Pregnancy	Depressed or failure to peak—ovarian failure
	Days 1–10: 4.3–18 ng/dl	15.9–66.6 pmol/L		
	Days 11–20: 7.5–19.6 ng/dl	27.8–72.5 pmol/L		
	Days 21–30: 13–20 ng/dl	48.1–74 pmol/L		
	Males: 2.5–7.5 ng/dl	9.3–27.8 pmol/L		
Ferritin—RIA	Males: 10–270 ng/ml	10–270 μg/L	Nephritis	Iron deficiency
	Females: 5–100 ng/ml	5–100 μg/L	Hemochromatosis	
			Certain neoplastic diseases	
			Acute myelogenous leukemia	
			Multiple myeloma	
Folic acid—RIA	4–16 ng/ml	9.1–36.3 nmol/L		Megaloblastic anemias of infancy and pregnancy
				Inadequate diet
				Liver disease
				Malabsorption syndrome
				Severe hemolytic anemia
Follicle stimulating hormone (FSH)—RIA	Females:		Menopause and primary ovarian failure	Pituitary failure
	Follicular phase: 5–20 mIU/ml	5–20 IU/L		
	Peak of middle cycle: 12–30 mIU/ml	12–30 IU/L		
	Luteinic phase: 5–15 mIU/ml	5–15 IU/L		
	Menopausal females: 40–200 mIU/ml	40–200 IU/L		
Galactose	<5 mg/dl	<0.28 mmol/L		Galactosemia
Gamma glutamyl transpeptidase	Males: <45 IU/L	45 U/L	Hepatobiliary disease	
	Females: <30 IU/L	30 U/L	Anicteric alcoholics	
			Drug therapy damage	
			Myocardial infarction	
			Renal infarction	
Gastrin—RIA	Fasting: 50–155 pg/ml	50–155 ng/L	Zollinger-Ellison syndrome	
	Postprandial: 80–170 pg/ml	80–170 ng/L	Peptic ulceration of the duodenum	
			Pernicious anemia	

(continued)

Reference Ranges—Serum, Plasma, and Whole Blood Chemistries (Continued)

Determination	Normal Adult Reference Range		Clinical Significance	
	Conventional Units	SI Units	Increased	Decreased
	Zollinger-Ellison syndrome: 200–over 2000 pg/ml	200–over 2000 ng/L		
	Pernicious anemia: 130–2260 pg/ml (mean 912)	130–2260 ng/L (mean 912)		
Glucose	Fasting: 60–110 mg/dl	3.3–6.05 mmol/L	Diabetes	Hyperinsulinism
	Postprandial (2 hr): 65–140 mg/dl	3.58–7.7 mmol/L	Nephritis	Hypothyroidism
			Hyperthyroidism	Late hyperpituitarism
			Early hyperpituitarism	Pernicious vomiting
			Cerebral lesions	Addison's disease
			Infections	Extensive hepatic damage
			Pregnancy	
			Uremia	
Glucose tolerance (oral)	Features of normal response:		(Flat or inverted curve)	(High or prolonged curve)
	1. Normal fasting between 60–110 mg/dl	3.3–6.05 mmol/L	Hyperinsulinism	Diabetes
	2. No sugar in urine		Adrenal cortical insufficiency (Addison's disease)	Hyperthyroidism
	3. Upper limits of normal:		Anterior pituitary hypofunction	Primary adrenal cortical tumor or hyperplasia
	Fasting = 125	6.88 mmol/L	Hypothyroidism	Severe anemia
	1 hour = 190	10.45 mmol/L	Sprue and celiac diseases	Certain central nervous system disorders
	2 hours = 140	7.70 mmol/L		
	3 hours = 125	6.88 mmol/L		
Glucose-6-phosphate dehydrogenase (red cells)	Screening: Decolorization in 20–100 min			Drug-induced hemolytic anemia
	Quantitative: 1.86–2.5 IU/ml RBC	1860–2500 U/L		Hemolytic disease of newborn
Glycoprotein (alpha-1-acid)	40–110 mg/dl	400–1100 mg/L	Neoplasm	
			Tuberculosis	
			Diabetes complicated by degenerative vascular disease	
			Pregnancy	
			Rheumatoid arthritis	
			Rheumatic fever	
			Infectious liver disease	
			Lupus erythematosus	
Growth hormone—RIA	<10 ng/ml	<10 mg/L	Acromegaly	Failure to stimulate with arginine or insulin—hypopituitarism
Haptoglobin	50–250 mg/dl	0.5–2.5 g/L	Pregnancy	Hemolytic anemia
			Estrogen therapy	Hemolytic blood transfusion reaction
			Chronic infections	
			Various inflammatory conditions	
Hemoglobin (plasma)	0.5–5 mg/dl	5–50 mg/L	Transfusion reactions	
			Paroxysmal nocturnal hemoglobinuria	
			Intravascular hemolysis	

(continued)

Reference Ranges—Serum, Plasma, and Whole Blood Chemistries (Continued)

Determination	Normal Adult Reference Range		Clinical Significance	
	Conventional Units	*SI Units*	*Increased*	*Decreased*
Hemoglobin A1 (glycohemoglobin)	Nondiabetics & diabetics whose control of glucose is: Good: 4.4%–8.2% Fair: 8.3%–9.2% Poor: >9.2%			
Hexosaminidase, total	Controls: 333–375 nM/ml/h Heterozygotes: 288–644 nM/ml/h Tay-Sachs disease: 284–1232 nM/ml/h Diabetics: 567–3560 nM/ml/h	333–375 μmol/L/h 288–644 μmol/L/h 284–1232 μmol/L/h 567–3560 μmol/L/h	Diabetes Tay-Sachs disease	
Hexosaminidase A	Controls: 49%–68% of total Heterozygotes: 26%–45% of total Tay-Sachs disease: 0%–4% of total Diabetics: 39%–59% of total	Fraction of total: 0.49–0.68 0.26–0.45 0–0.04 0.39–0.59		Tay-Sachs disease and heterozygotes
High-density lipoprotein cholesterol (HDL cholesterol)				HDL cholesterol is lower in patients with increased risk for coronary heart disease

Age (yr)	Males (mg/dl)	Females (mg/dl)	Males (mmol/L)	Females (mmol/L)
0–19	30–65	30–70	0.78–1.68	0.78–1.81
20–29	35–70	35–75	0.91–1.81	0.91–1.94
30–39	30–65	35–80	0.78–1.68	0.91–2.07
40–49	30–65	40–85	0.78–1.68	1.04–2.2
50–59	30–65	35–85	0.78–1.68	0.91–2.2
60–69	30–65	35–85	0.78–1.68	0.91–2.2

Determination	Conventional Units	SI Units	Increased	Decreased
17-Hydroxyprogesterone—RIA	Males: 0.4–4 ng/ml Females: 0.1–3.3 ng/ml Children: 0.1–0.5 ng/ml	1.2–12 nmol/L 0.3–10 nmol/L 0.3–1.5 nmol/L	Congenital adrenal hyperplasia Pregnancy Some cases of adrenal or ovarian adenomas	
Immunoglobulin A	Adults: 50–300 mg/ dl (in children the normal values are lower and vary with age)	0.5–3 g/L	Gamma A myeloma Wiskott-Aldrich syndrome Autoimmune disease Hepatic cirrhosis	Ataxia telangiectasis Agammaglobulinemia Hypogammaglobulinemia, transient Dysgammaglobulinemia Protein-losing enteropathies

(continued)

Reference Ranges—Serum, Plasma, and Whole Blood Chemistries (Continued)

Determination	Normal Adult Reference Range		Clinical Significance	
	Conventional Units	SI Units	Increased	Decreased
Immunoglobulin D	0–30 mg/dl	0–300 mg/L	IgD multiple myeloma Some patients with chronic infectious diseases	
Immunoglobulin E	20–740 ng/ml	20–740 μg/L	Allergic patients and those with parasitic infestations	
Immunoglobulin G	Adults: 635–1400 mg/dl	6.35–14 g/L	IgG myeloma Following hyperimmunization Autoimmune disease states Chronic infections	Congenital and acquired hypogammaglobulinemia IgA myelomas, Waldenstrom's (IgM) macroglobulinemia Some malabsorption syndromes Extensive protein loss
Immunoglobulin M	Adults: 40–280 mg/dl	0.4–2.8 g/L	Waldenstrom's macroglobulinemia Parasitic infections Hepatitis	Agammaglobulinemias Some IgG and IgA myelomas Chronic lymphatic leukemia
Insulin—RIA	5–25 μU/ml	0.2–1 μg/L	Insulinoma Acromegaly	Diabetes mellitus
Iron	65–170 μg/dl	11.6–30.4 μmol/L	Pernicious anemia Aplastic anemia Hemolytic anemia Hepatitis Hemochromatosis	Iron deficiency anemia
Iron-binding capacity	IBC: 150–235 μg/dl TIBC: 250–420 μg/dl % Saturation: 20–50	26.9–42.1 μmol/L 44.8–75.2 μmol/L Fraction of total ironbinding capacity: 0.2–0.5	Iron deficiency anemia Acute and chronic blood loss Hepatitis	Chronic infectious diseases Cirrhosis
Isocitric dehydrogenase	50–180 U	0.83–3 U/L	Hepatitis: cirrhosis Obstructive jaundice Metastatic carcinoma of the liver Megaloblastic anemia	
Lactic acid (whole blood)	Venous: 5–20 mg/dl Arterial: 3–7 mg/dl	0.6–2.2 mmol/L 0.3–0.8 mmol/L	Increased muscular activity Congestive heart failure Hemorrhage Shock Some varieties of metabolic acidosis Some febrile infections May be increased in severe liver disease	
Lactic dehydrogenase (LDH)	100–225 mU/ml	100–225 U/L	Untreated pernicious anemia Myocardial infarction Pulmonary infarction Liver disease	

(continued)

Reference Ranges—Serum, Plasma, and Whole Blood Chemistries (Continued)

Determination	Normal Adult Reference Range		Clinical Significance	
	Conventional Units	SI Units	Increased	Decreased
Lactic dehydrogenase isoenzymes				
Total lactic dehydrogenase	100–225 mU/ml	100–225 U/L Fraction of total LDH:	LDH-1 and LDH-2 are increased in myocardial infarction, megaloblastic anemia, and hemolytic anemia	
LDH-1	20%–35%	0.2–0.35		
LDH-2	25%–40%	0.25–0.4		
LDH-3	20%–30%	0.2–0.3		
LDH-4	0–20%	0–0.2	LDH-4 and LDH-5 are increased in pulmonary infarction, congestive heart failure, and liver disease	
LDH-5	0–25%	0–0.25		
Lead (whole blood)	Up to 40 μg/dl	Up to 2 μmol/L	Lead poisoning	
Leucine aminopeptidase	80–200 U/ml	19.2–48 U/L	Liver or biliary tract diseases Pancreatic disease Metastatic carcinoma of liver and pancreas Biliary obstruction	
Lipase	0.2–1.5 U/ml	55–417 U/L	Acute and chronic pancreatitis Biliary obstruction Cirrhosis Hepatitis Peptic ulcer	
Lipids, total	400–1000 mg/dl	4–10 g/L	Hypothyroidism Diabetes Nephrosis Glomerulonephritis Hyperlipoproteinemias	Hyperthyroidism

Lipoprotein Phenotype: Summary of Findings in the Primary Hyperlipoproteinemias

Type	Frequency	Appearance	Triglyceride	Cholesterol	Lipoprotein Staining				Secondary Causes
					Beta	Pre-Beta	Alpha	Chylomicrons	
Normal		Clear	Normal	Normal	Moderate	Zero to moderate	Moderate	Weak	
I	Very rare	Creamy	Markedly increased	Normal to moderately increased	Weak	Weak	Weak	Markedly increased	Dysglobulinemia
II	Common	Clear	Normal to slightly increased	Slightly to markedly increased	Strong	Zero to strong	Moderate	Weak	Hypothyroidism, myeloma, hepatic syndrome, macroglobulinemia, and high dietary cholesterol
III	Uncommon	Clear, cloudy, or milky	Increased	Increased	Broad intense band	Extends into beta	Moderate	Weak	

(continued)

Reference Ranges—Serum, Plasma, and Whole Blood Chemistries (Continued)

Determination	Normal Adult Reference Range		Clinical Significance	
	Conventional Units	*SI Units*	*Increased*	*Decreased*

Lipoprotein Phenotype: Summary of Findings in the Primary Hyperlipoproteinemias

Type	Frequency	Appearance	Triglyceride	Cholesterol	Lipoprotein Staining				Secondary Causes
					Beta	*Pre-Beta*	*Alpha*	*Chylomicrons*	
IV	Very common	Clear, cloudy, or milky	Slightly to markedly increased	Normal to slightly increased	Weak to moderate	Moderate to strong	Weak to moderate	Weak	Hypothyroidism, diabetes mellitus, pancreatitis, glycogen storage diseases, nephrotic syndrome, myeloma, pregnancy, and oral contraceptives
V	Rare	Cloudy to creamy	Markedly increased	Increased	Weak	Moderate	Weak	Strong	Diabetes mellitus, pancreatitis, and alcoholism

Type I and II are fat induced; types III and IV are carbohydrate induced; type V is fat and carbohydrate induced.

Determination	Conventional Units	SI Units	Increased	Decreased
Lithium	Usual maintenance level: 0.5–1 mEq/L	0.5–1 mmol/L		
Low-density lipoprotein cholesterol (LDL cholesterol)	Age (yr) mg/dl 0–19 50–170 20–29 60–170 30–39 70–190 40–49 80–190 50–59 80–210	mmol/L 1.30–4.40 1.55–4.40 1.80–4.92 2.07–4.92 2.07–5.44	LDL cholesterol is higher in patients with increased risk for coronary heart disease	
Luteinizing hormone—RIA	Males: 6–30 mIU/ml Females: Follicular phase: 2–3 miU/ml Ovulatory peak: 40–200 mIU/ml Luteal phase: 0–20 mIU/ml Postmenopausal: 35–120 mIU/ml	1.4–6.9 mg/L 0.5–6.9 mg/L 9.2–46 mg/L 0–5 mg/L 8–27.5 mg/L	Pituitary tumor Ovarian failure	Depressed or failure to peak—pituitary failure
Lysozyme (muramidase)	2.8–8 μg/ml	2.8–8 mg	Certain types of leukemia (acute monocytic leukemia) Inflammatory states and infections	Acute lymphocytic leukemia
Magnesium	1.3–2.4 mEq/L	0.7–1.2 mmol/L	Excess ingestion of magnesium-containing antacids	Chronic alcoholism Severe renal disease Diarrhea Defective growth
Manganese	0.04–1.4 μg/dl	72.9–255 nmol/L		
Mercury	Up to 10 μg/dl	Up to 0.5 μmol/L	Mercury poisoning	

(continued)

Reference Ranges—Serum, Plasma, and Whole Blood Chemistries (Continued)

| Determination | Normal Adult Reference Range | | Clinical Significance | |
	Conventional Units	SI Units	Increased	Decreased
Myoglobin—RIA	Up to 85 ng/ml	Up to 85 µg/ml	Myocardial infarction Muscle necrosis	
5′ Nucleotidase	3.2–11.6 IU/L	3.2–11.6 U/L	Hepatobiliary disease	
Osmolality	280–300 mOsm/kg	280–300 mmol/L	Useful in the study of electrolyte and water balance	Inappropriate secretion of antidiuretic hormone
Parathyroid hormone	160–350 pg/ml	160–350 ng/L	Hyperparathyroidism	
Phenylalanine	1.2–3.5 mg/dl 1st week 0.7–3.5 mg/dl thereafter	0.07–0.21 mmol/L 0.04–0.21 mmol/L	Phenylketonuria	
Phosphatase, acid, total	0–11 UL	0–11 UL	Carcinoma of prostate Advanced Paget's disease Hyperparathyroidism Gaucher's disease	
Phosphatase, acid, prostatic—RIA	0–10 ng/ml Borderline: 2.5–3.3 IU/L	0–10 µg/L	Carcinoma of prostate	
Phosphatase, alkaline	Adults: 30–115 mU/ml	30–115 µ/L	Conditions reflecting increased osteoblastic activity of bone Rickets Hyperparathyroidism Liver disease	
Phosphatase, alkaline, thermostable fraction	Thermostable fraction >35%: hepatic disease and combined disease with predominant hepatic component Thermostable fraction between 25% and 35% combined hepatic and skeletal disease Thermostable fraction <25%: skeletal disease with increased osteoblastic activity		Hepatic disease	
Phosphohexose isomerase	20–90 IU/L	20–90 U/L	Malignancy Disease of heart, liver, and skeletal muscles	
Phospholipids	125–300 mg/dl	1.25–3 g/L	Diabetes Nephritis	
Phosphorus, inorganic	2.5–4.5 mg/dl	0.8–1.45 mmol/L	Chronic nephritis Hypoparathyroidism	Hyperparathyroidism Vitamin D deficiency

(continued)

Reference Ranges—Serum, Plasma, and Whole Blood Chemistries (Continued)

Determination	Normal Adult Reference Range		Clinical Significance	
	Conventional Units	SI Units	Increased	Decreased
Potassium	3.8–5 mEq/L	3.8–5 mmol/L	Addison's disease Oliguria Anuria Tissue breakdown or hemolysis	Diabetic acidosis Diarrhea Vomiting
Progesterone—RIA	Follicular phase: up to 0.8 ng/ml Luteal phase: 10–20 ng/ml End of cycle: <1 ng/ml Pregnant: up to 50 ng/ml in 20th week	2.5 nmol/L 31.8–63.6 nmol/L <3 nmol/L Up to 160 nmol/L	Useful in evaluation of menstrual disorders and infertility and in the evaluation of placental function during pregnancies complicated by toxemia, diabetes mellitus, or threatened miscarriage	
Prolactin—RIA	6–24 ng/ml	6–24 μg/L	Pregnancy Functional or structural disorders of the hypothalamus Pituitary stalk section Pituitary tumors	
Protein, total Albumin Globulin	6–8 g/dl 3.5–5 g/dl 1.5–3 g/dl	60–80 g/L 35–50 g/L 15–30 g/L	Hemoconcentration Shock Multiple myeloma (globulin fraction) Chronic infections (globulin fraction) Liver disease (globulin)	Malnutrition Hemorrhage Loss of plasma from burns Proteinuria
Electrophoresis (cellulose acetate) Albumin Alpha-1 globulin Alpha-2 globulin Beta globulin Gamma globulin	3.5–5 g/dl 0.2–0.4 g/dl 0.6–1 g/dl 0.6–1.2 g/dl 0.7–1.5 g/dl	35–50 g/L 2–4 g/L 6–10 g/L 6–12 g/L 7–15 g/L		
Protoporphyrin erythrocyte (whole blood)	15–100 μg/dl	0.27–1.80 μmol/L	Lead toxicity Erythropoietic porphyria	
Pyridoxine	3.6–18 ng/ml			A wide spectrum of clinical conditions such as mental depression, peripheral neuropathy, anemia, neonatal seizures, and reactions to certain drug therapies
Pyruvic acid (whole blood)	0.3–0.7 mg/dl	34–80 μmol/L	Diabetes Severe thiamine deficiency Acute phase of some infections, possibly secondary to increased glycogenolysis and glycolysis	

(continued)

Reference Ranges—Serum, Plasma, and Whole Blood Chemistries (Continued)

Determination	Normal Adult Reference Range Conventional Units	SI Units	Clinical Significance Increased	Decreased
Renin (plasma)—RIA	Normal diet: Supine: 0.3–1.9 ng/ml/hr Upright: 0.6–3.6 ng/ml/hr Low salt diet: Supine: 0.9–4.5 ng/ml/hr Upright: 4.1–9.1 ng/ml/hr	0.08–0.52 ng/L/sec 0.16–1.00 μg/L/sec 0.25–1.25 μg/L/sec 1.13–2.53 μg/L/sec	Renovascular hypertension Malignant hypertension Untreated Addison's disease Primary salt-losing nephropathy Low-salt diet Diuretic therapy Hemorrhage	Frank primary aldosteronism Increased salt intake Salt-retaining steroid therapy Antidiuretic hormone therapy Blood transfusion
Sodium	135–145 mEq/L	135–145 mmol/L	Hemoconcentration Nephritis Pyloric obstruction	Alkali deficit Addison's disease Myxedema
Sulfate (inorganic)	0.5–1.5 mg/dl	0.05–0.15 mmol/L	Nephritis Nitrogen retention	
Testosterone—RIA	Females: 25–100 ng/dl Males: 300–800 ng/dl	0.9–3.5 nmol/L 10.5–28 nmol/L	Females: Polycystic ovary Virilizing tumors	Males: Orchidectomy for neoplastic disease of the prostate or breast Estrogen therapy Klinefelter's syndrome Hypopituitarism Hypogonadism Hepatic cirrhosis
T_3 (triiodothyronine) uptake	25%–35%	Relative uptake fraction: 0.25–0.35	Hyperthyroidism TBG deficiency Androgens and anabolic steroids	Hypothyroidism Pregnancy TBG excess Estrogens and antiovulatory drugs
T_3, total circulating—RIA	75–200 ng/dl	1.15–3.1 nmol/L	Pregnancy Hyperthyroidism	Hypothyroidism
T_4 (thyroxine)—RIA	4.5–11.5 μg/dl	58.5–150 nmol/L	Hyperthyroidism Thyroiditis Elevated thyroxine-binding proteins caused by oral contraceptives Pregnancy	Primary and pituitary hypothyroidism Idiopathic involvement Cases of diminished thyroxine-binding proteins caused by androgenic and anabolic steroids Hypoproteinemia Nephrotic syndrome
T_4, free	1–2.2 ng/dl	13–30 pmol/L	Euthyroid patients with normal free thyroxine levels may have abnormal T_3 and T_4 levels caused by drug preparations	
Thyroid-stimulating hormone (TSH)—RIA		0.3–5 m/IU/L	Hypothyroidism	Hyperthyroidism
Thyroid-binding globulin	10–26 μg/dl	100–260 μg/L	Hypothyroidism Pregnancy	Androgens and anabolic steroids

Reference Ranges—Serum, Plasma, and Whole Blood Chemistries (Continued)

Determination	Normal Adult Reference Range		Clinical Significance	
	Conventional Units	*SI Units*	*Increased*	*Decreased*
Transaminase, serum glutamic-oxaloacetate (SGOT, aspartate aminotransferase)	7–40 U/ml	4–20 U/L	Estrogen therapy Oral contraceptives Genetic and idiopathic Myocardial infarction Skeletal muscle disease Liver disease	Nephrotic syndrome Marked hypoproteinemia Hepatic disease
Transaminase, serum glutamic-pyruvic (SGPT, alanine aminotransferase)	10–40 U/ml	5–20 U/L	Same conditions as SGOT, but increase is more marked in liver disease than SGOT	
Transferrin	230–320 mg/dl	2.3–3.2 g/L	Pregnancy Iron-deficiency anemia due to hemorrhaging Acute hepatitis Polycythemia Oral contraceptives	Pernicious anemia in relapse Thalassemia and sickle cell anemia Chromatosis Neoplastic and hepatic diseases
Triglycerides	10–150 mg/dl	0.10–1.65 mmol/L	See lipoprotein phenotype table, pp. 1999–2000	
Tryptophan	1.4–3 mg/dl	68.6–147 nmol/L		Tryptophan-specific malabsorption syndrome
Tyrosine	0.5–4 mg/dl	27.6–220.8 mmol/L	Tyrosinosis	
Urea nitrogen (BUN)	10–20 mg/dl	3.6–7.2 mmol/L	Acute glomerulonephritis Obstructive uropathy Mercury poisoning Nephrotic syndrome	Severe hepatic failure Pregnancy
Uric acid	2.5–8 mg/dl	0.15–0.5 mmol/L	Gouty arthritis Acute leukemia Lymphomas treated by chemotherapy Toxemia of pregnancy	Xanthinuria Defective tubular reabsorption
Viscosity	1.4–1.8 relative to water at 37°C (98.6°F)		Patients with marked increases of the gamma globulins	
Vitamin A	50–220 μg/dl	1.75–7.7 μmol/L	Hypervitaminosis A	Vitamin A deficiency Celiac disease Sprue Obstructive jaundice Giardiasis Parenchymal hepatic disease
Vitamin B₁ (thiamine)	1.6–4 μg/dl	47.4–135.7 nmol/L		Anorexia Beriberi Polyneuropathy Cardiomyopathies

(continued)

Reference Ranges—Serum, Plasma, and Whole Blood Chemistries (Continued)

	Normal Adult Reference Range		Clinical Significance	
Determination	Conventional Units	SI Units	Increased	Decreased
Vitamin B$_6$ (pyridoxal phosphate)	3.6–18 ng/ml	14.6–72.8 nmol/L		Chronic alcoholism Malnutrition Uremia Neonatal seizures Malabsorption, such as celiac syndrome
Vitamin B$_{12}$—RIA	130–785 pg/ml	100–580 pmol/L	Hepatic cell damage and in association with the myeloproliferative disorders (the highest levels are encountered in myeloid leukemia)	Strict vegetarianism Alcoholism Pernicious anemia Total or partial gastrectomy Ileal resection Sprue and celiac disease Fish tapeworm infestation
Vitamin E	0.5–2 mg/dl	11.6–46.4 μmol/L		Vitamin E deficiency
Xylose absorption test	2 hr, 30–50 mg/dl	2–3.35 mmol/L		Malabsorption syndrome
Zinc	55–150 μg/dl	7.65–22.95 μmol/L	Zinc is essential for the growth and propagation of cell cultures and the functioning of several enzymes	

Reference Ranges—Urine Chemistry

	Normal Adult Reference Range		Clinical Significance	
Determination	Conventional Units	SI Units	Increased	Decreased
Acetone and acetoacetate	Zero		Uncontrolled diabetes Starvation	
Acid mucopolysaccharides	Negative		Hurler's syndrome Marfan's syndrome Morquio-Ulrich disease	

Aldosterone	Normal salt:
	  Normal:
	    4–20 μg/24 hr
	  Renovascular:
	    10–40 μg/24 hr
	  Tumor:
	    20–100 μg/24 hr
		
		11.1–55.5 nmol/24 hr
		
		27.7–111 nmol/24 hr
		
		55.4–227 nmol/24 hr
			Primary aldosteronism (adrenocortical tumor)
			Secondary aldosteronism
			Salt depletion
			Potassium loading
			ACTH in large doses
			Cardiac failure
			Cirrhosis with ascites formation
			Nephrosis
			Pregnancy	

(continued)

Reference Ranges—Urine Chemistry (Continued)

Determination	Normal Adult Reference Range		Clinical Significance	
	Conventional Units	SI Units	Increased	Decreased
Alpha amino nitrogen	50–200 mg/24 hr	3.6–14.3 mmol/24 hr	Leukemia Diabetes Phenylketonuria Other metabolic diseases	
Amylase	35–260 units excreted per hr	6.5–48.1 U/hr	Acute pancreatitis	
Arylsulfatase A	>2.4 U/ml			Metachromatic leukodystrophy
Bence-Jones protein	None detected		Myeloma	
Calcium	<150 mg/24 hr	<3.75 mmol/24 hr	Hyperparathyroidism Vitamin D intoxication Fanconi syndrome	Hypoparathyroidism Vitamin D deficiency

Catecholamines	Total:
	  0–275 µg/24 hr
	Epinephrine:
	  10%–40%
	Norepinephrine:
	  60%–90%
		0–275 µg/24 hr
		Fraction total: 0.10–8.4
		Fraction total: 0.60–0.90
			Pheochromocytoma
			Neuroblastoma	

Chorionic gonadotrophin, qualitative (pregnancy test)	Negative		Pregnancy Chorionepithelioma Hydatidiform mole	
Copper	20–70 µg/24 hr	0.32–1.12 µmol/24 hr	Wilson's disease Cirrhosis Nephrosis	
Coproporphyrin	50–300 µg/24 hr	0.075–0.45 µmol/24 hr	Poliomyelitis Lead poisoning Porphyria hepatica Porphyria erythropoietica Porphyria cutanea tarda	
Cortisol, free	20–90 µg/24 hr	55.2–248.4 nmol/day	Cushing's syndrome	
Creatine	0–200 mg/24 hr	0–1.52 mmol/24 hr	Muscular dystrophy Fever Carcinoma of liver Pregnancy Hyperthyroidism Myositis	
Creatinine	0.8–2 g/24 hr	7–17.6 mmol/24 hr	Typhoid fever Salmonella infections Tetanus	Muscular atrophy Anemia Advanced degeneration of kidneys Leukemia
Creatinine clearance	100–150 ml of blood cleared of creatinine per min	1.67–2.5 ml/sec		Measures glomerular filtration rate Renal diseases
Cystine and cysteine	10–100 mg/24 hr	0.08–0.83 mmol/24 hr	Cystinuria	
Delta aminolevulinic acid	0–0.54 mg/dl	0–40 µmol/L	Lead poisoning Porphyria hepatica Hepatitis Hepatic carcinoma	
11-Desoxycortisol	20–100 µg/24 hr	0.6–2.9 µmol/day	Hypertensive form of virilizing adrenal hyperplasia due to an 11-beta hydroxylase defect	

(continued)

Reference Ranges—Urine Chemistry (Continued)

Determination	Normal Adult Reference Range		Clinical Significance	
	Conventional Units	SI Units	Increased	Decreased
Estriol (placental)	Weeks of Pregnancy μm/24 hr	nmol/24 hr		Decreased values occur with fetal distress of many conditions, including preeclampsia, placental insufficiency, and poorly controlled diabetes mellitus
	12 <1	<3.5		
	16 2–7	7–24.5		
	20 4–9	14–32		
	24 6–13	21–45.5		
	28 8–22	28–77		
	32 12–43	42–150		
	36 14–45	49–158		
	40 19–46	66.5–160		
Estrogens, total (fluorometric)	Females: Onset of menstruation: 4–25 μg/24 hr Ovulation peak: 28 μg/24 hr Luteal peak: 22–105 μg/24 hr Menopausal: 1.4–19.6 μg/24 hr Males: 5–18 μg/24 hr	4–25 μg/24 hr 28 μg/24 hr 22–105 μg/24 hr 1.4–19.6 μg/24 hr 5–18 μg/24 hr	Hyperestrogenism due to gonadal or adrenal neoplasm	Primary or secondary amenorrhea
Etiocholanolone	Males: 1.9–6 mg/24 hr Females: 0.5–4 mg/24 hr	6.5–20.6 μmol/24 hr 1.7–13.8 μmol/24 hr	Adrenogenital syndrome Idiopathic hirsutism	
Follicle-stimulating hormone—RIA	Females: Follicular: 5–20 IU/24 hr Luteal: 5–15 IU/24 hr Midcycle: 15–60 IU/24 hr Menopausal: 50–100 IU/24 hr Males: 5–25 IU/24 hr	 5–20 IU/day 5–15 IU/day 15–60 IU/day 50–100 IU/day 5–25 IU/day	Menopause and primary ovarian failure	Pituitary failure
Glucose	Negative		Diabetes mellitus Pituitary disorders Intracranial pressure Lesion in floor of 4th ventricle	
Hemoglobin and myoglobin	Negative		Extensive burns Transfusion of incompatible blood Myoglobin increased in severe crushing injuries to muscles	
Homogentisic acid, qualitative	Negative		Alkaptonuria Ochronosis	
Homovanillic acid	Up to 15 mg/24 hr	Up to 82 μmol/day	Neuroblastoma	
17-hydroxycorticosteroids	2–10 mg/24 hr	5.5–27.5 μmol/day	Cushing's disease	Addison's disease Anterior pituitary hypofunction
5-Hydroxyindoleacetic acid, qualitative	Negative		Malignant carcinoid tumors	

(continued)

Reference Ranges—Urine Chemistry *(Continued)*

Determination	Normal Adult Reference Range		Clinical Significance	
	Conventional Units	*SI Units*	*Increased*	*Decreased*
Hydroxyproline	15–43 mg/24 hr	0.11–0.33 μmol/day	Paget's disease Fibrous dysplasia Osteomalacia Neoplastic bone disease Hyperparathyroidism	
17-Ketosteroids, total	Males: 10–22 mg/24 hr Females: 6–16 mg/24 hr	35–76 μmol/day 21–55 μmol/day	Interstitial cell tumor of testes Simple hirsutism, occasionally Adrenal hyperplasia Cushing's syndrome Adrenal cancer, virilism Arrhenoblastoma	Thyrotoxicosis Female hypogonadism Diabetes mellitus Hypertension Debilitating disease of mild to moderate severity Eunuchoidism Addison's disease Panhypopituitarism Myxedema Nephrosis
Lead	Up to 150 μg/24 hr	Up to 60 μmol/24 hr	Lead poisoning	

Luteinizing hormone	Males: 5–18 IU/24 hr
	Females:
	 Follicular phase:
	  2–25 IU/24 hr
	 Ovulatory peak:
	  30–95 IU/24 h
	 Luteal phase:
	  2–20 IU/24 hr
	 Postmenopausal:
	  40–110 IU/24 hr
		
		2–25 IU/day
		
		30–95 IU/day
		
		2–20 IU/day
		
		40–110 IU/day
			Pituitary tumor
			Ovarian failure
				Depressed or failure to peak—pituitary failure

Metanephrines, total	Less than 1.3 mg/24 hr	Less than 6.5 μmol/day	Pheochromocytoma; a few patients with pheochromocytoma may have elevated urinary metanephrines but normal catecholamines and VMA	
Osmolality	Males: 390–1090 mM/kg Females: 300–1090 mM/kg	390–1090 mmol/kg 300–1090 mmol/kg	Useful in the study of electrolyte and water balance	
Oxalate	Up to 40 mg/24 hr	Up to 456 μmol/day	Primary hyperoxaluria	
Phenylpyruvic acid qualitative	Negative		Phenylketonuria	
Phosphorus, inorganic	0.8–1.3 g/24 hr	26–42 mmol/24 hr	Hyperparathyroidism Vitamin D intoxication Paget's disease Metastatic neoplasm to bone	Hypoparathyroidism Vitamin D deficiency
Porphobilinogen, qualitative	Negative		Chronic lead poisoning Acute porphyria Liver disease	
Porphobilinogen, quantitative	0–1 mg/24 hr	0–4.4 μmol/24 hr	Acute porphyria Liver disease	

(continued)

Reference Ranges—Urine Chemistry (Continued)

| Determination | Normal Adult Reference Range | | Clinical Significance | |
	Conventional Units	SI Units	Increased	Decreased
Porphyrins, qualitative	Negative		See porphyrins, quantitative	
Porphyrins, quantitative (coproporphyrin and uroporphyrin)	Coproporphyrin: 50–160 μg/24 hr	0.075–0.24 μmol/24 hr	Porphyria hepatica Porphyria erythropoietica Porphyria cutanea tarda Lead poisoning (only coproporphyrin increased)	
	Uroporphyrin: up to 50 μg/24 hr	Up to 0.06 μmol/24 hr		
Potassium	40–65 mEq/24 hr	40–65 mmol/24 hr	Hemolysis	
Pregnanediol	Females:		Corpus luteum cysts	Placental dysfunction
	Proliferative phase:		When placental tissue remains in the uterus following parturition	Threatened abortion Intrauterine death
	0.5–1.5 mg/24 hr	1.6–4.8 μmol/24 hr		
	Luteal phase:		Some cases of adrenocortical tumors	
	2–7 mg/24 hr	6–22 μmol/24 hr		
	Menopause:			
	0.2–1 mg/24 hr	0.6–3.1 μmol/24 hr		

Pregnancy:

Weeks of Gestation	mg/24 hr	μmol/24 hr
10–12	5–15	15.6–47
12–18	5–25	15.6–78.0
18–24	15–33	47.0–103.0
24–28	20–42	62.4–131.0
28–32	27–47	84.2–146.6

Determination	Conventional Units	SI Units	Increased	Decreased
	Males: 0.1–2 mg/24 hr	0.3–6.2 μmol/24 hr		
Pregnanetriol	0.4–2.4 mg/24 hr	1.2–7.1 μmol/24 hr	Congenital adrenal androgenic hyperplasia	
Protein	Up to 100 mg/24 hr	Up to 100 mg/24 hr	Nephritis Cardiac failure Mercury poisoning Bence-Jones protein in multiple myeloma Febrile states Hematuria	
Sodium	130–200 mEq/24 hr	130–200 mmol/24 hr	Useful in detecting gross changes in water and salt balance	
Titratable acidity	20–40 mEq/24 hr	20–40 mmol/24 hr	Metabolic acidosis	Metabolic alkalosis
Urea nitrogen	9–16 gm/24 hr	0.32–0.57 mol/L	Excessive protein catabolism	Impaired kidney function
Uric acid	250–750 mg/24 hr	1.48–4.43 mmol/24 hr	Gout	Nephritis
Urobilinogen	Random urine: <0.25 mg/dl	<0.42 mol/24 hr	Liver and biliary tract disease	Complete or nearly complete biliary obstruction
	24-hour urine: up to 4 mg/24 hr	Up to 6.76 μmol/24 hr	Hemolytic anemias	Diarrhea Renal insufficiency
Uroporphyrins	Up to 50 μg/24 hr	Up to 0.06 μmol/24 hr	Porphyria	
Vanillylmandelic acid (VMA)	0.7–6.8 mg/24 hr	3.5–34.3 μmol/24 hr	Pheochromocytoma Neuroblastoma Coffee, tea, aspirin, bananas, and several different drugs	

(continued)

Reference Ranges—Urine Chemistry (Continued)

	Normal Adult Reference Range		Clinical Significance	
Determination	Conventional Units	SI Units	Increased	Decreased
Xylose absorption test (5 hour)	16%–33% of ingested xylose	Fraction abdorbed: 0.16–0.33		Malabsorption syndromes
Zinc	0.15–1.2 mg/24 hr	2.3–18.4 μmol/24 hr	Zinc is an essential nutritional element	

Reference Ranges—Cerebrospinal Fluid

	Normal Adult Reference Range		Clinical Significance	
Determination	Conventional Units	SI Units	Increased	Decreased
Albumin	15–30 mg/dl	150–300 mg/L	Certain neurologic disorders Lesion in the choroid plexus or blockage of the flow of CSF Damage to the blood–CNS barrier	
Cell count	0–5 mononuclear cells per mm^3	$0–5 \times 10^6$/L	Bacterial meningitis Neurosyphilis Anterior poliomyelitis Encephalitis lethargica	
Chloride	100–130 mEq/L	100–300 mmol/L	Uremia	Acute generalized meningitis Tuberculous meningitis
Glucose	50–75 mg/dl	2.75–4.13 mmol/L	Diabetes mellitus Diabetic coma Epidemic encephalitis Uremia	Acute meningitides Tuberculous meningitis Insulin shock
Glutamine	6–15 mg/dl	0.41–1 mmol/L	Hepatic encephalopathies, including Reye's syndrome Hepatic coma Cirrhosis	
IgG	0–6.6 mg/dl	0–66 mg/L	Damage to the blood–CNS barrier Multiple sclerosis Neurosyphilis Subacute sclerosing panencephalitis Chronic phases of CNS infections	
Lactic acid	<24 mg/dl	<2.7 mmol/L	Bacterial meningitis Hypocapnia Hydrocephalus Brain abscesses Cerebral ischemia	
Lactic dehydrogenase	1/10 that of serum	Activity fraction: 0.1 that of serum	CNS disease	
Protein: Lumbar Cisternal Ventricular	15–45 mg/dl 15–25 mg/dl 5–15 mg/dl	150–450 mg/L 150–250 mg/L 50–150 mg/L	Acute meningitides Tubercular meningitis Neurosyphilis Poliomyelitis Guillain-Barré syndrome	

(continued)

Reference Ranges—Cerebrospinal Fluid (Continued)

Determination	Normal Adult Reference Range		Clinical Significance	
	Conventional Units	SI Units	Increased	Decreased
Protein electrophoresis (cellulose acetate)	% of total:	Fraction:	An increase in the level of albumin alone can be the result of a lesion in the choroid plexus or a blockage of the flow of CSF. An elevated gamma globulin value with a normal albumin level has been reported in multiple sclerosis, neurosyphilis, subacute sclerosing panencephalitis, and the chronic phase of CNS infections. If the blood–CNS barrier has been damaged severely during the course of these diseases, the CSF albumin level may also be elevated.	
Prealbumin	3–7	0.03–0.07		
Albumin	56–74	0.56–0.74		
Alpha$_1$ globulin	2–6.5	0.02–0.065		
Alpha$_2$ globulin	3–12	0.03–0.12		
Beta globulin	8–18.5	0.08–0.185		
Gamma globulin	4–14	0.04–0.14		

Gastric Analysis

Determination	Normal Adult Reference Range		Clinical Significance	
	Conventional Units	SI Units	Increased	Decreased
pH	<2	<2		Pernicious anemia
Basal acid output	0–6 mEq/hr	0–6 mmol/hr	Peptic ulcer	Gastric carcinoma
Maximum acid	5–50 mEq/hr	5–40 mmol/hr	Zollinger-Ellison syndrome	Chronic atrophic gastritis Decreased normally with age

Miscellaneous Values

Determinations	Normal Value	Clinical Significance	
		Conventional Units	SI Units
Acetaminophen	0	Therapeutic level: 10–20 µg/ml	10–20 mg/L
Aminophylline (theophylline)	0	Therapeutic level: 10–20 µg/ml	10–20 mg/L
Bromide	0	Therapeutic level: 5–50 mg/dl	50–500 mg/L
Carbon monoxide	0%–2%	Symptoms with >20% saturation	
Chlordiazepoxide	0	Therapeutic level: 1–3 µg/ml	1–3 mg/L
Diazepam	0	Therapeutic level: 0.5–2.5 µg/dl	5–25 µg/L
Digitoxin	0	Therapeutic level: 5–30 ng/ml	5–30 µg/L
Digoxin	0	Therapeutic level: 0.5–2 ng/ml	0.5–2 µg/L
Ethanol	0%–0.01%	Legal intoxication level: 0.10% or above 0.3%–0.4%: marked intoxication 0.4%–0.5%: alcoholic stupor	

(continued)

Miscellaneous Values (Continued)

Determinations	Normal Value	Clinical Significance	
		Conventional Units	SI Units
Gentamicin	0	Therapeutic level: 4–10 μg/ml	4–10 mg/L
Methanol	0	May be fatal in concentration as low as 10 mg/dl	100 mg/L
Phenobarbital	0	Therapeutic level: 15–40 μg/ml	10–20 mg/L
Phenytoin	0	Therapeutic level: 10–20 μg/ml	10–20 mg/L
Primidone	0	Therapeutic level: 5–12 μg/ml	5–12 mg/L
Quinidine	0	Therapeutic level: 0.2–0.5 mg/dl	2–5 mg/L
Salicylate	0	Therapeutic level: 2–25 mg/dl	20–250 mg/L
		Toxic level: >30 mg/dl	300 mg/L
Sulfonamide	0	Therapeutic levels:	
		Sulfadiazine 8–15 mg/dl	80–150 mg/L
		Sulfaguanidine 3–5 mg/dl	30–50 mg/L
		Sulfamerazine 10–15 mg/dl	100–150 mg/L
		Sulfanilamide 10–15 mg/dl	100–150 mg/L

Index

Letters following page numbers indicate chart (*c*), figure (*f*), and table (*t*).

Prednisolone, in rheumatic disease, 1414t
Prednisone
  in Bell's palsy, 1756
  in breast cancer, 1307t
  in Hodgkin's disease, 805
  in rheumatic disease, 1414t
Preferred provider organizations, 11
Preganglionic fibers, of sympathetic nervous
    system, 1624, 1626
Pregnancy
  breast cancer and, 1308
  ectopic, 1255–1257, 1255f
  prevention of. See Contraception
Preload, 617–618
  in cardiac failure, 692
  after cardiac surgery, 722–723
Premature atrial contractions, 673–674, 674f
Premature ventricular contractions, 676, 676f
Premedication, before anesthesia, 411–412
Premenstrual syndrome, 1240, 1242–1243,
    1242f
Preoperative management, 401–414. See also
    specific procedure
  in ambulatory surgery, 468
  anxiety management in, 402–404, 410
  assessment in
    physical, 404–406
    psychosocial, 402–404
  body movement instruction in, 408c, 410
  breathing instruction in, 408c, 409–410
  in cardiac surgery, 718–720
  checklist for, 412, 413f
  cognitive control in, 410
  coughing instruction in, 408c, 409–410
  examples of, 399
  family assistance in, 412–413
  gerontologic considerations in, 406
  immediately before surgery, 411–412
  informed consent procedure in, 406–408,
    407t
  intestinal preparation in, 410
  nutritional measures in, 410
  pain control information in, 410
  patient education in, 408–410, 408c–409c
  preanesthetic medication in, 411–412
  skin preparation in, 410–411
  surgical indications and, 401–402, 402t
  in thoracic surgery, 545–546
  transportation in, 412
Preoperative phase, definition of, 400
Prerenal azotemia, 1136
Prerenal failure, 1136
Presbycusis, 175, 1594–1595
Presbyopia, 175, 1547–1548, 1551
Presenile dementia, 177
Pressure, tissue, measurement of, 1787, 1787f
Pressure-cycled ventilator, 534–535
Pressure ulcers
  assessment of, 237, 238c
  under cast, 1789f, 1792–1793
  gerontologic considerations in, 237
  in hip fracture surgery, 1839, 1844
  interventions for, 238–240, 239f
  in paraplegia, 1746
  risk factors for, 236–237, 236f, 237c
  in traction, 1800
Preventive ethics, 56–57, 59
Preventive health care. See Health promotion;
    Patient/health education
Priapism, 1341–1342
Prickly heat, 1463
Prima facie duty, 53
Primaquine, anemia induced by, 797
Primary nursing, 15–16
Primidone, in epilepsy, 1726t

PR interval
  in atrial fibrillation, 675, 675f
  in atrioventricular block, 681, 681f–682f
  in electrocardiography, 632, 632f
  in paroxysmal atrial tachycardia, 674, 674f
  in premature atrial contraction, 674, 674f
  in sinus bradycardia, 672, 672f
  in sinus tachycardia, 673, 673f
Prinzmetal's angina, 646c, 647
Priorities, in nursing process, 30, 32
Privacy, for elderly persons, 190
Probenecid, in gout, 1415t, 1433
Problem, in nursing diagnosis, 30
Problem-oriented record, 25–29
  guidelines for, 33, 35–36, 37c
"Problem patients," 146–148
Procainamide
  in CPR, 701t
  in malignant hyperthermia, 433t
Procaine
  as local anesthetic, 430t
  in spinal anesthesia, 429, 429t
Procarbazine, in Hodgkin's disease, 805
Procardia (nifedipine)
  in angina pectoris, 647
  in hypertension, 764t
Procidentia, 1273–1274, 1274f
Proctoscopy, 836–837
Procyclidine, in Parkinson's disease,
    1710–1711
Professional standards review organizations,
    10
Progesterone
  in ovarian cycle, 1239–1240, 1241f
  in premenstrual syndrome, 1240
Progesterone receptors, in breast cancer,
    1302–1303
Progestins, as oral contraceptives,
    1246–1247, 1247c
Progressive multifocal leukoencephalopathy,
    in AIDS, 1366
Progress notes, 33, 35–36, 37c
Prolactinoma, 1695
Proliferation stage, of immune response, 1353
Proliferative phase, of healing, 451, 451t
Promethazine, as narcotic potentiator, 264
Promotion, in carcinogenesis, 345
Pronation, definition of, 226c
Prone position, 225c
Propacil (propylthiouracil), in hyperthyroid-
    ism, 1087
Propranolol
  in angina pectoris, 647
  in esophageal varices, 1000, 1001t
  in hypertension, 761t–762t
  in migraine headache, 1693
Proprioception, assessment of, 1631
Proprioceptors, in ventilation control, 503
Propylthiouracil, in hyperthyroidism, 1087
Prostaglandin(s)
  in elective abortion, 1251
  in gastrointestinal regulation, 832t
  in hypersensitivity, 1390t, 1391
Prostaglandin inhibitors, in dysmenorrhea,
    1243
Prostatectomy, 1326–1332
  assessment in, 1326–1327
  complications of, 1329–1331
  perineal, 1326, 1327t, 1328f
  postoperative management in, 1329–1331
  preoperative management in, 1329
  in prostate cancer, 1332
  retropubic, 1326, 1327t, 1328f
  suprapubic, 1326, 1327t, 1328f
  transurethral, 1326, 1327t, 1328f
Prostate gland
  anatomy of, 1324, 1324f

  benign hyperplasia of, 1325–1326
  cancer of, 1332–1333, 1332t
    adrenalectomy in, 1102
    nursing care plan for, 1334–1337
  inflammation of, 1325
  removal of. See Prostatectomy
Prostate-specific antigen, in prostate cancer,
    1332
Prostatism, 1326
Prostatitis, 1325
Prostatodynia, 1325
Prosthesis. See also Implant(s)
  ambulation with, 235
  after amputation, 1849, 1849f, 1854
  for cardiac valves, 713–714, 714f
  hip. See Hip, total replacement of
  knee, 1811, 1811f
  in otosclerosis, 1606
  voice, 493, 493f
Prosthetist, on rehabilitation team, 218
Prostigmin (neostigmine), in myasthenia
    gravis, 1717
Protamine sulfate, in heparin reversal, 771
Protein
  in diabetic diet, 1029
  digestion of, 833
    enzymes for, 831t
  metabolism of, liver role in, 973
  plasma, 784–785
Protein-bound iodine test, 1080
Proteinuria
  definition of, 1138
  in nephrotic syndrome, 1186–1187
Prothrombin, deficiency of, bleeding in,
    810–811
Prothrombin complex, transfusion of,
    813–814, 814t
Prothrombin time test, 788c
Protozoan infections
  amebiasis, 1942–1943
  giardiasis, 1941–1942
  liver abscess, 1943
  malaria, 1940–1941
  sexually transmitted, 1913t
Provocative testing, for allergy, 1396
Pruritus
  in hematologic disorders, 787c
  in lice infestation, 1471–1472
  management of, 1463
  perianal, 1463
  relief of, 1454, 1456–1457
  in scabies, 1472–1473
  in tinea infections, 1469–1471, 1470t
  in vulvar cancer, 1281
Pseudarthrosis, in fracture healing, 1829
Pseudofolliculitis barbae, 1468
Pseudogout (calcium pyrophosphate
    dihydrate crystal deposition
    disease), 1433
Pseudomonas pneumonia, 562t–563t
Psilocybin, abuse of, 1976t–1977t
Psittacosis, 1936
Psoas sign, in appendicitis, 926
Psoralen, in psoriasis, 1476, 1477t
Psoriasis, 1474–1478
  assessment of, 1476
  clinical manifestations of, 1474, 1474f
  management of, 1475–1476, 1477t
  patient education on, 1476, 1478
  psychologic considerations in, 1475
Psoriatic arthritis, 1430
PSROs (professional standards review organi-
    zations), 10
Psychiatric emergencies, 1980–1981
Psychologic management, in emergency situ-
    ations, 1948–1949